西氏内科学

GOLDMAN-CECIL MEDICINE

西氏内科学
GOLDMAN-CECIL MEDICINE

第25版 · 第2卷

LEE GOLDMAN, MD

Harold and Margaret Hatch Professor
Executive Vice President and Dean of the
Faculties of Health Sciences and Medicine
Chief Executive, Columbia University Medical Center
Columbia University
New York, New York

ANDREW I. SCHAFER, MD

Professor of Medicine
Director, Richard T. Silver Center for Myeloproliferative Neoplasms
Weill Cornell Medical College
New York, New York

北京大学医学出版社

图书在版编目（CIP）数据

西氏内科学：第25版（精装版）：全2册 ：英文 ／（美）古德曼
(Goldman,L.)，（美）谢弗(Schafer,A.I.)主编．−北京：北京大学
医学出版社，2016.1
书名原文：GOLDMAN−CECIL MEDICINE
ISBN 978−7−5659−1282−5

Ⅰ．①西… Ⅱ．①古… ②谢… Ⅲ．①内科学−英文 Ⅳ．①R5

中国版本图书馆CIP数据核字(2015)第274005号

ELSEVIER

Elsevier (Singapore) Pte Ltd.
3 Killiney Road，#08-01 Winsland House I，Singapore 239519
Tel: (65) 6349-0200，Fax: (65) 6733-1817

西氏内科学（第25版）

原　　著：LEE GOLDMAN, ANDREW I. SCHAFER
出版发行：北京大学医学出版社
地　　址：（100191）北京市海淀区学院路38号　北京大学医学部院内
电　　话：发行部 010-82802230；图书邮购 010-82802495
网　　址：http://www.pumpress.com.cn
E-mail：booksale@bjmu.edu.cn
印　　刷：北京圣彩虹制版印刷技术有限公司
经　　销：新华书店
责任编辑：冯智勇　　责任印制：李　啸
开　　本：889mm×1194mm　1/16　印张：182　　字数：5533千字
版　　次：2016年1月第1版　2016年1月第1次印刷
书　　号：ISBN 978-7-5659-1282-5
定　　价：780.00元（全2卷）
版权所有，违者必究
（凡属质量问题请与本社发行部联系退换）

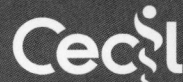

ASSOCIATE EDITORS

PREFACE

In the 90 years since the first edition of the *Cecil Textbook of Medicine* was published, almost everything we know about internal medicine has changed. Progress in medical science is now occurring at an ever-accelerating pace, and it is doing so within the framework of transformational changes in clinical practice and the delivery of health care at individual, social, and global levels. This textbook provides the latest medical knowledge in multiple formats that should appeal to students and seasoned practitioners regardless of how they prefer to access this rapidly changing information.

Even as *Cecil's* specific information has changed, however, we have remained true to the tradition of a comprehensive textbook of medicine that carefully explains the *why* (the underlying pathophysiology of disease) and the *how* (now expected to be evidence-based from randomized controlled trials and meta-analyses). Descriptions of physiology and pathophysiology include the latest genetic advances in a practical format that strives to be useful to the nonexpert. Medicine has entered an era when the acuity of illness and the limited time available to evaluate a patient have diminished the ability of physicians to satisfy their intellectual curiosity. As a result, the acquisition of information, quite easily achieved in this era, is often confused with knowledge. We have attempted to address this dilemma with a textbook that not only informs but also stimulates new questions and gives a glimpse of the future path to new knowledge. Grade A evidence is specifically highlighted in the text and referenced at the end of each chapter. In addition to the information provided in the textbook, the *Cecil* website supplies expanded content and functionality. In many cases, the full articles referenced in each chapter can be accessed from the *Cecil* website. The website is also continuously updated to incorporate subsequent Grade A information, other evidence, and new discoveries.

The sections for each organ system begin with a chapter that summarizes an approach to patients with key symptoms, signs, or laboratory abnormalities associated with dysfunction of that organ system. The text specifically provides clear, concise information regarding how a physician should approach more than 100 common symptoms, signs, and laboratory abnormalities, usually with a flow diagram, a table, or both for easy reference. In this way, *Cecil* remains a comprehensive text to guide diagnosis and therapy, not only for patients with suspected or known diseases but also for patients who may have undiagnosed abnormalities that require an initial evaluation.

Just as each edition brings new authors, it also reminds us of our gratitude to past editors and authors. Previous editors of *Cecil* include a short but remarkably distinguished group of leaders of American medicine: Russell Cecil, Paul Beeson, Walsh McDermott, James Wyngaarden, Lloyd H. Smith, Jr., Fred Plum, J. Claude Bennett, and Dennis Ausiello. As we welcome new associate editors—Mary K. Crow, James H. Doroshow, and Allen M. Spiegel—we also express our appreciation to William P. Arend, James O. Armitage, David R. Clemmons, and other associate editors from the previous editions on whose foundation we have built. Our returning associate editors—Jeffrey M. Drazen, Robert C. Griggs, Donald W. Landry, Wendy Levinson, Anil K. Rustgi, and W. Michael Scheld—continue to make critical contributions to the selection of authors and the review and approval of all manuscripts. The editors, however, are fully responsible for the book as well as the integration among chapters.

The tradition of *Cecil* is that all chapters are written by distinguished experts in each field. We are also most grateful for the editorial assistance in New York of Maribel Lim and Silva Sergenian. These individuals and others in our offices have shown extraordinary dedication and equanimity in working with authors and editors to manage the unending flow of manuscripts, figures, and permissions. We also thank Cassondra Andreychik, Ved Bhushan Arya, Cameron Harrison, Karen Krok, Robert J. Mentz, Gaétane Nocturne, Patrice Savard, Senthil Senniappan, Tejpratap Tiwari, and Sangeetha Venkatarajan, who contributed to various chapters, and we mourn the passing of Morton N. Swartz, MD, co-author of the chapter on "Meningitis: Bacterial, Viral, and Other" and Donald E. Low, MD, author of the chapter "Nonpneumococcal Streptococcal Infections, Rheumatic Fever." At Elsevier, we are most indebted to Kate Dimock and Maureen Iannuzzi, and also thank Maria Holman, Gabriela Benner, Cindy Thoms, Anne Altepeter, Linda McKinley, Paula Catalano, and Kristin Koehler, who have been critical to the planning and production process under the guidance of Mary Gatsch. Many of the clinical photographs were supplied by Charles D. Forbes and William F. Jackson, authors of *Color Atlas and Text of Clinical Medicine*, Third Edition, published in 2003 by Elsevier Science Ltd. We thank them for graciously permitting us to include their pictures in our book. We have been exposed to remarkable physicians in our lifetimes and would like to acknowledge the mentorship and support of several of those who exemplify this paradigm— Eugene Braunwald, Lloyd H. Smith, Jr., Frank Gardner, and William Castle. Finally, we would like to thank the Goldman family—Jill, Jeff, Abigail, Mira, Samuel, Daniel, Robyn, Tobin, and Dashel—and the Schafer family— Pauline, Eric, Melissa, Nathaniel, Pam, John, Evan, Samantha, Kate, and Sean, for their understanding of the time and focus required to edit a book that attempts to sustain the tradition of our predecessors and to meet the needs of today's physician.

LEE GOLDMAN, MD
ANDREW I. SCHAFER, MD

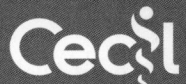

CONTRIBUTORS

Charles S. Abrams, MD
Professor of Medicine, Pathology, and Laboratory Medicine, University of Pennsylvania School of Medicine; Director, PENN-Chop Blood Center for Patient Care & Discovery, Hospital of the University of Pennsylvania, Philadelphia, Pennsylvania
Thrombocytopenia

Frank J. Accurso, MD
Professor of Pediatrics, University of Colorado School of Medicine; Attending Physician, Children's Hospital Colorado, Aurora, Colorado
Cystic Fibrosis

Ronald S. Adler, MD, PhD
Professor of Radiology, New York University School of Medicine; Department of Radiology, NYU Langone Medical Center, New York, New York
Imaging Studies in the Rheumatic Diseases

Cem Akin, MD, PhD
Associate Professor, Harvard Medical School; Attending Physician, Director, Mastocytosis Center, Brigham and Women's Hospital, Department of Medicine, Division of Rheumatology, Immunology, and Allergy, Boston, Massachusetts
Mastocytosis

Allen J. Aksamit, Jr., MD
Professor of Neurology, Mayo Clinic College of Medicine, Consultant in Neurology, Mayo Clinic, Rochester, Minnesota
Acute Viral Encephalitis

Qais Al-Awqati, MB ChB
Robert F. Loeb Professor of Medicine, Jay I. Meltzer Professor of Nephrology and Hypertension, Professor of Physiology and Cellular Biophysics, Division of Nephrology, Columbia University, College of Physicians and Surgeons, New York, New York
Structure and Function of the Kidneys

Ban Mishu Allos, MD
Associate Professor of Medicine, Division of Infectious Diseases, Associate Professor, Preventive Medicine, Vanderbilt University School of Medicine, Nashville, Tennessee
Campylobacter Infections

David Altshuler, MD, PhD
Professor of Genetics and of Medicine, Harvard Medical School, Massachusetts General Hospital; Professor of Biology (Adjunct), Massachusetts Institute of Technology, Boston and Cambridge, Massachusetts
The Inherited Basis of Common Diseases

Michael Aminoff, MD, DSc
Professor, Department of Neurology, University of California San Francisco, San Francisco, California
Approach to the Patient with Neurologic Disease

Jeffrey L. Anderson, MD
Professor of Internal Medicine, University of Utah School of Medicine; Vice-Chair for Research, Department of Internal Medicine, Associate Chief of Cardiology and Director of Cardiovascular Research, Intermountain Medical Center, Intermountain Healthcare, Salt Lake City, Utah
ST Segment Elevation Acute Myocardial Infarction and Complications of Myocardial Infarction

Larry J. Anderson, MD
Professor, Division of Infectious Disease, Department of Pediatrics, Emory University School of Medicine and Children's Healthcare of Atlanta, Atlanta, Georgia
Coronaviruses

Aśok C. Antony, MD
Chancellor's Professor of Medicine, Indiana University School of Medicine; Attending Physician, Indiana University Health Affiliated Hospitals and Richard L. Roudebush Veterans Affairs Medical Center, Indianapolis, Indiana
Megaloblastic Anemias

Gerald B. Appel, MD
Professor of Medicine, Division of Nephrology, Department of Medicine, Columbia University College of Physicians and Surgeons, New York, New York
Glomerular Disorders and Nephrotic Syndromes

Frederick R. Appelbaum, MD
Executive Vice President and Deputy Director, Fred Hutchinson Cancer Research Center; President, Seattle Cancer Care Alliance; Professor, Division of Medical Oncology, University of Washington School of Medicine, Seattle Washington
The Acute Leukemias

Suneel S. Apte, MBBS, DPhil
Staff, Cleveland Clinic Lerner College of Medicine at Case Western Reserve University, Cleveland, Ohio
Connective Tissue Structure and Function

James O. Armitage, MD
The Joe Shapiro Professor of Internal Medicine, University of Nebraska Medical Center, Omaha, Nebraska
Approach to the Patient with Lymphadenopathy and Splenomegaly; Non-Hodgkin Lymphomas

M. Amin Arnaout, MD
Professor of Medicine, Departments of Medicine and Developmental and Regenerative Biology, Harvard Medical School; Physician and Chief Emeritus, Division of Nephrology, Massachusetts General Hospital, Boston, Massachusetts
Cystic Kidney Diseases

Robert M. Arnold, MD
Leo H. Criep Professor of Clinical Care, Chief, Section of Palliative Care and Medical Ethics, University of Pittsburgh; Medical Director, UPMC Palliative and Supportive Care Institute, Pittsburgh, Pennsylvania
Care of Dying Patients and Their Families

David Atkins, MD, MPH
Director, Health Services Research and Development, Veterans Health Administration, Washington, D.C.
The Periodic Health Examination

John P. Atkinson, MD
Chief, Division of Rheumatology, Internal Medicine, Washington University School of Medicine in St. Louis, St. Louis, Missouri
Complement System in Disease

Bruce R. Bacon, MD
Endowed Chair in Gastroenterology, Professor of Internal Medicine, Co-Director, Saint Louis University Liver Center; Director, Saint Louis University Abdominal Transplant Center, Saint Louis University School of Medicine, St. Louis, Missouri
Iron Overload (Hemochromatosis)

Larry M. Baddour, MD
Professor of Medicine, Chair, Division of Infectious Diseases, Mayo Clinic, Rochester, Minnesota
Infective Endocarditis

Grover C. Bagby, MD
Professor of Medicine and Molecular and Medical Genetics, Knight Cancer Institute at Oregon Health and Science University and Portland VA Medical Center, Portland, Oregon
Aplastic Anemia and Related Bone Marrow Failure States

Barbara J. Bain, MBBS
Professor in Diagnostic Haematology, Imperial College London; Honorary Consultant Haematologist, St. Mary's Hospital, London, United Kingdom
The Peripheral Blood Smear

Dean F. Bajorin, MD
Attending Physician and Member, Medicine, Memorial Hospital, Memorial Sloan Kettering Cancer Center; Professor of Medicine, Weill Cornell Medical College, New York, New York
Tumors of the Kidney, Bladder, Ureters, and Renal Pelvis

Robert W. Baloh, MD
Professor of Neurology, University of California Los Angeles School of Medicine, Los Angeles, California
Neuro-Ophthalmology; Smell and Taste; Hearing and Equilibrium

Jonathan Barasch, MD, PhD
Professor of Medicine and Pathology and Cell Biology, Department of Medicine, Division of Nephrology, Columbia University College of Physicians & Surgeons, New York, New York
Structure and Function of the Kidneys

Richard L. Barbano, MD, PhD
Professor of Neurology, University of Rochester, Rochester, New York
Mechanical and Other Lesions of the Spine, Nerve Roots, and Spinal Cord

Elizabeth Barrett-Connor, MD
Professor of Community and Family Medicine, University of California San Diego, San Diego, California
Menopause

John R. Bartholomew, MD
Section Head, Vascular Medicine, Cardiovascular Medicine, Cleveland Clinic, Professor of Medicine, Cleveland Clinic Lerner College of Medicine of Case Western Reserve University, Cleveland, Ohio
Other Peripheral Arterial Diseases

Mary Barton, MD, MPP
Vice President, Performance Measurement, National Committee for Quality Assurance, Washington, D.C.
The Periodic Health Examination

Robert C. Basner, MD
Professor of Medicine, Columbia University Medical Center; Director, Columbia University Cardiopulmonary Sleep and Ventilatory Disorders Center, Columbia University College of Physicians and Surgeons, New York, New York
Obstructive Sleep Apnea

Stephen G. Baum, MD
Chairman of Medicine, Mount Sinai Beth Israel Hospital; Professor of Medicine and of Microbiology and Immunology, Albert Einstein College of Medicine, New York, New York
Mycoplasma Infections

Daniel G. Bausch, MD, MPH&TM
Associate Professor, Department of Tropical Medicine, Tulane University Health Sciences Center, New Orleans, Louisiana
Viral Hemorrhagic Fevers

Arnold S. Bayer, MD
Professor of Medicine, David Geffen School of Medicine at University of California Los Angeles; LA Biomedical Research Institute; Vice Chair for Academic Affairs, Department of Medicine, Harbor-UCLA Medical Center, Los Angeles, California
Infective Endocarditis

Hasan Bazari, MD
Associate Professor of Medicine, Harvard Medical School, Department of Medicine, Clinical Director, Nephrology, Program Director, Internal Medicine Residency Program, Massachusetts General Hospital, Boston, Massachusetts
Approach to the Patient with Renal Disease

John H. Beigel, MD
National Institute of Allergy and Infectious Diseases, National Institutes of Health, Bethesda, Maryland
Antiviral Therapy (Non-HIV)

George A. Beller, MD
Professor of Medicine, University of Virginia Health System, Charlottesville, Virginia
Noninvasive Cardiac Imaging

Robert M. Bennett, MD
Professor of Medicine, Oregon Health and Science University, Portland, Oregon
Fibromyalgia, Chronic Fatigue Syndrome, and Myofascial Pain

Joseph R. Berger, MD
Professor of Neurology, Chief of the Multiple Sclerosis Division, Department of Neurology, Perelman School of Medicine, University of Pennsylvania, Philadelphia, Pennsylvania
Cytomegalovirus, Epstein-Barr Virus, and Slow Virus Infections of the Central Nervous System; Neurologic Complications of Human Immunodeficiency Virus Infection; Brain Abscess and Parameningeal Infections

Paul D. Berk, MD
Professor of Medicine, Department of Medicine, Columbia University College of Physicians and Surgeons, New York, New York
Approach to the Patient with Jaundice or Abnormal Liver Tests

Nancy Berliner, MD
Professor of Medicine, Harvard Medical School; Chief, Division of Hematology, Brigham and Women's Hospital, Boston, Massachusetts
Leukocytosis and Leukopenia

James L. Bernat, MD
Louis and Ruth Frank Professor of Neuroscience, Professor of Neurology and Medicine, Geisel School of Medicine at Dartmouth, Hanover, New Hampshire; Department of Neurology, Dartmouth-Hitchcock Medical Center, Lebanon, New Hampshire
Coma, Vegetative State, and Brain Death

Philip J. Bierman, MD
Professor, Department of Internal Medicine, University of Nebraska Medical Center, Omaha, Nebraska
Approach to the Patient with Lymphadenopathy and Splenomegaly; Non-Hodgkin Lymphomas

Michael R. Bishop, MD
Professor of Medicine, Director, Hematopoietic Cellular Therapy Program, Section of Hematology and Oncology, Department of Medicine, University of Chicago, Chicago, Illinois
Hematopoietic Stem Cell Transplantation

Bruce R. Bistrian, MD, PhD, MPH
Professor of Medicine, Beth Israel Deaconess Medical Center; Professor of Medicine, Harvard Medical School, Boston, Massachusetts
Nutritional Assessment

Joseph J. Biundo, MD
Clinical Professor of Medicine, Tulane Medical Center, New Orleans, Louisiana
Bursitis, Tendinitis, and Other Periarticular Disorders and Sports Medicine

Adrian R. Black, PhD
Assistant Professor, Director of Tissue Sciences for the Eppley Institute, The Eppley Institute for Research in Cancer and Allied Diseases, University of Nebraska Medical Center, Omaha, Nebraska
Cancer Biology and Genetics

Charles D. Blanke, MD
Professor of Medicine, Oregon Health and Science University, Portland, Oregon
Neoplasms of the Small and Large Intestine

Joel N. Blankson, MD, PhD
Associate Professor, Johns Hopkins University School of Medicine, Baltimore, Maryland
Immunopathogenesis of Human Immunodeficiency Virus Infection

Martin J. Blaser, MD
Muriel and George Singer Professor of Medicine, Professor of Microbiology, Director, Human Microbiome Program, New York University Langone Medical Center, New York, New York
Acid Peptic Disease; Human Microbiome

William A. Blattner, MD
Professor and Associate Director, Institute of Human Virology, School of Medicine, University of Maryland; Professor of Medicine, School of Medicine, University of Maryland; Professor and Head, Division of Cancer Epidemiology, Department of Epidemiology and Public Health, School of Medicine, University of Maryland, Baltimore, Maryland
Retroviruses Other Than Human Immunodeficiency Virus

Thomas P. Bleck, MD
Professor of Neurological Sciences, Neurosurgery, Internal Medicine, and Anesthesiology, Associate Chief Medical Officer (Critical Care), Rush Medical College, Chicago, Illinois
Arboviruses Affecting the Central Nervous System

Joel A. Block, MD
The Willard L. Wood MD Professor and Director, Division of Rheumatology, Rush University Medical Center, Chicago, Illinois
Osteoarthritis

Henk Blom, MD
Laboratory of Clinical Biochemistry and Metabolism, Department of General Pediatrics, Adolescent Medicine and Neonatology, University Medical Centre Freiburg, Head of Laboratory/Clinical Biochemical Geneticist, Freiburg, Germany
Homocystinuria and Hyperhomocysteinemia

Olaf A. Bodamer, MD
Medical Genetics, University of Miami Hospital, Miami, Florida
Approach to Inborn Errors of Metabolism

William E. Boden, MD
Professor of Medicine, Albany Medical College; Chief of Medicine, Albany Stratton VA Medical Center; Vice-Chairman, Department of Medicine, Albany Medical Center, Albany, New York
Angina Pectoris and Stable Ischemic Heart Disease

Jean Bolognia, MD
Professor of Dermatology, Yale Medical School; Attending Physician, Yale-New Haven Hospital, New Haven, Connecticut
Infections, Hyperpigmentation and Hypopigmentation, Regional Dermatology, and Distinctive Lesions in Black Skin

Robert A. Bonomo, MD
Chief, Medical Service, Louis Stokes Cleveland VA Medical Center; Professor of Medicine, Pharmacology, Biochemistry, Molecular Biology, and Microbiology, Case Western Reserve University School of Medicine, Cleveland, Ohio
Diseases Caused by Acinetobacter and Stenotrophomonas Species

Larry Borish, MD
Professor of Medicine, Allergy, and Clinical Immunology, University of Virginia Health System, Charlottesville, Virgina
Allergic Rhinitis and Chronic Sinusitis

Patrick J. Bosque, MD
Associate Professor of Neurology, University of Colorado Denver School of Medicine; Neurologist, Denver Health Medical Center, Denver, Colorado
Prion Diseases

David J. Brenner, PhD, DSc
Higgins Professor of Radiation Biophysics, Center for Radiological Research, Columbia University Medical Center, New York, New York
Radiation Injury

Itzhak Brook, MD, MSc
Professor of Pediatrics and Medicine, Georgetown University, Georgetown University Medical Center, Washington, D.C.
Diseases Caused by Non–Spore-Forming Anaerobic Bacteria; Actinomycosis

Enrico Brunetti, MD
Assistant Professor of Infectious Diseases, University of Pavia; Attending Physician, Division of Infectious and Tropical Diseases, IRCCS San Matteo Hospital Foundation; Co-Director, WHO Collaborating Centre for Clinical Management of Cystic Echinococcosis, Pavia, Italy
Cestodes

David M. Buchner, MD, MPH
Shahid and Ann Carlson Khan Professor in Applied Health Sciences, Department of Kinesiology and Community Health, University of Illinois at Urbana-Champaign, Champaign, Illinois
Physical Activity

Pierre A. Buffet, MD, PhD
Research Unit Head, Erythrocyte Parasite Pathogenesis Research Team INSERM–University Paris 6, CIMI–Paris Research Center, University Pierre and Marie Curie; Associate Professor of Parasitology, Faculty of Medicine, University Pierre and Marie Curie, Pitié-Salpêtrière Hospital, Paris, France
Leishmaniasis

H. Franklin Bunn, MD
Professor of Medicine, Harvard Medical School; Physician, Brigham and Women's Hospital, Boston, Massachusetts
Approach to the Anemias

David A. Bushinsky, MD
John J. Kuiper Distinguished Professor of Medicine, Chief, Nephrology Division, University of Rochester School of Medicine; Associate Chair for Academic Affairs in Medicine, University of Rochester Medical Center, Rochester, New York
Nephrolithiasis

Vivian P. Bykerk, MD
Associate Professor of Medicine, Weill Cornell Medical College; Associate Attending Physician, Hospital for Special Surgery, New York, New York
Approach to the Patient with Rheumatic Disease

Peter A. Calabresi, MD
Professor of Neurology and Director of the Richard T. Johnson Division of Neuroimmunology and Neuroinfectious Diseases, Johns Hopkins University; Director of the Multiple Sclerosis Center, Johns Hopkins Hospital, Baltimore, Maryland
Multiple Sclerosis and Demyelinating Conditions of the Central Nervous System

David P. Calfee, MD, MS
Associate Professor of Medicine and Healthcare Policy and Research, Weill Cornell Medical College; Chief Hospital Epidemiologist, New York-Presbyterian Hospital/Weill Cornell Medical Center, New York, New York
Prevention and Control of Health Care–Associated Infections

Douglas Cameron, MD, MBA
Professor of Ophthalmology and Visual Neurosciences, University of Minnesota, Minneapolis, Minnesota
Diseases of the Visual System

Michael Camilleri, MD
Atherton and Winifred W. Bean Professor, Professor of Medicine, Pharmacology, and Physiology, College of Medicine, Mayo Clinic, Consultant, Division of Gastroenterology and Hepatology, Mayo Clinic, Rochester, Minnesota
Disorders of Gastrointestinal Motility

Grant W. Cannon, MD
Thomas E. and Rebecca D. Jeremy Presidential Endowed Chair for Arthritis Research, Associate Chief of Staff for Academic Affiliations, George E. Wahlen VA Medical Center, Salt Lake City, Utah
Immunosuppressing Drugs Including Corticosteroids

Maria Domenica Cappellini, MD
Professor of Internal Medicine, University of Milan, Fondazione IRCCS Ca' Granda Ospedale Maggiore Policlinico, University of Milan, Milan, Italy
The Thalassemias

Blase A. Carabello, MD
Professor of Medicine, Chairman, Department of Cardiology, Mount Sinai Beth Israel Heart Institute, New York, New York
Valvular Heart Disease

Edgar M. Carvalho, MD
Professor of Medicine and Clinical Immunology, Faculdade de Medicina da Bahia, Universidade Federal da Bahia and Escola Bahiana de Medicina e Saúde Pública, Salvador, Bahia, Brazil
Schistosomiasis (Bilharziasis)

William H. Catherino, MD, PhD
Professor and Research Head, Department of Obstetrics and Gynecology, Uniformed Services University of the Health Sciences Division of Reproductive Endocrinology and Infertility; Program in Reproductive and Adult Endocrinology, Eunice Kennedy Shriver National Institute of Child Health and Human Development, National Institutes of Health, Bethesda, Maryland
Ovaries and Development; Reproductive Endocrinology and Infertility

Jane A. Cauley, DrPH
Professor of Epidemiology, University of Pittsburgh Graduate School of Public Health, Vice Chair of the Department of Epidemiology, Pittsburgh, Pennsylvania
Epidemiology of Aging: Implications of the Aging of Society

Naga P. Chalasani, MD
David W. Crabb Professor and Director, Division of Gastroenterology and Hepatology, Indiana University School of Medicine, Indianapolis, Indiana
Alcoholic and Nonalcoholic Steatohepatitis

Henry F. Chambers, MD
Professor of Medicine, University of California San Francisco School of Medicine; Director, Clinical Research Services, Clinical and Translational Sciences Institute, San Francisco, California
Staphylococcal Infections

William P. Cheshire, Jr., MD
Professor of Neurology, Mayo Clinic, Jacksonville, Florida
Autonomic Disorders and Their Management

Ilseung Cho, MD, MS
Assistant Professor of Medicine, Division of Gastroenterology, Department of Medicine, New York University, New York, New York
Human Microbiome

Arun Chockalingam, PhD
Professor of Epidemiology and Global Health, Director, Office of Global Health Education and Training; Dalla Lana Faculty of Public Health, University of Toronto, Toronto, Ontario, Canada
Global Health

David C. Christiani, MD
Professor of Medicine, Harvard Medical School; Physician, Pulmonary and Critical Care, Massachusetts General Hospital; Elkan Blout Professor of Environmental Genetics, Environmental Health, Harvard School of Public Health, Boston, Massachusetts
Physical and Chemical Injuries of the Lung

David H. Chu, MD, PhD
Director, Contact Dermatitis, Division of Dermatology and Cutaneous Surgery, Scripps Clinic Medical Group, La Jolla, California
Structure and Function of the Skin

Theodore J. Cieslak, MD
Pediatric Infectious Diseases, Clinical Professor of Pediatrics, University of Texas Health Science Center at San Antonio; Department of Pediatrics, Fort Sam Houston, Texas
Bioterrorism

Carolyn Clancy, MD
Interim Under Secretary for Health, Veterans Administration, Washington, D.C.
Measuring Health and Health Care

David R. Clemmons, MD
Kenan Professor of Medicine, University of North Carolina School of Medicine; Attending Physician, Medicine, UNC Hospitals, Chapel Hill, North Carolina
Approach to the Patient with Endocrine Disease

David Cohen, MD
Professor of Medicine, Division of Nephrology; Medical Director, Kidney and Pancreas Transplantation, Columbia University Medical Center, New York, New York
Treatment of Irreversible Renal Failure

Jeffrey Cohen, MD
Chief, Laboratory of Infectious Diseases, National Institute of Allergy and Infectious Diseases, National Institutes of Health, Bethesda, Maryland
Varicella-Zoster Virus (Chickenpox, Shingles)

Myron S. Cohen, MD
Associate Vice Chancellor for Global Health, Director, UNC Institute for Global Health and Infectious Diseases, Chief, Division of Infectious Diseases, Yeargan-Bate Eminent Professor of Medicine, Microbiology, and Immunology and Epidemiology, Chapel Hill, North Carolina
Approach to the Patient with a Sexually Transmitted Infection; Prevention of Human Immunodeficiency Virus Infection

Steven P. Cohen, MD
Professor of Anesthesiology and Critical Care Medicine and Physical Medicine and Rehabilitation, Johns Hopkins School of Medicine, Baltimore, Maryland, and Uniformed Services University of the Health Sciences, Bethesda, Maryland; Director, Pain Research, Walter Reed National Military Medical Center, Bethesda, Maryland
Pain

Steven L. Cohn, MD
Professor of Clinical Medicine, University of Miami Miller School of Medicine; Medical Director, UHealth Preoperative Assessment Center; Director, Medical Consultation Service, University of Miami Hospital, Miami, Florida
Preoperative Evaluation

Robert Colebunders, MD
Emeritus Professor, Institute of Tropical Medicine, Antwerp, Belgium
Immune Reconstitution Inflammatory Syndrome in HIV/AIDS

Joseph M. Connors, MD
Clinical Professor, University of British Columbia; Clinical Director, BC Cancer Agency Centre for Lymphoid Cancer, Vancouver, British Columbia, Canada
Hodgkin Lymphoma

Deborah J. Cook, MD, MSc
Professor of Medicine, Clinical Epidemiology and Biostatistics, McMaster University, Hamilton, Ontario, Canada
Approach to the Patient in a Critical Care Setting

Kenneth H. Cowan, MD, PhD
Director, Fred & Pamela Buffett Cancer Center; Director, The Eppley Institute for Research in Cancer and Allied Diseases; Professor of Medicine, University of Nebraska Medical Center, Omaha, Nebraska
Cancer Biology and Genetics

Joseph Craft, MD
Paul B. Beeson Professor of Medicine and Immunobiology, Section Chief, Rheumatology, Program Director, Investigative Medicine, Department of Internal Medicine, Yale University School of Medicine, New Haven, Connecticut
The Adaptive Immune Systems

Jill Patricia Crandall, MD
Professor of Clinical Medicine, Division of Endocrinology and Diabetes Research Center, Albert Einstein College of Medicine, Bronx, New York
Diabetes Mellitus

Simon L. Croft, BSc, PhD
Professor of Parasitology, Faculty of Infectious and Tropical Diseases, London School of Hygiene and Tropical Medicine, London, United Kingdom
Leishmaniasis

Kristina Crothers, MD
Associate Professor, Department of Medicine, Division of Pulmonary and Critical Care, University of Washington School of Medicine, Seattle, Washington
Pulmonary Manifestations of Human Immunodeficiency Virus and Acquired Immunodeficiency Syndrome

Mary K. Crow, MD
Joseph P. Routh Professor of Rheumatic Diseases in Medicine, Weill Cornell Medical College; Physician in Chief and Benjamin M. Rosen Chair in Immunology and Inflammation Research, Hospital for Special Surgery, New York, New York
The Innate Immune Systems; Approach to the Patient with Rheumatic Disease; Systemic Lupus Erythematosus

John A. Crump, MB ChB, MD, DTM&H
McKinlay Professor of Global Health, Centre for International Health, University of Otago, Dunedin, New Zealand
Salmonella Infections (Including Enteric Fever)

Mark R. Cullen, MD
Professor of Medicine, Department of Medicine, Stanford University School of Medicine, Stanford, California
Principles of Occupational and Environmental Medicine

Charlotte Cunningham-Rundles, MD, PhD
Professor of Medicine and Pediatrics, Icahn School of Medicine at Mount Sinai, New York, New York
Primary Immunodeficiency Diseases

Inger K. Damon, MD, PhD
Director, Division of High Consequence Pathogens and Pathology, Centers for Disease Control and Prevention, Atlanta, Georgia
Smallpox, Monkeypox, and Other Poxvirus Infections

Troy E. Daniels, DDS, MS
Professor Emeritus of Oral Pathology and Pathology, University of California San Francisco, San Francisco, California
Diseases of the Mouth and Salivary Glands

Nancy E. Davidson, MD
Hillman Professor of Oncology, University of Pittsburgh; Director, University of Pittsburgh Cancer Institute and UPMC CancerCenter, Pittsburgh, Pennsylvania
Breast Cancer and Benign Breast Disorders

Lisa M. DeAngelis, MD
Chair, Department of Neurology, Memorial Sloan-Kettering Cancer Center; Professor of Neurology, Weill Cornell Medical College, New York, New York
Tumors of the Central Nervous System

Malcolm M. DeCamp, MD
Fowler McCormick Professor of Surgery, Feinberg School of Medicine, Northwestern University; Chief, Division of Thoracic Surgery, Northwestern Memorial Hospital, Chicago, Illinois
Interventional and Surgical Approaches to Lung Disease

Carlos del Rio, MD
Hubert Professor and Chair and Professor of Medicine, Hubert Department of Global Health, Rollins School of Public Health and Department of Medicine, Emory University School of Medicine, Atlanta, Georgia
Prevention of Human Immunodeficiency Virus Infection

Patricia A. Deuster, PhD, MPH
Professor and Director, Consortium for Health and Military Performance, Department of Military and Emergency Medicine, Uniformed Services University of the Health Sciences, Bethesda, Maryland
Rhabdomyolysis

Robert B. Diasio, MD
William J. and Charles H. Mayo Professor, Molecular Pharmacology and Experimental Therapeutics and Oncology, Mayo Clinic, Rochester, Minnesota
Principles of Drug Therapy

David J. Diemert, MD
Associate Professor, Department of Microbiology, Immunology, and Tropical Medicine, School of Medicine and Health Sciences, The George Washington University, Washington, D.C.
Intestinal Nematode Infections; Tissue Nematode Infections

Kathleen B. Digre, MD
Professor of Neurology, Ophthalmology, Director, Division of Headache and Neuro-Ophthalmology, University of Utah, Salt Lake City, Utah
Headaches and Other Head Pain

James H. Doroshow, MD
Bethesda, Maryland
Approach to the Patient with Cancer; Malignant Tumors of Bone, Sarcomas, and Other Soft Tissue Neoplasms

John M. Douglas, Jr., MD
Executive Director, Tri-County Health Department, Greenwood Village, Colorado
Papillomavirus

Jeffrey M. Drazen, MD
Distinguished Parker B. Francis Professor of Medicine, Harvard Medical School; Senior Physician, Brigham and Women's Hospital, Boston, Massachusetts
Asthma

Stephen C. Dreskin, MD, PhD
Professor of Medicine and Immunology, Division of Allergy and Clinical Immunology, Department of Medicine, University of Colorado Denver, School of Medicine, Aurora, Colorado
Urticaria and Angioedema

W. Lawrence Drew, MD, PhD
Professor Emeritus, Laboratory Medicine and Medicine, University of California San Francisco, San Francisco, California
Cytomegalovirus

George L. Drusano, MD
Professor and Director, Institute for Therapeutic Innovation, College of Medicine, University of Florida, Lake Nona, Florida
Antibacterial Chemotherapy

Thomas D. DuBose, Jr., MD
Emeritus Professor of Internal Medicine and Nephrology, Wake Forest School of Medicine, Winston-Salem, North Carolina
Vascular Disorders of the Kidney

F. Daniel Duffy, MD
Professor of Internal Medicine and Steve Landgarten Chair in Medical Leadership, School of Community Medicine, University of Oklahoma College of Medicine, Tulsa, Oklahoma
Counseling for Behavior Change

Herbert L. DuPont, MD, MACP
Mary W. Kelsey Chair and Director, Center for Infectious Diseases, University of Texas School of Public Health; H. Irving Schweppe Chair of Internal Medicine and Vice Chairman, Department of Medicine, Baylor College of Medicine; Chief of Internal Medicine, St. Luke's Hospital System, Houston, Texas
Approach to the Patient with Suspected Enteric Infection

Madeleine Duvic, MD
Professor and Deputy Chairman, Department of Dermatology, The University of Texas MD Anderson Cancer Center, Houston, Texas
Urticaria, Drug Hypersensitivity Rashes, Nodules and Tumors, and Atrophic Diseases

Kathryn M. Edwards, MD
Sarah H. Sell and Cornelius Vanderbilt Chair in Pediatrics, Vanderbilt University School of Medicine; Director, Vanderbilt Vaccine Research Program, Monroe Carrell Jr. Children's Hospital at Vanderbilt, Nashville, Tennessee
Parainfluenza Viral Disease

N. Lawrence Edwards, MD
Professor of Medicine, Vice Chairman, Department of Medicine, University of Florida; Chief, Section of Rheumatology, Medical Service, Malcom Randall Veterans Affairs Medical Center, Gainesville, Florida
Crystal Deposition Diseases

Lawrence H. Einhorn, MD
Distinguished Professor, Department of Medicine, Division of Hematology/Oncology, Livestrong Foundation Professor of Oncology, Indiana University School of Medicine, Indianapolis, Indiana
Testicular Cancer

Ronald J. Elin, MD, PhD
A.J. Miller Professor and Chairman, Department of Pathology and Laboratory Medicine, University of Louisville School of Medicine, Louisville, Kentucky
Reference Intervals and Laboratory Values

George M. Eliopoulos, MD
Professor of Medicine, Harvard Medical School; Physician, Division of Infectious Diseases, Beth Israel Deaconess Medical Center, Boston, Massachusetts
Principles of Anti-Infective Therapy

Perry Elliott, MD
Professor in Inherited Cardiovascular Disease, Institute of Cardiovascular Science, University College London, London, United Kingdom
Diseases of the Myocardium and Endocardium

Jerrold J. Ellner, MD
Professor of Medicine, Boston University School of Medicine; Chief, Section of Infectious Diseases, Boston Medical Center, Boston, Massachusetts
Tuberculosis

Dirk M. Elston, MD
Director, Ackerman Academy of Dermatopathology, New York, New York
Arthropods and Leeches

Ezekiel J. Emanuel, MD, PhD
Vice Provost for Global Initiatives, Diane V.S. Levy and Robert M. Levy University Professor, Chair, Department of Medical Ethics and Health Policy, University of Pennsylvania, Philadelphia, Pennsylvania
Bioethics in the Practice of Medicine

Joel D. Ernst, MD
Director, Division of Infectious Diseases and Immunology, Jeffrey Bergstein Professor of Medicine, Professor of Medicine, Pathology, and Microbiology, New York University School of Medicine; Attending Physician, New York University Langone Medical Center, New York, New York
Leprosy (Hansen Disease)

Gregory T. Everson, MD
Professor of Medicine, Director of Hepatology, University of Colorado School of Medicine, Aurora, Colorado
Hepatic Failure and Liver Transplantation

Amelia Evoli, MD
Associate Professor of Neurology, Catholic University, Agostino Gemelli University Hospital, Rome, Italy
Disorders of Neuromuscular Transmission

Douglas O. Faigel, MD
Professor of Medicine, Mayo Clinic, Chair, Division of Gastroenterology and Hepatology, Scottsdale, Arizona
Neoplasms of the Small and Large Intestine

Matthew E. Falagas, MD, MSc, DSc
Director, Alfa Institute of Biomedical Sciences, Athens, Greece; Adjunct Associate Professor of Medicine, Tufts University School of Medicine, Boston, Massachusetts; Chief, Department of Medicine and Infectious Diseases, Iaso General Hospital, Iaso Group, Athens, Greece
Pseudomonas and Related Gram-Negative Bacillary Infections

Gary W. Falk, MD, MS
Professor of Medicine, Division of Gastroenterology, University of Pennsylvania Perelman School of Medicine, Philadelphia, Pennsylvania
Diseases of the Esophagus

Gene Feder, MBBS, MD
Professor, Centre for Academic Primary Care, School of Social and Community Medicine, University of Bristol; General Practitioner, Helios Medical Centre, Bristol, United Kingdom
Intimate Partner Violence

David J. Feller-Kopman, MD
Director, Bronchoscopy and Interventional Pulmonology, Associate Professor of Medicine, The Johns Hopkins University, Baltimore, Maryland
Interventional and Surgical Approaches to Lung Disease

Gary S. Firestein, MD
Dean and Associate Vice Chancellor of Translational Medicine, University of California San Diego School of Medicine, La Jolla, California
Mechanisms of Inflammation and Tissue Repair

Glenn I. Fishman, MD
Director, Leon H. Charney Division of Cardiology, Vice-Chair for Research, Department of Medicine, William Goldring Professor of Medicine, New York University School of Medicine, New York, New York
Principles of Electrophysiology

Lee A. Fleisher, MD
Robert D. Dripps Professor and Chair, Anesthesiology and Critical Care, Professor of Medicine, University of Pennsylvania Perelman School of Medicine, Philadelphia, Pennsylvania
Overview of Anesthesia

Paul W. Flint, MD
Professor and Chair, Otolaryngology, Head and Neck Surgery, Oregon Health and Science University, Portland, Oregon
Throat Disorders

Evan L. Fogel, MD, MSc
Professor of Clinical Medicine, Indiana University School of Medicine, Indianapolis, Indiana
Diseases of the Gallbladder and Bile Ducts

Marsha D. Ford, MD
Adjunct Professor of Emergency Medicine, School of Medicine, University of North Carolina-Chapel Hill; Director, Carolinas Poison Center, Carolinas HealthCare System, Charlotte, North Carolina
Acute Poisoning

Chris E. Forsmark, MD
Professor of Medicine, Chief, Division of Gastroenterology, Hepatology, and Nutrition, University of Florida, Gainesville, Florida
Pancreatitis

Vance G. Fowler, Jr., MD, MHS
Professor of Medicine, Duke University Medical Center, Durham, North Carolina
Infective Endocarditis

Manuel A. Franco, MD, PhD
Director of Postgraduate Programs, School of Sciences, Pontificia Universidad Javeriana, Bogota, Colombia
Rotaviruses, Noroviruses, and Other Gastrointestinal Viruses

David O. Freedman, MD
Professor of Medicine and Microbiology, University of Alabama at Birmingham; Director, Gorgas Center for Geographic Medicine, Birmingham, Alabama
Approach to the Patient before and after Travel

Martyn A. French, MD
Professor in Clinical Immunology, School of Pathology and Laboratory Medicine, University of Western Australia, Perth, Australia
Immune Reconstitution Inflammatory Syndrome in HIV/AIDS

Karen Freund, MD, MPH
Professor of Medicine, Associate Director, Tufts Clinical and Translational Science Institute, Tufts University School of Medicine, Tufts Medical Center, Boston, Massachusetts
Approach to Women's Health

Cem Gabay, MD
Professor of Medicine, Head, Division of Rheumatology, University Hospitals of Geneva, Geneva, Switzerland
Biologic Agents

Kenneth L. Gage, PhD
Chief, Entomology and Ecology Activity, Centers for Disease Control and Prevention, Division of Vector-Borne Diseases, Bacterial Diseases Branch, Fort Collins, Colorado
Plague and Other Yersinia Infections

John N. Galgiani, MD
Professor of Medicine, Valley Fever Center for Excellence, University of Arizona, Tucson, Arizona
Coccidioidomycosis

Patrick G. Gallagher, MD
Professor of Pediatrics, Pathology, and Genetics, Yale University School of Medicine; Attending Physician, Yale–New Haven Hospital, New Haven, Connecticut
Hemolytic Anemias: Red Blood Cell Membrane and Metabolic Defects

Leonard Ganz, MD
Director of Cardiac Electrophysiology, Heritage Valley Health System, Beaver, Pennsylvania
Electrocardiography

Hasan Garan, MD
Director, Cardiac Electrophysiology, Dickinson W. Richards, Jr. Professor of Medicine, Columbia University Medical Center, New York, New York
Ventricular Arrhythmias

Guadalupe Garcia-Tsao, MD
Professor of Medicine, Yale University School of Medicine; Chief, Digestive Diseases, VA Connecticut Healthcare System, West Haven, Connecticut
Cirrhosis and Its Sequelae

William M. Geisler, MD, MPH
Professor of Medicine, University of Alabama at Birmingham, Birmingham, Alabama
Diseases Caused by Chlamydiae

Tony P. George, MD
Division of Brain and Therapeutics, Department of Psychiatry, University of Toronto; Schizophrenia Division, The Centre for Addiction and Mental Health, Toronto, Ontario, Canada
Nicotine and Tobacco

Lior Gepstein, MD, PhD
Edna and Jonathan Sohnis Professor in Medicine and Physiology,
Rappaport Faculty of Medicine and Research Institute, Technion–Israel
Institute of Technology, Rambam Health Care Campus, Haifa, Israel
Gene and Cell Therapy

Susan I. Gerber, MD
Team Lead, Respiratory Viruses/Picornaviruses, Division of Viral
Diseases/Epidemiology Branch, National Center for Immunization and
Respiratory Diseases, Centers for Disease Control and Prevention,
Atlanta, Georgia
Coronaviruses

Dale N. Gerding, MD
Professor of Medicine, Loyola University Chicago Stritch School of Medicine,
Research Physician, Edward Hines, Jr. VA Hospital, Hines, Illinois
Clostridial Infections

Morie A. Gertz, MD
Consultant, Division of Hematology, Mayo Clinic, Rochester, Minnesota;
Roland Seidler, Jr. Professor of the Art of Medicine in Honor of Michael
D. Brennan, MD, Professor of Medicine, Mayo Clinic, College of
Medicine, Rochester, Minnesota
Amyloidosis

Gordon D. Ginder, MD
Professor, Internal Medicine, Director, Massey Cancer Center, Virginia
Commonwealth University, Richmond, Virginia
Microcytic and Hypochromic Anemias

Jeffrey S. Ginsberg, MD
Professor of Medicine, McMaster University, Member of Thrombosis and
Atherosclerosis Research Institute, St. Joseph's Healthcare Hamilton,
Hamilton, Ontario, Canada
Peripheral Venous Disease

Geoffrey S. Ginsburg, MD, PhD
Director, Duke Center for Applied Genomics and Precision Medicine;
Professor of Medicine, Pathology and Biomedical Engineering, Duke
University, Durham, North Carolina
Applications of Molecular Technologies to Clinical Medicine

Michael Glogauer, DDS, PhD
Professor, Faculty of Dentistry, University of Toronto, Toronto, Ontario,
Canada
Disorders of Phagocyte Function

John W. Gnann, Jr., MD
Professor of Medicine, Department of Medicine, Division of Infectious
Diseases, Medical University of South Carolina, Charleston, South
Carolina
Mumps

Matthew R. Golden, MD, MPH
Professor of Medicine, University of Washington, Director, HIV/STD
Program, Public Health–Seattle & King County, Seattle, Washington
Neisseria Gonorrhoeae Infections

Lee Goldman, MD
Harold and Margaret Hatch Professor, Executive Vice President and Dean
of the Faculties of Health Sciences and Medicine, Chief Executive,
Columbia University Medical Center, Columbia University, New York,
New York
*Approach to Medicine, the Patient, and the Medical Profession: Medicine as a
Learned and Humane Profession; Approach to the Patient with Possible
Cardiovascular Disease*

Ellie J.C. Goldstein, MD
Clinical Professor of Medicine, David Geffen School of Medicine at
University of California Los Angeles, Los Angeles, California; Director,
R.M. Alden Research Laboratory, Santa Monica, California
Diseases Caused by Non–Spore-Forming Anaerobic Bacteria

Larry B. Goldstein, MD
Professor of Neurology, Director, Duke Stroke Center, Neurology, Duke
University; Staff Neurologist, Durham VA Medical Center, Durham,
North Carolina
Approach to Cerebrovascular Diseases; Ischemic Cerebrovascular Disease

Lawrence T. Goodnough, MD
Professor of Pathology and Medicine, Stanford University; Director,
Transfusion Service, Stanford University Medical Center, Stanford,
California
Transfusion Medicine

Eduardo H. Gotuzzo, MD
Professor of Medicine, Director, Alexander von Humboldt Tropical
Medicine Institute, Universidad Peruana Cayetano Heredia; Chief
Physician, Department of Infectious, Tropical, and Dermatologic
Diseases, National Hospital Cayetano Heredia, Lima, Peru
Cholera and Other Vibrio Infections; Liver, Intestinal, and Lung Fluke Infections

Deborah Grady, MD, MPH
Professor of Medicine, University of California San Francisco, San
Francisco, California
Menopause

Leslie C. Grammer, MD
Professor of Medicine, Northwestern University Feinberg School of
Medicine; Attending Physician, Northwestern Memorial Hospital,
Chicago, Illinois
Drug Allergy

F. Anthony Greco, MD
Medical Director, Sarah Cannon Cancer Center, Nashville, Tennessee
Cancer of Unknown Primary Origin

Harry B. Greenberg, MD
Professor, Departments of Medicine and Microbiology and Immunology,
Stanford University School of Medicine, Stanford, California
Rotaviruses, Noroviruses, and Other Gastrointestinal Viruses

Steven A. Greenberg, MD
Associate Professor of Neurology, Harvard Medical School; Associate
Neurologist, Brigham and Women's Hospital, Boston, Massachusetts
Inflammatory Myopathies

Robert C. Griggs, MD
Professor of Neurology, Medicine, Pediatrics, and Pathology and
Laboratory Medicine, University of Rochester School of Medicine and
Dentistry, Rochester, New York
Approach to the Patient with Neurologic Disease

Lev M. Grinberg, MD, PhD
Professor, Chief, Department of Pathology, Ural Medical University;
Chief Researcher of the Ural Scientific Research Institute of
Phthisiopulmonology, Chief Pathologist of Ekaterinburg, Ekaterinburg,
Russia
Anthrax

Daniel Grossman, MD
Vice President for Research, Ibis Reproductive Health, Oakland, California;
Assistant Clinical Professor, Bixby Center for Global Reproductive
Health, Department of Obstetrics, Gynecology and Reproductive
Sciences, University of California San Francisco, San Francisco,
California
Contraception

Lisa M. Guay-Woodford, MD
Hudson Professor of Pediatrics, The George Washington University;
Director, Center for Translational Science, Director, Clinical and
Translational Institute at Children's National, Children's National Health
System, Washington, D.C.
*Hereditary Nephropathies and Developmental Abnormalities of the Urinary
Tract*

Richard L. Guerrant, MD
Thomas H. Hunter Professor of International Medicine, Founding Director, Center for Global Health, Division of Infectious Diseases and International Health, University of Virginia School of Medicine, University of Virginia Health Sciences Center, Charlottesville, Virginia
Cryptosporidiosis

Roy M. Gulick, MD, MPH
Gladys and Roland Harrison Professor of Medicine, Medicine/Infectious Diseases, Weill Cornell Medical College; Attending Physician, New York–Presbyterian Hospital, New York, New York
Antiretroviral Therapy of HIV/AIDS

Klaus D. Hagspiel, MD
Professor of Radiology, Medicine, and Pediatrics, Chief, Noninvasive Cardiovascular Imaging, University of Virginia Health System, Charlottesville, Virginia
Noninvasive Cardiac Imaging

John D. Hainsworth, MD
Chief Scientific Officer, Sarah Cannon Research Institute, Nashville, Tennessee
Cancer of Unknown Primary Origin

Anders Hamsten, MD, PhD
Professor of Cardiovascular Diseases, Center for Molecular Medicine and Department of Cardiology, Karolinska University Hospital, Department of Medicine, Karolinska Institute, Stockholm, Sweden
Atherosclerosis, Thrombosis, and Vascular Biology

Kenneth R. Hande, MD
Professor of Medicine and Pharmacology, Vanderbilt/Ingram Cancer Center, Vanderbilt University School of Medicine, Nashville, Tennessee
Neuroendocrine Tumors and the Carcinoid Syndrome

H. Hunter Handsfield, MD
Professor Emeritus of Medicine, University of Washington Center for AIDS and STD, Seattle, Washington
Neisseria Gonorrhoeae Infections

Göran K. Hansson, MD, PhD
Professor of Cardiovascular Research, Center for Molecular Medicine at Karolinska University Hospital, Department of Medicine, Karolinska Institute, Stockholm, Sweden
Atherosclerosis, Thrombosis, and Vascular Biology

Raymond C. Harris, MD
Professor of Medicine, Ann and Roscoe R. Robinson Chair in Nephrology, Chief, Division of Nephrology, Vanderbilt University School of Medicine, Nashville, Tennessee
Diabetes and the Kidney

Stephen Crane Hauser, MD
Associate Professor of Medicine, Internal Medicine, Division of Gastroenterology and Hepatology, Mayo Clinic College of Medicine, Rochester, Minnesota
Vascular Diseases of the Gastrointestinal Tract

Frederick G. Hayden, MD
Stuart S. Richardson Professor of Clinical Virology and Professor of Medicine, University of Virginia School of Medicine; Staff Physician, University of Virginia Health System, Charlottesville, Virginia
Influenza

Douglas C. Heimburger, MD, MS
Professor of Medicine, Associate Director for Education and Training, Vanderbilt University School of Medicine, Vanderbilt Institute for Global Health, Nashville, Tennessee
Nutrition's Interface with Health and Disease

Erik L. Hewlett, MD
Professor of Medicine and of Microbiology, Immunology, and Cancer Biology, University of Virginia School of Medicine, University of Virginia Health System, Charlottesville, Virginia
Whooping Cough and Other Bordetella Infections

Richard J. Hift, PhD, MMed
School of Clinical Medicine, University of KwaZulu-Natal, Durban, South Africa
The Porphyrias

David R. Hill, MD, DTM&H
Professor of Medical Sciences, Director of Global Public Health, Frank H. Netter MD School of Medicine at Quinnipiac University, Hamden, Connecticut
Giardiasis

Nicholas S. Hill, MD
Professor of Medicine, Tufts University School of Medicine; Chief, Division of Pulmonary, Critical Care, and Sleep Medicine, Tufts Medical Center, Boston, Massachusetts
Respiratory Monitoring in Critical Care

L. David Hillis, MD
Professor and Chair, Department of Medicine, University of Texas Health Science Center at San Antonio, San Antonio, Texas
Acute Coronary Syndrome: Unstable Angina and Non-ST Elevation Myocardial Infarction

Jack Hirsh, CM, MD, DSc
Professor Emeritus, McMaster University, Hamilton, Ontario, Canada
Antithrombotic Therapy

Steven M. Holland, MD
Chief, Laboratory of Clinical Infectious Diseases, National Institute of Allergy and Infectious Diseases, National Institutes of Health, Bethesda, Maryland
The Nontuberculous Mycobacteria

Steven M. Hollenberg, MD
Professor of Medicine, Cooper Medical School of Rowan University; Director, Coronary Care Unit, Cooper University Hospital, Camden, New Jersey
Cardiogenic Shock

Edward W. Hook III, MD
Professor and Director, Division of Infectious Diseases, University of Alabama at Birmingham, Birmingham, Alabama
Granuloma Inguinale (Donovanosis); Syphilis; Nonsyphilitic Treponematoses

David J. Hunter, MBBS, MPH, ScD
Vincent L. Gregory Professor of Cancer Prevention, Harvard School of Public Health; Professor of Medicine, Harvard Medical School, Brigham and Women's Hospital, Boston, Massachusetts
The Epidemiology of Cancer

Khalid Hussain, MBChB, MD, MSc
Developmental Endocrinology Research Group, Clinical and Molecular Genetics Unit, Institute of Child Health, University College London, Department of Paediatric Endocrinology, Great Ormond Street Hospital for Children, London, United Kingdom
Hypoglycemia/Pancreatic Islet Cell Disorders

Steven E. Hyman, MD
Director, Stanley Center for Psychiatric Research, Broad Institute, Distinguished Service Professor of Stem Cell and Regenerative Biology, Harvard University, Cambridge, Massachusetts
Biology of Addiction

Michael C. Iannuzzi, MD, MBA
Chairman, Department of Internal Medicine, State University of New York Upstate Medical University, Syracuse, New York
Sarcoidosis

Robert D. Inman, MD
Professor of Medicine and Immunology, University of Toronto; Staff Rheumatologist, University Health Network, Toronto, Ontario, Canada
The Spondyloarthropathies

Sharon K. Inouye, MD, MPH
Professor of Medicine, Harvard Medical School; Director, Aging Brain Center, Institute for Aging Research, Hebrew SeniorLife, Boston, Massachusetts
Neuropsychiatric Aspects of Aging; Delirium or Acute Mental Status Change in the Older Patient

Geoffrey K. Isbister, MD, BSc
Associate Professor, Clinical Toxicologist, Calvary Mater Newcastle, Callaghan, Senior Research Academic, School of Medicine and Public Health, University of Newcastle, New South Wales, Australia
Envenomation

Michael G. Ison, MD, MS
Associate Professor in Medicine-Infectious Diseases and Surgery-Organ Transplantation, Northwestern University Feinberg School of Medicine, Chicago, Illinois
Adenovirus Diseases

Elias Jabbour, MD
Associate Professor, Department of Leukemia, Division of Medicine, The University of Texas MD Anderson Cancer Center, Houston, Texas
The Chronic Leukemias

Michael R. Jaff, DO
Professor of Medicine, Harvard Medical School, Chair, Institute for Heart, Vascular, and Stroke Care, Massachusetts General Hospital, Boston, Massachusetts
Other Peripheral Arterial Diseases

Joanna C. Jen, MD, PhD
Professor of Neurology, University of California Los Angeles School of Medicine, Los Angeles, California
Neuro-Ophthalmology; Smell and Taste; Hearing and Equilibrium

Dennis M. Jensen, MD
Professor of Medicine, David Geffen School of Medicine at University of California Los Angeles; Staff Physician, Medicine-GI, VA Greater Los Angeles Healthcare System; Key Investigator, Director, Human Studies Core & GI Hemostasis Research Unit, CURE Digestive Diseases Research Center, Los Angeles, California
Gastrointestinal Hemorrhage

Michael D. Jensen, MD
Professor of Medicine, Endocrine Research Unit, Director, Obesity Treatment Research Program, Mayo Clinic, Rochester, Minnesota
Obesity

Robert T. Jensen, MD
Chief, Cell Biology Section, Digestive Disease Branch, National Institute of Diabetes and Digestive and Kidney Diseases, National Institutes of Health, Clinical Center, Bethesda, Maryland
Pancreatic Neuroendocrine Tumors

Stuart Johnson, MD
Professor of Medicine, Loyola University Chicago Stritch School of Medicine; Associate Chief of Staff for Research, Edward Hines, Jr. VA Hospital, Hines, Illinois
Clostridial Infections

Richard C. Jordan, DDS, PhD
Professor of Oral Pathology, Pathology and Radiation Oncology, University of California San Francisco, San Francisco, California
Diseases of the Mouth and Salivary Glands

Ralph F. Józefowicz, MD
Professor, Neurology and Medicine, University of Rochester, Rochester, New York
Approach to the Patient with Neurologic Disease

Stephen G. Kaler, MD
Senior Investigator and Head, Section on Translational Neuroscience, Molecular Medicine Program, Eunice Kennedy Shriver National Institute of Child Health and Human Development, Bethesda, Maryland
Wilson Disease

Moses R. Kamya, MB ChB, MMed, MPH, PhD
Chairman, Department of Medicine, Makerere University College of Health Sciences, Kampala, Uganda
Malaria

Louise W. Kao, MD
Associate Professor of Emergency Medicine, Department of Emergency Medicine, Indiana University School of Medicine, Indianapolis, Indiana
Chronic Poisoning: Trace Metals and Others

Steven A. Kaplan, MD
E. Darracott Vaughan, Jr. Professor of Urology, Chief, Institute for Bladder and Prostate Health, Weill Cornell Medical College; Director, Iris Cantor Men's Health Center, NewYork–Presbyterian Hospital, New York, New York
Benign Prostatic Hyperplasia and Prostatitis

Daniel L. Kastner, MD, PhD
Scientific Director, National Human Genome Research Institute, National Institutes of Health, Bethesda, Maryland
The Systemic Autoinflammatory Diseases

Sekar Kathiresan, MD
Associate Professor in Medicine, Harvard Medical School; Director, Preventive Cardiology, Massachusetts General Hospital, Boston, Massachusetts
The Inherited Basis of Common Diseases

David A. Katzka, MD
Professor of and Consultant in Medicine, Gastroenterology, Mayo Clinic, Rochester, Minnesota
Diseases of the Esophagus

Debra K. Katzman, MD
Professor of Pediatrics, Senior Associate Scientist, The Research Institute, The Hospital for Sick Children and University of Toronto, Toronto, Ontario, Canada
Adolescent Medicine

Carol A. Kauffman, MD
Professor of Internal Medicine, University of Michigan Medical School; Chief, Infectious Diseases Section, Veterans Affairs Ann Arbor Healthcare System, Ann Arbor, Michigan
Histoplasmosis; Blastomycosis; Paracoccidioidomycosis; Cryptococcosis; Sporotrichosis; Candidiasis

Kenneth Kaushansky, MD
Senior Vice President for Health Sciences, Dean, School of Medicine, Stony Brook University, Stony Brook, New York
Hematopoiesis and Hematopoietic Growth Factors

Keith S. Kaye, MD, MPH
Professor of Medicine, Division of Infectious Diseases, Wayne State University School of Medicine, Detroit, Michigan
Diseases Caused by Acinetobacter and Stenotrophomonas Species

Armand Keating, MD
Professor of Medicine, Director, Division of Hematology, Epstein Chair in Cell Therapy and Transplantation, Professor, Institute of Biomaterials and Biomedical Engineering, University of Toronto, Toronto, Ontario, Canada
Hematopoietic Stem Cell Transplantation

Robin K. Kelley, MD
Assistant Professor of Medicine, University of California San Francisco, Helen Diller Family Comprehensive Cancer Center, San Francisco, California
Liver and Biliary Tract Cancers

Morton Kern, MD
Chief of Medicine, VA Long Beach Health Care System School of Medicine; Professor of Medicine, Associate Chief, Cardiology, University of California–Irvine, Irvine, California
Catheterization and Angiography

Gerald T. Keusch, MD
Professor of Medicine and International Health and Public Health, Boston University School of Medicine, Boston, Massachusetts
Shigellosis

Fadlo R. Khuri, MD
Professor and Chair, Hematology and Medical Oncology, Deputy Director, Winship Cancer Institute, Emory University, Atlanta, Georgia
Lung Cancer and Other Pulmonary Neoplasms

David H. Kim, MD
Vice Chair of Education, Professor of Radiology, Section of Abdominal Imaging, University of Wisconsin School of Medicine and Public Health, Madison, Wisconsin
Diagnostic Imaging Procedures in Gastroenterology

Matthew Kim, MD
Instructor of Medicine, Harvard Medical School; Associate Physician, Brigham and Women's Hospital, Boston, Massachusetts
Thyroid

Louis V. Kirchhoff, MD, MPH
Professor, Departments of Internal Medicine (Infectious Diseases) and Epidemiology, University of Iowa Health Care; Staff Physician, Medical Service, Department of Veterans Affairs Medical Center, Iowa City, Iowa
Chagas Disease

David S. Knopman, MD
Professor of Neurology, Mayo Clinic College of Medicine, Rochester, Minnesota
Regional Cerebral Dysfunction: Higher Mental Function; Alzheimer Disease and Other Dementias

Tamsin A. Knox, MD, MPH
Associate Professor of Medicine, Nutrition/Infection Unit, Tufts University School of Medicine, Boston, Massachusetts
Gastrointestinal Manifestions of HIV and AIDS

D.P. Kontoyiannis, MD, ScD
Professor, Department of Infectious Diseases, Infection Control and Employee Health, The University of Texas MD Anderson Cancer Center, Houston, Texas
Mucormycosis; Mycetoma

Barbara S. Koppel, MD
Professor of Clinical Neurology, New York Medical College, Chief of Neurology, Metropolitan Hospital Center, New York City Health and Hospital Corporation, New York, New York
Nutritional and Alcohol-Related Neurologic Disorders

Kevin M. Korenblat, MD
Associate Professor of Medicine, Department of Medicine, Washington University School of Medicine, St. Louis, Missouri
Approach to the Patient with Jaundice or Abnormal Liver Tests

Bruce R. Korf, MD, PhD
Wayne H. and Sara Crews Finley Chair in Medical Genetics, Professor and Chair, Department of Genetics, University of Alabama at Birmingham, Birmingham, Alabama
Principles of Genetics

Neil J. Korman, MD, PhD
Professor, Dermatology, Case Western Reserve University School of Medicine, University Hospitals Case Medical Center, Cleveland, Ohio
Macular, Papular, Vesiculobullous, and Pustular Diseases

Mark G. Kortepeter, MD, MPH
Associate Dean for Research, Associate Professor of Preventive Medicine and Medicine, Consultant to the Army Surgeon General for Biodefense; Office of the Dean, Edward Hébert School of Medicine, Uniformed Services University of the Health Sciences, Bethesda, Maryland
Bioterrorism

Joseph A. Kovacs, MD
Senior Investigator and Head, AIDS Section, Critical Care Medicine Department, National Institutes of Health, Bethesda, Maryland
Pneumocystis Pneumonia

Thomas O. Kovacs, MD
Professor of Medicine, Division of Digestive Diseases, David Geffen School of Medicine at University of California Los Angeles, Los Angeles, California
Gastrointestinal Hemorrhage

Monica Kraft, MD
Professor of Medicine, Duke University School of Medicine; Chief, Division of Pulmonary, Allergy, and Critical Care Medicine, Duke University Medical Center, Durham, North Carolina
Approach to the Patient with Respiratory Disease

Christopher M. Kramer, MD
Ruth C. Heede Professor of Cardiology, Professor of Radiology, Director, Cardiovascular Imaging Center, University of Virginia Health System, Charlottesville, Virginia
Noninvasive Cardiac Imaging

Donna M. Krasnewich, MD, PhD
Program Director, National Institute of General Medical Sciences, National Institutes of Health, Bethesda, Maryland
The Lysosomal Storage Diseases

Peter J. Krause, MD
Senior Research Scientist in Epidemiology, Medicine, and Pediatrics, Yale School of Public Health and Yale School of Medicine, New Haven, Connecticut
Babesiosis and Other Protozoan Diseases

John F. Kuemmerle, MD
Chair, Division of Gastroenterology, Hepatology, and Nutrition, Professor of Medicine, and Physiology and Biophysics, Center for Digestive Health, Virginia Commonwealth University, Richmond, Virginia
Inflammatory and Anatomic Diseases of the Intestine, Peritoneum, Mesentery, and Omentum

Ernst J. Kuipers, MD, PhD
Professor of Medicine, Department of Gastroenterology and Hepatology, Chief Executive Officer, Erasmus MC University Medical Center, Rotterdam, The Netherlands
Acid Peptic Disease

Paul W. Ladenson, MD
Professor of Medicine, Pathology, Oncology, and Radiology and Radiological Sciences, John Eager Howard Professor of Endocrinology and Metabolism, University Distinguished Service Professor, The Johns Hopkins University School of Medicine; Physician and Division Director, The Johns Hopkins Hospital, Baltimore, Maryland
Thyroid

Daniel Laheru, MD
Ian T. MacMillan Professorship in Clinical Pancreatic Research, Medical Oncology, Johns Hopkins University School of Medicine, Baltimore, Maryland
Pancreatic Cancer

Donald W. Landry, MD, PhD
Samuel Bard Professor of Medicine, Chair, Department of Medicine, Physician-in-Chief, NewYork-Presbyterian Hospital/Columbia University Medical Center, New York, New York
Approach to the Patient with Renal Disease

Anthony E. Lang, MD
Director, Division of Neurology, Jack Clark Chair for Research in Parkinson's Disease, University of Toronto; Director, Morton and Gloria Shulman Movement Disorders Clinic and the Edmond J. Safra Program in Parkinson's Disease and the Lily Safra Chair in Movement Disorders, Toronto Western Hospital, Toronto, Ontario, Canada
Parkinsonism; Other Movement Disorders

Richard A. Lange, MD, MBA
President and Dean, Paul L. Foster School of Medicine, Texas Tech University Health Sciences Center El Paso, El Paso, Texas
Acute Coronary Syndrome: Unstable Angina and Non-ST Elevation Myocardial Infarction

Frank A. Lederle, MD
Core Investigator, Center for Chronic Disease Outcomes Research, Minneapolis VA Medical Center; Professor of Medicine, University of Minnesota School of Medicine, Minneapolis, Minnesota
Diseases of the Aorta

Thomas H. Lee, MD, MSc
Senior Physician, Department of Medicine, Brigham and Women's Hospital; Chief Medical Officer, Press Ganey, Boston, Massachusetts
Using Data for Clinical Decisions

William M. Lee, MD
Professor of Internal Medicine, University of Texas Southwestern Medical Center, Dallas, Texas
Toxin- and Drug-Induced Liver Disease

James E. Leggett, MD
Associate Professor, Department of Medicine, Oregon Health and Science University; Infectious Diseases, Department of Medical Education, Providence Portland Medical Center, Portland, Oregon
Approach to Fever or Suspected Infection in the Normal Host

Stuart Levin, MD
Professor of Medicine, Emeritus Chairman, Department of Medicine, Rush University Medical Center, Chicago, Illinois
Zoonoses

Stephanie M. Levine, MD
Professor of Medicine, Division of Pulmonary Diseases and Critical Care Medicine, The University of Texas Health Science Center San Antonio, South Texas Veterans Health Care System, San Antonio, Texas
Alveolar Filling Disorders

Gary R. Lichtenstein, MD
Professor of Medicine, Perelman School of Medicine at the University of Pennsylvania, Director, Center for Inflammatory Bowel Disease, University of Pennsylvania, Philadelphia, Pennsylvania
Inflammatory Bowel Disease

Henry W. Lim, MD
Chairman and C.S. Livingood Chair, Department of Dermatology, Henry Ford Hospital; Senior Vice President for Academic Affairs, Henry Ford Health System, Detroit, Michigan
Eczemas, Photodermatoses, Papulosquamous (Including Fungal) Diseases, and Figurate Erythemas

Aldo A.M. Lima, MD, PhD
Professor of Medicine and Pharmacology, School of Medicine, Federal University of Ceará, Fortaleza, Ceará, Brazil
Cryptosporidiosis; Amebiasis

Geoffrey S.F. Ling, MD, PhD
Professor of Neurology, Uniformed Services University of the Health Sciences, Bethesda, Maryland
Traumatic Brain Injury and Spinal Cord Injury

William C. Little, MD
Patrick Lehan Professor of Cardiovascular Medicine, Chair, Department of Medicine, University of Mississippi Medical Center, Jackson, Mississippi
Pericardial Diseases

Donald M. Lloyd-Jones, MD, ScM
Senior Associate Dean, Chair, Department of Preventive Medicine, Eileen M. Foell Professor of Preventive Medicine and Medicine, Northwestern University Feinberg School of Medicine, Chicago, Illinois
Epidemiology of Cardiovascular Disease

Bennett Lorber, MD
Thomas M. Durant Professor of Medicine and Professor of Microbiology and Immunology, Temple University School of Medicine, Philadelphia, Pennsylvania
Listeriosis

Donald E. Low, MD†
Nonpneumococcal Streptococcal Infections, Rheumatic Fever

Daniel R. Lucey, MD, MPH
Adjunct Professor, Microbiology and Immunology, Georgetown University Medical Center, Washington, D.C.
Anthrax

James R. Lupski, MD, PhD
Cullen Professor of Molecular and Human Genetics, Professor of Pediatrics, Baylor College of Medicine and Texas Children's Hospital, Houston, Texas
Gene, Genomic, and Chromosomal Disorders

Jeffrey M. Lyness, MD
Senior Associate Dean for Academic Affairs, Professor of Psychiatry and Neurology, University of Rochester School of Medicine and Dentistry, Rochester, New York
Psychiatric Disorders in Medical Practice

Bruce W. Lytle, MD
Chair, Heart and Vascular Institute, Professor of Surgery, Thoracic and Cardiovascular Surgery, Cleveland Clinic, Cleveland, Ohio
Interventional and Surgical Treatment of Coronary Artery Disease

†Deceased.

C. Ronald MacKenzie, MD
Assistant Attending Physician, Department of Medicine-Rheumatology,
C. Ronald MacKenzie Chair in Ethics and Medicine, Hospital for Special
Surgery, Associate Professor of Clinical Medicine and Medical Ethics,
Weill Cornell Medical College of Cornell University, New York,
New York
Surgical Treatment of Joint Disease

Harriet L. MacMillan, MD, MSc
Professor, Departments of Psychiatry and Behavioural Neurosciences, and
Pediatrics, Chedoke Health Chair in Child Psychiatry, Offord Centre for
Child Studies, McMaster University, Hamilton, Ontario, Canada
Intimate Partner Violence

Robert D. Madoff, MD
Professor of Surgery, Stanley M. Goldberg, MD, Chair, Colon and Rectal
Surgery, University of Minnesota, Minneapolis, Minnesota
Diseases of the Rectum and Anus

Frank Maldarelli, MD, PhD
Head, Clinical Retrovirology Section, HIV Drug Resistance Program,
National Cancer Institute, National Institutes of Health, Bethesda,
Maryland
Biology of Human Immunodeficiency Viruses

Atul Malhotra, MD
Chief of Pulmonary and Critical Care, Kenneth M. Moser Professor of
Medicine, Director of Sleep Medicine, University of California San
Diego, La Jolla, California
Disorders of Ventilatory Control

Mark J. Manary, MD
Helene B. Roberson Professor of Pediatrics, Washington University School
of Medicine; Attending Physician, St. Louis Children's Hospital, St.
Louis, Missouri; Adjunct Professor, Children's Nutrition Research
Center, Baylor College of Medicine, Houston, Texas; Senior Lecturer in
Community Health, University of Malawi College of Medicine, Blantyre,
Malawi
Protein-Energy Malnutrition

Donna Mancini, MD
Professor of Medicine, Department of Medicine, Division of Cardiology,
Columbia University College of Physicians and Surgeons, Center for
Advanced Cardiac Care, Columbia University Medical Center, New
York, New York
Cardiac Transplantation

Lionel A. Mandell, MD
Professor of Medicine, Faculty of Health Sciences, McMaster University,
Hamilton, Ontario, Canada
Streptococcus Pneumoniae Infections

Peter Manu, MD
Professor of Medicine and Psychiatry, Hofstra North Shore–LIJ School of
Medicine at Hofstra University, Hempstead, New York; Adjunct
Professor of Clinical Medicine, Psychiatry and Behavioral Sciences,
Albert Einstein College of Medicine, Bronx, New York; Director of
Medical Services, Zucker Hillside Hospital, Glen Oaks, New York
Medical Consultation in Psychiatry

Ariane Marelli, MD, MPH
Professor of Medicine, McGill University, Director, McGill Adult Unit for
Congenital Heart Disease, Associate Director, Academic Affairs and
Research, Cardiology, McGill University Health Centre, Montreal,
Québec, Canada
Congenital Heart Disease in Adults

Xavier Mariette, MD, PhD
Professor, Rheumatology, Université Paris-Sud, AP-HP, Le Kremlin Bicêtre,
France
Sjögren Syndrome

Andrew R. Marks, MD
Wu Professor and Chair, Department of Physiology and Cellular
Biophysics, Founding Director, Helen and Clyde Wu Center for
Molecular Cardiology, Columbia University College of Physicians and
Surgeons, New York, New York
Cardiac Function and Circulatory Control

Kieren A. Marr, MD
Professor of Medicine and Oncology, The Johns Hopkins University,
Director, Transplant and Oncology Infectious Diseases, Baltimore,
Maryland
Approach to Fever and Suspected Infection in the Compromised Host

Thomas J. Marrie, MD
Dean, Faculty of Medicine, Dalhousie University; Professor of Medicine,
Capital District Health Authority, Halifax, Nova Scotia, Canada
Legionella Infections

Paul Martin, MD
Professor of Medicine and Chief, Division of Hepatology, Miller School of
Medicine, University of Miami, Miami, Florida
Approach to the Patient with Liver Disease

Joel B. Mason, MD
Professor of Medicine and Nutrition, Tufts University; Staff Physician,
Divisions of Gastroenterology and Clinical Nutrition, Tufts Medical
Center, Boston, Massachusetts
Vitamins, Trace Minerals, and Other Micronutrients

Henry Masur, MD
Chief, Critical Care Medicine Department, Clinical Center, National
Institutes of Health, Bethesda, Maryland
Infectious and Metabolic Complications of HIV and AIDS

Eric L. Matteson, MD, MPH
Professor of Medicine, Mayo Clinic College of Medicine, Consultant,
Divisions of Rheumatology and Epidemiology, Mayo Clinic, Rochester,
Minnesota
Infections of Bursae, Joints, and Bones

Michael A. Matthay, MD
Professor, Departments of Medicine and Anesthesia, University of
California San Francisco, San Francisco, California
Acute Respiratory Failure

Toby A. Maurer, MD
Professor of Dermatology, University of California San Francisco; Chief of
Dermatology, San Francisco General Hospital, San Francisco, California
Skin Manifestations in Patients with Human Immunodeficiency Virus Infection

Emeran A. Mayer, MD, PhD
Professor of Medicine, Physiology, and Psychiatry, Division of Digestive
Diseases, Department of Medicine, University of California Los Angeles,
Los Angeles, California
*Functional Gastrointestinal Disorders: Irritable Bowel Syndrome, Dyspepsia,
Chest Pain of Presumed Esophageal Origin, and Heartburn*

Stephan A. Mayer, MD
Director, Institute for Critical Care Medicine, Icahn School of Medicine at
Mount Sinai, New York, New York
Hemorrhagic Cerebrovascular Disease

Stephen A. McClave, MD
Professor of Medicine, Director of Clinical Nutrition, University of
Louisville School of Medicine, Louisville, Kentucky
Enteral Nutrition

F. Dennis McCool, MD
Professor of Medicine, The Warren Alpert Medical School of Brown
University; Medical Director of Sleep Center, Memorial Hospital of
Rhode Island, Pawtucket, Rhode Island
Diseases of the Diaphragm, Chest Wall, Pleura, and Mediastinum

Charles E. McCulloch, PhD
Professor of Biostatistics, Department of Epidemiology and Biostatistics, University of California San Francisco, San Francisco, California
Statistical Interpretation of Data

William J. McKenna, MD
Professor of Cardiology, Institute of Cardiovascular Science, University College London, London, United Kingdom
Diseases of the Myocardium and Endocardium

Vallerie McLaughlin, MD
Kim A. Eagle, MD, Endowed Professor of Cardiovascular Medicine, Director, Pulmonary Hypertension Program, University of Michigan, Ann Arbor, Michigan
Pulmonary Hypertension

John J.V. McMurray, MB, MD
Professor of Cardiology, Institute of Cardiovascular and Medical Sciences, University of Glasgow, Glasgow, Scotland, United Kingdom
Heart Failure: Management and Prognosis

Kenneth R. McQuaid, MD
Professor of Clinical Medicine, Marvin H. Sleisenger Endowed Chair, Vice Chairman, University of California San Francisco; Chief, Medical Services and Gastroenterology, San Francisco VA Medical Center, San Francisco, California
Approach to the Patient with Gastrointestinal Disease

Marc Michel, MD
Professor of Internal Medicine, Head of the Unit of Internal Medicine at Henri Mondor University Hospital, National Referral Center for Adult's Immune Cytopenias, Creteil, France
Autoimmune and Intravascular Hemolytic Anemias

Jonathan W. Mink, MD, PhD
Frederick A. Horner, MD Endowed Professor in Pediatric Neurology, Professor of Neurology, Neurobiology & Anatomy, Brain & Cognitive Sciences, and Pediatrics, Chief, Division of Child Neurology, Vice Chair, Department of Neurology, University of Rochester, Rochester, New York
Congenital, Developmental, and Neurocutaneous Disorders

William E. Mitch, MD
Gordon A. Cain Chair in Nephrology, Director of Nephrology, Baylor College of Medicine, Houston, Texas
Chronic Kidney Disease

Mark E. Molitch, MD
Martha Leland Sherwin Professor of Endocrinology, Division of Endocrinology, Metabolism, and Molecular Medicine, Northwestern University Feinberg School of Medicine, Chicago, Illinois
Neuroendocrinology and the Neuroendocrine System; Anterior Pituitary

Bruce A. Molitoris, MD
Professor of Medicine, and Cellular and Integrative Physiology Director, Indiana Center for Biological Microscopy, Indiana University, Indianapolis, Indiana
Acute Kidney Injury

Jose G. Montoya, MD
Professor of Medicine, Division of Infectious Disease and Geographic Medicine, Stanford University School of Medicine, Stanford, California; Director, Palo Alto Medical Foundation Toxoplasma Serology Laboratory, National Reference Center for the Study and Diagnosis of Toxoplasmosis, Palo Alto, California
Toxoplasmosis

Alison Morris, MD, MS
Associate Professor of Medicine, Clinical Translational Science, and Immunology, Division of Pulmonary, Allergy, and Critical Care Medicine, University of Pittsburgh School of Medicine, Pittsburgh, Pennsylvania
Pulmonary Manifestations of Human Immunodeficiency Virus and Acquired Immunodeficiency Syndrome

Ernest Moy, MD, MPH
Medical Officer, Center for Quality Improvement and Patient Safety Agency for Healthcare Research and Quality, Rockville, Maryland
Measuring Health and Health Care

Atis Muehlenbachs, MD, PhD
Infectious Diseases Pathology Branch, Centers for Disease Control and Prevention, Atlanta, Georgia
Leptospirosis

Andrew H. Murr, MD
Professor and Chairman, Roger Boles, MD Endowed Chair in Otolaryngology Education, Department of Otolaryngology-Head and Neck Surgery, University of California San Francisco School of Medicine, San Francisco, California
Approach to the Patient with Nose, Sinus, and Ear Disorders

Daniel M. Musher, MD
Professor of Medicine, Molecular Virology, and Microbiology, Distinguished Service Professor, Baylor College of Medicine, Infectious Disease Section, Michael E. DeBakey Veterans Affairs Medical Center, Houston, Texas
Overview of Pneumonia

Robert J. Myerburg, MD
Professor of Medicine and Physiology, Division of Cardiology, Department of Medicine, American Heart Association Chair in Cardiovascular Research, University of Miami Miller School of Medicine, Miami, Florida
Approach to Cardiac Arrest and Life-Threatening Arrhythmias

Sandesh C.S. Nagamani, MD
Assistant Professor, Department of Molecular and Human Genetics, Director, Clinic for Metabolic and Genetic Disorders of Bone, Baylor College of Medicine and Texas Children's Hospital, Houston, Texas
Gene, Genomic, and Chromosomal Disorders

Stanley J. Naides, MD
Medical Director and Interim Scientific Director, Immunology, Quest Diagnostics Nichols Institute, San Juan Capistrano, California
Arboviruses Causing Fever and Rash Syndromes

Yoshifumi Naka, MD, PhD
Professor of Surgery, Department of Surgery, Columbia University College of Physicians and Surgeons, New York, New York
Cardiac Transplantation

Theodore E. Nash, MD
Principal Investigator, Clinical Parasitology Section, Laboratory of Parasitic Diseases, National Institute of Allergy and Infectious Diseases, National Institutes of Health, Bethesda, Maryland
Giardiasis

Avindra Nath, MD
Chief, Section of Infections of the Nervous System, National Institute of Neurological Disorders and Stroke, National Institutes of Health, Bethesda, Maryland
Cytomegalovirus, Epstein-Barr Virus, and Slow Virus Infections of the Central Nervous System; Neurologic Complications of Human Immunodeficiency Virus Infection; Meningitis: Bacterial, Viral, and Other; Brain Abscess and Parameningeal Infections

Eric G. Neilson, MD
Vice President for Medical Affairs and Lewis Landsberg Dean, Northwestern University Feinberg School of Medicine, Northwestern Memorial Hospital, Chicago, Illinois
Tubulointerstitial Nephritis

Lawrence S. Neinstein, MD
Professor of Pediatrics and Medicine, Keck School of Medicine of USC; Executive Director, Engemann Student Health Center, Division Head of College Health, Assistant Provost, Student Health and Wellness, University of Southern California, Los Angeles, California
Adolescent Medicine

Lewis S. Nelson, MD
Professor of Emergency Medicine, Director, Fellowship in Medical Toxicology, New York University School of Medicine; Attending Physician, New York University Langone Medical Center and Bellevue Hospital Center, New York, New York
Acute Poisoning

Eric J. Nestler, MD, PhD
Nash Family Professor and Chair, Department of Neuroscience, Director, The Friedman Brain Institute, Icahn School of Medicine at Mount Sinai, New York, New York
Biology of Addiction

Anne B. Newman, MD, MPH
Professor of Epidemiology, The University of Pittsburgh Graduate School of Public Health; Chair, Department of Epidemiology, Director, University of Pittsburgh Center for Aging and Population Health, Pittsburgh, Pennsylvania
Epidemiology of Aging: Implications of the Aging of Society

Thomas B. Newman, MD, MPH
Professor, Epidemiology & Biostatistics and Pediatrics, University of California San Francisco, San Francisco, California
Statistical Interpretation of Data

William L. Nichols, MD
Associate Professor, Medicine and Laboratory Medicine, Mayo Clinic College of Medicine; Staff Physician, Special Coagulation Laboratory, Comprehensive Hemophilia Center, and Coagulation Clinic, Mayo Clinic, Rochester, Minnesota
Von Willebrand Disease and Hemorrhagic Abnormalities of Platelet and Vascular Function

Lindsay E. Nicolle, MD
Professor of Internal Medicine and Medical Microbiology, University of Manitoba, Health Sciences Centre, Winnipeg, Manitoba, Canada
Approach to the Patient with Urinary Tract Infection

Lynnette K. Nieman, MD
Senior Investigator, Program on Reproductive and Adult Endocrinology, Eunice Kennedy Shriver National Institute of Child Health and Human Development, Bethesda, Maryland
Approach to the Patient with Endocrine Disease; Adrenal Cortex; Polyglandular Disorders

Dennis E. Niewoehner, MD
Professor of Medicine, University of Minnesota; Staff Physician, Minneapolis Veterans Affairs Health Care System, Minneapolis, Minnesota
Chronic Obstructive Pulmonary Disease

S. Ragnar Norrby, MD, PhD
Director General, Swedish Institute for Infectious Disease Control, Solna, Sweden
Approach to the Patient with Urinary Tract Infection

Susan O'Brien, MD
Professor, Department of Leukemia, Division of Medicine, The University of Texas MD Anderson Cancer Center, Houston, Texas
The Chronic Leukemias

Christopher M. O'Connor, MD
Professor of Medicine and Chief, Division of Cardiology, Director, Duke Heart Center, Durham, North Carolina
Heart Failure: Pathophysiology and Diagnosis

Francis G. O'Connor, MD, MPH
Professor and Chair, Military and Emergency Medicine, Medical Director, Uniformed Services University Consortium for Health and Military Performance, Bethesda, Maryland
Disorders Due to Heat and Cold; Rhabdomyolysis

Patrick G. O'Connor, MD, MPH
Professor and Chief, General Internal Medicine, Yale University School of Medicine, New Haven, Connecticut
Alcohol Abuse and Dependence

James R. O'Dell, MD
Bruce Professor and Vice Chair of Internal Medicine, Chief, Division of Rheumatology, University of Nebraska Medical Center and Omaha VA Nebraska–Western Iowa Health Care System, Omaha, Nebraska
Rheumatoid Arthritis

Anne E. O'Donnell, MD
Professor of Medicine, Chief, Division of Pulmonary, Critical Care, and Sleep Medicine, Georgetown University Medical Center, Washington, D.C.
Bronchiectasis, Atelectasis, Cysts, and Localized Lung Disorders

Jae K. Oh, MD
Professor of Medicine, Director, Echocardiography Core Laboratory and Pericardial Clinic, Division of Cardiovascular Diseases, Co-Director, Integrated Cardiac Imaging, Division of Cardiovascular Diseases, Mayo Clinic, Rochester, Minnesota
Pericardial Diseases

Jeffrey E. Olgin, MD
Gallo-Chatterjee Distinguished Professor of Medicine, Chief, Division of Cardiology, Co-Director, Heart and Vascular Center, University of California San Francisco, San Francisco, California
Approach to the Patient with Suspected Arrhythmia

Walter A. Orenstein, MD
Professor of Medicine, Pediatrics, and Global Health, Emory University School of Medicine, Atlanta, Georgia
Immunization

Douglas R. Osmon, MD, MPH
Professor of Medicine, Mayo Clinic College of Medicine; Consultant, Division of Infectious Diseases, Mayo Clinic, Rochester, Minnesota
Infections of Bursae, Joints, and Bones

Catherine M. Otto, MD
J. Ward Kennedy-Hamilton Endowed Chair in Cardiology, Professor of Medicine, University of Washington School of Medicine; Director, Heart Valve Clinic, University of Washington Medical Center, Seattle, Washington
Echocardiography

Mark Papania, MD, MPH
Medical Epidemiologist, Division of Viral Diseases, Measles, Mumps, Rubella, and Herpes Virus Laboratory Branch, Centers for Disease Control and Prevention, Atlanta, Georgia
Measles

Peter G. Pappas, MD
Professor of Medicine, University of Alabama at Birmingham, Birmingham, Alabama
Dematiaceous Fungal Infections

Pankaj Jay Pasricha, MD
Director, The Johns Hopkins Center for Neurogastroenterology; Professor of Medicine and Neurosciences, The Johns Hopkins School of Medicine; Professor of Innovation Management, Johns Hopkins Carey Business School, Baltimore, Maryland
Gastrointestinal Endoscopy

David L. Paterson, MD
Professor of Medicine, University of Queensland Centre for Clinical Research, Royal Brisbane and Women's Hospital Campus, Brisbane, Queensland, Australia
Infections Due to Other Members of the Enterobacteriaceae, Including Management of Multidrug Resistant Strains

Carlo Patrono, MD
Professor and Chair of Pharmacology, Department of Pharmacology, Catholic University School of Medicine, Rome, Italy
Prostaglandin, Aspirin, and Related Compounds

Jean-Michel Pawlotsky, MD, PhD
Professor of Medicine, The University of Paris-Est; Director, National Reference Center for Viral Hepatitis B, C, and Delta and Department of Virology, Henri Mondor University Hospital; Director, Department of Molecular Virology and Immunology, Institut Mondor de Recherche Biomédicale, Créteil, France
Acute Viral Hepatitis; Chronic Viral and Autoimmune Hepatitis

Richard D. Pearson, MD
Professor of Medicine and Pathology, University of Virginia School of Medicine and University of Virginia Health System, Charlottesville, Virginia
Antiparasitic Therapy

Trish M. Perl, MD, MSc
Professor of Medicine and Pathology, The Johns Hopkins School of Medicine; Professor of Epidemiology, Johns Hopkins Bloomberg School of Public Health; Infectious Diseases Specialist and Senior Epidemiologist, The Johns Hopkins Hospital and Health System, Baltimore, Maryland
Enterococcal Infections

Adam Perlman, MD, MPH
Associate Professor, Department of Medicine, Duke University Medical Center; Executive Director, Duke Integrative Medicine, Duke University Health System, Durham, North Carolina
Complementary and Alternative Medicine

William A. Petri, Jr., MD, PhD
Wade Hampton Frost Professor, Departments of Medicine, Pathology, Microbiology, Immunology, and Cancer Biology, School of Medicine, University of Virginia; Chief, Division of Infectious Diseases and International Health, University of Virginia Hospitals, Charlottesville, Virginia
Relapsing Fever and Other Borrelia Infections; African Sleeping Sickness; Amebiasis

Marc A. Pfeffer, MD, PhD
Dzau Professor of Medicine, Harvard Medical School; Senior Physician, Cardiovascular Division, Brigham and Women's Hospital, Boston, Massachusetts
Heart Failure: Management and Prognosis

Perry J. Pickhardt, MD
Professor of Radiology and Chief, Gastrointestinal Imaging, Section of Abdominal Imaging, University of Wisconsin School of Medicine and Public Health, Madison, Wisconsin
Diagnostic Imaging Procedures in Gastroenterology

David S. Pisetsky, MD, PhD
Chief of Rheumatology, Medical Research Service, Durham VA Medical Center; Professor of Medicine and Immunology, Department of Medicine, Duke University Medical Center, Durham, North Carolina
Laboratory Testing in the Rheumatic Diseases

Marshall R. Posner, MD
Professor of Medicine, Director of Head and Neck Medical Oncology, Director of the Office of Cancer Clinical Trials, The Tisch Cancer Institute, Icahn School of Medicine at Mount Sinai, New York, New York
Head and Neck Cancer

Frank Powell, PhD
Professor of Medicine, Chief of Physiology, University of California San Diego, La Jolla, California
Disorders of Ventilatory Control

Reed E. Pyeritz, MD, PhD
William Smilow Professor of Medicine and Genetics and Vice Chair for Academic Affairs, Perelman School of Medicine at the University of Pennsylvania, Philadelphia, Pennsylvania
Inherited Diseases of Connective Tissue

Thomas C. Quinn, MD, MSc
Associate Director for International Research, Head, Section of International HIV/AIDS Research, Division of Intramural Research, National Institute of Allergy and Infectious Diseases, National Institutes of Health; Professor of Medicine, Pathology, International Health, Molecular Microbiology and Immunology, and Epidemiology, The Johns Hopkins Medical Institutions, Baltimore, Maryland
Epidemiology and Diagnosis of Human Immunodeficiency Virus Infection and Acquired Immunodeficiency Syndrome

Jai Radhakrishnan, MD, MS
Professor of Medicine, Division of Nephrology, Department of Medicine, Columbia University Medical Center; Associate Division Chief for Clinical Affairs, Division of Nephrology, New York-Presbyterian Hospital, New York, New York
Glomerular Disorders and Nephrotic Syndromes

Petros I. Rafailidis, MD, PhD, MSc
Senior Researcher, Alfa Institute of Biomedical Sciences, Attending Physician, Department of Medicine and Hematology, Athens Medical Center, Athens Medical Group, Athens, Greece
Pseudomonas and Related Gram-Negative Bacillary Infections

Ganesh Raghu, MD
Adjunct Professor of Medicine and Laboratory Medicine, University of Washington, Director, CENTER for Interstitial Lung Diseases at the University of Washington; Co-Director, Scleroderma Clinic, University of Washington Medical Center, Seattle, Washington
Interstitial Lung Disease

Margaret Ragni, MD, MPH
Professor of Medicine and Clinical Translational Science, Department of Hematology/Oncology, University of Pittsburgh Medical Center; Director, Hemophilia Center of Western Pennsylvania, Pittsburgh, Pennsylvania
Hemorrhagic Disorders: Coagulation Factor Deficiencies

Srinivasa N. Raja, MD
Professor of Anesthesiology and Neurology, Director, Division of Pain Medicine, The Johns Hopkins University School of Medicine, Baltimore, Maryland
Pain

S. Vincent Rajkumar, MD
Professor of Medicine, Division of Hematology, Mayo Clinic, Rochester, Minnesota
Plasma Cell Disorders

Stuart H. Ralston, MB ChB, MD
Professor of Rheumatology, Institute of Genetics and Molecular Medicine, Western General Hospital, The University of Edinburgh, Edinburgh, United Kingdom
Paget Disease of Bone

Didier Raoult, MD, PhD
Professor, Aix Marseille Université, Faculté de Médecine; Chief, Hôpital de la Timone, Fédération de Microbiologie Clinique, Marseille, France
Bartonella Infections; Rickettsial Infections

Robert W. Rebar, MD
Professor, Department of Obstetrics and Gynecology, Western Michigan University Homer Stryker MD School of Medicine, Kalamazoo, Michigan
Ovaries and Development; Reproductive Endocrinology and Infertility

Annette C. Reboli, MD
Founding Vice Dean, Professor of Medicine, Cooper Medical School of Rowan University, Cooper University Healthcare, Department of Medicine, Division of Infectious Diseases, Camden, New Jersey
Erysipelothrix Infections

K. Rajender Reddy, MD
Professor of Medicine, Professor of Medicine in Surgery, Perelman School of Medicine at the University of Pennsylvania; Director of Hepatology, Director, Viral Hepatitis Center, Hospital of the University of Pennsylvania, Philadelphia, Pennsylvania
Bacterial, Parasitic, Fungal, and Granulomatous Liver Diseases

Donald A. Redelmeier, MD
Professor of Medicine, University of Toronto; Senior Scientist and Staff Physician, Sunnybrook Health Sciences Centre, Toronto, Ontario, Canada
Postoperative Care and Complications

Susan E. Reef, MD
Centers for Disease Control and Prevention, Atlanta, Georgia
Rubella (German Measles)

Neil M. Resnick, MD
Thomas P. Detre Endowed Chair in Gerontology and Geriatric Medicine, Professor of Medicine and Division Chief, Geriatrics, Associate Director, University of Pittsburgh Institute on Aging, University of Pittsburgh; Chief, Division of Geriatric Medicine and Gerontology, University of Pittsburgh Medical Center, Pittsburgh, Pennsylvania
Incontinence

David B. Reuben, MD
Director, Multicampus Program in Geriatric Medicine and Gerontology; Chief, Division of Geriatrics, Archstone Professor of Medicine, David Geffen School of Medicine at University of California Los Angeles, Los Angeles, California
Geriatric Assessment

Emanuel P. Rivers, MD, MPH
Professor and Vice Chairman of Emergency Medicine, Wayne State University; Senior Staff Attending, Critical Care and Emergency Medicine, Henry Ford Hospital, Detroit, Michigan
Approach to the Patient with Shock

Joseph G. Rogers, MD
Professor of Medicine, Senior Vice Chief for Clinical Affairs, Division of Cardiology, Durham, North Carolina
Heart Failure: Pathophysiology and Diagnosis

Jean-Marc Rolain, PharmD, PhD
Professor, Institut Hospitalo-Universitaire Méditerranée-Infection, Aix-Marseille Université, Marseille, France
Bartonella Infections

José R. Romero, MD
Professor of Pediatrics, University of Arkansas for Medical Sciences, Horace C. Cabe Professor of Infectious Diseases; Director, Section of Pediatric Infectious Diseases, Arkansas Children's Hospital, Little Rock, Arkansas
Enteroviruses

Karen Rosene-Montella, MD
Professor and Vice Chair of Medicine, Director of Obstetric Medicine, The Warren Alpert Medical School of Brown University; Senior Vice President, Women's Services and Clinical Integration, Lifespan Health System, Providence, Rhode Island
Common Medical Problems in Pregnancy

Philip J. Rosenthal, MD
Professor, Department of Medicine, University of California San Francisco, San Francisco, California
Malaria

Marc E. Rothenberg, MD, PhD
Director, Division of Allergy and Immunology, Director, Cincinnati Center for Eosinophilic Disorders; Professor of Pediatrics, Cincinnati Children's Hospital Medical Center, University of Cincinnati College of Medicine, Cincinnati, Ohio
Eosinophilic Syndromes

James A. Russell, MD
Professor of Medicine, University of British Columbia; Associate Director, Intensive Care Unit, St. Paul's Hospital, Vancouver, British Columbia, Canada
Shock Syndromes Related to Sepsis

Anil K. Rustgi, MD
T. Grier Miller Professor of Medicine and Genetics, Chief of Gastroenterology, American Cancer Society; Professor, Perelman School of Medicine at the University of Pennsylvania, Philadelphia, Pennsylvania
Neoplasms of the Esophagus and Stomach

Daniel E. Rusyniak, MD
Professor of Emergency Medicine, Adjunct Professor of Neurology and Pharmacology and Toxicology, Department of Emergency Medicine, Indiana University School of Medicine, Indianapolis, Indiana
Chronic Poisoning: Trace Metals and Others

Robert A. Salata, MD
Professor and Executive Vice Chair, Department of Medicine, Chief, Division of Infectious Diseases and HIV Medicine, Case Western Reserve University, University Hospitals Case Medical Center, Cleveland, Ohio
Brucellosis

Jane E. Salmon, MD
Collette Kean Research Chair, Hospital for Special Surgery, Professor of Medicine, Weill Cornell Medical College, New York, New York
Mechanisms of Immune-Mediated Tissue Injury

Edsel Maurice T. Salvana, MD, DTM&H
Associate Professor of Medicine, Section of Infectious Diseases, Department of Medicine, Philippine General Hospital; Director, Institute of Molecular Biology and Biotechnology, National Institutes of Health, University of the Philippines Manila, Manila, Philippines
Brucellosis

Renato M. Santos, MD
Associate Professor, Cardiology, Wake Forest School of Medicine, Winston-Salem, North Carolina
Vascular Disorders of the Kidney

Michael N. Sawka, PhD
Professor, School of Applied Physiology, Georgia Institute of Technology, Atlanta, Georgia
Disorders Due to Heat and Cold

Paul D. Scanlon, MD
Professor of Medicine, Division of Pulmonary and Critical Care Medicine, Mayo Clinic, Rochester, Minnesota
Respiratory Function: Mechanisms and Testing

Carla Scanzello, MD, PhD
Assistant Professor of Medicine, Division of Rheumatology, Perelman School of Medicine at the University of Pennsylvania and Translational Musculoskeletal Research Center, Philadelphia Veterans Affairs Medical Center, Philadelphia, Pennsylvania
Osteoarthritis

Andrew I. Schafer, MD
Professor of Medicine, Director, Richard T. Silver Center for Myeloproliferative Neoplasms, Weill Cornell Medical College, New York, New York
Approach to Medicine, the Patient, and the Medical Profession: Medicine as a Learned and Humane Profession; Approach to the Patient with Bleeding and Thrombosis; Hemorrhagic Disorders: Disseminated Intravascular Coagulation, Liver Failure, and Vitamin K Deficiency; Thrombotic Disorders: Hypercoagulable States

William Schaffner, MD
Professor and Chair, Department of Preventive Medicine, Department of Health Policy; Professor of Medicine (Infectious Diseases), Vanderbilt University School of Medicine, Nashville, Tennessee
Tularemia and Other Francisella Infections

W. Michael Scheld, MD
Bayer-Gerald L. Mandell Professor of Infectious Diseases, Professor of Medicine, Clinical Professor of Neurosurgery, Director, Pfizer Initiative in International Health, University of Virginia Health System, Charlottesville, Virginia
Introduction to Microbial Disease: Host-Pathogen Interactions

Manuel Schiff, MD
Professor, Université Paris 7 Denis Diderot, Sorbonne Paris Cité, Head of Metabolic Unit/Reference Center for Inborn Errors of Metabolism, Robert Debré University Hospital, APHP, Paris, France
Homocystinuria and Hyperhomocysteinemia

Michael L. Schilsky, MD
Associate Professor, Medicine and Surgery, Yale University School of Medicine, New Haven, Connecticut
Wilson Disease

Robert T. Schooley, MD
Professor and Head, Division of Infectious Diseases, Executive Vice Chair for Academic Affairs, Department of Medicine, University of California San Diego, La Jolla, California
Epstein-Barr Virus Infection

David L. Schriger, MD, MPH
Professor, Department of Emergency Medicine, University of California Los Angeles, Los Angeles, California
Approach to the Patient with Abnormal Vital Signs

Steven A. Schroeder, MD
Distinguished Professor of Health and Healthcare and of Medicine, University of California San Francisco, San Francisco, California
Socioeconomic Issues in Medicine

Lynn M. Schuchter, MD
Professor of Medicine, University of Pennsylvania; Chief, Hematology/Oncology Division, Program Leader, Melanoma and Cutaneous Malignancies Program, Abramson Cancer Center, Hospital of the University of Pennsylvania, Philadelphia, Pennsylvania
Melanoma and Nonmelanoma Skin Cancers

Sam Schulman, MD, PhD
Professor, Division of Hematology and Thromboembolism, Director of Clinical Thromboembolism Program, Department of Medicine, McMaster University, Hamilton, Ontario, Canada
Antithrombotic Therapy

Lawrence B. Schwartz, MD, PhD
Charles and Evelyn Thomas Professor of Medicine, Internal Medicine, Virginia Commonwealth University, Richmond, Virginia
Systemic Anaphylaxis, Food Allergy, and Insect Sting Allergy

Carlos Seas, MD
Associate Professor of Medicine, Vice Director, Alexander von Humboldt Tropical Medicine Institute, Universidad Peruana Cayetano Heredia; Attending Physician, Department of Infectious, Tropical, and Dermatologic Diseases, National Hospital Cayetano Heredia, Lima, Peru
Cholera and Other Vibrio Infections

Steven A. Seifert, MD
Professor of Emergency Medicine, University of New Mexico School of Medicine, Medical Director, New Mexico Poison and Drug Information Center, University of New Mexico Health Sciences Center, Albuquerque, New Mexico
Envenomation

Julian L. Seifter, MD
Associate Professor of Medicine, Harvard Medical School; Senior Physician, Brigham and Women's Hospital, Boston, Massachusetts
Potassium Disorders; Acid-Base Disorders

Duygu Selcen, MD
Associate Professor of Neurology and Pediatrics, Department of Neurology, Mayo Clinic, Rochester, Minnesota
Muscle Diseases

Clay F. Semenkovich, MD
Herbert S. Gasser Professor and Chief, Division of Endocrinology, Metabolism and Lipid Research, Washington University School of Medicine, St. Louis, Missouri
Disorders of Lipid Metabolism

Carol E. Semrad, MD
Professor of Medicine, The University of Chicago Medicine, GI Section, Chicago, Illinois
Approach to the Patient with Diarrhea and Malabsorption

Harry Shamoon, MD
Professor of Medicine and Associate Dean for Clinical and Translational Research, Albert Einstein College of Medicine; Director, Harold and Muriel Block Institute for Clinical and Translational Research at Einstein and Montefiore, Bronx, New York
Diabetes Mellitus

James C. Shaw, MD
Associate Professor, Department of Medicine, University of Toronto; Head, Division of Dermatology, Department of Medicine, Women's College Hospital, Toronto, Ontario, Canada
Examination of the Skin and an Approach to Diagnosing Skin Diseases

Pamela J. Shaw, DBE, MBBS, MD
Professor of Neurology, University of Sheffield, Consultant Neurologist, Royal Hallamshire Hospital, Sheffield, United Kingdom
Amyotrophic Lateral Sclerosis and Other Motor Neuron Diseases

Robert L. Sheridan, MD
Associate Professor of Surgery, Burn Service Medical Director, Boston Shriners Hospital for Children, Massachusetts General Hospital, Division of Burns, Harvard Medical School, Boston, Massachusetts
Medical Aspects of Injuries and Burns

Stuart Sherman, MD
Professor of Medicine and Radiology, Director of ERCP, Indiana University School of Medicine, Indianapolis, Indiana
Diseases of the Gallbladder and Bile Ducts

Michael E. Shy, MD
Professor of Neurology, Pediatrics, and Physiology, University of Iowa, Iowa City, Iowa
Peripheral Neuropathies

Ellen Sidransky, MD
Chief, Section on Molecular Neurogenetics, Medical Genetics Branch, National Human Genome Research Institute, National Institutes of Health, Bethesda, Maryland
The Lysosomal Storage Diseases

Richard M. Siegel, MD, PhD
Clinical Director, National Institute of Arthritis, Musculoskeletal, and Skin Diseases, National Institutes of Health, Bethesda, Maryland
The Systemic Autoinflammatory Diseases

Robert F. Siliciano, MD, PhD
Professor, The Johns Hopkins University School of Medicine, Howard Hughes Medical Institute, Baltimore, Maryland
Immunopathogenesis of Human Immunodeficiency Virus Infection

Michael S. Simberkoff, MD
Chief of Staff, VA New York Harbor Healthcare System; Professor of Medicine, NYU School of Medicine, New York, New York
Haemophilus and Moraxella Infections

David L. Simel, MD, MHS
Professor of Medicine, Duke University; Chief, Medical Service, Durham Veterans Affairs Medical Center, Durham, North Carolina
Approach to the Patient: History and Physical Examination

Kamaljit Singh, MD
Associate Professor of Medicine, Attending Physician, Infectious Diseases, Rush University Medical Center, Chicago, Illinois
Zoonoses

Karl Skorecki, MD
Annie Chutick Professor in Medicine, Rappaport Faculty of Medicine and Research Institute, Technion–Israel Institute of Technology; Director, Medical and Research Development, Rambam Health Care Campus, Haifa, Israel
Gene and Cell Therapy; Disorders of Sodium and Water Homeostasis

Itzchak Slotki, MD
Associate Professor of Medicine, Hebrew University, Hadassah Medical School; Director, Division of Adult Nephrology, Shaare Zedek Medical Center, Jerusalem, Israel
Disorders of Sodium and Water Homeostasis

Arthur S. Slutsky, MD
Professor of Medicine, Surgery, and Biomedical Engineering, University of Toronto; Vice President (Research), St. Michael's Hospital, Keenan Research Centre, Li Ka Shing Knowledge Institute, Toronto, Ontario, Canada
Acute Respiratory Failure; Mechanical Ventilation

Eric J. Small, MD
Professor of Medicine and Urology, Deputy Director and Director of Clinical Sciences, Helen Diller Family Comprehensive Cancer Center; Chief, Division of Hematology and Oncology, University of California San Francisco School of Medicine, San Francisco, California
Prostate Cancer

Gerald W. Smetana, MD
Professor of Medicine, Harvard Medical School; Division of General Medicine and Primary Care, Beth Israel Deaconess Medical Center, Boston, Massachusetts
Principles of Medical Consultation

Frederick S. Southwick, MD
Professor of Medicine, Division of Infectious Diseases, University of Florida and VF Health, Gainesville, Florida
Nocardiosis

Allen M. Spiegel, MD
Dean, Albert Einstein College of Medicine, Bronx, New York
Principles of Endocrinology; Polyglandular Disorders

Robert F. Spiera, MD
Professor of Clinical Medicine, Weill Cornell Medical College; Director, Scleroderma, Vasculitis, and Myositis Center, The Hospital for Special Surgery, New York, New York
Polymyalgia Rheumatica and Temporal Arteritis

Stanley M. Spinola, MD
Professor and Chair, Department of Microbiology and Immunology, Professor of Medicine, Microbiology and Immunology, and Pathology and Laboratory Medicine, Indiana University School of Medicine, Indianapolis, Indiana
Chancroid

David Spriggs, MD
Head, Division of Solid Tumor Oncology, Department of Medicine, Memorial Sloan Kettering Cancer Center; Professor of Medicine, Department of Medicine, Weill Cornell Medical College, New York, New York
Gynecologic Cancers

Paweł Stankiewicz, MD, PhD
Department of Molecular and Human Genetics, Baylor College of Medicine, Houston, Texas
Gene, Genomic, and Chromosomal Disorders

Paul Stark, MD
Professor Emeritus, University of California San Diego; Chief of Cardiothoracic Radiology, VA San Diego Healthcare System, San Diego, California
Imaging in Pulmonary Disease

David P. Steensma, MD
Professor of Medicine, Harvard Medical School, Adult Leukemia Program, Dana-Farber Cancer Institute, Boston, Massachusetts
Myelodysplastic Syndrome

Martin H. Steinberg, MD
Professor of Medicine, Pediatrics, and Pathology and Laboratory Medicine, Boston University School of Medicine; Director, Center of Excellence in Sickle Cell Disease, Boston Medical Center, Boston, Massachusetts
Sickle Cell Disease and Other Hemoglobinopathies

Theodore S. Steiner, MD
Associate Professor, University of British Columbia; Associate Head, Division of Infectious Diseases, Vancouver General Hospital, Vancouver, British Columbia, Canada
Escherichia Coli Enteric Infections

David S. Stephens, MD
Stephen W. Schwarzmann Distinguished Professor of Medicine, Emory University School of Medicine and Woodruff Health Sciences Center, Atlanta, Georgia
Neisseria Meningitidis Infections

David A. Stevens, MD
Professor of Medicine, Stanford University Medical School; President, Principal Investigator, Infectious Diseases Research Laboratory, California Institute for Medical Research, San Jose and Stanford, California
Systemic Antifungal Agents

James K. Stoller, MD, MS
Chairman, Education Institute, Jean Wall Bennett Professor of Medicine, Cleveland Clinic Lerner College of Medicine; Staff, Respiratory Institute, Cleveland Clinic, Cleveland, Ohio
Respiratory Monitoring in Critical Care

John H. Stone, MD, MPH
Professor of Medicine, Director, Clinical Rheumatology, Harvard Medical School, Massachusetts General Hospital, Boston, Massachusetts
The Systemic Vasculitides

Richard M. Stone, MD
Professor of Medicine, Harvard Medical School, Clinical Director, Adult Leukemia Program, Dana-Farber Cancer Institute, Boston, Massachusetts
Myelodysplastic Syndrome

Raymond A. Strikas, MD, MPH
Education Team Lead, Immunization Services Division, National Center for Immunization and Respiratory Diseases, Centers for Disease Control and Prevention, Atlanta, Georgia
Immunization

Edwin P. Su, MD
Associate Professor of Clinical Orthopaedics, Orthopaedic Surgery, Weill Cornell University Medical College; Associate Attending Orthopaedic Surgeon, Adult Reconstruction and Joint Replacement, Hospital for Special Surgery, New York, New York
Surgical Treatment of Joint Disease

Roland W. Sutter, MD, MPH&TM
Coordinator, Research, Policy and Product Development, Polio Operations and Research Department, World Health Organization, Geneva, Switzerland
Diphtheria and Other Corynebacteria Infections

Ronald S. Swerdloff, MD
Professor of Medicine, David Geffen School of Medicine at University of California Los Angeles; Chief, Division of Endocrinology, Department of Medicine, Harbor-UCLA Medical Center, Torrance, California
The Testis and Male Hypogonadism, Infertility, and Sexual Dysfunction

Heidi Swygard, MD, MPH
Associate Professor of Medicine, University of North Carolina at Chapel Hill, Chapel Hill, North Carolina
Approach to the Patient with a Sexually Transmitted Infection

Megan Sykes, MD
Michael J. Friedlander Professor of Medicine, Director, Columbia Center for Translational Immunology, Columbia University Medical Center, New York, New York
Transplantation Immunology

Marian Tanofsky-Kraff, PhD
Associate Professor, Department of Medical and Clinical Psychology, Uniformed Services University of Health Sciences, Bethesda, Maryland
Eating Disorders

Susan M. Tarlo, MBBS
Professor of Medicine, Department of Medicine and Dalla Lana School of Public Health, University of Toronto, Respiratory Physician, University Health Network, Toronto Western Hospital and St. Michael's Hospital, Toronto, Ontario, Canada
Occupational Lung Disease

Victoria M. Taylor, MD, MPH
Professor of Medicine, University of Washington, Fred Hutchinson Cancer Research Center, Seattle, Washington
Cultural Context of Medicine

Ayalew Tefferi, MD
Professor of Medicine, Department of Hematology, Mayo Clinic, Rochester, Minnesota
Polycythemia Vera, Essential Thrombocythemia, and Primary Myelofibrosis

Paul S. Teirstein, MD
Chief of Cardiology, Department of Medicine, Scripps Clinic, La Jolla, California
Interventional and Surgical Treatment of Coronary Artery Disease

Sam R. Telford III, ScD
Professor, Tufts University Cummings School of Veterinary Medicine, North Grafton, Massachusetts
Babesiosis and Other Protozoan Diseases

Rajesh V. Thakker, MD
May Professor of Medicine, University of Oxford; Radcliffe Department of Clinical Medicine, OCDEM, Churchill Hospital, Headington, Oxford, United Kingdom
The Parathyroid Glands, Hypercalcemia, and Hypocalcemia

Antonella Tosti, MD
Professor of Clinical Dermatology, Department of Dermatology and Cutaneous Surgery, University of Miami, Miami, Florida
Diseases of Hair and Nails

Indi Trehan, MD, MPH, DTM&H
Assistant Professor of Pediatrics, Washington University School of Medicine; Attending Physician, St. Louis Children's Hospital, Barnes-Jewish Hospital, St. Louis, Missouri; Visiting Honorary Lecturer in Paediatrics and Child Health, University of Malawi College of Medicine; Consultant Paediatrician, Queen Elizabeth Central Hospital, Blantyre, Malawi
Protein-Energy Malnutrition

Ronald B. Turner, MD
Professor of Pediatrics, University of Virginia School of Medicine, Charlottesville, Virginia
The Common Cold

Thomas S. Uldrick, MD
Staff Clinician, HIV and AIDS Malignancy Branch, National Cancer Institute, Bethesda, Maryland
Hematology and Oncology in Patients with Human Immunodeficiency Virus Infection

Anthony M. Valeri, MD
Professor of Medicine, Columbia University Medical Center; Director, Hemodialysis, Medical Director, Kidney and Pancreas Transplantation, New York-Presbyterian Hospital (CUMC); Director, Hemodialysis, Columbia University Dialysis Center, New York, New York
Treatment of Irreversible Renal Failure

John Varga, MD
John and Nancy Hughes Professor of Medicine, Northwestern University Feinberg School of Medicine, Chicago, Illinois
Systemic Sclerosis (Scleroderma)

Bradley V. Vaughn, MD
Professor of Neurology, Department of Neurology, University of North Carolina, Chapel Hill, North Carolina
Disorders of Sleep

Alan P. Venook, MD
Professor of Medicine, University of California San Francisco, Helen Diller Family Comprehensive Cancer Center, San Francisco, California
Liver and Biliary Tract Cancers

Joseph G. Verbalis, MD
Professor of Medicine, Georgetown University; Chief, Endocrinology and Metabolism, Georgetown University Hospital, Washington, D.C.
Posterior Pituitary

Ronald G. Victor, MD
Professor of Medicine, Burns and Allen Chair in Cardiology Research, Director, Hypertension Center, Associate Director, The Heart Institute, Cedars-Sinai Medical Center, Los Angeles, California
Arterial Hypertension

Angela Vincent, MBBS
Professor of Neuroimmunology, University of Oxford; Honorary Consultant in Immunology, Oxford University Hospital Trust, Oxford, United Kingdom
Disorders of Neuromuscular Transmission

Robert M. Wachter, MD
Professor and Associate Chairman, Department of Medicine, University of California San Francisco, San Francisco, California
Quality of Care and Patient Safety

Edward H. Wagner, MD, MPH
Director Emeritus, MacColl Center for Health Care Innovation, Group Health Research Institute, Seattle, Washington
Comprehensive Chronic Disease Management

Edward E. Walsh, MD
Professor of Medicine, University of Rochester School of Medicine and Dentistry; Head, Infectious Diseases, Rochester General Hospital, Rochester, New York
Respiratory Syncytial Virus

Thomas J. Walsh, MD
Director, Transplantation-Oncology Infectious Diseases Program, Chief, Infectious Diseases Translational Research Laboratory, Professor of Medicine, Pediatrics, and Microbiology and Immunology, Weill Cornell Medical Center; Henry Schueler Foundation Scholar, Sharp Family Foundation Scholar in Pediatric Infectious Diseases, Adjunct Professor of Pathology, The Johns Hopkins University School of Medicine; Adjunct Professor of Medicine, The University of Maryland School of Medicine, Baltimore, Maryland
Aspergillosis

Jeremy D. Walston, MD
Raymond and Anna Lublin Professor of Geriatric Medicine and Gerontology, The Johns Hopkins University School of Medicine, Baltimore, Maryland
Common Clinical Sequelae of Aging

Christina Wang, MD
Professor of Medicine, David Geffen School of Medicine at University of California Los Angeles; Associate Director, UCLA Clinical and Translational Research Institute, Harbor-UCLA Medical Center, Torrance, California
The Testis and Male Hypogonadism, Infertility, and Sexual Dysfunction

Christine Wanke, MD
Professor of Medicine and Public Health, Director, Division of Nutrition and Infection, Associate Chair, Department of Public Health, Tufts University School of Medicine, Boston, Massachusetts
Gastrointestinal Manifestions of HIV and AIDS

Stephen I. Wasserman, MD
Professor of Medicine, University of California San Diego, La Jolla, California
Approach to the Patient with Allergic or Immunologic Disease

Thomas J. Weber, MD
Associate Professor, Medicine/Endocrinology, Duke University, Durham, North Carolina
Approach to the Patient with Metabolic Bone Disease; Osteoporosis

Heiner Wedemeyer, MD
Professor, Department of Gastroenterology, Hepatology, and Endocrinology, Hannover Medical School, Hannover, Germany
Acute Viral Hepatitis

Geoffrey A. Weinberg, MD
Professor of Pediatrics, University of Rochester School of Medicine and Dentistry; Director, Pediatric HIV Program, Golisano Children's Hospital at University of Rochester Medical Center, Rochester, New York
Parainfluenza Viral Disease

David A. Weinstein, MD, MMSc
Professor of Pediatric Endocrinology, Director, Glycogen Storage Disease Program, Division of Pediatric Endocrinology, University of Florida College of Medicine, Gainesville, Florida
Glycogen Storage Diseases

Robert S. Weinstein, MD
Professor of Medicine, Department of Medicine, University of Arkansas for Medical Sciences; Staff Endocrinologist, Department of Medicine, Central Arkansas Veterans Health Care System, Little Rock, Arkansas
Osteomalacia and Rickets

Roger D. Weiss, MD
Professor of Psychiatry, Harvard Medical School, Boston, Massachusetts; Chief, Division of Alcohol and Drug Abuse, McLean Hospital, Belmont, Massachusetts
Drug Abuse and Dependence

Martin Weisse, MD
Chair, Pediatrics, Tripler Army Medical Center, Honolulu, Hawaii; Professor, Pediatrics, Uniformed Services University of the Health Sciences, Bethesda, Maryland
Measles

Jeffrey I. Weitz, MD
Professor of Medicine and Biochemistry, McMaster University; Executive Director, Thrombosis and Atherosclerosis Research Institute, Hamilton, Ontario, Canada
Pulmonary Embolism

Samuel A. Wells, Jr., MD
Medical Oncology Branch, National Cancer Institute, National Institutes of Health, Bethesda, Maryland
Medullary Thyroid Carcinoma

Richard P. Wenzel, MD, MSc
Professor and Former Chairman, Internal Medicine, Virginia Commonwealth University, Richmond, Virginia
Acute Bronchitis and Tracheitis

Victoria P. Werth, MD
Professor of Dermatology and Medicine, Hospital of the University of Pennsylvania and Philadelphia Veterans Administration Medical Center; Chief, Dermatology Division, Philadelphia Veterans Administration Medical Center, Philadelphia, Pennsylvania
Principles of Therapy of Skin Diseases

Sterling G. West, MD, MACP
Professor of Medicine, University of Colorado School of Medicine; Associate Division Head for Clinical and Educational Affairs, University of Colorado Division of Rheumatology, Aurora, Colorado
Systemic Diseases in Which Arthritis Is a Feature

A. Clinton White, Jr., MD
Paul R. Stalnaker Distinguished Professor and Director, Infectious Disease Division, Department of Internal Medicine, University of Texas Medical Branch, Galveston, Texas
Cestodes

Christopher J. White, MD
Professor of Medicine, Ochsner Clinical School, University of Queensland School of Medicine; System Chairman of Cardiovascular Diseases, Ochsner Medical Center, New Orleans, Louisiana
Atherosclerotic Peripheral Arterial Disease; Electrophysiologic Interventional Procedures and Surgery

Perrin C. White, MD
Professor of Pediatrics, The Audry Newman Rapoport Distinguished Chair in Pediatric Endocrinology, University of Texas Southwestern Medical Center, Chief of Endocrinology, Children's Medical Center Dallas, Dallas, Texas
Disorders of Sexual Development

Richard J. Whitley, MD
Distinguished Professor of Pediatrics, Loeb Eminent Scholar Chair in Pediatrics, Professor of Pediatrics, Microbiology, Medicine, and Neurosurgery, The University of Alabama at Birmingham, Birmingham, Alabama
Herpes Simplex Virus Infections

Michael P. Whyte, MD
Professor of Medicine, Pediatrics, and Genetics, Division of Bone and Mineral Diseases, Washington University School of Medicine; Medical-Scientific Director, Center for Metabolic Bone Disease and Molecular Research, Shriners Hospital for Children, St. Louis, Missouri
Osteonecrosis, Osteosclerosis/Hyperostosis, and Other Disorders of Bone

Samuel Wiebe, MD, MSc
Professor of Clinical Neurosciences, University of Calgary; Co-Director, Calgary Epilepsy Program, Alberta Health Services, Foothills Medical Centre, Calgary, Alberta, Canada
The Epilepsies

Jeanine P. Wiener-Kronish, MD
Henry Isaiah Dorr Professor of Research and Teaching in Anaesthesia and Anesthestist-in-Chief, Department of Anesthesia, Critical Care and Pain Medicine, Massachusetts General Hospital/Harvard Medical School, Boston, Massachusetts
Overview of Anesthesia

Eelco F.M. Wijdicks, MD, PhD
Professor of Neurology, Division of Critical Care Neurology, Department of Neurology, Mayo Clinic, Rochester, Minnesota
Coma, Vegetative State, and Brain Death

David J. Wilber, MD
George M. Eisenberg Professor of Medicine, Loyola Stritch School of Medicine; Director, Division of Cardiology, Director, Clinical Electrophysiology, Loyola University Medical Center, Maywood, Illinois
Electrophysiologic Interventional Procedures and Surgery

Beverly Winikoff, MD, MPH
President, Gynuity Health Projects; Professor of Clinical Population and Family Health, Mailman School of Public Health, Columbia University, New York, New York
Contraception

Gary P. Wormser, MD
Professor of Medicine and Chief, Division of Infectious Diseases, Department of Medicine, New York Medical College, Valhalla, New York
Lyme Disease

Myron Yanoff, MD
Professor and Chair, Ophthalmology, Drexel University College of Medicine, Philadelphia, Pennsylvania
Diseases of the Visual System

Robert Yarchoan, MD
Branch Chief, HIV and AIDS Malignancy Branch, National Cancer Institute, Bethesda, Maryland
Hematology and Oncology in Patients with Human Immunodeficiency Virus Infection

Neal S. Young, MD
Chief, Hematology Branch, NHLBI and Director, Trans-NIH Center for Human Immunology, Autoimmunity, and Inflammation, National Institutes of Health, Bethesda, Maryland
Parvovirus

William F. Young, Jr., MD, MSc
Professor of Medicine, Mayo Clinic College of Medicine; Chair, Division of Endocrinology, Diabetes, Metabolism, and Nutrition, Mayo Clinic, Rochester, Minnesota
Adrenal Medulla, Catecholamines, and Pheochromocytoma

Alan S.L. Yu, MB, BChir
Harry Statland and Solon Summerfield Professor of Medicine, Director, Division of Nephrology and Hypertension and the Kidney Institute, University of Kansas Medical Center, Kansas City, Kansas
Disorders of Magnesium and Phosphorus

Sherif R. Zaki, MD, PhD
Chief, Infectious Diseases Pathology Branch, Centers for Disease Control and Prevention, Atlanta, Georgia
Leptospirosis

Mark L. Zeidel, MD
Herman L. Blumgart Professor of Medicine, Harvard Medical School; Physician-in-Chief and Chairman, Department of Medicine, Beth Israel Deaconess Medical Center, Boston, Massachusetts
Obstructive Uropathy

Thomas R. Ziegler, MD
Professor, Department of Medicine, Division of Endocrinology, Metabolism, and Lipids, Emory University School of Medicine, Atlanta, Georgia
Malnutrition, Nutritional Assessment, and Nutritional Support in Adult Hospitalized Patients

Peter Zimetbaum, MD
Associate Professor of Medicine, Harvard Medical School; Director of Clinical Cardiology, Beth Israel Deaconess Medical Center, Boston, Massachusetts
Cardiac Arrhythmias with Supraventricular Origin

CONTENTS

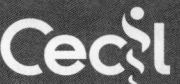

VOLUME II

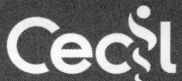

XVI

METABOLIC DISEASES

205

APPROACH TO INBORN ERRORS OF METABOLISM

OLAF A. BODAMER

DEFINITION

The term *metabolism* (Greek: *metabolé*, "change") refers to the network of chemical reactions that sustain the human organism through the digestion, absorption, transport, and utilization of nutrients. Inborn errors of metabolism are genetic disorders that affect these intrinsic metabolic pathways through deficiencies of enzymes, membrane transporter proteins, signaling peptides, or structural proteins. The resulting clinical phenotype follows a spectrum of different organ manifestations that may be progressive, fluctuating, or stationary in nature and may be manifested at any age. Any inborn error of metabolism can principally be manifested during adolescence or adulthood, although severe presentations are typically recognized during infancy and childhood.

HISTORY

Archibald Garrod pioneered the field of inborn errors of metabolism after recognizing alkaptonuria as one of the first metabolic conditions due to homozygosity of mutant alleles in 1902. He had the foresight to recognize the autosomal recessive inheritance of additional inborn errors of metabolism, including cystinuria, pentosuria, and albinism, and to speculate about "chemical individuality" as one of the driving forces of selection and evolution. However, it was not until the early 1950s that the deficiency of homogentisate 1,2-dioxygenase (HGD) was recognized as the underlying cause of alkaptonuria, and it took many more years to identify pathogenic mutations in the *HGD* gene.

The advent of novel analytical techniques led to the molecular and biochemical characterization of known inborn errors of metabolism and the delineation and recognition of new clinical phenotypes, some of which were previously not presumed to be due to inborn errors of metabolism. The completion of the first human genome in 2001 and the following "genomics" revolution laid the foundation for the successive identification of many additional inborn errors of metabolism through next-generation sequencing, bringing the total number of catalogued inborn errors of metabolism to more than 1500 (March 2014).

The initiation of population-based newborn screening in 1964 through Robert Guthrie resulted in its recognition as an important public health measure to prevent morbidity and mortality of inborn errors of metabolism. More than 4 million newborn infants are screened annually in the United States for 31 core conditions, including mostly inborn errors of metabolism. As a consequence, approximately 12,500 newborn infants are diagnosed each year through newborn screening. Rarely, mothers with an inborn error of metabolism are diagnosed through newborn screening of their infants subsequent to placental transfer of pathognomonic metabolites.

EPIDEMIOLOGY

Inborn errors of metabolism occur in all populations, although their incidence and prevalence rates may vary considerably because of differences in carrier rates. These variations are readily explained by the presence of founder mutations, for example, in individuals of Ashkenazi Jewish or Amish ancestry, or by an increased rate of parental consanguinity that leads to a relative increase in mutant allele frequency (Table 205-1). Knowledge of the increased carrier frequencies is instrumental for preconception genetic counseling and targeted carrier screening.

PATHOBIOLOGY

The complexity of human metabolism and its spatial relationship with the human proteome, genome, and methylome are poorly understood. Naturally occurring variants in human nucleotide sequences may or may not result in variation of amino acid sequences in peptides and proteins. It is now well established from whole exome and genome sequencing that individuals may carry in excess of 10,000 nucleotide variants; most variants are silent, *single-nucleotide polymorphic variants*. Up to 4% of variants may be pathogenic in

either recessive or dominant genes. These variants in particular will lead to functional changes in proteins that may render the affected individual susceptible to disease, increase the risk for undesired side effects on treatment with certain drugs, or increase the risk for genetic conditions in future generations.

Variation of human peptides and proteins is not merely explained through genomic sequence variation. Post-transcriptional alternative splicing will generate tissue-specific isoforms of proteins that are adapted to their functional needs through post-translational modification and conformational plasticity.

Genetics

Inborn errors of metabolism are monogenic conditions that follow autosomal recessive or dominant, X-linked recessive or dominant, or mitochondrial inheritance patterns. Of note is the existence of genetic or environmental modifiers that contribute to the interindividual and intrafamilial variability of phenotypic expression, although for most inborn errors of metabolism, these modifiers remain elusive. In case of mitochondrial inheritance, heteroplasmy (the random distribution and expression of mitochondrial mutations in different organs) may explain by itself the striking variability of clinical symptoms in mitochondrial conditions. The concept of synergistic heterozygosity (i.e., heterozygosity for pathogenic mutations affecting different enzymes simultaneously within the same pathway) may explain why some individuals with symptoms reminiscent of inborn errors of metabolism are not formally diagnosed.

Pathophysiology

The severity of any given inborn error of metabolism depends on the degree of enzyme deficiency and the complex interaction of the underlying pathogenic mutations, genetic modifiers, and environment. Hypomorphic mutations may not lead to overt disease until adulthood, whereas severe mutations in the same gene may lead to infantile-onset disease associated with significant morbidity and mortality. The underlying pathophysiologic mechanisms may contribute individually or in combination to the disease state (Table 205-2). Complete blockage of a catabolic pathway may result in accumulation of toxic substrates, activation of secondary minor pathways, or a relative shortage of downstream products. As a consequence, different organs may be affected by the same metabolic defect. An example is homocystinuria due to mutations in the gene for cystathionine β-synthase, which causes lens dislocation and intellectual disabilities and increases the risk for cardiovascular disease. Accumulation of homocysteine contributes to the vascular risk, whereas lack of the downstream product cysteine is an important factor in the dislocation of the lens through loosening of the zonular fibers (Table 205-3).

Clinical Phenotype

Inborn errors of metabolism typically affect multiple organs and, in more than 50% of cases, the central and peripheral nervous systems and muscles. One or more organ manifestations may dominate the clinical phenotype, although oligosymptomatic cases may occur. The clinical phenotype represents a continuous clinical spectrum ranging from the severe end, presenting during infancy, to the mild end of the spectrum, presenting during adolescence or adulthood. Some affected individuals may never come to medical attention because of almost complete absence of symptoms or atypical presentation. Recent data from newborn screening programs suggest much higher incidence rates for some inborn errors of metabolism due to the detection of a high rate of mild cases in which disease-related signs or symptoms may never develop. Some clinical signs are pathognomonic for an inborn error of metabolism, whereas others should raise the suspicion for the presence of an inborn error of metabolism (Table 205-4).

Classification

Inborn errors of metabolism can be classified on the basis of the underlying pathomechanism (see Table 205-2), the nature or localization of the protein involved (see Table 205-3), or the clinical phenotype (see Table 205-4). The most logical classification is based on the nature or localization of the affected protein and pathway.

INBORN ERRORS OF METABOLISM
Disorders of Protein Metabolism

These conditions are due to cytosolic or mitochondrial enzyme deficiencies affecting mostly catabolic pathways (Table 205-5). Disorders of protein

TABLE 205-1 INCIDENCE OF INBORN ERRORS OF METABOLISM

DISORDER	GENE	INCIDENCE*	CARRIER RATE	POPULATION
Familial hypercholesterolemia	LDLR	1 : 500	1 : 500	All
Phenylketonuria	PAH	1 : 4000 <1 : 120,000 1 : 15,000	1 : 32 <1 : 173 1 : 61	Ireland Finland, Japan United States
Gaucher's disease	GBA	1 : 20,000 1 : 450	1 : 71 1 : 11	United States† Ashkenazi Jews
Canavan's disease	ASPA	Unknown 1 : 6000	Unknown 1 : 39	United States Ashkenazi Jews
Glycogen storage disease IA	G6PC	1 : 100,000 1 : 1225	1 : 158 1 : 18	United States Ashkenazi Jews
Mucolipidosis IV	MCOLN1	Unknown 1 : 3000	Unknown 1 : 27	United States Ashkenazi Jews
Niemann-Pick disease A	SMPD1	<1 : 250,000 1 : 40,000	<1 : 250 1 : 100	United States Ashkenazi Jews
Tay-Sachs disease	HEXA	1 : 300,000 1 : 3500	1 : 274 1 : 30	United States Ashkenazi Jews

*Per live births.
†Includes Ashkenazi Jews.

TABLE 205-2 PATHOPHYSIOLOGIC MECHANISMS IN INBORN ERRORS OF METABOLISM

MECHANISM	DISORDER
Accumulation of toxic substrates through primary blockage of catabolic pathway	Organic acidopathies (MMA, PA) MSUD, tyrosinemia type I
Accumulation of nontoxic macromolecules through blockage of catabolic pathway	Lysosomal storage disorders (MPS)
Energy failure through primary blockage of pathway relevant for ATP synthesis	Fatty acid oxidation defects Glycogen storage disorder types I and III Respiratory chain enzyme deficiencies
Impairment of post-translational glycosylation	Congenital disorders of glycosylation
Deficiency of end product through primary blockage of anabolic pathway	Albinism, orotic aciduria, scurvy, disorders of creatine metabolism
Lack of detoxification through primary blockage of catabolic pathway	Urea cycle defects

ATP = adenosine triphosphate; MMA = methylmalonic aciduria; MPS = mucopolysaccharidoses; MSUD = maple syrup urine disease; PA = propionic aciduria.

TABLE 205-4 CHARACTERISTIC SIGNS OF INBORN ERRORS OF METABOLISM

ORGAN	CLINICAL SIGN	DISORDER
Eye (cornea)	Cornea verticillata	Fabry's disease
Skeletal system	Ochronosis, black urine	Alkaptonuria
Connective tissue	Carpal tunnel syndrome	MPS I, II, VI, and VII
Central nervous system	Ataxia	Respiratory chain enzyme deficiency
Muscle	Hypotonia	Pompe's disease, GSD V Disorders of creatine metabolism
Liver	Hepato(-spleno)megaly Fibrosis, cirrhosis	MPS I, II, VI, and VII GSD I, III GSD IV, IXb/c, LAL deficiency
Kidney	Renal insufficiency	Cystinosis, Fabry's disease
Skin	Angiokeratomas	Fabry's disease

GSD = glycogen storage disease; LAL = lysosomal acid lipase; MPS = mucopolysaccharidosis.

TABLE 205-3 SELECTED PROTEINS AND INBORN ERRORS OF METABOLISM

PROTEIN	LOCALIZATION	FUNCTION	DISORDER
Enzyme	Cytosolic	Urea production	Urea cycle defects
Enzyme	Mitochondrial	Fatty acid oxidation	Disorders of fatty acid oxidation
		ATP synthesis	Respiratory chain enzyme deficiencies
Transporter	Cellular membrane	Creatine transport Folic acid transport Carnitine transport	Creatine deficiency Folic acid deficiency CACT deficiency
	Mitochondrial membrane		
Transporter	Blood	Transport of cobalamin	Cobalamin deficiency

ATP = adenosine triphosphate; CACT = carnitine acylcarnitine translocase.

metabolism may also be due to defects of plasma membrane protein transport (Table 205-6).

PHENYLKETONURIA

Phenylalanine is an essential amino acid important for growth and production of thyroid hormone, neurotransmitters, and melanin. Phenylketonuria (PKU) is caused by deficiency of tetrahydrobiopterin (BH4)–dependent phenylalanine hydroxylase that catalyzes the conversion of phenylalanine to tyrosine. PKU may also be caused by deficiency of enzymes that are required for BH4 synthesis. PKU is one of the "traditional" inborn errors of metabolism and the first to be included in newborn screening programs, demonstrating that early diagnosis and continued therapy consistently result in normal intellectual development.[1]

TYROSINEMIA

There are three types of tyrosinemia due to different enzyme deficiencies within the catabolic pathway of tyrosine. Deficiency of fumarylacetoacetase in tyrosinemia type I leads to production of toxic byproducts of a minor pathway. These byproducts are primarily toxic to the liver, resulting in acute liver failure and renal Fanconi's tubulopathy if it is left untreated. Succinylacetone, one of the toxic byproducts, serves as a diagnostic metabolite. Tyrosinemia type II results in significant elevations of tyrosine concentration in all tissues, leading to painful corneal lesions, hyperkeratosis of the palms and soles, and mild intellectual disability.

MAPLE SYRUP URINE DISEASE

The clinical phenotype in maple syrup urine disease (MSUD) is due to accumulation of toxic compounds including oxoisocaproic acid resulting from deficiency of the branched-chain α-keto acid dehydrogenase complex. This multienzyme complex, similar to the pyruvate dehydrogenase complex, consists of four different subunits, E_{1a}, E_{1b}, E_2, and E_3. Deficiency of any subunit or a combination of subunits will cause MSUD. Mild forms of MSUD may

TABLE 205-5 DISORDERS OF PROTEIN METABOLISM

DISORDER	ENZYME DEFECT	METABOLITES	CLINICAL PHENOTYPE
Argininemia	Arginase	Arginine	Hyperammonemia, neurologic disease
Argininosuccinic aciduria	Argininosuccinate lyase	Argininosuccinate*	Hyperammonemia, liver cirrhosis
Citrullinemia	Argininosuccinate synthetase	Citrulline, orotic acid*	Hyperammonemia, liver cirrhosis
Homocystinuria	Cystathionine β-synthase	Homocysteine, methionine	Marfanoid habitus, intellectual disability, lens dislocation
Maple syrup urine disease	Branched-chain α-keto acid dehydrogenase complex	Alloisoleucine,* leucine, valine, isoleucine	Encephalopathy, ataxia, metabolic decompensation
Ornithine transcarbamylase deficiency	Ornithine transcarbamylase	Orotic acid,* ornithine, arginine	Severe hyperammonemia, X-linked inheritance
Phenylketonuria	Phenylalanine hydroxylase	Phenylalanine	Intellectual disability,[†] seizures[†]
Tyrosinemia type I	Fumarylacetoacetase	Succinylacetone,* tyrosine	Acute liver failure, tubulopathy
Tyrosinemia type II	Tyrosine aminotransferase	Tyrosine, phenylalanine	Corneal lesions, hyperkeratosis of the skin, mild intellectual disability

*Diagnostic compound.
[†]If untreated.

TABLE 205-6 INBORN ERRORS OF METABOLISM CAUSED BY DEFECTS IN PLASMA MEMBRANE TRANSPORTER PROTEINS

DISORDER	TISSUE AFFECTED	SUBSTRATE	MODE OF INHERITANCE	CLINICAL PHENOTYPE
Cobalamin malabsorption	Ileum	Cobalamin	Autosomal recessive	Pernicious anemia
Carnitine uptake deficiency	Kidney, small intestine	Carnitine	Autosomal recessive	Hypoglycemia, hypotonia
Cystic fibrosis	Apical epithelia	Chloride	Autosomal recessive	Pneumonia, ileus
Cystinuria	Kidney, small intestine	Cystine, lysine, arginine, ornithine	Autosomal recessive	Urolithiasis
Familial hypophosphatemic rickets	Kidney, small intestine	Phosphate	X-linked dominant	Rickets
Folate deficiency	Lymphocyte, erythrocyte	Methyltetrahydrofolate	Autosomal recessive	Aplastic anemia
GLUT1 deficiency	Blood-brain barrier, erythrocyte	Glucose	Autosomal recessive	Seizures, microcephaly
Hartnup's disease	Kidney, small intestine	Neutral amino acids	Autosomal recessive	Nicotinic acid deficiency
Hereditary renal hypouricemia	Kidney	Uric acid	Autosomal recessive	Urolithiasis
Hereditary spherocytosis	Erythrocyte	Sodium	Autosomal dominant or recessive	Hemolytic anemia
Iminoglycinuria	Kidney, small intestine	Glycine, proline, hydroxyproline	Autosomal recessive	Benign, pancreatitis?
Isolated lysinuria	Kidney, small intestine	Lysine	Autosomal recessive	Growth failure, seizures
Lysinuric protein intolerance	Kidney, liver, intestine	Lysine, arginine, ornithine	Autosomal recessive	Growth failure, intellectual disability, hyperammonemia
Renal glycosuria	Kidney	Glucose	Autosomal recessive	Benign
Renal tubular acidosis type 1	Distal renal tubule	H+ secretion, citrate, calcium	Autosomal dominant	Hypokalemia, growth failure, nephrocalcinosis
Renal tubular acidosis type 2	Proximal renal tubule	Bicarbonate	Autosomal recessive	Hyperchloremic metabolic acidosis

Modified from Elsas L II: Approach to inborn errors of metabolism. In: Goldman L, Schafer AI: Goldman's Cecil Medicine. 24th ed. Philadelphia: Elsevier Saunders; 2012:1340-1346.

present with fluctuating neurologic symptoms as well as episodes of ketoacidosis.

Disorders of the Urea Cycle

The role of the urea cycle is to convert ammonium as a byproduct of amino acid metabolism to nontoxic urea that is readily excreted in urine and to synthesize arginine and ornithine. Arginine is an important precursor for the nitric oxide pathway, and it is substrate for creatine/creatine phosphate synthesis. Several mitochondrial and cytosolic enzymes as well as transporters are required for the function of the urea cycle. Individuals with any of the disorders of the urea cycle are at risk for hyperammonemia during catabolic episodes when there is an increased rate of protein breakdown.[2] All conditions are inherited as an autosomal recessive trait with the exception of ornithine transcarbamylase deficiency, which is inherited as an X-linked recessive trait (see Table 205-5).

Disorders of Membrane Transport

Many inborn errors are due to mutations in genes encoding plasma membrane transporter proteins (see Table 205-6). These transporter proteins are responsible for the active transport of small molecules including vitamins, carnitine, glucose, amino acids, and electrolytes across different membranes. The blood-brain barrier plays a particular role in the protection and transport of nutrients to and from the central nervous system. GLUT1 facilitates the transport of glucose across many cellular membranes, including the blood-brain barrier. Deficiency of GLUT1 results in low cerebrospinal fluid glucose concentrations despite normal glucose levels in the blood, a circumstance that is used diagnostically. Affected individuals develop seizures that may be treated with ketone bodies. Other glucose transporters GLUT 2, 3, and 4 are expressed in the liver, kidneys, neurons, and skeletal and heart muscles, with more than one glucose transporter expressed by most cells.

Organic Acidurias

Organic acidurias are disorders due to mitochondrial enzyme deficiencies and accumulation of potentially toxic substrates, activation of alternative pathways, and lack of downstream products. Although the typical clinical presentation is during infancy or childhood, adult cases with mild or atypical symptoms have been reported in the medical literature. Although individuals with organic acidurias are at risk for metabolic decompensation during catabolic episodes, this risk is somewhat lower during adulthood (Table 205-7).

TABLE 205-7 ORGANIC ACIDURIAS

DISORDER	ENZYME DEFECT	INHERITANCE	URINE METABOLITES
Glutaric aciduria type I	Glutaryl-CoA dehydrogenase	Autosomal recessive	3-Hydroxyglutaric acid, glutaric acid
Holocarboxylase synthetase deficiency	Holocarboxylase synthetase	Autosomal recessive	β-Hydroxyisovaleric acid, β-methylcrotonylglycine, β-hydroxypropionic acid, 3-methylcitrate
Isobutyric aciduria	Isobutyryl-CoA dehydrogenase	Autosomal recessive	Isobutyric acid
Isovaleric aciduria	Isovaleryl-CoA dehydrogenase	Autosomal recessive	Isovaleric acid
Methylmalonic aciduria	Methylmalonyl-CoA dehydrogenase	Autosomal recessive	Methylmalonic acid
Mevalonic aciduria	Mevalonate kinase	Autosomal recessive	Mevalonic acid
Propionic aciduria	Propionyl-CoA carboxylase	Autosomal recessive	3-Methylcitrate, propionic acid, 3-hydroxypropionic acid

TABLE 205-8 INBORN ERRORS OF PEROXISOMES

DISORDER	GENE DEFECT	METABOLITES
Zellweger's spectrum	PEX 1,2,3,5,6,10,12,13,14,16,19,26; DLP1	Very long chain fatty acids, bile acids, phytanic and pipecolic acids, erythrocyte plasmalogen
Rhizomelic chondrodysplasia punctate type I	PEX 7	Phytanic acid, erythrocyte plasmalogen
X-linked adrenoleukodystrophy	ABCD1	Very long chain fatty acids
Acyl-CoA oxidase deficiency	ACOX1	Very long chain fatty acids
Methylacyl-CoA racemase deficiency	AMACR	Bile acid intermediates, phytanic and pristanic acids
Dihydroxyacetone phosphate acyltransferase deficiency	GNPAT	Erythrocyte plasmalogen
Refsum's disease	PHYH	Phytanic acid
Hyperoxaluria type I	AGXT	Oxalic acid

Lysosomal Storage Disorders

The lysosomal storage disorders comprise a heterogeneous group of more than 50 distinct disorders due to genetic defects in lysosomal enzymes and membrane proteins or transporters, resulting in lysosomal accumulation of specific substrates. The accumulation in tissues and organs is progressive, ultimately causing deterioration of cellular and tissue function. Many lysosomal disorders affect the central nervous system, and most patients have a decreased lifespan and significant morbidity. Lysosomal storage disorders may be categorized on the basis of the type of substrate stored. Disorders of glycosaminoglycan metabolism include the mucopolysaccharidoses (MPS): MPS I, Hurler's syndrome, Scheie's syndrome; MPS II, Hunter's syndrome; MPS IIIA-D, Sanfilippo's syndrome A-D; MPS IVA, IVB, Morquio's syndrome A and B; MPS VI, Maroteaux-Lamy syndrome; MPS VII, Sly's syndrome.[3] Disorders of ganglioside metabolism include Fabry's disease, Gaucher's disease, Niemann-Pick disease, Tay-Sachs disease, I-cell disease, fucosidosis, mannosidosis, sialidosis, and aspartylglycosaminuria. Danon's and Pompe's diseases are two lysosomal storage disorders resulting in storage of glycogen in different types of muscle cells.

Peroxisomal Disorders

Peroxisomes are cell organelles that are metabolically very active. They are the site of plasmalogen, cholesterol, and bile acid synthesis. Additional pathways include gluconeogenesis from amino acids, the formation of oxalic acid, and the breakdown of hydrogen peroxide, purines, polyamines, phytanic acid, pipecolic acid, and very long chain fatty acids. Disorders of peroxisomal metabolism may result in elevated very long chain fatty acids and phytanic and pipecolic acids but low plasmalogen concentrations (Table 205-8).

Disorders of Respiratory Chain Complexes

Thirteen proteins of the five different mitochondrial respiratory chain enzyme complexes are encoded in the mitochondrial gene, with the remainder being nuclear encoded. Complex II is entirely encoded by the nuclear genome. Disorders that affect any or a combination of the mitochondrial complexes will result in a broad clinical phenotype affecting multiple organs with marked intrafamilial and interfamilial variability due to heteroplasmy in case of mitochondrial inheritance.

Congenital Disorders of Glycosylation

Congenital disorders of glycosylation (CDG) are due to defects in proteins that are involved in post-translational glycosylation of peptides and proteins.

More than 30 different forms of CDG with a broad clinical spectrum affecting multiple organs are recognized. The traditional classification of CDG disorders is based on pathophysiologic considerations, whereas the newer classification uses the underlying molecular defects. Secondary changes in glycosylation pattern may be observed in galactosemia and hereditary fructose intolerance. The most common form of CDG, CDG type Ia, is due to deficiency in the PMM2 gene encoding phosphomannomutase. Most of the patients with CDG Ia present during infancy and childhood with developmental delay, severe infections, bleeding diathesis, and liver impairment, although older patients with milder phenotypes have been described.[4]

DIAGNOSIS

Biochemical and Molecular Testing

The path to a diagnosis of an inborn error of metabolism begins with ascertainment of the medical and family history as well as an in-depth clinical evaluation. The majority of inborn errors of metabolism can be diagnosed through analysis of small molecules (metabolites, peptides, and hormones) in appropriate body fluids (serum, whole blood, urine, and cerebrospinal fluid), followed by enzyme testing in tissues (dried whole blood, lymphocytes, leukocytes, fibroblasts, and muscle tissue). Tissue biopsies for histology and histochemistry are still of value in some cases. Selected metabolic tests for diagnosis of inborn errors of metabolism include analysis of amino acids in plasma, dried blood spots, urine, and cerebrospinal fluid; analysis of acylcarnitine species in plasma and dried blood spots; analysis of total and free carnitine in plasma and urine; analysis of succinylacetone in dried blood spots and urine; and analysis of orotic acid in plasma and urine.

Molecular confirmation is warranted for prediction of phenotype and is a prerequisite for family planning, including preimplantation diagnosis, prenatal testing, and carrier testing for the partner (Table 205-9).

Next-Generation Sequencing

The completion of the first draft sequence of the human genome in 2001 laid the foundation for a new era that came to fruition after the advent of next-generation sequencing technologies. Next-generation sequencing enables the rapid and accurate sequencing of whole human genomes and exomes that represent the 1 to 2% of the genome that is translated into proteins. The continuous refinement of next-generation sequencing technologies has led to a rapid decline of sequencing cost, thereby facilitating the sequencing of tens of thousands of individuals in both research and clinical settings.

Clinical whole exome or genome sequencing in CLIA- and CAP-accredited laboratories may aid in the diagnosis of rare mendelian disorders including

TABLE 205-9 DIAGNOSTIC TESTS FOR INBORN ERRORS OF METABOLISM

METABOLITE	BIOLOGIC MATRIX	METHOD	DISORDER
Amino acids	Plasma, urine, CSF	HPLC, MS-MS	Disorders of amino acid metabolism including PKU, MSUD, tyrosinemia, urea cycle defects, lysinuric protein intolerance
Organic acids	Urine, CSF	GC-MS	Organic acidopathies including MMA, PA, IVA Lactic acidosis, mitochondrial disorders including disorders of the Krebs cycle, respiratory chain enzymes, fatty acid oxidation defects
Acylcarnitine species	Plasma, DBS	MS-MS	Fatty acid oxidation defects, organic acidopathies
Total/free carnitine	Plasma, DBS, urine	MS-MS	Carnitine transporter deficiency, CPT I/II deficiencies (in conjunction with acylcarnitine species), secondary carnitine deficiency
Orotic acid	Plasma, urine	GC-MS, MS-MS	Orotic aciduria, OTC deficiency, citrullinemia type I
Succinylacetone	Plasma, DBS, urine	GC-MS	Tyrosinemia type I
Glycosaminoglycans	Urine	TLC, MS-MS	Mucopolysaccharidoses

CPT I/II = carnitine palmitoyltransferase I/II; CSF = cerebrospinal fluid; DBS = dried blood spots; GC-MS = gas chromatography–mass spectrometry; HPLC = high-pressure liquid chromatography; IVA = isovaleric aciduria; MMA = methylmalonic aciduria; MS-MS = tandem mass spectrometry; MSUD = maple syrup urine disease; OTC = ornithine transcarbamylase; PA = propionic aciduria; PKU = phenylketonuria; TLC = thin-layer chromatography.

TABLE 205-10 THERAPEUTIC STRATEGIES FOR INBORN ERRORS OF METABOLISM

LEVEL	THERAPEUTIC APPROACH	DISORDER
Gene	Solid organ transplantation	Urea cycle defects, tyrosinemia type I
	Stem cell transplantation	Adrenoleukodystrophy, MPS I, GSD IA (experimental)
	Gene therapy	Pompe's disease (phase I/II trial)
	Read-through therapy	Duchenne's muscular dystrophy (phase III), cystic fibrosis (phase III)
Enzyme	Recombinant enzyme infusion	Gaucher's, Pompe's, and Fabry's diseases; MPS I, II, IVA, VI
		Phenylketonuria (phase III)
	Chaperone	Fabry's and Pompe's diseases (phase III)
Substrate	Substrate reduction	Phenylketonuria, maple syrup urine disease
	Substrate inhibition	Gaucher's disease, Tay-Sachs disease

GSD IA = glycogen storage disease type IA; MPS I = mucopolysaccharidosis type I.

inborn errors of metabolism, provided all other diagnostic avenues are exhausted. Although sequencing may be relatively straightforward and inexpensive, analytical challenges remain. An individual may carry a large number of gene variants requiring a dedicated analytical pipeline to identify the pathogenic variants of interest. The diagnostic yield may be as high as 25% in preselected cases.[5]

TREATMENT Rx

The individual treatment strategy follows these general principles: enhancement of enzyme activity through cofactor administration; stabilization of enzyme structure through chaperone therapy; enzyme replacement therapy; reduction of substrate through dietary intervention; substrate inhibition through blockage of the reverse enzyme reaction; replacement of the affected organ (e.g., liver); and stem cell transplantation or therapy.[6,7] Other therapeutic approaches including "read-through" and gene therapies are in clinical trials. Read-through therapy refers to a small molecule (ataluren) that renders ribosomes less sensitive to premature stop codons and allows read-through. Ataluren has been tested in individuals with Duchenne's muscular dystrophy and cystic fibrosis due to nonsense mutations (Table 205-10).

The choice of therapy is guided by the underlying diagnosis, but additional factors warrant consideration. A curative approach may be preferred whenever possible, although this may be rarely an option in adults with inborn errors of metabolism, as in the case of bone marrow or stem cell transplantation in metachromatic leukodystrophy or X-linked adrenoleukodystrophy. Therapeutic agents that address central nervous system manifestations have to cross the blood-brain barrier to be effective, thereby limiting the use of larger molecules, including enzymes, for treatment of neurologic manifestations.

Individuals with inborn errors of metabolism should always be managed by a multidisciplinary team of biochemical geneticists, internists, and genetic counselors at a tertiary center with significant expertise in the management of these disorders. Ideally, a biochemical genetics laboratory to facilitate immediate sample testing should be on site.

Genetic Counseling

Genetic counseling through board-certified genetic counselors is an integral part of the evaluation and management of patients with any familial condition including complex inborn errors of metabolism. A three-generation family history and thorough medical history are the prerequisites for a focused clinical and diagnostic evaluation. Genetic counseling communicates the limitations and implications of genetic testing and associated test results to the patient and the family at large.

Enzyme Therapy

The therapeutic goal of enzyme therapy is to increase endogenous enzyme activity. Individuals with cofactor (vitamin)–responsive enzyme deficiencies may benefit from supraphysiologic doses of the respective vitamin. An example is BH4-responsive PKU due to mutations in the *PAH* gene affecting the binding site of phenylalanine hydroxylase (PAH); 20 mg/kg of BH4 will result in stabilization of the PAH through a chaperone-like effect and, as a consequence, increased PAH activity. Patients with BH4-responsive PKU will experience improved phenylalanine tolerance and metabolic control when taking BH4 supplementation.

Enzyme replacement therapy has been available for treatment of Gaucher's disease for more than 15 years. Initially, glucocerebrosidase, the enzyme deficient in Gaucher's disease, had been purified from human placentas and administered intravenously to affected patients. More recently, glucocerebrosidase has been overexpressed in Chinese hamster ovary cells and produced in large quantities in bioreactors. Recombinant enzyme replacement therapies are now available for Pompe's disease (α-glucosidase), Fabry's disease (α-galactosidase), mucopolysaccharidosis type I (α-iduronidase), mucopolysaccharidosis type II (α-iduronate sulfatase), mucopolysaccharidosis type IVA (galactosamine-6-sulfatase), and mucopolysaccharidosis type VI (arylsulfatase B). Additional enzyme therapies are currently in different phases of clinical trials (see Table 205-10).

Nutritional Therapy

The therapeutic goal of nutritional therapy is the correction of the metabolic imbalance through reduced substrate accumulation, promoting protein synthesis through anabolism and the prevention of episodes of metabolic decompensation. In addition, supplementation of a reduced product may be needed. An example is the therapy for PKU. The mainstay of its therapy is the reduction of phenylalanine intake through low-protein food and the simultaneous supplementation of phenylalanine-free amino acids for sustained growth and development. This regimen will reduce the phenylalanine levels in plasma and, most important, in the brain to nontoxic, nearly normal levels that facilitate age-appropriate intellectual development. On occasion, tyrosine supplementation is needed when tyrosine levels are low. Similar dietary strategies apply to other disorders of amino acid metabolism and organic acidopathies, although natural protein restriction may be more pronounced to reduce the risk for metabolic decompensation during a catabolic episode (intercurrent illness).

Another approach to reduce substrate accumulation is through inhibition of the reverse enzyme reaction that leads to substrate synthesis. This concept has been shown to be effective in reducing glucosylceramide in mild to moderate Gaucher's disease type I. Miglustat is an inhibitor of the enzyme glucosylceramide synthase that catalyzes the reverse direction of glucocerebrosidase, the enzyme that is deficient in Gaucher's disease type I.

Individuals with inborn errors of metabolism at risk for metabolic decompensation, such as urea cycle disorders, organic acidopathies, and disorders of fatty acid oxidation, should always carry an "emergency letter" detailing the diagnosis, symptoms of decompensation, emergency treatment, and contact information of the tertiary metabolic center.

Vitamin Therapy

There are a number of inborn errors of metabolism that affect transport or metabolism of vitamins. These conditions typically benefit from supraphysiologic doses of vitamins. An example is thiamine-responsive megaloblastic anemia, which is due to mutations in the thiamine transporter gene *SLC19A2*. Affected individuals develop sensorineural deafness, vision loss, diabetes mellitus, and megaloblastic anemia. Diabetes and anemia respond to high doses of thiamine. Other examples include disorders of vitamin B_{12} (cobalamin) absorption, transport, and metabolism and disorders of biotin and folic acid metabolism.

Organ, Bone Marrow, and Stem Cell Transplantation

Liver transplantation has been done in patients with tyrosinemia type I, urea cycle defects, methylmalonic aciduria, propionic aciduria, lysosomal lipase deficiency, and glycogen storage diseases affecting the liver. The effect of liver transplantation in these conditions is two-fold. First, metabolic control will be improved in those conditions in which the diseased liver is the main contributor to the overall lack of sufficient metabolic control. However, the intrinsic defect will not be corrected elsewhere after liver transplantation, and an affected individual may continue to have significant neurologic disease in methylmalonic aciduria, for example. Second, liver function will be restored in those conditions that lead to chronic liver disease, including liver fibrosis and cirrhosis, or in which there is a significant risk for malignant transformation. Kidney transplantation may be required in conditions that affect kidney function, as is the case in methylmalonic aciduria or cystinosis.

Bone marrow or stem cell transplantation has limited benefits in patients with inborn errors of metabolism. Examples include presymptomatic bone marrow or stem cell transplantation in severe mucopolysaccharidosis type I, metachromatic leukodystrophy, and X-linked adrenoleukodystrophy. Stem cell therapy is currently under investigation for glycogen storage disease type I.

GENERAL REFERENCES

For the General References and other additional features, please visit Expert Consult at https://expertconsult.inkling.com.

206

DISORDERS OF LIPID METABOLISM

CLAY F. SEMENKOVICH

As Western lifestyles become more pervasive, disorders of lipid metabolism remain among the most common problems faced by clinicians. Ischemic heart disease, the most common cause of global disability, is caused in part by abnormal lipids. Stroke, a common cause of death in the United States, is also related to disorders of lipid metabolism. Both are likely to dominate the clinical landscape of a world where obesity and diabetes are ubiquitous.

Appropriate management of common lipid disorders should be a part of the skill set for everyone who provides clinical care to adults.

COMPONENTS OF LIPID TRANSPORT

Cholesterol and Triglycerides

Cholesterol is a critical constituent of eukaryotic cell membranes and the precursor for the synthesis of steroid hormones such as cortisol, vitamin D, progestins, estradiol, and testosterone. Triglycerides carry fatty acids, nutrients that are used preferentially by muscle tissue and are especially important as an energy source in the fasting state. Because both cholesterol and triglycerides are essentially insoluble in water, the lipid transport system evolved to transport fats from one site to another through an aqueous environment.

Lipoproteins

Cholesterol and triglycerides are transported in lipoproteins (Table 206-1), spherical particles that differ in size and composition, depending on their site of origin. Each particle is composed of a central core consisting of cholesteryl esters (the product of an esterification reaction between the polar cholesterol molecule and a fatty acid) and triglycerides, both nonpolar compounds. Free cholesterol, phospholipids, and apolipoproteins are found on the particle surface.

Chylomicrons and their remnants are the largest lipoproteins. Produced by the intestine, these particles carry fats that are absorbed from the diet. Their residence time in the circulation after a meal is short, on the order of minutes in healthy people. Chylomicrons are large and light; that is, their density is low. Because fat floats on water, particles with high fat and low protein content have lower density. Very low density lipoprotein (VLDL) is a triglyceride-rich particle produced by the liver. The removal of triglycerides from VLDL converts this particle to intermediate-density lipoprotein (IDL), which is subsequently metabolized to yield low-density lipoprotein (LDL, known as bad cholesterol). A covalent modification of the apolipoprotein (apo) in LDL, apo B100, results in the formation of lipoprotein (a). High-density lipoprotein (HDL, or good cholesterol) is formed in the blood as a byproduct of the metabolism of triglyceride-rich lipoproteins and the acquisition of esterified cholesterol from peripheral tissues.

Apolipoproteins

Apolipoproteins are amphipathic molecules capable of interacting with both the lipids of the lipoprotein core and the aqueous environment of the plasma. They function as biochemical keys, allowing lipoprotein particles access to specific sites for the delivery, acceptance, or modification of lipids. Major apolipoproteins, their chromosomal locations with sequence accession numbers, and functions are shown in Table 206-2. Serum measurements of apolipoproteins may have clinical utility. For example, increased levels of apo B and decreased levels of apo AI are associated with vascular disease. Apo B48, specific for gut-derived particles, derives its name from the fact that it is about 48% of the size of apo B100. Apo B100 and apo B48 are products of the same gene, with B48 resulting from the post-transcriptional introduction of a premature stop codon in the apo B messenger RNA by apobec1, a cytidine deaminase. Apolipoproteins can be associated with well-defined disorders. For example, genetic variation at the lipoprotein (a) locus is associated with aortic valve calcification and clinical aortic stenosis.[1]

Receptors and Proteins

Several receptors and proteins required for normal lipid transport are listed in Table 206-3.

TABLE 206-1 LIPOPROTEIN CHARACTERISTICS

LIPOPROTEIN	APOLIPOPROTEIN CONTENT	MAJOR LIPIDS	SIZE (DIAMETER, nm)	DENSITY (g/mL)
Chylomicrons, chylomicron remnants	Apo B48, apo E, apo AI, apo AII, apo AIV, apo CII, apo CIII	Triglycerides from diet	80-500	≪1.006
VLDL	Apo B100, apo E, apo CII, apo CIII	Triglycerides from liver	30-80	<1.006
IDL	Apo B100, apo E	Cholesteryl esters, triglycerides	25-35	1.006-1.019
LDL	Apo B100	Cholesteryl esters	18-25	1.019-1.063
HDL	Apo AI, apo AII, apo AV	Cholesteryl esters, phospholipids	5-12	1.063-1.210
Lp(a)	Apo B100, apo(a)	Cholesteryl esters	~30	1.055-1.085

Apo = apolipoprotein; HDL = high-density lipoprotein; IDL = intermediate-density lipoprotein; LDL = low-density lipoprotein; Lp(a) = lipoprotein (a); VLDL = very low density lipoprotein.

TABLE 206-2 MAJOR APOLIPOPROTEINS

APOLIPOPROTEIN	CHROMOSOMAL LOCATION, GENBANK SEQUENCE IDENTIFICATION	FUNCTIONS
Apo B100	2p24-p23, M14162	Structural component of atherogenic lipoproteins (VLDL, IDL, LDL); VLDL secretion; ligand for LDL receptor; elevated levels associated with vascular disease
Apo B48	Same as apo B100	Chylomicron secretion from intestine
Apo E	19q13.31, K00396	Ligand for binding of triglyceride-rich particles to LDL receptor and LRP; potential roles in Alzheimer's disease and neuronal injury
Apo AI	11q23-q24, X02162	Structural component of HDL; activates LCAT; elevated levels associated with protection from vascular disease
Apo AII	1q21-Q23, NM_001643	Genetically and biochemically associated with familial combined hyperlipidemia
Apo AIV	11q23-qter, NM_000482	Potential role in regulating food intake
Apo AV	11q23, AF202889	Required for normal lipolysis of triglyceride-rich lipoproteins
Apo CII	19q13.2, X00568	Activator of LPL
Apo CIII	11q23-qter, X01388	Inhibitor of LPL
Apo (a)	6q26-q27, X06290	Covalent bond with apo B100 forms Lp(a) and renders particle resistant to uptake by LDL receptor; genetically and biochemically associated with valvular calcification and aortic stenosis

Apo = apolipoprotein; HDL = high-density lipoprotein; IDL = intermediate-density lipoprotein; LCAT = lecithin–cholesterol acyltransferase; LDL = low-density lipoprotein; Lp(a) = lipoprotein (a); LPL = lipoprotein lipase; LRP = LDL receptor–related protein; VLDL = very low density lipoprotein.

TABLE 206-3 IMPORTANT RECEPTORS AND PROTEINS IN LIPID TRANSPORT

PROTEIN	CHROMOSOMAL LOCATION, GENBANK SEQUENCE IDENTIFICATION	FUNCTIONS
LDL receptor	19p13.3, AY114155	Clearance of apo B100 and apo E–containing lipoproteins; activity increased by statin drugs; deficiency causes familial hypercholesterolemia
PCSK9	1p32.3, NC_000001.10	Degrades LDL receptor; deficiency decreases LDL levels
LDL receptor–related protein (LRP)	12Q13-Q14, NM_000014	Clearance of apo E–containing lipoproteins
Scavenger receptor B1 (SR-B1)	12q24.32, Z22555	HDL receptor
Lipoprotein lipase (LPL)	8p22, NM_000237	Rate limiting for triglyceride metabolism; deficiency causes chylomicronemia syndrome
Lecithin–cholesterol acyltransferase (LCAT)	16q22.1, NM_000229	Esterifies cholesterol in HDL to increase HDL cholesterol levels; deficiency decreases HDL levels
Cholesteryl ester transfer protein (CETP)	16q13, NM_000078	Exchanges cholesteryl ester in HDL for triglycerides in apo B–containing lipoproteins; deficiency increases HDL levels
ABCA1	9q31, AJ12376	Transfers cholesterol in tissues to nascent HDL particles; deficiency causes Tangier disease

ABCA1 = ATP-binding cassette A1; apo = apolipoprotein; HDL = high-density lipoprotein; LDL = low-density lipoprotein; PCSK9 = proprotein convertase subtilisin-like/kexin type 9.

Low-Density Lipoprotein Receptor

The LDL receptor mediates the removal of LDL as well as some VLDL and IDL particles by binding to apo B100 and apo E. The most important site of LDL receptor expression is the liver, where its regulation is controlled by sterol regulatory element–binding proteins (SREBPs). SREBPs are found in inactive forms in the endoplasmic reticulum. Cholesterol levels in the cell are sensed by SCAP (SREBP cleavage-activating protein), which interacts with SREBPs. SCAP is capable of transporting SREBPs to the Golgi and subsequently to a compartment where they are cleaved by proteases. These proteases result in the release of the SREBP N terminus, allowing this molecule to migrate to the nucleus to stimulate the expression of genes involved in cholesterol synthesis. When intracellular cholesterol levels are high, the SCAP/SREBP complex does not move to the Golgi, SREBPs are not processed, and cholesterol synthesis stops. When cholesterol levels are low, the SCAP/SREBP complex moves to the Golgi, SREBPs are converted to active forms, and genes important for cholesterol synthesis and acquisition (such as the LDL receptor) are transcribed. Statin drugs effectively lower cholesterol. They inhibit 3-hydroxy-3-methylglutaryl coenzyme A (HMG-CoA) reductase, the rate-limiting enzyme in cholesterol synthesis. When statins inhibit HMG-CoA reductase, intracellular cholesterol levels fall, SCAP shepherds SREBPs to the Golgi for activation, an active SREBP stimulates transcription of the LDL receptor gene, and increased levels of the LDL receptor protein on the surface of the hepatocyte bind and remove LDL particles from the circulation.

Proprotein Convertase Subtilisin-like/Kexin Type 9

Proprotein convertase subtilisin-like/kexin type 9 (PCSK9) is a secreted enzyme that binds to the LDL receptor and increases its degradation, resulting in elevated levels of LDL cholesterol. PCSK9 deficiency in humans is associated with low LDL levels and less atherosclerosis. Pharmacologic antagonism of PCSK9 strikingly lowers LDL cholesterol levels in humans treated with a statin.[2] Potential therapies targeting PCSK9 to affect clinical outcomes are being actively pursued.

Low-Density Lipoprotein Receptor–Related Protein

The LDL receptor–related protein (LRP), also called the chylomicron remnant receptor, participates in the removal of intestine-derived lipoproteins by interacting with apo E. Chylomicron remnants carry apo B48, which is missing the LDL receptor–binding domain, but these particles are also cleared by the LDL receptor through apo E binding.

Scavenger Receptor B1

Scavenger receptor B1 (SR-B1) is a protein expressed in liver that binds HDL. Unlike the LDL receptor that endocytoses LDL particles, the SR-B1 protein does not internalize HDL particles but instead facilitates the transfer of cholesteryl ester from HDL to the liver. Its genetic manipulation in mice has raised clinically relevant questions about the significance of elevated HDL levels. Inactivation of SR-B1 elevates HDL cholesterol levels but promotes atherosclerosis, presumably because of disruption of the transport of cholesterol from peripheral cells, where it can cause disease to the liver, where it is excreted. These results suggest that it is not the level of HDL but the flux of cholesterol through HDL that affords protection from vascular disease.

Lipoprotein Lipase

Lipoprotein lipase (LPL) is rate limiting for the metabolism of triglyceride-rich lipoproteins and is required for the generation of HDL particles because

HDL is absent from LPL-deficient mice. Deficient LPL activity thus provides a physiologic explanation for the common association between high triglyceride levels and low HDL cholesterol.

Niemann-Pick C1-like Protein

The Niemann-Pick C1-like protein (NPC1L1) in the small intestine and liver helps transport dietary cholesterol from the intestinal lumen to intestinal enterocytes. Heterozygous inactivating mutations of the *NPC1L1* gene are associated with 12-mg/dL lower LDL levels and a 50% lower risk of coronary disease.[3] Ezetimibe inhibits the NPC1L1 protein.

Lecithin–Cholesterol Acyltransferase

Lecithin–cholesterol acyltransferase (LCAT) is associated with HDL in the circulation, where it esterifies free cholesterol to form cholesteryl esters that are easily stored in the nonpolar core of the lipoprotein. LCAT deficiency, a rare disorder, is characterized by low HDL as well as by anemia and renal failure, clinical features probably related to disruption of normal membrane function by the accumulation of excess unesterified cholesterol.

Cholesteryl Ester Transfer Protein

Cholesteryl ester transfer protein (CETP) exchanges one molecule of cholesteryl ester in HDL for one molecule of triglyceride in apo B–containing particles such as VLDL. The resulting HDL particle is triglyceride enriched, enhancing its clearance (especially by an enzyme related to LPL, hepatic lipase) and lowering HDL. Inhibition of CETP activity increases HDL levels.

ATP-Binding Cassette A1

ATP-binding cassette A1 (ABCA1) is a cell membrane protein that mediates the transfer of cholesterol and phospholipids from cells to lipid-poor apo AI, a process that promotes HDL formation. ABCA1 in the liver contributes to the genesis of HDL, and overexpression of ABCA1 in macrophages may diminish atherosclerosis. Heterozygous ABCA1 deficiency is responsible for isolated low HDL cholesterol levels that occur in some families. Rare homozygotes for ABCA1 mutations have Tangier disease, characterized by the accumulation of cholesteryl esters in macrophages and resulting in distinctive features, including orange-yellow tonsils, neuropathy, and hepatosplenomegaly. HDL is very low to absent. Atherosclerosis is probably increased in these patients, but its extent may be moderated by concomitantly low LDL levels.

● EXOGENOUS LIPID METABOLISM

Animal products containing cholesterol and triglycerides are eaten regularly by most people. Dietary fats broken down in the gut into individual components are transported across cell membranes into the enterocyte, where they are re-esterified into cholesteryl ester and triglycerides, then packaged onto apo B48. These particles gain access to the plasma through the thoracic duct and acquire other apolipoproteins in part by transfer from HDL. These mature chylomicrons circulate to peripheral tissues. LPL, bound to the capillary endothelium in tissues such as adipose tissue and muscle, is activated by apo CII on chylomicrons, and fatty acids hydrolyzed from triglycerides by LPL are released and transported into adipose tissue for storage or into muscle for energy. This process also requires apo AV, an apolipoprotein transported in HDL that appears to facilitate the interaction between LPL and triglyceride-rich lipoproteins, as well as glycosylphosphatidylinositol-anchored high-density lipoprotein-binding protein 1 (GPIHBP1), a recently discovered protein that forms a platform for triglyceride metabolism at the endothelium.

Progressive hydrolysis of triglyceride converts chylomicrons into chylomicron remnants, which are enriched in cholesteryl esters. Chylomicron remnants are removed in the liver by species that bind apo E: LRP, the LDL receptor, and cell surface glycosaminoglycans. Chylomicrons are large, and it is unlikely that they contribute to atherosclerosis. Chylomicron remnants are small enough to enter the subendothelial space, where they are taken up by macrophages. Remnants are atherogenic and may promote atherosclerosis after meals. This process is missed by the standard practice of measuring fasting lipoproteins.

Chylomicrons are not soluble. Their presence causes the "tomato soup" appearance of blood drawn after a fatty meal. Because they are mostly triglycerides, they float to the top of serum that is refrigerated overnight, leaving a layer of "cream" on top of the sample. The detection of chylomicrons in fasting serum has clinical relevance because it indicates a risk for pancreatitis and other elements of the chylomicronemia syndrome.

● ENDOGENOUS LIPID METABOLISM

Fats deposited in the liver are metabolized into component lipid species, re-esterified as cholesteryl ester and triglycerides, and stored in hepatocytes or exported as lipoproteins (Fig. 206-1). The liver produces the triglyceride-rich VLDL. Its rate of production depends on the availability of triglycerides. Apo B100 is the major apolipoprotein of VLDL, but regulation of the apo B gene does not appear to control VLDL synthesis. Production of the apo B100 protein depends on its cotranslational stabilization. As the message is translated into protein, the presence of triglyceride stabilizes the peptide and allows the continued addition of amino acids. In the absence of triglycerides, the apo B molecule is degraded. The transfer of triglycerides to the growing apo B peptide is mediated by microsomal transfer protein (MTP). Mutations in MTP cause abetalipoproteinemia, a rare disease characterized by the absence of circulating apo B. In the absence of apo B, the metabolism of fat-soluble vitamins (normally carried in lipoproteins) is disrupted, and patients with abetalipoproteinemia suffer from multisystem defects, including severe neurologic dysfunction and retinopathy that are presumably caused by deficiency of vitamins E and A. Drugs that interfere with MTP function lower lipids but, not surprisingly, cause the accumulation of triglyceride in the liver. The apo B gene is normal in patients with abetalipoproteinemia. Mutations in the apo B gene cause another condition known as hypobetalipoproteinemia, caused by shortened forms of the apo B protein. Subjects with hypobetalipoproteinemia have very low but not absent levels of circulating lipids and appear to be healthy.

Nascent VLDL containing one apo B100 molecule per particle is secreted into the plasma, where it acquires apo E, apo CII, and apo CIII. In a process analogous to that occurring with chylomicrons, apo CII on VLDL activates LPL, and fatty acids hydrolyzed from triglycerides by LPL are released in capillary beds and transported into tissues. With continued hydrolysis, VLDL

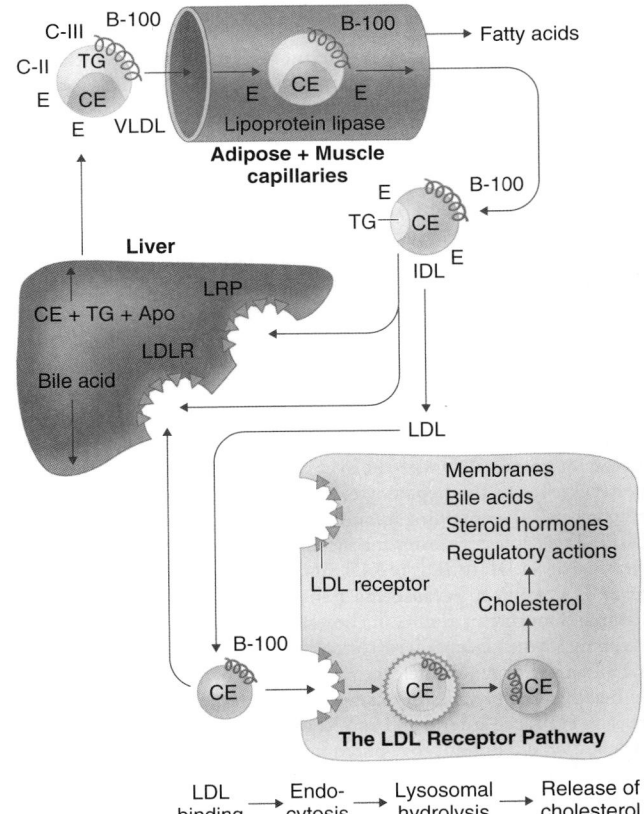

FIGURE 206-1. Endogenous lipid metabolism. In the liver, triglycerides (TG), cholesteryl esters (CE), and apolipoprotein B100 are packaged as very low density lipoprotein (VLDL) particles. TG is hydrolyzed by lipoprotein lipase to generate intermediate-density lipoprotein (IDL), which is further metabolized to generate low-density lipoprotein (LDL). This particle can be removed by the liver or by peripheral cells. Cholesterol derived from LDL regulates several processes and can be used for the synthesis of bile acids, steroid hormones, and cell membranes. LDLR = low-density lipoprotein receptor.

is converted to IDL, a cholesteryl ester–rich particle with an apolipoprotein complement of only apo B and apo E. These particles, like chylomicron remnants, are atherogenic. Unlike chylomicron remnants, IDLs are included in current management schemes because reporting of LDL cholesterol levels by most clinical laboratories includes IDL. IDL can be taken up by either the LRP or the LDL receptor in the liver. In the presence of a normal apo E molecule, IDLs are converted to LDL, consisting of one molecule of apo B100 per particle and cholesteryl esters with essentially no triglycerides. The majority of LDL is removed from the plasma by the LDL receptor pathway in the liver. LDL uptake is followed by migration of LDL particles to lysosomes, where cholesterol is released for (depending on the cell type) plasma membrane localization, bile acid synthesis, steroid hormone synthesis, and interaction with SCAP for the control of SREBP activation. Some LDL enters the subendothelial space of the vascular wall, where its modification by oxidation or other processes promotes its uptake by macrophages in atherosclerotic lesions.

Most VLDL particles are large and are not thought to promote vascular disease. Some small VLDL particles as well as IDL and LDL are atherogenic. Because VLDL is mostly triglyceride, patients with elevated fasting triglyceride levels have either increased numbers of VLDL particles or an increased triglyceride content in VLDL. LDL has a plasma half-life of 2 to 5 days. The detection of elevated fasting cholesterol levels usually reflects the presence of either increased numbers of LDL particles or increased cholesteryl ester in LDL. LDL also exists in a range of sizes. Small, dense LDL tends to occur in the setting of concomitant hypertriglyceridemia. This type of lipoprotein is thought to have greater atherogenic potential than larger LDL species, perhaps because of easy access to the vascular wall and greater susceptibility to oxidative modification. Lipoprotein particle size and number can be quantified by nuclear magnetic resonance techniques, but it is not clear that these data provide diagnostic advantages beyond the determination of total cholesterol, triglycerides, LDL cholesterol, and HDL cholesterol.

● REVERSE CHOLESTEROL TRANSPORT AND HIGH-DENSITY LIPOPROTEIN METABOLISM

Lipid metabolism is dynamic. Lipoprotein particles interact with the vasculature and with one another, exchanging surface materials, apolipoproteins, and nonpolar lipids. HDL is an important reservoir for components cast off during the metabolism of other lipoproteins as well as lipids discarded by cells. Nascent HDL is generated by the liver and intestine as a phospholipid disc containing apo AI and apo AII. It accepts unesterified (free) cholesterol and phospholipids shed from cells. This unesterified cholesterol is converted to cholesteryl ester by the action of LCAT and stored in the center of the disc, allowing it to become spherical. As the core triglycerides of VLDL are metabolized by LPL, the VLDL particle collapses, leaving redundant surface lipids (phospholipid in the form of lecithin and unesterified cholesterol) and excess apolipoproteins such as apo CII, apo CIII, and apo E, which are transferred to HDL.

Reverse cholesterol transport is the beneficial process by which cholesterol in peripheral cells, such as foam cells in an atherosclerotic lesion, is transported back to the liver for excretion. There are at least two well-defined pathways mediating this transfer (Fig. 206-2). First, after accepting cholesterol from peripheral cells and esterifying it through the action of LCAT, HDL can interact directly with the liver by binding to SR-B1 and transferring cholesteryl ester to the hepatocyte. Second, HDL can transfer cholesteryl ester to apo B100–containing lipoproteins such as VLDL through the action of CETP. This cholesteryl ester can ultimately be transported to the liver after conversion of VLDL to IDL to LDL and uptake by the LDL receptor. This pathway is not direct because the transfer of cholesteryl ester to apo B–containing lipoproteins results in cholesterol-enriched particles that may be taken up by foam cells in atherosclerotic plaques before being cleared by the liver. Humans with genetic defects in CETP have high HDL levels and appear to be healthy. The benefits of raising HDL with medications are uncertain. Increasing HDL cholesterol and apo AI through the use of the CETP inhibitor dalcetrapib did not improve outcomes in patients after an acute coronary syndrome.[4] Increasing HDL cholesterol through the use of niacin does not provide clinical benefit to patients with atherosclerotic vascular disease intensively treated with a statin.

● LIPID-ACTIVATED NUCLEAR RECEPTORS AND LIPID METABOLISM

Nuclear receptors are transcription factors that are activated by ligand binding to increase the expression of specific sets of genes. Several nuclear receptors

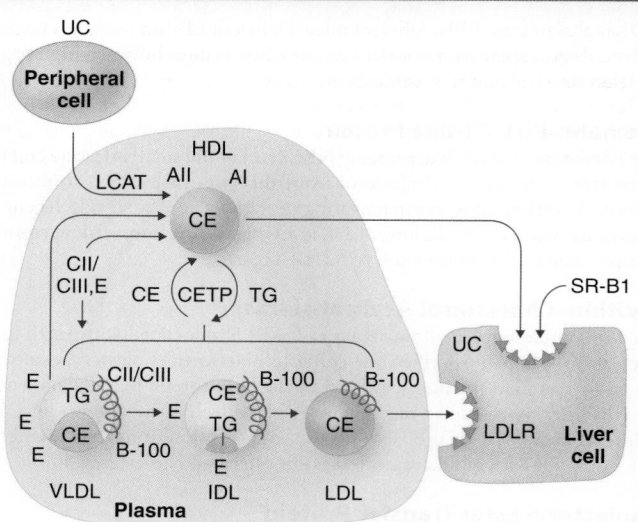

FIGURE 206-2. Reverse cholesterol transport and high-density lipoprotein (HDL) metabolism. Unesterified cholesterol (UC) in peripheral cells can be transferred to HDL and esterified by lecithin-cholesterol acyltransferase (LCAT). This cholesterol ester (CE) in HDL can be transferred to the liver directly through scavenger receptor B1 (SR-B1). Alternatively, it can be transferred to apolipoprotein B100–containing lipoproteins in exchange for triglycerides (TG) through the action of cholesteryl ester transfer protein (CETP). IDL = intermediate-density lipoprotein; LDL = low-density lipoprotein; LDLR = low-density lipoprotein receptor; VLDL = very low density lipoprotein.

are activated by lipids, play important roles in systemic lipid metabolism, and are current or potential targets of medications for altering lipids in patients.

Peroxisome proliferator-activated receptors (PPARs) are thought to be activated by fatty acids or their derivatives, such as phospholipids. There are at least three types: PPARα, PPARγ, and PPARδ. PPARα stimulates the expression of genes mediating fatty acid oxidation and those promoting the formation of HDL. Fibrate drugs such as gemfibrozil and fenofibrate work by activating PPARα. They lower triglycerides by accelerating the oxidation of fatty acids in the liver, so that less lipid is available for stabilizing apo B100 in VLDL secretion, and they elevate HDL by increasing the expression of apo AI, LPL, and other genes. PPARγ is expressed mostly in adipose tissue and macrophages. It increases the expression of genes promoting the development of fat tissue and appears to suppress chronic inflammation. Thiazolidinedione drugs such as pioglitazone work by activating PPARγ. They lower blood glucose concentration in people with diabetes by decreasing insulin resistance, a complex process that also results in multiple lipid effects, including lower triglycerides and higher HDL (expected to be beneficial) and higher LDL (expected to be detrimental). Their use is complicated by volume expansion and an increased risk of heart failure. PPARδ is expressed widely and has multiple effects, including increased fatty acid oxidation.

Two other nuclear receptors are activated by lipids and modulate lipid physiology. Liver X receptors (LXRα and LXRβ) are activated by oxidized derivatives of cholesterol. In the liver, they promote the synthesis of fatty acids and triglycerides in addition to stimulating both the conversion of cholesterol into bile acids and the excretion of bile acids into the gut. In the intestine, they suppress the absorption of cholesterol. The farnesoid X receptor (FXR) is activated by bile acids. FXR stimulates the secretion of bile acids into bile as well as the reabsorption of bile acids from the intestine.

Together, these receptors help orchestrate two important, futile cycles in lipid metabolism. In one, fatty acids exported from the liver (in the form of triglycerides within VLDL) and from the intestine (in chylomicron triglycerides) are released to peripheral tissues by the action of LPL. Some are taken up by muscle, where their activation of PPARα accelerates their oxidation in mitochondria, yielding adenosine triphosphate. Others enter adipose tissue, where they are re-esterified into triglycerides. From there, fatty acids are released in a process stimulated by catecholamines and glucagon. This process is complicated, involving hormone-sensitive lipase, adipose triglyceride lipase, and the remodeling of proteins that coat lipid droplets to alter their accessibility to lipases. After lipolysis, fatty acids bind to albumin and return to the liver, where they can fuel the production of more VLDL particles. Nicotinic acid improves lipids in part by blocking the release of fatty acids from adipose tissue through a process that is incompletely understood.

In another futile cycle, bile acids (formed from cholesterol and constituting the major pathway for the excretion of cholesterol from the body) are secreted into the intestine through events stimulated by LXR and FXR. Bile acids are reabsorbed in the terminal ileum. Treatment with bile acid sequestrants such as colesevelam interrupts this enterohepatic circulation, and the increased excretion of cholesterol (in the form of bile acids) depletes cholesterol content in the liver, leading to the induction of LDL receptors and thereby lowering circulating levels of LDL. This treatment also tends to elevate triglyceride levels, the result of de-repression of several processes mediated by FXR that decrease fatty acids and triglycerides. Through effects likely involving both LXR and FXR, colesevelam lowers blood glucose concentration in people with type 2 diabetes.

IMPORTANT CLINICAL DISORDERS OF LIPID METABOLISM

Familial Hypercholesterolemia

EPIDEMIOLOGY

Familial hypercholesterolemia (FH) is an autosomal dominant form of hypercholesterolemia caused by defects in LDL receptor activity. The majority of affected patients have mutations in the LDL receptor gene. Heterozygotes for LDL receptor mutations occur at a frequency of perhaps 1 in 500 in the population, but they account for up to 5% of premature myocardial infarctions (those occurring in men younger than 55 years and women younger than 65 years).

PATHOBIOLOGY

In addition to defects in the LDL receptor gene, other mutations can cause autosomal dominant hypercholesterolemia that is clinically indistinguishable from FH. These include familial defective apo B, caused by mutations that interfere with the ability of LDL to bind the LDL receptor, and variants in PCSK9.

CLINICAL MANIFESTATIONS

Total cholesterol levels are usually higher than 300 mg/dL, with LDL cholesterol levels higher than 200 mg/dL. Triglyceride levels are generally normal. Clinical features include thickening of the Achilles tendon as well as xanthomas at the extensor tendons of the knees and hands, reflecting the infiltration of lipid-laden macrophages at these sites. Clinically apparent tendon xanthomas may occur in a minority of patients with FH. Arthralgias are common, perhaps because of the presence of macrophage-mediated inflammation; these tend to improve with cholesterol lowering. Other features include xanthelasmas and corneal arcus, although the latter is also seen in elderly people and certain ethnic populations independent of cholesterol levels. Homozygotes (about 1 in 1 million) have total cholesterol levels in the range of 800 to 1000 mg/dL and usually do not survive to adulthood without liver transplantation to provide LDL receptors. Children and adolescents with this disease may develop aortic valve disease because of macrophage infiltration at the aortic origin.

The penetrance of cardiovascular events in heterozygous FH is variable. Some subjects present with sudden death or accelerated disease in their 20s, and others (generally women without other risk factors) survive beyond menopause without clinically evident disease.

TREATMENT   Rx

Treatment should address any associated risk factors for vascular disease, such as smoking, hypertension, and diabetes. Patients should be instructed in maintaining a diet low in saturated fat and cholesterol, and most require more than one cholesterol-lowering medication to achieve goals. It is not uncommon for FH patients to be treated with a statin drug, a bile acid sequestrant such as colesevelam, and nicotinic acid. Some with aggressive disease require LDL apheresis, which involves perfusing blood through a column that extracts apo B–containing lipoproteins. Lomitapide, an MTP inhibitor, was recently approved to treat homozygous FH. This agent prevents the assembly of apo B–containing lipoproteins, which allows improvement in circulating lipids in those who have LDL receptor deficiency and thus are unable to increase LDL receptor expression through the use of statins. A serious side effect of lomitapide is fatty liver. Mipomersen, an antisense oligonucleotide targeting apo B, was also recently approved to treat homozygous FH. Hepatic toxicity is also a concern with this agent. The exact role for these therapies is uncertain, and both require careful monitoring to ensure safe use.

Familial Combined Hyperlipidemia

EPIDEMIOLOGY

Familial combined hyperlipidemia is an autosomal dominant form of hyperlipidemia that is present in up to 2% of the general population. It accounts for as many as 20% of cases of premature coronary artery disease.

PATHOBIOLOGY

The specific molecular defect is uncertain. Familial combined hyperlipidemia also appears to be associated with the metabolic syndrome (Chapter 229). The disorder is characterized by the primary overproduction of apo B. VLDLs secreted by the liver are small. Small, dense LDLs, thought to be particularly atherogenic, accumulate. For a given concentration of LDL cholesterol, patients with familial combined hyperlipidemia have greater numbers of LDL particles and an increased apo B concentration.

DIAGNOSIS

The diagnosis is made in the setting of a family history of premature coronary disease with different lipid phenotypes combined in the same family. Affected family members may have elevated triglycerides, elevated LDL cholesterol, or both, or they may have hypertriglyceridemia with low HDL cholesterol. Lipid phenotypes commonly change over time.

Familial Hypertriglyceridemia

Familial hypertriglyceridemia is also a common autosomal dominant disorder, occurring in 1 to 2% of the general population. Affected family members have isolated elevated triglycerides. A unifying molecular mechanism is lacking. The phenotype is stable, with affected family members consistently showing isolated hypertriglyceridemia on repeated analyses. The disorder is characterized by primary overproduction of triglyceride. Lipoprotein particles tend to be large, consisting of increased amounts of triglyceride relative to apo B. For a given level of cholesterol, these patients have lower numbers of lipoprotein particles and a decreased apo B concentration. The relationship between this disorder and cardiovascular risk is uncertain. Affected kindreds do not appear to have a propensity for premature vascular disease, but these individuals are at risk for the chylomicronemia syndrome when an additional stimulus for hypertriglyceridemia, such as uncontrolled diabetes, is present.

Chylomicronemia Syndrome

PATHOBIOLOGY

This syndrome occurs when triglycerides are extremely elevated, usually higher than 2000 mg/dL. Individuals with homozygous defects in the *LPL* gene can present with the syndrome in infancy, although the penetrance of clinical sequelae is extremely variable. Some individuals suffer repeated episodes of the syndrome throughout life, whereas others with triglyceride levels consistently above 2000 mg/dL remain completely asymptomatic. The basis for the wide spectrum of symptoms despite similar degrees of severe hypertriglyceridemia is unknown. *LPL* gene therapy in the form of alipogene tiparvovec (the human *LPL* gene in an adeno-associated virus vector) was recently approved by the European Commission to treat patients with LPL deficiency. This represents the first gene therapy approved for use in the Western world. Other molecular defects responsible for the chylomicronemia syndrome include mutations in apo CII and apo AV.

Although defects in LPL, apo CII, and apo AV can cause the syndrome, the disorder is most likely to occur when patients with a common predisposition to hypertriglyceridemia (familial combined hyperlipidemia or familial hypertriglyceridemia) develop another defect associated with elevated triglycerides (such as uncontrolled diabetes, obesity, and treatment with glucocorticoids, estrogens, or other drugs).

CLINICAL MANIFESTATIONS

Clinical features include eruptive xanthomas (see Fig. 51-12) on the back, buttocks, knees, and elbows; lipemia retinalis (a white appearance of retinal blood vessels, usually seen with triglyceride levels >4000 mg/dL); severe abdominal pain and pancreatitis (which can be life-threatening); hepatosplenomegaly; dyspnea; lymphadenopathy; and neurologic dysfunction, such as memory loss and peripheral neuropathy.

DIAGNOSIS

Evaluation can be complicated by the presence of extreme hypertriglyceridemia, which interferes with the determination of amylase (pancreatic lipase should be measured when pancreatitis is suspected) and artifactually lowers serum glucose, sodium, and other analytes.

TREATMENT Rx

Treatment consists of intravenous hydration and other supportive care for pancreatitis, complete elimination of dietary fat (which usually causes striking decreases in lipids within 24 to 48 hours), and appropriate blood glucose control with insulin in the setting of diabetes.

Dysbetalipoproteinemia

This rare disorder is caused by a mutation in apo E. There are three common variants of the apo E protein: E2, E3 (considered normal), and E4. Subjects with one or more E4 alleles are at risk for Alzheimer's disease. Subjects with two E2 alleles are at risk for dysbetalipoproteinemia. The frequency of this genotype is about 1% in the general population, but dysbetalipoproteinemia is rare, requiring an additional poorly defined factor. Hypothyroidism is known to precipitate the disorder. Subjects classically present with equal elevations of triglycerides and cholesterol in the range of about 300 to 600 mg/dL and xanthomas, especially in the palmar creases of the hands. They are at substantial risk for coronary artery disease. Unlike patients with FH, patients with dysbetalipoproteinemia are also at risk for severe peripheral vascular disease. Atherosclerosis occurs in part because of the presence of elevated concentrations of chylomicron remnants, which are not removed normally because of the presence of apo E2, and IDL particles, which are not converted normally to LDL in the presence of apo E2. It is unknown why the remnants that accumulate in dysbetalipoproteinemia cause both peripheral vascular disease and coronary disease, whereas the LDL particles that accumulate in FH tend to cause only coronary disease.

Diabetic Dyslipidemia

PATHOBIOLOGY

Insulin is a critical regulator of lipid metabolism, and because diabetes represents impaired insulin signaling, lipid disorders are common in both type 1 and type 2 diabetes (Chapter 229). Hypertriglyceridemia is the hallmark of diabetic dyslipidemia. This is driven by two mechanisms. First, LPL is insulin dependent. In the absence of insulin or in the presence of insulin resistance, LPL enzyme activity is deficient, and triglyceride-rich lipoproteins cannot be metabolized appropriately. Second, insulin suppresses the release of free fatty acids from adipose tissue stores. Insulin deficiency or resistance results in unabated release of free fatty acids, and these return to the liver, where they stabilize apo B synthesis and increase VLDL production.

TREATMENT Rx

The lack of insulin in patients with type 1 diabetes causes diabetic ketoacidosis, in which elevated triglycerides can be severe and are corrected by reinstitution of insulin therapy (Chapter 229). Intensive insulin therapy in type 1 diabetes decreases triglycerides, LDL, and often lipoprotein (a). Patients gain weight with intensive insulin therapy, and increased adiposity tends to lower HDL levels, which may explain why HDL does not always increase in intensively treated type 1 patients. Patients with type 2 diabetes usually have increased triglycerides and decreased HDL. These abnormalities improve but seldom normalize with better glycemic control. Most of the improvement occurs with initial pharmacologic glucose-lowering therapy, regardless of its mechanism of action.

Diabetes is frequently classified as a secondary cause of lipid disorders. However, lipid abnormalities are intrinsic to diabetes, and people with diabetes who lack clinical evidence of vascular disease have the same risk for cardiovascular events as those with established coronary disease. Therefore, every person with diabetes should be evaluated for lipid disorders, and adequate control of lipid levels often requires treatment with a statin drug. In patients with diabetes, cholesterol-lowering therapy with a statin reduces major cardiovascular events on the basis of primary prevention trials[A1] as well as secondary prevention trials. Statin treatment should not be delayed while glycemic control is optimized.

● EVALUATION AND THERAPY OF LIPID DISORDERS

DIAGNOSIS

The initial evaluation should include a complete history and physical examination, with careful attention to potential secondary causes of lipid disorders (Table 206-4). Diabetes, obesity, hypothyroidism, and excess alcohol intake are probably the most common secondary contributors to abnormal lipid metabolism.

Among prescription medications, β-adrenergic blocking agents are frequent contributors to abnormal lipid profiles. These agents have proven beneficial effects after myocardial infarction but also tend to promote weight gain, to elevate triglycerides, and to decrease HDL. Many clinicians are using lower doses of these agents and relying on more lipid-neutral drugs (angiotensin-converting enzyme inhibitors and angiotensin receptor blockers) for blood pressure control.

It is now common for internists to encounter patients with human immunodeficiency virus (HIV) infection with hyperlipidemia. Some series estimate that more than half of HIV-infected patients treated with protease inhibitors for 2 years develop dyslipidemia, frequently with a redistribution of fat resembling that in genetic lipodystrophy syndromes (Chapter 389). Newer protease inhibitors appear to have fewer metabolic sequelae than older agents such as ritonavir. In addition to appropriate management of other risk factors, lipid-lowering therapy should be tailored to the ongoing HIV drug regimen. Pravastatin is least likely to interact with protease inhibitors but is less effective at lowering LDL cholesterol. Agents such as simvastatin that are substantially metabolized by the cytochrome P-450 3A4 system should not be used in patients treated with protease inhibitors because of delayed

TABLE 206-4	SECONDARY CAUSES OF LIPID DISORDERS
CONDITION OR MEDICATION	**COMMENTS**
Diabetes	Common contributor to dyslipidemia; abnormal lipids are seldom normalized by glycemic control alone
Obesity	Increased triglycerides and decreased HDL are common; LDL may be elevated in some and decrease with weight loss
Hypothyroidism	Thyroid hormone regulates multiple steps in lipid metabolism, including LDL receptor expression and LPL activity
Alcohol	Can cause hypertriglyceridemia in susceptible patients, but mild intake is linked to decreased risk of vascular disease
Renal disease	Increased LDL in nephrotic syndrome, hypertriglyceridemia in end-stage renal disease
Obstructive liver disease	Can be associated with very high cholesterol levels; some evidence that diseases such as primary biliary cirrhosis are not associated with increased vascular events despite dyslipidemia
Diuretics	Increased LDL with high doses; current practice of using low doses of thiazides decreases vascular events and has minimal effect on lipids
β-Adrenergic receptor blockers	Increased triglycerides and decreased HDL, probably by inhibiting LPL
Anabolic steroids	Can result in very low HDL (<10 mg/dL)
Estrogens	Exacerbate hypertriglyceridemia when given orally; this effect is not seen with topical estrogen therapy
Protease inhibitors	Increased triglycerides and decreased HDL, especially in the setting of HIV-associated lipodystrophy
Glucocorticoid excess	Increased triglycerides and decreased HDL, probably related to exacerbation of insulin resistance
Antipsychotics	Increased triglycerides and decreased HDL, probably related to increased adiposity and insulin resistance
Retinoids	Increased triglycerides
Systemic lupus erythematosus	Chronic inflammation may increase risk of vascular disease independent of effects on lipid metabolism
Acute intermittent porphyria	Many agents used to treat lipid disorders reported to provoke episodes of abdominal pain

HDL = high-density lipoprotein; HIV = human immunodeficiency virus; LDL = low-density lipoprotein; LPL = lipoprotein lipase.

clearance of the statin. PPARα agonists such as fenofibrate can be used to lower triglycerides, but the effects are limited because their clearance is accelerated by protease inhibitor treatment.

Antipsychotics have complex effects on metabolism. Some of the newer agents used to treat schizophrenia promote hyperlipidemia, obesity, and insulin resistance. Although therapeutic decisions should be based on psychiatric responses, substituting for agents with prominent metabolic side effects, such as olanzapine, can improve lipid profiles.

Laboratory Evaluation

After an 8- to 12-hour fast (tell patients that drinking water and other calorie-free beverages during this period is acceptable), total triglycerides, total cholesterol, HDL cholesterol, and LDL cholesterol should be measured. In most clinical laboratories, LDL cholesterol is still calculated by this formula: LDL = total cholesterol − HDL cholesterol − (triglycerides/5). This formula is not valid when triglyceride levels are higher than 400 mg/dL, however. It is also possible to measure LDL directly, which is sometimes useful for monitoring the therapeutic effects on LDL alone, and this determination does not require patients to fast. Excessive lipid determinations may not be helpful. Biologic and random variability in cholesterol levels is considerable, and for patients with levels that are 19 mg/dL or more below their goal, serial monitoring is more likely to detect false-positive than true-positive increases during a period of 3 years.

What constitutes "normal" lipid levels is unknown. Prior expert consensus panels have identified a normal triglyceride level as lower than 150 mg/dL. Values from 150 to 199 mg/dL are borderline high, 200 to 499 mg/dL is considered high, and above 500 mg/dL is very high. In patients with fasting triglyceride levels higher than 500 mg/dL, triglycerides are a primary target of therapy to decrease the risk of pancreatitis and chylomicronemia syndrome. These individuals should be managed in consultation with specialists in lipid disorders. Treatment usually involves a very low fat diet, an exercise program, a weight loss regimen in the setting of obesity, glycemic control in the setting of diabetes, and either nicotinic acid or a fibrate drug alone or in combination with fish oils.

Risk Assessment

In 2013, the American College of Cardiology and the American Heart Association released new guidelines for the treatment of cholesterol.[5,6] These recommendations differ from the recommendations of the National Cholesterol Education Program Adult Treatment Panel III report from 2002 in several important ways. Previously, the number of risk factors present was determined and used in conjunction with calculated risk to identify specific therapeutic goals for LDL cholesterol levels. Risk factors for coronary heart disease include smoking, hypertension (or treatment for hypertension), family history of premature coronary heart disease (younger than 55 years in men, 65 years in women), low HDL (<40 mg/dL), and age (older than 45 years in men, 55 years in women). These risk factors can still be useful in the evaluation and management of patients, but their use is de-emphasized in the most recent guidelines. Also de-emphasized is the notion of specific LDL targets. Previously, the LDL goal was lower than 100 mg/dL (or optionally lower than 70 mg/dL) in high-risk patients with known atherosclerotic cardiovascular disease. An alternative metric was non-HDL cholesterol. Goals for non-HDL cholesterol (calculated as total cholesterol minus HDL cholesterol) were 30 mg/dL higher than those for LDL. For example, in a high-risk patient with an LDL goal of less than 100 mg/dL, the corresponding non-HDL cholesterol goal was less than 130 mg/dL. These targets may still be useful in certain clinical settings, but they were not recommended in the most recent guidelines because their utility was not validated in randomized clinical trials.

The latest guidelines have not been uniformly endorsed by professional organizations representing those involved in the care of patients with lipid disorders. However, they are likely to influence clinical practice.[7] They are also subject to modifications as new data become available.

In short, the current American College of Cardiology/American Heart Association guidelines identify groups of individuals for which statin therapy is recommended and other groups for which statin therapy is not recommended. These are summarized in Table 206-5. High-intensity statin therapy to decrease LDL by 50% or more than with the use of higher doses of atorvastatin or rosuvastatin is recommended. Moderate-intensity therapy to decrease LDL by 30% to less than 50% with the use of lower doses of atorvastatin, rosuvastatin, or other statins is an option for patients who cannot tolerate high-intensity therapy or for patients with diabetes and a 10-year risk of atherosclerotic cardiovascular disease of less than 7.5%.

TABLE 206-5 TREATMENT RECOMMENDATIONS BASED ON 2013 ACC/AHA CHOLESTEROL TREATMENT GUIDELINES

STATIN THERAPY RECOMMENDED	STATIN THERAPY NOT RECOMMENDED
Patients with clinically evident atherosclerotic cardiovascular disease Adults with LDL cholesterol > 190 mg/dL Patients with type 1 or type 2 diabetes and LDL cholesterol ≥ 70 mg/dL Adults with LDL cholesterol ≥ 70 mg/dL and 10-year risk of atherosclerotic cardiovascular disease ≥ 7.5%*	Adults with end-stage renal disease Patients with NYHA class II, III, or IV heart failure Adults > 75 years of age without clinical evidence of atherosclerotic cardiovascular disease

*Determined by risk calculator found at *http://my.americanheart.org/cvriskcalculator.*
ACC/AHA = American College of Cardiology/American Heart Association; LDL = low-density lipoprotein; NYHA = New York Heart Association.

A risk calculator for estimating 10-year risk of atherosclerotic cardiovascular disease is found at *http://my.americanheart.org/cvriskcalculator.* This can be downloaded to devices such as smart phones, allowing the provision of individualized information to patients at the point of care.

TREATMENT Rx

General Measures
Intensive Lowering of Low-Density Lipoproteins
Many randomized clinical trials support the concept that intensive LDL lowering decreases cardiovascular event rates in patients with coronary heart disease and its equivalents.[A2] In the Heart Protection Study, those with an LDL level of less than 100 mg/dL benefited from further lowering of LDL with simvastatin. In the Pravastatin or Atorvastatin Evaluation and Infection Therapy trial, patients with acute coronary syndrome derived greater benefit with an LDL level of 62 mg/dL reached with atorvastatin than with an LDL level of 95 mg/dL reached with pravastatin. In the Treating to New Targets study, patients with stable coronary heart disease had fewer clinical events with an LDL level of 77 mg/dL on 80 mg of atorvastatin than with an LDL level of 101 mg/dL on 10 mg of atorvastatin. In the Incremental Decrease in End Points through Aggressive Lipid-Lowering study, patients with stable coronary heart disease with an LDL level of 81 mg/dL on 80 mg of atorvastatin had fewer events than those with an LDL level of 104 mg/dL on 20 mg of simvastatin. In healthy individuals with an LDL level less than 130 mg/dL and C-reactive protein level higher than 2 mg/dL, rosuvastatin (20 mg/day) reduced major cardiovascular events by 44% and all-cause mortality by 20%. Moderate-dose statin therapy increases the risk of diabetes by 2 persons per 1000 person-years, but it reduces the risk of cardiovascular events by 6.5 persons per 1000 person-years.[A3] The benefits of statin therapy exceed the diabetes hazard, even in patients at high risk for development of diabetes.[8]

Lifestyle Changes
Therapeutic lifestyle changes should be recommended as part of the treatment regimen. These include smoking cessation, weight reduction, exercise on most days of the week, reduced intake of dietary cholesterol to less than 200 mg/day, reduction of saturated fat to less than 7% of total calories, increased soluble fiber intake (to at least 10 g/day), and consumption of plant stanols or sterols (2 g/day). However, the role of these changes alone in reducing the risk of cardiovascular disease is unclear. In overweight or obese people with diabetes, an intensive lifestyle intervention did not decrease cardiovascular events.[9]

Medical Therapy
Medications commonly used to treat lipid disorders are listed in Table 206-6.

Statins
Statins are effective. An analysis of results from 90,000 participants in statin trials suggested that the 5-year incidence of cardiovascular events decreases by about 1% for each decrease of 2 mg/dL in LDL. The benefit appears to be independent of a patient's baseline lipid values.

Statins are safe, a notion confirmed in numerous studies during two decades. When statins were introduced, concerns were raised about the possibility of increased mortality with these agents due to noncardiovascular causes such as cancer. Eleven-year total follow-up of patients in the Heart Protection Study, a trial that compared simvastatin with placebo, confirmed long-term benefits with statin use without effects on noncardiovascular mortality or cancer incidence.[A4] In the entire Danish population, those using statins had reduced cancer mortality compared with those who never used statins for each of 13 different cancer types.[10]

TABLE 206-6 MEDICATIONS USED TO TREAT LIPID DISORDERS

CLASS	SIDE EFFECTS	LIPID EFFECTS	SPECIFIC AGENTS (DOSE)
Statins (HMG-CoA reductase inhibitors)	Mildly increased liver enzymes, myalgias without evidence of muscle disease, constipation, insomnia, rhabdomyolysis (rare)	↓↓LDL, 18-55% ↑HDL, 5-15% ↓TG, 7-30%	Simvastatin (20-40 mg/day) Atorvastatin (10-80 mg/day) Pravastatin (20-80 mg/day) Fluvastatin (20-80 mg/day) Lovastatin (20-80 mg/day) Rosuvastatin (10-40 mg/day) Pitavastatin (1-4 mg/day)
Nicotinic acid	Flushing, nausea, diarrhea, hyperglycemia, hyperuricemia, hepatotoxicity (rare)	↑↑HDL, 15-35% ↓↓TG, 20-50% ↓LDL, 5-25% ↓Lp(a), variable	Extended-release or crystalline niacin (1-2 g/day)
Fibrates	Mildly increased liver enzymes, dyspepsia, gallstones, hepatotoxicity (rare), rhabdomyolysis (rare)	↓↓TG, 20-90% ↑HDL, 10-20%	Gemfibrozil (1.2 g/day) Fenofibrate (34-200 mg/day)
Cholesterol absorption inhibitor	Hepatitis, abdominal pain, back pain, arthralgias	↓LDL, 18%	Ezetimibe (10 mg/day)
Bile acid sequestrants	Constipation, decreased absorption of some drugs	↓LDL, 15-30% ↑TG, variable ↑HDL, 3-5%	Colesevelam (2.5-3.75 g/day); this agent also approved for lowering glucose in type 2 diabetes Cholestyramine (4-16 g/day) Colestipol (2-16 g/day)
Fish oils	Eructation, dyspepsia	↓TG, variable ↑ LDL, variable	Omega-3-acid ethyl esters (variable)

HDL = high-density lipoprotein; HMG-CoA = 3-hydroxy-3-methylglutaryl coenzyme A; LDL = low-density lipoprotein; Lp(a) = lipoprotein (a); TG = triglyceride.

Statins are well tolerated. Up to 5% of patients have mildly elevated serum transaminases with therapy, which is usually asymptomatic and resolves spontaneously. Statins cause important liver injury in 1.2 per 100,000 users, usually 3 to 4 months after therapy is started. Atorvastatin is mostly associated with cholestatic liver injury, whereas hepatocellular injury is more common with simvastatin. Therapy should be discontinued if elevations exceed three times the upper limit of normal or if patients have symptoms of liver dysfunction (especially fatigue and weight loss). Rhabdomyolysis is rare and more likely in the setting of concurrent treatment with azole antifungals, erythromycin, cyclosporine, and several other agents. Common but generally mild side effects include constipation, abdominal pain, and difficulty sleeping. Some patients report cognitive difficulties with statins, but it is difficult to appreciate the exact role of statin use in the development of these symptoms.

A substantial minority of patients treated with statins develop myalgias without physical findings or laboratory evidence of muscle dysfunction. The cause of this side effect is unknown. Rarely, statins cause clinical myopathy, which may be related to genetic variations in the capacity to synthesize creatine.[11] Curiously, clinical trials have not documented a difference in muscle symptoms in statin-treated compared with placebo-treated subjects. Clinicians should not minimize the impact of statin intolerance on quality of life for people with lipid disorders. However, muscle aches and joint pain are experienced by all patients at some time, and these common symptoms are often incorrectly attributed to statins. It may be appropriate to consider hypothyroidism, vitamin D deficiency, rheumatologic disorders such as polymyalgia rheumatica, or depression in these patients. The problem may be resolved by stopping the medication, allowing symptoms to resolve, restarting at a much lower dose with gradual increases during weeks, and using a different statin. In one health care system, more than half of patients discontinued statins at least temporarily, 17% had statin-related events documented, and more than 90% of those who were rechallenged with a statin were still taking the medication 1 year later.[12]

Combinations of statins with other agents such as amlodipine and extended-release niacin can enhance compliance and decrease copayment costs.

Nicotinic Acid
Nicotinic acid is a B complex vitamin that in high doses lowers triglycerides, elevates HDL, and modestly lowers LDL. The most common side effect is flushing, which can be diminished with aspirin, by taking the medication with a small snack, and by avoiding hot beverages. It may be useful in patients with very high triglyceride levels who are at risk for pancreatitis. In those already achieving low levels of LDL with a statin, adding niacin does not improve clinical outcomes even though it lowers LDL and raises HDL, and it increases serious adverse events.[A5]

Fibrates
Fibrates lower triglycerides in patients with very high levels who are at risk for pancreatitis, especially those who cannot tolerate niacin. These drugs increase HDL but also tend to increase LDL in patients with high triglyceride levels. Fibrates in combination with a statin increase risk of rhabdomyolysis. In patients with type 2 diabetes, the addition of fenofibrate to simvastatin did not reduce cardiovascular end points compared with simvastatin alone.[13]

Other Agents
Ezetimibe lowers both LDL and triglycerides, with minimal effects on HDL. It is effective at achieving additional LDL lowering when it is used in combination with a statin. In a large randomized trial, the addition of 10 mg ezetimibe to high-dose statin therapy further reduced LDL from 70 mg/dL to 53 mg/dL and reduced adverse cardiovascular outcomes by an absolute 2% without adverse effects in patients who were stable after an acute coronary syndrome.[A6]

Proprotein convertase subtilisin/kexin type 9 (PCSK9), a serine protease that is produced primarily in the liver, controls levels of LDL cholesterol by binding to hepatic LDL receptors and promoting their degradation. PCSK9 antagonists lower LDL cholesterol levels by about 50% or more, regardless of whether they are added to diet therapy, statin therapy, or combined statin plus ezetimibe.[14] Ongoing clinical trials will assess whether they have an equivalent effect on cardiovascular outcomes.

Bile acid sequestrants lower LDL and decrease cardiovascular event rates. They are especially effective in combination with statins. Acceptance by patients is limited because of gastrointestinal side effects. These agents also tend to elevate triglycerides and decrease the absorption of some drugs. The sequestrant colesevelam may have less of an effect on the absorption of other drugs and has been demonstrated to lower glucose concentration in patients with type 2 diabetes.

Fish oils may be used as an adjunct in the therapy of patients with very high triglyceride levels. These omega-3 fatty acids, which occur naturally in cold-water fish, may work by activating PPARα. They may have beneficial effects on cardiovascular risk, but low-dose fish oil treatment of patients with diabetes or at risk for diabetes, most of whom were receiving statins, did not decrease cardiovascular events.[15]

PRIMARY PREVENTION
The results of clinical trials strongly support lipid lowering for secondary prevention, which is decreasing events in those with known disease. Data are less compelling for primary prevention, which is decreasing events in those without known disease. Use of a statin to lower lipids is clearly effective for primary prevention in at least three groups: patients with multiple risk factors, individuals with type 2 diabetes, and middle-aged and older people with relatively low LDL levels in the setting of elevated C-reactive protein. In the Anglo-Scandinavian Cardiac Outcomes Trial–Lipid-Lowering Arm, subjects with hypertension and at least three other risk factors had fewer events with an LDL level of 90 mg/dL achieved with atorvastatin than with an LDL level of about 130 mg/dL in control subjects. In the Collaborative Atorvastatin Diabetes Study, people with type 2 diabetes had fewer events with an LDL level of about 75 mg/dL achieved with atorvastatin compared with placebo-treated subjects with an LDL level of about 119 mg/dL. In the Justification for the Use of Statins in Prevention: An Intervention Trial Evaluating Rosuvastatin, men older than 50 years and women older than 60 years had fewer events and were less likely to die with an LDL level of about 55 mg/

dL achieved with rosuvastatin compared with placebo-treated subjects with an LDL level of about 108 mg/dL. An analysis of 18 primary trials involving more than 56,000 participants concluded that treatment of subjects with no evidence of cardiovascular disease with statins reduced all-cause mortality and vascular events with no evidence of excess adverse events.[A7]

The 2013 guidelines recommend statin therapy for primary prevention in individuals with an LDL cholesterol level above 190 mg/dl, those with diabetes, and those with a 10-year risk of atherosclerotic cardiovascular disease of at least 7.5% (see Table 206-5).

There does not appear to be a threshold effect of LDL on atherogenesis. In people with established coronary heart disease and those with diabetes, reaching very low LDL cholesterol levels is desirable. The absolute value at which maximal benefit is reached is unknown, and higher doses of statins are associated with more side effects (especially increased serum transaminases), but some analyses suggest that an LDL level of 40 mg/dL represents no increased risk of vascular disease.

Grade A References

A1. de Vries FM, Denig P, Pouwels KB, et al. Primary prevention of major cardiovascular and cerebrovascular events with statins in diabetic patients: a meta-analysis. *Drugs.* 2012;72:2365-2373.
A2. Mills EJ, O'Regan C, Eyawo O, et al. Intensive statin therapy compared with moderate dosing for prevention of cardiovascular events: a meta-analysis of >40,000 patients. *Eur Heart J.* 2011;32:1409-1415.
A3. Preiss D, Seshasai SR, Welsh P, et al. Risk of incident diabetes with intensive-dose compared with moderate-dose statin therapy: a meta-analysis. *JAMA.* 2011;305:2556-2564.
A4. Heart Protection Study Collaborative Group. Effects on 11-year mortality and morbidity of lowering LDL cholesterol with simvastatin for about 5 years in 20,536 high-risk individuals: a randomised controlled trial. *Lancet.* 2011;378:2013-2020.
A5. Landray MJ, Haynes R, Hopewell JC, et al. Effects of extended-release niacin with laropiprant in high-risk patients. *N Engl J Med.* 2014;371:203-212.
A6. Špinar J, Špinarová L, Vítovec J. IMProved Reduction of Outcomes: Vytorin Efficacy International Trial (studie IMPROVE-IT). *Vnitr Lek.* 2014;12:1095-1101.
A7. Taylor F, Huffman MD, Macedo AF, et al. Statins for the primary prevention of cardiovascular disease. *Cochrane Database Syst Rev.* 2013;1:CD004816.

GENERAL REFERENCES

For the General References and other additional features, please visit Expert Consult at https://expertconsult.inkling.com.

207

GLYCOGEN STORAGE DISEASES

DAVID A. WEINSTEIN

DEFINITION

Glycogen, a highly branched polymer of glucose, is the storage form of glucose in mammals. The major sites of glycogen deposition are skeletal muscle and liver. Several other tissues and organs, including the heart, smooth muscle, kidney, and intestine, are sites of glycogen synthesis that can be impaired in the glycogen storage diseases (GSDs).

EPIDEMIOLOGY

The overall frequency of the GSDs is approximately 1 case per 20,000 to 25,000 births. Sixteen distinct types have been identified, which are referred to either by the deficient enzyme or by a numbering system that reflects the historical sequence of their description. They are all uncommon and some are extremely rare. Six types account for approximately 97% of GSD cases: GSD I (25%), GSD II (15%), GSD III (24%), GSD IV (3%), and GSD VI and IX (30%). It is likely, however, that the mild forms of GSD are under-recognized.

PATHOBIOLOGY

Glucose transporter type 2 (GLUT2) predominates in the liver (and pancreatic beta cells) and has a high K_m ($\approx$15 to 20 mmol/L); consequently, the free glucose concentration in hepatocytes increases in direct proportion to the increase in plasma glucose concentration. Glucose is rapidly phosphorylated by glucokinase to form glucose 6-phosphate, which is converted to glucose 1-phosphate, the starting point for glycogen synthesis (Fig. 207-1). Hepatic glycogen synthase catalyzes the formation of α-1,4 linkages that elongate the chains of glucose molecules. A branching enzyme leads to formation of α-1,6 linkages at branch points along the chain. The concentration of GLUT4 in the plasma membrane of skeletal muscle increases markedly after exposure

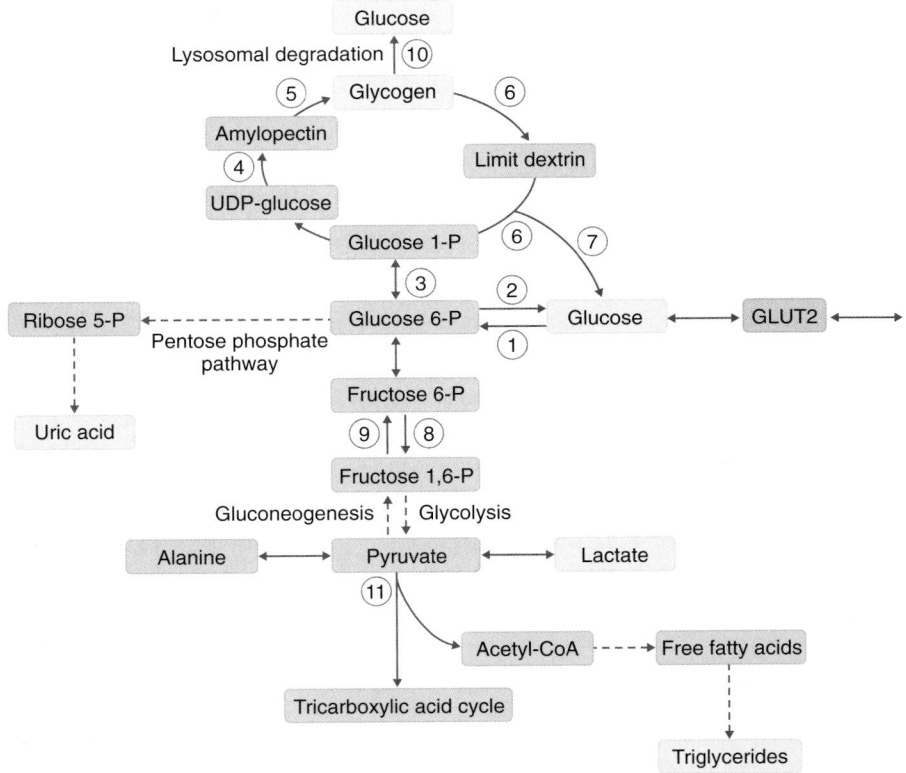

FIGURE 207-1. **Simplified scheme of glycogen synthesis and degradation in the liver.** Note that in skeletal muscle, GLUT4 transports glucose across the cell membrane and glucose-6-phosphatase is absent. UDP-glucose = uridine diphosphoglucose; 1, hexokinase/glucokinase; 2, glucose-6-phosphatase; 3, phosphoglucomutase; 4, glycogen synthase; 5, branching enzyme; 6, glycogen phosphorylase; 7, debranching enzyme; 8, phosphofructokinase; 9, fructose-1,6-bisphosphatase; 10, acid maltase; 11, pyruvate dehydrogenase.

to insulin and in response to exercise, resulting in increased glucose transport into skeletal muscle, where it is either oxidized to provide energy for contracting muscle or converted to glycogen.

In the intervals between meals and during the overnight fast, a cascade of enzymatic reactions (including adenylate cyclase, phosphorylase *b* kinase, and cyclic adenosine monophosphate–dependent protein kinase) activate hepatic glycogen phosphorylase, the rate-limiting enzyme in glycogenolysis, leading to the formation of glucose 6-phosphate. Glucose-6-phosphatase catalyzes the terminal reaction of both glycogenolysis and gluconeogenesis, the hydrolysis of glucose 6-phosphate, thereby allowing glucose to be released from the liver into the systemic circulation. This process is critically important for the maintenance of glucose homeostasis. Because muscle lacks glucose-6-phosphatase, it cannot release glucose for systemic use. Muscle glycogen is used to meet the energy requirement of contracting muscle and is a source of lactate, pyruvate, and alanine for gluconeogenesis early in starvation. The rate of glycogenolysis in muscle is most rapid during the first 5 to 10 minutes of exercise. As exercise continues and blood flow to muscle increases, blood-borne substrates (glucose and free fatty acids) become increasingly important sources of energy.

The GSDs or glycogenoses comprise several inherited disorders of glycogen synthesis or degradation. All are autosomal recessive with the exception of a subtype of GSD IX that is X-linked. The GSDs are caused by mutations in the genes that code for enzymes involved in the synthesis or degradation of glycogen and may involve the liver, skeletal muscle, and kidney. They are all characterized by an abnormal tissue concentration or structure (or both) of the glycogen molecule.

CLINICAL MANIFESTATIONS AND DIAGNOSIS

Hepatomegaly and hypoglycemia[1] are the principal clinical manifestations of the hepatic glycogenoses; muscle cramps, exercise intolerance, easy fatigability, and progressive weakness are the major manifestations of the muscle glycogenoses. Features of the most common GSDs are shown in Table 207-1. Molecular genetic testing performed on DNA extracted from blood or saliva is used to diagnose all the common forms of GSD.

TREATMENT   Rx

The goal of treatment of the hepatic forms of GSD is to prevent hypoglycemia and glucose counter-regulation. The specific details of therapy principally depend on whether normal gluconeogenesis can occur. In GSD I, abnormal glucose-6-phosphatase activity impairs both glycogenolysis and gluconeogenesis. In contrast, gluconeogenesis is intact in the other liver forms of GSD, allowing protein to be used as a substrate for endogenous glucose production. Fatty acid oxidation is also intact in all types of GSD except for GSD I, resulting in ketone formation during periods of hypoglycemia.[2]

TABLE 207-1   PRINCIPAL FEATURES OF THE COMMON GLYCOGEN STORAGE DISEASES

TYPE AND DEFECTIVE ENZYME	CHARACTERISTIC CLINICAL FEATURES	HIGH-RISK POPULATIONS	THERAPY
0 *Hepatic glycogen synthase*	Liver small or normal in size, fasting ketotic hypoglycemia, postprandial hyperglycemia and hyperlactatemia	French Canadian Italians	UCS, especially at bedtime, with high-protein diet
Ia *Glucose-6-phosphatase* *von Gierke's disease*	Hepatomegaly, failure to thrive, growth retardation, severe hypoglycemia, lactic acidosis, hyperuricemia, hyperlipidemia	Ashkenazi Jews Mexicans Chinese Japanese	UCS during the day and night or continuous overnight intragastric feeding
Ib *Glucose 6-phosphate transporter*	Same as type Ia; also neutropenia, recurrent bacterial infections, and inflammatory bowel disease	Native Americans Iranian Jews Italians	UCS as for Glycogen Storage Disease Ia; granulocyte colony-stimulating factor
II *Lysosomal acid maltase (α-glucosidase)* *Pompe's disease*	Infantile form is characterized by severe generalized hypotonia, muscle weakness, and hypertrophic cardiomyopathy leading to cardiorespiratory failure usually by 1 year of age. Skeletal myopathy with slowly progressing muscle weakness is the primary clinical manifestation of the juvenile- and adult-onset forms. Serum creatine kinase is markedly increased.	None	Intravenous enzyme replacement with recombinant human α-glucosidase
III *Debranching enzyme* *Cori's or Forbes' disease*	Hepatomegaly, moderate to severe ketotic hypoglycemia, muscle weakness and wasting, hypertrophic cardiomyopathy (IIIa), increased transaminases; without muscle involvement (IIIb)	Faroe Islanders First Nation (Canada) Indian subcontinent	High-protein diet with low-dose UCS supplementation
IV *Glycogen branching enzyme* *Andersen's disease*	A clinically heterogeneous disorder The typical presentation is liver disease in early childhood progressing to lethal cirrhosis. The less common neuromuscular presentation is distinguished by age at onset into 4 groups: perinatal, congenital, childhood, and adult.	None	No specific treatment Liver transplantation has resulted in decreased glycogen storage in heart and skeletal muscle.
V *Muscle glycogen phosphorylase* *McArdle's disease*	Symptoms usually begin in adolescence or early adulthood with exercise intolerance, fatigue, myalgia, muscle cramps, and muscle swelling. Transient myoglobinuria due to rhabdomyolysis may occur after exercise. Severe myoglobinuria may lead to acute renal failure. Later in adult life, persistent and progressive muscle weakness and atrophy with fatty replacement occur. Serum creatine kinase is increased.	None	High-protein diet (50% carbohydrate and 25-30% protein) Oral sucrose before sustained aerobic exercise may be beneficial.
VI *Hepatic glycogen phosphorylase* *Hers' disease*	Hepatomegaly; growth retardation; moderate ketotic hypoglycemia; increased serum transaminases, cholesterol, and triglycerides	Mennonites	UCS dosed to prevent hypoglycemia and ketosis
VII *Muscle phosphofructokinase* *Tarui's disease*	Manifested in childhood with fatigue, muscle cramps, exercise intolerance; rhabdomyolysis and myoglobinuria with strenuous exertion; increased serum creatine kinase; may have mild hemolytic anemia and mild hyperbilirubinemia; hyperuricemia	None	No specific treatment; avoid strenuous exercise
IX *Phosphorylase b kinase*	Hepatomegaly, mild ketotic hypoglycemia, growth retardation, increased serum transaminases, hypercholesterolemia, hypertriglyceridemia May be X-linked or autosomal recessive	None	UCS dosed to prevent hypoglycemia and ketosis; high-protein diet to normalize prealbumin

UCS = uncooked cornstarch.

Treatment of GSD I consists of providing a continuous dietary source of glucose to maintain blood glucose levels at 75 to 90 mg/dL before meals and overnight. Glucose concentrations must be maintained above 70 mg/dL to prevent counter-regulation, which causes shunting of glucose 6-phosphate into alternative pathways, resulting in hyperlactacidemia, hyperuricemia, and hypertriglyceridemia. In infants, continuous glucose can be provided by frequent feeds during the day and continuous intragastric feeds at night through a nasogastric or gastrostomy tube. Beginning at 6 to 12 months of age, uncooked cornstarch (UCS), which is slowly digested and absorbed into the circulation as glucose, can be used as an alternative method of continuously providing glucose. Initially, UCS is given every 3 hours. As children age and guided by the results of periodic blood glucose and lactate monitoring, the interval between feeds eventually is increased to 4 to 6 hours. An extended-release cornstarch preparation allows many older patients to sleep through the night without awakening.[3] Galactose and fructose must be restricted because they cannot be converted to glucose, and consumption of large quantities may exacerbate the biochemical derangements. Optimal care usually ameliorates all biochemical abnormalities; however, if optimal dietary management does not lower serum uric acid and triglycerides to acceptable levels, treatment with allopurinol and gemfibrozil, respectively, is indicated. Neutropenia (Chapter 167) in type Ib responds well to low-dose granulocyte colony-stimulating factor (G-CSF) therapy; however, untoward effects of G-CSF may include splenomegaly and very rare cases of leukemia.[4] The recommended starting dose (2.5 µg/kg/day) is therefore lower than in other conditions, and the lowest possible dose that prevents infections is used. An enterocolitis that resembles Crohn's disease (Chapter 141) occurs almost universally in GSD type Ib, and mesalamine (Pentasa) is the first-line therapy because small intestinal disease predominates.

Patients with the other forms of GSD use a high-protein diet (2 or 3 g/kg) supplemented with complex carbohydrates and UCS, which, typically, is administered every 6 to 8 hours to maintain glucose concentrations above 75 mg/dL. Because β-oxidation of fatty acids can occur in these forms of GSD, ketosis can develop rapidly and UCS doses are titrated to maintain a normal blood ketone concentration (<0.3 mmol/L). Protein dosing is aimed at normalization of total protein and prealbumin concentrations. Strict avoidance of fructose and sucrose is unnecessary; however, intake of simple sugars is still discouraged to avoid excessive storage of glycogen. This is particularly important in GSD III because excessive glycogen storage has been associated with worsening of the associated hypertrophic cardiomyopathy.[5]

Treatment of the muscle glycogenoses is shown in Table 207-1.

Prevention of Complications

Despite improvements in care, long-term complications are common in GSD I and III. There is increasing evidence, however, that complications can be delayed or even prevented with optimal metabolic control.[6] Hepatic adenomas can develop in patients with GSD I during adolescence or early adulthood and may gradually enlarge, undergo malignant transformation, or hemorrhage into the peritoneal cavity. Nephrocalcinosis and nephrolithiasis, caused by hypocitraturia, are also common and can be prevented by oral citrate supplementation. Maintenance of optimal metabolic control can prevent renal tubular dysfunction, focal segmental glomerulosclerosis, anemia, gout, and osteoporosis.[7,8]

In type III GSD, a hypertrophic cardiomyopathy can develop. The cardiac disease appears to be caused by overstorage of glycogen, and restriction of simple sugars and carbohydrates has resulted in normalization of cardiac function. Hepatic adenomas develop in 10% of patients, and hepatocellular cancer is rare. Most patients with type III do not have myopathic symptoms during childhood and early adulthood. Progressive myopathy can develop beginning in the teenage years, and it can become debilitating. A very high protein diet (3 or 4 g/kg) may slow the progression of the muscle disease.[2]

Short stature and osteoporosis are the only common complications in GSD 0, VI, and IX, but these can be prevented by maintenance of optimal metabolic control and avoidance of ketosis.[9] Cirrhosis has been described as a complication in untreated patients with GSD IX, but scarring may be prevented with treatment.[10]

The prognosis for all of the hepatic GSDs is now excellent. Almost all complications can be delayed or prevented with optimal metabolic control. Patients are doing well into adulthood, and pregnancies have now become routine.[11] Liver transplantation should be viewed as a treatment of last resort,[12] especially because gene therapy may be available for treatment of these disorders in the future.

The Association for Glycogen Storage Disease website (*http://www.agsdus.org*) provides basic information about the GSDs intended to be of use to people affected by one of the GSDs, their families, and other interested parties. Similar organizations exist in the United Kingdom, France, Spain, the Netherlands, Germany, Italy, Sweden, the Faroe Islands, Poland, and Russia.

For the General References and other additional features, please visit Expert Consult at https://expertconsult.inkling.com.

208

LYSOSOMAL STORAGE DISEASES

DONNA M. KRASNEWICH AND ELLEN SIDRANSKY

The lysosomal storage diseases encompass a group of more than 45 different inherited disorders, all sharing a defect in lysosomal function. Lysosomes are acidic, membrane-bound organelles present in the cytoplasm containing enzymes that degrade macromolecules. These disorders ensue when one or more of the hydrolytic enzymes are deficient or when essential lysosomal transporters, receptors, cofactors, or protective proteins are defective or lacking. Typically, complex macromolecules, including glycolipids, mucopolysaccharides, and glycoproteins are delivered to the lysosome, where they undergo sequential modification by a series of hydrolases. An enzymatic deficiency becomes clinically important when macromolecules accumulate owing to inadequate degradation. Different categories of defects resulting in lysosomal dysfunction are encountered in the lysosomal storage disorders; examples of each type are listed in Table 208-1.

Although most lysosomal storage disorders are rare, as a group their frequency is estimated to be 1 per 7000 to 8000 live births. This is an underestimate because milder or attenuated forms of these disorders are often not identified. All of the disorders have an autosomal recessive pattern of inheritance, with the exception of Fabry disease and Hunter's syndrome (mucopolysaccharidosis II), which are X-linked recessive, and Danon's disease, caused by mutations in the lysosome-associated membrane protein 2 (LAMP-2), which is inherited in an X-linked dominant manner. As a whole, these disorders are characterized by a vast spectrum of manifestations, often causing them to evade diagnosis. Many were traditionally classified into infantile, juvenile, and adult types on the basis of the patient's age at the onset of manifestations, but atypical presentations complicate these distinctions. Among the factors contributing to this phenotypic diversity are the amount of residual enzyme activity, the cellular localization of the enzyme, the genotype, and the genetic background of the affected individual as well as other genetic, environmental, and epigenetic influences.[1]

With the advent of new therapies for some of the lysosomal storage disorders, early establishment of the diagnosis is paramount. Suggestive clinical findings include coarse facial features; organomegaly; specific eye findings, including corneal clouding or a cherry red spot (of the macula); cytopenia; and skeletal abnormalities, notably dysostosis multiplex. Disorders associated with each of these findings are listed in Table 208-2. There should be a greater index of suspicion whenever these features occur in concert, the findings are progressive, there is developmental regression, or the patient appears dissimilar to other family members.

The diagnostic work-up includes a careful history, with analysis of the family pedigree and assessment of developmental milestones in childhood and adolescence. A family history of consanguinity, other affected siblings, multiple miscarriages, or early deaths can aid in making the diagnosis. Ethnicity can be a helpful clue because some of the lysosomal disorders occur with increased incidence in specific populations, such as Ashkenazi Jews (Gaucher disease type 1, Tay-Sachs' disease, mucolipidosis type IV) and Scandinavians (mannosidosis, aspartylglucosaminuria, Salla's disease, Gaucher disease type 3). On physical examination, special attention should be paid to head circumference, facial appearance, enlargement of the tongue, hepatosplenomegaly, skeletal manifestations (including kyphosis), broadening of the long bones, and stiffness of the joints. Skin evaluation may reveal angiokeratoma, especially around the umbilicus and in skin creases. The eye evaluation should include a funduscopic and slit-lamp examination as well as an assessment for atypical eye movements, which may be pathognomonic for disorders such as

TABLE 208-1 CLASSIFICATION OF LYSOSOMAL STORAGE DISORDERS BASED ON THE TYPE OF DEFECT*

SPHINGOLIPIDOSES

Fabry disease (α-galactosidase)
Farber disease (ceramidase)
GM₁ gangliosidosis/Landing's disease (β-galactosidase)
GM₂ gangliosidosis/Tay-Sachs' disease
Sandhoff's disease (α-hexosaminidases A and B)
Gaucher disease (glucocerebrosidase)
Niemann-Pick disease, types A and B (sphingomyelinase)
Metachromatic leukodystrophy (arylsulfatase A)
Krabbe's disease (β-galactocerebrosidase)

LIPID STORAGE DISORDERS

Wolman's disease (acid lipase)
Ceroid-lipofuscinosis, adult type, Kufs'/Parry's (CLN4, heterogeneous)

MUCOPOLYSACCHARIDOSES

Type I/Hurler's disease (α-L-iduronidase)
Type II/Hunter's disease (iduronate-2-sulfatase)
Type III/Sanfilippo's disease (four different enzymes in the degradation of heparan sulfate defining types A-D)
Type VI/Maroteaux-Lamy's disease (N-acetylgalactosamine-4-sulfatase)
Type VII/Sly's disease (α-glucuronidase)

OLIGOSACCHARIDOSES

Aspartylglucosaminuria (aspartylglucosaminidase)
Fucosidosis (α-fucosidase)
α-Mannosidosis (α-mannosidase)
Schindler's disease (α-N-acetylgalactosaminidase)
Sialidosis I (sialidase)
Sialidosis II/mucolipidosis I (sialidase)

MUCOLIPIDOSES

Mucolipidosis II/I-cell disease (N-acetylglucosaminylphosphotransferase)
Mucolipidosis III/pseudo-Hurler (N-acetylglucosaminylphosphotransferase)
Mucolipidosis IV (MCOLN1 mutation)

LYSOSOMAL GLYCOGEN STORAGE

Glycogenosis type II/Pompe's disease (α-1,4-glucosidase)

LYSOSOMAL TRANSPORT DISORDERS

Sialic acid storage disease/Salla's disease (sialin/SLC17A5)
Cystinosis (cystine transporter)
Niemann-Pick disease, type C (intracellular cholesterol transport)

MULTIPLE ENZYME DEFICIENCY

Galactosialidosis (β-galactosidase and sialidase)
Multiple sulfatase deficiency/Austin's disease (sulfatases)

*Full chapters describing each of these disorders are available in Valle D, Beaudet AL, Vogelstein B, et al, eds. The Online Metabolic and Molecular Bases of Inherited Disease. http://www.ommbid.com/OMMBID.

neuronopathic Gaucher disease and Niemann-Pick disease type C. Unexplained cardiomyopathy and cryptogenic stroke may be the initial presentation of Fabry's disease. A careful neurologic and cognitive evaluation can be fruitful because some of the later presentations include dementia and psychiatric manifestations.[2] Moreover, regression of milestones can provide an early diagnostic clue. Preliminary diagnostic studies include urine for thin-layer chromatography, blood count with smear for vacuolated white blood cells, skeletal radiography, and ophthalmologic examination.

For the most part, the diagnosis of a specific lysosomal storage disorder is made by assaying enzymatic activity in a blood sample or fibroblast cell line. A lysosomal panel, evaluating the activity of multiple lysosomal enzymes from the same sample, should be the first-tier test. If a lysosomal storage disorder is still suspected, a tissue biopsy, most often of the bone marrow or liver, can be considered, although this is rarely indicated. Most of the genes encoding the lysosomal enzymes have been identified, and mutation analysis is available. However, in most cases, there is vast genotypic heterogeneity, and mutation screening is useful only when a mutation has already been identified in a specific family or when specific mutations are known to be common in a specific ethnic group.

Improved care and new therapeutic modalities have transformed the natural history of several of these disorders. With patients' increased longevity, diseases that were once encountered only by pediatricians have now made their way to the offices of internists. Moreover, many of the classic complications are now avoided by early therapeutic interventions, such as

enzyme replacement therapy.[3] However, in some instances, prolonged longevity has unmasked unanticipated clinical manifestations. Physicians' increased awareness of the range of manifestations and presentations of lysosomal disorders may lessen the long delays in diagnosis that patients frequently describe. Lysosomal disorders encountered in adult patients are discussed here, with a focus on Gaucher disease and Fabry disease.[4] A brief discussion of specific disorders frequently diagnosed during adulthood as well as of childhood-onset lysosomal disorders that persist through adulthood is included.

GAUCHER DISEASE

PATHOBIOLOGY

Gaucher disease, the *autosomal* recessively inherited deficiency of the lysosomal enzyme glucocerebrosidase, is a disorder primarily of the reticuloendothelial system.[5] Lysosomes within macrophages become engorged with the substrate glucocerebroside, giving rise to the characteristic Gaucher cells, with a wrinkled-paper appearance resulting from intracytoplasmic substrate deposition. The accumulated glycolipid glucosylceramide is derived from the degradation of senescent leukocytes or erythrocyte membranes.

CLINICAL MANIFESTATIONS

Clinically, Gaucher disease has been divided into three types on the basis of the absence or presence and the rate of progression of neurologic involvement. Type 1, the non-neuronopathic form, is the most common type and can be manifested at any age. Type 2, the acute neuronopathic form, manifests before or shortly after birth and has a rapid and progressive course. Type 3 is the subacute neuronopathic form. The spectrum of manifestations encountered in this disorder ranges from asymptomatic octogenarians to infants who succumb in utero. Some patients defy classification into one of the three types. It is a pan-ethnic disorder, although type 1 Gaucher disease is more frequent among Ashkenazi Jews, in whom the carrier frequency is about 1 in 16; in contrast, the approximate carrier frequency in the general population is 1 in 100.

The gene encoding glucocerebrosidase (GBA1) is located on chromosome 1q21, and more than 300 different mutations have been found in patients. Several mutations are encountered with increased frequency in type 1 Gaucher disease; for example, among Ashkenazi Jews, mutation N370S is the most common allele. However, the mutations identified do not adequately account for the range of manifestations encountered.

In recent years, an association between Gaucher disease and parkinsonism (Chapter 409) has been reported.[6,7] Both patients with Gaucher disease and carriers of mutations in GBA1 have a higher incidence of Parkinson's disease and Lewy body disorders.[8] Studies in cohorts of patients with Parkinson's disease around the world demonstrate that they have a more than five-fold increased frequency of GBA1 mutations, rendering this the most common genetic risk factor for parkinsonism identified to date.

Commonly encountered symptoms in all types of Gaucher disease include easy bruisability, hepatomegaly, splenomegaly, chronic fatigue, and bone pain or pathologic fractures. Laboratory findings include anemia, thrombocytopenia, and elevations of ferritin, acid phosphatase, angiotensin-converting enzyme, and, at times, liver enzymes. Painless splenomegaly is the most common presentation in patients with type 1 Gaucher disease, and the spleen can be massively enlarged. Occasional patients have pulmonary involvement or pulmonary hypertension. Bone involvement is a significant cause of morbidity and can be manifested with extreme bone pain or pathologic fractures. Most patients have radiologic evidence of skeletal involvement, including the classic Erlenmeyer flask deformity of the distal end of the femur and osteopenia (Fig. 208-1A). Pathologic fractures (especially of the hip, ribs, or spine), lytic bone lesions, and osteoporosis may occur. Painful bone crises, episodes of bone infarcts, can last for weeks and may require aggressive pain management.

Type 2 disease, which is rare, is characterized by a rapid neurodegenerative course with extensive visceral involvement; death usually occurs within the first 2 years of life. The disease is diagnosed prenatally or in infancy and is associated with increased tone, strabismus, and organomegaly. Failure to thrive and compromised airway from laryngospasm are typical. Progressive psychomotor degeneration leads to death, usually secondary to an intercurrent respiratory infection and respiratory compromise.

Type 3 disease is clinically variable and is often noted in infancy or childhood. In addition to organomegaly and bone involvement, patients have abnormal horizontal eye movements, and some develop myoclonic epilepsy or neurodegenerative manifestations. A subgroup of patients has cardiac

TABLE 208-2 MANIFESTATIONS ENCOUNTERED IN DIFFERENT LYSOSOMAL STORAGE DISORDERS

FINDING	DISORDERS
Hepatosplenomegaly	GM$_1$ gangliosidosis, Niemann-Pick disease, Gaucher disease, Wolman's disease, fucosidosis, Pompe's disease, mannosidosis, multiple sulfatase deficiency, sialidosis, galactosialidosis, several mucopolysaccharidoses, cystinosis
Coarse facies	GM$_1$ gangliosidosis, fucosidosis, Pompe's disease, mannosidosis, multiple sulfatase deficiency, I-cell disease, several mucopolysaccharidoses, mucolipidosis II, sialic acid storage disease, aspartylglucosaminuria
Skeletal findings	GM$_1$ gangliosidosis, Gaucher disease, fucosidosis, mannosidosis, sialidosis, galactosialidosis, several mucopolysaccharidoses, I-cell disease, mucolipidosis III
Cherry red spot	Infantile forms of GM$_1$ gangliosidosis, Sandhoff's disease, Tay-Sachs' disease, Niemann-Pick disease, sialidosis, galactosialidosis, I-cell disease
Corneal clouding	GM$_1$ gangliosidosis, several mucopolysaccharidoses, mannosidosis, I-cell disease, mucolipidosis III and IV, multiple sulfatase deficiency, galactosialidosis
Cognitive impairment	GM$_1$ gangliosidosis, Sandhoff's disease, Tay-Sachs' disease, Niemann-Pick disease, Gaucher disease type 2, Wolman's disease, fucosidosis, mannosidosis, multiple sulfatase deficiency, sialidosis, galactosialidosis, several mucopolysaccharidoses, sialic acid storage disease, aspartylglucosaminuria, I-cell disease, mucolipidosis III and IV, Krabbe's disease, metachromatic leukodystrophy, neuronal ceroid lipofuscinosis

Hematologic
  Foam cells
  Granulated or vacuolated white blood cells
	GM$_1$ gangliosidosis, Niemann-Pick disease, Gaucher disease, acid lipase deficiency, fucosidosis
	Several mucopolysaccharidoses, sialidosis, galactosialidosis. neuronal ceroid-lipofuscinosis, Niemann-Pick disease, Wolman's disease, fucosidosis, mannosidosis, aspartylglucosaminuria, I-cell disease, mucolipidosis III, multiple sulfatase deficiency

Psychiatric or behavioral manifestations	Several mucopolysaccharidoses (especially Sanfilippo's), sialidosis, galactosialidosis, Fabry disease, mannosidosis, neuronal ceroid-lipofuscinosis, metachromatic leukodystrophy, Tay-Sachs' disease, Niemann-Pick disease, type C
Newborn presentations	Gaucher disease, type 2; GM$_1$ gangliosidosis; Krabbe's disease; Niemann-Pick disease, types A and C; mucopolysaccharidosis I, IVA, VII; Pompe's disease; sialidosis, types I and II; mucolipidosis, types I and II; Schindler's disease; Wolman's disease; infantile sialic acid storage disease; sialuria; Salla's disease; galactosialidosis; multiple sulfatase deficiency; prosaposin deficiency

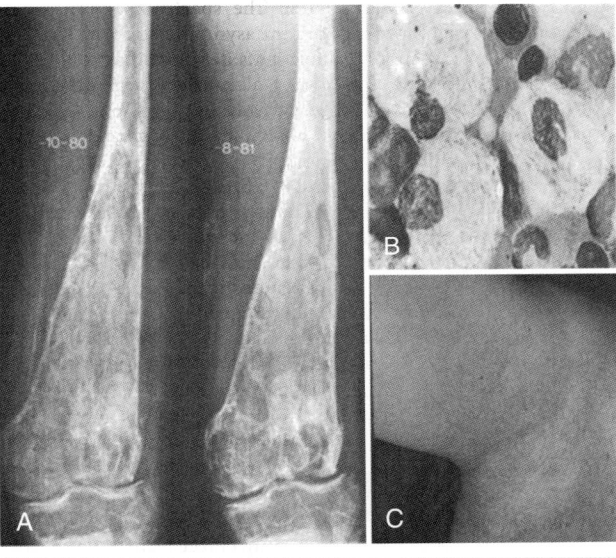

FIGURE 208-1. **A,** Radiographic image showing the Erlenmeyer flask deformity in Gaucher disease. There is cortical thinning and widening of the medullary cavity of the metaphysis and adjacent diaphysis. **B,** Gaucher cells—reticuloendothelial cells storing abnormal amounts of lipid. **C,** Angiokeratomas, the nonblanching punctate skin lesion in Fabry disease.

TABLE 208-3 SUGGESTIVE DIAGNOSTIC FEATURES IN ADULTHOOD FOR GAUCHER DISEASE AND FABRY DISEASE

GAUCHER DISEASE	FABRY DISEASE
Family member with Gaucher disease	Family history of Fabry disease
Hepatomegaly, splenomegaly (sometimes massive)	Cutaneous lesions of capillaries (angiokeratoma)
Frequent epistaxis	Hypohidrosis or heat intolerance
Easy bruising	Intermittent episodes of severe pain in the extremities (acroparesthesias)
Abnormal saccadic eye movements	Left ventricular hypertrophy of unknown etiology in young adulthood
Thrombocytopenia or anemia	Stroke of unknown etiology in young adulthood
Painful bone crisis	Chronic kidney disease of unknown etiology in young adulthood
Erlenmeyer flask deformity of the distal femur, aseptic necrosis of the femoral heads	Multiple renal sinus cysts discovered incidentally
Pathologic fractures, unexplained rib fracture	Female carriers may have more variable and less severe symptoms with later onset
Multiple myeloma	
Parkinsonism	
Elevated serum ferritin, angiotensin-converting enzyme, or tartrate-resistant acid phosphatase	

TREATMENT **Rx**

Enzyme replacement with recombinant glucocerebrosidase is available for the treatment of symptomatic patients with type 1 disease (Table 208-4). Studies show that anemia, thrombocytopenia, and organomegaly are reversed within 12 to 36 months with enzyme doses between 30 and 120 IU/kg given monthly. The treatment is ongoing, administered intravenously, and extremely expensive. Asymptomatic and mildly symptomatic adults do not always require treatment. Several companies are now marketing different forms of recombinantly produced enzyme. The enzyme does not cross the blood-brain barrier and does not alter the neurologic progression of patients with neuronopathic forms of Gaucher disease, but it can still be useful in alleviating visceral manifestations. It does not prevent the development of parkinsonism. Efforts are also under way to develop alternative therapies, including substrate reduction therapy, chemical chaperones, and gene therapy. One oral form of substrate reduction therapy, an iminosugar derivative, has been approved and is efficacious for some of the systemic manifestations of type 1 Gaucher disease. Useful supportive therapies include bisphosphonates for osteoporosis, orthopedic surgery for bone fractures, and palliative therapy and hydration for bone crises. Total or partial splenectomy, once commonly performed in patients with Gaucher disease, is now rarely indicated. Bone marrow transplantation (Chapter 178) has improved systemic but not neurologic manifestations.

calcifications, hydrocephalus, and other atypical manifestations, and all carry the mutation D409H in the *GBA1* gene.

DIAGNOSIS

Gaucher disease should be considered in the differential diagnosis of patients of all ages with unexplained organomegaly, easy bruisability, or bone pain (Table 208-3). The diagnosis can be made by demonstration of deficient glucocerebrosidase activity in leukocytes or cultured cells. In some populations, particularly Ashkenazi Jews, mutation analysis can be diagnostic as mutation N370S accounts for about 70% of mutant alleles. However, the presence of a highly homologous pseudogene sequence nearby can complicate molecular analyses. Bone marrow and liver biopsies show pathologic changes (Fig. 208-1B) but are not indicated for diagnosis. Carrier identification is best achieved by DNA testing when the mutant allele is known. Prenatal diagnosis is possible by determining the enzymatic activity or specific mutations in chorionic villi or cultured amniotic fluid cells.

TABLE 208-4	ENZYME REPLACEMENT THERAPY (ERT) FOR GAUCHER DISEASE AND FABRY DISEASE
GAUCHER DISEASE	**FABRY DISEASE**
ERT is a costly but effective intravenous therapy generally administered every other week for life.	ERT is costly, and there are not uniform recommendations for its use.
Decreased splenic and hepatic volumes and increases in hemoglobin levels and platelet counts should be expected in the first year of treatment.	On the basis of some current trials, hemizygous males with a low or undetectable level of α-galactosidase A should be treated with ERT, whether or not clinical features are present.
Asymptomatic and mildly symptomatic adults do not always require treatment.	On the basis of current trials, female carriers and atypically affected males with clinical features of Fabry disease should be treated with ERT.
ERT does not cross the blood-brain barrier and does not correct neurologic features of neuronopathic forms of Gaucher disease.	Other trials suggest that ERT should not be started in patients with proteinuria or reduced glomerular filtration rate unless there are other findings of Fabry disease.
ERT will not prevent the development of parkinsonism.	

FABRY DISEASE

PATHOBIOLOGY

Fabry disease, an X-linked inherited deficiency of the lysosomal enzyme α-galactosidase A, has intermediate penetrance in females and is considered a systemic vascular disorder. The disease incidence is about 1 in 117,000 live male births. Evidence suggests that 50% of females with Fabry disease are either asymptomatic or are not identified. This defect in the hydrolytic cleavage of the terminal molecule of galactose from glycolipids causes lysosomal accumulation of globotriaosylceramide and galabiosylceramide in many cell types. Lysosomal inclusions or lipid deposits can be seen in vascular cells, including both endothelial and smooth muscle cells; cardiac cells, such as endocardial cells, cardiomyocytes, and cardiac valves; kidney epithelial cells, including tubular and glomerular cells and podocytes; and nerve cells, including dorsal root ganglia and some central nervous system neurons.

The gene encoding α-galactosidase A, *GLA*, is located on Xq22.1. More than 431 mutations have been described, including missense/nonsense mutations, small deletions, large deletions, splice defects, and complex rearrangements. Most affected individuals have 2 to 25% residual activity, but the most severe form of Fabry disease has been correlated with complete absence of α-galactosidase A activity.

CLINICAL MANIFESTATIONS

Clinically, angiokeratomas (nonblanching, punctate, blue-black skin lesions), debilitating pain, and corneal opacities can occur in early childhood and may lead to the diagnosis. If the diagnosis is missed, the disease can result in progressive renal and cardiac deterioration. Patients have a propensity for ischemic stroke, sometimes in their 20s but more commonly in the fourth and fifth decades of life. As with many metabolic disorders, there is a spectrum of presentations that can mimic more common disorders, and many patients are undiagnosed.

Fabry disease typically manifests in childhood in classically affected males with episodes of extremity pain. Angiokeratomas develop in adolescence, followed by advancing renal disease during adulthood. The progressive cardiac and cerebrovascular involvement accounts for a majority of the deaths in adulthood associated with Fabry disease. X-linked inactivation and the penetrance of this X-linked disorder are reflected in the fact that approximately 90% of females carrying the mutation have symptoms,[9] although affected males show more significant clinical manifestations at an earlier age than heterozygous females do.

The majority of patients experience acroparesthesia, or a "Fabry crisis," characterized by excruciating, burning pain that may be either continuous or episodic. The pain typically affects the feet first, followed by the hands, and may be triggered by exercise, stress, and extremes in environmental temperatures. Abdominal or flank pain, simulating renal colic, may occur.

Angiokeratomas (Fig. 208-1C) are often the first sign of Fabry disease and may be accompanied by hypohidrosis. These classic skin lesions increase in number and size over time and are typically most dense between the umbilicus and the knees; however, they may occur anywhere, including the buccal mucosa. Ophthalmologic findings include conjunctival and retinal tortuosity and corneal opacities (cornea verticillata). Characteristic lenticular lesions are observed during slit-lamp examination and are present in affected males and female heterozygotes. Progressive hearing loss may also occur.

Renal involvement is common and is first manifested as proteinuria, followed by progressive renal insufficiency, with birefringent "Maltese crosses" sometimes seen in the urinary sediment. Chronic kidney disease is part of the natural history, and end-stage renal disease may develop in the second to fourth decades. Fabry disease should be considered when multiple renal sinus cysts are seen on an imaging study. As affected men and women age, cardiovascular findings may include ventricular hypertrophy, conduction defects, coronary artery disease, aortic and mitral valve insufficiency, and aortic root dilation. Furthermore, atypical Fabry disease can be manifested with concentric left ventricular hypertrophy and no other disease findings.[10] Cerebrovascular involvement, leading to transient ischemic attacks and stroke, occur in approximately 25% of patients, with a mean age at onset of 40 years.

Female carriers of this X-linked disorder tend to have more variable and less severe symptoms, with a later age at onset. Affected women may not have proteinuria, even with pronounced renal impairment, and in almost 40%, stroke is the initial presentation. Whereas angiokeratomas are not typically seen in affected women, half have hypohidrosis and heat intolerance. The initial stages of cardiomyopathy in affected women is generally 10 years later than the classic presentation in men and may be the only manifestation of Fabry disease.

DIAGNOSIS

Fabry disease should be considered in individuals with angiokeratoma, acroparesthesia, and corneal lesions as well as in individuals with cryptogenic strokes, idiopathic cardiomyopathy, or renal disease (Table 208-3). Men and women with left ventricular hypertrophy without any other explanation or with a family history of renal, cardiovascular, cerebrovascular, or skin issues should be screened for Fabry disease. Angiokeratoma should be differentiated from Fordyce's disease, benign angiokeratomas of the scrotum, and angiokeratoma circumscriptum. Angiokeratomas are also seen in other lysosomal disorders including mannosidosis, fucosidosis, sialidosis, and β-galactosidase and β-hexosaminidase deficiency. Corneal abnormalities are similar to those seen secondary to the use of chloroquine or amiodarone; exposure to silicone dust can result in similar renal findings.

A presumed diagnosis can be confirmed by low α-galactosidase activity in peripheral white blood cells or cultured skin fibroblasts. Levels below 20% of normal are considered diagnostic, and levels up to 35% of normal should be considered suggestive. *GLA* mutation analysis is available and is critical for confirmation in atypically presenting males and heterozygote females because random X chromosome inactivation may lead to only slightly reduced or normal enzyme activity.

TREATMENT ℞

Symptomatic treatment of the clinical manifestations of Fabry disease should follow standard medical care. Antiplatelet agents such as clopidogrel and aspirin or long-acting dipyridamole should be used for the prevention of strokes. Angiotensin-converting enzyme inhibitors and angiotensin receptor blockers are appropriate to manage hypertension and to preserve renal function. Kidney transplantation is effective in individuals with end-stage renal disease. Neuropathic pain can be treated with relatively low doses of antiepileptic medications, antidepressants, topical anesthetics, or pain relievers. Nonsteroidal anti-inflammatory agents should be avoided because of potential renal toxicity.

Enzyme replacement therapy has been available since 2001, and clinical trials suggest a modest benefit in modifying the natural course of the disease.[A1] Whereas there are no uniform recommendations, it is generally agreed that this therapy is appropriate for classically affected males, symptomatic females, and males with atypical disease (Table 208-4).[11]

OTHER LYSOSOMAL DISORDERS SEEN IN ADULTS

Metachromatic leukodystrophy, the deficiency of arylsulfatase A, results in the accumulation of sulfatides in the central and peripheral nervous systems, leading to demyelination of axons and peripheral nerves. It has a spectrum of manifestations, divided into childhood and adult variants. In both, gait disturbance and cognitive regression are seen. The adult form is associated with behavioral disturbances and dementia, often mistakenly resulting in a diagnosis of psychosis. Metachromatic leukodystrophy is a recognized underlying cause of psychiatric illness in adults, and prominent features include auditory hallucinations, bizarre delusions, behavioral changes, personality changes, disinhibition and disorganization in daily life, and catatonic posturing. The diagnosis can be especially difficult in these individuals. Other neurologic signs, such as dysarthria and spasticity, manifest later as the disease progresses. The diagnosis is made initially by demonstration of low arylsulfatase A activity. However, because there can be a pseudodeficiency, it must be confirmed by molecular diagnosis or the demonstration of the excretion of sulfatides in urine.

Tay-Sachs' disease, caused by β-hexosaminidase A deficiency, is characterized by an excessive accumulation of the fatty acid derivative ganglioside GM$_2$ in neurons. There are three clinical variants based on the age at onset: type 1, infantile acute; type 2, subacute (2 to 18 years); and type 3, late onset. The main features of the disease are neurologic and cognitive deterioration as well as blindness, the macular cherry red spot, and deafness. In patients with late-onset GM$_2$ gangliosidosis, psychiatric signs may manifest years before the appearance of motor findings. The most common psychiatric signs include acute psychosis, mania, and depression without psychosis. Either recurrent progressive psychosis, consistent with schizophrenia-hebephrenia, or major depression followed by psychotic features may occur. Dysarthria and progressive speech loss are also common. The disorder is diagnosed by measurement of β-hexosaminidase A activity in the serum or white blood cells in the presence of normal or elevated activity of the β-hexosaminidase B isoenzyme. In pregnant women or those taking oral contraceptives, the test should be performed only in leukocytes.

Niemann-Pick disease type C has a spectrum of features ranging from a rapidly progressive, fatal neonatal phenotype to an adult-onset chronic, neurodegenerative course. Progressive ataxia, vertical supranuclear ophthalmoplegia, dystonia, and dementia are variable. Hepatosplenomegaly is frequently encountered. The disorder results from an error in cellular trafficking of exogenous cholesterol, leading to lysosomal accumulation of unesterified cholesterol, and has been linked to mutations in the *NPC1* (95% of cases) and *NPC2* (5% of cases) genes. The diagnosis is made by demonstration of impaired cholesterol esterification in cultured fibroblasts, termed the Filipin test, or by molecular genetic testing for mutations. Glycosphingolipids and cholesterol accumulate in different tissues such as the liver, spleen, bone marrow, and brain. In adults, psychiatric manifestations are observed that are consistent with acute psychosis, paranoid delusions or schizophrenia with delusions, hallucinations, disorganized behavior, and aggressiveness. Miglustat (*N*-butyldeoxynojirimycin) has been shown in clinical trials to stabilize but not to prevent or reverse key neurologic findings.[12] Decisions about starting this therapy typically involve the team of physicians, parents, and caregivers of the affected individual.

Aspartylglucosaminuria, a disorder more common in Finland than elsewhere in the world, is an autosomal recessive defect in glycoprotein degradation characterized by a slow or progressive delay in psychomotor development. Delayed speech and motor defects are often accompanied by repeated upper respiratory infections. Patients typically achieve the developmental competency of a 5- to 6-year-old child at around puberty; subsequently, they may experience progressive deterioration, resulting in the severe cognitive impairment seen in adulthood. The characteristic coarse facial features, thick calvaria, and osteoporosis result from mild connective tissue transformation. About 20% of patients experience seizures during the later stages of the disease, resulting primarily from abnormalities in the differentiation between gray and white matter and delayed myelination. The diagnosis is made by the detection of elevated urine oligosaccharides and deficient aspartylglucosaminidase activity in leukocytes.

The *neuronal ceroid-lipofuscinoses* are divided into four major groups—infantile, classic late infantile, juvenile, and adult—reflecting the age at symptom onset and the appearance of storage material on electron microscopy. Although generally inherited in an autosomal recessive fashion, the adult type can be inherited as a dominant allele. These diseases are characterized clinically by visual impairment leading to blindness, gait abnormalities, seizures, dementia, and early death. They are a genetically heterogeneous group of progressive, hereditary neurodegenerative diseases with variable onset of clinical manifestations. To date, approximately 160 mutations causing neuronal ceroid-lipofuscinoses have been found in eight human genes, complicating genetic analysis. Symptoms result from deficiencies in palmitoyl-protein thioesterase 1 and tripeptidyl-peptidase 1. The diagnosis is based on diminished enzyme activity and molecular genetic testing and, in some cases, clinical findings and electron microscopy of biopsied tissues.

Accumulation of autofluorescent ceroid lipopigments is seen in the brain and other tissues. Adult patients may exhibit behavioral disturbances and cognitive decline, and parkinsonian features may be prominent.

Pompe's disease is discussed in Chapters 207 and 421.

The *mucopolysaccharidoses* (MPS) are a group of disorders resulting from defective lysosomal degradation of glycosaminoglycans. These chronic, progressive storage disorders show clinical manifestations that vary by type. Findings include coarse facial features, dysostosis multiplex, organomegaly, and neurologic manifestations with regression. All types are inherited in an autosomal recessive pattern except for MPS II/Hunter, which is X-linked. The mucopolysaccharidoses were once typically thought of as pediatric disorders, but with the advent of enzyme replacement therapy and the recognition of milder forms, more patients are reaching adulthood. Classically, patients with MPS type IS/Scheie, II/Hunter, III/Sanfilippo, IV/Morquio, and VI/Maroteaux-Lamy may have life expectancies beyond the pediatric years. Patients with MPS type IS may present with normal to short stature, normal intelligence, degenerative joint disease, corneal opacities, and cardiac valve lesions. Patients with MPS II/Hunter share the symptoms of MPS I/Hurler, except that airway involvement may be more significant in individuals with Hunter's syndrome, and the corneas are clear. Patients with MPS III/Sanfilippo have primarily central nervous system manifestations, with mild somatic involvement. They have progressive speech impairment, with the development of severe behavioral and sleep disturbances. Later they have an unrelenting loss of skills and deterioration into a vegetative state, with death in the third decade. Individuals with MPS IV have severe skeletal dysplasia, with normal intelligence in type A and a degenerative course in type B. Treatment is available in the form of enzyme replacement therapy for MPS IS, MPS II, and MPS IV, and enzyme therapies for other forms are in development. Medical management is type specific. In general, attention should focus on airway involvement resulting from progressive storage in the soft tissue of the upper airway and the need to optimize joint mobility and function by physical therapy. Patients with MPS I, II, and VI should be monitored for the development of cervical myelopathy due to dural thickening, which may lead to loss of endurance before ascending paralysis becomes apparent.[13]

Cystinosis is a lysosomal storage disorder with three clinical phenotypes: the most common infantile or nephropathic form, an intermediate or juvenile-onset form, and a benign form typically seen in adults and affecting primarily the eyes. Lysosomal cystine accumulation results from mutations in the gene *CTNS*, which codes for cystinosin, a lysosomal carrier protein. Individuals with the nephropathic form have lysosomal cystine accumulation leading to multiorgan system involvement, including progressive renal disease, corneal crystals, and effects on the thyroid, gonads, pancreas, muscle, and central nervous system. The adult form has only corneal crystals. Treatment is supportive and should include cysteamine, which is an oral medication that decreases cystine accumulation.[14] Cysteamine hydrochloride eyedrops dissolve corneal crystals and relieve photophobia.

Grade A Reference

A1. El Dib RP, Nascimento P, Pastores GM. Enzyme replacement therapy for Anderson-Fabry disease. *Cochrane Database Syst Rev.* 2013;2:CD006663.

GENERAL REFERENCES

For the General References and other additional features, please visit Expert Consult at https://expertconsult.inkling.com.

209

HOMOCYSTINURIA AND HYPERHOMOCYSTEINEMIA

MANUEL SCHIFF AND HENK BLOM

DEFINITION

Homocysteine is a nonprotein amino acid and is a key metabolic branch point metabolite between the trans-sulfuration and remethylation pathways of methionine metabolism. The many conditions associated with high homocysteine levels encompass a wide range of clinical manifestations. The normal level of plasma total homocysteine (tHcy) is below 15 μM. However, the threshold of tHcy above which a disorder of homocysteine metabolism should be suspected and a specific therapy should be initiated is around 50 μM.

Homocystinuria and hyperhomocysteinemia primarily include inherited disorders of homocysteine metabolism but can also involve acquired nutritional cobalamin (Cbl, vitamin B$_{12}$) or folate deficiencies. Severely elevated plasma levels of homocysteine are accompanied by homocystinuria as rare autosomal recessively inherited disorders that are associated with vascular, neurologic, ocular, and skeletal abnormalities. Lesser elevations of plasma homocysteine, without homocystinuria, occur in about 5 to 7% of the population; these individuals with hyperhomocysteinemia only do not have the clinical stigmata of homocystinuria but are at increased risk of atheroscle-

rotic cardiovascular disease (Chapter 52) and venous thromboembolism (Chapter 176).

Inherited disorders of homocysteine metabolism (Figs. 209-1 and 209-2) comprise *disorders of the trans-sulfuration pathway* with cystathionine β-synthase (CBS) deficiency (or classic homocystinuria) and *disorders of remethylation* of homocysteine to methionine. The latter include 5,10-methylenetetrahydrofolate reductase [MTHFR] deficiency and inherited disorders of cobalamin absorption, transport, and intracellular metabolism and the very rare congenital folate malabsorption disorder. Intracellular remethylation defects include disorders that all have defective methionine synthesis in common: MTHFR deficiency impairs methyltetrahydrofolate synthesis; defective lysosomal release of cobalamin (CblF and CblJ) and defects in cytosolic reduction and transport of hydroxocobalamin (CblC and CblD) impair the synthesis of both methylcobalamin and

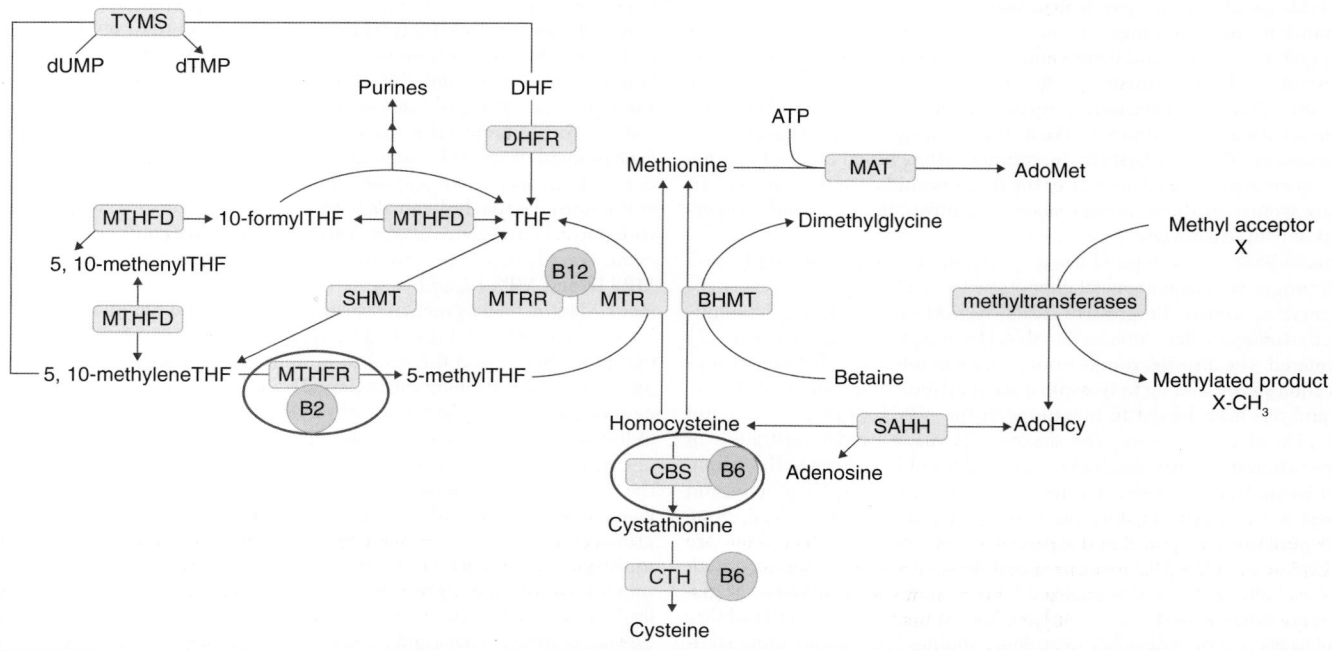

FIGURE 209-1. Homocysteine metabolism and the folate cycle. The two conditions leading to accumulation of homocysteine (CBS and MTHFR) are surrounded by a circle. AdoHcy = S-adenosylhomocysteine; AdoMet = S-adenosylmethionine; ATP = adenosine triphosphate; BHMT = betaine-homocysteine methyltransferase; CBS = cystathionine β-synthase; CTH = cystathionine γ-lyase; DHF = dihydrofolate; DHFR = dihydrofolate reductase; dTMP = deoxythymidine monophosphate; dUMP = deoxyuridine monophosphate; MAT = methionine-adenosyltransferase; MTHFD = methylenetetrahydrofolate dehydrogenase/methenyltetrahydrofolate cyclohydrolase/formyltetrahydrofolate synthetase; MTHFR = methylenetetrahydrofolate reductase; MTR = methionine synthase; MTRR = methionine synthase reductase; SAHH = S-adenosylhomocysteine hydrolase; SHMT = serine-hydroxymethyltransferase; THF = tetrahydrofolate; TYMS = thymidylate synthase.

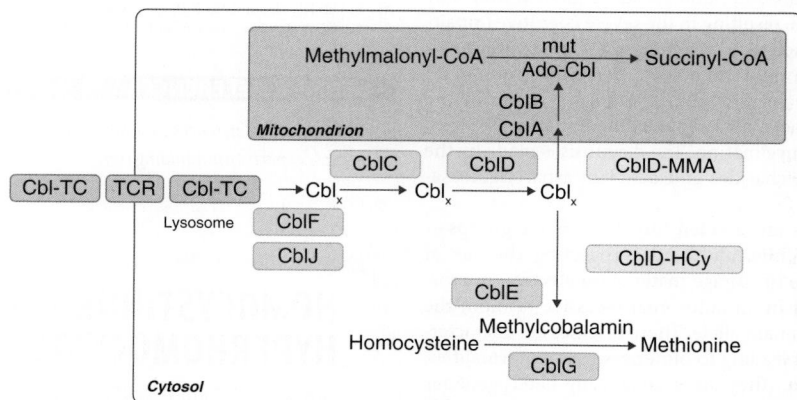

FIGURE 209-2. Intracellular cobalamin metabolism pathway and its defect. To date, 10 complementation group defects of the cobalamin pathway have been described. After binding to the transcobalamin receptor (TCR), cobalamin bound to TC enters the cell through lysosome-mediated endocytosis and is released through proteolysis. Export from the lysosome into the cytoplasm is defective in patients with the CblF and recently described CblJ defects. The steps in the cytosol after lysosomal release are defined by the complementation groups CblC and CblD. The exact form of cobalamin at this stage is unclear (as indicated by Cbl$_x$). In the cytosol, cobalamin is reductively methylated by methionine synthase reductase (CblE) to methylcobalamin, the cofactor for methionine synthase (CblG). After its transport into the mitochondrion, cobalamin is converted to adenosylcobalamin (Ado-Cbl), the cofactor for methylmalonyl–coenzyme A (CoA) mutase (mut), by cobalamin adenosyltransferase (CblB). The CblD defect can cause isolated methylmalonic aciduria (CblD-MMA complementation group), isolated homocystinuria (CblD-HCy), or both (CblD). In all these conditions with defective remethylation (TC and TC receptor deficiency, CblF, CblJ, CblC, CblD, CblD-HCy, CblE, and CblG defects), there is homocysteine accumulation due to dysfunction in methionine synthesis.

TABLE 209-1 GENETIC DEFECTS ASSOCIATED WITH HOMOCYSTINURIA

FUNCTIONAL DEFECT	COMMON NAME	ENZYME DEFECT	GENE	CHROMOSOME LOCUS
Trans-sulfuration	"Classic" homocystinuria	Cystathionine β-synthase	*CBS*	21q22.3
Remethylation	Folate-dependent homocystinuria	Methylenetetrahydrofolate reductase	*MTHFR*	1p36.3
	CblE	Methyltransferase reductase	*MTRR*	5p15.2-p15.3
	CblG	Methionine synthase	*MTR*	1q43
Cobalamin transport	TC-II	Transcobalamin	*TCN2*	22q11.2-qter
	CblF	Lysosomal B_{12} translocase	*LMBRD1*	6q13
Cobalamin processing	CblC	Intracellular cobalamin chaperone?	*MMACHC*	1p34.1
	CblD	Cobalamin reductase?	*MMADHC*	2q23.2
	CblJ	Cobalamin processing?	*ABCD4*	14q24.3

adenosylcobalamin; and isolated deficiencies of methionine synthase (CblE and CblG) are associated with defective methylcobalamin synthesis as well as the CblD-Hcy variant.

In CBS deficiency, in addition to severe elevations of plasma tHcy, plasma methionine level is also increased. In contrast, in remethylation disorders, the increased tHcy is accompanied by a low (or low-normal) level of methionine in plasma because of the ineffective conversion (remethylation) of homocysteine to methionine. Among the remethylation disorders, the cobalamin-processing (CblC) defect (the most frequent inherited disorder of intracellular cobalamin metabolism) and MTHFR deficiency are by far the most frequent, although in absolute numbers these disorders are still rare. Accordingly, this chapter focuses on CBS deficiency, CblC defect, and MTHFR deficiency.

EPIDEMIOLOGY
Prevalence and Incidence
The worldwide prevalence of CBS deficiency has been reported at 1 in 344,000. Minimum estimates of the incidence of CBS deficiency by newborn screening programs have ranged from 1 in 60,000 to 1 in 300,000 live births, varying with the population and the screening method. Estimates of its incidence in Europe have been in the area of 1 in 40,000, which corresponds to a carrier (heterozygote) frequency of about 1%, but studies screening for known mutations suggest that the prevalence may be more than twice that rate. Studies from the Middle Eastern countries have shown incidence rates as high as 1 in 1800. The incidence of severe homocysteine remethylation defects is probably less than 1 in 500,000 live births.

PATHOBIOLOGY
The homocysteine that accumulates (in both CBS deficiency and remethylation defects) is a multisystem toxic agent that exerts its effects either directly or indirectly through conversion to *S*-adenosylhomocysteine (see Fig. 209-1), which potentially inhibits many essential methyltransferases. Direct cellular homocysteine toxicity involves endothelial injury and neuronal cell death. The effects of homocysteine on vascular endothelium predispose to thrombosis that may occur at any age and affect arteries or veins of any size. Specifically in CBS deficiency, accumulation of homocysteine or cysteine deficiency induces modification of connective tissue proteins, possibly being the origin of the skeletal and ocular manifestations. These effects are probably related to fibrillin, which is a component of the matrix of periosteum and perichondrium, the major component of the zonular fibers of the ocular lens, and a protein singularly rich in cysteine. Fibrillin structure is affected by the linking of homocysteine to cysteine; as a result, some clinical features of homocystinuria overlap with fibrillin mutations (Marfan syndrome; Chapter 260).

Remethylation defects (CblC and MTHFR) result not only in severe elevations of homocysteine but also in a shortage of methionine, required for protein synthesis and *S*-adenosylmethionine generation. The latter causes, through this route, a further reduction of cellular methylation capacity in addition to the accumulation of *S*-adenosylhomocysteine, especially in the central nervous system. CblC defect is an inborn error of intracellular cobalamin metabolism due to defect of the methylmalonic aciduria and homocystinuria type C protein (*MMACHC*). After normal dietary intake, intestinal absorption, blood transport, and cellular uptake, cobalamin is delivered in the cytosol, where it becomes bound to MMACHC. This protein has been shown to catalyze dealkylation of alkylcobalamins, such as adenosylcobalamin and methylcobalamin, and the decyanation of cyanocobalamin.[1] In the absence of normal MMACHC, neither methylcobalamin (the cofactor of methionine synthase) nor adenosylcobalamin (the cofactor of methylmalonyl-

CoA mutase) is functional, leading to defects of the methionine synthase (remethylation defect) and methylmalonyl-CoA mutase (methylmalonic acid accumulation), respectively (see Fig. 209-2). In MTHFR deficiency, the methyl donor 5-methyltetrahydrofolate (5-methylTHF) cannot be produced, which secondarily impairs methionine synthase function and subsequent remethylation (see Fig. 209-2). The pathogenesis of MTHFR deficiency can be ascribed to homocysteine toxicity together with methionine cellular depletion. However, the pathophysiologic mechanism of the other remethylation defect, the CblC defect, remains incompletely understood. Toxic accumulation of methylmalonic acid in the CblC defect might play an additional role.

All these genetic disorders associated with homocystinuria are inherited in an autosomal recessive manner and are summarized in Table 209-1.

CLINICAL MANIFESTATIONS
CYSTATHIONINE β-SYNTHASE DEFICIENCY Affected individuals are normal at birth after an uneventful pregnancy and delivery. If untreated, they progressively develop the core clinical symptoms of CBS deficiency,[2] which involve four major organ systems.

CENTRAL NERVOUS SYSTEM Developmental delay and mental retardation affect about 60% of the patients to a variable degree of severity. Seizures, electroencephalographic abnormalities, and psychiatric disturbances have also been reported in approximately half of the cases. Focal neurologic signs may be a consequence of cerebrovascular accidents.

EYE Dislocation of the ocular lens (ectopia lentis), myopia, and glaucoma are frequent, severe, and characteristic complications. Retinal detachment and degeneration, optical atrophy, and cataracts may eventually appear. Myopia often precedes lens dislocation. Ectopia lentis is detected in most untreated patients from 5 to 10 years of age and in nearly all untreated patients by the end of the fourth decade. In children as well as in adults, it is often the clue to diagnosis. The dislocation is generally downward, whereas it is usually upward in Marfan syndrome. Once ectopia lentis has occurred, a peculiar trembling of the iris (iridodonesis) after eye or head movement may be evident.

SKELETON Osteoporosis is almost invariably detected, at least after childhood. Frequent consequences are scoliosis and a tendency toward pathologic fractures and vertebral collapse. Homocystinuric patients tend to be tall, with thinning and elongation (dolichostenomelia) of long bones near puberty, enlarged metaphyses and epiphyses (especially at the knees), and arachnodactyly, present in about half of the patients. Other bone deformities include genu valgum, pes cavus, and pectus carinatum or excavatum. Restricted joint mobility, particularly at the extremities, contrasts with the joint laxity observed in Marfan syndrome.

VASCULAR SYSTEM Thromboembolic complications, occurring in arteries and veins of all parts of the body, constitute the major cause of morbidity and mortality at any age. Because of the very low prevalence of arteriosclerosis and thrombosis in children or adolescents, homocystinurias should be excluded in any such case presenting with arterial or venous occlusive disease.

Two phenotypic variants are recognized, B_6-responsive homocystinuria and B_6-nonresponsive homocystinuria. B_6-responsive homocystinuria is usually milder than the nonresponsive variant.

Adult-Onset Clinical Presentation
The expression of all clinical symptoms is extremely variable and may be manifested during childhood but also during adulthood, even up to 60 years of age. Individuals are often tall and slender with a marfanoid habitus and are prone to osteoporosis. The main acute manifestation in adulthood is

cardiovascular disease. In all forms of inherited homocystinurias, isolated arterial and venous occlusive disease may be manifested at any age. Thromboembolism is the major cause of early death and morbidity. Adults can also present with isolated quick loss of diopter (refractive capacity), which is the most common symptom before diagnosis.

The IQ in individuals with untreated homocystinuria varies widely, from 10 to 138. In B_6-responsive untreated individuals, the mean IQ is 79 versus 57 for those who are B_6 nonresponsive. The neuropsychiatric symptoms (like schizophrenia or autism-like features) may remain apparently isolated, but a thorough clinical history and examination will often reveal associated features like marfanoid habitus, skeletal abnormalities, and lens dislocation.

Remethylation Disorders: CblC Defect and MTHFR Deficiency

Clinical signs of remethylation defects are mainly neurologic. Neonatal and early-onset patients exhibit acute neurologic distress. In childhood, patients exhibit nonspecific mental retardation often associated with acquired microcephaly. Without appropriate therapy, remethylation-defective patients may develop acute or rapidly progressive neurologic deterioration, sometimes leading to death. Adolescents and adults exhibit, after a period of normal development or mild developmental delay, a rapid mental or psychiatric deterioration. These patients may typically have signs of subacute combined degeneration of the cord. In addition, adults can be asymptomatic or present with isolated stroke.

In the CblC defect,[3-5] 5-methylTHF accumulates because of the block at methionine synthase (the 5-methylTHF trap), causing a functional cellular folate deficiency. This explains the hematologic manifestations (megaloblastic bone marrow leading to macrocytic anemia or pancytopenia) that are not present in MTHFR deficiency. In the CblC defect, severe (occasionally fatal) multisystem deterioration may occur. This includes hemolytic-uremic syndrome, cardiomyopathy, and interstitial pneumonia, which all share an identical pathologic hallmark (i.e., thrombotic microangiopathy). In addition, a peculiar and poorly understood retinopathy with nystagmus is often present.

Adult-Onset Clinical Presentation

Adult-onset CblC disease is less frequent than childhood onset and is dominated by neuropsychiatric manifestations such as ataxia, cognitive impairment, and psychosis. Hemolytic-uremic syndrome (even isolated) can also be present.

In MTHFR deficiency, the neuropsychiatric presentation is similar and can be subtle. Patients may remain asymptomatic or exhibit isolated arterial stroke.

In both remethylation defects, the neurologic disorder results in many signs similar to the late stage observed in childhood. Previously, most of these patients had either a normal or a mild developmental delay, and a striking

feature is the rapid mental deterioration occurring in the second decade of life accompanied by bouts of unexplained lethargy and a progressive cerebral, myelopathic, and neuropathic disorder with variable results on neurophysiologic investigations.

In both groups of inherited homocystinurias, isolated arterial and venous occlusive disease may be manifested at any age. Because of the very low incidence of arteriosclerosis and thrombosis in children or adolescents, homocystinurias should be excluded in any case in this age presenting with these clinical manifestations.

DIAGNOSIS

If homocystinuria is suspected clinically, plasma tHcy should be determined. If tHcy (normal values, 5-15 μM) is higher than 50 μM, determination of serum vitamin B_{12} and folate levels in both serum and red blood cells, plasma amino acids, and urinary organic acids (or plasma methylmalonic acid) is warranted. If tHcy is below 50 μM, the probability of a homocystinuria is minute. If plasma methionine is elevated or high-normal with low plasma cysteine, the plasma abnormalities point to CBS deficiency, whereas decreased or low-normal methionine and elevated tHcy point to remethylation defects. In the CblC defect, hematologic abnormalities with megaloblastic bone marrow maturation are observed along with normal vitamin B_{12} and folate blood levels. Nutritional vitamin B_{12} or folate deficiencies and other genetic causes of cobalamin and folate metabolism should also be considered in the differential diagnosis of remethylation defects.[6] It has to be kept in mind that CBS deficiency can cause secondary vitamin B_{12} and folate deficiency and remethylation defects can cause secondary folate deficiency. In MTHFR deficiency, folate levels (red blood cells or plasma) are usually low. Blood cell count with blood smear (looking for characteristics of vitamin B_{12} and folate deficiency), blood vitamin status, and metabolic biomarkers (tHcy, methionine, and methylmalonic acid) are usually enough to differentiate between the different forms of homocystinurias (Table 209-2). Definitive diagnosis can be confirmed at the molecular level by sequence analysis of the putative gene (see Table 209-1); if the molecular studies are not conclusive, functional studies can be performed in fibroblasts or lymphocytes.

TREATMENT

In 2015, general treatment guidelines will be available through the European Network and Registry for Homocystinurias and Methylation Defects website (http://www.e-hod.org). None of the treatment options are evidence based because of the rarity of these disorders.

Therapeutic Goals

The general therapeutic goal is to reduce tHcy accumulation and, for remethylation disorders, to bypass the remethylation defect, thereby

TABLE 209-2   CLINICAL FEATURES OF HOMOCYSTINURIAS

CLASS	BIOCHEMICAL FEATURES			CLINICAL FEATURES	
	tHcy	Meth	MMA	System	Signs
CBS deficiency	↑	↑	–	Ocular	Ectopia lentis, myopia, glaucoma, optic atrophy, retinal detachment
				Skeletal	Elongated and thinned bones, arachnodactyly, genu valgum, pectus malformation, scoliosis
				Vascular	Thromboembolic events (arterial or venous)
				Neurologic	Mental retardation in untreated cases, cerebrovascular thromboses, seizures Psychiatric disorders, personality disorder
MTHFR deficiency	↑	↓	–	Ocular	Ectopia lentis
				Vascular	Thromboses
				Neurologic	Variable: psychiatric to severe neurologic
Transcobalamin	↑	–/↓	+	Hematologic	Early-onset pancytopenia, macrocytosis
CblF, CblJ	↑	–/↓	+	Pansystemic	MMA, macrocytosis, stomatitis, congenital heart defects
CblC, CblD	↑	↓	+	Hematologic Neuropsychiatric Systemic (CblC)	Pancytopenia Hemolytic-uremic syndrome
CblE, CblG	↑	↓	–	Vascular Hematologic Neurologic	Thromboses Pancytopenia

Cbl = cobalamin; CBS = cystathionine β-synthase; Meth = plasma methionine; MMA = methylmalonic acid (urine or plasma); MTHFR = methylenetetrahydrofolate reductase; tHcy = total plasma homocysteine.

maintaining normal methionine and folate concentrations.[7] This should correct the hematologic abnormalities and ensure normal neurologic development or prevent further neurologic deterioration. Normalization of plasma tHcy levels would be ideal, but in practice, it is difficult if not impossible to achieve. However, the experience with CBS deficiency patients has shown that treatment can prevent further thromboembolic events even when the tHcy levels remain clearly above the normal range. Decreasing tHcy to 50 to 70 μM would therefore be a more reasonable goal in many patients with CBS deficiency as well as in those with remethylation disorders.

Available Treatment Options

To date, all the remethylation disorders are similarly treated with the combined supplementation of vitamin B_{12}, vitamin B_9 (folate), vitamin B_6 (pyridoxine), betaine, and methionine, although the dosage and route of administration may vary with the type of defect.

In CBS deficiency, therapy is more standardized with a longer experience available. It is based on (1) increasing residual CBS activity with the use of vitamin B_6 (in B_6-responsive patients); (2) decreasing the load on the affected pathway and replacing the deficient products by a low-methionine diet, limitation of natural proteins, amino acid mixture, special low-protein foods, and supplementation of cystine to increase cysteine; and (3) increasing remethylation to methionine with folate, vitamin B_{12}, and betaine to reduce tHcy accumulation.

Vitamin B_{12}

Vitamin B_{12} is the cofactor of methionine synthase. Its natural form, hydroxocobalamin, is more effective than the synthetic form cyanocobalamin. In CBS deficiency, hydroxocobalamin may be given orally (1 mg/day to 1 mg/week) according to the serum B_{12} level to prevent cobalamin deficiency.

In remethylation disorders, initial treatment includes daily parenteral administration of hydroxocobalamin (1 mg/day). If MTHFR deficiency is confirmed, switching to oral hydroxocobalamin (1 mg/day to 1 mg/week) or even stopping hydroxocobalamin supplementation may deserve discussion. Conversely, in CblC defect, lifelong high-dose intramuscular hydroxocobalamin injections are needed. The optimal interval between intramuscular injections remains to be determined, but recent data support the need for long-term daily doses.

Folate (Vitamin B_9)

Folate (vitamin B_9) is available in three different forms: folic acid, a stable synthetic form of the vitamin used, for example, in food fortification; folinic acid (5-formylTHF), the most stable form of the reduced and active vitamin; and 5-methylTHF (CH3-THF), the main natural and circulating form of the vitamin. A folinic acid formulation for parenteral administration is available for emergency treatment, whereas the other forms are available only for oral use. Whatever the disorder, folinic acid is more appropriate because it is the most stable reduced form, and folic acid may exacerbate cerebral CH3-THF deficiency, especially in MTHFR deficiency. In CBS deficiency, folinic acid should be given orally (1 to 5 mg/day) to avoid folate depletion. Moreover, folate repletion may be necessary to permit a pyridoxine response, which means that pyridoxine responsiveness should always be tested after potential folate depletion correction. In the CblC defect, long-term high-dose oral folinic supplementation is added to compensate for the methyl folate trap and to correct the hematologic abnormalities. The daily dose varies from 5 to 30 mg. The same folinic acid doses should be used in MTHFR deficiency.

Vitamin B_6 (Pyridoxine)

Vitamin B_6 (pyridoxine), through its action as the cofactor for CBS, is given orally in pharmaceutical doses in CBS-deficient patients to treat possible B_6-responsive individuals. There is no consensus on the dose and duration of B_6, which is usually given from 100 to 500 to 1000 mg/day during a period of several weeks, after which tHcy is determined to evaluate whether B_6 has been effective in normalizing (or even lowering) tHcy. As discussed before, B_6 should always be combined with folinic acid. In B_6-responsive patients, long-term therapy with pyridoxine and folate prevents further deterioration. In remethylation disorders, B_6 might theoretically enhance homocysteine removal and may be given at a low dose (50 to 100 mg/day).

For pyridoxine-responsive CBS-deficient patients, pyridoxine should be kept at the lowest dosage able to achieve adequate metabolic control. Because of reported high-dose pyridoxine toxicity on the nervous system, daily dosages higher than 400 to 500 mg/day in children and adults should probably be avoided for a long-term treatment. In pyridoxine-nonresponsive patients, a daily dosage of 50 to 100 mg of pyridoxine can be added to the treatment.

Betaine

Betaine is derived from choline and is a substrate for the enzyme betaine-homocysteine methyltransferase and therefore acts as a methyl donor (see Fig. 209-1). Oral betaine supplementation decreases homocysteine levels. Despite widespread use, there is little consensus on betaine dosage and frequency of administration. Case studies and early literature have used doses of 150 to 250 mg/kg/day in children and 5 to 10 g/day in adults, usually given two or three times daily. These early data were confirmed by pharmacokinetic studies (performed in CBS-deficient patients), which showed that above 200 mg/kg/day in two to three divided doses, there was no obvious benefit in lowering tHcy.

In CBS deficiency, the use of betaine is usually followed by an increase in plasma methionine and a fall in plasma tHcy. No harmful effects from raised methionine have been documented in patients receiving betaine therapy except one case of cerebral edema in a CBS patient with a plasma methionine level above 1000 μM. In B_6-nonresponsive early-treated patients, a low-methionine diet alone can be highly successful with good long-term outcomes, provided lifelong compliance is good. The clinical benefits of betaine are therefore questionable in compliant patients on a low-methionine diet. However, in some patients (especially when dietary compliance is a problem), betaine has been of benefit and may allow an increase in natural protein intake, thus improving the nutritional status.

In remethylation disorders, betaine increases systemic methionine levels and probably also methionine availability to the central nervous system, especially in patients with MTHFR deficiency. Early betaine treatment prevents mortality and allows normal psychomotor development in patients with severe MTHFR deficiency, highlighting the importance of timely recognition.[8] In the CblC defect, there are data reporting a synergistic action of hydroxocobalamin with betaine, lowering the tHcy level.

Oral Methionine

Oral methionine may also hold promise as an additional therapeutic measure in remethylation defects for several reasons. Cerebral methionine depletion is a key pathogenic factor. Added methionine might act synergistically with betaine by supplying intracellular methionine, and acute methionine loading does not lead to further homocysteine accumulation (with the attendant risk of thromboembolism). As a whole, whatever the remethylation defect, methionine depletion is rarely corrected by betaine therapy alone, whereas the association of methionine and betaine usually corrects methionine depletion.

PREVENTION

It is prudent to adopt measures to prevent additional risk of thrombosis, such as using long-term, low-dose aspirin and avoiding smoking and oral contraceptives. Nitrous oxide may also be relatively contraindicated because it can inhibit methionine synthase. Surgery poses serious risks but can be performed safely as long as attention is paid to the patient's hydration and coagulation status.

PROGNOSIS

In CBS deficiency, pyridoxine responsiveness generally correlates with higher residual enzyme activity, and the prognosis is significantly better than that for unresponsive cases, with or without treatment. Skeletal, ocular, vascular, and neurologic complications are all reduced with successful treatment. Without the early institution of treatment, the median IQ in a large outcome study was 57 for unresponsive patients and 78 for responsive patients. With early treatment, pyridoxine-unresponsive patients have a nearly normal median IQ. For patients who are responsive to and compliant with treatment, the prognosis for intellectual development is good, especially with diet alone. However, in case of poor adherence, significant elevations in tHcy generally persist, and some increased risk for vascular complications probably remains.

In the few MTHFR-deficient patients treated promptly in their neonatal period, the outcome is good with respect to the first years of neurologic development despite suboptimal metabolic control. If undiagnosed or untreated or late treated, these patients have a very poor outcome with severe impairments. In spite of some pathogenic similarity (intracellular methionine depletion due to impaired remethylation), CblC-defective patients have in general a particularly poor long-term outcome with multisystem involvement, thrombotic microangiopathy, and retinopathy.

GENERAL REFERENCES

For the General References and other additional features, please visit Expert Consult at https://expertconsult.inkling.com.

210

THE PORPHYRIAS

RICHARD J. HIFT

DEFINITION

The porphyrias are a group of eight disorders arising from disturbances in heme biosynthesis. Each disorder corresponds to abnormal activity of one of the enzymes that catalyze the heme biosynthetic pathway. Most porphyrias are genetic and heritable, with the exception of the sporadic form of porphyria cutanea tarda and rare instances of porphyria arising from acquired somatic mutations.

CLASSIFICATION

Approximately 90% of heme biosynthesis occurs within the erythron (specifically within erythroid precursors), leading to the production of heme for incorporation into hemoglobin. The remainder is synthesized in all other nucleated cells of the body, producing heme for incorporation into a number of vital hemoproteins. The liver is the predominant site of nonerythroid heme synthesis, with much of the product being incorporated into enzymes of the cytochrome P-450 (CYP) system.

Thus, the porphyrias may be classified into two categories, the erythropoietic and hepatic porphyrias. Disturbances in erythroid heme biosynthesis give rise to three forms of erythropoietic porphyria: congenital erythropoietic porphyria (CEP), erythropoietic protoporphyria (EPP), and X-linked protoporphyria (XLPP). Disturbances in nonerythroid heme biosynthesis give rise to five forms of hepatic porphyria: acute intermittent porphyria (AIP), variegate porphyria (VP), porphyria cutanea tarda (PCT), hereditary coproporphyria (HCP), and ALA dehydratase porphyria (ALADP).

A clinically applicable classification divides the porphyrias into another two cross-cutting groups (Table 210-1). The acute porphyrias are those characterized by the potential to develop the potentially fatal acute attack (AIP, VP, HCP, and ALADP). The nonacute porphyrias are accompanied predominantly by cutaneous manifestations (PCT, CEP, EPP, and XLPP).

EPIDEMIOLOGY

Each porphyria has a prevalence that may vary between populations, depending on local gene frequencies for the mutations that give rise to it. Assessment of prevalence is complicated by incomplete penetrance, difficulties in case ascertainment, and unevenness in the accuracy of biochemical diagnosis performed by different laboratories. The most accurate figures have recently been reported from Europe, where diagnostic laboratories in each country are centralized and linked into an international network. The network has reported a prevalence of 9.2 per million for EPP, 5.9 per million for AIP, and 3.2 per million for VP.[1] It is likely that the figures for North America will be broadly similar. PCT, which is environmentally induced and treatable, has an annual incidence exceeding 6 per million in Norway and nearly 4 per million in Sweden; its prevalence in the United States has been estimated at 4 per 100,000. HCP has a lower prevalence; the two autosomal recessive disorders, CEP and ALADP, are very rare, and experience is restricted to small case series and case reports.

AIP and VP may become prevalent in specific populations as a result of a founder effect, whereby a particular mutation spreads widely in an isolated population and becomes locally common. In northern Sweden, AIP has a prevalence estimated at 23 per million. In South Africa, VP has become the most common monogenetic disorder among the Dutch-descended immigrant population of South Africa, with a prevalence estimated at 1.2 per thousand of the white population.

PATHOBIOLOGY

The pathobiology of the porphyrias is easily understood by reference to the heme biosynthetic pathway (Fig. 210-1). There are slight differences between erythroid and nonerythroid heme synthesis. The initial step in the pathway is the synthesis of 5-aminolevulinate (ALA), catalyzed by the enzyme 5-aminolevulinate synthase (ALAS). The ubiquitous or housekeeping enzyme ALAS1 is strongly expressed in the liver and is encoded by the ALAS1 gene on chromosome 3. The erythroid form, ALAS2, is encoded by the ALAS2 gene on the X chromosome. The two genes share 73% homology.

TABLE 210-1 SUMMARY OF THE PORPHYRIAS

PORPHYRIA	KEY CLINICAL FEATURES AND LONG-TERM COMPLICATIONS	INHERITANCE
ACUTE PORPHYRIAS		
More Common		
Acute intermittent porphyria	Acute attacks Hypertension Renal failure Hepatocellular carcinoma	Autosomal dominant
Variegate porphyria	Vesiculo-erosive skin disease Acute attacks Hepatocellular carcinoma	Autosomal dominant
Less Common		
Hereditary coproporphyria	Vesiculo-erosive skin disease Acute attacks	Autosomal dominant
Rare		
ALA dehydratase porphyria	Acute attacks Neuropathy	Autosomal recessive
NONACUTE PORPHYRIAS		
More Common		
Porphyria cutanea tarda	Vesiculo-erosive skin disease Associated with iron loading, alcoholic liver disease, hepatitis C, HIV infection, renal failure, and other disorders	Acquired, sometimes on a background of an inherited mutation
*Erythropoietic protoporphyria	Immediate photosensitivity Cholelithiasis, liver disease	Autosomal recessive; frequently in association with a common polymorphism in the ferrochelatase gene
Rare		
*X-linked protoporphyria	Immediate photosensitivity Cholelithiasis, liver disease	X-linked
*Congenital erythropoietic porphyria	Vesiculo-erosive skin disease Severe photomutilation	Autosomal recessive

*The three forms of erythropoietic porphyria. The remainder are classified as hepatic porphyrias.

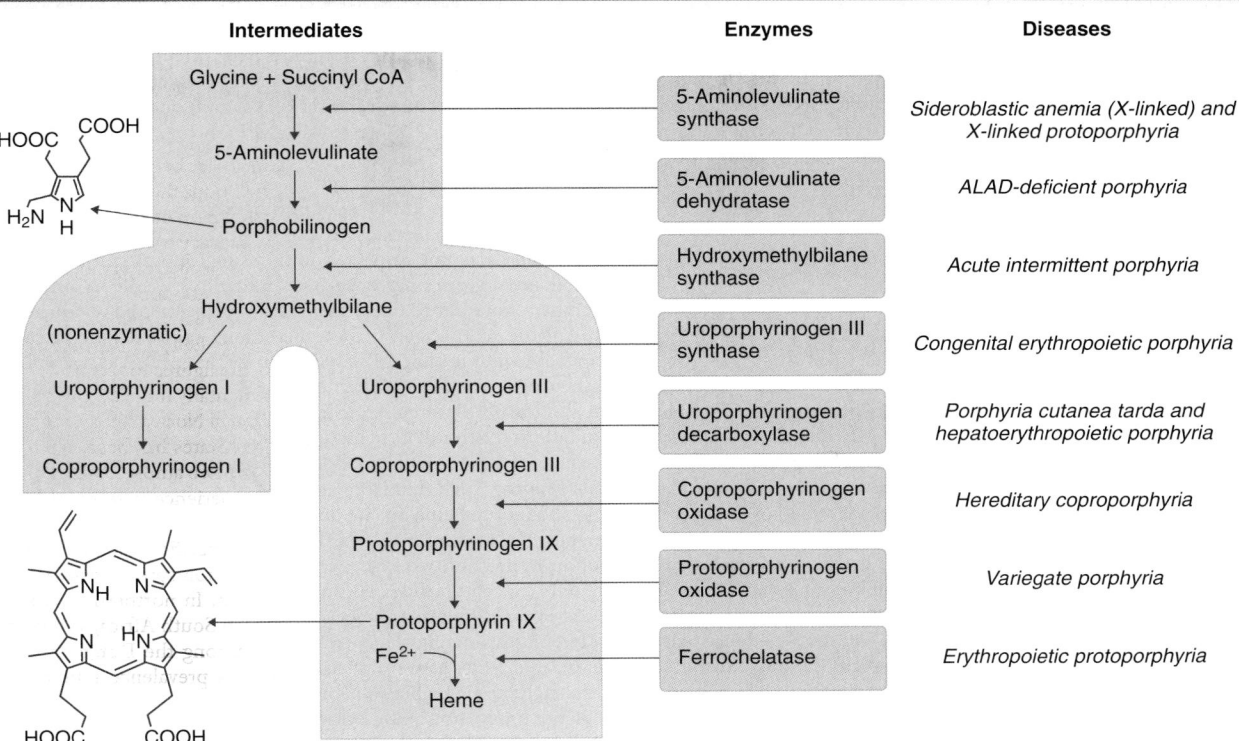

FIGURE 210-1. The heme biosynthetic pathway. Heme is synthesized through a series of porphyrin precursors and porphyrin intermediates, catalyzed by specific enzymes as indicated. The form of porphyria associated with abnormal enzyme function is shown on the right.

The remaining genes are common to both systems, although transcriptional variations lead to minor differences in size between the erythropoietic and hepatic forms of porphobilinogen synthase (previously known as ALA dehydratase), hydroxymethylbilane synthase, and uroporphyrinogen-III synthase.

Heme production is tightly coupled to heme requirement, and the flux of metabolites through the pathway is regulated by a process of negative feedback inhibition. The synthesis of ALA is the rate-limiting step in the pathway. In the liver, as heme use is increased (e.g., for incorporation into CYP), there is a reduction in a postulated hepatic regulatory free heme pool, the transcription of *ALAS1* is initiated, and ALAS1 activity increases. Conversely, when the requirement for heme drops, ALAS1 is repressed, leading to a reduction in porphyrin synthesis. Regulation in the erythropoietic system is somewhat different. Control is exercised through the binding of iron regulatory proteins to an iron response element in the 5′ region of the *ALAS2* mRNA. The extent of downregulation or upregulation of translation is controlled by the availability of iron.

The structure of the biochemical intermediates of heme biosynthesis as well as of the heme catabolic products biliverdin and bilirubin is shown in E-Figure 210-1. After ALAS-mediated synthesis, ALA is converted into porphobilinogen (PBG), which has a monopyrrolic ring structure. These two compounds, ALA and PBG, are classified as porphyrin precursors. Four PBG molecules are then combined to form the linear tetrapyrrole hydroxymethylbilane, which is then enzymatically cyclized by the enzyme uroporphyrinogen-III synthase, resulting in the tetrapyrrolic macrocycle uroporphyrinogen III. This is the first of a series of porphyrinogens. Spontaneous cyclization is possible but produces the series I isomer, which is not physiologic and is not further metabolized. Sequential modification of the porphyrinogen side chains results in the production of a sequence of porphyrinogens and their oxidized counterparts, the porphyrins. In the final step, iron is incorporated into the macrocycle, resulting in the functional heme molecule. The distinction between porphyrin precursors and porphyrins is important in diagnosis and in predicting the clinical presentation of each form of porphyria. The enzymes ALAS, coproporphyrinogen oxidase, protoporphyrinogen oxidase, and ferrochelatase are all mitochondrial, whereas the remaining enzymes are cytosolic. Heme synthesis therefore begins and ends in the mitochondrion, with intermediate metabolism occurring in the cytoplasm.

The porphyrin precursors and the initial porphyrins in the pathway are water soluble, circulate freely in the plasma, and are largely excreted in urine. The later porphyrins are hydrophobic, may be protein bound in the plasma, and undergo biliary excretion, eventually being excreted in the stool. The pattern of accumulation and excretion of precursors and porphyrins is exploited for the biochemical diagnosis of porphyrias and ultimately underlies the varying presentations of the acute and nonacute porphyrias. The acute attack is always associated with elevations in the precursors, and the acute porphyrias are therefore those in which such an accumulation occurs. Porphyrins are photosensitive molecules, and those forms of porphyria in which large amounts of porphyrin accumulate in plasma and skin have photosensitive skin disease as their major clinical presentation. In the nonacute porphyrias, the levels of precursors remain unchanged, accounting for the lack of acute attacks. Because porphyrins are typically elevated, they are manifested with skin disease alone. Two forms of porphyria, HCP and VP, may demonstrate both porphyrin elevation and a propensity to periodic elevation in the precursors; these porphyrias are therefore characterized by both skin disease and the risk of an acute attack.

Etiology
Acute Porphyrias
Acute Intermittent Porphyria
AIP is inherited as an autosomal dominant disorder. Because the enzyme block is early in the pathway, elevation of the precursors is characteristic and leads to a potential for development of the acute attack but not skin disease. Although an excess of nonphysiologic series I porphyrin isomers is typically observed in urine, this results from spontaneous cyclization of accumulated PBG, particularly in the bladder. Rare cases of homozygous AIP have been described.

Variegate Porphyria
VP is inherited as an autosomal dominant disorder. The *PPOX* gene is carried on chromosome 1. The number of known mutations approaches 200. Penetrance is estimated at approximately 37%. VP is associated with elevations in porphyrins, leading to photosensitivity, and also with acute attacks, during which phase of the illness the levels of precursors become markedly elevated. This has been ascribed to an allosteric inhibition of hydroxymethylbilane synthase by coproporphyrinogen and protoporphyrinogen, which accumulate in VP. Occasional cases of homozygous VP have been described. Such cases are either homozygous for mutations associated with some residual enzymatic activity or are compound heterozygotes, in which a mutation on one allele that results in complete loss of catalytic activity is accompanied on the other by a mutation associated with some residual catalytic activity. The homozygous state for mutations associated with complete loss of enzymatic activity is lethal.

Hereditary Coproporphyria

HCP is an autosomal dominant disorder. The *CPOX* gene is carried on chromosome 7, and more than 50 disease-associated mutations have been described. Both acute attacks and skin disease are encountered; the mechanism for the acute attack is similar to that of VP, with hydroxymethylbilane synthase being allosterically inhibited by accumulated coproporphyrinogen. Rare cases of homozygous HCP have been described.

ALA Dehydratase Porphyria

This is a rare autosomal recessive disorder, described in fewer than 10 cases. The *ALAD* gene is carried on chromosome 9.

Nonacute Porphyrias
Porphyria Cutanea Tarda

This disorder results from reduced activity of the enzyme uroporphyrinogen decarboxylase (UROD). PCT is unique among the porphyrias in that it is in most cases not inherited. Approximately 75% of patients present with sporadic PCT. In these cases, the *UROD* gene is normal, but patients will demonstrate a reduction in UROD activity. This is due to a chemically mediated inhibition of the enzyme. The inhibitor has been identified as uroporphomethene, an aberrant oxidative product of the normal substrate of the enzyme uroporphyrinogen. Sporadic PCT has a number of specific associations. First, nearly all cases are associated with some degree of hepatic iron loading. It is thought that the iron functions as an oxidant, facilitating the formation of the uroporphomethene inhibitor. Second, many cases will show evidence of liver dysfunction, commonly due to alcohol or hepatitis C viral infection. A number of other miscellaneous factors may also precipitate PCT, including HIV infection, estrogen exposure, renal failure, lymphoma, systemic lupus erythematosus, and toxins such as hexachlorobenzene. The relationship of viral infection and liver disease to PCT predisposition is not understood. It has been suggested that common factors may be downregulation of hepcidin, leading to iron overload, and increased oxidative stress, with these two factors potentiating the inhibitory mechanism.[2] An association with diabetes has also become evident. Reversal of the UROD inhibition results in biochemical and clinical remission.

In some cases, iron loading has been shown to relate directly to the inheritance of mutations in genes responsible for iron regulation. For example, the C282Y mutation in the *HFE* gene commonly found in white patients with hereditary hemochromatosis (Chapter 212) is over-represented in PCT. In other cases, the reason for the iron loading is less clear.

Approximately 25% of cases of PCT are classified as familial PCT. In these patients, an inherited mutation in a *UROD* allele can be shown. The resulting 50% reduction in UROD activity is not in itself sufficient to precipitate clinical expression. When disease does become clinically manifested, these patients commonly show evidence of the same precipitating factors described in sporadic PCT, but they may present at a younger age. Disease therefore results from a combination of an inherited mutation and environmental factors that result in inhibition of the remaining functional enzyme.

Rare cases of homozygous PCT have been described. These are known as hepatoerythropoietic porphyria and are manifested with severe photomutilation resembling that seen in CEP.

Erythropoietic Protoporphyria

EPP is inherited in a complex fashion. The *FECH* gene is carried on chromosome 18, and more than 100 disease-associated mutations have been reported. Molecular analysis demonstrates the presence of an inherited mutation on one allele resulting in reduced enzymatic activity. However, this is insufficient in its own right to result in clinical symptoms. A small proportion will be found to be homozygous, resulting in sufficiently reduced ferrochelatase activity for the disease to become clinically manifested. Approximately 94%, however, can be shown to have coinherited a *FECH* polymorphism, prevalent in white populations, that is associated with moderately reduced ferrochelatase activity. This *FECH**IVS3-48C low-expression allele is subject to aberrant splicing and decreased stability of the transcript, resulting in low expression. The gene frequency may reach 11% in European populations. The summative effect of the family-specific mutation and low-expression allele is sufficient to reduce ferrochelatase activities to a level below approximately 35%, at which stage the clinical syndrome may develop. In the strict sense, EPP is a recessive disorder, but the high prevalence of the low-expression allele in the population means that the compound heterozygous state occurs commonly in families carrying an EPP mutation. Thus, the prevalence is much higher than would typically be expected of an autosomal recessive

disorder; its inheritance has been described as pseudodominant. A recent study in North America of 155 unrelated patients reported that 136 carried the combination of a loss-of-function *FECH* mutation and the low-expression allele, whereas only three carried two loss-of-function mutations. The remaining 15 patients were shown to have XLPP.[3]

X-Linked Protoporphyria

This is the most recent form of porphyria to be identified. The clinical presentation is nearly identical to that of EPP, and its existence as an independent entity was not suspected until a subgroup of families with EPP were found not to carry ferrochelatase mutations. XLPP is associated with a number of mutations occurring in a sharply restricted region at the C terminus of the *ALAS2* gene. These mutations appear to modify an important control region leading to stabilization of the mRNA transcript or, possibly, enhanced access of succinyl coenzyme A to ALAS, either of which will result in abnormally elevated ALAS2 activity. These are therefore gain-of-function mutations that result in an increased flux of porphyrins through the erythroid heme biosynthetic pathway. Both ferrochelatase and iron availability become rate limiting, such that large amounts of protoporphyrin cannot be further metabolized to heme but are diverted to the plasma. Because the pathophysiologic mechanism for EPP is also dependent on the overproduction of protoporphyrin, the two disorders are nearly identical clinically. The *ALAS2* gene is carried on the X chromosome, making XLPP an X-linked disorder. Loss-of-function mutations in the *ALAS2* gene are responsible for X-linked sideroblastic anemia (Chapter 159), a condition unrelated to XLPP, that is associated with gain-of-function mutations. Erythrocyte protoporphyrin levels tend to be higher in patients with XLPP than in those with EPP, with a higher proportion being zinc chelated. Penetrance appears to be near 100%, and liver complications are more prevalent. Transmission is as expected of an X-linked disorder, one manifestation of which is the absence of father to son transmission.

Somatic Mutations

Very rarely, non-germline tissue-specific mutations may result in manifest porphyria. Cases of CEP, EPP, and VP have been described in neoplastic and paraneoplastic settings, such as myelodysplasia, myeloproliferative disorders, and hepatocellular carcinoma.

Pathogenesis
Photosensitivity

In those porphyrias associated with skin disease, porphyrins are found in high concentrations in plasma, skin, and blister fluid. Porphyrins are fluorescent. Stimulation by light results in an excitation of the porphyrin molecules, the promotion of electrons to a higher energy state, and the production of singlet oxygen. Relaxation to the ground state is accompanied by loss of energy manifesting as a radiation of red light. In the skin, this energy may be transferred to biologic molecules, resulting in oxidation of membrane lipids, polypeptides, and nucleic acids, thus accounting for the skin disease. The most potent wavelengths for porphyrin excitation lie within the ultraviolet spectrum, in the Soret band between 400 and 410 nm. Four additional absorption bands are present in the range of 500 to 700 nm; thus even visible light, against which most sunscreens are ineffective, is harmful to the skin in subjects with a cutaneous porphyria.

Pathologic examination will reveal epidermal bullae, duplication of basement membranes, and deposition of hyaline material, which appears to be associated with fibrin, immunoglobulins, and complement in and around the blood vessels of the dermis, suggesting that these vessels may be the principal target for light-induced injury.

Acute Attack

Elevated concentrations of the heme precursors ALA and PBG are always present in patients during the acute attack, and remission is commonly accompanied by a reduction in these concentrations. A causal role for either or both of these molecules has therefore long been suspected but never unequivocally proven. ALA is structurally similar to known neurotransmitters such as glutamine and γ-aminobutyric acid. Given the central role of nervous system dysfunction in the acute attack, it is suspected that ALA may be directly involved. Alternatively, it may serve as a proxy marker for some other as yet unidentified neurotoxin. An earlier contrasting hypothesis, that the neuropathy associated with an acute attack is mediated by intraneuronal heme deficiency, appears less likely because recent clinical experience has shown that liver transplantation cures AIP and VP and has induced acute attacks of porphyria in previously nonporphyric recipients who received an explanted porphyric liver as part of a domino transplant.

On histologic examination, nerve damage is characterized by axonal loss, although some degree of segmental demyelination may be present. There may be a reduction in intradermal nerve fiber density on skin biopsy. Skeletal muscle may show neurogenic atrophy. Nerve conduction studies, although not pathognomonic, tend to show a fairly characteristic pattern suggesting axonal neuropathy with relatively little evidence of demyelination. Upper limbs may be affected more than the lower limbs. Sensory nerves may be variably affected; electromyography initially shows a pattern of denervation, with widespread fibrillation, later replaced by a pattern of reinnervation marked by polyphasic motor unit potentials with increased amplitude and duration.

Induction of Porphyria

The block in porphyrin synthesis with consequent heme deficiency that characterizes all forms of porphyria does not appear to result in any direct clinical adverse effect. Although patients with CEP, EPP, and XLPP may be mildly anemic, this is in part secondary to hemolysis in CEP and iron deficiency in XLPP. In the acute porphyrias, hemoproteins such as CYP and tryptophan pyrrolase will reveal evidence of heme desaturation, again without obvious clinical consequences. The principal effect of the heme deficiency is the derepression of ALAS1, thus substantially increasing the flux of porphyrins through the pathway, accentuating the rate-limiting effect of the enzyme block and resulting in a significant overproduction of porphyrins and, possibly, precursors, which then result in the characteristic clinical syndromes. This mechanism is key to the understanding of the porphyrias.

The development of the acute attack is strongly associated with hyperinduction of ALAS1, typically by increased gene transcription in response to a reduction in free heme concentrations. Whereas the resultant increased activity of the heme biosynthetic pathway leads to an appropriate increase in heme levels in normal individuals, after which ALAS1 is suppressed, in patients with an acute porphyria, the defective enzyme is rate limiting; adequate heme concentrations are not reached, thereby leaving the pathway in a state of hyperinduction, and ALA and PBG accumulate in quantities sufficient to induce clinical symptoms. The most common precipitant of the acute attack is exposure to a number of drugs that share the ability to induce ALAS1. Such drugs are termed porphyrogenic.

This synthesis of CYP apoenzyme and heme is tightly correlated. The most powerfully porphyrogenic compounds include multifunctional inducers that induce multiple hepatic microsomal enzymes, those that induce the CYP3A and CYP2C9 subclasses, and those that are associated with irreversible mechanism-based inhibition of CYP. Such inhibition results in destruction of the enzyme, release of heme (which is then catabolized by heme oxygenase, leading to a reduction in the free heme pool), and consequently ALAS1 induction. These processes are mediated by nuclear receptors, particularly the constitutively active receptor and the pregnane xenobiotic receptor. Now that these mechanisms are understood, it is possible with high accuracy to predict which drugs are most likely to be porphyrogenic.

Calorie deprivation is known to induce porphyrin synthesis and even the acute attack, whereas glucose administration has a suppressive effect. This so-called glucose effect has been shown to be mediated by the transcriptional coactivator PGC-1α, which is induced when the liver shifts from the use of glucose as an energy substrate to β-fatty acid oxidation, activating the ALAS1 promoter and increasing heme synthesis.

Patients carrying a gene for an acute porphyria do not respond uniformly or predictably to drug exposure. Some patients will not respond at all, others may show some biochemical evidence of increased porphyrin production, and others will develop severe clinical symptoms. The reason for this variation in response or for the observation that acute attacks are extremely rare before puberty is not well understood. It is thought that the variability may result from the inheritance of polymorphisms in other genes responsible for drug metabolism, including cytochrome P-450, and possibly by metabolome-level variations, in other words, a complex interaction of genetic, biochemical, and hormonal interactions at a particular point in time. Similarly, the reason for the incomplete penetrance of many of the porphyrias is not yet understood; some 60% of patients carrying a gene for VP, for instance, fail to manifest biochemical or clinical evidence of disturbed porphyrin synthesis.

Women with AIP may show a pattern of regularly recurring attacks associated with the luteal phase of the menstrual cycle, although this is fortunately uncommon. It appears that endogenous hormone production is sufficient to stimulate ALAS and to cause an acute attack. Acute attacks have also been ascribed to calorie deprivation. Both stress and infection have been listed as possible inducers of the acute attack, although the evidence for this is weak.

CLINICAL MANIFESTATIONS

Patients with CEP, EPP, and the homozygous forms of the acute porphyrias usually present in childhood. This is an extremely rare occurrence in the three dominantly inherited acute porphyrias, in which both biochemical and clinical evidence of disease expression is typically delayed until after puberty. Although adult patients may present at any age, the first presentation is typically in the third decade.

Acute Porphyrias

The cardinal manifestation of the acute porphyrias is the acute attack. This metabolic crisis is characteristically manifested as severe, generalized abdominal pain, felt throughout the abdomen and sometimes in the lower back, buttocks, and thighs. The pain is severe and requires opioids for relief. It is not associated with peritonitis, and abdominal examination is typically unremarkable. There is autonomic overactivity manifested as hypertension, tachycardia, and gastrointestinal dysfunction, typically vomiting, constipation, and occasionally ileus.

Severe acute attacks are associated with a number of other features. Hyponatremia is common and when severe may lead to seizures and altered consciousness, particularly when hypotonic intravenous fluids are administered. Although often ascribed to the syndrome of inappropriate antidiuretic hormone (Chapter 116), the pattern of electrolyte excretion frequently suggests renal salt wasting, sometimes associated with marked urinary losses of potassium, calcium, and magnesium.

A severe, untreated acute attack may be complicated by a rapid-onset motor neuropathy, usually developing 24 hours or more after the onset of the abdominal pain. Very occasionally, a patient will present with neuropathy with a history of minimal or no abdominal pain; this may lead to a delay in suspecting porphyria as the cause. The neuropathy is typically symmetrical and may affect proximal muscles predominantly. Although motor signs predominate, there may be some sensory involvement in a central, so-called bathing suit distribution. The neuropathy may result in quadriparesis. Weakness of the respiratory muscles is common and may result in respiratory failure requiring ventilation. Once established, motor neuropathy typically requires months for recovery. Occasional patients may develop a prominent small-fiber neuropathy after attacks that is manifested with a generalized dysesthesia and hyperalgesia.

Cranial nerve or cerebellar involvement is occasionally noted, with facial and vagus nerve involvement in particular, although involvement of the trigeminal, hypoglossal, accessory, and oculomotor nerves has also been observed. The most extreme cases may develop the posterior reversible encephalopathy syndrome with radiologic evidence of reversible cerebral ischemia. On occasion, autonomic overactivity is so severe as to resemble a pheochromocytoma crisis (Chapter 228).

There is a widespread and unjustified misperception that psychiatric manifestations are a prominent part of the symptoms of the acute porphyrias. Claims that historical figures such as King George III of England and his relatives and Vincent van Gogh had porphyria all perpetuate the myth that AIP is associated with chronic insanity but are not supported by convincing evidence.[4] During the acute phase, the acute attack frequently is manifested with anxiety and sometimes with a short-lived psychotic episode, which reverses completely with remission of the attack. A statistical association with chronic anxiety and depression in patients with AIP has been shown. There is no association with chronic psychosis or a need for institutionalization.

The acute attack is more common in females than in males, is extremely rare before puberty, and becomes uncommon from the sixth decade onward. Pregnancy may precipitate acute attacks, but this is infrequent. Large studies suggest that there may be a slight increase in risk of perinatal death in women with the acute porphyrias; in a study of 136 deliveries, this did not reach statistical significance, but significance was shown when restricted to first pregnancies alone.[5]

The acute attack has become less common in recent decades as a result of earlier diagnosis and careful attention to its prevention. It is uncommon for a patient who has had an attack to suffer a recurrence once preventive measures have been instituted. Patients repeatedly exposed to porphyrogenic medication, including recreational drugs, may suffer recurrent acute attacks. A very small number of patients may show a course characterized by recurrent acute attacks of unknown etiology; this is particularly a feature of some young women with AIP. In some of these women, there is a clear relationship to the menstrual cycle. In the remainder, such an association is not obvious, and a vicious circle of recurrent attacks and hospitalizations becomes established. Such patients become severely debilitated and cachectic, show evidence of accumulating neuronal damage, experience a poor quality of life, and may ultimately die.

Other Manifestations

Patients with AIP are prone to develop chronic hypertension and renal dysfunction, probably due to chronic activation of the sympathetic nervous system. A strong and unexplained association between both AIP and VP and noncirrhotic hepatocellular carcinoma (Chapter 196) has been reported from several centers. Swedish patients with AIP older than 50 years have been shown to be at 86-fold increased risk of hepatocellular carcinoma.[6] The risk is significantly higher in women. There is evidence of an increased risk in VP as well, but surprisingly, such an association has not been seen in South Africa despite the frequency of VP in that population.

Homozygous Acute Porphyrias

Homozygous AIP is a serious disorder that may be associated with severe neurodevelopmental abnormalities, including porencephaly, psychomotor and developmental retardation, ataxia, epilepsy, cataracts, and a number of other neurologic manifestations. It is usually fatal in childhood. Homozygous VP is associated with skeletal dysmorphism, severe skin disease, nystagmus, seizures, a sensory neuropathy, and cognitive impairment. An association with cerebral demyelination, detectable on magnetic resonance imaging, has recently been described. Despite the severity of the symptoms, there is no appreciable early mortality, and for reasons as yet unknown, acute attacks are not a feature of homozygous VP. Homozygous HCP takes two forms: the first resembles homozygous VP with small stature, photosensitivity, psychomotor retardation, and neurologic defects; the second is manifested at birth with hemolytic anemia and severe jaundice. This variety is associated with specific mutations in the *CPOX* gene that specifically block an intermediate stage in the oxidation of coproporphyrinogen and protoporphyrinogen, resulting in the accumulation of a harderoporphyrinogen intermediate, and is known as harderoporphyria.

ALA Dehydratase Deficiency Porphyria

This is an extremely rare recessive disorder that may be manifested in either childhood or adulthood, depending on the severity of the phenotype, typically with chronic neuropathy, other neurologic symptoms, and acute attacks.

Vesiculo-erosive Skin Disease

The characteristic skin disease of VP, HCP, PCT, and CEP is described as vesiculo-erosive. Patients present with blistering and erosions, typically in response to minor skin trauma, in sun-exposed areas, particularly the dorsal surface of the hands and forearms, the face, and, if sun exposed, the nape of the neck and the dorsal surfaces of the feet. There is no immediate photosensitivity, and the changes develop insidiously. Therefore, patients frequently fail to make the association between sun exposure and skin damage. The lesions heal slowly, leaving a residuum of scarring and small, localized areas of hypopigmentation or hyperpigmentation (Fig. 210-2). Milia may be present, particularly on the dorsal surfaces of the hands and in the digital clefts.

It is unusual for the skin disease of VP and HCP to develop beyond this. Patients with PCT, however, may show marked facial hypertrichosis, hyperpigmentation, and sometimes alopecia. They may also develop thickening of the skin of the fingers and hands; these pseudosclerodermoid changes may occasionally lead to a misdiagnosis of localized scleroderma.

The most severe skin disease is characterized by marked photomutilation, including loss of skin appendages such as the nose, ears, and lips. This is seen in CEP and in hepatoerythropoietic porphyria. The skin disease of homozygous VP is marked by an accentuation of the features characteristic of heterozygous VP, alopecia and resorption of digits, which may be due to photo-osteolysis (Fig. 210-3) or, alternatively, may represent part of the skeletal dysmorphism characteristic of the disorder.

Porphyria Cutanea Tarda

PCT typically presents in middle-aged and older subjects who develop characteristic skin lesions in sun-exposed areas. Acute attacks are not a feature. Given the strong association with iron loading and liver disease, clinical and biochemical assessment commonly reveals evidence of increased iron storage, liver dysfunction, alcohol abuse, or renal dysfunction. In the less common

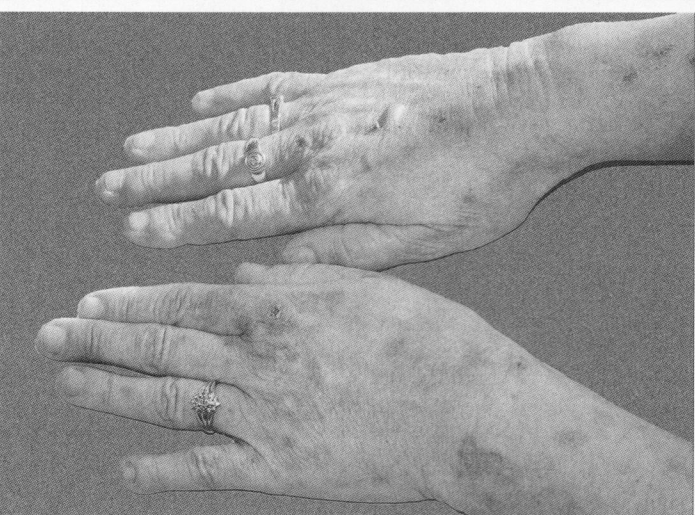

FIGURE 210-2. The hands in variegate porphyria. The characteristic lesions are bullae, shallow erosions that develop scabs and heal slowly, leaving areas of hypopigmentation and hyperpigmentation. The skin disease of porphyria cutanea tarda and hereditary coproporphyria is similar.

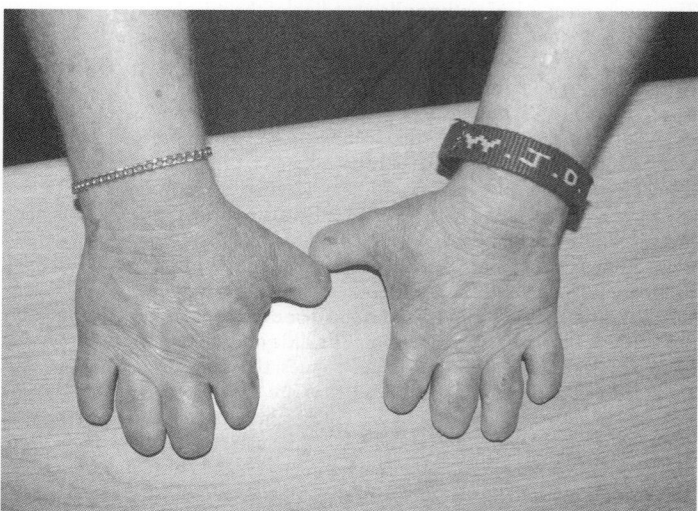

FIGURE 210-3. The hands of a patient with a homozygous form of variegate porphyria. In addition to the characteristic vesiculo-erosive skin lesions, there is marked brachydactyly, representing both photo-osteolysis and a skeletal developmental defect.

setting of HIV infection, systemic lupus erythematosus, or lymphoma, clinical evidence for these disorders will be present.

Congenital Erythropoietic Porphyria

This rare autosomal recessive disorder is associated with a spectrum of disease severity. Severely afflicted patients demonstrate photomutilation, with scarring, loss of skin appendages (such as ears, nose, lips, fingernails, and digits), ulcerative keratitis, and corneal scarring. A form of immediate photosensitivity after sunlight exposure and characteristic pink erythematous facial papules have been described.[7] Patients may show erythrodontia, osteodystrophy, hypercellular bone marrow, hemolytic anemia, and splenomegaly. Other patients are more mildly affected and may present later in life. The skin damage deteriorates progressively with increasing age. Impact on quality of life and psychosocial consequences may be severe. Prenatal cases presenting in utero with severe anemia associated with hydrops fetalis have been described. There is a variable genotype-phenotype correlation. Although some mutations tend to be associated with more severe disease, the severity may vary between patients even though they carry the same mutation. The most predictive features of a severe course are early age at onset and the presence of hematologic complications, particularly severe anemia and

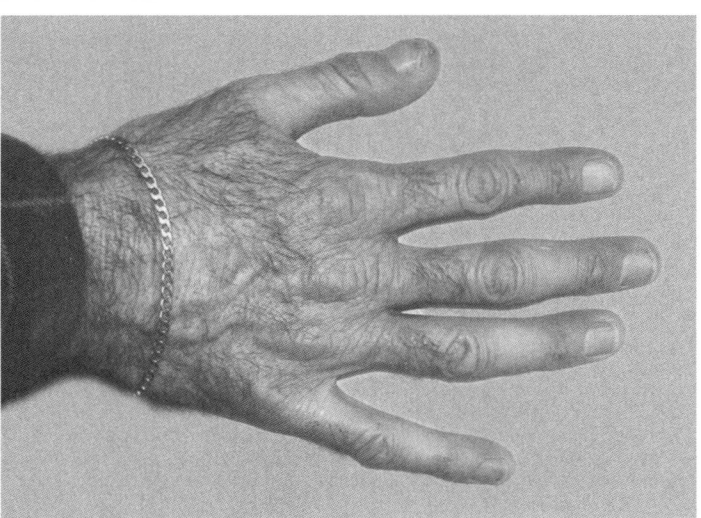

FIGURE 210-4. The hands in erythropoietic protoporphyria. There is thickening and grooving of the skin over the knuckles.

thrombocytopenia. One study has suggested that *ALAS2* acts as a modifier gene, with severity of phenotype being modulated by mutations in that gene.[8]

Skin Disease Associated with Immediate Photosensitivity
Erythropoietic Protoporphyria
Patients with EPP and XLPP do not manifest the typical vesiculo-erosive pattern of skin disease described before but develop a characteristic pattern of immediate photosensitivity. Patients will report that after a period of sun exposure, they develop severe discomfort and pain in sun-exposed areas. This may be associated with erythema and edema. The discomfort may take 24 to 48 hours to settle after cessation of sun exposure. The onset of the illness is often in childhood but diagnosis is frequently delayed, and the reason for a child's reluctance to remain outdoors is often not recognized immediately. Chronic skin changes are minimal and are usually limited to the development of a waxy thickening and grooving of the skin, typically over the bridge of the nose and over the knuckles (Fig. 210-4). A mild microcytic hypochromic anemia may be present. A subset of patients develop a condition known as seasonal palmar keratoderma; it has been shown that these patients carry homozygous or compound heterozygous ferrochelatase mutations.

Approximately 10% of patients with EPP will develop hepatobiliary disease secondary to the massive accumulation of protoporphyrin within the hepatocytes and biliary porphyrin excretion, typically with cholelithiasis secondary to elevated biliary porphyrin concentrations. Approximately 2% may present with severe and potentially life-threatening liver disease, including cirrhosis and liver failure.

X-Linked Protoporphyria
XLPP and EPP cannot for practical purposes be distinguished clinically. XLPP is likely to have a higher penetrance as well as a typical X-linked pattern of inheritance. Patients are more prone to liver disease than are those with EPP. Some patients will report a correlation between iron deficiency and severity of symptoms.

Other Settings
A transient immediate acute photosensitivity is occasionally observed in patients with VP as they emerge from an acute attack. This is sometimes associated with acute loss of fingernails. Some patients with CEP may manifest immediate photosensitivity in addition to the characteristic vesiculo-erosive skin response. Immediate photosensitivity is observed in some patients in whom the synthetic metalloporphyrin tin protoporphyrin was administered as a heme oxygenase inhibitor to prolong remission with repeated acute attacks of AIP. It is also noted in patients treated with ALA or synthetic porphyrin analogues as part of photodynamic therapy for cancer.

DIAGNOSIS
An accurate diagnosis is essential in the management of porphyria. Although the pattern of symptoms and skin manifestations may suggest the diagnosis,

a clinical diagnosis alone is notably inaccurate, given the varying and often nonspecific manifestations of the disorders as well as the inexperience of most physicians in dealing with them. A failure to diagnose the porphyrias may have serious consequences, with unnecessarily impaired quality of life and, in some, the potential for a possibly fatal acute attack. Conversely, it is not unusual for patients, typically with a history of frequent, unexplained abdominal pain, to be erroneously labeled as having an acute porphyria.

Biochemical Diagnosis
Biochemical analysis is central to the diagnosis and evaluation of the porphyrias. For AIP, hydroxymethylbilane synthase assays have been widely used but are now discouraged owing to their inaccuracy. Recent reports have highlighted the gain in diagnostic accuracy that results from restricting diagnostic testing for porphyria to a small number of national reference laboratories that analyze sufficient cases to develop expertise and that cooperate in a quality enhancement network.

The pattern of porphyrin accumulation in urine, stool, plasma, and erythrocytes that characterizes a specific porphyria forms the basis of diagnosis. In practice, this is complicated by the varying water solubility of the precursors and porphyrins, leading to differential patterns of accumulation in urine, stool, and plasma. It must be stressed that examination of urine alone may lead to both misdiagnosis and misclassification of the porphyria. Given the differential excretion of porphyrins, it is essential that testing include urine, stool, and plasma. Where an erythropoietic porphyria is suspected, an erythrocyte porphyrin analysis must be performed as well.

Porphyrin analysis is typically performed with a high-performance liquid chromatographic separation technique with fluorometric detection of the porphyrins. The series I and III isomers can be distinguished and the concentration of each individual porphyrin species quantitated by reference to standard specimens. Differentiation of isomers is particularly important in the identification of HCP. The erythropoietic porphyrias are easily confirmed by assessing the biochemical profile of porphyrins in erythrocytes.

A useful screening assessment is plasma fluorescence scanning. The fluorescence emission maximum varies between different porphyrins and with the extent of their protein binding. When it is subjected to ultraviolet light, a plasma sample will typically demonstrate an emission peak at approximately 630 nm in EPP, 625 nm in VP, and 619 nm in AIP, HCP, and PCT.

The acute attack is always associated with an elevation of the porphyrin precursors ALA and PBG. The first step in the assessment of the confirmation of an acute attack is therefore to submit urine for determination of these levels, specifically PBG. In the appropriate clinical setting, elevated levels are highly confirmatory; and conversely, when these are normal, the diagnosis must be reconsidered. Some laboratories are able to measure ALA and PBG in plasma, which may have a slight advantage in accuracy. For immediate use in the emergency setting, semiquantitative test kits that allow the identification of elevated urinary PBG concentrations without the use of specialized equipment have been developed. It is recommended that every emergency department have ready access to such a kit.

Genetic Testing
Given that the various porphyrias result from mutations in different genes and that within each porphyria, numerous family-specific mutations may give rise to the characteristic phenotype, molecular diagnosis is not well suited to the primary evaluation of a patient. No mutation-specific diagnostic test will exclude any form of porphyria other than the one specifically associated with that gene and that mutation. It is for this reason that biochemical analysis is recommended as the first step. Furthermore, whereas biochemical testing, by quantitating precursor and porphyrin levels, provides information on the degree of activity of the porphyria at a particular moment, molecular techniques do not. Once a biochemical diagnosis of porphyria has been made, the underlying mutation should be identified. Screening of family members for this mutation will then determine carrier status. This is particularly important in the case of the acute porphyrias, such that as-yet unaffected family members can practice risk avoidance, particularly in terms of their exposure to potentially porphyrogenic medication. Where there is a very high prevalence as a result of a founder effect, screening for that mutation may prove useful in preliminary assessment. This is the case in South Africa, where a single *PPOX* mutation, the R59W mutation, accounts for more than 95% of all cases of VP.

Differential Diagnosis
The differential diagnosis of an acute porphyria will include any cause of severe abdominal pain, including surgical emergencies. Forty percent of

children with hereditary tyrosinemia type I may develop a syndrome closely resembling the acute attack; this is mediated by the accumulation of succinylacetone, which is a potent inhibitor of 5-aminolevulinate dehydratase.

When patients present with a motor neuropathy or quadriparesis, other causes of neuropathy may be considered. The initial diagnosis in such cases is often the Guillain-Barré syndrome. A careful history may reveal a history of abdominal pain (although very occasionally this is absent), and neurophysiologic testing will show a pattern of axonal necrosis rather than demyelination. A biochemical analysis for porphyria will confirm the correct diagnosis.

The differential diagnosis of a typical vesiculo-erosive porphyria is limited. Other chronic bullous diseases will require exclusion. Epidermolysis bullosa is similar but is not restricted to sun-exposed areas. A common differential is pseudoporphyria, which may be found in association with end-stage renal or liver disease, with tanning bed use, or as a class of drug-induced skin reactions, particularly in response to nonsteroidal anti-inflammatory drugs, nalidixic acid or tetracycline, sulfur-containing diuretics, systemic retinoids, cyclosporine, and dapsone. The skin manifestations closely resemble a cutaneous porphyria. Despite the clinical similarity, there is no underlying enzymatic or genetic defect, and plasma porphyrin profiles are normal.

It is not uncommon for patients with liver disease to excrete elevated amounts of coproporphyrin in the urine. This is termed coproporphyrinuria. It represents a slight diversion of coproporphyrin excretion from bile to urine, is not related to any disturbance in heme biosynthesis, and is essentially irrelevant.

TREATMENT   Rx

Given the rarity of the porphyrias, the evidence for efficacy of therapy seldom reaches grade A status. In most instances, treatment recommendations are based on experience in small case series or on expert opinion.

Acute Porphyrias

It is essential that the physician treating the acute attack of porphyria have a clear concept of the disorder, what treatment is appropriate, and when and how it should be applied. It is therefore important for patients to be referred to a physician with experience in porphyria or to be managed in close cooperation with such an expert.

Supportive therapy includes opioid analgesia in doses sufficient to relieve the abdominal pain. This is severe, and physicians with little experience in porphyria will frequently underdose and may even disbelieve the patient's complaints, being misled by the lack of physical signs in the abdomen, even though this is typical of the acute attack. Morphine and newer opioids should be selected in preference to meperidine, given its addictive potential. It is essential that all porphyrogenic drugs or other potential precipitants be stopped or corrected, and no medication may be administered to the patient unless its safety in porphyria has been checked.

Patients may require antiemetics. Although β-blockers may assist in slowing the pulse and reducing blood pressure, these are rarely sufficiently elevated to require treatment in their own right. Furthermore, they settle rapidly once specific therapy is administered.

Electrolyte balance requires careful monitoring. Hyponatremia may be a problem, and hypotonic fluids, such as glucose, should not be administered in large volumes. Although carbohydrate loading has been shown to have a suppressive effect on porphyrin synthesis, its effect is minimal in comparison with heme therapy.

Specific Therapy

Administration of exogenous heme results in negative feedback inhibition of ALAS, resulting in a rapid reduction in porphyrin synthesis. Such therapy is effective, has been confirmed in a controlled trial,[A1] and is now the standard of care for the acute attack. The practical advantages have been three-fold: to shorten the period of symptoms for the patient; to shorten the course of the acute attack, allowing earlier discharge; and to prevent severe complications, such as encephalopathy and motor neuropathy. Although lyophilized hematin is effective, current practice is to administer heme arginate, a more stable compound. It is administered intravenously in a dose of 3 mg/kg daily for 4 days. The manufacturer recommends that the dose be reconstituted in 100 mL of a 0.9 % sodium chloride solution and infused into a large vein during at least 30 minutes. Some authorities suggest administration in human serum albumin as albumin has a buffering effect that may reduce the incidence of phlebitis at the site of infusion. There is also some evidence that administration in albumin may facilitate hepatic uptake. Typically, administration of heme arginate is followed within 24 hours by a reduction in symptoms, and after 72 hours the patient is usually symptom-free and may be discharged. Treatment during pregnancy has been shown to be safe.

It is essential that heme arginate be administered at an early stage of the acute attack. It will prevent but not reverse motor neuropathy. Once this has developed, the patient is committed to a lengthy period of hospitalization and rehabilitation.

Very rarely, patients present with a syndrome of severe, accelerated hypertension, tachycardia, and cerebral complications that may include coma, seizures, and the posterior reversible encephalopathy syndrome. This may resemble an uncontrolled pheochromocytoma. Administration of magnesium sulfate in association with combined α- and β-blockade is useful in controlling the autonomic overactivity while the attack is brought into remission with heme arginate. Recovery is usually complete.

Recurrent Attacks

Recurrent acute attacks are an uncommon manifestation of the acute porphyrias. A careful drug history is important in excluding exposure to porphyrogenic medication. Where a relationship between the attacks and the menstrual cycle is suspected, gonadal suppression with gonadotropin-releasing hormone agonists such as goserelin and buserelin may be attempted. In some patients, this is efficacious in aborting the pattern of recurrent attacks. In a small trial in 16 women, four responded with a complete cessation of symptoms, and 11 had some improvement. Because patients are at risk of osteoporosis after gonadal suppression, add-back hormonal therapy was attempted; estradiol and progesterone precipitated attacks in two and five of nine women, respectively.[9]

Some patients with a history of recurrent acute attacks have received prophylactic heme arginate at scheduled intervals, apparently with benefit in some. A permanent indwelling central venous catheter is often required for this. Currently, there is concern that frequent administration of heme arginate may induce heme oxygenase, leading to rapid catabolism of heme, thus initiating a vicious circle of reduction in hepatocyte free regulatory heme levels, ALAS1 induction, and increased porphyrin synthesis, promoting the development of another attack. Theoretically, this vicious circle might be ameliorated by the administration of heme oxygenase inhibitors, such as the metalloporphyrins like tin protoporphyrin, tin mesoporphyrin, and zinc mesoporphyrin. This has been attempted in a few patients and appeared to be of some short-term benefit, although it did not affect the overall outcome. Furthermore, exogenous hematin and heme arginate are iron rich, and patients receiving frequent courses of therapy may become iron overloaded. For these reasons, repetitive administration of heme arginate should be undertaken with extreme caution.

Orthotopic liver transplantation has now proved its value in the management of patients with recurrent acute attacks.[10] It is effectively curative in both AIP and VP, preventing further acute attacks. Transplantation should therefore be considered in any patient who develops a pattern of severe repetitive acute attacks, particularly when there is incomplete recovery between attacks, progressive disability, or severely impaired quality of life, and in patients for whom no causal factor amenable to removal or amelioration is identified.

Skin Disease

There is no specific therapy for vesiculo-erosive skin disease. Sun avoidance is central in management. This may require behavioral modification as well as careful attention to dress, wearing nontranslucent clothing to reduce the skin's ultraviolet exposure. Trauma to exposed areas should be minimized. Sunscreens may have a role but must prevent the transmission of both UVA and UVB wavelengths and preferably light at visible wavelengths as well. Zinc oxide is more effective than titanium dioxide. Although sunscreens containing micronized zinc oxide or titanium are translucent and cosmetically more acceptable, they reflect less light and therefore provide only partial protection. Nonmicronized pastes are more effective.

A number of photostable UVA filters are under development and may prove beneficial. Where skin disease is severe, as in CEP, consideration may be given to replacement of fluorescent lighting with other forms of illumination with lower short-wavelength light emission and the application of transparent film to windows, spectacles, and windshields to exclude the relevant wavelengths.

Established lesions should be carefully cleaned with nonastringent antiseptics. In our experience, aseptic lancing of bullae may hasten resolution. Where secondary infection is noted, topical or systemic antibiotics are indicated.

Porphyria Cutanea Tarda

PCT may be expected to remit once the precipitating factors have been removed. Therefore, alcohol use should be severely restricted. Hepatitis C, if present, should be treated. The reduction of hepatic iron stores is highly effective in the treatment of PCT. A common regimen is to carry out a 500-mL venesection (phlebotomy) fortnightly until iron parameters are in the low-normal range; this typically requires about 8 to 12 sessions. Intravenous and oral iron chelators are effective but are associated with more serious adverse effects than venesection. Patients with renal failure or conditions such as the myelodysplastic syndrome present a special problem as they are typically anemic. The drop in hemoglobin may be counteracted by administration of erythropoietin (erythropoiesis-stimulating agents), with the additional benefit of its effect in mobilizing iron from the liver. However, in our experience, careful venesection without erythropoietin has proved safe and effective, the hemoglobin level returning to its usual set point after each session.

Chloroquine has been shown in a trial to be as effective as venesection in inducing remission in PCT, with an efficacy similar to that of venesection.[11] By disrupting lysosomal structure, it allows the release of porphyrins stored in the liver into the plasma, from which they are cleared by the kidneys. Thus, it is common to see a transient increase in plasma porphyrins and worsening of skin disease in the first few weeks of therapy. Chloroquine must be used in low doses, typically 125 mg twice weekly, because larger, daily doses may result in a severe transaminitis. Units with experience in treating PCT tend to have their own preference for chloroquine therapy or venesection. Our practice has been to combine phlebotomy with chloroquine, and this has proved extremely satisfactory. Remission of PCT, once attained, is usually maintained for many years, although re-treatment may occasionally be necessary. There is some evidence that α-tocopherol may provide additional benefit when it is prescribed in association with standard therapy for PCT.

Reports have suggested that direct treatment of hepatitis C and HIV with antiviral agents has resulted in an improvement in PCT even in the absence of venesection or chloroquine therapy. Given the deleterious effects of iron overload, however, it would appear prudent to combine such treatment with iron-lowering therapy.

Erythropoietic Protoporphyria

A reduction in sun exposure is central to the management of EPP and requires behavioral change, attention to dress, and use of broad-spectrum sunscreens. A small proportion of patients appear to respond positively to the administration of β-carotene in doses sufficiently large to induce carotenodermia; however, despite a number of trials of varying quality, efficacy has not been convincingly proved.[12] If it is effective at all, it is not known whether the benefit is due to the light-reflecting effect of the increased skin pigmentation, to its antioxidant effects, or to a combination. Narrow-band UVB phototherapy has in some cases resulted in increased phototolerance. Treatment with slow-release subcutaneous implants of afamelanotide, a synthetic melanocyte-stimulating hormone analogue, has yielded encouraging results in preliminary clinical studies.[13] Such analogues induce the synthesis of both melanin and eumelanin, which absorbs and reflects radiation over a wider light spectrum. In addition to inducing hyperpigmentation, afamelanotide also has antioxidant properties that may be of some benefit.

Claims have been made for a number of interventions in terms of their utility in reducing the acute pain of EPP, including lotions, steroids, local anesthetics, antihistamines, water immersion, and ice packs. Although individual patients may feel that they are helped by one or another, a study has not shown a consistent benefit for any single intervention.

The liver disease found in association with EPP in a small proportion of patients constitutes a serious problem. Such patients require the care of an experienced hepatologist, and there are no clear guidelines in treatment. Administration of oral sorbents such as activated charcoal and cholestyramine, which interrupt hepatic porphyrin recycling, have yielded inconsistent results. Hypertransfusion and administration of heme arginate may suppress porphyrin synthesis but are not suitable for long-term use. Severely affected patients are candidates for orthotopic liver transplantation. Given that the viscera are porphyrin laden and prone to severe light-induced necrosis, careful preparation of the patient is necessary, and surgery has to be carried out with appropriately filtered operating lights. Severe motor neuropathy has proved to be an unexpected but not unusual complication of liver transplantation in EPP. After transplantation, protoporphyrin will reaccumulate in the liver. Consideration may therefore be given to performing combined bone marrow and liver transplantation.

Congenital Erythropoietic Porphyria

Light avoidance, with protection for both skin and eye, is essential. Afamelanotide has shown benefit in a single case. Given the hemolysis and resultant jaundice, neonates with CEP may be subjected to phototherapy, which may seriously damage the skin. Some patients require chronic transfusion for anemia and may benefit from splenectomy. CEP is often a severe disease, and successful autologous stem cell transplantation will prevent further disfigurement and inevitable psychosocial consequences. There is emerging consensus that young subjects with severe CEP should be offered stem cell transplantation.[14] It should be borne in mind that the phenotype of CEP is extremely variable. Currently, stem cell transplantation is reserved for patients with a mutation known to be associated with a severe phenotype and for those presenting at a younger age or with progressive severe hemolytic anemia or thrombocytopenia because these factors are predictive of a poor outcome. This will require an expert decision.

Investigational Therapies for the Porphyrias

Intravenous administration of recombinant hydroxymethylbilane synthase to patients with AIP was studied in a small series. Although it reduced plasma ALA and PBG levels, it was ineffective in treating symptoms; this was presumably due to limited access to the hepatocyte. Gene replacement, with a variety of vectors, is under active development and has shown promise in laboratory studies, particularly for the management of CEP and AIP. Gene silencing by RNA interference directed at ALAS1 mRNA to block ALAS1 induction in the acute porphyrias appears encouraging. Where the effect of a mutation is to reduce protein stability, interventions to improve stability may lead to improvement in enzyme concentration and activity. In CEP, laboratory studies suggest that administration of a proteosome inhibitor may improve UROS function where the enzyme deficiency is due to an unstable and rapidly degraded protein.[15]

Given the success of autologous stem cell transplantation in CEP and EPP and of liver transplantation in AIP and VP, experimental work on transplantation continues. A laboratory study suggesting that induced pluripotent stem cells are capable of correcting CEP was encouraging.[16] Hepatocyte transplantation has shown promise experimentally in the treatment of AIP and would have advantages over orthotopic liver transplantation.[17]

PREVENTION

Primary Prevention

Given that most of the porphyrias are genetically determined, there is currently no practical way in which these illnesses may be prevented. Diagnosis in utero by molecular methods for the identification of family-specific mutations is possible, and theoretically selective abortion would prevent transmission of the disease. In practice, however, this is not indicated. Only in a tiny minority of patients are the common acute porphyrias of sufficient severity to seriously impair the quality of the patient's life. Penetrance is incomplete, and even when the disease is clinically expressed, symptoms are not expected to develop until the end of the second decade. Termination of pregnancy is therefore inappropriate. Although patients with EPP may experience an impaired quality of life, few would argue that this is of a severity that would justify termination. The only situation in which it might be justified could be in CEP and in the homozygous acute porphyrias. However, these being recessive disorders, the incidence is extremely low, and these disorders are for practical purposes unforeseeable. The exception may be in cases of known consanguinity, in which the possibility of recessive inheritance is increased. Given that both familial and sporadic PCT tend to occur in association with disorders such as iron loading, hepatitis C, and alcoholic liver disease, treatment or avoidance of these conditions would be expected to reduce incidence.

Secondary Prevention

The most important aspect of prevention is anticipating and preventing or ameliorating the potential clinical effects and complications in the patient with known porphyria. In the acute porphyrias, interventions are directed at preventing the onset of the acute attacks. It is essential that the patient avoid exposure to any drug that might potentially be porphyrogenic. It is thus necessary that all gene carriers and the health professionals who care for them understand the absolute importance of consulting a drug safety database before taking or prescribing any medicinal agent. We recommend use of the European web-based database The Drug Database for Porphyria (http://www.drugs-porphyria.org) maintained by the Norwegian Porphyria Centre. Traditional drug safety lists are incomplete because the information on which they are based is typically obtained from clinical experience in porphyria and animal or tissue culture experiments and may therefore not be available for many drugs, particularly those that have come into use more recently. Second, the information derived from these sources is frequently poorly generalizable to the porphyric population at large, given the unreliability of some of the sources from which the information is derived, the extreme variability in response between individual patients, and the major differences in drug metabolism between species. The Drug Database for Porphyria, by contrast, is based on the prediction of porphyrogenicity on the grounds of metabolism and information is therefore available even before clinical experience has accumulated; preliminary analysis suggests that the predictions are highly reliable, and where a drug has been predicted to be safe, there have not as yet been any instances of clinical use resulting in an adverse effect.[18] The patient should wear a medical bracelet. Given the association of acute attacks with calorie deprivation, subjects with the acute porphyrias should avoid periods of low calorie intake.

Children with cutaneous porphyrias or those known to be a gene carrier for one of the adult-onset porphyrias with photocutaneous sensitivity, such as VP, should be encouraged to develop healthy habits of sun avoidance and sun protection before the onset of symptoms. Patients with established disease need to modify their behaviors and attend to their dress to limit sun exposure. In cases of extreme photosensitivity, filtering of natural and artificial light may be beneficial.

Patients with PCT should be screened for hemochromatosis-associated mutations. These may be of prognostic significance in family members in detecting and therefore treating hemochromatosis early.

PROGNOSIS

With few exceptions, the prognosis of all the porphyrias is good. PCT is treatable, and remission is expected once the precipitating factors, including iron overload, have been corrected. Patients with the acute porphyrias may expect a normal lifespan, provided the appropriate precautions are taken to prevent the acute attack or, should such an attack develop, it is appropriately treated at an early stage. The skin disease of porphyria is not life-threatening.

The prognosis is poor in those patients who present with a pattern of frequent, repeated attacks and do not respond to interventions intended to break the cycle. The course is frequently one of slow deterioration during several years and may ultimately be fatal. Such patients should be assessed for orthotopic liver transplantation. Patients with CEP are subject to severe photomutilation with serious psychosocial consequences and should be assessed for allogeneic stem cell transplantation. Patients with homozygous AIP are prone to severe developmental abnormalities and may die in childhood. By contrast, there appears to be no early mortality in patients with homozygous VP, although the photomutilation and neurodevelopmental effects will have psychosocial and educational consequences.

The prognosis for the individual acute attack is excellent, provided the condition is recognized, confirmed, and appropriately treated at an early stage before neuropathy has developed. Where the patient has developed quadriparesis, the prognosis for ultimate recovery is good with excellent supportive care, including assisted ventilation. Recovery to the point of independence and nearly full power may require a year of support and rehabilitation and is not always complete. Experience has shown that it is important to avoid further acute attacks during the period of convalescence and to treat them immediately and effectively should they develop to prevent a relapse in neuropathy.

Grade A Reference

A1. Herrick AL, McColl KE, Moore MR, et al. Controlled trial of haem arginate in acute hepatic porphyria. *Lancet.* 1989;1:1295-1297.

GENERAL REFERENCES

For the General References and other additional features, please visit Expert Consult at https://expertconsult.inkling.com.

211

WILSON DISEASE

STEPHEN G. KALER AND MICHAEL L. SCHILSKY

DEFINITION

Wilson disease is an autosomal recessive disorder of copper transport. Affected individuals accumulate abnormal levels of copper in the liver and later in the brain as a consequence of mutations in both alleles of the Wilson disease gene (*ATP7B*). The gene encodes a copper-transporting ATPase expressed primarily in the liver, where its major function is excretion of hepatic copper into the biliary tract. The clinical condition of hepatolenticular degeneration with associated cirrhosis was first described in 1912 by S.A.K. Wilson. There are wide differences between patients in the age at onset and the spectrum of symptoms.

EPIDEMIOLOGY

The incidence of Wilson disease, defined as the occurrence of new cases, is approximately 1 in 30,000 to 40,000 live births. For special populations in which consanguinity is common, the risk of autosomal recessive traits such as Wilson disease is higher. In the general population, the prevalence of heterozygous gene carriers (defined as the ratio of all individuals with one mutant *ATP7B* allele to the population at risk of harboring one) is estimated to be 1 in 90. Some consider this figure an underestimate, however, on the basis of recent population data of the frequency of *ATP7B* mutation in the United Kingdom.[1]

PATHOBIOLOGY

Individuals normally consume 1 to 3 mg of dietary copper daily, of which approximately 50% is absorbed through the gastrointestinal tract. Most diets contain adequate amounts of copper, and certain foods (e.g., shellfish, liver, mushrooms, chocolate, nuts) contain higher quantities. In normal homeostasis, copper is absorbed from the stomach and duodenum, where absorption at the apical surface of the enterocyte is mediated by a specific copper transporter, hCTR1. The Menkes disease gene (*ATP7A*), which encodes a copper-transporting ATPase with high homology to *ATP7B*, transports copper from intestinal epithelial cells into the blood stream, where it is bound by albumin or amino acids, carried to the liver and other organs and tissues, or excreted by the kidney. This last pathway represents a minor pathway for copper excretion, and adults excrete up to 40 µg of copper per day in the urine.

Within the liver, copper may be (1) incorporated into ceruloplasmin, a multifunctional 132-kD α_2-glycoprotein enzyme containing six or seven copper atoms per molecule; (2) used in the synthesis of other copper-requiring enzymes; (3) bound by metallothionein, a low-molecular-weight, cysteine-rich protein that provides a storage and detoxification depot for copper and other trace metal elements; or (4) excreted into the bile. Copper excreted into bile does not undergo enterohepatic recirculation and thus represents a pathway for copper excretion.

In Wilson disease, metallation of ceruloplasmin is usually reduced, reflecting impaired transport of copper into the trans-Golgi compartment, where glycoprotein processing and the copper acquisition by apoceruloplasmin occurs. This results in low circulating levels of holoceruloplasmin (the protein with its full complement of copper). Because ceruloplasmin accounts for 90% of circulating copper, total serum copper is also low in most Wilson disease patients. However, free copper (non–ceruloplasmin-bound) is abnormally elevated in untreated Wilson disease patients. The flaw in copper incorporation into ceruloplasmin does not cause hepatic copper accumulation in Wilson disease, as evidenced by patients with aceruloplasminemia, in whom complete absence of this protein is associated with normal hepatic copper content. Rather, it is the effect of mutant ATP7B to reduce biliary copper excretion that produces massive hepatic copper overload when the condition is unrecognized. If the diagnosis goes unrecognized, copper overload subsequently involves other tissues, including the brain, which is particularly sensitive to perturbations in trace metal homeostasis.

The brain concentrates copper and other heavy metals for metabolic use. Copper is important for brain development and function, and copper excess (as well as deficiency) can seriously affect brain function.[2] In brain, astrocytes are considered important regulators of copper homeostasis, and in Wilson disease, the occurrence of abnormal astrocytes is a typical neuropathologic feature.

CLINICAL MANIFESTATIONS

Presenting clinical features of Wilson disease include nonspecific liver disease (Fig. 211-1), neurologic abnormalities, psychiatric illness, hemolytic anemia, renal tubular Fanconi syndrome, and various skeletal abnormalities.

There is considerable variation in clinical presentation and phenotype in Wilson disease.[3,4] Age influences the specific presentation. Most individuals who present with liver disease are younger than 30 years, sometimes in the first decade of life, whereas those presenting with neurologic or psychiatric signs range in age from the first to the eighth decade of life. This reflects the sequence of events in the pathogenesis of this disease (see earlier discussion). However, regardless of clinical presentation, some degree of liver disease is invariably present.[5] In one series of 400 adult patients with Wilson disease, approximately 50% presented with neurologic and psychiatric symptoms, 20% with neurologic and hepatic symptoms, and 20% with purely hepatic symptoms.

In patients with neurologic presentations, abnormalities include speech difficulty (dysarthria), dystonia, rigidity, tremor or choreiform movements, abnormal gait, uncoordinated handwriting, and (rarely) a combined motor

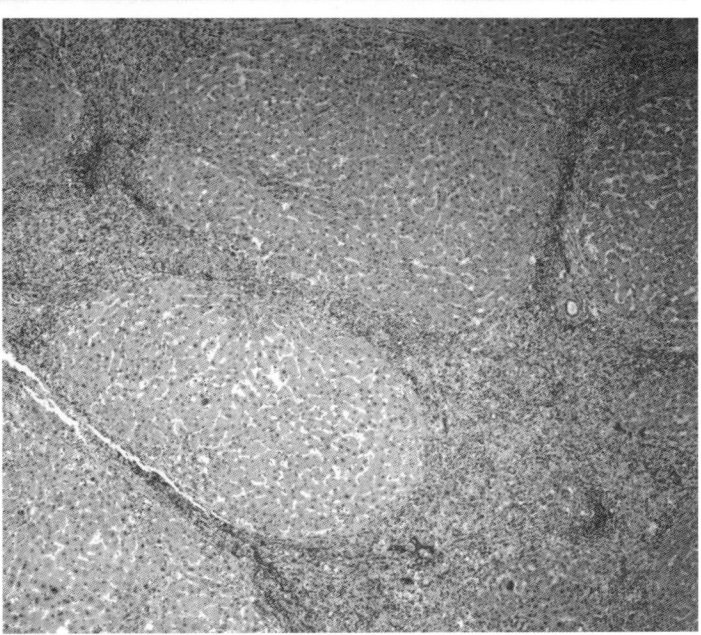

FIGURE 211-1. Hepatic cirrhosis in Wilson disease. (Image courtesy Kisha A. Mitchell, MD.)

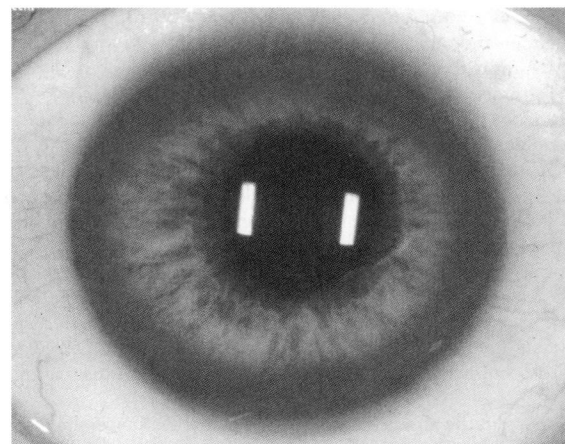

FIGURE 211-2. Kayser-Fleischer ring in a newly diagnosed patient with Wilson disease.

and sensory peripheral neuropathy.[6] Wilson disease may properly be classified as a movement disorder. The neurologic signs and symptoms reflect a predilection for involvement of the basal ganglia (e.g., caudate, putamen) in the brains of these individuals. Parkinson disease or other movement disorders may be mistakenly diagnosed.

In psychiatric presentations, changes in personality (irritability, anger, poor self-control), depression, and anxiety are common symptoms. Psychosis or bipolar disorder may also occur. Patients presenting with psychiatric symptoms are typically in their late teens or early 20s, a period during which substance abuse and schizophrenia are also prime diagnostic considerations. Wilson disease should be formally excluded in all teenagers and young adults with new-onset psychiatric signs, especially if results of liver function tests are abnormal or a family history of Wilson disease is noted.

In hepatic presentations, signs and symptoms include jaundice, hepatomegaly, edema, and ascites. Secondary endocrine effects of liver disease may include delayed puberty or amenorrhea. Viral hepatitis, autoimmune hepatitis, and cirrhosis are often initial diagnostic considerations in individuals with Wilson disease. Rare patients have Wilson disease concurrent with another liver disorder, and the diagnosis of Wilson disease is often delayed in these individuals as a consequence.

In addition to brain and liver, the eye is a primary site of copper deposition in Wilson disease, producing a benign but pathognomonic sign, the Kayser-Fleischer ring (Fig. 211-2). The Kayser-Fleischer ring is a golden to green-brown annular deposition of copper in the periphery of the cornea. This important diagnostic sign first appears as a superior crescent, then develops inferiorly and ultimately becomes circumferential. Slit-lamp examinations are required to detect rings in their early stage of formation. Copper can also accumulate in the lens and produce "sunflower" cataracts.

Approximately 95% of patients with neurologic signs manifest the Kayser-Fleischer ring, compared with approximately 50 to 65% of those with hepatic presentations. Copper chelation therapy, zinc treatment, and liver transplantation cause fading and even disappearance of corneal copper over time.

Hemolytic anemia resulting from the direct toxic effects of copper on red blood cell membranes has been observed in Wilson disease. This is usually associated with the release of massive quantities of hepatic copper into the circulation, a phenomenon that can be sudden and catastrophic due to the development of acute (fulminant) liver failure. On occasion, there may be bouts of hemolytic anemia unassociated with liver failure, but these individuals eventually develop progressive liver disease.

Renal dysfunction in Wilson disease is tubular in nature and leads to abnormal losses of amino acids, electrolytes, calcium, phosphorus, uric acid, and glucose. This effect is presumably related to direct copper toxicity or toxicity of copper complexes with metallothionein. High copper levels have

been noted previously in the kidneys of patients with Wilson disease. Treatment with copper chelation often improves the renal disturbances.

There can be skeletal effects of Wilson disease, including osteoporosis and rickets; these may be attributable to renal losses of calcium and phosphorus. Osteoarthritis primarily affecting the knees and wrists also occurs in Wilson disease patients and may involve excess copper deposition in the bone and cartilage.

DIAGNOSIS

Wilson disease should be considered in patients with liver disease without a clear etiology; in patients presenting with acute liver failure with associated hemolysis; in patients with neurologic and psychiatric disease, especially if there is concomitant liver disease; and in first-degree relatives of identified patients.

Laboratory findings that support the diagnosis include low levels of serum copper and serum ceruloplasmin, elevated urine copper excretion (>100 μg/24 hours), elevated hepatic transaminase levels, low serum albumin, elevated prothrombin time (international normalized ratio), aminoaciduria, low uric acid levels, and direct antiglobulin test (Coombs)–negative hemolytic anemia. Analysis of liver biopsy specimens for histologic features and copper content also can assist diagnosis; most patients have copper contents above 250 μg/g dry weight liver, although some may have values as low as 75 μg (normal, <40 μg). Clinical signs of the disease include the stigmata of chronic liver disease, neurologic signs and symptoms, and Kayser-Fleischer rings (possibly requiring slit-lamp examination for detection). A scoring system was developed by experts who attended an international meeting on Wilson disease in Leipzig that was designed to help determine if the diagnosis should be pursued further. This scoring system was the first to use biochemical, clinical, and molecular genetic data to give a cumulative score that would suggest further evaluation is needed or achievement of the diagnosis is accomplished; it has been used in a diagnostic algorithm developed by the European Association for the Study of the Liver.[7]

Molecular diagnostics for *ATP7B* mutations has been extremely helpful, especially for difficult to diagnose cases and for family screening, in which it may be used as first-line testing if the mutations in the proband have been identified.[8] Cost and the large numbers of mutations for *ATP7B* (now more than 500) have hampered use of genetic testing for all patients being considered for Wilson disease; however, technical advances will likely increase future use of this test.

Incorporation of a stable radioisotope, ^{64}Cu, into serum ceruloplasmin is a highly specific diagnostic test; patients with Wilson disease incorporate very little ^{64}Cu into ceruloplasmin. This test is particularly useful in patients thought to have Wilson disease despite normal ceruloplasmin levels, and it distinguishes affected individuals from heterozygotes. Clinical availability of this test, however, is limited.

Increased urinary excretion of copper (>100 μg/24 hours) is another easily performed and important diagnostic test for this disorder. Copper-free collection containers should be used. A variation involving serial urine copper measurements is the penicillamine "challenge," in which 500 mg of penicillamine is administered orally after collection of a baseline 24-hour urine specimen and repeated after 12 hours during the second 24-hour urine collection. A more than 10-fold increase in copper excretion is highly suggestive of Wilson disease.

Percutaneous needle liver biopsy for quantitative measurement of hepatic copper remains a useful test for the diagnosis of Wilson disease. As noted before, hepatic copper values higher than 250 μg/g of dry weight (normal, 20 to 50 μg/g dry weight) are characteristic of Wilson disease, although individuals with Wilson disease may have levels as low as 75 μg/g dry weight liver. Copper quantitation by inductively coupled plasma mass spectrometry or by atomic absorption spectrometry on dried and digested specimens is preferred to paraffin-embedded specimens, although paraffin-embedded specimens may be used when the diagnosis is considered retrospectively and adequate tissue was obtained. Histochemical staining of a liver biopsy specimen for copper by rhodanine may suggest Wilson disease but is less reliable.

In summary, in the absence of formal molecular evidence, the diagnosis of Wilson disease should be considered when at least two of the following are present: a positive family history, Kayser-Fleischer rings, Coombs-negative hemolytic anemia, low serum copper and ceruloplasmin levels, elevated hepatic copper content, increased 24-hour urine copper excretion, and positive penicillamine challenge result.[9,10]

TREATMENT Rx

Penicillamine contains a free thiol that binds copper and greatly enhances urinary excretion, thereby preventing copper overload and its effects. Faithful compliance with oral penicillamine treatment has enabled the good health of thousands of patients with Wilson disease worldwide during the past 50 years.[11,12] Pyridoxine (vitamin B_6) should be prescribed concomitantly to counter the vitamin B_6 deficiency that tends to develop with long-term penicillamine administration.

Certain individuals, about 20%, are intolerant of penicillamine. Significant side effects include hypersensitivity; nephrotoxicity; hematologic abnormalities; and a distinctive rash, elastosis perforans serpiginosa, that often involves the neck and axilla. Furthermore, in some patients with neurologic presentations, penicillamine treatment induces paradoxical worsening of the neurologic disease.

Even though penicillamine is the therapy with the longest experience, other pharmaceutical agents are available and may be considered for use as first-line drugs. For example, zinc acetate and triethylene tetramine dihydrochloride (trientine) are suitable alternative agents with somewhat less significant side effect profiles.

Oral zinc acetate also has proved highly effective in Wilson disease.[13] The mechanism involves decreased copper absorption by the intestine into the blood stream by induction of the copper storage protein metallothionein in intestinal epithelial cells. Zinc monotherapy has particular value in young, presymptomatic patients; in patients who are pregnant, given the possible fetal teratogenic effects of other compounds; and as maintenance therapy for patients. Whereas most patients do well with zinc therapy, 10 to 20% of users note dyspepsia, and a higher incidence of hepatic decompensation has been observed with long-term zinc therapy compared with chelation therapy. Another drawback to zinc is the relatively long time (4 to 6 months) needed to restore proper copper balance if zinc monotherapy is used in the initial stage of treatment.

Tetrathiomolybdate forms stable tripartite complexes with proteins and copper. This drug both decreases copper absorption and reduces circulating free copper. It is fast-acting and can restore normal copper balance within several weeks, compared with the several months required with other copper chelators or with zinc. Tetrathiomolybdate is especially appropriate for the initial treatment of patients with neurologic presentations on the basis of a completed clinical trial.[A1]

Regardless of the specific regimen chosen, treatment of Wilson disease is lifelong because noncompliance eventually leads to symptomatic disease or liver failure.[14]

Liver transplantation is a rare consideration in Wilson disease because the condition is typically responsive to medical therapy. It should be considered for patients presenting with acute liver failure due to Wilson disease or those presenting with end-stage liver disease with irreversible hepatic damage who are unlikely to respond to medical therapy. Long-term outcomes after transplantation for Wilson disease are excellent, and the disease does not recur in the transplanted organ.[15]

Apart from pharmacologic treatment, there are several other important considerations in the treatment of Wilson disease. These include dietary restriction of copper-containing foods, especially shellfish and liver, both of which are copper rich. The major sources of patients' drinking water should be tested for copper concentration and avoided if levels approach 1.3 mg/L,

which is the current maximum contaminant level goal (MCLG) established by the U.S. Environmental Protection Agency. The MCLG for copper in drinking water is set at a concentration at which no known or expected adverse health effects occur and for which there is an adequate margin of safety.

In newly diagnosed patients with neurologic manifestations, there is frequently a need for speech therapy and physical or occupational therapy and, for many others, psychological and genetic counseling.

Wilson Disease Heterozygotes

There is some debate about the risk of copper overload among individuals who are heterozygous carriers for Wilson disease. Even though Wilson disease is a classic autosomal recessive trait—that is, requiring two mutant alleles at the *ATP7B* locus for expression of the disease—a report from the U.S. National Academy of Sciences suggested that heterozygous carriers of Wilson disease may be a relatively sensitive population in terms of copper overload, particularly when dietary or drinking water copper exposure is higher than usual. Abnormally increased urinary copper excretion has been documented among some siblings of patients with Wilson disease, although genetic confirmation of the carrier or noncarrier status of these individuals was not available. Further patient and family studies are needed to formally address these questions.

PROGNOSIS

The prognosis in Wilson disease is generally favorable. Current therapeutic approaches can prevent, stabilize, or reverse most of the significant clinical signs and symptoms, including Kayser-Fleischer rings. However, if treatment is stopped, recurrence of symptoms and potentially fatal liver damage inevitably occurs.

FUTURE DIRECTIONS

Gene therapy for Wilson disease is a possibility. Because the Wilson copper transporter is expressed most prominently and functions most critically in the liver, this organ could be specifically targeted by the use of adenoviral or adeno-associated viral vectors (e.g., AAV8). Hepatocyte transplantation, an alternative to gene therapy, may also be applicable to the treatment of liver-specific metabolic disorders through therapeutic liver repopulation.

 Grade A Reference

A1. Brewer GJ, Askari F, Lorincz MT, et al. Treatment of Wilson disease with ammonium tetrathiomolybdate: IV, comparison of tetrathiomolybdate and trientine in a double-blind study of treatment of the neurologic presentation of Wilson disease. *Arch Neurol.* 2006;63:521-527.

GENERAL REFERENCES

For the General References and other additional features, please visit Expert Consult at https://expertconsult.inkling.com.

212

IRON OVERLOAD (HEMOCHROMATOSIS)

BRUCE R. BACON

DEFINITION AND EPIDEMIOLOGY

Hereditary hemochromatosis (HH) is a common inherited disorder of iron metabolism. The genetic abnormality responsible in most patients with typical HH is found in homozygous form in about 1 in 250 persons of northern European descent. It is characterized by an increase in iron absorption from the upper gastrointestinal tract, with subsequent tissue iron deposition in parenchymal cells of the liver, heart, pancreas, joints, and endocrine organs. The autosomal recessive inheritance pattern of HH was clearly shown in the 1970s, and the gene responsible for most cases of HH was identified in 1996 by investigators using a positional cloning technique.[1] The gene is called *HFE*

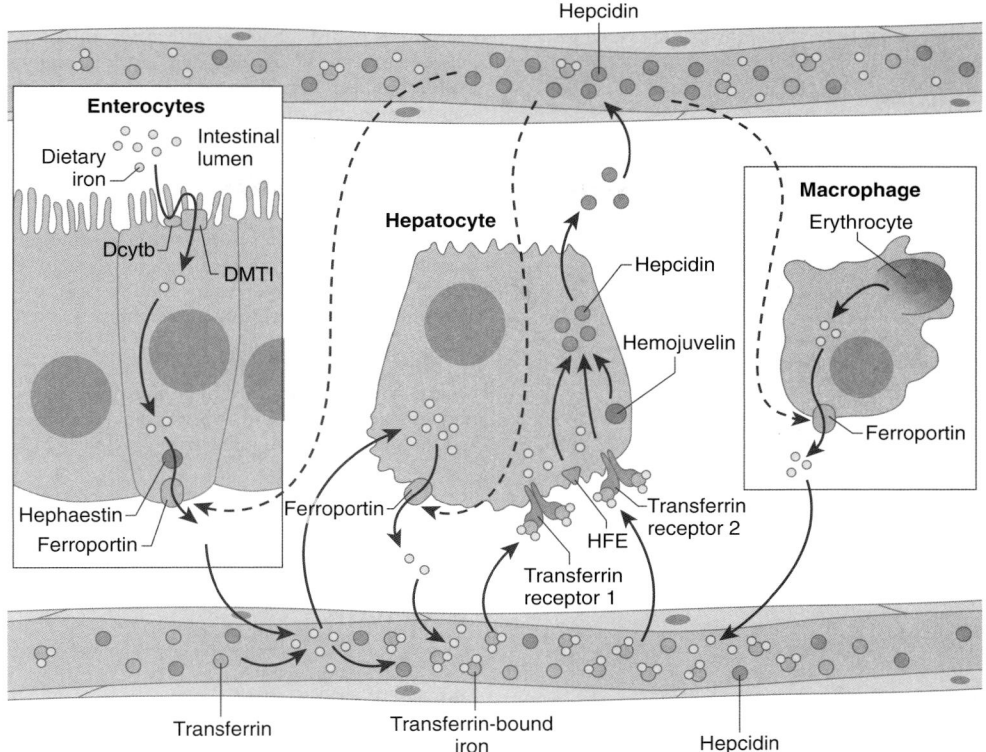

FIGURE 212-1. Orchestration of iron homeostasis. In the duodenal enterocyte, dietary iron is reduced to the ferrous state by duodenal ferric reductase (Dcytb), transported into the cell by divalent metal transporter 1 (DMT1), and released by way of ferroportin into the circulation. Hephaestin facilitates enterocyte iron release. Hepatocytes take up iron from the circulation either as free iron or as transferrin-bound iron (through transferrin receptors 1 and 2). Transferrin receptor 2 may serve as a sensor of circulating transferrin-bound iron, thereby influencing expression of the iron regulatory hormone hepcidin. The hepcidin response is also modulated by HFE and hemojuvelin. Hepcidin is secreted into the circulation, where it downregulates the ferroportin-mediated release of iron from enterocytes, macrophages, and hepatocytes (*dashed lines*). (From Fleming RE, Bacon BR. Orchestration of iron homeostasis. *N Engl J Med.* 2005;352:1741-1744.)

and encodes a novel major histocompatibility complex (MHC) class I–like molecule that binds with transferrin receptor (TfR) and affects hepcidin homeostasis (Fig. 212-1). Prospective population studies have demonstrated that only about 50 to 60% of patients who are homozygous for the major mutation found in *HFE* (called C282Y) have evidence of phenotypic expression of iron overload, and only a small percentage (<10%) go on to develop tissue damage from excess iron deposition. These findings of the highly variable penetrance of C282Y homozygosity have changed modern thinking about HH and must be considered when patients are evaluated for this disease in a physician's office and when national health policy for screening of this genetic disorder is developed.

The discovery of *HFE* has had a tremendous impact in a number of areas. The ability to accurately diagnose disorders of iron overload has been strengthened, family screening is improved, and the evaluation of patients with other forms of liver disease complicated by moderate to severe iron overload is possible. Furthermore, with the discovery of *HFE*, a considerable new body of knowledge about the mechanisms and regulation of iron absorption has been identified, both in the normal situation and in the pathologic condition seen when *HFE* mutations are present.

Classification of Iron Overload Syndromes

The term *hereditary hemochromatosis* should be reserved for inherited disorders of iron metabolism (see Fig. 212-1) that lead to tissue iron loading (Table 212-1). The most common form of this disease, *HFE*-related HH, is caused primarily by homozygosity for the C282Y mutation in the *HFE* gene. Other heritable forms of iron overload have also been recognized (non–*HFE*-related HH).[2,3] These include autosomal recessive forms of HH characterized by rapid iron accumulation and caused by mutations in the genes for hemojuvelin (*HJV*) and hepcidin (*HAMP*) (also called juvenile hemochromatosis); an autosomal dominant form of HH caused by mutations in the ferroportin gene; an autosomal recessive form of HH resulting from mutations in the gene for *TFR2* (*SLC40A1*); and rare forms of HH resulting from mutations in the *DMT1* gene or mutations in the portion of the ferritin gene

encoding the iron-responsive regulatory element. Some other types of iron overload may have a familial or inherited component, but the genes involved have not yet been identified. For example, African iron overload is a familial disorder of iron loading prevalent in sub-Saharan Africa that is exacerbated by the ingestion of an iron-rich home-brewed beer. However, iron overload can also occur in individuals who do not drink this beverage. A similar form of iron overload has been suggested in African Americans, and further study is necessary to clarify this condition. The degree of iron loading can be similar to that seen in *HFE*-related HH, but the cellular and lobular distribution of iron is different. In addition, a rare disorder termed congenital alloimmune hepatitis is responsible for most cases of neonatal iron overload and is characterized by a modest increase in hepatic iron accompanied by severe liver injury present at birth.

It has been recognized during the last several years that many patients who have *HFE*-linked hemochromatosis have no evidence of iron overload. With this in mind, four stages of HH have been described[4]:
1. Genetic predisposition with no phenotypic abnormality
2. Iron overload (approximately 2 to 5 g total body iron) without symptoms
3. Iron overload with mild or early symptoms
4. Iron overload with organ damage, such as cirrhosis

The ability to establish a genetic diagnosis has led to a much greater understanding of genotype-phenotype correlations.

Genetics and Pathophysiology of Hemochromatosis

Since the classic linkage studies of Simon and colleagues in the mid-1970s, it has been known that the gene for hemochromatosis is located in the human leukocyte antigen (HLA) region on chromosome 6. In 1996, a team of molecular geneticists using a positional cloning technique identified a candidate gene for HH, which is now called *HFE*. *HFE* codes for a novel MHC class I–like molecule, which, like all MHC proteins, requires interaction with β_2-microglobulin for normal presentation on the cell surface. Three principal missense mutations have been identified in *HFE*: one results in a change of cysteine at position 282 to tyrosine (Cys282 → Tyr, C282Y), the second

TABLE 212-1   CLASSIFICATION OF IRON OVERLOAD SYNDROMES

HEREDITARY HEMOCHROMATOSIS

HFE Related

C282Y/C282Y
C282Y/H63D
C282Y/S65C
Other mutations

Non–*HFE* Related

Hemojuvelin (*HJV*) mutations (autosomal recessive)
Hepcidin (*HAMP*) mutations (autosomal recessive)
Ferroportin (*SLC40A1*) mutations (autosomal dominant)
Transferrin receptor 2 (*TFR2*) mutations (autosomal recessive)
Divalent metal transporter 1 (*SLC11A2*) mutations (rare)
Ferritin regulatory mutations (rare)

Miscellaneous

African iron overload
Neonatal iron overload (rare)

SECONDARY IRON OVERLOAD

Anemia Caused by Ineffective Erythropoiesis

Thalassemia major
Sideroblastic anemias
Congenital dyserythropoietic anemias
Congenital atransferrinemia

Liver Disease

Alcoholic liver disease
Chronic viral hepatitis B and C
Porphyria cutanea tarda
Nonalcoholic steatohepatitis
After portacaval shunt

Miscellaneous

Transfusional iron overload
Excessive parenteral iron administration

results in a change of histidine at position 63 to aspartate (His63 → Asp, H63D), and the third results in a change of serine at position 65 to cysteine (Ser65 → Cys, S65C). A few other mutations have been identified in *HFE*, but their frequency is low and their clinical impact is limited. In the original studies, 83% of typical phenotypic HH patients were found to be homozygous for the C282Y mutation. Several other studies from around the world in predominantly white populations demonstrated that among patients with typical hemochromatosis, about 85 to 90% were homozygous for C282Y. Thus, about 10 to 15% of patients with typical phenotypic HH have some reason other than C282Y homozygosity for their iron overload.

Nearly all absorption of dietary iron occurs in the duodenum, where iron may be taken up either as ionic iron or as heme. Ionic iron requires reduction to the ferrous state, which is accomplished by the ferric reductases (e.g., duodenal ferric reductase), which are expressed on the luminal surface of duodenal enterocytes (see Fig. 212-1). This ferrous iron crosses the apical membrane through divalent metal transporter 1, and iron taken up by the enterocyte is either stored as ferritin or transferred across the basolateral membrane to the plasma. This latter process occurs by the iron transporter ferroportin and requires oxidation of iron to the ferric state by the ferroxidase hephaestin.[5] Hypoxia-inducible factor-2 (HIF-2α) regulates the expression of key genes involved in iron absorption and may be involved in the hyperabsorption of iron in the context of hepcidin deficiency in HH.[6]

Hepcidin is a 25–amino acid, liver-derived peptide that influences systemic iron status such that it is now considered to be the principal iron regulatory hormone (see Fig. 212-1). Dysregulation of hepcidin expression is thought to play a role in the pathogenesis of HH. Patients with *HFE*-related HH have low hepatic expression of hepcidin, as do *HFE* knockout mice, despite excess hepatic iron stores. Conversely, overexpression of hepcidin in *HFE* knockout mice prevents the HH phenotype. Iron-induced regulation of hepcidin expression involves a bone morphogenetic protein (BMP)–dependent signaling pathway. BMPs bind to specific receptors on hepatocytes, thereby triggering SMAD protein–dependent activation of hepcidin expression. Selective inhibition of BMP signaling abrogates iron-induced

upregulation of hepcidin. Hemojuvelin is a BMP coreceptor and facilitates the binding of BMP to its receptor; knockout of the hemojuvelin gene markedly decreases BMP signaling and hepcidin expression and causes iron overload. It has been hypothesized that *TFR2* in hepatocytes may act as an iron sensor. Mutations in *TFR2* cause a rare form of HH in humans, and *Tfr2* mutant mice have an HH phenotype. In HH, excess iron (both transferrin bound and non–transferrin bound) is avidly taken up by hepatocytes and stored. Iron stores increase to the point at which iron-induced oxidative damage occurs, resulting in cell injury and cell necrosis with phagocytosis by Kupffer cells. Iron-laden Kupffer cells become activated and produce profibrogenic cytokines (transforming growth factor-β, platelet-derived growth factor), which stimulate hepatic stellate cells to synthesize excess collagen and other matrix proteins. Increased fibrosis and then cirrhosis result.

CLINICAL MANIFESTATIONS

Several symptoms and clinical findings have been identified in patients with fully established HH, and all physicians should be aware of these symptoms and findings, which are summarized in Tables 212-2 and 212-3. Table 212-4

TABLE 212-2   SYMPTOMS IN PATIENTS WITH HEREDITARY HEMOCHROMATOSIS

ASYMPTOMATIC

Abnormalities of serum iron studies on routine screening chemistry panel
Abnormal liver test results
Identified by family screening
Identified by population screening

NONSPECIFIC SYSTEMIC SYMPTOMS

Weakness
Fatigue
Lethargy
Apathy
Weight loss

SPECIFIC ORGAN-RELATED SYMPTOMS

Abdominal pain (hepatomegaly)
Arthralgias (arthritis)
Symptoms of diabetes mellitus (pancreas)
Amenorrhea (cirrhosis)
Loss of libido, impotence (pituitary, cirrhosis)
Congestive heart failure symptoms (heart)
Arrhythmias (heart)

TABLE 212-3   PHYSICAL FINDINGS IN PATIENTS WITH HEREDITARY HEMOCHROMATOSIS

ASYMPTOMATIC

No physical findings
Hepatomegaly

SYMPTOMATIC

Liver

Hepatomegaly
Cutaneous stigmata of chronic liver disease
Splenomegaly
Signs of liver failure: ascites, encephalopathy

Joints

Arthritis
Joint swelling

Heart

Dilated cardiomyopathy
Congestive heart failure

Skin

Increased pigmentation

Endocrine

Testicular atrophy
Hypogonadism
Hypothyroidism

TABLE 212-4 LABORATORY FINDINGS IN PATIENTS WITH HEREDITARY HEMOCHROMATOSIS

MEASUREMENTS	NORMAL SUBJECTS	PATIENTS WITH HEREDITARY HEMOCHROMATOSIS	
		Asymptomatic	**Symptomatic**
BLOOD (FASTING)			
Serum iron level (µg/dL)	60-180	150-280	180-300
Serum transferrin level (mg/dL)	220-410	200-280	200-300
Transferrin saturation (%)	20-45	45-100	80-100
Serum ferritin level (ng/mL)			
Men	20-200	150-1000	500-6000
Women	15-150	120-1000	500-6000
GENETIC (*HFE* MUTATION ANALYSIS)			
C282Y/C282Y	wt/wt[†]	C282Y/C282Y	C282Y/C282Y
C282Y/H63D*	wt/wt	C282Y/H63D	C282Y/H63D
LIVER			
Hepatic iron concentration			
µg/g dry weight	300-1500	2000-10,000	8000-30,000
µmol/g dry weight	5-27	36-179	140-550
Hepatic iron index[†]	<1	1 to >1.9	>1.9
Liver histology			
Perls' Prussian blue stain	0, 1+	2+ to 4+	3+, 4+

*Compound heterozygote.
[†]Calculated by dividing the hepatic iron concentration (in µmol/g dry weight) by the age of the patient (in years). With the increased use of genetic testing in patients with iron overload, the specificity of the hepatic iron index has diminished.
[‡]wt/wt: wild type (normal).

summarizes the typical laboratory findings in symptomatic and asymptomatic patients with HH. Recent series have revealed that many asymptomatic patients who are C282Y homozygotes are now coming to medical attention because they are identified by family screening studies or population surveys or after abnormalities of iron studies are discovered on routine blood chemistry testing. It is ideal to identify patients who have some phenotypic expression with abnormal results of iron studies but no evidence of organ damage. Several large population screening studies have shown evidence of phenotypic expression with abnormal findings of iron studies in about 40 to 50% of C282Y homozygotes, but less than 10% of these individuals actually have signs and symptoms of the disease.

DIAGNOSIS

Because patients with genetic abnormalities can be identified before there is evidence of phenotypic expression, the method of diagnosing HH has undergone a change. The role of liver biopsy has lessened considerably with the advent of genetic testing. Nonetheless, some general principles should be acknowledged. If the diagnosis of HH is being considered, blood tests, including transferrin saturation (serum iron ÷ transferrin or total iron-binding capacity × 100%) and ferritin levels, should be obtained. Transferrin saturation does not need to be measured in the fasting state for reliable results to be obtained. In patients with symptoms (see Table 212-2), both these values are elevated; however, transferrin saturation is typically the earliest phenotypic marker of HH and may be elevated in young C282Y homozygotes with normal ferritin levels. Serum ferritin is sometimes elevated in other conditions in which there is no evidence of iron overload.[7] Confounding causes of high serum ferritin include alcohol consumption, metabolic syndrome, liver damage (acute or chronic), and more unusual disorders, such as Gaucher's disease and macrophage activation syndrome (hemophagocytic lymphohistiocytosis). Overall, about 90% of patients with hyperferritinemia do not have iron overload, which often remains unexplained. Thus, ferritin is relatively sensitive but not specific for iron overload.[8]

Magnetic resonance imaging is a fast and efficient noninvasive technique to assess and to monitor liver iron concentration. It is based on the accumulation of iron leading to signal loss in the liver, particularly with T2*-weighted sequences. Magnetic resonance sequences do lose accuracy, however, when the hepatic iron concentration is very high.

In the past, if an elevated transferrin saturation or ferritin level was identified, a liver biopsy would be performed to establish a diagnosis by histochemical iron stains and biochemical determination of the hepatic iron concentration with calculation of the hepatic iron index (HII). The HII is the patient's hepatic iron concentration (in µmol/g dry weight) divided by the patient's age in years. Previously, when the HII was higher than 1.9, the diagnosis of HH was established. Recent studies with genetic testing have shown that many (>50%) HH patients may have an HII of less than 1.9. Thus, the HII is no longer important in the diagnosis of HH.

Currently, when abnormalities of iron studies are identified, it is reasonable to proceed to genetic testing. Among individuals who are C282Y homozygotes or compound heterozygotes (C282Y/H63D), liver biopsy is reserved for those with elevated liver enzymes or ferritin levels above 1000 ng/mL (Fig. 212-2). Several studies have shown that advanced fibrosis or cirrhosis is not seen in HH patients when ferritin levels are below 1000 ng/mL or when liver enzymes are normal. Accordingly, as genetic testing has become more widely available, liver biopsy is less necessary.

When liver biopsy is performed, iron deposition is found preferentially in a periportal (acinar zone 1) region of the hepatic lobule, with a decrease in gradient in acinar zones 2 and 3. With significant iron loading, sinusoidal lining cell (Kupffer cell) iron deposition can be identified, and iron can be found in bile duct cells and in fibrous tissue in portal tracts or septa. In patients with secondary iron overload related to alcoholic liver disease or chronic viral hepatitis, iron deposition is typically in Kupffer cells as well as in hepatocytes, and it occurs in a panlobular (as opposed to a periportal) distribution. Histologic evaluation of iron-staining patterns provides information complementary to that obtained by traditional biochemical testing for iron overload along with genetic testing.

TREATMENT   Rx

Even though there have been advances in the molecular and cellular biologic understanding of HH, and although the impact of *HFE* mutation analysis on diagnosis has been significant, the treatment of HH remains simple, inexpensive, and safe. Patients should have therapeutic phlebotomy of 500 mL of whole blood (approximately 200 to 250 mg of iron, depending on the hemoglobin concentration) on a weekly basis, if tolerated. Therapeutic phlebotomy should be performed until iron-limited erythropoiesis develops, identified by failure of the hemoglobin level and hematocrit to recover before the next phlebotomy.[9] It is reasonable to monitor transferrin saturation and ferritin levels periodically (every 3 months) to predict the return of iron stores to normal and to provide encouragement to patients who are undergoing phlebotomy. Therapeutic phlebotomy should be continued until the ferritin level is into the normal range of 50 to 100 ng/mL. Transferrin saturation may still be elevated (> 50%) but should not dictate further phlebotomy.[10] It is not necessary for patients to become anemic or iron deficient—just depleted of excess iron stores. Some patients may require weekly phlebotomy for 1 year or longer. Others may be able to tolerate phlebotomy of only a half-unit of blood (250 mL) every other week. Once the initial *therapeutic* phlebotomy has been completed, most patients require *maintenance* phlebotomy, with 1 unit of blood removed every 2 to 3 months. This requirement is derived empirically, with the intent being to maintain a ferritin level between 50 and 100 ng/mL. Recognizing that HH subjects could constitute a safe source of blood for transfusion, the U.S. Food and Drug Administration now allows blood phlebotomized from HH donors to be used for transfusion as long as the phlebotomies are performed in authorized blood centers that comply with specific provisions for safeguard.[11]

With successful iron depletion, patients have an improved sense of well-being, right upper quadrant abdominal pain dissipates, liver test results improve, and diabetes may be easier to manage. Established cirrhosis, arthropathy, and testicular atrophy generally do not improve (Table 212-5).

Iron chelation therapy may be necessary for patients who are anemic and cannot tolerate phlebotomy. Parenteral infusions (administered either subcutaneously by an infusion pump or intravenously overnight through a port) of deferoxamine can be used. Ototoxicity and ocular toxicity are possible with deferoxamine, and appropriate monitoring should be performed. An orally administered iron chelator, deferasirox (Exjade), has been approved and is available for treatment of iron overload in patients with iron-loading anemias and HH.[12] This therapy is expensive and has potential for toxicity, but it is more convenient than phlebotomy. Minihepcidins that mimic hepcidin activity are being tested in laboratory animals as a possible future treatment of iron overload.[13]

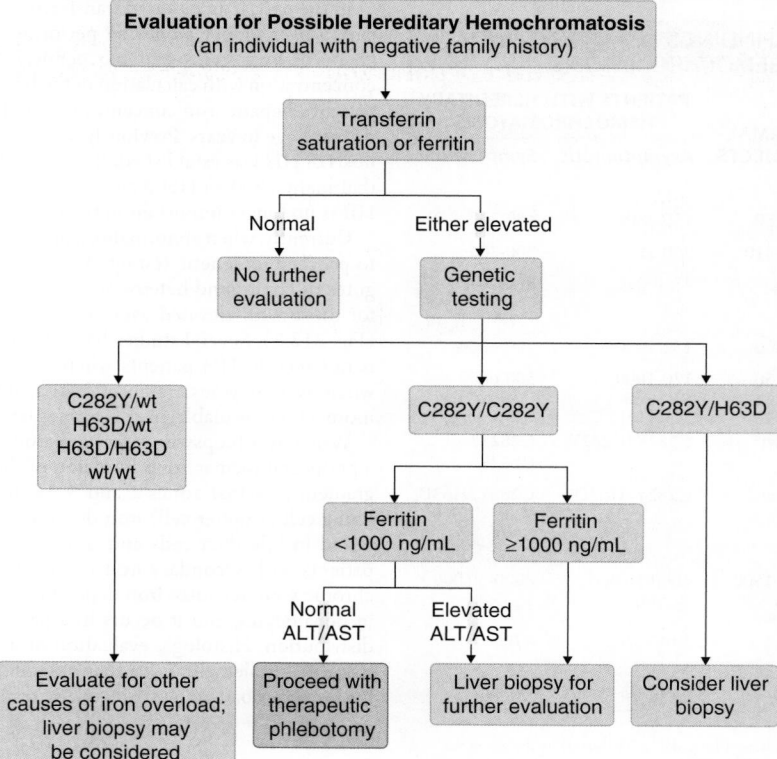

FIGURE 212-2. Algorithm for evaluation of possible hereditary hemochromatosis in a person with a negative family history. ALT = alanine transaminase; AST = aspartate transaminase.

TABLE 212-5 RESPONSE TO PHLEBOTOMY TREATMENT IN PATIENTS WITH HEREDITARY HEMOCHROMATOSIS

Reduction of tissue iron stores to normal
Improvement in survival if diagnosis is made and treatment is instituted before the development of cirrhosis and diabetes
Improvement in sense of well-being and energy level
Improvement in cardiac function
Improvement in controlling diabetes
Reduction in abdominal pain
Reduction in skin pigmentation
Normalization of elevated liver enzymes
Reversal of hepatic fibrosis
No reversal of established cirrhosis
Eliminates the risk of HH-related HCC if iron removal happens before the development of cirrhosis
Reduction in portal hypertension in patients with cirrhosis
No improvement in arthropathy
No reversal of testicular atrophy

HCC = hepatocellular cancer; HH = hereditary hemochromatosis.

PREVENTION

Family Screening

Once an HH proband is recognized, all first-degree relatives should be offered testing. In the past, HLA haplotyping was performed, but now *HFE* mutation analysis is recommended, along with the determination of transferrin saturation and ferritin levels. In probands with children, *HFE* mutation analysis is performed in the spouse to accurately predict the genotype in the child. If the spouse has either mutation, testing of the child is necessary, although the value and availability of genetic testing in children are debated. If an adult relative of a C282Y homozygote is identified and is either a C282Y homozygote or a compound heterozygote, and if results of blood iron studies are abnormal, a presumptive diagnosis can be made, and therapeutic phlebotomy can be initiated with the guidelines already discussed.

Population Screening

Because HH is a common disorder with a well-described treatment and a long latent period (i.e., time before disease occurs), some have suggested that it is an ideal candidate for population screening by genetic testing. However, studies have shown a less than expected phenotypic expression and a decreased number of patients with clinical manifestations of iron-mediated disease, raising questions about this recommendation. Initial results from a large National Institutes of Health–sponsored screening study in North America demonstrated a prevalence of C282Y homozygosity of 1 in 227 (Table 212-6). The C282Y homozygotes had higher ferritin levels than the general population, but 25% had normal ferritin levels. In screening for iron overload as opposed to screening for *HFE*-linked HH, transferrin saturation should be measured. In this situation, when abnormalities of iron studies are identified and the patient does not have a mutation in *HFE*, liver biopsy should be considered to clarify the situation relative to iron stores.

PROGNOSIS

If patients are identified, diagnosed, and treated[14] before the development of cirrhosis, their life expectancy is the same as that for an age- and sex-matched control population. If patients are not identified and treated before the development of cirrhosis, they are at risk for premature death from complications of diabetes, chronic liver disease, or hepatocellular cancer.[15] Treated cirrhotic patients are still at risk for hepatocellular cancer and should undergo surveillance abdominal imaging every 6 to 12 months.

Mutation Analysis in Patients with Liver Disease

Many patients with liver disease have abnormalities in serum parameters of iron metabolism. These abnormalities are more commonly seen in patients with hepatocellular liver diseases than in those with cholestatic liver diseases. Several clinical studies have shown that approximately 50% of patients with alcoholic liver disease, chronic viral hepatitis C, and nonalcoholic steatohepatitis (NASH) have abnormalities of serum iron studies. This abnormality is usually an elevation in serum ferritin, but elevated transferrin saturation is occasionally seen as well. When liver biopsy is performed, increased iron deposits can be seen, usually in a panlobular distribution, with iron in both hepatocytes and sinusoidal lining cells (Kupffer cells).

TABLE 212-6 PREVALENCE OF C282Y HOMOZYGOTES WITHOUT IRON OVERLOAD IN SCREENING STUDIES

POPULATION SAMPLE	COUNTRY	n	PREVALENCE OF HOMOZYGOTES	C282Y HOMOZYGOTES WITH A NORMAL FERRITIN LEVEL (%)
Electoral roll	New Zealand	1064	1 in 213	40
Primary care	United States	1653	1 in 276	50
Epidemiologic survey	Australia	3011	1 in 188	25
Blood donors	Canada	4211	1 in 327	81
General public	United States	41,038	1 in 270	33
Primary care	North America	44,082	1 in 227	25
General public	Australia	29,676	1 in 146	32
Total		124,636	1 in 240	41

Hepatic iron concentrations may be slightly increased or normal. When *HFE* mutations have been evaluated in patients with alcoholic liver disease, there has been no increased incidence of either C282Y or H63D (either heterozygote or homozygote) compared with control populations. Furthermore, there was no increase in *HFE* mutations in patients with alcoholic liver disease who had an increased amount of fibrosis. Thus, the abnormal iron studies frequently seen in patients with alcoholic liver disease are most likely due to mechanisms other than mutations in *HFE*.

In chronic hepatitis C, the relationship of abnormalities of iron studies and elevated hepatic iron concentration with a response to interferon monotherapy has been known for several years. Numerous studies have shown that patients who fail to respond to interferon monotherapy have a higher hepatic iron concentration than those who do respond. A corollary to this observation involves therapeutic phlebotomy to deplete iron stores in the hope of improving response to therapy. Reduction in iron stores by therapeutic phlebotomy does reduce elevated liver enzymes and has had some marginal beneficial effect on liver histologic features, but it does not have any virologic effects. When *HFE* mutation analysis has been investigated in patients with chronic hepatitis C, the frequency of C282Y and H63D has been equivalent to that in control populations. Most studies have shown that when *HFE* mutations are present, they correlate with increased iron stores seen histologically. Some studies have shown a synergistic effect with the development of fibrosis. At present, it is recommended that *HFE* mutation analysis be done when abnormalities of iron studies are seen in patients with chronic hepatitis C. Also, iron stains are typically performed on liver biopsy samples when biopsies are done to grade and to stage chronic hepatitis C. If iron stores are increased, it is reasonable to perform therapeutic phlebotomy to deplete excess iron stores before antiviral therapy is initiated.

In patients with NASH, several studies have provided conflicting results.[16] Some have shown an increase in *HFE* mutations in patients with NASH, and others have shown no difference from control populations. When there has been an increased prevalence of *HFE* mutations in NASH, there has been good correlation between abnormal serum parameters of iron and a correlation with hepatic iron concentration. Furthermore, some studies have shown an increase in fibrosis in NASH patients with *HFE* mutations. Finally, one study showed a reduction in elevated liver enzymes and improvement in parameters of insulin resistance in patients with NASH treated by phlebotomy to produce near iron deficiency. These observations suggest an interaction between the expression of fatty liver disease and iron metabolism.

Finally, in porphyria cutanea tarda (PCT), the relationship between abnormalities of iron metabolism and the role of therapeutic phlebotomy has been known for many years.[17] Also, it has recently been shown that as many as 70% of patients with PCT are infected with hepatitis C virus, and many patients with PCT drink excessive amounts of alcohol. An increased prevalence of *HFE* mutations has been shown in both European and American studies of PCT patients, and the use of phlebotomy to deplete excess iron stores is still recommended. Thus, *HFE* mutation analysis is of value in patients with PCT and may be of value in patients with chronic hepatitis C and NASH. It is probably not of value in patients with alcoholic liver disease.

GENERAL REFERENCES

For the General References and other additional features, please visit Expert Consult at https://expertconsult.inkling.com.

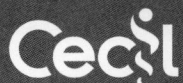

XVII

NUTRITIONAL DISEASES

213

NUTRITION'S INTERFACE WITH HEALTH AND DISEASE

DOUGLAS C. HEIMBURGER

⬤ OLD AND NEW PARADIGMS IN THE SCIENCE OF NUTRITION

Nutrition science was characterized by two major phases in the 20th century. During the first phase, nutrition scientists discovered, characterized, and synthesized the essential nutrients and described their deficiency syndromes in detail. The dietary requirements for these nutrients were estimated and periodically updated as recommended dietary allowances (RDAs). Beginning in 1997, the RDAs were reformulated in a series of volumes containing dietary reference intakes (DRIs); in addition to the recommended intakes judged to be sufficient to meet the nutrient requirements of nearly all healthy individuals, the DRIs include estimates of tolerable upper intake levels—that is, the highest intake levels likely not to pose any adverse health risks.

More fundamentally, the DRIs focus on accumulating evidence related to the relationships of diet and nutritional status to the diseases that plague Western societies, such as coronary heart disease (CHD), cancer, diabetes, and the other leading causes of death. DRIs recommend intake levels that not only prevent deficiencies but also may promote long-term health and disease prevention.

⬤ NUTRITION'S INFLUENCE ON MORTALITY AND MORBIDITY

Evidence of a Connection between Diet and Disease

It has been estimated that between 300,000 and 800,000 deaths per year could be prevented in the United States if Americans followed evidence-based dietary recommendations. Substantial additional benefits from reduced morbidity and enhanced functional status would also accrue. However, the causal connections between diet and chronic diseases are difficult to tease out of the complex network of other risk factors, including social and behavioral variables, so a wide variety of studies must be relied on to establish these connections with reasonable certainty.

Epidemiologic studies are unable to infer causal relationships and may be confounded by variables that have not been examined. They are also challenged by the difficulty of accurately assessing the diets of free-living individuals.

Animal and in vitro studies can overcome some of these drawbacks but may be confounded by experimental conditions that differ from those encountered by humans. A large number of prospective, randomized human intervention trials have been undertaken to test the effects of dietary change on risk for disease. However, even these trials are not always conclusive because of pitfalls associated with selecting study populations and isolating individual dietary factors.

Taken together, epidemiologic, animal, in vitro, and intervention studies are proving that human dietary habits contribute importantly to the pathogenesis of most of the major causes of death in developed countries.[1] In the recently published Global Burden of Disease Study 2010, 15 dietary risk factors and physical inactivity collectively accounted for 10% of global deaths and disability-adjusted life years.[2]

Diseases Influenced by Nutrition

Table 213-1 lists 8 of the top 15 causes of death in the United States that are influenced by nutrition. Five are strongly linked to dietary habits, and three are associated with alcohol abuse. The table also outlines dietary contributions to obesity, atherosclerosis, osteoporosis, diverticular disease, and neural tube defects. A meta-analysis indicates that vitamin D_3 supplementation reduces mortality in adults.[A1] Table 213-2 summarizes the 2010 Dietary Guidelines for Americans, and Table 213-3 compares dietary recommendations promulgated by professional societies for risk reduction and/or management of the major chronic diseases. The close agreement among these recommendations enhances their credibility.

Coronary Heart Disease

Nutritional influences on the leading cause of death in the United States, CHD, have been the subject of a great deal of research. The overall U.S. mortality rate from CHD peaked in the 1960s and, in a trend that initially surprised medical science, has declined steadily since then. Changes in lifestyle, including diet, are responsible for a substantial proportion of this decline. Elevated plasma low-density lipoprotein (LDL) cholesterol levels are a major risk factor for CHD and peripheral atherosclerosis, and they correlate strongly with dietary saturated fat intake and less strongly with cholesterol intake. Intake of both these substances in the United States is derived largely from foods of animal origin, such as meats, dairy products, and eggs. Attempts to produce less atherogenic substitutes for some of these foods have not always proved beneficial. For instance, hydrogenation of vegetable oils to create margarine and shortening results in the formation of *trans*-fatty acids, which affect serum cholesterol levels in a manner similar to—and are perhaps even worse than—the saturated fatty acids found in butter and lard. LDL cholesterol levels can be lowered modestly by increasing the intake of soluble fiber from legumes, fruits, vegetables, and flax seed, as well as by consuming proteins and isoflavones from soy foods. LDL must be oxidized before it induces injury to the arterial wall. Although adequate dietary levels of the antioxidant vitamins C and E and β-carotene have been shown to inhibit LDL oxidation, pharmacologic doses of these vitamins have not reduced CHD events when tested in randomized trials.[A2] In fact, pharmacologic doses of vitamin E (>400 IU/day) and other antioxidants have no benefit and may increase all-cause mortality.

Epidemiologic evidence suggests that fish consumption may reduce CHD risk, perhaps through the action of omega-3 fatty acids, but randomized trials have found no benefit from omega-3 supplementation.[A3] Evidence also indicates that moderate consumption of alcohol, especially wine, is associated with a decreased risk for CHD, possibly by increasing high-density lipoprotein (HDL) cholesterol levels, preventing the oxidation of LDL, or both. The polyphenols in red wine are also apparently beneficial. Traditional Mediterranean lifestyle patterns—with diets high in vegetables, fruits, olive oil, fish, nuts, complex grains and carbohydrates, and red wine, along with physical activity—are associated with reduced risks for cardiovascular disease.[A4,3] A conservative estimate suggests that moderate dietary modification by the U.S. population, consisting mainly of replacing saturated fats with complex carbohydrates, fiber, monounsaturated fats, and fish, could easily lead to a 10% reduction in serum cholesterol levels and a 20% or greater reduction in CHD.[4] The actual risk reduction could be much greater.

Cancer

Nutrients, non-nutritive dietary constituents, and nutritional status can influence the risk for cancer in a variety of ways. Nutrition interacts with each step of carcinogenesis (carcinogen activation and tumor initiation, promotion, and progression). Excess energy intake may favor the generation of free radicals and reduce the body's ability to detoxify carcinogens. By contrast, antioxidant nutrients scavenge free radicals and other (pre)carcinogens and may thereby inhibit their activation, their ability to initiate mutations, or both. Folic acid may improve a cell's ability to preserve, repair, and methylate its DNA, either preventing or reversing the tendency toward mutation. Folic acid supplementation, however, may increase the cancer risk in some individuals, so supplementation beyond the levels present in multivitamins is not advised.[A5] Obesity has emerged as a major risk factor for many cancers, perhaps by inducing insulin resistance and elevating serum levels of insulin, insulin-like growth factor, and related tumor-promoting hormones. Excessive alcohol intake also promotes tumor growth.

Lung Cancer

Evidence indicates that the number-one cancer killer, lung cancer (Chapter 191), is influenced by diet. Although the most important causal factor is cigarette smoking, consumption of fruits and vegetables is inversely associated with lung cancer risk in both smokers and nonsmokers. It is probable that both nutrients and the non-nutritive phytochemicals in fruits and vegetables are responsible for the protective effects. However, in view of the disappointing results of randomized trials of supplementation with β-carotene, which increased mortality from lung cancer and other causes, antioxidant supplements should not be used to reduce disease risk, especially in tobacco smokers.

Breast Cancer

The number-two cause of cancer deaths in women, breast cancer (Chapter 198), is positively associated with obesity, especially when excess adiposity is located predominantly in the abdomen, and with physical inactivity. The

TABLE 213-1 DIETARY INFLUENCES ON MAJOR CAUSES OF DEATH AND MORBIDITY IN THE UNITED STATES

CAUSE OF DEATH OR MORBIDITY	FACTORS ASSOCIATED WITH DECREASED RISK	FACTORS ASSOCIATED WITH INCREASED RISK
DEATH		
Heart disease	Intake of complex carbohydrates, particular fatty acids (e.g., monounsaturated, polyunsaturated, and omega-3 fatty acids from fish), soluble fiber, polyphenols, soy proteins, antioxidants (vitamins E and C, β-carotene, selenium), folic acid, moderate alcohol	Intake of saturated fat, cholesterol, excess calories, sodium; abdominal distribution of body fat
Cancer	Intake of fruits and vegetables (for β-carotene; vitamins A, C, D, and E; folic acid; calcium; selenium; phytochemicals), fiber	Intake of excess calories, fat, alcohol, red meat, salt- and nitrite-preserved meats, possibly grilled meats; abdominal distribution of body fat
Cerebrovascular disease	Intake of potassium, calcium, omega-3 fatty acids	Intake of sodium, alcohol (as with hypertension)
Accidents		Excess alcohol consumption
Diabetes mellitus	Intake of fiber	Intake of excess calories, fat, alcohol; abdominal distribution of body fat
Suicide		Excess alcohol consumption
Chronic liver disease and cirrhosis		Excess alcohol consumption
Hypertension and hypertensive renal disease	Intake of fruits and vegetables, potassium, calcium, magnesium, omega-3 fatty acids	Intake of sodium, alcohol, excess calories, total and saturated fat; abdominal distribution of body fat
MORBIDITY		
Obesity		Intake of excess calories and fat
Osteoporosis	Intake of calcium, vitamin D, vitamin K	Intake of excess vitamin A, sodium, protein
Diverticular disease, constipation	Intake of fiber	
Neural tube defects	Intake of folic acid	

TABLE 213-2 DIETARY GUIDELINES FOR AMERICANS, 2010: KEY RECOMMENDATIONS

BALANCING CALORIES TO MANAGE WEIGHT

Prevent and/or reduce overweight and obesity through improved eating and physical activity behaviors.
Control total calorie intake to manage body weight. For people who are overweight or obese, this will mean consuming fewer calories from foods and beverages.
Increase physical activity and reduce time spent in sedentary behaviors.
Maintain appropriate calorie balance during each stage of life—childhood, adolescence, adulthood, pregnancy and breast-feeding, and older age.

FOODS AND FOOD COMPONENTS TO REDUCE

Reduce daily sodium intake to less than 2300 milligrams (mg) and further reduce intake to 1500 mg among persons who are 51 years and older and those of any age who are African American or have hypertension, diabetes, or chronic kidney disease. The 1500-mg recommendation applies to about half of the U.S. population, including children and most adults.
Consume less than 10% of calories from saturated fatty acids by replacing them with monounsaturated and polyunsaturated fatty acids.
Consume less than 300 mg per day of dietary cholesterol.
Keep *trans*-fatty acid consumption as low as possible by limiting foods that contain synthetic sources of *trans* fats, such as partially hydrogenated oils, and by limiting other solid fats.
Reduce the intake of calories from solid fats and added sugars.
Limit the consumption of foods that contain refined grains, especially refined grain foods that contain solid fats, added sugars, and sodium.
If alcohol is consumed, it should be consumed in moderation—up to one drink per day for women and two drinks per day for men—and only by adults of legal drinking age.
Individuals should meet the following recommendations as part of a healthy eating pattern while staying within their calorie needs:
　Increase vegetable and fruit intake.
　Eat a variety of vegetables, especially dark-green and red and orange vegetables and beans and peas.
　Consume at least half of all grains as whole grains. Increase whole-grain intake by replacing refined grains with whole grains.
　Increase intake of fat-free or low-fat milk and milk products, such as milk, yogurt, cheese, or fortified soy beverages.
　Choose a variety of protein foods, which include seafood, lean meat and poultry, eggs, beans and peas, soy products, and unsalted nuts and seeds.
　Increase the amount and variety of seafood consumed by choosing seafood in place of some meat and poultry.
　Replace protein foods that are higher in solid fats with choices that are lower in solid fats and calories and/or are sources of oils.
　Use oils to replace solid fats where possible.
　Choose foods that provide more potassium, dietary fiber, calcium, and vitamin D, which are nutrients of concern in American diets. These foods include vegetables, fruits, whole grains, and milk and milk products.

BUILDING HEALTHY EATING PATTERNS

Select an eating pattern that meets nutrient needs over time at an appropriate calorie level.
Account for all foods and beverages consumed and assess how they fit within a total healthy eating pattern.
Follow food safety recommendations when preparing and eating foods to reduce the risk for food-borne illnesses.

RECOMMENDATIONS FOR SPECIFIC POPULATION GROUPS

Women Capable of Becoming Pregnant

Choose foods that supply heme iron, which is more readily absorbed by the body, additional iron sources, and enhancers of iron absorption such as vitamin C–rich foods.
Consume 400 μg per day of synthetic folic acid (from fortified foods and/or supplements) in addition to food forms of folate from a varied diet.

Women Who Are Pregnant or Breast-Feeding

Consume 8 to 12 ounces of seafood per week from a variety of seafood types.
Because of their high methyl mercury content, limit white (albacore) tuna to 6 ounces per week and do not eat the following four types of fish: tilefish, shark, swordfish, and king mackerel.
If pregnant, take an iron supplement, as recommended by an obstetrician or other health care provider.

Individuals Aged 50 Years and Older

Consume foods fortified with vitamin B_{12}, such as fortified cereals, or dietary supplements.

TABLE 213-3 DIETARY GUIDELINES PROMULGATED BY NATIONAL ORGANIZATIONS*

Indication or Objective	U.S. DEPARTMENT OF AGRICULTURE AND DEPARTMENT OF HEALTH AND HUMAN SERVICES: DIETARY GUIDELINES FOR AMERICANS (2010) *General Health Promotion and Disease Prevention*	NATIONAL CHOLESTEROL EDUCATION PROGRAM ADULT TREATMENT PANEL III: THERAPEUTIC LIFESTYLE CHANGE DIET (2002) *Elevated Cholesterol, Heart Disease Prevention*	NATIONAL HIGH BLOOD PRESSURE EDUCATION PROGRAM/JOINT NATIONAL COMMITTEE: 7 DIETARY APPROACHES TO STOP HYPERTENSION (DASH; 2006) *Prehypertension and Hypertension*	AMERICAN DIABETES ASSOCIATION (2004 AND 2012) *Diabetes Prevention and Treatment*	AMERICAN CANCER SOCIETY (2012) *Cancer prevention*
NUTRIENT/FOOD GROUP					
Total energy	Prevent and/or reduce overweight and obesity through improved eating and physical activity behaviors	Manage weight, increase physical activity	Reduce energy intake to lose weight if overweight	Reduced energy intake and modest weight loss can improve glycemia and insulin resistance and reduce risk for type 2 diabetes	Achieve and maintain a healthy weight throughout life. Choose foods and beverages in amounts that help achieve and maintain a healthy weight
Fruits and vegetables	Increase vegetable and fruit intake. Eat a variety of vegetables, especially dark-green and red and orange vegetables and beans and peas		8-10 servings/day		Consume a healthy diet, with an emphasis on plant foods. Eat at least 2.5 cups of vegetables and fruits each day
Meat	Choose a variety of protein foods, which include seafood, lean meat, and poultry (for more, see Protein). Choose seafood in place of some meat and poultry		≤6 servings/day		Limit consumption of processed and red meats
Dairy	Increase intake of fat-free or low-fat milk and milk products, such as milk, yogurt, cheese, or fortified soy beverages		2-3 servings/day of low-fat dairy		
Grains, fiber	Consume at least half of all grains as whole grains. Replace refined grains with whole grains	Consider increased viscous (soluble) fiber (10-25 g/day) and plant stanols/sterols (2 g/day) to enhance LDL lowering	6-8 servings of whole grains and whole-grain products	Achieve U.S. Dietary Guidelines recommendation	Choose whole grains instead of refined grain products
Fat	Replace protein foods that are higher in solid fats with choices that are lower in solid fats and calories and/or are sources of oils. Use oils to replace solid fats where possible	25-35% of daily energy intake	<27% of daily energy intake		The totality of the evidence does not support a relationship between total fat intake and cancer risk
Saturated fats	<10% of daily calories, by replacing them with MUFA and PUFA	<7% of daily energy intake	6% of daily energy intake	<7% of daily energy intake	
Polyunsaturated fats	Replace solid fats with PUFA	Up to 10% of daily energy intake		Up to 10% of daily energy intake	
Monounsaturated fats	Replace solid fats with MUFA	Up to 20% of daily energy intake		15-20% of daily energy intake; combination of MUFA and carbohydrates should equal 60-70% of total energy intake	
Trans-fats	Keep as low as possible	Intake should be kept low		Intake should be minimized	
Cholesterol	<300 mg/day	<200 mg/day	150 mg/day	<300 mg/day; those with LDL cholesterol ≥100 may benefit from lowering cholesterol intake to 200 mg/day	
Carbohydrates		50-60% of daily energy intake	55% of daily energy intake	Total amount of carbohydrate is more important than the source or type. Individualize the mix of carbohydrate, protein, and fat	
Sugar	Reduce added sugars			Sucrose and sucrose-containing foods do not need specific restriction by diabetic persons. Persons at risk for type 2 diabetes should limit sugar-sweetened beverages	

TABLE 213-3 DIETARY GUIDELINES PROMULGATED BY NATIONAL ORGANIZATIONS—cont'd

Indication or Objective	U.S. DEPARTMENT OF AGRICULTURE AND DEPARTMENT OF HEALTH AND HUMAN SERVICES: DIETARY GUIDELINES FOR AMERICANS (2010) *General Health Promotion and Disease Prevention*	NATIONAL CHOLESTEROL EDUCATION PROGRAM ADULT TREATMENT PANEL III: THERAPEUTIC LIFESTYLE CHANGE DIET (2002) *Elevated Cholesterol, Heart Disease Prevention*	NATIONAL HIGH BLOOD PRESSURE EDUCATION PROGRAM/JOINT NATIONAL COMMITTEE: 7 DIETARY APPROACHES TO STOP HYPERTENSION (DASH; 2006) *Prehypertension and Hypertension*	AMERICAN DIABETES ASSOCIATION (2004 AND 2012) *Diabetes Prevention and Treatment*	AMERICAN CANCER SOCIETY (2012) *Cancer prevention*
Protein	Choose a variety of protein foods, which include eggs, beans and peas, soy products, and unsalted nuts and seeds (for more, see Meat)	Approximately 15% of daily energy intake	18% of daily energy intake	10-20% of daily energy intake if renal function is normal	
Alcohol	Up to 2 drinks/day for men and up to 1 drink/day for women; persons in special circumstances (e.g., pregnancy, history of alcoholism) should abstain		<2 drinks/day for men and <1 drink/day for women	If individuals choose to drink, limit to 2 drinks/day for men and 1 drink/day for women, and take extra precautions to prevent hypoglycemia	Drink no more than 1 drink/day for women or 2 drinks/day for men
Sodium	Reduce daily sodium intake to less than 2300 mg, and further reduce intake to 1500 mg among persons who are 51 years and older or are members of special groups		<2400 mg/day	<2400 mg/day	
Potassium			4700 mg/day		
Calcium			1250 mg/day	1000-1500 mg/day	1000-1200 mg/day
Magnesium			500 mg/day		

*For further details, see the websites listed in this chapter.
LDL = low-density lipoprotein; MUFA = monounsaturated fatty acid; PUFA = polyunsaturated fatty acid.
Adapted from Heimburger DC, Ard JD, eds. *Handbook of Clinical Nutrition*, 4th ed. Philadelphia: Elsevier; 2006.

positive association between obesity and postmenopausal breast cancer has been attributed in part to the synthesis of estrogen (a risk factor for breast cancer) in adipose tissue. Epidemiologic evidence suggests that alcohol intake may also be a risk factor for this disease, particularly in women with lower intakes of folic acid.

Colorectal Cancer

Colorectal cancer (Chapter 193) is the third leading cause of cancer mortality in men and women. The risk for colorectal cancer correlates positively with the intake of red meat (especially when it is overcooked) and dietary fat and with obesity, and the risk correlates inversely with the intake of calcium and folic acid. Evidence regarding the effect of dietary fiber is somewhat equivocal, but the preponderance of evidence points to a protective effect; there is no evidence of harm. Higher physical activity is associated with a 30 to 50% lower risk for colon cancer.

Summary

The interaction of all these influences is powerful enough to suggest that diet and physical inactivity contribute to well over 35% of cancer deaths in Western countries. Even though no independent benefit has been found from dietary supplementation with potentially protective nutrients such as carotenoids, vitamins C and E,[A6][A7] folic acid, selenium,[A8] and fiber, they are all present in vegetables and fruits, and a liberal intake of fruits and vegetables is strongly recommended. A very large randomized trial indicated that lowering dietary fat intake did not reduce rates of breast cancer[A9] or colon cancer, but it is very likely that maintaining an appropriate body weight and being physically active can reduce cancer risks.

Hypertension

Elevated blood pressure (Chapter 67) is a major risk factor for stroke, CHD, heart failure, peripheral vascular disease, and renal disease. It is often associated with obesity, especially abdominal obesity, and weight reduction in obese hypertensive people generally leads to an improvement in blood pressure. Sodium restriction also usually reduces blood pressure levels. The Dietary Approaches to Stop Hypertension (DASH) diet, which is rich in fruits, vegetables, and low-fat dairy products and advocates a reduced satu-

rated and total fat content, can also decrease blood pressure levels; reducing one's sodium intake provides an additional benefit when included as part of the DASH diet.[5] Because alcohol intake elevates blood pressure, its use should be limited in hypertensive patients.

Diabetes Mellitus

Type 2 diabetes mellitus (Chapter 229) is strongly associated with obesity, especially abdominal obesity, so maintenance of a desirable body weight throughout life is of major importance in both preventing and treating type 2 diabetes. Sugar consumption does not lead to diabetes, except to the extent that it may promote weight gain. A focus on dietary carbohydrate restriction is no longer recommended for persons with type 2 diabetes; rather, a variety of dietary patterns, including low-carbohydrate, low-glycemic index, and Mediterranean diets, are effective in improving glycemic control and markers of cardiovascular disease risk.[A10] Because higher-fat diets tend to promote both obesity and CHD, for which diabetic patients are at high risk, dietary fat intake should be kept low. Alcohol can cause hypoglycemia, hyperglycemia, and increased triglyceride levels in diabetic patients, and its use should be limited. In both diabetic and nondiabetic people, excess alcohol intake is responsible for many deaths, particularly from accidents and liver disease, and it is a factor in some suicides.

Osteoporosis

Osteoporosis (Chapter 243) is influenced by several dietary factors. Inadequate calcium intake during adolescence can result in suboptimal peak bone mass in early adulthood, and during later life it can lead to accelerated bone loss, thereby increasing the risk for osteoporosis. Sodium and protein, which are consumed by Americans in greater quantities than required, may promote excess bone loss. Excessive supplementation with vitamin A reduces bone mass and increases fracture risk. Vitamin D, vitamin K, and magnesium assist in maintaining optimal bone mass.

Other Conditions
Obesity

The causes and health effects of obesity, the most prevalent nutritional disorder in the United States, are reviewed in Chapter 220. The metabolic

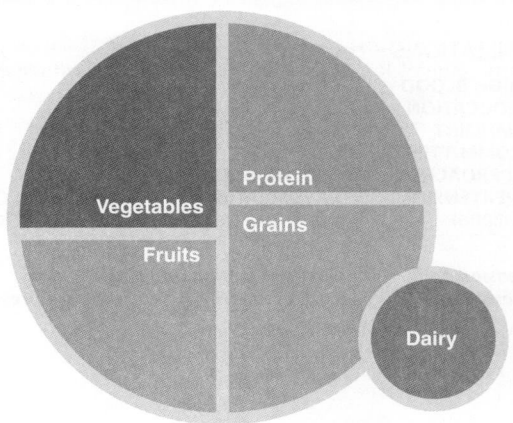

FIGURE 213-1. **U.S. Department of Agriculture's MyPlate. MyPlate illustrates that a substantial proportion of dietary intake should be derived from vegetables, fruits, and grains, as contrasted with many Americans' expectation that protein sources should dominate. For more information, see www.ChooseMyPlate.gov.**

syndrome, a constellation that includes obesity with an enlarged waist circumference; increased serum glucose, triglycerides, and blood pressure; and reduced HDL cholesterol, is strikingly prevalent in the United States and is a major risk factor for CHD, cancer, type 2 diabetes, and hypertension (Chapter 67).

Intestinal Diverticular Disease
Low dietary fiber intake causes constipation, and it is thought to be a cause of intestinal diverticular disease.

Congenital Neural Tube Defects
Inadequate maternal folic acid intake has been definitively proved to be a major risk factor for congenital neural tube defects such as spina bifida and myelomeningocele. For this reason, cereal and grain products have been fortified in the United States with folic acid since 1998.[6]

⬤ TRANSLATING EVIDENCE INTO DIETARY CHANGE

Thus, the evidence is strong that dietary habits can influence the incidence and severity of many incapacitating or lethal diseases in the United States. No justification exists for the belief that modification of the "usual" American diet is unnecessary or futile. The only questions are whether change is feasible and what is required to effect it. Various health agencies and the U.S. government have used public education, particularly the publication of dietary goals, as their primary means (see Table 213-3). The Department of Agriculture and the Department of Health and Human Services have developed and periodically revised the Dietary Guidelines for Americans (see Table 213-2) and a food guidance system, now called MyPlate (Fig. 213-1). MyPlate is part of a larger communications initiative based on the 2010 Dietary Guidelines for Americans to help consumers make better food choices. Although the practical application of nutritional genomics is not yet ready for routine clinical practice, it is an important, emerging science that may in the future be applied to nutrigenetic testing to provide dietary advice.[7]

Physicians can influence their patients' health by encouraging them to optimize their dietary habits and providing them with instructional materials and assistance from dietitians in making needed changes. A significant barrier to practical nutritional interventions could be removed if health insurers would reimburse dietitians' services.

ᴳʳᵃᵈᵉ Ⓐ Grade A References

A1. Bjelakovic G, Gluud LL, Nikolova D, et al. Vitamin D supplementation for prevention of mortality in adults. *Cochrane Database Syst Rev.* 2014;1:CD007470.

A2. Fortmann SP, Burda BU, Senger CA, et al. Vitamin and mineral supplements in the primary prevention of cardiovascular disease and cancer: An updated systematic evidence review for the U.S. Preventive Services Task Force. *Ann Intern Med.* 2013;159:824-834.

A3. Rees K, Hartley L, Flowers N, et al. "Mediterranean" dietary pattern for the primary prevention of cardiovascular disease. *Cochrane Database Syst Rev.* 2013;8:CD009825.

A4. Rizos EC, Ntzani EE, Bika E, et al. Association between omega-3 fatty acid supplementation and risk of major cardiovascular disease events: a systematic review and meta-analysis. *JAMA.* 2012;308:1024-1033.

A5. Ebbing M, Bønaa KH, Nygård O, et al. Cancer incidence and mortality after treatment with folic acid and vitamin B12. *JAMA.* 2009;302:2119-2126.

A6. Lin J, Cook NR, Albert C, et al. Vitamins C and E and beta carotene supplementation and cancer risk: a randomized controlled trial. *J Natl Cancer Inst.* 2009;101:14-23.

A7. Gaziano JM, Glynn RJ, Christen WG, et al. Vitamins E and C in the prevention of prostate and total cancer in men: the Physicians' Health Study II Randomized Controlled Trial. *JAMA.* 2009;301:52-62.

A8. Lippman SM, Klein EA, Goodman PJ, et al. Effect of selenium and vitamin E on risk of prostate cancer and other cancers: the Selenium and Vitamin E Cancer Prevention Trial (SELECT). *JAMA.* 2009;301:39-51.

A9. Thomson CA, Van Horn L, Caan BJ, et al. Cancer incidence and mortality during the intervention and postintervention periods of the Women's Health Initiative dietary modification trial. *Cancer Epidemiol Biomarkers Prev.* 2014;23:2924-2935.

A10. Ajala O, English P, Pinkney J. Systematic review and meta-analysis of different dietary approaches to the management of type 2 diabetes. *Am J Clin Nutr.* 2013;97:505-516.

GENERAL REFERENCES

For the General References and other additional features, please visit Expert Consult at https://expertconsult.inkling.com.

214

NUTRITIONAL ASSESSMENT
BRUCE R. BISTRIAN

⬤ GOALS AND IMPORTANCE OF NUTRITIONAL ASSESSMENT

Nutritional assessment in clinical medicine has three primary goals: to identify the presence and type of malnutrition, to define health-threatening obesity, and to devise suitable diets as prophylaxis against disease later in life. The focus of this chapter is on the diagnosis of protein-energy malnutrition because of its wide prevalence and major impact on disease outcome.[1,2] Other deficiency diseases are of much less relevance in that most occur in conjunction with protein-energy malnutrition or in specific disease states, such as thiamine deficiency in alcoholic liver disease and fat-soluble vitamin deficiency in malabsorptive states. The classic deficiency diseases, whether primary or secondary, are considered elsewhere in those chapters specifically dealing with the diseases mentioned here. The widespread availability of parenteral and enteral therapeutic measures since the mid-1980s that can provide adequate feeding regimens for virtually any disease condition makes a rudimentary knowledge of the pathophysiology of protein-energy malnutrition and its nutritional assessment essential for all primary care practitioners (Chapter 213).

⬤ CLINICAL NUTRITIONAL ASSESSMENT

Clinical assessment of protein nutritional status is based principally on the clinical history, physical examination including simple anthropometry, and measurement of the levels of several secretory proteins.

Clinical History

Although detailed dietary assessment can at times be helpful, in most circumstances physicians can safely limit their diet questions to whether patients have been following a prescribed diet, how much alcohol they drink, and whether they habitually take dietary supplements, including vitamins, minerals, and herbs. In ambulatory patients, the ability to maintain usual and adequate weight generally indicates that serious micronutrient deficiency is probably not the result of dietary inadequacy. Isolated vitamin deficiencies in the absence of weight loss or symptoms are rare, except perhaps for folate and vitamin B_{12} (Chapter 164). Although nutritional anemias do exist, as a consequence of strict vegetarian or vegan diets for vitamin B_{12}, or uncommonly today for folate except with extreme diets (as a result of widespread fortification of folate in food in developed countries), the role of dietary deficiency in anemias is limited in the absence of underlying disease, altered physiology (e.g., achlorhydria with aging), or weight loss. Only iron deficiency is a common cause of dietary anemia (Chapter 159). By contrast, full dietary assessment and diet prescriptions are likely to help patients with conditions such as fat malabsorption accompanied by weight loss, cramps, or diarrhea. Such evaluations are most effectively carried out by dietitians. Thus, detailed nutritional assessment of protein-energy malnutrition with secondary assessment of vitamin and mineral deficiencies is usually needed only when protein-energy malnutrition or a specific disorder known to interfere with nutrient metabolism coexists, such as celiac disease, pernicious anemia, or nutrient-drug interactions. Even then, the assessment should emphasize the likely deficiencies. For fat malabsorption (Chapter 140), one should check levels of the fat-soluble vitamins A, D, E, and K; important divalent and trivalent cations (calcium [Ca^{2+}], zinc [Zn^{2+}], magnesium [Mg^{2+}], and iron [Fe^{3+}]); and phosphorus and alkaline phosphatase. When ileal resection has occurred, serum vitamin B_{12} levels should be measured, and the potential for bile salt depletion should be considered. Weight loss resulting from short-gut syndrome should prompt assessment of the fat-soluble vitamins, folic acid, vitamin B_{12}, calcium, magnesium, phosphorus, zinc, and iron. At least initially, levels of the water-soluble vitamins likely to have clinical impact such as thiamine and ascorbic acid should be checked, but provision of the full complement of vitamins should be routine in the management of this condition. Measurements of body water status (weight, blood urea nitrogen, serum creatinine, serum sodium) and acid-base balance (serum carbon dioxide combining power, chloride and potassium, and urine and arterial pH) should be obtained if the diarrhea is profuse (Chapter 140).

Protein-energy malnutrition, as defined by significant weight loss of more than 5% or hypoalbuminemia, affects at least 25% of patients hospitalized for acute care and are secondary to the underlying disease in most instances. Many of these patients can benefit from nutritional support and require a thorough clinical nutritional assessment, including a dietary history, physical examination, and laboratory tests that serve to confirm clinical impressions. The history should list information about the timing and amount of weight loss, medical illnesses, medications, gastrointestinal symptoms (abdominal pain, diarrhea, dysphagia), diet habits (eating fewer than two meals per day, alcohol consumption, dietary supplement intake, dental status), social habits (eating alone, needing assistance in self-care), economic status (having enough money for food), and mental status, particularly the presence of depressive symptoms. A special focus should be reserved for elderly people, in whom protein-energy malnutrition secondary to these last factors is more common (Chapter 24).

Nutritional Support

Four factors principally determine the timing, need, and appropriateness of nutritional support: (1) the presence and severity of protein-energy malnutrition, defined primarily by degree of weight loss and weight-to-height ratio as a percentage of standard or body mass index (BMI); (2) the presence and severity of the systemic inflammatory response, defined principally by the serum albumin level but also by the presence of fever, leukocytosis, and increased band forms; (3) the actual or expected duration of inadequate nutritional intake; and (4) the prognosis of the underlying condition. Well-nourished individuals have a 7- to 10-day reserve of energy and protein to withstand a moderate systemic inflammatory response without adverse nutritional consequences. Greater degrees of systemic inflammatory response and preexisting protein-energy malnutrition dramatically shorten the period that semistarvation, defined as consuming less than 50% of the energy and protein needs, can be tolerated. An important corollary is that when energy intake is limited, protein requirements for optimal outcomes are increased such that a reduction in energy intake to 50% of needs nearly doubles the desirable intake for protein.

Weight Loss

A recent unintended weight loss of 10 lb, or more than 5% of usual weight, should prompt efforts to diagnose the underlying disorder or social circumstance. Weight loss alone does not distinguish the composition of tissue loss, which can range from 25 to 30% lean tissue in semistarvation alone to 50% lean tissue loss following semistarvation plus injury and as much as 75% of the weight loss with the severest forms of injury, severe sepsis, major body burns, severe closed head injury, and multiple trauma. Therefore, unintentional weight loss of more than 10 lb or more than 5% of usual weight indicates a need for thorough nutritional assessment. Weight loss in excess of 10% of usual weight should be considered to represent protein-energy malnutrition that will impair physiologic function, particularly muscle strength and endurance. Weight loss in excess of 20% should be considered severe protein-energy malnutrition that will substantially impair the function of most organ systems. If major elective surgery is planned (Chapter 431), such individuals would benefit from adequate feeding preoperatively for up to 7 days or at least early nutritional intervention postoperatively. If palliative or curative radiation therapy or systemic chemotherapy is planned, adequate feeding during therapy with the use of supplemental formulas, tube feeding, or parenteral

nutrition (in that order) is indicated, with enteral feeding preferred. However, if the weight loss represents end-stage systemic illness, commonly seen as a cachexia syndrome of loss of weight and muscle mass with symptoms of weakness (e.g., cancer; end-stage liver, renal, or lung disease; acquired immunodeficiency syndrome) for which no primary therapy is planned or is effective, invasive nutritional support is rarely indicated.

Physical Examination

Although the patient's external appearance and a check of the skin, eyes, mouth, hair, and nails often provide clues to the presence of nutritional abnormalities (Table 214-1), the physical findings of deficiency syndromes of vitamins, essential fatty acids, and trace metals are relatively insensitive and nonspecific. With respect to protein-energy malnutrition, only the marasmic form in which semistarvation is the principal mechanism and cachexia syndromes resulting from semistarvation and a mild systemic inflammatory response are evident at examination. Adult marasmus and cachexia, the more severe forms, can be defined as 15% or more of recent weight loss, a weight-to-height ratio lower than 85% of desirable weight, or a BMI of less than 17. Loss of subcutaneous fat and skeletal muscle is manifested by sunken temples, thin extremities, wasting of the muscles of the hand, and, rarely, edema. Although kwashiorkor in children is characterized by severe edema and a potbelly appearance from hepatomegaly and ascites, one rarely encounters these clinical signs in cases of hypoalbuminemic malnutrition that develops in the setting of systemic inflammation resulting from disease in industrialized societies. Significant hypoalbuminemia of less than 3.5 g/dL results from a systemic inflammatory response, often without the accompanying anthropometric changes for which nutritional support can help to improve outcome if the response is prolonged beyond a week. With severe injury and greater depression of serum albumin to the 2.4 g/dL level or lower, early feeding within the first 24 to 48 hours can improve outcome. A mixed picture of protein-energy malnutrition with weight loss and lean tissue loss with mild hypoalbuminemia (cachexia) is found with many chronic inflammatory conditions with end-stage systemic illness or the sarcopenia of aging.

Body Weight

The most useful element in the physical examination is body weight, which is expressed as a relative value to evaluate the patient in relation to the healthy population. Weight and height are easily obtained, and standards for comparison have been established (Table 214-2). Although newer standards are available, they reflect the increasing prevalence of obesity in the U.S. population. Use of the 1959 standards allows the same tables to be used to diagnose significant protein-energy malnutrition (<85% of desirable weight, which approximates the fifth percentile) and significant obesity, defined as obesity predisposing to excessive mortality risk (>130% of desirable weight or BMI of ≥30). Although severe protein-energy malnutrition often occurs at levels greater than 85% of desirable weight because of the greater likelihood of preexisting obesity, this condition is generally detected by percentage of weight loss or by upper arm anthropometry. Height can be measured in a reclining patient with a tape measure, and in certain situations the clinician may rely on the patient's history. The major confounding variable that limits the value of weight and height as an index of protein-energy malnutrition is the tendency for water retention with disease, and thus weight gain may not reflect an increase in lean body mass or protein content. Fluid retention is particularly a problem in patients with hypoalbuminemic malnutrition because of the effects of aldosterone, antidiuretic hormone, and insulin stimulated by the stress response, which causes sodium and fluid retention. Fluid retention, however, does not usually confound initial weight assessment in patients who are first seen at the physician's office, except in those patients with diseases such as cardiac failure, end-stage liver disease, and severe renal disease in whom the disturbance in water metabolism results from the underlying disease and not principally from the hormonal response to systemic inflammation.

Body Mass Index

The BMI, which is the weight in kilograms divided by the height in meters squared, has gained favor as a nutritional measure because of two valuable attributes. The measure is relatively independent of height, and the same standards apply to male and female patients. The following BMI values are used: normal nutrition, BMI of 20 to less than 30; significant protein-energy malnutrition, less than 18.5; overweight, from 25 to less than 30; and obesity, 30 or greater, with severe obesity defined as a BMI of 35 to less than 40, and morbid obesity as 40 and greater. Evidence from developing countries

TABLE 214-1 CLINICAL SIGNS AND SYMPTOMS OF NUTRITIONAL INADEQUACY IN ADULT PATIENTS

	CLINICAL SIGN OR SYMPTOM	NUTRIENT
General	Wasted, skinny appearance	Calorie
	Loss of appetite	Protein-energy, zinc
Skin	Psoriasiform rash, eczematous scaling	Zinc, vitamin A, essential fatty acids
	Pallor	Folate, iron, vitamin B_{12}, copper
	Follicular hyperkeratosis	Vitamin A, vitamin C
	Perifollicular petechiae	Vitamin C
	Flaking dermatitis	Protein-energy, niacin, riboflavin, zinc
	Bruising	Vitamin C, vitamin K
	Pigmentation changes	Niacin, protein-energy
	Scrotal dermatosis	Riboflavin
	Thickening and dryness of skin	Linoleic acid
Head	Temporal muscle wasting	Protein-energy
Hair	Sparse and thin, dyspigmented	Protein
	Easy to pull out	Protein
	Corkscrew hairs	Vitamin C
Eyes	History of night blindness (also impaired visual recovery after glare)	Vitamin A, zinc
	Photophobia, blurring, conjunctival inflammation	Riboflavin, vitamin A
	Corneal vascularization	Riboflavin
	Xerosis, Bitot's spots, keratomalacia	Vitamin A
Mouth	Glossitis	Riboflavin, niacin, folic acid, vitamin B_{12}, pyridoxine
	Bleeding gums	Vitamin C, riboflavin
	Cheilosis	Riboflavin, pyridoxine, niacin
	Angular stomatitis	Riboflavin, pyridoxine, niacin
	Hypogeusia	Zinc
	Tongue fissuring	Niacin
	Tongue atrophy	Riboflavin, niacin, iron
	Nasolabial seborrhea	Pyridoxine
Neck	Goiter	Iodine
	Parotid enlargement	Protein
Thorax	Thoracic rosary	Vitamin D
Abdomen	Diarrhea	Niacin, folate, vitamin B_{12}
	Distention	Protein-energy
	Hepatomegaly	Protein-energy
Extremities	Edema	Protein, thiamine
	Softening of bone	Vitamin D, calcium, phosphorus
	Bone tenderness	Vitamin D
	Bone ache, joint pain	Vitamin C
	Muscle wasting and weakness	Protein, calorie, vitamin D, selenium, sodium chloride
	Muscle tenderness, muscle pain	Thiamine
Nails	Spooning	Iron
	Transverse lines	Protein
Neurologic	Tetany	Calcium, magnesium
	Paresthesias	Thiamine, vitamin B_{12}
	Loss of reflexes, wristdrop, footdrop	Thiamine
	Loss of vibratory and position sense	Vitamin B_{12}
	Ataxia	Vitamin B_{12}
	Dementia, disorientation	Niacin
Blood	Anemia	Vitamin B_{12}, folate, iron, pyridoxine
	Hemolysis	Phosphorus, vitamin E

TABLE 214-2 DESIRABLE WEIGHT IN POUNDS IN RELATION TO HEIGHT FOR MEN AND WOMEN 25 YEARS OR OLDER*

MEN, MEDIUM FRAME				WOMEN, MEDIUM FRAME			
HEIGHT		WEIGHT (lb)		HEIGHT		WEIGHT (lb)	
Ft	In	Range	Midpoint	Ft	In	Range	Midpoint
				4	8	93-104	98.5
				4	9	95-107	101
				4	10	98-110	104
				4	11	101-113	107
				5	0	104-116	110
5	1	113-124	118.5	5	1	107-119	113
5	2	116-128	122	5	2	110-123	116.5
5	3	119-131	125	5	3	113-127	120
5	4	122-134	128	5	4	117-132	124.5
5	5	125-138	131.5	5	5	121-136	128.5
5	6	129-142	135.5	5	6	125-140	132.5
5	7	133-147	140	5	7	129-144	136.5
5	8	137-151	144	5	8	133-148	140.5
5	9	141-155	148	5	9	137-152	144.5
5	10	145-160	153	5	10	141-156	148.5
5	11	149-165	157				
6	0	153-170	161.5				
6	1	157-175	166				
6	2	162-180	171				
6	3	167-185	176				

*Corrected to nude weights and heights by assuming 1-inch heel for men, 2-inch heel for women, and indoor clothing weight of 5 and 3 lb for men and women, respectively.
Adapted from the *Metropolitan Life Insurance Company Statistical Bulletin*, 1959;4:1.

The principal value of the TSF measurement is to determine the arm muscle circumference (AMC) or arm muscle area.

$$AMC\,(cm) = arm\ circumference - (\pi)(TSF)[mm])/10$$

The AMC is a specific measure of protein-energy malnutrition if the fifth or tenth percentile is chosen as the cutoff point, and it is particularly valuable in patients with edematous states and in amputees, in whom weights are inaccurate or insensitive. The TSF and AMC measurements[3] are most useful in initially defining marasmic-type malnutrition or the mixed disorder. Many dietitians are skilled in upper arm anthropometry.

Serum Proteins

Despite many concerns, the serum albumin level remains the traditional standard for nutritional assessment by virtue of its extensive history and its continued use to separate the principal forms of protein-energy malnutrition. Hypoalbuminemia is a strong predictor of risk for morbidity and mortality[4] in both hospitalized and ambulatory patients. In almost all cases, except perhaps for hereditary analbuminemia, excessive loss secondary to nephrotic syndrome (Chapter 121), and, occasionally, protein-losing enteropathy, hypoalbuminemia identifies the recent or ongoing presence of a systemic inflammatory response. A value for serum albumin of less than 3.5 g/dL is considered to indicate a mild systemic inflammatory response, whereas a value of less than 2.4 g/dL represents a severe systemic inflammatory response, reflecting systemic inflammation that produces anorexia (limiting food intake) and increases protein catabolism and thus accelerates the development of protein-calorie malnutrition. With a half-life for albumin of 18 to 20 days and the fractional replacement rate of about 10% per day, the return of serum albumin to normal takes about 2 weeks of feeding when the stress response remits. Adequate feeding in the presence of systemic inflammation will not increase the serum albumin concentration, even though substantial nutritional benefit will occur in terms of wound healing and immune function. Levels of other proteins, such as transferrin, prealbumin, and retinol-binding protein, with respective half-lives of 7 days, 2 days, and half a day, also fall acutely with injury and respond more quickly when systemic inflammation remits. Serum transferrin also varies with iron status, however, and prealbumin and retinol-binding protein vary with dietary carbohydrate

suggests that the BMI is better correlated with outcome than are weight and height.

Upper Arm Anthropometry

Approximately 50% of body fat is subcutaneous. The use of skinfold calipers to define the triceps skinfold thickness (TSF) is the most practical technique to estimate body fat. Standards for skinfold measurement are available from the National Health and Nutrition Examination Surveys I and II and were derived from a probability sample of the U.S. population. Generally, a value lower than the fifth percentile is used to define abnormality (Table 214-3).

TABLE 214-3 FIFTH, TENTH, AND FIFTIETH PERCENTILES FOR TRICEPS SKINFOLD AND MID-UPPER ARM MUSCLE CIRCUMFERENCE OF U.S. MEN AND WOMEN FROM THE FIRST NATIONAL HEALTH AND NUTRITION EXAMINATION SURVEY

AGE GROUP	MUAMC (cm) PERCENTILE			TSF (mm) PERCENTILE		
	5th	10th	50th	5th	10th	50th
MEN						
18-74	23.8	24.8	27.9	4.5	6	11
18-24	23.5	24.4	27.2	4	5	9.5
25-34	24.2	25.3	28	4.5	5.5	12
35-44	25	25.6	28.7	5	6	12
45-54	24	24.9	28.1	5	6	11
55-64	22.8	24.4	27.9	5	6	11
65-74	22.5	23.7	26.9	4.5	5.5	11
WOMEN						
18-74	18.4	19	21.8	11	13	22
18-24	17.7	18.5	20.6	9.4	11	18
25-34	18.3	18.9	21.4	10.5	12	21
35-44	18.5	19.2	22	12	14	23
45-54	18.8	19.5	22.2	13	15	25
55-64	18.6	19.5	22.6	11	14	25
65-74	18.6	19.5	22.5	11.5	14	23

MUAMC = mid-upper arm muscle circumference; TSF = triceps skinfold.
From Bishop CW, Bowen PE, Ritchey SJ. Norms for nutritional assessment of American adults by upper arm anthropometry. *Am J Clin Nutr.* 1981;34:2530-2539.

and renal function. As a result, these proteins do not reliably identify the presence and severity of the systemic inflammatory response any better than does albumin, but they reflect the nutritional response more quickly when inflammation lessens.

Composite Screening Tools

Investigators have made numerous attempts to combine the various components of nutritional assessment, including clinical history, physical examination, anthropometry, and serum proteins, into a single score.[5] Some of the more widely used tools include the following: the Subjective Global Assessment,[6] which classifies patients as A, B, or C or as having normal, mild, or moderate malnutrition; the Nutritional Risk Index, which is based on weight loss and serum albumin only; and the more extensive evaluations with the Mini-Nutritional Assessment and Malnutrition Universal Screening Tool. A clear advantage of one technique over another has not been established.

● NUTRITIONAL THERAPY AND ITS ASSESSMENT

The same indices that are used in the baseline nutritional assessment can be used to assess response to therapy, provided certain points are kept in mind.

Assessing Lean Body Mass and Total Body Water

In a stressed, hospitalized patient receiving nutritional support, day-to-day weight changes generally reflect changes in fluid balance rather than energy balance. In an ambulatory setting, weight increases or decreases are most likely to reflect changes in protein nutritional status and body fat because the underlying illness is usually less severe. Even the most sensitive research methods for assessing changes in lean body mass, however, do not offer major improvements in diagnosis in the more seriously ill patients. Techniques that measure total body water, such as isotope dilution and underwater weighing, from which lean tissue is extrapolated, fail to account for the distortion in hydration of lean tissue with illness. Surrogate measures of total body protein to estimate lean tissues such as total body potassium measurement and dual x-ray absorptiometry do not adjust for differing body composition with disease. A newer method, single-frequency or multifrequency body impedance analysis, does show promise as a simple, accurate, noninvasive method[7] that may allow distinction between intracellular and extracellular water, with the former used to estimate lean tissue for an initial assessment. However, the inherent difficulties resulting from the greater disturbance of total body water in critically ill patients have not been overcome with this technique. Magnetic resonance imaging and total body nitrogen analysis are the most reliable tools for assessing the amount of lean tissue but are primarily useful for research purposes. The gold standard for assessing lean tissue is in vivo neutron activation analysis for nitrogen, but this is and will remain a research procedure. Combining clinically available, rapid techniques like dual x-ray absorptiometry scanning to assess body fat content with body impedance analysis[8] to measure total body water has shown some promise in estimating true lean tissue in critically ill patients.

Restoration of Lean Tissue

In an unstressed patient with the marasmic form of protein-calorie malnutrition, providing adequate energy and 1.2 to 1.5 g/kg protein should cause a positive nitrogen balance of 2 to 6 g/day (60 to 180 g lean tissue) and slow weight gain, depending on the extent of positive energy balance. For instance, a 300-kcal excess of intake over expenditure would provide approximately 120 g of lean tissue (100-kcal equivalent) in addition to 200 kcal (22 g) as fat, for a total of approximately 140 g, or approximately ⅓ pound of weight per day. Weight gains in excess of this number usually reflect sodium and thus water retention from the insulin stimulated by dietary carbohydrate. Such overhydration can be improved by reducing salt and limiting fluid intake. In patients with hypoalbuminemic malnutrition who are no longer stressed, a similar nutritional regimen will lead to a comparable gain of tissue, but weight change is often less as edema becomes mobilized, with normalization of serum albumin in 2 to 4 weeks and of retinol-binding protein, prealbumin, and transferrin more quickly. In stressed patients with hypoalbuminemic malnutrition, appropriate nutritional support often does not restore lean tissue but does improve other important functions, such as wound healing and immunocompetence. These are important treatment goals because they can improve the ultimate clinical outcome. Both the systemic inflammatory response and the limited activity level reduce the efficiency of skeletal muscle repletion, which represents 30% of body weight and 75% of actively metabolizing lean tissue. Functional testing of muscle strength and endurance, such as hand dynamometry, can be useful as a means of assessing this response but has not found wide clinical acceptance. Similarly, any reduction in other physiologic functions or impairment in the patient's ability to perform the usual activities of daily living will accentuate the consequences of protein-energy malnutrition. Cachexia syndromes reflect the loss of lean tissue with mild to moderate persistent inflammation due to an underlying chronic disease. Response to nutritional therapy is generally poor unless there is improvement or correction of the basic disease process.

Measures of Energy Expenditure and Caloric Need

Although caloric expenditure can now be reliably and easily measured with portable indirect calorimeters, estimated energy expenditure is sufficient in most clinical situations. The three components of total energy expenditure are basal energy expenditure (~55 to 65% of total energy expenditure), thermal effect of feeding (~10% of total energy expenditure), and activity energy expenditure (25 to 33%). An energy intake of 30 to 35 kcal/kg of body weight will maintain weight in most sedentary ambulatory patients, with adjustments upward or downward in 200- to 300-kcal increments as prompted by biweekly changes in weight. Although young, severely burned, or traumatized patients may require 35 to 40 kcal/kg in the acute phase to meet total energy expenditure, providing energy intakes principally as carbohydrates that exceed 35 kcal/kg substantially increases the likelihood of hyperglycemia. Evidence strongly implicates hyperglycemia in excess of 180 mg/dL as a major risk factor for nosocomial infection, thus emphasizing the importance of better glycemic control by the use of insulin infusions or by reducing the level of energy intake, or both. Most postoperative patients who require invasive nutritional support for mechanical or infectious complications usually require approximately 25 kcal/kg to meet energy needs and not more than 30 kcal/kg because of their older age and reduced activity and energy expenditure. Overfeeding should be avoided in such patients, and modest underfeeding for the first several weeks of acute illness may actually improve outcome in seriously ill patients.

The nutritional monitoring of the most critically ill patients[9] is primarily to assess how closely estimated nutritional needs are delivered on a daily basis, rather than any other presently defined nutritional marker beyond weight as an estimate of fluid status.[A1][A2] Early parenteral feeding is no better than enteral feeding.[A3] Moreover, it is yet to be determined how early the full feeding should begin (immediately or within 7 days) and what constitutes best feeding practice (hypocaloric feeding at 50 to 70% of estimated energy expenditure with higher protein of at least 1.5 g/kg, versus 100% of both energy and protein needs at least for the first several weeks of critical illness). The disadvantage of full feeding in critically ill patients is the greater risk for hyperglycemia and its increased infectious complications and greater fluid administration with its adverse consequences. Hypocaloric feeding appears to be as effective as full feeding for at least the first several weeks of critical illness. Measurement of energy expenditure by indirect calorimetry is generally reserved for the most severely marasmic patients, in whom estimates are often inaccurate, and for critically ill patients on prolonged mechanical ventilation or invasive nutritional support beyond several weeks, in whom provision of full energy needs may be beneficial.

Grade A References

A1. Casaer MP, Mesotten D, Hermans G, et al. Early versus late parenteral nutrition in critically ill adults. *N Engl J Med.* 2011;365:506-517.
A2. Heidegger CP, Berger MM, Graf S, et al. Optimisation of energy provision with supplemental parenteral nutrition in critically ill patients: a randomized controlled clinical trial. *Lancet.* 2013;381: 385-393.
A3. Harvey SE, Parrott F, Harrison DA, et al. Trial of the route of early nutritional support in critically ill adults. *N Engl J Med.* 2014;371:1673-1684.

GENERAL REFERENCES

For the General References and other additional features, please visit Expert Consult at https://expertconsult.inkling.com.

215

PROTEIN-ENERGY MALNUTRITION

MARK J. MANARY AND INDI TREHAN

DEFINITION

The term *protein-energy malnutrition* encompasses at least three distinct clinical syndromes. The first and most common, *stunting*, occurs throughout the developing world. It is a consequence of chronic macronutrient and micronutrient deficiency prenatally and during early childhood and is manifested as low birth weight and irreversible cognitive and physical stunting, including below normal weight and short stature in the first few years of life. In contrast to this chronic form of protein-energy malnutrition, a second manifestation takes the form of *acute malnutrition*, a primarily macronutrient deficiency. In its most severe forms, it includes kwashiorkor, marasmus (wasting), and marasmic kwashiorkor. The third syndrome is the wasting that occurs secondary to acute or chronic underlying illnesses such as renal or hepatic insufficiency, inflammatory bowel disease, malignancy, or a systemic infection such as HIV or tuberculosis.

EPIDEMIOLOGY

Global rates of stunting and acute malnutrition are difficult to quantify accurately, given the primarily rural populations where they mostly occur. Approximately 25% of children younger than 5 years are stunted worldwide, and another 8% suffer from marasmus. The number with kwashiorkor is unknown and underreported because of minimal high-quality surveillance data[1]; therapeutic feeding programs in southern Africa (the area with the highest prevalence) often report that 50 to 70% of cases of severe acute malnutrition have kwashiorkor rather than marasmus. It is estimated that some 15% of the total mortality for children younger than 5 years worldwide is attributable to stunting and that another 12% is attributable to wasting.[2]

Rates of secondary protein-energy malnutrition among those with medical and surgical illnesses vary widely and are a function of underlying disease processes, comorbidities, nutritional status before illness, and level of financial resources and social support. It is not unusual for malnutrition rates of 25 to 60% among hospitalized patients to be reported in the literature.

PATHOBIOLOGY

Most stunting in children occurs during the critical "1000 days" window between conception and 2 years of age, although there is some evidence that partial catch-up growth can occur in later childhood.[3] Maternal undernutrition contributes to low birth weight, which persists as underweight, short

stature, and cognitive stunting. Stunting also places children at elevated risk for acute malnutrition when challenged by food shortages or acute infections. Even children without prenatal stunting are at high risk for stunting and acute malnutrition when raised in impoverished environments. HIV infection and exposure, diarrhea, pneumonia, measles, and malaria are common in the developing world and can lead to anorexia with decreased dietary intake, increased energy expenditure, and poor nutrient absorption, placing the child at risk for stunting and acute malnutrition. The end of exclusive breastfeeding (whether prematurely or at the recommended 6 months of age) and the introduction of complementary feeding is also a high-risk period as the child ingests a variety of environmental pathogens and often suffers a relative loss of high-quality protein, lipids, and micronutrients.

Two major pathobiologic factors have been recently appreciated to contribute significantly to the development of protein-energy malnutrition in children.[4] The first is environmental enteric dysfunction (abbreviated EED, formerly "environmental enteropathy" or "tropical enteropathy"), endemic in children and adults throughout the developing world. It is characterized by blunted and atrophied intestinal villi, hyperplasia of the crypts, and lymphocytic infiltration of the lamina propria, histologically similar in many ways to celiac disease. EED appears to be a T-cell–mediated response to repeated environmental insults, such as gastrointestinal infections with a fecal-oral transmission pattern. The net effect of EED is an increase in intestinal permeability with bacterial and toxin translocation due to loss of tight junction integrity, impaired immune functioning, and malabsorption. EED is generally subclinical, predisposing children to growth faltering, and leaves them more susceptible to developing acute malnutrition. A second, related, risk factor for the development of acute malnutrition is a disturbed configuration of the intestinal microbiome, which fails to develop in an age-appropriate manner compared with unaffected children.[5,6] The ability to clinically identify these abnormalities in the microbiome and provide specific therapy is not yet available.

Secondary protein-energy malnutrition that occurs in the context of an underlying illness often results from a triad of decreased energy intake, malabsorption, and catabolic stressors. Virtually any chronic and/or critical illness can precipitate protein-energy malnutrition, but among the most common are cancer, HIV/AIDS, tuberculosis, inflammatory bowel disease, chronic kidney disease, chronic liver disease, and rheumatologic illnesses. The patient is in a state of net negative energy balance manifested by decreased weight and metabolic rate, accompanied to varying degrees by muscle wasting, depletion of fat stores, reduced cardiorespiratory capacity, skin thinning with easy breakdown and ulceration, hypothermia, immunodeficiency with impaired wound healing, and apathy.

The specific pathobiologic etiologies and risk factors for the development of this secondary protein-energy malnutrition are numerous. Primary among them is poor dietary intake as a result of nausea, anorexia, depression, poor dentition, and oral-motor weakness accompanying the underlying illness. Even nutrients that are ingested may not be absorbed, for example, because of reduced bile salt secretion leading to steatorrhea, pancreatic insufficiency, and damage to the intestinal mucosa in Crohn's disease. Systemic inflammation and oxidative stress are common in critical illness, cirrhosis, patients with HIV/AIDS and other infections, and hemodialysis patients, contributing to a catabolic state. In patients with chronic renal disease, altered amino acid homeostasis by the kidney, resistance to growth hormone and insulin-like growth factor-1, low testosterone levels, insulin resistance, and altered insulin signaling are all important factors in protein-energy wasting.[7] Patients with chronic liver disease often suffer from protein-energy malnutrition due to a combination of altered gut motility, dyspepsia, cholestasis with poor absorption of fat-soluble vitamins, small intestine bacterial overgrowth, a hypermetabolic state, inadequate hepatic protein synthesis, lack of glycogen reserves, and blood loss from varices and the intestinal lumen.

CLINICAL MANIFESTATIONS

Stunting manifests quite simply as short stature and underweight for age. Brain development, and thus head circumference, may also be small for age, although this is relatively proportional for overall body size.

Acute malnutrition manifests in at least three different forms. Children with wasting are emaciated and weak, having suffered significant weight loss in a relatively short period. The wasting often first manifests in the axilla and groin, progressing to the thighs and buttocks, and eventually visible in the face, which may take on an "old man" appearance. These children may appear apathetic but in fact may be quite inconsolable when approached. Wasting may be mild, moderate, or severe ("marasmus") (Fig. 215-1).

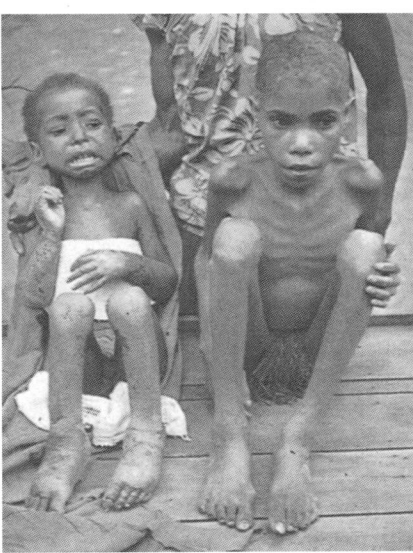

FIGURE 215-1. Kwashiorkor and marasmus in brothers. The younger brother, on the left, has kwashiorkor with generalized edema, skin changes, pale reddish yellow hair, and an unhappy expression. The older child, on the right, has marasmus, with generalized wasting, spindly arms and legs, and an apathetic expression. (From Peters W, Pasvol G, eds. *Tropical Medicine and Parasitology*, 5th ed. London: Mosby; 2002, Fig. 986.)

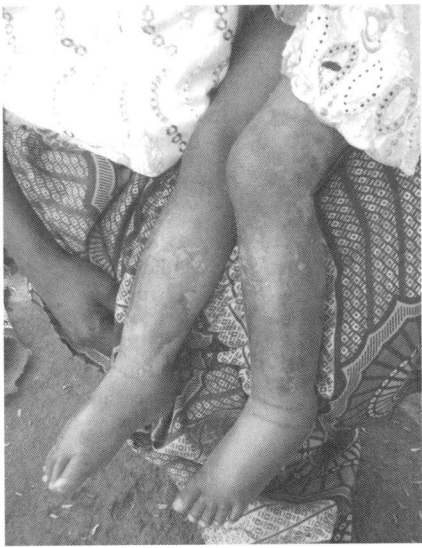

FIGURE 215-2. Edematous malnutrition or kwashiorkor.

The second form of acute malnutrition, edematous malnutrition or kwashiorkor, was classically described to occur when a child was weaned rapidly from the high-quality protein source that is breast milk, although this is not universal. Children with kwashiorkor have a weight that is generally low-to-average for their age. They present with bilateral peripheral edema that begins in the feet and progresses cephalad as it worsens. Despite what can be a relatively profound edema, they generally do not have ascites, nor is their illness a result of hepatic insufficiency or hypoalbuminemia. The skin may have patchy areas of "flaky paint" depigmentation, commonly with areas of breakdown and resultant infection (Fig. 215-2). The hair is often sparse, dry, brittle, and depigmented, appearing brown-yellow in children whose hair is normally black and thick.

Why some children in nearly identical living conditions develop marasmus while others develop kwashiorkor and most remain without acute malnutrition is not understood but does not appear to be a result of disparate protein intake; recent evidence suggests that alterations in the commensal intestinal microbiome may be responsible. Finally, children with marasmic

kwashiorkor have both the severe weight loss of marasmus and the edema of kwashiorkor. Compared with children with either syndrome alone, these children are generally the most ill with the poorest prognosis.

Protein-energy malnutrition in patients with severe or chronic underlying disease generally presents as low body-mass index (BMI) or with progressive weight loss.

Virtually every organ system and tissue type is starved of energy in all forms of protein-energy malnutrition, resulting in a homeostatic drive to adapt to the decreased energy available. Fat is increasingly used as the body's primary fuel source within the first few days, having replaced glucose, and ketosis quickly develops. Overall glucose production and protein breakdown decrease markedly, decreasing urea production and urinary fluid losses. The basal metabolic rate decreases, accompanied by hypothermia and easy fatiguing. As starvation continues, nearly all of the body's fat stores are depleted, and lean muscle tissue may be cut in half. In addition to decreased muscle mass, hypokalemia leads to rapid muscle fatigue. Cardiac muscle is not spared, potentially leading to bradycardia, decreased stroke volume, hypotension, and poor tissue perfusion. Intravascular volume may be diminished at the same time that cellular and capillary leakage increases, leading to generalized edema, particularly in kwashiorkor.

Pulmonary capacity is adversely affected because of decreased respiratory muscle mass and electrolyte disturbances. The skin and hair often atrophy, depigment, and break down, leaving the patient susceptible to cutaneous infections. Insulin and thyroid hormone levels decrease, and cortisol concentrations increase. A state of immunodeficiency develops as lymphoid tissues atrophy and cell-mediated immunity is diminished, placing the malnourished patient at high risk for opportunistic infections. Pancytopenia can occur as a result of bone marrow suppression. Prolonged malnutrition leads to deterioration of all portions of the gastrointestinal system, including atrophy and blunting of the intestinal villi (thereby complicating therapeutic feeding), impaired exocrine pancreatic function, and decreased gastric and biliary secretions. Hepatomegaly and fatty liver infiltration are seen. Except in cases in which renal pathology is the inciting pathway, kidney function is relatively well preserved until late in the course. Although the brain is preserved longer than other organs, cerebral atrophy is seen in acute malnutrition, and (often permanently) delayed cognitive development is a profound complication with lifelong consequences among survivors.

DIAGNOSIS

Careful anthropometry must be conducted to accurately evaluate any individual for protein-energy malnutrition. In the case of children, it can be particularly challenging to gain their cooperation for anthropometry. Precise measurements of height (to the nearest 0.5 cm or less), weight (to the nearest 100 g or less), mid-upper arm circumference (MUAC; to the nearest 2 mm or less), and an assessment of peripheral pitting edema should be performed. Standardized World Health Organization growth charts should be used for diagnosis and classification.[8]

A child is considered to have *moderate stunting* when the height-for-age Z-score (HAZ) lies between 2 and 3 standard deviations (SD) below the mean. *Severe stunting* is diagnosed when the HAZ is more than 3 SD below the mean. Familial short stature, hypothyroidism, growth hormone deficiency, and micronutrient deficiency are all on the differential diagnosis for a stunted child, although these will be relatively rare compared with stunting in the relevant epidemiologic context.

Moderate wasting is based on having a weight-for-height Z-score (WHZ) between 2 and 3 SD below the mean. *Severe wasting*, or marasmus, is based on a WHZ more than 3 SD below the mean. For children aged 6 to 59 months, the MUAC can also be used to diagnose wasting because a healthy minimum MUAC remains relatively constant throughout this age. In these children, MUAC cutoffs of 115 to 125 mm and of less than 115 mm are generally considered diagnostic for moderate and severe wasting, respectively. Most children diagnosed as wasted by WHZ and MUAC criteria will be the same, but there is a sizeable population that will only be diagnosed by one or the other criterion. Given that the population identified by MUAC is generally younger and at higher risk for death than the population identified by WHZ,[9] MUAC is preferred for identifying severely malnourished children. Nevertheless, if resources exist to screen children by WHZ in addition to MUAC, that strategy is most likely to identify all acutely wasted children. Congenital heart disease, severe diarrhea and dehydration, malabsorptive syndromes due to intestinal parasites, malaria, HIV/AIDS, and tuberculosis should be considered in the differential diagnosis of a child presenting with wasting. Still, if a child has wasting based on anthropometric criteria, nutritional rehabilitation needs to be provided while their underlying illness is addressed simultaneously.

The presence of edema in the appropriate clinical context, regardless of other anthropometric parameters, should prompt serious consideration of the diagnosis of kwashiorkor. Edema is most easily detected on the dorsum of the feet. The degree of edema is graded as 1+ if confined to the lower extremities, 2+ if additionally present on the upper extremities, and 3+ if extending to the face. The usual physiologic causes of edema, including underlying cardiac, hepatic, and renal diseases, should be considered in the differential diagnosis. In the rural impoverished populations where kwashiorkor is found, routine health care is also generally limited; thus, the possibilities of congenital or rheumatic heart disease, acute proliferative glomerulonephritis (postinfectious or post-streptococcal), profound anemia (from primary iron deficiency, severe malaria, or hookworm, among other causes), and tuberculosis should be considered. Nevertheless, for the overwhelming majority of children with edema presenting for care in these populations, kwashiorkor remains the leading diagnosis.

Secondary malnutrition due to underlying illness also requires careful anthropometry, with a BMI of less than 18.5 kg/m^2 representing moderate malnutrition and a BMI of less than 15 kg/m^2 representing severe protein-energy malnutrition. Even without a BMI this low, any significant weight loss, especially if associated with lean muscle loss in addition to depletion of fat stores, should prompt consideration of protein-energy malnutrition and necessitates an investigation into an underlying illness if one had not been previously identified. No reliable diagnostic tests are available to identify those with protein-energy malnutrition because serum markers such as albumin, prealbumin, and C-reactive protein are themselves acute phase reactants and nonspecific for this purpose.

TREATMENT   Rx

Studies of probiotics and antibiotics to treat environmental enteric dysfunction have not shown benefit.[A1] However, albendazole, zinc,[A2] and micronutrient supplementation have shown some benefit.[A3]

There is relatively little that can be done for a child with stunting because the physical and cognitive growth faltering suffered in the first "1000 days" is not likely to be amenable to therapy. These children remain at high risk for further stunting during childhood, although some degree of catch-up growth is possible in later childhood and adolescence, even without specific nutritional interventions. Attention should be directed to an overall improvement in their dietary quality and diversity, particularly with respect to increased protein intake. Exclusive breast-feeding until 6 months of age and continued breast-feeding with appropriate supplementary foods until at least 2 years of age should be encouraged whenever possible, except in the case of an HIV-infected mother. Routine health care, including immunizations, vitamin A

supplementation, and periodic deworming, should be ensured. In high-prevalence settings, HIV testing and treatment should be sought. Improvements in sanitary living conditions are likely to be the most beneficial.

Children with severe acute malnutrition have traditionally been managed as inpatients with fortified milk-based formulas as the key nutritional component of their overall care. A coordinated 10-step plan for the inpatient management of severe acute malnutrition has led to tremendous improvements in recovery and mortality rates (Fig. 215-3). Children are initially started on F-75 formula every 2 to 4 hours and then progress to F-100 as their appetite increases and they demonstrate that they are able to tolerate the solute load without severe diarrhea (Table 215-1).

However, the development and increasingly widespread availability of ready-to-use therapeutic food (RUTF), most often a fortified peanut paste, makes it preferable to treat children in community-based outpatient feeding programs instead, assuming that the child demonstrates a mental status and appetite conducive to feeding at home.[10] After ensuring that the child has an appetite and is not suffering from complications such as hypoglycemia, severe dehydration, respiratory distress, severe anemia, and high fevers, a test feeding of approximately 30 g RUTF is given under directly observed therapy. Most children will successfully complete this test feeding and can be discharged home with 1 to 2 weeks of 175 kcal/kg/day of RUTF. Anthropometry and clinical assessments are repeated at 1- to 2-week intervals; children are treated until their edema resolves and either their WHZ is no more than 2 SD below the mean or their MUAC reaches 125 mm (depending on whether they were diagnosed based on WHZ or MUAC criteria). Almost all children will recover within 8 to 12 weeks, with approximately half recovering by 4 to 6 weeks if the child is receiving all of the intended food and there are no interim complications. Any child not improving as expected should have a thorough social and medical assessment to evaluate whether they are being fed appropriately and whether any acute infectious complications have developed; inpatient care may be necessary in those situations.

Mortality and nutritional recovery outcomes from community-based programs are generally superior to those achieved by inpatient care, making this the current international standard of care[11] and relegating inpatient care only to those children with anorexia or medical complications or who are in an area where RUTF is not available. Outpatient care can be improved further with empirical antibiotic therapy for all patients because of the high risk for overwhelming sepsis and death.[A4] Integration of outpatient nutritional care into a complete package of routine health interventions, including linkage to HIV testing and treatment, will likely only improve outcomes further.

Patients with secondary protein-energy malnutrition should, first and foremost, have their underlying illness addressed because this is most likely to lead to long-term recovery of their nutritional status. Concomitantly, nutritional rehabilitation should be undertaken to prevent further energy losses and allow for recovery of damaged organic pathways. Fluid, electrolyte, and acid-base status should be corrected cautiously in the usual fashion. In general, enteral nutrition (Chapter 216) is preferred over parenteral, assuming the gastrointestinal tract is functioning adequately. Frequent small feedings or slow drip feedings may be necessary. Aggressive tube feeding or parenteral nutrition should be avoided in the early stages of rehabilitation because the

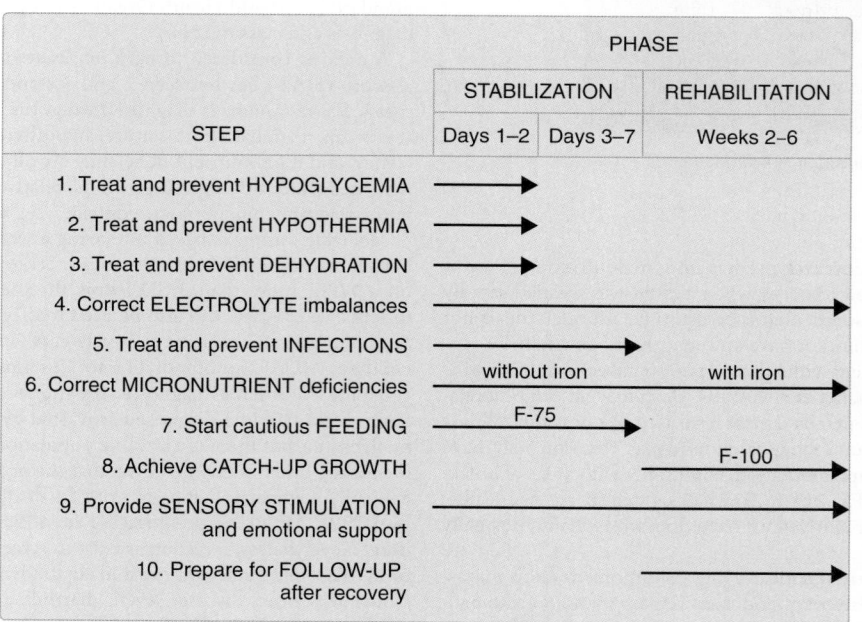

FIGURE 215-3. Ten-step inpatient management protocol for severe acute malnutrition. (Adapted from Ashworth A, Khanum S, Jackson A, Schofield C. *Guidelines for the Inpatient Treatment of Severely Malnourished Children.* Geneva: World Health Organization; 2003.)

TABLE 215-1	NUTRITIONAL COMPOSITION OF THERAPEUTIC FOODS FOR SEVERE ACUTE MALNUTRITION		
	F-75 (100 mL)	F-100 (100 mL)	RUTF (100 mg)
Energy (kcal)	75	100	543
Protein (g)	0.9	2.9	13.6
Lactose (g)	1.3	4.2	
Potassium (mg)	156	246	1111
Sodium (mg)	14	44	189
Magnesium (mg)	10.5	17.7	92
Zinc (mg)	2	2.3	14
Copper (mg)	0.25	0.25	1.78
Osmolarity (mOsm/L)	413	419	
% of total energy from protein	5	12	10-12
% of total energy from fat	36	53	45-60

RUTF = ready-to-use therapeutic food.

refeeding syndrome is a real danger in patients who are malnourished. Hypophosphatemia, hypokalemia, hypomagnesemia, hyperglycemia, fluid overload, muscular weakness, cardiac arrhythmias, and diarrhea are all possible with aggressive refeeding. Fluid status, glycemic status, and electrolyte levels should be monitored closely throughout the refeeding process.[12]

PREVENTION

Prevention of stunting and acute malnutrition remains one of the most challenging and elusive goals in global health, especially given the intergenerational effects of maternal malnutrition. Providing pregnant women with nutritional supplementation, intermittent malaria treatment, timely care for sexually transmitted infections, and comprehensive prenatal care shows some success in improving birth weights and decreasing premature delivery. Adherence to recommendations for exclusive breast-feeding for the first 6 months and continued breast-feeding for at least the first 2 years also shows profound benefit.[13] Early diagnosis and treatment of HIV in mothers and their infants is also beneficial.[14] Nevertheless, children in the developing world remain at high risk for stunting and acute malnutrition because of the relative lack of sanitation, high rates of food insecurity, spotty vaccination coverage, and limited access to medical care. Addressing these underlying societal factors may provide the most benefit to decreasing environmental enteric dysfunction, stunting, and acute malnutrition.

Close attention to the nutritional status of medical and surgical patients, with risk stratification based on BMI and weight trajectory, is necessary to limit the risk for protein-energy malnutrition in these patients as they are treated for their underlying illnesses. Optimizing nutritional status will aid in recovery from their primary conditions, and similarly recovery from the primary condition will improve benefit to overall nutritional status. Efforts to empirically provide extra protein, calories, and micronutrients during times of particular oxidative stress and catabolism will help limit weight loss and its adverse effects.

PROGNOSIS

The prognosis for stunted children generally remains poor because the physical and cognitive deficits they suffer are mostly carried with them throughout life,[15] despite some catch-up growth in later childhood and adolescence. Children who recover from an episode of severe acute malnutrition are somewhat more susceptible to further episodes over the next several months than their peers, although those with underlying illnesses such as HIV or tuberculosis remain at significantly elevated risk. The highest recovery rates in severe acute malnutrition treatment programs are approximately 90%, with about 4 to 5% mortality. Untreated, episodes of severe wasting carry an estimated 10%-20% mortality risk per month. Although many children will recover spontaneously, most will never return to their baseline nutritional status and fully thrive. Early childhood growth faltering may be linked to an increased risk for the metabolic syndrome as adults, contributing to the

double epidemic of childhood undernutrition and adult obesity being increasingly observed throughout the developing world.

 Grade A References

A1. Trehan I, Shulman RJ, Ou CN, et al. A randomized, double-blind, placebo-controlled trial of rifaximin, a nonabsorbable antibiotic, in the treatment of tropical enteropathy. *Am J Gastroenterol.* 2009;104:2326-2333.
A2. Ryan KN, Stephenson KB, Trehan I, et al. Oral zinc or albendazole ameliorates environmental enteropathy in Malawian children: a randomized controlled trial. *Clin Gastroenterol Hepatol.* 2014;12:1507-1513.
A3. Smith HE, Ryan KN, Stephenson KB, et al. Multiple micronutrient supplementation transiently ameliorates environmental enteropathy in Malawian children aged 12-35 months in a randomized controlled clinical trial. *J Nutr.* 2014;144:2059-2065.
A4. Trehan I, Goldbach HS, LaGrone LN, et al. Antibiotics as part of the management of severe acute malnutrition. *N Engl J Med.* 2013;368:425-435.

GENERAL REFERENCES

For the General References and other additional features, please visit Expert Consult at https://expertconsult.inkling.com.

216

ENTERAL NUTRITION

STEPHEN A. MCCLAVE

The benefit of nutrition therapy in the hospitalized patient is clearly related to the provision of early enteral nutrition (EN).[1] Outside the setting of intestinal failure or short bowel syndrome, a true benefit over providing parenteral nutrition (PN) is not clear, and its use should be determined on a case-by-case basis.[A1][A2] Providing early EN to the critically ill patient in the intensive care unit (ICU), on the other hand, exerts a beneficial physiologic effect that downregulates inflammation and improves patient outcome.[2] Because the gut is the largest immune organ in the body, the timing, volume, and content of nutrient that is infused into the lumen of the gut have a major impact on the level of oxidative stress, the tone of systemic immune responses, and the likelihood for complications. A window of opportunity exists shortly after admission to the ICU, during which placement of enteral access and initiation of feeding will improve patient outcome by reducing rates of infection, overall complications, organ failure, length of hospital stay, and, in some disease processes, even mortality.[3] Failure to utilize the gut in critical illness results in a different physiologic response, whereby the gut becomes a pro-inflammatory organ and outcome is worsened. Depending on the patient population, the window of opportunity for such modulation may be very narrow. Burns are considered "nutritional emergencies," in which the window of opportunity may be as short as 3 to 6 hours before increased permeability occurs. In other disease processes, such as pancreatitis or major elective operations, the window may be longer (i.e., 48 to 72 hours). At some point, the ability to modulate the immune system and contain gut barrier function begins to diminish. Preventing increases in permeability of the gut is easier than containment after barrier function is compromised. The main purpose of early EN in the hospitalized critically ill patient then is to maintain gut integrity and modulate systemic immunity. With time, provision of nutrients to prevent the deterioration of nutritional status and the development of malnutrition becomes increasingly important. Therefore, EN is indicated in any critically ill patient who is unable to eat and should be initiated as soon as the patient receives full volume resuscitation. If the patient is not critically ill, EN is indicated if the patient is anticipated to be unable to eat for more than 7 days. The only true contraindications to feeding are bowel ischemia, mechanical obstruction of the gut, and peritonitis. It is important for the clinician to realize that although ileus, pancreatitis, nausea, vomiting, and other such factors may make enteral feeding difficult, none is an absolute contraindication to providing EN.

PHYSIOLOGIC BENEFIT OF ENTERAL NUTRITION

The provision of EN maintains both the functional and structural integrity of the intestinal epithelium. Early EN stimulates intestinal contractility and

TABLE 216-1 COMPARISON OF PHYSIOLOGIC EFFECTS OF FEEDING VERSUS STARVATION

	ENTERAL FEEDING	STARVATION
Intestinal contractility	Increased	Decreased
Release of secretory IgA from gut	Increased	Decreased
Release of trophic agents (bile salts, gastrin)	Increased	Decreased
Splanchnic intestinal blood flow	Increased	Decreased
Luminal microbiota		
Organisms	Commensal	Pathogenic
Population	Normal	Overgrowth
Gut integrity and epithelial cell tight junctions	Intact	Permeable
Mass of GALT	Maintained	Diminished
Support of MALT at distant sites	Maintained	Diminished
Population of CD$_4$ helper lymphocytes emerging from gut into systemic circulation	T$_H$2 (anti-inflammatory)	T$_H$1 (pro-inflammatory)
Expression of adhesion molecules	MAdCAM	E-selectin
Cell line affected (pass out of vascular space)	GALT cells	Neutrophils

GALT = gut-associated lymphoid tissue; IgA = immunoglobulin A; MALT = mucosal-associated lymphoid tissue; MAdCAM = mucosal addressin adhesion molecule.

causes release of trophic substances such as bile salts, gastrin, bombesin, and motilin. Good contractility controls the overall number of bacteria within the lumen of the gut by peristaltic movement of organisms downstream. EN stimulates the release of secretory immunoglobulin A (IgA), which helps coat luminal bacteria and prevents their adherence to the epithelial wall (Table 216-1). EN stimulates blood flow to the gut and supports the mass of gut-associated lymphoid tissue (GALT). EN stimulates the production of T$_H$2 anti-inflammatory CD4 helper lymphocytes, which enter the systemic circulation and support immune function. Secretory immunoglobulin A (IgA)-producing immunocytes form mucosal-associated lymphoid tissue (MALT), which generates further production of secretory IgA. EN promotes the role of commensal bacteria, which provide *direct protection* by degrading bacterial toxins and *indirect protection* by preventing colonization of pathogenic organisms (such as *Pseudomonas aeruginosa*). By fermenting prebiotic fiber to short-chain fatty acids, commensal bacteria stimulate butyrate receptors in the colon, which further downregulates inflammation. EN also simulates the immune process of oral tolerance, which further supports the anti-inflammatory functions of T$_H$1 and T$_H$3 lymphocytes and the production of the anti-inflammatory agent transforming growth factor-β (TGF-β). The T$_H$2 cytokines that are produced in this process suppress the adhesion molecule E-selectin, which functions to trap neutrophils within the vasculature. T$_H$2 cytokines also stimulate the release of mucosal addressin cell adhesion molecule-1 (MAdCAM), which allows GALT cells to mobilize from the splanchnic circulation and return to the lamina propria of the gut.

In specific patient populations, the addition of certain pharmaconutrient agents to an enteral formula exerts a synergistic effect to the benefit already induced by standard enteral formula alone. The addition of arginine has a direct stimulant effect on immune function and thus may further support the T$_H$2 response, proliferation of lymphocytes, and secretory IgA-producing immunocytes created by the delivery of enteral feeding. The addition of antioxidants, particularly selenium, serves to decrease oxidative stress. Providing fat in the form of fish oil reduces stimulation of the inflammatory ligand toll-like receptor-4 (TLR-4) on macrophages, neutrophils, and adipocytes, reducing the production and generation of NFκ-B and tumor necrosis factor-β. Provision of fish oil generates alternative prostaglandins (PGE$_3$), leukotrienes (LTB$_5$), and thromboxane (TXA$_3$), which have a downregulatory effect on inflammatory mediators compared with the corresponding products of omega-6 fatty acids (PGE$_2$, LTB$_4$, TXA$_2$). Glutamine added to an enteral formula serves as an antioxidant and helps maintain gut integrity. Zinc has a direct effect on the zona occludens, maintaining tight junctions between the gut epithelial cells.

CONSEQUENCES OF NOT PROVIDING ENTERAL NUTRITION

For the critically ill patient, failure to provide enteral feeding generates a different physiologic response that is pro-inflammatory and is associated with worsened outcome. Increases in gut permeability allow activation of macrophages and neutrophils and upregulation of the innate immune responses. Engagement of the luminal bacteria by adherence to the gut epithelium with loss of barrier function adversely affects the acquired immune response, with stimulation and proliferation of T$_H$1 lymphocytes. Reduced contractility of the gut promotes bacterial overgrowth. Bacteria express virulence genes, which allow them to adhere to the epithelium. A contact-dependent activation of the epithelial cells results in the release of cytokines into the lymphatic channels. A gut-lung axis of inflammation is initiated, in which cytokines pass through the lymphatic channels and the thoracic duct to the systemic circulation and the capillary system of the lungs, promoting acute respiratory distress syndrome (ARDS) (Chapter 104) and pneumonia. The production of T$_H$1 cytokines stimulates the adhesion molecule E-selectin, which allows extravasation of activated neutrophils out of the vascular space and into the pulmonary alveoli. The same cytokines suppress the release of MAdCAM, which effectively traps GALT cells in the vascular space, preventing their return to the intestinal lamina propria. With the increases in gut permeability and the upregulation of immune responses, the gut becomes a pro-inflammatory organ and contributes its own component to the systemic inflammatory response syndrome (SIRS).

INITIATING ENTERAL FEEDING

In most cases, enteral access may be achieved quickly and easily by placing a nasogastric tube and initiating EN immediately after full volume resuscitation and attainment of hemodynamic stability. Although orogastric feeding may reduce the incidence of sinusitis compared with nasogastric feeding, it may be more difficult to secure a tube adequately that is protruding from the patient's mouth. Surprisingly, more than 95% of critically ill patients will tolerate gastric feeding despite risk for ileus and aspiration. Compared with small bowel feeding, gastric feeding tends to be initiated almost one full day sooner. Small bowel (postpyloric enteral) feeding quickly "catches up" such that the overall mean provision of calories and time to advancement to goal calories are the same between the two levels of feeding. Small bowel feeding does reduce the risk for aspiration but may not significantly reduce the incidence of pneumonia. Small bowel feeds are perceived to be tolerated better because residual volumes are lower compared with gastric feeding. Percutaneous access is required only in those patients anticipated to require tube feeding for longer than 4 weeks.

With initiation of feeding, it often is important to advance to goal as quickly as possible (within 24 to 36 hours).[4] For most patients, the goal of feeding is set by protein and calorie requirements. Accurate determination of caloric requirements helps avoid the danger of overfeeding. The caloric goal can be determined by weight-based equations, such as 25 kcal/kg/day, or by measuring requirements with indirect calorimetry. Protein requirements are best estimated again by weight-based equations, such as 1.2 to 1.5 g/kg/day, or by calculating nitrogen balance using measurement of urinary urea nitrogen excreted in 24 hours (protein requirement = 1 g urine urea nitrogen × 6.25 g protein/1 g N).

There are three clinical scenarios in which it may be appropriate to "permissively" underfeed the hospitalized patient. In obese critically ill patients, meeting protein requirements (estimated at 2.0 to 2.5 g/kg ideal body weight per day) while providing only 60 to 70% of caloric requirements may help mobilize fat stores while maintaining lean body mass.[5] In any patient placed on PN, providing 80% of caloric requirements over the first week of hospitalization helps avoid overfeeding, improves insulin sensitivity, and may increase the chance for an outcome benefit from the PN.[A3] In patient with ARDS, trophic feeds providing only 25% of caloric requirements over the first 6 days of hospitalization has been shown to have similar outcomes as full feeds.[A4]

However, patients at high nutritional risk should receive feeds as close to goal as possible. Nutrition risk is determined both by evidence of malnutrition (low body mass index, weight loss, or reduced nutrient intake before admission) and disease severity. Nutrition risk may be determined objectively by assessment tools such as the Nutrition Risk Score (NRS) 2002 and the Nutric Score.[6] Patients at high nutritional risk (NRS 2002 score ≥5 or Nutric Score ≥6) should receive at least 80% of goal feeds to obtain optimal benefit (and lowest mortality) from nutrition therapy.

Formula selection has been simplified with the advent of pharmaconutrient formulas. The initial decision in any critically ill patient concerns whether the individual is a candidate for an immune-modulating formula. Patients expected to benefit from an arginine-containing pharmaconutrient formula (compared with a standard formula) are those who require major elective gastrointestinal surgery (esophagectomy, gastrectomy, or pancreatectomy), patients who have experienced major trauma (with an Abdominal Trauma Index Score >20, especially with head injury), burn patients (total body surface area >30%), and patients with head and neck cancer.[A5] Critically ill patients who are septic or on mechanical ventilation have not been shown to benefit from use of an arginine-containing pharmaconutrient formula or from supplemental glutamine, omega-3 fatty acids, selenium, or antioxidants.[A6] As a result, a standard enteral formula providing 1.0 to 1.5 kcal/mL should be selected for most patients. The only other type of clinical scenario in which a specialty formula is required is when the patient demonstrates evidence of malassimilation (either maldigestion from pancreatic disease or malabsorption from compromise of small bowel absorption). In these patients, a formula composed of small peptides and medium-chain triglyceride oil or a fiber-containing formula should be initiated. Specialty formulas designed for specific organ failure are rarely indicated, owing to their increased expense and the fact that their use has not been shown to alter patient outcome.

After feeds are initiated, the clinician must assess tolerance of EN (Table 216-2). Patients should be assessed to make sure they have achieved adequate volume resuscitation before initiation. Evaluating gut motility is important in selecting the proper tube, the level of feeding within the gastrointestinal tract, and whether there is need for simultaneous gastric decompression while feeding into the small bowel. Adequate gastric contractility is indicated by a nasogastric output of less than 1200 mL/day. Small bowel contractility may be assessed by bowel distention, bowel sounds on physical examination, and air-fluid levels on abdominal radiograph. Colonic contractility is evaluated by passage of stool and flatus. In the absence of risk for ischemia (such as a patient who is hypotensive on pressor agents), ileus is not a contraindication to feeding. In fact, feeding will stimulate promotility agents such as bombesin and motilin. Clinicians should be encouraged to "feed an ileus." Rapid ramp-up in the rate of feeding is tolerated better than slow ramp-up, and enteral feeding protocols should be in place to prevent inappropriate cessation of feeding. The head of the patient's bed should be elevated 35 to 45 degrees, and oral hygiene with chlorhexidine mouthwash twice a day should be used to decrease the bacterial count in oropharyngeal secretions.

Physicians should have a low threshold for initiating prokinetic agents, should monitor laboratory tests to avoid the adverse effect of electrolyte abnormalities on motility, and in the future may use narcotic antagonists (a nonabsorbable methylnaltrexone or an intravenous μ-receptor antagonist, alvimopam) infused through the feeding tube to reverse the effects of any opioid narcotic in order to promote intestinal contractility. Promotility agents such as metoclopramide or erythromycin should be used with caution because they prolong QT intervals and thus may precipitate dysrhythmias.

Gastric residual volume (GRV) is a poor marker of gastric emptying and risk for aspiration. Raising the GRV cutoff level for cessation of feeds does not lead to increased aspiration, and lowering the number does not protect the patient from aspiration or pneumonia. Enteral feeding protocols should set the cutoff value for GRV somewhere between 400 and 500 mL, and feeds should not be stopped for the first GRV above this set point. After the first elevated GRV, the head of the bed should be elevated, the patient should be rolled over if possible into the right lateral decubitus position to promote gastric emptying, promotility agents should be considered, and the EN may be continued. In the absence of other signs of intolerance, the feedings should not be stopped for a single GRV above this cutoff point alone. Only after a second GRV is obtained above the cutoff level 4 hours later should feeds be stopped and the patient assessed further for evidence of intolerance. Eliminating use of GRV as a monitor has been shown surprisingly to increase delivery of EN without increases in aspiration, pneumonia, or any other adverse outcome.[A7]

COMPLICATIONS OF ENTERAL FEEDING

Aspiration is the most feared complication arising from provision of EN, but the ability of the clinician to monitor such events is limited. Studies using a very specific and very sensitive laboratory marker for aspiration (tracheal pepsin levels) have shown that most critically ill patients (>75%) show signs of aspiration, occurring at a frequency of 22 to 36% of bedside assessments done every 4 hours. These aspiration events are unwitnessed and unmeasurable by clinical parameters, but an increase in their frequency does correlate with increased risk for pneumonia.[7] Ironically, aspiration of bacteria-laden oropharyngeal secretions is more likely than aspiration of bacteria-laden gastric contents to cause pneumonia. Likelihood for developing pneumonia may be reduced in the high-risk patient by elevating the head of the bed, switching from bolus to continuous infusion, displacing the levels of feeds lower in the gastrointestinal tract below the ligament of Treitz, adding a prokinetic agent, initiating oral hygiene twice daily with chlorhexidine mouthwash, and adding simultaneous gastric decompression.

Tube occlusion occurs when acid from the stomach comes in contact with the formula in the tube and forms a clot. The best declogging agent is a Viokase pancreatic enzyme preparation combined with sodium bicarbonate tablets mixed in warm water. This combination is more than twice as effective as soft drinks or papain meat tenderizer. Failure to declog the tube with these agents may necessitate mechanical declogging with some kind of cytology brush, stylette, or commercial corkscrew device.

Although diarrhea is a frequent complaint in the ICU for patients on tube feeding, most cases represent low-volume incontinence. Although diarrhea in the ICU certainly creates a nursing problem, feeding does not need to be stopped. The most frequent cause of diarrhea in the ICU is the addition of sorbitol as a mixing agent for drugs infused through the feeding tube. Pseudomembranous colitis from Clostridium difficile occurs in less than 20% of patients (Chapter 296). Rarely, diarrhea is related to the osmolarity of the formula. Switching to a small peptide formula with medium-chain triglyceride oil or adding fiber to a formula often corrects the problem.

Bowel ischemia (Chapter 143) is a rare and unpredictable complication of enteral feeding. This complication is more often described in patients undergoing surgical placement of a small bowel feeding tube, but cases nonetheless have been shown to occur with nasoenteric feeding tubes. In the patient on EN who becomes hypotensive, feeds should be held if pressor therapy is being initiated, the dose of pressors are being increased, or a second or third agent is being added to the first. Feeds may be restarted in the hypotensive patient on pressor agents if they have been stable for 24 to 36 hours or the doses have already been reduced, or both. It is important to confirm adequate volume resuscitation, fiber should be avoided in these situations, and it may be safer to feed into the stomach than into the small bowel. Enteral feeding in the patient on pressor agents should be held for any sign of intolerance, such as increases in nasogastric output, sudden abdominal distention, new abdominal pain, or cessation of flatus and stool, because these may be the first signs of intestinal ischemia.

TABLE 216-2 ENTERAL NUTRITION (PROTOCOL FOR NASOGASTRIC FEEDING

1. Elevate head of bed 30 to 45 degrees at all times.
2. Scrutinize and correct electrolyte abnormalities (esp. K^+, Ca^{2+}, Mg^{2+}, and phosphorus).
3. Initiate proton pump inhibitor intravenously every 8 hours.
4. Place nasal bridle.
   - Place 12-French nasogastric tube into stomach.
   - Secure tube to bridle.
   - Confirm position by abdominal radiograph.
5. Initiate enteral nutrition (EN) feeds with small peptide/medium-chain triglycerides (MCT) oil formula full strength at 25 mL/hr.
   - Advance by 25 mL/hr every 12 hours as tolerated to goal.
   - State goal feeds: _____ kcal/day, infused at final rate _____ mL/hr.
6. Administer chlorhexidine mouthwash with good oral hygiene nursing care twice daily.
7. Check gastric residual volume (GRV) every 4 hours.
   - Return all contents <500 mL to the patient.
8. If GRV > 400 mL, initiate the following:
   - Continue EN at the current rate.
   - Turn patient to right lateral decubitus position if possible for 30 minutes.
   - Begin metoclopramide 10 mg IV every 6 hours (if patient is receiving opioid narcotics).
   - Begin naloxone, 8 mg in 10 mL saline per tube every 6 hours.
   - Recheck GRV in 4 hours.
9. Only if second GRV 4 hours later is >400 mL, hold EN.
   - Recheck GRV every 2 hours and restart EN when GRV is <400 mL.
   - If no other signs of intolerance, restart at same rate.
   - If other evidence of intolerance is present, consider reducing rate by 25 mL/hr when GRV <400 mL (or to baseline 25 mL/hr).
10. If tube in small bowel and GRV > 50 mL, recheck position of tube by abdominal radiograph. Consider switching to aspirate/feed nasojejunal tube.

One other complication that is seen even today in modern urban university-based hospitals is the *refeeding* syndrome,[8] a syndrome of sudden death associated with abrupt initiation of nutrition therapy. Potential candidates for refeeding syndrome are patients who have not been fed for more than 7 to 10 days, are already severely malnourished, require mechanical ventilation and are prone to hypercapnia, or have congestive heart failure. The mechanism of the refeeding syndrome is related to underlying cardiomyopathy and congestive heart failure, electrolyte shifts when the patient becomes anabolic, or volume overload from the feeding itself. Refeeding syndrome may be prevented by closely monitoring fluid volume, electrolytes, and caloric requirements, starting at a low rate of infusion with a mixed fuel substrate and advancing to goal slowly over 3 to 4 days.

CONCLUSION

The provision of early enteral feeding is one of the most important proactive therapeutic strategies that can favorably alter the outcome of critically ill patients through their course of hospitalization. A fairly narrow window of opportunity in time exists during which to initiate feeds in order to achieve attenuation of oxidative stress and modulate systemic immune responses. The timing, dose, and aspects of delivery of EN determine whether the patient receives the full benefit. The physiologic response seen from enteral feeding cannot be duplicated with parenteral nutrition or starvation. Instituting infusion protocols, improving clinician education (regarding issues such as ileus, GRVs, and perceived tolerance), and having the skills for deep jejunal placement of feeding tubes are all factors that promote the delivery of early EN in the ICU setting.

Grade A References

A1. Casaer MP, Mesotten D, Hermans G, et al. Early versus late parenteral nutrition in critically ill adults. *N Engl J Med.* 2011;365:506-517.

A2. Harvey SE, Parrott F, Harrison DA, et al. Trial of the route of early nutritional support in critically ill adults. *N Engl J Med.* 2014;371:1673-1684.

A3. Jiang H, Sun MW, Hefright B, et al. Efficacy of hypocaloric parenteral nutrition for surgical patients: a systematic review and meta-analysis. *Clin Nutr.* 2011;30:730-737.

A4. Rice TW, Wheeler AP, Thompson BT, et al. National Heart, Lung, and Blood Institute Acute Respiratory Distress Syndrome (ARDS) Clinical Trials Network. Initial trophic vs full enteral feeding in patients with acute lung injury: the EDEN randomized trial. *JAMA.* 2012;307:795-803.

A5. Drover JW, Dhaliwal R, Weitzel L, et al. Perioperative use of arginine-supplemented diets: a systematic review of the evidence. *J Am Coll Surg.* 2011;212:385-399.

A6. van Zanten AR, Sztark F, Kaisers UX, et al. High-protein enteral nutrition enriched with immune-modulating nutrients vs standard high-protein enteral nutrition and nosocomial infections in the ICU: a randomized clinical trial. *JAMA.* 2014;312:514-524.

A7. Reignier J, Mercier E, Le Gouge A, et al. Clinical Research in Intensive Care and Sepsis (CRICS) Group. Effect of not monitoring residual gastric volume on risk of ventilator-associated pneumonia in adults receiving mechanical ventilation and early enteral feeding: a randomized controlled trial. *JAMA.* 2013;309:249-256.

GENERAL REFERENCES

For the General References and other additional features, please visit Expert Consult at https://expertconsult.inkling.com.

217

MALNUTRITION, NUTRITIONAL ASSESSMENT, AND NUTRITIONAL SUPPORT IN ADULT HOSPITALIZED PATIENTS

THOMAS R. ZIEGLER

MALNUTRITION IN HOSPITALIZED PATIENTS

Numerous surveys conducted in developed countries in the 21st century continue to demonstrate the frequent rate of protein-energy malnutrition or depletion of specific micronutrients in patients with chronic illnesses and in those requiring elective or emergent hospital admission. Hospitalized patients commonly receive inadequate amounts of calories, protein, vitamins, and minerals during their stay, and ad libitum intake of prescribed diets is typically inadequate. Studies have shown that worsening of malnutrition during the hospital admission is common. This is a problem because adequate intake of essential macronutrients (energy, carbohydrate, protein/amino acids, and fats) and micronutrients (vitamins, minerals, and electrolytes) is critical for optimal cellular and organ structure and function, muscle mass, tissue repair, immune function, ambulatory capacity, and recovery of the patient. Significant erosion of lean body mass (predominantly derived from skeletal muscle) or deficiency of specific vitamins and minerals is variously associated with weakness and fatigue, increased rates of infection, impaired wound healing, and delayed convalescence. This relationship is especially apparent in those with chronic protein-energy malnutrition and body weight loss associated with illness (Chapters 215 and 216).

Patients with acute and chronic illnesses typically have experienced several days to several weeks or months of continuous or intermittent decreased food intake because of anorexia, gastrointestinal symptoms, depression or anxiety, and other medical factors. They may also have had food intake restricted because of surgical operations or diagnostic or therapeutic procedures and recovery from these. Some patients have abnormal nutrient losses due to diarrhea (e.g., with chronic malabsorptive and maldigestive disorders or infectious diarrhea), vomiting, polyuria (as in uncontrolled diabetes mellitus), wound drainage, dialysis, and other causes. Certain drugs, including corticosteroids, chemotherapeutic agents, antirejection drugs, and diuretics, are associated with skeletal muscle breakdown, gastrointestinal injury, and electrolyte or water-soluble vitamin losses, respectively. Bedrest or markedly decreased ambulation is common in outpatient and inpatient settings and in turn associated with skeletal muscle wasting and impaired protein synthesis. Catabolic and critical illnesses are associated with concomitantly increased blood concentrations of "counter-regulatory" hormones derived from the adrenal glands and pancreas (e.g., cortisol, catecholamines, glucagon); release of proinflammatory cytokines from stimulated immune, endothelial, and epithelial cells (interleukins 1, 6, and 8 and tumor necrosis factor-α); and peripheral tissue resistance to anabolic hormones (insulin and insulin-like growth factor-I). These hormonal and cytokine alterations serve to increase the availability of endogenous metabolic substrates critical for cellular and organ function, wound healing, and host survival (e.g., glucose through glycogenolysis and gluconeogenesis, amino acids through skeletal muscle breakdown, and free fatty acids through lipolysis). This combination of decreased nutrient intake and increased tissue nutrient losses, coupled with increased energy (calorie), protein, and micronutrient needs due to inflammation, infection, and cytokinemia, is responsible for the wasting and micronutrient depletion common in medical patients with acute and chronic illness. Common causes of protein-energy malnutrition and micronutrient depletion in medical patients are shown in Table 217-1. Obesity has become a widespread medical problem and is a form of malnutrition but is considered in detail elsewhere (Chapter 220).

NUTRITIONAL ASSESSMENT

Serial assessment of nutritional status is a critically important component of routine medical care (Chapter 214). The major objectives are to detect preexisting depletion of body protein, energy reserves, and micronutrients; to identify risk factors for malnutrition (see Table 217-1); and to take steps to prevent nutrient deficiencies, depletion of lean body mass, and loss of skeletal muscle. Unfortunately, there are still no practical "gold standard" tests that can be used as an index of general nutritional status. Blood concentrations of specific micronutrients (e.g., copper, zinc, thiamine, 25-hydroxyvitamin D, vitamin B_6, folate, vitamin B_{12}) and electrolytes (e.g., magnesium, potassium, phosphorus) are important to guide needs and repletion responses. Nutritional assessment (Chapter 214) involves an integration of multiple factors: medical and surgical history; type and severity of the acute or chronic underlying illness and anticipated medical and surgical course; fluid drainage sites and amounts; physical examination findings; history of body weight change (degree and temporal aspects); dietary intake pattern; use of nutritional supplements, including prior administration of specialized enteral nutrition (EN) or parenteral nutrition (PN); evaluation of current organ function and fluid status; and determination of selected vitamin, mineral, and electrolyte concentrations in blood. In the intensive care unit (ICU) setting, measured body weight typically reflects recent intravenous fluid administration and is typically much higher than recent "dry" or preoperative body weight, which is the best parameter to use.

TABLE 217-1	COMMON CAUSES OF PROTEIN-ENERGY MALNUTRITION AND MICRONUTRIENT DEPLETION IN MEDICAL PATIENTS WITH ACUTE OR CHRONIC ILLNESSES

- Decreased spontaneous food intake due to anorexia from chronic or acute illness, gastrointestinal symptoms (e.g., nausea, vomiting, abdominal pain), depression/anxiety
- Restricted food intake required for surgical operations or diagnostic/therapeutic procedures and gastrointestinal dysfunction that follows these
- Abnormal macronutrient and micronutrient losses from the body due to malabsorption (e.g., celiac sprue, short-gut syndrome, inflammatory bowel disease, cystic fibrosis, diarrhea), maldigestion (e.g., pancreatitis), emesis, polyuria (e.g., in diabetes), wound drainage, or renal replacement therapy
- Periods of increased energy expenditure (calorie needs), protein requirements, and micronutrient needs (e.g., critical illness, increased inflammation)
- Catabolic effects of counter-regulatory hormones (e.g., cortisol, catecholamines, glucagon), release of proinflammatory cytokines from stimulated immune cells and endothelial and epithelial cells (interleukins 1, 6, and 8 and tumor necrosis factor-α), and peripheral tissue resistance to the anabolic hormones insulin and insulin-like growth factor-I
- Bedrest, decreased ambulation, and chemical paralysis during mechanical ventilation (skeletal muscle wasting due to impaired protein synthesis)
- Administration of drugs that induce skeletal muscle breakdown, gastrointestinal injury, or electrolyte and water-soluble vitamin losses (e.g., corticosteroids, chemotherapeutic agents, diuretics, and antirejection regimens)
- Socioeconomic deprivation, inadequate caregivers, ambulation difficulties in the home setting
- Inadequate provision of calories, protein, and essential micronutrients (vitamins, minerals, and trace elements) during hospitalization

TABLE 217-2	CLINICAL MANIFESTATIONS OF SPECIFIC NUTRIENT DEFICIENCIES

PHYSICAL EXAMINATION SIGN OR SYMPTOM OF NUTRIENT DEPLETION	SPECIFIC NUTRIENT DEPLETED
Muscle and fat wasting, weakness	Calories, protein, combined calories and protein
Anorexia	Calories, protein
Glossitis (discolored, smooth, painful tongue)	Folate, vitamin B_{12}, niacin, riboflavin, thiamine, iron
Cheilosis, angular stomatitis	Riboflavin, niacin, folate, vitamin B_{12}
Symmetrical motor or sensory dysfunction, ataxia, nystagmus, heart failure, mental status changes or confusion	Thiamine (beriberi)
Peripheral edema	Thiamine (heart failure), protein (low oncotic pressure)
Loss of vibratory or position sense, fatigue	Vitamin B_{12}
Dermatitis (sun-exposed skin), diarrhea, dementia	Niacin (pellagra)
Bleeding gums, petechiae, ecchymosis	Vitamins C and K
Poor wound healing	Calories, protein, calories and protein, vitamin C, vitamin A, zinc, others
Bone pain	Vitamin D (osteomalacia)
Follicular hyperkeratosis, night blindness, Bitot's spots	Vitamin A
Flaky, whitish dermatitis	Essential fatty acid (linoleic, α-linolenic)
Hair sparse or easily pluckable	Zinc, protein
Pale skin, nail spooning (koilonychia)	Iron
Loss of taste; reddish dermatitis around nose, mouth, groin; hair loss	Zinc
Peripheral neuropathies, gait abnormalities, weakness, fatigue	Copper
Muscle pain, heart failure	Selenium
Paresthesias, carpal pedal spasm	Calcium, magnesium, phosphorus, or potassium

Note: Typically severe deficiency of specific nutrients (with depletion of initially tissue and later blood concentrations) has occurred before physical manifestations of deficiency.

Integration of the factors provides important information on whether patients are likely to be adequately nourished; to have mild, moderate, or severe protein-energy malnutrition; or to have depletion or deficiency of specific vitamins, minerals, or electrolytes. Patients with an involuntary body weight loss of 5 to 10% or more of their usual body weight in the previous few weeks or months, those weighing less than 90% of their ideal body weight, or those who have a body mass index less than 18.5 kg/m^2 should be carefully evaluated as these individuals are likely to be malnourished.

In hospitalized patients, especially those in the ICU, circulating concentrations of proteins (e.g., albumin, prealbumin) are generally low and not useful as protein nutritional status biomarkers, given their lack of specificity. Plasma concentrations of albumin and prealbumin typically fall during active inflammation or infection, in critical illness, and after traumatic injury (deceased synthesis by liver, catabolism of blood proteins) and are markedly affected by non-nutritional factors, including fluid status, capillary leak, decreased hepatic synthesis, and increased clearance from blood. Because of the long circulating half-life of albumin (18 to 21 days), concentrations in blood remain low despite adequate feeding and are slow to respond to nutritional repletion, irrespective of the other confounding factors noted before. Prealbumin has a much shorter circulating half-life than albumin (several days), and serial blood levels can be used as a general indicator of protein status in clinically stable outpatients. Table 217-2 illustrates physical examination findings that may be observed in association with depletion of specific nutrients.

Energy requirements can be estimated by standard equations, such as the Harris-Benedict equation, which incorporate the patient's age, gender, weight, and height to determine basal energy expenditure (BEE). Physical activity and the thermic effect of macronutrient administration can be added to the BEE to arrive at the energy prescription to maintain current body weight; this is estimated for most hospital patients and outpatients as 1.2 to 1.3 times BEE, unless the patient is sedated or at bedrest (common in the ICU), which decreases energy needs. The estimated maintenance energy requirement is approximately 1.3 times BEE in ambulatory subjects. Lower amounts of calories are now typically given in ICU patients (see later). Data obtained from a bedside metabolic cart machine (indirect calorimeter), which measures expired breath to determine oxygen consumption and carbon dioxide production, provide accurate actual energy expenditure in most settings and can be useful. A simple and relatively accurate method to estimate energy needs is simply to use 20 to 25 kcal/kg/day actual dry or ideal body weight in most patients. This assumes that the body weight used does not reflect intravenous fluid administration or capillary leak syndromes

(see earlier). In ICU patients, even lower calorie doses (equivalent to 15 to 20 kcal/kg dry weight/day) have been advocated by some on the basis of known complications of overfeeding (see later) and limited clinical outcome data as a function of energy dose. In clinically stable, malnourished, non-ICU patients who require nutritional repletion, higher doses of calories (up to 35 kcal/kg/day) appear to be generally well tolerated, as long as refeeding syndrome is avoided (see later). In obese subjects (defined for these calculations as >20 to 25% above ideal body weight), adjusted body weight should be used in the calculation of energy and protein needs by the following equation:

Adjusted body weight = current weight − ideal body weight (from standard tables or equations) × 0.25 + ideal body weight

Guidelines for protein/amino acid administration are given in Table 217-3. Studies in nonburned ICU patients indicate that protein loads of more than 2.0 g/kg/day are not efficiently used for protein synthesis and the excess may be oxidized and contribute to azotemia. In most catabolic patients requiring specialized feeding, a generally recommended protein dose is 1.5 g/kg/day in individuals with normal renal function. This is about twice the recommended dietary allowance for healthy adults of 0.8 g/kg/day. The administered protein dose should be adjusted downward as a function of the degree and tempo of azotemia (in the absence of dialysis therapy) and hyperbilirubinemia (see Table 217-3). This strategy takes into account the relative inability of catabolic patients to efficiently use exogenous nutrients and the knowledge that most protein and lean tissue repletion occurs in a period of several weeks to months during post-hospital convalescence. Adequate

TABLE 217-3 ESTIMATION OF PROTEIN/AMINO ACID REQUIREMENTS IN ADULT PATIENTS

CLINICAL CONDITION	PROTEIN/AMINO ACID DOSE (g/kg/day)*,†
Well nourished with acute illness	1.2-1.5
Malnourished or severe catabolic stress	1.5-2.0
Postoperative	1.2-1.5
Acute hepatic failure	0.6-1.2
Encephalopathy	0-0.6
Acute renal failure, not receiving renal replacement therapy	0.6-1.0
Renal failure, receiving renal replacement therapy	1.2-2.5

*Oral/enteral nutrient supplements and tube feedings contain either intact or partially hydrolyzed high-quality protein (typically casein, soy, or whey). Parenteral nutrition solutions for peripheral or central vein administration provide known essential L-amino acids combined with several nonessential amino acids. These may be limiting in certain conditionally essential amino acids (e.g., cysteine, taurine) in some clinical conditions.
†Limited data from randomized controlled trials on optimal protein/amino acid dosing in hospitalized patients are available.

TABLE 217-4 SOME CLINICAL INDICATIONS FOR SPECIALIZED ORAL/ENTERAL OR PARENTERAL NUTRITION SUPPORT

- Patient currently exhibits moderate to severe protein or protein-energy malnutrition or has evidence of specific deficiency of one or more essential micronutrients
- Patient with involuntary body weight loss of 5-10% or more of usual body weight in the previous few weeks or months, who weighs <90% of ideal body weight, or who has BMI <18.5 kg/m².
- Dietary food intake in hospital or outpatient setting likely to be <50% of needs for more than 5-10 days because of underlying illness
- Patient with severe catabolic stress (e.g., ICU care, serious infection) and adequate nutrient intake unlikely for >3-5 days
- After major gastrointestinal surgery or other major operations (e.g., hip replacement, partial organ resection)
- Medical illness associated with prolonged (>5-10 days) gastrointestinal dysfunction (diarrhea, nausea/vomiting, gastrointestinal bleeding, severe ileus, partial obstruction) or short-bowel syndrome, chronic/severe diarrhea, or other malabsorptive disorders
- Clinical settings in which adequate oral food intake may be contraindicated or otherwise significantly decreased, such as respiratory or other acute or severe organ failure, dementia, dysphagia, chemotherapy/irradiation, inflammatory bowel disease, pancreatitis, high-output enterocutaneous fistula, alcoholism, drug addiction
- Chronic obstructive lung disease, chronic infection, and other chronic inflammatory or catabolic disorders with documented poor nutrient intake or recent weight loss

BMI = body mass index; ICU = intensive care unit.

nonprotein energy is essential to allow amino acids to be effectively used for protein synthesis and to not be oxidized for energy (adenosine triphosphate) production. The nonprotein calorie-to-nitrogen ratio used in most centers now typically ranges from 75 : 1 to 125 : 1 (nitrogen = protein/6.25; thus, 75 to 125 nonprotein kilocalories for each 6.25 g of protein or amino acid administered). Highly catabolic patients in the ICU are typically given protein loads at the lower end of this range, assuming near-normal renal and hepatic function.

NUTRITIONAL SUPPORT

Table 217-4 lists common clinical scenarios in which specialized oral/EN or PN support may be indicated. In these settings, consultation with a multidisciplinary nutrition support team, if one is available, has been shown to reduce complications and costs and to increase the appropriate use of EN and PN in both academic and community medical centers.[1]

Oral nutrition supplementation includes provision of balanced oral diets of usual foods supplemented with complete liquid (or solid) nutrient products, protein supplements (e.g., hydrolyzed whey or casein powder that can be mixed with dietary beverages), high-potency multivitamin-mineral supplements, and specific micronutrients required to treat a diagnosed deficiency (e.g., zinc, copper, vitamin B_6, vitamin B_{12}, and vitamin D). Special supplements designed for patients with chronic renal failure featuring concentrated calories and low amounts of protein and electrolytes are available, as are a variety of formulations designed for other specific disease categories (see later). Several studies show that convalescence is enhanced with addition of one or two cans per day of complete liquid nutrient supplements to meals after stresses such as total hip replacement and gastrointestinal surgery. These provide calories, carbohydrate, high-quality protein, fat, and micronutrients; they are lactose and gluten free and may contain small peptides and medium-chain triglycerides to facilitate amino acid and fat absorption, respectively. Some formulations also contain soluble fiber or prebiotics (e.g., fructo-oligosaccharides) designed to decrease diarrhea. For patients who can tolerate oral medications, it is probably prudent to prescribe a potent oral multivitamin-mineral preparation, at least for several months, especially for those who either exhibit or are at risk for micronutrient depletion.

Administration of Enteral Tube Feeding

Patients with conditions outlined in Table 217-4 may have a functional gastrointestinal tract but may be unable to consume an adequate diet orally because of medical or surgical conditions (e.g., mechanically ventilated patients; those with pancreatitis, dementia, or dysphagia; and after trauma or burns). Although PN is commonly administered in these settings, this practice is not evidence based; academic guidelines strongly suggest that oral nutritional supplements or enteral tube feedings be used if specialized nutrition support is indicated in patients with a functional gastrointestinal tract ("if the gut works, use it"). On an individualized basis, aggressive nutrition support, including placement of feeding tubes, may not be desired by a competent patient or legally authorized representatives, such as in premorbid

states or terminal illness. In these cases, full discussion with the patient and family or representatives is required with regard to the plan for EN.

Detailed discussion of EN and enteral tube feeding is provided in Chapter 216.

Administration of Parenteral Nutrition

PN support includes administration of standard complete nutrient mixtures, which contain dextrose, L-amino acids, lipid emulsion, electrolytes, vitamins, and minerals (and certain medications as indicated, such as insulin or octreotide), given through either a peripheral or central vein. PN technically also includes parenteral administration of specific micronutrients or micronutrient combinations to replete a deficiency (e.g., thiamine, copper, electrolytes). Administration of complete PN therapy in patients with gastrointestinal tract dysfunction has become a standard of care in most hospitals and ICUs throughout the world, although use in individual institutions varies widely.[2,3] PN is life-saving in patients with intestinal failure (e.g., short-bowel syndrome); unfortunately, in patient subgroups with lesser degrees of intestinal failure, few objective data from properly designed, large, randomized controlled studies are available to determine the true efficacy of and optimal indications for PN.[4] The use of PN in ICUs in the United States declined during the past decade, with EN increasing coincidentally during the same time.[5]

Existing data indicate that PN does benefit patients with preexisting moderate to severe malnutrition or with critical illness by decreasing overall morbidity and possibly mortality compared with patients receiving inadequate EN or hydration (intravenous dextrose) therapy alone. An earlier meta-analysis of well-designed, intent-to-treat, randomized controlled trials in adult ICU patients showed that early PN and early EN (each started within 24 hours of ICU admission) were equivalent in terms of mortality, but PN was associated with decreased mortality compared with ICU patients who received delayed enteral feeding (begun >24 hours after admission).[A1] In this and earlier trials, however, PN use was associated with a higher rate of infection compared with enterally fed patients. Randomized controlled trials suggest that patient subtype and ability to tolerate EN can influence the clinical effects of different strategies for the timing of initiation of PN in critical illness. A consensus based on recent rigorous studies in critical illness is emerging that early PN is no better than early EN.[A2] PN should probably not be initiated until day 3 or 4 after ICU admission in patients unable to tolerate adequate EN.[A3][A4] The provision of early PN to critically ill adults with relative contraindications to early EN, compared with standard care, was recently found not to result in a difference in mortality at 60 days, fewer days of ventilation, or significantly shorter ICU stay or hospital days.[A5]

The basic principle in considering PN therapy is that the patient must be unable to achieve adequate nutrient intake by the enteral route. Compared with PN, EN is less expensive, probably maintains intestinal mucosal structure and function to a greater extent, is safer in terms of mechanical and metabolic complications (see later), and is associated with reduced rates of nosocomial infections. Thus, the enteral route of feeding should be used and advanced whenever possible and the amount of administered PN correspondingly reduced. Generally recognized indications for PN include the following:

- Patients with short-bowel syndrome or other conditions causing intestinal failure that prohibit adequate intake or absorption of enteral nutrients (e.g., motility disorders, obstruction, severe ileus, severe inflammatory bowel disease), especially in those with preexisting malnutrition
- Clinically stable patients in whom adequate enteral feeding (e.g., >50% of needs) is unlikely for 7 to 10 days because of any underlying illness
- Patients with severe catabolic stress requiring ICU care in whom adequate enteral nutrient intake is unlikely for more than 3 to 5 days

There is no reason to withhold PN in hospital patients for any time if they exhibit preexisting moderate to severe malnutrition and are deemed to be unlikely to meet their needs by the oral or enteral route.

Generally accepted contraindications to PN (that are largely not evidence based) include the following:

- The gastrointestinal tract is functional and access for enteral feeding is available
- PN is thought to be required for 5 days or less
- The patient cannot tolerate the extra intravenous fluid required for PN or has severe hyperglycemia or electrolyte abnormalities on the planned day of PN initiation
- The patient has uncontrolled blood stream infection or severe hemodynamic instability
- New placement of an intravenous line solely for PN poses undue risks on the basis of clinical judgment
- On an individualized basis when aggressive nutrition support is not desired by the competent patient or legally authorized representatives, such as in premorbid patients or those with terminal illness (full discussion with the patient and family or representatives is required)

PN can be delivered as either peripheral vein solutions or central vein solutions through percutaneous subclavian vein or internal jugular vein catheters for infusion into the superior vena cava (nontunneled in the hospital setting), subcutaneously tunneled central venous catheters (e.g., Hickman catheters) or central venous ports (for chronic home PN therapy), or peripherally inserted central venous catheters (PICC). Although data are limited, it is clearly preferable to manage patients requiring long-term central venous PN at home with a tunneled central venous catheter compared with a PICC line because of the higher rate of local complications (e.g., phlebitis, catheter breakage) and possibly catheter-associated infections with PICC lines.

A comparison of typical fluid, macronutrient, and micronutrient content of peripheral and central vein PN is shown in Table 217-5. To diminish the risk of phlebitis, typical peripheral vein PN solutions provide low concentrations of dextrose (5%; provides 3.4 kcal/g) and amino acids (<3.5 %; provides 4 kcal/g), with a large proportion of energy administration as fat emulsion (50 to 60% of total calories). Because fluid restriction or organ dysfunction often precludes use of large fluid volumes for PN, peripheral vein PN is generally not indicated in ICU patients or in patients with fluid overload or renal, hepatic, or cardiac failure. These solutions are most useful in stable patients who can tolerate the large fluid volumes required to meet amino acid and energy goals (usually 2.5 to 3 L/day) without providing excessive lipid.

Intravenous lipid emulsions (typically added to PN as a 20% soybean oil–based solution in the United States) provide both essential linoleic and α-linolenic fatty acids and energy (10 kcal/g); these are generally infused during a 24-hour period in the complete PN administration bag. The maximal recommended rate of fat emulsion infusion is approximately 1.0 g/kg/day. Most patients clear triglyceride from intravenous fat emulsion well from plasma. In some studies, larger doses of soybean oil–based fat emulsion were associated with proinflammatory and pro-oxidative effects and possibly immune suppression, presumably due to the high amount of omega-6 fatty acids derived from the linoleic fatty acid component. This has led to the approval and clinical availability of intravenous fish oil, olive oil/soybean oil, medium-chain triglyceride/soybean oil, and combinations of these formulations in Europe and other non-U.S. countries. An intravenous lipid emulsion of 80% olive oil/20% soybean oil was recently approved for use in adult PN

TABLE 217-5 COMPOSITION OF TYPICAL PARENTERAL NUTRITION SOLUTIONS

COMPONENT*	PERIPHERAL PN	CENTRAL PN
Volume (L/day)	2-3	1-1.5
Dextrose (%)	5	10-25
Amino acids (%)[†]	2.5-3.5	3-8
Lipid (%)[‡]	3.5-5.0	2.5-5.0
Sodium (mEq/L)	50-150	50-150
Potassium (mEq/L)	20-35	30-50
Phosphorus (mmol/L)	5-10	10-30
Magnesium (mEq/L)	8-10	10-20
Calcium (mEq/L)	2.5-5	2.5-5
Trace elements[§]		
Vitamins[§]		

*Electrolytes in parenteral nutrition (PN) are adjusted as indicated to maintain serially measured serum levels within the normal range. The percentage of sodium and potassium salts as chloride is increased to correct metabolic alkalosis, and the percentage of salts as acetate is increased to correct metabolic acidosis. Regular insulin is added to PN as needed to achieve blood glucose goals (separate intravenous insulin infusions are commonly required with hyperglycemia in intensive care unit settings).
[†]Provides all essential amino acids and several nonessential amino acids. Dose of amino acids is adjusted downward or upward to goal as a function of the degree of azotemia or hyperbilirubinemia in patients with renal and hepatic failure, respectively.
[‡]Lipid is given as soybean oil– or olive oil/soybean oil–based fat emulsion in the United States, Europe, and other non-U.S. countries; intravenous fish oil, olive oil, medium-chain triglycerides, and combinations of these are available for use in PN. Lipid is typically mixed with dextrose and amino acids in the same PN infusion bag ("all-in-one" solution).
[§]Trace elements added on a daily basis to peripheral vein and central vein PN are mixtures of chromium, copper, manganese, selenium, and zinc (can also be supplemented individually).
[§]Vitamins added on a daily basis to peripheral vein and central vein PN are mixtures of vitamins A, B_1 (thiamine), B_2 (riboflavin), B_3 (niacinamide), B_6 (pyridoxine), B_{12}, C, D, and E and biotin, folate, and pantothenic acid. Vitamin K is added on an individual basis (e.g., in patients with cirrhosis). Specific vitamins can also be supplemented individually.

in the United States. It is important to monitor blood triglyceride levels at baseline and then approximately weekly and as indicated to assess clearance of intravenous fat. Triglyceride levels should be maintained below 400 mg/dL to decrease the risk of pancreatitis or diminished pulmonary diffusion capacity in patients with severe chronic obstructive lung disease.

Central venous administration of PN allows higher concentrations of dextrose (3.4 kcal/g) and amino acids (4 kcal/g) to be delivered as hypertonic solutions, and thus lower amounts of fat emulsion are needed to reach calorie goals (see Table 217-5). Requirements for potassium, magnesium, and phosphorus are typically higher with central vein PN compared with peripheral vein PN because of the increased dextrose provided by insulin-mediated intracellular electrolyte shifts, use in anabolic pathways, glucose metabolism, and adenosine triphosphate production. The higher concentrations of dextrose and amino acids possible allow most patients to achieve calorie and amino acid goals with only 1 to 1.5 L/day of PN. In central vein PN, initial orders typically provide 60 to 70% of non–amino acid calories as dextrose and 30 to 40% of non–amino acid calories as fat emulsion. These percentages are adjusted as indicated on the basis of blood glucose and triglyceride levels, respectively. The dextrose amount in central vein PN should be reduced or regular insulin added to the PN bag to maintain blood glucose concentration within the desired range. Separate intravenous insulin infusions should usually be used in the ICU when patients receiving central vein PN develop hyperglycemia.[6]

Specific requirements for intravenous trace elements and vitamins have not been rigorously defined for patient subgroups, and therapy is directed at meeting published recommended doses that maintain blood levels in the normal range in most stable patients with standardized intravenous preparations (see Table 217-5). Several studies have shown that a significant proportion of ICU patients have low zinc, selenium, vitamin C, vitamin E, and vitamin D levels despite receiving specialized PN (or EN). Depletion of these essential nutrients may in turn impair antioxidant capacity, immunity, wound healing, and other important body functions. For example, zinc is known to be important for immune function, wound healing, protein synthesis, and gastrointestinal mucosal regeneration. Zinc (and other micronutrients, such as copper) should probably be increased in the PN of patients with burns, large wounds, significant gastrointestinal fluid losses, and other conditions if serum concentrations indicate low levels. This practical recommendation is not evidence based, however, because recent rigorous randomized trials in ICU patients administered large doses of selenium could not reproduce the positive clinical benefits observed in earlier smaller studies, and studies of zinc supplementation in the ICU setting have been inconclusive. Recent data suggest that thiamine depletion is not uncommon in patients receiving chronic diuretic therapy or in those with severe malabsorption.

Complications of Parenteral Nutrition

The most common complication of peripheral vein PN is local phlebitis due to the catheter. Alterations in blood electrolytes can be treated with adjustment of concentration in the peripheral PN prescription. Hypertriglyceridemia typically responds well to lowering of the total PN lipid dose. Central vein PN is associated with a much higher rate of mechanical, metabolic, and infectious complications than peripheral vein PN. Mechanical complications include those related to insertion of the central venous catheter (e.g., pneumothorax, hemothorax, malposition of the catheter, and thrombosis). Infectious complications include catheter-related blood stream infections and non–catheter-related infections by bacteria and fungal species that may in some cases be due to endogenous bacterial translocation from the gut lumen. The risk for these infections appears to be increased with use of non–subclavian vein central venous access (e.g., jugular, femoral veins) and multiple-use catheters with non-dedicated PN infusion ports used for additional purposes, such as blood drawing or medication administration. Poorly controlled blood glucose concentration (>140-180 mg/dL) is not uncommon in patients requiring central vein PN and is associated with an increased risk of nosocomial infection. Risk factors for hyperglycemia include poorly controlled blood glucose concentration at PN initiation; use of high dextrose concentrations (>10%) in the initial few days of PN administration or too rapid an increase in total dextrose load; insufficient exogenous insulin administration; inadequate monitoring of blood glucose responses to central vein PN administration; and administration of corticosteroids and vasopressor agents such as norepinephrine, which stimulate gluconeogenesis and cause insulin resistance.

Recent data also suggest that inadequate or no provision of the amino acid glutamine may increase infection risk in patients requiring PN. This amino acid appears to be conditionally essential in catabolic states and serves as an important fuel for immune cells and cells of the gut mucosa, among other potentially beneficial functions. A large number of animal studies and several human trials show that supplementation of glutamine in EN and PN enhances immunity, decreases hospital infections, and maintains indices of gut barrier function. Several expert panels now recommend that glutamine be routinely added to the PN in ICU patients, but this practice remains controversial because some studies show no benefit (or even harm) in certain patient subgroups, and an improvement in hospital mortality has not been documented.

Studies of nutrient use efficiency and metabolic complications in severely catabolic patients suggest that lower amounts of total energy and amino acid/protein should be administered than were routinely given in the past, particularly in unstable and ICU patients. High calorie, carbohydrate, amino acid, and fat loads (hyperalimentation) are easily administered by central vein PN but, if ordered by physicians, can induce severe metabolic complications, including carbon dioxide overproduction, azotemia, hyperglycemia, electrolyte alterations, and hepatic steatosis and injury (Table 217-6). Dextrose and lipid doses in PN should be advanced during several days after initiation; blood glucose concentration, electrolyte values, triglyceride levels, organ function test results, intake and output measurements, and the clinical course must be closely monitored.

Refeeding syndrome[7] with central vein PN administration is relatively common in patients at risk, including those with preexisting malnutrition, electrolyte depletion, or alcoholism, and after prolonged periods of intravenous hydration therapy (e.g., 5% dextrose) without nutrition support, all of which are common in hospitalized patients. Refeeding syndrome is mediated by administration of excessive intravenous dextrose (>150-250 g, such as given in 1 L of PN with 15-25% dextrose). This, in turn, markedly stimulates insulin release, which rapidly lowers blood potassium, magnesium, and especially phosphorus concentrations because of intracellular shift and use in carbohydrate metabolic pathways. Administration of high doses of carbohydrate also consumes thiamine, which is required as a cofactor for carbohy-

TABLE 217-6   SOME COMMON METABOLIC COMPLICATIONS OF PARENTERAL NUTRITION

PN ORDER PROBLEM	METABOLIC OR CLINICAL CONSEQUENCE
Excess kcal, CHO, fat	Abnormal liver function test results, hepatic steatosis
Excess CHO	Hypercapnia
Excess fluid, kcal, CHO, fat	Respiratory insufficiency
Excess amino acids	Azotemia
Excess sodium and fluid	Sodium and fluid retention
Excess CHO; inadequate insulin	Hyperglycemia-mediated immune cell dysfunction, infection
Inadequate or excessive electrolytes	Abnormal blood electrolyte levels
Excess fluid, kcal, sodium, CHO; inadequate electrolytes	Cardiac failure, arrhythmias
Excess CHO; inadequate electrolytes, thiamine	Refeeding syndrome

CHO = carbohydrate; kcal = calories; PN = parenteral nutrition.

drate metabolism and can precipitate symptoms of thiamine deficiency (see Table 217-2), especially in patients with poor thiamine nutrition at baseline. Hyperinsulinemia also tends to cause sodium and fluid retention at the level of the kidney. Together, fluid and sodium retention, the drop in blood electrolyte levels (which can cause arrhythmias), and hypermetabolism due to excessive calorie provision can result in heart failure, especially in patients with preexisting heart disease, as well as cardiac muscle atrophy due to prolonged protein-energy malnutrition. Prevention of refeeding syndrome requires vigilance to identify patients at risk; use of initially low PN dextrose concentrations; and empirical provision of higher doses of potassium, magnesium, and phosphorus based on current blood levels and renal function and supplemental thiamine (100 mg/day for 3 to 5 days).

For patients in whom home PN is indicated, primary physicians should consult with social service professionals to identify appropriate home care companies and nutrition support professionals to assess intravenous line access, metabolic status, and the home PN order and to arrange for follow-up care and monitoring of PN. It is important not to arrange for hasty hospital discharge in patients newly started on PN; obtaining appropriate venous access and monitoring of fluid and electrolyte status during a 2- to 3-day period are important aspects of care for most patients started on PN and imperative in those with severe malnutrition and those at risk for refeeding syndrome.

Grade A References

A1. Simpson F, Doig GS. Parenteral versus enteral nutrition in the critically ill patient: a meta-analysis of trials using the intention to treat principle. *Intensive Care Med.* 2005;31:12-23.
A2. Harvey SE, Parrott F, Harrison DA, et al. Trial of the route of early nutritional support in critically ill adults. *N Engl J Med.* 2014;371:1673-1684.
A3. Heidegger CP, Berger MM, Graf S, et al. Optimisation of energy provision with supplemental parenteral nutrition in critically ill patients: a randomised controlled clinical trial. *Lancet.* 2013;381:385-393.
A4. Casaer MP, Mesotten D, Hermans G, et al. Early versus late parenteral nutrition in critically ill adults. *N Engl J Med.* 2011;365:506-517.
A5. Doig GS, Simpson F, Sweetman EA, et al. Early parenteral nutrition in critically ill patients with short-term relative contraindications to early enteral nutrition: a randomized controlled trial. *JAMA.* 2013;309:2130-2138.
A6. Tao KM, Li XQ, Yang LQ, et al. Glutamine supplementation for critically ill adults. *Cochrane Database Syst Rev.* 2014;9:CD010050.

GENERAL REFERENCES

For the General References and other additional features, please visit Expert Consult at https://expertconsult.inkling.com.

218

VITAMINS, TRACE MINERALS, AND OTHER MICRONUTRIENTS

JOEL B. MASON

● MICRONUTRIENTS IN NUTRITIONAL SCIENCE

Dietary Requirements

Micronutrients are a diverse array of dietary components necessary to sustain health. The physiologic roles of micronutrients are as varied as their composition. Some micronutrients are used in enzymes as either coenzymes or prosthetic groups, others as biochemical substrates or hormones; in some instances, the functions are not well defined. Under normal circumstances, the average daily dietary intake for each micronutrient that is required to sustain normal physiologic functions is measured in milligrams or smaller quantities. In this manner, micronutrients are distinguished from macronutrients, which encompass carbohydrates, fats, and proteins as well as the macrominerals calcium, magnesium, and phosphorus.

Optimal Intake

For orderly homeostasis to proceed, most dietary nutrients must be ingested in quantities that are neither too small nor too great. Disorders may arise, therefore, when intake regularly falls outside of this physiologic window. The size of this physiologic window varies for each micronutrient and should be kept in mind, particularly in this era when the administration of large quantities of certain micronutrients is increasingly explored for possible therapeutic implications. The dietary requirement for a particular micronutrient is determined by many factors, only one of which is the amount needed to sustain those physiologic functions for which it is used (Table 218-1). The U.S. Institute of Medicine Food and Nutrition Board regularly updates dietary guidelines that define the quantity of each micronutrient that is "adequate to meet the known nutrient needs of practically all healthy persons." These *recommended dietary allowances* (RDAs) were most recently revised between 1998 and 2001, and the values for adults appear in Tables 218-2 and 218-3. Also established for the first time for each micronutrient were *tolerable upper limits* (TULs), which are the "maximal daily levels of oral intake likely to pose no adverse health risks." *Adequate intake,* the amount necessary to prevent a deficiency state, is not necessarily synonymous with *optimal intake.*

● TYPES AND FUNCTION OF MICRONUTRIENTS

Vitamins

Vitamins are categorized as either fat soluble (A, D, E, K) or water soluble (all the others), as shown in Table 218-2. This categorization remains physiologically meaningful. None of the fat-soluble vitamins appears to serve as a coenzyme. Intestinal absorption of the fat-soluble vitamins is primarily

through a micellar phase, and pathophysiologic conditions associated with fat malabsorption frequently are associated with selective deficiencies of the fat-soluble vitamins. In contrast, most of the functions of the water-soluble vitamins are as coenzymes, and they are not absorbed through the lipophilic phase in the intestine.

Trace Elements

Fifteen trace elements have been identified as essential for health: iron, zinc, copper, chromium, selenium, iodine, fluorine, manganese, molybdenum, cobalt, nickel, tin, silicon, vanadium, and arsenic (see Table 218-3), but only for the first 10 of these has compelling evidence indicated that they are essential nutrients in humans. Cobalt appears to be essential solely as a component of vitamin B_{12}, but an isolated deficiency state has never been described. Deficiency syndromes for several of the essential trace elements were not recognized until recently because of their exceedingly small requirements and because of the ubiquitous nature of these elements in foodstuffs. Only under exceptional circumstances, such as long-term reliance on total parenteral nutrition lacking these elements, have some of the deficiency syndromes been observed.

The biochemical functions of trace elements appear to be as components of prosthetic groups or as cofactors for enzymes. Determination of essential trace element status is problematic with the exception of iron. The low concentrations of these elements in body fluids and tissues, the finding that blood levels frequently do not correlate well with levels in the target tissues, and the fact that functional tests cannot be devised until their biochemical functions are better understood preclude an accurate laboratory method of assessing the adequacy of most trace elements.

Additional Compounds with Nutritional Relevance

Evidence indicates that humans also have an absolute requirement for the dietary component choline, which is a necessary precursor for acetylcholine and phospholipids and is needed to sustain normal levels of biologic methylation. To date, the most significant adverse effect of dietary inadequacy has been hepatic inflammation. Deficiency is nevertheless thought to be extremely rare, although pregnancy, and particularly lactation, increases the apparent requirement. Individuals whose long-term nutritional requirements are solely derived from total parenteral nutrition appear to be susceptible to choline deficiency. Both an RDA (425 mg, women; 550 mg, men) and a TUL (3.5 g) have now been established.

L-Carnitine is a dietary component that facilitates the transport of fatty acids into mitochondria, and a deficit therefore limits the fatty acid β-oxidation that occurs in those organelles.[1] Although no evidence exists for a dietary requirement in healthy children or adults, premature infants have very low stores of skeletal muscle carnitine. Therefore, preterm infants receiving parenteral nutrition without carnitine supplements appear to be a group at risk for deficiency. In clinical trials, parenteral supplementation of carnitine in such infants increases serum carnitine concentration, although it has not improved clinical end points in most studies. Similarly, it has been suggested that individuals on long-term hemodialysis and those dependent on total parenteral nutrition may also be susceptible to the clinical consequences of L-carnitine depletion, but convincing evidence is lacking.

● CONDITIONS THAT INCREASE REQUIRED DIETARY INTAKE

Many physiologic, pathophysiologic, and pharmacologic factors increase the dietary requirements for micronutrients (see Table 218-1), thereby enhancing the risk for development of a deficiency state.

Physiologic Factors

Stages of the life cycle frequently have a significant impact on the requirements of nutrients. Phases of rapid growth and development, such as in utero development, infancy, adolescence, and pregnancy, are associated with increases in the utilization of certain micronutrients on a per-kilogram basis.

Pregnancy

Requirements for most micronutrients are increased in pregnancy, but, proportionately, the observed increases in the maternal requirements for iron and folate are particularly great and are related to the rapid proliferation of the placental and fetal tissues. Periods of lactation are similarly associated with remarkable increases in requirements; a lactating woman experiences disproportionately large increases in her requirements for zinc and vitamins

Text continued on p. 1452

TABLE 218-1	FACTORS THAT DETERMINE DIETARY REQUIREMENT OF A MICRONUTRIENT

PHYSIOLOGIC FACTORS

Bioavailability: the proportion of a micronutrient that is ingested and is capable of being assimilated and used for physiologic purposes
Quantity required to fulfill physiologic roles
Extent to which the body can reuse the micronutrient
Distribution of nutrient in the body: storage compartments
Gender
Stage of life cycle: intrauterine development, childhood, adulthood, elder adulthood, pregnancy, lactation

PATHOPHYSIOLOGIC AND PHARMACOLOGIC FACTORS

Inborn errors of metabolism: variously affect assimilation, utilization, or excretion of micronutrients
Acquired disease states that alter the amounts required to sustain homeostasis (e.g., malabsorption, maldigestion, states that increase use)
Lifestyle habits: smoking, ethanol consumption
Drugs: may alter bioavailability or utilization

TABLE 218-2 VITAMINS AND THEIR FUNCTIONS

	BIOCHEMISTRY AND PHYSIOLOGY	DEFICIENCY [RDA*]	TOXICITY [TUL†]	ASSESSMENT OF STATUS
FAT-SOLUBLE VITAMINS				
Vitamin A	A family of the retinoid compounds, each member having biologic activity qualitatively similar to retinol. Carotenoids are structurally related to retinoids. Some carotenoids, most notably β-carotene, are metabolized into compounds with vitamin A activity and are therefore considered to be provitamin A compounds. Vitamin A is an integral component of rhodopsin and iodopsins, light-sensitive proteins in rod and cone cells in the retina. *Additional functions:* induction and maintenance of cellular differentiation in certain tissues; signal for appropriate morphogenesis in the developing embryo; maintenance of cell-mediated immunity. 1 µg of retinol = 3.33 IU of vitamin A.	Follicular hyperkeratosis and night blindness are early indicators. Conjunctival xerosis, degeneration of the cornea (keratomalacia), and dedifferentiation of rapidly proliferating epithelia are later indications of deficiency. *Bitot spots* (focal areas of the conjunctiva or cornea with foamy appearance) are an indication of xerosis. Blindness, due to corneal destruction and retinal dysfunction, ensues if left uncorrected. Increased susceptibility to infection is also a consequence. [F: 700 µg; M: 900 µg]	In adults, >150,000 µg may cause *acute* toxicity: fatal intracranial hypertension, skin exfoliation, and hepatocellular necrosis. *Chronic* toxicity may occur with habitual daily intake of >10,000 µg: alopecia, ataxia, bone and muscle pain, dermatitis, cheilitis, conjunctivitis, pseudotumor cerebri, hepatocellular necrosis, hyperlipidemia, and hyperostosis are common. Single, large doses of vitamin A (30,000 µg) or habitual intake of >4500 µg/day in early pregnancy can be teratogenic. Excessive intake of carotenoids causes a benign condition characterized by yellowish discoloration of the skin. Habitually large doses of canthaxanthin, a carotenoid, have the additional capability of inducing a retinopathy. [3000 µg]	Retinol concentration in the plasma and vitamin A concentrations in the milk and tears are reasonably accurate measures of adequate status. Toxicity is best assessed by elevated levels of retinyl esters in plasma. A quantitative measure of dark adaptation for night vision and electroretinography are useful functional tests.
Vitamin D	A group of sterol compounds whose parent structure is cholecalciferol (vitamin D_3) Cholecalciferol is formed in the skin from 7-dehydrocholesterol (provitamin D_3) by exposure to UVB radiation. A plant sterol, ergocalciferol (provitamin D_2), can be similarly converted into vitamin D_2 and has similar vitamin D activity. The vitamin undergoes sequential hydroxylations in the liver and kidney at the 25 and 1 positions, respectively, producing the most bioactive form of the vitamin, 1,25-dihydroxy vitamin D. Vitamin D maintains intracellular and extracellular concentrations of calcium and phosphate by enhancing intestinal absorption of the two ions and, in conjunction with PTH, promoting their mobilization from bone mineral. It retards proliferation and promotes differentiation in certain epithelia. Purported actions of vitamin D as an anti-diabetes, anti-inflammatory, and cancer preventive agent remain controversial and are under investigation. 1 µg = 40 IU.	Deficiency results in decreased mineralization of newly formed bone called *rickets* in childhood and *osteomalacia* in adults. Expansion of the epiphyseal growth plates and replacement of normal bone with unmineralized bone matrix are the cardinal features of rickets; the latter feature also characterizes osteomalacia. Deformity of bone and pathologic fractures occur. Decreased serum concentrations of calcium and phosphate may occur. [15 µg, ages 19-70 yr; 20 µg, age >70 yr]	Excess amounts result in abnormally high concentrations of calcium and phosphate in the serum; metastatic calcifications, renal damage, and altered mentation may occur. [100 µg for ages ≥9 yr]	The serum concentration of the major circulating metabolite, 25-hydroxyvitamin D, is the best indicator of systemic status except in advanced kidney disease (stages 4 and 5), in which the impairment of renal 1-hydroxylation results in disassociation of the mono- and dihydroxyvitamin concentrations. Measurement of the serum concentration of 1,25-dihydroxyvitamin D is then necessary.
Vitamin E	A group of at least 8 naturally occurring compounds, some of which are tocopherols and some of which are tocotrienols At present, the only dietary form that is thought to be biologically active in humans is α-tocopherol. Vitamin E acts as an antioxidant and free radical scavenger in lipophilic environments, most notably in cell membranes. It acts in conjunction with other antioxidants, such as selenium.	Deficiency due to dietary inadequacy is rare. It is usually seen in premature infants, individuals with fat malabsorption, and individuals with abetalipoproteinemia. Red blood cell fragility occurs and can produce a hemolytic anemia. Neuronal degeneration produces peripheral neuropathies, ophthalmoplegia, and destruction of posterior columns of spinal cord. Neurologic disease is frequently irreversible if deficiency is not corrected early enough. May contribute to the hemolytic anemia and retrolental fibroplasia seen in premature infants. Reported to suppress cell-mediated immunity [15 mg]	Depressed levels of vitamin K–dependent procoagulants and potentiation of oral anticoagulants have been reported, as has impaired WBC function. Doses of 800 mg/day have been reported to increase slightly the incidence of hemorrhagic stroke. [1000 mg]	Plasma or serum concentration of α-tocopherol is most commonly used. Additional accuracy is obtained by expressing this value per milligram of total plasma lipid. RBC peroxide hemolysis test is not entirely specific but is a useful functional measure of the antioxidant potential of cell membranes.

TABLE 218-2 VITAMINS AND THEIR FUNCTIONS—cont'd

	BIOCHEMISTRY AND PHYSIOLOGY	DEFICIENCY [RDA*]	TOXICITY [TUL†]	ASSESSMENT OF STATUS
Vitamin K	A family of naphthoquinone compounds with similar biologic activity. Phylloquinone (vitamin K_1) is derived from plants; a variety of menaquinones (vitamin K_2) are derived from bacterial and animal sources. Vitamin K serves as an essential cofactor in the post-translational γ-carboxylation of glutamic acid residues in many proteins. These proteins include several circulating procoagulants and anticoagulants as well as proteins in a variety of tissues.	Deficiency syndrome is uncommon except in breast-fed newborns, in whom it may cause "hemorrhagic disease of the newborn"; in adults with fat malabsorption or who are taking drugs that interfere with vitamin K metabolism (e.g., coumarin, phenytoin, broad-spectrum antibiotics); and in individuals taking large doses of vitamin E and anticoagulant drugs. Excessive hemorrhage is the usual manifestation. [F: 90 μg; M: 120 μg]	Rapid intravenous infusion of K_1 has been rarely associated with dyspnea, flushing, and cardiovascular collapse; this is likely related to the dispersing agents in the solution. Supplementation may interfere with coumarin-based anticoagulation. Pregnant women taking large amounts of the provitamin menadione may deliver infants with hemolytic anemia, hyperbilirubinemia, and kernicterus. [no TUL established]	Prothrombin time is typically used as a measure of functional K status; it is neither sensitive nor specific for vitamin K deficiency. Determination of fasting plasma vitamin K is an accurate indicator of status. Undercarboxylated plasma prothrombin is also an accurate metric, but only for detecting the deficient state, and is less widely available than plasma vitamin K.
WATER-SOLUBLE VITAMINS				
Thiamin (vitamin B_1)	A water-soluble compound containing substituted pyrimidine and thiazole rings and a hydroxyethyl side chain. The coenzyme form is thiamin pyrophosphate (TPP). Thiamin serves as a coenzyme in many α-ketoacid decarboxylation and transketolation reactions. Inadequate thiamin availability leads to impairments of these reactions, resulting in inadequate adenosine triphosphate synthesis and abnormal carbohydrate metabolism, respectively. It may have an additional role in neuronal conduction independent of the aforementioned actions.	Classic deficiency syndrome (beriberi) is described in Asian populations consuming a polished rice diet. Alcoholism, chronic renal dialysis, and persistent nausea and vomiting after bariatric surgery are also common precipitants. High carbohydrate intake increases need for B_1. *Mild deficiency*: irritability, fatigue, and headaches *More severe deficiency*: combinations of peripheral neuropathy, cardiovascular dysfunction, and cerebral dysfunction. Cardiovascular involvement (wet beriberi): congestive heart failure and low peripheral vascular resistance. Cerebral disease: nystagmus, ophthalmoplegia, and ataxia (Wernicke's encephalopathy); hallucinations, impaired short-term memory, and confabulation (Korsakoff's psychosis) Deficiency syndrome responds within 24 hr to parenteral thiamin but is partially or wholly irreversible after a certain stage. [F: 1.1 mg; M: 1.2 mg]	Excess intake is largely excreted in the urine, although parenteral doses of >400 mg/day are reported to cause lethargy, ataxia, and reduced tone of the gastrointestinal tract. [TUL not established]	The most effective measure of B_1 status is the erythrocyte transketolase activity coefficient, which measures enzyme activity before and after addition of exogenous TPP; RBCs from a deficient individual express a substantial increase in enzyme activity with addition of TPP. Thiamin concentrations in blood or urine are also used.
Riboflavin (vitamin B_2)	Consists of a substituted isoalloxazine ring with a ribitol side chain Riboflavin serves as a coenzyme for a diverse array of biochemical reactions. The primary coenzymatic forms are flavin mononucleotide and flavin adenine dinucleotide. Riboflavin holoenzymes participate in oxidation-reduction reactions in myriad metabolic pathways.	Deficiency is usually seen in conjunction with deficiencies of other B vitamins. Isolated deficiency of riboflavin produces hyperemia and edema of nasopharyngeal mucosa, cheilosis, angular stomatitis, glossitis, seborrheic dermatitis, and a normochromic, normocytic anemia. [F: 1.1; M: 1.3]	Toxicity is not reported in humans. [TUL not established]	The most common method of assessment is to determine the activity coefficient of glutathione reductase in RBCs (the test is invalid for individuals with glucose-6-phosphate dehydrogenase deficiency). Measurements of blood and urine concentrations are less desirable methods.

TABLE 218-2   VITAMINS AND THEIR FUNCTIONS—cont'd

	BIOCHEMISTRY AND PHYSIOLOGY	DEFICIENCY [RDA*]	TOXICITY [TUL†]	ASSESSMENT OF STATUS
Niacin (vitamin B₃)	Refers to nicotinic acid and the corresponding amide, nicotinamide The active coenzymic forms are composed of nicotinamide affixed to adenine dinucleotide, forming NAD or NADP. More than 200 apoenzymes use these compounds as electron acceptors or hydrogen donors, either as a coenzyme or as a co-substrate. The essential amino acid tryptophan is a precursor of niacin; 60 mg of dietary tryptophan yields approximately 1 mg of niacin. Dietary requirements thus depend partly on tryptophan intake. Requirement is often determined on basis of calorie intake (i.e., niacin equivalents/1000 kcal). Large doses of nicotinic acid (1.5-3 g/day) effectively lower low-density lipoprotein cholesterol and elevate high-density lipoprotein cholesterol.	*Pellagra* is the classic deficiency syndrome and is often seen in populations in which corn is the major source of energy; it is still endemic in parts of China, Africa, and India. Diarrhea, dementia (or associated symptoms of anxiety or insomnia), and a pigmented dermatitis that develops in sun-exposed areas are typical features. Glossitis, stomatitis, vaginitis, vertigo, and burning dysesthesias are early signs. It is reported occasionally to occur in carcinoid syndrome because tryptophan is diverted to other synthetic pathways. [F: 14 mg; M: 16 mg]	Human toxicity is known largely through studies examining hypolipidemic effects. Includes vasomotor phenomenon (flushing), hyperglycemia, parenchymal liver damage, and hyperuricemia. [35 mg]	Assessment of status is problematic; blood levels of the vitamin are not reliable. Measurement of urinary excretion of the niacin metabolites *N*-methylnicotinamide and 2-pyridone is thought to be the most effective means of assessment at present.
Vitamin B₆	Refers to several derivatives of pyridine, including pyridoxine, pyridoxal, and pyridoxamine, which are interconvertible in the body. The coenzymatic forms are pyridoxal-5-phosphate (PLP) and pyridoxamine-5-phosphate. As a coenzyme, B₆ is involved in many transamination reactions (and thereby in gluconeogenesis), in the synthesis of niacin from tryptophan, in the synthesis of several neurotransmitters, and in the synthesis of δ-aminolevulinic acid (and therefore in heme synthesis). It also has functions unrelated to coenzymatic activity: pyridoxal and PLP bind to hemoglobin and alter oxygen affinity; PLP also binds to steroid receptors, inhibiting receptor affinity to DNA and thereby modulating steroid activity.	Deficiency is usually seen in conjunction with other water-soluble vitamin deficiencies. Stomatitis, angular cheilosis, glossitis, irritability, depression, and confusion occur in moderate to severe depletion; normochromic, normocytic anemia has been reported in severe deficiency. Abnormalities on electroencephalography and, in infants, convulsions have also been observed. Some sideroblastic anemias respond to B₆ administration. Isoniazid, cycloserine, penicillamine, ethanol, and theophylline can inhibit B₆ metabolism. [Ages 19-50 yr: 1.3 mg; >50 yr: 1.5 mg for women, 1.7 mg for men]	Long-term use with doses exceeding 200 mg/day (in adults) may cause peripheral neuropathies and photosensitivity. [100 mg]	Many useful laboratory methods of assessment exist. The plasma or erythrocyte PLP levels are most common. Urinary excretion of xanthurenic acid after an oral tryptophan load and activity indices of RBC alanine or aspartate transaminase are functional measures of B₆-dependent enzyme activity.
Folate	A group of related pterin compounds More than 35 forms of the vitamin are found naturally. The fully oxidized form, folic acid, is not found in nature but is the pharmacologic form of the vitamin. All folate functions relate to its ability to transfer one-carbon groups. It is essential in the de novo synthesis of nucleotides and in the metabolism of several amino acids; it is an integral component for the regeneration of the "universal" methyl donor, *S*-adenosylmethionine. Inhibition of bacterial and cancer cell folate metabolism is the basis for the sulfonamide antibiotics and chemotherapeutic agents, such as methotrexate and 5-fluorouracil, respectively.	Women of childbearing age are most likely to be deficient. *Classic deficiency syndrome*: megaloblastic anemia, diarrhea. The hematopoietic cells in bone marrow become enlarged and have immature nuclei, reflecting ineffective DNA synthesis. The peripheral blood smear demonstrates macro-ovalocytes and polymorphonuclear leukocytes with an average of more than 3.5 nuclear lobes. Megaloblastic changes also occur in other epithelia that proliferate rapidly (e.g., oral mucosa and gastrointestinal tract, producing glossitis and diarrhea, respectively). Sulfasalazine and diphenytoin inhibit absorption and predispose to deficiency. [400 μg of dietary folate equivalents (DFE); 1 DFE = 1 μg food folate = 0.6 μg folic acid]	Doses >1000 μg/day may partially correct the anemia of B₁₂ deficiency and may therefore mask (and perhaps exacerbate) the associated neuropathy. Large doses are also reported to lower seizure threshold in individuals prone to seizures. Parenteral administration is rarely reported to cause allergic phenomena, which is probably due to dispersion agents. [1000 μg]	Serum folate measures short-term folate balance, whereas RBC folate is a better reflection of tissue status. Serum homocysteine rises early in deficiency but is nonspecific because B₁₂ or B₆ deficiency, renal insufficiency, and older age may also cause elevations.

TABLE 218-2 VITAMINS AND THEIR FUNCTIONS—cont'd

	BIOCHEMISTRY AND PHYSIOLOGY	DEFICIENCY [RDA*]	TOXICITY [TUL†]	ASSESSMENT OF STATUS
Vitamin C (ascorbic and dehydroascorbic acid)	Ascorbic acid readily oxidizes to dehydroascorbic acid in aqueous solution. Dehydroascorbic acid can be reduced in vivo, so it possesses vitamin C activity. Total vitamin C is therefore the sum of ascorbic and dehydroascorbic acid content. Vitamin C serves primarily as a biologic antioxidant in aqueous environments. Biosyntheses of collagen, carnitine, bile acids, and norepinephrine as well as proper functioning of the hepatic mixed-function oxygenase system depends on this property. Vitamin C in foodstuffs increases the intestinal absorption of nonheme iron.	Overt deficiency is uncommon in developed countries. The classic deficiency syndrome is *scurvy*: fatigue, depression, and widespread abnormalities in connective tissues, such as inflamed gingivae, petechiae, perifollicular hemorrhages, impaired wound healing, coiled hairs, hyperkeratosis, and bleeding into body cavities. In infants, defects in ossification and bone growth may occur. Tobacco smoking lowers plasma and leukocyte vitamin C levels. [F: 75 mg; M: 90 mg; increase requirement for cigarette smokers by 35 mg/day]	≥500 mg/day (in adults) may cause nausea and diarrhea. >1 g/day modestly increases risk for oxalate kidney stones. Supplementation may interfere with laboratory tests based on redox potential (e.g., fecal occult blood testing, serum cholesterol, and glucose). Withdrawal from chronic ingestion of high doses of vitamin C supplements should be done gradually because accommodation appears to occur, raising a concern of "rebound scurvy." [2 g]	Plasma ascorbic acid concentration reflects recent dietary intake, whereas WBC levels more closely reflect tissue stores. Women's plasma levels are approximately 20% higher than men's for any given dietary intake.
Vitamin B_{12}	A group of closely related cobalamin compounds composed of a corrin ring (with a cobalt atom in its center) connected to a ribonucleotide through an aminopropanol bridge. Microorganisms are the ultimate source of all naturally occurring B_{12}. The two active coenzyme forms are deoxyadenosylcobalamin and methylcobalamin. These coenzymes are needed for the synthesis of succinyl CoA, which is essential in lipid and carbohydrate metabolism, and for the synthesis of methionine. The synthesis of methionine is essential for amino acid metabolism, for purine and pyrimidine synthesis, for many methylation reactions, and for the intracellular retention of folates.	Dietary inadequacy is a rare cause of deficiency except in strict vegetarians. Most deficiencies arise from loss of intestinal absorption, which may occur with pernicious anemia, pancreatic insufficiency, atrophic gastritis, small bowel bacterial overgrowth, or ileal disease. Megaloblastic anemia and megaloblastic changes in other epithelia (see Folate) are the result of sustained depletion. Demyelination of peripheral nerves, posterior and lateral columns of spinal cord, and nerves within the brain may occur. Altered mentation, depression, and psychoses occur. Hematologic and neurologic complications may occur independently. Folate supplementation, in doses of 1000 µg/day, may partly correct the anemia, thereby masking (or perhaps exacerbating) the neuropathic complication. [2.4 µg]	A few allergic reactions have been reported to crystalline B_{12} preparations and are probably due to impurities, not the vitamin. [TUL not established]	Serum or plasma concentrations are generally accurate. Subtle deficiency with neurologic complications, as described in the Deficiency column, can best be established by concurrently measuring the concentration of plasma B_{12} and serum methylmalonic acid, which is a sensitive indicator of cellular deficiency.
Biotin	A bi-cyclic compound consisting of a ureido ring fused to a substituted tetrahydrothiophene ring. Endogenous synthesis by intestinal flora may contribute significantly to biotin nutriture. Most dietary biotin is linked to lysine, a compound called biotinyl lysine, or biocytin. The lysine must be hydrolyzed by an intestinal enzyme called biotinidase before intestinal absorption occurs. Biotin acts primarily as a coenzyme for several carboxylases; each holoenzyme catalyzes an adenosine triphosphate–dependent carbon dioxide transfer. The carboxylases are critical enzymes in carbohydrate and lipid metabolism.	Isolated deficiency is rare. Deficiency in humans has been produced by prolonged total parenteral nutrition lacking the vitamin and by ingestion of large quantities of raw egg white, which contains avidin, a protein that binds biotin with such high affinity that it renders it biounavailable. Alterations in mental status, myalgias, hyperesthesias, and anorexia occur. Later, a seborrheic dermatitis and alopecia develop. Deficiency is usually accompanied by lactic acidosis and organic aciduria. [30 µg]	Toxicity has not been reported in humans with doses as high as 60 mg/day in children. [TUL not established]	Plasma and urine concentrations of biotin are diminished in the deficient state. Elevated urine concentrations of methyl citrate, 3-methylcrotonylglycine, and 3-hydroxyisovalerate are also observed in deficiency.

TABLE 218-2 VITAMINS AND THEIR FUNCTIONS—cont'd

	BIOCHEMISTRY AND PHYSIOLOGY	DEFICIENCY [RDA*]	TOXICITY [TUL†]	ASSESSMENT OF STATUS
Pantothenic acid	Consists of pantoic acid linked to β-alanine through an amide bond Pantothenic acid is an essential component of CoA and phosphopantetheine, which are essential for synthesis and β-oxidation of fatty acids as well as for synthesis of cholesterol, steroid hormones, vitamins A and D, and other isoprenoid derivatives. CoA is also involved in the synthesis of several amino acids and δ-aminolevulinic acid, a precursor for the corrin ring of vitamin B_{12}, the porphyrin ring of heme, and of cytochromes. CoA is also necessary for the acetylation and fatty acid acylation of a variety of proteins.	Deficiency is rare; it has been reported only as a result of feeding of semisynthetic diets or an antagonist to the vitamin. Experimental, isolated deficiency in humans produces fatigue, abdominal pain, vomiting, insomnia, and paresthesias of the extremities. [5 mg]	In doses of 10 g/day, diarrhea is reported to occur. [TUL not established]	Whole blood and urine concentrations of pantothenate are indicators of status; serum levels are not thought to be accurate.

CoA = coenzyme A; NAD = nicotinamide adenine dinucleotide; NADP = nicotinamide adenine dinucleotide phosphate; PTH = parathyroid hormone; RBC = red blood cell; UVB = ultraviolet B; WBC = white blood cell.
*Recommended daily allowance (RDA) established for female (F) and male (M) adults by the U.S. Food and Nutrition Board, 1999-2001. In some instances, insufficient data exist to establish an RDA, in which case the adequate intake (AI) established by the board is listed.
†Tolerable upper limit (TUL) established for adults by the U.S. Food and Nutrition Board, 1999-2001.

TABLE 218-3 NUTRITIONAL TRACE ELEMENTS AND THEIR CLINICAL IMPLICATIONS

	BIOCHEMISTRY AND PHYSIOLOGY	DEFICIENCY [RDA*]	TOXICITY [TUL†]	ASSESSMENT OF STATUS
Chromium	Dietary chromium consists of both inorganic and organic forms. Its primary function in humans is to potentiate insulin action. It accomplishes this function as a circulating complex called *glucose tolerance factor*, thereby affecting carbohydrate, fat, and protein metabolism.	Deficiency in humans has been described only in long-term total parenteral nutrition (TPN) patients receiving insufficient chromium. Hyperglycemia or impaired glucose tolerance occurs. Elevated plasma free fatty acid concentrations, neuropathy, encephalopathy, and abnormalities in nitrogen metabolism are also reported. Whether supplemental chromium may improve glucose tolerance in glucose-intolerant individuals remains controversial. [F: 25 μg; M: 35 μg]	Toxicity after oral ingestion is uncommon and seems confined to gastric irritation. Airborne exposure may cause contact dermatitis, eczema, skin ulcers, and bronchogenic carcinoma. [no TUL established]	Plasma or serum concentration of chromium is a crude indicator of chromium status; it appears to be meaningful when the value is markedly above or below the normal range.
Copper	Copper is absorbed by a specific intestinal transport mechanism. It is carried to the liver, where it is bound to ceruloplasmin, which circulates systemically and delivers copper to target tissues in the body. Excretion of copper is largely through bile and then into the feces. Absorptive and excretory processes vary with the levels of dietary copper, providing a means of copper homeostasis. Copper serves as a component of many enzymes, including amine oxidases, ferroxidases, cytochrome *c* oxidase, dopamine β-hydroxylase, superoxide dismutase, and tyrosinase.	Dietary deficiency is rare; it has been observed in premature and low-birthweight infants fed exclusively on a cow's milk diet and in individuals on long-term TPN lacking copper. It has also been described after gastric bypass surgery and with chronic zinc supplementation. Clinical manifestations include depigmentation of skin and hair, myelopathy and other neurologic lesions, leukopenia, anemia, and skeletal abnormalities. Anemia arises from impaired utilization of iron and therefore often is manifested as a sideroblastic anemia. The peripheral smear and bone marrow may mimic myelodysplasia. A deficiency syndrome is also observed in Menkes' disease, a rare inherited condition associated with impaired copper utilization. [900 μg]	Acute copper toxicity has been described after excessive oral intake and with absorption of copper salts applied to burned skin. Milder manifestations include nausea, vomiting, epigastric pain, and diarrhea; coma and hepatic necrosis may ensue in severe cases. Toxicity may be seen with doses as low as 70 μg/kg/day. Chronic toxicity is also described. Wilson's disease is a rare, inherited disease associated with abnormally low ceruloplasmin levels and accumulation of copper in the liver and brain, eventually leading to damage to these two organs. [10 mg]	Practical methods to detect marginal deficiency are not available. Marked deficiency is reliably detected by diminished serum copper and ceruloplasmin concentrations as well as by low red blood cell superoxide dismutase activity.

TABLE 218-3 NUTRITIONAL TRACE ELEMENTS AND THEIR CLINICAL IMPLICATIONS—cont'd

	BIOCHEMISTRY AND PHYSIOLOGY	DEFICIENCY [RDA*]	TOXICITY [TUL†]	ASSESSMENT OF STATUS
Fluorine	Known more commonly by its ionic form, fluoride. Fluorine is incorporated into the crystalline structure of bone, thereby altering its physical characteristics.	Intake of <0.1 mg/day in infants and <0.5 mg/day in children is associated with an increased incidence of dental caries. Optimal intake in adults is between 1.5 and 4 mg/day. [F: 3 mg; M: 4 mg]	Acute ingestion of >30 mg/kg body weight is likely to cause death. Excessive chronic intake (0.1 mg/kg/day) leads to mottling of teeth (dental fluorosis), calcification of tendons and ligaments, and exostoses and may increase the brittleness of bones. [10 mg]	Estimates of intake and clinical assessment are used because no good laboratory test exists.
Iodine	Iodine is readily absorbed from the diet, concentrated in the thyroid, and integrated into the thyroid hormones thyroxine and triiodothyronine. These hormones circulate largely bound to thyroxine-binding globulin. They modulate resting energy expenditure and, in the developing human, growth and development.	In the absence of supplementation, populations relying primarily on food from soils with low iodine content have endemic iodine deficiency. Maternal iodine deficiency leads to fetal deficiency, which produces spontaneous abortions, stillbirths, hypothyroidism, cretinism, and dwarfism. Permanent cognitive deficits may result from iodine deficiency during the first 2 years of life. In the adult, compensatory hypertrophy of the thyroid (goiter) occurs along with varying degrees of hypothyroidism. [150 µg]	Large doses (>2 mg/day in adults) may induce hypothyroidism by blocking thyroid hormone synthesis. Supplementation with >100 mg/day to an individual who was formerly deficient occasionally induces hyperthyroidism. [1.1 mg]	Iodine status of a population can be estimated by the prevalence of goiter. Urinary excretion of iodine is an effective laboratory means of assessment. Thyroid-stimulating hormone blood level is an indirect and therefore not entirely specific means of assessment.
Iron	Conveys the capacity to participate in redox reactions to a number of metalloproteins, such as hemoglobin, myoglobin, cytochrome enzymes, and many oxidases and oxygenases. The primary storage form of iron is ferritin and, to a lesser degree, hemosiderin. Intestinal absorption is 15-20% for "heme" iron and 1-8% for iron contained in vegetables. Absorption of the latter form is enhanced by the ascorbic acid in foodstuffs; by poultry, fish, or beef; and by an iron-deficient state. It is decreased by phytate and tannins.	Iron deficiency is the most common micronutrient deficiency in the world. Women of childbearing age are the group at highest risk because of menstrual blood losses, pregnancy, and lactation. The classic deficiency syndrome is hypochromic, microcytic anemia. Glossitis and koilonychia ("spoon" nails) are also observed. Easy fatigability often is an early symptom, before anemia appears. In children, mild deficiency of insufficient severity to cause anemia is associated with behavioral disturbances and poor school performance. [postmenopausal F and M: 8 mg; premenopausal F: 18 mg]	Iron overload typically occurs when habitual dietary intake is extremely high, intestinal absorption is excessive, repeated parenteral administration occurs, or a combination of these factors exists. Excessive iron stores usually accumulate in the reticuloendothelial tissues and cause little damage (hemosiderosis). If overload continues, iron eventually begins to accumulate in tissues such as the hepatic parenchyma, pancreas, heart, and synovium, causing hemochromatosis (Chapter 212). Hereditary hemochromatosis results from homozygosity of a common recessive trait. Excessive intestinal absorption of iron is seen in homozygotes. [45 mg]	Negative iron balance initially leads to depletion of iron stores in the bone marrow; a bone marrow biopsy and the concentration of serum ferritin are accurate indicators of early depletion. As the severity of deficiency proceeds, serum iron (SI) decreases and total iron-binding capacity (TIBC) increases; an iron saturation (SI/TIBC) of <16% suggests iron deficiency. Microcytosis, hypochromia, and anemia ensue. Elevated levels of serum ferritin or an iron saturation of >60% suggest iron overload, although systemic inflammation elevates serum ferritin regardless of iron status.
Manganese	A component of several metalloenzymes. Most manganese is in mitochondria, where it is a component of manganese superoxide dismutase.	Manganese deficiency in the human has not been conclusively demonstrated. It is said to cause hypocholesterolemia, weight loss, hair and nail changes, dermatitis, and impaired synthesis of vitamin K–dependent proteins. [F: 1.8 mg; M: 2.3 mg]	Toxicity by oral ingestion is unknown in humans. Toxic inhalation causes hallucinations, other alterations in mentation, and extrapyramidal movement disorders. [11 mg]	Until the deficiency syndrome is better defined, an appropriate measure of status will be difficult to develop.
Molybdenum	A cofactor in several enzymes, most prominently xanthine oxidase and sulfite oxidase	A probable case of human deficiency is described as being secondary to parenteral administration of sulfite and resulted in hyperoxypurinemia, hypouricemia, and low sulfate excretion. [45 µg]	Toxicity not well described in humans, although it may interfere with copper metabolism at high doses. [2 mg]	Laboratory means of assessment are not meaningful until the deficiency syndrome is better described.

TABLE 218-3 NUTRITIONAL TRACE ELEMENTS AND THEIR CLINICAL IMPLICATIONS—cont'd

	BIOCHEMISTRY AND PHYSIOLOGY	DEFICIENCY [RDA*]	TOXICITY [TUL†]	ASSESSMENT OF STATUS
Selenium	Most dietary selenium is in the form of an amino acid complex. Nearly complete absorption of such forms occurs. Homeostasis is largely performed by the kidney, which regulates urinary excretion as a function of selenium status. Selenium is a component of several enzymes, most notably glutathione peroxidase and superoxide dismutase. These enzymes protect against oxidative and free radical damage of various cell structures. The antioxidant protection conveyed by selenium apparently operates in conjunction with vitamin E because deficiency of one seems to potentiate damage induced by a deficiency of the other. Selenium also participates in the enzymatic conversion of thyroxine to its more active metabolite, triiodothyronine.	Deficiency is rare in North America but has been observed in individuals on long-term TPN lacking selenium. Such individuals have myalgias or cardiomyopathies. Populations in some regions of the world, most notably some parts of China, have marginal intake of selenium. In these regions *Keshan's disease*, a condition characterized by cardiomyopathy, is endemic; it can be prevented (but not treated) by selenium supplementation. [55 μg]	Toxicity is associated with nausea, diarrhea, alterations in mental status, peripheral neuropathy, and loss of hair and nails; such symptoms were observed in adults who inadvertently consumed 27-2400 mg. [400 μg]	Erythrocyte glutathione peroxidase activity and plasma or whole blood selenium concentrations are the most commonly used methods of assessment. They are moderately accurate indicators of status.
Zinc	Intestinal absorption occurs by a specific process that is enhanced by pregnancy and corticosteroids and diminished by coingestion of phytates, phosphates, iron, copper, lead, or calcium. Diminished intake of zinc leads to an increased efficiency of absorption and decreased fecal excretion, providing a means of zinc homeostasis. Zinc is a component of more than 100 enzymes, among which are DNA polymerase, RNA polymerase, and transfer RNA synthetase.	Zinc deficiency has its most profound effect on rapidly proliferating tissues. *Mild deficiency:* growth retardation in children. *More severe deficiency:* growth arrest, teratogenicity, hypogonadism and infertility, dysgeusia, poor wound healing, diarrhea, dermatitis on the extremities and around orifices, glossitis, alopecia, corneal clouding, loss of dark adaptation, and behavioral changes. Impaired cellular immunity is observed. Excessive loss of gastrointestinal secretions through chronic diarrhea and fistulas may precipitate deficiency. *Acrodermatitis enteropathica* is a rare, recessively inherited disease in which intestinal absorption of zinc is impaired. [F: 8 mg; M: 11 mg]	Acute zinc toxicity can usually be induced by ingestion of >200 mg of zinc in a single day (in adults). It is manifested by epigastric pain, nausea, vomiting, and diarrhea. Hyperpnea, diaphoresis, and weakness may follow inhalation of zinc fumes. Copper and zinc compete for intestinal absorption: long-term ingestion of >25 mg/day of zinc may lead to copper deficiency. Long-term ingestion of >150 mg/day has been reported to cause gastric erosions, low high-density lipoprotein cholesterol levels, and impaired cellular immunity. [40 mg]	No accurate indicators of zinc status exist for routine clinical use. Plasma, red blood cell, and hair zinc concentrations are often misleading. Acute illness, in particular, is known to diminish plasma zinc levels, in part by inducing a shift of zinc out of the plasma compartment and into the liver. Functional tests that determine dark adaptation, taste acuity, and rate of wound healing lack specificity.

*Recommended daily allowance (RDA) established for female (F) and male (M) adults by the U.S. Food and Nutrition Board, 1999-2001. In some instances, insufficient data exist to establish an RDA, in which case the adequate intake (AI) established by the board is listed.
†Tolerable upper limit (TUL) established for adults by the U.S. Food and Nutrition Board, 1999-2001.

A, E, and C to meet the metabolic demands incurred by milk production in addition to the aforementioned needs observed in pregnancy.

Aside from its general role in supporting the rapid proliferation of placental and fetal tissues, folate plays a specific role in the prevention of particular birth defects. A 20 to 85% reduction in births complicated by neural tube defects (NTDs, i.e., spina bifida and anencephaly) has been realized by providing women with a daily supplement of folic acid in the form of supplements or fortified foods. The optimal dose is not well defined, but 200 to 400 μg/day clearly affords a substantial degree of protection. Populations with a high background rate of NTD births attain the largest reductions in NTDs from supplemental folate. However, because the nascent neural tube closes about day 20 after conception, the additional folate must be provided before this time to be effective.

Infancy
Infancy carries particular vulnerabilities to specific micronutrient inadequacies. Healthy infants in the United States are typically supplemented with vitamin K at birth and with iron and vitamin D during the course of the first year because of their particular susceptibility to deficiencies of these nutrients.

Women of Childbearing Age
The ability to maintain adequate iron status from menarche through menopause is compromised in women by the additional losses incurred by menstruation, pregnancy, and lactation. Therefore, it is not surprising that the population subset that almost invariably displays the highest rate of iron deficiency is women of childbearing age.

Elderly Persons
Specific dietary recommendations for elderly people have been formally incorporated into the recommended dietary allowances (RDA) because aging has an impact on the need for certain micronutrients. Vitamin B_{12} status declines significantly with aging, in large part because of the high prevalence of atrophic gastritis and its associated impairment in protein-bound vitamin B_{12} absorption.[2] Estimates suggest that 10 to 20% of the elderly population is at risk for clinically significant vitamin B_{12} deficiency. Consequently, elderly persons should consume some of their vitamin B_{12} requirement in the crystalline form rather than solely from the naturally occurring protein-bound forms found in food because absorption of the crystalline form is not impaired by atrophic gastritis. Elderly people also require greater quantities of vitamins B_6 and D to maintain health compared with younger adults, as reflected in

the new RDAs (see Table 218-2). For instance, the RDA of vitamin D in persons older than 70 years is now set at 20 μg/day (800 IU), as opposed to adults who are 70 years of age or younger, whose RDA is 15 μg/day.[3,4] This increased need appears to result from diminished cutaneous synthesis of vitamin D by senile skin and from decreased sun exposure, which appears to be particularly important in elders residing in institutional facilities. The need for crystalline vitamin B_{12} and for a quantity of vitamin D that is difficult to achieve without resorting to a supplement suggests that universal use of a daily supplement pill containing these nutrients would benefit elderly people. Widespread use of a multivitamin that contains a broad spectrum of micronutrients is more controversial, in part because of concerns about subtle toxicity. For example, elders with chronic renal failure appear to have a vulnerability to vitamin A toxicity, suggesting that use of supplements containing this vitamin is contraindicated.

PATHOPHYSIOLOGIC AND PHARMACOLOGIC FACTORS

Diseases of the Gastrointestinal Tract

Malabsorption and maldigestion predispose to multiple micronutrient deficiencies. Both fat- and water-soluble micronutrients (except vitamin B_{12}) are absorbed predominantly in the proximal small intestine. Therefore, diffuse mucosal diseases affecting the proximal portion of the gastrointestinal tract are likely to result in deficiencies. Even in the absence of mucosal disease of the proximal small intestine, extensive ileal disease, small bowel bacterial overgrowth, and chronic cholestasis can each interfere with the maintenance of adequate intraluminal conjugated bile acid concentrations and thereby impair absorption of fat-soluble vitamins. Maldigestion is usually the result of chronic pancreatitis. Untreated, it frequently causes malabsorption and deficiencies of fat-soluble vitamins. Vitamin B_{12} malabsorption can often be demonstrated in this setting, a result of inadequate R-protein digestion, but clinical vitamin B_{12} deficiency is rarely reported.

Inborn Errors of Metabolism

Myriad rare inborn errors of metabolism have been described for vitamins and minerals that impair an individual's ability to assimilate, to use, or to retain a particular micronutrient (Chapter 205). Such defects are usually partial and can often be overcome, to a certain extent, by administering doses of the nutrient that are several orders of magnitude greater than usually required. Suspicion for such defects should be entertained if a known defect exists in the family, a deficiency syndrome arises at birth or during infancy, or the deficiency syndrome is present despite adequate dietary intake and the absence of any disease that would impair the ability to assimilate the nutrient.

Medications

Long-term administration of many drugs may adversely affect micronutrient status. The manner in which drug-nutrient interactions occur varies; some of the more common mechanisms are outlined in Table 218-4. Some drugs exert their therapeutic effects by specifically inhibiting the actions of a micronutrient. Examples include coumarin, which inhibits γ-carboxylation reactions mediated by vitamin K, and methotrexate, which binds tightly to dihydrofolate reductase, thereby inhibiting folate metabolism.

Toxins

Tobacco smoking alters the metabolism of several vitamins, including folate and vitamins C and E. In large surveys, diminished plasma levels of folate and ascorbic acid have been observed in chronic smokers. Smoking is also associated with diminished levels of folate in cells of the oral mucosa, diminished ascorbic acid levels in leukocytes, and decreased concentrations of vitamin E in the alveolar fluid, findings providing evidence that many tissues can be affected by smoking and that the effect does not simply represent a shift of these micronutrients out of the plasma compartment.

ADVANCES IN NUTRITIONAL SCIENCE

New Frontiers in Marginal Deficiency States of Micronutrients

Does Optimal Intake of Micronutrients Optimize Health?

Updating the definition of a micronutrient deficiency and establishing recommended daily intakes that are consistent with the most recent evidence have proved difficult for several reasons. In some instances, a novel biochemical or physiologic role for a nutrient has been identified but the question that arises is whether optimization of such functions translates into optimization of health. For example, providing supplemental vitamin E to elderly individuals whose vitamin E status falls within normative standards enhances T-lymphocyte responsiveness; nevertheless, it is unclear whether this translates into diminished infection rates. Another difficult problem pertains to the use of micronutrients in supraphysiologic quantities that exceed all conventional concepts of what is necessary for health. Some micronutrients, when they are taken in large quantities, have effects on physiologic functions that impart apparent health benefits. The ingestion of gram quantities of niacin to reduce low-density lipoprotein (LDL) cholesterol is an example. Such physiologic effects are not observed at more conventional levels of intake and are therefore usually considered pharmacologic effects of the nutrient. Thus, the determination of optimal nutrient intake is highly dependent on which physiologic effect is sought. Furthermore, if only a segment of the population will benefit from supraphysiologic quantities of a nutrient, should dietary guidelines for the remainder of the population be established according to this effect?

Determining an adequate level of intake implies the existence of a means of measuring nutrient status. In seeking an appropriate measure of nutrient status, the diversity of function often makes it difficult to decide which measurement is the most germane. Tobacco smoking, for example, diminishes vitamin E levels in alveolar fluid but not in the serum. Thus, the concepts of localized nutrient deficiencies and tissue-specific requirements add an additional level of complexity to the determination of nutrient status.

Redefinition of Nutritional Requirements

Folate

An example of the complexities that have arisen in redefining the criteria for vitamin deficiencies and vitamin requirements is the water-soluble vitamin folate. In the past, guidelines regarding its necessary intake were straightforward because they were based solely on the prevention of megaloblastic anemia. Measurement of serum and erythrocyte folate concentrations was the most common means of assessing status, and maintaining these levels within accepted normative ranges provided assurance that folate status was adequate to prevent anemia. However, degrees of deficiency that are insufficient to cause anemia may still disturb normal biochemical and physiologic homeostasis and, in some instances, cause clinical disease. Clinical trials have demonstrated that women taking folic acid supplements at the time of conception have a markedly lower chance of delivering a baby with an NTD compared with women who are not folate supplemented but whose folate status falls within a conventionally accepted range. This observation compelled the U.S. government to mandate the fortification of flour, beginning in 1998. Present recommendations are that women of childbearing age consume 400 μg/day of folic acid in the form of supplements or fortified foods, although the dose-response curve of this effect is ill-defined.

Less than optimal intake of folate is also evidenced by an increase in serum homocysteine, an amino acid that is normally metabolized by a folate-dependent pathway. Before the federally mandated fortification of flour, the median intake of folate among adults was half of the present RDA, and a substantial minority of Americans had significantly elevated serum homocysteine levels. Elevated homocysteine is associated with the development of

TABLE 218-4	DRUG-MEDIATED EFFECTS ON MICRONUTRIENT STATUS: EXAMPLES	
DRUG	**NUTRIENT**	**MECHANISM OF INTERACTION**
Dextroamphetamine, fenfluramine, levodopa	Potentially all micronutrients	Induces anorexia
Cholestyramine	Vitamin D, folate	Adsorbs nutrient, decreases absorption
Omeprazole	Vitamin B_{12}	Modest bacterial overgrowth, decreases gastric acid, impairs absorption
Sulfasalazine	Folate	Impairs absorption and inhibits folate-dependent enzymes
Isoniazid	Pyridoxine	Impairs utilization of B_6
Nonsteroidal anti-inflammatory drugs	Iron	Gastrointestinal blood loss
Penicillamine	Zinc	Increases renal excretion

occlusive vascular disease and accelerated cognitive decline. In randomized clinical trials, however, supplementation with folate, vitamin B_{12}, and vitamin B_6 has shown no benefit against cardiovascular disease despite its ability to lower homocysteine levels.[A1] Such supplementation also has no clear benefit for cognitive function, except perhaps in patients with low baseline folate levels.[A2]

A compelling body of observations in both humans and animals has demonstrated that habitually low consumption of folate substantially increases the risk of colorectal cancer[5] and perhaps cancers of other organs, such as those of the breast and pancreas. This inverse relationship is observed even when folate status (or dietary intake) falls within the range of conventionally accepted normative values. This relationship has further complicated the determination of what constitutes an optimal intake of folate because the recent epidemiologic data suggest that about 500 μg constitutes the optimal daily intake for suppressing the risk of colon cancer. The issue is further confounded by observations, albeit controversial, suggesting that exceptionally high doses of supplemental folic acid among those who unknowingly harbor precancerous or cancerous lesions may paradoxically enhance the progression of these neoplasms,[6] thereby underscoring the potential for harm produced by taking a nutrient outside of its physiologic window.

The most recent update of the U.S. RDA for folate raised the value from 200 to 400 μg/day, citing both the prevention of anemia and optimization of serum homocysteine as criteria, and recommended that women capable of becoming pregnant consume an additional 400 μg/day in the form of supplements or fortified food. The issues surrounding the prevention of cardiovascular disease, cancer, and cognitive decline were not incorporated into that 1998 determination because the existing data at the time were inconclusive. However, future revisions of the RDAs may integrate some of this new knowledge. The potential for toxicity, the criterion for which was primarily linked to its ability to mask vitamin B_{12} deficiency, was dealt with by setting the TUL at 1000 μg/day of folic acid obtained from supplements and fortified foods in addition to that obtained from natural food sources (see Table 218-2).

Table 218-5 lists several examples of biochemical functions of vitamins that were not formerly recognized. As the clinical significance of each of these new roles is defined and as quantities of each vitamin needed to optimize such functions are determined, redefinition of the desirable range of vitamin status is likely to occur. Future efforts to refine appropriate dietary goals for each micronutrient will, however, need to take into consideration an important theme that is underscored by the previous discussion: the level of consumption of a particular micronutrient that conveys health benefits to one segment of the population is not necessarily beneficial, or even appropriate, for all segments of society.

Antioxidant and Free Radical Scavenging Vitamins and Provitamins

Vitamins A, C, and E as well as many of the carotenoids are effective antioxidants. In addition, vitamins C and E and some of the carotenoids can scavenge free radicals when these nutrients are taken in adequate quantities. Oxidation and free radical damage have been implicated as important contributors to common degenerative illnesses, such as atherosclerosis, cancer, cataracts, and retinal degeneration. Clinical trials to test the efficacy of antioxidant supplements have generally shown no benefit and in some instances

harm,[7] although growing evidence indicates that health benefits of such supplements can be realized in populations with marginal antioxidant status. Two large-scale clinical intervention trials with β-carotene supplements conducted in the 1990s reported increased rates of lung cancer among the recipients of the carotenoid. Subsequent mechanistic studies indicated that the large doses administered (20 to 30 mg/day) result in asymmetrical cleavage of the carotenoid into unnatural products that antagonize normal signaling pathways in the lung epithelium, whereas lower supplemental doses undergo symmetrical cleavage into two molecules of vitamin A, thereby protecting against neoplastic transformation.

LDL oxidized in vivo is atherogenic. Prevention of LDL oxidation, at least in animal models, retards the process of atherogenesis. Supplementation of human subjects with several times the RDA of α-tocopherol, and perhaps some of the other antioxidant micronutrients, is an effective means of preventing LDL oxidation. Human intervention trials with vitamin E or other antioxidant nutrients, however, have generally been unable to demonstrate clinical benefits in the reduction of cardiovascular events. There nevertheless has been a sizable reduction in cardiovascular events observed with vitamin E supplementation among populations of patients who are under exceptional oxidative stress, such as those with chronic renal failure and certain classes of diabetics, suggesting that it is only among select groups of individuals that a clinical benefit may be realized.

Epidemiologic studies indicate that occurrence of cancers of the oral cavity, lung, esophagus, and stomach (and perhaps the colorectum) is inversely related to dietary intake of fresh vegetables and fruits. Careful dissection of dietary data suggests that β-carotene and vitamin E content are strongly predictive components of these foodstuffs. High doses of vitamin A and some of its synthetic analogues (e.g., 13-cis-retinoic acid) can effectively reduce the recurrence of head and neck cancers, although hepatic toxicity is sometimes a limiting factor in such cancer preventive therapy. Similarly, these agents, as well as β-carotene or vitamin E, taken in large doses have been shown significantly to promote the regression of oral leukoplakia, a premalignant lesion. Daily supplementation with one to three times the U.S. RDA of β-carotene, selenium, and vitamin E has been shown to reduce the incidence of adenocarcinoma of the stomach in a region of China where the disease as well as marginal vitamin status is particularly prevalent. However, as mentioned earlier, trials conducted in developed Western countries have observed no diminution of lung cancer among smokers with daily supplementation of β-carotene and vitamin E.

Epidemiologic associations also suggest an inverse relationship between lens cataract or macular degeneration and the intake of vitamin C, vitamin E, and β-carotene. These common degenerative conditions of the eye are caused, at least in part, by photo-oxidation. Some evidence in animal models indicates that they can be retarded by supraphysiologic supplementation with vitamin C or E. When tested under the conditions of a rigorously conducted multicenter, controlled trial, daily supplementation with a combination of vitamin C, vitamin E, and β-carotene (with or without zinc) had no effects compared with placebo on the likelihood for development of cataracts. However, the combination that included zinc produced an approximately 30% decline in the progression of early macular degeneration to an advanced stage and the likelihood of moderate visual acuity loss.

Further investigation is necessary to define the circumstances more clearly under which antioxidant nutrients can be used to prevent or to treat chronic degenerative diseases.

Vitamin B_{12} and Neuropsychiatric Disease

Plasma vitamin B_{12} concentrations are considered to be an accurate indication of vitamin B_{12} status. Values greater than 150 pg/mL were thought, until recently, to exclude vitamin B_{12} deficiency as a cause of neurologic or psychiatric syndromes.[8] Recent observations now indicate that 7 to 10% of individuals who have plasma vitamin B_{12} values between 150 and 400 pg/mL may develop neuropsychiatric complications of vitamin B_{12} deficiency in the absence of any indications of megaloblastic anemia. Such individuals can be identified by the demonstration of an elevated level of methylmalonic acid in the blood that decreases to normal levels with parenteral vitamin B_{12} administration. An elevation in serum methylmalonic acid is both a sensitive and a specific indication of cellular vitamin B_{12} deficiency. An alternative approach is to administer several parenteral injections of vitamin B_{12} to an individual who has an otherwise unexplained neuropsychiatric syndrome and whose plasma vitamin B_{12} level falls in the range of 150 to 400 pg/mL. Awareness of this phenomenon is particularly important because it has become clear that atrophic gastritis, an asymptomatic condition that affects approximately

TABLE 218-5	NEWLY IDENTIFIED ROLES FOR VITAMINS	
VITAMIN OR PROVITAMIN	**CLASSIC ROLE**	**NEW ROLE**
β-Carotene	Pro-vitamin A	Antioxidant, free radical
Niacin	NAD/NADP coenzyme	Reduction of LDL, elevation of HDL cholesterol
Folate	Hematopoietic factor	Diminishes homocysteinemia
Vitamin A	Transduction of visual input in retina	Induction and maintenance of epithelial differentiation, signal in embryogenesis
Vitamin D	Regulator of calcium	Retards epithelial proliferation; promotes differentiation
Vitamin B_6	Coenzyme for transamination	Modulation of steroid activity

HDL = high-density lipoprotein; LDL = low-density lipoprotein; NAD = nicotinamide adenine dinucleotide; NADP = nicotinamide adenine dinucleotide phosphate.

30% of the elderly population, frequently produces a modest decrease in vitamin B_{12} status; similarly, long-term use of proton pump inhibitor drugs inhibits absorption and also increases the risk of clinically significant deficiency.[9]

Is Routine Multivitamin and Multimineral Supplementation Beneficial?

A common query by patients is whether regular use of a multivitamin or multimineral supplement is safe and efficacious in the maintenance of health. Although there is not a unanimous consensus about the "correct" answer to this question, the weight of available evidence indicates that for the general adult North American population, supplementation offers little or no benefit in regard to the prevention of the common chronic degenerative diseases, such as vascular disease, cancer, and dementia.[A3-A5] Although this apparent lack of efficacy has been notably contradicted by two clinical trials conducted in Western industrialized countries in which men taking multivitamins realized modest decreases in the incidence of cancer,[10] such benefits have not been substantiated by other investigations.

Although daily supplementation at the levels found in most multivitamin preparations probably presents no risk of harm, adverse health effects have been observed in several rigorously performed clinical trials in which long-term supplementation with micronutrients at levels that exceed the RDA (or conventional levels of dietary intake) by several-fold was examined. For example, an increased incidence of prostate cancer was observed in the SELECT trial, in which vitamin E was administered at a dose of 400 IU/day, and β-carotene supplementation resulted in an increased incidence of lung cancer among heavy smokers in the ATBC and CARET trials at doses of 20 to 30 mg/day.

This is not to say that health benefits cannot be realized from supplementation in select groups of individuals, although some thought needs to be exercised to determine which segments of the population should be targeted and what specific nutrients should be administered. Certainly, health benefits are likely in individuals whose dietary intake is chronically inadequate or in patients whose medical conditions are often complicated by micronutrient deficiencies, such as those on chronic renal dialysis or among individuals with marginally controlled intestinal malabsorption. The elderly frequently cannot achieve recommended intakes of vitamin D and calcium with diet alone, and therefore targeted supplementation with these nutrients is often indicated. Similarly, the high prevalence of atrophic gastritis among the elderly as well as the frequent use of proton pump inhibitor drugs each conspire to impair adequate vitamin B_{12} status.[11] Moreover, in many regions of the world, there continues to be a high prevalence of marginal micronutrient status among the general adult population, and in such areas widespread supplementation may be indicated; the Linxian trial in China, in which supplementation with a mixture of several antioxidant micronutrients led to a sizable decrease in gastric cancer, is one such example.

 Grade A References

A1. Clarke R, Halsey J, Lewington S, et al. Effects of lowering homocysteine levels with B vitamins on cardiovascular disease, cancer, and cause-specific mortality: meta-analysis of 8 randomized trials involving 37,485 individuals. *Arch Intern Med.* 2010;170:1622-1631.
A2. Balk EM, Raman G, Tatsioni A, et al. Vitamin B_6, B_{12}, and folic acid supplementation and cognitive function: a systematic review of randomized trials. *Arch Intern Med.* 2007;167:21-30.
A3. Fortmann S, Burda B, Senger C, et al. Vitamin and mineral supplements in the primary prevention of cardiovascular disease and cancer: an updated systematic evidence review for the U.S. Preventive Services Task Force. *Ann Intern Med.* 2013;159:824-834.
A4. Grodstein F, O'Brien J, Kang J, et al. Long-term multivitamin supplementation and cognitive function in men: a randomized trial. *Ann Intern Med.* 2013;159:806-814.
A5. Lamas G, Roineau R, Goertz C, et al. Oral high-dose multivitamins and minerals after myocardial infarction. A randomized trial. *Ann Intern Med.* 2013;159:797.

GENERAL REFERENCES

For the General References and other additional features, please visit Expert Consult at https://expertconsult.inkling.com.

219

EATING DISORDERS
MARIAN TANOFSKY-KRAFF

DEFINITION

Feeding and eating disorders are defined as syndromes "characterized by a persistent disturbance of eating or eating-related behavior that results in the altered consumption or absorption of food and that significantly impairs physical health or psychosocial functioning." The *Diagnostic and Statistical Manual of Mental Disorders*, fifth edition (DSM-5) defines anorexia nervosa (AN), bulimia nervosa (BN), and binge eating disorder (BED) as primary diagnoses in adolescents and adults. All other diagnoses are identified as Unspecified Feeding or Eating Disorder and represent presentations that do not meet the criteria for the primary eating disorders but nonetheless cause significant distress and impairment. The severity of each disorder is also specified as mild, moderate, severe, or extreme. Given the recent publication of the DSM-5, most empirical data available to date involve the criteria of the *Diagnostic and Statistical Manual of Mental Disorders*, fourth edition, text revision (DSM-IV-TR, published in 2000).

ANOREXIA NERVOSA

AN involves a restriction of "energy intake relative to requirements, leading to a significantly low body weight in the context of age, sex, developmental trajectory, and physical health."[1] Individuals with AN experience an intense fear of gaining weight or becoming fat, are overly concerned with weight or shape, and often may not recognize the seriousness of their low body weight. AN has two subtypes: restricting and binge-eating/purging. DSM-5 criteria for AN are listed in Table 219-1.

BULIMIA NERVOSA

A diagnosis of BN requires recurrent episodes of binge eating (i.e., the consumption of an unambiguously large amount of food given the context, accompanied by a sense of loss of control over eating). Episodes of binge eating co-occur with behaviors intended to compensate for energy consumed and to prevent weight gain, such as self-induced vomiting and fasting. Binge eating and compensatory behaviors must occur, on average, at least once a week for 3 months. The self-esteem of individuals with BN is excessively influenced by their body weight and shape. DSM-5 criteria for BN are outlined in Table 219-2.

BINGE EATING DISORDER

BED is characterized by recurrent episodes of binge eating in the absence of regular compensatory behaviors that are present in BN. The binge

TABLE 219-1 DSM-5 DIAGNOSTIC CRITERIA FOR ANOREXIA NERVOSA

A. Restriction of energy intake relative to requirements, leading to a significantly low body weight in the context of age, sex, developmental trajectory, and physical health. *Significantly low weight* is defined as a weight that is less than minimally normal or, for children and adolescents, less than minimally expected.
B. Intense fear of gaining weight or becoming fat, or persistent behavior that interferes with weight gain, even though at a significantly low weight.
C. Disturbance in the way in which one's body weight or shape is experienced, undue influence of body weight or shape on self-evaluation, or persistent lack of recognition of the seriousness of the current low body weight.
Specify whether:
Restricting type: During the last 3 months, the individual has not engaged in recurrent episodes of binge eating or purging behavior (i.e., self-induced vomiting or the misuse of laxatives, diuretics, or enemas). This subtype describes presentations in which weight loss is accomplished primarily through dieting, fasting, and/or excessive exercise.
Binge-eating/purging type: During the last 3 months, the individual has engaged in recurrent episodes of binge eating or purging behavior (i.e., self-induced vomiting or the misuse of laxatives, diuretics, or enemas).

From Diagnostic and Statistical Manual of Mental Disorders. 5th ed. Washington, DC: American Psychiatric Association; 2013.

TABLE 219-2 DSM-5 DIAGNOSTIC CRITERIA FOR BULIMIA NERVOSA

A. Recurrent episodes of binge eating. An episode of binge eating is characterized by both of the following:
  1. Eating, in a discrete period of time (e.g., within any 2-hour period), an amount of food that is definitely larger than most people would eat during a similar period of time and under similar circumstances.
  2. A sense of lack of control over eating during the episodes (e.g., a feeling that one cannot stop eating or control what or how much one is eating).
B. Recurrent inappropriate compensatory behavior in order to prevent weight gain, such as self-induced vomiting; misuse of laxatives, diuretics, enemas, or other medications; fasting; or excessive exercise.
C. The binge eating and inappropriate compensatory behaviors both occur, on average, at least once a week for 3 months.
D. Self-evaluation is unduly influenced by body shape and weight.
E. The disturbance does not occur exclusively during episodes of anorexia nervosa.

From Diagnostic and Statistical Manual of Mental Disorders. 5th ed. Washington, DC: American Psychiatric Association; 2013.

TABLE 219-3 DSM-5 DIAGNOSTIC CRITERIA FOR BINGE EATING DISORDER

A. Recurrent episodes of binge eating. An episode of binge eating is characterized by both of the following:
  1. Eating, in a discrete period of time (e.g., within any 2-hour period), an amount of food that is definitely larger than most people would eat during a similar period of time and under similar circumstances.
  2. A sense of lack of control over eating during the episodes (e.g., a feeling that one cannot stop eating or control what or how much one is eating).
B. The binge eating episodes are associated with three (or more) of the following:
  1. Eating much more rapidly than normal.
  2. Eating until feeling uncomfortably full.
  3. Eating large amounts of food when not feeling physically hungry.
  4. Eating alone because of feeling embarrassed by how much one is eating.
  5. Feeling disgusted with oneself, depressed, or very guilty afterward.
C. Marked distress regarding binge eating is present.
D. The binge eating occurs, on average, at least once a week for 3 months.
E. The binge eating is not associated with the recurrent use of inappropriate compensatory behavior as in bulimia nervosa and does not occur exclusively during the course of bulimia nervosa or anorexia nervosa.

From Diagnostic and Statistical Manual of Mental Disorders. 5th ed. Washington, DC: American Psychiatric Association; 2013.

episodes are distinguished by at least three associated characteristics, such as eating rapidly, eating until feeling uncomfortably full, and feeling disgust and guilt regarding the episodes. Individuals experience marked distress surrounding the binge episodes, and the binge eating episodes must occur, on average, at least once a week for 3 months. DSM-5 criteria for BED are listed in Table 219-3.

EPIDEMIOLOGY

Data suggest a lifetime prevalence of AN of approximately 0.6%, with higher rates among women (0.9%) compared with men (0.3%).[2] The lifetime prevalence of BN appears to be about 1%, with higher rates among women (1.5%) than among men (0.5%). The lifetime prevalence of BED is estimated at 3.5% for women and 2.0% for men. Among adolescents, lifetime prevalence estimates of AN, BN, and BED have been reported at 0.3%, 0.9%, and 1.6%, respectively.[3] Contrary to the view that eating disorders afflict only non-Hispanic white, affluent women, individuals of all races, ethnicities, and cultures are affected by these diagnoses.[4]

PATHOBIOLOGY

Research regarding the neuropathology of eating disorders is in nascent stages. Data suggest that several brain regions may be involved in and potentially interact in the manifestation of all eating disorders. Individuals with eating disorders appear to have brain function alterations in emotional/limbic, reward, and cognitive control circuits.[5] Fear circuitry networks involving the amygdala, anterior cingulate cortex, hippocampus, insula, striatum, and prefrontal cortex have demonstrated differential activation among individuals with eating disorders (with the majority of research in AN) compared with controls. Specifically, there tends to be a hyper-responsiveness in the limbic circuitry in response to potentially threatening cues, such as food and body weight/shape.

There also appear to be alterations in reward function in patients with AN, but the direction is unclear. By contrast, individuals with BN and BED consistently demonstrate hyper-responsivity in reward and somatosensory regions on exposure to food images. Data also suggest that individuals with eating disorders may have dysregulated frontal cortical cognitive neural networks acting in concert with regional reward systems.[6] Individuals with eating disorders have demonstrated impaired cognitive flexibility. Specific to BN, impulsivity and poor inhibitory control have also been reported.

Given the brain regions implicated in eating disorders, current studies have focused on the role of dopamine and serotonin in the manifestation of eating disorders. Individuals with AN appear to have impaired dopaminergic signaling, particularly in striatal circuits, that might contribute to altered reward and affect, decision making, and executive control as well as compulsivity and decreased food ingestion. Moreover, emerging clinical research suggests that striatal dopamine abnormalities exist in individuals with BN and BED. Because serotonin (5-hydroxytryptamine) 1A and 2A receptors and the serotonin transporter may play a part in symptoms of eating disorders, such as impulse control and associated mood symptoms, it is likely that interactions between the serotonin and dopaminergic systems contribute to eating disorders.

Risk Factors

Eating disorders develop as the result of multiple biological, psychological, and sociocultural factors. AN, BN, and BED aggregate in families, with estimates from twin studies suggesting that 40 to 60% of vulnerability for eating disorders is genetic. Studies have reported links between eating disorders and polymorphisms in the serotonin transporter gene (SLC6A4), the dopamine D_2 receptor (DRD2) gene, the μ_1 opioid receptor (OPRM1) gene, the fat mass and obesity-associated (FTO) gene, and the brain-derived neurotrophic factor (BDNF) gene. Although genetic linkage and association studies have implicated several susceptibility loci for AN, BN, and BED, specific genes that consistently lend vulnerability to eating disorders are less conclusive.[7]

Female sex, pediatric overweight, elevated shape and weight concerns, sexual abuse, trauma, and mood disorders have been identified as risk factors for all eating disorders. Personality-related variables, such as impulsivity and perfectionism, appear to be linked to eating disorders.[8] Importantly, internalization to the "thin ideal" (a sociocultural emphasis on shape and weight and a marked preference for a thin body type) with resulting weight and shape concerns has been proposed to contribute to eating disorder development, particularly among adolescents who are under strong influence from their peer and family environments. For example, parental overconcern about eating, shape, and weight as well as weight-related teasing by family members confers risk for eating disorders. Specific to BED, maltreatment, including teasing and bullying, and perceived stress are risk factors for the disorder.[9]

CLINICAL MANIFESTATIONS

Symptoms and Signs

For AN, physical symptoms and signs may include amenorrhea, constipation, cold intolerance, anemia, and lanugo hair. Reduced bone density is believed to predict the onset of premature osteopenia and osteoporosis. Health problems associated with malnutrition affect cardiovascular, gastrointestinal, reproductive, and endocrine systems. Individuals with AN frequently present with comorbid psychiatric disorders, including mood and anxiety disorders (e.g., social phobia, specific phobia, post-traumatic stress disorder), and high rates of suicidal ideation and behavior.

Individuals with BN present with signs and symptoms most commonly associated with purging behavior. These include dental enamel erosion secondary to vomiting, gastrointestinal symptoms, salivary gland hypertrophy, and electrolyte disturbances. Electrolyte abnormalities can have deleterious effects on the renal and cardiovascular systems. BN patients are at risk for cardiometabolic conditions (e.g., diabetes, stroke) as well as chronic pain. Metabolic acidosis can also occur in patients who are abusing laxatives as a result of the loss of bicarbonate from the bowel. Noninflammatory swelling of the salivary glands is a common clinical manifestation of BN. The most common psychiatric comorbidities in BN are major depressive disorder, anxiety disorders, substance use disorders, and disruptive behavioral disorders.

Individuals with BED are frequently overweight or obese. However, adults with BED are likely to report the development of diagnoses of metabolic syndrome components (e.g., dyslipidemia, hypertension, type 2 diabetes) after accounting for the contribution of body weight. The presence of BED may affect bariatric surgery outcome, resulting in less weight loss or more weight regain, but this is not a consistent finding. However, the presence of "loss of control" eating after surgery consistently predicts less weight loss or greater weight regain. Compared with obese adults without BED, those with the disorder experience significant impairment in a number of domains of psychosocial functioning, including a poorer quality of life and more impaired functioning in their home and social lives. Individuals with BED often have higher levels of disability, health problems, and work productivity impairment compared with obese and healthy controls without binge eating. With regard to comorbid psychiatric diagnoses, adults with BED experience Axis I psychiatric disorders at a rate comparable to (or higher than) that of individuals with AN or BN, including major depressive disorder, anxiety disorders, substance use disorders, and disruptive behavioral disorders.

Natural History

AN is typically manifested during adolescence, although the disorder can develop before puberty. BN frequently develops during later adolescence or early adulthood. BED is often manifested in adulthood, but adolescents also present with the disorder. Several retrospective and prospective studies report that binge and "out of control" eating occur as early as middle childhood.

Data on the natural course of eating disorders in the clear absence of treatment are limited. Eating disorders tend to exhibit a remitting and relapsing natural course across the lifespan, and there appear to be high rates of diagnostic crossover.[10] Treatment outcome data indicate that AN tends to transition to BN or an Unspecified Eating Disorder, and those with BN and BED tend to migrate from one to the other.

DIAGNOSIS

A number of structured, well-validated assessments for the diagnosis of eating disorders exist. These include but are not limited to the Structured Clinical Interview for the DSM and the Eating Disorder Examination. However, eating disorders are typically diagnosed by review of the patient's history, symptoms, and behaviors in an interview format. Evaluation of comorbid psychiatric problems, most notably mood, anxiety, substance use disorders, and disruptive behavioral disorders, is also required. Information should be gathered on interpersonal relationships, history of sexual and physical abuse, self-harm, and suicidal ideation or behavior. Family involvement is crucial, particularly for pediatric patients. A complete physical examination to assess body composition, vital signs, cardiovascular function, and hematologic and blood chemistry parameters is recommended for all patients.

TREATMENT Rx

Anorexia Nervosa

There is limited evidence on effective treatments for AN. For severely underweight patients, inpatient medical monitoring and supervised nutrition rehabilitation are required. The optimal setting (inpatient versus outpatient treatment) remains a subject of debate, and the evaluation of treatment costs in AN plays an important role in determining treatment. However, for pediatric patients, family-based psychotherapy, particularly during the early phases of the disorder, has demonstrated effectiveness.[11] Maudsley's family-based therapy involves both joint family sessions and simultaneous but independent patient/family intervention. Antidepressants (e.g., selective serotonin reuptake inhibitors) are associated with high rates of noncompliance, and compelling evidence of beneficial effects has not been found. The use of antipsychotic drugs has been explored, but results regarding their effectiveness remain nondefinitive.

Bulimia Nervosa

Cognitive-behavioral therapy (CBT) has been recognized as the treatment of choice for BN.[A1] Interpersonal psychotherapy (IPT) is also effective for the treatment of BN, particularly for those who are nonresponsive to CBT. There is growing support that pharmacotherapy may be helpful for some patients with BN. Antidepressants, especially selective serotonin reuptake inhibitors, are modestly effective for reducing binge eating in BN over the short and long term. Topiramate has consistently been shown to decrease binge eating in BN, but side effects may limit its usefulness. It is unclear whether combination therapy may be required for optimal outcomes.

Binge Eating Disorder

Psychological treatment for BED aims to reduce binge eating, weight and shape concerns, and prevent excess weight gain and/or induce modest weight loss. The psychotherapies most evaluated in clinical trials include CBT, IPT, behavioral weight loss, and CBT guided self-help (CBTgsh) approaches. CBT and IPT are first-line treatments. Given its cost-effectiveness, CBTgsh may be an optimal treatment option when specialist care is not available.[A2] With regard to pharmacologic treatment in BED, three medications or classes of medications have been studied in two or more placebo-controlled trials. Selective serotonin reuptake inhibitors, sibutramine, and topiramate all produce reductions in frequency of binge eating relative to placebo in short-term trials.[12] However, sibutramine has been withdrawn from the market, and topiramate is frequently associated with problematic cognitive effects, thus limiting its clinical utility.

PREVENTION

Whereas an increasing number of macro-level environmental public health initiatives have emerged (i.e., anti-dieting media campaigns and sanctions on advertising practices propagating an ideal of extreme thinness), few empirical data exist evaluating their efficacy. However, there are more data on individual, micro-level interventions aimed at reducing proximal eating disorder risk factors as well as current and distal eating pathology. Selected, interactive, multisession programs with adolescent girls may be more effective than universal, didactic, heterogeneous-sampled and single-session programs in reducing risk factors for eating disorder symptoms. For example, a dissonance-based program aimed at reducing eating disorder risk factors in adolescent girls has demonstrated effectiveness.

PROGNOSIS

Anorexia Nervosa

Remission rates vary widely for AN. Lower remission rates (29%) have been observed, particularly in studies with the shortest follow-up duration. However, most individuals with AN (approximately 76%) treated in outpatient settings will remit within 5 years after the initiation of treatment. Most individuals who do not achieve remission from AN during follow-up periods transition to a diagnosis of BN or an Unspecified Eating Disorder, which likely captures partial syndrome AN. Among psychiatric diagnoses, AN consistently has one of the highest mortality rates due to suicide, nutritional deficits, cardiac complications, and substance abuse.[13] The crude cumulative mortality rate is 2.8%, with longer duration of illness before receiving treatment and the need for inpatient treatment as negative prognostic indicators for AN.[14] Predictors of relapse include desiring a lower weight at the end of treatment and receiving treatment in a general (versus specialty) clinic.

Bulimia Nervosa

Similar to AN, most individuals with BN (70% or more) who receive treatment fully remit when assessed 5 to 20 years later, with remission rates being much lower (27 to 28%) at 1-year follow-up. If individuals with BN do not achieve remission within 5 years, however, they are likely to exhibit a chronic course of the illness. Mortality rates for BN range between 0 and 2%. Diagnostic crossover from BN to AN is relatively rare; yet, there is frequent diagnostic crossover between BN and BED, which may suggest a possible common psychological and/or biologic maintaining process. Negative prognostic indicators for BN include endorsement of greater psychiatric comorbidity, multiple impulsive behaviors (e.g., self-harm, substance use disorder), and a family history of alcohol abuse. Individuals who receive inpatient treatment or have a low motivation for engaging in treatment are more likely to relapse.

Binge Eating Disorder

A paucity of data exists on the long-term outcomes for BED patients. There are data to suggest that at 1 year after outpatient treatment, upwards of 80% of patients remit. In one clinical trial that examined 4-year outcomes, between 52 and 76% of individuals receiving psychological treatment for BED demonstrated remission from binge eating.[15] These preliminary data suggest that the prognostic trajectory may be similar to that of BN. Diagnostic crossover from BED to BN is high, whereas crossover to AN is relatively rare. Although examination of prognostic indicators for BED is in its early stages, patients reporting an undue influence of their body shape or weight on self-evaluation are less likely to have remission from binge eating at 12-month follow-up.[16] Rapid remission of binge eating has also been shown to be a positive prognostic indicator for binge remission.[17]

 Grade A References

A1. Lock J, Le Grange D, Agras WS, et al. Randomized clinical trial comparing family-based treatment with adolescent-focused individual therapy for adolescents with anorexia nervosa. *Arch Gen Psychiatry*. 2010;67:1025-1032.

A2. Poulsen S, Lunn S, Daniel SI, et al. A randomized controlled trial of psychoanalytic psychotherapy or cognitive-behavioral therapy for bulimia nervosa. *Am J Psychiatry*. 2014;171:109-116.

GENERAL REFERENCES

For the General References and other additional features, please visit Expert Consult at https://expertconsult.inkling.com.

220

OBESITY

MICHAEL D. JENSEN

Obesity is the most common nutritional disorder in the United States and directly or indirectly accounts for a significant portion of health-related expenses. The safest treatment approaches (lifestyle change and behavior modification) are not those commonly employed by physicians and require considerable time to implement. The recently released Guideline for the Management of Overweight and Obesity in Adults provides direction for clinicians for the treatment of obesity.

DEFINITION

The Guideline for the Management of Overweight and Obesity in Adults produced by the National Institutes of Health and the National Heart, Lung, and Blood Institute (NHLBI) and disseminated by the American College of Cardiology (ACC), the American Heart Association (AHA), and The Obesity Society (TOS) provides evidence-informed, scientifically based recommendations on evaluation and management of overweight and obesity.

Body mass index (BMI) continues to be the recommended approach to categorize weight relative to height for adults. BMI is calculated as weight (in kilograms) divided by height squared (in meters):

$$BMI = \frac{weight\ (kg)}{height^2\ (m^2)}$$

To calculate BMI with pounds and inches, the formula is modified as follows:

$$BMI = \frac{weight\ (lb)}{height^2\ (in^2)} \times 703$$

The guideline suggested that no changes are indicated in the weight classifications by BMI, which are summarized in Table 220-1. Individuals who are overweight (BMI of 25.0 to 29.9) may or may not be overfat. Some adults may be overweight because of increased muscle mass, which is a straightforward clinical observation. Although, in general, the risk for development of adiposity-related health problems increases continuously as the BMI exceeds 25, the new guideline continues to recommend the use of waist circumference measurements to discriminate among patients who may require more testing. Overweight and class I obese patients with a waist circumference in the high-risk category deserve a discussion of lifestyle issues as they relate to health and weight loss. Some individuals with a BMI of 27 to 29.9 develop serious metabolic complications that improve with weight loss and are candidates for more aggressive treatment, including pharmacotherapy if it is needed. Asian populations, in particular, are at risk for the typical metabolic complications of obesity at lower BMI and waist circumferences than those for whites, Hispanics, blacks, and Polynesians; the guideline for at-risk BMI in Asian populations is 23 to 24.

TABLE 220-1	CLASSIFICATION OF OVERWEIGHT AND OBESITY BY BODY MASS INDEX (BMI)	
	OBESITY CLASS	BMI (kg/m²)
Underweight		<18.5
Normal		18.5-24.9
Overweight		25.0-29.9
Obesity	I	30.0-34.9
Obesity	II	35.0-39.9
Extreme obesity	III	≥40

Jensen MD, Ryan DH, Apovian CM, et al. 2013 AHA/ACC/TOS guideline for the management of overweight and obesity in adults: a report of the American College of Cardiology/American Heart Association Task Force on Practice Guidelines and The Obesity Society. *J Am Coll Cardiol.* 2014;63:2985-3023.

The prevalence of comorbidities and risk of future morbidities increase considerably at a BMI of more than 30, the cut point for obesity. Obesity is divided into three classes, also depending on BMI (see Table 220-1). Treatment approaches may differ for those who are overweight and for different classes of obesity. For example, current U.S. Food and Drug Administration guidelines indicate that pharmacotherapy can be adjunct treatment for any class of obesity, even if medical complications are not present. Familiarity with the guidelines is important. Supervisory agencies and third-party payers use them to determine who is eligible for treatment benefits. Extreme obesity (BMI > 40) is one of the key features that would prompt consideration of a patient for bariatric surgery when medical treatments have failed. Patients with class II obesity (BMI of 35.0 to 39.9) may be considered for bariatric surgery if medical treatments have failed and if severe, life-threatening complications are present.

As noted, the new NHLBI/ACC/AHA/TOS guidelines continue to recommend waist circumference as an office assessment tool to help with the treatment decision-making process. The new guidelines suggest that the previous waist circumference cut points of more than 102 cm (40 inches) for men and more than 88 cm (35 inches) for women are indicators of increased metabolic risk. However, the report stated that the relationships between disease risk and waist circumference are continuous and progressive, with no obvious cut points. The recommendation is to measure waist circumference in overweight and class I obesity adults. Those adults with waist circumferences above the cut points deserve further evaluation to detect other cardiovascular disease risk factors. Adults with class II or class III obesity are at sufficiently high risk that waist circumference information does not appear to add valuable information. These definitions of overweight and obesity and of high-risk waist circumference are generally applicable to those of European and African descent, but lower values are recommended for those of Asian descent. The risks of metabolic abnormalities occur at lower BMI and lower waist circumference in these populations.

EPIDEMIOLOGY

Prevalence of Obesity

Although the number of overweight and obese adults in the United States has increased dramatically during the past 30 years, the increase in the prevalence is now slowing or leveling off.[1] In 2009-2010, the prevalence of obesity was 35.5% among adult men and 35.8% among adult women, with no significant change compared with 2003-2008. Approximately 60% of U.S. men and 51% of U.S. women are overweight or obese, although a greater percentage of women than men are obese. There are substantial differences in the prevalence of obesity by age, race, and socioeconomic status. The prevalence of obesity in adults tends to rise steadily from the ages of 20 to 60 years, decreasing in later years. It has been estimated that almost 75% of men aged 60 to 69 years in the United States have a BMI of more than 25. The increase in mean BMI with age is not as much of a threat to population health as is a similar increase in the BMI of younger populations. The lowest mortality rates for young adults are for a BMI in the lower part of the normal range (20.0 to 24.9), whereas the BMI associated with the lowest mortality rates is somewhat above 25 kg/m² for those in the 60s and 70s. Physicians should base their weight recommendations for individual patients on whether adverse health consequences associated with obesity are present.

The differences in overweight and obesity among African Americans, Mexican Americans, and European Americans are not subtle. African American women and Mexican Americans of both sexes have the highest rates of overweight and obesity in the United States. In interpreting these data, however, it is important to keep in mind that there is an inverse relationship between socioeconomic status and obesity, especially among women (Chapter 5). Women in lower socioeconomic classes are much more likely than those in higher socioeconomic classes to be obese. This association reduces but does not eliminate the racial differences in the prevalence of obesity. Whether the remaining racial differences in the prevalence of obesity are due to genetic, constitutional, or social factors is not yet known.

PATHOBIOLOGY

Etiology

Genetic and constitutional susceptibility to obesity are heavily influenced by the environment. Evidence from studies of twins adopted into different families indicates that within a given environment, a significant portion of the variation in weight is genetic.[2] That said, the remarkable increase in the prevalence of obesity in the United States during the past 3 decades is unlikely to be due to wholesale changes in the genetic makeup of Americans.

Genetic Aspects of Human Obesity

Although obesity susceptibility is a classic polygenic condition, there are also a number of syndromic and monogenic obesity syndromes. The long-recognized genetic defects resulting in obesity include Prader-Willi and Laurence-Moon-Biedl syndromes. More recently, rare monogenic forms of human obesity due to mutations in the leptin gene, the leptin receptor gene, and the melanocortin signaling system genes have been described. These gene mutations are most often associated with increased appetite rather than with reduced energy expenditure. Genome-wide association studies have reported a number of genes associated with higher BMI. Those that appear to predict the greatest amount of variance in BMI include the fat mass and obesity-associated (*FTO*) gene and the melanocortin-4 receptor (*MC4R*) gene. Other genes that have been reliably associated with obesity include *TMEM18*, *KCTD15*, *GNPDA2*, *SH2B1*, *MTCH2*, and *NEGR1*. Together, however, the combined effects of all the identified genetic contributions account for less than 1% of the variance in BMI. This emphasizes both the huge environmental effects and the polygenic nature of susceptibility to obesity.

Constitutional Influences on Obesity

A number of environmental factors can result in long-term, epigenetic effects on body weight regulation and the susceptibility to obesity-related health problems. These epigenetic effects are ascribed to processes that include changes in DNA methylation, acetylation, and chromatin remodeling. The effect of the intrauterine environment and the perinatal period on subsequent weight and health is best studied. Undernutrition in the last trimester of pregnancy and in the early postnatal period decreases the risk of adult obesity, although the low birthweight associated with undernutrition (or smoking) in late pregnancy also increases the risk of adulthood hypertension, abnormal glucose tolerance, and cardiovascular disease. In contrast, undernutrition limited to the first two trimesters of pregnancy is associated with an increased probability of adult obesity. The infants of diabetic mothers tend to be fatter than those of nondiabetic mothers, and children of diabetic mothers have a greater prevalence of obesity when they are 5 to 19 years old, independent of whether their mother is obese. Finally, intrauterine exposure to the diabetic environment results in an increased risk of diabetes mellitus and obesity in the offspring. Thus, the issue of the genes versus the environment in regard to obesity and metabolic complications of obesity is blurred in the intrauterine and perinatal time intervals. One of the striking and worrisome aspects of these metabolic effects is not only the long-term effects on the individual's weight regulation and health but also the suggestion that these traits can be passed on to future generations.

Environmental Contributors to Human Obesity

Dramatic changes in the environment of Western countries have occurred during the past 50 years, including reduced demands for physical activity and alterations in the food supply. These food supply changes appear to have either increased or prevented the expected decrease in energy intake that would be needed to match the reduced energy expenditure from physical activity.[3]

Food

A number of environmental factors can influence food intake (Table 220-2). Consuming energy-dense foods results in greater energy intake because adults tend to respond to food volume rather than to the energy content. This factor likely accounts for the association between high-fat diets and excess body weight; many high-fat foods are also energy dense. When humans consume diets that are high in fat but low in energy density, energy intake is not greater than would be expected on the basis of the energy density of the foods. Larger food portion size has also been shown to increase food intake. Given the trend in the United States to serve larger portions of food and beverage, this could contribute to greater obesity risk. Food variety can also affect energy intake. An increased variety of entrees, sweets, snacks, and carbohydrates in the diet is associated with an increase in body fatness and food intake. In contrast, an increase in the variety of vegetables available does not appear to increase energy intake and is not associated with increased body fatness. Other factors that may have broad population effects in the United States include the reduced costs of food, increased availability, and palatability. Finally, there is evidence that consumption of sugar-sweetened beverages, such as soft drinks and fruit juices, is not accompanied by a decrease in food intake to offset the extra energy intake. The implication is that some types of beverages will add to the energy intake during the day and promote weight gain.

A number of psychological factors also influence how the properties of food affect energy intake. Individuals vary with respect to their dietary restraint (the tendency to consciously limit food intake to control weight), their feelings of hunger, or their disinhibition (the tendency to overeat opportunistically). It has been proposed that interindividual differences in these factors modify how food variety and portion size affect the eating profile. The social context in which food is consumed and the emotional state of the individual also modulate food intake.

Physical Activity

Physical activity can be divided into three categories: (1) exercise (fitness- and sports-related activities); (2) work-related physical activity; and (3) non-exercise, nonemployment (spontaneous) activity. Tables are widely available that allow one to calculate energy expenditure on the basis of an individual's weight as well as the type and duration of exercise. Only about 20 to 30% of Americans engage in exercise at the recommended frequency, intensity, or duration that could be expected to have a protective effect on the development of obesity and other health problems, but this does not seem to have changed in recent decades. Recent data suggest that the amount of time spent in sedentary activities (e.g., watching television, using the computer) is an independent predictor of metabolic abnormalities associated with obesity over and above the effects of exercise. Thus, to the extent that reduced physical activity is contributing to the epidemic of obesity, it is likely that it is reduced employment-related and spontaneous physical activity that is changing.

Although it is becoming easier for individuals to measure the energy expended in nonexercise activity with step counters and electronic motion detection devices, there are insufficient longitudinal, population-based data to define the extent to which changes in this activity parameter have occurred. Certainly, employment-related physical activity has decreased with the advent of more automated systems in the workplace. One estimate suggests that between 1982 and 1992, energy expenditure at work decreased by about 50 kcal/day. The additional workplace changes since that time have probably reduced employment physical activity further.

The other component of nonexercise physical activity, the activities of daily living, has probably been reduced by the plethora of labor-saving conveniences (e.g., drive-through food and banking, escalators, remote controls, e-mail, online shopping) now available. Again, there are few hard data to assess how much of a change has actually occurred, although a reduction in daily walking trips and an increase in daily automobile trips have been documented.

There is a large amount of information on how differences in sedentary activity (television watching, video games, and computer use) relate to obesity and obesity complications. The evidence indicates that more time spent in sedentary pursuits is associated with an increased risk of overweight and obesity. The striking aspect to these studies is that the adverse effect of sedentary activities is independent of participation in traditional exercise activities.

Understanding the contributions of decreased work-related physical activity, decreases in activity of daily living, and increases in sedentary behavior can help the physician working with the patient to uncover patterns that may relate to weight gain. Physicians who are aware of these environmental factors are in a better position to help their obese patients identify which of these

TABLE 220-2	ENVIRONMENTAL FACTORS PROMOTING OBESITY	
DIETARY		**ACTIVITY**
↑ Energy density of foods		↑ Sedentary behavior
↑ Portion size		↓ Activities of daily living
↑ Variety*		↓ Employment physical activity
↑ Palatability		
↑ Availability		
↓ Cost		
↑ Caloric beverages (sugar-sweetened beverages)		

*Variety of sweets, snacks, and entrees.

environmental factors are contributing to the problem and to develop plans for intervention. In this regard, patients who regularly use step counters or other types of activity-monitoring devices will be better able to self-identify and modify their behavior to obtain sufficient physical activity.

Regulation of Body Weight and Energy Balance

The regulation of adult body weight is a well-balanced process. For example, the typical U.S. adult will take in and expend approximately 2000 to 3000 kcal/day. If there were a consistent error of even 1% in overconsumption of food, this would result in the gain of approximately 25 to 30 pounds of fat every 10 years, assuming no change in energy expenditure. It follows that most adults regulate their average energy balance with greater than 1% precision. There appears to be regulation of both energy intake and energy expenditure through conscious and unconscious processes.

The excess energy consumed by adults is generally stored as triglycerides in adipocytes. Humans continuously recruit new adipocytes from a large preadipocyte pool to replace dying adipocytes. Although the primary means by which abdominal adipose tissue mass expands is through increased fat cell size (adipocyte hypertrophy), this process can store only a limited amount of fat. Adults who gain leg fat accumulate more rather than larger adipocytes on average, resulting in a net increase in adipocyte number as more new adipocytes are created than needed to replace dying cells. Some adults recruit new adipocytes more readily than others do and thus gain weight more so from adipocyte hyperplasia (increased fat cell number) than from hypertrophy. Those who gain fat with large adipocytes, especially in association with an adipose tissue inflammatory response (greater numbers of classically activated macrophages and other immune cells), are more likely to be insulin resistant and to have signs of low-grade systemic inflammation (increased C-reactive protein, mildly elevated interleukin-6 and tumor necrosis factor).

Leptin, a cytokine family protein that is secreted almost exclusively by adipocytes, was the first identified adipose tissue hormone; it has been shown to have potent central nervous system effects on food intake in humans. Leptin also has other hypothalamic-pituitary functions and is proposed to have diverse peripheral physiologic actions. The leptin-deficient animal model of obesity, the *ob/ob* mouse, is severely obese, hyperphagic, hypometabolic, and sexually immature and has low levels of spontaneous activity. Administration of leptin to this animal corrects all of these defects. A few leptin-deficient humans (due to mutations in the leptin gene) have been identified. These children had very low plasma leptin concentrations, were hyperphagic and severely obese, and responded to exogenous leptin administration with dramatic weight loss, reduced food intake, and accelerated maturation of the pituitary-gonadal axis. Overwhelmingly, however, obese humans are not leptin deficient and in fact have high plasma leptin concentrations unless they are in a major negative energy balance circumstance. Because leptin is secreted as a function of percentage body fat, and because women have more body fat than men for any given BMI, they also have higher plasma leptin concentrations. Thus, screening for leptin deficiency is not warranted except in severe, hyperphagic obesity that begins in early childhood, is accompanied by sexual immaturity, and exists in the absence of other known causes (e.g., Prader-Willi syndrome).

Some animal models of genetic obesity (the *db/db* mouse and *fa/fa* rat) have defective leptin receptors, making them unresponsive to leptin. Although rare cases of obese humans with defective leptin receptor genes have been reported, again it appears that leptin resistance due to leptin receptor defects (or genetic post-receptor signaling abnormalities) is extremely uncommon. Clinical screening for leptin receptor mutations is not warranted, given that no treatment exists.

Energy Intake

Much of what has been learned about the biologic regulation of food intake has been from the study of animal models. These signals may affect different aspects of eating behavior. They can affect *hunger*, the compelling need or desire for food; *satiation*, the state of being satisfactorily full and unable to take on more; or *satiety*, the sense of no longer being hungry, a complex set of postprandial events that affect the interval to the next meal or the amount consumed at the next meal. Some of the signals that alter eating behavior affect one aspect and others affect multiple aspects. For example, ghrelin, a peptide produced by the stomach, increases hunger but does not appear to affect satiation or satiety. Cholecystokinin causes satiation but has no effect on satiety. Leptin appears to act on multiple pathways; leptin deficiency is associated with increased hunger and reduced satiation and satiety.

TABLE 220-3 SUGGESTED BIOLOGIC MODULATORS OF FOOD INTAKE

PERIPHERAL SIGNAL	PROPOSED EFFECT ON FOOD INTAKE
Vagal	–
Cholecystokinin	–
Apolipoprotein A-IV	–
Insulin	–
Peptide YY$_{3-36}$	–
Glucagon-like peptide 1	–
Other glucagon-related peptides	–
Leptin	+ when leptin ↓↓
Ghrelin	+
Tumor necrosis factor-α	–
Obestatin	–

TABLE 220-4 CENTRAL NERVOUS SYSTEM MODULATORS OF ENERGY BALANCE

CENTRAL ANABOLIC (↑ INTAKE)	CENTRAL CATABOLIC (↓ INTAKE)
Neuropeptide Y	α-Melanocyte-stimulating hormone
Agouti-related protein	Corticotropin-releasing hormone
Melanin-concentrating hormone	Thyrotropin-releasing hormone
Hypocretins and orexins	Cocaine- and amphetamine-regulated transcript
Galanin	Interleukin-1β
Norepinephrine	Urocortin
Endogenous endocannabinoids (anandamide and 2-arachidonoylglycerol)	Oxytocin
	Neurotensin
	Serotonin

Peripheral satiety signals act to inhibit further food intake at some point during meal consumption. Some of the signals reach the brain through the vagus nerve and some through the systemic circulation. Examples of the proposed factors modulating appetite are listed in Table 220-3. The compounds range from gut-derived (ghrelin, cholecystokinin, glucagon-like peptide 1) and pancreas-derived (insulin) hormones to peptides such as apolipoprotein A-IV, which is secreted with chylomicrons. The signals are thought to be triggered both by mechanical stimuli (e.g., the fullness of the stomach) and by the presence of nutrients in the jejunum and ileum.

The central nervous system regulation of food intake is becoming better understood. A number of neuropeptides, lipid derivatives, and monoamines have either anabolic (increased food intake with or without decreased energy expenditure) or catabolic (decreased food intake with or without increased energy expenditure) properties. A list of these molecules is provided in Table 220-4. Many of these compounds serve more than one function, such as regulation of hormone secretion (thyrotropin-releasing hormone and corticotropin-releasing hormone), wakefulness (norepinephrine), and behavior-reinforcing systems (endocannabinoids).

Energy Expenditure

There is a wide range of daily energy expenditure in adults, from less than 1400 kcal/day to more than 5000 kcal/day, with larger, more physically active individuals having the greatest energy needs. Typically, daily energy expenditure is divided into resting (or basal) metabolic rate, the thermic effect of food, and physical activity energy expenditure.

Basal Metabolic Rate

The basal metabolic rate (BMR) is the energy expenditure of lying still at rest, awake, in the overnight postabsorptive state. The resting metabolic rate (RMR) is similarly defined but is not necessarily measured before arising from bed. For most sedentary adult Americans, the RMR represents the major portion of energy expended during the day and may range from less than 1200 to more than 3000 kcal/day. Most (~80%) of the BMR can be explained by the amount of lean tissue an individual has. There are a number of formulas that can be used to estimate BMR. The Harris-Benedict formula (available through numerous online calculators) predicts BMR on the basis of height, weight, age, and sex and is accurate to within 10% in approximately 90% of adults with BMIs of 18.5 to 45 kg/m².

Not all components of lean tissue consume oxygen at the same relative rates. Visceral or splanchnic bed tissues account for about 25% of RMR but a much smaller proportion of body weight. The brain, which is only a small percentage of body weight, accounts for almost 15% of RMR. Likewise, the heart (~7%) and kidneys (~5 to 10%) account for greater portions of resting energy needs than their relative contribution to body mass. In contrast, resting muscle makes up 40 to 50% of lean tissue mass but accounts for only 25% of RMR. This contribution changes dramatically with exercise, however, at which time muscle can account for 80 to 90% of energy expenditure. Adipose tissue is a minor contributor to daily energy expenditure, consuming only approximately 3 kcal/kg of body fat per day.

Brown fat is adipose tissue that expresses large amounts of uncoupling protein-1, a protein that allows a mitochondrial membrane proton leak, resulting in heat release as opposed to chemical work from adenosine triphosphate—"uncoupling" of substrate oxidation from chemical or mechanical work. This thermogenic tissue was thought to be present only in human infants but has recently been shown to exist in adults.[4] Methods used to detect brown fat largely rely on ¹⁸F-fluorodeoxyglucose positron emission tomography scanning of humans exposed to cold. Lean adults are more likely than obese adults to have brown fat, and brown fat is more readily detectable after obese adults lose weight. Whether brown fat plays any meaningful role in thermogenesis is currently a matter of debate.

Although most of the RMR can be accounted for by the mass of lean tissue, there are also other, more subtle influences on RMR. Age, sex (women have slightly lower BMR even corrected for fat-free mass), and fat mass affect RMR. Small changes in BMR occur during the menstrual cycle (luteal phase > follicular phase). There is also evidence that heritable or family factors influence BMR, accounting for as much as 10% of the interindividual differences.

There are both obligatory and facultative components to RMR. With an energy-restricted diet, significant reductions in BMR relative to the amount of fat-free mass occur. Reductions in the production of triiodothyronine from thyroxine and the sympathetic nervous system drive are thought to contribute to this phenomenon. Likewise, during brief periods of overfeeding, RMR increases slightly above that which would be expected for the amount of lean tissue present.

It has been proposed that individuals with BMRs lower than predicted are at increased risk of future weight gain. Published data suggest that the relative risk is small, and clinical effort to identify such patients is not warranted. Measurement of BMR is sometimes helpful in the evaluation of patients who insist that they are unable to lose weight while following diets containing less than 1000 kcal/day. Almost without fail, if BMR is measured with a reliable instrument, it is substantially greater than the reported food intake. This underscores the fact that most adults are unreliable in assessing their own food intake.

The Thermic Effect of Food

An average of 10% of the energy content of food is expended in the process of digestion, absorption, and metabolism of nutrients. There is a significant interindividual variability in this value, however, ranging from a low of about 3% to a high of about 15% of meal calories that are "wasted" in the postprandial interval. The thermic effect of a meal is related to its carbohydrate and protein calorie content; the fat content has little stimulatory effect. Both obligatory (60 to 70%) and facultative (30 to 40%) components of the thermic effect of food have been identified. The obligatory components no doubt reflect the energy costs of digestion, absorption, and storage of nutrients. The two factors thought to play a role in the facultative component of the thermic effect of food are the postprandial insulin response and activation of the sympathetic nervous system. The thermic effect of food is somewhat lower in insulin-resistant and obese humans, but this has not been linked to future obesity.

Physical Activity Energy Expenditure

The energy expenditure of physical activity is a product of the amount of work done and the work efficiency of the individual. Tracking the total amount of physical activity that humans perform throughout the day is becoming easier with a variety of relatively inexpensive devices. By doing so, it is also possible to calculate the energy expended with published values for estimating the energy costs of work performed. Work units are expressed as metabolic equivalents (METs), a multiple of the RMR. If an individual's RMR is 1 kcal/minute (1440 kcal/day), a workload of 5 METs would be 5 kcal/minute. Although most sedentary individuals can work for only a limited amount of time at relatively low workloads, highly trained athletes can work at extremely high METs (>16) for extended periods. This is because athletes have both a greater peak work capacity (or maximal amount of calories or oxygen that can be consumed) and a higher lactate threshold. The lactate threshold is closely related to the level at which exercise begins to become so uncomfortable that it cannot be maintained much longer. The biochemical definition of lactate threshold describes the progressive rise in blood lactate concentrations observed during sufficiently high-intensity exercise. The lactate threshold may range from 50 to 90% of an individual's peak work capacity. Training raises the lactate threshold closer to the maximal workload and thus allows individuals to work at higher rates for longer periods. Thus, highly fit individuals can expend much greater amounts of energy per minute of exercise with less sense of discomfort than can obese, sedentary individuals who typically have low aerobic fitness and low lactate thresholds (sometimes on the order of 4 to 5 METs). The lactate threshold can be even lower in obese patients with type 2 diabetes, such that walking a mere 3 miles per hour can exceed their lactate threshold. Appreciation of the physical limitations of patients, which can usually be overcome with a carefully designed training program, is necessary to provide realistic activity recommendations.

Exercise (fitness- and sports-related activities) is commonly considered the main component of physical activity thermogenesis. Because most adults do not exercise at high levels or for a sufficient duration to expend a large amount of energy, focusing solely on "exercise" as the main component of physical activity will miss significant opportunities for improving energy balance. The benefits of and energy expended in nonexercise activity can be far greater than with exercise, given the limited amount of time and effort that most patients can commit to exercise.

Nonexercise activity thermogenesis (NEAT) is the calorie expense of performing all activities other than exercise- or employment-related and spontaneous activity. The range of observed NEAT under controlled (metabolic chamber) conditions has been less than 100 to more than 800 kcal/day. The energy expended from a physically demanding job or volitional exercise may or may not be offset by reductions in spontaneous (nonemployment) activity. For example, young adult men and women respond differently to 1 year of extra exercise; men lose weight and women do not, despite the absence of detectable change in food intake. Women must either reduce spontaneous activity in response to exercise or have subtle increases in food intake. It has also been shown that the variations in unconscious increases in NEAT relate strongly to the amount of fat gained in response to overeating. Low levels of NEAT have been reported to predict future weight gain in some populations, and there may be differences between lean and obese persons in the daily amount of NEAT, which could relate to differential tendencies to regulate weight.

Secondary Causes of Obesity
Medications

A number of medications cause weight gain in some or most of the patients for whom they are prescribed. Awareness of the medications that have this potential can facilitate weight loss treatment in some patients. Table 220-5 lists a number of medications that are associated with weight gain as well as alternative treatment approaches, if any, for the underlying condition.

Diseases

Less than 1% of obese patients have an underlying disease that can explain the development of their obesity. Endocrinopathies are the most common secondary cause of obesity. These include Cushing's syndrome (Chapter 227), hypothalamic damage resulting in overeating (most commonly after pituitary surgery), insulinoma (Chapter 230), and hypothyroidism (Chapter 226). A Cushing syndrome–like fat distribution is common; therefore, other physical or laboratory findings are the best clues to whether to test for this condition. These include the classic purple striae, thinning skin, easy bruising, proximal muscle weakness, and electrolyte abnormalities. Correction of Cushing's syndrome commonly results in substantial loss of excess body fat. Insulinoma is a rare tumor, and only a small portion of patients with

TABLE 220-5 PHARMACOLOGIC INFLUENCES IN WEIGHT GAIN AND ALTERNATIVE THERAPIES

DRUGS THAT MAY PROMOTE WEIGHT GAIN	ALTERNATIVE TREATMENTS: WEIGHT NEUTRAL OR WEIGHT LOSS

PSYCHIATRIC AND NEUROLOGIC MEDICATIONS
Antipsychotics: olanzapine, clozapine, risperidone, quetiapine, aripiprazole
Antidepressants
   Tricyclics: imipramine, amitriptyline
   Triazolopyridines: trazodone
   Serotonin reuptake inhibitors: paroxetine, fluoxetine, citalopram
Tetracyclics: mirtazapine
Monamine oxidase inhibitors
Antiepileptic drugs: gabapentin (higher doses), valproic acid, carbamazepine, divalproex
Mood stabilizers: lithium, carbamazepine, lamotrigine, gabapentin (higher doses)
	ALTERNATIVE PSYCHIATRIC AND NEUROLOGIC MEDICATIONS
	Ziprasidone
	Nortriptyline, bupropion, nefazodone, fluvoxamine, sertraline, duloxetine
	Topiramate, zonisamide (weight loss), lamotrigine (less weight gain)

STEROID HORMONES Progestational steroids Corticosteroids Hormonal contraceptives	**ALTERNATIVES TO STEROID HORMONES** Barrier methods, intrauterine device Nonsteroidal anti-inflammatory drugs
ANTIDIABETES AGENTS Insulin (most forms) Sulfonylureas Thiazolidinediones	**ALTERNATIVE ANTIDIABETES AGENTS** Metformin Acarbose, miglitol Exenatide Dipeptidyl peptidase 4 inhibitors Liraglutide Sodium-glucose co-transporter 2 inhibitors
ANTIHISTAMINES Commonly reported with older agents; also oxatomide, loratadine, and azelastine	**ALTERNATIVE TO ANTIHISTAMINES** Decongestants, mast cell stabilizers, antagonists of endogenous mediators of inflammation
ANTIHYPERTENSIVE AGENTS α-Adrenergic and β-adrenergic receptor blockers Calcium channel blockers: nisoldipine	**ALTERNATIVE ANTIHYPERTENSIVE AGENTS** Angiotensin-converting enzyme inhibitors Calcium channel blockers: most other agents Angiotensin receptor blockers Diuretics
HIGHLY ACTIVE ANTIRETROVIRAL THERAPY	

insulinoma develop obesity. The weight gain associated with hypothyroidism is largely due to fluid retention and resolves with thyroid hormone replacement. Unfortunately, successful treatment is not available for hyperphagia due to hypothalamic damage. Adult patients with growth hormone deficiency, most commonly after hypophysectomy, may lose excess body fat with growth hormone replacement therapy.

Psychosocial Aspects of Obesity

Sexual, physical, and emotional abuse, especially in women, can result in long-term adverse consequences, including obesity. The effects of the abuse tend to be most profound if it occurs in childhood and adolescence. These women may be severely obese, suffer from chronic depression, and experience a number of psychosomatic symptoms, particularly chronic gastrointestinal distress. Identifying these issues before initiation of weight loss programs is important because successful weight loss may actually aggravate the distress experienced by these women. In addition, appropriate referral for psychiatric help may be needed before initiation of treatment for obesity.

PATHOPHYSIOLOGY
Metabolic Complications of Obesity

A central or upper body fat distribution is more predictive than total fat mass of the metabolic complications of obesity. Adipose tissue release of free fatty acids (FFAs) and glycerol into the circulation through lipolysis provides 50 to 100% of daily energy needs. Adipose tissue lipolysis is regulated primarily by insulin (inhibition) and catecholamines (stimulation), although growth hormone, cortisol, and atrial natriuretic peptide also stimulate lipolysis. Upper body obesity is associated with several abnormalities of adipose tissue lipolysis, most remarkably with higher postprandial FFA release and concentrations; this abnormality is particularly evident in type 2 diabetes mellitus. Abnormally high FFA concentrations can contribute to a number of the metabolic complications of obesity.

Insulin Resistance

The term *insulin resistance* is typically used in referring to the ability of insulin to promote glucose uptake and to inhibit the release of glucose into the circulation. The primary site of insulin-stimulated glucose uptake, oxidation,

and storage is skeletal muscle. The principal site of glucose production is the liver. Insulin resistance initially leads to hyperinsulinemia and may eventually lead to the development of type 2 diabetes mellitus (Chapter 229).

The ability of insulin to promote glucose uptake, oxidation, and storage in muscle and to suppress plasma FFA concentrations is reduced in upper body obesity. High plasma FFA concentrations can induce a state of insulin resistance both in the muscle (glucose uptake) and in the liver (glucose release), independent of obesity. Thus, abnormal regulation of adipose tissue FFA export is a significant component of the development of insulin resistance. It is hypothesized that excess FFAs induce muscle insulin resistance by promoting increased synthesis of diacylglycerols and ceramides, both of which can interfere with the normal insulin signaling pathway.

Dysregulated production of a number of adipose-derived hormones, also called adipokines, is hypothesized to contribute to insulin resistance and the metabolic complications of obesity. Adiponectin, an adipocyte-derived hormone that improves insulin action, is secreted at reduced rates in obesity and diabetes. Increased production of resistin, interleukin-6, tumor necrosis factor, and retinol-binding protein-4 by adipose tissue has been linked to insulin resistance in animal models. We currently lack the experimental evidence from human studies to know what role adipokines play in the metabolic complications of obesity.

Islet Cell Failure and Type 2 Diabetes Mellitus

Type 2 diabetes usually results from defects in both insulin secretion and insulin action (Chapter 229). Many obese individuals are insulin resistant, yet only a subset will develop diabetes mellitus. It follows that those who develop type 2 diabetes develop pancreatic β-cell decompensation with subsequent hyperglycemia. Animal (rodent) studies have suggested that a process referred to as lipotoxicity is involved in pancreatic β-cell failure. In this model, increased FFAs are proposed to contribute to the insulin secretory abnormalities seen in obesity and ultimately to lead to β-cell failure. There is some evidence that elevated FFAs have adverse effects on islet β-cell function in humans. Another potential contributor to β-cell failure in obesity is the overproduction of islet amyloid polypeptide. This protein is co-secreted with insulin and, because of its tertiary structure, can form toxic amyloid deposits in β cells. Amyloid deposits have been found in the pancreatic islets obtained at autopsy from patients with type 2 diabetes mellitus.

Hypertension

Blood pressure can be increased by a number of mechanisms (Chapter 67). Increased circulating blood volume, abnormal vasoconstriction, decreased vascular relaxation, and increased cardiac output may all contribute to hypertension in obesity. The effect of hyperinsulinemia to increase renal sodium absorption may contribute to hypertension through increased circulating blood volume. Abnormalities of vascular resistance also contribute to the pathophysiologic process of obesity-related hypertension. Under some experimental conditions, elevated FFAs have been found to cause increased vasoconstriction and reduced nitric oxide–mediated vasorelaxation, similar to that seen in the metabolic syndrome. Some obese adults have increased sympathetic nervous system activity, which could contribute to obesity-associated hypertension. Finally, angiotensinogen (also produced by adipocytes) is a precursor of the vasoconstrictor angiotensin II and is proposed to contribute to elevated blood pressure.

Dyslipidemia

Upper body obesity and type 2 diabetes mellitus are associated with increased triglycerides, decreased high-density lipoprotein (HDL) cholesterol, and a high proportion of small, dense low-density lipoprotein (LDL) particles (Chapter 206). This dyslipidemia contributes to the increased cardiovascular risk observed in the metabolic syndrome. Fasting hypertriglyceridemia is caused by increased hepatic very low density lipoprotein (VLDL) secretion, which may be driven by increased delivery of FFAs to the liver coming from both visceral fat and upper body subcutaneous fat. The reduced HDL cholesterol concentrations and the increased small, dense LDL particle concentrations associated with upper body obesity are likely an indirect consequence of elevated triglyceride-rich VLDL. Increased cholesterol ester transfer protein activity and hepatic lipase activity can theoretically account for the atherogenic shifts in triglycerides and cholesterol between lipoproteins. Genetic influences play a significant role in the expression of these lipid abnormalities. Polymorphisms in the genes for apolipoprotein E, lipoprotein lipase, apolipoprotein B-100, and apolipoprotein A-II are correlated with increased triglycerides and decreased HDL.

Endocrine Manifestations of Obesity

Obesity is associated with abnormalities of the endocrine system, one of the most common being polycystic ovary syndrome. This syndrome (Chapter 236) is characterized by mild hirsutism and irregular menses or amenorrhea with anovulatory cycles. It is most commonly linked with obesity and often improves with weight loss and other treatments that improve insulin resistance. The insulin resistance associated with obesity may trigger the development of polycystic ovary syndrome in susceptible individuals. Whereas mild to moderate androgen overproduction is a feature of upper body obesity in women, obese men may suffer from mild to severe hypothalamic hypogonadism. This androgen deficiency improves with weight loss, and attempts to treat this condition with testosterone replacement offer little clinical benefit. There has been some concern that testosterone treatment of obese men may increase the risk of obstructive sleep apnea and perhaps even cardiovascular events. Although estrogens are not elevated in obese premenopausal women, they remain somewhat above postmenopausal levels in obese postmenopausal women. Serum growth hormone concentrations are commonly low in obese adults, but insulin-like growth factor-I concentrations are often normal, and growth hormone concentrations increase with weight loss. Treatment of these patients with growth hormone has been reported to worsen insulin resistance and glucose intolerance and cannot be justified, considering the costs and poor risk-to-benefit ratio.

Mechanical Complications of Obesity

The excess body weight associated with obesity is thought to be responsible for the increased prevalence of lower extremity degenerative joint disease. Extreme obesity can result in premature degenerative joint disease, and this may be especially difficult to treat surgically, given the greater stress on joint replacements. Severely obese individuals may also have problems with venous stasis, which is occasionally aggravated by right-sided heart failure (see later).

Obstructive Sleep Apnea and Sleep Restriction

Sleep apnea (Chapter 100) is common in severely obese patients, tending to be more prevalent in men and in women with an upper body/visceral obesity.

Sleep apnea is most likely explained by enlargement of upper airway soft tissue, resulting in collapse of the upper airways with inspiration during sleep. The obstruction leads to apneas, with hypoxemia, hypercarbia, and high catecholamine and endothelin levels. The frequent arousals to restore breathing result in poor sleep quality. Sleep apnea is associated with an increased risk of hypertension, and if sleep apnea is severe, it can lead to right-sided heart failure and sudden death. A history of daytime hypersomnolence, loud snoring, restless sleep, or morning headaches is suggestive of obstructive sleep apnea. Treatment of sleep apnea is important to improve cardiovascular risk, and the failure to recognize and to treat this complication may make weight loss intervention strategies much less successful.

Epidemiologic studies have linked short sleep duration and disruptions of circadian rhythm with increased risk of metabolic syndrome and diabetes. Experimentally induced sleep restriction combined with circadian disruption in humans led to decreased RMR and increased postprandial plasma glucose levels due to inadequate insulin secretion.

Cancer

The risk of breast cancer and endometrial cancer is increased in obese women (Chapter 180). It is thought that this may be due to the increased estrogen levels associated with obesity in the postmenopausal woman. Obese men also have a higher mortality of cancers of the prostate and colon. The reasons for this association are unknown.

Gastrointestinal Disorders

Gastroesophageal reflux disease and gallstones are more prevalent in obese patients. Likewise, fatty liver and nonalcoholic steatohepatitis (Chapter 152) are more common in obesity. Nonalcoholic steatohepatitis can eventually progress to life-threatening hepatic cirrhosis. Weight loss and interventions that improve insulin sensitivity have been shown to improve fatty liver and nonalcoholic steatohepatitis.

DIAGNOSIS
Evaluation of Obesity

In the office practice, obtaining height and weight allows calculation of BMI. For patients with a BMI above 25 and below 35, a second piece of information—the waist circumference—provides an added indicator as to whether the patient is at greater risk for adverse consequences (see earlier). Measurement of blood pressure (which may require a large blood pressure cuff) then provides a third item of health information at almost no cost. The presence or absence of dyslipidemia (HDL cholesterol < 45 mg/dL for women, HDL cholesterol < 35 mg/dL for men, or triglycerides > 150 mg/dL), hypertension, glucose intolerance and diabetes, and hyperuricemia should be documented. A history suggestive of sleep apnea should prompt a referral for overnight oximetry or a sleep disorder evaluation.

A review of the patient's lifestyle, including an assessment of physical activity level and eating habits, may help provide information about why the patient is obese. A family history of obesity, or long-standing obesity, provides evidence against a secondary cause of obesity. A careful medication history and social history may help the clinician identify precipitating factors that can be modified. By emphasizing the role of modifiable lifestyle factors that predispose to disease risk, as opposed to focusing solely on the patient's weight, it may be possible to initiate a conversation about weight/disease management in a less threatening manner from the patient's perspective.

Before a patient enters a weight management program, it is helpful to ensure that the patient is interested and ready to make lifestyle changes and has realistic goals and expectations. Patients who expect to lose large amounts of weight in a short time are virtually doomed to disappointment. Medical treatment programs, even if they include pharmacotherapy, struggle to routinely achieve sustained weight loss of more than 10%. Although this amount of weight loss is sufficient to markedly reduce the medical complications of obesity, disappointment with "only" 10% weight loss may cause patients to abandon a medically successful program. Helping the patient to understand that lifestyle changes resulting in achievable (10%) weight loss is a reasonable, initial goal can be one of the more challenging aspects for a physician.

It is sometimes necessary to delay entry into treatment programs if a patient is not ready to make lifestyle changes. In this case, a reasonable strategy is to remind the patient periodically of the potential health benefits of improved activity and eating habits. Once a willingness to make changes is apparent, treatment is more likely to succeed.

TREATMENT   Rx

Obesity represents an individual's response to the environment based on genetics and learned behavior and is best viewed as a chronic disease. Therefore, treatment must be considered a long-term issue, much like diabetes, hypertension, or dyslipidemia. Substantial weight loss can be induced through severe calorie restriction, but without approaches to ensure behavioral changes, body fat is invariably regained. To the extent that environmental factors contribute to a patient's overweight status, and to the extent that the macroenvironment is unlikely to change, patients must learn how to make permanent lifestyle changes (eating and activity behavior) to hope for permanent weight loss. Behavior modification approaches,[5] which can help patients recognize and circumvent environmental cues for sedentary behavior and overeating, can increase the likelihood that patients will accomplish these lifestyle changes.[A1] A randomized study has shown that intensive lifestyle intervention (as compared to only support and education) is associated with fewer hospitalizations, fewer medications, and lower health care costs in overweight or obese adults with type 2 diabetes.[A2]

Reducing energy intake is the most efficient and effective means to lose weight. For example, creating a 500 kcal/day deficit by reduced food intake will theoretically result in the loss of 1 pound of fat per week. Although possible, it is much more difficult to increase energy expenditure by 500 kcal/ week through exercise. Higher levels of physical activity can prevent weight gain (or weight regain after weight loss). Some patients are able to change eating and activity habits on their own, given the proper information, whereas others require formal or informal behavior modification interventions (see later) to help make these changes. In some instances, pharmacotherapy or surgery may be needed for treatment of obesity. A flow diagram on how to evaluate and to manage patients with overweight and obesity is presented in Figure 220-1.

Diet

Changes in eating habits must be permanent if weight loss is to be maintained. An experienced registered dietitian can be helpful in the evaluation of a patient's eating habits and will be able to provide the needed education. The diet history may identify eating behaviors that result in excess energy intake. Although it is important to address specific adverse eating behaviors, patients need to understand some general principles regarding diet. Reducing the energy density of food (most commonly accomplished by reducing dietary fat) can allow patients to feel satiated while consuming fewer calories. The NHLBI/ AHA/ACC/TOS obesity guideline[6] recommends that providers prescribe 1200 to 1500 kcal/day for women and 1500 to 1800 kcal/day for men. Alternatively, diets that produce an energy deficit of 500 to 750 kcal/day can be recommended. Because there appears to be no clear superiority of one diet over another with regard to weight loss,[A3] it is recommended that providers prescribe one of the evidence-based diets that restricts selected food types (e.g.,

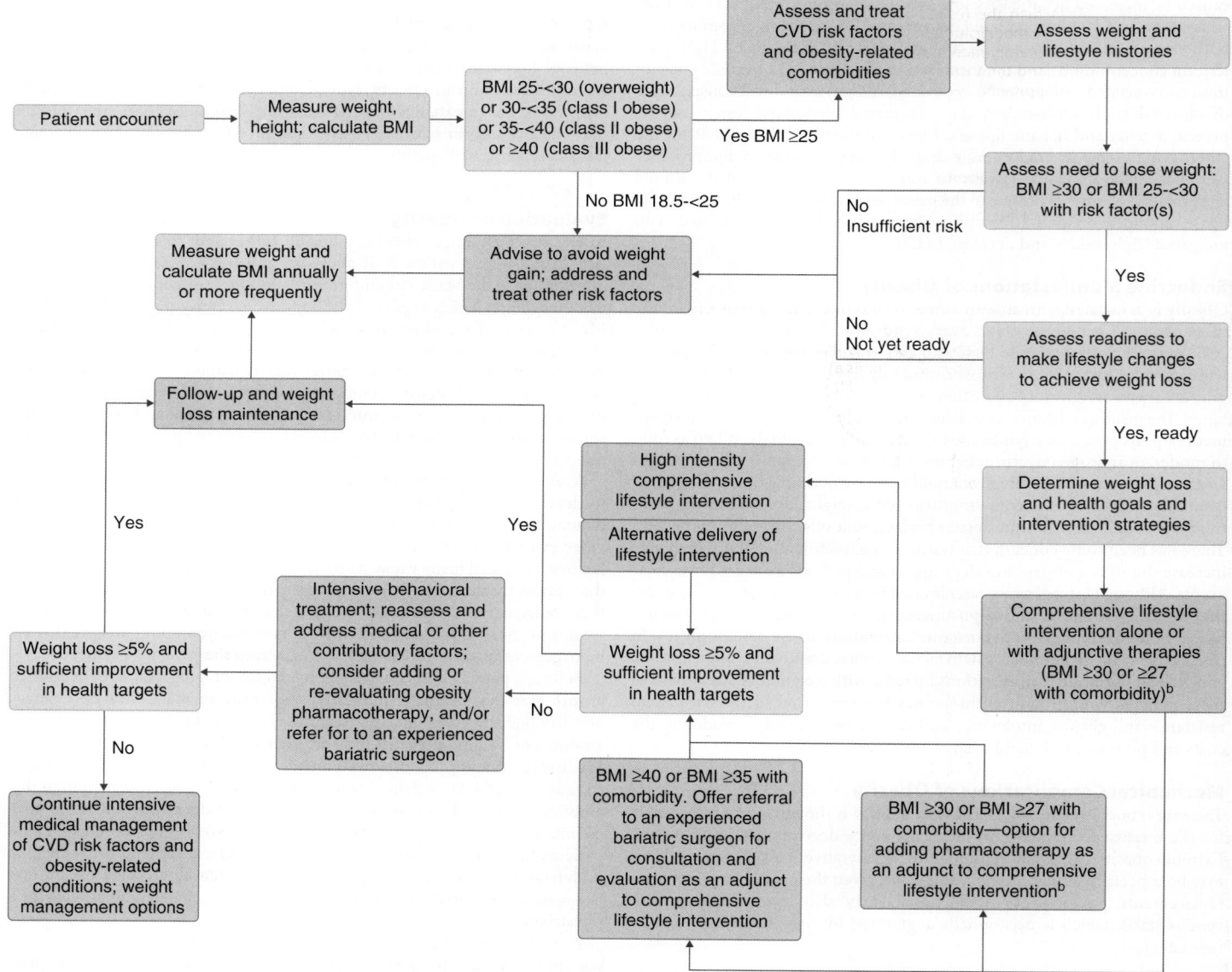

FIGURE 220-1. Flow diagram for the evaluation and management of overweight and obesity. BMI = body mass index; CVD = cardiovascular disease. [b]BMI cutpoint determined by the U.S. Food and Drug Administration (FDA) and listed on the package inserts of FDA-approved obesity medications. (Modified from Jensen MD, Ryan DH, Apovian CM, et al. 2013 AHA/ACC/TOS guideline for the management of overweight and obesity in adults: a report of the American College of Cardiology/American Heart Association Task Force on Practice Guidelines and The Obesity Society. *J Am Coll Cardiol.* 2014;63:2985-3023.)

high-carbohydrate foods, low-fiber foods, or high-fat foods) to create an energy deficit by reduced food intake as well as to address issues such as dyslipidemia, diabetes, and hypertension. Patients should be informed that consuming foods high in water and fiber (fruits, vegetables, legumes, and soups) can provide satiety without excess calories. Patients should be counseled to reduce the intake of beverages containing substantial calories, most often sugar-sweetened beverages. Finally, a regular pattern of eating should be encouraged.

New diets are continually being promoted with the promise of easy weight loss. A common feature of these diets is the claim that special properties of certain foods help people lose weight or are the cause of obesity. If followed, most of these diets result in weight loss because of a reduced energy intake. The reduced intake can be related to the monotony of the diet, and there have been no diets identified that cause persons to lose weight not in accordance with physiologic principles. Although a number of dietary approaches can be successful in promoting weight loss, if there is no peer-reviewed evidence for safety and success of new diets, a review by a dietitian for nutritional safety is warranted. The NHLBI/AHA/ACC/TOS obesity guideline concluded that many types of diets are able to help patients achieve long-term, medically significant weight loss. Thus, it may be less important what specific type of diet (DASH diet, Mediterranean diet, high-carbohydrate/low-fat or high-fat/low-carbohydrate diet) is recommended than for the patient to find dietary adherence to be relatively easy.[7] A comprehensive lifestyle intervention that includes a high-intensity, on-site behavioral intervention provides the best results.

Very low calorie diets (<800 calories per day) are still used to achieve accelerated weight loss. Because the long-term results of these diets are no better and sometimes worse than the results from the standard low-calorie diet combined with behavior modification, these diets are no longer commonly used. The expensive laboratory monitoring required for very low calorie diets without an improved long-term outcome raises questions about the costs versus benefits of this approach.

Physical Activity

A long-term increase in physical activity, either through the activities of daily living or through regular exercise, is key to preventing weight regain, thereby increasing the amount of successful, long-term weight loss.[A4] Unfortunately, many overweight and obese patients are unfit, being unable to walk even 1 mile continuously. It is not possible for most adults to expend a great deal of energy through exercise. For example, only about 100 kcal are expended by a 70-kg adult walking one mile. Losing weight solely by increasing exercise is impractical for most patients. However, increasing physical activity as a means of maintaining weight loss is an attainable goal for most patients.

Successful maintenance of weight loss requires that daily energy expenditure be an average of 80 to 90% above RMR. This is a considerable increase for most patients. For example, someone with an RMR of 1500 kcal/day would need to expend about 1000 kcal/day in physical activity to meet this target. Activities other than exercise are important means to achieve this goal. The most commonly applicable approach is by increasing the amount of walking done throughout the day.

The health benefits from regular physical activity over and above the effects on weight include lower cardiovascular and all-cause mortality as well as improved mood and cognition. The options for increasing physical activity include exercise (sports or fitness pursuits) and use of lifestyle approaches. Both methods can improve fitness and allow weight stability; however, persuading obese patients to become more active is not easy. Physicians can begin by asking patients about their current and past activity habits as well as what barriers they see to increasing physical activity. This accomplishes the goal of stimulating patients to think about the issue in a tactful manner. It can help to ask the patient what personal benefits are envisioned as a result of increasing the level of activity. If patients agree to begin an exercise or physical activity program, they will need to monitor their activity and set realistic goals for the amount of exercise they are going to achieve. The ready availability of step counters and electronic activity monitoring devices offers practical means for patients to track physical activity throughout the day and to assess the effects of changes in lifestyle on their activity level. Patients should be advised to acquire devices that have been shown to accurately count steps. Self-monitoring of how many steps are taken each day for 1 to 2 weeks can give patients a good sense of their baseline activity level. Many Americans take as few as 4000 to 5000 steps per day, whereas it may take as many as 15,000 to 17,000 steps per day to help those who have lost significant amounts of weight to maintain that lower weight. Gradually increasing the number of steps regularly taken during the day through a series of changes in habits (e.g., parking farther away, walking during work breaks) is more likely to result in long-term success for most persons than setting aside 2 hours or more for continuous walking.

Behavior Modification

Patients who are unable to make changes in eating activity habits on their own or with informal office counseling may benefit from referral to an

TABLE 220-6 INDICATIONS FOR PHARMACOLOGIC TREATMENT OF OBESITY

Body mass index > 27 kg/m^2

One or more complications or conditions that are likely to improve with weight loss

Previous failure of conservative treatment with behavioral intervention, diet, and exercise

Agree to 2- to 4-wk trial of making initial changes in diet and exercise before starting pharmacotherapy

Agree to continued treatment with diet, exercise, and behavioral modification while receiving pharmacologic treatment

Agree to periodic follow-up

Premenopausal women (able to have children) must use some form of contraception

Consider a pregnancy test on initiation of treatment if there is any possibility of pregnancy

No contraindications to the specific drug used for pharmacologic treatment

---

interventionist trained in behavior therapy. The goals are to help patients modify their eating, activity, and thinking habits that predispose to obesity and focus on specific pathways to achieve the goals. These pathways may include identifying and removing barriers to development of better eating or activity habits. Small, incremental, and consistent changes in behavior are encouraged. Self-monitoring of food and activity is considered a key feature to success because most obese patients underestimate food intake and overestimate exercise. Cognitive restructuring has been introduced as a way to help overcome the thought processes that can lead to failure of a weight management program. Patients are taught to identify, to challenge, and to correct self-defeating thoughts.

The best weight loss results are provided by in-person, high-intensity (≥14 sessions in 6 months) comprehensive behavioral interventions, which average an 8-kg (5 to 10% of body weight) loss in 6 months. Approaches that provide electronically delivered counseling (telephone or Internet), including some commercial programs, can also achieve weight loss, but generally less than with in-person delivery approaches. Commercial programs that have published their results in peer-reviewed journals are preferred. Physicians who refer patients to programs that offer intensive, comprehensive lifestyle interventions are encouraged to obtain outcomes data from those programs.

Pharmacotherapy

A limited number of drugs are currently available to help patients with weight loss.[8] Optimally, any medication for obesity treatment will be prescribed in the context of a comprehensive lifestyle intervention by providers knowledgeable in its use. Not all overweight or obese patients are candidates for pharmacologic treatment of obesity. Table 220-6 provides criteria that should help select patients for pharmacologic treatment. Because pharmacologic treatment of obesity exposes patients to some risks and expense, it is reasonable to require an objective benefit. A rational argument can be made that prioritization should be given to those with one or more medical complications or conditions that are likely to improve with weight loss. In prescribing antiobesity medications, it is important to set clear goals with respect to both weight loss and health benefits.

Currently Available Medications

The medications currently available for long-term use act through either appetite reduction or inhibition of pancreatic lipase, which results in fat maldigestion. Phentermine is approved only for short-term (3 months) use. Recent additions to the medications approved by the Food and Drug Administration for chronic treatment of obesity include lorcaserin, a selective serotonin 2C receptor agonist,[9] the combination of topiramate and phentermine (see later), and a combination of bupropion with naltrexone.[10] Because weight that is lost with pharmacotherapy (especially when it is used without a comprehensive program) is regained once the medication is discontinued, agents that are approved for long-term use are better therapeutic choices.

Orlistat at the typical dose of 120 mg three times daily with meals causes about 30% of dietary fat to be malabsorbed. As expected, adverse gastrointestinal side effects, such as oily spotting, abdominal pain, excess flatus, fecal urgency, and fatty or oily stools, are not uncommon. These side effects decrease over time, and the concomitant use of bulk-forming laxatives (e.g., psyllium, methylcellulose) can reduce these symptoms. A daily multivitamin is recommended for those receiving long-term orlistat therapy. It is not necessary to take orlistat if a nonfat meal is being consumed. Orlistat is now available as an over-the-counter medication. Orlistat improves the results of medical treatment programs that include diet, exercise, and behavior modification, resulting in almost twice as many patients achieving goal weight loss (10% of body weight).

The combination of phentermine and topiramate in an extended-release capsule is approved for chronic treatment of obesity. The highest dose (15 mg phentermine/92 mg controlled-release topiramate) resulted in an average of about 10% weight loss at 2 years (8% more than with placebo), with slightly more than half of patients achieving 10% weight loss and 15% of patients achieving 20% weight loss.[A5] As both components of this medication were previously approved (topiramate for seizures and migraine prevention), the side effects were most commonly upper respiratory tract infection, constipation, paresthesia, sinusitis, and dry mouth; the incidence of individual adverse effects diminishes significantly after the first year.

Lorcaserin inhibits the serotonin pathway in a manner similar to fenfluramine, but without the cardiac valvulopathy effects. Patients taking lorcaserin 10 mg/day for 1 year lost an average of 5.8 kg compared with 2.2 kg with placebo. At 1 year, 47% of patients treated with lorcaserin lost 5% or more of their body weight compared with 20% of the placebo group.[A6]

Combined bupropion and naltrexone addresses the issues of dopamine-induced gratification and addictive behavior. The drug results in an average weight loss comparable to other approved drugs, with few side effects and no abuse potential.

Success of Medical Therapy

It has been estimated that more than 95% of those embarking on self-diets or fad diets fail to maintain a significant weight loss for a time that would have meaningful health benefits. The published results from two commercial programs have shown better results. These commercial weight loss interventions provided a comprehensive intervention that was delivered in person and resulted in an average weight loss of 4.8 to 6.6 kg at 6 months in trials in which conventional foods were consumed and 6.6 to 10.1 kg at 12 months in trials in which prepared food was provided. Comprehensive weight management programs delivered at academic medical centers that employ behavior modification, dietary instruction, and physical activity can achieve equally or more impressive results. Average 1-year weight losses of about 10% can be achieved and maintained for 1 to 2 years, depending on the intensity of follow-up. The addition of medications, when indicated (see earlier), can produce even greater amounts of weight loss.

Bariatric Surgery

Surgical treatment can provide more weight loss than medications for class II and class III (see Table 220-1) obese patients with medical complications that could be expected to improve with successful weight loss, such as uncontrolled type 2 diabetes,[11] assuming past attempts at medical treatment have failed.[A7] Patients with a BMI of 35 to 40 with life-threatening complications can be considered, but more typically patients with a BMI higher than 40 and several complications are candidates for surgery. Because the risks and costs of surgical treatment are greater than for medical treatment, selection of patients who stand to obtain more potential benefit from surgery should optimize the risk-to-benefit ratio. Contraindications to surgery include active substance abuse, defined noncompliance or inability to comply with medical care, and schizophrenia, borderline personality disorder, or uncontrolled depression.

A multidisciplinary team, including a physician, dietitian, psychologist or psychiatrist with expertise in this area, and surgeon experienced in bariatric procedures, is important for optimal outcome. Defining realistic expectations is an important part of the evaluation process. Patients undergoing bariatric surgery are not likely to be reduced to their ideal body weight. Successful weight loss is typically defined as losing an average of 50 to 60% of excess body weight, which is a difficult criterion to explain to patients. An easier explanation is that most successful patients will achieve weight losses of 25 to 35% of body weight. Follow-up to support the necessary changes in long-term behavior is recommended to optimize weight loss outcomes.

A variety of bariatric surgical procedures have been used. The jejunoileal bypass, long abandoned because of complications that include liver failure, renal failure, and arthropathy, is typically encountered only in those who underwent bariatric surgery more than 3 decades ago and who present with these complications. Procedures that modify the capacity of the stomach (laparoscopic gastric banding and sleeve gastrectomy) but do not create malabsorption of nutrients are employed, but these are generally less effective than the Roux-en-Y gastric bypass in terms of long-term weight loss and outright surgical success. The partial pancreaticobiliary bypass, the very long limb Roux-en-Y gastric bypass, and the duodenal switch procedures create malabsorption that results in greater weight loss than with the standard Roux-en-Y gastric bypass. Unfortunately, the incidence of severe, even fatal vitamin and mineral deficiencies (Chapter 218) is much higher with these procedures. Laparoscopic approaches are now routinely employed for bariatric surgery as they have allowed the time of hospitalization to be reduced considerably and with lesser rates of incisional hernias compared with open procedures.

After surgery, almost all of the weight loss that occurs will happen during the first 1 to 2 years. Long-term (>5 year) success rates are outstanding in good

programs. Virtually all patients with successful weight loss will have a dramatic improvement in the medical complications of obesity. For these reasons, bariatric surgery has become an important tool in the treatment of severe, medically complicated obesity.

The results of the Roux-en-Y gastric bypass for treatment of morbid obesity have been favorable. Approximately 70% of patients achieve success as defined previously with this procedure. The mortality and morbidity (e.g., infection, anastomotic leak, wound dehiscence) of this procedure are low in centers with expertise, despite the high-risk population. Laparoscopic gastric banding, once popular because of the reduced short-term risk, is becoming less so as the inferior long-term weight loss results and late complications of band slippage, erosion, and weight regain become more apparent. Whether the sleeve gastrectomy results will more closely mimic gastric bypass or laparoscopic banding is not yet known. After any of the malabsorptive procedures, the patients require permanent follow-up specifically for adverse nutritional consequences.

The long-term follow-up of patients who have undergone gastric bypass surgery is needed to ensure adequate protein, calorie, vitamin, and mineral nutrition. Supplemental vitamin B_{12}, iron, and calcium are routinely added to standard multivitamins. The most common nutritional consequences of malabsorptive procedures are disorders of calcium and vitamin D metabolism, although many severely obese patients have low vitamin D levels even before surgery (Chapter 244). An increase in bone alkaline phosphatase may signal calcium or vitamin D deficiency. Low plasma vitamin D levels and low urinary calcium excretion should prompt aggressive replacement therapy. Iron deficiency, other fat-soluble vitamin deficiencies, and cases of copper deficiency occurring more than 5 to 10 years after surgery have been described. There have also been cases of pancreatogenous hypoglycemia that develop after bariatric surgical procedures. The symptoms are primarily postprandial and are occasionally severe enough to warrant partial pancreatectomy.

PREVENTION

The dramatic increase in the prevalence of obesity during the past few decades strongly suggests that preventive strategies are needed. Public health approaches that emphasize education have been almost uniformly unsuccessful at preventing weight gain or producing weight loss. Public health strategies that virtually impose behavior change are more successful in this regard. Unless widespread efforts are made to address the problem of obesity, it is likely that its prevalence and complications will become an ever-increasing health burden.

Grade A References

A1. Wadden TA, Butryn ML, Hong PS, et al. Behavioral treatment of obesity in patients encountered in primary care settings: a systematic review. *JAMA.* 2014;312:1779-1791.

A2. Espeland MA, Glick HA, Bertoni A, et al. Impact of an intensive lifestyle intervention on use and cost of medical services among overweight and obese adults with type 2 diabetes: the action for health in diabetes. *Diabetes Care.* 2014;37:2548-2556.

A3. Johnston BC, Kanters S, Bandayrel K, et al. Comparison of weight loss among named diet programs in overweight and obese adults: a meta-analysis. *JAMA.* 2014;312:923-933.

A4. Schwingshackl L, Dias S, Hoffmann G. Impact of long-term lifestyle programmes on weight loss and cardiovascular risk factors in overweight/obese participants: a systematic review and network meta-analysis. *Syst Rev.* 2014;3:130.

A5. Garvey WT, Ryan DH, Look M, et al. Two-year sustained weight loss and metabolic benefits with controlled-release phentermine/topiramate in obese and overweight adults (SEQUEL): a randomized, placebo-controlled, phase 3 extension study. *Am J Clin Nutr.* 2012;95:297-308.

A6. Smith SR, Weissman NJ, Anderson CM, et al. Behavioral Modification and Lorcaserin for Overweight and Obesity Management (BLOOM) Study Group. Multicenter, placebo-controlled trial of lorcaserin for weight management. *N Engl J Med.* 2010;363:245-256.

A7. Colquitt JL, Pickett K, Loveman E, et al. Surgery for weight loss in adults. *Cochrane Database Syst Rev.* 2014;8:CD003641.

GENERAL REFERENCES

For the General References and other additional features, please visit Expert Consult at https://expertconsult.inkling.com.

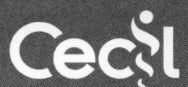

XVIII

ENDOCRINE DISEASES

APPROACH TO THE PATIENT WITH ENDOCRINE DISEASE

DAVID R. CLEMMONS AND LYNNETTE K. NIEMAN

Most endocrine disorders are due to either an excess or a deficiency of a hormone that is transported in the systemic circulation and therefore result in multiorgan manifestations. It is unusual for patients to present with a single isolated set of symptoms that are referable to only one organ system. Additionally, generalized nonspecific symptoms such as weakness, difficulty concentrating, lack of energy, and change in appetite occur commonly in patients with endocrine disorders. Often, a constellation of symptoms is required to point the clinician in the direction of the correct diagnosis, and single symptoms evaluated in isolation are rarely helpful even if one considers an exhaustive differential diagnosis (Table 221-1). Another important feature of the evaluation of patients presenting with endocrinologic disease is obtaining a good longitudinal history. The duration of exposure to a hormone excess or deficiency often dictates the severity of symptoms, and characterizing the symptomatic changes that occur over time can be very helpful in both selecting the tests to confirm the diagnosis and either substantiating the need for treatment or selecting the correct mode of treatment. Physical examination is helpful for confirming the likelihood of a diagnosis; for example, the presence of a symmetrically enlarged thyroid gland indicates that Graves disease is the most likely cause of hyperthyroidism. However, because of the accuracy and precision of modern endocrinologic testing, endocrine disorders sometimes are diagnosed in the absence of symptoms or signs of overt disease (e.g., hyperparathyroidism). In such instances, a thorough history and physical examination are still important because they establish that the patient is truly in the asymptomatic phase of the disease, and this is often helpful in determining whether therapy or observation is required. A careful temporal history of a symptomatic change may also be helpful in the differential diagnosis—for example, in ascertaining whether a thyroid mass is likely due to a hemorrhagic cyst (i.e., occurring suddenly) or is a thyroid adenoma that might have evolved over an extended period. A thorough general history and physical examination may help to establish the diagnosis of diseases that are associated with endocrinologic abnormalities, such as cancers that ectopically secrete hormones, or may help to exclude the likelihood of an endocrinologic etiology of a specific disease manifestation.

Precise genetic testing to establish the etiology of endocrinologic syndromes is becoming more prevalent; therefore, an accurate family history can be useful in determining the need for genetic testing and familial screening. A thorough evaluation of medication use is also mandatory. Some medications can clearly mask the symptoms of overt endocrine disease, such as β-blockers in hyperthyroidism, and others can exacerbate the findings, such as hydrochlorothiazide use in hyperparathyroidism. Often, specific medications will confound laboratory evaluation, such as diuretics in patients with hyperaldosteronism or antihypertensive drugs in patients being screened for pheochromocytoma. Appropriate withdrawal of the medication may be required to establish a firm diagnosis. Medications may also directly alter a laboratory test, such as use of oral contraceptives in attempting to diagnose hyperthyroidism or hypothyroidism. Finally, an accurate history of the specific complaint may be challenging. For example, in evaluating male sexual dysfunction, a corroborating history from the patient's partner is often necessary for verification.

COMMON SYMPTOMS OF ENDOCRINOLOGIC DISEASE

Generalized symptoms such as weakness and fatigue are prominent features of adrenal insufficiency, hyperthyroidism and hypothyroidism, hypopituitarism, and poorly controlled diabetes mellitus. Pain is an uncommon complaint in endocrinologic disorders and is usually only seen with acute endocrinologic emergencies, such as diabetic ketoacidosis or acute adrenal insufficiency (abdominal pain). Chronic pain seen in primary or secondary hyperparathyroidism due to bone reabsorption and in osteomalacia (Chapter 244) can occur in the shafts of the long bones. Symptoms of menstrual dysfunction are common in women with adrenal insufficiency, hypopituitarism,

Cushing's syndrome, hyperprolactinemia, hyperthyroidism, hypothyroidism, polycystic ovarian disease, and primary ovarian failure. Weakness and easy fatigability can be secondary to anemia, which is common in adrenal insufficiency, androgen deficiency, hypothyroidism, hyperparathyroidism, and panhypopituitarism.

The most common endocrine-related symptom of intestinal dysfunction is constipation. This occurs frequently in patients with diabetic autonomic neuropathy and in hypercalcemia, hypothyroidism, or pheochromocytoma. Diarrhea can be an early and prominent symptom in hyperthyroidism and metastatic carcinoid tumors. Fever, like abdominal pain, usually only occurs in endocrine emergencies, typically in severe adrenal insufficiency and very severe hyperthyroidism. Generalized hair loss not related to androgen excess occurs in hypothyroidism, hypopituitarism, and thyrotoxicosis. Typical male-pattern baldness can be a feature of hirsutism in women as well as Cushing's syndrome and acromegaly. Persistent recurrent headaches are a feature of expanding pituitary tumors, whereas episodic headaches occur frequently in patients with pheochromocytoma and hypoglycemia. Changes in libido are often present in patients with hyperthyroidism, hypopituitarism, hypogonadism, Cushing's syndrome, and poorly controlled diabetes mellitus. Polyuria and nocturia are features of both diabetes insipidus and diabetes mellitus and can also occur in severe hypercalcemia.

Weight gain is an early symptom of Cushing's syndrome and hypothyroidism. Weight loss accompanied by anorexia is common in adrenal insufficiency, metastatic hormone-producing tumors such as ectopic adrenocorticotropic (ACTH) hormone syndrome, type 1 diabetes mellitus, and panhypopituitarism. Weight loss with no change or an increase in appetite is common in hyperthyroidism (see Table 221-1). An important differential diagnostic issue in patients with weight loss is depression. Depression can occur concomitantly in patients with adrenal insufficiency, Cushing's syndrome, hypercalcemia, and hypothyroidism.

An important neuropsychiatric symptom is widening of mood swings—that is, an exaggeration of normal cyclothymic changes. This occurs in hyperthyroidism and Cushing's syndrome. A history of skin changes occurs with several endocrine disorders. Acanthosis nigricans occurs with severe obesity, polycystic ovarian disease, severe insulin resistance syndromes, Cushing's syndrome, and acromegaly. Acne is a symptom of androgen excess and occurs with androgen-producing tumors, polycystic ovarian disease, and Cushing's syndrome. Generalized hyperpigmentation occurs in Addison's disease and Nelson's syndrome. Dry skin is present in almost all patients with hypothyroidism. It also occurs in panhypopituitarism. In Cushing's syndrome, skin changes such as striae, plethora, and easy bruisability are common. Vitiligo occurs in association with several endocrine autoimmune diseases, most prominently with autoimmune thyroid disease and Addison's disease.

Assessment of any of these symptoms in isolation is unlikely to lead a clinician to the correct diagnosis. However, assessment of combinations of these symptoms (e.g., the combination of weight gain, constipation, cold intolerance, and dry skin in hypothyroidism) is likely to lead to the correct set of diagnostic decisions.

PHYSICAL EXAMINATION

Physical examination of a patient with a suspected endocrine disorder is extremely helpful in terms of confirming the significance of findings that were ascertained by a careful medical history (Table 221-2). Examination of the skin is important because endocrinopathies lead to skin changes that progress over time. These often occur early in the course of the illness and can be a major aid in making the correct diagnosis. Primary adrenal failure is usually accompanied by increased skin pigmentation, particularly over the creases of the palms and extensor surfaces. The oral mucosa is often hyperpigmented, which can be helpful in African Americans. Patients with Cushing's syndrome present with persistent facial plethora, acne, and characteristic striae, which are generally larger than 1 cm and exhibit a dark red to purplish hue. These are most common over the abdomen. The presence of axillary purpura is also suggestive of Cushing's syndrome and results from increased capillary fragility. Patients with acromegaly often present with excessive skin tags that increase in number over time and multiple types of benign skin tumors such as dermatofibromas and lipomas. The skin is also much thicker over the dorsum of the hand, and the amount of subcutaneous tissue in the palms is prominent. Patients with Cushing's syndrome have thinning of the skin over the forehead and around the eyes. Patients with hypothyroidism often present with evidence of hyperkeratosis, particularly over the extensor surfaces. Severe long-standing thyroid disease is also accompanied by myxedema of

TABLE 221-1 SYMPTOM CONSTELLATIONS SUGGESTING SPECIFIC ENDOCRINE DISORDERS

SYMPTOM CONSTELLATION	DIAGNOSIS
Weakness, fatigue, anorexia, loss of appetite, postural blood pressure changes	Adrenal insufficiency
Cold intolerance, dry skin, constipation, weight gain	Hypothyroidism
Fatigue, easy bruising, striae, proximal muscle weakness, central obesity, hypertension, acne	Cushing's syndrome
Weight loss, increased appetite, palpitations, tremor, emotional lability, diffuse hair thinning	Hyperthyroidism
Galactorrhea, amenorrhea, headaches	Prolactin-producing pituitary tumor
Weight loss, anorexia, loss of pubic and axillary hair	Hypopituitarism
Episodic palpitations, tremor, anxiety, headaches, sweating, weight loss	Pheochromocytoma
Episodic flushing, palpitations, abdominal cramping, and diarrhea	Carcinoid syndrome

TABLE 221-2 PHYSICAL SIGNS THAT SUGGEST SPECIFIC ENDOCRINE DISORDERS

Hyperpigmentation of palms, extensor surfaces, and buccal mucosa	Adrenal insufficiency
Facial plethora, moon facies, striae, purpura	Cushing's syndrome
Skin tags, acral enlargement, prognathism, orthodontia	Acromegaly
Proptosis, lid lag, symmetrically diffuse thyroid enlargement, hyperreflexia	Graves disease
Retinal microaneurysms, macular edema	Diabetic retinopathy
Short stature, web neck, loss of tears	Turner's syndrome
Shield-like chest, short fourth vertebra	Primary ovarian failure

the extremities, a specific skin finding of thickening of both the dermis and epidermis due to mucopolysaccharide accumulation. In contrast, patients with Graves disease present with thinning of the skin, but more prominently with skin that is moist and warm. Both adrenal insufficiency and hyperthyroidism or hypothyroidism can be associated with vitiligo. The nails in hyperthyroidism reveal onycholysis in cases of longer duration. Hair changes occur commonly with several endocrinopathies. In hypothyroidism, the hair becomes coarse, whereas in hyperthyroidism, diffuse thinning occurs. Long-standing hypothyroidism can be accompanied by loss of the lateral third of the eyebrow hair. Hirsutism with hair growth over the areolae and along the linea alba is present in patients with gonadal dysfunction or with hyperandrogenism due to polycystic ovarian disease or androgen-producing tumors. In contrast, patients with hypopituitarism or hypogonadism often present with loss of pubic and axillary hair.

The eye examination can be helpful in establishing the diagnosis of hyperthyroidism. Graves ophthalmopathy occurs in 40% of patients and presents with exophthalmos that can be unilateral. Extraocular movement assessment is important in patients with pituitary tumors because local expansion of these tumors can lead to third, fourth, or sixth nerve palsies, whereas compression of the optic tracts can cause the distinctive visual field defect of bitemporal hemianopsia. On neck examination, ascertainment of whether a goiter is smooth, symmetrical, and multinodular or a single nodule can be helpful in guiding further work-up in the evaluation of hyperthyroidism.

Cardiovascular evaluation is helpful for evaluating the severity and duration of endocrine illness. Patients with hyperthyroidism have evidence of increased sympathomimetic activity, including tachycardia, a widened pulse pressure, and prominent precordial activity. Flow murmurs may be heard as a result of increased cardiac output, and occasionally a bruit is easily heard on auscultation of the thyroid. In patients with hypothyroidism and Addison's disease, these findings are reversed. Specific cardiac abnormalities, such as coarctation of the aorta, may be present in patients with primary ovarian failure due to Turner's syndrome. Patients with pheochromocytoma often have a postural blood pressure change of greater than 20 mm Hg. Cardiomyopathy can be a feature of acromegaly. Hypertension is common in many endocrine disorders, including hypercalcemia, hyperparathyroidism, acromegaly, diabetes mellitus, obesity, Cushing's syndrome, primary aldosteronism, and pheochromocytoma.

Nearly all patients with acromegaly demonstrate evidence of hand and foot enlargement, a very unusual occurrence in adulthood. This often manifests as a history of changing ring size or shoe size and is easily demonstrable on physical examination. Patients with hyperthyroidism often have a significant hand tremor and evidence of peripheral bruits on auscultation. Evaluation of the extremities is also helpful in the differential diagnosis of metabolic bone disease. The presence of bowing of the legs can be found in either dietary or X-linked hypophosphatemic rickets. The presence of edema is usually an early sign of disorders of hormone-producing tumors that result in salt retention, including Cushing's syndrome and hyperaldosteronism. Measurement of upper to lower segment ratios and arm span is helpful in establishing the timing and onset of puberty in primary gonadal disorders.

Pelvic examination is a major aid to the differential diagnosis of ovarian disorders. Palpation may identify polycystic ovaries and suggest the absence of ovarian tissue. The absence of a uterus is important in the differential diagnosis of pseudohermaphroditism, and the evaluation of external genitalia can be important in establishing the presence of congenital adrenal hyperplasia. Vaginal dryness is a sign of severe estrogen deficiency, as is breast atrophy. Hyperprolactinemia often first manifests as the presence of expressible galactorrhea.

Neurologic changes can occur in a variety of diseases. Evaluation of the ability to detect monofilament or vibratory sensation is an important tool for evaluating the presence of diabetic neuropathy. The presence of peripheral motor nerve defects in diabetes is also an important presenting sign, as is the presence of a cranial nerve palsy, such as third nerve palsy. Funduscopic examination can reveal microaneurysms even in patients with undiagnosed type 2 diabetes, and this can be helpful for estimating antecedent duration of illness. Hyporeflexia with a delayed relaxation phase is one of the earliest physical changes in hypothyroidism and is prominent in most patients with clinically significant disease; hyperreflexia occurs in hyperthyroidism. Patients with Cushing's syndrome often have extreme proximal muscle weakness, and this occurs in severe long-standing hyperthyroidism. Midgut carcinoids frequently present with severe flushing and diarrhea. The skin characteristically has an unusual purplish hue, and this change typically lasts for the duration of the episode, about 20 to 30 minutes. Mental status changes occur frequently in patients with Cushing's syndrome, hyperthyroidism, and extreme hypercalcemia.

● LABORATORY EVALUATION

Patients with endocrinologic diseases are frequently diagnosed in an asymptomatic state as a result of abnormal radiologic evaluation or hormonal testing abnormalities.

The most common radiologic conundrums occur in patients who are noted incidentally to have small pituitary, thyroid, or adrenal masses. Although most of these patients generally do not have a hormonal dysfunction syndrome, proper evaluation to exclude the presence of a functionally active tumor is usually necessary. For pituitary tumors, the minimal evaluation would include measurements of a baseline serum prolactin level and, in cases with suggestive symptoms, of 24-hour urine free cortisol and of growth hormone after glucose suppression. In patients with incidentally found adrenal masses ("incidentalomas"),[1] important findings are a large tumor mass (i.e., >4 cm), hypertension or hypokalemia, and symptoms and signs of Cushing's syndrome. If any of these are present, appropriate evaluation to exclude hyperaldosteronism, Cushing's syndrome, and pheochromocytoma should be undertaken.

The sensitivity and specificity of hormonal testing have reached levels that have significantly changed the initial evaluation of patients for endocrine disorders. For example, screening of asymptomatic patients for thyroid disease, disorders of lipoprotein metabolism, and disorders of gonadal dysfunction are common and widespread.

Hormones are often measured using immunologic detection methods. Most measurements use blood or urine samples to detect the active hormone.

Occasionally, measurement of a metabolite of the active hormone, such as 25-hydroxycholecalciferol (a vitamin D metabolite), is more reliable than that of the parent hormone. Some hormones (e.g., thyroxine) have a very long half-life in plasma, and therefore a measurement at any time of day reflects the ability of the gland to produce that hormone. However, other hormones (e.g., growth hormone) are secreted episodically, and therefore a static measurement may or may not be indicative of hormone excess or deficiency. In these cases, suppression or stimulation testing is used to confirm the diagnosis. Usually, an exogenous substance (e.g., ACTH) is administered either orally or intravenously, and the production of the hormone (e.g., cortisol) by the gland is either stimulated or suppressed.

Many hormones are present in the circulation bound to binding proteins. With the exception of peptide hormones that circulate in the free (unbound) form, this can cause problems in interpretation: medications or concomitant illnesses can result in a major change in the concentration of the binding protein, which in turn alters the total hormone concentration. This problem can be obviated either by measuring the binding protein itself or by direct measurement of the free hormone, such as measurement of free thyroxine.[2] Free hormone measurements, however, can be less reliable than total hormone measurements; therefore, a decision sometimes needs to be made wherein the reliability of the assay is compared with the quality of the information that will be provided.

Often, static hormone measurements are used for screening—for example, morning cortisol in screening for the presence of hypoadrenalism. Subsequently, stimulation or suppression testing is used for confirmation of the diagnosis.[3] In some cases, plasma measurements are much less reliable than urinary testing (e.g., a single morning cortisol level to rule in or out the presence of Cushing's syndrome). In these cases, 24-hour urinary measurement of hormone is often required to document overproduction. Urinary assays have the advantage of providing integrative assessment over 24 hours and thus are less likely to be susceptible to errors due to episodic hormonal secretion over time. Occasionally, measurements of other substances, such as electrolytes or metabolites, are also informative for confirming the diagnosis. For example, measurement of 24-hour urinary calcium can be important in the differential diagnosis of hypercalcemia. Metabolites in the urine may be extremely important in the evaluation of adrenal disorders and in documentation of pheochromocytoma and carcinoid syndrome. Simultaneous measurements of two substances is extremely helpful in the diagnosis of some disorders. Measurement of simultaneous serum calcium and parathyroid hormone (PTH) is important for confirming the presence of hyperparathyroidism. Likewise, simultaneous measurement of blood glucose and insulin can be important in screening for the presence of an insulin-producing tumor. Indirect measurement of hormonal status can also be important; for example, measurement of insulin-like growth factor (IGF)-I, which is inducible by growth hormone (GH), provides an integrative measure of GH secretion. Similarly, measurement of hemoglobin A_{1c} provides an integrative measure of long-term blood sugar control in diabetes.

Imaging studies are commonly used in endocrine diagnosis. Magnetic resonance imaging and computed tomography are helpful in evaluating pituitary and adrenal masses. Scanning of the thyroid gland using radioactive iodine is useful for evaluation of the functional status of thyroid nodules and the functional activity of the thyroid gland as a whole.[4] Bone mineral density testing is now commonplace in screening of patients for osteoporosis and in the evaluation of patients with established fracture syndromes. Imaging can also be combined with hormonal measurements. Specifically, cannulation of the adrenal veins can be helpful in confirming the presence of functioning adrenal tumors such as aldosteronomas. Likewise, determining the location of tumors such as those producing PTH can often be confirmed by venous sampling procedures. Similarly, intraoperative measurements of hormones that change rapidly, such as intraoperative PTH, can help determine whether surgical removal of the hormone-secreting tumor has been adequate. The primary use of biopsy in endocrinologic diagnosis is fine-needle aspiration of the thyroid gland. This procedure can be done safely in the outpatient setting, often aided by ultrasound guidance. It is a highly accurate method for determining whether further diagnostic evaluation or therapeutic intervention is necessary.

GENETIC EVALUATION

Use of genetic testing in endocrinologic diagnosis has become much more commonplace. Polymerase chain reaction amplification of DNA obtained from peripheral blood cells is often used to determine the presence of a specific disorder. This has been extremely useful in differential diagnosis, for

determining prognosis, and for deciding whether family screening is required (e.g., in the presence of multiple endocrine neoplasia). Whether genetic testing is required is often dictated by whether this information is necessary to solve a differential diagnostic problem (e.g., disorders of vitamin D metabolism) or to decide whether more extensive surgery should be required (e.g., in pheochromocytoma) or whether family screening is necessary (e.g., in multiple endocrine neoplasia 2 syndrome).

EVALUATION OF THE RESPONSE OF AN ENDOCRINE DISEASE TO TREATMENT

Most hormone excess syndromes are treated surgically by removal of the particular endocrine gland or tumor that is oversecreting the hormone.[5] However, follow-up of these patients mandates that (1) it be established that the disease has truly been cured by the resection or (2) if residual disease is present, and (3) determining whether repeat operation is likely to be of benefit to the patient or some other means of treating the patient should be undertaken. These decisions generally need to be made in consultation with surgeons and radiotherapists. If an endocrine deficiency is present, hormone replacement therapy is most often used to correct the disorder. In some cases, the efficacy of substitution therapy can be measured directly by laboratory testing, such as measurement of thyroid-stimulating hormone during thyroxine replacement. In other cases (e.g., measurement of ACTH suppression during substitution therapy for adrenal insufficiency), testing could lead to misleading information and overtreatment of patients; therefore, a combination of return of symptoms and signs to normal, laboratory testing, and indirect tests (e.g., potassium, blood urea nitrogen, and creatinine in the case of adrenal insufficiency) is required to determine the adequacy of replacement therapy. Understanding the pharmacology of the particular synthetic hormone used is important for proper replacement therapy. For example, synthetic glucocorticoids vary greatly in their half-life, and therefore dosage and timing of administration are important issues for patients receiving these hormones. Some patients, such as those with hypopituitarism, require substitution with multiple hormones, and often these need to be coordinated (e.g., glucocorticoid dosage in a patient with panhypopituitarism is dependent on the dosage of thyroid hormone that is administered). Because monitoring thyroid-stimulating hormone is not useful in such patients, empirical substitution with both hormones is required to establish that the therapeutic regimen results in return of functional activity to normal. At times, the signs of hormone excesses may have to be treated with ancillary medications; for example, β-blockade may be useful in patients with hyperthyroidism, and both α- and β-blockade are often necessary in patients with pheochromocytoma. The etiology of osteoporosis is often unknown. In most cases, this disease is generally treated by administration of agents that inhibit bone reabsorption by a variety of mechanisms, including the bisphosphonates, estrogen replacement therapy, and calcitonin.

Hormones are also used throughout medicine for treatment of other disorders, and sometimes these treatments result in a hormone excess syndrome. The most common example is administration of high-dose glucocorticoid therapy for immune suppression resulting in Cushing's syndrome. Similarly, growth hormone may be administered to children with short stature who do not have GH deficiency. PTH is the only agent available for stimulation of an anabolic effect in bone; therefore, it is administered to patients with osteoporosis even though they do not have hypoparathyroidism. Octreotide acetate, a long-acting derivative of somatostatin, can be useful for controlling gastrointestinal symptoms in patients with neuroendocrine tumors. Supraphysiologic doses of progesterone are commonly used as contraceptives. Hormone antagonists are also used in both endocrine and nonendocrine disorders. Estrogen receptor antagonists are commonly used in breast cancer therapy, as are androgen receptor antagonists in prostate cancer therapy. Similarly, gonadotropin-releasing hormone agonists have been found to be useful in patients with prostate cancer that is metastatic to bone. Prostaglandin antagonists are commonly used in acute and chronic inflammatory disorders, and angiotensin receptor antagonists as well as renin antagonists are used in the treatment of hypertension, whether it is due to an endocrine or nonendocrine etiology. A comprehensive knowledge of the actions of these hormones can intelligently guide the proper use of these agents in treating nonendocrine disorders.

GENERAL REFERENCES

For the General References and other additional features, please visit Expert Consult at https://expertconsult.inkling.com.

222

PRINCIPLES OF ENDOCRINOLOGY

ALLEN M. SPIEGEL

INTRODUCTION

The principal manifestation of most endocrine diseases is over- or underse-cretion of one or more hormones, but the causes of endocrine disease are not unique to endocrinology as a subspecialty of medicine. Benign or malignant proliferation of endocrine cells, destruction of endocrine cells by autoim-mune, infectious, or other infiltrative processes, mutations in genes expressed by endocrine cells, and alterations in endocrine cell function caused by meta-bolic abnormalities or drugs are major causes of endocrine disease shared with diseases of other organ systems. If the causes of endocrine disease are not unique, there are nonetheless some general principles of endocrinology that define it as a medical subspecialty. These principles all derive from the study of hormones. Endocrinology was born with the recognition that certain cells secrete specific chemical entities—hormones—directly into the blood stream to act on specific distant targets. This immediately posed a series of questions: how are hormone synthesis and secretion regulated, how are hor-mones transported and metabolized, and how do hormones exert their actions on target tissues? This chapter will provide an overview of the answers to each of these questions and how they inform our current approach to the diagnosis and treatment of endocrine diseases.

WHAT IS A HORMONE?

The initial definition of a hormone was based on physiology rather than chemistry. Action on target cells reached via the blood stream was the opera-tive principle. Secretin, now known to be a peptide hormone secreted by enteroendocrine cells in the gastrointestinal lining and acting on pancreatic exocrine cells, was the first example.[1] In contrast to enteroendocrine cells dispersed in the gut lining with other cell types, discrete collections of hormone-secreting cells, endocrine glands such as the adrenals, gonads, thyroid, and parathyroids, were soon recognized and their hormonal secre-tions chemically characterized. We now know that peptides, steroids, and many other chemical substances fit the definition of a hormone.

Endocrine action, a hormone secreted into the blood stream acting at a distance, has been contrasted with *paracrine action*, a growth factor or other signaling molecule secreted from one cell and acting on adjacent cells, and *autocrine action*, a cell secreting a signaling molecule that acts on the same cell. The distinction between endocrine, paracrine, and autocrine actions is not sharp. In some cases, a factor such as parathyroid hormone–related peptide (PTHrP) that acts physiologically in paracrine fashion during normal bone development may act as an endocrine factor in the syndrome of humoral hypercalcemia of malignancy. The definition of what constitutes an endo-crine gland has also blurred. First came the discovery that specialized neurons could synthesize and secrete hormones directly into the blood stream, so-called neuroendocrine action, exemplified by vasopressin secretion by posterior pituitary cells. This contrasts with classic neuronal secretion of neurotransmitters into the synaptic cleft. With increasing recognition that many tissues secrete hormones (e.g., erythropoietin by the kidney and leptin and other adipokines by fat cells), the role of endocrine glands as the exclu-sive purveyors of hormonal secretions has diminished. This blurring of the boundaries between endocrinology and other medical specialties is a general phenomenon in which study of hormones has informed seemingly disparate fields. Radioimmunoassay, the concept of receptors, and other principles of signal transduction first elucidated in studying hormone action are now broadly applied in all fields of medicine.

REGULATION OF HORMONE SYNTHESIS AND SECRETION

There are two broad categories of hormone synthesis: (1) that responsible for synthesis of peptide hormones and (2) that responsible for synthesis of steroids, including the active form of vitamin D, thyroid hormones, catechol-amines, and other nonpeptide hormones. In the former category, hormone structure is encoded genetically. mRNA translation yields a protein precursor (pre-pro-hormone) that is generally cleaved through successive steps to yield the mature secreted product. Some protein precursors such as proopiomela-nocortin contain within them multiple hormonal products, adrenocortico-tropic hormone (ACTH), melanocyte-stimulating hormone (MSH), and endorphins in that example. In certain pathologic conditions, inappropriate immature hormone secretion occurs (e.g., excessive proinsulin secretion by insulinomas). Post-translational modifications occur for some hormones, such as disulfide bond formation for vasopressin and insulin, C-peptide cleav-age for insulin, and glycosylation of the pituitary glycoprotein hormones, thyroid-stimulating hormone (TSH), follicle-stimulating hormone (FSH), and luteinizing hormone (LH). Mutations in genes encoding peptide hor-mones can lead to disruption of normal hormone synthesis or secretion, a rare cause of hormone deficiency. Peptide hormones are typically stored in secretory granules, and they are secreted by exocytosis, a process regulated by Ca^{++} and other factors. For steroids and other nonpeptide hormones, hormone synthesis is accomplished by a series of enzymatic steps acting on precursors (cholesterol for steroid hormones; aromatic amino acids for thyroid hormones, catecholamines, and related compounds). Mutations in genes encoding enzymes responsible for one or more steps in hormone syn-thesis can lead to hormone deficiency.

Negative feedback regulation is the general principle that governs normal hormone synthesis and secretion. For endocrine glands whose growth and hormone secretion is stimulated by pituitary trophic hormones (gonads, adrenal cortex, thyroid), the hormone secreted by the gland acts directly on cognate pituitary trophic cells (e.g., cortisol acting on ACTH-secreting pitu-itary corticotrophs) to suppress hormone secretion (Fig. 222-1). Conversely, a physiologically meaningful reduction in target gland hormone secretion leads to increased pituitary trophic hormone secretion. In many other cases, negative feedback regulation operates without the pituitary as an intermedi-ate (e.g., PTH secretion from the parathyroid glands regulates extracellular Ca^{++} homeostasis, and Ca^{++} feeds back directly on parathyroid cells to regu-late PTH secretion). Chronic hormone deficiency with resultant loss of nega-tive feedback can lead to hypersecretion of the cognate trophic hormone and even to neoplastic proliferation of trophic hormone–secreting cells. Exam-ples include Nelson's syndrome in which corticotroph tumors form second-ary to adrenalectomy, and tertiary hyperparathyroidism in which parathyroid adenomas occur in the setting of chronic hypocalcemia. In some adrenal cortical disorders, hormone deficiency leading to loss of negative feedback of trophic hormone secretion causes pathologic hypersecretion of alternative steroid hormones. The various forms of congenital adrenal hyperplasia are caused by mutations in one of the several enzymes in the cortisol biosyn-thetic pathway. 21-Hydroxylase deficiency, the most common, can lead to virilization in female infants, with excessive adrenal androgen secretion caused by ACTH stimulation in the face of inability to synthesize cortisol. Inhibition of enzymatic steps in hormone synthesis, such as aromatase inhibi-tors to decrease estrogen formation in estrogen receptor–positive forms of breast cancer, may be an important therapeutic target.

Hormone hypersecretion syndromes in which excessive hormone secre-tion occurs in the face of "normal" levels of the factor that ordinarily sup-presses the cognate hormone are by definition caused by some intrinsic defect in negative feedback suppression. This may occur secondary to a neo-plastic proliferation of hormone-secreting cells, so that "basal" hormone secretion from the increased mass of cells exceeds physiologic levels. This may also be due to alterations in the intrinsic "set-point" for negative feedback suppression of hormone secretion. In practice, it may be impossible to dif-ferentiate these two mechanisms, and they are not mutually exclusive.

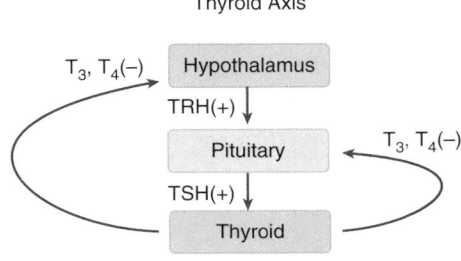

FIGURE 222-1. Hypothalamic-pituitary-thyroid axis illustrating negative feedback regulation. Following thyroid-stimulating hormone (TSH) secretion by the pituitary, the thyroid gland secretes T_3 and T_4, which feed back on the hypothalamus and pituitary to suppress further increases in thyrotropin-releasing hormone (TRH) and TSH secretion.

Hormone secretion is subject to many additional forms of regulation beyond simple negative feedback suppression. These include metabolic, neural, and other internal and environmental inputs. The temporal pattern of hormone secretion is often related to diurnal rhythms, as classically seen for cortisol, and also pulsatility. Changes in gonadotropin secretion during the menstrual cycle and during the course of puberty are striking examples of complex regulation of temporal patterns of hormone secretion.

HORMONE TRANSPORT AND METABOLISM

Most peptide hormones circulate as the free peptide, but insulin-like growth factor 1 (IGF-1) uniquely binds to a number of specialized binding proteins. Steroid and thyroid hormones are lipophilic molecules that circulate largely in protein-bound form. Specialized binding proteins for cortisol, androgens, estrogens, and thyroid hormones are selective for their cognate hormone. The free circulating hormone concentration is only a small fraction of the total hormone measured by routine analytic methods. Binding protein abnormalities can occur in liver disease, because most are synthesized by the liver. Thus, the determination of free as opposed to total plasma hormone concentration may be critical to accurate diagnosis in certain clinical conditions.

Hormone metabolism is another critical determinant of action for some hormones. For testosterone, thyroxine, and vitamin D, enzymatic conversion to more potent hormones—dihydrotestosterone formation in target tissues such as skin by 5-α reductase, thyroxine conversion to triiodothyronine by

deiodinases, and 1,25 dihydroxyvitamin D formation by sequential hydroxylations in the liver and kidney—are all critical to normal hormone action. Defects in these metabolic steps leads to impaired hormone action. Even some peptide hormones such as angiotensin must undergo enzymatic conversion from secreted precursor form to generate the active hormone.

MECHANISM OF HORMONE ACTION

The central question in hormone action is how a hormone circulating in the blood stream in minute concentrations recognizes its specific target cells and regulates physiologic processes within them. Research addressing this question over the past four decades defined receptors, previously a purely theoretical concept, in molecular terms. Receptors are highly selective molecules that bind their cognate hormones with high affinity and specificity. Two broad classes of receptors were identified: (1) cell surface receptors that typically span the plasma membrane one or more times (Fig. 222-2) and (2) so-called nuclear receptors that reside either in the nucleus or in the cytoplasm, with subsequent translocation to the nucleus[2] (Fig. 222-3).

Hormones regulate cellular physiologic processes such as secretion of hormones, enzymes, and other compounds, muscle contraction, growth, and proliferation. *Signal transduction* is the general term for the biochemical steps between hormone binding to receptor and alterations in cell physiology. Most peptide and protein hormones (e.g., insulin, growth hormone, ACTH) bind to cell surface receptors that can be classified according to the

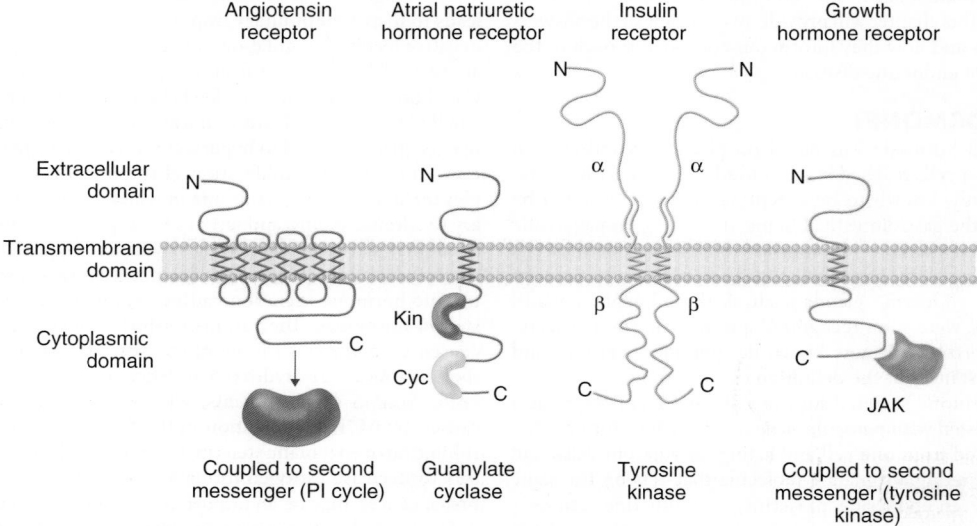

FIGURE 222-2. Structures of different types of peptide hormone receptors.

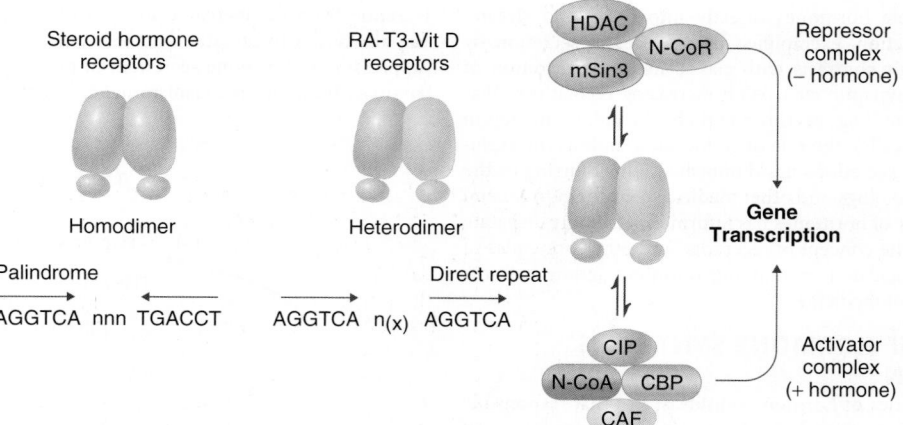

FIGURE 222-3. How steroid hormone receptors function. *Left,* Glucocorticoid receptor family members bind as homodimers to palindromic DNA sites. Thyroid hormone receptor family members bind primarily as heterodimers with retinoid X receptor to direct repeat DNA sites separated by varying numbers of base pairs. *Right,* As a result of hormone binding, repressor complexes dissociate and activator complexes bind to nuclear receptors. Repressor complexes contain histone deacetylase (HDAC), and activator complexes contain histone acetylase (CAF).

mechanism of signal transduction to which they are coupled (e.g., G protein–coupled[3] receptor tyrosine or serine kinase, JAK/STAT coupled; see Fig. 222-2). Cell surface receptors may generate "second messengers," which in turn regulate a kinase cascade. Receptor activation may have rapid effects such as exocytosis of secretory granules, but longer-term actions involving gene regulation may also be a consequence of second messenger and kinase cascade activation. Steroid and thyroid hormones and vitamin D bind to members of the nuclear receptor family. The latter act as "ligand-regulated" transcription factors to regulate gene expression (see Fig. 222-3).

Selectivity of hormone binding by receptors is not absolute. "Specificity spillover" is a clinically important phenomenon in which supraphysiologic concentrations of a hormone leads to binding and activation of a non-cognate receptor for a closely related hormone. Examples include: hypoglycemia seen with non–islet cell tumors secreting IGF-2, which binds to the insulin receptor[4]; skin hyperpigmentation in subjects with Addison's disease in whom excessive ACTH secretion activates the melanocortin receptor in melanocytes normally regulated by MSH; and hyperthyroidism in pregnant women with high human chorionic gonadotropin (HCG) concentrations activating the TSH receptor.

Genetic endocrine diseases include those caused by mutations in one component of a signal transduction pathway leading either to hormone "resistance" or hormone-independent activation (Tables 222-1 and 222-2). In the former, subjects present with apparent hormone deficiency, but direct hormone measurement reveals high concentrations of bioactive hormone that fails to act owing to target organ resistance. In the latter, patients present with apparent endocrine hyperfunction, but direct measurement reveals suppressed hormone concentration due to intact negative feedback. Loss-of-function mutations in receptors and in signaling intermediates such as G proteins have been identified in patients with hormone resistance. The converse, mutations that constitutively activate receptors or downstream signaling components,[5] have been identified in endocrine hyperactivity diseases such as familial male precocious puberty and familial nonautoimmune hyperthyroidism. Receptor inactivating mutations that lead to hormone-resistance diseases have been identified for both the cell surface and nuclear classes of receptors.

GENERAL REFERENCES

For the General References and other additional features, please visit Expert Consult at https://expertconsult.inkling.com.

223

NEUROENDOCRINOLOGY AND THE NEUROENDOCRINE SYSTEM

MARK E. MOLITCH

NEUROENDOCRINE REGULATION

Neuroendocrinology refers to the area of endocrinology in which the nervous system interacts with the endocrine system to link neural activity with metabolic and hormonal homeostatic activity. The neurohypophysial neurons originate from the paraventricular and supraoptic nuclei, traverse the hypothalamic-pituitary stalk, and release vasopressin and oxytocin from nerve endings in the posterior pituitary. The hypophysiotropic neurons localized in specific hypothalamic nuclei project their axons to the median eminence to secrete their peptide and bioamine releasing and inhibiting hormones into the proximal end of the hypothalamic-pituitary portal vessels (Fig. 223-1). The median eminence receives its blood supply from the superior hypophysial artery, which arborizes into a rich capillary bed. The capillary loops extend into the median eminence and coalesce to form the long portal veins that traverse the pituitary stalk and end in the pituitary. The neuroendocrine system operates through a series of feedback loops that regulate pituitary and target organ hormone levels. Target organ hormones can feed back at both the hypothalamic and the pituitary levels to complete the loop. The feedback loops can be perturbed, resulting in alterations of set points by such factors as length of day (circadian periodicity), stress, nutritional status, and systemic illness.

Hypophysiotropic Hormones
Regulation of pituitary hormones by the hypophysiotropic hormones is quite complex, in part because of the multiplicity of substances present in the hypothalamus that can affect pituitary hormone secretion and in part because of the redundancy and overlapping nature of the feedback loops alluded to earlier. In addition, some hypophysiotropic hormones exert effects on more than one pituitary hormone.

Thyrotropin-Releasing Hormone
The primary neuroendocrine functions of thyrotropin-releasing hormone (TRH) are to stimulate the synthesis and release of thyroid-stimulating hormone (TSH) and prolactin. In cases of hypothyroidism, the increased TRH synthesis and binding to the pituitary results in increased TSH and prolactin levels. Correction of the hypothyroidism with thyroid hormones decreases the elevated TSH and prolactin levels. Conversely, in cases of hyperthyroidism, TSH levels are markedly suppressed. Although TRH is the major regulator of TSH synthesis and secretion, the role of TRH as a physiologic prolactin-releasing factor (PRF) is unclear.

Gonadotropin-Releasing Hormone
Gonadotropin-releasing hormone (GnRH) is a 10–amino acid peptide; its neurons originate in the epithelium of the medial part of the olfactory

TABLE 222-1	DISEASES CAUSED BY G PROTEIN–COUPLED RECEPTOR LOSS-OF-FUNCTION MUTATIONS	
RECEPTOR	**DISEASE**	**INHERITANCE**
V2 vasopressin	Nephrogenic diabetes insipidus	X-linked
ACTH	Familial ACTH resistance	Autosomal recessive
GHRH	Familial GH deficiency	Autosomal recessive
GnRH	Hypogonadotropic hypogonadism	Autosomal recessive
GPR54	Hypogonadotropic hypogonadism	Autosomal recessive
Prokineticin receptor 2	Hypogonadotropic hypogonadism	Autosomal dominant*
FSH	Hypergonadotropic ovarian dysgenesis	Autosomal recessive
LH	Male pseudohermaphroditism	Autosomal recessive
TSH	Familial hypothyroidism	Autosomal recessive
Ca²⁺ sensing	Familial hypocalciuric hypercalcemia, neonatal severe primary hyperparathyroidism	Autosomal dominant Autosomal recessive
Melanocortin 4	Obesity	Autosomal recessive
PTH/PTHrP	Blomstrand chondrodysplasia	Autosomal recessive

*With incomplete penetrance
ACTH = Adrenocorticotropic hormone; FSH = follicle-stimulating hormone; GH = growth hormone; GHRH = growth hormone–releasing hormone; GnRH = gonadotropin-releasing hormone; LH = luteinizing hormone; PTH = parathyroid hormone; PTHrP = parathyroid hormone–related protein; TSH = thyroid-stimulating hormone.

TABLE 222-2	DISEASES CAUSED BY G PROTEIN–COUPLED RECEPTOR GAIN-OF-FUNCTION MUTATIONS	
RECEPTOR	**DISEASE**	**INHERITANCE**
LH	Familial male precocious puberty	Autosomal dominant
TSH	Sporadic hyperfunctional thyroid nodules	Noninherited (somatic)
TSH	Familial nonautoimmune hyperthyroidism	Autosomal dominant
Ca²⁺ sensing	Familial hypocalcemic hypercalciuria	Autosomal dominant
PTH/PTHrP	Jansen's metaphyseal chondrodysplasia	Autosomal dominant
V2 vasopressin	Nephrogenic inappropriate antidiuresis	Autosomal dominant

LH = Luteinizing hormone; PTH = parathyroid hormone; PTHrP = parathyroid hormone–related protein; TSH = thyroid-stimulating hormone.

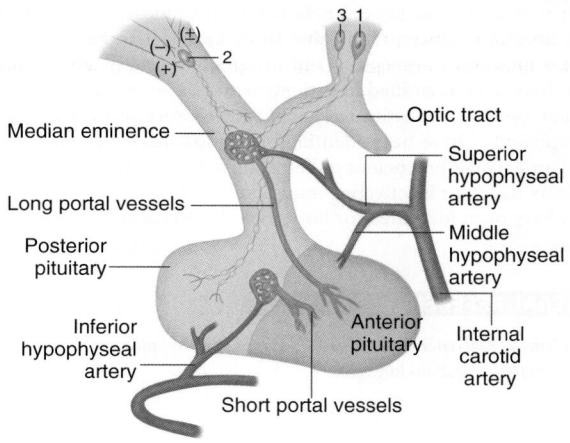

FIGURE 223-1. Neuroendocrine organization of the hypothalamus and pituitary gland. The posterior pituitary is fed by the inferior hypophyseal artery and the hypothalamus by the superior hypophyseal artery, both branches of the internal carotid artery. Most of the blood supply to the anterior pituitary is venous by way of the long portal vessels, which connect the portal capillary beds in the median eminence to the venous sinusoids in the anterior pituitary. Hypophysiotropic neuron 3 in the parvocellular division of the paraventricular nucleus and neuron 2 in the arcuate nucleus are shown to terminate in the median eminence on portal capillaries. These neurons of the tuberoinfundibular system secrete hypothalamic releasing and inhibiting hormones into the portal veins for conveyance to the anterior pituitary gland. Neuron 2 is innervated by monoaminergic neurons. Note that the multiple inputs to such neurons, using neuron 2 as an example, can be stimulatory, inhibitory, or neuromodulatory, in which another neuron may affect neurotransmitter release. Neuron 1 represents a peptidergic neuron originating in the magnocellular division of the paraventricular nucleus or supraoptic nucleus and projecting directly to the posterior pituitary by way of the hypothalamic-neurohypophyseal tract. (From Gay VL. The hypothalamus: physiology and clinical use of releasing factors. *Fertil Steril.* 1972;23:50-63, with permission of the American Society for Reproductive Medicine.)

placode. This origin of GnRH-producing neurons from olfactory epithelium is of clinical interest with respect to the entity of Kallmann's syndrome, in which GnRH deficiency is associated with agenesis of the olfactory bulbs. One form of Kallmann's syndrome is caused by loss of function of a protein (anosmin) that facilitates the embryologic migration of these GnRH-producing neurons. The primary function of GnRH is to stimulate the secretion of luteinizing hormone (LH) and follicle-stimulating hormone (FSH). Only one GnRH has been identified, and the differential secretion of LH and FSH is due to variations in sensitivity of the feedback effects of steroid and peptide hormones and variations in sensitivity to GnRH. GnRH pulsatile secretion directly increases its own receptor number, whereas continuous administration of GnRH is associated with a decrease. In women, positive and negative steroid hormone feedback regulation of the hypothalamic-pituitary-gonadal axis occurs at both the pituitary and hypothalamic levels, the hypothalamic effects being alteration of GnRH pulse amplitude and frequency, and the pituitary effects being modulation of the gonadotropin response to GnRH. In males, testosterone decreases GnRH pulsatile secretion, with a resultant decrease in gonadotropin pulse amplitude and frequency as well as a decreased gonadotropin response to exogenous GnRH.

The negative feedback effects of inhibin, a peptide produced by testicular Sertoli cells and ovarian granulosa cells, are predominantly on FSH at the pituitary, where inhibin causes a decrease in the sensitivity of gonadotrophs to GnRH. The related ovarian protein activin stimulates basal and GnRH-stimulated FSH synthesis and release from the pituitary, but its primary action is to facilitate the response of ovarian granulosa cells to FSH. Another gonadal peptide, follistatin, also inhibits the oophorectomy- and GnRH-induced rise in FSH selectively, primarily by binding to activin. These ovarian peptides are also found in the pituitary and may therefore have additional local effects on gonadotropin secretion.

GnRH has been administered with great success in pulsatile fashion to individuals with hypogonadotropic hypogonadism secondary to GnRH deficiency, leading to restoration of normal sexual function and fertility. Long-acting GnRH agonists have been used to downregulate GnRH receptors and gonadotropin secretion in a variety of conditions, including precocious puberty, prostate cancer, breast cancer, uterine fibroids, and endometriosis. Direct GnRH antagonists that compete for the GnRH receptor are used for similar conditions.

Somatostatin

Somatostatin (also known as somatotropin release inhibiting factor) inhibits GH secretion. The interaction of somatostatin and growth hormone–releasing hormone (GHRH) on GH secretion is complex. GH secretory episodes are associated with increased GHRH secretion, often accompanied by low somatostatin levels; the basal or trough GH levels are associated with low GHRH levels and more elevated somatostatin levels. Somatostatin also inhibits basal and stimulated TSH secretion. However, GH is about 10-fold more sensitive to inhibition by somatostatin than is TSH, suggesting that the physiologic role of somatostatin in inhibiting TSH secretion is limited. Somatostatin is also present in D cells of the pancreatic islets, the gut mucosa, and the myenteric neural plexus. Through paracrine and endocrine actions, it suppresses the secretion of insulin, glucagon, cholecystokinin, gastrin, secretin, vasoactive intestinal polypeptide (VIP), and other gastrointestinal hormones, as well as such functions as gastric acid secretion, gastric emptying, gallbladder contraction, and splanchnic blood flow. Analogues of somatostatin have been developed for the treatment of acromegaly, carcinoid tumors, VIP-secreting tumors, TSH-secreting pituitary tumors, and islet cell tumors.

Corticotropin-Releasing Hormone

Corticotropin-releasing hormone (CRH) releases adrenocorticotropic hormone (ACTH), β-endorphin, β-lipotropin, melanocyte-stimulating hormone (MSH), and other peptides generated from proopiomelanocortin (POMC) in equimolar amounts. CRH mediates 75% of the ACTH response to stress. The remaining 25% is due to vasopressin. CRH and vasopressin have synergistic effects on ACTH release. CRH and vasopressin are not always released coordinately, however, and stress selectively activates the vasopressin-containing subset of CRH neurons. Cortisol feeds back to decrease ACTH secretion at both the hypothalamic and the pituitary levels. ACTH and β-endorphin also feed back negatively to decrease CRH release by the hypothalamus. Central bioamines, opioids, and peptides influence CRH secretion. Monokines released by inflammatory tissue, such as interleukin (IL)-1, IL-6, and tumor necrosis factor (TNF)-α, stimulate the synthesis and release of CRH and vasopressin from the hypothalamus. The consequent increase in cortisol then reduces the intensity of the inflammatory response and release of these monokines, thus completing this inflammation-modulating feedback loop. CRH receptors are widely distributed in the brain, and increases in CRH are associated with activation of the sympathetic nervous system, suppression of the parasympathetic nervous system, stimulation of arousal, and increased learning performance. CRH may also be involved in the regulation of body weight; with overfeeding, increased leptin stimulates CRH, which causes decreased food intake and increased energy expenditure.

Biosynthetic human CRH has become available for clinical use. Its major utility is in the differential diagnosis of Cushing's disease versus ectopic ACTH syndrome, with the finding that patients with Cushing's disease respond with a greater than 35% increment, whereas those with ectopic ACTH secretion have a lesser response. If the results are equivocal, CRH testing during bilateral inferior petrosal sinus sampling for ACTH often provides additional discriminatory information.

Growth Hormone–Releasing Hormone

GHRH dose-dependently stimulates GH secretion. With repetitive administration, GHRH can cause the release of sufficient GH in children with GHRH deficiency to result in an increase in insulin-like growth factor (IGF)-I levels and an acceleration of growth. Both IGF-I and GH feed back negatively on GH secretion. This negative feedback results in both a decrease in GHRH and an increase in somatostatin. The feedback effect of IGF-I is clinically relevant, as documented by the high circulating GH levels that occur in IGF-I-deficient states such as renal insufficiency and cirrhosis. In children with mutations of the GH receptor resulting in their not being responsive to GH (GH insensitivity syndrome, also known as Laron-type dwarfism), IGF-I levels are very low and GH levels are correspondingly elevated.

Prolactin Inhibitory Factor

The inhibitory component of hypothalamic regulation of prolactin secretion predominates over the stimulatory component. Dopamine is the major physiologic prolactin inhibitory factor. It is likely that in most physiologic circumstances that cause a rise in prolactin (e.g., lactation), a simultaneous fall in dopamine occurs, along with a rise in a prolactin-releasing factor (PRF) such as VIP. Blockade of endogenous dopamine receptors by a variety of drugs, such as the antipsychotics, causes a rise in prolactin. Lesions that interrupt the basal hypothalamic neuronal pathways carrying dopamine to the median eminence or that interrupt portal blood flow, such as craniopharyngiomas or other large mass lesions, result in decreased dopamine reaching the pituitary and hyperprolactinemia.

Prolactin-Releasing Factor

A number of hypothalamic peptides other than TRH have also been shown to have PRF activity. VIP stimulates prolactin synthesis and release at concentrations found in hypothalamic-pituitary portal blood. Within the VIP precursor is another similarly sized peptide known as peptide histidine methionine, which also has PRF activity. The precise roles of VIP versus peptide histidine methionine are not clear. They appear to be of negligible physiologic importance in humans.

Endogenous Opioid Peptides

Most data now suggest a modest role for endogenous opioid peptides in neuroendocrine regulation. The endogenous opioid peptides have a common 5–amino acid sequence at their amino termini (Tyr-Gly-Gly-Phe-Met [or Leu]) that is important for their binding to endogenous opioid receptors and bioactivity. Three major opioid peptide receptors and three major groups of opioid peptides are recognized. The μ-receptor mediates most of the endocrine effects and analgesia. The primary peptide ligand for the μ-receptor is β-endorphin, which is derived from POMC. The δ-receptor mediates behavioral, analgesic, and some endocrine effects and has as its primary peptide ligands met- and leu-enkephalins, which are derived from proenkephalin A. It is much less well blocked by naloxone than is the μ-receptor. The κ-receptor mediates sedation and ataxia and binds primarily dynorphin and the neoendorphins. A fourth receptor has considerable sequence homology with the δ-receptor and binds to an endogenous 17–amino acid peptide called nociceptin (also known as orphanin FQ).

POMC is a 31-kD precursor peptide that harbors within it ACTH, β-lipotropin, and β-endorphin. POMC undergoes tissue-specific posttranslational processing. In the anterior pituitary, its major cleavage products are β-lipotropin and ACTH, with a significant proportion of β-lipotropin being further processed to β-endorphin. In the pituitary intermediate lobe, the major products are α-melanocyte stimulating hormone (α-MSH), corticotropin-like intermediate peptide, β-endorphin, and γ-lipotropin. Brain POMC, however, is processed primarily to β-endorphin, γ-lipotropin, and ACTH, with most of the ACTH being further processed to corticotropin-like intermediate peptide and α-MSH. The pentapeptide enkephalins are derived from the 28-kD precursor proenkephalin A. Neuronal perikarya containing the enkephalins are widely distributed throughout the brain. Dynorphin is a 17–amino acid peptide derived from a 28-kD precursor called proenkephalin B or prodynorphin. Shorter peptides called α- and β-neoendorphin, which have 10 and 9 amino acids, respectively, have also been isolated. These peptides react almost exclusively with the κ-receptor. Nociceptin is a 17–amino acid peptide derived from a κ precursor called prononociceptin. High concentrations of nociceptin and its receptor are present in the hypothalamus as well as in other areas of the brain that serve as the sources of monoamine neurotransmitters. In general, nociceptin appears to have an antiopioid or antinociceptive effect. The hypothalamus contains abundant opioid receptors. The effects of opioid peptides on anterior pituitary hormone secretion are produced through modulation of hypothalamic bioamines and hypophysiotropic factors.

The specific functions of the various opioid peptides and the opioid receptors are still not completely understood, although evidence links them to a number of body functions, including stress, mental illness, narcotic tolerance and dependence, eating, drinking, gastrointestinal function, learning, memory, reward, cardiovascular responses, respiration, thermoregulation, seizures, brain electrical activity, locomotor activity, pregnancy, and neuroimmune activity. Endogenous opioids have an inhibitory influence on gonadotropin secretion through action on GnRH secretion. Exogenous β-endorphin and enkephalin analogues increase serum GH and prolactin levels, but blockade of endogenous opioid pathways with naloxone does not alter basal or stimulated GH or prolactin levels. Opioids feed back negatively on ACTH and β-endorphin secretion, and naloxone can increase basal and stimulated ACTH levels. Overall, the effects of the endogenous opioids on normal physiologic regulation of the various pituitary hormones in humans is minimal. However, exogenous opioids in pharmacologic doses can impair GnRH and gonadotropin secretion, causing hypogonadism with reduced libido, sexual function, and fertility, and can also impair CRH and ACTH secretion, causing adrenal insufficiency.[1]

Central Nervous System Rhythms and Neuroendocrine Function

Pituitary hormones are secreted in a pulsatile fashion with a number of rhythms superimposed. The pulse amplitude of a pituitary hormone reflects the amount of releasing hormone and factors that alter sensitivity to that releasing hormone. Thus, the amplitude can be altered by the presence of inhibitory factors (e.g., GHRH versus somatostatin), nutritional factors, feedback effects of target organ hormones, and prior stimulation that depletes the releasable hormone pool. Pulse frequency is governed by the frequency of release of the hypophysiotropic factor, which is regulated by the hypothalamic pulse generator system.

The pituitary has an intrinsic rhythm of small amplitude with a frequency of every 2 to 10 minutes. Superimposed on this intrinsic rhythm is a rhythm caused by the pulsatile release of hypophysiotropic releasing factors, with or without the withdrawal of a corresponding inhibitory factor. Rhythms that are shorter than 1 day are referred to as ultradian rhythms. The next layer of rhythmicity is the circadian rhythm—that is, a rhythm with approximately 24-hour periodicity. These rhythms are usually synchronized with the 24-hour period by a periodic environmental cue such as the dark-light cycle. The suprachiasmatic nucleus functions as a circadian pacemaker and receives light-induced electrical impulses from the retina, transmitting those impulses to the pineal gland where they are converted to hormonal signals. Signals for a rhythm with a periodicity longer than 24 hours, an infradian rhythm, include the gravitational influence of the moon, which gives rise to the menstrual cycle.[2]

A number of factors may influence circadian and infradian rhythms. One of the most important is the sleep-wake cycle. GH, TSH, prolactin, ACTH, and pubertal LH secretion are all entrained more to the sleep-wake cycle than to the dark-light cycle. Each has an increase and maximal level that occur following sleep onset. The profound diurnal variation in cortisol and ACTH is often used as an index of "normality" of the system. Loss of this diurnal rhythm occurs with disordered regulation by CRH, which may be due to endogenous depression or excessive alcohol intake, or autonomous secretion of ACTH in Cushing's disease (Chapter 224). Loss of the diurnal rhythm of cortisol has been used as a diagnostic test for Cushing's syndrome.

Interesting changes occur in gonadotropin secretion as a child passes through puberty into adulthood. Early in puberty, the amplitude of the pulses increases during sleep at night, especially for LH, but in adulthood, this nocturnal rise is lost. In patients with anorexia nervosa, the pattern of gonadotropin secretion often reverts to this pubertal pattern. This phenomenon suggests that body composition may in some way affect regulation of the pulsatile secretion of gonadotropins. The percentage of body fat has been proposed as being important in the timing of the onset of puberty. Recent studies implicate leptin as the signal indicating this change in body composition.

⬤ NEUROENDOCRINE DISEASE
Diseases of the Hypothalamus

Diseases may affect the hypothalamus by discrete localization in the hypothalamus, being part of a generalized central nervous system (CNS) disease such as neurosarcoidosis, or indirectly by a process such as hydrocephalus (Table 223-1). Furthermore, hormonal changes mediated by functional alterations in hypothalamic regulation may occur in systemic illnesses.

The axons projecting to the median eminence that contain the various hypophysiotropic factors are concentrated in the basal portion of the hypothalamus. Thus, lesions located within this final common pathway might be expected to cause significant decreases in secretion of some or all of the pituitary hormones except prolactin, which may increase because of the elimination of tonic inhibition by dopamine. Diabetes insipidus (Chapter 225) may also occur. Symptoms resulting from hypothalamic dysfunction are related to the size of the lesion and consequently to the area of the hypothalamus involved, as well as to the rapidity of the increase in lesion size. Slowly growing lesions tend to cause problems of hormone dysregulation rather than dramatic symptoms. Large, slowly growing lesions may cause more acute problems, such as when a slight increment in growth eliminates the remaining vestiges of vasopressin or ACTH secretion. The best way of discerning lesions affecting the hypothalamus is by magnetic resonance imaging (MRI) with gadolinium enhancement, although computed tomographic (CT) scanning with intravenous contrast is also effective. Formal visual field testing may discern impingement of the optic nerves and chiasm by hypothalamic lesions. Detailed testing of hypothalamic-pituitary function may reveal evidence of functional hypothalamic disruption with great sensitivity.

TABLE 223-1 ETIOLOGY OF HYPOTHALAMIC DISEASE

NEONATES

Congenital embryopathic disorders: agenesis of the corpus callosum, cleft palate (HESX1)

Congenital disorders: isolated hormone and receptor mutations, combined pituitary hormone deficiency (PIT1, PROP1), Laurence-Moon-Bardet-Biedl syndrome, Prader-Labhart-Willi syndrome

Tumors: glioma, hemangioma

Trauma

Hydrocephalus, hydranencephaly, kernicterus

1 MONTH TO 2 YEARS

Tumors: glioma, especially optic glioma, hemangiomas

Infiltrative disease: Langerhans cell histiocytosis, meningitis

Hydrocephalus

2-10 YEARS

Tumors: craniopharyngioma, glioma, dysgerminoma, hamartoma, leukemia, ganglioneuroma, ependymoma, medulloblastoma

Infiltrative disease: Langerhans cell histiocytosis, meningitis, tuberculosis, encephalitis

Irradiation: for nasopharyngeal tumors, intracranial tumors, leukemia

Functional: psychosocial deprivation

10-25 YEARS

Congenital disorders: Kallmann's syndrome, gonadotropin-releasing hormone receptor defects

Tumors: craniopharyngioma, pituitary tumors, glioma, hamartoma, dysgerminoma, dermoid, lipoma, neuroblastoma

Trauma: subarachnoid hemorrhage, vascular aneurysm, arteriovenous malformation

Infiltrative diseases: Langerhans cell histiocytosis, sarcoidosis, tuberculosis, meningitis, encephalitis, leukemia

Chronic hydrocephalus or increased intracranial pressure

Functional: hypogonadotropic hypogonadism associated with weight loss, exercise

25-50 YEARS

Tumors: pituitary tumors, meningioma, craniopharyngioma, Rathke's cleft cyst, glioma, lymphoma, angioma, colloid cysts, ependymoma

Infiltrative diseases: sarcoidosis, Langerhans cell histiocytosis, tuberculosis, viral encephalitis

Subarachnoid hemorrhage, vascular aneurysms, arteriovenous malformation

Irradiation: for pituitary adenoma, nasopharyngeal tumors, intracranial tumors

Nutritional: Wernicke's disease

Functional: hypogonadotropic hypogonadism associated with weight loss, exercise

50 YEARS AND OLDER

Tumors: pituitary tumors, meningioma, craniopharyngioma, sarcoma, glioblastoma, lymphoma, colloid cysts, ependymoma

Vascular: infarct, subarachnoid hemorrhage, pituitary apoplexy, aneurysm

Irradiation: for pituitary adenoma, nasopharyngeal tumors, intracranial tumors

Infiltrative diseases: encephalitis, sarcoidosis, meningitis

Nutritional: Wernicke's disease

Modified from Plum F, Van Uitert R. Non-endocrine diseases of the hypothalamus. In: Reichlin S, Baldessarini RJ, Martin JB, eds. *The Hypothalamus.* New York: Raven Press; 1978:415.

CONGENITAL EMBRYOPATHIC DISORDERS

The most common embryopathic disorders to affect the hypothalamus are the midline cleft syndromes, which cause varying degrees of defects of midline structures, especially the optic and olfactory tracts, the septum pellucidum, the corpus callosum, the anterior commissure, the hypothalamus, and the pituitary. The clinical features of patients with midline cleft defects varies in severity from cyclopia to cleft lip and from isolated hypothalamic hormone defects to panhypopituitarism. The combination of absent septum pellucidum associated with optic nerve hypoplasia is referred to as septo-optic dysplasia and is associated with abnormalities of hypothalamic and other diencephalic structures. Some patients with septo-optic dysplasia and hypothalamic hypopituitarism have sexual precocity, presumably caused by a lack of inhibitory influences from other parts of the hypothalamus and intact GnRH-producing structures. Children with very mild midline cleft defects consisting of cleft lip, cleft palate, or both have an increased risk of GH and other pituitary hormone deficiencies. MRI studies of patients with "idiopathic" GH deficiency show absence of the infundibulum in nearly 50%.

Mutations responsible for these developmental defects are the subject of active investigation.[3] Mutations in the human HESX1, SOX2, SOX3, and OTX2 transcription factor genes cause agenesis of the corpus callosum and panhypopituitarism. Case reports of mutations in other transcription factors,

such as *Pitx2* (Rieger's syndrome) and *GLI2*, describe patients with varying brain and skull developmental abnormalities, along with varying degrees of hypopituitarism. Kallmann's syndrome is a condition characterized by anosmia or hyposmia and hypogonadotropic hypogonadism. The diagnosis is made by finding anosmia and low gonadotropin levels, and MRI will show absence or hypoplasia of the olfactory bulbs. The X-linked form of Kallmann's syndrome, representing about 85% of cases, is due to a gene defect (*KAL1*) resulting in loss of function of a protein called anosmin that facilitates the embryologic migration of GnRH-producing neurons from the olfactory placode to the hypothalamus and the olfactory nerves to the olfactory bulbs. Other genes implicated in Kallmann's syndrome include *PROK2, PROKR2, FGFR1,* and *FGF8*. The pituitary is usually intact in this condition, and treatment with pulsatile GnRH therapy or gonadotropins results in spermatogenesis and normal gonadal function. In some patients, other abnormalities may be present, including cerebellar ataxia, nerve deafness, color blindness, cleft lip and palate, disordered thirst, unilateral renal agenesis, synkinesia, dental agenesis, and skeletal anomalies such as syndactyly and polydactyly; these abnormalities tend to track with specific mutations of the genes outlined above.

TUMORS

The most common tumors affecting the hypothalamus are pituitary adenomas that have significant suprasellar extension. These tumors can cause varying degrees of hypopituitarism and hyperprolactinemia, either by compressing the normal pituitary or, more commonly, by affecting the pituitary stalk and mediobasal hypothalamus. Surprisingly, diabetes insipidus (Chapter 225) is a rare finding in patients with pituitary adenomas. In patients with normal or elevated prolactin levels, indicating a hypothalamic/stalk site of the lesion rather than pituitary destruction, pituitary function often returns following therapy.

Craniopharyngiomas are the next most common tumors affecting the hypothalamus.[4] Microscopically, craniopharyngiomas consist of cysts alternating with stratified squamous epithelium. The cyst fluid is usually thick and dark, and the material is often calcified. They arise from remnants of Rathke's pouch. A closely related lesion is Rathke's cleft cyst, which develops from the space between the anterior and rudimentary intermediate lobes. Rathke's cleft cysts are lined with cuboidal (as opposed to squamous) epithelium, and the cyst fluid is usually a white mucoid fluid. Craniopharyngiomas may be difficult to remove in their entirety, and postoperative radiation reduces recurrences. Rathke's cleft cysts less commonly recur. Craniopharyngiomas most commonly arise during childhood, but they may also occur in adults and even elderly people. These tumors come to attention because of mass effects, including headache, vomiting, visual disturbance, seizures, hypopituitarism, and polyuria. Some patients have galactorrhea, amenorrhea, and hyperprolactinemia, features suggestive of a prolactinoma. Careful endocrine testing reveals varying degrees of hypopituitarism in 50 to 75%, modest hyperprolactinemia in 25 to 50%, and often diabetes insipidus. Surgical extirpation of craniopharyngiomas commonly causes a worsening of pituitary function, often resulting in complete panhypopituitarism and diabetes insipidus because of stalk section, and may cause damage to the hypothalamic centers that regulate thirst, body temperature, and food intake, resulting in severe obesity. Recently, the technique of hypothalamic-sparing surgery for craniopharyngiomas has resulted in less obesity without increasing the recurrence rate.[5] Irradiation may also be helpful, especially in children.

Suprasellar dysgerminomas arise from primitive germ cells that have migrated to the CNS during fetal life and are structurally identical to germ cell tumors of the gonads. They most commonly occur in children, in whom they cause decreased growth because of hypopituitarism, as well as diabetes insipidus and visual problems. Hyperprolactinemia occurs in more than 50% of affected children, and 10% have precocious puberty from the production of human chorionic gonadotropin (HCG) by the tumor. The finding of an elevated HCG level in the spinal fluid may be diagnostic. As opposed to craniopharyngiomas, these tumors are very radiosensitive, and radiation therapy combined with chemotherapy is the preferred treatment.

A hypothalamic hamartoma is a nodule of growth of hypothalamic neurons, glia, and fiber bundles attached by a pedicle to the hypothalamus between the tuber cinereum and the mammillary bodies and extending into the basal cistern.[6] Asymptomatic hamartomas may be present in up to 20% of random autopsies; rarely, these lesions may enlarge and disrupt hypothalamic function because of compression of adjacent tissue. Less commonly, they may cause seizures, especially gelastic seizures. Some hamartomas can be associated with other congenital anomalies and mutations in the transcription factor gene *GLI3*. A variant of hamartoma consisting of similar tissue present within the anterior pituitary but without a neural attachment to the hypothalamus is called a choristoma or gangliocytoma. These neuronal tumors are of particular endocrine interest because they can produce hypophysiotropic hormones. A number of cases associated with precocious puberty have been reported in which the hamartomas produced GnRH. Successful treatment has been reported with surgery and with the administration of a long-acting GnRH analogue that suppresses gonadotropin secretion but does not affect the tumor itself. If the hamartoma does not cause other problems from mass effects, medical therapy with the GnRH analogue may be the best choice because surgery can be noncurative or even fatal. Some gangliocytomas have been reported that produce GHRH and acromegaly or CRH and Cushing's syndrome.

Other tumors and space-occupying lesions occurring in the suprasellar area include arachnoid cysts, meningiomas, gliomas, astrocytomas, chordomas, infundibulomas, cholesteatomas, neurofibromas, lipomas, and metastatic cancer (particularly from the breast and lung). Any such lesion may manifest as varying degrees of hypopituitarism, diabetes insipidus, and hyperprolactinemia, and surgical therapy often worsens the hormonal deficit and may cause other hypothalamic damage.

INFLAMMATORY AND INFILTRATIVE DISORDERS

CNS involvement in cases of sarcoidosis (Chapter 95) occurs in 1 to 5% of patients as determined on clinical grounds, and in up to 16% of cases at autopsy. Isolated CNS sarcoidosis is uncommon. When sarcoidosis does involve the CNS, the hypothalamus is involved in 10 to 20% of cases. Sarcoid granulomas can involve the hypothalamus, stalk, or pituitary and may be infiltrative or occur as a mass lesion.[7] The most common endocrine findings are varying degrees of hypopituitarism, diabetes insipidus, and hyperprolactinemia. Obesity secondary to hypothalamic involvement by sarcoidosis has also been reported. In patients with isolated CNS sarcoidosis, the diagnosis may be extremely difficult. Examination of cerebrospinal fluid usually shows elevated protein levels, low glucose levels, pleocytosis, and variable elevations of angiotensin-converting enzyme. However, biopsy is often necessary. Although corticosteroid therapy has been reported to at least partially reverse the thirst disorders, anterior pituitary hormone deficits usually do not respond.

Langerhans cell histiocytosis infiltration of the hypothalamus may cause diabetes insipidus, varying degrees of hypopituitarism, and hyperprolactinemia.[8] It is the most common cause of diabetes insipidus in children. Usually, this infiltration appears as a thickening of the pituitary stalk, but it may also appear as a mass lesion of the hypothalamus or pituitary (Fig. 223-2). Osteolytic lesions may be present in the jaw or mastoid, so radiographs of the jaw are a worthwhile part of the diagnostic evaluation of an unknown suprasellar mass or diabetes insipidus. Therapy consists of local surgery, focal irradiation, or chemotherapy with alkylating agents and high-dose corticosteroids.

Other infiltrative diseases (e.g., tuberculosis, lymphomas, fungal diseases) can also cause a progressive alteration in hypothalamic regulation of pituitary hormone secretion.

VASCULAR DISEASE

An enlarging aneurysm may manifest as a mass lesion of the hypothalamic-pituitary area and may cause hypopituitarism and visual field defects. Obviously, the distinction must be made before surgery. Tumors and aneurysms may also coexist, and careful radiologic evaluation with MRI is necessary to discern such association. Hypothalamic disease caused by vascular infarction is extremely rare. In the past several years, it has been found that subarachnoid hemorrhage may be associated with varying degrees of hypopituitarism in almost half of cases. On the other hand, diabetes insipidus is uncommon.

TRAUMA

Traumatic brain injury (TBI) (Chapter 399) can cause defects ranging from isolated ACTH deficiency to panhypopituitarism with diabetes insipidus. Within the first 72 hours of trauma, GH, LH, ACTH, TSH, and prolactin levels may actually be elevated in blood, perhaps because of acute release. These levels subsequently fall, and either pituitary function returns to normal or hypopituitarism develops. Overall, the frequency of hypopituitarism in TBI is less than in subarachnoid hemorrhage, occurring in about one fourth of surviving patients. In patients dying of head injury, damage to the hypothalamus, pituitary stalk, or anterior pituitary has been found in up to 86% of cases.[9] The paraventricular and supraoptic nuclei and median eminence are

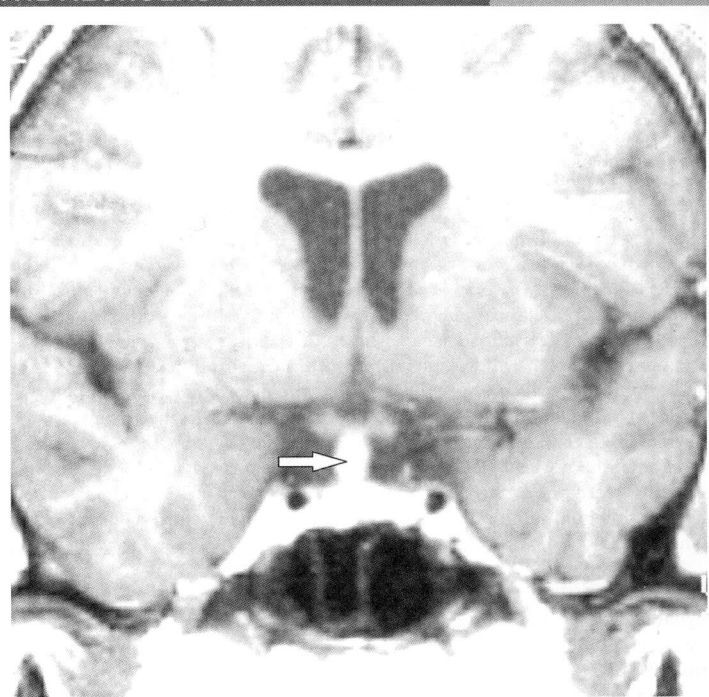

FIGURE 223-2. Thickened pituitary stalk in Langerhans cell histiocytosis. Magnetic resonance image of patient with Langerhans cell histiocytosis who manifested initially with amenorrhea, galactorrhea, and diabetes insipidus. Arrow points to the thickened pituitary stalk. (Reproduced with permission from Purdy LP, Molitch ME. Sudden onset of diabetes insipidus in an adolescent. *Endocr Trends.* 1998;5:1-7.)

particularly involved with microhemorrhages, hence the high frequency of panhypopituitarism with diabetes insipidus. With frontal injuries, the brain travels backward, but the pituitary cannot move; consequently, the pituitary stalk becomes avulsed, with interruption of the portal vessels. Most patients with head injury are hyperprolactinemic, which clinically confirms that the hypothalamus or stalk is the primary site of injury. In the past, pituitary function in patients with TBI and subarachnoid hemorrhage has not been assessed, and the role of untreated hypopituitarism in the long-term disability of such patients is unknown. Acute deficiency of ACTH/cortisol may be life-threatening. Therefore, cortisol levels should be monitored carefully in the hours and days after such events, and hypocortisolism treated with stress doses of glucocorticoids when necessary.

IRRADIATION

Whole-brain irradiation for intracranial neoplasms frequently results in hypothalamic dysfunction, as evidenced by endocrine abnormalities and behavioral changes. The most common endocrine abnormality is hyperprolactinemia, but hypopituitarism also occurs. When the radiotherapy is targeted to the hypothalamic area, hypopituitarism occurs even more frequently.[10] The frequency of loss of pituitary function is so high that all patients who have had their pituitary and hypothalamic areas irradiated must be monitored periodically for the purpose of detecting these deficits. However, the development of such deficiencies may take many years, so that yearly testing is warranted for up to 20 years. It appears that stereotactic irradiation using the gamma knife apparatus or a linear accelerator for pituitary and other parasellar tumors causes a risk of hypopituitarism similar to that of conventional irradiation.

Effects of Hypothalamic Disease on Pituitary Function

Hypothalamic disease can cause both pituitary hyperfunction and hypofunction in varying degrees of severity. Although severe disease can cause absolute deficiencies of the various hormones, milder disease may cause a subtle alteration in feedback loops and timing such that, for example, the integration of signals necessary for menstrual cycling is lost, with subsequent "hypothalamic" amenorrhea (Chapter 236). Furthermore, the hypothalamic defects may be interrelated. The rather common finding of hyperprolactinemia occurring with hypothalamic dysfunction causes a hypogonadotropic hypogonadism that is reversible when the elevated prolactin levels are brought down to normal. In many cases, no structural lesion can be found on MRI, and a functional defect caused by altered neurotransmitter regulation is invoked.

GROWTH HORMONE

Loss of normal GH secretion is the most common hormonal defect occurring with structural hypothalamic disease. About three fourths of cases with congenital idiopathic GH deficiency have a normal GH response to exogenous GHRH, which implies that the defect is probably disordered hypothalamic regulation. Defects in the gene for GHRH have not been found, but a rare form of GH deficiency has been found to be caused by a mutation in the GHRH receptor. A reversible form of idiopathic GH deficiency caused by inadequate parental care and affection is referred to as the emotional deprivation syndrome or psychosocial dwarfism. Restoration of a proper social environment for such a child results in prompt normalization of GH secretion and growth. It has been hypothesized that the disordered GH regulation is due to psychogenic alteration of the neurotransmitter balance necessary for normal GHRH and somatostatin secretion. Other systemic illnesses such as inflammatory bowel disease may also cause decreased GH secretion and growth; treatment of the systemic illness will correct the growth abnormality. Treatment of children and adults with GH deficiency is discussed in Chapter 224.

GONADOTROPINS
Hypothalamic Hypogonadism

The primary defect in this group of disorders is thought to involve the secretion of GnRH, with resultant impairment in pituitary gonadotropin secretion and gonadal function. The disorders causing these conditions may be primary (i.e., congenital) defects or acquired. Depending on the time of onset, they are manifested as either delayed puberty, interruption of pubertal progression, or loss of adult gonadal function. The lesions causing these disorders may cause loss of other hormones or may be isolated to GnRH. Loss of gonadotropin secretion as the result of hypothalamic structural damage is the second most common defect after GH deficiency. However, a substantial portion of these defects are due to hyperprolactinemia and are reversible with correction of the hyperprolactinemia. In some cases, the defect is idiopathic. Defects in the gene for GnRH have not been found, but mutations in the GnRH receptor do occur.

In children, if the disorder is limited to GnRH and the gonadotropins, prior growth and development are normal, but the growth spurt occurring at puberty is lost. Undescended testes are present in 50% of patients with GnRH deficiency, probably secondary to the absence of gonadotropins during fetal development. The most common congenital lesion causing prepubertal GnRH deficiency is Kallmann's syndrome, which affects 50% of males and 37% of females seen with isolated gonadotropin deficiency (see earlier). In patients with GnRH deficiency, replacement of GnRH through subcutaneous administration every 2 hours with a portable pump causes a rapid rise in LH and FSH, a rise in testosterone to normal, and the development of normal spermatogenesis. Similar approaches in women result in ovulatory cycles in 80%. The success of such therapy confirms the original hypothesis of a primary defect of GnRH secretion. In men, comparable results can be obtained with exogenous gonadotropins given three times per week and is much more practical. GnRH therapy is not successful in those with GnRH receptor mutations. Replacement with testosterone alone causes adequate androgenization but does not result in an increase in testicular size or in spermatogenesis.

Loss of formerly normal GnRH secretion in adults may be due to structural hypothalamic damage such as a tumor, a functional change unassociated with a detectable lesion, or hyperprolactinemia.[11] Structural disease must be excluded in such patients by CT or MRI. Most cases of functional hypogonadotropic hypogonadism occur in women, the most common causes being weight loss, excessive exercise, psychogenic stress, or systemic illness, but idiopathic forms occur as well. In some patients, exercise results in a loss of body fat not detected with total body weight measures, and it is unclear whether the hypogonadism is directly due to the loss of body fat or to the exercise per se. Studies of pulsatile gonadotropin secretion in such patients reveal absent pulses. Usually, the gonadotropin response to injected GnRH is normal. Regain of weight and stopping of the exercise result in resumption of normal gonadal function. Furthermore, the administration of leptin to such women results in a resumption of normal gonadotropin pulsatile secretion and ovulation, confirming the key role leptin has in mediating the influence of body energy stores on reproductive function.[12] However, in the idiopathic form, spontaneous resolution does not occur. Hyperprolactinemia

occurring postpubertally can also decrease GnRH and the pulsatile secretion of LH and FSH and thereby result in anovulation with oligomenorrhea and amenorrhea in women and impotence and infertility in men.

Two goals in the treatment of idiopathic functional hypogonadotropic amenorrhea are (1) restoration of a normal estrogen status to promote well-being and prevent osteoporosis and (2) facilitation of ovulation for fertility. The former can generally be achieved with cyclic estrogen and progesterone, whereas the latter may require clomiphene or GnRH or gonadotropin therapy. In men, similar goals may be achieved with testosterone or GnRH or gonadotropins.

Hypothalamic Hypergonadism (Precocious Puberty)

Precocious puberty is defined as the onset of puberty before the age of 8 years in girls or 9 years in boys. Pseudoprecocious puberty is that resulting from peripheral (gonadal or adrenal) causes. Central, "true," or GnRH-dependent precocious puberty is characterized by hormonal changes similar to those that occur at the time of normal puberty—that is, an increase in the pulsatile release of LH, an increase in the gonadotropin response to GnRH, and an increase in gonadal steroid secretion.[13] GnRH-dependent precocious puberty therefore represents premature activation of the GnRH pulse generator by a variety of lesions, or it may also be idiopathic. Only about 10% of cases of central precocious puberty occur in boys, but they tend to have more serious underlying disease. In boys with central GnRH-dependent precocious puberty, hypothalamic hamartomas account for 38% of cases, other CNS lesions represent 31%, familial disease accounts for 23%, and idiopathic disease accounts for only 8%. The picture is quite different in girls, however: hypothalamic hamartomas account for only 15% of cases, other CNS lesions represent 14%, the McCune-Albright syndrome (polyostotic fibrous dysplasia [Chapter 231]) accounts for 6%, and fully 65% are idiopathic. Dysgerminomas in the suprasellar or pineal region can produce HCG, which acts like LH in its stimulation of gonadal function. Usually, such tumors cause increased sex steroid formation but fail to cause ovulation.

Therapy for central GnRH-dependent precocious puberty consists of surgical removal of the tumor or medical therapy with a long-acting GnRH analogue, either in the form of monthly injections or yearly implants.[14] The latter can suppress gonadotropin and sex steroid hormone levels and cause a stabilization or even regression of secondary sex characteristics and a slowing of growth and bone maturation in most cases. When therapy is discontinued at the normal time of puberty, sex steroid levels increase, secondary sexual characteristics again develop, growth increases, and regular menses develop spontaneously.

PROLACTIN
Hypothalamic Hyperprolactinemia

Structural or infiltrative lesions of the hypothalamus, such as those discussed earlier, can decrease the amount of dopamine reaching the lactotrophs and thus cause modest hyperprolactinemia (usually < 100 ng/mL).[15] Because their therapy is quite different, it is very important to differentiate nonsecreting pituitary adenomas with extensive suprasellar extension causing prolactin elevations in this range from prolactin-secreting adenomas, which usually cause prolactin elevations 5 to 50 times higher. A peculiarity of some two-site immunoassays, referred to as the "hook effect," can sometimes cause a very high prolactin level to read falsely normal or just mildly elevated; a 1:100 dilution of the serum sample with saline will show the true level when the specimen is rerun. If there is any question about an assay being susceptible to the hook affect, in patients with very large tumors, prolactin should be measured undiluted and at 1:100 dilution to avoid this important spurious finding. A number of medications, antipsychotics in particular, can cause hyperprolactinemia, primarily by interfering with central catecholamines (Table 223-2).

Therapy is generally directed at the underlying cause. The hyperprolactinemia itself may impair gonadal function, so efforts may also be made to lower prolactin levels with dopamine agonists. Prolactin levels usually fall quite readily in such patients. Restoration of gonadal function is not automatic, however, because the primary hypothalamic lesion may also directly impair release of GnRH. In that circumstance, both dopamine agonists and sex steroid replacement may be necessary. When administration of psychotropic medications that cause the hyperprolactinemia cannot be stopped, dopamine agonists may be used but very rarely have been reported to exacerbate the psychosis. In such cases and in others in which fertility is not an issue, treatment with cyclic estrogen and progesterone replacement can be carried out safely.

TABLE 223-2 ETIOLOGIES OF HYPERPROLACTINEMIA

PITUITARY DISEASE

Prolactinomas
Acromegaly
Empty sella syndrome
Lymphocytic hypophysitis
Cushing's disease
Pituitary stalk section

HYPOTHALAMIC DISEASE

Craniopharyngiomas
Meningiomas
Dysgerminomas
Nonsecreting pituitary adenomas
Other tumors
Sarcoidosis
Langerhans cell histiocytosis
Neuraxis irradiation
Vascular

NEUROGENIC

Chest wall lesions
Spinal cord lesions
Breast stimulation

OTHER

Pregnancy
Hypothyroidism
Chronic renal failure
Cirrhosis
Pseudocyesis
Adrenal insufficiency
Idiopathic

MEDICATIONS

Antipsychotics
Atypical antipsychotics
Monoamine oxidase inhibitors
Tricyclic antidepressants
Reserpine
Methyldopa
Metoclopramide
Domperidone
Cocaine
Verapamil
Serotonin reuptake inhibitors

Modified from Molitch ME. Medication-induced hyperprolactinemia. *Mayo Clin Proc.* 2005;80:1050-1057.

Idiopathic Hyperprolactinemia

Idiopathic hyperprolactinemia is a diagnosis of exclusion. Prolactin levels in this condition are usually less than 100 ng/mL. In such cases, small pituitary or hypothalamic tumors could exist that are beyond the resolution of current imaging techniques, but when such patients are monitored for many years, it is very uncommon for tumors to later be visualized. Idiopathic hyperprolactinemia can cause amenorrhea, galactorrhea, impotence, infertility, and loss of libido, just as occurs with hyperprolactinemia of other causes, so the idiopathic hyperprolactinemia may need to be treated. Premature osteoporosis related to the estrogen deficiency may also occur. The only possible treatment is dopamine agonists, and these agents are successful in more than 90% of cases. Alternatively, cyclic estrogen and progesterone replacement may be given, but fertility will not be restored.

THYROID-STIMULATING HORMONE

Hypothalamic hypothyroidism is due to a central lesion that impairs the secretion of TRH, usually along with the loss of other hormones.[16] It occurs considerably less commonly than hypothalamic GH and gonadotropin deficiency. Defects in the gene for TRH have not been detected, but a case has been reported of a TRH receptor mutation causing hypothyroidism. TSH levels in this syndrome are generally normal or even slightly elevated. TSH in these patients is biologically less active than normal and binds to the TSH receptor less well because of altered glycosylation as a result of the TRH deficiency. Treatment is with L-thyroxine, and monitoring of therapy is done solely by measurement of free thyroxine (T_4) levels and not TSH levels.

ADRENOCORTICOTROPIC HORMONE

ACTH deficiency caused by hypothalamic lesions is uncommon.[17] It may occur with the loss of other hormones but may also appear as an isolated deficiency. The most common cause, of course, is prior suppression by exogenous or endogenous glucocorticoids. In the absence of CNS lesions or a history of trauma, many cases of isolated ACTH deficiency appear to be due to a pituitary autoimmune disorder. Treatment is with glucocorticoids; mineralocorticoids are not needed.

Effects of Hypothalamic Disease on Other Neurometabolic Functions

A number of functions that affect the internal milieu, in addition to anterior and posterior pituitary function, are regulated at least in part by the hypothalamus and include temperature control, behavior, consciousness, memory, sleep, food intake, and carbohydrate metabolism.

ALTERATIONS IN FOOD INTAKE

Hypothalamic Obesity

Destruction of the mediobasal hypothalamus will sometimes inhibit satiety and may result in hyperphagia and hypothalamic obesity.[18] The hyperphagia is due to destruction of noradrenergic fibers originating in the paraventricular nucleus and passing through the mediobasal hypothalamus. Because of their location, such lesions also usually produce hypopituitarism and diabetes insipidus. In a number of rare syndromes (Prader-Willi, Laurence-Moon-Biedl-Bardet) with obesity as a major characteristic, hypothalamic causes have been postulated but not proved.

Hypothalamic Anorexia

Lesions of the lateral hypothalamus, which destroy nigrostriatal dopaminergic fibers that pass through this area, produce hypophagia along with an increase in peripheral norepinephrine turnover and metabolic rate. This syndrome is very rare, probably owing to the requirement for bilateral lesions. The hormonal changes that occur in anorexia nervosa appear to all be secondary to the weight loss, and no evidence has been found for a primary hypothalamic disorder in this syndrome.

HYPERGLYCEMIA

Hypothalamic activation as part of the generalized response to stress can cause release of GH, prolactin, and ACTH, which serve as counter-regulatory hormones with respect to insulin. These hormones promote lipolysis, gluconeogenesis, and insulin resistance, resulting in glucose elevation. Of more importance in the acute response to stress, this hypothalamic response results in sympathetic activation with release of catecholamines that inhibit insulin secretion and stimulate glycogenolysis.

TEMPERATURE REGULATION

The anterior hypothalamus and preoptic area contain temperature-sensitive neurons that respond to internal temperature changes by initiating certain thermoregulatory responses necessary to restore a constant temperature. Measures that dissipate heat include cutaneous vasodilation, sweating, and panting, and measures that increase body heat include increasing metabolic heat production, shivering, and cutaneous vasoconstriction.

Rare patients have been reported with anterior hypothalamic lesions that cause paroxysmal or sustained hypothermia or hyperthermia from failure of these thermoregulatory activities. Some cases of paroxysmal hypothermia and hyperthermia respond to anticonvulsant medications, which suggests that the neuronal discharge effecting the temperature changes is seizure-like.

Poikilothermy results from an inability to dissipate or generate heat to keep the body temperature constant in the face of varying ambient temperatures. This condition results from bilateral lesions in the posterior hypothalamus and rostral mesencephalon, which are the areas responsible for the final integration of thermoregulatory neural efferents. Patients with this condition do not feel discomfort with temperature changes and are unaware of having a problem. Depending on the ambient temperature, they may experience life-threatening hypothermia or hyperthermia.

GENERAL REFERENCES

For the General References and other additional features, please visit Expert Consult at https://expertconsult.inkling.com.

ANTERIOR PITUITARY

MARK E. MOLITCH

ANATOMY AND EMBRYOLOGY

The pituitary is divided into anterior (adenohypophysis) and posterior (neurohypophysis) lobes. The optic chiasm, formed by the decussation of the optic nerves, is positioned directly above the pituitary gland. Specialized vascular structures located in the median eminence of the hypothalamus drain into portal veins that course down the pituitary stalk to join the sinusoidal capillaries of the anterior lobe. Hypothalamic hormones enter these capillaries and flow to the anterior pituitary (Fig. 224-1). Venous drainage from the anterior lobe is into the cavernous sinuses, which drain into the petrosal sinuses. The six major pituitary cell types include somatotrophs (growth hormone [GH] producing), lactotrophs (prolactin [PRL] producing), corticotrophs (adrenocorticotropic hormone [ACTH] producing), thyrotrophs (thyroid-stimulating hormone [TSH] producing), and gonadotrophs (follicle-stimulating hormone [FSH] and luteinizing hormone [LH] producing). Somatotrophs constitute 40 to 50% of anterior pituitary cells;

lactotrophs, 15 to 25%; corticotrophs, 10 to 20%; and gonadotrophs 10%. Only 5% of pituitary cells are thyrotrophs.

The pituitary is formed from the fusion of Rathke's pouch (which gives rise to the anterior pituitary) and a portion of the ventral diencephalon (which gives rise to the posterior pituitary). Several transcription factors are important in the development of the various types of pituitary cells. LHX3 and LHX4 are present in somatotrophs, lactotrophs, gonadotrophs and thyrotrophs, and mutations in these genes result in deficits of GH, PRL, TSH, and the gonadotropins, although the deficits with LHX4 mutations are more variable.[1] Mutations in *HESX1* usually are associated with dysplasia of the septum pellucidum and optic tracts, in addition to multiple pituitary hormone deficits. The transcription factor Pit-1 is produced in somatotrophs, lactotrophs, and thyrotrophs. Mutations in the *PIT1 (POU1F1)* gene prevent the development of these cells and cause deficiencies of GH, PRL, and TSH. This lineage relationship explains why some GH-producing tumors also secrete PRL, and some TSH-producing tumors co-secrete GH.[2] PROP-1, another transcription factor, is critical for the development of somatotrophs, lactotrophs, and thyrotrophs. Mutations in the *PROP1* gene result in deficiencies of GH, PRL, and TSH, and in some affected individuals there is delayed puberty. Combined pituitary hormone deficiency (GH, PRL, TSH) has an incidence of about 1 in 8000 births, and 10% have an affected relative. Between 25 and 50% of these cases are due to *PIT1* or *PROP1* mutations. Tpit is specific to corticotroph cells, and *TPIT* gene mutations cause isolated ACTH deficiency. Rare mutations in several other genes (*SOX 3, OTX2, FGF8,* and *GLI2*) have also been shown to cause hypopituitarism, and the list continues to grow.

RADIOLOGY OF THE PITUITARY

Magnetic resonance imaging (MRI) provides excellent resolution of the pituitary and surrounding cerebrospinal fluid (CSF) and vascular and central nervous system structures (Fig. 224-2).[3] There is less radiation exposure with MRI than with computed tomography (CT), allowing repeated imaging. However, bone structures are not as well defined by MRI compared with CT. On MRI, the normal anterior pituitary appears isointense with brain white matter, whereas the posterior pituitary exhibits high signal intensity ("bright spot"). The optic chiasm is readily identified because it is surrounded by hypodense areas. Pituitary adenomas typically appear hypointense on T1-weighted images and show less enhancement with gadolinium than surrounding normal tissue (Figs. 224-3 and 224-4). Focal hypodense areas are also seen in about one fourth of normal individuals, which may correspond to cysts or nonfunctioning small adenomas, emphasizing the importance of endocrine evaluation.

REGULATION OF THE PITUITARY AXIS

The pituitary gland integrates the influences of an array of positive and negative signals to modulate hormone secretion. PRL is the only major pituitary

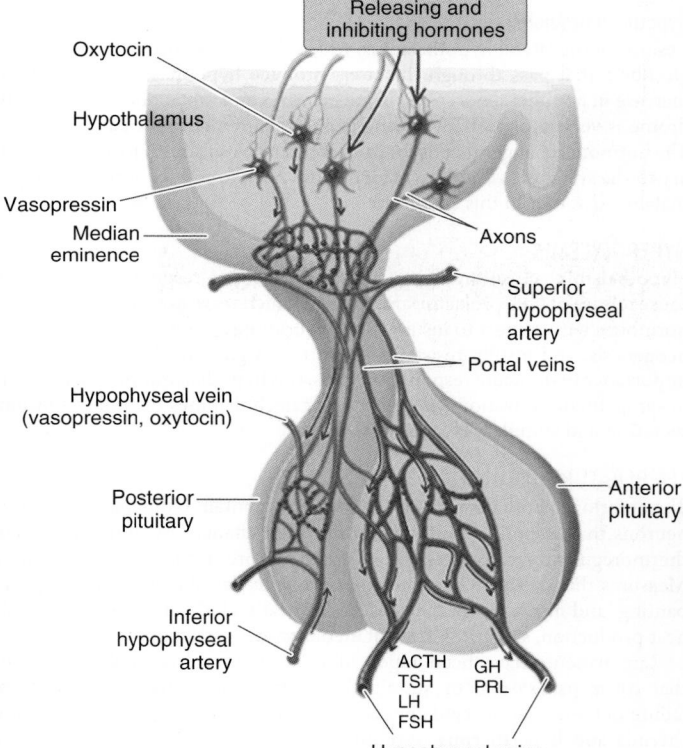

FIGURE 224-1. Structural-functional, humoral, endocrine, and neuroendocrine relationships within the hypothalamic-pituitary unit emphasize the unique and intimate interdependence of neural structures and hormone secretion with the circulation. Oxytocin and vasopressin neuron bodies located in the hypothalamus send axons through the pituitary stalk that terminate in the posterior pituitary, where they release oxytocin and vasopressin into blood vessels within the posterior pituitary. Hypothalamic neurons that produce growth hormone–releasing hormone, corticotropin-releasing hormone, thyrotropin-releasing hormone, and gonadotropin-releasing hormone send their axons through the median eminence to terminate and release their hormones into the hypophyseal-portal circulation. This network of blood vessels is located at the median eminence, which surrounds the pituitary stalk and penetrates into the anterior lobe of the pituitary. These hypothalamic neurohormones stimulate responsive anterior pituitary cells to secrete growth hormone (GH), adrenocorticotropic hormone (ACTH), thyroid-stimulating hormone (TSH), luteinizing hormone (LH), and follicle-stimulating hormone (FSH), respectively. Dopamine neurons reaching the median eminence are responsible for tonic inhibition of prolactin (PRL) secretion from the anterior pituitary, whereas somatostatin released from somatostatinergic neurons inhibit GH and TRH release. (From Melmed S. *The Pituitary.* 3rd ed. London: Elsevier; 2011.)

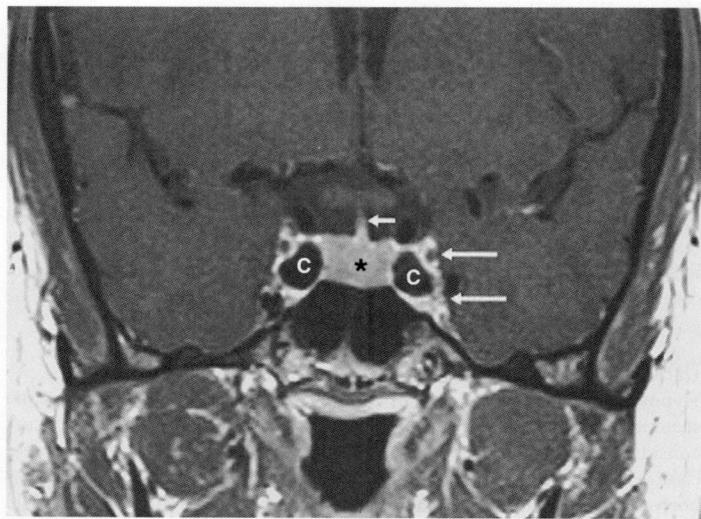

FIGURE 224-2. Magnetic resonance image of normal pituitary. Coronal postcontrast image shows homogeneously enhancing gland (*) and stalk (*short arrow*). Note the greater degree of contrast uptake in the cavernous sinuses, which contain the carotid arteries (C), easily depicted by their flow voids. Small hypointense dots (*long arrows*) are the cranial nerves within the cavernous sinuses. (From Melmed S. *The Pituitary.* 3rd ed. London: Elsevier; 2011.)

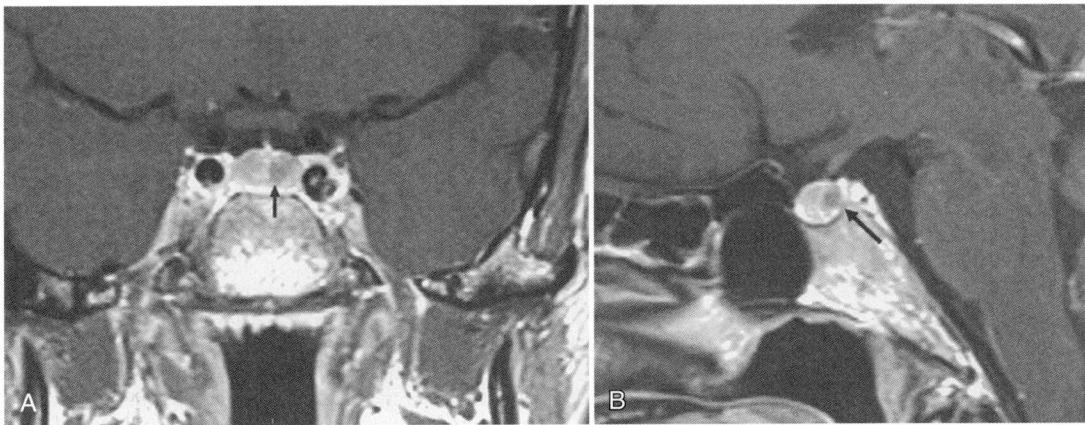

FIGURE 224-3. Magnetic resonance image showing a pituitary microadenoma. **(A)** Coronal and **(B)** sagittal T1-weighted images demonstrate a hypoenhancing lesion within the pituitary gland (*arrows*). (From Melmed S. *The Pituitary.* 3rd ed. London: Elsevier; 2011.)

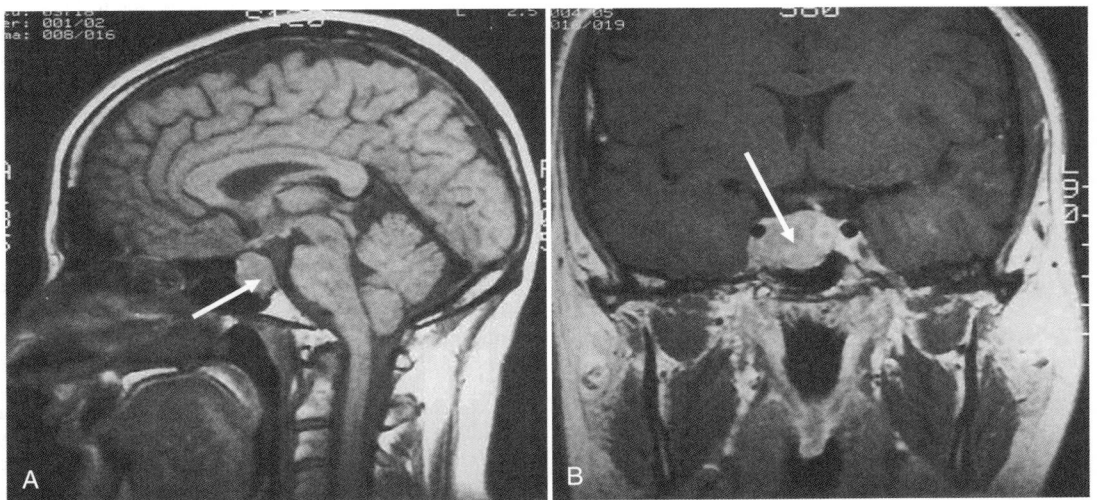

FIGURE 224-4. Magnetic resonance image showing a pituitary macroadenoma. Arrows point to the adenoma. **(A)** Sagittal view. **(B)** Coronal view.

hormone that is not subject to feedback inhibition by hormones produced in target tissues. It is controlled by positive and negative input from the hypothalamus, the latter being dominant.

The principles of feedback regulation are illustrated by the hypothalamic-pituitary-thyroid axis. Hypothalamic thyrotropin-releasing hormone (TRH) stimulates TSH secretion from the pituitary. TSH increases thyroid hormone secretion, which in turn suppresses hypothalamic TRH as well as pituitary TSH. A typical regulatory loop therefore has both positive (TRH, TSH) and negative (thyroxine [T_4], triiodothyronine [T_3]) components, allowing a high degree of control of hormone levels. The pituitary gland integrates positive TRH signals and the negative effects of thyroid hormone. The concept of feedback regulation is important not only for understanding pituitary physiology but also because it provides the basis for analyzing pituitary gland function using stimulation and suppression tests.

The feedback regulatory systems just described are superimposed on hormonal rhythms that are used for adaptation to the environment. Seasonal changes, the daily occurrence of the light-dark cycles, and stress have major impacts on the secretion of pituitary hormones (Chapter 2). Because many hormones are released in a pulsatile manner and in a rhythmic fashion, these characteristics of secretion should be considered when attempting to relate serum measurements to normal values. Although it is possible to characterize pulsatile patterns of hormone secretion using frequent blood sampling (every 10 minutes), this is not practical in a clinical setting. Alternative approaches include stimulation and suppression tests or the use of "integrated" measurements of hormone production, such as 24-hour urine free cortisol as an index of ACTH secretion, or insulin-like growth factor (IGF)-I as a biological marker of GH action.

HYPOPITUITARISM

Pituitary hormone deficiencies can be caused by loss of hypothalamic stimulation or by direct loss of pituitary function. When hypopituitarism is accompanied by diabetes insipidus or hyperprolactinemia, one should consider hypothalamic etiologies.

PATHOBIOLOGY

A variety of congenital and acquired causes of hypopituitarism have been described (Table 224-1). Congenital deficiencies of multiple pituitary hormones are often caused by mutations in the genes for the transcription factors mentioned previously (*HESX1, LHX3, PIT1, PROP1*). Gene mutations have been found at several steps leading to pituitary hormone secretion, including those for the hypophysiotropic releasing factor receptors for gonadotropin-releasing hormone (GnRH), growth hormone–releasing hormone (GHRH), and TRH; those for the pituitary hormone structures for GH, ACTH, and the β-subunits of FSH, TSH, and LH; and those for the target organ receptors for GH, ACTH, TSH, and LH. Mutations of the GH gene have been shown to be heterogeneous. Some are large deletions that are inherited in an autosomal recessive manner and involve genetic recombination between related DNA sequences in the duplicated GH gene cluster. Point mutations have also been described, and some of these can be inherited in an autosomal dominant manner. Mutations of the other types described earlier generally cause autosomal recessive forms of selective hormone deficiencies.

Neoplastic lesions, particularly pituitary macroadenomas, are the most common cause of acquired hypopituitarism. Pituitary adenomas cause hypopituitarism in several different ways. In some cases, there is direct destruction

TABLE 224-1   CAUSES OF HYPOPITUITARISM

GENETIC DEFECTS

Hypophysiotropic hormone gene defects
Hypophysiotropic hormone receptor gene defects
    GHRH receptor defect
    GnRH receptor defect
    TRH receptor defect
Pituitary hormone gene defects
    Gonadotropins: LH β- and FSH β-subunit gene defects
    GH: defects in GH gene
    Thyrotropin: defects in TSH β-subunit gene
    Multiple hormone (GH, PRL, TSH) defects due to mutation in *PIT1* and *PROP1* genes
Pituitary hormone receptor genetic defects
    GH receptor defects: GH insensitivity syndrome (Laron-type dwarfism)
    ACTH receptor defects: congenital insensitivity to ACTH
    LH receptor defects
    FSH receptor defects
    TSH receptor defects

CONGENITAL EMBRYOPATHIC DEFECTS

Anencephaly
Midline cleft defects: septo-optic dysplasia, basal encephalocele, cleft lip and palate
Pituitary aplasia
Kallmann's syndrome (GnRH defect with anosmia)

ACQUIRED DEFECTS

Tumors: pituitary adenomas, craniopharyngiomas, dysgerminomas, meningiomas, gliomas, metastatic tumors, hamartomas, Rathke's cleft cysts
Irradiation
Trauma: surgery, external blunt trauma
Empty sella syndrome
Vascular
    Pituitary apoplexy
    Sheehan syndrome
    Internal carotid aneurysm
    Vasculitis
    Subarachnoid hemorrhage
Inflammatory and infiltrative diseases
    Sarcoidosis
    Langerhans cell histiocytosis (histiocytosis X, eosinophilic granuloma)
    Tuberculosis, syphilis
    Meningitis
    Lymphocytic hypophysitis, infundibulohypophysitis
Metabolic
    Hemochromatosis
    Amyloidosis
    Critical illness
    Malnutrition
    Anorexia nervosa
    Psychosocial deprivation
Idiopathic

ACTH = adrenocorticotropic hormone; FSH = follicle-stimulating hormone; GH = growth hormone; GHRH = growth hormone releasing hormone; GnRH = gonadotropin-releasing hormone; LH = luteinizing hormone; PRL = prolactin; TRH = thyrotropin-releasing hormone; TSH = thyroid-stimulating hormone.

or compression of the normal pituitary. Compression of the pituitary stalk can impair blood supply to the pituitary as well as decrease input from hypothalamic hormones. Hemorrhage into tumors can lead to pituitary infarction. A mild degree of hyperprolactinemia (usually < 200 ng/mL) is characteristic of disorders that cause stalk compression, and hyperprolactinemia further impairs gonadotropin secretion. A variety of other neoplasms that occur near the sella, such as craniopharyngiomas, can also cause hypopituitarism (see Table 224-1).

Radiation causes hypopituitarism primarily because of its effects on hypothalamic function, although high-dose radiation (e.g., proton beam) can also cause direct pituitary damage. The sellar region is subjected to radiation in the treatment of pituitary adenomas, craniopharyngiomas, optic gliomas, meningiomas, dysgerminomas, and neoplasms of the oropharynx. The effects of radiation can be delayed several years, and patients at high risk should be evaluated yearly. Although GH and gonadotropin deficiencies develop first in most patients, ACTH or TSH deficiencies occasionally occur first, emphasizing the need to evaluate each of the major axes.

Empty sella syndrome can occur as a primary or as an acquired condition. It is caused by defects in the diaphragma sella that allow herniation of the arachnoid membrane into the hypophyseal fossa. In long-standing cases,

sellar enlargement occurs, probably because of persistent transmission of intracranial pressure. Imaging studies reveal the pituitary gland as a flattened rim of tissue along the floor of the sella. Primary empty sella occurs most commonly in women and may be associated with features of benign intracranial hypertension. Pituitary function is usually normal, but 10% have mild hyperprolactinemia, probably because of stretching of the pituitary stalk. Acquired forms may occur as a result of surgery, radiation, or pituitary infarction (usually of an adenoma).

Pituitary apoplexy is a syndrome caused by hemorrhage into a tumor, with associated infarction and leakage of the blood into the arachnoid space and resultant fever and stiff neck. When the hemorrhage is large, there can be mass effects, with headache and cranial nerve compression within the cavernous sinus. Asymptomatic infarctions are found in about 10 to 15% of pituitary adenomas. In the absence of a tumor, predispositions to apoplexy include trauma, pregnancy, anticoagulation, sickle cell anemia, and diabetes mellitus. Pituitary infarction in the peripartum period (Sheehan syndrome) is usually associated with significant obstetric hemorrhage and hypovolemia. Although Sheehan syndrome can manifest acutely with vascular collapse, it more commonly has a subacute manifestation consisting of postpartum inability to lactate, amenorrhea, and symptoms of adrenal insufficiency.

In lymphocytic hypophysitis, there is infiltration of the pituitary by lymphocytes and plasma cells, with destruction of the parenchyma; it is believed to have an autoimmune basis. The lesion is usually large, and patients present with either symptoms or signs of hypopituitarism or those of a mass lesion (i.e., visual field defects and headaches). Some patients may have mild hyperprolactinemia and diabetes insipidus. Almost all cases have been reported in women, and most present during or after pregnancy. Because of the presentation as a mass lesion during pregnancy, such lesions may be confused with prolactinomas. Mild PRL elevation points to a nonsecretory lesion rather than a prolactinoma. MRI cannot reliably differentiate pituitary adenoma from hypophysitis, although hypophysitis usually manifests with a diffuse enlargement of the pituitary that enhances, rather than as a focal lesion. Diagnosis is usually made by biopsy, but the lesion may be suspected clinically if it manifests during or just after pregnancy. Careful pituitary function testing is mandatory because many patients have died of adrenocortical insufficiency. Although the prognosis is not clear, a number of cases have resolved spontaneously. An entity with similar histologic findings involving the stalk and posterior pituitary, referred to as infundibuloneurohypophysitis, can cause diabetes insipidus. A third variant, panhypophysitis, involves both lobes of the pituitary. These last two forms occur in both sexes and are generally not associated with pregnancy. The causes and interrelationships between these entities remain unknown. In the past several years, secondary hypophysitis has been described in association with ipilimumab, a CTLA-4 blocking antibody used as an immunostimulant in some cancer chemotherapy regimens, and a plasmacytic infiltrative form in which the plasma cells produce antibodies of the IgG4 subclass.[4]

The pituitary may undergo damage because of iron deposition in patients with hemochromatosis (Chapter 212) and amyloid fibrils in patients with systemic amyloidosis (Chapter 188). Functional reversible hypopituitarism of varying degrees occurs in patients with severe systemic illness, severe psychosocial and emotional deprivation, and severe weight loss—particularly in those with anorexia nervosa.

DIAGNOSIS AND TREATMENT   Rx

The diagnosis of hypopituitarism rests on the stimulation tests that are summarized in Table 224-2. Therapy depends on the nature and severity of the hormone deficiencies as well as on the desired clinical end points. The goals are to replace hormones in a physiologic manner and to avoid the consequences of over-replacement. Examples of hormonal replacement paradigms are provided in Table 224-3. Adjustment of hormone doses is done primarily based on clinical findings; TSH levels are not helpful for adjusting thyroxine doses in patients with central hypothyroidism. Even when conventional hormone replacement (adrenal, thyroid, gonadal) is carried out appropriately, there is an approximately two-fold excess risk for death. Although untreated GH deficiency has been hypothesized to be the cause of this excess risk, this has not been proved. Other causes of death in this population include infections with inappropriate increase in steroid dose, and brain tumors related to prior irradiation.[5] The benefits of GH therapy are less clear than those of the other pituitary hormones and include improvements in body composition, bone, lipids, and quality of life; although there are few adverse effects, treatment involves daily injections.[6]

TABLE 224-2 TESTS OF PITUITARY INSUFFICIENCY

HORMONE	TEST	INTERPRETATION
Growth hormone (GH)	*Insulin tolerance test:* Regular insulin (0.05-0.15 U/kg) is given IV, and blood is drawn at −30, 0, 30, 45, 60, and 90 min for measurement of glucose and GH.	If hypoglycemia occurs (glucose < 40 mg/dL), GH should increase to > 5 μg/L.*
	Arginine-GHRH test: GHRH 1 μg/kg IV bolus followed by 30-min infusion of L-arginine (30 g)	Normal response is GH > 4.1 μg/L.
	Glucagon test: 1 mg IM with GH measurements at 0, 60, 90,120, 150, and 180 min	Normal response is GH > 3 μg/L.
Adrenocorticotropic hormone (ACTH)	*Insulin tolerance test:* Regular insulin (0.05-0.15 U/kg) is given IV, and blood is drawn at −30, 0, 30, 45, 60, and 90 min for measurement of glucose and cortisol.	If hypoglycemia occurs (glucose < 40 mg/dL), cortisol should increase by > 7 μg/dL or to > 20 μg/dL.
	CRH test: 1 μg/kg ovine CRH IV at 8 AM, with blood samples drawn at 0, 15, 30, 60, 90, and 120 min for measurement of ACTH and cortisol	In most normal individuals, the basal ACTH increases two- to four-fold and reaches a peak (20-100 pg/mL). ACTH responses may be delayed in cases of hypothalamic dysfunction. Cortisol levels usually reach 20-25 μg/dL.
	ACTH stimulation test: ACTH$_{1-24}$ (cosyntropin), 0.25 mg IM or IV. Cortisol is measured at 0, 30, and 60 min.	A normal response is cortisol > 18 μg/dL. In suspected hypothalamic-pituitary deficiency, a low-dose (1-μg) test may be more sensitive.
Thyroid-stimulating hormone (TSH)	*Basal thyroid function tests:* free T$_4$, free T$_3$, TSH	Low free thyroid hormone levels in the setting of TSH levels that are not appropriately increased
Luteinizing hormone (LH), follicle-stimulating hormone (FSH)	*Basal levels of LH, FSH, testosterone, estrogen*	Basal LH and FSH should be increased in postmenopausal women. Low testosterone levels in conjunction with low or low-normal LH and FSH are consistent with gonadotropin deficiency.

*Values are with polyclonal assays.
CRH = corticotropin-releasing hormone; GHRH = growth hormone–releasing hormone; IM = intramuscularly; IV = intravenously; T$_3$ = triiodothyronine; T$_4$ = thyroxine.

TABLE 224-3 HORMONAL REPLACEMENT THERAPY IN HYPOPITUITARISM*

PITUITARY AXIS	HORMONAL REPLACEMENTS
Growth hormone (GH)	In children, GH (0.25 mg/kg) SC daily. In adults, GH (0.3-1.2 mg) SC daily. Titrate dose to achieve IGF-I levels in middle to upper part of normal range. Women receiving oral estrogens require higher doses.
Prolactin	None
Adrenocorticotropic hormone–cortisol	Hydrocortisone (10-15 mg PO q AM; 5-10 mg PO q PM) or prednisone (2.5 mg PO q AM; 2.5 mg PO q PM). Dose adjusted on clinical basis. Stress dosing: 50-75 mg hydrocortisone IV q8h
Thyroid-stimulating hormone–thyroid	L-thyroxine (0.075-0.15 mg) PO daily
Gonadotropins–gonads	FSH and LH (or HCG) can be used to induce ovulation in women. HCG alone or with FSH can be used to induce spermatogenesis in men. In men, testosterone enanthate (100-300 mg) IM q1-3wk or testosterone cyclopentylpropionate (100-300 mg) IM q1-3wk. Testosterone transdermal patches can also be used (5 mg daily). Testosterone gel 5-10 g daily. In women, conjugated estrogens (0.625-1.25 mg) PO days 1-25 each month, cycled with medroxyprogesterone acetate (5-10 mg) PO days 15-25 each month. Low-dose contraceptive pills may also be used. Estrogen-containing transdermal patches are also available.
Posterior pituitary	Desmopressin, 0.05-0.2 mL (5-20 μg) intranasally once or twice daily, or tablets (0.1-0.4 mg q8-12h) or 0.5 mL (2 μg) SC

*Replacement therapy is dictated by the types of hormone deficiencies and by the clinical circumstances. In each case, the recommended preparations and doses are representative but need to be adjusted for individual patients. Other hormonal preparations are also available.
FSH = follicle-stimulating hormone; GnRH = gonadotropin-releasing hormone; HCG = human chorionic gonadotropin; IGF-I = insulin-like growth factor-I; IM = intramuscularly; LH = luteinizing hormone; PO, orally; SC = subcutaneously.

PITUITARY TUMORS

PATHOBIOLOGY

Pituitary tumors are classified according to the hormones they produce and their size: microadenomas, less than 10 mm in diameter; macroadenomas, more than 10 mm in diameter; and macroadenomas with extrasellar extension. In general, the levels of hormones produced by the tumors parallel the size of the tumors. The prevalence of the different types of pituitary adenomas, based on surgical data, is summarized in Table 224-4. Immunohistochemical studies using antibodies specific for each of the major pituitary hormones have been used to define tumor phenotype. Pituitary adenomas are rarely malignant but can be locally invasive.

Most pituitary tumors are monoclonal. This finding does not exclude a role for hormonal stimulation as a predisposing factor for somatic mutations, and the hormonal environment may also affect the rate of tumor growth (e.g., the growth of ACTH-secreting tumors following bilateral adrenalectomy). Supporting the concept that somatic mutations lead to pituitary tumorigenesis, a subset (35 to 40%) of somatotroph adenomas have activating mutations in the gene for the Gsα-subunit, resulting in two different amino acid (Arg201 and Glu227) substitutions.[7] Either mutation causes the Gsα-subunit to

stimulate adenylyl cyclase in a constitutive manner. The elevated intracellular cyclic adenosine monophosphate levels lead to increased cell growth as well as GH production. Mutations in other oncogenes, such as *ras, Rb,* and *p53,* are uncommon in pituitary tumors. Thus, the nature of the somatic mutations causing most pituitary tumors remains unknown.

At least five types of inherited predispositions to pituitary tumors are recognized. Patients with McCune-Albright syndrome (Chapter 231) occasionally develop pituitary adenomas as well as characteristic abnormalities in other tissues, particularly the ovary, bone, and thyroid. Interestingly, the McCune-Albright syndrome is also caused by mutations in the gene for the Gsα-subunit. However, the somatic mutations in McCune-Albright occur early during development, so that multiple tissues are affected. In multiple endocrine neoplasia type 1 (MEN 1) (Chapter 231), the menin gene is mutated, so that the predisposition to pituitary tumors is inherited in an autosomal dominant manner and occurs in conjunction with tumors of the parathyroid and pancreas.[8] Familial isolated pituitary adenoma (FIPA) syndrome is autosomal dominant and has low or variable penetrance. Germline mutations have been found in the gene for the aryl hydrocarbon receptor–interacting protein *(AIP),* which functions as a tumor suppressor. Such mutations have been found in about one third of FIPA families, most commonly

TABLE 224-4 PREVALENCE OF DIFFERENT TYPES OF PITUITARY ADENOMAS

TYPE OF PITUITARY ADENOMA	DISORDER	HORMONE PRODUCED	PREVALENCE (%)*
Somatotroph	Acromegaly and gigantism	Growth hormone	10-15
Lactotroph (prolactinoma)	Hypogonadism, galactorrhea	Prolactin	25-40
Corticotroph	Cushing's disease	Adrenocorticotropic hormone	10-15
Gonadotroph	Mass effects, hypopituitarism	Follicle-stimulating hormone and luteinizing hormone	15-20
Thyrotroph	Hyperthyroidism	Thyroid-stimulating hormone	<3
Nonfunctioning/ null cell	Mass effects, hypopituitarism	None	10-25

*The prevalence rates represent ranges described in several different large surgical series. Mixed tumors (e.g., growth hormone and prolactin) and plurihormonal adenomas are not shown. Rates vary depending on methods used to establish the diagnosis. Prolactinomas were underestimated in most recent pathologic series because they are largely managed medically. Most glycoprotein hormone–producing pituitary tumors were classified as nonfunctioning adenomas until the application of immunohistochemical studies.

in those with GH- and PRL-producing tumors. Carney's complex is an autosomal dominant condition consisting of pituitary adenomas, atrial myxomas, spotty skin pigmentation, and schwannomas. Primary pigmented nodular adrenocortical disease causing Cushing's syndrome occurs in about one third of patients with Carney's complex. The complex is caused by an inactivating mutation in the gene for the type 1A regulatory subunit of protein kinase A (PRKARIA).[7] The most recently discovered familial form involves mutations in the succinate dehydrogenase subunit genes, resulting in combinations of pituitary tumors and pheochromocytomas/paragangiomas.[9] In general, those tumors that arise as part of MEN 1 and FIPA tend to be more aggressive, occur at a younger age, and are less responsive to therapeutic interventions. It is now recommended that when a macroadenoma occurs in the context of a very young age or when there is a family history of pituitary or other endocrine tumors, that appropriate genetic screening be carried out.

CLINICAL MANIFESTATIONS

Many of the clinical manifestations of pituitary adenomas are related to the hypersecretion of hormones. However, the mass effects of the enlarging tumor can also lead to specific signs and symptoms (Chapter 189). Particularly in the case of nonfunctioning tumors or in those that produce gonadotropins, the primary clinical manifestations are related to effects of the tumor on surrounding structures.

Headaches are common in patients with macroadenomas and appear to be caused by expansion of the diaphragma sellae or by invasion of bone. The sudden onset of severe headache associated with nausea, vomiting, and altered consciousness can also be caused by hemorrhagic infarction with sudden enlargement of a pituitary adenoma. Severe cases require glucocorticoid treatment and possible surgical decompression.

Pituitary tumors that extend superiorly can affect visual fields. Expansion into the suprasellar region exerts pressure on the optic chiasm, usually in the central region where nerves emanating from the inferior and medial part of the retina (superior and temporal visual fields) cross, leading to bitemporal hemianopsia. Visual field loss is variable, however, and is affected by the location and flexibility of the chiasm as well as by the direction and extent of tumor growth.[10] Large tumors may invade the cavernous sinus or surround an optic nerve, leading to other patterns of visual field changes or loss of visual acuity. The tumor size and the direction and degree of extrasellar extension are best evaluated with MRI with gadolinium. If the tumor abuts the chiasm on MRI, formal visual field testing should be performed. Even long-standing visual loss may be reversible.

The normal pituitary is often compressed into a thin rim of tissue by large pituitary adenomas. Hypopituitarism probably results more from compression of the hypothalamic-pituitary stalk than from direct pressure on the normal pituitary. GH deficiency and hypogonadotropic hypogonadism are particularly common. Slightly elevated PRL levels (generally < 200 ng/mL) occur in cases of stalk compression because of diminished inhibition by

dopamine. It is important not to mistake such tumors for prolactinomas, because they will only rarely decrease in size in response to medical therapy with dopamine agonists, unlike prolactinomas, which commonly do. A peculiarity of some two-site immunoassays, referred to as the "hook effect," can sometimes cause a very high PRL level to read falsely normal or just mildly elevated; a 1:100 dilution of the serum sample with saline will show the true PRL level.[11] Preoperative hypopituitarism caused by a large pituitary mass is reversible in up to half of patients after surgical decompression.[9] Diabetes insipidus (vasopressin deficiency) is rarely caused by pituitary tumors and should raise the suspicion of a craniopharyngioma or other hypothalamic disorders.[12]

TREATMENT   Rx

Surgery

Except for prolactinomas, surgery is the primary mode of therapy for pituitary tumors that warrant intervention. Indications for surgery include reduction in hormone levels and decompression to relieve mass effects or prevent further tumor expansion. Currently, the transsphenoidal route, usually with an endoscopic endonasal approach, is used almost exclusively for decompression or extirpation of pituitary tumors.[13] Because of substantially greater morbidity, subfrontal craniotomy is reserved for patients with tumors that require extensive exploration of the suprasellar region and surrounding structures. In experienced hands, transsphenoidal surgery is effective, and complications are uncommon (<5% complication rate) but include CSF leak, hemorrhage, optic nerve injury, hypopituitarism, and sinusitis. Transient diabetes insipidus occurs in about 5% of patients after surgery but rarely persists long term. Mortality rates are less than 1%. Complication rates increase with increasing size of the tumor and when a craniotomy is performed.

Surgical cure rates are largely a function of the size and location of the pituitary mass. When stringent hormonal criteria are used to assess surgical success rates, 30 to 60% of macroadenomas are cured by transsphenoidal surgery, although considerable improvements in hormone levels or mass effects can be achieved. On the other hand, hormone hypersecretion by microadenomas can be corrected completely in 80 to 90% of patients, although the cure rates vary considerably at different institutions. Even with apparent surgical cure, 10 to 20% of tumors may recur over several years, resulting in a redevelopment of the hormone oversecretion syndrome.

Radiation Therapy

Irradiation is usually used as adjunctive therapy after surgery or in combination with medical therapy. Radiation has typically been administered over 5 weeks at a dose of 45 Gy using cobalt-60 or a linear accelerator. Proton beam therapy delivers very high doses of radiation within a localized region, but it is limited to intrasellar lesions and is not widely available. More recently, a radiation therapy technique referred to as stereotactic radiotherapy has been employed for many patients with pituitary tumors. With this technique, approximately the same dosage of radiation is administered as a single dose through multiple ports, using a computerized matching of irradiation to tumor geometry.[14] Response rates are slow (several years, but somewhat more rapid with stereotactic therapy). Complete remission is rarely achieved with any of these types of irradiation. Because the time to recurrence for most nonfunctioning macroadenomas is 5 to 10 years, and not all tumors recur, it is often reasonable to follow patients with imaging techniques, reserving irradiation for those with evidence of residual tumor or recurrence if no tumor was visible postoperatively.

Complications of irradiation are dose related but can also be idiosyncratic. Partial or complete hypopituitarism occurs in 50 to 70% of patients and is primarily due to hypothalamic injury. Conventional irradiation is associated with an increased risk for stroke. Second tumors occur in the radiation field in about 2% of patients over a 20-year period. Less common complications include optic nerve damage, brain necrosis, and cognitive dysfunction. Whether stereotactic radiotherapy will have similar rates of complications is at present unknown. Early studies show that hypopituitarism is developing at a rate similar to that seen with conventional therapy.

Medical Therapy

The emergence of medical therapies for pituitary tumors has dramatically affected patient management. The dopamine agonists bromocriptine and cabergoline have a primary role in the management of prolactinomas. They induce a rapid fall in PRL levels and, importantly, decrease tumor size. Dopamine agonists are also used in the management of acromegaly, although the GH responses and effects on tumor size are much less pronounced than in prolactinomas. Somatostatin analogues such as octreotide, lanreotide, and pasireotide act to suppress the secretion of a number of hormones, including GH, TSH, and ACTH and have been used to treat acromegaly, TSH-producing tumors, and Cushing's disease. Other medical therapy for Cushing's disease has primarily been directed toward inhibition of steroid biosynthesis; these drugs include ketoconazole, metyrapone, etomidate, and mitotane. Because of substantial side effects and because patients with Cushing's disease tend to escape from the cortisol-suppressing effects of these drugs, medical therapy is used primarily as an adjunctive treatment or to reduce cortisol levels preoperatively. Another new category of drugs to treat pituitary tumors includes the receptor blockers. Pegvisomant is a GH analogue with altered binding to the GH receptor that competitively inhibits GH binding to its receptor and is used in the treatment of acromegaly. Mifepristone can block the action of cortisol at its receptor and has been found to be effective for the treatment of Cushing's syndrome.

GROWTH HORMONE

The most important regulators of GH are the hypothalamic hormones: GHRH, which is stimulatory, and somatostatin, which is inhibitory. GH increases the production of IGF-I (formerly known as somatomedin C). The Gsα-subunit, which is coupled to the GHRH receptor, is one of the targets for activating mutations that lead to somatotroph adenomas.

IGF-I inhibits GH secretion, and it acts at both the pituitary and hypothalamic levels. In addition to reflecting GH action (primarily at the liver), serum IGF-I is also sensitive to nutritional and metabolic changes. In cases of starvation, anorexia nervosa, and poorly controlled diabetes, IGF-I levels are low, resulting in increased levels of GH. In cases of obesity, GH levels are low and GHRH responses are blunted, but IGF-I levels are generally normal and actually increase with increasing body mass index. Stress, exercise, and a variety of neurogenic stimuli also increase GH secretion. Estrogens stimulate GH secretion, but their effects are less pronounced than for PRL, and they inhibit the stimulatory effect of GH on IGF-I production.

Large bursts of GH secretion characteristically occur at night in association with slow-wave sleep. GH levels increase during puberty and decline gradually in adulthood. The amplitude of GH pulses is greater in women than in men, likely reflecting the effects of estrogens. Spontaneous GH pulses can reach 50 ng/mL; consequently, random GH levels can be quite variable. GH responses to GHRH are also variable even within an individual, owing to changes in endogenous somatostatin tone.

GH acts through a single transmembrane receptor that is structurally related to PRL and cytokine receptors. The GH molecule has two distinguishable receptor binding domains that allow it to contact two separate receptor molecules to induce receptor dimerization. Mutations in the gene for the GH receptor cause GH resistance and severe growth retardation, a condition referred to as the GH insensitivity syndrome (Laron-type dwarfism). In such patients, GH levels are elevated and IGF-I levels are low, reflecting the inability of the mutant receptor to transduce the GH signal. Mutations have also been found in signaling intermediates (e.g., the signal transducers of activators of transcription *STAT5b* gene) that mediate GH actions.

Many of the growth and metabolic effects of GH are transmitted indirectly through the actions of IGF-I. GH stimulates IGF-I production in most tissues, where it then exerts autocrine or paracrine effects. Circulating IGF-I is derived predominantly from the liver and is a useful marker of GH action because it has a longer half-life and integrates the effects of GH pulses. Although IGF-I levels are used in the diagnosis of acromegaly and to assess the integrity of the GH axis, factors other than GH (e.g., malnutrition) can alter IGF-I levels. IGF-I acts through widely distributed receptors that are structurally related to insulin receptors. In addition to its growth-promoting and anabolic effects, IGF-I also stimulates mitogenesis in many tissues. The bioactivity of IGF-I is itself modulated by six IGF-binding proteins (IGFBPs). These IGFBPs can inhibit or enhance IGF actions. IGFBP-3 is the major IGFBP in plasma; it is regulated by GH, and its levels generally parallel those of IGF-I.

GH has its major effects on linear growth but also influences a variety of metabolic pathways. Some of these effects are mediated by GH directly, whereas others are conferred by IGF-I. Although the relative roles of GH and IGF-I are debated, their actions are cooperative in many cases. The effects of GH on linear growth appear to be mediated largely by IGF-I, which has been used to stimulate growth in patients with the GH insensitivity syndrome. Linear growth in the fetus and neonate is not GH dependent, as illustrated by the fact that GH-deficient infants have normal birth lengths, although intrauterine IGF-I and IGF-II may be important for fetal growth independent of GH. In contrast, normal postnatal linear growth requires GH, as illustrated by the clinical manifestations of GH deficiency. GH and IGF-I act together to accelerate linear growth markedly, particularly at the time of puberty when sex steroids enhance GH and IGF-I levels.

GH also induces lipolysis and stimulates anabolic activity, including amino acid uptake and protein synthesis. As a result, it reduces body fat, increases lean body mass, and leads to positive nitrogen balance. These properties of GH are most strikingly seen in GH-deficient children who have undergone replacement. GH opposes many of the actions of insulin and can be considered diabetogenic. In diabetic individuals, nocturnal GH secretion accounts in large part for the so-called dawn phenomenon in which there is a decrease in glucose utilization, causing a tendency toward hyperglycemia.

Growth Hormone Deficiency
PATHOBIOLOGY
Causes of GH deficiency include hypothalamic-pituitary disorders, GHRH receptor mutations, GH gene mutations, combined pituitary hormone deficiencies, GH receptor mutations, IGF-I receptor mutations, radiation, and psychosocial deprivation (Chapter 223). Isolated idiopathic GH deficiency is the most common category, however, in children.

CLINICAL MANIFESTATIONS
The clinical manifestations of GH deficiency depend on the time of onset and the severity of hormone deficiency. Children with complete GH deficiency have slow linear growth rates (≈3 cm/year), and they rapidly fall below normal on standardized growth charts. GH-deficient children have normal skeletal proportions, and many have a pudgy, youthful appearance because of decreased lipolysis. Particularly in the setting of cortisol deficiency, there is a predisposition to hypoglycemia. Adults may acquire GH deficiency due to hypothalamic/pituitary disease such as tumors or infiltrative disease. Manifestations of adult GH deficiency include increased fat mass, decreased muscle mass, decreased bone mineral density, and decreased quality of life.

DIAGNOSIS
Basal GH does not provide a reliable measure of GH reserve, whereas low IGF-I is consistent with GH deficiency. However, not all patients documented to have GH deficiency by stimulation testing have IGF-I levels that are below the normal range. GH deficiency is assessed using insulin-induced hypoglycemia, which activates central nervous system pathways, leading to stimulation of both GH and ACTH secretion (see Table 224-2). The insulin tolerance test requires careful monitoring for symptoms of severe hypoglycemia, such as confusion or depressed consciousness. This test should be avoided in patients with seizure disorders or coronary artery disease. Insulin doses (0.1 to 0.15 U/kg) may need to be decreased if glucocorticoid deficiency is suspected or increased in conditions of insulin resistance (e.g., obesity). Alternatives to the insulin tolerance test for evaluation of GH are a combination of arginine and GHRH given intravenously or glucagon given intramuscularly.

TREATMENT   Rx

In children with well-documented GH deficiency, GH replacement is effective and is essential to increase final adult height. In a typical regimen, recombinant GH (0.025 mg/kg) is given daily as subcutaneous injections. The efficacy of GH treatment depends on when it is initiated as well as replacement of other hormone deficiencies, if they coexist. In the setting of multiple hormone deficiencies, replacement of thyroid hormone and cortisol is necessary for effective GH action. On the other hand, sex steroids lead to epiphyseal closure and limit linear growth. Consequently, GH is more effective before puberty; if exogenous sex steroids are given, low doses should be used. GH has also been shown to increase the final height of girls with Turner's syndrome (chromosomal XO state) (Chapter 236) and children with end-stage renal disease.

Only about one third of children with isolated idiopathic GH deficiency are found to be GH deficient when retested as adults. Thus, all such patients should be retested before GH therapy is continued or restarted unless they have proven molecular defects as the cause of their GH deficiency. Studies show that GH treatment can increase bone density[A1] and lean body mass, decrease fat mass, and improve the sense of well-being in adults with documented GH deficiency. In most studies, safety data for long-term GH administration show negligible adverse effects. Whether GH treatment in adults will affect the increased mortality rate associated with hypopituitarism remains to be seen. Adverse effects occur at lower doses in adults compared with children; a starting dose of 0.2 to 0.3 mg/day has been recommended, with gradual titration guided by clinical benefits, adverse effects, and IGF-I levels.

Growth Hormone Excess: Acromegaly and Gigantism

PATHOBIOLOGY

GH-producing pituitary tumors account for 10 to 15% of pituitary tumors (see Table 224-4). GH-producing tumors are frequently mixed tumors that secrete more than one hormone. PRL is produced in about 40% of somatotroph adenomas, and some patients may present because of symptoms due to the hyperprolactinemia (i.e., amenorrhea, galactorrhea, or both). Ectopic production of GHRH (usually carcinoid or pancreatic islets) is a well-documented but rare (<1%) cause of acromegaly that can result in somatotroph hyperplasia. Activating Gsα-subunit mutations occur in 35 to 40% of somatotroph adenomas. Molecular defects in the remaining 60 to 65% of somatotroph adenomas remain unidentified.

CLINICAL MANIFESTATIONS

Tumors that secrete GH cause acromegaly in adults and gigantism in children in whom GH excess occurs before epiphyseal closure. Acromegaly affects men and women with equal frequency and is most often recognized when patients are in their 30s or 40s, usually after a decade of GH excess. The most striking features of acromegaly usually involve the face, hands, and feet. The diagnosis is often suspected because of changes in facial appearance that include enlargement of the lower jaw (prognathism), the nose and lips, and the sinuses (causing frontal bossing) (Fig. 224-5). Oral cavity changes include malocclusion, increased spacing between the teeth, and enlargement of the tongue. A hollow, resonant voice is caused by changes in the vocal cords and the soft tissues of the hypopharynx. Sleep apnea may occur in patients with soft tissue obstruction of the pharynx but may also occur because of a central disorder. In addition to bony enlargement, there is a marked increase in the soft tissue of the hands and feet, leading to progressive increases in ring, glove, and shoe size. A moist, doughy, enveloping handshake is characteristic of acromegaly. Arthritis (hands, feet, hips, knees) is common (75%) and is caused by cartilage and synovial overgrowth. Some degree of carpal tunnel syndrome is seen in about half of patients. Skin changes include increased skinfolds, particularly over the brow and forehead. The skin is usually oily, owing to increased sebaceous activity and sweating. Skin tags are common, and their presence correlates with the presence of colonic polyps. Galactorrhea may be seen in women, and reproductive dysfunction occurs in both women and men when PRL levels are elevated. Headaches, visual field defects, and other neurologic symptoms depend on the location and extent of tumor growth.

Acromegaly causes a two- to three-fold increase in mortality rate.[15] Most of the increased mortality can be attributed to cardiovascular and cerebrovascular diseases and may be related to the increased prevalence of hypertension (25 to 35%) and diabetes mellitus (10 to 25%) in patients with acromegaly. There is evidence for cardiac hypertrophy in most patients, and symptomatic heart disease, consisting of coronary ischemia or congestive heart failure or both, occurs in 15 to 20% of patients. Sleep apnea may predispose patients to cardiac dysrhythmias. Some analyses have found an increased risk of premalignant polyps and colon cancer, and screening with colonoscopy is generally recommended. The disfigurement, metabolic complications, and increased mortality associated with acromegaly emphasize the importance of early diagnosis and implementation of appropriate therapy to lower the GH levels into the normal range.

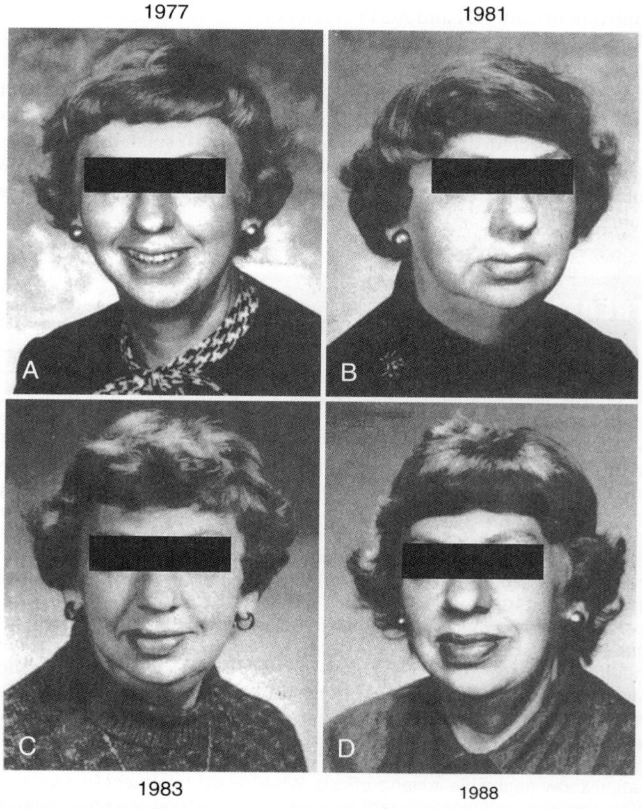

DIAGNOSIS

Because GH is secreted in a pulsatile manner and because the amplitude of normal GH pulses can be large (>50 ng/mL), random GH level measurements are not very useful in making the diagnosis of acromegaly. IGF-I levels provide an integrated index of GH production and provide a better screening test for acromegaly. IGF-I levels decrease with age, so normal ranges must be age adjusted. IGF-I levels correlate well with 24-hour GH production rates and with disease activity. The most standardized test for acromegaly is the glucose tolerance test (Table 224-5). In acromegaly, increased glucose levels fail to suppress GH levels to below 1 ng/mL with polyclonal antibody immunoassays and to levels below 0.4 ng/mL using newer monoclonal antibody two-site assays. Co-secretion of PRL should be evaluated. After the diagnosis of acromegaly is made, radiologic studies, preferably using MRI, should be used to evaluate the extent of tumor growth. Unlike in Cushing's disease and prolactinomas, most patients with acromegaly have macroadenomas.

FIGURE 224-5. Clinical features of acromegaly. Serial photographs of a 64-year-old woman with acromegaly. Over an 11-year period, there is a progressive coarsening of facial features, including enlargement of the nose and lips and development of prognathism. She also experienced hypertension, arthropathy, and enlargement of the hands (not shown). (From Molitch ME. Clinical manifestations of acromegaly. *Endocrinol Metab Clin North Am.* 1992;21:597-614.)

TREATMENT Rx

The goals of therapy are to reverse or prevent tumor mass effects and to reduce the long-term morbidity and mortality that result from excess GH production. Correction of the disorder prevents further physical disfigurement and can result in substantial resolution of soft tissue changes and improvements in metabolic derangements. Although reductions in GH levels are associated with improvements in symptoms, the ultimate goal is to achieve normal GH and IGF-I levels and to prevent tumor recurrence without incurring hypopituitarism.

Transsphenoidal surgery results in GH levels below 2.5 ng/mL in 80 to 90% of patients with microadenomas when performed by experienced neurosurgeons. This level, along with GH suppression below 1 ng/mL during an oral glucose tolerance test, and a normal IGF-I level have been associated with a normalization of the increased mortality of acromegaly. Patients with macroadenomas are less often cured by surgery (<30%) but usually have reductions in GH levels.

Medical therapies for acromegaly include: dopamine agonists such as cabergoline; somatostatin analogues such as octreotide, lanreotide, and pasireotide; and the GH receptor antagonist, pegvisomant. Although cabergoline can reduce GH and IGF-I levels in many patients, normal levels are achieved in only about one third. Long-acting preparations of octreotide, lanreotide, and especially pasireotide that can be given by intramuscular injection every 4 weeks reduce GH and IGF-I levels in almost all patients, with normal levels of IGF-I being achieved in about 50 to 60% of cases. A recent multicenter, randomized trial showed that the somatostatin analog pasireotide (long-acting release), at a dose of either 40 mg or 60 mg administered once every 28 days for 24 weeks, provides superior efficacy compared with continued treatment with octreotide or lanreotide, and could become the new standard pituitary-directed treatment in patients with acromegaly who are inadequately controlled with first-generation somatostatin analogs.[A2] Tumor size is reduced modestly in about one half of cases. Of those achieving normal levels of GH and IGF-I, about 10 to 20% can eventually be successfully withdrawn from treatment after several years. Somatostatin analogues are useful as adjunctive therapy in patients who are not cured by surgery or radiation and in some cases are used primarily when a surgical cure is not possible, such as in those with cavernous sinus invasion. Side effects of somatostatin analogues include diarrhea and increased risk of cholelithiasis, although cholecystitis and need for cholecystectomy are rare. Some patients experience additive beneficial effects from combining these two classes of medications while keeping the dose of each drug low enough to avoid adverse effects.

TABLE 224-5 SELECTED TESTS OF EXCESS PITUITARY FUNCTION

HORMONE	TEST	INTERPRETATION
Growth hormone (GH)	*Basal IGF-I* *Oral glucose suppression test:* after 75-g glucose load, GH is measured at −30, 0, 30, 60, 90, 120 min	Elevated IGF-I levels are consistent with acromegaly when interpreted in the context of age and nutritional status. GH should be suppressed to < 1 µg/L in normal persons with polyclonal radioimmunoassays; < 0.4 µg/L with two-site monoclonal assays. GH may paradoxically increase in acromegaly.
Prolactin	*Basal prolactin levels*	Elevated prolactin (>200 µg/L) is consistent with a prolactinoma. When prolactin levels are between 20 and 200 µg/L, other causes of hyperprolactinemia should be considered.
Adrenocorticotropic hormone (ACTH)	*Measurement of 24-hr urine free cortisol* *Midnight salivary cortisol:* special tubes with cotton pledgets available to collect saliva at 11 PM to midnight *Overnight dexamethasone suppression test:* dexamethasone (1 mg) PO at midnight, followed by 8 AM plasma cortisol *CRH test:* ovine CRH (1 µg/kg) is administered IV, and ACTH and cortisol are drawn at −15, 0, 15, 30, 60, 90, and 120 min. *Petrosal sinus ACTH sampling:* the inferior petrosal sinus is catheterized bilaterally, and plasma ACTH is compared with simultaneous peripheral samples. The sampling can be done in conjunction with CRH stimulation.	Elevated level is suggestive of Cushing's syndrome, but it has several other causes as well. In normal persons, the midnight salivary cortisol is very low because of the normal diurnal variation. In patients with Cushing's syndrome, the salivary cortisol is elevated. In normal persons, AM cortisol should be suppressed to < 5 µg/dL. Normal test excludes Cushing's syndrome. Other disorders can cause failure to suppress normally. In Cushing's disease, there is usually a 50% increase in ACTH and a 20% increase in cortisol. Adrenal adenoma is associated with suppressed ACTH. Ectopic ACTH is associated with high basal ACTH and cortisol levels that are not affected by CRH. In Cushing's disease, the ratio of ACTH in the petrosal sinus to the periphery is at least 2 basally and at least 3 after CRH. In ectopic ACTH, the ratio of petrosal sinus to peripheral level is < 1.5.
Thyroid-stimulating hormone (TSH)	*Basal thyroid function tests* *Free α-subunit level*	An inappropriate normal or elevated TSH in the setting of increased free thyroid hormone levels is consistent with a TSH-producing tumor or other causes of inappropriate TSH secretion. Elevated levels associated with inappropriately elevated TSH are suggestive of a TSH-producing tumor.
Follicle-stimulating hormone (FSH), luteinizing hormone (LH)	*Basal FSH, LH, testosterone*	Increased LH and testosterone levels in males are consistent with LH-secreting tumors. Elevated FSH and low-normal testosterone are suggestive of an FSH-producing tumor if primary gonadal failure is not present. In females, assessment of excess hormone secretion is difficult because of changes during the menstrual cycle and at menopause.

CRH = corticotropin-releasing hormone; IGF = insulin-like growth factor; TRH = thyrotropin-releasing hormone.

Pegvisomant is a biosynthetic GH analogue that prevents binding of GH to its receptor. It is capable of normalizing IGF-I levels in more than 90% of patients with corresponding clinical benefits, but it has no effects on the tumor itself. Pegvisomant is given by daily subcutaneous injection; although it generally has been held in reserve for patients not responding optimally to other treatment modalities, its high biochemical and clinical efficacy have led to increasing use now as initial medical therapy when tumors are not large. It has also been given in combination with somatostatin analogues. The most common adverse effect of pegvisomant is an increase in serum transaminase levels.

Radiation is not recommended as primary therapy for acromegaly because of the long time (5 to 10 years) required for reductions in GH levels and the high incidence of hypopituitarism and other complications. Adjunctive radiation therapy may be required for patients with macroadenomas when GH levels or mass effects persist after transsphenoidal surgery and medical therapy. Recent data suggest that stereotactic radiotherapy may be the most efficacious form of radiotherapy for acromegaly.

● PROLACTIN

PRL and GH appear to be derived from a common ancestral gene, which accounts for the similarities in their structures and some overlap in their functional properties. Although large-molecular-weight forms of PRL (due to binding to immunoglobulin [Ig]G, termed *macroprolactin*) react in radioimmunoassays, they have diminished biologic potency. Estrogen stimulates lactotroph proliferation, and their number is consequently greater in females than in males and during pregnancy (≈70% of pituitary cells).

Secretion of PRL is controlled by tonic inhibition by dopamine, which acts through D₂-type receptors on lactotrophs. PRL biosynthesis and secretion are stimulated by the hypothalamic peptides TRH and vasoactive intestinal peptide (VIP). Hypothyroidism causes increased TRH output and increased sensitivity of the lactotrophs to TRH and can result in hyperprolactinemia. Dopamine inhibition is the dominant influence for PRL

secretion; therefore, PRL is the one pituitary hormone that increases after pituitary stalk section. Secretion of PRL is pulsatile and increases with sleep, stress, chest wall stimulation, and pregnancy. PRL levels are usually less than 15 to 20 ng/mL in women and 10 to 15 ng/mL in men. The primary function of PRL is to induce and sustain lactation. During pregnancy, PRL levels increase, and in conjunction with other hormones (estrogens, progesterone, thyroid hormone, cortisol, and insulin), breast epithelium is stimulated to proliferate and milk synthesis is induced. High levels of estrogen and progesterone inhibit lactation during pregnancy, and their decline post partum permits lactation to occur. Neural pathways leading to the secretion of oxytocin provide the "let-down" reflex that induces lactation in response to suckling. Early in the postpartum period, PRL secretion is stimulated by suckling, but this response becomes damped with time as the frequency of suckling episodes decreases. PRL also suppresses gonadotropins. As a result, breast-feeding can suppress ovulation.

Prolactin Deficiency

PRL deficiency is rare and occurs primarily in the setting of combined hormone deficiencies. The only recognized consequence of PRL deficiency is the absence of postpartum lactation, and this scenario may be found with pituitary infarction occurring as a result of obstetric hemorrhage (Sheehan syndrome). No effects on breast development or other tissues have been described in PRL deficiency.

Hyperprolactinemia
PATHOBIOLOGY

Hyperprolactinemia can occur as a consequence of pharmacologic alterations in the pathways that control PRL secretion or of physiologic or metabolic effects on PRL production and clearance or as a neoplastic condition. Prolactinomas are neoplastic growths of lactotroph cells and are the most common type of pituitary adenoma (25 to 40%). Estrogen is a potent stimulus for lactotroph proliferation; however, there is no clear association between estrogens (e.g., oral contraceptive use) and the incidence of prolactinomas. However, the very high estrogen levels present during pregnancy may cause about 30% of large prolactinomas to increase in size. Diminished dopamine tone, such as may occur with prolonged treatment with antipsychotic agents, results in increased PRL but has not been shown to cause prolactinomas.

Microprolactinomas constitute the great majority of tumors in premenopausal women. In contrast, macroadenomas are more commonly seen in men and postmenopausal women. The predominance of smaller tumors in premenopausal women may be accounted for by an ascertainment bias, because elevated PRL levels in this group lead to clinical manifestations (amenorrhea, galactorrhea, or infertility). Subclinical prolactinomas exist in men and many older women, and about 5% of apparently normal individuals have PRL-positive microadenomas in autopsy series. Prolactinomas in children tend to be macroadenomas, possibly owing to an increased prevalence of *AIP* mutations (see earlier).

CLINICAL MANIFESTATIONS

Hyperprolactinemia causes galactorrhea and oligomenorrhea or amenorrhea in premenopausal women. Estrogen facilitates PRL-induced galactorrhea, which explains why it is less common in postmenopausal women. Amenorrhea is primarily a consequence of PRL suppression of GnRH, although PRL may also have inhibitory effects at the level of the pituitary and the gonad. Amenorrhea is associated with infertility, and PRL levels should be a routine part of the hormonal evaluation of infertility. Estrogen deficiency can cause decreased libido, vaginal dryness, and dyspareunia. Long-standing estrogen deficiency also leads to osteopenia in many women. Oral contraceptives may mask PRL-induced oligomenorrhea or amenorrhea that becomes apparent on their discontinuation. In postmenopausal women, prolactinomas are often identified because of mass effects rather than because of their hormonal effects.

In men, hyperprolactinemia causes hypogonadism with suppressed LH and FSH levels and low testosterone levels. Hypogonadism causes diminished libido, impotence, infertility, and rarely, gynecomastia or galactorrhea. Diminished libido may also reflect suppression of GnRH, because testosterone replacement is not as effective as suppression of hyperprolactinemia. Hyperprolactinemia is found in 1 to 2% of men being evaluated for sexual dysfunction.

DIAGNOSIS

There are four primary categories of causes of hyperprolactinemia that must be distinguished if the correct therapy is to be instituted: (1) physiologic or metabolic hyperprolactinemia, (2) pharmacologic hyperprolactinemia, (3) hypothalamic or pituitary stalk compression, and (4) prolactinoma (see Table 224-4).[16] With the exception of pregnancy and renal failure, physiologic causes of increased PRL result in minor elevations in PRL, usually less than 50 ng/mL. Primary hypothyroidism should be excluded as a cause of mild hyperprolactinemia. A careful drug history should be obtained in all patients with hyperprolactinemia because of the large number of agents that can stimulate PRL secretion. Psychotropic medications in particular can increase PRL, either by reducing dopamine production or by blocking its action. In most cases, the degree of hyperprolactinemia caused by drugs is less than 150 ng/mL. A variety of suprasellar and parasellar mass lesions cause hyperprolactinemia (generally between 20 and 100 ng/mL) because of compression of the hypothalamus or pituitary stalk. Unless there is very good evidence for physiologic or drug-induced hyperprolactinemia, even patients with mild hyperprolactinemia should be evaluated with MRI to distinguish among idiopathic hyperprolactinemia, microprolactinomas, and other large mass lesions that cause stalk compression resulting in decreased dopamine reaching the lactotrophs. However, specific caution is needed when some two-site assays are used, because patients with very high PRL levels may appear to have PRL levels that are normal or only modestly elevated, owing to the hook effect, in which the very high PRL levels saturate the antibodies in the assay. To avoid this problem, PRL levels should be remeasured at 1 : 100 dilution in patients with large macroadenomas (>3 cm) and normal to modestly elevated PRL levels, because PRL levels in samples with the hook effect will then increase dramatically. When no pituitary lesions are seen by radiographic studies and physiologic and pharmacologic causes of hyperprolactinemia cannot be identified, the diagnosis of idiopathic hyperprolactinemia is made. Idiopathic hyperprolactinemia may represent microprolactinomas too small to be detected accurately by imaging or altered hypothalamic regulation of PRL secretion. Whether such patients should be treated depends on the clinical effects of hyperprolactinemia. When followed for several years, few of these patients develop large tumors, only 10 to 15% show MRI evidence of microadenomas, and in one third of cases, the hyperprolactinemia resolves.

TREATMENT   Rx

The natural history of prolactinomas has been evaluated in several series. Although large prolactinomas evolve from smaller lesions, it is uncommon (≈7%) for microprolactinomas to progress to macroadenomas. Because of the slow rate of growth, it is reasonable to monitor patients with microprolactinomas without treatment by periodic measurement of PRL levels unless the hyperprolactinemia is causing symptoms that warrant therapy.

When hyperprolactinemia causes hypogonadism, osteopenia, or infertility, a dopamine agonist such as cabergoline or bromocriptine is the therapy of choice. Dopamine agonists normalize PRL levels and correct amenorrhea-galactorrhea in 80 to 90% of patients. Cabergoline is more effective, has fewer adverse effects than bromocriptine, and has the additional advantage in only having to be taken once or twice weekly. Bromocriptine must be started in low doses, with gradual increases to avoid side effects (nausea, dizziness, somnolence, and nasal stuffiness).

Cabergoline may cause a considerable reduction in tumor size in patients with macroprolactinomas (≈80 to 90% having > 50% reduction in tumor size), but such size reduction is seen in only about two thirds of patients treated with bromocriptine. Improvements in visual field defects can be seen in about 90% of patients with defects when treated with cabergoline. Thus, it is reasonable to use cabergoline as first-line therapy even in patients with visual field defects, so long as visual acuity is not threatened by rapid progression or recent tumor hemorrhage. Many patients treated with cabergoline whose tumors shrink to the point of nonvisualization on MRI and whose PRL levels are normal can maintain normal PRL levels and not experience tumor reexpansion after therapy has been tapered off. In some cases, prolactinomas appear to be resistant to a dopamine agonist. In these cases, switching from bromocriptine to cabergoline may be successful. Larger-than-standard doses (>2 mg/week) of cabergoline may be effective in normalizing PRL levels. The very high doses of cabergoline used in patients with Parkinson's disease have been associated with cardiac valvular abnormalities; such abnormalities have not been found with conventional doses of cabergoline used in patients with prolactinomas, but monitoring with echocardiography may be prudent in patients taking larger-than-standard doses. Alternatively, transsphenoidal surgery may be used. Although initial remission rates (80 to 90%) for transsphenoidal surgery of microprolactinomas are good, there is long-term recurrence in about 20% of patients. For macroprolactinomas, the initial remission rates with surgery are closer to 30%, with a similar recurrence rate. Radiation therapy, usually stereotactic, is reserved for patients with macroadenomas not responding to either medical or surgical treatment.

Dopamine agonist therapy for infertility, or when there is a possibility of pregnancy, deserves special consideration. These medications can induce ovulation in 80 to 90% of patients with hyperprolactinemia. Although neither bromocriptine nor cabergoline has been associated with congenital malformations, they should be stopped once pregnancy has been achieved. A form of barrier contraception is usually recommended until two to three regular menstrual cycles have occurred. Subsequently, pregnancy can be confirmed if a menstrual period is missed, allowing discontinuation of medication with exposure of the fetus to the drug for only 3 to 5 weeks. At present, the safety data for pregnancy outcome are more limited for cabergoline; therefore, some clinicians prefer bromocriptine when fertility is desired. Less than 3% of patients with microadenomas, but 23% of patients with macroadenomas, develop symptoms of tumor enlargement (headaches, visual field defects) during pregnancy (Fig. 224-6). If symptoms develop, MRI and formal visual field testing should be performed. If there is evidence of visual field compromise or tumor growth, dopamine agonist therapy should be restarted to shrink the tumor. PRL levels are not very useful because they are normally increased in pregnancy and an enlarging tumor may not cause PRL production to increase substantially. Because problems of tumor growth occur most often in patients with macroadenomas, consideration can also be given to the option of transsphenoidal decompression before pregnancy in women with large tumors, so long as fertility can be preserved. If the patient is far advanced in her gestation at the time tumor growth occurs, consideration could also be given to delivering the baby.

● ADRENOCORTICOTROPIC HORMONE

ACTH is a 39–amino acid peptide that is derived from a precursor polypeptide, proopiomelanocortin (POMC; 241 amino acids), which encodes several peptides, including ACTH and β-lipotropin (Chapter 223). The biologically active portion of ACTH resides within the first 18 of its 39 amino acids. However, because a synthetic peptide (cosyntropin) that includes the first 24 amino acids has a longer half-life, it is used clinically to assess adrenocortical function. In cases with neoplastic ectopic production of ACTH, the levels of precursor peptides or their processed products may be elevated.

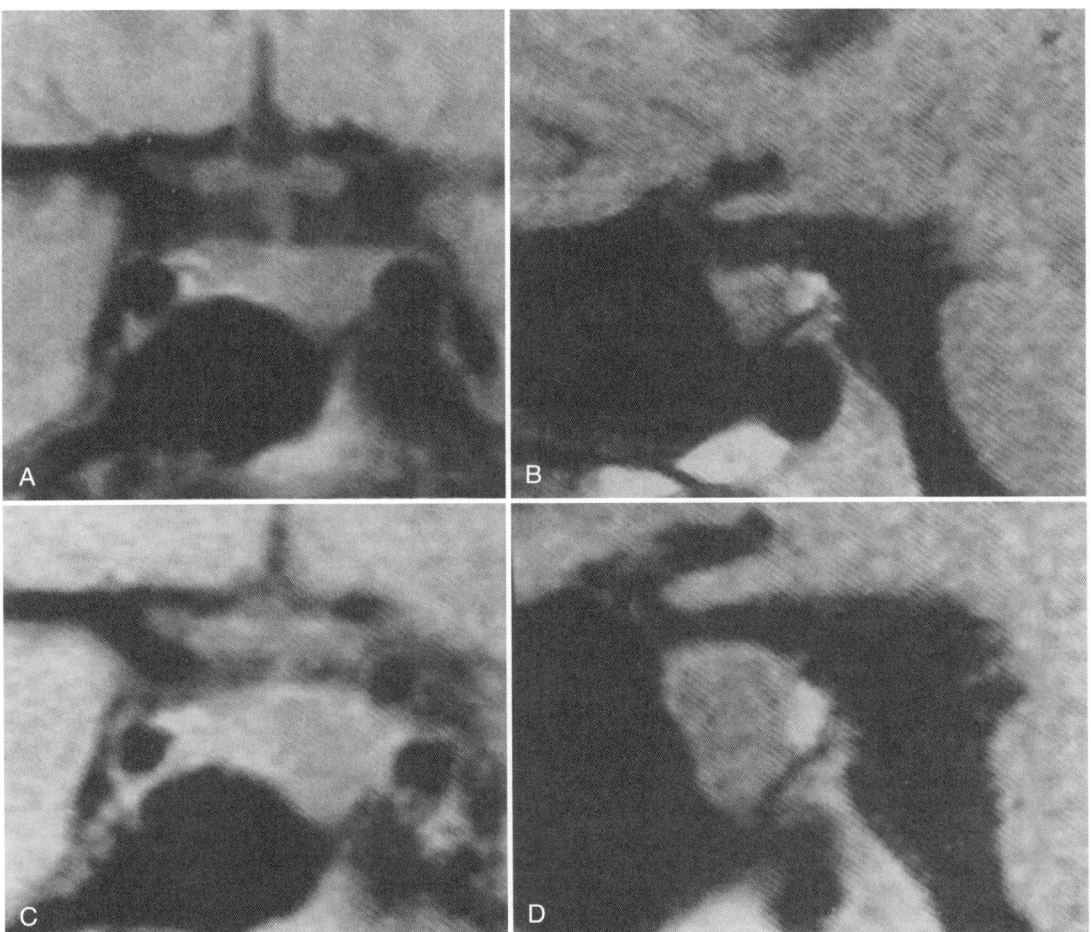

FIGURE 224-6. Magnetic resonance image showing enlargement of prolactinoma during pregnancy. *Above,* Coronal (**A**) and sagittal (**B**) views show intrasellar prolactin-secreting macroadenoma prior to conception. *Below,* Coronal (**C**) and sagittal (**D**) views show enlargement of the prolactinoma at 7 months' gestation. (From Molitch ME. Medical treatment of prolactinomas. *Endocrinol Metab Clin North Am.* 1999;28:143.)

The primary effect of ACTH is to stimulate the adrenal gland to produce cortisol. It also stimulates secretion of adrenal androgens and mineralocorticoids, although production of mineralocorticoids is controlled primarily through non–ACTH-dependent mechanisms (i.e., the renin-angiotensin system) (Chapter 227). Consequently, mineralocorticoid function is preserved in ACTH deficiency, in contrast to primary adrenal insufficiency, which is characterized by loss of glucocorticoid and mineralocorticoid function. Long-term stimulation by ACTH causes adrenal hyperplasia and enlargement. On the other hand, ACTH deficiency leads to adrenal atrophy.

Hypothalamic corticotropin-releasing hormone (CRH) is the most important stimulator of ACTH secretion. Chronic stimulation by CRH causes corticotroph cell hyperplasia, which can be seen in cases of ectopic CRH production. Cortisol inhibits ACTH secretion, blunts the ACTH response to CRH, and inhibits CRH production. After prolonged glucocorticoid suppression of the hypothalamic-pituitary-adrenal axis, the amount of endogenous CRH secretion appears to be rate limiting and can require several months to recover.

Plasma ACTH is secreted in discrete pulses (10 to 80 pg/mL), so random measurements are of little value. Most clinical tests are therefore based on levels of cortisol or its metabolites, which tend to integrate the effects of ACTH. ACTH and cortisol secretion exhibit marked diurnal rhythms, being greatest at night several hours after the initiation of sleep. Cortisol levels are highest in the early morning and reach a nadir in the late afternoon and evening. Patients with Cushing's disease lose or exhibit a blunted diurnal rhythm of ACTH and cortisol secretion. ACTH secretion can be stimulated by a variety of different forms of stress, including psychological stimuli such as fright, anticipation of athletic competition, or surgery. Depression is associated with activation of the hypothalamic-pituitary-adrenal axis and impaired dexamethasone suppressibility. Hypoglycemia induces ACTH

secretion through a central mechanism. The resulting increase in cortisol secretion represents one of several counter-regulatory mechanisms that increase glucose production. Insulin-induced hypoglycemia provides a mechanism for testing the integrity of the hypothalamic-pituitary-adrenal axis (see Table 224-2). Serious trauma and infection activate an array of cytokines that stimulate CRH and ACTH secretion. Because cortisol levels are often increased substantially in these circumstances, similar adjustments in cortisol replacement doses may be required in seriously ill patients with adrenal insufficiency.

Adrenocorticotropic Hormone Deficiency: Secondary Hypocortisolism

Secondary hypocortisolism causes symptoms of glucocorticoid deficiency, including nausea, vomiting, weakness, fatigue, fever, and hypotension. In addition to reduced levels of cortisol, abnormal laboratory test findings can include hyponatremia, hypoglycemia, and eosinophilia. Depending on its cause, the severity of cortisol deficiency in cases of secondary adrenal insufficiency is often not as marked as in primary adrenal insufficiency (Chapter 227). In addition, mineralocorticoid function is preserved in secondary adrenal deficiency. Consequently, the clinical manifestations of volume depletion are less pronounced, and hyperkalemia is not a feature of ACTH deficiency. Because ACTH levels are low, hyperpigmentation is not seen as in primary adrenal insufficiency. In women, reduced adrenal androgens can decrease libido and cause loss of axillary and pubic hair.

The most common cause of ACTH deficiency is treatment with exogenous glucocorticoids, which causes suppression of the hypothalamic-pituitary-adrenal axis. Sudden withdrawal of glucocorticoids or an increased requirement induced by the superimposition of severe illness can elicit symptoms of glucocorticoid deficiency. Congenital forms of ACTH deficiency are rare. When present, ACTH deficiency usually occurs in combination with the loss of other pituitary hormones, although acquired, isolated ACTH deficiency does occur, particularly in women with lymphocytic hypophysitis.

ACTH reserve is most often evaluated using the insulin tolerance test. Caution should be exercised before inducing hypoglycemia in patients with suspected adrenal insufficiency. Insulin-induced hypoglycemia stimulates central responses to neuroglycopenia (Chapter 230) and mimics some stresses that activate ACTH secretion. ACTH stimulation tests using $ACTH_{1-24}$ (cosyntropin) can accurately evaluate primary adrenocortical insufficiency but may less accurately assess secondary adrenal insufficiency. A variation of the ACTH stimulation test using the low dose of 1 μg has been found to be useful for diagnosing secondary adrenal insufficiency in some studies.

Deficiency of ACTH is treated by replacement with glucocorticoids. Doses need to be individualized and are based largely on clinical criteria in which symptoms of glucocorticoid deficiency are balanced against features of glucocorticoid excess. Typical amounts of hydrocortisone are in the range of 15 to 20 mg/day in divided doses. Such doses are usually doubled in the event of mild to moderate illness. Patients should wear MedicAlert tags and be instructed in the warning signs of cortisol deficiency: nausea, vomiting, abdominal pain, low-grade fever, fatigue, and postural dizziness. Emergency injection kits of hydrocortisone are frequently provided for home use in the event that vomiting precludes taking oral steroids, or for severe sudden stress (e.g., a fracture). Stress doses of steroids should be used during times of illness. Current recommendations call for doses in the range of 50 to 75 mg every 8 hours for severe stress. Mineralocorticoid replacement is not required in patients with ACTH deficiency.

Cushing's Disease

PATHOBIOLOGY

Cushing's disease results from a pituitary adenoma that causes excess production of ACTH. It should be distinguished from a variety of other causes of Cushing's syndrome (glucocorticoid excess), which include adrenal causes (adenomas, carcinomas) of cortisol excess, ectopic production of ACTH and CRH, and physiologic states that result in overproduction of cortisol. Cushing's disease accounts for 60 to 70% of cases of Cushing's syndrome. Ten to 15% of pituitary tumors secrete ACTH. Cushing's disease occurs about eight times more often in women than in men.

Most ACTH-producing pituitary neoplasms, like other pituitary tumors, are monoclonal, implying a primary defect in corticotroph cells. In addition, there are rare cases of corticotroph hyperplasia causing Cushing's syndrome that are secondary to CRH production by either adjacent CRH-producing intrasellar gangliocytomas or ectopic CRH-producing cancers. Most (80 to 90%) of the ACTH-secreting tumors are microadenomas at the time of diagnosis. The clinical features of cortisol excess may allow detection of corticotroph adenomas before they have grown to a larger size. High levels of cortisol may also restrain tumor growth. ACTH-secreting macroadenomas may be locally invasive.

CLINICAL MANIFESTATIONS

The clinical features of Cushing's disease are caused by the effects of excess glucocorticoids and by the hypersecretion of ACTH and other POMC peptide products. The severity of the features of Cushing's disease varies greatly and appears to reflect not only the level of free cortisol but also the duration of the disease and perhaps the sensitivity to glucocorticoid action. In florid cases of Cushing's disease (Fig. 224-7), the constellation of symptoms and physical features is readily recognized. Early in the disease or in mild cases, it can be challenging to distinguish the clinical features of Cushing's disease from similar traits that are seen in the normal population. Clinical suspicion is of paramount importance. On the other hand, one must be discriminating and not formally evaluate everyone with obesity, hypertension, and glucose intolerance. Of the many features listed in Table 224-6, some are relatively specific for Cushing's disease. For example, the centripetal distribution of fat with the characteristic "buffalo hump," "moon facies," and deposition of fat in the supraclavicular area but not in the extremities is much more specific than generalized obesity. Striae that are wide (>1 cm) and purple reflect steroid-induced thinning of the dermis and can be distinguished from the more common "stretch marks." Numerous spontaneous ecchymoses also occur because of thinning of the skin and capillary fragility. Proximal muscle weakness represents another manifestation of glucocorticoid excess. Osteopenia and hypokalemia, when present, provide objective evidence consistent with ACTH excess. Hypokalemia results from the effects of ACTH on mineralocorticoid production but also from the ability of high levels of cortisol to saturate 11β-dehydrogenase, an enzyme in the kidney that

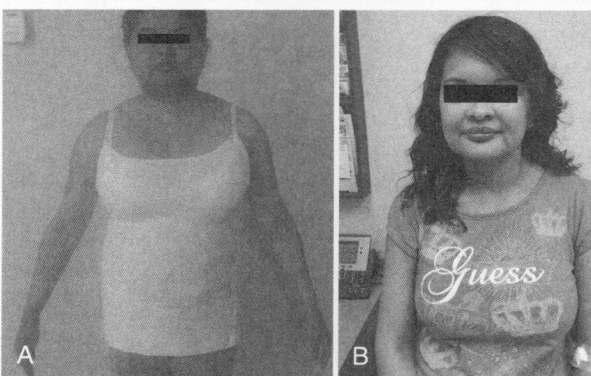

FIGURE 224-7. **(A)** This 30 year old woman initially presented with a three year history of increasing facial hair, facial rounding, abdominal obesity, hypertension, diabetes, and oligomenorrhea. She had no muscle weakness or pigmented striae. **(B)** Following successful transsphenoidal resection of her ACTH-secreting microadenoma, she had a dramatic improvement in her clinical appearance with resolution of her diabetes and hypertension.

TABLE 224-6   CLINICAL FEATURES OF CUSHING'S DISEASE
GENERAL
Obesity (centripetal distribution)
"Moon facies" and mild proptosis
Increased supraclavicular fat and "buffalo hump"
Hypertension
SKIN
Hyperpigmentation
Facial plethora
Hirsutism
Violaceous striae and thin skin
Capillary fragility and easy bruising
Acne
Edema
MUSCULOSKELETAL
Muscle weakness (proximal)
Osteoporosis and back pain
REPRODUCTIVE
Decreased libido
Oligomenorrhea and amenorrhea
NEUROPSYCHIATRIC
Depression
Irritability and emotional lability
Psychosis
METABOLIC
Hypokalemia and alkalosis
Hypercalciuria and renal stones
Glucose intolerance or diabetes mellitus
Impaired wound healing
Impaired resistance to infection
Granulocytosis and lymphopenia
TUMOR MASS EFFECTS
Headache
Visual field loss
Hypopituitarism

inactivates cortisol. As a result, cortisol can "spill over" and act on mineralocorticoid receptors in the distal tubule. The hyperpigmentation associated with Cushing's disease is not as striking as that seen in Addison's disease or in ectopic ACTH syndrome, but in association with other findings, it should raise the suspicion of Cushing's disease and help distinguish it from adrenal causes of hypercortisolemia. Hirsutism and acne are caused by increased production of adrenal androgens and are more prominent in patients with Cushing's disease than in those with adrenal adenomas, in whom glucocorticoids tend to be the predominant product. Oligomenorrhea and amenorrhea probably have several causes, including androgen effects on the reproductive axis and glucocorticoid inhibition of GnRH, which may also account for diminished libido. Hypertension and glucose intolerance are caused by glucocorticoid excess. Immunosuppression, venous thrombo-

TABLE 224-7 TESTS USED IN THE DIFFERENTIAL DIAGNOSIS OF CUSHING'S SYNDROME*

ETIOLOGY	OVERNIGHT DEXAMETHASONE SUPPRESSION TEST	PLASMA ACTH	CORTICOTROPIN-RELEASING HORMONE STIMULATION OF ACTH	PETROSAL-TO-PERIPHERAL ACTH RATIO
Normal	Suppression	Normal	Normal	
Pituitary	No suppression	Normal or high	Normal or increased	>2
Ectopic	No suppression	High or normal	No response	<1.5
Adrenal	No suppression	Low	No response	

*Classic responses are indicated. Certain cases of ectopic adrenocorticotropic hormone (ACTH) production are suppressed by high-dose dexamethasone (not shown in this Table) or are stimulated by corticotropin-releasing hormone. In these cases, petrosal sinus sampling is the most reliable method for distinguishing pituitary and ectopic sources of ACTH.

embolism, opportunistic infections, and impaired wound healing can lead to considerable morbidity and mortality.[17] Neuropsychiatric symptoms, including depression, can be prominent effects of Cushing's disease. Suicide occurs with increased frequency in patients who receive no treatment for Cushing's disease.

DIAGNOSIS

The screening tests and differential diagnosis of Cushing's syndrome represent one of the greatest diagnostic challenges in endocrinology (Chapter 227). The first step is to determine whether a patient truly has cortisol excess. After confirmation of Cushing's syndrome, one must distinguish among (1) adrenal causes of cortisol excess, (2) pituitary causes of ACTH excess (Cushing's disease), (3) ectopic sources of ACTH, and (4) ectopic CRH (Table 224-7).

In screening for hypercortisolism, random cortisol levels are not useful because of diurnal variation of the hormone. The overnight dexamethasone test has been the most widely used screening test (see Table 224-5). A normal result of the dexamethasone test excludes Cushing's syndrome. It should be noted, however, that abnormal overnight dexamethasone suppression can be seen in up to 30% of hospitalized patients and in many patients with depression or during alcohol withdrawal. An elevated 24-hour urine free cortisol value provides an alternative or additional screening test for hypercortisolism. Often, two sequential specimens are collected because of day-to-day variations in hormone production. The sensitivity and specificity of urinary free cortisol measurements are greater than those of the overnight dexamethasone suppression test, particularly in hospitalized patients. A third test takes advantage of the observation that there is a loss of diurnal variation of cortisol levels in all forms of Cushing's syndrome. This test consists of finding elevation of a midnight cortisol level in the saliva. Kits are available for patients to obtain a late-night salivary cortisol sample. The sensitivity and specificity of late-night salivary cortisol measurements are very high, and this test now has become the one most commonly used by endocrinologists.

After demonstrating that cortisol excess is present, the next step is to determine the source of excess ACTH or cortisol. This is done by measuring an ACTH level along with a cortisol level, with primary adrenal disease causing suppressed ACTH levels. The classic approach of performing a low-dose, followed by a high-dose, dexamethasone suppression test has been largely abandoned (see Tables 224-5 and 224-7). The high-dose dexamethasone test is one of several means to to discriminate between pituitary and ectopic causes of ACTH-dependent Cushing's syndrome (see Table 224-7). Pituitary and ectopic causes of Cushing's disease are both ACTH dependent but respond differently to high-dose dexamethasone. Pituitary adenomas have an altered set point for glucocorticoid inhibition but retain a partial ability to respond to high-dose dexamethasone. The exact criteria for dexamethasone suppression in the high-dose test are debated. In most cases of ACTH-producing pituitary adenomas, urinary free cortisol is suppressed below 90% of baseline during the high-dose dexamethasone test.

The ectopic ACTH syndrome should be suspected in patients with known malignancies, particularly small-cell carcinoma of the lung; bronchial, thymic, or gastrointestinal carcinoids; islet cell tumors; and medullary carcinoma of the thyroid, among others. Plasma ACTH levels are often very high (>200 pg/mL) and can be associated with hyperpigmentation. Clinical features of Cushing's syndrome may be altered by the rapid onset of extreme hypercortisolemia coincident with elements of tumor cachexia. Pronounced weakness, fluid retention, glucose intolerance, hypokalemia, and poor skin integrity are often seen. Ectopic ACTH syndrome is readily recognized in its classic form. However, a subset of tumors, particularly carcinoids (Chapter 232), exhibit dexamethasone suppression that is similar to that seen with pituitary adenomas. When suspected, carcinoids can sometimes be detected by CT or MRI, but many are too small to be seen even with these techniques.

Because of these exceptions to the high-dose dexamethasone test, a variety of procedures have been devised in an attempt to further distinguish ectopic and pituitary dependent sources of ACTH. CRH testing may also prove useful, with pituitary tumors exhibiting an increase in ACTH and tumors making ACTH ectopically having little or no response.

In recent years, inferior petrosal sinus sampling has been used to distinguish pituitary and ectopic sources of ACTH when the source of ACTH is not obvious based on the clinical circumstances, biochemical evaluation, and imaging studies. This test requires an experienced radiologist for safe and effective catheterization of the petrosal sinuses. Blood samples are taken simultaneously from the left and right petrosal sinuses and from the periphery before and after CRH stimulation. In the case of ACTH-producing pituitary adenomas, there is a gradient in ACTH levels between the central and peripheral blood specimens. When clinical and biochemical studies suggest the presence of a pituitary adenoma, pituitary imaging should be performed using CT or MRI. Most ACTH-secreting pituitary adenomas are small, and scans are normal in more than half of patients.

TREATMENT Rx

The efficacy of transsphenoidal surgery for Cushing's disease is greatly aided by making the correct diagnosis preoperatively. In experienced hands, surgical cures of ACTH-producing microadenomas occur in 75 to 90% of patients undergoing a first operation. As in other pituitary tumors, complete remissions with macroadenomas are much less common. In the event of surgical remission or cure, postoperative hypocortisolism is to be expected because of suppression of the hypothalamic-pituitary axis. After coverage for steroid withdrawal in the postoperative period, cortisol replacement should gradually be decreased to allow recovery of the hypothalamic-pituitary-adrenal axis; recovery may take up to 1 year.

If transsphenoidal surgery is unsuccessful, reoperation may be indicated and can result in remission in up to 50% of patients[18]; in this circumstance, consideration should be given to performing a total hypophysectomy at reoperation. If transsphenoidal surgery cannot be performed or has failed, alternative forms of therapy should be used to prevent the long-term consequences of hypercortisolism.[19] Pituitary irradiation is often the second line of treatment for Cushing's disease. It is more efficacious in children and in younger patients, but even in older adults, remissions can be achieved in about 50% within 2 years. To prevent the continued ravages of hypercortisolism during this period, however, concomitant medical therapy (see later) is usually given. Bilateral adrenalectomy represents another alternative for patients with severe hypercortisolism after transsphenoidal surgery. It rapidly and effectively lowers cortisol levels but is associated with relatively high morbidity and mortality rates (as high as 5%) because of the associated metabolic and immune system alterations caused by hypercortisolism. The morbidity has been reduced in recent years by introduction of the laparoscopic approach. After adrenalectomy, patients must be maintained on glucocorticoids and mineralocorticoids and are at risk for the development of Nelson syndrome (see later).

Medical therapy for Cushing's disease has its primary role in preparation for surgery or control of hypercortisolism following unsuccessful surgery. It may also be used during the interval when radiation therapy is taking effect (Fig. 224-8). The antifungal agent ketoconazole is effective in decreasing glucocorticoid biosynthesis and also inhibits ACTH secretion, so it has been the most common medical therapy used; it has hepatotoxicity and is not actually approved for use for Cushing's syndrome. Other drugs that interfere with cortisol synthesis (e.g., mitotane, etomidate, metyrapone) have been used less commonly. In a few small studies, cabergoline has also been shown to cause a normalization of cortisol levels in about one third of patients with Cushing's disease, although it has not been approved for this indication. Recently, two new drugs have been approved for the treatment of Cushing's disease. Mifepristone is a progesterone receptor blocker that also is a glucocorticoid receptor blocker and is highly effective in improving clinical signs and symptoms of Cushing's syndrome; because of its mechanism of action, with

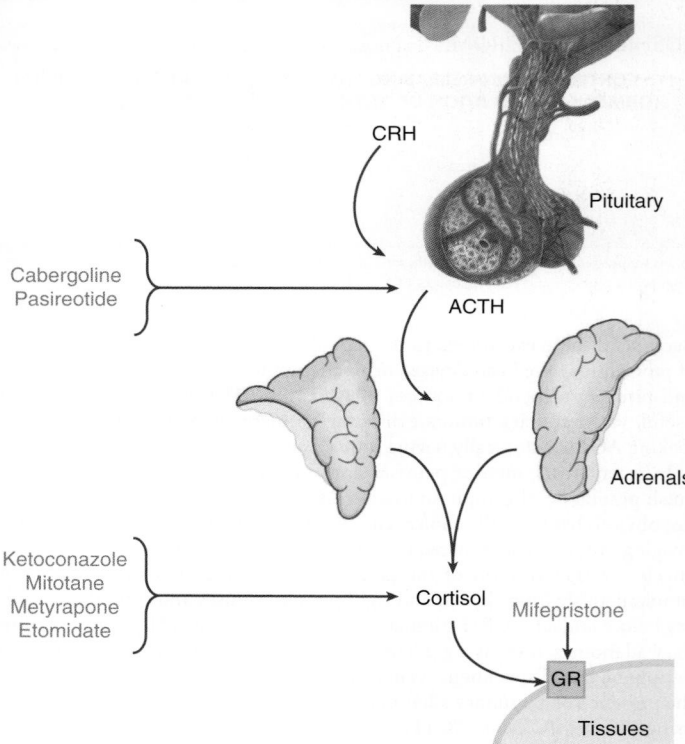

FIGURE 224-8. **Medical therapies for Cushing's disease.** Cabergoline and pasireotide act to decrease ACTH secretion from the corticotroph tumor. Several drugs (ketoconazole, metyrapone, mitotane, etomidate) work at the adrenal level to decrease cortisol synthesis. Mitotane works at the adrenal level by blocking cortisol action at the glucocorticoid receptor. ACTH = adrenocorticotropic hormone; CRH = corticotropin-releasing hormone; GR = glucocorticoid receptor. (Adapted from Petersenn S. Medical management of Cushing's disease. In: Swearingen B, Biller BMK (eds) Endocrine updates vol. 31: Cushing's disease. 2011, Springer, New York, pp 167–182, Figure 1. As adapted from Petersenn S, Endocrine Updates, 2011, Springer Science+Business Media B.V.)

treatment, cortisol and ACTH levels actually rise while the clinical signs improve. The higher levels of cortisol may "spill over" to the mineralocorticoid receptor, causing a blood pressure rise and hypokalemia. Symptoms of glucocorticoid withdrawal and even adrenal insufficiency may occur. Blockade of the progesterone receptor by mifepristone may cause menorrhagia. Pasireotide is a somatostatin receptor analog that has much greater activity on corticotroph adenomas than other somatostatin analogs because it has additional activity at the somatostatin-5 receptor. A large multicenter study has recently shown clinical and biochemical efficacy in patients with Cushing's disease[A3]; the major adverse effect is hyperglycemia and a worsening of preexisting diabetes mellitus. This worsening of glucose levels is likely due to a reduction in insulin and glucagon-like peptide (GLP)-1 levels.

Nelson Syndrome

Nelson syndrome was initially described as the appearance of a pituitary adenoma after bilateral adrenalectomy. In addition to an enlarging pituitary mass, the syndrome is characterized by very high ACTH levels and hyperpigmentation. It is caused by a preexisting ACTH-producing tumor that grows in the absence of feedback inhibition by high levels of glucocorticoids. The incidence of clinically significant Nelson syndrome after adrenalectomy for Cushing's disease varies from 10 to 50% in different series.[20] Patients with Cushing's disease who have undergone adrenalectomy should be followed with imaging studies and plasma ACTH levels, because tumors that cause Nelson syndrome can be very aggressive. When there is evidence of mass effects or rapid growth, transsphenoidal surgery should be performed. Postoperative irradiation may provide additional benefit, although it appears to be less efficacious than in other ACTH-producing adenomas. In theory, Nelson syndrome could also occur in patients being treated with mifepristone, and such patients should also be monitored with periodic pituitary MRI scans, although short-term follow-up data are reassuring at this point.

GONADOTROPINS (FOLLICLE-STIMULATING HORMONE AND LUTEINIZING HORMONE)

The pituitary glycoprotein hormones include FSH, LH, and TSH. Chorionic gonadotropin, which is structurally very similar to LH, is made in the placenta. Each of the glycoprotein hormones has a specific β-subunit that forms a noncovalently bound dimer with the common α-subunit. The α- and β-subunits each undergo glycosylation, which is important for correct hormone folding, intracellular transport, and secretion. Glycosylation is also required for biologic activity, presumably because of effects on the tertiary structure of the hormones. The gonadotropins are involved in sexual differentiation, sex steroid production, and gametogenesis. The regulation and physiologic roles of gonadotropins are quite different in males and females.

In males, receptors for FSH are located on Sertoli cells and seminiferous tubules, whereas LH receptors are located on Leydig cells in the testis. LH stimulates androgen production by the Leydig cells. FSH is involved primarily in sperm maturation in the seminiferous tubules. Thus, FSH and LH act together to induce spermatogenesis (Chapter 234).

In females, ovarian FSH receptors are located on granulosa cells, where they induce enzymes involved in estrogen biosynthesis. LH receptors are located predominantly on thecal cells in the ovary and stimulate the production of ovarian androgens and steroid precursors that are transported to granulosa cells for aromatization to estrogens. The pattern of FSH and LH secretion during the menstrual cycle results in follicular recruitment and maturation (largely FSH mediated), followed by ovulation (largely LH mediated) and steroid production by the corpus luteum (Chapter 235).

Gonadotropin secretion is regulated primarily by the hypothalamic decapeptide GnRH. The gonadotroph cell is exquisitely sensitive to the pattern of GnRH stimulation. Continuous, rather than pulsatile, exposure to GnRH causes gonadotroph desensitization and suppression of LH and FSH. Gonadotroph sensitivity to GnRH is modulated by sex steroids and probably other hypothalamic peptides such as neuropeptide Y. Increased GnRH secretion, in combination with a higher density of GnRH receptors and rising estradiol concentrations, accounts in part for the dramatic release of gonadotropins that induces ovulation.

Hypogonadotropic Hypogonadism

CLINICAL MANIFESTATIONS AND DIAGNOSIS

Clinical features of hypogonadotropic hypogonadism in women are primarily due to estrogen deficiency and include breast atrophy, vaginal dryness, and diminished libido. Hot flashes are uncommon, in contrast to postmenopausal estrogen deficiency. In premenopausal women, normal menstrual cycles provide evidence for an intact hypothalamic-pituitary-gonadal axis. LH and FSH levels should be increased in postmenopausal women, and normal levels may indicate deficiency. Hypogonadism in men causes decreased libido and sexual function. In men, low testosterone without elevation of LH and FSH is consistent with impaired hypothalamic-pituitary reserve. GnRH stimulation can distinguish hypothalamic and pituitary deficiency but may require multiple injections to prime the pituitary.

A congenital form of hypogonadotropic hypogonadism is caused by deficiency of GnRH, which in turn causes deficiencies of LH and FSH. When associated with anosmia (absent sense of smell), the condition is referred to as Kallmann's syndrome (Chapter 223).

Secondary hypogonadotropic hypogonadism is relatively common. In most cases, it is reversible and is caused by weight loss, anorexia nervosa, stress, heavy exercise, or severe illness. Reversible forms of secondary hypogonadotropic hypogonadism are caused by GnRH deficiency and are more common in women than men.

A variety of pathologic conditions can cause secondary hypogonadotropic hypogonadism, often in association with deficiencies of other pituitary hormones (see Table 224-1). These include hypothalamic lesions and central nervous system irradiation. Pituitary tumors can suppress gonadotropins because of stalk compression and disruption of pulsatile GnRH input, as well as by direct destruction of normal pituitary tissue. Hyperprolactinemia can suppress GnRH and lead to reduced gonadotropin levels.

In contrast to the aforementioned causes of hypogonadotropic hypogonadism that result from GnRH deficiency, primary deficiencies of LH and FSH are uncommon. An acquired form of isolated gonadotropin deficiency is rarely encountered and may have an autoimmune basis. Mutations in the *LHβ* or *FSHβ* genes have been described in case reports and cause selective loss of individual gonadotropins. Inactivating mutations in the GnRH receptor and the LH and FSH receptors causing hypogonadotropic hypogonadism have also been reported.

In premenopausal women, preparations of estrogen and progestins should be used for hormonal replacement and to allow cyclical growth of the endometrium. Pulsatile GnRH (for GnRH-deficient patients) has been given to induce ovulation and fertility but is not commonly used at present. Gonadotropin injections are more commonly used when fertility is desired. Testosterone can be replaced in men, using intramuscular injections that are given at 2- to 4-week intervals. Doses and the intervals between injections should be adjusted on an individual basis using libido and testosterone levels before the next injection as a guide. Oral preparations of androgens should be avoided because of hepatotoxicity. Transdermal patch and gel preparations are also available and maintain more stable testosterone levels but are more expensive. With gels, care has to be used to prevent exposure of the partner or children. Although induction of spermatogenesis can be achieved using pulsatile GnRH (for GnRH-deficient patients), injections of gonadotropins are more commonly used.

Pulsatile GnRH has been used to induce puberty and fertility in both males and females with Kallmann's syndrome and other forms of GnRH deficiency, but more commonly, injections of gonadotropins are used.

Secondary hypogonadotropic hypogonadism is ideally treated by correcting the underlying cause.[21] Many women have a discrete threshold for weight or exercise level that will cause loss of menstrual periods. When it is not possible to correct the underlying abnormality, hormonal replacement can be used in women for protection against osteopenia and to cycle the endometrium. Permanent idiopathic hypogonadotropic hypogonadism can also occur in both sexes and will require hormone replacement.

Follicle-Stimulating Hormone– and Luteinizing Hormone–Producing Tumors

PATHOBIOLOGY

The majority (70 to 80%) of pituitary tumors classified previously as nonfunctioning adenomas can be shown to produce low levels of intact glycoprotein hormones or their uncombined α- or β-subunits. Biosynthetic defects in the tumor cells account for relatively inefficient hormone secretion as well as the propensity to produce uncombined subunits. FSH is produced more commonly than LH. Elevated levels of free α-subunits are noted more often than increased free β-subunits.

CLINICAL MANIFESTATIONS

Gonadotropin-producing tumors are somewhat more common in men than women and increase in prevalence with age. FSH- and LH-producing tumors do not usually cause a characteristic hormone excess syndrome. The tumors, typically large macroadenomas, present as clinically nonfunctioning tumors with symptoms and signs related to local mass effects. Visual field loss is found in more than 70% of patients. Many are detected incidentally by CT and MRI performed for unrelated indications. Symptoms of hypogonadism with loss of libido are also common. Men with predominantly FSH-secreting tumors may present with testicular enlargement from hypertrophy of the seminiferous tubules but may also be hypogonadal due to low levels of testosterone. These patients must be distinguished from those with primary hypogonadism due to testicular dysfunction. Tumors that primarily secrete LH are rare but can cause increased testosterone levels. Premenopausal women with gonadotropin-producing tumors may experience menstrual irregularity or secondary hypogonadism. Postmenopausal women often show reduced gonadotropin levels because the mass effects of the gonadotropin-producing tumors cause stalk compression, impairing GnRH stimulation of gonadotropins from normal pituitary cells.

DIAGNOSIS

Because of the absence of a clinical syndrome in most patients, almost all gonadotropin-producing pituitary tumors are diagnosed by postoperative immunohistochemistry, because they had presented with mass effects. There is no particular clinical benefit to distinguish whether a nonfunctioning adenoma is truly a gonadotroph adenoma. Some patients can have moderately elevated PRL levels that are caused by tumor mass effects. It is important to distinguish this group from patients with true prolactinomas. As noted earlier, many women, including those in the postmenopausal group, have

paradoxically low gonadotropin levels. Thus, the absence of elevated gonadotropins does not exclude the diagnosis of a gonadotropin-producing tumor.

Because the major symptoms of the gonadotropin-producing tumors are due to extrasellar extension and local mass effects, the main aim of treatment is reduction in tumor size. Complete or partial reversal of visual field defects and hypopituitarism can be accomplished by surgery unless these conditions have been of long standing. Transsphenoidal surgery is rarely curative, however, because of the large size of the tumors. Patients with significant residual tumor may benefit from radiation therapy. Because most tumors are slow growing, when no tumor is visible postoperatively by MRI, the patient may be followed with yearly monitoring for tumor recurrence, using visual fields and CT or MRI. If tumor markers such as free α- or β-subunit levels are available, they can also be used to monitor tumor function. When follow-up studies show tumor regrowth, repeat surgery, radiation therapy, or both are indicated. Medical therapy with dopamine agonists and somatostatin analogues has been successful in only a minority of patients.

THYROID-STIMULATING HORMONE

Like the other glycoprotein hormones, TSH is a heterodimer composed of the common α-subunit and the unique TSH β-subunit. Normal levels of TSH range from 0.4 to 4.0 μU/mL. The detection limit for current TSH assays is less than 0.01 μU/mL, allowing measurement of suppressed TSH levels in patients with hyperthyroidism. TSH controls thyroid hormone (T_4 and T_3) synthesis and secretion from the thyroid gland. Hypothalamic TRH stimulates TSH synthesis and secretion. Somatostatin and dopamine can inhibit TSH secretion, but their roles in normal physiology have not been clearly elucidated. Thyroid hormones have an inhibitory effect on the production of TRH and TSH and constitute a powerful negative feedback loop acting at both the hypothalamic and pituitary levels. Secretion of TSH is pulsatile, but the amplitude of the pulses is relatively small and does not create the difficulties in measurement of TSH that are encountered with measurements of other pituitary hormones. Because of the integrated nature of the hypothalamic-pituitary-thyroid axis, thyroid function tests are best interpreted when concentrations of TSH, free T_4, and free T_3 levels are known. Except in conditions of secondary hypothyroidism or TSH-secreting pituitary tumors (see later), TSH levels provide an excellent screening test for thyroid dysfunction.

Central Hypothyroidism

Central forms of hypothyroidism are due to loss of either TSH or TRH.[22] Three different types of congenital TSH deficiency are caused by genetic mutations. One type involves mutations in the *TSHβ* gene. A second involves mutations in *PIT1*, which causes combined deficiencies of GH, PRL, and TSH (see earlier). A third involves a mutation in the gene for TRH. Acquired central forms of hypothyroidism are usually associated with other pituitary hormone deficiencies, and usually there is no goiter because of low TSH levels.

Tests for TSH deficiency are best performed by analyzing free T_4 levels in combination with TSH. Low free T_4 without elevated TSH is consistent with central hypothyroidism. In some patients with hypothalamic disease, the TSH level is partially elevated in the presence of low levels of free T_4, but the bioactivity of the TSH is reduced. Central forms of hypothyroidism must be distinguished from the sick-euthyroid condition (Chapter 226). Laboratory tests in the sick-euthyroid syndrome progress through several phases but can include prolonged periods when both TSH and free thyroid hormone levels are low. It can be very difficult in these patients to exclude central hypothyroidism unequivocally. In addition to the clinical setting in which thyroid function tests are measured, the presence of normal thyroid function tests before the illness and the absence of known hypothalamic or pituitary disease make true central hypothyroidism unlikely. Increased levels of reverse T_3 are suggestive of sick-euthyroidism, and free T_4 may be in the normal or low-normal range in sick-euthyroid patients. When TSH deficiency is documented, thyroid hormone is replaced using daily doses of L-thyroxine (0.05 to 0.15 mg/day). Because TSH cannot be used as an end point, one monitors the patient clinically and with serum levels of free T_4 and T_3.

Thyroid-Stimulating Hormone–Secreting Tumors

TSH-secreting tumors are rare and account for between 1 and 3% of pituitary tumors. A recent analysis from Sweden showed that the prevalence was only

2.8 per 1 million.[23] As many as 45% of TSH-producing tumors are plurihormonal. GH and PRL are co-secreted most often, perhaps reflecting the common cellular lineage for thyrotrophs, somatotrophs, and lactotrophs. Long-standing severe hypothyroidism can cause thyrotroph hyperplasia and pituitary enlargement. These hyperplastic masses regress with thyroid hormone replacement therapy, however. Most true TSH-producing tumors are relatively autonomous and respond weakly, if at all, to TRH stimulation or thyroid hormone suppression.

TSH-secreting tumors are usually macroadenomas by the time a diagnosis has been made. Consequently, many patients exhibit mass effects of the tumor, as well as hyperthyroidism. The clinical features of TSH-secreting tumors resemble those of Graves' disease, except that features of autoimmunity (e.g., ophthalmopathy) are absent. Circulating levels of T_4 and T_3 range widely but can be elevated as much as two- to three-fold. Diffuse goiter is present in most patients with TSH-producing tumors, and the 24-hour uptake of radioiodine is elevated.

Because feedback inhibition of TSH is impaired in TSH-producing tumors, TSH levels are inappropriately elevated in the presence of high levels of T_4 and T_3. TSH levels produced by tumors range from the low-normal range to as high as 500 μU/mL, but most levels are minimally elevated. Most TSH-producing tumors (>80%) secrete excess free α-subunit, and its assessment can be very useful in confirming the diagnosis. Thus, the diagnosis can usually be made by demonstrating that a hyperthyroid patient has a detectable serum TSH level associated with excess secretion of the free α-subunit. The finding of a mass lesion on CT or MRI confirms the diagnosis. Several other causes of inappropriate TSH secretion should be considered, including resistance to thyroid hormone and familial dysalbuminemic hyperthyroxinemia and other disorders that alter serum thyroid hormone binding proteins.

TREATMENT   Rx

The goals of therapy are to treat the underlying TSH-secreting tumor and to correct the hyperthyroidism. Transsphenoidal surgery alone is rarely curative because of the large size of most tumors, but it can alleviate mass effects and lower TSH levels. As in other large pituitary tumors, adjunctive irradiation may be required to control tumor growth. Somatostatin analogues have been used as adjunctive medical therapy, and they decrease TSH and α-subunit levels in about 80% of patients with TSH-secreting tumors, but consistent effects on tumor growth have not been demonstrated. Hyperthyroidism caused by TSH-secreting tumors can also be treated using antithyroid drugs or radioiodine.

CLINICALLY NONFUNCTIONING PITUITARY TUMORS

Most clinically nonfunctioning adenomas can be shown to produce low levels of the free α-subunit, free β-subunits of FSH and LH, and intact FSH and LH when analyzed by immunocytochemistry or messenger RNA expression. A smaller fraction can be shown to produce low levels of other pituitary hormones, particularly ACTH or GH, that escaped detection based on routine endocrine testing.[24] Even with detailed analyses of hormone production, a subset (10 to 20%) of nonfunctioning adenomas does not appear to produce any of the known pituitary hormones.

The clinical features and management of nonfunctioning tumors are similar to those for gonadotropin-producing tumors. The major signs and symptoms result from tumor mass effects that cause visual field defects, headache and other neurologic symptoms, and hypopituitarism. Transsphenoidal surgery is the primary mode of treatment, with a goal of debulking the tumor to relieve mass effects. Because there are no serum tumor markers, patients must be followed by CT or MRI in conjunction with visual field tests.

Some pituitary tumors are discovered as incidental findings on CT or MRI scans that were done for other reasons.[25] Such tumors should be screened for hormone oversecretion with measurement of PRL, IGF-I, and a midnight salivary cortisol or an overnight dexamethasone suppression test, but most will be found to be nonfunctioning. If the tumor abuts the optic chiasm, a formal visual field examination should be performed. Over several years, about 10% of incidental microadenomas and 20% of macroadenomas enlarge. Indications for surgery include compression of the optic chiasm, with or without visual field defects and significant tumor enlargement. Hypopituitarism is also a relative indication for surgery (Fig. e224-1). In the absence of these indications for surgery, it is reasonable to follow such patients with MRI scans to look for size change at yearly intervals initially and then at less frequent intervals.

Grade A References

A1. Barake M, Klibanski A, Tritos NA. Effects of recombinant human growth hormone therapy on bone mineral density in adults with growth hormone deficiency: a meta-analysis. *J Clin Endocrinol Metab.* 2014;99:852-860.
A2. Gadelha MR, Bronstein MD, Brue T, et al. Pasireotide versus continued treatment with octreotide or lanreotide in patients with inadequately controlled acromegaly (PAOLA): a randomised, phase 3 trial. *Lancet Diabetes Endocrinol.* 2014;2:875-884.
A3. Colao A, Petersenn S, Newell-Price J, et al. A 12-month phase 3 study of pasireotide in Cushing's disease. *N Engl J Med.* 2012;366:914-924.

GENERAL REFERENCES

For the General References and other additional features, please visit Expert Consult at https://expertconsult.inkling.com.

225

POSTERIOR PITUITARY

JOSEPH G. VERBALIS

ANATOMY AND HORMONE SYNTHESIS

The hormones of the posterior pituitary, vasopressin and oxytocin, are synthesized in specialized neurons in the hypothalamus, the neurohypophysial neurons. These neurons, notable for their large size, are termed *magnocellular neurons.* In the hypothalamus, the magnocellular neurons are clustered in the paired paraventricular and supraoptic nuclei (Fig. 225-1). Vasopressin and oxytocin are also synthesized in parvicellular (i.e., small cell) neurons of the paraventricular nuclei, and vasopressin (but not oxytocin) is also synthesized in the suprachiasmatic nucleus.

Transcription of vasopressin and oxytocin messenger RNA and translation of the vasopressin and oxytocin prohormones occur entirely in the cell bodies of the neurohypophysial neurons. The prohormones provasopressin and pro-oxytocin are packaged along with processing enzymes into neurosecretory granules that are transported out of the perikaryon of the neurohypophysial neurons via microtubules and down the long axons that form the supraopticohypophysial tract, which terminates in the posterior pituitary. During transport, the processing enzymes cleave provasopressin into vasopressin (9 amino acids), vasopressin-neurophysin (95 amino acids), and vasopressin glycopeptide, or copeptin (39 amino acids). Pro-oxytocin is similarly cleaved to oxytocin (which differs from vasopressin by only two of nine amino acids) and oxytocin-neurophysin. The neurophysins form neurophysin-hormone complexes that stabilize the hormones. Stimulatory (e.g., glutamatergic, cholinergic, and angiotensin) neurotransmitter terminals and inhibitory (e.g., γ-aminobutyric acid and noradrenergic) neurotransmitter terminals control the release of vasopressin through the activity of synaptic contacts on the neurohypophyseal cell bodies. Physiologic release of vasopressin or oxytocin into the general circulation occurs at the level of the posterior pituitary, where, in response to an action potential, intracellular calcium is increased and causes the neurosecretory granules to fuse with the axon membrane, thereby releasing each hormone into the general circulation. Although each of the other prohormone fragments are released into the circulation, vasopressin and oxytocin are the only biologically active components of the prohormones. Factors that stimulate the release of neurohypophysial hormones also stimulate their synthesis. Because synthesis is delayed, maintenance of a large store of hormone in the posterior pituitary is essential to enable the instantaneous release of each hormone that is necessary following acute hemorrhage (vasopressin) or during parturition (oxytocin). In most species, sufficient vasopressin is stored in the posterior pituitary to support maximal antidiuresis for several days and to maintain baseline levels of antidiuresis for weeks.

Vasopressin

Vasopressin and Regulation of Osmolality

The primary physiologic action of vasopressin is its function as a water-retaining hormone. The central sensing system (osmostat) for controlling the release of vasopressin is anatomically discrete, located in a small area of the hypothalamus just anterior to the third ventricle (see Fig. 225-1). The

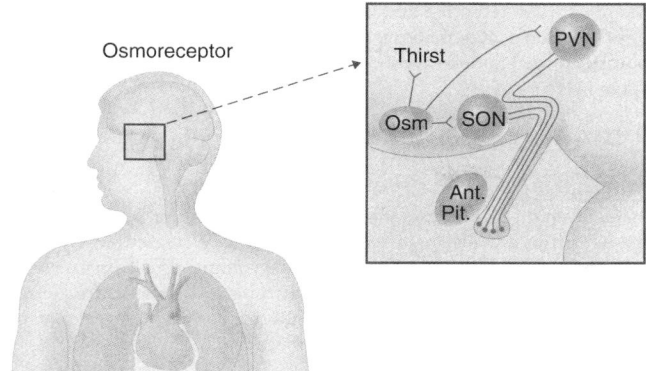

FIGURE 225-1. Sagittal view of the head, demonstrating the position of the neuro-hypophysis. The magnocellular neurons are clustered in two paraventricular nuclei (PVN) and two supraoptic nuclei (SON). Only one nucleus of each pair is illustrated. The supraoptic nuclei are lateral to the edge of the optic chiasm, whereas the paraventricular nuclei are central along the wall of the third ventricle. The axons of the four nuclei combine to form the supraopticohypophysial tract as they course through the pituitary stalk to their storage terminals in the posterior pituitary. The osmostat (Osm) is in the hypothalamus anterior to the third ventricle; the thirst center (Thirst) is distributed across different brain areas. Ant. Pit. = anterior pituitary. (From Buonocore CM, Robinson AG. Diagnosis and management of diabetes insipidus during medical emergencies. *Endocrinol Metab Clin North Am.* 1993;22:411-423.)

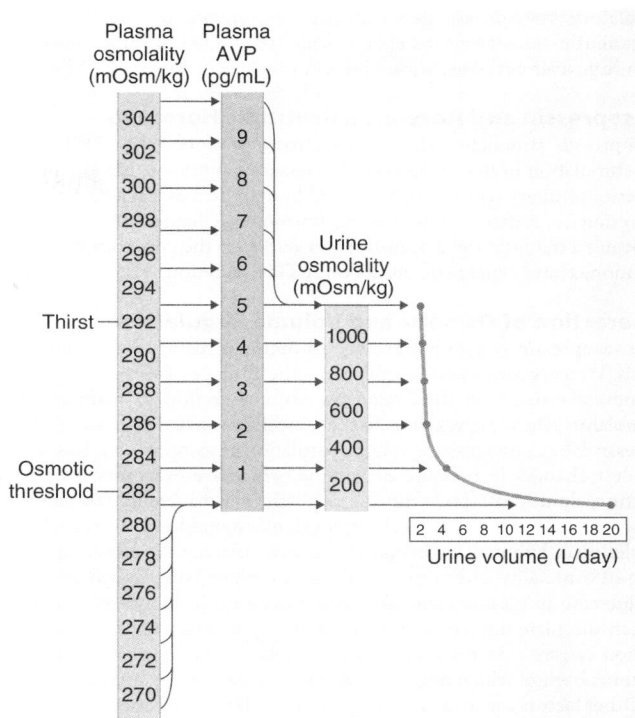

FIGURE 225-2. Idealized schematic of the normal physiologic relationships among plasma osmolality, plasma vasopressin (AVP), urine osmolality, and urine volume. The entire physiologic range of urine osmolality occurs with plasma vasopressin levels from 0 to 5 pg/mL. Increases in plasma osmolality above approximately 290 to 295 mOsm/kg H_2O result in increases in plasma vasopressin but no further concentration of the urine, which is limited by the maximal osmolality in the inner medulla. The relation of volume (calculated on the basis of a constant osmolar load) is inversely exponential to the other parameters. Because of this relationship, urine volume does not change substantially until there is nearly absent vasopressin secretion, after which urine volume increases dramatically. (Calculated from formulas presented in Robertson GL, Shelton RL, Athar S. The osmoregulation of vasopressin. *Kidney Int.* 1976;10:25-37. Figure drawn by J.G. Verbalis, Georgetown University, Washington, DC.)

osmostat controls the release of vasopressin to cause water retention and also stimulates thirst to cause water repletion.

Osmotic regulation of vasopressin release and osmotic regulation of thirst are usually tightly coupled, but they can be dissociated under pathologic conditions. The primary extracellular osmolyte to which the osmoreceptor responds is sodium. Under normal physiologic conditions, glucose and urea cross neuron cell membranes and do not stimulate the release of vasopressin. Although basal osmolality in normal subjects ranges between 280 and 295 mOsm/kg H_2O, extracellular fluid osmolality for each individual is maintained within narrow ranges. Increases in plasma osmolality as small as 1 to 2% are sufficient to stimulate vasopressin release. Basal plasma levels of vasopressin are generally 0.5 to 2 pg/mL, which maintains urine osmolality above plasma osmolality and urine volume in the range of 2 to 3 L/day. When vasopressin levels are suppressed below 0.5 pg/mL, maximal urine osmolality decreases to below 100 mOsm/kg H_2O, and a free water diuresis (or "aquaresis") ensues at levels that approach 800 to 1000 mL/hour (18 to 24 L/day). Increases in plasma osmolality cause a linear increase in plasma vasopressin and a corresponding linear increase in urine osmolality. At a plasma osmolality of approximately 295 mOsm/kg H_2O, urine osmolality is maximally concentrated to 1000 to 1200 mOsm/kg H_2O. Thus, the entire physiologic range of urine osmolality is accomplished by relatively small changes in plasma vasopressin levels of 0 to 5 pg/mL (Fig. 225-2).

To maintain fluid balance, water must be not only conserved but also consumed to replace insensible water losses and obligate urine output. Thirst is not stimulated until a somewhat higher plasma osmolality (5 to 10 mOsm/kg H_2O) than the threshold for release of vasopressin. Most humans derive sufficient water from habitual fluid intake and catabolism of food to maintain plasma osmolality below the threshold that activates thirst. Therefore, under normal physiologic conditions, water balance (and hence plasma osmolality) is regulated more by secretion of vasopressin than by thirst. However, with severe degrees of dehydration, thirst is essential to restore body water deficits.

Vasopressin acts on the V$_2$ subtype of vasopressin receptors in the collecting duct principal cells of the kidney to cause water retention, or antidiuresis. Vasopressin V$_2$ receptors are G protein–coupled receptors that activate adenylate cyclase, with subsequent increased intracellular cyclic adenosine monophosphate (cAMP) levels upon ligand activation of the receptor. The increased cAMP initiates the movement of aquaporin-2 (AQP2) water channels to the apical (luminal) membrane of the collecting duct cells. These channels allow facilitated rapid transport of water from the collecting duct lumen into the principal cell along osmotic gradients. The water then exits the cell through the basolateral membrane into the kidney medullary circulation through constitutively expressed aquaporin-3 and aquaporin-4 water channels.[1] This entire process is termed *antidiuresis*. In the absence of vasopressin, the AQP2 channels are reinternalized from the apical membrane into subapical vesicles. This prevents active reabsorption of water from

the collecting duct lumen, resulting in diuresis. In addition to this rapid "shuttling" of the AQP2 channels to regulate water reabsorption on a minute-to-minute basis, vasopressin also acts through the V$_2$ receptors to regulate long-term stores of AQP2—that is, increased vasopressin stimulates AQP2 synthesis, and the absence of vasopressin results in decreased AQP2 synthesis. The hypertonic medullary interstitium is the determinant of the maximal concentration of the urine, which is in equilibrium with the osmolality of the inner medulla of the kidney under conditions of maximal antidiuresis (Chapter 115).

Vasopressin and Pressure and Volume Regulation

High-pressure baroreceptors are located in the aorta and carotid sinus, and low-pressure baroreceptors are located in the right and left atria. Decreases in blood pressure or intravascular volume stimulate vasopressin release, whereas situations that increase blood volume or left atrial pressure (e.g., negative-pressure breathing) decrease the secretion of vasopressin. The release of vasopressin in response to changes in volume or pressure is much less sensitive than the release in response to osmoreceptors; generally a 10 to 15% reduction in blood volume or pressure is needed to stimulate the release of vasopressin. However, once arterial pressure falls below this threshold, the stimulated response is exponential resulting in plasma levels of vasopressin that are markedly greater than those resulting from osmotic stimulation.

The pressor effects of vasopressin are mediated through a separate vasopressin receptor subtype, the V$_{1a}$ receptors, located on vascular smooth muscle. The relatively insensitive regulation of vasopressin secretion by changes in volume and pressure and the modest role of vasopressin to regulate blood pressure are consistent with the notion that regulation of sodium homeostasis by the renin-angiotensin-aldosterone system (Chapter 227) is more important for controlling extracellular and blood volume than is the regulation of water homeostasis. However, the pressor effects of vasopressin to increase blood pressure can become prominent when other blood pressure regulatory systems are deficient (e.g., autonomic neuropathy or renin-angiotensin-aldosterone system blockade) or in states of pathologic vasodilation (e.g., liver cirrhosis, septic shock).

Vasopressin and Adrenocorticotropic Hormone

Vasopressin stimulates adrenocorticotropic hormone (ACTH) secretion via stimulation of the vasopressin V_{1b} receptor subtypes that are located on anterior pituitary corticotroph cells. Although the major regulator of ACTH secretion is corticotropin-releasing hormone (Chapter 224), vasopressin activates a different signal transduction system in the corticotrophs, so these hormones have synergistic effects on ACTH secretion.

Interaction of Osmotic and Volume Regulation

The vasopressin system has evolved to optimize mammalian water homeostasis. Water is consumed as available in the absence of stimulated thirst, and vasopressin secretion then regulates water excretion to maintain plasma osmolality. Thirst serves as a backup mechanism if dehydration becomes excessive. Because pressure-volume regulation of vasopressin is less sensitive, modest changes in pressure or volume, which are exacerbated by upright posture, do not interfere with the regulation of osmolality. Yet the pressor effect of high vasopressin levels serves to maintain blood pressure if volume depletion or hypotension becomes excessive. Usually, the physiologic regulation of osmolality and pressure-volume are synergistic. Dehydration causes an increase in plasma osmolality and a decrease in blood volume, both of which stimulate the release of vasopressin. Conversely, excess fluid administration causes a decrease in plasma osmolality and an expansion of blood volume, both of which inhibit vasopressin secretion.

Other factors can also modulate osmotic release and action of vasopressin. With volume expansion, natriuretic factors such as atrial natriuretic peptide and brain natriuretic peptide are released from atrial myocytes and act at the kidney to induce a natriuresis. Brain natriuretic peptide is also synthesized in the hypothalamus, where it may act to decrease vasopressin secretion. During pregnancy, there is a decrease of plasma osmolality by approximately 10 mOsm/kg H_2O as a result of a resetting of the osmostat for vasopressin secretion, and the osmostat for thirst is reset downward in parallel. These effects appear to be mediated by the placental hormone relaxin.

Abnormalities in water and electrolyte balance are common in the elderly. This is due in part to age-related changes in body volume (as much as a 50% decrease in total body water occurs in those older than 75 years) and renal function. The elderly also have a decreased sense of thirst. Although there is a normal or even increased ability to secrete vasopressin with age, there is a decreased ability to achieve either maximal urine concentration to retain water or maximal dilution of urine to excrete water. Consequently, the elderly are particularly prone to both hypernatremia or hyponatremia with diseases that affect water balance or from the drugs used to treat various diseases.[2]

Oxytocin

Prolactin is the main hormone necessary for milk production, but oxytocin is essential for milk secretion. Suckling stimulates tactile receptors, producing an afferent signal to the hypothalamus that causes a synchronized release of oxytocin from the posterior pituitary. Oxytocin binds to oxytocin receptors in the breast and induces contraction of myoepithelial cells around the alveoli and ductules to eject milk. In addition, upregulation of uterine oxytocin receptors dramatically increases uterine smooth muscle contractions in response to oxytocin secretion at the end of pregnancy. The greatest release of oxytocin occurs with, not before, delivery of the infant, probably secondary to stretching of the vaginal wall. Because transgenic mice lacking either oxytocin or oxytocin receptors have normal parturition, oxytocin release may be more important to induce uterine contraction to inhibit blood loss after delivery than to initiate parturition. No pathologic syndromes of either increased or decreased secretion of oxytocin have yet been defined, but experimental studies have implicated oxytocin in maternal and affiliative behavior as well as bone formation.[3] However, because of the structural similarity between vasopressin and oxytocin, at high plasma levels oxytocin can activate vasopressin receptors, and vasopressin can activate oxytocin receptors, both of which can have pathologic consequences.

● SYNDROME OF INAPPROPRIATE ANTIDIURETIC HORMONE SECRETION

Excess secretion of vasopressin can be caused by abnormally regulated secretion from the posterior pituitary, or by ectopic synthesis and secretion of vasopressin by tumors. Osmotically inappropriate secretion of vasopressin causes renal water retention and volume expansion of body fluids, with consequent dilutional hyponatremia. This disorder is called the syndrome of inappropriate antidiuretic hormone secretion (SIADH) and is discussed in Chapter 116.

● DIABETES INSIPIDUS

DEFINITION

Diabetes insipidus is the excretion of a large volume of hypotonic insipid (tasteless) urine, usually manifested by polyuria (increased urination) and polydipsia (increased thirst).[4] The large urine volume, usually in excess of 50 to 60 mL/kg/day, must be distinguished from an increased frequency of small urine volumes and from large volumes of isotonic or hypertonic urine, both of which have different clinical significance.

PATHOBIOLOGY

Five pathophysiologic mechanisms must be considered in the differential diagnosis of diabetes insipidus.

1. Central diabetes insipidus is caused by the inability of the hypothalamus–posterior pituitary to secrete (and usually to synthesize) vasopressin in response to increased osmolality. No concentration of the dilute glomerular filtrate takes place in the renal collecting duct, and consequently, a large volume of hypotonic (i.e., dilute) urine is excreted. This produces a secondary increase in serum osmolality, with stimulation of thirst and secondary polydipsia. Levels of vasopressin in plasma are unmeasurable or inappropriately low for the plasma osmolality.

2. Nephrogenic diabetes insipidus is caused by the inability of an otherwise normal kidney to respond to vasopressin. As in hypothalamic (central) diabetes insipidus, the dilute glomerular filtrate entering the collecting duct is excreted as a large volume of hypotonic urine. The rise in plasma osmolality that occurs stimulates thirst and produces polydipsia. Unlike central diabetes insipidus, however, measured levels of vasopressin in plasma are high or appropriate for plasma osmolality.

3. Gestational diabetes insipidus is a rare condition produced by elevated levels or activity of placental cystine aminopeptidase (oxytocinase or vasopressinase) during pregnancy. The rapid destruction of vasopressin produces diabetes insipidus with polyuria and secondary stimulation of thirst with polydipsia. Because of the circulating vasopressinase, plasma vasopressin levels usually cannot be measured.

4. Primary polydipsia is a disorder of excess fluid ingestion rather than of vasopressin secretion or activity. Excessive ingested water produces a mild decrease in plasma osmolality that shuts off the secretion of vasopressin. In the absence of vasopressin action on the kidney, urine does not become concentrated, and a large volume of hypotonic urine is excreted. The amount of vasopressin in plasma is unmeasurable or low but is appropriate for the low plasma osmolality.

5. Osmoreceptor dysfunction is a variant of central diabetes insipidus in which the neurohypophysis is intact, but the osmoreceptive cells in the anterior hypothalamus have been damaged (see Fig. 225-1). Because the osmoreceptor cells are necessary for osmotically stimulated vasopressin secretion, the patient manifests polyuria. However, because the osmoreceptor cells also control thirst, these patients do not have polydipsia. As a result, they are characterized by elevated serum sodium levels and plasma osmolalities. For this reason, this disorder has also been called essential hypernatremia and adipsic hypernatremia, in recognition of the profound thirst deficits found in most of the affected patients.

Although the pathophysiologic mechanisms for each of these five disorders are distinct, patients in the first four categories usually manifest polyuria and polydipsia, and the serum sodium level is usually normal because an intact thirst mechanism is sufficiently sensitive to maintain water homeostasis in the first three disorders, and the normal kidney has sufficient capacity to excrete the excess water load in the fourth. The fifth category of osmoreceptor dysfunction is the exception, owing to a defective thirst mechanism leading to hypernatremia.

CLINICAL MANIFESTATIONS

Central Diabetes Insipidus

The sudden appearance of hypotonic polyuria[5] after transcranial surgery in the area of the hypothalamus or after head trauma with basal skull fracture and hypothalamic damage obviously suggests the diagnosis of central diabetes insipidus.[6] In these situations, if the patient is unconscious and unable to recognize thirst, hypernatremia is a common accompaniment. However, even in patients with more insidious progression of a specific disease or in patients with idiopathic central diabetes insipidus, the onset of polyuria is often relatively abrupt and occurs over several days or weeks. Most patients do not notice polyuria until urine volume exceeds 4 L/day, and as illustrated in Figure 225-2, urine volume does not exceed 4 L/day until the ability to concentrate the urine is severely limited and plasma vasopressin is nearly absent. As few as 10 to 15% of the normal number of vasopressinergic neurons in the hypothalamus is sufficient to maintain an asymptomatic urine volume, but the further loss of just a small number of these neurons produces a rapid increase in urine volume and symptomatic polyuria. Urine volume seldom exceeds the amount of dilute fluid delivered to the collecting duct ($\approx$18 to 24 L in humans); in many cases, urine volume is significantly less because patients voluntarily restrict fluid intake, which causes some mild volume contraction and increased proximal tubular reabsorption of fluid. Patients often express a preference for cold liquids, which are more effective in assuaging thirst. Both thirst and increased urine output persist through the night, impairing sleep. Patients with partial central diabetes insipidus have some ability to secrete vasopressin, but this secretion is markedly attenuated at normal levels of plasma osmolality. Therefore, these patients often have symptoms and urine volume similar to those of patients with complete central diabetes insipidus. Because most patients with central diabetes insipidus have sufficient thirst to drink fluid to match urine output, few laboratory abnormalities are present at the time of initial evaluation. The serum sodium level can be in the high-normal range, whereas the blood urea nitrogen level can be low secondary to the large urine volume. Uric acid is relatively high because of the modest volume contraction and lack of action of vasopressin on V_{1a} receptors in the kidney, which stimulate the clearance of uric acid. Uric acid levels greater than 5 mg/dL can distinguish diabetes insipidus from primary polydipsia.

Osmoreceptor Dysfunction

A variant of central diabetes insipidus is the syndrome of osmoreceptor dysfunction. Physiologic maneuvers demonstrate that when patients are euvolemic, an increase in plasma osmolality produces neither secretion of vasopressin nor a sensation of thirst. However, vasopressin is still synthesized by the hypothalamus and stored in the posterior pituitary, because stimulation of baroreceptors by hypovolemia or hypotension results in the prompt secretion of vasopressin; the kidney is responsive because vasopressin release by volume receptor stimulation causes urinary concentration. Because patients lack thirst, they are chronically dehydrated, often with markedly increased serum sodium levels. However, it is the dehydration-induced volume depletion, not the increased osmolality, that eventually stimulates the secretion of vasopressin. The volume of urine output depends on the degree of dehydration-induced secretion of vasopressin. If sufficient fluid replacement is given to return extracellular fluid volume to normal, these patients are unable to regulate vasopressin by osmolality and again become polyuric, thereby manifesting their underlying central diabetes insipidus. Lesions that cause osmoreceptor dysfunction are similar to lesions that can cause central diabetes insipidus, but in contrast to central diabetes insipidus these lesions usually occur more rostrally in the hypothalamus, consistent with the anterior hypothalamic location of the primary osmoreceptor cells (see Fig. 15-2). One lesion that is unique to this disorder is an anterior communicating cerebral artery aneurysm, particularly following resection of the aneurysm.

Central diabetes insipidus can be inherited as an autosomal dominant disease that is typically characterized by an asymptomatic infancy and an onset later in childhood. Most genetic defects are either in the signal peptide of the pre-prohormone or in the neurophysin portion of the prohormone.[7] Mutations involving the vasopressin sequence itself are few. Most cases are believed to result from disruption of cleavage from the signal peptide or abnormal folding of the neurophysin, which slows trafficking of the mutant prohormone through the endoplasmic reticulum, leading to neuronal cell dysfunction and/or death. Because this is a cumulative process, this explains the later onset of central diabetes insipidus with these types of mutations.

Myxedema and adrenal insufficiency both impair the ability to excrete free water by renal mechanisms. The simultaneous occurrence of either of these diseases with central diabetes insipidus (as can occur with a tumor of the hypothalamus or pituitary) can decrease an otherwise large urine output, thereby masking the symptoms of diabetes insipidus. Replacement treatment for the anterior pituitary deficiency, especially glucocorticoids, can then cause a sudden and massive excretion of dilute urine. Similarly, the onset of either hypothyroidism or adrenal insufficiency during the course of diabetes insipidus can decrease the need for vasopressin replacement and in some cases can even cause hyponatremia. Central diabetes insipidus occurs commonly in patients with severe brain ischemia, and is often indicative of

brain death. Treatment of the diabetes insipidus along with any coexistent anterior pituitary hormone deficiencies can be used to preserve donor organs in such cases.

Nephrogenic Diabetes Insipidus

Nephrogenic diabetes insipidus is caused by mutations of the vasopressin V_2 receptor or the vasopressin-induced water channel AQP2, or by impairments in the signal transduction system linking V_2 receptor activation and AQP2 membrane insertion. Familial nephrogenic diabetes insipidus is a rare disease, most cases of which (>90%) are due to mutations of the V_2 receptor. More than 100 different V_2 receptor mutations have been described and can be classified into several different general categories based on differences in transport of the mutant receptor to the cell surface and vasopressin binding or stimulation of adenylate cyclase. Because the gene for the V_2 receptor is located on the X chromosome, this is an X-linked recessive disease. Symptoms are noted only in affected males, who often present with vomiting, constipation, failure to thrive, fever, and polyuria during the first week of life. Hypernatremia with a hypotonic urine is typically present. The phenotype is similar in the less than 10% of patients with mutations of the AQP2 water channel, but because the AQP2 gene is located on chromosome 12, mutations cause autosomal recessive disease; consequently, consanguinity and a family history of the disease in men and women is common, and this disorder should be suspected when the proband is female.[8]

Nephrogenic diabetes insipidus can also be acquired during treatment with certain drugs such as demeclocycline (which can be used to treat inappropriate secretion of vasopressin), lithium carbonate (used to treat bipolar disorders), and fluoride (previously used in fluorocarbon anesthetics), and from electrolyte abnormalities such as severe hypokalemia and hypercalcemia. All causes of acquired nephrogenic diabetes insipidus have in common the decreased synthesis and function of AQP2 due to impaired vasopressin signaling from V_2 receptor binding and activation. Other diseases of the kidney can produce polyuria and inability to concentrate the urine secondary to altered renal medullary blood flow or to other disorders that inhibit maintenance of the hyperosmolar concentrating gradient in the inner medulla. Renal manifestations of such disorders (e.g., sickle cell disease, sarcoidosis, pyelonephritis, multiple myeloma, analgesic nephropathy) are discussed in Chapter 121.

Gestational Diabetes Insipidus

In pregnancy, there is an increased metabolism of vasopressin due to cystine aminopeptidase (oxytocinase or vasopressinase), an enzyme that degrades oxytocin and prevents premature uterine contractions. Normally, this is compensated for by increased synthesis and secretion of vasopressin. Rarely, women with normal regulation of vasopressin develop diabetes insipidus because of markedly elevated levels of vasopressinase. Some of these patients have accompanying preeclampsia, acute fatty liver, and coagulopathies, but causal relations between diabetes insipidus and these abnormalities have not been identified. In general, diabetes insipidus does not persist after the pregnancy ends and does not recur in subsequent normal pregnancies.[9]

Polyuria can also manifest in patients who have limited vasopressin reserve (partial central diabetes insipidus) or who respond poorly to vasopressin action (compensated nephrogenic diabetes insipidus). Treatment may be required only during the pregnancy, and the patient often returns to her previous baseline function without the need for therapy when the pregnancy ends. Less commonly, central diabetes insipidus of another cause first becomes symptomatic during pregnancy and then persists afterward, following the usual course of diabetes insipidus.

Primary Polydipsia

Excessive fluid intake also causes hypotonic polyuria and, by definition, polydipsia. This disorder must be differentiated from the various causes of diabetes insipidus. Despite normal pituitary and kidney function, patients with this disorder share many characteristics of both central diabetes insipidus (vasopressin secretion is suppressed as a result of decreased plasma osmolality) and nephrogenic diabetes insipidus (kidney AQP2 expression is decreased as a result of suppressed plasma vasopressin levels). Many different names have been used for this excessive fluid intake, including dipsogenic diabetes insipidus, but primary polydipsia remains the best descriptor to avoid confusing this order with diabetes insipidus as classically defined.

Primary polydipsia is sometimes due to a severe mental illness such as schizophrenia, mania, or obsessive-compulsive disorder, in which case it is called psychogenic polydipsia. These patients usually deny true thirst and attribute their polydipsia to bizarre motives, such as a need to cleanse the body of poisons. The incidence in psychiatric hospitals can be as high as 40%, and there is no obvious explanation for the polydipsia. Primary polydipsia can also be caused by an abnormality in the osmoregulatory control of thirst, in which case it is called dipsogenic diabetes insipidus. These patients have no overt psychiatric illness and invariably attribute their polydipsia to a nearly constant thirst. Dipsogenic diabetes insipidus is usually idiopathic, but it can also be secondary to organic structural lesions in the hypothalamus identical to those causing central diabetes insipidus, such as neurosarcoidosis of the hypothalamus, tuberculous meningitis, multiple sclerosis, or trauma. Consequently, all polydipsic patients should be evaluated with magnetic resonance imaging (MRI) of the brain before it is concluded that excessive water intake is due to an idiopathic or psychiatric cause. Primary polydipsia can also be produced by diseases or drugs that cause a dry mouth, or by any peripheral disorder causing marked elevations of renin or angiotensin.

Finally, primary polydipsia is sometimes caused by physicians, nurses, lay practitioners, or health writers who recommend a high fluid intake for valid (e.g., recurrent nephrolithiasis) or unsubstantiated health reasons. These patients lack overt signs of mental illness, but they also deny thirst and usually attribute their polydipsia to habits acquired from years of adherence to a drinking regimen. Laboratory studies in these patients are generally normal, although the serum sodium concentration is sometimes at the low end of the normal range, and the level of uric acid is lower than in patients with other forms of diabetes insipidus.

DIAGNOSIS
Physiologic Diagnosis
Diabetes insipidus should be considered in all patients presenting with significant polyuria, defined as urine output greater than 50 mL/kg/day. Although osmotic diuresis secondary to hyperglycemia, intravenous contrast agents, or renal injury is a more common clinical cause of polyuria, the medical history, an isotonic urine osmolality, and routine clinical laboratory tests generally distinguish these disorders from diabetes insipidus. A diagnosis of diabetes insipidus can be made when urine osmolality is inappropriately low in the presence of an elevated plasma osmolality as a result of increased serum sodium concentration. These criteria are sometimes met at the initial examination, especially in cases of acute diabetes insipidus occurring after trauma or surgery with inadequate fluid replacement. In such patients with hypernatremia and hypotonic urine osmolality with normal renal function, one need only administer a vasopressin agonist to differentiate central diabetes insipidus, in which a renal response with decreased urine volume and increased urine osmolality occurs, from nephrogenic diabetes insipidus, in which a subnormal renal response is seen. Sometimes in the postoperative state, a water diuresis occurs as a result of water retention during the surgical procedure. Vasopressin is normally secreted in response to surgical stress, causing fluid administered intravenously during the procedure to be retained. During recovery, vasopressin levels fall, and a diuresis of the retained fluid occurs. In this case, the serum sodium level is almost always normal; however, if additional fluid is administered to match the urine output, persistent polyuria can be mistaken for diabetes insipidus. In this situation, the physician should decrease the rate of fluid administered and follow the urine output and serum sodium level. If the urine output decreases and the serum sodium level remains normal, no treatment is necessary; if serum sodium rises above the normal range and the urine remains hypotonic, diabetes insipidus is likely, and the response to a vasopressin agonist can ascertain the type (central versus nephrogenic).

Most outpatients with diabetes insipidus are not hypernatremic, because the polydipsia produced by a normal thirst response is generally sufficient to maintain water homeostasis. Instead, they present with polyuria, polydipsia, and a normal sodium level. In these patients, further testing is necessary to increase serum osmolality and then measure the plasma vasopressin level or the urinary response to an administered vasopressin agonist. The best described test is the water deprivation test (Fig. 225-3),[10] which should be carried out under controlled observation in the hospital or an appropriately equipped outpatient area. The exact timing of the test depends on the patient's symptoms. If the patient has marked polyuria during the night, it is best to begin the test during the day because the patient may become overly dehydrated overnight. However, if the patient has only two or three episodes of nocturia per night, it is best to begin the test in the evening so that the major part of the dehydration takes place when the patient is asleep. In either case, the patient is weighed at the beginning of the test, and all subsequent fluids are withheld. The volume and osmolality of all excreted urine are measured, and the patient is reweighed after each liter of urine output. When three

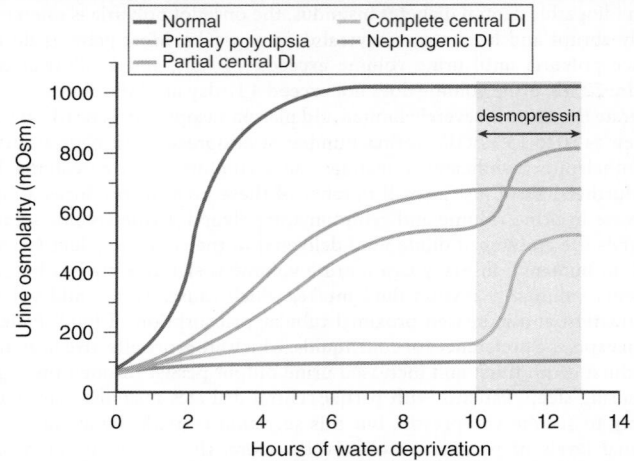

FIGURE 225-3. Responses to the water deprivation test to differentiate various types of diabetes insipidus (DI) and primary polydipsia (as described by Miller M, Dalakos T, Moses AM, et al. Recognition of partial defects in antidiuretic hormone secretion. *Ann Intern Med.* 1970;73:721-729). The response to dehydration reaches a plateau, and the subsequent change in urine osmolality in response to administered desmopressin is illustrated. See the discussion in the text.

consecutive urine samples have an osmolality differing by no more than 10% and the patient has lost at least 2% of body weight, a blood sample is obtained for the measurement of serum osmolality, sodium, and plasma vasopressin. The patient is then given 2 μg of desmopressin intravenously or intramuscularly and observed for an additional 2 hours.

Adults with normal vasopressin secretion concentrate their urine to greater than 800 mOsm/kg H_2O and have less than a 10% increase in urine osmolality in response to administered desmopressin. Patients with complete central diabetes insipidus have minimal concentration of the urine with dehydration, and a marked increase in urine osmolality (usually >50%) in response to administered desmopressin. Patients with nephrogenic diabetes insipidus usually have no increase in urine concentration in response to administered desmopressin, although in some cases of acquired nephrogenic diabetes insipidus, some increased urinary concentration (but generally < 10%) can occur. Nephrogenic diabetes insipidus is best distinguished from central diabetes insipidus by the measurement of vasopressin in plasma; plasma vasopressin levels are elevated in cases of nephrogenic diabetes insipidus, especially after dehydration.

In patients with partial central diabetes insipidus and patients with primary polydipsia, the urine is often somewhat concentrated in response to dehydration, but not to the maximum of a normal person. The chronically reduced level of vasopressin downregulates the synthesis of AQP2 water channels, and the large urine volume, regardless of cause, washes out the medullary osmotic gradient that is the determinant of maximal urine concentration. When desmopressin is administered, patients with partial central diabetes insipidus have a further increase (usually > 10% but < 50%) in urine osmolality, whereas most patients with primary polydipsia have no further increase (i.e., <10%). However, the reliability of distinguishing between these two disorders by the water deprivation test is suboptimal. Some patients with primary polydipsia may not become sufficiently dehydrated to secrete maximal vasopressin and hence have an increase in urine osmolality in response to administered desmopressin. Alternatively, some patients with partial central diabetes insipidus can become sufficiently dehydrated that their maximal concentration of urine is reached during the test, and no further concentration is seen with administered desmopressin. Plasma vasopressin levels at the end of dehydration are better at discriminating between these two disorders, but only at high serum sodium concentrations (i.e., >145 mmol/L). Consequently, some investigators recommend a limited infusion of hypertonic (3%) sodium chloride solution to achieve these elevated levels if they are not achieved by the water deprivation itself. Measurement of the C-terminal fragment of the vasopressin prohormone copeptin may be a better surrogate measure of vasopressin secretion.[11]

In some difficult cases, the response to treatment with a vasopressin agonist can be a useful aid to diagnosis. If a decrease in polyuria and thirst with maintenance of normal serum sodium concentration occurs, a diagnosis of partial central diabetes insipidus is likely; however, if polydipsia persists and hyponatremia develops, a diagnosis of primary polydipsia is confirmed.

Etiologic Diagnosis

If the water deprivation test confirms that inadequate vasopressin secretion is responsible for the polyuria, the underlying cause must be determined. MRI of the hypothalamic-pituitary area is the most important diagnostic tool in these cases. The three areas of interest are the immediate suprasellar region of the hypothalamus, the pituitary stalk, and the posterior pituitary within the sella turcica (see the earlier discussion of anatomy). Most slow-growing tumors confined to the sella do not cause diabetes insipidus. To cause central diabetes insipidus, tumors in the hypothalamic area immediately above the sella must be either sufficiently large to destroy 80 to 90% of the vasopressin cells or located where the paths of the four nuclear groups converge at the origin of the pituitary stalk, just above the diaphragma sellae. Primary tumors, especially craniopharyngioma and suprasellar germinoma, metastatic tumors, and infiltrative diseases can also cause diabetes insipidus by infiltration of the pituitary stalk, which is then thickened (i.e., >2 mm) on MRI. On T1-weighted MRI, the vasopressin and oxytocin stored in neurosecretory granules in the posterior pituitary are visualized as a bright spot in the sella turcica. Most but not all normal subjects have this bright spot (it is absent more frequently in elderly and dehydrated patients); in most but not all patients with central diabetes insipidus, the bright spot is absent. Thickening of the stalk and absence of the bright spot are therefore especially suggestive of a hypothalamic disease process.[12]

Tumors that cause central diabetes insipidus are most often benign primary intracranial tumors such as craniopharyngioma, ependymoma (suprasellar germinoma), and pinealoma, which arise in the third ventricle. Primary tumors of the anterior pituitary (Chapter 224) cause diabetes insipidus only when substantial suprasellar extension is present. However, rapidly growing intrasellar lesions, such as metastases from carcinomas of the lung, breast, and melanoma or hemorrhage into pituitary adenomas, can cause diabetes insipidus because there is insufficient time for the vasopressin axons to adapt by releasing vasopressin from the hypothalamus. Metastases to the hypothalamus can also destroy the supraopticohypophysial tract and produce diabetes insipidus. Granulomatous diseases, such as Langerhans cell histiocytosis, sarcoidosis, tuberculosis, and leukemic infiltrates and lymphomas of the hypothalamus, can cause diabetes insipidus by destroying vasopressin cells. In such patients, the diagnosis is usually suspected on the basis of peripheral manifestations of the respective diseases. Lymphocytic infundibuloneurohypophysitis is an autoimmune disease similar to lymphocytic hypophysitis of the anterior pituitary (Chapter 224) in which lymphocytes infiltrate the neurohypophysis to produce diabetes insipidus. The hallmarks of this process are a thickened pituitary stalk and an absence of the pituitary bright spot in a patient with the abrupt onset of polyuria and polydipsia, particularly a postpartum female. The diagnosis was originally demonstrated by pituitary biopsy, but now is more commonly made by regression of the thickened stalk with continued MRI follow-up. When no specific cause is identified, the diagnosis of exclusion is idiopathic diabetes insipidus; but most such cases are probably caused by an autoimmune disease, and other autoimmune diseases, including anterior pituitary hypophysitis,[13] are often recognized in affected patients. When central nervous system disease is suspected but not diagnosed by MRI or general physical examination, cerebrospinal fluid obtained by lumbar puncture may be helpful in identifying tumor cells or markers of tumors or inflammatory processes (e.g., elevated angiotensin-converting enzyme levels with neurosarcoidosis, elevated β-HCG levels with germinomas). A family history suggestive of diabetes insipidus should be investigated with genetic testing for inherited mutations in the vasopressin or vasopressin receptor genes depending on the site of the defect.

TREATMENT Rx

Because excess excretion of water is the primary manifestation of diabetes insipidus, water replacement in adequate quantities avoids the metabolic complications of all forms of this disease. However, oral or intravenous administration of the volume of fluid required to replace the often large urinary losses in diabetes insipidus is difficult and inconvenient. The goal of therapy is therefore to reduce the amount of polyuria and polydipsia to a tolerable level while avoiding overtreatment, which can produce water retention and hyponatremia.

Central Diabetes Insipidus

The best therapeutic agent for the treatment of central diabetes insipidus is the vasopressin agonist desmopressin.[14] Desmopressin is different from vasopressin in that the amino group of the N-terminal cystine residue has been removed to prolong the duration of action, and D-arginine has been substituted for L-arginine in position 8 to decrease the vasopressor effects. At therapeutic dosages, this agent acts primarily on V_2 or antidiuretic receptors, with minimal activity at V_{1a} or pressor receptors. Desmopressin is available as tablets of 0.1 or 0.2 mg for oral administration and in either a spray bottle that delivers a fixed dose of 10 μg in 100 μL or a bottle with a rhinal catheter that can deliver 50 to 200 μL (5 to 20 μg) for intranasal administration. When therapy is initiated, it is generally best to begin with a low dose (e.g., half of a 0.1-mg tablet, 5 μg by the rhinal tube, or a single 100 μL spray of 10 μg) at bedtime to allow the patient to sleep through the night, and then determine the duration of action by quantifying the polyuria the next day. The duration of action of a single dose varies from 6 to 24 hours, but in most patients, a good therapeutic response can be achieved on an every-12-hour schedule for the nasal spray or an 8- or 12-hour schedule for the tablets. Desmopressin is also available for parenteral use in 1-mL vials of 4 μg/mL. Parenteral administration is especially useful postoperatively or when a patient is unable to take the nasal preparation. In hospitalized patients, some physicians add vasopressin directly to a crystalloid solution to infuse doses in the range of 0.25 to 2.7 mIU/kg/hour to cause modest but persistent urinary concentration as a treatment of diabetes insipidus. With any form of desmopressin administration, serum sodium levels should be monitored regularly to prevent the development of hyponatremia.[15]

Osmoreceptor Dysfunction

Because the diabetes insipidus of patients with osmoreceptor dysfunction is central, they respond to desmopressin as do patients with central diabetes insipidus. However, because of their thirst defect, this is usually not sufficient to maintain normal plasma osmolality. Consequently, they must be given a "prescription" for amounts of fluids to be consumed each 24 hours in order to maintain normal serum sodium levels and plasma osmolalities. This must be individualized to each patient because overconsumption of fluid coupled with desmopressin administration can produce severe hyponatremia. Body weights using an accurate scale is useful as a guide to preventing under- or overhydration, but frequent monitoring of serum sodium levels is usually necessary as well.

Nephrogenic Diabetes Insipidus

Although most patients with nephrogenic diabetes insipidus do not respond to desmopressin, a small number have a partial response to higher doses (e.g., 10 to 20 μg subcutaneously or intranasally). For the majority of patients who have no response to desmopressin, some orally administered pharmacologic agents are also useful in treating nephrogenic diabetes insipidus. Thiazide diuretics cause sodium depletion and volume contraction and decrease urine volume by increasing proximal tubular reabsorption of glomerular filtrate. Prostaglandin synthase inhibitors (e.g., indomethacin) block the action of prostaglandin E to inhibit the action of vasopressin on the kidney. Chlorothiazide, amiloride, and prostaglandin synthase inhibitors are useful to reduce polyuria in nephrogenic diabetes insipidus. However, none of these agents has been approved by the U.S. Food and Drug Administration for the treatment of diabetes insipidus; therefore, the prescribing physician should be aware of potential toxicities and side effects. In cases of drug-induced nephrogenic diabetes insipidus, the most direct therapy is discontinuation of the offending agent, if possible. Symptomatic nephrogenic diabetes insipidus is usually treated with a thiazide diuretic, which is enhanced by coadministration of the potassium-sparing diuretic amiloride. Amiloride can be especially beneficial in cases of nephrogenic diabetes insipidus induced by lithium, because the drug decreases the entrance of lithium into cells in the distal tubule. When diuretics are used to treat nephrogenic diabetes insipidus, special attention should be paid to the possibility that the induced dehydration may increase the concentration of other drugs.

Gestational Diabetes Insipidus

During pregnancy, vasopressinase increases the metabolism of vasopressin but not of desmopressin, so desmopressin is the drug of choice for these patients. The vasopressinase activity subsides by a few weeks after delivery, and patients with the onset of partial diabetes insipidus during pregnancy may become asymptomatic after delivery. An additional advantage of desmopressin is that it has little action on the oxytocin receptors of the uterus. During pregnancy, normal plasma osmolality decreases by approximately 10 mOsm/kg H$_2$O because of changes in serum sodium, so pregnant patients with diabetes insipidus require only enough desmopressin to maintain the serum sodium at this lower level.

Correction of Hyperosmolality

Some situations require special attention during therapy. Rarely, if patients with diabetes insipidus are unable to drink or are given a hypertonic solution, severe hypernatremia can develop acutely. Osmotic equilibrium with the intracellular water of neurons and glia produces shrinking of the brain. The brain is in a closed vault (i.e., the skull), and when the brain shrinks, traction on the vasculature of the central nervous system can cause the rupture of blood vessels and subarachnoid or intracerebral hemorrhage. If the hypernatremia persists for a longer time, the neurons accommodate by producing organic osmolytes (previously called idiogenic osmoles), which limit the amount of brain shrinkage. Once this adaptation has occurred, a too-rapid lowering of osmolality in the extracellular fluid will produce a shift of water into the brain and cause cerebral edema. In this situation, desmopressin can be administered to produce constant antidiuresis, and the amount of water given can be regulated to decrease osmolality by no more than approximately 12 mEq/L every 24 hours. Postoperatively or after head trauma, diabetes insipidus can be transient (see Prognosis), and the need for long-term maintenance therapy cannot be immediately established.

PROGNOSIS

The prognosis of properly treated diabetes insipidus is excellent. If nephrogenic diabetes insipidus is diagnosed and treated early, intracranial calcification and mental retardation do not occur. When the diabetes insipidus is secondary to a recognized disease process, that disease generally determines the ultimate prognosis. In some specific clinical situations, the course is different and characteristic. The development of diabetes insipidus after surgical or traumatic injury to the neurohypophysis can follow any of several well-defined patterns (Fig. 225-4). In some patients, polyuria develops 1 to 4 days after injury and resolves spontaneously. Less often, the diabetes insipidus is permanent and continues indefinitely. Most interestingly, one can see a "triphasic" response that has been well described after pituitary stalk transection. The first phase of diabetes insipidus is due to axon shock and lack of function of the damaged neurons. This phase lasts several hours to several days and is followed by a second, antidiuretic phase that is due to the uncontrolled release of vasopressin from the disconnected and degenerating posterior pituitary or from the remaining severed neurons. Overly aggressive administration of fluids during this second phase does not suppress the

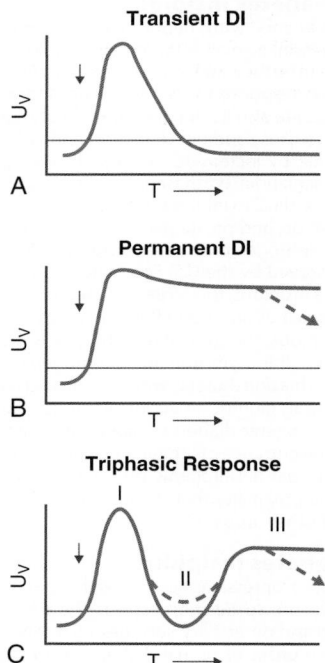

FIGURE 225-4. A to C, Diagrammatic summary of the major patterns of postoperative and post-traumatic diabetes insipidus (DI). The abscissa represents time (T) after the initial injury (*arrow*); the ordinate represents urinary volume (Uv) relative to a hypothetical "normal" urine output of 2 to 3 L/24 hours (*solid line*). See the discussion in the text. During the triphasic response (C), uncontrolled release of vasopressin from the disconnected or damaged posterior pituitary gland causes an antidiuresis that can lead to water retention and a dilutional hyponatremia. Diabetes insipidus returns as the third phase after the stored hormone in the posterior pituitary has been depleted. (From Verbalis JG, Robinson AG, Moses AM. Postoperative and post-traumatic diabetes insipidus. In: Czernichow AP, Robinson A, eds. *Diabetes Insipidus in Man: Frontiers of Hormone Research.* Basel: S Karger; 1985:247.)

uncontrolled vasopressin release from the damaged neurohypophysis and can lead to hyponatremia. The antidiuresis can last 2 to 14 days, after which diabetes insipidus recurs after depletion of vasopressin from the degenerating posterior pituitary gland (third phase). Transient hyponatremia without preceding or subsequent diabetes insipidus has been reported after transsphenoidal surgery for pituitary microadenomas.

Once a deficiency of vasopressin secretion has been present for more than a few weeks, it rarely improves, even if the underlying cause of the neurohypophysial destruction is eliminated. The major exception to this is postoperative diabetes insipidus, in which spontaneous resolution is the rule. Although recovery from diabetes insipidus that persists more than several weeks postoperatively is less common, and is uncommon after 1 year of continued diabetes insipidus, well-documented cases of recovery as long as 10 years after the initiating event have been reported. Potential return of function is a reason to occasionally withhold therapy during long-term treatment. Diabetes insipidus should not be considered idiopathic until at least 4 years of follow-up. During this interval, annual computed tomography or MRI is indicated to search for a tumor or infiltrative process that may not have been detected at the initial examination.

GENERAL REFERENCES

For the General References and other additional features, please visit Expert Consult at https://expertconsult.inkling.com.

226

THYROID

MATTHEW KIM AND PAUL W. LADENSON

The adult thyroid gland contains two lobes that wrap along the anterolateral aspects of the trachea, midway between the thyroid cartilage and the suprasternal notch. Each lobe is demarcated into upper, middle, and lower poles. The right and left lobes are connected by an isthmus on the anterior aspect of the trachea just below the cricoid cartilage. The normal terminus of the thyroglossal duct can persist as a pyramidal lobe, which is often palpably enlarged in diffuse thyroid disorders such as autoimmune thyroiditis and Graves disease.

With thyroid enlargement, the attachment of the sternothyroid muscle to the trachea limits upward expansion of the lobes, but further lateral, posterior, and downward growth may lead the gland to extend into the superior mediastinum, compressing the trachea and veins at the thoracic outlet. The parathyroid glands usually lie behind the superior and inferior poles of the thyroid lobes. The recurrent laryngeal nerves course upward along the tracheoesophageal groove, from which branches pass behind each thyroid lobe to innervate the larynx.

Thyroid tissue is composed of clustered spherical follicles, each containing a single layer of follicular epithelial cells known as thyrocytes that surround a lumen containing colloid. The principal component of colloid is thyroglobulin, a thyrocyte-specific protein. Parafollicular C cells, which are derived from neural crest tissue and produce calcitonin, are widely dispersed between follicles.

PHYSIOLOGY
Thyroid Hormone Synthesis and Secretion

Dietary iodine in the form of iodide (I^-) or iodate (IO_3^-) is absorbed by the gastrointestinal tract and distributed in the extracellular fluid. Daily iodine intake in the United States equals or exceeds the recommended daily intake of 150 μg because of the widespread use of iodized salt and iodate preservatives in baked goods. Circulating iodide is actively transported into the thyrocyte by the sodium-iodide symporter. Within the thyrocyte, iodide is rapidly oxidized by H_2O_2 in a reaction catalyzed by thyroid peroxidase. The reactive intermediate formed is covalently bound to tyrosyl residues present in thyroglobulin to generate monoiodotyrosine and diiodotyrosine residues through a process known as organification. Thyroid peroxidase also catalyzes the coupling of the monoiodotyrosine and diiodotyrosine residues to generate thyroxine (T_4) and triiodothyronine (T_3) residues in thyroglobulin, which is secreted into the follicular lumen. Thyroglobulin is then pinocytosed at the apical membrane, and T_4 and T_3 are secreted after proteolysis of thyroglobulin. In the normal state, approximately 100 μg of T_4 and 5 μg of T_3 are directly released into the circulation each day. Pharmacologic amounts of iodine inhibit iodide trapping, organification, and release of the thyroid hormones. Lithium can also block thyroid hormone release.

Thyroid Hormone Transport and Metabolism

Circulating thyroid hormones are more than 99% bound to three classes of plasma proteins. Thyroxine-binding globulin (TBG) functions as the principal transport protein. Thyroxine-binding prealbumin (also known as transthyretin) and albumin make lesser contributions to T_4 and T_3 transport in blood. Pregnancy and exposure to pharmacologic doses of estrogens can increase the TBG level, as can hepatitis, familial TBG excess, and certain medications including 5-fluorouracil, tamoxifen, and methadone. Conversely, decreased TBG levels may occur with systemic illness, severe hepatic disease, nephrotic syndrome, and treatment with androgens, glucocorticoids, and slow-release nicotinic acid. Whereas total T_4 and T_3 levels rise and fall with changes in TBG, free T_4 and T_3 levels remain constant. Familial dysalbuminemic hyperthyroxinemia is an autosomal dominant disorder characterized by the production of an albumin fraction that binds T_4 with a higher-than-normal affinity. Affected individuals may present with high total T_4 levels with an inappropriately normal thyroid-stimulating hormone (TSH), and with normal free T_4 when this is measured by equilibrium dialysis.

The receptor binding and biologic activity of T_3 is eight-fold greater than that of T_4. More than 80% of the T_3 present in target tissues is derived from T_4 through the action of deiodinase enzymes that remove an outer-ring iodine, converting T_4 to T_3, generating the pool of T_3 in target tissues, and contributing to T_3 in the circulation. The type 2 deiodinase is present in the pituitary gland and brain, whereas type 1 deiodinase predominates in other peripheral tissues such as the liver and kidney. Activity of these deiodinases may be inhibited by systemic illness, iodide-containing compounds (e.g., amiodarone, radiocontrast agents), glucocorticoid therapy, and selenium deficiency. T_4 can also be converted by inner-ring deiodination to biologically inactive reverse T_3 (rT_3) by type 1 deiodinase and the type 3 deiodinase present in glial cells of the central nervous system. It deactivates thyroid hormone by inner-ring monodeiodination, a process that converts T_4 to inactive reverse T_3 (rT_3) and T_3 to inactive diiodothyronine (T_2). Type 3 deiodinase is also expressed in placenta, accounting for the increased thyroxine dose requirement in pregnant women.

Control of Thyroid Function

The growth of thyroid tissue and the production of thyroid hormones are controlled by the hypothalamus and the pituitary gland. Thyrotropin-releasing hormone (TRH) is a tripeptide synthesized by the hypothalamus and transported to the pituitary gland by the hypothalamic-pituitary portal system, where it binds to receptors on thyrotrophic cells, stimulating the synthesis and secretion of TSH (thyrotropin). TSH is a heterodimeric glycoprotein composed of a unique β-subunit coupled to an α-subunit identical to that present in follicle-stimulating hormone, luteinizing hormone, and chorionic gonadotropin (CG). It is transported in the circulation to the thyroid gland, where it binds to the TSH receptor on thyrocytes. The binding of TSH to the TSH receptor stimulates thyrocyte growth and all of the steps in synthesis and secretion of thyroid hormone. Circulating T_4 and T_3 exert negative feedback at the levels of both the hypothalamus and the pituitary gland, inhibiting the synthesis and secretion of TRH and TSH, respectively.

Thyroid Hormone Action

Thyroid hormone binds receptors that are members of the nuclear receptor superfamily, regulating expression of thyroid hormone–responsive genes. Isoforms of the thyroid hormone receptors (α_1, β_1, and β_2) bind to a specific hexameric oligonucleotide sequence in the transcriptional regulatory region of thyroid hormone–responsive genes. For example, in liver, T_3 increases expression of the low-density lipoprotein (LDL) receptor, resulting in accelerated LDL cholesterol clearance. In myocardium, T_3 increases myocyte contractility and relaxation by promoting expression of alpha myosin heavy chain and sarcoplasmic reticulum adenosine triphosphatase (ATPase), respectively. In the cardiac conducting system, T_3 increases the heart rate by accelerating sinoatrial node depolarization and repolarization. Other physiologic effects of thyroid hormone include increases in basal metabolic rate, mental alertness, ventilatory drive, gastrointestinal motility, and bone turnover. During fetal development, thyroid hormone plays critical roles in brain development and skeletal maturation.

DIAGNOSIS

Physical Examination

Examination of the thyroid begins with inspection of the lower anterior portion of the neck to check for diffuse or asymmetrical gland enlargement, tracheal deviation, lymphadenopathy, and jugular venous distention. Palpation can be performed by an anterior or posterior approach. Anterior palpation can be performed by using the thumb of one hand to locate the isthmus of the gland beneath the cricoid cartilage. The right lobe of the thyroid gland can be palpated by placing the left thumb along the left side of the trachea to displace the contralateral lobe, using the tips of the fingers of the right hand medial to the right sternocleidomastoid muscle at the level of the isthmus, and using the pads of the fingers of the right hand to define, while the patient swallows, the characteristics of that thyroid lobe (i.e., its size, firmness, contour, mobility, and potential tenderness). The maneuver is reversed to examine the left lobe.

Laboratory Findings

TSH and Thyroid Hormone Levels

The serum TSH level is a sensitive indicator of primary thyroid gland dysfunction. Contemporary TSH immunoassays permit accurate detection of all common causes of thyroid hormone deficiency and excess. Indeed, TSH levels even become abnormal when patients' thyroid hormone levels remain within broad reference ranges, conditions termed *subclinical hypothyroidism* and *subclinical thyrotoxicosis*. In most patients with primary thyroid gland dysfunction, measurement of a single TSH level permits an accurate classification of the thyroid status. Limitations of TSH testing occur when there is TSH-mediated secondary thyroid dysfunction, reduced biologic activity of T_3 or TSH itself, temporary disequilibrium of the hypothalamic-pituitary-thyroid axis, or analytic problems affecting the TSH immunoassay. A longitudinal community-based cohort study has documented that aging is associated with increased serum TSH concentrations with no change in free T_4 levels.[1] These findings suggest that the TSH increase in many elderly individuals arises from age-related alteration in the TSH set point or reduced TSH bioactivity, rather than occult thyroid disease.

Measurements of serum T_4 and T_3 levels confirm the significance of an abnormal TSH level, define the severity of thyroid dysfunction, and provide a clue to the underlying cause. Whereas assays that measure total T_4 and T_3 levels are accurate, their results do not distinguish between large plasma protein–bound and free fractions of each hormone. Consequently, congenital and acquired derangements of TBG (and, less commonly, transthyretin and albumin) can alter the total, but not the free T_4 and T_3 levels. These conditions can be misdiagnosed as abnormal thyroid function unless a discordance in TSH is noted or one of these underlying conditions is suspected (Tables 226-1 and 226-2). There are several methods of estimating unbound T_4 and T_3 levels. Free T_4 and free T_3 immunoassays are now widely employed for this purpose and yield reliable results in common conditions that alter plasma protein levels, such as estrogen-induced TBG excess. Free T_4 measurement after equilibrium dialysis of serum is the most accurate approach, but it is technically demanding and less readily available.

Other Laboratory Tests

Measurement of thyroid autoantibody titers can be useful in the evaluation of thyroid dysfunction. Antithyroid peroxidase and antithyroglobulin antibody titers can confirm the diagnosis of autoimmune thyroiditis. TSH receptor binding and stimulating immunoglobulin levels can be used to confirm the diagnosis of Graves disease. The erythrocyte sedimentation rate (ESR) can be helpful in the diagnosis of subacute thyroiditis. Serum thyroglobulin and calcitonin levels are used as tumor markers when observing patients treated for differentiated and medullary thyroid cancers, respectively.

Imaging

Anatomic Imaging

Ultrasonography provides images that characterize the thyroid gland's size, symmetry, texture, vascularity, and structural abnormalities including solid nodules, simple cysts, and partially cystic nodules. Diffuse heterogeneity suggests autoimmune thyroiditis. Certain characteristics of nodules—including their number, echogenicity, capsular regularity, vascularity, and patterns of calcification—alter the probability of malignancy but rarely confirm or

TABLE 226-1 CAUSES OF EUTHYROID HYPERTHYROXINEMIA (INCREASED TOTAL T₄, NORMAL TSH, NORMAL FREE T₄)

Increased synthesis of thyroxine-binding globulin
  Pregnancy
  Hepatitis
  Acute intermittent porphyria
  Drugs
    Estrogens
    Tamoxifen
    Raloxifene
    Methadone
    5-Fluorouracil
Increased binding of thyroid hormone to albumin
  Familial dysalbuminemic hyperthyroxinemia
Increased binding of thyroid hormone to transthyretin
  Hereditary variants
  Pancreatic neuroendocrine tumors

T_4 = thyroxine; TSH = thyroid-stimulating hormone.

TABLE 226-2 CAUSES OF EUTHYROID HYPOTHYROXINEMIA (DECREASED TOTAL T₄, NORMAL TSH, NORMAL FREE T₄)

Increased metabolism of thyroid hormone
  Drugs
    Phenytoin
    Phenobarbital
    Carbamazepine
    Rifampin
Decreased synthesis of thyroxine-binding globulin
  Severe liver disease
  Malnutrition
  Drugs
    Androgens
    Danazol
    L-Asparaginase
Increased clearance of thyroxine-binding globulin
  Nephrotic syndrome
  Protein-losing enteropathy
Decreased binding of thyroid hormone to thyroxine-binding globulin
  Drugs
    Salicylates (high dose)
    Phenytoin (high dose)
    Furosemide (intravenous)

T_4 = thyroxine; TSH = thyroid-stimulating hormone.

TABLE 226-3 ETIOLOGIES OF HYPOTHYROIDISM

PRIMARY HYPOTHYROIDISM

Insufficient functioning thyroid tissue
  Congenital absence of thyroid tissue
  Autoimmune destruction of thyroid tissue
    Autoimmune thyroiditis (Hashimoto's thyroiditis)
  Surgical removal of thyroid tissue
  Radioablation of thyroid tissue by radioactive iodine or external beam radiation
  Infiltrative destruction of thyroid tissue
    Hemochromatosis
    Scleroderma
    Amyloidosis
Impaired thyroid hormone synthesis
  Iodine deficiency
  Congenital enzymatic defects that disrupt thyroid hormone synthesis
  Drug-mediated inhibition of thyroid hormone production and release
    Thionamides
    Amiodarone
    Lithium
    Aminoglutethimide
    Certain tyrosine kinase inhibitors (e.g., sunitinib)

SECONDARY HYPOTHYROIDISM

Insufficient secretion of TRH or TSH
  Hypothalamic disorders
    Tumor (lymphoma, germinoma, glioma)
    Irradiation
    Inflammation (sarcoidosis, vasculitis)
  Hypopituitarism
    Mass lesions
    Pituitary surgery
    Pituitary radiation
    Hemorrhagic apoplexy (Sheehan syndrome)
    Infiltration (hemochromatosis, tuberculosis, fungal infection)
    Lymphocytic hypophysitis
Thyroid hormone resistance syndrome

index of the gland's activity. Typically, technetium pertechnetate uptake at 20 minutes ranges from 0.5 to 3%, whereas radioiodine uptake at 24 hours ranges from 8 to 28%. These fractional thyroid uptakes can be useful in the differential diagnosis of thyrotoxicosis. Radioiodine uptake values are also used to calculate effective ^{131}I doses to be administered for the treatment of hyperthyroidism and thyroid cancer.

HYPOTHYROIDISM

DEFINITION

Primary hypothyroidism (termed *myxedema* when it is severe) refers to hormone deficiency caused by intrinsic thyroid gland dysfunction that disrupts the synthesis and secretion of T_4 and T_3 (Table 226-3). Overt primary hypothyroidism is characterized by an elevated TSH level (usually > 10 mIU/L) in conjunction with a free T_4 level below the lower limit of the reference range. In subclinical hypothyroidism, the TSH level is only modestly elevated; the free T_4 level remains in the low-normal to normal range.

Secondary or central hypothyroidism refers to deficient thyroid gland function that is the result of inadequate stimulation by TSH. This is due in turn to production of either insufficient or inactive TSH from a number of congenital or acquired pituitary and hypothalamic disorders (Chapter 224).

EPIDEMIOLOGY

Primary hypothyroidism is common, occurring in 5% of individuals. Mild hypothyroidism is present in as many as 15% of older adults. Hypothyroidism is more common in women. It is more prevalent among whites and Latin Americans. Secondary hypothyroidism is rare, representing less than 1% of cases.

PATHOBIOLOGY

Dietary iodine deficiency is a cause of primary hypothyroidism in regions where this micronutrient deficiency exists and is uncorrected by iodine supplementation. The most common cause of primary hypothyroidism in developed countries is autoimmune (or Hashimoto's) thyroiditis, a condition in which defective immune tolerance leads to inflammatory destruction of thyroid tissue and impaired gland function.[2] The condition is characterized by a lymphocytic infiltrate and fibrosis. Circulating antithyroid

exclude thyroid cancer with certainty. Imaging of surrounding structures may identify cervical lymphadenopathy not detectable on physical examination.

The value of computed tomography (CT) and magnetic resonance imaging (MRI) lies in their ability to delineate tracheal deviation, narrowing, and substernal extension of the thyroid into the mediastinum. Cervical CT scanning can also help define and localize regional lymphadenopathy. Positron emission tomography (PET) plays a role in the localization of metastatic thyroid cancer.

Functional Imaging

Radionuclide scanning takes advantage of the fact that gamma ray–emitting tracers transported into thyrocytes by the sodium-iodide symporter can generate images that reflect the regional activity of thyroid tissue. Technetium-99m (^{99m}Tc) and iodine-123 (^{123}I) are commonly used for this purpose. ^{99m}Tc-pertechnetate is rapidly trapped by thyrocytes, and scans obtained using this tracer can be acquired 20 to 30 minutes after injection. ^{123}I and ^{131}I thyroid scans generate images that more precisely reflect thyroid tissue function—for example, indicating whether a nodule is hypofunctioning (cold), hyperfunctioning (hot), or equivalent in function to extranodular tissue (warm). However, radionuclide imaging no longer plays a central role in the differential diagnosis of most thyroid nodules. When needed, ^{123}I is the preferred tracer because of its lower thyroidal and whole body radiation dose.

Thyroid Uptake

The fraction of an administered radioactive iodine or technetium dose taken up and retained by the thyroid gland during a defined period represents an antibodies directed against thyroid peroxidase and thyroglobulin are markers of the disease, but glandular inflammation is principally the result of altered T-cell-mediated immunity. There is a genetic predisposition to the condition, with linkage studies suggesting a polygenic basis. Patients with autoimmune thyroiditis may have other endocrine and nonendocrine autoimmune disorders. It may be a component of the type 2 polyglandular autoimmune syndrome associated with autoimmune adrenal insufficiency and type 1 diabetes mellitus. It is less commonly a component of the type 1 syndrome, which includes adrenal insufficiency, hypoparathyroidism, and chronic mucocutaneous candidiasis (Chapter 231). Other nonendocrine autoimmune conditions associated with autoimmune thyroiditis include atrophic gastritis, pernicious anemia, systemic sclerosis, Sjögren's syndrome, celiac disease, and vitiligo. Individuals treated with the immunomodulatory agent interferon-α may develop autoimmune thyroiditis with transient or permanent hypothyroidism.

Surgical resection of the thyroid gland predictably leads to hypothyroidism. Radioactive iodine therapy for treatment of hyperthyroidism commonly destroys sufficient thyroid tissue to cause postablative hypothyroidism. External beam radiation therapy for head and neck cancer can also cause thyroid gland failure. Exposure to pharmacologic and radiocontrast agents that contain large amounts of iodine (e.g., amiodarone, radiocontrast dyes, some expectorants, topical disinfectants) can disrupt thyroid hormone production. Lithium inhibits secretion of T_4 and T_3, leading to hypothyroidism in 10% of treated patients. Other pharmacologic agents reported to cause hypothyroidism include stavudine, thalidomide, lenalidomide, imatinib, sunitinib, sorafenib, motesanib, bexarotene, ipilimumab, and aminoglutethimide.

There are a number of other rare causes of primary hypothyroidism (see Table 226-3). Congenital hypothyroidism can be due to agenesis or dysgenesis of the thyroid gland or to mutations in genes encoding the enzymes catalyzing thyroid hormone synthesis. Infiltrative disorders that can disrupt thyroid function include hemochromatosis, amyloidosis, systemic sclerosis, and invasive fibrous thyroiditis (also known as Riedel's thyroiditis). The thyroid gland inflammation that occurs with subacute thyroiditis and painless (postpartum) thyroiditis causes transient hypothyroidism from which most patients recover. Consumptive hypothyroidism can occur in individuals with hemangiomas expressing the type 3 deiodinase, which converts T_4 to biologically inactive reverse T_3.

Secondary or central hypothyroidism may be caused by a number of disorders that impair normal hypothalamic or pituitary control of the thyroid gland (Chapter 224). Infiltrative disorders affecting the hypothalamus that can interfere with TRH secretion include sarcoidosis, hemochromatosis, and histiocytosis. Masses that impinge on the pituitary stalk can impede TRH delivery through the hypophyseal portal system. Compression of thyrotrophic cells by pituitary adenomas and other masses in the sella turcica can inhibit synthesis and secretion of TSH. Surgery and radiation therapy to treat pituitary adenomas can destroy thyrotrophic cells, leading to secondary hypothyroidism that develops as a component of panhypopituitarism. Other disorders associated with secondary hypothyroidism include lymphocytic hypophysitis, pituitary metastases from primary malignant neoplasms,

apoplexy, infarction caused by hemorrhage at the time of delivery in women (also known as Sheehan syndrome [Chapter 224]), and head trauma.

Symptoms and Signs
Symptoms of hypothyroidism include fatigue, lethargy, weight gain despite poor appetite, cold intolerance, hoarseness, constipation, weakness, myalgias, arthralgias, paresthesias, dry skin, and hair loss. Females may develop precocious puberty, menorrhagia, amenorrhea, and galactorrhea. Affected individuals may experience depressed mood with limited initiative and sociability. Cognitive deficits can range from mild lapses in memory to delirium, dementia, seizures, and coma. The nonspecific nature of most of these symptoms makes it difficult to determine which patients presenting with them have hypothyroidism rather than other causes. Furthermore, in most cases, hypothyroidism is insidious in onset, making its recognition difficult. Symptoms that are new, progressive, or present in combination are more likely to be due to hypothyroidism.

The physical findings associated with hypothyroidism vary according to the age at onset and disease severity. Children may present with delayed linear growth despite weight gain, precocious or delayed puberty, and pseudohypertrophy of muscle. Adults can present with bradycardia, diastolic hypertension, and mild hypothermia. The skin may be coarse, dry, yellow, and cool to the touch as a result of peripheral vasoconstriction. Diffuse thinning of scalp hair accompanied by thinning of the lateral eyebrows may occur. The nails may become brittle. Examination of the chest may reveal distant heart sounds. The extremities may reveal diffuse nonpitting edema caused by the deposition of glycosaminoglycans. Neurologic examination may reveal slow, dysarthric speech and diffuse slowing of deep tendon reflexes with a marked delay in the terminal relaxation phase.

Examination of the neck may reveal a range of findings. Healed cervical incisional scars in this region may indicate a history of surgical resection of thyroid tissue. In autoimmune thyroiditis, the thyroid gland may be normal in size, diffusely enlarged, or atrophic to the degree it may be difficult to palpate at all. It may be soft and smooth with a lobular texture, or firm and irregular with a variegated nodular texture.

Other Routine Test Abnormalities
Routine blood tests may reveal anemia (which is typically macrocytic), hyponatremia, hypoglycemia, and elevated creatine phosphokinase, prolactin, homocysteine, triglyceride, and total and LDL cholesterol levels. Electrocardiography may show sinus bradycardia with low voltage in the limb leads. Chest radiography may show a widened cardiac silhouette, and echocardiography may confirm a pericardial effusion.

Suspected primary hypothyroidism is confirmed by an elevated TSH level (Fig. 226-1). Established reference ranges for TSH levels typically extend from 0.5 to 4.5 mIU/L. However, the distribution of values within this range is skewed toward the lower half, such that the mean TSH level in adults is

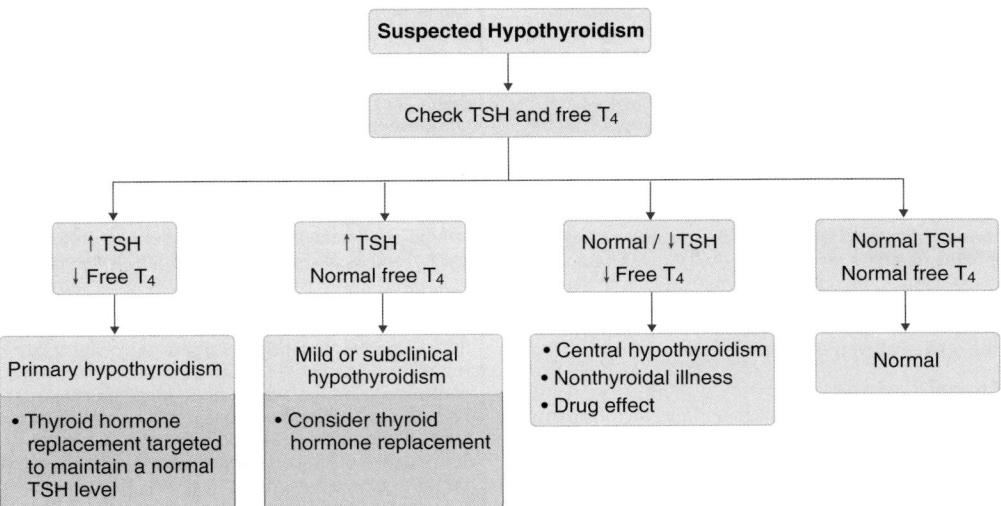

FIGURE 226-1. Laboratory assessment of suspected hypothyroidism. TSH = thyroid-stimulating hormone.

1.5 mIU/L. Measurement of the free T_4 level confirms the diagnosis of primary hypothyroidism and characterizes its severity. A low free T_4 level in conjunction with a persistently elevated TSH level represents overt primary hypothyroidism, whereas a low-normal free T_4 level with an elevated TSH level is termed *mild* or *subclinical primary hypothyroidism*. Other uncommon causes of isolated TSH elevation should be considered in appropriate settings, including recovery from severe systemic illness, renal failure, and adrenal insufficiency.

The underlying cause of primary hypothyroidism is usually clinically obvious, and laboratory testing is unnecessary in most cases. When confirmation is required (e.g., to convince a patient the condition is permanent), serum antithyroid antibodies may be assessed. Measurement of thyroid peroxidase antibody is a more sensitive test than thyroglobulin antibody for this purpose. However, 10% of patients with histologically documented autoimmune thyroiditis have no circulating antithyroid antibodies.

When clinical findings such as the presence of a sellar mass, previous pituitary surgery or irradiation, or other pituitary axis hormone deficiencies suggest the possibility of secondary hypothyroidism, the TSH level cannot be relied on to provide an accurate index of thyroid function. In these settings, the serum free T_4 level must be assessed, and a low or even low-normal free T_4 level can confirm the diagnosis. The TSH level in patients with secondary hypothyroidism can be low, normal, or even modestly elevated.

TREATMENT   Rx

The goals of thyroid hormone replacement therapy are straightforward: to replace endogenous thyroid hormone production, to avoid iatrogenic thyrotoxicosis, and (rarely) to treat systemic complications of severe hypothyroidism. Levothyroxine sodium (hereafter thyroxine) is the hormonal preparation of choice.[3] Thyroxine has a number of favorable pharmacokinetic characteristics. It is well absorbed, and its plasma protein binding gives it a 7-day half-life, permitting daily dosing. Thyroxine is physiologically deiodinated to the more biologically active T_3 in peripheral tissues. However, thyroxine has a narrow therapeutic index, and doses differing by as little as 12% can have clinical consequences. Tablets of multiple dose strengths ranging from 25 to 300 µg are available. Regulatory standards ensure pharmaceutical equivalence in terms of mass of thyroxine, but bioavailability may differ by as much as 12% among different preparations. Consequently, adherence to a single thyroxine formulation is advisable.

The optimal dose of thyroxine for replacement therapy is related to lean body weight, with most adults requiring a daily dose of approximately 1.8 µg/kg. The dose requirement for elderly adults is typically lower (e.g., 1 µg/kg/day) because of slower metabolic clearance. Patients with postsurgical or postablative hypothyroidism usually require a higher daily dose than patients with autoimmune thyroiditis, who may have some residual gland function. Patients with coexisting malabsorptive disorders may require higher and variable doses. Certain medications, mineral supplements, and foods can interfere with thyroxine absorption, including ferrous sulfate, calcium carbonate, aluminum hydroxide, sucralfate, cholestyramine, and soy-containing foods (Table 226-4). Thyroxine doses should be separated from these substances by 8 hours or longer.

Thyroxine dose requirements may increase as a result of accelerated metabolic clearance in several circumstances. Patients with nephrotic syndrome and other systemic illnesses that lead to rapid clearance of thyroid hormone require higher daily doses. Dose requirements increase by an average of 75% in most pregnant women as a result of placental deiodinative metabolism of thyroxine.[4] Simultaneous treatment with phenytoin, phenobarbital, carbamazepine, or rifampin also typically accelerates thyroxine metabolism.

Most adults without known or suspected coronary artery disease can be started on a full replacement dose of thyroxine. The initial dose can be calculated on the basis of the patient's weight and age, rounding down to the nearest available dose strength. For patients with primary hypothyroidism, adequacy of thyroxine therapy can be assessed by TSH measurement 4 to 6 weeks after therapy is started. The target TSH level for most treated individuals should be the lower half of the reference range (i.e., 0.5 to 2.0 mIU/L). Once an adequate dose has been established, the TSH level should be checked annually. In patients with secondary hypothyroidism, the serum free T_4 level should be monitored 2 to 4 weeks after the thyroxine dose is started or adjusted, with a target free T_4 level in the upper half of the reference range.

Management of Complications

Complications of thyroxine therapy are limited to iatrogenic thyrotoxicosis and, rarely, adverse effects of restoring euthyroidism. Typical symptoms and signs of thyrotoxicosis usually accompany significant degrees of overtreatment. However, even a modestly excessive thyroxine dose can induce bone mineral loss, especially in postmenopausal women, and it can increase the risk of atrial fibrillation in older individuals. In patients with underlying coronary

---

TABLE 226-4   INTERFERENCE WITH THYROXINE REPLACEMENT THERAPY

FACTORS CONTRIBUTING TO UNDERREPLACEMENT

Inadequate prescribed dose
Limited compliance
Decreased absorption due to ingestion of agents that bind thyroxine
  Ferrous sulfate
  Calcium carbonate
  Aluminum hydroxide
  Sucralfate
  Cholestyramine
  Soy protein
Increased metabolism of thyroxine
  Pregnancy
  Drugs
    Phenytoin
    Phenobarbital
    Carbamazepine
    Rifampin
Diminishing residual thyroid function
Changing formulations

FACTORS CONTRIBUTING TO OVERREPLACEMENT

Excessive prescribed dose
Factitious ingestion of additional doses
Decreased metabolism of thyroxine due to aging
Increasing residual thyroid function
Changing formulations

---

artery disease, the positive chronotropic and inotropic effects of thyroxine may exacerbate myocardial ischemia.[5] Consequently, adults with known or suspected ischemic heart disease should be started on a low dose that is titrated upward in small increments once tolerance is ensured (e.g., starting with 25 µg daily, then increasing the dose by 12.5 to 25 µg every 4 to 6 weeks). In some cases, β-blocker therapy may need to be intensified to counter the induction of myocardial ischemia. However, deliberate suboptimal dosing of thyroxine should be avoided. If necessary, coronary revascularization may be required before euthyroidism can be fully restored. Coexisting adrenal insufficiency associated with hypopituitarism or the type 2 polyglandular autoimmune syndrome may be unmasked when cortisol clearance is accelerated by a return to the euthyroid state. Other adverse effects that infrequently occur with thyroxine therapy include transient hair loss, acute sympathomimetic symptoms that resolve with dose reduction and slow advancement, and pseudotumor cerebri in children.

A minority of patients with thyroxine-treated hypothyroidism continue to report bothersome symptoms despite biochemical evidence of adequate thyroid hormone replacement. Several randomized clinical trials have shown that combinations of T_3 and T_4—in the form of desiccated thyroid or synthetic thyroid hormone preparations—are not superior to T_4 alone. [A1]

Subclinical and Mild Hypothyroidism

Whether individuals diagnosed with subclinical hypothyroidism (i.e., an elevated or high-normal TSH level with a free T_4 level within the reference range) benefit from thyroxine therapy remains controversial.[6] In practice, many providers opt for a trial of therapy in mildly hypothyroid patients who are symptomatic, have underlying hypercholesterolemia, or have a high likelihood of progressing to overt hypothyroidism. Predictors of progressive thyroid failure include age older than 65 years, TSH level higher than 10 mIU/L, and the presence of circulating thyroid autoantibodies, indicating underlying autoimmune thyroiditis.

Myxedema Coma

Severe hypothyroidism can culminate in myxedema coma, a life-threatening condition characterized by hypothermia, bradycardia, hypotension, altered mental status, and multisystem organ failure. Risk factors include advanced age, poor access to health care, and other underlying major organ system diseases. Most patients have severe and long-standing thyroid hormone deficiency. Treatment should include thyroxine (1.8 µg/kg/day, with or without a 500-µg loading dose). Some experts advocate coadministration of triiodothyronine in divided doses to compensate for impaired conversion of T_4 to T_3. No controlled trials have been performed to evaluate the relative benefits and risks of these different approaches. Glucocorticoids should be administered in stress doses after a cosyntropin stimulation test has been performed to check for evidence of concomitant adrenal insufficiency (Chapter 227). Care should be taken to avoid exposure to potent sedative or analgesic agents that may exacerbate altered mental status. Hypothermia should be treated with external warming to reduce the risk of circulatory collapse.

Nonthyroidal Illness

In patients with severe nonthyroidal illness, a characteristic constellation of thyroid function test changes occurs that often appears to be consistent with hypothyroidism (see Fig. 226-1).[7] The T_3 level usually declines as a result of decreased extrathyroidal T_4-to-T_3 conversion. With increasingly severe disease, total T_4 and free T_4 levels also decline. TSH levels are usually low to low-normal. During the course of recovery, the TSH level can rise above the upper limit of the normal range, producing a profile that can be mistaken for primary hypothyroidism. Clinical correlation is essential to assess thyroid function in severely ill patients (e.g., a history of preexisting thyroid or pituitary disease, the presence of a goiter, or features suggesting other elements of hypopituitarism). Because no benefit of thyroid hormone treatment has been shown for these patients, observation with retesting 6 to 8 weeks after recovery is the preferred approach.

THYROTOXICOSIS

DEFINITION AND EPIDEMIOLOGY

Thyrotoxicosis is a systemic syndrome caused by exposure to excessive thyroid hormone (Table 226-5). Its prevalence is 1 in 2000 adults, affecting 1% of all individuals during the course of their lifetime.

PATHOBIOLOGY

Thyrotoxicosis is the result of excessive circulating and tissue effects of thyroid hormone. Strictly speaking, hyperthyroidism refers to those forms of thyrotoxicosis that are caused by excessive production of thyroid hormone by the thyroid gland due to a thyrotropic stimulus or autonomous thyroid tissue function (see Table 226-5). In Graves disease, the most common cause of hyperthyroidism, the thyroid gland is stimulated by autoantibodies that bind to and activate the TSH receptor. Excessive secretion of TSH causes hyperthyroidism in patients with rare TSH-secreting pituitary adenomas (Chapter 224). CG, a glycoprotein with high TSH homology, can cause transient gestational hyperthyroidism during pregnancy, when a choriocarcinoma or a germ cell tumor produces variant forms of HCG that are more active or when mutant TSH receptors bind HCG more avidly, as occurs in familial gestational thyrotoxicosis.

Autonomous production of thyroid hormone occurs when thyrocytes function independently of TSH receptor activation. This can occur as a result of growth of a benign functioning thyroid adenoma or growth of multiple autonomously functioning nodules forming a toxic multinodular goiter. In rare cases, it can occur when patients with well-differentiated thyroid cancer present with functioning metastases. In some toxic adenomas, somatic

TABLE 226-5 ETIOLOGIES OF THYROTOXICOSIS

HYPERTHYROIDISM

Antibody-mediated stimulation of thyroid tissue
  Graves disease
Autonomously functioning thyroid tissue
  Toxic multinodular goiter
  Toxic adenoma
  Iodine exposure
Autonomously functioning heterotopic thyroid tissue
  Struma ovarii
  Metastatic differentiated thyroid cancer
Excessive secretion of TSH
  TSH-secreting pituitary adenoma

NONHYPERTHYROID THYROTOXICOSIS

Ingestion of exogenous thyroid hormone
  Pharmacologic
    Levothyroxine
    Liothyronine
    Combination preparations
  Nonpharmacologic
    Dietary supplements
    Improperly processed meat products
Inflammation causing release of endogenous thyroid hormone
  Subacute thyroiditis
  Autoimmune thyroiditis

TSH = thyroid-stimulating hormone.

mutations in the TSH receptor gene lead to constitutive activation. In patients whose thyroid glands have the potential for autonomous function, exposure to excessive amounts of iodine in the form of amiodarone or iodinated contrast agents can provoke hyperthyroidism.

Transient thyrotoxicosis can also be caused by inflammatory conditions that release an excessive amount of thyroid hormone stored in the gland (see the section on thyroiditis). These include subacute thyroiditis, which is believed to be caused by a viral infection; acute or suppurative thyroiditis, caused by bacterial infection; radiation-induced thyroiditis; and pharmacologic thyroiditis (e.g., due to amiodarone). Autoimmunity can also provoke an inflammatory thyroiditis that causes transient thyrotoxicosis. This commonly occurs in the setting of lymphocytic thyroiditis (also known as silent, painless, or postpartum thyroiditis). It rarely occurs in the setting of autoimmune thyroiditis (also known as Hashimoto's thyroiditis).

In rare cases, excess thyroid hormone can be secreted by ectopic thyroid tissue located anywhere from the base of the tongue to the mediastinum, or by heterotopic thyroid tissue that develops as part of an ovarian teratoma (a condition known as struma ovarii).

Thyrotoxicosis can also be caused by ingestion of excessive amounts of thyroid hormone. This is most often the result of the prescription of excessive doses of pharmacologic preparations of thyroid hormone, but it can rarely be due to surreptitious or accidental ingestion.

CLINICAL MANIFESTATIONS

Symptoms and Signs

The classic symptoms of thyrotoxicosis include weight loss despite a hearty appetite, heat intolerance, palpitations, tremor, and hyperdefecation (increased frequency of formed bowel movements). Thyrotoxicosis can escape early detection because of its presentation with common nonspecific symptoms such as fatigue, insomnia, anxiety, irritability, weakness, atypical chest pain, or dyspnea on exertion. Delayed recognition may also occur when atypical symptoms such as headache, weight loss, periodic paralysis, or nausea and vomiting dominate the clinical picture. Elderly patients may present with apathetic thyrotoxicosis typified by weight loss and the absence of sympathomimetic symptoms and signs.

Signs of thyrotoxicosis include resting tachycardia, systolic hypertension with a widened pulse pressure, warm moist skin with a velvety texture, onycholysis, and a staring gaze with lid lag (noted to be present when a rim of sclera is visible between the upper eyelid and the superior margin of the iris on downward gaze). Cardiac examination may reveal a prominent apical impulse and a systolic flow murmur. Neurologic findings may include a restless, impatient demeanor, pressured speech, proximal muscle weakness, distal hand tremor, and brisk deep-tendon reflexes.

Clinical findings often provide clues to the underlying cause.[8] In Graves disease, the gland is diffusely enlarged with a smooth or slightly lobulated contour, and may manifest an audible bruit or palpable thrill. Thyroid ophthalmopathy and dermopathy are also unique to Graves disease. In patients with toxic nodular goiter, one or more discrete nodules may be appreciated. In subacute thyroiditis, the gland is modestly enlarged, extremely tender, and firm. A history of recent pregnancy suggests possible painless thyroiditis. Recent exposure to amiodarone, other iodine-containing compounds, interferon-α, or pharmacologic preparations of thyroid hormone may suggest the characteristic forms of thyrotoxicosis associated with these agents.

Graves Disease

DEFINITION

Graves disease is an autoimmune disorder characterized by a variable combination of hyperthyroidism, ophthalmopathy (also known as thyroid eye disease), and dermopathy.

EPIDEMIOLOGY

Graves disease is more common among women, but it also affects men. It can develop at any time during life, but the onset most often occurs between 30 and 60 years of age.

PATHOBIOLOGY

The proximate cause of hyperthyroidism in Graves disease is the production of thyroid-stimulating immunoglobulins that bind to and activate the TSH receptor, promoting thyroid hormone secretion and gland growth. Thyrotropin (TSH) receptor antibodies of the stimulating variety are the hallmark of hyperthyroidism in Graves disease. Other thyroid autoantibodies commonly identified in the setting of Graves disease include thyroid peroxidase antibodies, thyroglobulin antibodies, and TSH receptor antibodies. Although the fundamental cause of Graves disease remains unknown, a genetic predisposition is implicated by a higher incidence in monozygotic twins and first-degree relatives of affected individuals. Environmental factors implicated in triggering the onset of Graves disease include exposure to cigarette smoke, high dietary iodine intake, and perhaps stressful life events and certain antecedent infections.

CLINICAL MANIFESTATIONS

Affected individuals usually present with thyrotoxicosis and a thyroid gland that is diffusely enlarged with a rubbery consistency, smooth contour, definable pyramidal lobe, and audible bruit or palpable thrill due to increased blood flow. When it is clinically evident, thyroid eye disease usually presents within a few months of onset. In rare cases, it may develop long before, long after, or without any biochemical confirmation of hyperthyroidism.

PROGNOSIS

The hyperthyroidism associated with this condition often follows a persistent and progressive course, but one fourth of patients with Graves disease demonstrate spontaneous disease remission.

OPHTHALMOPATHY

DEFINITION

Thyroid eye disease is a distinctive disorder characterized by inflammation and swelling of the extraocular muscles and orbital fat, eyelid retraction, periorbital edema, episcleral vascular injection, conjunctival swelling (chemosis), and proptosis (also called exophthalmos).[9] Swelling of soft tissues within the confines of the orbits precipitated by fibroblast growth and inflammatory cell infiltrate can cause proptosis, entrapment of extraocular muscles, and compression of the optic nerve.

CLINICAL MANIFESTATIONS

Affected individuals typically complain of a change in eye appearance, ocular irritation, foreign body sensation, dryness, and ironically, excessive tearing. More severe involvement may cause exposure keratitis with corneal ulceration, diplopia, and blurred vision. On examination, patients may have a staring gaze, a rim of sclera visible between the upper eyelid and the superior margin of the iris during downward gaze (lid lag), signs of conjunctival inflammation, periorbital edema, and abnormalities of conjugate gaze, color vision, and visual acuity (Fig. 226-2). The precise degree of proptosis can be measured with an exophthalmometer. Orbital imaging with CT scanning or ultrasonography can confirm the diagnosis, which must sometimes be distinguished from other causes of bilateral and unilateral proptosis.

TREATMENT   Rx

Treatment of mild thyroid eye disease focuses on protecting the cornea from exposure and desiccation with moisturizing drops and ointment, glasses, and sometimes taping the eyelids closed at bedtime. Selenium supplementation may help to relieve some of the symptoms associated with active inflammation in mild to moderate cases.[A2] High-dose systemic glucocorticoid therapy can attenuate orbital inflammation in more severe cases. Orbital irradiation may be helpful in controlling inflammatory symptoms in some patients. Persistent corneal exposure, diplopia, altered vision due to optic nerve compression, and cosmetic issues may require surgery to decompress the orbits and readjust the extraocular muscles. Immunosuppressive agents and plasmapheresis have been used in severely affected patients, with anecdotal success.

DERMOPATHY

Infiltrative dermopathy, the least common aspect of Graves disease, is precipitated by the deposition of glycosaminoglycans in the dermis of the skin. Affected individuals usually present with mildly pruritic, orange peel–like thickening of the skin along the anterior aspects of the shins, known as pretibial myxedema. The dorsal aspects of the feet and fingers, the extensor surface of the elbows, and the face are more rarely affected.

The diagnosis can be confirmed by skin biopsy. Treatment of early infiltrative dermopathy with topical glucocorticoids under an occlusive wrap may limit its progression. Treatments involving the use of intradermal or systemic glucocorticoids, long-acting somatostatin analogues, and even surgical resection of soft tissue have demonstrated limited success.

Toxic Adenoma

A toxic adenoma is a solitary, autonomously functioning thyroid neoplasm that synthesizes and secretes excessive amounts of thyroid hormone independent of TSH stimulation. These neoplasms are almost always benign. Most grow large enough to be palpated by the time they present with thyrotoxicosis. Somatic gene mutations causing constitutive activation of the TSH receptor and the α-subunit of the stimulatory guanine nucleotide binding protein ($G_s\alpha$) have been identified in a subset of toxic adenomas. Hyperthyroidism caused by a toxic adenoma does not remit spontaneously, except in unusual cases complicated by hemorrhagic infarction of the neoplasm.

Toxic Multinodular Goiter

A toxic multinodular goiter is composed of multiple autonomously functioning thyroid nodules that synthesize and secrete excessive amounts of thyroid hormone. In some patients with nontoxic multinodular goiters, hyperthyroidism can be precipitated by exposure to excessive amounts of iodine. Most affected individuals have a goiter with multiple palpable thyroid nodules. Progressive enlargement may go undetected when there is substernal extension of nodular tissue. Toxic multinodular goiters are more common among older individuals.

TSH-Secreting Pituitary Adenoma

TSH-secreting pituitary adenomas represent less than 1% of all functioning pituitary tumors (Chapter 224). Patients may present with typical clinical manifestations of thyrotoxicosis, a diffuse goiter, symptoms and signs precipitated by an expanding sellar mass, syndromes associated with co-secretion of other anterior pituitary hormones (growth hormone, prolactin, or adrenocorticotropic hormone), or symptoms and signs of hypopituitarism. The key to suspecting the condition is usually recognition of an inappropriately nonsuppressed TSH level in a patient with thyrotoxicosis. The diagnosis is confirmed in most cases when laboratory testing reveals an elevated circulating level of the pituitary glycoprotein α-subunit in conjunction with a radiographically definable sellar mass.

DIAGNOSIS
Laboratory Findings

Abnormalities detected in routinely ordered laboratory tests are often the first clues to the presence of thyrotoxicosis. Thyrotoxic patients may have hypercalcemia or hypercalciuria, increased alkaline phosphatase levels, modestly elevated transaminase levels, and low or declining total and LDL

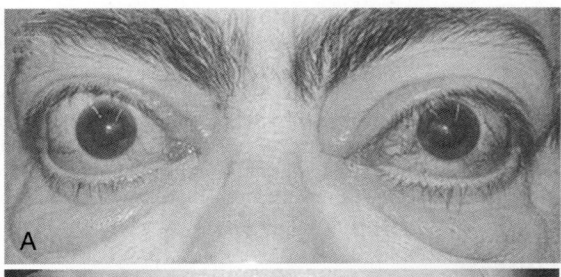

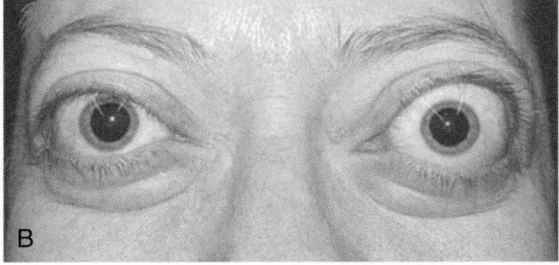

FIGURE 226-2. Graves ophthalmopathy. **A,** A 59-year-old woman with excess proptosis, moderate eyelid edema, and erythema with moderate eyelid retraction affecting all four eyelids. Conjunctival chemosis (edema) and erythema with bilateral edema of the caruncles, with prolapse of the right caruncle, are evident. **B,** A 40-year-old woman with excess proptosis, minimal bilateral injection, and chemosis with slight erythema of the eyelids. On slit lamp examination, she also had evidence of moderate superior limbic keratoconjunctivitis. (From Bahn RS. Graves' ophthalmopathy. *N Engl J Med.* 2010;362:726-738. Copyright 2010, Massachusetts Medical Society. All rights reserved.)

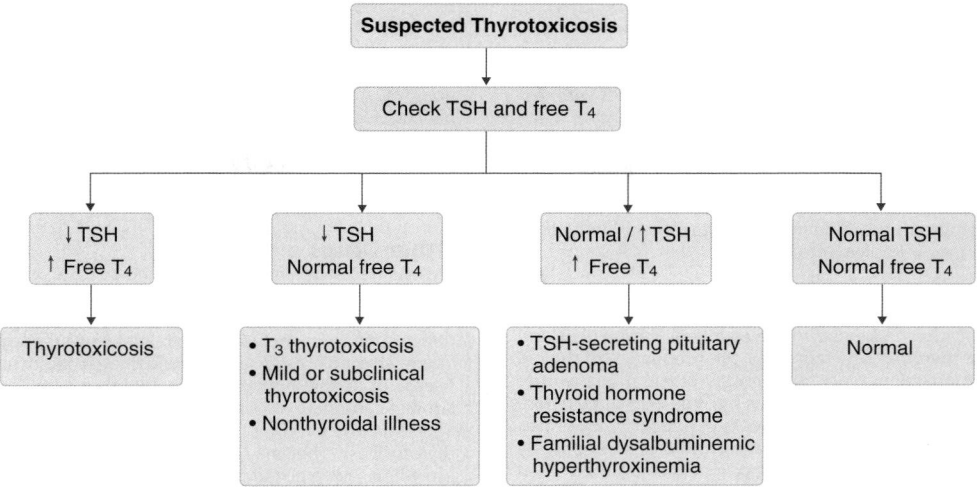

FIGURE 226-3. Laboratory assessment of suspected thyrotoxicosis. TSH = thyroid-stimulating hormone.

cholesterol levels. When they are measured, ferritin and angiotensin-converting enzyme levels are often increased. Electrocardiography typically reveals resting sinus tachycardia or atrial tachyarrhythmias, particularly atrial fibrillation with a rapid ventricular response. In severe cases, chest radiography may reveal cardiomegaly.

In most patients with suspected thyrotoxicosis, the diagnosis can be confirmed by measurement of a TSH level (Fig. 226-3). Sensitive TSH immunoassays with a detection limit of less than 0.02 mIU/L can accurately discriminate between clearly suppressed TSH levels, characteristic of all common forms of thyrotoxicosis, and mildly suppressed levels that fall just beneath the reference range, as may occur in otherwise sick individuals. Only the rare conditions associated with TSH-mediated hyperthyroidism (TSH-secreting pituitary tumors and isolated pituitary resistance to thyroid hormone) lack TSH suppression when testing for thyrotoxicosis. Measurement of serum free T_4 and T_3 levels confirms the diagnosis of thyrotoxicosis, defines its severity, and occasionally provides a clue to its underlying cause. Overt thyrotoxicosis is characterized by free T_4 or T_3 levels above the upper limit of the reference range, whereas mild or subclinical thyrotoxicosis is characterized by a suppressed TSH level with free T_4 and T_3 levels within the normal reference range. When only the free T_4 or T_3 concentrations are elevated, the terms T_4 *toxicosis* and T_3 *toxicosis* are applied, respectively.

Differential Diagnosis

Once thyrotoxicosis is confirmed, it is important to define its underlying cause to determine the most appropriate course of treatment. The relative degrees of T_4 and T_3 elevation sometimes can be helpful. Predominantly T_3 toxicosis is typical of Graves disease and can also occur with toxic nodular goiter. In contrast, predominantly T_4 toxicosis is more typical of subacute or painless thyroiditis. T_4 toxicosis is also more common in patients with iodine-induced hyperthyroidism.

Other laboratory tests are sometimes helpful in differential diagnosis. Antithyrotropin-receptor antibodies are pathognomonic of Graves disease. Levels of antithyrotropin-receptor antibodies are especially high in thyroid dermopathy and correlate positively with the clinical features and prognosis of Graves ophthalmopathy. An elevated ESR is typically seen in subacute thyroiditis.

Imaging studies can be helpful for the differential diagnosis. The fractional thyroidal uptake of radiotracer by the thyroid and its distribution in the gland on scintigraphic scanning often helps establish a definitive diagnosis (Table 226-6). Thyroid ultrasonography can confirm the presence of solitary or multiple thyroid nodules. Chest radiography and CT scanning may help delineate a substernal goiter.

TREATMENT Rx

Selection of the most effective treatment for a specific condition causing thyrotoxicosis requires an understanding of the underlying pathophysiologic process and natural history.[A3] For example, toxic multinodular goiter does not

TABLE 226-6 RADIOGRAPHIC EVALUATION OF SUSPECTED THYROTOXICOSIS

ETIOLOGY	FRACTIONAL 24-HOUR RADIOIODINE UPTAKE (%)	THYROID SCAN APPEARANCE
Graves disease	35-95	Diffuse increased homogeneous uptake; visible pyramidal lobe extending from isthmus
Toxic adenoma	20-60	Solitary focus of intense uptake; suppression of uptake in remainder of thyroid
Toxic multinodular goiter	20-60	Patchy heterogeneous foci of increased uptake interspersed with regions of diminished uptake
Subacute thyroiditis	0-2	Minimal to absent uptake
Autoimmune thyroiditis	0-2	Minimal to absent uptake; patchy heterogeneous uptake during recovery
Iodine-induced hyperthyroidism	0-2	Minimal to absent uptake
Exogenous thyroid hormone intoxication	0-2	Minimal to absent uptake
Metastatic differentiated thyroid cancer	0-5	Focal uptake in metastases
TSH-secreting pituitary adenoma	30-80	Diffuse increased homogeneous uptake

TSH = thyroid-stimulating hormone.

remit and requires definitive radioiodine treatment or surgery; subacute thyroiditis subsides spontaneously and requires only temporizing symptomatic therapy.

β-Blockers

β-Blockers help alleviate the sympathomimetic manifestations of thyrotoxicosis, regardless of the underlying cause. Palpitations, tremor, and anxiety can often be promptly controlled. However, other clinical features of thyrotoxicosis, including weight loss, heat intolerance, and fatigue, are not ameliorated by these agents. In thyrotoxic patients with marked sinus tachycardia or atrial fibrillation with a rapid ventricular response rate, β-blockers can be used as rate-controlling agents. Propranolol also partially inhibits extrathyroidal conversion of T_4 to T_3, which may be of added benefit in patients with severe thyrotoxicosis.

Propranolol can be started at a dose of 20 to 40 mg every 8 hours and titrated upward to a maximal daily dose of 240 mg on the basis of symptom control. Sustained-release propranolol or longer-acting β-blockers, such as metoprolol and atenolol, can also be used. β-Blockers should be used with caution in thyrotoxic patients with a history of obstructive pulmonary disease, Raynaud's phenomenon, or heart failure. Esmolol can be used when a short-acting parenteral agent is required for heart rate control in patients with thyrotoxic heart failure.

For patients with transient forms of thyrotoxicosis (subacute thyroiditis, autoimmune thyroiditis, or exogenous thyroid hormone intoxication), a β-blocker may be the only treatment required. In patients with more sustained conditions, such as Graves disease or toxic nodular goiter, β-blockers provide prompt initial relief of symptoms while definitive treatment with antithyroid drugs, radioiodine, or surgery is implemented.

Antithyroid Drugs

The thionamides inhibit thyroid hormone biosynthesis by competitively inhibiting iodine organification and iodotyrosine coupling. These agents are used for the treatment of thyrotoxicosis caused by overproduction of thyroid hormones. Because the thionamides block only new thyroid hormone synthesis, glandular stores of preexisting thyroid hormone must be exhausted before they are fully effective. This may require 3 to 8 weeks in patients with Graves disease or toxic multinodular goiter. Although antithyroid drugs can provide long-term control of hyperthyroidism, they are most appropriately used when there is a possibility that the underlying condition will remit, as in Graves disease, or when thyrotoxicosis must be attenuated before radioiodine treatment or surgery.

Two thionamide agents are currently available: methimazole and propylthiouracil. Methimazole can be taken as a single daily dose because of its longer half-life and higher effective intrathyroidal concentration. This can bolster patients' adherence and drug effectiveness. Propylthiouracil also inhibits extrathyroidal conversion of T_4 to T_3, an effect that may be beneficial in patients with severe complicated thyrotoxicosis. Propylthiouracil is preferred for pregnant hyperthyroid women in the first trimester because methimazole has been rarely associated with the congenital anomalies of choanal atresia and cutis aplasia.[10] However, the shorter half-life of propylthiouracil necessitates its administration three or four times daily. Furthermore, risk of severe hepatotoxicity associated with the use of propylthiouracil has prompted the recommendation that methimazole be the first-line antithyroid drug to treat hyperthyroidism in children and adults, including women after the first trimester of pregnancy.[A4]

For patients with mild to moderate hyperthyroidism, methimazole is usually started at a dose of 10 to 30 mg once daily and increased to as much as 90 mg daily. For patients with more severe hyperthyroidism, thyrotoxicosis complicated by cardiac disease, or concomitant pregnancy, propylthiouracil can be started at a dose of 50 to 200 mg every 6 to 8 hours. Methimazole can be given rectally if necessary. The anticipated duration of treatment depends on the underlying cause. In patients with toxic multinodular goiter, antithyroid drugs are generally used only to restore euthyroidism in anticipation of definitive therapy. An effective dose can be continued for 6 to 24 months in a patient with Graves disease, before it is tapered off to determine whether there has been a remission of the patient's autoimmune thyroid disease. Patients most likely to respond are those who present with mild clinical and biochemical hyperthyroidism, a small thyroid gland, and no active ophthalmopathy.

Patients treated with antithyroid drugs should have thyroid function tests checked every 3 to 12 weeks during dose titration to monitor for iatrogenic hypothyroidism. Common side effects include rash, pruritus, fever, and arthralgias, which affect 5% of thionamide-treated patients. Agranulocytosis and hepatitis are rare but potentially fatal adverse reactions to thionamide medications. Their presentations are relatively sudden in onset and unpredictable. Monitoring of leukocyte counts and liver function test results is not useful as a preventive measure. Patients who are prescribed antithyroid drugs should be cautioned about manifestations of these adverse reactions and should be instructed to discontinue treatment and seek medical attention if they develop a high fever, pharyngitis, jaundice, or abdominal pain.

Radioactive Iodine

The selective uptake and concentration of iodide in thyrocytes permits the use of radioactive iodine to treat hyperthyroidism.[11] Once it is concentrated in the gland after oral administration, ^{131}I destroys thyroid tissue and controls hyperthyroidism, usually within 1 to 2 months. The dose of ^{131}I can be calculated on the basis of the fractional uptake of radioiodine, but the outcome of dosimetry is not superior to that achieved with the administration of empirical doses. Patients can be treated on an outpatient basis, with precautions taken to prevent exposure of others. Approximately three quarters of patients are cured with a single dose of radioiodine.

The principal side effect of radioactive iodine therapy is postablative hypothyroidism, which develops in most individuals receiving treatment for Graves disease and in a lesser proportion of patients treated for toxic nodular goiter. Lifelong monitoring of thyroid function is required because patients develop postablative hypothyroidism at a rate of 3% per year. Another less common complication is a transient exacerbation of thyrotoxicosis, which occurs in one quarter of patients during the first month after treatment as a result of radiation thyroiditis. Long-term follow-up studies have shown that radioiodine-treated patients with Graves disease do not have any greater risk of thyroid cancer or other malignant neoplasms. However, hyperthyroid children and adolescents treated with radioactive iodine are more likely to develop benign nodules. Among hyperthyroid women treated with radioiodine, the incidences of infertility, spontaneous abortion, and children with birth defects are not increased. Diagnostic or therapeutic radioactive iodine is contraindicated in women during pregnancy, and treated women should avoid pregnancy until euthyroidism has been confirmed 3 to 6 months after administration of a dose.

Other Drugs

Saturated solution of potassium iodide (SSKI) or Lugol's solution transiently inhibit the synthesis and release of thyroid hormone from the gland. They may be used to accelerate recovery after radioactive iodine treatment, to prepare patients for thyroidectomy, and to augment other treatments used to control severe thyrotoxicosis (see later). Iodinated radiocontrast agents inhibit the release of thyroid hormone while blocking peripheral conversion of T_4 to T_3. Lithium carbonate also inhibits the release of thyroid hormone. Rarely, these agents are used in combination with thionamides to treat patients with severe thyrotoxicosis. They may also help provide temporary control of hyperthyroidism when severe allergies preclude the continued use of thionamides. Cholestyramine can be used to bind thyroid hormone in the gut to interrupt enterohepatic circulation in cases of suspected exogenous thyroid hormone intoxication.

Surgery

Surgery has a limited role because of its potential to injure the adjacent recurrent laryngeal nerves and parathyroid glands. Resection of a toxic adenoma by lobectomy is curative and often preserves sufficient normal thyroid tissue for euthyroidism to be maintained. Consequently, it is often recommended in younger individuals. Toxic multinodular goiters causing compressive symptoms or cosmetic disfigurement may be appropriately managed with surgical resection. Although surgery is seldom recommended in the United States for the treatment of hyperthyroid Graves disease, it may be appropriate when other modalities are contraindicated, such as when there has been an adverse reaction to an antithyroid drug in pregnancy, when a thyroid nodule is thought to be malignant, or when hyperparathyroidism also requires surgical intervention.

Specific Treatment Scenarios

Pregnancy

Pregnant patients with hyperthyroidism present special challenges. Diagnosis requires a careful assessment of symptoms, especially heat intolerance, palpitations, and vomiting, which also occur during normal pregnancy. The serum total T_4 level is elevated because of increased TBG, and the TSH level can be suppressed in the first trimester as a result of HCG-mediated thyroid stimulation. Diagnostic radionuclide imaging studies are contraindicated. After diagnostic confirmation, hyperthyroidism must be treated because it is associated with an increased risk of spontaneous abortion, premature labor, low birth weight, and toxemia. β-Blockers should be used only transiently to control severe symptoms. Propylthiouracil is the preferred thionamide for treatment of Graves disease during the first trimester of pregnancy, because it crosses the placenta less readily than methimazole and because methimazole has been rarely linked to congenital malformations (i.e., choanal atresia and cutis aplasia). However, owing to the risk of very rare but potentially fatal propylthiouracil-related hepatitis, methimazole is preferred after the first trimester. Because Graves disease often remits later in pregnancy, antithyroid drug dose requirements often decline as gestation progresses. Measurement of maternal thyroid-stimulating immunoglobulin levels can help predict the risk of an infant developing neonatal Graves disease.

Subclinical and Mild Hyperthyroidism

Patients with subclinical or mild hyperthyroidism (i.e., a suppressed serum TSH with normal free T_4 and T_3 levels) may have symptoms that justify treatment. In patients with a serum TSH level suppressed to less than 0.1 mIU/L, bone mineral loss can lead to osteoporosis, particularly in postmenopausal women. Atrial fibrillation occurs more commonly in mildly hyperthyroid patients aged 60 years and older with TSH suppression below normal. It is less clear, however, whether younger asymptomatic patients with modestly suppressed TSH levels (e.g., 0.1 to 0.5 mIU/L) require anything more than periodic monitoring.

Thyrotoxic Crisis

Thyrotoxic crisis, also known as thyroid storm, is a potentially life-threatening syndrome that is usually the end result of severe and sustained thyrotoxicosis. It can affect patients with other medical conditions that render them vulnerable to the cardiovascular, neuropsychiatric, and gastrointestinal effects of exposure to excessive amounts of thyroid hormone. Thyrotoxic crisis typically develops in the setting of inadequately treated Graves disease and may be precipitated by intercurrent illness, surgery, or treatment with radioactive iodine. Affected individuals present with fever, atrial tachyarrhythmias, congestive heart failure, nausea and vomiting, diarrhea, and seizures. Mental status changes can include agitation, delirium, psychosis, and coma. Prompt recognition and treatment in a monitored setting are crucial. A multifaceted treatment regimen should incorporate antipyretics, β-blockers, thionamides, iodinated contrast agents, and glucocorticoids, as well as aggressive evaluation and management of underlying medical problems.

THYROIDITIS
Subacute (de Quervain's) Thyroiditis
PATHOBIOLOGY
Transient thyrotoxicosis results from the uncontrolled release of thyroid hormone from the inflamed gland. After 2 to 8 weeks, when the supply of stored hormone is exhausted, thyrotoxicosis resolves spontaneously. Hypothyroidism ensues because the gland's biosynthetic capabilities remain impaired. This is also transient (lasting ≈ 1 month), with subsequent restoration of normal thyroid function in most patients.

CLINICAL MANIFESTATIONS
Subacute thyroiditis is characterized by painful enlargement of the thyroid, systemic inflammatory symptoms, and transient thyrotoxicosis that is often followed by transient hypothyroidism. The histologic pattern shows inflammatory cell infiltrates that are believed to be the result of a viral infection. Many patients with subacute thyroiditis report antecedent upper respiratory infections.

Patients usually present with pain localized to the thyroid or radiating to the throat, ears, or jaw. Constitutional symptoms, including fever, chills, sweats, and malaise, are often present. On occasion, these inflammatory features may dominate the presentation. Examination of the thyroid typically reveals an exquisitely tender, modestly enlarged, and woody, hard gland.

DIAGNOSIS
Differential Diagnosis
The differential diagnosis of thyroid pain must be considered in the evaluation of patients presenting with pain and tenderness localized to the lower anterior neck. In addition to subacute thyroiditis, potential causes of thyroid pain include acute (suppurative) thyroiditis, hemorrhage into an existing thyroid nodule, and rapid growth of anaplastic thyroid cancer, diffusely infiltrating thyroid cancer, or thyroid lymphoma.

Laboratory Findings
Laboratory testing in patients with subacute thyroiditis reveals a profile of overt thyrotoxicosis. Elevated T_4 levels are usually proportionately higher than T_3 levels. Patients typically have an elevated ESR during the acute phase. The fractional uptake of radioiodine is typically less than 2% at 24 hours (see Table 226-6).

TREATMENT   Rx
High-dose aspirin or naproxen sodium can be used to treat thyroid pain and systemic inflammatory symptoms. Patients who fail to respond may require glucocorticoid therapy, but it must be tapered over several weeks to prevent a relapse, prolonging the overall course of the illness. Symptoms ascribed to transient thyrotoxicosis may respond to treatment with a β-blocker continued for a limited course of 1 to 3 weeks. Patients who progress to symptomatic hypothyroidism may need short-term thyroxine replacement therapy, but most do not require long-term thyroid hormone replacement.

Lymphocytic (Postpartum, Painless, Silent) Thyroiditis
EPIDEMIOLOGY
Lymphocytic thyroiditis occurs most commonly in postpartum women, affecting as many as 6% of women 2 to 12 months after delivery or termination. Rarely, this condition occurs in non-postpartum women or in men. Predisposing factors include a history of previous episodes of postpartum thyroiditis, type 1 diabetes mellitus, and circulating antithyroid autoantibodies.

PATHOBIOLOGY
This painless inflammation of the thyroid gland can cause transient thyrotoxicosis followed by transient or persistent hypothyroidism. Each of these phases of thyroid dysfunction typically lasts 2 to 8 weeks. This condition is believed to reflect transient autoimmunity.

DIAGNOSIS
The diagnosis of lymphocytic thyroiditis is often overlooked when nonspecific symptoms of thyrotoxicosis (e.g., weight loss, insomnia, anxiety) or hypothyroidism (e.g., fatigue, depression) are misinterpreted as common postpartum complaints. The thyroid gland is nontender and either normal in size or modestly enlarged. Once it is considered, a diagnosis of lymphocytic thyroiditis can be readily confirmed or excluded by laboratory testing, which reveals a suppressed TSH level during phases of thyrotoxicosis and an elevated TSH level during phases of hypothyroidism. This condition must be distinguished from Graves disease, which can also present in the same time frame after delivery. Relative degrees of T_4 and T_3 elevation can sometimes provide a clue to which condition is present; lymphocytic thyroiditis is typically characterized by predominant increases in T_4 levels. Fractional uptake of radioiodine is either absent or very low in the setting of lymphocytic thyroiditis, whereas it is increased in active Graves disease (see Table 226-6).

TREATMENT
Lymphocytic thyroiditis can often be managed with reassurance and observation alone. Symptomatic thyrotoxicosis can be treated with a course of β-blocker therapy. Overt hypothyroidism may require short-term thyroxine replacement.

PROGNOSIS
Most patients with lymphocytic thyroiditis eventually return to a euthyroid state, but 25% develop persistent hypothyroidism due to classic autoimmune thyroiditis.

Acute (Suppurative) Thyroiditis
Infection of the thyroid gland is a rare condition that typically presents with severe thyroid pain, fever, and other systemic manifestations of infection. Bacterial infection of thyroid tissue can be the result of direct spread of gram-positive or gram-negative pathogens through fistulas communicating with the piriform sinus or the skin. Hematogenous spread of bacterial, mycobacterial, fungal, or parasitic organisms, especially *Pneumocystis carinii*, can occur in immunocompromised individuals. On examination, affected patients are typically febrile, with asymmetrical swelling of a thyroid that is tender, warm, and fluctuant to firm in consistency beneath erythematous skin. Ultrasonography may reveal an abscess that can be aspirated to identify a pathogen. Patients with suppurative thyroiditis require prompt treatment with appropriate antibiotics. Surgical drainage of abscesses may be required.

Other Forms of Thyroiditis
Certain drugs can cause thyroid gland inflammation. Amiodarone can produce a painless thyroiditis associated with thyrotoxicosis. Whenever possible, this should be distinguished from the iodine-induced form of thyrotoxicosis that can also be associated with amiodarone therapy. The former is optimally treated with glucocorticoid therapy, whereas the latter is managed with antithyroid drugs.[12] Interferon-α can provoke a painless thyroiditis associated with transient thyrotoxicosis. This must be differentiated from interferon-α–induced Graves disease; the former is managed with β-blockers and the latter with antithyroid drugs.

Riedel's thyroiditis or struma is characterized by fibrotic replacement of the thyroid, with adherence and infiltration of adjacent structures that causes local compressive symptoms. In this idiopathic condition, the thyroid is substantially enlarged, hardened, and fixed. Affected patients may also develop mediastinal and retroperitoneal fibrosis, sclerosing cholangitis, or orbital pseudotumor. Diagnosis requires open biopsy. Surgical excision is difficult or impossible. Glucocorticoid therapy and tamoxifen therapy have been anecdotally reported to be effective.

GOITER

DEFINITION

Goiters can be classified as diffuse or nodular, nontoxic or toxic (i.e., associated with thyroid hormone overproduction), and benign or malignant. Thyroid enlargement can be the result of thyrocyte proliferation stimulated by circulating factors (e.g., TSH and thyroid-stimulating autoantibodies), infiltration of the gland by inflammatory or malignant cells, or benign or malignant neoplastic changes within the gland itself. In a patient with a goiter, three clinical issues must be considered: enlargement causing local compressive or cosmetic concern, gland hyperfunction or hypofunction, and potential malignancy.

EPIDEMIOLOGY

Dietary iodine deficiency represents the most common cause of goiter worldwide. It is encountered in the United States only among immigrants from iodine-deficient regions. Younger patients present with diffuse or simple goiters that shrink in response to adequate iodine supplementation. In older individuals, iodine-deficient goiters become multinodular and do not decrease in size with iodine repletion. Excessive iodine exposure can provoke thyrotoxicosis in these patients.

PATHOBIOLOGY

Benign multinodular goiter or adenoma can be the result of genetic defects that lead to dyshormonogenesis, including mutations in the thyroglobulin, thyroid peroxidase, dual oxidase, and pendrin genes. Similarly, exposure to goitrogenic substances in foodstuffs, water, or drugs (e.g., lithium carbonate) that inhibit the normal steps in thyroid hormone synthesis can lead to goiter. In most patients, the underlying cause is unknown.

Autoimmune thyroiditis typically produces a modest goiter as a result of glandular infiltration with lymphocytes, inflammatory changes in thyrocytes, and fibrosis. The hypothyroid state caused by autoimmune thyroiditis results in increased TSH, which further stimulates thyroid enlargement. Graves disease is also characterized by diffuse thyroid enlargement due to the action of thyroid-stimulating immunoglobulins. Other forms of thyroiditis can present with goitrous enlargement of the thyroid gland, including subacute, lymphocytic, and acute (suppurative) thyroiditis (see earlier sections).

Malignant neoplasms that involve the gland diffusely, including thyroid lymphoma and infiltrative papillary, medullary, and anaplastic thyroid cancers, may present as rapidly enlarging goiters (see later sections). Affected patients often experience local pain and symptoms related to tumor expansion.

DIAGNOSIS

Clinical Examination

The first step in evaluating a suspected goiter is to confirm whether neck swelling represents enlargement of the thyroid. Redundant skin and subcutaneous fat in the lower anterior neck can be mistaken for an enlarged thyroid. These findings can usually be distinguished from true thyroid enlargement by palpating a normal thyroid beneath the misleading soft tissue and by observing that the fullness does not rise and fall with deglutition. Ultrasonography may help resolve uncertainty.

A patient's history can provide important clues to the underlying cause. A childhood social history may confirm previous iodine deficiency. Symptoms of hypothyroidism may suggest autoimmune thyroiditis, whereas clinical evidence of thyrotoxicosis may suggest Graves disease or toxic multinodular goiter. Clinical findings may lead to recognition of one of the various forms of thyroiditis (e.g., pain in subacute thyroiditis or postpartum status in lymphocytic thyroiditis). Symptoms suggesting the invasion of adjacent structures may raise concerns about malignant disease or Riedel's thyroiditis.

On examination, diffuse enlargement favors one of the forms of thyroiditis, Graves disease, or a diffusely infiltrating malignant neoplasm. Nodular enlargement is more likely to reflect a benign multinodular goiter or malignant neoplasm. The precise size of the gland should be documented. Dysphonia, tracheal deviation, cervical lymphadenopathy, and venous engorgement in the neck should be noted. Subtotal obstruction of the thoracic outlet may be revealed by having the patient touch his or her hands together above the head (Pemberton's maneuver) while checking for signs of facial plethora and cervical venous distention.

Laboratory Findings

A TSH level determines whether there is primary hypothyroidism or thyrotoxicosis. Elevated antithyroid peroxidase antibody titers can confirm suspected autoimmune thyroiditis. In asymptomatic patients with a modest diffuse goiter, no further evaluation may be indicated. Other blood tests (e.g., ESR for subacute thyroiditis or calcitonin for medullary thyroid cancer) can be useful when clinical clues suggest specific diagnoses.

Imaging

Cervical ultrasonography is the best imaging technique to define the character and extent of a goiter limited to the neck. It can help determine whether a goiter is diffuse or nodular, whether the thyroid is impinging on other cervical structures, and whether lymphadenopathy is present. Ultrasonography is also essential for guidance of fine-needle aspiration for cytologic differential diagnosis (see later). When a goiter extends posteriorly or beneath the sternal notch into the thorax, CT or MRI may be required. The administration of iodine-containing radiocontrast dye should generally be avoided in the evaluation of patients with goiters, because the stable iodide load may interfere with subsequent radioiodine imaging or therapy. Thyroid radionuclide uptake studies with ^{99m}Tc pertechnetate or ^{123}I can help characterize the functional status of the gland. Radionuclide scanning can help determine the cause of a goiter and whether a superior mediastinal mass is thyroid tissue. Barium swallow radiographs with fixed-diameter markers and pulmonary function testing with flow-volume loops can help determine whether symptoms are directly related to compression of the esophagus or trachea, respectively. Laryngoscopy is useful to evaluate vocal cord function in patients with potential recurrent laryngeal nerve involvement.

TREATMENT   Rx

Once thyroid dysfunction and malignant disease have been excluded, asymptomatic patients with goiters can be observed with periodic clinical assessment. Ultrasonography can be relied on as a reproducible technique for monitoring the size of an enlarged thyroid gland. Thyroxine therapy to suppress TSH levels is effective in shrinking goiters in only a minority of patients. Furthermore, chronic thyroid hormone treatment carries the risks of symptomatic thyrotoxicosis, atrial fibrillation, and bone mineral loss.

Patients with benign multinodular goiters causing local compressive symptoms or cosmetic concerns can be treated with surgery or radioactive iodine therapy. Surgery is often preferred when a patient has substantial gland enlargement causing compressive complications, especially when there is substernal extension of the goiter or acute obstructive symptoms. When surgery is contraindicated by the patient's health status, radioactive iodine therapy has been shown to reduce goiter size by an average of 50% over 12 to 24 months.

THYROID NODULES

EPIDEMIOLOGY

Thyroid nodules are common, being detected by palpation in 6% of women and 2% of men. Contemporary high-resolution ultrasonography identifies thyroid nodules in as many as 50% of all adults. Although the majority of these represent small, benign adenomatoid nodules or cysts, 5 to 10% of thyroid nodules are malignant. Less commonly, thyroid nodules are clinical problems by virtue of being hyperfunctioning or causing local compressive symptoms or cosmetic dissatisfaction.

DIAGNOSIS

Thyroid nodules can be noted by the patient or their physician in the absence of any other complaints.[13] It is also common for thyroid nodules to be detected incidentally on imaging procedures, such as carotid ultrasonography and cervical spine CT or MRI. Symptoms of compression or invasion of adjacent tissues suggest that a nodule may be malignant. These include pain in the lower anterior neck, cough or dyspnea due to tracheal compression, hemoptysis due to tracheal invasion, dysphonia due to recurrent laryngeal nerve encasement, and dysphagia or odynophagia due to esophageal compression. Certain other symptoms and signs lead to the consideration of specific underlying conditions. A toxic adenoma should be suspected in a patient with a thyroid nodule and the classic clinical manifestations of thyrotoxicosis. Hypothyroid symptoms and signs suggest autoimmune thyroiditis with asymmetrical thyroid enlargement. Hypercalcitoninemia associated with the metastatic spread of medullary thyroid cancer can cause pruritus, flushing, and diarrhea. The clinical assessment should also include symptoms and signs related to common sites of thyroid cancer metastasis, such as chest pain, dyspnea, bone pain, and neurologic findings. Thyroid nodules rarely can be due to metastasis from other primary malignant neoplasms including kidney, colon, and breast cancers.

History

A special predisposition to thyroid cancer is suggested by a personal history of therapeutic neck irradiation in childhood. Family history can be informative if relatives have had medullary or papillary thyroid cancers, which are familial in 50% and 10% of cases, respectively. The possibility of medullary thyroid cancer should also be considered when there is a personal or family history of clinical problems associated with multiple endocrine neoplasia type 2 (MEN 2) syndromes, including hyperparathyroidism and pheochromocytoma (Chapter 231).

Physical Examination

Physical examination of a thyroid nodule should seek to define its size, consistency, surface texture, mobility, and tenderness. The presence of malignant disease is suggested by fixation and ipsilateral regional adenopathy or vocal cord paresis. Multinodularity of the gland may reflect benign nodular goiter, but it is not sufficiently reassuring to dispense with further diagnostic testing.[14] This is particularly true for a so-called dominant nodule that is larger, enlarging faster, or more symptomatic than others present in the thyroid.

Laboratory Findings

Routine laboratory testing includes measurement of TSH levels to identify patients with hyperthyroidism or hypothyroidism. When the TSH level is low or undetectable, the possibility of a benign autonomously functioning toxic adenoma can be pursued with radionuclide thyroid scanning (see Table 226-6). If an elevated TSH level indicates primary hypothyroidism, antithyroid peroxidase antibody titers can confirm whether the patient has autoimmune thyroiditis. Ultrasonography can distinguish asymmetrical enlargement caused by autoimmune thyroiditis from a discrete nodule. Calcitonin levels should be measured in patients with a known or suspected family history of MEN 2 or familial medullary thyroid cancer. Serum thyroglobulin measurement is not helpful in distinguishing benign from malignant thyroid abnormalities.

Imaging

Cervical ultrasonography helps confirm that a mass is within the thyroid, accurately defines its size, classifies it as cystic or solid, and determines whether additional nodules are present. Ultrasonography occasionally reveals other suspicious findings in nodules, such as fine calcifications, irregular nodule borders, and cervical adenopathy.

Radionuclide scanning with radioiodine or technetium pertechnetate is helpful only in selected cases. In patients with a thyroid nodule and a suppressed TSH level, scanning can confirm that the nodule is hyperfunctioning or "hot," in which case biopsy is usually not required.

Invasive Evaluation
Fine-Needle Aspiration Biopsy

Fine-needle aspiration biopsy is the most accurate test to exclude or confirm malignant disease in patients with a nodule and a normal TSH level (Fig. 226-4). Most solid nodules and complex cysts larger than 1.0 to 1.5 cm in diameter should be sampled. Although aspiration can be directed by palpation alone when a nodule is readily definable, ultrasonography provides more certain guidance for the sampling of poorly localized lesions, often revealing additional nodules that should be assessed.

The cytologic assessment of aspirated material must first confirm that there is adequate material for assessment (e.g., 6 clumps of 10 cells on 2 slides). Biopsies with inadequate specimens, which are more common in cystic lesions, must be repeated. Ultrasonographic guidance and on-site preliminary cytologic assessment can improve the yield of biopsy. In accordance with the Bethesda System for Reporting Thyroid Cytopathology, a sampled nodule can be categorized as benign, atypical, suspicious for a follicular neoplasm, suspicious for malignancy, or malignant (Table 226-7).[15]

Benign nodules typically yield samples containing clusters of normal-appearing follicular epithelial cells with colloid. Pure colloid cysts may have scant epithelium. This classification is highly accurate, with a false-negative rate of less than 3% in sonographically directed biopsy specimens, and surgical resection is not required. In most cases, conservative observation based on yearly clinical or sonographic reassessment can be recommended. Further enlargement during observation (i.e., >20% increase in two of three dimensions) should prompt a repeat biopsy. Surgical resection should be considered if a cytologically benign nodule continues to grow, causing compressive symptoms or cosmetic disfigurement.

Cytologic material classified as malignant typically contains abundant epithelial cells with atypical nuclear features, overlapping, and scant or absent colloid. This is also a highly reliable finding, with 98% of such lesions found to be thyroid cancers on subsequent resection. Consequently, bilateral thyroidectomy is indicated in patients without contraindications to operation. Samples that contain sparser quantities of epithelial cells with similar atypical nuclear features may be classified as suspicious for malignancy. Approximately 75% of nodules in this category represent thyroid cancers.

One in five biopsies yields adequate but diagnostically indeterminate cytologic material.[16] Specific findings that classify an indeterminate nodule as suspicious for a follicular neoplasm include abundant follicular or Hürthle cells in microfollicles with little or no colloid and minor degrees of nuclear atypia, potentially indicative of papillary cancer. Although the majority of such indeterminate nodules are benign follicular adenomas, 15 to 30% are thyroid carcinomas. Biopsy samples that reveal nuclear or architectural features considered to be abnormal but not clearly suspicious for malignancy or a follicular neoplasm are classified as demonstrating atypia of undetermined significance. Nodules that initially fall into this category have been estimated to harbor malignancy at rates ranging from 5 to 25%. Repeat sampling may provide a more specific diagnosis to guide further management in 75% of cases.

Definitive determination of whether a suspicious or atypical nodule represents a focus of malignancy requires surgery targeted to remove either the lobe of the thyroid containing the nodule or the entire gland for surgical pathologic examination. Unilateral thyroid lobectomy has the advantage of a lower incidence of surgical complications and postoperative hypothyroidism when the lesion is benign, but it necessitates a subsequent completion thyroidectomy for most patients who prove to have cancer.

Molecular diagnostic testing is available to reduce the number of surgeries performed in patients with cytologically indeterminate nodules, approximately 75% of which prove to be histopathologically benign. There are two general strategies: (1) testing aspirated material for oncogenic mutations associated with thyroid malignancies and (2) gene expression classifier microarrays designed to identify benign nodules. For a typical population of cytologically indeterminate nodule patients with a prevalence of thyroid cancer of 20 to 35%, the negative predictive value of oncogenic testing and gene expression classification have been shown to be approximately 85% and 95%, respectively. For patients with no clinical features of malignancy, particularly middle-aged or older women with multinodular glands in whom the prevalence of malignancy is 5% or less, vigilant observation with serial sonography is an alternative.

THYROID CANCER

Cancers of the thyroid gland have a spectrum of behavior that ranges from incidentally detected and clinically inconsequential microcarcinomas to aggressive and virtually untreatable anaplastic malignant neoplasms. When thyroid cancer is diagnosed early, treatment is effective for most types. Most thyroid cancers present as thyroid nodules that are either asymptomatic or associated with local cervical symptoms or adenopathy. Less often, thyroid cancers first present with manifestations of metastatic disease, such as a pulmonary mass or bone pain.

Papillary and Follicular (Epithelial) Thyroid Carcinomas

Papillary and follicular thyroid cancers arise from follicular epithelium and often retain responsiveness to TSH, produce thyroglobulin, and concentrate iodide. They are distinguished by their histopathologic appearances and characteristic patterns of progression. Hürthle cell carcinoma of the thyroid is composed of thyrocytes with abundant mitochondria-laden cytoplasm, and behaves like a follicular thyroid cancer, although it typically does not have iodine-concentrating ability.

EPIDEMIOLOGY

Approximately 60,000 new cases of thyroid cancer are diagnosed annually in the United States. Thyroid cancer is three times more common in women, in

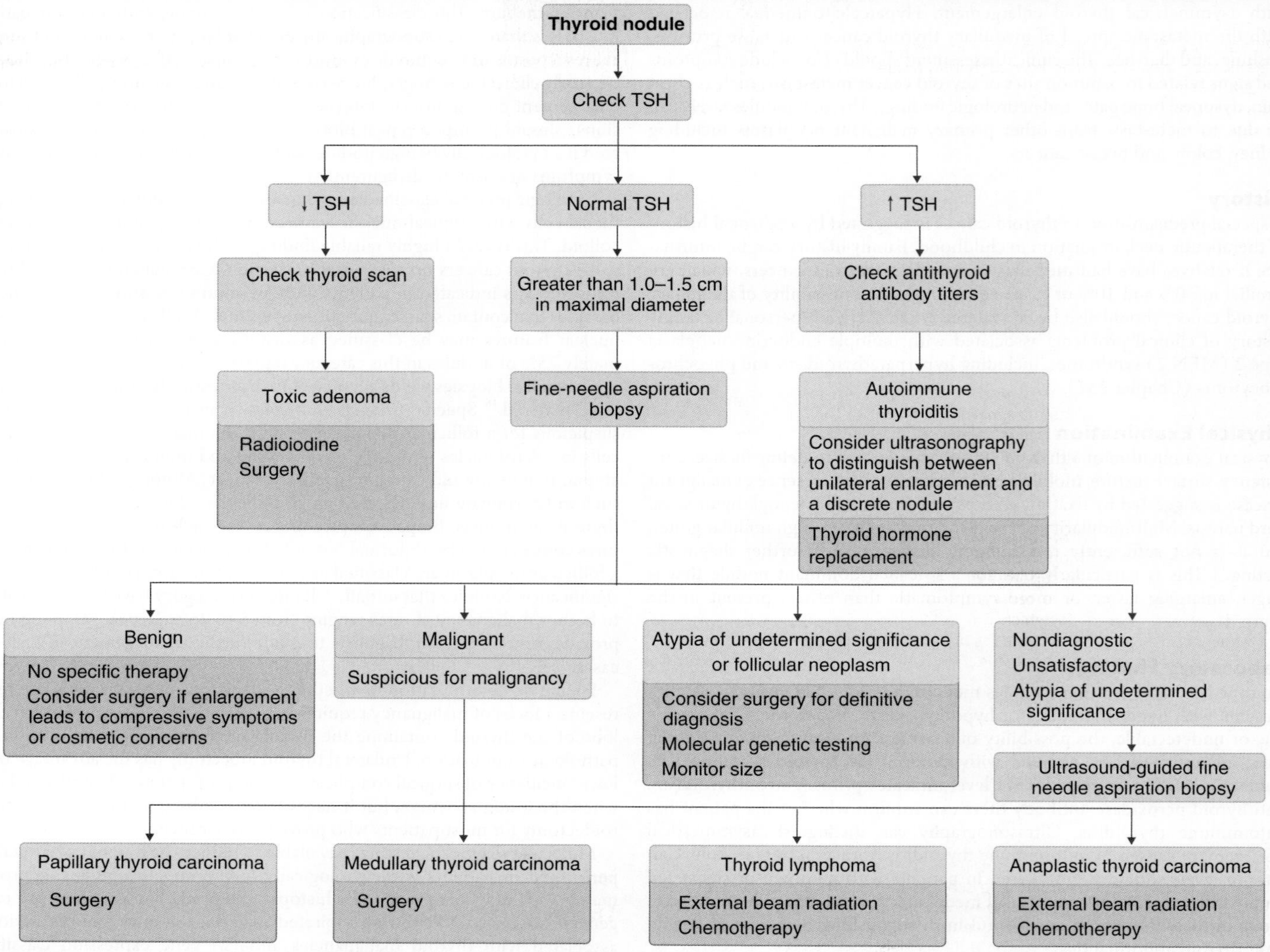

```
                          ┌──────────────────┐
                          │  Thyroid nodule  │
                          └────────┬─────────┘
                          ┌────────▼─────────┐
                          │    Check TSH     │
                          └────────┬─────────┘
        ┌──────────────────────────┼──────────────────────────┐
   ┌────▼────┐               ┌──────▼──────┐              ┌────▼────┐
   │ ↓ TSH   │               │ Normal TSH  │              │ ↑ TSH   │
   └────┬────┘               └──────┬──────┘              └────┬────┘
```

↓ TSH	Normal TSH	↑ TSH
Check thyroid scan	**Greater than 1.0–1.5 cm in maximal diameter**	**Check antithyroid antibody titers**
Toxic adenoma Radioiodine Surgery	**Fine-needle aspiration biopsy**	**Autoimmune thyroiditis** Consider ultrasonography to distinguish between unilateral enlargement and a discrete nodule Thyroid hormone replacement

Benign	Malignant	Atypia of undetermined significance or follicular neoplasm	Nondiagnostic Unsatisfactory Atypia of undetermined significance
No specific therapy Consider surgery if enlargement leads to compressive symptoms or cosmetic concerns	Suspicious for malignancy	Consider surgery for definitive diagnosis Molecular genetic testing Monitor size	Ultrasound-guided fine needle aspiration biopsy

Papillary thyroid carcinoma	Medullary thyroid carcinoma	Thyroid lymphoma	Anaplastic thyroid carcinoma
Surgery	Surgery	External beam radiation Chemotherapy	External beam radiation Chemotherapy

FIGURE 226-4. Evaluation of a thyroid nodule. TSH = thyroid-stimulating hormone.

TABLE 226-7 BETHESDA SYSTEM FOR REPORTING CYTOPATHOLOGY

CYTOLOGIC DIAGNOSIS	RISK OF MALIGNANCY
Benign	0-3%
Atypia of undetermined significance	20-25%
Suspicious for a follicular neoplasm	15-30%
Suspicious for malignancy	60-77%
Malignant	97-99%

Diagnostic categories associated with risk of malignancy.
Adapted from Bongiovanny M, Spitale A, Faquin WC, et al. The Bethesda System for Reporting Thyroid Cytopathology: a meta-analysis. *Acta Cytol.* 2012;56:333-339.

radioiodine exposure after nuclear incidents. A substantial body of evidence now implicates *RET/PTC* and *BRAF* gene mutations that activate the MAP kinase signaling pathway in the pathogenesis and progression of papillary thyroid cancer. Most papillary thyroid carcinomas are slow growing and either remain confined to the gland or metastasize to cervical lymph nodes. Papillary microcarcinomas are a common incidental pathologic finding in 5% of thyroid glands excised for other reasons. However, papillary thyroid carcinomas can be more aggressive, with extension into adjacent tissues, extensive nodal involvement, and distant metastatic spread, most commonly to the lungs. Such aggressive behavior is, in general, more common in older patients.

Follicular and Hürthle cell thyroid carcinomas account for 9% of all thyroid cancers. When these tumors show histologic evidence of invading only the tumor capsule, they are termed *minimally invasive* and generally behave like papillary thyroid carcinomas. However, follicular and Hürthle cell carcinomas with vascular invasion are more likely to be associated with distant metastatic disease, which most commonly involves the lungs and skeleton.

whom its incidence is currently rising faster than that of any other malignancy. There are estimated to be 450,000 U.S. thyroid cancer survivors who require lifelong follow-up for recurrence. Papillary thyroid carcinoma is the most common form of thyroid cancer, representing 90% of cases. The mean age at diagnosis is 45 years, but papillary thyroid carcinoma does occur in children and increases in incidence with age.

PATHOBIOLOGY

Irradiation of the thyroid gland in childhood is a risk factor, as evidenced by the epidemics of thyroid cancer that have followed both external beam radiation therapy for benign childhood conditions (e.g., tonsillitis and acne) and

TREATMENT Rx

Treatment of epithelial thyroid cancer entails surgery, often followed by radioiodine ablation of remnant thyroid tissue. Total or near-total thyroidectomy with selective central compartment lymph node resection is usually the appropriate initial surgical procedure. Thyroid surgery can be complicated by hypoparathyroidism or recurrent laryngeal nerve injury, which causes hoarseness if it is unilateral and airway obstruction if it is bilateral. The rationale for bilateral surgery is the frequent presence of bilateral disease in papillary thyroid cancer and the lower risk of recurrence after bilateral gland removal. In addition, there is greater accuracy in detecting residual disease after the eradication of all remaining normal thyroid tissue.

A prospective cohort study of a national database of 30-day follow-up of patients undergoing thyroidectomy (for cancer or other indications) documented the increased risk of major pulmonary, cardiac, and infectious complications in the elderly. Elderly patients (65 to 79 years old) are twice as likely, and the most elderly (80 years or older) are 5 times as likely as young patients (16 to 64 years old) to have major systematic complications.[17]

Follow-up

Postoperatively, ^{131}I administration after TSH stimulation can be employed to ablate the small amount of normal thyroid tissue that usually remains after surgery. This tissue, if it is not destroyed, leaves patients with circulating thyroglobulin and iodine-concentrating tissue on whole body scanning, decreasing the accuracy of these tests to identify residual disease. In controlled but nonrandomized trials, radioiodine has been associated with a lower rate of tumor recurrence in patients with advanced disease (stages 3 and 4) at presentation (see later), but there is no demonstrated clinical benefit of adjunctive radioiodine therapy for patients with lower stages of disease. TSH stimulation of residual thyroid tissue, which is essential for effective radioiodine therapy, can be accomplished either by the temporary withdrawal of thyroid hormone therapy to promote endogenous TSH production or by the administration of recombinant thyrotropin, which avoids the morbidity of hypothyroidism.

Thyroxine therapy is appropriate for all patients with treated thyroid cancer, regardless of the extent of surgery and whether they received radioiodine ablative therapy. In addition to providing thyroid hormone replacement, thyroxine can be adjusted to suppress the patient's circulating TSH level to the low or low-normal range to reduce the likelihood of tumor recurrence. In determining the extent to which the TSH level should be suppressed, the patient's risk of cancer recurrence must be balanced against potential thyrotoxic complications such as bone mineral loss in postmenopausal women and atrial fibrillation in older patients.

Long-term monitoring of patients entails periodic clinical assessment, measurement of serum thyroglobulin levels, radioiodine imaging in the early postoperative phase, and occasional use of ultrasonography. Clinically, patients should be assessed for local neck symptoms or recurrent cervical masses, as well as for optimization of thyroid hormone therapy. For patients with treated epithelial thyroid cancers, thyroglobulin is a more specific tumor marker if all remaining normal thyroid tissue has been ablated. For patients with undetectable thyroglobulin levels on TSH-suppressive thyroid hormone therapy, thyroglobulin measurement after recombinant TSH stimulation can sometimes reveal residual disease. Radioiodine scanning after TSH stimulation can be helpful in patients who have previously undergone radioiodine ablation, but once radioiodine imaging is negative, it offers little or no advantage over measurement of stimulated thyroglobulin levels. This is particularly true in recurrent papillary thyroid cancers, which often lose the ability to concentrate iodine. Unfortunately, thyroglobulin testing is impossible in the 20% of patients who have circulating thyroglobulin autoantibodies that interfere with thyroglobulin immunoassays. Because most epithelial thyroid cancer recurrences are in cervical nodes or soft tissues, ultrasonography is useful for postoperative monitoring, particularly in patients who presented with extensive cervical disease or who have persistently detectable serum thyroglobulin. CT scanning of the chest should be employed to detect intrathoracic disease in patients whose findings suggest recurrence outside the neck. In patients with substantial detectable thyroglobulin levels (>10 ng/mL) and negative findings on standard imaging studies, PET scanning can identify sites of residual disease in more than 50% of patients.

Localization of recurrent cervical disease is usually an indication for comprehensive compartmental neck dissection. Distant and nonresectable metastases that are iodine avid, which occur more commonly in patients with invasive follicular thyroid cancer, can be treated with repeated doses of [131]I. Symptomatic hilar node and bone metastases can be treated palliatively with external beam radiation therapy. Surgery can be employed for isolated metastatic disease sites. Conventional chemotherapy has limited efficacy in the treatment of differentiated thyroid cancer, but newer biologic agents targeting the molecular pathways involved in the pathogenesis of thyroid cancer hold promise.[18] For example, the multikinase inhibitor sorafenib was shown in a phase 3 trial to double progression free survival to almost 11 months in patients with metastatic non–iodine avid epithelial thyroid cancers and shrink disease sites in 12% of patients.[A6] Another multikinase inhibitor, vandetanib, is also effective against locally advanced or metastatic differentiated thyroid cancer.[A7] However, multikinase inhibitors commonly have adverse effects, and because they are only tumoristatic must be used continuously.

PROGNOSIS

The TNM (tumor, node, metastasis) staging system is commonly used to stage epithelial thyroid cancers. In addition to tumor size, extent of node involvement, and presence of distant metastatic disease, the age of the patient at presentation is an important predictor of outcome. Patients younger than 45 years have a better prognosis than older individuals. The overall age-adjusted 10-year survival rates for patients with papillary and follicular thyroid cancer are 98% and 92%, respectively. However, disease recurrence is relatively common, occurring in approximately one third of patients with papillary thyroid cancer. Consequently, patients with treated thyroid cancer must be monitored for recurrent disease.

Medullary Thyroid Carcinoma

Patients with medullary thyroid cancer (Chapter 246) typically present with a thyroid nodule, cervical adenopathy, distant disease, or symptoms of flushing, diarrhea, and pruritus when the circulating calcitonin level is markedly elevated. Features of the other elements of MEN 2a (e.g., hypertension) or MEN 2b (e.g., marfanoid habitus, submucosal neuromas) should be sought.

Anaplastic Thyroid Carcinoma

Anaplastic thyroid carcinoma is a rare, histologically undifferentiated, clinically aggressive malignant neoplasm that typically arises in older patients, one fourth of whom present with evidence of a preceding differentiated thyroid cancer. Affected patients present with a rapidly enlarging mass in the anterior or lateral neck associated with pain, tenderness, and compressive symptoms including dysphagia, dysphonia, and stridorous dyspnea. Fine-needle aspiration biopsy of the mass usually yields large, pleomorphic, undifferentiated cells, but open surgical biopsy is sometimes required to confirm the diagnosis.

Most cases are unresectable at presentation because of invasion of cervical structures. Surgery is not curative and should aim to secure the patient's airway. A percutaneous gastrostomy tube is often placed to ensure adequate nutrition in the face of esophageal impingement. Conventional therapy consisting of combined external beam radiation therapy and chemotherapy with doxorubicin with or without cisplatin produces an initial response in 25% of patients. Rare patients with disease limited to the neck may have extended survival, but almost all patients relapse within a few months and succumb to their disease, with median survival ranging from 3 to 7 months. Current research is focused on the use of targeted antiangiogenic agents to treat unresponsive disease.

Thyroid Lymphoma

Lymphoma rarely arises in the thyroid gland, typically presenting in older persons as a rapidly enlarging and painful diffuse goiter. Patients often have a preceding history of autoimmune thyroiditis. The diagnosis is further suspected when fine-needle aspiration biopsy yields abundant lymphocytes without other cellular features of autoimmune thyroiditis. Immunohistochemical staining and flow cytometry of sampled material can characterize a monoclonal lymphocyte population. Surgical biopsy is sometimes required to establish the diagnosis. In 50% of cases, lymphoma is primary to the thyroid gland, and it is usually an intermediate-grade non-Hodgkin's–type lymphoma (Chapter 185).

Surgical resection of the thyroid is usually not indicated, but elective tracheostomy may be required if tracheal compression is imminent. Most patients respond to treatment with combined external beam radiation therapy and chemotherapy. Disease-free survival rates vary with the disease stage at diagnosis and the initial response to combination therapy.

 Grade A References

A1. McDermott MT. Does combination T4 and T3 therapy make sense? *Endocr Pract.* 2012;18: 750-757.

A2. Marcocci C, Kahaly GJ, Krassas GE, et al. Selenium and the course of mild Graves' orbitopathy. *N Engl J Med.* 2011;364:1920-1931.

A3. Bahn Chair RS, Burch HB, Cooper DS, et al. Hyperthyroidism and other causes of thyrotoxicosis: management guidelines of the American Thyroid Association and American Association of Clinical Endocrinologists. *Thyroid.* 2011;21:593-646.

A4. Stagnaro-Green A, Abalovich M, Alexander E, et al. Guidelines of the American Thyroid Association for the diagnosis and management of thyroid disease during pregnancy and postpartum. *Thyroid.* 2011;21:1081-1125.

A5. Smallridge RC, Ain KB, Asa SL, et al. American Thyroid Association guidelines for management of patients with anaplastic thyroid cancer. *Thyroid.* 2012;22:1104-1139.

A6. Brose MS, Nutting CM, Jarzab B, et al. Sorafenib in radioactive iodine-refractory, locally advanced or metastatic differentiated thyroid cancer: a randomised, double-blind, phase 3 trial. *Lancet.* 2014; 384:319-328.

A7. Leboulleux S, Bastholt L, Krause T, et al. Vandetanib in locally advanced or metastatic differentiated thyroid cancer: a randomised, double-blind, phase 2 trial. *Lancet Oncol.* 2012;13: 897-905.

GENERAL REFERENCES

For the General References and other additional features, please visit Expert Consult at https://expertconsult.inkling.com.

227

ADRENAL CORTEX

LYNNETTE K. NIEMAN

The adrenal glands weigh 6 to 8 g in adults (Fig. 227-1). Each contains a cortex, which makes steroid hormones, and a medulla, which produces catecholamines. Diseases of the adrenal medulla are discussed in Chapter 228. In the adrenal cortex, production of the three major classes of steroids occurs in specific zones: the outermost layer, the glomerulosa, produces mineralocorticoids, primarily aldosterone; the middle layer, the fasciculata, produces glucocorticoids, primarily cortisol; the innermost layer, the reticularis, produces adrenal "androgens," primarily dehydroepiandrosterone (DHEA) and its sulfated conjugate (DHEA-S) (Fig. 227-2). This division reflects the fact that certain critical enzymes are restricted to specific zones, resulting in the ability or inability to synthesize specific end products.

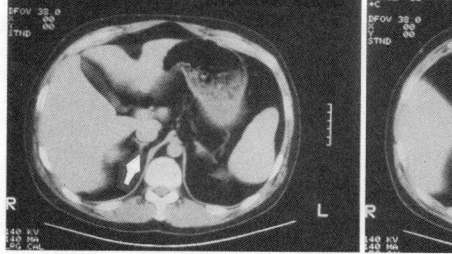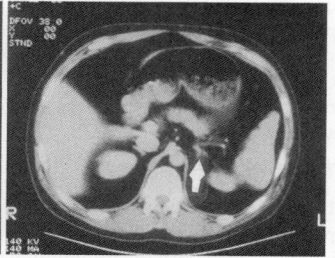

FIGURE 227-1. Magnetic resonance images of the abdomen showing the position and relative size of the normal adrenal glands.

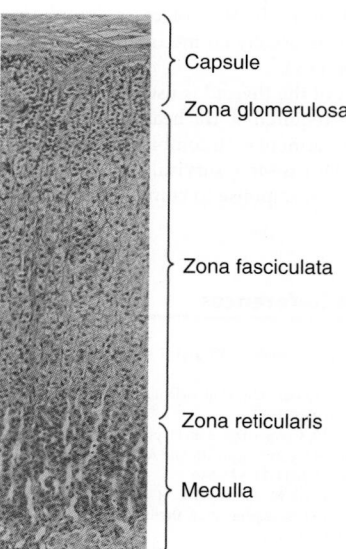

- Capsule
- Zona glomerulosa
- Zona fasciculata
- Zona reticularis
- Medulla

FIGURE 227-2. Histologic section through a normal adult adrenal gland showing the progression (from outside to inside) of the zona glomerulosa, zona fasciculata, zona reticularis, and medulla.

FUNCTION

The actions and regulation of these steroid classes differ. Mineralocorticoids act through the renal mineralocorticoid receptor to promote the reabsorption of sodium and the secretion of potassium. In addition to this classic action, mineralocorticoids have important action on the vasculature and may exacerbate the metabolic syndrome.[1] Aldosterone secretion is stimulated primarily by hyperkalemia and angiotensin II (which itself is stimulated by hypovolemia and excess renin). These agents increase the production of aldosterone synthase to restore homeostasis through this feedback loop. Aldosterone production is stimulated to a much smaller degree by adrenocorticotropic hormone (ACTH).

Cortisol and other glucocorticoids act through the glucocorticoid receptor type 2 and its isoforms. The actions of this class of steroids are much broader, including effects on carbohydrate handling, lipid and calcium metabolism, and the immune and nervous systems. Cortisol production is regulated primarily by ACTH, which is secreted in a circadian rhythm in response to corticotropin-releasing hormone (CRH) so that cortisol levels are highest in the morning and fall to a nadir around midnight. Cortisol coordinates ACTH production through negative feedback at the pituitary (ACTH) and hypothalamus (CRH). Vasopressin secretion also plays a role in stimulating ACTH release.

DHEA and DHEA-S are the most abundant products of the adrenal gland. They exert their estrogenic and androgenic effects as prohormones, being converted to estrogens and testosterone in the peripheral tissues and activating the androgen and estrogen receptors. There is no known regulator of DHEA synthesis, but its production declines with age.

DISORDERS OF ADRENAL FUNCTION

Most disorders of the adrenal cortex reflect overproduction or underproduction of the products of a single synthetic zone—cortisol, aldosterone, or testosterone or estrogen (Fig. 227-3). The congenital adrenal hyperplasias are an exception and are manifested with both overproduction and underproduction. Abnormal secretion is suggested by clinical features of each disorder and is reflected in plasma or urine levels of the relevant hormones or by the consequent increases or decreases in feedback systems, which form the basis of the biochemical diagnostic tests.

Glucocorticoid Excess: Cushing Syndrome

CLINICAL MANIFESTATIONS

Cushing syndrome is a symptom complex that reflects excessive tissue exposure to cortisol. Classic features of Cushing syndrome include weight gain, plethora, hypertension, and striae (Table 227-1). Not all patients have all features; the number and severity of features correlate roughly with the duration and severity of hypercortisolism. Because many of the signs and symptoms are nonspecific, the diagnosis may be confused with psychiatric disorders, polycystic ovary syndrome, the metabolic syndrome, simple obesity, fibromyalgia, or acute illness. However, because worsening hypercortisolism may precipitate hypertension, glucose intolerance, infections, psychiatric disturbances, impaired cognition, and hypercoagulability, it is important to identify this treatable disorder to prevent its associated morbidity and mortality.[2]

Changes in mood and cognition are useful markers of hypercortisolism. These include irritability, crying, and restlessness; depressed mood; decreased libido; insomnia; anxiety; and decreased concentration and impaired memory.

DIAGNOSIS

Clinical Examination

Cushing syndrome screening is most likely to be positive in the presence of signs that are typical of glucocorticoid excess, such as abnormal fat distribution in the supraclavicular and temporal fossae, proximal muscle weakness, wide (>1 cm) purple striae, and new irritability, decreased cognition, and decreased short-term memory. Testing is indicated when clinical features have progressed over time. For example, oligomenorrhea is more suggestive of Cushing syndrome if a woman previously had regular menses. Serial seven subtractions and recall of three cities (or objects) are useful bedside strategies to identify deficits in cognition and memory.

Laboratory Findings

Exogenous administration of glucocorticoid should be excluded before screening for endogenous Cushing syndrome. In the absence of pseudo-Cushing states (see later), at least two different screening test results should

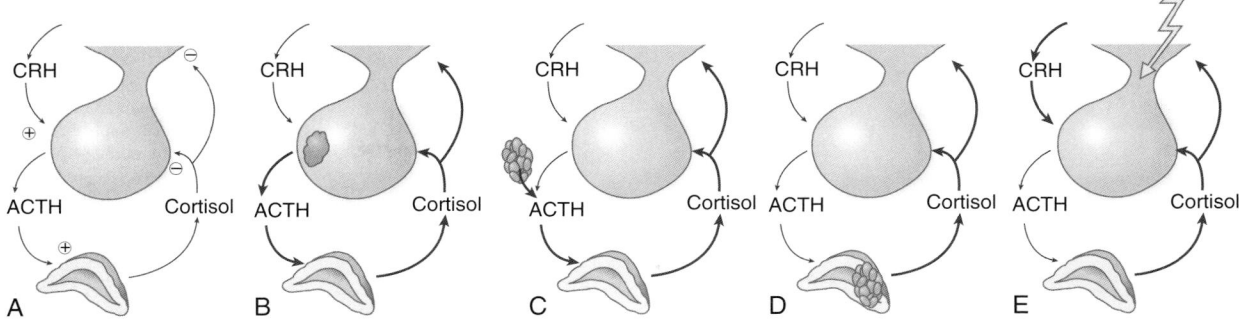

FIGURE 227-3. Physiology of the adrenal axis in health, Cushing syndrome, and pseudo-Cushing states. **A,** In healthy individuals, cortisol production is stimulated by the increased hypothalamic release of corticotropin-releasing hormone (CRH), which then travels down the pituitary stalk to stimulate adrenocorticotropic hormone (ACTH) secretion and release by corticotropes. Circulating ACTH stimulates adrenal gland production and secretion of cortisol. Cortisol then functions in a negative feedback mechanism to inhibit both CRH and ACTH. **B,** In Cushing disease, a pituitary tumor releases excessive amounts of ACTH, which results in increased cortisol secretion by the adrenal glands. **C,** In ectopic ACTH secretion, a nonpituitary ACTH-secreting tumor releases excessive amounts of ACTH, which results in increased cortisol secretion by the adrenal glands. **D,** In ACTH-independent adrenal forms of Cushing syndrome, the adrenal tumor autonomously releases excess amounts of cortisol. In all forms of Cushing syndrome, the negative feedback effects of excessive cortisol inhibit endogenous CRH and ACTH secretion, so that circulating ACTH levels reflect the underlying tumor (levels are normal or increased) or independent cortisol production (levels are suppressed). **E,** In pseudo-Cushing states, central stimulation increases CRH secretion, which in turn increases ACTH and hence cortisol production. In this setting, the negative feedback effects of excessive cortisol inhibit endogenous CRH and ACTH secretion, so that cortisol levels are ultimately constrained, albeit at an increased level.

TABLE 227-1 THE FREQUENCY OF CLINICAL SIGNS AND SYMPTOMS OF CUSHING SYNDROME

SIGN OR SYMPTOM	PERCENTAGE
Decreased libido in men and women	100
Obesity or weight gain	97
Plethora	94
Round face	88
Menstrual changes	84
Hirsutism	81
Hypertension	74
Ecchymoses	62
Lethargy, depression	62
Striae	56
Weakness	56
Electrocardiographic changes or atherosclerosis	55
Dorsal fat pad	54
Edema	50
Abnormal glucose tolerance	50
Osteopenia or fracture	50
Headache	47
Backache	43
Recurrent infections	25
Abdominal pain	21
Acne	21
Female balding	13

be abnormal to establish the diagnosis. Tests for the differential diagnosis of Cushing syndrome should not be used to make the diagnosis. Figure 227-4 is the Endocrine Society's recommended algorithm for testing of patients suspected of having Cushing syndrome.[3]

Urine, Saliva, and Serum Cortisol Measurements

Urine free cortisol (UFC) excretion during 24 hours is a good screening test. Specific, structurally based assay techniques, such as high-performance liquid chromatography and tandem mass spectrometry, are the "gold standard." The upper-normal limit of these tests is much lower and more specific than that of antibody-based assays, in which other steroids may cross-react. This cross-reactivity may be an advantage in screening for hypercortisolism.

UFC excretion also may be increased in the so-called *pseudo-Cushing states,* including psychiatric disorders (depression, anxiety disorder, obsessive-compulsive disorder), chronic pain, severe exercise, alcoholism, uncontrolled diabetes, and morbid obesity. Here, it is hypothesized that higher brain pathways stimulate CRH release and activation of the entire hypothalamic-pituitary-adrenal axis (see Fig. 227-3E). Cortisol negative feedback inhibition on CRH and pituitary ACTH release restrains the resulting hypercortisoluria to less than four-fold greater than normal. Thus, Cushing syndrome cannot be diagnosed with certainty unless values reach this threshold. Conversely, patients with Cushing syndrome may have normal UFC excretion because of mild or intermittent hypercortisolism or altered renal metabolism of cortisol. If UFC is only mildly elevated and clinical features are minimal, it is best to treat any pseudo-Cushing state and to remeasure UFC excretion with the expectation that it will normalize. Alternatively, if UFC values are normal but clinical suspicion is high, repeated measurement might disclose intermittent hypercortisolism.

Measurement of plasma cortisol at midnight distinguishes pseudo-Cushing states from Cushing syndrome with 95% diagnostic accuracy; a level greater than 7.5 µg/dL is required for the diagnosis of Cushing syndrome. Measurement of salivary cortisol at bedtime or at midnight works as well, is more convenient, and may be the best screening test in patients with mild or intermittent hypercortisolism.[4,5] However, the criteria for its interpretation differ, so each assay must be validated before it is used for this purpose.

Dexamethasone Suppression Tests

The dexamethasone suppression test is a simple screening test that takes advantage of the negative feedback effect of glucocorticoids to reduce ACTH (and hence serum cortisol). Dexamethasone 1 mg is given orally between 11:00 PM and midnight, and plasma cortisol is measured between 8:00 and 9:00 the next morning. The test has an 8% false-negative rate in patients with Cushing disease and a 30% false-positive rate in chronic illness, obesity, psychiatric disorders, and normal individuals. As a result, Cushing syndrome cannot be diagnosed by this test alone unless the result is extremely abnormal.

The 2-day, 2-mg dexamethasone suppression test discriminates patients with a pseudo-Cushing state if plasma cortisol end points of less than 1.4 or 2.2 µg/dL are used. Dexamethasone 500 µg is given orally every 6 hours for eight doses, and plasma cortisol is measured 2 hours after the last dose. The test has excellent sensitivity (90 to 100%) and specificity (97 to 100%) for discriminating Cushing syndrome, but it is costly and requires excellent compliance of the patient. The immediate subsequent administration of CRH (1 µg per kilogram of body weight intravenously) and the measurement of cortisol 15 minutes later increased the sensitivity and specificity to 100% in a small study of patients, with values above 1.4 µg/dL indicating Cushing syndrome. Although this combined dexamethasone-CRH test has high diagnostic accuracy, it has the same disadvantages as the 2-day dexamethasone suppression test and the added cost of CRH testing. Because of these drawbacks, these tests are usually reserved for patients with ambiguous or confusing results on other screening tests. CRH is available commercially (Acthrel), with Food and Drug Administration–approved labeling for the differential diagnosis of Cushing syndrome. Its use in the dexamethasone-CRH test is an off-label use.

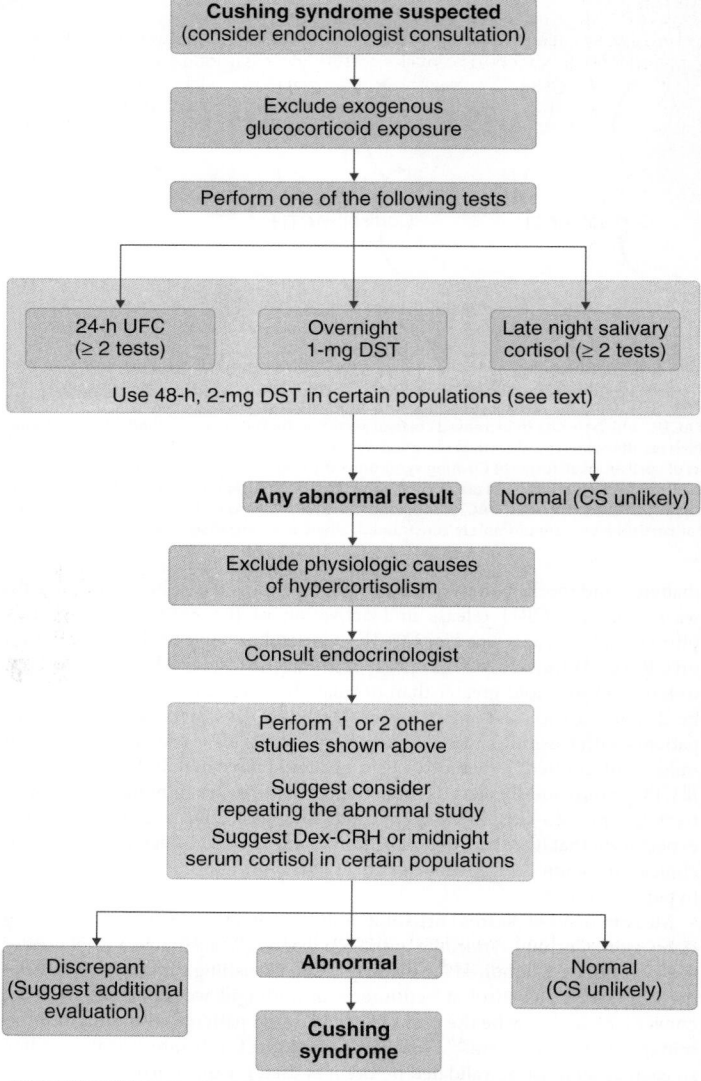

FIGURE 227-4. Algorithm for testing of patients suspected of having Cushing syndrome (CS). All statements are recommendations except for those prefaced by "suggest". Diagnostic criteria that suggest Cushing syndrome are urine free cortisol (UFC) greater than the normal range for the assay, serum cortisol greater than 1.8 μg/dL (50 nmol/liter) after 1 mg dexamethasone (1-mg DST), and late-night salivary cortisol greater than 145 ng/dL (4 nmol/liter). Dex-CRH = dexamethasone–corticotropin-releasing hormone test; DST = dexamethasone suppression test. (Reprinted with permission from Nieman LK, Biller BM, Findling JW, et al. The diagnosis of Cushing syndrome: an Endocrine Society clinical practice guideline. *J Clin Endocrinol Metab.* 2008;93:1526-1540.)

TABLE 227-2	ETIOLOGY OF CUSHING SYNDROME
EXOGENOUS	**ENDOGENOUS**
Most common cause of Cushing syndrome:	ACTH independent—autonomous adrenal activation (20% of all cases)
Glucocorticoid or ACTH driven	Adrenal adenoma (40-50%)
May be factitious or iatrogenic	Adrenal carcinoma (40-50%)
	Primary pigmented nodular adrenal disease
	McCune-Albright syndrome
	Massive macronodular adrenal disease
	Gastric inhibitory polypeptide or food induced
	ACTH dependent—adrenal activation by excessive ACTH (80% of all cases)
	Corticotrope adenoma (80%)
	Ectopic ACTH secretion (20%)
	Ectopic CRH secretion (rare)

ACTH = adrenocorticotropic hormone; CRH = corticotropin-releasing hormone.

result, patients must be queried closely about exogenous steroid administration, recognizing that parenteral, inhaled, and topical steroids can all cause glucocorticoid excess. Patients with endogenous Cushing syndrome and low ACTH concentrations should undergo adrenal imaging to identify the site of adrenal abnormality. Nonautonomous adrenal tissue atrophies when ACTH support is subnormal. Because of this, the common ACTH-independent forms of Cushing syndrome—adrenal adenoma and carcinoma—are manifested as a unilateral adrenal mass, with atrophy of the adjacent and contralateral tissue on magnetic resonance imaging or computed tomography.

Bilateral forms of primary adrenal disease are rare and may be manifested with small or large adrenal nodules.[6] Primary pigmented nodular adrenal disease occurs primarily in children and young adults and is characterized by small to normal-sized adrenal glands containing small (<5 mm) black-brown cortical nodules. About half of these patients have additional features, termed *Carney complex*, which are often inherited in an autosomal dominant fashion. The clinical features of Carney complex include myxomas of the skin, breast, and heart; spotty pigmentation, such as lentigines and blue nevi; and other endocrine overactivity, such as acromegaly and testicular tumors. Some of these patients have mutations leading to a truncated form of protein kinase A regulatory 1α subunit. The resultant increase in protein kinase A activation by cyclic adenosine monophosphate presumably allows tumor formation. Bilateral nodular hyperplasia with Cushing syndrome can occur in the setting of *McCune-Albright syndrome*, mostly in infants or children. Massive macronodular adrenal disease generally is manifested after the age of 40 years with huge adrenal glands and aberrant expression of "illicit" receptors for various ligands (gastric inhibitory polypeptide, β-adrenergic, vasopressin), which presumably mediates autonomous cortisol production.

A normal or elevated plasma ACTH level (>15 pg/mL; 3.3 pmol/L) is consistent with an ACTH-producing tumor.[7] Intermediate ACTH concentrations between 5 and 15 pg/mL (1.1 to 3.3 pmol/L) in a two-site sandwich assay are not diagnostic. In these patients, suboptimal cortisol responses to CRH stimulation may identify the minority of cases of ACTH-independent Cushing syndrome with borderline basal ACTH values. In addition, a suppressed plasma DHEA-S value supports the diagnosis of an ACTH-independent disorder.

Cushing disease,[8] an ACTH-secreting pituitary adenoma, is the most common cause of Cushing syndrome. It is more common in women than in men (6 : 1 ratio), with a mean age at onset in the fourth decade. ACTH also may be secreted ectopically by a variety of neuroendocrine tumors, as shown in Table 227-3.

Pituitary magnetic resonance imaging shows a tumor in only about 40 to 50% of patients with Cushing disease, but it is obtained routinely in patients with ACTH-dependent disease to exclude a macroadenoma or abnormal anatomy before petrosal sinus sampling or surgery. A pituitary lesion less than 6 mm is seen in up to 10% of healthy individuals and so does not always indicate Cushing disease. Biochemical tests must be used to distinguish among the ACTH-dependent causes of Cushing syndrome, and they must be performed after a 6- to 8-week period of sustained hypercortisolism sufficient to suppress normal corticotrope function.

Inferior petrosal sinus sampling is the best test to distinguish between a pituitary and an ectopic source of excess ACTH; worldwide, the overall

Any dexamethasone test may give false results in patients with abnormal metabolic clearance of the drug. Agents that induce the cytochrome P-450 CYP3A4 enzymes (alcohol, rifampin, phenytoin, phenobarbital) increase dexamethasone clearance, whereas renal or hepatic failure decreases it. Measurement of a dexamethasone level can determine whether its clearance has been altered.

Differential Diagnosis

The causes of endogenous Cushing syndrome can be divided broadly into ACTH-dependent (80%) and ACTH-independent (20%) forms (Table 227-2). Hypercortisolism from autonomously functioning adrenal tumors suppresses ACTH, whereas in primary disorders of ACTH excess, the adrenal glands respond to tumor-derived ACTH. Plasma ACTH concentration distinguishes between these causes. ACTH is usually less than 10 pg/mL in primary adrenal disorders but is also suppressed by exogenous steroids, whether they are prescribed intentionally (iatrogenic Cushing syndrome) or taken factitiously. Patients in the latter group often have had multiple surgical procedures and do not reveal that they are self-administering steroids. As a

TABLE 227-3 THE INCIDENCE AND TYPES OF TUMORS CAUSING THE SYNDROME OF ECTOPIC ACTH SECRETION

TUMOR TYPE	PERCENTAGE
Carcinoma of lung (small cell or oat cell)	19-50
Carcinoid of bronchus	2-37
Carcinoid of thymus	8-12
Pancreatic tumors, carcinoid and islet cell	4-12
Pheochromocytoma, neuroblastoma, ganglioma, paraganglioma	5-12
Medullary carcinoma of the thyroid	0-5
Miscellaneous*	<1

*Miscellaneous tumors reported to secrete ACTH in 1 to 10 cases include carcinoma of the ovary, prostate, breast, thyroid, kidney, salivary glands, testes, gallbladder, esophagus, and appendix; gastric carcinoid and renal carcinoid; acute myeloblastic leukemia; melanoma; and cloacogenic carcinoma of the anal canal.
ACTH = adrenocorticotropic hormone.

sensitivity and specificity are about 94%. The test involves catheterization of a peripheral vein and also the petrosal sinuses draining the pituitary gland; simultaneous measurement of ACTH levels at each site before and 3, 5, and 10 minutes after administration of CRH; and calculation of the central-to-peripheral ACTH ratio at each time point. Ratios of more than 2 before CRH administration or more than 3 after CRH administration are consistent with Cushing disease.

Although it is accurate in experienced hands, inferior petrosal sinus sampling carries a small risk of stroke, is expensive, and is not widely available. Other tests, such as the CRH test and the 8-mg dexamethasone suppression test, may be useful if both responses indicate Cushing disease. In this setting, the likelihood of ectopic ACTH secretion is low. However, the diagnosis is not clear if both responses are negative or if they are mixed.

If endocrine tests suggest ectopic ACTH secretion, imaging is obtained to localize the tumor. Computed tomography and magnetic resonance imaging of the chest are the best initial screens because these tumors are most often in the thoracic cavity. Octreotide scintigraphy is a useful adjunctive test. Measurement of serum calcitonin and gastrin and measurement of plasma or urine catecholamines may identify medullary carcinoma of the thyroid, gastrinoma, and pheochromocytoma. The process can be repeated every 6 to 12 months; tumors that make ACTH ectopically have a spectrum of malignant potential, and annual screening should continue, regardless of treatment for hypercortisolism.

TREATMENT Rx

Surgical Therapy

The optimal treatment of Cushing syndrome is surgical resection of the lesion that is producing excessive ACTH or cortisol. In ACTH-dependent Cushing syndrome, if this is unsuccessful or cannot be done, bilateral adrenalectomy is an option.

Transsphenoidal resection of a microadenoma is the optimal therapy for a patient with Cushing disease, with up to a 90% chance of cure in the hands of an experienced neurosurgeon. A successful outcome is less likely if the initial surgery is not curative, in cases of recurrence, and for macroadenomas. Controversy exists about the criteria for remission; although a low postoperative cortisol level is encouraging, it does not preclude later recurrence. If recurrence develops, additional resection or alternative therapy should be considered.

Patients with ectopic ACTH secretion can be cured if the tumor can be removed and is not metastatic. Otherwise, adrenalectomy or medical therapy is chosen (see later). Adrenalectomy is appropriate when the patient cannot tolerate the medical toxicity, cost, or adverse psychological effects of long-term medical therapy and monitoring; when rapid correction of hypercortisolism is needed; or if maximal daily doses of ketoconazole (1600 mg) and metyrapone (2 g) given in combination do not render the patient eucortisolemic.

Nonmalignant primary adrenal causes of Cushing syndrome are cured by resection of the abnormal tissue. Laparoscopy is the preferred approach. Surgery is the mainstay in the treatment of adrenal cancer; multiple operations may be needed to resect primary lesions, local recurrences, and hepatic, thoracic, and intracranial metastases. Adjuvant adrenolytic therapy with mitotane may provide a chemotherapeutic benefit.

Radiation Therapy

Radiation therapy to the pituitary gland, with adjunctive therapy with steroidogenesis inhibitors to normalize cortisol levels, is a good option for patients with Cushing disease who cannot undergo surgery, for those in whom the risk of Nelson syndrome (Chapter 224) is deemed great, and for those with recurrent disease. This is usually delivered in 200-rad daily increments to a total dose of 4500 cGy. The disadvantage of radiation therapy is the length of time needed for a full response—up to 10 years—and the possibility of hypopituitarism. There is less experience with high-energy radiosurgery, such as the gamma knife, which has the advantage of requiring only one or two treatments. Adrenalectomy is preferable if rapid normalization of hypercortisolism is needed, and this option may be chosen by patients who have concerns about radiation-induced hypopituitarism and loss of reproductive function.

Medical Therapy

Medical therapy can also be used for patients with occult ectopic ACTH-secreting tumors or in combination with pituitary irradiation to treat Cushing disease.

Medical therapy with steroidogenesis inhibitors alone is rarely appropriate for Cushing disease because it requires close monitoring and adjustment of dose. Cabergoline or pasireotide may normalize UFC in 40% and 20% of patients, respectively. [A1] There are limited data on the long-term efficacy of any medical therapy in Cushing disease.

For advanced adrenocortical carcinoma, rates of response and progression-free survival but not overall survival are significantly better with first-line therapy using a combination of etoposide (100 mg/m² on days 2 to 4), doxorubicin (40 mg/m² on day 1), and cisplatin (40 mg/m² on days 3 and 4) plus oral mitotane (to achieve a blood level of 14 to 20 mg/L) than with streptozocin plus mitotane as first-line therapy, with similar rates of toxic events. [A2]

Mineralocorticoid Excess

DIAGNOSIS

Patients with mineralocorticoid excess often have few clinical symptoms apart from fatigue and muscle weakness or cramps related to hypokalemia. Most often the condition is suspected because of hypertension, especially if it occurs at an early age in association with spontaneous hypokalemia or is difficult to control.[9] Mineralocorticoid excess can result from primary adrenal disease, in which aldosterone (or another mineralocorticoid) is produced autonomously (and renin levels are low), or it may be due to nonadrenal causes as a result of elevated renin values, which stimulate aldosterone secretion. The latter situations include states of contracted arterial intravascular volume, such as congestive heart failure or cirrhosis with ascites, decreased renal arterial blood flow, and tumor production of renin (Table 227-4).

RENIN-INDEPENDENT MINERALOCORTICOID EXCESS

DIAGNOSIS

Although most of these conditions result from excessive aldosterone production by one or both adrenal glands, excessive production of other mineralocorticoids or constitutive activation of the renal sodium channel must be excluded. In these latter conditions, both aldosterone and renin values are low, resulting in the so-called syndrome of apparent mineralocorticoid excess. In this setting, diagnostic information is obtained by history (licorice ingestion) or measurement of other mineralocorticoids (see Table 227-4).

Primary hyperaldosteronism is diagnosed when there is an increased ratio (>20) of morning aldosterone to plasma renin activity (Fig. 227-5). One of four tests (usually salt loading) is used to confirm primary hyperaldosteronism by demonstrating a lack of aldosterone suppression.[10]

Differential Diagnosis

Having made the diagnosis of aldosterone-dependent mineralocorticoid excess, one must differentiate between the two most common adrenal causes—hyperplasia and adenoma—after excluding potential rare causes of hyperaldosteronism. Two rare autosomal dominant forms of familial hyperaldosteronism are type 1, a glucocorticoid-suppressible hyperaldosteronism, and type 2. Familial hyperaldosteronism type 1 is caused by a genetic swap of the promoter for CYP11B1 (11β-hydroxylase) with that of CYP11B2 (aldosterone synthase), forming a chimeric gene in which ACTH stimulates aldosterone synthase. It should be suspected in the setting of familial disease, particularly if there is a history of early-onset cardiovascular events, and is confirmed by gene testing (see http://www.brighamandwomens.org/Departments_and_Services/medicine/services/endocrine/Services/gra/default.aspx). The genetic abnormality in familial hyperaldosteronism

TABLE 227-4   CAUSES OF MINERALOCORTICOID EXCESS

PRIMARY HYPERALDOSTERONISM: HIGH ALDOSTERONE, LOW RENIN

Aldosterone-producing adenomas (30-50%)
Bilateral zona glomerulosa hyperplasia
Familial hyperaldosteronism
    Type 1: glucocorticoid-remediable hyperaldosteronism—this results from
    formation of a chimeric gene containing the regulator portion of 11β-hydroxylase
    (normally regulated by ACTH) and the synthetic region of aldosterone synthase;
    as a result, ACTH stimulates aldosterone synthase and hence aldosterone
    production
    Type 2: adrenal adenomas or hyperplasia expressed in a familial pattern
    Type 3: caused by mutant KCNJ5, often younger and more severe than Type 2
Aldosterone-producing adrenal carcinoma
Ectopic aldosterone secretion (rare): kidney, ovary

SECONDARY HYPERALDOSTERONISM: HIGH ALDOSTERONE, HIGH RENIN

Renovascular hypertension and aortic stenosis
Diuretic use
Renin-secreting tumors
Severe cardiac failure

APPARENT MINERALOCORTICOID EXCESS: LOW ALDOSTERONE, LOW RENIN

Licorice ingestion: licorice (candy or flavored tobacco) containing glycyrrhetinic acid
    (or similar compounds such as carbenoxolone) inhibits renal 11β-hydroxysteroid
    dehydrogenase type 2, reducing cortisol conversion to cortisone and enabling
    cortisol to act as an endogenous mineralocorticoid
Severe hypercortisolism: similar in mechanism to licorice ingestion; very high
    cortisol levels are thought to overwhelm the ability of 11β-hydroxysteroid
    dehydrogenase type 2 to convert cortisol to cortisone in the kidney; cortisol itself
    then acts as a potent mineralocorticoid
Liddle's syndrome: mutation of the β or γ subunit of the collecting tubule sodium
    channel leads to a constitutive increase in sodium reabsorption and potassium
    excretion
11β-Hydroxylase deficiency form of congenital adrenal hyperplasia: 11-deoxycortisol
    accumulates because of an inability to convert it to cortisol
17-Hydroxylase deficiency form of congenital adrenal hyperplasia:
    deoxycorticosterone and corticosterone are increased

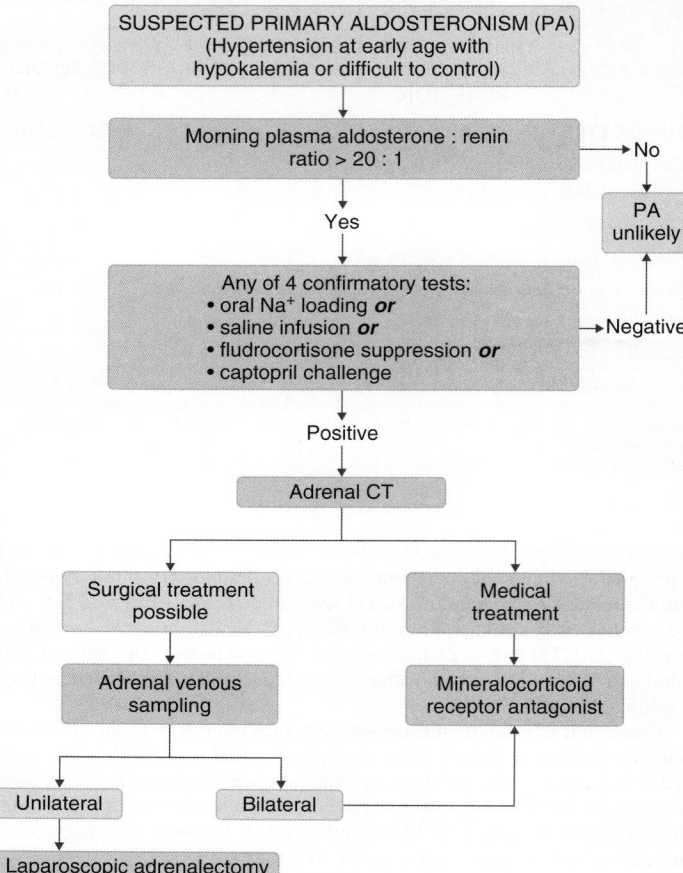

FIGURE 227-5. Algorithm for the detection, confirmation, subtype testing, and treatment of primary aldosteronism (PA). We recommend the case detection of PA in patient groups with relatively high prevalence of PA. These include patients with moderate, severe, or resistant hypertension; spontaneous or diuretic-induced hypokalemia; hypertension with adrenal incidentaloma; or a family history of early-onset hypertension or cerebrovascular accident at a young age (<40 years). We recommend use of the plasma aldosterone-to-renin ratio (ARR) to detect cases of PA in these patient groups. We recommend that patients with a positive ARR undergo testing, using any of four confirmatory tests, to definitively confirm or exclude the diagnosis. We recommend that all patients with PA undergo an adrenal computed tomography (CT) scan as the initial study in subtype testing and to exclude adrenocortical carcinoma. When surgical treatment is practicable and desired by the patient, the distinction between unilateral and bilateral adrenal disease should be made by adrenal venous sampling (AVS). We recommend that treatment by unilateral laparoscopic adrenalectomy be offered to patients with AVS-documented unilateral aldosterone-producing adenoma. If a patient is unable or unwilling to undergo surgery, we recommend medical treatment with a mineralocorticoid receptor (MR) antagonist. In patients with PA due to bilateral adrenal disease, we recommend medical treatment with an MR antagonist. In patients with confirmed PA who have a family history of PA or of strokes at young age (<40 years), or with onset of hypertension earlier than at 20 years of age, we suggest genetic testing for glucocorticoid-remediable aldosteronism. In patients with glucocorticoid-remediable aldosteronism, we recommend the use of the lowest dose of glucocorticoid receptor agonist that can normalize blood pressure and serum potassium levels. (Reprinted, with slight modification of text, from Funder JW, Carey RM, Fardella C, et al. Case detection, diagnosis, and treatment of patients with primary aldosteronism: an Endocrine Society clinical practice guideline. *J Clin Endocrinol Metab.* 2008;93:3266-3281.)

type 2 is not known; its clinical presentation is similar to sporadic hyperaldosteronism. Recent studies demonstrate rare germline mutations of a potassium channel in familial hyperalsosteronism, and somatic adrenal mutations in about 40% of patients.

For the more common conditions, adrenal computed tomography scans may show nonfunctioning nodules and falsely suggest an adenoma.[11] The responses to physiologic maneuvers, such as upright posture, and salt loading with oral or intravenous sodium tend to be preserved in patients with hyperplasia, but there is significant overlap among groups of patients. The best diagnostic test involves the measurement of cortisol and aldosterone in bilateral adrenal venous effluent and a peripheral vein before and during an ACTH infusion. Cortisol is used to evaluate catheter placement in the adrenal veins, as levels from the two sides should be similar. When an adenoma is present, the aldosterone-to-cortisol ratio on one side is usually at least five-fold greater than the other, which may be similar to the periphery, indicating suppression. Bilateral hyperplasia tends to produce similar values on each side.

TREATMENT   **Rx**

Treatment of primary hyperaldosteronism includes laparoscopic resection for adenomas.[12] Afterward, hypokalemia generally resolves, but hypertension persists in up to 65% of patients. A mineralocorticoid antagonist, spironolactone or eplerenone, is used to treat patients unable to undergo surgery or those with hyperplasia. Eplerenone is a more selective mineralocorticoid antagonist (with fewer side effects of sexual dysfunction and gynecomastia compared with spironolactone). A sodium channel blocker (e.g., amiloride) may be helpful, and antihypertensive agents are continued as needed.

Androgen Excess
DEFINITION

Women with excess circulating androgens or increased sensitivity to androgens present with complaints of hirsutism, acne, and anovulation or

infertility. When testosterone is secreted in great excess, women may virilize and exhibit a deepened voice, clitorimegaly, masculinized body habitus, and alopecia.

DIAGNOSIS

The adrenal causes of hyperandrogenism—congenital adrenal hyperplasia, Cushing disease, adrenal cancer, and androgen-producing adrenal adenoma—are uncommon. Most women have no clear-cut cause (idiopathic hirsutism) or polycystic ovary syndrome. Rarely, androgen-secreting ovarian tumors, hyperprolactinemia, glucocorticoid resistance, or exogenous drugs cause hyperandrogenism. Patients with an adrenal source of hyperandrogenism usually have increased serum levels of DHEA, DHEA-S, or androstenedione, in contrast to the testosterone excess that is more typical of an ovarian source. DHEA and DHEA-S are weak androgens that can be converted locally to testosterone in the hair follicles. Because DHEA and DHEA-S levels decline throughout adult life, these values must be interpreted within age-specific normal ranges. Although a tumor is more likely if DHEA-S is greater than 500 μg/dL or testosterone is greater than 200 ng/mL, it is not excluded at lower levels.

Imaging identifies nearly all adrenal tumors but may miss a small intraovarian one. UFC may be elevated in patients with virilizing adrenal carcinoma or Cushing disease (see earlier) and in those with glucocorticoid resistance. By contrast, androgen-secreting adrenal adenomas do not have glucocorticoid excess. In women suspected of having nonclassic forms of congenital adrenal hyperplasia, precursor and product hormones should be measured before and after ACTH to confirm the diagnosis.

TREATMENT Rx

Treatment of adrenal causes of hyperandrogenism varies according to the disorder. Classic congenital adrenal hyperplasia is treated by glucocorticoids to normalize ACTH and hence androgen levels (typically, dexamethasone 0.125 to 0.375 mg at bedtime). The nonclassic forms respond well to oral contraceptive or antiandrogen treatment, with dexamethasone reserved for ovulation induction. Surgery with adjunctive medical treatment may be used in adrenal carcinoma (see earlier).

Mixed Mineralocorticoid and Glucocorticoid Deficiency: Adrenal Insufficiency

PATHOBIOLOGY
Primary Adrenal Insufficiency
Autoimmune Destruction
Autoimmune destruction is the most common cause of primary adrenal insufficiency in industrialized countries and may occur alone or, rarely, in association with autoimmune polyglandular syndromes. These syndromes tend to be manifested either in childhood (type 1), in association with hypoparathyroidism and mucocutaneous candidiasis, or in adulthood (type 2), in association with insulin-dependent diabetes mellitus, autoimmune thyroid disease, alopecia areata, or vitiligo. The glands are small on imaging.

Adrenoleukodystrophy
Adrenoleukodystrophy, a rare (1 in 25,000) X-linked condition, is characterized by a deficiency of peroxisomal membrane adrenoleukodystrophy protein, which transports activated acyl-coenzyme A derivates into the peroxisomes, where they are shortened by β-oxidation. This deficiency results in the accumulation of very long chain fatty acids in the central nervous system and other tissues and increased plasma $C_{26:0}$ fatty acids. Incomplete penetrance of the genetic defect and variable accumulation of very long chain fatty acids in the adrenal gland, brain, testis, and liver account for the clinical phenotypes, which differ by age and presentation.[13]

Replacement of Adrenal Tissue
Infections cause about 15% of primary adrenal insufficiency. Typical infections include tuberculosis and systemic fungal diseases (histoplasmosis, coccidioidomycosis, blastomycosis), in which the adrenal tissue is replaced by caseating granulomas. End-stage AIDS-associated opportunistic infections, such as cytomegalovirus or *Mycobacterium avium-intracellulare*, may reduce adrenal function. Adrenal tissue may be replaced by bilateral metastases (most commonly primary carcinoma of the lung, breast, kidney, or gut) or primary lymphoma, although adrenal insufficiency is uncommon. Intraadrenal hemorrhage may also lead to insufficient steroidogenesis. Hemorrhage typically occurs in a stressed, hospitalized patient receiving long-term prophylactic anticoagulation and is often accompanied by back pain. The adrenal glands tend to be large on imaging.

Congenital Adrenal Hyperplasias
The congenital adrenal hyperplasias[14] are a disparate group of diseases caused by a genetic deficiency of one of the enzymes needed for adrenal steroidogenesis. Patients with nearly complete deficiency of an enzyme required for cortisol synthesis present in infancy with adrenal insufficiency and salt-wasting crisis. This is most problematic in patients with mutation of the 21-hydroxylase (*CYP21A2*) or 11β-hydroxylase (*CYP11B1*) gene. The increase in ACTH levels caused by cortisol deficiency drives the intact steroidogenic pathways so that there is excessive production of the steroids just proximal to the enzymatic block—17-hydroxyprogesterone and 11-deoxycortisol, respectively, in 21-hydroxylase and 11β-hydroxylase deficiency. The increased levels of precursor steroids enable increased adrenal androgen synthesis, so that severely affected girls may be virilized in utero. Girls and women with nonclassic congenital adrenal hyperplasia present later. They have greater enzyme activity, so that cortisol production is adequate, but increased ACTH levels cause hyperandrogenism.

Rare Causes
Other rare causes of primary adrenal insufficiency include ACTH resistance, congenital adrenal hypoplasia, Smith-Lemli-Opitz syndrome, and amyloidosis. Patients with primary adrenal insufficiency should undergo further evaluation to determine its cause (Table 227-5). Detection of antibodies to 21-hydroxylase identifies nearly all patients with idiopathic disease. In a male with negative results, measurement of plasma $C_{26:0}$ fatty acids will detect adrenoleukodystrophy. Taken together, this strategy identifies the cause in

TABLE 227-5 CAUSES OF ADRENAL INSUFFICIENCY AND ANCILLARY TESTS

SPECIFIC CAUSES	SUGGESTIVE CLINICAL FEATURES	USEFUL ANCILLARY TESTS
Primary adrenal insufficiency	Hyperpigmentation, orthostatic hypotension	Hyperkalemia, elevated ACTH
Idiopathic autoimmune destruction	Most common cause (80%) in developed countries; with or without other endocrinopathies, as below	Antibodies to 21-hydroxylase are present; on imaging, adrenal glands are small
Polyglandular failure type 1	Hypoparathyroidism, mucocutaneous candidiasis, vitiligo; age <20 years	
Polyglandular failure type 2	Insulin-dependent diabetes, autoimmune thyroid disease, alopecia areata, vitiligo; age >40 years	On imaging, adrenal glands are small
Infections: tuberculosis, systemic fungal diseases, AIDS-associated opportunistic infections (e.g., cytomegalovirus)	15% of patients in U.S. series	Adrenal glands tend to be large on CT and may be calcified
Space-occupying adrenal lesions	Metastases from carcinoma of lung, breast, kidney, gut; lymphoma or hemorrhage (heparin use)	Abnormal shape of adrenal glands on CT; evidence of hemorrhage
Bilateral adrenalectomy or treatment with steroidogenesis inhibitors		Ketoconazole, mitotane, aminoglutethimide, trilostane, and metyrapone reduce cortisol levels
Adrenoleukodystrophy	X-linked—screen males; in childhood, cognitive and gait disturbances; in adults, spastic paraparesis	Deficiency of peroxisomal very long chain acyl-coenzyme A synthetase leads to elevated plasma $C_{26:0}$ fatty acid levels
Secondary adrenal insufficiency		
Suppression of the adrenal axis by exogenous or endogenous glucocorticoids	Medication history; history of Cushing syndrome	Adrenal glands are small on imaging
Structural lesions of the hypothalamus or pituitary gland (tumors, destruction by infiltrating disorders, x-irradiation, and lymphocytic hypophysitis)	Other pituitary deficiencies	Adrenal glands are normal or small on imaging; MRI or CT may show pituitary or hypothalamic lesion
Isolated ACTH deficiency		
Head trauma		

ACTH = adrenocorticotropic hormone; AIDS = acquired immunodeficiency syndrome; CT = computed tomography; MRI = magnetic resonance imaging.

nearly all adult patients with idiopathic adrenal insufficiency. Patients with autoimmune disease should be tested for other endocrine deficiencies, and those with adrenoleukodystrophy require neurologic evaluation.

Secondary Adrenal Insufficiency
Suppression of the Pituitary Axis

Suppression of the hypothalamic-pituitary-adrenal axis by exogenous or endogenous glucocorticoids is the most common cause of secondary adrenal insufficiency. This phenomenon depends on the dose, duration, and schedule of glucocorticoid administration. Thus, adrenal suppression is unusual with "replacement" doses of glucocorticoid that are roughly equivalent to daily production (e.g., total daily doses of 20 mg hydrocortisone, 5 mg prednisone, or 0.3 to 0.5 mg dexamethasone). At higher doses, adrenal suppression is usually not seen until after 3 weeks of administration, and a single morning administration is less suppressive than are divided doses given during the day. When potentially suppressive doses of glucocorticoids are stopped, symptoms of adrenal insufficiency may occur within 48 hours, and the entire axis may not recover for up to 18 months. During this time, the patient should receive replacement glucocorticoid treatment or supplemental steroids at times of physiologic stress, depending on the degree of impairment (see later).

Lesions of the Hypothalamus or Pituitary

Secondary adrenal insufficiency also may result from structural lesions of the hypothalamus or pituitary gland that interfere with CRH production or transport or with corticotrope function. These causes include tumors, trauma, destruction by infiltrating disorders, x-irradiation, and lymphocytic hypophysitis. In general, these are not reversible conditions. Patients with secondary adrenal insufficiency not ascribed to glucocorticoid use should undergo imaging of the pituitary and hypothalamus to exclude a structural or infiltrating lesion as well as tests of other pituitary function to exclude additional deficiencies.

CLINICAL MANIFESTATIONS

The clinical presentation of adrenal insufficiency reflects the cause and duration of this uncommon condition. Primary adrenal insufficiency eventually destroys the entire adrenal cortex, with loss of both glucocorticoid and mineralocorticoid activity. By contrast, secondary adrenal insufficiency reflects an inability of the hypothalamic-pituitary unit to deliver CRH or ACTH, thus reducing trophic support to otherwise normal glands. As a result, only cortisol production decreases because mineralocorticoid production is not very ACTH dependent (Fig. 227-6).

The characteristic clinical presentation of acute primary adrenal insufficiency includes orthostatic hypotension, agitation, confusion, circulatory collapse, abdominal pain, and fever.[15] These features are most likely to be caused by hemorrhage, metastasis, or acute infection and can lead to death if not treated. In contrast, the typical history and clinical findings of chronic primary adrenal insufficiency include a longer history of malaise, fatigue, anorexia, weight loss, joint and back pain, and darkening of the skin (especially in the creases of the hands, extensor surfaces, recent scars, buccal and vaginal mucosa, and nipples). Patients may crave salt and may develop unusual food preferences, such as drinking the brine from pickles. Associated biochemical features for both acute and chronic presentations include hyponatremia, hypoglycemia, hyperkalemia, unexplained eosinophilia, and mild prerenal azotemia.

Chronic secondary adrenal insufficiency is manifested in a similar way, but without hyperpigmentation or mineralocorticoid abnormalities.

DIAGNOSIS

Biochemical testing confirms the diagnosis of adrenal insufficiency. A morning serum cortisol measurement is an inexpensive but relatively insensitive screening test for adrenal insufficiency in patients who are not acutely ill. The diagnosis is virtually excluded by values greater than 19 µg/dL (524 nmol/L) and is likely if the value is less than 3 µg/dL (83 nmol/L). However, both healthy individuals and patients with adrenal insufficiency may have indeterminate results (3 to 19 µg/dL) that require additional evaluation.

Patients with acute adrenal insufficiency should be evaluated for sepsis, adrenal metastases, and hemorrhage. Imaging of the glands and other testing may reveal an infectious cause. In acute adrenal insufficiency, a serum cortisol value is generally inappropriately normal or subnormal in the setting of hypotension, in which cortisol values are usually well above 18 µg/dL.

There is controversy about the best test to diagnose chronic adrenal insufficiency. Many use the cortisol response to exogenous ACTH as a gold

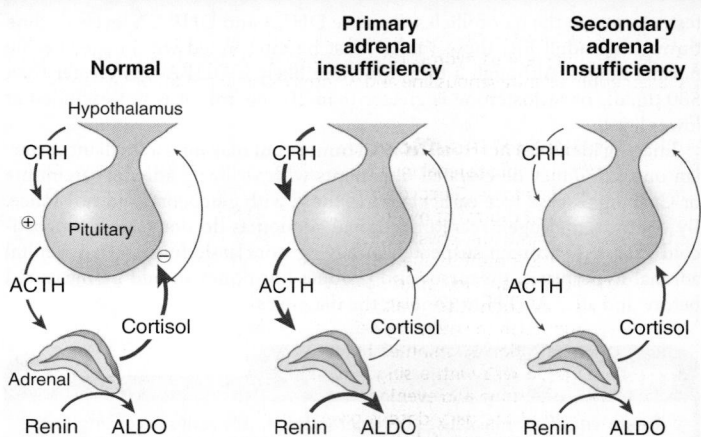

Normal   **Primary adrenal insufficiency**   **Secondary adrenal insufficiency**

FIGURE 227-6. Physiology of the adrenal axis in health, primary adrenal insufficiency, and secondary adrenal insufficiency. *In healthy individuals* (Normal), cortisol production is stimulated by the increased hypothalamic release of corticotropin-releasing hormone (CRH), which then travels down the pituitary stalk to stimulate adrenocorticotropic hormone (ACTH) secretion and release by corticotropes. Circulating ACTH stimulates adrenal gland production and secretion of cortisol. Cortisol then functions in a negative feedback mechanism to inhibit both CRH and ACTH. *In patients with primary adrenal insufficiency,* destruction or replacement of the entire adrenal cortex results in decreased cortisol, aldosterone, and dehydroepiandrosterone (DHEA, not shown) secretion by the adrenal glands. As a result of decreased cortisol negative feedback, the normal hypothalamus and pituitary gland increase CRH and ACTH secretion. The decreased aldosterone levels lead to an increase in renin levels. *In patients with secondary adrenal insufficiency,* ACTH or CRH secretion is reduced because of destruction or replacement of the hypothalamus or pituitary gland or because of disruption of the pituitary stalk. The decreased ACTH stimulation results in decreased cortisol (and, not shown, DHEA) secretion by the adrenal glands. Aldosterone production is only slightly affected by ACTH stimulation, and levels remain normal. The abnormal hypothalamus and pituitary gland do not increase CRH and ACTH secretion in response to the decreased cortisol negative feedback.

standard test of adrenal steroidogenic ability. In the classic test, 250 µg of ACTH (1-24, cosyntropin) is given intravenously at any time of day. This dose of ACTH is a maximal stimulus to the adrenal gland, so that the serum cortisol level measured 30 to 60 minutes later is greater than 18 µg/dL. Lower values indicate adrenal insufficiency. Insulin-induced hypoglycemia, metyrapone stimulation, and lower doses of ACTH stimulation have been proposed as better tests for patients with mild or recent secondary adrenal insufficiency, who may respond to pharmacologic doses of ACTH. None of these is ideal. Also, because there is no commercial formulation of ACTH for lower-dose tests, the product must be diluted on site, leading to concerns about the accuracy of the administered dose and the validity of results. Metyrapone has limited availability in the United States.

Cerebral adrenoleukodystrophy, presenting in childhood, is characterized by cognitive and gait disturbances; the adult form, adrenomyeloneuropathy, is characterized by spinal cord and peripheral nerve demyelination. In both forms, the accumulation of very long chain fatty acids in the adrenal cortex alters membrane function and inhibits signal transduction by ACTH. Because a substantial minority of patients in both groups present first with adrenal insufficiency, boys and young men with adrenal insufficiency should be screened for adrenoleukodystrophy.

Differential Diagnosis

Primary and secondary adrenal insufficiency can be distinguished by measurement of plasma ACTH. In primary adrenal insufficiency, ACTH levels are generally above the normal range and may exceed the normal range before the cortisol response to exogenous ACTH stimulation is subnormal. In addition, hyperkalemia and elevated renin values are characteristic of primary but not of secondary adrenal insufficiency, which is identified by a suppressed or inappropriately normal ACTH level.

TREATMENT   Rx

Acute Adrenal Insufficiency

In suspected acute adrenal insufficiency, hydrocortisone is the treatment of choice because it has both glucocorticoid and mineralocorticoid activity.

Treatment with intravenous saline for volume expansion, glucose for hypoglycemia, and intravenous hydrocortisone (100 mg) is started immediately after placement of an intravenous line and withdrawal of blood for documentation of the cortisol value.

Chronic Adrenal Insufficiency

Therapy for chronic adrenal insufficiency[16] aims to provide the physiologic replacement of steroids. Glucocorticoid replacement is achieved by administration of 10 to 12 mg/m² of hydrocortisone daily in one to three oral doses, attempting to mimic the physiologic diurnal variation of cortisol concentrations. Hydrocortisone offers the advantage of multiple-dose tablets, which allows fine adjustment and splitting of the daily dose. Ideally, the morning dose is given as soon after waking as possible; for individuals who feel extremely fatigued in the morning before the agent is absorbed, a strategy of taking the medication 30 minutes before arising may be helpful. Although many patients do well with a single dose, others complain of pronounced fatigue in the afternoon and evening. For them, a split-dose regimen, in which about one third of the daily dose is given around 4:00 PM or two afternoon doses are given, may be useful.

Other glucocorticoids may be used for daily replacement therapy. Prednisone, 5 to 7.5 mg daily, has the advantage of a long half-life and may be particularly helpful in patients with afternoon or evening fatigue. Dexamethasone may be used, but because of variable interindividual metabolism, it is difficult to recommend a specific replacement dose; in addition, few options for fixed doses are available, so it is difficult to adjust the dose.

Patients with primary adrenal insufficiency should be encouraged to salt their food and not to limit salt intake. Nearly all patients also require a mineralocorticoid, such as fludrocortisone 50 to 300 µg/day. The dose is adjusted until plasma renin activity is normal. If a mineralocorticoid is not given, the dose of hydrocortisone or other steroid with mineralocorticoid activity is often mistakenly increased to reduce an "unwell" feeling or hyperkalemia or salt craving. However, if a supraphysiologic dose is given, the patient becomes cushingoid.

Patients with primary adrenal insufficiency also have decreased serum DHEA levels. Controversy exists about its replacement. A meta-analysis concluded that there is insufficient evidence to support its routine use in these patients.[A3]

Ensuring Proper Dosing
Education of the Patient

All patients receiving chronic glucocorticoid replacement therapy should be instructed that they must take the glucocorticoids as prescribed and that failure to take or to absorb the medication will lead to adrenal crisis and possibly death. They should wear medical information bracelets or necklaces that identify this requirement. It is important to educate patients and their families about glucocorticoid adjustment during physiologic stress conditions, including the emergency administration of intramuscular glucocorticoid by means of a kit containing prefilled syringes with injectable steroid.

Dosing for Stress

The daily oral glucocorticoid dose is usually doubled for "stressful" physiologic conditions, such as fever, nausea, and diarrhea, although there are few data to support this strategy. In addition, this practice may lead to chronic overmedication by the patient because of a liberal interpretation of what constitutes physical stress. Thus, education about when and how to change the dose of steroid should be reinforced periodically, preferably with written material, and the dangers of excessive steroid use should be emphasized. If the patient is vomiting, has severe diarrhea, or has collapsed, intramuscular glucocorticoids should be given before transport to a medical facility.

The glucocorticoid dose is increased in proportion to the amount of stress. Thus, during maximally stressful situations (e.g., adrenal crisis, major surgery, trauma, labor and delivery), the daily hydrocortisone dose is 100 to 300 mg. Few data support the need for this supraphysiologic dose, but the safety of not following this practice has not been established. The dose may be tapered by 50% per day if the patient is clinically stable. For more moderate stress, such as that of cholecystectomy, 75 to 100 mg of hydrocortisone is given on the day of surgery, and the dose is tapered more rapidly. Patients undergoing minimal stress, such as tooth extraction or short operative orthopedic procedures, may not require any additional supplementation.

Assessment to Ensure Proper Dosing

Clinical assessment is the best way to judge whether the glucocorticoid dose is correct. Symptoms of adrenal insufficiency improve with adequate therapy. The development of cushingoid features or osteopenia suggests frank or subtle overreplacement, respectively, and the presence of adrenal insufficiency symptoms (fatigue, anorexia, weight loss) suggests underreplacement. In women, DHEA replacement increases testosterone levels, so that hirsutism, acne, or other signs of androgen excess may suggest overreplacement. In primary adrenal insufficiency, adequate hormone replacement results in plasma ACTH levels that decrease but remain elevated, in the range of 100 to 200 pg/mL. Renin values, however, normalize completely and may be used to

judge the adequacy of mineralocorticoid replacement. Although hydrocortisone is metabolized to cortisol, plasma cortisol values should not be used to monitor therapy because clearance from the blood stream is rapid, and circulating values are low for most of the day. UFC does not reflect adequate replacement; the increase in plasma cortisol levels after a single daily dose may exceed corticosteroid-binding globulin capacity, resulting in excessive urine levels and overestimation of integrated cortisol levels.

Mineralocorticoid Deficiency

Hypoaldosteronism may be classified as a low-normal or a high renin state on the basis of plasma renin activity after 4 hours of upright posture. Renin deficiency is the most common cause of hypoaldosteronism, occurring most often in older patients with mild, nonoliguric renal disease who often have insulin-dependent diabetes and potentially diabetic nephropathy. Indomethacin and other prostaglandin synthesis inhibitors as well as autonomic dysfunction associated with prolonged bedrest can also result in hyporeninemic hypoaldosteronism.

CLINICAL MANIFESTATIONS

There are few clinical features associated with mineralocorticoid deficiency; as a result, it is usually suspected when laboratory results reveal hyperkalemia, hyponatremia, and a mild metabolic alkalosis. If glucocorticoid deficiency is excluded, isolated hypoaldosteronism is established if the circulating level of aldosterone is inappropriately low.

High renin states of hypoaldosteronism include congenital adrenal hyperplasias with mineralocorticoid deficiency and primary adrenal insufficiency when it is treated with pure glucocorticoid replacement.

Treatment of these conditions involves sodium replacement with at least 10 mEq/kg/day, roughly equivalent to the 4 g of sodium chloride found in a typical diet in the United States. For individuals who do not maintain such a diet (often the elderly or the young), fludrocortisone can be given at the same doses used in primary adrenal insufficiency.

Grade A References

A1. Colao A, Petersenn S, Newell-Price J, et al. A 12-month phase 3 study of pasireotide in Cushing disease. N Engl J Med. 2012;366:914-924.

A2. Fassnacht M, Terzolo M, Allolio B, et al. Combination chemotherapy in advanced adrenocortical carcinoma. N Engl J Med. 2012;366:2189-2197.

A3. Alkatib AA, Cosma M, Elamin MB, et al. A systematic review and meta-analysis of randomized placebo-controlled trials of DHEA treatment effects on quality of life in women with adrenal insufficiency. J Clin Endocrinol Metab. 2009;94:3676-3681.

GENERAL REFERENCES

For the General References and other additional features, please visit Expert Consult at https://expertconsult.inkling.com.

228

ADRENAL MEDULLA, CATECHOLAMINES, AND PHEOCHROMOCYTOMA

WILLIAM F. YOUNG, JR.

ADRENAL MEDULLA AND CATECHOLAMINES

The adrenal medulla occupies the central portion of the adrenal gland. Adrenomedullary cells are called chromaffin cells (they stain brown with chromium salts). Chromaffin cells differentiate in the center of the adrenal gland in response to cortisol; some chromaffin cells also migrate to form paraganglia. The largest cluster of chromaffin cells outside the adrenal medulla is near the level of the inferior mesenteric artery and is referred to as the organ of Zuckerkandl.

The term *catecholamine* refers to substances that contain catechol (*o*-dihydroxybenzene) and a side chain with an amino group—the catechol

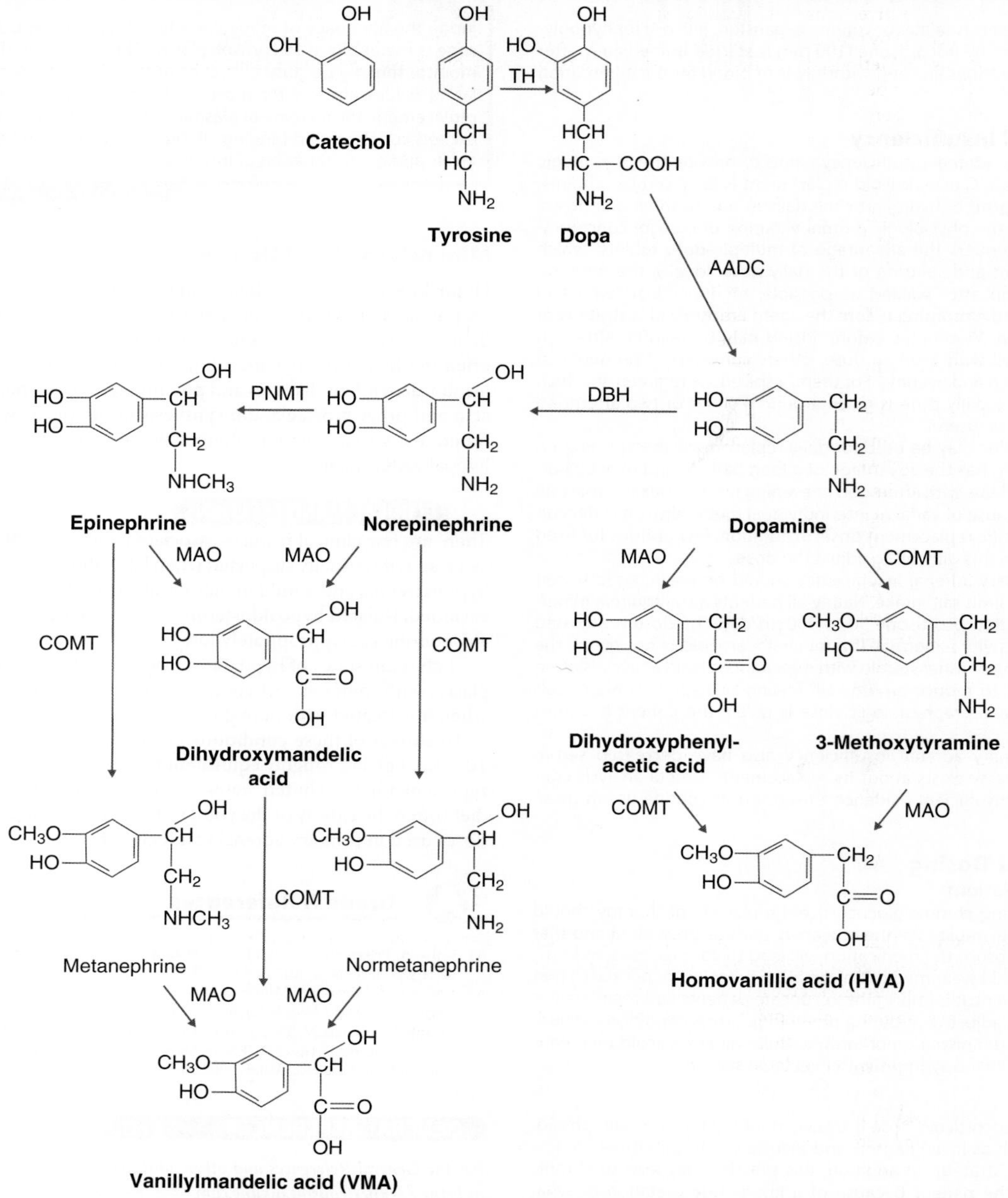

FIGURE 228-1. Biosynthetic and metabolic pathways for catecholamines. The term *catecholamine* comes from the catechol (*o*-dihydroxybenzene) structure and a side chain with an amino group—the catechol nucleus (*top left*). Tyrosine is converted to 3,4-dihydroxyphenylalanine (dopa) in the rate-limiting step by tyrosine hydroxylase (TH). Aromatic L-amino acid decarboxylase (AADC) converts dopa to dopamine. Dopamine is hydroxylated to norepinephrine by dopamine β-hydroxylase (DBH). Norepinephrine is converted to epinephrine by phenylethanolamine *N*-methyltransferase (PNMT); cortisol serves as a cofactor for PNMT, and this is why epinephrine-secreting pheochromocytomas are almost exclusively localized to the adrenal medulla. Metabolism of catecholamines occurs through two enzymatic pathways. Catechol-*O*-methyltransferase (COMT) converts epinephrine to metanephrine and norepinephrine to normetanephrine by meta-*O*-methylation. Metanephrine and normetanephrine are oxidized by monoamine oxidase (MAO) to vanillylmandelic acid by oxidative deamination. Monoamine oxidase also may oxidize epinephrine and norepinephrine to dihydroxymandelic acid, which is then converted by catechol-*O*-methyltransferase to vanillylmandelic acid. Dopamine is also metabolized by monoamine oxidase and catechol-*O*-methyltransferase, with the final metabolite homovanillic acid.

nucleus (Fig. 228-1). Epinephrine is synthesized and stored in the adrenal medulla and released into the systemic circulation. Norepinephrine is synthesized and stored not only in the adrenal medulla but also in the peripheral sympathetic nerves. Dopamine, the precursor of norepinephrine, is found in the adrenal medulla and peripheral sympathetic nerves.

Catecholamines affect many cardiovascular and metabolic processes, including increasing the heart rate, blood pressure, myocardial contractility, and cardiac conduction velocity. Specific receptors mediate the biologic actions. The three types of adrenergic receptors are α, β, and DA; their receptor subtypes are α_1, α_2, β_1, β_2, β_3, DA_1, and DA_2. The α_1 subtype is a postsynaptic receptor that mediates vascular and smooth muscle contraction; stimulation causes vasoconstriction and increased blood pressure. The α_2-receptors are located on presynaptic sympathetic nerve endings and, when activated, inhibit the release of norepinephrine; stimulation causes suppres-

sion in central sympathetic outflow and decreased blood pressure. Stimulation of the β_1-receptor causes positive inotropic and chronotropic effects on the heart, increased renin secretion in the kidney, and lipolysis in adipocytes as well as bronchodilation, vasodilation in skeletal muscle, glycogenolysis, and increased release of norepinephrine from sympathetic nerve terminals. The β_3-receptor regulates energy expenditure and lipolysis. DA_1 receptors are localized to the cerebral, renal, mesenteric, and coronary vasculature; stimulation causes vasodilation in these vascular beds. DA_2 receptors are presynaptic and localized to sympathetic nerve endings, sympathetic ganglia, and brain; stimulation inhibits the release of norepinephrine, inhibits ganglionic transmission, and inhibits prolactin release.

Catecholamines are synthesized from tyrosine by a process of hydroxylation and decarboxylation (see Fig. 228-1). Tyrosine is derived from ingested food or synthesized from phenylalanine in the liver, and it enters neurons and chromaffin cells by active transport. Tyrosine is converted to 3,4-dihydroxyphenylalanine (dopa) by tyrosine hydroxylase, the rate-limiting step in catecholamine synthesis. α-Methyl-p-tyrosine (metyrosine) is a tyrosine hydroxylase inhibitor that may be used therapeutically in patients with catecholamine-secreting tumors. Aromatic L-amino acid decarboxylase catalyzes the decarboxylation of dopa to dopamine. Dopamine is actively transported into granulated vesicles to be hydroxylated to norepinephrine by the dopamine β-hydroxylase. These reactions occur in the synaptic vesicle of adrenergic neurons and the chromaffin cells of the adrenal medulla. In the adrenal medulla, norepinephrine is released from the granule into the cytoplasm, where phenylethanolamine N-methyltransferase converts it to epinephrine. Expression of phenylethanolamine N-methyltransferase is positively regulated by glucocorticoids. Thus, catecholamine-secreting tumors that secrete primarily epinephrine are localized to the adrenal medulla. In normal adrenal medullary tissue, approximately 80% of the catecholamine released is epinephrine.

The biologic half-life of circulating catecholamines is between 10 and 100 seconds. Thus, plasma concentrations of catecholamines fluctuate widely. Catecholamines are removed from the circulation by either reuptake by sympathetic nerve terminals or metabolism through two enzyme pathways (see Fig. 228-1), followed by sulfate conjugation and renal excretion. Almost 90% of catecholamines released at sympathetic synapses are taken up locally by the nerve endings (uptake 1). Uptake 1 can be blocked by cocaine, tricyclic antidepressants, and phenothiazine. Extraneuronal tissues also take up catecholamines (uptake 2). Most of these catecholamines are metabolized by catechol-O-methyltransferase. Metanephrine and normetanephrine are oxidized by monoamine oxidase to vanillylmandelic acid by oxidative deamination. Monoamine oxidase may also oxidize epinephrine and norepinephrine to 3,4-dihydroxymandelic acid, which is then converted by catechol-O-methyltransferase to vanillylmandelic acid. In the storage vesicle, norepinephrine is protected from metabolism by monoamine oxidase. Monoamine oxidase and catechol-O-methyltransferase metabolize dopamine to homovanillic acid (see Fig. 228-1).

PHEOCHROMOCYTOMA AND PARAGANGLIOMA

DEFINITION

Catecholamine-secreting tumors that arise from chromaffin cells of the adrenal medulla and the sympathetic ganglia are referred to as pheochromocytomas and extra-adrenal catecholamine-secreting paragangliomas, respectively. Because the tumors have similar clinical presentations and are treated with similar approaches, many clinicians use the term *pheochromocytoma* to refer to both entities. However, the distinction between pheochromocytoma and paraganglioma is an important one because there are differences in the risk for associated neoplasms, risk for malignant transformation, and type of genetic testing that should be considered.

EPIDEMIOLOGY

Catecholamine-secreting tumors are rare; the annual incidence is 2 to 8 cases per million people. Nevertheless, it is important to suspect, confirm, localize, and resect these tumors. The associated hypertension is curable with surgical removal of the tumor, a risk of lethal paroxysm exists, and at least 10% of the tumors are malignant. Approximately 30% of cases are familial, so detection of this tumor in the proband may result in early diagnosis in other family members.

PATHOBIOLOGY
Genetics

Approximately 30% of patients with catecholamine-secreting tumors have germline mutations (inherited mutations present in all cells of the body) in genes associated with the genetic disease.[1] Hereditary catecholamine-secreting tumors typically are manifested at a younger age than sporadic neoplasms are. Sporadic pheochromocytoma is typically diagnosed on the basis of symptoms or incidental discovery on computed imaging, whereas syndromic pheochromocytoma and paraganglioma are frequently diagnosed earlier in the course of disease because of biochemical surveillance or genetic testing.

Multiple Endocrine Neoplasia

Multiple endocrine neoplasia (MEN) type 2A is an autosomal dominant disorder (Chapters 231 and 246). The phenotype includes adrenal pheochromocytoma in 50% (usually bilateral and may be asynchronous),

medullary carcinoma of the thyroid in 100%, hyperparathyroidism in 20 to 30%, and cutaneous lichen amyloidosis in 5%.[2] Medullary carcinoma of the thyroid is usually detected before pheochromocytoma. Numerous activating mutations in the RET proto-oncogene have been documented in persons with MEN type 2A (these are described in detail in Chapter 246).

MEN type 2B is also an autosomal dominant disorder, and it represents approximately 5% of all MEN type 2 cases. The phenotype includes pheochromocytoma in 50% (usually bilateral), aggressive medullary carcinoma of the thyroid in 100%, mucosal neuromas (typically involving the tongue, lips, and eyelids) in most patients, thickened corneal nerves, intestinal ganglioneuromatosis, and marfanoid body habitus. MEN 2B–associated tumors are caused by mutations in the RET protein's intracellular domain, as described in detail in Chapter 246.

Von Hippel–Lindau Disease

Von Hippel–Lindau (VHL) disease is an autosomal dominant disorder characterized by pheochromocytoma (frequently bilateral), paraganglioma (mediastinal, abdominal, pelvic), hemangioblastoma (involving the cerebellum, spinal cord, or brain stem), retinal angioma, clear cell renal cell carcinoma, pancreatic neuroendocrine tumor, endolymphatic sac tumor of the middle ear, serous cystadenoma of the pancreas, and papillary cystadenoma of the epididymis and broad ligament.[3] Pheochromocytoma occurs in about 10 to 20% of patients with VHL disease. Nearly 100% of patients have an identifiable gene mutation (VHL tumor suppressor gene). Certain missense mutations appear to be associated with a "pheochromocytoma only" presentation of VHL disease.

Neurofibromatosis

Neurofibromatosis type 1 (NF1) is an autosomal dominant disorder characterized by neurofibromas, multiple café au lait spots, axillary and inguinal freckling, iris hamartomas (Lisch nodules), bone abnormalities, central nervous system gliomas, pheochromocytoma and paraganglioma, macrocephaly, and cognitive deficits. The expression of these features is variable. Approximately 2% of patients with NF1 develop catecholamine-secreting tumors; in these patients, the tumor is usually a solitary benign adrenal pheochromocytoma, occasionally bilateral adrenal pheochromocytomas, and rarely an abdominal paraganglioma. Inactivating NF1 mutations cause the disorder (NF1 tumor suppressor gene).

Familial Paraganglioma

Familial paraganglioma is an autosomal dominant disorder characterized by paragangliomas that are located in the skull base and neck, thorax, abdomen, and pelvis. Most cases of familial paraganglioma are caused by mutations in the succinate dehydrogenase (SDH; succinate:ubiquinone oxidoreductase) subunit genes (SDHB, SDHC, SDHD, SDHAF2, SDHA), which compose portions of mitochondrial complex II. Inactivating germline mutations in SDHD have been identified in multigenerational families with head and neck parasympathetic paragangliomas that are usually nonfunctional and occasionally in those with adrenal pheochromocytoma. In patients with SDHD mutations, penetrance depends on the mutation's parent of origin. Hence, the disease does not manifest when the mutation is inherited from the mother but is highly penetrant when it is inherited from the father. This phenomenon is known as maternal imprinting. Multiple cofactors are required for normal activity of the SDH complex, including flavin adenine dinucleotide (FAD) in the SDH1 subunit. FAD is covalently attached to Sdh1, and deletion of SDHAF2 causes a complete loss of FAD cofactor attachment (flavination) of Sdh1. Germline loss-of-function mutations in the SDHAF2 gene, located on chromosome 11q13.1, have been associated with disease in a family with hereditary paraganglioma. Like families with mutations in SDHD, those with mutations in SDHAF2 also exhibit maternal imprinting and parasympathetic paragangliomas that typically occur in the skull base and neck. Inactivating mutations in the tumor suppressor gene SDHB, located on chromosome 1p35-36, are associated with paragangliomas in the abdomen, pelvis, and mediastinum. Adrenal pheochromocytomas may also be found in patients with SDHB mutations. Patients with SDHB mutations have an increased risk for malignant paraganglioma.

Genetic Testing

Since 1990, 15 different pheochromocytoma and paraganglioma susceptibility genes have been reported: NF1, RET, VHL, SDHD, SDHC, SDHB, EGLN1/PHD2, KIF1B, SDHAF2, IDH1, TMEM127, SDHA, MAX, HIF2A, and FH gene encoding fumarate hydratase.[4,5]

Genetic testing should be considered if a patient has one or more of the following: paraganglioma, bilateral adrenal pheochromocytomas, unilateral adrenal pheochromocytoma and a family history of pheochromocytoma or paraganglioma, onset of unilateral adrenal pheochromocytoma at a young age (before 45 years), or other clinical findings suggestive of one of the previously discussed syndromic disorders.[6] Genetic testing can be complex; testing of one family member has implications for related individuals.[7] Genetic counseling is recommended to help families understand the implications of genetic test results; to coordinate the testing of at-risk individuals; and to help families work through the psychosocial issues that may arise before, during, or after the testing process. A list of clinically approved molecular genetic diagnostic laboratories is available at www.genetests.org.

CLINICAL MANIFESTATIONS

Catecholamine-secreting tumors occur with equal frequency in men and women, primarily in the third, fourth, and fifth decades of life. These tumors are rare in children; when discovered, they may be multifocal and associated with a hereditary syndrome. When symptoms are present, they are due to the pharmacologic effects of excess concentrations of circulating catecholamines (Table 228-1). The resulting hypertension may be sustained (in approximately half of patients) or paroxysmal (in approximately a third of patients). The remaining patients have normal blood pressure. Episodic symptoms may occur in spells, or paroxysms, that can be extremely variable in presentation but typically include forceful heartbeat, pallor, tremor, headache, and diaphoresis.[8] The spell may start with the sensation of a "rush" in the chest and a sense of shortness of breath, followed by a "pounding" heartbeat in the chest that typically progresses to a throbbing headache. Peripheral vasoconstriction with a spell results in cool or cold hands and feet and facial pallor. Increased sense of body heat and sweating are common symptoms that occur toward the end of the spell. Spells may be spontaneous or precipitated by postural change, anxiety, medications (e.g., metoclopramide, β-adrenergic inhibitors, anesthetic agents), exercise, or maneuvers that increase intra-abdominal pressure (e.g., change in position, lifting, defecation, exercise, colonoscopy, pregnancy, trauma). Although the types of spells experienced by patients are highly variable, spells tend to be stereotypical for each patient. Spells may occur multiple times a day or as infrequently as once a month. The typical duration of a pheochromocytoma spell is 15 to 20 minutes, but it may be much shorter or last several hours. The clinician must recognize that most patients with spells do not have a pheochromocytoma.

Additional clinical signs of catecholamine-secreting tumors include hypertensive retinopathy, orthostatic hypotension, angina, nausea, constipation (megacolon may be the presenting symptom), hyperglycemia, diabetes mellitus, hypercalcemia, Raynaud's phenomenon, livedo reticularis, erythrocytosis, and mass effects from the tumor. Fasting hyperglycemia and diabetes mellitus are caused in part by the α-adrenergic inhibition of insulin release. Painless hematuria and paroxysmal attacks induced by micturition and defecation are associated with urinary bladder paragangliomas. Some of the co-secreted hormones that may dominate the clinical presentation include corticotropin (Cushing's syndrome), parathyroid hormone–related peptide (hypercalcemia), vasopressin (syndrome of inappropriate antidiuretic hormone secretion), vasoactive intestinal peptide (watery diarrhea), and growth hormone–releasing hormone (acromegaly) (see Table 228-1). Cardiomyopathy and congestive heart failure are the symptomatic presentations of pheochromocytoma that are most frequently unrecognized by clinicians. Cardiomyopathy, whether dilated or hypertrophic, may be totally reversible with tumor resection. Some patients with pheochromocytoma may be asymptomatic despite high circulating levels of catecholamines, probably reflecting adrenergic receptor desensitization related to chronic stimulation.

Symptomatic pheochromocytomas are localized to the adrenal glands, with an average diameter of 4.5 cm (Fig. 228-2). Paragangliomas are found where there is chromaffin tissue: along the para-aortic sympathetic chain, within the organs of Zuckerkandl (at the origin of the inferior mesenteric artery), in the wall of the urinary bladder, and along the sympathetic chain in the neck or mediastinum. Paragangliomas in the head and neck region (e.g., carotid body tumors, glomus tumors, chemodectomas) usually arise from parasympathetic tissue and typically do not hypersecrete catecholamines and metanephrines, whereas paragangliomas in the mediastinum, abdomen, and pelvis usually arise from sympathetic chromaffin tissue and usually do hypersecrete catecholamines and metanephrines.

DIAGNOSIS
Differential Diagnosis

Numerous disorders can cause signs and symptoms that may lead the clinician to test for pheochromocytoma. These disorders span much of medicine and include endocrine disorders (e.g., primary hypogonadism), cardiovascular disorders (e.g., idiopathic orthostatic hypotension), psychological

TABLE 228-1	SIGNS AND SYMPTOMS ASSOCIATED WITH CATECHOLAMINE-SECRETING TUMORS

SPELL RELATED

Anxiety and fear of impending death
Diaphoresis
Dyspnea
Epigastric and chest pain
Headache
Hypertension
Nausea and vomiting
Pallor
Palpitation (forceful heartbeat)
Tremor

CHRONIC

Anxiety and fear of impending death
Cold hands and feet
Congestive heart failure—dilated or hypertrophic cardiomyopathy
Constipation
Diaphoresis
Dyspnea
Ectopic hormone secretion–dependent symptoms (e.g., CRH/ACTH, GHRH, PTH-RP, VIP)
Epigastric and chest pain
Fatigue
Fever
General increase in sweating
Grade II to IV retinopathy
Headache
Hyperglycemia
Hypertension
Nausea and vomiting
Orthostatic hypotension
Painless hematuria (associated with urinary bladder paraganglioma)
Pallor
Palpitation (forceful heartbeat)
Tremor
Weight loss

NOT TYPICAL OF PHEOCHROMOCYTOMA

Flushing

ACTH = adrenocorticotropic hormone; CRH = corticotropin-releasing hormone; GHRH = growth hormone–releasing hormone; PTH-RP = parathyroid hormone–related peptide; VIP = vasoactive intestinal polypeptide.
Modified from Young WF Jr. Pheochromocytoma: 1926-1993. *Trends Endocrinol Metab.* 1993;4:122-127.

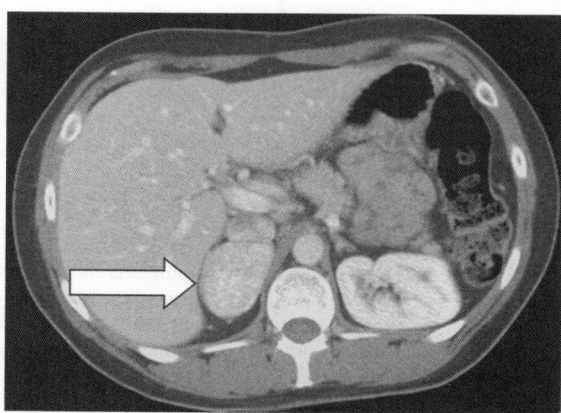

FIGURE 228-2. Contrast-enhanced computed tomography of the abdomen in a 32-year-old second-year medical student with the peripartum discovery of a pheochromocytoma. The plasma fractionated metanephrines were abnormal: metanephrine, 0.19 nmol/L (normal, <0.5 nmol/L); normetanephrine, 28.6 nmol/L (normal, <0.9 nmol/L). The 24-hour urine values were abnormal: norepinephrine, 781 μg (normal, <170 μg); epinephrine, 2.4 μg (normal, <35 μg); dopamine, 197 μg (normal, <700 μg); metanephrine, 117 μg (normal, <400 μg); normetanephrine, 8760 μg (normal, <900 μg). The axial image shows a typical 5-cm heterogeneously enhancing right adrenal mass, consistent with pheochromocytoma (*arrow*). After α- and β-adrenergic blockade, a 5.3 × 5.0 × 2.0-cm, 40-g pheochromocytoma was removed laparoscopically.

disorders (e.g., panic disorder), pharmacologic causes (e.g., withdrawal from an adrenergic inhibitor), neurologic disorders (e.g., postural orthostatic tachycardia syndrome), and miscellaneous disorders (e.g., mast cell disease). Indeed, most patients tested for pheochromocytoma do not have it. In addition, fractionated catecholamines and metanephrines may be elevated in several clinical scenarios: withdrawal from medications or drugs (e.g., clonidine, alcohol), any acute illness (e.g., subarachnoid hemorrhage, migraine headache, preeclampsia), and administration of many drugs and medications (e.g., tricyclic antidepressants, levodopa, cocaine, phencyclidine, lysergic acid diethylamide, amphetamines, ephedrine, pseudoephedrine, phenylpropanolamine, isoproterenol) (Table 228-2).

Pheochromocytoma should be suspected in patients who have one or more of the following: hyperadrenergic spells (e.g., self-limited episodes of nonexertional palpitations, diaphoresis, headache, tremor, or pallor); resistant hypertension; a familial syndrome that predisposes to catecholamine-secreting tumors (e.g., MEN type 2, NF1, VHL disease); a family history of pheochromocytoma or a history of a resected pheochromocytoma and a present history of recurrent hypertension or spells; an incidentally discovered adrenal mass; hypertension and diabetes; pressor response during anesthesia, surgery, or angiography; onset of hypertension at a young age (before 20 years); and idiopathic dilated cardiomyopathy.

Laboratory Findings

The diagnosis must be confirmed biochemically by increased concentrations of fractionated metanephrines in the plasma or fractionated catecholamines and metanephrines in a 24-hour urine collection (Fig. 228-3).[9] Most laboratories now measure fractionated catecholamines (dopamine, norepinephrine, and epinephrine) and metanephrines (metanephrine and normetanephrine)

by high-performance liquid chromatography with electrochemical detection or tandem mass spectroscopy.[10] These techniques have overcome the problems with fluorometric analysis (e.g., false-positive results caused by α-methyldopa, labetalol, sotalol, and imaging contrast agents). One of the most reliable methods of identifying catecholamine-secreting tumors is measurement of fractionated metanephrines and catecholamines in a 24-hour urine collection (sensitivity, 98%; specificity, 98%).[11] If clinical suspicion is high, plasma fractionated metanephrines should also be measured. Some groups have advocated the measurement of plasma fractionated metanephrines as a first-line test for pheochromocytoma; the predictive value of a

TABLE 228-2	MEDICATIONS THAT MAY INCREASE MEASURED LEVELS OF CATECHOLAMINES AND METANEPHRINES
Tricyclic antidepressants (including cyclobenzaprine)	
Levodopa	
Drugs containing adrenergic receptor agonists (e.g., decongestants)	
Amphetamines	
Buspirone and antipsychotic agents	
Prochlorperazine	
Reserpine	
Withdrawal from clonidine and other drugs	
Ethanol	

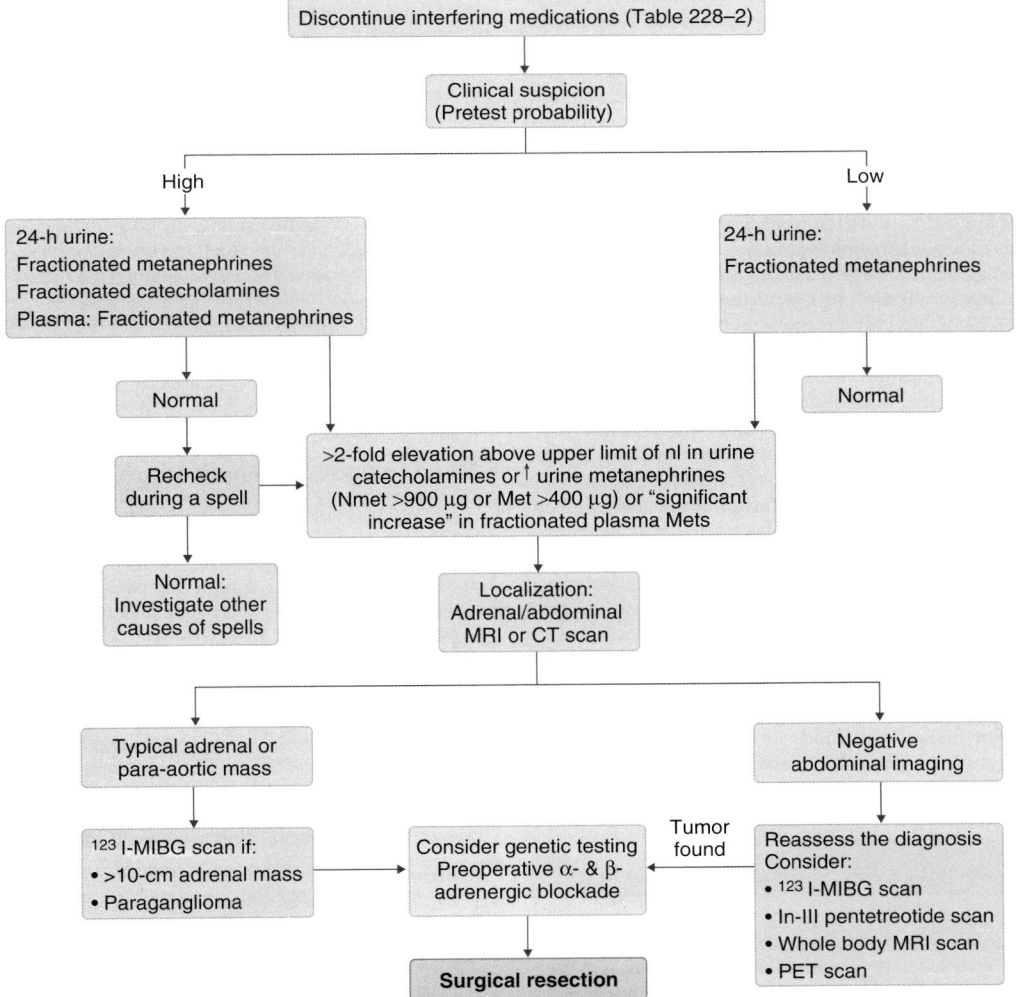

FIGURE 228-3. Evaluation and treatment of catecholamine-secreting tumors. Clinical suspicion is triggered by the following: paroxysmal symptoms (especially hypertension); hypertension that is intermittent, unusually labile, or resistant to treatment; family history of pheochromocytoma or associated conditions; or incidentally discovered adrenal mass. The details are discussed in the text. CT = computed tomography; ^{123}I-MIBG = ^{123}I-metaiodobenzylguanidine; Met = metanephrine; MRI = magnetic resonance imaging; nl = normal; Nmet = normetanephrine; PET = positron emission tomography. (Modified from Young WF Jr. Pheochromocytoma: 1926-1993. *Trends Endocrinol Metab.* 1993;4:122.)

negative test result is extremely high, and the finding of normal plasma fractionated metanephrines excludes pheochromocytoma, except in patients with early preclinical disease and those with strictly dopamine-secreting neoplasms.[12] A plasma test is also attractive because of its simplicity. Although measurement of plasma fractionated metanephrines has a sensitivity of 96 to 100%, the specificity is poor at only 85 to 89%; the specificity falls to 77% in patients older than 60 years. It has been estimated that 97% of patients with hypertension seen in a tertiary care clinic who have abnormal plasma fractionated metanephrine measurements do not have pheochromocytoma. This high false-positive rate results in excessive health care expenditures because of subsequent imaging as well as potentially inappropriate surgery. Thus, plasma fractionated metanephrines lack the necessary specificity to be recommended as a first-line test; this measurement is reserved for cases in which the index of suspicion is high. However, measurement of plasma fractionated metanephrines is a good first-line test for children, in whom it is difficult to obtain a complete 24-hour urine collection.

The index of suspicion for pheochromocytoma should be high (see Fig. 228-3) in patients with the clinical scenarios described earlier and in those with an incidentally discovered adrenal mass that has imaging characteristics consistent with pheochromocytoma. These include increased baseline computed tomography (CT) Hounsfield unit density (e.g., >20 HU), marked enhancement with intravenous contrast medium on CT, high signal intensity on T2-weighted magnetic resonance imaging (MRI), cystic and hemorrhagic changes, bilaterality, and large size (>4 cm) (see later).

Although it is preferable for patients not to receive any medications during the diagnostic evaluation, treatment with most medications can be continued. Tricyclic antidepressants interfere most frequently with the interpretation of fractionated catecholamines and metanephrines. For the effective detection of catecholamine-secreting tumors, treatment with tricyclic antidepressants and other psychoactive agents listed in Table 228-2 should be tapered and discontinued at least 2 weeks before any hormonal assessments. Furthermore, catecholamine secretion may be appropriately increased in situations of physical stress or illness (e.g., stroke, myocardial infarction, congestive heart failure, obstructive sleep apnea). Therefore, the clinical circumstances under which catecholamines and metanephrines are measured must be assessed in each case.

Imaging

Localization studies should not be initiated until biochemical studies have confirmed the diagnosis of a catecholamine-secreting tumor (see Fig. 228-3). Computer-assisted imaging of the adrenal glands and abdomen with CT or MRI should be the first localization test (sensitivity, >95%; specificity, >65%). Approximately 85% of these tumors are found in the adrenal glands, and 95% are found in the abdomen. If the results of abdominal imaging are normal, scintigraphic localization with ^{123}I-labeled metaiodobenzylguanidine (^{123}I-MIBG) is indicated (see Fig. 228-3). This radiopharmaceutical agent accumulates preferentially in catecholamine-producing tumors (sensitivity, 88%; specificity, 94%). If a typical (<10 cm) unilateral adrenal pheochromocytoma is found on CT or MRI, ^{123}I-MIBG scintigraphy is superfluous, and the results may even cause confusion. If the adrenal pheochromocytoma is larger than 10 cm in diameter or if a paraganglioma is identified on CT or MRI, ^{123}I-MIBG scintigraphy is indicated because the patient has an increased risk of malignant disease and additional paragangliomas.[18]F-Fluorodeoxyglucose positron emission tomography is an excellent imaging modality to detect metastatic disease.[13,14]

Other localizing procedures that can be used but are rarely required include computer-assisted imaging of the chest and neck as well as somatostatin receptor imaging with [^{111}In]pentetreotide (see Fig. 228-3). Because of marked gradients between the adrenal glands in non-pheochromocytoma patients, adrenal venous sampling for catecholamines is not helpful in the investigation of adrenal pheochromocytoma.

TREATMENT   Rx

Medical Therapy

Some form of preoperative pharmacologic preparation is indicated for all patients with catecholamine-secreting neoplasms. However, no randomized controlled trials have compared the different approaches. Combined α- and β-adrenergic blockade is one approach to control blood pressure and to prevent intraoperative hypertensive crises. α-Adrenergic blockade should be started 7 to 10 days preoperatively to normalize blood pressure and to expand

the contracted blood volume. A longer duration of preoperative α-adrenergic blockade is indicated in patients with recent myocardial infarction, catecholamine cardiomyopathy, and catecholamine-induced vasculitis. Blood pressure should be monitored with the patient in the seated and standing positions twice daily. Target blood pressure is less than 120/80 mm Hg (seated), with systolic blood pressure greater than 90 mm Hg (standing); both targets should be modified on the basis of the patient's age and comorbid disease. On the second or third day of α-adrenergic blockade, patients are encouraged to start a diet high in sodium content (≥5000 mg daily) because of the catecholamine-induced volume contraction and the orthostasis associated with α-adrenergic blockade. This degree of volume expansion may be contraindicated in patients with congestive heart failure or renal insufficiency. After adequate α-adrenergic blockade has been achieved, β-adrenergic blockade is initiated, which typically occurs 2 or 3 days preoperatively.

Phenoxybenzamine is the preferred drug to control blood pressure and arrhythmia preoperatively.[15] It is an irreversible, long-acting, nonspecific α-adrenergic blocking agent. The initial dosage is 10 mg once or twice daily, and the dose is increased by 10 to 20 mg in divided doses every 2 or 3 days as needed to control blood pressure and spells. The final dosage of phenoxybenzamine is typically between 20 and 100 mg daily.

The β-adrenergic antagonist should be administered only after α-adrenergic blockade is effective; with β-adrenergic blockade alone, hypertension may be more severe from the unopposed α-adrenergic stimulation. Preoperative β-adrenergic blockade is indicated to control the tachycardia associated with both the high concentrations of circulating catecholamines and the α-adrenergic blockade. The clinician should exercise caution if the patient is asthmatic or has congestive heart failure. Chronic catecholamine excess can produce a cardiomyopathy that may become evident with the initiation of β-adrenergic blockade, resulting in acute pulmonary edema. Therefore, the β-adrenergic blocker should be administered cautiously and at a low dose. Other agents that may be used to prepare the patient with pheochromocytoma for surgery include α-methyl-*p*-tyrosine (metyrosine) and calcium-channel blockers. Acute hypertensive crises may occur before or during an operation, and they should be treated with intravenous sodium nitroprusside, phentolamine, or nicardipine.

Surgical Therapy

The treatment of choice for pheochromocytoma is complete surgical resection. Surgical survival rates are 98 to 100% and are highly dependent on the skill of the endocrinologist–endocrine surgeon–anesthesiologist team. Careful preoperative pharmacologic preparation is crucial for successful treatment. Most catecholamine-secreting tumors are benign and can be totally excised. Tumor excision usually cures hypertension.

In the past, an anterior midline abdominal surgical approach was generally used to resect adrenal pheochromocytoma. However, the laparoscopic approach to the adrenal gland is currently the procedure of choice for a solitary intra-adrenal pheochromocytoma smaller than 8 cm in diameter.[16] Laparoscopic adrenalectomy for pheochromocytoma should be converted to open adrenalectomy in cases of difficult dissection, invasion, adhesions, or an inexperienced surgeon. An anterior midline abdominal surgical approach is indicated for abdominal paragangliomas. The midline abdomen should be inspected carefully. Paragangliomas of the neck, chest, and urinary bladder require specialized approaches.

Management of Complications

Hypotension may occur during and after surgical resection of the pheochromocytoma, and it should be treated with fluids and colloids and then intravenous pressor agents if necessary. Postoperative hypotension is less frequent in patients who have had adequate preoperative α-adrenergic blockade and volume expansion. If both adrenal glands were manipulated during surgery, adrenocortical insufficiency should be considered a potential cause of postoperative hypotension. Because hypoglycemia can occur in the immediate postoperative period, blood glucose levels should be monitored, and intravenous fluids should contain 5% dextrose.

Approximately 1 to 2 weeks after surgery, fractionated catecholamines and metanephrines should be measured by collection of a 24-hour urine specimen. If the levels are normal, resection of the pheochromocytoma should be considered complete. Increased levels of fractionated catecholamines and metanephrines detected postoperatively are consistent with residual tumor due to either a second primary lesion or occult metastases. Common sites of metastasis include lymph nodes, liver, lung, and bone.

Follow-up

The 24-hour urinary excretion of fractionated catecholamines and metanephrines or plasma fractionated metanephrines should be checked annually for life. Annual biochemical testing assesses for metastatic disease, tumor recurrence in the adrenal bed, or delayed appearance of multiple primary tumors. Follow-up CT or MRI is not needed unless the metanephrine or catecholamine levels become elevated or the original tumor was associated with minimal or no catecholamine or metanephrine excess.

MALIGNANT PHEOCHROMOCYTOMA AND PARAGANGLIOMA

Distinguishing between benign and malignant catecholamine-secreting tumors is difficult on the basis of clinical, biochemical, or histopathologic characteristics. Malignant disease is rare in patients with an adrenal familial syndrome but common in those with familial paraganglioma caused by mutations in *SDHB*. Although the 5-year survival rate for patients with malignant pheochromocytoma is less than 50%, the prognosis is variable[17]; approximately 50% of patients have an indolent form of the disease, with a life expectancy of more than 20 years, and the other 50% have rapidly progressive disease, with death occurring 1 to 5 years after diagnosis. The clinician should assess the pace of the malignant disease and base the level of therapy on the aggressiveness of the tumor's behavior. A multimodality, multidisciplinary, individualized approach is indicated to control catecholamine-dependent symptoms, local mass effects, and overall tumor burden.

PHEOCHROMOCYTOMA IN PREGNANCY

Pheochromocytoma in pregnancy can cause the death of both the fetus and the mother. The approach to the biochemical diagnosis is the same as for nonpregnant patients. MRI without gadolinium enhancement is the preferred imaging modality.[123]I-MIBG scintigraphy is contraindicated. The treatment of hypertensive crises is the same as for nonpregnant patients, except that nitroprusside should be avoided. Although the most appropriate management is debated, adrenal pheochromocytomas should be removed promptly after α- and β-adrenergic blockade if the diagnosis is made during the first two trimesters of pregnancy.[18] The preoperative preparation is the same as for nonpregnant patients. If the pregnancy is in the third trimester, one operation is recommended for cesarean delivery and removal of the adrenal pheochromocytoma at the same time. Spontaneous labor and delivery should be avoided. The management of catecholamine-secreting paragangliomas in pregnancy may require modification of these guidelines, depending on tumor location.

GENERAL REFERENCES

For the General References and other additional features, please visit Expert Consult at https://expertconsult.inkling.com.

229

DIABETES MELLITUS

JILL CRANDALL AND HARRY SHAMOON

Diabetes mellitus is a chronic disorder characterized by abnormal metabolic regulation as well as by the potential for vascular and neuropathic complications. Diabetes comprises a cluster of heterogeneous disorders with elevated blood glucose levels as a common diagnostic feature; however, as genetic and molecular studies have suggested, it is likely that the cluster includes many subcategories, each of which requires tailored prevention, diagnosis, and treatment approaches. Depending on the context in which the patient presents, diabetes can be an acute life-threatening condition, a pregnancy-associated disorder, or a gradually evolving chronic disorder that carries with it secondary complications that may be ultimately more debilitating than hyperglycemia. Other factors make diabetes an unusual clinical challenge, including the need for active participation by patients in their treatment, the varying presentations across the age spectrum, and the unstable and evolving clinical presentation. Because the severity of the underlying metabolic defects does not remain static, diabetes management always requires changes in treatment according to the stage of the disease. These patterns of evolution are superimposed on the phenotypes at presentation and depend on a host of factors including age, sex, race, societal setting, and others.

It is now established that diabetes-related vascular and neuropathic complications stem from imperfect treatment of the metabolic disturbances, defined principally by hyperglycemia. There is also evidence that genetic factors may predispose or protect individual patients from the deleterious effects of hyperglycemia. Regardless of the specific subtype of diabetes, all

TABLE 229-1	CLASSIFICATION OF DIABETES	
	TYPE 1	**TYPE 2**
Age at onset	Childhood or early adulthood, but can be manifested at any age	Middle age or older, but can be manifested in obese children and adolescents
Family history/genetic factors	Genetic risk defined, but most cases are sporadic	Strong genetic component, polygenic in most cases
Environmental triggers	Largely unknown	Obesity, sedentary lifestyle
Requirement for insulin therapy	Universal	Variable
Frequency among people with diabetes	5-10%	~90%
Associated disorders	Autoimmunity, especially thyroid, other endocrine disorders	Hypertension, dyslipidemia, metabolic syndrome, polycystic ovary syndrome

have in common some degree of insulin deficiency; insulin deficiency may be absolute, as in type 1 diabetes, or a relative deficit with coexisting insulin resistance, as in type 2 diabetes. Deficient insulin is the primary driver of impaired fuel homeostasis, whereas hyperglycemia plays the dominant role in disease-related complications. Major strides in our understanding of diabetes have been made during the last 40 years, with accompanying additions to the diagnostic and treatment armamentarium.

DEFINITIONS

Despite the heterogeneity of phenotypes, it is possible to generally classify diabetes into two major subgroups, type 1 (previously referred to as juvenile-onset or insulin-dependent diabetes) and type 2 (previously referred to as adult-onset or non–insulin-dependent diabetes). The major clinical features of type 1 and type 2 are shown in Table 229-1 and are described in detail in the corresponding sections later.

In addition to these two large categories, diabetes may occur in association with other disorders, with use of certain medications, or, rarely, as a result of a specific genetic mutation, such as maturity-onset diabetes of youth (MODY).

Diabetes Associated with Other Disorders or Syndromes

Diabetes may occur as part of several inherited syndromes, including the Turner, Klinefelter, Prader-Willi, Down, and Wolfram syndromes, among others. The genetic and metabolic defects involved are heterogeneous but usually result in impaired β-cell function. The obesity (and resulting insulin resistance) associated with many of these syndromes also contributes. Diseases of the exocrine pancreas, such as pancreatitis, pancreatic cancer, hemochromatosis, and cystic fibrosis, can be accompanied by impaired pancreatic endocrine function, leading to insulin-deficient diabetes. Several endocrinopathies that are associated with insulin resistance, including acromegaly, Cushing syndrome, and pheochromocytoma, may result in impaired glucose tolerance or frank diabetes in predisposed individuals. Viral infections, such as congenital rubella and cytomegalovirus, may cause diabetes by β-cell destruction. Finally, hyperglycemia may be associated with the use of certain drugs, including those that worsen insulin resistance (e.g., glucocorticoids, nicotinic acid, thiazide diuretics) and those that impair β-cell function (e.g., pentamidine, diazoxide, interferon gamma).

Diagnostic Criteria for Diabetes

Diabetes is diagnosed on the basis of one of several criteria, including fasting plasma glucose concentration, plasma glucose concentration after a standard 75-g oral glucose challenge (oral glucose tolerance test), and percentage of glycosylated hemoglobin (HbA_{1c}) (Table 229-2). In most cases, abnormal results require a confirmatory test, but diabetes can be diagnosed in the presence of unequivocal hyperglycemia (casual plasma glucose concentration > 200 mg/dL) and typical symptoms of polyuria, polydipsia, and weight loss.

Because plasma glucose levels exist on a continuum, the selection of a specific diagnostic threshold is in some respects arbitrary. Current criteria are based on the plasma glucose or HbA_{1c} level above which the risk of diabetes-specific microvascular complications (e.g., retinopathy) is perceptibly

TABLE 229-2 DIAGNOSTIC CRITERIA FOR DIABETES

	NORMAL	IMPAIRED (PRE-DIABETES)	DIABETES
Fasting glucose concentration (mg/dL)	<100	100-125	≥126
OGTT 2-hour glucose concentration (mg/dL)	<140	140-199	≥200
HbA$_{1c}$ (%)	<5.7	5.7-6.4	≥6.5

OGTT = oral glucose tolerance test.
Modified from American Diabetes Association. Standards of medical care in diabetes—2014. *Diabetes Care.* 2015;38(Suppl 1):S8-S16.

TABLE 229-3 THE RELATIONSHIP BETWEEN HbA$_{1c}$ AND ESTIMATED AVERAGE GLUCOSE LEVELS DURING THE PRECEDING 3 MONTHS

HbA$_{1c}$ (%)	ESTIMATED AVERAGE GLUCOSE LEVEL	
	mg/dL	*mmol/L*
5	97	5.4
6	126	7.0
7	154	8.6
8	183	10.2
9	212	11.8
10	240	13.4
11	269	14.9
12	298	16.5

From Nathan DM, Kuenen J, Borg R, et al. Translating the A1c assay into estimated average glucose values. *Diabetes Care.* 2008;31:1473-1478.

increased. In situations of altered red blood cell turnover or certain hemoglobinopathies, HbA$_{1c}$ may not accurately reflect mean plasma glucose levels (see later section on glycosylated hemoglobin), and direct glucose measurement should be used. Separate glucose criteria exist for the diagnosis of gestational diabetes (see section on gestational diabetes under clinical manifestations of type 2 diabetes).

States of impaired glucose regulation, not meeting the criteria for diabetes, have also been defined (fasting glucose concentration of 100 to 125 mg/dL, 2-hour glucose concentration of 140 to 199 mg/dL, or HbA$_{1c}$ level of 5.7 to 6.4%). Individuals in these categories are at increased risk for diabetes, although not all will progress and some may revert to normal glucose regulation. Impaired glucose tolerance (oral glucose tolerance test 2-hour glucose concentration of 140 to 199 mg/dL) has also been associated with increased risk of atherosclerotic cardiovascular disease (CVD), which may be independent of future development of diabetes.

Glycosylated Hemoglobin

Measurements of glycosylated hemoglobin have been in clinical use since the 1980s as a means of assessing glucose control in patients with diabetes and more recently for the diagnosis of diabetes and pre-diabetic states. Hemoglobin A$_{1c}$ (HbA$_{1c}$) is formed by the nonenzymatic glycosylation of hemoglobin, and its percentage reflects the exposure of the hemoglobin A molecule to glucose during the lifespan of red blood cells (~120 days). Thus, HbA$_{1c}$ has a predictable (but nonlinear) relationship with mean plasma glucose levels during the preceding 3 to 4 months, although more recent exposure (preceding 4 weeks) contributes relatively more to the percentage of glycosylation. The relationship between HbA$_{1c}$ and mean glucose levels was initially based on data obtained from the Diabetes Control and Complications Trial (DCCT) and recently updated on the basis of data obtained from studies using continuous glucose monitoring in ambulatory individuals, including those with and without diabetes (Table 229-3).

Although several different types of assays (e.g., affinity chromatography, immunoassay) are used to measure HbA$_{1c}$, most methods have been harmonized to a common standard and generally allow results from different laboratories to be used interchangeably. HbA$_{1c}$ results may be influenced by a number of factors, including conditions that alter red cell survival (e.g., hemolytic anemia) or cause interference with a specific assay. In these situations, measurement of fructosamine (glycosylated serum proteins) or glycated albumin, both of which reflect mean glucose levels during the preceding 2 to 3 weeks, may provide more accurate assessment of recent glucose levels. However, these assays have not been as well standardized, and the relationship with mean plasma glucose levels is less well established (Table 229-4).

PATHOBIOLOGY OF DIABETES

Figure 229-1 summarizes the effects of insulin deficiency on body fuel metabolism.

Given the dominant role of insulin in carbohydrate metabolism, it is not surprising that its availability and effectiveness play a role in every form of diabetes. However, because many other diabetogenic factors can be invoked and there is interdependence of many of these homeostatic mechanisms, teasing out their individual contributions is virtually impossible in any given patient.

Normal insulin physiology is orchestrated in a complex dynamic involving metabolic fuels, neurotransmitters, and other hormones. Insulin is synthesized as preproinsulin in the ribosomes of the rough endoplasmic reticulum of pancreatic islet β cells and is then converted to proinsulin, which in turn

TABLE 229-4 CONDITIONS THAT MAY AFFECT MEASUREMENT OR INTERPRETATION OF HbA$_{1c}$

MECHANISM OF HbA$_{1c}$ INTERFERENCE	CONDITION OR DISEASE	EFFECT ON HbA$_{1c}$
Reduced red cell lifespan	Hemolytic anemia Acute blood loss Hypersplenism	Falsely low
Increased red cell lifespan	Iron deficiency anemia	Falsely high
Altered glycation	High-dose vitamin supplementation (vitamins A and C)	Falsely low
Assay interference	Hemoglobins S, G, D, C, E Hemoglobin F	Falsely high Falsely low
Miscellaneous	Chronic renal disease Chronic liver disease Red cell transfusion African ancestry	Falsely high Falsely low Falsely low or high Falsely high

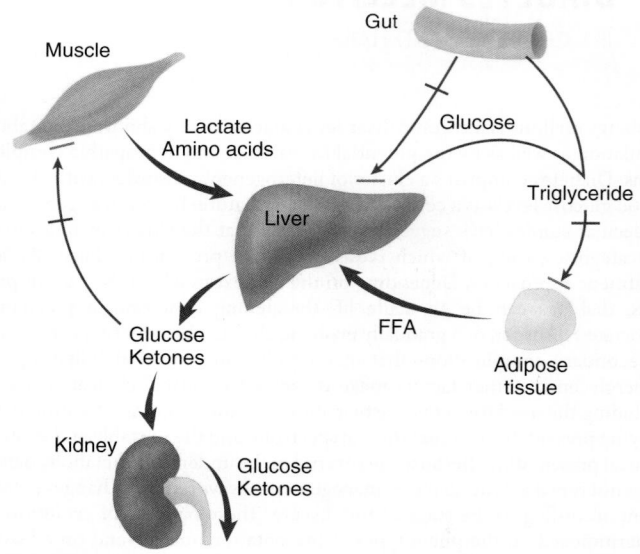

FIGURE 229-1. Effects of insulin deficiency on body fuel metabolism. Lack of insulin leads to mobilization of substrates for gluconeogenesis and ketogenesis from muscle and adipose tissue, accelerated production of glucose and ketones by the liver, and impaired removal of endogenous and exogenous fuels by insulin-responsive tissues. The net results are severe hyperglycemia and hyperketonemia that overwhelm renal removal mechanisms. FFA = free fatty acids.

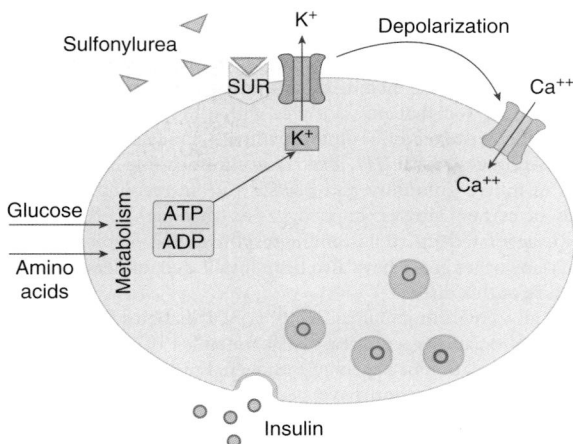

FIGURE 229-2. Nutrient regulation of insulin secretion. Glucose is taken up by the β cell through the GLUT2 glucose transporter and is metabolized (initially through phosphorylation by the glucokinase to glucose 6-phosphate). This leads to an increase in intracellular ATP (and an increase in the cytoplasmic ATP/ADP ratio), which causes closure of the ATP-dependent potassium channel, followed by membrane depolarization and the subsequent opening of voltage-gated calcium channels. The influx of calcium mobilizes the insulin secretory granules to fuse with the cell membrane and to release insulin into the extracellular fluid. The sulfonylurea 1 receptor (SUR1) is a component of the ATP-dependent potassium channel. ADP = adenosine diphosphate; ATP = adenosine triphosphate.

TABLE 229-5	THE METABOLIC EFFECTS OF INSULIN	
METABOLIC EFFECT	**STIMULATED BY INSULIN**	**INHIBITED BY INSULIN**
Carbohydrate metabolism	Glucose transport Glycolysis Glycogen synthesis	Glycogen breakdown Gluconeogenesis
Protein metabolism	Amino acid transport Protein synthesis	Protein breakdown
Lipid metabolism	Triglyceride uptake Lipogenesis	Lipolysis Fatty acid oxidation

is transported to the Golgi apparatus, where it is packaged into secretory granules. Proinsulin is cleaved into equimolar amounts of insulin and a connecting segment (C-peptide) in the secretory granules. The stimulation of insulin secretion results in release of equimolar quantities of insulin and C-peptide (as well as a small amount of proinsulin) into the hepatic portal vein. Whereas a large proportion of insulin is bound to its hepatic receptor and metabolized in its "first pass" through the liver, C-peptide is much less prone to hepatic metabolism and is a better reflection of insulin secretion, although it is quantitatively of limited usefulness in the clinical diagnosis or treatment of diabetes.

The principal regulator of insulin secretion is glucose. The process of β-cell insulin secretion is shown schematically in Figure 229-2. Glucose is taken up by the β cells through the GLUT2 glucose transporter system and then phosphorylated to glucose 6-phosphate by an islet-specific glucokinase. Thus, glucokinase can be considered the "glucose sensor" of the β cell; mutations in this enzyme can lead to a specific diabetes syndrome (MODY2), and there is evidence of its role in common forms of type 2 diabetes. The conversion of glucose to glucose 6-phosphate results in a sequential increase in intracellular adenosine triphosphate (ATP), closing of the ATP-dependent potassium (K_{ATP}) channels in the β-cell membrane, membrane depolarization and influx of calcium, migration of the insulin secretory granules to the cell membrane and their fusion with the membrane, and finally release of insulin into the extracellular fluid. The K_{ATP} channel is made up of the sulfonylurea 1 receptor (SUR1) and an inward potassium channel subunit, Kir6.2. Mutations in either the SUR1 gene or the Kir6.2 gene lead to loss of K_{ATP} activity; as a result, the cell is depolarized, resulting in chronic release of insulin and a syndrome termed *persistent hyperinsulinemic hypoglycemia of infancy*. Mutations in Kir6.2 and SUR1 have also been identified in patients with permanent neonatal diabetes mellitus; treatment with sulfonylurea can normalize insulin secretion in these patients.

The magnitude of the insulin secretory response is determined by the level of blood glucose as well as by the mode of glucose entry. Compared with intravenous administration of glucose, higher insulin levels are produced when glucose is taken up orally because of the simultaneous release of gut-derived incretins that include glucagon-like peptide 1 (GLP-1) and glucose-dependent insulinotropic peptide (GIP), both of which augment insulin secretion. In fact, drugs that mimic or enhance this incretin effect are useful in the treatment of type 2 diabetes.

Rapid increases in blood glucose concentration (e.g., after intravenous administration of glucose) cause a spike of insulin secretion that peaks within a few minutes and declines quickly (so-called first-phase insulin secretion). With more persistent elevations of plasma glucose concentration, insulin secretion is sustained (so-called second-phase insulin secretion). The earliest

pathophysiologic indicator of defective β-cell function may be the loss of first-phase secretion of insulin, which precedes by years the decline in insulin secretory reserve sufficient to lead to overt glucose intolerance or diabetes.

Insulin Action

The actions of insulin on its principal target organs (i.e., muscle, fat, liver) have complex and coordinated effects on the metabolism of carbohydrates, proteins, and lipids and are mediated by its interaction with the insulin receptor. Insulin receptor signaling through insulin receptor substrate 1 and phosphatidylinositol 3-kinase is a major pathway in the mediation of insulin-stimulated glucose transport, notably by stimulating the translocation of the glucose transporter GLUT4 to the cell membrane. This pathway is also responsible for the vasodilator effects of insulin (through increased expression of endothelial nitric oxide synthase), which may contribute to glucose utilization by increasing nutrient delivery to tissues. Defects in these intracellular signaling pathways are an important cause of impaired insulin action, or "insulin resistance" (see section on impaired insulin action [insulin resistance] under pathobiology of type 2 diabetes).

The overall actions of insulin tend to promote uptake and storage of nutrients in the fed state and release of nutrients from body stores in the fasting state, as summarized in Table 229-5.

In the *postprandial period*, rising glucose levels simultaneously trigger insulin secretion and suppress glucagon release. The resulting rise in the insulin-to-glucagon ratio increases hepatic glycogen synthesis and inhibits release of glucose from the liver. Insulin stimulates glucose uptake into skeletal muscle and adipose tissue, promoting the synthesis of protein and triglycerides. In the *fasting state*, declining glucose levels inhibit insulin release, thereby increasing glycogenolysis and gluconeogenesis and the resulting delivery of glucose into the circulation. In states of absolute or relative insulin deficiency, inadequate basal insulin levels allow unrestrained hepatic glucose production, which results in fasting hyperglycemia. Inadequate insulin in the fed state impedes peripheral (predominantly skeletal muscle) glucose uptake, thereby contributing to postprandial hyperglycemia. Impaired suppression of hepatic glucose production also contributes to postprandial hyperglycemia in patients with diabetes (see also the section on type 2 diabetes).

TYPE 1 DIABETES

EPIDEMIOLOGY

Type 1 diabetes may be manifested at any age but most typically appears in childhood, especially around puberty. However, new cases of type 1 diabetes can appear at any time in life, and in the United States, approximately 30% of patients are diagnosed after young adulthood.[1]

Worldwide, the incidence of type 1 diabetes varies 50- to 100-fold, with the highest rates occurring in individuals of northern European descent. Both sexes are equally affected in childhood, but men are affected more commonly in early adult life. The incidence of childhood type 1 diabetes is rising rapidly in all populations, especially in the age group younger than 5 years, with a doubling time of less than 20 years in Europe. The increasing incidence of type 1 diabetes suggests a major environmental contribution, but the role of specific pathogenic factors remains largely unsettled. The distinction between type 1 and type 2 diabetes can become blurred in later life, and the true lifetime incidence of the condition is therefore unknown.

In Europe, the highest rates of childhood diabetes are found in Scandinavia, with an incidence for children from birth to 14 years of age ranging from 57/100,000 per year in Finland to 4/100,000 in Macedonia. In the United States, the overall annual incidence in youths is about 19/100,000. Prevalence rates are strikingly different among ethnic groups living in the same geographic region, probably because of genetic differences in susceptibility to the disease. Early-onset diabetes carries a higher familial risk, and affected fathers are more likely to transmit type 1 diabetes to their offspring than affected mothers are, with risks being 6 to 9% and 1 to 3%, respectively.

Given that the United States does not have a systematic health registry and that its population is multiethnic, previous estimates of the prevalence and incidence of type 1 diabetes have been based on extrapolations from limited cohorts. The SEARCH for Diabetes in Youth multicenter study (funded by the Centers for Disease Control and Prevention and the National Institutes of Health) examined diabetes among children and adolescents in the United States. During 2008-2009, an estimated 18,436 people younger than 20 years in the United States were newly diagnosed with type 1 diabetes annually, and 5089 people younger than 20 years were newly diagnosed with type 2 diabetes annually. For those younger than 10 years, new cases of type 1 far outweighed type 2 (22.2/100,000 per year for type 1 diabetes vs. 0.8/100,000 for type 2 diabetes). Among youth aged 10 years or older, the rate of new cases of type 1 was about double that of type 2 (21.9/100,000 per year for type 1 diabetes vs. 11.0/100,000 for type 2 diabetes). Non-Hispanic white youth had the highest rate of new cases of type 1 diabetes in all age groups. Diabetes incidence rates by age and race/ethnicity are summarized in Figure 229-3.

Higher body mass index (BMI) is associated with younger age at diagnosis of type 1 diabetes, but this appears to be the case only in children with already compromised β-cell function. In addition, low birth weight may be a factor in accelerating the onset of type 1 diabetes, suggesting that the intrauterine environment may be an important determinant of age at onset for type 1 diabetes.

PATHOBIOLOGY

In type 1 diabetes, a complex interplay of genetic, environmental, and autoimmune factors selectively targets insulin-producing β cells and ultimately produces complete β-cell destruction. The role of genetic factors in type 1 diabetes has long been appreciated, emphasized by familial clustering with other autoimmune endocrine disorders and by concordance rates in identical twins of 30 to 40%. Because these concordance rates are not as high as in type 2 diabetes (i.e., >80%), environmental factors must clearly play a major role. Although the presence of an environmental trigger for type 1 diabetes is highly likely, even identical twins do not express identical T-cell receptor and immunoglobulin genes; as a result, total concordance might not be expected. Siblings who are HLA identical to the proband have a 12 to 15% risk for development of diabetes by the age of 20 years.

Although many of the genes linked to type 1 diabetes have yet to be identified, some are known. HLA genes, located on the short arm of chromosome 6, contribute about 50% of genetic susceptibility to type 1 diabetes. Two HLA class II haplotypes, DR4-DQ8 and DR3-DQ2, are present in about 90% of children with type 1 diabetes. The genotype containing both haplotypes carries the highest risk of diabetes (about 5%) and is most commonly seen in early-onset disease. In contrast, the DR15-DQ6 haplotype is highly protective, being found in only 1% of children with type 1 diabetes in contrast to 20% in the general population. HLA susceptibility haplotypes are overrepresented in adult-onset type 1, but at lower frequency than in classic type 1 diabetes in youth. Other genes likely contribute to the genetic susceptibility to type 1 diabetes. These include the insulin gene (on chromosome 11) and a number of other loci that are associated with other autoimmune conditions, suggesting the existence of common pathways predisposing to loss of self-tolerance. Another gene, *IFIH1*, located on chromosome 2, encodes a protein involved in innate immunity and plays a role in recognition of the RNA genomes of certain viruses. It is suggested that high IFIH1 levels might provoke exaggerated antiviral immune responses that predispose to autoimmunity. Many other genes have also been implicated, underscoring the polygenic nature of this disease.

Historically, environmental causes of type 1 diabetes focused on viruses because of associations with seasonal pandemics of infections and rarely because of the isolation of a specific pathogen. Epidemics of mumps, rubella, and coxsackievirus infection have been associated with an increased frequency of type 1 diabetes. Moreover, specific and convincing rare examples of virus-induced diabetes have been reported. However, it is believed that virus-mediated β-cell damage is not responsible for the massive destruction of β cells but that it triggers an autoimmune response in genetically predisposed individuals. Thus, viruses may contain molecules that resemble a β-cell protein, and viral infection could thus nullify self-tolerance and trigger autoimmune responses.

It has long been recognized that about 80% of patients with new-onset type 1 diabetes have antibodies directed against various islet cell proteins, including insulin, glutamic acid decarboxylase (GAD65 and GAD67), and the secretory granule protein islet cell antigen 512 (IA-2). These antibody biomarkers have been important tools for studying the potential for early identification and prevention of total β-cell destruction in individuals susceptible to type 1 diabetes. Until the mid-1980s, it was mistakenly surmised that the autoimmune destruction of β-cells was mediated by these antibodies rather than their being epiphenomena, as is now understood. Rather, β-cell destruction is mediated by a variety of cytokines or by direct T-lymphocyte activity that causes apoptosis or cellular destruction. Both animal models and human pathologic studies have established that islet-targeted inflammatory cell infiltrates (termed insulitis) that are composed of CD8+ and CD4+ T cells, macrophages, and B cells are linked to the onset of diabetes. Over time, the islets become completely devoid of β cells and inflammatory infiltrates; α, δ, and pancreatic polypeptide cells are left intact, thus illustrating the specificity of the autoimmune attack on β cells.

A critical role for T cells is suggested by studies involving pancreatic transplantation in identical twins. Monozygotic twins with diabetes who received kidney and pancreas grafts from their nondiabetic, genetically identical siblings required little or no therapeutic immunosuppression. However, these patients eventually experienced a resumption of insulitis, with the subsequent recurrence of diabetes. Evidence implicating T cells in diabetes autoimmunity also derives from clinical trials using immunosuppressive drugs. Drugs such as cyclosporine or antibodies directed against a component of the T-cell receptor (anti-CD3) or that alter antigen presentation by B cells (anti-CD20) slow the progression of recent-onset diabetes, but this effect is not sustained if immunosuppression is withdrawn.

CLINICAL MANIFESTATIONS

It has been clearly established that type 1 diabetes has a long preclinical phase, best described in Figure 229-4. At the time of clinical diagnosis, about 10 to 20% of the original β-cell mass may still be functional. In most cases, overt hyperglycemia (and ketosis if it is present) may be precipitated by an unrelated medical illness or stress placed on an already-limited islet reserve, thus triggering the diagnosis. Typically, symptomatic hyperglycemia, manifested by polyuria, polydipsia, weight loss, and fatigue, occurs abruptly in an otherwise healthy child or young adult. For a minority of patients, the initial presentation may be diabetic ketoacidosis (DKA), which can occur if there is a delay in recognizing the symptoms of diabetes. Whereas the disease has an increased incidence in the winter months, classically attributed to respiratory viral infections, this seasonal pattern may be the result of illness-associated counter-regulatory hormones that drive hyperglycemia in individuals with already compromised β-cell function. Similarly, the coincidence of type 1 diabetes with puberty has been attributed to insulin resistance associated with increases in sex and growth hormone secretion.

The diagnosis of diabetes is made according to glucose criteria (see Table 229-2). Measurement of anti–glutamic acid decarboxylase antibodies is sometimes performed, but the determination of type 1 etiology is generally

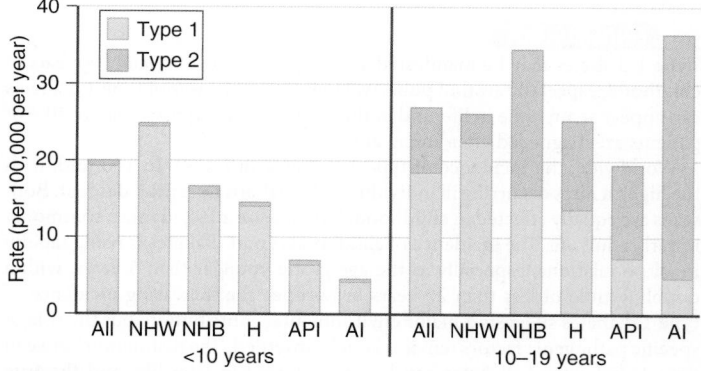

FIGURE 229-3. Rate of new cases of type 1 and type 2 diabetes among people younger than 20 years in the United States, by age and race/ethnicity, 2008-2009. AI = American Indians; API = Asian/Pacific Islander Americans; H = Hispanics/Latinos; NHB = non-Hispanic blacks; NHW = non-Hispanic whites. (From Centers for Disease Control and Prevention. *National Diabetes Statistics Report: Estimates of Diabetes and Its Burden in the United States, 2014.* Atlanta, GA: US Department of Health and Human Services; 2014. Source: SEARCH for Diabetes in Youth Study).

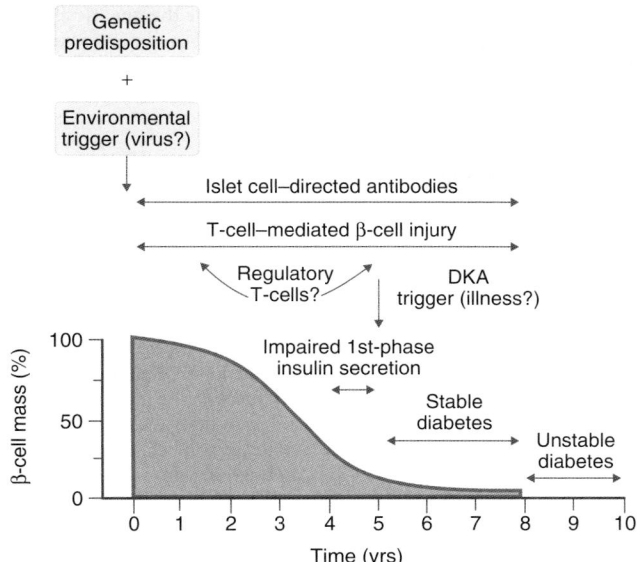

FIGURE 229-4. Summary of the sequence of events that lead to pancreatic β-cell loss and ultimately to the clinical evolution of type 1 diabetes. DKA = diabetic ketoacidosis.

TABLE 229-6 INSULIN PREPARATIONS

TYPE OF INSULIN	ONSET OF ACTION	PEAK EFFECT	DURATION OF ACTION
BASAL INSULIN			
Glargine	~ 2 hours	None	~ 24 hours
Detemir	~ 2 hours	3-9 hours	6-24 hours
Degludec	~ 2 hours	None	~ 40 hours
NPH/NPL	~ 2 hours	6-12 hours	14-24 hours
PRANDIAL INSULIN			
Lispro, aspart, glulisine	5 to 15 minutes	45-75 minutes	2-4 hours
Regular	~ 30 minutes	2-4 hours	5-8 hours

NPH = neutral protamine Hagedorn; NPL = neutral protamine lispro.

made on clinical grounds. After initiation of insulin therapy and stabilization of plasma glucose levels, the patient may experience a period of weeks to months of relatively mild and easily controlled hyperglycemia. This so-called honeymoon phase of type 1 diabetes results from transient improvement in β-cell function and reflects the phenomenon of severe but not total β-cell destruction with ongoing (albeit reduced) insulin secretion. Ultimately, patients with type 1 diabetes experience progressive decline in insulin production, generally to undetectable levels after a few years. However, with highly sensitive C-peptide assays, low levels of insulin production have been detected in some patients with long-standing type 1 diabetes and are associated with more stable glycemic control and reduced risk of vascular complications.[2] In patients with onset of type 1 diabetes in adulthood, the clinical presentation may follow a more indolent course (termed latent autoimmune diabetes in adults), perhaps because β-cell mass declines at a slower pace. In fact, type 1 diabetes may be misdiagnosed as type 2 in many of these patients until the progression of insulin deficiency reveals the phenotype of permanent and complete insulin dependence.

TREATMENT Rx

The key to successful treatment of type 1 diabetes is to achieve physiologic insulin replacement, that is, to replicate the normal and tightly regulated relationship between plasma glucose and insulin secretion. Although current technology can only mimic this normal physiology, substantial progress has been made to permit maintenance of relative euglycemia by many patients. Successful glucose management requires substantial commitment by the patient and health care practitioner.

Insulin Therapy

All patients with type 1 diabetes require insulin treatment to maintain life. The approach to insulin replacement in type 1 diabetes requires consideration of both basal insulin requirements (insulin required to maintain homeostasis in the fasting state) and insulin required for the influx of nutrients that occurs with meals. A variety of insulin preparations are available, which differ by their pattern of absorption after subcutaneous injection. Most currently used insulin preparations are analogues of human insulin that have been modified (usually by changing one or more amino acids) to alter pharmacokinetics to speed or to delay absorption (Table 229-6).

Patients with type 1 diabetes are treated with both a long-acting "basal" insulin and a shorter-acting "prandial" insulin at mealtime, by a multiple daily insulin injection regimen or a continuous subcutaneous insulin infusion pump. Typically, the daily insulin requirement for patients with type 1 diabetes is between 0.3 and 1.0 unit/kg/day, with half given as basal insulin and the remainder divided into pre-meal boluses. Prandial insulin doses are determined by meal carbohydrate content plus a "correction factor" if glucose is

elevated before the meal. For example, a common approach is to use 1 unit for every 10 to 15 g of meal carbohydrate plus a correction factor of 1 unit to lower plasma glucose concentration by 20 to 50 mg/dL. However, insulin requirements are influenced by a number of factors (e.g., age, body size, insulin sensitivity) and vary substantially among patients; therefore, these algorithms need to be individualized. A number of mobile phone applications and computer programs are available to assist patients with dose calculation. Critical to the success of physiologic insulin replacement is the need for the patient to monitor blood glucose concentration, generally several times a day (see later).

A continuous subcutaneous insulin infusion pump using a short-acting insulin analogue can be programmed to deliver both a basal infusion and a preprandial bolus. Most insulin pumps contain an insulin reservoir attached by thin flexible tubing to a very small catheter that is inserted subcutaneously by the patient and changed every 2 or 3 days to avoid local inflammation and fibrosis, which can interfere with insulin absorption. The basal insulin delivery rate can be programmed to vary throughout the day and may be especially useful to prevent hyperglycemia associated with the "dawn phenomenon" (rising blood glucose levels in the early morning hours, thought largely to be due to increased growth hormone secretion). Most insulin pumps can be programmed to calculate prandial insulin doses, based on pre-meal glucose level and meal carbohydrate content, which is entered by the patient. However, in the event of pump malfunction, metabolic decompensation, including DKA, can develop within several hours because there is no subcutaneous reservoir of long-acting insulin. Successful use of an insulin pump requires a motivated and educated patient plus the support of a specialized diabetes team, including a certified diabetes educator. When it is used appropriately, continuous subcutaneous insulin infusion provides patients with maximal lifestyle flexibility and the best chance to achieve near-normal blood glucose levels. **A1**

Some patients who find adherence to a multiple injection or insulin pump regimen difficult can be treated with premixed "biphasic" insulin combinations, for example, a mixture of NPH and regular insulin given twice daily. This approach may be appropriate for patients with recent onset of type 1 diabetes who still maintain some endogenous insulin production. However, for most patients, this regimen is rarely optimal because it lacks flexibility and often increases the risk of hypoglycemia.

Diet and Lifestyle Treatment

In type 1 diabetes, the focus of dietary planning is on accurate estimation of meal carbohydrate content to allow appropriate prandial insulin dosing. This can be approached by promotion of "carbohydrate consistency" from meal to meal and the use of relatively fixed pre-meal insulin dosing. A more flexible approach is for the patient to learn "carbohydrate counting," which specifies an insulin dose per amount of carbohydrate in the meal. With either approach, patients need to monitor the nutrient content of their meals. Avoidance of concentrated sweets and other high-carbohydrate meals, including those with a high "glycemic index," tends to facilitate accurate insulin dosing and to minimize postprandial glycemic excursions. In contrast to type 2 diabetes, most patients with type 1 diabetes are not overweight or obese, and calorie restriction is neither required nor helpful. A variety of eating patterns are considered acceptable, and recommendations for a "heart healthy" diet (low in saturated fat and cholesterol) are the same as for the general population.[3]

Glucose Self-monitoring

Successful management of type 1 diabetes requires consistent self-monitoring of blood glucose concentration by the patient or caregiver several times a day. Small portable meters with disposable strips are easy to use and reasonably accurate in most ambulatory care settings. Frequent testing (i.e., before meals and at bedtime) allows appropriate prandial insulin dosing and correction of unexpected hyperglycemia as well as detection or confirmation of hypoglycemia. Most current meters store a large number of readings, which can be downloaded to a computer for analysis by the patient and health care team. Subcutaneous glucose monitors that provide continuous reading of interstitial glucose levels are available and are most commonly used in conjunction with an insulin pump. These monitors are most useful to determine glucose patterns and can be programmed to sound an alarm when the glucose level exceeds a preset range or rate of change. However, the accuracy of current monitors is such that they cannot replace conventional blood glucose monitoring for immediate treatment decisions. Research is progressing in the development of a "closed loop" system combining an insulin pump with a highly accurate continuous glucose monitor, allowing adjustments of insulin dosing without direct input of the patient. The first such device has received Food and Drug Administration approval for patients older than 16 years, but experience with this approach remains limited.

Patients with type 1 diabetes should be instructed to test urine ketones (with a reagent strip) in situations in which blood glucose concentration is unexpectedly and persistently elevated, especially if it is accompanied by symptoms suggestive of DKA (see section on diabetic ketoacidosis under hyperglycemic states in acute metabolic complications of diabetes). Small or trace amounts of urinary ketones are not cause for concern, but moderate or large amounts may indicate the onset of DKA and should prompt the patient to seek urgent medical attention.

Whole Pancreas and Islet Cell Transplantation

The ultimate goal of a "cure" of type 1 diabetes could most likely be achieved by successful transplantation of insulin-producing β cells. Whole pancreas transplantation has been performed for more than two decades and has a reasonable success rate, with 5-year graft survival rates of about 70%. However, the surgical procedure is complicated, and lifelong immunosuppression is required, as with any organ transplant. For these reasons, pancreas transplantation is generally reserved for patients who already have or are concurrently receiving a kidney transplant. In the absence of indications for kidney transplantation, pancreas-alone transplantation may be considered for patients who have a history of frequent, acute and severe metabolic complications (especially severe hypoglycemia) or severe and incapacitating psychosocial problems related to insulin therapy. Pancreatic islet cell transplants hold significant potential advantages over whole-gland transplants. However, at this time, islet cell transplantation is an experimental procedure, also requiring systemic immunosuppression, and is performed only within the setting of controlled research studies.

PREVENTION OF TYPE 1 DIABETES

Given that type 1 diabetes is an immunologically mediated disease, it has long been supposed that immune intervention should alter its natural history and perhaps even prevent it altogether. Furthermore, the significant heritability of type 1 diabetes suggests that treatment could target only susceptible individuals, and the existence of known biomarkers (antibodies that reflect disease activity as well as levels of insulin or C-peptide that reflect islet function) also lends credence to experimental immunologic treatments. Unfortunately, however, the major challenge for most immunologic interventions has been their lack of specificity for immune-mediated insulitis or the risks of spillover immune suppression in otherwise healthy persons. Given the experimental nature of all the tested therapies, we provide only a brief overview here.[4]

Prevention of type 1 diabetes can theoretically be undertaken at three stages: (1) in susceptible individuals before there is evidence of immune attack against islet cells (primary prevention); (2) in nondiabetic people who already have evidence of immune activation (antibodies, insulin defects) to prevent progression to actual diabetes (secondary prevention); and (3) in newly diagnosed patients in whom the goal is to slow the β-cell destructive process (tertiary prevention).

Avoidance of putative environmental triggers of islet autoimmunity (e.g., cow's milk) is one approach, and dietary supplementation with nutrients that may diminish islet autoimmunity (e.g., omega-3 fatty acids or vitamin D) has been attempted. On the basis of positive results of an earlier small cohort study, the first large trial of primary prevention by removal of cow's milk from the infant diet was initiated in 2002 and is expected to be completed in 2017. Secondary prevention trials have also been undertaken with oral, inhaled, or injected insulin and with nicotinamide, but the results have been equivocal. There are secondary prevention studies with teplizumab (an FcR-nonbinding anti-CD32 monoclonal antibody) and with abatacept (a costimulation modulator) under way. Several tertiary prevention studies (i.e., after the diagnosis of diabetes) have been published. Nonspecific immune interventions, such as cyclosporine, demonstrate that immunotherapy can indeed rescue β cells

from ongoing destruction, but it is not an acceptable therapeutic alternative given that it preserves β-cell function only transiently and carries heightened risks of adverse effects, such as nephropathy. Anti-CD3 antibodies currently appear more promising and are being evaluated in clinical trials.

PROGNOSIS

Substantial progress has been made in recent decades in improving the prognosis for patients affected by type 1 diabetes. This is largely due to adoption of more intensive glucose control and more effective nonglycemic treatment of early stages of renal disease and retinopathy. Data from long-term follow-up of the intensively treated DCCT cohort showed that after 30 years' duration of diabetes, rates of serious diabetes complications were substantially lower than in historical controls, and less than 1% became blind, required renal replacement, or had an amputation due to diabetes. In the absence of renal disease, life expectancy for type 1 patients in the United States is comparable to that of the general population.[5] However, the mortality rate of all type 1 diabetic patients from age 35 onward is about twice as high as in nondiabetics even if the HgbA$_{1c}$ level is 6.9% or lower and becomes progressively higher for HgbA$_{1c}$ levels above 7.9%.[6] Analysis of nationally representative hospitalization and registry data has shown large reductions in the incidence of a broad spectrum of diabetes-related complications between 1990 and 2010 in the U.S. population of adults with diabetes; however, despite the substantial decline in the rates of diabetes-related complications in the past two decades, a large burden of disease persists because of the continued increase in the prevalence of diabetes.[7]

TYPE 2 DIABETES

EPIDEMIOLOGY

Type 2 diabetes is one of the most common chronic diseases, affecting more than 25 million people in the United States and an estimated 366 million worldwide. The prevalence of type 2 diabetes has been increasing in the United States, from approximately 3% of the population in 1995 to more than 9% in 2012. This increase is in part due to demographic shifts (i.e., the aging of the population), but incidence rates are also increasing and parallel the rise of overweight and obesity as well as increasingly sedentary lifestyles. A similar pattern is observed globally, with projections of 550 million (approximately half undiagnosed) to be affected by 2030. Although type 2 diabetes is being increasingly recognized in obese adolescents and young adults, older age remains a major risk factor for type 2 diabetes. More than one quarter of adults aged 65 years and older have diabetes, and another 50% have glucose or HbA$_{1c}$ levels in the impaired or pre-diabetic range. Type 2 diabetes in the United States is more common among some racial and ethnic groups, with prevalence rates highest among non-Hispanic blacks (13%), Hispanics (12%), and American Indians (16%) and lowest among non-Hispanic whites (7%). Individuals from the Indian subcontinent (i.e., India, Pakistan, Bangladesh) and the Pacific Islands (e.g., Hawaii, Nauru, Samoa) also have high rates of type 2 diabetes. In general, men and women have about equal prevalence of type 2 diabetes.

PATHOBIOLOGY

Type 2 diabetes is characterized by variable defects in both insulin secretion and insulin action.[8] The underlying metabolic phenotype of type 2 diabetes is distinctly heterogeneous among individuals with the disease; some have a more pronounced defect in insulin secretion, and others have greater resistance to insulin action. The metabolic profile also varies within a given patient over time, as insulin secretion progressively declines with longer duration of disease. Although heterogeneous, type 2 diabetes is characterized in all cases by inadequate insulin secretion for the prevailing glucose level and degree of insulin sensitivity.

Impaired Insulin Secretion

The relative insulin deficiency characteristic of type 2 diabetes appears to be a consequence of both functional (i.e., reduced responsiveness to secretagogues) and quantitative (i.e., reduction in β-cell mass) factors. Insulin secretory capacity is difficult to directly measure in humans, but reductions of β-cell mass up to 60% are estimated to occur in type 2 diabetes. However, this alone is insufficient to explain insulin deficiency in type 2 diabetes, as evidenced by the observation that 50% surgical pancreatectomy does not lead to hyperglycemia in otherwise healthy individuals. Classic studies in diabetic patients have demonstrated failure of insulin secretion in response to glucose but a normal response to the amino acid arginine, providing further evidence for the presence of a functional defect specific to glucose sensing. Abnormalities in the usual pulsatile and oscillatory patterns of insulin secretion and inefficient insulin biosynthesis have also been demonstrated in type 2 diabetes. For example, abnormal peptide processing results in increased secretion of intact proinsulin, which serves as a useful biomarker of future diabetes risk. Increased accumulation of amyloid also occurs within diabetic islets and may contribute to impaired secretory function. Ultimately, the β-cell defects in type 2 diabetes appear to be multifactorial, in part genetically determined (see later) but also influenced by environmental exposure, for example, to high levels of circulating glucose (glucotoxicity) and lipids (lipotoxicity). In addition, the β-cell defects are not static but worsen with increasing duration of diabetes.

Impaired Insulin Action (Insulin Resistance)
Resistance to the metabolic effects of insulin is also a characteristic although variable feature of type 2 diabetes. Hyperinsulinemia, thought to be a compensatory response to impaired insulin action, can be demonstrated in patients with pre-diabetes and in many patients with established type 2 diabetes, particularly early in its course. More precise techniques to measure insulin action (e.g., the euglycemic hyperinsulinemic clamp) have demonstrated resistance to insulin action primarily in peripheral tissues (reduced capacity to stimulate glucose uptake in muscle and fat) but also in the liver (reduced capacity of insulin to suppress hepatic glucose production). Insulin resistance is closely associated with obesity (see later) but also has genetic determinants, reflected by the observation that some obese patients do not have severe insulin resistance. Insulin resistance frequently occurs as part of a constellation of features, termed the metabolic syndrome, which include hypertension, abdominal obesity, dyslipidemia, glucose intolerance, and increased cardiovascular risk. Insulin resistance is also a common feature of the polycystic ovary syndrome.

There are multiple molecular mechanisms that can lead to resistance to physiologic insulin action, including pre-receptor defects (e.g., an abnormal insulin molecule) and abnormal insulin receptors (e.g., due to gene mutations). However, common forms of insulin resistance that occur in association with type 2 diabetes are generally due to post-receptor defects, that is, abnormalities in intracellular signaling. In insulin target tissues, signaling through the phosphatidylinositol 3-kinase pathway is responsible for translocation of the glucose transporter GLUT4, which is necessary for uptake of glucose into the cell. Several defects in this pathway have been described in humans with insulin resistance, including abnormalities in insulin receptor substrate 1 and protein kinase B/Akt2. Some specific gene mutations associated with insulin resistance have been identified, but insulin resistance may also be acquired as a consequence of obesity (see later), increases in circulating free fatty acids, certain medications (e.g., glucocorticoids, niacin), and inflammatory states.

Evidence from natural history and genetic association studies (see later) indicates that defects in either insulin action or insulin secretion can remain clinically silent. For example, insulin resistance can induce compensatory hyperinsulinemia, which early in the course of the disease is sufficient to maintain euglycemia. However, in individuals with inherited or acquired defects in β-cell function, this compensation ultimately fails and hyperglycemia ensues. Viewed another way, a subclinical β-cell defect may remain silent in the setting of normal insulin sensitivity but be manifested as hyperglycemia when acquired insulin resistance develops because of weight gain, aging, or some other factor. A unifying theory that explains the coexistence of defects in both insulin action and insulin secretion is appealing but so far elusive.

Genetics
The evidence for familial aggregation of type 2 diabetes is substantial and supports the presence of an important genetic influence. An individual with one parent with type 2 diabetes has a lifetime risk for development of type 2 diabetes of approximately 40%, with risk increasing to approximately 70% if both parents are affected. Further, the concordance rate among monozygotic twins is as high as 70%. The greater risk of type 2 diabetes among certain racial and ethnic groups also supports an important genetic component. The overall heritability of type 2 diabetes is estimated to be between 25 and 50%, although the specific gene or genes ultimately responsible for common forms of type 2 diabetes have not been established.[9]

Single-Gene Mutations Linked to Type 2 Diabetes Phenotype
A number of syndromes, termed maturity-onset diabetes of youth (MODY), characterized by impaired β-cell function have been recognized and linked

	MUTATION	METABOLIC DEFECT	CLINICAL PHENOTYPE
MODY 2	Glucokinase	Decreased β-cell sensitivity to glucose	Mild nonprogressive hyperglycemia, may not require pharmacologic treatment; diabetes complications rare
MODY 3	Hepatic nuclear factor 1α	Abnormal regulation of β-cell gene transcription	Mild hyperglycemia, may be progressive; renal glycosuria; increased sensitivity to sulfonylurea drugs; susceptibility to microvascular complications

TABLE 229-7 SINGLE-GENE MUTATIONS RESPONSIBLE FOR THE MORE COMMON FORMS OF MATURITY-ONSET DIABETES OF YOUTH (MODY)

to specific single-gene mutations. The phenotypes vary with the mutation but generally include early onset of relatively mild hyperglycemia in nonobese children or young adults and an autosomal dominant pattern of inheritance. Although not common (representing 1 to 3% of diabetes cases worldwide), their discovery has provided insight into the role of β-cell function in the more common forms of type 2 diabetes. MODY 2 is associated with a mutation of glucokinase, which acts as a glucose sensor within the β cell. In this case, higher levels of glucose are required to stimulate release of insulin from the β cell. MODY 3 is due to a mutation of the gene for hepatic nuclear factor 1α, which is involved in early pancreatic development and in the regulation of insulin gene expression. Other MODY forms (1, 4, 5, 6) are much less common, having been described in only a few families (Table 229-7).

Other examples of single-gene mutations associated with specific diabetes syndromes include activating mutations of *KCNJ11* (encoding a portion of the β-cell sulfonylurea receptor), which causes severe neonatal diabetes, and *WFS1*, which encodes a protein that is defective in Wolfram syndrome (diabetes insipidus, diabetes mellitus, optic atrophy, and deafness).

Polygenic, Common Type 2 Diabetes
Common forms of type 2 diabetes are likely polygenic and multifactorial and represent a complex interaction between genes and environment. In the past several years, more than 50 genetic risk loci for common forms of type 2 diabetes have been identified by genome-wide association studies, but collectively these explain only about 15% of the heritability of the disorder. The gene with the strongest effect size to date (odds ratio for diabetes, 1.4), *TCF7L2*, is associated with reduced insulin secretion, as are the majority of other recognized gene variants. Others include a β-cell zinc transporter (ZnT-8; odds ratio, 1.15), the sulfonylurea receptor (*KCNJ11*; odds ratio, 1.1), and melatonin receptor 1B (*MTNR1B*; odds ratio, 1.10). A smaller number of gene variants associated with insulin resistance have been identified and include genes encoding peroxisome proliferator-activated receptor γ (odds ratio, 1.20) and insulin receptor substrate 1 (odds ratio, 1.10). Sequence variants in *SLC16A11*, a gene involved in intracellular lipid metabolism, were discovered to be a relatively common risk allele (odds ratio, 1.29) in Mexican populations. Current knowledge about genetic variants associated with type 2 diabetes risk is not useful for clinical disease prediction, offering no advantage to simple clinical tools based on traditional risk factors.

There is emerging evidence that epigenetic changes may play an important role in development of type 2 diabetes. Epidemiologic studies suggest that "metabolic programming" may occur in utero, with both fetal starvation and fetal overnutrition predisposing to diabetes in adult life. One example comes from experience with the Pima Indians, who have an extremely high prevalence of type 2 diabetes. Children born to mothers who were diabetic during their pregnancy had higher rates of adult diabetes than did children born to the same mothers before they became diabetic, suggesting that intrauterine exposure can have long-lasting metabolic effects. Studies of DNA methylation in animal models support this hypothesis, although human epigenome-wide studies are just now being conducted. Conversely, maternal undernutrition is associated with diabetes in offspring. Low birth weight has been linked to predisposition to CVD and diabetes in adulthood. According to the widely cited Barker hypothesis, nutrient deficiency in utero (e.g., due to maternal starvation or placental insufficiency) impairs development of the endocrine pancreas, leading to inadequate insulin production later in life.[10] The available data suggest that maternal nutrition may play an important role in metabolic programming, resulting in increased diabetes susceptibility in adulthood.

Obesity

The presence of overweight or obesity (Chapter 220) substantially increases the risk for type 2 diabetes and likely accounts for the dramatic increase in diabetes prevalence during the past several decades. In fact, the presence of overweight or obesity is the single most important clinical predictor of type 2 diabetes, particularly for young or middle-aged individuals. The relationship between BMI and type 2 diabetes is linear, and increased risk can be observed even within the BMI range defined as normal ($<25 \text{ kg/m}^2$). Related factors, such as sedentary lifestyle and diet (increased consumption of foods with high glycemic load, increased *trans* and saturated fat), may also contribute to diabetes risk, independent of BMI. Distribution of body fat also plays an important role, with visceral adiposity (as assessed by waist circumference or waist-to-hip ratio) being a particularly strong diabetes risk factor in Asian populations, who tend to develop type 2 diabetes at a lower BMI than some other racial or ethnic groups do. Ectopic accumulation of adipose tissue in the liver, often manifested as nonalcoholic fatty liver disease, is also strongly associated with increased diabetes risk.

The increase in adipose tissue mass impairs insulin action by a number of proposed mechanisms, including alterations in fatty acid metabolism, accumulation of triglycerides in the liver, and low-grade systemic inflammation. Adipose tissue macrophages produce proinflammatory cytokines, including tumor necrosis factor-α and interleukin-6, which can interfere with insulin signaling. Obesity is also associated with reduced levels of the fat-derived peptide adiponectin, which exhibits both anti-inflammatory and insulin-sensitizing properties. The increase of circulating free fatty acids that is characteristic of obese states can interfere with insulin action in skeletal muscle and liver, and increased intramyocellular lipid is also associated with insulin resistance. Further, increased lipid accumulation in pancreatic islets may lead to impaired insulin secretion. Interestingly, some obese individuals have apparently normal insulin sensitivity and glucose metabolism, sometimes referred to as the obesity paradox. The mechanisms that may protect someone from the diabetogenic effects of excess adiposity are not known, but intact cardiorespiratory fitness may play a role.

CLINICAL MANIFESTATIONS

Typical Type 2 Diabetes

The classic hyperglycemic symptoms of polyuria, polydipsia, and weight loss occur when the renal threshold for glucose reabsorption (~180 mg/dL) is exceeded and glycosuria with osmotic diuresis occurs. Therefore, patients may have plasma glucose concentration that is elevated but below this threshold, for years if not for decades, before specific symptoms appear. In the current era, many patients are found to have diabetes during routine screening or in the course of investigation for another disorder (typically, CVD). The initial presentation for some patients may be severe decompensated hyperglycemia, with profound dehydration, electrolyte imbalance, and plasma glucose levels of 400 mg/dL or higher, with the most striking examples being hyperosmolar hyperglycemic state (HHS) and DKA (see corresponding sections later).

A key feature of type 2 diabetes is that the metabolic defects are not static but tend to worsen over time. A patient early in the course of type 2 diabetes may maintain acceptable glucose control with simple dietary modification and modest weight loss. For many patients, these measures alone fail over time, and combinations of oral medications and often insulin therapy become necessary to control blood glucose levels.

Although the defining clinical feature of type 2 diabetes is hyperglycemia, it is actually the vascular complications of the disorder that cause the greatest morbidity and mortality. For a minority of patients, the initial clinical presentation of diabetes may be the presence of diabetic microvascular complications (retinopathy, neuropathy, nephropathy), which usually indicates many years of unrecognized hyperglycemia. More typical is the insidious onset of symptomatic microvascular complications after many years of diabetes, especially if it is poorly controlled.

Atypical Diabetes

DKA may be the initial clinical presentation for a minority of patients with type 2 diabetes, who subsequently recover β-cell function and do not require insulin treatment. This entity, referred to as ketosis-prone type 2 or Flatbush diabetes (named for the New York City neighborhood where it was first described), appears to be more common among African Americans and some other ethnic minorities. These patients typically lack markers of β-cell autoimmunity and have a strong family history of type 2 diabetes. Once the initial episode of DKA is treated and glucose levels stabilize, patients may have near-normoglycemic remissions lasting many years. The pathogenesis of this form of diabetes is not clear, but a unique β-cell predisposition to glucose desensitization ("glucose toxicity") has been proposed.

Gestational Diabetes

Diabetes that appears for the first time during pregnancy and typically regresses after delivery is termed gestational diabetes (Chapter 239). Women who develop gestational diabetes usually have risk factors including overweight or obesity, older age (>30 years), and a family history of type 2 diabetes. The majority will develop permanent type 2 diabetes during their lifetime. Hormonal changes (increases in placental lactogen, estrogen, progesterone) induce insulin resistance during pregnancy and may uncover latent β-cell defects in predisposed women. Babies born to mothers with diabetes mellitus are at risk for a number of adverse outcomes, especially macrosomia but also preterm birth, neonatal hypoglycemia, and hyperbilirubinemia. Routine screening, with an oral glucose tolerance test, of all pregnant women at 24 to 28 weeks of gestation is currently recommended. Because glucose levels tend to be lower than in the nonpregnant state, separate criteria have been developed for the diagnosis of diabetes in pregnancy. These include the presence of any of the following: fasting glucose concentration of 92 mg/dL or higher; glucose concentration of 180 mg/dL or higher at 1 hour or 153 mg/dL or higher at 2 hours after a 75-g oral glucose load. Aggressive glycemic control has been shown to reduce adverse pregnancy outcomes, including macrosomia and traumatic delivery, although its effects on long-term outcomes in offspring have not been established. Medical nutrition therapy is recommended for all women with gestational diabetes, with emphasis on moderate carbohydrate intake and avoidance of excessive weight gain. If diet modification is inadequate to maintain euglycemia, insulin has historically been considered first-line pharmacologic treatment for gestational diabetes. Oral diabetic medications, including glyburide and metformin, are increasingly being used to treat gestational diabetes, although they are not approved for this indication by the U.S. Food and Drug Administration. After delivery, women with gestational diabetes should continue to be observed for the development of type 2 diabetes.

TREATMENT

Effective treatment of type 2 diabetes is uniquely challenging because it encompasses management of lifestyle factors (including diet, exercise, and weight control), use of multiple oral or injectable medications, self-monitoring of blood glucose concentration, and surveillance and treatment for acute and chronic diabetic complications. The active participation of the patient in this complex program is critical for successful diabetes management, and many patients benefit from participation in a program of diabetes self-management education.

Goals of Therapy Including Glucose Targets

The primary goals of diabetes management are to prevent symptomatic hyperglycemia and hypoglycemia and to prevent the vascular complications associated with diabetes (see later section on chronic vascular complications). Intensive glycemic control (near-normoglycemia) has been shown to reduce microvascular and neuropathic complications of diabetes but not CVD or mortality.[A2] The current consensus view is that lowering of the HbA$_{1c}$ level to 7% or below is an appropriate goal for most patients with diabetes. More stringent glycemic control (HbA$_{1c}$ level close to the normal range) may be appropriate for some individuals (e.g., young patients with short duration of disease) if it can be achieved without excessive hypoglycemia. Conversely, less stringent goals may be suitable for patients with established vasculopathy, significant comorbidities, or reduced life expectancy. Generally accepted targets for fasting and postprandial glucose levels are 70 to 130 mg/dL and less than 180 mg/dL, respectively. Glycemic targets during pregnancy are different, in part because plasma glucose levels normally are lower during pregnancy and because of the risk of adverse fetal outcomes with even modest hyperglycemia (Table 229-8).

Diet and Lifestyle Management

Dietary recommendations for patients with type 2 diabetes have varied over the years and in the past included strict avoidance of sugars and the use

TABLE 229-8 RECOMMENDED GLYCEMIC TARGETS FOR ADULTS WITH DIABETES

	FASTING GLUCOSE LEVEL	POSTPRANDIAL GLUCOSE LEVEL	HbA$_{1c}$
Nonpregnant adults	70-130 mg/dL	<180 mg/dL	<7%
Gestational diabetes	≤95 mg/dL	<140 mg/dL (1 hour after meal) or <120 mg/dL (2 hours after meal)	—
Pre–gestational diabetes	60-99 mg/dL	100-129 mg/dL	<6%

Modified from American Diabetes Association. Standards of medical care in diabetes—2014. *Diabetes Care.* 2015;38(Suppl 1):S33-S40.

of specific diet plans (e.g., "exchange systems") that provided prescribed amounts of carbohydrate, fat, and protein. Current approaches for most patients focus on calorie restriction to achieve and to maintain modest (approximately 5 to 10% of body weight) weight loss, moderate carbohydrate intake, and avoidance of concentrated sweets and foods high in saturated fats and cholesterol. An optimal macronutrient distribution for patients with type 2 diabetes has not been established, and individualization of nutrition plans, depending on such factors as renal function, weight status, and the patient's preference, is recommended. Evidence suggests that a low-fat, low-carbohydrate (Atkins-type) diet and a Mediterranean-type diet can each be effective in promoting weight loss and improving glucose control in patients with diabetes. Moderate alcohol consumption is not prohibited, with the proper consideration of calorie intake (7 kcal/g) and hypoglycemia risk if alcohol is consumed without food, particularly in insulin-treated patients. Referral to a registered dietitian for medical nutrition therapy should be considered for patients newly diagnosed with type 2 diabetes and those who are not achieving glycemic or weight targets.

Regular exercise is an important but often overlooked component of diabetes management. Both aerobic exercise and resistance training can improve blood glucose control, even in the absence of significant weight change. Current recommendations are for a minimum of 150 minutes per week of moderate-intensity physical activity, such as brisk walking, biking, or swimming, and muscle-strengthening exercises two or three times per week. Assessment of cardiovascular status before beginning of an exercise program should be considered for selected patients, but routine screening (e.g., with an exercise stress test) of asymptomatic patients is not recommended. The presence of some diabetic complications may require restriction of certain activities. For example, in patients with proliferative retinopathy, vigorous aerobic or resistance exercise could precipitate retinal hemorrhage or detachment. The presence of significant sensory loss due to peripheral neuropathy can increase the risk of foot injury, including skin ulceration and Charcot joint destruction. Use of proper footwear and careful foot inspection are recommended, and avoidance of weight-bearing exercise may be required for high-risk patients. Finally, exercise-induced hypoglycemia can occur in patients treated with insulin or some secretagogues (i.e., sulfonylureas) and may require adjustment of the medication regimen or added carbohydrate before exercise.

Bariatric Surgery

Weight loss is considered the cornerstone for treatment of patients with type 2 diabetes, the majority of whom are overweight or obese. It has been clearly shown to improve glucose control. As expected, diabetic patients who undergo bariatric (weight reduction) surgery (Chapter 220) also show improvement in glucose control, which in some cases is dramatic. Improvements in glycemia often occur almost immediately after surgery, before significant weight loss has occurred, and appear to be related to changes in gut hormones (including GLP-1 and GIP) or bile acid metabolism. Many patients are able to discontinue diabetes medications, and diabetes remission rates above 50% have been reported. Among obese patients with uncontrolled type 2 diabetes, 3 years of intensive medical therapy plus bariatric surgery was reported to result in glycemic control in significantly more patients than did medical therapy alone; bodyweight, use of glucose-lowering medications, and quality of life also showed more favorable results at 3 years in the surgical groups. [A3]

Pharmacologic Therapy

Although weight control and nutrition form the foundation of effective management, most patients with type 2 diabetes will require use of pharmacologic agents, often multiple, to maintain recommended levels of glycemic control. During the last two decades, several new classes of drugs, targeting different metabolic pathways, have become available for treatment of type 2 diabetes. However, some of the most effective drugs are the oldest, and the long-term safety profile of newer agents remains to be established. Medications can be broadly categorized as those that enhance insulin availability (insulin and insulin secretagogues), those that enhance insulin action, or a miscellaneous group with other targets. Insulin therapy is also covered later and in the section on type 1 diabetes.

Insulin Sensitizers
Metformin

The biguanide drug metformin is the most widely used antidiabetic medication and is considered preferred initial therapy for patients with type 2 diabetes. The pleiotropic effects of metformin are thought to be mediated primarily through inhibition of mitochondrial complex 1 (i.e., effects on mitochondrial oxidative phosphorylation and cellular energy charge) and, in part, through regulation of the activity of 5′-adenosine monophosphate–activated protein kinase and the mammalian target of rapamycin. Metformin lowers glucose levels primarily through suppression of hepatic glucose production, but it also may enhance insulin sensitivity (improved insulin-mediated glucose uptake) and limit intestinal glucose absorption. Modest and sustained weight loss (~2 to 4 kg) is common with metformin.[11] Metformin is used orally twice a day, and extended-release forms are available for once-daily dosing. Hypoglycemia occurs rarely if at all with metformin monotherapy. The most common adverse effect is gastrointestinal intolerance (dyspepsia, diarrhea), which can be minimized by slow upward dose titration. Vitamin B$_{12}$ malabsorption, leading to clinical B$_{12}$ deficiency, has also been reported. The occurrence of lactic acidosis is the most serious although rare adverse effect, which occurs almost exclusively in patients with renal insufficiency and another precipitating factor, such as sepsis or shock. Renal function should be monitored periodically; metformin must be used with caution in those with an estimated glomerular filtration rate (GFR) of 45 mL/minute or lower and should be discontinued for an estimated GFR of 30 mL/minute or lower. Unique among available antidiabetic therapies, metformin was shown to reduce cardiovascular and all-cause mortality in the U.K. Prospective Diabetes Study (UKPDS), which adds to its appeal as a first-line agent. Metformin has also been used for diabetes prevention and for treatment of polycystic ovary syndrome.

Thiazolidinediones

The thiazolidinediones, which include rosiglitazone and pioglitazone, improve insulin-mediated glucose uptake and reduce hepatic glucose production. They bind to a nuclear receptor, peroxisome proliferator-activated receptor γ, and thus regulate the transcription of a variety of genes involved in carbohydrate and lipid metabolism. Thiazolidinedione therapy has pronounced effects on adipose tissue, reducing lipolysis, increasing fat mass, and causing redistribution of fat away from visceral to subcutaneous depots. Increases in circulating adiponectin, an adipokine with insulin-sensitizing and anti-inflammatory properties, may also play a role in the glucose-lowering effect of these drugs. Thiazolidinediones are given orally in once-a-day dosing. Common adverse effects include weight gain and fluid retention, including precipitation or worsening of congestive heart failure. Also reported have been an increase in fractures in postmenopausal women and increased risk of bladder cancer. The potential cardiovascular toxicity of rosiglitazone remains controversial, and its use has been restricted in many countries; these effects have not been observed for pioglitazone.

Insulin Secretagogues
Sulfonylureas

The sulfonylurea class of insulin secretagogues is among the oldest available oral antidiabetes drugs. Sulfonylureas currently in common use include glipizide, glyburide, and glimepiride; older sulfonylureas (chlorpropamide, tolbutamide) are still sometimes used outside of the United States. Their mechanism of action is to bind to the ATP-sensitive potassium channel in the β-cell membrane (at a site termed the sulfonylurea receptor), resulting in membrane depolarization and, ultimately, release of insulin from preformed secretory granules. Therefore, the presence of a sufficient mass of intact β cells is required for efficacy of these drugs. They can be used as monotherapy or in combination with other drugs. The major adverse effect of sulfonylureas is their potential to cause hypoglycemia because insulin secretion occurs regardless of ambient plasma glucose. Modest weight gain is also common. Results of a study conducted in the 1970s (University Group Diabetes Program) suggested that sulfonylurea drugs may increase the risk of cardiovascular events and mortality. These findings were not confirmed in other trials, but the issue remains controversial. Despite this, sulfonylureas are among the most widely used antidiabetic medications.

Glinides

Repaglinide and nateglinide are chemically distinct non-sulfonylurea insulin secretagogues that also bind to the ATP-sensitive potassium channel in the β-cell membrane. Their onset and duration of action are much shorter than those of sulfonylureas, and the frequency of fasting hypoglycemia may be less. They are administered orally before each meal, making them somewhat less convenient than medications with a single daily dose but potentially providing an advantage for patients with inconsistent meal timing or content.

Incretin-Based Therapies/GLP-1 Agonists

Exenatide and liraglutide are analogues of the endogenous incretin hormone GLP-1 and stimulate insulin secretion by binding to GLP-1 receptors on β cells. These drugs augment glucose-stimulated insulin secretion and thus have less potential to cause hypoglycemia than sulfonylureas and glinides do. They also suppress hepatic glucose production (by reduction of glucagon secretion), delay gastric emptying, and suppress appetite, resulting in modest weight loss for many patients. GLP-1 agonists are given by injection once or twice a day, and a weekly long-acting formulation is also available. Major adverse effects include gastrointestinal intolerance (nausea and vomiting), which can be minimized by initiation with a low dose and gradual titration. An increased risk of acute pancreatitis has been reported with GLP-1 agonists (and DPP-4 inhibitors; see later), but the magnitude of the risk is uncertain and requires additional research. An increase in C-cell hyperplasia and medullary thyroid cancer was found in laboratory animals, although the relevance of this to humans is unclear.

Incretin-Based Therapies/DPP-4 Inhibitors

Inhibitors of dipeptidyl peptidase 4 (DPP-4), a ubiquitous serine protease, work by preventing the breakdown of endogenous GLP-1, thus prolonging its effects. DPP-4 inhibitors, including sitagliptin, saxagliptin, and linagliptin, are given orally in a single daily dose. Similar to GLP-1 agonists, they rarely cause hypoglycemia, but they are generally weight neutral and cause fewer gastrointestinal side effects. Concern about potential risk of pancreatitis and medullary thyroid cancer has also been raised but unconfirmed.

Other Pharmacologic Agents
SGLT2 Inhibitors

Canagliflozin and dapagliflozin are inhibitors of the sodium glucose cotransporter 2 (SGLT2) in the proximal renal tubule. This inhibition prevents the reabsorption of filtered glucose and results in glycosuria, which is accompanied by mild osmotic diuresis and modest weight loss. Experience to date with SGLT2 inhibitors is limited, and little is known about long-term efficacy and toxicity. The most common adverse effect is an increase in mycotic genital infections; hyperkalemia, urinary tract infections, and reductions in blood pressure have also been reported.

α-Glucosidase Inhibitors

Acarbose and miglitol are inhibitors of α-glucosidase enzymes in the intestinal lumen that are required for the breakdown and absorption of complex carbohydrates. Use of α-glucosidase inhibitors slows carbohydrate absorption in the small intestine, thus delaying the systemic delivery of glucose in the postprandial period and allowing better coordination with sluggish endogenous insulin secretion. α-Glucosidase inhibitors are given with meals, are weight neutral, and do not cause hypoglycemia when used as monotherapy. The major limiting factor for α-glucosidase inhibitor use is gastrointestinal side effects, predominantly flatulence and bloating due to the action of colonic bacteria on intestinal contents. Extremely slow dose titration may overcome this effect, but many patients cannot or will not tolerate these symptoms.

Pramlintide

Pramlintide is an analogue of the peptide amylin, which is co-secreted from the β cell along with insulin. The primary effects of pramlintide are to suppress hepatic glucose production in the postprandial period and to delay gastric emptying. Pramlintide is given by injection at mealtime and is approved for use in insulin-treated patients. Mild nausea and anorexia are common, which results in modest weight loss in some patients.

Bromocriptine

The dopamine agonist bromocriptine has been in use for many years as a therapy for Parkinson's disease and hyperprolactinemia. It was observed to have a glucose-lowering effect and has been approved as an antidiabetic drug. Its mechanism of action is thought to be through reduction in sympathetic nervous system activation, resulting in lower rates of hepatic glucose production and lipolysis. Its glucose-lowering effect is modest, and adverse effects (nausea, dizziness, weakness) are common.

Colesevelam

The bile acid–binding resin colesevelam was originally approved as a cholesterol-lowering drug and was also discovered to have a glucose-lowering effect. The mechanism of its antidiabetic action is not well understood but may involve enhanced availability of incretin hormones, including GLP-1. Colesevelam treatment requires two- or three-times-daily dosing and is accompanied by gastrointestinal side effects, notably constipation. The drug has a modest low-density lipoprotein (LDL)–lowering effect, but increases in triglycerides are common and may be limiting for some patients.

Insulin Therapy

Insulin treatment can be considered for patients with type 2 diabetes at any point in the course of the disorder, although typically it is used after "failure" of oral or other noninsulin therapies. Insulin may also be preferred therapy in specific situations, such as during hospitalizations (especially in the perioperative period) or in pregnancy. In contrast to patients with type 1 diabetes, patients with type 2 diabetes may be adequately controlled with basal insulin alone or in combination with other antidiabetic medications. Basal insulin is frequently used in combination with oral medications (e.g., metformin, DPP-4 inhibitors) or GLP-1 agonists (exenatide, liraglutide). However, reflecting the heterogeneity of type 2 diabetes, some patients may require physiologic insulin replacement similar to that used in type 1 diabetes, and insulin pump therapy is a safe and valuable option in patients who otherwise require multiple daily injections.[A4] Daily insulin requirements tend to be higher for patients with type 2 compared with type 1 diabetes, reflecting the existence of insulin resistance. Information about available insulin preparations and insulin regimens is provided in the section on insulin therapy under type 1 diabetes earlier and in Table 229-6.

Treatment Algorithms

Use of multidrug regimens is common in type 2 diabetes, and algorithms have been developed to guide therapy; however, the current evidence base to support these recommendations is limited. There is general agreement that metformin should be initial therapy for most patients and that subsequent drugs (when needed) are added to but do not replace metformin. The choice of a specific drug combination is driven by a number of factors, including efficacy, cost, side effect profile (e.g., hypoglycemia, weight gain), and preference of the patient (Fig. 229-5).

Metabolic Monitoring

Ongoing assessment of glycemic control is necessary to ensure optimal outcomes in patients with diabetes. Measurement of HbA$_{1c}$, which reflects mean glucose levels during the preceding 2- to 3-month period, should be performed routinely in all patients with diabetes, beginning at diagnosis and periodically thereafter. Quarterly tests should be done for patients whose therapy has been recently changed or who are not meeting glycemic goals. More stable patients can be tested twice a year. Self-monitoring of blood glucose levels is recommended for all patients using insulin and may be useful for any patient trying to achieve target glucose control. Monitoring for the development of vascular complications is addressed in the later section on chronic vascular complications.

Inpatient Management

Management of blood glucose levels during hospitalization is increasingly recognized as an important clinical issue, especially because 40 to 70% of hospitalized patients carry a concomitant diagnosis of diabetes. Frequently, diabetes is not the reason for admission, and attention to glucose management is secondary to other more critical medical problems. However, both hyperglycemia and hypoglycemia are associated with adverse outcomes in hospitalized patients, which has stimulated the development of algorithms and guidelines for inpatient glucose management, although the evidence base to support them is limited. Obviously, all patients with type 1 diabetes require continued insulin use during hospitalization.

Critically Ill Patients

After initial enthusiasm for intensive glucose control (maintenance of near-normoglycemia) for critically ill patients, more recent evidence suggests that it may be harmful, particularly when it is accompanied by hypoglycemia.[A5] Current guidelines recommend intravenous administration of insulin for critically ill patients in intensive care settings, with a goal of maintaining plasma glucose concentration between 140 and 180 mg/dL.[12] Application of standardized infusion protocols, which include frequent glucose monitoring, is recommended.

Non–Critically Ill Patients

The evidence base to support specific treatment guidelines for non–critically ill hospitalized patients is weak because this has not been systematically studied in randomized trials. However, there is agreement that subcutaneous administration of insulin is the preferred therapy to control glucose for most hospitalized (non–critically ill) patients with diabetes. Generally accepted targets are below 140 mg/dL for fasting glucose concentration and below 180 mg/dL for random or postprandial glucose concentration, if this can be achieved with minimal hypoglycemia risk. The patient's status needs to be reassessed frequently and insulin doses adjusted as needed to maintain target glucose levels. Use of basal insulin (see Table 229-6) is sufficient for many type 2 patients, but some may require the addition of prandial or corrective doses of short-acting insulin. However, prolonged dependence on insulin "sliding scales" to manage hyperglycemia should be avoided as this is rarely successful and carries increased risk of hypoglycemia. For stable patients who are eating consistent meals and those nearing hospital

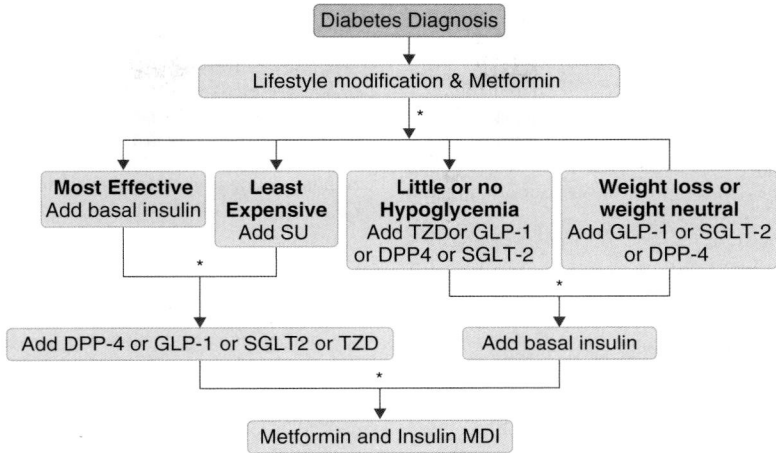

FIGURE 229-5. Algorithm for pharmacologic treatment of type 2 diabetes. DPP-4 = dipeptidyl peptidase 4; DPP-4-i = DPP-4 inhibitor; GLP-1 = glucagon-like peptide 1; GLP-1-RA = GLP-1 receptor agonist; HbA₁c = glycosylated hemoglobin; TZD = thiazolidinedione.

discharge, resumption of their usual oral or noninsulin injectable medications can be considered. Most patients with type 1 diabetes can be managed with their usual insulin injection regimen during hospitalization, but extra attention should be paid to hypoglycemia risk due to missed or delayed meals. Insulin pump therapy can be continued during hospitalization if the patient is able to direct its use and hospital personnel are sufficiently familiar with this form of treatment.

PREVENTION OF TYPE 2 DIABETES

The substantial burden, both human and societal, that accompanies type 2 diabetes and the difficulty in treating it effectively once it has developed make it an appropriate target for prevention. Further, the existence of a defined state of increased risk, pre-diabetes (i.e., impaired glucose tolerance and impaired fasting glucose), allows identification of patients who are most likely to benefit. Interventions that have been studied to date include lifestyle change (i.e., weight loss and exercise) and several antidiabetic medications.

Lifestyle Change

The largest and longest diabetes prevention study to date was the Diabetes Prevention Program, conducted in the United States beginning in the 1990s. Individuals at high risk for type 2 diabetes on the basis of the presence of overweight or obesity and pre-diabetic hyperglycemia (fasting glucose concentration of 95 to 125 mg/dL and 2-hour glucose concentration of 140 to 199 mg/dL) were randomly assigned to an intensive lifestyle program or a medication arm (metformin vs. placebo) and observed for a mean of 3 years. The lifestyle intervention stressed modest weight reduction (minimum 7% of body weight) with a reduced fat, hypocalorie diet and moderate-intensity physical activity for 150 minutes/week. Incident diabetes (determined by oral glucose tolerance test) was reduced by 58% compared with placebo, although the risk reduction was somewhat diminished (34%) with longer-term follow-up of the cohort. Successful weight loss was the major predictor of diabetes prevention, with every kilogram of weight loss reducing diabetes risk by 16%. Similar findings were reported from other studies, including the Finnish Diabetes Prevention Study. Even among individuals who did not lose weight, achieving the physical activity goal was associated with lower diabetes risk.

Medication

Several classes of antidiabetic drugs have been studied for diabetes prevention, including metformin, which reduced the risk of diabetes by 31% in the Diabetes Prevention Program. In smaller studies, the α-glucosidase inhibitor acarbose showed modest reduction in diabetes risk (~25%). The thiazolidinediones (e.g., troglitazone and rosiglitazone) have also shown diabetes prevention effects but are not widely used for this purpose because of concerns about their long-term safety. None of these drugs is approved by the Food and Drug Administration for diabetes prevention.

Recommendations

Lifestyle modification and metformin can both be recommended for individuals at high risk of diabetes. Candidates for prevention include those with defined glucose abnormalities (impaired glucose tolerance, impaired fasting glucose) and those with overweight or obesity plus an additional risk factor, such as family history of diabetes. The curriculum for the lifestyle intervention used in the Diabetes Prevention Program is available online (http://www.bsc.gwu.edu/dpp/lifestyle/dpp_part.html) and has been widely implemented in community settings, including the YMCA. Both lifestyle modification and metformin have shown positive effects on cardiovascular risk factors, but whether interventions to prevent diabetes will result in lower rates of microvascular or macrovascular complications remains to be determined.

Screening for Type 2 Diabetes

Individuals with risk factors for type 2 diabetes should be considered for screening for diabetes and impaired glucose regulation. This is especially important given that hyperglycemia can be present for years without specific symptoms and up to 30% of people with diabetes in the United States are undiagnosed. Screening will also allow identification of people with pre-diabetes, who may benefit from prevention interventions (Table 229-9).

Diabetes screening may be conducted with HbA₁c level, fasting glucose concentration, or oral glucose tolerance test, with the choice of test depending on the clinical setting and the preference of the patient. Screening should also be considered for asymptomatic children with BMI above the 85th percentile for age and sex plus any two of the following risk factors: family history of type 2 diabetes, high-risk race/ethnicity, or evidence of insulin resistance or features associated with insulin resistance (acanthosis nigricans, hypertension, dyslipidemia, polycystic ovary syndrome, or small-for-gestational-age birth weight). Pregnant women with risk factors for diabetes should be screened for undiagnosed diabetes at the first prenatal visit. Otherwise, a 75-g oral glucose tolerance test should be performed at 24 to 28 weeks of gestation to detect gestational diabetes.

PROGNOSIS

Type 2 diabetes is a chronic and, in most cases, progressive condition with potentially serious health consequences. However, it is also uniquely sensitive to modification of nutritional and lifestyle factors, which has been shown to be effective for both prevention and treatment of diabetes. Further, several classes of effective antihyperglycemic medications are available. There is substantial evidence that early intervention with a multifactorial approach to achieve and to maintain metabolic control, plus aggressive control of CVD

TABLE 229-9 CRITERIA FOR DIABETES SCREENING IN ASYMPTOMATIC ADULTS

Testing should be considered for any adult who is overweight (BMI >25 kg/m^2) and has at least one additional risk factor:

- Physical inactivity
- First-degree relative with type 2 diabetes
- High-risk race/ethnicity (e.g., African American, Latino, Native American, Asian American, Pacific Islander)
- Women with history of gestational diabetes or who delivered a baby weighing > 9 lb
- Hypertension
- HDL cholesterol < 35 mg/dL or triglyceride level > 250 mg/dL
- Women with polycystic ovary syndrome
- Clinical conditions associated with insulin resistance (e.g., severe obesity, acanthosis nigricans)

In the absence of the above risk factors, testing should begin at the age of 45 years. If results are normal, screening should be repeated at least at 3-year intervals.

BMI = body mass index; HDL = high-density lipoprotein.
Modified from American Diabetes Association. Standards of medical care in diabetes—2014. *Diabetes Care.* 2015;38(Suppl 1):S8-S16.

TABLE 229-10 CLASSIFICATION OF IATROGENIC HYPOGLYCEMIA IN TREATED DIABETIC PATIENTS

	CLINICAL FEATURES
Severe hypoglycemia	Episode with neurocognitive impairment that requires another person to administer treatment
Documented symptomatic hypoglycemia	Measured glucose concentration ≤70 mg/dL that coincides with sympathoadrenal or neurologic symptoms. Episode is self-managed.
Asymptomatic hypoglycemia	Measured glucose concentration ≤70 mg/dL, but without concomitant symptoms. Absence of symptoms may be due to hypoglycemia unawareness or hypoglycemia-associated autonomic failure.
Pseudo-hypoglycemia	Typical hypoglycemia symptoms, but with measured glucose concentration >70 mg/dL. Symptoms may be caused by resetting of counter-regulatory system in the setting of chronic poor glucose control.

risk factors, will substantially reduce the burden of diabetes complications and improve quality of life.[A7]

ACUTE METABOLIC COMPLICATIONS OF DIABETES

Hypoglycemia

Iatrogenic hypoglycemia in people with diabetes is the most frequent cause of low blood glucose concentration. Hypoglycemia (Chapter 230) affects the daily lives of persons with diabetes and can have a dramatic effect on quality of life. It can induce great fear, preclude comfortable engagement in routine activities (e.g., driving, uninterrupted sleep), and lead both patient and clinician to set higher glycemic targets and hence worse metabolic control. Thus, hypoglycemia continues to be a major limiting factor in the treatment of diabetes with most medications, particularly the use of insulin.[13]

Whereas insulin-stimulatory drugs (e.g., sulfonylureas) and parenteral insulin are the primary causes of drug-induced iatrogenic hypoglycemia, underlying defects in some parts of the counter-regulatory cascade contribute to the greater frequency and potential morbidity and mortality of hypoglycemia among patients with diabetes. The normal counter-regulatory response to hypoglycemia and the typical adrenergic and neuroglycopenic hypoglycemia symptoms are described in Chapter 230.

The threshold plasma glucose value that results in hypoglycemic symptoms is not constant; it is lower after recent antecedent hypoglycemia and higher in patients with poor glycemic control. However, there is general consensus that a self-monitored glucose level of 70 mg/dL or lower is a value that should alert the patient or caregiver, regardless of the presence of symptoms. A more detailed classification system to describe hypoglycemia has been established and widely adopted in research settings (Table 229-10).

However, these distinctions are not commonly used in clinical practice, and the severity of symptoms is often confused with severity of the actual prevailing physiologic state. Thus, a patient may feel intense symptoms at a glucose level of 50 to 60 mg/dL, for which there is no evidence of cognitive impairment or imminent danger, whereas potentially dangerous plasma glucose levels in the range of 20 to 40 mg/dL might go unappreciated owing to lack of classical symptoms. This also has implications for the epidemiology of hypoglycemia; most studies have reliably ascertained only the rates of severe hypoglycemia because other episodes are less likely to be documented. In type 1 diabetes, the DCCT reported 62 severe hypoglycemic episodes per 100 patient-years, although the actual risk may be higher in clinical settings. An episode of severe hypoglycemia can be the immediate cause of death in patients with type 1 diabetes, with recently reported mortality rates ranging from 4 to 10%. There remains uncertainty about the temporal relationship between hypoglycemia and death, and although prolonged episodes of very low circulating glucose (<15 mg/dL) can cause brain death, episodes of fatal hypoglycemia may be due to other mechanisms, such as ventricular arrhythmias. Episodes of severe hypoglycemia are much less common in patients with type 2 diabetes (see later).

In patients with treated diabetes, the initiation of the hypoglycemic event is due to mismatching of prevailing insulin levels to the underlying physiologic state of the individual. Thus, even absent overt insulin overdosage, factors such as missed meals, exercise, recent weight loss, alcohol, or insulin-sensitizing drugs create this mismatch and may set the plasma glucose concentration on a downward trajectory. In addition, the counter-regulatory systems that normally would counteract the decline of glucose to dangerous levels may be impaired. In patients with type 1 diabetes, glucagon release during hypoglycemia may become impaired shortly after the onset of diabetes, although glucagon is still secreted in response to other secretagogues, suggesting the presence of a functional defect. Epinephrine release during hypoglycemia also becomes progressively defective in type 1 diabetes; it is not triggered until the plasma glucose level is lower, and the maximal concentration of epinephrine released is significantly reduced. This decrease in epinephrine response during hypoglycemia is accompanied by an attenuated autonomic neural response, which results in the clinical syndrome of *impaired awareness of hypoglycemia*. Without autonomic symptoms, mild hypoglycemia may proceed unnoticed to more advanced and dangerous phases. Patients who have both impaired awareness of hypoglycemia and defective counter-regulation are at the greatest risk for development of severe hypoglycemia.

Hypoglycemia-associated autonomic failure in type 1 diabetes apparently results from antecedent episodes of mild hypoglycemia that further degrade the counter-regulatory response. In experiments in people without diabetes, recurrent or recent episodes of hypoglycemia are associated with reduced autonomic (epinephrine and norepinephrine), symptomatic, and cognitive functional responses to subsequent episodes of hypoglycemia, impairing the endogenous defense mechanisms and the clinical signs required for hypoglycemia detection. Because patients with type 1 diabetes already have a reduced counter-regulatory response, hypoglycemia-associated autonomic failure may play a role in the vicious circle of hypoglycemia begetting hypoglycemia. Meticulous avoidance of hypoglycemia is the only current approach proven to improve the epinephrine response and to reverse impaired awareness of hypoglycemia.

Compared with type 1 diabetes, type 2 diabetes is associated with a much lower risk of hypoglycemia. However, hypoglycemia remains a major clinical problem in this population. Episodes of severe hypoglycemia become progressively more common in patients with longer duration of type 2 diabetes, due in part to progressive β-cell failure and increased dependence on pharmacologic treatments. Use of sulfonylureas accounts for a substantial proportion of cases of drug-induced hypoglycemia, and severe episodes characterized by coma have been reported with all the agents in common use. The hypoglycemic potential of an agent is related to its potency, its plasma and biologic half-lives, its metabolism, and the concomitant use of other drugs. For example, liver disease prolongs the hypoglycemic actions of glyburide and glipizide because these drugs are partially metabolized in the liver. Similarly, renal disease may prolong the action of insulin (due to impaired insulin clearance) or potentiate the effects of hypoglycemic drugs by other mechanisms. Other antidiabetic agents, such as metformin, thiazolidinediones, and incretin-based drugs, have been associated with measureable albeit lower risks of hypoglycemia; however, symptomatic hypoglycemia is rare unless these drugs are used in combination with insulin. The elderly are at particularly high risk for iatrogenic hypoglycemia because the intensity of adrenergic symptoms may be reduced and hypoglycemia-induced cognitive impairment greater.

CLINICAL APPROACH TO HYPOGLYCEMIA PREVENTION AND TREATMENT

Rx

Patients with diabetes need to be well informed about the symptoms of hypoglycemia and the factors that predispose to its occurrence: meal timing and content, exercise, and the expected time course of the drugs in use (especially insulin). Patients should also be made aware that the accuracy of some home glucose meters may be reduced in the hypoglycemia range and that the typical sympathoadrenal symptoms may wane during years of diabetes. A history of recurrent hypoglycemia should be carefully evaluated and attempts made to determine whether the patient had experienced events that went unrecognized. For example, reports of unexplained night sweats or a clouded mental state on arising in the morning may be due to nocturnal hypoglycemia and should be investigated. Patients should be encouraged to document episodes of hypoglycemia and to contact the care team if they have unexpected or more frequent episodes.

Table 229-11 lists several risk factors for severe hypoglycemia. Patients with these characteristics require greater vigilance, both in selection of treatment regimen and in the recognition and treatment of acute episodes.

Most mild or moderate episodes of hypoglycemia can be self-treated by ingestion of fast-acting carbohydrates such as glucose tablets, glucose gels, or food (juices, soft drinks, or a meal). The suggested amount of carbohydrate to be ingested is about 15 g, which will increase the plasma glucose concentration by about 15 mg/dL. Importantly, foods that are rich in fat delay glucose absorption and are thus less effective. If plasma glucose levels are still below 70 mg/dL and if symptoms have not abated after 15 minutes, the patient should take an additional 15 g of carbohydrate. Because the glycemic response to oral glucose is relatively transient, ingestion of a snack or a meal shortly after correction of hypoglycemia is recommended.

Parenteral treatment of hypoglycemia is recommended if the patient is unwilling or unable to ingest carbohydrates (e.g., due to impaired mental status) or if a patient has sulfonylurea- induced hypoglycemia (which may be prolonged). Intravenous administration of glucose (25 g) is the preferred treatment of hypoglycemia. Parenteral glucagon (1 mg subcutaneously) is an alternative, especially in patients with type 1 diabetes who may have to be treated by family members for severe hypoglycemia. Because glucagon stimulates secretion of insulin in addition to promoting glucose production, it is less effective in patients with type 2 diabetes.

Nocturnal hypoglycemia may be a particular problem for patients with type 1 diabetes. It may be asymptomatic and unsuspected because plasma glucose concentration is rarely measured during the night. Risk factors for nocturnal hypoglycemia include increased physical activity in the last 24 hours, certain insulin regimens (e.g., use of NPH or regular insulin), meal content (e.g., the amount of fat), and alcohol consumption. In addition, sleep is associated with a decrease in the autonomic response to hypoglycemia. Currently, the only practical approaches to detection of nocturnal hypoglycemia are regular nocturnal (3 AM) self-monitoring or the use of continuous glucose monitors with alarm features. Some patients with nocturnal hypoglycemia present with sleep disturbances, morning headache, chronic fatigue, or depression. Children in particular may present with seizures or enuresis. Strategies to prevent nocturnal hypoglycemia include eating "long-acting" bedtime snacks (slowly absorbed carbohydrate, such as uncooked cornstarch) and regular monitoring of blood glucose concentration at bedtime. The bedtime glucose level has been reported to be highly predictive of subsequent development of hypoglycemia during sleep.

Hyperglycemic States

DKA and HHS are the most serious acute hyperglycemic complications of diabetes. DKA is typically associated with severe insulin-deficient states (i.e., type 1 diabetes). It may also occur rarely in type 2 diabetes under conditions of extreme stress, such as major infection or trauma or as a presentation of a variant of type 2 diabetes (ketosis-prone or Flatbush diabetes). On the other hand, HHS typically occurs in patients with type 2 diabetes. However, the distinction between the two clinical scenarios is sometimes blurred (e.g., patients with HHS may present with ketosis and acidosis), and these states may be considered as parts of the spectrum of severe metabolic decompensation. Despite aggressive treatment, mortality rates remain high for both conditions, approaching 5% for DKA and 15% for HHS. Mortality is associated with the extremes of age (i.e., the very young and the elderly) and comorbidities but, importantly, with the severity of the precipitating illness or event. Thus, in addition to correction of fluid and electrolyte imbalance and administration of insulin, treatment also includes prompt recognition of and therapy for any precipitating illness or event. A list of precipitating conditions commonly associated with DKA and HHS is shown in Table 229-12.

PATHOBIOLOGY

The pathogenesis of DKA and HHS mirrors the underlying respective forms of diabetes. The three fundamental biochemical features of DKA—hyperglycemia, ketosis, and acidosis—result from the combined effects of deficient circulating insulin and counter-regulatory hormone excess. This hormonal milieu promotes the delivery of substrates from muscle (amino acids, lactate, pyruvate) and adipose tissue (free fatty acids, glycerol) to the liver, where they are converted to glucose or to ketone bodies (β-hydroxybutyrate, acetoacetate, acetone). Glucose and ketones are thus released into the circulation at greater rates than their utilization, resulting in severe hyperglycemia (>250 mg/dL), ketoacidosis (arterial pH <7.30), and an osmotic diuresis that promotes dehydration and electrolyte loss. In HHS, despite comparable elevations of glucagon, the presence of some endogenous insulin modulates the ketosis even though the plasma glucose concentration in HHS typically exceeds 600 mg/dL, whereas in DKA it is usually more than 250 mg/dL.

In both states, fluid depletion plays a major role in causing dramatic elevations in circulating glucose. Indeed, the hyperosmolality accompanying DKA and HHS is best linked to the patient's level of neural and cognitive function, and treatment of both conditions depends on restoration of fluid balance. Finally, other factors have been invoked, including other hormones (such as epinephrine, growth hormone, and cortisol), proinflammatory cytokines (such as tumor necrosis factor-α, interleukin-1β, interleukin-6, and interleukin-8), and lipid peroxidation markers as well as plasminogen activator inhibitor 1 and C-reactive protein. Whether all these factors are simply "stress markers" reflecting the disordered metabolic state or true pathogenetic factors remains uncertain.

TABLE 229-11 RISK FACTORS FOR SEVERE HYPOGLYCEMIA IN PATIENTS WITH DIABETES

Youth (children)
Elderly taking sulfonylurea drugs or insulin
Altered consciousness
Ethanol use
Strenuous exercise in the previous 24 hours
Recent antecedent hypoglycemia
Use of pentamidine, quinine, or nonselective β-blocker drugs
Concomitant illnesses, such as sepsis, or hepatic, renal, or cardiac failure
Type 1 diabetes with history of recurrent severe hypoglycemia
Recent rapid improvement in HbA$_{1c}$ into the normal range

TABLE 229-12 PRECIPITANTS OF DIABETIC KETOACIDOSIS AND HYPEROSMOLAR HYPERGLYCEMIC STATE

MOST COMMON

Inadequate insulin treatment or noncompliance
New-onset diabetes
Infections
Myocardial infarction

OTHER PRECIPITATING FACTORS

Cerebrovascular accident
Acute pulmonary embolism
Acute pancreatitis
Intestinal or mesenteric thrombosis
Alcohol intoxication
Endocrinopathies: Cushing syndrome, thyrotoxicosis, acromegaly
Severe burns, hyperthermia, hypothermia
Drugs: clozapine, olanzapine, cocaine, lithium, sympathomimetics, corticosteroids, thiazide diuretics

DIABETIC KETOACIDOSIS

CLINICAL MANIFESTATIONS

DKA (Chapter 118) may signal the onset of type 1 diabetes, but changes in medical practice in the developed world during the past several decades have enhanced earlier diagnosis of type 1 diabetes, and now the majority of childhood cases are detected and treated before ketoacidosis occurs. Thus, DKA is more frequently seen in those with established diabetes, usually in the setting of coexisting illness or poor adherence. For example, a patient may be unable to maintain adequate hydration during an illness, such as a viral gastroenteritis, and may mistakenly omit insulin because of inability to eat. A key component of a diabetes treatment program is education in "sick-day" rules focused on home-based prevention of DKA (e.g., frequent blood glucose monitoring, serum or urine ketone testing, fluid intake, determination of insulin dosing or delivery problems). Behavioral factors may also be involved; some younger patients may omit insulin deliberately to promote weight loss or to call attention to a dysfunctional home situation. This should be suspected in cases of recurrent episodes of DKA.

The clinical history of DKA typically involves deterioration during several hours to days, with progressive polyuria, polydipsia, and other symptoms of hyperglycemia. Other common clinical features are weakness, lethargy, nausea, and anorexia. Nonlocalizing upper abdominal pain in the setting of DKA can mimic an acute abdomen. Reduced motility of the gastrointestinal tract or, in severe cases, paralytic ileus may further contribute to diagnostic confusion. Nausea and vomiting are symptoms that indicate the need for in-hospital treatment because they preclude oral fluid intake. Physical findings in DKA are mainly secondary to dehydration, hyperosmolality, and acidosis; these include dry skin and mucous membranes, reduced jugular venous pressure, tachycardia, orthostatic hypotension, depressed mental function, and deep, rapid respirations (Kussmaul breathing).

DIAGNOSIS

In DKA, glucose levels may vary from modestly elevated to more than 1000 mg/dL, serum bicarbonate concentration drops below 18 mEq/L, and there is an excess anion gap that is generally proportional to the decrease in serum bicarbonate (Table 229-13). Hyperchloremia may be superimposed if the patient maintains an adequate GFR and is able to exchange keto acids for chloride in the kidney. The degree of depression of arterial pH depends largely on respiratory compensation. In mild cases, the pH may range from 7.20 to 7.30; in severe cases, it can fall below 7.00. On occasion, a degree of superimposed metabolic alkalosis (e.g., caused by vomiting or diuretic use) may obscure the true severity of the ketoacidosis. An anion gap out of proportion to the fall of bicarbonate should suggest this possibility. Other laboratory abnormalities commonly seen in DKA include a reduced measured serum sodium concentration (due to hyperosmolarity and the resulting osmotic shift of intracellular water into the intravascular space), prerenal azotemia, and elevated serum amylase. The last is usually of nonpancreatic origin and can lead to an erroneous diagnosis of pancreatitis. Normal, elevated, or reduced concentrations of potassium, phosphate, and magnesium may exist when DKA is diagnosed; however, large deficits of these electrolytes invariably accompany the osmotic diuresis and become readily apparent during the course of treatment. The serum triglyceride concentration is frequently elevated, a reflection of deranged lipid metabolism in the setting of insulin deficiency. The white blood cell count is typically elevated; the hemoglobin and hematocrit may be elevated, reflecting volume contraction.

Special care should be taken in interpreting serum or urine ketone results. Because quantitative measurements of β-hydroxybutyrate and acetoacetate are not readily available, rapid diagnosis usually requires qualitative assessment of serum ketones by the use of serum dilutions and reagent strips (e.g., Ketostix) or tablets (e.g., Acetest), which depend on a nitroprusside reaction with acetoacetate. However, acetone reacts weakly with nitroprusside, and β-hydroxybutyrate does not react at all; thus, the results of qualitative testing for ketones can be misleadingly low. Furthermore, because of the presence of intracellular acidosis, β-hydroxybutyrate levels are often much higher than acetoacetate levels, which may further conceal the true degree of ketoacidosis. Conversely, after insulin therapy is begun, the nitroprusside reaction may give the "false" impression of sustained ketoacidosis for hours or even days. This results because nonacidic acetone is slowly cleared from the circulation and also because, as acidosis improves, β-hydroxybutyrate is converted to acetoacetate, giving the false impression that ketosis is worsening.

TREATMENT Rx

An overview of the treatment of DKA and HHS is shown in Figure 229-6.

In the early hours of treatment, the primary considerations are to restore intravascular volume, to correct tissue hypoperfusion, and to restore insulin sensitivity. With DKA, large total body deficits of water (5 to 10 L), sodium (5 to 10 mEq/kg), and other electrolytes may exist (Chapter 118). These losses are even more profound in HHS, which typically develops during a longer time. Although water loss usually exceeds the loss of sodium, it is almost always preferable to begin fluid replacement with isotonic normal saline (0.9% NaCl solution) for efficient intravascular volume restoration. Fluid replacement regimens vary, but it is common to administer 1 L of normal saline within the first hour, followed by a continuous infusion with either 0.45% NaCl or 0.9% NaCl, depending on the corrected serum sodium concentration, the patient's hemodynamic status, and the clinical assessment of tissue perfusion. Likewise, the rate of infusion (commonly 250 to 500 mL/hour) should be adjusted according to both biochemical responses and the age and clinical status of the patient (e.g., oliguria or underlying CVD). In children, isotonic solutions are generally preferred because they are less likely than hypotonic solutions to accelerate water shifts into the intracellular space and contribute to cerebral edema. As the blood glucose concentration falls below 250 mg/dL, dextrose should be added to intravenous fluids to avoid later insulin-induced hypoglycemia because continued insulin delivery may be required to correct the persistent acidemia.

Although insulin resistance is present in both DKA and HHS, supraphysiologic doses of insulin are unnecessary and are more likely to provoke hypokalemia, hypophosphatemia, and delayed hypoglycemia. A typical insulin replacement regimen uses an intravenous bolus of 0.15 U/kg of rapid-acting (e.g., regular) insulin, followed by 0.1 U/kg/hour thereafter. Intravenous administration is the most predictable way to deliver insulin to target tissues, particularly in severely hypovolemic patients with reduced peripheral blood flow. If intravenous administration is not possible, intramuscular or subcutaneous routes of administration can be used. It is ideal if blood glucose levels fall at a steady and predictable rate (50 to 75 mg/dL/hour), so it is important to monitor blood glucose levels hourly during insulin therapy to ensure an appropriate rate of decline. Blood glucose levels should not fall too rapidly, especially in young children, in whom accelerated correction of plasma glucose concentrations has been associated with cerebral edema.

After a stable blood glucose level of 150 to 250 mg/dL is achieved, with resolution of the anion gap acidosis, subcutaneous administration of insulin can be started and the intravenous insulin infusion discontinued. With DKA, it is important to overlap the intravenous and subcutaneous routes by at least 1 to 2 hours to avoid the rebound ketoacidosis if insulin levels drop precipitously. After stabilization, and with resumption of oral food intake, long-term

CRITERION	MILD DKA	MODERATE DKA	SEVERE DKA	HHS
Plasma glucose concentration (mg/dL)	≥250	≥250	≥250	≥600
Effective serum osmolality (mOsm/kg)	Variable	Variable	Variable	≥320
Urine or serum ketones (nitroprusside reaction)	Positive	Positive	Positive	Negative to small
Arterial pH	7.25-7.30	7.00-7.24	<7.00	>7.30
Serum bicarbonate (mEq/L)	15-18	10-15	<10	>15
Anion gap (mEq/L)	>10	>12	>12	Variable, usually <12
Typical mental status	Alert	Drowsy	Stupor or coma	Stupor or coma

TABLE 229-13 DIAGNOSTIC CRITERIA FOR DIABETIC KETOACIDOSIS (DKA) AND HYPEROSMOLAR HYPERGLYCEMIC STATE (HHS)

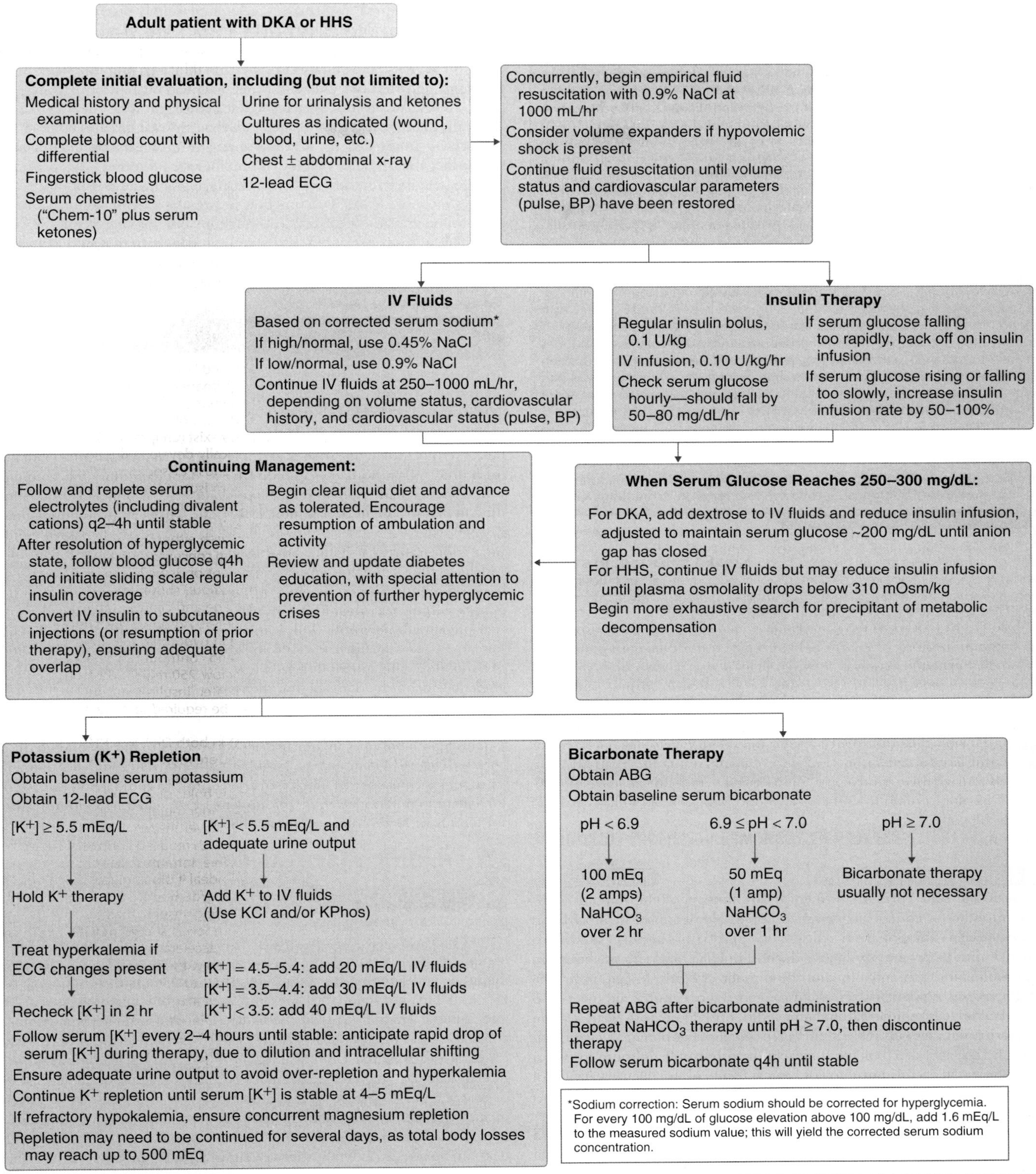

Adult patient with DKA or HHS

Complete initial evaluation, including (but not limited to):

Medical history and physical examination

Complete blood count with differential

Fingerstick blood glucose

Serum chemistries ("Chem-10" plus serum ketones)

Urine for urinalysis and ketones

Cultures as indicated (wound, blood, urine, etc.)

Chest ± abdominal x-ray

12-lead ECG

Concurrently, begin empirical fluid resuscitation with 0.9% NaCl at 1000 mL/hr

Consider volume expanders if hypovolemic shock is present

Continue fluid resuscitation until volume status and cardiovascular parameters (pulse, BP) have been restored

IV Fluids

Based on corrected serum sodium*

If high/normal, use 0.45% NaCl

If low/normal, use 0.9% NaCl

Continue IV fluids at 250–1000 mL/hr, depending on volume status, cardiovascular history, and cardiovascular status (pulse, BP)

Insulin Therapy

Regular insulin bolus, 0.1 U/kg

IV infusion, 0.10 U/kg/hr

Check serum glucose hourly—should fall by 50–80 mg/dL/hr

If serum glucose falling too rapidly, back off on insulin infusion

If serum glucose rising or falling too slowly, increase insulin infusion rate by 50–100%

Continuing Management:

Follow and replete serum electrolytes (including divalent cations) q2–4h until stable

After resolution of hyperglycemic state, follow blood glucose q4h and initiate sliding scale regular insulin coverage

Convert IV insulin to subcutaneous injections (or resumption of prior therapy), ensuring adequate overlap

Begin clear liquid diet and advance as tolerated. Encourage resumption of ambulation and activity

Review and update diabetes education, with special attention to prevention of further hyperglycemic crises

When Serum Glucose Reaches 250–300 mg/dL:

For DKA, add dextrose to IV fluids and reduce insulin infusion, adjusted to maintain serum glucose ~200 mg/dL until anion gap has closed

For HHS, continue IV fluids but may reduce insulin infusion until plasma osmolality drops below 310 mOsm/kg

Begin more exhaustive search for precipitant of metabolic decompensation

Potassium (K⁺) Repletion

Obtain baseline serum potassium

Obtain 12-lead ECG

[K⁺] ≥ 5.5 mEq/L

Hold K⁺ therapy

Treat hyperkalemia if ECG changes present

Recheck [K⁺] in 2 hr

[K⁺] < 5.5 mEq/L and adequate urine output

Add K⁺ to IV fluids (Use KCl and/or KPhos)

[K⁺] = 4.5–5.4: add 20 mEq/L IV fluids

[K⁺] = 3.5–4.4: add 30 mEq/L IV fluids

[K⁺] < 3.5: add 40 mEq/L IV fluids

Follow serum [K⁺] every 2–4 hours until stable: anticipate rapid drop of serum [K⁺] during therapy, due to dilution and intracellular shifting

Ensure adequate urine output to avoid over-repletion and hyperkalemia

Continue K⁺ repletion until serum [K⁺] is stable at 4–5 mEq/L

If refractory hypokalemia, ensure concurrent magnesium repletion

Repletion may need to be continued for several days, as total body losses may reach up to 500 mEq

Bicarbonate Therapy

Obtain ABG

Obtain baseline serum bicarbonate

pH < 6.9

100 mEq (2 amps) NaHCO₃ over 2 hr

6.9 ≤ pH < 7.0

50 mEq (1 amp) NaHCO₃ over 1 hr

pH ≥ 7.0

Bicarbonate therapy usually not necessary

Repeat ABG after bicarbonate administration

Repeat NaHCO₃ therapy until pH ≥ 7.0, then discontinue therapy

Follow serum bicarbonate q4h until stable

*Sodium correction: Serum sodium should be corrected for hyperglycemia. For every 100 mg/dL of glucose elevation above 100 mg/dL, add 1.6 mEq/L to the measured sodium value; this will yield the corrected serum sodium concentration.

FIGURE 229-6. Management of diabetic ketoacidosis (DKA) and hyperosmolar hyperglycemic syndrome (HHS). ABG = arterial blood gas; BP = blood pressure; ECG = electrocardiogram; IV = intravenous.

medical management should be initiated (or resumed), with both long-acting and short-acting insulins, to approximate the desired outpatient regimen. A temporary "regular insulin sliding scale" should be avoided because such therapy is reactive to hyperglycemia and the swings in glycemia will not allow safe discharge of the patient. The eventual dosage and frequency of insulin depend on multiple factors, including body weight, comorbidity, insulin sensitivity, and effectiveness of prior therapeutic regimens.

Potassium replacement is usually required in DKA. Overt hypokalemia can result in muscle weakness, cramps, and nausea; both hyperkalemia and hypokalemia are associated with cardiac arrhythmias. Even absent severe hypokalemia, patients have a significant total body potassium deficit (about 3 to 7 mEq/kg), and measured serum potassium levels may be normal or high as acidosis and renal failure can mask the potassium deficiency. As insulin is infused, potassium will move into the intracellular space, further lowering serum potassium to levels that may trigger life-threatening arrhythmias. In addition, fluid replacement causes extracellular dilution of potassium, leading to improved renal perfusion and increased urinary potassium excretion. Thus, potassium replacement should be initiated as soon as it is established that the patient is not in renal failure. A low potassium level (<3.5 mEq/L) requires prompt treatment with up to 40 mEq/hour, whereas "normal" serum levels (3.5 to 5.0 mEq/L) call for less aggressive repletion of potassium (10 to 30 mEq/hour), assuming adequate urine output. In patients who may have lost potassium for additional reasons, such as diuretic use or gastrointestinal loss, there will be need for greater potassium supplementation.

In the majority of patients with mild to moderate DKA, keto acids clear spontaneously with standard therapeutic measures, and correction of the pH with alkali (as bicarbonate) is unnecessary. Suppression of lipolysis by insulin reduces free fatty acid flux to the liver and blocks ketogenesis, and circulating keto acids are then cleared or oxidized, with subsequent regeneration of bicarbonate and restoration of arterial pH. However, in cases of severe acidosis (pH <6.9 to 7.0), bicarbonate administration may be indicated if the clinical picture dictates (e.g., hypotension that is unresponsive to fluids, cardiac dysfunction, respiratory exhaustion). Bicarbonate therapy should be used with caution and only at the minimal doses required to stabilize the patient because it can further provoke hypokalemia. In addition, by causing a sudden left shift of the dissociation curve for oxyhemoglobin, bicarbonate may impair oxygen delivery to the tissues. Therefore, if alkali therapy is given, small amounts should be administered slowly: 50 mEq of $NaHCO_3$ during 1 hour for arterial pH 6.9 to 7.0, and 100 mEq during 2 hours for pH below 6.9. After bicarbonate administration, arterial pH (and serum potassium levels) should be rechecked every 2 hours, and alkaline therapy should be discontinued when the pH rises above 7.0.

In the setting of DKA, phosphate losses average 3 to 7 mmol/kg; magnesium losses reach 1 to 2 mEq/kg. Phosphate is shifted extracellularly during hyperosmolar states, so initial serum levels may be falsely elevated and may drop rapidly during therapy. Complications of hypophosphatemia generally occur at serum levels below 1.0 mg/dL and include respiratory and skeletal muscle weakness, impaired cardiac systolic performance, and hemolytic anemia. Phosphate repletion should be used in patients with serum phosphate levels below 1.0 mg/dL and in patients with evidence of cardiac or respiratory compromise, hypoxia, or hemolytic anemia. An effective means of replacing phosphate is to replace one third to one half of the potassium losses (discussed previously) as potassium phosphate. In severe hypophosphatemia, cautious intravenous administration of additional small amounts of potassium phosphate may be necessary. Because of calcium binding, hypocalcemic tetany may complicate phosphate therapy unless magnesium supplements are also provided; for this reason, serum calcium, phosphate, and magnesium levels should be monitored during any phosphate infusion.

HYPEROSMOLAR HYPERGLYCEMIC SYNDROME

CLINICAL MANIFESTATIONS

The metabolic state formerly known as the hyperglycemic hyperosmolar nonketotic state or coma has been renamed the *hyperosmolar hyperglycemic syndrome* (HHS) to highlight two important points: (1) ketosis (and acidosis) may in fact be present to varying degrees in HHS, and (2) alterations in sensorium most commonly occur in the absence of coma. In fact, only 10% of HHS patients present with frank coma, and an equal percentage show no signs whatsoever of mental status change. Major risk factors for HHS include older age (most cases occur in patients aged 65 years and older) and impaired cognition (i.e., impaired ability to recognize thirst or to obtain access to water).

As shown in Table 229-13, the hallmarks of the HHS are severe hyperosmolarity (>320 mOsm/L) and hyperglycemia (>600 mg/dL). Severe hyperglycemia occurs because patients cannot consume enough liquid to keep pace with a vigorous osmotic diuresis. The resulting impairment in renal function eventually further reduces glucose excretion through the kidney, leading to remarkable blood glucose elevations, sometimes exceeding 1000 mg/dL. In contrast to DKA, even though glucose concentrations are generally higher, severe acidosis and ketosis are usually absent in the HHS. This is probably explained by the presence of some residual insulin secretory capacity that is sufficient to suppress lipolysis and to avoid significant keto acid production. However, some type 2 patients with depressed endogenous insulin secretion may be unable to suppress ketone production fully in the face of elevated counter-regulatory hormones produced by physical illness. However, because HHS patients have higher portal vein insulin concentrations than do patients with DKA, keto acid production by the liver is quantitatively less, yielding only mild acidosis. In the HHS, in the absence of

concurrent acid-base disturbances, arterial pH rarely drops below 7.30, and serum bicarbonate levels typically do not fall below 18 mEq/L.

In the HHS, clinical severity and levels of consciousness generally correlate with the severity and duration of hyperosmolarity. Clinical signs indicate profound dehydration; gastrointestinal symptoms are seen less frequently than in DKA. A variety of often reversible neurologic abnormalities may exist, including grand mal or focal seizures, extensor plantar reflexes, aphasia, hemisensory or motor deficits, and worsening of a preexisting organic mental syndrome. The laboratory picture is dominated by the effects of uncontrolled diabetes and dehydration; renal function is impaired, hemoglobin and hematocrit are elevated, and liver function test results may be abnormal because of baseline hepatic steatosis. Although severe hyperglycemia would be expected to lower measured serum sodium concentration, it is not uncommon to see normal or even elevated sodium levels because of the severity of dehydration. The serum osmolarity can be measured directly or estimated.

TREATMENT   Rx

The approach to treatment of HHS is similar to that of DKA and requires aggressive management of fluids and electrolytes (see Fig. 229-6). Importantly, patients with HHS tend to have more dramatic volume contraction, and by definition, acidosis is not present or is minimal in degree. It is important to volume resuscitate the patient adequately before insulin is administered because intracellular fluid shifts that occur as glucose levels are reduced may worsen systemic tissue perfusion. In fact, glucose levels usually drop substantially with hydration alone, in part because of improved renal perfusion, thus promoting glycosuria. Coadministration of dextrose along with insulin, as is recommended in patients with DKA to allow ketones to clear and the acidosis to resolve, is rarely required. Further, because recurrent acidosis is less of a concern, patients may be transitioned directly from insulin infusion to subcutaneous injections. Because altered mental status (and, in some cases, coma) is a frequent feature of HHS, attention should be paid to respiratory status and appropriate airway protection. A diligent search for underlying precipitating illness should be made, keeping in mind that the typical HHS patient is elderly and may well have overt or subclinical CVD. The presence of impaired cardiac function, also more common among the elderly, needs to be considered in the management of intravenous fluid resuscitation.

After resolution of the HHS episode, some patients may ultimately be able to be managed with oral agents alone. However, the development of HHS signifies a significant degree of insulin deficiency. As a consequence, it is always best to prescribe insulin injections before the patient is discharged and to reserve judgment about the appropriateness of using oral agents until the patient's progress can be monitored and reassessed in the outpatient setting.

CHRONIC VASCULAR COMPLICATIONS

EPIDEMIOLOGY

The major clinical burden associated with long-standing diabetes is the development of vascular disease, which includes characteristic microvascular complications (retinopathy, nephropathy, neuropathy) and accelerated medium- and large-vessel atherosclerosis. Diabetes is the leading cause of kidney failure, nontraumatic lower limb amputations, and new cases of blindness among adults in the United States. Diabetes is also a major cause of coronary heart disease, heart failure, and stroke and is the seventh leading cause of death in the United States. The microvascular complications are directly linked to hyperglycemia, with both the duration of diabetes and the degree of glucose elevation constituting the major risk factors. Other factors, including genetic susceptibility, smoking, and concomitant conditions like hypertension, also contribute to the risk of complications (Fig. 229-7). Diabetic microvascular complications occur in both type 1 and type 2 diabetes; given that most patients with type 1 diabetes develop it when younger, they may face greater lifetime risk of complications.

The central role for hyperglycemia in the development of diabetic complications was long suspected and ultimately confirmed by the landmark DCCT, which was reported in 1993.[14] In this study, 1441 adolescents and younger adults with type 1 diabetes were randomly assigned to conventional treatment designed to avoid symptomatic hypoglycemia or hyperglycemia (standard therapy at the time) or to an experimental treatment group designed to achieve near-normoglycemia. The experimental group received intensive management with multiple daily insulin injections or use of a continuous subcutaneous insulin pump; frequent self-monitored blood glucose determinations; and adoption of detailed algorithms to guide the patient in determining insulin dosing in response to meals, glucose, and exercise. During the course of the study, mean HbA_{1c} levels were 7.2% in the intensive group compared with 9% for the conventional treatment group. The unequivocal DCCT results showed substantially lower rates of retinopathy, nephropathy, and neuropathy in the intensively treated group and led to major changes in the approach to diabetes treatment in the United States and worldwide. Results of the UKPDS, conducted in a cohort of recently diagnosed patients with type 2 diabetes, later confirmed the benefits of more intensive glucose control in the prevention of microvascular complications. These and other studies have provided convincing evidence that hyperglycemia is the driving force behind diabetic microvascular disease. Indeed, the long-term follow-up studies of the DCCT cohort showed that the benefits seen in the intensively treated group persisted for at least a decade after the study ended, even after HbA_{1c} levels between the two treatment groups converged, suggesting that the mechanisms underlying microvascular complications are conditioned by the prevailing metabolic milieu.

PATHOBIOLOGY

The cellular and molecular mechanisms that mediate hyperglycemic tissue damage are complex and still being elucidated. We now know that multiple interrelated pathways are involved, including four that have received the most attention as key mediators of vasculopathy (Fig. 229-8).

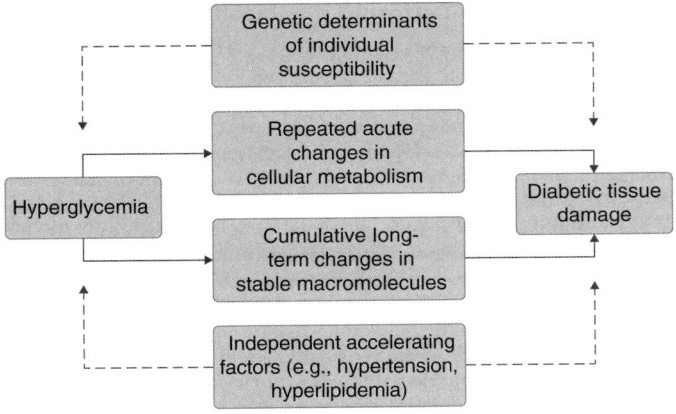

FIGURE 229-7. Factors related to the pathogenesis of diabetes complications. (From Brownlee M. The pathobiology of diabetic complications: a unifying mechanism. *Diabetes*. 2005;54:1615-1625.)

Advanced Glycation End Products

Advanced glycation end products (AGEs) are a heterogeneous group of compounds that form by the nonenzymatic interaction of glucose with amino groups on proteins. This process occurs continuously in vivo but is markedly accelerated in the presence of hyperglycemia. Indeed, the HbA_{1c} test to monitor the chronic level of glycemia was the result of observations of the glycosylation of subfractions of adult hemoglobin. Levels of AGEs in serum and tissues (e.g., skin collagen) correlate with diabetic vascular complications and mean glucose levels over time. AGEs can alter the properties and function of long-lived proteins, such as collagen and elastin, leading to vascular stiffness and increases in basement membrane thickness. AGE binding to specific cell surface receptors (e.g., receptors for AGE, RAGE), particularly on macrophages and endothelial cells, stimulates activation of signaling cascades that promote inflammation and oxidative stress. For example, AGE-RAGE interaction activates the transcription factor NF-κB, leading to multiple pathologic changes in gene expression. Further, AGEs formed intracellularly alter the function of many important cellular proteins. Studies in animal models provide strong evidence that AGE formation is a key process mediating hyperglycemic damage. However, to date, studies of anti-AGE compounds (e.g., aminoguanidine) have failed to demonstrate efficacy in preventing or ameliorating diabetic complications in humans.

Increased Polyol Pathway Flux

Metabolism of glucose through the aldose reductase pathway is generally minor because this enzyme has a low affinity for glucose. However, in the setting of intracellular hyperglycemia (most likely to occur in tissues that cannot downregulate glucose uptake, such as neurons and endothelial cells), there is increased flux through this pathway, leading to an accumulation of osmotically active sorbitol within the cell. Increased cellular osmolarity occurs, along with an increase in redox stress due to depletion of the reduced form of nicotinamide adenine dinucleotide phosphate and reduced glutathione. Inhibitors of aldose reductase have been proposed as a therapeutic strategy to reduce diabetic complications. Current evidence from clinical trials does not support their use, but this remains an active area of research.

Activation of Protein Kinase C

Intracellular hyperglycemia leads to increased de novo synthesis of diacylglycerol, which is a major activator of the protein kinase C family of enzymes. Activation of protein kinase C initiates a complex network of intracellular signaling that alters gene expression and results in enhanced angiogenesis, vasoconstriction, vascular permeability (by increases in vascular endothelial growth factor), cytokine activation, and extracellular matrix expansion. These alterations in cellular function have been linked to the development of

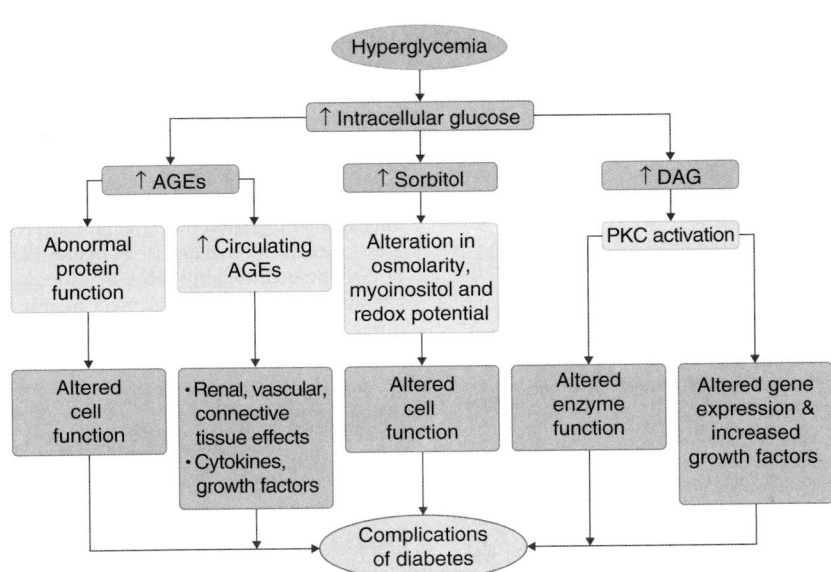

FIGURE 229-8. Proposed mechanisms of hyperglycemia-induced vascular complications. See text for discussion. AGEs = advanced glycation end products; DAG = diacylglycerol; PKC = protein kinase C.

microvascular complications (especially retinopathy) and atherosclerosis. Inhibitors of specific protein kinase C isoforms are being studied in clinical trials as agents specific for diabetic retinopathy and macular edema.

Increased Hexosamine Pathway Flux

In the setting of hyperglycemia and excess fatty acid oxidation, there is also increased flux of glucose through the hexosamine pathway, leading to increases in glucosamine 6-phosphate and ultimately post-translational modification of certain cytoplasmic and nuclear proteins. Associated with this are increases in expression of key genes, including those for transforming growth factor (α and β_1) and plasminogen activator inhibitor 1, and inhibition of endothelial nitric oxide synthase activity. Whereas the pathway has been linked to defective insulin action, its role in specific complications remains unclear.

These multiple and complex pathways are not mutually exclusive but are interconnected and may have a common antecedent process, which is overproduction of superoxide by the mitochondrial electron transport chain. Superoxide generates the production of other reactive oxygen species that can lead to cellular damage in a variety of ways. Data from animal models support the possibility that correction of diabetes-induced superoxide overproduction will have positive downstream effects on the various pathways leading to hyperglycemic tissue damage, but this remains to be confirmed in human studies.

Microvascular Complications

DIABETIC RETINOPATHY

Diabetic retinopathy (Chapter 423) is a highly prevalent, pathognomonic, microvascular complication, eventually affecting more than 50% of patients with long-term diabetes, although it causes vision impairment less frequently. The occurrence of vision loss due to diabetic retinopathy has declined during the past few decades as glucose and blood pressure control have improved in the population with diabetes. Nonetheless, it remains an important cause of preventable blindness, especially among patients with poor metabolic control. Both vascular and neural tissues in the retina are affected by chronic hyperglycemia. Early changes include the loss of retinal supporting cells (pericytes), basement membrane thickening, and retinal blood flow changes. Damaged retinal capillaries leak protein, red blood cells, and lipids, leading to retinal edema. Chronic retinal hypoxia (due to capillary occlusion) promotes neovascularization; these new vessels are abnormal and prone to rupture. Retinal hemorrhage, inflammation, and scarring can ultimately lead to traction retinal detachment and permanent vision loss (Table 229-14).

Diabetic retinopathy can be detected by dilated funduscopy, with early signs being the presence of microaneurysms, exudates, and intraretinal hemorrhages. Additional tests, including fluorescein angiography and ocular coherence tomography, are helpful to detect abnormal vessel permeability and macular edema, which can threaten vision. Regular screening by an eye care specialist (an ophthalmologist or optometrist) is recommended for all patients with diabetes because significant and potentially vision-threatening retinopathy can be present in the absence of any symptoms. Screening should begin at diabetes diagnosis for patients with type 2 diabetes because hyperglycemia has typically been present for years before it is recognized clinically. For patients with type 1 diabetes, screening can begin at 5 years after diagnosis or after puberty for childhood onset. Because retinopathy can progress rapidly during pregnancy, screening and follow-up should be more aggressive during this time (Table 229-15).

As with other diabetic complications, intensive glycemic control can prevent diabetic retinopathy and delay its progression but has limited effects on advanced retinal disease. Blood pressure control is also important to prevent worsening of retinopathy; there is some evidence that renin-angiotensin system (RAS) blockers may be especially beneficial.

Treatment of diabetic retinopathy (Chapter 423) includes laser photocoagulation, which can ablate abnormal vessels (thus reducing the risk of hemorrhage) and treat macular edema. Laser photocoagulation can be focal (to treat clinically significant macular edema or nonproliferative diabetic retinopathy) or panretinal (to treat severe nonproliferative diabetic retinopathy or proliferative diabetic retinopathy). Vitrectomy is a surgical procedure to remove hemorrhage and scar tissue that is obscuring vision. Nonsurgical therapies include intravitreal injection of glucocorticoids or anti–vascular endothelial growth factor monoclonal antibodies (e.g., ranibizumab) to treat macular edema.[A8] The established efficacy of retinopathy treatment, particularly photocoagulation, in preventing vision loss provides strong justification for routine retinopathy screening. There is evidence that treatment with fenofibrate reduces the progression of retinopathy,[A9] although the medication has not been approved for this indication in the United States. In addition to its well-known effects on lipid metabolism, fenofibrate appears to have significant anti-inflammatory, antiangiogenic, and antioxidant properties that are relevant to retinal disease. The presence of retinopathy is not considered a contraindication to the use of aspirin for CVD prevention.

Other eye conditions also affect patients with diabetes. Transient osmotically induced refractive error is common, especially at the time of diabetes diagnosis, but resolves with glucose control. Age-related eye conditions, such as cataracts and glaucoma, tend to occur at younger ages among diabetic patients. Diplopia and other gaze disorders due to acute mononeuropathy involving the cranial nerves (typically III or VI) are also more common in diabetes.

DIABETIC NEPHROPATHY

Diabetic nephropathy (Chapter 125) remains the most common single cause of end-stage renal failure, accounting for up to 50% of the cases in Western societies. Further, despite advances in the management of glucose and hypertension, the prevalence of chronic kidney disease among patients with diabetes has not declined in the past several decades. Overall, 20 to 30% of type 1 and type 2 diabetic patients develop evidence of nephropathy, although fewer type 2 patients progress to end-stage renal disease (ESRD). This may be because of competing mortality from CVD, with fewer surviving to ESRD. However, because of their much greater frequency in the population, the majority of diabetic patients presenting for treatment of ESRD (dialysis or transplantation) have type 2 diabetes. The major risk factor for the development of diabetic neuropathy is the duration and severity of hyperglycemia, but there is evidence for variation in genetic susceptibility. For example, African Americans and individuals with a family history of diabetic or nondiabetic renal disease are at higher risk for diabetic nephropathy. An insertion/deletion polymorphism in the gene encoding angiotensin-converting enzyme (ACE) has been widely reported to be associated with increased risk of diabetic nephropathy, but variants in genes involved in the polyol pathway, lipid metabolism, inflammatory cytokines, angiogenesis, and oxidative stress have also been identified.

Diabetic nephropathy develops during many years to decades, with a prolonged "silent" period before clinical detection, followed by more rapid progression to overt renal disease (Chapter 125). In the classic view, the hallmark of diabetic nephropathy is the development of proteinuria, which is due to alteration in glomerular basement membrane permeability and increases in intraglomerular pressure. The first clinical evidence of incipient nephropathy is the development of albuminuria, which is quantitatively minor at first

TABLE 229-14	CLASSIFICATION OF DIABETIC RETINOPATHY
	CLINICAL FEATURES
Mild NPDR	At least one microaneurysm
Moderate NPDR	Microaneurysms, intraretinal (blot) hemorrhage, soft exudates, venous beading, intraretinal microvascular abnormalities
Severe NPDR	More extensive intraretinal hemorrhages (>20 in each of four quadrants) *or* venous beading in at least two quadrants *or* prominent intraretinal microvascular abnormalities
PDR	Neovascularization and/or vitreous or pre-retinal hemorrhage; traction retinal detachment
Clinically significant macular edema	Retinal thickening or hard exudates approaching or involving the center of the macula

NPDR = nonproliferative diabetic retinopathy; PDR = proliferative diabetic retinopathy.

TABLE 229-15	RECOMMENDED INTERVALS FOR DIABETIC RETINOPATHY SCREENING	
DIABETES TYPE	**FIRST EXAMINATION**	**FOLLOW-UP**
Type 1	5 years after diagnosis	Annual
Type 2	At time of diagnosis	Annual
Established diabetes during pregnancy	Before or soon after conception	At least every 3 months

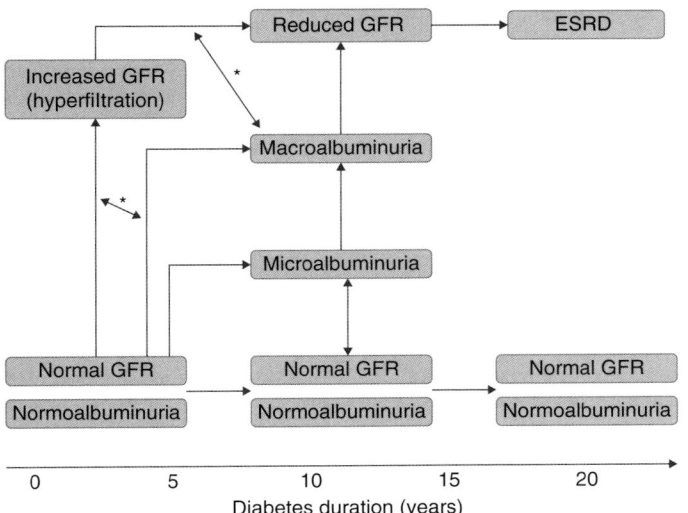

FIGURE 229-9. Development of diabetic nephropathy. See text for discussion. GFR = glomerular filtration rate; ESRD = end-stage renal disease. *GFR and albuminuria may progress independently of each other, i.e., patients may have micro- or macroalbuminuria even though their GFR is normal or even slightly elevated. However, macroalbuminuria is usually associated with reduced GFR, and is a strong risk for progressive ESRD. (From Boger CA, Sedor JR. GWAS of diabetic nephropathy: is the GENIE out of the bottle? *PLoS Genet.* 2012;8:e1002.)

(microalbuminuria, urine albumin-to-creatinine ratio of 30 to 300 mg/g) and then progresses to overt proteinuria, sometimes in the nephrotic range (>2 g/day). During the microalbuminuria phase, GFR is preserved but begins to decline in parallel with increasing proteinuria, leading to ESRD 5 to 15 years after the first detection of abnormal albumin excretion. However, recent evidence suggests that chronic kidney disease in diabetes is more heterogeneous than previously thought, with some patients progressing to advanced stages of chronic kidney disease in the absence of albuminuria (Fig. 229-9). Nonalbuminuric diabetic kidney disease appears more likely to occur in older patients with type 2 diabetes and may reflect, in part, the concurrence of multiple renal risk factors, including hypertension, obesity, and dyslipidemia. Further, microalbuminuria does not inevitably progress, with some patients regressing to normal or maintaining small but stable amounts of albuminuria. However, persistent and increasing albuminuria is a marker of high risk for progression to clinical nephropathy. Pathologic changes that are typical of diabetic nephropathy include an increase in glomerular basement membrane thickness and increased accumulation of extracellular matrix leading to mesangial expansion and the classic Kimmelstiel-Wilson nodular lesion.

Patients with diabetes should be screened annually for renal involvement (Chapter 125) by measurement of albumin on a spot urine sample with a sensitive immunoassay to detect microalbuminuria and by measurement of serum creatinine for calculation of estimated GFR. The finding of moderately increased urine albumin-to-creatinine ratio (30 to 300 mg albumin per gram of creatinine) should be confirmed on two of three repeated tests because transient increases are not uncommon but may not be clinically important. Data from the DCCT and other studies provide strong evidence that aggressive glycemic control can prevent the development of diabetic nephropathy and can retard the progression of microalbuminuria. However, there is little evidence that glycemic control can modulate the course once clinical albuminuria (>300 mg/day) and declining GFR occur. Central to the treatment of patients with albuminuria (micro or clinical) is intensive blood pressure control, preferentially by blockade of the RAS. Both ACE inhibitors and angiotensin receptor blockers have been shown to delay the progression of diabetic nephropathy and are recommended for patients with albuminuria even in the absence of hypertension. Despite initial enthusiasm, combined ACE inhibitor and angiotensin receptor blocker therapy is not recommended because of high rates of hyperkalemia and acute renal injury. In hypertensive patients, other drugs, such as calcium-channel blockers, diuretics, and β-blockers, can be used as additional therapy if needed to achieve adequate blood pressure control. There is little evidence to support use of RAS blockade in diabetic patients who are normotensive and normoalbuminuric, although there may be a therapeutic rationale for use of these agents in patients who cannot achieve adequate glycemic control. Dietary protein restriction has been recommended in the past for patients with nephropathy, but recent trials have been unable to demonstrate an effect of a low-protein diet on the rate of deterioration of GFR.[15]

DIABETIC NEUROPATHY

Diabetic neuropathy (Chapter 420) is a common complication of diabetes, with an estimated lifetime prevalence of about 50%. Diabetic neuropathy can be manifested in a variety of syndromes, including radiculoplexopathy and autonomic neuropathy, but the most common form is a characteristic distal symmetrical polyneuropathy (DSP), resulting from large-fiber nerve damage. Despite its high prevalence, there is no distinct neuropathic symptom or lesion that is specific to diabetes, and separation of diabetic neuropathy from other causes of nerve damage can be problematic. As for other microvascular complications, the etiology of DSP is attributed to hyperglycemic damage, as demonstrated by the dramatic 60% reduction in neuropathy in the intensive treatment group in the DCCT study. However, the possibility that the pathogenesis of DSP may differ in type 2 diabetes, with dyslipidemia and insulin resistance also contributing, has recently emerged. Support for this view comes from largely negative neuropathy results of clinical trials of intensive glucose control in type 2 diabetes (e.g., Action to Control Cardiovascular Risk in Diabetes [ACCORD] trial, VA Cooperative study) and the observation that the prevalence of DSP is already increased in the setting of prediabetes and the metabolic syndrome.

The clinical manifestations of DSP include symptoms of pain, paresthesias, and numbness that typically begin in the feet and progress more proximally in a "stocking and glove" distribution (Chapter 420). For some patients, neuropathic pain can be severe and disabling, resulting in a major reduction in quality of life. Loss of sensation, which may not be noticed by the patient, constitutes an important risk factor for falls due to gait instability. Ulceration, uncontrolled infection, and amputation can also occur from altered foot mechanics and inability to perceive repetitive trauma or other foot injury. DSP can be diagnosed by the presence of classic symptoms and by loss of ability to perceive pressure from a nylon (Semmes-Weinstein) monofilament. Additional tests, such as nerve conduction studies or electromyography, are occasionally indicated to distinguish DSP from radiculopathy. Current treatment options are mostly limited to control of metabolic risk factors (i.e., glucose, lipids) and symptoms, although some agents in clinical trials (e.g., aldose reductase inhibitors) show some promise. The chronic pain of DSP can be difficult to manage. Available therapies include tricyclic antidepressants, serotonin-norepinephrine reuptake inhibitors, anticonvulsants (such as gabapentin and pregabalin), and opioids.

Other forms of diabetic nerve damage (Chapter 420)[16] include small-fiber predominant neuropathy, radiculoplexopathy (diabetic amyotrophy), noncompressive radiculopathy, and mononeuritis multiplex. Autonomic neuropathy can be manifested as gastroparesis, urinary retention, erectile dysfunction, sudomotor dysfunction (typically anhidrosis of the extremities with or without hyperhidrosis of the trunk), cardiac arrhythmias, and disturbance of gut motility (diabetic diarrhea or constipation). Cardiac autonomic neuropathy is an especially ominous form of diabetic autonomic neuropathy. Typical clinical manifestations of cardiac autonomic neuropathy include resting tachycardia, diminished heart rate variability, and orthostatic blood pressure changes. Patients with cardiac autonomic neuropathy are at high risk for myocardial infarction, congestive heart failure, and sudden cardiac death.

DIABETIC FOOT

The combination of sensory impairment due to peripheral neuropathy and reduced tissue perfusion due to large-vessel atherosclerosis (peripheral arterial disease) or microvascular dysfunction can result in ulceration, infection, and ultimately lower extremity amputation. A typical case involves development of an ulceration (often surrounded by callus formation) on the plantar surface of the foot, often underneath the metatarsal heads. Ulceration can be slow to heal because of repetitive trauma from walking and impaired blood flow; hyperglycemia may also impair wound healing by effects on white blood cell migration and function. In the absence of protective sensation, an infection may fester for weeks and eventually invade the bone, leading to osteomyelitis. Altered foot mechanics can also lead to repeated (and usually undetected) fractures that destroy normal foot architecture and result in the classic Charcot foot deformity.

For many patients, foot amputation is the most feared diabetic complication; fortunately, it can be prevented in most cases but requires vigilance on the part of the patient and health care team. Routine foot examination, especially for patients who have evidence of sensory loss, should be performed at every medical visit, and patients should be instructed to inspect their feet daily for cracks, fissures, ulcers, or inflammation. Patients should avoid walking barefoot (even at home) and should wear protective covering (avoid sandals) outside. Thermal injuries can be prevented by avoiding use of heating pads or hot-water bottles on the feet. Referral to a foot care specialist should be considered for patients with sensory loss, foot deformity, extensive callus formation, and nonhealing ulcers. Ulcers are treated with aggressive débridement of necrotic tissue and systemic antibiotics (guided by culture of infected tissue) if infection is present. Pressure "off-loading" by use of special shoes, orthotics, or application of total contact casts may be necessary to allow healing. Additional treatments include use of topical platelet-derived growth factor, bioengineered skin substitutes, hyperbaric oxygen, and negative-pressure wound therapy, although none of these has shown conclusive evidence of effectiveness in promoting wound healing.

OTHER ASSOCIATED CONDITIONS

Although not traditionally recognized as diabetic complications, there are a number of disorders that are increased in frequency or severity in patients with diabetes and that have a plausible or established relationship with hyperglycemia. These include periodontal disease, Alzheimer dementia, and musculoskeletal disorders, such as limited joint mobility, adhesive capsulitis, Dupuytren contracture, and trigger finger (flexor tenosynovitis). Patients with poorly controlled diabetes are widely thought to have increased susceptibility to infection, particularly with fungal pathogens. Defects in immune function (impaired neutrophil chemotaxis) have been described in diabetes, but whether this occurs in reasonably controlled diabetes or contributes to clinical infection is unclear. The incidence of osteoporotic fractures appears to be increased in women with diabetes, despite the presence of normal or even increased bone density. There is also emerging evidence that the frequency of some cancers (e.g., pancreatic, endometrial, colorectal, breast) is increased among people with diabetes.

Cardiovascular Disease in Diabetes

Atherosclerotic CVD is the major cause of morbidity and mortality for patients with diabetes and contributes substantially to its economic costs. The clinical and pathologic features of CVD in diabetes are generally not distinguishable from those occurring in nondiabetic individuals, but they are manifested at an earlier age, are more aggressive, and are associated with mortality rates that are two to four times higher in patients with diabetes (Chapter 52). This increased CVD risk is true for both type 1 and type 2 diabetes, with CVD in type 1 diabetes being strongly associated with concurrent presence of renal disease. Diabetes is also an important risk factor for peripheral vascular disease and stroke, which carries greater mortality risk than in nondiabetic patients.

PATHOBIOLOGY OF CARDIOVASCULAR DISEASE IN DIABETES

The pathogenesis of atherosclerotic CVD in diabetes is complex and multifactorial, with several mechanisms playing key roles. *Metabolic factors*, including hyperglycemia, insulin resistance, dyslipidemia, and increases in circulating free fatty acids, contribute to atherosclerotic plaque formation. Increases in *oxidation and glycoxidation* of lipoproteins increase their atherogenicity and enhance foam cell formation. *Endothelial dysfunction*, an early event in the development of atherosclerosis, has been described in association with several metabolic syndrome components, including hyperglycemia, insulin resistance, hypertension, and dyslipidemia. Systemic *inflammation*, which contributes to accelerated plaque formation, is increased in diabetes and obesity as a consequence of increased cytokine production by adipose tissue. Finally, diabetes is characterized by a *prothrombotic* state due to enhanced platelet reactivity and alterations in coagulation factors, including increased circulating levels of fibrinogen and plasminogen activator inhibitor 1.

DIABETIC CARDIOMYOPATHY AND HEART FAILURE

Diabetic cardiomyopathy is defined as alterations in cardiac structure and function that are not directly attributable to coronary artery disease or hypertension (Chapters 58 and 59). Characteristic features include cardiac hypertrophy, left ventricular dysfunction (diastolic may precede systolic), and altered myocardial metabolism. Diabetes is a recognized risk factor for the development of heart failure, even in the absence of atherosclerotic heart disease. For example, in the Framingham Heart Study, the frequency of heart failure was twice in diabetic men and five times in diabetic women compared with age-matched controls and persisted despite correction for hypertension,

obesity, dyslipidemia, and coronary artery disease. Increased activation of the renin-angiotensin-aldosterone system and formation of AGEs are thought to contribute to myocardial fibrosis and stiffness, and altered substrate utilization (preferential use of free fatty acids) can promote myocyte dysfunction by enhanced production of reactive oxygen species and other mechanisms. Characteristic changes in myocardial function and structure were reported in type 1 diabetes in the DCCT and Epidemiology of Diabetes Interventions and Complications (EDIC) study and were related to long-term glycemic control.

PREVENTION OF CARDIOVASCULAR DISEASE IN DIABETES

Aggressive control of CVD risk factors is recommended for most patients with diabetes, keeping in mind that the presence of diabetes is considered the risk equivalent of a prior myocardial infarction by most risk assessment algorithms (e.g., Framingham risk score, Adult Treatment Panel III Report of the National Cholesterol Education Program). Assessment of blood pressure, lipid profile, and smoking status should be included as part of routine diabetes care. Determination of the optimal targets for risk factor control has been the subject of several large randomized trials, which have informed consensus guidelines.

GLUCOSE CONTROL

Hyperglycemia is a major risk for atherosclerotic CVD. In population-based studies including diabetic and nondiabetic cohorts, HbA_{1c} has been reported as an independent predictor of all-cause and CVD mortality, and among individuals with diabetes, every 1% rise in HbA_{1c} is associated with a 30% increase in all-cause mortality and a 40% increase in CVD mortality. Compelling evidence for the benefit of intensive glucose control in patients with type 1 diabetes was shown in the DCCT/EDIC study, in which CVD events were reduced by 58%. However, in type 2 diabetes, hyperglycemia occurs in the setting of multiple other CVD risk factors, including hypertension, dyslipidemia, and obesity, which also contribute to risk, so the contribution of glucose control is unclear. Several large clinical trials in patients with type 2 diabetes have failed to show that control of hyperglycemia has important effects on CVD outcomes (see later), highlighting the complex pathogenesis of vascular disease in diabetes. Similarly, an intensive lifestyle program designed to achieve weight loss and exercise goals also failed to demonstrate significant effects on CVD outcomes in type 2 diabetes patients.[A11]

The strongest evidence in favor of intensive glucose control comes from the long-term follow-up of the UKPDS, which demonstrated 15% reduction in myocardial infarction and 13% reduction in all-cause mortality in the intensive versus conventional treatment group. More recently, in the ACCORD trial, an intensive treatment arm, designed to maintain HbA_{1c} below 6%, was compared with conventional treatment with HbA_{1c} goal of 7.5% in a cohort of type 2 diabetes patients at high risk for CVD. This trial was stopped early because of unexpected increased mortality, largely CVD related, in the intensive treatment group. The reasons for increased mortality with intensive treatment are not known for certain, but increased frequency and severity of hypoglycemia or the toxicity of specific drugs or combinations has been proposed. Secondary analysis of ACCORD data showed a reduction in nonfatal myocardial infarction in the intensive treatment group, leading to speculation that some patients might still benefit. Other studies designed to address this, including the VA Cooperative Study and ADVANCE, also failed to show CVD benefit for intensive glucose control.[A12] These trials differed somewhat in patient characteristics, HbA_{1c} goal, and specific treatment regimens, and the largely negative results stimulated controversy. However, some consensus views have emerged[17]: (1) in the current era of effective treatment of other CVD risk factors (i.e., with statins, RAS blockers, antiplatelet therapy), the additional benefits of intensive glycemic control are modest at best; (2) patients with long-standing diabetes or established CVD are least likely to benefit from intensive glucose lowering; (3) the benefits of glucose lowering in the prevention of microvascular complications provide an independent rationale for strict glucose control for many patients; and (4) specific glycemic targets should be individualized according to the patient's characteristics (e.g., comorbidities, life expectancy, hypoglycemia risk) and preferences.

HYPERTENSION

Hypertension (Chapter 67) is a common comorbidity in diabetes, affecting the majority of patients with type 2 diabetes, and constitutes an important modifiable CVD risk factor. Further, in even the earliest stages of diabetic nephropathy (i.e., microalbuminuria), hypertension is further accelerated. In type 1 diabetes, hypertension is generally the result of concurrent renal disease, with both contributing to CVD risk. The importance of blood pressure control in reducing CVD events as well as microvascular outcomes in patients with diabetes was established by several major trials, including the UKPDS, Systolic Hypertension in the Elderly Program (SHEP), Hypertension Optimal Treatment (HOT) study, and others. However, analysis of these and other trials failed to show evidence of improved outcomes (i.e., in myocardial infarction or mortality) with systolic blood pressure targets of 130 mm Hg or lower. An even more aggressive target systolic blood pressure of less than 120 mm Hg was shown to be of no additional benefit in reducing CVD events in the ACCORD trial. The current consensus is that blood pressure goals should be less stringent than previously recommended. The Eighth Joint National Committee (JNC8) guidelines recommend a blood pressure goal of less than 140/90 mm Hg for all patients younger than 60 years, regardless of diabetes or renal status, and less than 150/90 mm Hg for patients 60 years and older.[18] Other guidelines, including those from the American Diabetes Association (ADA), suggest a blood pressure target of less than 140/80 mm Hg for patients with diabetes but with the further recommendation that a lower target may be considered for younger patients if it can be achieved without excessive treatment burden. However, many of these recommendations are based on expert opinion rather than on evidence from randomized trials, and some uncertainty remains.

The choice of antihypertensive agent has also received considerable study, which is complicated by the fact that many patients will require treatment with two or more drugs to achieve target blood pressure. ACE inhibitors and angiotensin receptor blockers are generally considered first-line therapy for patients with diabetes, in part on the basis of their demonstrated renoprotective benefits. In addition, results from several randomized trials, including the Heart Outcomes Protection Study (HOPE), Fosinopril versus Amlodipine Cardiovascular Events Trial (FACET), and Appropriate Blood Pressure Control in Diabetes (ABCD), indicated improved cardiovascular outcomes with ACE inhibitors compared with other antihypertensive drugs, although this was not the case for the UKPDS, in which β-blockers were equally effective. Calcium-channel blockers and low-dose diuretics are also recommended as add-on therapy if needed to achieve blood pressure targets. Use of β-blockers should be considered in the setting of established CVD because of their proven benefits in patients with prior myocardial infarction and congestive heart failure. However, β-blockers should be used with caution in patients at high risk for hypoglycemia because they may blunt the autonomic warning symptoms associated with low glucose concentration. Both β-blockers and thiazide diuretics have been reported to increase the risk for development of diabetes, although there is little evidence for significant deterioration of glycemic control in patients with diabetes.

DYSLIPIDEMIA

The characteristic dyslipidemia of type 2 diabetes and insulin-resistant states, which includes low levels of high-density lipoprotein (HDL) cholesterol, elevated triglycerides, and small dense LDL particles, is highly atherogenic (Chapter 206). LDLs also are prone to oxidative modification in the setting of hyperglycemia, which enhances their atherogenicity. There is substantial clinical trial evidence to support lowering of LDL cholesterol levels with statin drugs in the majority of patients with diabetes older than 40 years. These findings come from trials limited to diabetes (Collaborative Atorvastatin Diabetes Study [CARDS]) and to diabetes subset analysis of larger trials (Heart Protection Study), all of which report similar CVD benefits of statin therapy among diabetics and nondiabetics. ADA recommendations are for target LDL levels of less than 100 mg/dL for most adult patients with diabetes and less than 70 mg/dL for diabetic patients with established CVD or multiple risk factors. Recent guidelines from the American Heart Association (AHA) and American College of Cardiology (ACC) have focused on CVD risk stratification to determine the need for and intensity of statin therapy.[19] With this approach, virtually all patients with diabetes (aged 40 to 75 years) would be candidates for statin therapy, regardless of baseline level of LDL cholesterol. Diabetic patients with established atherosclerotic CVD or estimated 10-year CVD risk of more than 7.5% would receive high-intensity statin treatment (regimens sufficient to lower LDL cholesterol >50% from untreated baseline); all others would be considered for moderate-intensity treatment (lowering of LDL cholesterol 30 to <50%). The evidence base to support these new recommendations is considered relatively strong. Although the ADA and the AHA/ACC guidelines differ in structure, ultimately the recommendations for most patients with diabetes will be similar with either approach.

Recent observations from several trials (e.g., JUPITER) and observational cohort studies of an increase in incident diabetes with statin therapy have generated concern, although the risk appears to be small in magnitude (hazard ratio, ~1.2) and is outweighed by the substantial benefits of CVD protection.[20] Clinically relevant effects of statins on glucose control among established diabetics have not been reported. In patients intolerant of statins, nicotinic acid (niacin) can be used, although CVD outcome trials have been disappointing despite substantial improvement in lipid parameters, including lowering of LDL cholesterol and increasing of HDL cholesterol levels. Further, nicotinic acid may worsen insulin resistance and glycemic control in some patients. Bile acid sequestrants, such as colesevelam or cholestyramine, can also be used but may exacerbate the hypertriglyceridemia characteristic of diabetic dyslipidemia.

In contrast to the definitive benefits of LDL lowering, there is less evidence that pharmacologic treatment of hypertriglyceridemia or of low HDL cholesterol levels reduces CVD risk. This may be in part due to the lesser efficacy of available drugs to alter these lipid subfractions. Trials with fibrate derivatives (gemfibrozil and fenofibrate) have yielded mixed results, and the addition of fenofibrate to a statin did not reduce the rate of major CVD events compared with statin alone in the ACCORD trial. Because most statins have some triglyceride-lowering effect, maximizing statin dose should be considered for patients with high triglyceride levels. Lifestyle factors are also effective, including weight loss and dietary modification (reduced fat diet, avoidance of alcohol). Omega-3 fatty acid supplementation is another option to lower triglyceride levels, although CVD outcome data are lacking. Pharmacologic treatment (i.e., with fibrates or fish oil supplements) of severe hypertriglyceridemia (triglyceride level >1000 mg/dL) is indicated to prevent acute pancreatitis.

ANTIPLATELET THERAPY

Prophylactic aspirin therapy is widely used for prevention of cardiovascular events in high-risk patients (i.e., those with prior myocardial infarction or stroke), with reported risk reductions of about 12% (Chapter 38). Results from clinical trials in patients with diabetes suggest that aspirin may be somewhat less effective for CVD prevention than in patients without diabetes, although this has not been a consistent finding. Current guidelines recommend aspirin therapy for diabetic patients with a prior CVD event (secondary prevention) or with increased CVD risk (10-year risk of >10%). This includes most men older than 50 years or women older than 60 years who also have one or more additional CVD risk factors: smoking, hypertension, albuminuria, dyslipidemia, or family history of CVD. For patients at lower CVD risk, the potential adverse effects from bleeding may outweigh the potential benefits, and routine use is not recommended. The optimal dose (balancing thrombosis prevention with the risk of bleeding) of aspirin has not been established and may differ according to patient characteristics, but 75 to 162 mg/day is commonly recommended. For high-risk patients who are unable to tolerate aspirin, clopidogrel is an effective alternative.

TREATMENT OF ESTABLISHED CARDIOVASCULAR DISEASE IN DIABETES Rx

In general, treatment of clinically established CVD, including acute coronary syndromes and stable angina, is similar in diabetic and nondiabetic patients. There is some evidence that ischemic symptoms may be less intense, atypical, or absent in diabetic patients, leading to higher rates of "silent" myocardial infarction. However, a strategy of screening for ischemic heart disease, by exercise stress testing, in asymptomatic patients did not result in lower event rates or improved outcomes. Therefore, current recommendations are for coronary artery disease screening in patients with symptoms suggestive of ischemia.

The role of intravenous insulin (with or without potassium and glucose infusion) in the setting of acute myocardial infarction has been considered in a few studies. In the Diabetes and Insulin-Glucose Infusion in Acute Myocardial Infarction (DIGAMI) study, acute myocardial infarction patients with diabetes were treated with standard therapy or with insulin infusion during the first 48 hours, followed by continued insulin use after hospital discharge. Mortality after 1 year was reduced by 30% in the insulin-treated group. However, the implications of these results have been debated because factors other than insulin treatment differed between the two groups (i.e., sulfonylureas were routinely used in the standard therapy group but withdrawn from the insulin group). These findings subsequently were not confirmed in a follow-up study, and this approach has largely been abandoned.

Several studies have addressed the roles of medical therapy and revascularization in diabetic patients with coronary artery disease. Among them, the Bypass Angioplasty Revascularization Investigation 2 Diabetes (BARI 2D) study demonstrated that a policy of medical management (including aggressive risk factor modification) was as effective as early revascularization in diabetic patients with stable angina. In the Future Revascularization Evaluation in Patients with Diabetes Mellitus: Optimal Management of Multivessel Disease (FREEDOM) trial, diabetic patients with multivessel coronary disease had better outcome (reduced rates of death from any cause or nonfatal myocardial infarction) with coronary bypass surgery compared with percutaneous intervention with drug-eluting stents, although strokes were more frequent in the surgical group.

Grade A References

A1. Misso ML, Egberts KJ, Page M, et al. Continuous subcutaneous insulin infusion (CSII) versus multiple insulin injections for type 1 diabetes mellitus. *Cochrane Databse Syst Rev.* 2010;1: CD005103.

A2. Hemmingsen B, Lunc S, Gluud C, et al. Targeting intensive glycaemic control versus targeting conventional glycaemic control for type 2 diabetes mellitus. *Cochrane Database Syst Rev.* 2013;11:CD008143.

A3. Schauer PR, Bhatt DL, Kirwan JP, et al. Bariatric surgery versus intensive medical therapy for diabetes—3 year outcomes. *N Engl J Med.* 2014;370:2002-2013.

A4. Reznik Y, Cohen O, Aronson R, et al. Insulin pump treatment compared with multiple daily injections for treatment of type 2 diabetes (OpT2mise): a randomised open-label controlled trial. *Lancet.* 2014;384:1265-1272.

A5. Finfer S, Liu B, Chittock DR, et al. The NICE-SUGAR Study Investigators. Hypoglycemia and risk of death in critically ill patients. *N Engl J Med.* 2012;367:1108-1118.

A6. Diabetes Prevention Program Research Group. 10-year follow-up of diabetes incidence and weight loss in the Diabetes Prevention Program Outcomes Study. *Lancet.* 2009;374:1677-1686.

A7. Gaede P, Lund-Andersen H, Parving HH, et al. Effect of a multifactorial intervention on mortality in type 2 diabetes. *N Engl J Med.* 2008;358:580-591.

A8. Nguyen Q, Brown D, Marcus D, et al. Ranibizumab for diabetic macular edema: results from 2 phase III randomized trials: RISE and RIDE. *Ophthalmology.* 2012;119:789-801.

A9. Keech AC, Mitchell P, Summanen PA, et al. Effect of fenofibrate on the need for laser treatment for diabetic retinopathy (FIELD study): a randomized controlled trial. *Lancet.* 2007;370: 1687-1697.

A10. Fried L, Emanuele N, Zhang J, et al. Combined angiotensin inhibition for the treatment of diabetic nephropathy. *N Engl J Med.* 2013;369:1892-1903.

A11. Wing RR, Bolin P, Brancati FL, et al. Cardiovascular effects of intensive lifestyle intervention in type 2 diabetes. *N Engl J Med.* 2013;369:145-154.

A12. Zoungas S, Chalmers J, Neal B, et al. Follow-up of blood-pressure lowering and glucose control in type 2 diabetes. *N Engl J Med.* 2014;371:1392-1406.

GENERAL REFERENCES

For the General References and other additional features, please visit Expert Consult at https://expertconsult.inkling.com.

230

HYPOGLYCEMIA AND PANCREATIC ISLET CELL DISORDERS

KHALID HUSSAIN

DEFINITIONS

Hypoglycemia is one of the most common biochemical abnormalities observed in clinical practice. It is a biochemical finding and not a diagnosis. Hypoglycemic disorders are more common in neonates, infants and children as compared to adults. Inappropriately treated hypoglycemia can have severe consequences, including seizures, permanent brain injury, or death. This is especially the case in neonates with persistent forms of hypoglycemia, who are at high risk of brain injury from delays in diagnosis and effective therapy.

Hypoglycemic disorders in neonates, infants, and children differ from adults in important aspects. First, they are most often due to congenital or genetic disorders, such as disorders of insulin secretion, as well as a range of metabolic and endocrine diseases. Second, during a transitional period of 1

to 3 days after birth, low plasma glucose concentrations are common in normal neonates, which makes it difficult to identify the minority who have a persistent hypoglycemia disorder or a genetic hypoglycemia disorder. Third, the importance of early recognition and treatment of such persistent hypoglycemia disorders in neonates is emphasized by reports that developmental handicap, which might have been avoidable by early recognition and treatment, occurs in 25 to 50% of cases with congenital hyperinsulinism.[1]

There is no absolute number that defines hypoglycemia in adults and in children. The current adult recommendations define clinical hypoglycemia as a plasma (or serum) glucose concentration low enough to cause symptoms and/or signs, including impairment of brain function. Because the clinical manifestations and symptoms of hypoglycemia are nonspecific, it is therefore not possible to state a single plasma glucose concentration that categorically defines hypoglycemia. The measured plasma or serum glucose concentration may be low owing to an artifact (e.g., when the blood sample is collected in a tube that does not contain an inhibitor of glycolysis and when separation of the plasma or serum from the formed elements is delayed).

For these reasons, guidelines in adults emphasize the value of Whipple triad for confirming hypoglycemia: (1) symptoms and/or signs compatible with hypoglycemia, (2) a low measured plasma glucose concentration, and (3) resolution of symptoms and signs when glucose concentrations are raised. Because circulating fuels such as ketone bodies can be used by the brain, lower plasma glucose concentrations can occur in healthy individuals, particularly in women and children, without symptoms or signs during extended fasting. Therefore, for all of these reasons, it is not possible to state a single plasma glucose concentration that categorically defines hypoglycemia.

The aim of this chapter is to outline the physiologic and biochemical changes associated with maintenance of a normal blood glucose level, describe the role of the counter-regulatory hormones, review the different hypoglycemia disorders observed in adults and children, and then finally discuss the various management strategies.

PATHOBIOLOGY

Physiologic and Biochemical Changes During Fasting and Feeding

Overview

Plasma glucose concentration is tightly controlled by a balance between glucose production and utilization. Glucose is derived from three sources: (1) intestinal absorption that follows digestion of dietary carbohydrates; (2) glycogenolysis, the breakdown of glycogen, which is the polymerized storage form of glucose; and (3) gluconeogenesis, the formation of glucose from precursors including lactate (and pyruvate), amino acids (especially alanine and glutamine), and to a lesser extent, glycerol. Normally, there is tight coordination between rates of endogenous glucose influx into the circulation and glucose efflux out of the circulation into insulin-dependent tissues (skeletal muscle, adipose tissue, and liver). This coordination, despite periods of feeding and fasting, maintains the plasma glucose concentration in a relatively narrow range between 70 and 110 mg/dL (3.8 to 6 mmol/L). Figure 230-1 shows an outline of glucose physiology.

Glucose is an obligate metabolic fuel for the brain under physiologic conditions. Unlike other body tissues, the brain cannot oxidize fatty acids, and neither can it synthesize/store glucose for later use. It is dependent on a continuous supply of glucose from the circulation. Given the vital importance of brain function and the above circumstances, it is not surprising that physiologic mechanisms have evolved for the maintenance of plasma glucose concentrations.

Changes During Fasting

During fasting, the basal rate of glucose output by the liver is precisely matched to glucose uptake by various body tissues. They average 2.2 mg/kg/minute in healthy adults after an overnight fast. In infants, these rates are much higher (≈6 mg/kg/minute) because of their greater brain mass relative to their body weight. The brain is responsible for nearly two thirds of basal glucose utilization. The remaining one third is used by red blood cells, renal medulla, and to some extent muscle and fat.

Hepatic glucose production results from a combination of glycogenolysis and gluconeogenesis. Endogenous glucose production is also contributed by gluconeogenesis in the kidneys. Breakdown of stored hepatic glycogen is a readily available source of free glucose. However, in an average adult, this process can only provide less than an 8-hour supply of free glucose. (In infants, this may provide only 4 hours of free glucose.) Considering this

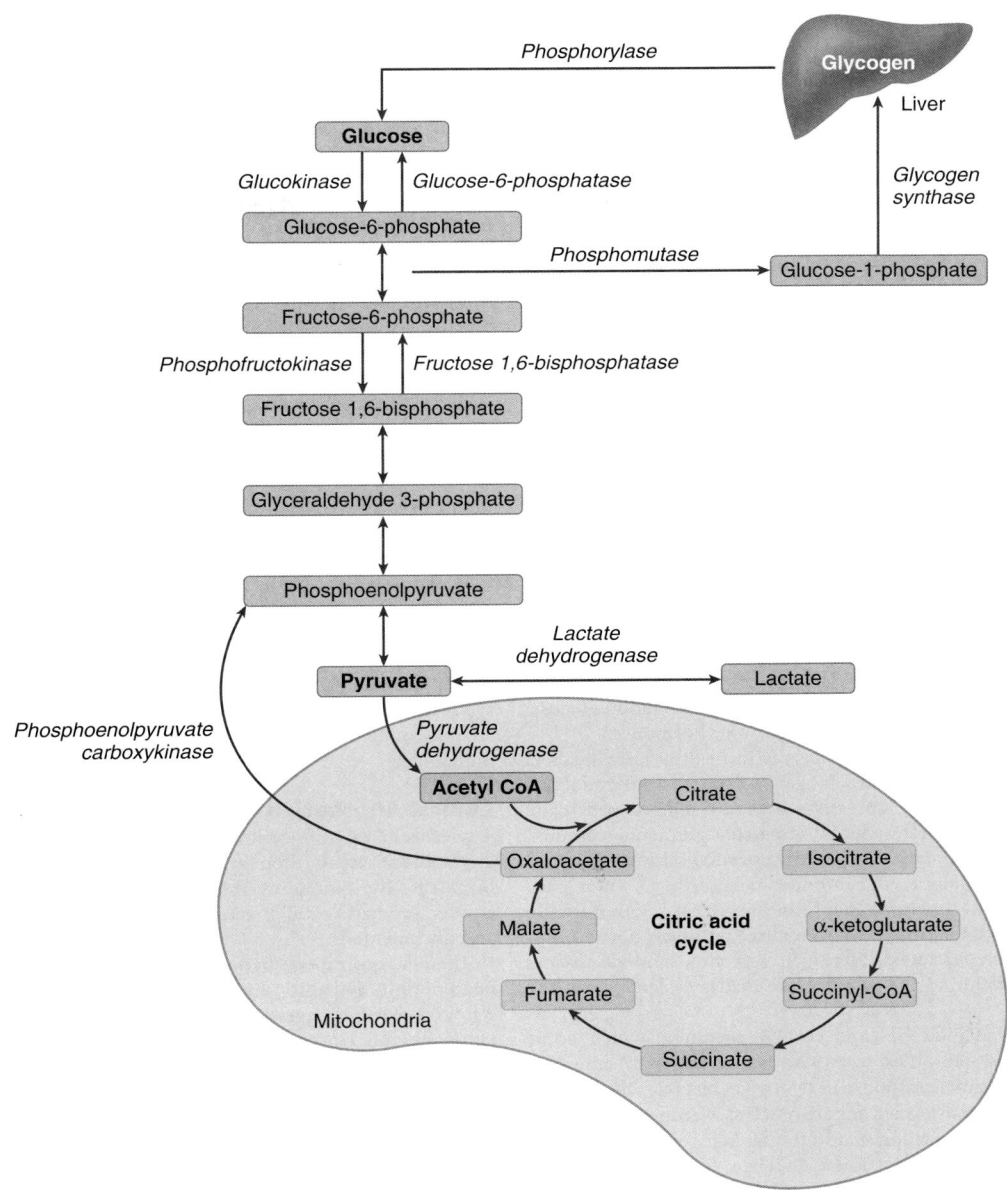

FIGURE 230-1. Outline of the biochemical pathways involved in glucose physiology.

limited capacity of glycogenolysis, gluconeogenesis is very important in supporting hepatic glycogen stores during an overnight fast.

Gluconeogenesis uses a number of key enzymes: pyruvate carboxylase, phosphoenolpyruvate carboxykinase (PEPCK), and fructose-1,6-bisphosphatase and its precursors, including lactate, alanine, glutamine, glycerol, and pyruvate. Muscle and adipose tissue, which utilize glucose in the fed state, respond to prolonged fasting by reducing their glucose uptake virtually to zero and satisfying their energy requirements by the β-oxidation of fatty acids. Additionally, through the process of proteolysis, muscle tissue provides amino acids to the liver to serve as gluconeogenic precursors for net glucose formation. Changes in the hormonal milieu during fasting (suppressed insulin and elevated counter-regulatory hormones) stimulate ketogenesis. Ketones become a major source of fuel for the brain when glucose utilization by the brain declines. This results in a decrease in the rate of gluconeogenesis required to maintain the plasma glucose concentration and hence in diminished protein wasting.

Changes During Feeding
After a meal, glucose absorption into the circulation increases glucose concentrations, which stimulates secretion of insulin from the pancreatic β-cells and suppresses secretion of glucagon from the pancreatic α-cells. This change

in the hormonal milieu switches off endogenous hepatic glucose production and accelerates glucose utilization by liver, muscle, and adipose tissue. Glucose concentration then returns gradually to the postabsorptive level, at which endogenous glucose production is equal to the glucose uptake by peripheral tissues.

Counter-Regulatory Hormonal Responses to Hypoglycemia
The counter-regulatory hormones play a key role in the maintenance of normal blood glucose concentration.[2] If counter-regulation is intact, hypoglycemia (irrespective of the cause) will result in a decrease in insulin secretion and an increase in glucagon, epinephrine, norepinephrine, cortisol, and growth hormone (GH) secretion. Glucagon secretion increases rapidly in response to hypoglycemia, and studies have shown that the glucagon response is the primary essential defense mechanism against acute hypoglycemia. GH and cortisol have numerous effects on glucose metabolism, including increasing the rate of gluconeogenesis and antagonizing the effects of insulin. In adults, the glycemic thresholds for the activation of glucose counter-regulatory hormones such as GH and cortisol lie within or just below the physiologic blood glucose concentration and slightly higher than the threshold for symptoms. This suggests that GH and cortisol secretion increase in response to blood glucose concentrations within the normoglycemic range,

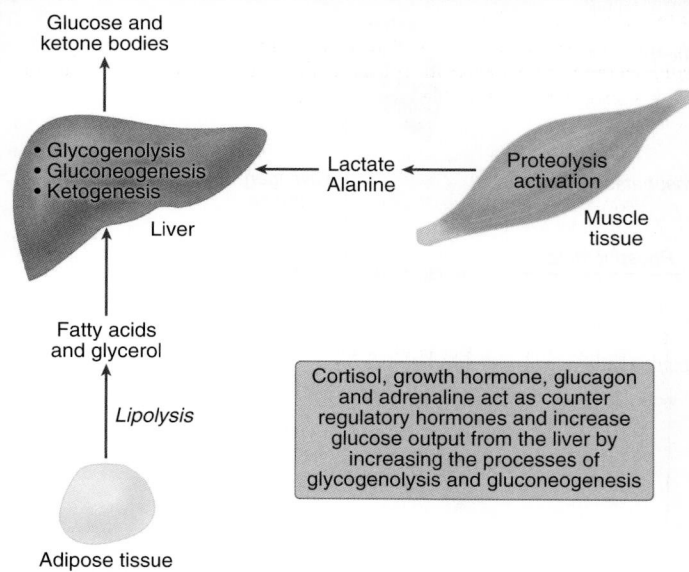

FIGURE 230-2. The role of the counter-regulatory hormones, glycogenolysis, gluconeogenesis, and lipolysis in glucose physiology.

and these increases are inversely proportional to the nadir in blood glucose. Figure 230-2 outlines the role of the counter-regulatory hormones.

Insulin secretion from β-cells of the pancreas in healthy individuals is inhibited as blood glucose concentration falls below 72 mg/dL (4.0 mmol/L). As insulin secretion is reduced, the repressive effect of insulin on pancreatic α-cell function is removed, thereby rapidly increasing glucagon secretion. Glucagon acts on the liver to increase hepatic glycogenolysis and gluconeogenesis. When the blood glucose concentration falls further (≈68 mg/dL [3.8 mmol/L]), epinephrine and norepinephrine are released both from the adrenals and directly into interstitial fluid from nerve terminals, further suppressing insulin secretion, increasing glucagon secretion, and decreasing peripheral glucose utilization in the muscle and increasing lipolysis in the adipose tissues.

Additional responses include GH and cortisol secretion, which occur below a blood glucose concentration of around 66 mg/dL (≈3.7 mmol/L) and are initiators of the adaptive response to hypoglycemia (e.g., during prolonged starvation); glucose-raising actions are much slower in onset (several hours). These hormone responses stimulate lipolysis, ketogenesis, and gluconeogenesis. Permissive amounts of cortisol and GH are required for a normal hepatic response to glucagon and epinephrine. In healthy individuals, this system ensures that hypoglycemia is rarely experienced and would only occur during starvation or ultra-endurance sports. Drugs or diseases that inhibit counter-regulatory secretion or action predispose patients to hypoglycemia.

Activation of counter-regulation depends on effective detection of falling blood glucose levels. This is achieved by the complex integration of various glucose-sensing systems in both the periphery and central nervous system.[3] Fluctuations in peripheral glucose levels are detected by glucose-sensing neurons in the oral cavity, gut, portal/mesenteric vein (PMV), and carotid body. PMV neurons detect changes in blood glucose prior to entry into the liver from the gut. This information is then relayed through the vagus nerve and spinal cord to the hindbrain and then to the hypothalamus. In addition, the hypothalamus, because of its location adjacent to the third ventricle and median eminence, may sample factors from peripheral circulation, including glucose, as well as hormones such as insulin and leptin. Although a complex network of glucose sensors has been described in the central nervous system and peripherally, the brain appears to have the dominant role during hypoglycemia and, specifically, the ventromedial region of the hypothalamus (VMH). VMH neurons contain the same glucose-sensing mechanisms (e.g., glucokinase, ATP-sensitive K+ channels) as found in pancreatic β-cells.

CLINICAL MANIFESTATIONS
Symptoms of Hypoglycemia
The symptoms of hypoglycemia reflect the responses of the brain to a decrease in the blood glucose level; such symptoms may be nonspecific and

vague, especially in the childhood period. Children may not be able to communicate their hypoglycemic symptoms. The symptoms of hypoglycemia may be categorized into two main groups: (1) those that arise as a result of the central nervous system being deprived of glucose (neuroglycopenic) and (2) symptoms arising from the perception of physiologic changes caused by the central nervous system–mediated sympatho-adrenal discharge triggered by hypoglycemia (neurogenic or autonomic).[4] The neurogenic symptoms of hypoglycemia are largely the result of sympathetic neural, rather than adrenomedullary, activation.

Neuroglycopenic symptoms (e.g., dizziness, confusion, tiredness, difficulty with speaking, headache, inability to concentrate, coma, and seizures) arise from the failure of brain function itself and are caused by deficient supply of glucose to the brain.[5] Neurogenic symptoms include both adrenergic responses (catecholamine-mediated symptoms such as palpitations, tremor, and anxiety) and cholinergic responses (acetylcholine-mediated symptoms such as sweating, hunger, paresthesias). Awareness of hypoglycemia chiefly depends on perception of the central and peripheral effects of neurogenic (as opposed to neuroglycopenic) responses to hypoglycemia.

In nondiabetic adults during acute insulin-induced hypoglycemia, autonomic symptoms become apparent at a threshold of approximately 60 mg/dL (3.3 mmol/L), and impairment of brain function manifested by neuroglycopenic symptoms occurs at a threshold of approximately 50 mg/dL (2.8 mmol/L) in arterialized venous blood (venous levels would be ≈ 3 mg/dL [0.16 mmol/L] less). However, in patients with recurrent hypoglycemia, the glycemic thresholds for responses to hypoglycemia are reset at a lower plasma glucose concentration. The glucose thresholds for the activation of neuroglycopenic and autonomic symptoms in children are not as clearly defined as in adults. The symptoms and signs of hypoglycemia are not influenced by the rate of blood glucose decline in nondiabetic individuals.

Clinical Approach to the Patient with Hypoglycemia
A careful clinical history, description of symptoms, physical examination, and a systematic step-by-step approach are the cornerstones of establishing a diagnosis. The symptoms of hypoglycemia may be very nonspecific, hence any symptomatic child or adult must have the blood glucose level measured and documented.

The relationship of a hypoglycemic episode to the most recent meal can be important diagnostically. Hypoglycemia occurring after a short fast (2 to 3 hours) may be suggestive of hyperinsulinism or glycogen storage disease. Hypoglycemia occurring after a long fast (12 to 14 hours) may suggest a disorder of gluconeogenesis. Postprandial hypoglycemia may indicate galactosemia, hereditary fructose intolerance, dumping syndrome, insulinoma, insulin autoimmune syndrome, and noninsulinoma pancreatogenous hypoglycemia syndrome. In both children and adults, a clear documentation of the medication history is important.

DIAGNOSIS
After the clinical history has been taken and the examination completed, a diagnostic cascade of appropriate tests is necessary. These may be guided in the context of the most common causes of hypoglycemia as listed in Table 230-1.

The current adult recommendations[6] state that evaluation and management of hypoglycemia should only be undertaken in patients in whom Whipple's triad—symptoms, signs, or both consistent with hypoglycemia, a low plasma glucose concentration, and resolution of those symptoms or signs after the plasma glucose concentration is raised—is documented. However, this does not apply to children for the reasons discussed earlier.

Causes of Hypoglycemia
Hypoglycemia is more common in the childhood period than in adults and can be due to a large number of causes. Table 230-1 summarizes the differential diagnosis of hypoglycemia.

Hypoglycemia Due to Excess Production of Hormones
Inappropriate and excess production of certain hormones can lead to hypoglycemia. The two most common conditions associated with excess production of a hormone are hyperinsulinemic hypoglycemia (HH) and non–islet cell tumor hypoglycemia (NICTH) or IGF-2-oma (insulin-like growth factor–secreting tumor). Inappropriate production of insulin can either lead to fasting hypoglycemia or postprandial hypoglycemia.

TABLE 230-1 DIFFERENTIAL DIAGNOSIS OF HYPOGLYCEMIA*

HYPERINSULINEMIC HYPOGLYCEMIA (INCLUDING POSTPRANDIAL)

Transient: infant of diabetic mother, perinatal asphyxia, Rhesus disease, intrauterine growth retardation, Beckwith-Wiedemann syndrome
Congenital: *ABCC8, KCNJ11*, **GCK**, GDH, HADH, HNF4A, **SLC16A1**
Dumping syndrome
Insulin receptor mutations and antibodies
Insulinoma
Noninsulinoma pancreatogenous hypoglycemia (adults)
Gastric bypass surgery for morbid obesity
Non–islet cell tumor hypoglycemia (NICTH) or IGF-2-oma
Insulin autoimmune syndrome
Insulin factitious hypoglycemia

HORMONAL DEFICIENCY/RESISTANCE

Adrenocorticotropic hormone
Cortisol
Growth hormone
Glucagon†
Adrenaline†

DEFECTS IN HEPATIC GLYCOGEN RELEASE/STORAGE

Glycogen storage diseases: **glucose-6-phosphatase, amylo-1,6-glucosidase deficiency**, liver phosphorylase deficiency, glycogen storage disease type 0

DEFECTS IN GLUCONEOGENESIS

Fructose-1,6-bisphosphatase deficiency, phosphoenolpyruvate carboxykinase deficiency, pyruvate carboxylase deficiency

CARNITINE METABOLISM

Carnitine deficiency (primary and secondary)
Carnitine palmitoyltransferase deficiency (CPT 1 and 2)
Carnitine transporter defects

FATTY ACID OXIDATION

Medium-chain acyl-CoA dehydrogenase (MCAD) deficiency
Very long-chain acyl-CoA dehydrogenase (VLCAD) deficiency
Short-chain acyl-CoA dehydrogenase (SCAD) deficiency
Long/short-chain L-3-hydroxyacyl-CoA (L/SCHAD) deficiency

DEFECTS IN KETONE BODY SYNTHESIS/UTILIZATION

HMG-CoA synthase deficiency, HMG-CoA lyase deficiency
Succinyl-CoA: 3-oxoacid-CoA transferase (SCOT) deficiency

METABOLIC CONDITIONS (COMMON ONES)

Organic acidemias (propionic, methylmalonic)
Maple syrup urine disease, galactosemia, fructosemia, tyrosinemia
Hereditary fructose intolerance
Mitochondrial respiratory chain complex deficiencies
Congenital disorders of glycosylation (CGD)

DRUG INDUCED

Sulfonylureas
Insulin
β-Blockers
Salicylates
Alcohol
Quinine
Haloperidol
Pentamidine
Levofloxacin
Methadone
Disopyramide
Indomethacin
Cibenzoline
Gatifloxacin

MISCELLANEOUS CAUSES (MECHANISM[S] NOT CLEAR)

Idiopathic ketotic hypoglycemia (diagnosis of exclusion)
Infections (sepsis, malaria), congenital heart disease

*Boldface indicates more common in adults.
†No human case yet reported with glucagon or adrenaline deficiency.
HMG = 3-hydroxy-3-methylglutaryl; IGF = insulin-like growth factor.

Hyperinsulinemic Hypoglycemia

HH is a heterogeneous group of disorders characterized by unregulated insulin secretion from pancreatic β-cells. In the face of hypoglycemia, patients have inappropriately detectable serum insulin levels, low ketone bodies, and low fatty acids and show a glycemic response to glucagon.[7]

Congenital Forms of Hyperinsulinemic Hypoglycemia

In patients with congenital forms of HH, mutations in the key genes (*ABCC8, KCNJ11, GLUD1, GCK, HADH, SLC16A1, HNF4A, HNF1A*, and *UCP2*) regulating insulin secretion have been identified.[8] Children with inactivating mutations in the genes *ABCC8* and *KCNJ11* present with the most severe forms of congenital HH, typically in the newborn period. Hyperinsulinism-hyperammonemia syndrome due to activating mutations in the *GLUD1* gene and activating mutations in the *GCK* gene, leading to HH, have both been described in adults as well as children. Exercise-induced HH due to activating mutations in the *SLC16A1* gene has also been recognized in adults.

Insulinoma

An insulinoma is the commonest cause of endogenous HH in adults. Insulinomas have the highest incidence in the fifth and sixth decades.[9] Insulinomas are insulin-secreting tumors of pancreatic origin, with an incidence of 1 to 4 per million. The majority (90%) of them are benign, solitary, intrapancreatic and less than 2 cm in diameter. Classically, symptoms become evident in the fasting state or following exercise. However, it is now known that insulinoma can also present with postprandial symptoms. Diagnosis is based on findings of abnormal serum levels of insulin and C-peptide (also proinsulin) at the time of fasting hypoglycemia. An insulinoma can occur either in isolation or in association with multiple endocrine neoplasia type 1 (MEN 1), with a lifetime prevalence of 10% among adults carrying mutations in *MEN1* (Chapter 231). Around 6% of insulinomas occur in patients with MEN 1, and most insulinomas are benign, but 5 to 10% are malignant.

Postprandial Hyperinsulinemic Hypoglycemia

Postprandial hyperinsulinemic hypoglycemia (PPHH) refers to hypoglycemia within a few hours of meal ingestion, secondary to inappropriate insulin secretion in response to a meal. If PPHH is clinically suspected, then an oral glucose tolerance test (OGTT) or a mixed-meal provocation test is performed. (See later in section "Investigations for Hypoglycemia.") A physiologic dip in the blood glucose level seen in OGTT might lead to misdiagnosis. However, corresponding biochemical evidence of endogenous HH and symptoms of neuroglycopenia during a hypoglycemic episode would help distinguish between pathologic PPHH and reactive hypoglycemia. A decrease of more than 108 mg/dL (6 mmol/L) between peak and nadir blood glucose during OGTT has been used as a diagnostic criterion for dumping syndrome in adults.

DUMPING SYNDROME. Dumping syndrome seen in infants after Nissen fundoplication is a classic example of PPHH. Precipitous emptying of hyperosmolar carbohydrate-containing solutions into the small bowel results in rapid glucose absorption, hyperglycemia, and reactive hypoglycemia. These children also tend to have abnormally exaggerated secretion of glucagon-like peptide-1 (GLP-1), which may contribute to the exaggerated insulin surge and resultant hypoglycemia.[10]

INSULIN AUTOIMMUNE SYNDROME. Insulin autoimmune syndrome, or Hirata's disease, is a rare condition characterized by HH associated with high titers of antibodies to endogenous insulin in the absence of pathologic abnormalities of pancreatic islets and prior exposure to exogenous insulin. The disease is extremely uncommon in Western countries. Insulin autoimmune syndrome affects men and women equally and is seen more frequently in patients older than 40 years. The binding kinetics of endogenous insulin by the antibodies are thought to lead to physiologically inappropriate levels of bioavailable insulin, causing either hyper- or hypoglycemia.

In this syndrome, the insulin levels are markedly elevated, usually above 100 mU/L. After a meal or glucose load, these patients often demonstrate initial hyperglycemia, followed by hypoglycemia a few hours later. The hyperglycemia is caused by the anti-insulin antibodies that bind the insulin secreted in response to rising blood glucose levels after a meal. This binding reduces the bioavailability of the secreted insulin to the receptors in the liver and peripheral tissues, resulting in hyperglycemia and further insulin secretion. As blood glucose concentrations begin to decrease and insulin secretion declines, the insulin bound to the antibodies is released, resulting in inappropriately high free insulin concentrations for the blood glucose, causing hypoglycemia.

PPHH IN PATIENTS WITH INSULIN-RECEPTOR MUTATIONS. PPHH has been described in patients who carried a heterozygote mutation (Arg-1174Gln) in the insulin-receptor gene. Hyperinsulinism seems to be associated with decreased degradation rather than increased secretion of insulin, as evidenced by increased fasting levels of serum insulin despite normal levels of serum C-peptide and reduced clearance of exogenous insulin during clamp studies.

PPHH AFTER GASTRIC BYPASS SURGERY. A consequence of the obesity epidemic is the increasing use of gastric bypass surgery for patients with severe, medically complicated obesity (Chapter 220), which has led to a number of reports of postprandial HH.[11] In a review of the Swedish Bariatric Surgery registry, the incidence of hospitalization for hypoglycemia in post–gastric bypass patients was reported as less than 1%.

A number of different explanations have been suggested to explain hypoglycemia post gastric bypass surgery. This can either be a manifestation of dumping syndrome or improved insulin sensitivity following weight loss unmasking an underlying hyperinsulinemia syndrome. The hypoglycemia could also be due to an effect on the enteroinsular axis induced by the diversion of nutrients into the small intestine.

The principal reason seems to be enhanced postprandial insulin secretion, thought to be due primarily to increased secretion of glucose-dependent insulinotropic polypeptide (GIP) and especially GLP-1. GLP-1 levels are now well documented to be increased two- to five-fold after gastric bypass. The elevations of incretins tend to be seen early, even as early as 2 days after gastric bypass, and levels may decline as substantial weight loss and normalization of insulin sensitivity occurs. In patients with PPHH, elevated levels of GIP and GLP-1 persist for years after surgery.

Increased postprandial insulin secretion by incretins is mediated by islet cell hypertrophy and hyperplasia. Both GIP and GLP-1 have been implicated in increasing pancreatic β-cell mass in rodent models. GLP-1 regulates islet growth by inducing the expression of the transcription factor pancreatic-duodenum homeobox-1 (PDX-1).

Overexpression of IGF-2 and IGF-1 receptor alpha (IGF1Rα) have been found in pancreatic tissue removed from patients with persistent PPHH after gastric bypass surgery as compared to controls. These findings are suggestive of the role of growth factors in islet hyperfunction seen in post–gastric bypass patients.

NONINSULINOMA PANCREATOGENOUS HYPOGLYCEMIA SYNDROME. Noninsulinoma pancreatogenous hypoglycemia syndrome (NIPHS) is characterized by postprandial neuroglycopenia in the presence of negative prolonged fasting tests and negative perioperative localization studies for insulinoma.[12] However, in some patients the selective arterial calcium stimulation test is positive, with the histology of the resected pancreas showing nesidioblastosis. The underlying genetic basis of NIPHS is not known.

These patients are negative for *ABCC8/KCNJ11* mutations and show islet hypertrophy histologically (as observed in diffuse congenital HH).

Immunohistologic studies of the resected pancreatic tissue have failed to show an increased rate of proliferation of β-cells or abnormal synthesis and/or processing of either proinsulin or amylin. Neither has there been any evidence of overexpression of pancreatic differentiation factors, PDX-1, and Nkx-6.1, nor the calcium-sensing receptor (CaSR).

Insulin Factitious Hypoglycemia

Hypoglycemia can also be induced pharmacologically, either intentionally as a diagnostic tool, accidentally as a complication of the treatment of diabetes mellitus, or as a consequence of poisoning either with insulin itself or with drugs (e.g., sulfonylureas) that stimulate insulin release. Whenever severe hypoglycemia occurs with documented hyperinsulinism, the possibility of Munchausen's syndrome by proxy should be considered in children. The possibility of malicious administration of insulin or an oral sulfonylurea should always be suspected in cases of sudden onset of hypoglycemia in a previously healthy individual. In the case of insulin administration, the clue in the biochemistry will be a raised insulin level accompanied by normal C-peptide.

Non–Islet Cell Tumor Hypoglycemia, or IGF-2-oma

NICTH, or IGF-2-oma, denotes the syndrome of hypoglycemia produced by or associated with any neoplasm other than an insulinoma. These are usually tumors of mesenchymal and epithelial origin (including hepatomas, fibromas, and fibrosarcomas). The underlying mechanism of hypoglycemia in nearly all patients with this syndrome is overproduction of IGF-2 by the tumor, which includes mature IGF-2 and incompletely processed forms of IGF-2, referred to collectively as "big" IGF-2.[13] The elevated IGF-2–related peptides mimic the fasting hypoglycemia characteristic of patients with insulin-producing islet cell tumors. Rarely, markedly elevated IGF-2 levels produce somatic changes suggestive of acromegaly. Typically, the elevated IGF-2 levels are associated with suppressed plasma levels of insulin, IGF-1, and GH.

Hypoglycemia Due to Hormone Deficiency

Deficiency of glucagon, adrenaline, GH, and cortisol can cause hypoglycemia. Glucagon and adrenaline deficiency is extremely rare, and so far no true human, genetically proven defects in glucagon and adrenaline deficiency have been described. Children and adults can present with hypoglycemia due to deficiency of various hormones. This might be either in isolation (e.g., isolated GH, adrenocorticotropic hormone [ACTH], or cortisol deficiency) or in combination with other hormones, such as in patients with hypopituitarism. The etiology of the hypoglycemia resulting from cortisol and GH deficiency is due to a combination of factors, including reduced gluconeogenic substrate availability (decreased mobilization of fats and proteins) and increased glucose utilization due to increased insulin sensitivity of tissues in the absence of these two hormones.

Acquired hypopituitarism may result from tumors (most commonly craniopharyngioma), radiation, infection, hydrocephalus, vascular anomalies, and trauma. Addison disease (AD) results from adrenal cortex hypofunction/dysfunction, with deficient production of glucocorticoids, mineralocorticoids, and androgens, and with high levels of both ACTH and plasma renin activity (Chapter 227). Autoimmune AD is the most frequent etiologic form in adult patients, accounting for about 80% of cases, followed by post-tuberculosis AD in 10 to 15%; the remaining 5% of cases are due to vascular, neoplastic, or rare genetic forms.

The markers of autoimmune AD are adrenal cortex (ACA) or 21-hydroxylase autoantibodies (21-OHAbs), and they are present at diagnosis in more than 90% of cases. In autoimmune AD, the adrenal cortex is infiltrated by lymphocytes and plasma cells, and the glands are sclerotic and reduced in volume. Autoimmune AD occurs mainly in middle-aged women, alone or associated with other (clinical, subclinical, or potential) autoimmune diseases, giving rise to various forms of autoimmune polyglandular syndrome. Replacement therapy with gluco- and mineralocorticoids is life-saving for patients with chronic adrenal insufficiency.

Hypoglycemia Due to Defects in Hepatic Glycogen Release/Storage

Glucose-6-phosphatase deficiency (glycogen storage disease [GSD] type I, Von Gierke disease) is the commonest of the glycogen storage diseases causing hypoglycemia (Chapter 207). Deficiency of this enzyme results in the inability to release free glucose from glucose-6-phosphate, with resultant hepatomegaly due to stored glycogen. These children and adults present with recurrent hypoglycemia associated with lactic acidosis, hyperuricemia, and hyperlipidemia.[14] The two other glycogen storage diseases causing hypoglycemia are due to deficiencies of the enzymes amylo-1,6-glucosidase (GSD type III) and liver phosphorylase (GSD type VI). The clinical and biochemical features of GSD-III subjects are quite heterogeneous.

Hypoglycemia Due to Defects in Gluconeogenesis

Gluconeogenesis, or the formation of glucose from mainly lactate/pyruvate, glycerol, glutamine, and alanine, plays an essential role in the maintenance of normoglycemia during fasting. Inborn deficiencies are known in each of the four enzymes of the glycolytic-gluconeogenic pathway that ensure a unidirectional flux from pyruvate to glucose: pyruvate carboxylase, phosphoenolpyruvate carboxykinase (PEPCK), fructose-1,6-bisphosphatase, and glucose-6-phosphatase. Gluconeogenesis can essentially be viewed as a reversal of glycolysis but with a few important differences. Patients with defects in gluconeogenesis present with fasting hypoglycemia and lactic acidosis. Pyruvate carboxylase deficiency may lead to a more widespread clinical presentation, with lactic acidosis, severe mental and developmental retardation, and proximal renal tubular acidosis.

Hypoglycemia Due to Disorders of Carnitine Metabolism and Defects of Fatty Acid Oxidation

Serious clinical consequences may occur if fatty acid oxidation (FAO) is impaired, including hypoglycemic seizures, muscle damage, cardiomyopathy, metabolic acidosis, and liver dysfunction. Fatty acids are taken up by hepatocytes and muscle, where they are subsequently activated to their coenzyme A (CoA) esters. FAO disorders are individually rare, but they are collectively common because of the number of different enzymes affected. When defects occur in fatty acid degradation, excess acylcarnitine intermediates accumulate in the tissues, including heart, liver, and skeletal muscle, which can lead to organ dysfunction. The diversion of acyl-CoA intermediates into β-oxidation results in accumulation of toxic dicarboxylic acids. Acylcarnitines that spill into the blood provide a marker for diagnosis.

Primary carnitine deficiency is an autosomal recessive disorder of fatty acid oxidation that can present at different ages with hypoketotic hypoglycemia and cardiomyopathy and/or skeletal myopathy (Chapter 205). This disease is suspected based on reduced levels of carnitine in plasma and confirmed by measurement of carnitine transport in the patient's fibroblasts. Carnitine transport is markedly reduced (usually < 5% of normal) in fibroblasts from patients with primary carnitine deficiency. Patients with the hepatic isoform of carnitine palmityltransferase (CPT)-1 deficiency present with hypoketotic hypoglycemia in the neonatal period.

The commonest disorder of fatty acid β-oxidation is medium-chain acyl-CoA dehydrogenase (MCAD) deficiency, an autosomal recessive disease presenting in children who are typically asymptomatic except during times of fasting and metabolic stress, usually associated with a viral illness, when they present with fasting nonketotic hypoglycemia; if undiagnosed, 20 to 25% of affected patients will die during the first episode.

Metabolic Diseases
Hypoglycemia can also be due to a number of metabolic conditions (Chapter 205), including galactosemia, fructosemia, tyrosinemia, organic acidemias, maple syrup urine disease, glutaric aciduria type II, and in mitochondrial respiratory chain defects. Hereditary fructose intolerance, caused by catalytic deficiency of aldolase B (fructose-1,6-phosphate aldolase), is a recessively inherited condition in which affected homozygotes develop hypoglycemia and severe abdominal symptoms after taking foods containing fructose and cognate sugars. Continued ingestion of noxious sugars leads to hepatic and renal injury and growth retardation.

Noninsulinoma Islet Cell Tumors
Islet cell tumors present an important challenge to the clinician because of their protean manifestations and potential lethality. These tumors can be clinically silent or active (functioning). Early diagnosis is essential and depends on recognition of the classic and variant clinical syndromes followed by confirmation of elevated peptide levels by radioimmunoassay.[15] Glucagonoma, gastrinoma, VIPoma (VIP = vasoactive intestinal peptide), somatostatinoma, and ACTHoma are functioning tumors that may occur in isolation but can also be part of MEN 1 syndrome (Chapter 231) and von Hippel-Lindau disease (Chapter 417).

Tumor marker measurement gives useful information for the follow-up and management of patients with noninsulinoma islet cell tumors (neuroendocrine tumors). The currently used tumor markers are neuron-specific enolase (NSE) and chromogranin A (CgA). The clinical accuracy of these biomarkers depends on histotype and disease extent. CgA is thought to be the optimal marker for most neuroendocrine tumors, because it is independent of the biological characteristics of the tumor.

Glucagonoma
Glucagonomas are α-cell tumors that, when they are active, produce a syndrome characterized by necrolytic migratory erythema, diabetes mellitus, weight loss, anemia, glossitis, thromboembolism, neuropsychiatric disturbances, and hyperglucagonemia. Tumor characterization is made by computed tomography (CT) and/or pancreatic endoscopic ultrasonic and indium-labeled octreoscan. The diagnosis is established by documenting the presence of hyperglucagonemia, with diagnostic levels being generally above 500 pg/mL (normal, <120). It is important to remember that other diseases can also cause hyperglucagonemia, including cirrhosis, pancreatitis, diabetes mellitus, prolonged fasting, sepsis, burns, renal failure, acromegaly, and familial hyperglucagonemia. Surgery is the main component of treatment, in some cases in association with chemotherapy.

Gastrinoma
Gastrinomas are uncommon tumors of the endocrine system, occurring within the pancreas and duodenum. Overproduction of the hormone gastrin by these tumors produces a sustained increase in gastric acid secretion, leading to complications of peptic ulceration known as the Zollinger-Ellison syndrome (ZES). Gastrinomas can occur sporadically or in a familial pattern as a component of the MEN 1 syndrome. Gastrinomas have the potential to metastasize to regional lymph nodes, the liver, and other distant sites.

VIPoma
VIPoma is very rare, with 80% of these tumors originating from the pancreas, mostly in the tail. The majority of cases are sporadic. About 50 to 60% of cases have metastasized by the time the diagnosis is made. Most patients have secretory watery diarrhea, resulting in electrolyte disturbances, such as hypokalemia, hypophosphatemia, hypomagnesemia, and metabolic acidosis (Verner-Morrison syndrome, pancreatic cholera, WDHA syndrome). Hypochlorhydria or achlorhydria occurs in 75% of cases, owing to the inhibition of gastric acid production by VIP. Hyperchloremic acidosis can also occur as a result of low bicarbonate levels from severe intestinal loss. Occasionally, hypercalcemia, glucose intolerance, and hypotension may be present. The VIP level is elevated in almost all cases, but it can also be normal between episodes of diarrhea.

Somatostatinoma
Somatostatinomas are rare neuroendocrine tumors with an incidence of 1 in 40 million. These unusual tumors arise predominantly in the pancreas and peripancreatic duodenum, and patients often present with nonspecific symptoms. Rarely, patients present with somatostatinoma syndrome (diabetes, gallstones, and steatorrhea) when the tumor is secretory.

Investigations for Hypoglycemia
From the clinical history, description of symptoms, and physical examination, there might be important clues to the underlying cause of hypoglycemia, and the investigations can then be tailored to the particular cause. However, in some cases the clinical history and physical examination may not provide any clues, and in these cases the patient will need to be investigated more extensively.

Reagent strips in combination with a reflectance meter are the most common method of measuring bedside blood glucose levels. However, it is important to remember that these should be used only as a guide (they can be inaccurate), and the blood glucose concentration should always be checked in the laboratory. Whole-blood glucose is approximately 15% lower than serum glucose levels because of the lower glucose content and intracellular water content of the red cells. Glucose concentrations in venous blood are 10% lower than arterial blood. The blood sample for glucose measurement should be collected in a fluoride container to inhibit glycolysis. It should also be analyzed immediately because, even in the presence of fluoride, the blood glucose concentration will decrease over time.

In an ideal situation, the blood glucose level should be measured at the time of a spontaneous episode of hypoglycemia, and samples for plasma glucose, insulin, C-peptide, proinsulin, and β-hydroxybutyrate concentrations and toxicology screen for oral hypoglycemic agents taken. The blood glucose must be considered in the context of the whole fuel economy and in the light of concurrent hormone concentrations. However, this is not always possible, and patients may require further tests (e.g., fasting, mixed-meal, or provocation testing) to unravel the cause of the hypoglycemia. The various tests used for eliciting hypoglycemia in adults and children are described next. Table 230-2 shows the routine baseline investigations that should be performed in children and adults presenting with hypoglycemia.

TABLE 230-2	ROUTINE BASELINE INVESTIGATIONS IN PATIENTS WITH SUSPECTED HYPOGLYCEMIA	
BLOOD		**URINE**
Glucose		Ketones
Insulin		Reducing substances
Cortisol		Organic acids
Lactate		
Growth hormone		
Nonesterified fatty acids		
3β-Hydroxybutyrate		
Carnitine (free and total)		
Blood spot acylcarnitine		
Ammonia		

TABLE 230-3 PROTOCOL FOR 72-HOUR FAST IN ADULTS

1. Start the fast from the last ingestion of a meal. Stop all medications that might interfere with test.
2. The patient can drink water during the test.
3. The patient must be active during waking hours.
4. Measure plasma glucose, insulin, C-peptide, and β-hydroxybutyrate (on the same venipuncture specimen) every 6 hours until plasma glucose reaches 60 mg/dL (3.3 mM). Then measure every 1 to 2 hours.
5. End the fast when the plasma glucose is 45 mg/dL (2.5 mM) and the patient has symptoms or signs of hypoglycemia, or plasma glucose is 55 mg/dL if Whipple triad had been demonstrated previously.
6. At the end of the fast, measure plasma glucose, insulin, C-peptide, β-hydroxybutyrate, and sulfonylurea (on the same venipuncture specimen). Then inject glucagon, 1 mg intravenously, and measure plasma glucose every 10 minutes three times. Once the fast is completed, allow the patient to eat normally.

Adapted from Cryer PE, Axelrod L, Grossman AB, et al. Evaluation and management of adult hypoglycemic disorders: an Endocrine Society clinical practice guideline. *J Clin Endocrinol Metab.* 2009;94:709-728.

TABLE 230-4 SUGGESTED PROTOCOL FOR A MIXED-MEAL DIAGNOSTIC TEST IN ADULTS

1. Fast patient overnight. Stop all medications that might interfere with test.
2. Use a mixed meal similar to one that causes patient to experience symptoms.
3. Collect samples for plasma glucose, insulin, C-peptide, and proinsulin before ingestion and every 30 minutes through 300 minutes after meal ingestion.
4. Observe the patient for symptoms and/or signs of hypoglycemia, and ask the patient to keep a written log of all symptoms, timed from the start of meal ingestion.
5. The mixed-meal test should be interpreted on the basis of laboratory measured plasma glucose concentrations, not those estimated with a point-of-care glucose monitor. If it is judged necessary to treat before 300 minutes because of severe symptoms, obtain samples for all the following *before* administering carbohydrates: plasma insulin, C-peptide, and proinsulin (sent for analysis only in those samples in which plasma glucose is < 60 mg/dL [3.3 mmol/L]), and a measurement of oral hypoglycemic agents. If Whipple triad is demonstrated, antibodies to insulin should also be measured.

Adapted from Cryer PE, Axelrod L, Grossman AB, et al. Evaluation and management of adult hypoglycemic disorders: an Endocrine Society clinical practice guideline. *J Clin Endocrinol Metab.* 2009;94:709-728.

Fasting Tests

Controlled fasting tests are important procedures for eliciting the cause of hypoglycemia in both children and adults. In adults it is recommended that a prolonged supervised (72-hour) fast be conducted in a standardized fashion (Table 230-3). During the fast, if patients have any signs or symptoms of hypoglycemia, with a documented low blood glucose level, the fast should be terminated. It is currently recommended that the fast not be prolonged beyond 72 hours if patients do not have any symptoms or signs of hypoglycemia and no documentation of low blood glucose. Monitoring for symptoms or signs of hypoglycemia during the fast is essential because patients may experience some symptoms but have serum glucose levels higher than the hypoglycemic range. In some healthy women (thin and lean) and men, blood glucose levels may drop to 40 mg/dL (2.2 mmol/L) during prolonged fasting. Some patients have lower glycemic thresholds without symptoms or signs of hypoglycemia.

In an adult patient where Whipple triad has been demonstrated, the 72-hour fast may be terminated if the plasma glucose concentration is 55 mg/dL (3 mmol/L) or less. The interpretation of serum insulin, C-peptide, and proinsulin during the 72-hour fast will depend on the concurrent plasma glucose concentration. Pancreatic β-cell insulin secretion becomes undetectable in healthy persons when the plasma glucose concentration is down to 55 mg/dL (3 mmol/L). Most patients with an insulinoma become hypoglycemic before 72 hours. However, continuation of the fast to 72 hours is necessary to rule out the likelihood of organic hypoglycemia.

HH in adults is characterized by plasma insulin concentrations of 3 μU/mL or greater (C-peptide of 200 pmol/L or more and proinsulin 5 pmol/L or more). Insulinoma patients have plasma insulin concentrations that rarely exceed 100 μU/mL, and plasma insulin levels greater than 1000 μU/mL suggest exogenous insulin administration or the presence of insulin antibodies. In the childhood period, any detectable plasma insulin in the presence of hypoglycemia is inappropriate and is highly suggestive of HH.

Measurement of the plasma β-hydroxybutyrate concentration is used as a surrogate marker of insulin action at the end of the 72-hour fast in healthy adult individuals and when Whipple triad is fulfilled in patients during a diagnostic fast. In patients with HH, because of the suppressive action of insulin on ketogenesis, plasma concentrations of β-hydroxybutyrate are typically less than 2.7 mmol/L. This is in contrast to healthy individuals, who will show a progressive rise in the concentration of β-hydroxybutyrate during the 72-hour test. If a value above 2.7 mmol/L is documented at any time point in the fast, the test can be terminated. In the childhood period, there is no clear-cut plasma level of β-hydroxybutyrate that can be used to confirm HH.

Another useful marker of insulin action in both adults and children is the glycemic increment in response to an intravenous/intramuscular injection of glucagon (1-mg dose in adults). Patients with HH will have increased glycogen stores, and giving glucagon will result in glycogenolysis. A positive response is defined as a maximal increment at least 25 mg/dL (1.3 mmol/L) greater than the terminal fasting serum glucose.

During the 72-hour prolonged fast, blood should also be collected for measurement of plasma sulfonylureas and meglitinides if the patient develops hypoglycemia. Sulfonylureas stimulate pancreatic β-cell insulin and C-peptide secretion, and the biochemical pattern is similar to that of an insulinoma.

Mixed-Meal Test

A mixed-meal test is performed in patients in whom there is a history suggestive of neuroglycopenic symptoms for up to 5 hours after food ingestion (Table 230-4). A positive test is defined as the onset of neuroglycopenic symptoms in association a documented low blood glucose level (e.g., ≤50 mg/dL). In postprandial HH, plasma insulin and C-peptide levels might be inappropriately elevated. Neuroglycopenic symptoms after a meal are reported in patients with insulinoma, patients with NIPHS, and patients who have undergone surgery for obesity.

The combination of a positive mixed-meal test and a negative 72-hour fast may occur in a patient with insulinoma or with NIPHS. The 5-hour oral glucose tolerance test should not be used as a diagnostic test for hypoglycemia, because a substantial percentage of healthy persons may have a serum glucose concentration of 50 mg/dL (2.7 mmol/L) or less.

Insulin Antibodies

Insulin autoimmune syndrome (IAS) is an uncommon cause of HH characterized by autoantibodies to endogenous insulin in individuals without previous exposure to exogenous insulin. IAS is the third leading cause of spontaneous hypoglycemia in Japan, and is increasingly being recognized worldwide in non-Asian populations. In patients with insulin autoimmune hypoglycemia from the spontaneous generation of insulin antibodies, such antibodies may be monoclonal or polyclonal and are present in very high titers, in contrast to the much lower titers in insulin-treated diabetes. It is important to test for the presence of insulin antibodies, because even low titers—which may have no diagnostic significance—may cause spurious results of the assay for insulin. Hypoglycemia due to IAS typically occurs in the fasting period but can occur postprandially as well.

Radiologic Investigations

Noninvasive imaging procedures such as CT and magnetic resonance imaging (MRI) are used when a diagnosis of insulinoma has been made to localize the source of pathologic insulin secretion. Invasive modalities, such as endoscopic ultrasonography (EUS) and arterial stimulation venous sampling (ASVS), are highly accurate in the preoperative localization of insulinomas and have frequently been shown to be superior to noninvasive localization techniques.[16] Intraoperative manual palpation of the pancreas by an experienced surgeon and intraoperative ultrasonography are both sensitive methods with which to finalize the location of insulinomas.

The sensitivity of transabdominal ultrasonography in the localization of insulinomas is poor (ranging from 9% to 64%). However, insulinomas demonstrate characteristic features when imaged with both CT and MRI, and the sensitivity of these techniques is 33 to 64% and 40 to 90%, respectively. The sensitivity and specificity of MRI is generally superior to that of CT, as is the detection of extrapancreatic extensions. Insulinomas generally demonstrate low signal intensity on T1-weighted images and high signal intensity on T2-weighted images.

Invasive modalities such as EUS and ASVS have been shown to be highly accurate in the preoperative localization of insulinomas and have frequently been shown to be superior to noninvasive localization techniques. EUS is currently the test of choice in most Western centers, with reported detection rates of 86.6 to 92.3%.

ASVS has greatly facilitated the precise regionalization of insulinomas smaller than 2 cm, which noninvasive techniques like ultrasonography, CT, and MRI often fail to localize. This test requires access to intra-abdominal vessels, including the right hepatic vein, splenic artery, gastroduodenal artery, and superior mesenteric artery. A two- to three-fold increase in insulin concentration in the right hepatic vein in response to calcium injection into one or more of the arteries supplying the pancreas suggests that the region served by that artery may harbor abnormally functioning β-cells, whether from insulinoma or islet hypertrophy or nesidioblastosis. Calcium injection will stimulate a brisk response of insulin, C-peptide, and proinsulin simultaneously, and the magnitude of increase of both insulin and C-peptide appears to be correlated well with the degree of differentiation of the tumor cells.

Insulinomas have been shown to express GLP-1R in high density, and GLP-1R imaging has been used in a few patients for insulinoma localization. Fluorine-18-L-dihydroxyphenylalanine (18F-DOPA) positron emission tomography (PET) has also been used in localizing neuroendocrine tumors. In children with congenital HH, 18F-DOPA PET/CT is the gold standard for localizing focal lesions prior to surgery. 18F-DOPA PET has been found to be useful in some patients with insulinoma who had negative CT, MRI, and ultrasound results.

The positive responses to selective arterial calcium stimulation in some patients with NIPHS, despite negative radiologic localizing studies, establish that this technique should be performed in all adults with HH of unknown etiology.

Protein/Leucine Sensitivity Testing

Protein sensitivity is observed in some patients with congenital HH. Typically, mutations in the genes *ABCC8/KCNJ11*, *GDH*, and *HADH* lead to protein-induced hypoglycemia. These patients will demonstrate severe hypoglycemia in response to a protein or leucine load.

Exercise Test

In some patients, exercise can trigger unregulated insulin secretion. This is referred to as exercise-induced hyperinsulinism. Promoter-activating mutations induce expression of the *SLC16A1* gene in β-cells, where this gene is not usually transcribed, permitting pyruvate uptake and pyruvate-stimulated insulin release despite ensuing hypoglycemia. A physical exercise test will identify this group of patients.

Genetic Studies

Genetic testing should be undertaken in children who have been diagnosed with congenital HH and other causes of hypoglycemia that might have a genetic basis. Mutation in the genes *ABCC8/KCNJ11* is the commonest cause of medically unresponsive congenital HH. All patients with insulinoma and noninsulinoma islet cell tumors should be tested for mutations in the *MEN1* gene.

TREATMENT   Rx

The correct management of hypoglycemia will depend on the underlying cause. Therefore, establishing the correct diagnosis is fundamentally important in both children and adults.

Emergency Management

Acute management of hypoglycemia involves giving a bolus of intravenous glucose (in adults a bolus of 50% dextrose) to correct the blood glucose level. This will then need to be followed by an infusion of 10% dextrose to maintain normoglycemia. Glucagon can be used in the emergency management of hypoglycemia (in emergency, give 1 mg stat intramuscularly). Glucagon can cause rebound hypoglycemia, so the patient will need blood glucose monitoring after the administration of glucagon.

Management of Specific Causes of Hypoglycemia

The long-term management of hypoglycemia depends on the underlying cause. Below is a summary of the management of the different types of hypoglycemia.

Hyperinsulinemic Hypoglycemia

Diazoxide (5 to 20 mg/kg/day given orally three times daily) is the first-line medical therapy in children and adults with HH. Fluid retention is a major side effect. Diazoxide may be combined with a diuretic to reduce the side effect of fluid retention. Second-line therapies include the use of octreotide (5 to

35 µg/kg/day as an infusion or injection 3 or 4 times daily) and glucagon (1 to 10 µg/kg/hour given as a subcutaneous or intravenous infusion).

For adult patients with insulinoma, pancreatectomy is the treatment of choice.[17] However, there are reports of insulinoma in adults responding to therapy with diazoxide and octreotide (including long-acting octreotide). The mTOR inhibitor everolimus has been reported to be effective in controlling hypoglycemia in patients with malignant insulinomas or those who cannot undergo surgical resection. Adult patients with PPHH after gastric bypass surgery can be treated with diazoxide and octreotide, but some will require pancreatectomy.[18] The insulin autoimmune syndrome will respond to therapy with glucocorticoids, but some patients have responded to diazoxide and octreotide. NICTH or IGF-2-oma patients will require resection of the primary tumor.

Hypoglycemia Due to Hormonal Deficiencies

Adult patients and children with GH and cortisol deficiency will require replacement therapy with recombinant GH and hydrocortisone (prednisolone), respectively. Replacement therapy with gluco- and mineralocorticoids can be life-saving in patients with adrenal insufficiency.

Hypoglycemia Due to Glycogen Storage Diseases

Patients with hypoglycemia due to disorders of hepatic glycogen storage and release need to avoid prolonged periods of fasting. Children will require overnight continuous feeding. Raw, uncooked cornstarch is commonly used as a slow-release source of glucose and helps with prolonging the period of fasting.

Hypoglycemia Due to Defects in Fatty Acid Oxidation, Disorders of Gluconeogenesis, and Disorders of Ketone Body Metabolism

Principles similar to those already discussed also apply to these patients. However, patients with fatty acid oxidation disorders should have carnitine supplementation.

GENERAL REFERENCES

For the General References and other additional features, please visit Expert Consult at https://expertconsult.inkling.com.

231

POLYGLANDULAR DISORDERS

LYNNETTE K. NIEMAN AND ALLEN M. SPIEGEL

DEFINITION AND CLINICAL SIGNIFICANCE

Polyglandular syndromes are disorders in which there is dysfunction and pathology of more than one endocrine gland. These disorders can be classified into (a) neoplastic syndromes in which there is abnormal endocrine cell proliferation, and often, but not invariably, hormone hypersecretion, and (b) into autoimmune syndromes in which there is evidence of immune destruction of endocrine cells, often resulting in hypofunction and reduced hormone secretion. Both the neoplastic and autoimmune polyglandular syndromes often have nonendocrine manifestations that are relatively syndrome specific.

With few exceptions, the polyglandular syndromes are due to germline mutations of key growth regulatory genes (neoplastic syndromes) or immune regulatory genes (autoimmune syndromes).[1] It is important to recognize these disorders and differentiate them from sporadic single–endocrine gland diseases for several reasons. First, recognition of a specific polyglandular syndrome should alert the clinician to look for other endocrine and extra-endocrine manifestations of the syndrome. Although some patients will present with multiple endocrine gland manifestations, some will initially present with only a single endocrine gland affected. Careful family history and screening for other endocrine and characteristic extra-endocrine manifestations is needed in such cases. Second, treatment of polyglandular disease may differ from treatment of individual gland disease. Third, because of the

TABLE 231-1 POLYGLANDULAR NEOPLASIA SYNDROMES

SYNDROME	GENETIC BASIS*	ENDOCRINE TUMORS	NONENDOCRINE FEATURES
MEN 1	MEN1	Parathyroid Anterior pituitary Pancreatic islet	Subcutaneous lipomas Skin collagenomas
MEN 2 (A and B)	RET	Medullary thyroid cancer Pheochromocytoma Parathyroid (2A)	Mucosal neuromas (2B) Megacolon (2B)
MEN 4	CDNK1B	Anterior pituitary Parathyroid	Renal tumors
Carney complex	PKAR1A	Adrenal cortex Anterior pituitary Thyroid	Atrial myxomas Skin lentigines
von Hippel-Lindau disease	VHL	Pheochromocytoma Pancreatic islet	Renal cell cancer CNS hemangioblastoma
McCune-Albright syndrome	GNAS (mosaic)	Thyroid Anterior pituitary Adrenal cortex Gonads	Fibrous dysplasia Café au lait skin lesions

*With the exception of McCune-Albright, all syndromes are caused by heterozygous germline mutations of the gene listed and show autosomal dominant inheritance.
CA = cancer; CNS = central nervous system.

genetic basis of most of these syndromes, taking a careful family history and, in some cases, screening other family members to allow disease prevention in affected individuals is indicated.

This chapter discusses the best-characterized polyglandular disorders. Other chapters on the anterior pituitary (Chapter 224), thyroid (Chapter 226), adrenal cortex (Chapter 227), adrenal medulla (Chapter 228), pancreatic islets (Chapters 195 and 230), and parathyroids (Chapter 245) should be consulted for more detailed discussion of the diseases of individual glands.

NEOPLASTIC SYNDROMES

Six distinct neoplastic syndromes involve more than one endocrine gland. These include multiple endocrine neoplasia type 1 (MEN 1), multiple endocrine neoplasia types 2A (MEN 2) and 2B (sometimes referred to as MEN 3), multiple endocrine neoplasia type 4 (MEN 4), Carney complex,[2] von Hippel-Lindau disease (VHL), and McCune-Albright syndrome (MAS) (Table 231-1).[3] All but the latter are caused by heterozygous germline mutations and are inherited in autosomal dominant fashion. The genes responsible for MEN 1 and 4, Carney complex, and von Hippel-Lindau disease act as tumor suppressor genes. Germline loss-of-function mutations in one allele are followed by somatic mutations inactivating the second normal allele, leading to tumorigenesis. The basis for the tissue-specific expression of both the endocrine and extra-endocrine manifestations of these syndromes is not well understood, but the germline nature of the mutation and the expression of the affected gene in more than one endocrine gland explains the polyglandular aspect of the disorder. MEN 2A and B, in contrast, are caused by germline activating mutations of an oncogene, RET. The pattern of expression of this gene, involving chromaffin cells, helps explain the specific clinical manifestations. McCune-Albright syndrome is caused by a somatic rather than germline mutation that constitutively activates the ubiquitously expressed GNAS gene. This mutation, which may occur early in embryogenesis, leads to unregulated cyclic adenosine monophosphate (cAMP) formation in affected cells. The resultant mosaic distribution of the mutant gene helps explain the pleiotropic manifestations of the disease.

Patients with polyglandular neoplastic syndromes typically present with their respective endocrine tumors at a younger age than patients with single-gland sporadic endocrine tumors. Treatment of the polyglandular neoplastic syndromes, both in terms of the neoplastic component and the hormone hypersecretion, poses greater challenges than treatment of individual endocrine tumors.[4] For disorders with high risk of fatal cancer, such as medullary thyroid cancer in MEN 2, early genetic diagnosis and prophylactic surgical removal of the thyroid is indicated.[5] In other disorders such as MEN 1 and Carney complex, less aggressive approaches such as selective tumor resection and pharmacologic treatment to reduce hormone hypersecretion may be more appropriate. More detailed discussion of the clinical features, diagnosis, and treatment of these neoplastic syndromes may be found in other chapters

TABLE 231-2 CLINICAL FEATURES OF AUTOIMMUNE POLYGLANDULAR SYNDROMES

FEATURE	TYPE 1	TYPE 2
Mucocutaneous candidiasis	Very common	Not seen
Hypoparathyroidism	Common	Rare
Addison's disease	Common	Common
Primary hypogonadism	Common	Occurs
Autoimmune thyroid disease	Rare	Common
Autoimmune diabetes	Occurs	Common
Hypophysitis	Occurs	Occurs
Autoimmune hepatitis	Occurs	Not seen
Pernicious anemia	Occurs	Occurs
Vitiligo	Occurs	Occurs
Malabsorption syndrome	Occurs	Occurs as celiac disease
Alopecia	Common	Occurs
Myasthenia gravis	Not seen	Occurs
Keratopathy	Common	Not seen
Tympanic membrane calcification	Common	Not seen
Inheritance	Autosomal recessive	HLA association
Age at onset	Usually childhood	Usually adulthood

HLA = human leukocyte antigen.

(MEN 1 in Chapter 245; MEN 2 and 3 in Chapter 246; McCune-Albright syndrome in Chapters 233 and 235).

AUTOIMMUNE SYNDROMES

Organ-specific autoimmune disease, characterized by lymphocytic infiltration and organ-specific autoantibodies, commonly results in endocrine hypofunction. Not uncommonly, however, disorders of more than one endocrine gland appear in families or individual patients. Characteristic patterns of disease presentation and genetic inheritance allow the definition of two syndromes with overlapping manifestations (Table 231-2).[6]

Autoimmune Polyglandular Syndrome Type 1

DEFINITION

Autoimmune polyglandular syndrome (APS) type 1 is a rare disease that is also known as autoimmune polyendocrinopathy, candidiasis, and ectodermal dystrophy syndrome. It typically manifests in early childhood.

PATHOGENESIS

APS type 1 is an autosomal recessive disorder caused by a variety of inactivating mutations in the gene encoding autoimmune regulator-1 (AIRE-1),[7] which controls the expression of autoantigens by medullary epithelial cells of the thymus. These antigens are also expressed in peripheral tissues. Their expression in the thymus is important for negative selection (elimination) of autoreactive T cells, which underlies the development of (self-) tolerance. These autoreactive T cells escape to the periphery in the absence of AIRE, and if activated, induce autoimmune destruction of the specific tissue. The appearance of organ-specific autoantibodies precedes disease presentation and predicts the development of specific end-organ damage. The role of these antibodies is unknown, however.

CLINICAL MANIFESTATIONS

Mucocutaneous candidiasis (Chapter 338) occurs in virtually all patients and is usually the first manifestation of disease. Hypoparathyroidism and Addison's disease are the most common endocrine manifestations; each of these diseases occurs in 70 to 80% of patients. Hypoparathyroidism usually precedes Addison's disease; both diseases typically manifest before age 15 years. Premature ovarian failure (in 60% of affected women) usually presents as secondary amenorrhea; testicular failure occurs less frequently. Insulin-dependent diabetes mellitus occurs in 12% of patients, usually in adulthood; hypothyroidism is uncommon.

Nonendocrine components of this syndrome, in addition to the mucocutaneous candidiasis, include alopecia, vitiligo, corneal opacities, autoimmune hepatitis, enamel hypoplasia of teeth, tympanic membrane calcification, nail dystrophy that correlates only loosely with obvious candidiasis, parietal cell atrophy and vitamin B_{12} malabsorption, and more general intestinal malabsorption with steatorrhea. Asplenism, with Howell-Jolly bodies on peripheral blood smears (Chapter 157), has been noted in several patients. Each of the disease components should be sought when any patient presents with hypoparathyroidism, primary adrenal insufficiency, or mucocutaneous candidiasis.[8]

TREATMENT **Rx**

The hypoparathyroidism is treated, like the sporadic disease, with oral calcium and 1,25-dihydroxyvitamin D, although variable intestinal malabsorption can present a particular therapeutic challenge. The candidiasis can be satisfactorily controlled with ketoconazole. Primary adrenal insufficiency is treated with glucocorticoid and mineralocorticoid replacement.

PROGNOSIS

The prognosis of the variably expressed hormonal disorders is similar to that of their sporadic counterparts. When the diagnosis of APS type 1 is made, surveys for other components of the syndrome can allow earlier treatment than would otherwise occur.

Autoimmune Polyglandular Syndrome Type 2
PATHOGENESIS

APS type 2 is usually inherited in families with characteristic (normal) variants of genes that regulate the presentation of antigens to T cells and subsequent T-cell function. The most common genetic locus associated with this syndrome is the human leukocyte antigen (HLA) locus, particularly the B8, DR3, and D4 alleles.[9] The HLA associations do not predict disease absolutely, even in identical twins, so environmental factors must contribute to disease presentation. Abnormal expression of the gene encoding cytotoxic T-lymphocyte antigen-4 (CTLA-4) can also predispose to APS type 2. The protein tyrosine phosphatase nonreceptor type 22 gene that encodes the lymphoid tyrosine phosphatase opposes signaling from the activated T-cell receptor. A variant of this gene is enriched in families with both type 1 diabetes mellitus and autoimmune thyroid disease. Genome-wide association studies have identified a large number of genes associated with type 1 diabetes. Although this approach has not yet been used for APS type 2, it seems likely that many of the genes identified in these studies will prove relevant because a large fraction of them appear to influence immune responsiveness.

CLINICAL MANIFESTATIONS

APS type 2 is considerably more common than type 1 and typically manifests in the fourth decade of life. Insulin-dependent diabetes mellitus and thyroid dysfunction, either autoimmune hypothyroidism or Graves disease, are the most frequent manifestations. Addison's disease (Chapter 227) is the third major endocrine component of this disorder. Although most patients who present with autoimmune diabetes or thyroid disease have clinical involvement of only one gland, many patients with autoimmune Addison's disease develop clinically evident disease in other endocrine glands. Less common components of the type 2 APS include primary hypogonadism and hypophysitis. Pernicious anemia, vitiligo, celiac disease, alopecia, and myasthenia gravis are also associated with this syndrome.

Organ-specific antibodies appear before clinical disease and predict subsequent disease. The role of these antibodies in organ hypofunction has not been established, however.

TREATMENT **Rx**

The treatment of each component of this syndrome is identical to the treatment of each disorder in isolation, although possible clustering of diseases must be kept in mind during the evaluation and follow-up of all patients with each individual component disorder. Thyroid hormone therapy can precipitate symptoms of adrenal insufficiency in patients with both disorders. Consequently, a careful history (including family history), physical examination, and a low threshold for specific laboratory testing for adrenal insufficiency should be part of the evaluation of every patient with autoimmune hypothyroidism. Further, combinations of hypothyroidism, adrenal insufficiency, and hypogonadism can mimic hypopituitarism, although specific hormonal testing (Chapter 224) can easily distinguish these disorders. Because multiple components of the syndrome can appear asynchronously, periodic evaluation for the early appearance of additional disease components is indicated.

PROGNOSIS

The prognosis of the individual components of APS type 2 is the same as for the sporadic versions of each component.

GENERAL REFERENCES

For the General References and other additional features, please visit Expert Consult at https://expertconsult.inkling.com.

232
NEUROENDOCRINE TUMORS AND THE CARCINOID SYNDROME

KENNETH R. HANDE

NEUROENDOCRINE TUMORS: DESCRIPTION, INCIDENCE, AND PRESENTATION

Neuroendocrine tumors are cancers that arise from enterochromaffin cells found throughout the body. A "carcinoid tumor" implies a well-differentiated neuroendocrine tumor and excludes high-grade or poorly differentiated neuroendocrine tumors. Although several classification systems for neuroendocrine tumors currently exist, there has been a shift away from the term *carcinoid tumor* in favor of the term *well-differentiated neuroendocrine tumor*.[1]

Well-differentiated neuroendocrine tumors, or carcinoids, occur most often in the lung (30% of all carcinoid tumors), small intestine (25%), rectum (15%), appendix (10%), and stomach (5%) but may be seen in many other organs. Typical well-differentiated neuroendocrine tumors demonstrate a histologic pattern of dense nests of cells of uniform size and nuclear appearance that contain secretory granules. The neurosecretory granules contain various amines such as 5-hydroxytryptamine (serotonin), peptides, tachykinins, and prostaglandins. Low-grade neuroendocrine tumors have a low mutation rate compared to most neoplasms. Mutations in key oncogenic pathways, such as the PI3K/AKT/mTOR pathway, have been identified.[2] The incidence of carcinoid tumors (2 to 5 per 100,000 population) has been increasing over the past 20 years.[3] Because carcinoid tumors are relatively slow growing, their prevalence is actually greater than that of esophageal, gastric, or pancreatic cancers. Carcinoid tumors may be associated with multiple endocrine neoplasia type 1 (MEN 1) syndrome (Chapter 231). Thymic carcinoid tumors present in patients with MEN 1 portend a worse prognosis.[4]

Patients with neuroendocrine tumors present either with symptoms related to tumor mass or symptoms resulting from the release of biologically active peptides into blood. Abdominal pain from a tumor mass or bowel obstruction related to the desmoplastic reaction in the surrounding mesentery is a common presenting symptom. The desmoplastic reaction is believed to develop in response to the secretion of growth factors such as platelet-derived growth factor, insulin-like growth factor, epidermal growth factor, and transforming growth factor-β. Infrequently, primary tumors cause hemoptysis or gastrointestinal bleeding. Hepatomegaly may be noted at diagnosis. Other patients may present with symptoms related to the systemic release of peptides from tumor cells, referred to as the carcinoid syndrome.

THE CARCINOID SYNDROME

The term *carcinoid syndrome* refers to the systemic signs and symptoms resulting from the release of neuroendocrine mediators by some carcinoid tumors. Cutaneous flushing, diarrhea, and cardiac valvular lesions are the most common manifestations of the carcinoid syndrome. Only 8 to 10% of all neuroendocrine tumors are associated with the carcinoid syndrome, usually ileal carcinoids with hepatic metastases. Carcinoids from different primary sites possess unique clinical characteristics. Carcinoid tumors arising from organs of the embryonic foregut (e.g., bronchus, stomach, pancreas, and thyroid) are infrequently associated with the carcinoid syndrome; carcinoids from the distal large intestine may metastasize but do not exhibit endocrine effects.

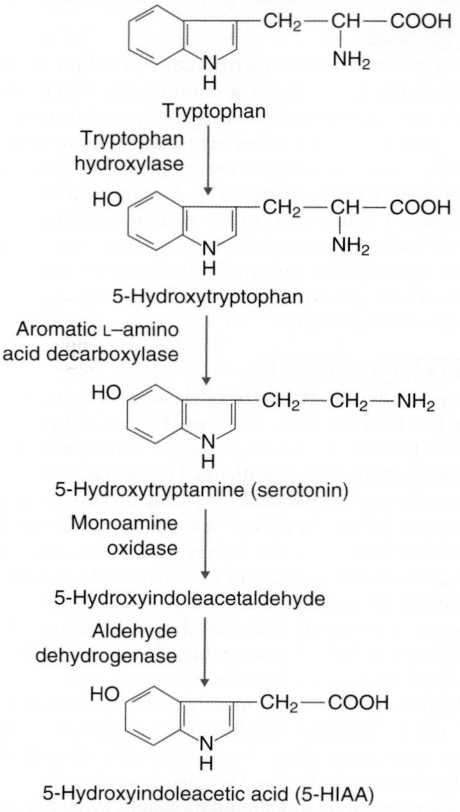

PATHOPHYSIOLOGY OF THE CARCINOID SYNDROME

The carcinoid syndrome results from the production of a variety of biologically active substances by the neuroendocrine tumor cells, including serotonin, tachykinins, histamine, and prostaglandins. Most low-grade neuroendocrine tumors contain the enzyme tryptophan hydroxylase, which catalyzes the formation of 5-hydroxytryptophan (5-HTP) from tryptophan (Fig. 232-1). The typical ileal carcinoid tumor also contains aromatic L-amino-acid decarboxylase, which catalyzes the conversion of 5-HTP to 5-hydroxytryptamine (5-HT or serotonin). Following its release, serotonin is oxidized to 5-hydroxyindoleacetaldehyde and rapidly converted to 5-hydroxyindoleacetic acid (5-HIAA) by aldehyde dehydrogenase. This acid is excreted into the urine, and almost all circulating serotonin can be accounted for as urinary 5-HIAA. Tachykinins are also stored in neuroendocrine tumors. Of these, neuropeptide K, neurokinins A and B, and substance P have been identified in tumors and blood from patients with the carcinoid syndrome. Some carcinoid tumors, particularly those of gastric origin, release excessive amounts of histamine. Secretion of a variety of prostaglandins by carcinoids has also been demonstrated. Neuroendocrine tumors, particularly of the thymus and lung, have been associated with ectopic production of adrenocorticotropic hormone and growth hormone–releasing hormone.

Serotonin contributes to the intestinal hypermotility and diarrhea associated with the carcinoid syndrome. A secondary effect of serotonin overproduction occurs when a large fraction of dietary tryptophan is shunted into the hydroxylation pathway, leaving less tryptophan available for the formation of nicotinic acid and protein. When urinary excretion of 5-HIAA exceeds 100 mg/day, low levels of plasma tryptophan and evidence of nicotinic acid deficiency (pellagra) can be seen. The interaction of serotonin with platelets and the cardiac endothelium is considered the cause of carcinoid heart disease. This hypothesis is supported by the finding of valvular heart disease in patients who took appetite suppressants, such as fenfluramine, that release serotonin. The risk of valvular heart disease in patients with the carcinoid syndrome is correlated with the amount of 5-HIAA excreted in the urine.

Most evidence points to the tachykinins as mediators of the carcinoid flush. Tachykinins are known vasodilators. Tachykinin levels are increased during pentagastrin-induced flushing; when pentagastrin-induced flushing is inhibited by somatostatin, the rise in tachykinin levels is also blocked. Serotonin does not appear to be the mediator of flushing. Flushing attacks can be attributed to histamine in certain gastric carcinoids. Flushing can be triggered

FIGURE 232-1. Synthesis and degradation of serotonin.

by catecholamines, and this probably accounts for the association of flushing with exercise and emotional stimuli. Injection of isoproterenol or pentagastrin can also trigger flushing, an action that may explain the provocation of flushes by eating in some patients. The carcinoid syndrome occurs when mediators produced by the tumor and normally metabolized by the liver escape into the systemic circulation. Thus, most patients with the carcinoid syndrome have hepatic metastasis.

CLINICAL MANIFESTATIONS OF THE CARCINOID SYNDROME

VASODILATOR PAROXYSMS. Cutaneous flushing, which occurs in 80% of patients with the carcinoid syndrome, is the most common clinical feature. The typical flush is dark red to violaceous and involves the head, neck, and upper trunk (blush area). The flush usually lasts for 30 seconds to 3 minutes. Neuroendocrine tumors of the foregut produce a slightly different flush, characteristically bright salmon pink to red. Prolonged flushing attacks may be associated with lacrimation and periorbital edema. The flush may be accompanied by tachycardia. The blood pressure usually falls or does not change. A rise in blood pressure during flushing is rare, and the carcinoid syndrome is not a cause of sustained hypertension. Flushing may be provoked by excitement, exertion, eating, and ethanol ingestion. In patients with the bronchial carcinoid variant, flushing may last for hours. In addition to paroxysms of cutaneous vasodilatation, some patients develop telangiectasias, which are most marked in the malar area. These patients may have the characteristic features of rosacea.

GASTROINTESTINAL SYMPTOMS. Intestinal hypermotility with borborygmi and cramping occurs in 50 to 70% of patients with the carcinoid syndrome. Explosive secretory diarrhea may occur, although chronic diarrhea with a secretory component is more common. When diarrhea is severe, malabsorption may occur. Gastrointestinal transit times through the small and large bowel are two- to six-fold faster than in physiologically normal patients.

PELLAGRA. Tryptophan is normally used to form nicotinic acid. In patients with the carcinoid syndrome, up to 60% of dietary tryptophan may be used to form 5-HTP and 5-HT. Nicotinic acid levels are occasionally depleted, resulting in symptoms of pellagra (dermatitis, diarrhea, and dementia) (Chapter 218).

CARDIAC MANIFESTATIONS. Symptomatic valvular heart disease is present in 15 to 20% of patients with the carcinoid syndrome (Chapter 60). Up to 50% of patients have echocardiographic evidence of heart disease.[5] Plaque-like thickening of the endocardium of the valvular cusps and cardiac chambers occurs primarily on the right side of the heart but may rarely involve the left side (<10%). Lesions of the tricuspid valve (usually regurgitation) are present in 65% of patients with carcinoid heart disease, and pulmonic valvular disease (again, usually regurgitation) is seen in 20%.

OTHER SYMPTOMS. Generalized fatigue and debilitation are underappreciated features of the carcinoid syndrome. Bronchoconstriction, usually most pronounced during flushing attacks, is a less common feature of the syndrome, but when it occurs it may be severe. Attacks of severe and sustained flushing with life-threatening hemodynamic compromise and bronchoconstriction are referred to as carcinoid crisis. Precipitating factors include anesthesia, surgery, tumor necrosis, and catecholamine infusion. Cognitive impairment has also been associated with the carcinoid syndrome.[6]

DIAGNOSIS

When all its clinical features are present, the carcinoid syndrome is easily recognized. The diagnosis also must be considered when any one of its clinical manifestations is present. The diagnostic hallmark consists of overproduction of 5-hydroxyindoles accompanied by increased excretion of urinary 5-HIAA in a patient with a biopsy-proven carcinoid tumor. Normally, excretion of 5-HIAA does not exceed 10 mg/day. Ingestion of foods containing serotonin may complicate the biochemical diagnosis of the carcinoid syndrome; bananas, walnuts, and certain other foods contain enough serotonin to produce abnormally elevated urinary excretion of 5-HIAA after their ingestion. Selected drugs (e.g., guaifenesin, acetaminophen) may also falsely elevate urinary 5-HIAA measurements. When dietary 5-hydroxyindoles are excluded, urinary excretion of 25 mg/day of 5-HIAA is diagnostic of the carcinoid syndrome. Elevation in the range of 9 to 25 mg/day may be seen with the carcinoid syndrome, nontropical sprue, vomiting, or acute intestinal obstruction. Measurement of serotonin in blood or platelets is of interest but has less diagnostic value than assay of the major metabolite of serotonin in the urine. Plasma chromogranin A concentrations are often elevated in carcinoid patients, including those who do not have the carcinoid syndrome, and may serve as a marker of tumor mass. The diagnostic value of plasma chromogranin A is relatively low, however, because this substance is increased in patients with renal failure, atrophic gastritis, and patients taking proton pump inhibitors. Assessment of the extent and localization of both primary and metastatic tumor is aided by computed tomography of the abdomen and chest and by imaging with radionuclide-labeled somatostatin receptor ligands.

The typical carcinoid syndrome usually results from tumors of midgut origin, which almost invariably secrete serotonin. In contrast, tumors arising from the embryonic foregut have a lower serotonin content and may secrete 5-HTP. Patients with gastric carcinoids may exhibit unique flushing, beginning as bright, patchy erythema with sharply delineated serpentine borders that coalesce as the blush heightens. Food ingestion is especially likely to produce flushes. With carcinoid tumors arising from the bronchus, attacks of flushing tend to be prolonged and severe and may be associated with periorbital edema, excessive lacrimation and salivation, hypotension, tachycardia, anxiety, and tremulousness. This group is therapeutically unique in that severe flushes can sometimes be prevented by corticosteroids.

Differential Diagnosis of the Carcinoid Syndrome

Attacks of flushing in a patient with normal urinary excretion of 5-HIAA raise other diagnostic possibilities. Systemic mastocyte activation disorders, including systemic mastocytosis (Chapter 255) and idiopathic anaphylaxis (Chapter 253), produce flushing and diarrhea and should be considered when 5-HIAA excretion is not elevated. Flushing also occurs in genetically predisposed individuals following ethanol ingestion, in the postmenopausal state (Chapter 240), and in conjunction with other neuroendocrine tumors such as VIPomas and medullary carcinomas of the thyroid.

Somatostatin Analogues

More than 80% of neuroendocrine tumors have somatostatin receptors on the cell surface. Somatostatin can bind to these receptors and prevent flushing and other endocrine symptoms. The development of analogues of somatostatin with longer biologic half-lives than the native hormone has made subcutaneous and intramuscular administration feasible and has been a major advance in the treatment of these patients.

Roughly 70% of patients with carcinoid syndrome have a 50% or greater reduction in the frequency of diarrhea and/or flushing with the use of octreotide, one of the somatostatin analogs. Therapy is usually associated with a decrease in urinary 5-HIAA excretion and in plasma tachykinin levels. With the improvement of endocrine symptoms and fatigue, a considerable improvement in quality of life may be achieved. Symptom control with octreotide can be durable, with 50 to 60% of patients continuing to have improvement in symptoms of diarrhea and flushing following 12 months of therapy.[7] Long-acting somatostatin analogues (octreotide LAR and lanreotide) have been developed, permitting once-monthly dosing. Two to 4 weeks may be required to achieve steady-state levels of octreotide following administration of octreotide LAR, during which time supplementation with subcutaneous octreotide may be needed. Octreotide is generally well tolerated. However, it may suppress pancreatic exocrine function, causing steatorrhea, abnormal glucose control, and inhibition of the release of cholecystokinin. Hyperglycemia, symptomatic cholelithiasis, steatorrhea, and hypoglycemia are seen in 9, 15, 3, and 2% of patients, respectively. Octreotide should be used to prevent carcinoid crises that accompany the massive release of mediators that may occur during operative procedures. In patients with histamine-secreting gastric neuroendocrine tumors, blockade of both histamine (H_1) and H_2 receptors ameliorates flushing. In patients receiving octreotide, regression in tumor mass is uncommon. However, octreotide slows the growth rate of low-grade neuroendocrine tumors. With octreotide therapy, disease stability is seen in 65% of patients at 6-month follow-up, compared to only 35% of patients not receiving octreotide.[A1]

Surgery

Early diagnosis of the carcinoid syndrome leads to complete surgical cure in the few neuroendocrine tumors that release their humoral mediators directly into the systemic circulation (e.g., bronchial carcinoids). In contrast, tumors that release humoral substances into the portal circulation usually produce the syndrome only after hepatic metastases occur. Given the slow growth rate of low-grade neuroendocrine tumors, effective reduction in tumor mass can ameliorate morbidity and improve quality of life even after metastases have occurred. In selected patients, this goal can be achieved by surgical debulking of tumor, including partial hepatectomy for unilobar metastases, excision of large superficial hepatic metastases, and removal of the primary tumor and regional lymph nodes. In selected series,[8] over 90% of patients report symptom relief from pain and/or carcinoid syndrome following cytoreductive surgery (50 to 70%, complete relief). Median time to recurrence of symptoms is 3 years, and overall survival is greater than 5 years. Elective cholecystectomy during the surgical intervention prevents cholelithiasis that may result from octreotide treatment. Because the blood supply of hepatic metastases is largely arterial, percutaneous embolization of the hepatic arterial supply to the most involved hepatic lobe can shrink inoperable hepatic metastases; however, the procedure carries a risk of serious complications, with mortality of up to 6%.[9] In selected series, 90% of patients report improvement in symptoms for an average of 2 years' duration. Median survival in embolized patients has been 24 to 30 months. Valve replacement surgery is indicated in severe disease, in which it can usually improve life expectancy (Chapter 60).[10]

Chemotherapy

In contrast to high-grade, poorly differentiated neuroendocrine cancers, chemotherapy with single or combination cytotoxic agents rarely produces tumor regression in low-grade neuroendocrine tumors. However, recent studies suggest that several drugs, including the antiangiogenic agents bevacizumab and sunitinib and the mTOR inhibitor everolimus, may slow the growth rate of low-grade neuroendocrine tumors. In a randomized double-blind placebo-controlled study,[A2] 10 mg/day of everolimus increased progression-free survival from 11 months in control patients to 16 months (hazard ratio, 0.77). No overall survival advantage was noted, however, and stomatitis, rash, fatigue, and diarrhea are noted treatment side effects. For patients who exhibit tumor progression or whose clinical syndrome has failed to improve following cytoreduction and octreotide, everolimus may be considered for palliative therapy.

TREATMENT Rx

Treatment of the carcinoid syndrome is directed toward pharmacologic therapy for humorally mediated symptoms and at measures designed to reduce the tumor mass.

PROGNOSIS

The metastatic potential of localized carcinoid tumors correlates with tumor size, location, and histologic grade. Even when metastatic, typical neuroendocrine tumors generally have a slow rate of growth, and many patients survive for years after metastatic disease is recognized. Prior to development of therapies for the carcinoid syndrome, morbidity resulted from the endocrine manifestations of the tumor. However, with current therapy, symptoms of the carcinoid syndrome can usually be controlled. Death from typical neuroendocrine tumors is usually caused by complications associated with tumor growth, such as bowel obstruction or hepatic failure. A concerted strategy consisting of removal of the primary tumor, reduction in tumor bulk, and administration of octreotide can lead to considerable amelioration of symptoms, improvement in the quality of life, reduction in the release of the humoral substances that engender cardiac lesions, and prolongation of survival.[11] The median survival of patients with metastatic neuroendocrine tumors and the carcinoid syndrome now exceeds 5 years in carefully managed patients, with patients having small bowel primaries living longer than those with lung or colon primaries.

Grade A References

A1. Rinke A, Muller HH, Schade-Brittinger C, et al. Placebo-controlled, double-blind, prospective, randomized study of the effect of octreotide LAR in the control of tumor growth in patients with metastatic neuroendocrine midgut tumors: a report from the PROMID study group. *J Clin Oncol.* 2009;27:4656-4663.

A2. Pavel ME, Hainsworth JD, Baudin E, et al. Everolimus plus octreotide long-acting repeatable for the treatment of advanced neuroendocrine tumors associated with carcinoid syndrome (RADIANT-2): a randomized, placebo-controlled trial. *Lancet.* 2011;378:2005-2012.

GENERAL REFERENCES

For the General References and other additional features, please visit Expert Consult at https://expertconsult.inkling.com.

233

DISORDERS OF SEXUAL DEVELOPMENT

PERRIN C. WHITE

DEFINITION

This chapter reviews the concepts underlying the initial evaluation and management of patients with disorders of sexual development (DSD). By definition, such an individual has lack of concordance of various aspects of gender. These include chromosomal sex (46,XX, 46,XY, or other), gonadal or reproductive sex (ovaries, fallopian tubes, and uterus vs. testes, seminal vesicles, prostate gland, and ejaculatory ducts), genital sex (vagina and clitoris vs. scrotum and penis), and gender-specific behavior. Depending on chromosomal sex, most patients can be classified as incompletely masculinized 46,XY males, virilized 46,XX females, and patients with abnormalities of sex chromosomes, such as those with mixed gonadal dysgenesis. (In the past, 46,XY and 46,XX DSD patients were referred to as male and female pseudohermaphrodites, respectively, but these terms are no longer preferred.) Many conditions can cause DSD (Table 233-1).

Normal Sexual Differentiation
Gonadal Differentiation

At 5 to 6 weeks' gestation, the gonadal primordia (gonadal ridges) develop from the coelomic epithelium overlying the medial surface of the mesonephros (primitive kidneys; Fig. 233-1). These primitive gonads are identical in both sexes. Germ cells form at 3 to 4 weeks' gestation and migrate through the gut mesentery into the gonads at this early bipotential stage. Whether germ cells are directed toward male or female gametogenesis depends largely on the environment generated by surrounding somatic cells rather than on factors intrinsic to the germ cells.

During the seventh week, XY male gonads begin to differentiate under the influence of testis-determining genes.[1,2] The first to be expressed is *SRY*, the key gene on the Y chromosome controlling male differentiation, which initiates the development of Sertoli cells. Sertoli cells surround germ cells to form testis cords, which nourish primordial germ cells and direct them into the pathway for male gametogenesis. Recruitment of endothelial cells leads to development of a testis-specific vasculature that is required for normal organization of the testis.

TABLE 233-1	DISORDERS OF SEXUAL DEVELOPMENT*

VIRILIZATION OR SEX REVERSAL IN XX FEMALES

Virilizing forms of congenital adrenal hyperplasia
   21-Hydroxylase deficiency (1 : 16,000 births) [*CYP21*]: salt-wasting or simple virilizing forms
   11β-Hydroxylase deficiency [*CYP11B1*]
   3β-Hydroxysteroid dehydrogenase deficiency [*HSD3B2*]
   Cytochrome P-450 oxidoreductase deficiency (also has a maternal effect) [*POR*]
Maternal or exogenous androgens
   Drugs (danazol, progestins)
   Luteoma
   Aromatase deficiency [*CYP19*]
   Transcription factor mutations
Mutations in genes affecting gonadal differentiation
   SRY (translocation to X)
   SOX9 (duplication)
   WT1 (Denys-Drash syndrome)
Structural/idiopathic

UNDERVIRILIZATION OR SEX REVERSAL IN XY MALES

Biosynthetic defects
   Lipoid adrenal hyperplasia [*STAR*]
   17α-Hydroxylase/17,20 lyase [*CYP17*]
   3β-Hydroxysteroid dehydrogenase [*HSD3B2*]
   17-Ketosteroid reductase [*HSD17B3*]
   5α-Reductase [*SRD5A2*]
   Cytochrome P-450 oxidoreductase deficiency [*POR*]
   Smith-Lemli-Opitz syndrome (1 : 20,000) [*DHCR7*]
Androgen insensitivity (1 : 20,000) [*AR*]: complete or partial
Luteinizing hormone insensitivity [*LHR*]
Mutations in genes affecting gonadal differentiation
   SRY
   SOX9 (campomelic dysplasia)
   SF1 (sometimes associated with adrenal hypoplasia)
   WT1 (WAGR and Denys-Drash syndromes)
   DAX1 or WNT4 duplications
   DHH (associated with peripheral neuropathy)
   ATRX (X-linked α-thalassemia and mental retardation)
Exposure to 5α-reductase inhibitors, other endocrine disruptors

MICROPENIS

Panhypopituitarism [including *PROP1* mutations]
Septo-optic dysplasia [including *HESX* mutations]
Hypogonadotropic hypogonadism
   Kallmann syndrome [*KAL1*]
   Prader-Willi syndrome [paternal chromosome 15q11 deletion]
   Adrenal hypoplasia congenita [*DAX1*]
Vanishing testes (may also cause ambiguous genitalia)

OTHER SYNDROMES AFFECTING REPRODUCTIVE SYSTEMS

Chromosomal aneuploidy
   Turner syndrome (1 : 2500): 45,X; 45,X/46,XX mosaics; 46,XXr; 46,XXq–
   Klinefelter's syndrome (1 : 1000): 47,XXY
   Mixed gonadal dysgenesis (1 : 20,000): 45,X/46,XY; 45,X/47,XXY
   Other: Trisomy 13, trisomy 18, triploidy, 4p–, 13q–
Persistent müllerian duct syndrome in XY males
   Type 1 [*AMH*]
   Type 2 [*AMHR2*]
Mayer-Rokitansky-Küster-Hauser syndrome (vaginal atresia) (1 : 6000)

*Frequencies of relatively common (at least 1:20,000) diseases are noted in parentheses. When causative genetic mutations have been identified, the affected locus is noted in square brackets. WAGR = Wilms' tumor, aniridia, genitourinary abnormalities or gonadoblastoma, and mental retardation.

Steroidogenic cells develop from the mesonephros and migrate into the developing adrenal cortex and testis at 8 weeks. In the testis, they become Leydig cells, which secrete the testosterone required for subsequent male reproductive development. In the first trimester, testosterone secretion is mainly under the control of human chorionic gonadotropin (HCG); it subsequently requires luteinizing hormone (LH) secreted by the fetal anterior pituitary.

Ovaries are recognizable at approximately 10 weeks. The signaling molecule WNT4 plays an active role in ovarian development, repressing expression of testis-specific genes and vascular development.[3] Germ cells in the ovary continue into the first meiotic prophase beginning at 12 weeks' gestation and continuing until 7 months' gestation.

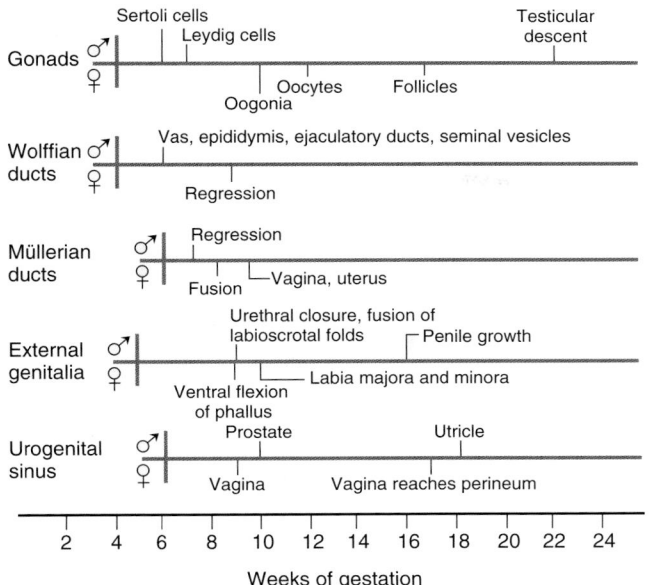

FIGURE 233-1. Time course of prenatal sexual differentiation in male and female fetuses. (Modified from Barthold JS, Gonzalez R. Intersex states. In: Gonzales ET, Bauer SB, eds. *Pediatric Urology Practice*. Philadelphia: Lippincott Williams & Wilkins; 1999.)

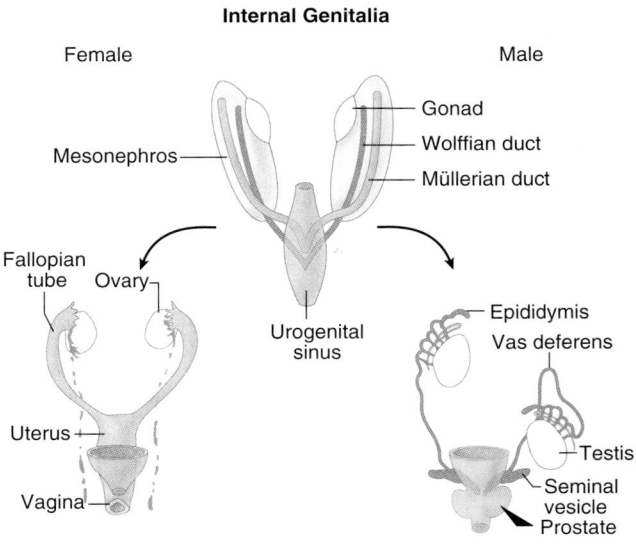

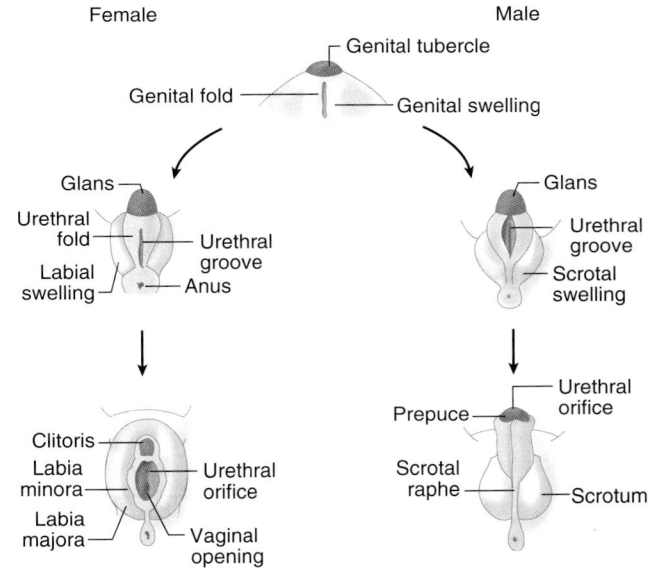

FIGURE 233-2. Differentiation of the internal and external genitalia of the human fetus. (Modified from Griffen JE, Ojeda SR, eds. *Textbook of Endocrine Physiology*. New York: Oxford University Press; 1996.)

Development of Male and Female Internal Reproductive Tracts

The reproductive tracts are derived from intermediate mesoderm. The male reproductive tract develops from the mesonephric (wolffian) ducts, and the female reproductive tract develops from the paramesonephric (müllerian) ducts (Fig. 233-2). Both sets of ducts are present in normal embryos.

Development of wolffian or müllerian structures depends on the presence or absence of normally functioning testes. The Sertoli cells secrete antimüllerian hormone (AMH, also termed müllerian inhibiting substance) starting when the testes differentiate.[4] Expression of AMH is controlled by several transcription factors: SF1 and WT1 (Wilms' tumor locus) synergize to promote transcription, whereas DAX1 antagonizes it. The overall effect of AMH is to induce regression of müllerian structures between 8 and 12 weeks' gestation. In its absence, development of the müllerian ducts proceeds, and the female internal structures (fallopian tubes, uterus, cervix, and upper vagina) are formed.

Development of the structures derived from the wolffian ducts, including the epididymis, ductus deferens, ejaculatory ducts, and seminiferous tubules, requires high local concentrations of testosterone secreted from Leydig cells of the testis beginning at approximately 7 weeks' gestation. In the absence of testosterone, wolffian ducts regress. Levels of testosterone in the circulation are insufficient to develop wolffian structures. Thus, in conditions in which the gonads develop asymmetrically (e.g., true hermaphroditism or mixed gonadal dysgenesis; see later), wolffian structures develop asymmetrically as well. Development of wolffian structures requires an intact androgen receptor.

Development of the External Genitalia

External genital structures are also bipotential in early gestation and consist of the genital tubercle, genital folds (later, urethral-labial folds), and genital swelling (later, labioscrotal folds) (see Fig. 233-2). Differentiation to male genitalia occurs from approximately 8 to 14 weeks' gestation under the influence of dihydrotestosterone, which must interact with an intact androgen receptor. The genital tubercle becomes the glans penis; the genital folds fuse to become the shaft of the penis and penile urethra, and the labioscrotal folds (derived from the genital swelling) fuse to become the scrotum. Without androgens, these structures become the clitoris, labia minora, and labia majora, respectively.

Normal Gonadal and Adrenal Steroidogenesis

Many forms of genital ambiguity result from defects in steroid biosynthesis in the testes or adrenal cortex or from defective steroid metabolism in the placenta or in target tissues[5] (Fig. 233-3).

Steroid biosynthesis in the testes and adrenals begins with the importation of cholesterol into mitochondria, a highly regulated process controlled largely by the steroidogenic acute regulatory (StAR) protein; levels of StAR are controlled within the adrenals by adrenocorticotropic hormone (ACTH) and within the testis by HCG during the first trimester and by LH later in pregnancy.

Within mitochondria, the side chain of cholesterol is cleaved between carbons 20 and 22 by the cholesterol side-chain cleavage enzyme (cholesterol desmolase, CYP11A), a cytochrome P-450 enzyme. The product is pregnenolone, which is transported to the endoplasmic reticulum. Some pregnenolone is converted by 17α-hydroxylase (CYP17) to 17-hydroxypregnenolone. Both 17-hydroxypregnenolone and the remaining pregnenolone are converted by 3β-hydroxysteroid dehydrogenase (HSD3B2) to 17-hydroxyprogesterone and progesterone, respectively. The side chain of 17-hydroxypregnenolone is cleaved by the 17,20-lyase activity of CYP17 to dehydroepiandrosterone (DHEA). DHEA may also be converted to androstenedione by HSD3B2.

All the preceding steps can occur in the adrenal cortex, in Leydig cells of the testis, and (after puberty) in theca cells of ovarian follicles. Subsequent

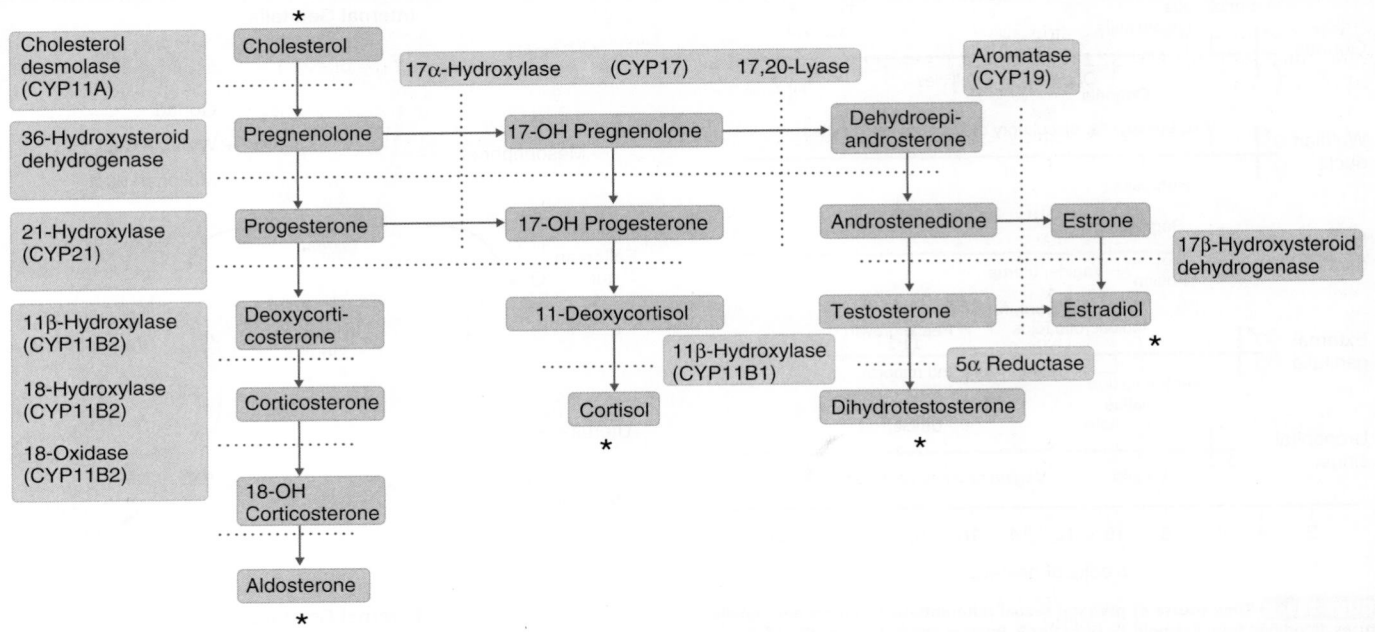

FIGURE 233-3. Steroidogenesis. Pathways for the synthesis of progesterone and mineralocorticoids (aldosterone), glucocorticoids (cortisol), androgens (testosterone and dihydrotestosterone), and estrogens (estradiol) are arranged from left to right. The enzymatic activities catalyzing each bioconversion are written in boxes. For those activities mediated by specific cytochrome P-450 subsets, the systematic name of the enzyme (CYP followed by a number) is listed in parentheses. CYP11B2 and CYP17 have multiple activities. *For an expanded version of this image, including planar structures for cholesterol and the end products of each pathway, see E-Figure 233-1.

biosynthetic steps are specific to different glands. In the adrenal cortex, 17-hydroxyprogesterone is converted by 21-hydroxylase (CYP21, a microsomal P-450) to 11-deoxycortisol, which is then converted in mitochondria to cortisol by 11β-hydroxylase (CYP11B1). Additionally, progesterone is converted to deoxycorticosterone by CYP21, which is then converted to aldosterone by aldosterone synthase (CYP11B2).

In Leydig cells of the testis, androstenedione is converted to testosterone by 17-ketosteroid reductase (17β-hydroxysteroid dehydrogenase type 3 [HSD17B3]); the same reaction occurs in theca cells of the ovary, catalyzed by 17β-hydroxysteroid dehydrogenase type 1 (HSD17B1). In granulosa cells of the ovary (after puberty), androstenedione and testosterone are converted by aromatase (CYP19) to estrone and estradiol, respectively. In skin of the developing male external genitalia, steroid 5α-reductase (SRD5A2) converts testosterone to a more potent androgen, dihydrotestosterone.

The placenta is a steroid-synthesizing and steroid-metabolizing tissue as well; it has high steroid sulfatase activity that converts DHEA sulfate from the fetal adrenal gland back to DHEA. This is then successively converted by 3β-hydroxysteroid dehydrogenase type 1 (HSD3B1) and aromatase (CYP19) to androstenedione and estrone, respectively, which are then converted to estradiol by HSD17B1.

DEFECTS OF SEX DIFFERENTIATION
Defects of Steroidogenesis

PATHOBIOLOGY

Genital ambiguity in genetic females is usually the result of exposure to excessive levels of androgens. Virilizing congenital adrenal hyperplasia (CAH), the most common cause of genital ambiguity in female infants, occurs in 1 in 16,000 births.[6]

Conversely, severe deficiencies of androgens, if present early in gestation, cause ambiguous or female-appearing external genitalia in male infants. Usually, müllerian structures such as the uterus, cervix, and upper vagina are not present because the testes are able to secrete müllerian inhibitory substance. Thus, individuals with these conditions have a short vagina ending in a blind pouch.

CONGENITAL ADRENAL HYPERPLASIA
The fundamental defect among patients with any form of CAH is inadequate synthesis of cortisol (see Fig. 233-3). Inefficient cortisol synthesis signals the

hypothalamus and pituitary to increase corticotropin-releasing hormone and ACTH, respectively (Chapter 223). Consequently, the adrenal glands become hyperplastic, and steroid precursors accumulate proximal to the block in biosynthesis. In some conditions, these precursors can be converted to androgens.

Lipoid Hyperplasia
Lipoid hyperplasia results from mutations in the *STAR* gene. Cholesterol is not imported efficiently into mitochondria and thus accumulates in cells. Steroid biosynthesis is drastically reduced because of the lack of substrate, and the lipid accumulation quickly kills steroid-synthesizing cells in both the adrenals and the testes. Thus, affected male patients are born as phenotypically female because they cannot synthesize testosterone. Affected female patients may undergo transient spontaneous puberty because human ovarian granulosa cells do not synthesize steroid hormones (and thus do not accumulate cholesterol) until puberty. Both sexes have adrenal insufficiency and are unable to synthesize either cortisol or aldosterone.

17α-Hydroxylase/17,20 Lyase Deficiency
Severe mutations in the *CYP17* gene prevent the synthesis of any sex hormones. Affected male patients have female-appearing external genitalia but have no müllerian structures because the testes synthesize AMH. Affected female patients remain sexually infantile without hormone replacement. Milder mutations result in ambiguous genitalia in male patients. Although cortisol synthesis is also abolished, even severely affected individuals are able to synthesize corticosterone, an active glucocorticoid, as well as aldosterone. Thus, they do not develop adrenal insufficiency. On the contrary, they secrete excessive amounts of deoxycorticosterone, which has mineralocorticoid activity, and are therefore prone to develop hypertension.

Whereas most *CYP17* mutations affect both the hydroxylase and lyase activities, rare mutations can affect the lyase activity alone. Additionally, mutations in genes other than *CYP17* can have the same phenotype as 17,20, lyase deficiency (i.e., deficient androgen synthesis with normal cortisol synthesis). These include an accessory electron transfer protein, cytochrome b$_5$, and mutations in the genes for two aldo-keto reductases, AKR1C2 and AKR1C4. These AKR1C isozymes normally catalyze 3α-hydroxysteroid dehydrogenase activity, which allows synthesis of the potent androgen, dihydrotestosterone, through an alternative "backdoor" biosynthetic pathway that does not include testosterone as an intermediate.

3β-Hydroxysteroid Dehydrogenase Deficiency

Severe mutations in the *HSD3B2* gene prevent the synthesis of aldosterone, cortisol, testosterone, and estrogens. Because DHEA, a weak androgen, is synthesized and secreted at high levels, some degree of phallic growth is present. Thus, affected male patients have severely ambiguous genitalia, but affected female patients may have clitorimegaly. Both sexes develop adrenal insufficiency if they are untreated.

Because many children with premature adrenarche (early development of axillary and pubic hair), as well as many women with polycystic ovary syndrome, have elevated levels of DHEA, it was once thought that such individuals could have a mild form of HSD3B2 deficiency. However, mutations in *HSD3B2* are rarely if ever found in such individuals, who instead have an imbalance in the relative levels of HSD3B2 and CYP17 activity within the adrenal cortex.

21-Hydroxylase Deficiency

More than 90% of cases of CAH are caused by 21-hydroxylase deficiency resulting from mutations in the *CYP21* (or *CYP21A2*) gene. *CYP21* and a highly homologous pseudogene, *CYP21P (or CYP21A1P),* are located within the major histocompatibility complex on chromosome 6p21.3, a genomic region noteworthy for a high rate of recombination. More than 90% of all mutations are the result of intergenic recombination between *CYP21* and *CYP21P*. Most are transfers of deleterious mutations from *CYP21P* to *CYP21*, whereas 20% are net deletions of *CYP21* resulting from unequal meiotic crossover.

In patients with 21-hydroxylase deficiency, the adrenals produce excess 17-hydroxyprogesterone, 17-hydroxypregnenolone, and progesterone, which are further metabolized to DHEA and androstenedione. Once secreted, these substances are further metabolized to active androgens (testosterone and dihydrotestosterone) and, to a lesser extent, to estrogens (estrone and estradiol).

Adrenal secretion of excess androgen precursors does not significantly affect male sexual differentiation. In affected female patients, the urogenital sinus is in the process of septation when the fetal adrenal begins to produce excess androgens, which function to prevent the formation of separate vaginal and urethral canals. Further adrenal-derived androgens interact with androgen receptors in genital skin and induce clitoral enlargement, promote fusion of the labial folds, and cause rostral migration of the urethral/vaginal perineal orifice. However, internal wolffian structures such as the prostate gland and spermatic ducts are usually not virilized, presumably because development of the wolffian ducts requires markedly higher local concentrations of testosterone than the external genitalia. Nevertheless, severely affected female patients occasionally have some development of typically male internal genital structures.

Thus, the typical result in severely affected girls is ambiguous or male-appearing external genitalia with perineal hypospadias and chordee, but without palpable testes (Fig. 233-4). The severity of virilization is often quantitated using a five-point scale developed by Prader (Fig. 233-5). Not all female patients with classic CAH develop the same degree of genital ambiguity. One could speculate that the physical signs of androgen excess depend not only on direct adrenal secretion of androgen precursors but also on the efficiency with which such hormones are converted to more potent products, such as dihydrotestosterone, by peripheral enzymes such as 5α-reductase. Additionally, the concentration and transcriptional activity of androgen receptors may play a role in determining genital phenotype.

Most patients (75%) cannot synthesize sufficient aldosterone to maintain sodium balance and are termed *salt wasters*. These patients are predisposed to episodic and potentially life-threatening hyponatremic dehydration. Patients with sufficient aldosterone production to prevent salt wasting and who have signs of prenatal virilization and/or markedly increased production of hormonal substrates of 21-hydroxylase (e.g., 17-hydroxyprogesterone) are termed *simple virilizers*.

11β-Hydroxylase Deficiency

Patients with 11β-hydroxylase deficiency have mutations in the *CYP11B1* gene. They have elevated levels of deoxycorticosterone and 11-deoxycortisol, as well as earlier cortisol precursors such as 17-hydroxyprogesterone. These patients secrete excess adrenal androgens, with consequences similar to those

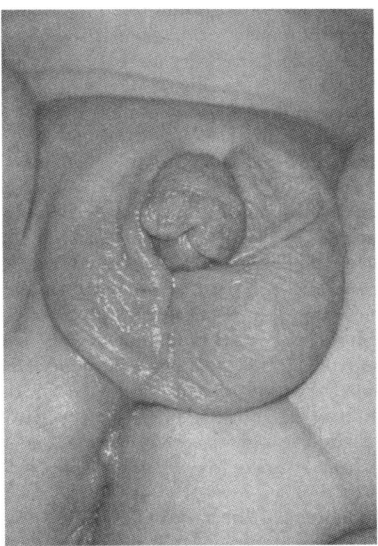

FIGURE 233-4. Virilized external genitalia in a female infant with congenital adrenal hyperplasia caused by 21-hydroxylase deficiency. No gonads are present in the scrotum.

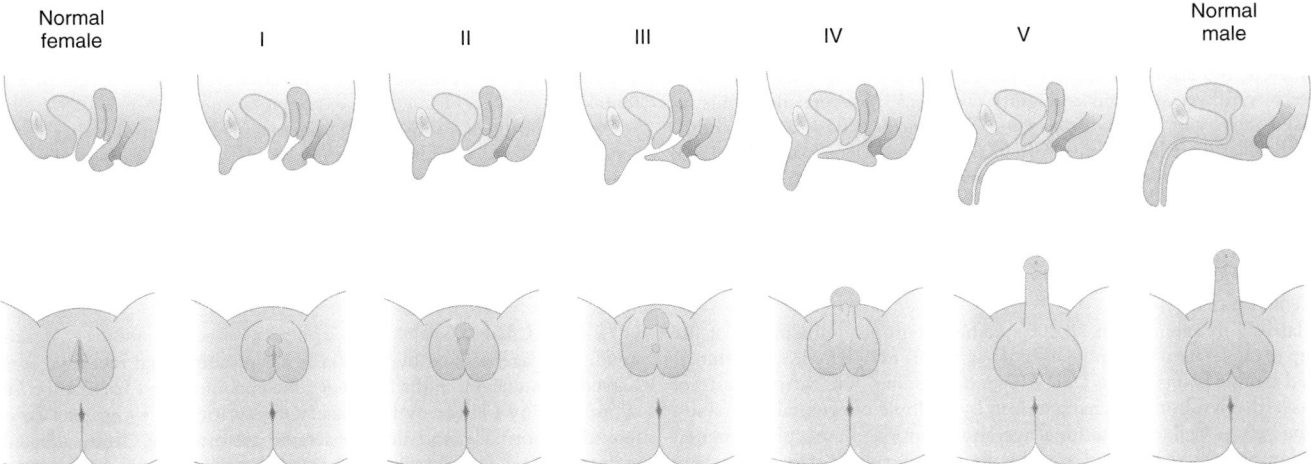

FIGURE 233-5. Abnormal differentiation of the urogenital sinus and external genitalia. Schematic representations of normal female and male anatomy flank a series of schematics illustrating different degrees of virilization of females, graded using the scale developed by Prader. The uterus (*shaded*) persists in virilized females even when the external genitalia have a completely masculine appearance (Prader grade V). (Modified from Prader A. Der Genitalbefund beim Pseudohermaphroditismus femininus der kengenitalen adrenogenitalen Syndroms. *Helv Paediatr Acta.* 1954;9:231-248.)

seen in 21-hydroxylase deficiency. However, patients with 11β-hydroxylase deficiency synthesize aldosterone normally and do not have problems with salt wasting. Instead, they are likely to become hypertensive as a result of elevated levels of deoxycorticosterone and its metabolites.

DEFECTS OF ANDROGEN BIOSYNTHESIS

Lipoid hyperplasia, 17-hydroxylase/17,20 lyase deficiency, and HSD3B2 deficiency affect the biosynthesis of both corticosteroids and sex hormones. In contrast, two enzymatic defects affect only androgen biosynthesis. They have similar phenotypes. Affected male patients are born with ambiguous genitalia, but they virilize at puberty and often reassign themselves to a male gender if they were raised as females. They have absent müllerian structures as a result of the secretion of AMH by the testes.

17-Ketosteroid Reductase (17-Hydroxysteroid Dehydrogenase 3) Deficiency

This disorder is caused by mutations in the HSD17B3 gene. Although testosterone is not synthesized well, androstenedione, an active androgen, is synthesized. Because several other isozymes have 17-ketosteroid reductase activity in other tissues, some testosterone is invariably synthesized, especially at puberty, when circulating levels of androstenedione increase.

5α-Reductase Deficiency

Patients with 5α-reductase deficiency resulting from mutations in the SRD5A2 gene synthesize entirely normal amounts of testosterone, but they cannot synthesize adequate amounts of dihydrotestosterone, the most potent naturally occurring androgen. This enzyme is not expressed at high levels in the testes (circulating levels of dihydrotestosterone are relatively low); instead, it is expressed in genital skin. Internal wolffian structures do not require this enzyme and are intact; high testosterone levels at puberty induce significant phallic growth without 5α-reductase activity.

OTHER DEFECTS OF STEROIDOGENESIS

Aromatase Deficiency

Mutations in CYP19 cause aromatase deficiency in both the fetus and the placenta. The placenta can convert DHEA sulfate to androstenedione and testosterone normally, but it cannot convert these androgens to estrone and estradiol. These androgens accumulate in both the fetal and maternal circulations and virilize both the mother and the affected fetus if it is female. Affected male infants are phenotypically normal. Affected female patients virilize further at puberty if they are untreated. The lack of aromatase activity within bone leads to tall stature in both sexes (because estrogens are required to close the growth plates) and later to osteoporosis.

Cytochrome P-450 Oxidoreductase Deficiency

This deficiency is one form of Antley-Bixler syndrome, which is characterized by skeletal anomalies and craniosynostosis; most patients also have ambiguous genitalia associated with mutations in the POR gene. Antley-Bixler syndrome without genital abnormalities is caused by mutations in the FGF receptor (FGFR2) gene.

Because this disorder affects the activity of all microsomal cytochrome P-450 subsets, complete deficiency of cytochrome P-450 oxidoreductase (POR) is lethal, and identified mutations in humans yield POR with partial activity. POR mutations may cause skeletal anomalies by interfering with cholesterol synthesis. Genital ambiguity is caused by several mechanisms. Decreased activity of 17α-hydroxylase/17,20 lyase (CYP17) affects androgen synthesis and leads to undervirilization in males. Conversely, decreased activity of 21-hydroxylase (CYP21) can virilize affected females. These two deficiencies also can cause adrenal insufficiency. Finally, decreased activity of placental aromatase (CYP19) virilizes both the mother and the affected fetus (if female).

Smith-Lemli-Opitz Syndrome

This relatively frequent (1 in 20,000 northern Europeans) disorder of the final step of cholesterol biosynthesis (conversion from 7-dehydrocholesterol) is caused by mutations in the DHCR7 gene encoding 7-dehydrocholesterol reductase. The syndrome is characterized by multiple congenital anomalies, including being small for gestational age, short stature, microcephaly, mental retardation, aggressive behavior, seizures, hypotonia, polydactyly, cleft palate, cardiac defects, lung hypoplasia, and renal anomalies. Male patients have ambiguous genitalia. The range of clinical severity is wide and depends on the nature of the mutations. Pathogenetic mechanisms for the ambiguous genitalia may include insufficient provision of cholesterol for steroid hormone biosynthesis or toxic effects of the precursor, 7-dehydrocholesterol, on steroidogenic cells.

MATERNAL CONDITIONS AFFECTING THE FETUS

LUTEOMA OF PREGNANCY

Luteomas are the most common causes of maternal virilization during pregnancy. They often occur bilaterally. Although many luteomas are discovered incidentally during cesarean sections or postpartum tubal ligations, one fourth of mothers virilize during the latter half of pregnancy, and half of female infants born to these mothers also exhibit signs of virilization, most typically clitorimegaly and labial fusion. Spontaneous regression of the luteoma generally begins within days after delivery.

DRUG EXPOSURE

Depending on the agent, maternal drug exposure may affect either male or female fetuses. Females may be virilized by androgens such as 19-nor-testosterone or progestins administered to prevent spontaneous abortion. Undervirilized males can be born to women exposed to 5α-reductase inhibitors such as finasteride. The antifungal agent fluconazole can inhibit many cytochrome P-450 enzymes and can lead to a condition closely resembling Antley-Bixler syndrome.

The synthetic estrogen diethylstilbestrol was used several decades ago to prevent spontaneous abortion (it was actually ineffective for this purpose). Males exposed to this agent in utero were born with testicular hypoplasia, cryptorchidism, hypospadias, and/or microphallus. Females had uterine, cervical, and vaginal abnormalities and an increased risk for clear cell adenocarcinoma of the vagina. Considering that many cases of genital ambiguity are idiopathic, it is likely that additional endocrine disruptors in the environment have not yet been identified.[7]

HORMONE INSENSITIVITY SYNDROMES AND OTHER HORMONE DEFICIENCIES

ANDROGEN INSENSITIVITY

Males normally carry a single copy of the X-linked androgen receptor (AR) gene.[8] Thus, a single mutation can completely inactivate the receptor in males and lead to complete androgen insensitivity (formerly termed testicular feminization syndrome). This is one of the most frequent forms of 46,XY DSD, occurring in approximately 1 in 20,000 male births.[9]

Patients with the complete form of androgen insensitivity have normal female external genitalia. Unless suspicion is raised by prior knowledge of the infant's karyotype, the condition is rarely discovered before puberty unless the testes are palpated in the groin or labia on routine examination. Because the testes secrete AMH, müllerian structures are absent, including the uterus, fallopian tubes, and cervix. Thus, the vagina is usually shallow and ends blindly. Wolffian structures are also absent. The testes may be located in the abdomen or in the labia majora and do not undergo spermatogenesis. AMH levels are elevated during the first year and (if the testes have not been removed) after puberty. Testosterone and LH levels in infancy and at puberty are elevated as a result of defective feedback regulation caused by androgen resistance at the level of the hypothalamus.

At puberty, pubic and axillary hair is scant or absent. Testosterone can be aromatized to estradiol by CYP19 in breast fat, and estrogen receptors are unaffected in this condition. Thus, breast development is that of a normal female.

Partial androgen insensitivity (Reifenstein's syndrome) is characterized by a variable degree of genital ambiguity, and both virilization and breast development occur at puberty. Mild androgen insensitivity also can occur with a male phenotype, with gynecomastia and infertility as the sole manifestations. Mutations in the androgen receptor are not detected in many mild cases, which may result from defects in other transcription factors affecting actions of the receptor.

LEYDIG CELL AGENESIS

Leydig cell agenesis or hypoplasia is a rare autosomal recessive syndrome caused by mutations in the LHGCR gene encoding the LH receptor. Without stimulation by LH (or by HCG early in gestation), Leydig cells do not differentiate normally and do not secrete testosterone. Thus, affected male infants are born with female-appearing or ambiguous external genitalia. Müllerian structures are absent because of unaffected secretion of AMH by Sertoli cells. LH levels are high in infancy and at puberty, and they respond normally to gonadotropin-releasing hormone, whereas testosterone levels are low and do not respond to stimulation by HCG. Affected females are phenotypically normal but may have oligomenorrhea resulting from primary ovarian dysfunction.

PERSISTENT MÜLLERIAN DUCT SYNDROME

Persistent müllerian duct syndrome (PMDS) is a rare autosomal recessive condition that results from mutations in the genes for either AMH (PMDS type I) or the AMH receptor (*AMHR2* gene, PMDS type II). The two are distinguished clinically by low or absent AMH levels in patients with AMH mutations and by AMH levels in the high-normal range in those with AMH receptor mutations.

Affected male patients have unimpaired testosterone secretion and thus have normal external genitalia and wolffian structures. However, the lack of AMH action prevents regression of müllerian structures, so these patients also retain a uterus and fallopian tubes. These structures are often closely approximated to the vas deferens. The müllerian structures are usually dragged into the inguinal canal by the descending testes. However, these structures typically prevent the testes from descending into the scrotum and thus cause bilateral inguinal hernias (with the uterus on one side) and bilateral or occasionally unilateral cryptorchidism. The condition is usually discovered only at surgery. Fertility in affected patients may be normal or impaired, with an increased risk for malignant disease in undescended testes left in the abdomen.

HYPOGONADOTROPIC HYPOGONADISM

Milder or later appearing deficiencies of androgen biosynthesis (after 13 to 14 weeks) may allow complete fusion of the labioscrotal folds and normal positioning of the urethral meatus, but subsequent growth of the phallus is suboptimal. Such individuals have a micropenis. The most common cause is lack of gonadotropin (specifically, LH) secretion; even when LH is lacking, early male development is normal because testosterone secretion is controlled mostly by HCG during the first trimester.

Defective LH and follicle-stimulating hormone secretion can result when the neurons that normally secrete gonadotropin-releasing hormone fail to migrate into the hypothalamus.[10] This condition, *Kallmann syndrome,* is most often X-linked, resulting from mutations in the *KAL1* gene. It is often associated with anosmia. Other conditions that affect hypothalamic development and cause hypogonadotropic hypogonadism include *Prader-Willi syndrome,* which is a result of paternal deletions, methylation defects, and maternal uniparental disomy of imprinted loci on chromosome 15q12. Children with this syndrome have a characteristic appearance consisting of a narrow bitemporal diameter, almond-shaped eyes with an antimongoloid slant, and small hands and feet. They typically have marked hypotonia as infants, with subsequent moderate developmental delay and slow somatic growth. Hypothalamic obesity develops during childhood. Patients with adrenal hypoplasia congenita resulting from mutations in the DAX1 transcription factor have defective development of the ventromedial hypothalamus and consequent hypogonadotropic hypogonadism, associated with adrenal insufficiency that typically manifests with aldosterone deficiency and salt wasting. Steroidogenic factor-1 (SF-1), encoded by the *NR5A1* gene, is an orphan nuclear receptor that is critical for the development and function of the adrenal glands, gonads, pituitary gonadotropes, ventromedial nucleus of the hypothalamus, and male sexual differentiation. Heterozygous null mutations or homozygous milder mutations have been identified mainly among undervirilized 46,XY individuals and 46,XX women with premature ovarian failure. Only a minority have adrenal insufficiency.

Hypogonadotropic hypogonadism often results from failure of the entire anterior pituitary gland, or particular cellular populations therein, to develop.[11] Pituitary gland abnormalities can be associated with other midline defects, including hypoplasia of the optic nerves and the septum pellucidum, a condition termed *septo-optic dysplasia.* Associated pituitary hormone deficiencies may include growth hormone, ACTH, and thyroid-stimulating hormone. These deficiencies may manifest in the neonatal period as hypoglycemia or hypothyroidism (detected by newborn screening programs). Optic nerve dysfunction is difficult to detect by routine examination in the neonatal period, but it causes a characteristic wandering nystagmus after a few months of age.

Although panhypopituitarism is most often sporadic, mutations in transcription factors controlling pituitary development have been documented (Chapter 224), particularly PROP1, and septo-optic dysplasia has been associated with mutations in the *HESX* gene. Rarely, mutations in the gene encoding the β-subunit of LH may yield a phenotype similar to hypogonadotropic hypogonadism.

⬤ OTHER GENETIC CONDITIONS

ANEUPLOIDY OF SEX CHROMOSOMES

Turner Syndrome

Patients with Turner syndrome have normal female external genitalia and a normal uterus and fallopian tubes, but they have dysgenetic streak ovaries.[12] Most fetuses with Turner syndrome spontaneously abort, but the incidence in live births is approximately 1 in 2500. Classically, the karyotype is 45,X, but many patients retain an abnormal second X chromosome or even a fragment of a Y chromosome lacking *SRY.* Other patients are mosaic for 46,XX and 45,X cells and may have relatively mild phenotypes.

Untreated patients are short. Many have typical dysmorphic features, including lymphedema of the neck at birth, webbed neck, low posterior hairline, increased carrying angle of the arms, shield chest with widely spaced nipples, low-set ears, and micrognathia. Patients typically have primary amenorrhea and are infertile, but they occasionally have menarche followed by premature ovarian failure.

Klinefelter's Syndrome

In this condition, male patients have normal development of the penis and scrotum, but the testes are small and firm. Patients tend to be tall. At adolescence, gynecomastia is frequent. Signs of testosterone deficiency occur in most affected adults, and most have azoospermia. The usual karyotype is 47,XXY. Hormonal findings include elevated gonadotropin levels and a decreased serum testosterone concentration. Klinefelter's syndrome is a common disorder that occurs in 1 in 500 to 1000 men.

Mixed Gonadal Dysgenesis

Mixed gonadal dysgenesis, a frequent cause of sexual ambiguity, occurs in approximately 1 in 20,000 births.[13] The karyotype is usually mosaic 45,X/46,XY. Gonadal pathologic features can vary from fibrous streaks indistinguishable from those in Turner syndrome to normally developed testes and a normal male phenotype. Typically, patients have a testis on one side and a fibrous streak on the other. Some patients may have a Turner-like phenotype. A fallopian tube is usually present on the side of the streak gonad. Leydig cell function, evaluated by testosterone response to HCG, and Sertoli cell function, evaluated by serum AMH levels, vary from poor to normal.

XX MALE SYNDROME

Males with a 46,XX karyotype have normal external and internal male genitalia; however, they resemble patients with Klinefelter's syndrome in that they have small testes, azoospermia, and infertility. Translocation of the *SRY* gene to the X chromosome is detected in 75 to 90% of sporadic cases; this can occur because the gene is located very near the pseudoautosomal region, where the short arms of the X and Y chromosomes are homologous and meiotic recombination is possible. Duplication of the SOX9 transcription factor may be responsible for some familial cases of XX sex reversal.

XY FEMALE SYNDROMES

Patients with pure XY gonadal dysgenesis (Swyer syndrome) have a normal female phenotype, including a uterus and fallopian tubes, but they have streak gonads. These patients are free of Turner-like malformations and attain normal height. Mutations of the *SRY* gene have been identified in 15% of cases. Unlike 45,X patients with Turner syndrome, these patients have an increased risk for gonadoblastoma.

Similar phenotypes result from duplication of the region of the X chromosome containing the *DAX1* gene, from duplication of the *WNT4* gene, or from haploinsufficiency of the SF1 transcription factor (see earlier). XY sex reversal also can result from mutations in the SOX9 transcription factor associated with campomelic dysplasia, a form of dwarfism. Mutations of DHH cause XY gonadal dysgenesis, associated with peripheral neuropathy.

Some 46,XY patients with absent gonads have various degrees of sexual ambiguity and no müllerian derivatives. The implication that some testicular tissue was functional at least up to 10 weeks' gestation and subsequently regressed led to the name *fetal testicular regression syndrome.* Testicular regression may occur in late pregnancy or even postnatally; these fully virilized male patients have isolated anorchia.

VAGINAL ATRESIA

Mayer-Rokitansky-Küster-Hauser syndrome refers to aplasia of the uterus and upper vagina, occurring in approximately 1 in 5000 women. In approximately one third of cases, it occurs along with other abnormalities including unilateral renal aplasia, and cervicothoracic somite dysplasia (MURCS association). The genetic basis is unknown in most cases. Rare affected individuals have heterozygous mutations of *WNT4*; such patients usually have clinical and biochemical signs of androgen excess.

TRUE HERMAPHRODITISM (OVOTESTICULAR DISORDER OF SEXUAL DEVELOPMENT)

True hermaphroditism (ovotesticular DSD), a rare and usually sporadic disorder, is defined as the coexistence of seminiferous tubules and ovarian follicles. Most patients have an ovotestis with either an ovary or a testis on the opposite side; a gonad in the scrotum is usually a testis but may be an ovotestis.

The genitalia are usually ambiguous, but they may appear completely masculine or feminine. The anatomy of the internal reproductive tract depends on the nature of the gonads, particularly whether they secrete AMH. A uterus or uterine horn is present in 90% of cases. Testosterone response to HCG is variable, and AMH levels are usually low. Most patients experience breast development, ovulation, and even menstruation at puberty; pregnancy and successful childbirth are possible if selective removal of testicular tissue is feasible. Unless sex of rearing has already been chosen, male gender assignment should be restricted to patients with no uterus and descended testicular tissue because the latter is usually dysgenetic and prone to malignant degeneration. Most patients with ovotesticular DSD have a 46,XX karyotype. Despite the presence of testicular tissue, they usually lack *SRY*; this suggests that the condition is the result of constitutive activation of a gene normally triggered by *SRY*.

● MANAGEMENT OF INDIVIDUALS WITH DISORDERS OF SEXUAL DEVELOPMENT: GENDER ROLE AND IDENTITY

The influence of prenatal sex steroid exposure or epigenetic changes in the estrogen receptor[14] on personality is controversial.[15] In considering this question, it is important to distinguish among gender role, sexual orientation, and gender identity.

Gender Role

Gender role refers to gender-stereotyped behaviors, such as the choice of toys by young children. For example, parents of young girls with CAH often report that their daughters prefer to play with trucks rather than dolls and tend to be tomboyish later in childhood. Decreased interest in maternal behavior, beginning with infrequent doll play in early childhood and extending to lack of interest in child rearing in older girls and women, occurs frequently.

Sexual Orientation

Sexual orientation refers to homosexual versus heterosexual preferences. In many studies, a significant minority of women with CAH have been actively homosexual or bisexual or have had an increased tendency toward homoerotic fantasies. These characteristics occur more frequently in women with the salt-wasting form of 21-hydroxylase deficiency, suggesting that they are a consequence of prenatal exposure of the brain to androgens. However, the vast majority of both male and female homosexuals have no identifiable endocrinologic abnormality.

Gender Identity

Gender identity refers to self-identification as male or female. Gender self-reassignment back to male has been reported in cases of male patients with penile trauma or exstrophy of the bladder who were raised as girls. This may also occur in 46,XY patients with disorders of sexual development (DSD) raised as girls, especially in cases of 5α-reductase or 17-ketosteroid reductase deficiencies, in which the brain may be exposed to high circulating levels of androgens. Self-reassignment to the male gender is unusual in women with CAH. When it occurs, it may be related to delays in gender assignment or genital surgery or to inadequate suppression of adrenal androgens with glucocorticoid therapy.

Transgendered individuals rarely have identifiable hormonal abnormalities; nonhormonal mechanisms governing gender identity are poorly understood. Gender identity disorders are much more likely to occur in both identical twins than in fraternal twins, suggesting a high degree of heritability. Neuroanatomic studies suggest that the bed nucleus of the stria terminalis is larger in males and female-to-male transsexuals and smaller in females and

male-to-female transsexuals. Similar findings involving other sexually dimorphic brain regions have been identified by MRI. Thus, gender identity disorder may be considered a brain-limited form of DSD.

▶ DIAGNOSIS

Management of a child born with ambiguous genitalia presents a difficult challenge to medical personnel.[16] It is important to refrain from assigning sex until diagnostic information can be gathered. Usually, test results can be obtained within 24 to 48 hours and parents can be advised about the child's chromosomal and gonadal sex and the anatomy of internal sexual structures.

In addition, the physician must keep in mind that DSD may be associated with life-threatening biochemical or anatomic abnormalities. In particular, the most common cause of severely masculinized external genitalia in females, the salt-wasting form of CAH resulting from steroid 21-hydroxylase deficiency, may cause hyponatremia, hyperkalemia, hypovolemia, and shock. In contrast, male patients with ambiguous genitalia may have lipoid adrenal hyperplasia or a salt-wasting form of 3/3-hydroxysteroid dehydrogenase (HSD3B2) deficiency. Males with micropenis may have panhypopituitarism; in this case they are at risk for significant hypoglycemia and hyponatremia resulting from low cortisol (because of low ACTH) and low growth hormone levels, or they may have adrenal hypoplasia congenita, in which case they could have adrenal insufficiency. Finally, patients with ambiguous genitalia are at increased risk for renal anomalies, or they may have chromosomal syndromes with other associated anomalies.

History

The gestational history should concentrate on potential exposure to agents that could interfere with normal sexual differentiation. For a female infant with virilized genitalia, these include progestational agents, whereas the mother of a male with incompletely masculinized genitalia may have been exposed to a 5α-reductase inhibitor through her husband's use of such an agent for male pattern baldness or prostate enlargement. It should be determined whether amniocentesis and karyotyping have been performed. A family history should elicit similar cases of genital ambiguity or cases of sudden death, which could raise suspicion of undiagnosed salt-wasting CAH or adrenal hypoplasia congenita.

Physical Examination

The physical examination should document the size of the phallus (clitoris or penis), the degree of chordee (ventral bowing of the phallus), and the extent of fusion of the labioscrotal folds. The urethral meatus should be identified, and there must be careful palpation for gonads in the inguinal canals and labia or scrotum. Bilateral cryptorchidism, even if an isolated finding in a phenotypic male patient, should always lead to evaluation for a possible DSD.

Biochemical Evaluation of the Virilized Female

The minimal diagnostic tests should include measurement of basal serum 17-hydroxyprogesterone, androstenedione, and testosterone. Preferably, a complete profile of adrenocortical hormones is obtained before and 1 hour after stimulation of the adrenal cortex with 125 to 250 μg of cosyntropin (ACTH$_{1-24}$). These assays should be deferred until after the first 24 hours of life. They will identify potential defects in adrenal steroidogenesis (i.e., CAH); 21-hydroxylase deficiency is identified by elevations in 17-hydroxyprogesterone, whereas 11-deoxycortisol and 11-deoxycorticosterone are high in 11β-hydroxylase deficiency.

Biochemical Evaluation of the Undervirilized Male

In 46,XY DSD patients, it is necessary to test adrenal and gonadal function as well as extragonadal androgen metabolism. With regard to adrenal defects, 11-deoxycorticosterone and the ratio of pregnenolone to 17-hydroxypregnenolone are high in 17α-hydroxylase deficiency, 17-hydroxypregnenolone and DHEA are high in HSD3B2 deficiency, and all steroids are low in lipoid hyperplasia.

Defects in gonadal steroidogenesis are best evaluated after stimulation with HCG (1500 IU intramuscularly on days 1, 3, and 5, with blood drawn on day 6). However, 17-hydroxylase and HSD3B2 deficiencies affect both the gonads and the adrenal cortex and thus are often diagnosed by cosyntropin stimulation testing. Low levels of all androgen precursors suggest lipoid hyperplasia, 17α-hydroxylase/17,20 lyase deficiency, or a generalized defect in testicular function, such as the vanishing testes syndrome (testicular regression-syndrome) or gonadotropin insensitivity. A high ratio of androstenedione to testosterone is indicative of 17-ketosteroid reductase (HSD17B3) deficiency, and a high ratio of testosterone to dihydrotestosterone is diagnostic of 5α-reductase deficiency. The diagnosis of androgen insensitivity syndrome is suspected when a 46,XY patient has ambiguous or female-appearing external genitalia despite normal or high circulating levels of testosterone and dihydrotestosterone.

Gonadal Biopsies

Patients with mixed gonadal dysgenesis, true hermaphroditism, or unclear diagnoses should undergo bilateral gonadal biopsies (histology of the two gonads is often not identical). Dysgenetic gonads have a high potential for malignant transformation and usually need to be removed in childhood.

TREATMENT Rx

Initial Medical Management

Patients with CAH resulting from 21-hydroxylase or HSD3B2 deficiencies or those with lipoid hyperplasia or adrenal hypoplasia congenita require replacement of both glucocorticoids and mineralocorticoids, usually with hydrocortisone (15 to 20 mg/m^2/day in divided doses) and fludrocortisone (usually 0.1 mg/day, but as much as 0.4 mg/day in neonates with salt-wasting crises). Neonates with severe salt losses may require sodium chloride supplementation (≤8 mEq/kg/day). Patients with 11β-hydroxylase or 17α-hydroxylase deficiencies have normal aldosterone biosynthesis and usually require only glucocorticoids. Patients with panhypopituitarism usually require treatment with hydrocortisone, thyroxine, and growth hormone.

All male infants with ambiguous genitalia or micropenis in whom rearing as a boy is contemplated should have a 3- or 4-month therapeutic trial of monthly depot testosterone injections (25 mg) to attempt to increase the size of the phallus during infancy. This treatment may improve social acceptability of the genitalia later in childhood and adolescence and may make reconstructive surgery easier. In cases of suspected partial androgen insensitivity, this treatment also documents the degree to which the patient is androgen responsive and thus may provide useful information about whether rearing as a boy is feasible. Higher doses of testosterone (75 mg every 4 weeks) may be used under these circumstances.

Considerations Related to Sex Assignment

In large medical centers, a team consisting of a neonatologist, a pediatric endocrinologist, a urologist, and preferably an experienced social worker and/or child psychiatrist or psychologist should promptly review the early diagnostic data and make a recommendation to the family as to the sex of rearing and any medical or surgical treatments. These recommendations should be based on both current knowledge of psychosexual development in DSD individuals and the feasibility of surgical treatment (see later).[17]

In general, the recommended sex assignment should be that of the genetic/gonadal sex, if for no other reason than to retain the possibility of reproductive function. This is especially true for female infants with CAH who have normal internal genital structures and the potential for childbearing. An exception may be considered in a genetically female infant with completely male-appearing genitalia, especially if the child has been raised as a boy for more than a few months. Such children need to be castrated at puberty to avoid feminization.

Conversely, genetic male infants with completely female-appearing external genitalia (usually resulting from complete androgen insensitivity syndrome, but also seen with severe testosterone biosynthetic defects) should be raised as female because the potential for reconstruction of male genitalia is poor. They, too, need to be castrated by early adulthood to avoid malignant transformation of the testes. However, male infants with 17-ketosteroid reductase or 5α-reductase deficiency should usually be reared as boys because they have normal levels of androstenedione or testosterone, respectively, and often virilize significantly at puberty. Indeed, many of these patients reassign themselves to the male gender when they are made aware of the diagnosis. The same considerations pertain to male patients with normal testosterone biosynthesis who have penile trauma or anatomic abnormalities such as bladder exstrophy.

Recommendations for sex assignment are to some extent culture specific. In cultures that value boys over girls, parents may strongly resist rearing a female infant with ambiguous genitalia as a girl, and many girls with severely virilized external genitalia will be raised as boys.

Surgical Management
Surgery for Ambiguous Genitalia

Whether, how, and when to intervene surgically in the correction of genital anomalies are the subject of continuing debate. Some adult patients with DSD conditions are unhappy with their gender assignments or surgical outcomes. Some physicians advocate postponing cosmetic genital surgery until the

affected individual is able to provide informed consent, thus keeping all the options open if the adult patient wishes to function sexually with abnormal genitalia that nevertheless have sensation undiminished by surgery or chooses to reassign his or her gender. Declining or postponing surgery should not be confused with raising the child with an indeterminate gender, a concept currently well outside the mainstream. The option of deferring surgery should always be presented as part of the informed consent process. Nevertheless, most parents want their child to look as "normal" as possible, and they often resist suggestions to postpone genital surgery.

In addressing this question, it is best to consider the various general types of genital surgery separately. The greatest change in practice over the past few decades probably pertains to male infants with ambiguous (but not completely female) external genitalia. Physicians are far less likely to recommend that such patients be reared as female because it is now recognized that many of these patients reassign themselves as male at puberty. Thus, the ambiguous genitalia in such patients should rarely be "corrected" to female. On the contrary, surgical techniques for hypospadias repair have advanced significantly, and reconstruction of male genitalia is attempted more often, particularly if the infant responds to a course of testosterone with significant phallic growth.

Surgery for female infants with ambiguous genitalia may need to address an enlarged clitoris, the lack of a vaginal introitus, and the presence of a urogenital sinus. The clitoris is normally prominent in many infant girls. Even when enlarged in a girl with virilizing CAH, the clitoris can be prevented from growing larger with adequate suppression of adrenal androgens by glucocorticoids, and it will become less prominent as the patient grows. Thus, mild-to-moderate clitorimegaly is often best managed without surgery. When clitoroplasty is attempted, one must keep in mind the important role of clitoral sensation in the female sexual response. Such surgery must be performed only by experienced operators with scrupulous attention to the preservation of clitoral innervation.

Consensus is still lacking regarding the best age for vaginoplasty. Although many surgeons advocate a first procedure in infancy, it is difficult to maintain a functionally adequate introitus in the absence of estrogen exposure and mechanical dilation (with dilators or through sexual intercourse), and many patients require reoperation as young adults. Conversely, many women with atresia of the upper vagina (owing to complete androgen insensitivity or Mayer-Rokitansky-Küster-Hauser syndromes) can use dilators to lengthen the vagina without the need for surgery.

There is a dearth of large longitudinal studies comparing outcomes in patients who have had early genital surgery versus those who have had no surgery or surgery in adolescence. According to self-assessment surveys among sexually active women with CAH who have had genital surgery, most are able to have satisfactory sexual intercourse. As surgical and medical treatment regimens have improved in recent years, more women with CAH have successfully conceived spontaneously, completed pregnancies, and given birth. Most often, delivery is by cesarean section because of an inadequate introitus, but vaginal delivery is possible in some cases.

Hypospadias repair is usually begun in the first year of life, after testosterone treatment (if necessary to increase phallic size). Depending on the degree of hypospadias, more than one surgical procedure may be required.

Removal of Intra-abdominal Testes in 46,XY Patients with Disorders of Sexual Development

Intra-abdominal testes are at increasing risk for malignant transformation over time. In a boy with cryptorchidism who is being reared as male, orchiopexy should be performed as quickly as possible; this also maximizes the possibility of fertility when the underlying condition does not preclude it. Dysgenetic gonads that cannot be brought into the scrotum should be removed soon after diagnosis because the risk for malignant transformation in childhood is relatively high.

There is a lack of consensus regarding nondysgenetic testes in severely undervirilized genetic male infants in whom rearing as female is planned. In patients with complete androgen insensitivity or complete defects in testosterone biosynthesis, no possibility of fertility exists, and so there seems to be no reason to retain the testes. Conversely, the risk for malignant transformation in such gonads is low before puberty, and patients with complete androgen insensitivity can undergo spontaneous breast development at puberty. At that time, patients themselves can assent or consent to gonadectomy, which can usually be accomplished laparoscopically. This is of particular importance in genetic male patients with partial androgen insensitivity or incomplete defects of testosterone biosynthesis, because such patients may eventually desire a male gender role.

Patients with persistent müllerian duct syndrome have a reduced but still appreciable potential for fertility, and virilization is unaffected. Thus, the testes should be removed only if they cannot be brought into the scrotum. Because the müllerian and wolffian structures are closely approximated in these patients, surgical excision of the uterus and fallopian tubes may result in ischemic and/or traumatic damage to the vas deferens and testes; thus, salpingectomy and hysterectomy are indicated only in patients whose müllerian structures limit intrascrotal placement of the testes.

Space does not permit extensive discussion of surgical management of transgendered adults; options for male-to-female transsexuals include genitoplasty and, for those who did not have hormonal management during adolescence (see the next section), breast augmentation, body contouring, and facial and/or laryngeal surgery to produce a more feminine appearance. Female-to-male transsexuals often desire breast reduction surgery or complete mastectomies.

Treatment of Transgendered Individuals

Children and Adolescents

Transgendered individuals should be treated by multidisciplinary teams that can provide psychosocial evaluation and support.[18,19] Prepubertal children do not require medical management. The majority of such children do not persist in their identification with the opposite sex, although many will be homosexual as adults. Persistently transgendered children may develop significant gender dysphoria (distress at functioning in their natal gender) when puberty commences and are at increased risk for self-injury and suicide as adolescence progresses. If at all possible, such children should be allowed to function in the desired gender role. The current standard of care in many centers for children who have lived in a transgendered role for at least 6 months is to delay pubertal progression until mid-adolescence (~16 years old), with use of gonadotropin-releasing hormone (GnRH) agonists such as leuprolide depot injections or histrelin (Supprelin) implants. This will prevent the development of secondary sexual characteristics that may be distressing to the patient and may present cosmetic barriers to functioning in the desired, non-natal gender. These include breast enlargement, widened hips, and gynecoid adipose distribution in natal females or penile enlargement, facial and body hair, laryngeal enlargement and deep voice, and prominent jaw in natal males.

When the patient is confirmed in the desired gender role (e.g., by living completely in that role for at least 1 year), treatment may begin with the appropriate sex hormones. In high doses, such treatment will itself suppress gonadotropin secretion, and the GnRH agonist may be discontinued. Female-to-male transsexuals can be treated with depot testosterone whereas male-to-female transsexuals can be treated with parental forms of estradiol. Oral estrogen preparations should be avoided because they tend to increase production of clotting factors by the liver and may thus increase the risk for thromboembolism.

Adults

The medical treatment of transgendered adults follows the same principles as for adolescents, except that because secondary sexual characteristics have already developed, prolonged treatment with GnRH agonists is unnecessary. However, continuing such treatment in male-to-female transsexuals permits use of much lower estradiol doses with a concomitant reduction in the risks associated with high dose estrogen treatment. Nevertheless, cost represents a barrier to the long term use of GnRH agonists.

Prenatal Diagnosis and Treatment

Many conditions causing ambiguous genitalia can be detected by karyotyping of chorionic villus samples (for chromosomal abnormalities) or by direct molecular genetic testing. In most cases, this information is useful only for counseling purposes. In the case of virilizing forms of CAH (particularly 21-hydroxylase deficiency), the mother of an affected female fetus can take dexamethasone (20 μg/kg/day), which can cross the placenta and suppress the fetal adrenal gland, thus reducing the secretion of androgens and ameliorating virilization of the external genitalia. To be most effective, this treatment should be started by the sixth week of gestation, before the sex or genotype of the fetus is known. Thus, seven unaffected or male fetuses must be treated with dexamethasone to avoid genital ambiguity in one affected female, until chorionic villus sampling can be performed. Although effective in reducing prenatal virilization, this dose of dexamethasone can cause Cushing syndrome in the mother, and the long-term sequelae in the fetus are not known. Recent consensus statements suggest that this treatment be used only under approved research protocols that allow for case registries and long-term follow-up.

Psychosocial Support

Families of patients with DSD should be assessed for emotional health, initially by the pediatrician and/or pediatric endocrinologist. Parents should be offered psychological counseling soon after the diagnosis is made. Intermittent assessment of family functioning may be a useful tool in predicting future problems. As children mature, they should repeatedly be informed about their condition by parents and physicians in a sensitive and age-appropriate manner. When psychotherapy is undertaken, medical and psychiatric caregivers should communicate with each other so both are aware of the patient's and family's status. Unfortunately, many locales lack mental health professionals with experience in counseling patients with DSD and their families.

Although the psychosexual development of individuals with DSD cannot be predicted with confidence, patients' families should receive anticipatory

counseling. For example, counseling of parents of girls affected with CAH should address the high likelihood that such girls will exhibit tomboyish behavior, masculine play preferences, and perhaps, when older, a preference for a career over domestic activities. The endocrinologist and/or mental health professional (depending on inclination and experience) caring for the adolescents with DSDs should address sexual orientation, both fantasized and actual. For example, some women with CAH are most comfortable as homosexuals; such individuals should receive appropriate psychosocial support. Adult patients also should be made aware of relevant patient advocacy groups.

GENERAL REFERENCES

For the General References and other additional features, please visit Expert Consult at https://expertconsult.inkling.com.

234

THE TESTIS AND MALE HYPOGONADISM, INFERTILITY, AND SEXUAL DYSFUNCTION

RONALD S. SWERDLOFF AND CHRISTINA WANG

PHYSIOLOGY

The testis is a bifunctional organ serving as the site of sex steroid (i.e., testosterone) synthesis and sperm production in the male. Androgens and their metabolites (including estrogens) also act on nonreproductive organs and serve essential roles in muscles, adipose tissues, bones, metabolism, and brain functions.

The male reproductive axis consists of six main components: (1) extra-hypothalamic central nervous system (CNS), (2) hypothalamus, (3) pituitary, (4) testes, (5) sex steroid–sensitive end organs, and (6) sites of androgen transport and metabolism (Fig. 234-1). The components of this system function in an integrated fashion to control the concentrations of circulating gonadal steroids required for normal male sexual development

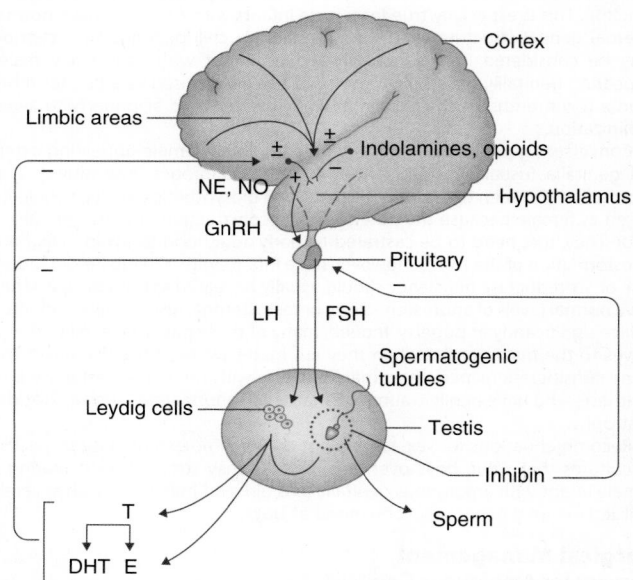

FIGURE 234-1. **The hypothalamic-pituitary-gonadal axis in the male.** DHT = dihydrotestosterone; E = estrogen; FSH = follicle-stimulating hormone; GnRH = gonadotropin-releasing hormone; LH = luteinizing hormone; NE = norepinephrine; NO = nitric oxide; T = testosterone.

and function and for androgen- and estrogen-mediated metabolic effects on critical end organs. The reproductive axis is also responsible for normal germ cell development and maturation. Accessory sexual organs, including the epididymides, seminal vesicles, and prostate gland, are important for sperm maturation (epididymis) and seminal fluid production. An anatomically functional sperm transport and ejaculatory system are necessary to ensure male fertility.

Hypothalamic-Pituitary Function

The hypothalamus is responsible for the normal pulsatile secretion of gonadotropin-releasing hormone (GnRH) (Chapter 224). The pulsatile release of GnRH provides the signals for the timing of the release of luteinizing hormone (LH) and follicle-stimulating hormone (FSH), which occurs every 60 to 90 minutes in men. The secretion of GnRH is regulated by neuronal input from higher cognitive and sensory centers and by circulating levels of sex steroids and peptide hormones such as prolactin and leptin (Chapter 223). Testosterone or its metabolic products (i.e., estradiol and dihydrotestosterone [DHT]) inhibit the secretion and release of GnRH, LH, and FSH. Prolactin is also a potent inhibitor of GnRH secretion.

Both LH and FSH consist of two subunits (α and β). Both subunits are required for biologic activity; the subunits can be detected in serum and may be increased in certain pathologic conditions (e.g., α-subunit elevations in gonadotropin-secreting pituitary adenomas). LH has a shorter half-life than FSH. Feedback regulation of LH and FSH secretion also occurs at the pituitary, with testosterone, DHT, and estrogens inhibiting the synthesis or release of both gonadotropins. The circulating testicular peptide inhibin, produced by Sertoli cells, also selectively inhibits FSH. LH and FSH act on the testes through specific cell surface receptors on the Leydig and Sertoli cells, respectively.

Testosterone

The testis is a complex organ consisting of (1) seminiferous tubules containing Sertoli cells and germ cells and (2) the interstitium, which contains the steroid-secreting (Leydig) cells. Leydig cells synthesize steroid hormones under the regulation of LH. The LH receptors on the cell surface of the Leydig cells lead to G protein–, adenyl cyclase–, and cyclic adenosine monophosphate–mediated activation of steroid biosynthesis.

Testosterone is the principal male hormone secreted by the testes; approximately 5 to 10 mg/day is produced in adult men. Testosterone synthesis occurs in the human testes through either the Δ^4 or the predominant Δ^5 pathway. The enzymatic rate-limiting steps in the process are the LH-inducible steroid acute regulatory (StAR) protein and the conversion of cholesterol to pregnenolone by the cholesterol side-chain cleavage enzyme P450SCC (Fig. 234-2).

Testosterone circulates mainly bound to two plasma proteins: sex hormone–binding globulin (SHBG) and albumin. In young adult men, approximately 54% of testosterone is bound to albumin, 44% is bound to SHBG, and 2 to 3% is unbound. Bioavailable testosterone refers to the sum of albumin-bound and free testosterone and is measured by separating SHBG-bound testosterone from total testosterone. Serum SHBG levels are increased in hyperestrogenemic states, hyperthyroidism, aging, phenytoin treatment, anorexia nervosa, and prolonged stress. SHBG levels are lowered in hyperandrogenic states (endogenous and exogenous as in androgen treatment), obesity, acromegaly, and hypothyroidism. In most instances, measurement of serum total testosterone provides biochemical support for the diagnosis of androgen deficiency. In conditions with abnormal SHBG levels, however, the total testosterone measurement may be misleading, and measurement of non–SHBG-bound testosterone may allow better interpretation of the active testosterone levels. This can be done by direct measurement of free testosterone by the equilibrium dialysis method, measurement of bioavailable testosterone, or calculation of the free testosterone by a formula requiring the serum testosterone and SHBG concentrations. Most guidelines recommend against measurement of free testosterone by a "direct" or analogue displacement method because of lack of accuracy traceable to a standard.

Testosterone exerts its effects either through direct action or after conversion to DHT by two separate 5α-reductase isozymes (1 and 2) or to estradiol by the aromatase enzyme (Fig. 234-3). Thus, testosterone can act directly on the androgen receptor or as a precursor for DHT, which also binds efficiently to the androgen receptor. Different tissues have coactivators or coinhibitors that modify the action of the androgen-receptor complex, providing tissue selectivity and amplification. Testosterone also can serve as a precursor for estradiol in some tissues, and after conversion, estrogen binds the estrogen receptors (α or β) to induce its effects. Various end organs differ in their 5α-reductase isoenzyme and aromatase concentrations and/or activity. Congenital and acquired defects in these two enzymes, as well as in the estrogen and androgen receptors, result in distinct syndromes with characteristic phenotypes that are experiments in nature and provide understanding of the actions of specific receptors and enzyme activities (Chapter 233).

Spermatogenesis

The spermatogenic compartment of the testis consists of the Sertoli and germ cells that are intimately interactive with the interstitial compartment. The Sertoli cells bridge the entire space between the basement membrane and the lumen of the tubules. They are the target of androgenic and FSH stimulation of spermatogenesis and also the source of a multitude of paracrine regulators of spermatogenesis (e.g., inhibin, activin, growth factors, cytokines).

Germ cell development and maturation depend on the proper hormonal (FSH) and paracrine (testosterone) milieu. Both testosterone and FSH stimulate progression of spermatogonia to mature spermatozoa, limit the amount of germ cell death (apoptosis), and regulate sperm release from the germinal epithelium.

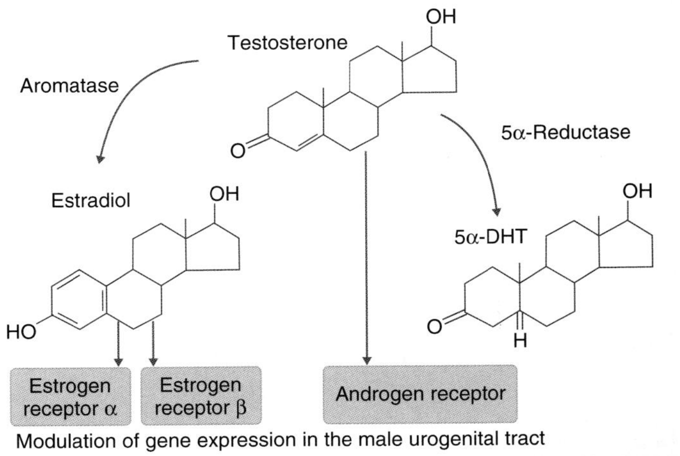

Testosterone Synthesis in the Testis

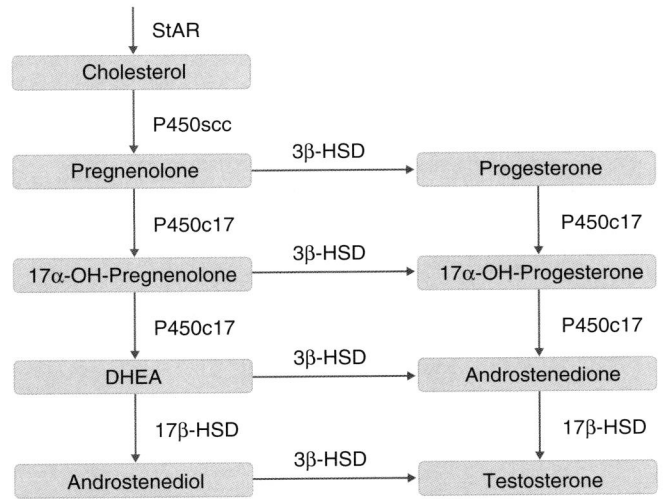

FIGURE 234-2. The steroid acute regulatory (*StAR*) protein mobilizes cholesterol from cellular stores to the mitochondria. Intratesticular steroidogenic pathways for the synthesis of testosterone. Although both the Δ^5 (*left*) and Δ^4 (*right*) pathways exist, the Δ^5 pathway predominates in the testis. DHEA = dehydroepiandrosterone; HSD = hydroxysteroid dehydrogenase.

FIGURE 234-3. Testosterone action is mediated directly (androgen receptor), after conversion to estradiol (estrogen receptor α or β), or after conversion to dihydrotestosterone (DHT; androgen receptor). (From Kuiper GCJM, Carlquist M, Gustafsson JA. Estrogen is a male and female hormone. *Sci Med.* 1998;5:36-45.)

After spermatogenesis is completed, mature spermatozoa are released into the excretory system and travel through the rete testes and epididymis, where they become functionally mature and acquire fertilizing capacity before traversing the vas deferens. The seminal fluid gains constituents from the seminal vesicles, prostate, and bulbourethral glands before ejaculation.

Sexual Function and Erectile Physiology

Sexual function in men requires normal sexual desire (libido) and erectile, ejaculatory, and orgasmic capacity. The process is complex, involving cognitive, sensory, hormonal, autonomic neuronal, and penile vascular integrative actions for normal function. Defects can occur at multiple levels.

The brain is the integrative center of the sexual response system. It processes sensory input and hormonal signals to create the hypothalamic neuronal message that traverses the spinal cord to the T9-12 sympathetic and sacral parasympathetic outflow tracts. The nonadrenergic, noncholinergic autonomic plexus nerves initiate vasodilation of the cavernosal arterial and corpora cavernosal sinusoids of the penis through the release of local vasodilators (e.g., nitric oxide and vasoactive intestinal peptide) from the vascular endothelium and the sinusoidal smooth muscle cells of the sinusoids (Fig. 234-4). Nitric oxide produces smooth muscle dilation by the generation of cyclic guanosine monophosphate (cGMP) and the modification of calcium flux. The neurogenic mechanisms leading to vasodilation of the cavernosal arterioles and sinusoids lead to a rapid increase in penile blood flow and expansion of the vascular channels; this, in turn, inhibits venous return through compression of the venous channels against the tunica albuginea and limits venous drainage.

Testosterone's primary effect on erectile function is to enhance libido. Testosterone also increases penile nitric oxide synthase activity and enhances smooth muscle cell growth. Sexual desire and fantasy are highly sensitive to testosterone, explaining the preservation of erectile capacity in many men with partial androgen deficiency.[1]

Physiology in Development and Aging
Reproductive Axis Development during Childhood and Puberty
Adrenarche and Puberty

Adrenarche occurs at approximately 7 or 8 years of age when the zona reticularis of the adrenal gland undergoes maturation, leading to increased secretion of androstenedione, dehydroepiandrosterone (DHEA), and DHEA sulfate (DHEA-S). The process is under the control of adrenocorticotropic hormone, not LH or FSH. Androstenedione and DHEA are technically androgenic prehormones, and the prepubertal growth spurt, as well as the early development of pubic and axillary hair, are mediated to a great extent by the conversion of these precursors to testosterone and DHT in peripheral tissues.

Initiation of puberty is determined by an increase in the pulsatile pattern of hypothalamic GnRH secretion. This is marked by nocturnal bursts of LH secretion. As puberty progresses, feedback sensitivity of the hypothalamus and pituitary to circulating steroids lessens, thus increasing the secretion of gonadotropins. The increasing concentrations of intratesticular testosterone and circulating FSH stimulate the Sertoli cell to produce factors leading to the maturation of spermatogenesis. The majority of the extratesticular end-organ events of puberty are secondary to the increased testosterone and its metabolic products (DHT and estradiol) (Table 234-1). The penis and scrotum grow and become pigmented. As spermatogenesis advances, the testes increase in size from 1 to 2 mL at the outset of puberty to 15 to 35 mL in adulthood. There is a progressive increase in facial, axillary, chest, abdominal, thigh, and pubic hair; frontal scalp hair regresses, and the voice deepens (Fig. 234-5). Genital and sexual hair development and temporal scalp hair regression require DHT. The increased levels of sex steroids result in closure of the epiphysis and achievement of adult height.

Aberrations of Timing of Puberty

Delayed puberty, more common in boys than in girls, is usually defined as a temporary form of hypothalamic hypogonadotropic hypogonadism in which sexual development has not begun by age 13.5 years. Height age (the age

TABLE 234-1	PUBERTAL STAGES IN BOYS	
STAGE	**PUBIC HAIR**	**GENITAL**
1	Absence of pubic hair	Childlike penis, testes, and scrotum (testes 2 mL)
2	Sparse, lightly pigmented hair mainly at base of penis	Scrotum enlarged with early rugation and pigmentation; testes begin to enlarge (3-5 mL)
3	Hair becomes coarse, darker, more curled, and more extensive	Penis has grown in length and diameter; testes now 8-10 mL; scrotum more rugated
4	Hair adult in quality, but distribution does not include medial aspect of thighs	Penis further enlarged, with development of glans; scrotum and testes (10-13 mL) further enlarged
5	Hair is adult and extends to thighs	Penis and scrotum fully adult; testes ≥ 15 mL

Modified from Marshall WA, Tanner JM. Variation in pattern of pubertal changes in boys. *Arch Dis Child.* 1970;45:13-23.

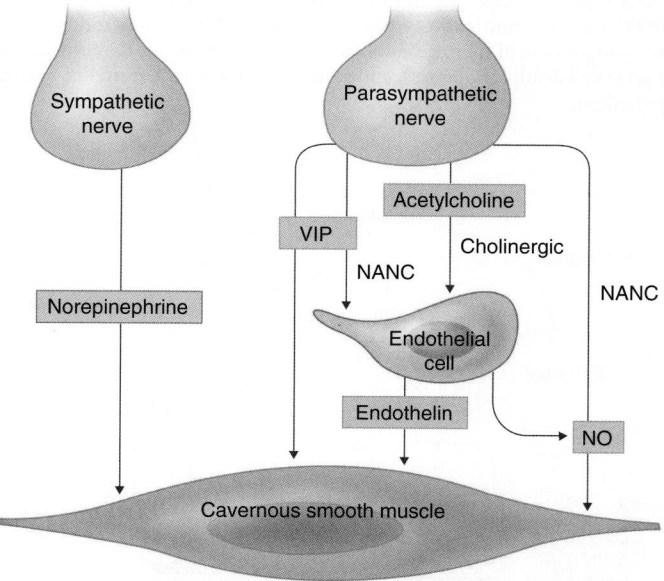

FIGURE 234-4. The interaction among cholinergic, adrenergic, and nonadrenergic, noncholinergic (*NANC*) neuronal pathways and their contribution to penile smooth muscle contraction and dilation (*arrows*). NO = nitric oxide; VIP = vasoactive intestinal polypeptide. (From Lue TF. Physiology of penile erection and pathophysiology of erectile dysfunction and priapism. In: Walsh P, Retick A, Vaughn E, Wein A, eds. *Campbell's Urology,* 7th ed. Philadelphia: WB Saunders; 1998:1164.)

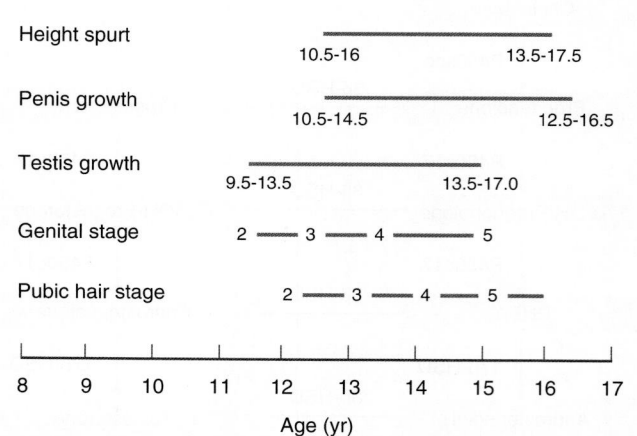

FIGURE 234-5. Diagram of the timing of the various components of puberty. The range of ages at which each parameter begins and is completed is shown for each bar. These data were obtained from European children 40 years ago. Since then, there may be a slight trend for an earlier onset of puberty. (From Marshall WA, Tanner JM. Variations in the pattern of pubertal changes in boys. *Arch Dis Child.* 1970;45:13-23.)

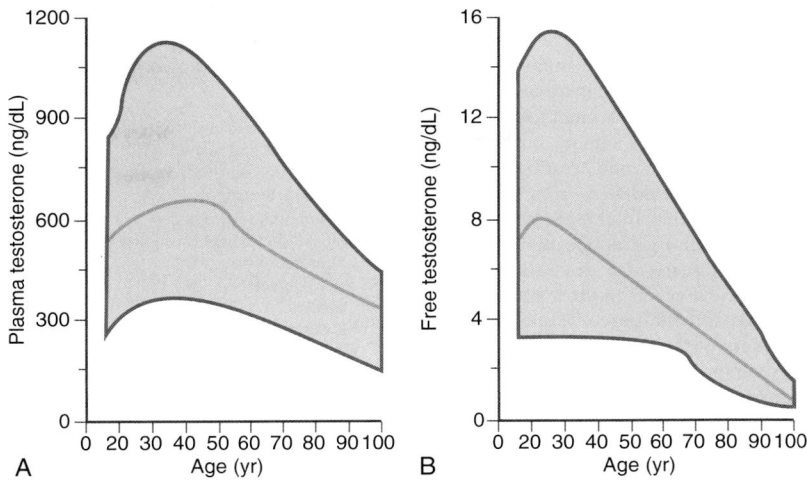

FIGURE 234-6. Relationship between plasma testosterone (A) and free testosterone (B) levels and age in normal males. (From Baker HWG, Berger HG, DeKretser DM, et al. Changes in the pituitary-testicular system with age. *Clin Endocrinol.* 1996;5:349-372.)

representative of 50% of normal children at the patient's height) is delayed with respect to chronologic age, but it is concordant with bone age. Once initiated, puberty is normally completed within 4.5 years. The majority of boys with delayed development eventually attain full sexual adulthood. There is often a family history of a parent or sibling being a "late bloomer." The *GPR54* gene encodes a kisspeptin-responsive G protein–coupled receptor whose absence results in hypogonadotropic hypogonadism resulting from impaired secretion of GnRH. Careful documentation of changing physical findings and measurement of serum LH, FSH, and testosterone concentrations may provide valuable clues to the beginning of puberty. An increase in testicular size to more than 3 mL usually heralds other signs of pubertal onset. Inquiring and testing for hyposmia or anosmia and other midline defects may indicate a common variant of congenital hypogonadotropic hypogonadism (Kallmann's syndrome). The decision to institute early treatment depends on the perceived degree of psychological stress associated with the maturational delay. The major concern is early fusion of the epiphyses induced by treatment with testosterone, which compromises optimal height; however, with proper dosing and monitoring of bone age, this is unusual. In adolescent boys with delayed puberty and low levels of gonadotropins, periodic withdrawal of treatment is used to determine whether spontaneous puberty has occurred. Many adult men diagnosed with and treated as adolescents for a presumed diagnosis of hypogonadotropic hypogonadism achieve normal reproductive function when they discontinue therapy.

Precocious puberty in boys is defined as the onset of pubertal (genital and secondary sexual) development before 9 years of age. Sexual precocity can be subcategorized as true (complete and incomplete) isosexual precocious puberty and pseudo–precocious puberty. The distinction is that true precocious puberty is associated with increases in GnRH-stimulated LH and FSH secretion (hypothalamic-pituitary origin), whereas pseudo–precocious puberty is independent of GnRH stimulation of LH and FSH secretion. True precocious puberty in boys is often associated with CNS disease (two thirds of boys), including hypothalamic tumors, cysts, inflammatory conditions, and seizure disorders. Diagnostic findings include sexual precocity, inappropriately elevated serum LH levels, and associated elevations of testosterone. Magnetic resonance imaging can localize most lesions. Another cause of central precocious puberty is human chorionic gonadotropin secretory germinomas (testicular, hepatic, hypothalamic, or pineal tumors). Pseudo–precocious puberty is characterized by increased testosterone with suppressed LH. Causes of pseudo–precocious puberty include congenital virilizing adrenal hyperplasia, testicular testosterone-secreting neoplasms, and constitutively active LH receptor mutations; the latter condition results in uncontrolled testosterone secretion (testotoxicosis). Treatment of true precocious puberty is removal or correction (with surgery or radiation therapy) of the CNS lesion, if possible, and treatment with GnRH analogues to temporarily suppress LH and FSH secretion. Treatment of pseudo–precocious puberty depends on the cause but includes glucocorticoids for congenital virilizing adrenal hyperplasia and ketoconazole (to suppress steroidogenesis), with or without antiandrogens (e.g., spironolactone, flutamide).

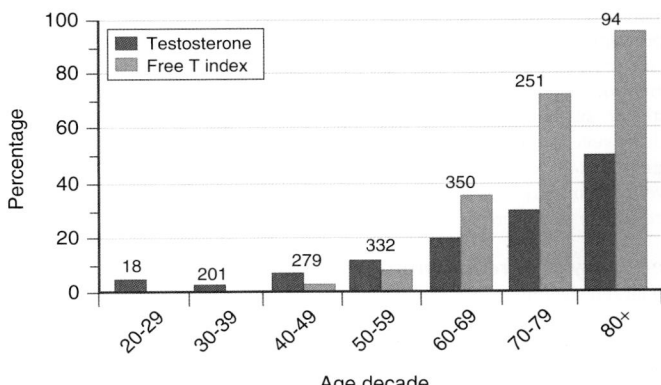

FIGURE 234-7. Hypogonadism in aging men. Bar height indicates the percentage of men in each 10-year interval, from the third to the ninth decades, with at least one testosterone value in the hypogonadal range. The criteria used for these determinations are total testosterone less than 11.3 nmol/L (325 ng/dL) and testosterone and sex hormone–binding globulin (free T index) less than 0.153 nmol/nmol. The numbers above each pair of bars indicate the number of men studied in the corresponding decade. The fraction of men who are hypogonadal increases progressively after age 50 years by either criterion. More men are hypogonadal by free T index than by total testosterone after 50 years, and there seems to be a progressively greater difference, with increasing age, between the two criteria.

Male Senescence: Decreased Testosterone and Other Anabolic Hormones

Testosterone Deficiency in the Elderly

Blood concentrations of testosterone, other anabolic hormones (e.g., growth hormone), and prehormones (e.g., DHEA, DHEA-S) are significantly lower in older men than in young adult men. Both total and bioavailable or free serum testosterone levels progressively decrease with aging (Fig. 234-6). The percentage decline in serum testosterone has been estimated as 1 to 2% per year. Serum SHBG levels also rise with age in men, resulting in a higher percentage of circulating testosterone that is tightly bound and less bioavailable. Between 20 and 80% of men older than 70 years have blood levels of bioavailable or free testosterone below the normal range for young adults (Fig. 234-7). Many older men with serum testosterone below the young adult reference range do not complain of symptoms attributable to low testosterone. In men between 30 and 70 years of age the crude prevalence rate of symptomatic testosterone deficiency has been estimated to be approximately 6%. Low testosterone levels are associated with comorbidities such as obesity, metabolic syndrome, and the commonest symptoms associated with low total or free testosterone in older men are sexual symptoms.[2]

Many of the effects of low testosterone levels in aging men are similar to those observed in younger hypogonadal men. These include decreases in libido, erectile function, muscle mass, muscle strength, bone mass, and impaired mood and sense of well-being. Older men have increased body fat, particularly visceral fat. The benefits of testosterone treatment for symptomatic older men with low serum testosterone levels remain controversial. Recommendations on the diagnosis, investigation, and treatment of late-onset hypogonadism are available but lack evidence from large-scale randomized, controlled national or international intervention studies. A randomized trial of testosterone versus placebo gel application in elderly men with a high prevalence of chronic disease was discontinued early because of an increased risk for cardiovascular events in those receiving testosterone, but the small size of the trial and the unique population prevented broader inferences about the safety of the testosterone therapy.[A1] In a more recent study of men in the Veterans Administration health system who underwent coronary angiography and had low serum testosterone levels, the use of the testosterone therapy was found to be associated with increased risk for adverse outcomes.[3] Beneficial effects of testosterone replacement have been demonstrated in elderly men with relatively low serum testosterone levels. Testosterone replacement therapy (up to 3 years) decreases fat mass, increases lean body mass, improves strength, and increases bone mineral density in older men.[A2] In larger, more recent studies of treatment with testosterone improved muscle strength and physical function were found in frail elderly men.[A3,4] Erectile dysfunction in older men is usually multifactorial (see later), with impaired penile vasodilatory function a predominant factor in many cases. Thus testosterone replacement therapy in older men may enhance libido but often does not improve erectile dysfunction. At present, testosterone treatment is not recommended for men with or suspected of having prostate cancer, moderate-to-severe heart failure, severe and uncorrected sleep apnea, or high red blood cell mass. A digital rectal examination should be performed, prostate-specific antigen level determined, and symptoms of severe urinary tract obstruction evaluated before testosterone treatment is instituted.[5]

Deficiency of Adrenal Androgen in Older Men
A marked decline in the circulating levels of adrenal androgens, especially DHEA and DHEA-S, has been recognized in elderly men and women (Chapter 234). Serum levels of DHEA and DHEA-S peak at approximately the third decade of life and then decline at about 2% per year, resulting in levels 10 to 20% of baseline by 80 years of age. DHEA is a precursor to androgens such as testosterone and DHT. Studies have shown that the oral administration of 50 mg of DHEA to older men raises serum DHEA and DHEA-S concentrations to the levels found in young men without changing serum levels of testosterone, with no beneficial effects on quality of life, sexual function, mood, body composition, or exercise capacity. In the United States, DHEA is available without prescription as a health supplement and is widely used, making large-scale multicenter, prospective, placebo-controlled trials difficult to perform.

MALE HYPOGONADISM

DEFINITION
Hypogonadism (androgen deficiency) is diagnosed in men with consistent symptoms and signs and unequivocally low circulating levels of testosterone.[6] Most men with more severe androgen deficiency have very low intratesticular testosterone concentrations and are infertile. Primary hypogonadism indicates that the abnormality originates in the testis; it is characterized by increased serum LH and FSH levels. Secondary hypogonadism indicates a defect at the hypothalamus or pituitary, resulting in decreased gonadotropins (LH, FSH, or both). Combined primary and secondary hypogonadism occurs in aging and in a number of systemic diseases, such as alcoholism, liver disease, metabolic syndrome, type 2 diabetes mellitus, human immunodeficiency virus (HIV) infection, hemochromatosis, and sickle cell disease. Obesity leads to low total and free testosterone levels. Greater decreases are seen in the total testosterone level because obesity not only decreases testosterone secretion but also lowers SHBG levels. Decreased androgen action with normal or elevated testosterone levels, mimicking androgen deficiency, may occur in patients with androgen receptor defects (androgen resistance), postreceptor signaling abnormalities, and inability to convert testosterone to the active metabolite DHT (5α-reductase abnormalities).

Many of the causes of primary and secondary hypogonadism are listed in Tables 234-2 and 234-3 (see also Chapter 233).

TABLE 234-2 CAUSES OF PRIMARY TESTICULAR FAILURE AND END-ORGAN RESISTANCE

Congenital disorders
  Chromosome disorders
  Klinefelter's and related syndromes (e.g., XXY, XXY/XY, XYY, XX males)
  Testosterone biosynthetic enzyme defects
  Myotonic dystrophy
Developmental disorders
  Prenatal diethylstilbestrol syndrome
  Cryptorchidism
Acquired defects
  Orchitis
  Mumps and other viruses
  Granulomatous disease (e.g., tuberculosis, leprosy)
  Human immunodeficiency virus infection
  Infiltrative disease (e.g., hemochromatosis, amyloidosis)
  Surgical, traumatic injuries, torsion of testis
  Irradiation
Toxins (e.g., alcohol, fungicides, insecticides, heavy metals, cottonseed oil, DDT, other environmental "endocrine disruptors")
Drugs
  Cytotoxic agents
  Inhibitors of testosterone synthesis and antiandrogens (e.g., ketoconazole, cimetidine, flutamide, cyproterone, spironolactone)
  Ethanol, opioids, other recreational drugs
Autoimmune testicular failure
  Isolated
  Associated with other organ-specific disorders (e.g., Addison's disease, Hashimoto's thyroiditis, insulin-dependent diabetes)
Androgen resistance syndromes
5α-Reductase deficiency
Systemic diseases* (e.g., cirrhosis, chronic renal failure, sickle cell disease, acquired immunodeficiency syndrome, amyloidosis)
Aging*

*Systemic diseases and aging produce a mixed pattern of testicular and hypothalamic-pituitary dysfunction.

TABLE 234-3 CAUSES OF HYPOGONADOTROPIC HYPOGONADISM

IDIOPATHIC OR CONGENITAL

Isolated deficiency of gonadotropin-releasing hormone
  With anosmia (Kallmann's syndrome)
  With other abnormalities (Prader-Willi syndrome, Laurence-Moon-Biedl syndrome, basal encephalocele)
Partial deficiency of gonadotropin-releasing hormone (fertile eunuch syndrome)
Multiple hypothalamic and pituitary hormone deficiency
Pituitary hypoplasia or aplasia

ACQUIRED

Traumatic brain injury, after surgery or irradiation
Neoplastic
Pituitary adenoma (prolactinoma, other functional and nonfunctional tumors)
Craniopharyngioma, germinoma, glioma, leukemia, lymphoma
Pituitary infarction, carotid aneurysm
Infiltrative and infectious diseases of hypothalamus and pituitary (sarcoidosis, tuberculosis, coccidioidomycosis, histoplasmosis, syphilis, abscess, histiocytosis X, hemochromatosis)
Autoimmune hypophysitis
Aging and systemic diseases*
Obesity
Malnutrition
Anorexia nervosa, starvation, renal failure, liver failure
Exogenous hormones and drugs
Antiandrogens, estrogens and antiestrogens, progestogens, glucocorticoids, cimetidine, spironolactone, digoxin, drug-induced hyperprolactinemia (metoclopramide, tranquilizers, antihypertensives)

*Aging and systemic diseases produce a mixed pattern of central and testicular dysfunction.

CLINICAL MANIFESTATIONS
History
The medical history should focus on testicular descent, pubertal development, shaving frequency, changes in body hair, and present and past systemic illnesses. A complete sexual history includes changes in libido, erectile and

ejaculatory functions, frequency of masturbation, coital activity, and fertility (including that of present and previous partners). Information should be obtained on previous orchitis, sinopulmonary complaints, sexually transmitted diseases, human immunodeficiency virus (HIV) status, genitourinary infections, and previous surgical procedures that might affect the reproductive tract (e.g., vasectomy, hernia repair, prostatectomy, varicocele ligation). Social history includes tobacco and alcohol intake. Medication and self-prescribed drug history includes recreational drugs; opioids; anabolic steroids; 5α-reductase inhibitors; and psychiatric, antihypertensive, antiandrogenic, cytotoxic, and alternative medicine therapies; environmental toxins; and exposure to heat (including saunas and Jacuzzis) and irradiation.

Physical Examination

The general physical examination is supplemented by height and span measurements; characterization of facial, pubic, and body hair distribution; presence of acne and facial wrinkling; breast examination for gynecomastia; assessment of muscle mass and adiposity; measurement of penile length and urethral meatus localization; digital rectal prostate examination; and visual field assessment if secondary hypogonadism is suspected. The scrotal examination should include an assessment of midline fusion (e.g., bifid scrotum, hypospadias); testicular size and consistency; presence of intratesticular masses; abnormalities of the epididymis; bilateral presence of vas deferens; and varicoceles, hydroceles, or hernias. Normal testicular size ranges from 3.6 to 5.5 cm in length, 2.1 to 3.2 cm in width, and 15 to 35 mL in volume in white and black men. Asian men have a slightly smaller mean testicular size. A decrease in testicular volume usually implies decreased spermatogenic cells because the seminiferous tubules account for more than 80% of testicular volume.

Laboratory Studies

Because there is a strong diurnal rhythm in testosterone secretion in young men (highest in the morning), testosterone, LH, and FSH are routinely determined from morning blood samples. There is a broad range of reference values of these hormones due partly to measurement variability but also influenced by the selection criteria for the reference population. Most hospital laboratories used immunoassay methods to measure serum testosterone, which may lack precision at low serum testosterone levels. Recent studies suggest that methods using liquid or gas chromatography and mass spectrometry may give more accurate results even at very low serum testosterone levels. Elevated LH and FSH levels distinguish primary from secondary hypogonadism (both have low serum testosterone levels), but many older men with low serum testosterone levels have normal LH concentrations. Serum prolactin levels should be measured in all low testosterone, low LH cases (hypogonadotropic hypogonadism) and in men with known pituitary mass lesions, or galactorrhea. DHT is measured in cases of abnormal differentiation of the genitalia and when 5α-reductase deficiency is suspected. Serum estradiol should be measured in cases of gynecomastia. Assessment of other testosterone precursors and products may be required in special circumstances, including suspected congenital enzyme defects. The semen analysis is the "cornerstone" of the laboratory examination for male infertility.

Primary Testicular Hypogonadism

Primary hypogonadism refers to a condition of androgen deficiency with or without infertility in which the pathologic process lies at the testis level. A list of common causes is given in Table 234-2.

CONGENITAL DEFECTS

The commonest congenital defect is due to chromosomal abnormalities (Klinefelter's syndrome), and other causes are listed in Table 234-2 and described in Chapter 233.

ACQUIRED DEFECTS
Mumps, Orchitis, Leprosy, Human Immunodeficiency Virus Infection, and Hemochromatosis

After puberty, mumps (Chapter 369) is associated with clinical orchitis in 25% of cases, and 60% of those affected become infertile. During acute orchitis, the testes are inflamed, painful, and swollen. This is followed by a gradual decrease in size. The testes may return to normal size and function, or they may atrophy. Spermatogenic defects occur more often and earlier than Leydig cell dysfunction. Thus, patients with postorchitic infertility may have normal testosterone and LH levels with increased serum FSH levels.

Over time, elevations in LH and lower serum testosterone levels may appear. Leprosy (Chapter 326) also may cause orchitis and gonadal insufficiency. HIV infection is often associated with hypogonadism, which can be either hypogonadotropic or hypergonadotropic. Hemochromatosis (Chapter 212) may affect the hypothalamus-pituitary, as well as act directly on the testis.

Trauma

The exposed position of the testes in the scrotum makes them particularly susceptible to injury. Surgical injury during scrotal surgery for hernia, varicocele, and vasectomy can result in permanent testicular damage.

Irradiation

Exposure of the testes to irradiation in the treatment of malignant diseases produces testicular germ cell, and less commonly, Leydig cell damage.

DRUGS AND TOXINS

Chemotherapy, in particular alkylating agents such as cyclophosphamide, busulfan, frequently leads to irreversible germ cell damage. Heavy metals (lead, cadmium) and cottonseed oil (gossypol) cause damage to the germ cells. Leydig cells are relatively less susceptible to most chemotherapeutic drugs than are Sertoli and germ cells. Some medications may interfere with testosterone biosynthesis (e.g., ketoconazole, spironolactone) or action (e.g., cyproterone, flutamide). Ethanol, independent of its role in causing liver disease, inhibits testosterone biosynthesis. Marijuana, heroin, methadone, medroxyprogesterone acetate, other progestins, and estrogens lower testosterone, mainly by decreasing LH. Medical treatment with androgens such as testosterone, DHT, and synthetic anabolic steroids or their illicit use (e.g., in athletes, bodybuilders) lowers serum LH and FSH and sperm counts. Serum testosterone levels are low after the use of DHT and synthetic anabolic agents. Environmental toxins such as fungicides and insecticides (e.g., DBCP, metabolites of DDT, vinclozolin) and byproducts of the plastics industry (e.g., phthalates, bisphenol A) are called "endocrine disruptors" because these chemicals may have either weak estrogenic or antiandrogenic effects and have been shown to cause testicular dysgenesis in male offspring when administered in large doses to pregnant female rodents. Data linking "endocrine disruptors" to male reproductive dysfunction in humans are principally associations studies and do not prove causality.[7]

AUTOIMMUNE TESTICULAR FAILURE

Antibodies against the microsomal fraction of the Leydig cells may occur either as an isolated disorder or as part of a multiglandular disorder (Chapter 231) involving, to variable degrees, the thyroid, pituitary, adrenals, pancreas, and other organs.

ANDROGEN RESISTANCE (ANDROGEN-SENSITIVE END-ORGAN DEFICIENCY)

Certain conditions have clinical phenotypes mimicking testosterone deficiency in the absence of lowered testosterone levels. These androgen-resistant states may be drug-induced (antiandrogens) or genetic sensitive defects in the androgen receptor, congenital or acquired post–androgen receptor signaling defects, or 5α-reductase deficiency (Chapter 233).

Hypogonadism Associated with Systemic Diseases

Abnormalities of the hypothalamic-pituitary-testicular axis occur in a number of systemic diseases, including liver failure, renal failure, severe malnutrition, sickle cell anemia, advanced malignant disease, severe obesity, metabolic syndrome, type 2 diabetes, cystic fibrosis, and amyloidosis, as well as in those on chronic hemodialysis. The effects of cirrhosis of the liver on testicular function are complex and may be either independent of or associated with the direct toxic effects of the continued use of alcohol. Gynecomastia, testicular atrophy, and impotence are concomitant signs of cirrhosis. Decreased spermatogenesis with peritubular fibrosis occurs in 50% of cases. Estradiol levels are usually elevated. This results in an increased ratio of serum estradiol to testosterone, often associated with gynecomastia. In sickle cell anemia and thalassemia major, boys may have impaired sexual maturation, and men are often infertile. Diabetes and obesity are two major factors in hypogonadism. Emerging data show that type 2 diabetes is associated with low blood testosterone levels mainly as a result of hypothalamic-pituitary dysfunction; the decrease in serum testosterone correlates with the degree of hyperglycemia.

Secondary Gonadal Insufficiency (Hypogonadotropic Hypogonadism)

CONGENITAL HYPOGONADOTROPIC HYPOGONADISM

Hypogonadotropic hypogonadism represents a deficiency in the secretion of gonadotropins (LH and FSH) because of an intrinsic or functional abnormality in the hypothalamus or pituitary glands (see earlier and Chapter 233). Such disorders result in secondary Leydig cell dysfunction (see Table 234-3). The clinical manifestations depend on the age of the patient at the onset of the disorder.

ACQUIRED HYPOGONADOTROPIC DISORDERS AND FUNCTIONAL DISORDERS

Anorexia Nervosa and Weight Loss

Anorexia nervosa (Chapter 219) and weight loss are examples of functional defects resulting in low serum testosterone levels. Men and women with anorexia nervosa present with manifestations of hypogonadotropic hypogonadism. Starvation also may reduce gonadotropic secretion. Strenuous exercise has minimal effects on testicular function in men.

Stress and Illness

Severe stress (e.g., surgery, trauma) and systemic illness also lower gonadotropin and testosterone levels. Organic hypothalamic-pituitary disorders include neoplastic, granulomatous, infiltrative, and post-traumatic lesions in the region of the hypothalamus and pituitary.

Pituitary Tumors

Prolactinomas manifest differently in men than in women (Chapter 224). In men, these tumors are usually large (>1 cm in diameter; macroadenomas) by the time they are detected. Male patients with prolactin-secreting macroadenomas usually present with hypogonadism, erectile dysfunction, and visual manifestations from suprasellar extension. In small tumors, hypogonadotropic hypogonadism may be due to suppressive effects on GnRH described earlier, but in large tumors, it also may be due to a mass effect damaging the non-neoplastic gonadotrophs.

Large non–prolactin-secreting pituitary tumors (growth hormone, adrenocorticotropic hormone, glycopeptide, and null cell) also may produce gonadotropin insufficiency from damage to the adjacent normal pituitary gland (Chapter 224), resulting in decreased serum LH and testosterone levels.

DIAGNOSIS

The diagnosis is based on clinical symptoms and signs and a reduced serum testosterone level. The normal range of serum total testosterone in a young adult male population varies across different laboratories but should be in the general range of 300 to 1000 ng/dL (10-35 nmol/L). Accurate measurements of testosterone in the severely hypogonadal range are best done by gas or liquid chromatography followed by tandem mass spectrometry. Total testosterone measurements may be misleading indicators of Leydig cell secretory status in conditions in which SHBG levels are abnormal (see earlier section). In these circumstances, a measurement of free testosterone (by an equilibrium dialysis method), bioavailable testosterone (consisting of free plus albumin bound), or calculated free testosterone (by total testosterone and SHBG measurements) may be useful.

The following rules on measurement of serum testosterone apply to most young and middle-aged men thought to have hypogonadism. If a morning serum total testosterone level is repeatedly below 230 ng/dL (8 nmol/L), and he has symptoms or signs compatible with low testosterone state, the patient is probably hypogonadal, and testosterone replacement is indicated. If the serum testosterone level is between 230 and 320 ng/dL with normal serum LH levels, the patient may or may not be clinically hypogonadal and androgen replacement may not improve the symptoms (e.g., sexual dysfunction). Thus, when serum total testosterone is borderline and LH is not increased, one of the measurements of bioactive testosterone is indicated (e.g., free testosterone). The guidelines for men older than 60 years are less certain. Because SHBG levels are often increased, total testosterone levels may overestimate the biologically active forms. A serum total testosterone level above 350 to 400 ng/dL indicates that hypogonadism is very unlikely to be the cause of the symptoms, and the clinician should look for other etiologies for the symptoms.

TREATMENT Rx

The main medical indication for androgen replacement therapy is male hypogonadism (Table 234-4). In approximately 10% of men with idiopathic hypogonadism reversed by testosterone therapy, the reversal is sustained after therapy is stopped. This suggests that some patients with low serum testosterone may have a transient cause of the deficiency. Administration of testosterone to elderly men with low-normal testosterone concentrations increases lean body mass and decreases fat mass. There are insufficient data to judge whether testosterone treatment will improve functional status or cognition. Carefully designed studies of the efficacy of testosterone treatment in older men are ongoing.

Absolute contraindications to androgen replacement therapy include carcinoma of the prostate and the male breast. Androgens should be used with caution in older men with an enlarged prostate and urinary symptoms, elevated hematocrit, and sleep-related breathing disorders. The various methods of delivering testosterone treatment are shown in Table 234-5.

TABLE 234-4   INDICATIONS FOR ANDROGEN THERAPY

Androgen deficiency (hypogonadism)
Microphallus (neonatal)
Delayed puberty in boys
Elderly men with low total or bioavailable or free testosterone levels and symptoms
Angioneurotic edema
Other possible uses or under investigation
　Hormonal male contraception
　Sarcopenia associated with cancer, human immunodeficiency virus infection,
　　chronic infection, frailty in older men and women
　Hypoactive sexual disorder in postmenopausal women

TABLE 234-5   ANDROGEN PREPARATIONS

ROUTE	PREPARATION	DOSE AND FREQUENCY OF ADMINISTRATION
Oral*	Testosterone undecenoate (not available in United States; available in Canada, Mexico, Europe, Asia)	40-80 mg PO two or three times daily
Buccal	Transbuccal testosterone, mucoadhesive tablets (Striant)	30 mg two times daily
Injection	Testosterone enanthate and cypionate	100 mg/wk IM or 150-200 mg IM every 2-3 wk
	Testosterone undecanoate (not available in United States)	750-1000 mg IM every 10-12 wk
Implant	Testosterone implants	75-mg pellets (in United States), 6-10 inserted once every 4-6 months
Transdermal	Scrotal patch	One patch delivering testosterone 4 or 6/day
	Nonscrotal patch Androderm	Two patches, each delivering testosterone 2.5 mg/day; or one patch delivering testosterone 5 mg/day
	Testoderm TTS	One patch delivering testosterone 5 mg/day
Transdermal gels	AndroGel or Testogel; Testim; Axiron; Fortesta	1 to 2% gel applied once daily delivering 50-100 mg testosterone on skin and 5 to 10 mg to body

*Oral modified 17α-alkylated androgens such as methyltestosterone, fluoxymesterone, oxymetholone, stanozolol, and oxandrolone are not recommended for the treatment of androgen-deficient states because of potential hepatotoxicity and adverse effects on serum lipids.
IM = intramuscularly; PO = orally.

Testosterone esters, such as testosterone enanthate (or cypionate) injections, are widely used in the United States and throughout the world. The recommended dose is 150 to 200 mg administered intramuscularly once every 2 to 3 weeks. Testosterone undecenoate injections administered every 10 to 12 weeks are available in many parts of the world but not yet in the United States.

Modified 17α-alkylated androgens (methyltestosterone and many anabolic steroids), which are available in oral preparations, are not recommended as androgen replacement. These agents may lead to abnormalities in liver function, marked decreases in high-density lipoprotein cholesterol, and increases in total cholesterol levels compared with the testosterone esters. Oral testosterone undecanoate capsules have been available for over 20 years in many parts of the world but not in the United States. Transbuccal delivery of testosterone by mucoadhesive tablets (30 mg applied twice daily) results in physiologic-range testosterone levels through direct absorption into the systemic circulation, thus avoiding first-pass effects on the liver. The tablets may be dislodged from the buccal mucous membrane. Other oral formulations are in clinical trials in the United States.

Implants (pellets) of crystalline testosterone are available for chronic treatment of hypogonadism. Serum testosterone levels are maintained in the physiologic range for 4 to 6 months. Implants are not usually used but are gaining some popularity with urologists in the United States; they are widely used in Australia and the United Kingdom.

Transdermal testosterone delivery through skin patches and gels have been available in the United States for over 15 years. The nonscrotal patches deliver 5 mg/day of testosterone, which is the physiologic production rate. These patches deliver levels of testosterone within the normal range but have a high incidence of skin irritability (redness, swelling, and blisters). Hydroalcoholic and nonalcoholic testosterone gels have been developed for transdermal application and have become the most widely used testosterone formulations in the United States. The usual dosage is 50 to 100 mg of 1, 1.62, and 2% testosterone gel applied daily to the skin, delivering 5 to 10 mg of testosterone to the body. This results in a more consistent serum concentration and causes little skin irritation. Transfer from the user to others is possible during routine use and may be a concern if there is close skin contact with women and children. Protective clothing or a shower is necessary to avoid transferring testosterone through skin-to-skin contact.

Table 234-6 shows the benefits and potential side effects of androgen treatment. In hypogonadal men, androgen replacement leads to the development and maintenance of secondary sexual characteristics. Testosterone has important anabolic effects on muscle and bone and improves libido and sexual dysfunction. It has less effect on erectile dysfunction. It has no major short-term effects on prostate tissue.[8] Epidemiologic studies indicate that lower testosterone is a risk factor for cardiovascular disease. Many small studies have shown benefit or no effect of cardiovascular disease but more recent studies suggest testosterone replacement may increase the risk for cardiovascular events in elderly men, especially those who are frail and have multiple comorbidties.[9]

TABLE 234-6   ANDROGEN THERAPY: RISKS VERSUS BENEFITS

BENEFITS	RISKS
Development or maintenance of secondary sex characteristics	Fluid retention
Improved libido and sexual function	Gynecomastia
Increased muscle mass and strength	Acne, oily skin
Increased bone mineral density	Increased hematocrit
Decreased body and visceral fat	Decreased high-density lipoprotein cholesterol (oral 17α-alkylated agents produce the greatest effect)
Improved mood	
Effect on cognition (?)	Sleep apnea
Effect on vitality and quality of life (?)	Aggressive behavior (?)
Decreased cardiovascular disease risk (epidemiologic studies); clinical study no benefits/risk	Prostate disease
	Benign prostatic hyperplasia (?)
	Carcinoma of prostate (aggravate existing cancer)
	Increased cardiovascular adverse events in one study in frail elderly men with multiple comorbid conditions

MALE INFERTILITY

DEFINITION

Infertility is defined as the failure of a couple to achieve pregnancy after at least 1 year of frequent unprotected intercourse. If a pregnancy has not occurred after 3 years, infertility will most likely persist without medical treatment.

EPIDEMIOLOGY

Studies in the United States and Europe showed a 1-year prevalence of infertility in 15% of couples. The prevalence in developing countries is likely to be higher because of the higher prevalence of genital tract infection. Of subfertility cases, 30 to 35% can be attributed to predominantly female factors, 25 to 30% to male factors, and 25 to 30% to problems in both partners.

PATHOBIOLOGY

Hypothalamic-pituitary disorders are infrequent causes of male infertility and are discussed in the section on hypogonadism and androgen deficiency. Testicular disorders are the most frequent identifiable cause of infertility (see Table 234-2). Y chromosome microdeletions are increasingly recognized as a genetic cause of azoospermia and severe oligozoospermia. Up to 25% of infertile men have microdeletions in the long arm of the Y chromosome, many of which map to the Yq11 region of the chromosome, which is called the azoospermic factor (AZF). Mutations in the AZF a and b regions are associated with azoospermia, whereas mutations of AFZc region may be associated with oligozoospermia.[10]

DIAGNOSIS

The approach to the diagnosis of an infertile couple includes management of both the male and the female partner (Figs. 234-8 and 234-9).

Examination of the ejaculate is the cornerstone for the investigation of an infertile man (Table 234-7). Semen samples are collected at the physician's office or at home, preferably after 2 to 7 days of abstinence from ejaculatory activity. The generally accepted reference values for a semen analysis are given in Table 234-8. A normal sperm concentration is greater than 15 million/mL, with a total sperm number greater than 39 million per ejaculate; however, men with lower sperm counts can be fertile. More than 40% of the spermatozoa should be motile, and more than 32% should demonstrate a progressive motility pattern. Using strict criteria to assess sperm morphology, the percentage of morphologically normal forms should be above 4%. There is considerable overlap in the semen quality of fertile and subfertile men. Low sperm concentration and/or poor sperm morphology are associated with lower chances of natural conception in the female partner. In patients with abnormal semen analyses, measurements of serum FSH, LH, and testosterone are indicated (see Fig. 234-7). Elevated FSH levels usually indicate severe germinal epithelium damage. A decreased serum inhibin B level also reflects poor Sertoli cell function and may indicate spermatogenic dysfunction. Elevated serum LH and FSH concentrations together with a low serum testosterone level indicate pantesticular failure leading to hypogonadism and infertility. Low serum FSH, LH, and testosterone concentrations suggest hypothalamic-pituitary dysfunction; serum prolactin should be measured, and additional investigations may be required. A low sperm concentration and suppressed LH level with an increased, normal, or low serum testosterone level (without clinical manifestations of androgen deficiency) may suggest exogenous androgen use. The hormonal pattern in androgen insensitivity (an uncommon cause of male infertility) is elevated LH, normal FSH, and high-normal to increased serum testosterone levels. Normal hormonal parameters in azoospermic (no sperm in the ejaculate) men with normal-sized testes may suggest congenital or acquired obstruction in the epididymis or vas deferens.

TREATMENT   Rx

An algorithmic approach to the treatment of male infertility is illustrated in Figures 234-8 and 234-9. The principles of managing male infertility can be summarized as follows. (1) Men with mild-to-moderate oligozoospermia, with or without decreased sperm motility and some impairment of motility, are

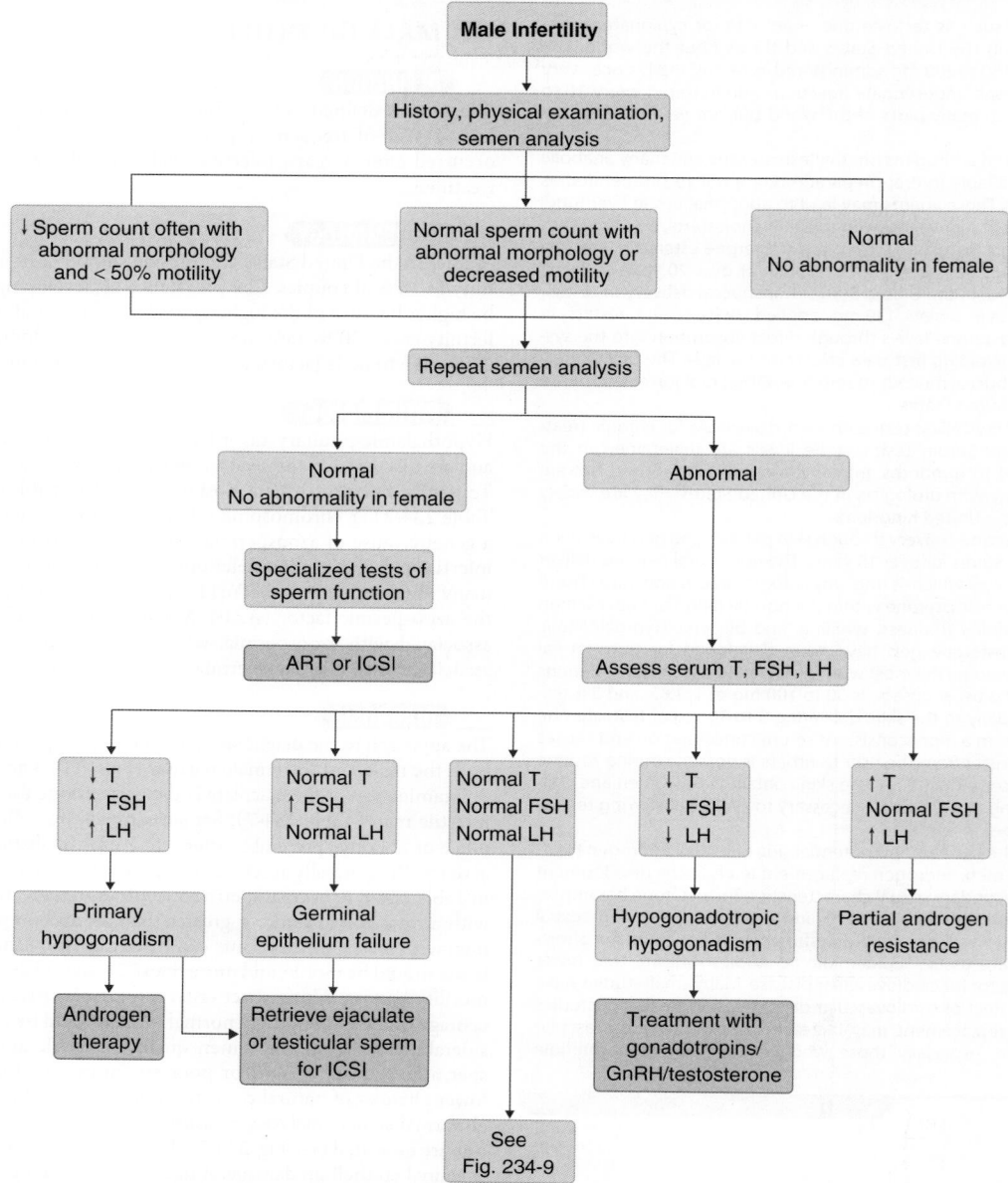

FIGURE 234-8. Algorithmic approach to the diagnosis and treatment of male infertility. ART = assisted reproductive technology; FSH = follicle-stimulating hormone; GnRH = gonadotropin-releasing hormone; ICSI = intracytoplasmic sperm injection; LH = serum luteinizing hormone; T = serum testosterone.

subfertile rather than infertile. Spontaneous pregnancies can occur in this group. (2) Reliable pharmaceutical treatment is limited to the 1 to 2% of infertile men with gonadotropin insufficiency. (3) Assisted reproductive technologies, including in vitro fertilization and intracytoplasmic sperm injection, have dramatically improved pregnancy rates. (4) In male factor infertility azoospermia (absence of sperm in the ejaculate) may occur in men with obstruction of the ejaculatory system. In these patients, in vitro fertilization and intracytoplasmic sperm injection after either percutaneous epididymal sperm extraction or microsurgical epididymal sperm extraction are highly successful. (5) Azoospermia resulting from impaired spermatogenesis may not be a sterile state, because sperm may be present within the testes. These sperm can be extracted, and intracytoplasmic sperm injection can be performed with good success, even in patients with Klinefelter's syndrome.

SEXUAL DYSFUNCTION

Sexual dysfunction can be divided into four main categories: (1) loss of desire (libido), (2) erectile dysfunction, (3) ejaculatory insufficiency, and (4) anorgasmic states.

Decreased Libido

Loss of libido refers to a reduction in sexual interest, initiative, and frequency and intensity of responses to internal or external erotic stimuli. Causal factors include psychogenic factors, CNS disease, androgen deficiency and resistance, and side effects from medications (e.g., antihypertensives, psychotropics, alcohol, narcotics, dopamine blockers, antiandrogens, and possibly 5α-reductase inhibitors). Treatment is directed toward the causal mechanism.

Ejaculatory Failure and Impaired Orgasm

Ejaculatory insufficiency refers to absent or reduced seminal emission or impaired ejaculatory contraction. It is usually associated with neurologic conditions and medication therapy. An anorgasmic state is a distressing but relatively uncommon condition in men in which the normal process of erection and ejaculation occurs in the absence of the subjective sensation of pleasure initiated at the time of emission and ejaculation. Premature ejaculation is the most common form of male sexual dysfunction. Estimates of prevalence vary, but 25 to 30% seems to be a reasonable estimate. The recently published *Diagnostic and Statistical Manual of Mental Disorders-5 (2013)* defines premature ejaculation as ejaculation occurring within approximately 1 minute of vaginal penetration before the person wishes it on 75% of occasions for at least 6 months and causing personal distress. The

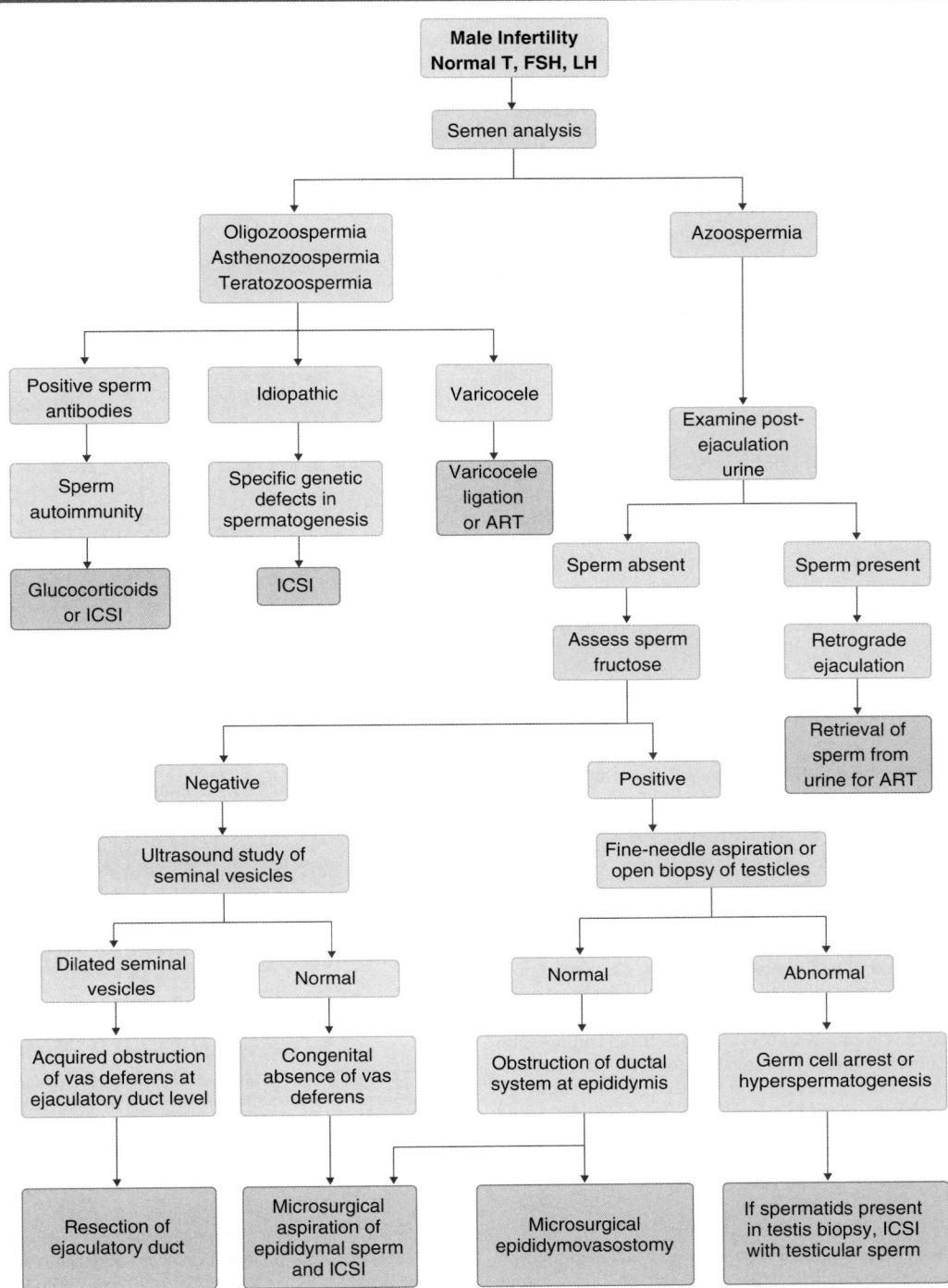

FIGURE 234-9. Algorithmic approach to the diagnosis and treatment of male infertility in patients with normal serum hormone concentrations. ART = assisted reproductive technology; FSH = follicle-stimulating hormone; ICSI = intracytoplasmic sperm injection; LH = serum luteinizing hormone; T = serum testosterone.

pathobiology of premature ejaculation is unknown. It may be associated with marked distress or interpersonal difficulty and is not a direct effect of substance abuse such as opiate withdrawal. The diagnosis is based mainly on sexual history and includes assessment of intravaginal ejaculatory latency time, perceived control, distress, and interpersonal difficulty. The first-line treatment is with selective serotonin reuptake inhibitors or a serotonin transporter inhibitor (e.g., dapoxetine 60 mg as on-demand therapy)[A3] together with behavioral therapy and relationship counseling. Topical anesthetic creams can be used as alternatives.[11]

Erectile Dysfunction
DEFINITION
Erectile dysfunction can be defined as a man's inability to obtain rigidity sufficient to permit coitus of adequate duration to satisfy himself and his partner.

EPIDEMIOLOGY
Current estimates suggest that 10 to 15% of all American men suffer from erectile dysfunction, with the incidence progressively increased as men become older. Data from the Massachusetts Aging Study report that 52% of men 40 to 70 years of age experience some degree of erectile dysfunction. The prevalence of erectile dysfunction is even higher in men with type 2 diabetes mellitus and after radical prostatectomy for prostate cancer. Recent epidemiologic studies in the United States and Europe in men between 50 to 80 years indicate that erectile dysfunction is associated with lower urinary tract obstructive symptoms/benign prostatic hyperplasia.

PATHOBIOLOGY
The causes of erectile dysfunction are many, but they can generally be categorized as follows: vasculogenic, psychological, endocrine, neurologic,

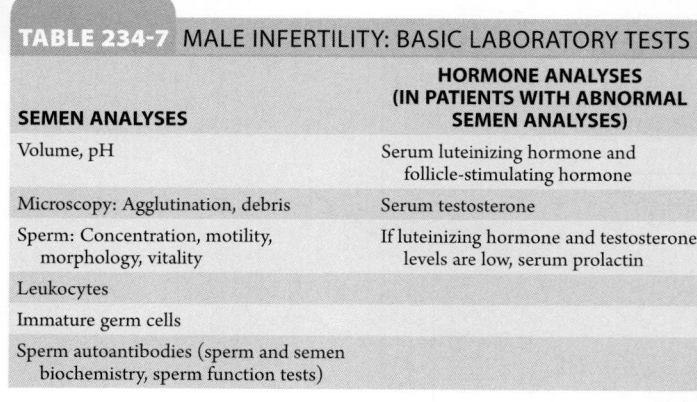

TABLE 234-7 MALE INFERTILITY: BASIC LABORATORY TESTS

SEMEN ANALYSES	HORMONE ANALYSES (IN PATIENTS WITH ABNORMAL SEMEN ANALYSES)
Volume, pH	Serum luteinizing hormone and follicle-stimulating hormone
Microscopy: Agglutination, debris	Serum testosterone
Sperm: Concentration, motility, morphology, vitality	If luteinizing hormone and testosterone levels are low, serum prolactin
Leukocytes	
Immature germ cells	
Sperm autoantibodies (sperm and semen biochemistry, sperm function tests)	

TABLE 234-8 SEMEN ANALYSIS: REFERENCE RANGE FROM FERTILE MEN*

PARAMETER	REFERENCE RANGE
Semen volume	>1.5 mL
Sperm	
Concentration	>15 million/mL
Total count	>39 million/ejaculate
Motility	>40% motile
	>32% progressively motile
Morphology	>4% normal[+]
Vitality (live)	>58%
Leukocytes	<1 million/mL

*Men whose partners had a time-to-pregnancy of ≤12 months were chosen to provide reference distributions for semen parameters.
[+]This value is based on the strict criteria for assessing sperm morphology in studies using in vitro fertilization as an end point.

iatrogenic (post–radical prostatectomy), drug related, systemic illness, and aging. Erectile dysfunction is common in older men, despite normal serum testosterone levels; this effect appears to be the result of impaired penile vasodilatory capacity as a result of endothelial dysfunction. Decreased non-adrenergic, noncholinergic nerve activity and reduced production of nitric oxide by endothelial cells result in decreased cavernous smooth muscle relaxation, decreased filling of the cavernous sinusoids, and reduced compression of the venous plexus against the tunica lead to failure of erection. Men presenting with erectile dysfunction share common risk factors with cardiovascular disease (smoking, obesity, metabolic syndrome, hyperlipidemia, and type 2 diabetes mellitus).[12] Recent evidence indicates that men presenting with mild erectile dysfunction should be assessed for cardiovascular disease, particularly when other risk factors are present.

DIAGNOSIS

The diagnosis of erectile dysfunction is based mainly on a detailed medical and sexual history of the patient and his partner when available. The history may reveal the underlying cause or other common disorders associated with erectile dysfunction. Physical examination should focus on genitourinary, cardiovascular, endocrine, and neurologic systems. Prostate examination is important because erectile dysfunction is commonly associated with symptomatic benign prostatic hyperplasia. Laboratory tests should include a morning serum testosterone, and, if indicated, prostate-specific antigen, fasting glucose (or hemoglobin A_{1C}), and cholesterol. Specific diagnostic tests are rarely required.

TREATMENT   Rx

The treatment of erectile dysfunction is to find the cause and treat the cause if found.[13] Symptoms can be effectively treated by the oral administration of penile-selective phosphodiesterase-5 inhibitors (sildenafil, vardenafil, tadalafil).[A5] A treatment algorithm for erectile dysfunction is given in Fig. 234-10. Lifestyle interventions reduce obesity and improve erectile function.[14] Combined androgen deficiency with decreased libido and decreased penile responsiveness resulting from impaired nitric oxide synthase activity may be

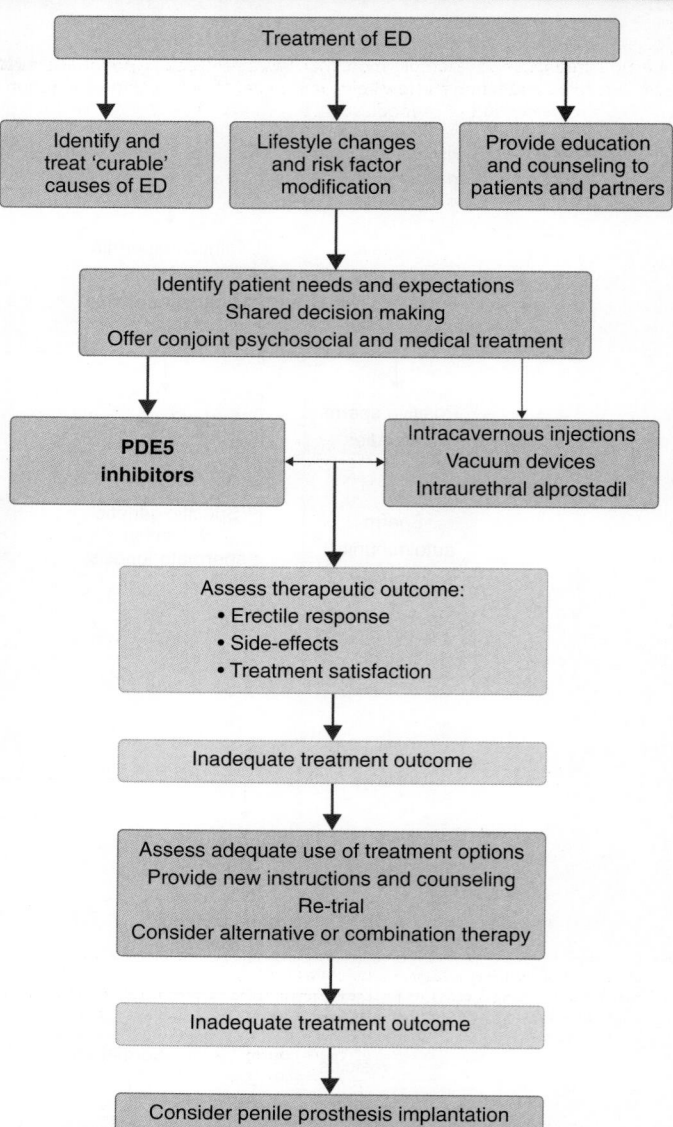

FIGURE 234-10. Treatment algorithm for erectile dysfunction (*ED*). PDE5 = cyclic GMP phosphodiesterase-5. (Reprinted with permission from Hatzimouratidis K, Amar E, Eardley I, et al. Guidelines on male sexual dysfunction: erectile dysfunction and premature ejaculation. *Eur Urol.* 2010;57:804-814. 2015 update: http://uroweb.org/guideline/male-sexual-dysfunction/. Accessed March 26, 2015.)

common in elderly men. With the availability of effective penile vasodilatory medications to ensure erectile capacity, complaints of diminished libido can be effectively treated with androgen supplementation.

Medical Therapy
Oral Medications

Oral and selective inhibitors of cGMP phosphodiesterase-5 (the primary phosphodiesterase in the penile cavernosal tissue) are effective for at least 60% of men. Inhibition of phosphodiesterase-5 causes persistence of normally (sexually) stimulated cGMP in the corpora cavernosa, resulting in protracted cavernosal tumescence and rigidity. Patients with diabetes mellitus, spinal cord injuries, prostatic surgery, and pelvic irradiation also benefit, but with a somewhat lower response rate. The usual starting dose of sildenafil is 50 mg, increasing in 25-mg increments up to 100 mg. Because of its mechanism of action, sildenafil is used on demand with recommended administration 20 to 60 minutes before intercourse. Two other potent phosphodiesterase-5 inhibitors (vardenafil and tadalafil) are widely used for the treatment of erectile dysfunction and appear to be equally effective. Vardenafil (5, 10, and 20 mg) has a relatively longer duration of action (4 to 6 hours), and tadalafil (10 or 20 mg) has an even longer duration of action (up to 36 hours). Randomized controlled trials showed that daily administration of tadalafil (5 mg) improved erectile function compared to on-demand treatment. Daily dosing of tadalafil is well tolerated and effective. Thus, daily dosing starting with 2.5 mg of tadalafil may be an alternative to on-demand administration if intercourse is expected to be more frequent—for example, more than twice per week. Hypogonadal men with erectile dysfunction and low libido may benefit from combined treatment with testosterone and phosphodiesterase-5 inhibitors (PDE-5). However, the addition of testosterone to sildenafil does not further improve erectile dysfunction.[A6] PDE-5 inhibitors should not be administered with nitrates because the accumulation of cGMP may result in lowering of blood pressure and hypotension. PDE-5 inhibitors also may interact with antihypertensive agents, including α-blockers, resulting in orthostatic hypotension.

Intracavernosal Injection

Second-line treatment of erectile dysfunction involves intracavernosal injection with vasodilators such as prostaglandin E₁ (Alprostadil) alone or with other vasodilators (papaverine, phentolamine) These medications are injected into the cavernosal space with a 27- to 30-gauge needle and may be useful in men who are refractory to oral agents. The main side effects of penile injections are pain and cavernosal fibrosis which usually resolves after discontinuation of injections. Presence of tunica fibrosis may suggest early Peyronie's disease,[15] and injections should be stopped. The intraurethral prostaglandin E₁ suppository alprostadil is believed to work locally on the corpora cavernosa as a vasodilatory agent. The suppository is apparently successful in improving erectile function in 30 to 66% of cases.

Penile Prostheses

Surgical implantation of penile prostheses that include inflatable and malleable devices are the third line of treatment for men who prefer a permanent solution of their problem or for those who do not respond to other therapies.

Grade A References

A1. Basaria S, Coviello AD, Travison TG, et al. Adverse events associated with testosterone administration. *N Engl J Med.* 2010;363:109-122.

A2. Corona G, Rastrelli G, Giagulli VA, et al. Dehydroepiandrosterone supplementation in elderly men: a meta-analysis study of placebo-controlled trials. *J Clin Endocrinol Metab.* 2013;98:3615-3626.

A3. Srinivas-Shankar U, Roberts SA, Connolly MJ, et al. Effects of testosterone on muscle strength, physical function, body composition, and quality of life in intermediate-frail and frail elderly men: a randomized, double-blind, placebo-controlled study. *J Clin Endocrinol Metab.* 2010;95:639-650.

A4. De Hong C, Ren LL, Yu H, et al. The role of dapoxetine hydrochloride on-demand for the treatment of men with premature ejaculation. *Sci Rep.* 2014;4:7269.

A5. Yuan J, Zhang R, Yang Z, et al. Comparative effectiveness and safety of oral phosphodiesterase type 5 inhibitors for erectile dysfunction: a systematic review and network meta-analysis. *Eur Urol.* 2013;63:902-912.

A6. Spitzer M, Basaria S, Travison TG, et al. Effect of testosterone replacement on response to sildenafil citrate in men with erectile dysfunction: a parallel, randomized trial. *Ann Intern Med.* 2012;157:681-691.

GENERAL REFERENCES

For the General References and other additional features, please visit Expert Consult at https://expertconsult.inkling.com.

235

OVARIES AND PUBERTAL DEVELOPMENT

ROBERT W. REBAR AND WILLIAM H. CATHERINO

DEFINITION

The ovaries or female gonads episodically release female gametes (oocytes or eggs) and secrete sex steroid hormones, principally androstenedione, estradiol, and progesterone. Oocytes are released only during the adult reproductive years, when sex steroid secretion is also greatest, but the ovaries are physiologically active throughout life.

Sex steroids affect the growth, differentiation, and function of a variety of tissues and organs throughout the body; therefore, abnormalities of the ovaries and of sex steroid secretion should be recognized by all physicians. A rational approach to the diagnosis and treatment of reproductive disorders in women requires an understanding of the functions of the ovaries and of their most important unit, the follicle, throughout life.

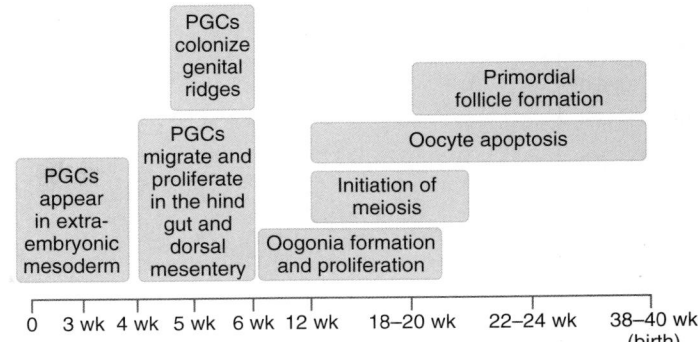

FIGURE 235-1. Diagram illustrating the developmental timetable of the major events that ultimately lead to the formation of primordial follicles during the process of human ovary organogenesis. PGC = primordial germ cell.

PHYSIOLOGY

Embryology

Embryogenesis and Differentiation

Organogenesis of the ovaries occurs during fetal life. Ovarian cells are derived from two different sources: (1) primordial germ cells (PGCs) originate at a site outside the prospective gonads, and (2) somatic cells differentiate from the coelomic epithelium and gonadal mesenchyme. In females, PGCs become oocytes, whereas somatic cells differentiate into a variety of cell types, including granulosa, theca, and vascular cells.

PGCs in the human embryo can be distinguished at the gastrula stage (Fig. 235-1). Shortly after formation, PGCs migrate through the dorsal mesentery to the genital ridges. Chemotaxis plays a role in directing PGCs to the gonads. During migration, PGCs proliferate in response to growth factors, most notably Kit ligand. The importance of Kit is demonstrated by the finding that loss-of-function mutations result in a paucity of PGCs, which in turn results in premature ovarian failure.

The genital ridges are characterized by a thickening of the coelomic epithelium and underlying primary mesenchyme. Initially, the gonads are sexually indifferent. Male gonadal differentiation is triggered by the Y chromosome–encoded testis-determining factor SRY. SRY expression results in the differentiation of Sertoli cells and the secretion of müllerian-inhibiting substance, which induces regression of the müllerian ducts. Testicular interstitial cells differentiate into Leydig cells, which secrete testosterone, which in turn stimulates wolffian duct development. In the female, the absence of müllerian-inhibiting substance and testosterone and the activation of the WNT4 pathway leads to the degeneration of the wolffian ducts and the development of the müllerian ducts.[1,2] Thus, the development of the ovaries and female reproductive system is considered a "default" pathway.

When PGCs enter the genital ridges, they begin gametogenesis (see Fig. 235-1). In females, this process is termed *oogenesis* and involves the differentiation of PGCs into oogonia and oocytes. When sex-specific differentiation of the ovary commences, the inactive X chromosome in the PGCs becomes active. This denotes the formation of mitotically active oogonia. The importance of two functional X chromosomes during oogenesis is emphasized by the fact that 45,X females lack oocytes and undergo premature menopause.

After repeated mitosis, oogonia initiate meiosis and become oocytes (see Fig. 235-1). At approximately the same time, granulosa cells differentiate within the gonadal mesenchyme and establish intimate associations with oocytes. Oocytes that become surrounded by granulosa cells stop meiosis after diplotene, and the bivalents enter an interphase state known as dictyotene. If an oocyte is not surrounded by granulosa cells, meiosis continues to diakinesis, and the oocyte dies by apoptosis, although this may not always be true.[3] Granulosa cells, therefore, are critical for oocyte survival. The majority of oocytes die during fetal ovary development (Fig. 235-2), apparently from a lack of contact with granulosa cells.

With further development, the oocyte–granulosa cell complex becomes a primordial follicle. This occurs between the sixth and ninth months of gestation (Fig. 235-3). A primordial follicle consists of a single layer of squamous granulosa cells, a small (about 15 μm in diameter) dictyotene oocyte, and a thin basal lamina (see Fig. 235-3). In the human female, all potential future eggs have entered diplotene of meiosis at the time of birth.

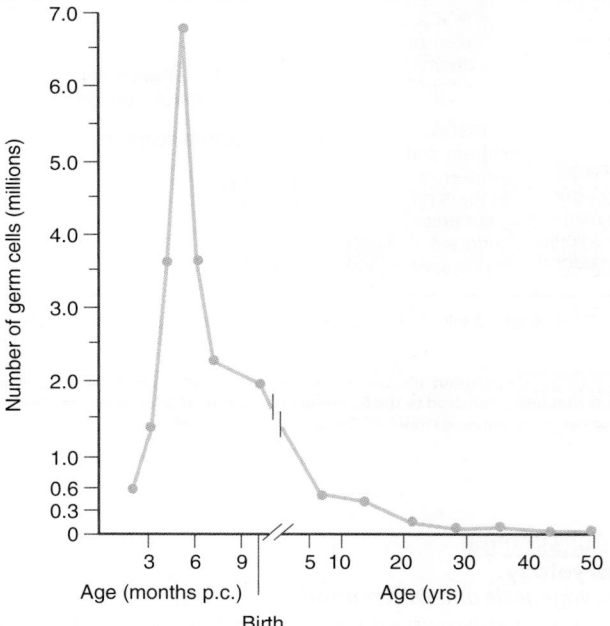

FIGURE 235-2. Changes in the total number of germ cells in the human ovaries during aging. At early to mid-gestation, the number of germ cells increases to almost 7 million; shortly thereafter, the number declines rapidly to about 2 million at birth. The number continues to decline until no oocytes are detected at 50 years of age. p.c. = Post conception. (From Baker TG. Radiosensitivity of mammalian oocytes with particular reference to the human female. *Am J Obstet Gynecol.* 1971;110:746-761.)

Anatomy

The Adult Ovary

The ovaries, which normally measure 2.5 to 5.0 cm long, 1.5 to 3.0 cm wide, and 0.6 to 1.5 cm thick in adults, are organized into two principal parts. A central zone, the medulla, is surrounded by a prominent peripheral zone, the cortex (Fig. 235-4). Growing follicles at different stages of development are present in the cortex. Typically, one follicle per cycle reaches maturity and ovulates its ovum. After ovulation, the follicle transforms into a corpus luteum. The corpus luteum of the cycle lasts for about 14 days, after which it dies and becomes a nodule of dense connective tissue, the corpus albicans (see Fig. 235-4).

The medulla is composed of loose connective tissue with numerous blood vessels and associated nerves. The arterial supply to the ovary originates from two principal sources: the ovarian artery and the uterine artery. These two vessels, which enter the medulla from opposite directions, form an anastomotic trunk and become a common vessel called the ramus ovaricus artery. This artery gives rise to a series of primary branches (spiral arteries) that enter the hilum. In the hilum, numerous secondary and tertiary branches are given off to supply the medulla and the follicles and luteal tissue in the cortex (see Fig. 235-4). The hilum also contains the hilus cells (see Fig. 235-4), which, like the testicular Leydig cells, contain Reinke crystals and secrete testosterone. The physiologic role of the hilus cells is still unknown.

Ovarian Function in Childhood and Puberty

Physical Changes at Puberty

Puberty extends from the earliest signs of sexual maturation until the attainment of physical, mental, and emotional maturity. Pubertal changes in girls result directly or indirectly from maturation of the hypothalamic-pituitary-ovarian (HPO) unit.[4] Human puberty is characterized hormonally by a resetting of the negative gonadal steroid feedback loop, the establishment of new circadian and ultradian (frequent) gonadotropin rhythms, and the acquisition in the female of a positive estrogen feedback loop controlling the menstrual cycle as interdependent expressions of the gonadotropins and ovarian steroids. In girls, pubertal development generally occurs between 7 and 14 years of age. The age at onset and the rate of progress through puberty are variable and depend on genetic, socioeconomic, nutritional, physical, and psychological factors. It appears that there are racial differences in the onset of pubertal development. In the United States, development begins earlier in African American than in white girls.

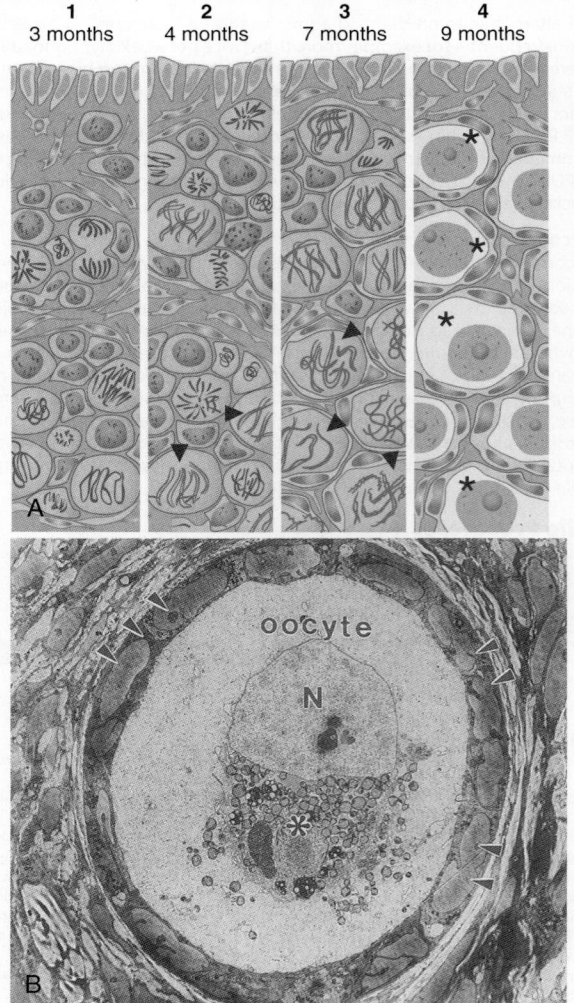

FIGURE 235-3. A, Drawing showing gametogenesis in the human fetal ovary leading to the formation of primordial follicles. At 3 months (1), oogonia divide mitotically. At 4 months (2), some oogonia deep within the cortical cords enter meiosis *(arrowheads)*. At 7 months (3), the cords are no longer distinct, and all germ cells are in meiotic prophase I. At 9 months (4), some oocytes become associated with granulosa cells and appear as primordial follicles *(asterisks)*. B, Electron micrograph of human primordial follicle. Granulosa cells *(arrowheads)*, oocyte nucleus (N), and Balbiani's body *(asterisk)* are shown. (From Erickson GF. The ovary: basic principles and concepts. In: Felig P, Baxter JD, Broadus AE, et al, eds. *Endocrinology and Metabolism*, 3rd ed. New York: McGraw-Hill; 1995.)

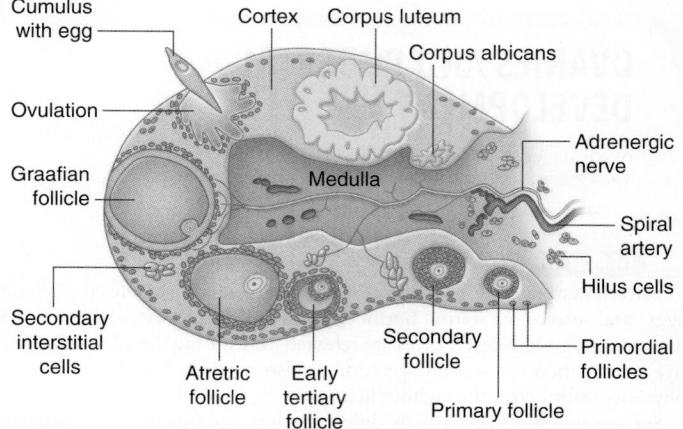

FIGURE 235-4. Diagram showing the anatomy of the human ovary during the reproductive years. Developing follicles and the corpus luteum are located in the cortex; the hilus cells, autonomic nerves, and spiral arteries are present in the medulla. (From Erickson GF. The ovary: basic principles and concepts. In: Felig P, Baxter JD, Broadus AE, et al, eds. *Endocrinology and Metabolism*, 3rd ed. New York: McGraw-Hill; 1995.)

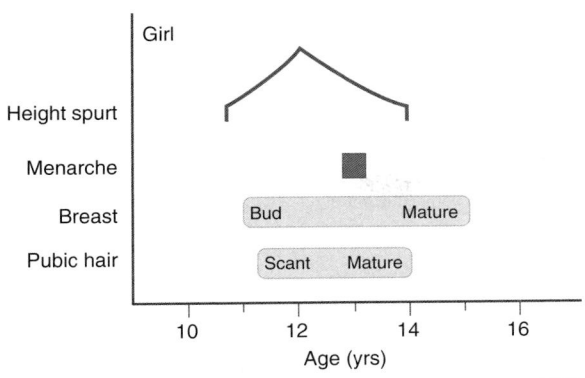

FIGURE 235-5. Temporal sequence of events for the "average" girl during puberty. (From Rebar RW. Practical evaluation of hormonal status. In: Yen SSC, Jaffe RB, Barbieri RL, eds. *Reproductive Endocrinology: Physiology, Pathophysiology, and Clinical Management,* 4th ed. Philadelphia: WB Saunders; 1999:710.)

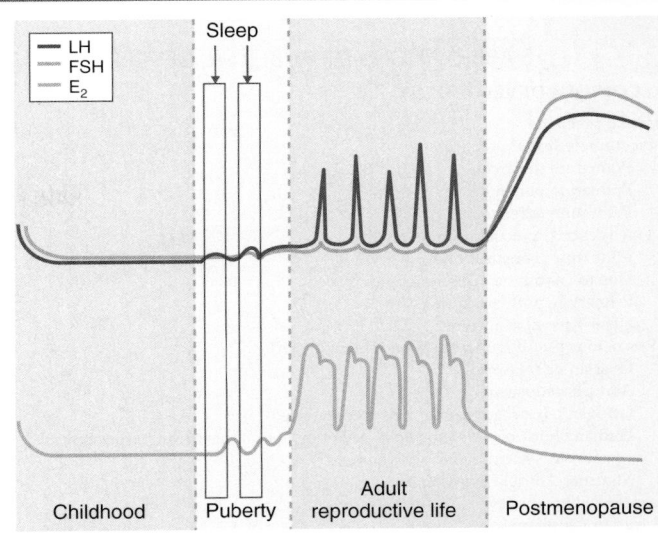

FIGURE 235-6. The changing patterns of luteinizing hormone (LH), follicle-stimulating hormone (FSH), and estradiol (E₂) concentrations in peripheral blood throughout the life of a woman. Not shown is the fact that both LH and FSH are secreted in a pulsatile fashion. The pubertal period has been expanded to illustrate the sleep-associated increases in LH and FSH followed by morning increases in E₂ that are observed during puberty. (Reprinted with permission from Endocrine and Metabolism Continuing Education Quality Control Program, 1982. Copyright American Association for Clinical Chemistry Inc.)

Physical changes occur in an orderly sequence during a definite time frame in puberty (Fig. 235-5).[5] Breast budding in girls is usually the first pubertal change, followed shortly by the appearance of pubic hair, with menarche occurring late in pubertal development. The time from breast budding (mean age of 10.0 years in white girls and 8.9 years in African Americans) to menarche is 2 years. Breast development results from increasing ovarian estrogen production, and pubic and axillary hair results from increasing androgen production. Estrogens are required for the growth of pubic hair as well.

The ovarian sex steroids join with growth hormone and adrenal androgens to produce the adolescent growth spurt. Peak growth velocity is achieved relatively early, with little growth observed after menarche. It has been estimated that more than 50 genes play roles in determining final adult height. It is now clear that estrogen, and not testosterone, is the primary hormone mediating pubertal bone growth in both males and females. Lean body mass, skeletal mass, and body fat are equal in prepubertal boys and girls, but by maturity, women have twice as much body fat as men and less lean body mass and skeletal mass as a result of differences in sex steroid secretion. Estrogens are necessary for the normal formation, mineralization, and maturation of bones. Well-established standards exist for determining whether bone age is appropriate for chronologic age, typically by examining radiographs of the bones of the wrist. Estrogen deficiencies retard, and excesses advance, bone age in relation to chronologic age.

Hormonal Changes

The ovaries function even in early childhood. Low levels of luteinizing hormone (LH) and follicle-stimulating hormone (FSH) are normally present, and these levels increase if the ovaries are removed before puberty, just as they do later in life, indicating the exquisite sensitivity of the hypothalamic-pituitary unit to extremely low circulating sex steroid levels. As puberty nears, there is a progressive decrease in sensitivity of the hypothalamic-pituitary unit to sex steroids, leading to the increased secretion of pituitary gonadotropins, stimulation of sex steroid output, and development of secondary sex characteristics. Increased secretion of both LH and FSH initially occurs at night with sleep and is associated with increased estradiol secretion the next morning (Fig. 235-6). As is true for most hormones, LH and FSH are secreted in an episodic or pulsatile rather than a continuous fashion. Later in puberty, secretion of LH and FSH is increased throughout the 24-hour period, except during the early follicular phase, when nighttime increases still occur. Basal levels of estradiol, the major estrogen secreted by the ovaries, increase throughout puberty. A "critical body mass" may be required for positive estrogen feedback and ovulation. During the first 2 years after menarche, up to 90% of menstrual cycles may be anovulatory because of a delay in synchronization of the HPO axis.

⬤ ABERRATIONS IN PUBERTAL DEVELOPMENT

Abnormalities of pubertal development can be divided into four major categories (Table 235-1):

1. Precocious puberty represents any pubertal changes before age 9 years in white girls and before age 8 years in African American girls. This remains controversial. Some clinicians believe evaluation is warranted only if pubertal development begins before age 7 years in white girls and 6 years in African American girls. A compromise may involve careful screening by history and physical examination of girls with early-onset puberty, looking for central nervous system (CNS) symptoms, behavioral concerns, and any other abnormal findings that might warrant further evaluation. The nearer pubertal development begins to the mean age of puberty onset, the less likely it is to have a pathologic basis. Precocious development is isosexual when it is common to the phenotypic sex of the individual and heterosexual when the development is characteristic of the opposite sex. True or central precocious puberty is due to premature maturation of the hypothalamic-pituitary axis. In the absence of increased hypothalamic-pituitary activity, precocious pseudopuberty exists.

2. Delayed (or interrupted) puberty is defined as the absence of any secondary sex characteristics by age 13 years, the absence of menarche by age 16 years, or the passage of 5 years or more from breast budding to menarche.

3. Asynchronous pubertal development occurs when there is deviation from the normal pattern of pubertal development.

4. Heterosexual pubertal development occurs at the appropriate time but has some features characteristic of the opposite sex.

Precocious Puberty

▶ DIAGNOSIS

The overall incidence of precocious puberty has been estimated at 1 in 5000 to 10,000 children. About 10 times as many girls as boys are affected.

Differential Diagnosis

The temporal sequence in which the signs and symptoms of sex steroid hormone excess appear is most important. *Incomplete isosexual precocious puberty* indicates premature development of only a single pubertal feature. If breast budding occurs before age 8 years in the absence of any other development, the diagnosis may be *premature thelarche.* Premature thelarche is believed to be due to transient increases in estrogen secretion or increased breast sensitivity to the small quantities of circulating estrogens present before puberty. Simple ovarian cysts may be present in some girls with this disorder and may be due in some cases to the same genetic abnormality found in girls with McCune-Albright syndrome (Chapters 231 and 248). If pubic or axillary hair develops alone and persists, *premature pubarche* and *adrenarche* must be considered. These abnormalities are associated with slight increases in adrenal androgen secretion but not with clitorimegaly or other signs of virilization. These syndromes require no treatment, and affected girls typically begin true puberty at the usual age. Careful follow-up is required to distinguish these disorders from true precocious puberty.

TABLE 235-1   ABERRATIONS OF PUBERTAL DEVELOPMENT

PRECOCIOUS DEVELOPMENT

Isosexual precocity
  Incomplete sexual precocity
    Premature thelarche
    Premature pubarche
    Premature adrenarche
  True (central) precocious puberty
    Idiopathic (constitutional)
    Due to central nervous system lesions
    Primary hypothyroidism
    Silver-Russell syndrome
  Precocious pseudopuberty (of peripheral origin)
    Ovarian neoplasms
    Adrenal neoplasms
    Iatrogenic (estrogen-containing preparations)
    Human chorionic gonadotropin–secreting neoplasms distinct from central nervous system and ovarian tumors
    McCune-Albright syndrome
Heterosexual precocity
  Ovarian neoplasms
  Adrenal neoplasms
  Congenital adrenal hyperplasia
  Other rare disorders of sexual differentiation

DELAYED PUBERTAL DEVELOPMENT*

Anatomic abnormalities
  Mayer-Rokitansky-Küster-Hauser syndrome
  Distal genital tract obstruction
    Transverse vaginal septum
    Imperforate hymen
    Vaginal agenesis
Hypergonadotropic hypogonadism (FSH >30-40 mIU/mL)
  Gonadal dysgenesis
    With stigmata of Turner syndrome
    Pure (46,XX or 46,XY)
    Mixed
  Ovarian failure with normal ovarian development
    Genetic disorders
    Autoimmune disorders
    Gonadotropin receptor or postreceptor defects (resistant ovary or Savage's syndrome?)
    Enzymatic defects (17α-hydroxylase deficiency, galactosemia)
    Physical causes
      Irradiation
      Chemotherapeutic agents
      Viral agents
    Idiopathic

Hypogonadotropic or normogonadotropic hypogonadism (LH and FSH <10 mIU/mL, or LH and FSH 6-25 mIU/mL with at least one being <10 mIU/mL)
  Isolated gonadotropin deficiency
  In association with midline defects (Kallmann's syndrome)
    Independent of associated disorders
  Neoplasms of the hypothalamic-pituitary axis
    Craniopharyngiomas
    Pituitary tumors
    Others
  Infiltrative processes (Langerhans-type histiocytosis)
  Idiopathic hypopituitarism
  "Hypothalamic" forms of amenorrhea
    Psychogenic
    Exercise associated
    Associated with malnutrition
    Anorexia nervosa
  Miscellaneous disorders
    Prader-Labhart-Willi syndrome
    Laurence-Moon-Bardet-Biedl syndrome
    Primary hypothyroidism
Constitutional delayed puberty

ASYNCHRONOUS PUBERTAL DEVELOPMENT

Incomplete forms of androgen insensitivity
Complete forms of androgen insensitivity

HETEROSEXUAL PUBERTAL DEVELOPMENT

Polycystic ovary syndrome
Congenital adrenal hyperplasia (female pseudohermaphroditism)
  21-Hydroxylase deficiency
  11β-Hydroxylase deficiency
  3β-ol-Hydroxysteroid dehydrogenase deficiency
Male pseudohermaphroditism due to 5α-reductase deficiency
Male pseudohermaphroditism due to partial androgen insensitivity
Mixed gonadal dysgenesis
Androgen-producing neoplasms
  Ovarian
  Adrenal
Cushing's syndrome

*No development by age 13 yr, absence of menarche by age 15 yr, or passage of ≥5 yr from breast budding without menarche.
FSH = follicle-stimulating hormone; LH = luteinizing hormone.

When precocious development is isosexual, the purpose of the evaluation is to determine whether the cause is central (true precocious puberty) or peripheral, in which case it is considered gonadotropin-releasing hormone (GnRH)–independent precocious puberty or precocious pseudopuberty. Careful questioning of the patient and her parents may indicate the inadvertent ingestion or absorption of sex steroids (iatrogenic or factitious). As many as 20% of individuals with true precocious puberty have one of several organic brain diseases, including any of several neoplasms, tuberous sclerosis, neurofibromatosis, encephalitis, meningitis, vascular malformations, and hydrocephalus. Because of the seriousness of intracranial lesions, girls with precocious puberty must have radiographic evaluation of the CNS, most effectively by magnetic resonance imaging (MRI). In at least 75% of girls with true precocious puberty, however, no cause is identified (idiopathic or constitutional).

The physical examination may also provide critical information about the cause of the precocious development. Cutaneous café au lait spots, facial asymmetry, polyostotic fibrous dysplasia and other skeletal abnormalities, cranial nerve deficits, and multiple ovarian follicular cysts suggest McCune-Albright syndrome (Chapters 231 and 248) in a girl with precocious development. It is now known that various clones of cells in the endocrine glands of girls with this disorder function autonomously with respect to cyclic adenosine monophosphate production as a consequence of a mutation within exon 8 of the *GNAS* gene, encoding the G$_s$ protein α–subunit. This same mutation probably accounts for the bone lesions and café au lait hyperpigmentation.

Other endocrine cells may be similarly affected and lead to pituitary adenomas (usually secreting growth hormone), hyperthyroidism, and, rarely, adrenal hyperplasia.

Studies on the etiologic causes for precocious puberty are ongoing. Heterozygous mutations in the paternal *MKRN3* gene are a diagnosable cause of familial central precocious puberty.[6] Another molecule, kisspeptin, is involved in pubertal development. Kisspeptin and its receptor GPR54 are essential regulators of GnRH-induced gonadotropin secretion and pubertal onset. Activation results in stimulation of the HPO axis, and elevated kisspeptin levels are associated with precocious puberty. Additionally, kisspeptin loss-of-function mutations result in normosmic idiopathic hypogonadotropic hypogonadism.

Abdominal and rectal examination may reveal a mass, suggesting an adrenal or ovarian tumor. Because palpable ovarian cysts may rarely develop before ovulation in true precocious puberty, the presence of a mass does not confirm the diagnosis of precocious pseudopuberty.

When vaginal bleeding is the only sign of development, the diagnosis of sexual precocity should be suspect. Common causes of bleeding in this age group include irritation from a vaginal infection or foreign body, sexual assault, prolapse of the urethral meatus, and ingestion of estrogen-containing medications (most commonly, oral contraceptive preparations). A vaginal or cervical neoplasm is also a rare possibility. Thus, vaginal bleeding requires a vaginal examination, which is often best performed with the patient under anesthesia, before further evaluation is undertaken.

Heterosexual precocity in an apparent prepubertal female is almost always due to congenital adrenal hyperplasia or to an androgen-secreting adrenal or ovarian neoplasm. Only rarely must another disorder of sexual differentiation be considered (Chapter 233). It is important to examine the external genitalia carefully because congenital adrenal hyperplasia is usually associated with some degree of sexual ambiguity.

Excessive androgens produced endogenously by abnormal fetal adrenal glands in utero or diffusing across the placenta to the fetus from the mother can virilize the external genitalia and result in female pseudohermaphroditism. The extent of virilization varies from only an enlarged clitoris to sexual ambiguity sufficient to make gender assignment difficult.

Excessive maternal androgen secretion, typically from an ovarian or adrenal neoplasm, can lead to virilization of a female fetus. This occurs very rarely because of the great capacity of the placenta to aromatize naturally occurring androgens to estrogens. Virilization of a female fetus is much more likely to occur if a pregnant woman has ingested a synthetic steroid preparation with androgenic properties because synthetic compounds generally cannot be aromatized.

Excessive androgen secretion beginning in utero is usually associated with defective cortisol synthesis. As a consequence, pituitary corticotropin secretion is increased, resulting in congenital adrenal hyperplasia and excessive androgen secretion. The three different enzyme defects in the steroidogenic pathway that can lead to virilization of the female fetus are described in Chapter 233. The most common form of congenital adrenal hyperplasia is 21-hydroxylase deficiency, accounting for the disorder in more than 90% of affected individuals. The defect may vary from partial to complete deficiency of the enzyme.

Diagnostic Tests
Measurement of Peptide and Steroid Hormones
Increased levels of immunoreactive human chorionic gonadotropin (HCG) may suggest an HCG-secreting neoplasm, most commonly an ovarian teratoma or dysgerminoma. In such cases, the HCG, which is antigenically and biologically similar to LH, stimulates ovarian steroid secretion and pseudopubertal development. Because even specific LH immunoassays show some cross-reactivity with HCG, values for serum LH may be elevated in individuals with HCG-secreting tumors. Immunoreactive HCG is always elevated in the presence of such tumors. Levels and ratios of FSH and LH typical of pubertal as opposed to prepubertal girls help in the diagnosis of true precocious puberty. Timed urine collections rather than blood samples can be used to measure gonadotropin secretion if necessary. The use of exogenous GnRH to stimulate endogenous LH and FSH secretion can help differentiate gonadotropin-dependent from gonadotropin-independent precocious puberty and is regarded as the "gold standard" in the diagnosis of central precocious puberty.[7] If GnRH is not available, a GnRH analogue can be substituted. Excessively high circulating levels of estrogen (>100 pg estradiol) suggest an estrogen-producing neoplasm or a functioning ovarian cyst. High levels of serum testosterone suggest an ovarian source of excess androgen in girls with heterosexual development, whereas increased levels of dehydroepiandrosterone or its sulfate (the principal precursors of 17-ketosteroids) suggest an adrenal source. High levels of serum 17-hydroxyprogesterone imply congenital adrenal hyperplasia secondary to 21-hydroxylase deficiency, whereas high levels of serum 11-deoxycortisol imply an 11β-hydroxylase deficiency (Chapter 233). In congenital adrenal hyperplasia, these hormone levels should decrease promptly after the oral administration of suppressive doses of dexamethasone. Suppression in response to exogenous corticoids occurs much less consistently in individuals with adrenal cortical adenomas and carcinomas (Chapter 227) and rarely in those with ovarian androgen-secreting neoplasms.

Additional Studies
Imaging of the CNS is the most important test if true precocious puberty is present or if there are any neurologic deficits. Ultrasonography of the adrenals and ovaries or computed tomography (CT) of the adrenals may be indicated to confirm clinical suspicions. In girls with ovarian or adrenal neoplasms, the tumor can almost always be localized radiographically. Catheterization of the ovarian and adrenal veins and measurements of the effluent steroids from each gland should be pursued only when CT, ultrasonography, or MRI fails to identify a suspected neoplasm. Radiographic estimation of bone age is also indicated and serves as a useful tool to follow the results of treatment.

TREATMENT [Rx]

Treatment of precocious puberty should be initiated promptly so that the patient's ultimate height is not compromised as a result of sex steroid–induced premature epiphyseal closure and to prevent or attenuate emotional disturbances in the patient and her parents.[8]

GnRH analogues are now the preferred therapy for suppressing gonadotropin secretion, and they also may prevent early bone maturation. No randomized trials have been conducted, but there is universal acknowledgment that GnRH analogues increase ultimate adult height in girls presenting before 6 years of age. Two unresolved issues are whether to initiate treatment with GnRH analogues in girls between 6 and 8 years of age and at what age to stop treatment. In addition, some data suggest that metformin may prevent hirsutism and oligomenorrhea in the teenage years when started in 8- to 12-year-old girls with a history of low-normal birth weight and precocious puberty,[A1] although these findings have not been confirmed by other groups. The analogues are not effective in children with McCune-Albright syndrome, and ketoconazole and testolactone have been only marginally successful. Aqueous depot medroxyprogesterone acetate (100 to 200 mg intramuscularly every 2 to 4 weeks) also may be used to suppress gonadotropin secretion; however, it does not always prevent premature epiphyseal closure and the resultant short stature. Effective treatment appears to improve fertility in adult life.[9]

Individuals with CNS or steroid-secreting neoplasms must undergo therapy appropriate for the particular lesion. Girls with congenital adrenal hyperplasia are appropriately managed with glucocorticoids (plus mineralocorticoids when indicated), as outlined in Chapter 233.

Delayed Puberty

Girls who have no evidence of thelarche by age 13 years or who fail to undergo menarche by age 15 years have delayed puberty and should be evaluated.[10] Ovarian failure, congenital absence of the uterus and vagina, and constitutional delay constitute about two thirds of cases in large series. Because of the anxiety generated by delayed puberty, some evaluation is always indicated regardless of the age of the patient.

When pubertal development progresses normally but menstruation does not begin, an abnormality in the genital tract should be considered. Congenital malformations of the müllerian ducts are uncommon, occurring in 0.02% of all women. Most do not cause amenorrhea, and many do not impair reproduction. The anomalies associated with amenorrhea vary in severity from an imperforate hymen to complete aplasia of all müllerian duct derivatives, with vaginal atresia. Although aplasia generally involves all the müllerian duct derivatives, defects may involve only a single part of the distal genital tract. Family aggregates of the most common disorders of müllerian differentiation in females—müllerian aplasia and incomplete müllerian fusion—do occur and are best explained by polygenic or multifactorial inheritance. It is clear that the HOX genes, a family of regulatory genes that encode transcription factors, are essential for proper development of the müllerian tract.

A müllerian duct anomaly is suggested by (1) normal levels of serum gonadotropins and steroids, (2) an abnormal outflow tract, (3) a history of cyclic abdominal pain with or without a palpable mass, and (4) normal development of secondary sex characteristics. Normal ovarian function still induces endometrial growth and shedding after menarche if the uterus is normal. In the absence of a normal outflow tract, however, the menstrual effluent is retained and may or may not escape into the abdominal cavity. Free in the abdominal cavity, the effluent may cause endometriosis. Constrained to the uterine cavity, the effluent causes hematometra and a large abdominal mass. In the absence of a mass or cyclic pain, karyotyping is indicated in girls with evidence of an abnormal genital tract to rule out disorders of sexual differentiation (Chapter 233). Such disorders, however, almost never occur together with completely normal pubertal development. In girls with a normal karyotype and a genital tract anomaly, examination under anesthesia and diagnostic laparoscopy should be undertaken to delineate the extent of the defect. When the abnormality consists of an imperforate hymen or transverse vaginal septum only, surgical restoration can be accomplished relatively simply. Attempts to provide an outflow tract for the uterus should not be undertaken if there is no cervix because of the high risk for recurrent pelvic infection. Even with a functional cervix, the construction of an outflow tract that permits successful pregnancy is unlikely. A functional vagina can be constructed surgically or by the daily use of ever-larger dilators. To prevent shrinkage and scarring, surgery should be deferred until the patient is willing to use dilators on a daily basis or she is about to become sexually active.

Other causes of delayed puberty and primary amenorrhea are the same as those that cause amenorrhea in older women (Chapter 236). When no apparent cause of delayed development is found, constitutional delayed puberty must be entertained as a diagnosis of exclusion.[11] A strong family history of delayed maturation supports this presumption. Small doses of estrogen can be administered to induce some pubertal development, but this may obscure a pathologic cause of the delay and may compromise linear growth and ultimate height.[12]

Asynchronous Pubertal Development

Asynchronous pubertal development is characteristic of male pseudohermaphroditism due to androgen insensitivity, especially complete testicular feminization. This syndrome of androgen insensitivity is inherited as either an X-linked recessive trait or a sex-limited autosomal dominant trait. Despite the presence of intra-abdominal or inguinal testes, there is complete failure of virilization. Affected individuals develop breasts (but only to Tanner stage 3) and a typical female habitus with unambiguous female external genitalia, but with the absence of internal female structures and generally only a foreshortened, blind-ending vagina. Little or no pubic and axillary hair develops. The karyotype is 46,XY in these individuals. Circulating testosterone levels are equivalent to or higher than those found in normal men, LH levels are elevated, and FSH levels are normal compared with those in menstruating women. For a more detailed description, see Chapter 233.

Heterosexual Pubertal Development
POLYCYSTIC OVARY SYNDROME

Polycystic ovary syndrome (PCOS), by far the most common cause of heterosexual pubertal development, is associated with the development of some secondary sex features characteristic of males at the normal age of puberty. Feminization occurs in affected girls, and they develop normal breasts and a typical female habitus, but masculinization also occurs (in contrast, girls with congenital adrenal hyperplasia generally show little if any female development at puberty). A heterogeneous syndrome, PCOS typically begins at or near puberty with hirsutism and irregular menses from the time of menarche. Many girls who develop PCOS are overweight in childhood, and obesity is clearly a risk factor. It now appears that many girls who develop PCOS have alterations in insulin signaling.[13] Menarche may be delayed in a few cases, so young women may present with primary amenorrhea. Basal LH levels tend to be somewhat elevated in perhaps two thirds of cases, and circulating levels of all androgens are moderately elevated. Some degree of insulin resistance is commonly present as well, and hypercholesterolemia may predispose to cardiovascular disease later in life. This is discussed more completely in Chapter 236.

CONGENITAL ADRENAL HYPERPLASIA

Congenital adrenal hyperplasia is generally diagnosed before puberty, and heterosexual precocious pseudopuberty is typical. However, if the defect is mild and changes to the external genitalia are minimal, masculinization may occur at the expected age of puberty. This attenuated or nonclassic form of 21-hydroxylase deficiency seems to occur in families with a strong history of hirsutism. Affected girls generally have some defeminization, with flattening of the breasts, severe hirsutism, relatively short stature, and obesity. For a more detailed description, see Chapter 233.

MIXED GONADAL DYSGENESIS

Mixed gonadal dysgenesis designates asymmetrical gonadal development, with a germ cell tumor or a testis on one side and an undifferentiated streak, rudimentary gonad, or no gonad on the other. The extent of genital virilization before puberty is variable in this rare disorder. Most individuals are reared as girls, in whom virilization occurs at puberty; some may note breast development as well. Affected individuals generally have a mosaic karyotype, with 45,X/46,XY being most common. Short stature and other stigmata associated with a 45,X karyotype in Turner syndrome are less common in patients with tumors than in patients with testes. Gonadectomy is indicated in all individuals with a Y chromosome to eliminate the increased neoplastic potential of such dysgenetic gonads and in all patients in whom virilization occurs at puberty to remove the source of androgen. Estrogen replacement therapy is warranted after gonadectomy. Other causes of male pseudohermaphroditism associated with heterosexual pubertal development are described in Chapter 233.

OTHER CAUSES

An androgen-producing adrenal neoplasm or Cushing's syndrome may occur rarely during the pubertal years and lead to heterosexual development (Chapter 227).

Grade A Reference

A1. Ibáñez L, López-Bermejo A, Díaz M, et al. Early metformin therapy (age 8-12 years) in girls with precocious pubarche to reduce hirsutism, androgen excess, and oligomenorrhea in adolescence. J Clin Endocrinol Metab. 2011;96:E1262-E1267.

GENERAL REFERENCES

For the General References and other additional features, please visit Expert Consult at https://expertconsult.inkling.com.

236

REPRODUCTIVE ENDOCRINOLOGY AND INFERTILITY

ROBERT W. REBAR AND WILLIAM H. CATHERINO

THE NORMAL MENSTRUAL CYCLE

Between menarche and menopause, the reproductive organs of normal women undergo a series of closely coordinated changes at monthly intervals that constitute the normal menstrual cycle. The menstrual cycle is the expression of the coordinated interactions of the hypothalamic-pituitary-ovarian axis, with associated changes in the target tissues (endometrium, cervix, vagina) of the reproductive tract.

A menstrual cycle begins with the first day of genital bleeding (day 1; menses) and ends just before the next menstrual period. The median menstrual cycle length is 28 days but normally ranges from 21 to 35 days. Menstrual cycles vary most in the years immediately after menarche and preceding menopause, partly because of an increase in anovulatory cycles. Irregularities in menstrual cycle length may be caused by changes in diet, exercise, emotional disturbances, parturition, or abortion. The menstrual cycle has three distinct phases: follicular, ovulatory, and luteal.

Follicular (Preovulatory) Phase

The follicular phase begins with the first day of bleeding and extends to the day before the preovulatory luteinizing hormone (LH) surge. A rise in serum follicle-stimulating hormone (FSH) begins in the late luteal phase of the previous menstrual cycle and continues into the early follicular phase. This initiates development of a group of follicles (Fig. 236-1). The preovulatory follicle destined for ovulation is selected from this cohort. After the early follicular phase, FSH levels fall, and LH levels rise slowly. About 7 days before the preovulatory LH surge, estradiol and estrone increase until the day before the LH surge. The divergence in LH and FSH levels may be related to secretion of inhibin B, which inhibits the release of FSH. Several days before the LH surge, plasma androgens begin to increase. They peak on the day of the LH surge. Progesterone does not increase until just before the LH surge onset.

Ovulatory Phase

During this phase, the ovum is released from the mature graafian follicle about 32 to 34 hours after the preovulatory LH surge. The ovulatory phase extends from 1 day before the LH surge to 1 day after the LH surge (see Fig. 236-1). Some women experience unilateral pelvic pain near the time of ovulation, termed *mittelschmerz*, which occurs before or after ovulation. During the ovulatory phase, a rapid rise in plasma LH in response to positive estrogen feedback leads to ovulation. As peak LH levels are reached, estradiol levels drop, but progesterone levels increase.

Luteal (Postovulatory) Phase

The luteal phase is about 14 days in length and ends with the onset of menses (see Fig. 236-1). This phase includes the functional lifespan of the corpus

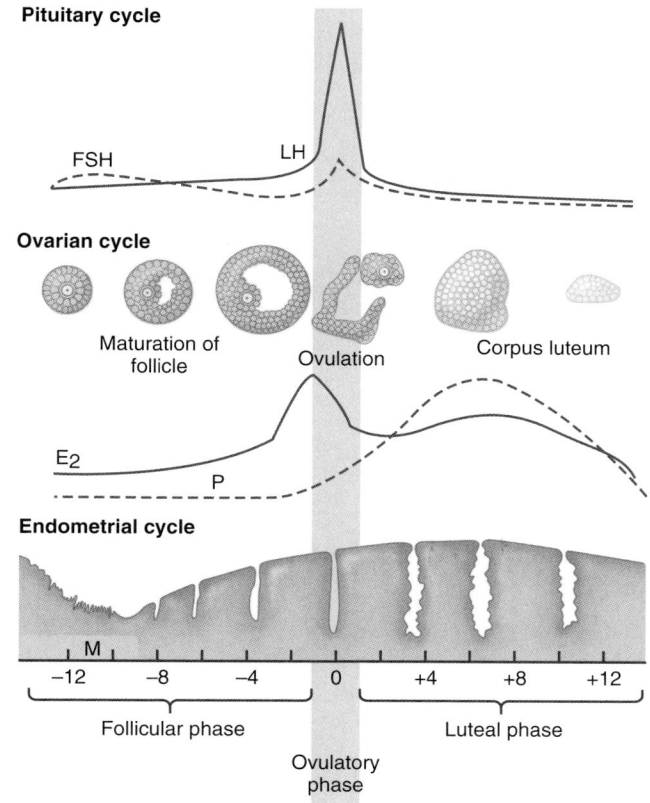

Pituitary cycle

FSH LH

Ovarian cycle

Maturation of
follicle

Ovulation

Corpus luteum

E₂

P

Endometrial cycle

M

−12 −8 −4 0 +4 +8 +12

Follicular phase Luteal phase

Ovulatory
phase

FIGURE 236-1. The idealized cyclic changes observed in gonadotropins, estradiol (E₂), progesterone (P), and uterine endometrium during the normal menstrual cycle. The data are centered on the day of the luteinizing hormone (LH) surge (day 0). Days of menstrual bleeding are indicated by M. FSH = follicle-stimulating hormone; LH = luteinizing hormone. (From Endocrine and Metabolism Continuing Education Quality Control Program, 1982. Copyright American Association for Clinical Chemistry, Inc.)

luteum, which supports the released ovum by secreting progesterone. Progesterone secretion increases up to 8 days after the LH surge. Smaller increases in 17α-hydroxyprogesterone, estradiol, and estrone occur. Progesterone decreases before menses unless the ovum is fertilized and pregnancy results. A serum progesterone level higher than 3 ng/mL 1 week before menses is probably diagnostic of ovulation.

CYCLIC CHANGES IN TARGET ORGANS

Endometrium

The endometrium undergoes histologic and cytologic changes that culminate with menstrual bleeding when the corpus luteum ceases to secrete progesterone (see Fig. 236-1). The basal layer of the endometrium then regenerates the superficial layer of compact epithelial cells lining the uterine cavity and an intermediate layer of spongiosa. Both superficial layers are shed at menstruation. Endometrial glands proliferate under the influence of estrogen, and the mucosa thickens. In the luteal phase, the glands become coiled and secretory, with increased vascularity and edema of the stroma. When estradiol and progesterone decline, the stroma becomes edematous, endometrial and blood vessel necrosis occurs, and bleeding ensues. Local release of prostaglandins may initiate vasospasm with ischemic necrosis and uterine contractions that accompany menstrual flow. Prostaglandin synthetase inhibitors can relieve menstrual cramping. The histologic changes are characteristic; therefore, endometrial biopsies can be used to characterize the stage of the cycle and to assess the tissue response to gonadal steroids.

Cervix and Cervical Mucus

During the follicular phase, cervical vascularity, congestion, and edema increase as a result of estrogen. Cervical mucus increases in quantity (10- to 30-fold) and in elasticity. So-called ferning becomes prominent. Progesterone stimulates cervical mucus thickening and loss of elasticity and ability to fern. These characteristics are useful in evaluating the stage of the cycle and the amount of estrogen present.

Vagina

Low estrogen is associated with pale, thin vaginal epithelium. As estrogens rise, the number of cornified epithelial cells increases. Subsequently, progesterone decreases the percentage of cornified cells and increases the number of precornified intermediate cells. There is also increased cellular debris and clumping of shed desquamated cells. Histologic changes in the vaginal epithelium are sensitive indicators of estrogen status.

Ovary

The ovaries produce a single dominant graafian follicle that grows and develops to the preovulatory stage during the follicular phase. This process is brought about by the combined actions of FSH and LH on the follicle wall to increase estradiol biosynthesis. The LH surge acts on the preovulatory follicle to cause the secretion of the mature fertilizable oocyte. After ovulation, the follicle wall transforms into the corpus luteum, which produces progesterone and estradiol. If implantation does not occur, the corpus luteum undergoes luteolysis and stops hormone production. In the late luteal phase, another dominant follicle develops, and a new menstrual cycle begins.

Chronology of Folliculogenesis

The preovulatory follicle begins its development when a primordial follicle is recruited into the pool of growing follicles. There are two major phases of folliculogenesis: the preantral (gonadotropin-independent) and the antral (gonadotropin-dependent) periods. The first phase is characterized by growth of the oocyte and granulosa proliferation. Preantral folliculogenesis proceeds slowly, requiring at least 300 days. During the second phase, granulosa and theca cells proliferate, and the antrum enlarges. The graafian follicle increases relatively rapidly as it develops. The mature graafian follicle that will ovulate requires 40 to 50 days to complete the antral phase.

Selection

The dominant follicle is selected from a cohort at the end of the luteal phase of the previous menstrual cycle. The selected follicle requires 20 days to develop to the ovulatory stage.

Shortly after the midluteal phase of the cycle, the granulosa cells show a sharp increase in the rate of mitosis. The first indication of selection is that the granulosa cells continue dividing at a high rate. As a consequence of the high and sustained mitotic rate and the progressive accumulation of follicular fluid, the dominant follicle undergoes remarkable growth. The increase in plasma FSH levels that begins at the end of luteal phase and continues through the early follicular phase evokes follicle selection. The concentration of FSH in the follicular fluid of the healthy (dominant) follicle increases but does not increase in the nondominant atretic follicles. The manner in which this selective increase in FSH is controlled is unknown. More than 99.9% of all follicles are not selected and undergo atresia.

Mechanism of Follicle-Stimulating Hormone Action

FSH exerts its influence on follicle growth and development by stimulating granulosa cell mitosis and cytodifferentiation. FSH activates high-affinity receptors on the granulosa cell. The binding event is transduced into an intracellular signal through the cyclic adenosine monophosphate (cAMP)-dependent protein kinase A signal transduction pathway. This leads to an increase in cell number and cytodifferentiation.

The granulosa cells in the chosen follicle continue to divide at a relatively rapid rate throughout the follicular phase of the cycle, increasing from 1×10^6 cells to 50×10^6 cells at ovulation. FSH induces granulosa cytodifferentiation in the dominant follicle. Expression of cytochrome P-450 aromatase (P450arom) is induced by FSH. The temporal pattern of expression of P450arom determines when and how much estradiol is produced. FSH also induces the expression of LH receptors. This is delayed until the dominant follicle is fully differentiated at day 12. The large number of LH receptors in the granulosa cells is essential for the LH surge to trigger ovulation. The terminal differentiation of the granulosa cells is characterized by the accumulation of other FSH-regulated gene products, including inhibin B, activin, and follistatin.

Mechanism of Luteinizing Hormone Action

The primary function of LH in follicle development is to stimulate androgen production by the theca interstitial cells. LH binds to LH-human chorionic gonadotropin (HCG) receptors located on theca cells, which interact with G proteins and activate adenylate cyclase, leading to the synthesis of cAMP, which stimulates gene expression through protein kinase A. This leads to increased conversion of cholesterol to androstenedione. Theca cells express insulin receptors, and insulin stimulates theca androgen production. The crosstalk between the insulin and LH receptor signaling is clinically relevant because of the relationship between hyperinsulinemia and hyperandrogenism in women.

One of the most important consequences of FSH and LH action on the dominant follicle is the production of estradiol. This physiologically important process is called the *two-gonadotropin, two-cell concept* of follicular estrogen production.

Ovulation

At midpoint in the menstrual cycle, the preovulatory surges of LH and FSH act on the preovulatory follicle to initiate the events leading to ovulation. The LH surge induces meiotic maturation, a process that converts the oocyte into a fertilizable egg arrested at the second meiotic metaphase. During meiotic maturation, the granulosa cells next to the oocyte are stimulated by FSH to undergo cumulus expansion. This is a prerequisite for the oocyte's pickup and transport by the oviduct. The LH surge also stimulates production of proteolytic enzymes in the vicinity of the presumptive stigma. This process requires the LH stimulation of progesterone and prostaglandins, which are obligatory for stigma formation. After 36 hours, the fertilizable egg and surrounding cumulus cells are secreted through the stigma.

Luteogenesis

Ovulation leads to changes in the granulosa and theca cells of the ovulated follicle that result in increased production of progesterone and estradiol during the first week of the luteal phase. This event, termed *luteinization*, is important for the formation and development of a secretory endometrium. Three major physiologic mechanisms are responsible for luteinization: removal of luteinization inhibitors; secretion of LH by the pituitary; and delivery of high levels of cholesterol. The induction of StAR, P450c22, and 3β-hydroxysteroid dehydrogenase in the granulosa lutein cells leads to progesterone production by the corpus luteum. The two-cell, two-gonadotropin mechanism is responsible for estradiol production. If implantation does not occur, the corpus luteum initiates luteolysis, leading to decreases in progesterone, estradiol, and apoptosis. When luteolysis occurs, another dominant follicle is selected, and a new menstrual cycle begins.

Neuroendocrine Regulation of the Ovaries

Neurons containing various peptide hormones that can release or inhibit secretion of the gonadotropins are found in the hypothalamus (Chapter 223). Cells containing gonadotropin-releasing hormone (GnRH) occur in the arcuate nucleus, median eminence, and preoptic area. Axons from these neurons run in the tuberoinfundibular tract and terminate on capillaries within the median eminence, allowing delivery of their products to the anterior pituitary gland. Neurotransmitters, including norepinephrine, dopamine, and serotonin, as well as neuromodulators, such as endogenous opiates and prostaglandins, influence secretion of GnRH. Estrogens and androgens bind to cells in the hypothalamus and the anterior pituitary, and progestins bind to cells in the hypothalamus, to influence hypothalamic-pituitary regulation of ovarian function.

GnRH is secreted in a pulsatile fashion and is responsible for pulsatile release of gonadotropins. Pulsatile gonadotropin release accounts for the pulsatile secretion of sex steroids from the ovaries. The ovarian sex steroids feed back on the hypothalamic-pituitary unit to modulate both the frequency and amplitude of the gonadotropin pulse (Fig. 236-2). Gonadotropin pulses vary throughout the menstrual cycle. Pulses occur at approximately 60- to 90-minute intervals in the follicular phase and at intervals of 180 minutes in the luteal phase.

Gonadal steroids can exert both negative and positive feedback effects on gonadotropin secretion. 17β-Estradiol is the most potent inhibitor of gonadotropin secretion. For women to ovulate, estradiol must also elicit a positive feedback effect on gonadotropin release. The feedback effects are both time and dose dependent. In the normal menstrual cycle, the positive feedback action of estradiol leading to the LH surge is preceded by a period when lower estradiol levels are present.

It appears that the ovary is the "clock" for the timing of ovulation, with the hypothalamus stimulating pulsatile release of the gonadotropins. The follicle complex and corpus luteum develop in response to gonadotropin stimulation. For appropriate ovarian regulation of reproductive function in women,

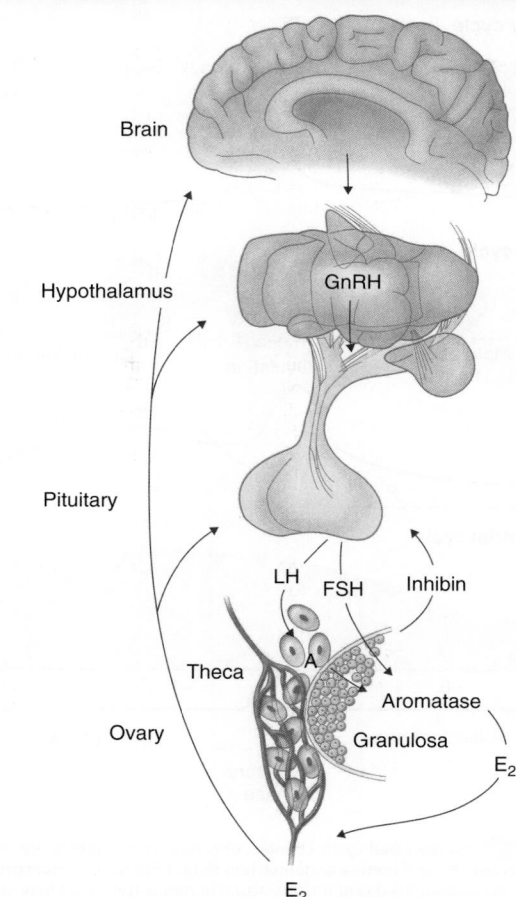

FIGURE 236-2. The hypothalamic-pituitary-ovarian axis in the regulation of follicular maturation and steroidogenesis. A = androgens; E_2 = estradiol; FSH = follicle-stimulating hormone; GnRH = gonadotropin-releasing hormone; LH = luteinizing hormone. (Modified from Endocrine and Metabolism Continuing Education Quality Control Program, 1982. Copyright American Association for Clinical Chemistry, Inc.)

three biologic characteristics are necessary: an appropriate balance and sequence of negative and positive feedback actions; differential feedback effects on the release of LH and FSH; and local intraovarian controls on follicular growth and maturation.

⬤ ABNORMALITIES OF THE REPRODUCTIVE YEARS
Dysmenorrhea and Endometriosis

DEFINITION

Dysmenorrhea, defined as painful menstruation, affects about 50% of postpubertal women[1] and can be classified as primary or secondary. *Endometriosis*, which may result in dysmenorrhea, infertility, and dyspareunia (i.e., painful intercourse), is the ectopic occurrence of endometrial tissue, most commonly within the abdominal cavity but sometimes in surgical scars, on the vulva, in the umbilicus, and elsewhere.[2]

PATHOBIOLOGY

Primary dysmenorrhea occurs only in ovulatory cycles. Prostaglandins produce dysmenorrhea by initiating painful, exaggerated uterine contractions and myometrial ischemia. Associated systemic symptoms include nausea, diarrhea, headache, and emotional changes. In secondary dysmenorrhea, there is a pathologic cause, with endometriosis being the most common. Other causes include pelvic inflammatory disease; congenital abnormalities, such as atresia of a portion of the distal genital tract and cystic duplication of the paramesonephric ducts; and cervical stenosis. Recent studies suggest the possibility that the pain of endometriosis is caused by the presence of nerve fibers within ectopic endometrium.

TREATMENT Rx

Prostaglandin synthetase inhibitors (Chapter 37), such as naproxen, ibuprofen, mefenamic acid, and indomethacin, are used to treat primary dysmenorrhea.[3] If the dysmenorrhea persists, addition of an oral contraceptive to inhibit ovulation and limit prostaglandin release is generally effective. In cases in which the pelvic pain remains intractable, additional evaluation is warranted. If thorough evaluation of the gastrointestinal and urinary tracts fails to reveal a definitive cause, examination under anesthesia and diagnostic laparoscopy may be indicated.

If endometriosis is diagnosed at laparoscopy, treatment varies according to the severity of the disease and the goals of the patient regarding fertility.[4] It may be possible to fulgurate implants or to lyse adhesions. Available data do not demonstrate a benefit of excision over ablation at the time of initial diagnosis as the preferred approach to controlling symptoms.[A1] From this point onward, efforts should be directed toward treating endometriosis medically, with additional surgery deferred until infertility (if present) becomes manifest.[A2] Medical therapy can consist of continuous suppression with oral contraceptives, progestins (oral, injectable, or implantable), or GnRH analogues or danazol for 3 to 6 months. GnRH analogues are currently the most frequently used form of medical suppressive therapy.[A3] After a course of treatment, use of oral contraceptive agents should probably be continued until fertility is desired. Conservative surgical resection of endometriotic tissue should almost always be deferred until it is established as the cause of infertility. Surgery may be required, however, for continuing severe pain, severe endometriosis, or large ovarian cysts containing endometriosis (endometriomas). If symptoms continue despite adequate treatment or if psychological overlay is suspected, psychiatric evaluation may be indicated. Medical causes of dysmenorrhea, however, should be eliminated first.

Premenstrual Syndrome

DEFINITION

Premenstrual syndrome (PMS), also known as *premenstrual tension*, is a complex of physical and emotional symptoms that occur repetitively in a cyclic fashion before menstruation and that diminish or disappear with menstruation.[5]

DIAGNOSIS

The cyclic symptoms typically are sufficiently severe to interfere with some aspects of life. More than 150 different symptoms are now thought to vary with the menstrual cycle (Table 236-1). Estimates of the prevalence of PMS range from 25 to 100%. The *Diagnostic and Statistical Manual of Mental Disorders* (DSM-5) classifies severe PMS as premenstrual dysphoric disorder (PMDD). For most women, PMS is merely annoying; severe PMS (or PMDD) causes serious difficulties for 3 to 5% of women of reproductive age. The diagnosis of both PMS and PMDD is best established by requiring patients to keep prospective daily records of symptoms during a 2- to 3-month period. Less than 50% of women complaining of PMS are found to have the syndrome when such records are examined.

TABLE 236-1 COMMON SYMPTOMS OF CYCLIC PREMENSTRUAL SYNDROME

SOMATIC SYMPTOMS	
Abdominal bloating	Constipation or diarrhea
Acne	Headache
Alcohol intolerance	Peripheral edema
Breast engorgement and tenderness	Weight gain
Clumsiness	

EMOTIONAL AND MENTAL SYMPTOMS	
Anxiety	Insomnia
Change in libido	Irritability
Depression	Lethargy
Fatigue	Mood swings
Food cravings (especially salt and sugar)	Panic attacks
Hostility	Paranoia
Inability to concentrate	Violence toward self and others
Increased appetite	Withdrawal from others

Most women seek help for PMS in their 30s after 10 or more years of symptoms. Many report that their symptoms began at menarche; approximately half state that symptoms followed childbirth. Severity and duration of symptoms are often reported to increase after each successive pregnancy and to become more severe with advancing age. Women with severe long-standing PMS almost always describe associated psychological reactions, including social difficulties, such as marital discord, difficulty relating to their children, difficulty maintaining friendships, and withdrawal from social activities.

TREATMENT Rx

General Measures

The cause of PMS is unknown, and patients should be informed that no one therapy has been effective in all women. Women with mild premenstrual symptoms often benefit from simple changes in lifestyle, including daily mild aerobic exercise; reduction in intake of caffeine-containing beverages, salt, and refined sugar, particularly in the luteal phase; stress reduction; and adequate rest.

Medical Therapy

Women with more severe PMS may benefit from symptomatic treatment. Continuous oral contraceptives have inconsistent but generally positive therapeutic benefit.[6] Bromocriptine (generally 2.5 mg twice a day) or danazol (100 to 400 mg/day in two divided doses) may be given continuously for relief of mastalgia (breast pain), although this use is not listed in the manufacturer's directive or approved by the U.S. Food and Drug Administration (FDA), and efficacy has not been documented by rigorous randomized trials. Prostaglandin synthetase inhibitors may help reduce dysmenorrhea and may alleviate headaches. Mild sedatives and tranquilizers may help reduce insomnia and anxiety. Low doses of fluoxetine (20 mg) and other selective serotonin reuptake inhibitors, administered either daily or for the last 2 weeks of each menstrual cycle, are highly effective in reducing the emotional symptoms associated with PMS.[A4] Mild diuretics (especially spironolactone at doses up to 100 mg each morning) may benefit cyclic edema.

Natural progesterone, given in the form of vaginal suppositories, has been used, but results of double-blind placebo-controlled trials show no efficacy.[A5] Likewise, the value of large quantities of multiple vitamins or of oil of evening primrose, containing the essential fatty acid γ-linolenic acid, a precursor of prostaglandins, is unsubstantiated.

Surgical Therapy

Because PMS requires the occurrence of cyclic ovulation, oophorectomy is occasionally considered for patients with particularly intractable symptoms. However, oophorectomy may create new problems related to estrogen deficiency for women with PMS treated in this permanent fashion. Several trials employing a GnRH agonist together with exogenous steroids have been described as reducing PMS. Whether such therapy can be used in the long term remains to be determined.

Abnormal Uterine Bleeding

DIAGNOSIS

Differential Diagnosis

Because there is considerable confusion about terminology of abnormal uterine bleeding, it is important to determine just what is being included in any term used other than *abnormal uterine bleeding*.[7] Postmenarchal bleeding in adolescents secondary to immaturity of the hypothalamic-pituitary-ovarian axis (resulting in anovulation) accounts for about 20% of cases, and perimenopausal bleeding consequent to incipient ovarian failure constitutes more than half.

The causes of abnormal uterine bleeding in the reproductive years include complications from the use of oral contraceptives; complications of pregnancy, especially threatened, incomplete, or missed miscarriages and ectopic pregnancy; coagulation disorders, most commonly idiopathic thrombocytopenic purpura (Chapter 172) and von Willebrand disease (Chapter 173); and pelvic disease, such as intrauterine polyps, leiomyomas, and tumors of the vagina and cervix. Clear cell adenocarcinoma of the vagina or cervix (Chapter 199) may occur in women exposed to diethylstilbestrol during fetal life. Affected women may also have congenital abnormalities of the upper vagina, cervix, and uterus. Women with a history of diethylstilbestrol exposure should be reassured that the incidence of malignant change is extremely low. Trauma (coital or otherwise), foreign bodies, systemic illnesses including various endocrinopathies (e.g., diabetes mellitus, hypothyroidism and hyperthyroidism, Cushing's syndrome, and Addison's disease), leukemia, and renal disease may also be associated with abnormal bleeding as the presenting manifestation.

Abnormal uterine bleeding with no demonstrable organic genital or extragenital cause (75% of cases) is most frequently associated with anovulation and is appropriately termed *anovulatory* (sometimes termed *dysfunctional*) *bleeding*. Most anovulatory bleeding is due to either estrogen withdrawal or estrogen breakthrough bleeding. In anovulatory women, estrogen stimulates the endometrium unopposed by progesterone. The endometrium proliferates, becomes thicker, and may shed irregularly. Anovulatory bleeding tends to occur at less frequent intervals, and organic lesions tend to cause bleeding more frequently than cyclic menses.

Clinical Evaluation

All cases of abnormal bleeding should be evaluated, beginning with a thorough history emphasizing the amount and duration of blood loss. Prospective charting of the days on which bleeding occurs may be required to evaluate the bleeding pattern. Complications of pregnancy or a bleeding diathesis must always be ruled out.

The findings on physical examination (including the Papanicolaou smear) are normal in anovulatory bleeding except for signs of anemia in the more severe cases. Laboratory tests should include a complete blood count, platelet count, coagulation studies, thyroid function tests, and fasting blood glucose concentration. Anovulatory bleeding must be a diagnosis of exclusion, with management depending on the age of the patient and the extent of the bleeding. A sample of the endometrium should be obtained by biopsy or by dilation and curettage from all women older than 35 years and from those at increased risk for endometrial carcinoma because of prolonged anovulatory bleeding.

TREATMENT   Rx

Even profuse bleeding in hemodynamically stable anovulatory women can almost always be successfully treated by the administration of one combination oral contraceptive pill every 6 hours for 5 to 7 days, although this use is not listed in the manufacturer's directive or approved by the FDA. Bleeding should cease within 24 hours, but patients should be warned to expect heavy bleeding 2 to 4 days after therapy is stopped. If anemia is profound, blood transfusion may be necessary. If the bleeding continues despite therapy, curettage can be carried out. Recurrence can be prevented by giving the patient combination oral contraceptive agents cyclically if pregnancy is not desired. If pregnancy is desired, ovulation can be induced.

Acute episodes of anovulatory bleeding can also be treated with conjugated estrogens administered intravenously (25 mg every 4 hours for up to three doses) until bleeding ceases, although this use is not listed in the manufacturer's directive or approved by the FDA. Progestin therapy (medroxyprogesterone acetate, 5 to 10 mg orally for 10 days) should be started simultaneously. Withdrawal bleeding occurs after cessation of therapy, and the patient can then be treated with oral contraceptive agents for at least three cycles.

For individuals with anovulatory bleeding without an episode of profuse bleeding, treatment with cyclic oral contraceptive agents or progestin can be provided unless pregnancy is desired, in which case ovulation must be induced.

Endometrial ablation by any of several methods is being used increasingly to treat persistent bleeding. However, ablation is not 100% effective, and medical management remains the first line of therapy for most women. Hysterectomy may be an appropriate choice for a small number of women.

Amenorrhea

DEFINITION

Amenorrhea is the absence of menstruation for 3 months or more in women with past menses (secondary amenorrhea) or the absence of menarche by the age of 15 years regardless of the absence or presence of secondary sex characteristics (primary amenorrhea).[8]

PATHOBIOLOGY

If an intact genital outflow tract exists and there is no primary disease of the uterus, amenorrhea is a sign of failure of the hypothalamic-pituitary-ovarian axis to produce cyclically the hormones necessary for menses. Amenorrhea is physiologic in the prepubertal girl, during pregnancy and early in lactation, and after menopause. At any other time, it is pathologic and demands evaluation. Use of the term *postpill amenorrhea* to refer to failure to resume menses within 3 months of discontinuation of oral contraceptives is inappropriate. Women so affected should be evaluated in the same manner as any woman with amenorrhea. Similarly, individuals with menses occurring at infrequent intervals of more than 40 days or having fewer than nine menses per year, termed *oligomenorrhea*, should be evaluated identically to women with amenorrhea.

DIAGNOSIS

Clinical Evaluation

In patients with amenorrhea, even subtle hormonal abnormalities may lead to signs and symptoms. Breast development indicates exposure to estrogens, and the presence of pubic and axillary hair indicates androgenic stimulation.

Patients should be questioned especially closely for evidence of psychological disturbances, dietary and exercise habits, lifestyle, environmental stresses, family history of genetic anomalies, abnormal growth and development, and signs of hyperandrogenism, including hirsutism, temporal balding, deepening of the voice, increased muscle mass, clitorimegaly, and increased libido, and signs of defeminization, including decreasing breast size and vaginal atrophy. Any history of galactorrhea should be determined. A history of symptoms related to thyroid and adrenal dysfunction should also be sought (Chapters 224, 226, and 227).

The physical examination should focus on the evaluation of body dimensions and habitus, extent and distribution of body hair, breast development and secretions, and genitalia. In normal adult women, the arm span is similar to the height; in hypogonadal women, the span is generally more than 5 cm greater than the height. The distribution and quantity of body hair should be considered in view of the family history. The extent of any hirsutism should be recorded, preferably by photographs. Other signs of virilization should be sought carefully. Breast development should be graded according to the method of Tanner (Table 236-2).[9] Breast secretion should be sought by applying pressure to the breasts while the patient is seated. Any secretion should be examined microscopically for the presence of perfectly round fat globules of varying size, which indicate galactorrhea. Finally, the female genitalia should be examined carefully because they are such sensitive indicators of the hormonal milieu. The Tanner stage of pubic hair development should be noted (see Table 236-2).

Because the sensitivity of the genitalia to androgens decreases onward from early in fetal development, the extent of any virilization is important. Fusion of the labia and enlargement of the clitoris with or without formation

TABLE 236-2   CRITERIA FOR DISTINGUISHING TANNER STAGES 1 TO 5 DURING PUBERTAL MATURATION

TANNER STAGE	BREAST	PUBIC HAIR
1 (Prepubertal)	No palpable glandular tissue or pigmentation of areola; elevation of areola only	No pubic hair; short, fine vellus hair only
2	Glandular tissue palpable with elevation of breast and areola together as a small mound; areolar diameter increased	Sparse, long, pigmented terminal hair chiefly along the labia majora
3	Further enlargement without separation of breast and areola; although more darkly pigmented, areola still pale and immature; nipple generally at or above midplane of breast tissue when individual is seated upright	Dark, coarse, curly hair, extending sparsely over mons
4	Secondary mound of areola and papilla above breast	Adult-type hair, abundant but limited to mons and labia
5 (Adult)	Recession of areola to contour of breast; development of Montgomery's glands and ducts on areola; further pigmentation of areola; nipple generally below midplane of breast tissue when individual is seated upright; maturation independent of breast size	Adult-type hair in quantity and distribution; spread to inner aspects of the thighs in most racial groups

Data from Ross GT. Disorders of the ovary and female reproductive tract. In: Wilson JD, Foster DW, eds. *Textbook of Endocrinology*, 7th ed. Philadelphia: WB Saunders; 1985:206; Speroff L, Glass RH, Kase N. *Clinical Gynecologic Endocrinology and Infertility*, 3rd ed. Baltimore: Williams & Wilkins; 1983:377; and Kustin J, Rebar RW. Menstrual disorders in the adolescent age group. *Primary Care*. 1987;14:139-166.

of a penile urethra are observed in women exposed to androgens during the first 3 months of fetal development (Chapter 233). Significant clitorimegaly in the absence of other signs of sexual ambiguity and in the presence of other signs of virilization requires marked androgenic stimulation and strongly implicates an androgen-secreting neoplasm. The development of the labia minora in postpubertal women indicates the influence of estrogens. Overt anomalies of the distal genital tract and any evidence of obstruction to the escape of menstrual blood should be sought. Under the influence of estrogen, the vaginal mucosa changes during sexual maturation from a tissue with a shiny, bright red appearance with sparse, thin secretions to a dull, gray-pink rugated surface with copious, thick secretions.

The history and physical examination quickly differentiate among several causes of amenorrhea (Table 236-3). The various disorders of sexual differentiation and the other anatomic causes are often apparent on inspection. Distal genital tract obstruction should be identified at the time of pelvic examination even if the specific abnormality is not obvious. The physical stigmata of Turner's syndrome, discussed subsequently, generally make the diagnosis simple. Any sexual ambiguity indicates the need for chromosomal analysis and the measurement of 17α-hydroxyprogesterone to rule out congenital adrenal hyperplasia. Pregnancy and gestational trophoblastic disease may be diagnosed by measurement of HCG. The possibility of intrauterine synechiae or adhesions (Asherman's syndrome) must be considered in individuals in whom amenorrhea develops after curettage or endometritis. Tuberculous endometritis, especially in younger women, may also lead to this disorder. Without hormonal measurements, it may be impossible to distinguish between individuals with chronic anovulation, in whom hypothalamic-pituitary-ovarian function is insufficiently coordinated to produce cyclic ovulation, and those with ovarian failure. However, it is generally possible to form a clinical impression about the cause of the amenorrhea. It can be noted whether the patient has absence of, incomplete, or complete development of secondary sex characteristics. The presence of excess body hair or galactorrhea may provide clinical evidence of the pathogenesis of the amenorrhea. Signs and symptoms of adrenal or thyroid dysfunction may be important as well. Administration of a progestin (typically medroxyprogesterone acetate, 5 to 10 mg given orally for 5 to 10 days, or progesterone in oil, 100 mg given intramuscularly) has been advocated to assess the level of endogenous estrogen. This test is of limited value, however, because almost half the young women with premature ovarian failure experience withdrawal bleeding in response to progestin.

To ascertain whether the outflow tract is intact, an orally active estrogen, such as 2.5 mg of conjugated estrogen daily for 21 days, with 5 to 10 mg of oral medroxyprogesterone acetate for the last 5 to 10 days, is administered. Withdrawal bleeding should occur if the endometrium is normal. Still, hysterosalpingography and hysteroscopy may be required for the diagnosis of Asherman's syndrome because some patients with a normal endometrium

TABLE 236-3 CAUSES OF AMENORRHEA

ANATOMIC CAUSES

Pregnancy
Various disorders of sexual differentiation
  Distal genital tract obstruction (müllerian agenesis or dysgenesis)
  Gonadal dysgenesis*
  Ambiguity of external genitalia (male and female pseudohermaphroditism)
Intrauterine adhesions (Asherman's syndrome)
Gestational trophoblastic disease

CHRONIC ANOVULATION

Due to CNS-hypothalamic-pituitary dysfunction
With inappropriate steroid feedback (e.g., polycystic ovary syndrome)
Due to thyroid or adrenal disorders

OVARIAN "FAILURE"

Menopause
Genetic abnormalities
Physical and environmental causes (e.g., chemotherapeutic agents, irradiation)
Autoimmune disorders
Idiopathic

*Gonadal dysgenesis may be viewed as both a disorder of sexual differentiation and a form of gonadal "failure."
CNS = central nervous system.

may not have a withdraw bleed due to obstruction of the cervical os by scar tissue.

Laboratory Findings

Basal levels of FSH, prolactin, and thyroid-stimulating hormone (TSH) should be measured in all amenorrheic and oligomenorrheic women to confirm the clinical impression (Fig. 236-3).[10]

Increased TSH levels with or without increased levels of prolactin imply primary hypothyroidism, and further evaluation for this disorder is indicated (Chapter 226). Although hypothyroidism commonly results in anovulation, amenorrhea occurs in only some hypothyroid women. Menorrhagia and oligomenorrhea may occur as well. The sensitive immunoassays for TSH permit identification of women with hyperthyroidism as well because TSH levels are suppressed in those individuals.

If the prolactin concentration is minimally increased and the TSH level is normal, measurement of the prolactin concentration should be repeated before more extensive evaluation is undertaken because prolactin levels are increased by nonspecific stressful stimuli, sleep, and food ingestion. Prolactin levels may be elevated in as many as one third of women with amenorrhea.

Increased FSH levels (generally >30 mIU/mL) imply ovarian failure and require further evaluation. Incipient ovarian failure should be considered in any woman with basal FSH levels of 15 mIU/mL or higher other than during the midcycle LH surge. Many clinicians believe that chromosomal evaluation is indicated in all individuals with elevated FSH levels before age 40 years, and it is certainly indicated if hypergonadotropic amenorrhea begins before age 30 years.

If FSH levels are low or normal, the measurement of total testosterone levels may be helpful whether or not there is any evidence of hirsutism or virilization. Hyperandrogenic women need not be hirsute because some have relative insensitivity of the hair follicles to androgens. Mildly increased levels of testosterone (and perhaps dehydroepiandrosterone sulfate as well) suggest polycystic ovary syndrome (PCOS). However, total circulating androgen levels need not be elevated because of the alterations in metabolic clearance rate and sex hormone–binding globulin that are present in PCOS. Consequently, some clinicians prefer to measure circulating free testosterone levels.

Circulating levels of LH and FSH may aid in differentiation of PCOS from hypothalamic-pituitary dysfunction. LH levels are often elevated in PCOS so that the ratio of LH to FSH is increased; however, LH levels may be identical to those observed in normal women in the follicular phase. In contrast, levels of LH and FSH are normal or slightly reduced in hypothalamic-pituitary dysfunction. There is some overlap between women with "polycystic ovarian–like" disorders and those with hypothalamic-pituitary dysfunction. Radiographic assessment of the sella turcica is indicated in all amenorrheic women in whom both LH and FSH levels are consistently low (both <10 mIU/mL) to exclude a pituitary or parapituitary neoplasm (Chapter 224). Other pituitary functions should be evaluated in any individual with significantly impaired LH and FSH secretion. Both total testosterone and dehydroepiandrosterone sulfate levels should be measured in hirsute or virilized women. Testosterone levels greater than 200 ng/dL should lead to investigation for an androgen-producing neoplasm, most likely of ovarian origin. Dehydroepiandrosterone sulfate greater than 7.0 μg/mL should lead to evaluation for an adrenal neoplasm, and levels between 5.0 and 7.0 μg/mL should lead to evaluation for adult-onset congenital adrenal hyperplasia.

Hypergonadotropic Amenorrhea (Presumptive Ovarian Failure, Primary Hypogonadism, Primary Ovarian Insufficiency)

DIAGNOSIS

Differential Diagnosis

Gonadal failure may begin at any time during embryonic or postnatal development and may result from many causes. Normally, the ovaries fail at menopause, when virtually no functioning follicles remain. However, premature loss of oocytes before the age of 40 years may occur and lead to premature ovarian failure. Circulating gonadotropin levels increase whenever ovarian failure occurs because of decreased negative estrogen feedback to the hypothalamic-pituitary unit.

PATHOBIOLOGY

There are several causes for premature ovarian failure, including genetic causes (a growing list that includes karyotypic abnormalities, single gene

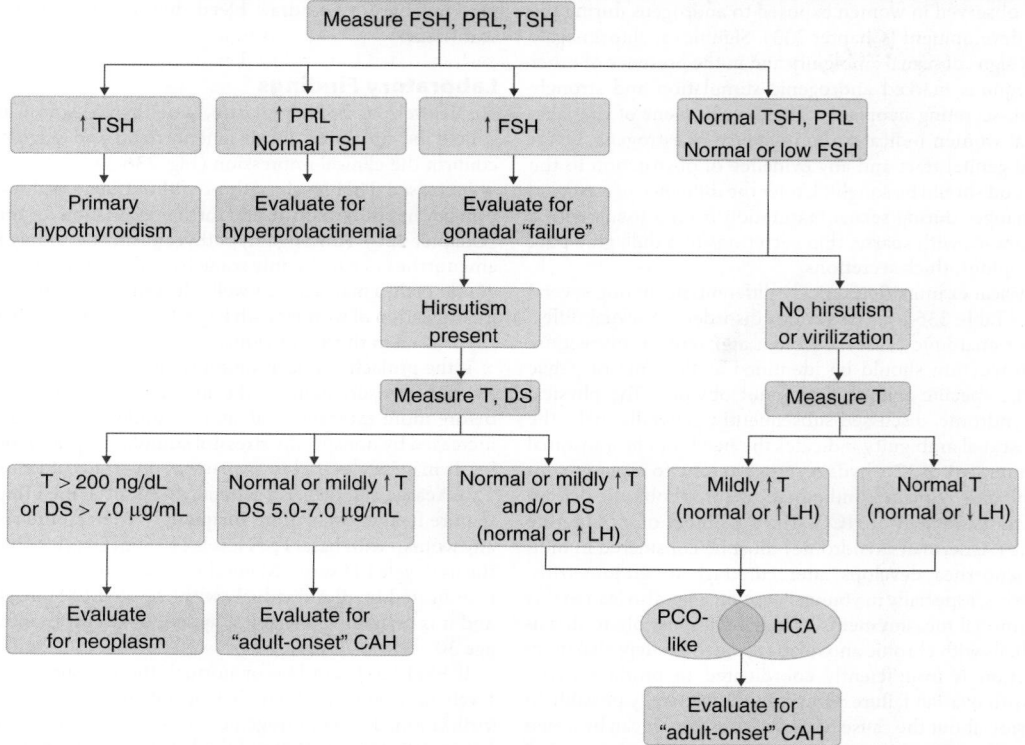

FIGURE 236-3. Biochemical evaluation of amenorrhea. This schema must be considered an adjunct to the clinical evaluation of the patient. See text for details. CAH = congenital adrenal hyperplasia; DS = dehydroepiandrosterone sulfate; FSH = follicle-stimulating hormone; HCA = hypothalamic chronic anovulation; LH = luteinizing hormone; PCO-like = polycystic ovarian syndrome–like; PRL = prolactin; T = testosterone; TSH = thyroid-stimulating hormone.

mutations, and complex multifactorial polygenic inheritance), physical and environmental causes, and autoimmune disturbances. In addition, there may be families in which menopause begins earlier than the expected age without any further pathologic cause.

Genetic Abnormalities

Several pathologic conditions with dysgenetic gonads involve elevated gonadotropin levels and amenorrhea as well as abnormalities of the X chromosome. The term *gonadal dysgenesis* refers to individuals with undifferentiated streak gonads without any association with either extragonadal stigmata or sex chromosome aberrations. Because individuals with gonadal dysgenesis have the normal complement of oocytes at 20 weeks of fetal age but virtually none by birth, this disorder is a form of premature ovarian failure.

Turner's Syndrome

Turner's syndrome (also see Chapter 233) describes patients with streak gonads composed of fibrous stroma and four cardinal features: a female phenotype; sexual infantilism; short stature; and several physical abnormalities, sometimes including webbed neck, low-set ears, multiple pigmented nevi, double eyelashes, micrognathia, epicanthal folds, shieldlike chest with microthelia, short fourth metacarpals, increased carrying angle of the arms, and certain renal and cardiovascular defects (most commonly coarctation of the aorta and aortic stenosis) (Fig. 236-4).[11] The diagnosis can sometimes be made at birth because of unexplained lymphedema of the hands and feet. The syndrome is associated with an abnormality of sex chromosome number, morphology, or both. Most commonly, the second sex chromosome is absent (45,X). Turner's syndrome is the single most common chromosome disorder in humans, but more than 95% of such fetuses are aborted, and the incidence in newborns is approximately 1 in 3000 to 5000. Chromosome breakage and mosaicism occur as well. In mosaic individuals with a normal 46,XX cell line, sufficient follicles may persist postnatally to initiate pubertal changes and to cause ovulation so that pregnancy is possible. Deletions of the X-chromosome–linked *SHOX* gene explain many of the dysmorphic skeletal features that are present, including the short stature. It is believed that the number of phenotypic findings may be related to the percentage of cells that are 45,X. There also may be an effect of imprinting with the variation in phenotype partly explained by the parental origin of the one remaining X chromosome.

Pure Gonadal Dysgenesis

Pure gonadal dysgenesis is the term given to phenotypically female individuals with streak gonads who are of normal stature and have none of the physical stigmata associated with Turner's syndrome. Such individuals have either a 46,XX or 46,XY karyotype. The 46,XX defect may be inherited as an autosomal recessive, with 10% having associated nerve deafness. The 46,XY defect may be inherited as an X-linked recessive, with clitorimegaly occurring in 10 to 15% and gonadal tumors developing in 25% if the gonads are not removed.

Mutations in the X Chromosome Associated with Premature Ovarian Failure

Several regions of the X chromosome are now recognized to contain mutations in genes that may result in premature ovarian failure. Of particular note is the fragile X mental retardation (*FMR1*) gene. More than 5% of women with 46,XX spontaneous premature ovarian failure have mutations of the *FMR1* gene. This risk is increased if there is a family history of premature ovarian failure. A family history of fragile X syndrome, unexplained mental retardation, dementia, developmental delay of a child, or tremor-ataxia syndrome is reason for genetic counseling. Mutations in the *FMR1* gene are known to be associated with a neurodegenerative disorder. Women with mutations in the *FMR1* gene are at risk for having a child with mental retardation, should they be one of the 6 to 8% of women with premature ovarian failure who conceive spontaneously. For *FMR1*, a CGG repeat sequence occurs, with up to 60 repeats being normal. Expansion to more than 200 repeats leads to the fragile X syndrome, with the high level of repeats causing hypermethylation of the gene promoter and silencing of the gene. Female carriers of the permutation have an unstable intermediate number of repeats (i.e., 60 to 199) and the predisposition for premature ovarian failure.

Trisomy X

Trisomy X (46,XXX karyotype) is also associated with premature menopause, although many such individuals have normal reproductive lives. Premature menopause can also occur in mosaic individuals with cell lines with excess X chromosomes. When gonadal abnormalities occur in women with excess X chromosomes, they seem to occur after ovarian differentiation so that some ovarian function is possible. Only later in life do such women develop secondary amenorrhea and premature ovarian failure.

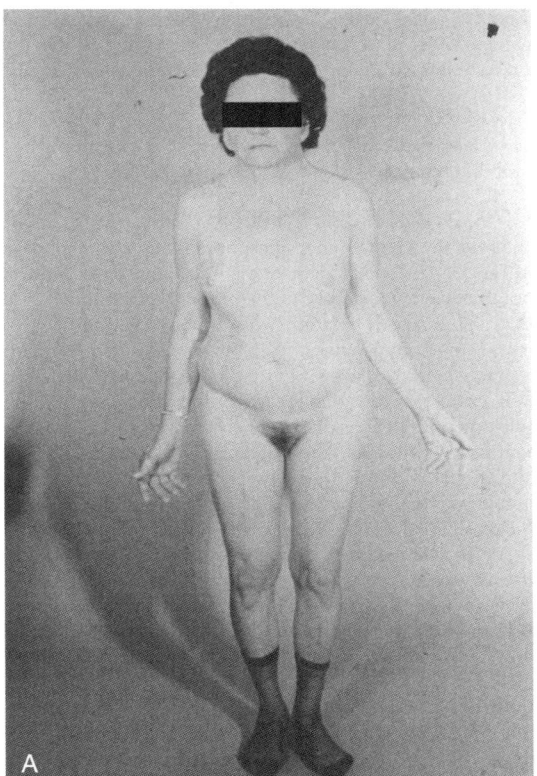

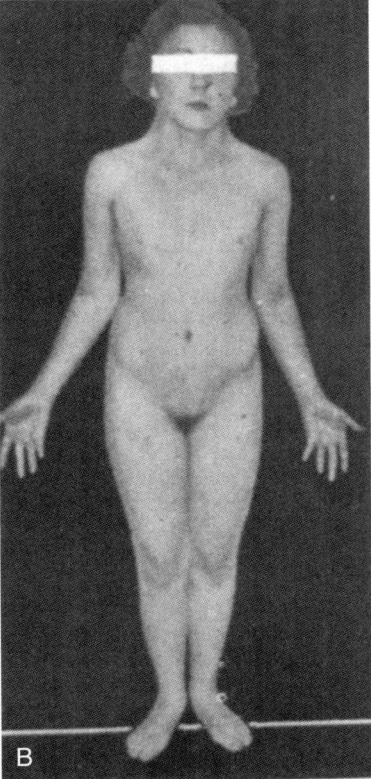

FIGURE 236-4. Adult with Turner's syndrome. This woman was seen at age 56 years by the author of the chapter (Dr. Rebar), and was case number 2, an adolescent at that time, in the original publication of Dr. Henry Turner describing the syndrome.

Known Genetic Alterations of Specific Genes

In girls with the rare syndrome of 17α-hydroxylase deficiency involving *p450c17* who survive until the expected age of puberty, sexual infantilism and primary amenorrhea occur together with elevated levels of gonadotropins (also see Chapter 233). Defects in the 20,22-lyase (*p450scc*) or aromatase

(*p450arom*) enzymes may also lead to ovarian failure. Women with galactosemia also experience ovarian failure early in life, even when a galactose-restricted diet is introduced early in infancy.

Mutations of several autosomal genes result in premature ovarian failure. Included in this growing list are mutations involving *FSHR* (the FSH receptor gene), *FOXL2* (a forkhead transcription factor associated with the blepharophimosis-ptosis-epicanthus inversus syndrome), *INHA* (the inhibin-α gene), *E1F2B* (a family of genes associated with central nervous system leukodystrophy and ovarian failure), *PMM2* (the gene for phosphomannomutase), *GALT* (the gene for galactose-1-phosphate uridyltransferase), and *AIRE* (leading to the autoimmune polyendocrinopathy-candidiasis-ectodermal dystrophy syndrome). Myotonic dystrophy (Chapter 421) is caused by an autosomal triple repeat mutation, like the fragile X syndrome, that is similarly associated with premature loss of germ cells from the ovary. The list of mutations associated with early ovarian failure continues to increase as the function of more genes is determined.

Mutations Involving Reproductive Hormones, Their Receptors, and Action

The resistant ovary (Savage's) syndrome occurs in young amenorrheic women who have elevated peripheral gonadotropin concentrations, normal (although immature) follicles present on ovarian biopsy, 46,XX karyotype with no evidence of mosaicism, fully developed secondary sex characteristics, and ovarian resistance to stimulation with human menopausal or pituitary gonadotropins. At least some of these women have mutations in the FSH receptor. It is probably inappropriate to use the term "resistant ovary syndrome" because it is likely that this is a heterogeneous disorder due to various genetic mutations.

Other Causes
Physical and Environmental

Irradiation and chemotherapeutic agents used to treat various malignant diseases may also cause premature ovarian failure. Ovulation and cyclic menses return in some of these patients even after prolonged intervals of hypergonadotropic amenorrhea associated with signs and symptoms of profound hypoestrogenism. In general, the younger the individual at the time of treatment, the less likely is she to have permanent ovarian failure after the completion of therapy. Rarely, mumps affects the ovaries and causes ovarian failure.

Autoimmune Disorders

Premature ovarian failure may occur in conjunction with a variety of autoimmune disorders. The most well-known syndrome (autoimmune polyglandular syndrome type 1) involves hypoadrenalism, hypoparathyroidism, and mucocutaneous candidiasis together with ovarian failure (Chapter 231). Testing for adrenal antibodies by indirect immunofluorescence will identify the 4% of women with spontaneous premature ovarian failure who have steroidogenic cell autoimmunity and are at risk for adrenal insufficiency. Thyroiditis is the most commonly associated abnormality. Antibodies to the FSH receptor have been identified in a few cases. These associations make it mandatory to rule out other potentially life-threatening endocrinopathies in young women with hypergonadotropic amenorrhea.

TREATMENT

Women with hypergonadotropic amenorrhea and ovarian failure should be treated identically whether or not they have signs of hypoestrogenism or desire pregnancy. Counseling and psychological support are indicated in women in whom the diagnosis of premature ovarian failure is made. Ovarian biopsy is not indicated to document the existence of follicles because only a small portion of each ovary can be sampled and because pregnancies have resulted in patients who had biopsy samples devoid of follicles. Estrogen replacement is warranted to prevent the accelerated bone loss known to occur in affected women (Chapter 243). The estrogen should be given sequentially with a progestin to prevent endometrial hyperplasia. Young women with ovarian failure may require twice as much estrogen as postmenopausal women for relief of signs and symptoms of hypoestrogenism. Inexplicably, women with premature ovarian failure may conceive while taking exogenous estrogen, even in the form of oral contraceptive agents, at the same rate as those not taking estrogen, so barrier contraception should be discussed if pregnancy is not desired.

Women with hypergonadotropic amenorrhea are rarely able to become pregnant. It is not clear why pregnancy may rarely occur in such women, but the pregnancy and delivery rate is 6 to 8%. Infertility treatment of young women with hypergonadotropic amenorrhea involves hormone replacement to mimic the normal menstrual cycle and embryo transfer by use of donor oocytes. Whether women with gonadal dysgenesis should be offered pregnancy by use of donor oocytes is now the subject of debate because a markedly increased incidence of aortic rupture during pregnancy secondary to medial necrosis has been documented.

Women with Turner's syndrome contemplating pregnancy should be counseled regarding the risks. The coordination of health care of adult women with Turner's syndrome often falls to the endocrinologist because many of the complications of the disease are endocrinologic: hypothyroidism, diabetes, hypertension, obesity, osteoporosis, and hypogonadism. However, guidelines have been published about the surveillance of other multisystem conditions for which Turner's syndrome patients are at risk, including significant psychosocial problems, congenital heart disease, deafness, and gastrointestinal and hepatic disorders.

CHRONIC ANOVULATION

Chronic anovulation, the most frequent form of amenorrhea encountered in women of reproductive age, implies that functional ovarian follicles remain and that cyclic ovulation can be induced with appropriate therapy (Table 236-4). The cause of the anovulation should be determined. The pathophysiologic bases for several forms of anovulation are unknown, but the anovulation can be interrupted transiently by nonspecific induction of ovulation in most affected women. Anovulation can result in either amenorrhea or irregular (generally less frequent) menses.

Hypothalamic Chronic Anovulation

DEFINITION

Hypothalamic chronic anovulation (HCA) represents a heterogeneous group of disorders with similar manifestations. Emotional and physical stress,

TABLE 236-4 CAUSES OF CHRONIC ANOVULATION

Chronic anovulation of hypothalamic-pituitary origin
  Hypothalamic chronic anovulation
    Psychogenic
    Exercise associated
    Associated with diet, weight loss, or malnutrition
    Anorexia nervosa and bulimia
    Pseudocyesis
  Forms of isolated (idiopathic) hypogonadotropic hypogonadism (including Kallmann's syndrome)
  Due to hypothalamic-pituitary damage
    Pituitary and parapituitary tumors
    Empty sella syndrome
    Following surgery
    Following irradiation
    Following trauma
    Following infection
    Following infarction
  Idiopathic hypopituitarism
  Hypothalamic-pituitary dysfunction or failure with hyperprolactinemia (multiple causes)
  Due to systemic diseases
Chronic anovulation due to inappropriate feedback (i.e., polycystic ovary syndrome)
  Excessive extraglandular estrogen production (i.e., obesity)
  Abnormal buffering involving sex hormone–binding globulin (including liver disease)
  Functional androgen excess (adrenal or ovarian)
  Neoplasms producing androgens or estrogens
  Neoplasms producing chorionic gonadotropin
Chronic anovulation due to other endocrine and metabolic disorders
  Adrenal hyperfunction
    Cushing's syndrome
    Congenital adrenal hyperplasia (female pseudohermaphroditism)
  Thyroid dysfunction
    Hyperthyroidism
    Hypothyroidism
  Prolactin or growth hormone excess
    Hypothalamic dysfunction
    Pituitary dysfunction (microadenomas and macroadenomas)
    Drug induced
  Malnutrition

excessive exercise, nutritional deficiencies, weight loss, reduced body fat, and other unrecognized factors may contribute in varying proportions to the anovulation. Women with HCA have normal neuroanatomic findings.

ANOREXIA NERVOSA
Individuals with amenorrhea and significant weight loss should be examined for the possibility of anorexia nervosa (Chapter 219).

ISOLATED HYPOGONADOTROPIC HYPOGONADISM
Affected individuals have absence of spontaneous pubertal development. Most have functional GnRH deficiency, but some have abnormalities of gonadotropin deficiency localized to the pituitary gland.

Kallmann's syndrome is a familial disorder consisting of gonadotropin deficiency, anosmia or hyposmia, and color blindness in men or, more rarely, in women (Chapter 223). Partial or complete agenesis of the olfactory bulb is present on autopsy, accounting for use of the term *olfactogenital dysplasia*. Isolated gonadotropin deficiency in the absence of anosmia occurs as well. Sexual infantilism with a eunuchoid habitus is the clinical hallmark of this disorder, but moderate breast development may occur. Circulating LH and FSH levels are low but almost always detectable. Mutations in *KAL1*, *FGFR1*, *FGF8*, *PROK2*, *ROKR2*, *HS6ST1*, *WDR11*, or *CHD7* have been identified in a minority of patients with Kallmann's syndrome. Ovulation induction requires use of exogenous gonadotropins and HCG or pulsatile GnRH. Estrogen replacement therapy is indicated in these women until pregnancy is desired. It may not be possible to distinguish between partial isolated gonadotropin deficiency and functional HCA in all cases.

HYPOPITUITARISM
Hypopituitarism may be obvious on cursory inspection or sufficiently subtle to require endocrine testing (Chapter 224). The clinical presentation depends on the age at onset, the cause, and the nutritional status of the individual. Failure of development of secondary sex characteristics must always raise the question of hypopituitarism. Ovulation can be induced successfully with exogenous gonadotropins when pregnancy is desired and after the hypopituitarism is treated appropriately. Replacement therapy with estrogen is indicated.

HYPERPROLACTINEMIA
Galactorrhea associated with hyperprolactinemia, whatever the cause, almost always occurs together with amenorrhea caused by hypothalamic-pituitary dysfunction or failure. Many conditions can cause excess prolactin secretion (Chapter 224). A prolactinoma must be excluded. Hirsutism may be observed occasionally in association with amenorrhea-galactorrhea and hyperprolactinemia. Elevated levels of the adrenal androgens dehydroepiandrosterone and dehydroepiandrosterone sulfate may be observed and may account for the polycystic-type ovaries present in some hyperprolactinemic women.

FAILURE OF THE HYPOTHALAMIC-PITUITARY UNIT
The hypothalamic-pituitary unit may also fail to function normally in a number of stressful, debilitating, systemic illnesses that interfere with somatic growth and development. Chronic renal failure, liver disease, and diabetes mellitus are the most prominent examples.

DIAGNOSIS

Abrupt cessation of menses in women younger than 30 years who have no anatomic abnormalities of the hypothalamic-pituitary-ovarian axis and no other endocrine disturbances suggests a diagnosis of HCA. Affected individuals tend to be bright, educated, and engaged in intellectual occupations and may well give a history of psychosexual problems and socioenvironmental trauma. HCA is characterized by low to normal levels of gonadotropins and relative hypoestrogenism. Rarely, however, do affected women present with signs and symptoms of estrogen deficiency. It is important to rule out a central lesion as the cause of the hypogonadotropic hypogonadism in women who appear to have HCA.

TREATMENT   **Rx**

Psychological counseling or a change in lifestyle, especially for women engaged in strenuous exercise programs, may be effective in inducing cyclic ovulation and menses in women with functional HCA. Cognitive behavior therapy is effective in a proportion of women with functional HCA. For women desiring pregnancy, ovulation can also be induced with clomiphene citrate (50 to 100 mg/day for 5 days beginning on the third to fifth day of withdrawal bleeding). Treatment with exogenous gonadotropins to induce follicular maturation followed by HCG to induce follicular rupture may be effective in women who do not ovulate in response to clomiphene. Because women with HCA have low circulating levels of leptin, investigators have given recombinant leptin and documented that ovulation may resume in some affected women. Given the heterogeneous nature of the disorder, it is not surprising that exogenous leptin is not effective in all women.

Most physicians advocate the use of exogenous gonadal steroids to prevent osteoporosis. A regimen can consist of daily oral conjugated or esterified estrogens (0.625 to 1.25 mg), ethinyl estradiol (20 µg), or micronized estradiol-17β (1 to 2 mg) or transdermal estradiol-17β (0.05 to 0.10 mg) daily, with oral medroxyprogesterone acetate (5 to 10 mg) added for the first 12 to 14 days of each month. Sexually active women can be given oral contraceptive agents as an alternative. If steroid therapy is administered, patients must be informed that the amenorrhea will probably be present when therapy is discontinued. Other physicians believe that only periodic observation is indicated, with barrier methods of contraception recommended for fertility control. Adequate ingestion of calcium should be ensured regardless of therapy. Contraception is needed for sexually active women with HCA because the functional defect is mild in these disorders and may resolve spontaneously at any time, with ovulation occurring before any episode of menstruation.

Chronic Anovulation Related to Inappropriate Feedback

DEFINITION

PCOS is a heterogeneous disorder in which there is considerable clinical and biochemical variability among affected individuals. (See PCOS as the most common cause of heterosexual pubertal development in Chapter 235.) PCOS is currently considered to exist in women with any two of the following: (1) oligo-ovulation or anovulation, (2) hyperandrogenism, or (3) polycystic ovaries on ultrasound, and in whom other etiologies have been eliminated. PCOS is the classic disorder in which the amenorrhea or oligomenorrhea results from inappropriate feedback of gonadal steroids from the ovaries.

PATHOBIOLOGY

Current evidence suggests that the hypothalamic-pituitary unit is intact and that a functional derangement, perhaps involving insulin-like growth factors (IGFs) such as IGF-I within the ovary, results in abnormal gonadotropin secretion. PCOS is characterized by insulin resistance and compensatory hyperinsulinemia. (See association between PCOS, insulin resistance, and obesity in Chapter 220.) The insulin resistance has been found in affected women of many racial and ethnic groups, implying that it is a universal characteristic and that a common defect may be present. There is increasing evidence of specific genetic abnormalities in some women with PCOS.

CLINICAL MANIFESTATIONS

Although patients usually present with amenorrhea, hirsutism, and obesity, affected women may instead complain of irregular and profuse uterine bleeding, may not have hirsutism, and may be of normal weight (Fig. 236-5). Excess androgen from any source or increased extraglandular conversion of androgens to estrogens can lead to the typical findings of PCOS. Included are such diverse disorders as Cushing's syndrome, mild congenital adrenal hyperplasia, virilizing tumors of adrenal or ovarian origin, hyperthyroidism and hypothyroidism, obesity, and primary PCOS with no other recognizable cause.

In the primary syndrome, the irregular menses, mild obesity, and hirsutism begin during puberty and typically become more severe with time, although there is increasing evidence of improvement in the years just before menopause. Obesity alone can lead to a polycystic ovarian–like syndrome, with the degree of obesity required to cause anovulation varying widely. The increase in the prevalence of obesity is leading to an increased prevalence of PCOS. All such patients are well estrogenized regardless of whether they present with primary or secondary amenorrhea or dysfunctional bleeding. LH concentrations tend to be elevated, with relatively low and constant FSH levels, but both may be in the normal range for the follicular phase of the menstrual cycle. Levels of most circulating androgens, especially testosterone, tend to be mildly elevated.

DIAGNOSIS

After exclusion of other etiologies, two of the following three are required for diagnosis of PCOS: (1) hyperandrogenism (clinical or biochemical);

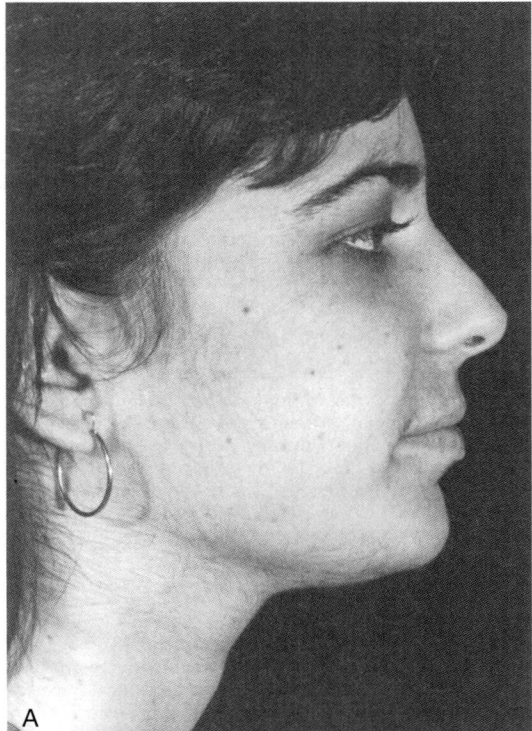

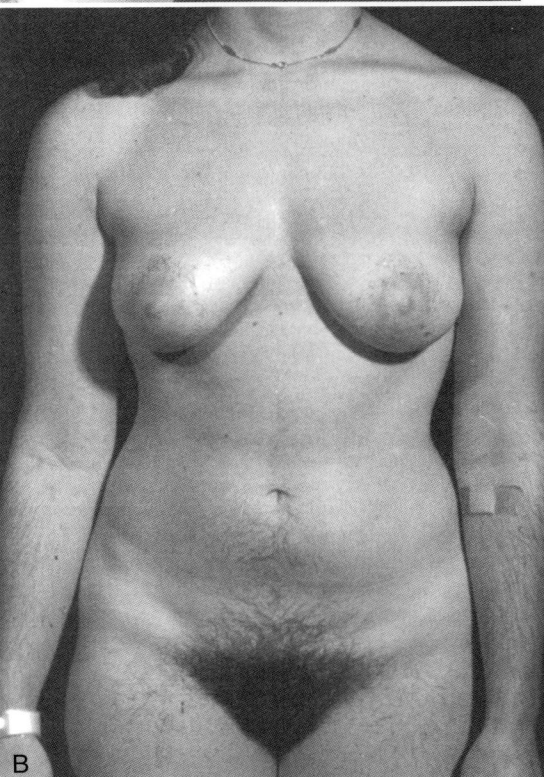

FIGURE 236-5. Adult with polycystic ovary syndrome (PCOS). This 28-year-old woman with documented PCOS had elevated luteinizing hormone levels, irregular menses, and hirsutism since puberty. Note the increased hair in the midline extending up to and above the umbilicus. Other findings (which are not necessarily abnormal) are periareolar hair and hypertrichosis of the arms.

(2) oligo-ovulation or anovulation; (3) polycystic ovaries on ultrasound examination or at surgery.[12]

This definition is confusing to clinicians because it implies that hirsute women with polycystic ovaries on ultrasound examination who ovulate regularly should be considered to have PCOS. Moreover, it is clear that polycystic ovaries may be identified on ultrasound examination in normal women. In any case, the aim of the diagnostic evaluation is to rule out any causes (such as neoplasms) that require definitive therapy. Hirsutism should be evaluated as detailed in Chapter 442.

A particularly severely affected subset of women present with marked obesity, anovulation, mild glucose intolerance with high levels of circulating insulin, acanthosis nigricans, hyperuricemia, severe hirsutism, and elevated circulating androgen levels. These women have hyperthecosis of the ovaries, in which the androgen-producing cells in the stromal, hilar, and thecal regions are increased greatly in number. Hyperthecosis should probably be viewed as a part of the spectrum of disorders constituting PCOS.

TREATMENT Rx

Patients generally require therapy for hirsutism, for induction of ovulation if pregnancy is desired, and for prevention of estrogen-induced endometrial hyperplasia and cancer. No ideal therapy exists; the therapeutic approach must be individualized. The risks for metabolic syndrome, cardiovascular disease, and diabetes mellitus are increased in women with PCOS, at least in part because of the increased androgens and insulin resistance. Moreover, many women have elevated cholesterol levels.

Medical Therapy

In the anovulatory woman not desiring pregnancy who is not hirsute, therapy with intermittent progestin administration (e.g., medroxyprogesterone acetate, 5 to 10 mg orally for 10 to 14 days each month) or oral contraceptives can be provided to reduce the increased risk for endometrial carcinoma that is present in such a woman with unopposed estrogen. All women using intermittent progestin administration should be cautioned about the need for effective contraception if they are sexually active because these agents do not inhibit ovulation when they are administered intermittently.

Improvements in insulin sensitivity in women with polycystic ovaries, either through lifestyle changes (i.e., exercise and diet) or through pharmacologic intervention, consistently result in improvements in the reproductive and metabolic abnormalities. Resumption of ovulation may occur in up to 60 to 70% of affected women.

The longest and largest published experiences with any agent that improves insulin sensitivity in PCOS is with metformin, a biguanide that functions primarily by suppressing hepatic gluconeogenesis and also improves insulin sensitivity.[A6] Its use in PCOS leads to reductions in insulin and androgen levels and resumption of menses in some women. Divided doses of 1500 to 2000 mg/day have proved effective.

Some clinicians advocate giving metformin to all women with polycystic ovaries, whereas others would administer such an agent only to those with documented insulin resistance. Some clinicians also advocate giving metformin first to women who desire pregnancy and then adding an agent to induce ovulation if the metformin proves ineffective. These agents are not approved for use in pregnant women or for the induction of ovulation.

Treatment Considering Pregnancy

Oral contraceptive agents are the first line of therapy for hirsute anovulatory woman not desiring pregnancy and offer protection from endometrial hyperplasia. In women with PCOS desiring pregnancy, clomiphene citrate or letrozole can be used to induce ovulation.[A7][A8] Letrozole is not approved for this use by the FDA, but a large multicenter randomized trial has demonstrated its superiority to clomiphene in obese women with PCOS.[A9] About 75 to 80% conceive with such therapy. In addition to insulin-sensitizing agents, other possible methods of inducing ovulation include use of exogenous gonadotropins and HCG, and laparoscopic ovarian surgery with multiple punctures of the ovary by diathermy or laser. A large clinical trial documented that clomiphene citrate is more effective than metformin in inducing ovulation and resulting in pregnancy; there was no further improvement when the two agents were used concurrently.[A10]

Surgical Treatment

Laparoscopic ovarian surgery can achieve unifollicular ovulation or make it easier for medical ovulation induction but increases the risk for development of ovarian adhesions (themselves leading to infertility). It may be successful in a small subset of women with PCOS who are geographically removed from good medical care.

Chronic Anovulation Related to Other Endocrine and Metabolic Disorders

Adrenal hyperfunction appears to cause chronic anovulation by inducing a polycystic ovarian-like syndrome secondary to increased adrenal androgen secretion. Both hyperthyroidism and hypothyroidism are associated with a variety of menstrual disturbances, including dysfunctional uterine bleeding and amenorrhea as a result of alterations in the metabolism of androgens and estrogens. These metabolic changes in turn result in inappropriate steroid feedback and chronic anovulation.

Luteinized Unruptured Follicle Syndrome

The luteinized unruptured follicle syndrome refers to the development of a dominant follicle without its subsequent disruption and release of the ovum. The abnormality can be diagnosed by ultrasonography or by the absence of evidence of ovulation when the ovary is viewed at laparoscopy. The disorder occurs infrequently and is not a significant cause of infertility. Menstrual cycles in which no ovum is released are characterized by presumptive evidence of ovulation, including biphasic basal body temperatures, secretory endometrium, normal LH surge, and normal progesterone production in the luteal phase.

Luteal Phase Dysfunction

PATHOBIOLOGY

Progesterone secretion in the luteal phase may be reduced in duration (termed *luteal phase insufficiency*) or in amount (termed *luteal phase inadequacy*). More rarely, the endometrium may be unable to respond to secreted progesterone because of the absence of progesterone receptors. These disorders represent causes of infertility (because of inability of fertilized ova to implant) in less than 5% of infertile couples. Abnormalities of the follicular phase, especially in the frequency of gonadotropin pulses, may account for most luteal phase defects. Luteal phase defects may also occur sporadically in normally ovulating women.

DIAGNOSIS

Luteal phase dysfunction may be associated with several clinical entities, including mild or intermittent hyperprolactinemia, strenuous physical exercise, inadequately treated 21-hydroxylase deficiency, and recurrent miscarriage. Luteal dysfunction occurs more commonly at the extremes of reproductive life and in the first menstrual cycles after full-term delivery, abortion, or discontinuation of oral contraceptives. It may also occur during ovulatory cycles induced with clomiphene citrate or exogenous gonadotropins and HCG.

TREATMENT Rx

Treatment of luteal dysfunction is controversial. Any underlying defect should be treated. If subsequent luteal function depends on prior follicular development, modification of follicular development with either clomiphene citrate (25 to 100 mg daily by mouth for 5 days beginning on cycle day 3 to 5) or FSH (75 to 300 IU intramuscularly for 3 to 5 days beginning on cycle day 3 to 5) can be used; HCG (2500 to 5000 IU intramuscularly at 2- to 3-day intervals beginning with the shift in basal body temperature) or progesterone (12.5 mg intramuscularly in oil daily or 25 mg twice a day as rectal or vaginal suppositories) can be used as well. Bromocriptine may correct the abnormality in individuals with hyperprolactinemia. Synthetic progestational agents should not be used to treat luteal phase defects because of their possible association with congenital anomalies. Furthermore, the synthetic progestins produce an abnormal endometrium. None of these agents has been shown to increase the pregnancy rate.

INFERTILITY

DEFINITION

The World Health Organization (WHO) has defined *infertility* as "a disease of the reproductive system defined by the failure to achieve a clinical pregnancy after 12 months or more of regular unprotected sexual intercourse." *Sterility* is total inability to reproduce. More than 10% of couples in the United States seek medical assistance for infertility.

The requirements for pregnancy to occur are several:
- The male must produce adequate numbers of normal, motile spermatozoa.
- The male must be capable of ejaculating the sperm through a patent ductal system.
- The sperm must be able to traverse an unobstructed female reproductive tract.
- The female must ovulate and release an ovum.

TABLE 236-5 CAUSES OF INFERTILITY AND THEIR APPROXIMATE INCIDENCE (WHERE AVAILABLE)*

Male factors (40%)
  Decreased production of spermatozoa
    Varicocele
    Testicular failure
    Endocrine disorders
    Cryptorchidism
    Stress, smoking, caffeine, nicotine, recreational drugs
  Ductal obstruction
    Epididymal (after infection)
    Congenital absence of vas deferens
    Ejaculatory duct (after infection)
    After vasectomy
  Inability to deliver sperm into vagina
    Ejaculatory disturbances
    Hypospadias
    Sexual problems (i.e., impotence), medical or psychological
  Abnormal semen
    Infection
    Abnormal volume
    Abnormal viscosity
  Immunologic factors
    Sperm-immobilizing antibodies
    Sperm-agglutinating antibodies

Female factors
  Fallopian tube disease (20-30%)
    Pelvic inflammatory disease or puerperal infection
    Congenital anomalies
    Endometriosis
    Secondary to past peritonitis of nongenital origin
  Amenorrhea and anovulation (15%)
  Minor ovulatory disturbances (<5%)
  Cervical and uterine factors (10%)
    Leiomyomas and polyps
    Uterine anomalies
    Intrauterine synechiae (Asherman's syndrome)
    Destroyed endocervical glands (after surgery or after infection)
  Vaginal factors (<5%)
    Congenital absence of vagina
    Imperforate hymen
    Vaginismus
    Vaginitis
  Immunologic factors (<5%)
    Sperm-immobilizing antibodies
    Sperm-agglutinating antibodies
  Nutritional and metabolic factors (5%)
    Thyroid disorders
    Diabetes mellitus
    Severe nutritional disturbances

Idiopathic or unexplained (<10%)

*World Health Organization definition of infertility: ≥12 months of regular unprotected sexual intercourse. In about one third of couples, more than one cause contributes to the infertility.

- The sperm must be able to fertilize the ovum.
- The fertilized ovum must be capable of developing and implanting in appropriately prepared endometrium.

In approximately 40% of cases, infertility is caused by the male (Table 236-5). In one third of couples, more than one cause contributes to the infertility.

Peak age for fertility in the female is 25 years. For nulliparous women of this age, the average time during which unprotected intercourse occurs until conception is 5.3 months. For parous women, the average duration of intercourse until conception is 2.7 months. The reproductive performance of couples is influenced by the ages of the female and male partners, the frequency of intercourse, and the length of time the couple has been attempting to conceive. There is a decline in both female and male reproductive performance after the age of 25 years.

DIAGNOSIS

Couples who complain of infertility merit evaluation regardless of the length of infertility. Evaluation is warranted in all women after 12 months and in women 35 years of age or older after 6 months of regular unprotected intercourse.

The evaluation begins with a detailed history obtained from both partners and physical examinations of both individuals. If possible, the couple should be seen together. Each couple should be questioned together and separately because separate interviews may uncover information that would not be imparted in the presence of the partner.

Initial evaluation for infertility includes assessment of semen; documentation of ovulation by basal body temperature, serum progesterone determination 6 to 8 days before menses, serum thyroid hormone, or (rarely) endometrial biopsy less than 3 days before onset of menses; and evaluation of the female genital tract by hysterosalpingography or sonohysterography. Diagnostic laparoscopy with tubal dye instillation may be performed if results of all previous tests are normal because 30 to 50% of women are found to have endometriosis or tubal disease on surgical evaluation; alternatively, patients with initial normal findings may be merely treated as having idiopathic infertility.

TREATMENT Rx

Treatment must be predicated on the findings of the infertility evaluation. Abnormalities of sperm are difficult disorders to treat. Low sperm count or poor motility is best treated either by donor insemination or in vitro fertilization with intracytoplasmic injection of a single viable sperm into each oocyte. Obstruction of the fallopian tubes may be amenable to surgical intervention, but success rates are often greater with in vitro fertilization. Endometriosis causing infertility may be treated by surgery or various suppressive drugs as indicated; however, here, too, in vitro fertilization may be indicated.

Induction of ovulation is one of the most successful therapies when used in anovulatory women.

Induction of ovulation should never be attempted until serious disorders precluding pregnancy are ruled out or treated. Furthermore, ovulation induction should not be used in women with ovarian failure because they are unresponsive to any form of ovulation induction.

Clomiphene citrate is the agent that usually induces ovulation most easily. Clomiphene should be used in individuals without hyperprolactinemia who have the ability to release LH and FSH. A typical course of clomiphene therapy is begun on the third to fifth days after either spontaneous or induced uterine bleeding. The initial dosage is 50 mg daily for 5 days. Clomiphene appears to act as an antiestrogen and stimulates gonadotropin secretion by the pituitary gland to initiate follicular development. If ovulation is not achieved in the first cycle of treatment, the daily dosage is increased to 100 mg. If ovulation is still not achieved, dosage is increased in a stepwise fashion in 50-mg increments to a maximum of 200 to 250 mg daily for 5 days. The highest dose should be continued for 3 to 6 months before the patient is regarded as unresponsive to clomiphene. The quantity of drug and the length of time that it can be used, as suggested here, are greater than those recommended by the manufacturers and the FDA but conform to published series. Despite absence of FDA approval, letrozole is being used increasingly in place of clomiphene.

The ovulatory surge of LH may occur 5 to 12 days (average, 7 days) after the completion of the last day of clomiphene treatment. Couples are advised to have intercourse every other day during this interval. Ovulation can be documented by monitoring changes in basal body temperature or preferably by measuring serum progesterone 14 days after the last clomiphene dose. Menses should occur after 3 weeks. Withdrawal bleeding with progestin can be induced if the patient fails to bleed within 4 weeks of therapy and if a serum HCG level documents that the patient is not pregnant. Testing the urine for an LH surge may also be useful in timing ovulation.

Some clinicians give 5000 to 10,000 IU of HCG intramuscularly 7 days after the last day of clomiphene therapy to trigger ovulation, but this approach has not been established to increase effectiveness. The administration of HCG, however, does serve to time ovulation and may be helpful in selected couples. Ovulation can be expected to occur approximately 36 hours after HCG administration.

Of appropriately selected patients, 75 to 80% ovulate, and 40 to 50% can be expected to become pregnant. About 15% of pregnancies can be expected with each ovulatory cycle. The multiple pregnancy rate is about 8%, with almost all being twins. The incidence of congenital anomalies is not increased. Side effects of clomiphene are uncommon and rarely serious. The most serious ones include vasomotor flushes (10%), abdominal discomfort (5%), breast tenderness (2%), nausea and vomiting (2%), visual symptoms (1.5%), and headache (1%). Ovarian enlargement may occur but is rare (5%). Concern has been raised about the potential for clomiphene to increase the risk for epithelial ovarian cancer. The bulk of the evidence now indicates that clomiphene does not increase this risk.

The addition of dexamethasone, 0.5 mg orally at bedtime, to blunt the nighttime secretion of adrenocorticotropic hormone may be useful in hyperandrogenic women who fail to ovulate in response to clomiphene. Other individuals who do not respond to clomiphene typically require exogenous gonadotropins and HCG or perhaps pulsatile GnRH to induce ovulation.

Both bromocriptine and cabergoline are effective in inducing ovulation in hyperprolactinemic women. The drug should be stopped when pregnancy is confirmed. Ovulatory menses and pregnancy are achieved in about 80% of patients with galactorrhea and hyperprolactinemia. Most women with prolactin-secreting pituitary tumors remain asymptomatic during pregnancy. It is rare for a patient with either a microadenoma or a macroadenoma to develop a problem related to the tumor that affects either the mother or the fetus during pregnancy. Monitoring during pregnancy need consist only of questioning the patient about the development of visual symptoms and headaches. Formal assessment of visual fields and computed tomography or magnetic resonance imaging should be carried out in any patient experiencing suggestive symptoms. Symptoms generally abate with institution of therapy with a dopamine agonist. No adverse effects of dopamine agonists on fetuses or pregnancies have been reported. Concerns have been raised that ergot-derived dopamine agonists, in the large doses used in the treatment of Parkinson disease, may increase the risk for cardiac valve regurgitation. Although there is no evidence of risk in women treated with much lower doses for hyperprolactinemia, they should be counseled about this potential side effect.

Several preparations of purified and synthetic biochemically engineered gonadotropins for use for induction of ovulation now exist. Synthetic preparations consist entirely of FSH, whereas most purified preparations contain some LH as well. Each vial typically contains 75 IU of gonadotropin. Individuals with gonadotropin deficiency require a preparation containing some LH. Exogenous gonadotropins are typically administered at doses of two to four vials (intramuscularly or subcutaneously, depending on the preparation) for 5 to 12 days to achieve follicular development as monitored by ultrasonography and serum or urinary estradiol concentrations; HCG, 5000 to 10,000 IU, is administered as a single intramuscular dose when follicular maturation is apparent. The HCG should be withheld if more than three follicles mature together. GnRH analogues are now being used to suppress endogenous follicular activity before initiation of therapy with exogenous gonadotropins and continued until HCG is given in older women and those with poor responses to exogenous gonadotropins. Use of the analogues necessitates administration of larger doses of exogenous gonadotropins. Success rates, however, appear to be somewhat improved with this combined therapy. Because of the expense and the complication rate, thorough evaluation should be carried out to exclude other causes of infertility before exogenous gonadotropins and HCG are used. Ovulation can be induced in almost 100% of patients, but pregnancy occurs in only 50 to 70%. There is no increased risk for congenital anomalies with exogenous gonadotropins and HCG. The rate of multiple pregnancies with exogenous gonadotropins and HCG may approach 30%, with 5% being triplets or more.

Ovarian hyperstimulation (*ovarian hyperstimulation syndrome*, or OHSS) is the major side effect and may be life-threatening. The ovaries enlarge remarkably, and multiple follicle cysts, stromal edema, and multiple corpora lutea are present. There is a shift of fluid from the intravascular space into the abdominal cavity with resultant hypovolemia and hemoconcentration. The cause of the ascites is unknown. The most serious complications of OHSS may include thromboembolism, renal failure, adult respiratory distress syndrome, and hemorrhage from ovarian rupture. Treatment is conservative, with monitoring of fluid and electrolyte status. Pelvic examinations should not be performed for fear of rupturing the ovaries. The hyperstimulation generally resolves slowly during about 7 days but lasts longer if the cycle results in pregnancy.

Clomiphene citrate or exogenous gonadotropins together with intrauterine insemination of spermatozoa may be used in women with unexplained infertility as so-called controlled ovarian hyperstimulation (COH). The intent is to stimulate several oocytes to be ovulated, but multiple (sometimes high-order) gestations are a significant risk. A randomized trial has noted that the risk for multiple gestation and the costs are reduced if COH with gonadotropins is not used and patients are advanced immediately to treatment by in vitro fertilization.

Assisted Reproductive Technologies

The assisted reproductive technologies, in which by definition both eggs and sperm are handled outside of the body, are being used commonly to treat infertile couples with tubal disease, endometriosis, oligospermia and azoospermia, sperm antibodies, and unexplained infertility. The procedure consists of in vitro fertilization and several variants. In vitro fertilization involves ovarian hyperstimulation, oocyte retrieval, fertilization, embryo culture, and embryo transfer. Ovarian hyperstimulation with clomiphene citrate and exogenous gonadotropins, gonadotropins alone, or a GnRH agonist or antagonist plus gonadotropins typically causes 1 to 20 oocytes to mature, depending on the patient's age and ovarian "reserve." After follicular growth is judged sufficient by ultrasound examination, HCG is given to induce final follicular maturation. About 34 hours after HCG administration, the oocytes are retrieved by direct needle puncture of each follicle, usually transvaginally with ultrasound guidance. The oocytes are then inseminated in vitro with washed sperm, or a single sperm is injected directly into a single egg (so-called intracytoplasmic sperm injection). The embryos are cultured for about 40 to 120 hours, after which one or more embryos are transferred to the uterine cavity. Embryos may

be cultured to the blastocyst stage (at 120 hours) before transfer. Additional embryos can be frozen in liquid nitrogen for transfer in a subsequent natural cycle. The success rate is most dependent on the age of the woman. In the United States, the percentage of cycles resulting in live births ranges from 40.1% in women younger than 35 years to 12.2% in women aged 41 to 42 years. Approximately 30% are twins and 1% are triplets or higher-order multiples.

It is now possible to test the early embryo for genetic abnormalities by removal of either a single cell (i.e., blastomere) or a polar body from the embryo in vitro and testing it with probes by fluorescent in situ hybridization, with the assistance of polymerase chain reaction, or most recently by comparative genomic hybridization. Identification of normal and abnormal embryos allows only normal embryos to be transferred in families with recognized and testable genetic abnormalities.

● SEXUAL FUNCTION AND DYSFUNCTION

Sexual Function

▶ DEFINITION

Sexual responses historically have been divided into four phases: excitement, plateau, orgasm, and resolution. With sexual arousal and excitement, vasocongestion and muscle tension increase progressively, primarily in the genital region, manifested by vaginal lubrication in the female. The lubrication is due to formation of a transudate in the vagina. Sexual excitement is initiated by any of a variety of psychogenic or somatogenic sexual stimuli and must be reinforced to result in orgasm. With continued stimulation, the excitement phase increases in intensity into a plateau phase during which a high state of sexual interest is maintained. The plateau phase may be short or long, and it is from this phase that an individual can shift to orgasm. The orgasmic phase tends to be brief and is characterized by rapid release from the developed vasocongestion and muscle tension. The orgasmic release is also known as the climax because peak psychological and physical intensity is achieved and there is an attendant feeling of satisfaction. Copious secretions and transudate may flow during orgasm in women. Characteristic genital and extragenital responses occur during these phases. Estrogens magnify the sexual responses, but responses may occur in estrogen-deficient women. For women, these changes occur in the breasts and in the pudendal region and are variable from one response cycle to another. For some women, excitement proceeds quickly through plateau to orgasm, and orgasm is explosive and accompanied by vocalization and involuntary contractions of the pelvic skeletal muscles. For other women, the responses are slow in building, controlled in amplitude, and long lasting. For a few women, orgasm never occurs; for many, it is intermittently absent.

The somatic sensate focus enabling orgasmic release is variable and may include stimulation of the breasts, vagina, or clitoris. The psychological aspect of coitus may involve concentration on the current partner or act or fantasies about other times and persons. Although orgasms may vary in physiologic intensity, what is important is psychological satisfaction. Satisfaction for both men and women may be had without orgasm.

Many clinicians have noted several limitations of this traditional human sex response cycle. Many clinicians and researchers see the cycle as circular with stimuli of different types leading to arousal. Clinicians in this field now have extended this theory to include desire and arousal. Women seek sexual experiences for intimacy as well as for sexual gratification. Women may be receptive to or seek out sexual stimuli to enhance intimacy. Biologic and psychological factors contribute to the processing of these stimuli and can enhance arousal and desire simultaneously.

Sexual Dysfunction

Women may seek consultation because of disturbances in normal sexual arousal or orgasm.[13] Such sexual dysfunction may be due to either organic or functional disturbances.

A variety of diseases affecting neurologic function, including diabetes mellitus and multiple sclerosis, may prevent sexual arousal. So, too, may local pelvic disorders, such as endometriosis and vaginitis, which cause dyspareunia and lead to sexual avoidance. Estrogen deficiency causing vaginal atrophy and dyspareunia is a relatively common cause of sexual dysfunction. Debilitating systemic diseases such as malignant disease may also affect sexual function indirectly.

In many cases, the cause of sexual dysfunction is psychological.[14] For instance, vaginismus involves involuntary contractions of the muscles surrounding the introitus and leads to dyspareunia. It is a conditioned response engendered by a previous real or imagined traumatic sexual experience. Feelings of guilt (caused by incest or rape, as examples), of inadequacy (caused by hysterectomy or mastectomy), or of depression or anxiety may lead to failure to be aroused. Failure to achieve orgasm may be viewed as a dysfunction if the woman is frustrated or dissatisfied.

TREATMENT Rx

Treatment of sexual dysfunction should eliminate functional causes and provide the patient, often together with her partner, with appropriate psychological counseling.[15] Behavioral modification is effective in treating many women with psychological sexual dysfunction. In one randomized trial, self-reported sexual satisfaction was increased in women treated with testosterone.[16] However, dosing guidelines are not clear, and the therapy cannot be considered standard care based on current evidence.

Grade A References

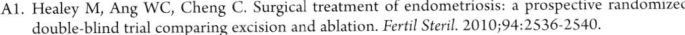

A1. Healey M, Ang WC, Cheng C. Surgical treatment of endometriosis: a prospective randomized double-blind trial comparing excision and ablation. *Fertil Steril.* 2010;94:2536-2540.

A2. Alkatout I, Mettler L, Beteta C, et al. Combined surgical and hormonal therapy for endometriosis is the most effective treatment: prospective, randomized, controlled trial. *J Minim Invasive Gynecol.* 2013;20:473-481.

A3. Guzick DS, Huang LS, Broadman BA, et al. Randomized trial of leuprolide versus continuous oral contraceptives in the treatment of endometriosis-associated pelvic pain. *Fertil Steril.* 2011;95:1568-1573.

A4. Marjoribanks J, Brown J, O'Brien PM, et al. Selective serotonin reuptake inhibitors for premenstrual syndrome. *Cochrane Database Syst Rev.* 2013;6:CD001396.

A5. Ford O, Lethaby A, Roberst H, et al. Progesterone for premenstrual syndrome. *Cochrane Database Syst Rev.* 2012;3:CD003415.

A6. Kjøtrød SB, Carlsen SM, Rsmussen PE, et al. Use of metformin before and during assisted reproductive technology in non-obese young infertile women with polycystic ovary syndrome: a prospective, randomized, double-blind, multi-centre study. *Hum Reprod.* 2011;26:2045-2053.

A7. Roy KK, Baruah J, Singla S, et al. A prospective randomized trial comparing the efficacy of letrozole and clomiphene citrate in induction of ovulation in polycystic ovarian syndrome. *J Hum Reprod Sci.* 2012;5:20-25.

A8. Badawy A, Gibreal A. Clomiphene citrate versus tamoxifen for ovulation induction in women with PCOS: a prospective randomized trial. *Eur J Obstet Gynecol Reprod Biol.* 2011;159:151-154.

A9. Legro RS, Brzyski RG, Diamond MP, et al. Letrozole versus clomiphene for infertility in the polycystic ovary syndrome. *N Engl J Med.* 2014;371:119-129.

A10. Legro RS, Barnhart HX, Schlaff WD, et al. Clomiphene, metformin, or both for infertility in the polycystic ovary syndrome. *N Engl J Med.* 2007;356:551-566.

GENERAL REFERENCES

For the General References and other additional features, please visit Expert Consult at https://expertconsult.inkling.com.

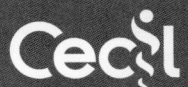

XIX

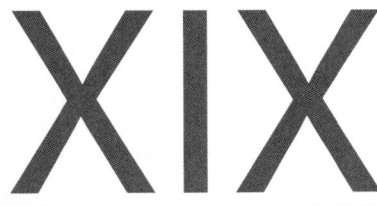

WOMEN'S HEALTH

237

APPROACH TO WOMEN'S HEALTH

KAREN FREUND

An approach to the care of women must go beyond an understanding of differences in the incidence of disease between men and women. Providers need to consider the impact of sex differences (those based on genetic and hormonal differences) and gender differences (those attributable to the roles men and women are ascribed in society). Therapeutic decisions should take into account both genetic and environmental differences in the presentation of disease and the effectiveness of therapeutic options, the patient's reproductive life stage, comorbidities, and social and cultural contexts of care. Empirical evidence about care for women has expanded since 1994, when the National Institutes of Health required the inclusion of women as research subjects. The increased number of women participating in clinical research, coupled with initiatives through the Office on Research and Women's Health, has led to a broad expansion of knowledge; however, there is a continued need for gender-specific analyses of data to evaluate the impact of any therapeutic intervention.

● LIFESPAN GROUPS

Many important women's health issues are linked to the social, psychological, and biologic context at certain ages and stages of life. When considering both preventive care and common causes of mortality and morbidity, these lifespan stages provide a context for organizing care (Table 237-1).

For most women, young adulthood (15 to 44 years) is marked by social transitions in family structure, such as forming one's own family and parenting, and entering the work force. Mortality rates are low, and health visits can focus on behavioral decisions that will influence the risk for future disease, such as those pertaining to sexual behavior, smoking, alcohol and drug use, diet, and exercise. Major sources of morbidity include intentional and unintentional injury, including interpersonal violence (Chapter 241) and motor vehicle crashes. HIV is a leading cause of morbidity and mortality in this age group. Depression and anxiety are common in this and all life stages. Reproductive issues are considered in most therapeutic decisions.

The middle years (ages 45 to 65 years) continue to be influenced by behavioral decisions, especially diet, exercise, and alcohol and substance use. The social context includes role changes as children reach adulthood; caregiving responsibilities are for dependent children and possibly grandchildren, as well as aging parents. The menopausal transition may be accompanied by new symptomatic concerns. Common causes of morbidity, including diabetes and obesity, now reflect earlier behavioral decisions. Cancer is the leading cause of mortality.

Health issues in older women (65+ years) may occur in the context of loss of function and independence, and because women commonly survive their male partners, they are more likely at this stage of life to be single and possibly more isolated. Cardiovascular disease is the major cause of mortality, followed by cancer, cerebrovascular disease, chronic obstructive lung disease, and pneumonia. Loss of independence is related to cognitive decline, osteoarthritis, osteoporotic fractures, and incontinence.

● HEALTH DISPARITIES AMONG WOMEN

It is critical to consider the racial and ethnic differences in outcomes for most common causes of mortality and morbidity when addressing the health status of women. American women with a minority racial or ethnic affiliation, including those of African descent (whether born in the United States or abroad), women from many Asian and Pacific Island nations, Native Americans, and women of Latino background, share poorer outcomes for a wide variety of conditions. This broad finding of poorer outcomes across many diverse ethnic and racial groups points away from specific genetic differences in these populations and toward social determinants of health. Minority racial and ethnic affiliation is correlated with lower educational attainment, lower income, residence in neighborhoods with higher crime and more environmental health hazards, less access to comprehensive health insurance, and less access to care even when insured. Common recommendations for health promotion, including a diet low in fats and processed sugars and high in whole grains, fruits, and vegetables, along with regular exercise, such as walking, may be difficult to follow in high-crime neighborhoods or in those without markets offering a variety of affordable, nutritious food options. Barriers to health care access and poor adherence to medical therapy are more common in low-income women. For instance, they may have difficulty scheduling appointments that do not interfere with their work schedules or unpaid time off from clerical or service jobs. The need to care for dependent children or elders may interfere with women's ability to address their own health care needs. Lack of health literacy and cultural barriers can create additional barriers (Chapter 5).

● COMMON CAUSES OF MORTALITY IN WOMEN

Cardiovascular Disease

Cardiovascular disease (CVD; Chapter 52) is the overall leading cause of death in women. However, because CVD-related death occurs most often in women older than 65 years, its impact is often under-recognized or underestimated. Racial ethnicity plays a large role in the risk for CVD; African American women have much higher rates of CVD and death from CVD than any other racial or ethnic group, and Latinas and Asian women also have higher rates of CVD and CVD death than white populations.

The incidence rate of CVD in women lags 10 years behind that of men from ages 40 through 70 years; that is, a 65-year-old woman has a similar risk to a 55-year-old man. There is no abrupt increase in CVD risk at menopause in women, suggesting that menopausal changes in estrogen or progesterone do not account for this sex difference. Furthermore, randomized clinical trials have confirmed that hormone therapy in women does not prevent CVD and is not indicated for CVD prevention.[A1] Re-analysis of the Women's Health Initiative confirmed the increased risk for CVD *with* hormone therapy, even when treatment is initiated within 10 years of menopause.[1] There has been some controversy about the impact of calcium supplementation for bone and health on increased risk for myocardial infarction, but not CVD deaths. However, most observational studies do not find an association in women, and calcium and vitamin D supplementation are still recommended for women regardless of CVD risk (Chapter 243).[2-4] Other risk factors for CVD in women are the same as those in men: elevated lipids, lack of physical activity, obesity, smoking, hypertension, and diabetes. Women with diabetes have the same risk for CVD as men of the same age with diabetes. Because smoking rates in current cohorts of young women continue to increase, cigarette smoking continues to be an important behavioral risk factor for CVD, especially in younger women, American Indian women, and women with low incomes and low educational attainment. The incidence of many known risk factors, including obesity, hypertension, and hypercholesterolemia, is greater in African American women than in white women. Furthermore, data suggest that women are less likely to receive risk factor reduction therapy, reflecting an inertia caused by misperception by clinicians and patients of heart disease risk.

The presentation of coronary disease in women differs from that in men. Although chest pain is the most common presentation in women, atypical and noncardiac pain is a more common presentation in women than in men, and fewer women have typical chest tightness or pressure as their presenting complaint. For this and other reasons, there are delays in seeking and provision of emergency care at all steps from home to arrival to hospital for women compared with men, which can limit some therapeutic options and increase the severity of disease complications, including congestive heart failure.

The guidelines for the management of lipid disorders (Chapter 206) do not differ per se by gender, but do account for gender differences in the risk models used to guide therapy. The decision to begin statin therapy is based on the absolute low-density lipoprotein (LDL) level as well as age and the presence of diabetes. High intensity statin therapy is recommended for women with clinical vascular disease under age 75 years, for primary prevention when LDL is greater than 190 mg/dL, or for women with a 10 year calculated risk of atherosclerotic cardiovascular disease greater than 7.5%.

Medical management is similar for men and women with acute coronary syndromes, including unstable angina and acute myocardial infarction (Chapter 72). The use of aspirin, β-blockers, angiotensin-converting enzyme (ACE) inhibitors, heparin, and thrombolytic therapy and recommendations for noninvasive testing are the same for women and men. Randomized controlled trial data show that low-risk women with unstable angina or non–ST segment elevation myocardial infarction do not benefit from early revascularization and that medical management is indicated.[A2]

TABLE 237-1 IMPORTANT HEALTH ISSUES FOR WOMEN THROUGH THE LIFESPAN

ISSUE	AGES		
	15-44 yr	**45-65 yr**	**65+ yr**
Behavioral issues	Risk behaviors Sexual behavior Smoking Alcohol and drug use Exercise Diet	Risk behaviors Smoking Alcohol and drug use Exercise Diet	Risk behaviors Smoking Exercise
Social roles	Entering work force Relationship transitions Parenting	Caregiving to several generations Transitions in family and work environments	Losses and social isolation
Reproductive issues	Reproductive health issues	Menopause transition	
Injury	Intentional and unintentional interpersonal violence Motor vehicle crashes		Falls
Common causes of mortality and morbidity	Depression Anxiety HIV/AIDS	Cancer Obesity Diabetes Depression Anxiety	Cardiovascular disease Cancer Cognitive decline Osteoporosis Osteoarthritis Incontinence Depression Anxiety

Type 2 Diabetes

The rates of type 2 diabetes (Chapter 229) continue to rise, with a greater risk in women who are overweight or obese and physically inactive. Rates are higher in many racial and ethnic groups than among white women, including African Americans, Asians, Native Americans, and Latinas. No randomized clinical trials to date on low- to moderate-risk populations have shown a mortality benefit of screening, and most guidelines do not currently recommend universal screening. Screening women for known risk factors (e.g., hypertension [blood pressure >130/85 mm Hg], obesity, family history) is recommended by some. For women who develop gestational diabetes (Chapter 239), the risk of developing type 2 diabetes later in life increases five-fold; therefore, screening with hemoglobin A_{1C} 6 to 12 weeks postpartum and every 3 years thereafter is recommended by some.

The incidence of diabetes is rising in women at younger ages, with significant perinatal implications. Ongoing discussion of fertility control and family planning is critical in diabetic women with childbearing potential. Tight glycemic control before conception and through the first trimester is critical to reduce the risk for birth anomalies, and it is important later in pregnancy to reduce the risk for adverse fetal events, including macrosomia (large for gestational age) and preterm birth (Chapter 239). Ideally, women planning a pregnancy should switch from oral agents to insulin, with home glucose monitoring for tight control (Table 237-2).

Cancer

Cancer is the leading cause of death in women 40 through 65 years, and it is the leading cause of years of life lost in women younger than 65. Breast cancer (Chapter 198) is the most common type of cancer and the second leading cause of cancer death in women, although most women who develop breast cancer do survive. Studies indicate that many women significantly overestimate their personal risk for the disease. The lack of understanding of the cause of most breast cancers and the limitations of the imaging modalities used as screening tests have hampered efforts at breast cancer control. Recent data suggesting overdiagnosis of breast cancer, especially in women 40 to 50 years of age, has prompted growing interest in joint decision making regarding screening in this age group.[5] After decades of an increasing incidence of breast cancer in the United States, incidence rates have fallen in the past 12 years. The cause of this decline is not understood; reduced use of postmenopausal

hormone therapy and recent declines in screening rates have both been implicated.

Lung cancer (Chapter 191) is now the leading cause of cancer death in women, and rates continue to rise, commensurate with the number of women who took up smoking in the 1940s and 1950s and the lower rates of smoking cessation in women compared with men. Most lung cancers are smoking related, although women are more likely than men to have lung cancers that are not tobacco related. Low-dose chest tomography has been shown to reduce death from lung cancer in those with greater than a 30 pack-year smoking history who are current smokers or quit within the previous 15 years; the harms of are false-positive scans and potential overdiagnosis.[A3] The National Lung Screening Trial enrolled 41% women but has not at this time provided any gender-specific analyses. An analysis based on quintiles of lung cancer risk, including sex, showed female sex associated with a lower risk for cancer. This subanalysis suggests that women may benefit from screening less than men, independent of pack years of smoking. Because of the harms of screening, smoking cessation efforts continue to be recommended as the most effective strategy to prevent lung cancer.

Colorectal cancer (Chapter 193) has a similar incidence in both women and men. Testing for occult blood in the stool using fecal immunochemical test, sigmoidoscopy, and colonoscopy is effective at detecting precancerous lesions and thereby reducing rates of both new cancers and later stage disease.

Ovarian cancer (Chapter 199) is relatively rare, with 21,500 cases in the United States annually, but mortality is high owing to its presentation at late stages in most cases. Lower abdominal or pelvic pain, urinary symptoms, and changes in bowel habits are nonspecific and common in many women, limiting the ability to detect this cancer at an early stage. There is no effective screening test for women at average risk, and screening pelvic examination is no longer recommended in asymptomatic women.[6] CA-125 has both low sensitivity and low specificity, with normal levels in early-stage disease and elevations with nonmalignant ovarian pathology. One randomized clinical trial of average-risk women showed no benefit of mortality and increased harms in terms of false-positive studies and complications due to operative procedures.[A4] While awaiting the results of another large randomized controlled trial, current recommendations are to consider genetic counseling and testing for women with a family history of ovarian cancer.

The greatest recent advance in cancer prevention is the development of vaccines against the most carcinogenic subtypes of human papillomavirus (HPV) associated with cervical cancer (Chapters 199 and 373) and anal cancer. The vaccine has the potential to reduce significant morbidity caused by the management of premalignant lesions, including the risk for cervical incompetence and preterm labor. Vaccine rates in the United States are low, especially in minority communities. Despite this, there is evidence of reduced HPV prevalence since the vaccine became available. Although concern of tacit approval resulting in increased sexual activity among young adolescents has been cited by parents as a reason to delaying vaccination, evidence does not demonstrate this concern to be founded. Guidelines now suggest delaying Pap test screening in women until age 21 years and increasing the screening interval to every 2 years in women aged 20 to 29 years and to every 3 to 5 years in women aged 30 years and older if previous screening has demonstrated no high-risk subtypes of the HPV and negative HPV serology.[7] Pap tests are not recommended for women after hysterectomy for nonmalignant indications, or for women older than 65 years with adequate recent screening and no high-risk factors.

Osteoporosis

Hip fracture due to osteoporosis (Chapter 243) is one of the major causes of disability, loss of independence, and mortality in older women. Osteoporosis prevention through calcium and vitamin D intake and weight-bearing exercise begins at puberty and extends throughout adulthood. Women require a calcium intake of 1000 mg/day, increasing to 1300 mg in puberty and breastfeeding and 1200 mg after menopause, in order to maintain the structural strength of bone. Vitamin D is a necessary element for the absorption of calcium (Chapter 218), and it is available through direct sun exposure or vitamin D supplementation of milk (not most other dairy products) and some juices. Epidemiologic data suggest widespread vitamin D deficiency in women in the United States. This is attributed to low levels of dietary replacement, decreased sun exposure with the use of sunscreens, and lack of vitamin D production in the skin (even with sun exposure) in northern climates during the winter months. Screening for a single baseline serum 25-hydroxyvitamin D level can provide women with useful information about the adequacy of their diets, with levels above 20 ng/mL considered

TABLE 237-2 PREFERRED MEDICATIONS FOR WOMEN OF REPRODUCTIVE POTENTIAL

COMMON CONDITIONS IN WOMEN OF REPRODUCTIVE POTENTIAL	ISSUES TO BE AWARE OF	PREFERRED MEDICATIONS OR GROUPS OF MEDICATIONS
Depression	Must consider effects of untreated depression on mother and infant	Avoid newer medications when older drugs with more information are available SSRIs are generally considered safe; fluoxetine has most safety data
Anxiety	Commonly associated with depression in women	Benzodiazepines generally considered safe
GERD	No data on harmful effects of either H$_2$-blockers or PPIs Misoprostol is contraindicated; can cause miscarriage, fetal death, congenital anomalies	Calcium-containing antacids are first-line therapy H$_2$-blockers preferred over PPIs
Acne	Oral isotretinoin and topical tazarotene are contraindicated owing to congenital defects	Most other topical agents are considered classes B and C
Asthma	Extensive data on safety of common drug categories: benefit ratios far exceed risk in treating women	Cortisone inhalers Systemic prednisone for flares Short- and long-acting bronchodilators
Seizure disorders	Difficult to separate effects of medication from effects of seizure on fetal development All agents associated with some increased risk for fetal abnormality (4-8%, compared with 1-2% in general population). Valproate and phenobarbital with highest risks	Monotherapy at lowest doses recommended Avoid medication changes in first trimester Folate supplementation in preconception period
Hypertension (not preeclampsia)	ACE inhibitors and ARBs are contraindicated in pregnancy; possibly associated with cardiovascular and neurologic anomalies in first trimester; may cause abnormalities in renal hemodynamics in third trimester Most data suggest thiazide diuretics are safe if stable use before pregnancy	β-blockers, especially labetalol, and methyldopa are first-lines choices Calcium-channel blockers are also considered safe
Lipid disorders	Circulating lipid levels are elevated with pregnancy and breast-feeding.	No medications during pregnancy; ideally, stop statins before conception
Analgesics for fever and pain management	Controversy about whether NSAIDs slightly increase risk for miscarriage in first trimester	Acetaminophen preferred; aspirin also considered safe
Headache	Controversy about whether NSAIDs slightly increase risk for miscarriage in first trimester	Acetaminophen preferred; aspirin also considered safe
Diabetes	First-generation sulfonylureas contraindicated in pregnancy; may cause fetal hyperinsulinemia and birth defects	Conversion to insulin during planned preconception period Insulin, metformin, and glyburide preferred in women of childbearing potential
Autoimmune conditions	Must weigh benefits of immunosuppressive use against potential risks to both mother and infant Methotrexate is contraindicated in pregnancy because it induces miscarriage No data on safety or risk for TNF and IL-1 inhibitors	Prednisone generally considered safe in pregnancy Azathioprine, sulfasalazine, cyclosporine, and hydroxychloroquine generally preferred if required
Tobacco control	Cigarette smoking has known harmful effects on fetus In one small randomized controlled trial, nicotine replacement was associated with reduced levels of nicotine and improved birth outcomes Bupropion is linked with reports of some fetal anomalies	Try nonpharmacologic approaches to cessation first Short course of nicotine replacement likely better for fetus than smoking
Polycystic ovarian disease	Metformin can restore ovulatory cycles; use with contraception	
Bacterial infections	Tetracyclines accumulate in fetal bone and teeth Sulfa drugs may increase risk for neural tube defects with use in first trimester and kernicterus with use in third trimester Trimethoprim interferes with folic acid metabolism Streptomycin and kanamycin associated with bilateral deafness	Penicillins, cephalosporins, erythromycin, azithromycin

ACE = angiotensin-converting enzyme; ARB = angiotensin receptor blocker; GERD = gastroesophageal reflux disease; IL-1 = interleukin-1; NSAID = nonsteroidal anti-inflammatory drug; PPI = proton pump inhibitor; SSRI = selective serotonin re-uptake inhibitor; TNF = tumor necrosis factor.

sufficient or ideal. Daily replacement of vitamin D of 600 IU is recommended for women, with 800 IU recommended after age 70 years.

Although no long-term outcome data exist on the benefits of dual-energy x-ray absorptiometry (DXA) screening (DEXA bone densitometry), most guidelines recommend DXA screening at age 65 years in women, and in women ages 50 to 65 year who have one risk factor (smoking, family history, body mass index < 22, or alcohol use). An algorithm to assess risk for bone fracture based on DXA and individual risk factors is available through the World Health Organization and can guide decision making on preventive therapy.[8] Long-term estrogen therapy is not recommended for osteoporosis prevention. Complications from bisphosphonate therapy include gastroesophageal erosions, preventable in most women with weekly doses on an empty stomach while sitting upright for 30 minutes. Rare but debilitating jaw osteonecrosis (Chapter 248) has been seen in women with and without risk factors, such as dental disease. Raloxifene, a selective estrogen receptor

modulator, has the benefits of preventing osteoporosis while reducing breast cancer risk without increasing the risk for CVD; it has been underused as a preventive agent.

COMMON CAUSES OF MORBIDITY IN WOMEN
Obesity

Obesity rates continue to rise, and the prevalence of obesity is higher in women than men, especially among minority and low-income women (Chapter 220). The rates of increase in obesity in women have doubled from 1976-80, when it was at 17%, to the rate of 35% in 2007-10. Dietary reduction in calories and increased caloric output with aerobic exercise are the short- and long-term strategies for care. Studies suggest that no single diet is superior to others, and many common diet strategies can reduce weight. Increasing activity during the course of one's daily routine is as effective as shorter intervals of more strenuous activity. The most effective programs include a combination of behavioral therapy, either individually or in groups, to address behavioral patterns in food intake, and with diet and exercise. Weight loss targets of 1 to 2 lb/week and a total loss of up to 5 to 10% of body weight are realistic goals. Even modest changes in weight and modest increases in physical activity reduce morbidity and mortality on a population basis.

Exercise and diet changes are difficult for many people to achieve, for a wide variety of reasons. The physical environment may not be conducive to physical activity owing to the sedentary nature of most workplaces, the lack of safe areas to exercise, and architectural design features, such as the lack of easy access to stairs instead of elevators. The use of prepared foods and the consumption of fast foods, high in fat and calories and low in nutritional content, increase the risk for obesity.

There are currently no evidence-based interventions to support weight reduction in the setting of a brief office visit. Most guidelines focus on assessing body mass index (BMI) in all women and recommending weight reduction with diet restriction and exercise, including behavioral therapy to support these behavioral changes. Orlistat and sibutramine are U.S. Food and Drug Administration (FDA)-approved medications with moderate weight reduction efficacy that should be used in conjunction with an exercise and diet program, and not as sole therapy. For obese women with a BMI greater than 40, or those with a BMI greater than 35 and major comorbidities such as diabetes, sleep apnea, or osteoarthritis, bariatric surgery (Chapter 220) is indicated after other weight loss methods have failed. Bariatric surgery leads to short- and long-term benefits in multiple comorbidities and reduced mortality because of improvements in comorbidities. Critical to the success of this intervention is a team approach, with psychological assessment and diet and exercise programs beginning before and continuing after surgery. Management of obesity in general is discussed in detail in Chapter 220.

Depression

Major depression and other related disorders, including dysthymia, predominate in women (Chapter 434). Multiple short screening tools have been developed to identify depression. Women with depression are highly likely to come to the attention of the health care system. Depression is a significant comorbidity in many chronic medical conditions. Somatic complaints are a common presentation of depressive disorders. All specialties are likely to see patients with unexplained symptoms, such as chest pain, headache, abdominal pain, and other complaints. It is critical to include depression as either a primary or a secondary diagnosis and to treat depression as part of the overall management plan.

Anxiety Disorders

Anxiety disorders also predominate in women. They commonly coexist with depressive disorders. Anxiety disorders, including post-traumatic stress disorder, may be a consequence of violence against women, which often remains unidentified (Chapter 241). Benzodiazepines have been demonstrated to be safe and effective in trials for short-term use. Selective serotonin re-uptake inhibitors (SSRIs) and behavioral therapies are effective for the long-term management of anxiety disorders.

Osteoarthritis

Osteoarthritis (Chapter 262) is one of the most common causes of morbidity and functional status limitation, especially as women age. Assessment of pain and functional status is at the core of management. Physical and occupational therapy to restore functional status is a critical component of care. Joint replacement (Chapter 276) should be considered and recommended when functional status interferes with activities of daily living and supportive care and other symptom management strategies are ineffective.

Smoking

Tobacco use, most commonly cigarette smoking, continues to be one of the major preventable causes of morbidity and mortality in women (Chapter 32). Although there has been much progress in smoking cessation efforts, lower income women and younger women continue to start smoking and fail to quit smoking at high rates. Health care providers can achieve 1 to 2% smoking cessation rates by asking all patients about their smoking status and making a simple statement encouraging smokers to quit. Further gains in smoking cessation are possible with targeted counseling, which involves assessing the patient's stage of readiness to change and providing counseling relevant to that stage.

Nicotine replacement is equally effective in women and men. Smokers with a physiologic addiction to nicotine (those who smoke more than one pack daily or smoke within 20 minutes of awakening) benefit the most from nicotine replacement. Many women report weight gain as a major barrier to smoking cessation. Chapter 32 describes approaches to smoking cessation in detail.

Alcohol Use and Substance Use

Alcohol dependence is estimated in 5% of women; however, this is underrecognized in clinical practice (Chapter 33). It is well established that lower amounts of alcohol cause alcohol-related liver and other disease in women compared with men and increases the risk for breast cancer. Also worrisome is the frequency of binge drinking (defined as four drinks or more at a sitting) by women, with reports that one in eight women drink with this pattern, with risk for poor judgment in personal safety.

Although women in general have lower rates of most substance abuse than men, they have similar rates of nonmedical use of narcotic medications (about 2% of population), a problem that has more than doubled in the past decade, and narcotic overdose deaths have increased five-fold in women in the same timeframe. Current recommendations include specific training for all prescribing physicians; in addition, all nononcology patients who are prescribed more than 30 days of narcotics should be part of a narcotics program, with signed consent on risks and benefits, agreement to obtain medications from a single practice source, and agreement to monitoring, including random pill counts and drug testing, for the presence of the prescribed medication and the absence of other medications.[9]

Alcohol abuse and dependence and drug abuse and dependence are described and discussed in detail in Chapters 33 and 34, respectively.

Incontinence

Urinary incontinence (Chapter 26) is a frequently overlooked cause of major functional status limitations in middle-aged and older women. As many as half of affected women underreport this problem to their physicians and alter their lifestyles to adapt to the problem, including reducing fluid intake, avoiding activities that exacerbate the problem, and restricting travel where access to facilities is uncertain. There are two broad categories of incontinence—stress incontinence and urge incontinence—although women commonly have aspects of both types. Stress incontinence is defined as leaking with increases in intra-abdominal pressure, such as occurs with sneezing or coughing as well as running or walking. The most common reasons are pelvic floor laxity, often from childbirth. Kegel exercises are frequently recommended but are of limited value. A number of surgical procedures are available to address this condition. Less invasive procedures may be tried first, including the fitting of a vaginal pessary or periurethral injections with biodegradable materials such as collagen or with nonbiodegradable materials. Urge incontinence, described as detrusor muscle instability, results in the urge to void with low volumes. Anticholinergic medications and bladder training are both effective. Urodynamic evaluation should be considered if the history does not clearly identify a cause. The problem of incontinence is discussed in more detail in Chapter 26.

HIV Disease

The risk factors for HIV disease in women are heterosexual contact in 80% of new cases and injection drug use in 20%. HIV continues to affect minority women disproportionately, with 61% of incident cases affecting African American women. Incidence rates remain lower in women than in men, with only 27% of incident cases affecting women; in large part, this is due to the fact that male-to-male sexual contact continues to account for 72% of new cases in men. However, the absolute number of new infections from heterosexual contact is twice as high in women as it is in men. Women with HIV/AIDS continue to have poorer survival than men, despite the availability of antiretroviral therapies. There are no data of differential effectiveness of therapy by gender, and there are no gender-specific recommendations regarding timing and type of antiretroviral therapy. Some data suggest that women are less likely than men to adhere to an antiretroviral therapy regimen. The gender difference in therapy adherence was associated with caring for dependent children in one study, suggesting that women's caregiving roles may be a barrier to their own care. Cervical and anal dysplasia and cancer are more common among women with HIV than those without. Therefore, annual Pap tests are recommended for all women with HIV infection, even in the absence of positive HPV testing. There is insufficient evidence to support anal screening for dysplasia, but providers should be aware of the increased risk and perform an external examination for evidence of lesions.

Prophylaxis and management of complications of HIV/AIDS are discussed in detail in Chapter 389, and other aspects of HIV/AIDS are covered in individual chapters in Section XXIV.

REPRODUCTIVE HEALTH ISSUES

All providers caring for women with reproductive potential should consider the reproductive implications of preventive and therapeutic decisions. With half of all pregnancies in the United States unplanned, providers should routinely inquire about contraceptive practices and consider these in their care plans.

All primary care providers should be comfortable counseling patients about contraceptive choices and prescribing oral contraceptives. The absolute contraindications to oral contraceptives are a personal history of CVD, thromboembolic disease, migraine headache with aura, and gynecologic or breast cancer. A family history of cancer is not considered a contraindication; in fact, data suggest that the use of oral contraceptives decreases the risk for both endometrial and ovarian cancer. Smoking while using oral contraceptives increases the risk for thromboembolic events in all women, but especially in those older than 30 years. Oral contraceptive use is considered safe in nonsmoking women until menopause. Although factor V Leiden and other thrombophilias (Chapter 176) have been associated with an increased risk for deep vein thrombosis in those taking oral contraceptives, the absolute risk to any woman is still very low; therefore, screening for this and other genetic thrombophilias is not indicated. Preexisting hypertension is a relative contraindication to oral contraceptive use. Some women develop elevated blood pressures on oral contraceptives; therefore, blood pressure should be monitored at 3 months after starting the drug and then annually.

Providers should consider the reproductive implications of all chronic medications in women of reproductive potential (Chapter 239). Given that the teratogenic effects of medications may occur during the first trimester and before an initial obstetric assessment, the principle when choosing chronic medications for women during their reproductive years is to select those with the greatest safety profile during the first trimester of pregnancy.[10] Table 237-2 outlines common drug categories and recommendations for use in pregnancy.

Antidepressant medications deserve particular attention because of the conflicting data regarding their use in pregnancy.[11] Some initial reports suggested that antidepressants, especially paroxetine, were associated with congenital defects, preterm birth, and neonatology mortality. However, in studies that are able to assess whether prescriptions were filled or not and account for severity of depression and other risk factors of birth defects, specifically smoking, the risks from antidepressants are no greater than in the overall population. For women who wish to take no medication during pregnancy, the recommendation is to gradually reduce the dosage over the course of several weeks and not to abruptly stop taking the medication. The risk for untreated depression during pregnancy and the risk for postpartum depression to the woman and her infant are substantial. Therefore, treatment goals should be to provide adequate and even increased dosing to prevent the worsening of depression during this period and to provide close surveillance of women, whether or not they stop antidepressant medications.

Grade A References

A1. Rossouw JE, Anderson GL, Prentice RL, et al; Writing Group for the Women's Health Initiative Investigators. Risks and benefits of estrogen plus progestin in healthy postmenopausal women: principal results from the Women's Health Initiative randomized controlled trial. *JAMA.* 2002;288: 321-333.
A2. O'Donoghue M, Boden WE, Braunwald E, et al. Early invasive vs conservative treatment strategies in women and men with unstable angina and non–ST-segment elevation myocardial infarction: a meta-analysis. *JAMA.* 2008;300:71-80.
A3. Kovalchik SA, Tammemagi M, Berg CD, et al. Targeting of low-dose CT screening according to the risk of lung-cancer death. *N Engl J Med.* 2013;369:245-254.
A4. Buys SS, Partridge E, Black A, et al. Effect of screening on ovarian cancer mortality: the Prostate, Lung, Colorectal and Ovarian (PLCO) Cancer Screening Randomized Controlled Trial. *JAMA.* 2011;305:2295-2303.

GENERAL REFERENCES

For the General References and other additional features, please visit Expert Consult at https://expertconsult.inkling.com.

238

CONTRACEPTION

BEVERLY WINIKOFF AND DANIEL GROSSMAN

CONTRACEPTIVE USE

Contraception enables men and women to avoid unwanted fertility by preventing pregnancy. Methods can be classified in many different ways. Some classification schemes distinguish among mechanisms (e.g., barriers to the encounter of sperm and ovum versus methods that prevent ovulation); other categories emphasize the timing of use (at the time of intercourse versus ongoing); still other classifications focus on the permanence of the method (sterilization, which is intended as a permanent method, long-acting methods that last for years, and short-term methods that depend on the behavior of the user periodically, every day or at every exposure to pregnancy). There are advantages and disadvantages of each contraceptive method. These advantages and disadvantages should be thoroughly explained so that the individual or couple will choose the most acceptable method that suits their lifestyles and will be used most effectively. Because medical contraindications to individual methods are uncommon among young women, in most cases the choice of contraceptive method depends most on the user's preferences.

In the United States, about 62 million women are in the reproductive age group (15 to 44 years), and about 38 million (62%) are using a method of contraception.[1] Of the remainder, most were either noncontraceptively sterile (about 2%), pregnant or trying to conceive (8%), or never sexually active or had no recent sexual activity (19%). About 8% of women were sexually active in the prior 3 months but were not using a method of contraception. About 50% of U.S. pregnancies are unintended,[2] and more than half of such pregnancies occur in women who are not practicing contraception.[3]

In the United States in 2006 to 2010, the most common methods of fertility prevention were oral contraceptives (OCs) and female sterilization, used by 17.1% and 16.5% of women aged 15 to 44 years, respectively.[4] Next in frequency of use was the male condom (10.2%), followed by male sterilization (6.2%). The injectable progestin was used by 2.4%. However, the intrauterine device (IUD), the most effective method of reversible contraception, was used by only 3.5%, although this is about three times higher than the proportion using an IUD in 2002. Between 1982 and 2006 to 2010, there was a marked decrease in diaphragm use and an increase in condom use.

Contraceptive Effectiveness

Despite an increased use of contraceptive methods by U.S. women since 1982, about half of pregnancies are unintended, meaning they are either mistimed or unwanted. Of the 6.6 million pregnancies that occurred in the United States in 2006 (the most recent data available), 49% were unintended, and 43% of these pregnancies were terminated by elective abortion. Of the women with an unintended pregnancy, 50% stated they were using a method of contraception in the month they conceived. In recent years, teen pregnancy rates have declined, and women aged 18 to 24 years have the highest unintended pregnancy rates. Poor women and those who are unmarried and living with a partner have significantly higher rates of unintended pregnancy compared with women with higher incomes and those who are married or not living with a partner. Research has identified a variety of factors associated with nonuse of contraception or gaps in use, including side effects (both experienced and feared), not liking a method, personal or religious reasons, and barriers to access, including difficulty obtaining a prescription or the method itself, and high cost of a method.

The most pressing need worldwide is that the highly effective contraceptive methods already available should be affordable to most of the population and also that these methods should fulfill the needs of women of different ages and with different reproductive requirements.[5]

Perfect Use versus Typical Use

The terms *perfect use* and *typical use* describe different aspects of the effectiveness of the various contraceptive methods. Perfect use refers to use of the method as intended and covering all acts of exposure to pregnancy. So, for user-dependent methods such as oral pills or condoms, for example, this measure can only be applied to situations in which the user reliably uses the method every day or at every act of intercourse. Perfect use is a measure of the maximum possible efficacy of the method. *Typical use,* on the other hand, is a measure of how effective methods are when used as a group of people under study actually use them. These rates may be considerably lower than perfect use rates, especially if there is the possibility of not using the method at every intercourse or in other ways not using the method as intended. Methods used at the time of coitus have higher failure rates than OCs, implants, injections, IUDs, and sterilization. IUDs, implants, and sterilization have lower failure rates than pills, patches, and injections because they act over a long period of time, and there is nothing a user needs to do to keep using them. Table 238-1 illustrates the differences in failure rates among the contraception methods under conditions of perfect and typical use.

Cumulative failure rates for use of long-acting methods are low. The effectiveness of long-acting reversible contraception is superior to that of contraceptive pills, patch, or ring and is not altered in adolescents and young women.[6] The cumulative failure rates of all types of tubal sterilization are 1.31% during the first 5 years after the procedure and 1.85% after 10 years;

rates are higher for tubal fulguration and lower for segmental resection. The cumulative pregnancy rate for 5 years' use of the levonorgestrel-releasing IUD is 0.5%, and for 10 years' use of the copper T380 IUD, it is 1.7%.

The World Health Organization has developed a chart that nicely represents the actual use (typical) failure rates of most contraceptives, dividing them into three main classes of effectiveness (Figure 238-1).

Contraindications, Risks, and Benefits

Most contraceptives can be used safely by most people, but some conditions or concomitant medications are considered contraindications to use. The U.S. Centers for Disease Control and Prevention have developed evidence-based Medical Eligibility Criteria (MEC) for contraceptive use, based on a similar document developed by the World Health Organization.[7,8] The MEC categorizes conditions or medications into four groups for each contraceptive method: 1—no restriction on use; 2—advantages of use generally outweigh theoretical or proven risks; 3—theoretical or proven risks generally outweigh advantages of using the method; and 4—the condition represents an

TABLE 238-1 PERCENTAGE OF WOMEN EXPERIENCING AN UNINTENDED PREGNANCY DURING THE FIRST YEAR OF TYPICAL USE AND THE FIRST YEAR OF PERFECT USE OF CONTRACEPTION AND THE PERCENTAGE CONTINUING USE AT THE END OF THE FIRST YEAR—UNITED STATES

METHOD	WOMEN EXPERIENCING AN UNINTENDED PREGNANCY WITHIN THE FIRST YEAR OF USE (%)		WOMEN CONTINUING USE AT 1 YEAR (%)[‡]
	TYPICAL USE*	PERFECT USE[†]	
No method[§]	85	85	—
Spermicides[‖]	28	18	42
Fertility awareness–based methods[¶]	24	—	47
Standard-days method	—	5	—
Two-day method	—	4	—
Ovulation method	—	3	—
Symptothermal method	—	0.4	—
Withdrawal	22	4	46
Sponge			
Parous women	24	20	36
Nulliparous women	12	9	
Condom**			
Female	21	5	41
Male	18	2	43
Diaphragm[††]	12	6	57
Combined pill and progestin-only pill	9	0.3	67
Evra patch	9	0.3	67
NuvaRing	9	0.3	67
Depo-Provera	6	0.2	56
Intrauterine devices			
Paragard (copper containing)	0.8	0.6	78
Mirena (levonorgestrel releasing)	0.2	0.2	80
Implanon	0.05	0.05	84
Female sterilization	0.5	0.5	100
Male sterilization	0.15	0.10	100
Lactational amenorrhea method[‡‡]	—	—	—

*Among typical couples who initiate use of a method (not necessarily for the first time), the percentage who experience an accidental pregnancy during the first year if they do not stop use for any other reason. Estimates of the probability of pregnancy during the first year of typical use for spermicides and the diaphragm are taken from the 1995 National Survey Growth (NSFG) and corrected for underreporting of abortion; estimates for fertility awareness-based methods, withdrawal, the male condom, the pill, and Depo-Provera are taken from the 1995-2002 NSFG corrected for underreporting of abortion.

[†]Among couples who initiate use of a method (not necessarily for the first time) and who use it perfectly (both consistently and correctly), the percentage who experience an accidental pregnancy during the first year if they do not stop use for any other reason.

[‡]Among couples attempting to avoid pregnancy, the percentage who continues to use a method for 1 year.

[§]The percentage who become pregnant in the second and third columns are based on data from populations in which contraception is not used and from women who cease using contraception to become pregnant. Among such populations, approximately 89% become pregnant within 1 year. This estimate was lowered slightly (to 85%) to represent the percentage who would become pregnant within 1 year among women not relying on reversible methods of contraception if they abandoned contraception altogether.

[‖]Foams, creams, gels, vaginal suppositories, and vaginal film.

[¶]The ovulation and 2-day methods are based on evaluation of cervical mucus. The standard-days method avoids intercourse on cycle days 8 to 19. The symptothermal method is a double-check method based on evaluation of cervical mucus to determine the first fertile day and evaluation of cervical mucus and temperature to determine the last fertile day.

**Without spermicides.

[††]With spermicidal cream or jelly.

[‡‡]This is a highly effective, temporary method of contraception. However, to maintain effective protection against pregnancy, another method of contraception must be used as soon as menstruation resumes, the frequency of duration of breast-feeds is reduced, bottle-feeds are introduced, or the baby reaches age 6 months.

Adapted from Trussell J. Contraceptive failure in the United States. *Contraception.* 2011;83:397-404.

Effectiveness of Family Planning Methods

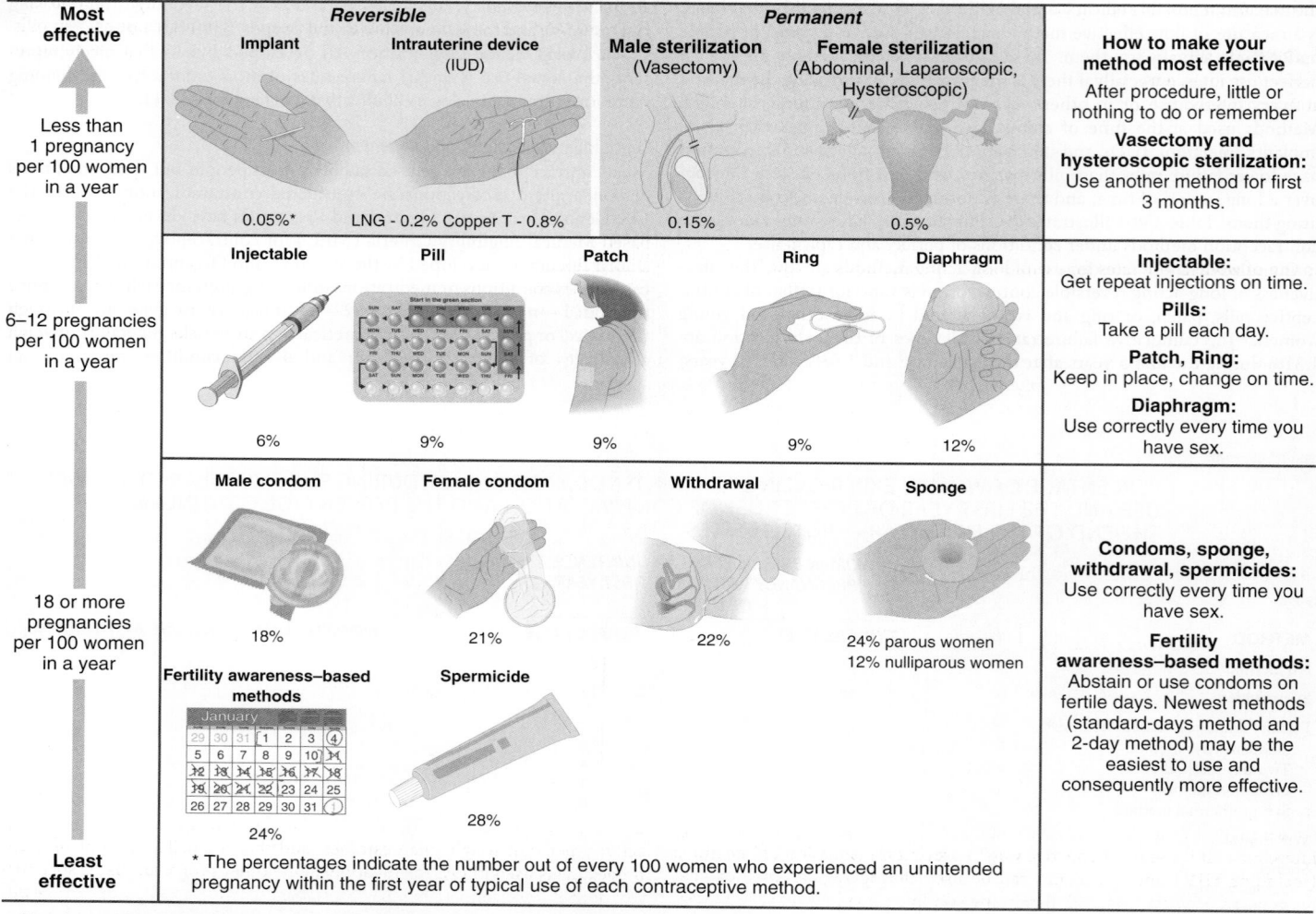

Most effective ↑		*Reversible*		*Permanent*	
	Implant	Intrauterine device (IUD)	Male sterilization (Vasectomy)	Female sterilization (Abdominal, Laparoscopic, Hysteroscopic)	**How to make your method most effective**

Most effective ↑

Less than 1 pregnancy per 100 women in a year

Reversible

Implant 0.05%*

Intrauterine device (IUD) LNG - 0.2% Copper T - 0.8%

Permanent

Male sterilization (Vasectomy) 0.15%

Female sterilization (Abdominal, Laparoscopic, Hysteroscopic) 0.5%

How to make your method most effective

After procedure, little or nothing to do or remember

Vasectomy and hysteroscopic sterilization: Use another method for first 3 months.

6–12 pregnancies per 100 women in a year

Injectable 6%

Pill 9%

Patch 9%

Ring 9%

Diaphragm 12%

Injectable: Get repeat injections on time.

Pills: Take a pill each day.

Patch, Ring: Keep in place, change on time.

Diaphragm: Use correctly every time you have sex.

18 or more pregnancies per 100 women in a year

Male condom 18%

Female condom 21%

Withdrawal 22%

Sponge 24% parous women 12% nulliparous women

Fertility awareness–based methods 24%

Spermicide 28%

Condoms, sponge, withdrawal, spermicides: Use correctly every time you have sex.

Fertility awareness–based methods: Abstain or use condoms on fertile days. Newest methods (standard-days method and 2-day method) may be the easiest to use and consequently more effective.

Least effective

* The percentages indicate the number out of every 100 women who experienced an unintended pregnancy within the first year of typical use of each contraceptive method.

Condoms should always be used to reduce the risk for sexually transmitted infections.

Other Methods of Contraceptions

Lactational Amenorrhea Method: LAM is a highly effective, temporary method of contraception.

Emergency contraception: Emergency contraceptive pills or a copper IUD after unprotected intercourse substantially reduces risk for pregnancy.

FIGURE 238-1. Detailed chart of the effectiveness of family planning methods with instructions for subjects. (Adapted from World Health Organization (WHO) Department of Reproductive Health and Research, Johns Hopkins Bloomberg School of Public Health/Center for Communication Programs (CCP), Knowledge for Health Project. *Family Planning: A Global Handbook for Providers.* 2011 updates. Baltimore, Geneva: CCP and WHO; 2011, and Trussell J. Contraceptive failure in the United States. *Contraception.* 2011;83:397-404.)

unacceptable health risk if the method is used. For conditions that represent relative contraindications (MEC category 3), it is important to recognize that pregnancy may also be risky, and if the method is the best choice to avoid an unintended pregnancy, it may be worth the risk.

In addition to preventing unintended pregnancy, many contraceptive methods have additional benefits. Some of the most significant noncontraceptive benefits include the reduced risk for transmission of HIV and other sexually transmitted infections associated with the use of male and female condoms, as well as the reduction in dysmenorrhea and menorrhagia associated with the use of combined hormonal contraception.

● TYPES OF CONTRACEPTIVES

Natural Methods

Methods that rely on the natural infertility of different times in the menstrual or life cycle are often called "natural" methods. These methods are not really more natural than other methods, because they involve disruptions in the "natural" desire for sexual intimacy; however, they do not rely on any specific external technologies to create a state of low fertility potential. Because male sperm can live only 5 days in the female genital tract and female ova have a lifespan of only about 24 hours, the window for fertilization is only 5 to 6 days each month. In theory, if couples avoid unprotected intercourse on those 5 to 6 days, the potential for pregnancy is markedly reduced. The calendar

method counts the days of the cycle to predict fertile and infertile days, and the symptothermal method relies on the calendar plus the biologic signals of impending ovulation (changes in vaginal mucus) and of ovulation itself (rise in basal body temperature) to enhance prediction of "safe" days for intercourse. Breast-feeding in the postpartum period also lowers fertility and is considered another natural method of contraception. Exclusive breast-feeding during the first 6 months after a birth provides a good level of protection against pregnancy. However, once a baby is older than 6 months or if foods other than breast milk become part of the infant's diet, then a woman is at much higher risk for ovulation and possible pregnancy.

Withdrawal, or coitus interruptus, when the penis is removed from the vagina before ejaculation, is a commonly used method, with up to 60% of women reporting ever using it. Although the method can be effective with perfect use, with a pregnancy rate of only 4% in the first year of use, failure is much more common in typical use. A recent study reported that among U.S. women aged 15 to 24 years using withdrawal as their primary method, 21% experienced an unintended pregnancy, which was a significantly higher pregnancy rate than that among users of other contraceptive methods.

Barriers

Barrier methods are so called because their mechanism of action is to impose a chemical or physical barrier between ovum and sperm so that fertilization is not possible. Barrier methods include spermicides, diaphragm, and male and female condoms, among others.

Spermicides
All spermicidal agents contain a surfactant (in U.S. products this chemical is nonoxynol-9) that immobilizes or kills sperm on contact. The spermicidal products are available in foams, creams, and vaginal suppositories that need to be placed into the vagina before each coital act—and reapplied even if coital acts follow immediately after each other. The typical-use effectiveness of spermicides as a sole contraceptive is among the lowest of modern methods (about 28% of women using the method report an unintended pregnancy during 1 year of use.) There is no increased risk for birth defects in the off-spring of women who conceive while using spermicides.

Diaphragm
A diaphragm is a dome-shaped latex or silicone device with a flexible rim that seals off the upper genital tract from contact with deposited semen. It is usually used with a spermicide applied inside and around the rim. The device must be fitted by a health care provider using the largest size that does not cause discomfort or undue pressure on the vagina. The woman will need to insert the diaphragm before every act of intercourse. It should be left in place for 6 hours after intercourse, but should not be left in place for more than 24 hours because it may cause ulceration of the vaginal epithelium. In actual use, the diaphragm is more effective than other barrier methods (12% unintended pregnancy rate in first year of use) and provides contraceptive protection almost as well as hormonal pills in actual use. Diaphragm size for any one woman may change after a birth, miscarriage or abortion after 14 weeks, abdominal/pelvic surgery, or a change in weight of more than 20%. The diaphragm may provide some protection against gonorrhea and *Chlamydia* infection, but not against HIV and herpes. A condom is recommended if infection is a concern. Diaphragm users have an increased risk for urinary tract infection.

Male Condom
The male condom is one of the oldest contraceptives known. It is safe, easy to use, and widely available. The modern version is a stretchy latex or plastic sheath that fits over the erect penis and captures the man's ejaculate during intercourse. It is the most effective way to prevent transmission of infections (including HIV) during sex and can be used during vaginal, oral, or anal intercourse. However, natural membrane condoms (made from sheep intestine) do not prevent sexually transmitted infections. Condoms can be used for protection against infection even if another method is used for protection against pregnancy. If the condom is used alone for contraception, in typical use about 18% of women will experience an unintended pregnancy in 1 year. For optimum protection, the condom must be used at every sex act and requires the active participation of the man. Lubricants containing oil-based products may weaken latex condoms and should not be used with them; water-based lubricants (K-Y jelly is one) are safe to use. The male condom causes no side effects except possible irritation or allergy.

Female Condom
The female condom is a soft, loose-fitting prelubricated pouch with two flexible polyurethane rings, one at each end. The smaller ring at the closed end is inserted well into the vagina, creating a barrier to sperm. The larger ring remains outside the vagina, covering the vulva and providing additional protection. The female condom can be inserted before beginning sexual activity and left in place for a longer time than the male condom after ejaculation occurs. Because polyurethane is stronger than the latex used in most male condoms, the female condom is less likely to rupture. Both polyurethane and latex prevent virus transmission and should reduce the risk for acquiring HIV infection.

Hormonal (Steroidal) Contraception
Contraception using steroid hormones has been available since the 1960s. The use of hormones (or derivatives/analogues of hormones) that occur naturally in the female reproductive cycle can alter the reproductive system so that ovulation does not occur or so that physical factors (such as mucus production, tubal motility, and endometrial thickness) that enhance the probability of fertilization or implantation are altered. All modern hormonal formulations are made from synthetic steroids. The hormones are either a combination of an estrogen and a progestin or, in some formulations, a progestin alone. There are two major types of synthetic progestins: derivatives

of 19-nortestosterone (which are used in OCs) and derivatives of 17α-acetoxyprogesterone (pregnanes). Pregnanes are structurally related to progesterone and are used in injectable contraceptives, but are not used in pills.

After the discontinuation of hormonal contraceptives, the rate of return of fertility is slightly lower for users of OCs than for users of barrier methods—but faster than for users of Depo-Provera. OCs do not cause permanent infertility or adversely affect pregnancies that occur after their discontinuation. OCs are not teratogenic if they are accidentally ingested during pregnancy.

From the user's point of view, the main differences are route of administration, length of action, how much attention the user needs to pay to the administration of the drug, and side effects. All these methods are very effective, and if used consistently they have very low pregnancy rates. Even with typical use, they are among the more effective methods, although, with the exception of the implants, they are less effective than sterilization or the IUD. The most commonly used of these methods is the OC ("the pill"), which was also the first hormonal contraceptive and the one most widely used globally.

Oral Contraceptives
There are three major types of OC formulations: fixed-dose combination, combination phasic, and daily progestin. The combination formulations are the most widely used and most effective. They consist of tablets containing both an estrogen and a progestin, usually given continuously for 3 weeks. Generally, no steroids are given for the fourth week. Three types of pills provide active tablets for 24 days, with 4 days of inactive tablets. Other types provide active tablets for 84 days followed by 7 days without active tablets or with a low dose of estrogen to allow withdrawal bleeding. The endometrium usually begins to slough 1 to 3 days after steroid ingestion is stopped, causing withdrawal bleeding, which usually lasts 3 to 4 days (and which users interpret as menstrual bleeding). The uterine blood loss with OC use averages about 25 mL per cycle, less than the 35 mL average for ovulatory cycles.

Three estrogens (ethinyl estradiol and its 3-methyl ether, mestranol, as well as one agent with estradiol valerate) are used in combined OCs. They are combined with one of two major types of 19-nortestosterone progestins—estranes and gonanes—both of which have androgenic activity. The estranes currently used in several OCs are norethindrone and its acetates, norethindrone acetate, and ethynodiol diacetate. Gonanes have greater progestational activity per unit weight than estranes, and thus a smaller amount of these progestins is used in OC formulations. One other progestin that is structurally related to spironolactone has been formulated in an OC. This progestin is called drospirenone and has antimineralocorticoid and antiandrogenic actions as well as progestational activity without androgenic activity. There are also daily progestin-only formulations that include norethindrone, levonorgestrel, or desogestrel.

Combined OCs, which contain both estrogen and progestin, consistently inhibit the midcycle gonadotropin surge and thus prevent ovulation. The progestin-only formulation has a lower dose of progestin than the combined agents and does not consistently inhibit ovulation, even though it is ingested every day. Progestin-only pills containing desogestrel appear to more consistently inhibit ovulation than other progestin-only formulations. Both combined OCs and progestin-only formulations also act on the cervical mucus and tubal motility to interfere with sperm transport. Progestins also alter the endometrium so that if fertilization occurs, implantation may be prevented. For contraceptive effectiveness to be maintained with the combination formulations, it is important that the pill-free interval be limited to no more than 7 days. This is made easier to remember by inclusion of placebo pills in the packet for the 7 hormone-free days. Continuous or extended cycle combined OCs seem to be an equally safe option for women who prefer it.[A1]

Side Effects
The synthetic steroids in OC formulations have many metabolic effects in addition to their contraceptive actions. These effects can cause the more common, less serious side effects as well as the rare, serious complications. The magnitude of these effects is directly related to the dosage and potency of the steroids in the formulations.

The most frequent symptoms produced by the estrogen component include nausea, breast tenderness, and fluid retention (bloating). The progestins can produce certain androgenic effects, such as weight gain, acne, and depression. But because estrogens decrease sebum production, women who have acne may experience improvement in their symptoms. Insufficient estrogen, too much progestin, or a combination of both may result in unscheduled (breakthrough) bleeding. This problem is more common with formulations containing 20 μg of estrogen than with those containing 30 to 35 μg and is increased in women who also smoke cigarettes. Shortening the pill-free interval to 3 or 4 days may decrease the incidence of unscheduled bleeding with low-estrogen formulations.

The synthetic estrogens used in OCs cause an increase in the hepatic production of several proteins. Some of the proteins that are increased by ethinyl estradiol, such as factors V, VIII, and X and fibrinogen, have the potential to enhance thrombosis (see later), and an increase in angiotensinogen levels may elevate blood pressure in some users. The incidence of both venous and arterial thrombosis is higher with 50-μg estrogen formulations than with those with 20 to 35 μg of estrogen. Blood pressure should be followed in all users of combined OCs and the drug discontinued if there is a clinically significant increase. The progestins do not affect protein synthesis except to reduce levels of sex hormone–binding globulin.

High-progestin formulations have an adverse effect on the lipid profile. However, estrogen has a beneficial effect on the arterial wall and on serum lipids, so users of these agents do not have an increased risk for cardiovascular disease. The newer combination formulations with less androgenic progestins have a more favorable effect on the lipid profile. The effect of OCs on glucose metabolism is directly related to the dose, potency, and type of progestin. Although high-progestin formulations caused peripheral insulin resistance, the low-progestin formulations in current use do not significantly alter levels of glucose, insulin, or glucagon after a glucose load.

Complications and Risk Factors

Thrombosis

The background rate of venous thrombosis and embolism in women of reproductive age is about 3 per 10,000 woman years. Women of reproductive age who are not pregnant or using OCs experience thrombosis at a rate of 1.9 to 3.7 per 10,000 woman years. Among users of OCs, the relative risk is 3.5 (95% confidence interval, 2.9 to 4.3) compared with nonusers, but less than the rate of 5 to 20 per 10,000 woman years that occurs in association with pregnancy.[A7] The risk for venous thrombosis and embolism is higher for women using OCs with 50 μg of ethinyl estradiol than for those using 30 to 35 μg. In the presence of an inherited hypercoagulable state (Chapter 176), the risk for venous thrombosis is increased several-fold. Screening for coagulation deficiencies before women are started on OCs is not recommended unless the individual has a personal or significant family history of thrombotic events. Women with known inherited or acquired thrombogenic conditions should not use estrogen-containing steroid contraceptives in pills, rings, or patches because each of these agents has thrombogenic effects. Some epidemiologic studies have found that the risk for venous thromboembolism is greater in individuals ingesting OCs with the newer, less androgenic progestins than those containing levonorgestrel with the same amount of estrogen. However, other studies have reported that the risk is similar with formulations containing these two types of progestins. These studies are all observational and thus subject to bias.

Myocardial Infarction and Stroke

Myocardial infarction is rare among women of reproductive age, with a rate of 10.1 per 100,000 person years in a recent Danish cohort. Although the absolute risks for myocardial infarction and thrombotic stroke associated with the use of hormonal contraception were found to be low, the risk was increased by a factor of 0.9 to 1.7 with OCs that included ethinyl estradiol at a dose of 20 μg and by a factor of 1.3 to 2.3 with those that included ethinyl estradiol at a dose of 30 to 40 μg, with relatively small differences in risk according to progestin type. The use of high-dose OCs by women who smoke cigarettes increases the risk for myocardial infarction by about 10-fold. Therefore, combination OCs should not be prescribed to women older than 35 years who smoke cigarettes or use alternate forms of nicotine. Epidemiologic studies indicate that use of low-dose OCs by nonsmoking women without hypertension is not associated with a significantly increased incidence of either myocardial infarction or either hemorrhagic or thrombotic stroke.

Cancers of the Reproductive System

An analysis of worldwide epidemiologic data in 1988 showed that the risk for breast cancer diagnosis was increased by about 25% in young women who were currently using OCs, but this increased risk was no longer present 10 years or more after they stopped using OCs. Several studies have reported that use of OCs by women with a family history of breast cancer does not increase their risk for developing breast cancer. A large study of women aged 35 to 64 years in the United States reported that there was no significantly increased risk for breast cancer among current and former OC users compared with women who had not used OCs. A very large cohort study in Great Britain of OC users and aged-matched nonusers was initiated in 1968. Data accumulated until 2004 showed a similar incidence of breast cancer in both groups.[A3]

The epidemiologic data are conflicting regarding OC use and the risk for invasive cervical cancer or cervical intraepithelial neoplasia. Most well-controlled studies indicate that there is no change in risk for cervical intraepithelial neoplasia with OC use. The single most comprehensive study now indicates a significant increase in the risk for cervical cancer among OC users that increases with duration of use and declines with interval since last use.

Several studies have shown that the use of OCs has a protective effect against endometrial cancer. Moreover, the decrease in risk persists for many years after OCs are stopped. This protective effect is related to duration of use, increasing from a 20% reduction with 1 year of use to a 60% reduction with 4 years of use. The level of protection declines with time after use is stopped.

In addition, OCs reduce the risk for development of epithelial ovarian cancer as well as cancers with low malignant potential. The magnitude of the decrease in risk is directly related to the duration of OC use, increasing from about a 40% reduction with 4 years of use to a 60% reduction with 12 years of use. The protective effect continues for at least 20 years after the use of OCs ends. As with endometrial cancer, the protective effect occurs only in women of low parity (fewer than four), who are at greatest risk for this type of cancer.

Studies have reported that OCs significantly reduce the risk for development of colorectal cancer by about 20%.

Benign Hepatocellular Adenoma

The development of a benign hepatocellular adenoma was a rare occurrence in long-term users of high-dose OCs containing mestranol, but it is not increased by use of ethinyl estradiol OCs. There is no increased risk for liver cancer associated with OC use.

Contraindications

OCs can be prescribed for most women of reproductive age. According to the MEC, several conditions are considered absolute contraindications to use of combined hormonal contraceptives (category 4), including smoking 15 cigarettes or more per day, at age 35 or older, and severe hypertension, among others. There is no evidence that individuals with asymptomatic mitral valve prolapse should avoid using OCs. The presence of migraine headaches without aura is also not a contraindication to OC use, but if aura is present, combination OCs should not be prescribed because of a possible increased risk for stroke. OC use does not increase the risk for development of malignant melanoma or prolactin-secreting pituitary adenomas.

Management of OC Therapy

If a healthy woman has no contraindications to OC use, it is unnecessary to perform any laboratory tests, including cervical cytology, before she uses them. A pelvic examination is not required. Starting pills on the day of the visit is associated with better long-term use of the method. There is no reason to discontinue OC use unless pregnancy is desired. Intermittent discontinuation is unnecessary and puts women at risk for an unwanted pregnancy.

Although synthetic sex steroids can retard the biotransformation of certain drugs (e.g., phenazone and meperidine) as a result of substrate competition, such interference is usually not important clinically. However, some drugs can interfere clinically with the action of OCs by inducing liver enzymes that convert the steroids to more polar and less biologically active metabolites. These drugs include barbiturates, sulfonamides, cyclophosphamide, griseofulvin, and rifampin. There is a high incidence of OC failure in women ingesting rifampin as well as systemic griseofulvin, and neither should be given concurrently with OCs. Products containing St. John's wort reduce contraceptive effectiveness and cause breakthrough bleeding. Women taking certain medications for epilepsy should be treated with 50-μg estrogen formulations because many antiepileptic medications lower ethinyl estradiol levels and cause breakthrough bleeding, which may cause premature discontinuation of use.

Because of their many health benefits, including reduction in risk for endometrial and ovarian cancer and induction of regular cyclic uterine bleeding, OC use can be continued until menopause in normotensive, nonsmoking women without contraindications.

A common clinical question is what to do if a pill is missed. The standard advice for combined OCs is to take the first missed pill as soon as possible and take the remaining pills at the usual time, even if it means taking two pills in one day (discarding any additional missed pills). If two or more pills are missed, take the most recent missed pill as soon as possible, continue taking the remaining pills at the usual time, even if it means taking two or more pills on the same day, and use back up contraception (e.g., condoms) or avoid sexual intercourse until pills have been taken for at least 7 consecutive days. If pills were missed in the last week of hormonal pills (third week of cycle), omit the hormone-free interval and start a new pack the next day. Emergency contraception should be considered. Vomiting and diarrhea for up to 48 hours should be considered as one missed pill; vomiting and diarrhea for more than 48 hours should be treated as two or more missed pills. For norethindrone-containing progestin-only pills, a pill is considered "missed" if it is more than 3 hours late.

Emergency Contraception

There is now a way that a women can avoid pregnancy even after unprotected sex acts. The method is termed *emergency contraception* because it should be used as early as possible after the unprotected sex. A formulation of 1500 µg (1.5 mg) levonorgestrel in a single tablet prevents about 85% of expected pregnancies, if used within 72 hours after coitus.[9,10] Another recently approved agent for emergency contraception is the selective progesterone receptor modulator ulipristal acetate given as a single 30-mg dose. This agent is as effective as levonorgestrel and is effective for 5 days after intercourse.[A4]

Transdermal and Intravaginal Steroid Contraceptives
Transdermal Patch

In the United States, there is one transdermal contraceptive patch that contains both estrogen and progestin (Ortho Evra). The patch has an area of 20 cm^2 and delivers 150 µg of the progestin norelgestromin, the active metabolite of norgestimate, and 20 µg of ethinyl estradiol daily. It may be applied to the buttocks, lower abdomen, upper arm, or upper torso (but not the breasts). The patch should be removed after 7 days and a new patch applied to a different area of skin. A woman using this method uses three patches sequentially, each for 7 days. After the third patch is removed, she waits 7 days before starting her next patch, thus mimicking the 28-day combined OC cycle (21 hormone days, followed by 7 hormone-free days, during which withdrawal bleeding occurs). Because the patch does not require daily attention, adherence with the patch is somewhat higher than with OCs. Contraceptive efficacy, bleeding patterns, and side effects are similar to those associated with OCs, and the contraindications are similar. Although the effectiveness of the patch may be decreased among women weighing more than 90 kg, there does not appear to be an association between pregnancy risk and body mass index (BMI). For all combined hormonal contraceptives, a BMI of 30 kg/m^2 or greater is considered category 2 (benefits of use outweigh potential risks) by the MEC.

Intravaginal Ring

Another option for nonoral hormonal contraception is the vaginal ring (NuvaRing in the United States). This soft, flexible ring measures 58 mm in diameter and is 4 mm thick. The ring is composed of ethinyl vinyl acetate and contains the progestin etonogestrel, a major metabolite of desogestrel, and ethinyl estradiol. The ring is inserted and removed by the woman herself. There is no "wrong" position or placement of the ring as long as it is inside the vagina. Each ring is left in place for 3 weeks, after which time it is removed for 1 week to allow withdrawal bleeding. Each day, 120 µg of etonogestrel and 15 µg of ethinyl estradiol are released from the ring, and bleeding with the ring in place is uncommon. Contraceptive efficacy and side effects are similar to those of combined OCs, as are contraindications. Women may keep the ring in place during intercourse, or it can be safely removed for up to 3 hours and then reinserted. Tampons may also be used concurrently with the ring without affecting efficacy.

Injectable Steroid Contraceptives
Constituents and Use

Although several types of injectable steroid formulations are in use for contraception throughout the world, currently the only injectable available in the United States is depot medroxyprogesterone acetate (DMPA). The initial formulation of this contraceptive was administered as an intramuscular injection of 1 mL of an aqueous suspension containing 150 mg of crystalline medroxyprogesterone acetate once every 3 months. A recently developed formulation that is administered subcutaneously (DMPA-SC) contains 104 mg of DMPA in 0.65 mL of solution. This lower dose formulation has a

lower peak medroxyprogesterone acetate concentration than DMPA and a long duration of action that suppresses ovulation for at least 13 weeks and is not affected by body mass. The formulation for subcutaneous administration allows the possibility for women to self-inject the medication. Other injectable contraceptives include norethindrone enanthate, given in a dose of 200 mg every 2 months, and several once-a-month injections of combinations of different progestins and estrogens.

DMPA has a low failure rate, 0.1% at 1 year and 0.4% at 2 years. The major contraceptive action of DMPA is inhibition of ovulation, and it also impedes sperm transport by thickening cervical mucus. With DMPA and DMPA-SC, serum medroxyprogesterone levels rapidly increase to contraceptively effective blood levels (>0.5 ng/mL) within 24 hours after the injection. With DMPA, medroxyprogesterone levels plateau for about 3 months, after which there is a gradual decline until levels become undetectable 7 to 9 months after the injection. With DMPA-SC, medroxyprogesterone levels steadily decline after the initial peak and reach 0.2 ng/mL 3 to 4 months after the injection.

Side Effects

With both formulations, mean endogenous estradiol levels remain above the postmenopausal range (40 to 60 pg/mL), and symptoms of estrogen deficiency do not occur. Although DMPA may decrease bone mineral density during use, it is unnecessary to measure bone mineral density or to administer bone antiresorptive agents in DMPA users because the bone loss is temporary and reversible after stopping DMPA.

Because of the lag time it takes to clear DMPA from the circulation, resumption of ovulation is delayed for a variable time after the last injection. It may take as long as 1 year for ovulatory cycles to return. After this initial delay, fecundity resumes at a rate similar to that found after discontinuation of a barrier contraceptive.

The major side effect of DMPA is complete disruption of the menstrual cycle. Because this formulation contains only a progestin, without an estrogen, endometrial integrity is not maintained, and usually light uterine bleeding occurs at irregular and unpredictable intervals. As duration of therapy increases, the incidence of frequent bleeding steadily declines and the incidence of amenorrhea steadily increases so that at the end of 2 years, about 70% of users are amenorrheic. Because the major reason for discontinuance of all progestin-injectable contraceptives is menstrual irregularity, several combined progestin-estrogen injectables that are given once monthly and produce regular withdrawal bleeding have been developed, but these are not available in the United States.

Most DMPA users gain between 1.5 and 4 kg in their first year of use and continue to gain weight thereafter. If weight gain occurs, calorie intake should be decreased. Because there is no estrogen in DMPA, its use does not cause hypertension or thromboembolism. DMPA use is associated with a reduction in seizures among women with epilepsy, as well as a reduction in painful crises among women with sickle cell disease.

Subdermal Implants
Constituents and Use

The only subdermal implant currently available in the United States is a single 4-cm by 2-mm ethylene vinyl acetate rod containing 68 µg of etonogestrel, the active metabolite of desogestrel (Implanon or Nexplanon, which is radiopaque). It provides effective contraception for 3 years. The rod is packaged in a disposable metal trocar inserter and does not require a skin incision for insertion, only for removal. Ovulation is inhibited by the circulating etonogestrel levels, and no pregnancies were reported in three large clinical trials. As with other progestin-only implants, irregular bleeding is the most common clinical complaint. Because implants are not user dependent, the typical-use and perfect-use failure rates are identical and very low, making this method essentially as effective as IUDs and sterilization. Another subdermal implant, Jadelle, consists of two 4.3-cm rods each containing 75 mg of levonorgestrel and is approved for 5 years of contraception; it is not yet available in the United States.

Intrauterine Devices

Two options for intrauterine contraception are available in the United States: the copper-containing IUD and the levonorgestrel intrauterine system (LNG-IUS). Both methods are exceedingly effective with perfect- and typical-use failure rates of less than 1%.

The copper T380A IUD is approved for use in the United States for 10 years and maintains its high levels of effectiveness for at least 12 years. The

LNG-IUS is approved for 5 years of use, and it releases a dose of 20 μg of levonorgestrel from the device into the endometrial cavity each day. This causes atrophy of the endometrial lining, which markedly reduces the amount of uterine bleeding, and it is approved to treat menorrhagia. A newer LNG-containing IUD recently became available in the United States that is smaller and designed for use by nulliparous women.

The main mechanism of action for copper IUD is spermicidal. This effect is caused by a local sterile leukocytic response produced by the copper as well as the plastic IUD. The levonorgestrel-releasing IUD acts mainly by preventing transport of spermatozoa through the cervical mucus and thus preventing fertilization of the ovum. In addition, some women do not ovulate because of the systemic absorption of levonorgestrel. After removal of each type of IUD, the inflammatory reaction rapidly disappears, and resumption of fertility is prompt.

The main difference between the two IUDs is the menstrual bleeding pattern. With the copper IUD, women generally continue to have a regular menstrual period, which may be associated with more pain and heavier bleeding. With the LNG-IUS, irregular bleeding is common in the first 4 to 6 months of use, but after that time, most women develop amenorrhea.

Both IUDs can be easily inserted by any clinician who has been trained. No special tests are needed routinely before insertion, and if it is reasonably certain that the woman is not pregnant, the IUD may be inserted on the same day she presents requesting it. It is not necessary to wait for the next menstrual period. Almost all women, including nulliparous and young women, are considered good candidates for the IUD. Uterine perforation is a rare complication of IUD insertion, occurring in less than 0.1% of cases. Spontaneous expulsion of the IUD after insertion is also rare and happens in less than 5% of users. An IUD may be safely inserted immediately after a delivery or abortion, although the expulsion rate may be slightly higher.[A5]

Development of acute salpingitis more than 1 month after insertion of the IUD is due to infection with a sexually transmitted pathogen and is unrelated to the presence of the device. All IUD-related upper genital tract infections occur only during the insertion process. If there is clinical suspicion that cervicitis is present, an endocervical test for chlamydia and gonorrhea should be performed and the insertion delayed until negative results are obtained. It is not recommended to administer antibiotics routinely with IUD insertion.

Sterilization

Considering both tubal ligations for women and vasectomy for men, sterilization is the most common contraceptive method used by couples in the United States. Female sterilization may be performed transabdominally, such as at the time of cesarean delivery; through a minilaparotomy incision immediately postpartum; laparoscopically; or hysteroscopically. Both laparoscopic tubal ligation and hysteroscopic sterilization may be performed as outpatient procedures. Hysteroscopic tubal occlusion using the Essure device requires evaluation with a hysterosalpingogram 3 months after the procedure to confirm tubal occlusion.

Vasectomy is a simple outpatient procedure that can be performed under local anesthesia. Although many men are concerned about the possibility, sexual function is not affected by vasectomy. There are often programs that support contraceptive services for low-income women, but it is often more difficult for low-income men to access vasectomy.

Grade A References

A1. Edelman A, Micks E, Gallo MF, et al. Continuous or extended cycle vs. cyclic use of combined hormonal contraceptives for contraception. *Cochrane Database Syst Rev.* 2014;7:CD004695.
A2. Stegeman BH, de Bastos M, Rosendaal FR, et al. Different combined oral contraceptives and the risk of venous thrombosis: systematic review and network meta-analysis. *BMJ.* 2013;347:f5298.
A3. Vessey M, Yeates D. Oral contraceptive use and cancer: final report from the Oxford-Family Planning Association contraceptive study. *Contraception.* 2013;88:678-683.
A4. Piaggio G, Kapp N, von Hertzen H. Effect on pregnancy rates of the delay in the administration of levonorgestrel for emergency contraception: a combined analysis of four WHO trails. *Contraception.* 2011;84:35-39.
A5. Hohmann HL, Reeves MF, Chen BA, et al. Immediate versus delayed insertion of the levonorgestrel-releasing intrauterine device following dilation and evacuation: a randomized controlled trial. *Contraception.* 2012;85:240-245.

GENERAL REFERENCES

For the General References and other additional features, please visit Expert Consult at https://expertconsult.inkling.com.

239

COMMON MEDICAL PROBLEMS IN PREGNANCY

KAREN ROSENE-MONTELLA

There are 62 million women of childbearing age in the United States, 85% of whom will give birth by the age of 44 years. The majority of these women will not have obtained preventive health services in any given year, and more than half the pregnancies will be unplanned or unintended. At least 25% will enter pregnancy with a chronic medical illness, and more than half will be overweight or obese, making the role of the internist paramount in maternal health. In the most recent Confidential Enquiry into maternal mortality in the United Kingdom, more than half of all women who died of direct or indirect causes were overweight or obese, and more than 15% of all deaths were in morbidly obese women. Sixteen percent of pregnant women have depression in the perinatal period, and depression rates are even higher in those with chronic illnesses, such as diabetes and asthma.

By the time pregnant patients are seen by their obstetricians, most major teratogenic abnormalities have already occurred (Fig. 239-1), and the window of opportunity to enter pregnancy in a quiescent disease state, on the safest possible medication profile, may have passed. For this reason, internists caring for women of childbearing age have a unique responsibility to provide preconception care at a time when interventions will be of maximum benefit to both the fetus and the mother. Table 239-1 describes preconception interventions for women with chronic medical illnesses.

The basic principles involved in the care of pregnant patients with medical disorders are reviewed here, followed by a more detailed discussion of certain medical conditions, selected because of their contribution to maternal mortality or because of the frequency with which they occur.

BASIC PRINCIPLES

Pregnancy is associated with significant but normal physiologic changes that have an impact on the diagnosis and management of disease states and the pharmacokinetics of most drugs (Table 239-2).[1] The physiologic changes required during pregnancy may stress the woman's ability to adapt, particularly in the presence of an underlying disease. The mother's response to pregnancy often unmasks diseases or predicts future risk, so pregnancy is an opportunity to identify women at risk for other non–pregnancy-related illnesses. For example, gestational diabetes is predictive of an increased risk for type 2 diabetes; preeclampsia is predictive of increased risk for ischemic heart disease and stroke[2]; and thrombosis, late fetal loss, or preeclampsia may unmask an underlying thrombophilia.

Fetal well-being depends on maternal well-being. Although there is often thought to be a dichotomy between maternal and fetal needs, they are usually one and the same. The fetus is dependent on maternal perfusion, oxygenation, and nutrition. Thus, more harm may be done by withholding necessary treatments and investigations from pregnant women than by providing them. Uninvestigated symptoms lead to the progression of untreated disease, and untreated maternal disease compromises fetal safety, growth, and development. The major cause of asthma exacerbations and seizures during pregnancy is abrupt discontinuation of medications, exposing the fetus to hypoxemia and acidosis in an effort to save the fetus from drug exposure. A population analysis of prescriptions for asthma medications in The Netherlands showed that prescriptions for controller medications decreased by 30% during the first months of pregnancy.[3] In the U.K. Confidential Enquiry, in more than half the cases of maternal death from pulmonary embolism, failure to make the diagnosis was due to the unfounded fear that diagnostic testing would be harmful to the fetus. Most diagnostic imaging can be used safely in pregnancy. The effects of radiation in utero depend on both the gestational age at exposure and the level of exposure. Recommendations on fetal exposure from the National Commission on Radiation Protection are summarized in Table 239-3. Radiation exposure from specific diagnostic tests is provided in Table 239-4.

The effect of contrast agents is related to the bioavailability of iodine, and there is concern about the impact on the fetal thyroid. Iodine availability is extremely low, and single-dose exposures, even if they are high, are unlikely

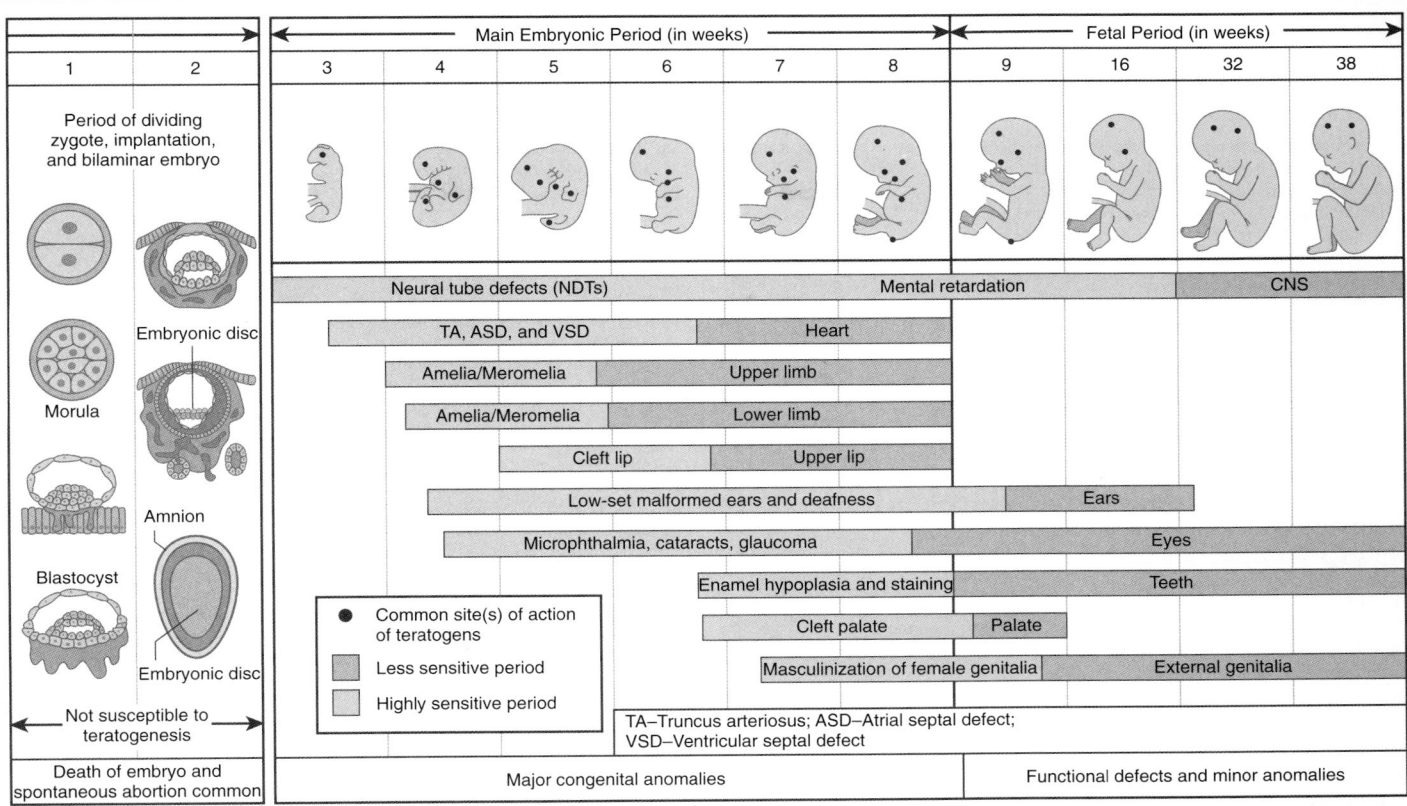

FIGURE 239-1. The developing fetus. CNS = central nervous system. (From Moore K. The Developing Human: Clinically Oriented Embryology. Philadelphia: WB Saunders; 1982, with permission from Annals of Internal Medicine.)

to be harmful. Therefore, contrast agents may be used when necessary. There are limited data on gadolinium, so the current recommendation is to avoid gadolinium exposure if possible.

The use of medications to treat pregnant women requires a rational risk-benefit analysis and a good understanding of the maternal indications. It is helpful to view treatment as justifiable or not justifiable rather than as safe or not safe. It is important to consider whether the condition is self-limited or harmless, what the maternal and fetal consequences of discontinuing a medication will be, and the safety data for the drug. U.S. Food and Drug Administration categories may be misleading and often do not include adequate data for a proper risk-benefit analysis. Resources such as the Teratology Information Service, found at http://depts.washington.edu/terisweb/teris, offer more complete information.

The list of known human teratogens is small and includes warfarin, cyclophosphamide, diethylstilbestrol, lithium, thalidomide, penicillamine, isotretinoin, methotrexate, acetazolamide, and the antiepileptic drugs phenytoin, carbamazepine, phenobarbital, and valproic acid. Of the antiepileptic drugs, valproate has the most significant data, and it is the only antiepileptic drug for which discontinuation during pregnancy is recommended if there is an effective alternative.[4] Angiotensin-converting enzyme (ACE) inhibitors and angiotensin II receptor blockers (ARBs) should be added to this list on the basis of data confirming that first-trimester exposure is associated with fetal renal agenesis and renal failure. Tetracyclines should be avoided because of later effects on fetal teeth and bone.

⬤ HYPERTENSIVE DISORDERS OF PREGNANCY

DEFINITION

Hypertension in pregnancy is defined as a blood pressure (BP) of 140/90 mm Hg or higher. It is defined as chronic hypertension when it predates pregnancy, is diagnosed before 20 weeks' gestation, or persists post partum. Transient late or gestational hypertension occurs toward term and resolves post partum in the absence of any other signs or symptoms of preeclampsia.

EPIDEMIOLOGY

Chronic hypertension is the most common medical condition encountered in women of childbearing age. The incidence is increasing parallel to the increase in obesity, insulin resistance, and pregnancies in women older than 30 years. Hypertension complicates 5 to 8% of pregnancies and is associated with a 20% risk for the development of preeclampsia.

PATHOBIOLOGY

Systemic arterial BP decreases by 10 to 15 mm Hg during normal pregnancy, with a greater fall in diastolic than in systolic pressures, probably because of the decreased sensitivity to angiotensin II that has been demonstrated in pregnant women. BP begins to fall in the first trimester, reaching a nadir toward the end of the second trimester and returning toward baseline at term. This decrease may be exaggerated in women with chronic hypertension, making the diagnosis of chronic hypertension difficult during pregnancy and affecting both diagnostic and therapeutic considerations.

DIAGNOSIS

The diagnosis of hypertension relies simply on a BP measurement, in the sitting position at the level of the heart, of 140/90 mm Hg or higher on two occasions 6 hours apart. Later in pregnancy, inferior vena cava compression by the gravid uterus may lower BP substantially in the supine position, so it is critical to measure maternal BP in the sitting position. The initial evaluation should document target organ damage (such as left ventricular hypertrophy), renal disease (creatinine concentration, urinalysis, and potassium concentration), and retinopathy so that a baseline is established. Consideration of secondary causes is necessary in this young population (Chapter 67), but the diagnosis of secondary causes of hypertension is complicated by normal pregnancy-related changes.[5] The diagnosis of Cushing's syndrome is complicated by increased levels of cortisol and the placental production of adrenocorticotropic hormone and corticotropin-releasing hormone, so the best test is a 24-hour urine free cortisol measurement with higher pregnancy-specific reference ranges. Primary hyperaldosteronism (Chapter 227) may also be

TABLE 239-1 PRECONCEPTION INTERVENTIONS FOR WOMEN WITH MEDICAL ILLNESSES

TYPE 1 AND TYPE 2 DIABETES

Discuss importance of a normal hemoglobin A_{1c} before conception and importance of using contraception until that is achieved

Evaluate for microvascular complications

    Obtain remission for proliferative retinopathy

    Emphasize need to discontinue ACE inhibitor after first missed period

Discontinue thiazolidinediones and statins

Consider change to insulin therapy for type 2 diabetic patients on oral agents unless using metformin for ovulation induction in PCOS

Discuss probable need to reduce insulin dose in first trimester

THYROID DISEASE

Screen for hypothyroidism in women at risk

Normalize TSH and free T_4 before pregnancy

Counsel women taking levothyroxine on probable need to increase dose soon after conception

Diagnose cause of hyperthyroidism and consider ablative therapy for women with Graves' disease requiring high doses of PTU

CHRONIC HYPERTENSION/RENAL DISEASE

Rule out secondary causes of hypertension if appropriate

Evaluate extent of end-organ disease

Quantify GFR and proteinuria

Discuss drugs of choice for hypertension and replace ACE inhibitor

Discuss risk of superimposed preeclampsia and use of low-dose aspirin for women at significant risk of preeclampsia

THROMBOEMBOLIC DISEASE

Consider evaluation for congenital or acquired thrombophilias in women with previous VTE, previous poor obstetric outcome, or family history

Discuss risks of warfarin in pregnancy, need to discontinue warfarin by 4-6 weeks' gestation, and conversion to unfractionated or low-molecular-weight heparin

Discuss options to combined oral contraceptives

EPILEPSY

Determine whether patient is a candidate for withdrawal of antiepileptic drugs

Consider monotherapy with most effective agent at lowest dose possible

Prescribe folate at 1 to 4 mg/day

Discuss possible ineffectiveness of low-dose contraceptives with phenobarbital, phenytoin, and carbamazepine

Consider discontinuing valproate

CARDIAC DISEASE

Obtain baseline echocardiography if congenital disease, stenotic lesion, or pulmonary hypertension suspected

Evaluate for coronary artery disease in women with multiple risk factors

ASTHMA

Verify patient's asthma action plan and peak flowmeter use

Discuss relative safety of all asthma medications except leukotriene modifiers

SYSTEMIC LUPUS ERYTHEMATOSUS AND AUTOIMMUNE DISEASE

Evaluate for renal and cardiopulmonary disease and antiphospholipid, anti-Ro, anti-La antibodies

Avoid pregnancy if disease is active

Discuss relative safety of most immunosuppressants

ACE = angiotensin-converting enzyme; GFR = glomerular filtration rate; PCOS = polycystic ovary syndrome; PTU = propylthiouracil; T_4 = thyroxine; TSH = thyroid-stimulating hormone; VTE = venous thromboembolism.
From Rosene-Montella K, Keely EJ, Lee RV, Barbour LA, eds. *Medical Care of the Pregnant Patient.* 2nd ed. Philadelphia: ACP Press/American College of Physicians; 2008.

TABLE 239-2 NORMAL PHYSIOLOGIC CHANGES IN PREGNANCY

CARDIAC

Cardiac output increased 40%

Blood volume increased 30-50%

Heart rate increased 10-20 beats/min

Blood pressure decreased 10-15 mm Hg

ECG changes related to widened thorax, dextrorotation of heart, elevation of diaphragm

PULMONARY

Upper airway hyperemia and glandular hyperactivity leading to increased edema and friability

Nasal congestion, gestational rhinitis, snoring

Difficult airway management and failed intubation

Minute ventilation increased (owing to an increase in tidal volume, *not* respiratory rate, which remains unchanged), which leads to relative respiratory alkalosis (pH 7.4-7.45)

    Normal Pao_2 100-105 mm Hg

    Normal $Paco_2$ 28-32 mm Hg

RENAL

Increased GFR to 150-180 mL/min/1.73 m^2

Normal serum creatinine concentration <0.8 mg/dL

Increased renal excretion of bicarbonate, limiting buffering capacity in patients who become acidotic

Decreased oncotic pressure

ALTERED PHARMACOKINETICS

Increased renal and hepatic clearance of drugs

Altered absorption

Altered protein binding

Increased volume of distribution

ECG = electrocardiogram; GFR = glomerular filtration rate.
These physiologic changes generally progress throughout gestation.

TABLE 239-3 NATIONAL COMMISSION ON RADIATION PROTECTION (NCRP) RECOMMENDED PREGNANCY EXPOSURES

TOTAL EXPOSURE DURING PREGNANCY (rad)	NCRP RECOMMENDATIONS
≤5	Acceptable; low likelihood of problems
5-10	Low risk for problems
10-15 (at ≤8 wk gestation)	Higher risk; consideration of termination
>15	Termination of pregnancy recommended

From Rosene-Montella K, Keely EJ, Lee RV, Barbour LA, eds. *Medical Care of the Pregnant Patient.* 2nd ed. Philadelphia: ACP Press/American College of Physicians; 2008.

TABLE 239-4 RADIATION EXPOSURE

STUDY	RADIATION EXPOSURE (rad)
Chest radiography	<0.001
Lung scan	0.01-0.02 ventilation 0.01-0.03 perfusion
Pulmonary angiography	<0.050 by brachial route 0.2-0.3 by femoral route
CT angiography	0.2-0.3
Ultrasound	None
MRI, MRA, MRV	None
Upper gastrointestinal series	0.1
Lumbar spine series	0.9
Barium enema	1
Complete IVP	0.5
Head CT	<0.01
CT of abdomen	2.0-3.0

CT = computed tomography; IVP = intravenous pyelography; MRA = magnetic resonance angiography; MRI = magnetic resonance imaging; MRV = magnetic resonance venography.

difficult to diagnose in the face of normal pregnancy-related elevations in plasma renin activity and aldosterone and because progesterone ameliorates both the hypertensive and the kaliuretic effects of aldosterone. Primary hyperaldosteronism should be strongly considered in any patient with chronic hypertension in whom there is a marked increase in BP toward term or post partum. Pheochromocytoma (Chapter 228) is associated with a high maternal and fetal mortality rate, in large part owing to a delay in diagnosis. Both magnetic resonance imaging and magnetic resonance angiography (which do not require gadolinium) can be used safely in pregnancy to evaluate the adrenal glands and renal arteries.

TREATMENT   Rx

Patients previously receiving drug therapy can often discontinue antihypertensives and restart them when BP gradually rises to prepregnant values toward term. It is difficult to determine whether rising BP represents a normal physiologic return to earlier pressure or the development of preeclampsia. Baseline preeclampsia laboratory tests (see later), very close follow-up, and comanagement with the patient's obstetrician are required. Patients with good BP control may prefer to continue safe medications or switch to another regimen. The drugs for which there is grade A evidence of efficacy and safety are methyldopa and labetalol (Table 67-5). Nifedipine, hydralazine, and other β-blockers, especially those with intrinsic sympathomimetic activity, have also been studied and are acceptable second- and third-line agents.

Dosing should take into consideration the increase in renal and hepatic clearance and the increased volume of distribution, which may require higher doses or narrowed dosing intervals during pregnancy. ACE inhibitors and ARBs should be discontinued at the diagnosis of pregnancy because of their teratogenicity and their association with fetal and neonatal renal agenesis and renal failure even when they are used later in gestation.

The goal of antihypertensive therapy in pregnancy is not clear. Most consensus recommendations, which address fetal concerns and short-term maternal safety only, recommend keeping BP below 160/100 mm Hg. Given the long-term maternal data, most centers prefer to keep maternal BP, particularly in patients with diabetes or renal disease, below 140/90 mm Hg. Consensus recommendations agree that maintaining BP above 120/80 mm Hg is necessary to preserve placental perfusion. There is no evidence that salt restriction or dietary changes improve BP control in pregnancy, and weight loss is not recommended. Likewise, there is no evidence that BP control decreases the risk of preeclampsia. It is important to obtain baseline preeclampsia laboratory tests (complete blood count, platelet count, creatinine concentration, uric acid level, aspartate transaminase level, urinalysis) in all patients with hypertension, given the 20% risk of preeclampsia, and low-dose aspirin and calcium supplementation should be considered to prevent preeclampsia (see later). Fetal monitoring with serial ultrasound for growth and amniotic fluid volume, nonstress testing (fetal heart rate acceleration in response to movement) once or twice a week after 32 weeks, and consideration of Doppler flow velocimetry are recommended.

Most antihypertensives are safe for breast-feeding, which should be encouraged. Hydrochlorothiazides, α-methyldopa, nifedipine, acebutolol, and metoprolol are all approved by the American Academy of Pediatricians. There is no evidence that hydrochlorothiazides affect milk volume. There is evidence that propranolol and atenolol are concentrated in breast milk, so they should be avoided. Enalapril and captopril are the preferred ACE inhibitors in breast-feeding women, but it may be prudent to delay ACE inhibitors for the first few weeks of the baby's life and for mothers of premature babies, given the adverse pregnancy data.

PROGNOSIS

Hypertension may increase the risk of placental abruption, intrauterine growth restriction (IUGR), and low-birthweight babies. The major risk, however, is its contribution to the risk for preeclampsia and the associated increase in perinatal morbidity and mortality. In addition, chronic hypertension in patients with other comorbidities significantly increases the risk for maternal and fetal complications[6] (Table 239-5).

Women who develop hypertension during pregnancy are at increased lifetime risk for the development of chronic hypertension, even if the BP normalizes post partum.[7]

● PREECLAMPSIA

DEFINITION

Preeclampsia is a multisystem disorder defined as BP of 140/90 mm Hg or higher, accompanied by proteinuria of more than 300 mg/24 hours after the 20th week of gestation in a previously normotensive patient. When it is diagnosed in a patient with preexisting chronic hypertension, it is referred to as chronic hypertension with superimposed preeclampsia.

A urine protein-creatinine ratio of at least 0.3 may become a criterion for proteinuria, but the American College of Obstetricians and Gynecologists has not yet added this to the definition. Edema and hyperreflexia are no longer considered diagnostic criteria, and the 30 mm Hg increase in systolic pressure or 15 mm Hg increase in diastolic pressure has been dropped from the criteria for hypertension. Severe preeclampsia is defined as the presence of one of the following symptoms or signs with preeclampsia: systolic BP of 160 mm Hg or higher, or diastolic BP of 110 mm Hg or higher, on two occasions at least 6 hours apart; proteinuria of more than 5 g in a 24-hour period; pulmonary edema; oliguria (<400 mL in 24 hours); persistent headaches; epigastric pain or impaired liver function; thrombocytopenia; and IUGR.

EPIDEMIOLOGY

Preeclampsia complicates 6 to 8% of pregnancies worldwide. Preeclampsia/eclampsia is a leading cause of maternal mortality in the developing world and continues to contribute to maternal mortality in the United States despite the availability of antihypertensives and antiseizure medications. In the United States, preeclampsia is believed to be responsible for 15% of premature deliveries and 17.6% of maternal deaths. Worldwide, preeclampsia and eclampsia are estimated to be responsible for approximately 14% of maternal deaths per year (50,000 to 75,000).

Primigravida and multigravida women with new partners are at increased risk, suggesting a role for paternal antigens. Additional risk factors include prior history of preeclampsia, black race, diabetes or insulin resistance, obesity, systemic lupus erythematosus (SLE), renal disease, hypertension, thrombophilia, obesity, molar pregnancy, multiple gestation, and extremes of age (younger than 20 years or older than 40 years).

PATHOBIOLOGY

Preeclampsia is a disorder of abnormal placentation that begins early in gestation, well before its manifestations are clinically apparent. In normal pregnancy, uterine spiral arteries undergo remodeling when they are invaded by fetal cytotrophoblastic cells, resulting in an adhesion receptor switch from cells with characteristics of epithelial cells to cells with the phenotype of endothelial cells. This leads to the transformation of previously narrow, high-resistance maternal uterine blood vessels into dilated, high-capacitance blood vessels. The proximal portions of the spiral arteries are further dilated by the hormonal effects of estrogen and progesterone, resulting in an overall increase in uterine blood flow from 45 mL/minute during menstruation to 750 mL/minute at term. In preeclampsia, this cell switching does not occur, and the fetal cells' only superficial invasion into maternal vasculature results in limited placental perfusion. As the pregnancy progresses, abnormal placentation produces relative hypoxia and ischemia as this compromised uterine blood flow cannot keep up with the growing demands of the fetus and the placenta. The result is diffuse endothelial dysfunction that is manifested as the clinical syndrome of preeclampsia (Fig. 239-2).

Recent work on the potential mechanism of the endothelial dysfunction that underlies this disease state has focused on the imbalance between pro-angiogenic and anti-angiogenic factors, arising from studies showing elevated concentrations of placental soluble film-like tyrosine kinase 1 in the plasma of women with preeclampsia. This protein prevents the interaction of placental growth factor and vascular endothelial growth factor with endothelial receptors, inducing endothelial dysfunction. A placenta-derived soluble transforming growth factor-β coreceptor, soluble endoglin, is elevated in the sera of patients with preeclampsia, inducing vascular permeability and hypertension; the degree of elevation correlates with disease severity, and levels fall after delivery. Additional factors currently being studied include ADAM12 trophoblast and angiogenesis markers, pregnancy-associated plasma protein A, placental protein 13, and placental growth factor.[8] To date, no definitive predictive model has been established. Current studies to address both the cause of and the mechanism linking preeclampsia and the risk of cardiovascular disease are ongoing and focus on endothelial dysfunction.[9]

DIAGNOSIS

The diagnosis of preeclampsia depends on a BP of 140/90 mm Hg or higher and proteinuria of more than 300 mg/24 hours after 20 weeks' gestation. Eclampsia is diagnosed when a patient with preeclampsia has a seizure. Additional abnormalities that contribute to the diagnosis include hyperuricemia, hemoconcentration, elevated creatinine or liver function test results, and thrombocytopenia. The HELLP syndrome (hemolysis, elevated liver enzymes, and low platelets) (Chapter 172) is likely to be a more severe form of preeclampsia. The diagnosis of severe preeclampsia depends on the criteria previously listed.

Diagnostic evaluation should include a careful history, asking about headache, visual complaints, epigastric pain, weight gain, and edema and reviewing the presence of risk factors. The physical examination should include a careful neurologic examination, looking for funduscopic changes (retinal vasospasm, edema, or hemorrhage) or hyperreflexia, and examination for any

TABLE 239-5 ODDS RATIOS FOR FETAL AND MATERNAL COMPLICATIONS: 1995-2008

VARIABLE	PREGESTATIONAL DIABETES		CHRONIC RENAL DISEASE		COLLAGEN VASCULAR DISEASE		THYROID DISORDERS	
	With Chronic Hypertension	*Without Chronic Hypertension*	*With Chronic Hypertension*	*Without Chronic Hypertension*	*With Chronic Hypertension*	*Without Chronic Hypertension*	*With Chronic Hypertension*	*Without Chronic Hypertension*
FETAL OUTCOMES								
Stillbirth[a]	4.30 (3.81-4.85)	3.05 (2.88-3.23)	7.29 (5.59-9.52)	1.74 (1.51-2.02)	7.42 (5.37-10.25)	2.74 (2.35-3.20)	1.86 (1.48-2.33)	0.98 (0.92-1.05)
Poor fetal growth[a]	2.66 (2.40-2.94)	1.20 (1.14-1.27)	7.94 (6.67-9.44)	2.29 (2.12-2.49)	7.99 (6.44-9.91)	3.87 (3.55-4.22)	3.59 (3.20-4.02)	1.29 (1.25-1.34)
Spontaneous delivery <37 wk gestation[a]	4.88 (4.63-5.15)	2.90 (2.83-2.98)	8.60 (7.64-9.67)	2.25 (2.15-2.35)	7.19 (6.22-8.30)	3.15 (2.98-3.33)	3.24 (3.02-3.48)	1.24 (1.21-1.27)
MATERNAL OUTCOMES								
Preeclampsia[a]	13.96 (13.29-14.66)	3.80 (3.69-3.91)	27.87 (24.85-31.25)	3.28 (3.10-3.47)	17.41 (15.09-20.09)	2.96 (2.76-3.18)	9.74 (9.15-10.35)	1.38 (1.35-1.42)
Stroke/cerebrovascular complications[a]	7.14 (4.90-10.40)	1.85 (1.41-2.44)	13.73 (6.63-28.44)	3.52 (2.34-5.31)	23.00 (11.47-46.14)	7.60 (5.26-10.97)	3.87 (2.07-7.23)	1.58 (1.29-1.94)
Acute renal failure[a]	35.41 (28.39-44.16)	4.43 (3.57-5.48)	253.4 (199.5-321.9)	62.40 (54.37-71.63)	191.5 (141.4-259.4)	12.60 (8.88-17.88)	14.17 (9.65-20.82)	1.27 (0.97-1.65)
Pulmonary edema[a]	11.97 (7.86-18.24)	4.01 (3.07-5.25)	23.29 (10.32-52.56)	9.06 (5.84-14.06)	15.52 (4.92-48.95)	6.08 (3.46-10.69)	9.85 (5.64-17.19)	1.54 (1.16-2.05)
Ventilation[a]	11.87 (9.22-15.26)	3.34 (2.80-4.00)	19.29 (11.36-32.76)	8.25 (6.43-10.60)	26.20 (15.04-45.63)	11.09 (8.46-14.52)	5.71 (3.69-8.86)	1.84 (1.55-2.18)
Cesarean delivery[b]	5.75 (5.46-6.05)	3.33 (3.26-3.41)	5.73 (5.03-6.53)	1.74 (1.68-1.81)	4.38 (3.74-5.12)	1.89 (1.80-1.98)	3.16 (2.97-3.36)	1.27 (1.25-1.29)
Length of stay >6 days[c]	14.74 (13.68-15.89)	5.34 (5.09-5.60)	42.16 (36.78-48.32)	6.52 (6.12-6.95)	30.29 (25.45-36.04)	6.18 (5.69-6.71)	8.40 (7.60-9.28)	1.77 (1.71-1.84)
In-hospital mortality[a]	6.02 (2.71-13.40)	2.58 (1.59-4.17)	27.02 (8.72-83.73)	6.88 (3.56-13.29)	88.81 (41.90-188.2)	23.81 (14.67-38.66)	1.74 (0.24-12.40)	1.72 (1.06-2.77)

For each analysis, reference group was delivery admissions without chronic hypertension and without comorbidity of interest. Admissions with chronic hypertension but without comorbidity of interest were included as a group in each analysis. Because of similarity of estimates of association in these groups to those obtained when analyzing effect of overall chronic hypertension, results are not shown.

[a]Adjusted for multiple birth, year of study, insurance status, region, and age.

[b]Adjusted for previous cesarean delivery, multiple birth, year of study, insurance status, region, and age.

[c]Adjusted for disposition status, admission status, multiple birth, year of study, insurance status, region, and age.

From Bateman BT, Bansil P, Hernandez-Diaz S, et al. Prevalence, trends, and outcomes of chronic hypertension: a nationwide sample of delivery admissions. *Am J Obstet Gynecol* 2012;206:134.e1-134.e8, 2012.

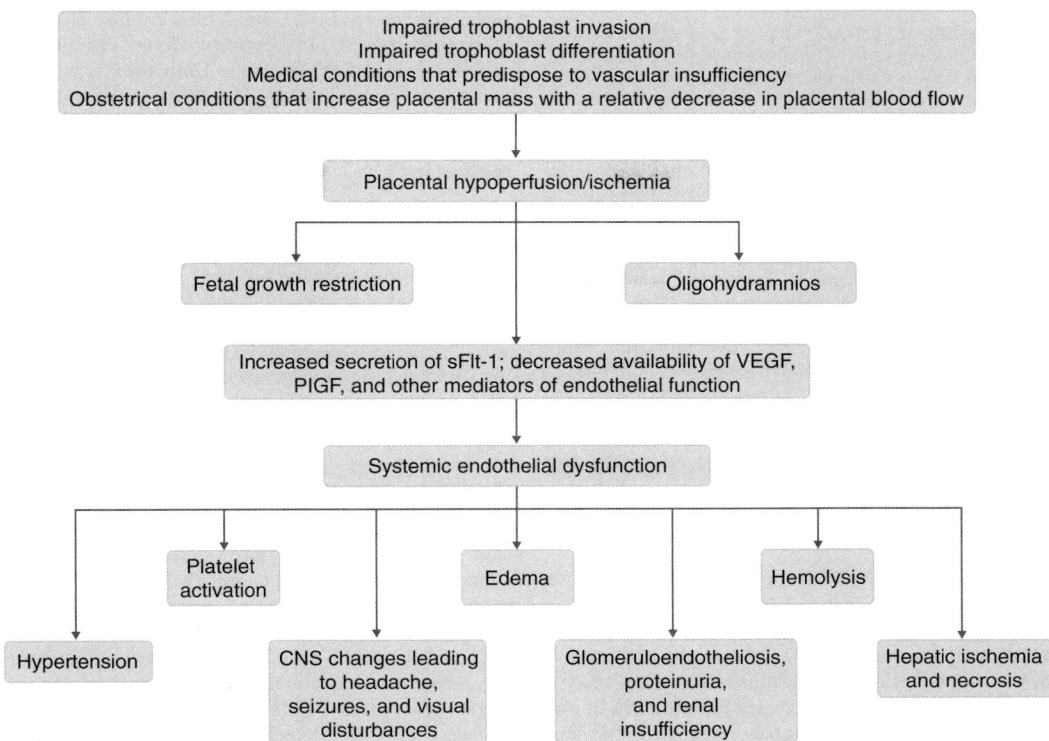

FIGURE 239-2. Model for the pathogenesis of preeclampsia. CNS = central nervous system; PlGF = placental growth factor; sFlt-1 = soluble film-like tyrosine kinase; VEGF = vascular endothelial growth factor. (From Rosene-Montella K, Keely EJ, Lee RV, Barbour LA, eds. *Medical Care of the Pregnant Patient.* 2nd ed. Philadelphia: ACP Press/American College of Physicians; 2008.)

focal findings suggestive of mass effect, hepatic tenderness, and edema. Laboratory testing for preeclampsia includes a complete blood count, platelet count, urine protein-creatinine ratio or 24-hour urine protein, liver function tests, creatinine concentration, and uric acid level. Additional evaluation includes fetal testing and close maternal monitoring for life-threatening consequences, such as severe hypertension, seizures, pulmonary edema, cerebral hemorrhage, hepatic infarction or rupture, disseminated intravascular coagulation, and renal failure.

Currently, diagnosis depends on development of the full clinical syndrome, but earlier diagnosis may be possible on the basis of biomarkers. It is likely that a combined model that looks at soluble endoglin, soluble film-like tyrosine kinase 1, pregnancy-associated plasma protein A, ADAM12, and placental growth factor concentrations will be a better prediction instrument before 20 weeks' gestation than any individual marker.

The differential diagnosis of each individual manifestation of preeclampsia is broad, so the diagnosis centers on the constellation of signs and symptoms that suggest preeclampsia. The clinical conditions that can mimic preeclampsia include SLE with nephritis (Chapter 266), thrombotic thrombocytopenic purpura, and hemolytic-uremic syndrome (Chapter 172). Differentiation of preeclampsia from a flare of SLE with nephritis (Chapter 266) is difficult because both can cause hypertension, proteinuria, thrombocytopenia, and rises in serum creatinine concentration. The differential diagnostic features that favor SLE include falling serum complement levels, rising anti-DNA antibodies, and extrarenal manifestations of SLE such as rash and arthralgias. The proteinuria and hypertension in preeclampsia are more likely to be of sudden onset.

TREATMENT   Rx

Once it occurs, the only known treatment of preeclampsia is delivery as soon as it is obstetrically feasible. Nevertheless, preeclampsia can be manifested post partum, and both preeclampsia and eclampsia have been reported up to 21 days after delivery. Management of preeclampsia includes treatment of hypertension, seizure prophylaxis, and limitation of fluids due to the risk of pulmonary edema. Treatment of severe hypertension in preeclampsia is reviewed in Table 239-6. Magnesium sulfate is recommended as first-line treatment of eclampsia as well as for prophylaxis against eclampsia in women with

TABLE 239-6 TREATMENT OF SEVERE HYPERTENSION IN PREECLAMPTIC PATIENTS

MEDICATION	ONSET AND DURATION OF ACTION	ACUTE DOSING FOR SEVERE HYPERTENSION	MAINTENANCE DOSE
Labetalol	Begins to work in 5-10 min Lasts 3-6 hr	Given as a series of boluses until BP reaches the desired level: 10 mg IV push; then in 10 min, 20 mg IV push; then in 10 min, 40 mg IV push; then in 10 min, 80 mg IV push; then in 10 min, 80 mg IV push, up to a total dose of no more than 300 mg Follow with PO labetalol or labetalol drip	100-200 mg PO bid-tid (100-600 mg bid-tid; maximum 2400 mg/day) IV infusion 0.5-2.0 mg/min (labetalol comes in vials of 100 mg/20 mL) Put 5 vials (100 mL) labetalol into 150 mL IV fluid (D₅W, LR, or NS) to get a solution of 2 mg/mL; start at 15 mL/hr (0.5 mg/min); titrate up to as high as 60 mL/hr (2 mg/min)
Nifedipine	Begins to work in <30 min Lasts 4-5 hr	10-20 mg PO q30min to a maximum of 50 mg	10-20 mg PO tid of short-acting nifedipine or 30-120 mg once daily of long-acting formulation
Hydralazine	Begins to work in 10-20 min Lasts for 3-6 hr	2.5-10 mg IV q30min	Start at 10 mg PO qid; can be gradually increased to 50 mg PO qid

BP = blood pressure; D₅W = dextrose 5% in water (solution); LR = lactated Ringer's (solution); NS = normal saline.
From Rosene-Montella K, Keely EJ, Lee RV, Barbour LA, eds. *Medical Care of the Pregnant Patient.* 2nd ed. Philadelphia: ACP Press/American College of Physicians; 2008.

severe and nonsevere preeclampsia.[A2] Phenytoin and benzodiazepines should not be used for eclampsia prophylaxis or treatment unless there is a contraindication to magnesium sulfate or it is ineffective. There is evidence from two randomized controlled trials that magnesium is superior to phenytoin for the prevention of both primary seizures and recurrent seizures in eclampsia.

Treatment of acute seizures in eclampsia includes airway protection, fetal monitoring, magnesium, BP control, and benzodiazepines as needed to stop seizures acutely. Treatment of severe hypertension is as outlined in Table 239-6.

Severe maternal manifestations of preeclampsia that may warrant early delivery include seizure, renal failure, severe hypertension, severe thrombocytopenia or hemolysis, aspartate transaminase or alanine transaminase elevation of more than two to three times normal, pulmonary edema, retinal hemorrhage, and other symptoms suggestive of end-organ damage (headache, visual disturbance, epigastric or right upper quadrant pain). Fetal indications for delivery may include significant IUGR, oligohydramnios, and nonreassuring fetal testing. Women with preeclampsia before 34 weeks' gestation should receive a corticosteroid that crosses the placenta, such as betamethasone or dexamethasone, to accelerate fetal lung maturation.

PREVENTION

Multiple trials of antihypertensives, antioxidant supplementation with vitamins C and E, magnesium,[A3] protein or salt restriction, fish oil, and other dietary changes have failed to prevent preeclampsia. Low-dose aspirin in high-risk populations is the only intervention with data to support a positive effect. Initial trials showed limited effects, but a subsequent meta-analysis found that low-dose aspirin (<100 mg/day) decreases both the risk of preeclampsia and fetal and neonatal deaths.[A4] We recommend aspirin 81 mg/day in all patients with risk factors for preeclampsia. Trials of calcium supplementation have shown conflicting results, but given the inverse relationship between dietary calcium intake and BP in the general population, calcium supplementation of at least 1 g/day is recommended for women with a low dietary intake of calcium (<600 mg/day). An alternative to supplementation may be to increase dietary calcium by eating three or four servings per day of dairy products (assuming 250 to 300 mg of calcium per serving).

PROGNOSIS

Women who have had preeclampsia are at increased risk of heart disease, stroke, and cardiovascular death. Preeclampsia is also a marker for increased risk of end-stage renal disease. One year after delivery, preeclampsia patients observed longitudinally by Smith and colleagues had evidence of increased insulin resistance, BP, cholesterol, and triglycerides, which may be the first manifestations of the metabolic syndrome. The same group recently reported on the calculated 10-year, 30-year, and lifetime risk of cardiovascular disease in this cohort.[10] The 10-year, 30-year, and lifetime risk for development of cardiovascular disease was 18.2% versus 1.7%, 31.3% versus 5.1%, and 41.4% versus 17.8% in matched controls who did not have preeclampsia. It is unclear whether there is a shared pathogenesis, an unmasking of already established disease, or a contribution to the development of disease. It is possible that preexisting abnormal endothelial function predisposes to renal and vascular disease later in life and is, in fact, the same abnormality that disturbs implantation, resulting in preeclampsia and fetal loss. It is also possible that preeclampsia itself contributes to the later development of disease.

Continuing care beyond 6 weeks post partum is strongly recommended. Women with a history of severe preeclampsia should be screened for preexisting hypertension, underlying renal disease, thrombophilia, and possibly secondary causes of hypertension. They should also be informed of the risk for preeclampsia in subsequent pregnancies, particularly if the birth interval is less than 2 years or more than 10 years. Women who are overweight should be advised to normalize their body mass index before another pregnancy and to reduce long-term risk. Both women with preexisting hypertension and those whose BP normalizes are likely to benefit from an overall assessment of cardiovascular risk that includes a lipid profile, smoking cessation, and early interventions to reduce risk.

DEEP VENOUS THROMBOSIS, PULMONARY EMBOLISM, AND THROMBOPHILIA
(Chapters 81, 98, and 176)

Pulmonary embolism (PE) is the leading medical cause of maternal mortality in the developed world. It was responsible for 30% of direct maternal deaths in the most recent U.K. Confidential Enquiry. Despite our best efforts, mortality rates from PE in pregnancy have not changed in more than 2 decades, and the incidence of PE in the United States is rising, likely owing to the increase in obesity and cesarean deliveries. Current strategies to reduce risk from PE must address the widespread use of appropriate prophylaxis, early detection of venous thromboembolism (VTE), and prompt, safe, and effective therapy.[11]

EPIDEMIOLOGY

More than half of the VTE events in women younger than 40 years occur in association with pregnancy. VTE is 10 times more common in pregnant than in nonpregnant women of comparable age. It occurs in 5 to 12 of 10,000 pregnancies ante partum and in 3 to 7 of 10,000 post partum. The risk of VTE with pregnancy is increased by the presence of additional risk factors, including prolonged bedrest, cesarean section, preeclampsia, three or more children, smoking, obesity, previous superficial thrombophlebitis, previous VTE, thrombophilia, and family history of VTE.

PATHOBIOLOGY

Pregnancy is a hypercoagulable state (Chapter 176) characterized by venous stasis, maternal prothrombotic imbalance in which activation of the coagulation system exceeds the fibrinolytic response progressively through the course of pregnancy, and endothelial disruption. Venous stasis occurs as a result of progesterone-induced venodilation early in pregnancy and is later increased by the compressive effects of the gravid uterus. Compression of the left iliac vein by the right iliac artery further increases venous stasis on the left, which may explain the finding that more than 90% of cases of deep venous thrombosis (DVT) in pregnancy occur in the left leg. Endothelial damage occurs with preeclampsia and with both vaginal and operative delivery, further contributing to VTE risk.

Genetic and Acquired Thrombophilias

A positive family history for VTE (possibly a marker for thrombophilia) or a known thrombophilia significantly increases the risk for VTE in pregnancy (see Chapter 176). The best-described genetic thrombophilias include deficiencies in protein C, protein S, and antithrombin III, all of which appear to have autosomal dominant inheritance with variable penetrance, and the presence of the single-gene mutations factor V Leiden and prothrombin G202010. Of these, antithrombin-deficient homozygotes (rare) and compound heterozygotes have the highest risk of VTE in pregnancy. The thrombophilias have also been associated with obstetric complications, including IUGR, abruption, both early and late pregnancy loss, and preeclampsia (early, severe, or recurrent). The antiphospholipid antibody syndrome is the major acquired thrombophilia for which there are compelling pregnancy data supporting a link with both thrombosis risk and obstetric complications as well as the use of thromboprophylaxis to prevent poor obstetric outcome (Chapter 176). A large international, multicenter trial, the Thrombophilia in Pregnancy Prophylaxis Study, is currently under way, randomizing patients with thrombophilias and adverse pregnancy outcomes to surveillance versus thromboprophylaxis. Preliminary data analysis has failed to demonstrate efficacy of thromboprophylaxis for the prevention of the adverse pregnancy outcomes described before, and the most recent American College of Obstetricians and Gynecologists technical bulletin recommends against prophylaxis for prevention of adverse pregnancy outcome in patients with thrombophilias other than the antiphospholipid antibody syndrome.[12]

DIAGNOSIS

The diagnosis of VTE during pregnancy is complicated by both normal pregnancy-related physiologic changes and the reluctance to use diagnostic imaging in pregnancy. Clinical signs are unreliable, and leg swelling and complaints of dyspnea are common during pregnancy, making it difficult to decide when to investigate for VTE. The finding that 90% of DVT occurs in the left leg led to the observation that the combination of symptoms in the left leg, calf circumference difference of 2 cm or more, and first-trimester presentation (when leg swelling is less likely) is highly predictive of DVT. Most DVTs occur ante partum, and events are evenly distributed throughout gestation. The majority of fatal PEs in most studies occurred in the postpartum period, so vigilance is required for a prolonged period after delivery. Diagnosis of DVT requires compression ultrasonography that includes the iliac veins and the inferior vena cava at the level of the liver (Chapter 81). It also requires repeated compression ultrasonography if study findings are normal but there is high pretest probability and continuing symptoms. In patients with suspected iliac or pelvic vein thrombosis and normal findings on ultrasound studies, magnetic resonance imaging or magnetic resonance venography is recommended.

The diagnosis of PE is even more of a problem, given the frequency of dyspnea, the likelihood of normal oxygenation in young patients with no underlying cardiopulmonary disease, and the more invasive nature of diagnostic testing. Arterial blood gas analysis is not helpful; the A-a gradient was normal in 60% of pregnant patients with documented PE in a retrospective review done at two centers.

The radiation exposure from imaging required for the diagnosis of PE is well below that allowed by the National Commission on Radiation Protection (see Table 239-3), so testing should never be withheld out of concern for fetal exposure. Ventilation-perfusion (V/Q) scanning is still the diagnostic test of choice in most centers outside the United States. It is better validated in pregnancy, involves no administration of contrast material, and has good negative predictive value in normal scans and in low-probability scans when it is paired with leg studies. If V/Q is used, it must be understood that there is still a significant risk of PE in patients with scans interpreted to be "intermediate" and "indeterminate," so additional testing is required in those cases. Computed tomography angiography has replaced V/Q scanning in most U.S. centers on the basis of its use in the nonpregnant population. The technique is dependent on cardiac output and plasma volume, both of which are increased during pregnancy. This may lead to poor opacification of the vessels, causing artifacts to be read as filling defects or the failure to visualize clots, so the technique must be adjusted for pregnancy. It is a sensitive, cost-effective test that offers an alternative diagnosis in 25 to 40% of cases, and it is preferred if there is an abnormality on the chest radiograph. It is well tolerated and has a shorter breath-holding time than V/Q scans, so it is also preferred in unstable patients, especially if an alternative diagnosis is suspected. Computed tomography angiography exposes the maternal breast to 2 to 3.5 rad, and exposure of the breast to 1 rad increases the lifetime risk of breast cancer by 13%. The use of breast shields decreases this exposure by about 50% without compromising the integrity of the test, so breast shields are strongly recommended.

The role of D-dimer testing in pregnancy has not yet been elucidated because D-dimer is elevated during normal pregnancy. It may have some use for its negative predictive value, but studies are inadequate to recommend its use at this time.

TREATMENT   Rx

The safety of unfractionated heparin (UFH) and low-molecular-weight heparin (LMWH) (Chapter 38) for the fetus is well established, so they are the drugs of choice for both the treatment and the prevention of VTE. Warfarin is a teratogen that crosses the placenta and has been associated with fetal bleeding and central nervous system abnormalities later in gestation, so it is not used for this indication in pregnancy. Initial treatment of VTE in the pregnant patient is either intravenous UFH, followed by subcutaneous UFH or LMWH, or an initial adjusted dose of LMWH that is then continued; both are acceptable.

LMWH causes a lower incidence of heparin-induced thrombocytopenia (Chapter 172) and less osteoporosis, so, given the prolonged exposure during pregnancy, it is the preferred agent. The 2012 American College of Chest Physicians consensus guidelines now recommend LMWH as the preferred agent in pregnancy.[13] The same consensus conference suggests limiting the use of fondaparinux and parenteral direct thrombin inhibitors to patients with severe allergic reactions to heparin (e.g., heparin-induced thrombocytopenia) who cannot receive danaparoid. The use of oral direct thrombin and anti-Xa inhibitors is not recommended (Table 239-7). LMWH has increased bioavailability, but the ease of administration in pregnancy is mitigated by the need for twice-daily dosing and frequent monitoring. Dosing requirements increase with increasing gestation, so it is necessary to follow anti-Xa levels. Because LMWH has limited reversibility with protamine and because it has been associated with epidural hematomas in nonpregnant patients given spinal or epidural anesthesia, most centers recommend a switch to UFH by 34 to 36 weeks. This allows patients the option of epidural anesthesia for delivery, and in the event of an emergent delivery before holding of anticoagulation, UFH can be reversed with protamine. Specific treatment recommendations are outlined in Table 239-8.

PREVENTION

The overall recurrence risk of VTE during pregnancy ranges from 5 to 20%, depending in part on the circumstances of the index clot. Patients with a previous idiopathic VTE (while not pregnant) or a secondary VTE that occurred during a previous pregnancy or while taking oral contraceptives and patients with a positive family history of or identified thrombophilia are at the highest risk. The thrombophilias with the highest recurrence risk are the antiphospholipid antibody syndrome and homozygosity or compound heterozygosity with more than one mutation and antithrombin deficiency. Thromboprophylaxis is required in all these groups, and its intensity is related to the severity of the risk (see Table 239-8). The lowest risk of recurrence, based on retrospective data, appears to be in patients without a family history of thrombophilia in whom the previous VTE occurred in association with a transient risk factor other than pregnancy or oral contraceptive use. The American College of Chest Physicians consensus guidelines now suggest surveillance with postpartum thromboprophylaxis in this group, but many U.S. centers would also offer antepartum thromboprophylaxis. Prophylaxis should be continued for at least 6 to 8 weeks post partum, when the hemostatic changes of pregnancy return to prepregnant values. Additional groups that should be considered for thromboprophylaxis are patients who have undergone cesarean section, particularly if they have an additional risk factor for VTE, and patients on prolonged bedrest. Patients receiving continued prophylactic or treatment doses post partum have the option of switching to warfarin, which is safe in breast-feeding women.

PROGNOSIS

VTE during pregnancy may be the first manifestation of a hypercoagulable state, as pregnancy acts as a "stress test" for thrombophilia. Fifty percent of initial episodes of VTE in women younger than 40 years are manifested in association with pregnancy. A thrombophilia evaluation is indicated in all patients who present with VTE during pregnancy to assess long-term maternal and family risk and to guide future secondary prophylaxis recommendations. Patients with an identified thrombophilia and an adverse pregnancy outcome may be at risk for a similar outcome in a subsequent pregnancy and should be counseled about this risk and considered for thromboprophylaxis.

Patients who have had DVT during pregnancy have a high risk of postphlebitic syndrome and venous insufficiency. Two randomized controlled trials demonstrated a 50% risk reduction in symptoms of post-thrombotic syndrome when compression stockings were used within 1 month of diagnosis and continued for a minimum of 1 year after diagnosis.

ASTHMA (Chapter 87)

Maintaining adequate control of asthma during pregnancy is important for both maternal and fetal outcome. Asthma may be associated with increased perinatal mortality, preterm birth, IUGR, gestational diabetes, and preeclampsia. Well-controlled asthma reduces the likelihood of these adverse outcomes to baseline, so it is safer for both mother and fetus to treat maternal asthma than to allow exacerbations to occur.

EPIDEMIOLOGY

Asthma is the most common respiratory disease in pregnancy. It affects 3.7 to 8.4% of pregnancies in the United States and 12 to 13% of pregnancies in Australia and the United Kingdom. Approximately 10% of U.S. women of reproductive age have asthma, and the rates of asthma reported during labor and delivery have doubled during the last decade.

Effect of Pregnancy on Asthma

The course of asthma in pregnancy is unpredictable, and most studies have found that a third of patients improve, a third worsen, and a third stay the same. The most likely predictor in any individual patient is her course during a previous pregnancy. In most studies, the majority of exacerbations occurred between 17 and 32 weeks, with some improvement reported by 36 weeks' gestation. Patients with mild asthma do well during labor and delivery, but almost 50% of patients with severe asthma worsen during labor and delivery. Risk factors for exacerbations include severe asthma, poor compliance with medications (especially inhaled corticosteroids), obesity, viral infections, rhinitis, gastroesophageal reflux, and poor prenatal care. The highest morbidity and mortality are reported in African American patients.

Effect of Asthma on Pregnancy

Pregnancy and perinatal outcome are improved when asthma is well controlled. Poorly controlled asthma increases the risk of spontaneous abortion,

TABLE 239-7 SAFETY AND PHARMACOKINETICS OF ANTICOAGULANTS IN PREGNANCY

	UFH	LMWH	SEMISYNTHETIC HEPARINOIDS (DANAPAROID)	SYNTHETIC HEPARINS AND FACTOR Xa INHIBITOR (FONDAPARINUX, RIVAROXABAN)	THROMBIN INHIBITORS (RECOMBINANT HIRUDINS)	THROMBIN INHIBITORS (ARGATROBAN, DABIGATRAN)	WARFARIN (COUMADIN)
Monitoring	aPTT	Anti-Xa level	Anti-Xa level	Anti-Xa level	aPTT	aPTT	INR
Half-life	1.5 hr	Enoxaparin: 4.5-7 hr; Tinzaparin: 3-4 hr; Dalteparin: 3-5 hr. All prolonged in renal impairment	24 hr. Prolonged in severe renal impairment	17-21 hr. Prolonged in severe renal impairment	Lepirudin: 1.3 hr; Bivalirudin: 25 min; Desirudin: 2 hr. All prolonged in renal impairment	Argatroban: 39-51 min; Dabigatran: 12-17 hr. All prolonged in renal impairment	20-60 hr
Clearance	Liver, reticuloendothelial system	Liver. 40% urine excretion	Plasma. Urine excretion	Metabolism unknown. Urine excretion	Lepirudin: metabolism unknown, 48% urine excretion. Bivalirudin: plasma (80%); urine (20%) excretion. Desirudin: kidney	Argatroban: liver; urine and fecal excretion. Dabigatran: liver; urine excretion	Liver. 92% urine excretion
Safety	Does not cross the placenta. No known risk of teratogenicity	Enoxaparin, tinzaparin, and dalteparin: do not appear to cross the placenta and are not believed to increase risk of birth defects on the basis of animal studies and some human studies outcomes.	No longer available in the United States. Many case reports of use of danaparoid in pregnancy in various doses and duration have shown successful pregnancy outcomes.	Fondaparinux: on the basis of experimental animal studies, use of fondaparinux in pregnancy is not expected to increase the risk of malformations. Small amounts cross the placenta, but clinical significance of such is unknown. Rivaroxaban: postimplantation pregnancy loss, increased fetal toxicity, and maternal hemorrhagic complications have been observed in animal studies. There are no adequate and well-controlled human studies.	Lepirudin: on the basis of experimental animal studies, it is not expected to increase the risk of congenital malformations, although it is known to cross rat placenta. Case reports of its use during various times of pregnancy did not show adverse events in exposed neonates. Bivalirudin: no epidemiologic studies of congenital anomalies among infants born to women treated with bivalirudin during pregnancy have been reported. Desirudin: teratogenic effects were observed in some animal reproductive studies.	Argatroban: did not produce malformations in rats and rabbits, but dosing was low compared with human therapeutic dose levels. Few case reports describing its use during pregnancy with no adverse newborn outcomes. Dabigatran: adverse events were observed in some animal reproductive studies. There are no adequate and well-controlled studies in pregnant women.	Warfarin crosses the placental barrier. Risk of birth defect with early exposure; potential for fatal hemorrhage to the fetus in utero.
Lactation	Safe	Enoxaparin: excretions in milk unknown. Tinzaparin, dalteparin: no data available	Little or no danaparoid appears in breast milk and would likely be inactivated in infant's stomach	Fondaparinux: appears in rat milk. Possible adverse effects of exposure through milk have not been described. Rivaroxaban: no data available	Lepirudin: in one case report, it was used during lactation without adverse events. It was not detectable in milk. Bivalirudin and desirudin: no data available	Argatroban, dabigatran: no data available	Safe
Administration	SC and IV	SC and IV	SC and IV	Fondaparinux: IV; Rivaroxaban: PO	IV	Argatroban: IV; Dabigatran: PO	PO

aPTT = activated partial thromboplastin time; INR = international normalized ratio; LMWH = low-molecular-weight heparin; UFH = unfractionated heparin.

From Mazer J, Zouein J, Bourjeily G. Treatment of pulmonary embolism in pregnancy. *US Respir Dis.* 2012;8:30-35.

TABLE 239-8 TREATMENT OF VENOUS THROMBOEMBOLISM IN PREGNANCY: ANTEPARTUM ANTICOAGULATION

| DRUG | PROPHYLAXIS | | AGGRESSIVE PROPHYLAXIS | | FULL TREATMENT |
	First 20 Weeks	20-37 Weeks	First 20 Weeks	20 Weeks to Term	
Dalteparin	5000 U/day	5000 U q12h	100 U/kg/day	100 U/kg/day	100 U/kg q12h with anti-Xa monitoring
Enoxaparin	30 mg/day	30 mg q12h	1 mg/kg/day	1 mg/kg/day	1 mg/kg q12h with anti-Xa monitoring
Tinzaparin	4500 U/day	4500 U q12h	88 U/kg/day	88 U/kg/day	88 U/kg q12h with anti-Xa monitoring
Heparin	Alternative if LMWH unaffordable: 750 U bid first 20 wk; 10,000 U bid wk 20-37		Alternative if LMWH unaffordable: 10,000 U bid to achieve anti-Xa level of 0.1-0.3 U/mL		Adjusted to mid-interval anti-Xa of 0.35-0.67 with q12h SC injections

LMWH = low-molecular-weight heparin.
Modified from Bourjeily G, Rosene-Montella K, eds. Venous thromboembolism in pregnancy. In: *Pulmonary Problems in Pregnancy, Respiratory Medicine.* New York: Humana Press; 2009.

low birthweight, IUGR, and cesarean section. Preterm delivery, gestational diabetes, and preeclampsia have also been associated with poorly controlled asthma, but it is unclear how systemic steroids contribute to these complications. Systemic steroids have been associated with an increased risk of premature rupture of membranes, preeclampsia, prematurity and low birthweight, and gestational diabetes. A retrospective study suggested that some complications may increase even in patients with mild asthma or asthma in good control.

PATHOBIOLOGY

The normal physiologic changes of pregnancy may contribute to variations in asthma severity. Factors contributing to the worsening of asthma include gastroesophageal reflux disease and rhinitis or sinusitis, triggers for asthma that are common during pregnancy. Gastroesophageal reflux may be manifested initially during pregnancy or worsen in patients with preexisting reflux owing to both hormonal and mechanical effects. Progesterone acts as a smooth muscle dilator that reduces lower esophageal sphincter pressure and contributes to delayed gastric emptying. Later in gestation, uterine enlargement further contributes to gastric displacement and increased reflux. Rhinitis and sinusitis clearly contribute to asthma exacerbations in nonpregnant patients. Gestational rhinitis related to hormonal effects is present in most pregnant women, and its behavior seems to parallel that of asthma. Bacterial sinusitis is five to six times more common in pregnancy and should be treated aggressively.

Hormonal effects on the airway may also contribute to asthma status. There is a progressive increase in serum cortisol and estradiol, which affects the quality of mucus production, and in progesterone, which decreases smooth muscle contractility and thereby causes airway dilation and improves minute ventilation. Immunologic factors during normal pregnancy may also contribute to the course of asthma. There is a suppression of cell-mediated immunity, with a predominant T_H2 environment and high interleukin-5 and tumor necrosis factor messenger RNA. In pregnant women with asthma (not receiving inhaled corticosteroid therapy), the T_H2/T_H1 ratio is even higher, possibly contributing to exacerbations.

The mechanism by which asthma exacerbations affect perinatal outcome is probably related to chronic maternal hypoxia, with consequent placental dysfunction and decreased uteroplacental flow, which contributes to decreased fetal growth. Poorly controlled asthma increases low birthweight 2.5-fold. Relative placental ischemia in asthma, particularly in disease that was poorly controlled before conception, is likely the link to an increased risk for preeclampsia. Placentas from women with asthma show a change in response to vasodilators and constrictors in vitro, similar to that seen in preeclampsia.

DIAGNOSIS

The diagnosis of asthma during pregnancy is the same as in the nonpregnant state (Chapter 87): normal forced expiratory volume in 1 second (FEV_1)/forced vital capacity on baseline pulmonary function tests with an obstructive physiology during exacerbations that is reversible either spontaneously or with medications. Airway hyperresponsiveness, as demonstrated by a methacholine challenge causing a 20% drop in FEV_1 from baseline, is also useful for diagnosis in pregnancy. Asthma severity in pregnancy is classified the same as in nonpregnant patients by the new classification of asthma severity that incorporates short-acting β-agonist use. The new classification includes both the level of impairment (daytime and nighttime frequency, quality of life and interference with normal activities, lung function) and the risk of exacerbations based on frequency and severity of prior exacerbations.

Differential Diagnosis

Dyspnea of pregnancy is a benign condition that often occurs later in pregnancy and is characterized by an increased awareness of the work of breathing that is disturbing for many patients. It is not likely to be acute, occurs less with rest, and should not interfere with normal daily activities. Dyspnea of pregnancy should not be accompanied by an increase in respiratory rate, wheezing, or hypoxia. It is important to consider pulmonary edema in any pregnant patient complaining of shortness of breath (Chapter 69). Pregnancy-related causes of pulmonary edema and acute respiratory distress syndrome include tocolytics (drugs that slow contractions), preeclampsia, gastric aspiration, amniotic fluid embolism, sepsis (related to pyelonephritis, chorioamnionitis, septic abortion), abruption, and obstetric hemorrhage. Cardiac causes should be suspected when pulmonary edema is manifested at the peak of blood volume (28 to 32 weeks), when occult valvular disease (Chapter 75) is most likely to be unmasked. Additional cardiac considerations are peripartum cardiomyopathy, preeclampsia, and ischemic heart disease, which in pregnancy may also be caused by coronary dissection.

TREATMENT ℞

Management of asthma during pregnancy does not differ greatly from that of the nonpregnant patient (Chapter 87).[15] However, normal arterial carbon dioxide pressure ($PaCO_2$) in pregnancy is 28 to 32 mm Hg, so a tachypneic pregnant patient with a $PaCO_2$ above this range may be in impending respiratory failure. Minute ventilation in pregnancy increases by an increase in tidal volume, but respiratory rate is unchanged by pregnancy, so tachypnea is always an abnormal finding.

The goal of asthma therapy during pregnancy is to maintain adequate control to ensure maternal and fetal health. It is always safer for pregnant women with asthma to be treated with asthma medications than to experience symptoms and exacerbations.[A5] Careful monitoring during all prenatal visits, preferably with spirometry, and stepped-up therapy are required both for maternal asthma control and to ensure appropriate oxygenation of the fetus. Maternal arterial oxygen saturation should be maintained at 95% or more, or the arterial oxygen pressure (PaO_2) should be maintained at 80 mm Hg or more, to maintain fetal oxygenation. E-Figure 239-1 outlines the classification of asthma and care for pregnant patients with asthma. More detailed recommendations for the home management of exacerbations and for hospitalization and emergency care for pregnant patients can be found in the *National Asthma Education and Prevention Program Working Group Report for Managing Asthma During Pregnancy.*

Albuterol is the preferred short-acting β-agonist because it has an excellent safety profile and the most data related to safety during human pregnancy. Inhaled corticosteroids are the preferred medication for long-term control. Budesonide is the preferred inhaled corticosteroid solely because of the amount of reassuring data on its use in pregnant patients. There are, however, no adverse data on the other inhaled corticosteroids. Data on the effectiveness and safety of long-acting β-agonists during pregnancy are limited, although it is reasonable to assume that they have a safety profile similar to that of albuterol. Salmeterol is the preferred agent, based only on its longer availability and lack of reports of adverse outcomes in exposed pregnancies. Cromolyn has an excellent safety profile but has limited effectiveness compared with inhaled corticosteroids.

Minimal published reports are available on the use of leukotriene receptor antagonists during pregnancy; however, animal safety data are reassuring. Current guidelines do not recommend leukotriene receptor antagonists because of the limited data, unless a patient's asthma was well controlled with this type of drug before pregnancy.

Intranasal corticosteroids are recommended for the treatment of allergic rhinitis (Chapter 251), given the limited systemic effect. The current nonsedating antihistamines of choice are loratadine and cetirizine.

Patients at risk for fatal asthma are those with a large bronchodilator response, overreliance on short-acting bronchodilators, marked circadian variation in lung function, history of hospitalization or intubation, and frequent systemic steroid use. There are specific considerations based on pregnancy physiology in pregnant patients who may require airway intubation. Pregnant patients have a low functional residual capacity and oxygen reserve, a more profound response to sedatives, airway edema, and larger airways. Intubation failure is much higher in pregnant women, so intubation should be performed by the most experienced professional available.

Breast-feeding should be encouraged in all patients with asthma as there is some evidence that it decreases atopy in offspring. Data are conflicting regarding the development of asthma in offspring.

DIABETES (Chapter 229)

Diabetes affects 1.85 million women of reproductive age, and it is estimated that preconception management could reduce the risk for 113,000 births per year. All women of reproductive age with diabetes should be counseled about the relationship between glucose control and congenital anomalies. Hyperglycemia is a teratogen, and the incidence of congenital anomalies is directly related to the hemoglobin A_{1c} level at conception (Fig. 239-3). The anomaly rate was as high as 11% in women without preconception care, including cardiac anomalies, neural tube defects, and sacral agenesis. The single most important contribution an internist can make to the prevention of congenital anomalies is to address pregnancy risk with all women of childbearing age with diabetes. The responsibility to normalize hemoglobin A_{1c} before conception falls to the medical care provider; once pregnancy is diagnosed and the patient is seen by her obstetrician, the teratogenic effects of glucose have already occurred.

DEFINITION

Gestational diabetes mellitus (GDM) is defined as glucose intolerance that first occurs or is first identified during pregnancy. Either type 1 or type 2 diabetes in a pregnant patient is referred to as preexisting or pregestational diabetes.

EPIDEMIOLOGY

The frequency of GDM is rising in the United States; it now occurs in 4 to 14% of all pregnancies, depending on the patient's characteristics. The epidemic of type 2 diabetes has resulted in a higher prevalence at a younger age; in the United States, there has been a 70% increase in the prevalence of diabetes in the 30- to 39-year-old age group versus 33% overall. The proportion of women with type 2 versus type 1 pregestational diabetes has also increased, from 26% in 1980 to 65% in 2000, and it is still increasing. The perinatal morbidity and mortality associated with type 2 diabetes is at least as great as that associated with type 1 during pregnancy.

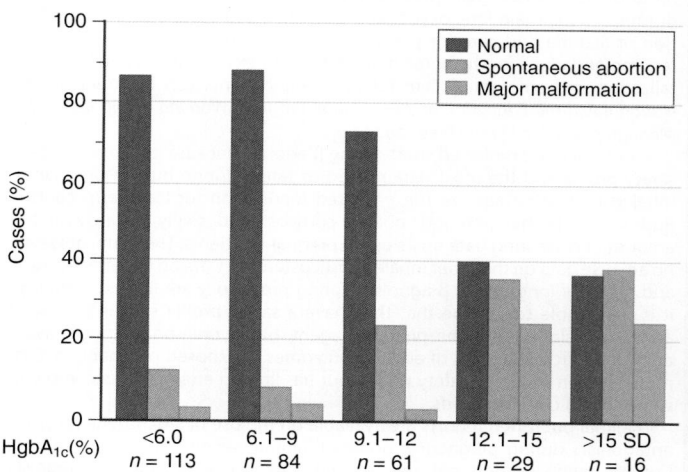

FIGURE 239-3. Relationship of hemoglobin A_{1c} (HgbA$_{1c}$), congenital anomalies, and spontaneous abortion.

PATHOBIOLOGY

Type 1 diabetes is caused by autoimmune destruction of pancreatic beta cells, resulting in an absolute insulin deficiency. Ninety percent of cases are diagnosed before the age of 25 years and are often associated with other autoimmune illnesses or a family history of autoimmune illness, including thyroid disorders, Addison's disease, and celiac disease. Type 2 diabetes is part of the metabolic syndrome, which includes insulin resistance, hyperinsulinemia, dyslipidemia, abdominal obesity, and hypertension with premature atherosclerosis; it probably has a genetic component. GDM may also be a manifestation of the metabolic syndrome, unmasked by the insulin-resistant state of pregnancy. Patients with GDM have a 50% chance for development of type 2 diabetes in the ensuing 5 to 10 years and a long-term risk of approximately 70%.

Pregnancy is a state of accelerated starvation and marked insulin resistance. Lower fasting glucose levels are seen early in the first trimester, and nocturnal hypoglycemia is common. There is blunted hypoglycemic awareness due to decreased epinephrine and norepinephrine release, with falls in blood glucose concentration and increased ketogenesis, resulting in an increased risk for diabetic ketoacidosis. Insulin requirements may decrease 20% in weeks 7 to 12 but then gradually rise later in gestation, such that insulin doses need to be increased by 16 weeks' gestation. Marked insulin resistance is related to the presence of elevated levels of cortisol, prolactin, human placental lactogen, and human placental growth hormone. Insulin sensitivity is decreased by about 50% in the third trimester, resulting in increased serum insulin and postprandial glucose levels, explaining the timing of the onset of GDM.

DIAGNOSIS

The diagnosis of pregestational diabetes is based on the finding of a fasting blood glucose level of more than 125 mg/dL or a 2-hour or random blood glucose level of 200 mg/dL or more. The American Diabetes Association recently added a hemoglobin A_{1c} level of 6.5% or higher as an acceptable alternative diagnostic criterion. GDM is based on the results of a blood glucose screen after a 50-g glucose challenge test (≥140 mg/dL), followed by a 3-hour confirmatory 100-g oral glucose tolerance test. Positive results are any two of the following: fasting, 95 mg/dL or more; 1 hour, 180 mg/dL; 2 hours, 155 mg/dL; and 3 hours, 140 mg/dL. It may be difficult to distinguish between GDM and type 2 diabetes that was not diagnosed before pregnancy. Elevated fasting glucose levels before 24 weeks' gestation and elevated hemoglobin A_{1c} are both suggestive of type 2 diabetes. Any diabetes diagnosed during pregnancy is referred to as GDM; if it persists post partum, it is reclassified as type 2.

TREATMENT Rx

Dietary recommendations are for 30 kcal/kg, with 40 to 50% carbohydrates, divided into three meals and three snacks. Aerobic exercise may decrease insulin resistance and reduce maternal glucose levels and may be an effective adjunct to diet in patients with GDM. Adjustment of medications should include the discontinuation of ACE inhibitors, ARBs, and statins and the institution of folate and prenatal vitamins. An assessment of baseline disease status in all patients with diabetes should include hemoglobin A_{1c}, ophthalmologic examination, electrocardiogram, assessment of urine protein excretion, serum creatinine concentration, and thyroid-stimulating hormone level. Baseline preeclampsia laboratory studies are also recommended.

The fetal assessment plan includes ultrasound to confirm dates and viability; this is done by the patient's obstetric care provider. There will also be a quad screen, looking for serum markers that suggest neural tube defects or Down syndrome; an ultrasound nuchal translucency and a level 2 ultrasound to assess for congenital anomalies; and a fetal echocardiogram.

Control of Blood Glucose

The goal of treatment for pregestational diabetes is the best hemoglobin A_{1c} level possible, without excessive hypoglycemia. This is achieved by frequent insulin adjustments and self-monitoring of blood glucose level at least four times a day. The specific goals for both GDM and pregestational diabetes are fasting glucose concentration of 65 to 95 mg/dL, 1-hour postprandial glucose concentration of less than 140 mg/dL, and 2-hour glucose concentration of less than 120 mg/dL. This is best achieved by multiple doses of insulin, including basal, intermediate, and long-acting insulin, with preprandial bolus rapid-acting insulin to cover the anticipated carbohydrate load. This regimen requires self-monitoring of blood glucose levels six or seven times a day, so it may be difficult to comply with. Further, the risk of serious hypoglycemia may limit these glycemic targets, particularly in women with type 1 diabetes. Extreme vigilance is required to avoid serious hypoglycemia, particularly in weeks 7 to 12, when insulin requirements are the lowest during pregnancy.[16] In patients with decreased glycemic awareness, the risk of night-time hypoglycemia is significant, and patients' partners should be counseled about this risk.

Insulin analogues are being used with increasing frequency. Of the rapid-acting analogues, there are data that lispro does not cross the placenta; there are no data yet on aspart. Although long-acting glargine is being used in pregnancy, its placental transfer is unknown, and there are theoretical concerns about its binding to the insulin-like growth factor receptor and its mito-genic potential.

Of the oral agents for which there are data, glyburide is safe and effica-cious in women with GDM, and it is more efficacious than metformin in this setting. [A6] Oral agents are less useful with significant insulin resistance and type 2 diabetes, so insulin continues to be the "gold standard" in this group. Metformin does not appear to increase the risk of congenital anomalies or spontaneous abortion, but it does cross the placenta. Women with polycystic ovary syndrome treated with metformin may regain their fertility and should be advised to use contraception. Recent trials support the safety of metfor-min in the second and third trimesters. In the United States, metformin is not yet recommended for the treatment of type 2 diabetes in pregnancy or for GDM. There are inadequate pregnancy data for the meglitinides and glitazones.

Maternal and Fetal Monitoring

During pregnancy, increased vigilance and continual assessment for the development of complications, including hypertension, preeclampsia, wors-ening nephropathy, and retinopathy, are required. The incidence of retinopa-thy in pregnant women with type 1 and type 2 diabetes is 34 to 50% and 3 to 5%, respectively. Nephropathy is found in 4% of diabetic pregnancies and is associated with increased maternal and perinatal morbidity. Most studies agree that pregnancy may accelerate the progression of nephropathy, but the reversibility of this complication is unclear. Most studies show a worsening of retinopathy in pregnant patients similar to that occurring during the same period in nonpregnant patients. The level of severity of retinopathy before pregnancy is most predictive of worsening during pregnancy, and treatment is recommended before conception.

Labor and Delivery

During labor and delivery, tight glucose control is necessary to avoid neo-natal hypoglycemia due to hyperinsulinemia at birth. The goal is to maintain serum glucose levels of 72 to 144 mg/dL. The use of an insulin drip with dex-trose infusion in active labor is recommended. Immediately after delivery, insulin requirements decrease to prepregnancy levels. Insulin needs should be one half to two thirds prepregnancy requirements, with a further decreased need found in breast-feeding patients.

Postpartum Considerations

Fifteen percent to 25% of type 1 diabetics develop postpartum thyroiditis, so all patients require postpartum measurements of thyroid-stimulating hormone and follow-up for 6 months. Other postpartum recommendations are to restart ACE inhibitors and to monitor closely for infection. It is impor-tant to discuss diabetes prevention in the offspring and to address con-traception. It is most important to recommend an effective contraceptive method that is acceptable to the patient. Oral estrogens can increase triglyc-erides, and both oral and injectable progesterone-only contraceptives may increase insulin resistance. Low-dose combined oral contraceptives and the progesterone-releasing intrauterine device appear to have little effect on glucose.

Insulin is acceptable in breast-feeding women, and limited data suggest that glyburide and metformin are safe as well. One small study found that glyburide is not excreted in breast milk and that metformin is excreted in a small amount that is probably not clinically significant.

PROGNOSIS AND COMPLICATIONS

The maternal complications of diabetes may be affected by pregnancy and may affect the course of the pregnancy. Patients with nephropathy experience an increase in proteinuria and a risk for progression of renal disease, especially if the serum creatinine concentration is more than 1.4 mg/dL. There is an increased risk for hypertension, which is seen in 30% of patients during the first trimester and 75% of patients by the third trimester. Autonomic neuropa-thy may worsen, as manifested by increasing gastroparesis, orthostatic hypo-tension, and decreased hypoglycemic awareness. Patients with long-standing diabetes may need to be evaluated for ischemic heart disease, which may impair the heart's ability to meet the cardiovascular demands of pregnancy. Pregnant patients are also at risk for hyperlipidemia and for preeclampsia. Diabetes increases the risk for operative delivery and for infections, the most common of which are wound, urinary tract, and respiratory.

Diabetic ketoacidosis may be precipitated by steroid use for fetal lung maturity, hyperemesis, infection, and noncompliance with insulin regimens. Acidosis may occur more quickly and at lower glucose levels in pregnant than in nonpregnant patients. There is a high fetal mortality associated with dia-betic ketoacidosis (9 to 10%), and patients should be monitored in an inten-sive care setting.

Fetal and Neonatal Effects (Fig. 239-4)

There is an increased risk of spontaneous abortion, fetal loss, congenital anomalies, preeclampsia, and preterm delivery in patients with diabetes. Poor

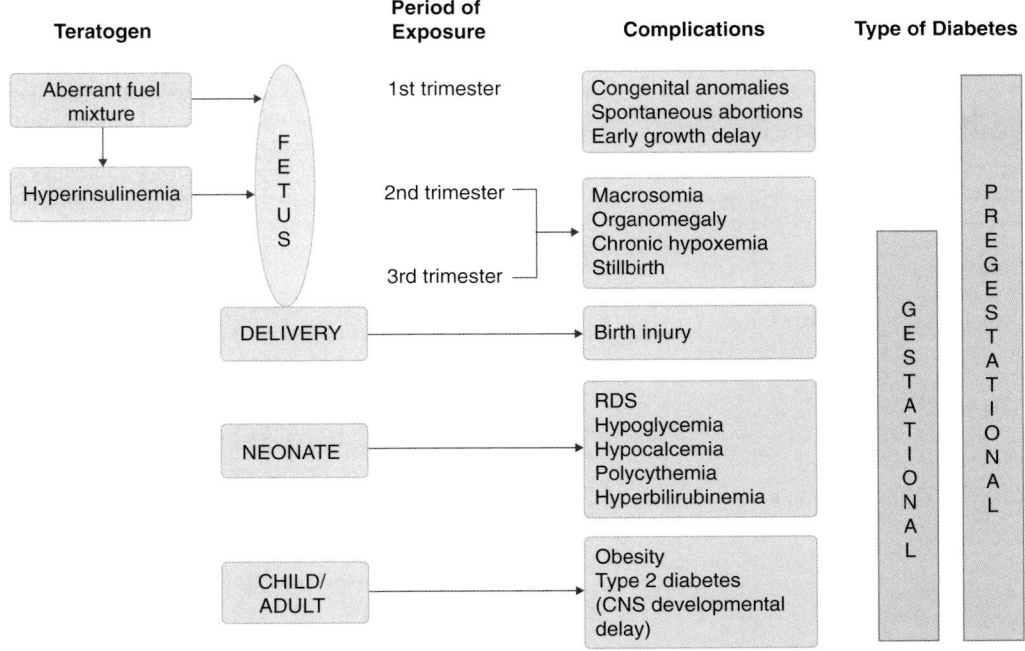

FIGURE 239-4. Fetal, neonatal, and childhood effects of exposure to hyperglycemia. CNS = central nervous system; RDS = respiratory distress syndrome.

glycemic control during pregnancy, especially in type 2 diabetes and GDM, is also associated with macrosomia (baby weighing >4000 g) and fetal intraventricular septal hypertrophy. Poor control is also associated with the effects of maternal vascular and renal disease and ketoacidosis, which include fetal loss, preeclampsia, and low birthweight. A study looking at differences in causes of pregnancy loss in type 1 and type 2 diabetic mothers compared the placental histology of patients with type 1 and type 2 diabetes and found an increase in histologic infarcts in type 2, suggesting a vascular rather than a glycemic cause of pregnancy complications and signs of abnormal development of placentas from patients with type 1 disease.[17]

Neonatal complications include respiratory distress syndrome, hypoglycemia, hypocalcemia, cardiac hypertrophy, hyperbilirubinemia, and polycythemia. The risk of hypoglycemia may be ameliorated by careful control of maternal glucose concentration during labor and delivery. Normalization of maternal glucose concentration prevents hyperinsulinemia in the fetus and mitigates the risk of neonatal hypoglycemia.

Maternal Effects
GDM is a marker for type 2 diabetes; 50% of patients will develop type 2 diabetes within 7 to 10 years, and overall, 70% will develop the disease. Patients who have had GDM need directed testing at their 6-week postpartum visit, annual screening, and recommendations for lifestyle modification and cardiovascular risk reduction. Offspring of patients with GDM and type 2 diabetes are at increased risk for obesity and glucose intolerance.

● LIVER DISEASE IN PREGNANCY
Liver disease found during pregnancy may be unique to pregnancy, represent underlying liver disease unmasked during pregnancy, or develop during pregnancy. Most liver function test results are unchanged by pregnancy with the exception of an increase in alkaline phosphatase (which is produced by the placenta), an increase in fibrinogen, and a decrease in serum albumin.

Table 239-9 outlines pregnancy-related liver disease. This discussion focuses on diseases unique to pregnancy and those diseases for which there are specific management considerations during pregnancy.

Liver Diseases Unique to Pregnancy
INTRAHEPATIC CHOLESTASIS OF PREGNANCY (OBSTETRIC CHOLESTASIS)
DIAGNOSIS
Intrahepatic cholestasis of pregnancy (ICP) or obstetric cholestasis affects 0.5 to 2% of pregnant women, although in Bolivia and Chile, rates of 4 to 28% have been observed. ICP is manifested most commonly in the late second or third trimester with intense pruritus accompanied by an increase in serum bile acids and often transaminases and prothrombin time. ICP is likely to be a metabolic disease of multifactorial etiology characterized in most cases by a genetic variation in the biliary transporters and receptors that govern bile acid homeostasis.[18] It is more common in patients with underlying hepatitis C, so it is important to screen all patients with hepatitis C serology. ICP is

TABLE 239-9   LIVER DISEASE AND PREGNANCY

UNIQUE TO PREGNANCY

Acute fatty liver of pregnancy
HELLP syndrome (hemolysis, elevated liver enzymes, and low platelets)
Hyperemesis gravidarum
Intrahepatic cholestasis of pregnancy
Preeclampsia and eclampsia

INCREASED INCIDENCE DURING PREGNANCY

Budd-Chiari syndrome
Drug-induced hepatotoxicity
Gallstones
Liver transplantation
Sepsis
Viral hepatitis

UNDERLYING CONDITION THAT MAY BE REVEALED

Autoimmune hepatitis
Cirrhosis
Hepatitis B and C
Primary biliary cirrhosis
Primary sclerosing cholangitis
Wilson's disease

Modified from Mufti AR, Reau N. Liver disease in pregnancy. *Clin Liver Dis.* 2012;16:247-269.

associated with preterm labor, meconium staining, fetal hypoxia, and sudden fetal demise.

TREATMENT   Rx
Because no antenatal testing has been able to predict those patients at risk for fetal demise, consensus guidelines recommend delivery at 37 to 38 weeks of gestation in patients with a significant elevation in serum bile acids (≥40 μmol/L). The treatment of choice is ursodeoxycholic acid at 10 to 15 mg/kg, which leads to both symptomatic and biochemical improvement. There are no studies demonstrating a beneficial effect on pregnancy outcome.

PREECLAMPSIA AND ECLAMPSIA
As discussed before, preeclampsia can be associated with liver abnormalities including liver edema and infarction, subcapsular hematoma, liver laceration, and HELLP syndrome (hemolysis, elevated liver enzymes, and low platelets).

HYPEREMESIS GRAVIDARUM
Hyperemesis gravidarum, defined as severe persistent nausea and vomiting of pregnancy with weight loss, ketosis, or dehydration, can be associated with transaminase elevations in 50 to 60% of cases.

TREATMENT   Rx
Treatment is supportive with rehydration, antiemetics, and vitamin replacement,[19] often requiring hospitalization. Oral fluid repletion can often be accomplished as indwelling intravenous catheters have been associated with a significant risk of thrombosis and of infections. Hyperemesis gravidarum is usually a reversible condition with no permanent liver damage.

ACUTE FATTY LIVER OF PREGNANCY
DIAGNOSIS
Acute fatty liver of pregnancy is a rare condition that is estimated to occur in 5 per 100,000 pregnancies. It most commonly is manifested in the third trimester and post partum; in its most severe form, it can be associated with fulminant liver failure and the need for liver transplantation. Maternal mortality rates were earlier thought to be as high as 20%, but a more recent U.K. study found a 2% maternal and 11% perinatal mortality rate. The Swansea criteria have recently been validated as a diagnostic tool for the diagnosis of acute fatty liver of pregnancy (Table 239-10).

PROGNOSIS
The maternal mortality rate has been estimated at 18%. Acute fatty liver of pregnancy is associated with an inherited defect in mitochondrial fatty acid B oxidation. The defect results in accumulation of toxic metabolites produced by the fetus and placenta that, after entering the maternal circulation, are deposited in maternal liver. Diagnosis is clinical, based on the constellations of findings described in Table 239-10. Liver function abnormalities can be severe, and hypoglycemia is a poor prognostic sign. Anyone with evidence of liver failure should be seen at a transplant center as early in the course as possible.

TABLE 239-10   SWANSEA DIAGNOSTIC CRITERIA FOR ACUTE FATTY LIVER OF PREGNANCY

Six or more of the following features in the absence of another explanation:

• Vomiting	• Leukocytosis
• Abdominal pain	• Ascites or bright liver on ultrasound scan
• Polydipsia/polyuria	• Elevated transaminases
• Encephalopathy	• Elevated ammonia
• Elevated bilirubin	• Renal impairment
• Hypoglycemia	• Coagulopathy
• Elevated urate	• Microvesicular steatosis on liver biopsy

From Ch'ng CL, Morgan M, Hainsworth I, et al. Prospective study of liver dysfunction in pregnancy in Southwest Wales. *Gut.* 2002;51:876-880.

Preexisting or New-Onset Liver Disease during Pregnancy

The major importance of recognition of underlying liver disease in pregnancy is both for maternal health and for those diseases in which lack of treatment results in a high rate of vertical transmission to the fetus or neonate.

VIRAL HEPATITIS

Hepatitis C virus (HCV) infection (Chapter 148) has become an increasingly important and prevalent issue in pregnancy; maternal to child HCV vertical transmission rates are 5 to 10% and as high as 22% with HIV coinfection. New screening guidelines will lead to more universal screening in this age group. The mode of delivery does not have an impact on vertical transmission rates. The higher the viral load and the longer the duration of ruptured membranes, the higher the risk of transmission. Infection with hepatitis E virus and herpes simplex virus is much more likely to be severe in pregnant women. Particularly in the third trimester, it can be associated with fulminant disease and high maternal and perinatal mortality. All pregnant patients with new-onset hepatitis should also be screened for cytomegalovirus and Epstein-Barr virus.

TREATMENT   Rx

All pregnant women in the United States are screened for hepatitis B virus (HBV) with hepatitis B surface antigen (Chapter 148). All neonates born to positive mothers are treated with hepatitis B immune globulin within 12 hours of birth and given their first dose of HBV vaccine at birth. This regimen is less effective in mothers with a high viral load or in the presence of hepatitis B e antigen positivity.

Fetal risks involved in the use of interferon during pregnancy outweigh its benefits. All current oral anti-HBV drugs (including lamivudine, entecavir, and adefovir) are categorized as Food and Drug Administration pregnancy category C, except telbivudine and tenofovir, which are pregnancy category B drugs.[20] Vertical transmission of HCV occurs, but data supporting recommendations for prevention are limited. Both ribavirin and interferon are contraindicated during pregnancy.

CHRONIC LIVER DISEASE

Chronic liver disease may be associated with anovulation, amenorrhea, and infertility. Thus, it is unusual to see pregnant patients with significant liver decompensation and cirrhosis. Patients with portal hypertension, autoimmune hepatitis, Wilson's disease, hepatic masses, and successful liver transplantation will be seen during pregnancy.

TREATMENT   Rx

The management of these patients requires an understanding of their course in pregnancy and a recognition of the importance of continuing prepregnant treatment.

Portal hypertension (Chapter 153) of any cause will be affected by the increase in blood volume during pregnancy, requiring careful follow-up and management of esophageal varices and splenic artery aneurysm. β-Blockers should be continued, and baseline endoscopy should be done early to consider banding of larger varices.

Autoimmune hepatitis (Chapter 149) improves dramatically with immunosuppression, so many women regain fertility with treatment.[21] Immunosuppression with steroids and azathioprine should be continued to avoid relapse and progression of disease. The cholestasis associated with primary biliary cirrhosis can be treated with ursodeoxycholic acid as outlined for ICP.

Similar to women with autoimmune hepatitis, patients with treated Wilson's disease (Chapter 211) regain fertility. Chelation therapy should be continued as discontinuation is associated with marked rises in copper levels and can lead to fulminant liver failure.

Hepatic masses are most commonly benign adenomas, focal nodular hyperplasia, or hemangiomas in women of childbearing age. Careful follow-up of these estrogen-sensitive masses is important because enlargement and hemorrhage may be complications of pregnancy.

● SUMMARY

Women of childbearing age with chronic medical conditions benefit greatly from preconception counseling and interventions that address control of their disease and safety of their medications. Pregnant patients with acute or chronic medical illnesses require a multidisciplinary team that understands the maternal and fetal risks related to both the underlying illness and untreated disease. Pregnancy is a window of opportunity to address maternal health, and the maternal response to pregnancy may be predictive of future risk. The 6-week postpartum visit, rather than being the end of pregnancy care, should represent the beginning of a woman's long-term health care.

Grade A References

A1. Koopmans CM, Bijlenga D, Groen H, et al. Induction of labour versus expectant monitoring for gestational hypertension or mild pre-eclampsia after 36 weeks' gestation (HYPITAT): a multicentre, open-label randomised controlled trial. *Lancet.* 2009;374:979-988.

A2. Belfort MA, Anthony J, Saade GR, et al. A comparison of magnesium sulfate and nimodipine for the prevention of eclampsia. *N Engl J Med.* 2003;348:304-341.

A3. Roberts JM, Myatt L, Spong CY, et al. Vitamins C and E to prevent complications of pregnancy-associated hypertension. *N Engl J Med.* 2010;362:1282-1291.

A4. Henderson JT, Whitlock EP, O'Connor E, et al. Low-dose aspirin for prevention of morbidity and mortality from preeclampsia: a systematic evidence review for the U.S. Preventive Services Task Force. *Ann Intern Med.* 2014;160:695-703.

A5. Bain E, Pierides KL, Clifton VL, et al. Interventions for managing asthma in pregnancy. *Cochrane Database Syst Rev.* 2014;10:CD010660.

A6. Moore LE, Clokey D, Rappaport VJ, et al. Metformin compared with glyburide in gestational diabetes: a randomized controlled trial. *Obstet Gynecol.* 2010;115:55-59.

GENERAL REFERENCES

For the General References and other additional features, please visit Expert Consult at https://expertconsult.inkling.com.

240

MENOPAUSE

DEBORAH GRADY AND ELIZABETH BARRETT-CONNOR

DEFINITION

All healthy women transition from a reproductive or premenopausal period marked by regular ovulation and cyclic menstrual bleeding to a postmenopausal period marked by infertility and amenorrhea (Fig. 240-1). The onset of the menopausal transition is generally marked by subtle shortening in the length of the menstrual cycle and changes in the duration or amount of menstrual flow. As the menopausal transition progresses, menstrual cycles are missed until complete amenorrhea occurs, but the pattern of missed cycles is not predictable. Amenorrhea for a few months is not a good indicator of menopause because one half to three fourths of middle-aged women who are amenorrheic for 6 months resume cycles. Thus, menopause is typically defined retrospectively after 12 months of amenorrhea.

EPIDEMIOLOGY

The menopausal transition usually begins in the middle to late 40s and lasts approximately 4 years, with menopause occurring at a median age of 51 years and ranging from approximately 45 to 57 years. Age at menopause has not changed significantly during the past century. However, a gradual increase in life expectancy to the low 80s now means that the average woman is postmenopausal for more than one third of her life. Age at menopause does not vary significantly by race or ethnicity, but on average, cigarette smokers experience menopause approximately 2 years earlier than nonsmokers do.

BIOLOGY

During the early menopausal transition, estrogen levels are generally normal (50 to 200 pg/mL, depending on the stage of the menstrual cycle) or even slightly elevated, whereas the levels of follicle-stimulating hormone (FSH) and luteinizing hormone (LH) begin to increase (see Fig. 240-1). As the menopause transition progresses, estrogen levels fall markedly, and FSH continues to increase. After menopause, women do not ovulate, and their ovaries do not produce estradiol or progesterone. However, a small amount of estrogen may be produced by metabolism of adrenal steroids to estradiol in peripheral fat tissue. In the early postmenopausal period, mean estradiol

	Reproductive			Menopause Transition		Postmenopause	
Reproductive stage	Early	Peak	Late	Early	Late	Early	Late
				Perimenopause			
Menstrual cycle	Variable or regular	Regular		Cycle length variable, 1 or 2 missed cycles per year	3 or more missed cycles	None	
Age (duration)	Puberty to mid-40s			Mid-40s to mid-50s (4 yr)		Mean of 51 years to death	
Steroid hormones	Estradiol 50 to 200 pg/mL			Same or slightly higher		40 pg/mL	0-15 pg/mL
	Testosterone 400 pg/mL			Same		same	same
Pituitary hormones	FSH 10 mIU/mL day 2-4			Same or higher		>100 mIU/mL	
	LH 10 mIU/mL day 2-4			Same or higher		>100 mIU/mL	

FIGURE 240-1. Stages of the menopause transition. FSH = follicle-stimulating hormone; LH = luteinizing hormone.

levels average approximately 40 pg/mL, and they fall to less than 15 pg/mL in the late postmenopausal period. Depending on the measurement method, estradiol is unmeasurable in approximately 15 to 30% of older postmenopausal women. After menopause, testosterone levels may fall slightly but are generally similar to premenopausal levels.

It is not clear what causes menopause, but two leading theories have been proposed.[1] Age-related depletion of ovarian follicles may lead to decreased production of estrogen and inhibin and may thus cause altered hypothalamic-pituitary feedback that results in menopause. Alternatively, age-related changes in hypothalamic production of gonadotropin-releasing hormone and subsequent effects on FSH and LH may be responsible for the increased rate of loss of ovarian follicles, declining ovarian function, and menopause.

MENOPAUSAL SYMPTOMS

Menopause is a positive occurrence in the life of many women. It marks the end of cyclic bleeding and the need for birth control. It occurs at an age when children generally have become independent adults, thereby reducing family and child care responsibilities. Conversely, menopause is a notable sign of aging in cultures that value youth. In addition, it often occurs with other stresses, such as caring for elderly or ill parents. Women in the menopausal transition commonly report a wide variety of symptoms, including hot flushes, night sweats, vaginal dryness, trouble sleeping, sexual dysfunction, depression, anxiety, labile mood, memory loss, fatigue, headache, joint pains, weight gain, and urinary incontinence.

Only vasomotor symptoms, vaginal dryness, and sleep disturbance are consistently associated with the menopausal transition. Other reported symptoms may result from aging or stress associated with menopause. Some symptoms, such as depression, anxiety, memory loss, and fatigue, may be the consequence of frequent hot flushes or poor sleep.

Vasomotor Symptoms
DEFINITION

Vasomotor symptoms include hot flushes, chills, and sweats.[2] A hot flush is a sudden feeling of warmth, generally most intense over the face, neck, and chest. The duration is variable, but it averages approximately 4 minutes. It is often accompanied by sweating that can be profuse and followed by a chill.

EPIDEMIOLOGY

The prevalence of hot flushes is maximal in the late menopausal transition, occurring in approximately 50% of women (Fig. 240-2).[3] However, prevalence varies markedly, depending on the definition of flushing (any flushing, daily flushing, troublesome flushing) and the population studied. Lower prevalence is reported among women in China, Japan, and other Asian countries. The reason for this variation is not clear, but investigators have suggested that it may result from differences in biology, cultural influences on

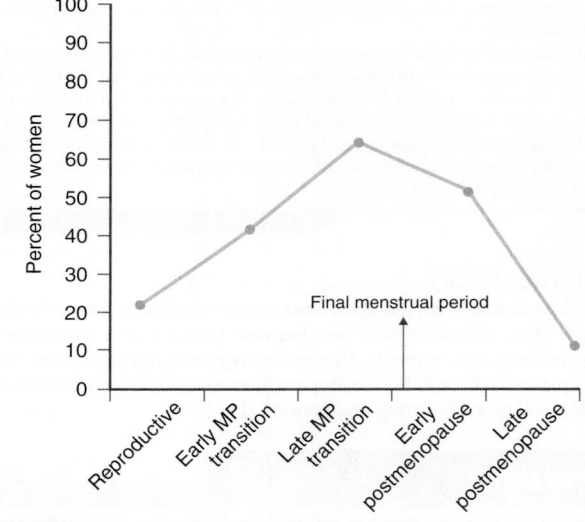

FIGURE 240-2. Prevalence of hot flushes during the menopause (MP) transition.

experiencing or reporting flushes, or diet and lifestyle. In the United States, flushes are more common in African American and Latina women and less common in Chinese and Japanese women compared with white women. Approximately 15% of women with menopausal symptoms consult a physician.

Cigarette smoking increases the likelihood of flushing, but other potential risk factors, including surgical menopause, physical activity, body mass index, alcohol consumption, and socioeconomic status, have been inconsistently associated with hot flushes. Currently, there is no way to predict whether an individual woman will suffer from hot flushes.

In most women, hot flushes are transient. Approximately 50% of women report resolution of symptoms within a few years, and symptoms resolve in about 90% within 8 years. However, some women continue to have frequent and severe flushes many years after menopause. Approximately 10% of women in their middle to late 60s report significant flushing. It is not clear why flushes persist for many years in some women and resolve in others.

PATHOBIOLOGY

Thermoregulation is abnormal in menopausal women with hot flushes. Body temperature is regulated by inducing vasodilation and sweating to release heat and vasoconstriction and shivering to conserve heat. Thermoregulation is complex and depends on central stimuli from the anterior hypothalamus and local changes in cutaneous vasoconstriction or dilation (Chapters 223 and 418). A hot flush is similar to a heat dissipation response because both result in vasodilation, sweating, and reduction in core body temperature. The mechanism of altered thermoregulation is not clear. The acute vasodilation associated with hot flushes is preceded by a marked increase in skin sympathetic activity, which mediates vasodilation by a number of substances including nitric oxide, vasoactive intestinal peptide, prostaglandins, and substance P. Local blockade of skin sympathetic activity prevents vasodilation, as does local blockade of nitric oxide.

One theory suggests that abnormalities in central nervous system adrenergic neurotransmission cause hot flushes. This theory is supported by studies showing that systemic administration of yohimbine, an α_2-adrenergic antagonist that increases norepinephrine release, provokes hot flushes, whereas administration of clonidine, an α_2-adrenergic agonist that decreases norepinephrine release, reduces the frequency of hot flushes. Alternatively, some evidence indicates that changes in serotonergic neurotransmission could cause hot flushes. Lower estrogen levels are associated with lower levels of serotonin (5-hydroxytryptamine) in blood, resulting in increased sensitivity of 5-hydroxytryptamine type 2A receptors in the hypothalamus. Stimulation of these receptors can alter the thermoregulatory set point in animals. Mild stressors, such as heat and anxiety, cause a brief release of 5-hydroxytryptamine that may stimulate central 5-hydroxytryptamine type 2A receptors, lower the thermoregulatory set point, and cause flushing. This hypothesis is supported by the finding that drugs that increase central serotonin levels are modestly effective in the treatment of hot flushes.

Estrogen treatment effectively relieves hot flushes, but the exact role of estrogen in flushing is not clear. Fluctuations in estrogen levels in an individual woman do not correlate with the onset of flushes. Prepubertal girls with very low levels of endogenous estrogen, premenopausal women with marked fluctuations in estrogen during the menstrual cycle, and most postmenopausal women with low, constant levels of estradiol do not experience flushing. However, women with gonadal dysgenesis (Chapter 233) who are treated with estrogen for several months experience flushing when treatment is discontinued. Thus, withdrawal of estrogen, rather than the absolute estrogen level, appears to play a key role in the etiology of hot flushes.

In addition to changes in estradiol, menopause is associated with multiple other hormonal changes. In the Study of Women's Health Across the Nation, a large cohort study in the United States, lower estradiol was associated with flushing in middle-aged women in univariate models. However, higher FSH was the only measure independently associated with flushing after multivariate adjustment for other hormone levels. Hot flushes correlate with pulsatile increases in LH, but suppression of LH with gonadotropin-releasing hormone agonists does not eliminate flushing. Androgens may also play a role because men who are treated with androgen deprivation therapy for prostate cancer frequently report flushing.

DIAGNOSIS

Vasomotor symptoms are classic manifestations of the menopause transition, and the diagnosis is generally obvious from a woman's age and description of the symptoms. No abnormal physical findings are associated with hot flushes. Estradiol, FSH, and LH levels may be in the normal premenopausal range during the menopausal transition (see Fig. 240-1). A woman in her middle 40s to middle 50s who complains of classic hot flushes does not require any specific physical or laboratory evaluation unless there is good reason to suspect another cause of flushing (Table 240-1). However, an FSH determination may be helpful in assessing the risk for pregnancy. A woman

TABLE 240-1 DIFFERENTIAL DIAGNOSIS OF HOT FLUSHES

Alcohol consumption
Carcinoid syndrome
Dumping syndrome
Hyperthyroidism
Narcotic withdrawal
Pheochromocytoma
Medications
   Aromatase inhibitors
   Gonadotropin-releasing hormone agonists or antagonists
   Nicotinic acid
   Nitrates
   Selective estrogen receptor modulators (tamoxifen and raloxifene)

in her middle 40s to middle 50s with an FSH level obtained on the third day after menses that is higher than 20 IU/L is at very low risk of becoming pregnant.

TREATMENT Rx

Because self-reported frequency and severity of hot flushes improve markedly with placebo, conclusive evidence of efficacy of treatments requires randomized, blinded trials.

General Measures
Behavioral and Alternative Therapies
Many women have mild flushes and obtain adequate relief with simple measures such as lowering ambient temperature and wearing lighter clothing. Weight loss has been shown to improve hot flashes, but moderate exercise does not alleviate flushing.

There is no convincing evidence that acupuncture, yoga, Chinese herbs, dong quai, evening primrose oil, ginseng, kava, omega-3 fatty acids, or red clover extract improves hot flushes, although a more recent trial found that, among health sedentary menopausal women, yoga appears to improve menopausal quality of lie.[A1] Evidence regarding black cohosh is mixed but primarily negative. Multiple trials have been performed with different phytoestrogen preparations. Although some of these studies have reported benefit, the weight of evidence, especially from good-quality trials with blinded comparisons, suggests little benefit. One trial of vitamin E supplementation found an improvement in flushes, but the decrease was only one hot flush per day. Many women prefer alternative medications because they believe that these treatments are harmless, but phytoestrogens and possibly black cohosh bind estrogen receptors and theoretically could cause adverse outcomes similar to those observed with estrogen. No studies of these preparations have been of adequate size or duration to document safety.

Medical Therapy
Estrogens
Multiple randomized trials have demonstrated that estrogen markedly improves the frequency and severity of hot flushes.[4,5] All types, preparations, and routes of administration of estrogen are effective, reducing the frequency of hot flushes 60 to 95%, depending on the dose. Higher doses of estrogen may control symptoms more rapidly but are also associated with a higher rate of side effects, including uterine bleeding, breast tenderness, and headache.

At similar biologically active doses, oral and transdermal estrogens are approximately equally effective for treatment of vasomotor symptoms. Oral estrogens undergo first-pass metabolism in the liver that results in changes in hepatic proteins and enzymes. Hepatic effects are responsible for the beneficial effects of estrogen on lipoproteins (reduced low-density lipoprotein cholesterol and increased high-density lipoprotein cholesterol) but may also cause adverse effects, such as increases in clotting factors. The transdermal route may be safer because it minimizes these changes.

Many estrogen preparations are approved for treatment of vasomotor symptoms (Table 240-2).[6] To individualize treatment, physicians should become familiar with several of these preparations.

Treatment with estrogen alone markedly increases the risk for uterine hyperplasia and cancer. The risk for endometrial abnormalities appears not to be increased with the use of vaginal estrogens that deliver low systemic doses, especially if they are used only a few times per week, as is generally recommended (Table 240-3).

Adding a progestin to the estrogen regimen prevents the increased risk for uterine cancer. For this reason, a woman with a uterus who takes estrogen should also be given a progestin.[7] There is no reason to add progestins to the hormone regimen in women who have had a hysterectomy. Several progestins are approved by the U.S. Food and Drug Administration (FDA) for this purpose and are available to add to estrogen or in preparations combined with estrogen (see Table 240-2). Two general approaches are used in prescribing progestins to protect the endometrium. Sequential therapy (estrogen given daily with a progestin added on the last 10 to 14 days of a 28-day cycle) results in endometrial shedding and cyclic bleeding resembling a menstrual period in approximately 80% of women. To avoid monthly menstruation-like bleeding, the progestin may be added to estrogen every 3 to 6 months. However, data regarding the safety of this "long cycle" approach to prevent endometrial hyperplasia are mixed, and women using this regimen should undergo vaginal ultrasound or endometrial biopsy if they experience abnormal vaginal bleeding.

Alternatively, the progestin can be added to the estrogen every day. This continuous regimen results in endometrial atrophy and unpredictable uterine spotting or bleeding that can be difficult for the woman to anticipate and manage. Bleeding occurs in approximately 80% of women in the first 6 months of continuous treatment. Amenorrhea becomes common with prolonged use, but some women continue to bleed or spot for many years.

The most commonly used progestins in sequential regimens in women using standard doses of estrogens (0.625 mg oral conjugated estrogens, 1 mg

TABLE 240-2   ESTROGEN AND PROGESTIN PREPARATIONS FOR TREATMENT OF MENOPAUSAL VASOMOTOR SYMPTOMS

HORMONES	GENERIC NAME	BRAND NAME	DOSE (mg/day)
ESTROGENS*			
Oral	Conjugated estrogens	Premarin	0.3, 0.45, **0.625**, 0.9, 1.25
	17β-Estradiol	Estrace/ generics	0.5, **1.0**, 2.0
Transdermal	17β-Estradiol	Alora patch[†]	0.025, **0.05**, 0.075, 0.1
		Climara patch[‡]	0.025, 0.0375, **0.05**, 0.075, 0.1
		Menostar patch[‡]	0.014
		Evamist spray	1.53/spray
		Elestrin gel	0.025/pump
Vaginal	Estradiol acetate	Femring vaginal ring[§]	0.05, 0.10
	0.05, 0.1		
PROGESTINS			
Oral	Medroxyprogesterone acetate	Provera/ generics	2.5, 5.0, 10.0
	Micronized progesterone	Prometrium	100, 200 (in peanut oil)
Vaginal	Progesterone	Prochieve 4%	45 every other day
COMBINATION PREPARATIONS			
Oral sequential[‖]	Conjugated estrogens and medroxyprogesterone acetate	Premphase	0.625 + 5.0
Oral continuous[¶]	Conjugated estrogens and medroxyprogesterone acetate	Prempro	0.625 + 2.5 or 5.0; 0.45 + 2.5 or 1.5; 0.3 + 1.5
	17β-Estradiol and norethindrone acetate	Activella	1.0 + 0.5; 0.5 + 0.1
	Conjugated estrogens and bazedoxifene	Duavee	0.45 + 20
Transdermal continuous[¶]	17β-Estradiol and levonorgestrel	Climara Pro[†]	0.045 + 0.015
	17β-Estradiol and norethindrone acetate	CombiPatch[†]	0.05 + 0.14 or 0.25

*Approximately equivalent doses of estrogens are shown in **bold**.
[†]Patch applied twice per week.
[‡]Patch applied once per week.
[§]Vaginal ring inserted every 90 days; note that Femring, as opposed to the vaginal preparations listed in Table 240-3, delivers systemic levels of estrogen and should be opposed by a progestin in women with a uterus.
[‖]Each pill contains estrogen days 1 to 14 and estrogen with progestin days 15 to 28.
[¶]Each pill or patch contains estrogen and progestin.

TABLE 240-3   ESTROGEN VAGINAL PREPARATIONS FOR TREATMENT OF VAGINAL DRYNESS*

PREPARATION	GENERIC NAME	BRAND NAME	DOSE
Vaginal cream	Conjugated estrogens	Premarin	0.625 mg/2 g cream: 2 g/day for 2 wk, then 1-2 g 2 to 3 times/wk
	17β-Estradiol	Estrace	0.1 mg/2 g cream: 2 g/day for 2 wk, then 1-2 g 2 to 3 times/wk
Vaginal tablet	Estradiol hemihydrate	Vagifem	0.025 mg tablet: 1 tablet/day for 2 wk, then 1 tablet twice/wk
Vaginal ring	17β-Estradiol	Estring[†]	0.0075 mg/day

*Most oral, transdermal, and vaginal products listed in Table 240-2 for treatment of vasomotor symptoms are also approved for treatment of vaginal dryness.
[†]Vaginal ring is inserted every 90 days.

TABLE 240-4   RESULTS OF THE WOMEN'S HEALTH INITIATIVE RANDOMIZED TRIALS OF THE EFFECTS OF POSTMENOPAUSAL HORMONE THERAPY ON DISEASE OUTCOMES

	RELATIVE RISK AND 95% CONFIDENCE INTERVAL	
OUTCOMES	*Estrogen and Progestin**	*Estrogen*[†]
Coronary heart disease events	1.29 (1.02-1.63)	0.91 (0.75-1.12)
Stroke	1.41 (1.07-1.85)	1.39 (1.10-1.77)
Pulmonary embolism	2.13 (1.39-3.25)	1.34 (0.87-2.06)
Breast cancer	1.26 (1.00-1.59)	0.77 (0.59-1.01)
Colon cancer	0.63 (0.43-0.92)	1.08 (0.75-1.55)
Hip fracture	0.66 (0.45-0.98)	0.61 (0.41-0.91)
Dementia	2.05 (1.21-3.48)	1.49 (0.83-2.66)
Death	0.98 (0.82-1.18)	1.04 (0.88-1.22)

*Results of the Women's Health Initiative estrogen plus progestin randomized trial: 16,608 postmenopausal women without hysterectomy randomized to 0.625 mg conjugated estrogen plus 2.5 mg medroxyprogesterone acetate per day or identical placebo and observed for 5.2 years.
[†]Results of the Women's Health Initiative estrogen-only randomized trial: 10,739 postmenopausal women with hysterectomy randomized to 0.625 mg conjugated estrogen per day or identical placebo and observed for 6.8 years.

oral estradiol, or 0.05 mg transdermal estradiol) are medroxyprogesterone acetate 5 mg and micronized progesterone 200 mg for 10 to 14 days per month. Continuous regimens generally include about half these progestin doses given daily. In some situations, it may be slightly less costly to prescribe estrogen and progestins separately, but the convenience of taking a single pill and the assurance that the estrogen is adequately opposed by progestin make combination preparations preferable.

A combination of conjugated equine estrogens (0.45 mg) and bazedoxifene (20 mg) has been approved by the FDA for treatment of hot flashes in women with a uterus. Bazedoxifene is a selective estrogen receptor modulator that, like progestin, appears to block the carcinogenic effects of estrogen on the uterus. In clinical trials, conjugated estrogens plus bazedoxifene reduced the frequency of hot flashes about 80%, improved dyspareunia, and increased bone density with few side effects. [A2] Studies of up to 2 years have not identified other important adverse effects, such as endometrial cancer, breast cancer, venous thromboembolic events, or stroke, but experience with this preparation is limited.

The use of "bioidentical hormones" is based on the concept that estrogens (estradiol, estrone, and estriol) and progestins (progesterone) made from plant products are identical to women's endogenous hormones and therefore more natural, safe, and effective than FDA-approved hormone preparations. Bioidentical hormone therapy often uses doses and combinations of steroid hormones guided by the patient's symptoms or serum hormone levels, and prescriptions are generally filled by Internet-based compounding pharmacies. There is little scientific rationale for the mixtures and ratios of hormones employed, and there are no adequate clinical trial data to support the safety or efficacy of these regimens, some of which include very large doses of estradiol. Bioidentical hormones are not approved by the FDA for treatment of menopausal symptoms.

Side Effects and Risks of Postmenopausal Hormone Therapy

Estrogen is generally well tolerated, but it may cause headache (especially in women with a history of migraine) and breast tenderness. Added progestins tend to make these side effects more severe and also cause uterine bleeding.

The effects of hormone therapy on disease outcomes have been evaluated among postmenopausal women in the Women's Health Initiative (WHI) randomized trials (Table 240-4). Both estrogen and estrogen in combination with progestin reduced the risk for hip fracture by 35 to 40%. Neither estrogen alone nor estrogen with a progestin reduced the risk for coronary events, and both increased the risk for stroke by approximately 40%.

Compared with estrogen alone, added progestin appears to increase the risk for coronary events, pulmonary embolism, breast cancer, and dementia (Table 240-4). This finding suggests that adding a progestin should be avoided, but treatment with unopposed estrogen in women with a uterus markedly increases the risk for uterine hyperplasia and cancer as well as the rate of gynecologic procedures and hysterectomy. Replacing progestins with the selective estrogen receptor modulator bazedoxifene is a novel approach to blocking the carcinogenic effects of estrogen on the uterus, but at this time bazedoxifene has not been proved to be safer than progestins.

The excess risk of any one of the adverse events listed in Table 240-4 in the WHI trials was about 2 per 1000 women treated for 1 year with estrogen in combination with progestin (about 4 per 1000 per year in women older than

65 years if dementia is included) and 1 stroke per 1000 women treated with unopposed estrogen.[A3] These risks are relatively small, but they cumulate such that treatment for 5 years is associated with an excess risk of 1 event per 100 women treated with estrogen in combination with progestin and 3 strokes per 1000 women treated with unopposed estrogen. Given these potential harms and the availability of other effective and safe drugs for prevention of osteoporotic fractures, postmenopausal hormone therapy currently has no role for prevention of disease, especially in older women.

The average age of women enrolled in the WHI trials was 63 years. In contrast, most women who use hormone therapy for treatment of hot flashes are generally in their 50s. Subgroup analyses by age from the WHI trials that include women who took hormone therapy for 5 to 7 years show that the *relative* risk for any adverse event among women who took estrogen plus progestin was similar for younger (50 to 59 years) and older (70 to 79 years) women; but given the lower rate of events in younger women, the *absolute* increase in the rate of any major adverse event in the younger women was about 1 per 1000 per year, compared with 4 per 1000 per year for older women. Among women who took estrogen alone, the *relative* risk was lower in younger women than in older women, and the *absolute* rate of adverse events was decreased by 2 per 1000 per year in the younger women compared with an increase of 5 per 1000 per year in the older women. These data suggest that the risk for women in their 50s taking estrogen plus progestin for a few years for the treatment of hot flashes is very low, and there may be no risk associated with taking estrogen alone.

Despite these findings, hormone therapy is relatively contraindicated in women with a history of stroke, breast cancer, or venous thromboembolic events and should be avoided in women at high risk for these conditions.

Stopping Hormone Therapy

Given the possible adverse effects of hormone therapy, current guidelines recommend that women use the lowest effective dose for the shortest time necessary. Vasomotor symptoms improve or resolve spontaneously within a few years of onset in most women, suggesting that most should be able to discontinue hormone therapy within a few years of starting. Women using hormone therapy for treatment of symptoms should stop every 6 to 12 months to determine whether symptoms have improved to the point that treatment is no longer needed. A small percentage of women are unable to stop hormone therapy because vasomotor symptoms persist for many years.

Women experiencing intolerable symptoms after stopping hormone treatment can be told to resume therapy and either to begin a slow taper or to wait 6 months before trying again to stop. Tapering can be accomplished by decreasing the dose of hormone therapy, but it may be easier to decrease the number of days per week that hormone therapy is used. The *dose taper* involves progressively reducing the dose of hormone therapy, for example, by reducing the dose of conjugated estrogens from 0.625 mg/day to 0.45 to 0.3 mg/day and then discontinuing therapy. If changing to a lower dose is associated with tolerable symptoms, the next reduction in dose should not occur until symptoms improve, which may require 3 to 6 months in some women. The *day taper* involves decreasing the number of days per week of hormone therapy use and effectively decreasing the weekly dose. For example, therapy with the same dose may be continued, but only Monday through Friday. If this reduced weekly dose is tolerated, therapy may be discontinued on Friday, and so on. As with the dose taper, if symptoms develop, the weekly dose should be maintained until symptoms improve. Both these approaches to tapering can require many months or even years until therapy is discontinued. The day taper has the advantages of allowing smaller reductions in weekly dose, ensuring that the estrogen dose is appropriately opposed by a progestin in women using continuous therapy, and does not require multiple new prescriptions for different doses of hormone therapy. For women who cannot tolerate even a slow taper, the value of symptom relief likely outweighs the risks of hormone therapy.

Other Prescription Drugs

The progestins megestrol and medroxyprogesterone acetate are effective for the treatment of hot flushes, but they have frequent side effects, and progestin use was associated with increased risk for adverse effects in the WHI trials. Several selective serotonin and serotonin-norepinephrine reuptake inhibitors and gabapentin have been studied (Table 240-5). Paroxetine[A4] and escitalopram[A5] reduce the frequency of hot flashes by about 0.5 to 1 hot flash per day more than placebo; these drugs have side effects typical of selective serotonin reuptake inhibitors. Low-dose paroxetine mesylate (7.5 mg/day) reduces hot flash frequency by about 1 hot flash per day more than placebo, and side effects were uncommon.[A6] This is the only nonhormonal drug currently approved by the FDA for the treatment of hot flashes. In a randomized, double-blinded trial, the efficacy of low-dose oral estradiol (0.5 mg daily) was found to be only slightly superior to that of the serotonin-norepinephrine reuptake inhibitor venlafaxine (extended release, 75 mg daily) in alleviating vasomotor symptoms.[A7] Gabapentin also has only modest efficacy (reducing the frequency of hot flashes by 0.5 to 1 hot flash per day more than placebo) but is associated with dizziness, somnolence, headache, and nausea. Extended-release gabapentin has been studied in three phase III randomized trials, but results have not been published and the drug was not approved by the FDA

for treatment of hot flashes. Clinical trials of these prescription drugs have generally lasted only 3 months and have not been adequately large or prolonged to detect uncommon adverse effects.

Summary of Approach to Treatment of Vasomotor Symptoms

Women with mild vasomotor symptoms may find adequate relief by wearing layered clothing and keeping the home and bedroom cool. Women with moderate symptoms may choose a low dose of estrogen or a nonestrogen therapy. Low-dose paroxetine is modestly effective, has the best side effect profile of the nonhormonal drugs, and is approved by the FDA for this indication. For women with severe symptoms, hormone therapy is the most effective treatment.

Vaginal Symptoms

EPIDEMIOLOGY

The prevalence of vaginal dryness, discomfort, itching, and dyspareunia increases as women transition through the menopause. Up to 30% of perimenopausal and early postmenopausal women and a higher proportion of older menopausal women express these complaints. Urologic symptoms, including urgency, frequency, dysuria, and incontinence, are not clearly correlated with the menopause transition.

PATHOBIOLOGY

Vaginal symptoms generally correlate with findings (often called vaginal atrophy) including pallor, dryness, friability, and decreased rugosity of the vaginal mucosa. Vaginal fluid in premenopausal women is acidic, ranging from a pH of approximately 4.5 to 5.5 with mild alkalinization to approximately 6.0 before ovulation. Acidity is produced by proton excretion from the vaginal epithelial cells and by metabolism of glycogen stored in vaginal epithelial cells by *Lactobacillus* species, the normal vaginal flora. The acid environment of the vagina inhibits growth of *Escherichia coli* and other enteric gram-negative bacteria that are a potential cause of urinary tract infections. Vaginal pH can easily be measured from lateral vaginal wall fluid.

In postmenopausal women, vaginal pH is generally neutral, and the predominant flora are often *E. coli* and other gram-negative bacteria. This appears to occur because estrogen deficiency associated with menopause causes vaginal epithelial cell dysfunction, including decreased storage of glycogen, less ability to acidify the vaginal fluid, and lowered production of vaginal lubrication. Vaginal epithelial cells, which are primarily superficial and intermediate cells in premenopausal women, shift to predominantly immature parabasal cells in postmenopausal women. Treatment with estrogen improves or relieves vaginal dryness, lowers vaginal pH, and increases the proportion of superficial cells in the vaginal epithelium.

DIAGNOSIS

Diagnosis is primarily based on typical complaints of vaginal dryness, discomfort, itching, or dyspareunia in women undergoing the menopause transition or older postmenopausal women. Pelvic examination should be performed to exclude other causes of symptoms, including infections, lesions, and trauma. Physical findings of vaginal dryness, pallor, friability, and vaginal pH above 5.5 support the diagnosis. Cytologic examination of the proportion of superficial, intermediate, and parabasal cells from a scraping of the lateral vaginal wall (vaginal maturation index) showing primarily parabasal cells also supports the diagnosis. In clinical practice, measurement of pH and vaginal maturation index are not necessary to make the diagnosis.

TREATMENT   Rx

Some women with mild dyspareunia may obtain adequate relief with over-the-counter vaginal lubricants used as needed for sexual intercourse.[8] Over-the-counter vaginal moisturizers, such as Replens (a bioadhesive polycarbophil vaginal gel used daily or three times per week), have been shown to improve vaginal symptoms and findings. Estrogen therapy is highly effective.[9] Topical therapy is efficacious[10] and is preferred because it generally results in smaller increases in systemic estrogen levels than with oral or transdermal therapy.[A8] Estrogen vaginal creams, tablets, and rings approved for treatment of vaginal dryness are listed in Table 240-3.

Most clinicians do not add a progestin to protect the uterus in women treated with vaginal estrogen, but evidence to support the uterine safety of vaginal estrogen is limited to short-term studies. Low-dose, intermittent

TABLE 240-5 EVIDENCE FROM RANDOMIZED, CONTROLLED CLINICAL TRIALS OF THE EFFICACY OF NONESTROGEN DRUGS FOR TREATMENT OF MENOPAUSAL HOT FLUSHES

TREATMENT	EVIDENCE OF BENEFIT	COMMENTS	REFERENCES	SIDE EFFECTS*
ANTIDEPRESSANTS				
Citalopram	No	No benefit of 30 mg citalopram compared with placebo	Suvanto-Luukkonen E, Koivunen R, Sundstrom H, et al. *Menopause.* 2005;12:18-26.	Selective serotonin reuptake inhibitors citalopram, escitalopram, fluoxetine, paroxetine, and sertraline: nausea, vomiting, diarrhea, insomnia or somnolence, anxiety, decreased libido, dry mouth, worsening depression, mania, suicidality, serotonin syndrome, withdrawal syndrome, and possible decreased tamoxifen effectiveness
Escitalopram	Yes	Among generally healthy women, frequency of hot flushes reduced 47% with escitalopram 10 to 20 mg/day compared with 33% with placebo	Freeman EW, Guthrie KA, Caan B, et al. *JAMA.* 2011;305:267-274.	
Fluoxetine	Mixed	Among breast cancer survivors, frequency of hot flushes reduced 50% with fluoxetine 20 mg/day compared with 36% with placebo No benefit among women with breast cancer treated with 30 mg fluoxetine compared with placebo	Loprinzi CL, Sloan JA, Perez EA, et al. *J Clin Oncol.* 2002:20:1578-1583. Suvanto-Luukkonen E, Koivunen R, Sundstrom H, et al. *Menopause.* 2005;12:18-26.	
Paroxetine	Yes	Among generally healthy women, frequency of hot flushes reduced 62% with 12.5 mg and 65% with 25 mg paroxetine CR compared with 38% in placebo In a crossover trial in which 81% of participants had a history of breast cancer, paroxetine 10 mg reduced hot flush frequency by 41% compared with 14% with placebo, and paroxetine 20 mg reduced hot flush frequency by 52% compared with 27% placebo In 2 similarly designed trials of 7.5 mg of paroxetine mesylate daily compared with placebo, paroxetine reduced the frequency of hot flashes by about 1 hot flash per day more than placebo	Steans V, Beebe KL, Lyengar M, et al. *JAMA.* 2003;289:2827-2834. Stearns V, Slack R, Greep N, et al. *J Clin Oncol.* 2005;23:6919-6930. Simon JA, Portman DJ, Kaunitz AM, et al. *Menopause.* 2013;20:1027-1035.	
Sertraline	No	Among women with a history of breast cancer, no benefit of treatment with 50 mg of sertraline compared with placebo Among generally healthy women, no benefit of 100 mg of sertraline compared with placebo	Kimmick GG, Lovato J, McQuellon R, et al. *Breast J.* 2006;12:114-122. Grady D, Cohen B, Tice J, et al. *Obstet Gynecol.* 2007;109:823-830.	
Venlafaxine	Mixed	Among breast cancer survivors, frequency of hot flushes reduced 61% with 75 or 150 mg venlafaxine compared with 27% placebo Among women without breast cancer, no effect on frequency of flushes with 75 mg venlafaxine, but women treated with venlafaxine were more likely to report that flushes improved compared with placebo	Loprinzi CL, Kugler JW, Sloan JA, et al. *Lancet.* 2003;356:2059-2063. Evans ML, Pritts E, Vittinghoff E, et al. *Obstet Gynecol.* 2005;105:161-166.	In addition to the side effects noted above, the selective serotonin-norepinephrine reuptake inhibitors venlafaxine and desvenlafaxine can also cause hypertension.
Desvenlafaxine	Yes	Meta-analysis of the results of 6 randomized trials showed that treatment with 100 to 150 mg of desvenlafaxine per day reduces the frequency of hot flashes by 0.3 to 0.5 more than with placebo	Umland EM, Falconieri L. *Int J Womens Health.* 2012;4:305-319.	
ANTIHYPERTENSIVES				
Clonidine	Mixed	Small trials suggest little or no benefit	Nelson HD, Haney E, Humphrey L, et al. AHRQ Publication No. 05-E016-2. Rockville, MD: Agency for Healthcare Research and Quality; 2005. Goldberg RM, Loprinzi CL, O'Fallon JR, et al. *J Clin Oncol.* 1994;12:155-158. Pandya KJ, Raubertas RF, Flynn PJ, et al. *Ann Intern Med.* 2000;132:78-93.	α-Adrenergic antagonists clonidine and methyldopa: dry mouth, drowsiness, dizziness, hypotension, rebound hypertension
Methyldopa	No		Nelson HD, Haney E, Humphrey L, et al. AHRQ Publication No. 05-E016-2. Rockville, MD: Agency for Healthcare Research and Quality; 2005.	

TABLE 240-5 EVIDENCE FROM RANDOMIZED, CONTROLLED CLINICAL TRIALS OF THE EFFICACY OF NONESTROGEN DRUGS FOR TREATMENT OF MENOPAUSAL HOT FLUSHES—cont'd

TREATMENT	EVIDENCE OF BENEFIT	COMMENTS	REFERENCES	SIDE EFFECTS*
HORMONES				
Medroxyprogesterone acetate	Yes	Frequency of hot flushes was reduced 74% with 20 mg medroxyprogesterone acetate compared with 26% with placebo	Schiff I, Tulchinsky D, Cramer D, et al. *JAMA.* 1980;244:1443-1445.	Progestins medroxyprogesterone and megestrol: nausea, vomiting, constipation, somnolence, depression, breast tenderness, uterine bleeding; possible increased risk for venous thromboembolism, cardiovascular events, and breast cancer
Megestrol	Yes	Among breast cancer survivors, frequency of hot flushes reduced 74% with 20 mg megestrol twice a day compared with 27% with placebo	Loprinzi CL, Michalak JC, Quella SK, et al. *N Engl J Med.* 1994;331:347-352.	
OTHER DRUGS				
Gabapentin	Yes	Among healthy women, frequency of hot flushes was reduced 45% with gabapentin 300 mg three times/day compared with 29% with placebo	Guttuso TJ, Kurlan R, McDermott MP, et al. *Obstet Gynecol.* 2003;101:337-345.	Nausea, vomiting, somnolence, dizziness, rash, ataxia, fatigue, leukopenia
		Frequency of hot flushes was reduced 31% more than with placebo among breast cancer survivors	Pandya JK, Morrow GR, Rosco JA, et al. *Lancet.* 2005;366:818-824.	

*Side effects were reported in clinical trials of the therapy or from Epocrates RX drug reference (available at http://www.epocrates.com).

treatment (e.g., 1 to 2 g conjugated estrogen cream or 0.025 mg estradiol tablet twice a week) results in small increases in systemic estrogen levels that appear not to cause endometrial stimulation. However, full-dose daily treatment has been shown to increase estradiol levels to 50 pg/mL or higher in approximately half of treated women and has been associated with uterine bleeding and hyperplasia.

Ospemifene, an oral selective estrogen receptor modulator, is approved by the FDA for the treatment of menopausal vaginal dryness and dyspareunia. Treatment with 60 mg once daily reduces the bothersomeness of vaginal symptoms about 10 to 15% more than placebo does, but it is associated with hot flashes, urinary tract infection, and vaginal infections.[A9] Small studies of up to 1 year have not shown increased risk of endometrial cancer, breast cancer, venous thromboembolic events, or stroke, but because ospemifene is a selective estrogen agonist, these potential adverse effects are of concern.

Sleep Disturbance

The prevalence of self-reported sleep disturbance increases from about 40% of premenopausal women to approximately 60% of postmenopausal women. Sleep disturbances, including trouble falling asleep and early awakening, are reported by menopausal women, but awakening during the night appears to be most bothersome.

The etiology of sleep disturbance associated with menopause is unclear. Postmenopausal women with hot flushes are more likely to report sleep disturbance than are those without flushes, and women commonly report that they are awakened by hot flushes. However, studies using polysomnography find that nocturnal hot flushes do not consistently occur at the same time as sleep disturbance. Thus, disturbed sleep appears to be part of a menopausal syndrome, but it may not be caused by flushing.

Menopause-related sleep disturbance can be treated by standard approaches to sleep hygiene and prescription medications. Both oral and transdermal estrogen preparations improve sleep in perimenopausal and postmenopausal women with hot flushes.

Grade A References

A1. Reed SD, Guthrie KA, Newton KM, et al. Menopausal quality of life: RCT of yoga, exercise, and omega-3 supplements. *Am J Obstet Gynecol.* 2014;210:244.e1-244.e11.
A2. Pinkerton JV, Utian WH, Constantine GD, et al. Relief of vasomotor symptoms with the tissue-selective estrogen complex containing bazedoxifene/conjugated estrogens: a randomized, controlled trial. *Menopause.* 2009;16:1116-1124.
A3. Manson JE, Chlebowski RT, Stefanick ML, et al. Menopausal hormone therapy and health outcomes during the intervention and extended poststopping phases of the Women's Health Initiative randomized trials. *JAMA.* 2013;310:1353-1368.
A4. Simon JA, Portman DJ, Kaunitz AM, et al. Low-dose paroxetine 7.5 mg for menopausal vasomotor symptoms: two randomized controlled trials. *Menopause.* 2013;20:1027-1035.
A5. Freeman EW, Guthrie KA, Caan B, et al. Efficacy of escitalopram for hot flashes in healthy menopausal women: a randomized controlled trial. *JAMA.* 2011;305:267-274.
A6. Hayes LP, Carroll DG, Kelley KW. Use of gabapentin for the management of natural or surgical menopausal hot flashes. *Ann Pharmacother.* 2011;45:388-394.
A7. Joffe H, Guthrie KA, LaCroix AZ, et al. Low-dose estradiol and the serotonin-norepinephrine reuptake inhibitor venlafaxine for vasomotor symptoms: a randomized clinical trial. *JAMA Intern Med.* 2014;174:1058-1066.
A8. Suckling J, Lethaby A, Kennedy R. Local oestrogen for vaginal atrophy in postmenopausal women. *Cochrane Database Syst Rev.* 2006;4:CD001500.
A9. Portman DJ, Bachmann GA, Simon JA. Ospemifene, a novel selective estrogen receptor modulator for treating dyspareunia associated with postmenopausal vulvar and vaginal atrophy. *Menopause.* 2013;20:623-630.

GENERAL REFERENCES

For the General References and other additional features, please visit Expert Consult at https://expertconsult.inkling.com.

241

INTIMATE PARTNER VIOLENCE

GENE FEDER AND HARRIET L. MACMILLAN

DEFINITION

Intimate partner violence (IPV) is defined as any behavior within an intimate relationship or ex-relationship that causes physical, psychological, or sexual harm. This includes physical aggression, such as hitting, kicking, and beating; psychological violence, such as intimidation and constant humiliation; various controlling behaviors, such as isolation from family and friends, monitoring of movements, financial control, and restricting access to services; and sexual violence, including forced intercourse and other sexual coercion. Lifetime prevalence of isolated violent acts within relationships is comparable for men and women, but repeated coercive, sexual, or severe physical violence is perpetrated largely against women by men. Although IPV also occurs in same-sex relationships, research evidence on the health consequences of IPV and the care of survivors is largely confined to women in heterosexual relationships.

Historically, there has been the stereotype of a male batterer as one who uses severe, repeated, and unilateral violence against a nonviolent female victim. It is now recognized that *bilateral violence* is a common form of IPV, even though the overwhelming burden of morbidity and mortality related to IPV is experienced by women. Bilateral violence, sometimes referred to as *common couple violence,* is considered less severe than the pattern of abuse known as *battering* or *intimate terrorism,* a severe and escalating form of IPV characterized by threats, terrorization, multiple forms of abuse, and controlling behavior on the part of the abuser. Current research suggests that women rarely subject men to battering.

IPV is a risk factor for a wide range of medical and psychiatric conditions and therefore can be understood as an epidemiologic exposure. Yet violence perpetrated by an intimate partner or ex-partner is essentially a violation of human rights and a preventable psychosocial issue that needs to be addressed through social and educational policies.

EPIDEMIOLOGY

The prevalence of IPV against women varies internationally but is universally high, comparable to that of chronic conditions like diabetes and asthma. The most robust comparative study (24,097 women from 15 sites in 10 countries), conducted by the World Health Organization, found a lifetime prevalence of physical violence, sexual violence, or both ranging from 15 to 71%.[1] Prevalence of physical or sexual violence during the past year ranged from 15 to 54%. In all sites but one, women were more at risk for violence from a partner or ex-partner than from violence by other people. A systematic review that included data from 66 countries found that one in seven homicides globally are committed by an intimate partner; this figure is six times higher for female homicides compared with male homicides.[2]

Causation

Several theories about the causes of IPV have been proposed over the years. Social learning theory suggests that IPV is a learned behavior. The fact that male perpetrators and female victims are more likely to report histories of exposure to violence in childhood supports this theory. However, most individuals exposed to violence in childhood do not go on to commit violence as adults, and not all abusers have violent upbringings. Furthermore, the link between poor parenting generally, including neglect, and subsequent IPV in adulthood suggests that the effect is not simply one of modeling abusive behavior. Exposure to rejecting or neglectful parenting is associated with adverse effects on intrapersonal (e.g., poor self-worth) and interpersonal development that are associated with IPV.

A feminist perspective views IPV against women as a form of social control that results from society's patriarchal structure leading to inequality in power relationships between men and women. Lending support to this perspective is the finding that IPV appears to be less common in more democratic and less economically polarized societies. Although IPV occurs more often in contexts in which there is support for male authority in the family and women have less access to economic security, it is not clear why some individuals are more likely than others to be violent under such conditions.

With regard to psychological theory, there are conflicting views about the association between IPV and psychopathology. Some researchers argue that abusive males have deficits in one or more coping mechanisms, anger control, and communication skills, whereas others suggest that IPV results from dysfunctional interactional patterns between partners. Because types of IPV are not the same for all couples, there are likely to be multiple causes for its occurrence. Most of the research has focused on factors associated with increased risk of men abusing women (Table 241-1)[3]; however, whether these factors are "causal" is unknown.

CLINICAL MANIFESTATIONS

The information in this section pertains to female patients because most of the research examining clinical manifestations associated with IPV exposure has focused on women. However, studies of male victims suggest that they also experience increased risk for poor health as well as chronic physical and emotional health problems and injuries.[4]

Patients seldom present with a chief complaint of IPV. Injuries are the most obvious manifestation; a clinician should have increased suspicion for IPV if there are multiple injuries, the presenting history of injuries is not consistent with the physical examination, and there is a delay in seeking medical care for injuries. Patients exposed to physical violence may present with injuries that vary from minor abrasions to life-threatening trauma. Although there can be overlap between injuries resulting from IPV and injuries from other causes, the former typically involve trauma to the head, face, and neck, whereas the latter are more typically injuries of the extremities.[5] Multiple

TABLE 241-1	FACTORS ASSOCIATED WITH A MAN'S RISK FOR ABUSING HIS PARTNER		
INDIVIDUAL	**RELATIONSHIP**	**COMMUNITY**	**SOCIETAL**
Young age	Poor family functioning	Weak community sanctions against intimate partner violence	Traditional gender norms
Heavy drinking	Marital instability	Poverty	Social norms supportive of violence
Depression	Marital conflict	Economic inequality	
Personality disorders	Male dominance	Low social capital	
Low academic achievement	Economic stress		
Low income			
Exposure to violence in childhood			

Modified from World Health Organization: World Report on Violence and Health. Geneva: World Health Organization; 2002.

facial injuries are suggestive of IPV rather than of other causes, and those that are more specific for IPV include zygomatic complex fractures, orbital blow-out fractures, and perforated tympanic membrane. Although facial injuries are the most common injuries associated with IPV, they have low specificity. Musculoskeletal injuries are considered the second most common type of injuries, including sprains, fractures, and dislocations.[6] Blunt-force trauma to the forearms should raise suspicion of IPV because these can occur when trying to block being struck.

Victims of IPV often experience multiple mechanisms of injury; being struck by a hand is the most common, followed by use of a household object. Injuries from weapons such as knives and guns are far less common (<1%) but are associated with higher risk for mortality. Strangulation also occurs frequently,[7] but less is known about the types of clinical manifestations that result from this form of IPV. Other injuries that raise suspicion of IPV include fractures of the spine or trunk, bites, hair pulling, and open wounds. Those exposed to sexual abuse may show signs of trauma to the genital area, but sexual assault is associated with signs of injury in less than one third of cases.

Most victims of IPV presenting to health care settings do not have signs of obvious trauma but rather have a constellation of overlapping physical and mental health problems. A patient presenting with vague signs and symptoms or chronic somatic complaints, including pain, suggests the possibility of IPV. Other behaviors that suggest IPV include delay in seeking medical care, multiple cancellations of medical appointments, and noncompliance with vital medications (e.g., insulin).

There are no systematic reviews of studies on the overall physical health consequences of IPV, but an overview of studies reported increased rates of chronic physical conditions, particularly gynecologic, gastrointestinal, and nervous system disorders, as well as increased cardiovascular risk, although most of the studies were small and poorly adjusted for other risk factors. The overview also found that women with a history of abuse, particularly physical and sexual violence, were more likely to experience chronic pain and nonspecific symptoms, although an association between abuse and number of physical symptoms is also found in women who experience emotional abuse without any physical abuse. The World Health Organization study reported significant associations between women's lifetime experiences of partner violence and self-reported poor health and specific health problems in the previous 4 weeks, such as difficulty in walking, difficulty with daily activities, pain, memory loss, dizziness, and vaginal discharge. Other physical conditions that should raise suspicion of IPV include chronic gynecologic or gastrointestinal symptoms, such as irritable bowel syndrome and chronic pelvic pain. It should not be assumed, however, that there is a specific association of functional disorders, such as irritable bowel syndrome and fibromyalgia, over and above the greater reporting of physical syndromes in general. IPV exposure is associated with an increased risk for sexually transmitted infections, including human papillomavirus.

Exposure to any type of IPV can be associated with a wide range of emotional and behavioral symptoms[8]; depression and post-traumatic stress disorder (PTSD) are the two most commonly associated emotional conditions, but other anxiety disorders and substance abuse are also associated with IPV exposure. In the World Health Organization study, women who reported IPV at least once in their life reported three to four times more emotional distress, suicidal thoughts, and suicide attempts than nonabused women. There is strong evidence of increased risk for depression, anxiety, substance abuse, and PTSD, with longitudinal studies reporting increased morbidity after violence. A recent meta-analysis examining the association between IPV against adult women and depressive conditions found a 2- to 3-fold increase in risk of major depressive disorder and a 1.5- to 2-fold increased risk of postpartum depression and elevated depressive symptoms.[9] The cross-sectional design of most studies examining associated impairment precludes conclusions about the causal role of IPV in these conditions, but the few published longitudinal studies show the onset or worsening of depression, PTSD, and substance abuse *after* exposure to IPV.

Pregnant women deserve special mention because IPV can threaten the health of both mother and fetus. Injury patterns during pregnancy are more likely to be central, including blunt trauma to the head, torso, abdomen, breasts, and genitalia. Abuse directed to the abdomen may lead to poor pregnancy outcomes and perinatal death. Although the evidence regarding a direct association between IPV in pregnancy and low birthweight has been conflicting, the increased risk for preterm birth as well as other factors, such as psychosocial stress, may play a role in adverse outcomes for infants, but more investigation is required.

Although it is beyond the scope of this chapter, there is increasing recognition that children's exposure to IPV shows a significant association with children's internalizing and externalizing problems, including trauma symptoms, developmental delay, educational problems, and long-term mental health conditions.[10]

Identification

Despite some guidelines recommending universal screening for IPV, randomized controlled trials have shown that although such screening increases the identification of women with IPV, it has not been shown to improve women's health outcomes or to reduce the occurrence of IPV.[A1-A3] Consistent with the World Health Organization guidelines referred to before, IPV screening is not recommended for women of any age group.[11] However, it is important to be alert to the signs and symptoms associated with IPV, including those associated with the broad range of physical and mental health conditions referred to previously, and for clinicians to have a low threshold for asking about abuse. Indicators that suggest a higher likelihood of IPV include symptoms of depression, somatization, and PTSD in the female patient and a history of alcohol or drug abuse and unemployment in the male partner (or ex-partner). It is important, when asking about exposure to IPV, to do so privately, with no one else present, including a child (beyond infancy) or partner. If the inquiry or response is overheard, it could put the patient at risk for further IPV. A meta-analysis of qualitative studies of women's expectations and experiences reported that when the topic of IPV is raised, patients want questioning that is nonjudgmental, compassionate, and caring.[11] Women want to be asked about IPV with confidentiality ensured but do not want to be pressured to disclose. In some jurisdictions, however, disclosure of IPV when a patient has children in the home can lead to mandatory reporting to child protection services. It is important that patients be advised about the limits of confidentiality before being asked about IPV exposure.

Possible questions to ask if IPV is suspected include the following:
Sometimes partners or ex-partners use physical force. Has this ever happened to you?
Have you felt humiliated or emotionally harmed by your partner or ex-partner?
Are you now or have you ever been afraid of your partner or ex-partner?
Have you ever been physically threatened or hurt by your partner or ex-partner?
Have you been forced to have any kind of sexual activity by your partner or ex-partner?
Has your partner or ex-partner ever tried to control your behavior, for example, control where you go or whom you see?

The initial clinical response when IPV is identified should include validation of the experience (e.g., everyone deserves to feel safe at home), affirmation that violence is unacceptable, and expression of support. The clinician needs to acknowledge the complexity of IPV and respect the patient's individual concerns and decisions. The assessment should include an evaluation of safety; the patient should be asked if it is safe for her (or him or any children) to return home. The following are examples of safety considerations:
Has the frequency or severity of the violence increased?
Is the partner or ex-partner obsessed with the patient?
How safe does she (he) feel?
Does the partner or ex-partner have a weapon or access to one?
Has she (he) been threatened with a weapon?

Although a general discussion of gun violence is beyond the scope of this chapter, having firearms in the home is associated with an increased risk for homicide associated with IPV. Another predictor of domestic homicide is threats of deadly violence.

TREATMENT Rx

Inquiry and Disclosure

The initial response of clinicians to the disclosure of IPV by female patients, whether the disclosure is spontaneous or the result of clinical inquiry, is crucial in gaining trust and is the basis of further management. IPV is a highly stigmatized condition, akin to sexually transmitted infection or substance abuse, with the added dimension of risk for further harm from breach of confidentiality. A number of qualitative studies of women's expectations and experiences (847 informants) reported consistent messages about how clinicians can respond appropriately to disclosure. *Before disclosure or questioning,* they should understand the problem, including knowing about the available community services and appropriate referral systems; ensure that the clinical environment is supportive, welcoming, and non-threatening; place brochures and posters in the clinical setting; try to ensure continuity of care; assure abused women about matters of privacy, safety, and confidentiality; be alert to the signs of abuse and raise the matter when indicated; use verbal and nonverbal communication skills to develop trust; and be compassionate, supportive, and respectful toward abused women. *When the topic of IPV is raised,* they should be nonjudgmental, compassionate, and caring when questioning about abuse; be confident and comfortable asking about domestic violence; not pressure women to disclose abuse because simply raising the topic may be helpful to women; ask about abuse during the course of several interviews because a woman may disclose abuse at a later date; ensure that the environment is private and confidential; and provide time. *Immediate response to disclosure* should be nonjudgmental, with compassion, support, and belief of experiences; acknowledge the complexity of the problem and respect the woman's unique concerns and decisions; put the needs identified by the woman first and help ensure that social and psychological needs are met; take time to listen, to provide information, and to offer referrals to specialist help; validate her experiences, challenge assumptions, and provide encouragement; and respond to any concerns about safety. *Response in later interactions* should be patient and supportive, allowing her to progress at her own therapeutic pace; understand the chronicity of the problem and provide follow-up and continued support; respect the woman's wishes and not pressure her into making any decisions; be nonjudgmental if a woman does not follow up with referrals immediately; and give abused women an opportunity to disclose abuse at a later date.

Referral Services and Advocacy

Beyond their initial response and managing the medical sequelae of abuse, most generalists have neither the expertise nor the capacity to meet the specific needs of women experiencing IPV, which include legal, financial, housing, and safety needs. A key step, particularly in the context of current or recent violence, is an offer of referral to some sort of specialist support. Two main types of services have been evaluated: advocacy programs and psychological interventions (individual or group based). In general, advocates engage with individual clients who are being abused, aiming to empower them and linking them to community services. Core activities of advocacy include provision of legal, housing, and financial advice; facilitation of access to and use of community resources, such as refuges (shelters, safe houses) and emergency housing; and provision of safety planning advice. Advocates can also provide ongoing support and informal counseling. A Cochrane review of 10 randomized controlled trials (1527 participants) of domestic violence advocacy concluded that there was equivocal evidence that advocacy for women recruited in domestic violence shelters (refuges) had a beneficial effect on their physical and psychosocial well-being and was unable to draw any conclusions for women receiving advocacy in or referred from health care settings.[A4] A broader systematic review that included all controlled studies of domestic violence advocacy concluded that most showed a reduction in abuse, increased social support, and improved quality of life as well as increased use of safety behaviors and accessing of community resources.[A5] Only two of the studies had participants referred from health care settings. Clinicians should be able to refer patients to specialist IPV advocacy and are more likely to ask about abuse if they have the support of these services. If such services are not immediately available, shelters and refuges often provide these kinds of services for women both in residences and on an outreach basis.

Individual and Group Psychological Interventions

A systematic review of controlled studies of psychological interventions for survivors of IPV identified 17 studies, 7 of individual and 10 of group interventions. There was a wide range of individual psychological interventions that

TABLE 241-2 SUMMARY OF SELECT INTIMATE PARTNER VIOLENCE RECOMMENDATIONS FROM THE WORLD HEALTH ORGANIZATION

CATEGORY	RECOMMENDATION	QUALITY OF EVIDENCE	STRENGTH OF RECOMMENDATION
Woman-centered care	Women who disclose any form of violence by an intimate partner (or other family member) should be offered immediate support by clinicians, at a minimum. If clinicians are unable to provide this first-line support, they should ensure that someone else (within their health care setting or another that is easily accessible) is immediately available to do so.	Indirect	Strong
Identification of survivors	Universal screening is not recommended.	Low-moderate	Conditional
	Ask about exposure to IPV when assessing conditions that may be caused or complicated by abuse.	Indirect	Strong
	Written information about IPV should be available in all health care settings.	No relevant evidence	Conditional
Care for survivors	Women with preexisting diagnosed or IPV-related mental disorders should receive mental health delivered by health care professionals with a good understanding of violence against women.	Indirect	Strong
	Cognitive-behavioral therapy or eye movement desensitization and reprocessing interventions, delivered by health care professionals with a good understanding of violence against women, should be offered to women with post-traumatic stress disorder who are no longer experiencing violence.	Low-moderate	Strong
	Women who have spent at least 1 night in a shelter, refuge, or safe house should be offered a structured program of advocacy, support, and/or empowerment.	Low	Conditional
	For children who are exposed to IPV at home, a psychotherapeutic intervention should be offered.	Moderate	Conditional
Training of clinicians	Training at prequalification level in first-line support for women who have experienced IPV should be given to clinicians (in particular physicians, nurses, and midwives).	Very low	Strong
	Clinicians offering care to women should receive in-service training integrated with training on managing sexual assault.	Low-moderate	Strong
Health care policy	Care for women experiencing IPV should be integrated into existing health services rather than as a stand-alone service.	Very low	Strong
Mandatory reporting	Mandatory reporting to the police by clinicians is not recommended; clinicians should offer to report the incident to the appropriate authorities (including the police) if the woman wants this and is aware of her rights.	Very low	Strong

IPV = intimate partner violence. (From Feder G, Wathen CN, MacMillan HL. An evidence-based response to intimate partner violence: WHO guidelines. *JAMA* 2013;310:479-480.)

demonstrated improvements in psychological outcomes, including depression, PTSD, and self-esteem. Well-executed trials of individual cognitive therapy–based interventions for women with PTSD who were no longer experiencing violence provided reasonable evidence for this intervention, but this cannot be extrapolated to women still in an abusive relationship.[A6][A7] All the studies of group psychological interventions showed improvement in one or more psychological or mental health outcomes, but with the exception of one study, they were poorly conducted. Consequently, the effectiveness of this type of intervention remains uncertain, particularly for women who are still experiencing IPV.

Treatment of Abuser and Couple Therapy

Although the assessment and treatment of the abuser should be carried out by mental health professionals with expertise in this area, it can be helpful for general clinicians to have some awareness of the effects of treatment. The evidence for batterer treatment is mixed, with the better-designed studies generally indicating little or no benefit or potential harm (i.e., increased recidivism).[A8] To date, there is insufficient evidence to recommend specific treatment for those committing IPV. The evidence for couple therapy is mixed, with trial-level evidence indicating no benefit in a military sample.[A9] Most authors caution that these couple therapy programs are not safe for many abused women, particularly those experiencing "intimate terrorism." Furthermore, when abusers are enrolled in treatment programs, it is important that women be provided with concurrent advocacy and support. There is some evidence to suggest that permanent, but not temporary, civil protection orders may be effective in reducing future violence.

PREVENTION

From a public health perspective, primary prevention of IPV is desirable, although most of the available research focuses on the health care response to the survivors of IPV, both while a woman is still exposed to abuse (secondary prevention) and when she is experiencing the long-term health problems associated with IPV (tertiary prevention).

Efforts aimed at primary prevention of IPV through educational programs have generally focused on changes in attitude, knowledge, skills, or self-reports of dating (relationship) violence. No studies to date have measured physical or emotional health outcomes. A meta-analysis assessed the efficacy of interventions aimed at preventing dating or relationship violence in adolescents and young adults; such violence is often considered a precursor to

IPV in adulthood.[A10] The authors concluded that there was no evidence that the interventions were effective in improving attitudes, behaviors, or skills related to relationship violence or in reducing episodes of relationship violence; there was a small improvement in knowledge about relationships. However, given that there was substantial heterogeneity between the studies, and that when those studies considered at high risk of selection bias were excluded, the only remaining study showed no effect on knowledge, the overall conclusion was no evidence of effect for the interventions.

There is no clinical trial evidence for the effectiveness of interventions provided in general medical settings with the aim of secondary prevention. A systematic review concluded that there is insufficient evidence to determine the effectiveness of interventions in preventing IPV against pregnant women.[A11] However, an advocacy and empowerment program in antenatal clinics reduced psychological and minor physical violence,[A12] and a program for pregnant African American women based on individual counseling sessions reduced violence and improved pregnancy outcomes.[A13] Within an Australian family medicine setting, there was equivocal benefit in terms of mental health and safety of a brief counseling intervention delivered by physicians.[A14] Outside of health care settings, intensive advocacy (12 hours or more duration) may reduce physical abuse among women leaving shelters or refuges after 12 to 24 months of follow-up, but not for shorter or longer follow-up. There is evidence that a training and support program for primary care clinicians improves identification of women experiencing abuse and referral to advocacy services.[A15] The World Health Organization has published guidelines for the health care response to IPV with recommendations linked to the current evidence base. Table 241-2 outlines the key recommendations related to prevention of IPV and treatment of conditions associated with exposure to IPV. Particularly noteworthy are the recommendation on training for clinicians in first-line support to women who have disclosed IPV and the recommendations against screening and mandatory reporting.

PROGNOSIS

The prognosis of IPV with and without intervention is uncertain. Trials of interventions have small samples and short follow-up, and most have substantial attrition of participants. As far as the "natural history" of the condition is concerned, cohort studies are rare, and cross-sectional studies are potentially misleading. In a 3-year follow-up of participants who received an advocacy intervention after leaving a shelter, 36% had been assaulted by their original partner or a new partner in the 6 months before the interview. The difference in re-victimization at 2 years between intervention and control arms did not persist, but there was still a significant difference in quality of life and social support among women receiving advocacy. In a U.S. cohort study, 44% of participants were still being abused after 3½ years.

Grade A References

A1. MacMillan HL, Wathen CN, Jamieson E, et al. Screening for intimate partner violence in health care settings: a randomized trial. *JAMA*. 2009;302:493-501.

A2. Klevens J, Kee R, Trick W, et al. Effect of screening for partner violence on women's quality of life: a randomized controlled trial. *JAMA*. 2012;308:681-689.

A3. O'Doherty LJ, Taft A, Hegarty K, et al. Screening women for intimate partner violence in health-care settings: abridged Cochrane systematic review and meta-analysis. *BMJ*. 2014;348:g2913.

A4. Ramsay J, Carter Y, Davidson L, et al. Advocacy interventions to reduce or eliminate violence and promote the physical and psychosocial well-being of women who experience intimate partner abuse. *Cochrane Database Syst Rev*. 2009;3:CD005043.

A5. Feder G, Ramsay J, Dunne D, et al. How far does screening women for domestic (partner) violence in different health-care settings meet criteria for a screening programme? Systematic reviews of nine UK National Screening Committee criteria. *Health Technol Assess*. 2009;13:iii-iv, xi-xiii, 1-113, 137-347.

A6. Kubany ES, Hill EE, Owens JA, et al. Cognitive trauma therapy for battered women with PTSD (CTT-BW). *J Consult Clin Psychol*. 2004;72:3-18.

A7. Tirado-Munoz J, Gilchrist G, Farre M, et al. The efficacy of cognitive behavioural therapy and advocacy interventions for women who have experienced intimate partner violence: a systematic review and meta-analysis. *Ann Med*. 2014;46:567-586.

A8. Babcock JC, Green CE, Robie C. Does batterers' treatment work? A meta-analytic review of domestic violence treatment. *Clin Psychol Rev*. 2004;23:1023-1053.

A9. Dunford FW. The San Diego Navy experiment: an assessment of interventions for men who assault their wives. *J Consult Clin Psychol*. 2000;68:468-476.

A10. Fellmeth GLT, Heffernan C, Nurse J, et al. Educational and skills-based interventions for preventing relationship and dating violence in adolescents and young adults. *Cochrane Database Syst Rev*. 2013;6:CD004534.

A11. Jahanfar S, Janssen PA, Howard LM, et al. Interventions for preventing or reducing domestic violence against pregnant women. *Cochrane Database Syst Rev*. 2013;2:CD009414.

A12. Tiwari A, Leung WC, Leung TW, et al. A randomised controlled trial of empowerment training for Chinese abused pregnant women in Hong Kong. *Br J Obstet Gynaecol*. 2005;112:1249-1256.

A13. Kiely M, El-Mohandes AA, El-Khorazaty MN, et al. An integrated intervention to reduce intimate partner violence in pregnancy: a randomized controlled trial. *Obstet Gynecol*. 2010;115:273-283.

A14. Hegarty K, O'Doherty L, Taft A, et al. Screening and counselling in the primary care setting for women who have experienced intimate partner violence (WEAVE): a cluster randomised controlled trial. *Lancet*. 2013;382:249-258.

A15. Feder G, Davies RA, Baird K, et al. Identification and Referral to Improve Safety (IRIS) of women experiencing domestic violence with a primary care training and support programme: a cluster randomised controlled trial. *Lancet*. 2011;378:1788-1795.

GENERAL REFERENCES

For the General References and other additional features, please visit Expert Consult at https://expertconsult.inkling.com.

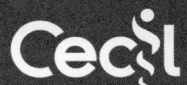

XX

DISEASES OF BONE AND MINERAL METABOLISM

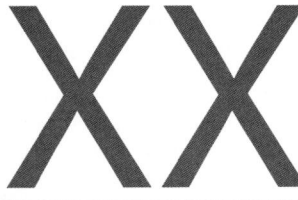

242

APPROACH TO THE PATIENT WITH METABOLIC BONE DISEASE

THOMAS J. WEBER

DIAGNOSIS

History

Patients with metabolic bone disease may present to the clinician in a number of ways, ranging from no symptoms to disabling musculoskeletal pain, depending on the nature of the underlying disorder. The most common conditions, osteoporosis and primary hyperparathyroidism, encompass a clinical spectrum that ranges from asymptomatic (diagnosed by low bone density and an elevated serum calcium, respectively)[1] to severe disease (fractures and bone pain). Less common conditions, such as osteomalacia, have more predictable presentations. In osteoporosis, fractures of the long bones (humerus, distal forearm, femur, and tibia) are clearly evident, whereas fractures at other sites (vertebrae, ribs, pelvis) may not be (see later and Chapter 243).[2] Patients with osteomalacia may complain of deep bone pain or aches, although often it is difficult for them to distinguish such pain from muscular pain. They may also report proximal muscle weakness that impairs their ability to ascend stairs. Vitamin D deficiency, the most common cause of osteomalacia, may confer similar bone and muscle complaints as well. In hyperparathyroidism, either self-reported or elicited fatigue may be a common complaint, along with mildly impaired cognition and memory. A history of recurrent nephrolithiasis is a hallmark of symptomatic primary hyperparathyroidism.

Physical Examination

Patients may exhibit physical clues to their skeletal condition. Height loss of more than 2 inches from a self-reported maximum, measured accurately with a calibrated stadiometer, may suggest the presence of vertebral compression fractures, which are clinically silent in up to three fourths of patients. Corresponding thoracic kyphosis may be present, and tenderness to palpation or percussion over the spinous process may suggest a recent vertebral fracture. Thoracic kyphosis will also impart quantifiable physical characteristics, including decreased and increased rib-pelvis and wall-occiput distances, respectively, which may be followed clinically in patients and significantly predict the presence of vertebral fractures. The method for the rib-pelvis distance measurement is illustrated in Figure 242-1. The wall-occiput distance is the space between the wall and the occiput of the head when a patient stands straight with the heel, buttocks, and back against the wall: it reflects the degree of kyphosis. Patients may also exhibit signs of secondary causes of osteoporosis (e.g., blue sclerae with osteogenesis imperfecta, goiter and

proptosis with hyperthyroidism, facial plethora and purple striae with Cushing's syndrome). Patients with Paget's disease may have a skeletal deformity and warmth over the affected sites. Patients with osteomalacia often have tenderness to palpation over the tibia or other long bones due to expansion of the subperiosteal space by undermineralized osteoid with nerve irritation. These patients may also have a wide-based, "waddling" gait due to pain. Hyperparathyroid patients may have flank tenderness if active nephrolithiasis is present and can rarely have corneal calcification if hypercalcemia is severe and longstanding. Such patients rarely have a palpable parathyroid adenoma. If present, however, a diagnosis of parathyroid carcinoma should be entertained.

Laboratory and Radiologic Investigations

Laboratory studies are a useful adjunct in the evaluation of metabolic bone disease, although their specificity depends somewhat on the disease in question. In particular, studies performed in the work-up of osteoporosis are generally not solely diagnostic but rather are supportive of secondary etiologies that may contribute to bone loss. Examples include thyroid-stimulating hormone, 25(OH)D, and testosterone levels (Table 242-1). In addition to a cursory work-up as detailed, additional investigations may also be indicated as clinically indicated and in individuals with a greater dual-energy x-ray absorptiometry (DXA) bone density deficit than expected for age (see later and Chapter 243).[3] In contrast, the diagnosis of other conditions is more securely based on abnormal studies, such as alkaline phosphatase (elevated in Pagets disease and depressed in hypophosphatasia) and parathyroid hormone (elevated in hyperparathyroidism). More sophisticated studies that target a specific diagnosis should be based on the history and examination (i.e., genetic testing for osteogenesis imperfecta). Bone turnover markers, which are cellular products of bone formation and resorption that can be measured in the blood and urine of patients, may provide noninvasive information on skeletal turnover (i.e., high or low) but cannot be used for diagnosis. They also have unacceptable biologic and measurement variability that precludes their clinical usefulness at this time.

Radiologic studies are critical to the diagnosis and management of these patients. Because the most common clinical event is fracture, plain radiographs of the involved skeletal sites are often indicated.[4] It is important to note that radiographs are relatively insensitive in identifying stress fractures and may also lag behind a frank fracture by hours or days. As such, additional, more sensitive modalities may be employed, including computed tomography and magnetic resonance imaging, to confirm a fracture. These studies also reveal characteristic patterns of skeletal involvement in certain conditions (i.e., Paget's disease). Whole body bone scintigraphy with the radioisotope techneticum-99m is the most sensitive tool to identify an active skeletal process but is nonspecific as to the nature of the underlying process (e.g., fracture, infection, malignancy). Perhaps most widely used and critical to management of osteoporosis is bone mineral density (BMD) testing, generally by DXA. As detailed in Chapter 243, DXA is a low-radiation, noninvasive examination of the spine, proximal femur, and distal forearm that may be used to identify and subsequently follow the treatment response to pharmacologic or conservative therapies. Finally, although rarely needed, tetracycline-labeled, transcortical bone biopsy of the iliac crest, with subsequent histomorphometic analysis, may be useful in the management of patients. Bone biopsy, which is generally performed by an orthopedic surgeon under conscious sedation, may be indicated to best guide management in patients with excessive bone fragility that cannot be adequately characterized by noninvasive means (e.g., patients with renal osteodystrophy, suspected osteomalacia, fractures with normal BMD by DXA).

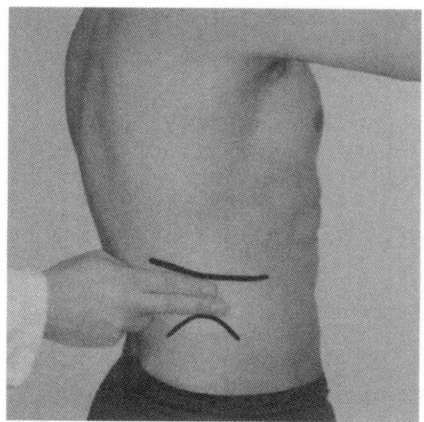

FIGURE 242-1. Method of assessing rib-pelvis distance. While standing behind the subject, the examiner holds his or her hands vertically and places them into the space between the inferior margin of the ribs and the superior surface of the pelvis in the mid-axillary line. The vertical distance is then measured in fingerbreadths.

TABLE 242-1 LABORATORY WORK-UP OF OSTEOPOROSIS

ALL OSTEOPOROSIS/OSTEOPENIA PATIENTS	AS CLINICALLY INDICATED
Serum creatinine, calcium, total protein, albumin, phosphorus, alkaline phosphatase, liver function tests	Serum and urine protein electrophoresis (SPEP and UPEP) (if total protein-to-albumin ratio is >2.0)
Complete blood count	Intact parathyroid hormone
Thyroid-stimulating hormone	24-Hour urine cortisol
24-Hour urine calcium and creatinine	Celiac panel (antigliadin/antiendomyseal antibodies)
Serum 25(OH)D	Fasting morning testosterone (men)

TREATMENT Rx

Management of patients with metabolic bone disease is generally directed by the disease process, although there are some unifying aspects of treatment. Adequate intake of calcium and vitamin D, usually through a combination of diet and supplements, is recommended for patients with osteoporosis. High-dose vitamin D is indicated for low-vitamin D–related osteomalacia, and phosphorus in combination with vitamin D analogues (i.e., calcitriol) is necessary to heal osteomalacia and facilitate normal longitudinal growth in children and adolescents with certain osteomalacic conditions (e.g., X-linked hypophosphatemic rickets or X-linked hypophosphatemia). Weight bearing and resistive exercise are also advisable for osteoporotic patients, although physical therapy consultation may be indicated in patients at high risk for fracture (previous fractures, frequent falls). Pharmacotherapy with oral and parenteral bisphosphonates is frontline therapy for patients with both osteoporosis and Paget's disease because of the anticatabolic effect on excessive osteoclastic bone resorption that underlies these diseases. In addition, other antiresorptive drugs, such as raloxifene and denosumab, are approved for the treatment of osteoporosis. Parenteral bisphosphonates and denosumab also are effective in combating malignancy-related bone disease (e.g., metastatic breast cancer, multiple myeloma). Finally, the anabolic bone agent teriparatide, a recombinant parathyroid hormone analogue, is useful in "building" bone density and reducing fracture risk in patients with severe osteoporosis, defined as very low BMD, high fracture risk, and/or multiple fractures. Newer drugs in development that target more recently identified aspects of bone physiology (e.g., the Wnt pathway in bone formation), as well as specific derangements in less common diseases (e.g. FGF-23 antibody in X-linked hypophosphatemia), will necessarily further improve the management of patients with metabolic bone disease.

GENERAL REFERENCES

For the General References and other additional features, please visit Expert Consult at https://expertconsult.inkling.com.

243

OSTEOPOROSIS

THOMAS J. WEBER

DEFINITION

Osteoporosis is defined as a skeletal disorder characterized by compromised bone strength predisposing to an increased risk for fracture. The pertinent clinical outcomes of this disease include fractures, bone pain, height loss, and physical deformity. This definition was developed by the National Institutes of Health in 2000 to help clinicians better diagnose and treat patients with the disease. The concept of bone strength is central to understanding the disorder because patients who suffer an osteoporotic or fragility fracture may or may not have osteoporosis by bone mineral density (BMD) criteria. The World Health Organization defines osteoporosis as a BMD that is equal to or greater than 2 standard deviations (SD) below that of an average individual at peak bone mass (generally age 20 to 30 years, depending on the measured skeletal site). However, it is well established that most fragility fractures, which are defined as fractures occurring from the energy imparted from a fall from a standing height or less, occur in individuals who have low (osteopenia) or even normal BMD. (Osteopenia, or low bone density, is defined as a BMD between −1.0 and −2.5 SD below young average normal.) This observation is consistent with the lack of a specific BMD threshold for fracture. Given these observations, it is clear that other factors must also significantly influence fracture risk. Certainly, falls and traumatic injuries are a significant, independent risk factor for fractures. Excluding falls and trauma, however, studies to date have also identified qualitative factors that are integral to bone strength, including skeletal microarchitecture, bone turnover, damage accumulation (e.g., microfractures), and pattern or degree of mineralization. Newer technologies are currently in development to improve our under-

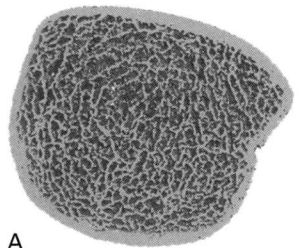 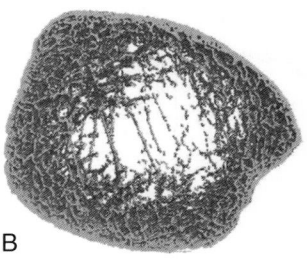

FIGURE 243-1. High-resolution peripheral computed tomography (Xtreme CT) of distal tibia in subject with normal bone mineral density (A) and severe osteoporosis (B). The deterioration in trabecular architecture with reduced trabecular number, trabecular thinning, increased trabecular spacing, generalized cortical thinning, and increased cortical porosity is readily appreciable in the osteoporotic subject. (From Griffith JF, Genant HK. New advances in imaging osteoporosis and its complications. *Endocrine.* 2012;42:39-51.)

standing of how these qualitative changes in bone compromise skeletal strength, including high-resolution peripheral quantitative computed tomography (HR-pQCT) and high-resolution magnetic resonance imagine (MRI) (Fig. 243-1).[1] Although promising, these newer techniques are not widely available. More important, they have not enhanced fracture prediction to date over known risk factors and BMD. Indeed, the availability and widespread application of Internet-based fracture prediction tools such as FRAX, which incorporate independent, additive clinical risk factors for fracture with or without hip BMD, are currently the best approach for identifying individuals at risk for and most likely to benefit from treatment to prevent fragility fractures.

EPIDEMIOLOGY

Approximately half of white women will develop an osteoporosis-related fracture in their lifetime, which is greater than their risk for breast cancer, heart attack, and stroke combined. In addition, one in five men will also fracture.[2] More than 2 million fractures occur annually in the United States, at an estimated total direct cost of $17 billion. Nearly three fourths of them occur in women, with most occurring in white women. Nonetheless, there are no ethnic exclusions to developing the disorder. The most common site of osteoporotic fracture is the spine, accounting for more than 750,000 fractures annually. Fractures of the proximal femur, which disproportionately confer a greater cost than other osteoporotic fractures, account for 14% of incident fractures but nearly three fourths of costs. Additional sites of fracture include the distal forearm, proximal humerus, and pelvis, with the latter two more commonly occurring in elderly people. The risk for fracture increases markedly with age, although the pattern of fracture risk does differ by skeletal site. The risk of Colles fractures increases until the mid-60s and then plateaus, whereas the risk for hip fractures increases exponentially in woman after the age of 65 years. Vertebral fracture risk rises earlier than that of hip, although many spine fractures are not clinically apparent and only identified through radiographic assessment. Although clinically silent, such fractures do confer a significant independent risk for future fractures, particularly if they are of recent occurrence.[3] Men also ascribe to an age-independent increase in fracture risk, although the increase in incidence generally lags at least 5 to 10 years behind that of women (Fig. 243-2). The reason for the gender-based difference in fracture incidence is likely related to anatomic differences because although men and woman have similar volumetric bone density at a given skeletal site, bone size is larger in men than in women and confers an independent mechanical protection against fracture. Nonetheless, the independent contribution of age to fracture risk necessarily predicts a higher morbidity and cost related to osteoporosis in men as well as women, with an increase in the United States alone by the year 2025 to greater than 3 million fractures with an associated annual cost of $25.3 billion.

There are also significant ethnic and geographic differences in the rate of osteoporotic fractures. African Americans have a lower lifetime risk for osteoporotic fracture, approximately roughly half that of whites. Differences in bone size, bone microarchitecture (thicker trabeculae in blacks), body composition, calcium absorption in youth, and life expectancy are potential reasons for this observation. Asian Americans and Hispanics have a fracture risk that is intermediate between that of whites and blacks, despite the fact that the former have a BMD that generally approximates that of whites.

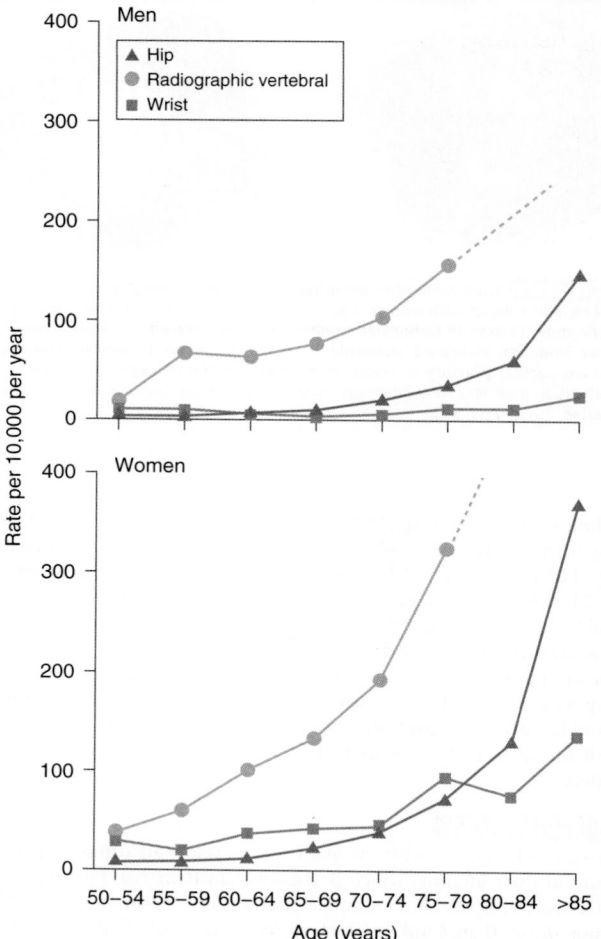

FIGURE 243-2. Age-specific and sex-specific incidence of radiographic vertebral, hip, and distal forearm fractures. (Data derived from European Prospective Osteoporosis Study and General Practice Research Database; from Sambrook P, Cooper C. Osteoporosis. *Lancet.* 2006;367:2010-2018.)

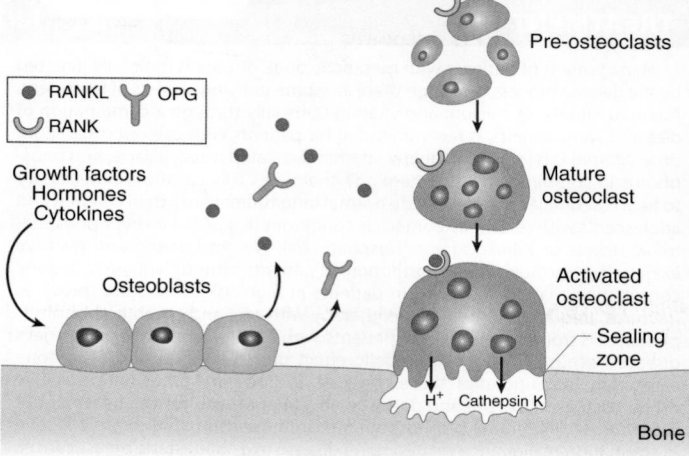

FIGURE 243-3. RANKL expressed by osteoblast lineage cells binds to RANK on the surface of pre-osteoclasts and mature osteoclasts, resulting in increased bone resorption through an increase in osteoclast differentiation, activity, and survival. Osteoprotogerin (OPG) is a "decoy receptor," also produced by osteoblasts, that binds to RANKL, preventing RANKL binding to RANK and thereby inhibiting osteoclastic bone resorption. It is the balance of RANKL and OPG that determines the ultimate rate of bone resorption. (Adapted from Lewiecki EM. New targets for intervention in the treatment of postmenopausal osteoporosis. *Nat Rev Rheumatol.* 2011;7:631-638.)

Indeed, the risk for hip fracture in U.S. Asian men and women is actually equal to or lower than that of U.S. blacks. The U.S. data are consistent with the global experience as well because hip fracture rates in China are lower than those observed in the United States, despite similar bone density at the hip. Differences in hip geometry, physical activity, and diet have been proposed as possible explanations. Despite this, rates of hip fracture have actually been increasing in the Far East, while declining in the United States for unclear reasons. Changing patterns of nutrition and physical activity could be responsible for the former, although the latter observation remains heretofore unexplained.

PATHOBIOLOGY
Normal Bone Biology

BMD in adults is determined by the magnitude of bone acquisition during adolescence and young adulthood, and the rate of bone loss that ensues thereafter. These processes are generally referred to as bone modeling and remodeling. Heritable factors, including gender and ethnicity, account for 60 to 80% of the variability in skeletal development, including peak bone mass, bone size, and bone geometry, although nutrition, lifestyle, and other factors also have a significant impact. Peak bone mass is achieved in most individuals by the early to late 20s and differs in timing by skeletal site (age 18 to 20 years for proximal femur, 25 to 30 years for spine). Modeling of the skeleton occurs during this time and represents a true increase in bone mass and bone size through endochondral ossification of the axial skeleton and periosteal apposition of the appendicular skeleton.

To best understand the underlying pathophysiology of osteoporosis, one must first appreciate the concept of bone remodeling. Skeletal remodeling is

a finely orchestrated process of bone resorption and subsequent formation. It is a necessary physiologic function that results in repair of damaged bone and redistribution of the skeleton to adapt to changes in mechanical stress and to provide calcium to the systemic circulation for critical cellular processes. Recent evidence suggests that the osteocyte, which accounts for 90 to 95% of all bone cells, is the critical cell that regulates both resorption and formation. Osteocytes are derived from osteoblasts that are embedded within the bone matrix. During this maturation phase, this "osteoid-osteocyte" cell actively secretes and calcifies bone matrix material. In addition, mature osteocytes within bone contain dendritic processes that may directly regulate osteoblast recruitment and bone formation. Recent studies also suggest that mature osteocytes may form new bone within their lacunae. In addition, osteocytes produce proteins that regulate mineralization, including positive (PHEX, DMP-1) and negative (FGF-23) factors.

Osteocytes also regulate bone resorption, both directly through apoptosis proximate to skeletal microcracks or fatigue damage in need of repair and indirectly through enhancement of pre-osteoblast or mesenchymal stromal cell (MSC) development. (MSCs may also develop into adipocytes, chondrocytes, and muscle cells, depending on developmental stimuli.) These events result in the production, expression, and release of cytokines critical to osteoclast recruitment and development, including interleukin-1 (IL-1), interleukin-6 (IL-6), osteoprotogerin (OPG), and receptor activator of nuclear factor-κB ligand (RANKL). The cognate receptor for RANKL, RANK, is expressed on the surface of the developing and mature osteoclast, which itself is a derivative of cells of the monocyte-macrophage lineage. RANKL is a critical determinant of osteoclast recruitment, development, and survival, such that disruption of RANKL signaling results in high bone density fragility disorders (e.g., osteopetrosis). OPG, which is also produced by pre-osteoblasts, is a decoy receptor for RANK that binds to RANKL, preventing RANKL binding to RANK and thereby serving as an endogenous suppresser of osteoclast function. In essence, RANKL/OPG represent a "yin/yang" paradigm in which osteoclast biology and bone resorption are intricately regulated and controlled (Fig. 243-3).

Factors Affecting Peak Bone Mass and Remodeling

As mentioned, peak bone mass is achieved by the third decade. Longitudinal studies in children and adolescents suggest that hormonal, physical activity, nutritional, and genetic factors are all important in this process. Hereditary influence is the most important determinant and to date the least well understood. Growth hormone and sex hormones play critical roles in growth of the appendicular (long bones) and axial (vertebrae) skeleton, with the former maturing earlier than the latter (end of puberty vs. young adulthood). Males

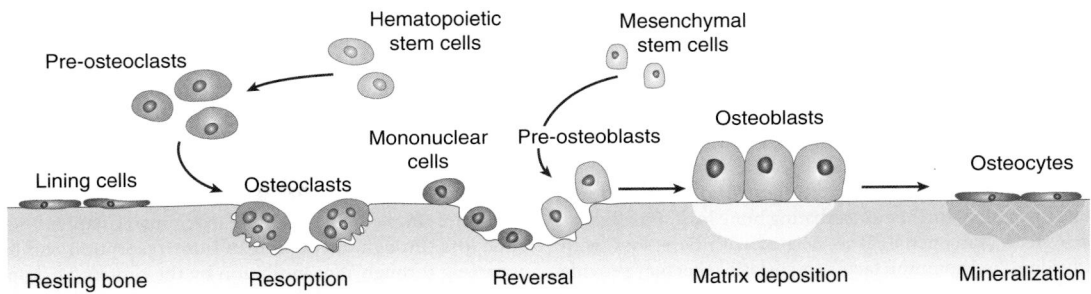

FIGURE 243-4. The basic multicellular unit (BMU) moving across the bone tissue. First, 10 to 20 osteoclasts resorb old or damaged tissue; then they recruit 1000 to 2000 osteoblasts, which produce new bone matrix. The BMU moves at a speed of 20 to 40 µm/day and survives for up to 6 months. (From Kapinas K, Delany AM. MicroRNA biogenesis and regulation of bone remodeling. *Arthritis Res Ther.* 2011;13:220.)

have larger bones as a result of greater periosteal (outer surface of bone) expansion of bone than occurs in females. Current evidence supports a positive effect of exercise and loading on bone size and mineral density, although a subsequent potential antifracture benefit later in adult life is not proved. Poor nutrition and concomitant disease may also affect bone accrual, primarily through delayed pubertal onset and progression, although studies do support a potential for "catch-up" growth, which depends on the degree of insult and timing of resolution.

Although these factors are all important, genetic factors appear to account for 60 to 80% of the variance in peak BMD. Genome-wide association studies have identified 62 distinct loci that are significantly associated with BMD.[4] Three known obligatory pathways of bone metabolism were identified by genome-wide association studies, namely Wnt, RANK-RANKL-OPG, and endochondral ossification. The RANK pathway was discussed previously. The Wnt signaling pathway is obligatory for bone formation, owing to its role in osteoblast proliferation and differentiation. It was initially discovered through study on kindreds with high bone mass and the osteoporosis pseudoganglioma syndrome, who have, respectively, activating and inactivating mutations in the Wnt pathway receptor LRP5. Endochondral ossification, a process that involves the cartilage growth plate and subsequent ossification of the cartilaginous skeleton, is dependent on transcription factors (SOX6, RUNX2) and proteins (parathyroid hormone–related peptide, bone sialoprotein 2, and osteopontin) that are necessary for the development of the cartilage growth plate, bone matrix mineralization, and osteoblast differentiation. Indeed, the first two pathways are already the target of existing and developing therapies for osteoporosis. Despite these advances, our understanding of the relationship between genes and bone mass accrual remains poor, as evidenced by the fact that less than 6% of the variance in femoral neck BMD is explained by the loci identified in genome-wide association studies.

In adults, bone remodeling is a physiologic process through which skeletal repair and adaption to changes in biomechanical stress occur. The basic multicellular unit (BMU), which is composed of bone-resorbing osteoclasts, bone-forming osteoblasts, bone lining cells, and embedded osteocytes, is the cellular apparatus that facilitates remodeling (Fig. 243-4). After the age of 30 years, this process is reasonably matched, resulting in rates of bone loss of only 0.3 to 0.5% per year from the third through fifth decades of life. As individuals age, mismatches in bone remodeling, either due to reduced formation, increased resorption, or a combination of both, result in greater rates of bone loss. Biologic changes, such as menopause and aging, systemic disease, personal vices, and medications (most notably glucocorticoids), may contribute to this imbalance. In addition, there is evidence that genetic factors also influence rates of bone loss and fracture. Although not as robust an influence as on peak BMD, twin and family-based studies suggest that genetic factors contribute roughly 30 to 50% of the variance in rates of bone loss at the spine, hip, and forearm. However, studies attempting to identify specific genes that are associated with accelerated rates of bone loss have been inconsistent to date, including ones that have identified the collagen gene (*COL1A1*), vitamin D receptor gene (*VDR*), estrogen receptor-1 gene (*ESR1*), interleukin-6 (IL-6), and the apoprotein AOE*4 allele as potential candidates. This inconsistency may be due to insufficient data sets that do not have repeated measures of bone density. Interestingly, there is a fairly robust heritability of menarche and menopausal onset, perhaps paralleling the

observations on *ESR1* and IL-6 (whose production is suppressed by estrogen) and supporting hormonal pathways as a potential target of genetically mediated bone loss.

Although a better understanding of the genetic influences on bone mass accrual and subsequent loss is critically needed, it is perhaps more important to extend these analyses to the pertinent clinical outcome in this disease—fracture. This is further supported given the previously described significant unexplained variance between BMD and fracture risk. Unfortunately, such work to date has yielded disappointing results, likely in part because the heritability of fracture risk diminishes significantly with aging. In addition, the contributions of individual genetic variants to fracture risk are quite small and potentially falsely negative when studied. Nonetheless, there is preliminary evidence that simulated genetic profiling using a large number of variants could increase the discriminatory value of existing fracture prediction models and significantly re-stratify individuals in need of or not requiring antifracture therapies.[5]

Mechanisms of Bone Loss
"Natural" and Aging-Related Bone Loss
As noted previously, net bone loss during adult life is expected, although the rate of bone loss accelerates during the latter decades because of a number of factors. Perhaps most important for women, rates of bone loss increase substantially in the perimenopausal and early postmenopausal years, amounting to losses of 1 to 5% per year. Unfortunately, there are currently no biologic markers that help determine which women a priori are "rapid losers." Bone loss is slower in obese women, likely because of higher estrogen levels afforded by production through aromatization in adipose tissue. A decline in circulating estrogen is primarily responsible for bone loss following both natural and surgical menopause, which is mediated primarily through upregulation of cytokines (most notably RANKL) and a resultant increase in the number, activity, and depth of osteoclast-mediated bone resorption sites. In addition, OPG production is diminished, further amplifying bone resorption, although estrogen replacement can restore OPG production while reducing RANKL expression and thereby help mitigate bone loss during this period. Although bone resorption and formation do occur sequentially during this period, resorption outpaces formation because of potentiation of the former aided by the release of soluble cytokines, resulting in a significant uncoupling of bone remodeling and accelerated bone loss. Fortunately, this phase of rapid bone loss is typically limited to 5 to 7 years in most women.

Current evidence supports a key role in bone loss for reduced estrogen levels in men, perhaps owing to reduced aromatase activity in fat tissue. Decline in circulating insulin-like growth factor-I levels also occurs with aging, which may inhibit the production of MSCs and pre-osteoblasts, in addition to limiting periosteal bone expansion. The latter is a normal adaptive process to aging that increases bone size, more so in men than in women, somewhat attenuating the observed increase in fracture risk with aging. Bone loss in later decades also is caused by lower 25-hydroxy vitamin D (25[OH]D) levels, related to restricted sun exposure and a reduced capacity to generate pre–vitamin D in the skin with aging, as well as limited intake of vitamin D and calcium. Indeed, more than 75% in individuals in the United States are either vitamin D deficient or insufficient (25[OH]D < 30 ng/mL). Low vitamin D results in secondary hyperparathyroidism, which accelerates cortical bone loss, as well as likely increasing the risk for falls. Increase in bone marrow adiposity is also inversely and significantly correlated with aging-related bone loss. This process likely reduces bone formation through the production of fewer osteoblast precursors, which share a common mesenchymal stem cell lineage with adipocytes. It is also likely the result of increased activation of the nuclear receptor peroxisome proliferator activator receptor-γ (PPARG), which commits stem cells toward adipocyte and away from osteoblast differentiation. Additionally, fat-derived adipokines (adiponectin and leptin) may negatively affect bone remodeling through a "bone-fat" connection by reducing bone formation, further exacerbating bone loss.[6] Finally, loss of weight and muscle mass (sarcopenia) is associated with bone loss, with evidence of a recently identified common factor (myostatin) that may provide insights on this muscle-bone interaction.[7]

Secondary Causes and Clinical Impact of Bone Loss

Bone loss also occurs as a result of secondary processes, such as diseases and medications. In fact, such processes are identifiable in more than one fourth of individuals with osteoporosis and may be more likely with greater degrees of skeletal deficit. A list of secondary causes of osteoporosis, based on a systems-based approach, is detailed in Table 243-1. As expected, endocrine

TABLE 243-1	SECONDARY CAUSES OF OSTEOPOROSIS
ENDOCRINE DISORDERS	
Hypogonadism: female and male	
Hypercortisolism: endogenous and exogenous	
Hyperthyroidism	
Hyperparathyroidism	
Idiopathic hypercalciuria	
Diabetes mellitus: type 1 and type 2	
NUTRITIONAL AND GASTROINTESTINAL DISORDERS	
Malabsorption: celiac disease, gastrointestinal bypass	
Vitamin D deficiency	
Cirrhosis (including primary biliary cirrhosis)	
Pancreatic insufficiency	
Inflammatory bowel disease	
Cystic fibrosis	
Anorexia nervosa, bulimia	
HEMATOLOGIC AND ONCOLOGIC DISORDERS	
Multiple myeloma	
Hemolytic anemia	
Hemoglobinopathies: thalassemia, sickle cell	
Myeloproliferative neoplasms	
Skeletal metastases	
Pompe's disease	
Mastocytosis	
CONNECTIVE TISSUE AND METABOLIC DISORDERS	
Osteogenesis imperfecta	
Ehlers-Danlos syndrome	
Marfan syndrome	
Homocystinuria	
Gaucher's disease	
Pompe's disease	
MEDICATIONS	
Glucocorticoids	
Thyroxine (excessive)	
Antiepileptics	
Heparin	
Gonadotropin-releasing hormone agonists	
Depo-Provera	
Immunosuppressants: tacrolimus, cyclosporine	
Chemotherapy	
Selective serotonin reuptake inhibitors*	
Proton pump inhibitors*	
Thiazolidinediones*	
Alcohol	
MISCELLANEOUS	
Rheumatoid arthritis	
Immobilization	
Juvenile osteoporosis	
Pregnancy-associated osteoporosis	

*Association based.

disorders, including hypogonadism and Cushing's syndrome, predominate. Nonetheless, bone loss in several conditions is mediated indirectly through attendant effects on vitamin D metabolism (e.g., malabsorption, chronic liver disease) and is the case with certain medications as well (antiepileptic drugs phenytoin and phenobarbital). In the case of vitamin D deficiency, undermineralization of bone may confound the clinical picture of bone loss and should be considered first before initiation of bone active medications (see later). Rarely, malignancies can be the principal cause of osteoporosis, with the best example being multiple myeloma (Chapter 187). Myeloma causes bone loss through uncoupling of bone resorption and formation, the latter occurring through Wnt inhibition by the protein Dickopf. Medications also cause bone loss through both osteoclastic activation and osteoblastic inhibition. Reduced bone formation is the mechanism by which glucocorticoids cause bone loss, both through exogenous administration and exogenous overproduction. Previous work has confirmed reduced osteoblast and osteocyte function and survival as the principal mechanism of glucocorticoid-induced osteoporosis. Anorexia nervosa likely interferes with the anabolic effect of insulin-like growth factor-I on bone. Alcohol excess appears to suppress osteoblast function, perhaps both directly and indirectly through associated malnutrition, but it may also possibly cause bone loss through hypogonadism, which results in accelerated turnover. Finally, relatively rare connective tissue disorders, such as osteogenesis imperfecta and Marfan syndrome, increase skeletal fragility by means of disturbances in the skeletal matrix and mechanical integrity rather than altered bone remodeling.

The resulting clinical impact of bone loss and the persistence of effect depend on a number of factors, both potentially modifiable and nonmodifiable. The age at which bone loss occurs (e.g., young adult vs. 80-year-old) affects the ability to recover BMD with resolution or treatment of the condition (younger people have more robust recovery than elderly people) and also appears to hold for conditions of accelerated bone resorption (e.g., immobilization) or reduced bone formation (e.g., glucocorticoids). Predicated on and paralleling this observation, BMD response to treatment is generally more pronounced in individuals with higher rates of bone turnover, likely reflecting to some extent a "filling in" of bone remodeling space. Menopausal stage in women also influences rate of bone loss as described previously, with greater rates of decline occurring within the first 5 to 7 years of cessation of menses (Chapter 240). Concomitant vitamin D deficiency and resulting secondary hyperparathyroidism also potentiate rates of BMD loss, particularly in elderly people; it is thought to be a major contributing factor to the increase in hip fracture incidence in this group. Tobacco and alcohol overuse may also accelerate bone loss, owing to global effects that include reduced sex hormones, altered calcium metabolism, and weight loss and frailty, resulting in uncoupled bone remodeling. Therefore, a distinct appreciation of the clinical context is critical to defining an appropriate diagnostic and treatment approach to patients with osteoporosis.

CLINICAL MANIFESTATIONS

Historically, osteoporosis was diagnosed in an individual presenting with a low trauma or fragility fracture, typically of the vertebrae or hips. Classic representations of women with the so-called dowager's hump or kyphotic deformity were common depictions of the disease. Currently, however, the disease is appreciated both for its clinical and subclinical manifestations, because of both the advent of bone density testing and the appreciation that many vertebral fractures are clinically silent. This approach is akin to paradigms that identify a surrogate marker for both diagnosis and risk stratification, such as hypertension for stroke and hyperlipidemia for myocardial infarction.

A history of fragility fracture is strongly suggestive of osteoporosis, although there is evidence that a history of high trauma fractures also identifies persons with low BMD and those at higher risk for low-trauma fractures. The National Osteoporosis Foundation considers fractures of the spine, proximal femur, distal forearm, and proximal humerus "major" osteoporotic fractures, although other skeletal sites are also prone to fragility fractures. These include the pelvis, ribs, and proximal tibia, although there is controversy about whether ankle fractures should be considered as such. Fractures of the spine are generally from the mid-thoracic region through the lower lumbar region, with the greatest frequency at T11 through L2.[8] Patient often present after a fall or a spinal flexion-loading event in which they may hear a "pop" and complain of sharp midline back pain that may radiate to the flanks. Patients may also present with complaints of back "tiredness," which is improved with sitting or lying down. This symptom is likely related to paraspinal weakness or spasm from abnormal spinal curvature that occurs with chronic vertebral compression. Back pain may commonly be related to other pathology, such as degenerative disc and spine disease that is concomitantly present. This is important to note because low bone mass in and of itself does not cause pain, unless it is due to osteomalacia (see later). Vertebral fractures may occur without acute symptoms as well, as noted later. In contrast, nonvertebral fracture events are always clinically evident. Hip fractures generally occur with falls, although they may rarely occur with limited force such as twisting.

Physical examination may also indicate the presence of osteoporosis and associated fractures, as well as potentially identifying underlying secondary processes contributing to the disease. Measured height loss, best confirmed using a calibrated device such as a stadiometer, of greater than 4 cm since young adult maximum height is suggestive of prior vertebral fractures. Height loss also occurs with scoliosis and aging (approximately ⅓ inch of height is lost per decade after age 50 years). A kyphotic deformity of the upper thoracic spine may be present, although it is important to distinguish it from accentuated cervical lordosis with associated prominence of T1. Spinal tenderness to palpation and percussion can occur with an acute vertebral compression fracture. Palpable tenderness of the long bones may suggest underlying osteomalacia instead, due to periosteal expansion and nerve irritation. Reduced rib-pelvis and increased wall-occiput distances are correlated with vertebral fractures as well.

In addition to the history and physical examination, radiologic findings may identify the presence of osteoporosis, sometimes somewhat surreptitiously. Plain films can detect bone loss by means of accentuation of vertical striations on spine radiographs that represent loss of horizontal trabeculae, although this generally indicates BMD loss of at least 25% or more. Kyphosis and compression fractures may be present, and patients often are unaware of the deformities because nearly three fourths of such fractures occur without acute pain. Furthermore, radiologic reporting of these fractures is inconsistent, suggesting that, if possible, the clinician review available digitized lateral chest radiographs and even lateral scout films often available from computed tomography (CT) to identify such fractures (Fig. 243-5). This is critical for optimal management, given the aforementioned risk conferred by previous fractures on future fracture events. The degree of compression fracture is also important because more severe fractures (>25% vertebral height loss) appear to better predict future fractures, as do nonvertebral fractures. When fractures are suspected, CT and MRI may be used, given that plain radiographs have a lower sensitivity acutely and with stress fractures. MRI also can be used to define a vertebral fracture with persistent swelling and edema based on T2 characteristics, potentially identifying patients who could benefit from vertebroplasty or kyphoplasty (see later). Finally, whole body bone scintigraphy is the most sensitive test for fracture but can be falsely positive because of inflammation, infection, or tumor and usually is positive for 6 to 12 months after a fracture event.

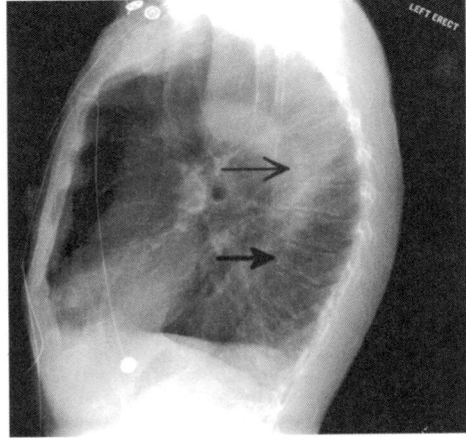

FIGURE 243-5. Incidental vertebral compression fractures on chest radiograph. Lateral radiograph of the chest of a 74-year-old man studied for cough. No relevant pulmonary abnormality was noted on the frontal radiograph (not shown). Examination of the thoracic spine shows the presence of a mild anterior wedge compression fracture of T9 (*thick arrow*) and moderate anterior wedge fracture of T6 (*thin arrow*). Neither fracture was reported on the radiographic report.

DIAGNOSIS

Although a recent fragility fracture is a reasonable basis for diagnosis of osteoporosis, other skeletal conditions should also be entertained, including inherited and acquired osteomalacias and pathologic fracture due to malignancy. These disorders can often be distinguished by history and physical examination, although additional investigations may be required. This distinction is critical because therapies may differ greatly between disorders. Most patients with osteoporosis are diagnosed on the basis of BMD measurement, generally by dual-energy x-ray absorptiometry (DXA). DXA is a low-radiation-based radiologic measurement of the areal bone density (g/cm^2) of the lumbar spine, proximal femur, and distal radius. Osteoporosis can be diagnosed if the BMD of a postmenopausal woman or man older than 50 years is more than 2.5 SD below young average normal (T score ≤ −2.5). A T score between −1.0 and −2.5 is considered low bone density or osteopenia, and a Z score (age-matched BMD) in premenopausal women and men younger than 50 years that is more than 2 SD below that of an a average age-matched individual is considered low bone density for age. BMD is an independent predictor of fracture risk, such that the relative risk for fracture increases by 1.5- to 2-fold for each 1 SD decrease in T score. In addition, fracture risk increases exponentially below a T score of −2.5. Furthermore, BMD of the femoral neck may be used in fracture prediction models such as FRAX to better define an individual's risk for subsequent fracture (see later). In addition to DXA, other modalities are also used to diagnose osteoporosis, including quantitative CT of the spine (QCT) and wrist and tibia (pQCT), finger DXA, and ultrasound of the calcaneus or wrist. Measurement of BMD by all of these techniques has been shown to globally predict fractures, akin to DXA. QCT and pQCT provide additional information on cortical and trabecular bone compartments but are accompanied by higher radiation exposure and poorer reproducibility compared with DXA. Ultrasound is radiation free and easy to operate but is less sensitive in diagnosing osteoporosis and does not measure change in a reliable fashion in response to age or treatment, making it useful as a screening modality but not for longitudinal care.

Although DXA is an effective diagnostic tool, several potential limitations and caveats need to be considered by the clinician. First, DXA cannot distinguish between low bone density and undermineralized bone matrix, the latter of which occurs in osteomalacia (Chapter 244). BMD may also be quite disparate between regions, perhaps in more than one third of individuals. This inconsistency results from a number of factors, including differences in bone composition (predominantly trabecular bone in the spine and cortical bone in the one-third radius) with resultant variations in rates of bone loss due to aging and disease (vertebral bone loss with menopause and glucocorticoid use versus cortical bone loss in hyperparathyroidism). Degenerative changes due to aging, such as facet osteoarthritis and aortic calcification, may artifactually raise spine BMD value. Given these considerations, the lowest skeletal site should be used for diagnosis. Finally, BMD should be measured longitudinally on the same DXA machine if possible, because of intermachine and intermanufacturer differences that may confound the ability to validly measure change over time. Despite these caveats, DXA remains the best method to diagnose and manage osteoporosis by bone density testing.

Despite its utility, bone density has been limited historically in optimally predicting fracture risk in individual patients. In addition, BMD does not take into account clinical factors that independently predict fracture. Under this premise, fracture prediction models have been developed that combine BMD and risk factors to better stratify fracture risk. The best known and most widely used of these prediction models is FRAX. FRAX was developed by the World Health Organization in collaboration with national and international osteoporosis foundations as an Internet-based computer algorithm that defines a person's 10-year risk for hip and major osteoporotic fracture (hip, clinical spine, forearm, and proximal humerus all combined). The model uses country-specific data on clinical risk factors and femoral neck BMD to calculate fracture probability and is available as a web-based tool that can be used by clinicians with their patients to assist in making informed decisions on osteoporosis management (http://www.shef.ac.uk/FRAX/). FRAX can be also be used to define country-specific recommended diagnostic and treatment thresholds. An example of this is the National Osteoporosis Foundation guidance that 10-year risks equal to or exceeding 3 and 20% for hip and major fracture risk, respectively, warrant consideration of pharmacologic treatment, which is based on cost-effective analyses in the United States. Furthermore, the number needed to treat (NNT) can be determined to best inform patients of their expected risk and benefit of treatment (e.g., bisphosphonate use roughly reduces hip fracture risk by half, or from 10 to 5%, with NNT of 1/0.05, or 20 patients treated to prevent one hip fracture). Despite its utility and ease of use, FRAX does have limitations. These include inability to use patients who are not treatment naïve, underestimation of fracture risk in those with disparately lower BMD in the spine than hip, absence of fall history/fall risk in the model, and the use of fixed clinical risk factors. Modifications have been suggested for the latest guidelines, including adjusting FRAX score up or down based on glucocorticoid dose. In addition, although fracture risk calculators that incorporate fall risk are available (e.g., from the Garvan Institute), they do not include the competing risk of mortality as FRAX does. As such, FRAX should be viewed, not as a perfect, but rather as a complementary tool to BMD in best defining a person's risk for fracture and candidacy for pharmacologic intervention.

Finally, all patients presenting with osteoporosis require an assessment for secondary causes of bone loss, given that 20 to 25% of women and perhaps an even greater portion of men will have identifiable additional etiologies that may contribute to bone loss (see Table 243-1). Most patients will have had routine chemistry, hematology, and thyroid studies as part of their annual examination. The 25(OH)D level should be measured in all patients for multiple reasons, as previously discussed. Additional investigations may also be considered, as directed by the clinical history and physical examination. In addition, a greater degree of BMD deficit (i.e., lower Z score) indicates a need for more extensive testing, given the greater likelihood of secondary causes being present. Bone turnover markers (BTMs) are serum and urinary products of bone formation or resorption that can also be used to assist in management. Available tests include bone-specific alkaline phosphatase, osteocalcin, type I procollagen amino-terminal propeptide, and type I procollagen carboxy-terminal propeptide as formation markers, and serum and urine C- and N-terminal peptides of type I collagen as resorption markers, among others. Their use is predicated on studies showing that high bone turnover increases fracture risk independent of BMD. In addition, fracture risk reduction correlates well with reduction in bone turnover based on clinical trials with anticatabolic agents. Nonetheless, their clinical utility has been tempered to date by several issues. First, there is significant biologic variability due to nonmodifiable (e.g., age, gender, underlying comorbid disease, medications) and modifiable (e.g., time of day, food intake, presence of fracture) factors that limit the ability to detect meaningful change over time in an individual patient. Second, optimal specimen processing is required for valid results and interpretation. Finally, and perhaps in part secondary to these issues and others, evidence to date does not demonstrate significant benefit of BTMs in individual patients in securely predicting bone density increase, fracture risk reduction, or cost effectiveness through patient feedback and improved adherence. Therefore, at present, BTMs should not be used in routine clinical practice, although they could help inform management in more complicated cases of metabolic bone disease.[9]

PREVENTION AND TREATMENT   Rx

Calcium

Adequate intake of calcium is critical to the optimal accumulation and maintenance of bone mineral density. Calcium supplementation has meaningful impact on BMD and fracture risk reduction, although the latter is much less certain. BMD is modestly improved by 1 to 2%, although evidence of a definitive reduction in hip and nonvertebral fracture risk when given without vitamin D is lacking at present, although previous studies have suggested a trend toward vertebral fracture risk reduction. Given the established increase in rate of nephrolithiasis and a possible, albeit unproven, potential increase in nonfatal cardiac events with higher dose calcium supplementation, it would seem prudent to recommend that adults with osteoporosis obtain 1200 to 1500 mg of calcium from a combination of supplements and dietary sources.

Vitamin D

Appropriate circulating levels of 25(OH)D are necessary for optimal intestinal absorption of calcium and skeletal accrual and maintenance. Despite this, a significant proportion of children and adults have vitamin D levels that would be deemed insufficient (i.e., 25[OH]D < 20 ng/mL). Data in adults with osteoporosis confirm a benefit of vitamin D supplementation for fracture risk reduction, although the effect is dependent on the patient population and the amount of supplementation. Doses of 400 to 800 IU of vitamin D combined with 1000 mg of calcium reduce the risk for hip fracture in postmenopausal women and men aged 65 years and older, although the benefit is less certain for community-dwelling individuals than for those in assisted living centers.[A1] In addition, it appears that a 25(OH)D level of at least 30 ng/mL is needed to reduce the risk for hip fracture,[A2] although there is some controversy over this recommendation based on the results of other meta-analyses with likely different methodologies. In addition, a daily vitamin D intake of at least 800 IU also reduces the risk for falls, likely by improving muscle strength and reducing body sway.[A3] It should be noted that the recent U.S. Preventive Services Task Force recommendation against the use of calcium and vitamin D[10] was based on the general U.S. population and does not pertain to patients with osteoporosis. Finally, although activated vitamin D analogues such as calcitriol and α-calcidiol have been shown to reduce fracture risk, they are generally not indicated based on unacceptable risk for hypercalcemia. The exception to use of vitamin D analogues is possibly patients with stage 3 and 4 chronic kidney disease, wherein treatment of secondary hyperparathyroidism could provide skeletal benefit.

Exercise and Lifestyle

Physical activity is also a critical element of osteoporosis management, which can be indirectly inferred based on the known profound effects of decreased gravitational force (i.e., immobilization, paraplegia, weightlessness in space) on inducing bone loss. Physical activity likely also confers additional benefits through enhanced muscle strength, improved cardiovascular status, and reduction in fall risk. Meta-analysis confirmed a modest benefit of exercise on lumbar spine (mean difference = 0.85%) and trochanteric BMD (mean difference = 1.03%) in postmenopausal women compared with placebo, although it did not show significant changes in femoral neck or total hip BMD.[A4] However, studies to date have not confirmed an improvement in bone strength with exercise in this patient group. Studies concerning middle-aged and older men are much more limited in number and quality, although preliminary evidence suggests that resistance training with or without impact-loading activities has the greatest BMD benefit. Importantly, although none of the aforementioned studies have demonstrated a clear antifracture benefit from exercise, there are abundant data that multiple targeted exercise interventions do reduce either the risk for falling (Tai Chi) or both the rate and risk for falling (group and home-based exercise programs),[A5] which is most likely an inciting event in older patients incurring an osteoporotic fracture. Finally, modification of aberrant lifestyles is also indicated in patients with osteoporosis, especially tobacco cessation and moderation of caffeine, carbonated beverage, and alcohol intake. Data are lacking, however, on whether these reduce overall fracture risk.

Medications

There is robust evidence that pharmacologic therapy significantly reduces the risk for osteoporotic fracture in a clinically meaningful and cost-effective manner.[11] Medications approved for osteoporosis can be classified based on their mechanism of action: anticatabolic (i.e., antiresorptive) and anabolic (i.e., bone building).

Anticatabolic Agents

Anticatabolic medications, or antiresorptive as they were more commonly known, inhibit osteoclast recruitment, function, and/or survival, resulting in reductions in skeletal turnover and bone loss. These agents, depending on the potency and persistence of bone effect, reduce the number of new activation sites (BMUs) and the bone remodeling space, thereby improving BMD while strengthening the skeletal microstructure and reducing fracture risk.

Bisphosphonates

Bisphosphonates (BPs) are the most widely prescribed and used medications for the treatment of osteoporosis, owing in large part to good tolerability and an ability to dose them infrequently (from once weekly to once yearly, depending on the drug). BPs are chemically engineered analogues of the naturally occurring molecule pyrophosphate in which a carbon is substituted for an oxygen. As a result, BPs have an extremely high affinity for hydroxyapatite crystals within bone. After incorporation into bone, BPs are taken up by osteoclasts and thereafter inhibit cellular attachment, function, and survival. The carbon side-chain molecules largely determine skeletal affinity and potency of BP effect. The first-generation BP etidronate, which is not approved in the United States for treatment of osteoporosis, is the least potent agent of the class. It must also be given in an interrupted fashion for 2 weeks every 3 months owing to the potential to cause focal osteomalacia, and it may cause lower gastrointestinal symptoms (i.e., abdominal pain and diarrhea). Nonetheless, it is has been shown to reduce the risk for vertebral but not nonvertebral nor hip fractures.

Three oral bisphosphonates are approved by the U.S. Food and Drug Administration (FDA) and currently available in the United States: alendronate, risedronate, and ibandronate, in order of time since initial FDA approval. All three drugs are also available as generic preparations, although some differences do exist between the brand name and generic drugs in regard to the

TABLE 243-2 STRENGTH OF EVIDENCE FOR THE REDUCTION OF RISK FOR FRACTURE TYPES WITH PHARMACOTHERAPY IN WOMEN WITH POSTMENOPAUSAL OSTEOPOROSIS

	FRACTURE SKELETAL SITES			
	VERTEBRAL	**NONVERTEBRAL**	**HIP**	**WRIST**
Alendronate	• • •	• • •	• • •	•
Ibandronate	• • •	• •	•	▮
Risedronate	• • •	• • •	• • •	•
Zoledronate	• • •	• • •	• • •	▮
Denosumab	• • •	• • •	• • •	▮
Teriparatide	• • •	• •	•	▮
Raloxifene	• • •	▮	▮	▮

Strength of evidence symbol legend: ▮ = insufficient strength of evidence; • = low strength of evidence; • • = moderate strength of evidence; • • • = high strength of evidence.
(Adapted with permission from Levis S, Theodore G. Summary of AHRQ's comparative effectiveness review of treatment to prevent fractures in men and women with low bone density or osteoporosis: update of the 2007 report. *J Manag Care Pharm.* 2012;18[4 Suppl B]:S1-S15, discussion S13.)

inactive excipients. The oral BPS may be administered once weekly (alendronate and risedronate) or once monthly (risedronate and ibandronate), fasting in the morning with water only, and the patient must remain fasting in a sitting or standing position for 30 to 60 minutes after the dose. Recently, a delayed-release formulation of risedronate (Atelvia) was approved that may be taken immediately after breakfast. The most common side effect is precipitation or aggravation of gastroesophageal reflux, although most patients tolerate the drugs without difficulty. In light of this side effect and a potential risk for esophageal irritation and ulceration, these drugs are contraindicated in patients with functional or anatomic disorders of esophageal transit (i.e., esophageal stricture, achalasia). All three drugs significantly reduce the risk for vertebral fractures, although high-strength evidence for hip and nonvertebral fracture risk reduction exists for alendronate and risedronate but not ibandronate (Table 243-2).[A6] In addition, studies confirm a persistent BMD and likely antifracture benefit after 5 years of therapy.

Parenteral BPs are also approved and available for osteoporosis treatment, although they should be considered second line to oral BPs based on overall risk-benefit assessment in most osteoporotic patients. They may be considered for use in patients with contraindications to oral BPs (e.g., esophageal disease, inability to sit upright and/or fast after dose), documented or expected poor adherence to oral BPs, or failure to respond to oral BPs or other FDA-approved therapies (recurrent fractures, declining BMD). Zoledronic acid, 5 mg once yearly, and ibandronate, 3 mg quarterly, may be given, although high-strength evidence would favor the use of zoledronic acid, given its unequivocal effect on spine, hip, and nonvertebral fracture risk reduction.[A6] Intriguingly, zoledronic acid has also been shown to reduce mortality in women and men following a low-trauma hip fracture,[A7] although the mechanism of the mortality benefit is unknown. Finally, BMD remains stable and the antifracture effect likely persists for 3 years after three annual doses of zoledronic acid.[A8] Both drugs are associated with an approximately 15 to 20% likelihood of a flu-like reaction, typically consisting of fever, arthralgias, and myalgias, usually limited to the first infusion, and generally lasting 24 to 48 hours, although symptoms lasting weeks to months have rarely been reported to the FDA. Both drugs confer a higher risk as well for delayed healing of exposed bone in the oral cavity compared with oral BPs (see later).

Rare, considerably more serious adverse effects have been associated with both oral and intravenous BPs. Osteonecrosis of the jaw, which is defined as exposed bone within the oral cavity for more than 8 weeks following an invasive dental procedure (e.g., tooth extraction, dental implant) or spontaneous tooth loss, occurs in roughly 1 in 10,000 to 100,000 patients treated with oral BPs, although it likely occurs in 1 in 1000 to 10,000 in intravenous BP–treated patients with osteoporosis. Current evidence suggests that microbial biofilm formation on an acellular bone surface, perhaps facilitated by BPs and the non-BP drug denosumab (see later), may be operative in the development of this disorder. As such, patients on intravenous BPs should maintain optimal oral hygiene and consider a BP holiday or delay in dose if invasive oral procedures are planned. Atypical femoral fractures have also been recently described in patients on long-term bisphosphonate therapy, generally after 5 years or more of treatment. Patients will typically have prodromal thigh or groin pain, which is referable to a stress fracture of a thickened lateral femoral cortex, inferior to the greater trochanter. These fractures can be bilateral in

nature and may be identified radiographically with plain films, MRI, or CT. These patients are at risk for low-trauma, severe, oblique, "chalk-stick" fractures, which often represent orthopedic repair and healing challenges. Fortunately, the estimated prevalence of atypical femoral fractures is low (~1 in 5,000 to 10,000). Nonetheless, the severe manifestations of osteonecrosis of the jaw and atypical femoral fractures make it prudent for clinicians to consider a BP drug holiday, particularly given strong evidence of continued benefit on discontinuation.

Selective Estrogen Receptor Modulators

Selective estrogen receptor modulators (SERMs) are compounds that bind to the estrogen receptor and thereby influence bone and reproductive biology. As with estrogen (see later), SERMs are anticatabolic agents in bone, acting through a reduction in cytokines (RANKL, tumor necrosis factor-α) that engender osteoclast activation and function. Raloxifene is the only FDA-approved drug for prevention and treatment of osteoporosis in menopausal women, although the breast cancer drug tamoxifen likely has skeletal benefits as well. Both drugs have antiestrogenic effects in the breast and are FDA approved for the prevention of breast cancer in high-risk patients. Raloxifene does reduce the risk for vertebral fractures by approximately 30 to 50% but does not reduce the risk for hip and nonvertebral fractures. This antifracture profile positions it as an alternative to bisphosphonates in postmenopausal women with osteopenia and a relatively low risk for hip and other nonspine fractures. The most common side effects include hot flushes and leg cramps in about 10 to 15% and about 5% of patients, respectively. SERMs also increase the risk for deep vein thrombosis, with an absolute risk of roughly 1 in 400, akin to that seen with oral estrogen replacement therapy (ERT). Raloxifene has also been associated with an increased risk for fatal stroke in women at higher baseline risk for stroke, likely precluding its general consideration in women older than 65 years.

Estrogen

ERT, either alone or in combination with a progestin in women with an intact uterus, had historically been a frontline agent in the management of osteoporosis in postmenopausal women (Chapter 240). ERT prevents bone loss if administered to women at menopause and significantly increases BMD by approximately 3 to 5% in woman who are well into their menopausal years. Although lower doses of estrogen may have skeletal benefits, more standard doses of estrogen (0.625 mg of conjugated equine estrogen and 1.0 mg of ethinyl estradiol) have been proved efficacious. Long-term estrogen therapy reduces the risk for all clinical fractures by about 27%, based on the available moderate-quality evidence.[A9] ERT is also the most efficacious agent available for treatment of vasomotor symptoms. These data notwithstanding, ERT is associated with an increased risk for stroke (34% increase),[A9] and the use of continuous combined hormone replacement therapy (HRT) confers an unacceptable greater global risk than benefit in woman initiating HRT, based on the results of the Woman's Health Initiative. These results, however, may not be applicable to the younger postmenopausal population, based on differences in cardiovascular risk, although data confirming this are currently lacking. Both ERT and HRT are also associated with a two- to three-fold increase in the risk for venous thromboembolic disease. Therefore, ERT/HRT is recommended only for postmenopausal women at significant risk for fracture for whom other antifracture therapies are unsuitable.

Denosumab

As detailed previously, increased osteoclast activation through the RANKL pathway is a key mechanism through which bone loss occurs in menopause and other osteoporotic conditions. Intuitively, a therapy that targets this process directly would be desirable. Denosumab is a fully human monoclonal antibody to RANKL that is FDA approved for the treatment of osteoporosis in postmenopausal women and in men, as well as for individuals with breast and prostate cancer to reduce bone loss associated with hormonal deprivation therapy. It is administered twice yearly as a subcutaneous injection in the clinic and clearly reduces the risk for spine, hip, and nonvertebral fractures.[A10] Denosumab does not undergo hepatic or renal metabolism and thus can potentially be used in patients with more advanced renal dysfunction, unlike BPs. In contrast to BPs, it is reversible, such that robust bone loss ensues once the medication is stopped. Denosumab is well tolerated in clinical studies, although a higher incidence of skin conditions (eczema and erysipelas) and infections, including serious infections that required hospitalization, were observed in drug- versus placebo-treated subjects. Therefore, the drug is likely not suitable for patients on immunosuppressant therapy who are at higher baseline risk for infection.

Anabolic Agents

Although anticatabolic drugs are effective at retarding bone loss and reducing fracture risk, anabolic or "bone-building" drugs would be preferred. Teriparatide (TPTD) is a recombinant human parathyroid hormone analogue that encompasses amino acids 1 to 34 and was approved by the FDA in 2002. Given as a self-administered once-daily subcutaneous injection, TPTD is truly anabolic based on robust increases in bone density (~10% over 2 years in the lumbar spine) and bone formation as determined by bone biopsies and other sophisticated imaging studies. More important, TPTD significantly reduces the risk for vertebral and nonvertebral fractures by approximately two thirds and one half, respectively. Because bone resorption increases along with bone formation, bone loss generally ensues on cessation of therapy, necessitating the initiation of an anticatabolic bone drug to preserve the increase in BMD facilitated by TPTD. Finally, although it is plausible to consider that a combination of TPTD and an anticatabolic drug is more beneficial than either drug alone, evidence from randomized controlled trials to date has failed to confirm this. Recent studies, however, suggest that the combination of TPTD and denosumab may have a truly synergistic effect on BMD.

TPTD is more expensive than other treatments for osteoporosis, although it is generally covered by insurance in patients who have severe osteoporosis (based on BMD and/or fracture risk) and who cannot tolerate or have contraindications to other antifracture agents. The drug is generally well tolerated, with the most common adverse effects being dizziness and leg cramps. TPTD has a black box warning, based on the fact that toxicology studies in rats revealed an increase in risk for osteosarcoma in animals treated with suprapharmacologic doses of the drug, particularly in growing animals. Given this, the drug is contra-indicated for patients who are at a higher baseline risk for osteosarcoma, including patients with Paget disease and previous therapeutic radiotherapy, as well as younger individuals with open epiphyses. Fortunately, there has not been an observed increase in the rate of osteosarcoma in teriparatide treated patients above that expected in the general population to date.

Other Therapies and Treatment Considerations
Currently Available and Emerging Therapies

Nasal calcitonin is FDA approved and available at the time of this writing for treatment of postmenopausal osteoporosis, although it is widely considered the weakest antifracture agent based on marginal vertebral fracture benefit. In addition, recent human studies have suggested a possible link to cancer, potentially further limiting its clinical utility and future availability in the United States. Strontium ranelate is approved in Europe for the treatment of osteoporosis and may have a dual proformation-anticatabolic effect on bone. It has been shown to reduce the risk for vertebral and nonvertebral fractures, as well as clinical osteoporotic fractures.[A11] It is not available for use in the United States, and alternative forms of strontium salts cannot be assumed to be effective as well. In addition, BMD by DXA cannot be followed in patients on strontium because of artifactual increases in BMD related to the incorporation into bone of the strontium salt.

Emerging therapies on the horizon will likely provide additional tools to treat this debilitating disease, including new anticatabolic agents (e.g., cathepsin K inhibitors) and new anabolic therapies (e.g., sclerostin antibody). Odanacatib is an oral, small molecule that reversibly inhibits cathepsin K, which is produced by activated osteoclasts and primarily is responsible for the breakdown of type 1 collagen. Odanacatib also does not significantly suppress bone formation, perhaps "uncoupling" bone turnover in a favorable fashion to potentiate improvements in BMD. Sclerostin is a naturally occurring inhibitor of the Wnt pathway and bone formation, and preliminary clinical studies do confirm a significant anabolic effect and BMD increase with intermittent administration of a monoclonal antibody to sclerostin.[A12] Interestingly, unlike TPTD, inhibition of sclerostin does not appear to stimulate bone resorption, potentially affording greater and more persistent gains in BMD. Ongoing and future clinical studies are needed to confirm an antifracture benefit of this compound.

Glucocorticoid-Induced and Male Osteoporosis

As detailed previously, glucocorticoids are a major cause of and the most common etiology of medication-related secondary osteoporosis. Glucocorticoids are prescribed for a number of common inflammatory conditions, often in a chronic, long-term manner. They are potent suppressors of bone formation and at higher doses likely increase bone resorption, principally through central suppression of sex steroid production. This resultant "uncoupling" of bone turnover can result in dramatic declines in BMD within the first 6 months of starting therapy. In addition to bone loss, there is good evidence to support that individuals on glucocorticoids may fracture at a higher level on BMD compared with non-glucocorticoid-treated patients. Fracture rates are increased as well with doses of prednisone as low as 2.5 mg per day, although the increase in risk appears to attenuate with glucocorticoid discontinuation. The treatment approach to glucocorticoid-induced osteoporosis is similar to osteoporosis in general, with the exception that attempts should be made to reduce the steroid dose to as low as the underlying treated disease will permit.[12] Calcium and vitamin D are important adjuncts but are insufficient to prevent bone loss or fractures. Although not clearly evidence-based, replacement of deficient sex steroids is a reasonable strategy in younger individuals who are at lower risk for fracture. The BPs alendronate, risedronate, and zoledronic acid are FDA approved for glucocorticoid-induced osteoporosis in

women and men, although the established benefit is based primarily on BMD improvement. A more logical and indeed superior treatment of glucocorticoid-induced osteoporosis is TPTD, which as an anabolic drug more directly addresses the primary mechanism of bone loss in glucocorticoid-induced osteoporosis: osteoblast inhibition. TPTD is FDA approved for treatment of glucocorticoid-induced osteoporosis in women and men and is superior to alendronate in improving BMD and vertebral fracture risk reduction.[A13] Although the drug was used for 36 months in this head-to-head trial, treatment is advised for no more than 24 months based on previously mentioned safety considerations.

Male osteoporosis historically has been under-recognized and underappreciated by primary care clinicians and patients alike, although the current data support a significantly more prevalent and clinically significant disorder. More than 2 million men in the United States have osteoporosis, and one in four men older than 50 years will suffer a fragility fracture in their remaining lifetime. Roughly 30% of vertebral and hip fractures combined occur in men, and these are the more common fractures in older men. In addition, men have a substantially higher mortality after hip fracture compared with women. As in women, aging, low body weight, and prior fragility fractures are independent predictors of fracture. In some contradistinction to women, however, osteoporosis in men is more commonly multifactorial in etiology, with the most common secondary causes being excess glucocorticoids, hypogonadism, and alcohol overuse. Despite these associations and others (current smoking, history of falls), there is not at present sufficient evidence to warrant use of a specific testing or screening strategy to identify men at higher risk for fracture. The laboratory work-up of male osteoporosis is similar to that for women, with the exception of a morning fasting testosterone level. Idiopathic osteoporosis may also occur, particularly in younger men with no discernable cause. Genetic factors may well be important in these men, with studies suggesting an association with lower production and circulating levels of estrogen. As in women, primary treatment of male osteoporosis is targeted at lifestyle changes, adequate nutrition (calcium and vitamin D), and exercise. Bisphosphonates (oral and intravenous), denosumab, and TPTD are all effective at improving BMD in men. Although more limited in scope, antifracture efficacy is evident for denosumab in men with prostate cancer on androgen deprivation therapy. True antifracture efficacy for the other agents is either less convincing or absent, based on the paucity of randomized controlled trial data, although this should not be construed as a reason not to treat. Testosterone replacement of men with significant biochemical hypogonadism (total T score < 200 ng/dL) does improve bone density, although data on fracture risk reduction are lacking. In older men (>50 years) at a substantial risk for fracture based on history and risk factors, androgen replacement should be considered second line behind the aforementioned other therapies, based on overall risk-benefit and lack-of-fracture data.

Vertebroplasty and Kyphoplasty and Low-Intensity Vibration

Although often clinically silent, vertebral fractures may cause acute and severe back pain. In addition, up to one third of vertebral fractures remain chronically painful, perhaps related to incomplete healing or instability of the fracture. Over the past decade, vertebroplasty and kyphoplasty have been developed and advanced to reduce the morbidity associated with acute spine fractures. These invasive procedures introduce, through the spinal pedicles, a cement-like substance (polymethylmethacrylate) to the compressed vertebral body, with (kyphoplasty) or without (vertebroplasty) use of saline-infused balloon tamps that permit a few millimeters of elevation of the vertebral end plates. Initial randomized trials suggested a benefit of vertebroplasty over conservative management in patients with acute vertebral fractures, although a recent meta-analysis of patient-level data from two randomized controlled trials did not confirm this finding.[A14] Additionally, there may be a concern about fracture of adjacent vertebrae following the procedure, reinforcing the need for further, adequately powered and designed clinical trials.

Low-intensity vibration is also under active investigation as an anticatabolic and possibly anabolic intervention for osteoporosis. Animal studies using low-intensity vibration appears to show enhanced osteoblast and hindered osteoclast development, thereby "coupling" bone remodeling. Clinical studies suggest a modest but significant BMD benefit in postmenopausal women and other groups (children with cerebral palsy, adults on prolonged bed rest), although further studies are needed to confirm a true clinical and ideally antifracture benefit of this intervention.

PROGNOSIS

It stands to reason that, based on the information and data discussed previously, the burden incurred by individual patients and society as a whole can be significantly lessened through a combination of diagnostic, preventive, and therapeutic interventions. Although there is no true "cure" for osteoporosis, current pharmacotherapies reduce the risk for fracture roughly by half.

This reduction is critical because there is robust evidence to suggest an independent increase in mortality after an osteoporotic fracture, including fractures of the spine, humerus, tibia, and pelvis, as well as the proximal femur. Moreover, available data, primarily from randomized controlled trials with bisphosphonates, confirm a statistically significant reduction in death with pharmacologic treatment of osteoporosis, although the mechanism of this effect is not known.[13] These data further underscore the importance of identifying and treating patients with osteoporosis.

Grade A References

A1. Avenell A, Gillespie WJ, Gillespie LD, et al. Vitamin D and vitamin D analogues for preventing fractures associated with involutional and post-menopausal osteoporosis. *Cochrane Database Syst Rev.* 2014;14:CD000227.

A2. Bischoff-Ferrari HA, Willett WC, Wong JB, et al. Prevention of nonvertebral fractures with oral vitamin D and dose dependency: a meta-analysis of randomized controlled trials. *Arch Intern Med.* 2009;169:551-561.

A3. Bischoff-Ferrari HA, Dawson-Hughes B, Staehelin HB, et al. Fall prevention with supplemental and active forms of vitamin D: a meta-analysis of randomised controlled trials. *BMJ.* 2009;339:b3692.

A4. Howe TE, Shea B, Dawson LJ, et al. Exercise for preventing and treating osteoporosis in postmenopausal women. *Cochrane Database Syst Rev.* 2011;7:CD000333.

A5. Gillespie LD, Robertson MC, Gillespie WJ, et al. Interventions for preventing falls in older people living in the community. *Cochrane Database Syst Rev.* 2012;9:CD007146.

A6. Levis S, Theodore G. Summary of AHRQ's comparative effectiveness review of treatment to prevent fractures in men and women with low bone density or osteoporosis: update of the 2007 report. *J Manag Care Pharm.* 2012;18:S1-S15.

A7. Lyles KW, Colon-Emeric CS, Magaziner JS, et al. Zoledronic acid and clinical fractures and mortality after hip fracture. *N Engl J Med.* 2007;357:1799-1809.

A8. Black DM, Rein IR, Boonen S, et al. The effect of 3 versus 6 years of zoledronic acid treatment of osteoporosis: a randomized extension to the HORIZON-Pivotal Fracture Trial (PFT). *J Bone Miner Res.* 2012;27:243-254.

A9. Marjoribanks J, Farguhar C, Roberts H, et al. Long term hormone therapy for perimenopausal and postmenopausal women. *Cochrane Database Syst Rev.* 2012;7:CD004143.

A10. Cummings SR, Ensrud K, Delmas PD, et al. Denosumab for prevention of fractures in postmenopausal women with osteoporosis. *N Engl J Med.* 2009;361:756-765.

A11. Kanis JA, Johansson H, Oden A, et al. A meta-analysis of the effect of strontium ranelate on the risk of vertebral and non-vertebral fracture in postmenopausal osteoporosis and the interaction with FRAX(®). *Osteoporos Int.* 2011;22:2347-2355.

A12. McClung MR, Grauer A, Boonen S, et al. Romosozumab in postmenopausal women with low bone mineral density. *N Engl J Med.* 2014;370:412-420.

A13. Saag KG, Zanchetta JR, Devogelaer JP, et al. Effects of teriparatide versus alendronate for treating glucocorticoid-induced osteoporosis: thirty-six-month results of a randomized, double-blind, controlled trial. *Arthritis Rheum.* 2009;60:3346-3355.

A14. Staples MP, Kallmes DF, Comstock BA, et al. Effectiveness of vertebroplasty using individual patient data from two randomised placebo controlled trials: meta-analysis. *BMJ.* 2011;343:d3952.

GENERAL REFERENCES

For the General References and other additional features, please visit Expert Consult at https://expertconsult.inkling.com.

244

OSTEOMALACIA AND RICKETS

ROBERT S. WEINSTEIN

DEFINITION

Rickets refers to impaired mineralization of the cartilaginous growth plate and abnormal endochondral bone formation and therefore cannot occur in adults after epiphyseal closure.[1] Osteomalacia, literally meaning softening of bone, refers to defective or delayed mineralization of the organic matrix of bone, or osteoid, at the interface between calcified bone and osteoid, and may occur at any age. Both rickets and osteomalacia may be present in a growing child, but defective mineralization can cause only osteomalacia in adults; therefore, this chapter will focus on osteomalacia. Despite advances in our understanding of vitamin D metabolism and the increased sensitivity of measurements of serum 25-hydroxyvitamin D, osteomalacia remains a common and frequently overlooked disorder in the world. Optimal therapy requires precise identification of the etiology of the abnormal mineralization, which may present a problem because there are numerous causes (Table 244-1). However, after a correct diagnosis is made, therapy is usually gratifying and often spectacular. Early recognition of osteomalacia depends on familiarity

TABLE 244-1 CAUSES OF OSTEOMALACIA

VITAMIN D DEFICIENCY

Dietary deprivation and lack of sunlight exposure

VITAMIN D MALABSORPTION

Postgastrectomy
Gastric bypass for obesity
Gluten enteropathy
Small bowel disease or resection
Pancreatic insufficiency
Cholestyramine therapy for cholestatic liver disease
Laxative abuse

IMPAIRED 1-HYDROXYLATION OF 25-HYDROXYVITAMIN D

Vitamin D–dependent rickets type I
X-linked hypophosphatemia
Autosomal dominant hypophosphatemic rickets/osteomalacia
Oncogenic osteomalacia

IMPAIRED TARGET-ORGAN RESPONSE TO 1,25-DIHYDROXYVITAMIN D

Vitamin D–dependent rickets type II

HYPOPHOSPHATEMIA

X-linked hypophosphatemia
Autosomal dominant hypophosphatemic rickets/osteomalacia
Sporadic hypophosphatemia
Fibrous dysplasia
Oncogenic osteomalacia
Antacid-induced osteomalacia
Chronic metabolic acidosis
Paraproteinemia
Saccharated ferric oxide
Tenofovir
Cadmium

INHIBITORS OF MINERALIZATION

Etidronate
Fluoride
Aluminum
Iron

MISCELLANEOUS

Hypophosphatasia
Axial osteomalacia
Fibrogenesis imperfecta ossium

with the typical clinical manifestations and settings. It is helpful to appreciate that the bone disease almost always manifests in the same manner regardless of the cause of the osteomalacia.

EPIDEMIOLOGY

About 20% of North American women receiving treatment for osteoporosis have 25-hydroxyvitamin D levels below 20 ng/mL (adequate values are greater than 30 ng/mL), and 8% have levels below 15 ng/mL. This indicates that, at the least, impaired bone mineralization could be a confounding factor in their osteoporosis treatment and, at worst, osteomalacia is the correct diagnosis (a defect in mineralization) rather than osteoporosis (a reduced amount of normally mineralized bone). An inadequate response to the bisphosphonate treatment commonly used for postmenopausal osteoporosis is four times more likely when 25-hydroxyvitamin D levels are subnormal than when the levels are above 30 ng/mL.[2] Vitamin D deficiency is more common in elderly people, especially in nonaffluent people during the winter, at higher latitudes, and with low sun exposure. Vitamin D deficiency is also commonly found in medical inpatients, institutionalized patients, and postmenopausal women with acute hip fracture.[3]

The prevalence of osteomalacia due to vitamin D deficiency varies with the referral source. The disorder is far more frequent when patients are referred from geriatricians, gastroenterologists (osteomalacia may be found in up to 30% of patients with gastric surgery or bypass for obesity), nursing homes, or orthopedists concerned about symmetrical or nonhealing fractures. The most common hypophosphatemic osteomalacia is the inherited disease X-linked hypophosphatemia (XLH), but affected adults infrequently present to internists and then only when troubled by severe bone pain or nonunion of fractures.

PATHOBIOLOGY

A review of normal bone remodeling and the mineralization of osteoid (bone matrix) serves as a background to understand the abnormal mineralization characteristic of osteomalacia. Bone remodeling or turnover is carried out by teams of juxtaposed osteoclasts and osteoblasts, comprising temporary anatomical structures known as basic multicellular units (BMUs). In cortical bone, the BMUs drill tunnels or "cutting cones" through the compact tissue; whereas in spongy, cancellous bone, they gouge across the trabecular surface, forming serpiginous trenches. Bone turnover begins by conversion of a quiescent skeletal surface to a remodeling site, a process referred to as *activation*. Activation involves proliferation of new blood vessels needed to bring recruited osteoclast progenitors to the remodeling site and retraction of the flat, pavement-like bone-lining cells that cover the quiescent surfaces to expose the mineralized bone surface. The recruited cells become multinucleated osteoclasts, which attach to the newly exposed bone surface with a ring of contractile proteins sealing off a subosteoclastic resorption compartment. Lysosomal enzymes, hydrogen ions, and collagenase are secreted through the microvilli of the ruffled underside border of the osteoclasts, and these chemicals begin to excavate a resorption cavity. The osteoclasts remove both the bone mineral and matrix. It is a misunderstanding to attribute to these cells or to metabolic acidosis the ability to remove only the mineral, leaving behind demineralized osteoid. Demineralized bone in vivo is a misnomer. Demineralized or decalcified bone only occurs when bones are placed in acid (1N HCl) or chelating solutions (ethylenediaminetetraacetate, or EDTA). Osteoclasts are motile cells, capable of resorbing more than just the cavity within which they are identified. After an osteoclast digs a cavity, it may detach from bone and move on to a new resorption site or die by apoptosis and be quickly removed by phagocytes. When the osteoclasts have moved on, osteoblasts assemble to reconstitute the previously resorbed cavity with new bone. In any established BMU, both events are happening at the same time; bone formation begins to occur while bone resorption advances.

Between the end of bone resorption and the beginning of bone formation is the reversal phase, when mononuclear phagocytes smooth out the jagged erosion bays. During this phase, the old bone is coated by a thin layer of cement substance, a collagen- and mineral-poor matrix rich in glycosaminoglycans, glycoproteins, and acid phosphatase, to which the new osteoblasts attach. In adults, new osteoblasts assemble only at sites where osteoclasts have recently been eroding bone; a phenomenon referred to as *coupling*. The arrival of the osteoblasts in the right place at the right time and in sufficient numbers to reconstitute the cavity is referred to as *remodeling balance* and is likely due to proportional production of osteoblasts and osteoclasts in the bone marrow, release of osteoblast-recruiting substances from the resorbed bone, and chemotaxis by the cement substances. As osteoblasts complete their bone matrix synthesis and move away from the cement line, they gradually flatten. Some osteoblasts become bone-lining cells, and some become osteocytes, but as many as 65% of the osteoblasts that originally assembled at the remodeling site die by apoptosis. It is the balance between cell proliferation and apoptosis that determines the amount of work performed by these cells.

Normally, up to 70% of the mineralization of the osteoid deposited by the osteoblasts starts within 4 to 12 days and proceeds at about 1 μm per day; but in osteomalacia, mineral deposition in the osteoid slows or stops completely, while the osteoblasts continue to make osteoid, which then accumulates in excessive amounts. Therefore, normal osteoid width is about 4 to 12 μm, but in osteomalacia, the osteoid width may become dramatically augmented. Depending on the extent of the delay in mineralization, overt osteomalacia may take many years to develop. In normal subjects, further mineralization proceeds slowly over months to years and at the cost of displacement of the water in the hydroxyapatite crystals, resulting in a modest increase in brittleness and the eventual need for another round of remodeling. Even though 1 million BMUs are undergoing remodeling every day, bone mass in a healthy adult is preserved thanks to a remarkably tight balance between the amount of bone resorbed and the amount formed during each cycle of remodeling. By this means, the adult skeleton is almost completely regenerated every 10 years.

Mineralization requires the availability of sufficient calcium and phosphorus at the remodeling site, the presence of a normal bone collagen matrix, the absence of inhibitors of mineralization, and an adequate amount of skeletal alkaline phosphatase activity. Defects in these requirements are the cause of most forms of osteomalacia. Deficiency of vitamin D per se has traditionally been incriminated as the cause of the osteomalacia, but today, considerable evidence indicates that the abnormal mineralization associated with vitamin

D deficiency depends more on the deficiency of calcium and phosphorus than the absence of a direct effect of vitamin D on bone cells. The primary function of vitamin D is to provide adequate levels of calcium and phosphorus by increasing their intestinal absorption. Chronic metabolic acidosis has also been identified as a cause of osteomalacia, but evidence suggests that the bone disease associated with chronic metabolic acidosis is primarily due to the associated hypophosphatemia.

CLINICAL MANIFESTATIONS

The clinical presentation of osteomalacia depends on three overlapping manifestations: those due to the underlying disorder, such as gastrointestinal disease or surgery (especially troublesome are gastric resection, stapling or bypass for obesity, and intestinal malabsorption); those due to hypocalcemia or hypophosphatemia; and those directly due to the bone disease. The most common symptoms and signs are bone pain, muscle weakness, and bone tenderness. The bone pain is usually nonspecific and poorly localized. Because of the paucity of findings, the pain is often attributed to rheumatism or neurosis. It may be worse at night and after sudden movements such as turning in bed or the change from sitting to standing. Most often, the pain is in the lower back, pelvis and legs and is worse on weight bearing, resulting in a characteristic flat-footed, springless, waddling gait made worse by proximal muscle weakness. The gait has been referred to as "mother penguin's walk." Patients may complain that they can only climb stairs by pulling themselves up with the hand rail or rise from sitting in a chair or on the toilet by using their hands to push off. The decrease in strength is usually far greater than the degree of muscle wasting. Fasciculations are absent, and both reflexes and sensation remain normal. The bulbar, facial, and ocular muscles are always spared. However, muscle weakness is conspicuously absent when the osteomalacia is due to X-linked hypophosphatemia (see Table 244-1). Often, bone tenderness can be elicited by rib cage compression or pressing on the tibiae, wrists, pubic rami, or iliac crests. Hypocalcemia is usually mild to moderate but, rarely, can be severe enough to present with paresthesias, muscle cramps, a positive Chvostek's sign, or seizures. If the osteomalacia is mistaken for osteoporosis and treatment is started with a bisphosphonate, the patient may experience new-onset paresthesias, muscle cramps, and palpitations. This not uncommon scenario occurs because the antiresorptive treatment interferes with the compensatory secondary hyperparathyroidism and aggravates the hypocalcemia.

DIAGNOSIS

Biochemical changes depend on the stage of the disease and its etiology. In vitamin D deficiency, hypophosphatemia precedes and is more severe than the hypocalcemia because of the secondary or compensatory hyperparathyroidism (Chapter 245) that almost invariably accompanies the disorder by the time that osteomalacia has occurred. In malabsorption, hypomagnesemia may contribute to the hypocalcemia, and hypoalbuminemia may lead to a spurious diagnosis of hypocalcemia. Increased serum alkaline phosphatase activity is classically associated with osteomalacia due to vitamin D deficiency but is not an early or reliable clue because some patients may have normal or borderline levels. The serum 25-hydroxyvitamin D levels are often less than 10 to 15 ng/mL. In contrast, serum 1,25-dihydroxyvitamin D levels are usually elevated because of the concomitant hyperparathyroidism and do not contribute to the diagnosis of osteomalacia except in the rare abnormalities of vitamin D resistance (when 1,25-dihydroxyvitamin D levels may be extraordinarily high) or when 1-hydroxylation is defective (and 1,25-dihydroxyvitamin D levels are low). Quite a different pattern occurs with the inherited disease hypophosphatasia: serum 25-hydroxyvitamin D and calcium are normal, phosphorus and vitamin B_6 levels are high normal or frankly elevated, and alkaline phosphatase activity is below the normal range.[4]

Radiographic findings may be absent with early osteomalacia, and only blurred margins of the cancellous bone with thin cortices may be noted. The presence of bilateral, thin (2 to 3 mm), radiolucent bands known as *pseudofractures* (Fig. 244-1) found perpendicular to the periosteal surface in ribs, pubic and ischial rami, the neck of the femur, and metatarsals and below the glenoid fossa on the outer border of the scapulae are generally considered to be pathognomonic of osteomalacia, but this classical radiographic sign is infrequent today. Rarely, it may be seen in disorders lacking excessive osteoid. These pseudofractures (sometimes called *Looser's zones* or *Milkman's fractures*) show increased uptake on bone scans (Fig. 244-2) and may lead to an inappropriate search for a primary malignancy. Bone mineral density T scores are often −3 or −4, with the radial diaphyseal density lower than that of the lumbar spine or total proximal femur.

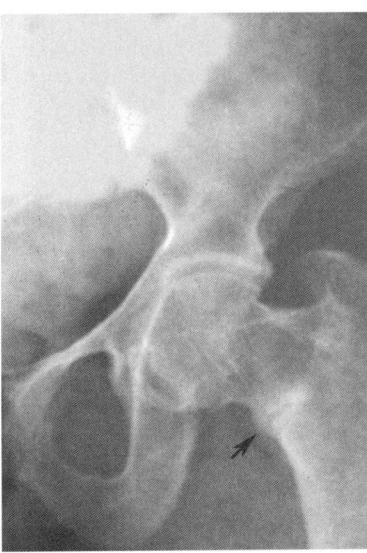

FIGURE 244-1. Radiographic evidence of a pseudofracture of the femoral neck is suspicious for osteomalacia *(arrow)*.

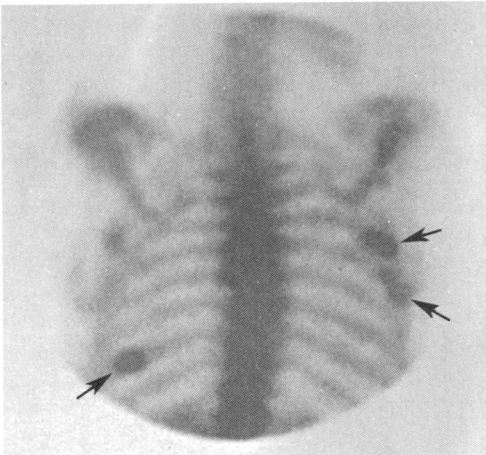

FIGURE 244-2. In osteomalacia, focal increased uptake of radionuclide on a bone scan may erroneously suggest metastatic disease *(arrows)*.

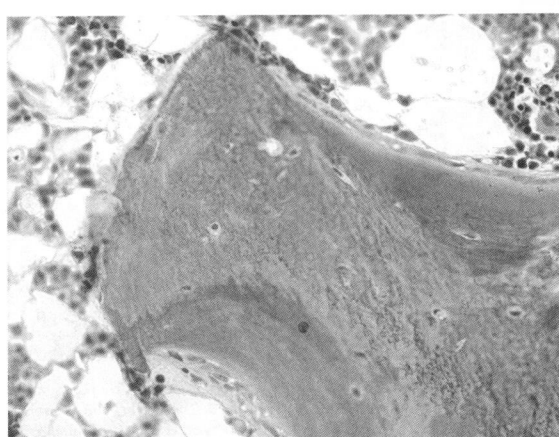

FIGURE 244-3. An undecalcified bone biopsy specimen shows the characteristic abundant osteoid and flattened osteoblasts of osteomalacia (normally mineralized bone is *blue* and osteoid is *red*).

Although characteristic clinical, radiographic, and biochemical findings may suggest osteomalacia, the absence of these findings cannot exclude the diagnosis. Quantitative histologic examination of undecalcified bone is, therefore, required to establish the unequivocal presence of osteomalacia (Fig. 244-3). Rigorous kinetic criteria for the histologic recognition of osteomalacia are necessary to preserve the traditional clinical, biochemical, and therapeutic connotations of the term. Therefore, a review of the quantitative bone histologic findings or histomorphometry in osteomalacia is useful.[5] The histomorphometric diagnosis of osteomalacia requires the simultaneous presence of three findings: (1) excessive osteoid (osteoid area >10% of the cancellous bone area; normal is <4%), (2) augmentation of the osteoid width (>15 µm; normal is 4 to 12 µm), (3) and prolongation of the mineralization lag time (>100 days; normal is 9 to 20 days), as determined by the osteoid width divided by the distance between and linear extent of double tetracycline labels observed in the bone after the patient receives two time-spaced courses of oral tetracycline. Tetracycline is deposited early in the course of hydroxyapatite crystal formation and generates bright stripes at the interface of mineralized bone and osteoid when viewed with fluorescent microscopy. If the two time-spaced courses of tetracycline (1 g/day for 3 days) are separated by a 14-day interval, the rate of mineralization (µm/day) can be calculated by measuring the average distance between the double labels divided by the number of days between the two courses. When the double labels are numerous and widely spaced, mineralization is intact and excess osteoid must

be due to increased bone turnover. A paucity of tetracycline labels that are narrowly spaced indicates that if excessive osteoid is present, it must be due to the delayed or ceased mineralization of osteomalacia (Fig. 244-4).

Therefore, it follows that excessive osteoid can occur from two distinct mechanisms. Osteomalacia is the consequence of defective mineralization, while osteoid production continues. However, osteoid will also accumulate with accelerated bone formation if the rate of osteoid deposition exceeds the rate of mineralization, as occurs in states of greatly increased bone turnover, such as hyperparathyroidism (Chapter 245), Paget's disease (Chapter 247), or thyrotoxicosis (Chapter 226). Even though osteoblasts in osteomalacia are usually sparse and flattened, whereas they are numerous, plump, and cuboidal with high bone turnover, these two groups of disorders can only be reliably distinguished with the use of tetracycline markers. The treatment of increased bone turnover and of defective mineralization is completely different, which is why the three histomorphometric criteria are necessary. Additionally, evaluation of each of the criteria in isolation has limitations. Regarding the first requirement, a small increase in the osteoid area relative to the total bone area may occur in osteoporosis, with a decrease in the amount of mineralized bone. In the second requirement, wide osteoid seams may be seen in some specimens obtained from patients with severe secondary hyperparathyroidism, such as those on maintenance hemodialysis therapy (Chapter 131). In the third requirement, reduced mineral appositional rate and increased mineralization lag time are nonspecific indices of impaired matrix synthesis by osteoblasts, as is often found in patients with involutional osteoporosis. Only when all three requirements are fulfilled is the diagnosis of osteomalacia irrefutable.

Several presumed causes of osteomalacia (anticonvulsant drugs, metabolic acidosis without hypophosphatemia, pseudohypoparathyroidism, and chronic renal failure) have not fulfilled all of these requirements and primarily represent secondary hyperparathyroidism. Patients with the nephrotic syndrome lose albumin and vitamin D metabolites in the urine, but evidence indicates that serum ionized calcium and parathyroid hormone levels are normal and metabolic bone disease in adults with the nephrotic syndrome is absent. Muscle weakness and bone pain are significantly more common in patients in whom the rigorous histologic diagnosis of osteomalacia has been proved. However, bone biopsy is not always necessary to be reasonably certain of the diagnosis. When biopsy is necessary, the local pathologist must be familiar with the processing of undecalcified bone specimens and plastic embedding; otherwise, the best solution is to refer the patient to a histomorphometry center for biopsy. This ensures satisfactory communication between the clinician, operator, and pathologist and is the best insurance against the incomplete, broken, fragmented, or accidentally decalcified bone specimens. Such referral may be indispensable in the evaluation of a patient with unusually painful disease or progressive loss of bone mineral density, particularly when the results of the physical examination, radiographs, and biochemical findings are ambiguous. Biopsy may also be indicated in patients with unexplained chronic hypophosphatemia.

The best approach is to avoid overlooking the diagnosis of osteomalacia by maintaining a high degree of suspicion in the typical clinical settings.[6] This is especially important because osteomalacia can usually be successfully

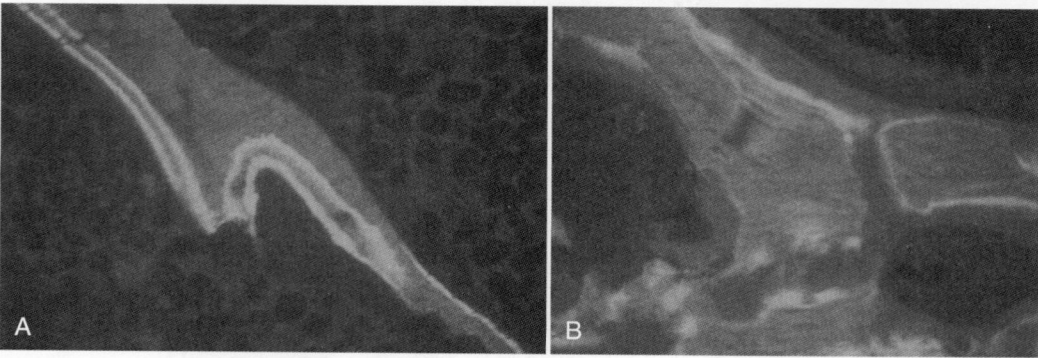

FIGURE 244-4. Histomorphometric diagnosis of osteomalacia by fluorescence imaging of double tetracycline labeling. **A**, Tetracycline double labels are numerous, discrete, and widely spaced, as is typical of intact mineralization. **B**, The tetracycline labels are mostly single despite the administration of two time-spaced doses of oral tetracycline, indicating that mineralization must be delayed or ceased, as is typical of osteomalacia.

treated. An investigation for osteomalacia is indicated in elderly patients with bone pain and muscle weakness, in patients with gastric surgery and low bone mineral density or bone pain, and in patients with persistent hypophosphatemia. Unexplained elevations of the serum alkaline phosphatase activity are usually due to drugs (e.g., anticonvulsants, anabolic steroids, phenothiazines, or antibiotics) or Paget's disease of bone (Chapter 247) but rarely may be the only biochemical clue to osteomalacia in a patient with variable skeletal discomfort. Bilateral or slowly healing fractures also warrant an investigation for osteomalacia.

TREATMENT Rx

Understanding of the treatment of osteomalacia is facilitated by dividing the disease into four subgroups. The *first subgroup* is osteomalacia due to disorders of vitamin D absorption or metabolism; the *second* is osteomalacia due to chronic hypophosphatemia. Most patients with osteomalacia will be in these first two subgroups. Treatment of osteomalacia caused by these two subgroups is discussed in detail in the next two sections. The *third subgroup* includes osteomalacia caused by inhibitors of mineralization, such as etidronate (the first oral bisphosphonate, now rarely used in North America); high doses of fluoride; accumulation of a skeletal burden of aluminum from water used for dialysis or as a contaminate in solutions used for parenteral nutrition (now rarely seen); iron overload as in thalassemia; and cadmium, which induces the proximal tubular lesion of Fanconi's syndrome and causes osteomalacia due to the resultant hypophosphatemia. The *fourth subgroup* includes miscellaneous causes of osteomalacia that lack specific therapy but are fortunately quite rare. This last subgroup includes the variable forms of the heritable disorder hypophosphatasia, caused by a deficiency of the tissue-nonspecific (liver, bone, kidney) isoenzyme of alkaline phosphatase (although, therapeutic trials have shown that enzyme replacement is effective); axial osteomalacia, a sporadic osteosclerotic disorder primarily affecting middle-aged men and presenting with mild to moderate pain in the spine and pelvis (but without fractures), apparently due to the production of an abnormal and poorly mineralized bone matrix by osteoblasts; and fibrogenesis imperfecta ossium, another sporadic disorder presenting with intractable bone pain and fractures, mainly in middle-aged men and women and apparently also due to production of an abnormal bone matrix lacking the normal collagen birefringence by osteoblasts. In axial osteomalacia and fibrogenesis imperfecta ossium, serum calcium, phosphorus, and vitamin D levels are normal, but serum alkaline phosphates activity may be increased. General measures for this last subgroup include routine nutritional advice and avoidance of further bone loss due to postmenopausal or involutional osteoporosis. High-dose vitamin D therapy in these disorders has caused nephrocalcinosis, nephrolithiasis, and renal insufficiency and must be avoided.

Osteomalacia Due to Vitamin D Disorders

Iron deficiency anemia, hypocalcemia, weight loss, glossitis, or pruritic rash and bone discomfort in a patient with low bone mineral density point to celiac disease even without gastrointestinal symptoms. These signs suggest the need to test for immunoglobulin A antiendomysial and antitissue transglutaminase antibodies. Cholestyramine therapy for cholestatic liver disease may increase malabsorption of vitamin D by binding bile salts. Laxative abuse may cause osteomalacia and severe resistance to vitamin D supplementation, including treatment with calcitriol. Advice on nutrition and sun exposure, discontinuation of offending drugs, adherence to a gluten-free diet, and pancreatic enzyme replacement may cure the mineralization defect in mild cases without the need for additional treatment.

Patients with severe disease will usually require vitamin D and calcium supplementation. Replacement doses depend on the serum 25-hydroxyvitamin

*If not >30 ng/mL after 10 weeks, exclude malabsorption, gluten enteropathy, and noncompliance. High-quality cholecalciferol, free from gluten, dairy, egg, fish nuts, soy, or artificial colors can be obtained from †BIOTECH at 1-800-345-1199. Weekly tanning bed treatments may be used if oral vitamin therapy fails or a switch to the more costly calcitriol may be necessary. 25(OH)D = 25-hydroxyvitamin D.

TABLE 244-2 VITAMIN D PREPARATIONS FOR TREATMENT OF OSTEOMALACIA

	VITAMIN D₃ (CHOLECALCIFEROL)	CALCITRIOL (1,25[OH]₂D₃)
Trade names	Calciferol, BIOTECH†	Calcitriol
Dosage form	Caps: 50,000 units = 1.25 mg	Caps: 0.25 and 0.50 μg
Dosage:		0.50-2.0 μg/day
If serum 25(OH)D = 20 to 30 ng/mL	50,000 units once a week × 10 weeks* and once a month thereafter	
If serum 25(OH)D = 10 to 20 ng/mL	50,000 units twice a week × 10 weeks* and twice a month thereafter	
If serum 25(OH)D = less than 10 ng/mL	50,000 units three times a week × 10 weeks* and three times a month thereafter	
Dosage in resistant cases	Up to 50,000 units per day	5-20 μg/day
Time to reach maximum effects	4-10 weeks	3-7 days
Persistence of effects after cessation	6-30 weeks	3-7 days
Cost in U.S.	$40/100 capsules of 50,000 units	$130/100 capsules of 0.25 μg $150/100 capsules of 0.5 μg

D level, as shown in Table 244-2. Because pharmacologic doses of any vitamin D preparation carry the risk for vitamin D intoxication, increases in the dose must be made carefully. The interval between increments in dosage should be at least the time required to reach maximal effects plus about 50%. However, experience with the doses given in Table 244-2 indicates that serum 25-hydroxyvitamin D levels rarely reach 80 to 100 ng/mL. Vitamin D intoxication is unlikely even with of levels of 200 to 250 ng/mL. The goal is to raise the serum 25-hydoxyvitamin D level well above 30 ng/mL and restore the elevated parathyroid hormone concentration to normal without hypercalcemia or hypercalciuria. Urinary calcium excretion should be monitored when treatment has normalized the serum calcium level. The urinary calcium-to-creatinine ratio (mg/mg) should be kept below 0.22. Approximately 1 to 1.5 g/day of oral elemental calcium is a reasonable initial dose. Frequent small doses (three times a day) are more effective and tolerable than fewer larger ones, and the absorbability of calcium supplements is enhanced with meals. Most patient do well using the calcium preparations used for osteoporosis, such as calcium carbonate (40% calcium as in Os-Cal or the equivalent) or calcium citrate (21% calcium as in Caltrate or the equivalent). Some patients who cannot tolerate calcium carbonate or citrate experience fewer adverse gastrointestinal symptoms with the use of the chocolate or coffee-flavored formulations known as Viactiv (500 mg calcium per tablet). The vitamin D content of these calcium supplements is trivial in the treatment of osteomalacia.

In patients with malabsorption, vitamin D requirements may increase during periods of increased diarrhea, and calcitriol may be easier for these patients to absorb. Its rapid onset of action and disappearance after cessation add to the safety of treatment, albeit at far greater cost. Calcium, phosphorus, potassium, magnesium, multivitamins, and gonadal steroids may also be beneficial in patients with malabsorption. Some patients do not tolerate any form of oral vitamin D, and the parenteral ergocalciferol preparations in North America are ineffective. These patients can be improved, although not restored to normal, by the use of weekly tanning bed treatments to areas of their bodies not normally exposed to the sun, an attempt to minimize solar-induced skin cancer. Calcitriol is the drug of choice in patients with the autosomal recessive disease, vitamin D–dependent rickets type I, in which the 1α-hydoxylase enzyme necessary to convert 25-hydroxyvitamin D to 1,25-dihydroxyvitamin D is deficient. In vitamin D–dependent rickets type II, another rare autosomal recessive disease presenting with alopecia, diminished target sensitivity to 1,25-dihydroxyvitamin D may require extraordinarily high doses of calcitriol. If oral treatment fails, nocturnal infusions of calcium and phosphorus have been successful, providing additional evidence that the osteomalacia is due to inadequate calcium and phosphorus rather than the defect in vitamin D metabolism.

An increase in the serum alkaline phosphatase activity (the healing "flare") and a small increase in the serum and urine calcium levels are the earliest signs of effective treatment. Thereafter, the serum alkaline phosphatase activity level falls progressively as healing occurs. At the start of therapy, serum calcium levels should be measured at weekly intervals. If hypoalbuminemia is present, serum ionized calcium determinations are more useful. When therapy appears stabilized, biweekly or monthly intervals are usually sufficient for the first 3 or 4 months, but even with long-term therapy, measurements should be at least two to three times a year. In some patients with severe osteomalacia, bone pain and paresthesias may increase and the serum calcium levels decrease during the first few weeks of therapy. This is due to the increased skeletal avidity for mineral during healing and indicates the need for additional calcium supplementation.

Osteomalacia Due to Hypophosphatemia

Therapy of chronic hypophosphatemia is aimed at maintaining normal concentrations of serum phosphorus without inducing secondary hyperparathyroidism or nephrocalcinosis. This considerably difficult task requires divided doses of phosphorus supplements (1 to 3 g/day) and calcitriol (1 to 4 μg/day) to increase the absorption of phosphorus and try to prevent the increase in parathyroid hormone (Tables 244-2 and 244-3). If phosphorus-induced secondary hyperparathyroidism develops, the phosphorus supplements are rapidly excreted, and therapy thus is not only futile but also causes the additional bone disease of hyperparathyroidism. Baseline and yearly renal ultrasound examinations are necessary to recognize early nephrocalcinosis or nephrolithiasis.

X-linked hypophosphatemia (XLH) is the most common cause of chronic hypophosphatemia, and the presence of a positive family history, pediatric onset, and bowed legs usually substantiates the diagnosis. Treatment with an anti-FG23 antibody can raise serum phosphorus and 1,25 vitamin D levels,[A1] although the long-term benefits are not yet known. However, some hypophosphatemic patients have an autosomal dominant family history and present in adulthood with osteomalacia but without lower extremity deformities. Like patients affected with XLH, these patients may present with bone pain, pseudofractures, and high-normal or frankly elevated levels of fibroblast growth factor 23 (FGF23), a phosphaturic protein that interferes with 1-hydroxylation of 25-hydroxyvitamin D.[7] Patients with autosomal dominant hypophosphatemic osteomalacia (ADHR) appear to acquire the renal phosphate losses in adolescence or adulthood, whereas other patients with ADHR may lose the

defect as they age. A diagnostic problem arises when a patient with chronic hypophosphatemia presents without a positive family history or bowed legs because this presentation resembles that of patients with oncogenic osteomalacia. This disorder is associated with a variety of small, hard to find, benign mesenchymal tumors that secrete FGF23.[8,9] The muscle pain, weakness, fractures, and osteomalacia characteristic of this syndrome are due to hypophosphatemia made worse by inappropriately low levels of 1,25-dihydroxy vitamin D. Oncogenic osteomalacia is also treated with phosphorus supplementation and calcitriol until the offending tumor can be located and resected. Improved tumor localization has been reported with positron emission tomography and computed tomography.[9-11] Surgical correction of deformities should be postponed until medical management achieves persistently normal levels of calcium, phosphorus, and alkaline phosphatase activity. An exception to this rule is an acute fracture of the femoral neck. Prompt surgical repair may be essential to avoid osteonecrosis. Oncogenic osteomalacia rarely occurs with malignant tumors that secrete FGF23, but unless surgical resection is complete, the osteomalacia will persist. Recent evidence suggests that tumors in surgically difficult locations may be treated by radiofrequency ablation.[12] Antacid-induced hypophosphatemia due to the ingestion of large quantities of phosphate-binding antacids has become rare with the increased availability of proton pump inhibitors but still occurs occasionally.

PREVENTION

Advice about vitamin D supplementation should help to prevent osteomalacia caused by vitamin D deficiency, but this has proved to be difficult because routine supplements may be inadequate and compliance with nutritional supplements is poor. The optimal vitamin D supplementation dosage is not clear, but most bone and mineral problems are avoided by 50,000 units of ergocalciferol given once monthly. Notable exceptions occur in patients with celiac disease, gastric surgery, or bypass for obesity, who often require much larger amounts (see Table 244-2). In patients with osteomalacia due to hypophosphatemia, the need for phosphorus supplementation may be lifelong. Rare exceptions occur in oncogenic osteomalacia if complete surgical removal or destruction of the tumor is accomplished.

PROGNOSIS

The response to appropriate treatment in most forms of osteomalacia is usually excellent. Improvements in bone pain and muscle weakness usually occur within 2 or 3 months, and healing of skeletal lesions occurs within 6 to 18 months. Depending on the quantity of excess osteoid, repeat bone mineral density determinations may show as much as 20% gains at the lumbar spine and total proximal femur. However, bone density at the radial diaphysis may not improve because of the irreversible loss of cortical bone resulting from prolonged secondary hyperparathyroidism. Furthermore, if decreased bone volume is present in addition to excess osteoid, skeletal recovery may be incomplete, and the risk for fractures may remain increased.

 Grade A Reference

A1. Carpenter TO, Imel EA, Ruppe MD, et al. Randomized trial of the anti-FGF23 antibody KRN23 in X-linked hypophosphatemia. *J Clin Invest.* 2014;124:1587-1597.

GENERAL REFERENCES

For the General References and other additional features, please visit Expert Consult at https://expertconsult.inkling.com.

245

THE PARATHYROID GLANDS, HYPERCALCEMIA AND HYPOCALCEMIA

RAJESH V. THAKKER

CALCIUM METABOLISM

A healthy adult body has a total of 1 kg of calcium; about 99% of this is present within the crystal structure of bone mineral, and less than 1% is in soluble form in the extracellular and intracellular fluid compartments. In the extracellular fluid compartment (ECF), about half of the total calcium is

| | TABLE 244-3 | PHOSPHATE PREPARATIONS FOR TREATMENT OF OSTEOMALACIA |

PREPARATION	TABLET MARKINGS AND SHAPE	SODIUM CONTENT (mEq)	POTASSIUM CONTENT (mEq)	AMOUNT THAT CONTAINS 1 GRAM OF ELEMENTAL PHOSPHORUS
Neutra-Phos	0	28.5	28.5	4 unit dose caps*
Neutra-Phos-K	0	0	57.0	4 unit dose caps*
K-Phos Neutral	"Beach 11-25" oblong	50.4	4.6	4 tabs
K-Phos Original	"Beach 1111" round	0	33.0	9 tabs

*Each unit dose cap is reconstituted with 75 mL of water, fruit juice, or cola, and this formulation is preferred by children. The unit dose cap contains the powder concentrate and is not to be swallowed undiluted. Adults prefer the K-Phos Neutral tablets.

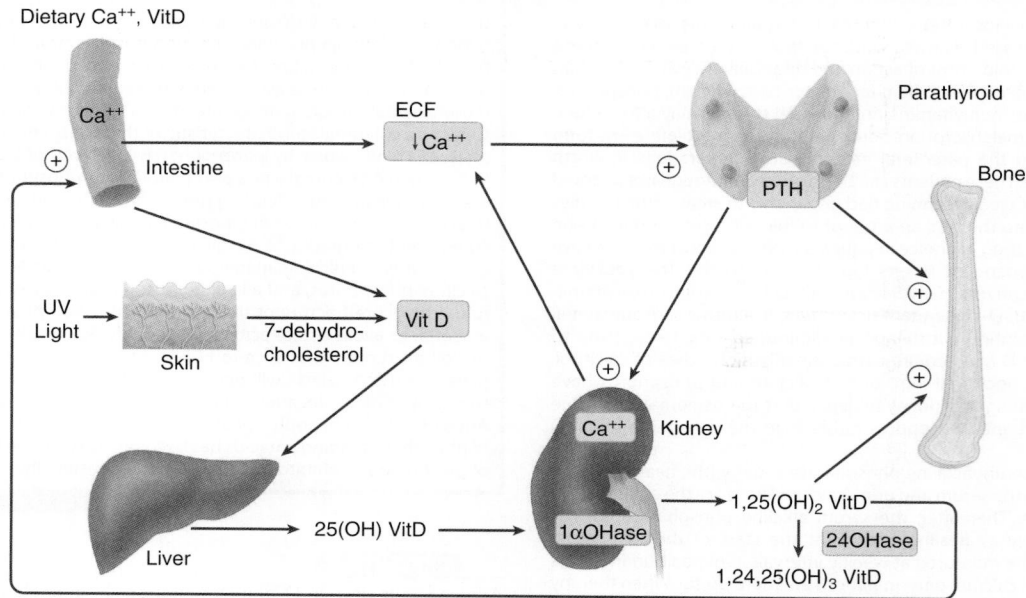

FIGURE 245-1. Regulation of extracellular fluid (ECF) calcium (Ca^{2+}) by parathyroid hormone (PTH) action on kidney, bone, and intestine. A decrease in ECF Ca^{2+} is sensed by the calcium-sensing receptor (see Fig. 245-2), and this leads to an increase in PTH secretion and a reduction in PTH degradation. The increased circulating PTH predominantly acts directly on kidney and bone that possess the PTH receptor (PTHR, Fig. 245-2). The skeletal effects of PTH are to increase (+) osteoclastic bone reabsorption. However, because osteoclasts do not have PTHRs, this action is mediated by the osteoblasts, which do have PTHRs and in response release cytokines and factors in turn that activate osteoclasts. In the kidney, PTH stimulates (+) the 1α-hydroxylase (1αOHase) to increase the conversion of 25-hydroxyvitamin D [25(OH)VitD] to the active metabolite 1,25-dihydroxyvitamin D [1,25(OH)$_2$VitD]. In addition, PTH increases (+) the reabsorption of Ca^{2+} from the renal distal tubule and inhibits the reabsorption of phosphate from the proximal tubule, thereby leading to hypercalcemia and hypophosphatemia. PTH also inhibits Na$^+$, H$^+$ antiporter activity and bicarbonate reabsorption, thereby causing a mild hyperchloremic acidosis. The elevated 1,25(OH)$_2$VitD acts on the intestine to increase (+) absorption of dietary calcium and phosphate. It is important to note that PTH does not appear to have a direct action on the gut. Thus, in response to hypocalcemia and the increase in PTH secretion, all of these direct and indirect actions of PTH on the kidney, bone, and intestine will help to increase ECF Ca^{2+}, which in turn will act through the calcium-sensing receptor to decrease PTH secretion. (From Thakker RV, Bringhurst FR, Jüppner HH. Regulation of calcium homeostasis and genetic disorders that affect calcium metabolism. In: Jameson JL, De Groot LJ, giudice LC, et al., eds. *Endocrinology: Adult & Pediatric.* 7th ed. Philadelphia: Saunders; 2016.)

ionized, and the rest is principally bound to albumin or complexed with counter-ions. Ionized calcium in the ECF plays an important role in many physiologic pathways, including muscle contraction, secretion of neurotransmitters and hormones, and coagulation pathways. Ionized serum calcium concentrations range from 4.65 to 5.25 mg/dL (1.16 to 1.31 mmol/L), and the total serum calcium concentration ranges from 8.5 to 10.5 mg/dL (2.12 to 2.62 mmol/L).[1] However, the usual 2 : 1 ratio of total to ionized calcium may be disturbed by disorders such as metabolic acidosis, which reduces calcium binding by proteins, or by changes in protein concentration, caused by cirrhosis, dehydration, venous stasis, or multiple myeloma1. In view of this, total serum calcium concentrations are adjusted, or "corrected," to a reference albumin concentration: the actual total serum calcium value is adjusted by adding or subtracting 0.8 mg/dL (0.016 mmol/L) for every 1 g/dL (1 g/L) of albumin below or above a reference albumin concentration of 4 g/dL (40 g/L), respectively.

The control of body calcium involves a balance between the amounts that are absorbed from the gut, deposited into bone and into cells, and excreted from the kidney (Fig. 245-1).[2] This fine balance, involving three organs, is chiefly under the control of parathyroid hormone (PTH), which is synthesized and secreted by the parathyroid glands. Hypocalcemia leads to an increased secretion of PTH, whereas hypercalcemia results in diminished PTH secretion. Regulation of extracellular calcium takes place through complex interactions (Fig. 245-2) at the target organs of the major calcium-regulating hormone, PTH, and vitamin D and its active metabolites, 1,25-dihydroxyvitamin D (1,25[OH]$_2$D).

● PARATHYROID GLANDS, PARATHYROID HORMONE, *PTH* GENE, AND PARATHYROID HORMONE ACTIONS

Parathyroid Glands

There are usually four parathyroid glands, which are located in close proximity to the superior and inferior poles of the lobes of the thyroid gland. The superior parathyroids are derived from the endoderm of the embryonic fourth pharyngeal pouches, and the inferior parathyroids are derived with the thymus from the endoderm of the third pharyngeal pouches. Extra parathyroid glands are commonly found in aberrant locations along this migrating

path and also within the thymus and thyroid. Parathyroid cells express a G protein–coupled receptor (GPCR), referred to as the *calcium-sensing receptor* (CaSR), that detects changes in extracellular calcium and leads to alterations in PTH secretions.[3] For example, activation of the CaSR, which is also expressed in renal tubular cells, as a result of elevated extracellular calcium concentrations causes G protein–dependent stimulation of phospholipase C activity through Gαq and Gα11, which leads to accumulation of inositol 1,4,5-trisphosphate and an increase in intracellular calcium concentrations.[4] These changes, in turn, lead to reduced circulating PTH concentrations and increased urinary calcium excretion. Disorders of the parathyroid glands may cause hypercalcemia or hypocalcemia, and these can be classified according to whether they arise from an excess of PTH, its deficiency, or insensitivity to its effects (Table 245-1; see Fig. 245-2).

Parathyroid Hormone and *PTH* Gene

The mature PTH peptide is encoded by the *PTH* gene and secreted from the parathyroid chief cells as an 84–amino acid peptide; however, when the *PTH* mRNA is first translated, it is as pre-proPTH peptide. The "pre" sequence consists of a 25–amino acid signal peptide (leader sequence) that is responsible for directing the nascent peptide into the endoplasmic reticulum to be packaged for secretion from the cell. The "pro" sequence is 6 amino acids in length and, although its function is less well defined than that of the "pre" sequence, is also essential for correct PTH processing and secretion. After the 84–amino acid mature PTH peptide is secreted from the parathyroid cell, it is cleared from the circulation with a short half-life of about 2 minutes, by nonsaturable hepatic uptake and renal excretion.

Parathyroid Hormone Actions

PTH shares a receptor with PTH-related peptide (PTHrP); this PTH/PTHrP receptor (see Fig. 245-2) is a member of a subgroup of the G protein–coupled receptor family.[5] PTH/PTHrP receptors are expressed in kidney and bone, where PTH is its predominant agonist, and thus PTH acts directly on kidney and bone cells and indirectly on intestinal cells (see Fig. 245-1) to enhance renal calcium reabsorption, release stored calcium in bones into the ECF, and increase gut calcium absorption, respectively. Expression of the PTH/PTHrP receptor also occurs in the brain, heart, skin, lung, liver, and testis, where it mediates the actions of PTHrP. Mutations

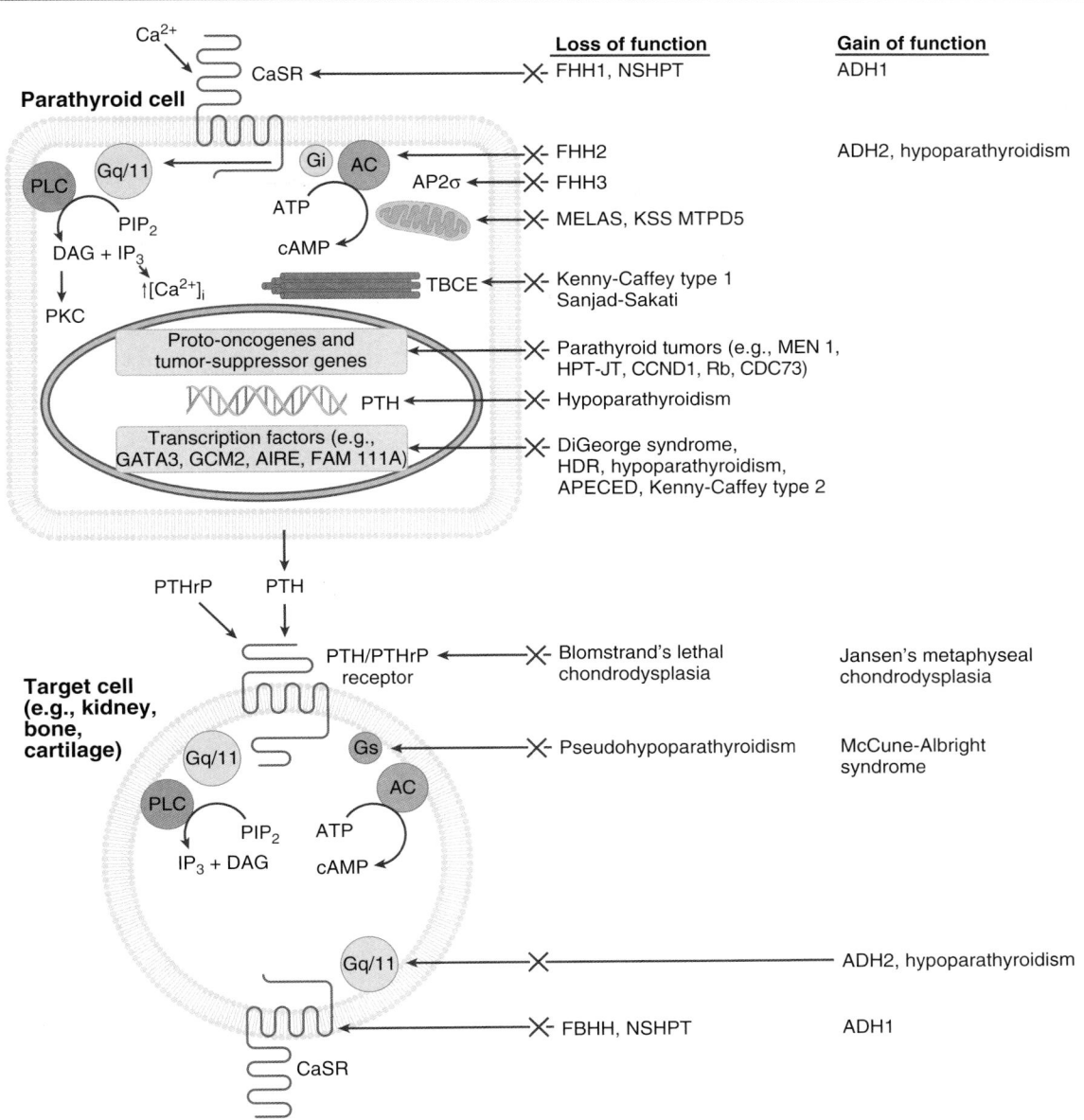

FIGURE 245-2. Schematic representation of some of the components involved in calcium homeostasis. Alterations in extracellular calcium are detected by the calcium-sensing receptor (CaSR), which is a 1078–amino acid G protein–coupled receptor. The PTH/PTHrP receptor, which mediates the actions of PTH and PTHrP, is also a G protein–coupled receptor. Thus, Ca^{2+}, PTH, and PTHrP involve G protein–coupled signaling pathways, and interaction with their specific receptors can lead to activation of Gs, Gi, and Gq, respectively. Gs stimulates adenylcyclase (AC), which catalyzes the formation of cyclic adenosine monophosphate (cAMP) from adenosine triphosphate (ATP). Gi inhibits AC activity. cAMP stimulates protein kinase A (PKA), which phosphorylates cell-specific substrates. Activation of Gq stimulates phospholipase C (PLC), which catalyzes the hydrolysis of the phosphoinositide (PIP$_2$) to inositol triphosphate (IP$_3$), which then increases intracellular calcium, and diacylglycerol (DAG), activating protein kinase C (PKC). These proximal signals modulate downstream pathways, which result in specific physiologic effects. Loss of function in several genes, shown with their respective sites of action on the right, has been identified in specific disorders of calcium homeostasis (also see Table 245-1). (From Thakker RV, Bringhurst FR, Jüppner H. Regulation of calcium homeostasis and genetic disorders that affect calcium metabolism. In: Jameson JL, De Groot LJ, giudice LC, et al., eds. *Endocrinology: Adult & Pediatric.* 7th ed. Philadelphia: Saunders; 2016.)

involving the genes that encode these proteins and receptors in this calcium-regulating pathway (see Fig. 245-2) are associated with hypercalcemic and hypocalcemic disorders (see Table 245-1).

Renal Actions

Calcium is absorbed at multiple sites and by different mechanisms, which include passive paracellular or active transcellular transport, along the renal tubule.[2] The renal actions of PTH are to (1) stimulate activity of the proximal tubular cell 1α-hydroxylase; (2) increase reabsorption of calcium by the cells of the distal tubule, connecting tubules and the thick ascending loop of Henle (TAL); and (3) inhibit phosphate reabsorption by proximal tubular cells (see Fig. 245-1). PTH increases the formation of biologically active 1,25(OH)$_2$D from its precursor 25-OH-D by stimulating the activity of the renal 1α-hydroxylase and inhibiting the 24-hydroxylase, which metabolizes 1,25(OH)$_2$D to the inactive 24,25(OH)$_2$D form (see Fig. 245-1). PTH regulates calcium reabsorption by distal tubular cells by upregulating expression

of the transient receptor potential vanilloid 5 (TRPV5), thereby promoting calcium entry into the cell, and increasing calbindin-D28K expression to enhance transcellular calcium reabsorption by increased buffering of subapical Ca^{2+} ions. In the TAL, PTH may increase active transcellular transport of calcium, as well as paracellular calcium transport, by augmenting the transepithelial voltage gradient. Phosphate transport in proximal tubular cells is mediated by the luminal membrane sodium-phosphate cotransporters 2a and 2c (NPT2a and NPT2c), and PTH actions lead to internalization and degradation of NPT2a and NPT2c, thereby resulting in decreased reabsorption of phosphate.

Skeletal Actions

PTH acts directly on osteoblasts and indirectly on osteoclasts to increase their numbers and activity, thereby enhancing bone turnover and release of stored calcium. Thus, PTH increases the size of the osteoblast precursor pool, increases the bone-forming activity of mature osteoblasts, and stimulates

TABLE 245-1 PARATHYROID DISEASES AND THEIR CHROMOSOMAL LOCATIONS

METABOLIC ABNORMALITY	DISEASE	INHERITANCE	GENE/GENE PRODUCT	CHROMOSOMAL LOCATION
HYPERCALCEMIA				
	Multiple endocrine neoplasia type 1	Autosomal dominant	MENIN	11q13
	Multiple endocrine neoplasia type 2	Autosomal dominant	*RET*	10q11.2
	Hereditary hyperparathyroidism and jaw tumors (HPT-JT)	Autosomal dominant	PARAFIBROMIN	1q31.2
	Sporadic hyperparathyroidism	Sporadic	*PRAD1/CCND1*	11q13
			Retinoblastoma	13q14
			Unknown	1p32-pter
	Parathyroid carcinoma	Autosomal dominant or sporadic	PARAFIBROMIN	1q31.2
			Retinoblastoma	13q14
	Familial benign hypercalcemia (FBH)			
	FBH1	Autosomal dominant	*CaSR*	3q 21.1
	FBH2	Autosomal dominant	Gα11	19p13
	FBH3	Autosomal dominant	*AP2S1*	19p13
	Neonatal severe hyperparathyroidism (NSHPT)	Autosomal recessive or autosomal dominant	*CaSR*	3q21.1
	Jansen's disease	Autosomal dominant	PTHR/PTHrP receptor	3p21.3
	Williams syndrome	Autosomal dominant	*Elastin, LIMK* (and other genes)	7q11.23
	Infantile hypercalcemia	Autosomal recessive	CYP24A	20q13.2-q13.3
	McCune-Albright syndrome	Mutations during early embryonic development?	Gsα	20q13.3
HYPOCALCEMIA				
	Isolated hypoparathyroidism	Autosomal dominant	*PTH, GCMB*	11p15*
		Autosomal recessive	*PTH, GCMB*	11p15*, 6p24.2
		X-linked recessive	SOX3	Xq26–27
	Autosomal dominant hypocalcemia type 1 (ADH1)	Autosomal dominant	*CaSR*	3q21.1
	Autosomal dominant hypocalcemia type 2 (ADH2)	Autosomal dominant	Gα11	19p13
	Hypoparathyroidism associated with polyglandular autoimmune syndrome (APECED)	Autosomal recessive	*AIRE-1*	21q22.3
	Hypoparathyroidism associated with Kearns-Sayre and MELAS	Maternal	Mitochondrial genome	
	Hypoparathyroidism associated with complex congenital syndromes			
	DiGeorge syndrome	Autosomal dominant	*TBX1*	22q11.2/10p
	HDR syndrome	Autosomal dominant	GATA3	10p15
	Blomstrand's lethal chondrodysplasia	Autosomal recessive	PTHR/PTHrP receptor	3p21.3
	Kenney-Caffey syndrome type 1, Sanjad-Sakati syndrome	Autosomal dominant	TBCE	1q42.3
	Kenney-Caffey syndrome type 2	Autosomal recessive	*FAMIIIA*	11q12.1
	Barakat syndrome	Autosomal recessive†	Unknown	?
	Lymphedema	Autosomal recessive	Unknown	?
	Nephropathy, nerve deafness	Autosomal dominant†	Unknown	?
	Nerve deafness without renal dysplasia	Autosomal dominant	Unknown?	?
	Pseudohypoparathyroidism (type 1a)	Autosomal dominant parentally imprinted	*GNAS exons 1-3*	20q13.3
	Pseudohypoparathyroidism (type 1b)	Autosomal dominant parentally imprinted	*GNAS* Upstream deletion	20q13.3

HDR = hypoparathyroidism, deafness, and renal dysplasia; MELAS = mitochondrial encephalopathy, stroke-like episodes, and lactic acidosis; ? = location not known.
*Mutations of PTH gene are identified only in some families.
†Most likely inheritance.

osteoblasts to release cytokines such as colony-stimulating factor 1 and receptor activator of nuclear factor-κB (NF-κB) ligand (RANKL), which stimulate the formation of new osteoclasts and activate mature osteoclasts. PTH also inhibits osteoblast production of osteoprotegrin (OPG), which is a soluble decoy receptor for RANKL that inhibits osteoclast development. Calcium transport involves TRPV4 and TRPV5 in bone cells; TRPV4 regulates intracellular calcium concentrations in osteoblasts and osteoclasts, whereas TRPV5, expressed in osteoclasts, participates to remove the mineral bone matrix.[2] The net result of persistent elevations of PTH is linked to an increase in osteoclast activity more than osteoblast activity, hence liberating the stores of calcium to the ECF (see Fig. 245-1).

Intestinal Actions
Calcium is absorbed throughout the intestine by passive paracellular routes and active transcellular routes, which involve TRPV6 and calbindin D9K. PTH exerts indirect actions on intestinal calcium absorption by increasing the circulating $1,25(OH)_2D$ concentrations (see Fig. 245-1). The increased $1,25(OH)_2D$ concentrations increase TRPV6 expression, which facilitates enhanced calcium entry into the cell from the lumen, and cytosolic calbindin D9K expression, which facilitates transcellular transport of calcium.

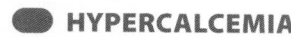 **HYPERCALCEMIA**

DEFINITION
Hypercalcemia is defined as a serum calcium concentration greater than 2 standard deviations above the normal mean, and this is usually a total serum calcium above 10.5 mg/dL (2.62 mmol/L) and an ionized serum calcium of above 5.25 mg/dL (1.31 mmol/L). There is no formal grading system for defining the severity of hypercalcemia, but mild, moderate, and severe hypercalcemia is generally considered for total serum calcium concentrations less than 12 mg/dL (3 mmol/L), between 12 and 14 mg/dL (3 to 3.5 mmol/L), and greater than 14 mg/dL (3.50 mmol/L), respectively.

PATHOBIOLOGY
Hypercalcemia may arise through one of three mechanisms: increased bone resorption, increased gastrointestinal absorption of calcium, and decreased renal calcium excretion (see Fig. 245-1). For example, lytic bone metastases cause increased bone resorption; thiazide diuretics lead to a decrease in calcium excretion; and excessive PTH will either directly or indirectly, by increasing $1,25(OH)_2D$ production, stimulate bone resorption and calcium

absorption from the gut and renal tubules.[6] The causes of hypercalcemia may be classified according to whether serum PTH concentrations are elevated (i.e., primary or tertiary hyperparathyroidism due to parathyroid tumors) or reduced (i.e., not due to parathyroid tumors but instead to an excessive production of PTHrP by a cancer; a defect in the PTH receptor, for example, the PTH/PTHrP receptor; an excess production of downstream mediators, for example, 1,25(OH)$_2$D; or an altered set point in the calcium-sensing receptor) (Table 245-2; see Fig. 245-2). Primary hyperparathyroidism and malignancy are the most common causes and account for more than 90% of patients with hypercalcemia. Detailed clinical history and examination will usually help to differentiate between these two diagnoses. In primary hyperparathyroidism, the hypercalcemia is often less than 12 mg/dL (3 mmol/L), asymptomatic, and may have been present for months or years. If symptoms, such as nephrolithiasis, are present, then they have usually been present for several months. However, in malignancy, the patients are usually acutely ill, often with neurologic symptoms; the hypercalcemia is more than 12 mg/dL (3 mmol/L); and the cancer (e.g., lung, breast, or myeloma) is often readily apparent. Hypercalcemia from causes other than primary hyperparathyroidism or malignancy may also occur (see Table 245-2), and a careful history (e.g., for vitamin D ingestion, drugs, renal disease) and examination (e.g., for thyrotoxicosis, adrenal disease, granulomatous diseases), together with appropriate investigations (Table 245-3; Fig. 245-3), are essential for establishing the diagnosis.

CLINICAL MANIFESTATIONS AND DIAGNOSIS

The clinical presentation of hypercalcemia varies from a mild, asymptomatic, biochemical abnormality detected during routine screening to a life-threatening medical emergency. In general, the presence or absence of symptoms correlates with the severity and rapidity of onset of the hypercalcemia.

Thus, symptoms do not usually develop when serum calcium is below 12 mg/dL (3 mmol/L) and are invariably present when the hypercalcemia exceeds 14 mg/dL (3.5 mmol/L). However, there is a considerable variability, and some patients may be symptomatic with mild hypercalcemia. Although there are many causes of hypercalcemia (see Table 245-2), the signs and symptoms of hypercalcemia are similar, regardless of etiology. Indeed, the clinical manifestations of hypercalcemia involve several organ systems that include the renal, musculoskeletal, gastrointestinal, neurologic, and cardiac systems (Table 245-4), and many of these have been referred to as "moans, groans, pains, and stones." Investigations should be directed at confirming the presence of hypercalcemia and establishing the cause (Table 245-5; see Table 245-3).

TABLE 245-2 CAUSES OF HYPERCALCEMIA

HIGH PARATHYROID HORMONE LEVELS

Primary hyperparathyroidism* (adenoma, hyperplasia, or carcinoma): nonfamilial or familial, e.g., MEN 1, MEN 2, HPT-JT, FIHP
Tertiary hyperparathyroidism (hyperplasia or adenoma in chronic renal failure)

LOW PARATHYROID HORMONE LEVELS

Malignancy*
  Primary
  • Parathyroid hormone–related peptide (PTHrP): carcinoma of lung, esophagus, renal cell, ovary, and bladder
  • Excess production of 1,25(OH)$_2$D (lymphoma)
  Secondary
  • Lytic bone metastases* (multiple myeloma* and breast carcinoma*)
  • Other location, ectopic factors (e.g., cytokines)
Excess vitamin D
  Exogenous vitamin D toxicity by parent D compound, 25(OH) vitamin D$_3$, or 1,25(OH)$_2$ vitamin D$_3$ in vitamin preparations, cod liver oil, herbal medicines
  Endogenous production of 25(OH) vitamin D$_3$—Williams syndrome
  Endogenous production of 1,25(OH)$_2$ vitamin D$_3$, e.g., granulomatous disorders (sarcoidosis, HIV, TB, histoplasmosis, coccidioidomycosis, leprosy), lymphoma, and infantile hypercalcemia
Drugs
  Thiazide diuretics
  Lithium
  Total parenteral nutrition
  Estrogens/antiestrogens, testosterone
  Milk-alkali syndrome
  Vitamin A toxicity
  Aluminum intoxication (in chronic renal failure)
  Aminophylline
Nonparathyroid endocrine disorders
  Thyrotoxicosis
  Pheochromocytoma
  Acute adrenal insufficiency
  Vasoactive intestinal polypeptide hormone producing tumor (VIPoma)
  Immobilization

INAPPROPRIATE PARATHYROID HORMONE LEVELS DUE TO ALTERED SET POINT

Familial benign hypocalciuric hypercalcemia (FBH or FHH)

*Most common causes.
FIHP = familial isolated hyperparathyroidism; HIV = human immunodeficiency virus; HPT-JT = hyperparathyroidism with jaw tumors; MEN = multiple endocrine neoplasia; TB = tuberculosis.

TABLE 245-3 PRELIMINARY INVESTIGATIONS FOR HYPERCALCEMIA

BLOOD

× 2-3 estimations of serum calcium, phosphate, albumin, urea and electrolytes, creatinine, alkaline phosphatase, liver function tests
Parathyroid hormone
Complete blood count
Electrophoretic protein strip or serum protein electrophoresis
25-OH-D$_3$ (and if indicated, 1,25[OH]$_2$D$_3$)
Thyroid function tests
Magnesium
Parathyroid hormone–related peptide (if malignancy suspected)

URINE

× 2-3 estimations of 24-hr urinary calcium and creatinine clearance, and clearance ratios
Imaging
  Chest radiograph
  Radiograph of hands
  Ultrasound of kidneys

TABLE 245-4 CLINICAL FEATURES OF HYPERCALCEMIA

Renal
  Stones (nephrolithiasis) and nephrocalcinosis, polyuria, polydipsia
Musculoskeletal
  Bone pain, osteopenia, fractures, muscular weakness, especially proximal myopathy
Gastrointestinal
  Nausea, vomiting, lack of appetite, constipation, peptic ulcers, and pancreatitis
Neurologic
  Tiredness, lethargy, inability to concentrate, increased sleepiness, depression, confusion, coma
Cardiac
  Bradycardia, first-degree atrioventricular block, arrhythmias, shortened QT interval

TABLE 245-5 SUMMARY OF GUIDELINES FOR PARATHYROID SURGERY IN PRIMARY HYPERPARATHYROIDISM PATIENTS

Surgery* recommended if patient meets any one of the following criteria:
  • Serum calcium >1 mg/dL (0.25 mmol/L) above upper limit of normal
  • Any complication of primary hyperparathyroidism (e.g., nephrolithiasis† or bone erosions of osteitis fibrosa cystica)
  • An episode of acute primary hyperparathyroidism with life-threatening hypercalcemia
  • Significant reduction in creatinine clearance (i.e., <60 mL/min)
  • Reduction in bone mineral density (i.e., T score <−2.5, and/or previous fracture fragility)
  • Age <50 years

*Surgery is also indicated in patients for whom medical surveillance is neither desired nor possible.
†Some physicians still regard marked hypercalciuria (>9 mmol/L per 24 hr or >400 mg/24 hr) as an indication for surgery.
Adapted from Bilezikian JP, Khan AA, Potts JT Jr. Guidelines for the management of asymptomatic primary hyperparathyroidism: summary statement from the third international workshop. *J Clin Endocrinol Metab.* 2009;94:335-339.

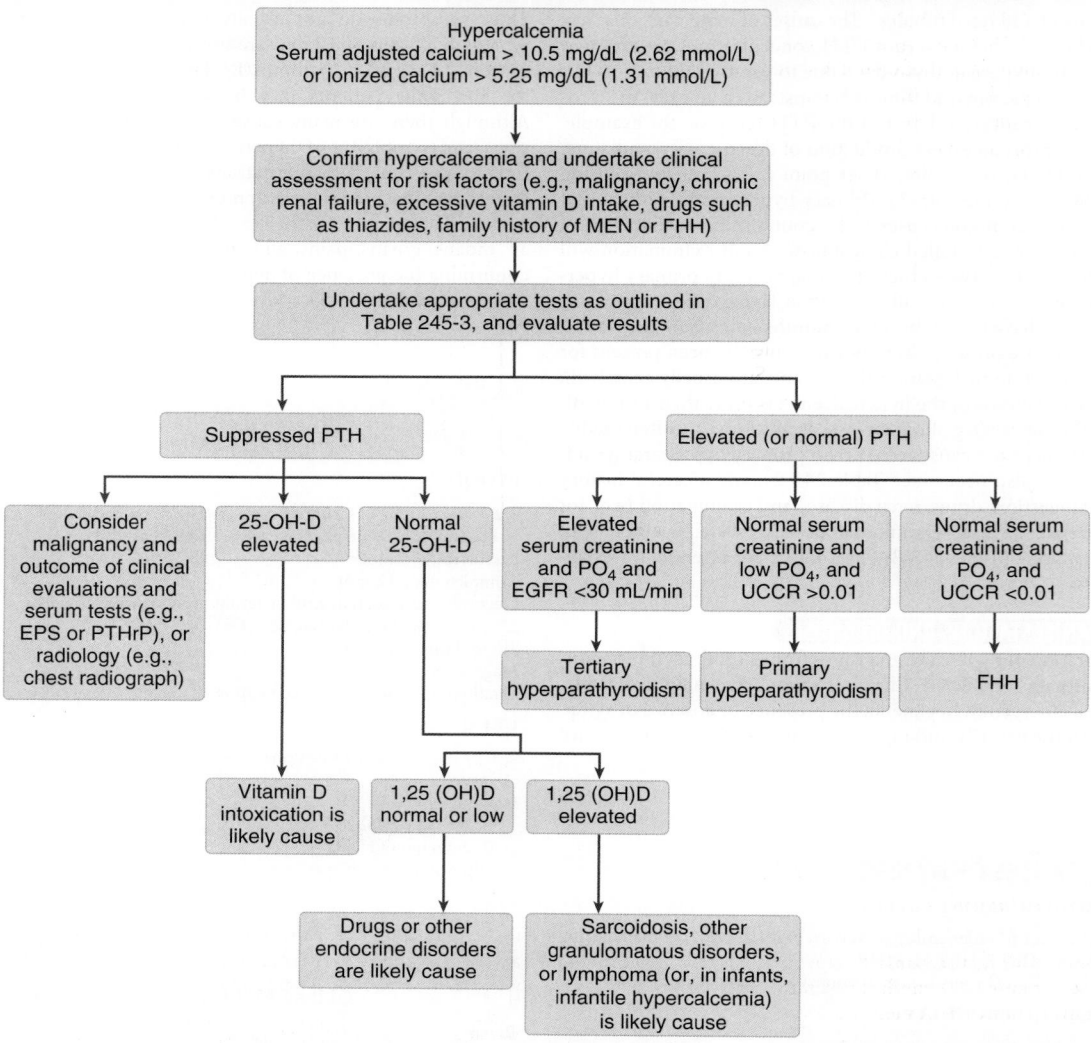

FIGURE 245-3. Clinical approach to the investigation of causes of hypercalcemia. $1,25(OH)_2D$ = 1,25-dihydroxyvitamin D; 25-OH-D = 25-hydroxyvitamin D; EGFR = estimated glomerular filtration rate; EPS = electrophoretic strip (serum protein electrophoresis); FHH = familial hypocalciuric hypercalcemia; MEN = multiple endocrine neoplasia; PTH = parathyroid hormone; PTHrP = parathyroid hormone–related peptide; UCCR = 24-hour urinary calcium clearance–to–creatinine clearance ratio.

TREATMENT Rx

The treatment of hypercalcemia depends on the severity of the hypercalcemia and the presence of symptoms. Thus, asymptomatic patients with mild hypercalcemia do not usually need urgent treatment, whereas patients with severe hypercalcemia would require treatment regardless of symptoms, and patients with moderate hypercalcemia would require urgent treatment if symptomatic. Before instituting treatment, it is always important to consider the underlying causes (see Table 245-2) and to initiate investigations (see Table 245-3). In addition, drugs such as thiazides and vitamin D compounds, which cause hypercalcemia, should be discontinued and, if appropriate, dietary calcium restricted.

The acute management of hypercalcemia involves general measures to enhance hydration and diuresis and specific measures using drugs to lower serum calcium. Dehydration due to hypercalcemic symptoms, such as anorexia, nausea, vomiting, and polyuria because of defective urinary concentration, is very common, and patients may require 5 to 10 liters of 0.9% sodium chloride over a 24- to 48-hour period. This vigorous hydration with normal saline may lower serum calcium by 1 to 3 mg/dL (0.25 to 0.75 mmol/L); it enhances urinary calcium excretion by increasing glomerular filtration and reducing proximal and distal renal tubular reabsorption of calcium and sodium. This saline diuresis may need adjuvant therapy with a loop diuretic (e.g., furosemide, 10 to 20 mg), as necessary to control complications due to volume overload, especially in elderly patients and those with impaired cardiovascular and renal function. Note that excessive use of furosemide before intravascular volume has been restored may worsen the hypercalcemia by exacerbating volume depletion. Saline diuresis may lead to hypokalemia, hypomagnesemia, and electrolyte imbalance, which will need correction.

If saline diuresis is not successful, particularly if the hypercalcemia is very severe, then more specific measures, such dialysis and/or drugs, will be required. The drugs of choice are pamidronate and zoledronic acid, which are potent bisphosphonates, but these should not be used if the hypercalcemia is due to primary or tertiary hyperparathyroidism. Recommended treatments are to administer pamidronate (15-60 mg, depending on serum calcium concentration, in a single IV infusion or in divided doses, depending upon renal function and responses, over 2-4 days; maximum of 90 mg per treatment course) or zoledronic acid (4 mg as single IV infusion). Other bisphosphonates (e.g., etidronate and clodronate) and other agents, such as mithramycin, calcitonin, and gallium nitrate, have also been used in the past. Glucocorticoid therapy (e.g., hydrocortisone, 120 mg/day in three divided doses, in adults) is particularly effective when the hypercalcemia is mediated by the actions of $1,25(OH)_2D$, for example in granulomatous disease or lymphoma, or myeloma. Dialysis using a low or zero calcium dialysate should be considered if these treatments are not effective or if the patient has renal failure. When the acute management of hypercalcemia has been completed, appropriate treatment for the underlying cause needs to be undertaken.

HYPERPARATHYROIDISM

DEFINITION

Hyperparathyroidism is characterized by high concentrations of serum immunoreactive PTH, and three types, referred to as primary, secondary, and tertiary, are recognized. Primary and tertiary hyperparathyroidism are associated with hypercalcemia (see Table 245-2), whereas secondary hyperparathyroidism is associated with hypocalcemia (see later). Primary hyperparathyroidism usually occurs as an isolated nonsyndromic endocrinopathy and less commonly as part of complex syndromic disorders such as the multiple endocrine neoplasia (MEN)[7] and hyperparathyroidism with jaw tumors (HPT-JT). Syndromic and nonsyndromic forms of primary hyperparathyroidism may also occur as hereditary (i.e., familial), usually autosomal dominant disorders, or they may occur as nonfamilial (i.e., sporadic) diseases. Tertiary hyperparathyroidism usually arises in association with chronic renal failure.

Primary Hyperparathyroidism

EPIDEMIOLOGY

Primary hyperparathyroidism, which affects 3 in 1000 adults, is one of the two most common causes of hypercalcemia and is due to an excessive secretion of PTH from one or more parathyroid tumors. Studies have estimated that the global prevalence of parathyroid tumors is 4 million. Primary hyperparathyroidism usually occurs as a nonsyndromic isolated endocrinopathy, between the ages of 40 and 65 years, and is three times more common in females than males.

PATHOBIOLOGY

Eighty percent of patients with primary hyperparathyroidism will have a solitary parathyroid adenoma, and 15 to 20% of patients will have hyperplasia involving all four parathyroid glands. Parathyroid carcinoma occurs in less than 0.5% of patients with primary hyperparathyroidism. The underlying causes of primary hyperparathyroidism are largely unknown. However, more than 10% of patients with clinically nonfamilial primary hyperparathyroidism occurring before 45 years of age have a germline mutation in 1 of 11 genes, including those of MEN 1 (*MEN1*), cell division cycle 73 (*CDC73*), and *CaSR*. In addition, studies of nonfamilial sporadic parathyroid adenomas have shown that 35% to 50% have somatic mutation of the *MEN1* gene; 15% have overexpression of cyclin D1; and more than 85% have an abnormality of the Wnt/β-catenin pathway.[8,9]

CLINICAL MANIFESTATIONS

Many patients with primary hyperparathyroidism are asymptomatic, and the hypercalcemia, which is usually mild, is detected by chance at the time of biochemical screening for other reasons.[10,11] However, it is important to note that nearly half the patients have subtle neuromuscular symptoms such as fatigue and weakness, and this becomes apparent only in retrospect after a successful parathyroidectomy.

Symptomatic hypercalcemia (see Table 245-4) predominantly affects the skeletal, renal, and gastrointestinal systems; peptic ulcers and pancreatitis may develop. The skeletal changes of osteitis fibrosa cystica due to subperiosteal resorption of the distal phalanges, tapering of the distal clavicles, a salt-and-pepper appearance of the skull, bone cysts, and brown tumors of the long bones are now identified in less than 5% of patients. However, osteopenia, as assessed by bone mineral density, occurs in 25% of patients. Renal stone disease (nephrolithiasis and nephrocalcinosis) occurs in 20% of patients, and hypercalciuria occurs in 30% of patients; renal impairment may complicate this disease.

DIAGNOSIS

In the presence of hypercalcemia, the finding of elevated circulating PTH concentrations establishes the diagnosis because PTH is elevated in approximately 90% of patients with primary hyperparathyroidism, who invariably have hypercalcemia (see Fig. 245-3). However, it is important to make sure that the immunoradiometric (IRMA) and immunochemiluminometric (ICMA) assays for PTH are being used to measure the intact molecule, rather than the older radioimmunoassays, which were not as reliable. The only other hypercalcemic disorders in which PTH may occasionally be elevated are those related to familial benign hypocalciuric hypercalcemia (FBH or FHH), immobilization, or lithium or thiazide use (see Table 245-2), and a careful history and a cessation of drug use helps to exclude these possibilities.[12,13] The hypercalcemia of primary hyperparathyroidism, unlike that of malignancy or granulomatous disease, is usually not suppressible by a 10-day course of oral hydrocortisone (120 mg/day given in three divided doses). This test, referred to as the *steroid suppression test*, was previously used to differentiate primary hyperparathyroidism from other causes of hypercalcemia; however, with the advent of more reliable PTH assays, this test is rarely used now. About one third of patients with primary hyperparathyroidism have a low serum phosphate level (see Fig. 245-3), and in the others, it is in the lower

range of normal. In addition, some patients have a small increase in serum chloride concentration and a concomitant decrease in bicarbonate concentration. Serum alkaline phosphatase activity may be elevated in some patients, and urinary calcium excretion is increased in 30% of patients. The circulating $1,25(OH)_2D$ concentration is elevated in some patients with primary hyperparathyroidism, although it is not of diagnostic value because it is also elevated in other hypercalcemic disorders such as sarcoidosis and lymphomas (see Fig. 245-3). The serum 25-OH-D concentration is within the normal range. Densitometric scanning is of use in detecting early skeletal changes. Patients with primary hyperparathyroidism develop reduced bone mineral densities (osteopenia) primarily of the cortical bone (e.g., distal third of forearm) rather than the cancellous bone (e.g., lumbar spine). The hip bones, which are an equal mixture of cortical and cancellous bone, show intermediate reductions in bone mineral density. Overall, the risk for bone fractures in patients with mild primary hyperparathyroidism is similar to those in matched, normal controls. However, successful parathyoidectomy does lead to an increase in bone mineral density over a 6- to 12-month period, and this continues for up to 10 years. Indeed, bone mineral density measurements are used in the evaluation of patients with primary hyperparathyroidism and in deciding on conservative as opposed to surgical management (see Table 245-5).

Preoperative localization to define the sites of the parathyroid tumors may be undertaken.[14] The noninvasive tests consist of ultrasonography, computed tomography (CT), magnetic resonance imaging (MRI), and scintigraphy with technetium-99m sestamibi. Sestamibi scintigraphy has now become established as the best and most convenient localization test; this can be performed with CT techniques (e.g., single-photon emission computed tomography [SPECT]) to give a three-dimensional image with greater anatomic resolution. It is important to note that there is an appreciable incidence of false-positive rates with all the noninvasive localization procedures, so a confirmation using two methods is preferable. Invasive localization tests consist of arteriography and selective venous sampling for PTH in the veins draining the thyroidal region. These tests are time consuming, expensive, difficult, and dependent on the skill of the radiologist. It is generally accepted that these preoperative localization tests are indicated in those patients who have had previous neck surgery. However, their role in patients who have not had prior surgery remains to be established, and at present, the preferences and expertise of the local medical, radiology, and surgery teams usually determine the use of venous sampling procedures.

TREATMENT   Rx

Parathyroidectomy, which is the definitive cure, is a generally successful and safe procedure if undertaken by an experienced surgeon. There have also been major advances in surgery that have facilitated a surgical approach to be undertaken under local, as opposed to general, anesthesia. An example of this is the use of minimally invasive parathyroidectomy (MIP) in the patient with single gland disease that has been successfully localized by the combined use of sestamibi scintigraphy and ultrasonography. Surgery is recommended for symptomatic patients and for those who have skeletal and renal complications (see Table 245-5). Complications of parathyroid surgery include damage to the recurrent laryngeal nerve and permanent hypoparathyroidism. However, the decision to recommend surgery may be difficult in asymptomatic patients, who may constitute more than 50% of patients with primary hyperparathyroidism. The natural history of primary hyperparathyroidism in most patients is to progress slowly or not at all. For example, among asymptomatic patients, only 25% have progressive disease, which is usually manifested as a decrease in bone mineral density during a 10-year period. This has led to a controversy regarding the indications for surgery, and guidelines have been provided by the Third International Workshop (2008) on the Management of Asymptomatic Primary Hyperparathyroidism (see Table 245-5). However, these guidelines may not exclusively influence the decision for or against surgery, and a careful evaluation and assessment of the risks and benefits is considered by most medical and surgical teams in conjunction with the patient. Clearly, some patients will not wish to continue living with a curable disease and will prefer surgery despite the guidelines (see Table 245-5), whereas other patients will decline surgery, despite having guideline indications for surgery, because they may have coexisting medical conditions that make them feel that the risks for surgery are too great.

Patients who do not undergo parathyroidectomy should be evaluated clinically and also monitored for serum calcium, creatinine, and PTH at 12-month intervals, and for bone mineral density at 12- to 24-month intervals. In addition, the following medical guidelines are recommended. First, they should avoid dehydration and remain ambulant. Second, the dietary intake of calcium should be moderate, that is, at or below 1000 mg/day, and thiazide diuretics should be avoided. Finally, they should avoid herbal and tonic remedies that may contain vitamin D or vitamin A. Drugs that have been used for the treatment of primary hyperparathyroidism include oral phosphate, estrogens, or selective estrogen receptor modulators (SERMs) in postmenopausal women; bisphosphonates; and the calcimimetic, cinacalcet. Phosphate is not used because of concerns related to soft tissue ectopic calcification. Estrogens and SERMs (e.g., raloxifene) do increase bone density in postmenopausal women with primary hyperparathyroidism, but they have only small effects on the serum calcium and PTH concentrations. The bisphosphonates (e.g., alendronate and zoledronic acid) inhibit bone resorption and reduce serum calcium. However, these effects are not sustained. In a randomized, double-blind, placebo-controlled clinical trial, cinacalcet was effective in lowering serum calcium concentrations to normal values and reducing PTH levels in patients with primary hyperparathyroidism.[A1] These effects were maintained with long-term treatment without major adverse effects. Bone mineral density in the treated patients remained unchanged, but there was a reduction in biochemical markers for bone resorption and formation. Cinacalcet may therefore represent an effective nonsurgical treatment for the management of primary hyperparathyroidism. Daily high dose (70 mg or 2800U) cholecalciferol also can decrease PTH and improve bone density when used for 6 months before and after parathyroidectomy.[A2]

FAMILIAL PRIMARY HYPERPARATHYROIDISM

Primary hyperparathyroidism is most frequently encountered as a nonfamilial (sporadic) disorder. However, approximately 10% of patients with primary hyperparathyroidism have a hereditary form that may either be part of the MEN 1, MEN 2, MEN 3, and MEN 4 syndromes or part of the HPT-JT syndrome. In addition, hereditary primary hyperparathyroidism may develop as a solitary endocrinopathy, and this has also been referred to as familial isolated hyperparathyroidism (FIHP). Patients with these familial forms of primary hyperparathyroidism, including the MEN syndromes, have important differences from those developing nonfamilial forms; these include an earlier age of onset (20 to 25 years versus 55 years) and an equal male-to-female ratio (1:1 versus 1:3). In addition, MEN syndromes are associated with the occurrence of multiple parathyroid tumors, rather than the solitary parathyroid adenomas typically found in the sporadic form; and HPT-JT is associated with occurrence of parathyroid carcinoma in 15% of patients. This has implications for the treatment of parathyroid tumors in patients with these disorders. Thus, minimally invasive parathyroidectomy is an unsuitable approach in MEN patients because of multigland disease, and patients with HPT-JT are likely to require earlier surgery because of the higher risk for parathyroid carcinoma. Investigations of the hereditary and sporadic forms of primary HPT have helped to identify some of the genes and chromosomal regions that are involved in the etiology of parathyroid tumors (see Table 245-1 and Fig. 245-2). FIHP has been reported in several kindreds, and some have been shown to harbor mutations of the MEN1, CDC73, or CaSR genes. The familial syndromes associated with parathyroid tumors include MEN 1, MEN 2, MEN 3, and MEN 4. They are reviewed in detail in Chapter 231.

HYPERPARATHYROIDISM—JAW TUMOR SYNDROME

The HPT-JT syndrome is an autosomal dominant disorder characterized by the occurrence of parathyroid tumors, which may be carcinomas in approximately 15% of patients, and ossifying fibromas that usually affect the maxilla or mandible. In addition, some patients may also develop Wilms' tumors, renal cysts, renal hamartomas, renal cortical adenomas, papillary renal cell carcinomas, uterine tumors that may be malignant, pancreatic adenocarcinomas, testicular mixed germ cell tumors with a major seminoma component, and Hurthle cell thyroid adenomas. Mutations of the CDC73 gene, which is located on chromosome 1q31.2 and encodes a 531–amino acid protein, parafibromin, cause HPT-JT. Parafibromin has been shown to be associated with the human homologue of the Paf1 protein complex, which interacts with RNA polymerase II, and as part of this protein complex, parafibromin may regulate post-transcriptional events and histone modification. Patients with nonfamilial parathyroid carcinomas frequently harbor germline CDC73 mutations.

UREMIC HYPERPARATHYROIDISM
PATHOBIOLOGY

Serum PTH levels rise in response to hypocalcemia, and this secondary hyperparathyroidism usually resolves with treatment of the underlying cause of hypocalcemia (Table 245-6). However, in chronic renal failure (Chapter

TABLE 245-6   CAUSES OF HYPOCALCEMIA

LOW PARATHYROID HORMONE LEVELS (HYPOPARATHYROIDISM)

Parathyroid agenesis
  Isolated or part of complex developmental anomaly (e.g., DiGeorge syndrome)
Parathyroid destruction
  Surgery*
  Radiation
  Infiltration by metastases or systemic disease (e.g., hemochromatosis, amyloidosis, sarcoidosis, Wilson's disease, thalassemia)
Autoimmune
  Isolated
  Polyglandular (type 1)
Reduced parathyroid function (i.e., parathyroid hormone secretion)
  Parathyroid hormone gene defects
  Hypomagnesemia*
  Neonatal hypocalcemia (may be associated with maternal hypercalcemia)
  Hungry bone disease (postparathyroidectomy)
  Calcium-sensing receptor or Gα11 mutations

HIGH PARATHYROID HORMONE LEVELS (SECONDARY HYPERPARATHYROIDISM)

Vitamin D deficiency*
  As a result of nutritional lack,* malabsorption,* liver disease, or vitamin D receptor defects
  Inadequate production of active vitamin D (1,25[OH]$_2$D) as a result of chronic renal failure*
Vitamin D resistance (rickets)
  As a result of renal tubular dysfunction (Fanconi's syndrome) or vitamin D receptor defects
Parathyroid hormone resistance
  (e.g., pseudohypoparathyroidism, hypomagnesemia)
Drugs
  Calcium chelators (e.g., citrated blood transfusions, phosphate—cow's milk is rich in phosphate)
  Inhibitors of bone resorption (e.g., bisphosphonates, calcitonin, plicamycin)
  Altered vitamin D metabolism (e.g., phenytoin, ketoconazole)
  Foscarnet
Miscellaneous
  Acute pancreatitis
  Acute rhabdomyolysis
  Massive tumor lysis
  Osteoblastic metastases (e.g., from prostate or breast carcinoma)
  Toxic shock syndrome
  Hyperventilation

*Most common causes.

130), the secondary hyperparathyroidism may persist for a longer time, and eventually the parathyroid cells gain an autonomous function, secreting excessive PTH despite hypercalcemia; this state is referred to as tertiary hyperparathyroidism (see Table 245-2). The cause of progression from the early, presumably polyclonal, secondary hyperplasia of the parathyroids to the later, presumably monoclonal, tumors is not understood and appears to involve genes other than those involved in the etiologies of the sporadic and familial forms of primary hyperparathyroidism (see Table 245-2).

CLINICAL MANIFESTATIONS AND TREATMENT   Rx

In chronic renal failure, the ensuing phosphate retention and decreased production of 1,25(OH)$_2$D result in hypocalcemia and secondary hyperparathyroidism. This combination of biochemical abnormalities results in a severe bone disease that shows combined features of hyperparathyroidism and vitamin D deficiency (i.e., osteomalacia). Thus, in renal osteodystrophy, bone erosions and osteomalacia are simultaneously observed. Treatment is based on correcting the hypocalcemia, for example, with oral administration of calcium salts, which also ameliorates the hyperphosphatemia by chelating phosphate in the intestines, and with calcitriol (1,25[OH]$_2$D). The use of the most appropriate phosphate binder is not well established, but it is clear that aluminum-containing compounds are to be avoided. Aluminum in these preparations and as a contaminant of dialysis solutions contributed in the recent past to the osteomalacic osseous disease and other aspects of metal toxicity in patients with renal failure (e.g., hypochromic anemia and encephalopathy). Early treatment of the metabolic disturbance will prevent or delay the onset of severe secondary hyperparathyroidism and tertiary hyperparathyroidism, which requires parathyroidectomy. For patients who have end-stage renal failure and are on dialysis, cinacalcet, the allosteric activator of the CaSR, can be used to treat the severe secondary hyperparathyroidism. Cinacalcet will reduce the PTH concentrations and may also have an antiproliferative effect.

DISORDERS AND SYNDROMES ASSOCIATED WITH HYPERCALCEMIA

Endocrine Causes of Hypercalcemia Other than Hyperparathyroidism

Several nonparathyroid disorders (see Table 245-2) are associated with hypercalcemia, and these include thyrotoxicosis, pheochromocytoma, Addison's disease, vasoactive intestinal polypeptide hormone producing tumor (VIPomas), familial benign hypocalciuric hypercalcemia, Jansen's disease, and Williams syndrome.

THYROTOXICOSIS

Mild hypercalcemia (<12 mg/dL, or 3 mmol/L)) frequently accompanies thyrotoxicosis, which leads to increased bone turnover and resorption. The hypercalcemia may respond to treatment with β-adrenergic blockers.

FAMILIAL BENIGN HYPOCALCIURIC HYPERCALCEMIA

Familial benign hypercalcemia (FBH), which is also referred to as familial hypocalciuric hypercalcemia (FHH), is an autosomal dominant disorder characterized by lifelong asymptomatic hypercalcemia in association with an inappropriately low urinary calcium excretion (i.e., calcium clearance–to–creatinine clearance ratio (CCR) <0.01), and normal circulating PTH concentrations in 80% of patients. Hypermagnesemia is also typically present. Although most patients with FBH are asymptomatic, chondrocalcinosis and acute pancreatitis have occasionally been observed. Patients with FHH have been misdiagnosed as having primary hyperparathyroidism because 20% of FHH patients may have elevated plasma PTH concentrations. In addition, 20% of FHH patients may have a CCR greater than 0.01 and therefore be indistinguishable from patients with primary hyperparathyroidism. Moreover, low CCRs are observed in patients with primary hyperparathyroidism who have vitamin D deficiency or renal insufficiency or are of African American origin. It is important to distinguish FHH patients from those with primary hyperparathyroidism because the hypercalcemia in FHH is generally benign and does not result in sequelae (see Table 245-4). Moreover, parathyroidectomy does not correct the hypercalcemia in FHH. Mutational analysis may help in identifying FHH patients from those with primary hyperparathyroidism.

FHH is genetically heterogenous, with three reported variants—FHH1, FHH2 and FHH3—whose loci are on chromosomes 3q21.1, 19p, and 19q13, respectively (see Table 245-1). FHH1 is due to heterozygous loss-of-function mutations of the CaSR, which is a GPCR that signals through $G\alpha q$ and $G\alpha 11$. The human CaSR, a 1078–amino acid cell surface GPCR encoded by the *CaSR* gene located on chromosome 3q21.1, is expressed in parathyroid cells, thyroid cells, and kidney (see Fig. 245-2). Approximately two thirds of FHH kindreds have unique heterozygous mutations of the CaSR, and expression studies of these mutations have demonstrated a loss of CaSR function whereby there is an increase in the calcium ion–dependent set point for PTH release from the parathyroid cell. FHH2 is due to loss-of-function mutations in the G-protein subunit $\alpha 11$ ($G\alpha 11$) (see Fig. 245-2), which decrease the sensitivity of cells expressing the CaSR, probably by impairing the release of guanosine diphosphate. Such $G\alpha 11$ loss-of-function mutations may occur in less than 5% of FHH patients.

FHH3 is due to loss-of-function mutations of the adaptor protein 2 (AP2) sigma subunit (AP2σ) (see Fig. 245-2). AP2 is a central component of clathrin-coated vesicles (CCVs) and is pivotal in clathrin-mediated endocytosis, which internalizes plasma membrane constituents such as GPCRs. AP2 is a heterotetramer of α, β, μ, and σ subunits and links clathrin to vesicle membranes and binds to tyrosine- and dileucine-based motifs of membrane-associated cargo proteins. The FHH3-associated AP2σ mutations, which all involve an Arg15 residue that forms key contacts with the dileucine-based motifs of CCV cargo proteins, result in a decreased sensitivity of CaSR-expressing cells to extracellular calcium and reduced CaSR endocytosis, probably through loss of interaction with a C-terminal CaSR dileucine-based

motif, whose disruption also decreases intracellular signaling. Such AP2σ loss-of-function mutations occur in more than 5% of FHH patients. FHH1, FHH2, and FHH3 have similar clinical features, and thus genetic analysis is required to identify the relevant mutations.

AUTOIMMUNE HYPOCALCIURIC HYPERCALCEMIA

Some patients, who have the clinical features of FHH1, but not CaSR mutations, may have autoimmune hypocalciuric hypercalcemia (AHH). Such patients may have multiple clinical autoimmune manifestations, including antithyroid, antigliadin, or antiendomyseal antibodies. These patients were shown to have circulating antibodies to the extracellular domain of the CaSR, and these antibodies stimulated PTH release from dispersed human parathyroid cells in vitro, probably by inhibiting the activation of the CaSR by extracellular calcium. The effects of treatment with glucocorticoids have been variable, with the hypercalcemia responding in one patient but not in another. Thus, AHH is a condition of extracellular calcium-sensing that should be considered in FHH1 patients who do not have CaSR mutations.

NEONATAL SEVERE PRIMARY HYPERPARATHYROIDISM

Neonatal severe primary hyperparathyroidism (NSHPT) is defined as symptomatic hypercalcemia with skeletal manifestations of hyperparathyroidism in the first 6 months of life.[5] NSHPT children often present in the first few days or weeks of life with failure to thrive, dehydration, hypotonia, constipation, rib cage deformities, and multiple fractures due to bony undermineralization. Children with NSHPT often have life-threatening hypercalcemia and require urgent parathyroidectomy, which corrects the PTH-dependent hypercalcemia and bone demineralization. FBH or FHH is due to heterozygous inactivating mutations of the CaSR, and NSHPT is often associated with inactivating homozygous CaSR mutations when the children are from consanguineous parents with FHH1 (see Fig. 245-2). However, NSHPT has also been observed in children for whom one parent had clinically apparent FBH, and many other NSHPT patients appear to be sporadic; that is, both parents have normal serum calcium concentrations. In such NSHPT patients with heterozygous CaSR mutations, the mutant CaSR may exert a dominant negative action on the normal CaSR.

JANSEN'S DISEASE

Jansen's disease is an autosomal dominant disease that is characterized by short-limbed dwarfism due to metaphyseal chondrodysplasia and severe hypercalcemia and hypophosphatemia despite normal or undetectable serum levels of PTH. These abnormalities are associated with activating mutations of the PTH receptor (see Fig. 245-2), and thus this represents a PTH-independent activation of the PTH receptor (PTHR).

WILLIAMS SYNDROME

Williams syndrome is an autosomal dominant disorder characterized by supravalvular aortic stenosis, elfin-like facies, psychomotor retardation, and infantile hypercalcemia. The underlying abnormality causing hypercalcemia, which affects 5 to 50% of patients, remains unknown, but abnormal $1,25(OH)_2D_3$ metabolism and decreased calcitonin production have been implicated, although no abnormality has been consistently demonstrated. Hemizygosity due to a microdeletion of chromosome 7q11.23 involving the *ELASTIN* and *LIM-KINASE* genes, which may explain the respective cardiovascular and neurologic features, have been reported in Williams syndrome patients. However, the calcitonin receptor gene, located on chromosome 7q21 and close to the region deleted in Williams syndrome, was not involved in the deletion found in four patients with Williams syndrome, indicating that it is unlikely to be implicated in the hypercalcemia of such children. Another, as yet uncharacterized gene that is within this contiguously deleted region is likely to be involved to explain the abnormalities of calcium metabolism.

INFANTILE HYPERCALCEMIA

Infantile hypercalcemia is associated with failure to thrive and is characterized by severe hypercalcemia, hypercalciuria, and nephrocalcinosis and elevated circulating $1,25(OH)_2D$ concentrations. Some infants with this disorder have homozygous or compound heterozygous mutations of the gene encoding the 24-hydroxylase (CYP24A1) enzyme, which metabolizes the active $1,25(OH)_2D$ to the inactive $1,24,25(OH)_3D$ form (see Fig. 245-1).

Malignancy

Hypercalcemia may occur in 20 to 30% of patients with a malignancy, and this is usually due to increased bone resorption, which may either be directly due to skeletal metastases or indirectly due to tumor production of a humoral factor that stimulates osteoclastic bone resorption (Chapter 179). The cancers that typically metastasize to produce lytic bone lesions are from the breast, lymphomas, or multiple myeloma (see Table 245-2). The associated osteolysis, mediated by recruitment and activation of osteoclasts, involves cytokines. Denosumab, a humanized neutralizing monoclonal antibody to RANKL, may be used to prevent the recruitment and activation of osteoclasts. The cancers that are typically associated with the humoral hypercalcemia of malignancy (HHM) are squamous carcinomas of the lung, esophagus, cervix, vulva, skin, head, or neck, but other types from the kidney, bladder, ovary, and breast may also occur. HHM accounts for up to 80% of patients with malignancy-associated hypercalcemia. The most common factor causing HHM is PTHrP, which can be measured in the serum by immunoassay. However, these assays are relatively insensitive, and the failure to detect serum PTHrP does not exclude the diagnosis of HHM. Patients with HHM generally have hypercalcemia associated with lower or undetectable serum PTH levels, marked hypercalcemia, and a reduced plasma $1,25(OH)_2D$ level. Therapy of HHM is aimed at (1) reducing the tumor load by surgery, radiotherapy, and/or chemotherapy; (2) reducing osteoclastic bone resorption by use of bisphosphonates (e.g., zoledronate) calcitonin or denosumab; and (3) increasing renal calcium clearance by a saline diuresis.

Granulomatous Disorders

Several granulomatous disorders are associated with hypercalcemia (see Table 245-2), and this is invariably associated with elevated circulating concentrations of $1,25(OH)_2D$, which is due to extrarenal synthesis. Sarcoidosis is the most frequently encountered granulomatous disorder associated with hypercalcemia; 10% of patients with sarcoidosis have hypercalcemia, and about half become hypercalciuric. The finding of raised serum angiotensin-converting enzyme (ACE) activity may help confirm the diagnosis. Glucocorticoids (e.g., 40 to 60 mg of prednisolone) decrease $1,25(OH)_2D$ production and restore the calcium concentration to normal. Failure to achieve normal serum calcium concentrations within 10 days of glucocorticoid therapy (e.g., hydrocortisone, 40 mg three times per day), the steroid suppression test, should suggest the coexistence of another cause for the hypercalcemia, such as primary hyperparathyroidism or malignancy.

Drugs

Several drugs (see Table 245-2) can cause hypercalcemia by different mechanisms. Compounds containing vitamins D and A are common and frequently associated with hypercalcemia. The use of thiazide diuretics is often associated with hypercalcemia. The hypercalcemia appears to be largely renal in origin because thiazides enhance distal renal tubular calcium reabsorption. Hypercalcemia reverses rapidly with discontinuation of the drug.

The milk-alkali syndrome was first described in the 1930s, generally in the context of ulcer treatment with large quantities of milk together with sodium bicarbonate. Today, the responsible agent is usually calcium carbonate, although consumption of large quantities of dairy products (milk, cheese, and yogurt) may still contribute. Classic features include moderate to severe hypercalcemia with alkalosis and renal impairment. The amount of calcium ingested by patients with this syndrome is usually 5 to 15 g/day. Treatment consists of (1) discontinuing the ingestion of the calcium containing compounds and antacids; (2) rehydration; and (3) saline diuresis.

● HYPOCALCEMIA

DEFINITION

Hypocalcemia is defined as a serum calcium concentration below the lower limit of normal range, and this is usually an ionized serum calcium below 4.65 mg/dL (1.16 mmol/L) and a total serum calcium below 8.5 mg/dL (2.12 mmol/L). Mild hypocalcemia is defined as a total serum calcium of 8 to 8.5 mg/dL (2 to 2.12 mmol/L) and severe hypocalcemia as a total serum calcium below 7.6 mg/dL (1.9 mmol/L).

PATHOBIOLOGY

Hypocalcemia (see Table 245-6) can be classified by cause, according to whether serum PTH concentrations are low (i.e., hypoparathyroid disorders) or high (i.e., disorders associated with secondary hyperparathyroidism). Hypocalcemia is most commonly caused by hypoparathyroidism, a deficiency or abnormal metabolism of vitamin D, acute or chronic renal failure, or hypomagnesemia. Hypocalcemic diseases (see Table 245-6) may arise because of a destruction of the parathyroid glands, failure of parathyroid

TABLE 245-7 HYPOCALCEMIC CLINICAL FEATURES OF NEUROMUSCULAR IRRITABILITY

Paresthesia, usually of fingers, toes, and circumoral regions
Tetany, carpopedal spasm, muscle cramps
Chvostek's sign*
Trousseau's sign†
Seizures of all types (i.e., focal or petit mal, grand mal, or syncope)
Prolonged QT interval on electrocardiogram
Laryngospasm
Bronchospasm

*Chvostek's sign is twitching of the circumoral muscles in response to gentle tapping of the facial nerve just anterior to the ear; it may be present in 10% of normal individuals.
†Trousseau's sign is carpal spasm elicited by inflation of a blood pressure cuff to 20 mm Hg above the patient's systolic blood pressure for 3 minute.

gland development, or reduced PTH secretion or PTH-mediated actions in target tissues. Thus, these diseases may be classified as being due to a deficiency of PTH, a defect in the PTH receptor (i.e., the PTH/PTHrP receptor), or insensitivity to PTH caused by defects downstream of the PTH/PTHrP receptor (see Fig. 245-2). The diseases may also be classified as being part of the hypoparathyroid disorders, of the CaSR abnormalities, or of the pseudohypoparathyroid disorders.

CLINICAL MANIFESTATIONS AND DIAGNOSIS

The clinical presentation of hypocalcemia ranges from an asymptomatic biochemical abnormality to a severe, life-threatening condition. In mild hypocalcemia, patients may be asymptomatic. Those with more severe and long-term hypocalcemia may develop acute symptoms of neuromuscular irritability (Table 245-7), ectopic calcification (e.g., in the basal ganglia, which may be associated with extrapyramidal neurological symptoms), subcapsular cataract, papilledema, and abnormal dentition. Investigations should be directed at confirming the presence of hypocalcemia and establishing the cause (Fig. 245-4).

In hypoparathyroidism, serum calcium is low, phosphate is high, and PTH is undetectable; renal function and concentrations of the 25-hydroxy and 1,25-dihydroxy metabolites of vitamin D are usually normal (see Fig. 245-4). The features of pseudohypoparathyroidism are similar to those of hypoparathyroidism except for PTH, which is markedly increased.[15] In chronic renal failure, which is the most common cause of hypocalcemia, phosphate is high, and alkaline phosphatase, creatinine, and PTH are elevated; $25-OH-D_3$ is normal, and $1,25(OH)_2D_3$ is low (see Fig. 245-1). In vitamin D deficiency osteomalacia, serum calcium and phosphate are low, alkaline phosphatase and PTH are elevated, renal function is normal, and $25-OH-D_3$ is low (see Fig. 245-4). The most frequent artifactual cause of hypocalcemia is hypoalbuminemia, such as occurs in liver disease or the nephrotic syndrome.

TREATMENT   Rx

Acute Hypocalcemia

The management of acute hypocalcemia depends on the severity of the hypocalcemia, the rapidity with which it developed, and the degree of neuromuscular irritability (see Table 245-7). Treatment should be given to symptomatic patients (e.g., with seizures or tetany) and asymptomatic patients with a serum calcium of less than 7.6 mg/dL (1.90 mmol/L) who are at high risk for developing complications. The preferred treatment for acute symptomatic hypocalcemia is calcium gluconate, 10 mL 10% w/v (2.20 mmol of calcium) intravenous, diluted in 50 mL of 5% dextrose or 0.9% sodium chloride and given by slow injection (>5 minutes); this can be repeated as required to control symptoms. Serum calcium concentrations should be assessed regularly. Continuing hypocalcemia may be managed acutely by administration of a calcium gluconate infusion; for example, dilute 10 ampules of calcium gluconate, 10 mL 10% w/v (22 mmol of calcium), in 1 liter of 5% dextrose or 0.9% sodium chloride, start infusion at 50 mL/hour, and titrate to maintain serum calcium concentrations in the normal range. Generally, 1.2 to 1.6 mg/kg (0.3 to 0.4 mmol/kg) of elemental calcium infused over 4 to 6 hours increases serum calcium by 2 to 3 mg/dL (0.5 to 0.75 mmol/L). If hypocalcemia is likely to persist, oral vitamin D therapy (see later) should also be administered. In hypocalcemic patients who are also hypomagnesemic, the hypomagnesemia must be corrected before the hypocalcemia will resolve. This may occur in the postparathyroidectomy period or in patients with severe malabsorption, for example, those with established celiac disease (Chapter 140).

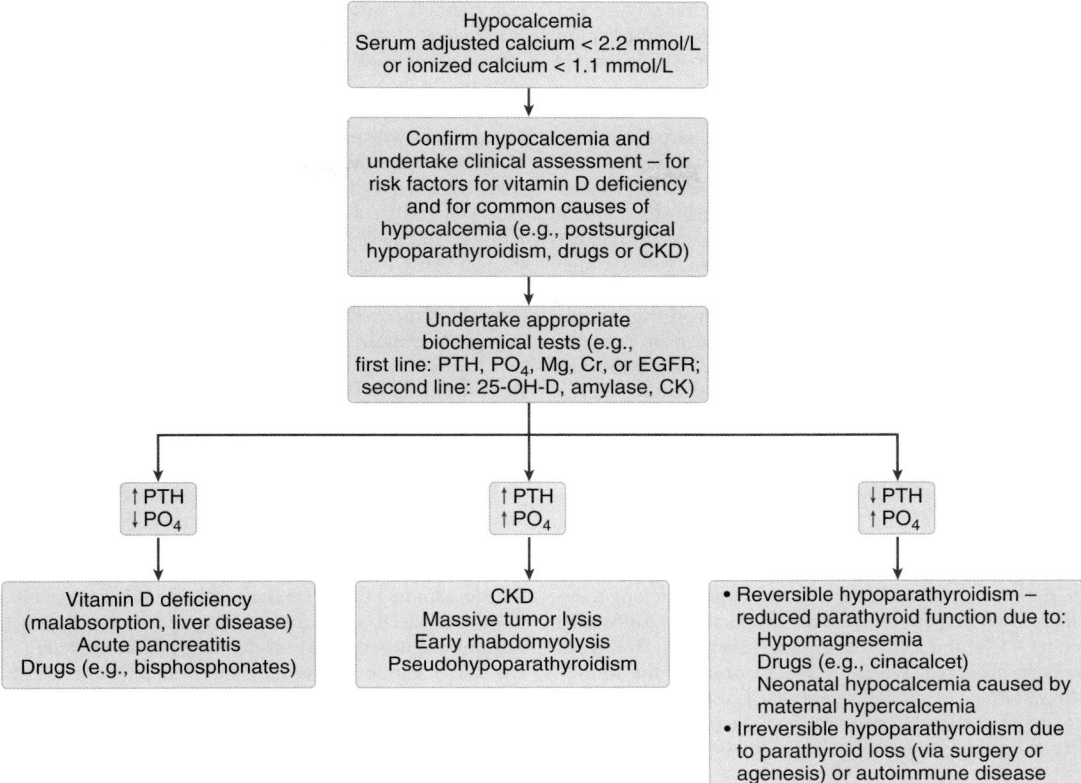

FIGURE 245-4. Clinical approach to investigation of causes of hypocalcemia. 25-OH-D = 25-hydroxyvitamin D; CK = creatinine kinase ; CKD = chronic kidney disease; Cr = creatinine; EGFR = estimated glomerular filtration rate; PTH = parathyroid hormone.

Chronic Hypocalcemia

The two main agents available for the treatment of chronic (long-term) hypocalcemia are supplemental calcium, about 10 to 20 mmol calcium every 6 to 12 hours, and vitamin D preparations. Patients with hypoparathyroidism seldom require calcium supplements after the early stages of stabilization with vitamin D. A variety of vitamin D preparations have been used. These include vitamin D_3 (cholecalciferol) or vitamin D_2 (ergocalciferol), 10,000 to 50,000 units (0.25 to 1.25 mg/day); dihydrotachysterol (now seldom used), 0.25 to 1.25 mg/day; alfacalcidol (1α-hydroxycholecalciferol), 0.25 to 1 μg/day; and calcitriol (1,25-dihydroxy cholecalciferol), 0.25 to 2 μg/day. In children, these preparations are prescribed in doses based on body weight. Cholecalciferol and ergocalciferol are the least expensive preparations but have the longest durations of action and may result in prolonged toxicity; however, they are the preparations of choice for treating hypocalcemia associated with vitamin D deficiency (see Table 245-6). The other preparations, which do not require renal 1α-hydroxylation, have the advantage of shorter half-lives and thereby minimize the risk for prolonged toxicity. For treatment of hypocalcemia due to hypoparathyroidism or chronic renal failure, calcitriol is the drug of choice because it is the active metabolite and, unlike alfacalcidol, does not require hepatic 25-hydroxylation. Close monitoring (at about 1- to 2-week intervals) of the patient's serum and urine calcium concentrations are required initially, and 3- to 6-month intervals are appropriate once stabilization is achieved. The aim is to avoid hypercalcemia, hypercalciuria, nephrolithiasis, and renal failure. It should be noted that hypercalciuria may occur in the absence of hypercalcemia. The use of PTH (1-84) in hypoparathyroid patients has been reported to be associated with improvement in the biochemical and skeletal indices, as well as in mental and physical health.[16]

HYPOPARATHYROIDISM

DEFINITION

Hypoparathyroidism is characterized by hypocalcemia and hyperphosphatemia, which are the result of a deficiency in PTH secretion or action.[17] Serum concentrations of immunoreactive PTH are low or undetectable, and the concentrations of $1,25(OH)_2D_3$ are usually in the low-normal to low range, but alkaline phosphatase activity is unchanged (see Fig. 245-4). The daily

urinary excretion of calcium is reduced, although the fractional excretion of calcium is increased. Nephrogenous cyclic adenosine monophosphate (cAMP) excretion is low, and renal tubular reabsorption of phosphate is elevated. Urinary cAMP, plasma cAMP, and urinary phosphate excretion increase markedly after administration of exogenous bioactive PTH (Chase-Aurbach and Ellsworth-Howard tests).

PATHOBIOLOGY

Hypoparathyroidism may result from agenesis (e.g., DiGeorge syndrome) or destruction of the parathyroid glands (e.g., following neck surgery, in autoimmune diseases), from reduced secretion of PTH (e.g., neonatal hypocalcemia or hypomagnesemia), or from resistance to PTH (which may occur as a primary disorder (e.g., pseudohypoparathyroidism or secondary to hypomagnesemia) (see Table 245-6). In addition, hypoparathyroidism may occur as an inherited syndromic disorder (see Table 245-1) that may either be part of a complex congenital defect (e.g., DiGeorge syndrome) or part of a polyglandular autoimmune disorder (see Table 245-6 and Fig. 245-2). Hypoparathyroidism may also occur as a nonsyndromic solitary endocrinopathy, which has been referred to as isolated or idiopathic hypoparathyroidism. Familial occurrences of isolated hypoparathyroidism with autosomal dominant, autosomal recessive, and X-linked recessive inheritances have been established.

Isolated Hypoparathyroidism

Isolated hypoparathyroidism may either be inherited or acquired by damage to the parathyroids at surgery, by infiltrating metastases, or by systemic disease (see Table 245-6).

ACQUIRED FORMS OF HYPOPARATHYROIDISM

Hypoparathyroidism may occur after neck surgery, after irradiation, or because of infiltration by metastases or systemic disease, for example, hemochromatosis, amyloidosis, sarcoidosis, Wilson's disease, or thalassemia (see Table 245-6). Surgical damage to the parathyroids occurs most commonly after a radical neck dissection, such as for laryngeal or esophageal carcinoma treatment, after a total thyroid resection, or after repeated parathyroidectomies for polyglandular disease (e.g., in MEN 1 or MEN 2, discussed previously). Hypocalcemic symptoms begin 12 to 24 hours after surgery and may need treatment with oral or intravenous calcium. Parathyroid function often returns, but persistent hypocalcemia requires treatment with vitamin D preparations.

Neonatal hypoparathyroidism resulting in hypocalcemia may occur in the infant of a mother with hypercalcemia caused by primary hyperparathyroidism (see Table 245-6). Maternal hypercalcemia results in increased calcium delivery to the fetus, and this fetal hypercalcemia suppresses fetal PTH secretion. Postpartum, the infant's suppressed parathyroids are unable to maintain normocalcemia. The disorder is usually self-limited, but occasionally therapy may be required. In addition, the feeding of cow's milk, which has a high phosphate content, to infants may result in hypocalcemia in some children.

Functional hypoparathyroidism may result from severe hypomagnesemia (<0.4 mmol/L), which may be due to a severe intestinal malabsorption disorder (e.g., Crohn's disease) or a renal tubular disorder (see Table 245-6). It is associated with hypoparathyroidism because magnesium is required for the release of PTH from the parathyroid gland and also for PTH action through adenyl cyclase. Magnesium chloride, 35 to 50 mmol intravenously in 1 liter of 5% glucose or other isotonic solution given over 12 to 24 hours, may be repeatedly required to restore normomagnesemia.

INHERITED HYPOPARATHYROIDISM

Patients with inherited forms of hypoparathyroidism may develop hypocalcemic seizures in the neonatal or infantile periods and require lifelong treatment with oral vitamin D preparations, such as calcitriol. Autosomal dominant, autosomal recessive, and X-linked recessive inheritances for hypoparathyroidism have been observed (see Table 245-1). Some of the autosomal forms are due to mutations of the *PTH* gene, the CaSR (see later), the Gα11 subunit (see later), and the transcriptional factor *GCMB* (glial cells missing B). The X-linked forms likely alter regulation of SOX3 (see Fig. 245-4).

Autosomal Dominant Hypocalcemia Type 1 and Type 2

Autosomal dominant hypocalcemia type 1 (ADH1) is characterized by lifelong mild or severe hypocalcemia in association with normal serum PTH concentrations in about 40% of patients or low serum PTH concentrations in about 60% of patients. Serum phosphate and magnesium concentrations may be elevated or low, respectively. Approximately 50% of ADH1 patients have asymptomatic hypocalcemia, and the remaining 50% may experience paresthesia, muscle cramps, carpopedal spasms, and seizures, which may be associated with a febrile illness. In addition, about 10% of ADH1 patients may have absolute hypercalciuria, which may be associated with nephrocalcinosis and kidney stones in 35% of patients. Vitamin D preparations and calcium supplementation to correct the hypocalcemia may worsen the hypercalciuria and lead to renal impairment. Basal ganglia or ectopic calcification may be found in more than 35% of patients. About 20% of ADH1 patients do not have a previously reported family history because they have de novo mutations. ADH1 is due to gain-of-function mutations of the CaSR (see Table 245-1 and Fig. 245-2). ADH2 is due to gain-of-function mutations of the Gα11 subunit, and ADH2 patients appear to have clinical features that are similar to those in ADH1 patients.

Complex Syndromes Associated with Hypoparathyroidism

Hypoparathyroidism may occur as part of a complex syndrome that may be associated with either a congenital developmental anomaly or an autoimmune syndrome. The congenital developmental anomalies associated with hypoparathyroidism, which occurs in 1 in 4000 live births, include DiGeorge syndrome, hypoparathyroidism, deafness, and renal anomalies (HDR) syndrome, Kenney-Caffey and Barakat syndromes, and also syndromes associated with either lymphedema or dysmorphic features and growth failure (see Table 245-1 and Fig. 245-2).

POLYGLANDULAR AUTOIMMUNE HYPOPARATHYROIDISM

Polyglandular autoimmune hypoparathyroidism comprises hypoparathyroidism, Addison's disease, candidiasis, and two or three of the following: type 1 diabetes mellitus, primary hypogonadism, autoimmune thyroid disease, pernicious anemia, chronic active hepatitis, steatorrhoea (malabsorption), alopecia (totalis or areata), and vitiligo. The disorder has also been referred to as either the autoimmune polyendocrinopathy candidiasis ectodermal dystrophy (APECED) syndrome or the polyglandular autoimmune type 1 syndrome (see Table 245-1). Antibodies directed against the adrenal, thyroid, and parathyroid glands are detected in the sera of some patients. The polyglandular autoimmune type 2 syndrome is characterized by adrenal insufficiency, type 1 diabetes mellitus, and thyroid disease and does not involve hypoparathyroidism. APECED, which has an autosomal recessive inheritance, has a high incidence in Finland and among Iranian Jews. The *APECED* gene, which has been located to chromosome 21q22.3, encodes a 545–amino acid protein that contains motifs associated with a transcriptional factor and includes two zinc-finger motifs, a proline-rich region, and three LXXLL motifs. The gene is referred to as *AIRE* (autoimmune regulator) (see Fig. 245-2). Four *AIRE* mutations are commonly found in APECED families, and these likely abolish the E3 ubiquitin ligase activity of the AIRE1 protein. AIRE1 has been shown to regulate the elimination of organ-specific T cells in the thymus, and APECED is likely to be caused by a failure of this specialized mechanism for deleting forbidden T cells and establishing immunologic tolerance.

AUTOIMMUNE ACQUIRED HYPOPARATHYROIDISM

Twenty percent of patients who had acquired hypoparathyroidism (AH) in association with autoimmune hypothyroidism were found to have autoantibodies to the extracellular domain of the CaSR (see Table 245-1 and Fig. 245-2). The CaSR autoantibodies did not persist for long; 72% of patients who had AH for less than 5 years had detectable CaSR autoantibodies, whereas only 14% of patients with AH for more than 5 years had such autoantibodies. The majority of the patients who had CaSR autoantibodies were female, a finding that is similar to that found in other autoantibody-mediated diseases. Indeed, a few acquired hypoparathyroidism patients have also had features of autoimmune polyglandular syndrome type 1. The epitopes for the anti-CaSR antibodies were localized to the N terminal of the extracellular domain of the receptor. These findings establish that the CaSR is an autoantigen in acquired hypoparathyroidism.

DIGEORGE SYNDROME

Patients with the DiGeorge syndrome suffer from neonatal hypoparathyroidism, T-cell immunodeficiency, congenital heart defects, and deformities of the ear, nose, and mouth (e.g., cleft lip and/or palate). Children with DiGeorge syndrome often die from infections related to the immunodeficiency. The disorder arises from a congenital failure in the development of the derivatives of the third and fourth pharyngeal pouches with resulting absence or hypoplasia of the parathyroids and thymus. Most cases are sporadic, but an autosomal dominant inheritance of DiGeorge syndrome has been observed, and an association between the syndrome and an unbalanced translocation and deletions involving chromosome 22q11.2 has also been reported (see Table 245-1). In some patients, deletions of another locus on chromosome 10p13-p14 have been observed in association with DiGeorge syndrome, and this is referred to as DGS2, whereas patients with the 22q11.2 deletions are referred to as having DGS1. Studies of the DGS1 deleted region on chromosome 22q11.2 have revealed four genes (*RNEX40*, *NEX2.2-NEX3*, *UDFIL*, and *TBX1*) to be involved. However, point mutations in DGS1 patients have been detected only in the *TBX1* gene, and *TBX1* is now considered to be the gene causing DGS1 (see Table 245-1 and Fig. 245-2). *TBX1* encodes a DNA-binding transcriptional factor, of the T-BOX family, that is known to have an important role in vertebrate and invertebrate organogenesis and pattern formation. The *TBX1* gene is deleted in approximately 96% of all DGS1 patients, and some of those without deletions have been shown to harbor mutations of *TBX1*.

HYPOPARATHYROIDISM, DEAFNESS, AND RENAL ANOMALIES SYNDROME

HDR syndrome is an autosomal dominant disorder in which patients often have asymptomatic hypocalcemia with undetectable or inappropriately normal serum concentrations of PTH. Bilateral, symmetrical, sensorineural deafness involving all frequencies occurs, and the renal abnormalities consist mainly of bilateral cysts that compress the glomeruli and tubules and lead to renal impairment. Cytogenetic abnormalities involving chromosome 10p14-10pter were identified in HDR patients, and HDR patients have deletions or mutations of the zinc-finger transcription factor *GATA3* (see Table 245-1 and Fig. 245-2).

MITOCHONDRIAL DISORDERS ASSOCIATED WITH HYPOPARATHYROIDISM

Hypoparathyroidism has been reported to occur in three disorders associated with mitochondrial dysfunction: Kearns-Sayre syndrome, MELAS syndrome, and a mitochondrial trifunctional protein deficiency syndrome (MTPDS) (see Table 245-1 and Fig. 245-2). Kearns-Sayre syndrome is characterized by progressive external ophthalmoplegia and pigmentary

TABLE 245-8   CLINICAL, BIOCHEMICAL, AND GENETIC FEATURES OF HYPOPARATHYROID AND PSEUDOHYPOPARATHYROID DISORDERS

		PSEUDOHYPOPARATHYROIDISM				
	HYPOPARATHYROIDISM	PHP 1a	PPHP	PHP 1b	PHP 1c	PHP 2
AHO manifestations	No	Yes	Yes	No	Yes	No
Serum calcium	↓	↓	N	↓	↓	↓
Serum PO₄	↑	↑	N	↑	↑	↑
Serum PTH	↓	↑	N	↑	↑	↑
Response to PTH:						
Urinary cAMP* (Chase-Aurbach test)	↑	↓	↑	↓	↓	↑
Urinary PO₄ (Ellsworth-Howard test)	↑	↓	↑	↓	↓	↓
Gsα activity	N	↓	↓	N	N	N
Inheritance	AD, AR, X	AD	AD	AD	AD	Sporadic
Molecular defect	PTH, CaSR, GATA3, Gcm2, others	GNAS1	GNAS1	GNAS1†	?Adenyl cyclase	?cAMP targets
Other hormonal resistance	No	Yes	No	No	Yes	No

↓ = decreased; ↑ = increased; ? = presumed, but not proved; AD = autosomal dominant; AHO = Albright's hereditary osteodystrophy; AR = autosomal recessive; N = normal; PHP = pseudoparathyroidism; PPHP = pseudopseudoparathyroidism; PTH = parathyroid hormone; X = X-linked.
*Plasma cyclic adenosine monophosphate (cAMP) responses are similar to those of urinary cAMP.
†Involves deletions that are located upstream of GNAS1.

retinopathy before the age of 20 years and is often associated with heart block or cardiomyopathy. MELAS syndrome consists of a childhood onset of mitochondrial encephalopathy, lactic acidosis, and stroke-like episodes. In addition, varying degrees of proximal myopathy can be seen in both conditions. Both Kearns-Sayre and MELAS syndromes have been reported to occur with type 1 diabetes mellitus and hypoparathyroidism, and mitochondrial gene abnormalities have been identified in some patients. Mitochondrial trifunctional protein deficiency is a disorder of fatty acid oxidation that is associated with peripheral neuropathy, pigmentary retinopathy, and acute fatty liver degeneration in pregnant women who carry an affected fetus. Hypoparathyroidism has been observed in one patient with trifunctional protein deficiency.

KENNEY-CAFFEY, SANJAD-SAKATI, AND KIRK-RICHARDSON SYNDROMES

Hypoparathyroidism has been reported to occur in more than 50% of patients with Kenney-Caffey syndrome, which is associated with short stature, osteosclerosis, cortical thickening of the long bones, delayed closure of the anterior fontanel, basal ganglia calcification, nanophthalmos, and hyperopia. Parathyroid tissue could not be found in a detailed postmortem examination of one patient, and this suggests that hypoparathyroidism may be due to an embryologic defect of parathyroid development. In Kirk-Richardson and Sanjad-Sakati syndromes, which are similar, hypoparathyroidism is associated with severe growth failure and dysmorphic features. This has been reported in patients of Middle Eastern origin whose parents were consanguineous, indicating that these are autosomal recessive disorders. Molecular genetic investigations have identified mutations of the tubulin-specific chaperone (*TBCE*), located on chromosome 1q42-q43, to be associated with the Kenney-Caffey type 1 and Sanjad-Sakati syndromes (see Table 245-1 and Fig. 245-2). *TBCE* encodes one of several chaperone proteins required for the proper folding of α-tubulin subunits and the formation of αβ-tubulin heterodimers. Kenney-Caffey type 2 syndrome is due to mutations of a member of the family with sequence similarity 111 of gene (*FAM111A*), located on chromosome 11q12.1.

PSEUDOHYPOPARATHYROIDISM

Patients with pseudohypoparathyroidism (PHP), which may be inherited as an autosomal dominant disorder, are characterized by hypocalcemia and hyperphosphatemia due to PTH resistance rather than PTH deficiency (see Table 245-6). Five variants are recognized on the basis of biochemical and somatic features (Table 245-8), and three of these—PHP type 1a (PHP 1a), PHP type 1b (PHP 1b), and pseudopseudohypoparathyroidism (PPHP)—will be reviewed in further detail. Patients with PHP 1a exhibit PTH resistance (hypocalcemia, hyperphosphatemia, elevated serum PTH, and an absence of an increase in serum and urinary cAMP and urinary phosphate

following intravenous human PTH infusion), together with the features of Albright's hereditary osteodystrophy (AHO), which includes short stature, obesity, subcutaneous calcification, mental retardation, round faces, dental hypoplasia, and brachydactyly (i.e., shortening of the metacarpals, particularly the third, fourth, and fifth). In addition to brachydactyly, other skeletal abnormalities of the long bones and shortening of the metatarsals may occur. Patients with PHP 1b exhibit PTH resistance only and do not have the somatic features of AHO, whereas patients with PPHP exhibit the somatic features of AHO in the absence of PTH resistance. The absence of a normal rise in urinary excretion of cAMP after an infusion of PTH in PHP 1a indicated a defect at some site of the PTH receptor–adenyl cyclase system (see Fig. 245-2). This receptor system is regulated by at least two G proteins, one of which stimulates (Gsα) and another of which inhibits (Giα) the activity of the membrane-bound enzyme that catalyses the formation of the intracellular second messenger cAMP. Patients with PHP 1a may also show resistance to other hormones, such as thyroid-stimulating hormone, follicle-stimulating hormone, and luteinizing hormone, that act through GPCRs. Inactivating mutations of the Gsα gene (referred to as *GNAS1*), which is located on chromosome 20q13.2, have been identified in PHP 1a and PPHP patients (see Table 245-1 and Fig. 245-2). However, *GNAS1* mutations do not fully explain the PHP 1a or PPHP phenotypes, and studies of PHP 1a and PPHP that occurred within the same kindred revealed that the hormonal resistance is parentally imprinted. Thus, PHP 1a occurs in a child only when the mutation is inherited from a mother affected with either PHP 1a or PPHP; and PPHP occurs in a child only when the mutation is inherited from a father affected with either PHP 1a or PPHP. PHP 1b is due to deletions that are located upstream of the *GNAS1* gene. Moreover, in affected individuals, the deletion involved the maternal allele, whereas its occurrence on the paternal allele resulted in unaffected healthy carriers. This is consistent with parental imprinting of the *GNAS1* abnormality causing PHP 1b.

 Grade A References

A1. Peacock M, Bilezikian JP, Bolognese MA, et al. Cinacalcet HCl reduces hypercalcemia in primary hyperparathyroidism across a wide spectrum of disease severity. *J Clin Endocrinol Metab.* 2011;96:E9-E18.

A2. Rolighed L, Rejnmark L, Sikjaer T, et al. Vitamin D treatment in primary hyperparathyroidism: a randomized placebo controlled trial. *J Clin Endocrinol Metab.* 2014;99:1072-1080.

GENERAL REFERENCES

For the General References and other additional features, please visit Expert Consult at https://expertconsult.inkling.com.

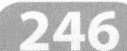

MEDULLARY THYROID CARCINOMA

SAMUEL A. WELLS, JR.

MEDULLARY THYROID CARCINOMA

DEFINITION

Medullary thyroid carcinoma (MTC) is an uncommon cancer that arises from the neural crest—derived C cells of the thyroid gland.

EPIDEMIOLOGY

MTC accounts for 5% of thyroid cancers, and there will be approximately 3000 new cases in the United States in 2015. MTC occurs either sporadically (75% of cases) or as part of the multiple endocrine neoplasia (MEN) syndromes, MEN 2A (Online Mendelian Inheritance in Man [OMIM] #171400) or MEN 2B (OMIM #162300), or the related syndrome familial medullary thyroid carcinoma (FMTC) (OMIM #155240).[1] The incidence of MEN 2A and FMTC combined is approximately 1 in 100,000 live births, whereas the incidence of MEN 2B is approximately 1 in 2,000,000 live births.

PATHOBIOLOGY

As the lateral thyroid complex closes during embryogenesis, the C cells are incorporated within the middle and upper portions of the thyroid lobes. Because of its anatomic location, MTC is classified as a thyroid tumor; however, considering its origin from the neural crest rather than the thyroid follicular cells, it is a neuroendocrine tumor. Sporadic MTC occurs as a solitary tumor in one thyroid lobe, whereas hereditary MTC develops in both thyroid lobes and is multicentric. In patients with hereditary MTC, the first manifestation of a C-cell disorder is C-cell hyperplasia (CCH) that progresses over time to microinvasive MTC and then to invasive MTC.[2]

The C-cell mass is much greater in the thyroid glands of men than in women, which accounts for the higher serum calcitonin levels seen in men compared with women.

The C cells have diverse biosynthetic activity and secrete calcitonin (CTN) and carcinoembryonic antigen (CEA), which are excellent serum markers for the presence of a C-cell disorder. CTN was once thought to be important in calcium homeostasis; however, its physiologic importance has been called into question. The RET protooncogene encodes a single-pass transmembrane receptor of the tyrosine kinase family of proteins. At several stages of development, it is expressed in cells derived from the branchial arches (parathyroids), the neural crest (brain, parasympathetic and sympathetic ganglia, thyroid C cells, adrenal medulla, and enteric ganglia), and the urogenital system. Activating, germline point mutations in RET are present in virtually all hereditary MTCs, and somatic RET mutations are present in approximately half of sporadic MTCs.[3,4] Recently, it was discovered that somatic mutations in HRAS, KRAS, and rarely NRAS are present in sporadic MTCs and are almost always mutually exclusive with the presence of somatic RET mutations.[5]

Approximately 75 RET mutations have been reported in association with MEN 2A, MEN 2B, and FMTC. The mutations for MEN 2A and FMTC are located in exons 5, 8, 10, 11, 13, 14, 15, and 16. The mutations for MEN 2A are mostly located in the extracellular, cysteine-rich region of exon 10 (including codons 609, 611, 618, and 620) and exon 11 (including codons 630 and 634). Approximately 85% of the mutations associated with MEN 2A involve RET codon 634, about half of which are C634R RET mutations. The RET mutations in MEN 2B cause constitutive activation, which alters substrate specificity, presumably owing to a conformational change in the binding pocket of the kinase. Approximately 95% of mutations causing MEN 2B are in codon M918T, and 5% are in codon A883F. Rare cases of MEN 2B are caused by double somatic RET mutations involving codon V804M and either codon Y806C, S904C, or E805K.

In 50% of patients with MEN 2B and 10% of patients with MEN 2A and FMTC, the disease arises de novo. In such founder cases, the de novo mutation almost always derives from the paternal allele.[6]

CLINICAL MANIFESTATIONS

The peak incidence of sporadic MTC is in the fifth decade of life, and most patients present with a solitary thyroid nodule and lymph node metastases. Clinically, the tumors are more aggressive than papillary thyroid carcinoma

TABLE 246-1	CLINICAL MANIFESTATIONS OF MULTIPLE ENDOCRINE NEOPLASIA 2A, 2B, AND FAMILIAL MEDULLARY THYROID CARCINOMA

MULTIPLE ENDOCRINE NEOPLASIA (MEN) 2A

Medullary thyroid carcinoma (~100%)
Pheochromocytoma (incidence of 50% in families with a *RET* codon 634 germline mutation but less in families with other *RET* codon mutations)
Hyperparathyroidism (incidence of 30% in families with a *RET* codon 634 germline mutation but less in families with other *RET* codon mutations.)

VARIANTS OF MEN 2A

MEN 2A with cutaneous lichen amyloidosis (almost always associated with a *RET* codon 634 germline mutation.)
MEN 2A with Hirschsprung disease (most common in families with *RET* germline mutation most commonly involving codon 620)

FAMILIAL MEDULLARY THYROID CARCINOMA (FMTC)

Since the original description of this syndrome, there has been confusion about the designation FMTC. Most clinicians now consider it a variant of MEN 2A.

MEN 2B

Medullary thyroid carcinoma (~100%)
Pheochromocytoma (50%)
Mucosal neuroma, ganglioneuromatosis, marfanoid habitus, colonic abnormalities, characteristic physical appearance (~100%)

and follicular thyroid carcinoma but less aggressive than anaplastic thyroid carcinoma (Chapter 226). The 10-year survival rate is 75%. In the expectation of detecting MTC at any early stage, clinicians in Europe evaluate serum CTN levels in patients with thyroid nodules who have no history of hereditary MTC. The detection rate of MTC is less than 0.5%, however, and clinicians in the United States have not adopted this practice. The clinical manifestations of MEN 2A, MEN 2B, and FMTC are listed in Table 246-1.

MEN 2A (80% of cases), MEN 2B (5% of cases), and FMTC (15% of cases) are inherited as autosomal dominant traits with near-complete penetrance and, in the cases of MEN 2A and MEN 2B, variable expressivity. Approximately 50% of patients with MEN 2A (and a codon 634 mutation) develop pheochromocytomas (Chapters 228 and 231), the frequency being much lower in association with mutations in codons 609, 611, 618, and 620.[7] Before the availability of biochemical and genetic screening in families with MEN 2A, the most frequent cause of death was pheochromocytoma, not MTC. The deaths occurred most often in patients during childbirth or interventional procedures. Thus, pheochromocytoma must be excluded in patients with a confirmed or presumptive diagnosis of hereditary MTC (Chapter 228). With rare exceptions, the pheochromocytoma should be excised first in patients who also have MTC.

Parathyroid hyperplasia occurs in up to 30% of patients with MEN 2A and is usually associated with a *RET* codon 634 mutation. The disease is frequently asymptomatic, with the only abnormality being an elevated serum calcium concentration.[8]

Patients with MEN 2A may also develop cutaneous lichen amyloidosis (CLA) or Hirschsprung disease (HD).[9] CLA occurs in about 25% of patients and involves the interscapular region of the back, corresponding to dermatomes T2 through T6. Pruritus, the dominant symptom, leads to repetitive scratching and secondary skin changes characterized by the deposition of amyloid. The lesion may be evident in infancy, thus serving as a precursor marker of MEN 2A. Cutaneous lichen amyloidosis is almost always associated with a *RET* codon 634 mutation.

HD, manifested by the absence of intrinsic ganglion cells in the distal gastrointestinal tract, has been reported in 30 or more families with MEN 2A or FMTC and is associated with mutations in *RET* exon 10 involving codons 609 (15%), 611 (4%), 618 (30%), and 620 (50%). In functional studies, the cell surface expression of *RET* with these codon mutations is lower than that found with a codon 634 mutation. This suggests a novel mechanism whereby the specified *RET* mutations have low transforming activity, which is sufficient to trigger the development of MTC and pheochromocytoma, yet is insufficient to stimulate differentiation of intestinal ganglion cells. It is also of interest that 50% of patients with familial HD and 30% of patients with sporadic HD have germline *RET* mutations.

Patients with MEN 2B develop mucosal neuromas, ganglioneuromatosis throughout the aerodigestive tract, hypotonia, skeletal malformations, and medullated corneal nerves. They also develop colonic dysfunction manifested by abdominal pain and occasionally intestinal obstruction. Patients have a characteristic physical appearance, which may not be evident early in life. The failure to diagnose MEN 2B at a young age can be catastrophic because MTC is often evident soon after birth, and regional or distant metastases occur soon thereafter. The MTC associated with MEN 2B is much more aggressive than that occurring with MEN 2A or FMTC. The primary basis for the difference is that MEN 2B mutations are associated with significantly higher basal kinase activity compared with mutations in MEN 2A and FMTC. Patients with FMTC develop only MTC, which, relative to the tumors in patients with MEN 2A and MEN 2B, is slow growing. Many clinicians consider FMTC a variant of MEN 2A.

DIAGNOSIS

The measurement of serum levels of CTN, either in the basal state or following the intravenous administration of the secretagogues calcium, pentagastrin, or both, was initially the primary method of establishing the diagnosis of a C-cell disorder. With the discovery that MEN 2A, MEN 2B, and FMTC are caused by mutations in the *RET* protooncogene, direct DNA analysis became the method of choice for identifying affected family members who had inherited a mutated *RET* allele. At present, the determination of CTN is primarily used to detect persistent or recurrent MTC following thyroidectomy or to evaluate response to therapy in patients with regional or metastatic disease. As we have learned more about the variable clinical expression of MEN 2A in families with the identical *RET* mutation, however, the measurement of basal and stimulated serum CTN levels has assumed importance in timing early thyroidectomy in young family members with *RET* mutations.[10] The two-site, two-step, chemiluminescent, immunometric assay that is highly specific for monomeric CTN is the preferred method for quantitating serum CTN levels.

At present, direct DNA analysis of RET has become the preferred method of detecting *RET* mutations in families with hereditary MTC. The Gene Tests directory currently lists 63 laboratories that perform DNA analysis for *RET* mutations (http://www.genetests.org). Almost all laboratories use direct sequence analysis to evaluate mutations in exons 10, 11, 13, 14, 15, and 16, and some laboratories include exon 8. If no mutations are found in these exons, the entire coding region of *RET* can be sequenced. It is important to perform direct DNA analysis for *RET* mutations in all patients with presumed sporadic MTC because approximately 7% of them will have hereditary MTC. A diagnosis of hereditary MTC in this setting mandates a different treatment strategy for the patient, as well as his family members, who should be offered the opportunity for clinical evaluation and genetic testing.

TREATMENT Rx

The primary treatment for patients with MTC, whether sporadic or hereditary, is total thyroidectomy. Resection of lymph nodes in the central compartment is included in all adults and in children with MEN 2B but is excluded in outwardly normal youngsters with MEN 2A and FMTC who are undergoing early thyroidectomy based on directed DNA analysis. If enlarged cervical lymph nodes are evident on preoperative ultrasound examination or at the time of thyroidectomy, the involved anatomic nodal compartment should also be resected. During the thyroidectomy, great care must be taken to preserve the parathyroid glands, the recurrent laryngeal nerves, and the external branch of the superior laryngeal nerve. Postoperatively, serum calcitonin is normal in only 10% of patients with node-positive disease compared with 60% of patients with node-negative disease. Many patients with regional lymph node metastases have a good prognosis, however, with 5- and 10-year survival rates of 80 and 70%, respectively.

Repeat neck operation following initial thyroidectomy is indicated in patients with complications from recurrent tumor compressing or invading vital structures, such as the spinal cord, airway, or esophagus. Also, patients who have intractable diarrhea due to markedly elevated tumor hormone secretions, presumably CTN, may obtain symptom relief by tumor debulking. Patients who develop persistent or recurrent MTC following thyroidectomy, as indicated by elevated serum levels of CTN or CEA, are also candidates for reoperation; however, the benefit of such surgical procedures is open to question because there are no long-term data on quality of life and survival. Rarely, patients with MTC develop Cushing syndrome (Chapter 227) due to the inappropriate secretion of adrenocorticotrophic hormone (ACTH) or corticotropin-releasing hormone. Such patients have advanced disease, and bilateral adrenalectomy may be required if steroidogenesis inhibitors are ineffective. Inappropriate secretion of ACTH is a poor prognostic sign, associated with an average survival of 2 years.

The treatment of pheochromocytoma is adrenalectomy, as described in Chapter 228. Hyperparathyroidism (Chapter 245) is managed by either subtotal parathyroidectomy or total parathyroidectomy with heterotopic autotransplantation.

For patients with locally advanced or metastatic MTC, single-agent or combined chemotherapeutic regimens have been minimally effective, being characterized by low response rates of short duration. External beam radiotherapy is indicated primarily for the treatment of localized metastases, primarily of the central nervous system or bone.

With the demonstration that the tyrosine kinase inhibitor imatinib induced remissions in patients with chronic myelogenous leukemia and gastrointestinal stromal tumors, there was hope that similar molecular targeted therapeutics (MTTs) would be developed for other solid tumors, including MTC. In a recent prospective, randomized, placebo-controlled, double-blind, phase III trial, patients treated with the MTT vandetanib had a significantly prolonged progression-free survival compared with placebo.[A1] On the basis of this study, the U.S. Food and Drug Administration (FDA) approved vandetanib for the treatment of patients with advanced MTC.[11] The FDA also recently approved a second MTT, cabozantinib,[12] based on similar results of a phase III trial.[A2] Thus, effective systemic therapies are available for patients with advanced MTC, and additional studies of other MTTs have recently been initiated.

PREVENTION

In patients with a hereditary cancer syndrome, the removal of an organ destined to become malignant should be considered in the light of five factors. There should be (1) near-complete penetrance of the mutated gene, (2) a reliable method of detecting family members who have inherited a mutated allele, (3) minimal morbidity associated with removal of the organ at risk, (4) excellent replacement therapy for the function of the removed organ, and (5) a reliable method for determining whether the operative procedure has been curative. Few hereditary malignancies meet all of these criteria; fortunately, MEN 2A, MEN 2B, and FMTC meet each of them. Young members of kindred with hereditary MTC who are found to have a mutated *RET* allele on genetic screening have the greatest likelihood of being cured by early thyroidectomy. Surgeons in several countries have reported success with this operative procedure, and the question is no longer should it be done but at what age.

The Consensus Committee of the 7th International Workshop on MEN, the National Comprehensive Cancer Network, and the American Thyroid Association have all proposed guidelines for the timing of prophylactic thyroidectomy in patients with MEN 2A, MEN 2B, and FMTC[13]. The recommendations of the three groups are similar, in that children with MEN 2B (or with mutations in codons 918 or 882) should have thyroidectomy at the time of diagnosis, even during the first months of life. Children with MEN 2A and mutations in codons 611, 618, 620, or 634 should have the thyroid removed at or before 5 years of age. In children with mutations in other *RET* codons, the recommended timing of thyroidectomy is less clear but is generally between 5 and 10 years of age.

PROGNOSIS

Several factors portend an adverse outcome in patients with MTC.[14] Poor prognosis is associated with older age, advanced disease at the time of diagnosis of a large primary tumor, lymph node metastases, markedly elevated serum levels of CTN and CEA preoperatively, extrathyroidal invasion of the trachea or soft tissues, and distant metastases. Patients with MEN 2B and patients with MEN 2A who have *RET* mutations in codon 634 have a poorer prognosis than those with *RET* mutations in other codons. Also, in patients with sporadic MTC, the presence of a *RET M918T* mutation, compared with other codon mutations, is associated with a more aggressive tumor and a poor prognosis. Patients apparently cured by thyroidectomy are followed at 6-month intervals with measurement of serum levels of CTN and CEA. The doubling times of serum CTN are especially useful in predicting the course of the disease. CTN doubling times of less than 6 months (compared with those greater than 24 months) are associated with a very poor prognosis.

Grade A References

A1. Wells SA Jr, Robinson BG, Gagel RF, et al. Vandetanib in patients with locally advanced or metastatic medullary thyroid cancer: a randomized, double-blind phase III trial. *J Clin Oncol.* 2012;30:134-141.

A2. Elisei R, Schlumberger MJ, Müller SP, et al. Cabozantinib in progressive medullary thyroid cancer. *J Clin Oncol.* 2013;31:3639-3646.

GENERAL REFERENCES

For the General References and other additional features, please visit Expert Consult at https://expertconsult.inkling.com.

247

PAGET DISEASE OF BONE

STUART H. RALSTON

DEFINITION

Paget disease of bone is a disorder of skeleton characterized by increased and disorganized bone remodeling affecting one or more skeletal sites. Affected bones enlarge, become deformed, and are at increased risk for pathologic fractures

EPIDEMIOLOGY

The population prevalence of Paget disease is about 1% in the United States and 2% in the United Kingdom. It is also common in Western Europe and in people of European descent who have migrated to other parts of the world. Paget disease is rare in Scandinavians, Africans, and Asians. These differences are thought to have a genetic basis and to be caused by founder mutations that occurred in Europeans many centuries ago with subsequent spread to the rest of the world through emigration. Paget disease is strongly related to age; in the United Kingdom, the incidence is 0.3 to 0.5 per 10,000 person years in those aged 55 to 59 years but doubles in frequency each decade thereafter to reach an incidence of 5.4 per 10,000 person years in women and 7.6 per 10,000 person years in men in those 85 years and older. The prevalence and severity of Paget disease have diminished in most countries over the past 25 years.[1] The causes are unclear, but suggested explanations include influx of migrants from low prevalence areas in some populations, improved nutrition, a more sedentary lifestyle with a reduction in skeletal injuries, and reduced exposure to infections.[2]

PATHOBIOLOGY

Susceptibility to Paget disease seems to be genetically determined, but environmental factors also play a key role in regulating onset and severity of the disease. The importance of genetics is emphasized by the fact that between 15 and 40% of patients have a positive family history and that the risk for developing Paget disease in a first-degree relative of a patient is about seven-fold higher than in the general population.[3] In many families, the disease is transmitted in an autosomal dominant manner, although penetrance is incomplete. The most important susceptibility gene for classical Paget disease is *SQSTM1*. Mutations of *SQSTM1* are present in up to 40% of patients with a family history and 5 to 10% of people with sporadic disease. The *SQSTM1* gene encodes a protein called p62 that is involved in regulating signal transduction downstream of the receptor activator of nuclear factor κB (RANK), which plays a critical role in regulating osteoclastogenesis when activated by RANK ligand (RANKL) (Fig. 247-1). The disease-causing mutations cluster in the ubiquitin-associated domain and have the effect of upregulating nuclear factor κB (NFκB) signaling and stimulating osteoclastogenesis by complex mechanisms that are reviewed in detail elsewhere. Genome-wide association

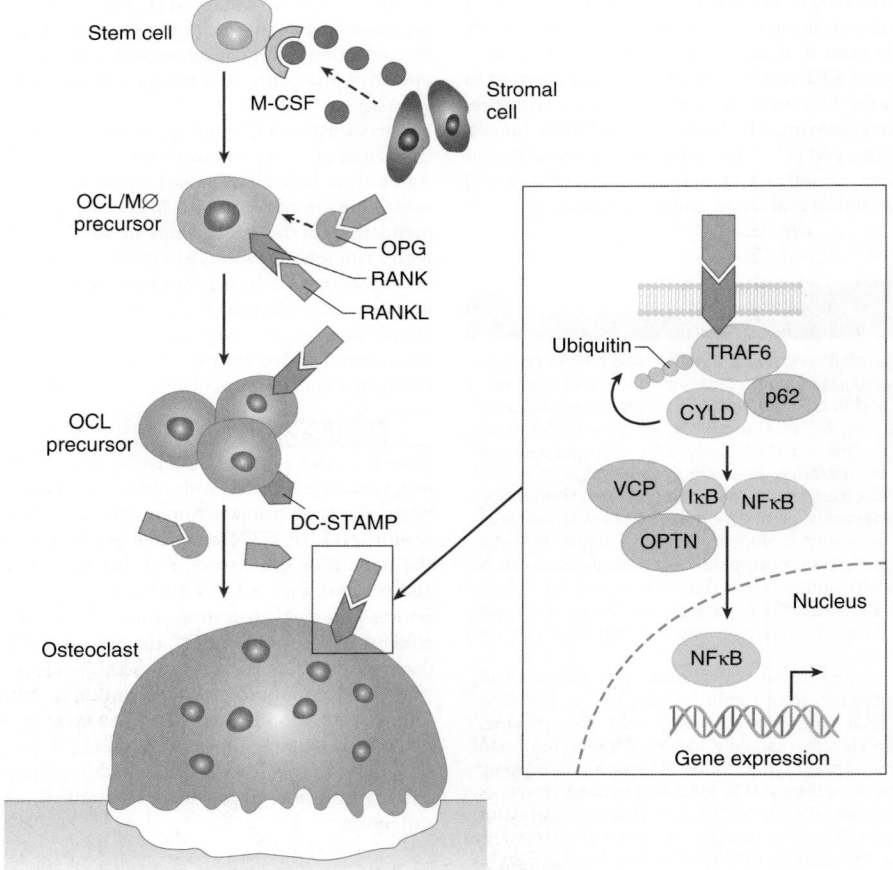

FIGURE 247-1. Regulators of osteoclast dysfunction in Paget disease. Some of the key molecules that have been implicated in the pathogenesis of Paget disease are illustrated. Macrophage colony-stimulating factor (M-CSF) encoded by *CSF1* is required for differentiation of stem cells to the osteoclast/macrophage (OCL/MØ) lineage. Osteoclast differentiation and activity are enhanced when RANK (encoded by *TNFRSF11A*) is activated by RANKL but inhibited by OPG (encoded by *TNFRSF11B*). Fusion of osteoclast precursors to form mature osteoclasts requires DC-STAMP (encoded by *TM7SF4*). Within the cell *(inset)*, p62 (encoded by *SQSTM1*) is required for signal transduction downstream of the RANK receptor and is also involved in regulating autophagy. Both VCP (encoded by *VCP*) and OPTN (encoded by *OPTN*) also play a role in regulating NFκB signaling and autophagy.

TABLE 247-1 GENES THAT PREDISPOSE TO PAGET DISEASE–LIKE SYNDROMES

SYNDROME	GENE (PROTEIN)	GENE FUNCTION	INHERITANCE/MUTATION	CLINICAL FEATURES
Familial expansile osteolysis Early-onset familial Paget disease of bone Expansile skeletal hyperplasia	*TNFRSF11A* (RANK)	Enhances osteoclast differentiation and bone resorption	Autosomal dominant Insertion mutations exon 1	Onset during adolescence, extensive bone lesions, deafness, tooth loss.
Juvenile Paget disease	*TNFRSF11B* (OPG)	Inhibits osteoclast differentiation and bone resorption	Autosomal recessive Various loss of function mutations	Onset during childhood, extensive bone lesions, deafness, fractures, deformity, premature cardiovascular disease
Inclusion body myopathy, Paget disease, and frontotemporal dementia	*VCP* (p97)	Multiple cellular functions, including roles in NFκB signaling and autophagy	Autosomal dominant Loss of function mutations in UBA domain	Onset during 3rd-4th decades, with myopathy, Paget disease, and dementia occurring during 5th-6th decades

studies have identified seven other loci that predispose to Paget disease, which individually increase the risk between 1.4 and 1.7 fold.[4,5] These loci have additive effects such that individuals who carry several predisposing alleles have a substantially increased risk for developing Paget disease. Many of these loci lie close to genes that play key roles in osteoclast function, including *CSF1*, which encodes macrophage colony-stimulating factor (M-CSF); *TNFRSF11A*, which encodes RANK; *TM7SF4*, which encodes DC-STAMP; and *OPTN*, which encodes optineurin (see Fig. 247-1). Several inherited diseases with clinical features overlapping with those of Paget disease have also been described (Table 247-1). These syndromes are also caused by mutations in genes that regulate osteoclast function.

Under normal circumstances, bone is renewed and repaired in an orderly and tightly regulated fashion through the process of bone remodeling. The bone remodeling process is highly abnormal in Paget disease. Osteoclasts are increased in number, larger than normal, and hypernucleated. Some contain nuclear inclusion bodies. These were originally thought to be paramyxovirus nucleocapsids, but it has been suggested more recently that they may be aggregates of un-degraded proteins caused by defects in the autophagy pathway. Bone formation is also markedly increased, but the amount of new bone that is formed greatly exceeds that which has been removed by osteoclast activity, leading to enlargement and deformity of affected bones (Fig. 247-2). The bone that is formed is laid down in a disorganized fashion (woven bone) and has impaired mechanical strength. Other features include increased vascularity and marrow fibrosis. The focal nature of Paget disease remains a puzzle. Suggested explanations include the occurrence of somatic mutations in affected bones, which locally increase osteoclast activity, or excessive mechanical loading or skeletal injuries early in life, which by causing microdamage act as a focus for localized increases in bone remodeling.

CLINICAL MANIFESTATIONS

It has been estimated that between 7 and 16% of patients with Paget disease come to medical attention, and the presentation is highly variable.[6] Many patients are asymptomatic, and Paget disease is detected as the result of a raised serum alkaline phosphatase (ALP) or an abnormal radiograph in patients who are being investigated for another reason. In those that do present clinically, symptoms that are attributable to Paget disease are observed in about 75% of cases. The most common is pain, which can be due to either increased bone turnover or a complication such as osteoarthritis, spinal stenosis, pseudofractures, or nerve compression syndromes. Deafness may occur in patients with skull involvement, but this is usually conductive rather than due to auditory nerve compression. Osteosarcoma occurs in less than 0.5% of cases but should be suspected in patients who experience a sudden increase in bone pain or swelling of an affected site. Other, rare complications include obstructive hydrocephalus, high-output cardiac failure, and hypercalcemia in patients who are immobilized. The risk for cardiovascular disease is increased in patients with Paget disease compared with age- and gender-matched controls, probably owing to an increased prevalence of vascular calcification. Most patients have no clinical signs but some present with bone deformity (see Fig. 247-2) or warmth of the skin overlying an affected bone.

DIAGNOSIS

The diagnosis can usually be made by radiograph, which shows the typical features of focal osteolysis with coarsening of the trabecular pattern, bone expansion, and cortical thickening (see Fig. 247-2). Occasionally, the disease

may be predominantly lytic in nature (see Fig. 247-2). The most sensitive way of defining the extent of Paget disease is a radionuclide bone scan in which tracer uptake is intensely increased at affected sites (see Fig. 247-2). Imaging with magnetic resonance imaging and computed tomography is not usually required unless complications such as spinal stenosis or osteosarcoma are suspected. Laboratory testing should include assessment of renal function, calcium, albumin, alkaline phosphatase (ALP), and 25(OH)D levels; liver function should be assessed to rule out the possibility that elevations in ALP are of hepatic origin. Typically, Paget disease presents with an elevation in ALP with otherwise normal biochemistries, but normal levels of ALP do not exclude the diagnosis. Vitamin D deficiency is a common finding but most likely reflects the fact that Paget disease predominantly affects older people in whom vitamin D deficiency is prevalent. Specialized markers such as bone-specific ALP or procollagen type 1 N-terminal propeptide can be useful in patients with coexisting liver disease but otherwise offer no advantage over total ALP in diagnosis and assessing treatment response. Susceptibility to Paget disease can be assessed in relatives of affected patients by genetic testing for *SQSTM1* mutations, although this is not commonly performed in routine clinical practice.

The differential diagnosis includes hyperostosis frontalis interna (a benign condition characterized by osteosclerosis of the frontal bones of the skull), fibrous dysplasia, pustulotic arthro-osteitis (which can present with mixed osteosclerotic and osteolytic lesions of the clavicle and ribs),[7] and osteosclerotic metastases, particularly from carcinoma of the prostate. Usually, Paget disease can be distinguished from these conditions biochemically and through imaging, but occasionally, biopsy of an affected site may be required.

Treatment

The most common indication for medical treatment of Paget disease is bone pain localized to an affected site.[8] Although such pain may be caused by increased metabolic activity, other causes may also be operative, including nerve compression syndromes, pseudofractures, secondary osteoarthritis, and other musculoskeletal conditions. Careful assessment of the patient is therefore necessary to decide on the most appropriate treatment. Bone pain caused by increased metabolic activity is localized to the affected site and is usually accompanied by a raised ALP level. It is common to encounter patients in whom pain occurs in the presence of coexisting osteoarthritis, bone deformity, or other musculoskeletal conditions. In such cases, it can be difficult to be sure about the origin of the pain, and many clinicians give a therapeutic trial of bisphosphonates. If the pain responds, then one can assume it was due to increased metabolic activity; if it does not, further evaluation should be undertaken to identify the cause and treat the patient appropriately. Pseudofractures represent a distinct management problem. These are areas of focal osteolysis that traverse the lateral cortex of weight-bearing bones of the lower limbs. Some remain stable for prolonged periods without causing symptoms; others regress spontaneously; and others progress to pathologic fracture, often in association with a localized increase in pain at the affected site.[9]

Bisphosphonates

Bisphosphonates are the drugs of first choice for the treatment of pain that is thought to be due to increased metabolic activity. Nowadays, nitrogen-containing bisphosphonates (aminobisphosphonates) are used in preference to older bisphosphonates because of their greater potency (Table 247-2).

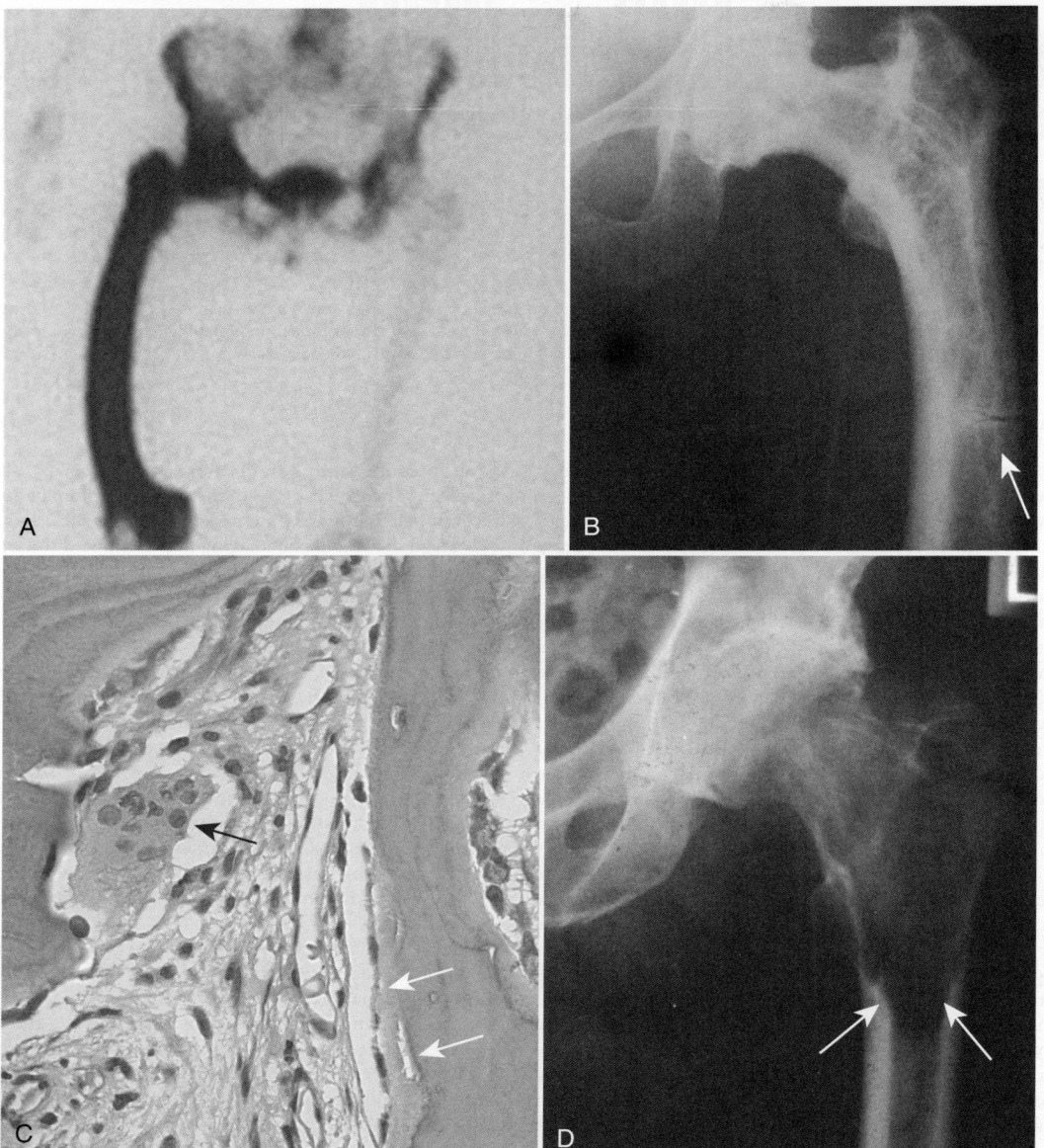

FIGURE 247-2. Radiographic and histologic features of Paget disease. **A,** Radionuclide bone scan image showing intense tracer uptake, typical of Paget disease of bone (PDB) in the right femur. **B,** Radiograph of an affected left femur showing bone expansion with mixed osteolytic/osteosclerotic areas and loss of normal trabecular pattern. A pseudofracture is visible in the lateral cortex *(arrow)*. **C,** Histologic features from a hematoxylin and eosin stained section. A large osteoclast is visible *(black arrow)* close to an area of new bone formation *(white arrows)*. There is extensive marrow fibrosis. Irregular cement lines typical of woven bone are apparent to the right of section. **D,** Predominantly lytic Paget disease of the left femur. The lytic area involves the intertrochanteric region and extends down the femoral shaft *(white arrows)*.

Placebo controlled trials have shown that most bisphosphonates are effective at improving bone pain in Paget disease. Superiority of aminobisphosphonates over etidronate and tiludronate at suppressing ALP levels has been demonstrated, but with little difference in the response of pain. There are limited data comparing different aminobisphosphonates. In an open-label study comparing pamidronate 180 mg intravenously in unit doses of 30 mg weekly or 60 mg alternate weeks to oral alendronate 40 mg daily given in 3-monthly blocks over a 2-year period, there were no significant differences in the proportion of patients who achieved normal levels of ALP (86 and 91% respectively) or in symptomatic response.[A1] Another study that compared a single infusion of 5 mg zoledronic acid with oral risedronate 30 mg daily for 2 months showed significant superiority of zoledronic acid in lowering ALP. Those randomized to zoledronic acid had greater improvement in some domains of health-related quality of life, but the differences between groups were small (1 to 2 points) and below the threshold of 5 points, which is considered clinically significant.[A2] Another randomized trial compared the effects of giving repeated course of bisphosphonates (mainly risedronate) with the aim of normalizing ALP (intensive treatment), with therapy primarily aimed at

controlling symptoms (symptomatic therapy) in Paget disease.[A3] This showed no difference in response of pain, quality of life, or complications between the groups, indicating that trying to restore ALP to normal confers no clinical advantage in most patients with Paget disease.

After initiation of bisphosphonate therapy, levels of ALP start to fall within about 10 days and reach a nadir between 3 and 6 months. Levels of ALP can remain suppressed for many months or years thereafter, particularly with zoledronic acid. Symptoms can improve while ALP levels are still falling, and good clinical responses are often observed in patients whose ALP levels are not restored to normal.

Intravenous bisphosphonates can cause transient bone pain, myalgia, headache, nausea, pyrexia, and fatigue within 1 to 3 days of the infusion in about 25% of cases (acute phase response). These symptoms can be ameliorated by acetaminophen given before and for a few days after the infusion, but they almost always subside within 7 days even without treatment. The acute phase response is much less common after second and subsequent infusions. Hypocalcemia may occur, particularly in patients with substantial elevations in bone turnover and vitamin D deficiency. The risk can be

TABLE 247-2	BISPHOSPHONATES USED IN THE TREATMENT OF PAGET DISEASE	
DRUG	**DOSE**	**COMMON ADVERSE EFFECTS**
Oral		
Etidronate*	400 mg/day orally for 3-6 mo	Diarrhea, nausea, abdominal pain
Tiludronate	400 mg/day orally for 3 mo	Diarrhea, nausea, dyspepsia
Risedronate	30 mg/day orally for 2 mo	Dyspepsia, esophagitis
Alendronic acid†	40 mg/day orally for 6 mo	Dyspepsia, esophagitis
Intravenous		
Pamidronate	180 mg IV in unit doses of 30 mg weekly or 60 mg alternate weeks	Acute phase response, hypocalcemia
Zoledronic acid	5 mg IV	Acute phase response, hypocalcemia

*Now seldom used.
†Not licensed in the United Kingdom or Europe for Paget disease. Etidronate, pamidronate, tiludronate, and risedronate should be avoided if estimated glomerular filtration rate (eGFR) <30; zoledronic acid and alendronic acid should be avoided if eGFR <35.

minimized by correcting vitamin D deficiency before treatment and providing calcium and vitamin D supplements for the first 1 or 2 weeks after the infusion.

Patients taking oral bisphosphonates must fast for 30 minutes (risedronate, alendronate) or 120 minutes (etidronate, tiludronate) before and after dosing to achieve adequate absorption. The most common adverse effects are dyspepsia (risedronate and alendronic acid) and diarrhea (tiludronate and etidronate). Other rare side effects of bisphosphonates include uveitis, skin rashes, atrial fibrillation, and osteonecrosis of the jaw, as well as atypical subtrochanteric fractures. Bisphosphonates can cause kidney injury and are contraindicated in patients with significant renal impairment.

Other Drug Treatments

Analgesics, anti-inflammatory drugs, and antineuropathic agents are often required in patients with Paget disease, particularly when there is coexisting osteoarthritis or a nerve compression syndrome. Calcitonin can improve bone pain due to metabolic activity in Paget disease but is seldom used except in patients for whom bisphosphonates are contraindicated. Adverse effects such as nausea and flushing can be problematic, and resistance may develop owing to the formation of neutralizing antibodies. Anecdotal reports suggest that the osteoclast inhibitor denosumab may also be effective at reducing ALP levels in Paget disease of bone, but it is not licensed for this indication.

Nonpharmacologic Treatments

Nonpharmacologic approaches (acupuncture, physiotherapy, hydrotherapy, and transcutaneous electrical nerve stimulation) are often used to control pain, but their effectiveness has not been specifically investigated in controlled trials. Clinical experience suggests that specific problems such as limb shortening and deformity can be helped by aids and devices such as walking sticks and shoe raises.

Monitoring Disease Activity and the Effects of Treatment

Metabolic activity and the response to treatment is typically assessed by measuring ALP, although levels can be normal in patients with localized disease that is metabolically active. Further courses of treatment should be considered in patients with recurrent or persistent pain in whom ALP levels remain or become elevated.

Surgery

Orthopedic surgery may be required for the management of coexisting osteoarthritis, pseudofractures, fractures, bone deformity, and spinal stenosis. Osteotomy is performed infrequently, but analyses of small cases series have reported good results in about 60% of patients. Surgery is much more frequently required to repair fractures and to replace joints that are affected by osteoarthritis. Surgical treatment of Paget disease can be technically challenging because of deformity, osteosclerosis, and increased vascularity, but evidence from case series indicate that fractures through pagetic bone heal normally and that joint replacement surgery has a good outcome. It has been suggested that a bisphosphonate should be given before orthopedic and spinal surgery with the aim of reducing operative blood loss, but the effectiveness of this has not been studied. There is a theoretical concern that previous bisphosphonate therapy might impair fracture union and bone repair, but there is little evidence to suggest that this is a problem in clinical practice.[10] Orthopedic surgery may also be required in patients who develop osteosarcoma, but the prognosis is poor even with aggressive operative treatment.

The prognosis of Paget disease is highly variable. Some patients remain completely asymptomatic throughout life, but those that present clinically frequently have complications and have a significant reduction in quality of life. [A3] Although modern bisphosphonates are highly effective at suppressing bone turnover in Paget disease,[11] they have not as yet been shown to alter the natural history of the disease or prevent complications. Disease severity and extent can be predicted by genotyping for *SQSTM1* mutations and other risk alleles, and studies are currently in progress to determine whether genetic testing can be combined with prophylactic bisphosphonate therapy to prevent or delay the onset of disease.

 Grade A References

A1. Walsh JP, Ward LC, Stewart GO, et al. A randomized clinical trial comparing oral alendronate and intravenous pamidronate for the treatment of Paget disease of bone. *Bone.* 2004;34:747-754.
A2. Reid IR, Miller P, Lyles K. Comparison of a single infusion of zoledronic acid with risedronate for Paget disease. *N Engl J Med.* 2005;353:898-908.
A3. Langston AL, Campbell MK, Fraser WD, et al. Randomised trial of intensive bisphosphonate treatment versus symptomatic management in Paget disease of bone. *J Bone Miner Res.* 2010;25:20-31.

GENERAL REFERENCES

For the General References and other additional features, please visit Expert Consult at https://expertconsult.inkling.com.

248

OSTEONECROSIS, OSTEOSCLEROSIS/HYPEROSTOSIS, AND OTHER DISORDERS OF BONE

MICHAEL P. WHYTE

OSTEONECROSIS

DEFINITION

Osteonecrosis (aseptic, avascular, or ischemic necrosis of bone) refers to skeletal infarction. Bone infarcts may be asymptomatic, cause self-limited discomfort, or engender painful collapse of subarticular bone that leads to joint destruction.

PATHOBIOLOGY AND PATHOGENESIS

Many conditions are associated with osteonecrosis (Table 248-1). In adults, the most common causes are ethanol abuse and long-term glucocorticoid therapy, both of which have dose-dependent effects.

Skeletal infarction may result from blood vessel destruction (e.g., joint dislocation, fracture), obstruction (e.g., thromboemboli, sickle cell disease, fat emboli, caisson disease), or, hypothetically, compression from local expansion of fatty tissue (e.g., ethanol abuse, glucocorticoid treatment, diabetes mellitus). However, symptoms may not occur unless, weeks later, resorption of dead bone during skeletal repair leads to pathologic fracture. Certain skeletal sites (often subarticular) are predisposed to osteonecrosis,

TABLE 248-1 CAUSES OF ISCHEMIC NECROSIS OF CARTILAGE AND BONE

Endocrine/metabolic
   Ethanol abuse
   Glucocorticoid therapy
   Cushing disease
   Diabetes mellitus
   Hyperuricemia
   Osteomalacia
   Hyperlipidemia
   Bone antiresorptive therapy (osteonecrosis of the jaw)
Storage diseases (e.g., Gaucher disease)
Hemoglobinopathies (e.g., sickle cell disease)
Trauma (e.g., dislocation, fracture)
Human immunodeficiency virus (HIV) infection
Dysbaric conditions (e.g., caisson disease)
Collagen vascular disorders
Irradiation
Pancreatitis
Organ transplantation
Hemodialysis
Burns
Intravascular coagulation
Idiopathic, familial
Pregnancy

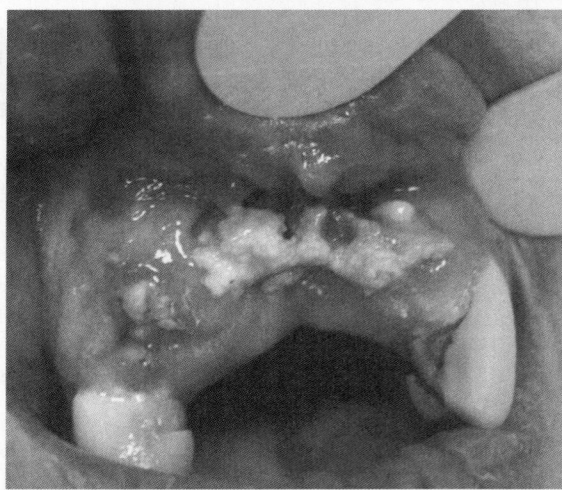

FIGURE 248-1. Exposed dead bone characterizes osteonecrosis of the jaw.

but the locations differ for traumatic and nontraumatic processes and for children and adults. *Osteochondrosis* refers to necrosis of ossification centers; more than 50 eponymic types have been recorded. The susceptibility of children to osteochondrosis and its pathogenesis are poorly understood. At all ages, however, the femoral head is especially prone to infarction. Nontraumatic osteonecrosis commonly affects the humeral head, femoral condyles, distal end of the tibia, and talus. Although the pathogenesis is uncertain, administration of potent bone antiresorptive agents, especially to patients with malignant disease, has been associated with osteonecrosis of the jaw (Fig. 248-1).[1]

CLINICAL MANIFESTATIONS

Pain occurs acutely if there is skeletal collapse. Chronic arthralgia results from desquamated necrotic tissue and articular destruction.

DIAGNOSIS

Magnetic resonance imaging that demonstrates bone marrow edema is especially sensitive for detection of early osteonecrosis. Bone scintigraphy discloses skeletal reconstitution with or without fracture. Relatively late in the pathologic process, radiographs first show patchy areas of osteopenia and osteosclerosis that reflect skeletal repair. A linear subchondral radiolucency (crescent sign) indicates bone collapse.

TREATMENT   Rx

Non–weight bearing is advisable for the affected limb. Decompression by trephine insertion is used at some sites. Arthrotomy to remove debris, transpositional osteotomy, arthroplasty, or joint replacement may be necessary.

OSTEOSCLEROSIS/HYPEROSTOSIS

Many conditions are associated with radiographic evidence of increased bone density. Skeletal dysplasias, metabolic disturbances, and various other disorders can cause generalized or focal increases in bone mass (Table 248-2). Aberrations in skeletal growth, modeling (shaping), or remodeling (turnover) may be at fault. *Osteosclerosis* refers to thickening of trabecular (spongy, cancellous) bone. *Hyperostosis* describes widening of cortical (compact) bone. Increases in trabecular bone, cortical bone, or both may augment skeletal density.

Osteosclerosis

Neoplastic, hematologic, and metabolic disorders may preferentially cause sclerosis in trabecular bone because it houses marrow and remodels more rapidly than cortical bone.

TABLE 248-2 DISORDERS THAT CAUSE DENSE BONES

DYSPLASIAS

Central osteosclerosis with ectodermal dysplasia
Craniodiaphyseal dysplasia
Craniometaphyseal dysplasia
Dysosteosclerosis
Endosteal hyperostosis
   van Buchem disease
   Sclerosteosis
   Worth type (LRP5 activation)
Frontometaphyseal dysplasia
Infantile cortical hyperostosis (Caffey disease)
Juvenile Paget disease
Lenz-Majewski syndrome
Melorheostosis
Metaphyseal dysplasia (Pyle disease)
Mixed sclerosing bone dystrophy
Oculodento-osseous dysplasia
Osteodysplasia of Melnick and Needles
Osteopathia striata
Osteopetrosis (several types)
Osteopoikilosis
Progressive diaphyseal dysplasia (Engelmann disease)
Pyknodysostosis

METABOLIC CONDITIONS

Carbonic anhydrase II deficiency
Fluorosis
Heavy metal poisoning
Hepatitis C–associated osteosclerosis
Hyperparathyroidism, hypoparathyroidism, pseudohypoparathyroidism
Hypervitaminosis A, D
Hypophosphatemic rickets or osteomalacia
Milk-alkali syndrome
Renal osteodystrophy

OTHER DISORDERS

Axial osteomalacia
Fibrogenesis imperfecta ossium
Ionizing radiation
Lymphoma
Mastocytosis
Multiple myeloma
Myelofibrosis
Osteomyelitis
Osteonecrosis
Paget bone disease
Sarcoidosis
Skeletal metastases
Tuberous sclerosis

From Whyte MP. Skeletal disorders characterized by osteosclerosis or hyperostosis. In: Avioli LV, Krane SM, eds. *Metabolic Bone Disease.* 3rd ed. San Diego: Academic Press; 1998.

FIBROGENESIS IMPERFECTA OSSIUM

DEFINITION

This rare, sporadic condition features generalized osteopenia, but coarsening of the remaining trabeculae places it among disorders that manifest osteosclerosis.

PATHOBIOLOGY

The cause is unknown. Subperiosteal bone formation and collagen synthesis in nonosseous tissues seem to be normal.

CLINICAL MANIFESTATIONS

Intractable skeletal pain typically begins gradually during middle age or later and then rapidly increases with a debilitating course and eventual immobility. Spontaneous fractures are a prominent complication. Physical examination reveals marked bone tenderness.

DIAGNOSIS

On radiography, only the skull is spared. Initially, osteopenia and a slightly abnormal appearance of trabecular bone are noted. Subsequently, the changes suggest osteomalacia. Corticomedullary junctions become indistinct as compact bone is replaced by an abnormal cancellous pattern. Generalized osteopenia causes the remaining spongy bone to appear coarse and dense, in a fishnet pattern of mixed lytic and sclerotic areas. Alkaline phosphatase activity in serum is increased.

The skeletal lesion is a localized form of osteomalacia that varies considerably in severity from area to area.

Hyperostosis
PROGRESSIVE DIAPHYSEAL DYSPLASIA (CAMURATI-ENGELMANN DISEASE)

PATHOBIOLOGY

Progressive diaphyseal dysplasia (Camurati-Engelmann disease) affects all races and is inherited as an autosomal dominant trait with variable expressivity. New bone formation gradually envelops both the periosteal and endosteal surfaces of long bone diaphyses. In patients with severe disease, osteosclerosis also occurs in the axial skeleton.

Mutations alter the gene that encodes transforming growth factor-β1. Osteoblast differentiation may be deranged.

CLINICAL MANIFESTATIONS

During childhood, limping or a broad-based, waddling gait is noted. Muscular dystrophy can be diagnosed erroneously. Severely affected individuals may have a characteristic body habitus featuring an enlarged head with a prominent forehead, proptosis, and thin limbs with little subcutaneous fat or muscle mass and tender, thickened bones. Cranial nerve palsies and raised intracranial pressure can occur. Some patients have hepatosplenomegaly and Raynaud phenomenon. Symptoms may remit after puberty.

DIAGNOSIS

Irregular hyperostosis of the diaphyses of the major long bones slowly develops as a result of periosteal and endosteal new bone formation. The femur and tibia are most commonly affected. Metaphyses may be involved. The age at onset, rate of progression, and severity are variable. Clinical, radiographic, and bone scan findings are generally concordant. Serum alkaline phosphatase activity, biochemical markers of skeletal turnover, and erythrocyte sedimentation rate may be elevated. Histopathologic study reveals newly formed woven bone that matures and becomes incorporated into cortical bone. Electron microscopy of muscle may show myopathic changes and vascular abnormalities.

TREATMENT ℞

Glucocorticoid therapy (typically a low dose of prednisone on alternate days) can relieve bone pain and may normalize skeletal histology. Bisphosphonates are sometimes useful.

ENDOSTEAL HYPEROSTOSIS

PATHOBIOLOGY

Sclerosteosis and van Buchem disease, autosomal recessive disorders, are the most severe types of endosteal hyperostosis. Sclerosteosis is caused by deactivating mutations in a gene called *SOST*. Van Buchem disease involves a deletion downstream of *SOST*. Enhanced osteoblast activity from sclerostin deficiency, with failure of osteoclasts to compensate for the increased bone formation, leads to the skeletal changes.

CLINICAL MANIFESTATIONS

Sclerosteosis (cortical hyperostosis with syndactyly) occurs primarily in individuals of Dutch ancestry. The gender distribution appears to be equal. Patients are tall and heavy beginning in childhood; have a prominent, square mandible; and are deaf and experience facial nerve palsy from cranial nerve entrapment. Raised intracranial pressure and headache may reflect a small cranial cavity that can shorten life expectancy. Van Buchem disease causes progressive asymmetrical enlargement of the jaw during puberty. Patients may be symptom free, or, beginning as early as infancy, they may have recurrent facial nerve palsy, deafness, and optic atrophy from narrowing of cranial foramina. Long bones may hurt with applied pressure but are strong.

DIAGNOSIS

In sclerosteosis, the skeleton is radiographically normal in early childhood except for syndactyly, which is common and most often involves the index and third fingers. Progressive bone thickening widens the skull and causes prognathism. Osteosclerosis involves the skull base, facial bones, vertebrae, pelvis, and ribs. Endosteal thickening homogeneously widens diaphyseal cortices and narrows medullary canals. Computed tomography has shown fusion of ossicles and narrowing of the internal auditory canals and cochlear aqueducts. Serum alkaline phosphatase activity can be increased from enhanced bone formation.

TREATMENT ℞

Surgical decompression of narrowed foramina may alleviate cranial nerve palsies.

PACHYDERMOPERIOSTOSIS

PATHOBIOLOGY

Pachydermoperiostosis (hypertrophic osteoarthropathy, primary or idiopathic) is an autosomal dominant disorder that features clubbing of the digits, hyperhidrosis with thickening of the skin (especially of the face), and periosteal new bone formation, most prominently in the distal ends of the limbs. Not all patients manifest all three principal features.[2] A loss-of-function mutation is found in the gene that encodes 15-hydroxyprostaglandin dehydrogenase. Autosomal recessive inheritance also seems to occur.

CLINICAL MANIFESTATIONS

Men seem to be more severely affected than women, and blacks are affected more commonly than whites. Symptoms typically begin during adolescence, intensify during the next decade, but then become quiescent. Arthralgia and fatigue are common. Stiffness and limited mobility occur in both the appendicular and the axial skeleton. Clubbing, with slowly progressive enlargement of the hands and feet, results in a pawlike appearance. Cutaneous changes include thickening, furrowing, pitting, and oiliness, especially of the scalp and face.

DIAGNOSIS

Periostitis thickens the distal portions of the tibia, fibula, radius, and ulna. Clubbing is obvious, and acro-osteolysis can occur. Periosteal proliferation is exuberant, with an irregular texture, and it often involves the epiphyses, whereas secondary hypertrophic osteoarthropathy (pulmonary or otherwise) typically causes a smooth and undulating periosteal reaction. Ankylosis of the joints, especially in the hands and feet, may trouble older patients. Bone scanning reveals symmetrical, diffuse, regular uptake along the cortical margins of long bones, especially in the legs—the double stripe sign.

TREATMENT ℞

Patients with painful synovial effusions may respond to nonsteroidal anti-inflammatory drugs. Contractures or neurovascular compression by osteosclerotic lesions may require surgical intervention.

● OSTEOSCLEROSIS WITH HYPEROSTOSIS
Osteopetrosis

DEFINITION

Osteopetrosis (marble bone disease) is a group of rare disorders characterized by an increase in bone mass due to dysfunction in or lack of osteoclasts during growth. There are two major clinical categories: the autosomal recessive or "malignant" type, which often results in death by early childhood if untreated; and the autosomal dominant or "benign" type, which causes lesser complications. Autosomal recessive types can also feature intermediate severity, neuronal storage disease, or renal tubular acidosis with cerebral calcification due to carbonic anhydrase II deficiency. Bisphosphonate-induced osteopetrosis has been reported.

PATHOGENESIS

The defective gene causing autosomal dominant osteopetrosis encodes a chloride channel important for osteoclast activity. Bi-allelic mutations in this gene, or ones that encode components of a vacuolar proton pump, result in malignant osteopetrosis. Carbonic anhydrase II deficiency is caused by deactivating mutations in the gene that encodes this isoenzyme. Especially rare autosomal recessive cases involve deficient osteoclastogenesis from loss-of-function mutations within the genes for either receptor activator of nuclear factor κB (RANK) or its ligand (RANKL).

Histopathologic studies show that all true forms of osteopetrosis feature profound deficiency of osteoclast action. Bone embedded primary spongiosa (calcified cartilage deposited during endochondral bone formation) persists away from growth plates and constitutes the pathognomonic finding. Defective endosteal bone resorption impairs the formation of marrow space. Quiescent skeletal remodeling leads to bone fragility from the diminished interconnection of osteons and the delayed conversion of immature (woven) bone to mature (compact) bone. Neuronal storage disease (ceroid-lipofuscin) may reflect a lysosomal defect. Deficient superoxide production (necessary for bone resorption) has been considered a pathogenetic factor.

CLINICAL MANIFESTATIONS

Malignant osteopetrosis can be manifested during infancy as nasal "stuffiness" from underdeveloped mastoid and paranasal sinuses. Small cranial foramina may cause optic, oculomotor, or facial nerve palsy. Failure to thrive, delayed dentition, and fractures are common. Hypersplenism and recurrent infection, bruising, and bleeding reflect myelophthisis. Short stature, large head, frontal bossing, nystagmus, hepatosplenomegaly, and genu valgum are characteristic physical features. Untreated children usually die during the first decade of life of hemorrhage, pneumonia, severe anemia, or sepsis. Benign osteopetrosis can cause fracture, facial palsy, deafness, mandibular osteomyelitis, bone marrow failure, impaired vision, psychomotor delay, carpal tunnel syndrome, or osteoarthritis. Carbonic anhydrase II deficiency can cause failure to thrive, fracture, developmental delay, mental subnormality, and short stature. Cerebral calcification develops during childhood, but defective skeletal modeling and osteosclerosis may resolve. Both proximal and distal renal tubular acidosis have been described.

DIAGNOSIS

A generalized increase in bone density is the radiographic hallmark of osteopetrosis. In severe disease, modeling defects in long bones produce an "Erlenmeyer flask" deformity (Fig. 248-2). Alternating dense and lucent bands commonly occur in the metaphyses and pelvis. The cranium is usually thickened and dense, especially at the base, and the paranasal and mastoid sinuses are underpneumatized. Vertebrae may show, on a lateral view, a "bone-in-bone" (endobone) configuration or end-plate sclerosis causing a "rugger jersey" appearance. Skeletal scintigraphy can disclose fractures and osteomyelitis. Magnetic resonance imaging helps monitor the response to bone marrow transplantation.

Serum levels of acid phosphatase and creatine kinase (brain isoenzyme) are often increased. In malignant osteopetrosis, hypocalcemia with secondary hyperparathyroidism and elevated serum concentrations of calcitriol can accompany radiographic changes that resemble rickets. In benign osteopetrosis, biochemical indices of mineral homeostasis are typically unremarkable, although serum parathyroid hormone levels may be elevated.

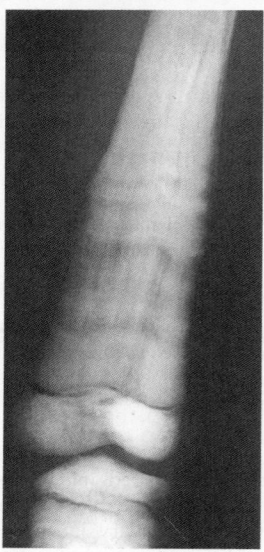

FIGURE 248-2. Osteopetrosis. Anteroposterior radiograph of the distal end of the femur shows a widened metadiaphyseal region, with characteristic alternating dense and lucent bands. (From Whyte MP, Murphy WA. Osteopetrosis and other sclerosing bone disorders. In: Avioli LV, Krane SM, eds. *Metabolic Bone Disease.* 2nd ed. Philadelphia: WB Saunders; 1990.)

TREATMENT   Rx

Because the origin, molecular pathogenesis, prognosis, and treatment of the more than 10 types of osteopetrosis can differ, precise diagnosis is crucial.[3] Now, commercially available mutation analysis can delineate most patients. For the malignant form, prompt use of human leukocyte antigen–identical bone marrow transplantation to supply functional osteoclasts has remarkably benefited some children. Calcium-deficient diets have been tried but may be limited by hypocalcemia and rickets and have uncertain efficacy. Pharmacologic doses of calcitriol (1,25-dihydroxyvitamin D_3) administered orally, together with dietary calcium restriction (to prevent hypercalciuria and hypercalcemia) or human interferon-γ, believed to enhance superoxide production, have reportedly stimulated osteoclast activity. Prednisone alone or with a low-calcium, high-phosphate diet can sometimes be effective. Glucocorticoid therapy stabilizes pancytopenia and hepatosplenomegaly. Hyperbaric oxygenation helps treat osteomyelitis. Surgical decompression of optic and facial nerves can be beneficial.

Pyknodysostosis
EPIDEMIOLOGY

Pyknodysostosis is believed to have affected French impressionist painter Henri de Toulouse-Lautrec (1864-1901). Most descriptions have come from Europe and the United States, but the disorder seems to be especially common in Japan.

PATHOBIOLOGY

This autosomal recessive condition is caused by loss-of-function mutations in *CTSK*, the gene that encodes cathepsin K.[4] Consequently, bone collagen degradation and skeletal turnover are diminished. In chondrocytes and osteoblasts, abnormal inclusions have been described.

CLINICAL MANIFESTATIONS

Characteristic features of pyknodysostosis seen during infancy or early childhood are relatively large cranium, fronto-occipital prominence, proptosis, bluish sclerae, beaked and pointed nose, small facies and chin, obtuse mandibular angle, high-arched palate, dental malocclusion with retention of primary teeth, and disproportionate short stature. Cranial sutures remain open. Fingers are short and clubbed from acro-osteolysis or aplasia of the terminal phalanges, and the hands are small and square. Repeated fractures cause knock-knee deformity. Mental retardation is noted in approximately 10% of patients. Adult height ranges from 4 feet 3 inches to 4 feet 11 inches. Life expectancy can be shortened by recurrent respiratory infections and right-sided heart failure from chronic upper airway obstruction secondary to micrognathia.

DIAGNOSIS

Osteosclerosis is uniform, first becoming apparent in childhood and increasing with age. Skeletal modeling defects do not occur, although long bones appear to have thick cortices because of narrow medullary canals. Clavicles are gracile and hypoplastic at their lateral segments. The calvarum and base of the skull are sclerotic, orbital ridges are dense, and wormian bones are present.

TREATMENT   Rx

No effective medical therapy has been documented. Fractures of the long bones usually mend satisfactorily. Internal fixation of long bones is formidable because of their narrow medullary space and bone hardness. Tooth extraction is difficult. Osteomyelitis of the mandible may require antibiotic, surgical, or hyperbaric therapy.

Hepatitis C–Associated Osteosclerosis

Rarely, achy and tender limbs develop periodically in individuals who are infected with hepatitis C virus. Radiographic studies reveal a marked generalized increase in bone mass from osteosclerosis and hyperostosis. Disturbances in the insulin-like growth factor system may explain the enhanced bone formation. Calcitonin or bisphosphonate therapy to slow bone turnover or antiviral treatment has benefited some patients.

● FOCAL OSTEOSCLEROSIS/HYPEROSTOSIS
Osteopoikilosis

Osteopoikilosis ("spotted bones") is generally a radiographic curiosity due to a deactivating mutation of the *LEMD3* gene transmitted as a highly penetrant autosomal dominant trait. The bone lesions are usually asymptomatic. However, incorrect diagnosis may lead to confusion with serious conditions, including metastatic disease.[5] Some patients have connective tissue nevi called *dermatofibrosis lenticularis disseminata* (or Buschke-Ollendorff syndrome). On radiologic examination, numerous small, round or oval foci of bone sclerosis appear in cancellous bone in the tarsal, carpal, pelvic, and metaepiphyseal regions of tubular bones.

Osteopathia Striata

This finding is usually an autosomal dominant curiosity of asymptomatic linear striations in the metaphyseal regions of long bones and in the ilium. However, two clinically important X-linked dominant disorders with osteopathia striata affect predominantly females: osteopathia striata with cranial sclerosis due to mutation of the *WTX* gene[6]; and osteopathia striata with widespread linear areas of dermal hypoplasia and various bone defects in the limbs due to mutation of the *PORCN* gene (Goltz's syndrome).

Melorheostosis
DEFINITION

Melorheostosis is a sporadic disorder that features bone changes with the appearance of wax that has dripped down a candle. No mendelian basis has been established. The anatomic distribution suggests a postzygotic segmentary defect.

CLINICAL MANIFESTATIONS

Monomelic involvement is usually noted; bilateral disease is generally asymmetrical. Cutaneous changes over affected bones are common (e.g., linear scleroderma-like areas and hypertrichosis) and often appear before the hyperostosis. Symptoms typically begin during childhood, with pain and stiffness as the major complaints. Joints may become contracted and deformed from ectopic bone. Leg length inequality results from soft tissue contractures and premature fusion of epiphyses. Skeletal changes seem to progress most rapidly throughout childhood. During adult life, melorheostosis may or may not gradually spread, but pain is especially common.

DIAGNOSIS

As seen radiographically, irregular, dense, eccentric periosteal and endosteal hyperostosis affects a single bone or several adjacent bones. The lower limbs

are most commonly involved. Endosteal thickening predominates during infancy and childhood, and periosteal new bone formation is prominent during adulthood. Ectopic bone formation may occur, particularly near joints.

TREATMENT   Rx

Surgical correction of contractures is difficult. Recurrent deformity is common.

Mixed Sclerosing Bone Dystrophy

This typically sporadic disorder features combinations of osteopoikilosis, osteopathia striata, melorheostosis, cranial sclerosis, and other skeletal aberrations in one individual. Complications derive from the specific types of osteosclerosis or hyperostosis, such as nerve palsy with cranial sclerosis and bone pain with melorheostosis.

● OTHER DISORDERS OF BONE
Fibrous Dysplasia

This sporadic developmental disorder features one or more expansile fibrous lesions within bone. Polyostotic disease is typically seen before the age of 10 years; monostotic disease begins in adolescence or early adulthood. *McCune-Albright syndrome* refers to polyostotic fibrous dysplasia, cafe au lait spots (Fig. 248-3), and endocrine hyperfunction.[7]

PATHOBIOLOGY

Fibrous dysplasia and McCune-Albright syndrome are caused by postzygotic mosaicism for an activating mutation in the gene that encodes the α subunit of the receptor subunit/adenylate cyclase–coupling G protein, *GNAS*. Imperfect bone forms because mesenchymal cells do not fully differentiate to osteoblasts.

CLINICAL MANIFESTATIONS

Monostotic fibrous dysplasia is more common than polyostotic disease. The skull and long bones are affected most often. The skeletal lesions can deform bones, cause fractures, and occasionally entrap nerves. Sarcomatous degeneration is rare (<1%) but typically occurs within the facial bones or femur and is more frequent with polyostotic disease. Pregnancy may reactivate quiescent lesions. McCune-Albright syndrome usually causes pseudo–precocious puberty in girls. Less commonly, one sees pseudo–precocious puberty in boys. There can also be thyrotoxicosis, Cushing's disease,

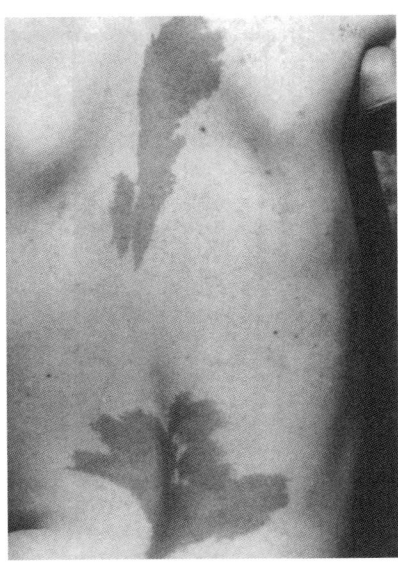

FIGURE 248-3. McCune-Albright syndrome. Typical rough-border ("coast of Maine"), pigmented cafe au lait spots. (From Whyte MP. Metabolic and dysplastic disorders. In: Coe FL, Favus MJ, eds. *Disorders of Bone and Mineral Metabolism*. New York: Raven Press; 1992.)

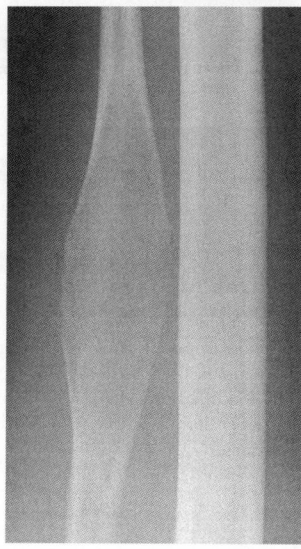

FIGURE 248-4. Fibrous dysplasia. A characteristic expansile lesion with a ground-glass appearance has caused thinning of the cortex in the mid-diaphysis of the fibula. (From Whyte MP. Fibrous dysplasia. In: Favus MJ, ed. *Primer on the Metabolic Bone Diseases and Disorders of Mineral Metabolism.* 3rd ed. Philadelphia: Lippincott-Raven; 1996.)

acromegaly, hyperprolactinemia, or hyperparathyroidism. In some patients, acquired renal phosphate wasting causes hypophosphatemic rickets or osteomalacia.

DIAGNOSIS

The skeletal lesions have a characteristic radiographic appearance. In the long bones, they are found in either the metaphysis or diaphysis, typically are well defined with thin cortices, and have a ground-glass appearance (Fig. 248-4). With aging, the defects can become lobulated, with trabeculated areas of radiolucency.

TREATMENT Rx

In patients with mild disease, bone lesions may not expand. In severe cases, individual defects can progress, and new ones may appear, during childhood. Spontaneous healing does not occur, but pathologic fractures generally mend well. Stress fractures, however, can be difficult to detect and to treat. When the skull is involved, nerve compression may require surgical intervention. In McCune-Albright syndrome, search for and pharmacologic control of associated endocrinopathies are often important. Bone antiresorptive treatment has helped some patients.

Hereditary Multiple Exostoses

This relatively common, highly penetrant, autosomal dominant disorder features irregular bone excrescences that protrude from expanded metaphyses. Mutations have been identified in the *EXT1* and *EXT2* genes. Osteocartilaginous exostoses arise from growth plates and increase in size until linear growth ceases. Lesions may or may not become detached from the parent bone. Their structure is relatively unremarkable, with an outer cortex and an inner spongiosa. Disability results primarily from limb length discrepancies when linear bone growth suffers at the expense of transverse expansion. Compression of nerves, the spinal cord, or the vascular system occurs occasionally. Sarcomatous degeneration (0.5 to 2% of patients) should be suspected when an exostosis enlarges rapidly, especially in an adult.

Enchondromatosis (Dyschondroplasia, Ollier Disease)

This sporadic disorder features cartilaginous masses within the trabecular bone that arise from growth plates. The condition begins in childhood with localized swelling and interferes with linear bone growth. At puberty, expansion of cartilage masses ceases, and these lesions can be replaced by mature bone. Enchondromas appear radiographically as lucent defects in flat bones or in metaphyses of tubular bones, often with central calcific stippling. When enchondromatosis occurs together with multiple hemangiomas (Maffucci syndrome), the enchondromas or hemangiomas undergo malignant transformation in 15% of cases. Ollier disease and Maffucci syndrome are caused by somatic mosaic mutations in the *IDH1* and *IDH2* genes.

Achondroplasia

Chondrodystrophies are disorders of cartilage growth that result in disproportionate short stature. Achondroplasia is the most common. A defect occurs in the gene that encodes fibroblast growth factor receptor type 3; 80% of cases are the result of new autosomal dominant mutations, which are more prevalent with increasing paternal age. Short tubular bones form because of abnormal endochondral ossification in the limbs. In the chondrocranium, membranous ossification is undisturbed; hence the skull vault is normal. However, the cranial base and foramen magnum are small. The head is large, with frontal bossing and midface hypoplasia. Lumbar lordosis is greatly exaggerated, and the spinal canal narrows from the upper to lower segments of the vertebral column. This disturbance is revealed radiographically by a decreasing interpediculate distance. The trunk length is relatively normal, but the limbs show rhizomelic shortening, and the hands have a trident configuration. The long bones appear massive because of their disproportionately normal width. Growth plates are not grossly disorganized, and chondrocytes appear normal. Complications can include hydrocephalus and compression of the brain stem, spinal cord, or nerve roots. Minimal impingement by a disc or osteophyte on the small spinal canal can cause neurologic disturbances.[8] Despite these problems, achondroplasia is compatible with good health and a normal lifespan.

GENERAL REFERENCES

For the General References and other additional features, please visit Expert Consult at https://expertconsult.inkling.com.

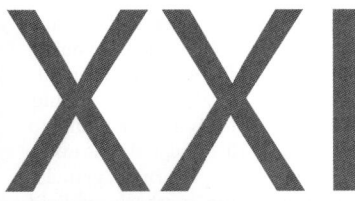

XXI

DISEASES OF ALLERGY AND CLINICAL IMMUNOLOGY

249

APPROACH TO THE PATIENT WITH ALLERGIC OR IMMUNOLOGIC DISEASE

STEPHEN I. WASSERMAN

Allergic diseases and disorders of the immune system affect multiple organ systems and may arise in a variety of manners. The reader is directed to Section VII for a detailed discussion of the immune system and specific autoimmune and acquired immune disorders. This chapter addresses allergic disorders, the most common manifestation of immune system dysfunction, and primary immune deficiencies, which are uncommon manifestations of immune dysfunction. For clarity, these two issues are treated separately.

ALLERGIC DISEASE

DEFINITION

Allergic disorders are common, and their prevalence is increasing, particularly in urbanized, Western societies. It is said that allergic diseases are the most common disorders seen by primary care physicians. Moreover, even in nonallergic patients, consideration of allergy frequently enters the differential diagnosis of a problem under consideration. Therefore, an appreciation of how to approach the diagnosis and treatment of allergic patients is of major importance to the practice of internal medicine. Allergic disorders are those caused by the interaction of a sensitized host (one who has made immunoglobulin E [IgE] antibody recognizing a specific antigen) with a specific allergen. Not all patients possessing specific IgE antibody react adversely on interaction with the allergen, and such individuals are sensitized but not allergic. The primary allergic conditions are seasonal allergic rhinoconjunctivitis (hay fever), perennial allergic rhinitis/sinusitis, asthma, anaphylaxis (especially secondary to foods, medications, and hymenopteran stings), urticaria or angioedema, atopic dermatitis (eczema), and food allergy.

EPIDEMIOLOGY

It is currently estimated that more than 50% of the population is atopic (i.e., able to mount an IgE immune response and to exhibit an immediate positive prick-puncture hypersensitivity response to common aeroallergens). Clinically, 10 to 20% of the general population will develop allergic rhinoconjunctivitis, 5 to 7% will have active asthma, and 20% will experience urticaria at some time. The incidence of allergic rhinitis and asthma is increasing worldwide and most rapidly in those areas with prior low incidence of these disorders.

The increase in allergic diseases noted in the past two decades is thought to result from better hygienic conditions, decreases in infant and childhood infections, and increasingly sedentary and indoor lifestyle with its attendant exposures to indoor allergens and risk for obesity. These changes appear to be associated with a less effective activation of the innate immune system, thereby altering the protective maturation of the acquired immune system. The immune bias in utero and in infancy is toward a type 2 helper T-lymphocyte (T_H2)–directed immune response, which is the immune pathway required for the expression of allergic disease. Ineffective generation of regulatory T lymphocytes underlies the genesis and persistence of allergy. It is therefore postulated that without sufficient early childhood immunologic exposure (e.g., with infection) to induce a switch to an effective and protective T_H1 immune response, allergic disease is more likely to emerge during childhood. Substantial epidemiologic evidence has been gathered to support this concept, now termed the hygiene hypothesis. Thus, allergy is more prevalent in individuals of higher socioeconomic status, among those living in urban areas, in less polluted communities (e.g., western Germany), in first-born children compared with later siblings, in multiply immunized individuals, and in those free of mycobacterial disease. Conversely, children living on farms, in rural communities, and in more highly polluted areas as well as children with mycobacterial infection and those who have experienced multiple early childhood infections are less likely to develop allergic disorders. A concentration-effect relationship appears to exist between exposure to endotoxin (as a marker for hygiene) and the incidence of allergic sensitization. Low and very high levels of exposure to endotoxin are associated with abnormal immune maturation and allergic expression, whereas moderate levels of exposure predispose to a nonallergic phenotype.

PATHOBIOLOGY

The persistence or aberrant activation of T_H2 lymphocytes leads to the generation of cytokines (e.g., interleukins-4, -5, -13), which stimulate B-lymphocyte synthesis of IgE antibody and the production of eosinophilic polymorphonuclear leukocytes. The expression of allergic disorders results from the interaction of a specific allergen with allergen-reactive IgE bound to high-affinity receptors on mast cells and basophils. This interaction leads to the activation of these target cells and to their release of preformed, granule-associated mediators (exemplified by histamine); the synthesis of lipid mediators from membrane lipids (sulfidopeptide leukotrienes); and the transcription and secretion of cytokines, including tumor necrosis factor-α and interleukins-4, -5, and -13. These mediators directly induce smooth muscle contraction, vascular dilation, and endothelial leakage; they also cause vascular adhesion molecule expression, and they attract and activate inflammatory leukocytes, particularly CD4$^+$ T lymphocytes, basophils, and eosinophils. These and other IgE-dependent mediators are thought to be responsible for stimulating smooth muscle proliferation and tissue remodeling.

DIAGNOSIS

Allergy is a systemic immune disorder, so its expression can be multifocal. It is essential to remember this fact when examining a patient with suspected allergic problems because a focus on only the major presenting symptom may be insufficient to identify all the pertinent medical issues in a given patient.

History

Allergic disease has a high degree of heritability, with a great degree of concordance in identical twins. The risk of expressing allergic disease is highest if both parents are atopic. The inheritance of specific manifestations of allergy and of the specific allergen to which a patient is sensitized is less simple. Often, the diagnosis of allergic disorders is straightforward and can be made by asking about the nature of the patient's complaints, when and where reactions occur, and what exposures the patient believes are relevant to symptom induction or exacerbation (Table 249-1).

Seasonal and Perennial Rhinitis

Patients with seasonal and perennial rhinitis (Chapter 251) commonly present with complaints of itchy nose and palate; sneezing; watery rhinorrhea; itching, watery, and burning eyes; and nasal obstruction, which, when severe, may cause anosmia. In the evaluation of possible causes of seasonal rhinoconjunctivitis or sinusitis, the time of the year when symptoms occur is pertinent. Symptoms may be associated with the pollination of trees (early spring), grasses (late spring and summer), or weeds (fall). Important geographic differences exist in allergen concentration and exposure; for example, there is little ragweed in the western United States, and the grasses present in New England and Florida are quite different. In some patients with perennial symptoms, the multiple overlapping pollen seasons are responsible for their symptoms. However, indoor exposures at home, school, work, or recreational sites to furred animals, dust mites or insects, and mold should be addressed in the search for additional causes of perennial symptoms. Mold and mites are to be expected in humid environments, and mites are nearly ubiquitous in bedding and in homes with pets, carpeting, and overstuffed furnishings. Additional occupational or recreational exposures may be pertinent in selected situations (e.g., bakers, health care workers, food handlers, horse fanciers, laboratory animal handlers) in which specific inciting allergens may be identified. Because many patients with rhinitis have concomitant asthma, it is important to obtain information about the presence of this disease in patients with rhinitis. The concurrence of asthma and rhinitis has led to the concept of a "single airway" in which insults/responses in one part of the airway (i.e., upper) may be reflected in the other (i.e., lower).

Asthma

Patients with asthma (Chapter 87) may present with cough or wheeze with dyspnea, which is reversible spontaneously or with treatment. In addition to the association with rhinitis, the influence of exercise, exposure to tobacco smoke, effect of respiratory infection (particularly viral), occupational exposures (e.g., ≤30% of atopic animal handlers develop asthma), and medication use (e.g., β-adrenergic blocking drugs) are pertinent. Because most patients with asthma have concurrent rhinitis, it is essential that the physician evaluate this issue in all asthmatic patients. Wheezing may accompany other

TABLE 249-1 SYMPTOMS, SIGNS, AND TREATMENT OF ALLERGIC DISEASE

SYMPTOMS AND SIGNS	APPROACH TO TREATMENT
SYMPTOMS	
Cutaneous: itch, rash	H_1-antihistamine
Ocular: gritty sensation, itch	Topical H_1-antihistamine or mast cell stabilizing agent
Upper respiratory: palatal pruritus, clear rhinorrhea, sneeze, nasal obstruction	Topical corticosteroid, oral H_1-antihistamine, leukotriene receptor antagonist, topical nasal H_1-antihistamine
Lower respiratory: wheeze, cough, dyspnea	β_2-Agonist, inhaled corticosteroid, inhaled β_2-agonist, leukotriene receptor antagonist, oral methylxanthine, parenteral corticosteroid, parenteral anti-IgE
Gastrointestinal: nausea, vomiting, cramping pain	Epinephrine (if caused by anaphylaxis), oral corticosteroid, oral cromolyn
SIGNS	
Cutaneous: flushing, urticaria, angioedema, eczema	
Ocular: conjunctival erythema, chemosis	
Upper respiratory: pallor, edema, clear rhinorrhea, polyps	
Lower respiratory: wheeze	

disorders, including pulmonary edema in congestive heart failure and pulmonary embolic disease.

Urticaria and Angioedema

Patients with urticaria (Chapter 252) describe pruritic, erythematous cutaneous lesions with regular or irregular borders occurring anywhere on the body; they may vary in size from small (1×1 mm) to extremely large. Skin lesions are often preceded by intense intertriginous pruritus and erythema. Individual urticarial lesions generally persist for a few hours and rarely last for more than 24 hours.[1] However, many disorders can cause a sensation of itching; for more on skin and systemic diseases associated with pruritus (see Chapter 436). Angioedema (Chapter 252) is most frequently appreciated in the face, hands, and other soft tissues and is generally accompanied by symptoms of stretching, tingling, and tightness of the skin rather than by pruritus. Lesions, especially in the face, typically last 24 to 36 hours. Although most cases of urticaria or angioedema are not IgE-allergen mediated (particularly in chronic urticaria), it is important to identify foods and medications used by patients with acute urticaria or angioedema, particularly those substances ingested within 2 to 4 hours of the development of lesions, and to inquire about insect stings. Chronic urticaria is less often IgE mediated; questions about medications, especially nonsteroidal anti-inflammatory drugs, recent infection (especially with Epstein-Barr virus), and the presence of autoantibodies to the IgE receptor must be addressed. Approximately one half to two thirds of patients with such autoantibodies also have antibodies to thyroid antigens. In angioedema, the use of angiotensin-converting enzyme inhibitors must be sought, with special attention to those of African American heritage. Atopic dermatitis is another allergic cutaneous disorder in which patients complain of intense pruritus, especially in flexural surfaces. In adults, foods (IgE mediated) and cutaneous infection with *Staphylococcus aureus* (superantigen mediated) are the most commonly identified precipitating events for atopic dermatitis.

Anaphylaxis

Anaphylaxis (Chapter 253) is the most important allergic emergency and is potentially fatal. It is an acute allergic response associated with cutaneous (urticaria, angioedema, flushing), respiratory (laryngeal edema, asthma), cardiovascular (arrhythmia, hypotension, extravascular fluid loss), gastrointestinal (nausea, vomiting, abdominal pain, diarrhea), and nonspecific symptoms (metallic taste, sense of impending doom) that may occur singly or together. Historical information of note includes all medications, foods, and other encounters occurring within 2 hours of the reaction. Epidemiologic data suggest that foods (especially peanuts, tree nuts, shellfish, milk, and eggs), hymenopteran stings, and medications (antibiotics, muscle relaxants, radiocontrast media) are the most frequently identified causes of this important problem. Patients with elevated basal tryptase levels are at increased risk

for anaphylaxis, especially with hymenopteran stings, and all patients suffering anaphylaxis after such an exposure should have baseline tryptase determined; if it is elevated, appropriate follow-up evaluation for occult mast cell disorders should be undertaken.

Food Allergy

Patients presenting with food allergy[2] often complain of oral pruritus and nausea, vomiting, diarrhea, and abdominal pain. Eczema, urticaria, and anaphylaxis, as noted previously, may also be consequences of food allergy. In general, allergic symptoms consequent to foods occur within minutes to 2 hours of ingestion of the causative food; delayed symptoms are unlikely to be mediated by an IgE-allergen interaction. Eosinophilic esophagitis has recently been added to the list of disorders in which food allergy is thought to play a role. Other symptoms attributable to foods are less easily explained by allergic mechanisms and are termed food intolerance.

Physical Examination

The physical examination of a patient with suspected allergic disease should emphasize the organ systems pertinent to the patient's complaints. The skin should be examined for the presence of urticarial or angioedematous lesions and for signs of atopic dermatitis, including flexural papules, excoriations, and lichenification. Keratosis pilaris, particularly on the outer aspect of the upper arm, commonly accompanies atopic dermatitis. Urticaria typically consists of small, pink, irregular lesions that blanch on pressure and then clear, leaving normal skin. In a patient with urticaria, a simple test for dermatographism should be undertaken. Angioedematous lesions are larger, more diffuse, and pale, and they are found most often on the face and in acral areas.

The eyes, ears, nose, and throat should be examined in all patients thought to have allergic disease, particularly those whose symptoms suggest seasonal or perennial allergic rhinoconjunctivitis-sinusitis or asthma. In allergic disease, the conjunctivae are often injected and may be edematous. "Cobblestoning" of the epithelium may be present. The periorbital tissues may be swollen and darkened. Examination of the nares may show pale and edematous nasal mucous membranes and swollen turbinates, and polyps may be seen. Secretions, generally clear, may be seen in the nasal passages or in the posterior pharynx. Such secretions generally contain copious numbers of eosinophils (see later), and their absence is a point against an allergic cause. Fever and discolored secretions, particularly those that are thick and yellow or green, in the presence of neutrophilic polymorphonuclear leukocytes suggest infection. Percussion over the maxillary or frontal sinuses may elicit tenderness in acute sinusitis. In chronic sinusitis, the physical examination may be unrevealing. In acute otitis media, patients may have erythema and bulging or perforation of the tympanic membrane, with fluid in the canal; in chronic cases, the drum may be scarred and retracted. Alteration in airborne conduction may be noted as well.

Patients with acute asthma may display tachypnea and auditory wheezes, and they may be unable to speak in full sentences because of shortness of breath. Use of accessory muscles of respiration and evidence of cyanosis should be sought. Examination of the chest includes inspection for evidence of chronic hyperinflation and auscultation for wheezing (which, if unilateral, may suggest a foreign body or tumor). In mild asthma, the examination findings may be normal, or the only physical finding may be wheezing on forced expiration and a slight prolongation of the expiratory phase.

Patients experiencing acute anaphylaxis usually demonstrate flushing, and concomitant urticaria and angioedema are often present. Assessment of vital signs may disclose hypotension and tachycardia. In some situations, hoarseness or stridor related to laryngeal edema or wheezing secondary to asthma can be identified. Hyperactive bowel sounds may be noted. Progressive hypoxia and cyanosis may ensue. In severe anaphylaxis, cardiovascular collapse secondary to hypoxia and hypotension may result in death.

Laboratory Evaluation

In the evaluation of patients with allergic disorders, the laboratory may be of assistance in both the identification and the quantification of specific organ dysfunction as well as in the assessment of the presence and specificity of IgE antibody.[3]

Assessment of Total and Allergen-Specific Immunoglobulin E

Essentially all (>95%) IgE antibody is bound to specific high-affinity receptors on tissue mast cells and circulating peripheral blood basophils. The small amount of free serum IgE antibody circulates in nanogram quantities and can be identified only with techniques of sufficient sensitivity. A large proportion

TABLE 249-2   ADVANTAGES AND DISADVANTAGES OF DIFFERENT ALLERGY TESTING METHODS

METHOD	PATIENT SELECTION	CLINICAL ADVANTAGES	CLINICAL DISADVANTAGES
Skin testing	Clinical indication suggesting allergic disease	Rapid (15-30 min) turnaround Sensitive and specific; prick-puncture for aeroallergens; prick-puncture followed by intradermal testing for drugs, sera, and venoms	Patient must not be taking H_1-antihistamine agents for 5-7 days Not interpretable in the presence of dermatographism Requires sufficient normal skin to enable testing
In vitro testing	Clinical indication suggesting allergic disease	Antihistamine therapy not contraindicated Dermatographism not a problem Sensitive and specific; equal to prick-puncture skin testing	Requires blood to be drawn Slow turnaround (7-14 days)

of IgE in a given individual may be directed toward a single antigen. Therefore, total IgE levels may be normal in the presence of allergic disease, and the measurement of total serum IgE is rarely of help in making a diagnosis. In a few situations, such as adult atopic dermatitis or allergic bronchopulmonary aspergillosis, measurement of total serum IgE levels may provide insight into disease severity or risk of disease exacerbation.

Of more importance is the identification of allergen-specific IgE in a patient with suspected allergic disease (Table 249-2).[4] Such specific IgE may be identified in vitro or in vivo. A search for allergen-specific IgE is particularly useful in the evaluation of patients with suspected allergic rhinitis, asthma, eczema, food reactions, and anaphylaxis. In vitro assessment is similar to the quantification of total IgE, except the initial capture reagent bound to a solid phase is a specific allergen from pollen, mold, insect, venom, food, or other material. Development of the assay is identical to that used to quantify total IgE, and results are generally reported in a semiquantitative manner. The magnitude of the reaction is weakly correlated with the expression of allergy, although for certain foods, more precise correlative data exist on the risk of allergy and the amount of allergen-specific IgE detected. To assess allergen-specific IgE in vivo, a minute quantity of the allergen in question is introduced into the skin by a prick-puncture technique, and the cutaneous response is assessed 15 to 30 minutes thereafter. A positive response is one in which a wheal and flare at least 2 mm larger than that caused by a saline control occur at the injection site. In vivo tests are rapid and inexpensive; their use requires the absence of dermatographism, that patients not be taking antihistamine medications, and that patients exhibit a positive response to a control with histamine. In some situations (e.g., penicillin allergy or hymenopteran sting), a more diluted allergen is injected intradermally, and the wheal and flare response is assessed similarly. The presence of allergen-specific IgE antibody and a clear temporal correlation between exposure to allergen and genesis of symptoms are required to conclude that a patient is allergic to a specific allergen. In the absence of symptoms, a patient with allergen-specific IgE is termed sensitized but not allergic.

Specific in vivo challenge tests can also be used to identify allergen responsiveness. Such tests in the presence of specific IgE antibody may be useful in research settings, or they may be used clinically to clarify the exact relationship between exposure and symptoms. The tests can be dangerous, however, because they introduce the allergen to which the patient is presumed allergic. In the case of food allergy, such challenges are best done in a double-blind and placebo-controlled manner; they may be useful to distinguish allergy from sensitization or to eliminate a suspect food from consideration. However, food challenge tests are unnecessary in the case of anaphylaxis and a positive test response for IgE antibody to the putative allergen. Because many patients falsely believe that foods are responsible for their symptoms, such double-blind challenges may be useful in directing patients' concerns to more productive areas. Inhalation tests employing specific allergens or chemicals have been helpful in elucidating some cases of occupational allergy or asthma.

Other Laboratory Aids in Allergic Disease

In a patient with acute asthma, chest radiographs generally demonstrate hyperinflation. In some instances, evidence of bronchiectasis may be present, a finding that raises the specter of allergic bronchopulmonary aspergillosis. The presence of a tumor or radiopaque foreign body may be noted on a chest radiograph and should be sought in a patient with unilateral localized wheezing. In the examination of a patient with asthma, assessment of both airflow and volumes can provide a clear picture of the severity of asthma and its response to treatment. Flow-volume loops can also identify the presence of vocal cord dysfunction or tracheomalacia. When patients with airway obstruction are evaluated, their response to an inhaled β_2-adrenergic agonist medication (or a short-acting anticholinergic agent) can be helpful in eluci-

dating the reversible nature of their disorder. A large majority of asthmatic patients exhibiting bronchoconstriction display a bronchodilatory response to the inhalation of such agents. In suspected cases of asthma in which pulmonary function is normal, a histamine or methacholine challenge can be performed. These agents take advantage of the nonspecific bronchial hyperresponsiveness that is characteristic of patients with asthma. Failure to develop bronchoconstriction on inhalation of either of these agents strongly argues against the diagnosis of asthma.

Other laboratory tools may be of clinical benefit in the identification and classification of allergic disorders. Audiometry may clarify the degree of hearing loss caused by otitis media in a patient with allergic rhinitis. When sinusitis is suspected, computed tomography of the sinuses provides the most complete image and has the highest degree of sensitivity for the identification of mucosal thickening, opacification of air spaces, and presence of polyps and bone erosions. Computed tomography is particularly useful in the examination of the ethmoid and sphenoid sinuses, which are often affected in chronic allergic disease and are difficult to assess on physical examination or with plain radiographs. Imaging studies are not indicated, however, in most cases of acute sinusitis.

The quantification of blood, sputum, nasal mucus, or tissue eosinophilia and the response to corticosteroid therapy are useful correlates in the identification and management of allergic disease. The quantification of tryptase, a mast cell–specific protease with a serum half-life of 2 hours, can assist in the diagnosis of anaphylaxis if it is performed on serum or plasma obtained within hours of a systemic response with associated hypotension. Quantification of exhaled nitric oxide has been used to assess airways inflammation in asthma and primarily reflects eosinophilic inflammation.

IMMUNOLOGIC DISEASE

EPIDEMIOLOGY

Diseases related to disordered immune function (immunodeficiency) are far less common than allergic disorders.[5] The most frequent is IgA deficiency, which occurs in approximately 1 in 1000 individuals and is often asymptomatic. Next most frequent are disorders of B and T lymphocytes, such as common variable hypogammaglobulinemia, and other disorders, including DiGeorge syndrome and severe combined immunodeficiency (Chapter 250). Much less common are defects in neutrophil function or complement.

DIAGNOSIS

The clinical expression of immunodeficiency disorders is primarily infection, related to impaired host defense. Thus, the diagnosis of suspected immunodeficiency involves the evaluation of recurrent, persistent, severe, unusual, and otherwise unexplained infections. Many but not all immune disorders arise in early childhood, and with improved management, many patients presenting in childhood live into adulthood. It is important for the general internist and internal medicine subspecialist to be cognizant of the presentation of these disorders.

History

The most important historical information includes the following: age at onset of the problem in question; family history of frequent infection or death at an early age from infection; number, site, and type of infections; and presence of other physical abnormalities (Table 249-3). The earlier the onset of infections, the more severe the immune defect is likely to be. T-lymphocyte defects, with or without B-cell deficiencies, usually are manifested in the first 3 to 5 months of life, whereas B-cell function is supported by maternal antibody until after 6 months of age. Many of the immune disorders are X-linked,

TABLE 249-3 KEY POINTS REGARDING IMMUNOLOGIC DISORDERS

ANTIBODY DEFICIENCY DISORDERS

Onset after 6 months of age
Recurrent respiratory infection
Infection with bacteria, especially encapsulated organisms
Absence of isohemagglutinins
Evaluation of B-cell function, not numbers

CELLULAR IMMUNE DEFECTS

Onset before 6 months of age
Recurrent viral, fungal, or parasitic (opportunistic) infection
Defective delayed hypersensitivity skin responses
Malabsorption or diarrhea

COMPLEMENT DEFICIENCIES

Recurrent bacterial infection
Recurrent neisserial infection (deficiency of late components)
Associated rheumatic disorder (especially systemic lupus erythematosus)

FACTORS SUGGESTING NEUTROPHIL DYSFUNCTION

Late separation of umbilical cord
Persistent neutrophilic leukocytosis
Recurrent or persistent gingivitis or periodontitis
Recurrent bacterial infection with granuloma formation

and a careful family history is critical in such situations. Infection-related death of a patient's male sibling or the patient's mother should lead to the search for such an X-linked disorder.

In a patient with a T-cell disorder, viral, fungal, mycobacterial, and other opportunistic infections (*Pneumocystis jiroveci, Toxoplasma gondii*) are most commonly noted, and live virus vaccination may be associated with disseminated and progressive viral disease. Persistent thrush, diarrhea, malabsorption, and failure to thrive occurring in early childhood may suggest the presence of T-cell abnormalities.

In B-cell or antibody deficiency, pyogenic bacterial infections predominate, particularly infections involving encapsulated microorganisms. Such infections usually affect the upper and lower respiratory tract and the skin and are severe, recurrent, and often persistent. Infections with unusual organisms, with unexpected complications, or involving multiple sites (lung, sinus, joint, bone, or meninges, with abscess formation or sepsis) should raise the index of suspicion. In adults, the most common disorder in this class is termed common variable immunodeficiency.

As in any patient with infection, information should be sought about exposure to ill individuals or to irritants such as tobacco smoke, the hygiene of the environment to which the patient has been exposed, and the presence of an anatomic abnormality or allergy that could predispose to infection.

Physical Examination

Physical examination beyond that necessary to assess the extent and severity of a particular infection should focus on immune organs. Assessment of tonsillar tissue and determination of the presence and size of lymph nodes, spleen, and liver are important. Patients with common variable immunodeficiency often present with hepatosplenomegaly and lymph node hyperplasia, whereas in X-linked hypogammaglobulinemia, lymph tissue is absent. Telangiectasia (ataxia-telangiectasia), cardiac defects (DiGeorge syndrome), chronic eczema (Wiskott-Aldrich syndrome), and chronic periodontitis (neutrophil defects) all suggest immunodeficiency syndromes.

Laboratory Evaluation

The proper use of the laboratory is essential to elucidate a suspected immunodeficiency disorder.[6] Screening tests appropriate to the generalist's initial approach include complete blood count, total neutrophil and lymphocyte enumeration, quantitative immunoglobulin levels, and assessment of isohemagglutinins (especially when common variable immunodeficiency is suspected). In some situations, quantification of IgG subclasses may be warranted to identify a specific subclass deficiency. In considering T-lymphocyte defects, it is important to enumerate total T cells and specific T-cell subsets. Delayed hypersensitivity skin testing to recall antigens is also helpful in assessing cellular immunity. When neutrophil defects are suspected, a nitroblue tetrazolium test or measurement of phagocytic potency can be performed. Complement defects are best addressed by obtaining a CH_{50} level. CH_{50} is the amount of the patient's serum required to cause lysis of 50% of

test erythrocytes. It is compared with the amount of pooled normal serum required to cause the same degree of lysis. Tests for specific individual components of complement, or of complement regulatory proteins, can also be obtained under special circumstances (e.g., late complement components in patients with recurrent *Neisseria* species infection).

Additional tests of antibody production in response to defined stimuli, including vaccinations, may be helpful when selective antibody deficiency is suspected or when borderline immunoglobulin levels are encountered in the presence of frequent infection. In some situations, assessment of T-cell proliferation to mitogens or antigen may be of benefit. Further testing might include the assessment of natural killer-cell function and the production of cytokines by activated lymphocytes. In general, such additional laboratory tests should be performed in consultation with an expert in immune disorders.

GENERAL REFERENCES

For the General References and other additional features, please visit Expert Consult at https://expertconsult.inkling.com.

250

PRIMARY IMMUNODEFICIENCY DISEASES

CHARLOTTE CUNNINGHAM-RUNDLES

Since the descriptions of the first genetic immune defects, severe combined immunodeficiency (SCID) and X-linked agammaglobulinemia (XLA), in the 1940s, the number of known primary immune defects (175+) has expanded exponentially.[1] To keep pace, every few years the International Union of Immunological Societies has compiled these defects into eight general categories: T- and B-cell combined defects, B-cell/antibody defects, complement disorders, phagocyte defects, defects with syndromic features, diseases of immune dysregulation, autoinflammatory syndromes, and defects of innate immunity (Table 250-1).[2] Autoinflammatory syndromes are covered in Chapter 261. In this chapter, our current understanding of these other primary immune defects is considered with emphasis on immune defects found in adults. Complement and phagocyte disorders are discussed in more detail in Chapters 50 and 169, respectively.

AN APPROACH TO EVALUATION OF THE IMMUNE SYSTEM

Because of the numbers and types of immune deficiency, recognition of the many clinical phenotypes can be difficult, leading in many cases to a delayed diagnosis. The spectrum of immune defects found in populations varies with the age of the patient and with the combined T- and B-cell immune defects, defects of phagocyte function, defects with syndromic features, defects of immune dysregulation, and innate defects; selected infections are more commonly recognized in childhood, whereas defects of complement and antibody production are more characteristic of adults. However, there are many exceptions to this general observation; in addition, even if an immune defect has been diagnosed in childhood, adequate treatment has allowed these patients to increasingly appear in the offices of internists and adult specialists.

For most patients, the first symptom of an immune defect is a series of relatively common infections, particularly involving the respiratory tract. These may include chronic sinusitis, otitis, and bacterial pneumonia. For adults with immune defects, infections are likely to last longer, are likely to require additional courses of antibiotics, and tend to recur. Infections may lead to additional complications or procedures, such as empyema after bacterial pneumonia or the need for myringotomy tubes in an adult with chronic otitis. For infants and children, chronic infections lead to poor appetite and an obvious failure to grow normally; for adults, some weight loss may occur, but it is less apparent. Because of lack of immunity, shingles (Chapter 375) is relatively common in patients with T-cell defects or lack of antibody. Other common clinical presentations include acute gastrointestinal infections with characteristic organisms such as *Giardia* (Chapter 351) and chronic intestinal inflammatory diseases with weight loss and malabsorption (Chapter 140). General guidelines to approach the laboratory evaluation of the main immune defects outlined in this chapter, based on clinical presentations,[3] are provided in Table 250-2. Flow charts of the work-up of immune defects in Table 250-1, based on clinical phenotypes, have been published.[4]

TABLE 250-1 CATEGORIES OF PRIMARY IMMUNODEFICIENCY DISEASES

T- and B-cell combined deficiencies
Antibody deficiencies
Complement disorders
Phagocyte defects
Well-defined defects with syndromic features
Immune dysregulation syndromes
Autoinflammatory defects
Defects of innate immunity

T- AND B-CELL COMBINED DEFECTS

DEFINITION

Combined immune defects are diseases in which both the T- and B-cell compartments are greatly impaired. With the very early onset and severe nature of these defects, this group contains all forms of SCID and other syndromes in which both T- and B-cell limbs of the immune system are markedly abnormal.

EPIDEMIOLOGY

The incidence of SCID has undergone a downward revision from the estimated 1 : 100,00 a few years ago because of newborn screening, currently performed for about half of all newborns in the United States.[5] The aggregate incidence of these forms, listed in Table 250-3, appears to be about 1 : 54,000. When the larger spectrum of combined immune defects is also included, the incidence is likely to be higher.

PATHOBIOLOGY AND GENETICS

The hallmark of combined defects is that they eliminate or greatly impair T-cell development, in most cases leading to profound lymphopenia. Infants

TABLE 250-2 CLINICAL PRESENTATION AND EVALUATION OF THE IMMUNE SYSTEM

CLINICAL PRESENTATION	DEFECTS	IMMUNE DEFECTS	CONDITIONS	LABORATORY TESTING
Recurrent or chronic bacterial, viral, or fungal infections Opportunistic infections	Cell-mediated immunity	Impaired killing of intracellular organisms Impaired viral immunity Hypogammaglobulinemia	SCID	Absolute lymphocyte count Enumeration of T cells and T-cell subsets Proliferative tests for T-cell function
Bacterial infections Viral infections Autoimmunity Inflammatory diseases Enteropathy Giardiasis	B cells	Hypogammaglobulinemia Impaired bacterial killing Impaired clearance of virus or toxins	Hypogammaglobulinemia Agammaglobulinemia IgA deficiency CVID IgG subclass defects Antibody deficiency	Enumeration of B cells Serum IgG, IgA, and IgM Antibody testing (i.e., tetanus, diphtheria) Vaccine challenge and antibody testing (pneumococcal vaccine)
Bacterial infections Susceptibility to meningococcal disease Autoimmunity Angioedema	Complement	Impaired opsonization Impaired bacterial killing Lack of clearance of immune complexes	Complement C2 deficiency Other complement defects HAE	CH_{50} AH_{50} Measuring individual components C1 inhibitor protein and function
Bacterial infections Poor skin healing Fungal infections Stomatitis Periodontal disease	Phagocytic cells	Impaired neutrophil mobilization Impaired opsonization Impaired bacterial killing	Chronic neutropenia Cyclic neutropenia Autoimmune neutropenia LAD CGD	Absolute neutrophil counts Neutrophil oxidative burst examined by dihydrorhodamine test by flow cytometry Examination of the blood smear Antineutrophil antibodies

CGD = chronic granulomatous disease; CVID = combined variable immunodeficiency; HAE = hereditary angioedema; LAD = leukocyte adhesion deficiency; SCID = severe combined immunodeficiency.

TABLE 250-3 EXAMPLES OF COMBINED IMMUNE DEFECTS

SCID TYPE	GENES	INHERITANCE	LABORATORY FEATURES	DISEASE AND COMPLICATIONS
Defects of V(D)J recombination	*RAG1, RAG2* ARTEMIS DNA-PKcs	AR	Very low lymphocyte numbers with loss of T and B cells; hypogammaglobulinemia	Severe infections, failure to thrive; leaky versions may have autoreactive T cells (Omenn syndrome)
Adenosine deaminase deficiency	Adenosine deaminase	AR	Variably low lymphocyte numbers with loss of T and B cells; also decreased NK cells; hypogammaglobulinemia	Severe infections, failure to thrive; often with costochondral junction flaring, neurologic features, hearing impairment, lung and liver manifestations
X-linked SCID	Common γ chain of cytokine receptors	XL	Low lymphocyte numbers with loss of T cells; B cells present; markedly decreased NK cells; hypogammaglobulinemia	Severe infections, failure to thrive; leaky cases may present with low T or NK cells or Omenn syndrome
JAK3 deficiency	*JAK3*	AR	Low lymphocyte numbers with loss of T cells; B cells present; hypogammaglobulinemia	Severe infections, failure to thrive; leaky cases may present with variable T or NK cells
IL-7 deficiency	α chain of the IL-7 receptor	AR	Low lymphocyte numbers with loss of T cells; B cells present; normal NK cells; hypogammaglobulinemia	Severe infections, failure to thrive; leaky cases may present with low T or NK cells or Omenn syndrome
T-cell receptor chain defects	γ-, ε-, and ζ-chain mutations	AR	Low lymphocyte numbers due to loss of T cells; normal B and NK cells; hypogammaglobulinemia	Severe infections, failure to thrive; leaky cases may present with low T or NK cells or Omenn syndrome

AR = autosomal recessive; DNA-PKcs = DNA-dependent protein kinase catalytic subunits; IL-7 = interleukin-7; JAK3 = Janus kinase 3; NK = natural killer; SCID = severe combined immunodeficiency; XL = X-linked.

with defects that affect the formation of T- and B-cell receptors, such as defects of the recombinase activating genes *RAG1* and *RAG2*, which impair VDJ recombination, have few if any T and B cells. Similarly, other defects of DNA recombination or repair genes (ARTEMIS, DNA-PKcs) will have a similar phenotype. When T-cell immunity is absent, B cells may be present, but they will have no function. This is the case for the most common form of SCID, the X-linked form, due to mutations in the cytokine γ chain, the signaling component of six cytokine receptors: interleukin (IL)–2, IL-4, IL-7, IL-9, IL-15, and IL-21. Similarly, defects of the *JAK3* gene, downstream from the cytokine γ chain, or of the IL-7 receptor itself lead to a similar immune profile.

CLINICAL MANIFESTATIONS

With loss of both essential limbs of the adaptive immune system, infants with combined immune defects have severe and recurrent infections due to bacteria, viruses, and fungi. Other common features include diarrhea, dermatitis, and failure to thrive. Clinically, most patients present before the age of 3 months, but there is a significant number of exceptions as infants may present later, although still usually in the first year of life. Without intervention, SCID usually results in severe infections and death by the age of 2 years. In some cases, the immune defect is such that a few T cells can develop, but these are often self-reactive; these cases are often termed leaky SCID. When the presentation of these cases includes rashes and evidence of autoimmunity, infants are said to have Omenn syndrome.

DIAGNOSIS

Newborns normally have an absolute lymphocyte count of 4000/mm³ or higher. Thus, the first measure in suspected SCID is the complete blood count; most infants have significant lymphopenia. When the clinical manifestations suggest SCID, a flow cytometer panel is used to enumerate T, B, and NK cells; this will also suggest genes that may be responsible. Further genetic testing can be done, but only after stem cell transplant approaches have been launched.[6] A number of states have recently introduced newborn screening for SCID, based on standard blood spot (Guthrie) cards to determine if the DNA signature of new T cells emigrating from the infant thymus can be detected in normal numbers. This method has been shown to be both highly sensitive and specific and is likely to be universally adopted.

TREATMENT AND PROGNOSIS

Without immune reconstitution, infants with SCID will die, and prompt recognition is essential. Early reconstitution with stem cells from human leukocyte antigen (HLA)–matched bone marrow or mobilized peripheral blood is mandatory. When the diagnosis is made early and no severe infections have occurred, hematopoietic stem cell transplantation (HSCT; Chapter 178) is likely to be curative in 90% of cases. Gene therapy in some cases is gaining a new role and will likely lead to additional options in the future.

ANTIBODY DEFECTS

DEFINITION

The antibody defects are due to loss of B-cell development, loss of production of one or more of the immunoglobulin (Ig) isotypes, or loss of functional antibody production.

EPIDEMIOLOGY

As a group, antibody defects are the most prevalent immune defects and are found in patients of all ages. Selective IgA deficiency is most common in patients of white background, but the incidence varies with the population studied from 1:400 to more than 1:10,000. IgA deficiency is found in 1:400 in Finland but much less commonly in African Americans or Asians (1:14,000 or fewer). Common variable immune deficiency (CVID) has an estimated incidence of 1 in 50,000; IgG subclass or selective antibody defects are also common, but the incidence is unknown.

PATHOBIOLOGY AND CLINICAL MANIFESTATIONS

Whereas the genetic causes have been elucidated for many of the combined forms of immune deficiency, the genes are not yet known for many of the more common B-cell defects (Table 250-4). Antibody defects can be considered in three main forms: B cells are absent; B cells are present but one or more immunoglobulin isotypes is not made; and B cells and immunoglobulin levels are normal but the produced immunoglobulins have no function.

Lack of B Cells Leading to Agammaglobulinemia

The first severe antibody defect described was the X-linked form of agammaglobulinemia (XLA). The gene affected, a tyrosine kinase (BTK) located on the X chromosome, is essential for downstream signaling from the B-cell receptor. Without these signals, B cells do not survive, leading to profound hypogammaglobulinemia. The incidence of this disease is approximately 1 in 100,000. The main clinical manifestations appear in the first year of life, but males may come to clinical attention later, in some cases not until the second decade. Whereas X-linked inheritance is a central feature, the family history may or may not be positive because of de novo mutations. Infections are usually bacterial, generally with encapsulated organisms like *Streptococcus pneumoniae, Haemophilus influenzae, Staphylococcus aureus,* and *Pseudomonas* species. A particular propensity for *Mycoplasma* infections in XLA has been long noted; these may occur in joints or the urinary tract and can be difficult to diagnose as appropriate culture techniques are not widely available.

In addition to XLA, there are other genetic forms of agammaglobulinemia. These are gene defects of the B-cell receptor itself, such as the μ heavy chain, the surrogate light chain λ5, Igα, and Igβ. Similarly, mutations in signaling proteins immediately downstream from the B-cell receptor lead to the same outcome, with loss of all B cells. As these genes are not on the X chromosome, these defects, although rare, are found in both sexes.

Good Syndrome

A special case of agammaglobulinemia with loss of B cells in adults is a poorly understood immune defect associated with thymomas (Good syndrome). This appears to be a secondary immune defect, but it is important to include it here as the loss of B cells, with either agammaglobulinemia or hypogammaglobulinemia, leads to many of the same infectious manifestations as with the other profound antibody defects. Quite rare, Good syndrome occurs in adults, most often after the age of 40 years, and includes an increased incidence of opportunistic infections, such as *Pneumocystis jiroveci, Candida* infections with nail or other cutaneous involvement, viral infections, and inflammatory complications such as lichen planus. The connection between thymoma, loss of B-cell function, and the unusual infections remains unclear.

Hypogammaglobulinemia with B cells
Common Variable Immune Deficiency

Patients with CVID have varying degrees of hypogammaglobulinemia ranging from almost total loss of immunoglobulins to more modest reductions of IgG and IgA or IgM. From the clinical point of view, CVID is a noteworthy disorder as it is relatively common (1:25,000 to 1:50,000), has a later onset than other immune defects (generally between the ages of 20 and 40 years), and has a highly heterogeneous clinical presentation. Delays in diagnosis are common. Before diagnosis, about 80% of subjects with CVID will have had one or more episodes of pneumonia, sometimes leading to empyema. Over time, bronchiectasis may develop. The bacterial species most commonly found include *S. pneumoniae, H. influenzae, S. aureus,* and *Mycoplasma* species. The gastrointestinal tract is not uncommonly involved; this may be infectious (e.g., *Giardia, Campylobacter,* norovirus) or inflammatory, including lymphoid hyperplasia and forms of inflammatory bowel disease leading to malabsorption. However, a biopsy will show loss of plasma cells in the gastrointestinal mucosa. About one quarter of subjects with CVID have autoimmune conditions such as thrombocytopenia, hemolytic anemia, achlorhydria, pernicious anemia, and granulomatous disease suggesting sarcoidosis.[7] Clinically, lymphadenopathy is common, and splenomegaly is noted in 28%. Malignant disease is also increased, usually B-cell lymphomas, but other cancers appear more common as well. In the past decade, some of the gene mutations responsible for a minority of these cases have been discovered and are included in Table 250-4. However, at this time, most subjects with hypogammaglobulinemia do not have a known gene defect.

Hyperimmunoglobulin M Syndromes

The hyperimmunoglobulin M (hyper-IgM) syndromes are defects in which there is a loss of isotype switch; that is, whereas B cells do produce IgM, they do not secrete IgG or IgA. The prototypic form is the X-linked version in which an essential T-cell activation receptor, the CD40 ligand encoded on the X chromosome, is missing or nonfunctional. Mutations in the gene for its receptor partner, the CD40 on B cells, lead to a similar defect. Several

TABLE 250-4 EXAMPLES OF ANTIBODY DEFECTS

TYPE	GENES	INHERITANCE	LABORATORY FEATURES	DISEASE AND COMPLICATIONS
ABSENT B CELLS: SEVERE REDUCTIONS IN IgG, IgA, AND IgM				
X-linked agammaglobulinemia	Bruton tyrosine kinase	XL	IgG, IgA, and IgM are very low or absent	Severe bacterial infections
Autosomal forms of agammaglobulinemia	Defects of the B-cell receptor or its signaling pathways; λ5, Igα, Igβ	AR	IgG, IgA, and IgM are very low or absent	Severe bacterial infections
Good syndrome	Unknown	Unknown	Variable hypogammaglobulinemia	Associated with thymoma; may have opportunistic infections
B CELLS PRESENT BUT LOW SERUM IgG, IgA, AND/OR IgM				
Common variable immune deficiency	Unknown	Unknown	Low IgG, IgA and/or IgM	Bacterial infections and other inflammatory complications
ICOS deficiency	ICOS	AR	Low IgG, IgA and/or IgM	Recurrent infections; autoimmunity
Defects of the B-cell receptor	CD19, CD81, CD20, CD21	AR	Low IgG, IgA and/or IgM	Recurrent infections
Defects of other B-cell receptors	TACI, BAFFr, TWEAK	AD and sporadic	Variably low IgG, IgA and/or IgM; antibody defects	Recurrent infections and autoimmunity; variable clinical expression
B CELLS PRESENT: SEVERE REDUCTION IN SERUM IgG AND IgA BUT NORMAL OR ELEVATED IgM				
X-linked hyper-IgM syndrome	CD40 ligand	XL	IgG and IgA decreased; IgM may be normal or increased; B-cell numbers may be normal or increased	Bacterial and opportunistic infections, neutropenia, autoimmune disease
CD40 deficiency	CD40	AR	Low IgG and IgA; normal or increased IgM	Bacterial and opportunistic infections, neutropenia, autoimmune disease
Defects of DNA recombination	AID and UNG	AR	IgG and IgA decreased; IgM increased	Bacterial infections; enlarged lymph nodes and germinal centers
B CELLS PRESENT: ISOTYPE DEFICIENCIES				
Selective IgA deficiency	Unknown	Unknown	IgA absent	Usually asymptomatic; allergies and autoimmunity may be more common
IgA with IgG subclass deficiency	Unknown	Unknown	Reduced IgA with decrease in one or more IgG subclass	Infections in some with loss of antibody
IgG subclass deficiency	Unknown	Unknown	Reduction in one or more IgG subclass	Asymptomatic in many; infections in some with loss of antibody
B CELLS PRESENT: NORMAL IgG, IgA, AND IgM				
Antibody deficiency	Unknown	Unknown	Normal serum immunoglobulins but no vaccine responses to protein and carbohydrate antigens or vaccines	May lead to recurrent infections

AD = autosomal dominant; AR = autosomal recessive; ICOS = inducible T-cell costimulator; XL = X-linked.

other genetic defects lead to a similar immunologic phenotype, including defects of the gene for enzyme activation-induced cytidine deaminase (*AICDA*) and uracil-DNA glycosylase, both important for DNA recombination. The complications of the hyper-IgM syndromes include bacterial infections, autoimmunity, and enteropathy similar to CVID but also *P. jiroveci* pneumonia, neutropenia, and unusual cancers. A predilection to infections with *Cryptosporidium* has been noted in hyper-IgM syndromes, which unfortunately can lead to irreversible liver disease.

IgA Deficiency
Selective IgA deficiency (IgA <7 mg/dL with other isotypes normal) is the most common of the primary immunodeficiency disorders, but most subjects are asymptomatic. Lack of infections in most subjects is generally ascribed to the overlapping and compensatory role of other immune functions, but this is not clearly understood. However, allergies, autoimmunity, increased serum IgE, asthma, rheumatoid arthritis, gluten intolerance, and inflammatory bowel disease are found more commonly in selective IgA-deficient subjects than in other populations.[8] Presumably owing to the loss of secretory IgA, *Giardia* infections may occur (Chapter 351). The treatments used in subjects with IgA deficiency are based on the clinical conditions found. Some subjects with IgA deficiency are IgG2 and IgG4 deficient, with loss of antibacterial antibody leading to severe infections and, in some cases, chronic lung disease.

IgG Subclass Defects
Another variable immune deficiency is represented by the IgG subclass defects. The incidence of these is difficult to determine, partly because

laboratory normal ranges vary. The clinical consequences depend on how much antibody function is lost. Whereas there are structural differences in IgG isotypes, their functional roles have considerable overlap; thus, the importance of isotype defects can be controversial, especially if loss of antibody is not demonstrable. In adults, IgG3 deficiency appears to be the most common but is likely to have no significance. However, low IgG2 or IgG4, most often found in subjects with selective IgA deficiency, may lead to a profound deficiency of antibody production, especially to carbohydrate antigens such as contained in the pneumococcal vaccine.

Antibody Deficiency with Normal Immunoglobulins
More complex and heterogeneous is the loosely described defect termed antibody deficiency with normal serum immunoglobulins. The incidence is unknown; all ages are affected, but in general, children younger than 5 years are not included to allow transient forms of physiologic immune deficiency to resolve. Although B cells are present and there are normal levels of IgG, IgA, and IgM, these subjects do not form protective levels of serum antibodies after having an infection exposure or vaccination with protein or carbohydrate vaccines. In the most severe cases, even strong immunogens such as herpes zoster or tetanus vaccines are ineffective; in milder cases, the pneumococcal vaccine does not result in titers of antibody considered sufficient for protection.

DIAGNOSIS
The diagnosis of antibody defects is based on the laboratory tests of numbers of B cells, the serum immunoglobulin levels (IgG, IgA, and IgM), and an evaluation of a panel of vaccine responses to determine the levels of functional

antibody.[9] If B cells are absent and the levels of immunoglobulins are very low, further antibody testing is not required. For a young male with a family history of males with immune deficiency, the diagnosis of XLA or hyper-IgM can be investigated by flow cytometer (to determine numbers of B cells for XLA) or by genetic tests (hyper-IgM). For older subjects (generally older than 45 years), a thymoma may be sought by chest computed tomography, which may show a mass in the mediastinum. Most subjects with hypogammaglobulinemia will be found to have B cells in peripheral blood and some amount of serum IgG, IgA, or IgM. In these cases, the loss of functional antibody should be tested by commercial laboratories to determine if protective titers of antibody to common vaccine antigens (i.e., tetanus, diphtheria, *H. influenzae*, and pneumococci) can be detected. In some cases, revaccination may be needed to determine if a response occurs (tested again in 4 to 6 weeks). Most authorities use the laboratory-stipulated protective ranges for protein vaccines and for pneumococcal vaccination, usually 1.3 μg/mL for individual serotypes. When high levels of B cells are found in adults, the possibility of a clonal B-cell expansion should be considered (e.g., chronic lymphocytic leukemia). For subjects with IgG subclass defects or normal immunoglobulins levels, the use of a panel of antibody titers is also recommended to have a clear understanding of immune competence or immune defect.

TREATMENT Rx

The essential treatment of significant IgG antibody defects is intravenous or subcutaneous immune globulin, usually given in doses of 400 to 600 mg/kg body weight per month. The intravenous forms are usually given every 3 or 4 weeks, the subcutaneous forms weekly or biweekly, depending on body weight. Indwelling ports are not required and are discouraged. Most patients also require occasional courses of antibiotics, chosen on the basis of culture results, at intervals dictated by clinical events. Referring to Table 250-4, the defects that require IgG replacement are those in which B cells are absent (XLA, other agammaglobulinemias, the hyper-IgM syndromes, IgG subclass defects with demonstrable loss of antibody function, and some cases of loss of antibody with normal immunoglobulins). Subjects with IgA deficiency do not require immune globulin replacement unless there is clear loss of antibody. For unclear reasons, some of the antibody defects have an increased incidence of autoimmune or inflammatory complications. These require treatments commonly prescribed for immunocompetent subjects but with a view to minimizing courses of immune suppressants. Immune cytopenias may be treated with rituximab with some success; splenectomy is to be avoided. As many subjects with antibody defects have experienced one or more bouts of pneumonia, lung functions may be abnormal and intermittent or prophylactic antibiotics required, but there is no consensus on the medications, dose, or intervals to use.

PROGNOSIS

The prognosis for subjects with antibody defects is variable and depends on the degree of the defect, the response to treatment, whether organ damage has occurred, and whether other complications develop. Subjects with loss of B cells have a pure B-cell defect; when they are diagnosed and treated early with sufficient immune globulin, the prognosis appears excellent. Subjects with selective IgA deficiency can be indistinguishable from age-matched healthy peers. CVID subjects with varying degrees of hypogammaglobulinemia ranging from almost total loss of immunoglobulins to more modest reductions of IgG and IgA or IgM often have additional complications, in some cases because the diagnosis has been delayed and pulmonary or other damage has occurred. Chronic lung disease, lymphoid hyperplasia, and gastrointestinal enteropathy may be difficult to treat, leading to increased morbidity. Improved survival to prior years is likely overall in CVID, but the inflammatory complications still present additional challenges.[10] For subjects with IgG subclass defects or antibody deficiency, with immune reconstitution if required, no increased morbidity or mortality is expected.

● COMPLEMENT DISORDERS

DEFINITION

The complement system is a network of proteins that both amplify and control many actions of the immune system. It is generally considered to have three main branches, the classical, alternative, and lectin pathways; deficiencies of individual components lead to increased susceptibility to infections, autoimmunity, and inflammatory diseases (Table 250-5). For further details of these disorders, see Chapter 50.

EPIDEMIOLOGY

Complement C2 deficiency is found in 1 : 10,000 white subjects and usually in subjects with a conserved major histocompatibility complex haplotype due to a founder defect; more than 95% of C2-deficient individuals are homozygous for the same *C2* mutation. The other complement component defects are rare but found in unequal distribution in selected populations; C6 deficiency is more common in persons of African descent and C9 deficiency in Asians, with an estimated incidence of 0.036 to 0.095%. Disorders of members of these pathways are discussed here; deficiency of C1 inhibitor is discussed separately.

PATHOBIOLOGY

The classical pathway is triggered by interaction of the Fc portion of an IgG1, IgG2, IgG3, or IgM antibody with C1q, which subsequently engages C1r,

TABLE 250-5 EXAMPLES OF COMPLEMENT DEFECTS

TYPE	GENES	INHERITANCE	LABORATORY FEATURES	ALTERED FUNCTIONS	DISEASE AND COMPLICATIONS
C1q, C1r, C1s deficiency	*C1qA, C1qB, C1qC; C1r, C1s*	AR	Absent CH_{50} hemolytic activity	Loss of early complement activation; impaired dissolution of immune complexes; impaired clearance of apoptotic cells	Bacterial infections; SLE-like syndrome, rheumatoid disease, multiple autoimmune diseases, infections
C4 deficiency	*C4A* and *C4B*	AR	Absent CH_{50} hemolytic activity	Loss of early complement activation	Bacterial infections
C2 deficiency	*C2*	AR	Absent CH_{50} hemolytic activity	Loss of early complement activation	Bacterial infections; SLE-like syndrome, vasculitis, early atherosclerosis, polymyositis, glomerulonephritis
C3 deficiency	*C3*	AR	Absent CH_{50} hemolytic activity	Loss of classical and alternative pathways of complement activation	Life-threatening pyogenic infections; SLE-like disease; glomerulonephritis; atypical hemolytic-uremic syndrome
C5, C6, C7, C8 deficiency	*C5*	AR	Absent CH_{50} hemolytic activity	Loss of complement activation	Neisserial infections, SLE
C9 deficiency	*C9*	AR	Reduced CH_{50} and AP_{50} hemolytic activity	Partial loss of complement activation	Some *Neisseria* infections
C1 inhibitor deficiency	C1 inhibitor	AD	Activation of complement; low levels of C4 and C2	Loss of regulation of activities of complement C1	Angioedema

AD = autosomal dominant; AR = autosomal recessive; SLE = systemic lupus erythematosus.

C1s, C2, and C3, leading to activation of C4, C5, C6, C7, C8, C9, resulting in lysis of bacteria (discussed in Chapter 50). As opsonization of bacteria is essential for antibody function, patients with these defects have infections similar to those of subjects with loss of immunoglobulin. The alternative pathway is activated in an antibody-independent manner and involves opsonization of bacteria with subsequent involvement of C3 and the alternative pathway. The lectin pathway includes other serum binding proteins that coat bacteria or fungi, leading to downstream complement activation and the assembly of the membrane attack complex, the C7, C8, C9 components responsible for microbial lysis. The genes of the complement system are located on many chromosomes, and in general, the defects are autosomal recessive in inheritance, with one exception, defects of X-linked properdin. In addition to the three pathways of activation, the complement system also includes an even larger number of control proteins that, when genetically defective, also lead to severe infections, hemolytic-uremic syndrome, severe eclampsia, glomerulonephritis, thrombosis, and macular degeneration, which are outside the scope of this chapter.

CLINICAL MANIFESTATIONS

With genetic loss of the classical and alternative pathways, severe bacterial infections are likely; this is particularly true of subjects with defects of C3, which lies at the convergence of the three pathways. For unclear reasons, with loss of C6, C7, C8, and C9 or properdin, *Neisseria gonorrhoeae* or *Neisseria meningitidis* infections are more common. More complex but equally potent is the role that the complement proteins play in immune regulation. With loss of the early components of the classical system, C1q, C1r , C1s, C2, and C4, autoimmunity, especially systemic lupus erythematosus, is common; this complication is estimated at 93% for subjects with defects of C1q and 75% for defects of C4. Complement is important for clearing immune complexes and possibly apoptotic cells, potentially explaining this observation.

DIAGNOSIS

Deficiencies of complement are diagnosed by testing total serum hemolytic complement (CH_{50}) and the alternative hemolytic complement (AP_{50}). The CH_{50} tests for deficiencies in the classical pathway by determining whether the patient's serum can lyse antibody-coated sheep erythrocytes; this will be zero if the proteins of the classical pathway are defective. The AP_{50} tests for alternative pathway activity. Further testing usually includes measurement and function of individual serum complement proteins to determine the most applicable diagnosis. (Note that the most common reason for low levels in CH_{50} and AP_{50} is improper blood handling.)

TREATMENT   Rx

There are no treatments for complement deficiencies. Whereas loss of these classical components may lead to severe clinical consequences, for C2 in particular but also for C4 and C5-C9, there may be no history of illness. Prompt antibiotic therapy for acute infections and control of autoimmunity are the important therapeutics. However, periodic immunizations with pneumococcal, *H. influenzae*, and meningococcal vaccines may be helpful to boost antibody titers to enhance bacterial clearance.

PROGNOSIS

The prognosis of complement defects is highly variable because of the clinical complications; also, most of these defects have been found in healthy subjects. However, for defects of the classical pathway, prompt recognition and treatment of bacterial infections and possibly preemptive vaccination with appropriate vaccines would be important. The prognosis for subjects with autoimmunity will depend on disease manifestation and response to treatment. Whereas C2 deficiency is commonly viewed as usually asymptomatic, some data suggest a higher incidence of premature arteriosclerotic heart disease.

C1 INHIBITOR DEFICIENCY

DEFINITION

C1inhibitor (C1 INH) deficiency is discussed in detail in Chapter 252. It is classified as either genetic or acquired. The genetic form is called hereditary angioedema (HAE), due to mutations of C1 INH, inherited as an autosomal dominant trait. However, approximately 25% of patients with HAE have a

spontaneous mutation in C1 INH, with no family history. C1 INH defects are classified as type I, due to loss of C1 INH protein, or type II, in which the protein is present but nonfunctional. Another inherited, estrogen-dependent form of HAE due to mutations in factor XII has also been recognized. The acquired form of C1 INH deficiency may be due to interfering autoantibodies and often clinically resembles the genetic forms, except that it usually is manifested later in life.

PATHOBIOLOGY AND GENETICS

Defects of C1 INH are inherited as autosomal dominant traits, but the outcome in families may vary considerably, from no angioedema in some members to frequent episodes in others. The C1 INH protein is the main regulator of the early activation steps of the classical complement pathway. It binds to and inactivates C1r and C1s in the C1 complex of the classical pathway, and when insufficient amounts are present, the classical pathway can be activated. C1 INH protein also inhibits proteases in the bradykinin pathways, increasing bradykinin production and leading to angioedema. With loss of C1 INH activity, fluid leaks from the vascular endothelium, leading to localized edema.

CLINICAL MANIFESTATIONS

A diagnosis of C1 INH deficiency is suggested by a history of recurrent attacks of angioedema or in some cases (25%) episodes of recurrent abdominal pain due to edema. The edema is nonpitting, nonpruritic, and localized to one regional area, such as the lips and mouth, hands, genitals, or abdomen, leading to concern for acute colitis or appendicitis. The presence of urticaria with angioedema suggests an IgE-mediated process and is not typical. As these defects are inherited as autosomal dominant defects, a family history is likely but not always identified. The hereditary forms usually become clinically apparent in early adolescence, but angioedema may occur before or after, with the first episode appearing first in adult life. Attacks may be preceded by "prodromes" of erythema, nausea, or a tingling sensation. Although the cause of an attack onset may often be unpredictable, there are certain triggers of HAE, including dental work, accidents, surgery, emotional stress, and infection. Unlike allergic angioedema, angioedema from C1 INH deficiency does not respond to treatment with antihistamines or corticosteroids and resolves slowly during 3 to 5 days. Selected medications (estrogen and angiotensin-converting enzyme inhibitors) can exacerbate or cause attacks and are to be avoided.

DIAGNOSIS

The diagnosis is suggested by a low serum C4 level. In HAE I, there is low C1 INH protein; in HAE II, there is normal C1 INH protein but a low function. The acquired form is suggested by a decreased C4 level, low C1 INH protein and function, and decreased C1q. A diagnosis of this form should prompt further evaluation of an underlying malignant or autoimmune disease. Blood tests for either HAE or the acquired form should be repeated to confirm the diagnosis because falsely low C1 INH function levels may result from improper handling of blood.

TREATMENT   Rx

The treatment of hereditary C1 INH deficiency includes management of the attacks and prophylaxis against angioedema. These are described in Chapter 252.

PHAGOCYTE DEFECTS

DEFINITION

Abnormalities of the phagocytic system are presented in detail in Chapters 167 and 169. They are categorized as neutropenia, abnormal neutrophil morphology, defective cell adhesion and migration, or defective microbial killing. Neutropenia (Chapter 167) is defined as counts of less than 1000×10^9/L.

EPIDEMIOLOGY

Whereas neutropenia is a common laboratory finding (due to conditions described in Chapter 167), genetic defects impairing neutrophil development, adhesion, locomotion, or intracellular killing are rare. The most common is chronic granulomatous disease (CGD), with an estimated incidence of 1 : 100,000 to 1 : 200,000.

PATHOBIOLOGY AND GENETICS

Circulating neutrophils are attracted to sites of inflammation by complement components C5a, chemokines, and bacterial byproducts, but traveling to these sites requires migration through capillaries and into tissues. The best known diseases in which neutrophil adhesion is impaired are the leukocyte adhesion defects (LAD types 1, 2, and 3), discussed in Chapter 169. Other defects of neutrophil motility include juvenile periodontitis, Shwachman-Diamond syndrome, and the Chédiak-Higashi syndrome.

About two thirds of patients with CGD are males as they have defects in an X-linked gene encoding $gp91^{phox}$. Autosomal defects in $p47^{phox}$ are the next most common form, occurring in 20% of patients and often due to the same deletion. Other autosomal forms are due to defects in the gene encoding the $p22^{phox}$ or $p67^{phox}$ subunits (about 5% each).

CLINICAL MANIFESTATIONS

The genetic neutrophil disorders have specific clinical associations: delayed separation of the umbilical cord and poor wound healing in LAD-1; growth delay, mental retardation, and Bombay blood group in LAD-2; peripheral nerve conduction defects, pigmentary dilution with partial oculocutaneous albinism, easy bruising, and risk of hemophagocytic disease in Chédiak-Higashi syndrome; and pancreatic insufficiency (fat malabsorption), growth failure, and skeletal abnormalities in Shwachman-Diamond syndrome. For both Shwachman-Diamond syndrome and the severe congenital neutropenias, there is a risk for development of myelodysplastic disease and leukemia.

The clinical manifestations of CGD usually include bacterial or fungal infections. Males with the X-linked form will generally present in the first decade of life, whereas subjects with autosomal forms may have a later onset of symptoms (into the second decade). Regardless of the genetic cause, most patients with CGD will have one or more episodes of pneumonia; the most common causes of infection are *Staphylococcus, Burkholderia cepacia, Klebsiella, Aspergillus, Serratia,* and *Nocardia* species. Common clinical manifestations include acute or chronic lymphadenitis, colitis leading to recurrent diarrhea, *Staphylococus* liver abscess, osteomyelitis, and rectal abscess. Patients with CGD are also prone to infections with unusual organisms, for example, *Chromobacterium violaceum, Trichosporon inkin, Francisella philomiragia,* and *Granulibacter bethesdensis.* For this reason, exposure to contaminated water or decaying plant material (compost, mulch) presents significant risk to subjects with CGD.

DIAGNOSIS

The differential diagnosis of neutropenia is presented in Table 167-4; the genetic diagnosis of congenital neutropenia syndromes, in Table 167-5; and a diagnostic approach to suspected phagocyte defects, in Figure 169-4.

TREATMENT

The management of patients with neutropenia is discussed in Chapter 167. The treatment of CGD is summarized in Chapter 169.

WELL-DEFINED DEFECTS WITH SYNDROMIC FEATURES

Another group of primary immune defects are those that have distinctive systemic characteristics, aside from the obvious abnormities in the immune system (Table 250-6). The best known of these are the Wiskott-Aldrich syndrome, ataxia-telangiectasia, DiGeorge syndrome, hyperimmunoglobulin E (Buckley-Job) syndrome, and cartilage-hair hypoplasia. As these are distinct from each other, they are discussed separately.

Wiskott-Aldrich Syndrome

DEFINITION AND EPIDEMIOLOGY

Wiskott-Aldrich syndrome (WAS) is a rare X-linked recessive disease characterized by eczema, thrombocytopenia, and immune deficiency. WAS is rare, estimated as 1 and 10 cases per million males. Ethnic differences are not known.

PATHOBIOLOGY AND CLINICAL MANIFESTATIONS

WAS is inherited as an X-linked disease, and the main manifestations in early childhood include eczema, chronic thrombocytopenia sometimes leading to bloody diarrhea, and immune deficiency with recurrent infections.[11] Not uncommonly, autoimmunity or inflammatory disease including autoimmune hemolytic anemia, splenomegaly, arthritis, inflammatory bowel disease, and vasculitis appear. There is a clear increase in the incidence of lymphoma in WAS. The syndrome is caused by mutations in the *WAS* gene, which codes for the protein called WASP, an intracellular cytoplasmic scaffold protein important for the activation and mobility of all blood cells. WASP is involved in actin polymerization and in establishing an interface between immune cells (the immune synapse). Partly depending on the location of the

---

TABLE 250-6 WELL-DEFINED DEFECTS OF IMMUNITY WITH SYNDROMIC FEATURES

TYPE	GENES	INHERITANCE	LABORATORY FEATURES	ALTERED FUNCTIONS	DISEASE AND COMPLICATIONS
Wiskott-Aldrich syndrome	*WAS*	XL	Thrombocytopenia, small platelets	Impaired cell activation, mobility	Eczema; lymphoma; autoimmune disease; bacterial and viral infections
Ataxia-telangiectasia	*ATM*	AR	Some have IgA deficiency; IgG defects, lymphopenia in some	Impaired DNA double-stranded break repair	Ataxia; telangiectasia; pulmonary infections; lymphoreticular and other malignant neoplasms; increased α-fetoprotein; x-ray sensitivity
DiGeorge anomaly	22q11.2 deletion; rarely a deletion in 10p	De novo (majority) or AD	Lymphopenia; low T-cell numbers; large deletion in chromosome 22 on fluorescence in situ hybridization	Impaired T-cell immunity	Cardiac abnormalities; hypoparathyroidism, abnormal facies
Hyper-IgE syndrome (Buckley-Job syndrome)	*STAT3*	AD, de novo	Eosinophilia, high IgE	Loss of normal cytokine activation, defective IL-17	Bacterial infections; eczema, distinctive facial features, osteoporosis , fractures, scoliosis, delay of shedding primary teeth, hyperextensible joints, candidiasis
Cartilage-hair hypoplasia	*RMRP*	AR	Lymphopenia, low T-cell numbers	Impaired processing of mitochondrial RNA	Short-limbed dwarfism, sparse hair, celiac disease, Hirschsprung disease, bone marrow failure, autoimmunity, susceptibility to lymphoma

AD = autosomal dominant; AR = autosomal recessive; IL = interleukin; XL = X-linked.

mutation in the *WAS* gene, milder versions are known, leading to X-linked thrombocytopenia in some cohorts. Another, much rarer version leads to X-linked neutropenia.

DIAGNOSIS

The diagnosis is commonly made in the first few years of life in males with the characteristic symptoms of eczema with thrombocytopenia leading to petechiae. Typically, IgM levels are low, whereas IgA (and sometimes IgE) levels are increased. Platelet sizes are smaller than normal, and clot retraction is poor. Family history may include male relatives with WAS or thrombocytopenia. The diagnosis can be suggested by lack of the WAS protein as detected by flow cytometry in reference laboratories, but definitive diagnosis requires gene testing.

TREATMENT   Rx

Treatment strategies in WAS are diverse and usually considered on a case-by-case basis. Conservative management includes prophylactic antibiotics, immunization with conjugated polysaccharide vaccines, and intravenous or subcutaneous immune goblin for subjects with repeated infections. For eczema, standard measures are used (Chapter 438). For significant thrombocytopenia (Chapter 172), splenectomy has been performed but is discouraged as lifelong post-splenectomy sepsis poses a significant risk. For these subjects, lifelong antibiotic prophylaxis is mandatory. Platelet transfusions should be reserved for active bleeding that cannot be managed with usual methods (e.g., aminocaproic acid) and avoided for subjects for whom transplantation is considered. Autoimmunity can be difficult to control, and immune suppression should be used with caution. Treatment of lymphomas is by standard regimens (Chapter 185). Definitive treatment is by HSCT, which has proved successful in many subjects. Trials with gene therapy are also ongoing.

PROGNOSIS

The prognosis in WAS is highly heterogeneous. Some have mild thrombocytopenia leading to occasional nose bleeds, whereas other subjects have inflammatory disease or other complications that require additional, sometimes intensive medical management. HSCT (Chapter 178) offers a cure, but this is best done early and requires careful matching and standard protocols.

Ataxia-Telangiectasia

DEFINITION AND EPIDEMIOLOGY

Ataxia-telangiectasia (AT) is a rare neurodegenerative disease that leads to cerebellar atrophy, skin telangiectasia, and immune defects. AT is estimated to occur in 1 in 40,000 to 100,000 but is more common in selected isolated populations. Sexes are affected equally.

PATHOBIOLOGY

AT is due to recessive mutations in the gene that encodes the ATM protein, important in both cell division and DNA repair. With the loss of the ATM protein, DNA breakage cannot be repaired, leading to cell death.

CLINICAL MANIFESTATIONS

The clinical manifestations include progressive difficulty in walking, with ataxia beginning around the age of 5 years. Skin telangiectasias develop on the bulbar conjunctiva and behind the ears. The immune defects include IgA deficiency, IgG subclass defects, and cellular defects leading to recurring pulmonary infections and lung damage in some. Subjects with AT have radiosensitivity, and the development of lymphomas is common with increasing age.

DIAGNOSIS

The diagnosis can usually be made by the characteristic clinical phenotype, coupled with an increase in α-fetoprotein in the blood. Radiosensitivity can be assessed in vitro in fibroblast cell lines. Definitive diagnosis is by *ATM* gene sequencing.

TREATMENT AND PROGNOSIS   Rx

Treatment for AT includes supportive measures and physical therapy as needed. The life expectancy for subjects with AT varies greatly, but most live into early adulthood.

DiGeorge Syndrome

DEFINITION AND EPIDEMIOLOGY

DiGeorge syndrome is an autosomal dominant defect and one of the members of the 22q11.2 deletion syndrome that includes velocardiofacial syndrome, conotruncal anomaly face syndrome, congenital thymic aplasia, and thymic hypoplasia. DiGeorge syndrome is one of the most common of the immune defects, estimated at 1 : 4000. Sexes are affected equally.

PATHOBIOLOGY AND CLINICAL MANIFESTATIONS

Although it is classified as an immune defect because of thymic hypoplasia or aplasia, patients with DiGeorge syndrome are likely also to have congenital heart disease, cleft palate or pharyngeal closure defects, characteristic facies, hypocalcemia due to parathyroid insufficiency, and learning disability. The more common cardiac defects include tetralogy of Fallot, interrupted aortic arch, ventricular septal defects, vascular rings, and anomalous return of brachial arteries. The mnemonic CATCH-22 has been applied: cardiac issues, abnormal facies, thymic aplasia, cleft palate, and hypocalcemia. With loss of thymic tissue, cellular immunity is mildly to moderately impaired, leading to recurrent infections. Hypogammaglobulinemia is not uncommon and may be associated with autoimmune cytopenias, especially thrombocytopenia.[12]

DIAGNOSIS

The diagnosis of DiGeorge syndrome for most patients is based on the genetic test fluorescence in situ hybridization, which detects the loss of the 22q11.2 gene segment or, more rarely, a loss of 10p14-p13. However, about 10% do not have a gene defect but have the syndrome due to maternal diabetes, fetal alcohol syndrome, or prenatal exposure to isotretinoin (Accutane).

TREATMENT

Treatment of DiGeorge syndrome is based on individual need and may require cardiac surgery, cleft palate repair, and calcium and vitamin D supplementation if hypocalcemia is found. Some subjects are hypothyroid, requiring thyroid supplementation. The immune defect in DiGeorge syndrome varies widely, from complete loss of thymic development with no circulating T cells to normal T-cell numbers. For most, the thymus is hypoplastic, and whereas the level of T cells may be subnormal for age, sufficient T-cell function remains and no specific treatment is needed. Withholding of live viral vaccines may not be necessary as reports of ill effects are rare and the protection afforded is likely to outweigh any risk . For complete loss of the thymus, thymic transplantation, HSCT, or, for some, infusion of HLA-matched peripheral T cells can supply sufficient reconstitution.

PROGNOSIS

For most subjects, the prognosis depends on the concomitant medical issues, such as results of cardiac surgery, surgical repair of cleft palate, management of swallowing difficulties, and resources to enhance muscle strength and to overcome speech impediments and learning disabilities. For most, the T-cell defect is a minor component and a normal lifespan is likely; but with age, autoimmunity may become more prominent.

Hyperimmunoglobulin E Syndrome

DEFINITION

Hyperimmunoglobulin E syndrome (HIES), also called Buckley-Job syndrome, is an immune deficiency syndrome characterized by eczema, skin and lung abscesses, hyperextensible joints and recurrent bone fractures, distinctive coarse facies, eosinophilia, and high levels of serum IgE.

PATHOBIOLOGY AND CLINICAL MANIFESTATIONS

Most but not all patients with HIES have an autosomal dominant defect in the gene *STAT3* encoding a transcription factor, signal transducer and activator of transcription 3. After activation by selected cytokines and growth factors, STAT3 protein is phosphorylated and translocated to the cell nucleus. Whereas loss of STAT3 signaling affects many cellular processes, the syndrome itself is often clinically recognizable from the characteristic clinical findings of eczema, recurrent skin boils, unusual facies with tubular nose, cyst-forming pneumonias often due to *S. aureus*, and increased serum IgE. Other common manifestations include a rash in the newborn period; mucocutaneous candidiasis; and skeletal abnormalities, such as scoliosis, osteoporosis, fractures with minimal trauma, and delayed shedding of primary teeth.

Features of the HIES syndrome have been found in a few patients with rare autosomal recessive defects in genes encoding tyrosine kinase 2 (Tyk2) and dedicator of cytokinesis 8 (DOCK8), but in both of these, viral infections are also prominent.

DIAGNOSIS

The diagnosis can be strongly suspected on clinical grounds, but a useful scoring system composed of a composite of laboratory and clinical characteristics has been shown to aid in the dissection of hyperimmunoglobulin E subjects from other subjects with high serum IgE levels, for example, severely atopic subjects. IgE levels may range from 1000 to 40,000 IU or more; some references note that IgE levels may normalize in older subjects. Eosinophilia is common. However, a definitive diagnosis is best confirmed by identifying a *STAT3* mutation.

TREATMENT Rx

There is no definitive treatment for HIES syndrome. Because of the propensity for staphylococcal infections, prophylaxis with appropriate antibiotics (trimethoprim-sulfamethoxazole, 5 mg/kg/day trimethoprim divided twice daily) is commonly used, along with oral antifungals such as itraconazole, 100 mg daily for patients aged <13 years or weighing <50 kg; 200 mg daily for those aged >13 years or weighing >50 kg. Surgical drainage of abscesses is also important, but wound healing may be poor. Skin care for eczema may include bleach baths to reduce bacterial burden and antihistamines to control pruritus. Optimization of calcium and vitamin D levels may be useful to strengthen bones.

PROGNOSIS

HIES is a lifelong disease, and infections or complications require individual care. With increasing age, increased respiratory dysfunction is likely. Recent reports note vascular, especially arterial, abnormalities, which are important to define.

Cartilage-Hair Hypoplasia

DEFINITION AND EPIDEMIOLOGY

Cartilage-hair hypoplasia (CHH) is a rare autosomal recessive form of short-limbed dwarfism associated with a variable cellular immune deficiency. In the Old Order Amish population, CHH affects 1 in 1300 newborns; for those of Finnish descent, the incidence is about 1 in 20,000. A common point mutation in the gene is prevalent in the particularly affected populations.

PATHOBIOLOGY AND CLINICAL MANIFESTATIONS

The genetic defect in CHH is in the *RMRP* gene, which encodes the RNA in a mitochondrial RNA-processing endoribonuclease that helps copy mitochondrial DNA and process ribosomal RNA. In CHH, the encoded RNA is unstable, leading to skeletal dysplasia, sparse hair, and the predominantly T-cell deficiency disease. For unclear reasons, the cellular defect is varied, ranging from mildly impaired immunity to severe defects requiring HSCT. Other clinical features of CHH include short stature, anemia, autoimmunity, celiac disease, Hirschsprung disease, and several cancers including lymphoma.

DIAGNOSIS

The diagnosis can be suspected by inheritance patterns and clinical phenotype, but definitive diagnosis is made by genetic sequencing of the *RMRP* gene.

TREATMENT AND PROGNOSIS Rx

For patients with severe T-cell defects and infections (essentially SCID phenotype) suggesting a significantly impaired immune system, HSCT is required. Aside from the cellular defect, treatment is directed at the other presenting clinical issues. The prognosis of CHH is varied, and the prognosis depends on the depth of the cellular defect, the therapies required, and the associated clinical complications. As the defect is so variable, normal lifespans may be achieved.

IMMUNE DYSREGULATION SYNDROMES

Clustered into a separate set of immunodeficiency diseases are syndromes that have immune dysregulation as a main theme. These mostly monogenic diseases have in common lymphoid proliferation, immune activation, and inflammatory or autoimmune complications. These include the hemophagocytic lymphohistiocytosis (HLH) diseases (Chapter 169), the lymphoproliferative syndromes linked to Epstein-Barr virus (EBV) infection, autoimmune polyendocrinopathy–candidiasis–ectodermal dystrophy (APECED), autoimmune lymphoproliferative syndromes (ALPS), and defects of T-regulatory cells (Table 250-7).

EPIDEMIOLOGY

The estimated incidence of the genetic HLH syndromes is 1 : 50,000; the incidence of X-linked lymphoproliferative disease is 1 to 3 in 1,000,000; and the incidence of APECED is high in Finland (1 in 25,000) and in Sardinians and Iranian Jews (1 in 9000) but otherwise much rarer. The incidence of ALPS and defects of T-regulatory cells is unknown.

PATHOBIOLOGY AND CLINICAL MANIFESTATIONS

HLH is a form of extreme and potentially life-threatening immune activation. It is further discussed under the section Hemophagocytic Lymphohistiocytosis and Macrophage Activation Syndrome in Chapter 169. There are two forms: genetic, due to mutations in genes that control cellular cytotoxicity; and secondary, due to acute viral illnesses, autoimmune activation, or underlying malignant disease.[13] The familial form is a heterogeneous autosomal recessive disorder due to mutations in one of five genes essential for control of T-cell cytotoxicity. Immune activation leads to expansion of poorly controlled cytotoxic T cells and macrophages, leading to the release of interferon (IFN)-γ, IL-1, IL-6, and IL-10. Patients have high fevers, cytopenias, liver dysfunction, coagulopathy, and sometimes neurologic symptoms. HLH may be fatal unless it is treated with aggressive measures and may require HSCT. Life-threatening accelerated immune activation syndromes are also characteristic of other genetic defects that impair cytotoxicity, such as the Chédiak-Higashi syndrome.

Monogenic defects leading to impaired immunity to EBV produce another group of immune dysregulation syndromes. The first described (and the most common, 70 to 80%) is the X-linked proliferative disorder (XLP) due to mutations of the X-linked gene *SH2D1A*, which encodes the gene *SAP*, a signaling lymphocytic activation molecule (SLAM)–associated protein. Other genetic causes for loss of control of EBV are due to mutations in *XIAP* (20 to 30%) or, rarely, *ITK* and *CD27*. XLP and *XIAP* are on the X chromosome; the other defects are inherited as autosomal recessive traits. In each case, infection with EBV leads to an acute illness with lymphoproliferation, progressive but variable hypogammaglobulinemia, and lymphoma in *XLP*, *ITP*, and *CD27* defects. A unifying theme of these syndromes is loss of function of NK-T cells, a subset of T cells important in viral immunity.

A unique member of the genetic immune dysregulation diseases is APECED or autoimmune polyglandular syndrome type 1 (Chapter 231). Whereas the clinical presentation is usually due to endocrine disease (hypoparathyroidism, Addison disease, hypogonadism, and secondary amenorrhea), the disease is caused by loss of thymic recognition of self-antigens due to mutations in the autoimmune regulator gene (*AIRE*).[14] Chronic mucocutaneous candidiasis is common, probably due to circulating anticytokine antibodies (interferon and IL-17). The transcription factor encoded by the *AIRE* gene, found in thymic epithelial cells, is involved in the early negative selection of cells with autoimmune potential. Clinically, cutaneous candidiasis or the endocrine defect may be the first sign of the syndrome; for unclear reasons, chronic diarrhea with malabsorption is also common. Other autoimmune complications may include hepatitis, alopecia, vitiligo, diabetes mellitus, anemia, and pernicious anemia.

Defects in lymphocyte apoptosis lead to another form of immune dysregulation; in these subjects, because of impaired death of lymphocytes, lymph nodes and spleen enlarge and autoimmunity, especially thrombocytopenia and hemolytic anemia, occur. Together, these are commonly referred to as ALPS. The most common of these defects are due to autosomal dominant mutations in the *FAS* gene, which encodes the important FAS death receptor, and less commonly in FAS ligand. Both are dominant but have variable penetrance. Much less common forms of autoimmune lymphoproliferation are due to mutations in caspase 10 or even more rarely the oncogenes *KRAS* and *NRAS* or protein kinase Cδ.[15]

TABLE 250-7 DISEASES OF IMMUNE DYSREGULATION

TYPE	GENES	INHERITANCE	LABORATORY FEATURES	ALTERED FUNCTION	DISEASE AND COMPLICATIONS
Familial hemophagocytic lymphohistiocytosis syndromes	PRF1, UNC13D, STX11, and STXBP2	AR	Anemia, neutropenia, thrombocytopenia, abnormal liver functions, high ferritin and serum IL-2 receptor, hemophagocytosis in bone marrow and liver	Decreased to absent NK cells and cytotoxic activities	Fever, hepatosplenomegaly, cytopenias, hemophagocytic lymphohistiocytosis, neurologic disease in some
Chédiak-Higashi syndrome	LYST	AR	Neutrophils with giant inclusions; hair: pigment clumps	Impaired chemotaxis	Partial albinism, recurrent infections, late-onset primary encephalopathy, increased lymphoma risk
Lymphoproliferative syndromes	SAP, XIAP (ITK, CD27)	XL, AR	Epstein-Barr virus infection; decreased NK cells and CD8+ CTL activation; deficient NK-T cells; anemia; hypogammaglobulinemia in some	Loss of function of NK-T cells leading to impaired viral control	Clinical and immunologic features triggered by Epstein-Barr virus infection; lymphoproliferation, lymphoma
Autoimmune polyendocrinopathy–candidiasis–ectodermal dystrophy	AIRE	AR	Endocrine dysfunction; hepatitis	Loss of thymic self-tolerance	Autoimmunity leading to hypoparathyroidism, hypothyroidism, diabetes, adrenal and gonadal dysfunction; cutaneous candidiasis; hepatitis
Autoimmune lymphoproliferative syndrome	FAS, FAS ligand; (caspase 10; KRAS; NRAS; protein kinase Cδ)	AD	Increased double-negative T cells (CD4⁻/CD8⁻), increased serum B₁₂	Defects in lymphocyte apoptosis	Splenomegaly, lymphadenopathy, autoimmune cytopenias; increased risk of lymphoma
Genetic defects of T-regulatory cells	FOXP3 (CD25, STAT5B and ITCH, STAT1)	XL, AR	Diabetes, anemia, eosinophilia, high serum IgE, hyperglobulinemia, loss of FOXP3 expression in the XL form	Lack of (or impaired function of) CD4+, CD25+, FOXP3+ regulatory T cells (Tregs)	Enteropathy, dermatitis, eczema, early-onset diabetes, thyroiditis, hemolytic anemia, thrombocytopenia, elevated IgE and IgA

AD = autosomal dominant; AR = autosomal recessive; CTL = cytotoxic T lymphocyte; IL = interleukin; XL = X-linked.

The defects of T-regulatory cells are the final member of this set of genetic defects leading to loss of regulation.[16] The first to be described was the immune dysregulation, polyendocrinopathy, enteropathy, X-linked (IPEX) syndrome, a generally lethal disease in males, characterized by early-onset insulin-dependent diabetes mellitus, enteropathy with severe diarrhea, and eczema-like dermatitis. Other manifestations include anemia, thrombocytopenia, and neutropenia as well as liver or kidney autoimmune disease. The defect is generally due to mutations of the X chromosome forkhead box protein 3 (FOXP3) gene, a gene essential for the development of regulatory T cells. However, other genetic defects may lead to a similar clinical syndrome.[16]

DIAGNOSIS

The diagnosis of these syndromes may be suspected from the clinical manifestations, family history, and laboratory grounds, but genetic validation is required for definitive diagnosis.

TREATMENT   Rx

For the HLH diseases and related syndromes, prompt immune suppression by established protocols and intense supportive care are necessary. For the genetic forms, HSCT is often required. The lymphoproliferative syndromes associated with EBV are similar in that prompt supportive care is required and transplantation is potentially curative. Rituximab has been used in these defects to reduce B-cell numbers and EBV burden if infection occurs. Treatment of the cytopenias in ALPS includes corticosteroids, rapamycin, and other agents. For unclear reasons, rituximab may lead to permanent hypogammaglobulinemia in ALPS, and splenectomy is to be avoided. Patients with APECED usually require endocrine and possibly nutritional management as well as treatment for cutaneous candidiasis. For the defects of T-regulatory cells due to mutations in IPEX, HSCT is the only curative measure.

PROGNOSIS

The diseases of immune dysregulation have a varied prognosis. For the genetic HLH syndromes, EBV-related lymphoproliferative diseases, and IPEX, immune reconstitution is required. Because of the broad spectrum of manifestations for ALPS and APECED, management of the clinical issues may be sufficient.

DEFECTS OF INNATE IMMUNITY THAT LEAD TO SELECTED INFECTIONS

DEFINITION

As opposed to the adaptive immune system (in which a previous exposure is required to form immune memory; Chapter 46), many components of the immune system function quickly with no pre-exposure. These components of the innate immune system (Chapter 45) include, for example, complement, phagocytic cells, and natural killer cells. Screening of large populations for selected microbial diseases has revealed a number of novel defects of innate immunity. Some of these defects are discussed here (Table 250-8).

PATHOBIOLOGY AND CLINICAL MANIFESTATIONS

Innate defects appear to be rare and the incidence is not known. One of the first recognized was anhidrotic ectodermal dysplasia with immunodeficiency, a syndrome due to mutations in the IKBKG gene that encodes nuclear factor κB (NF-κB) essential modulator (NEMO). This is an X-linked disease and was first assigned to the category of hyper-IgM syndromes. However, the actual phenotype is broad due to impairment of NEMO, which is essential for both cytokine and toll-like receptor signaling pathways. Impairment in this gene leads to severe bacterial infections and mycobacterial disease as well as to the characteristics of ectodermal dysplasia: sparse hair, abnormal tooth development, and lack of sweat glands. After NEMO defects were recognized, a series of other genetic defects in toll-like receptors and their signaling

TABLE 250-8 EXAMPLES OF DISEASES OF INNATE IMMUNITY

DISEASE	GENES	INHERITANCE	LABORATORY FEATURES	ALTERED FUNCTION	ASSOCIATED FEATURES
Anhidrotic ectodermal dysplasia with immunodeficiency	NEMO (IKBKG), IKBA	XL, AD	Variable hypogammaglobulinemia for NEMO with increased IgM in some; lack of antibody response to polysaccharides	Defective NF-κB signaling pathway	Bacterial and mycobacterial infections Ectodermal dysplasia, hair loss, heat intolerance due to loss of sweat glands Tooth abnormalities
IRAK4 deficiency	IRAK4	AR	Impaired cytokine responses to toll receptor activators	Defective TIR-IRAK signaling pathway	Bacterial infections, especially Staphylococcus and S. pneumoniae
MyD88 deficiency	MYD88	AR	Impaired cytokine responses to toll receptor activators	Defective TIR-MyD88 signaling pathway	Bacterial infections, especially Staphylococcus and S. pneumoniae
Herpes simplex encephalitis	TLR3 UNC93B1 TRAF3	AD AR	Impaired cytokine responses to TLR3 activators	Defective IFN-α, IFN-β, and IFN-γ induction	Herpes simplex virus 1 encephalitis
Predisposition to fungal diseases	CARD9	AR	Fungal cultures positive	Defective CARD9 signaling pathway	Invasive candidiasis and other fungal diseases
Chronic mucocutaneous candidiasis	IL17RA IL17F STAT1	AR, AD	Fungal cultures positive	Defective IL-17R signaling pathways	Mucocutaneous candidiasis
IL-12, IL-23 receptor deficiency	IL12RB IL12 IL23	AR	Mycobacterial cultures positive	Defective cytokine receptor binding and signaling	Mycobacterial and salmonella infections
IFN-γ receptors 1 and 2 deficiency	IFNGR1 IFNGR2	AR	Mycobacterial cultures positive	Defective IFN-γ binding and signaling	Mycobacterial and salmonella infections
GATA2 deficiency	GATA2	AR, AD	Multilineage cytopenias; very low monocyte numbers		Infections with mycobacteria, papillomaviruses, histoplasmosis, alveolar proteinosis, but also myelodysplasia and leukemias

AD = autosomal dominant; AR = autosomal recessive; IFN = interferon; IL = interleukin; IL-17R = interleukin-17 receptor; NF-κB = nuclear factor-κB; TIR = intracytoplasmic Toll and IL-1 receptor; TLR = toll-like receptor; XL = X-linked.

pathways have been recognized, for example, autosomal recessive defects in IRAK4 and MyD88, both of which lead to severe pneumococcal and staphylococcal infections. In contrast, effects of the TLR3 pathway lead to early herpes simplex encephalitis. Much more clinically heterogeneous are the genetic defects that lead to chronic mucocutaneous candidiasis. These defects may be autosomal dominant or recessive and lead to simple onychomycosis in some to invasive fungal infections in others. Patients of any age may have defects in these pathways. The pathogenesis of some of these includes genes that disrupt the dectin-1 pathway. Dectin-1 is a surface lectin receptor that recognizes the β1-3 glucan of fungi; downstream mutations in CARD9 impair the secretion of IL-17A, IL-17F, and IL-22, cytokines that are essential in fungal clearance.[17]

A separate and unique category of innate defects are the cytokine/receptor mutations that impair the functions of cytokines IL-12, IL-23, and IFN-γ, which are needed for control of mycobacterial and other intracellular infections, such as salmonella. Chronic mycobacterial infections may also occur in patients with autosomal recessive mutations in the gene for signal transducer and activator of transcription 1 (STAT1), a gene downstream of both IFN-γ and IFN-α receptors. However, as the functions of both cytokines are impaired, these patients may also have severe viral or fungal infections. On the other hand, dominant (activating) mutations in STAT1 may lead to simple cutaneous candidiasis or more complex clinical outcomes in others. More complex is the syndrome of GATA2 deficiency, in which mycobacterial disease may also develop, but other organisms (papillomaviruses, fungi) and serious complications (cytopenias, myelodysplasia, pulmonary alveolar proteinosis, peripheral edema) may be foremost. Whereas GATA2 defects are dominantly inherited, members of the same family with the same mutations may have very different clinical manifestations.

DIAGNOSIS

The diagnosis of innate defects is first based on exclusion of other causes and then confirmed by genetic testing. The family history may be helpful, but for patients with mutations in STAT1 or GATA2, although dominant inheritance is likely, the extreme range of clinical phenotypes may obscure easy recognition.

TREATMENT AND PROGNOSIS   Rx

The treatment of innate defects includes antimicrobial therapy to clear active infections and, probably, relevant prophylactic therapy on an ongoing basis. For the more severe defects, HSCT is required.

GENERAL REFERENCES

For the General References and other additional features, please visit Expert Consult at https://expertconsult.inkling.com.

251

ALLERGIC RHINITIS AND CHRONIC SINUSITIS

LARRY BORISH

ALLERGIC RHINITIS

Allergic rhinitis (AR) refers to the nasal and ocular symptoms that result from an inflammatory hypersensitivity reaction to aeroallergens deposited on the nasal mucosa and conjunctiva.

EPIDEMIOLOGY

AR, the most common chronic disease in the United States, affects between 10 and 30% of adults and up to 40% of children. Each year, nearly 80 million people in the United States experience 7 days or more of nasal or ocular symptoms as a result of AR. Although it is not a severe disorder, the socioeconomic costs of AR are substantial. AR is one of the chief reasons for visiting a primary care physician; it adversely affects work productivity and school performance, and it limits socialization. The impact of AR also reflects its association with a variety of comorbid conditions, including asthma (Chapter 87), acute and chronic sinusitis, nasal polyposis, secretory otitis media, and sleep disorders. Adequately addressing AR requires a thorough understanding of its pathophysiology, its relation to these comorbid conditions, and the effects of various therapeutic options on AR and its associated comorbidities.

PATHOBIOLOGY

Airborne Allergens

Allergic respiratory diseases result from a hypersensitivity immune reaction to airborne allergens. These include the pollens and molds that are responsible for seasonal AR (SAR) and the indoor allergens, such as dust mites, indoor molds, and animal proteins, that are responsible for perennial AR (PAR) (Table 251-1).

In any area, the specific pollens that are likely to cause symptoms can be predicted from the number of days a pollen is airborne in large numbers. All these pollens use a wind-borne mechanism to achieve fertilization. Insect-borne pollens, specifically those produced by flowers, are not significantly airborne and therefore are not inhaled in sufficient concentrations to generate immune responses. In the United States, grass pollens (May to June) and ragweed (mid-August to October) are the most important causes of SAR. Tree pollens vary locally but typically start in late February and continue through April. The major trees implicated in allergy include birch in the North, oak in the mid-Atlantic region, live oak in the South, and mountain cedar in the Southwest. In addition to pollens, outdoor molds, particularly *Alternaria* and *Cladosporium*, can produce symptoms. These molds have variable seasons, depending on the weather; high levels of airborne fungi may be common at any time between March and October. In recent years, climate change has influenced both the length and the region of pollen seasons.

PAR may occur year-round, but the term is applied to any rhinitis that does not have a clearly defined seasonal association. The most common causes include (1) indoor fungi, which are related to periods of high indoor humidity; (2) animal danders, particularly cats, but rodents (mice, rats, guinea pigs, ferrets, hamsters), rabbits, dogs, and birds may also be significant; (3) dust mites of the genus *Dermatophagoides*, which grow in bedding and pillows and are semiseasonal, with maximal levels from August to December; and (4) other insects (the best studied is the cockroach, but gypsy moths, crickets, ladybugs, spiders, and beetles may be locally important). Dust mites and cats produce the most important indoor allergens. Dust mites grow well only with a relative humidity higher than 50%. Dust mite allergy is probably relevant in all areas with more than 6 humid months in the year.

Immunoglobulin E, Mast Cell, and Basophil Activation

The traditional view is that AR is caused by the triggering of mast cell degranulation resulting from the cross-linking of surface-bound immunoglobulin (Ig) E molecules by the aeroallergen. As with all antibody-mediated immune responses, the initial exposure to the antigen results in B-lymphocyte secretion of low-affinity IgM antibodies. Subsequent exposure to the allergen in genetically predisposed subjects leads to a secondary immune response characterized by the isotype switch to IgE. The specific mechanisms underlying isotype switching to IgE are controversial, including the exact location where this occurs and the extent to which this requires an IgG intermediate. Similarly, the relative production of IgE-producing long-lived B cells or plasma cells is very poorly understood, although experience with bee stings and drug allergy suggests ongoing IgE synthesis for up to 10 years after an isolated allergenic exposure.[1] The resulting release of IgE antibodies into the circulation does not cause allergic symptoms; only after these IgE antibodies bind to their high-affinity receptors on basophils and mast cells do symptoms develop with subsequent allergen exposure. It takes the cross-linking of approximately 300 IgE receptors and cells to stimulate degranulation; therefore, and with the large number of mast cells scattered through virtually all tissues, it often requires several allergy seasons before sufficient numbers of allergen-specific IgE molecules are present on the surface of a given mast cell to drive its degranulation. This means that the development of symptomatic AR is a protracted process, generally requiring at least three or four exposures. As a result, SAR is generally not observed in children until they are approximately 4 years of age. Similarly, in adults, symptomatic responses to local allergens may not develop until approximately 4 years after moving to a region. PAR, however, can develop much faster.

Within minutes of allergen exposure, IgE-sensitized mast cells degranulate and release preformed and newly synthesized mediators, including histamine, proteases (tryptase and chymase), cysteinyl leukotrienes, prostaglandins, platelet-activating factor, and cytokines. Some of these mediators produce the characteristic early-phase symptoms of AR, namely, sneezing, pruritus, rhinorrhea, and, to some extent, congestion. Other mediators stimulate infiltration of the nasal mucosa with inflammatory cells, including basophils, eosinophils, neutrophils, additional mast cells, and mononuclear cells. This infiltration of inflammatory cells and their subsequent release of a secondary wave of mediators sustain the inflammatory reaction and produce the late-phase response of AR. This slowly developing inflammatory response is characterized primarily by nasal congestion. The inflammation that develops during the course of an allergy season is associated with an approximately 10-fold increase in the number of mast cells present in nasal epithelial and submucosal tissue. This reflects the migration of preexisting mast cells into the epithelium and the differentiation and influx of newly synthesized mast cells under the influence of cytokine growth factors. During the course of chronic allergen stimulation, these mast cells also display increased *priming*, which reflects increases in the number of IgE receptors and surface-bound IgE as well as enhancement of signal transduction pathways. As a result, as the allergen season progresses, less and less allergen (engagement of fewer and fewer IgE receptors) is required to trigger mast cell degranulation.

Antigen-Presenting Cell and Helper T-Lymphocyte Activation

In addition to their interaction with mast cells, allergens behave like any other foreign antigen and are processed and presented by antigen-presenting cells

TABLE 251-1	ALLERGENS CAUSING ALLERGIC RHINITIS	
COMMON NAME		**SEASON**
SEASONAL ALLERGENS		
Trees		
Birch		March–May
Cottonwood		April–May
Elm		February–May
Cedar		March–May
Oak		May–June
Maple		March–May
Grasses		
Kentucky blue		Mid-May–June
Timothy		Mid-May–June
Orchard		Mid-May–June
Sweet vernal		Mid-May–June
Fescue		Mid-May–June
Bermuda		Mid-May–June
Weeds		
Ragweed		August–September
Kochia		July–September
Russian thistle		July–September
Sage		July–September
Marsh elder		July–September
English plantain		July–September
Outdoor Molds		
Alternaria		Spring–fall
Cladosporium		Spring–fall
PERENNIAL ALLERGENS		
Household Allergens		
Cockroaches (German and American)		
Dust mites: *Dermatophagoides farinae, D. pteronyssinus, Blomia tropicalis*		More active in summer and humid months
Other insects (spiders, ladybugs)		
Animals		
Cats		
Dogs		
Other pets (guinea pigs, ferrets, hamsters, horses)		
Rodents		
Indoor Molds		
Aspergillus		
Cladosporium		
Penicillium		

to helper T (T$_H$) lymphocytes. Activation of these antigen-presenting cells, including mononuclear phagocytic cells, B lymphocytes, and especially dendritic cells, is an important source of cytokines, especially those associated with innate immunity, such as interleukin (IL)–1, IL-6, and tumor necrosis factor-α (TNF-α). Recent understanding of the molecular mimicry of allergens has increasingly expanded our understanding of the role of pathogen-associated molecular patterns receptors in dendritic cell activation, such as the engagement of toll-like receptor 4 by *Dermatophagoides* and similarly engagement of the lectin receptor dectin-2 by *Aspergillus*.[2] Engagement of these receptors promotes an inflammatory response to these otherwise innocuous inhaled particles. With the ensuing development of allergic inflammation, there is an increased presence of B cells expressing allergen-specific surface immunoglobulin and dendritic cells expressing surface-bound IgE. These antibodies can function as receptors that "capture" allergen and increase these cells' effectiveness in antigen processing. The newly activated T lymphocytes tend to resemble T$_H$2 cells, characterized by the production of IL-4, IL-5, IL-9, IL-13, and granulocyte-macrophage colony-stimulating factor (GM-CSF). These cytokines are also major components of the inflammatory response in AR and contribute to the increased production, recruitment, and activation of eosinophils, mast cells, and basophils. A milieu rich in IL-4 and IL-13 drives the IgE isotype switch and contributes to the further production of allergen-specific IgE. IL-13 also drives the metaplastic differentiation of nasal epithelial cells into goblet cells that are characterized not only by production of mucus but, importantly, also by chemokines such as CCL5, CCL11, CCL24, and CCL26 that further mediate basophil and eosinophil chemotaxis.

Innate Lymphoid Type 2 Cells as Additional Sources of Type 2 Signature Cytokines
An additional cell type, the type 2 innate lymphoid cell (ILC2), having features of NK cells and sharing with the NK cell the absence of a T-cell receptor, has recently been defined and distinguished by its secretion of preformed IL-5 and IL-13.[3] ILC2s can be activated through several pathways, but it is increasingly appreciated that nasal epithelial cells themselves respond to allergens to secrete two cytokines, IL-25 and IL-33, that are central to this process. This cellular mechanism defines a pathway linking allergen engagement of receptors on epithelium that drives their secretion of IL-25 and IL-33, leading in turn to an allergic inflammatory milieu driven by ILC2–derived IL-5 and IL-13. This provides a parallel pathway for development of allergen-induced inflammation that does not require engagement of the adaptive immune system (i.e., allergen-specific IgE or allergen-targeting T effector cells).

Through these mechanisms, during the seasonal course of allergen exposure, rhinitis evolves and becomes more dependent on mediators associated with the infiltration of eosinophils, basophils, neutrophils, mononuclear cells, and T$_H$ lymphocytes as well as the increasingly primed mast cells. The symptoms of acute rhinitis, such as sneezing, itching, and rhinorrhea, largely reflect vasoactive mediator release, especially histamine. As SAR or PAR persists, however, these infiltrating cells continue to produce cytokines and other inflammatory mediators, leading to mucus hypersecretion, tissue edema, goblet cell hyperplasia, and tissue damage that become the primary sources of allergy patients' symptoms. As the role of histamine diminishes with AR progression (discussed later), antihistamines become less and less effective.

Eosinophils represent an important component of the inflammation that develops in AR. Eosinophils release a wide variety of proinflammatory mediators, including cysteinyl leukotrienes (leukotrienes C4, D4, and E4), eosinophil cationic protein, eosinophil peroxidase, major basic protein, IL-3, IL-4, interferon-γ, GM-CSF, and platelet-activating factor. Eosinophil-derived mediators are major components of the chronic allergic response and produce many of the symptoms of AR, especially nasal congestion. The natural history of AR is for symptoms to worsen inexorably during several weeks in the presence of ongoing allergen exposure. Symptoms often do not peak until well after the peak in pollen counts, and then they persist after pollen counts have declined. These observations reflect the time frame of the onset of nasal inflammation and tissue damage. The influx of eosinophils into the nasal mucosa correlates with the development and progression of symptoms. In summary, the natural history of AR represents an evolution from an acute, primarily mast cell–mediated process that is responsive to antihistamines to a chronic inflammatory process that is primarily eosinophil mediated and is much less responsive to antihistamines.

CLINICAL MANIFESTATIONS
The diagnosis of AR is based on a history of sneezing, which is often paroxysmal; rhinorrhea with clear, watery secretions; nasal congestion; and itching

in the nares and palate. These symptoms are generally associated with allergic conjunctivitis manifested by ocular itching, lacrimation, and conjunctival injection. Severe conjunctivitis is less common in PAR than in SAR. The best explanation for this difference is that pollen grains affect the eyes when they are blown into them. With the exception of cat-derived allergens, which have a strong tendency to remain airborne, indoor allergens including those derived from dog and dust mites are less likely to be blown into the eyes because these allergens are on heavy particles that do not remain airborne. Instead, these indoor aeroallergens are drawn into the nose by breathing.

What is less well appreciated—in the literature but certainly not in AR sufferers—is that AR is a systemic disease associated with circulating activated T lymphocytes and mononuclear phagocytic cells. The activation of these cells is demonstrated by their production of cytokines associated with innate immunity, such as IL-1, TNF-α, and IL-6. These cytokines are responsible for the lethargy, fatigue, arthralgias, myalgias, and cognitive impairment that frequently accompany AR. These systemic symptoms, which are often the chief complaints of allergy sufferers, contribute to a diminished quality of life and are often severe enough to make normal activities difficult, including work or school.[4] Although fever is not a feature of AR, it is intriguing that the lay term for this condition is *hay fever*, a designation reflecting the pronounced influenza-like nature of this disease.

DIAGNOSIS
AR is primarily a clinical diagnosis based on symptoms and exposure history. It is a complex genetic disorder, and affected patients generally give a positive family history. Vasoactive mediators induce glandular secretions and vascular leakage along with engorgement of capacitance nasal venous sinusoids. Physical examination therefore reveals the nasal mucosa to be cyanotic and swollen, with clear secretions. Smears of nasal secretions (Hansel stains) are seldom required, but when they are performed, they typically reveal eosinophils.

The diagnosis of AR is confirmed by the demonstration of specific IgE antibodies reactive to the relevant allergen through either positive allergy skin test responses or IgE immunoassays. Identification of the specific triggering allergen is essential for the institution of appropriate environmental controls. Prick skin testing is safe, specific, and rapid, and it is the diagnostic test of choice for identifying relevant allergens. A positive intradermal test response in the presence of a negative prick skin test response is often a false-positive result. Intradermal testing is therefore rarely indicated and is associated with potentially life-threatening systemic reactions. If prick skin testing is not available or if the test cannot be performed (e.g., in patients with eczema or dermatographism or in those using antihistamines or antipsychotic agents), IgE immunoassays are an appropriate alternative. As with prick skin tests, positive IgE immunoassays correlate with symptoms caused by natural exposure, establish the diagnosis of AR, and can form the basis for environmental therapy; these assays should therefore be used extensively by primary care physicians who manage patients with AR. However, a negative IgE immunoassay with a strong clinical suspicion suggests the need for referral.

Differential Diagnosis
Other causes of rhinitis are shown in Table 251-2. The approach to patients with sneezing and rhinorrhea is illustrated in Figure 251-1.

Viral rhinitis may be difficult to distinguish from SAR. Viral rhinitis is not associated with the release of mast cell mediators. The main mediators present in nasal secretions from patients with the common cold are kinins; histamine and cysteinyl leukotrienes are less prevalent. In contrast to the pervasive eosinophilia in AR, infectious rhinitis is defined by the presence of polymorphonuclear leukocytes, reflecting in large part the secretion of IL-8 by infected epithelium. The presence of these different mediators is in keeping with the observation that pruritus, paroxysmal sneezing, and clear secretions help distinguish SAR from viral rhinitis, along with the distinct recurrent, seasonal nature of SAR. Viral rhinitis produces thicker, purulent secretions, with neutrophils present on the nasal smear. Conjunctival symptoms are less pronounced, and on physical examination, the nasal mucosa is erythematous and swollen.

Hormonal influences that may produce chronic nasal congestion and rhinorrhea include hypothyroidism, birth control pill use, pregnancy, and menopause. Abuse of topical nasal decongestants (e.g., oxymetazoline), with chronic reflex vasodilation, has historically been the most common cause of rhinitis medicamentosa; however, cocaine and nasal narcotic abuse is another frequent cause of this condition. Chronic unilateral nasal blockage suggests an anatomic defect, typically a deviated or fractured septum, but such blockage can also result from polyps, foreign bodies, and tumors, which can be malignant. This history necessitates referral for rhinoscopy and possibly computed tomography (CT) of the nose and sinuses. Nasal septum deviation is an unlikely cause of bilateral nasal congestion, and

surgical therapy has little role in the treatment of rhinitis that is producing symptomatic congestion.

An abnormal neurogenic response to irritants (e.g., cold air, pollutants, cigarette smoke, strong odors, alcohol, foods) is the predominant feature of vasomotor rhinitis. This disorder is characterized by nasal autonomic nerve dysfunction. Patients with vasomotor rhinitis typically have chronic nasal congestion and posterior pharyngeal drainage, but they lack the paroxysmal sneezing, rhinorrhea, pruritus, conjunctivitis, and systemic complaints typical of patients with AR. In addition, eosinophils are absent in their nasal mucus. Topical antihistamines (nasal azelastine, olopatadine) are often effective in vasomotor rhinitis. Patients with this condition also respond to therapy with topical corticosteroids but also to atropine (nasal ipratropium).

An increasingly recognized cause of perennial nasal congestion and posterior pharyngeal drainage that often occurs in association with cough and hoarseness can be ascribed to laryngopharyngeal reflux. These patients are often otherwise asymptomatic from ("silent") gastroesophageal reflux, making recognition challenging. Intra-arytenoid erythema on laryngoscopy is traditionally ascribed to reflux; however, the specificity of this finding has never been determined, and other causes of chronic cough may produce identical findings. Because symptoms may not resolve until after several months of aggressive reflux treatment and because proton pump inhibitors by themselves may not prevent reflux of digestive enzymes (e.g., pepsin) or other stomach-derived irritants, proper diagnosis can be daunting. More recent techniques, including esophageal impedance testing and laryngeal smears for pepsin, are promising diagnostic advances.

Chronic sinusitis (see next section) with or without nasal polyposis can produce a spectrum of symptoms, including rhinorrhea, mucopurulent posterior pharyngeal drainage, and nasal congestion, that can be mistaken for PAR. However, chronic sinusitis, particularly when it is eosinophilic (discussed later), is often asymptomatic, and a reduced or absent sense of smell may be the only complaint. In contrast to acute (infectious) sinusitis, headaches are an unusual manifestation of either perennial rhinitis (allergic or nonallergic) or chronic sinusitis, and virtually all patients who complain of "sinus headaches" suffer from atypical migraines or other headache syndromes.[5] Atypical migraines routinely produce headaches that occur in a bilateral distribution involving the maxillary or ophthalmic branches of the

TABLE 251-2 DIFFERENTIAL DIAGNOSIS OF RHINITIS

ALLERGIC

Seasonal allergic rhinitis (SAR)
Perennial allergic rhinitis (PAR)

INFLAMMATORY

Infectious rhinitis (viral)
Nonallergic rhinitis with eosinophilia syndrome (NARES)
Chronic sinusitis with or without nasal polyposis
Laryngopharyngeal reflux

HORMONAL

Pregnancy, oral contraceptives, perimenopause
Hypothyroidism
Hyperthyroidism

RHINITIS MEDICAMENTOSA

Topical or, less commonly, oral decongestants
Antihypertensives
Antidepressants
Cocaine

VASOMOTOR

Irritant induced (pollution, cigarette smoke)
Cold air induced
Gustatory (food induced)

ANATOMIC

Nasal septal deviation
Tumor, neoplasm
Foreign body
Cerebrospinal fluid leak
Atrophic (postsurgical or trauma)

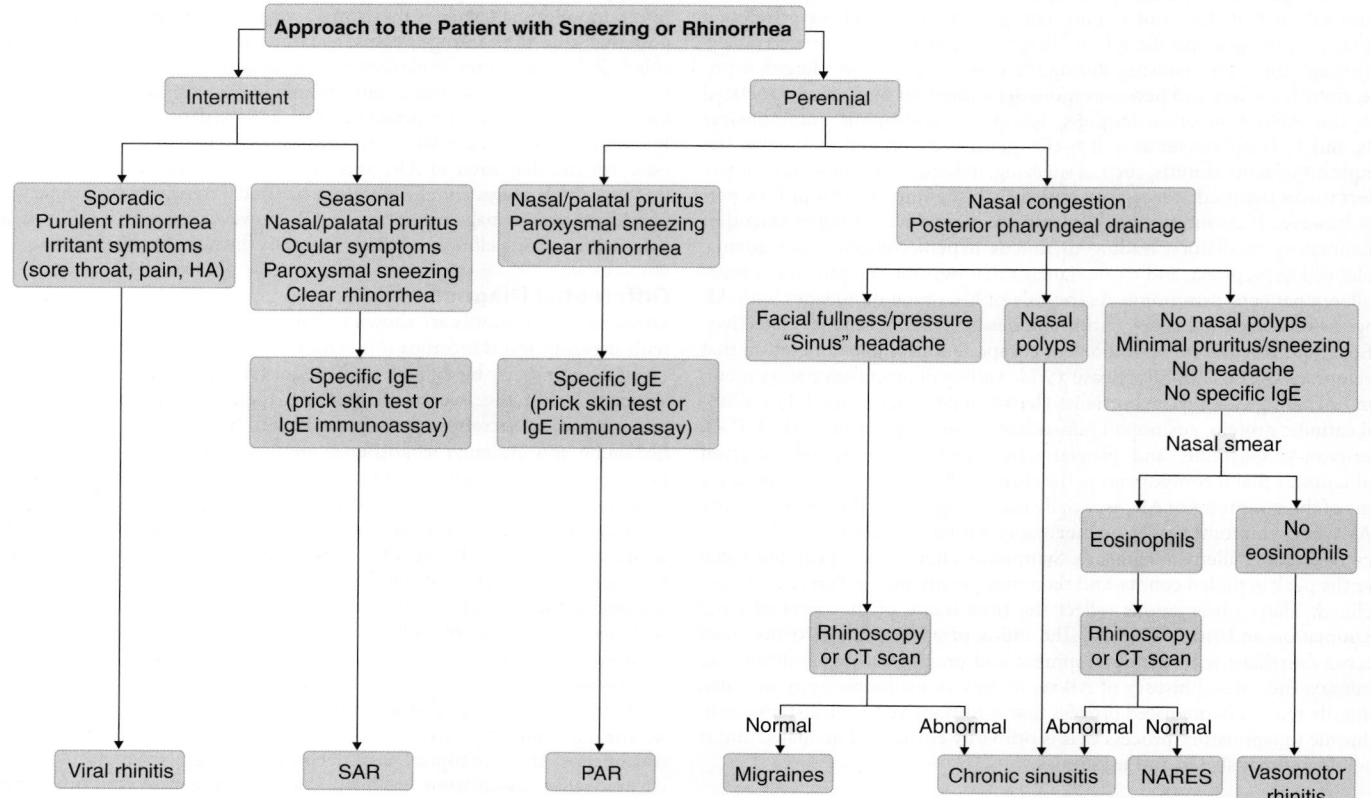

FIGURE 251-1. Approach to the patient with rhinitis symptoms. CT = computed tomography; HA = headache; IgE = immunoglobulin E; NARES = nonallergic rhinitis with eosinophilia syndrome; PAR = perennial allergic rhinitis; SAR = seasonal allergic rhinitis.

trigeminal nerve; this distribution, especially when it is combined with vasomotor symptoms such as nasal congestion, rhinorrhea, and conjunctival injection, often leads to misdiagnosis as chronic sinusitis or rhinitis. This complex becomes even more confusing with the recognition that vasoactive mediators released in association with allergic (or nonallergic) rhinitis (e.g., histamine) can trigger migraines. Because of this overlap in symptoms among chronic sinusitis, perennial rhinitis, and atypical migraines and their synergistic influences on each other, objective evaluation with either CT or rhinoscopy is usually required to establish the diagnosis of chronic sinusitis.

Atrophic rhinitis is characterized by atrophy of the nasal epithelium and is associated with complaints of nasal congestion and a perceived bad odor. It is observed in elderly patients, but the most common cause is devascularization secondary to nasal surgery or trauma.

Finally, a nonallergic nasal disease characterized by prominent eosinophilic inflammation has been described and termed non-AR with eosinophilia syndrome (NARES). On further analysis, many of these patients prove to have chronic sinusitis and nasal polyps. Patients with NARES present with symptoms similar to those of vasomotor rhinitis. NARES is diagnosed by performing a nasal smear (Hansel stain) for eosinophils; however, a CT scan or rhinoscopy is required to rule out chronic sinusitis or nasal polyposis because these conditions may be minimally symptomatic. In contrast to vasomotor rhinitis, NARES is more responsive to intranasal cromolyn and intranasal corticosteroids.

⬤ CHRONIC SINUSITIS

Chronic sinusitis represents many disease processes, including those caused by chronic bacterial infections, cystic fibrosis, immotile cilia syndrome, immune deficiencies, nonspecific inflammation, hypersensitivity to colonized fungi (allergic fungal sinusitis), aspirin-exacerbated respiratory disease (Samter's triad), and a disorder termed chronic hyperplastic eosinophilic sinusitis (CHES) (Table 251-3).[6] In the absence of immunodeficiency or cystic fibrosis, infection is a *very* unusual cause of chronic sinusitis. Noneosinophilic forms of chronic sinusitis most often reflect congenital anatomic variants or acquired nasal disorders (e.g., allergic rhinitis) that lead to ostial occlusion, with the secondary development of frequent, protracted acute infections. This ultimately produces tissue remodeling within the sinuses (with or, more often, without nasal polyps). These patients typically respond to surgical interventions that address the underlying anatomic precipitant.

CHES, which more often occurs in association with nasal polyposis, is an inflammatory disorder characterized by the accumulation of eosinophils, fibroblasts, mast cells, other stromal cells, and T_H2-like lymphocytes along with goblet cell metaplasia and mucous gland hypertrophy. The prominent accumulation of eosinophils, however, is the diagnostic feature of this condition. The inflamed tissue expresses cytokines responsible for eosinophil hematopoiesis (IL-5), survival (IL-3, IL-5, and GM-CSF), recruitment (CCL11 [eotaxin]), and activation (CCL11, CCL5 [RANTES], IL-3, IL-4, IL-5, GM-CSF, and TNF-α). This histologic appearance and immune profile of CHES bears striking similarity to asthma. Indeed, approximately half of patients with CHES have asthma, and virtually all asthmatics have some component of CHES. Together, these observations suggest that CHES and asthma are similar diseases affecting the upper and lower portions of the airway (the "unified" airway concept). Whereas surgery may be a useful therapeutic adjuvant, as with asthma, treatment requires lifelong anti-inflammatory therapy. Therapies useful in asthma, such as topical corticosteroids and biotherapeutics that target IgE and IL-5, also appear useful in CHES.[7,8]

PREVENTION
Avoidance and Environmental Control

When it is feasible, avoidance or elimination of the source of the allergen is the treatment of choice for patients with AR. Avoidance studies in AR are limited, and the amount of allergen reduction needed to alleviate symptoms is unknown. Avoidance studies in asthma (Chapter 87) provide compelling evidence of a beneficial effect on bronchial hyperreactivity, symptom severity, and need for β-agonist rescue therapy.

Dust mite avoidance involves four principles: (1) remove reservoirs for mite growth (i.e., use allergen-impermeable mattress and pillow covers), (2) keep the relative humidity lower than 50%, (3) wash bedding in hot water (130° F) to kill mites, and (4) wear a simple mask when dust is being disturbed. Many of the measures suggested for mites are also helpful for fungi, especially dehumidification. Windows, shower curtains, and indoor plants are important sites for fungal growth and can be treated with mild fungicides (dilute household bleach).

In some houses, and particularly urban apartment blocks, large numbers of cockroaches are present, and IgE sensitivity is common. Although it may be difficult to kill cockroaches in an apartment, it is usually possible to keep a house clear of cockroaches by using chemical sprays and traps. Care must be taken in using chemical sprays because they can be an irritant to asthmatic patients.

Air-conditioning with closed windows is useful for reducing seasonal allergens, and the dehumidification provided by air-conditioning also mitigates the mite and indoor mold load.

Pets, especially cats, are the most preventable source of allergic diseases. Animal dander accumulates in houses during a prolonged period and takes many months to eliminate after the pet is removed. Although it is difficult to persuade patients to get rid of their animals, it may be possible to move the pet outside into the garage or to restrict the pet's access to certain parts of the house. Dogs kept outside and allowed into the house only occasionally do not appear to be an important cause of symptoms. Cat allergy is a much more serious problem because a single cat can deposit a huge concentration of allergen, and cat allergen remains airborne for prolonged periods. Cat owners, in turn, deposit sufficient concentrations of allergen in classrooms and work environments to induce symptoms in their allergic colleagues. The dominant rodent allergen is a urinary protein, and rodents, like cats, can deposit large quantities of allergen in a house.

TABLE 251-3	HETEROGENEITY OF CHRONIC SINUSITIS
PHENOTYPE	**CHARACTERISTIC**
Infectious	Very unusual as a cause of chronic sinusitis Occurs in association with cystic fibrosis, immune deficiency, ciliary dyskinesia
Inflammatory	Reflects remodeling secondary to frequent, recurrent acute sinusitis Develops secondary to anatomic obstruction of the sinus ostia; often resolves after surgical correction Pathologic examination demonstrates dense collagen fibrils, goblet cell metaplasia, and glandular hypertrophy and a chronic mononuclear infiltrate, with or without neutrophils Bacterial biofilms contribute to presence and severity Less often associated with nasal polyps
Hyperplastic eosinophilic	Prominent eosinophilic infiltrate with systemic eosinophilia Pathologic examination demonstrates edema, sub-basement thickening Frequent association with allergies and asthma Usually associated with nasal polyps
Allergic fungal	Often unilateral; presents as expansive, dense infiltrate on CT scan Associated with elevated total IgE and specific IgE to colonizing fungi
Aspirin-exacerbated respiratory disease (Samter's triad)	Intense eosinophilic infiltrate Usually associated with nasal polyps and asthma Exacerbations of upper and lower respiratory disease (asthma) after ingestion of aspirin and nonselective COX1 inhibitors

COX1 = cyclooxygenase 1; CT = computed tomography; IgE = immunoglobulin E.

TREATMENT   Rx

Although avoidance interventions can reduce allergen levels, they often fail to produce clinically significant improvement. As a result, pharmacotherapy is frequently required.

Antihistamines

Antihistamines are the oldest drugs used to treat AR and are considered first-line therapy. Antihistamines compete with histamine for the H_1-receptor sites that contribute to sneezing, itching, rhinorrhea, and conjunctivitis. Oral antihistamines ameliorate these symptoms of AR but generally do not improve nasal congestion. They also inhibit mast cell activation as manifested by diminished histamine, cysteinyl leukotrienes, and mast cell tryptase secretion. First-generation antihistamines cross the blood-brain barrier and have significant sedative and anticholinergic effects. In addition to causing sleepiness, they interfere with school, work, driving, or use of machinery, and as such, the use of these drugs is no longer recommended. Second-generation antihistamines have a longer duration of action, do not cross the blood-brain barrier, and are nonsedating. These agents include cetirizine, levocetirizine, fexofenadine, descarboxyloratadine, and loratadine. Although less sedating than their parent compound hydroxyzine, cetirizine and levocetirizine may occasionally produce sedation. The intranasal antihistamines azelastine and olopatadine have a more rapid onset of action than oral antihistamines, and reflecting the high local concentrations they are able to achieve, they do have decongestant efficacy. They are also distinguished from oral antihistamines in being effective for nonallergic forms of rhinitis. No studies have convincingly demonstrated the superiority of one antihistamine over another.

As discussed earlier, the role of histamine diminishes during the course of an allergy season or with PAR, making antihistamines less effective. Antihistamines are effective for acute allergic reactions that are mediated predominantly by mast cell–derived histamine; as such, they are most beneficial in patients with intermittent allergen exposures, such as occasional outdoor exposure during pollen season. In patients with continuous allergen exposures, however, such as PAR caused by indoor allergens or after several days of continuous exposure to seasonal allergens, these drugs often prove to be little better than placebo.

Decongestants

Decongestants such as pseudoephedrine treat nasal stuffiness but are mild stimulants and even in oral formulations may produce rebound congestion and headaches. These drugs are usually used in combination with antihistamines to control the full spectrum of AR symptoms. Antihistamines and decongestants alone generally do not provide satisfactory relief in patients with moderate to severe AR.

Leukotriene Modifiers

Leukotriene modifiers (zileuton, zafirlukast, montelukast) have a confirmed efficacy in AR that is comparable to that of antihistamines but do significantly improve sneezing, rhinorrhea, nasal congestion, ocular symptoms, and quality of life in patients with both SAR and PAR. This efficacy reflects the presence and importance of these proinflammatory vasoactive mediators in AR.

Nasal Cromolyn

Nasal cromolyn stabilizes mast cells and mediates additional anti-inflammatory activities. Although it is not as effective as intranasal corticosteroids, cromolyn provides relief in patients with mild to moderate symptoms. The value of cromolyn is mitigated by the need for frequent doses (four times/day), a lack of efficacy in approximately 30 to 40% of recipients, and the superior efficacy of intranasal corticosteroids in controlled studies. Cromolyn may be especially useful preventively (e.g., immediately before cat exposure). Ocular cromolyn has been especially useful in the treatment of allergic conjunctivitis. No significant side effects are associated with its use.

Intranasal Corticosteroids

Intranasal corticosteroids (fluticasone [Flonase, Veramyst], beclomethasone [Qnasl], triamcinolone [Nasacort], flunisolide [Nasarel], budesonide [Rhinocort], mometasone [Nasonex], and ciclesonide [Omnaris]) are the most effective AR treatments and are considered the treatments of choice for patients with moderate to severe SAR or PAR.[A1] Comparative studies of antihistamines and intranasal corticosteroids consistently favor the corticosteroids.[A2] In well-performed placebo-controlled studies, intranasal corticosteroids provided a 50 to 90% reduction in symptoms (compared with 20 to 30% for antihistamines). In contrast to oral antihistamines, topical corticosteroids reduce nasal congestion in addition to relieving itching, rhinorrhea, sneezing, and allergic conjunctivitis.[9] Few studies have directly addressed the influence of corticosteroids on the systemic effects of AR—including missed work and school, poor productivity, reduced cognition, and fatigue—that are often the dominant complaints of patients with AR; however, intranasal corticosteroids significantly improve quality of life, reflecting relief from these complaints. Although they are slower in onset than antihistamines, intranasal corticosteroids produce some clinical improvement as quickly as 6 to 8 hours and achieve full effectiveness after several days.

Topical corticosteroid therapy does not inhibit IgE synthesis or mast cell degranulation, traditionally considered the two determinants for the development of AR. However, corticosteroids do inhibit T-lymphocyte proliferation, chemokine and cytokine production, recruitment of eosinophils and basophils, mucus secretion, vascular permeability, and mast cell proliferation. Intranasal corticosteroid use is therefore associated with diminished nasal eosinophilia, mast cell numbers, and cytokine expression. The efficacy of intranasal corticosteroids emphasizes the importance of these nonhistamine mechanisms to the pathophysiologic process of AR.

Several intranasal corticosteroid preparations are currently available and differ according to dose, approval age, and propellant (Table 251-4). No studies have demonstrated superior efficacy for any of the nasal corticosteroid preparations. Clinical experience with asthma (Chapter 87) suggests that patients

TABLE 251-4   INTRANASAL CORTICOSTEROIDS*

GENERIC NAME	DOSE (PER ACTUATION)	MINIMUM APPROVED AGE	USUAL DOSING
Beclomethasone AQ	42 µg	6 yr	Twice daily
Beclomethasone HFA	80 µg	12 yr	Once daily
Flunisolide	25 µg	6 yr	Twice daily
Triamcinolone	55 µg	2 yr	Once daily
Budesonide	32 µg	6 yr	Twice daily
Fluticasone furoate	27.5 µg	2 yr	Once daily
Fluticasone propionate	50 µg	4 yr	Once daily
Mometasone	50 µg	2 yr	Once daily
Ciclesonide	50 µg	6 yr	Once daily
Ciclesonide HFA	37 µg	12 yr	Once daily

*Intranasal corticosteroids are generally administered at 2 sprays per nostril.

refractory to one intranasal corticosteroid may be switched to a higher-potency corticosteroid; however, the best evidence is that all these agents are comparably valuable when patients are willing to comply with their use. Choices should be based primarily on the patient's preference.

There is no convincing evidence of clinically significant systemic absorption or systemic side effects from intranasal corticosteroids. Given these drugs' hydrophobicity, local metabolism, and lack of absorption from lung tissue, clinically meaningful systemic absorption from the nasal passages is unlikely. Intranasal corticosteroids, even at greater than recommended doses, do not significantly suppress serum or urinary cortisol levels. There is a small but statistically significant effect on short-term growth velocity in children with PAR but minimal or no impact on ultimate adult height. Nasal corticosteroids cause minimal topical side effects, including local irritation, dryness, and epistaxis. Nasal perforation has been reported, but primarily in the setting of underlying devascularization (previous trauma, surgery, or cocaine abuse).

Immunotherapy

The clinical efficacy of subcutaneous immunotherapy for AR caused by grass, ragweed, many other pollens, cat and dog dander, and dust mites has been categorically established in innumerable well-designed, controlled studies.[10] Immunotherapy decreases the severity of AR, reduces the need for pharmacotherapy, and significantly improves quality of life. In patients with severe AR and conjunctivitis poorly controlled by antihistamines and intranasal corticosteroids, immunotherapy can reduce allergen sensitivity by more than 10-fold as well as significantly decrease total symptoms and reduce total antiallergic drug use. Efficacy depends on delivery of the correct antigen, regular injections for 3 to 5 years, and administration of an adequate dose of the allergen (10 to 15 µg, a dose much higher than that used historically).

Immunotherapy is indicated primarily in patients with refractory rhinitis or in those experiencing unacceptable side effects from standard medications. Because intranasal corticosteroids are not universally effective and do not provide complete relief in all patients, consideration of immunotherapy is necessary. In addition, despite the excellent safety profile of intranasal corticosteroids, many patients are reluctant to use them. Patients should normally go through at least one full pollen season before considering immunotherapy. Immunotherapy is the only treatment that produces long-term immune modulation. Both avoidance and pharmacotherapy are effective only if they are sustained. The effects of immunotherapy, in contrast, persist for many years after a 3- to 5-year course of treatment has been discontinued, and they could be lifelong. As such, a 5-year course of immunotherapy has cost advantages over lifelong pharmacotherapy. Many patients are attracted to immunotherapy by this potential for long-term immune modulation, remission of symptoms, and ability to discontinue daily pharmacotherapy.

Immunotherapy is associated with a small risk of fatal anaphylaxis (about 3 fatalities/year in the United States, of 2 million people receiving this form of treatment). Because of this risk, immunotherapy must be administered only in a facility where resuscitation equipment and trained personnel are available. Asthmatic patients are uniquely at risk for fatal anaphylaxis, so immunotherapy should be recommended with caution in these patients.

Because of the risk for anaphylaxis and the inconvenience of having to receive subcutaneous immunotherapy in a facility where evaluation and treatment of anaphylaxis are available, there is increasing enthusiasm for alternative forms of immunotherapy, specifically, sublingual immunotherapy. Sublingual immunotherapy has been extensively studied and proved to provide significant clinical benefit along with reduced need for pharmacologic therapy for numerous allergens including grass, ragweed, and dust mites.[A3-A6] In comparison to subcutaneous administration, sublingual immunotherapy is sufficiently safe to permit home administration. As with subcutaneous immunotherapy, long-term clinical benefits are observed after it is discontinued, although recurrences are common after 5 to 10 years. Whereas few direct comparative studies have been performed, the preponderance of evidence suggests that subcutaneous immunotherapy does provide greater and longer lasting benefits.[11]

Summary

Many patients have multiple antigen sensitivities, and specific immunotherapy at effective doses may not be practical. Furthermore, immunotherapy has poor efficacy for many antigens, such as molds. These issues have led to a search for new immune-based therapies capable of attenuating allergic inflammation. Many experimental approaches being developed for asthma, including various anticytokine therapies, may have efficacy for AR.

In general, however, currently available therapies provide adequate relief for virtually all AR sufferers. The persistence of nasal symptoms in the face of adequate AR-directed pharmacotherapies should suggest the diagnosis of an alternative form of rhinitis (see Fig. 251-1) or the presence of sinusitis or—especially if headaches are present—atypical migraines and rebound headaches. Given the high frequency of AR in the population (and the even higher prevalence of allergic sensitization), treatment becomes particularly challenging when a patient presents with nonallergic nasal symptoms and either concomitant AR or clinically innocuous allergic sensitization (positive skin test responses or IgE immunoassays) occurring in the absence of actual AR.

Grade A References

A1. Zalmanovici Trestioreanu A, Yaphe J. Intranasal steroids for acute sinusitis. *Cochrane Database Syst Rev.* 2013;12:CD005149.
A2. Glacy J, Putnam K, Godfrey S, et al. Treatments for Seasonal Allergic Rhinitis [Internet]. Rockville (MD): Agency for Healthcare Research and Quality (US); 2013. Report No.: 13-EHC098-EF.
A3. Aasbjerg K, Backer V, Lund G, et al. Immunological comparison of allergen immunotherapy tablet treatment and subcutaneous immunotherapy against grass allergy. *Clin Exp Allergy.* 2014;44: 417-428.
A4. Creticos PS, Maloney J, Bernstein DI, et al. Randomized controlled trial of a ragweed allergy immunotherapy tablet in North American and European adults. *J Allergy Clin Immunol.* 2013;131: 1342-1349.
A5. Wang DH, Chen L, Cheng L, et al. Fast onset of action of sublingual immunotherapy in house dust mite–induced allergic rhinitis: a multicenter, double-blind, placebo-controlled trial. *Laryngoscope.* 2013;123:1334-1340.
A6. Lin SY, Erekosima N, Kim JM, et al. Sublingual immunotherapy for the treatment of allergic rhinoconjunctivitis and asthma: a systematic review. *JAMA.* 2013;309:1278-1288.

GENERAL REFERENCES

For the General References and other additional features, please visit Expert Consult at https://expertconsult.inkling.com.

252

URTICARIA AND ANGIOEDEMA

STEPHEN C. DRESKIN

● URTICARIA

Urticaria (hives) consists of pruritic, edematous, erythematous, blanching papules that are round or oval; have pale, raised centers (wheals); are several millimeters to a few centimeters in size; and are transient, lasting minutes to days (Fig. 252-1). Angioedema appears as a brawny, nonpitting edema, typically without well-defined margins and without erythema. Angioedema can be accompanied by a sense of burning, pressure, or aching but not pruritus; it is distinguished from other edematous states by its frequent involvement of the lips, tongue, eyelids, hands, feet, or genitalia and its rare occurrence in dependent areas of the body. Episodes (daily or almost daily symptoms) of recurrent hives or angioedema during a period of less than 6 weeks are considered acute, and those lasting longer are said to be chronic. Patients typically present with urticaria alone or urticaria with angioedema. Rarely, patients present with angioedema alone, and this becomes a diagnostic dilemma because angioedema as an isolated finding may be due to activation

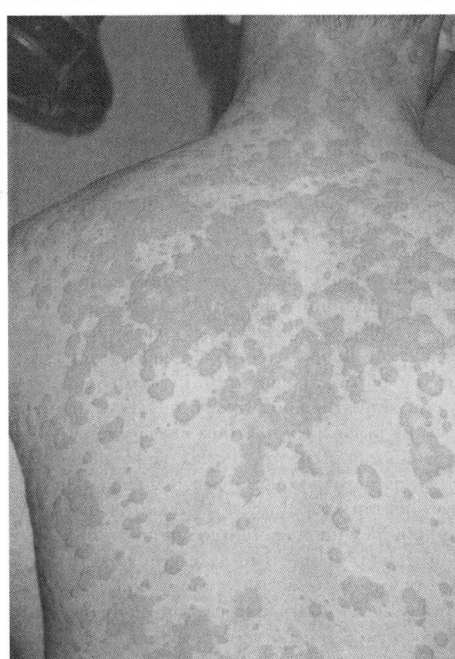

FIGURE 252-1. Extensive urticaria. Many presentations are more subtle. (From Roitt I, Brostoff J, Male D, eds. Immunology. 6th ed. London: Mosby; 2001.)

of the kinin system or may be due to activation of mast cells (see later). The terms *urticaria* and *urticaria/angioedema* are used interchangeably here to refer to illnesses characterized by urticaria or angioedema in which mast cells are activated.

EPIDEMIOLOGY

Urticaria/angioedema occurs in 15 to 25% of individuals at some time during their lives and can affect both genders and all races. Acute urticaria is more common in young adults and children. Chronic urticaria is more common in adults, affecting women (75% of cases) more often than men.[1]

PATHOBIOLOGY

Mast cells, the primary effector cells in urticaria/angioedema, are found in high numbers throughout the body, particularly within the subcutaneous tissue. After activation of mast cells, there is a rapid (<10 minutes) release of histamine, leukotriene C_4, and prostaglandin D_2, leading to vasodilation, subcutaneous and intradermal leakage of plasma from postcapillary venules, and pruritus. In addition, there is the delayed (4 to 8 hours) production and secretion of inflammatory cytokines such as tumor necrosis factor-α, interleukin-4, and interleukin-5, leading to an inflammatory infiltrate and perpetuation of longer-lived lesions. Angioedema is formed by a similar extravasation of fluid, not superficially in the skin but in deeper dermal and subdermal sites.

Lesions of acute urticaria typically show subcutaneous edema with widened dermal papillae, swollen collagen fibers, and rare inflammatory cells. Most episodes of acute urticaria/angioedema are caused by immediate hypersensitivity reactions to drugs or foods or result from inflammatory processes initiated by viral illnesses. The most common drugs that cause acute urticaria/angioedema are penicillins, sulfonamides, muscle relaxants, diuretics, and nonsteroidal anti-inflammatory drugs (NSAIDs), although any drug acting as a hapten can generate an allergic response. The predominant allergenic foods are milk, eggs, and peanuts for children and peanuts, tree nuts, fish, and shellfish for adults, although sensitization can occur to many other foods as well. These allergens cross-link immunoglobulin (Ig) E bound to the high-affinity receptor for IgE (FcεRI), leading to activation of mast cells. Some drugs (e.g., opioids, vancomycin, NSAIDs) and radiocontrast dye can activate mast cells by an IgE-independent (pseudoallergic) mechanism. Ingestion of fish contaminated with bacteria that produce histamine leads to hives as part of a toxic reaction to the histamine (scombroid food poisoning).

Lesions of chronic urticaria are characterized by similar edematous findings, with the addition of a dense perivascular inflammatory infiltrate consisting of CD4⁻ and CD8⁺ T lymphocytes, eosinophils, basophils, and neutrophils. A minority of patients exhibit urticarial vasculitis, with lesions characterized by vascular destruction with leukocytoclasis.

The largest subgroup of chronic urticaria/angioedema is idiopathic urticaria, accounting for approximately 70 to 80% of cases. Recently, an effort has been made to replace the term *chronic idiopathic urticaria* with the more descriptive term *chronic spontaneous urticaria*. These patients have symptoms in the absence of a specific physical trigger, allergen exposure, or coexistent disease. Half the patients with idiopathic urticaria have evidence of autoimmunity based on the presence of IgG antibodies that can cross-link FcεRI or antithyroid antibodies. Some experts consider these patients to have a separate entity called autoimmune urticaria, whereas others consider these patients to have idiopathic urticaria with evidence of autoimmunity.[2]

Physical stimuli activate mast cells by unknown mechanisms and account for about 20 to 30% of cases of chronic urticaria. The most common of the physical urticarias is dermographism (also called dermatographism), in which wheals can be "written on the skin" by simple stroking or scratching. Cholinergic urticaria is a physical urticaria in which the trigger leading to mast cell activation is related to cholinergic stimuli occurring after exposure to heat or after exercise. Other physical stimuli can cause urticaria, including cold, solar radiation, pressure, vibration, and water. Cold-induced urticaria is rarely caused by cryoglobulins. Cold-induced urticaria needs to be distinguished from the cryopyrin-associated periodic fever syndromes that include familial cold autoinflammatory syndrome and the Muckle-Wells syndrome (see later and Chapter 261).

In approximately 1-2% of patients with chronic urticaria/angioedema, symptoms appear to be caused by ingestants (e.g., foods, medications, dietary supplements), contactants (e.g., soaps, detergents, cosmetics, hair or nail products, latex), concomitant infections, hormonal changes, or systemic illnesses. A food must be consumed regularly to cause chronic urticaria. Wheat is rarely found to be a trigger. Multicellular parasites (e.g., those causing strongyloidiasis or filariasis) elicit strong IgE responses and are important causes of chronic urticaria in endemic areas. Rare patients report that their urticaria occurs only during menses or is worsened by menses. Although hormonal variation often is associated with worsening of urticaria, a detailed history may reveal ingestion of NSAIDs taken for uterine cramping. Chronic urticaria/angioedema can be associated with flares of rheumatic conditions, other autoimmune conditions (including Hashimoto thyroiditis), or neoplastic conditions. Occult neoplasia is exceedingly unlikely to be the cause of chronic urticaria.

CLINICAL MANIFESTATIONS

Patients often report that the first sensation of urticaria is poorly localized pruritus that quickly develops into the typical lesions of urticaria. The intensity of the pruritus varies from a minor inconvenience to an unbearable sensation that can lead to self-inflicted abrasion of the skin. Groups of hives often appear together during a short period, and episodes of hives can come in waves starting several times a day. Patients with cholinergic urticaria usually have a distinctive clinical presentation of diffuse urticarial lesions measuring a few millimeters in diameter on exertion sufficient to cause sweating. The pruritus is particularly intense, and all the symptoms are generally limited to the skin. A self-rated quality-of-life survey of patients with chronic urticaria revealed dramatic impairment in terms of loss of sleep, fatigue, and emotional discomfort. Angioedema can originate near a wheal or independently in other parts of the body. Symptoms vary from minor discomfort to an intense sense of pressure and may lead to other symptoms, such as severe shortness of breath if there is compromise of the airway. Rarely, patients report angioedema beginning 4 to 6 hours after application of local pressure, and this is called delayed pressure urticaria. This is a debilitating condition that is often difficult to treat.

DIAGNOSIS

The first episode of acute urticaria/angioedema may occur in the absence of an identifiable stimulus. If hives occur 5 to 30 minutes after ingestion of a drug or a food, the patient often can identify the association. If a physician is consulted, the best approach is to take a careful history, with attention to ingestants and intercurrent illnesses. Unnecessary drugs and food supplements should be discontinued, and any recently added medication should be changed to a structurally different agent. Most often, no causative agent is identified, and the hives are treated symptomatically (see the later discussion) for days or weeks before they resolve spontaneously.

TABLE 252-1   CLASSIFICATION OF URTICARIA AND ANGIOEDEMA

I. Acute urticaria/angioedema
  A. Hypersensitivity reactions
    1. Drug allergy
    2. Food allergy
    3. Insect allergy
  B. Idiopathic
  C. Pseudoallergic reactions
    1. Drugs
    2. Radiocontrast dye
  D. Toxic reactions
  E. Immune complex
    1. Serum sickness
    2. Transfusion related
    3. Postviral
II. Chronic urticaria/angioedema
  A. Idiopathic
    1. Autoantibody associated
      a. Anti-IgE receptor (FcεRI)
      b. Anti-IgE
      c. Antithyroid
      d. Other
    2. Not associated with autoantibodies
  B. Physical
    1. Dermographism
    2. Cholinergic
    3. Delayed pressure
    4. Solar
    5. Cold
    6. Vibratory
    7. Aquagenic
  C. Immune complex
    1. Urticarial vasculitis
    2. Collagen vascular disease associated
III. Urticaria pigmentosa and systemic mastocytosis
IV. Complement-related and kinin-mediated angioedema
  A. Hereditary angioedema
  B. Acquired angioedema
  C. Angiotensin-converting enzyme inhibitor–induced angioedema
  D. Renin inhibitor–induced angioedema
V. Urticaria pigmentosa and systemic mastocytosis

Differential Diagnosis

The differential diagnosis of chronic urticaria/angioedema includes the subgroups of urticaria discussed earlier: idiopathic, autoimmune, physical, ingestant mediated, and associated with a variety of systemic illnesses.[3] Other conditions that can be confused with chronic urticaria/angioedema include diffuse pruritus complicated by dermographism, flushing disorders, urticarial vasculitis, urticaria pigmentosa, systemic mastocytosis, exercise-induced anaphylaxis, exercise-induced food-associated anaphylaxis, idiopathic anaphylaxis, hereditary angioedema, acquired angioedema, and angioedema associated with angiotensin-converting enzyme (ACE) inhibitors (Table 252-1).

Approximately 95% of patients with urticaria/angioedema are not reacting to an ingestant and do not have another illness that is causing their hives. However, it is sometimes difficult for patients (and some physicians) to accept this fact, prompting an extensive, invasive, expensive, and unnecessary investigation. The best "test" to identify patients with a specific underlying cause (i.e., physical trigger, autoimmune condition, allergen, or systemic disease) is a careful and detailed history and physical examination by a specialist knowledgeable in urticarial disease.

A good place to begin is by excluding possible physical triggers. Specific tests are available to establish the diagnosis of most physical urticarias, including scratching the skin and exposing the skin to heat, ice, vibration, pressure, ultraviolet radiation, or water. Cold urticaria must be distinguished from cryopyrin-associated periodic fever syndromes that are characterized by a cold-induced papular rash (not urticaria) and are now classified in the family of hereditary periodic fever syndromes. Solar urticaria must be distinguished from other types of light sensitivity, including metabolic abnormalities (e.g., erythrogenic porphyria) and photosensitivity due to drugs.

Even though foods and drugs are infrequent causes of chronic urticaria, many patients focus on ingestants and are not satisfied until these causes are ruled out. As in the evaluation of acute urticaria, the patient should discontinue all food supplements and medications that are not absolutely necessary and, if possible, change essential medications to structurally unrelated compounds. The patient then keeps a food diary to identify suspect foods that can be eliminated. Some allergists use skin tests with foods to identify "suspects" (Chapter 249), but this approach is unproven. For highly motivated patients, 2 weeks of a severely restricted diet, often based on lamb and rice, is recommended. Antihistamines and other medications used to control the urticaria must be discontinued. If the urticaria resolves, it is critical to reintroduce foods in a controlled fashion to identify the specific food causing the urticaria and to reinstate a healthy diet.

Chronic infections, including sinus infection, dental abscess, *Helicobacter pylori* gastric infection, cholecystitis, onychomycosis, and tinea pedis, have been associated with urticaria. Case reports indicate the resolution of urticaria after treatment of these infections, although rigorous proof of an association is lacking. The natural history of chronic urticaria probably accounts for coincidental spontaneous improvement after treatment of these conditions, at least in some cases.

Laboratory evaluation in a patient with typical urticaria should always include a complete blood count with differential, basic metabolic panel, liver enzymes, and urinalysis. Specialists are not in full agreement about the necessity of additional laboratory testing. Levels of thyroid-stimulating hormone and antithyroid antibodies may be measured in otherwise euthyroid-appearing patients to screen for subclinical Hashimoto thyroiditis. Skin tests for immediate hypersensitivity to foods may be ordered for patients with a suggestive history. Some specialists order no screening tests at all. As in vitro tests for anti-FcεRI autoantibodies have become more widely available, some specialists will perform this test. A positive test response for anti-FcεRI autoantibodies is useful because this reassures the patient that the urticaria is being driven by an internal process and is not caused by an ingestant or occult illness. Other tests should be ordered only as a result of positive findings in the history and physical examination.[4]

Although it is not routinely indicated in every case of chronic urticaria, a skin biopsy can provide useful information. The most common indication for this procedure is to rule out urticarial vasculitis when the hives are more painful than pruritic, last longer than 24 hours, or leave discolored skin. The presence of vascular destruction, fibrinoid necrosis, and immune complex deposition on microscopic examination (including immunofluorescence) should lead to a consideration of the specific causes of urticarial vasculitis (e.g., systemic lupus erythematosus) and the rapid initiation of more aggressive treatment.

Primary mast cell disorders rarely manifest as chronic urticaria (Chapter 255). Systemic mastocytosis is a very rare condition characterized by increased numbers of atypical mast cells in the bone marrow, skin, and other organs. Levels of tryptase (an enzyme specific for mast cells) are usually elevated in the serum. This condition is frequently accompanied by episodic flushing, urticaria pigmentosa, prominent gastrointestinal symptoms, neuropsychiatric symptoms, or recurrent anaphylaxis. Urticaria pigmentosa is characterized by distinctive pigmented cutaneous lesions containing nests of mast cells and is not easily confused with urticaria/angioedema.

Hereditary angioedema, acquired angioedema, and angioedema associated with ACE inhibitors are discussed later in this chapter. Briefly, these syndromes are characterized by episodic swelling without urticaria and are best identified by a careful history, physical examination, and focused laboratory evaluation.[5] An approach to the evaluation and treatment of patients with urticaria or angioedema is summarized in Figure 252-2.

On occasion, a brief course of corticosteroids is warranted to control severe symptoms. Epinephrine (0.3 mL of 1:1000 intramuscularly) quickly (but transiently) reverses the signs and symptoms of urticaria and angioedema. Patients who have experienced potentially life-threatening angioedema or anaphylaxis should have ready access to self-injectable epinephrine and be knowledgeable about its indications, administration, and brief duration of action. β-Blockers not only can aggravate urticaria but also can interfere with the action of epinephrine. NSAIDs and codeine can lead to IgE-independent mast cell activation. These medications should be discontinued if it is clinically safe to do so.

H_1 antihistamines are also the cornerstone of therapy for chronic urticaria/angioedema but are frequently inadequate to control symptoms. Certain H_1 antihistamines have been proposed as "preferred" for particular subtypes of chronic urticaria, such as hydroxyzine (25 to 50 mg three to four times daily) for cholinergic urticaria or cyproheptadine (2 to 4 mg every 6 hours) for cold-induced urticaria. Some have advocated using multiple H_1 antihistamines, changing or "rotating" agents, or using them in dosages well above those approved by U.S. Food and Drug Administration (FDA) labeling procedures.[6]

Approximately 15% of histamine receptors in the skin are of the H_2 subtype; therefore, the addition of an H_2 antihistamine, such as ranitidine (150 mg twice daily) or famotidine (20 mg twice daily), is a logical adjunct to H_1 antihistamine therapy, providing additional clinical benefit. The tricyclic antidepressant doxepin (10 to 100 mg nightly at bedtime) has highly potent H_1 and H_2 antihistamine activity, with an H_1-receptor affinity almost 800 times that of diphenhydramine and an H_2-receptor affinity 6 times that of cimetidine, but its use can be limited by significant sedation and its tendency to stimulate the appetite, leading to significant gain of weight.

Symptoms often persist despite the use of maximal or supramaximal doses of antihistamines. This is not surprising, considering the number of vasoactive and pruritogenic mediators released by mast cells, of which histamine is only one. Antileukotriene medications, such as montelukast (10 mg/day) or zafirlukast (20 mg twice daily), can be added to antihistamines, with some success. Especially severe symptoms may require systemic corticosteroids (prednisone 10 to 60 mg/day) to achieve symptomatic control, but strong concerns about side effects limit their usefulness.

Refractory symptoms have been treated with a wide variety of other medications. Some of these medications (adrenergic agents, calcium-channel blockers) are thought to decrease the ability of mast cells to release mediators. Others drugs are anti-inflammatory (hydroxychloroquine, sulfasalazine, dapsone, colchicine), immunomodulatory (cyclosporine, tacrolimus, mycophenolate), or antimetabolic (azathioprine, cyclophosphamide, methotrexate). Other treatments of refractory autoimmune chronic urticaria include intravenous immune globulin, plasmapheresis, and omalizumab (anti-IgE).

Evidence-Based Treatments

Multiple randomized, placebo-controlled studies of chronic urticaria/angioedema have shown the efficacy of both sedating and nonsedating antihistamines.[7] If sedating antihistamines must be used, doxepin is more effective than diphenhydramine, but it must be titrated carefully to avoid significant sedation. H_2-receptor antagonists alone are ineffective, but a meta-analysis of four studies with a total of 144 subjects demonstrated that they are effective when combined with H_1-receptor antagonists.[A1] Prednisone is generally accepted as a mainstay of therapy in difficult cases but has not been formally studied. Cyclosporine (4 mg/kg/day) was shown to be effective in a randomized, placebo-controlled, parallel study of 30 patients with autoimmune urticaria.[8] Leukotriene C_4 receptor antagonists (montelukast, zafirlukast) do not provide any incremental benefit when added to an antihistamine. Omalizumab (a humanized monoclonal antibody that binds and inactivates IgE; 300 mg SQ every 4 weeks) has been shown to be effective in a large randomized placebo-controlled trial.[A2] Although well characterized by described in case studies and used by experts, sulfasalazine, hydroxychloroquine, dapsone, colchicine, methotrexate, azathioprine, and intravenous gamma globulin are immunomodulatory agents that appear to be effective but have not been formally studied.

TREATMENT Rx

Acute urticaria is usually self-limited and responds well to histamine$_1$ (H_1)–type antihistamines. Antihistamines work better if they are taken prophylactically rather than after histamine has been released and is bound to the receptor. Patients often self-medicate with or are prescribed diphenhydramine (25 to 50 mg every 6 hours) or hydroxyzine (25 to 50 mg every 6 hours), but they may experience significant sedation. Second-generation antihistamines such as cetirizine (10 mg nightly at bedtime), fexofenadine (180 mg/day), and loratadine (10 mg/day) are much better tolerated and can be effective, although doses up to four times the standard doses are sometimes necessary.

PREVENTION

It is essential to encourage patients with chronic urticaria to accept the chronicity of their illness and to focus on achieving reasonable symptomatic control with effective treatments that cause the fewest side effects. Many patients with physical urticaria can learn to avoid or to minimize triggers. The few patients for whom chronic urticaria is a feature of systemic illness may find relief if the underlying condition is appropriately treated. An excellent example is that chronic urticaria in patients with clinically apparent thyroid disease often resolves once the thyroid disease is treated. For many patients, other factors that exacerbate their specific symptoms can be identified, including stress or anxiety, hormonal fluctuations, aspirin and other NSAIDs,

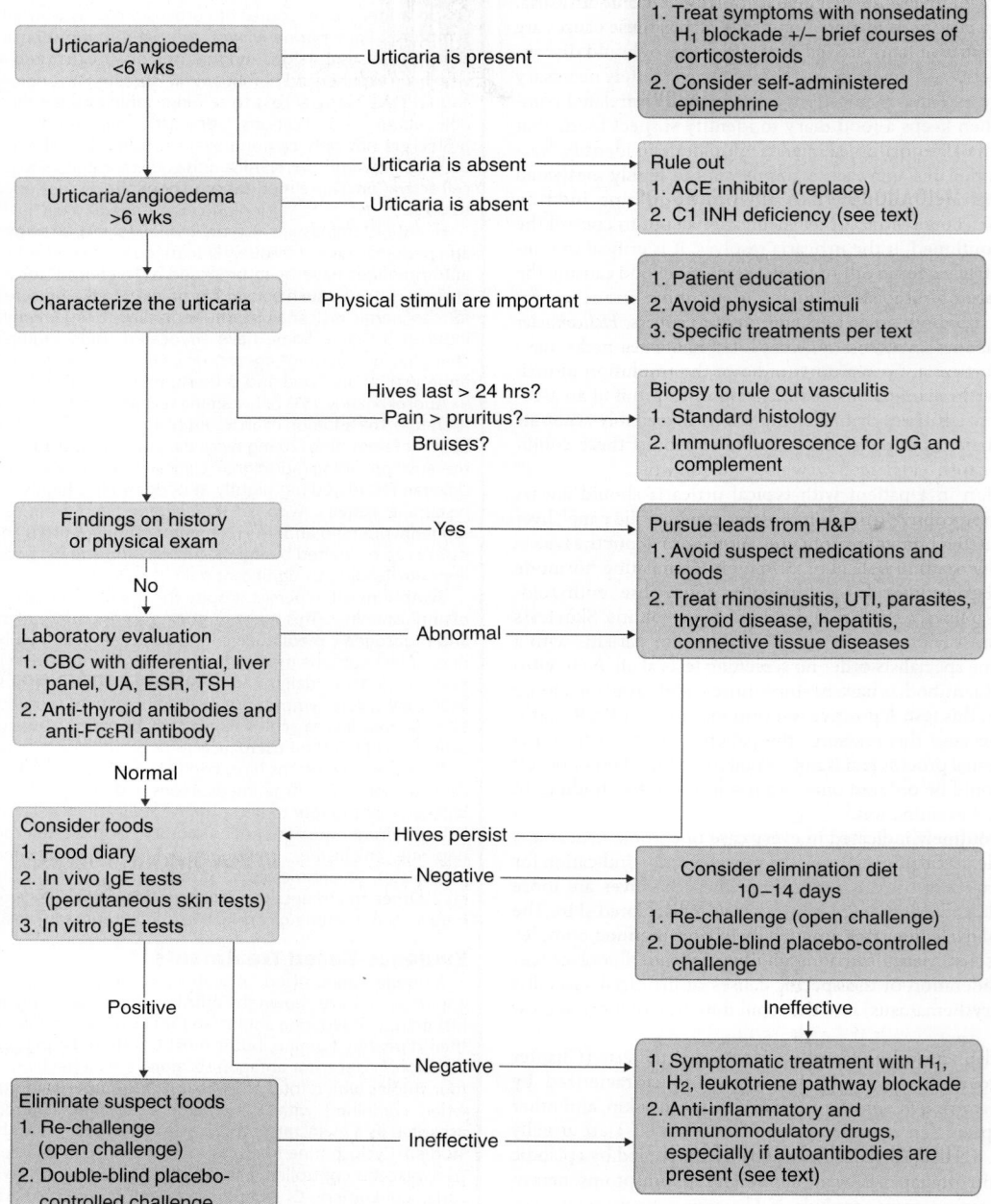

FIGURE 252-2. Evaluation and treatment of urticaria/angioedema. Treatment of urticaria with or without angioedema (AE) can be similar. However, treatment of AE without urticaria depends on the cause. If the AE is caused by an angiotensin-converting enzyme (ACE) inhibitor, discontinuation of the medication is required. Treatment of AE caused by a deficiency or dysfunction of C1 inhibitor (C1 INH) is discussed in the text. Idiopathic AE often responds to treatments described for urticaria/angioedema. CBC = complete blood count; ESR = erythrocyte sedimentation rate; FcεRI = high-affinity receptor for IgE; H & P = history and physical examination; H_1 = histamine$_1$-receptor antagonist; H_2 = histamine$_2$-receptor antagonist; IgE = immunoglobulin E; IgG = immunoglobulin G; TSH = thyroid-stimulating hormone; UA = urinalysis; UTI = urinary tract infection.

and agents that cause cutaneous vasodilation (e.g., alcohol, hot baths or showers, exercise, heated waterbeds). Psychosocial stress is a commonly reported trigger of worsening symptoms. A plausible biochemical mechanism may include increased release of cutaneous neuropeptides known to lower the threshold for mast cell degranulation.

PROGNOSIS

The prognosis for most patients with chronic urticaria/angioedema is excellent. Spontaneous resolution occurs within 12 months in 50% of patients and within 5 years in an additional 20%. However, 10 to 20% of patients, particularly those with physical or autoimmune urticaria, continue to have symptoms for as long as 20 years. Patients who had one episode of chronic urticaria that lasted for months or years and then resolved may experience one or more similar recurrences later in life.

FUTURE DIRECTIONS

The current trend in the treatment of urticaria/angioedema is to use multiple antihistamines and other agents that block the actions of the mediators produced by mast cells. In the near future, it is likely that patients will be treated earlier with anti-inflammatory and immunomodulatory drugs. Some agents under development for asthma and rhinitis may be useful for the treatment of urticaria/angioedema, including 5-lipoxygenase inhibitors, prostaglandin D$_2$-receptor antagonists, and more potent nonsedating antihistamines. Agents that decrease the sensitivity of mast cells to degranulation, such as phosphodiesterase 4 inhibitors and spleen tyrosine kinase (Syk) inhibitors, may also find a role in the treatment of this condition. In spite of the fact that chronic urticaria/angioedema is not thought to be an IgE-mediated disease, as mentioned before, omalizumab (anti-IgE) has been shown to be very effective. This may be due to unexpected effects of IgE on mast cell activation. This finding could have a significant impact on future therapies.[9]

HEREDITARY ANGIOEDEMA AND RELATED DISEASES

DEFINITION

Hereditary angioedema (HAE) and related illnesses are characterized by recurrent attacks of angioedema mediated by vasoactive peptides such as bradykinin.[10]

EPIDEMIOLOGY

HAE affects approximately 1 in 50,000 people. It is an autosomal dominant disease and therefore affects 50% of offspring of both genders. Frequently, a history of several generations with this disease is obtained, but new mutations do occur, and a negative family history is not uncommon. Acquired angioedema (AAE) is more common, affecting older persons who often have a monoclonal gammopathy or a malignant disease such as lymphoma. Angioedema associated with ACE inhibitors occurs in 0.1 to 0.2% of treated patients.[11]

PATHOBIOLOGY

HAE and AAE are caused by either low levels or abnormal function of a regulatory protein in the plasma, C1 inhibitor (C1 INH deficiency), which exerts control of the complement, fibrinolytic, and kinin-generating pathways. Because there is one normal gene, levels of C1 INH are detectable but, because of the abnormal gene, are not sufficient to control the generation of kinins. The C1 esterase enzyme, when activated, cleaves two complement products, C4 and C2. Without proper inhibition, this leads to low levels of circulating C4 and C2. C1 INH is also a critical modulator of the bradykinin pathway, and decreased C1 INH function leads to increased levels of bradykinin. Increased generation of bradykinin, not mediators from mast cells or activation of complement, leads to capillary leakage and angioedema. Changes in levels of C4 and C2, although not important in the pathophysiologic mechanism of the disease, are useful diagnostically.[12]

In HAE type I (85% of patients), the abnormal gene does not produce C1 INH. In HAE type II (15%), an antigenically detectable C1 INH protein is produced, but it is not functional. In HAE type III (very rare), C1 INH is present and functional, but there is a yet-to-be-defined abnormality in the generation of vasoactive compounds. In AAE, unknown factors activate C1 and deplete the C1 INH activity in plasma, or there is an autoantibody to C1 INH that interferes with its function. ACE inhibitor–associated angioedema is due to unintended inhibition of the enzyme that inactivates bradykinin; the complement pathway is unaffected.

CLINICAL MANIFESTATIONS

Children with HAE can have attacks shortly after birth, but these tend to be mild. For most patients, the severity of the attacks worsens at puberty, with episodes of swelling that can affect any external body surface, including the genitalia. Mucosal surfaces are also affected, and patients can have life-threatening swelling of the uvula and posterior pharynx, leading to asphyxiation. Swelling of the submucosa of the gastrointestinal tract can cause symptoms of an "acute abdomen," leading to unnecessary exploratory laparotomy. About half of patients report that trauma, particularly trauma associated with local pressure, precipitates an attack, and about half note an increased frequency of attacks during times of emotional stress. Attacks in patients with AAE are clinically similar to those in patients with HAE. In patients taking ACE inhibitors, angioedema may be manifested as severe swelling or simply as a chronic cough beginning days to months after ACE inhibitor therapy is initiated.

DIAGNOSIS

The best tests to support the diagnosis of HAE or AAE are measurements of C1 INH levels, C1 INH function, and C4 levels, particularly during an attack. The distinguishing features of AAE are onset later in life and the presence of a malignant disease or paraproteinemia. However, in addition to having low levels of C2 and C4, patients with AAE can have profound depressions in the level of C1, a protein that is commonly normal in HAE. Patients with ACE inhibitor–associated angioedema can present within hours after initiation of therapy or after many months and even years. The angioedema seen in urticaria/angioedema is distinctive in that it is usually associated with a pruritic urticarial rash, laboratory evaluation is normal, there is no history of

treatment with an ACE inhibitor, and it responds to antihistamines, steroids, and epinephrine.

TREATMENT ℞

Acute Attacks of Hereditary Angioedema
C1 INH concentrate purified from human plasma (Berinert; 20 units/kg intravenously), icatibant, a bradykinin receptor 2 antagonist (Firazyr; 30 mg SC), and ecallantide, a kallikrein inhibitor (Kalbitor; 30 mg SQ), are all FDA approved for acute attacks of HAE. If these agents are not available, treatment of angioedema of the airway should include racemic epinephrine (1:1000) delivered in the airway by nebulization and by intramuscular injections (0.2 to 0.3 mL of 1:1000 at intervals of 20 to 30 minutes). The addition of antihistamine for sedation may be helpful. Treating physicians must be prepared to perform nasotracheal intubation, preferably in the operating room under conditions in which tracheostomy can be performed if needed. Acute attacks can be terminated by administration of 2 units of fresh-frozen plasma (FFP) to supply the missing C1 INH; but in rare instances, patients may become more edematous, presumably reflecting the increased availability of substrates for the generation of kinins. Therefore, although FFP can be useful for treatment of non–life-threatening acute attacks, it is not recommended for life-threatening laryngeal edema.[13]

Long-term Treatment of Hereditary Angioedema
Attenuated androgens, such as danazol (50 to 200 mg up to twice daily), increase the production of C1 INH and lead to a marked amelioration of symptoms in patients with HAE. Masculinizing side effects are usually mild but can be problematic. These drugs are absolutely contraindicated in pregnancy. C1 INH concentrate (Cinryze; 1000 units IV every 3 to 4 days) is approved for long-term treatment. Many patients with relatively mild disease or infrequent attacks are treated with "on-demand" therapy with either C1 INH, icatibant, or ecallantide.[14]

Prophylaxis
Patients should be treated prophylactically before dental work or other procedures that involve trauma to tissue. Those treated with attenuated androgens, antifibrinolytic agents, FFP (2 units intravenously), or C1 INH concentrate (500 units subcutaneously) have fewer attacks.

Acquired Angioedema
Treatment of AAE is similar to that of HAE, but definitive treatment requires amelioration of the underlying disease.

ACE Inhibitor–Associated Angioedema
Treatment of angioedema associated with the use of an ACE inhibitor includes antihistamines, epinephrine, or both, as appropriate, and discontinuation of the ACE inhibitor. The direct renin inhibitor aliskiren is also associated with a significant risk of angioedema. Rare patients develop angioedema when taking angiotension receptor blockers. These patients are more likely to have idiopathic angioedema than angioedema due to the angiotension receptor blocker.

Evidence-Based Treatments
Current therapy for HAE in the United States includes both prophylactic treatment and on-demand, patient-centered treatment of attacks. Prophylactic administration of anabolic steroids and of C1 INH concentrate[A3] has been shown in a double-blind, placebo-controlled trial to significantly reduce the number of acute attacks. On-demand treatment for acute attacks has been shown to be effective with C1 INH,[A4] icatibant,[A5,A6] and ecallantide.[A7] Ecallantide provides only marginal benefit for treating acute ACE inhibitor-induced angioedema in the emergency department setting.[A8]

PROGNOSIS

The long-term outlook for patients with HAE is largely dependent on the phenotype of the illness (frequency of laryngeal attacks), the ability of the patient to tolerate attenuated androgens, and the patient's access to C1 INH concentrate, icatibant, or ecallantide. Repeated use of these medications for recurrent acute episodes appears to be safe and effective.[15] For most patients, life expectancy should be normal. AAE usually resolves with treatment of the underlying condition, but the ultimate prognosis depends on the nature of that illness. Angioedema associated with the use of an ACE inhibitor can be fatal but usually resolves after the medication is removed.

FUTURE DIRECTIONS

In the last several years, there has been dramatic progress in the availability of medication for HAE.[16] In the near future, the focus will be on tailoring therapy to individual patients and controlling costs.

Grade A References

A1. Fedorowicz Z, van Zuren EJ, Hu N. Histamine H$_2$-receptor antagonists for urticaria. *Cochrane Database Syst Rev.* 2012;3:CD008596.

A2. Maurer M, Rosen K, Hsieh HJ, et al. Omalizumab for the treatment of chronic idiopathic or spontaneous urticaria. *N Engl J Med.* 2013;368:924-935.

A3. Zuraw BL, Busse PJ, White M, et al. Nanofiltered C1 inhibitor concentrate for treatment of hereditary angioedema. *N Engl J Med.* 2010;363:513-522.

A4. Riedl MA, Bernstein JA, Li H, et al. Recombinant human C1-esterase inhibitor relieves symptoms of hereditary angioedema attacks: phase 3, randomized, placebo-controlled trial. *Ann Allergy Asthma Immunol.* 2014;112:163-169.

A5. Cicardi M, Banerji A, Bracho F, et al. Icatibant, a new bradykinin-receptor antagonist, in hereditary angioedema. *N Engl J Med.* 2010;363:532-541.

A6. Lumry WR, Li HH, Levy RJ, et al. Randomized placebo-controlled trial of the bradykinin B$_2$ receptor antagonist icatibant for the treatment of acute attacks of hereditary angioedema: the FAST-3 trial. *Ann Allergy Asthma Immunol.* 2011;107:529-537.

A7. Cicardi M, Levy RJ, McNeil DL, et al. Ecallantide for the treatment of acute attacks in hereditary angioedema. *N Engl J Med.* 2010;363:523-531.

A8. Lewis LM, Graffeo C, Crosley P, et al. Ecallantide for the acute treatment of angiotensin-converting enzyme inhibitor-induced angioedema: a multicenter, randomized, controlled trial. *Ann Emerg Med.* 2014;65:204-213.

GENERAL REFERENCES

For the General References and other additional features, please visit Expert Consult at https://expertconsult.inkling.com.

253

SYSTEMIC ANAPHYLAXIS, FOOD ALLERGY, AND INSECT STING ALLERGY

LAWRENCE B. SCHWARTZ

DEFINITION

Systemic anaphylaxis, a form of immediate hypersensitivity, arises when mast cells and possibly basophils are provoked to secrete mediators with potent vasoactive and smooth muscle contractile activities that evoke a systemic response. Although mast cells in any organ system may be involved, depending on the distribution of the instigating stimulus, the principal targets are the cardiovascular, cutaneous, respiratory, and gastrointestinal systems, sites where mast cells are most abundant. Systemic anaphylaxis can occur when these cells are activated by allergen that binds immunoglobulin E (IgE), or classic immediate hypersensitivity, and by alternative pathways.

EPIDEMIOLOGY

Assessments of the annual incidence of systemic anaphylaxis and the prevalence of those at risk for systemic anaphylaxis are compromised by imprecise diagnostic measures. Approximately 1500 to 2000 deaths in the United States per year are attributed to systemic anaphylaxis. The incidence of nonfatal cases has been estimated to be between 10 and 100 cases per 100,000 person-years. A random public telephone survey of 1000 adults conducted in 2011, designed to estimate the lifetime prevalence of systemic anaphylaxis, elicited a positive personal history in 7.7% of the participants, which was lowered to 1.6% using stringent criteria based on severity (hospitalization and "felt their life was in danger") and at least two organ systems being involved, including either respiratory or cardiovascular or both.[1] In children and adolescents,[2] because food allergy is more common, the incidence of anaphylaxis is likely to be higher. A separate survey of about 1000 at-risk patients also was conducted, focusing on subjects who had a history of some type of generalized allergic reaction, identifying systemic anaphylaxis in about one third. In both public and patient surveys, respiratory or cutaneous symptoms each occurred in more than 50%, whereas cardiovascular, neurologic, or gastrointestinal symptoms were recognized in less than 50%. Among patients, medications were the most common trigger, followed by insect stings, foods, environmental allergens, and latex, but the list of offending agents was lengthy and in some cases was unknown. About half of the reactions occurred at home, 14% at a hospital or clinic, and 6 to 7% at a family member's or friend's home, at work, or at a restaurant. Among adolescents, it has been estimated that one

in four first-time reactions occurs outside the home, and therefore training of school and college staff also is essential.[2] Antibiotics and radiocontrast media are the most common triggers in hospitals. In the perioperative setting, systemic anaphylactic reactions occur with a frequency of about 1 in 3500, muscle relaxants being the most common, but antibiotics, latex, induction drugs, and other drugs can also be the culprit.[3]

Anaphylaxis to foods and insect stings each account for about 100 deaths per year. Most fatal anaphylactic reactions to injected venom proteins begin within 30 minutes after the sting. Most fatal food and insect sting reactions and many drug reactions are preceded by a mild immediate hypersensitivity reaction to the same allergen. Recognition of these earlier events as an important risk factor for future fatal anaphylaxis should lead to implementation of an action plan to prevent and deal with such reactions.

Food allergy is found in about 6% of children younger than 3 years of age and in half that percentage of adults, and these individuals are at risk for food-induced anaphylaxis. Most children lose their allergic sensitivities to cow's milk, egg, wheat, or soy by 5 years of age, whereas sensitivities to peanut, tree nuts, or seafood are typically long lasting. About 20% of children lose peanut sensitivity by school age, but a small portion of these regain peanut sensitivity later in life, particularly if they continue to avoid this food.

Latex provokes anaphylaxis in a small but significant group of individuals, particularly patients who have undergone multiple surgical procedures early in life, such as those with spina bifida or congenital urinary tract disorders, and those with frequent exposure later in life, such as medical personnel. Estimates of the prevalence of latex hypersensitivity range from 1 to 6% in the general population and about 10% among regularly exposed health care workers. Over a 5-year period, the U.S. Food and Drug Administration (FDA) collected approximately 1100 reports of latex-induced anaphylaxis, including 15 deaths. Elimination of powder latex gloves and availability of nonlatex gloves has diminished the prevalence of this problem. Contact hypersensitivity is diagnosed by patch testing, and immediate hypersensitivity by latex-specific IgE tests performed in vitro. Latex allergen skin test reagents have not yet received FDA approval.

PATHOBIOLOGY
Etiology

The mediators produced by activated mast cells and basophils initiate many of the signs and symptoms of anaphylaxis. These cells constitutively express the high-affinity receptor for IgE, FcεRI, on their cell surfaces. Consequently, these cells will always be armed with antigen-specific IgE, which is produced by sensitive individuals and enables cells to respond to antigens that aggregate IgE-FcεRI complexes on their surfaces. Therapeutic interventions aim to prevent the activation of these cells and to block the production or actions of their mediators. Cells other than mast cells and basophils also undoubtedly participate in systemic anaphylaxis, particularly those expressing FcεRI. Eosinophils, monocytes, antigen-presenting cells, and epithelial cells may be induced to express this receptor and thereby affect the intensity, duration, or character of anaphylactic reactions.

Most IgE-dependent mast cell activation events occur at local sites and result in local disease. For example, allergic conjunctivitis, allergic rhinitis, or allergic asthma typically occurs when allergen lands on the corresponding mucosal surface of a sensitive individual and diffuses into the tissue where mast cells reside. Systemic anaphylaxis presumably requires the allergen (or nonallergen agonist) to distribute systemically to activate mast cells at remote sites. This is more likely to occur when allergen is administered parenterally and is less likely after oral ingestion, inhalation, or cutaneous or ocular topical contact. Activation of mast cells in perivascular locations should have the greatest effect on systemic vascular responses. Additionally, the responsiveness of various organ systems to mast cell mediators may be influenced by local factors. Although mediators released at one tissue site could, in theory, spill into the circulation and affect remote sites, most vasoactive mediators are rapidly metabolized.

Allergens

The most common allergens causing systemic anaphylactic reactions include drugs, insect venoms, foods, radiocontrast media, allergen immunotherapy injections, and latex (Table 253-1). Most allergens are typically proteins or glycoproteins that serve as complete antigens, having at least two epitopes recognized by different IgE antibodies, and thereby capable of eliciting immediate hypersensitivity reactions in a sensitized subject without further processing. The protease activity of some allergens, such as house dust mite Der

TABLE 253-1 CAUSES OF SYSTEMIC ANAPHYLAXIS

IgE-MEDIATED	NON-IgE-MEDIATED
Insect stings	Aspirin
Foods	Radiocontrast media
Drugs	Exercise
Latex	Narcotics, vancomycin
Allergen extracts	Autoimmune
	Idiopathic

IgE = immunoglobulin E.

p1, may facilitate their penetration at mucosal sites. Others have lipid-binding domains, such as Der p2, that increase their antigenic potency. Anaphylactic reactions to a humanized monoclonal antibody, cetuximab, can occur on first exposure, owing to IgE against a nonhuman carbohydrate moiety, alpha-gal, which was made by the animal cells and conjugated to the recombinant humanized antibody being expressed. This IgE antibody seems to form against alpha-gal in tick secretions, also causing delayed (3 to 6 hours) anaphylactic reactions after ingestion of red meats, which contain alpha-gal.

In contrast to complete antigens, most drugs act as haptens. They become covalently linked to self-proteins in the circulation, in tissues or on cells, emerging as multivalent allergens. Multivalency is important for immediate hypersensitivity because cross-linking of at least two IgE molecules on the surface of cells aggregates FcεRI molecules, which then transmit an activating signal into the cell. Monovalent antigens fail to elicit mediator release because they bind IgE molecules without cross-linking them.

An allergen exposure must lead to sensitization before an immediate hypersensitivity reaction can occur. This process, which takes at least 1 week, involves antigen processing by antigen-presenting cells, which then present peptide antigens to T_H2 cells (helper T lymphocytes), which in turn select, nurture, and instruct allergen-specific B cells to switch from production of allergen-specific IgM or IgG to IgE. Production of interleukin-4 (IL-4) or IL-13 by T_H2 cells and binding of T_H2 CD40 ligand to B-cell CD40 are essential for this antibody class switch. Consequently, anaphylaxis does not typically occur on first exposure to an allergen (sensitization phase) because the antigen is likely gone by the time antigen-specific IgE is made, but it may occur after subsequent exposures.

Food

Most cases of *food-induced anaphylaxis* in children occur in response to egg, peanut, cow's milk, wheat, or soy, whereas peanuts, tree nuts, and seafood account for most reactions in adults. Reactions to seeds such as sesame seem to be growing in importance, and a variety of different foods have proved to be important allergens in specific individuals. Some patients have the *oral allergy syndrome*, which typically occurs in subjects sensitive to pollen allergens, their pollen-specific IgE cross-reacting to certain food allergens, such as ragweed with melon or birch with peach or apple. Also, the food epitopes involved are typically conformational (rather than linear), are therefore more easily destroyed by heating (cooking), by acid in the stomach, or by proteases in the intestines, and thus rarely progress to systemic reactions.

Food allergy-associated exercise-dependent anaphylaxis occurs when a sensitive subject exercises within several hours after eating the food to which they are sensitive, but not when eating the food without exercise. Shrimp and wheat are most commonly implicated. Exercise appears to increase intestinal permeability to food antigens, which then enter into the systemic circulation. Aspirin and nonsteroidal anti-inflammatory drugs (NSAIDs) also act to increase intestinal permeability. Avoiding the implicated food for 4 to 6 hours before exercise is recommended.

Insect Sting

Hymenoptera families primarily responsible for anaphylactic reactions include the Apidae (honey bees and bumble bees), Vespidae (hornets, yellow jackets, and paper wasps), and Formicidae (fire ants). Major allergens of honeybees include phospholipase A_2 (Api m 1), hyaluronidase (Api m 2), and melitin (Api m 4). Bumblebee venom proteins exhibit immunologic cross-reactivity with those of the honeybee, even though melitin is lacking. Vespid venoms cross-react among themselves and include proteins named antigen 5, phospholipase, and hyaluronidase, the latter allergen cross-reacting with bee hyaluronidase. Fire ant venom toxicity is caused principally by various alkaloids, which are not allergenic. Immediate hypersensitivity

reactions to fire ant venom target a phospholipase that cross-reacts with the comparable vespid enzyme and various other proteins that are unique antigens. Allergens in fire ant venom cross-react with those in scorpion venom. A person may exhibit an anaphylactic reaction on first exposure to an insect's sting if previously sensitized to cross-reactive venom from a different insect. In contrast to stinging insects, allergens from biting insects of the Diptera order (mosquitoes, gnats, midges, true flies) are salivary in origin and do not cross-react with Hymenoptera venom allergens. Anaphylaxis to these salivary proteins appears to be uncommon, but precise epidemiologic data are problematic because people are often unaware of an ongoing mosquito bite, and commercial diagnostic reagents of high quality are not yet available.

Latex

Latex allergens are derived from the rubber tree, *Hevea brasiliensis*. Irritant dermatitis is the most frequent contact reaction and does not involve acquired immunity. Contact hypersensitivity, which results from cell-mediated immunity to haptenic chemicals added to latex during processing, produces a poison ivy–like local reaction that may appear the day after a sensitive subject is exposed. In contrast, immediate hypersensitivity occurs when IgE is made against proteins naturally found in this plant-derived product. Cutaneous (elastic materials), mucosal or intravascular (catheters), oral (balloon), and inhaled (powdered latex gloves) routes of exposure have been well documented and generally elicit signs and symptoms within minutes of exposure. IgE-mediated cross-reactivities between latex proteins and allergens in certain fresh foods such as banana, chestnut, avocado, kiwi, peach, bell pepper, and tomato have been reported and may necessitate avoidance of these foods.

Non–IgE-Dependent Agonists

Most foreign agents that trigger non–IgE-dependent anaphylaxis do not require antigen processing and can elicit a mast cell activation response on first exposure. These include radiocontrast dyes, narcotics such as codeine and morphine, and vancomycin (see Table 253-1). The dose and rate of administration and individual variations in sensitivity are determinants of severity. For radiocontrast dyes, media of low ionic strength and iso-osmolarity are less likely than those of high ionic strength and hyperosmolarity to elicit a systemic reaction. Vancomycin produces a non–IgE-dependent mast cell activation event known as *red man syndrome*, typically involving flushing and sometimes urticaria, but without cardiovascular compromise unless infused too rapidly; and these reactions usually can be avoided by reducing the rate of administration of the antibiotic, thereby reducing peak levels.

Endogenous mast cell activators include neuropeptides such as substance P, neurokinin A, calcitonin gene–related peptide, and the complement anaphylatoxins C3a and C5a. Whether a magnitude of mast cell activation sufficient to cause systemic anaphylaxis can result from endogenous secretion or generation of these peptides by themselves is unproved. For example, an anaphylactic shock–like syndrome occurred in hemodialysis patients exposed to a contaminated hemodialysis membrane that was associated with complement activation without detectable mast cell activation, and infusion of heparin contaminated with oversulfated chondroitin sulfate caused shock by activating the contact pathway and presumably generating bradykinin.

Aspirin and NSAIDs

Aspirin hypersensitivity typically manifests as either a respiratory or a cardiovascular reaction, although sometimes overlap is observed.[4] Respiratory reactions include bronchospasm, nasal congestion, and rhinorrhea and may extend beyond the respiratory tract to include abdominal cramping, watery diarrhea, and urticaria. Cardiovascular reactions that are identical clinically to allergen-induced systemic anaphylaxis and shock also can occur. In most cases, such reactions appear to be pharmacologically (not IgE) mediated, and in sensitive subjects they can occur in response to any of the cyclooxygenase 1 (COX1) inhibitors. Although cyclooxygenase inhibitors may shunt arachidonic acid metabolism to the lipoxygenase pathway, a mechanism to explain mast cell activation has not yet emerged. COX2-selective inhibitors appear to be relatively safe in aspirin-intolerant asthmatic patients but may still cause cardiovascular reactions in those who present with this manifestation. Less commonly, sensitivity occurs to only one of the drugs within this class and is caused by IgE against an associated unique chemical moiety on that particular drug. Human mast cells also express the low-affinity IgG receptor, FcγRIIa, which when aggregated by IgG immune complexes is capable of activating mast cells, and, at least in theory, may contribute to some episodes of anaphylaxis.[5]

Physical Stimuli

Physical stimuli may precipitate systemic anaphylaxis in certain individuals. Episodes can occur in response to exercise, heat, solar radiation, vibration, pressure, or cold. Exercise-dependent anaphylaxis is sometimes associated with ingestion of any food, regardless if sensitivity to the food can be documented, occurring within several hours of ingestion, and it might be avoided by delaying exercise until several hours after eating.

Autoimmunity and Activating Kit Mutations

Some patients experience spontaneous bouts of anaphylaxis without an obvious stimulus. Those with systemic mastocytosis (Chapter 255) are particularly prone to systemic anaphylaxis, perhaps because they have too many mast cells and because the mast cells they do have harbor a somatically acquired activating mutation of Kit tyrosine kinase that primes their activation status.[6] A corollary of this is that systemic anaphylaxis to an insect sting may be a presenting manifestation of mastocytosis, particularly if a baseline serum tryptase level is elevated (see later).[7] A related disorder, *mast cell activation syndrome*, includes patients with clonal mast cell disease, reflected by these same Kit mutations, who have recurrent bouts of anaphylaxis, but who either do or do not meet diagnostic criteria for systemic mastocytosis.[8] A cohort of patients, described in 2014, had elevated baseline serum tryptase levels, atopy and connective tissue disorders, and either spontaneous anaphylaxis or anaphylaxis triggered by heat, exercise, vibration, emotional stress, nonspecific foods, or minor physical trauma, inheriting this phenotype in an autosomal dominant pattern, but having no discernible mutations in their *c-Kit* gene, suggesting that mutation in other genes might increase the risk for anaphylaxis.

Some cases of chronic urticaria are known to be associated with IgG and IgM antibodies against FcεRI or IgE.[9] In such cases, complement activation leading to the generation of complement anaphylatoxins at the surface of mast cells has been postulated to synergize with FcεRI-mediated activation. These reactions may occur preferentially in the skin because of the expression of anaphylatoxin receptors on the type of mast cell that predominates in the skin but not on the type that predominates in lung. An analogous, albeit speculative, autoimmune process might activate mast cells localized in blood vessel walls, the result being anaphylaxis.

Autoimmune progesterone-mediated anaphylaxis, *catamenial anaphylaxis*, which tends to occur just before menses, is uncommon but well documented and may respond to medical or surgical interventions that prevent menses.[10]

Pathophysiology

Mast cells participate in both acquired and innate forms of immunity (Chapter 255). They develop in peripheral tissues from bone marrow progenitors, primarily under the influence of stem cell factor, the ligand for the tyrosine kinase receptor called Kit. Armed with allergen-specific IgE, mast cells are activated by multivalent allergens that cross-link IgE and aggregate FcεRI molecules on the cell surface. This may be important in the defense against certain parasites that elicit a strong IgE response. Experiments performed in rodents suggest that mast cells can be directly activated by microbial products, leading to the secretion of mediators that recruit neutrophils. This innate immune response may restrain bacterial dissemination until a more potent acquired immune response develops. Activation of mast cells by endogenous peptides such as substance P or calcitonin gene–related peptide may influence basic biologic processes such as wound healing and angiogenesis. Whether human mast cells have a critical, nonredundant role in these biologic and immunologic processes remains controversial. However, their central role in immediate hypersensitivity is clear.

Mediators released by mast cells include preformed mediators stored in secretory granules, some of which are preferentially or exclusively made by mast cells, newly generated lipid products, which are not precise biomarkers for mast cells and include metabolites of arachidonic acid, and an array of cytokines and chemokines. Histamine, formed from histidine by histidine decarboxylase, is the sole biogenic amine stored in all granules of human mast cells and basophils. Histamine released by mast cells or basophils diffuses freely and interacts with H_1, H_2, H_3, and H_4 receptors. H_1 receptors are found on endothelial cells, smooth muscle cells, and sensory nerves; when stimulated, bronchial and gastrointestinal smooth muscle contraction, vascular smooth muscle relaxation, increased permeability of postcapillary venules, coronary artery vasoconstriction, and pruritus can occur—signs and symptoms often associated with systemic anaphylaxis. In the central nervous system (CNS), blockade of H_1 receptors appears to cause drowsiness. H_2 receptors reside on gastric parietal cells and at lower levels on inflammatory cells, bronchial epithelium, and endothelium and in the CNS. H_2-receptor–mediated increased acid production in the stomach may occur transiently during systemic anaphylaxis, but it is more likely to become clinically significant if histamine levels are chronically elevated, as occurs with systemic mastocytosis. H_3 receptors are found primarily on cells in the CNS. H_4 receptors are found on hematopoietic cells, such as mast cells, basophils, eosinophils and lymphocytes, and may modulate certain aspects of inflammation, such as eosinophil recruitment, as well as pruritus. Histamine, after its secretion from mast cells and basophils, is rapidly metabolized to inactive methylhistamine and methylimidazole acetic acid.

Prostaglandin D_2 (PGD_2) is the principal COX-catalyzed product of arachidonic acid secreted by activated mast cells, but it is not made by basophils. It binds to the G protein–coupled receptors, CRTH2 and DP. Both COX1 and COX2 are involved in PGD_2 production by mast cells. Consequently, a COX inhibitor that is bipotent might be better than one that is selective at blocking PGD_2-mediated responses during anaphylaxis, which may include hypotension, bronchospasm, inhibition of platelet aggregation, and prolonged asymptomatic cutaneous erythema.

Leukotriene C_4 (LTC_4) is released by both mast cells and basophils after its formation from arachidonic acid and glutathione; its formation is sequentially catalyzed first by 5-lipoxygenase together with 5-lipoxygenase–activating protein and then by LTC synthase. Conversion to LTD_4 and LTE_4, which also are bioactive, occurs in the extracellular space. These sulfidopeptide leukotrienes bind to the G protein–coupled receptors cysteinyl leukotriene 1 ($CysLT_1$), on bronchial smooth muscle, epithelial and endothelial cells, and leukocytes, and $CysLT_2$, on vascular smooth muscle, endothelial and epithelial cells, leukocytes, and heart muscle. LTE_4 may have selective affinity for the P2Y receptor, gpr99. Sulfidopeptide leukotrienes cause bronchoconstriction, mucus secretion, eosinophil recruitment, vasopermeability, diminished cardiac contractility, vasoconstriction of coronary and peripheral arteries, vasodilation of venules, and a burning cutaneous wheal-and-flare response. Antagonists of $CysLT_1$ (montelukast, zafirlukast), but not of $CysLT_2$, as well as a 5-lipoxygenase inhibitor (zileuton), are currently available to patients.

Platelet-activating factor (PAF) is generated from 2-lyso-glycero-3-phosphorylcholine when an acetyl group is placed on the sn-2 carbon of glycerol by acetyltransferase. PAF activates platelets but also is a potent vasoactive mediator that enhances vasodilation and vasopermeability and a smooth muscle constrictor that is capable of inducing bronchospasm. PAF is generated by both mast cells and basophils, as well as by other cell types. Elevated levels of PAF and low levels of circulating PAF acetylhydrolase, which converts PAF back to inactive lyso-PAF by removing the sn-2 acetyl moiety, have been associated with more severe food-induced systemic anaphylaxis. Sphingosine-1-phosphate (S1P) is generated from sphingosine by sphingosine kinase in activated mast cells, as well as in other cell types, and may enhance the vascular response during systemic anaphylaxis.

Mast cells also are the sole or principal source of heparin proteoglycan and certain proteases. All express β-tryptase, and a subset also expresses chymase, mast cell carboxypeptidase, and cathepsin G (like neutrophils and monocytes). Mast cells that express only tryptase are called MC_T cells; those that also express the other proteases are called MC_{TC} cells. Mature tryptase is stored in the secretory granules of all mast cells and is released during degranulation of activated cells; acute levels in serum serve as a clinical biomarker for mast cell activation. In contrast, precursor forms of tryptase (protryptase) are spontaneously secreted by mast cells at rest; baseline levels in serum reflect the total body burden of mast cells, serve as a minor diagnostic criterion for systemic mastocytosis, and serve as a biomarker for anaphylactic risk in allergen-sensitized subjects. MC_{TC} but not MC_T cells express CD88, the C5a receptor, and therefore are activated by complement C5a. Basophils are relatively deficient in these proteases but likewise express CD88.

Cytokines (tumor necrosis factor-α [TNF-α]; IL-4, -5, -6, -8, -13, and 16; granulocyte-macrophage colony-stimulating factor [GM-CSF]; basic fibroblast growth factor [bFGF]; vascular endothelial growth factor [VEGF]) and chemokines (IL-8, monocyte chemotactic protein-1, monocyte inflammatory protein-1α) represent another dimension of the mediators released by mast cells and basophils. Although these mediators are not selectively produced by these cell types, their vasoactive and inflammatory potential could affect the severity and duration of anaphylaxis. As selective antagonists of the relevant cytokines and chemokines become available and are tested for therapeutic benefits, the roles of these mediators in the pathogenesis of anaphylaxis will be better understood.

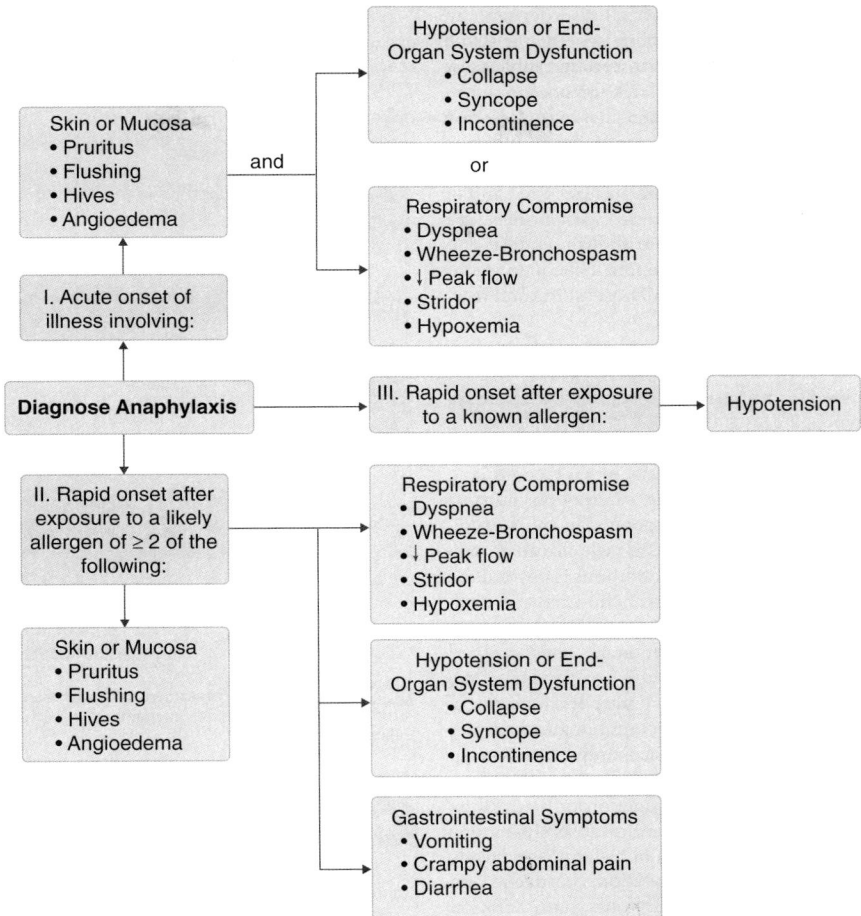

FIGURE 253-1. **Clinical diagnosis of systemic anaphylaxis.** Acute onset of systemic anaphylaxis in the apparent absence of allergen exposure means that the signs and symptoms develop over minutes to several hours, while rapid onset after exposure to a likely or known allergen means that these signs and symptoms begin to occur within minutes to several hours after that exposure. This is based on the Second National Institute of Allergy and Infectious Disease/Food Allergy and Anaphylaxis Network Symposium (From Sampson HA, Muñoz-Furlong A, Campbell RL, et al. Second symposium on the definition and management of anaphylaxis: summary report—second National Institute of Allergy and Infectious Disease/Food Allergy and Anaphylaxis Network symposium. *J Allergy Clin Immunol.* 2006;117:391-397).

DIAGNOSIS

Systemic anaphylaxis can be diagnosed clinically in real time by consensus criteria outlined in Figure 253-1.[11-13] Acute onset of cutaneous signs of immediate hypersensitivity along with either hypotension or respiratory compromise in the apparent absence of allergen exposure, rapid onset of hypersensitivity signs involving at least two organs from among cutaneous, gastrointestinal, respiratory and cardiovascular systems after exposure to a likely allergen, or rapid onset of hypotension after exposure to a known allergen can be used to diagnose systemic anaphylaxis—which sometimes can be precisely confirmed in the laboratory by demonstration of antigen-specific IgE (sensitization) and an acute serum level of total (mature plus pro) tryptase (mast cell activation) that is greater than a baseline level obtained at least 24 hours after all signs and symptoms have resolved. Skin testing or in vitro measurements of antigen-specific IgE should be delayed for at least 2 weeks after the precipitating event to prevent false-negative results. Insect venom allergies also have been assessed by experimental sting challenges, but these are not recommended for routine evaluations. For food allergies, larger wheal-and-flare responses to prick skin tests and higher IgE titers to specific allergens are associated with more severe reactions. Oral food challenges are performed under certain circumstances, taking care to minimize the risk for systemic anaphylaxis. These food-allergic reactions involve IgE sensitization and IgE-dependent mechanisms and should be distinguished from a variety of other types of adverse food reactions, including lactose intolerance due to a deficiency in lactase, food-induced enterocolitis in infants (in reaction to cow's milk, soy, or grains), and celiac disease associated with ingestion of gluten in wheat and other grains.

An increased level of total tryptase in acute (over baseline) serum, which peaks 15 to 60 minutes after the onset of the signs or symptoms of anaphylaxis and then declines with a half-life of about 2 hours (normal baseline levels ranging from 1 to 11 ng/mL), indicates that mast cell activation has occurred. During a study of experimental insect sting–induced anaphylaxis, the increased level of tryptase correlated closely with the drop in mean arterial pressure, indicating that the magnitude of mast cell activation is a primary determinant of clinical severity. Although an increased serum total tryptase level during putative systemic anaphylaxis may be useful for distinguishing anaphylaxis from other conditions in the differential diagnosis, elevations may not be detected after anaphylaxis triggered by food ingestion, or, in general, if anaphylactic severity is either modest (no hypotension) or local (laryngeal edema), or if the acute sample was collected outside of the optimal time. Whether there are anaphylactic IgE-dependent pathways that do not require mast cell activation, but instead involve basophil activation, is unknown but has been considered for anaphylaxis triggered by food allergen ingestion. Plasma histamine, because it is rapidly metabolized, is not as practical as serum or plasma tryptase for detecting anaphylaxis. However, urinary histamine or methylhistamine levels also may reflect overall levels of released histamine, accumulating in urine during anaphylaxis and stored in the bladder until micturition; but levels are affected by ingested histamine-containing foods, histamine-producing mucosal bacteria, and variability in histamine metabolism. PGD$_2$, which is made by several cell types, including activated mast cells, is rapidly metabolized to PGF$_{2\alpha}$, and urinary levels of this metabolite should be elevated in urine formed during anaphylaxis.

An elevated baseline level of serum total tryptase also appears to be a risk factor for increasing severity of insect venom-mediated systemic anaphylaxis, perhaps in part because of an underlying clonal mast cell disorder with an activating c-kit mutation. Future studies will determine whether baseline serum tryptase levels should guide therapy for venom-sensitive subjects as well as those with other allergic sensitivities. Other risk factors for severe systemic anaphylaxis include a prior allergic event to that allergen and having high blood pressure, particularly if being treated with nonspecific β-blockers or angiotensin-converting enzyme (ACE) inhibitors.

Low serum levels of PAF acetyl hydrolase, which metabolizes PAF, and of ACE, which metabolizes bradykinin, have been associated with more severe food-induced systemic anaphylaxis. Whether slow metabolism of PAF and bradykinin might allow these mediators to play a role in such reactions and whether mediator-specific therapies would be clinically useful in such reactions remain to be determined.

Differential Diagnosis

Anaphylaxis should be distinguished from a variety of disorders with overlapping presentations. Vasovagal syncope causes diaphoresis, nausea, hypotension, and bradycardia, but without urticaria and tachycardia. Flushing disorders may be benign and unrelated to anaphylaxis, or they could be a manifestation of pathologic conditions such as the carcinoid syndrome (Chapter 232), with which urticaria and profound hypotension are not typically associated, or pheochromocytoma (Chapter 228), which causes episodic hypertension. Precise detection of these latter conditions is beyond the scope of this chapter. Panic attacks and vocal cord dysfunction can be a challenge to distinguish from anaphylaxis, especially by history alone, but nevertheless must be considered. Acute attacks of hereditary and acquired angioedema (Chapter 252) caused by C1 esterase inhibitor deficiency are not associated with pruritus or urticaria and persist longer than attacks of anaphylaxis. Shock due to complement activation by contaminated hemodialysis tubing, leading to the generation of C3a and C5a anaphylatoxins, or to activation of the contact system by an oversulfated chondroitin sulfate contaminant in heparin preparations, leading to the production of bradykinin, can occur without involving mast cell activation. Scombroidosis (histamine fish poisoning) occurs 5 to 90 minutes after ingestion of histamine, typically in poorly stored fish, and manifests with flushing, palpitations, headache, and gastrointestinal symptoms. The condition lasts several hours, both duration and severity depending on the amount of histamine ingested, and usually responds to H_1-receptor and H_2-receptor antihistamines, but occasionally requires epinephrine and intravenous fluids. Acute serum sickness, various cell activation syndromes, endotoxin-mediated septic shock, and superantigen-mediated toxic shock syndromes manifest with fever, which is not characteristic of anaphylaxis by itself. Also, hypoglycemia, seizure, and primary pulmonary or cardiac events should be considered.

In some cases, systemic anaphylaxis occurs together with another disorder. For example, a 65-year-old man, after being stung by a wasp, complained of dizziness and shortness of breath, was hypotensive with urticaria, and responded to treatment with intramuscular epinephrine, but also complained of chest pressure; electrocardiography indicated an inferior wall infarction. Acute serum levels of both tryptase and cardiac enzymes were elevated, indicating that both anaphylaxis and myocardial infarction had occurred.

Systemic mastocytosis (Chapter 255) is an important condition to consider in the setting of anaphylaxis. In adults, a somatic activating mutation in the gene for Kit in mast cell progenitors results in an excessive body burden of mast cells. The disease may regress spontaneously in children with this disorder, but this is uncommon in adults. Patients with too many mast cells are at increased risk for anaphylaxis, and anaphylaxis may be a presenting manifestation of systemic mastocytosis. For example, anaphylaxis in response to an insect sting, particularly in the absence of venom-specific IgE (due to direct mast cell agonists), should raise the possibility of systemic mastocytosis. Diagnostic tests for systemic mastocytosis might include a lesional skin biopsy when urticaria pigmentosa is suspected and a bone marrow biopsy, each stained for mast cells by antitryptase and anti-Kit (CD117) immunohistochemistry. Findings of mast cell granulomas (major criterion) and numerous spindle-shaped mast cells (minor criterion) in the bone marrow biopsy, along with mast cells that express CD2 or CD25, a D816V Kit mutation, and an elevated baseline level of serum total tryptase (>20 ng/mL) during a clinically quiescent interval (minor criteria) are used to diagnose systemic mastocytosis. One major and one minor, or three minor, criteria are recommended by the World Health Organization for diagnosis. Mast cell activation syndrome can be diagnosed when spontaneous anaphylaxis occurs in association with only two of these minor criteria.

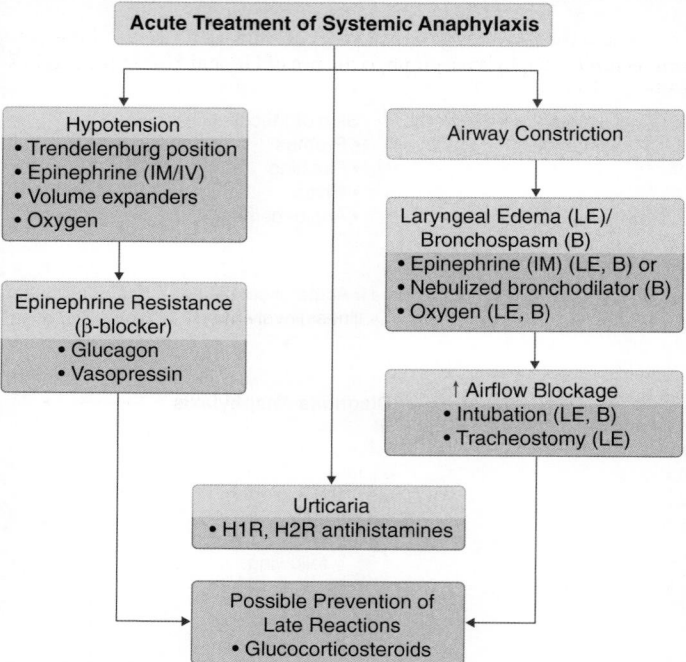

FIGURE 253-2. Acute treatment of systemic anaphylaxis. B = bronchospasm; H1R = histamine-1 receptor; H2R = histamine-2 receptor; IM = intramuscular; LE = laryngeal edema.

TREATMENT   Rx

Fatal outcomes in anaphylaxis are principally the result of either airway constriction or hypotension. Accordingly, the acute treatment of systemic anaphylaxis requires that airway patency, blood pressure, and cardiac status be addressed (Fig. 253-2).[14] Epinephrine, intubation, tracheostomy, volume expanders, and vasopressors may be needed. Patients exhibiting any signs or symptoms of hypotension should immediately assume the Trendelenburg position, which may prevent progression to anaphylactic shock or what has been called in postmortem examinations the *empty ventricle syndrome*—because almost all hypotensive anaphylactic deaths are preceded by syncope occurring in a sitting or upright posture. Epinephrine injected intramuscularly into the thigh (0.2 to 0.5 mg for adults, 0.01 mg/kg up to 0.3 mg for children, repeated every 5 to 30 minutes as indicated) is the most critical drug to administer, the earlier during the course of an anaphylactic event the better. Alternatively, intravenous administration of a solution of epinephrine (1 mg/100 mL solution starting at 30 to 100 mL/hour) and titrated to the lowest effective rate of infusion can be considered. Epinephrine relaxes bronchial smooth muscle and improves vasomotor tone and vasopermeability, thereby counteracting bronchospasm, hypotension, and tissue edema. However, the benefits of epinephrine need to be weighed against its disadvantages in elderly subjects and in those with cerebrovascular or coronary artery disease, hypertension, diabetes, hyperthyroidism, cardiomyopathy, or narrow-angle glaucoma, in whom adverse events such as myocardial infarction, stroke, or pulmonary edema can be precipitated. Also, patients taking a β-blocker may be resistant to epinephrine; in such a case, glucagon (1 to 5 mg/hour intravenously [IV] in adults or 20-30 mcg/kg in children, in each case administered over 5 min or vasopressin (2 to 40 IU IV in adults) may be used. Oxygen should be administered by nasal cannula. Inhaled bronchodilators can relieve bronchospasm. Parenteral administration of H_1-receptor (diphenhydramine, 1 to 2 mg/kg up to 50 mg) and H_2-receptor (ranitidine, 50 mg in adults and 1 mg/kg in children, in each case administered IV over 5 minutes) antihistamines may prevent progression of some of the signs and symptoms, particularly urticaria and pruritus, but is not likely to reverse hypotension or tissue edema. Prednisone (20 mg orally) or Solu-Medrol (40 mg IV) may reduce the risk for a protracted reaction or the late phase of biphasic anaphylaxis but is unlikely to be of benefit acutely.

PREVENTION

Patients who have experienced an anaphylactic reaction are at greatest risk for another episode. Such individuals should wear a Medic-Alert bracelet and be instructed in the use of epinephrine (e.g., EpiPen), which they should carry. Avoidance of nonspecific β-blockers and ACE inhibitors is recommended because either may worsen the severity of an anaphylactic episode, and β-blockers might interfere with β-agonist treatment. In subjects with recurrent anaphylaxis, prophylactic use of H_1- and H_2-receptor antihistamines is beneficial. A leukotriene antagonist and cyclooxygenase inhibitor theoretically would provide additional benefit, but this has not been well studied. Finally, cyclosporine (3 to 5mg/kg per day) might be considered in difficult cases of recurrent anaphylaxis because of its ability to inhibit mast cell activation in vitro and in vivo in chronic urticaria. Omalizumab neutralizes free IgE, and anecdotal reports show benefit in controlling both urticaria and spontaneous episodes of anaphylaxis in mastocytosis patients, but it is not currently approved by the FDA for this indication. Glucocorticosteroids do not inhibit mast cell activation in vitro or immediate skin test responses to allergens in vivo but nevertheless may be beneficial in selected patients with recurrent anaphylaxis.

Specific anaphylactic syndromes have unique considerations. Anti-IgE therapy in peanut-allergic subjects can increase the threshold of sensitivity, on average, from the equivalent of half a peanut to almost nine peanuts.[A1] Insect venom sensitivity can be selectively treated by venom immunotherapy,[A2] dramatically decreasing the risk for anaphylaxis in response to future stings.[15] Reactions to radiocontrast media can be prevented or attenuated by prior administration of prednisone and H_1- and H_2-receptor antihistamines. Patients who are hypersensitive to penicillin should avoid β-lactam antibiotics in general but can be desensitized if an antibiotic in this class is critically needed (e.g., penicillin for neurosyphilis). However, desensitization is temporary; after the drug has cleared, sensitivity is likely to return. Catamenial anaphylaxis may respond to the luteinizing hormone–releasing hormone analog, Lupron, to oophorectomy, or to conjugated estrogens. Patients with systemic mastocytosis, in addition to prophylactic pharmacologic measures, should avoid using direct mast cell agonists such as codeine, morphine, and vancomycin. Aspirin-intolerant subjects can be desensitized but then must continue to ingest a daily dose of aspirin to maintain their desensitization status, thereby benefiting from better asthma control and regression of any nasal polyps that might be present. Food- and latex-sensitive subjects must practice avoidance of the provocative agent, although preliminary data with anti-IgE neutralization therapy and oral immunotherapy indicate that these measures might provide some protection against small inadvertent food allergen exposures. Future research should yield more effective and long-lasting interventions that reduce anaphylactic risk (including better desensitization regimens) and that more effectively reverse the signs and symptoms of this potentially fatal disorder.

Grade A References

A1. Anagnostou K, Islam S, King Y, et al. Assessing the efficacy of oral immunotherapy for the desensitisation of peanut allergy in children (STOP II): a phase 2 randomised controlled trial. *Lancet.* 2014;383:1297-1304.
A2. Boyle RJ, Elremeli M, Hockenhull J, et al. Venom immunotherapy for preventing allergic reactions to insect stings. *Cochrane Database Syst Rev.* 2012;10:CD008838.

GENERAL REFERENCES

For the General References and other additional features, please visit Expert Consult at https://expertconsult.inkling.com.

254

DRUG ALLERGY

LESLIE C. GRAMMER

DEFINITION

Adverse drug reactions (ADRs) are recognized as an important public health problem as they result in both morbidity and mortality. An ADR is defined by the World Health Organization as an unintended, noxious response to a drug that occurs at a dose usually prescribed for human patients. The classic pharmacologic definition of ADRs by Rawlins and Thompson separates these into two major types: type A reactions, which are predictable and dose

dependent; and type B reactions, which are unpredictable and not dose dependent. Type B reactions account for 10 to 25% of all ADRs and include drug allergy. The World Health Organization Nomenclature Review Committee defines *drug allergy* as a hypersensitivity reaction for which a definite immunologic mechanism, either a B-cell–mediated (antibody) or a T-cell–mediated process, is documented. Most published epidemiologic studies refer to ADRs in general and not to drug allergy specifically because the demonstration of drug-specific B-cell–mediated or T-cell–mediated mechanisms is often difficult, and the immunologic culprit may be a drug metabolite.

EPIDEMIOLOGY

Drug allergy is responsible for significant mortality, morbidity, and socioeconomic costs that are probably underestimated. Current data must be evaluated carefully because they involve different populations, different definitions of ADRs and drug allergy, and different methodologies, especially in terms of data analysis. The Boston Collaborative Drug Surveillance Program collected information on all ADRs in 4031 hospitalized patients during a period of 6 months. An incidence of 6.1% was reported, of which 42% were severe; 1% of the severe reactions resulted in the patient's death. Using an automatic detection system in a Salt Lake City hospital, Claussen and coinvestigators identified 731 ADRs among 36,653 hospitalized patients. Of note, only 12.3% of these were reported by physicians in the hospital. In a meta-analysis of 33 U.S. prospective studies from 1966 to 1996, Lazarou reported that 15% of hospitalized patients experienced ADRs and that the frequency of drug-related hospital admissions varied from 3 to 6%. Most other subsequent studies reported similar data.[1] Epidemiologic information on drug allergy in nonhospitalized people and in the general population is even more limited and is confined mainly to studies of antibiotics.

Risk Factors

Some risk factors have been identified for the development of drug allergy.[2] Certain drugs more commonly cause adverse reactions, and some drugs lead to more severe reactions (Table 254-1). The dosage and route of administration of a drug can also be risk factors; intermittent, repeated administrations of a drug can be more sensitizing than uninterrupted therapy. Drug allergy is more commonly reported in women and in patients with HIV infection[3] or reactivation of some herpes viruses. Some ethnic groups appear to be more prone to certain ADRs. For example, white Americans are at a higher risk than other ethnic groups for hypersensitivity reactions to abacavir, a reverse transcriptase inhibitor. For drug allergy caused by angiotensin-converting enzyme inhibitors, the more vulnerable population is African American.

In the United States, approximately 10% of individuals who seek health care have a history of penicillin allergy. However, if tested with an appropriate panel of skin tests, less than 10% of those individuals would be deemed to have a penicillin allergy. Individuals with a positive history and negative skin test results tolerate penicillin-type antibiotics at the same rate as the general population with a negative history; in addition, there is a very low rate of resensitization.

TABLE 254-1	DRUGS FREQUENTLY IMPLICATED IN ALLERGIC DRUG REACTIONS
Allopurinol	
Amiodarone	
Antiarrhythmic drugs (procainamide, quinidine)	
Antibiotics (β-lactams, sulfas, nitrofurans)	
Anticonvulsants (hydantoin, phenobarbital, carbamazepine)	
Antihypertensive agents (angiotensin-converting enzyme inhibitors)	
Antipsychotic tranquilizers	
Antisera (antitoxins, antivirals)	
Antituberculous drugs (isoniazid, rifampicin)	
Aspirin and nonsteroidal anti-inflammatory drugs	
Biologics (monoclonal antibodies such as anti–tumor necrosis factor and other recombinant DNA protein products)	
Chemotherapy agents (cisplatin, doxorubicin, taxanes)	
Enzymes (L-asparaginase, streptokinase, chymopapain)	
Heavy metals (gold salts)	
Muscle relaxants (rocuronium, succinylcholine)	
Radiocontrast media	
Vaccines (egg protein, gelatin)	

PATHOBIOLOGY

Hypersensitivity reactions to drugs can be classified according to the type of immunologic reaction, as originally described by Gell and Coombs with later modifications by Janeway, Kay, and Pichler. An immunologic response to any antigen may be diverse and the resulting reaction complex; drugs are no exception. Drugs that are more frequent perpetrators of significant allergy are listed in Table 254-1.

Most pharmacologic agents are simple structures with a molecular mass of less than 1000 D. Alone, they are unable to induce hypersensitivity-type immunologic responses. However, most of these agents have the ability to covalently bind to proteins and form hapten-carrier complexes, with the low-molecular-weight agent acting as the hapten and the protein being the carrier. Hapten-carrier complexes can induce immunologic responses, with most responses being directed at the hapten. In addition to low-molecular-weight drugs acting as haptens, there is evidence that they may activate immune receptors by binding to them directly. This is known as the pharmacologic interaction with immune receptors (or the p-I) concept.[4]

A well-known example of a low-molecular-weight agent is penicillin. Benzylpenicillin has a molecular mass of approximately 300 D and is metabolized into a penicilloyl hapten moiety. The penicilloyl moiety, which constitutes about 95% of all penicillin metabolites, is referred to as the major determinant because it is the major metabolite in terms of quantity. It has been conjugated to poly-D-lysine to form penicilloyl-polylysine, which is now commercially available as Pre-Pen (ALK-Abelló, Round Rock, TX) for skin testing. The other 5% of penicillin metabolites are referred to as the minor determinants. Although they are minor in quantity, these determinants actually cause most of the immediate-type anaphylactic reactions, whereas the major determinant is associated with later and less severe reactions. Minor determinant reagents have never been commercially available in the United States. Penicillin skin testing[5] is not widely used by U.S. physicians; annually, only 40,000 doses of the major determinant are sold.

In contrast to simple low-molecular-weight drugs, therapeutic agents that are proteins with a molecular mass exceeding 5000 D can be recognized by the human immune system and can result in sensitization and hypersensitivity reactions on subsequent exposure. Because these proteins are complete antigens, they can be used as skin testing reagents or as antigens or allergens in in vitro assays. Included among therapeutic protein reagents that reportedly cause hypersensitivity are antithymocyte globulin (rabbit or equine), streptokinase, latex, and vaccines such as tetanus toxoid. Biologics, including monoclonal antibodies, are increasingly recognized causes of drug hypersensitivity. As anticipated, murine antibodies are most immunogenic, followed by chimeric and then humanized monoclonals. Unexpectedly, a variety of human recombinant proteins, including insulin and fully human monoclonal antibodies, can cause hypersensitivity reactions. In addition to hypersensitivity reactions, biologics such as monoclonal antibodies can cause other immunologic reactions (Chapter 36). One such reaction is the *cytokine release syndrome*, in which high cytokine levels result in systemic symptoms, including fever, arthralgia, and capillary leak; interleukin-2 is the original biologic agent in which this was described.[6] Immune imbalance is another immunologic reaction, exemplified by anti–tumor necrosis factor therapy that results in immune dysregulation consisting of increased susceptibility to infection or autoimmunity.

CLINICAL MANIFESTATIONS

The clinical manifestations of drug allergy often include a dermatologic component (Chapter 440). It is estimated that 80 to 90% of drug allergies result in one of the following cutaneous manifestations: exanthematous or morbilliform eruption; urticaria, angioedema, or both; contact dermatitis; fixed drug eruption; erythema multiforme–like eruption; or photosensitivity.[7] Severe cutaneous adverse reactions (SCARs) are generally induced by drugs and encompass the conditions of Stevens-Johnson syndrome and toxic epidermal necrolysis; drug-induced eosinophilia and systemic syndrome, also known as drug-induced hypersensitivity syndrome; and acute generalized exanthematous pustulosis. These conditions, although rare, cause significant morbidity and even mortality, which is why it is important for the treating physician to promptly recognize SCARs and to discontinue implicated drugs. Some features of SCARs that distinguish them from nonserious cutaneous reactions include involvement of other organs (e.g., liver, kidneys); fever; eosinophilia; mucosal involvement; and lesions that are painful, blistering, or pustular.

DIAGNOSIS

The diagnosis of drug allergy may be simple if a patient has recently started therapy with a single agent known to cause hypersensitivity, such as a β-lactam antibiotic. In contrast, in a hospitalized patient in whom multiple drugs have been started and stopped, identifying the offending drug may be difficult, requiring a complete and exhaustive history along with a physical examination. It also requires compatible clinical manifestations and temporal relationships. In vitro tests are rarely useful clinically. In vivo testing, such as cutaneous tests and provocative test dosing, may be indicated in some situations.

Differential Diagnosis

To distinguish drug allergy from other ADRs, several criteria are helpful.[8] Allergic reactions occur in a tiny fraction of individuals who receive the drug, and they cannot be predicted. The observed clinical effects do not resemble known pharmacologic actions of the drug. In the absence of prior exposure to the drug, allergic or hypersensitivity symptoms rarely appear before 1 week of continuous therapy. In general, drugs used consistently for several months or longer are rarely responsible.

Drug allergy often resembles other allergic or hypersensitivity reactions, such as anaphylaxis, urticaria, and serum sickness–like illness. Although most drug reactions include cutaneous manifestations, some involve only other organ systems, for example, pulmonary infiltrates with eosinophilia, hepatitis, and acute interstitial nephritis. A list of drugs that cause organ-specific reactions is provided in Table 254-2. Drug-specific antibodies or T-cell receptors have been identified that react with the suspected drugs or relevant drug metabolites. As with ADRs in general, the reaction often subsides after the drug is discontinued. However, a hypersensitivity reaction may persist or

TABLE 254-2 ORGAN-SPECIFIC REACTIONS AND IMPLICATED DRUGS

REACTION	IMPLICATED DRUG
PULMONARY MANIFESTATIONS	
Pulmonary infiltrates with eosinophilia	Minocycline, nitrofurantoin
Pneumonitis and fibrosis	Bleomycin, amiodarone
Noncardiogenic pulmonary edema	Hydrochlorothiazide, cocaine, heroin, methadone
AUTOIMMUNE MANIFESTATIONS	
Drug-induced lupus	Hydralazine, procainamide
DRUG-INDUCED IMMUNE CYTOPENIAS	
Thrombocytopenia	Quinidine, gold salts, sulfonamides, heparin
Hemolytic anemia	Penicillin, methyldopa
Agranulocytosis	Sulfonamides, propylthiouracil, quinidine, procainamide, phenytoin
HEPATIC MANIFESTATIONS	
Cholestasis	Aminosalicylic acid, dapsone
Hepatocellular damage	Phenothiazines, erythromycin
Mixed pattern	Halothane, isoniazid, diclofenac
	Phenytoin, sulfonamides
RENAL MANIFESTATIONS	
Nephrotic syndrome	Gold salts, captopril, NSAIDs, penicillamine
Acute interstitial nephritis	β-Lactam antibiotics, NSAIDs, sulfonamides
LYMPHOID SYSTEM MANIFESTATIONS	
Pseudolymphoma	Phenytoin
Infectious mononucleosis–like syndrome	Aminosalicylic acid, dapsone
CARDIAC MANIFESTATIONS	Sulfonamides, β-lactam antibiotics
NEUROLOGIC MANIFESTATIONS	
Peripheral neuritis	Colchicine, nitrofurantoin, sulfonamides

NSAIDs = nonsteroidal anti-inflammatory drugs.

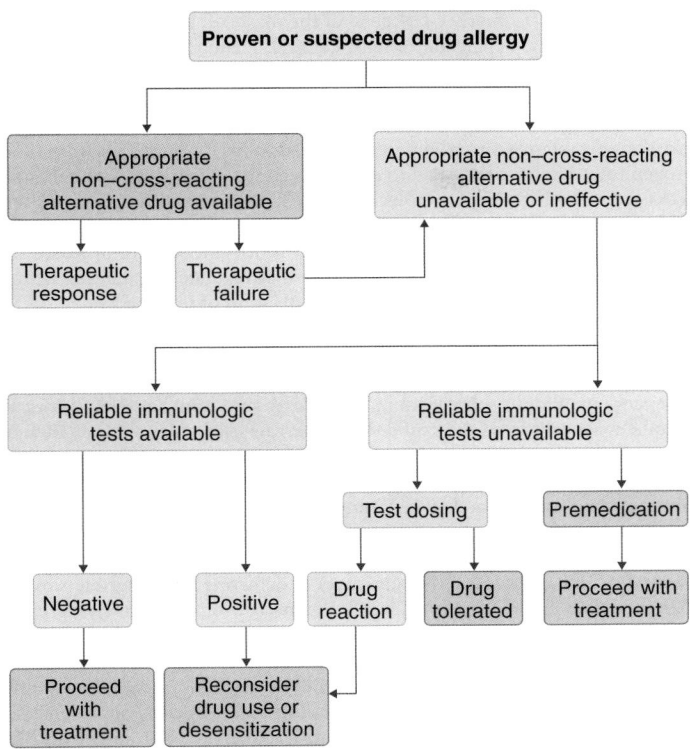

FIGURE 254-1. Guidelines for the treatment of patients with a history of drug allergy. In patients with a suspected or known drug allergy, the first choice is to use an appropriate non–cross-reacting drug. If such a drug is not available, or if the patient does not respond to it, further evaluation is based on the availability of a reliable immunologic test to detect drug hypersensitivity.

TABLE 254-3	RISK OF ANAPHYLACTIC REACTION TO PENICILLIN OR OTHER PHARMACOTHERAPEUTIC AGENTS	
FACTOR	**LOW RISK**	**HIGH RISK**
Onset of previous reaction	>24 hr	<30 min
Signs and symptoms of previous reaction	Morbilliform eruption Urticaria alone	Life-threatening symptoms: hypotension, upper airway angioedema, bronchospasm
Time elapsed since previous reaction	>20 yr	<1 yr

even intensify because of the formation of drug metabolites, which act as haptens and bind to carrier proteins such as human serum albumin.

TREATMENT   Rx

Evidence-Based Treatments

There is a paucity of evidence-based information regarding drug allergy, a disease that is generally iatrogenic. One study evaluated HIV patients who previously had an adverse reaction to cotrimoxazole; it was concluded that desensitization resulted in fewer adverse reactions and fewer treatment discontinuations in patients with a previous history of mild or moderate hypersensitivity.[A1] A second study, evaluating treatment for toxic epidermal necrolysis, concluded that there are no randomized controlled trials of the most commonly used therapies (i.e., systemic steroids, cyclosporine, intravenous immune globulins).

There are published clinical guidelines for the management of infusion-related hypersensitivity reactions caused by the administration of chemotherapeutic or biologic therapy. These guidelines were developed as part of a performance improvement initiative and resulted in a standardized approach to the management and reporting of ADRs.

PREVENTION

Although the outcome of ADRs is generally favorable, prevention is the obvious goal. The physician should prescribe medications only if they are clinically appropriate and, if possible, should avoid drugs that are known to produce significant hypersensitivity reactions (see Table 254-1). Before starting a medication, the patient should be asked about prior ADRs to the medication or to other pharmacologically related medications. If appropriate, oral administration is probably preferable to parenteral administration; anaphylaxis is less likely, as is sensitization. Protocols for skin testing to foreign antisera and for management of medication hypersensitivity reactions (e.g., premedication, test dosing, desensitization) are available.[9,10] Therapeutic guidelines regarding treatment of the most important and common ADRs are also reviewed in those references.[11] A general algorithm is provided in Figure 254-1.

The risk of an anaphylactic reaction to a drug such as penicillin is a function of the history of onset, severity, and proximity (Table 254-3). If an individual experienced an immediate-type reaction that was rapid in onset, involved life-threatening symptoms or signs, and occurred relatively recently, that individual is at high risk for a severe anaphylactic reaction on subsequent exposure.

Even with a negative Pre-Pen skin test result, a patient could have reactivity against minor determinants; therefore, the approach to a patient who needs a β-lactam antibiotic depends on the risk as listed in Table 254-3. Risks and benefits should be thoroughly discussed and documented. In a high-risk individual, cautious test dosing can be performed. If a reaction occurs, desensitization can be considered if the clinical risks and benefits so warrant.

PROGNOSIS

Most drug allergies involve cutaneous eruptions that are self-limited and resolve shortly after the offending agent has been discontinued. However, severe, life-threatening reactions occur in approximately 1 in every 1000 hospitalized patients. SCARs are especially likely to cause morbidity and mortality. In 1998, the death rate for hospitalized Medicare patients was 20% higher in those who experienced an ADR. The proportion of ADRs that were allergic reactions was not determined in this study, but it can be estimated at about one fifth. The incidence of adverse cutaneous reactions to drugs is higher in women than in men. There is also an increased incidence of ADRs in the elderly.

One of the most severe reactions associated with drug allergy is anaphylactic shock (Chapter 253). It is usually immunoglobulin E (IgE) mediated, but it may occur with non–IgE-mediated reactions to drugs such as nonsteroidal anti-inflammatory drugs or radiocontrast media. It is estimated that approximately 1500 people die annually in the United States owing to anaphylaxis from medications. In the United Kingdom, drugs are the leading cause of anaphylactic fatalities.

FUTURE DIRECTIONS

Pharmacogenomics will be an important method of identifying those individuals at risk for a significant allergic reaction to a given drug.[12] Human leukocyte antigen (HLA) genotyping can reportedly identify individuals who are at increased risk for drug hypersensitivity. For example, individuals with HLA-B*5701 are at greater risk for a drug hypersensitivity reaction to abacavir, an HIV transcriptase inhibitor. Severe cutaneous adverse reactions to allopurinol are highly associated with the genetic marker HLA-B*5801. In patients of Asian ancestry, HLA-B*1508 is highly associated with development of Stevens-Johnson syndrome if carbamazepine is prescribed. Why this genetic variant is not a risk factor in patients of African or European ancestry is unclear.[13] Other avenues by which susceptible individuals may be identified include polymorphisms in genes for immune recognition molecules, drug-metabolizing enzymes, and macromolecular adduct repair systems.

Grade A Reference

A1. Lin D, Li WK, Rieder MJ. Cotrimoxazole for prophylaxis or treatment of opportunistic infections of HIV/AIDS in patients with previous history of hypersensitivity to cotrimoxazole. *Cochrane Database Syst Rev.* 2007;2:CD005646.

GENERAL REFERENCES

For the General References and other additional features, please visit Expert Consult at https://expertconsult.inkling.com.

255

MASTOCYTOSIS
CEM AKIN

DEFINITION

Mastocytosis is a heterogeneous group of disorders characterized by pathologic accumulation of mast cells in tissues such as skin and bone marrow. According to the classification of the World Health Organization (WHO), based on clinical presentation and pathologic findings, there are seven distinct categories of mastocytosis (Table 255-1). The term *cutaneous mastocytosis* describes skin disease alone without any evidence of internal organ involvement, whereas the term *systemic mastocytosis* describes the disorder when it involves internal organs (most commonly the bone marrow) with or without skin disease.

EPIDEMIOLOGY

Mastocytosis can be diagnosed at any age.[1] Pediatric-onset and adult-onset forms are distinguished on the basis of the age of the patient at initial diagnosis. These forms display differences in their clinical course, molecular pathology, and prognosis. The most common clinical scenario leading to diagnosis in the pediatric population is a child presenting with skin lesions of cutaneous mastocytosis within the first year of life. Patients with a later onset of skin lesions are more likely to have systemic mastocytosis, as are most patients with adult-onset mastocytosis. The disease has been diagnosed in all ethnic populations. Estimates of the prevalence of patients with cutaneous mastocytosis range from 1 in 500 to 1 in 8000 patients presenting in dermatology clinics. The prevalence of systemic mastocytosis is more difficult to estimate because the diagnosis requires biopsy of an involved tissue and a high degree of clinical suspicion, especially if skin lesions are absent. Systemic mastocytosis is likely to be underdiagnosed, considering the fact that there are neither physical examination findings nor routine hematologic or chemistry laboratory abnormalities specifically associated with the disease. Consequently, it is not unusual to encounter several years' delay after the onset of symptoms in many patients before a diagnosis of mastocytosis is reached. The disease is sporadic, although rare cases of familial occurrence have been described.

PATHOBIOLOGY
Pathogenesis

The pathogenesis of mastocytosis involves the accumulation of mast cells in tissues, with mediators released by activated mast cells. The primary reason for the increased mast cell numbers in tissues appears to be defective apoptosis rather than uncontrolled proliferation. It is unusual to see increased mitotic activity in biopsy specimens from patients with mastocytosis, and, in most patients, the disease follows an indolent course. Tissue microenvironment and altered chemotaxis may also contribute to the final level of tissue mast cell burden.

Genetics

Mast cells are derived from hematopoietic progenitors (Chapter 156). Systemic mastocytosis is associated with somatic gain-of-function point muta-

tions in the *KIT* (formerly *c-kit*) gene of the mast cell progenitor, leading to a clonal neoplastic expansion of mast cells. *KIT* encodes a transmembrane receptor (Kit) whose intracellular portion functions as a tyrosine kinase enzyme. The extracellular portion of Kit binds the cytokine stem cell factor (SCF or Kit ligand). The interaction between SCF and Kit provides the single most important growth and differentiation stimulus for mast cells from their progenitors. Under physiologic conditions, homodimeric SCF binds and cross-links two Kit receptor molecules, which leads to autophosphorylation of the tyrosine amino acids of the intracellular portion of the Kit molecule. Phosphorylated tyrosine residues in turn act as docking sites for downstream adaptor and signal transduction molecules that regulate the differentiation, proliferation, chemotaxis, and functional activation of mast cells.

The most common mutation reported in mastocytosis[2] involves codon 816 in *KIT* (located in exon 17), resulting in the replacement of an aspartic acid by a valine residue (D816V) in the Kit protein, leading to ligand-independent autophosphorylation. The D816V mutation has been shown in lesional mast cells from the skin or bone marrow tissue of more than 90% of adults and approximately 40% of pediatric patients with mastocytosis. Another 40% of pediatric patients carry *KIT* mutations in other exons, most commonly in exons 8 and 9. *KIT* mutations can be demonstrated in non–mast cell hematopoietic lineages in advanced variants of systemic mastocytosis, similar to the multilineage involvement observed in myeloproliferative neoplasms (Chapter 166). The sensitivity of detecting the mutation is much higher when a lesional tissue such as bone marrow or skin is analyzed compared with peripheral blood. Other pathogenetic factors, some yet to be determined, appear to be responsible for the final disease phenotype because the presence of the D816V *KIT* mutation alone does not explain the remarkable heterogeneity in the clinical presentation and prognosis of the disease. Molecular aberrations in *TET2*, *SRSF2*, *ASXL1*, *CBL*, *RUNX1*, and *DNMT3A* were the other most frequently identified mutations in advanced forms of systemic mastocytosis. In advanced systemic mastocytosis, most patients carry three or more mutations.

CLINICAL MANIFESTATIONS
Symptoms

The symptoms of mastocytosis are primarily related to the release of mast cell mediators and rarely by the destructive infiltration of mast cells into tissues. Mast cell activation results in the release of various preformed mediators stored in mast cell granules, de novo synthesis of sulfidopeptide leukotrienes such as LTC_4 and prostaglandins (mostly PGD_2) from membrane lipids, and cytokine synthesis. Preformed mediators stored in mast cell granules include histamine; proteases such as tryptase, chymase, and carboxypeptidase A; and proteoglycans such as heparin and chondroitin sulfate. Vasoactive mediators such as histamine, LTC_4, and PGD_2 at local or distant tissues cause vasodilation, which may lead to flushing, tachycardia, hypotension, presyncope, and syncope. Histamine also causes pruritus and stimulates gastric acid hypersecretion from parietal cells. Mast cells are rich sources of cytokines. Elevated serum levels of tumor necrosis factor-α and interleukin-6 have been found in patients with mastocytosis and may contribute to the pathophysiologic process of fatigue and accelerated osteoporosis observed in some patients. Rare aggressive categories of mastocytosis may be associated with an extensive destructive infiltration of mast cells into tissues such as the gastrointestinal tract, which may result in malabsorption, and the liver, which may cause portal fibrosis with associated portal hypertension.

Mast cell activation and mediator release may occur after triggers, such as temperature changes (e.g., hot showers), exercise, ingestion of alcohol or spicy foods, emotional stress, insect stings, and exposure to certain drugs (such as opioid analgesics, nonsteroidal anti-inflammatory drugs, or muscle relaxants), and sometimes spontaneously without an obvious trigger. The prevalence of atopic disease in patients with mastocytosis is similar to that in the general population, and the serum immunoglobulin E (IgE) level is often found to be low. However, patients with anaphylactic sensitivity to hymenoptera venoms appear to have a disproportionately high incidence of mastocytosis.[3]

Mastocytosis is a disease with protean clinical manifestations. Although in some patients the only complaint is the cosmetic appearance of urticaria pigmentosa lesions, others suffer from frequent episodes of vascular instability or have life-threatening hematologic disease. In general, patients with mastocytosis belong to one of two broad categories, according to the site of tissue involvement: those with cutaneous disease alone, or those with systemic disease with or without skin involvement. Cutaneous mastocytosis (i.e., disease limited to the skin in the absence of internal organ involvement)

TABLE 255-1	WORLD HEALTH ORGANIZATION CLASSIFICATION OF MASTOCYTOSIS

Cutaneous mastocytosis
Indolent systemic mastocytosis
Systemic mastocytosis with associated clonal hematologic non–mast cell lineage disease
Aggressive systemic mastocytosis
Mast cell leukemia
Mast cell sarcoma
Extracutaneous mastocytoma

From Horny HP, Metcalfe DD, Bennett JM, et al. Mastocytosis. In: Swerdlow SH, Campo E, Harris NL, et al, eds. WHO Classification of Tumours of Haematopoietic and Lymphoid Tissues. Lyon, France: IARC Press; 2008:54-63.

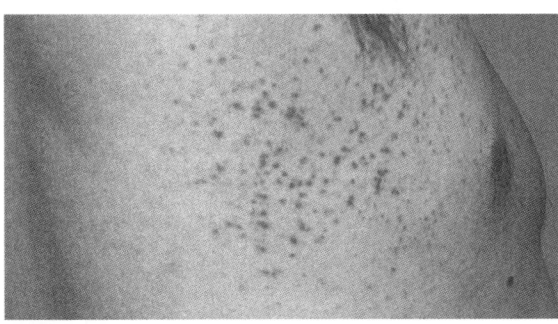

FIGURE 255-1. Urticaria pigmentosa.

is commonly diagnosed in children within the first year of life, whereas systemic mastocytosis is mostly diagnosed in adults by a bone marrow biopsy and aspirate.

Cutaneous Manifestations

Maculopapular skin lesions of urticaria pigmentosa are the most common presentation of cutaneous mastocytosis (Fig. 255-1). They are also present in 50 to 90% of patients with systemic mastocytosis, depending on the disease category. Remarkably different in appearance from urticaria or hives, lesions of urticaria pigmentosa are fixed, tan- to salmon-colored lesions varying in size from a few millimeters to a few centimeters. They are most prominently observed on the trunk and extremities and tend to spare the face and the sun-exposed areas of the skin, although facial involvement may be seen in children. Blistering of the lesions may occur in children in the first 3 years of life. The lesions are generally not pruritic at rest but may urticate after exposure to a number of triggers (see Pathobiology). Many patients note that the skin lesions become more prominent after exposure to heat or after physical irritation such as rubbing. The lesions may be found concentrated in skin areas that are prone to irritation, such as the axillae and groin.

Uncommon presentations of cutaneous mastocytosis include mastocytomas, diffuse cutaneous mastocytosis, and telangiectasia macularis eruptiva perstans (TMEP). Mastocytomas are benign and generally solitary mast cell tumors, although they have been known to precede urticaria pigmentosa lesions in some cases. They occur almost exclusively in children, and physical irritation of the lesion may result in generalized flushing and other symptoms of mast cell mediator release. Diffuse cutaneous mastocytosis is another form of skin involvement seen exclusively in children. It is characterized by diffuse thickening of the skin and appendages with a peau d'orange appearance without individual urticaria pigmentosa lesions. TMEP is a rare form of cutaneous mastocytosis characterized by the presence of diffuse telangiectatic macules. Because TMEP lesions are generally seen in the presence of urticaria pigmentosa, there is debate about whether TMEP represents a distinct form of cutaneous mastocytosis.

Patients with cutaneous mastocytosis may manifest systemic symptoms, such as abdominal pain, diarrhea, and flushing.

Systemic Manifestations

Symptoms caused by mast cell degranulation may be experienced as brief, recurrent, and self-limited episodes with multiorgan manifestations or as chronic complaints during a prolonged time course. A typical mast cell degranulation episode may variably involve flushing, conjunctival hyperemia, nausea, vomiting, abdominal cramping, diarrhea, tachycardia, and lightheadedness. Hypotension may develop, and the episode may progress to full loss of consciousness in some patients. Therefore, mastocytosis should be ruled out in all patients with recurrent anaphylaxis before a diagnosis of idiopathic anaphylaxis can be made.[4] Tryptase, a protease stored in mast cell granules, may be elevated above the patient's baseline level in the serum or plasma if it is measured within 3 hours after the onset of the episode in patients with suspected mast cell degranulation or anaphylaxis, regardless of the cause. Angioedema, hives, and wheezing are uncommon in mastocytosis, in contrast to idiopathic anaphylaxis. Flushing usually involves the face and upper chest area. A consistent trigger can be identified in only a small number of patients (see Pathobiology). The episodes usually last 30 minutes to a few hours. Hypotensive episodes can be life-threatening, particularly in the presence of comorbidities, such as cardiac or pulmonary disease. Systemic mastocytosis should be suspected in all patients with systemic reactions to hymenoptera stings, especially those involving hypotensive syncope or near-syncope.

Gastrointestinal Symptoms

Gastrointestinal symptoms are observed in more than 50% of patients with mastocytosis. Epigastric pain, lower abdominal cramping, nausea, vomiting, or diarrhea can occur episodically in the context of an acute mast cell degranulation episode or on a chronic basis. Gastric acid hypersecretion induced by mast cell–derived histamine may lead to esophagitis, gastritis, and peptic ulcer disease, although measurements of basal acid output have shown great variability in different studies, ranging from hypersecretion in the range of Zollinger-Ellison syndrome to achlorhydria. Mucosal edema, thickened gastric or duodenal mucosal folds, or nodular lesions may be observed in radiographic or endoscopic evaluations. Diarrhea alternating with constipation may be seen. Severe persistent diarrhea may be complicated by clinically significant malabsorption in patients with aggressive systemic mastocytosis. Hematochezia, hematemesis, and melena are uncommon symptoms and should prompt endoscopic evaluation to rule out coexisting disease. Mast cells are constituents of the normal lamina propria in gastrointestinal mucosa, and their numbers may be increased in inflammatory states affecting the gastrointestinal tract. However, quantitation of mast cell numbers in gastrointestinal biopsy specimens is generally not helpful, and diagnosis of mast cell disease by a gastrointestinal biopsy, solely based on increased mast cell numbers without evidence for other WHO criteria, should be avoided. Mild to moderate hepatomegaly with or without abnormalities in serum transaminases may be observed, although portal hypertension and ascites are rare and indicate the presence of advanced categories of mastocytosis. Jaundice and findings on cholangiography resembling those of primary sclerosing cholangitis have been reported in some patients.

Musculoskeletal Symptoms

Musculoskeletal pain is common in patients with mastocytosis and is mostly caused by soft tissue pain resembling fibromyalgia. Accelerated osteoporosis may be seen in a subgroup of patients, particularly those with other risk factors, such as postmenopausal women, and those receiving glucocorticoid therapy. Pathologic compression fractures may be the initial finding in some patients.[5] A bone densitometry measurement should be recommended as part of the standard evaluation of women with mastocytosis and of any patient with a history of pathologic fractures. Radiographic abnormalities have been reported in up to 75% of patients with mastocytosis. In addition to generalized osteoporosis, bone surveys may show a mixture of sclerotic or lytic lesions, and skeletal scintigraphy may reveal focal or diffuse radiotracer uptake.

Hematologic Manifestations

Peripheral blood abnormalities have been noted in up to 50% of patients with systemic mastocytosis. Mild normochromic normocytic anemia is the most common abnormality, followed by thrombocytopenia, eosinophilia, monocytosis, and leukopenia. Eosinophilia in mastocytosis rarely causes organ damage, as is observed in chronic eosinophilic leukemia or idiopathic hypereosinophilic syndrome (Chapter 170). It is important to differentiate a primary eosinophilic disorder from mastocytosis with eosinophilia. Some cases of chronic eosinophilic leukemia are associated with the *FIP1L1-PDGFRA* fusion gene and respond to the drug imatinib, whereas systemic mastocytosis is associated with codon 816 point mutations of the *KIT* gene, which confers resistance to this drug.

Approximately 20% of patients with systemic mastocytosis have been reported to display evidence of another clonal non–mast cell hematologic disease. Non–mast cell clonal hematologic neoplasms associated with mastocytosis are commonly myeloid in nature (myeloproliferative neoplasms, myelodysplastic syndromes, or myeloid leukemias) but may also involve lymphoproliferative disorders, such as lymphomas, myelomas, and lymphocytic leukemias.

DIAGNOSIS

The diagnosis and classification of mastocytosis are carried out according to the guidelines published by the WHO. A suggested algorithm for the diagnosis of mastocytosis is shown in Figure 255-2.

Cutaneous Mastocytosis

Diagnosis of cutaneous mastocytosis is made by observing the typical hyperpigmented maculopapular lesions of urticaria pigmentosa and is confirmed

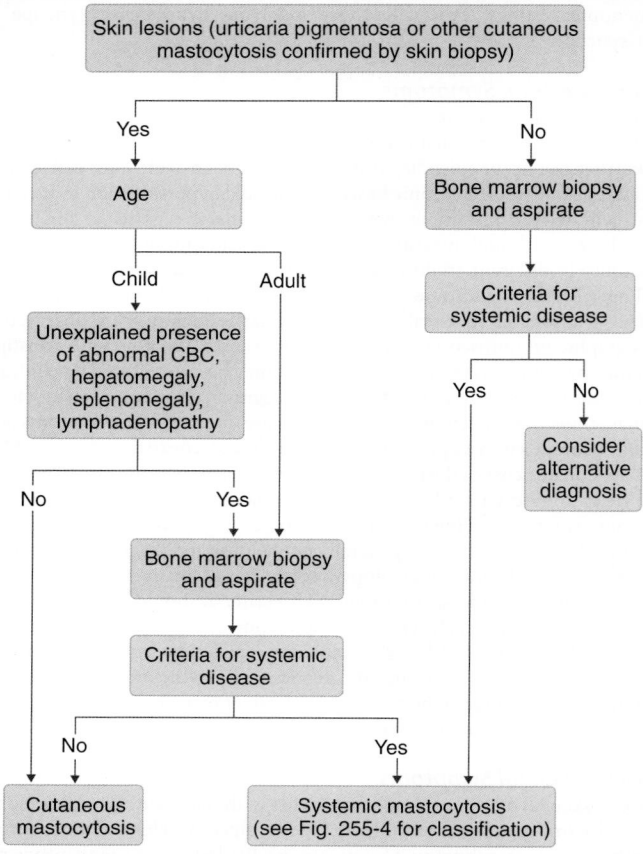

FIGURE 255-2. Suggested diagnostic algorithm for mastocytosis. CBC = complete blood count.

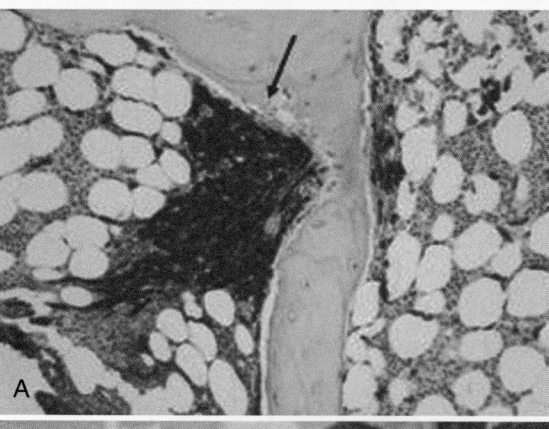

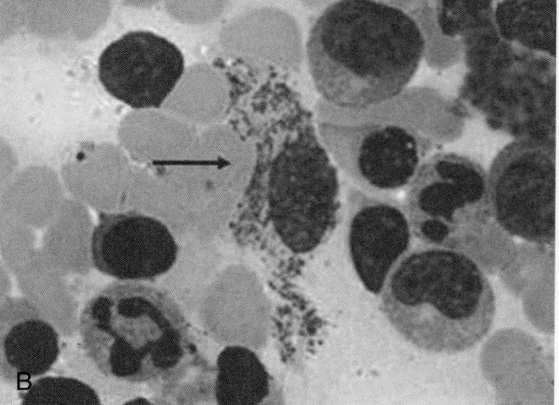

FIGURE 255-3. Diagnostic findings in the bone marrow biopsy specimen and aspirate smear. A, Characteristic mast cell aggregates on tryptase staining (major criterion) in biopsy section (*arrow*). B, Mast cells with atypical spindle shapes in aspirate smear (*arrow*).

by skin biopsy, which shows infiltration of mast cells in the upper dermis, particularly in perivascular locations. Mild increases in mast cell numbers can be observed in inflammatory and neoplastic skin diseases, and establishing a diagnosis of cutaneous mastocytosis by a blind skin biopsy or biopsy of a lesion that does not have the typical appearance of urticaria pigmentosa should be avoided. A localized wheal-and-flare reaction limited to the lesional skin within a few minutes after rubbing or scratching of the skin is known as Darier's sign. Diagnosis of urticaria pigmentosa in adults should always prompt investigation of possible systemic mastocytosis.

Systemic Mastocytosis
Biopsy
The recommended diagnostic procedure to evaluate the presence of WHO diagnostic criteria for systemic disease (discussed later) is a bone marrow biopsy and aspiration. This procedure is recommended for all patients with adult-onset urticaria pigmentosa, patients with recurrent symptoms suggestive of mast cell degranulation (such as flushing and hypotension accompanied by abdominal complaints), patients with unexplained osteoporosis, and patients with suspected hematologic disease (see Clinical Manifestations). Children with an onset of lesions within the first year of life usually do not require a bone marrow biopsy unless they have abnormal blood counts, lymphadenopathy, hepatomegaly, or splenomegaly. Children with late-onset skin lesions and those who experience persistence of urticaria pigmentosa into adulthood should be considered for diagnostic evaluation for systemic disease.

World Health Organization Diagnostic Criteria
WHO guidelines for diagnosis of systemic mastocytosis consist of one major and four minor criteria (Table 255-2). Presence of the major criterion with at least one minor criterion, or demonstration of three minor criteria in the absence of the major criterion, is needed to establish a diagnosis of systemic mastocytosis and to distinguish it from reactive mast cell hyperplasia. The major diagnostic criterion is the presence of multifocal, dense aggregates of 15 or more mast cells in bone marrow or other extracutaneous tissue biopsy

TABLE 255-2	WORLD HEALTH ORGANIZATION DIAGNOSTIC CRITERIA FOR SYSTEMIC MASTOCYTOSIS

MAJOR

Multifocal, dense infiltrates of mast cells consisting of 15 or more mast cells in aggregates detected in sections of bone marrow and/or other extracutaneous organs, confirmed by tryptase immunohistochemistry or other special stains

MINOR

More than 25% of mast cells in biopsy sections or bone marrow aspirate smears showing spindle shape or atypical morphology

Detection of a *KIT* codon 816 point mutation in bone marrow, blood, or other extracutaneous organs

Expression of CD2 and/or CD25 by mast cells in bone marrow, blood, or extracutaneous organs

Persistent elevation of serum total tryptase >20 ng/mL*

*Criterion not valid if there is an associated clonal myeloid disorder.
From Horny HP, Metcalfe DD, Bennett JM, et al. Mastocytosis. In: Swerdlow SH, Campo E, Harris NL, et al, eds. WHO Classification of Tumours of Haematopoietic and Lymphoid Tissues. Lyon, France: IARC Press; 2008:54-63.

sections (Fig. 255-3A). Such clusters are frequently observed around blood vessels and next to bone trabeculae in bone marrow biopsy sections. Immunohistochemical staining for tryptase is the recommended method for visualization of mast cells. Routine hematoxylin and eosin or metachromatic stains such as toluidine blue are not sufficiently sensitive to demonstrate subtle mast cell infiltrates or abnormal morphologic features of mast cells within the infiltrates in decalcified bone marrow biopsy sections.

Mast cell morphology in bone marrow provides important clues to the diagnosis of systemic mastocytosis. Bone marrow mast cells in systemic mastocytosis often display atypical morphology, such as an elongated (spindle) shape, hypogranularity, and an eccentric or lobulated nucleus (Fig. 255-3B). These atypical mast cells are usually observed in close association with bone marrow spicules in the aspirate smear. Mast cells in mast cell leukemia (MCL) may be very sparsely granulated.

Flow cytometric analysis of the mast cells in a bone marrow aspirate, when it is performed appropriately, is a sensitive diagnostic aid. The mean percentage of mast cells in a healthy bone marrow aspirate is approximately 0.02%, and it does not exceed 1% in most patients with mastocytosis. Therefore, to visualize the mast cell population correctly, the total cell numbers analyzed by flow cytometry should be significantly higher than those in other, more routine evaluations (e.g., leukemia phenotyping). The characteristic flow cytometric finding of systemic mastocytosis is the aberrant expression of CD25 or CD2 on CD117+ mast cells. CD25 is more sensitive than CD2 as CD2 may be absent or weakly expressed in some cases of advanced mastocytosis. Aberrant CD25 expression can also be demonstrated by immunohistochemical staining of bone marrow biopsy specimens.[6] Serum tryptase level may be elevated in patients with mastocytosis.[7] Currently available commercial tryptase immunoassays measure levels of total tryptase, the sum of mature tryptase, and tryptase precursors. Mature tryptase enzyme is a serine protease stored in mast cell granules and is transiently elevated in serum or plasma after mast cell degranulation episodes, such as anaphylaxis. In contrast, tryptase precursor proenzymes (α and β protryptases) are constitutively secreted outside the cell, and their serum levels at baseline correlate with mast cell burden. The median serum tryptase level in a healthy population is approximately 5 ng/mL. A serum tryptase level higher than 20 ng/mL raises suspicion for systemic mastocytosis in the appropriate clinical setting. A normal tryptase level does not rule out a diagnosis of mastocytosis, and increased tryptase levels can be seen in other conditions, such as myelodysplastic syndromes, acute myeloid leukemias, chronic eosinophilic leukemia, and chronic renal insufficiency. Metabolites of histamine, such as N-methylhistamine, and prostaglandin D_2 can be elevated in a 24-hour urine specimen but are neither more sensitive nor more specific than the baseline serum tryptase measurement in mastocytosis.

Demonstration of a codon 816 *KIT* mutation (D816V) may be necessary to fulfill the diagnostic criteria in patients lacking the major criterion (see Pathobiology).[8] Examination of lesional tissues, such as skin and bone marrow, affords the highest sensitivity. Codon 816 *KIT* mutations have been detected in a variety of other neoplastic diseases, such as core binding factor acute myeloid leukemias, sinonasal lymphomas, and seminomas, in addition to mastocytosis.

A rare histologic variant with clustering of mature round mast cells without CD25 expression termed well-differentiated systemic mastocytosis has been described. These patients generally have a history of childhood-onset mastocytosis without the D816V *KIT* mutation and therefore may respond to imatinib as opposed to those with typical systemic mastocytosis carrying the D816V mutation (see Treatment).

World Health Organization Disease Categories

Each patient diagnosed with mastocytosis should be assigned a category of disease according to the WHO classification (see Table 255-1). *Cutaneous mastocytosis* in the absence of bone marrow and internal organ involvement is the most common category in patients with pediatric-onset disease.

Systemic mastocytosis is divided into the categories of indolent systemic mastocytosis, systemic mastocytosis with associated clonal hematologic non–mast cell lineage disease (SM-AHNMD), aggressive systemic mastocytosis, and MCL. An algorithm for classification of systemic mastocytosis is presented in Figure 255-4. *Indolent systemic mastocytosis* is the most common category in adults. Patients in this category usually have a normal life expectancy compared with age-matched general populations, although they experience symptoms related to release of mast cell mediators.[9] Indolent systemic mastocytosis follows a persistent course, and progression to a more advanced category is unusual (<5% of cases). *SM-AHNMD* is the second most common category in adults, and a non–mast cell hematologic disease is usually diagnosed at the time that the diagnosis of mastocytosis is made. Therefore, bone marrow biopsy and aspirate specimens should be carefully evaluated for the presence of other hematologic disease in every patient with newly diagnosed systemic mastocytosis. *Aggressive systemic mastocytosis* is a rare category characterized by the presence of organ dysfunction resulting from destructive mast cell infiltration. Aggressive systemic mastocytosis may involve the hematopoietic, gastrointestinal, and skeletal systems in the form of cytopenias, hypersplenism, malabsorption with weight loss, hepatomegaly with portal hypertension and ascites, and large osteolytic lesions with pathologic fractures; these constitute so-called C-findings as defined by the WHO criteria. MCL is characterized by 10% or more mast cells in the peripheral

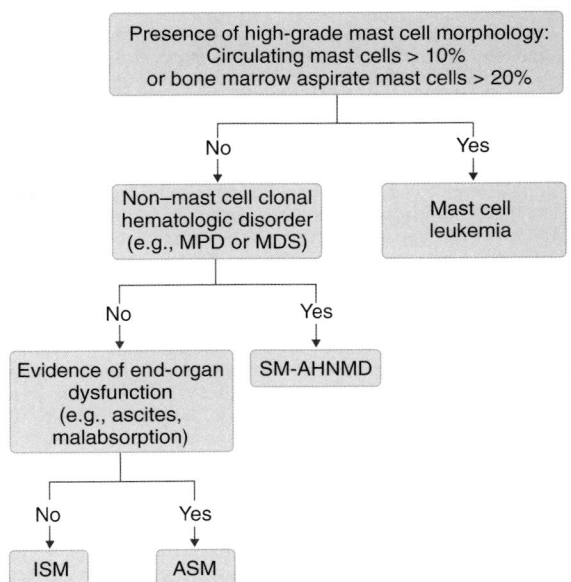

FIGURE 255-4. An algorithm for classification of systemic mastocytosis. ASM = aggressive systemic mastocytosis; ISM = indolent systemic mastocytosis; MDS = myelodysplastic syndromes; MPD = myeloproliferative disorders (neoplasms); SM-AHNMD = systemic mastocytosis with associated clonal hematologic non–mast cell lineage disease.

circulation or 20% or more mast cells in bone marrow aspirate smears, or both. To diagnose MCL, the mast cell percentage in bone marrow aspirate smears should be assessed in an area of the slide that is sufficiently distant from the spicules. *Mast cell sarcoma* and *extracutaneous mastocytoma* are rare diagnoses characterized by malignant and benign solid mast cell collections, respectively.

There is a subset of patients with recurrent idiopathic or hymenoptera venom–induced anaphylaxis who have evidence of clonal mast cells carrying the D816V *KIT* mutation or aberrantly expressing surface CD25, without fully meeting the WHO diagnostic criteria and without displaying urticaria pigmentosa skin lesions. Such patients are provisionally referred to as having a monoclonal mast cell activation syndrome.

TREATMENT

The major goal of treatment for all categories of mastocytosis is symptom control. A reduction in mast cell numbers is considered only in disease categories with a poor prognosis (i.e., SM-AHNMD, aggressive systemic mastocytosis, MCL, and mast cell sarcoma).[10,11] Current treatment modalities have not been shown to change the natural course of the disease.[12]

Medical Therapy

Patients with cutaneous and indolent systemic mastocytosis are treated symptomatically. Pruritus in mastocytosis usually responds to scheduled doses of histamine₁-receptor blocker antihistamines, such as fexofenadine or cetirizine. Sedating antihistamines, such as hydroxyzine or diphenhydramine, may be used before bedtime. Photochemotherapy (oral psoralen plus ultraviolet A) or phototherapy may be helpful in patients with refractory pruritus; it results in symptomatic improvement and temporary fading of the pigmented skin lesions in up to 50% of patients. The side effects of phototherapy, including increased risk of skin cancer, should be taken into account when this treatment is considered.

Histamine₂-receptor blocker antihistamines, such as ranitidine or famotidine, are usually prescribed as a first-line treatment for patients with gastrointestinal complaints, such as heartburn, nausea, and abdominal pain. Proton pump inhibitors may be added in patients whose abdominal symptoms are refractory to histamine₂-receptor blockers. Oral cromolyn sodium (adult dose, 200 mg four times daily) has been effective in reducing abdominal pain, diarrhea, nausea, vomiting, and pruritus in various studies, although the beneficial effects are variable among patients. Finally, low to moderate doses of systemic glucocorticoids can be beneficial in unusual cases of aggressive mastocytosis presenting with recalcitrant diarrhea associated with malabsorption or hepatomegaly with ascites.

Cysteinyl leukotrienes, such as LTC_4, that are produced after mast cell activation are thought to contribute to symptoms in mastocytosis. Therefore, drugs targeting the synthesis or receptor binding of leukotrienes are usually added to the treatment regimens of patients who derive suboptimal relief of itching and abdominal pain from histamine receptor–blocking therapy. However, there have been no controlled studies evaluating the clinical efficacy of this class of drugs in patients with mastocytosis.

Self-administered epinephrine should be considered for all patients even if they do not have any history of hypotensive or anaphylactic episodes resulting in presyncope or syncope from acute mast cell degranulation. These episodes should be treated like systemic anaphylaxis (Chapter 253).

Cytoreductive therapy, considered in aggressive disease variants associated with poor prognosis, has yielded disappointing results thus far. Some patients with recurrent life-threatening episodes of mast cell mediator release unresponsive to conventional therapy may also be candidates for cytoreductive therapy after careful consideration of risks and benefits. Approaches to cytoreductive treatment of mastocytosis have included interferon alfa-2b and the nucleoside analogue 2-chlorodeoxyadenosine. Interferon alfa-2b (0.5 to 5 million units, three to five times per week), alone or with prednisone, has been reported to partially improve clinical and laboratory abnormalities in approximately 50% of patients with aggressive systemic mastocytosis, patients with osteoporosis and pathologic fractures, and patients with recalcitrant recurrent anaphylaxis, although complete histopathologic and molecular remissions appear to be rare. Interferon alfa is difficult to tolerate because of its many side effects, including influenza-like symptoms, bone pain, and depression. A regimen of 2-chlorodeoxyadenosine (0.10 to 0.17 mg/kg/day for 5 days, repeated at intervals of 4 to 8 weeks) has been reported to result in partial and transient responses in patients with advanced categories of disease in case reports and small series. MCL usually is treated with polychemotherapy as acute myeloid leukemia (Chapter 183), although a successful treatment regimen has not yet been identified.

Imatinib, a tyrosine kinase inhibitor with activity against wild-type *KIT*, *PDGFR*, and *abl*, has been effective in a small number of patients without D816V *KIT* mutation or with the *FIP1L1-PDGFRA* fusion gene, who present with chronic eosinophilic leukemia (Chapter 170) with a modest increase in bone marrow mast cells. However, most patients with mastocytosis have the D816V *KIT* mutation, which confers resistance to imatinib, and therefore are not appropriate candidates for this therapy.[13]

Ancillary and Other Therapies

Avoidance of the triggers of mast cell degranulation is an important adjunct to the pharmacologic treatment of symptoms. These show remarkable individual variation among patients (see Pathobiology), and the individual medical history can be helpful in identifying such triggers. General anesthesia and surgery impose an additional risk to patients with mastocytosis because several agents that are used perioperatively, such as muscle relaxants, opioid analgesics, and nonsteroidal anti-inflammatory drugs, can induce acute mast cell degranulation. Prior surgical and anesthesia records should be obtained if available, and an appropriate strategy for the anesthetic management of the patient should be determined, with close communication involving the patient, anesthesiologist, surgeon, and an allergist.

Non–mast cell clonal hematologic disorders associated with mastocytosis should be treated according to the standard-of-care guidelines for those disorders, regardless of the presence of mastocytosis. Bone marrow transplantation (Chapter 178) has yielded variable results for the treatment of mast cell disease, and occasional cases resulting in complete remission have been reported.

Venom immunotherapy is recommended for those with a history of systemic reactions to hymenoptera who have evidence of IgE-mediated sensitization (by blood or skin allergy testing). Most experts recommend the duration of the therapy to be indefinite as fatalities have been reported after discontinuation of immunotherapy.

Because of the high prevalence of osteoporosis and pathologic bone fractures in mastocytosis, bone densitometry should be considered a standard diagnostic procedure in adult patients with mastocytosis. If osteoporosis is detected, it should be treated per standard recommendations (Chapter 243).

PROGNOSIS

The prognosis for mastocytosis varies by the category of disease. At least 50% of patients with pediatric-onset cutaneous mastocytosis have complete resolution of the disease by adolescence, and the great majority of the rest of those patients experience improvement or fading of the skin lesions. Indolent systemic mastocytosis is a persistent disease but has a good prognosis without a decrease in life expectancy, and progression to a more aggressive disease category is rare.[14] Factors associated with poorer prognosis have been reported as the absence of urticaria pigmentosa, older age at onset of symptoms, elevated serum lactate dehydrogenase or alkaline phosphatase, thrombocytopenia, anemia, peripheral blood smear abnormalities, and detectability of the D816V *KIT* mutation in peripheral blood. The prognosis for SM-AHNMD is determined by the prognosis for the associated hematologic disorder. Aggressive systemic mastocytosis and MCL have poor prognoses, with median survival times of less than 3 years and less than 1 year, respectively.

GENERAL REFERENCES

For the General References and other additional features, please visit Expert Consult at https://expertconsult.inkling.com.

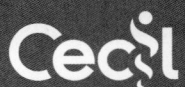

XXII

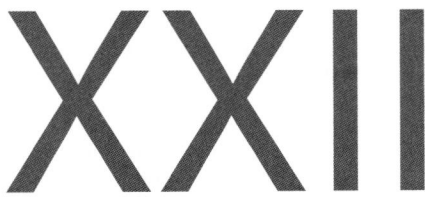

RHEUMATIC DISEASES

256

APPROACH TO THE PATIENT WITH RHEUMATIC DISEASE

VIVIAN P. BYKERK AND MARY K. CROW

Rheumatic diseases are common and an important cause of reduced quality of life, increased comorbidity, and reduced life expectancy. They incur a significant socioeconomic burden and warrant expertise on the part of all physicians who treat patients. This chapter provides a framework to approach the evaluation of patients who present with signs and symptoms suggesting a rheumatic disease. An algorithmic approach is provided that allows the physician to incorporate presenting features, patient characteristics, anatomic structures, along with diagnostic tests, to facilitate a diagnosis and treatment plan.

DEFINITION AND CATEGORIZATION

Rheumatic diseases are disorders of connective tissue in which general or localized inflammation frequently manifests as pain attributable to peripheral joints, the spine, or muscles. Systemic features such as stiffness, fever, or weight loss and a multitude of extramusculoskeletal features, ranging from skin rashes to renal dysfunction, often accompany rheumatic diseases. In most cases, the basic underlying pathology is understood, although this is less true of pain disorders appearing alone or accompanying a rheumatic disease (Chapter 30). For most rheumatic disorders, the underlying molecular mechanisms through which environmental triggers and genetic susceptibility factors collaborate to result in a particular rheumatic disease in an individual remain to be fully elucidated. These diseases can be broadly considered as those that are primarily degenerative, with inflammation occurring secondarily, and those in which inflammation is the primary mediator of the disease. In the latter, the pathogenesis can be mediated through aberrant immune responses or as a result of metabolic abnormalities.

Histopathology

Rheumatic diseases are often also termed *connective tissue diseases*, understandably, because connective tissue is the most abundant tissue in the body supporting and connecting other tissues and organs. Loose and dense connective tissues include cellular components and extracellular matrix. Loose connective tissue fills spaces between muscle sheaths, encases blood and lymphatic vessels, and holds fibroblasts that synthesize collagen fibers. It includes reticular fibers that provide the skeleton of muscle cells, nerves, and capillaries. Dense connective tissue supports the body's soft tissues and includes more collagen fibers and fewer cells. It is found in the dermis, joint capsules, cartilage, bone, and fascia of muscles, and it forms tendons, ligaments, and points of connection where these insert into bone (aponeurosis). Cells included in connective tissue may be wandering, such as mast cells or macrophages, or resident cells, such as fibroblasts, fibrocytes, and reticular cells. Fibroblasts are responsible for synthesizing collagen, elastic reticular fibers, and ground substance of extracellular matrix, including tissue fluids and collagen fibers. Importantly, connective tissue is integrated with cells associated with the body's defense system: lymphocytes, plasma cells, macrophages, dendritic cells, and eosinophils. The close proximity of connective tissue to blood vessels and cells of the immune system provides the setting for a group of disorders that are mediated by impaired immune system regulation and disruptions of the vascular system.

Classification of Rheumatic Diseases

More than 100 types of rheumatic diseases have been described. Although these can be considered to be based primarily on one of two degenerative or inflammatory overarching processes, one can further subdivide rheumatic diseases as follows (and also outlined in Table 256-1): (1) those associated with degeneration of connective tissues attributable to (a) trauma, (b) structural/mechanical imbalances, or (3) inherent early demise of cellular components; (2) those associated with systemic autoimmunity,[1] often linked with measurable autoantibodies that can manifest primarily with (a) synovitis, (b) widespread organ involvement, (c) inflamed blood vessels, or (d) inflammation of muscle; (3) other inflammatory connective tissue diseases

involving more dense tissues, not associated with the formation of autoantibodies and hence termed *seronegative rheumatic diseases* or *spondyloarthropathies*; (4) diseases in which inflammation of the vasculature, particularly small, medium, or large arteries, is the predominant feature; (5) autoinflammatory diseases that can be associated with crystal deposition or genetic mutations involving cytokine pathways; and (6) pain syndromes that must often be considered in the context of these diseases, in which some appear to be comorbid and closely linked to the underlying rheumatic disease, such as diffuse pain associated with Sjögren's syndrome, hypermobility of connective tissue, or those regional pain syndromes that are anatomically linked to mechanical disruption. Patients presenting with generalized pain syndromes require investigation to exclude a connective tissue disease. Increasingly, genotypes have been identified that are associated with diseases that fall into each of these categories, and in some cases specific immunologic pathways have allowed grouping of a set of rheumatic diseases previously considered more distinct.

Mimics of rheumatic diseases exist, and clinicians need to be mindful of considering these when evaluating a patient for a rheumatic disease. For instance, arthropathies and syndromes resembling a rheumatic disease can occur in the settings of both infection and malignancy. Autoimmune phenomena are increasingly being recognized in the setting of malignancy.[2] Red flags for each need to be considered in the assessment of a patient for possible rheumatic disease.

No classification of rheumatic disease can completely explain its genesis. However, considering these in a classification schema can aid in the approach to a patient in whom these disorders are being considered (see Table 256-1).

EPIDEMIOLOGY

Although connective tissue diseases can generally be categorized as noted in Table 256-1, in adults there are six prototypical rheumatic diseases most often assessed and managed by rheumatologists: rheumatoid arthritis (RA), systemic lupus erythematosus (SLE), systemic sclerosis (SSc), spondyloarthropathies (SpA) (primarily ankylosing spondylitis [AS]), Sjögren's syndrome (SS), and vasculitis. These diseases are ubiquitous throughout the world (Table 256-2) and for the most part have a similar incidence and prevalence throughout the globe. Each is associated with differing immune aberrations and mechanisms of inflammatory damage, although the cause and reasons for chronicity still remain unknown. Autoimmune rheumatic diseases are also among the leading causes of death and morbidity in the industrial world, in part related to associated comorbid diseases, particularly comorbid cardiovascular disease. They contribute to a significant socioeconomic burden. Increasing evidence points to risks for their genesis relating to environmental factors, socioeconomic factors, and exposure to infectious agents, ultraviolet radiation, and pollutants. Smoking, in particular, has been associated with an increased risk for SLE and RA in genetically susceptible individuals in Western cultures. Effects of migration elucidate some of these risks. For instance, Africans who migrate far away from their native environmental and cultural origins appear to have an increased susceptibility to SLE. Also, reports have linked occupational exposures, such as silica dust, mercury, pesticides, solvents, and metals, to an increased risk for SLE and RA.

In some cases, geographic clusters of rare autoimmune disease argue for specific genetic determinants. For example, with SSc, higher incidence, prevalence, and mortality rates have been reported in African American populations compared with white populations, and the prevalence has been reported as higher in southern Europe, particularly Italy (prevalence of 7 to 33 per 100,000). Additionally, social and demographic factors may contribute to the epidemiology of rheumatic diseases. For example, the prevalence of SLE is reported as very high in Georgia, United States, whereas the prevalence of AS is rare in malaria endemic regions where HLA-B27 genotypes are rare. Inflammatory arthropathies, including RA and AS, have a higher prevalence in North American Native populations.

CLINICAL MANIFESTATIONS

It is important to understand the potential clinical manifestations and natural history of rheumatic diseases. Primary care and hospital-based health care providers are often the first to evaluate a patient with an evolving rheumatic disease, and they need to be attuned to the presenting features to make a timely diagnosis. In many cases, the presentation could signal a life- or organ-threatening condition. Evaluation of constitutional, systemic and joint symptoms should always include rheumatic disease in the differential diagnosis.

TABLE 256-1 COMMON RHEUMATIC DISEASES BROADLY CLASSIFIED ACCORDING TO PATHOGENESIS

DEGENERATIVE DISEASES OF BONES AND JOINTS	SYSTEMIC AUTOIMMUNE DISEASES	SERONEGATIVE SPONDYLOARTHROPATHIES	VASCULAR RHEUMATIC DISEASES	AUTOINFLAMMATORY DISEASES	PAIN DISORDERS
Osteoarthritis	Rheumatoid arthritis	Ankylosing spondylitis	ANCA- associated vasculitis	Adult-onset Still's disease	Regional myofascial pain syndromes
DISH	Systemic lupus erythematosus	Psoriatic arthritis	Temporal artery vasculitis	Crystal diseases	Tendonitis/bursitis
Degenerative disc disease	Sjögren's syndrome	Reactive arthritis	Polymyalgia rheumatica	Pediatric periodic fever syndromes	Adhesive capsulitis
Spinal stenosis	Inflammatory myopathies (polymyositis, dermatomyositis)	Enteropathic arthritis	Behçet's disease		Reflex sympathetic dystrophy
Osteoporosis	Systemic sclerosis				Pain with hypermobility syndromes
					Fibromyalgia*

*The only pain disorder that has not been associated primarily with inflammation.
ANCA = antineutrophil cytoplasmic antibody; DISH = diffuse idiopathic sclerosing hyperostosis (also linked to metabolic factors, including elevated growth hormone).

TABLE 256-2 WORLDWIDE PREVALENCE* AND INCIDENCE OF RHEUMATIC DISEASES ASSOCIATED WITH AUTOIMMUNITY

DISEASE	NORTH AMERICA	CENTRAL AMERICA	SOUTH AMERICA	EUROPE	MIDDLE EAST	ASIA	SUB SAHARAN AFRICA	AUSTRALIA
RA	600-1000 (40)	400-2000	100-500	200-900 (2-7)	200-1500	100-800 (40-90)	Rare - 900	2000
SLE	20-60 (2-7)	50-60 (5)	N/A	20-70 (2-7)	N/A	20-70 (3)	Rare	20-80 (11)
SSc	13-28	N/A	N/A	<10-15 (<2)	N/A	<10	N/A	23 (2)
SpA	50-130 (7)	N/A	N/A	100-850 (2-9)	500	10-240	Rare	N/A
SS	320 (4)	N/A	N/A	200-600 (4-5)	N/A	330-700 (China)	N/A	N/A

*Prevalence (annual incidence) per 100,000 by world regions.
RA = rheumatoid arthritis; SLE = systemic lupus erythematosus; SpA = spondyloarthropathy (primarily ankylosing spondylitis); SS = Sjögren's syndrome; SSc = systemic sclerosis.
Data from Shapira Y, Agmon-Levin N, Shoenfeld Y. Geoepidemiology of autoimmune rheumatic diseases. *Nat Rev Rheumatol.* 2010;6(8):468-476; and Chaaya M, Slim ZN, Habib RR, et al. High burden of rheumatic diseases in Lebanon: a COPCORD study. *Int J Rheum Dis.* 2012;15(2):136-143.

Joint Symptoms as a Common Presenting Feature

Almost all rheumatic diseases can manifest with joint-related symptoms as a significant and frequently presenting feature. This can include symptoms of pain, stiffness, swelling, and erythema, as in the case of autoinflammatory diseases such as gout or pseudogout. The pattern of joint involvement, particularly duration and timing of maximal symptoms, can help the health care provider identify patients who present with spondyloarthropathy or any inflammatory arthritis, regardless of pathogenetic classification. For instance, joint pain that is worse in the morning, is associated with prolonged stiffness, and improves with activity is a classic presentation of inflammatory pain. On the contrary, pain that is worse with activity, better with rest, and associated with a very short period of stiffness signals that the category is degenerative. Location provides a clue to broad classification. Patients describing "pain all over" may have a primary pain syndrome. However pain with an inflammatory pattern localized to the spine or an enthesis (site of ligament insertion) is more likely to indicate a seronegative spondyloarthropathy. A patient noting an inflammatory pattern of symptoms in small joints of the hands and feet suggests the presence of one of the autoimmune rheumatic diseases associated with either a positive antinuclear antibody (ANA) or rheumatoid factor (RF). Thus, joint symptom patterns become central to the evaluation of any rheumatic disease.

Nonspecific Clinical Presentations

All of the rheumatic diseases can be associated with joint involvement. However, joint symptoms are not always present in many of these diseases. Thus, a working knowledge of other patterns of presentation is important. Fever or cutaneous manifestations, including rashes, are common in vasculitis and in the presentation of SLE. Sicca symptoms are pathognomonic of Sjögren's syndrome. Both Sjögren's syndrome and inflammation of blood vessels can occur concurrently in patients with SLE. Systemic features such as myalgias or fatigue are common to almost all rheumatic diseases regardless of their classification, whereas true weakness may be the only presenting complaint of an inflammatory myopathy. Renal involvement is common to seropositive systemic autoimmune diseases and vasculitis and can present with anasarca if proteinuria is severe or prolonged. Consequently, specific and nonspecific features associated with various connective tissue diseases must be identified to correctly develop a differential diagnosis that fits within the classification described in Table 256-1. Features may present sequentially over time; thus, rheumatic diseases from more than one category must often be considered in a patient whose disease has not yet been diagnosed, leaving the patient with a label of a nonspecific or undifferentiated connective tissue disease. Most rheumatic diseases have specific classification criteria. When these are not yet met, features are considered in the context of the broad classifications, and terms such as *undifferentiated inflammatory polyarthritis* or *undifferentiated spondyloarthropathy* may be used in the interim to aid in diagnosis and management. When a patient's disease is not yet diagnosed, investigations and monitoring over time, as indicated in Figure 256-1, can help to ultimately identify an emerging rheumatic disease.

Cutaneous Manifestations

Although cutaneous manifestations are frequent in patients with seropositive autoimmune diseases, particularly SLE, they are important manifestations of all autoimmune diseases. A nonblanching purpuric rash can indicate a vasculitis, and rashes involving specific extensor regions are common to dermatomyositis. In cases of SLE or dermatomyositis, rashes are triggered or worsened by exposure to ultraviolet light and occur in a light-exposed distribution. Rashes of vasculitic origin can indicate either the presence of an autoimmune disease such as SLE or an inflammatory vascular disease such as antineutrophil cytoplasmic antibody (ANCA)-associated vasculitis. These tend to be present for days and are often palpable, and a tissue biopsy of the lesions will be very helpful in diagnosis. Rashes can be transient. In adult-onset Still's disease (an adult form of systemic inflammatory arthritis classified as an autoinflammatory disease), patients present with daily spiking fevers, peaking late in the day, associated with a salmon-colored evanescent blanching rash lasting only 1 to 2 hours. The specific location of a rash aids in diagnosis. A facial rash that spares the nasolabial folds is classic for lupus. A rash that does not spare the nasolabial folds suggests rosacea. Psoriasis is almost always present in psoriatic arthritis (a spondyloarthropathy variant). Although psoriasis is often widespread, involving extensor surfaces, it can be missed if there

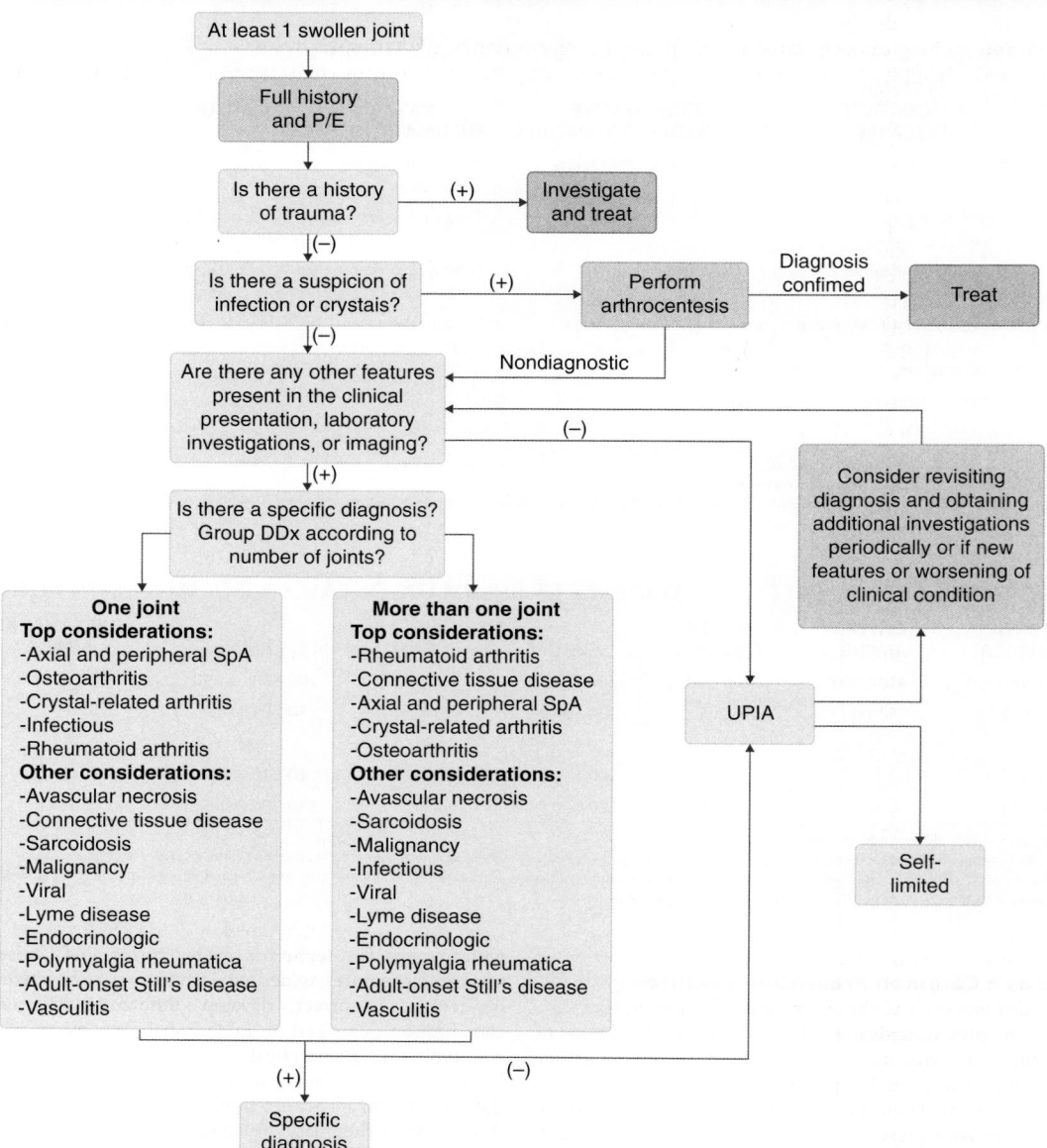

FIGURE 256-1. Algorithm for identification of undifferentiated peripheral inflammatory arthritis. Recommended minimum investigations in all patients: rheumatoid factor and/or anti–citrullinated peptide antibodies, erythrocyte sedimentation rate and/or C-reactive protein, complete blood count, and radiographs of affected joints. DDx = differential diagnosis; P/E = physical examination; SpA = spondyloarthritis; UPIA = undifferentiated peripheral inflammatory arthritis. (From: Hazlewood G, Aletthaha D, Carmona L, et al. Algorithm for identification of undifferentiated peripheral inflammatory arthritis: a multinational collaboration through the 3e initiative. *J Rheumatol Suppl.* 2011;87:54-58.)

are very few lesions or if it is located in areas that are not easily seen (intertriginous regions, such as in the ear, umbilicus, buttock creases, or scalp) or if it only involves the nails. The rash of psoriasis can be seen in any of the variants of the spondyloarthropathies. Occasionally RA will manifest with nodules over the extensor surfaces or rashes in the same areas, but this is increasingly rare. However, the presence of nodules over extensor surfaces may also indicate gouty tophi. In SSc, distal tightening of the skin, presence of telangiectasias, and digital ulcers can be seen. These should also be sought in the context of Raynaud's syndrome, characterized by vascular spasm in the hands.

Pattern of Onset of Rheumatic Diseases by Category

Most rheumatic diseases appear spontaneously and often insidiously or with a subacute onset. Not all will manifest with all typical features at the time of presentation, and a diagnosis can take time to make as defining features present themselves. Almost all rheumatic diseases have had classification criteria published that account for the typical and specific features of the disease (these are detailed in other chapters). Although classification criteria are generally published to ensure homogenous recruitment of participants in research studies, they can also aid in diagnosis. However, a diagnosis can be made without meeting all classification criteria because some features of a rheumatic disease are highly specific and are not associated with other diseases. For example, SLE is the only disease that presents with a classic malar rash and a particular autoantibody, anti-Sm, in the serum.

The natural history of each rheumatic disease is related to the severity of presentation, the specific additional organs that become involved, and the development of comorbidities. RA may present with one or two swollen joints or pain in the forefoot. However, when the patient has a high titer of anti–cyclic citrullinated peptide antibody (ACPA), an autoantibody associated with development of erosive joint disease, the diagnosis can be made quickly and treatment initiated early. Autoimmune and vascular rheumatic diseases are associated with high morbidity and mortality when left untreated, and efforts to investigate for all manifestations early on are warranted.

Degenerative Rheumatic Diseases

These refer to rheumatic diseases commonly associated with advancing age. Degenerative joint disease (DJD) is usually thought to include osteoarthritis (OA) and degenerative disc disease (DDD). DJD is heralded by breakdown of articular collagenous structures (cartilage or intervertebral discs) and development of bony hypertrophy. Controversy remains as to which occurs first. As collagenous structures degrade, associated inflammation commonly occurs. Resultant pain from varying causes contributes to immobility, secondary comorbidities, and disability. DJD represents, by far, the most common of the rheumatic diseases and is described in detail in Chapter 262. In general, these diseases are not associated with rashes or nonspecific constitutional symptoms.

Autoimmune Rheumatic Diseases

These diseases include SLE, RA, SSc, primary Sjögren's syndrome, idiopathic inflammatory myositis, and the systemic vasculitides. They involve multiple organ systems, are heterogeneous in clinical manifestations,[3] and are associated with and partially characterized by autoantibodies that can be measured in the serum (Tables 256-3 and 256-4). Many of these diseases affect females more than males. Most striking is SLE (Chapter 266), which affects 8 to 10 women for every 1 man and typically has its onset in the childbearing years. As noted, cutaneous manifestations, sicca symptoms (of dry eyes or mouth), mucosal ulceration, fevers, alopecia, and Raynaud's syndrome are common and often described by patients. These occur alone or in addition to symptoms affecting the joints and muscles. RA (Chapter 264) has a female-to-male ratio of approximately 3 : 1 and typically has its onset in the later adult decades, with symmetrical arthritis the classic presenting feature. Specific to SSc (Chapter 267), often referred to as scleroderma, are symptoms of skin tightness in the extremities. This is often associated initially with swelling of the digits, followed by tightness of the hands and ultimately tightness of the skin. In addition, skin tightness can involve the face, arms, and in the case of diffuse SSc, trunk, back, and legs. Although these diseases can present classically, facilitating rapid diagnosis, features can overlap. For instance, Sjögren's syndrome (Chapter 268), with prototypical sicca symptoms and autoantibodies, can occur concurrently in SLE and RA. Autoimmune vasculitides and SLE can share similar organ system manifestations, including those involving the lungs, kidneys, skin, and nervous systems. Most can have constitutional disturbance, arthralgia and arthritis, and myalgias. Overlap of symptoms expands the differential diagnosis, and a clear distinction is often not readily apparent, even after serologic testing. Tissue biopsy may help to provide a definitive answer.

Spondyloarthropathies

AS (Chapter 265) is more common in males than females. Localization of symptoms to the back, sacroiliac joints, and large lower extremity joints can be used to differentiate AS from RA. The typical presence of psoriatic skin lesions in patients with psoriatic arthritis can be a distinguishing feature from RA.

Forms of Vasculitis

There are many vasculitis syndromes, and these are generally grouped based on vessel size (Chapter 270). Some are classified as such though not always proved to be of vascular origin. Polymyalgia rheumatica (PMR) (Chapter 271) is a common inflammatory rheumatic disease of the elderly and shares many pathogenetic and epidemiologic features with giant cell arteritis (GCA), a form of older-onset vasculitis.[4] Patients complain of aching around the neck and bilateral involvement of the shoulder and hip girdles, along with significant stiffness that is most problematic in the morning. Symptom onset can be abrupt or insidious over weeks to months. The diagnosis of PMR is primarily clinical, although diagnostic criteria have been suggested, based on the typical clinical presentation and laboratory evidence of acute-phase reactants. Mimics of PMR can include elderly onset RA; thus, tests to exclude this may be indicated. More important, when considering PMR, always consider GCA, often involving inflammation of the temporal arteries, because the consequences of this disease can be damaging and severe, sometimes leading to blindness.

Autoinflammatory Diseases

Rare autoinflammatory diseases that are based on mutations in genes involved in inflammatory pathways are typically diagnosed in children and are covered in detail in Chapter 261. Gout (Chapter 273) is common in middle-aged and older men and may be increasing in prevalence. Exquisitely painful joint erythema and swelling are presenting features. Tophi that might be confused with rheumatoid nodules can be seen.

Pain and Pain Syndromes

Pain (also see Chapter 30) is a common and nonspecific, but very important, symptom central to nearly all rheumatic diseases. Pain is the key presenting feature of joint disease as perceived by the patient. In regional pain syndromes, the distribution of pain is the key clue to the diagnosis. Diffuse pain without evidence of underlying pathology associated with inordinate levels of fatigue, difficulty coping, and intricately detailed descriptions of pain using colorful analogies herald fibromyalgia (Chapter 274). Fibromyalgia is defined as widespread pain involving right and left sides and upper and lower extremities, as well as the neck and back. Most pain syndromes are regional pain syndromes. For instance, a regional pain syndrome relating to a mechanical neck and shoulder syndrome will result in the patient having pain in the involved neck and shoulder but also the trapezius, upper chest, and lower arm and hand. A large proportion of patients presenting with musculoskeletal pain will have regional pain relating to muscular imbalances with or without underlying degenerative arthritis, tendinopathy, or enthesopathy. As an

---

TABLE 256-3 CLUES TO DIAGNOSIS FOR EACH CATEGORY OF RHEUMATIC DISEASE

DEGENERATIVE DISEASES OF BONES AND JOINTS	SYSTEMIC AUTOIMMUNE DISEASES	SERONEGATIVE SPONDYLOARTHROPATHIES	VASCULAR RHEUMATIC DISEASES	AUTOINFLAMMATORY DISEASES	PAIN DISORDERS
Investigate if persistent symptoms >6 wk or failure of conservative measures (physical therapy, acetaminophen, NSAIDs). If at risk for bone loss and possible fragility fracture, consider osteoporosis.	Frequently associated with inflammatory joint pain and/or swelling with or without constitutional symptoms and other organ involvement. Perform ANA, RF, ESR, CRP.	Consider if psoriasis is present, or if back pain has inflammatory features; consider when known associated nonarticular features are present (e.g., uveitis, inflammatory bowel disease, urethritis, enthesitis, dactylitis).	Consider in all situations in which infarction of tissue has occurred or vasculitic rashes, pulmonary hemorrhage, or acute or subacute renal syndromes are present.	All can present with fever. In children, these are usually genetically determined syndromes mediated through interleukin-1 or TNF-α. In adults, consider crystal diseases.	Consider in situations in which pain is in excess of findings, with history of resolved trauma or repetitive strain, referred pain symptoms, diffuse pain, or colorful descriptions of pain.
INITIAL INVESTIGATIVE APPROACH TO CONFIRM SUSPECTED RHEUMATIC DISEASE IN EACH CATEGORY					
Image specific region giving rise to persistent pain (consider pain may be referred). If osteoporosis is a concern, perform BMD and investigate for metabolic bone diseases.	Investigations should specifically target suspected diseases, e.g., perform CPK if weakness or myalgia; anti-CCP (ACPA) if possible RA; ANA, dsDNA, C3, C4, ENA if possible SLE.	Imaging of sacroiliac (SI) joints (radiographs if long-standing symptoms, MRI if more recent onset). HLAB27 testing if inflammatory back pain or SI pain most predominant, clinical suspicion high for inflammatory back pain, but imaging is negative.	ANCA Anti-PR3 Anti-MPO Acute phase reactants (ESR, CRP) Tissue sampling of involved organs to facilitate pathophysiologic classification.	For suspected crystal disease, perform aspiration of synovial fluid or tophus and examine under polarized light microscopy.	Usually a diagnosis of exclusion. In reflex sympathetic dystrophy, tendonitis or enthesitis, specific physical findings and imaging can facilitate diagnosis.

ACPA = anti–citrullinated peptide antibodies; ANA = antinuclear antibodies; ANCA = antinuclear cytoplasmic antibodies; anti-CCP = anti–cyclic citrullinated peptide; anti-MPO = anti-myeloperoxidase; anti-PR3 = anti-proteinase-3; BMD = bone mineral density scan; CPK = creatinine phosphokinase; CRP = C-reactive protein; dsDNA = anti-double-stranded DNA; ENA = antibodies to extractable nuclear antigens (e.g., Ro, La, Sm, RNP, Scl70, Jo-1); ESR = erythrocyte sedimentation rate; MRI = magnetic resonance imaging; NSAIDs = nonsteroidal anti-inflammatory drugs; RF = rheumatoid factor; SLE = systemic lupus erythematosus; TNF-α = tumor necrosis factor-α.

TABLE 256-4 AUTOANTIBODIES ASSOCIATED WITH SPECIFIC FEATURES OF SEROPOSITIVE SYSTEMIC AUTOIMMUNE DISEASES

	ANTIBODY PREVALENCE	MAIN CLINICAL MANIFESTATIONS AND ASSOCIATIONS
SLE		
Double-stranded DNA	70-80	Kidney disease, skin disease
Nucleosomes	60-90	Kidney disease, skin disease
Smith	10-30	Kidney disease
Small nuclear ribonucleoproteins (spliceosomes, U1-RNP, 70kD, A, C)	15-25	Raynaud's syndrome, puffy fingers, myositis, and hypergammaglobulinemia
N-methyl-D-aspartate receptor	33-50	CNS lupus
Phospholipids (cardiolipin, β2 GP1, prothrombin)	20-30	Thrombosis, pregnancy loss, thickened heart valve disease, and livedo reticularis
α-Actinin	20	Kidney disease
Ribosomes P0, P1, P2	4-12	Hepatic, CNS manifestations (psychosis)
C1q	40-50	Kidney disease, associated with disease activity
SLE AND SJÖGREN'S SYNDROME		
Ro/SSA	30-40	Kidney disease in SLE in the absence of anti-La/SSB, skin disease in SLE and photosensitivity; congenital heart block and neonatal lupus erythematosus, sicca symptoms; subacute cutaneous lupus, hypergammaglobulinemia, leukopenia; interstitial nephritis and increased risk for non-Hodgkin's lymphoma in patients with Sjögren's syndrome
La/SSB	15-20	Congenital heart block and neonatal lupus erythematosus, sicca symptoms; photosensitivity, subacute cutaneous lupus erythematosus, hypergammaglobulinemia, leukopenia; increased risk for increased non-Hodgkin's lymphoma in patients with Sjögren's syndrome
α-Fodrine	46-100 in Sjögren's syndrome and 30 in SLE	Sicca symptoms
IDIOPATHIC INFLAMMATORY MYOSITIS		
Jo-1, Pl-7, Pl-12, OJ, EJ	20-30	Antisynthetase syndrome
Signal recognition particle	2-8	Necrotizing myopathy
Mi-2	8-12 in idiopathic inflammatory myositis, 15-20 dermatomyositis	Dermatomyositis and idiopathic inflammatory myositis
TRIM33	10-30 of dermatomyositis	Dermatomyositis, malignancy
U1-RNP/U2-RNP	8-15	Mixed connective tissue more commonly than system lupus erythematosus, systemic sclerosis, and undifferentiated connective tissue disorder
PM/Scl	12-16	Dermatomyositis and systemic sclerosis overlap, systemic sclerosis, and dermatomyositis
Ku	1-7	Myositis overlap, SLE, idiopathic inflammatory myositis, and systemic sclerosis
CADM-140/anti-MDA-5 antibody (clinically amyopathic dermatomyositis/antimelanoma-differentiation-associated gene 5)	Infrequent	Amyopathic dermatomyositis (53%) with interstitial disease
SYSTEMIC SCLEROSIS		
Centromere	15-40	Limited systemic sclerosis, pulmonary hypertension
Scl-70/topoisomerase	10-40	Diffuse cutaneous systemic sclerosis, pulmonary fibrosis
RNA polymerase III	5-25	Diffuse cutaneous systemic sclerosis, renal crisis, pulmonary hypertension
AUTOANTIBODIES WITHOUT DISEASE SPECIFICITY		
Rheumatoid factor	30-40, 90-95, and 10-20	SLE, Sjögren's syndrome, and myositis
Antibodies against proteasome subunits	40-60, 50-60, and 40	Idiopathic inflammatory myositis, SLE, and Sjögren's syndrome

CNS = central nervous system; SLE = systemic lupus erythematosus.
From Goldblatt F, O'Neill SG. Clinical aspects of autoimmune rheumatic diseases. *Lancet*. 2013;382(9894):797-808.

example, pain syndromes in the trapezial region, referring down the arm to the deltoid and even forearm, can be multifactorial and associated with a combination of muscular spasm, underlying degenerative arthritis in the cervical spine or rotator cuff impingement, not infrequently relating to repetitive activities. Pain in an extremity after trauma or surgery associated with a cold extremity is suggestive of reflex sympathetic dystrophy. The etiology of these will become apparent with a careful history of the pain, along with a medical history, physical examination, and exclusion of "red flags" or factors that indicate an underlying organic pathology. Pain in the setting of a history of malignancy should suggest the possibility of metastases. A tick bite may indicate prior Lyme disease. Most pain syndromes warrant a full medical evaluation before making a definitive diagnosis.

DIFFERENTIAL DIAGNOSIS AND DIAGNOSTIC EVALUATION:

A comprehensive history is needed to complete an evaluation of a patient with a rheumatic disease. In addition to considering age and gender, a patient's personal history, including marital status, occupation, and psychosocial factors, helps to elucidate a patient's diagnosis, prognosis, and treatment options. Clues helpful in making a diagnosis of one of the rheumatic diseases are summarized in Table 256-3.

Assessing clinical signs and symptoms is the cornerstone of diagnosis. Most rheumatic disorders will present with symptoms that involve, or seem to involve, joints. This can be limited to pain involving a specific joint or group of joints or periarticular structures. Querying the patient to determine the pattern of symptoms—whether pain, swelling, or stiffness associated with joints—is key to narrowing the differential diagnosis of a rheumatic disease. Joint symptoms may have inflammatory features such as prolonged stiffness, pain at rest, or noninflammatory and mechanical features, such as instability or giving way, locking, or increased symptoms with use. Patterns of joint involvement—whether primarily small joints of the hands, wrist, and feet; large joints of the elbows, knees, ankles, or "root" (shoulders or hips); or spinal involvement—will help to narrow down the possible diagnoses. Moreover, questions regarding recent illnesses, exposure to possible infectious pathogens, and presence or absence of systemic features such as fever, fatigue, or weight loss will provide important clues. Appreciation of signs and symptoms indicating extra-articular features, particularly cutaneous, pulmonary, renal, neurologic, or vascular manifestations, will not only help to facilitate a diagnosis but aid in prognosis and an understanding of the needed intensity of therapy.

The presence of one rheumatic disease can be associated with comorbid manifestations unrelated to connective tissue. For example, myocardial infarction is more common in many patients with rheumatic diseases. Immobility or treatment-related factors leading to obesity can increase risks for diabetes and lower joint degeneration.

Factors in the Medical History that Contribute to Diagnosis and Prognosis
Age and Gender
Certain rheumatic diseases typically manifest in childhood. These include genetically based disorders such as hemophilia, associated with arthritis, and a number of autoinflammatory conditions that are by definition childhood diseases. Juvenile idiopathic arthritis refers to forms of arthritis in which the onset occurs before the age of 16 years. Autoimmune rheumatic diseases, and inflammatory rheumatic diseases such as spondyloarthropathies, RA, and SLE, can begin in young adulthood, whereas degenerative conditions such as OA rarely do and more often begin to manifest in the middle and late middle years. The peak onset of RA occurs in the late middle years, although onset can occur at almost any time in life. Elderly people are more prone to OA and PMR, but the latter has a wide differential diagnosis and should be considered at all ages. Autoimmune diseases are more common in women, whereas spondyloarthropathies can be equally common in men and women. Gouty arthritis is more common in men and rarely attacks women before menopause.

Occupation and Recreation
Occupation and recreational activities may give rise to physical and psychological stresses. The demands of a patient's occupation need to be understood, particularly when repetitive activities may contribute to the development of DJD or to regional pain syndromes. Similarly, trauma from sports, including prior injuries, can be significant contributors to DJD.

Family History
It is important to obtain a complete family history because autoimmune diseases, spondyloarthropathies, and gout occur with an increased incidence in families. It is common to see family pedigrees in which different forms of autoimmunity occur throughout a family. This does not mean that any one autoimmune disease has specific heritability. Also, generalized OA that involves the hands and other joints commonly runs in families.

Concomitant Medication Use
Concomitant medications may contribute to the genesis of a rheumatic disease. For example, diuretics can increase hyperuricemia and risk for gouty arthritis. Minocycline can be associated with lupus-like presentations. Antibiotics in the fluoroquinolone class have been associated with enthesopathies. A full medication history needs to be considered in the assessment of patients with rheumatic diseases.

Habits and Social Circumstances
Smoking has increasingly been associated with RA and SLE. Also, poor socioeconomic circumstances and psychosocial or physical stress may contribute to the severity of symptoms and should be considered in planning management strategies. Similarly, patients of different ethnic and cultural origins may have differences in their ability to describe symptoms and in preferences around treatment choices.

Onset and Evolution of Symptoms
Knowledge of the pattern of onset, location, and evolution of symptoms is essential to make an accurate diagnosis of a rheumatic disease. Symptoms that develop over hours to days typically suggest an inflammatory, or possibly an infectious or traumatic, process. When they persist for more than 6 weeks, symptom onset is considered subacute, and the disease chronic. Early in the presentation of some rheumatic diseases, the symptoms can be intermittent or palindromic before becoming constant. Sudden onset of joint pain and swelling, particularly involving one or a few joints, should be considered to be due to an infectious or crystalline etiology during the course of investigation.

Pain and Stiffness
Pain assessment should include a description of its onset, constancy/chronicity, severity, quality, factors that trigger or improve it, and location and radiation of the pain. Stiffness, often described as tightness or linked to difficulty with movement or function, should be determined in terms of location (e.g., is it in a particular joint or more diffuse) and timing and duration (e.g., occurring after a period of rest). Stiffness that resolves in 10 to 15 minutes is more characteristic of OA. In inflammatory disease, stiffness typically lasts longer, often at least 1 hour and even all day.

Joint Involvement
The distribution of joint involvement is key to making a diagnosis of a rheumatic disease. Monoarthritis describes symptoms in a single joint; oligoarthritis (or pauciarthritis) refers to symptoms in two to four joints; and polyarthritis indicates involvement of at least five joints. Peripheral arthritis involves an extremity, whereas spinal involvement is termed *axial disease*. Symmetrical as opposed to asymmetrical peripheral joint disease is more commonly associated with autoimmune rheumatic disorders, whereas asymmetrical arthritis can be associated with spondyloarthropathies or OA. Similarly, predominant small joint involvement is more typical in RA or SLE, whereas large joint involvement is classic for spondyloarthropathies. In addition the presence of associated enthesitis and axial symptoms herald spondyloarthropathy. Joint or spine symptoms associated with inflammatory causes often include predominance of symptoms in the morning, associated with stiffness for more than 60 minutes, worsening with rest, and improvement over the day and with activity. Joint or spine symptoms associated with degenerative joint disease typically worsen with activity, are often worse later in the day, and associated with stiffness, and typically resolve quickly over 15 to 30 minutes. Joint pain is usually felt at the joints (exceptions include shoulder pain, felt over the deltoid, and hip pain, felt in the groin). Joint pain from degenerative or inflammatory causes can vary in severity. Most patients will describe joint pain as aching and rarely rate the pain higher than 8/10 on an ascending severity scale. Pain relating to localized myofascial pain syndromes, including tendinopathies and enthesopathies, may be described as being close to joints, and being worse with specific movements. In people suffering from generalized pain syndromes, pain is often rated very highly (10/10), is poorly localized, involving upper and lower body regions, with descriptions including qualifiers to impress the severity of the pain ("like a truck ran over me").

It is also important to distinguish between arthralgia (subjective joint pain without objective signs) and arthritis, where pain and tenderness are associated with objective signs of joint swelling and warmth (synovitis), deformity, or limitation of movement. Objective findings on physical examination must be identified for a diagnosis of arthritis to be made.

Function
Function is commonly compromised in patients with rheumatic disease. Although this can be related to fatigue or muscular weakness, in the case of rheumatic disorders in which there is no articular involvement, most commonly functional impairment is related to joint involvement. Function should be assessed in terms of a patient's ability to perform activities of daily living, work, and participation. Validated questionnaires of function are available to identify functional limitations.

Physical Examination
Essential Concepts
A complete examination by a physician is required to identify and classify a rheumatic disease. This should include an assessment of temperature, body mass index, affect, pain behaviors, gait, and posture, as well as examination of the scalp, skin, eyes, lymph nodes, cardiovascular system, lungs, abdomen, joints, spine, and skeletal muscles. A systematic joint examination is key to the rheumatic disease examination and should include all regions, with comparisons of right and left sides. The pattern of joint involvement, including symmetry, and axial versus peripheral involvement, should be recorded. Use

of a joint diagram (homunculus) helps to track joint involvement. The joint examination should include documentation of the presence or absence of tenderness, periarticular wasting, erythema, swelling, limitation in range of motion (ROM), sites of prior surgery and trauma, and joint deformity, allowing for comparison over time and between different examiners. Using a four-step systematic approach to joint examination facilitates a thorough examination. This should include (1) inspection (looking for asymmetry, erythema, swelling, and deformity), (2) palpation (feeling for tenderness, specifically joint line tenderness, warmth, synovial thickening and effusion, bony hypertrophy, and crepitus), (3) ROM (both actively and passively for each joint), and (4) special tests specific to each joint or region. A complete examination should also consider relevant possible extra-articular manifestations.

Examples of Musculoskeletal Findings that Help to Classify a Rheumatic Disease

When considering the joint examination, a finding of redness (erythema) can indicate more acute and/or severe inflammation. The presence of erythema is more typically seen in the case of infection or crystalline arthritis. Joint warmth also signifies underlying inflammation. Joint swelling, a definitive sign of joint inflammation or arthritis, may indicate the presence of a joint effusion (excess synovial fluid) representing inflammation of the synovial membrane (synovitis). All rheumatic diseases short of specific pain syndromes can present with synovitis. Palpable bony thickening around a joint indicates swelling related to osteophytes, which is characteristic of OA. Crepitus feels like a grinding sensation under the examiner's hand during active or passive joint motion. Fine or velvety crepitus may indicate chronic proliferative synovitis, whereas coarse crepitus may indicate either roughening of the cartilage surface or complete loss of hyaline cartilage. Joint damage may manifest as loss of cartilage or bony hypertrophy. In some diseases such as RA, psoriatic arthritis, or Jaccoud's arthropathy (a form of SLE-related deforming arthropathy) deformity occurs as a result of joint subluxation or contracture related to nature's forces on joints and tendons and where chronic synovitis has caused joint capsule distension, ligamentous laxity, tendon rupture, or contracture.

Assessing Range of Motion

Both active and passive ROM should be assessed to appreciate joint function. Generally, active ROM is assessed first by asking patients to demonstrate full ROM of a joint; active ROM requires intact strength, innervation, muscle and tendon function, and joint mobility. Passive ROM is assessed by the examiner and for the most part assesses joint mobility or in some cases ligament or tendon impingement. First, assessing active ROM enables the examiner to appreciate potential areas of pain and where to examine carefully. If mobility is full on passive ROM, other causes can be considered for loss of mobility.

Establishing a Diagnosis

The findings from a thorough history and physical examination can be used to guide an appropriate set of investigations. Table 256-3 and Figure 256-1 provide clinical clues that are helpful in establishing a diagnosis based on the broad classifications in Table 256-1. By using the algorithm and Table 256-3, clinicians can develop a more parsimonious differential diagnosis and use investigations that will help to confirm the suspected diagnosis.

Laboratory and Imaging in Rheumatic Diseases

Identifying the presence of specific laboratory or imaging features can support a diagnosis and aid in specific classification of a rheumatic disease.[5] For example, in vasculitis, testing ANCAs or imaging the vascular tree of an involved area is key to establishing a diagnosis. Similarly, in seronegative spondyloarthropathies, imaging of the sacroiliac joint using radiographs when symptoms are sustained, or MRI if the disease is of more recent onset, is key. Radiographs and MRIs of specific joint areas in DJD not only help establish diagnosis but also aid in staging the disease. In the case of RA, testing of rheumatoid factor and ACPA is critical. When considering other prototypical seropositive systemic rheumatic diseases, the list of potential autoantibodies is much longer, and depending on the degree of difficulty in making the diagnosis, or appreciating the extent of disease and associated organ involvement, many of these can be considered for testing. These are listed in Table 256-4. It should be noted that no test alone should be used to diagnose a rheumatic disease, but rather that the tests should support the diagnosis.

TREATMENT   Rx

The treatment approaches to each rheumatic disease are highlighted in detail in the following chapters. Therapeutic approaches to degenerative rheumatic diseases continue to involve control of symptoms with either nonsteroidal anti-inflammatory drugs or analgesics. Additionally, physical modalities and injections of glucocorticoids (GCs) or other agents are employed to manage symptoms. When these conservative approaches fail, orthopedic surgery is often indicated. However, the approach to systemic and inflammatory rheumatic diseases usually requires more intense or immune-modulatory therapies. GCs are a major component of treatment regimens, particularly when organs are at risk for damage, when other agents take time to become fully effective, and in situations in which there are no alternative options for therapy. However, GCs are not without risk, and these should be discussed with each patient. Depending on the disease, GC-sparing therapies are usually initiated, the potency of which is tailored to the severity and risk for the illness itself. For example, SLE patients presenting with only a rash or synovitis may receive hydroxychloroquine, whereas patients with renal disease may receive mycophenolate mofetil, cyclophosphamide, or other therapies to most effectively treat that disease manifestation. Similarly in RA, patients presenting with high-titer ACPA levels, a high swollen joint count, and erosions on baseline radiographs of the hands and feet may receive rapidly escalating doses of methotrexate with or without other disease-modifying antirheumatic drugs and earlier use of tumor necrosis factor inhibitors. Specific approaches and GC-sparing therapies will be outlined in chapters addressing each rheumatic disease. In almost all rheumatic diseases, GCs are used as transitional therapy with a view to tapering these and using them again only for disease exacerbations.

● SUMMARY

A broad-based set of rheumatic disease classifications can provide an overall construct for consideration of a multitude of possible rheumatic diseases. When the classifications are based on pathogenic mechanisms as well as clinical features, this facilitates identification of specific symptoms and signs and guides a further line of investigation. Although all rheumatic diseases will not fit within this classification, a systematic and directed analysis will accelerate achieving the correct diagnosis of the patient.

GENERAL REFERENCES

For the General References and other additional features, please visit Expert Consult at https://expertconsult.inkling.com.

257

LABORATORY TESTING IN THE RHEUMATIC DISEASES

DAVID S. PISETSKY

The rheumatic diseases are a heterogeneous group of conditions that result from diverse pathophysiologic mechanisms and involve the musculoskeletal system as well as other organs. These conditions range from mild, diffuse joint and muscle pain to severe life-threatening kidney failure and stroke. Although the rheumatic diseases have many origins, immune disturbances resulting in local and systemic inflammation are frequently the underlying basis for disease manifestations. The approach to diagnosis therefore entails a wide array of laboratory tests to assess functional disturbances of individual organs and their relationship to inflammation and autoimmunity.

Laboratory testing in patients with rheumatic disease involves determination of biomarkers of the following kinds: antecedent (risk for disease); screening (subclinical disease); diagnostic (overt disease); staging (disease severity or activity); and prognostic (disease course, response to therapy, monitoring therapy). Some tests are useful in all contexts, although others have more specific uses related to their performance characteristics, specificity, and pattern of expression during disease. In view of the increasing efficacy of treatment for diseases such as rheumatoid arthritis (RA) and the availability of more specific serologic assays for early diagnosis, laboratory screening may be important to improve outcomes further by identifying individuals who have symptoms (e.g., arthralgias) that could represent the first manifestations of disease (preclinical autoimmunity); serologic screening could also be useful in identifying individuals at risk for disease (e.g., siblings or first-degree relatives). In general, the assessment of damage relies on specific tests of end-organ function or structure rather than process markers. Distinguishing activity from damage is important in patient management, especially with respect to the use of therapies associated with toxicity. In many diseases, prognosis can reflect ongoing disease activity as well as damage from past disease activity and effects of treatment, with laboratory testing needed to assess these various processes.

MARKERS OF INFLAMMATION

For many patients, the initial goal of evaluation is to determine the presence of inflammation. Inflammation is the body's response to injury and is characterized by a cascade of cellular and molecular events that arise irrespective of stimulus or locale (Chapter 48). The immediate response to inflammatory stimuli is termed the *acute phase response* and includes a set of proteins produced primarily in the liver in response to cytokines such as interleukin-6 (IL-6), tumor necrosis factor-α (TNF-α), and IL-1. These cytokines are produced by macrophages and dendritic cells after stimulation of pattern recognition receptors (PRRs) that include both toll-like receptors (TLRs) and other non-TLR sensing systems that trigger a system called the *inflammasome*; PRRs recognize intracellular as well as extracellular bacterial and viral products as well as large and small (e.g., adenosine triphosphate, uric acid) molecules released from damaged cells. The result is stimulation of innate immunity (Chapters 46 and 48). Many proteins in the acute phase response show large increases in serum levels, although some show a reduction. Because the levels of these proteins can increase dramatically in magnitude, they provide a sensitive and powerful set of markers for inflammation, whether induced by infection, trauma, or autoimmunity.

Of the proteins stimulated during the acute phase response, C-reactive protein (CRP) has received the most attention as a marker of inflammation in both rheumatic and nonrheumatic diseases. CRP is a member of the pentraxin family; although its function is not fully known, its ability to bind to phosphocholine suggests a scavenger function to eliminate bacterial products or damaged cells and to attenuate the consequences of infection or tissue injury.[1] Other molecules, such as serum amyloid protein (SAP), fibrinogen, and complement, also show marked elevations in levels during the acute phase response, signifying a broad-based effort at host defense.

The CRP level provides a very useful measure of inflammation and can convey information for categorization of a clinical process (e.g., inflammatory versus noninflammatory arthritis) as well as assessment of disease activity or prognosis (e.g., activity of RA or likelihood of joint erosion). The advantage of measuring CRP in the blood, rather than cytokines, is that the protein levels are much higher. Furthermore, CRP levels remain elevated for a longer period (days) than do cytokines; the latter may appear only transiently in the blood and thereby evade detection. The levels of CRP are in part determined by genetic factors, with baseline values important in determining the significance of any increases that can be associated with disease activity. Although CRP testing is commonly performed to assess the risk for atherosclerosis, a frequent complication of systemic rheumatic disease, the application of this screening in a patient with an inflammatory condition must take into account the various determinants of this marker, especially during active disease.

Another simple laboratory test reflecting the acute phase response is the erythrocyte sedimentation rate (ESR). In this test, commonly called the *sed rate*, anticoagulated blood is drawn into a long, thin tube and allowed to settle under the influence of gravity for 1 hour. The distance the blood falls depends on a number of factors, including the concentration of serum proteins such as immunoglobulins and fibrinogen, an acute phase reactant. The sedimentation rate is nonspecific with respect to disease association and also depends on the age and gender of the person. The upper limits of normal vary between women and men. Other simple laboratory tests point to an acute phase response. For example, patients with inflammation frequently exhibit a leukocytosis or thrombocytosis, most likely reflecting the action of cytokines and other mediators, including glucocorticoids, during this process. With chronic inflammation, anemia of chronic disease can also occur, with the hematocrit, in conjunction with the white blood cell and platelet counts, pointing to the presence of an inflammatory process. In this regard, in systemic lupus erythematosus (SLE), lymphopenia, thrombocytopenia, and low CRP values often characterize active disease, with the discordance between laboratory and clinical findings a clue to diagnosis.

LABORATORY EVALUATION OF MUSCULOSKELETAL DISEASE

The most common presentation of musculoskeletal disease is pain in and around the joints in association with functional impairment. Collectively, diseases causing joint symptoms are called arthritis, implying inflammation. The extent of inflammation in these diseases varies markedly, however, with some forms such as osteoarthritis (Chapter 262) showing only limited evidence of inflammation either locally or systemically.

Arthritis results from many different diseases and occurs in various patterns defined by the number and size of joints affected, symmetry, and involvement of the axial as well as peripheral joints. For each pattern (e.g., chronic polyarthritis), a key issue in diagnosis concerns its place in the spectrum of inflammatory versus noninflammatory arthritis. Furthermore, although many diseases can cause arthritis, their prevalence varies enormously, with osteoarthritis or degenerative joint disease being the most common form of noninflammatory arthritis and RA the most common form of inflammatory arthritis.

The differential diagnosis of arthritis is based on a comprehensive history and physical examination to assess symptoms suggesting inflammation (e.g., morning stiffness and fatigue), the presence of synovitis, and results of laboratory tests indicative of inflammation. Of these tests, the ESR and CRP are nonspecific indicators of inflammation. Depending on the stage of disease and prior therapy of the patient, however, both the CRP and ESR may not be elevated at the time of an initial evaluation because many treatments, especially those directed against cytokines, can effectively reduce the acute phase response; multiplex assays of various other mediators may allow assessment of disease activity in this circumstance. Two autoantibody tests, rheumatoid factor (RF) and antibodies to citrullinated proteins, provide more specific diagnostic information. Given the demographics of inflammatory arthritis, testing for antinuclear antibodies is often part of this evaluation as well.

Rheumatoid Factor

RF comprises a family of specificities that bind to the immunoglobulin G (IgG) molecule. These RFs target primarily the constant region or Fc portion of IgG, reacting with antigenic determinants that are most likely conformational in origin. IgM RFs are the most abundant of these antibodies and have been easiest to measure, using agglutination assays with red blood cells or latex beads coated with IgG. More recently, enzyme-linked immunosorbent assay (ELISA) and nephelometry have been used to detect RFs.

RFs occur in approximately 80% of patients with RA (Chapter 264) and represent one criterion for the classification or diagnosis of this disease. Furthermore, high levels of RFs are often associated with a worse prognosis, the occurrence of joint erosion as measured by radiographs, and deformity. Despite these associations, RFs occur in the sera of patients with a wide range of autoimmune and inflammatory diseases as well as in normal individuals, especially with age (Table 257-1). The frequent occurrence of RFs may reflect their etiology and role in innate immune responses to promote the binding of IgG to antigen by Fc cross-linking. Although RFs may occur in many settings other than RA, depending on the pretest probability, the test nevertheless remains useful in the evaluation of patients with inflammatory arthritis.

Antibodies to Citrullinated Proteins

Antibodies to citrullinated proteins are other autoantibody specificities important in the diagnosis of RA (Chapter 264). Citrulline is a post-translational modification of the amino acid arginine that results from deimidation. This chemical reaction is catalyzed by the enzyme peptidylarginine deiminase (PAD) and may occur in the setting of inflammation; the function of this modification is unknown. Citrullination can affect many different proteins, creating antigenic sites on proteins that include vimentin, enolase, and filaggrin.[2]

Although antibodies are directed to citrullinated residues on intact proteins, they can be conveniently measured using synthetic peptides containing citrulline. Among these synthetic antigens, a citrulline-containing protein with a cyclic structure provides sensitive and specific assays in an ELISA format. Antibodies directed to this type of antigen are known as anti-CCP (cyclic citrullinated peptide) and can be formally distinguished from antibodies to the citrullinated proteins themselves (ACPA, or anti–citrullinated protein antibodies); The term *anti-CCP* is commonly used for these

TABLE 257-1 RHEUMATIC DISEASES AND NONRHEUMATIC CONDITIONS ASSOCIATED WITH A POSITIVE RHEUMATOID FACTOR

DISEASES	FREQUENCY
Rheumatoid arthritis	50-90%
Systemic lupus erythematosus	15-35%
Sjögren's syndrome	75-95%
Systemic sclerosis	20-30%
Polymyositis/dermatomyositis	5-10%
Cryoglobulinemia	40-100%
Mixed connective tissue disease	50-60%
Aging (>70 yr)	10-25%
Infection	
Bacterial endocarditis	25-50%
Liver disease	15-40%
Tuberculosis	8%
Syphilis	Up to 13%
Parasitic diseases	20-90%
Leprosy	5-58%
Viral infection	15-65%
Pulmonary disease	
Sarcoidosis	3-33%
Interstitial pulmonary fibrosis	10-50%
Silicosis	30-50%
Asbestosis	30%
Miscellaneous diseases	
Primary biliary cirrhosis	45-70%
Malignancy	5-25%

Modified from Shmerling RH, Delbanco TL. The rheumatoid factor: an analysis of clinical utility. *Am J Med.* 1991;91:530.

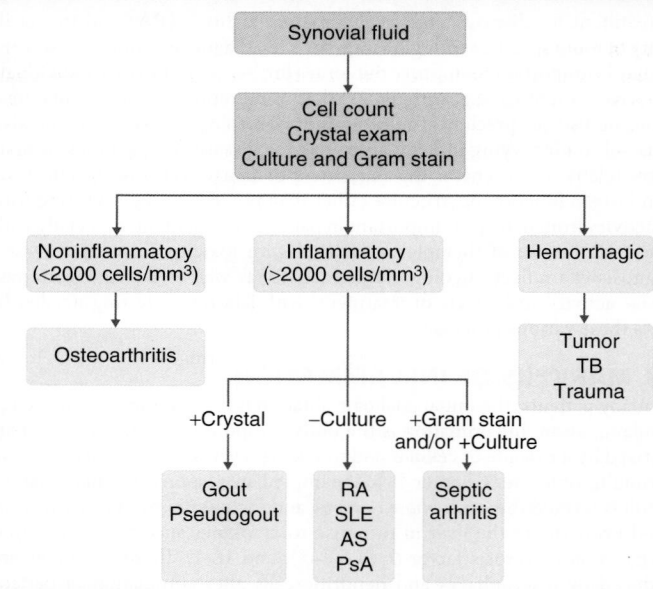

FIGURE 257-1. Algorithm for analysis of joint fluid. Examples of inflammatory arthritis are indicated, although many conditions can produce these findings. AS = ankylosing spondylitis; PsA = psoriatic arthritis; RA = rheumatoid arthritis; SLE = systemic lupus erythematosus; TB = tuberculosis.

specificities, although it is not formally synonymous with ACPA. ACPA can be assessed by a variety of analytic techniques using as antigens both modified proteins as well as arrays of peptides. For detection of anti-CCP antibodies, the formulation of peptides has changed over the years as designated by assay generation. Furthermore, among commercially available assays, results of assays can vary, making it important to know the performance characteristics of assays in interpreting the results of testing.

Anti-CCP antibodies are highly associated with RA and represent a criterion in the classification of patients with this disease.[3] Depending on the assay, these antibodies occur in 60 to 70% of patients with RA and uncommonly in those with other forms of inflammatory arthritis, making their presence important in diagnosis. Significantly, anti-CCP antibodies can occur before the onset of other signs and symptoms of RA, suggesting utility for screening of at-risk patients. In addition, in patients with arthralgias without clinical evidence of synovitis by examination, the presence of anti-CCP may predict the development of subsequent arthritis. Thus, because of the specificity of anti-CCP for RA, the presence of these antibodies in patients with early signs and symptoms of disease may indicate the diagnosis of RA and allow more prompt initiation of therapy before disease is fully manifest. In this regard, although RA can occur in the absence of anti-CCP antibodies, the presence of these antibodies may define disease subsets that differ in etiology, clinical course, and response to therapy.

Joint Fluid Analysis

Analysis of joint fluid can provide decisive data in the evaluation of arthritis and, in some instances, a definitive diagnosis. This analysis is essential in the setting of acute monoarthritis to investigate the possibility of infection; for chronic forms of arthritis, joint fluid should be analyzed if there is uncertainty about the diagnosis and involvement of one joint out of proportion to others. Joint aspiration is a sterile procedure performed with a local anesthetic. Although fluid can be analyzed by tests to assess viscosity and mucin content, the cell count, examination of crystals, and stains and cultures to evaluate infection are the most informative.

On the basis of cell counts, joint fluids can be categorized into four main types: noninflammatory, inflammatory, septic, and hemorrhagic. A noninflammatory fluid has fewer than 2000 cells/mm³ with mononuclear cell predominance. An inflammatory fluid has more than 2000 cells/mm³, with 50,000 cells/mm³ frequently used as the upper limit for this type of fluid. In an inflammatory fluid, polymorphonuclear cells predominate. A septic fluid is an inflammatory fluid in which culture or staining for microorganisms demonstrates infection. Suspicion of infection is especially high for fluids with cell counts greater than 50,000/mm³. However, crystal-induced arthritis can produce cell counts of this magnitude, and an infected fluid can have counts below this level. Hemorrhagic fluids have red cell predominance that can approximate that of blood.

In the setting of an acute monoarthritis, crystal-induced disease is much more common than infection, with the presence of crystals demonstrated by polarization microscopy. With this technique, monosodium urate crystals in gout appear needle shaped and are negatively birefringent. In contrast, calcium pyrophosphate dihydrate crystals in pseudogout are rhomboidal in shape and are weakly positively birefringent. Infection can coexist with crystal-induced disease, necessitating microbiologic evaluation even when crystals are found. Hemorrhagic fluids can also result from infection, although their presence suggests malignancy or trauma. Figure 257-1 provides an algorithm for the analysis of joint fluid.

Depending on the clinical findings and the results of initial laboratory testing, other studies may be performed to investigate less common diagnostic possibilities such as metabolic disease or malignancy. The laboratory evaluation of inflammatory arthritis may also include serologic tests for infections such as Lyme disease, HIV infection, or hepatitis.

● LABORATORY EVALUATION OF SYSTEMIC INFLAMMATORY DISEASE

Among rheumatic diseases, some are characterized by severe systemic inflammation that can cause organ-threatening and life-threatening manifestations. These diseases can have arthritis as a component and presenting complaint, although the prominence of extra-articular manifestations, especially as they develop over time and involve organs such as the kidney, points to their systemic nature. These diseases can be categorized on the basis of clinical, serologic, and pathologic findings, with the presence of vasculitis, irrespective of blood vessel size, providing a unifying feature in disease classification.

The terms *connective tissue disease* (CTD) and *collagen vascular disease* are both used to denote a group of diseases that includes RA, SLE, Sjögren syndrome, polymyositis, dermatomyositis, and progressive systemic sclerosis. Diseases in this group can share common or overlapping clinical features, especially early in their course, when their presentations may be similar. In this stage of disease, the condition may be called *undifferentiated CTD*, with serologic markers sometimes predictive of the eventual diagnosis.

Antinuclear Antibodies

The expression of antibodies to components of the cell nucleus (antinuclear antibodies, or ANAs) is characteristic of CTD and is essentially invariable in patients with SLE (Chapter 266). These antibodies target a host of nuclear macromolecules, including DNA, RNA, and proteins as well as complexes of proteins with nucleic acid. These antigens are ubiquitously expressed in cells and subserve critical processes related to chromosomal structure, cell division, transcription, and translation. The basis for the antigenicity of these molecules is unknown, although DNA and RNA both have intrinsic immunologic activities and can stimulate cytokine production through action on both TLR and non-TLR PRRs, especially when in the form of immune complexes. Furthermore, these antigens may undergo post-translation modification as well as enzymatic cleavage reactions during cell death, perhaps increasing their immunogenicity.

ANAs are commonly measured by immunofluorescence (IF) assays in which sera are incubated with tissue culture cells (e.g., Hep2 cells) fixed to a glass slide. Antibody binding is revealed by fluorescence microscopy after incubation of the slide with a fluoresceinated anti-immunoglobulin reagent. Results are reported in terms of the pattern of fluorescence as well as the end-point titer of sera at which fluorescence can be observed. The patterns of binding differ depending on the location of the particular macromolecular target, although a few patterns predominate. These patterns include homogeneous, rim, nucleolar, and speckled; in addition, ANA tests can detect antibodies to cytoplasmic antigens. Despite some disease associations, these patterns do not have diagnostic significance. Table 257-2 presents a list of major ANAs with their pattern and disease associations.

A major limitation in the assays of ANAs concerns the frequency of positive reactivity in the sera of otherwise normal individuals who lack evidence of a CTD. Depending on the titer for screening, the sera of as many as 20% of normal individuals express reactivity in the IF ANA test.[4] The basis of this reactivity, which occurs more commonly in women than men, is not well understood, although it may reflect a predisposition to autoimmunity that is manifest in ANA production in the absence of other immunopathologic disturbances for the complete development of a CTD. Because ANA testing is often performed to evaluate nonspecific complaints such as arthralgias, fatigue, and fever, a positive test must be interpreted with caution and not used as proof of a CTD in the absence of correlative clinical or laboratory findings.

Because of detailed biochemical studies, the molecular identity of many ANAs is now known, allowing for the development of specific immunochemical assays using technologies that can eliminate the need for visual inspection of a slide stained for fluorescence. These tests (e.g., ELISA) can be performed individually, although multiplex assays provide simultaneous assessment of multiple specificities. With multiplex assays, a version of the ANA test can be generated by measuring antibodies to a select set of more commonly targeted autoantigens, with positive binding to any one antigen considered indicative of a positive value for an ANA. Because sera of patients with SLE and other systemic inflammatory diseases contain numerous ANAs, focus on a limited set of specificities may fail to detect some positive sera. In addition, because immunochemical assays may detect low levels of antibody binding, the significance of this reactivity is not certain. Thus, although multiplex assays are operationally easier than conventional ANA testing by immunofluorescent staining, in clinical situations, the IF assay remains an important laboratory test for patient evaluation.

Among many ANA specificities now identified, only a few are performed routinely because of their value for diagnosis and prognosis. For certain CTDs, diagnosis can be readily determined from clinical findings or other laboratory tests. In these instances, the ANA determination provides confirmatory information as well as clues to the occurrence of certain clinical manifestations.

Antibodies to DNA

Antibodies to DNA (anti-DNA) are serologic markers of SLE and represent a criterion in the classification of patients with this disease (Chapter 266). These antibodies bind sites on both single-stranded (ss) and double-stranded (ds) DNA, although anti-dsDNA antibodies are more specific for SLE and therefore routinely measured. Although these antibodies can bind free DNA, DNA in the cell occurs in association with histones to form a structure called the *nucleosome*, with DNA wrapped around a histone core. Anti-DNA may therefore be considered a subset of antibodies to nucleosomes, with nucleosomes probably serving as the driving antigen for this response.[5]

In clinical practice, the measurement of anti-DNA antibodies is an important element in the evaluation of patients with a broad array of clinical complaints, given the heterogeneity and multisystemic nature of SLE. Anti-DNA determinations, in addition to their value in diagnosis, also convey prognostic information and serve as an index of disease activity. The association with disease activity appears strongest with glomerulonephritis, most likely because of the role of DNA–anti-DNA immune complexes in immunopathogenesis. The association of anti-DNA antibodies with other disease manifestations is less certain, limiting the use of this marker as a measure of overall disease activity. The presence of anti-DNA may nevertheless be important in assessing likelihood of response to therapies such as belimumab (anti-BLyS or anti-BAFF), an agent indicated for treatment of patients with active disease as evidenced by the presence of either anti-DNA antibodies or a positive test for ANA.

Several immunochemical approaches can be used to detect anti-DNA antibodies, although solid-phase ELISA assays are convenient and sensitive and eliminate the need for radioactivity. The assays vary in regard to the spectrum of anti-DNA antibodies detected, and results between assays may not

TABLE 257-2 SELECTED ANTINUCLEAR ANTIBODIES AND RHEUMATIC DISEASES

DISEASE PATTERN	ANTIBODY	ANTIGEN	ASSOCIATION
Homogeneous	Antihistone	Histones H1, H2A, H2B, H3, H4	Drug-induced lupus (>95%)
Rim	Anti-double-stranded DNA	Double-stranded DNA	SLE (50%)
Speckled	Anti-Sm	snRNP proteins	SLE (30%)
	Anti-U1-RNP	U1 snRNP proteins	SLE (30%); MCTD (>95%)
	Anti-Ro (SS-A)	Two proteins complexed to small RNAs Y1-Y5	SLE (30%); Sjögren syndrome (70-80%)
	Anti-La (SS-B)	Single protein plus RNA polymerase III transcript	SLE (15%); Sjögren syndrome (50-70%)
	Anti-Ku	DNA binding protein	SLE (10%)
	Anti-SCL-70	DNA topoisomerase I	PSS (40-70%); CREST (10-20%)
Nucleolar	Anti-PM-Scl	Nucleolar protein complex	PSS (3%); PM (8%)
	Anti-Mi-2	Nuclear protein complex	DM (15-20%)
	Anti-RNA polymerase	Subunits of RNA polymerase I	PSS (4%)
Dividing cell	Anticentromere	Centromere/kinetochore protein	CREST (80%); PSS (30%)
	Antiproliferating cell nuclear antigen	Auxiliary protein of DNA polymerase δ	SLE (3%)
Cytoplasmic	Anti-Jo-1	Histidyl tRNA synthetase	ILD in PM/DM (18-25%)
	Anti-PL-7	Threonyl tRNA synthetase	PM/DM (3%)
	Anti-PL-12	Alanyl tRNA synthetase	PM (4%)
	Anti-SRP	Signal recognition particle	SLE (10%)
	Anti-ribosomal P	Large ribosomal subunit	PM/DM (3%)

CREST = calcinosis, Raynaud phenomenon, esophageal dysmotility, sclerodactyly, and telangiectasia; DM = dermatomyositis; ILD = interstitial lung disease; MCTD = mixed connective tissue disease; PM = polymyositis; PSS = progressive systemic sclerosis (diffuse scleroderma); SLE = systemic lupus erythematosus; snRNP = small nuclear ribonucleoprotein; tRNA = transfer RNA.

correlate.[6] Nevertheless, for each assay, the dynamic range for testing is large. With treatment and disease quiescence, anti-DNA antibodies may essentially disappear; with flare, levels may increase dramatically. This property distinguishes anti-DNA antibodies from other ANAs in SLE, levels of which tend to be more consistent over time.

As is the case for other ANAs, the appearance of anti-DNA antibodies in the serum may precede other manifestations of SLE, suggesting vigilance if these antibodies are present in patients who have symptoms that suggest a CTD but lack other evidence to establish a firm diagnosis.

Other Antinuclear Antibodies

Anti-Sm and anti-RNP antibodies are related specificities that commonly occur together in the sera of patients with SLE, a phenomenon called *linkage*. These antibodies bind proteins on subcellular particles called *snRNPs* (small nuclear ribonucleoproteins) that are composed of a set of proteins and uridine-rich RNAs. Anti-Sm and anti-RNP antibodies differ in protein specificity and in the ability to cause immunoprecipitation of the bound RNA molecules. Anti-Sm antibodies occur only in patients with SLE and represent a serologic marker in disease classification. In contrast, anti-RNP antibodies can appear in the sera of patients with other clinical presentations and, in the absence of anti-Sm, may characterize patients with overlapping CTD features, so-called mixed CTD or MCTD. In SLE, the frequencies of anti-Sm and anti-RNP antibodies vary among racial and ethnic groups, although a clear association with particular clinical manifestations has not been established.

Anti-Ro and anti-La antibodies (or anti-SS-A and anti-SS-B), another set of linked ANAs, are directed to protein-RNA complexes that are involved in cellular metabolism of RNA. These antibodies are expressed more widely in patients with CTD and appear in the sera of patients with SLE, RA, and Sjögren's syndrome, among others. Assessment of these antibodies is important because of their association with the neonatal lupus syndrome, which results from the transplacental passage of antibodies and causes congenital heart block as well as rash in the neonate. Although both Sm/RNP and Ro/La are complexes of proteins and RNA, these antibodies appear to be expressed by different patient subsets, suggesting distinct mechanisms of induction and clinical associations.[7]

Although ANAs are directed to ubiquitous antigens, they nevertheless are expressed in disease-specific patterns and may show association with particular organ-specific manifestations. These associations include anti–ribosomal P antibodies with central nervous systemic involvement in SLE, antibodies to DNA topoisomerase 1 (anti-SCL-70) with progressive systemic sclerosis (diffuse scleroderma), antibodies to centromeres with CREST syndrome (calcinosis, Raynaud phenomenon, esophageal dysmotility, sclerodactyly, and telangiectasia), and antibodies to histidyl transfer RNA synthetase (anti-Jo-1) with interstitial lung disease in scleroderma (Chapter 267). In inflammatory myopathies, the presence of certain autoantibodies may be associated with particular patterns of disease, with antibodies to the enzyme 3-hydroxy-3-methylglutaryl-coenzyme A (HMG-CoA) reductase present in a syndrome of necrotizing myositis; the syndrome can occur in patients treated with statins, which can inhibit the enzyme.[8]

In addition to their association with specific disease manifestations, antibodies to both DNA- and RNA-binding proteins such as Sm and RNP may contribute to overall immune dysregulation in patients with autoimmune disease because of their formation of immune complexes containing DNA or RNA. These complexes can stimulate the production of type 1 interferon by triggering both TLR and non-TLR nucleic acid sensors as well as other cellular receptors (e.g., Fc receptors). Because immunoassays of interferon with patient sera are limited, the presence of interferon is observed more clearly in the pattern of gene expression known as the interferon signature in peripheral blood cells. This signature can be assessed by both microarray assays and measurement of more limited sets of messenger RNA molecules that are induced by interferon. Because antibodies to RNA-binding proteins in particular may promote this pattern, the serologic assay of these ANAs may allow assessment of the likelihood of both nonspecific and specific immunologic disturbances.[9]

Antibodies to Phospholipids

Originally defined by their effects on in vitro clotting tests, antibodies to phospholipids (APLs) are associated with in vivo thrombosis and have been termed *lupus anticoagulants* (LACs). Patients with these antibodies display a clinical condition, termed the *antiphospholipid antibody syndrome*, which is characterized by arterial or venous thrombosis, thrombocytopenia, and first-trimester spontaneous abortions (Chapter 176). This syndrome may occur by itself or in the context of SLE, where it may contribute to the acceleration

of atherosclerosis, premature stroke, and myocardial infarction. The laboratory evaluation of this condition involves specific assays of antibodies to phospholipids and related proteins as well as functional assays of clotting. Because expression of these antibodies may vary over time, testing must be performed on more than one occasion at least 6 weeks apart. Furthermore, the results of immunochemical and functional assays may not be congruent because they are likely related to the heterogeneity of antibodies.

The serology of APLs is complicated because it is related to the nature of the antigenic targets as well as heterogeneity among patients.[10,11] These antigens include phospholipids such as cardiolipin. Cardiolipin, however, can bind to the protein β_2-glycoprotein 1, which is also a target for antibodies in this condition. Serologic evaluation thus involves assays with a complex of cardiolipin and $\beta2$-glycoprotein 1 as well as $\beta2$-glcycoprotein in an ELISA format using reagents to measure IgG and IgM. The association of antibodies with thrombosis appears strongest with IgG antibodies; determination of the IgA isotype may also be informative depending on the results of IgG and IgM assays. ELISAs for these antibodies are not yet standardized, making it important to specify assay features related to quantitation such as cutoff values used to define positivity and values that are considered significant.

Functional assays for LACs involve tests directed at inhibition of in vitro clotting (e.g., activated partial thromboplastin time, dilute Russell viper venom time), recognizing the discordance between in vivo thrombosis and in vitro anticoagulation. Functional assays to detect lupus anticoagulants involve a mixing step in which patient plasma is mixed with normal plasma to determine the presence of an inhibitor (i.e., an antibody) as opposed to a deficiency state. The mechanisms by which antibodies to phospholipids and related proteins may cause thrombosis in vivo are unknown, although these antibodies may interact with the surface of cells (e.g., endothelium) to promote a prothrombotic state. Assessing the likelihood of the syndrome is best accomplished by considering results of both the immunoassays and functional assays in the context of the individual patient because both factors may promote thrombotic events.

Complement

Assessment of the complement system can provide valuable information on the activity of diseases in which immune complex deposition may promote inflammation and tissue injury (Chapter 50). This system involves a large number of proteins that function in enzyme cascades to generate degradation products that amplify immunologic reactions and promote the destruction or removal of foreign organisms as well as damaged cells. In the setting of SLE and in certain forms of vasculitis and glomerulonephritis, immune complexes activate complement to promote local inflammation. This activation can be measured in terms of the total complement level in the blood by functional assays of hemolytic activity; by measurement of individual complement components such as C3 and C4, whose levels are reduced by cleavage during activation; by measurement of split products of cleaved complement components; and by measurement of complement fragments bound to red blood cells during complement activation. Proteins of the complement system are acute phase reactants and can increase with inflammation, including active disease. Correspondingly, low levels may reflect inherited complement deficiency rather than consumption; genetic deficiency of C1q, for example, is highly associated with SLE.

Antineutrophil Cytoplasmic Antibodies

Antineutrophil cytoplasmic antibodies (ANCAs) are autoantibodies that react to determinants in the neutrophil and occur prominently in patients with certain forms of necrotizing vasculitis or rapidly progressive glomerulonephritis. Reflecting the serology, conditions have been called ANCA-associated vasculitis (AAV). Two main forms of ANCA have been distinguished on the basis of the target antigens and pattern of immunofluorescence staining of fixed neutrophils: PR3-ANCA (C-ANCA), which reacts with proteinase-3 (PR3), and MPO-ANCA (P-ANCA), which reacts with myeloperoxidase (MPO). By immunofluorescence, PR3-ANCA shows staining in the cytoplasm; staining by MPO-ANCA localizes in the perinuclear area. ANCAs to other proteins have also been identified, but these may also occur in conditions other than vasculitis.

In the evaluation of severe, multisystem inflammatory disease, ANCA testing is important to evaluate diagnostic possibilities.[12] ANCAs occur in association with varying clinical manifestations in patients with AAV and help define patterns of clinical involvement in terms of organ system involvement as well as histopathology (e.g., presence of granulomatous inflammation). PR3-ANCA occurs commonly in patients with granulomatosis with polyangiitis (GPA, formerly called Wegener granulomatosis) as well eosinophilic granulomatosis with polyangiitis (EGPA, formerly called Churg-Strauss disease); MPO-ANCA marks the course of vasculitis caused by microscopic polyangiitis.[13] Although there is overlap between serology and clinical features, PR3-ANCA occurs commonly in patients with upper airway disease, whereas MPO-ANA occurs commonly patients with patients with rapidly progressive renal disease (Chapter 270).

In patients with ANCA-associated glomerulonephritis, the kidney lacks evidence of immune deposits, as indicated by the lack of staining for immunoglobulins or complement. Kidney disease of this kind is termed *pauci-immune glomerulonephritis*. Although ANCA testing is useful in initial diagnosis, its role for assessing disease activity is less certain. Occasionally, in patients who are desperately ill and cannot tolerate a lung or kidney biopsy, the presence of an ANCA can be used as preliminary evidence for diagnosis to allow the initiation of immunosuppressive therapy. ANCA testing is also useful for assessing the likelihood for relapse because patients who express PR3-ANCA appear at risk for recurrent disease.

Cryoglobulins

Cryoglobulins are serum immunoglobulins that precipitate in the cold and promote the pathogenesis of systemic inflammatory disease through tissue deposition. The presence of a cryoglobulin is detected by allowing blood, collected warm, to remain cool at 2° to 4° C for 1 or more days. After centrifugation, the amount of cryoprecipitate is measured and expressed as a cryocrit. In the preanalytical phase, it is important that the blood remain at a temperature of 37° C during all steps from drawing the blood from the patient to separation of the serum fraction after coagulation. Thermos flasks with preheated sand or water and other special devices are available to keep the blood tubes at 37° C during transport. If these steps are not taken, cryoprecipitation at even room temperature may already occur before separation of the serum from the blood cells, possibly resulting in false-negative results.[14]

Subsequent analysis of the cryoprecipitate by immunochemical assays allows determination of its components. Cryoglobulins can be classified into three main types on the basis of their composition: (1) single, or type I; (2) mixed, type II; and (3) mixed, type III. A type I cryoglobulin consists of only a monoclonal immunoglobulin that precipitates in the cold. A mixed-type cryoglobulin contains RFs bound to polyclonal IgG to form an immune complex. In type II cryoglobulins, the IgM RF is monoclonal, and in type III, the IgM RF is polyclonal.

Type I cryoglobulins occur in patients with lymphoproliferative disorders such as Waldenström macroglobulinemia, multiple myeloma, or chronic lymphocytic lymphoma (Chapters 184 and 187). In contrast, patients with mixed cryoglobulins can present with a wide range of signs and symptoms resulting from vasculitis. These manifestations include purpura (a sign of leukocytoclastic vasculitis), weakness, arthritis, and neuropathy, representing a syndrome known as *essential mixed cryoglobulinemia*. Most patients with this condition have infection with hepatitis C virus, with viral components present in the complexes. These patients have serologic evidence of this infection as well as manifestations attributable to the underlying liver disease. As in the case of other CTDs and systemic inflammatory diseases, the evaluation of patients with essential mixed cryoglobulinemia demands attention to the entire patient and the impact of disease on multiple organs.

GENERAL REFERENCES

For the General References and other additional features, please visit Expert Consult at https://expertconsult.inkling.com.

258

IMAGING STUDIES IN THE RHEUMATIC DISEASES

RONALD S. ADLER

Historically, rheumatic disorders have been well characterized by conventional imaging. In as much as these disorders often manifest in characteristic distributions and present with specific alterations in the appendicular or axial skeleton and adjacent soft tissues, radiographic evaluation has been sufficient to both characterize the abnormalities as well as provide a relatively small number of differential possibilities as to the specific disease. The most well-studied example is rheumatoid arthritis (RA) in which symmetric involvement of the metacarpophalangeal joints, uniform joint space narrowing, periarticular osteopenia, and juxta-articular erosions along the "bare areas" are pathognomonic.

The development of new therapeutic alternatives for the inflammatory arthritides, so-called disease-modifying antirheumatic drugs (DMARDs), and chondroprotective strategies in the case of osteoarthrosis, require methods to diagnose these diseases at an earlier stage, characterize the degree of inflammation, and provide a useful metric to assess therapeutic response.[1] Indeed, it has become necessary to assess for possible joint and soft tissue abnormalities before irreversible tissue damage, the latter often being the case when the radiographic findings are abnormal. Fortunately, the requirement to achieve earlier diagnosis has paralleled advances in imaging. Ultrasonography and magnetic resonance imaging (MRI) have largely supplanted conventional radiographic evaluation in the imaging work-up of patients with suspected rheumatologic disorders and negative radiographs.[2,3] The term *molecular imaging* has been applied, particularly in the case of MRI and positron emission tomography (PET), in as much as these modalities reflect local tissue environment or metabolic activity.

● RADIOGRAPHIC EVALUATION

Radiographic evaluation is among the first studies ordered in patients with a suspected rheumatologic disorder. In the current digital era, conventional analog-based radiographs have been largely replaced by computed radiography. Images are usually displayed on workstations with high-resolution monitors within the context of a picture archiving system (PACS). Digital radiographs are of high spatial resolution but relatively poor soft tissue contrast. These images are amenable to a variety of image processing schemes, resulting in enhanced definition of the cortical surfaces and cancellous bone, which may be of value in displaying subtle erosions.

It is important to recognize that radiographs are projection images. To detect an abnormality, it may be necessary to view a joint or other structure at a specific angle. For instance, subtle erosions may only be apparent when viewed tangentially as opposed to en face. It is therefore necessary to have specific image protocols in order to optimally display the joint, cortical surface, or soft tissue structure. Most radiographic evaluations contain at least two orthogonal projections. The addition of an oblique view or other specialized projection may be necessary to address a specific clinical question.

The nature and distribution of joint space narrowing, presence of osteopenia, new bone formation, soft tissue swelling, soft tissue calcification, chondrocalcinosis, presence and nature of erosions, and assessment for joint malalignment may allow a specific diagnosis and help determine the severity of disease (Fig. 258-1). For instance, the presence of a juxta-articular erosion extending over an adjacent area of slightly hyperdense soft tissue swelling in the setting of normal bone mineralization with maintenance of the adjacent joint space is diagnostic of gout, in contrast to RA noted earlier. The seronegative arthritides, such as psoriatic arthritis, have a characteristic appearance in the small joints of the hand and feet, including a predilection for distal joints, asymmetry, and appositional new bone formation.

Table 258-1 summarizes some of the features of several of the more common diseases that may be encountered in clinical practice.

Finally, radiographs provide a direct means for needle localization during percutaneous procedures, predominantly joint injections, aspirations, and some biopsies. These are generally performed while imaging in real time (fluoroscopy) using short bursts of low-intensity x-rays enhanced through an image intensifier. Injection of joints under fluoroscopic guidance provides a convenient means to ensure intra-articular deposition of therapeutic agent or for diagnostic aspiration. Intra-articular location is verified by injection of a small amount of a standard iodinated contrast material. Arthrography using fluoroscopic guidance can be used as a primary diagnostic tool, but this application has largely been replaced by intra-articular injection of contrast followed by computed tomography (CT) or MRI.

For some procedures, CT may be preferable, depending on the location of the abnormality. The principal disadvantages of fluoroscopy relate to the use of ionizing radiation and poor soft tissue contrast. The latter becomes important with needle placements near neurovascular structures that may be potentially compromised by poor position. CT allows greater control over needle placement at the cost of greater levels of radiation exposure. Ultrasonography has replaced fluoroscopy and CT for a large number of percutaneous procedures. MRI provides another method to perform a variety of procedures without the necessity of ionizing radiation. These options will be discussed in greater detail below.

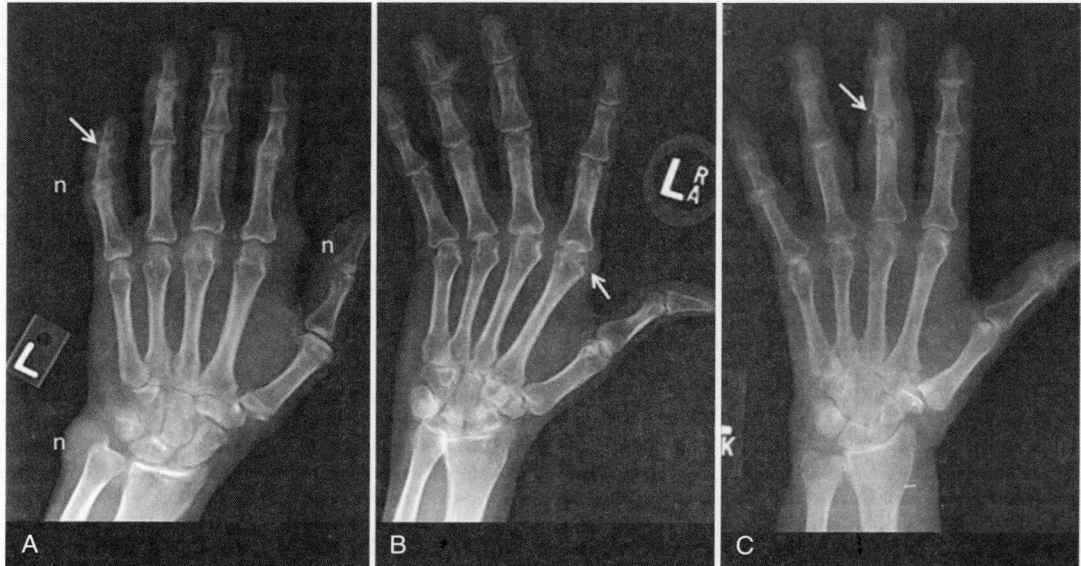

FIGURE 258-1. **Three hands with different diagnoses. A, Gout.** Radiograph of the left hand showing multiple dense soft tissue nodules (n) with multiple small erosions affecting the ulnar styloid, triquetrum and fifth ray. A large erosion (arrow) at the fifth distal interphalangeal (DIP) joint demonstrates bone formation extending circumferentially about the adjacent tophaceous deposit typical of an overhanging edge. Bone mineralization and joint spaces are preserved. **B, Rheumatoid arthritis.** There is ulnar deviation of the second through fifth metacarpophalangeal (MCP) joints with uniform joint space loss involving the MCP joints and the carpus. The DIP joints are spared. Periarticular demineralization is present with small erosions along the radiovolar aspect of the second (arrow) MCP joint. **C, Osteoarthrosis.** Soft tissue swelling affecting the third digit with joint space narrowing and bone production affecting the DIP joints, third and fifth proximal interphalangeal (PIP) joints, basal joint of the thumb, and scaphotrapeziotrapezoid joint. There are subchondral cystic changes at the third PIP joint having an erosive character (arrow). Mineralization is preserved, as are the radiocarpal and MCP joint spaces.

TABLE 258-1   DISTINGUISHING RADIOGRAPHIC FEATURES OF SEVERAL COMMON RHEUMATIC DISEASES

CONDITION	COMMON SITES	DISTRIBUTION	RADIOGRAPHIC FEATURES
Rheumatoid arthritis	Hands: MCP, PIP; wrists: intercarpal, DRUJ, ulnar styloid; feet: fifth MTP, cervical spine (atlantoaxial, apophyseal)	Bilateral, symmetric, polyarticular	Periarticular osteopenia, periarticular swelling, subluxations (e.g., ulnar, volar), uniform joint space loss, erosions (bare areas)
Osteoarthritis (primary)	Hands (DIP), wrists (basal joint, STT),feet (first MTP), hips (superolateral), knees (medial), spine (discs, facet, apophyseal, uncovertebral)	Symmetric, weight-bearing joints	Normal or increased density, nonuniform joint space loss, subchondral sclerosis, cysts, bone formation (osteophytes) Spine–disc space narrowing, end plate sclerosis and bone formation
Psoriatic arthritis	Hands (DIP, terminal tufts), feet (IP joints), entheses (calcaneus: plantar, posterior), spine, sacroiliac joints	Asymmetric (single ray), polyarticular, segmental (intervertebral, apophyseal)	Normal or increased density, periosteal bone formation, soft tissue swelling, ankylosis (SI joints), thick hyperostosis spine (nonmarginal syndesmophytes), juxta- and periarticular erosions
Ankylosing spondylitis	Spine, SI joints, fibrous joints (pubic symphysis), entheses (adductor origin), rhizomelic joints (hips, shoulders)	Symmetric, continuous (may affect entire spine-bamboo spine)	Normal or increased density, erosions (spine squaring, shining corner) with superimposed bone formation (ankylosis: SI), thin (marginal) syndesmophytes
Gout	Feet (first MTP), other damaged joints, elbow, knee, hindfoot	Asymmetric, extensor surfaces (elbow), abnormal joints (e.g., osteoarthritic joints)	Normal joint space, normal or increased density, dense soft tissue nodules (tophi), para-articular and subchondral erosions with bone formation along tophi (overhanging edge)
Calcium pyrophosphate dihydrate crystal deposition disease	Hands (second, third MCP), wrists (radiocarpal), TFC, knees (lateral compartment and patella-femoral, menisci)	Symmetric, fibrocartilaginous joints	Normal or increased density, hypertrophic bone formation, subchondral or periarticular cysts, chondrocalcinosis (hyaline, fibrocartilage), periarticular, peritendinous, periligamentous calcification
Infection	Any joint, pyogenic, TB	Monoarticular (mostly), any joint	Pyogenic (osteopenia; 8-10 days), joint space widened (early), joint space loss (rapid development), soft tissue swelling, erosions (both sides of joint), sequestra, periostitis, TB (joint space and mineralization may be preserved), juxta-articular erosions, spine–disc space loss and end plate erosion

DIP = distal interphalangeal; DRUJ = distal radial ulnar joint; IP = interphalangeal; MCP = metacarpophalangeal; MTP = metatarsophalangeal; PIP = proximal interphalangeal; SI = sacroiliac;
STT = scaphotrapezotraphezoid; TB = tuberculosis; TFC = triangular fibrocartilage.

COMPUTED TOMOGRAPHY

Computed tomography provides a two-dimensional map of tissue attenuation obtained from external x-ray source(s) located on a rotating gantry, whose radiation is detected by a series of detectors opposite the source. The current generation of CT scanners uses multiple detectors (16, 32, 64, and so on), allowing rapid image acquisition that can be displayed in a single plane in real time (CT-fluoroscopy) or as extremely thin section contiguous or overlapping acquisitions in the axial plane. The acquired images can be reconstructed in multiple planes with equivalent (isotropic) resolution elements (voxels) or as a three-dimensional rendering. Some scanners use dual energy sources, taking advantage of differences in the attenuation characteristics of various tissues at different energies. This has received greatest attention in the setting of gout, enabling a definitive diagnosis as well as depicting tophaceous deposits in anatomic locations not conducive to radiographs or ultrasound.[4]

Computed tomography allows the best assessment of trabecular and cortical bone, providing an excellent means to assess fractures and erosions, the presence of new bone formation (e.g., fracture callus), and degenerative or inflammatory arthritis. Soft tissue mineralization can likewise be well characterized, providing important information as to its etiology. Joints that are difficult to assess on radiographs, including the sacroiliac, temporomandibular, wrist, and sternoclavicular joints, are well seen on CT (Fig. 258-2).

Computed tomography generally has poor soft tissue contrast. Nevertheless, it is still very useful in performing a number of guided procedures because of its tomographic nature and rapid image acquisition capability. Improved soft tissue contrast can be obtained with use of iodinated contrast material. A number of soft tissue tumors, inflammatory synovitis, and infectious processes display pathologic enhancement after contrast administration. CT can likewise be used to produce angiographic displays (CTA) when used in combination with contrast, providing exquisite detail of central and peripheral vascular disease, including in patients with suspected vasculitis. These agents are typically administered intravenously following well-defined enhancement characteristics. CTA has become the method of choice in evaluating patients with suspected pulmonary embolism. Likewise, contrast agents may be used to improve intra-articular contrast (CT arthrography), currently the method of choice in assessing internal derangement in the postoperative shoulder, knee, and so on and in patients who are unable to undergo MRI (e.g., those with claustrophobia, aneurysm clips, or cardiac pacemakers). Imaging of cartilage and soft tissue abnormalities usually depends on pathologic imbibition of contrast material, indicative of degeneration or tearing. A limitation of this approach resides in the fact that some abnormalities may remain occult. An example is the inability to detect a bursal-sided rotator cuff tear after shoulder CT arthrography.

The radiation dose from CT can be high, especially when using the newer scanners. This is most significant when one is looking to minimize exposure, such as in children, requiring protocols specifically designed for the pediatric population. Intravenous (IV) use of iodinated contrast agents are contraindicated in patients with impaired renal function or history of allergic reaction. Nonionic agents can diminish the associated risks but still should be used with caution.

ULTRASONOGRAPHY

Ultrasound imaging takes advantage of the near uniform speed of sound and predictable attenuation characteristics of sound propagation in soft tissue. In general, anatomic images derive from specular surfaces whose dimensions exceed the ultrasound wavelength; inherent noise (speckle) within the image derives from small scatterers, smaller than the resolution element of the transducer. Modern ultrasound equipment contains various methods to reduce speckle in the image, resulting in a more anatomic rendition of the soft tissues. Rapid image acquisition and processing enables ultrasonography to be performed in real time (≈30 frames per second). Ultrasonography is also conducive to evaluation of blood flow from which estimates of flow velocity can be obtained through the Doppler equation. Doppler information is typically reported by either continuously estimating velocity at a specific depth (spectral Doppler) or through a color encoded two-dimensional map (color or power Doppler).

There is great appeal for using ultrasonography in patients with rheumatic disorders. There is no ionizing radiation, and it is real time, inexpensive, relatively portable, and well tolerated. Historically, however, ultrasonography has played only a limited role in the diagnostic assessment and treatment of patients with suspected musculoskeletal abnormalities, being used to differentiate fluid-filled from solid masses. The detection of a Baker cyst in the knee or the presence of a joint effusion constituted two major applications. There has also been limited application of ultrasonography to perform image-guided aspirations and biopsies. Within the United States, in particular, the development of MRI further limited the musculoskeletal applications of ultrasonography.

With the development of linear high-frequency small parts transducers; new imaging capabilities of ultrasound scanners; and the evolution of a new class of compact, portable (laptop) ultrasound units that have excellent image quality, the role of ultrasonography has dramatically changed in recent years.[5,6] These new applications have paralleled the development of new classes of DMARDs for which diagnosis of inflammatory synovitis prior to joint destruction is optimal.

The current generation of ultrasound scanners enables examination of the small joints of the hands and feet, allowing early detection of synovitis (Fig. 258-3). Typically, a 10-MHz or higher frequency linear transducer is used. The displacement of the joint capsule by hypoechoic (dark) soft tissue that displays vascularity on Doppler imaging or is incompressible with direct pressure by the transducer is characteristic, allowing differentiation of synovitis from an effusion. In addition to the detection of synovitis, ultrasonography has been shown to be more sensitive than conventional radiographs in the detection of erosions. Erosions appear as discrete irregular discontinuities

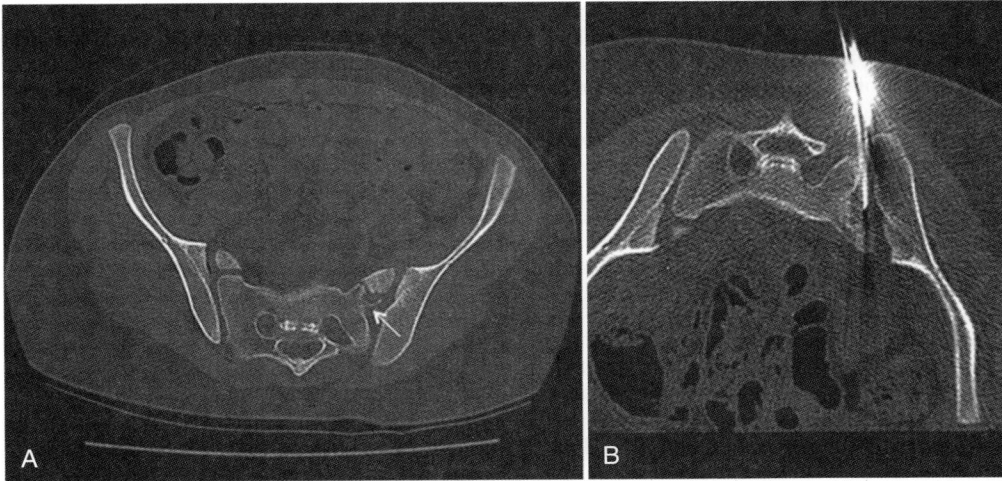

FIGURE 258-2. Infectious sacroiliitis in a 12-year-old boy with a 2-week history of back and left hip pain. A, Axial computed tomography (CT) image of the pelvis at the level of the sacroiliac joints (SIs) photographed using window settings optimized for bone detail. There is clear asymmetry in the two SI joints, with the left appearing more irregular. The cortical margins of the left sacral ala are less distinct and there is an isolated bone fragment (*arrow*) surrounded by soft tissue suspicious for a sequestrum. B, CT-guided aspiration of the left SI joint confirmed an infectious origin.

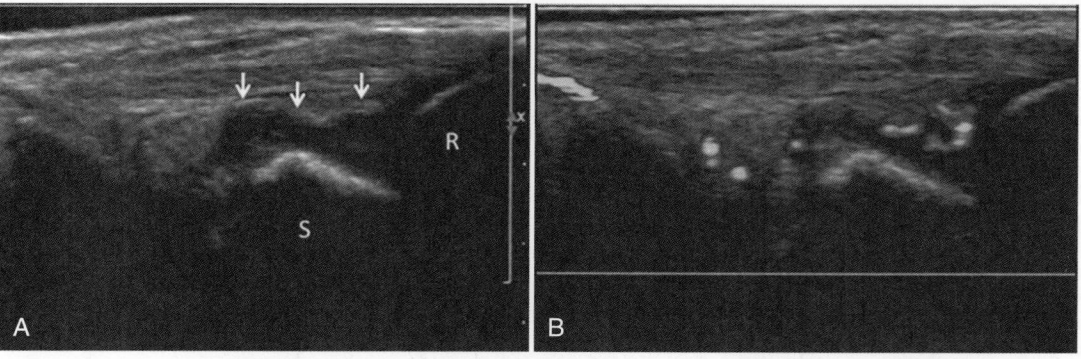

FIGURE 258-3. Synovitis on ultrasonography in a female patient with normal hand radiographs. **A,** Gray-scale ultrasound image obtained along the dorsal aspect of the radioscaphoid joint shows hypoechoic soft tissue (*arrows*) distending the dorsal recess. The cortical margins of the scaphoid (S) and radius (R) appear as bright reflectors on ultrasonography. **B,** Power Doppler image depicts the marked vascularity (*red color hues*) of the soft tissue illustrating the level of disease activity.

in the normally smooth hyperechoic (bright), reflecting cortical surfaces, often seen in continuity with adjacent inflammatory soft tissue. There is some variation in the appearance of synovitis among various arthritides. The distribution, presence, or lack of symmetry and other concomitant findings may be necessary to obtain a specific diagnosis.

The level of vascularity on color-flow imaging can reflect active inflammation, correlating with clinical and biochemical parameters. A parametric image encoding either mean Doppler shift (color Doppler) or amplitude (power Doppler) is typically used as a standard Doppler map. Both maps can be used to detect abnormal levels of vascularity. Whereas power Doppler provides an indirect measure of the number of moving scatterers within the region being scanned, color Doppler provides a velocity map, and therefore is more subject to artifact (angle dependence and sampling errors). When combined with color-flow imaging, the activity of the synovitis can be estimated. Ultrasound contrast agents can depict capillary flow, resulting in significantly improved detection sensitivity of synovial inflammation, and are used extensively in Europe. They constitute microbubble agents encased in a lipid or polysaccharide shell that can be instilled as either bolus or constant infusion, with the shell being metabolized in the liver and the gas exhaled in the lungs. These agents have biological half-lives on the order of minutes and are best suited to examining target joints. Contrast agents have received Food and Drug Administration approval for cardiovascular applications and therefore can only be used off label for the assessment of synovitis.

Articular and fibrocartilage have characteristic appearances on ultrasonography. Whereas the former appears as a thin hypoechoic band paralleling the articular surface, fibrocartilage appears hyperechoic. Chondrocalcinosis appears as discrete hyperechoic foci with the substance of the cartilage, in which case its presence is suggestive of calcium pyrophosphate deposition disease. Calcification along the margin of the articular cartilage gives rise to the double-line sign seen in gout.

Tendons and muscles have characteristic appearances on ultrasonography. The presence of tendinosis, tendon tears, muscle edema or inflammation, atrophy, and tears can be diagnosed. Ultrasonography is very sensitive, although not specific, for the detection of small amounts of calcification or ossification. It is an excellent method to assess for calcific peritendinitis and to provide guidance for treatment. Abnormal fluid distention of synovial lined structures can be assessed and treated under ultrasound guidance. Ultrasonography is an excellent modality to provide image guidance for therapeutic aspiration and injection of small and large joints, tendon sheaths, and cysts (e.g., bursae, ganglion, paralabral cysts, hematomas, abscesses,) (Fig. 258-4). The real-time capability of ultrasonography is useful to demonstrate the presence of subluxations or painful snapping, to document the distribution of injected material, and to assess adhesions. Ultrasonography is considered the method of choice to detect foreign bodies.

Nerves also have a characteristic appearance on ultrasonography. In cross-section, a nerve often has a "cluster of grapes" appearance, with nerve fascicles appearing hypoechoic and surrounded by hyperechoic endo- and epineural fat. In long axis, nerves display a characteristic tram-track appearance. Ultrasonography has been shown to be useful in the diagnosis and treatment of carpal tunnel syndrome and cubital tunnel syndrome. It is an excellent modality to assess for the presence of posttraumatic or postsurgical and interdigital neuromas and to provide image guidance for treatment, including therapeutic injections and ablative therapy.

Although ultrasonography is well suited to the evaluation of superficial structures, it is less well suited to deep structures. Frequency and penetration are reciprocally related: the higher the frequency, the better the axial resolution but poorer the degree of penetration. A 15-MHz linear transducer would work well in the hand but not in the hip. Examination of a hip might require a 5-MHz transducer and curved transducer geometry with reduced image quality. Excessive abdominal fat can further limit acoustic penetration and distort the ultrasound beam, limiting image quality. Diagnostic ultrasonography does not penetrate bone, resulting in limited acoustic access to joint structures. In some instances, soft tissue contrast can be poor. An inexperienced scanner may find ligaments and tendinous insertions difficult to differentiate from adjacent fibrofatty structures.

● MAGNETIC RESONANCE IMAGING

The natural abundance of hydrogen in biological systems and an inherent property of hydrogen, called *spin*, form the basis of conventional MRI. When placed in a strong magnetic field, protons tend to align themselves along the direction of the field. Magnetic field strengths are specified as Tesla and can be variable between clinical scanners. The majority of scanners in clinical usage vary between 1 and 3 Tesla. Application of a radiofrequency (RF) pulse to the system of protons induces the spins to rotate away from the direction of the field, during which time they precess about the direction of the magnetic field at a characteristic frequency, called the Larmor frequency. When the RF pulse is turned off, the spins relax toward their initial state determined by two tissue-dependent relaxation times, T1 and T2, which vary with field strength. T1 (also known as the spin-lattice relaxation) and T2 (or the transverse relaxation time) along with proton density are the principal determinants of signal intensity. The image can emphasize either the T1 or T2 characteristics of the tissue, impacting tissue contrast. Different tissues have varying appearance often based of levels of fat and water content, reflected by their inherent T1 and T2 relaxation times. Tissue morphology is often characterized by their appearance on T1-weighted or proton density images: tendon, muscle, fat, marrow, cortical bone, articular, and fibrocartilage have characteristic appearances. Many pathologic states, alternatively, are characterized by increased mobile water or effective T2 lengthening. Examples include soft tissue edema, inflammatory infiltrates, and neoplasm (Fig. 258-5). Images that emphasize T2 contrast are therefore helpful to display most pathologic states. Selective maps of T2 have been used to characterize the state of articular cartilage in early degenerative disease.[7] Other cartilage specific properties that relate to water content, glycosaminoglycan (GAG) content, and integrity of collagen architecture can be assessed using T2 and other parametric maps that can be derived from the MR data (Fig. 258-6).

The widely used contrast for MRI studies is a neutral, hydrophilic salt of the gadolinium chelate, gadolinium diethylenetriamine-penta-acetic acid (Gd-DTPA). Gadolinium can be injected intravenously or directly into the joint. IV injection (indirect magnetic resonance arthrography) carries the contrast in the vascular system to areas of hyperemia and inflammation (Fig. 258-7). It can be used for assessment of synovial activity in inflammatory joint diseases.[8] Gadolinium is taken up in inflamed synovium and is able to demonstrate thickened pannus. The slope of the early time-signal intensity curve provides a measure of tissue perfusion and can quantify inflammatory activity. Contrast material excreted into the synovial fluid provides excellent depiction of intra-articular structures and can be used in lieu of arthrographic

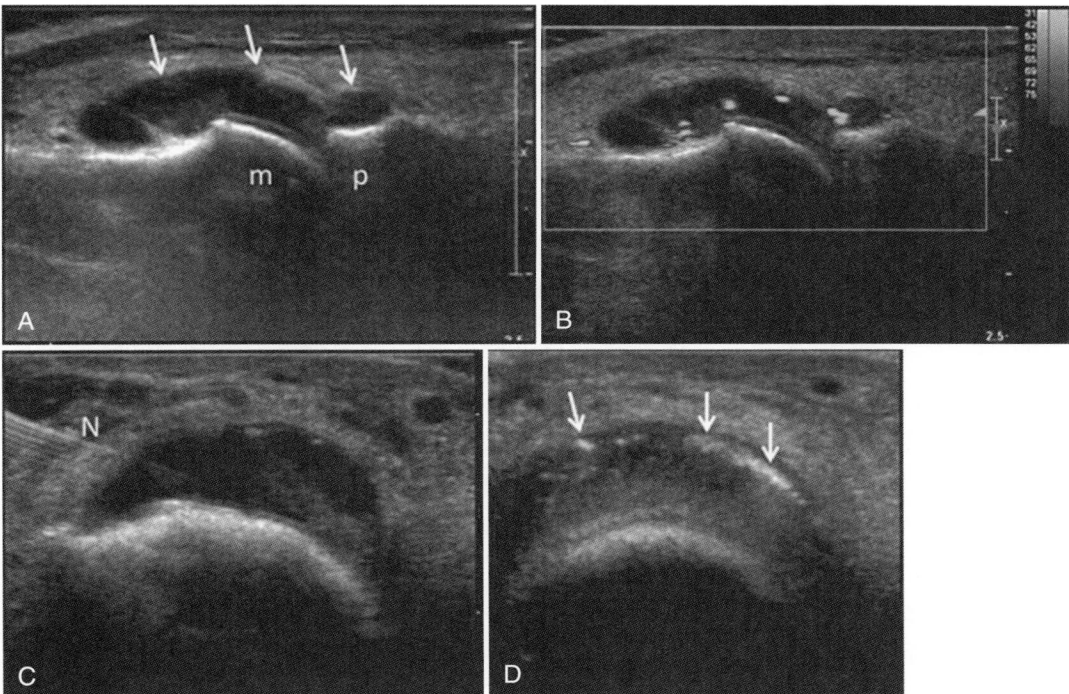

FIGURE 258-4. Ultrasound-guided therapy in the first metatarsophalangeal (MTP) joint of a patient with pain and swelling. **A,** Longitudinal gray scale image of the dorsal recess of the first MTP joint. Fluid and soft tissue distend the joint capsule (*arrows*). The metatarsal (m) and proximal phalanx (p) are labeled. Note that a thin hypoechoic (dark) band parallels the surface of the metatarsal head, corresponding to the overlying articular cartilage. **B,** Increased vascularity (*red color hues*) demonstrated on power Doppler imaging within the dorsal recess reflects the level of disease activity. **C,** Transverse gray scale ultrasound image shows a needle (N) within the distended dorsal recess from which several drops of synovial fluid were aspirated followed by therapeutic injection. **D,** Postinjection transverse ultrasonography depicts low level echoes (small echogenic foci within dorsal recess) and microbubbles (*arrows*) within the distended joint capsule from injected material. Whereas microbubbles aggregate along the nondependent portion of the distended joint capsule, injected material tends to settle to the deep portion of the recess.

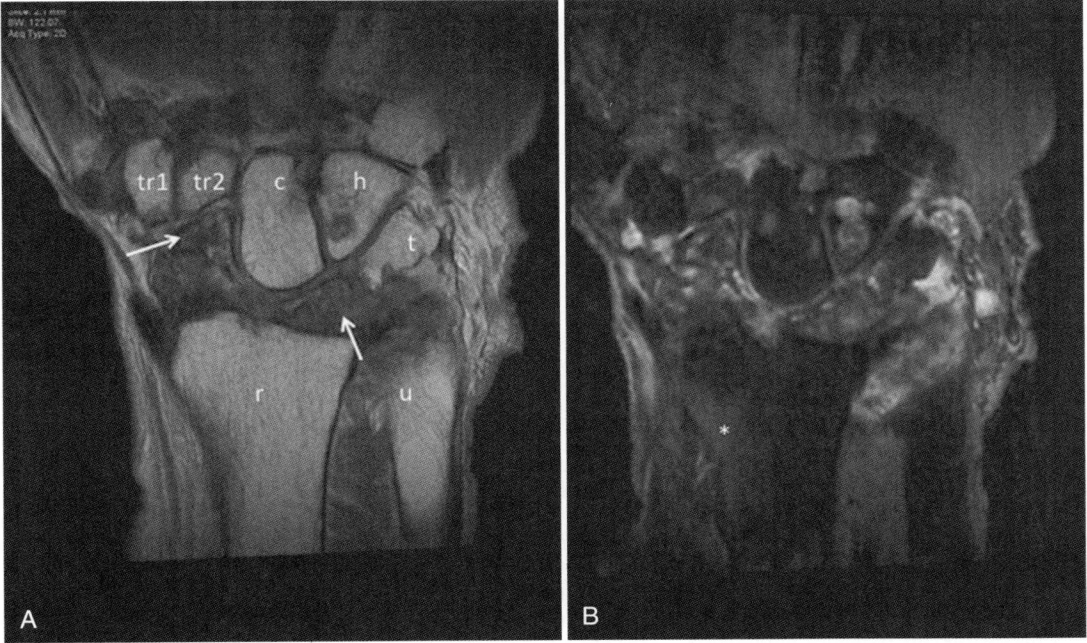

FIGURE 258-5. Magnetic resonance image of the right wrist in a female patient with advanced rheumatoid arthritis. **A,** Proton density coronal image shows loss of normally bright marrow signal within the scaphoid and lunate bones (*arrows*). The proximal scaphoid is eroded, and the lunate appears deformed and translocated and volarly tilted (not shown), giving rise to its triangular appearance. The distal ulna (u) is poorly visualized because of a large erosion. Intermediate-intensity material (appears dark gray) within the carpus and distal radioulnar joint is difficult to separate from the distal ulna, lunate, and scaphoid. The triquetrum (t), hamate (h), trapezium (tr1) and trapezoid (tr2), capitate (c), and radius (r) are labeled. **B,** Fluid-sensitive coronal image emphasizing T2 relaxation demonstrates increased signal intensity (bright) within the inflammatory pannus, compatible with increase in mobile water associated with inflammation. Increased signal intensity is evident within the lunate, scaphoid, and distal ulna, including focal areas within the distal row of carpal bones, corresponding to small erosions. Diffuse increased signal within the distal radius likely reflects reactive marrow edema (*asterisk*).

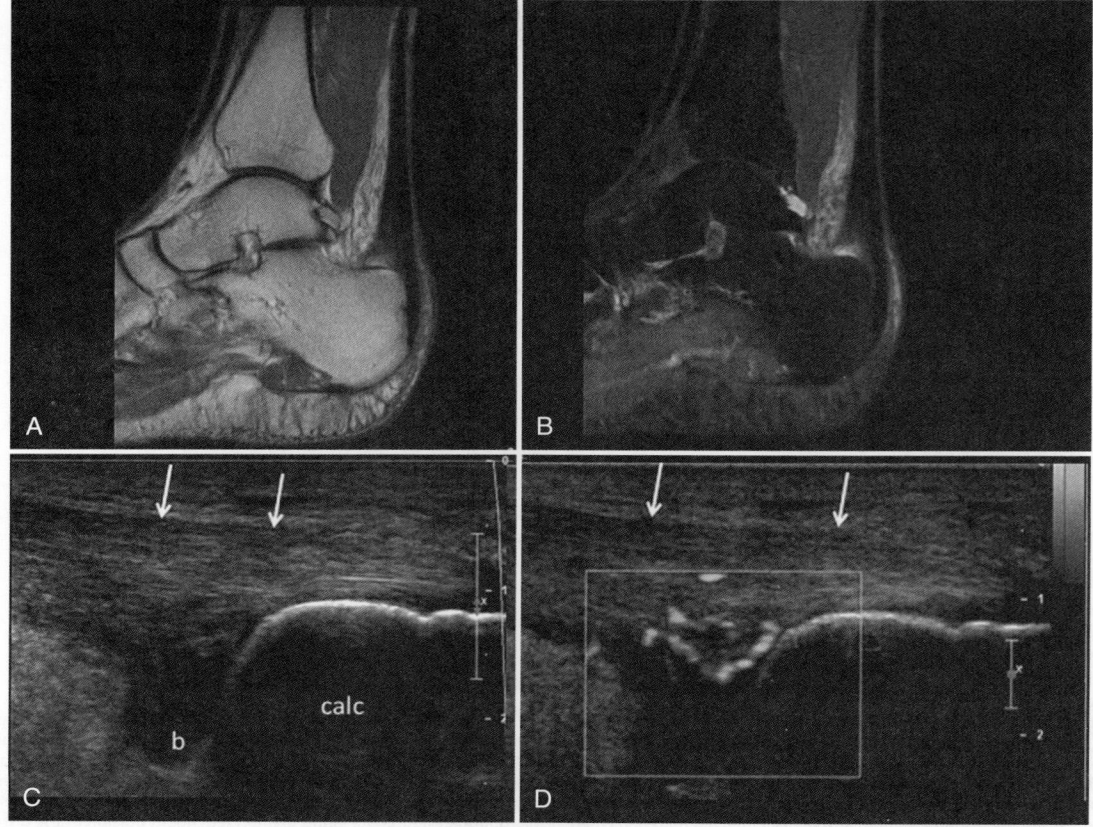

FIGURE 258-6. Imaging of the soft tissues in a patient with retrocalcaneal pain demonstrating complementary nature of magnetic resonance imaging and ultrasonography. Whereas the proton-density sagittal image (A) emphasizes anatomic detail, the fluid-sensitive image (B) depicts thickening and increased signal intensity within the distal Achilles tendon, reflecting tendinosis, retrocalcaneal bursitis, or a tear of the deep surface of the tendon. Surrounding increased signal intensity (bright areas) within the adjacent soft tissue reflects adjacent soft tissue edema. Long-axis gray scale (C) and power Doppler (D) images of the same patient obtained when the patient presented for ultrasound-guided therapeutic injection. The tendon (*arrows*) is inhomogeneous. A prominent hypoechoic collection deep to the tendon is compatible with retrocalcaneal bursitis (b). There is prominent increased vascularity on power Doppler imaging at the margin of the bursa and tendon. The calcaneus (calc) is labeled.

direct techniques. In glycosaminoglycan (GAG) -depleted cartilage, there can be delayed uptake of contrast into the cartilage, which would normally be inhibited by the negatively charged GAG molecules.

Patients with renal disease who receive IV injection of gadolinium can develop nephrogenic systemic fibrosis (NSF). (Also see the section Nephrogenic Systemic Fibrosis in Chapter 267.) When the kidney cannot sufficiently clear out the gadolinium, it produces fibrosis of many tissues, including the skin, muscle, heart, nerves, and pleura. To date, NSF has been seen only in patients who have been given IV gadolinium with acute or chronic renal insufficiency. The changes in the skin with NSF are usually bilateral and symmetrical, primarily involving the extremities and the trunk. These changes can mimic systemic sclerosis but, unlike that disease, the face is usually spared. If renal function improves, the skin lesions may stabilize or get better, although in some patients, the process progresses, affecting mobility and causing severe pain.

Injection of dilute gadolinium into the joint (direct magnetic resonance arthrography) is helpful for outlining structures to determine whether there is morphologic damage. Injection is usually performed either under fluoroscopic or ultrasound guidance. This technique is particularly effective for visualization of small structures such as the labrum of the hip or shoulder if there is no joint effusion. It is also helpful for demonstrating breakdown of soft tissue structures that normally prevent communication between joint compartments such as the rotator cuff, triangular fibrocartilage of the wrist, and ligaments in the various joints. Newer techniques that enable image acquisition in near real time as well as the development of MR-compatible needles now permit a variety of percutaneous procedures to be performed directly under MR guidance.

● SCINTIGRAPHY

Scintigraphy by its nature represents physiologic imaging because it derives from labeling physiologically occurring substances with a gamma-emitting radionuclide and uses detectors in the form of gamma cameras arranged in a planar or circumferential configuration to determine the distribution of radionuclide within the tissue. Scintigraphy can provide a global assessment of abnormal tracer update or can be performed using a targeted approach (Fig. 258-8). Images often provide high tissue contrast but are of relatively poor spatial resolution. Commonly used agents vary from tagged red blood cells to assess blood flow; agents that reflect bone metabolism (technetium-99m methylene diphosphate [Tc-MDP]); agents that reflect glucose metabolism (18-fluorine deoxy-glucose [18-FDG]), in the case of PET ; and agents that concentrate at sites of inflammation, such as autologous white blood cells labeled with ^{111}In (Indium) and ^{67}Ga-citrate (gallium). Clinical applications include detection of a variety of malignancies, osteomyelitis, vascular graft infection, multifocal infectious disease, inflammatory diseases such as RA, vasculitis, inflammatory bowel disease, sarcoidosis, fever of unknown origin, and infection of joint prostheses.

Traditional nuclear medicine involves use of single gamma photon emissions as a product of nuclear decay. The information can be displayed using planar imaging through a single (or multiple) pinhole camera or displayed tomographically in a manner similar to CT (single-photon emission computed tomography [SPECT]). Bone scintigraphy uses Tc-MDP as the radioactive tracer. The isotope goes to areas of high bone turnover and vascular flow as well as areas of calcium or bone deposition. Three-phase bone scans are obtained at different intervals after injection, reflecting the early vascular phase, the intermediate blood pool phase, and the late phase. Each phase allows for further characterization of the disease process. Abnormal tracer uptake is seen in areas of inflammation, infection, neoplasm, osteonecrosis, and fracture. The scan is most useful to identify the location of lesions within the skeleton but is nonspecific.

Positron emission tomography scans use the appearance of two simultaneously produced 511-KEV gamma rays after annihilation of a positron and electron pair to localize the distribution of radionuclide. The

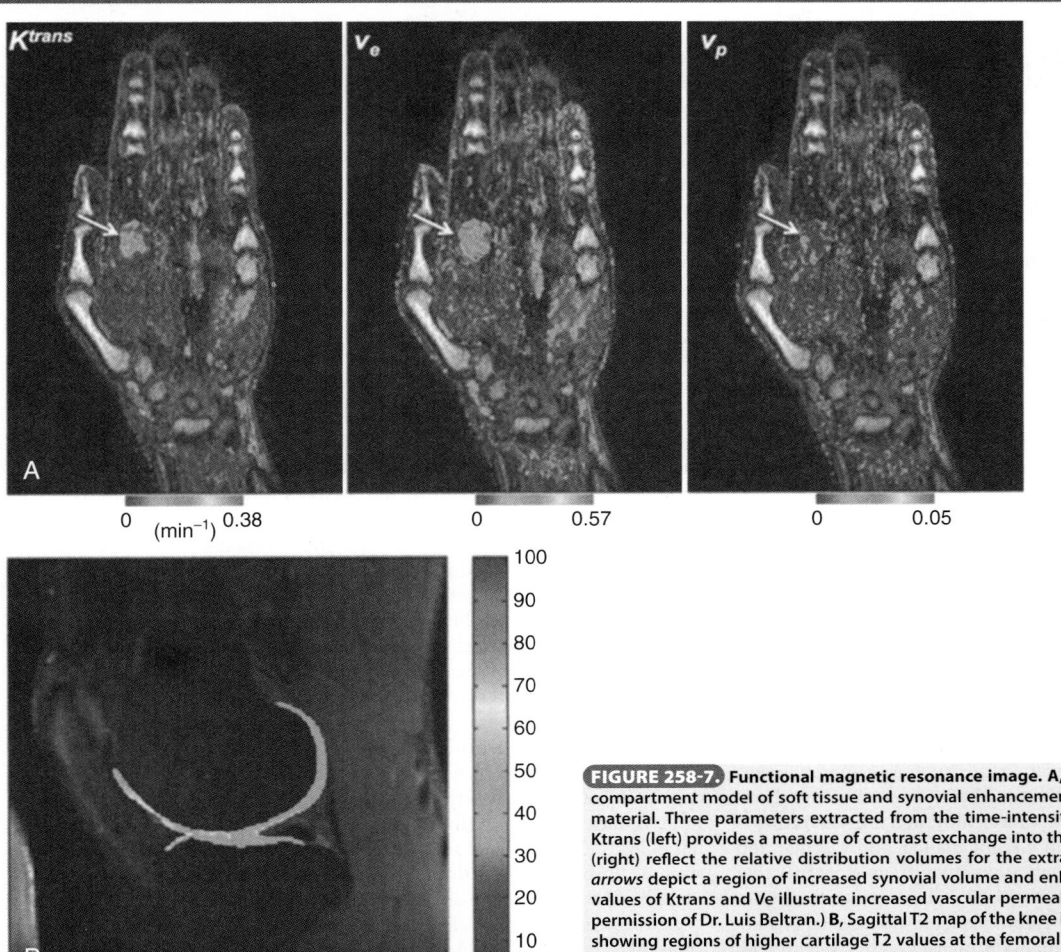

FIGURE 258-7. Functional magnetic resonance image. **A,** Parametric image derived from fitting a two-compartment model of soft tissue and synovial enhancement after intravenous administration of contrast material. Three parameters extracted from the time-intensity curves are displayed as parametric images: Ktrans (left) provides a measure of contrast exchange into the extravascular soft tissues; Ve (center) and Vp (right) reflect the relative distribution volumes for the extravascular space and plasma, respectively. The *arrows* depict a region of increased synovial volume and enhancement at the second MCP joint. Increased values of Ktrans and Ve illustrate increased vascular permeability at the site of inflammation. (Printed with permission of Dr. Luis Beltran.) **B,** Sagittal T2 map of the knee in which relative T2 relaxation is color encoded, showing regions of higher cartilage T2 values at the femoral condyle and tibial plateau. This reflects alterations in cartilage collagen architecture and water content and possibly early osteoarthritis. (Printed with permission of Dr. Gregory Chang.)

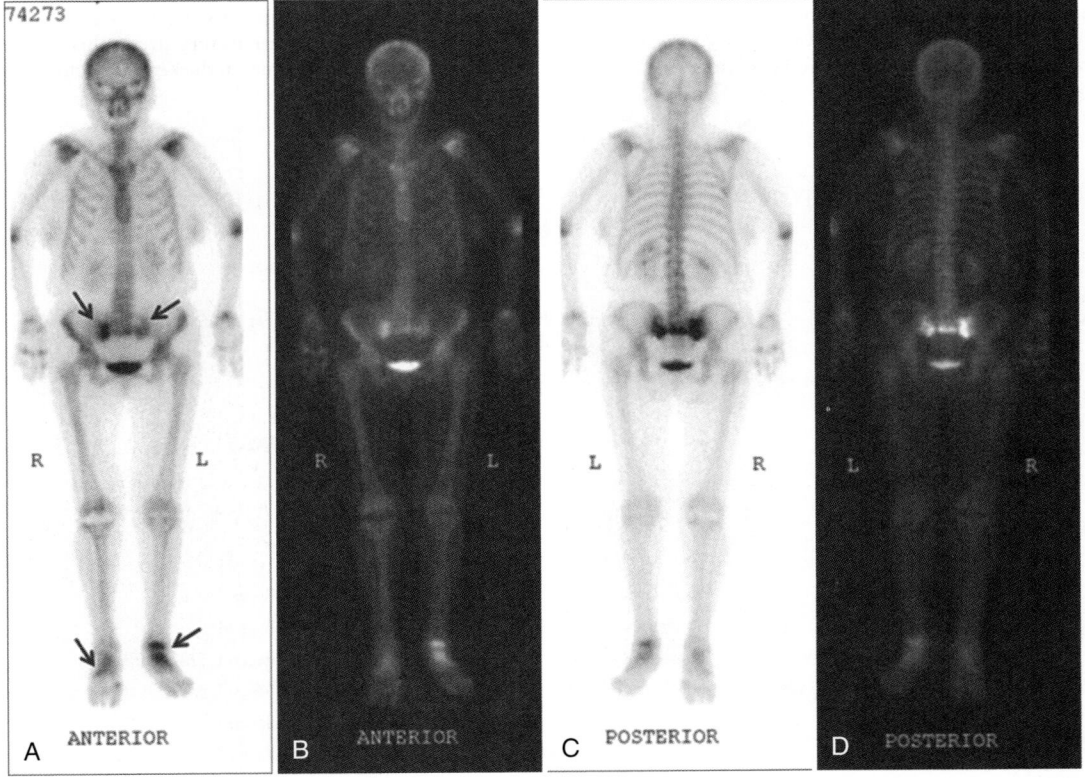

FIGURE 258-8. Rectilinear bone scan in a patient with back pain. Anterior (A) and posterior (B) delayed rimages of the axial and appendicular skeleton demonstrate increased tracer uptake in the region of the sacral ala, left ankle, and right midfoot (*arrows*). Follow-up radiographs confirmed the presence of bilateral sacral ala fractures. Note that the central pooling of tracer in the expected location of the urinary bladder is normal. Bone scans provide a sensitive but nonspecific method to evaluate the appendicular and axial skeletal. Increased uptake in the feet in this patient was attributed to degenerative change.

near-simultaneous detection of the photons (coincidence counting) provides an estimate of source tracer concentration. Newer PET scanners are often used in combination with either CT or MRI to achieve improved spatial registration, allow accurate estimates of soft tissue attenuation, provide high-quality anatomic images, and quantify metabolic activity.[9] Combined PET-CT or PET-MRI provides high-resolution images of abnormal metabolic activity and may ultimately provide the most definitive maps of inflammatory activity in patients with rheumatic disease.[10] Early results to date have been promising and are expected to provide sensitive evaluation of the response to DMARDs in patients with inflammatory arthritis.

GENERAL REFERENCES

For the General References and other additional features, please visit Expert Consult at https://expertconsult.inkling.com.

259

CONNECTIVE TISSUE STRUCTURE AND FUNCTION

SUNEEL S. APTE

Connective tissues are those having a primary mechanical or structural role. They are typically skeletal or osteoarticular tissues such as bone, cartilage, tendon, ligament, fascia, intervertebral disc, and joint-associated structures such as synovium and fibrocartilaginous menisci, although adipose tissue is also included (Table 259-1). However, all viscera, glands, and vascular and nervous tissue contain varying amounts of connective tissue elements that maintain proper spatial relationships between their cells, organize them into functional units, and provide an internal fibrous skeleton or external protective capsule. These connective tissue elements primarily comprise extracellular matrix (ECM), which is organized as a basement membrane or an interstitial matrix. Examples include elastic fibers in the aorta and lung that mediate stretch and recoil, glomerular basement membrane that participates in filtration, and the fibrous endoskeleton that connects the heart valves and transmits myocardial contraction. Indeed, heart valves and chordae tendinae have regional structural similarities to cartilage and tendons.

In addition to their structural role, connective tissues are involved in storage and activation of growth factors, cytokines, and morphogens. Some connective tissue molecules mediate inflammation when released as intact molecules, or may acquire new properties as proteolytically derived fragments (matrikines).[1] Connective tissues such as bone, cartilage, and tendon harbor mesenchymal stem-like cells (MSC) that undergo expansion and differentiation during growth, repair, and regeneration and are therapeutically valuable. Bone contributes to calcium and phosphate homeostasis. A broad perspective on connective tissue is thus crucial for understanding the complex clinical presentation of inherited connective tissue disorders, pathways of tissue repair and regeneration, and pathogenesis of degenerative and autoimmune conditions.

CONNECTIVE TISSUE CELLS, THEIR EXTRACELLULAR MATRIX AND TISSUE-SPECIFIC BIOMECHANICS

Connective tissues comprise cells, typically derived from mesoderm, or in the craniofacial region, derived from the neural crest, and the ECM they secrete and assemble around them. Unique morphologic and biosynthetic properties of the differentiated cells specify osteoblasts, osteoclasts, and osteocytes (in bone); chondrocytes (in cartilage); and tenocytes (in tendons), as well as mixed phenotypes such as cells of fibrocartilage (in the intervertebral disc, some tendon and ligament insertions, and joint menisci). Chondrocytes alter their biosynthetic profile as they terminally differentiate into hypertrophic chondrocytes in growth plate cartilage, downregulating aggrecan and collagen II expression and synthesizing collagen X as a specialized product.[2] As the growth plate transitions into bone, the hypertrophic cells die, blood vessels invade the cartilage, and the cartilage matrix is gradually replaced by bone. Fibroblasts, which secrete collagens as a major product, are the dominant cells in tendons, fascia, ligaments, and dermis. The abundant ECM of connective tissues is their major defining characteristic, but in other tissues and organs, fibroblasts are relatively quiescent, and the interstitial ECM is less organized and not as abundant. However, under appropriate stimuli, fibroblasts transition to highly contractile, biosynthetically active myofibroblasts, which are associated with hypertrophic scars and fibrosis.

During embryonic development, undifferentiated connective tissue cells (mesenchymal cells) produce a hydrated, loose, provisional ECM optimal for migration, branching, and folding of individual cells and cell collectives, such as epithelial sheets. As embryogenesis progresses, provisional ECM is remodeled by matrix-degrading proteinases and replaced by specialized connective tissues whose mechanical properties[3] are better suited to weight bearing, locomotion, and increased circulatory stress. This requirement for increased mechanical strength is not met in the severest forms of inherited connective

TABLE 259-1 DIVERSITY OF CONNECTIVE TISSUES

STRUCTURE	FUNCTION	CELLS	KEY MATRIX COMPONENTS
Adipose tissue	Energy metabolism Physical protection	Adipocytes, fibroblasts, endothelial cells	Collagen I, collagen III, microfibrils, collagen IV, laminin
Basement membranes	Epithelial support Cell polarity Filtration barrier Cell barrier Transparency (lens)	Epithelial and endothelial cells, myotubes, adipocytes, lens fibers	Collagen IV, laminin, nidogens, perlecan
Bone	Structural support Hematopoiesis Mineral storage	Osteoblasts, osteoclasts, osteocytes	Collagen I, osteocalcin, bone sialoprotein, hydroxyapatite
Cartilage	Bone growth Joint motion Load transmission	Chondrocytes	Collagen II, aggrecan
Dermis	Elasticity and resiliency	Fibroblasts	Collagen I, elastin
Ligament	Connects bone to bone	Fibroblasts	Collagen I, SLRPs
Tendon	Connects muscle to bone	Fibroblasts	Collagen I, SLRPs, fibrillins
Visceral stroma	Internal scaffold and capsule	Fibroblasts	Collagen I, collagen III, versican, fibronectin
Synovium	Produces synovial fluid	Fibroblasts, macrophages	Collagen I, collagen III
Vessel wall	Barrier, elastic recoil	Endothelium, vascular smooth muscle cells	Collagen III, collagen IV, elastin, fibrillins, fibulins, versican

SLRP = small leucine repeat-rich protein.

tissue disorders affecting the vasculature, bone, or cartilage, with neonatal, juvenile, or early adult mortality resulting.

Connective tissues continually sense and adapt to their mechanical environment. The anabolic response of many connective tissues to optimal levels of mechanical stress is now recognized as a crucial, remediable determinant of health. This concept is embodied in Wolff's law of bone remodeling, which states that bone remodels in response to the mechanical loads imposed on it. The composition of specific connective tissues reflects adaptations in response to their mechanical environment or requirements for other specialized functions. For example, articular cartilage and other hyaline cartilages comprise proteoglycan aggregates that exert a swelling pressure and a network of collagen II fibrils that restrain them, contributing to compressive strength and shock absorption.[4] The superficial zone of articular cartilage, in contrast, in enriched in collagenous fibrils that are arranged parallel to the surface to resist shear forces. A mucinous glycoprotein, lubricin, present on the joint surfaces, ensures the low coefficient of friction of synovial joints. In tendons, the major ECM component is collagen I, which has high tensile strength, but in bone, a composite of collagen I and calcium hydroxyapatite provides tensile and compressive strength. The contractile apparatus of skeletal muscle is connected by the dystrophin–glycoprotein complex to the muscle basement membrane and via hierarchical assemblies of interstitial matrix (endomysium, perimysium, and epimysium) to tendons and ultimately to bone, thus efficiently transmitting muscle contraction forces.[5] In the intervertebral disc, the nucleus pulposus is rich in aggrecan, which exerts a swelling pressure that is constrained by the surrounding concentric lamellae of fibrillar collagen in the annulus fibrosus. This composite structure absorbs vertical loads on the spine while limiting deformation of the nucleus pulposus. The interfaces between different connective tissues show structured transitions, highlighted by fibrocartilage present at tendon insertion sites and by Sharpey fibers, which seamlessly integrate perimysial collagen of muscle fibers with collagen in bone. In knee menisci, the cells and ECM of the inner third are cartilaginous, with abundant proteoglycans. Whereas the cells of the outer third, which is vascular and connected to ligaments, are fibroblastic, with corresponding predominance of fibrillar collagens, the cells and ECM in the middle third have an intermediate fibrochondrocyte phenotype.

⬤ MAJOR EXTRACELLULAR MATRIX COMPONENTS

Extracellular matrix comprises collagens; the glycosaminoglycan (GAG) hyaluronan (HA); proteoglycans; a variety of glycoproteins; phosphoproteins (especially in bones and teeth); and matricellular proteins such as thrombospondin, tenascin, and periostin, which regulate cellular functions via ECM but do not have a structural role. The distribution of ECM molecules and macromolecules is tightly regulated to achieve specific microenvironments that control proliferation, differentiation, polarity, and migration of cells and provide niches for postnatal stem cells. Collagens, the most abundant proteins of the body, comprise several distinct molecules, each containing at least one triple-helical domain composed of αchains having a repeating Gly-X-Y sequence. Twenty-eight different collagen types are formed from the products of more than 40 genes encoding collagen α chains. The presence of glycine, the smallest amino acid, at every third position, permits triple-helix formation; the amino acid proline, which is frequently modified to form hydroxyproline at the Y position, ensures stability of the triple helix. Fibrillar collagens (e.g., types I-III, V, XI) have long triple-helical (collagenous) regions, so they form rodlike structures. Whereas collagen I, the most widely distributed and abundant, is a heterotrimer comprising two α1(I) chains and an α2(I) chain, collagen II and III are homotrimers of α1(II) and α1(III) chains, respectively. Mutations of either collagen I chain cause the majority of cases of osteogenesis imperfect (Chapter 260) and infrequently can also cause rare subtypes of Ehlers-Danlos syndrome (EDS) (Chapter 260). The triple helices of nonfibrillar collagens are shorter and interspersed with interruptions of the Gly-X-Y sequence or noncollagenous domains that introduce flexible regions. Collagen XIII, XVII, XXIII, and XXV are transmembrane proteins. Fibrillar collagens are synthesized as procollagens having bulky terminal propeptides. The folding of the triple helix occurs intracellularly and is propagated from the C- to the N-terminus to form homo- or heterotrimeric triple helices. The propeptides are subsequently excised by specific proteinases, resulting in rodlike tropocollagen that can be assembled into tightly packed, quarter-staggered fibrils. Failure to remove the N-propeptide of collagen I impairs fibril assembly and leads to a specific type of EDS with severe skin fragility (type VIIc or dermatosparactic type). Whereas collagen I is the major component of bone, dermis, tendons, ligaments, and the sclera of the eye, collagen III is abundant in the skin, lung, and vasculature, explaining

the association of genes encoding these collagens with osteogenesis imperfecta and vascular EDS (also known as type IV). Collagen II, together with minor amounts of collagen IX and collagen XI, predominates in cartilage, ocular vitreous and the nucleus pulposus of the intervertebral disc, and mutations of either of these collagen genes can cause the Stickler syndrome (triad of cartilage, eye, and hearing anomalies). Collagen fibrils can consist of more than one collagen type; for instance, collagen V is found in heterotypic fibrils with collagen I and is required for nucleation of fibrillogenesis to form large collagen I fibrils.

Basement membranes are formed from collagen IV, with significant content of laminins, nidogens, and the heparin sulfate proteoglycan perlecan, which is also an important constituent of cartilage. Basement membranes have crucial roles in regulating molecular transport, such as in glomerular filtration, and in establishment and maintenance of epithelial polarity. Collagen VI is widely distributed as beaded microfibrils that form pericellular matrices in fibroblasts and, alongside collagen VII anchoring fibrils, connect basement membranes to interstitial ECM. Hyaluronan, a polymer with repeating disaccharide units, can achieve a molecular weight in the millions of Daltons. It is a key component of cartilage matrix, pericellular matrix of many cell types, and a mediator of inflammation. Proteoglycans are characterized by covalent attachment of glycosaminoglycans, such as chondroitin, heparan, and keratan sulfate, to a core protein. Aggrecan and versican are large chondroitin sulfate proteoglycans that form giant aggregates with hyaluronan in chondrocytes or nucleus pulposus cells and fibroblasts, respectively. On the other hand, some small leucine repeat-rich proteins (SLRPs) such as decorin, biglycan, and lumican are proteoglycans that may have only one or two glycosaminoglycan chains. This class of molecules, which also includes fibromodulin, interacts with collagen fibrils to cross-link them and regulate fibril diameter. They have been shown to bind transforming growth factor β (TGF-β) and, when released from connective tissue, to provide danger signals to the immune system. During connective tissue healing, fibrin and fibronectin provide a transitional ECM permissive for cell migration, differentiation, and other aspects of the repair process.

Elastic fibers are formed by coacervation of a soluble precursor named tropoelastin. Elastic fiber assembly is guided by tissue microfibrils that are formed from three large glycoproteins named fibrillins.[6] Fibrillin-1 is abundant in the aorta, ocular zonule, and perichondrium of bone and is mutated in Marfan syndrome (Chapter 260), resulting in aneurysms, ectopia lentis, and skeletal overgrowth. Fibrillin-2 mutations cause Beals syndrome, with skeletal overgrowth and limb contractures as major features but typically, not severe cardiac or eye problems. The elastic fiber-microfibril network additionally contains versican, microfibril-associated glycoproteins, latent TGF-β–binding proteins, and fibulins. Cutis laxa, which primarily affects the skin but can also involve vasculature and internal organs, can be caused by mutations affecting elastin and fibulin-5.

Most ECM molecules undergo one or more posttranslational modifications. These include enzymatic formation of intra- and interchain disulfide bonds, phosphorylation, and several kinds of glycosylation, including addition of N- and O-linked sugars or glycosaminoglycans such as chondroitin, keratan, or heparan sulfate. Whereas N-linked sugars on some proteins are essential for protein folding and secretion, glycosaminoglycan (GAG) chains provide crucial biophysical properties (such as of aggrecan) and mediate intermolecular interactions. During its biosynthesis, collagen undergoes lysyl and prolyl hydroxylation. Some lysyl and hydroxylysyl residues are modified extracellularly by lysyl oxidase and form stable cross-links between adjacent collagen molecules, which strengthens bone, tendons, and skin.[7] Gene defects affecting collagen-modifying enzymes or subunits of the molecular complexes they operate in lead to various recessive forms of osteogenesis imperfecta or EDS. L-Ascorbic acid is a cofactor for lysyl hydroxylase and prolyl hydroxylase and stimulates procollagen synthesis. Its nutritional deficiency leads to scurvy by reducing collagen synthesis, triple-helical stability, and tropocollagen cross-linking. Lathyrism (a now rarely seen neurotoxic disease) is caused by excess ingestion of β-aminopropionitrile, which inhibits lysyl oxidase–mediated formation of lysine aldehydes, which are the precursors of the major collagen and elastin cross-links, and leads to connective tissue fragility. Copper is a required cofactor for lysyl oxidase, and its deficiency can also lead to lathyrism.

⬤ CELL-MATRIX INTERACTIONS IN CONNECTIVE TISSUE REGULATION

Cellular ECM receptors mediate cell-matrix interactions that ensure force transmission from cells to ECM[8]; the dynamic reciprocity between cells and

ECM is crucial for environmental sensing and adaptive responses. Receptors provide feedback to the cells regarding the quality, content, or mechanical properties of the matrix (outside-in signaling) to generate appropriate responses, including cell proliferation or migration, or lead to altered ECM synthesis or degradation. Alternatively, cytoplasmic signals may alter cell-matrix interactions (inside-out signaling). Integrins are a large group of heterodimeric receptors with distinct binding preferences that comprise α and β subunits having short cytoplasmic domains. Integrins are crucial for fibronectin assembly, which in turn substantially influences assembly of collagen, fibrillins, and TGF-β activation. Intracellular signals activate integrins to promote high-affinity binding to ECM proteins, and binding of ECM proteins via specific integrin-binding motifs such as Arg-Gly-Asp initiates clustering of cell adhesion complexes and intracellular signaling that, among diverse effects, may elicit the production of inflammatory cytokines. Integrin $\alpha v \beta 6$ transmits cellular traction to matrix-bound latent TGF-β, exposing the active growth factor. Because osteoclast attachment to and spreading on bone surfaces is dependent on $\alpha_v \beta_3$, it is being targeted for treatment of osteoporosis (Chapter 243) using chemical antagonists or blocking antibodies. Syndecans are transmembrane heparan sulfate proteoglycans that work as coreceptors alongside high-affinity ECM receptors such as integrins. Discoidin domain receptors are receptor tyrosine kinases activated by binding to native triple-helical collagen.[9] DDR1 and DDR2 bind to fibrillar collagens I-III and collagen V. Collagen IV activates DDR1 but not DDR2, whereas collagen X activates DDR2. With their extended structure, extensive post-translational modification, and exposure of numerous binding sites, ECM molecules such as collagens, fibrillins, and the classical cell-binding protein fibronectin bind to multiple receptor types. Among several hyaluronan-binding molecules on the cell surface, including hyaluronan synthases, CD44 is a major hyaluronan receptor with a role in assembling the pericellular matrix and in inflammation.

EXTRACELLULAR MATRIX NETWORKS AND CONNECTIVE TISSUE DISORDERS

Extracellular matrix molecules and macromolecules are assembled to form higher order (supramolecular) complexes and networks whose varied composition and geometry further diversify connective tissues. These are exemplified by parallel arrays of extensively cross-linked collagen fibrils conferring high tensile strength to tendons, ligaments, and bone, by the multidirectional or "basket-weave" arrangement of collagen in dermis, both permitting and constraining multiaxial mobility, and by the concentric elastic lamellae and crimped collagen in the aorta that regulate hemodynamics. In the eye, orthogonally oriented collagen fibrils in corneal stroma and the lattice-like structure of collagen VIII in the Descemet membrane allow transparency and are crucial for normal vision.

Cartilage and nucleus pulposus ECM comprises large aggregates of hyaluronan and aggrecan, with hundreds of aggrecan molecules attached to each hyaluronan polymer via their N-terminal domain, leaving the C-terminal domain free for interactions with fibrillins, fibulins, and other ECM networks. Each aggrecan molecule has approximately 100 chondroitin sulfate chains and several keratan sulfate chains. Their high fixed-charge density creates an osmotic environment that favors water retention and restricts water flux in cartilage. Through the attachment of hyaluronan to cell-surface receptors, the aggrecan–hyaluronan network is retained by the chondrocyte as a conspicuous pericellular matrix (or glycocalyx). In connective tissue cells other than chondrocytes, pericellular matrices use versican or heparin sulfate proteoglycans instead of aggrecan. The pericellular matrix occupies the crucial interface between cells and their environment and influences cell behavior. It is a provisional ECM in microcosm because it is metabolically more active than further removed matrix, which is more stable. Some interstitial collagen and elastin can be stable for decades.

Connective tissue disorders arise from inborn defects affecting cells or ECM, as well as cellular dysfunction caused by repetitive injury, inflammation, or metabolic or aging processes. Because ECM is such a crucial component of connective tissues, most inherited and acquired connective tissue disorders result from mutant ECM molecules, insufficient but essentially normal matrix (e.g., osteoporosis), or excess or inappropriately deposited matrix (e.g., adhesions, fibrosis, and scleroderma). Osteoarthritis (OA) involves all structures that form the joint, including the synovium and subchondral bone, and appears to result from a combination of genetic and nongenetic factors (Chapter 262). OA of the hip and hands has a stronger genetic component than OA of the knee. Because the function of cartilage is to absorb impact and distribute it to bone without aberrant loading of joint

structures, variations in genes that affect joint congruity and alignment or cartilage or meniscal integrity could predispose to OA. For instance, variations in genes encoding cartilage ECM components mutated in chondrodysplasias (Chapter 205), such as collagen II, IX, cartilage oligomeric protein, or matrilins, have been associated with early-onset OA, suggesting a genetic link and a spectrum extending from OA predisposition at the milder end to severe chondrodysplasia. Another genetic link is with the mechanisms that influence the formation of joints, correlating with the association between joint malalignment and OA. Variations in genes associated with the TGF-β superfamily pathway, including *GDF5* (encoding a morphogen required for joint development), *ASPN* (encoding an ECM protein that binds TGFβ), and SMAD3 (encoding a cytoplasm-nucleus signaling intermediary), are associated with OA.[10] Factors that affect load distribution across joints, such as ligament and meniscal tears or hip dysplasia, predispose to OA. Cartilage breakdown in arthritis is not caused by wear and tear but by altered cell-matrix interactions that lead to enzymatic digestion. Loss of aggrecan, followed by loss of SLRPs and other molecules from the surface of collagen fibrils, are initial changes that render collagen fibrils susceptible to destruction by collagenases. The loss of articular cartilage collagen II is thought to constitute an irreversible change in joint disease. Whatever the original insult, the response of chondrocytes or synovium can lead to a vicious cycle of joint destruction because the cells may respond by producing excess ECM and ECM-degrading proteases, with release of both intact and fragmented molecules that may further potentiate inflammation. Rodent immune arthritis models have revealed a role for the alternative complement pathway in arthritis, and cartilage proteins and their fragments released by proteolytic breakdown can have complex effects on the complement pathways that lead to both activation and suppression.

Cell-matrix interactions are profoundly affected in muscular dystrophies (Chapter 421), revealing a continuum that is essential for force transmission from the cytoskeleton to interstitial matrix. Mutations affecting components of the dystrophin–glycoprotein complex including dystroglycan, a receptor that connects muscle cytoskeleton to laminin in the muscle basement membrane, muscle basement membrane (laminin and collagen IV), and collagen VI filaments in ECM, cause a variety of muscular dystrophies. Specific adhesion complexes such as hemidesmosomes in the epidermis mediate anchorage to basement membranes and underlying interstitial ECM. Autoantibodies against collagen XVII and VII, or laminin 5 mutations, affect major components of these complexes and lead to blistering skin diseases (Chapter 439).

PROTEASES AND CONNECTIVE TISSUE TURNOVER

Reflecting continuous adaptation to their environment, connective tissues have intrinsic mechanisms that ensure ECM renewal (i.e., through coupled synthesis and degradation). ECM molecules are substrates for several proteinase classes, chiefly matrix metalloproteinases (MMPs), astacin MMPs such as BMP1 and tolloids, cathepsins, and A disintegrin-like and metalloproteinase domain with thrombospondin type 1 repeats (ADAMTS).[11] Although these proteases are typically considered to be catabolic, some are also essential for the maturation of precursor proteins, such as ADAMTS2, which excises the amino-propeptide of procollagen I, II, and III and is defective in EDS, dermatosparactic type. BMP1, which excises the C-propeptides of procollagen I, II, and III and cleaves lysyl oxidase and several other proteins, is deficient in a type of recessive osteogenesis imperfecta. Although most MMPs are secreted, a class of membrane-type MMPs is cell-surface bound. Most MMPs require proteolytic activation by other MMPs or serine proteinases such as plasmin and furin, and are inhibited by tissue inhibitors of MMPs (TIMPs) and α_2-macroglobulin. Whereas MT1-MMP is crucial for collagen I proteolysis in bone, MMP-13 has been implicated as a major collagen II degrading enzyme in arthritis. Cell surface MMPs such as MT1-MMP and A disintegrin-like and MMPs (ADAM) are responsible for ectodomain shedding of ECM receptors, cell-surface cytokines and cytokine receptors, together regulating a variety of inflammatory and oncogenic situations. ADAMTS4 and ADAMTS5, also known as aggrecanase-1 and -2, respectively, are principal aggrecan-degrading proteases implicated in OA and, together with MMP-13, are potential drug targets in this disorder. However, MMPs, ADAMs, and ADAMTSs have structurally similar catalytic domains and zinc and calcium-dependent proteolytic mechanisms, which renders selective inhibition of any single proteinase from these classes challenging. Indeed, a major side effect of MMP inhibitors used in clinical trials for cancer was connective tissue stiffness and inflammation, presumably resulting from reduced physiological turnover of collagen and other

ECM proteins. Among other proteinases, cathepsin K produced by osteoclasts is active at acidic pH, unlike MMPs, and therefore efficiently digests bone collagen in the acidic osteoclast–bone interface. Neutrophil elastase (a serine proteinase), MMP-9, and MMP-12 (metalloelastase) can degrade elastin. Proteolysis of ECM proteins can release bioactive fragments (matrikines) such as endostatin (from collagen XVIII) or endorepellin (from perlecan), which are antiangiogenic; some fibronectin fragments released in OA are proinflammatory. Hydroxyproline antibodies that recognize ECM-fragments with specific cleaved ends (neoepitope antibodies), as well as cross-linked collagen fragments released by proteolytic activity, are useful biomarkers of bone and cartilage turnover.

AGING OF CONNECTIVE TISSUE

Some visible hallmarks of aging result not only from cellular senescence but also reduced ECM synthesis and increased catabolism, as well as greater connective tissue fragility. This leads, for example, to reduced bone mass or osteoporosis; thinning and loss of elastic properties of dermal ECM, which are visible as wrinkles and sagging skin; reduced volume of intervertebral discs; and increased capillary fragility. Loss of HA and GAGs reduces tissue hydration and of collagen and elastin reduces tensile strength and elasticity, respectively. Products of ECM proteolysis stimulate cells to release free radicals and cytokines that further accelerate ECM breakdown or lead to cell death. Extrinsic factors such as sunburn and ultraviolet irradiation induce cytokines that accelerate this process. In addition, aging collagen can be cross-linked by the Maillard reaction, especially when glucose levels are high, resulting in its modification by advanced glycation end products (AGE), which renders it inflexible, alters the rate of turnover, and affects binding to matrix receptors.[12] AGE binding to a cellular receptor has been shown to lead to cellular dysfunction, oxidative stress, and inflammation.

In summary, connective tissue provides the framework of the musculoskeletal system and a structural scaffold for internal organs while serving as a reservoir for growth factors, cytokines, and stem-like precursor cells. Inherited connective tissue disorders have the potential to disturb these functions in specific ways. Acquired disorders such as OA and fibrosis reflect perturbation of diverse physiological networks and pathways, with altered cell-matrix interactions at the center.

GENERAL REFERENCES

For the General References and other additional features, please visit Expert Consult at https://expertconsult.inkling.com.

260

INHERITED DISEASES OF CONNECTIVE TISSUE

REED E. PYERITZ

MUCOPOLYSACCHARIDOSES

DEFINITION

Proteoglycans are ubiquitous components of the extracellular matrix (ECM) and the surfaces of cells, and they are among the largest and most complex of human molecules. Proteoglycans consist of a protein core to which are covalently bound glycosaminoglycans (GAGs; formerly called mucopolysaccharides) of several types: dermatan sulfate, heparan sulfate, keratan sulfate, and chondroitin sulfate. These four polymeric molecules are cleaved from their protein core in lysosomes; then they, plus hyaluronan (a GAG lacking a protein core), are catabolized further in lysosomes in a stepwise fashion by more than a dozen enzymes. Genetic defects in any one of these enzymes lead to the accumulation of GAG metabolites in lysosomes, with profound disruption of cellular physiology. The phenotypes resulting from deficiencies of these catabolic enzymes are termed *mucopolysaccharidoses* (MPSs) and are classified into seven types (Table 260-1). Several additional storage disorders, termed *mucolipidoses* (MLs), are caused by a genetic defect in posttranslational modification of lysosomal enzymes and share features with the MPSs.

EPIDEMIOLOGY

All MPS disorders are rare, each with an incidence of one or fewer cases per 100,000 births, and are without ethnic predilection.

PATHOBIOLOGY

With the exception of MPS II (Hunter syndrome), which is X-linked, each of these disorders is autosomal recessive. All MPSs are caused by deficiency of a single lysosomal enzyme responsible for a specific step in GAG metabolism. Catabolism of GAG proceeds normally until the step requiring the defective enzyme, when further normal metabolism halts. Although a minor degree of nonspecific breakdown occurs, resulting in urinary excretion of cleaved GAG that can be useful diagnostically, the accumulation of GAG within lysosomes of cells of mesenchymal origin; endothelium; and, in most cases, neurons causes widespread, progressive cellular dysfunction and clinical effects. Lysosomal enzymes are targeted to lysosomes by posttranslational addition of mannose 6-phosphate. Deficiency of the phosphotransferase that catalyzes the first step in this reaction results in an inability to catabolize any GAG molecules. The catabolic enzymes, which normally would be transported into lysosomes, instead are secreted from the cell and are found in unusually high concentrations in plasma, providing one diagnostic test for MLs.[1]

Pathology

All pathologic manifestations of MPS and ML disorders worsen with age, and some are present from early developmental stages. Gross anatomic hallmarks are hepatosplenomegaly, marked skeletal alterations (termed *dysostosis multiplex*)[2] that result in short stature and thoracic cage deformity, thickening and narrowing of airways and arteries, and coarsening of facial features. Although mental retardation is a prominent feature of some of these conditions, the brain may show only ventriculomegaly secondary to communicating hydrocephalus. On microscopy, mesenchymal cells show a cytoplasm full of apparently empty vacuoles; these are lysosomes from which GAG has been removed by fixation. Cells cultured from patients show greatly enlarged lysosomes filled with granular material. In the severe form of ML, dense inclusions are present, which gave rise to the common name, *I-cell disease*.

CLINICAL MANIFESTATIONS

Each of the disorders in Table 260-1 shows a wide spectrum of clinical severity. This wide spectrum has led to a classification that gives the impression of separate disorders within some of the MPS and ML types, but these represent the apparent ends of the continuum. Some of the disorders result in death by adolescence (Hurler syndrome, severe Hunter syndrome, ML II), but others are commonly compatible with survival to adulthood. The latter group of disorders is emphasized here.

The milder end of the MPS I spectrum, Scheie syndrome, may not be diagnosed until adulthood; patients present with stiffened joints, corneal clouding and glaucoma, carpal tunnel syndrome, and aortic valvular disease. Stature and intelligence are not affected. The main health risks are valvular involvement, thickening of meninges that can produce a myelopathy, and thickening of the upper airways that can produce obstructive symptoms and sleep apnea.

The milder form of MPS II, Hunter syndrome, is distinctive because it is X-linked (affecting males almost exclusively), and the cornea shows little overt clouding. Cervical myelopathy, obstructive airway disease, and cor pulmonale are important concerns. A combined conductive and neurosensory hearing loss is common.

Neither MPS IV (Morquio syndrome) nor MPS VI (Maroteaux-Lamy syndrome) affects intelligence. Both syndromes often are associated with severe skeletal changes, which are distinct radiographically but produce similar problems of kyphoscoliosis, pectus carinatum, restrictive lung disease, severe short stature, and joint degeneration. Cervical myelopathy resulting from a thickened dura is common to both disorders and is accentuated by odontoid hypoplasia in MPS IV. Thickening of the aortic and mitral valves may produce severe dysfunction necessitating their replacement. General anesthesia is especially hazardous because of the narrow upper and middle airways and cervical instability.

Patients with ML III (pseudo-Hurler polydystrophy) resemble patients with MPS VI but often have mild to moderate mental retardation. Aortic regurgitation is common.

TABLE 260-1 MUCOPOLYSACCHARIDOSES AND MUCOLIPIDOSES

TYPE	EPONYM OR COMMON NAME	CLINICAL FEATURES	INHERITANCE	OMIM*	ENZYMATIC DEFECT
MPS IH	Hurler syndrome	DM and short stature; MR; corneal clouding; HS; heart disease; death in childhood	AR	252800	α-L-iduronidase
MPS IS	Scheie syndrome	Coarse facies; stiff joints, corneal clouding; aortic valve disease; normal intelligence and lifespan	AR	252800	α-L-iduronidase
MPS II	Hunter syndrome	Severe form: coarse facies, DM and short stature, HS; MR; no corneal clouding; death by late adolescence Mild form: coarse facies, short stature; normal intelligence; survival to adulthood	XL	309900	Iduronate sulfatase
MPS IIIA	Sanfilippo A	Severe MR and hyperactivity; mild somatic changes	AR	252900	Heparan N-sulfatase
MPS IIIB	Sanfilippo B	Same as MPS IIIA	AR	252920	α-N-acetylglucosaminidase
MPS IIIC	Sanfilippo C	Same as MPS IIIA	AR	252930	Acetyl-coenzyme A: α-glucosaminide acetyltransferase
MPS IIID	Sanfilippo D	Same as MPS IIIA	AR	252940	N-acetylglucosamine 6-sulfatase
MPS IVA	Morquio A	Short stature and distinct skeletal dysplasia with odontoid hypoplasia and myelopathy; corneal clouding; normal intelligence; valvular heart disease	AR	253000	Galactose 6-sulfatase
MPS IVB	Morquio B	Same as MPS IVA	AR	253010	β-Galactosidase
MPS VI	Maroteaux-Lamy	DM and short stature; corneal clouding; normal intelligence; aortic stenosis; leukocyte inclusions; hydrocephalus in severe form	AR	253200	N-acetylgalactosamine
MPS VII	Sly syndrome	DM; HS; widely variable, including MR	AR	253220	β-Glucuronidase
MPS IX	—	Short stature; periarticular soft tissue masses	AR	601492	Hyaluronidase
ML II	I-cell disease	Similar to but more severe than MPS IH but with cellular inclusions; no mucopolysacchariduria	AR	252500	UDP-N-acetylglucosamine: lysosomal enzyme N-acetylglucosaminyl-1- phosphotransferase
ML III	Pseudo-Hurler polydystrophy	Short stature and mild DM; stiff joints, mild MR; survival to adulthood	AR	252500	Same as ML II arthropathy, coarse facies; variable but milder

*Entries in Online Mendelian Inheritance in Man, OMIM. McKusick-Nathans Institute of Genetic Medicine. Baltimore: Johns Hopkins University. http://omim.org.
AR = autosomal recessive; DM = dysostosis multiplex; HS = hepatosplenomegaly; MR= mental retardation; XL = X-linked.

DIAGNOSIS

Differential Diagnosis

Diagnosis of these conditions is difficult in young children, before most of the clinical features have progressed, but should be considered in any person with hepatosplenomegaly and coarsening of the facial features. Evaluation requires a pedigree analysis, ophthalmologic examination, skeletal radiographic survey, echocardiography, and analysis of the urine for excretion of GAGs. Often the specific MPS is evident from radiographs, the presence or absence of corneal clouding, and the pattern of mucopolysacchariduria. Enzymatic analysis of leukocytes confirms the diagnosis. Patients with MLs do not show mucopolysacchariduria but have marked elevation of all the GAG catabolic lysosomal enzymes in plasma.

TREATMENT   Rx

Ventriculoperitoneal shunting is necessary if intracranial pressure is elevated. Close attention to hearing and visual problems is essential throughout life. Many adults with MPS or ML require surgery for carpal tunnel syndrome. Cardiovascular surgery for valvular or coronary disease may be necessary. All use of anesthesia is high risk because of the narrow airways and, in the case of MPS IV, atlantoaxial instability. For patients who remain ambulatory, selective joint replacement can be beneficial. Because of the morbidity associated with thoracic cage deformity, consideration should be given to stabilizing the spinal deformity before it becomes severe.

Replacement of the deficient enzyme via intravenous infusion is being studied for most of the MPS disorders. Laronidase (Aldurazyme) has been approved in the United States for treatment of MPS I. An infusion every 2 weeks for 1 year in adolescent and adult patients resulted in substantial reduction in hepatosplenomegaly and modest improvement in pulmonary function, sleep apnea, and joint mobility. Whether early institution of therapy in young children modulates mental retardation in the Hurler variant of MPS I is uncertain. Galsulfase (Naglazyme) has been approved for the treatment of MPS VI, in which somatic rather than neurologic problems predominate. Bone marrow transplantation has been attempted in many of the MPS disorders, with mixed success. The earlier transplantation occurs, the better the outcome

in terms of somatic problems, but prevention of mental retardation has not occurred. Current recommendations based on consensus in Europe calls for hematopoietic stem cell transplantation for patients with Hurler syndrome before the age of 2.5 years. Enzyme replacement should be started in all patients when diagnosed.[3]

MARFAN SYNDROME

DEFINITION

Marfan syndrome is an autosomal dominant, pleiotropic disorder caused by defects in the principal component of the extracellular microfibril, the large glycoprotein fibrillin-1. The disease manifestations occur in multiple systems, especially the eye, skeleton, heart, aorta, lung, and integument. Notable features include dislocation of the ocular lens, tall stature with particularly long limbs and digits, deformity of the thoracic cage from pectus carinatum or excavatum with abnormal curvature of the spine, mitral and tricuspid valve prolapse, dilation of the sinuses of Valsalva and predisposition to aortic dissection, spontaneous pneumothorax, abnormal skin stretch marks, hernias, and dural ectasia. If untreated, patients often die before 30 or 40 years of age from aortic dissection or congestive heart failure.

EPIDEMIOLOGY

Marfan syndrome is a common Mendelian disorder, with an estimated incidence of about one per 5000 births. Marfan syndrome is found throughout the world, without ethnic or geographic predilection.

PATHOBIOLOGY

Pathogenesis

Mutations in *FBN1*, which maps to human chromosome 15q21.1 and encodes fibrillin-1, cause Marfan syndrome and related connective tissue disorders. More than 1000 distinct mutations have been found, and few occur in more than one family. Patients are heterozygous for mutations in *FBN1*, leading to autosomal dominant inheritance. Extracellular microfibrils are polymers of many fibrillin-1 molecules and are ubiquitous in the ECM of most tissues. Latent transforming growth factor β (TGF-β) binding protein, which keeps the cytokine inactive, bears striking homology to regions of fibrillin. Abnormalities of either the quality or the quantity of microfibrils disrupt normal signaling by TGF-β, especially during embryonic development and postnatal growth. Studies in mice engineered to harbor human mutations in *FBN1* showed that excessive TGF-β signaling causes abnormal lung septation (the precursor to pneumothorax), mitral valve prolapse, muscular hypoplasia, and aortic dilatation. This fundamental shift in understanding of the pathogenesis of Marfan syndrome has suggested novel therapies, such as with small molecules that affect the activity of TGF-β or its downstream signaling.

The features of Marfan syndrome are highly variable, even among relatives who share the same mutation in *FBN1*. This variability persists after accounting for the effects of age. Men tend to be affected more severely, for unclear reasons.

Pathology

The features of Marfan syndrome are age dependent. Some severely affected infants have flagrant features and often die of mitral regurgitation and heart failure despite aggressive management. At the other end of the clinical spectrum, Marfan syndrome merges with several related disorders, and patients may not come to medical attention, let alone receive a definitive diagnosis, until adulthood.

None of the gross or microscopic pathologic changes is specific for Marfan syndrome. The medial degeneration of the aortic wall, characterized by disarray and fragmentation of the elastic fibers and increased proteoglycan (often inappropriately termed *cystic medial necrosis*) also can be seen in other disorders and in older people with hypertension. Aortic dissection (Chapter 78) usually begins just superior to the aortic valve (type A) and often progresses to the bifurcation. Death usually results from retrograde dissection and hemopericardium. About 10% of dissections begin in the descending thoracic aorta (type B).

CLINICAL MANIFESTATIONS

The lens tends to be displaced superiorly, and usually the zonules remain intact. The retina is at increased risk of detachment, especially in patients who are highly myopic. Tubular bones overgrow, accounting for the disproportionate tall stature (dolichostenomelia), long digits (arachnodactyly), and sternal deformity. Ligaments may be lax, causing scoliosis and joint hypermobility. Alternatively, congenital contractures are common, especially of the elbows. The palate typically is highly arched, and the dentition can be crowded and maloccluded. Mitral valve prolapse occurs in about 80% of cases, and the valve leaflets become progressively thickened (myxomatous on histopathology) (Chapter 75). The mitral annulus may dilate and calcify. Aortic root dilation begins in the sinuses of Valsalva and progresses with age, albeit at highly variable rates (Chapter 78).[4] Most males with Marfan syndrome have an aortic root dimension above the upper limit of normal for their body surface area by adolescence. Some females show a slower progression and may have a root diameter near the upper limit of normal well into adulthood. The dilation usually does not involve the distal ascending aorta. Spontaneous pneumothorax, resulting from rupture of apical blebs, occurs in about 5% of patients. Stretch marks (striae atrophicae) occur over areas of flexural stress, such as the shoulders, breasts, and lower back. The neural canal in the lumbosacral region is enlarged in most people with Marfan syndrome; this may be visible on plain radiographs, especially if the neuroforamina are widened. Imaging by computed tomography or magnetic resonance imaging is diagnostic and should be used in patients with back pain and radicular symptoms. Dural ectasia progresses with age; large anterior meningoceles in the pelvis are a severe manifestation.[5] Simple cysts in the liver and kidneys are common, increase with age, and seldom cause clinical problems. Sleep apnea is of increased frequency in adults.[6]

DIAGNOSIS

Differential Diagnosis

The conditions that overlap clinically and genetically with Marfan syndrome include familial aortic aneurysm, familial ectopia lentis, mitral valve prolapse, mild aortic dilation, striae, skeleton (MASS) phenotype (which includes many families with mitral valve prolapse syndrome), and Loeys-Dietz syndrome. Most of these conditions are diagnosed clinically, so differentiating among them is arbitrary. A careful family history is essential to this process. Molecular genetic testing has a limited role. However, if the mutation in

FBN1 is known in a family, analysis of DNA can be used effectively for presymptomatic or prenatal diagnosis. Loeys-Dietz syndrome, which is associated with generalized arterial tortuosity and susceptibility to dissection, is caused by mutation in either of two receptors for TGF-β, *TGFBR1* and *TGFBR2*, and molecular analysis is clinically available.

A question of Marfan syndrome arises most commonly in tall, lanky adolescents who have several minor skeletal features, nearsightedness, and athletic desires. A detailed ophthalmologic examination with full pupillary dilation and a transthoracic echocardiogram are essential components in the evaluation. If these test results are negative and no one in the family has a history of Marfan syndrome or aortic dissection, the patient probably can be reassured.[7]

TREATMENT Rx

Life expectancy for those with Marfan syndrome has improved markedly, to the point that many patients can expect survival to advanced years. All patients should be seen at least annually by a physician who manages the overall care. Most patients require annual ophthalmologic and cardiologic consultation and orthopedic consultation as required by specific problems. Lens subluxation often requires surgical correction.[8] A number of studies, but only one randomized clinical trial, support the prophylactic use of β-adrenergic blockade from an early age to slow the rate of aortic root dilation and protect against aortic dissection. Based on studies of the Marfan mouse, therapies that interfere with excess signaling through pathways mediated by TGF-β are being studied in human clinical trials. One large European trial suggested a benefit of the angiotensin receptor blocker losartan on aortic root dilatation rate,[A3] but a large international trial found no benefit of losartan compared with atenolol.[A2] Prophylactic surgical repair of the aortic root has had the greatest beneficial impact. The composite graft, involving a prosthetic valve in a Dacron tube and implantation of the coronary ostia into the graft, was the first approach to produce markedly improved survival in these patients. More recently, replacement of the aneurysm and preservation of the native aortic valve have shown promise and should be considered first.[9,10] For adults, aortic root surgery should be strongly considered when the maximal aortic diameter reaches 45 mm, and a family history of aortic dissection should prompt earlier repair (Chapter 78).

EHLERS-DANLOS SYNDROMES

DEFINITION

The Ehlers-Danlos syndromes (EDSs) are clinically variable and genetically heterogeneous. Diagnoses still are based largely on the bedside examination. The unifying themes among these disorders are fragility of tissues, joint hypermobility, and skin hyperextensibility.[11]

EPIDEMIOLOGY

No accurate data exist, but an incidence of about one in 5000 births is a reasonable estimate of how many individuals qualify for one of the EDS diagnoses. Each type represents something of a clinical spectrum, with the mild end merging with what might be considered normal variation. Just as the diagnostic criteria are arbitrary, so would be any determination of prevalence based on phenotypic criteria. The extent to which normal variation in joint hypermobility, skin elasticity, and tissue fragility represents genetic variation at loci that encode collagen or other ECM genes requires considerable research.

PATHOBIOLOGY

Pathogenesis

Defects in collagen and other proteins in the ECM of various tissues underlie all forms of EDS that have been elucidated so far. The specific mutations occur in a variety of genes, with the effect of altering the structure, synthesis, posttranslational modifications, or stability of the collagens involved. The known molecular defects are listed in Table 260-2.

Pathology

Few findings in the routine pathologic evaluation distinguish among the various types of EDS or even distinguish individual types from normal. Thickness of the dermis is decreased in some forms, especially the vascular type, and the walls of arteries are reduced in thickness in this type. By electron microscopy, the classic, hypermobile, and kyphoscoliotic types have abnormal collagen fibers, especially when viewed in cross section (variable and often increased fiber diameter with an irregular outline). In the vascular type,

TABLE 260-2 EHLERS-DANLOS SYNDROMES

TYPE	FORMER NAME	CLINICAL FEATURES*	INHERITANCE	OMIM†	MOLECULAR DEFECT
Classic	EDS I and II	Joint hypermobility; skin hyperextensibility; atrophic scars; smooth, velvety skin; subcutaneous spheroids	AD	130000 130010	Structure of type V collagen caused by mutations in COL5A1 or COL5A2
Hypermobility	EDS III	Joint hypermobility; some skin hyperextensibility, with or without a smooth, velvety texture	AD AR	130020 225320	? Tenascin-X (TNX)
Vascular	EDS IV	Thin skin; easy bruising; pinched nose; acrogeria; rupture of large- and medium-caliber arteries, uterus, and large bowel	AD	130050 (225350) (225360)	Deficient type III collagen (COL3A1)
Kyphoscoliotic	EDS VI	Joint hypermobility; congenital, progressive rupture; scoliosis; scleral fragility with globe rupture; tissue fragility, aortic dilation, MVP	AR	225400	Deficiency of lysyl hydroxylase
Arthrochalasis	EDS VII A	Joint hypermobility, severe, with subluxations, congenital hip dislocation; and skin hyperextensibility; tissue fragility	AD	130060	No cleavage of amino terminus of type I procollagen caused by mutations in COL1A1 or COL1A2
Dermatosparaxis	EDS VII C	Severe skin fragility; decreased skin elasticity, easy bruising; hernias; premature rupture of fetal membranes	AR	225410	No cleavage of amino terminus of type I procollagen caused by deficiency of peptidase
Unclassified types	EDS V	Classic features	XL	305200	?
	EDS VIII	Classic features and periodontal disease	AD	130080	?
	EDS X	Mild classic features, MVP	?	225310	?
	EDS XI	Joint instability	AD	147900	?
	EDS IX	Classic features; occipital horns	XL	309400	Allelic to Menkes syndrome
	EDS, progeroid form	Classic features and premature aging	AR	130700	Deficiency of galactosyltransferase I

*Listed in order of diagnostic importance.
†Entries in Online Mendelian Inheritance in Man, OMIM. McKusick-Nathans Institute of Genetic Medicine. Baltimore: Johns Hopkins University. http://omim.org.
AD = autosomal dominant; AR = autosomal recessive; EDS = Ehlers-Danlos syndrome; MVP = mitral valve prolapse; XL = X-linked.

some patients have dilated endoplasmic reticulum consistent with aberrant secretion of type III collagen molecules.

CLINICAL MANIFESTATIONS

The major and minor features of each EDS are detailed in Table 260-2. Infants with classic EDS often are born prematurely by 4 to 8 weeks because of rupture of fetal membranes. Diagnosis of the vascular and kyphoscoliotic types is important because of their cardiovascular features. The vascular type, previously termed *EDS IV*, is characterized by spontaneous rupture of large arteries and hollow organs, especially the colon and uterus, and pneumothorax. Because these events carry considerable morbidity, life expectancy is reduced, on average, by more than half. During pregnancy, women with this form of EDS are especially vulnerable to rupture of major arteries and the uterus. In the kyphoscoliotic type, aortic root dilation and aortic regurgitation can develop. Patients with most forms of EDS are prone to develop mitral valve prolapse, and progression to mitral regurgitation (Chapter 75) occurs more often than in the common form of mitral valve prolapse.

DIAGNOSIS
Differential Diagnosis

By carefully adherence to the clinical features shown in Table 260-2 and judicious use of laboratory tests, the various defined types of EDS can be differentiated. Many specific non-EDS syndromes need to be excluded. The kyphoscoliotic type of EDS in infants shares some features with severe Marfan syndrome. Patients with Larsen syndrome may resemble patients with the arthrochalasis type of EDS. The skin redundancy and loss of elasticity of the dermatosparaxis type of EDS is reminiscent of autosomal dominant cutis laxa, which is not associated with easy bruising or tissue fragility.

The most difficult decision is whether any diagnosis of EDS is warranted. Patients who have only joint hypermobility without skin changes should not be labeled with EDS; a diagnosis of familial joint hypermobility might be more appropriate. Familial joint instability involves a predisposition to dislocations of major joints that is rare in most types of EDS except for arthrochalasis.

TREATMENT Rx

Management of most skin and joint problems should be conservative and preventive. Sutures need to be placed with careful attention to approximating the margins and avoiding tension; removable sutures should be left in place for twice the usual time. Most instances of joint hypermobility and pain in EDS do not require surgical treatment. Benefit often is derived from physical therapy designed to strengthen the muscles that provide support for the loose ligaments. All patients should receive genetic counseling about the mode of inheritance and their risk of having children affected with EDS. The possibility of prenatal diagnosis exists for all of the EDS types with defined molecular or biochemical defects.

The vascular type of EDS requires particular surgical care; the ruptured arteries are difficult to repair because of the pronounced vascular fragility. Experienced vascular surgeons are having some success with prophylactic repair of vessels deemed to be at risk of dissection or rupture.[12] One clinical trial suggested improved outcomes with prophylactic β-adrenergic blockade.[A3] Rupture of the bowel is a surgical emergency. Because the risk of uterine and vascular rupture is especially high during pregnancy in women with the vascular form, affected women should be advised that there is a substantial risk of death related to pregnancy and delivery. Patients should be advised to avoid contact sports and to treat blood pressure elevations aggressively. Arteriography and arterial lines should be avoided if possible. Biochemical and genetic screening holds the potential for reassuring relatives at risk that they do not have a defect in type III collagen.

The kyphoscoliotic type of EDS may improve with large doses of vitamin C (1-4 g/day) because ascorbate is a cofactor for the enzyme that is deficient. No other metabolic or genetic therapy is effective in other forms of EDS.

OSTEOGENESIS IMPERFECTA SYNDROMES

DEFINITION

The heterogeneous group of disorders called *osteogenesis imperfecta* (OI) includes, at one end of the severity spectrum, a type that is lethal prenatally or in the neonatal period and, at the other, such mild features that distinguishing affected individuals from the general population is difficult. The unifying feature is hereditary osteopenia (insufficient bone), with primary defects in the protein matrix in bone and other tissues. The clinical syndromes all involve osteoporosis with liability to fracture (Chapter 243).

EPIDEMIOLOGY

No careful epidemiologic study has been performed, and the milder forms of type I OI merge with the phenotypes of familial osteoporosis, fracture

TABLE 260-3 OSTEOGENESIS IMPERFECTA

TYPE	CLINICAL FEATURES	INHERITANCE	OMIM*	BASIC DEFECTS
I	Fractures variable in number; little deformity; stature normal or nearly so; blue sclerae; hearing loss common but not always present; DI uncommon	AD	166200	Typically, one nonfunctional *COL1A1* allele
II	Lethal in utero or shortly after birth; many fractures at birth typically involving ribs (may appear "beaded") and other long bones; little calvaria; pulmonary hypertension	AD	166210	*COL1A1* or *COL1A2*: substitution of glycyl residues; occasionally deletions of a portion of the triple-helical domain
		AR	259400	Deletion in *COL1A2* plus a nonfunctional allele
III	Fractures common, but long bones progressively deform starting in utero; stature markedly reduced; sclerae often blue but become lighter with age; DI and hearing loss common	AD	259420	One single amino acid substitution
		AR (rare)	259440	Two mutations in *COL1A1* and/or *COL1A2* (rarely)
IV	Fractures common; stature usually reduced; bone deformity common but rarely severe; scleral hue normal to grayish; hearing loss variable; DI common	AD	166220	Point mutations in *COL1A1* or *COL1A2*
			166240	Exon skipping mutations in *COL1A2*
V	Similar to type IV without DI or blue sclerae; fractures develop hyperplastic callus; calcification of the interosseous membrane between the radius and ulna	AD	610967	?
VI	Similar to type IV without DI, blue sclerae or Wormian bones; excess osteoid present in bone	?	610968	?
VII	Similar to types II or III with fractures at birth, blue sclerae, no DI; presence of rhizomelic limb shortening and coxa vara	AR	610682	Mutations in *CRTAP*
VIII	Similar to types II or III with fractures at birth	AR	610915	Mutations in *LEPRE1*
IX	Similar to types II or III with fractures at birth	AR	259440	Mutations in *PPIB*

*Entries in Online Mendelian Inheritance in Man, OMIM. McKusick-Nathans Institute of Genetic Medicine. Baltimore: Johns Hopkins University. http://omim.org.
AD = autosomal dominant; AR = autosomal recessive; DI = dentinogenesis imperfecta.

susceptibility, and joint hypermobility found in the general population. A crude estimate of the overall prevalence of OI is one to two per 20,000 births. The neonatal lethal form (type II), which is almost always caused by a new mutation in a parental gamete, has an incidence of about one in 50,000 births.

PATHOBIOLOGY
Pathogenesis
Most patients in whom mutations have been found usually have defects in the two genes that encode the procollagen chains of type I collagen, *COL1A1* and *COL1A2*. Type I collagen is composed of two $\alpha1(I)$ and one $\alpha2(I)$ procollagen chains; the mature fiber requires considerable posttranslational modification, which occurs appropriately only if the three procollagen chains have intertwined to form a triple helix that is perfect and completed at the right speed. A mutation that affects formation of the triple helix, such as substitution of one of the mandatory glycine residues that occurs at every third position, also has adverse effects on the modifications that render the molecule capable of forming effective mature fibers. As a result, a single nucleotide change resulting in a missense mutation can have profound effects on the ECM and produce a severe condition.[13] Alternatively, and at first glance paradoxically, a mutation that eliminates an entire allele, or at least production of any product capable of intertwining with normal procollagen chains, has a much milder effect on the ECM and on the severity of OI. Examples of the most common classes of mutations are shown in Table 260-3. Hundreds of mutations have been described. Patients with mutations in *COL1A1* or *COL1A2* are heterozygous, and thus the most common forms of OI are inherited as autosomal dominant traits. Several autosomal recessive forms of OI occur because of mutations in genes that encode enzymes that process type I collagen into mature fibrils.[14]

Pathology
Other than the gross pathology associated with the clinical manifestations, the most characteristic pathology is a primary reduction in bone matrix with secondary undermineralization.

CLINICAL MANIFESTATIONS
The major phenotypic features of OI are shown in Table 260-3. Among the most common forms, the most severe type is type II, followed in decreasing order by types III, IV, and I. In type II, infants either are stillborn or die soon after birth of pulmonary failure secondary to the small thorax, which usually is compromised further by myriad rib fractures. A few infants have

survived for at least a few years but require enormous attention to their medical needs.

Type III OI may be confused with type II at birth, but survival alone helps make the distinction. Bony deformity is pronounced and not necessarily caused by fractures. Mobility is impaired, and most patients require a wheelchair at an early age. Stature may be severely compromised. Because of progressive vertebral column deformity and rib fractures, restrictive lung disease is a common problem as patients age; many die of pulmonary complications. Basilar impression causing compression of the brain stem and the craniocervical junction can produce central sleep apnea, headache, and upper motor neuron signs.

Patients with type IV OI generally have reduced stature, some bony deformity, and abnormal teeth that are opalescent and wear easily (dentinogenesis imperfecta). As in type I OI, the tendency to fracture is highest in childhood and lessens with adolescence. A distinguishing characteristic of type IV OI is a normal scleral hue.

Type I OI is probably the most common form and is associated with a bluish or blue-gray scleral hue. People with type I OI who also have dentinogenesis imperfecta tend to have more severe skeletal problems. The risk of fracture diminishes during adulthood but reemerges as a major concern for women after menopause. Hearing impairment in all forms of OI is common and age related, being rare before adolescence. The deficits are of either a mixed or a predominantly conductive form.

The recessive forms of OI (types VI-IX) range in severity from type IV to type II and may have distinctive radiologic or histopathologic findings.

DIAGNOSIS
Differential Diagnosis
The range of diagnostic possibilities in a person with multiple fractures largely depends on age. In infancy, the genetic conditions hypophosphatasia, severe osteochondrodysplasias (e.g., achondrogenesis and forms of spondyloepiphyseal dysplasia), and Menkes syndrome need to be excluded when a diagnosis of type II or type III OI is considered. The radiographic features eventually become entirely diagnostic, but often the neonatologist has to arrive at a definitive answer in short order. Analysis of serum alkaline phosphatase and copper can be helpful. In childhood, the most common situation leading to consideration of a mild form of OI is child abuse. In this situation, the pattern of fracture is usually distinct, and bone mineralization should be normal if the child is the object of nonaccidental or repeated accidental trauma. Abnormal scleral hue, dentinogenesis imperfecta, and wormian bones (microfractures along the cranial sutures) all support the diagnosis of

OI. The legal and child-protective systems often request exclusion of OI by analysis of collagen production from cultured skin fibroblasts or analysis of DNA for a mutation.

In older children, the disorder idiopathic juvenile osteoporosis should be considered in any patient seen initially with repeated fractures. Many osteochondrodysplasias are associated with short stature, skeletal deformity, and a tendency to fracture. Pyknodysostosis and osteopetrosis are associated with sclerotic bones rather than osteoporotic ones. In adulthood, early-onset osteoporosis may be confused with OI (Chapter 243). Mutations in type I collagen also cause familial osteoporosis, and the skeletal phenotypes merge; patients with true OI may have scleral, hearing, or dental abnormalities and a positive family history.

Analysis of the specific enzymes defective in the recessive forms of OI is useful for establishing the diagnosis and enabling reproductive counseling and prenatal diagnosis if desired.

TREATMENT   Rx

Management of the skeletal complications largely depends on orthopedic, physical, and occupational therapy approaches. Risedronate (2.5 or 5 mg daily) increases bone mineral density and reduces both first and recurrent fractures in children with OI. The long-term goals are for the patient to maintain function and independence as an individual. These goals can be advanced in some patients by judicious use of intramedullary rods in the long bones of the legs; if mobility and especially ambulation can be maintained, the demineralization associated with inactivity can be avoided.

Unaffected parents of a child with OI and all affected individuals should have genetic counseling. For the parents of a child with type II OI, the possibility of germinal mosaicism (which has been well documented in this condition) should not be overlooked. If one parent has a "new" mutation in one of the type I procollagen genes and multiple gonadal cells carry this mutation, the risk of recurrence in future children is not negligible. If the mutation in the affected child can be defined, the risk of recurrence can be quantified (through molecular analysis of sperm) if the mutation arose in the father.

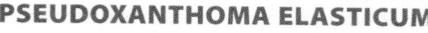

PSEUDOXANTHOMA ELASTICUM

DEFINITION

Pseudoxanthoma elasticum (PXE) is a heritable disorder of connective tissue with pleiotropic manifestations wherever elastic fibers are found but primarily in the skin, eye, and vasculature.[15] Life expectancy is reduced, on average, because of a predisposition to myocardial infarction and gastrointestinal hemorrhage.

EPIDEMIOLOGY

The exact frequency of PXE is unknown, but it is probably underdiagnosed. Rough approximations suggest a prevalence of one in 25,000 to 100,000 births. Males and females are equally affected, although women are more likely to seek medical attention out of concern for the skin changes.

PATHOBIOLOGY
Pathogenesis

In most families, PXE occurs as an autosomal recessive trait, which means, given relatively small sibships, that many patients will have no affected relatives. Apparent autosomal dominant inheritance may reflect expression in occasional heterozygotes. The gene for PXE maps to human chromosome 16 and encodes one of the adenosine triphosphate (ATP)-binding cassette transporters (*ABCC6*). Because of the prominent histopathologic feature of calcification of elastic tissue, this gene may be important in calcium homeostasis. It is unclear, however, whether calcification is a primary or a secondary phenomenon in PXE.

Pathology

The hallmark of PXE, and an important diagnostic clue, is the histopathologic finding of hyperproliferated elastic fibers in the mid-dermis; these fibers become fragmented, clumped, and calcified. An arteriolar sclerosis develops in the media of muscular arteries and arterioles; the lumen may become progressively and concentrically narrowed. Alternatively, microaneurysms can form. Thickening of the endocardium, especially in the atria, develops in some patients. In the eye, Bruch membrane becomes calcified and fragmented.

CLINICAL MANIFESTATIONS

Because of the pleiotropic nature of PXE, the diagnosis initially may be suspected by any of a variety of clinicians, especially dermatologists, ophthalmologists, cardiologists, and gastroenterologists. The condition gains its name from the dermatologic feature of yellowish papules that appear at areas of flexural stress, especially the neck, groin, and popliteal and cubital fossae; in periumbilical regions; and on the buccal mucosa. The appearance of affected skin has been likened to that of a "plucked chicken." Over time, affected areas coalesce and become thickened.

Changes in the eye begin as a generalized, subtle, mottled pattern in the retina (peau d'orange) and progress to the characteristic angioid streaks. The latter changes are not specific for PXE and can be seen in diabetes mellitus, sickle cell disease, and a variety of other conditions. Streaks represent breaks in Bruch's membrane, an elastic lamina that lies between the retinal vasculature and the choroid. Spontaneous hemorrhages, especially those involving the macula, lead to progressive visual loss.[16]

Involvement of arteries of various calibers produces problems because of occlusion and hemorrhage.[17] The lifetime risk of serious gastrointestinal hemorrhage from any site, but especially the stomach, is about 10%. Hypertension is relatively common, in part because of involvement of the renal vasculature. Progressive occlusion of peripheral arteries leads to absence of pulses; acral ischemia is rare because of the development of collaterals. The risk for stroke, myocardial infarction, abdominal angina, and intermittent claudication is increased independent of other risk factors. Impaired left ventricular function is common in adults.

DIAGNOSIS
Differential Diagnosis

Whole exome sequencing is an efficient and sensitive way to make the diagnosis.[18] An acquired form of PXE has been reported and is also of unclear etiology. This form is difficult to differentiate from a sporadic case in a family because of heterozygosity in the parents, but it tends to affect only the skin. As suggested by the name, the cutaneous features of PXE need to be differentiated from those of true xanthoma, which results from a disorder of lipid metabolism (Chapter 206). The dermatologic manifestations need to be differentiated from those of Miescher elastoma, elastic tissue nevi (Buschke-Ollendorff syndrome), and solar elastosis.

TREATMENT   Rx

No cure for or means of preventing PXE is known. In many instances, careful attention to the ocular features by a retinal specialist experienced in PXE can delay but not prevent loss of vision. The risk of gastrointestinal hemorrhage suggests that patients should avoid gastric irritants such as aspirin, nonsteroidal anti-inflammatory drugs, and excessive alcohol. Stool should be checked regularly for occult blood, and angiography may be necessary to detect the source of bleeding. All standard risk factors for atherosclerosis should be managed aggressively. Complaints of chest pain should prompt a rigorous investigation for coronary artery disease. Angioplasty has not been reported to be effective, and the coronary lesions tend to be diffuse. Coronary artery bypass graft surgery has been performed, but long-term results have not been reported. It may be theoretically advantageous to use vein grafts rather than the internal mammary artery for bypass. The excessive wrinkling and pseudoxanthoma in exposed areas can be ameliorated by plastic surgery.

FUTURE DIRECTIONS

Each of these disorders poses special considerations in clinical diagnosis, utility of molecular testing, genetic counseling, and management. For the storage disorders, the clinical utility of enzyme replacement therapy is actively being pursued by several pharmaceutical companies. For several of the other conditions, somatic stem cell therapy offers some promise but is years away from routine clinical use. In Marfan syndrome, clinical trials of drugs that modulate activity of TGF-β are underway. Additionally, close medical management for individuals detected as being at heightened risk for cardiovascular, skeletal, and ocular complications will remain a mainstay.

 Grade A References

A1. Groenink M, den Hartog AW, Franken R, et al. Losartan reduces aortic dilatation rate in adults with Marfan syndrome: a randomized controlled trial. *Eur Heart J.* 2013;34:3491-3500.

A2. Lacro RV, Dietz HC, Sleeper LA, et al. Atenolol versus losartan in children and young adults with Marfan's syndrome. *N Engl J Med.* 2014;371:2061-2071.

A3. Ong KT, Perdu J, De Backer J, et al. Effect of celiprolol on prevention of cardiovascular events in vascular Ehlers-Danlos syndrome: a prospective, randomized, open, blinded-endpoints trial. *Lancet.* 2010;376:1476-1484.

A4. Bishop N, Adami S, Ahmed SF, et al. Risedronate in children with osteogenesis imperfecta: a randomised, double-blind, placebo-controlled trial. *Lancet.* 2013;382:1424-1432.

GENERAL REFERENCES

For the General References and other additional features, please visit Expert Consult at https://expertconsult.inkling.com.

261

THE SYSTEMIC AUTOINFLAMMATORY DISEASES

RICHARD M. SIEGEL AND DANIEL L. KASTNER

DEFINITION

The systemic autoinflammatory diseases (Table 261-1) are a group of illnesses characterized by seemingly unprovoked inflammation, without evidence of high-titer autoantibodies or antigen-specific T cells, thus distinguishing them from the more classic autoimmune diseases. The first conditions recognized as autoinflammatory were the hereditary recurrent fevers, a group of mendelian disorders characterized by episodic or fluctuating degrees of fever and localized inflammation. The scope of autoinflammatory disease has been broadened to include other heritable illnesses, including disorders in which purulent or granulomatous inflammation predominates, as well as inherited disorders of the complement system (Chapter 50).[1-6] In addition, in numerous autoinflammatory conditions, some of which manifest in childhood and others that occur later in life, there is a complex interaction of genetic susceptibilities and environmental factors. These illnesses include systemic-onset juvenile idiopathic arthritis (Still's disease), Behçet's disease, and even the crystalline arthritides. Recent advances in the genetics and pathophysiology of the inherited autoinflammatory diseases suggest that these conditions are inborn errors of innate immunity, the phylogenetically more primitive part of the immune system that uses germline membrane and intracellular receptors expressed in granulocytes and macrophages to mount the body's first line of defense against pathogens (Chapters 45 and 48).

HEREDITARY RECURRENT FEVER SYNDROMES
Familial Mediterranean Fever

DEFINITION

Familial Mediterranean fever (FMF) is a recessively inherited illness that typically manifests with 12- to 72-hour episodes of fever and localized serosal, synovial, or cutaneous inflammation. Between attacks, patients usually feel completely well, although biochemical evidence of inflammation may remain, and some patients eventually develop systemic amyloidosis. Before the identification of the causative gene, FMF was defined purely clinically; clinical features remain an important part of the diagnosis, because some patients with typical disease have only one, or sometimes no, demonstrable mutation in *MEFV*, the only known causative gene.

EPIDEMIOLOGY

FMF is most common in individuals of Jewish, Arab, Armenian, Turkish, and Italian ancestry. The frequency of asymptomatic carriers of a single *MEFV* mutation in these populations is as high as 1 in 5, a finding that suggests a selective advantage for heterozygotes. With genetic testing, FMF is now frequently recognized in both Ashkenazi (eastern European) and non-Ashkenazi Jewish populations, as well as in Mediterranean populations previously thought not to be at risk. Mutation-positive individuals with typical symptoms have been documented worldwide. FMF usually manifests in childhood, sometimes even in infancy, although approximately 10% of patients experience their first attack as adults; infrequently, FMF first occurs in persons older than 40 years.

PATHOBIOLOGY

MEFV, the gene for FMF, was identified by positional cloning in 1997. It encodes a 781–amino acid protein denoted pyrin (or marenostrin) that is expressed in granulocytes, monocytes, and dendritic cells, as well as in peritoneal, synovial, and dermal fibroblasts. The N-terminal 92 amino acids of pyrin are the prototype for a motif, the PYRIN domain, that is involved in protein-protein interactions; this domain defines a family of more than 20 human proteins, including pyrin itself, involved in the regulation of cytokine production (particularly the interleukin-1 [IL-1] family), nuclear factor kappa B (NF-κB) activation, and apoptosis. More than 50 FMF-associated mutations in pyrin have been identified, many of which reside in the C-terminal domain encoded by exon 10 of *MEFV*. An even larger number of variants of unknown significance have been described in individual patients with a spectrum of inflammatory phenotypes.

CLINICAL MANIFESTATIONS

Episodes of FMF are more properly termed recurrent than periodic, and some patients associate attacks with psychological stress or physical exertion. Women of childbearing age sometimes experience their attacks with menses, with remissions during pregnancy. Some patients are unaware of fever during the attacks, but it is almost always observed when sought.

Serosal involvement in FMF is usually peritoneal or pleural. Abdominal attacks are the most frequent, and they may vary from mild discomfort to frank peritonitis, with boardlike rigidity, direct and rebound tenderness, and air-fluid levels on upright films of the abdomen. Regardless of the severity of the abdominal attack, constipation is much more common than diarrhea. When a laparotomy or laparoscopy is performed during an attack, a small amount of sterile exudate rich in polymorphonuclear leukocytes is found. Except for serosal inflammation, the appendix is normal. Repeated abdominal attacks may cause peritoneal adhesions, but ascites is rare. Pleurisy, usually unilateral, may accompany abdominal pain, or it may occur independently. Physical findings, if present, may include diminished breath sounds and a pleural friction rub, whereas x-ray films may show a small effusion or atelectasis. With multiple attacks, pleural thickening may develop. Symptomatic nonuremic pericardial involvement in FMF has been reported but is unusual.

In adults, the arthritis of FMF typically manifests as monoarticular involvement of the knee, hip, or ankle, and attacks of arthritis may persist for up to 1 week at a time. In children, oligoarticular or polyarticular joint involvement may occur. Large joint effusions are sometimes present, and the synovial fluid may have as many as 100,000 leukocytes/mm^3. In approximately 5% of patients who are not treated with prophylactic colchicine, chronic arthritis (usually of the hip or knee) may develop, often necessitating joint replacement surgery. Regardless of colchicine treatment or a particular human leukocyte antigen (HLA-B27) status, some patients with FMF develop sacroiliitis. Arthralgia without frank arthritis is common in FMF.

Cutaneous manifestations of FMF tend to be less common than serosal or synovial involvement. The characteristic skin lesion of FMF is erysipeloid erythema, a painful, demarcated erythematous area most often seen on the lower leg, ankle, or dorsum of the foot. This rash may occur independently, or it may accompany an episode of arthritis. Histologically, a mixed perivascular cellular infiltrate is seen. Other acute manifestations of FMF include unilateral scrotal inflammation (the tunica vaginalis is an embryologic remnant of the peritoneal membrane) and myalgia, either with fever or, especially in children, without fever and induced by vigorous exercise. Various forms of vasculitis also have been associated with FMF; Henoch-Schönlein purpura may occur in children with FMF; less frequently, polyarteritis nodosa is seen.

COMPLICATIONS

Before the widespread use of colchicine prophylaxis, systemic AA amyloidosis (Chapter 188) was a frequent complication of FMF, caused by the ectopic deposition of a misfolded fragment of serum amyloid A (SAA), an acute phase reactant, in the gastrointestinal tract, kidneys, spleen, lung, testes, and adrenals. Malabsorption and nephrotic proteinuria leading to renal failure are the most common manifestations of AA amyloidosis. Cardiomyopathy is less common, and neuropathy and arthropathy are rare. Several risk factors for amyloidosis development in FMF have been identified, including late diagnosis of FMF, colchicine noncompliance, male gender, and specific

TABLE 261-1   SYSTEMIC AUTOINFLAMMATORY DISEASES: A PARTIAL LISTING

INHERITED AUTOINFLAMMATORY DISEASES	INHERITANCE/ETIOLOGY	GENES OR RISK FACTORS	OMIM*
HEREDITARY RECURRENT FEVER SYNDROMES			
Familial Mediterranean fever (FMF)	Autosomal recessive	MEFV[†]	249100
Tumor necrosis factor receptor–associated periodic syndrome (TRAPS)	Autosomal dominant	TNFRSF1A[†]	142680
Hyperimmunoglobulinemia D with periodic fever syndrome (HIDS)	Autosomal recessive	MVK[†]	260920
Familial cold autoinflammatory syndrome (FCAS)	Autosomal dominant	NLRP3 (formerly CIAS1)[†]	120100
Muckle-Wells syndrome (MWS)	Autosomal dominant	NLRP3 (formerly CIAS1)[†]	191900
Neonatal-onset multisystem inflammatory disease (NOMID)/chronic infantile neurologic cutaneous and articular (CINCA) syndrome	Sporadic, autosomal dominant	NLRP3 (formerly CIAS1)[†]	607115
GRANULOMATOUS DISORDERS			
Granulomatous inflammatory arthritis, dermatitis, and uveitis (Blau's syndrome)	Autosomal dominant	NOD2/CARD15[†]	186580
Early-onset sarcoidosis	Sporadic, autosomal dominant	NOD2/CARD15[†]	609464
Crohn's disease	Complex inheritance	NOD2/CARD15[†]	266600
PYOGENIC DISORDERS			
Syndrome of pyogenic arthritis with pyoderma gangrenosum and acne (PAPA)	Autosomal dominant	PSTPIP1[†]	604416
AUTOINFLAMMATORY DISORDERS OF SKIN AND BONE			
Deficiency of interleukin-1 receptor antagonist (DIRA)	Autosomal recessive	IL1RN	612852
Chronic recurrent multifocal osteomyelitis (CRMO)	Sporadic, autosomal recessive	LPIN2,[†] when associated with congenital dyserythropoietic anemia (Majeed syndrome)	259680
Synovitis acne pustulosis hyperostosis osteitis syndrome (SAPHO)	Idiopathic	—	—
COMPLEMENT DISORDERS			
Hereditary angioedema	Autosomal dominant	C1NH	106100
Hemolytic-uremic syndrome	Autosomal dominant, sporadic	HF1 (complement factor H)	235400
Age-related macular degeneration	Complex inheritance	HF1 (complement factor H)	603075
OTHER AUTOINFLAMMATORY SYNDROMES			
Syndrome of periodic fever with aphthous stomatitis, pharyngitis, and cervical adenopathy (PFAPA)	Idiopathic	—	—
Autoinflammation, lipodystrophy, and dermatosis syndrome (Nakajo-Nishimura syndrome, JMP syndrome, CANDLE syndrome)	Autosomal recessive	PSMB8	256040
Systemic-onset juvenile idiopathic arthritis (SOJIA)	Complex inheritance	IL-6, MIF polymorphisms	604302
Adult-onset Still's disease	Idiopathic	—	—
Schnitzler's syndrome	Idiopathic	—	—
Behçet's disease	Complex inheritance	HLA-B51, polymorphisms in IL10, IL23R, CCR1, STAT4, KLRC4, ERAP1, MEFV, TLR4	109650
Crystalline arthropathies	Complex inheritance	SLC2A9/GLUT9, ABCG2	—

*Online Mendelian Inheritance in Man, an online catalogue of genetic disorders, available at http://www.ncbi.nlm.nih.gov/entrez/query.fcgi?db=OMIM. Accessed September 29, 2014.
[†]An updated list of disease-associated mutations is available online at http://fmf.igh.cnrs.fr/infevers. Accessed September 29, 2014.

genotypes of the MEFV and SAA genes. Amyloidosis in FMF is less common in the United States than in the Middle East. Abdominal fat aspirates are much less sensitive than rectal or renal biopsy in detecting the amyloidosis of FMF. The latter procedure may be preferred, because of the increasing recognition of nonamyloid glomerular disease in FMF. With early diagnosis, aggressive suppression of the acute phase response with colchicine or adjunctive agents may lead to improvement, but for patients with renal failure, early renal transplantation is preferred.

DIAGNOSIS

Based on a simple recessive model of inheritance, two mutations in MEFV, in trans, should be identified to establish the genetic diagnosis of FMF. Nevertheless, the interpretation of genetic testing is complicated by complex alleles consisting of various combinations of mutations in cis, as well as by the observations that as many as one third of patients with clinically typical FMF have only one demonstrable mutation in MEFV, and a few patients with typical disease have no identifiable MEFV mutations. These latter two findings suggest that, under some circumstances, one MEFV mutation may be sufficient for symptoms or that additional genes for FMF exist.

For these reasons, clinical data remain an essential part of the diagnosis of FMF, and genetic testing plays an adjunctive role in settings in which clinical experience is limited.[7] Clinical criteria emphasize attack duration (12 to 72 hours); recurrence of symptoms (three or more episodes); documented fever (rectal temperature > 38° C); painful manifestations in the abdomen, chest,

joints, or skin; and the absence of other causative factors. The differential diagnosis includes the other hereditary recurrent fever syndromes (Table 261-2), as well as other conditions specific to the clinical setting. For patients with recurrent abdominal pain, considerations include gynecologic disorders, porphyria (Chapter 210; which can be distinguished by hypertension during attacks, dominant inheritance, and urine porphyrins), and hereditary angioedema (Chapter 252; which usually does not cause fever). The syndrome of periodic fever with aphthous stomatitis, pharyngitis, and cervical adenopathy is probably the most common cause of unexplained recurrent fever in children and is also included in the differential diagnosis. In patients presenting primarily with recurrent monoarthritis, joint aspiration for cultures and crystals may aid in excluding bacterial and crystalline arthritis, respectively.

Still's disease in children (systemic-onset juvenile idiopathic arthritis) and adults (adult-onset Still's disease) is also considered in the differential diagnosis. Adult-onset Still's disease[8] (see Table 261-1) is an uncommon autoinflammatory condition of unknown cause that is not considered to be hereditary. It is characterized by spiking fever, an evanescent salmon-pink maculopapular rash, arthritis, and neutrophilic leukocytosis. It can be clinically distinguished from FMF by the pattern of fever (intermittent quotidian in Still's disease vs. discrete episodes in FMF), the pattern of arthritis (chronic polyarthritis vs. intermittent monoarthritis), the characteristic skin involvement (evanescent rash vs. erysipeloid erythema), and the presence of lymphadenopathy (more common in Still's disease).

TABLE 261-2 CLINICAL FEATURES OF SELECTED HEREDITARY RECURRENT FEVER SYNDROMES

CLINICAL FEATURE	FMF	TRAPS	HIDS	FCAS	MWS	NOMID/CINCA
Typical ethnicity	Arab, Armenian, Italian, Jewish, Turkish	Any ethnicity	Dutch, other North European	European	European	Any
Attack duration	12-72 hr	Days to weeks	3-7 days	12-24 hr	1-2 days	Continuous, with flares
Abdominal attacks	Sterile peritonitis, constipation more often than diarrhea	Severe pain, vomiting, peritonitis	Sterile peritonitis, diarrhea, rarely constipation	Nausea	Abdominal pain	Not common
Pleural attacks	Common	Common	Rare	Not seen	Rare	Rare
Joint/bone involvement	Monoarthritis, rarely protracted arthritis in knee or hip	Arthritis in large joints, arthralgia	Arthralgia, symmetrical polyarthritis	Polyarthralgia	Polyarthralgia, oligoarthritis, clubbing	Epiphyseal overgrowth, contractures, intermittent or chronic arthritis, clubbing
Skin rash	Erysipeloid erythema on lower leg, ankle, foot	Migratory rash, underlying myalgia	Diffuse maculopapular rash, urticaria	Cold-induced urticaria-like rash	Urticaria-like rash	Urticaria-like rash
Lymphatic involvement	Splenomegaly, occasional lymphadenopathy	Splenomegaly, occasional lymphadenopathy	Cervical adenopathy in children	Not seen	Rare	Hepatosplenomegaly, adenopathy
Neurologic involvement	Aseptic meningitis?	Controversial	Headache	Headache	Sensorineural deafness	Sensorineural deafness, chronic aseptic meningitis, intellectual disability, headache
Ophthalmologic involvement	Rare	Conjunctivitis, periorbital edema, rarely uveitis	Uncommon	Conjunctivitis	Conjunctivitis, episcleritis	Uveitis, conjunctivitis, progressive vision loss
Vasculitis	Henoch-Schönlein purpura (HSP), polyarteritis nodosa	HSP, lymphocytic vasculitis	Cutaneous vasculitis common, rarely HSP	Not seen	Not seen	Occasional
Systemic amyloidosis	Risk depends on *MEFV* and *SAA* genotypes; more common in Middle East	Occurs in ~10%; risk increased with cysteine mutations	Rare	Rare	Occurs in ~25%	May develop in some, usually in adulthood

FCAS = familial cold autoinflammatory syndrome; FMF = familial Mediterranean fever; HIDS = hyperimmunoglobulinemia D with periodic fever syndrome; MWS = Muckle-Wells syndrome; NOMID/CINCA = neonatal-onset multisystem inflammatory disease/chronic infantile neurologic cutaneous and articular syndrome; TRAPS = tumor necrosis factor receptor–associated periodic syndrome.

TREATMENT Rx

The mainstay of therapy for FMF is daily oral colchicine, which can prevent both acute attacks of FMF and the development of systemic amyloidosis. Colchicine probably works by several mechanisms, including its effects on inhibiting leukocyte adhesion and modulating cytokine production. In adults, the therapeutic dose is 1.2 to 1.8 mg/day, and nearly 90% of patients note significant improvement at this dose. The major side effects are gastrointestinal, and they can usually be minimized by gradually increasing the dosage and avoiding milk products in patients who develop lactose intolerance. Most experts continue to prescribe colchicine to patients during pregnancy, with the recommendation that amniocentesis be performed to exclude trisomy 21, for which there may be a slightly increased risk. Use of colchicine in lactating women is considered safe. Intravenous colchicine should be used with extreme caution, if at all, in FMF, because fatal toxicity has been reported in patients already receiving oral colchicine who are given the drug intravenously. IL-1 inhibitors[9] may be effective in patients who are poorly responsive to colchicine or who cannot tolerate therapeutic doses.

Tumor Necrosis Factor Receptor–Associated Periodic Syndrome

DEFINITION

Worldwide, the tumor necrosis factor (TNF) receptor–associated periodic syndrome (TRAPS) is the second most frequently diagnosed hereditary recurrent fever syndrome, behind FMF. TRAPS is defined by recurrent episodes of fever and localized inflammation, in many ways resembling FMF, but differing in key details (noted later) and caused by mutations in the 55-kD receptor for TNF (TNFRSF1A, TNFR1, p55, CD120a). Whereas a positive genetic test is not necessary to diagnose FMF, the diagnosis of TRAPS requires the identification of a TNF receptor mutation. One of the first well-characterized families with what was later defined as TRAPS was of Irish ancestry, and the condition was termed *familial Hibernian fever* to emphasize

the ethnic background and clinical differences from FMF. However, with the discovery of TNF receptor mutations in families of other ancestries, the ethnically neutral TRAPS nomenclature was proposed.

PATHOBIOLOGY

The p55 TNF receptor is composed of four cysteine-rich extracellular domains, a transmembrane region, and an intracellular death domain. To date, nearly all of the more than 90 mutations described are in the extracellular domains and approximately one third are missense substitutions of cysteine residues that abolish highly conserved disulfide bonds. The initial description of TRAPS documented a defect in activation-induced ectodomain cleavage of the p55 receptor in patients with the C52F *TNFRSF1A* mutation, possibly leading to a defect in homeostasis by impaired downregulation of membrane receptors and diminished shedding of potentially antagonistic soluble receptor molecules. More recent studies indicate a more complex pathogenetic picture, because not all mutant receptors exhibit this shedding defect. Additional mechanisms by which p55 mutations may lead to autoinflammation include impaired leukocyte apoptosis and impaired intracellular receptor trafficking, with possible constitutive activation of mitogen-activated protein (MAP) kinases by intracellular aggregates of mutant receptors.[10]

DIAGNOSIS

Although genetic testing is necessary for the diagnosis of TRAPS, certain clinical clues can help distinguish TRAPS from FMF. These include ethnicity (FMF is seen predominantly in Mediterranean and Middle Eastern populations, whereas TRAPS has a more widespread distribution), mode of inheritance (autosomal recessive in FMF, dominant in TRAPS), and duration of attacks, which tends to be longer in TRAPS and sometimes approaches continuous symptoms. The rash of FMF is typically erysipeloid erythema on the lower extremity, whereas patients with TRAPS often have a distinctive erythematous rash, often with underlying myalgia, which may migrate on the trunk or centrifugally on the extremities. Ocular involvement, with periorbital edema, conjunctivitis, and occasionally even uveitis, is observed in

TRAPS but not in FMF. Finally, whereas colchicine is much more effective than corticosteroids in FMF, the opposite is true in TRAPS. Nevertheless, aside from the difference in duration and susceptibility to pharmacologic intervention, the abdominal, pleural, synovial, and even scrotal manifestations of the two diseases are rather similar. The usual age of onset for TRAPS is also in childhood, and systemic AA amyloidosis is seen in approximately 10% of untreated patients with TRAPS. As in FMF, life expectancy in TRAPS is normal in patients whose disease is not complicated by amyloidosis.

As noted earlier, the diagnosis of TRAPS is established by the identification of *TNFRSF1A* mutations in the appropriate clinical setting. One variant, the substitution of glutamine for arginine at residue 92 (R92Q), is present in more than 1% of whites and may be associated with a broader spectrum of symptoms than is typically seen in TRAPS, including early inflammatory arthritis or, in some cases, no symptoms at all. The substitution of lysine for proline at residue 46 (P46L) is common among African American patients with TRAPS and is associated with a receptor shedding defect, but it is also seen among healthy African American controls. These findings establish a "gray zone" for the diagnosis of TRAPS and emphasize the potential role of polymorphisms in the recurrent fever genes in other more common phenotypes.

TREATMENT   Rx

The treatment of TRAPS depends on the frequency and severity of attacks. Patients with relatively infrequent, mild episodes may respond to nonsteroidal anti-inflammatory drugs (NSAIDs). Patients with more severe attacks that occur infrequently may be treated with corticosteroids, although increasing doses may be required as the episodes become more frequent and toxicities may become limiting. For patients with severe attacks occurring once a month or more frequently, treatment with etanercept, the soluble p75 TNF receptor:Fc fusion protein, may be warranted. This may be a unique effect of etanercept, because there is anecdotal evidence that monoclonal antibodies against TNF may actually exacerbate TRAPS. Consistent with a model implicating multiple cytokines in the pathogenesis of TRAPS, IL-1 inhibitors have also been found effective in TRAPS.[11]

INTERLEUKIN-1–ASSOCIATED AUTOINFLAMMATORY DISEASES

The IL-1–associated autoinflammatory diseases are linked by markedly increased expression or cellular responsiveness to this cytokine, and dramatic resolution of symptoms with IL-1 blockade. Interleukin-1α and Interleukin-1β (IL-1α and IL-1β) are structurally related cytokines released from cells triggered by a number of inflammatory stimuli, such as lipopolysaccharide. They mediate inflammatory responses by binding to a common receptor that is present on the surface of a wide variety of cell types and signals to activate inflammatory genes through the nuclear factor kappa B (NF-κB) transcription factor complex. IL-1 is part of a larger family of cytokines including IL-18, IL-33, and IL-36, which bind to related receptors and share the property of not having a characteristic signal peptide that normally targets cytokines to secretory vesicles. Because of this, IL-1 family cytokines may be secreted only by dead or dying cells, functioning as molecular markers of cellular stress, which can trigger beneficial inflammatory responses to infection and injury. IL-1β and IL-18 are unique in that they are not biologically active until cleaved by the protease caspase-1. Caspase-1 is itself activated in cytoplasmic protein complexes containing various sensor proteins such as NLRP3, and the adapter protein ASC. These complexes are referred to as *inflammasomes* because of their ability to trigger IL-1–mediated inflammation. Autoinflammatory diseases caused by mutations in genes encoding proteins that process or sense IL-1 are described later.

Cryopyrin-Associated Periodic Syndromes: The Cryopyrinopathies

Three rare, recurrent febrile disorders usually beginning early in life have been associated with mutations in *NLRP3* (formerly *CIAS1*), the gene encoding a protein variously named cryopyrin, NLRP3, NALP3, PYPAF1, or CATER-PILLER 1.1, a key component of the NLRP3 inflammasome that activates caspase-1. These disorders are referred to as cryopyrinopathies or cryopyrin-associated periodic syndromes (CAPS). The least severe clinical phenotype is familial cold autoinflammatory syndrome (FCAS; formerly called familial cold urticaria), which is dominantly inherited and is notable for day-long attacks of chills, fever, headache, diffuse urticarial skin rash, arthralgia, and

conjunctivitis, precipitated by generalized cold exposure. Amyloidosis is rare in FCAS. Of intermediate severity is Muckle-Wells syndrome (MWS), also dominantly inherited, in which 1- to 2-day episodes of chills, fever, urticarial rash, limb pain, and arthritis occur independently of cold exposure. Sensorineural hearing loss is common in MWS, and systemic amyloidosis also may occur. The most severe *NLRP3*-associated phenotype is neonatal-onset multisystem inflammatory disease (NOMID), known in Europe as chronic infantile neurologic cutaneous and articular (CINCA) syndrome. It is usually sporadic owing to the reduced reproductive fitness of most affected individuals. Fever and constitutional symptoms occur almost daily, often from birth, with generalized urticarial skin rash, a peculiar arthropathy characterized by epiphyseal overgrowth of the long bones, and central nervous system (CNS) involvement that includes chronic aseptic meningitis, uveitis, and cochlear inflammation, which may lead to intellectual disability, blindness, and deafness. In all three cryopyrinopathies, the rash is not true urticaria because there is a neutrophilic rather than a mast cell infiltrate and serum histamine levels are normal.

The protein mutated in all three disorders is NLRP3, a critical component of the eponymous NLRP3 inflammasome, which serves as an intracellular scaffold for the processing of IL-1β. The alternative name of this protein, cryopyrin, refers to its aminoterminal PYRIN domain, the basis for a structural and functional relationship to the protein mutated in FMF. Disease-associated cryopyrin mutations are thought to decrease the threshold for inflammasome activation, thereby increasing IL-1β production. The discovery that the NLRP3 inflammasome is also necessary for IL-1β production in response to crystalline forms of monosodium urate and calcium pyrophosphate connected the pathophysiology of these rare autoinflammatory diseases to crystal-induced arthritis (Chapter 273), which shares some clinical features, such as episodic, self-limited attacks, with autoinflammatory diseases.

Because there are patients with FCAS, MWS, and NOMID/CINCA without demonstrable *NLRP3* mutations, these diagnoses remain clinical, although genetic testing serves as a valuable adjunct and has greatly increased the recognition of all three conditions. Deep sequencing has identified somatic *NLRP3* mutations in some patients with symptoms consistent with CAPS who are negative for mutations by standard genetic testing. In addition, overlap syndromes that are intermediate between FCAS and MWS and between MWS and NOMID/CINCA have been reported.

TREATMENT   Rx

Blockade with anakinra, a recombinant IL-1 receptor antagonist, is effective in controlling fever and acute phase reactants in all three cryopyrinopathies, and longitudinal analysis of a large series of patients at the National Institutes of Health showed that long-term treatment with anakinra markedly decreased CNS inflammation and end-organ damage in NOMID/CINCA, which led to the regulatory approval of anakinra for the treatment of this condition in the United States and Europe. Recent studies have also documented the efficacy of rilonacept, another soluble IL-1 blocker, and canakinumab, a monoclonal antibody against IL-1β, in FCAS and MWS, although these agents may be less effective against NOMID/CINCA because of reduced penetration into the CNS. The efficacy of canakinumab suggests that the major biologic effect of cryopyrin in humans is mediated through IL-1β rather than by IL-1α or other distinct inflammatory pathways.

Deficiency of Interleukin-1 Receptor Antagonist

Deficiency of the IL-1 receptor antagonist (DIRA) is characterized by the neonatal onset of a pustular skin rash, multifocal osteomyelitis, periostitis, and, rarely, vasculitis.[12] Fever is not a prominent finding, although acute phase reactants are markedly elevated. DIRA is caused by recessively inherited loss-of-function mutations in *IL1RN*, which encodes the IL-1 receptor antagonist (IL-1Ra). Patients usually present within the first 2 weeks of life with skin lesions ranging from discrete crops of pustules to generalized severe pustulosis or ichthyosiform lesions. Histologic examination demonstrates extensive neutrophilic infiltrates in the dermis and epidermis. Typical radiographic findings include multifocal osteolytic lesions, periosteal elevation of the long bones, heterotopic ossification of the proximal femurs, and widening of the anterior rib ends. Bone biopsies demonstrate sterile purulent osteomyelitis, fibrosis, and sclerosis. To date, five different *IL1RN* mutations have been identified, three of which are truncating point mutations that drastically reduce IL-1Ra messenger RNA and protein levels. The fourth is a 15bp in-frame deletion, and the fifth is a 175-kilobase genomic deletion in chromosome 2q that subsumes *IL1RN* and five other genes in the IL-1 family. In DIRA, the lack of IL-1Ra leads to unopposed IL-1β and IL-1α signaling, whereas in the cryopyrinopathies, *NLRP3* mutations lead to inflammasome activation and increased IL-1β production. DIRA patients respond dramatically to anakinra, a recombinant form of the protein they lack.

OTHER INHERITED SYSTEMIC AUTOINFLAMMATORY DISEASES

Syndrome of Pyogenic Arthritis with Pyoderma Gangrenosum and Acne

The syndrome of pyogenic arthritis with pyoderma gangrenosum and acne (PAPA) is a rare, dominantly inherited autoinflammatory disease characterized by intermittent episodes of sterile pyogenic arthritis, pyoderma gangrenosum, and severe cystic acne. It is caused by mutations in proline-serine-threonine phosphatase–interacting protein 1 (PSTPIP1), also known as CD2BP1. PSTPIP1 is a cytoskeletal protein that interacts with certain other proteins involved in the immune response, including CD2; the Wiskott-Aldrich syndrome protein (WASP); a phosphatase denoted PTP-PEST; and pyrin, the FMF protein. PAPA mutations abrogate the binding of PSTPIP1 to PTP-PEST, leading to hyperphosphorylation of PSTPIP1 and increased binding to pyrin. Both in patients and in cell lines, this finding is associated with markedly increased IL-1β production. Early in life, PAPA tends to present with monoarticular or pauciarticular pyogenic arthritis, sometimes induced by trauma. In the absence of treatment, arthritis may progress to severe joint damage and ankylosis. As patients reach puberty, skin manifestations begin to predominate, including disfiguring cystic acne. Pathergy also may develop, and extensive pyoderma gangrenosum may require opiates for pain control. The diagnosis of PAPA syndrome is made by documenting *PSTPIP1* mutations in the appropriate clinical setting. High doses of corticosteroids have been used in PAPA, with varying success, and patients with arthritis sometimes require aspiration, intra-articular corticosteroids, or open drainage. Newer investigational approaches for PAPA syndrome focus on the use of targeted cytokine inhibitors. Anecdotal evidence supports the use of anakinra for the arthritis and monoclonal anti-TNF antibodies for the pyoderma gangrenosum of PAPA.

Granulomatous Inflammatory Arthritis, Dermatitis, and Uveitis (Blau's Syndrome)

Blau's syndrome is a rare, dominantly inherited illness characterized by the following features: early-onset granulomatous synovitis often complicated by cyst formation and camptodactyly (flexion contractures of the fingers and toes); granulomatous anterior and posterior uveitis, sometimes causing retinal detachment, glaucoma, cataracts, and blindness; and an intermittent papular rash with noncaseating granulomas. Lung or other visceral involvement is generally not present. However, visceral involvement of the liver and spleen is observed in early-onset sarcoidosis (Chapter 95), which is phenotypically quite similar to Blau's syndrome. Both Blau's syndrome and some cases of early-onset sarcoidosis are caused by mutations in *NOD2/CARD15*. Distinct variants of *NOD2/CARD15* have been associated with susceptibility to Crohn's disease, which manifests as granulomatous inflammation of the gastrointestinal tract (Chapter 141). The protein encoded by this gene is thought to be an intracellular sensor of bacterial products. Crohn's disease–associated mutations in the ligand-binding, leucine-rich repeat region of the protein may alter responses to bacterial products in the gastrointestinal tract to cause inflammation, whereas Blau's syndrome mutations in the nucleotide binding domain may lead to constitutive extraintestinal inflammation. Topical and systemic corticosteroids are currently the mainstay of treatment of Blau's syndrome. There are case reports of the efficacy of TNF and IL-1 inhibitors in this disease.

Hyperimmunoglobulinemia D with Periodic Fever Syndrome

Hyperimmunoglobulinemia D with periodic fever syndrome (HIDS) was first described in 1984 as an FMF-like illness seen in six patients of Dutch ancestry. Besides the difference in ethnicity, a key distinction was the observation of extremely high levels of immunoglobulin D (IgD) in the serum of these patients, thus prompting the HIDS nomenclature. HIDS is now recognized in a broader ethnic distribution, although northern Europeans still predominate. Overall, HIDS is still quite rare. Family studies documented autosomal recessive inheritance. In 1999, patients with HIDS were found to have mutations in *MVK*, which encodes the mevalonate kinase enzyme

involved in the biosynthesis of cholesterol and nonsterol isoprenes. Enzyme activity in patients is markedly reduced, but not absent. The elevated immunoglobulin D (IgD) levels seen in HIDS appear to be an epiphenomenon and do not correlate with disease severity either among patients or in a given patient over time, although IgD may contribute to the release of proinflammatory cytokines in vitro. Moreover, modest elevations of IgD are seen in several inflammatory conditions, including chronic infections, and can be observed in other hereditary recurrent fever syndromes. Up to 20% of patients (particularly young children) with typical recurrent fevers and *MVK* mutations have normal serum IgD levels. Current data suggest that isoprenoid deficiency may play a more important pathogenic role in the pathophysiology of HIDS. In vitro studies suggest that isoprenoid deficiency may lead to excessive IL-1β production, and increased body temperature can further decrease mevalonate kinase enzymatic activity, thereby creating a vicious circle in which infection or immunization can precipitate HIDS attacks. One of the well-recognized clinical characteristics of HIDS is the provocation of attacks by immunizations. Other distinguishing clinical features include a very early age of onset (average age, 6 months), a duration of attacks intermediate between FMF and TRAPS (3 to 7 days), prominent cervical lymphadenopathy during attacks, polyarticular joint involvement, a diffuse maculopapular rash, the predominance of diarrhea over constipation with abdominal attacks, and the infrequency of pleuritic attacks or systemic amyloidosis.

The diagnosis of HIDS can be established in a patient with recurrent episodes of fever and typical associated findings by documenting either two mutations in *MVK* or elevated levels of mevalonic acid, the substrate for mevalonate kinase, in the urine during attacks. Approximately 10% of patients with otherwise typical disease have only a single identifiable *MVK* mutation. The significance of elevated IgD without genetic or biochemical findings remains unknown. NSAIDs or corticosteroids are sometimes useful in the treatment of the arthritic manifestations of HIDS. Colchicine is generally not effective. Numerous agents are investigational in HIDS, including the statins, TNF inhibitors, and IL-1 inhibitors. Patients with HIDS have a normal lifespan, and attacks may become somewhat less frequent in adulthood.

Proteasome-Associated Systemic Inflammatory Diseases

Recently, a constellation of diseases have been described linked to recessive loss of function mutations in *PSMB8*, which encodes the β5i subunit of the proteasome, also known as LMP7. An autosomal recessive syndrome in adults characterized by recurrent fevers, progressive lipodystrophy, joint contractures, and cardiac manifestations was linked to homozygous missense mutations in *PSMB8*.[13] Patients with a pediatric syndrome termed CANDLE (chronic atypical neutrophilic dermatosis with lipodystrophy and elevated temperature) were found to have homozygous missense and nonsense mutations in *PSMB8*, with some patients having only one known *PSMB8* mutation. It is not yet clear whether these syndromes represent identical diseases related to loss of function of β5i. The β5i proteasome subunit is one of the subunits that that are induced in immune cells through immune stimuli such as interferons, altering the proteasome so that it more efficiently processes peptides for antigen presentation to T cells. However, there is no indication of a T cell component to this disease, and studies have shown that the β5i proteasome subunit can be expressed in nonimmune cells such as adipocytes. A striking interferon transcriptional signature, similar to that seen in systemic lupus erythematosus, was observed in circulating blood cells from patients with CANDLE. Defective degradation of proteins in cells lacking β5i may result in buildup of ubiquitinated proteins, which somehow triggers interferon production, or PSMB8 deficiency may enhance interferon signaling by stabilizing components of the interferon signal transduction machinery that are negatively regulated by ubiquitin-proteasome degradation. Whichever the mechanisms, the link to interferon hyperactivity suggests that blocking interferons with antibodies or inhibitors of interferon signal transcution may be effective in the therapy of CANDLE and possibly other PSMB8-associated syndromes.

New Autoinflammatory Syndromes and the Promise of Whole-Exome Sequencing

Recent years have seen a dramatic acceleration in the pace of discovery of new mendelian inflammatory diseases as a result of the availability of whole-exome sequencing, which allows unbiased identification of disease-causing mutations in protein coding sequences, although it should be noted that accurate clinical description of these syndromes is as important as the genetic tools for identification of new syndromes. These discoveries have confirmed the role of gene products in human inflammation that were identified in other animal model systems and identified new genes and proteins not previously thought to be involved in the regulation of inflammation. Early-onset, apparently sporadic, cases of inflammatory syndromes have often turned out to be due to de novo mutations in a child when screened against parental DNA. For example, inherited gain-of-function mutations in *CARD14,* encoding an adapter protein in innate immune sensing, cause dominantly inherited familial psoriasis, and a more severe gain-of-function de novo mutation in the same gene caused infantile-onset severe pustular psoriasis. Recessive mutations causing systemic autoinflammatory disease also have been identified by whole-exome sequencing from just a few families. Recent examples of novel diseases discovered through these methods include a syndrome characterized by fevers, early-onset strokes, and vasculopathy or frank vasculitis caused by autosomal recessive mutations in *CECR1,* encoding adenosine deaminase 2 (ADA2), a serum protein with newly recognized effects on macrophage differentiation and vascular development.[14] Recessive mutations in *HOIL1* that impair the addition of linear ubiquitin chains to receptor signaling complexes cause a complex syndrome marked by autoinflammation and immunodeficiency and intramuscular glycogen deposition. Gain-of-function mutations in *PLCG2,* encoding phospholipase Cγ2, an enzyme with essential functions in B-cell receptor and Fc Rceptor signaling, cause a dominantly inherited autoinflammatory syndrome characterized by blistering skin lesions, bronchiolitis, arthralgia, ocular inflammation, and enterocolitis in the absence of autoantibodies.

GENERAL REFERENCES

For the General References and other additional features, please visit Expert Consult at https://expertconsult.inkling.com.

262

OSTEOARTHRITIS

JOEL A. BLOCK AND CARLA SCANZELLO

DEFINITION

Osteoarthritis (OA) is a heterogeneous disease that has many names, including degenerative joint disease and osteoarthrosis. It is a joint disease characterized clinically by pain and functional loss. Although local inflammation of involved joints is common, OA is not associated with a systemic inflammatory process, in contrast to other arthritides. It is the most common form of arthritis and accounts for the overwhelming majority of arthritis cases, and its prevalence is expected to rise dramatically during the next 20 years as global populations age. OA is often neglected either because it is not a fatal disease or because many physicians assume it is a normal part of aging and is not inherently treatable. Yet it results in vast direct medical costs and significant loss of work; it is the leading indication for total joint replacement and is a leading cause of work disability. Formal definitions of OA have evolved as our understanding of pathophysiology has progressed. Whereas it conventionally had been considered primarily a degenerative process of cartilage, it is now clear that OA involves the entire joint. Thus, a modern definition of OA is a *painful* degenerative process involving progressive deterioration of all joint structures and remodeling of subchondral bone that is not primarily inflammatory. It is important to distinguish true OA from asymptomatic structural degeneration of joints that is virtually universal during normal aging.

EPIDEMIOLOGY

As an age-related disease, OA prevalence has risen substantially with the aging population of the developed world; an estimated 27 million people had physician-diagnosed OA in the United States in 2005, increased from 21 million a decade earlier, and this number is expected to reach 67 million patients with clinically significant OA by 2030. For epidemiologic studies, OA is often defined radiographically by the presence of osteophytes, joint space narrowing, and subchondral sclerosis. However, a substantial number

of individuals have these x-ray changes but remain clinically asymptomatic. Thus, estimates of OA prevalence vary widely depending on whether one is assessing *radiographic* or *symptomatic* OA. In either case, the lifetime risk is exceedingly high. There is general concordance among epidemiologic studies across North American, Asian, and European populations that the prevalence of radiographic OA in the knees, hips, and hands is quite low before age 45 and increases dramatically with aging, with most people having x-ray evidence of OA in at least one joint by the seventh decade. Symptomatic knee OA affects between 7% and 17% of those older than 44 years, with rates increasing with age; women have higher prevalence than men, and African Americans have higher prevalence than white Americans. Symptomatic hip OA is less prevalent than knee OA, with overall rates between 6.7% and 9.7% among those over age 44; as with knee OA, prevalence is higher among the elderly, women, and African Americans.[1] Symptomatic hand OA affects at least 6.8% of those older than 25, occurring in women more than two-fold more frequently than in men. Hand OA may be less common in African Americans than in white Americans.

Risk factors for the development of OA and for specific joint involvement have been extensively studied. Among nonmodifiable risk factors, the strongest is aging. This is true both for radiographic changes of OA and for symptomatic involvement. In addition, female sex is a risk for prevalence and severity of OA, especially after menopause. There is a significant heritable component, particularly for hand OA and hip OA. This component is estimated at 48 to 65% for so-called generalized OA characterized by osteophytes of the distal interphalangeal joints (Heberden nodes) or the proximal interphalangeal joints (Bouchard's nodes).

Modifiable OA risk factors may provide clues for preventive strategies. The most important of these is obesity, which alone confers an approximately three-fold increased risk for incident OA. Occupational and lifestyle activities that involve repeated trauma or excessive loading may be associated with increased risk for OA. These include chronic squatting, bending, and lifting such as by warehouse workers and laborers, who have increased knee involvement, and, classically, pneumatic drill operators who develop OA of the wrist and elbow. Significant trauma, such as major knee or ankle injury, is strongly associated with subsequent development of OA in the injured joint. Aberrant loading of joints is an important risk factor for the development and progression of OA. For example, excessive loading of the knee has been observed to result in significantly increased risk for progression to advanced knee OA. In addition, joint alignment is an important parameter in OA, and malalignment at the knee is among the strongest predictors of OA progression.[2]

PATHOBIOLOGY

Although degeneration of articular cartilage is a central common pathway in OA, multiple joint and periarticular tissues are compromised and contribute to clinical manifestations. Pathologic changes in synovium, ligaments, supporting musculature, and fibrocartilagenous structures such as the menisci in the knee are common.[3] Unlike autoimmune arthritides, OA does not affect extra-articular organs. However, the chronic pain of OA involves both the peripheral and central nervous system (CNS) and OA-related disability degrades the general physical and mental health of the patient. Appreciation of the global effects of OA has important implications for current and future treatment approaches.

Tissues Central to the Osteoarthritis Process
Cartilage
The hallmark of osteoarthritis is progressive deterioration of articular cartilage. Normal articular cartilage distributes loads across joint surfaces and allows for almost frictionless joint motion. These functions are furnished by the extracellular matrix, which accounts for more than 90% of the tissue volume and is organized by a network of collagen type II fibers, which provides tensile strength, entrapping aggrecan complexes, a proteoglycan that confers compressive stiffness and resilience (Fig. 262-1A and C). There is one major cell type, the chondrocyte, that synthesizes these matrix components. In mature cartilage, turnover of extracellular matrix molecules, particularly collagen type II, is slow.

Cartilage change in OA begins with swelling of the matrix, then progresses through stages of surface roughening, fibrillation, fissuring, and eventually full-thickness erosion. These are accompanied by activation of chondrocytes to increase synthesis of proteolytic enzymes that degrade matrix.[4] Matrix metalloproteinase-13 (MMP-13; collagenase-3) plays a central role in collagen type II degradation, while ADAMTS-4 and -5 (a disintegrin and metalloproteinase with thrombospondin motifs-4 and -5) proteases are important

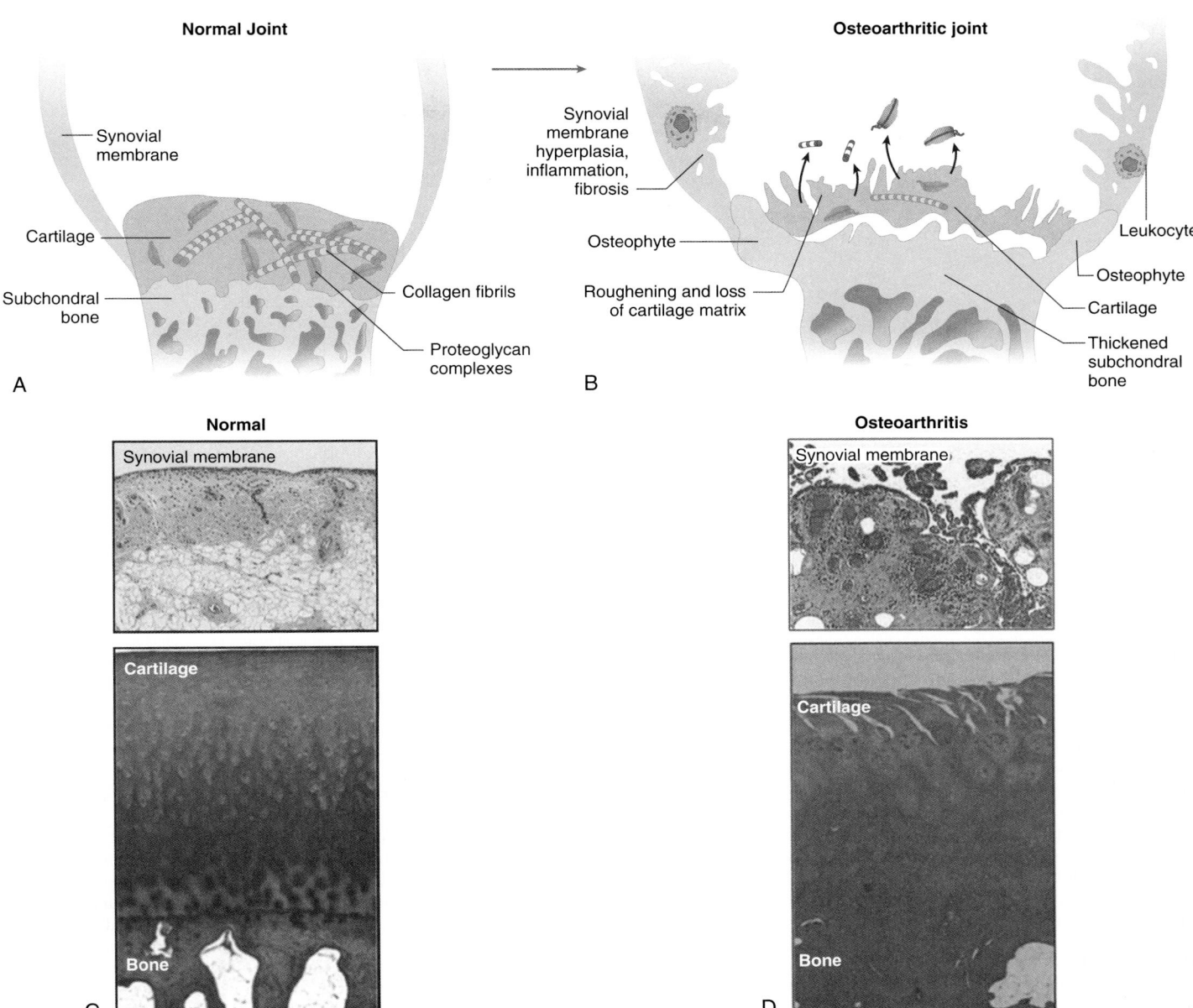

FIGURE 262-1. Pathologic features of osteoarthritic joint tissues. A, Features of a normal adult synovial joint. Healthy adult articular cartilage is characterized by a smooth surface and extracellular matrix (ECM) composed of a collagen type II fibrillar network and large proteoglycan complexes. The ECM is produced and maintained by the cellular components of cartilage, chondrocytes. The subchondral bone consists of a thin cortical layer and underlying trabecular bone. The synovial membrane lines the joint capsule and attaches at the cartilage-bone interface. In the normal state, it consists of a lining layer 1 or 2 cells thick, with underlying vascularized loose connective tissue. B, Typical changes to tissues seen in osteoarthritis (OA). Enzymatic activities (ADAMTS-4,5 and MMP-13 in particular) cleave proteoglycan and collagen components of the ECM, leading to loss of these molecules from the matrix. As the process advances, the articular cartilage thins and fibrillates and eventually fissures down to the underlying bone. Simultaneously, a remodeling response in the bone is observed. Thickening of the cortical subchondral bone layer occurs, and new bone growth at the margins appears as osteophytes. The synovial membrane changes observed in OA patients include lining layer hyperplasia, inflammation in the form of leukocyte infiltration, and fibrosis which can be seen to varying degrees. Photomicrographs of human joint tissues showing these features are depicted in C (normal tissues) and D (OA tissues). (C and D courtesy of Edward F. DiCarlo, MD. Hospital for Special Surgery, New York, NY).

for loss of aggrecan, but other enzymes participate (see Fig. 262-1B and D). Concomitantly, the activated chondrocytes proliferate to form clonal clusters and produce inflammatory mediators, including interleukin-1α and β, (IL-1α and IL-1β), IL-6, tumor necrosis factor-α (TNF-α) and nitric oxide (NO), which accelerate the degradative cycle and stimulate chondrocyte apoptosis. Thus, both cellular *and* molecular components of cartilage are lost as the process progresses.[5]

Bone
The cortical bone underlying articular cartilage (subchondral bone) supports load-bearing and transmits mechanical signals to articular chondrocytes. In OA, there is increased remodeling, likely in response to abnormal biome-

chanical loading. This may result in thinning (attrition) and reduced bone density, leading to subchondral cyst formation in early disease, but progresses to subchondral sclerosis as bone formation outpaces resorption (see Fig. 262-1B and D).[6] Remodeling at joint margins and entheses results in osteophytes (bone spurs). An important role for the growth factors transforming growth factor-β (TGF-β) and bone morphogenetic protein-2 (BMP-2) in driving osteophyte formation has been demonstrated in animal models.

Synovium
Synovial involvement in OA is more variable than in rheumatoid arthritis, but low-grade synovitis, characterized by infiltration of macrophages and lymphocytes, increased vascularity, synovial lining hyperplasia, and fibrosis,

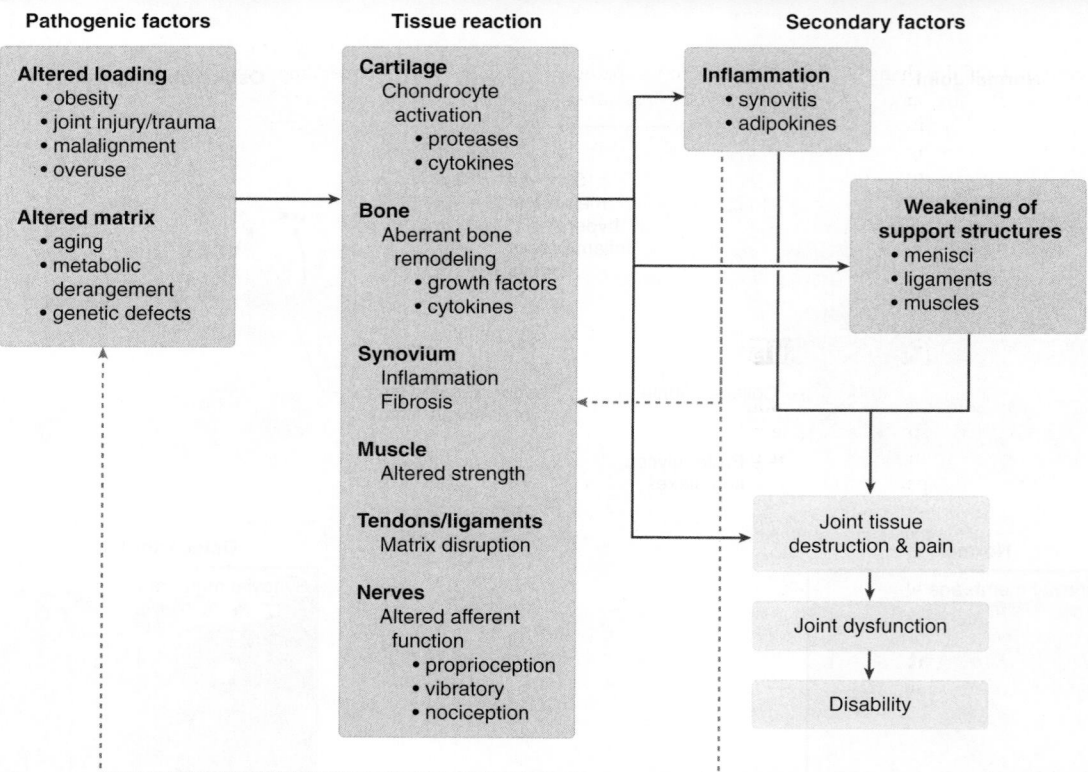

FIGURE 262-2. Schematic of the pathophysiology of osteoarthritis. A variety of stimuli can alter biomechanical loading patterns of joint tissues or exert biologic pressure on the extracellular matrix. These result in specific responses in the various joint tissues. Aided by secondary factors, these lead to tissue degeneration, pain, and ultimately joint dysfunction.

is common and occurs in up to 75% of patients (see Fig. 262-1B and D). Although this synovial reaction is likely a secondary response to molecular breakdown products present in the OA joint, it results in release of cytokines (e.g., IL-6, TNF-α), chemokines (IL-8, monocyte chemoattractant protein 1 [MCP-1], C-C motif chemokine 19 [CCL19]), enzymatic mediators of cartilage catabolism, and growth factors involved in bone remodeling, and when present it is associated with more severe symptoms and possibly more rapid progression of cartilage degradation.[7]

Menisci and Ligaments

Traumatic and athletic injuries to the menisci and ligaments are known risk factors for incident OA. However, meniscal and ligamentous abnormalities are common in patients with OA even without injury and are detectable in 80% and 30% (respectively) of patients undergoing magnetic resonance imaging (MRI). These structures are sensitive to the same inflammatory and enzymatic mediators that promote cartilage deterioration in OA, and their compromise promotes degenerative injuries, accelerated cartilage erosion, joint instability, and mechanical symptoms (i.e., locking or catching).

Muscles

Periarticular muscle weakness and atrophy are characteristic of hip and knee OA. Such weakness is associated with altered gait kinematics and pathologic joint loading, but it remains unclear whether this is a cause or an effect of OA.

Peripheral and Central Nervous System

Somatosensory deficits associated with neuromuscular function, including proprioceptive and widespread vibratory deficits, have been described.[8] Also, patients with OA exhibit signs of peripheral and CNS sensitization in the form of hyperalgesia and allodynia. Inflammatory mediators (e.g., MCP-1) and growth factors (e.g., nerve growth factor [NGF]) have been implicated in pain pathways in OA.[9] Additional work is necessary to fully understand the mechanisms leading to symptomatic OA, but pain in OA is clearly multifactorial, involving the peripheral and the central nervous systems in addition to joint tissues and inflammation.

Pathogenic Factors (Fig. 262-2)
Biomechanics

Aberrant loading of joints mediates evolution of structural joint degeneration and may contribute to initiation of the process. This is evident in the high risk that malalignment of the knee carries for knee OA progression. Weight-bearing regions of OA joints bear greater loads during ambulation than normal, and these loading patterns have been shown to be predictive of subsequent progression of lower extremity joint disease longitudinally. Mechanistically, abnormal biomechanical loading promotes pathologic activation of chondrocytes and bone remodeling, and may be precipitated by joint injury, congenital dysplasias, malalignment, joint instability (e.g., in the setting of aging or heritable connective tissue diseases), and abnormal neuromuscular control (e.g., neuropathic diseases), each of which is a risk factor for OA.

Metabolic Factors

Several metabolic conditions, including alkaptonuria, acromegaly, hemochromotosis, and the metabolic syndrome, among others, predispose individuals to early OA, though they have different mechanisms and disease patterns. In the metabolic syndrome, obesity increases loads on weight-bearing joints, but its association with OA of non–weight-bearing joints in the hands suggests a nonmechanical etiology as well. A possible mechanism may be related to the overproduction of adipokines, IL-6, and leptin leading to chronic low-grade systemic inflammation that may potentiate molecular deterioration of joint tissues and contribute to joint symptoms.[10]

Genetic Factors

Rare single-gene defects may lead to early or aggressive OA. Heritable defects in the collagen II gene have occasionally been described in families with chondrodysplasias, as have lubricin defects. However, variations in multiple genes are likely implicated in the majority of OA cases. Genome-wide association studies have identified polymorphisms in genes involved in proliferation, skeletal development (e.g., GDF5), and regulation of body weight associated with risk for radiographic knee and hip OA.[11] Additional polymorphisms have been associated with pain in OA (e.g., PACE4 and TRPV1).

Aging

Aging-related molecular and cellular changes likely contribute to OA pathogenesis.[12] Modifications of extracellular matrix components, such as accumulation of advanced-glycation end products, and carboxylation associated with oxidative-stress, occur with advancing age. These can alter protein folding, weaken tissues, and increase susceptibility to proteolytic cleavage. Age-related changes to chondrocytes and other cells include the "senescence-associated secretory phenotype" associated with decreased proliferative capacity but increased secretory activity that may promote abnormal chondrocyte responses to injury and aberrant loading. Nonetheless, the link between aging-related changes and symptoms remains poorly understood.

CLINICAL MANIFESTATIONS OF OSTEOARTHRITIS

Symptoms

Pain is the most prominent symptom of OA. Although often limited to affected joints, it can become widespread over time.[13] The quality of pain experienced is variable, ranging from "aching" joint pain to less localized periarticular or radiating pain. OA pain is typically worsened by joint use while stiffness is exacerbated by prolonged inactivity. Morning stiffness may occur but is brief, lasting less than 30 minutes. Other symptoms include joint instability, limitation of motion, locking, and a grinding feeling with motion. Symptom severity varies over time, but with advanced disease, pain becomes persistent and can disturb sleep.

Patterns of Joint Involvement

The joint pattern may help distinguish OA from other forms of arthritis (Fig. 262-3).

Lower Extremities

The large weight-bearing joints (knees and hips) are most commonly affected. Knee OA encompasses any of the three compartments. The medial compartment is involved in the majority of patients and may lead to varus (bow-legged) deformity. Lateral compartment OA may result in valgus (knock-kneed) deformity, and patellofemoral OA typically causes pain exacerbated by descending stairs. Meniscal or ligamentous degeneration often accompanies OA and exacerbates knee instability. Effusions, synovial (Baker's) cysts, and anserine or prepatellar bursitis may be present and cause additional pain. Hip OA often begins with restricted internal rotation and progresses to limited motion in all directions and limb length discrepancy. Pain is felt in the groin area and may radiate to the anterior thigh and knee and be confused with knee pain. It also must be differentiated from lateral thigh pain, which more likely originates from other structures (e.g., trochanteric bursa, illiotibial band, lumbar spine). In the foot, OA typically involves the first metatarsophalangeal joint, resulting in bunion deformity.

Spine

Spinal OA typically involves the lumbar and cervical regions, affecting the apophyseal (facet) and uncovertebral (joints of Luschka) joints. Low-grade inflammation and bone remodeling can lead to local pain, and nerve root compression by osteophytes causes radicular, radiating pain. Degenerative disc disease often coexists with spinal OA, and together they contribute to spinal stenosis causing muscle weakness, paresthesias, and numbness. In severe cases, cord impingement with myelopathy may result.

Upper Extremities

The small joints of the hands are most commonly affected, specifically the distal and proximal interphalangeal joints (DIPs and PIPs) and first carpometacarpal (CMC) joints. Osteophytosis of DIPs and PIPs leads to bony, palpable Heberden and Bouchard nodes, respectively. This pattern is more common in white women and is termed *primary generalized OA*. Patients may experience difficulty grasping, opening jars, buttoning clothes, and turning doorknobs. Erosive or inflammatory OA is a less common but distinct subset in which erosions develop in the DIPs and PIPs, and the patient experiences repeated episodes of acute inflammatory symptoms.

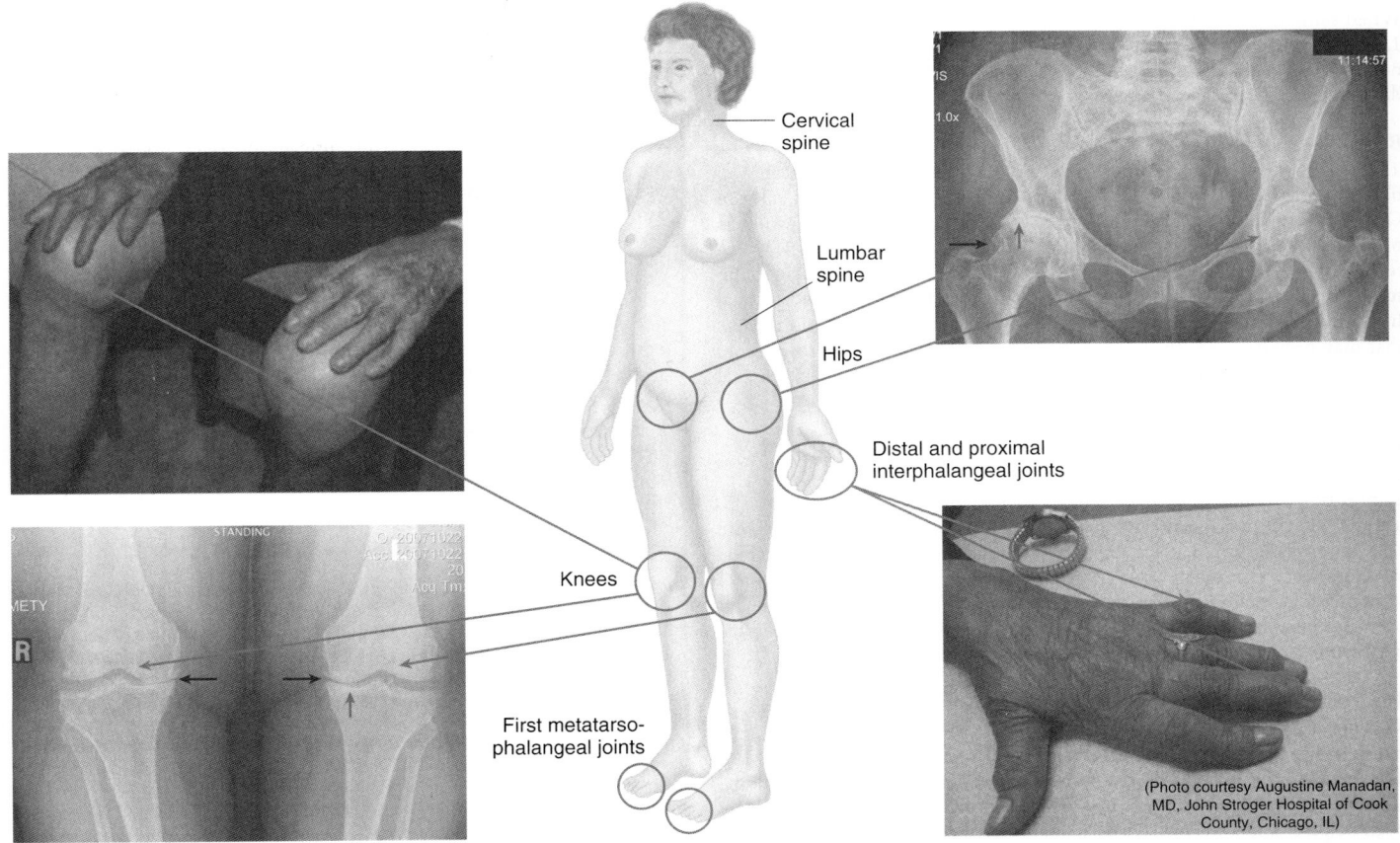

FIGURE 262-3. Commonly affected joints in osteoarthritis. Joints in which symptomatic osteoarthritis typically develops are depicted in the whole-body drawing in the center. The distal and proximal interphalangeal joints of the hands characteristically exhibit palpable bony bumps (*right lower panel*). Synovial effusions and bony outgrowths, or osteophytes, may be visualized in the knee (*left upper panel*), and radiographic involvement of the knee (*left lower panel*) or of the hip (*right upper panel*) shows characteristic features of joint space narrowing, osteophytes (*black arrows*), and subchondral sclerosis (*blue arrows*).

DIAGNOSIS

The diagnosis of OA depends primarily on the clinical presentation; unlike other rheumatic diseases, imaging and laboratory analysis have relatively small roles in diagnosis. Because OA primarily affects tissues of the joint and does not involve systemic inflammation, laboratory tests are more useful for excluding competing diagnoses than for establishing an OA diagnosis.

Physical Examination

When cartilage surfaces become roughened, crepitus (palpable or audible crackling) may be detected by physical examination. As cartilage is further compromised, small fragments can dislodge and, if sufficiently large, may restrict joint motion and cause locking.

Osteophytes can be palpated in superficial joints as bony projections and may result in deformities. Their growth is sometimes inflammatory, with erythema, tenderness, and swelling. Heberden and Bouchard nodes of the DIP and PIP joints, respectively, are typical, but squaring of the first CMC joint and palpable knee osteophytes are also common. These deformities may eventually restrict joint range of motion. Classically, severe joint inflammation is not appreciated; however, effusions are common and may cause mild joint warmth.

Laboratory Evaluation

Blood Tests

OA is limited to joints; thus, tests of systemic inflammation and those that assess critical organ function are generally normal. These include the sedimentation rate, conventional C-reactive protein, and other acute phase reactants, as well as the blood count and the comprehensive metabolic panel. Nonetheless, OA is prevalent among the elderly and concomitant diseases may confound the interpretation of laboratory testing. Tests for autoantibodies are unremarkable, though low-titer detection of nonspecific rheumatoid factors and antinuclear antibody (ANA) may be seen in the normal aging population.

Synovial Fluid

When sampled, synovial fluid total leukocyte counts are typically less than 1500 to 2000 cells/mm^3 with a predominance of lymphocytes rather than neutrophils. Incidental findings of crystals, such as calcium pyrophosphate dihydrate, or of cartilage fragments may sometimes be observed.

Biomarkers

There has been an aggressive search for macromolecules measurable in blood, synovial fluid, or urine that provide prognostic or diagnostic value in OA. A variety of macromolecules, typically breakdown or cleavage products of cartilage or bone matrix, have been identified that have a statistical correlation with OA progression or pain. The OA Initiative is an ongoing longitudinal study of several thousand individuals, spearheaded by the National Institutes of Health, to identify novel body fluid and imaging biomarkers that may provide predictive information about OA onset and progression. But no biomarkers have yet been demonstrated to be useful for clinical evaluation.

Imaging

Radiography

Conventional radiography is the mainstay for imaging OA. Characteristic features include narrowed joint space, osteophytes, and subchondral bone sclerosis (see Fig. 262-3). Not all patients have all three features, and there is an imperfect relationship between radiographic appearance and clinical symptoms. Disease progression can be monitored by longitudinal imaging, both by qualitative grading and by quantitative assessment of joint space narrowing.

Magnetic Resonance Imaging

MRI provides the most detailed images of joint structures and, in contrast to radiography, detects subtle defects of articular cartilage.[14] In addition, MRI detects subchondral bone marrow lesions that are associated with symptomatic disease. MRI remains predominantly a research tool in OA, where it has been helpful in identifying soft tissue pathologic conditions and measuring early cartilage pathology; clinically, it has little role in routine OA evaluation and management. MRI is often used in OA to exclude other potential sources of pain, such as degenerative menisci, ligamentous tears, and other intraarticular pathology.

Ultrasonography

Although operator dependent, careful ultrasonography reveals outstanding details of joint structure and does not expose the patient to ionizing radiation. It may identify osteophytes undetectable by standard radiography, and articular cartilage lesions can often be observed. Its primary use, though, may be to detect local synovitis that is prevalent in OA; it remains unclear whether it can play a significant role in diagnosis.

Radionuclide Imaging

Whereas radioisotope scanning formerly had utility in OA, it has been largely supplanted by more sensitive and specific modalities for detecting articular pathology.

TREATMENT Rx

Many physicians persist in counseling their symptomatic patients that there is nothing to be done, and that OA is an inevitable sign of "getting old." Although no interventions have been demonstrated to alter the natural history of structural joint degeneration, symptomatic OA is not inevitable, and many strategies provide relief and maintain function among those with even advanced OA.[15] Patient education and support are critical; self-help programs alone have been shown to improve outcomes in OA. Patients should be provided thorough information about the natural course of OA, their role in disease management, and appropriate expectations. In general, the goals of OA therapy are similar to the treatment of any disease—to maintain or restore function, relieve symptoms, and prevent disease progression.

Maintenance of Function

Strategies to retain function and independence in patients with OA include ambulatory assistive devices, such as canes and walkers, which provide stability in addition to reducing loading across arthritic joints. Motorized carts can assist individuals with severe knee or hip OA to retain independence in the community. Physical therapy can help to retain strength and range of motion, and occupational therapy can provide customized assist devices and braces. Whenever possible, counseling on weight loss for overweight or obese patients should be provided as weight loss can improve both pain and function.[A1]

Symptom Palliation

A variety of strategies can provide effective pain palliation in OA. These include physical measures, medical therapy, and surgical interventions.[16]

Physical Measures

Exercise is especially important in OA, both to improve function and to palliate pain.[17] Exercises aimed at strengthening muscles surrounding affected joints are of value physiologically and have been consistently demonstrated to provide significant pain relief. Patients should be encouraged to exercise regularly and may benefit from physical therapy for instruction in appropriate strength training and to improve and maintain range of motion. During painful flares and immediately after exertion, application of heat or ice to affected joints can be useful.

Pain may be mediated by aberrant biomechanical loading. Therefore, canes and walkers, which significantly reduce loads across the knee during gait, can reduce pain and improve stability. Similarly, unloading knee braces, when tolerated, may provide palliation for knee OA.

Medication

Most patients will need more pain relief than is provided by physical measures. Among the elderly, choice of medication is often influenced by comorbidities. Topical agents may reduce risk for of systemic adverse effects and are appropriate when only a few joints are symptomatic. Topical capsaicin has been approved for knee OA; its use requires frequent application and careful handwashing after contact. Topical nonsteroidal anti-inflammatory drugs (NSAIDs) are available, including salicylic acid and diclofenac.

When physical measures and topical agents are insufficient, oral analgesics are used. Many specialty organizations, including the American College of Rheumatology,[18] suggest that acetaminophen may be beneficial, especially among patients with contraindications to NSAIDs such as renal dysfunction or cardiac disease. Nonetheless, acetaminophen may not be effective for long-term analgesia and chronic use carries its own potential toxicities, including liver damage and hypertension. Therefore, acetaminophen may be most properly used for short-term flares of OA pain, typically lasting no more than a few weeks. Approved alternatives to acetaminophen include tramadol and opiates, which though demonstrated to relieve OA pain, also substantially increase morbidity among the elderly, especially the risk for traumatic falls. Finally, neuroactive agents are widely used for OA pain. One such medication, duloxetine hydrochloride, a serotonin and norepinephrine reuptake inhibitor (SNRI), received U.S. Food and Drug Administration approval in 2010 for the treatment of musculoskeletal pain, including OA, based on positive results in clinical trials.[A2]

NSAIDs have been demonstrated to be effective for OA pain and may maintain efficacy for years.[A3] These medications remain the mainstay of OA medical therapy, but are not an option for many patients with renal, cardiac, or gastrointestinal conditions. Proton pump inhibitors or misoprostol can provide gastric protection in middle-aged and elderly patients and those at risk for gastrointestinal bleeding. Cyclooxygenase-2 inhibitors also may be used; in the United States, celecoxib is the only representative of this class available. Six weeks of low-dose oral prednisolone (7.5 mg daily) is also effective, and its benefits can persist for at least another six weeks.[A4]

Intra-articular Therapy

Intra-articular glucocorticoids may provide short-term relief of OA pain, often lasting months.[A5] Their use is limited to three or four times per year in any single joint because of theoretical concerns of toxicity to articular cartilage. A variety of hyaluronan derivatives are available for injection to relieve OA pain, but controversy exists as to whether they are more effective than placebo. Originally developed to supplement viscosity of synovial fluid in an attempt to improve articular lubrication, residence time in the joint is too brief to have this effect.

Surgical Approaches

Joint replacement surgery restores function and relives pain in the majority of patients and is the most important therapeutic advance in OA treatment to date (Chapter 276). It should be reserved for those in whom pain or joint dysfunction significantly limits normal life activities despite optimal medical and physical management. The presence of advanced structural degeneration of the joints alone, without severe symptoms, should not be an indication for arthroplasty. Knees and hips are most frequently replaced, but good results are now obtained in other joints as well. The durability of joint prostheses is limited, so joint replacement surgery should be delayed in younger patients when practical. Aside from total joint replacement, there are a variety of temporizing strategies that may be used in joints that have less severe structural degeneration, including realignment osteotomy in the knee and hemiarthroplasty.

Delay of Disease Progression

There has been extensive effort to identify disease-modifying OA drugs (DMOADS) that would retard disease progression and affect OA morbidity. To date, no true DMOADs have been identified, although investigation continues into agents targeting cartilage and joint tissue metabolism and inflammation. There remains optimism that as the mechanism of joint degeneration becomes more fully elucidated, rational drug discovery may identify effective DMOADs. In addition, tissue engineering approaches and mesenchymal stem cell technology may permit the development of functional joint tissue replacement in the future. Current cartilage replacement techniques are not indicated for OA treatment, but are restricted to patients with isolated chondral defects.

Biomechanically Active Approaches

OA progression is at least partly mediated by aberrant loading of joints, so improving loading patterns should affect structural progression. At present, no approaches to alter loading have yet been shown to substantially affect OA progression, but specialized footwear, gait modifications, and mechanically derived exercise regimens are under active investigation.

Complementary and Alternative Approaches

Similar to what occurs with other chronic pain conditions, the overwhelming majority of patients with OA try complementary approaches (Chapter 39). Among the more popular are glucosamine, chondroitin, and acupuncture. None has been clearly demonstrated to substantially retard joint degeneration and independently funded trials have been negative, but many patients feel pain improvement. In any blinded study of OA pain, a substantial placebo response is typically observed. Many complementary approaches have been systematically studied, and controversy remains regarding the incremental pain relief provided by these modalities over that obtained with placebo. Regardless, many of these approaches can be safely used by individual patients who derive relief from them.

PROGNOSIS

Once structural joint damage is present, it is likely to progress, although at variable rates. Slowly progressive structural disease in the absence of severe symptoms may never require surgical intervention, whereas rapidly progressive symptomatic disease might prompt early intervention. The causes of this variability remain unclear, but several factors may contribute to an individual's prognosis. Female gender, obesity, and pain severity are associated with both the incidence and progression of radiographic knee OA, and joint malalignment (varus or valgus) is a strong predictor of progression. Symptomatically, MRI or sonographically detected synovial thickening or effusion may predict progressive cartilage defects and pain severity. In the hip, joint shape is predictive of radiographic progression, as is meniscal pathology (tears,

extrusion, and maceration). MRI-identified subchondral bone marrow lesions are associated with pain severity and progressive cartilage loss.

PREVENTION

No current treatments substantially alter OA progression, but some strategies reduce the risk for development of OA and ameliorate symptomatic progression. Obesity may be the most modifiable of the strong OA risk factors. Weight loss in adulthood reduces the risk for incident radiographic and symptomatic OA and reduces pain severity in patients who already have OA.[A6] Exercise is an important component of weight strategies and ameliorates pain, but specific types of exercise have not yet shown consistent preventive effects. Strategies to decrease joint injuries in young athletes are critical to reducing post-traumatic OA,[19] and proper conditioning has been shown to reduce knee injuries among female soccer players.[A7] New insights into the biology and biomechanics of OA in the coming years may be expected to yield novel strategies to prevent the onset and progression of the disease.

Grade A References

A1. Bliddal H, Leeds AR, Stigsgaard L, et al. Weight loss as treatment for knee osteoarthritis symptoms in obese patients: 1-year results from a randomised controlled trial. *Ann Rheum Dis.* 2011;70: 1798-1803.

A2. Chappell AS, Ossanna MJ, Liu-Seifert H, et al. Duloxetine, a centrally acting analgesic, in the treatment of patients with osteoarthritis knee pain: a 13-week, randomized, placebo-controlled trial. *Pain.* 2009;146:253-260.

A3. Chou R, McDonagh MS, Nakamoto E, et al. Analgesics for osteoarthritis: an update of the 2006 Comparative Effectiveness Review. Agency for Healthcare Research and Quality (US); 2011. Report No.: 11(12)-EHC076-EF.

A4. Abou-Raya A, Abou-Raya S, Khadrawi T, et al. Effect of low-dose oral prednisolone on symptoms and systemic inflammation in older adults with moderate to severe knee osteoarthritis: a randomized placebo-controlled trial. *J Rheumatol.* 2014;41:53-59.

A5. Yavuz U, Sokucu S, Albayrak A, et al. Efficacy comparisons of the intraarticular steroidal agents in the patients with knee osteoarthritis. *Rheumatol Int.* 2012;32:3391-3396.

A6. Messier SP, Mihalko SL, Legault C, et al. Effects of intensive diet and exercise on knee joint loads, inflammation, and clinical outcomes among overweight and obese adults with knee osteoarthritis: the IDEA randomized clinical trial. *JAMA.* 2013;310:1263-1273.

A7. Steffen K, Emery CA, Romiti M, et al. High adherence to a neuromuscular injury prevention programme (FIFA 11+) improves functional balance and reduces injury risk in Canadian youth female football players: a cluster randomised trial. *Br J Sports Med.* 2013;47:794-802.

GENERAL REFERENCES

For the General References and other additional features, please visit Expert Consult at https://expertconsult.inkling.com.

263

BURSITIS, TENDINITIS, AND OTHER PERIARTICULAR DISORDERS AND SPORTS MEDICINE

JOSEPH J. BIUNDO

DEFINITION

An array of painful and sometimes disabling musculoskeletal syndromes exist that are not articular in origin but arise from tendons and bursae. These conditions are referred to by various names, in addition to *tendinitis* and *bursitis*, including the terms *nonarticular rheumatism, soft tissue diseases, regional rheumatic pain syndromes, overuse syndromes,* and *repetitive use syndromes* (Tables 263-1 and 263-2). These entities are often ignored, misdiagnosed as arthritis, or attributed to the aging process; awareness of the existence of these conditions and knowledge of basic musculoskeletal anatomy (Figs. 263-1 and 263-2) are the fundamental requirements for diagnosis. This knowledge is coupled with brief but specific physical diagnosis techniques. The accurate diagnosis and successful treatment of these conditions is gratifying to the clinician because many people can be relieved of their chronic painful syndromes.

Various terms regarding tendon injuries are used and may be confusing. The main term used is *tendinitis*. *Tendinosis* has been proposed as the correct terminology because there are degenerative changes in the tendon but very few inflammatory cells. In addition, fatty mucoid degeneration and hyaline

TABLE 263-1   MUSCULOSKELETAL CONDITIONS BY ETIOLOGY

TENDINITIS	TENDON RUPTURE	BURSITIS
Rotator cuff	Rotator cuff	Subacromial
Bicipital	Bicipital	Olecranon
Volar flexor	Quadriceps	Trochanteric
de Quervain	Patellar	Ischial
Patellar	Posterior tibialis	Iliopsoas
Posterior tibialis	Achilles	Pes anserine
Achilles		Prepatellar
Epicondylitis		Retrocalcaneal

TABLE 263-2   TENDINITIS AND BURSITIS CONDITIONS BY REGION

SHOULDER

Rotator cuff tendinitis
Rotator cuff tear
Bicipital tendinitis
Subacromial bursitis
Adhesive capsulitis

ELBOW

Olecranon bursitis
Medial epicondylitis
Lateral epicondylitis

WRIST AND HAND

de Quervain's tenosynovitis
Volar flexor tenosynovitis
Ganglion

HIP

Trochanteric bursitis
Iliopsoas bursitis
Ischial bursitis
Coccydynia

KNEE

Prepatellar bursitis
Pes anserine bursitis
Popliteal cyst (Baker's cyst)
Patellar tendinitis
Patellar/quadriceps tendon tear

ANKLE AND FOOT

Achilles tendinitis
Achilles tendon tear
Posterior tibial tendinitis
Posterior tibial tendon tear
Retrocalcaneal bursitis
Plantar fasciitis

features occur in these tendon syndromes. These tendon conditions are described by some as a *tendinopathy* because use of this term avoids the need to decide whether inflammation is a factor. Also, tendons may *rupture* or *tear*, partially or completely. The term *tendon insufficiency* is used when the tendon is stretched or is partially or even completely torn. The terms *tenosynovitis* and *peritendinitis* refer to an inflammatory response of the tenosynovium or peritendon, respectively.

Tendon syndromes are basically "overuse" injuries. Tendinitis may occur when the tendon repeatedly bears more load than it can withstand. This may result from excessively high loads across normal tendons or from normal loads across degenerated tendons. In addition to load and repetitiveness, tendon changes resulting from immobility and from aging may play a role, as may the use of certain medications such as fluoroquinolones and corticosteroids.[1]

Bursae are closed sacs lined by a synovial membrane and serve as a cushion. They are located between tendon and bone, tendon and tendon, or bone and skin and allow smooth gliding between these structures. A bursa, which normally has a small amount of bursal fluid, can become inflamed from trauma or overuse, or become infected, producing a bursitis. When this occurs, some swelling and pain of the bursa may be present.

EPIDEMIOLOGY

The incidence of the nonarticular syndromes of bursitis and tendinitis is high. They are more common than both rheumatoid arthritis (RA) and systemic lupus erythematosus (SLE). For example, the incidence of shoulder pain, largely a result of rotator cuff tendinitis and rotator cuff tear, was approximately 20% in a population older than 70 years of age.

DIAGNOSIS

A precise history is needed to identify the conditions present, and more than one syndrome can occur concomitantly. A working knowledge of regional anatomy and an approach that uses a regional differential diagnosis will help in obtaining a specific diagnosis. A complete neuromusculoskeletal examination should be performed, emphasizing careful palpation, passive range of motion (ROM), and active ROM alone or sometimes with resistance. Systemic and infectious causes must be considered. Diagnostic ultrasonography and magnetic resonance imaging (MRI) are sometimes useful in confirming a diagnosis.

TREATMENT   Rx

Treatment of tendinitis and bursitis includes use of nonsteroidal anti-inflammatory drugs (NSAIDs), relative rest of the injured site, stretching and strengthening exercises, friction massage, use of modalities (heat, ice, and ultrasound), splinting, corticosteroid injections,[A1] and surgery. A comprehensive management of these regional syndromes should be undertaken, rather than relying on oral medications alone. The causative aspects should be evaluated, and activity modification should be advised as needed. The goals of therapeutic exercise are to increase flexibility by stretching, increase muscle strength by resistive exercises, and improve muscle endurance by some repetitive regimen. Caution should be exerted in performing corticosteroid injections; the injections should not be placed into the tendon proper, but rather into the peritendinous sheath. The injected solution should be placed beneath the subcutaneous tissue, to avoid skin and subcutaneous fat atrophy, and

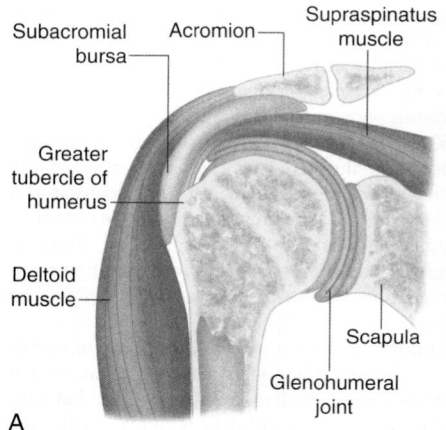

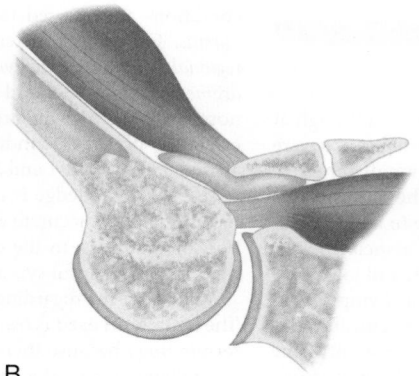

FIGURE 263-1. Relationship of subacromial bursa (shown in *blue*) to supraspinatus muscle and acromion process. **A,** In the position of adduction of the humerus. To show this bursa more clearly, the synovial membrane of the glenohumeral joint is not shown in *blue*. **B,** In the position of abduction of the humerus, the acromion impinges on the subacromial bursa and the insertion of the supraspinatus tendon. (From Polley HF, Hunder GG, eds. *Rheumatologic Interviewing and Physical Examination of the Joints,* 2nd ed. Philadelphia: WB Saunders; 1978:65.)

A   B

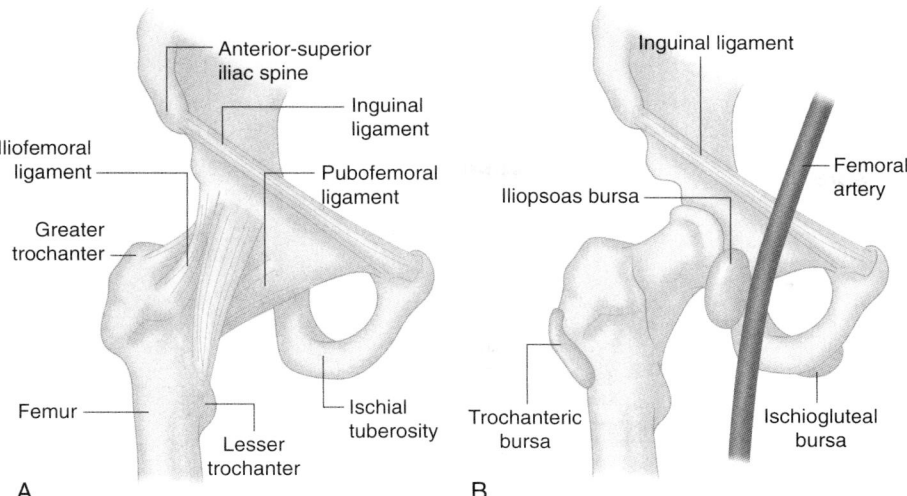

FIGURE 263-2. Musculoskeletal anatomy of the hip. A, Anterior aspect of the hip joint and bony structures. B, Relationship of the distended iliopsoas, trochanteric, and ischiogluteal bursae (shown in *blue*) to the hip joint and adjacent structures. (From Polley HF, Hunder GG, eds. *Rheumatologic Interviewing and Physical Examination of the Joints,* 2nd ed. Philadelphia: WB Saunders; 1978:183.)

injections should not be given too frequently, to avoid the possibility of weakening and rupture of the tendon. The accuracy of injections may be improved with concomitant use of diagnostic ultrasonography to assist with determining the correct needle site. Also, fluoroscopically guided injections can be used to increase accuracy.

SPORTS MEDICINE INJURIES

An overlap exists between commonly occurring conditions of tendinitis and bursitis and those attributed to sports injuries (Table 263-3). For example, lateral epicondylitis, frequently referred to as *tennis elbow,* occurs more commonly secondary to non–sports-related causes. In contradistinction, iliotibial band syndrome is usually related to sports. Other entities that occur more often in relation to sports include ligamentous knee injuries, patellar tendinitis, ankle sprains, turf toe, and acromioclavicular separations. It is important in both categories to know the anatomy and biomechanics of the condition, so as to better diagnose and treat the problem. Sports-related injuries are helped with the classic RICE treatment, consisting of *r*est, *i*ce, *c*ompression, and *e*levation. Often, anti-inflammatory and analgesic drugs are used. However, there is less use of corticosteroid injections in athletic injuries than in routine cases of tendinitis and bursitis.

DISORDERS OF THE SHOULDER REGION

Shoulder pain is one of the most common musculoskeletal complaints in people older than 40 years of age. In younger people, athletic injuries are a frequent source of such pain.

Rotator cuff tendinitis, or impingement syndrome, is the most common cause of shoulder pain.[2] Tendinitis (and not bursitis) is the primary cause of pain, but secondary involvement of the subacromial bursa occurs in some cases. The condition may be acute or chronic and may or may not be associated with calcific deposits within the tendon. The key finding is pain in the rotator cuff on active abduction, especially between 60 and 120 degrees, and sometimes when lowering the arm. In more severe cases, pain may begin on initial abduction and continue throughout the ROM. Typically, chronic rotator cuff tendinitis manifests as an ache in the shoulder, usually over the lateral deltoid, and occurs with various movements, especially abduction and internal rotation. Other symptoms include difficulty in dressing oneself and night pain because of difficulty in positioning the shoulders. The physical findings include pain and loss of active abduction and internal rotation, less pain on passive motion, tenderness of the area of supraspinatus insertion, and a positive impingement sign (Fig. 263-3, Neer's sign, which is pain occurring in forced flexion.[3] The causes of rotator cuff tendinitis are multifactorial, but relative overuse, especially from overhead activity causing impingement of the rotator cuff, is commonly implicated. Treatment consists of rest and modalities such as hot packs, ultrasound, or cold applications, with specific ROM exercises as soon as tolerated. NSAIDs are often beneficial, but the most frequent treatment is injection of a depot corticosteroid[A2] into the subacromial bursa, the floor of which is contiguous with the rotator cuff. Disodium ethylenediaminetetraacetic acid (EDTA) administered by phonophoresis and mesotherapy to patients with calcific tendinitis of the shoulder

TABLE 263-3 ADDITIONAL SPORTS-RELATED CONDITIONS

SHOULDER

Acromioclavicular separation
Glenoid labial tear (SLAP lesion)
Glenohumeral instability with dislocation

ELBOW

Triceps tendinopathy
Little League elbow (apophysitis)
Distal biceps tendinitis

WRIST AND HAND

Gamekeeper's thumb (skier's thumb)
Mallet finger (baseball finger)
Extensor carpi ulnaris tendinitis
Rupture of flexor digitorum profundus tendon
Injury to triangular fibrocartilage

HIP

Adductor strain (groin pull)
Hip pointer
Hamstring strain

KNEE

Anterior cruciate tear
Posterior cruciate tear
Medial collateral ligament tear/strain
Lateral collateral ligament tear/strain
Popliteal tendinitis
Medial and lateral meniscal tears
Patellar tendinitis
Iliotibial band syndrome

ANKLE AND FOOT

Ankle sprain
Turf toe
Stress fracture

has been found to be effective in pain reduction, improvement in shoulder function, and disappearance of calcifications.[A3] Extracorporeal shock wave therapy can also be beneficial for chronic calcific tendinitis.[A4]

In a rotator cuff tear, an acute tear after trauma is usually easily recognized. The trauma may be superimposed on an already degenerative and possibly even partially torn cuff. In cases of trauma resulting in a ruptured cuff, fracture of the humeral head and dislocation of the joint also should be considered. However, most patients with a tear recall no trauma. In these cases, degeneration of the rotator cuff occurs gradually, resulting ultimately in a complete tear. Rotator cuff tears are classified as small (≤1 cm), medium (1 to 3 cm), large (3 to 5 cm), or massive (>5 cm). Shoulder pain, weakness on abduction, and loss of motion occur in varying degrees, ranging from severe pain and mild weakness to no pain and marked weakness. A positive drop-arm sign with inability to maintain actively 90 degrees of passive shoulder abduction may be present in patients with large or massive tears. Small complete tears

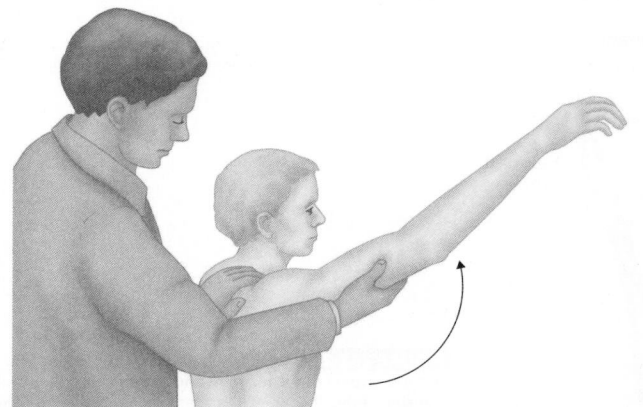

FIGURE 263-3. The impingement sign is elicited by forced forward elevation of the arm. Pain results as the greater tuberosity impinges on the acromion. The examiner's hand prevents scapular rotation. This maneuver may be positive in other periarticular disorders. (From Neer CS II. Impingement lesions. *Clin Orthop.* 1983;173:70-77.)

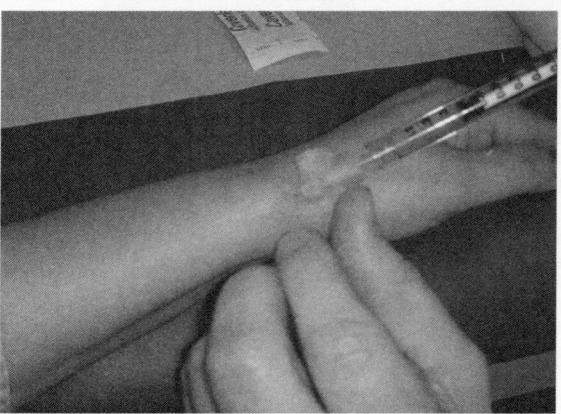

FIGURE 263-4. Injection of de Quervain tenosynovitis.

and incomplete tears of the rotator cuff are treated conservatively with rest, physical therapy, and NSAIDs. Although its role has not yet been established by careful studies, a subacromial injection of a corticosteroid may relieve pain. Surgical repair may be indicated in younger patients.

Bicipital tendinitis is manifested by pain, most often in the anterior region of the shoulder and occasionally more diffusely. The pain may be acute but is usually chronic and is related to impingement of the biceps tendon by the acromion. Tenosynovitis of the long head of the biceps is present, and the tendon may be frayed and fibrotic. Palpation over the bicipital groove reveals localized tenderness. The patient's response should be compared with the response to palpation of the opposite side (i.e., tendon with normal tenderness). Pain may be reproduced over the bicipital tendon in some cases by supination of the forearm against resistance (Yergason's sign), shoulder flexion against resistance (Speed's test), or extension of the shoulder. Treatment of bicipital tendinitis consists of rest, hot packs, ultrasound, and, as pain subsides, passive and then active ROM exercises. NSAIDs may be helpful, and occasionally a small amount of corticosteroid carefully injected into the tendon sheath may be of benefit. Rupture of the biceps tendon can occur at the superior edge of the bicipital groove, producing a characteristic bulbous enlargement of the lateral half of the muscle belly.

Adhesive capsulitis (frozen shoulder) is associated with generalized pain and tenderness and severe loss of active and passive motion in all planes. It is rare before 40 years of age but may occur secondary to any type of shoulder problem. However, not every stiff and painful shoulder is necessarily adhesive capsulitis. Inflammatory arthritis and diabetes can cause adhesive capsulitis. Additional factors such as immobility, low pain threshold, depression, and neglect or improper initial treatment also favor the development of a frozen shoulder. Many cases, however, are idiopathic. The joint capsule adheres to the anatomic neck, and the axillary fold binds to itself, causing restricted motion. The capsule becomes thickened and contracted. Arthrography can help confirm this diagnosis by showing a decrease in volume of the shoulder joint capsule. Oral steroids improve pain and range of motion in the short term, but a frozen shoulder is probably best treated with a comprehensive program involving NSAIDs and corticosteroid injections into the glenohumeral joint and the subacromial bursa. Physical therapy consists of ice packs, ultrasound, transcutaneous electrical nerve stimulation, and gentle ROM exercises, beginning with pendulum exercises and wall climbing with the fingers and progressing to active ROM and strengthening exercises.

DISORDERS OF THE ELBOW REGION

Olecranon bursitis occurs frequently and involves the subcutaneous olecranon bursa, either secondary to trauma or as an idiopathic condition. The bursa is characteristically swollen and tender on pressure, but pain may be minimal and usually no motion is lost. Aspiration may yield clear or blood-tinged fluid with a low viscosity or grossly hemorrhagic fluid. Inflammatory olecranon bursitis may be caused by gout, RA, or calcium pyrophosphate deposition disease, and infection can also cause a bursitis. Aspiration alone and protection from trauma are usually sufficient to resolve the condition. A small dose of corticosteroid may be injected into the bursa. With septic olecranon bursitis, localized erythema is the major clue. Heat, pain, and a positive culture are also frequently present.

Lateral epicondylitis, or tennis elbow, is a common condition in those who overuse their arms.[4] Localized tenderness directly over or slightly anterior to the lateral epicondyle is the hallmark of this disorder. Pain may occur during handshakes, while lifting a briefcase, or with other similar activities. Probably less than 10% of patients actually acquire lateral epicondylitis through playing tennis. Job and recreational activities, including gardening and athletics, are the usual causes. Pathologically, the condition consists of degeneration of the common extensor tendon, particularly of the extensor carpi radialis brevis tendon.[5] Treatment is aimed at altering activities and preventing overuse of the forearm musculature. Ice packs, heat, and NSAIDs are of some benefit. A forearm brace also can be used. A local corticosteroid injection with a 25-gauge needle over the lateral epicondyle often produces satisfactory initial relief. Isometric strengthening is important as the initial part of a rehabilitation program.

Medial epicondylitis, or golfer's elbow, which mainly involves the flexor carpi radialis, is less common and less disabling than lateral epicondylitis. Local pain and tenderness over the medial epicondyle are present, and resistance to wrist flexion exacerbates the pain.

DISORDERS OF THE WRIST AND HAND

A ganglion is a cystic swelling that arises from a joint or tendon sheath and occurs most commonly over the dorsum of the wrist. It is synovial lined and contains thick, jelly-like fluid. Ganglia apparently develop secondary to trauma or prolonged wrist extension. Usually, the only symptom is swelling, but occasionally a large ganglion produces discomfort on wrist extension.

De Quervain's tenosynovitis may result from repetitive activity that involves pinching with the thumb while moving the wrist. The symptoms are pain, tenderness, and occasionally swelling over the radial styloid. Pathologic findings include inflammation and narrowing of the tendon sheath around the abductor pollicis longus and extensor pollicis brevis. A positive Finkelstein test result is usually seen; pain increases when the thumb is folded across the palm and the fingers are flexed over the thumb as the examiner passively deviates the wrist toward the ulnar side. However, this test also may be positive in patients with osteoarthritis (OA) of the first carpometacarpal joint and must be differentiated from this common condition. Treatment involves splinting, local corticosteroid injection (Fig. 263-4), and NSAIDs as indicated. Rarely, surgical removal of the inflamed tenosynovium is needed.

Volar flexor tenosynovitis consists of inflammation of the tendon sheaths of the flexor digitorum superficialis and flexor digitorum profundus tendons in the palm. It is extremely common but often unrecognized. Pain in the palm is felt on finger flexion, but in some cases the pain radiates to the proximal interphalangeal (PIP) and metacarpophalangeal (MCP) joints on the dorsal side, misleading the examiner. The diagnosis is made by palpation and identification of localized tenderness and swelling of the volar tendon sheaths. The middle and index fingers are most commonly involved, but the ring and little fingers also can be affected. Often a nodule composed of fibrous tissue can be palpated in the palm just proximal to the MCP joint on the volar side. The nodule interferes with the normal tendon gliding and can cause a triggering or locking, which may be intermittent and may produce an uncomfortable sensation. Similar involvement can occur at the flexor tendon of the thumb. The most common cause is overuse trauma of the hands from gripping with increased pull on the flexor tendons. It may be part of inflammatory conditions, such as RA, psoriatic arthritis, or apatite crystal deposition disease. It is seen frequently in conjunction with OA of the hands. Injection of a long-acting steroid into the tendon sheath usually relieves the problem, although surgery on the tendon sheath may be needed in unremitting cases.

Gamekeeper's thumb (skier's thumb) is caused by trauma to the thumb resulting in instability of the first MCP joint. This instability is due to laxity or rupture of the ulnar collateral ligament. It is treated by immobilization, but surgical repair may be necessary.

Avulsion of flexor digitorum profundus (jersey finger) may result from trauma, usually in football, when a player grabs onto a jersey. The distal phalanx, usually the fourth, is hyperextended while the digitorum profundus is contracting maximally. The avulsion of the tendon results in an inability to flex the distal phalanx of that digit. Surgery is required to correct the problem.

DISORDERS OF THE HIP REGION

Although trochanteric bursitis is common, it frequently goes undiagnosed. It occurs predominantly in middle-aged to elderly people, and somewhat more often in women. The main symptom is aching over the trochanteric area and lateral thigh. Walking, various hip movements, and lying on the involved hip may intensify the pain. Onset may be acute, but more often it is gradual, with symptoms lasting for months. In chronic cases, the patient may fail to locate or describe the pain adequately, or the physician may fail to note the symptoms or interpret them correctly. Occasionally, the pain has a pseudoradiculopathic quality, radiating down the lateral aspect of the thigh. In a few cases, the pain is so severe that the patient cannot walk and complains of diffuse pain of the entire thigh. The best way to diagnose trochanteric bursitis is to palpate over the trochanteric area and elicit point tenderness. In addition to specific pain on deep pressure over the trochanter, other tender points may be noted throughout the lateral aspect of the thigh muscle. Pain may be worse with external rotation and abduction against resistance. Although bursitis has historically been described as the principal problem, the condition may actually arise at the insertions of the gluteus medius and gluteus minimus tendons.[6] Local trauma and degeneration play a role in the pathogenesis, leading to tendinosis and/or tendon tears. Conditions that may contribute to trochanteric bursitis, apparently by adding stress to the area, include OA of the lumbar spine or of the hip, leg-length discrepancy, and scoliosis. Treatment consists of local injection of depot corticosteroid using a 22-gauge, 3.5-inch needle to ensure that the bursal area is reached (Fig. 263-5). NSAIDs, weight loss, and strengthening and stretching of the gluteus medius muscle and iliotibial band help in management.

Coccydynia is manifested by pain in the coccyx area when pressure is applied to the area. This most notably occurs on sitting. The patient squirms from buttock to buttock to relieve the pressure and consequent pain and often chooses to sit on a cushion. The symptoms may be chronic and severe. The condition may relate to a fall on the coccyx, dropping to a hard chair when sitting, or some related trauma to the coccyx. However, at times no obvious cause can be detected. Women are much more frequently affected, perhaps because the lordosis that often occurs in women exposes the coccyx to more trauma. The diagnosis is confirmed by finding localized tenderness over the coccyx on palpation. A plain x-ray film can be obtained to exclude a fracture or dislocation of the coccyx. Treatment with a local injection of 1 mL of a long-acting corticosteroid and 2 mL of a 2% lidocaine solution is usually very effective. The exact nature of the pathology of coccydynia has not been studied, but it is presumed to be a bone bruise.

In iliopsoas bursitis, groin and anterior thigh pain are present and worsen on passive hip hyperextension and sometimes on flexion, especially with resistance. Tenderness is palpable over an involved bursa. The patient may hold the hip in flexion and external rotation to eliminate pain and may limp to prevent hyperextension of the hip. The iliopsoas bursa lies behind the iliopsoas muscle, anterior to the hip joint and lateral to the femoral vessels. It communicates with the hip in 15% of cases. The diagnosis is more apparent if a cystic mass is seen (~30% of cases); however, other causes of cystic swelling in the femoral area must first be excluded. A bursal mass can cause femoral venous obstruction or femoral nerve compression. As with most cases of bursitis, acute or recurrent trauma and inflammatory conditions such as RA may lead to iliopsoas bursitis (also called *iliopectineal bursitis*). Iliopsoas tendinitis may overlap with the bursitis or occur independently in a similar clinical picture. The diagnosis is confirmed by plain x-ray with injection of a contrast medium into the bursa, or by ultrasonography, computed tomography, or MRI. Iliopsoas bursitis/tendinitis usually responds to conservative treatment including physical therapy and corticosteroid injections. With recurrent involvement, excision of the bursa may be necessary.

Ischial or ischiogluteal bursitis is caused by trauma or by prolonged sitting on hard surfaces, as evidenced by the name *weaver's bottom*. Pain is often exquisite when sitting or lying down. The hamstring muscles originate from the ischial tuberosity, and the ischiogluteal bursa is superficial to the tuberosity. Because the bursa is superficial to the tuberosity, separating the gluteus maximus from the tuberosity, the pain may radiate down the back of the thigh. Point tenderness over the ischial tuberosity is present. Use of cushions, hamstring stretching, and local injection of a corticosteroid are helpful.

DISORDERS OF THE KNEE REGION

Anserine bursitis is seen predominantly in overweight, middle-aged to elderly women with large legs and OA of the knees. The symptoms are pain and tenderness over the medial aspect of the knee approximately 2 inches below the joint margin, with the pain worsened by climbing stairs. The pes anserinus (Latin for "goose foot") is composed of the conjoined tendons of the sartorius, gracilis, and semitendinosus muscles. The bursa extends between the above tendons and the tibial collateral ligament. Tendinitis of these tendons, rather than bursitis, is the predominate cause of the syndrome. The diagnosis is made by eliciting exquisite tenderness over the bursal area. Anserine bursitis is often overlooked because it frequently occurs concomitantly with OA of the knee, which, when present, is the assumed cause of pain; however, in some cases of dual involvement, anserine bursitis is the principal source of pain. The treatment is rest, stretching of the adductor and quadriceps muscles, and a corticosteroid injection into the bursa and tendon insertion site.

Prepatellar bursitis manifests as a swelling superficial to the kneecap and results from trauma such as frequent kneeling, leading to the name *housemaid's knee*. The prepatellar bursa lies anterior to the lower half of the patella and the upper half of the patellar ligament. The pain is generally slight unless pressure is applied directly over the bursa. The infrapatellar bursa, which lies between the patellar ligament and the tibia, is also subject to trauma and swelling. Chronic prepatellar bursitis can be treated by protecting the knee from the irritating trauma.

Patellar tendinitis (jumper's knee) is seen predominantly in athletes engaging in activities such as repetitive running, jumping, or kicking. Pain and tenderness are present over the patellar tendon.

Iliotibial band syndrome manifests by lateral knee pain caused by friction between the iliotibial band and the lateral femoral condyle. It is an overuse injury and is seen in runners, cyclists, and other athletes performing repetitive knee flexion activities.

Popliteal cysts,[7] also known as Baker's cysts, are not uncommon, and the clinician should be well aware of the possibility of their dissection or rupture. A cystic swelling behind the knee with mild or no discomfort can be the only initial finding. With further distention of the cyst, however, a greater awareness and discomfort are experienced, particularly on full flexion or extension. The cyst is best seen when the patient is standing and examined from behind. Any knee disease having a synovial effusion can develop into a popliteal cyst. Popliteal cysts are most common secondary to RA, OA, or internal derangements of the knee. There are a few reported cases secondary to gout and Reiter's syndrome. A syndrome of pseudothrombophlebitis may occur as a result of cyst dissection into the calf or actual rupture of the cyst. Findings include diffuse swelling of the calf, pain, and sometimes erythema and edema of the ankle. An ultrasound or arthrogram of the knee confirms both the cyst and the possible dissection or rupture. A cyst related to an inflammatory arthritis is treated by injection of a depot corticosteroid into the knee joint, and possibly into the cyst itself, which usually resolves the problem. If the cyst results from OA or an internal derangement of the knee, surgical repair of the underlying joint lesion is usually necessary to prevent a recurrence of the cyst.

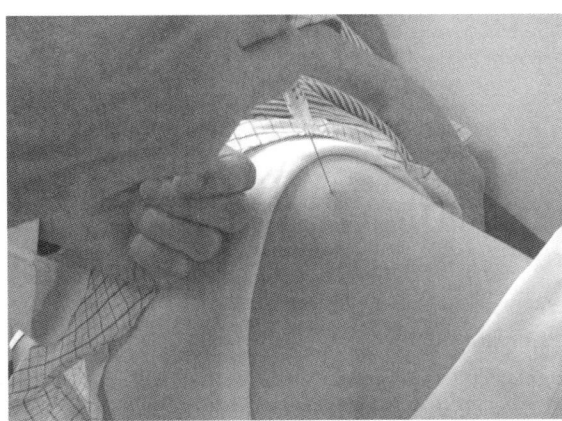

FIGURE 263-5. Injection of trochanteric bursitis.

In the knee area, tendon ruptures may occur, and quadriceps tendon rupture is involved approximately 50% of the time; otherwise, patellar tendon rupture occurs. Quadriceps tendon rupture is generally caused by sudden violent contractions of the quadriceps muscle when the knee is flexed. A hemarthrosis of the knee joint may follow. Patients with chronic renal failure, RA, hyperparathyroidism, or gout and patients with SLE taking steroids have been reported to have spontaneous ruptures of the quadriceps tendon. The patient experiences a sudden sharp pain and cannot extend the leg. X-ray studies may show a high-riding patella. The tendon is usually found to be degenerated, and surgical repair is often indicated. Rupture of the patellar tendon has been associated with a specific episode of trauma, repetitive trauma from sporting activities, and systemic diseases.

Meniscal tears are common causes of knee "locking" and pain. Physical examination may show pain, with or without clicking, when the hip and knee are bent to 90°. Magnetic resonance imaging is the diagnostic test of choice. Physical therapy is often as effective as surgery.[A5][A6]

⬤ DISORDERS OF THE ANKLE AND FOOT REGION

Achilles tendinitis usually results from trauma, athletic overactivity, or improperly fitting shoes with a stiff heel counter, but it also can be caused by inflammatory conditions such as ankylosing spondylitis, Reiter's syndrome, gout, RA, and calcium pyrophosphate dihydrate crystal deposition disease.[9] Pain, swelling, and tenderness occur over the Achilles tendon at its attachment and in the area proximal to the attachment. Crepitus on motion and pain on dorsiflexion may be present. Management includes NSAIDs, rest, shoe corrections, heel lift, gentle stretching, and sometimes a splint with slight plantar flexion. Local injection of platelet-rich plasma (PRP) has become an increasingly used treatment for releasing growth factors into degenerative tendons; however, more recent randomized, placebo-controlled trials for treatment of chronic Achilles and other tendinopathies have found PRP injections to be ineffective in improving pain and activity.[A7] The Achilles tendon is vulnerable to rupture when involved with tendinitis, and treatment with a corticosteroid injection could increase this possibility.

Achilles tendon rupture is well known and occurs with a sudden onset of pain during forced dorsiflexion. An audible snap may be heard, followed by difficulty in walking and standing on toes. Swelling and edema over the area usually develop. Diagnosis can be made with the Thompson test, in which the patient kneels on a chair with the feet extending over the edge and the examiner squeezes the calf and pushes toward the knee. Normally this produces plantar flexion, but in a ruptured tendon, no plantar flexion occurs. Achilles tendon rupture usually occurs during athletic events or with trauma from jumps or falls. The tendon is more prone to tear in people with preexisting Achilles tendon disease and in those taking corticosteroids. Orthopedic consultation should be obtained, and immobilization or surgery may be selected, depending on the situation.

For acute, severe ankle sprain, a below-knee cast or Aircast produces a faster recovery than a tubular compression bandage, but there is no difference in outcomes at 9 months.[A8] Plantar fasciitis, which is seen primarily in persons between 40 and 60 years of age, is characterized by pain in the plantar area of the heel. The onset may be gradual, or it may occur with trauma or overuse from some activity, such as athletics, prolonged walking, using improper shoes, or striking the heel with some force. Plantar fasciitis may be idiopathic; it also is likely to be present in younger patients with spondyloarthritis (Chapter 265). The pain characteristically occurs in the morning on arising and is most severe for the first few steps. After an initial improvement, the pain may worsen later in the day, especially after prolonged standing or walking. The pain is burning, aching, and occasionally lancinating. Palpation typically reveals tenderness anteromedially on the medial calcaneal tubercle at the origin of the plantar fascia. Treatment includes relative rest with a reduction in stressful activities, NSAIDs, use of heel pad or heel cup orthosis, arch support, and stretching of the heel cord and plantar fascia. A local corticosteroid injection, using a 25-gauge needle, is often of help.

In posterior tibial tendinitis, pain and tenderness occur just posterior to the medial malleolus; it can be caused by trauma, excessive pronation, RA, or spondyloarthropathy. Extension and flexion may be normal, but pain is present on resisted inversion or passive eversion. The discomfort is usually worse after athletic activity, and swelling and localized tenderness may be present. Treatment usually includes rest, NSAIDs, and possibly a local injection of corticosteroid. Immobilization with a splint is sometimes needed.

Posterior tibialis tendon rupture, which is not commonly recognized, is a cause of progressive flat foot. It can result from trauma, chronic tendon degeneration, or RA. An insidious onset of pain and tenderness may be noted along the course of the tendon just distal to the medial malleolus, along with swelling medial to the hind foot. The unilateral deformity of hind foot valgus and forefoot abduction is an important finding. The forefoot abduction can best be seen from behind; more toes are seen from this position than would be seen normally. The result of the single heel rise test is positive when the patient is unable to rise onto the ball of the affected foot while the contralateral foot is off the floor. Treatment usually includes rest, NSAIDs, and possibly an orthosis. Surgical repair of the tendon is sometimes indicated. Manifestations of retrocalcaneal bursitis include pain at the back of the heel, tenderness of the area anterior to the Achilles tendon, and pain on dorsiflexion. Local swelling is present, with bulging on the medial and lateral aspects of the tendon. Retrocalcaneal bursitis, also called sub-Achilles bursitis, may coexist with Achilles tendinitis, and distinguishing the two is sometimes difficult. This condition may be secondary to RA, spondylitis, a reactive arthritis, gout, or trauma.

Turf toe is an injury of the big toe originally described during play on artificial turf. It results from hyperextension of the first metatarsophalangeal (MTP) joint when a fixed, dorsiflexed foot is forced into the ground. The plantar capsular ligament may be sprained or torn.

Stress fracture is also known as march fracture or fatigue fracture because it was first associated with spontaneous fracture after long marches in army recruits. Pain, swelling, tenderness, and occasionally erythema develop over the metatarsal area, usually without any clear history of trauma. On questioning, however, the episode of spontaneous pain related to onset of the fracture can be identified in some cases. The neck of the second metatarsal bone is most frequently involved, but the third metatarsal is also a site of fracture. Aside from prolonged marching, other athletic events with overactivity, including jogging, are common causes. Stress fractures may be seen in patients with RA and in elderly people. The difficulty in diagnosing stress fractures is that the initial x-ray films usually show no abnormalities or, at most, only a faint fracture line. A repeat x-ray examination several weeks later shows healing with callus formation. Bone scans aid the early diagnosis of stress fractures by showing an increase in uptake over the fracture site. Usually these fractures heal spontaneously, and rest and strapping of the foot are helpful. Occasionally, a cast is needed.

Grade A References

A1. Coombes BK, Bisset L, Vicenzino B. Efficacy and safety of corticosteroid injections and other injections for management of tendinopathy: a systematic review of randomised controlled trials. *Lancet.* 2010;376:1751-1767.

A2. Rhon DI, Boyles RB, Cleland JA. One-year outcome of subacromial corticosteroid injection compared with manual physical therapy for the management of the unilateral shoulder impingement syndrome: a pragmatic randomized trial. *Ann Intern Med.* 2014;161:161-169.

A3. Cacchio A, De Blasis E, Desiati P, et al. Effectiveness of treatment of calcific tendinitis of the shoulder by disodium EDTA. *Arthritis Rheum.* 2009;61:84-91.

A4. Bannuru RR, Flavin NE, Vaysbrot E, et al. High-energy extracorporeal shock-wave therapy for treating chronic calcific tendinitis of the shoulder: a systematic review. *Ann Intern Med.* 2014;160:542-549.

A5. Katz JN, Brophy RH, Chaisson CE, et al. Surgery versus physical therapy for a meniscal tear and osteoarthritis. *N Engl J Med.* 2013;368:1675-1684.

A6. Sihvonen R, Paavola M, Malmivaara A, et al. Arthroscopic partial meniscectomy versus sham surgery for a degenerative meniscal tear. *N Engl J Med.* 2013;369:2515-2524.

A7. Moraes VY, Lenza M, Tamaoki MJ, et al. Platelet-rich therapies for musculoskeletal soft tissue injuries. *Cochrane Database Syst Rev.* 2014;4:CD010071.

A8. Lamb SE, Marsh JL, Hutton JL, et al. Mechanical supports for acute, severe ankle sprain: a pragmatic multicentre, randomised controlled trial. *Lancet.* 2009;373:575-581.

GENERAL REFERENCES

For the General References and other additional features, please visit Expert Consult at https://expertconsult.inkling.com.

264

RHEUMATOID ARTHRITIS

JAMES R. O'DELL

DEFINITION

Rheumatoid arthritis (RA) is a chronic systemic inflammatory disease of unknown etiology that primarily targets synovial tissues. It is relatively common, with a prevalence of slightly less than 1% in adults all over the world. RA shortens survival and significantly affects quality of life in many patients. Essentially all patients exhibit some systemic features such as fatigue, low-grade fevers, anemia, and elevations of acute phase reactants (erythrocyte sedimentation rate [ESR] or C-reactive protein [CRP]). This systemic inflammation is believed to be responsible for vascular endothelial damage and a marked increased risk for coronary artery disease and congestive heart failure in patients with RA.[1] However, the primary target of RA is the synovium and it is responsible for most of the protean clinical features. Synovial tissues proliferate in an uncontrolled fashion, resulting in excess fluid production, destruction of cartilage, erosion of marginal bone, and stretching and damage of the tendons and ligaments.

In the past two decades, the treatment of RA has changed dramatically. Current therapeutic strategies should result in over 50% of patients achieving clinical remissions with treatment with appropriate disease-modifying antirheumatic drugs (DMARD) or combinations of DMARDs.

EPIDEMIOLOGY

RA is present all over the world, with a prevalence of 0.5 to 1% of adults and with some differences in certain population groups. For reasons that are still unclear, the prevalence in women is two or three times greater than that in men. RA can occur at any age, but onset before the age of 45 years in men is uncommon. The relatively few well-done inception cohorts suggest that the yearly incidence of RA is approximately 40 per 100,000 for women and about half that for men. These figures vary significantly based on the age of the cohort. The best available data suggest that the incidence of RA in women increases with age until approximately 60 years of age and then plateaus. The incidence rate is much lower in young men, approximately one third that in women, but increases steadily with age and approaches that of women older than 65 years. Because the incidence of RA increases or is stable with age and RA is a lifelong disease, the prevalence of RA increases with each decade. Recent data suggest that the incidence of RA, particularly rheumatoid factor (RF)-negative RA, may be decreasing. The reasons for this are unclear, but, if elucidated, they could provide valuable insights into the etiology and pathogenesis of RA and might allow the implementation of strategies to prevent clinical disease.

RA has a significant genetic component; therefore, it is not surprising that RA is reportedly very unusual in certain populations and more common in others. Most notably, cohorts have been described in rural Nigeria in which no individuals are affected with RA; in contrast, a prevalence of RA of 5% has been found in some studies of Chippewa, Yakima, and Inuit Native American tribes.

PATHOBIOLOGY

Genetics

Genetics play a significant role in determining both the risk for developing RA and the severity of the disease.[2] Twin studies reveal a concordance rate for RA that averages 15% for monozygotic twins and approximately 5% for dizygotic twins. These data in monozygotic twins simultaneously reveal both the significance of genetic factors and the fact that they are clearly not the only important factor, or else the concordance rate would approach unity.

It has been clearly shown that RA is a multigene disease with important contributions from both human leukocyte antigen (HLA) and non-HLA genes. The association of certain HLA alleles, specifically HLA-DR4, with an increased risk for developing RA and of having more severe disease has long been recognized. This association is explained by a particular amino acid sequence in the third hypervariable region on the DRβ1 chain. HLA-DR molecules are present on the surface of antigen-presenting cells and allow T cells to recognize antigen in the context of DR. Hypervariable regions on the DR molecule are particularly important for antigen recognition. The amino acid sequence associated with RA has been called the *shared epitope* or the *at-risk allele*. It has been shown by a number of investigators that patients with the shared epitope have more severe RA and more extra-articular manifestations than those who are negative. Furthermore, individuals with two copies of the shared epitope, particularly those with HLA-DR4, have a further increased risk for the development of severe RA. This association with a particular antigen recognition site may ultimately aid understanding of the antigen or antigens that are important for triggering RA. Proteins in which arginine has been converted to citrulline are bound with greater avidity by the shared epitope. The importance of certain DRβ1 alleles in RA supports the concept that T cells are integrally involved in the pathogenesis.

Population-based studies have suggested that only 30 to 50% of the genetic risk for RA is explained by genes located in the HLA region. A functional polymorphism for the gene that encodes intracellular protein tyrosine phosphatase nonreceptor 22 *(PTPN22)* has been reproducibly associated with RA and a number of other autoimmune diseases, including type 1 diabetes, systemic lupus erythematosus, Graves' disease, and Hashimoto's thyroiditis. Genome-wide association studies have identified at least 80 other candidate genes associated with RA, including polymorphisms for signal transducer and activator of transcription (STAT4), tumor necrosis factor receptor–associated factor 1 (TRAF-1), and CD40. To complicate things further, HLA-DRB1 03 is associated with lower titers of anti–citrullinated peptide antigen (ACPA) antibodies but is associated with increased risk for cyclic citrullinated peptide–negative RA.

The shared epitope is present in approximately 25 to 35% of the white population, but the chance of developing RA among individuals who carry this allele is only approximately 1 in 25. Therefore, despite identifying the most important genetic risk factor for RA, this test has little or no clinical utility. The role of epigenetics in RA is currently receiving attention and may provide important insights.

Etiology

Clearly, other factors, in addition to genetics, are active in precipitating or triggering RA. RA appears to require the complex interaction of genetic and environmental factors with the immune system and ultimately in the synovial tissues throughout the body (Fig. 264-1).[3] Sera collected before the development of clinical RA show that immunologic changes predate clinical manifestations by years. Autoantibodies, particularly ACPA antibodies and rheumatoid factor (RF), are present in the sera of many individuals 5 to 10 years before the clinical onset of disease. By following cohorts of people at high risk for RA, investigators are learning much about these early immunologic changes and ultimately it is hoped about the triggers for the disease.

The use of oral contraceptives has been associated with a decrease in the incidence of RA; because the effect appears to be strongest for oral contraceptives that have high estrogen content, it is postulated that estrogen is responsible for this protective effect. Studies that have tried to address the question of postmenopausal estrogen use and its effect on RA have yielded conflicting results.

Smoking has long been associated with a significant increase in the risk for developing RA, but more recently it has been shown that this is true only for ACPA-positive patients and is not associated with ACPA-negative disease. Furthermore, smoking appears to be a risk factor for RA only in those patients who are positive for shared epitope. Purported triggers for RA in addition to smoking have included bacteria (*Mycobacteria, Streptococcus, Mycoplasma, Escherichia coli, Helicobacter pylori*), viruses (rubella, Epstein-Barr virus, parvovirus), and periodontal disease.

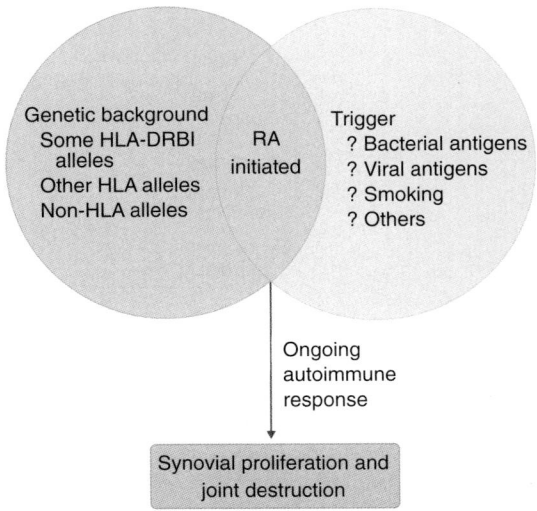

FIGURE 264-1. Initiation of rheumatoid arthritis (RA). HLA = human leukocyte antigen.

Pathogenesis

The pathogenesis of RA is complex, and there are almost certainly multiple triggering mechanisms, including but not limited to smoking, infection, molecular mimicry, immune complexes, altered T-cell repertoire, and T-cell reactivity. Furthermore, it is likely that the triggers may be different based on the genetic background. As mentioned previously, smoking is a well-known trigger for some individuals but appears to be a risk factor only in those patients who possess the shared epitope.

Rheumatic fever, reactive arthritis (formerly known as *Reiter's syndrome*), and, more recently, Lyme arthritis are examples of arthritic syndromes for which infectious triggers have clearly been demonstrated, but these triggering agents are often difficult or impossible to isolate at the time when the arthritic syndromes occur. Many other examples exist in animal models of arthritis, including syndromes induced by mycobacteria and streptococci. Reactive arthritis (Chapter 265) has clearly been shown to occur when any one of a myriad of different but specific infectious triggers is presented to a specific location in the body (the gastrointestinal or genitourinary tract) of individuals with a certain genetic background, in most cases HLA-B27. Additionally, in this syndrome, the age and gender of the individual and hence the maturity of the immune system may be critical in the development of clinical disease, which occurs primarily between the ages of 15 and 40 years in males. Once unraveled, the pathophysiology of RA is likely to be similarly complex.

Despite the absence of clear evidence linking any infectious agent to RA, it is widely believed that ultimately an important triggering role will be elucidated for infectious or other environmental agents. Once triggers for RA are identified, strategies for prevention can be addressed, but this information may not help individuals with established disease. Possibly infections involving the innate immune system are causative in an early subclinical phase of the rheumatoid disease process, with the agents being absent once clinical disease develops.

The relative roles of the cellular versus the humoral immune system in the initiation and perpetuation of RA are much debated; both appear to be important. Most likely, the mechanisms of initiation of the disease process are different from those that perpetuate the chronic disease. T cells, particularly of the activated T_H1 and T_H17 types, appear to predominate in synovial tissues. These T cells, presumably activated by some as yet unknown antigen presented by macrophages, B cells, or synoviocytes in the context of HLA-DR, secrete cytokines that drive further synovial proliferation. It is believed by many that, although RA may initially be triggered by exogenous antigens, the process, once initiated, may be perpetuated by autoantigens. Macrophage-derived cytokines, particularly interleukin-1 (IL-1) and tumor necrosis factor-α (TNF-α), play central roles in this ongoing inflammatory process. As definitive proof, biologic products directed against these cytokines have shown significant efficacy in the treatment of RA.

The humoral immune system also plays a role. RF has long been a serologic marker of RA and is well known to correlate with more severe disease, including erosions of bone, and with the presence of extra-articular features. The reason that RF is produced in excess and the exact role that it plays remain elusive. RF production may increase complement activation and result in the release of lysosomal enzymes, kinins, and oxygen free radicals. ACPA antibodies exhibit a high specificity (95 to 99%) for RA, although their sensitivity for RA with currently available assays is only approximately 70%. Even though both RF and ACPA antibodies also correlate with more aggressive erosive disease, this link is strongest for ACPA antibodies.

Pathology

The synovial tissues are the primary target of the autoimmune inflammatory process that is RA; the reason for this remains elusive. However, the generalized inflammation of RA also involves the vascular endothelium and results in significant premature atherosclerosis. Once RA is initiated, the synovial tissues throughout the body become the site of a complex interaction of T cells, B cells, macrophages, and synovial cells (Fig. 264-2). The resultant proliferation of the synovial tissues (synovitis) causes the production of excessive amounts of synovial fluid and the infiltration of pannus into adjacent bone and cartilage. Synovitis results in the destruction of cartilage and marginal bone and in the stretching or rupture of the joint capsule or tendons and ligaments. In patients, these effects are manifested by the deformities (Fig. 264-3) and disabilities that make up the clinical picture of RA.

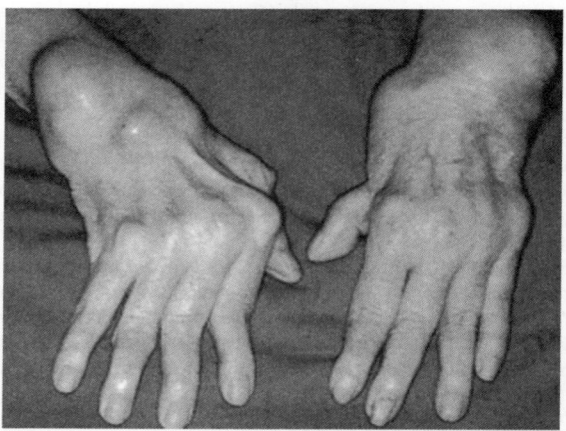

FIGURE 264-3. Severe advanced rheumatoid arthritis of the hands. There is massive tendon swelling over the dorsal surface of both wrists, severe muscle wasting, ulnar deviation of the metacarpophalangeal joints, and swan-neck deformity of the fingers. (From Forbes CD, Jackson WF. *Color Atlas and Text of Clinical Medicine,* 3rd ed. London: Mosby; 2003.)

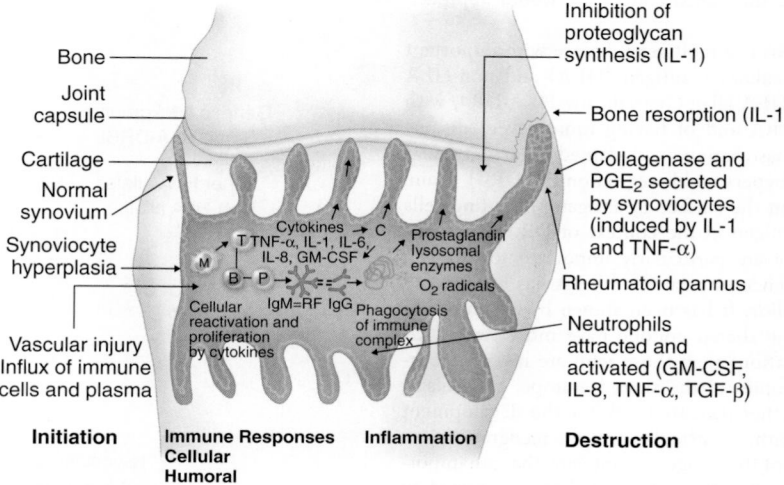

FIGURE 264-2. Events involved in the pathogenesis of rheumatoid synovitis (progressing from *left* to *right*). B = B lymphocyte; C = complement; GM-CSF = granulocyte-macrophage colony-stimulating factor; IgG, IgM = immunoglobulin G, M; IL = interleukin; M = macrophage; P = plasma cell; PGE$_2$ = prostaglandin E$_2$; RF = rheumatoid factor; T = T lymphocyte; TGF-β = transforming growth factor-β; TNF-α = tumor necrosis factor-α.

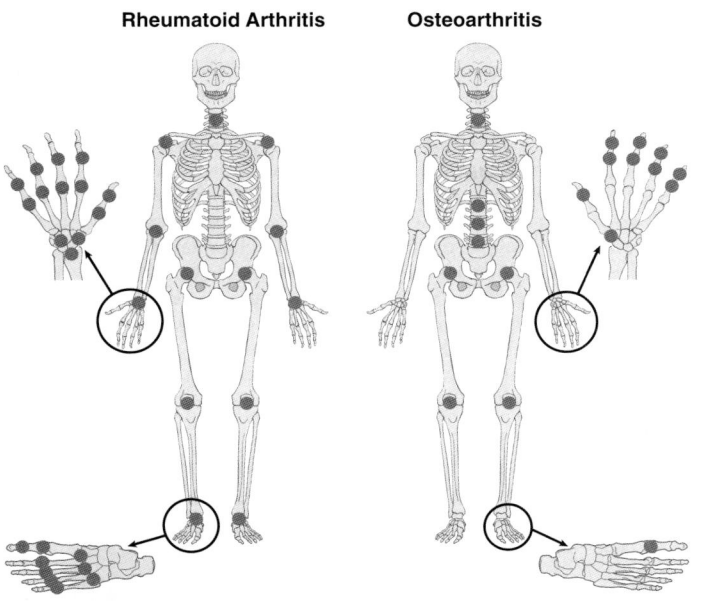

Rheumatoid Arthritis **Osteoarthritis**

FIGURE 264-4. Distribution of involved joints in the two most common forms of arthritis: rheumatoid arthritis and osteoarthritis. *Shaded circles* are shown over the involved joint areas.

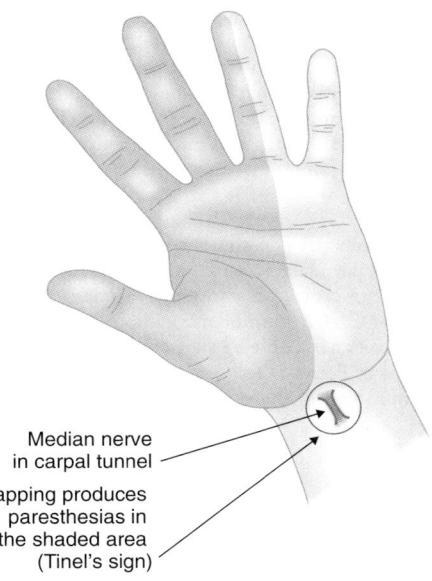

Median nerve in carpal tunnel

Tapping produces paresthesias in the shaded area (Tinel's sign)

FIGURE 264-5. Carpal tunnel syndrome. Distribution of pain and/or paresthesias (*shaded area*) when the median nerve is compressed by swelling in the wrist (carpal tunnel).

CLINICAL MANIFESTATIONS
Articular Manifestations

RA can affect any of the synovial (diarthrodial) joints (Fig. 264-4). Most commonly, the disease starts in the metacarpophalangeal (MCP), proximal interphalangeal (PIP), and metatarsophalangeal (MTP) joints, followed by the wrists, knees, elbows, ankles, hips, and shoulders, in roughly that order. Early treatment limits the joints involved. Less commonly, and usually later, RA may involve the temporomandibular, cricoarytenoid, and sternoclavicular joints. RA may involve the upper part of the cervical spine, particularly the C1-C2 articulation, but, unlike the spondyloarthropathies (Chapter 265), it does not involve the rest of the spine. RA patients are at an increased risk for osteoporosis (Chapter 243), and this risk should be considered and dealt with early.

Hands

The hands are a major site of involvement, and a significant portion of the disability that RA causes is because of damage and dysfunction of the hands. Typically disease starts with swelling of the PIPs and MCPs. The distal interphalangeal (DIP) joints are almost never involved; significant involvement of the DIP joints should suggest the possibility of a different diagnosis (i.e., osteoarthritis or psoriatic arthritis). Figure 264-3 illustrates the classic ulnar deviation of the MCP joints and swan-neck deformities (hyperextension of the PIP joints) that are commonly seen in late disease. Boutonnière (or buttonhole) deformities also occur as a result of hyperflexion of the PIP joints. If the clinical disease remains active, hand function deteriorates. Sudden loss of function of individual fingers may occur as a result of tendon rupture, which requires the expertise of a hand surgeon to repair.

Feet

Feet, particularly the MTP joints, are involved early in most patients with RA. Radiographic erosions occur at least as early in the feet as in the hands. Subluxation of the toes is common and leads to the dual problem of breakdown of the skin and ulcers on the top of the toes and malalignment of the MTP heads. Painful ambulation develops owing to loss of the cushioning pads that usually protect the heads of the MTP joints.

Wrists

The wrist joints are involved in most patients with RA; radial deviation is the rule, and patients with severe involvement may progress to volar subluxation. Even early in the course of the disease, synovial proliferation in and around the wrists may compress the median nerve, causing carpal tunnel syndrome (Fig. 264-5). Later, this synovial proliferation may invade tendons and lead to rupture of extensor tendons.

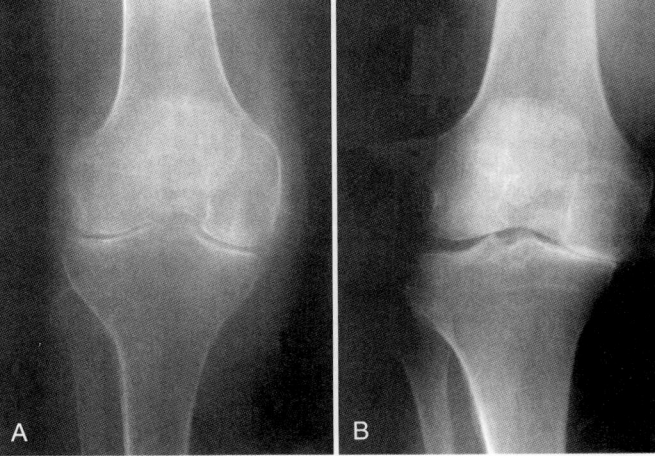

FIGURE 264-6. Radiographs of the knees in the two most common forms of arthritis: rheumatoid arthritis and osteoarthritis. **A,** Severe involvement in rheumatoid arthritis, with almost complete symmetrical loss of joint space in both the medial and the lateral compartments, but with little subchondral sclerosis or osteophyte formation. **B,** Typical osteoarthritis, with severe, near-total loss of joint space of one compartment and a normal or actually increased joint space of the other compartment. Note also the significant subchondral sclerosis in the involved area, typical of osteoarthritis.

Large Joints

Involvement of knees, ankles, elbows, hips, and shoulders is common. Characteristically, the whole joint surface is involved in a symmetrical fashion. Therefore, RA is symmetrical not only from one side of the body to the other but also within the individual joint. In the case of the knee (Fig. 264-6A), the medial and lateral compartments are both severely narrowed in RA; in contrast, in patients with osteoarthritis (see Fig. 264-6B) typically only one compartment of the knee is involved.

Synovial cysts may occur around any of the joints (large or small), and they occasionally manifest as soft, fluctuant masses that present diagnostic challenges. When the knee produces excess synovial fluid, it may accumulate in the popliteal space (popliteal or Baker's cyst). These cysts can cause problems by pressing on the popliteal nerve, artery, or veins. Baker's cysts may dissect into the tissues of the calf (usually posteriorly), or they may rupture into the upper calf. Dissection may produce only minor symptoms, such as a feeling of fullness; rupture of the cyst with extravasation of the inflammatory content produces significant pain and swelling and may be confused with thrombophlebitis, the so-called pseudothrombophlebitis syndrome. Ultrasonography of the popliteal fossa and calf is useful to establish the correct diagnosis and rule out thrombophlebitis, which may be precipitated by popliteal cysts. Treatment of popliteal or any other cyst should be directed at interrupting the inflammatory process through an intra-articular injection of corticosteroid into the associated joint.

Neck

Although most of the axial skeleton is spared in RA, the cervical spine is commonly involved, particularly the C1-C2 articulation. Bony erosions and ligament damage can occur in this area and may lead to subluxation. Most often, subluxation at C1-C2 is minor and without accompanying symptoms; patients and caregivers need only be cautious and avoid actively forcing the neck into positions of flexion. Occasionally, subluxation at C1-C2 is severe and leads to compromise of the cervical cord with symptoms and in some cases death.

Other Joints

Wherever synovial tissue exists, RA can cause problems. The temporomandibular, cricoarytenoid, and sternoclavicular joints are examples of other joints that may be involved in RA. The cricoarytenoid joint is responsible for abduction and adduction of the vocal cords. Involvement of this joint may lead to a feeling of fullness in the throat, to hoarseness, and, rarely, when the cords are essentially fused in a closed position, to a syndrome of acute respiratory distress with or without stridor. In this latter situation, emergent tracheotomy may be life-saving.

Extra-Articular Manifestations

Systemic features of RA such as fatigue, weight loss, and low-grade fevers occur frequently. As with all the other extra-articular features, they are more common in those patients who possess RF or ACPA antibodies or both (Table 264-1) and respond to treatment of the RA.

Skin

Subcutaneous nodules are seen in approximately one fifth of patients with RA, almost exclusively in those who are RF positive. Patients with nodules who are RF negative should be carefully scrutinized for a different diagnosis, such as chronic tophaceous gout. Nodules may occur almost anywhere (e.g., lungs, heart, eye), but most commonly they occur subcutaneously on extensor surfaces (particularly the forearms) (Fig. 264-7), over joints, or over pressure points. Rheumatoid nodules are firm on examination, usually are not tender, have a characteristic histologic picture, and are thought to be initiated by small vessel vasculitis. A syndrome of increased nodulosis, despite good control of the joint disease, has been described with methotrexate therapy (Fig. 264-8).

Small vessel vasculitis,[4] manifested as digital infarcts or leukocytoclastic vasculitis, may occur in RA (Fig. 264-9) and should prompt more aggressive DMARD treatment. A vasculitis of small and medium arteries that is indistinguishable from polyarteritis nodosa also can be seen with RA and requires aggressive systemic therapy. Finally, pyoderma gangrenosum occurs with increased frequency in association with RA.

Cardiovascular Involvement

Cardiac involvement directly related to RA is uncommon; however, patients with RA have a significantly increased morbidity and mortality from coronary artery disease and congestive heart failure. A meta-analysis of observational studies has shown that the risk for incident cardiovascular disease is increased by 48% in patients with RA compared with that in the general population. The reasons are not clear, but chronic inflammation appears to be the major cause. Some of the medications used to treat RA and a sedentary lifestyle may be additional risk factors for the development of coronary artery disease. Pericardial effusions are common in RA (50% by echocardiography) but usually are asymptomatic. Rarely, long-standing pericardial disease may result in a fibrinous pericarditis, and patients may present clinically with constrictive pericarditis (Chapter 77). A population-based inception cohort of patients with RA in Olmstead County, Minnesota, has shown an increased incidence of venous thromboembolism compared with subjects without RA.

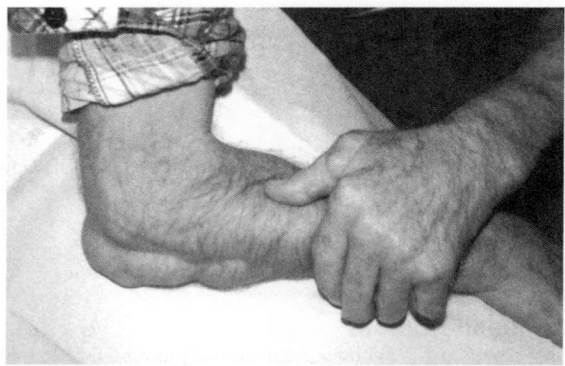

FIGURE 264-7. **Rheumatoid nodules.** Large rheumatoid nodules are seen in a classic location along the extensor surface of the forearm and in the olecranon bursa.

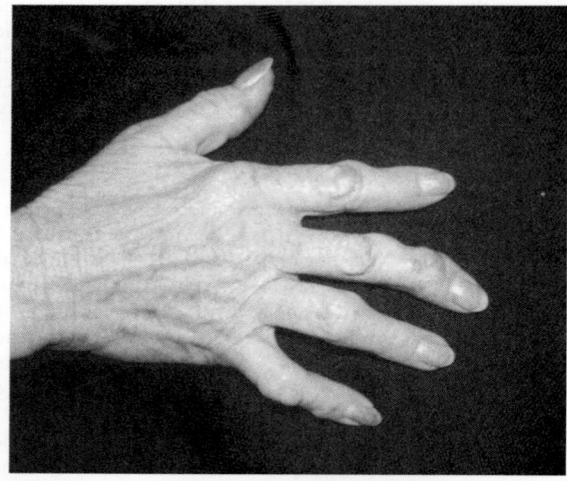

FIGURE 264-8. **Rheumatoid nodulosis.** In this patient, multiple rheumatoid nodules are present over joints. In some cases, nodules may dominate the clinical picture. Rarely, this may be seen as a side effect of methotrexate therapy.

TABLE 264-1	EXTRA-ARTICULAR MANIFESTATIONS OF RHEUMATOID ARTHRITIS
Skin	Nodules, fragility, vasculitis, pyoderma gangrenosum
Heart	Pericarditis, premature atherosclerosis, vasculitis, valve disease, and valve ring nodules
Lung	Pleural effusions, interstitial lung disease, bronchiolitis obliterans, rheumatoid nodules, vasculitis
Eye	Keratoconjunctivitis sicca, episcleritis, scleritis, scleromalacia perforans, peripheral ulcerative keratopathy
Neurologic	Entrapment neuropathy, cervical myelopathy, mononeuritis multiplex (vasculitis), peripheral neuropathy
Hematopoietic	Anemia, thrombocytosis, lymphadenopathy, Felty's syndrome
Kidney	Amyloidosis, vasculitis
Bone	Osteopenia

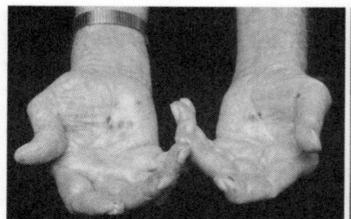 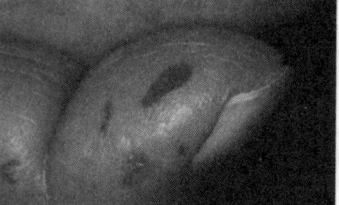

FIGURE 264-9. **Small vessel vasculitis.** A and B, Rheumatoid vasculitis with small brown infarcts of palms and fingers in chronic rheumatoid arthritis. (Courtesy Dr. Martin Lidsky, Houston, TX.)

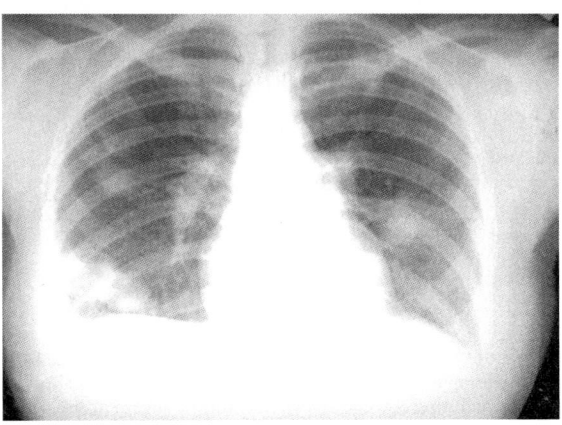

FIGURE 264-10. Rheumatoid nodules in the lung. Chest radiograph demonstrates discrete rheumatoid nodules in both right and left lower lobes. (Courtesy Dr. Martin Lidsky, Houston, TX.)

TABLE 264-2	CLASSIFICATION CRITERIA FOR RHEUMATOID ARTHRITIS*

Morning stiffness (≥1 hr)
Swelling (soft tissue) of three or more joints
Swelling (soft tissue) of hand joints (PIP, MCP, or wrist)
Symmetrical swelling (soft tissue)
Subcutaneous nodules
Serum rheumatoid factor
Erosions and/or periarticular osteopenia in hand or wrist joints seen on radiograph

*Criteria 1 through 4 must have been continuously present for 6 wk or longer, and criteria 2 through 5 must be observed by a physician. A classification of rheumatoid arthritis requires that 4 of the 7 criteria be fulfilled.
MCP = metacarpophalangeal; PIP = proximal interphalangeal.

Pulmonary Manifestations

Pulmonary manifestations of RA include pleural effusions, rheumatoid nodules, and parenchymal lung disease (Chapters 84 and 92). Pleural effusions occur more commonly in men and are usually small and asymptomatic. Of interest, pleural fluid in RA is characterized by low levels of glucose and low pH and, therefore, may at times be confused with empyema. Rheumatoid nodules may occur in the lung, especially in men (Fig. 264-10); these are usually solid but may calcify, cavitate, or become infected. Rarely, pulmonary nodules rupture and produce a pneumothorax. If patients with RA are exposed to coal or silica dust, diffuse nodular densities may occur (Caplan's syndrome). Differentiating rheumatoid nodules from lung cancer can be problematic, particularly if the lesion is solitary. Therefore, the presence of pulmonary nodules in a patient with RA should precipitate an aggressive diagnostic evaluation.

Diffuse interstitial fibrosis occurs in RA and may progress to a honeycomb appearance on radiography with increasing dyspnea. Rarely, bronchiolitis obliterans can be seen, with or without organizing pneumonia.

Ophthalmologic Manifestations

The most common manifestation of RA in the eye is keratoconjunctivitis sicca (dry eyes) from secondary Sjögren's syndrome (Chapter 268). Patients may have associated xerostomia (dry mouth), parotid gland swelling, or, occasionally, lymphadenopathy. Scleritis also can occur and may be painful, with progression to thinning of the sclera, with deep pigment showing through on physical examination, and may progress to perforation (scleromalacia perforans). Rarely, tendonitis of the superior oblique muscles can result in double vision (Brown's syndrome).

Neurologic Manifestations

Peripheral nerve entrapment syndromes, including carpal tunnel syndrome (median nerve at the wrist), and tarsal tunnel syndrome (anterior tibial nerve at the ankle), are common in RA. Vasculitis can lead to a stocking and glove neuropathy or mononeuritis multiplex, both of which may require aggressive therapy. Subluxations at C1-C2 may produce myelopathy. Rheumatoid nodules in the central nervous system have been described but are rare and usually asymptomatic.

Felty's Syndrome

Felty's syndrome is the triad of RA, splenomegaly, and neutropenia. This complication is seen in patients with severe, RF/ACPA-positive disease and may be accompanied by hepatomegaly, thrombocytopenia, lymphadenopathy, and fevers. Most patients with Felty's syndrome do not require special therapy; instead, treatment should be directed toward their severe RA. If severe neutropenia (Chapter 167) exists (<500 cells/μL) and is accompanied by recurrent bacterial infections or chronic, nonhealing leg ulcers, splenectomy may rarely be indicated.

Some patients with RA, who were previously thought to have Felty's syndrome, have peripheral white blood cell counts dominated by large granular lymphocytes with almost complete absence of neutrophils. This condition is known as the *large granular lymphocyte syndrome* and is thought to be a variant of T-cell leukemia. In the setting of RA, this syndrome has a good prognosis, with the neutropenia often responding dramatically to methotrexate therapy.

Clinical Course

Although the presentation is variable, most patients with RA have insidious onset of pain, stiffness, or swelling in multiple small joints over the course of weeks to months. Systemic features such as fatigue, low-grade fevers, and weight loss also may be present. Less commonly, the onset can be fulminant, occurring almost overnight, or patients may exhibit persistent monoarthritis or oligoarthritis for prolonged periods before manifesting the more typical pattern of joint involvement. Rarely, particularly men, develop extra-articular features of RA before the joint problems appear.

The distribution of involved joints is a critical clue to the underlying diagnosis. The joints that are involved in RA at presentation are variable; typically, the symptoms start in the small joints of the hands (PIP and MCP joints) and in the toes (MTP joints). Importantly, RA usually spares the DIP joints and the small joints of the toes (see Fig. 264-4). Later, RA moves, or some would say "metastasizes," to larger joints: wrists, knees, elbows, ankles, hips, and shoulders (roughly in that order). Although the patient's history of joint symptoms (arthralgia) is important, the diagnosis of RA requires the presence of inflammation (swelling, warmth, or both) on examination of the joints.

Morning stiffness is a hallmark of inflammatory arthritis and is a prominent feature of RA. Patients with RA are characteristically at their worst in the morning or after prolonged periods of rest. This stiffness in and around joints often lasts for hours, and quantifying it is one way to measure improvement. Stiffness is relieved by warmth and activity, and reducing or eliminating joint stiffness is a clear goal of therapy.

DIAGNOSIS

All current treatment paradigms for RA stress the early and aggressive use of DMARDs. Therefore, the importance of accurate early diagnosis of RA cannot be overemphasized. There is no one single finding on physical examination or laboratory testing that is pathognomonic of RA. Instead, the diagnosis of RA requires a collection of historical and physical features, as well as an alert and informed clinician.

Classification

There are currently two classification systems for RA: one designed for clinical use and one designed for studies. Table 264-2 lists the current clinical classification for RA; although designed for classification, these criteria are widely used as a diagnostic aid. The first five criteria are all clinical; in other words, they are established by physical examination or by talking with the patient. Only the last two criteria require laboratory tests or radiographs. The first four criteria must be present for at least 6 weeks before a diagnosis of RA should be made. This caveat is important, because a host of conditions, including many virus-related syndromes, can cause self-limited polyarthritis syndromes that look identical to RA, including at times the presence of RF. Such conditions usually last only 2 to 3 weeks. New classification criteria for RA have been developed for use in clinical trials and, although less specific, improve early classification.[5] These American College of Rheumatology/ European League Against Rheumatism criteria do not require 6 weeks of disease and give significant weight to the presence of high-titer RF or ACPA positivity. The presence of ACPA antibodies, even in the first few weeks of an inflammatory arthritis, is strongly suggestive of ongoing aggressive RA.[6]

TABLE 264-3 DIFFERENTIAL DIAGNOSIS OF RHEUMATOID ARTHRITIS

DISORDER	SUBCUTANEOUS NODULES	RHEUMATOID FACTOR
Viral arthritis (hepatitis B and C, parvovirus, rubella, others)	–	±
Bacterial endocarditis	±	+
Rheumatic fever	+	–
Sarcoidosis	+	+
Reactive arthritis	–	–
Psoriatic arthritis	–	–
Systemic lupus erythematosus	±	+
Primary Sjögren's syndrome	–	+
Chronic tophus gout	+	–
Calcium pyrophosphate disease	–	–
Polymyalgia rheumatica	–	–
Osteoarthritis (erosive)	–	–

– = Not present; + = frequently present; ± = occasionally present.

TABLE 264-4 KEYS TO OPTIMIZE OUTCOME OF TREATMENT OF RHEUMATOID ARTHRITIS

Early, accurate diagnosis
Early DMARD therapy
Strive for remission in all patients
Monitor carefully for treatment toxicities
Consider and treat comorbid conditions*

*Important comorbid conditions include cardiovascular disease, increased susceptibility to infections, and osteoporosis.
DMARD = disease-modifying antirheumatic drug.

remitting RF-negative symmetrical synovitis with pitting edema (the so-called RS3PE syndrome) and paraneoplastic syndromes should be considered. Chronic tophaceous gout also may mimic severe nodular RA. Hypothyroidism not only causes many rheumatic manifestations but also occurs commonly in conjunction with RA and, therefore, should be kept in mind.

Laboratory Findings

Historically, the most characteristic laboratory abnormality in RA is the presence of RF, which is found in approximately 80% of patients. RF was first described in the 1930s and is an antibody that recognizes the Fc portion of immunoglobulin G as its antigen. The presence of RF is strongly associated with more severe articular disease, as well as with essentially all the extra-articular features previously discussed. Importantly, RF is seen in association with many diseases other than RA, particularly in disease processes that provide chronic stimulation of the immune system (Table 264-3). ACPA antibodies, found in approximately 75% of patients with RA, have a high specificity (93 to 98%), are often present before clinical disease is diagnosed, and are associated with aggressive erosive disease. Approximately 15% of RA patients are negative for both RF and ACPA (seronegative). RA is associated with many other autoantibodies, including antinuclear antibodies (~30%) and antineutrophil cytoplasmic antibodies, particularly of the perinuclear type (~30%) (Chapter 257).

Most patients with RA have an anemia of chronic disease, and the degree is proportional to the activity of the disease. Therapy that controls the disease will normalize the hemoglobin levels. Other causes of anemia should also be considered in RA, particularly iron deficiency anemia from gastrointestinal blood loss. Thrombocytosis is common, with platelet counts returning to normal as the inflammation is controlled. Acute phase reactants such as ESR and CRP levels parallel the activity of the disease, and their persistent elevation portends a poor prognosis in terms of both joint destruction and mortality. White blood cell counts may be elevated, normal, or, in the case of Felty's syndrome, profoundly depressed. Eosinophilia is present in some patients with RA.

Synovial fluid in RA is characterized by white blood cell counts in the range of 5000 to 100,000/mm³, with approximately two thirds of the cells being polymorphonuclear leukocytes. There are no synovial fluid findings that are pathognomonic of RA.

Differential Diagnosis

The accurate diagnosis of RA early in its course, although challenging, is critical if patients are to benefit maximally from therapeutic intervention. Once disease has been present and active for years and the characteristic deformities and radiographic changes have occurred, the diagnosis is all too obvious. Once RA has progressed to that point, deformities may no longer be amenable to medical therapy.

Many diseases can mimic RA (see Table 264-3). Early in the course of disease, self-limited viral syndromes need to be considered, especially hepatitis B and C, parvovirus, rubella (infection or vaccination), and Epstein-Barr virus. At any time, systemic lupus erythematosus, psoriatic arthritis, and reactive arthritis may present differential diagnostic challenges. In the case of these three mimics, a targeted history and examination to elucidate their associated clinical features, such as rashes, oral ulcers, nail changes, dactylitis, urethritis, and renal, pulmonary, gastrointestinal, or ophthalmologic involvement, is critical. Especially in elderly patients with fulminant-onset RA,

TREATMENT Rx

General Measures

RA is a lifelong disease process that has no known cure; the diagnosis is made based on clinical criteria, and many different options exist for treatment. These factors magnify the importance of the patient-physician relationship and place a premium on the art rather than the science of medicine. Optimal care for patients with RA requires effective ongoing interactions between primary care physicians and rheumatologists, and, in some cases, physical therapists, occupational therapists, and orthopedic surgeons.[7] Because of the serious nature of the disease, the rapid introduction of new treatments, and the need for expertise in monitoring these therapies, all patients with RA should be evaluated early and followed closely by a rheumatologist.

The goal of therapy is disease remission (Table 264-4) or very low disease activity.[8] When RA is treated early, remission is possible in over 50% of patients. However, remissions require the ongoing use of DMARDs and are not always durable. Essentially all patients with RA should be treated with DMARDs.[9,10] Some combination of nonsteroidal anti-inflammatory drugs (NSAIDs), steroids, and DMARDs is necessary in many patients. In many patients with RA, combinations of different DMARDs (conventional and biologic) are necessary for optimal control.[A1] Therapy should be escalated rapidly to ensure maximal suppression of disease while minimizing toxicity and expense. Patients with RA should be educated about their disease and its treatment. Patients should have an opportunity to spend time with physical therapists and occupational therapists to learn about range-of-motion exercises, joint protection, and assistive devices.

Medical Therapy

In the treatment of RA, three types of medical therapies are used: NSAIDs, glucocorticoids, and DMARDs (both conventional and biologic). Initial therapy should always include a DMARD.

Nonsteroidal Anti-inflammatory Drugs

NSAIDs are important for the symptomatic relief they provide to patients with RA; however, they play only a minor role in altering the underlying disease process (Chapter 37). Therefore, NSAIDs should rarely, if ever, be used to treat RA without the concomitant use of DMARDs. Many clinicians waste valuable time switching from one NSAID to another before starting DMARD therapy.

Much has been written about the gastrointestinal toxicity of NSAIDs, and these concerns are particularly relevant to patients with RA, who often have significant risk factors, including age and concomitant steroid use. Therefore, cyclooxygenase-2 (COX2)-selective agents have been a popular choice for patients with RA. The evidence linking these agents to increased cardiovascular toxicity has been particularly troubling for patients with RA, who are already at high risk for myocardial infarction. Therefore, if COX2-selective agents are used, they should be kept at a low dose. Consideration should be given to low-dose aspirin prophylaxis in RA, but this may increase the gastrointestinal toxicity of NSAIDs. The use of concomitant misoprostol or proton pump inhibitors should be considered in all patients with RA who are taking NSAIDs. Additionally, the potential for NSAIDs to decrease renal blood flow and to increase blood pressure should be kept in mind.

Glucocorticoids

Glucocorticoids have had a significant role in the treatment of RA for more than half a century (Chapter 35). Indeed, RA was chosen as the first disease to be treated with this new therapy, partly because it was thought that RA was

TABLE 264-5 GUIDELINES FOR USE OF GLUCOCORTICOIDS

Avoid use of glucocorticoids without DMARDs
Prednisone, >10 mg/day, is rarely indicated for articular disease
Taper to the lowest effective dose
Use as "bridge therapy" until DMARD therapy is effective
Remember prophylaxis against osteoporosis

DMARD = disease-modifying antirheumatic drug.

TABLE 264-6 CAVEATS FOR MONITORING DISEASE-MODIFYING ANTIRHEUMATIC DRUG THERAPIES*

MEDICATION	CAVEATS
Prednisone	Use as bridge to effective DMARD therapy. Prophylaxis for osteoporosis? (see Table 264-5)
Hydroxychloroquine	Keep dosage lower than 6.5 mg/kg/day. Yearly eye checkup by ophthalmologist
Sulfasalazine	CBC for neutropenia, initially every month, then every 6 mo
Methotrexate	CBC and SGOT/SGPT every 8-12 wk when dose is stable. Many toxicities respond to folic acid or small dose reduction. If pneumonitis, stop and do not restart. Decreasing renal function may precipitate toxicities. Absolute contraindication in pregnancy
Leflunomide	CBC and SGOT/SGPT every 4-8 wk; long half-life may require cholestyramine washout; absolute contraindication in pregnancy
TNF inhibitors	If fevers or infectious symptoms of any kind, stop until symptoms resolve; aggressively work up and treat possible infections. May precipitate congestive heart failure, demyelinating syndromes, or lupus-like syndromes

*Patients receiving DMARDs, both conventional and biologic, should be monitored by a rheumatologist.
CBC = complete blood count; DMARD = disease-modifying antirheumatic drug; SGOT = serum glutamate oxaloacetate transaminase (aspartate aminotransferase); SGPT = serum glutamate pyruvate transaminase (alanine aminotransferase); TNF = tumor necrosis factor.

a disease of glucocorticoid deficiency (an issue that remains unresolved). As was the case with the first patient treated in 1948, glucocorticoids are dramatically and rapidly effective in patients with RA. Not only are glucocorticoids useful for symptomatic improvement but they also significantly decrease the radiographic progression of RA.[A2] However, the toxicities of long-term therapy are extensive and potentially devastating. Therefore, the optimal use of these drugs requires an understanding of several principles (Table 264-5).

Glucocorticoids remain among the most potent anti-inflammatory treatments available; for this reason, and because of their rapid onset of action, they are ideally suited to help control the inflammation in RA while the much slower-acting DMARDs are starting to work. Prednisone, the most commonly used glucocorticoid, should rarely be used in doses higher than 10 mg/day to treat the stiffness and articular manifestations of RA. At this dose at the start of methotrexate-based treatment, the addition of prednisone reduces erosive joint damage, disease activity, physical disability, and the use of biologic treatment at 2 years. The dose should be slowly tapered to the lowest effective dose, and the concomitant DMARD therapy should be adjusted to make this possible. Glucocorticoids should rarely, if ever, be used to treat RA without concomitant DMARD therapy. The paradigm is to shut off inflammation rapidly with glucocorticoids and then to taper them as the DMARD is taking effect ("bridge therapy"). In all patients receiving glucocorticoids, strong measures should be taken to prevent osteoporosis. Bisphosphonates have been shown to be particularly effective in this regard but are contraindicated in women of childbearing age. Higher doses of glucocorticoids may be necessary to treat extra-articular manifestations, especially vasculitis and scleritis.

Disease-Modifying Antirheumatic Drugs

DMARDs are a group of medications that have the ability to halt the disease process in the synovium and to modify or change the disabling potential of RA. These drugs have the ability to halt or slow the radiographic progression of RA.

Conventional Disease-Modifying Antirheumatic Drugs

Included in this group of medications are methotrexate, sulfasalazine, gold, antimalarials (hydroxychloroquine [Plaquenil] and others), leflunomide (Arava), azathioprine (Imuran), minocycline, and the newly approved tofacitinib (Xeljanz). It is critically important that clinicians and patients understand that conventional DMARDs take 2 to 6 months to exert their maximal effect, and all require some monitoring (Table 264-6). Therefore, other measures, such as glucocorticoid therapy, may be needed to control the disease while these medications are starting to work.

These DMARDs have been shown to be effective in treating both early and more advanced RA. Until additional research elucidates factors that allow selection of the best initial therapy for each patient, the choice will depend on patient and physician concerns about toxicity and monitoring issues, as well as the activity of disease and presence of comorbid conditions. The critical issue is not which DMARD to start first but rather getting the DMARD therapy started early in the disease process.

Methotrexate

Methotrexate is the preferred initial DMARD of most rheumatologists, in part because patients have a more durable response, and because, with correct monitoring, serious toxicities are rare.[A3] Methotrexate is dramatically effective in slowing radiographic progression and is usually given orally in doses ranging from 5 to 30 mg/week as a single dose. This once-per-week administration is worthy of emphasis; prior experience with daily therapy in psoriasis has demonstrated the importance of allowing the liver time to recover between doses. Oral absorption of methotrexate is variable; subcutaneous injections of methotrexate may be effective if oral treatment is not. Side effects of methotrexate include oral ulcers, nausea, hepatotoxicity, bone marrow suppression, and pneumonitis. With the exception of pneumonitis, these toxicities respond to dose adjustments. Monitoring of blood counts and liver blood tests (albumin and aspartate aminotransaminase [SGOT] or alanine aminotransferase [SGPT]) should be done every 4 to 8 weeks initially and, when stable, every 3 months thereafter, with adjustments in the dose of methotrexate as needed. Renal function is critical for clearance of methotrexate; previously stable patients may experience severe toxicities if renal function deteriorates. Pneumonitis, although rare, is less predictable and can be fatal, particularly if the methotrexate is not stopped or is restarted. Folic acid, 1 to 4 mg/day, can significantly decrease most methotrexate toxicities without interfering with efficacy. If methotrexate alone does not sufficiently control

disease, it is combined with other DMARDs.[A4] Methotrexate in combination with virtually any of the other DMARDs (conventional or biologic) has been shown to be more effective than either drug alone.

Leflunomide

Leflunomide, a pyrimidine antagonist, has a very long half-life and is most commonly started at 10 to 20 mg/day orally. Diarrhea is the most common toxicity and responds to dose reduction, and doses of leflunomide of 10 to 20 mg three to five times per week are frequently used. Also, because of the long half-life and teratogenic potential of leflunomide, women wishing to become pregnant who have previously received leflunomide, even if therapy was stopped years ago, should have blood levels drawn. If toxicity occurs or if pregnancy is being considered, leflunomide can be rapidly eliminated from the body by treatment with cholestyramine. Laboratory monitoring for hematologic and hepatic toxicity should be done during treatment with leflunomide, as recommended for methotrexate.

Antimalarial Drugs

The antimalarial drugs hydroxychloroquine (Plaquenil) and chloroquine are frequently used for the treatment of RA. They have the least toxicity of any of the DMARDs and do not require monitoring of blood tests. Yearly monitoring by an ophthalmologist after 5 years of therapy is recommended to detect any signs of retinal toxicity (rare). Hydroxychloroquine is the most commonly used preparation and is given orally at 200 to 400 mg/day. These drugs are frequently used in combination with other DMARDs, particularly methotrexate. Hydroxychloroquine decreases cholesterol levels and has recently been shown to decrease the incidence of diabetes in patients with RA.

Sulfasalazine

Sulfasalazine is an effective treatment when given in doses of 1 to 3 g/day. Monitoring of blood counts, particularly white blood cell counts, in the first 6 months is recommended. Sulfasalazine and hydroxychloroquine are often combined with methotrexate, a regimen referred to as triple therapy.

Minocycline

Minocycline 100 mg twice daily has been shown to be an effective treatment for RA, particularly when used in early, RF-positive disease. Chronic therapy (>2 years) with minocycline may lead to cutaneous hyperpigmentation. Minocycline has been associated with drug-induced lupus.

Gold

Gold, the oldest DMARD, is effective but cumbersome and is currently rarely used.

Tofacitinib

Tofacitinib (Xeljanz) has been recently approved for the treatment of RA in the United States. It is the first Jak kinase inhibitor to be approved for RA. It is given orally at a dose of 5 mg twice daily, and complete blood count and liver function tests should be monitored. Additional toxicity concerns include infections, including tuberculosis, and malignancies. Tofacitinib has been shown to be effective as initial DMARD therapy,[A5] when combined with methotrexate in patients who have had incomplete responses to methotrexate, and in patients who have failed TNF inhibitors. Tofacitinib has not yet been approved in Europe.

Biologic Disease-Modifying Antirheumatic Drugs

Recent research has continued to elucidate the central role that cytokines, most notably TNF-α, IL-1 and IL-6, play in the pathophysiology of RA (Chapter 36). This led directly to the development and clinical use of biologic agents directed against TNF-α[11] (etanercept [Enbrel], infliximab [Remicade], adalimumab [Humira], golimumab [Simponi], and certolizumab [Cimzia]), IL-1 (anakinra [Kineret]), and IL-6 (tocilizumab [Actemra]). Additionally, monoclonal antibodies that deplete B cells (anti-CD20, rituximab [Rituxan]) and that block the second signal for T cell activation (abatacept [Orencia]) are effective agents in the treatment of RA. All patients with RA receiving biologic therapies should be monitored by a rheumatologist, and their physicians should be aware of the risk for infections that are often atypical.[12] All the biologics, when combined with methotrexate, have been shown to decrease disease activity and slow radiographic progression in patients with RA with active disease despite methotrexate.[A6] Early treatment with abatacept plus methotrexate was shown to result in greater sustainable clinical, functional, and radiographic benefits than methotrexate alone, with acceptable safety and tolerability, in early erosive RA. Currently, biologic agents should not be used in combination with each other because all studies to date have shown a significant increase in infections. See Chapter 36 for further details on the use of biologic agents in the treatment of RA.

The Order of Therapy in Rheumatoid Arthritis

Several randomized double-blind trials have elucidated the order of therapy in RA. The Treatment of Early Aggressive Rheumatoid Arthritis (TEAR) trial nicely showed that initial therapy with methotrexate in patients with poor-prognosis RA was not inferior at 2 years to initial combinations of either conventional DMARDs or the combination of methotrexate and etanercept.[A7] The Rheumatoid Arthritis: Comparison of Active Therapies (RACAT) trial has also shown that in those patients who are not controlled on methotrexate alone, the strategy of initially adding sulfasalazine and hydroxychloroquine to methotrexate (triple therapy) was not inferior to the addition of etanercept to methotrexate.[A8] Therefore, because of the huge economic advantages, the typical RA patient should be started on methotrexate monotherapy, and, if not controlled after 3 months on maximum methotrexate, advanced to triple therapy. If the patient does not achieve adequate control after 3 to 6 months on triple therapy, either a TNF inhibitor or abatacept should be added to methotrexate.

Treatment of Underlying Conditions

Optimal care of patients with RA requires recognition of the associated comorbid conditions, including an increased risk for cardiovascular death, osteoporosis, infections (especially pneumonia), and certain cancers.

Cardiovascular Disease

Increasingly, cardiovascular disease is being recognized as the cause of much of the excess mortality in RA. Various factors contribute to this mortality, including sedentary lifestyle and glucocorticoid therapy. However, a strong association between chronic inflammation and cardiovascular disease has been identified, and it is likely that this may be the most significant factor. Therapies that control RA earlier and better can be expected to decrease cardiovascular morbidity and mortality. Both methotrexate and TNF inhibitors have been shown to decrease cardiovascular mortality in RA. Clinicians should consider RA a risk factor for cardiovascular disease and should aggressively address other cardiovascular risk factors (Chapter 52) in their patients with RA.[13]

Other Associated Diseases

Osteoporosis is common in patients with RA, and early treatment results in long-term dividends. Patients with RA are at an increased risk for infections, and some forms of treatment further increase this risk. Patients should be cautioned to seek medical attention early for even minor symptoms suggestive of infection, especially if receiving biologic therapy. All patients with RA should receive a pneumococcal vaccine at appropriate intervals and yearly influenza vaccinations. Finally, patients with RA have an increased risk for lymphoma. Occasionally, B-cell lymphoma is associated with immunosuppression and regress after immunosuppression is discontinued. Patients with RA have significantly decreased risk of developing colon cancer. This is thought to be secondary to chronic inhibition of COX by NSAIDs.

RA is not a benign disease and is not limited to the joints. Once established, RA is a lifelong progressive disease that produces significant morbidity in most patients and premature mortality in many. Long-term studies have

found that 50% of patients with RA have had to stop working after 10 years (~10 times the average rate). Patients who are RF or ACPA positive and those who are positive for the shared epitope have a worse prognosis, with more erosions and more extra-articular disease (see Table 264-1). Once deformities are found on examination or erosions on radiography, the damage is largely irreversible. It has been clearly shown that erosions occur in most patients in the first 1 to 2 years and that the rate of radiographic damage can be affected by early therapy. A recent cohort study has shown that the aggressive use of disease-modifying agents and the introduction of biologic agents have been associated with substantial reductions in disability. Therefore, early DMARD therapy is critical. Although limited long-term data are available, the current information strongly suggests that patients have the opportunity to benefit greatly if the newer principles of therapy are practiced.

FUTURE DIRECTIONS

Significant advances in the effective treatment of RA have come from an understanding of the cytokine imbalance that accompanies this disease. Much research is focused on the further development of biologic products to modulate this balance. There remains a critical need for a cytokine thermostat that would allow titration of the desired cytokine balance to control disease without altering critical immune functions.

Even with existing therapies, there are many different effective options for patients with RA. The challenge for the clinician is to pick the right option for each patient. Few data are currently available to aid in this choice, and the establishment of parameters, genetic or otherwise, that would allow selection of the best initial option for each patient would be a major breakthrough. Finally, elucidation of the trigger or triggers for RA may allow the development of strategies to prevent the onset of clinical disease.

Grade A References

A1. Goekoop-Ruiterman YP, de Vries-Bouwstra JK, Allaart CF, et al. Comparison of treatment strategies in early rheumatoid arthritis: a randomized trial. *Ann Intern Med.* 2007;146:406-415.

A2. Bakker MF, Jacobs JW, Welsing PM, et al. Low-dose prednisone inclusion in a methotrexate-based, tight control strategy for early rheumatoid arthritis: a randomized trial. *Ann Intern Med.* 2012;156:329-339.

A3. Lopez-Olivo MA, Siddhanamatha HR, Shea B, et al. Methotrexate for treating rheumatoid arthritis. *Cochrane Database Syst Rev.* 2014;6:CD000957.

A4. Moreland LW, O'Dell JR, Paulus HE, et al. TEAR Investigators. A randomized comparative effectiveness study of oral triple therapy versus etanercept plus methotrexate in early aggressive rheumatoid arthritis. *Arthritis Rheum.* 2012;64:2824-2835.

A5. Lee EB, Fleischmann R, Hall S, et al. Tofacitinib versus methotrexate in rheumatoid arthritis. *N Engl J Med.* 2014;370:2377-2386.

A6. Nam JL, Ramiro S, Gaujoux-Viala C, et al. Efficacy of biological disease-modifying antirheumatic drugs: a systematic literature review informing the 2013 update of the EULAR recommendations for the management of rheumatoid arthritis. *Ann Rheum Dis.* 2014;73:516-528.

A7. O'Dell JR, Curtis JR, Mikuls TR, et al. Validation of the methotrexate-first strategy in patients with early, poor-prognosis rheumatoid arthritis: results from a two-year randomized, double-blind trial. *Arthritis Rheum.* 2013;65:1985-1994.

A8. O'Dell JR, Mikuls TR, Taylor TH, et al. Therapies for active rheumatoid arthritis after methotrexate failure. *N Engl J Med.* 2013;369:307-318.

GENERAL REFERENCES

For the General References and other additional features, please visit Expert Consult at https://expertconsult.inkling.com.

265

THE SPONDYLOARTHROPATHIES

ROBERT D. INMAN

COMMON FEATURES OF SPONDYLOARTHRITIS

DEFINITION

Spondyloarthritis (SpA) encompasses a group of clinical syndromes that are linked in terms of disease manifestations and genetic susceptibility. The

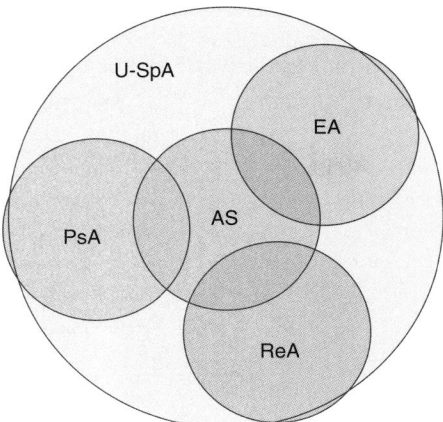

FIGURE 265-1. Schematic relationships among the different spondyloarthritis (SpA) subsets. Ankylosing spondylitis (AS), considered the classic SpA, encompasses the essential features of this family of diseases. AS may overlap with psoriatic arthritis (PsA), enteropathic arthritis (EA), or reactive arthritis (ReA). Many patients have clinical features of SpA that do not meet the diagnostic criteria for any of the four defined subsets. Such cases are termed *undifferentiated SpA* (U-SpA).

TABLE 265-1	ASAS CLASSIFICATION CRITERIA FOR AXIAL SPONDYLOARTHRITIS	
Sacroiliitis* *Plus* ≥SpA feature†	OR	HLA-B27 *Plus* ≥2 other SpA features†
*Sacroiliitis (x-rays or MRI)		†SpA features:
• Definite radiographic sacroiliitis according to modified New York criteria (see Table 265-3) *Or* • Active (acute) inflammation on MRI highly suggestive of sacroiliitis associated with SpA		• IBP • Arthritis • Enthesitis (heel) • Dactylitis • Psoriasis • Crohn's disease/ulcerative colitis • Good response to NSAIDs • Family history of SpA • Elevated CRP • HLA-827

ASAS = Assessment in Spondyloarthritis International Society; CRP = C-reactive protein; IBP = inflammatory back pain; MRI = magnetic resonance imaging; NSAIDs = nonsteroidal anti-inflammatory drugs; SpA = spondyloarthritis.

clinical subsets most commonly recognized are ankylosing spondylitis (AS), reactive arthritis (ReA), psoriatic arthritis (PsA), and enteropathic arthritis (EA) (Fig. 265-1). In addition, a sizable number of patients do not fit into one of these distinct diagnostic categories but share some of the common clinical features described in this chapter. This syndrome is termed *undifferentiated spondyloarthritis* (USpA); it may evolve over time into a classic pattern such as AS, or it may retain an undifferentiated pattern in long-term follow-up studies.

PATHOBIOLOGY

Family studies involving multiple individuals with SpA have emphasized some of the common features among the four distinct subsets. The impression from such studies is that there is a shared common path of immunogenetic susceptibility, with further genetic and environmental influences that lead to characteristic clinical subsets. Thus, EA may occur in one such family, but in another family the disease may be PsA. In this sense, the subsets of SpA seem to "breed true." It should be recognized, however, that some distinct clinical features can be very similar in their manifestations (e.g., guttate psoriasis and keratoderma blennorrhagicum), making simple discrimination difficult.

CLINICAL MANIFESTATIONS

There are several common features in the clinical subsets of SpA that serve to both link them with and distinguish them from the other major contributor to chronic polyarthritis—rheumatoid arthritis (RA) (Chapter 264). SpA has a strong predilection for the spine, in particular the sacroiliac joints. There is a shared tendency for new bone formation at sites of chronic inflammation, with joint ankylosis as a consequence. When peripheral arthritis occurs, it is commonly in the lower extremity and asymmetrical. There is a predilection for involvement at sites of tendon insertion into bone (entheses), so enthesitis is one of the most specific clinical manifestations of SpA. Theories postulating the basis for this target organ involvement have invoked biomechanical factors, innervation, local vascularity, and bone marrow–derived inflammatory mediators, but the precise mechanism remains incompletely defined. Whatever the reason, inflammation in the enthesis and contiguous subchondral bone is a characteristic feature of this form of arthritis, and the appearance of this inflammation on magnetic resonance imaging (MRI) is distinct enough to be increasingly used for diagnostic purposes, particularly when the x-rays are not diagnostic.

A predilection for ocular inflammation, particularly acute anterior uveitis, is a common feature of SpA. Indeed, some investigators consider anterior uveitis to be a feature of SpA in its own right because it may occur in the same susceptible population of patients even in the absence of joint involvement, and it may have a unique genetic predisposition. Finally, all SpA subsets have an association with the class I human leukocyte antigen (HLA) allele B27, with the strength of the association varying somewhat among them. Newer genetic risk associations such as *IL23R*, which are shared between SpA, pso-

riatic arthritis, and inflammatory bowel disease (IBD), further link the clinical subsets of SpA.

DIAGNOSIS

Increasingly, diagnostic criteria (Table 265-1 [Assessment in Spondyloarthritis International Society criteria]) are emphasizing the common clinical features—namely, inflammatory spinal pain or asymmetrical lower extremity synovitis. Several distinct features differentiate SpA from RA, the other main contributor to the differential diagnosis of chronic polyarthritis (Table 265-2). These features include sex predilection, HLA association, pattern of joint involvement, and presence of rheumatoid factor, which becomes the serologic distinction between seropositive disease (RA) and seronegative disease (SpA).

At the level of joint histopathology, sites of chronic inflammation in RA are associated with erosions, but in SpA such sites are associated with new bone formation. This distinction suggests a fundamental difference in the cytokine profile in the microenvironment of the joint, but this issue has not been resolved, and the mediators of neo-ossification await identification. Dysregulation of the wnt/β-catenin pathway may play a key role in the ankylosing process. Synovial histopathology in SpA is characterized by abundant neutrophils, macrophages, and hypervascularity, whereas in RA the prominent features are lymphoid aggregates, dendritic cells, lining cell hyperplasia, and citrullinated proteins. These differences suggest that SpA reflects a fundamental alteration in innate immunity, whereas RA reflects dysregulation of adaptive immunity.

TREATMENT   Rx

General Measures

SpA necessitates a global approach to management in which education of patients is the cornerstone.[1-3] Because the typical onset is during young adulthood, these patients may experience significant frustration or depression if their acute arthritis evolves into a chronic disease that significantly impairs their functional capabilities and quality of life. A clinician managing patients with SpA should be aware that these psychosocial aspects are an important part of the burden of illness. Similarly, there may be important implications for the workplace, particularly if a job demands significant bending or twisting. It is important to include the mechanical demands of the workplace in the global assessment of patients with SpA.

Exercise is an important part of the treatment plan for patients with AS.[4] Generally, high-impact sports should be avoided, whereas swimming is an ideal exercise. Stretching to maintain mobility and maintenance of posture should be emphasized, and an experienced physiotherapist can greatly assist in instructing patients in daily exercises. Long car trips and air travel should include periodic stretching. Sleep position should emphasize a straight back position rather than one curled on the side. Deep breathing exercises and avoidance of smoking should be stressed.

One key area of concern for patients is prognosis, because SpAs, particularly ReA, often occur in young, active individuals for whom athletic activity is a

TABLE 265-2 DIFFERENTIAL DIAGNOSIS OF CHRONIC POLYARTHRITIS

FEATURE	RHEUMATOID ARTHRITIS	ANKYLOSING SPONDYLITIS	ENTEROPATHIC ARTHRITIS	PSORIATIC ARTHRITIS	REACTIVE ARTHRITIS
Male-female ratio	1:3	3:1	1:1	1:1	10:1
HLA association	DR4	B27	B27 (axial)	B27 (axial)	B27
Joint pattern	Symmetrical, peripheral	Axial	Axial and peripheral	Axial and asymmetrical, peripheral	Axial and asymmetrical, peripheral
Sacroiliac	0	Symmetrical	Symmetrical	Asymmetrical	Asymmetrical
Syndesmophyte	0	Smooth, marginal	Smooth, marginal	Coarse, nonmarginal	Coarse, nonmarginal
Eye	Scleritis	Iritis	+/−	0	Iritis and conjunctivitis
Skin	Vasculitis	0	0	Psoriasis	Keratoderma
Rheumatoid factor	>80%	0	0	0	0

HLA = human leukocyte antigen.

priority. There is general recognition that ReA has a greater propensity for chronicity than was previously appreciated, and this should temper an overly optimistic projection of the disease's natural history. At the 5-year follow-up of a cohort of patients with *Salmonella*-induced ReA, two thirds continued to have subjective complaints, and one third demonstrated objective changes in their joints. The variability in prognosis for the large group of patients falling into the USpA group is perplexing. At present, there is a lack of reliable predictors of progression in patients with this heterogeneous cluster of articular and extra-articular features.

Medical Therapy
Nonsteroidal Anti-inflammatory Drugs
In general, joint inflammation in SpA improves significantly after the introduction of nonsteroidal anti-inflammatory drugs (NSAIDs). Indomethacin and diclofenac (up to 150 mg/day in divided doses) or naproxen (up to 1000 mg/day in divided doses) are generally well tolerated in this population. These agents have to be used with caution in EA because of concern about exacerbating possible underlying IBD. In the case of AS, the goal with anti-inflammatory treatment is to achieve sufficient relief of pain and stiffness to allow an active, sustained program of exercise and physical activity that maintains posture and improves quality of life. Some studies have suggested that NSAIDs have disease-modifying capability, but this effect appears to be restricted to those patients with elevated C-reactive protein (CRP) or erythrocyte sedimentation rate (ESR).

Corticosteroids
The response to the intra-articular injection of steroids in the peripheral joints of patients with SpA is often neither as dramatic nor as sustained as in those with RA. Corticosteroid injection into the sacroiliac joints is usually performed under imaging guidance (fluoroscopy or computed tomography [CT]). One study found that such injections resulted in a good response in 79% of patients and that the improvement could persist for many months. Systemic corticosteroids (either orally or via an intravenous bolus protocol) have been used for severe symptomatic flares, but there are few controlled trials to validate their effectiveness. The goal should be prompt tapering of the dose when symptomatic control is achieved. The recognition that osteoporosis (Chapter 243) is a significant problem in AS provides further impetus to use corticosteroids sparingly. Topical steroids are usually effective for the treatment of the mucous membrane and skin manifestations of ReA. For uveitis, topical corticosteroid eye drops are an integral component of management, and treatment should be monitored jointly with an ophthalmologist.

Sulfasalazine
Randomized placebo-controlled trials have provided some support for the use of sulfasalazine (SSZ), particularly in PsA. Three 36-week randomized double-blind multicenter studies of patients with AS, PsA, and ReA, respectively, were undertaken to compare SSZ (2 g/day) with placebo in each case. An analysis of these studies stratified the patients into those having axial disease and those having peripheral disease. In patients with only axial disease, response criteria were met equally in the SSZ group and the placebo group. In patients with peripheral arthritis, significantly superior responses were seen with SSZ: 59% of the SSZ group and 43% of the placebo group responded (*P* < .0005).[A1] These findings are useful in guiding the selection of patients for SSZ treatment. A recent study comparing SSZ with etanercept in AS demonstrated the superiority of tumor necrosis factor (TNF) inhibitor therapy with respect to symptomatic improvement as well as MRI evidence of inflammation.[A1]

Methotrexate
Concurrent with the widespread use of methotrexate (MTX) in patients with RA, there has been increasing use of MTX in patients with SpA, but responses

have been good only for peripheral joint disease. There is no evidence that MTX is effective for the spinal inflammation characteristic of AS, nor is there evidence that MTX changes the course of axial involvement in AS. Experience with long-term MTX therapy in patients with PsA has increased, although there has been little in the way of randomized controlled trials. Long-term follow-up may be required to resolve whether MTX has a joint-sparing effect in PsA.

Disease-Modifying Agents
There have been additional therapeutic approaches to the control of PsA. The clinical impression of leflunomide therapy has been positive, in general, although there are few formal trials to validate this impression. The mechanism of action of disease-modifying antirheumatic drugs (DMARDs) in SpA has not been resolved. The response of SpA patients to SSZ may be attributable to the antibiotic moiety of this compound (sulfapyridine) or to the anti-inflammatory moiety (5-aminosalicylic acid).

Antibiotic Therapy
The current concept of the pathogenesis of ReA postulates that a bacterial infection, usually gastrointestinal (GI) or genitourinary (GU), is the triggering event in an immunogenetically susceptible host. For the other subsets of SpA, there is less compelling evidence that infection plays a causal role. It is sound clinical practice to treat any culture-proven chlamydial urethritis in conjunction with treatment of the sexual partner. For this indication, a single 1-g dose of azithromycin is as effective as doxycycline 100 mg twice a day for 7 days. The role of antibiotics in the management of ReA has been controversial. A meta-analysis concluded that there is little evidence for efficacy of antibiotic therapy in ReA.[A2] But a recent report compared rifampin/azithromycin, rifampin/doxycycline, and placebo for chronic *Chlamydia*-induced ReA and observed that tender and swollen joint counts responded more significantly to the combination antibiotics than to placebo.[A3] The precise role of antibiotics in chronic post-*Chlamydia* ReA has not yet been determined.

Anti–Tumor Necrosis Factor Therapy
The pathogenic role of immunomodulatory cytokines in the pathogenesis of SpA has remained unresolved, but the advent of biologic agents has changed the landscape for SpA.[5,6] Biologic agents such as monoclonal antibodies to TNF-α (infliximab, adalimumab, golimumab) or the soluble TNF receptor (etanercept) have been used in the treatment of SpA. So far, these four anti-TNF agents have been comparably effective in trials of AS and PsA.[A4-A7] These studies have generally reported a prompt response in clinical outcome measures and in laboratory indicators of inflammation, and MRI evaluations have shown improvement in local inflammation in the sacroiliac joints and spine. The anti-TNF treatments have been well tolerated, with no significant incidence of serious adverse events, but patients appear to relapse when treatment is discontinued. Experience with longer-term treatment with anti-TNF agents has been encouraging with regard to the persistence of the therapeutic effect and the infrequency of late adverse events. These biologic agents have been shown to retard radiographic progression in PsA, and a recent report suggests a similar effect in AS.[7] Additional data using MRI may be helpful in assessing the capacity for these agents to alter the long-term outcomes of AS structurally as well as functionally.

● GENETIC SUSCEPTIBILITY
Recent genome-wide association studies in AS have identified additional genetic markers of susceptibility for AS. Polymorphisms in the *IL-23R* gene are associated with AS, and these particular variants are the same as those seen in IBD and psoriasis.[8] Thus the clinical convergence of these different diseases, well known to clinicians, now appears to have a common genetic

element. Polymorphisms in the endoplasmic reticulum aminopeptidase (ERAP) gene constitute the strongest genetic risk factor for AS after HLA-B27,[9] and the association with AS is restricted to HLA-B27+ AS patients, suggesting a gene-gene interaction. ERAP plays a key role in trimming peptides in the endoplasmic reticulum before loading these peptide complexes onto a nascent class I MHC molecule. This finding continues to attribute a central role to MHC class I peptide presentation in the pathogenesis of AS. With larger numbers studied, the list of candidate genes conferring susceptibility to AS has now extended to more than 20, but the odds ratio for any one gene is modest, with the notable exception of HLA-B27.

It is believed that the prevalence of AS in various parts of the world closely parallels the prevalence of B27 in that population, and in general, this pattern is valid. What introduces complexity into this concept is the recognition that there are more than 30 subtypes of B27. HLA-B2705 is regarded as the primordial subtype, with variability developing over time on the basis of alterations in genomic DNA. Some subtypes, notably B2706 and B2709, do not seem to confer increased susceptibility to the development of AS. This observation has led to a search for "arthritogenic peptides" that are presented by the disease-associated subtypes such as B2705 and B2704, but not by the non–disease-associated subtypes. To date, no simple peptide-susceptibility relationship has been demonstrated, but this is an important clue to the pathogenic role of B27, and studies are ongoing to explore this relationship. Recent studies have suggested that certain B27 subtypes have specific interactions with ERAP, which might fundamentally alter MHC structure and function.

Genome-wide screening studies of multiplex families with SpAs, particularly AS, are ongoing in several countries to identify other genes involved in the predisposition to these diseases. The strongest association of SpA to date remains with the HLA complex, so at least in familial AS, B27 may to a certain extent be necessary (but not sufficient) to confer disease susceptibility. MRI studies in asymptomatic B27-positive individuals indicate that there is a much higher prevalence of sacroiliitis than previously recognized, and studies are continuing to define that prevalence and indeed the prevalence of SpAs in the general population. Some investigators have concluded that SpA is as common as RA.

CLINICAL SUBSETS OF THE SPONDYLOARTHROPATHIES
Ankylosing Spondylitis

EPIDEMIOLOGY

AS is the most common inflammatory disorder of the axial skeleton.[10] The following is a useful rule of thumb: AS occurs in 0.2% of the general population, in 2% of the B27-positive population, and in 20% of B27-positive individuals with an affected family member. There is a male preponderance in the disease, with the male-to-female ratio ranging from 2.5 : 1 to 5 : 1; however, recent epidemiologic studies have found more female involvement than these earlier estimates indicate. The basis for the gender bias has not been resolved. It is held, however, that AS is underrecognized in women, perhaps because of milder axial disease and a more delayed disease onset, but alternative diagnoses of pelvic and low back pain in women may hinder clinician awareness of the disease in female patients.

CLINICAL MANIFESTATIONS

AS typically begins in young adulthood, but symptoms may arise in adolescence or earlier. Up to 15% of children with juvenile idiopathic arthritis are classified as having juvenile AS. Such children may have a pauciarticular pattern, with a predilection for the tarsal joints and frequently minimal spinal complaints. During the adolescent years there is an increasing prevalence of radiographic sacroiliitis, with a significant proportion of patients manifesting this feature by the end of the teenage years. At the other end of the age spectrum, a small number of patients with late-onset AS may have sacroiliitis and oligoarthritis. The axial involvement and asymmetrical lower extremity involvement may serve to differentiate such patients from those with late-onset RA, although there may be overlapping clinical features. Recent studies indicate that the rate of radiographic progression may be less in juvenile-onset AS than in adult-onset AS.

The classic manifestation of AS is the onset of low back pain that persists for more than 3 months, is accompanied by early-morning stiffness, and is typically improved by exercise but not by rest (Table 265-3). Some studies would include a response to NSAID therapy as an additional feature differentiating AS from mechanical low back pain. Back pain that awakens the

TABLE 265-3 MODIFIED NEW YORK CRITERIA FOR ANKYLOSING SPONDYLITIS (1984)

CLINICAL CRITERIA

Low back pain and stiffness for > 3 mo that improve with exercise but are not relieved by rest

Limitation of motion of the lumbar spine in both sagittal and frontal planes

Limitation of chest expansion

RADIOLOGIC CRITERIA

Sacroiliitis: grade ≥ 2 bilateral or grade 3 or 4 unilateral

GRADING

Definite AS if the radiologic criterion is associated with at least one clinical variable

Probable AS if:
  The three clinical criteria are present
  The radiologic criterion is present without the clinical criteria

AS = ankylosing spondylitis.

patient from sleep is often a clue to inflammatory back pain that may have been misdiagnosed as the pain of degenerative disc disease, the latter being a much more common cause of low back pain in the population at large. The pain typically occurs in the region of the sacroiliac joints, with or without slight radiation to the buttock area. Midthoracic pain and cervical pain, particularly at night, are less common but strongly suggest inflammatory back pain when they occur. Fatigue is also a suggestive symptom and is often a major concern for the typical young male patient who has a high functional target in terms of sports and recreation. If the inflammation is inadequately controlled, there is increasing stiffness that may persist most of the day, as well as progressive loss of mobility and flexibility.

Peripheral oligoarthritis is seen in up to 30% of patients with AS. Typically, it is an asymmetrical oligoarthritis with a predilection for the lower extremities. It is important to ask about concurrent or previous tendinitis (e.g., Achilles tendinitis) or heel pain (e.g., plantar fasciitis), because either may reflect an enthesitis that is part of the clinical picture. Involvement of the hip can occur at any point in the course of AS and can follow a course to joint destruction. A hip flexion contracture on this basis may contribute to increasing stoop on standing and walking, which may otherwise be attributed to spinal involvement in the disease.

Extra-articular features most commonly involve the eye. Ocular involvement may occur in up to 40% of AS patients, most typically acute anterior uveitis (iritis). The uveitis often manifests as a slight impairment in visual acuity, with accompanying photophobia and eye pain. Typically, it is unilateral and recurrent. IBD and psoriasis occur in approximately 10% of AS cohorts. Less common manifestations include aortic insufficiency, cardiac conduction defects, and pulmonary fibrosis.

DIAGNOSIS
Physical Examination

Physical examination of the spine characteristically indicates restricted movement, which in the early stages may reflect paraspinal muscle spasm in part; late in the course it reflects ankylosis of the zygapophyseal joints and syndesmophyte bridging of the vertebral bodies. Forward flexion is restricted and can be monitored by Schober's test. This test is used to measure mobility in the lower part of the back: with the patient standing upright, a 10-cm span is marked from the fifth lumbar vertebra upward. On maximal forward flexion, the distance between the marks is remeasured. With normal spinal mobility, the flexed distance should register as 15 cm or an increment of 5 cm. Thoracic involvement is measured in chest expansion, with the chest circumference at maximal inspiration being more than 5 cm greater than the circumference at maximal expiration. Changes in cervical mobility can be measured as the occiput-to-wall distance, with the patient's heels against the wall as the patient attempts to touch the back of the head to the wall. Restricted spinal mobility early in the course of the disease may best be detected by lateral spinal flexion, measured as the difference in the finger-to-floor distance when standing erect compared with maximal bending to the side. Inflammation in the sacroiliac joint may be reflected by joint line tenderness to direct pressure or by the FABERE test (for Flexion, ABduction, External Rotation, and Extension) or Gaenslen maneuver. In the former, the patient lies supine while the examiner flexes and externally rotates the hip. In the latter, the examiner extends the hip by letting the leg dangle off the side of the examining table. In both cases, stress is placed on the sacroiliac joint and may reproduce the back pain if it derives from this site.

Laboratory Findings

Laboratory tests in the evaluation of inflammatory back pain are relatively nonspecific. The ESR and CRP are typically elevated, but normal levels do not exclude inflammatory back pain, and the degree of elevation is typically less than would be seen in acute RA. Anemia of chronic disease may be observed if the condition is long-standing. HLA-B27 is rarely the definitive factor for diagnosis, and the false-positive and false-negative rates have already been discussed; however, in the setting of characteristic back symptoms, the test has reasonably high sensitivity and specificity.

Imaging

Radiographic assessment is important for confirmation of disease, but early in the course there may be no radiographic changes in the sacroiliac joints. If the clinician has a high index of suspicion in such cases, MRI may improve the sensitivity of the plain radiograph because inflammatory changes on MRI predate radiographic changes.[11,12] When ordering x-rays, specific views of the sacroiliac joints can be requested. A routine anteroposterior pelvic radiograph is generally the standard diagnostic x-ray. The classic findings are bilateral changes in the sacroiliac joints (Fig. 265-2). Abnormalities include erosions in the joint line, pseudowidening, subchondral sclerosis, and, finally, ankylosis, reflecting complete bony replacement of the sacroiliac joints.

Radiographs of the spine may reveal squaring of the vertebral bodies (loss of the normal anterior concavity of the lumbar vertebra) and "shiny corners" (subchondral sclerosis at the upper edge of the vertebral body), both of which are manifestations of enthesitis. Syndesmophytes, which represent marginal bridging of the vertebrae (Figs. 265-3 and 265-4), eventually develop and make the diagnosis clear. Because ankylosis of the apophyseal joints may occur without syndesmophyte formation, it is important to assess the posterior joints on the lateral lumbosacral spine views, as well as the anterior margin of the vertebrae. Eventually, the changes may result in a "bamboo spine," so called because the bridging syndesmophytes can mimic the appearance of bamboo. It is now appreciated that osteoporosis (Chapter 243) is a significant feature of AS, probably reflecting both the local chronic inflammation and the abnormal biomechanical loading of the vertebrae as the disease progresses.

Differential Diagnosis

The differential diagnosis of AS includes the following: osteitis condensans ilii; diffuse idiopathic skeletal hyperostosis (DISH); the syndrome of synovitis, acne, pustulosis, hyperostosis, and osteomyelitis (SAPHO); and some induced hyperostotic states (vitamin A intoxication, fluorosis). New bone formation occurs in degenerative disc disease, but the bulky horizontal appearance of osteophytes is usually easily distinguished from that of syndesmophytes, and narrowing of the disc space is not a feature of AS. Osteoarthritis of the sacroiliac joint has recently been recognized as having a higher prevalence than previously appreciated.

The clinical course and severity of AS are highly variable. Inflammatory back pain and stiffness dominate the picture in the early stages, whereas chronic pain and deformity may develop over time. In both early and late phases of the disease, there may be a significant impact on work disability and quality of life. In only a minority of patients does the full-blown picture of a bamboo spine eventually develop, but there are few variables that can reliably aid in prognosticating the course. At present, the strongest predictor of new syndesmophyte formation is the presence of syndesmophytes at baseline. In AS patients in whom new, refractory spinal pain develops, an intervertebral fracture should be considered, which can occur after only minimal trauma.

Additional late complications may include cauda equina syndrome, osteoporotic compression fractures, spondylodiscitis, and restrictive lung disease.

Reactive Arthritis

DEFINITION

ReA is an aseptic arthritis that occurs subsequent to an extra-articular infection, most typically of the GI or GU tract. In the GI tract, the key pathogens

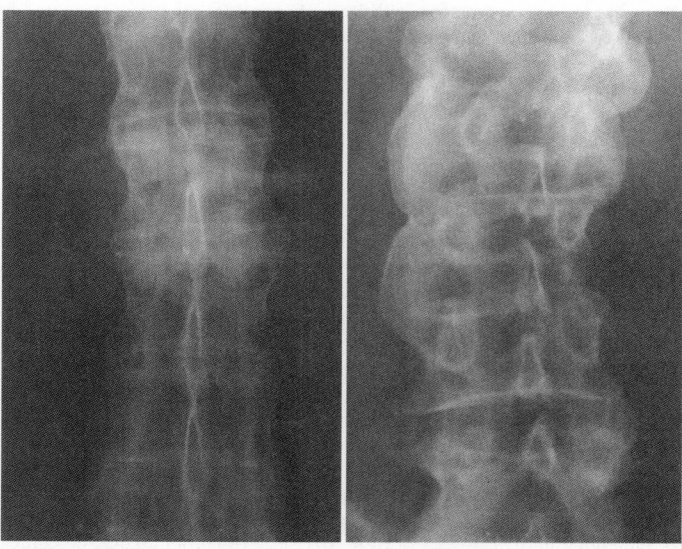

FIGURE 265-3. *Left,* Lumbar spondylitis in ankylosing spondylitis, with symmetrical marginal bridging syndesmophytes and calcification of the spinal ligament. *Right,* The bulky, nonmarginal, asymmetrical syndesmophytes of reactive arthritis with lumbar spondylitis.

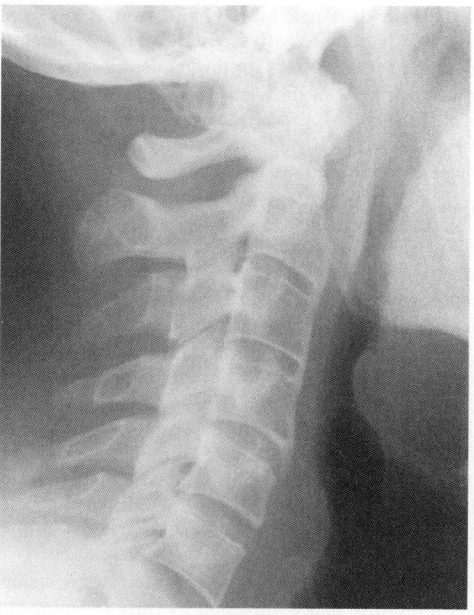

FIGURE 265-4. A 34-year-old man who has had ankylosing spondylitis for 9 years and neck pain. Radiographs demonstrate narrowing of the C2-C3 apophyseal joints posteriorly and anterior bridging marginal syndesmophytes extending from C2 to C5.

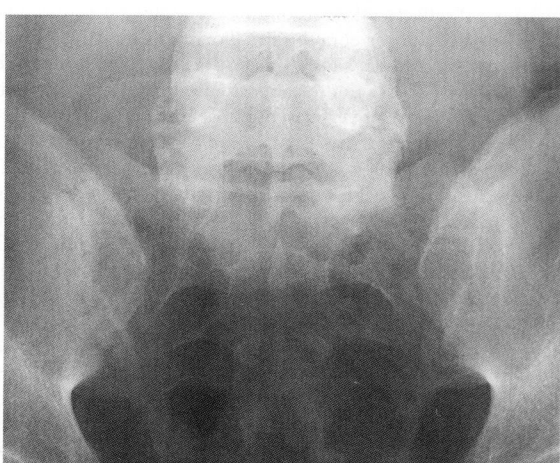

FIGURE 265-2. Bilaterally symmetrical sacroiliitis in ankylosing spondylitis.

are *Salmonella typhimurium, Yersinia enterocolitica, Shigella flexneri,* and *Campylobacter jejuni.* In the GU tract, *Chlamydia trachomatis* is the most common offender.

EPIDEMIOLOGY

The true incidence and prevalence of ReA are not well defined. In epidemics involving *Salmonella* (Chapter 308) or *Yersinia* (Chapter 312), it is estimated that ReA develops in 2 to 7% of infected individuals but in as many as 20% of B27-positive infected individuals. In such epidemic studies, B27 confers risk not only for the onset of arthritis but also for axial involvement and chronicity. Genetic variants in toll-like receptor 2 (TLR-2) are associated with acute ReA, thus implicating host innate immunity as central in ReA. The variability in the rate of ReA is determined by the heterogeneity of the cohorts reported, which introduces confounding variables of different genetic backgrounds in the population and different species of pathogens. Even in the setting of an epidemic point source outbreak, the inoculum varies widely among the exposed individuals, and the genetic makeup of the population at risk (e.g., the prevalence of B27) may differ greatly among different studies. Case ascertainment and relative risk are even more difficult to determine for post-*Chlamydia* ReA. Young adults in the United States have a high prevalence of asymptomatic *Chlamydia* carriage in the GU tract, and establishing a causal link between *Chlamydia* and synovitis can be difficult. Nevertheless, it is with *Chlamydia* that ReA has been most intensively studied.

PATHOBIOLOGY

Although immunofluorescence studies have identified bacterial antigens in the joints of patients with ReA after both GI and GU infections, it is primarily in post-*Chlamydia* ReA that results of polymerase chain reaction studies on synovial tissues have most consistently been positive, suggesting that viable *Chlamydia* may persist in the joints of such patients, albeit in a metabolically altered state.

Typically, the onset of arthritis occurs 1 to 3 weeks after the GI or GU infection, but the temporal details are often difficult to define precisely.

Although the definition of aseptic arthritis after an extra-articular infection may include a broader range of pathogens (e.g., *Chlamydia pneumoniae*), sites of infection (e.g., streptococcal pharyngitis), and types of infections (e.g., *Giardia* infections of the GI tract), these clinical scenarios have not generally been included in the category of ReA. They lack the other associated clinical features of the SpA group of diseases, and they lack an association with B27.

DIAGNOSIS

The pattern of joint involvement in ReA is one of asymmetrical oligoarthritis with a predilection for the lower extremity, a pattern shared by most SpA syndromes. Enthesitis may present as Achilles tendinitis or plantar fasciitis. Dactylitis, appearing as a sausage digit, may also be seen. Dactylitis is the net result of inflammatory changes affecting the joint capsule, entheses, periarticular structures, and periosteal bone. Sacroiliitis may be seen in the acute phase, but radiographic changes are seen largely in patients with a more chronic course.[13]

When ReA is accompanied by certain extra-articular features such as urethritis, conjunctivitis, or mucocutaneous lesions, the term *Reiter's syndrome* has been applied historically, but it is no longer in common use. The urethritis may manifest as dysuria or discharge, and the rash as circinate balanitis, which appears as vesicles or shallow ulcerations on the glans penis. Painless lingual or oral ulcerations may also be seen. The fact that the cervicitis may be less symptomatic could partially account for the underdiagnosis in women. The classic skin manifestation of ReA is keratoderma blennorrhagicum, a painless papulosquamous eruption on the palms or soles (Fig. 265-5). Occasionally, nail dystrophy with pitting and onycholysis or subungual keratosis can be seen. The conjunctivitis can be bilateral and painful; in contrast, the acute anterior uveitis that can also be seen in this setting tends to be less painful and unilateral.

Radiographic changes of ReA can be seen in the involved peripheral joints, with early findings consisting of soft tissue swelling and juxta-articular osteopenia. Areas of periostitis and new bone formation may develop in peripheral joints. When changes in the sacroiliac joints are seen, they are typically asymmetrical (Fig. 265-6), in contrast to the symmetrical pattern seen in AS. In the chronic phase, syndesmophytes may develop, but they are described as bulky, nonmarginal, often asymmetrical formations that differ from the classic syndesmophytes of AS. The frequency with which ReA evolves into bona fide AS has not been determined definitively.

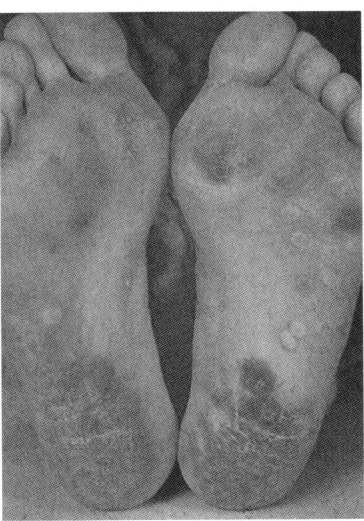

FIGURE 265-5. Keratoderma blennorrhagicum of the feet in reactive arthritis.

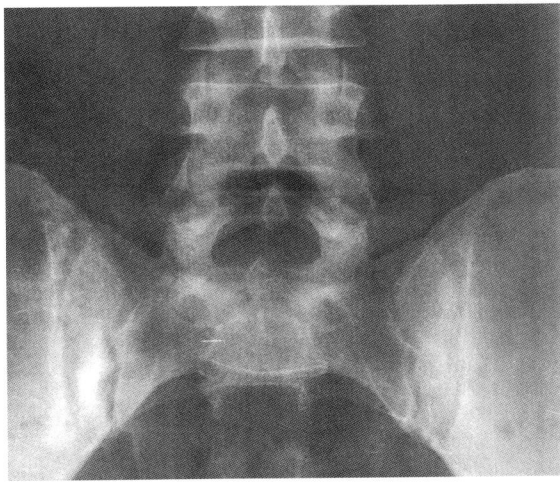

FIGURE 265-6. Bilaterally asymmetrical sacroiliitis in reactive arthritis. Erosions, pseudowidening, and ileal sclerosis are present.

Differential Diagnosis

The most important differential diagnosis for such reactive arthropathies is septic arthritis. Both *Yersinia* and *Salmonella* can cause septic arthritis, so an appropriate culture of synovial fluid should precede the diagnosis of ReA whenever possible. The course of ReA is variable, and few prognostic markers are available for the clinician to predict the course in an individual case. The majority of patients have an initial episode lasting 2 to 3 months, but synovitis may persist for a year or longer. In one 5-year follow-up of a point source cohort of post-*Salmonella* ReA, 20% of patients had ongoing inflammatory joint disease, and some degree of functional disability was observed in 30% of patients 5 years after the onset of disease.

REACTIVE ARTHRITIS AND HUMAN IMMUNODEFICIENCY VIRUS

An aggressive form of SpA may be seen in patients who are concomitantly infected with HIV.[14] There is no increased frequency of ReA in patients with HIV, but HIV may alter the course of these arthropathies, with a tendency for a more aggressive and more refractory joint disease. Aggressive skin and joint disease may be seen in patients in whom PsA develops in the setting of HIV infection. Most North American patients with the HIV-ReA constellation are B27 positive, but studies of comparable patients in Africa have found a sizable B27-negative component in such patients. The arthritis in these patients falls into two clinical patterns: (1) an additive, asymmetrical polyarthritis or (2) an intermittent oligoarthritis that most commonly affects the lower extremities. Enthesitis, fasciitis, conjunctivitis, and urethritis can all be seen in such patients. Sacroiliitis can occur, although extensive spinal syndesmophyte formation is not common.

Psoriatic Arthritis

EPIDEMIOLOGY

PsA develops in 5 to 7% of patients with psoriasis. Although most cases arise in patients with established cutaneous disease, some patients (particularly children) have arthritis that antedates the appearance of the skin lesions.[15] Although the extent of psoriatic skin disease correlates poorly with the development of arthritis, the risk for PsA increases with a family history of SpA. The age at onset can range from 30 to 55 years, with an equal predilection for PsA in women and men. Psoriatic spondylitis has a slight male preponderance. Two large prospective studies suggest that obesity is a significant risk factor for psoriatic arthritis.[16,17]

PATHOBIOLOGY

The genetic associations with PsA are complex. Psoriasis itself is associated with several HLA loci; some B alleles have been reported, but the dominant element is HLA-Cw6. HLA-B39 and HLA-B27 have been associated with sacroiliitis and axial involvement. No etiologic agent has been proved in PsA, although some investigators have proposed that the disease process represents ReA in response to cutaneous bacteria. The histopathology of the synovitis of PsA is comparable to that of the other forms of SpA, with the absence of the local production of immunoglobulin and rheumatoid factor differentiating this disease from RA. There is the potential for aggressive osteolysis, fibrous ankylosis, and heterotopic new bone formation to occur in PsA. As mentioned earlier, the coexistence of HIV and PsA seems to set the stage for an aggressive course of joint destruction in some patients.

DIAGNOSIS

PsA has a variable manifestation and disease course, but several clinical patterns have been identified in prospectively monitored cohorts of patients. The clinical subsets are not mutually exclusive, nor are they static over time. The most common form, which affects 30 to 50% of patients, is an asymmetrical oligoarthritis that may involve both large and small joints. Dactylitis, arising as sausage digits, can be seen in fingers and toes and actually represents an enthesitis. In the second subset there is selective targeting of the distal interphalangeal joints, seen in 10 to 15% of patients. These changes are strongly associated with nail dystrophy, of which the features are onycholysis, subungual keratosis, pitting, and oil drop–like staining (Fig. 265-7). The third subset (15 to 30% of patients) has a symmetrical polyarthritis that mimics RA in many ways, except for the absence of rheumatoid nodules and rheumatoid factor. The fourth clinical variant is psoriatic spondylitis, which occurs in 20% of patients; 50% of such patients are B27 positive. Finally, arthritis mutilans (5% of patients) is a destructive, erosive arthritis that affects large and small joints and can be associated with marked deformities and significant disability.

Radiographic changes in PsA involve soft tissue swelling (particularly in the case of dactylitis), erosions, and periostitis. Axial involvement may lead to the appearance of asymmetrical sacroiliitis with syndesmophytes that are bulky, asymmetrical, and nonmarginal. The classic "pencil-in-cup" deformity may be seen in patients with distal interphalangeal joint disease or arthritis mutilans. Acro-osteolysis is noted in a minority of patients and reflects an aggressive erosive process.

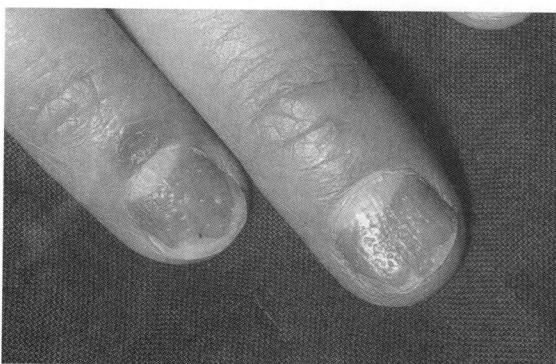

FIGURE 265-7. Nail pitting in psoriasis. The pits are more discrete and regular compared with pits affecting the nail plate in dermatitis.

Differential Diagnosis

The diagnosis of PsA depends on finding the typical skin or nail changes in association with one of the articular variants described previously. The differential diagnosis for the skin lesions can include seborrheic dermatitis, dyshidrotic eczema, fungal infection, keratoderma blennorrhagicum, and palmoplantar pustulosis.

TREATMENT   Rx

Patients typically receive aggressive treatment for psoriasis (Chapter 438). The advent of biologic agents has had a major impact on the treatment of PsA. The anti-TNF agents have been studied most extensively, indicating the efficacy of infliximab, etanercept, adalimumab, and golimumab. In a phase III randomized placebo-controlled trial, treatment of psoriatic arthritis with subcutaneous golimumab (50 mg to 100 mg every 4 weeks) inhibited the progression of structural damage and demonstrated continued clinical efficacy and safety through 1 year.[A8] In a study of patients with PsA, ustekinumab, a monoclonal antibody against interleukin-12/23, was well tolerated, reduced the extent and severity of psoriasis, and was safe.[A9] Brodalumab, a human monoclonal antibody against interleukin-17 receptor A (IL17RA), significantly improved response rates among patients with PsA in a phase 2 randomized, double-blind, placebo-controlled study.[A10] The European League Against Rheumatism in 2012 published recommendations for the management of PsA with systemic and local (nontopical) symptomatic and disease-modifying antirheumatic drugs. They suggest nonsteroidal anti-inflammatory drugs to relieve musculoskeletal signs and symptoms; treatment with disease-modifying drugs such as methotrexate, sulfasalazine, or leflunomide in patients with swollen joints, structural damage in the presence of inflammation, or clinically relevant extraarticular manifestations; and anti-TNF agents in patients with active enthesitis and/or dactylitis and insufficient response to other medications. Patients should be switched to another anti-TNF agent if the first is not successful.

Enteropathic Arthritis

DEFINITION

EA refers to the arthritis associated with Crohn's disease (CD) or ulcerative colitis (UC) (Chapter 141; Table 265-4).

PATHOBIOLOGY

All extraenteric manifestations, including arthritis, occur more commonly in CD than in UC. Peripheral arthritis occurs in 10 to 20% of CD patients and in 2 to 7% of UC patients. This pattern of arthritis occurs more commonly in patients with other extraenteric features (e.g., erythema nodosum, iritis). It is typically an inflammatory nonerosive polyarthritis, predominantly of large joints. In general, the clinical activity of the peripheral arthritis parallels the

TABLE 265-4	ENTEROPATHIC ARTHRITIS	
FEATURE	**PERIPHERAL ARTHRITIS**	**SACROILIITIS, SPONDYLITIS**
CROHN'S DISEASE (CD)		
Frequency in CD	10-20%	2-7%
HLA-B27 associated	No	Yes
Pattern	Transient, symmetrical	Chronic
Course	Related to activity of CD	Unrelated to activity of CD
Effect of surgery	Remission of arthritis uncommon	No effect
Effect of anti-TNF therapy	Effective	Effective
ULCERATIVE COLITIS (UC)		
Frequency in UC	5-10%	2-7%
HLA-B27 associated	No	Yes
Pattern	Transient	Chronic
Course	More common in pancolitis than in proctitis; related to activity of UC	Unrelated
Effect of surgery	Remission of arthritis	No effect

HLA = human leukocyte antigen; TNF = tumor necrosis factor.

activity of the gut inflammation, and measures that control the GI disease usually control the joint disease as well. The peripheral arthritis of EA is not associated with B27. As mentioned earlier, IBD and AS share genetic susceptibility associated with numerous genes.

In contrast, the sacroiliitis or spondylitis of EA follows a pattern in which the joint inflammation waxes and wanes independently of the bowel inflammation. Axial disease occurs in 2 to 7% of both CD and UC patients. HLA-B27 is found in 50% of patients with axial arthritis. The course tends to be chronic, as opposed to the transient course of peripheral arthritis.

The association of bowel inflammation and arthritis is supported by ileocolonoscopic studies in which subclinical inflammation of the bowel has been demonstrated in diseases covering the entire spectrum of SpAs. Histologic evaluation demonstrates that changes of acute ileitis are seen in postdysenteric ReA, whereas chronic inflammatory changes are more likely to be seen in patients with AS. As mentioned earlier, the abnormalities in the bowel of B27 transgenic rats have strong similarity to the lesions of CD, and a germfree environment minimizes inflammatory changes in both the gut and the joints. This finding argues that altered bowel permeability, with enhanced bacteremia or antigenemia, may provide the link in both cases.

DIAGNOSIS

It is important to recognize that the musculoskeletal features of EA may precede any GI symptoms or signs. Conversely, the diarrhea preceding the onset of peripheral or axial arthritis in a young patient could just as likely represent a food-borne pathogen (e.g., *Salmonella*, *Yersinia*), with secondary ReA as IBD and accompanying EA. In the initial assessment of such a patient, it is important to carry out careful and complete stool cultures. If the GI symptoms persist, diagnostic colonoscopy is often required to resolve the issue.

Undifferentiated Spondyloarthritis

Despite careful clinical and radiographic assessment, there are still a substantial number of patients who do not fall into one of the classic diagnostic subsets of SpA outlined previously. These patients are often defined as having USpA with peripheral enthesitis, asymmetrical arthritis or sacroiliitis, or iritis in the absence of identifiable antecedent infection or concurrent IBD or psoriasis. The natural history of USpA has not been well defined, and case heterogeneity and diagnostic dilemmas plague a systematic or multicenter approach to the problem. When the clinical course is examined, a number of patients may finally meet the diagnostic criteria for AS, but many retain a distinct USpA pattern for prolonged periods.[18]

 Grade A References

A1. Braun J, van der Horst-Bruinsma F, Huang F, et al. Clinical efficacy and safety of etanercept versus sulfasalazine in ankylosing spondylitis patients: a randomized, double-blind study (ASCEND Trial). *Arthritis Rheum.* 2011;63:1543-1551.

A2. Barber CE, Kim J, Inman RD, et al. Antibiotics for treatment of reactive arthritis: a systematic review and metaanalysis. *J Rheumatol.* 2013;40:916-928.

A3. Carter JD, Espinoza LR, Inman RD, et al. Combination antibiotics as a treatment for chronic *Chlamydia*-induced reactive arthritis: a double-blind, placebo-controlled, prospective trial. *Arthritis Rheum.* 2010;62:1298-1307.

A4. Inman RD, Davis JC, van der Heijde D, et al. Efficacy and safety of golimumab in patients with ankylosing spondylitis: results of the randomized, double-blind, placebo-controlled GO-RAISE trial. *Arthritis Rheum.* 2008;58:3402-3412.

A5. Sieper J, Lenaerts J, Wollenhaupt J, et al. Efficacy and safety of infliximab plus naproxen versus naproxen alone in patients with early, active axial spondyloarthritis: results from the double-blind, placebo-controlled INFAST study, Part 1. *Ann Rheum Dis.* 2014;73:101-107.

A6. Dougados M, van der Heijde D, Sieper J, et al. Symptomatic efficacy of etanercept and its effects on objective signs of inflammation in early nonradiographic axial spondyloarthritis: a multicenter, randomized, double-blind, placebo-controlled trial. *Arthritis Rheum.* 2014;66:2091-2102.

A7. Song IH, Hermann KG, Haibel H, et al. Consistently good clinical response in patients with early axial spondyloarthritis after 3 years of continuous treatment with etanercept: longterm data of the ESTHER trial. *J Rheumatol.* 2014;41:2034-2040.

A8. Kavanaugh A, van der Heijde D, McInnes IB, et al. Golimumab in psoriatic arthritis. One-year clinical efficacy, radiographic, and safety results from a phase III, randomized, placebo-controlled trial. *Arthritis Rheum.* 2012;64:2504-2517.

A9. Gottlieb A, Menter A, Mendelsohn A, et al. Ustekinumab, a human interleukin 12/23 monoclonal antibody, for psoriatic arthritis: randomised, double-blind, placebo-controlled, crossover trial. *Lancet.* 2009;373:633-640.

A10. Mease PJ, Genovese MC, Greenwald MW, et al. Brodalumab, an anti-IL17RA monoclonal antibody, in psoriatic arthritis. *N Engl J Med.* 2014;370:2295-2306.

GENERAL REFERENCES

For the General References and other additional features, please visit Expert Consult at https://expertconsult.inkling.com.

266

SYSTEMIC LUPUS ERYTHEMATOSUS

MARY K. CROW

DEFINITION

Systemic lupus erythematosus (SLE) is a multisystemic autoimmune disease that results from immune system–mediated tissue damage. Manifestations of SLE can involve the skin, joints, kidney, central nervous system (CNS), cardiovascular system, serosal membranes, and the hematologic and immune systems. The disease is highly heterogeneous, with individual patients manifesting variable combinations of clinical features. In most patients with SLE, the disease is characterized by a waxing and waning clinical course, although some demonstrate a pattern of chronic activity. The molecular triggers of the disease are not known, but the pathogenesis is understood to involve the production of autoantibodies exhibiting multiple specificities, with reactivity with nucleic acid–binding proteins being a common feature. Immune complexes, along with immune system cells and soluble mediators, generate inflammation and tissue damage. Therapeutic approaches generally involve immunosuppression.

EPIDEMIOLOGY

A notable feature of SLE is that it occurs much more frequently in females than in males. Like Hashimoto's thyroiditis and Sjögren's syndrome, the female-to-male ratio is approximately 8 : 1 to 10 : 1 in adults, and most cases are diagnosed between the ages of 15 and 44 years. In children and women older than 55, the ratio is closer to 2 : 1. The prevalence of SLE in the United States is estimated to be approximately 73 per 100,000, and the incidence of new cases is 5.5 per 100,000 per year. The prevalence, severity, and characteristics of disease differ in different ethnic groups, with SLE being 2.3-fold more frequent in African Americans than in the white population. The severity of disease is also greater in Hispanic individuals than in whites, although data for Hispanic populations are less abundant. Asians may also have a higher prevalence of disease than whites. Recent studies of lupus in minority populations indicate that socioeconomic factors are major contributors to the increased prevalence and severity of disease in African Americans and Hispanic Americans.

PATHOBIOLOGY

Current understanding of lupus pathogenesis incorporates roles for genetic susceptibility based on a threshold model involving multiple genes[1]; environmental triggers, including microbial infection, sunlight, and certain drugs; and altered immune system function. Recent advances in immunology have focused attention on the mechanisms that account for innate immune system activation.[2] At least some of the genetic and environmental contributions to lupus are likely to promote innate immune system activation and subsequent autoimmunity. Others may contribute to inflammation and tissue damage. Induction of cellular stress responses, including oxidative modification of cell proteins, is of current interest as a mechanism that links environmental triggers to altered immune function.

Murine models have proved useful in identifying genes that could contribute to lupus susceptibility or define patterns of disease. Production of autoantibodies characteristic of SLE and development of nephritis and accelerated death have been demonstrated in numerous murine strains in which immune system genes have been modified. In most cases, no alterations have been noted in the homologous human genes. The ease of induction of lupus-like disease in murine models suggests that there are numerous possible pathogenic paths that might lead to the clinical manifestations of lupus. It is not known which of these molecular pathways is responsible for human SLE, although mediators of the immune response to viral infection, particularly components of the type I interferon response, are associated with lupus in both murine and human systems and are likely to be important in disease pathogenesis.[3]

Genetics

An important role for a genetic contribution to lupus susceptibility is suggested by the high concordance of disease in monozygotic twins (14 to 57%).

Genes that might account for increased lupus susceptibility or severity include those encoding components of the complement pathway, including C1q, C2, and C4A. Impaired production of these early complement components may decrease the clearance of apoptotic cells, thereby augmenting the pool of available autoantigens, or decrease the solubility of immune complexes. Polymorphic variants in components of the toll-like receptor (TLR) pathways that regulate type I interferon production, including interferon regulatory factor 5 (IRF5), have been associated with a diagnosis of SLE and increased plasma interferon activity in some populations. Association of SLE with the major histocompatibility complex (MHC) class II alleles human leukocyte antigen (HLA)-DR2 and HLA-DR3 has been documented in many studies and is most striking in patients expressing particular autoantibody specificities. Polymorphisms in the Fc receptor genes FCGR2A and FCGR3A have been associated with SLE nephritis, possibly based on altered clearance of immune complexes. Variants of the PTPN22 gene, which encodes a phosphatase that regulates T-cell activation, are also associated with SLE. Genome-wide association studies have expanded the list of lupus-associated gene variants to include regulators of innate immune system activation (TNFAIP3, ITGAM, IRAK1) and signaling molecules important in lymphocyte activation (STAT4, BANK1, BLK, and LYN). Rare mutations in genes encoding proteins that regulate nucleic acid integrity and degradation, including TREX1, encoding a DNase; SAMHD1, a triphosphohydrolase; RNASEH2A, B and C; and ADAR, an RNA-specific adenosine deaminase, have been documented in some patients with a lupus-like syndrome called Aicardi-Goutieres syndrome, characterized by skin lesions, CNS disease, autoantibodies, and high levels of interferon. Mutations in these genes have also been documented in rare patients with SLE and have provided new insights into the likely contribution of endogenous nucleic acids to innate immune system activation and lupus pathogenesis.[4] The available data suggest a common theme: the genes that have been associated with lupus confer either increased activation or impaired regulation of the innate or adaptive immune responses, with increased type I interferon often observed in association with the risk genotype.

Environmental Triggers

Several classes of potential environmental triggers for lupus have been studied.[5] Although the female preponderance of SLE implies a role for hormonal factors in the disease, recent concepts describe a possible contribution of epigenetic modification or dosage effects of the X chromosome as accounting for at least some of the sex skewing. A role for microbial triggers—particularly viral infection—has been postulated, consistent with the constitutional symptoms that often characterize the earliest stage of the disease. Epstein-Barr virus has garnered particular interest among investigators, because the frequency of previous infection in SLE patients is significantly higher than in the general population (99 vs. 94%). Evidence of exposure to other viruses, including cytomegalovirus, is equivalent between SLE patients and healthy control subjects. Ultraviolet light exposure is a well-described trigger of lupus flares. Possible mechanisms include DNA damage, induction of cellular stress responses, and induction of apoptosis of skin cells, which result in concentration of nucleic acids and associated proteins in cell membrane blebs and increased processing by antigen-presenting cells. Data also support an association between current tobacco use and anti–double-stranded DNA antibodies and lupus disease activity. Certain drugs, including procainamide and hydralazine, can induce a lupus-like syndrome, but the symptoms usually abate after discontinuing use of the drug. These agents may promote demethylation of DNA, thereby altering gene expression and potentially increasing the availability of immunostimulatory DNA. Sulfa antibiotics have been reported to induce lupus flare in some patients. Administration of recombinant interferon-α to patients with hematologic malignancies or hepatitis C infection has been associated with induction of a lupus-like syndrome. In addition, anti–tumor necrosis factor agents have induced lupus autoantibodies and occasionally clinical lupus in patients with rheumatoid arthritis.

Immunologic Triggers

Genetic and environmental factors that increase the probability of development of SLE are likely to act on the immune system to induce autoimmunity and consequent tissue inflammation and damage. In addition to mechanisms that increase the availability of self-antigens (such as ultraviolet light), altered expression of gene products that mediate or regulate apoptosis, or impaired clearance of apoptotic debris, results in generalized activation of the immune system and contributes to autoimmunity in lupus. In parallel with the events

that account for effective immune responses directed at exogenous microbes, the autoimmunity that occurs in SLE patients is likely to require activation of both innate and adaptive immune responses. The innate immune response is first activated by common molecular patterns expressed on the microbe and results in augmented antigen-presenting cell capacity and successful generation of an antigen-specific adaptive immune response. The characterization of the TLR family of pattern recognition receptors has provided new understanding of the mechanisms through which the innate immune system is activated by exogenous and endogenous stimuli, including nucleic acid–containing immune complexes, and promotes induction of a self-directed adaptive immune response.[6]

Type I Interferon

Recent studies of gene expression in peripheral blood mononuclear cells of SLE patients using microarray technology have demonstrated that activation of genes regulated by type I interferon is a common feature in patients with active disease and may represent innate immune system activation. Interferon (IFN)-α may be responsible for many of the immunologic alterations that have been observed in SLE and is identified as a potential therapeutic target. Immune complexes containing DNA or RNA are postulated to contribute to the production of type I interferon in SLE. Demethylated CpG-rich DNA or RNA associated with nucleic acid–binding proteins can activate plasmacytoid dendritic cells and other immune system cells through TLRs and thereby result in the production of type I interferon (IFN-α or IFN-β) and other proinflammatory cytokines. Diverse effects of type I interferon on immune system function are consistent with the altered immune responses observed in SLE patients, including maturation of dendritic cells, increased immunoglobulin class switching to mature immunoglobulin isotypes (immunoglobulin [Ig]G and IgA), and induction of soluble mediators that increase B-cell differentiation and inflammatory responses, such as B-lymphocyte stimulator (BLyS) and IFN-γ.[7] Induction of an immunostimulatory microenvironment by IFN-α may support the development of a humoral immune response directed at self-antigens, particularly intracellular particles that contain nucleic acids and nucleic acid–binding proteins. It is not known why some individuals initiate immune system activation directed at self-antigens and others do not. In addition to its effects on immune system function, type I interferon has been associated with altered endothelial cell function and may contribute to the development of atherosclerotic vascular pathology in patients with lupus.[8]

Autoantibodies

The most characteristic lupus autoantibodies target intracellular particles containing both nucleic acid and nucleic acid–binding proteins. Understanding the significance of induction of these particular autoantibody specificities may provide clues to the etiology of SLE. A recent analysis of the spectrum of autoantibodies present in the sera of individuals in whom SLE is later diagnosed has suggested that autoantibodies reactive with certain RNA-binding proteins, including the Ro protein, occur early in the preclinical stage of the disease, along with a positive antinuclear antibody (ANA) test. These are often followed by anti-DNA antibodies and, finally, by the development of antibodies specific for the spliceosomal proteins Smith (Sm) and ribonucleoprotein (RNP) at approximately the time of diagnosis (Fig. 266-1). These observations suggest that individuals who demonstrate progression from humoral immunity targeting proteins associated with RNA to antibodies that bind DNA and other specificities are those in whom sufficient autoimmunity develops to manifest clinical symptoms. Approximately one third of SLE patients have autoantibodies reactive with phospholipids or the proteins associated with them, particularly β_2-glycoprotein I (β_2GPI). These autoantibody specificities can also be present independently of SLE in primary antiphospholipid antibody syndrome (Chapter 174).

Immune Complexes and Complement

Tissue and organ damage in SLE is mediated by the deposition or in situ formation of immune complexes and subsequent complement activation and inflammation. The complement system (Chapter 50), composed of more than 30 proteins that act in concert to protect the host against invading organisms, initiates inflammation and tissue injury. Complement activation promotes chemotaxis of inflammatory cells and generates proteolytic fragments that enhance phagocytosis by neutrophils and monocytes. The classic pathway is activated when antibodies bind to antigen and generate potent effectors. Alternative pathway activation mechanisms differ in that they are initiated by the binding of spontaneously activated complement components

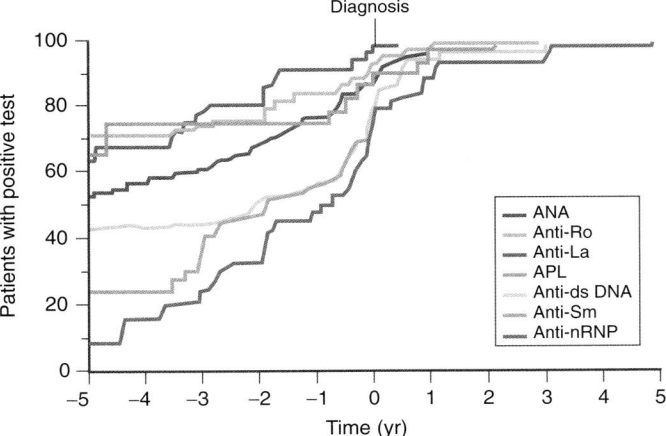

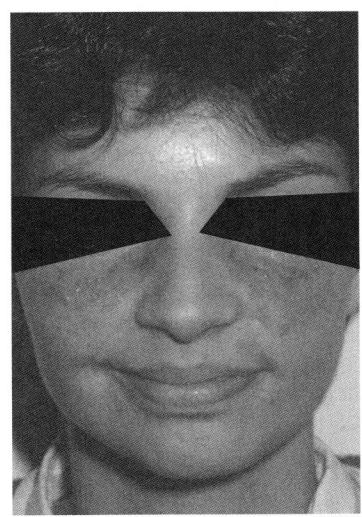

FIGURE 266-1. Proportion of patients with positive antibody tests relative to the time of diagnosis or appearance of the first clinical manifestation of systemic lupus erythematosus (SLE). For each autoantibody, the proportion of patients testing positive relative to the time of diagnosis or to the time of appearance of the first clinical criterion was assessed. In analyses of the time from antibody development to the diagnosis of SLE, antinuclear antibodies (ANAs) appeared significantly earlier than anti-Sm antibodies and antinuclear ribonucleoprotein (anti-nRNP) antibodies, but not significantly earlier than anti-Ro, anti-La, antiphospholipid (APL), or anti–double-stranded DNA antibodies (anti-dsDNA). (From Arbuckle MR, McClain MT, Rubertone MV, et al. Development of autoantibodies before the clinical onset of systemic lupus erythematosus. *N Engl J Med.* 2003;349:16.)

FIGURE 266-2. Malar rash in a patient with systemic lupus erythematosus. Note that the rash does not cross the nasolabial fold. (From Gladman DD, Urowitz MB. Systemic lupus erythematosus: clinical features. In: Klippel JH, Dieppe PA, eds. *Rheumatology.* 2nd ed. London: Mosby; 1998.)

TABLE 266-1 CLINICAL MANIFESTATIONS OF SYSTEMIC LUPUS ERYTHEMATOSUS

MANIFESTATION	APPROXIMATE FREQUENCY (%)
Cutaneous	88
Arthritis/arthralgias	76
Neuropsychiatric	66
Pleurisy/pericarditis	63
Anemia	57
Raynaud's phenomenon	44
Vasculitis	43
Atherosclerosis	37
Nephritis	31
Thrombocytopenia	30
Sensorimotor neuropathy	28
Cardiac valvar disease	18
Pulmonary alveolar hemorrhage	12
Pancreatitis	10
Myositis	5
Myocarditis	5

to the surfaces of pathogens or self-tissues. C3a, an anaphylatoxin that binds to receptors on leukocytes and other cells, causes activation and release of inflammatory mediators. C5a is a potent soluble inflammatory, anaphylatoxic, and chemotactic molecule that promotes recruitment and activation of neutrophils and monocytes and mediates endothelial cell activation through its receptor. The release of reactive oxygen and nitrogen intermediates is an additional mechanism that contributes to tissue damage.

Tissues targeted by immune system activity in lupus include the skin, where immune complexes and complement are deposited in a linear pattern (as demonstrated in the lupus band test, in which deposited antibodies are identified by a fluorescent tag), the glomeruli, and heart valves. Antibodies reactive with hippocampal neurons in the brain can mediate excitotoxic death. Immune and inflammatory mechanisms responsible for the vasculopathy of lupus are multifactorial and not clearly defined. Microvascular damage is observed in splenic arteries and is characterized by the typical onion-skin pattern of concentric connective tissue deposition. In addition to vascular damage mediated by inflammation, thrombosis, including microthrombi, contributes to ischemia and cell necrosis in the brain and other organs.

CLINICAL MANIFESTATIONS

Symptoms and Signs
Constitutional Symptoms
SLE is a disease that involves virtually all components of the immune system and can be accompanied by constitutional symptoms similar to those seen in the setting of microbial infection. Fatigue, headaches, weight loss, and fevers are common, along with generalized arthralgias, myalgias, and lymphadenopathy. The level of activity of lupus typically follows a pattern of flares and remissions, although some patients sustain active disease for prolonged periods. Careful monitoring for the development of major organ system disease is important to ensure timely adjustments in medical therapy.

Cutaneous and Mucous Membranes
The skin and mucous membranes are affected in most lupus patients (Table 266-1). The erythematous facial rash with a butterfly distribution across the malar and nasal prominences and sparing of the nasolabial folds is the classic rash of SLE and is seen in 30 to 60% of patients (Fig. 266-2). The butterfly rash is often triggered by sun exposure, but photosensitivity can also be demonstrated diffusely in other areas of the body.

The discoid skin lesions are erythematous plaques with central scarring and may be covered with scale. These lesions are seen in about 25% of patients, involve the scalp or the face and ears, and may be associated with alopecia. Discoid lesions can be present in the absence of systemic

manifestations of SLE (discoid lupus). In addition to the scarring alopecia of discoid lupus, more transient alopecia may be a clinical sign of increased disease activity and is associated with apoptosis of cells in the hair follicle.

Inflammation of the deep dermis and subcutaneous fat can result in lupus panniculitis, with firm painful nodules that sometimes adhere to the epidermis, causing irregularities in the superficial skin. Subacute cutaneous lupus erythematosus is seen in sun-exposed areas and can involve erythematous plaques or psoriasiform lesions. It is associated with autoantibodies to the Ro (SSA) RNA-binding protein. Mucosal ulcerations, especially of the buccal mucosa and upper palate, result from mucositis and are typical of SLE. Manifestations of vasculopathy are also common in SLE, including arteriolar spasm or infarcts in the nail folds, a diffuse lacey pattern over the skin described as livedo reticularis, and petechial-purpuric or urticarial lesions on the extremities. Vasculopathy in SLE is often associated with the presence of antiphospholipid antibodies.

Musculoskeletal System
Arthralgias and nonerosive arthritis are among the most common clinical features of SLE and are experienced by more than 85% of patients. The

proximal interphalangeal and metacarpophalangeal joints of the hand are most commonly symptomatic, along with the knees and wrists. In some patients (≈10%), deformities resulting from damage to periarticular tissue can occur, a condition termed *Jaccoud arthropathy*. The heavy use of corticosteroids in many lupus patients can be accompanied by the development of osteoporosis, including osteoporotic fractures or osteonecrosis, most commonly of the hips, although the underlying vasculopathy can also contribute to joint damage.

Inflammation of the muscles with elevated creatine phosphokinase can occur rarely in SLE, and myopathy may be observed as a consequence of corticosteroid therapy. Fibromyalgia, characterized by painful trigger points at characteristic locations, commonly accompanies SLE and can contribute to fatigue and depression.

Renal System

Kidney involvement in SLE is common, with 74% of patients being affected at some time in the course of disease, and is a poor prognostic indicator. Renal pathology is generally attributed to the deposition of circulating immune complexes or in situ formation of these complexes in glomeruli and results in the activation of complement and subsequent recruitment of inflammatory cells. In addition to glomerular inflammation, necrosis, and scarring, renal pathology is characterized by vascular lesions, including thrombotic microangiopathy and extraglomerular vasculitis. Tubulointerstitial disease, including infiltration of the interstitium with mononuclear cells, tubular atrophy, and interstitial fibrosis, is increasingly recognized as associated with a poor prognosis for persistent nephritis and renal survival. Hypertension may be a consequence of significant renal involvement.

Most cases of lupus nephritis present a complex immunopathologic picture, but in general, the pattern of renal disease reflects the site of deposition of immunoglobulins and the quality of the effector mechanisms they induce. Mesangial deposition of immunoglobulin induces mesangial cell proliferation and is associated with microscopic hematuria and mild proteinuria (Fig. 266-3). Subendothelial deposition of immune complexes results in proliferative and exudative inflammation, together with hematuria, mild to moderate proteinuria, and reduced glomerular filtration rate. Subepithelial deposition of immune complexes adjacent to podocytes and along the glomerular basement membrane can result in membranous nephritis with nephrotic-range proteinuria. In addition, antiphospholipid antibodies may support the development of thrombotic or inflammatory vascular lesions within or external to glomeruli.

A World Health Organization classification of lupus nephritis lesions was first published in 1975, with subsequent revisions. These classifications were reviewed and rigorously reexamined in the revised International Society of Nephrology and Renal Pathology Society classification criteria for lupus glomerulonephritis (GN) (Table 121-7 in Chapter 121). Class I and II GN involves mesangial deposition of immune complexes (class I without and class II with mesangial hypercellularity); class III describes focal GN involving less than 50% of total glomeruli; class IV includes diffuse GN involving 50% or more of glomeruli; class V designates membranous lupus nephritis; and class VI is characterized by advanced sclerotic lesions. Classes III and IV have subdivisions for active and sclerotic lesions, and class IV also has subdivisions for segmental and global involvement. Pathologic diagnosis should include descriptions of tubulointerstitial and vascular disease as well as glomerular involvement.

The prognosis of class I and class II disease is usually good, whereas class IV, the most common form of lupus nephritis, has the worst prognosis, particularly when the serum creatinine level is elevated at the time of diagnosis. Class V nephritis occurs in 10 to 20% of patients, and the implication for long-term outcome depends on the degree of proteinuria, with mild proteinuria having a good prognosis and nephrotic syndrome with chronic edema having a more negative prognosis. It should be noted that renal veins can occasionally become involved with thrombosis, which then also contributes to nephrotic syndrome. This complication can be evaluated by renal ultrasound (Chapter 121).

Cardiovascular System

Pericarditis and valve nodules were among the first clinical manifestations described in SLE. It is only recently that the extent of premature atherosclerotic disease has been well documented. Pericarditis (Chapter 77) is the most common cardiac manifestation, but it is sometimes recognized only on imaging studies or at autopsy. It is a component of the generalized serositis that is often a feature of SLE and is associated with local autoantibodies and

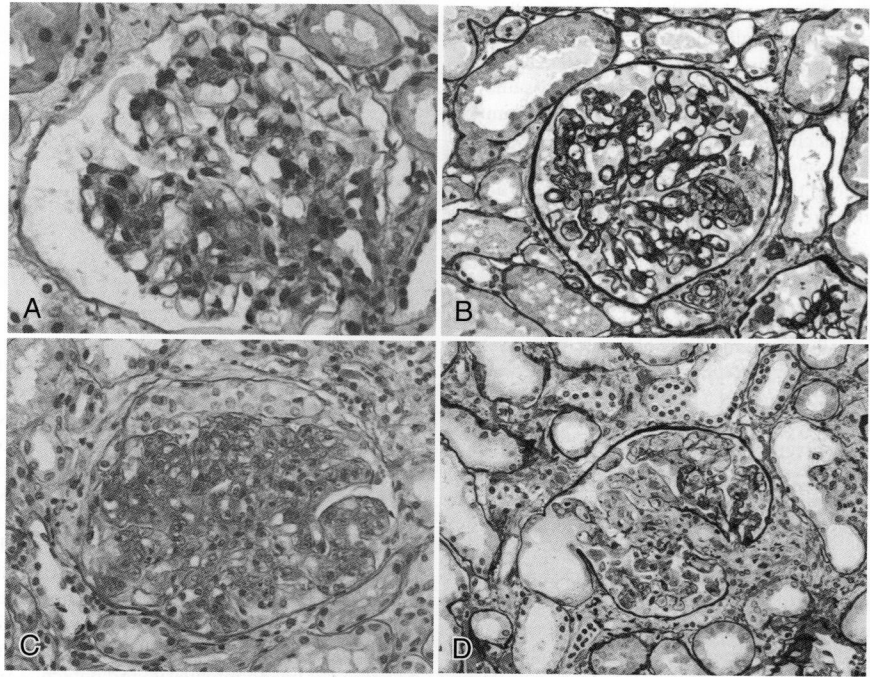

FIGURE 266-3. Histopathology of lupus nephritis. **A,** Lupus nephritis class II. A light micrograph of a glomerulus shows mild mesangial hypercellularity (periodic acid–Schiff). **B,** Lupus nephritis class III (A). Light micrograph showing a glomerulus with segmental endocapillary hypercellularity, mesangial hypercellularity, capillary wall thickening, and early segmental capillary necrosis (methenamine silver). **C,** Lupus nephritis class IV-G (A/C). A glomerulus manifests global endocapillary proliferation, leukocyte influx and apoptotic bodies, double contours, crescent formation with tubular transformation, early sclerosis, and disruption of Bowman's capsule (periodic acid–Schiff). **D,** Thrombotic microangiopathy in a patient with systemic lupus erythematosus and circulating anticoagulant. A glomerulus shows severe capillary and arteriolar thrombosis, endothelial cell swelling and necrosis, neutrophil influx, and stasis of erythrocytes. No signs of immune deposits were found (methenamine silver). (From Wenning JJ, D'Agati VD, Schwartz MM, et al. The classification of glomerulonephritis in systemic lupus erythematosus revisited. *J Am Soc Nephrol.* 2004;15:241.)

immune complexes. Pericarditis is usually manifested as substernal chest pain that is improved by bending forward and can be exacerbated by inspiration or coughing. The symptoms and effusions associated with pericarditis are quite responsive to moderate-dose (20 to 30 mg/day of prednisone) corticosteroid treatment.

Structural valve abnormalities in SLE range from sterile nodules (originally described by Libman and Sacks) to nonspecific valve thickening (Chapter 75). The nodules are immobile and usually located on the atrial side of the mitral valve and sometimes on the arterial side of the aortic valve. Right-sided lesions are rare. These structural changes may in some cases result in valvular regurgitation. Although valve nodules are detected in most patients with SLE at autopsy, clinically significant valvular heart disease is much less common (1 to 18%). The verrucous valvular lesions of Libman and Sacks are most likely inflammatory in nature and may be associated with the presence of antiphospholipid antibodies.

Premature and accelerated atherosclerosis is prevalent in lupus patients, and preclinical atherosclerotic carotid plaque has been documented in 37% of SLE patients as opposed to 15% of age- and sex-matched controls. Traditional cardiovascular risk factors apply, but the diagnosis of SLE is itself a significant risk factor for premature atherosclerosis (Chapter 70). Among the lupus-related mechanisms that confer additional risk for atherosclerosis, IFN-α and oxidative modification of lipid-associated proteins contribute to the accumulation of vascular damage.[9] Mortality from atherosclerosis may be up to 10 times greater in patients with SLE than in age- and sex-matched controls.

Although not specific to SLE, Raynaud's phenomenon (Chapter 80), characterized by episodic vasospasm and occlusion of the digital arteries in response to cold and emotional stress, is a feature in up to 60% of SLE patients and contributes to pain and sometimes necrosis of the distal ends of extremities. The character of the digits classically changes from pallor to cyanosis and then to rubor as vascular perfusion becomes impaired and then reperfusion ensues. In addition, small arteries, arterioles, and capillaries can be affected by vasculitis and fibrinoid necrosis, with clinical manifestations that include periungual telangiectases, abdominal pain, and neuropsychiatric symptoms.

Pulmonary System

Pleuritis is the most frequent manifestation of pulmonary involvement in SLE and occurs in about 30% of patients at some point in their disease course. Pleuritis is characterized by pain on respiration and exudative effusions (Chapter 99). Parenchymal disease is less common but may be based on several distinct mechanisms, including pneumonitis in the absence of documented infection and sometimes involving alveolar hemorrhage (in up to 12% of patients), pulmonary embolism secondary to venous thrombosis, or pulmonary hypertension with increased pulmonary resistance and impaired diffusing capacity.

Neuropsychiatric Involvement

Clinical features of SLE that involve the nervous system include both neurologic and psychiatric manifestations. The central and peripheral nervous systems can be affected by the disease. The American College of Rheumatology has identified 19 neuropsychiatric syndromes that can be associated with SLE, and validation of these neuropsychiatric findings has been substantiated in several independent studies. The most common manifestations that are probably attributable to SLE cerebritis include cognitive dysfunction, present in 17 to 66% of SLE patients; psychosis or mood disorder, the former reported in up to 8% of patients; cerebrovascular disease in 5 to 18% of patients; and seizures, present in 6 to 51% of patients. Headaches are also common. Because none of these CNS manifestations is found exclusively in SLE, it can be difficult to be certain that a neuropsychiatric complaint or symptom should be attributed to SLE.

Evaluation of neuropsychiatric lupus depends on a careful clinical history and physical and laboratory examinations and, in some cases, imaging studies and analysis of cerebrospinal fluid to rule out infection. Magnetic resonance imaging is useful for detecting intracranial abnormalities, which are seen in 19 to 70% of patients and include white matter lesions, cerebral infarction, venous sinus thrombosis, and sometimes atrophy. More sophisticated imaging techniques such as magnetic resonance angiography and magnetic resonance spectroscopy can be used to assess cerebral blood flow or neuronal metabolism.

Cranial nerve and ocular involvement, most likely based on vasculopathy and focal ischemia, can sometimes affect vision. Ocular examination of the retina can reveal cotton-wool spots as a result of retinal ischemia or necrosis. Although rare, transverse myelopathy, frequently associated with antiphospholipid antibodies, can have devastating consequences, including paraplegia. Sensorimotor neuropathies, often asymmetrical, are more common (up to 28%) and are based on damage to small nerve fibers with vasculopathy in the small arteries that supply the nerve fibers.

As is the case with lupus nephritis, the pathophysiologic mechanisms that account for the neuropsychiatric manifestations of SLE are diverse and complex. Recent data suggest that autoantibodies cross-reactive with neuronal cell surface glutamate receptors and DNA may mediate excitotoxic death of neurons and are proposed to contribute to cognitive dysfunction. Antibodies directed against ribosomal P protein have also been associated with neuropsychiatric lupus, and antiphospholipid antibodies can contribute to a procoagulant state, vascular thrombosis, and cerebral ischemia. Cerebral vasculopathy has been clearly demonstrated by angiographic and pathologic studies. Noninflammatory small vessel vasculopathy is the most common lesion and can be associated with microinfarcts. Inflammatory mediators, including the cytokines interleukin (IL)-6 and IFN-α, and matrix metalloproteinases may also contribute to the neuropsychiatric manifestations of SLE.

Gastrointestinal System

Although uncommon, vasculitis of the gastrointestinal tract or mesentery can result in pain and bowel necrosis. Less common than pleuritis and pericarditis, peritonitis can manifest as peritoneal effusion and abdominal pain. Pancreatitis occurs in less than 10% of patients but may also be due to vascular pathology. Lupoid hepatitis, a syndrome that was named for the presence of positive ANAs in patients with chronic active hepatitis, is a misnomer because elevated transaminases are only rarely seen in lupus patients.

Lymphadenopathy

About one third of SLE patients demonstrate diffuse lymphadenopathy at some time during the course of their disease. The nodes are often nontender, and lymphoma is sometimes considered in the differential diagnosis. Biopsy usually reveals follicular hyperplasia, although some histopathologic findings appear similar to the histiocytic necrotizing lymphadenitis that is a feature of Kikuchi's disease, a self-limited syndrome characterized by fever and lymphadenopathy. Recent multicenter studies have determined the frequency of malignancies in patients with SLE and have found a significant increase in hematologic malignancies, particularly non-Hodgkin's lymphoma. Splenomegaly is sometimes seen in SLE, and spleen pathology is characterized by a classic onion-skin histology that appears as concentric circles of collagen matrix surrounding splenic arteries and arterioles.

Hematologic System

In addition to autoantibody specificities that are fairly specific for SLE (anti-DNA, anti-Sm), antibodies that target each of the cellular blood elements are also common. Anemia is present in about 50% of patients and is multifactorial. It can be associated with a positive Coombs test or microangiopathic hemolysis (Chapter 160) or reflect chronic disease (normochromic, normocytic) (Chapter 158). Leukopenia, particularly lymphopenia, is observed, with the lymphocyte count decreasing in the setting of increased disease activity. Antibodies that bind to lymphocytes and neutrophils have been described, and an increased tendency for lymphocytes to undergo spontaneous apoptosis may contribute to lymphopenia. Idiopathic thrombocytopenic purpura (Chapter 172) can be an early manifestation of SLE, and thrombocytopenia induced by antiplatelet autoantibodies can sometimes lead to a life-threatening risk for hemorrhage. Autoantibodies to clotting factors can also occur and contribute to impaired clot formation and hemorrhage.

Lupus Pregnancy and Neonatal Lupus

Whether pregnancy increases the likelihood of lupus exacerbation has been debated, with differences on this point presented by different investigators. However, abundant data indicate that patients with SLE have worse fetal outcomes than healthy individuals.[10] Gestational hypertension, fetal growth restriction, and fetal distress are increased in patients with SLE and may lead to fetal loss or premature delivery. Preeclampsia can contribute to a poor outcome in both the mother and fetus and can be difficult to distinguish from a lupus flare associated with lupus nephritis.

Neonatal lupus is a distinct entity that can occur in infants of mothers with or without a diagnosis of SLE.[11] The syndrome is characterized by cutaneous lesions and congenital heart block in the infant and the presence of antibodies

TABLE 266-2 UPDATE OF THE 1982 REVISED CRITERIA FOR CLASSIFICATION OF SYSTEMIC LUPUS ERYTHEMATOSUS

CRITERION*	DEFINITION
1. Malar rash	Fixed erythema, flat or raised, over the malar eminences that tends to spare the nasolabial folds
2. Discoid rash	Erythematous raised patches with adherent keratotic scaling and follicular plugging; atrophic scarring may occur in older lesions
3. Photosensitivity	Rash as a result of unusual reaction to sunlight, by history or physician observation
4. Oral ulcers	Oral or nasopharyngeal ulceration, usually painless, observed by a physician
5. Arthritis	Nonerosive arthritis involving 2 or more peripheral joints and characterized by tenderness, swelling, or effusion
6. Serositis	A. Pleuritis—convincing history of pleuritic pain or rubbing heard by a physician or evidence of pleural effusion _or_ B. Pericarditis—documented by electrocardiography, a rub, or evidence of pericardial effusion
7. Renal disorder	A. Persistent proteinuria > 0.5 g/day or > 3+ if quantitation is not performed _or_ B. Cellular casts—may be red cell, hemoglobin, granular, tubular, or mixed
8. Neurologic disorder	A. Seizures—in the absence of offending drugs or known metabolic derangements (e.g., uremia, ketoacidosis, electrolyte imbalance) _or_ B. Psychosis—in the absence of offending drugs or known metabolic derangements (e.g., uremia, ketoacidosis, electrolyte imbalance)
9. Hematologic disorder	A. Hemolytic anemia—with reticulocytosis _or_ B. Leukopenia—<4000/mm^3 total on 2 or more occasions _or_ C. Lymphopenia—<1500/mm^3 on 2 or more occasions _or_ D. Thrombocytopenia—<100,000/mm^3 in the absence of offending drugs
10. Immunologic disorder	A. Deleted in 1997 update B. Anti-DNA: antibody to native DNA in abnormal titer _or_ C. Anti-Sm: presence of antibody to Sm nuclear antigen _or_ D. Positive finding of antiphospholipid antibodies based on (1) an abnormal serum level of immunoglobulin (Ig)G or IgM anticardiolipin antibodies, (2) a positive test for lupus anticoagulant using a standard method, or (3) a false-positive serologic test for syphilis known to be positive for at least 6 months and confirmed by _Treponema pallidum_ immobilization or the fluorescent treponemal antibody absorption test (modified in the 1997 update)
11. Antinuclear antibody	An abnormal titer of antinuclear antibody by immunofluorescence or an equivalent assay at any point in time and in the absence of drugs known to be associated with "drug-induced lupus" syndrome

*The proposed classification is based on 11 criteria. For the purpose of identifying patients in clinical studies, a person shall be said to have systemic lupus erythematosus if any 4 or more of the 11 criteria are present, serially or simultaneously, during any interval of observation.
Modified from Tan EM, Cohen AS, Fries JF, et al. The 1982 revised criteria for the classification of systemic lupus erythematosus. _Arthritis Rheum._ 1982;25:1271.

to the Ro (SSA) or La (SSB) RNA-binding proteins (or both) in the mother. Mortality in babies with a congenital heart block is 15 to 31%. Deposition of anti-Ro IgG in the fetal heart, indicative of transplacental transfer of maternal autoantibody, and dense connective tissue encompassing the conduction system have been demonstrated in autopsy specimens. Prenatal testing of lupus mothers for the presence of anti-Ro and anti-La antibodies is appropriate, and careful monitoring with fetal echocardiography starting at week 16 of pregnancy can detect conduction defects. Fluorinated corticosteroids such as dexamethasone have been effective in reversing heart block in some cases. The role of hydroxychloroquine in prevention of neonatal lupus manifestations is under investigation.

Antiphospholipid Antibody Syndrome

Antiphospholipid antibodies represent a distinct class of autoantibodies that are seen in about one third of SLE patients but can also be present in individuals who do not carry a diagnosis of SLE (Chapter 171). Although these antibodies were initially thought to be specific for phospholipids exposed in cell membranes, particularly after "flipping" of the membranes of apoptotic cells, extensive data support their primary reactivity with phospholipid-binding proteins, particularly β_2GPI. Whether in primary antiphospholipid syndrome or in SLE, antiphospholipid antibodies have been associated with venous and arterial thromboses.[12] In addition to vascular thromboses, clinical manifestations of antiphospholipid syndrome include thrombotic microangiopathic glomerular disease, cardiac valve lesions, livedo reticularis, thrombocytopenia, hemolytic anemia, and CNS disease. Recent data indicate that these autoantibodies can contribute to fetal loss and growth restriction by binding to the placenta, activating the complement system, and inducing inflammation. Catastrophic antiphospholipid syndrome, triggered by the acute onset of multisystemic (three or more organs) thrombosis, is resistant to anticoagulation treatment and is fatal in approximately 50% of cases.[13]

DIAGNOSIS
Classification

Criteria for the classification of patients with SLE for the purpose of clinical studies were developed by the American College of Rheumatology, with the most recent full revision published in 1982 and an update published in 1997 (Table 266-2). The criteria include 11 features that encompass manifestations of skin and mucosal involvement, arthritis, serositis, renal disorder, neurologic disorder, hematologic disorder, immunologic disorder, and an abnormal titer in the ANA test, with at least four criteria required for classification as SLE. ANA has low specificity but strengthens the sensitivity of the criteria because it is positive in virtually all lupus patients. These criteria are not intended for use as diagnostic criteria, because more than 50% of patients with SLE do not meet four criteria at any point in time, although all do meet these criteria at some point during the course of the disease. The criteria are useful in reminding the clinician of the most characteristic features of SLE, but a careful history with detailed review of systems and triggering factors, as well as a family history, is essential in raising suspicion for a diagnosis of SLE. Because drugs can trigger a lupus-like syndrome, a careful drug history should be taken. Procainamide and hydralazine present the greatest risk for development of lupus, with quinidine, isoniazid, minocycline, and recombinant interferon-α presenting a lower risk. At the onset of clinical symptoms, the diagnosis of SLE can be uncertain because many of the systemic manifestations of lupus can mimic other conditions, particularly viral infections or malignancy, and only some of the typical clinical symptoms may be expressed at any one point in time. Important features of SLE are its multisystemic nature and characteristic serology. The differential diagnosis of SLE includes other rheumatic disorders, such as rheumatoid arthritis and vasculitis; infections, including gonococcal arthritis, parvovirus B19, and mononucleosis; inflammatory bowel disease; thrombotic thrombocytopenic purpura; drug reactions; and malignancies, particularly lymphoma. It should be recognized that the clinical manifestations of lupus can demonstrate overlap with those of other autoimmune rheumatic diseases and can evolve over time. Many genetic, environmental, and immunologic factors associated with lupus are also associated with other systemic autoimmune diseases, often contributing to a complex clinical picture.

Laboratory Findings

Laboratory tests can be very helpful in supporting the diagnosis of SLE. All cellular elements of blood can be affected in lupus, so the complete blood count is an essential test that aids in diagnosis and management. A prolonged activated partial thromboplastin time (aPTT) can indicate the presence of pathogenic antiphospholipid antibodies (Chapter 171). These antibodies are also associated with a false-positive result in the serologic test for syphilis, an observation that is mainly of historical interest.

Evaluation of renal disease in SLE includes urinalysis with microscopic analysis of urine sediment, serum blood urea nitrogen and creatinine, and 24-hour urine collection (or alternatively, spot urine protein-to-creatinine ratio) for estimation of protein and creatinine clearance. Low serum albumin would be consistent with persistent proteinuria and membranous GN, whereas red and white blood cell casts in the urinary sediment suggest proliferative GN. Although a renal biopsy is usually performed only when the result may influence therapeutic decisions, pathologic classification of the features of renal disease can provide prognostic information.

The erythrocyte sedimentation rate (ESR), although a very nonspecific indicator of systemic inflammation, is often monitored and in many patients can provide an indication of disease activity. Interestingly, C-reactive protein, an acute phase reactant, is relatively uninformative in SLE because it is often low in comparison to an ESR performed on the same occasion.

Assaying and monitoring characteristic lupus serologic tests can strongly support the diagnosis of SLE and, in some cases, can assist in the assessment of disease activity. The ANA test is positive in virtually all patients and does not need to be repeated once it has been documented to be positive (Table 266-3). Anti–double-stranded DNA antibodies are common in SLE, and some studies have found that monitoring their titer can be useful in assessing the activity of lupus nephritis. Autoantibodies specific for proteins that associate with nucleic acids in intracellular particles are present in many patients and can provide support for a diagnosis of SLE. Anti-Sm antibodies are highly specific for SLE and, along with anti-RNP antibodies, react with the spliceosome particle. Anti-Ro (SSA) and anti-La (SSB) antibodies are specific for proteins in an RNA-containing particle and are common in patients with Sjögren's syndrome and in mothers of babies with neonatal lupus, as well as being a feature of SLE. It is useful to document the presence of anti-Sm, anti-RNP, anti-Ro, and anti-La antibodies when the diagnosis of SLE is being made, but the titers of these autoantibodies are not helpful in monitoring disease activity.

Proteins of the complement system are activated by immune complexes, such as those that form in patients with SLE. The activation products that result from enzymatic cleavage of the complement components promote inflammation directly by binding to cell surface receptors on mononuclear phagocytes, and indirectly by acting as chemotactic agents to recruit inflammatory cells. Decreased levels of two of the more stable complement components, C3 and C4, are typically measured in serum, and decreased C3 and C4 levels are often indicators of enhanced consumption and increased disease activity. Some laboratories also use a functional measure of total hemolytic complement activity (CH_{50}).

It is the global picture provided by a careful history, physical examination, and blood, urine, and serologic data that supports a diagnosis of SLE. It should be recognized that there is considerable heterogeneity among patients and that different combinations of clinical features will characterize any one individual. As is the case with many systemic diseases, infection and some malignancies may have a similar picture and should be included in the differential until the diagnosis of SLE is secure.

TABLE 266-3 AUTOANTIBODIES ASSOCIATED WITH SYSTEMIC LUPUS ERYTHEMATOSUS

TARGET ANTIGEN	APPROXIMATE FREQUENCY
Nuclear antigens	99
dsDNA	70
Sm	38
RNP (U1-RNP)	33
Ro (SSA)	49
La (SSB)	35
Phospholipids	21
Ribosomal P	10

TREATMENT Rx

Although current knowledge of genetic risk factors for SLE is not sufficient to predict those in whom the disease will develop, once the diagnosis has been made, regular counseling and education are fundamental to the treatment of SLE patients. Patients should be advised to avoid known triggers of disease exacerbation, such as ultraviolet light, and should be instructed regarding the need for adequate rest. Pregnancy should be undertaken with caution and with careful monitoring. Lupus patients can be informed that data indicate that oral contraceptive agents[A1] and estrogen replacement therapy[A2] do not contribute to disease exacerbations.

Conventional Medical Therapy

Clinical manifestations of lupus that do not involve major organ systems can often be managed with nonsteroidal anti-inflammatory drugs, low-dose corticosteroids, and antimalarials. Corticosteroids (Chapter 35) are immunosuppressive agents that modulate many functions of lymphocytes and monocytes, including the production of proinflammatory cytokines. Oral prednisone in doses ranging from 5 to 30 mg daily is effective in treating constitutional symptoms, arthralgias, pericarditis and pleuritis, and skin disease. Topical corticosteroids are sometimes applied to cutaneous lesions. Although effective, corticosteroids also have toxicities that add to the morbidity associated with lupus. The broad immunosuppression mediated by these drugs contributes to the susceptibility to infection that is an inherent feature of SLE. Osteonecrosis, osteoporotic fractures, posterior subcapsular cataracts, diabetes, myopathy, hypertension, hypoadrenalism, and emotional disturbance are additional deleterious effects of corticosteroids.

Antimalarial agents, most commonly hydroxychloroquine administered at 200 to 400 mg/day, have long been used to control skin involvement and arthralgias and are now routinely used in most lupus patients. An important Canadian study demonstrating an increased frequency of disease flare in patients who discontinued hydroxychloroquine contributed to its recent use in lupus for a broader range of clinical manifestations. Hydroxychloroquine has been associated with a decreased incidence of thrombosis, a mechanism that could affect vasculopathy and end-organ damage. An additional potential mechanism of action implicates the TLR pathway, which is responsible for activation of the innate immune response.[14] The effects of antimalarial agents on acidification of the intracellular vesicles where TLRs associate with their ligands may inhibit immune cell activation mediated by stimulatory nucleic acids. Antimalarials are well tolerated. Because they can rarely cause eye toxicity, ophthalmologic examinations should precede initiation of therapy and take place every 6 to 12 months.

Management of Serious Organ-System Disease

For more serious disease, particularly active nephritis, CNS disease, or systemic vasculitis, prednisone at 60 mg daily or 1 g of intravenous methylprednisolone administered daily for 3 days can sometimes gain control of disease activity. In many situations, additional immunosuppressive, cytotoxic, or biologic therapies are required. Because lupus nephritis is the most common severe clinical organ-system manifestation of SLE, an algorithm describing guidelines for medical management of lupus nephritis developed by a Task Force Panel assembled by the American College of Rheumatology is useful (Fig. 266-4).[15] A similar approach can be applied to other serious clinical disease flares. Lupus flares involving rapid decompensation of renal function, CNS disease (including seizures, strokes, or psychosis), or widespread vasculitis or vasculopathy can be life-threatening and must be recognized and treated early and aggressively.[16] Careful attention to monitoring for concurrent or superimposed infection is an important priority during management of a severe lupus flare, and distinguishing sepsis from active lupus or catastrophic antiphospholipid syndrome can be a particular challenge. In general, cyclophosphamide is added to high-dose corticosteroid therapy in the setting of severe flare, although mycophenolate mofetil has gained increased use in situations where the physician or patient wishes to avoid the potential toxicities associated with cyclophosphamide.[A3][A4] Randomized controlled studies have investigated options for maintaining improvement in those patients who respond to induction therapy in the setting of lupus nephritis flare, with current data favoring mycophenolate mofetil over azathioprine.[A5][A6] One biologic agent, belimumab, a monoclonal antibody reactive with BLyS, has been approved by the U.S. Food and Drug Administration (FDA) for treatment of active autoantibody-positive SLE in conjunction with standard therapies, but belimumab has not yet been tested in patients with lupus nephritis or other severe manifestations of lupus. Agents used in management of lupus are reviewed below.

Immunosuppressive Agents
Alkylating Agents

Approximately 33% of lupus patients receive cytotoxic therapy during the course of their disease. Cyclophosphamide is a cytotoxic agent that has been one of the more reliable and studied treatments for severe organ system manifestations of lupus, particularly lupus nephritis and CNS involvement.

Induction Therapy: Class III/IV

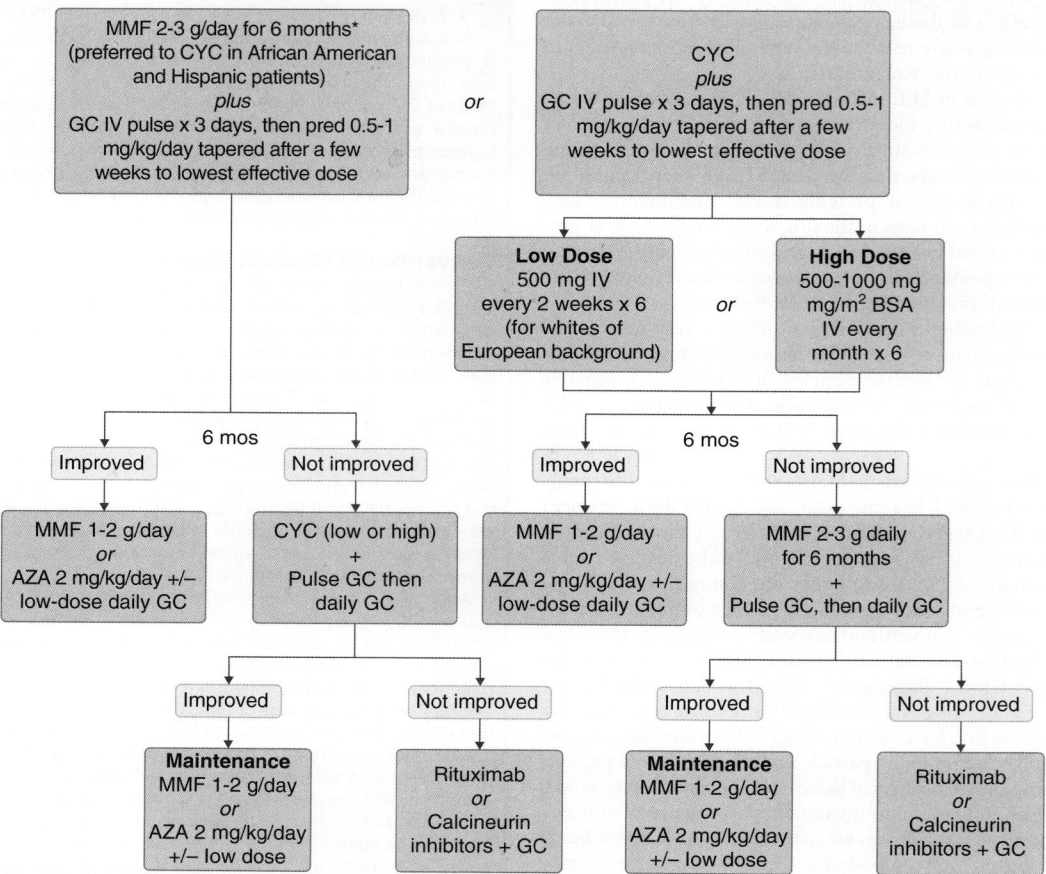

FIGURE 266-4. **Algorithm for induction therapy for lupus nephritis.** Guidelines developed by the Task Force Panel of the American College of Rheumatology for management of class III/IV lupus nephritis. Refer to reference 15 for guidelines for management of class III/IV lupus nephritis with crescents and class V membranous lupus nephritis without prolifera- tive changes and nephrotic range proteinuria. *The Task Force Panel preferred MMF over CYC in patients who desire to preserve fertility. AZA = azathioprine; BSA = body surface area; CYC = cyclophosphamide; GC = glucocorticoid; IV = intravenous; MMF = mycophenolate mofetil; pred = prednisone. (From Hahn BH, McMahon MA, Wilkinson A, et al. American College of Rheumatology guidelines for screening, treatment, and management of lupus nephritis. *Arthritis Care Res (Hoboken).* 2012;64:797-808.)

Studies performed at the National Institutes of Health in the 1980s led to recommendations of a standard regimen of cyclophosphamide, 0.5 to 1 g/m^2 body surface area administered intravenously monthly for 6 months, followed by quarterly doses through 2 years. Cyclophosphamide is usually given with oral prednisone in tapering doses or sometimes with pulse methylprednisolone. Although this regimen is often effective in controlling GN, overall patient survival has not been demonstrated to be increased, and cyclophosphamide is associated with significant toxicity, including cytopenia, infection, gonadal failure, and malignancy. Recent clinical studies have included modified immunosuppressive regimens, such as a 6-month induction followed by maintenance with less toxic immunosuppressive agents, including azathioprine or, even better, mycophenolate mofetil (MMF). Cyclophosphamide is relatively contraindicated in pregnant women.

Purine Synthesis Inhibitors

Azathioprine has been used for the treatment of lupus nephritis and as a steroid-sparing agent in SLE for many years. Azathioprine inhibits DNA synthesis and inhibits key signaling pathways in T lymphocytes. Azathioprine is commonly dosed at 2 to 3 mg/kg/day administered as a tablet. Toxicities of azathioprine target the bone marrow (and result in cytopenias) as well as the liver, occasionally resulting in transaminitis. Its use is rarely associated with non-Hodgkin's lymphoma (Chapter 185). It has been used safely in pregnant women.

MMF is an inhibitor that binds to the isoform of inosine monophosphate dehydrogenase that mediates purine synthesis in activated lymphocytes. It has a good track record of utility in inhibiting allograft rejection. Recent clinical trials have compared MMF with intravenous cyclophosphamide for induction therapy in lupus nephritis; the results demonstrated equivalence of MMF and cyclophosphamide in patients with lupus nephritis.[A7] In a randomized trial, MMF (1 g twice daily) was more effective than azathioprine for the maintenance treatment of lupus nephritis, with treatment failure rates reduced from 32 to 16%.[A8]

Methotrexate

Methotrexate is a folate antagonist that is commonly used in rheumatoid arthritis. A double-blind randomized placebo-controlled trial of oral methotrexate (15 to 25 mg/week for 6 months) in SLE controlled disease and allowed tapering of prednisone. The most responsive clinical manifestations were cutaneous and articular.

Ancillary and Other Therapies

Intravenous Gamma Globulin

Although positive data from controlled trials of intravenous gamma globulin are not available, case reports and clinical experience indicate that administration of pooled IgG fractions can sometimes be efficacious in gaining control of lupus disease activity that is refractory to other therapies. A common regimen is 2 g/kg in divided doses over a 3- to 5-day period. Several mechanisms have been proposed for this therapy, including blockade of Fc receptors, modulation of lymphocyte function through Fc receptors, increased catabolism of pathogenic immunoglobulin, and actions of the anti-idiotype antibody that is a component of the administered IgG.

Plasmapheresis

Removal of pathogenic antibodies and immune complexes is the goal of plasmapheresis, but there are scant data supporting the utility of this therapy. Nonetheless, plasmapheresis has been occasionally useful in lupus patients with life-threatening complications in which the clinical manifestations can be clearly attributed to pathogenic autoantibodies. In particular, plasmapheresis has been effective in cases of thrombotic thrombocytopenic purpura associated with SLE (Chapter 172).

Biologic Therapies

Biologic therapies (Chapter 36) are being actively investigated in clinical trials, but only one agent has been successful as yet in phase III studies. Belimumab, a monoclonal antibody, blocks a B-cell survival and differentiation signal. At a dose of 1 mg/kg or 10 mg/kg intravenously on days 1 and 28 and then every 28 days for 48 weeks, belimumab reduced disease activity by both validated measures and physician global assessment and decreased autoantibody levels.[A9] In a second study, belimumab at a dose of 10 mg/kg administered intravenously on days 0, 14, and 28 and then every 28 days, the currently recommended regimen, for 72 weeks, added to standard therapy, significantly improved response rate, disease activity, and severe flares, and was generally well tolerated in SLE.[A10] The clinical settings that are most appropriate for the use of belimumab, which was approved by the FDA, will be determined by future clinical trials and clinical experience. Additional agents under investigation target B cells, T-cell activation, and cytokines.[17] Rituximab, a monoclonal antibody specific for the cell surface B-cell molecule CD20, is approved for use in B-cell lymphomas and has been used in some patients with SLE who are poorly responsive to other therapies. Rituximab depletes B cells, often for many months, and may limit T-cell activation by eliminating activated B cells that can serve as antigen-presenting cells. However, controlled clinical trials of rituximab in lupus have not shown efficacy. In a randomized double-blind placebo-controlled phase III trial in patients with active proliferative lupus nephritis, rituximab therapy led to more responders and greater reductions in anti-dsDNA and C3/C4 levels, but did not improve clinical outcomes after 1 year of treatment.[A11] Other agents that block B-cell survival and differentiation factors or target B-cell surface molecules are under study. T-cell targets include CD28 and inducible costimulator (ICOS), a T-cell surface molecule in the same molecular family as CD28 and CTLA4. Blockade of T-cell activation by CTLA4-Ig, a soluble inhibitor of CD28 ligation, or inhibition of ICOS-ICOS ligand interaction might inhibit B-cell differentiation in the germinal center. Monoclonal antibodies specific for most isoforms of IFN-α are under study and represent a rational approach in view of the strong genetic and immunologic role of type I interferon in many SLE patients.[18] IL-6 and IFN-γ represent additional cytokine targets under study.

Adjunctive Therapies

In addition to controlling autoimmunity and inflammation in SLE, it is essential to control hypertension adequately when it occurs. In those with lupus nephritis, treatment with an angiotensin inhibitor or an angiotensin receptor blocker reduces intraglomerular pressure, thus reducing proteinuria. In patients with a history of thrombosis, who will usually have antiphospholipid antibodies, long-term warfarin is recommended. The potential use of statins in lupus is of interest because those agents have anti-inflammatory as well as lipid lowering effects, but statins have not yet been shown efficacious in controlling lupus disease activity in controlled trials. The role of vitamin D supplementation in lupus is under study.

Future Directions

Recent advances in basic immunology, together with detailed molecular and clinical characterization of cohorts of SLE patients, have directed attention to the role adjuvant-like factors play in activating the innate immune response through TLRs. The primary triggers of that response are not known, but abundant data support production of type I interferon as an important consequence of immune activation that has an impact on many aspects of lymphocyte function, probably including induction of self-antigen–specific immune responses. In addition to the biologic therapies currently under study that target T and B lymphocytes, future therapies may be designed that can inhibit TLR activation, signaling components downstream from TLRs, cytoplasmic sensors of stimulatory nucleic acids, or type I interferon itself. Recognition that the complement system is an essential contributor to inflammation triggered by antiphospholipid antibodies, as well as by immune complexes, provides additional targets that might be inhibited therapeutically and limit tissue damage. Continued investigation of the genetic and environmental factors that contribute to disease susceptibility may permit identification of individuals at risk for the development of SLE and may elucidate the primary stimuli that lead to autoimmunity. Identification of informative biomarkers that reflect or even predict disease flares would improve medical management of lupus patients.

PROGNOSIS

Although survival of patients with a diagnosis of SLE is good, lupus remains a disease that is potentially fatal. SLE demonstrates a bimodal pattern of death, with deaths within the first year attributable to active lupus and infection and late deaths attributable to atherosclerotic cardiovascular disease. Recent cohort studies have estimated 5-year survival rates greater than 90%, with improvement in medical management probably contributing to improved outcomes, as opposed to earlier studies, and 85% survival rates at 10 years. However, once a diagnosis of SLE has been made, prolonged remission is rare. Of 702 patients registered in a lupus clinic in Canada, 6.5% achieved complete remission (score of 0 on the SLE Disease Activity Index), and only 1.7% maintained remission for at least 5 years with no treatment.

The presence of any permanent organ damage within the first year after a diagnosis of SLE is associated with poorer survival at 10 years (a 75 vs. 95% rate in those without permanent organ damage). Regarding renal outcome, an elevated level of serum creatinine at the time of diagnosis has been correlated with an adverse outcome.

Recent studies of minority populations in the United States have indicated that predictors of high lupus disease activity include Hispanic Texan and African American ethnicities, lack of health insurance, and poor social support. African admixture and anti–double-stranded DNA antibodies also predicted high levels of disease activity, as did previous disease activity.

Data from a multicenter study of nearly 10,000 patients has supported an increased risk for hematologic malignancies in SLE patients, particularly non-Hodgkin's lymphoma. Prognostic factors for an adverse fetal outcome in pregnant lupus mothers are maternal renal disease and hypertension.

Grade A References

A1. Petri M, Kim MY, Kalunian KC, et al. Combined oral contraceptives in women with systemic lupus erythematosus. *N Engl J Med.* 2005;353:2550-2558.

A2. Sanchez-Guerrero J, Gonzalez-Perez M, Durand-Carbajal M, et al. Menopause hormonal therapy in women with systemic lupus erythematosus. *Arthritis Rheum.* 2007;56:3070-3079.

A3. Houssiau FA, Vasconcelos C, D'Crus D, et al. The 10-year follow-up data of the Euro-Lupus Nephritis Trial comparing low-dose and high-dose intravenous cyclophosphamide. *Ann Rheum Dis.* 2010;69:61-64.

A4. Arends S, Grootscholten C, Derksen RH, et al., Dutch Working Party on systemic lupus erythematosus. Long-term follow-up of a randomised controlled trial of azathioprine/methylprednisolone versus cyclophosphamide in patients with proliferative lupus nephritis. *Ann Rheum Dis.* 2012;71:966-973.

A5. Houssiau FA, D'Cruz D, Sangle S, et al. MAINTAIN Nephritis Trial Group. Azathioprine versus mycophenolate mofetil for long-term immunosuppression in lupus nephritis: results from the MAINTAIN Nephritis Trial. *Ann Rheum Dis.* 2010;69:2083-2089.

A6. Feng L, Deng J, Huo DM, et al. Mycophenolate mofetil versus azathioprine as maintenance therapy for lupus nephritis: a meta-analysis. *Nephrology (Carlton).* 2013;18:104-110.

A7. Appel GB, Contreras G, Dooley MA, et al. Mycophenolate mofetil versus cyclophosphamide for induction treatment of lupus nephritis. *J Am Soc Nephrol.* 2009;20:1103-1112.

A8. Dooley MA, Jayne D, Ginzler EM, et al. Mycophenolate versus azathioprine as maintenance therapy for lupus nephritis. *N Engl J Med.* 2011;365:1886-1895.

A9. Navarra SV, Guzmán RM, Gallacher AE, et al. Efficacy and safety of belimumab in patients with active systemic lupus erythematosus: a randomised, placebo-controlled, phase 3 trial. *Lancet.* 2011;377:721-731.

A10. Furie R, Petri M, Zamani O, et al. A phase III, randomized, placebo-controlled study of belimumab, a monoclonal antibody that inhibits B lymphocyte stimulator, in patients with systemic lupus erythematosus. *Arthritis Rheum.* 2011;63:3918-3930.

A11. Rovin BH, Furie R, Latinis K, et al. Efficacy and safety of rituximab in patients with active proliferative lupus nephritis. *Arthritis Rheum.* 2012;64:1215-1226.

GENERAL REFERENCES

For the General References and other additional features, please visit Expert Consult at https://expertconsult.inkling.com.

267

SYSTEMIC SCLEROSIS (SCLERODERMA)

JOHN VARGA

DEFINITION

Systemic sclerosis (SSc) is a chronic autoimmune connective tissue disease of unknown cause. Although middle-aged women are most commonly affected, SSc can occur at any age and is associated with considerable morbidity and increased mortality. The disease shows marked clinical heterogeneity, has protean clinical manifestations, and commonly follows a progressive course.[1] The hallmark of SSc is thickening and hardening of the skin (scleroderma), but in most patients the lungs, gastrointestinal (GI) tract, kidneys, and heart are also affected. In its earliest stages, SSc is associated with prominent inflammation and autoimmunity and altered microvascular function. Over time, progressive structural alterations in small blood vessels and fibrosis in multiple organs cause organ failure. Although there is no approved disease-modifying therapy for SSc, current treatment strategies can control symptoms, slow disease progression, improve quality of life, and prolong survival. The presence of scleroderma (hard skin) distinguishes SSc from other autoimmune and rheumatic diseases, but skin induration also features prominently in localized forms of scleroderma and multiple unrelated conditions (Table 267-1).

Classification

Systemic Sclerosis

SSc is clinically classified into two subsets: diffuse cutaneous SSc (dcSSc) and limited cutaneous SSc (lcSSc), defined by the pattern of skin involvement and associated with distinct clinical and laboratory manifestations and natural history (Table 267-2). In lcSSc, skin involvement is restricted to the fingers, toes, distal extremities, and face; proximal extremities and the trunk are spared. Diffuse cutaneous SSc is characterized by involvement of the skin proximal to the elbows and knees, including the trunk, along with the distal extremities. In patients with lcSSc, Raynaud phenomenon commonly precedes other disease manifestations. In contrast to lcSSc, dcSSc is generally rapidly progressive and may be complicated by early pulmonary fibrosis, accelerated hypertension, and acute renal failure. The constellation of calcinosis cutis, Raynaud phenomenon, esophageal dysmotility, sclerodactyly (scleroderma of the fingers), and telangiectasia in a subset of patients with lcSSc is termed *CREST syndrome*. Patients with CREST generally follow an indolent course and have a relatively good prognosis. Raynaud phenomenon and other characteristic clinical and laboratory findings of SSc in the absence of obvious skin thickening is the hallmark of SSc sine scleroderma.

TABLE 267-1 CONDITIONS WITH SCLERODERMA-LIKE SKIN INDURATION

Systemic sclerosis (SSc)
   Limited cutaneous SSc
   Diffuse cutaneous SSc
Localized scleroderma
   Morphea (plaque, guttate, generalized)
   Pansclerotic morphea
   Linear scleroderma, "coup de sabre"
Scleredema and diabetic scleredema
Scleromyxedema (papular mucinosis)
Nephrogenic fibrosing syndrome (nephrogenic systemic fibrosis)
Chronic graft-versus-host disease
Diffuse fasciitis with eosinophilia (Shulman disease, eosinophilic fasciitis)
Eosinophilia-myalgia syndrome
Chemically induced scleroderma-like conditions
   • Vinyl chloride–induced disease, other solvents
   • Pentazocine-induced skin fibrosis
   • Other drug associations
Paraneoplastic syndrome

TABLE 267-2 CLASSIFICATION OF SYSTEMIC SCLEROSIS

CHARACTERISTIC FEATURES	LIMITED CUTANEOUS SYSTEMIC SCLEROSIS	DIFFUSE CUTANEOUS SYSTEMIC SCLEROSIS
Skin induration	Limited to fingers, distal to elbows, face; progression slow	Diffuse: fingers, extremities, face, trunk; progression rapid; tendon friction rubs
Raynaud phenomenon	Precedes skin involvement; often severe; associated with critical ischemia	Onset occurs coincident with or subsequent to skin involvement
Pulmonary fibrosis	Occasional, moderately severe	Frequent, early, can be progressive and severe
Pulmonary arterial hypertension	Frequent, late, may be isolated	Occasional, commonly in association with pulmonary fibrosis
Scleroderma renal crisis	Very rare	Occurs in up to 15%; early
Calcinosis cutis	Frequent, prominent	Infrequent
Characteristic autoantibodies	Anticentromere	Antitopoisomerase I (Scl-70), anti-RNA polymerase III

Mixed Connective Tissue Disorder

Mixed connective tissue disorder (MCTD) is an overlap syndrome first described in 1971 that is characterized by features of systemic lupus erythematosus (SLE), SSc, and myositis, all occurring in the same patient. In the early phase, most patients have Raynaud phenomenon in association with edema of the hands and evidence of inflammatory muscle disease. Over time, these patients sequentially manifest other features of connective tissue diseases, including pericarditis, esophageal dysmotility, sclerodactyly, neuropathy, and pulmonary arterial hypertension (PAH). Erosive arthritis does not occur. On the other hand, some patients develop acute renal involvement similar to scleroderma renal crisis. In the early stage of this disorder, it is often difficult to predict whether the patient will progress to develop a distinct connective tissue disease such as SSc or SLE or will be ultimately diagnosed with MCTD. A diagnostic hallmark of MCTD is the presence in the serum of a highly characteristic autoantibody specificity against U1-ribonuclear protein (U1-RNP). Most MCTD patients have a very high titer (often > 1 : 1000) of anti-U1-RNP autoantibody. Some of the features of MCTD might respond to corticosteroid therapy. Overall, patients with MCTD generally have a better prognosis than those with SSc.

Localized Scleroderma

Localized scleroderma refers to a family of generally benign skin conditions primarily affecting children. These conditions are characterized by discreet areas of skin induration in the absence of Raynaud phenomenon or systemic involvement. Lesional skin is discolored and indurated and histologically may be indistinguishable from SSc. Localized scleroderma has multiple distinct forms. When it occurs as single or multiple solitary patches of induration, it is called morphea. When these patches coalesce, the condition is called generalized morphea. The lesions are generally asymmetrical in distribution and spare the digits. Some individuals have extensive and disabling induration (pansclerotic morphea). Induration may follow in a linear distribution, most commonly on the lower extremities (linear scleroderma). In children, linear scleroderma can be complicated by growth retardation and joint contractures.

EPIDEMIOLOGY

SSc is a sporadic disease with a worldwide distribution. The incidence is 9 to 19 cases per million per year, with an estimated 100,000 cases in the United States. Studies from several countries suggest that the incidence of SSc may be increasing. Like other connective tissue diseases, SSc shows a marked female predominance, particularly in the childbearing years. The peak age of onset is 30 to 50 years for both the limited and diffuse cutaneous forms. African Americans have a higher incidence and an earlier age of disease onset compared to whites, and are more likely to have the diffuse cutaneous form of SSc associated with interstitial lung involvement and a worse prognosis.

Etiology and Environmental and Occupational Exposures

Although the cause of SSc is unknown, the onset is commonly ascribed to an interplay between environmental factors and genetic susceptibility. Suspected environmental triggers include occupational, dietary, medical, and lifestyle exposures, and possibly certain infectious agents. Because some SSc autoantibodies cross-react with certain virus-associated epitopes, molecular mimicry has been proposed as a possible pathogenetic link between viral infection and SSc.

Epidemic outbreaks of SSc-like syndromes have been linked with toxic exposures. A Spanish outbreak of toxic oil syndrome in the 1980s affected more than 20,000 individuals. The syndrome was characterized by chronic skin induration and neuropathy, and the outbreak was linked to ingestion of contaminated rapeseed oils used for cooking. An outbreak of eosinophilia-myalgia syndrome (EMS) a decade later was linked to ingestion of over-the-counter L-tryptophan dietary supplements used for insomnia, weight loss, and other indications. The syndrome was characterized by peripheral blood eosinophilia and severe myalgia in the acute stage, followed by intractable scleroderma-like diffuse skin induration. Neither toxic oil syndrome nor EMS was associated with Raynaud phenomenon or SSc-specific autoantibodies.

Occupational exposures tentatively linked with SSc include silica (in miners), polyvinyl chloride, epoxy resins, and aromatic hydrocarbons including toluene and trichloroethylene. Certain drugs, including bleomycin, pentazocine, hormone replacement therapy, cocaine, and appetite suppressants, have been linked with SSc or PAH. Although earlier studies implied a possible association of SSc with silicone breast implants, large-scale epidemiologic investigations failed to establish an increased risk.

Genetic Factors

A genetic contribution to SSc susceptibility is indicated by the fact that 1.6% of patients have a first-degree relative with SSc, a prevalence rate substantially higher than in the general population (0.026). Indeed, a family history is the strongest identified risk factor for SSc. Moreover, patients with SSc are more likely to have first-degree relatives with Raynaud phenomenon and interstitial lung disease, as well as other autoimmune diseases including multiple sclerosis, rheumatoid arthritis, and thyroiditis. Genomewide association and candidate-gene studies in SSc have identified association with multiple HLA loci, as well as non-HLA loci including *STAT4*, *IRF4*, *PTPN22*, *TNIP-1*, *IRAK1*, *CD247*, and *BANK1*, each of which encodes genes involved in immune regulation or autoimmunity. Moreover, most of these SSc-associated risk alleles are also linked with other autoimmune diseases, especially SLE.

PATHOBIOLOGY

The protean clinical and pathologic manifestations of SSc reflect a complex underlying pathobiology encompassing three interrelated cardinal processes: autoimmunity and inflammation, vascular injury and obliteration, and fibrosis and excessive matrix accumulation in multiple tissues and organs (Fig. 267-1).[2] This canonical triad is operative to a greater or lesser extent in all patients with SSc, and their variable relative contribution of each process to the individual phenotype account for the observed disease heterogeneity.

Pathology

The distinguishing pathologic hallmark of SSc is the constellation of capillary loss (rarefaction) and obliterative vasculopathy coexisting with fibrosis in the skin and internal organs. In early-stage disease, perivascular inflammation can be detected in multiple organs before the appearance of fibrosis. The vascular lesion is characterized by intimal proliferation in the small and medium-sized arteries, resulting in luminal narrowing and obliteration.[3] In later-stage SSc, fibrosis is prominent in the skin, lungs, GI tract, heart, tendon sheath, perifascicular tissue surrounding skeletal muscle, and some endocrine organs.[4] Accumulation of connective tissue rich in collagens, fibronectin, cartilage oligomeric matrix protein (COMP), and proteoglycans disrupts normal architecture, resulting in functional impairment of affected organs.

In the skin, dermal collagen deposition causes obliteration of the hair follicles, sweat glands, and other adnexae, as well as invasion of the subjacent adipose layer with entrapment of fat cells. The epidermis is atrophic, and the rete pegs are effaced. In late-stage disease, there is a paucity of vascular and lymphatic endothelium. In the lungs, the interstitium and alveolar spaces are infiltrated with inflammatory cells in early disease. With progression, interstitial fibrosis and vascular damage, often coexisting within the same lesions, dominate the pathologic picture. The most common histologic pattern in SSc-associated lung disease is nonspecific interstitial pneumonitis (NSIP). Progressive thickening of the alveolar septae results in obliteration of the air spaces, honeycombing, and loss of pulmonary blood vessels.

Intimal thickening of the pulmonary arteries (Fig. 267-2), best seen with elastin stain, underlies PAH (Chapter 68). These vascular lesions resemble those of, but are distinct from, idiopathic PAH, but the hallmark plexiform lesions are uncommon in SSc. In the GI tract, pathologic changes can be found at any level from the mouth to the rectum. Fibrosis of the lamina propria and submucosa with atrophy of the muscular layers are prominent in the lower esophagus, whereas striated muscle in the upper third of the esophagus is generally spared (Chapter 138). Replacement of the normal gut architecture leads to disordered peristaltic activity with gastroesophageal reflux and dysmotility, gastroparesis, and small bowel obstruction. Chronic reflux

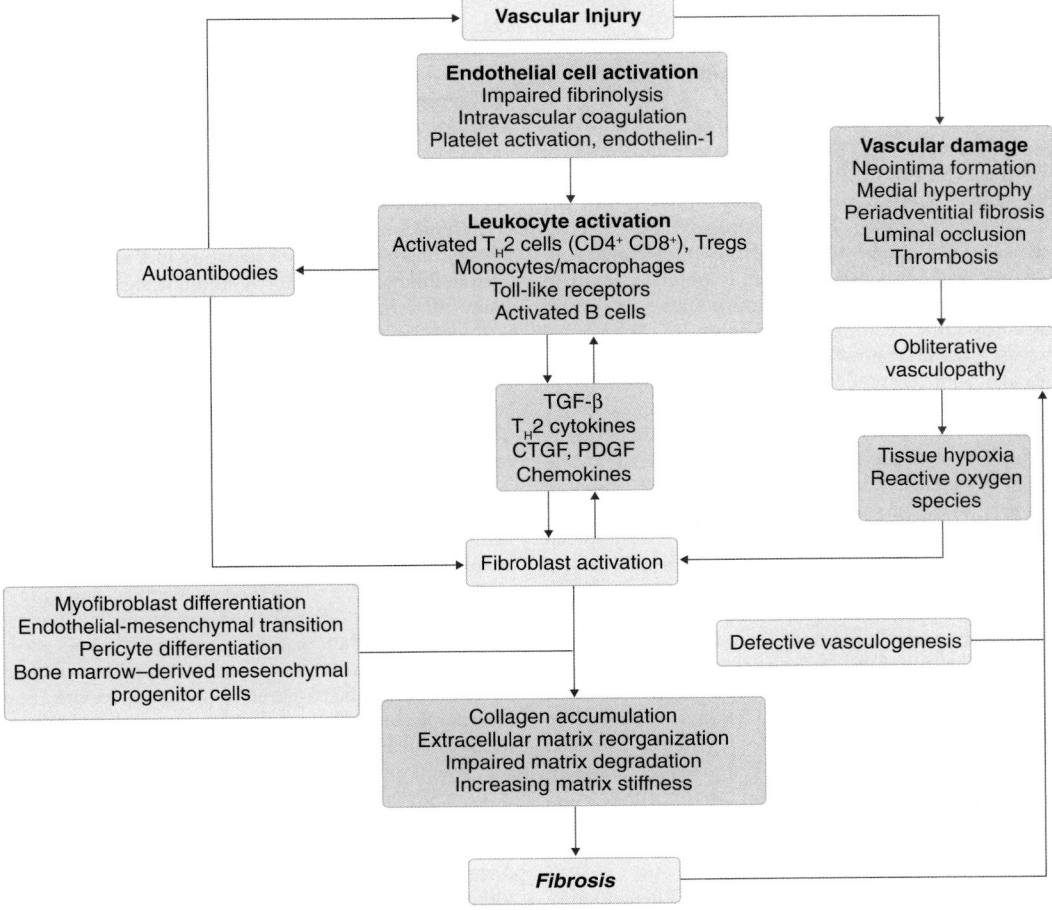

FIGURE 267-1. The pathogenetic triad of systemic sclerosis: vasculopathy, autoimmunity, fibrosis. Initial endothelial injury in a genetically susceptible individual leads to vascular damage, inflammation, and autoimmunity. The inflammatory and immune responses initiate fibroblast activation, resulting in intractable fibrosis. Vasculopathy, loss of microvasculature, and reduced blood flow result in ischemia and generation of reactive oxygen species that contribute to and further aggravate vascular damage, tissue fibrosis, and atrophy. CTGF = connective tissue growth factor; PDGF = platelet-derived growth factor; TGF-β = transforming growth factor-β.

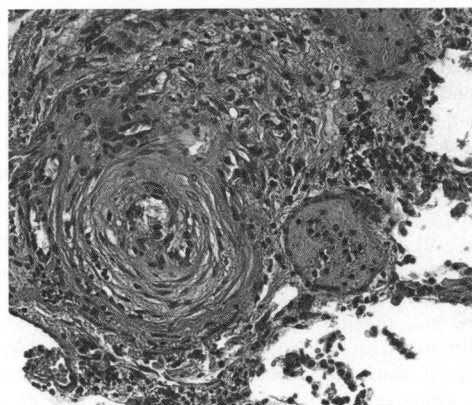

FIGURE 267-2. Pulmonary artery obliterative vasculopathy. Striking intimal hyperplasia and narrowing of the lumen of a small pulmonary artery, coexisting with interstitial pulmonary fibrosis, in a patient with diffuse cutaneous systemic sclerosis.

TABLE 267-3	CHARACTERISTIC AUTOANTIBODIES IN SYSTEMIC SCLEROSIS	
AUTOANTIBODY (FREQUENCY IN SSc)	**SYSTEMIC SCLEROSIS SUBSET**	**CLINICAL ASSOCIATION**
Topoisomerase-I (10-40%)	Diffuse cutaneous (less commonly limited)	Tendon friction rubs, ILD, cardiac involvement, scleroderma renal crisis; isolated PAH rare
Centromere (15-40%)	Limited cutaneous	Digital ischemia, calcinosis cutis, isolated PAH, PBC; severe ILD and scleroderma renal crisis rare
RNA polymerase III (4-25%)	Diffuse cutaneous	Extensive skin involvement; tendon friction rubs, scleroderma renal crisis, increased cancer risk
U3-RNP/fibrillarin (1-5%)	Diffuse cutaneous	PAH, ILD, myositis
Th/To (1-7%)	Limited cutaneous	ILD, isolated PAH
PM/Scl (0-6%)	Limited cutaneous	Calcinosis, myositis, arthritis
U1-RNP (5-35%)	MCTD	Severe PAH, myositis

ILD = interstitial lung disease; MCTD = mixed connective tissue disease; PAH = pulmonary arterial hypertension, PBC = primary biliary cirrhosis.

is associated with esophageal inflammation, ulcerations, stricture formation, and Barrett metaplasia.

Pathologic changes in the heart are common in SSc, with involvement of the myocardium and pericardium. Characteristic microvascular lesions include concentric intimal hypertrophy and luminal narrowing. Contraction band necrosis reflecting ischemia-reperfusion injury in the myocardium is prominent and may be accompanied by patchy myocardial fibrosis. In the kidneys, noninflammatory lesions occur in the interlobular arteries. Scleroderma renal crisis (Chapter 125) is associated with striking changes in small renal arteries, with reduplication of elastic lamina, marked intimal proliferation, and concentric narrowing of the lumen giving rise to the onion-skin appearance, frequently accompanied by thrombosis and microangiopathic hemolysis.[5]

Pathophysiologic Triad: Vasculopathy, Immune Dysregulation, and Fibrosis
Vasculopathy
Vascular injury is an early and presumably primary event in pathogenesis of SSc. It effects primarily the small and medium-sized arteries and arterioles in multiple vascular beds and accounts for major clinical complications. The initial vascular endothelial injury might be caused by viruses and other infectious agents, oxygen radicals, circulating cytotoxic factors, complement activation, or autoantibodies. Endothelial cell injury and apoptosis result in altered production of endothelium-derived vasodilatory (nitric oxide and prostacyclin) and vasoconstricting (endothelin-1) molecules. Endothelial dysfunction causes increased vascular permeability associated with upregulation of adhesion molecules with transendothelial leukocyte diapedesis, as well as platelet aggregation, activation of intravascular coagulation, defective fibrinolysis, and thrombosis. Small blood vessels show intimal hyperplasia with thickening and reduplication of the basement membrane. In the vascular media, myointimal cells proliferate, whereas the adventitial layers develop fibrosis; the net result is progressive narrowing and obliteration of capillaries, arterioles, and even large vessels. Impaired blood flow results in widespread tissue ischemia, which is a potent stimulus for fibrogenesis. Recurrent ischemia-reperfusion is associated with the generation of reactive oxygen species that further damage the endothelium. Paradoxically, despite the presence of tissue hypoxia and sometimes dramatically elevated levels of angiogenic factors, compensatory vasculogenesis is impaired owing to reduced production, mobilization, or maturation of endothelial progenitor cells. The combination of widespread capillary loss, obliterative vasculopathy of small and medium-sized arteries, and failure to regenerate damaged blood vessels are hallmarks of SSc that underlie Raynaud phenomenon, ischemic digital ulcers, cutaneous telangiectasia, PAH, and other major vascular manifestations.

Raynaud Phenomenon
The earliest and most common vascular complication of SSc, Raynaud phenomenon, reflects abnormal thermal regulation of blood flow and can precede other disease manifestations by years.[6] Raynaud phenomenon in SSc is characterized by autonomic and peripheral nervous system changes leading to impaired production of calcitonin gene–related peptide from sensory afferent nerves and heightened sensitivity of α_2-adrenergic receptors on vascular smooth muscle cells. In contrast to primary Raynaud phenomenon, a common and relatively benign condition, Raynaud phenomenon in SSc is generally progressive and complicated by vascular remodeling with irreversible structural changes that result in tissue damage.

Inflammation and Autoimmunity
Cellular Immunity
Immune dysregulation is a hallmark SSc shares with other autoimmune diseases. In early SSc, activated T cells, B cells, and monocyte-macrophages accumulate in lesional tissues. Recent studies employing genomewide transcriptional profiling indicate that a subset of SSc patients demonstrate a strong inflammatory gene signature in their lesional skin, with evidence of activated innate and adaptive immune signaling and elevated expression of many inflammatory chemokines and cytokines.

Infiltrating $CD4^+$ T cells display restricted TcR receptor signatures indicative of their oligoclonal expansion in response to unknown antigens. Moreover, these T cells show T_H2 polarization with secretion of interleukin (IL)-4, IL-13, and IL-21, and low levels of interferon (IFN)-γ. T_H2 cytokines induce TGF-β and promote the synthesis of collagen and other extracellular matrix molecules. Increased levels of IL-17 detected in the serum suggest a role for T_H17 cells in SSc. The frequency of circulating regulatory T cells is elevated, but their immunosuppressive function appears to be defective. Myeloid dendritic cells show abnormally high secretion of inflammatory cytokines and chemokines such as CXCL.[7] Moreover, in response to thymic stromal lymphopoietin (TSLP), which is elevated in SSc, dendritic cells contribute to the persistence of the T_H2-polarized profibrotic immune response. Macrophages show evidence of alternative activation associated with pathologic fibrogenesis. In SSc, aberrant innate immune responses in dendritic cells and tissue fibroblasts might be triggered by damage-associated nucleic acids and matrix macromolecules. These responses are mediated through toll-like receptors (TLRs) and are likely to contribute to autoimmunity and progressive fibrosis.[8] The elevated expression of type I interferon-regulated genes (IFN signature) in SSc is consistent with innate immune activation and may contribute to vascular injury.

Autoantibodies and B Cells
Although circulating autoantibodies have well-established clinical utility in SSc as diagnostic and prognostic markers, their role in driving pathogenesis and tissue damage remains speculative. In addition to antinuclear antibodies (ANAs) that are detected in virtually all patients with SSc, a number of highly disease-specific and mutually exclusive autoantibodies occur (Table 267-3).

Most SSc-specific autoantibodies are directed against intracellular proteins, such as topoisomerase-I, centromere, and RNA polymerases I and III. Recent studies identified autoantibodies in SSc that are directed against endothelial cell or myenteric neuron epitopes, or recognize cell surface receptors (platelet-derived growth factor receptor [PDGFR], angiotensin II receptor, and muscarinic-3-acetylcholine receptor), and appear to directly contribute to vascular injury, intestinal wall atrophy and dysmotility, or tissue fibrosis. B cells are implicated in mediating both the autoimmune and fibrotic components of SSc. In addition to their role in antibody production, B cells also present antigen, produce IL-6 and other profibrotic cytokines, and modulate the function of T cells and dendritic cells. Gene expression profiling of SSc skin biopsies has identified messenger RNA expression signatures characteristic of B-cell activation.

Fibrosis

Fibrosis of the skin and multiple internal organs is the distinguishing feature of SSc. It characteristically follows, and is thought to be a consequence of, inflammation and vascular injury. Fibrosis is characterized by replacement of normal tissue architecture with a collagen-rich extracellular matrix that is secreted by resident fibroblasts and myofibroblasts.[9] Under physiologic conditions, these mesenchymal cells undergo controlled activation triggered by TGF-β, IL-6, PDGF, hypoxia, oxygen radicals, and other factors. Fibroblasts proliferate, migrate, synthesize and secrete collagens and extracellular matrix, and transdifferentiate into contractile myofibroblasts, enabling them to repair damaged tissue with full regeneration. When this tightly regulated wound healing program becomes sustained and amplified, excessive scar tissue formation ensues, leading to intractable fibrosis.

Effector Cells in Fibrosis

Myofibroblasts are mesenchymal cells with both smooth muscle cell–like contractile and biosynthetic properties. Myofibroblasts appear transiently in wounds, where they contribute to healing through production of collagen and TGF-β and contraction of the surrounding extracellular matrix. In SSc, activated myofibroblasts accumulate in lesional tissue and persist there because of one of three pathways: (1) in situ activation of quiescent resident fibroblasts, (2) through transdifferentiation from damaged epithelial cells, endothelial cells, or pericytes, or (3) by migration and terminal differentiation of bone marrow–derived mesenchymal progenitor cells.

CLINICAL MANIFESTATIONS

Overview

Multiple organs are affected in SSc, but the frequency, tempo, and severity of their involvement show substantial patient-to-patient variability. Patients with dcSSc characteristically develop extensive skin induration associated with early and progressive internal organ involvement. In contrast, patients with lcSSc commonly present with long-standing Raynaud phenomenon, skin changes limited to the distal extremities and face, and indolent progression of internal organ disease. However, patients with SSc frequently defy easy subclassification, or show an overlap of typical SSc features coexisting with clinical and laboratory evidence of another autoimmune disease such as polymyositis, Sjögren syndrome, polyarthritis, or SLE.

Initial Clinical Presentation
Diffuse Cutaneous Systemic Sclerosis

Patients with dcSSc typically present with soft tissue swelling, erythema, and pruritus, often accompanied by fatigue, stiffness, and malaise. Although

arthralgia, muscle weakness, and carpal tunnel syndrome are common, Raynaud phenomenon may not be present until later in the disease. In the ensuing weeks to months, the inflammatory edematous phase evolves into a chronic "fibrotic" phase with skin induration accompanied by hyperpigmentation, loss of body hair, and impaired sweating. The wrists, elbows, shoulders, knees, and ankles become stiff owing to fibrosis of the joint structures. Advancing skin changes are commonly accompanied by onset of internal organ involvement that is most rapidly progressive during the initial 4 years from disease onset. The risk for new organ involvement declines thereafter.

Limited Cutaneous Systemic Sclerosis

In lcSSc, the diagnosis is generally made at a more advanced stage of the disease. These patients give a history of long-standing Raynaud phenomenon, sometimes complicated by ischemic ulcerations at the fingertips. The course of disease is indolent, with delayed onset and slow progression of gastroesophageal reflux, telangiectasia, or cutaneous calcinosis. Vascular manifestations of lcSSc tend to be more pronounced compared with dcSSc, and digital ischemia, cutaneous telangiectasia, and progressive PAH are frequent late manifestations. In contrast, scleroderma renal crisis is uncommon in lcSSc.

Organ Involvement
Skin

Skin thickening, the distinguishing hallmark of SSc, typically starts in the fingers and advances in a centripetal pattern from distal to proximal extremities. The skin becomes hyperpigmented, but dark-skinned individuals may develop vitiligo-like hypopigmentation or "salt-and-pepper" changes, most prominently on the upper back and chest. Obliteration of eccrine sweat glands and sebaceous glands results in decreased sweating and oil secretion, causing dry and itchy skin. The face may assume a characteristic appearance with a beaklike nose, thinning and retraction of the lips, fine wrinkles (radial furrowing) around the mouth, and occasionally a masklike facies due to reduced mobility of the eyelids, cheeks, and mouth (Fig. 267-3). Decreased oral aperture (microstomia) interferes with eating and oral hygiene.

In patients with long-standing SSc, the skin is atrophic and tethered to the subcutaneous tissue. Telangiectasias are prominent on the face, hands, lips, and oral mucosa. They resemble the skin lesions of hereditary hemorrhagic telangiectasia and are due to dilatation of postcapillary venules in the upper dermis. Breakdown of atrophic skin leads to painful ulcerations at the extensor surfaces of the interphalangeal joints, fingertips, and bony prominences such as the elbows and malleoli. Ulcers may become secondarily infected, resulting in osteomyelitis. Ischemic fingertip ulcerations heal slowly and give rise to characteristic digital tip "pits." Ischemic soft tissue loss at the fingertips is associated with resorption of the terminal phalanges (acroosteolysis) (Fig. 267-4).

Calcium deposits composed of calcium hydroxyapatite crystals develop in the skin and soft tissues. These deposits, varying in size from tiny punctate lesions to large conglomerate masses, can be readily visualized on plain radiographs. Frequent locations include the finger pads, extensor surfaces of the forearms, and olecranon and prepatellar bursae. Calcific deposits can ulcerate through the overlying skin, producing drainage of chalky white material, pain, and local inflammation.

Raynaud Phenomenon

Raynaud phenomenon (Chapter 80) is an episodic vasoconstriction in the digits that occurs in virtually all patients with SSc.[8] Typical attacks start with

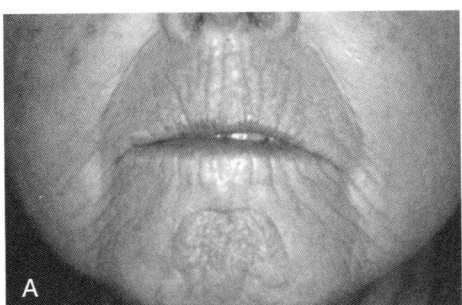
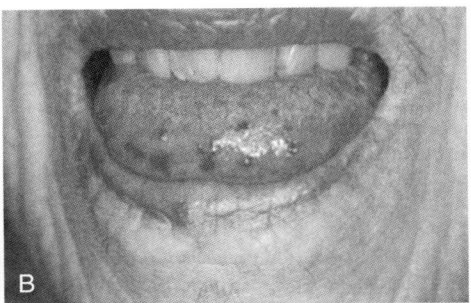

FIGURE 267-3. Facial features in systemic sclerosis. **A,** Perioral furrowing. Note vertical lines of furrowing around the mouth in a patient with diffuse cutaneous systemic sclerosis. **B,** Telangiectasia on the lips and tongue in a patient with long-standing limited cutaneous systemic sclerosis.

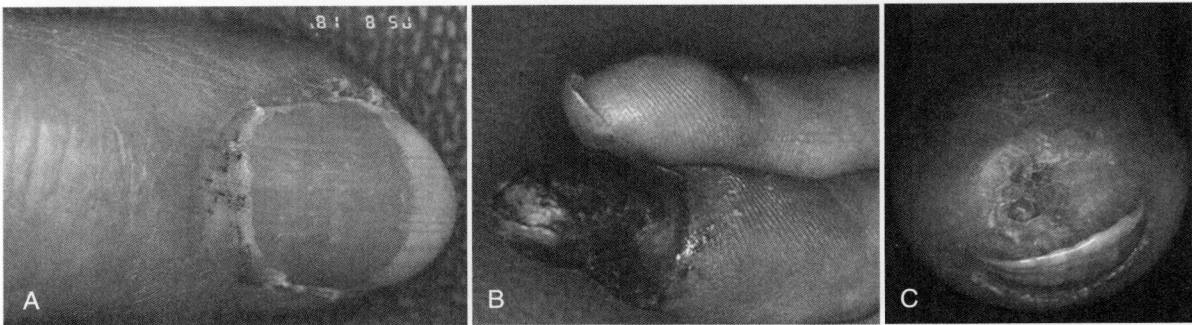

FIGURE 267-4. Vascular complications of systemic sclerosis in the fingers. **A,** Nailfold microvascular changes. **B,** Digital infarction. Sharply demarcated necrosis of the fingertip in a patient with limited cutaneous systemic sclerosis associated with severe Raynaud phenomenon. **C,** Digital tip ulceration and pitting.

pallor (vasoconstriction) followed by cyanosis (ischemia) and erythema (reperfusion), commonly triggered by exposure to cold or emotional stress. Primary Raynaud phenomenon, a benign condition representing an exaggerated physiologic response to cold, occurs in 3 to 5% of the population and is more frequent in women. Secondary Raynaud phenomenon occurs in SSc but also other connective tissue diseases, hematologic and endocrine conditions, and occupational disorders, and with the use of β-blockers and anticancer drugs such as cisplatin and bleomycin.

Distinguishing primary from secondary Raynaud phenomenon can present a challenge. Secondary Raynaud phenomenon typically develops at an older age (>30 years), tends to be more severe, and is frequently complicated by critical ischemia. Nailfold capillaroscopy allows cutaneous capillaries to be viewed under a drop of immersion oil using an ophthalmoscope. Patients with primary Raynaud phenomenon have normal nailfold capillaries that appear as regularly spaced parallel vascular loops, whereas in SSc, capillaries are distorted with widened and irregular loops, dilated lumen, and areas of vascular "dropout."

Gastrointestinal Involvement

GI tract involvement is very common in both lcSSc and dcSSc and may be the presenting manifestation of the disease. A pathologic picture of smooth muscle atrophy and obliterative small vessel vasculopathy with or without fibrosis is seen throughout the length of the GI tract, causing altered peristaltic activity and consequent complications. Severe intestinal involvement and malnutrition are associated with high mortality.

Upper Gastrointestinal Tract

Oropharyngeal manifestations of SSc include xerostomia, reduced oral aperture, periodontal disease, and resorption of the mandibular condyles. The frenulum of the tongue may be shortened. The most frequently affected GI organ is the esophagus. Gastroesophageal reflux is associated with heartburn, regurgitation, and dysphagia but can also be asymptomatic (Chapter 138). Reduced lower esophageal sphincter pressure resulting in gastroesophageal reflux frequently coexists with impaired esophageal clearance of refluxed gastric contents due to diminished motility in the distal two thirds of the esophagus. Delayed gastric emptying further aggravates the problem. On high-resolution computed tomography (HRCT) of the chest, the esophagus is dilated and shows intraluminal air. Endoscopy may show severe erosive esophagitis in patients with minimal reflux symptoms. Esophageal strictures and Barrett esophagus (Chapter 138) can complicate long-standing reflux. Because Barrett esophagus is associated with an increased risk for adenocarcinoma, SSc patients require periodic endoscopy with mucosal biopsy. Hoarseness and chronic cough may be extraesophageal manifestations of gastroesophageal reflux disease (GERD). Chronic microaspiration of gastric contents may aggravate underlying interstitial lung disease. A distinct pattern of interstitial lung disease called centrilobular fibrosis, associated with esophageal dilatation and chronic gastroesophageal reflux, is occasionally seen in SSc.

Stomach

Gastroparesis contributes to delayed gastric emptying with early satiety, abdominal distention, and aggravated reflux symptoms. Gastric vascular ectasia (GAVE) develops in 5% of patients and is equally prevalent in limited and diffuse cutaneous disease. On endoscopy, parallel longitudinal mucosal folds resembling the stripes of a watermelon are seen in the antrum. The

histologic features of dilated thrombosed mucosal capillaries and fibromuscular dysplasia of the lamina propria reflect the diffuse small vessel vasculopathy of SSc. Patients with GAVE may develop recurrent GI bleeding and typically present with unexplained iron deficiency anemia.

Lower Gastrointestinal Tract

Impaired small bowel motility in SSc can cause chronic diarrhea due to bacterial overgrowth. Fat and protein malabsorption, vitamin B_{12} and D deficiency, and malnutrition may ensue and are associated with high mortality. Malabsorption is diagnosed by hydrogen breath test or 14C-D-xylose test, and serum prealbumin (transthyretin) is useful to monitor malnutrition (Chapter 140). Disturbed intestinal motor function can also cause recurrent episodes of intestinal pseudo-obstruction with acute abdominal pain, nausea, and vomiting. Differentiating pseudo-obstruction, which responds to supportive care and intravenous nutritional supplementation, from mechanical bowel obstruction is a difficult diagnostic challenge. Colonic and anorectal involvement causing constipation, rectal prolapse, and fecal incontinence is frequent and is the source of much distress. In late-stage SSc, wide-mouth colonic sacculations can occur and cause perforation and bleeding. An occasional radiologic finding is pneumatosis cystoides intestinalis due to air trapping in the bowel wall. These lesions can rupture and cause pneumoperitoneum. The liver is rarely affected in SSc. However, primary biliary cirrhosis associated with antimitochondrial antibodies may occur.

Lung Involvement

The two major forms of lung involvement in SSc are interstitial lung disease and PAH, with many patients developing both. Less frequent pulmonary manifestations include aspiration pneumonitis complicating gastroesophageal reflux, pulmonary hemorrhage, obliterative bronchiolitis, pleural reactions, restrictive ventilatory disease due to chest wall fibrosis, spontaneous pneumothorax, and drug-induced lung toxicity. The incidence of lung cancer, particularly bronchoalveolar carcinoma (Chapter 191), is increased.

Interstitial Lung Disease

Interstitial lung disease (Chapter 92) in SSc can remain asymptomatic until quite advanced.[10] The most frequent presenting symptoms are exertional dyspnea, fatigue, and reduced exercise tolerance. A chronic dry cough may be present. Physical examination may reveal "Velcro" crackles at the lung bases. Pulmonary function testing (Chapter 85) is a sensitive method for detecting early interstitial lung disease. The most common abnormalities are reductions in forced vital capacity (FVC) or single breath diffusing capacity (D_{LCO}). However, a reduction in D_{LCO} that is significantly out of proportion to the reduction in FVC (FVC/D_{LCO} ratio > 1.6) suggests pulmonary vascular disease.

Evidence of interstitial lung disease can be found in almost all patients with SSc and is clinically significant in up to 50%. Risk factors include male sex, African American race, diffuse skin involvement, severe gastroesophageal reflux, and the presence of topoisomerase-I autoantibodies. The most rapid progression in interstitial lung disease occurs within the first 3 years of the disease.

Chest radiography is useful for ruling out infection and other causes of pulmonary involvement but is relatively insensitive for detection of early interstitial lung disease. In contrast, HRCT is highly sensitive (Chapter 84). Prominent HRCT findings include reticular linear interstitial opacities, predominantly in the lower lobe periphery, occurring in isolation or in combination with ground-glass opacification. Additional findings include mediastinal lymphadenopathy and, rarely, honeycombing. The extent of lung disease on initial HRCT correlates with progression and prognosis of interstitial lung disease and may provide useful information regarding the need for initiating therapy. Bronchoalveolar lavage (Chapter 85) may be indicated for ruling out occult infection. Lung biopsy is rarely useful.

Pulmonary Arterial Hypertension
Approximately 15% of SSc patients develop PAH, defined as a mean pulmonary arterial pressure of 25 mm Hg or greater, with a pulmonary capillary wedge pressure of 15 mm Hg or less (Chapter 68). In the setting of SSc, PAH can occur as an isolated abnormality (World Health Organization [WHO] group I), or coexist with interstitial lung disease (WHO group III). Although the natural history of SSc-associated PAH is variable, patients generally follow a progressive downhill course, with development of right heart failure and increased mortality. Risk factors for SSc-associated PAH include limited cutaneous disease, older age of disease onset, severe Raynaud phenomenon, large number of cutaneous telangiectasias, and anticentromere, U1-RNP, U3-RNP (fibrillarin), Th/To, B23, and β_2-glycoprotein I autoantibodies.

The initial symptoms of PAH are exertional dyspnea and reduced exercise capacity, but early-stage disease is often clinically silent. With progression, angina, syncope, and symptoms and signs of right-sided heart failure develop. Physical examination shows tachypnea, a prominent pulmonic S_2 heart sound, palpable right ventricular heave, elevated jugular venous pressure, and dependent edema. Pulmonary arterial systolic pressures above 40 mm Hg (determined by Doppler echocardiography) suggest PAH, as does an isolated low DLCO or a FVC/DLCO ratio over 1.6. Right heart catheterization is required for confirming the diagnosis of PAH, assessing its severity, and evaluating ventricular function. The serum levels of N-terminal brain natriuretic peptide (NT-pro-BNP) are elevated in PAH and correlate with severity and survival.

Kidney Involvement
Scleroderma renal crisis is an uncommon but life-threatening acute complication of SSc, but chronic and indolent kidney disease also occurs.

Scleroderma Renal Crisis
Scleroderma renal crisis, the most dreaded complication of SSc, develops in 10 to 15% of patients, almost always within 4 years of disease onset.[11] Prior to the advent of angiotensin-converting enzyme (ACE)-inhibiting drugs in the 1980s, scleroderma renal crisis was invariably fatal, often within weeks. The pathogenesis involves obliterative vasculopathy and luminal narrowing of the renal arcuate arteries. Progressive reduction in renal blood flow, aggravated by vasospasm, leads to juxtaglomerular hyperplasia and increased renin secretion, with further renal vasoconstriction resulting in a vicious cycle that culminates in malignant hypertension (Chapters 67 and 125).

Scleroderma renal crisis is a medical emergency. Although most patients present with abrupt onset of hypertension and progressive renal insufficiency, in some cases the blood pressure remains normal or only modestly elevated. Normotensive renal crisis is associated with a poor outcome. Hypertensive encephalopathy and retinopathy, pericarditis, and arrhythmias may complicate scleroderma renal crisis. Urinalysis shows mild proteinuria, granular casts, and microscopic hematuria. When thrombocytopenia and microangiopathic hemolysis with fragmented red blood cells are detected, the diagnosis of thrombotic thrombocytopenic purpura (Chapter 172) is sometimes entertained. In many patients, oliguric renal failure develops over a period of weeks. Kidney biopsy can be useful for diagnosis and prognosis, but the characteristic lesions of intimal and medial proliferation and luminal narrowing are indistinguishable from the changes of accelerated hypertension.

Risk factors for scleroderma renal crisis include early-stage disease, rapidly progressive skin involvement and the presence of tendon friction rubs, African American race, male sex, and autoantibodies to RNA polymerases I and III. In contrast, the presence of anticentromere antibodies is associated with a low risk for scleroderma renal crisis. Pericardial effusion, new-onset anemia, and thrombocytopenia may be harbingers of impending scleroderma renal crisis, and a history of recent corticosteroid use is associated with a more than 10-fold increased risk. Accordingly, SSc patients with early and progressive cutaneous disease should be counseled to determine their blood pressure daily. In these patients, corticosteroids should be used only when absolutely required, and at low doses.

Once scleroderma renal crisis sets in, hospitalization and prompt initiation of short-acting ACE inhibitors is essential. The goal is adequate blood pressure control before the onset of renal failure. Despite appropriate timely intervention, more than half of patients with scleroderma renal crisis require hemodialysis, although some of these ultimately recover sufficient renal function to be able to discontinue hemodialysis. Oliguria or a serum creatinine level higher than 3 mg/dL at presentation predict poor outcome. The "prophylactic" use of ACE inhibitors to prevent scleroderma renal crisis is associated with a worse outcome and is not recommended.

Chronic Kidney Disease
Kidney biopsies in patients with SSc commonly show chronic changes including reduplication of elastic fibers, sclerosed glomeruli, tubular atrophy, and interstitial fibrosis. In one study, abnormal renal function or proteinuria was detected in more than one third of patients, none of whom progressed to end-stage renal disease. Rarely, glomerulonephritis associated with lupus serologies or antineutrophil cytoplasmic antibody–positive renal vasculitis occurs.

Cardiac Involvement
Cardiac involvement is frequently detected using sensitive diagnostic tools but is commonly clinically silent. Clinical cardiac involvement is more frequently seen in patients with dcSSc; it generally develops early in the course of the disease and is a poor prognostic factor. The endocardium, myocardium, and pericardium may be affected separately or together. Clinical manifestations include tachyarrhythmias, conduction abnormalities, valvular regurgitation, diastolic heart failure, and pericardial effusion. Systemic and pulmonary arterial hypertension, as well as lung and renal involvement, also affect the heart. Conventional echocardiography has a low sensitivity for detecting SSc heart involvement. Tissue Doppler echocardiography, single-photon emission computed tomography, and especially cardiac magnetic resonance imaging (cMRI) reveal a high prevalence of myocardial abnormalities such as abnormal ventricular relaxation and reversible perfusion defects. An elevated level of serum NT-pro-BNP is a sensitive marker for increased pulmonary artery pressure but may also indicate primary cardiac involvement. Myocarditis can develop in association with muscle inflammation. Pericardial effusion develops in more than 15% of SSc patients but is rarely significant.

Musculoskeletal Complications
Carpal tunnel syndrome (Chapter 420) occurs frequently and may be a presenting manifestation of SSc. Joint mobility is progressively impaired, especially in the hands. Large joint contractures can be accompanied by audible or palpable tendon friction rubs that are caused by extensive fibrosis and adhesion of the tendon sheaths and fascial planes at the affected joint. The presence of tendon friction rubs often signals aggressive disease. Frank joint inflammation is uncommon in SSc; however, erosive polyarthritis in the hands can occur. Muscle weakness may be a sign of deconditioning, disuse atrophy, and malnutrition. Less commonly, inflammatory myositis indistinguishable from idiopathic polymyositis (Chapter 269) occurs in early disease. A noninflammatory myopathy characterized by atrophy and fibrosis in the absence of elevated muscle enzyme levels may occur in late disease. Bone resorption affects the distal tufts of terminal phalanges (acro-osteolysis), mandibular condyles, ribs, and distal clavicles.

Other Clinical Manifestations
In addition to microangiopathy, involvement of larger blood vessels (>100 μm) is common in SSc. Manifestations of macrovascular disease include occlusion of the digital and ulnar arteries, leading to ischemic ulcerations and even loss of digits or limbs. Epidemiologic studies indicate increased risk of coronary artery disease in patients with SSc. Dry eyes and dry mouth are common in SSc, but in contrast to Sjögren syndrome (Chapter 268), salivary gland biopsy in such cases shows fibrosis rather than focal lymphocytic infiltration. Hypothyroidism due to thyroid fibrosis is common and may be associated with antithyroid autoantibodies. Although the brain and central nervous system are generally spared in SSc, autonomic neuropathy, as well as a primarily sensory neuropathy of the trigeminal nerve due to fibrosis or vasculopathy, can occur. Pregnancy in women with active SSc is associated with an increased rate of adverse fetal outcomes. Furthermore, cardiopulmonary involvement might worsen during pregnancy, and scleroderma renal crisis can occur. Inability to attain or maintain penile erection is due to vascular insufficiency and fibrosis; the problem is frequent and may be the presenting disease manifestation in males with SSc.

Systemic Sclerosis and Cancer

Patients with SSc have an increased risk of cancer. In these patients, lung cancer and esophageal adenocarcinoma typically occur in the setting of long-standing interstitial lung disease or GERD, and chronic inflammation and tissue repair may be contributing factors. In contrast, breast, lung, and ovarian carcinoma and lymphoma in SSc tend to occur in close temporal association with the clinical onset of SSc and are often associated with anti-RNA polymerase III antibodies. In these cases, SSc might be a paraneoplastic syndrome that is triggered by the antitumor immune response.

DIAGNOSIS

Skin induration in the fingers or proximally (associated with Raynaud phenomenon) and characteristic visceral organ manifestations are sufficient to establish the diagnosis of SSc. Occasionally, diagnostic full-thickness skin biopsy may be required for ruling out scleroderma mimics such as scleredema, scleromyxedema, or nephrogenic systemic fibrosis (see Table 267-1). Primary Raynaud phenomenon is differentiated from SSc by normal-appearing nailfold capillaries and absence of autoantibodies. Diagnosing SSc can be difficult in the early stages of the disease because initial symptoms and findings are often nonspecific and can be mistaken for rheumatoid arthritis, SLE, myositis, or undifferentiated connective tissue disease. Rarely, patients with SSc first present with accelerated hypertension or GI bleeding caused by watermelon stomach as the initial manifestation.

Laboratory Features

Anemia is common and may reflect chronic inflammation, GI bleeding from gastric vascular ectasia, erosive gastritis or chronic esophagitis, or folate and vitamin B_{12} deficiency due to small bowel bacterial overgrowth and malabsorption. Microangiopathic hemolytic anemia (Chapter 160) caused by mechanical trauma and red blood cell fragmentation is a hallmark of scleroderma renal crisis. In contrast to other connective tissue diseases, the erythrocyte sedimentation rate and C-reactive protein generally show only modest elevation. Monitoring serum levels of prealbumin and vitamin K is useful in patients with small bowel bacterial overgrowth and malabsorption.

Antinuclear autoantibodies (ANAs) are present in virtually all patients with SSc and can be detected at, or even prior to, disease onset. Autoantibodies specific for SSc are described in Table 267-3. Anticentromere antibodies are associated with PAH, but cardiac involvement, significant pulmonary fibrosis, or scleroderma renal crisis occurs only rarely in these patients. Topoisomerase-I antibody positivity is associated with reduced survival, whereas anticentromere antibody–positive patients have improved survival compared with those without this antibody. Antibodies to RNA polymerase III (recognized based on its speckled immunofluorescence pattern) are associated with increased risk for scleroderma renal crisis. Antibodies to β_2-glycoprotein I are not specific but in SSc identify increased risk for critical ischemia.

TREATMENT AND PREVENTION   Rx

With the exception of ACE inhibitors for scleroderma renal crisis, no therapy to date has been shown to significantly alter the natural history of SSc. In contrast, organ-based treatments are effective in alleviating symptoms and slowing progression of the cumulative organ damage. A significant reduction in disease-related mortality has occurred during the past 25 years. Treatment must be tailored to each patient's unique needs. Because of the marked heterogeneity in clinical presentation, a thorough and individualized baseline evaluation is paramount. Optimal management incorporates the following principles: prompt diagnosis, accurate classification and risk stratification, early recognition and assessment of organ-based complications, and monitoring progression, disease activity, and response to therapy. Management of complications should be proactive, with regular screening and initiation of appropriate intervention at the earliest possible opportunity. Given the multisystemic nature of SSc, an integrated team-based management approach, typically at specialized medical centers, is desirable. The team should incorporate appropriate medical specialists. Patients are empowered by learning about potential complications, therapeutic options, and the natural history of their disease.

Disease-Modifying Therapy
Immunosuppressive Agents

Immunosuppressive agents that are highly effective in the treatment of other connective tissue diseases have generally shown modest or no benefit in SSc.[12] Corticosteroids may alleviate stiffness and aching in early-stage dcSSc

but do not slow the progression of skin or internal organ involvement and are associated with an increased risk for scleroderma renal crisis. Therefore, corticosteroids should be avoided if possible; when absolutely necessary, they should be given at the lowest dose possible and for brief periods only.

Cyclophosphamide was shown to reduce the progression of symptomatic interstitial lung disease in early SSc.[A1][A2] Compared with placebo, patients treated with oral cyclophosphamide showed stabilization and, rarely, modest improvement in respiratory symptoms, pulmonary function, and abnormalities on chest HRCT after 1 year of treatment, but these benefits were short-lived. The use of cyclophosphamide in SSc needs to be balanced against its potential for side effects, including bone marrow suppression, opportunistic infections, hemorrhagic cystitis, bladder cancer, and premature ovarian failure.

In small clinical trials, methotrexate was associated with a modest improvement in skin involvement. Mycophenolate mofetil treatment was shown to improve skin involvement and stabilize lung disease. There is some support in the literature for the use of immunomodulatory agents and interventions including rituximab, intravenous immunoglobulin, and extracorporeal photopheresis for the treatment of SSc. Recent reports suggest that rituximab might be effective in ameliorating skin and lung involvement. In patients with severe SSc who fail to respond to other treatments (Chapter 178), autologous hematopoietic stem cell transplantation (HSCT) improves long term, event-free survival despite an increased treatment-related mortality in the first year.[A3] Because of this potential morbidity and mortality and its substantial cost, HSCT is presently considered an investigational therapy for SSc.

Antifibrotic Therapy

Because tissue fibrosis causes progressive and irreversible organ damage, drugs that block or slow the fibrotic process represent a rational approach to therapy. D-Penicillamine has been extensively used as an antifibrotic agent. In retrospective studies, D-penicillamine stabilized and improved skin induration, prevented new internal organ involvement, and improved survival. However, in a randomized controlled clinical trial, there was no difference in the extent of skin involvement between patients treated with standard-dose (750 mg/day) or very low-dose (125 mg every other day) D-penicillamine. Minocycline, bosentan, recombinant relaxin, interferon-γ, and inhibitors of tumor necrosis factor are putative antifibrotic agents that have failed to show meaningful benefit in SSc clinical trials. Small-molecule inhibitors of protein tyrosine kinases used in malignancies (e.g., imatinib, nilotinib, and dasatinib) block signaling by TGF-β and PDGF and thereby prevent fibrotic responses in vitro and in vivo. These agents are currently in clinical trials for SSc.

Treatment of Organ-Specific Complications
Gastrointestinal Complications

Because significant gastroesophageal reflux may occur in the absence of symptoms, all patients with SSc should be treated for this complication. Proton pump inhibitors may need to be given in relatively high doses and for prolonged periods, and patients should be instructed to elevate the head of the bed and eat frequent small meals. Recurrent GI bleeding due to GAVE can be treated with laser or argon plasma photocoagulation. Bacterial overgrowth due to small bowel hypomotility causes bloating and diarrhea and may lead to malabsorption, weight loss, and malnutrition. Treatment with short courses of rotating broad-spectrum antibiotics such as metronidazole, erythromycin, and tetracycline can eradicate bacterial overgrowth, but many patients relapse when antibiotics are stopped. In patients with malnutrition but intact small bowel function, enteral nutrition via a jejunostomy can be effective. In others, total parenteral nutrition may be indicated. Refractory hypomotility of the small bowel may respond to subcutaneous octreotide injections. Anorectal complications may respond to sacral neuromodulation.

Vascular Therapy and Raynaud Phenomenon

The goal of therapy is to reduce the frequency and duration of vasospastic episodes, prevent ischemic complications and enhance their healing, and slow the progression of obliterative vasculopathy. Patients should dress warmly, minimize cold exposure, and avoid drugs that could precipitate or exacerbate vasospastic episodes. Calcium-channel blockers such as nifedipine and diltiazem are used commonly for Raynaud's phenomenon but show only moderate benefit, and their use is often limited by side effects (palpitations, dependent edema, light-headedness). ACE inhibitors do not reduce the frequency or severity of episodes, but angiotensin II receptor blockers such as losartan are effective and generally well tolerated. Patients with severe Raynaud phenomenon require α_1-adrenergic receptor blockers (e.g., prazosin), 5-phosphodiesterase inhibitors (e.g., sildenafil), topical nitroglycerine, or intravenous prostaglandins. Low-dose aspirin and dipyridamole prevent platelet aggregation and may have a role as adjunctive agents but must be used with caution in light of the risk of bleeding from GAVE lesions. The endothelin-1 receptor antagonist bosentan reduces development of new ischemic ulcers. Intravenous prostacyclin infusion, local injections of botulinum toxin, and digital sympathectomy are options for some patients with critical digital ischemia. Patients with ischemic digital ulcerations may require surgical débridement, especially if necrotic tissue is present. Empirical long-term therapy with statins and antioxidants may slow the progression of vascular damage.

Pulmonary Arterial Hypertension

All patients with SSc should be screened for PAH at initial evaluation, and those at high risk on a yearly basis. Treatment for symptomatic PAH should be started with an endothelin-1 receptor antagonist or a 5-phosphodiesterase inhibitor. Diuretics, oral anticoagulation, and digoxin may be used when appropriate. If hypoxemia is documented, supplemental oxygen should be given. If clinical response is inadequate, 5-phosphodiesterase inhibitors may be used in combination with endothelin-1 receptor antagonists. Prostacyclin analogues can be administered intravenously, by continuous subcutaneous infusion, or by frequent inhalations. Lung transplantation remains an option for selected patients with SSc-associated PAH who fail medical therapy.

Treatment and Prevention of Scleroderma Renal Crisis

Prompt recognition of impending or early scleroderma renal crisis is essential. Because patients with early-stage SSc and progressive skin involvement are at highest risk, they should monitor their blood pressure daily and report significant alterations immediately. Corticosteroids should be used only when absolutely necessary and at the lowest possible doses. When scleroderma renal crisis occurs, patients should be hospitalized and treatment with short-acting ACE inhibitors started immediately to achieve prompt blood pressure normalization. There is no evidence that "prophylactic" use of ACE inhibitors can prevent the development of scleroderma renal crisis or ameliorate its severity. Although up to two thirds of patients who develop renal crisis require dialysis, delayed recovery of renal function can occur. Kidney transplantation is appropriate for patients unable to discontinue dialysis after 2 years. Survival with renal transplantation in SSc is comparable to that in other connective tissue diseases, and recurrence of scleroderma renal crisis is rare.

Skin Care

Skin involvement in early SSc is inflammatory and can be controlled with systemic antihistamines or short-term low-dose corticosteroids. Because of the increased risk for scleroderma renal crisis, blood pressure should be carefully monitored. Cyclophosphamide, methotrexate, D-penicillamine, and mycophenolate have been associated with modest improvement in skin induration in early-stage SSc. Skin dryness can be managed with the use of hydrophilic ointments and emollient bath oils. Fingertip ulcerations should be protected by occlusive dressing to promote healing and prevent infection. Infected skin ulcers are treated with topical or oral antibiotics and may necessitate surgical débridement. No medical therapy has been shown to be effective in preventing soft tissue calcification or in promoting its dissolution, and surgical therapy is only occasionally effective.

PROGNOSIS AND NATURAL HISTORY

Patients with dcSSc have a more rapidly progressive course, greater internal organ involvement, and worse prognosis compared to those with lcSSc. However, the outcome of the disease is difficult to predict.

Early inflammatory symptoms of dcSSc such as fatigue, edema, arthralgia, and pruritus commonly subside after 2 to 4 years, and skin thickening reaches a plateau followed by slow regression, which characteristically occurs in an order that is the reverse of initial involvement, with softening on the trunk followed by proximal and finally the distal extremities. Sclerodactyly and finger contractures generally persist. Relapse or recurrence of skin thickening is rare. Visceral organ involvement develops and progresses most rapidly during the initial 2 to 4 years of the disease. New organ involvement rarely occurs once the skin involvement has plateaued. Similarly, scleroderma renal crisis almost invariably occurs within the first 4 years of disease. In patients with lcSSc, Raynaud phenomenon may precede other disease manifestations by years or even decades, and visceral organ complications such as PAH and primary biliary cirrhosis generally occur late in the course of the disease.

Age- and gender-adjusted mortality rates in patients with SSc are more than five-fold higher than in the general population. The 10-year survival rate is 55% for patients with dcSSc and 75% for patients with lcSSc. Survival correlates with the extent of skin involvement, which represents a surrogate for visceral organ involvement. The leading causes of death are pulmonary fibrosis, PAH, severe GI involvement, and cardiac disease. Markers of poor prognosis include male sex, African American race, older age of disease onset, low body mass index, extensive skin thickening with truncal involvement, and evidence of significant or progressive visceral organ involvement. Autoantibodies to topoisomerase-I or absence of anticentromere antibodies are markers of poor prognosis. In one study, SSc patients who had extensive skin involvement, vital capacity less than 55% of predicted, significant GI involvement, and clinically evident cardiac involvement or scleroderma renal crisis

had a less than 40% 10-year survival. The severity of PAH is correlated with mortality, and SSc patients with a mean pulmonary arterial pressure of 45 mm Hg or higher had a 33% 3-year survival rate. In scleroderma renal crisis, therapy with ACE inhibitors has had a dramatic effect on survival, increasing from less than 10% at 1 year in the pre-ACE inhibitor era to better than 70% 3-year survival at the present time.

NEPHROGENIC SYSTEMIC FIBROSIS

Nephrogenic systemic fibrosis (NSF) is a novel complication of renal insufficiency with certain clinical features resembling SSc.[13] The condition was initially described in 2000 and is now recognized as an emerging problem in patients with chronic renal failure. It is estimated that 2% of patients on long-term hemodialysis might develop NSF. Originally considered a purely dermatologic scleromyxedema-like condition and termed *nephrogenic fibrosing dermatopathy*, NSF is now recognized to be associated with visceral organ involvement and is therefore more accurately termed *nephrogenic systemic fibrosis*. The cutaneous manifestations of NSF share histopathologic and clinical features with other scleroderma-spectrum disorders, notably fasciitis and scleromyxedema. In most patients with NSF, the condition develops while undergoing long-term dialysis. However, no association with a particular route or type of renal replacement therapy has been demonstrated. Furthermore, NSF has also been described in patients who have never received dialysis. Histologic hallmarks include cutaneous fibrosis with mucin deposition and accumulation of spindle-shaped cells, including numerous CD34-positive cells, in the lesional skin.

The clinical hallmark of NSF is thickening and "woody" tightness of skin over the lower and, less commonly, upper extremities and contractures at large joints. A link between NSF and exposure to gadolinium-containing MRI contrast agents was suggested in 2006, leading to a warning by the U.S. Food and Drug Administration regarding the use of these agents in patients with renal insufficiency. This was followed by a substantial decline in the incidence of NSF. The course of NSF is generally progressive, and the prognosis is poor. Some patients show improvement with adjustment to renal replacement therapy, and others respond to renal transplantation. Anecdotal reports describe treatment with phototherapy, imatinib mesylate, and immunosuppressive agents. However, in most patients with NSF, the induration is resistant to therapy and leads to progressive induration, joint contractures, and reduced mobility.

The topic of immunoglobulin (Ig)G4-related disease is discussed in Chapter 275.

Grade A References

A1. Tashkin DP, Celli B, Senn S, et al. Cyclophosphamide versus placebo in scleroderma lung disease. *N Engl J Med.* 2006;354:2655-2666.

A2. Hoyles RK, Ellis RW, Wellsbury J, et al. A multicenter, prospective, randomized, double-blind, placebo-controlled trial of corticosteroids and intravenous cyclophosphamide followed by oral azathioprine for the treatment of pulmonary fibrosis in scleroderma. *Arthritis Rheum.* 2006;54:3962-3970.

A3. van Laar JM, Farge D, Sont JK, et al. Autologous hematopoietic stem cell transplantation vs intravenous pulse cyclophosphamide in diffuse cutaneous systemic sclerosis: a randomized clinical trial. *JAMA.* 2014;311:2490-2498.

GENERAL REFERENCES

For the General References and other additional features, please visit Expert Consult at https://expertconsult.inkling.com.

268

SJÖGREN SYNDROME

XAVIER MARIETTE

DEFINITION

Sjögren syndrome (SS) is a systemic autoimmune disease characterized by lymphocytic infiltrates of salivary and tear glands, leading to oral and ocular dryness, and by autoantibody secretion. It can be encountered either alone (primary Sjögren syndrome [pSS]) or in the presence of other systemic autoimmune diseases (secondary Sjögren syndrome [sSS]) like rheumatoid arthritis (RA), systemic lupus erythematosus (SLE), inflammatory myositis, and systemic sclerosis. SS in the setting of RA usually follows RA diagnosis by many years and is mainly manifested by keratoconjunctivitis sicca, with systemic features being rather uncommon. Associated with other systemic autoimmune disease, the presentation of sSS is very close to pSS. Of note, pSS may be also associated with organ-specific systemic autoimmune disease, such as autoimmune thyroiditis and primary biliary cirrhosis.

EPIDEMIOLOGY

Primary SS is a common disease that affects 0.1 to 0.6% of the general adult female population.[1] A higher prevalence of the disease has been reported (0.5 to 2%), but this must be considered with caution because the reported prevalence of SS depends on the classification criteria used in the various studies, and the prevalence of sicca symptoms in the general population is high. Conversely, in recent studies with strict criteria, a lower prevalence has been found: 1.02 per 10,000 adults.[2] Primary SS has a female preponderance (female-to-male ratio at least 9 : 1). The age peak of the disease occurs after menopause in the mid-50s.

PATHOPHYSIOLOGY

Recent years have witnessed major advances in the pathophysiologic mechanisms of the disease. Several studies have confirmed the role of innate immunity, genetics, and B-cell activation and the relation between abnormalities in them.

The presence of an interferon (IFN) signature has been shown both in salivary glands and blood.[3] Plasmacytoid dendritic cells, the professional cells secreting type 1 IFN, are present within the glands. Type 2 IFN-dependent genes can be overexpressed in salivary glands. Natural killer (NK) cells, another actor of innate immunity able to secrete type 2 IFN are present in salivary glands of patients and play a role in the disease.[4]

In line with this IFN signature, multiple viral agents have been incriminated as etiologic factors for either the development or the modulation of SS; these include Epstein-Barr virus, retroviruses, and coxsackieviruses, but in all cases the data remain controversial.[5]

The genetics of pSS is now better understood with the reports of two genome-wide association studies (GWAS).[6] Like in other systemic autoimmune diseases, HLA is the most important region associated with the disease, and especially HLA-DR3-DQ1 in patients with autoantibodies. Interestingly, other genes associated with the disease are involved in the IFN response. These include IFN regulatory factor 5 (IRF-5), a pivotal transcription factor in the type 1 IFN pathway, and signal transducer and activator of transcription 4 (STAT-4), and IL-12A, involved in the type 2 IFN pathway. Other genes found to be associated with the disease are TNIP1, playing a role in control of nuclear factor (NF)-κB activation, and CXCR5, involved in germinal center formation.

The presence of ectopic salivary gland germinal centers demonstrates the importance of B-cell activation in pSS. Different cytokines may explain this B-cell activation. Several studies have focused on the role of BAFF (B-cell activating factor of the tumor necrosis factor [TNF] family), a cytokine that promotes B-cell maturation, proliferation, and survival. It has been shown that BAFF is enhanced in sera and in salivary glands from pSS patients. Interestingly, BAFF can be secreted by salivary gland epithelial cells, the target of autoimmunity, after stimulation by the innate immune system (type 1 or type 2 IFN, or viral infections). Thus, this cytokine is likely to be a link between innate immunity and autoimmunity.

The current hypothetical scenario for the development of pSS is based on the successive activation of innate and adaptive immune systems (Fig. 268-1). Environmental factors such as viral infections or hormonal imbalance may act at the initial stage of the disease by activating epithelial cells. This epithelial cell activation is promoted in patients who carry susceptibility factors in the genes for IFN pathway proteins. These patients experience a greater degree of IFN pathway activation, which leads to BAFF overproduction,

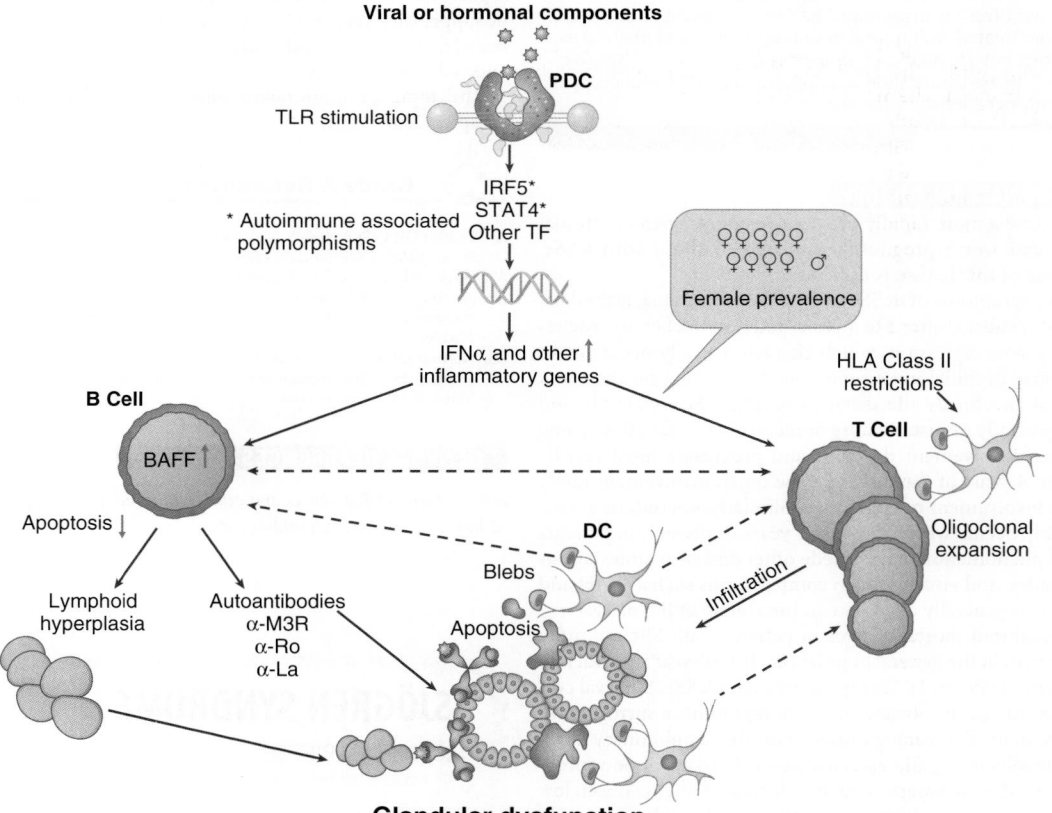

FIGURE 268-1. Hypothetical scenario for development of primary Sjögren syndrome. An environmental factor (e.g., virus) causes epithelial cell and dendritic cell (DC) activation. Plasmacytoid DCs are also activated by immune complexes, promoting interferon (IFN) pathway activation, which leads to BAFF overproduction and to B- and T-cell activation. B-cell activation leads to autoantibody production within germinal center–like structures. Interleukin-12 secreted by myeloid DCs leads to natural killer cell and T-helper 1 activation, which promotes tissue damage and IFN-γ production. IFN-α and IFN-γ enhance BAFF secretion. Epithelial cells release autoantigens that participate in immune complex formation and perpetuate the vicious cycle of immune system overactivation. BAFF = B-cell activating factor of the tumor necrosis factor family; IRF5 = interferon regulatory factor 5; PDC = plasmacytoid dendritic cell; STAT4 = signal transducer and activator of transcription 4; TF = transcription factors; TLR = toll-like receptors.

B- and T-cell activation, and secretion of autoantibodies, especially in predisposed patients. These autoantibodies constitute immune complexes that participate in the maintenance of IFN-α production. Altogether, these steps promote a vicious cycle of immune system activation leading to tissue damage.

CLINICAL MANIFESTATIONS

Glandular

Decreased salivary secretion results in mouth dryness and increased incidence of oral infections, mucosal friability, and dental caries due to loss of the lubricating, buffering, and antimicrobial capacities of saliva.[7] Fungal infections (primarily candidiasis) are also common. Parotid salivary gland or other major salivary gland enlargement can also occur. Persistent enlargement should be carefully followed, however, to exclude bacterial superinfection and, more importantly, the development of lymphoma.

Decreased lacrimal flow and impaired lacrimal composition lead to damage of the corneal and conjunctival epithelia, a condition known as keratoconjunctivitis sicca. As a result of keratoconjunctivitis sicca, SS patients might experience foreign-body sensation, grittiness, irritation, photosensitivity, and thick rope-like secretions at the inner canthus, all leading to increased discomfort and possibly visual impairment, with considerable functional disability. Furthermore, ocular complications include corneal ulceration and scarring, bacterial keratitis, and eyelid infections that require continuous ophthalmologic care and treatment.

Systemic

In addition to the sicca features, systemic manifestations occur in approximately 20 to 30% of pSS patients. Of note, it has been increasingly appreciated that the extraglandular manifestations in SS can be divided into two major types according to the underlying pathophysiologic mechanism. Thus, lymphocytic infiltration of the epithelia of organs beyond the exocrine glands (e.g., renal, liver, and bronchial epithelial cells) results in interstitial nephritis, autoimmune cholangitis, and obstructive bronchiolitis, respectively. These clinical features seem to appear early and usually have a benign course. On the other hand, immune complex deposition as a result of the ongoing B-cell hyperreactivity can give rise to the extraepithelial manifestations—palpable purpura, glomerulonephritis, interstitial pneumonitis, and peripheral neuropathy—that are linked to increased morbidity and risk for lymphoma development. The main systemic manifestations are listed in Table 268-1. Peripheral neuropathy may occur through various mechanisms. Vasculitis may be present with cryoglobulinemia, leading to both sensory and motor symptoms. More frequently, pure sensory neuropathy is present, sometimes purely ataxic and sometimes in the form of small-fiber neuropathy. This latter entity is difficult to diagnose because clinical and electromyographic examinations are normal. The diagnosis may be made by skin biopsy showing rarefaction of sensory small fibers.

Sjögren Syndrome and Non-Hodgkin Lymphomas

Chronic polyclonal B-cell activation is commonly present in pSS, which may explain why this autoimmune disease has the strongest association with the development of B-cell lymphoma (relative risk, 15 to 20). More recent studies have estimated this risk at a lower level: 6 in Denmark and Sweden, 7 in Taiwan, and 9 in Norway.

Lymphomas complicating pSS have specific features (Chapter 185). They are mostly B-cell non-Hodgkin lymphomas with a predominance of low-grade, marginal-zone histologic type. Mucosal localization is predominant, notably as mucosa-associated lymphoid tissue (MALT) lymphomas. Interestingly, lymphomas often develop in organs where pSS is active, such as salivary glands.

In the setting of SS, chronic autoimmune B-cell activation plays the major role in the lymphomagenesis process, and the identified predictors of lymphoma development in pSS are in line with this phenomenon. The main clinical predictors are permanent swelling of salivary glands, splenomegaly, lymphadenopathy, and palpable purpura. The main biological predictors are positivity of rheumatoid factor (RF), cryoglobulinemia, lymphopenia (especially CD4 lymphopenia), low complement levels, and a monoclonal component in serum or urine. Three novel predictive factors for lymphoma development have been recently described: (1) the presence of ectopic germinal centers associated with the occurrence of lymphoma in pSS patients[8]; (2) demonstration that BAFF levels are increased in pSS patients with current or previous lymphoma compared with patients without lymphoma[9]; (3) abnormalities of the gene TNFAIP3 coding for the A20 protein that regulates NF-κB activation, found in up to 77% of MALT lymphomas

TABLE 268-1 EXTRAGLANDULAR MANIFESTATIONS OF PRIMARY SJÖGREN SYNDROME

CONSTITUTIONAL SYMPTOMS

Fatigue
Low-grade fever

SKIN AND VASCULAR

Small vessel vasculitis
Raynaud phenomenon
Photosensitivity reactions similar to subacute cutaneous systemic lupus erythematosus
Xerosis

UPPER AND LOWER AIRWAYS

Pyogenic sialoadenitis or parotitis
Interstitial pneumonitis or fibrosis
Chronic bronchitis
Bronchiectasis
Bronchiolitis obliterans with organizing pneumonia
Chronic obstructive pulmonary disease

MUSCULOSKELETAL

Polyarthralgia, polyarthritis
Myopathy, polymyositis

RENAL

Type I renal tubular acidosis
Tubular interstitial nephritis
Glomerulonephritis

NEUROLOGIC

Peripheral motor sensory neuropathy
Pure sensory neuropathy (including pure ataxic neuropathy)
Small fiber sensitive neuropathy
Multiple sclerosis–like focal lesions
Spinal cord dysfunction, including transverse myelitis

NEOPLASIA

Lymphadenopathy, MALT (mucosa-associated lymphoid tissue) lymphoma

complicating pSS.[10] In half of the cases, TNFAIP3 mutations or deletions occur within lymphoma cells; in the other 50%, they involve germline TNFAIP3 mutations with functional consequences.

Laboratory Findings

The most common serologic finding in pSS is hypergammaglobulinemia. The elevated γ-globulins contain several autoantibodies directed against non–organ-specific antigens, such as RF and antinuclear antibody (ANA). Specific ANA, anti-SSA/Ro, and anti-SSB/La antibodies are present in 60 to 80% and 30 to 40% of patients, respectively, and anti-SSB/La is never present without anti-SSA/Ro. Of note, the presence of anti-SSA/Ro, possibly with anti-SSB/La, may mediate complete heart block of newborns owing to cross-mimicry between specific fetal myocardial antigens and epitopes of the SSA/Ro-SSB/La complex.

Anemia of chronic inflammation and high erythrocyte sedimentation rates (due to hypergammaglobulinemia) are frequently encountered, whereas C-reactive protein levels are usually within normal limits. Cytopenias (most frequently lymphopenia and neutropenia) can also occur. In the setting of interstitial nephritis, the presence of hypokalemic, hyperchloremic acidosis might reveal distal renal tubular acidosis.

A monoclonal immunoglobulin can be detected in 10 to 15% of patients with SS, depending on the technique used. Approximately 20% of patients with SS have cryoglobulins in their sera. Complement levels may be decreased, especially C4. This low C4 level may be either genetically determined or secondary to consumption (in immune complexes or cryoglobulinemia).

DIAGNOSIS

Differential Diagnosis

The definition of pSS had suffered for a long time from the absence of accurate and consensus-driven diagnostic criteria. This is important because the patients' main symptoms (dryness, fatigue, and pain) are frequent in the general population. They can be caused by numerous drugs (Table 268-2), anxiety and/or depression, other comorbidities, or aging (Table 268-3). Sarcoidosis can mimic the clinical picture of SS. However, in sarcoidosis minor salivary gland biopsy reveals noncaseating granulomas, and autoantibodies

TABLE 268-2 DRUGS AND TOXINS THAT MIGHT DECREASE LACRIMAL AND SALIVARY SECRETION

STRONG EFFECT	MODERATE EFFECT
Atropine, atropinic antiparkinsonian drugs, anticholinergic antihistaminic drugs	β-Adrenergic blockers
Antidepressants: imipraminic (amitriptyline) and inhibitors of monoamine oxidase	α-Adrenergic blockers
Neuroleptics	Calcium channel blockers
Morphine, codeine, tramadol	Benzodiazepines
A-type botulinum toxin	Inhibitors of serotonin reuptake (very slight effect)
Class IA antiarrhythmic (disopyramide)	H₁ antihistaminic drugs
Isotretinoin	Diuretics
Toxins and psychotropic drugs: tobacco, ecstasy, cannabis, cocaine	Some antiretroviral drugs

TABLE 268-3 THE DIFFERENT CAUSES OF SICCA SYMPTOMS

Drugs, particularly psychotropic drugs (see Table 268-2)
Aging, postmenopausal estrogen deficiency
Prolonged use of contact lenses
Fibromyalgia and chronic fatigue syndrome
Anxiodepressive syndromes
Head and neck radiotherapy
Diabetes (uncontrolled)
Severe hyperlipidemia
Amyloidosis
Sarcoidosis
Lymphoma
Graft-versus-host disease
Some viral infections (HIV, HCV, HTVL-1)
IgG4-related sialoadenitis
Sjögren syndrome

HCV = hepatitis C virus; HIV = human immunodeficiency virus; HTVL-1 = human T-lymphocytic virus-1.

are typically absent. Other SS mimickers include chronic graft-versus-host disease, amyloidosis, infection with viruses such as HIV, human T-lymphocytic virus-I (HTLV-I), and hepatitis C virus (HCV), and IgG4-related disease (Chapter 275). The latter disease is important in the differential diagnosis of SS. It more often involves men with salivary or lacrimal gland enlargement (previously called Mickuliz disease) with previous organ-specific autoimmune disease (like autoimmune pancreatitis) without anti-SSA/SSB antibodies. Sicca symptoms without salivary lymphoid infiltrate and without anti-SSA/SSB antibodies may be part of the fibromyalgia syndrome (Chapter 274), and several acronyms have been proposed for designating these patients: sicca asthenia polyalgia syndrome (SAPS) or dry eyes and mouth syndrome (DEMS).

Diagnostic Criteria

International agreement has established a definition of SS based on the American-European Consensus Group (AECG) criteria, which require the presence of either focal lymphocytic infiltrates in minor salivary glands with a focus score of 1 or more, or anti-SSA/SSB autoantibodies (Table 268-4). A new set of preliminary criteria for SS classification was proposed by an expert consensus panel (American College of Rheumatology [ACR]-Sjögren International Collaborative Clinical Alliance [SICCA]). According to these criteria, classification of an individual as a pSS patient requires the presence of two out of three of the following objective items: (1) a positive serum test for anti-Ro/SSA and/or anti-La/SSB antibodies, or positive rheumatoid factor (RF) and antinuclear antibody (ANA) (titer > 1: 320); (2) presence of keratoconjunctivitis sicca, defined by an ocular staining score over 3; and (3) presence of focal lymphocytic sialoadenitis, defined by a focus score of 1 focus/4 mm² or above in a labial salivary gland biopsy.[11]

Assessment of Activity of the Disease

An international expert group recently set up an SS activity score under the umbrella of the European League Against Rheumatism (EULAR). Two indices have been developed: (1) a patient-administered questionnaire to assess subjective features, the EULAR Sjögren Syndrome Patient Reported Index (ESSPRI), based on three different visual analogic scores: dryness,

TABLE 268-4 CLASSIFICATION CRITERIA FOR SJÖGREN SYNDROME

I. OCULAR SYMPTOMS

Positive response to at least one of these three questions:
1. Have you had daily, persistent, troublesome dry eyes for more than 3 months?
2. Do you have a recurrent sensation of sand or gravel in the eyes?
3. Do you use tear substitutes more than three times a day?

II. ORAL SYMPTOMS

Positive response to at least one of these three questions:
1. Have you had a daily feeling of dry mouth for more than 3 months?
2. Have you had recurrent or persistently swollen salivary glands as an adult?
3. Do you frequently drink liquids to aid in swallowing dry food?

III. OCULAR SIGNS

Objective evidence of ocular involvement, defined as a positive result in at least one of the following two tests:
1. Schirmer test (≤5 mm in 5 min)
2. Rose bengal score (≥4 according to van Bijsterveld scoring system)

IV. HISTOPATHOLOGY

Focus score ≥1 in a minor salivary gland biopsy specimen (a focus is defined as an agglomerate of at least 50 mononuclear cells; the focus score is defined by the number of foci in 4 mm² of glandular tissue)

V. SALIVARY GLAND INVOLVEMENT

Objective evidence of salivary gland involvement, defined by a positive result in at least one of the following three diagnostic tests:
1. Salivary scintigraphy
2. Parotid sialography
3. Unstimulated salivary flow (≤1.5 mL in 15 min)

VI. AUTOANTIBODIES

Presence in the serum of the following autoantibodies: antibodies to Ro (SSA) or La (SSB) antigens, or both

RULES FOR CLASSIFICATION

In patients without any potentially associated disease, primary Sjögren syndrome is diagnosed if:
    Four of six criteria are met, including IV or VI; _or_
    Three of four criteria from III, IV, V, and VI are met
For secondary Sjögren syndrome, criteria I or II plus any two from criteria III, IV, and V should be met

EXCLUSION CRITERIA

Preexisting lymphoma, AIDS, sarcoidosis, graft-versus-host disease, past head and neck radiation treatment, use of anticholinergic drugs, and hepatitis C

From Vitali C, Bombardieri S, Jonsson R, et al. Classification criteria for Sjögren syndrome: a revised version of the European criteria proposed by the American-European Consensus Group. *Ann Rheum Dis.* 2002;61:554-558.

fatigue, and limb pain[12]; and (2) a systemic activity index to assess systemic complications, the EULAR Sjögren Syndrome Disease Activity Index (ESSDAI).[13] The latter index comprises 12 domains with 3 or 4 levels of activity for each domain. Determination of the threshold of moderate activity as well as the minimal clinically important improvement is in progress, with the objective to base inclusion criteria and primary end-points of future clinical studies on ESSDAI levels.

TREATMENT

Symptomatic Treatment

A recent systematic review of the literature confirms benefits for muscarinic agonists (pilocarpine hydrochloride and more recently cevimeline hydrochloride) for sicca features (oral dryness and, to a lesser extent, ocular dryness).[A1] Topical cyclosporine collyrium (0.05%) also was effective for moderate or severe ocular dryness and inflammation in a randomized controlled trial versus placebo, as were 0.1% clobetasone butyrate eyedrops.[A2] Environmental measures (avoidance of hot air heating systems or excessive air conditioning, use of a humidifier, appropriate glasses to protect the eye from evaporating air flow) and "little means" (sugar-free chewing gums, regular water drinking, salivary substitutes) might be useful. Regular dental examinations and oral hygiene are crucial for reducing subsequent oral health issues (i.e., caries and periodontal disease associated with xerostomia). To treat pain, simple analgesics should be used first, particularly acetaminophen/paracetamol, which does not cause dryness.

Immunomodulatory Drugs

To date, no immunomodulatory drug has proved efficacious in pSS. Severe organ manifestations of pSS have to be treated in accordance with treatment modalities used in SLE or other connective tissue diseases. Randomized trials have assessed hydroxychloroquine in pSS and failed to demonstrate any clinical efficacy.[A3] In spite of these negative results on clinical outcomes, hydroxychloroquine is frequently used in pSS, especially to treat arthralgia with or without synovitis or purpura. Controlled studies are needed to assess the use of methotrexate, leflunomide, mycophenolate sodium, azathioprine, and cyclosporine. Intravenous gamma globulin (IVIG) has been used in the treatment of SS-associated sensorimotor neuropathies or non-ataxic sensory neuropathy without any necrotizing vasculitis.

Biologics

Two randomized controlled trials (RCT) of infliximab and etanercept did not show any efficacy of TNF-blocker agents in pSS on a composite primary outcome including limb pain, fatigue, and dryness visual analogue scales (VAS).[A4] B-cell targeting appears to be a promising strategy in pSS. Three randomized controlled trials assessed efficacy of the monoclonal anti-CD20 antibody (rituximab). In the first one, a significant improvement from baseline in a fatigue VAS was observed in the rituximab group but not in the placebo group.[A5] In the second one, rituximab demonstrated significant efficacy compared to placebo in improving stimulated salivary flow, the primary end-point, but also oral and ocular dryness, fatigue VAS, and systemic complications.[A6] In the third study, the composite primary end-point, using 4 VAS, was achieved at 6 weeks but not at 6 months.[A7] Lastly, recent data derived from the French Autoimmune and Rituximab (AIR) registry, including 78 pSS patients with mainly systemic manifestations, suggested the efficacy of rituximab on systemic manifestations in approximately two thirds of the patients.[14] Overall, rituximab seems to be useful in cases of persistent parotid swelling or systemic complications, especially in cryoglobulinemia-induced vasculitis. Inhibitors of BAFF, especially the anti-BAFF monoclonal antibody belimumab (which is approved in SLE), has been used in pSS in a first open phase 2 study, with promising results.[15]

FUTURE DIRECTIONS

SS is a model of autoimmune disease, because it can be primary or associated with other autoimmune diseases; it represents autoimmunity where the risk of lymphoma is most important. SS is the autoimmune disease for which the target tissue of autoimmunity is the most easily available, with the lip biopsy being necessary for diagnosis. Recent progress in pathophysiology has emphasized a number of similarities with SLE that support consideration of SS as a sort of lupus of the mucosa. Even if the pathogenetic mechanisms of the disease remain largely unknown, improved knowledge of the effector mechanisms will allow identification of new targets for future therapy. Moreover, with the recently validated composite activity scores of ESSPRI and ESSDAI, the tools are now available to begin new clinical trials with novel drugs for this disease that will improve the poor quality of life currently associated with it.

Grade A References

A1. Ramos-Casals M, Tzioufas AG, Stone JH, et al. Treatment of primary Sjögren syndrome: a systematic review. *JAMA.* 2010;304:452-460.

A2. Aragona P, Spinella R, Rania L, et al. Safety and efficacy of 0.1% clobetasone butyrate eyedrops in the treatment of dry eye in Sjogren syndrome. *Eur J Ophthalmol.* 2013;23:368-376.

A3. Gottenberg JE, Ravaud P, Puechal X, et al. Effects of hydroxychloroquine on symptomatic improvement in primary Sjogren syndrome: the JOQUER randomized clinical trial. *JAMA.* 2014;312:249-258.

A4. Mariette X, Ravaud P, Steinfeld S, et al. Inefficacy of infliximab in primary Sjögren's syndrome: results of the randomized, controlled Trial of Remicade in Primary Sjogren's Syndrome (TRIPSS). *Arthritis Rheum.* 2004;50:1270-1276.

A5. Dass S, Bowman SJ, Vital EM, et al. Reduction of fatigue in Sjögren syndrome with rituximab: results of a randomised, double-blind, placebo-controlled pilot study. *Ann Rheum Dis.* 2008;67:1541-1544.

A6. Meijer JM, Meiners PM, Vissink A, et al. Effectiveness of rituximab treatment in primary Sjögren syndrome: a randomized, double-blind, placebo-controlled trial. *Arthritis Rheum.* 2010;62:960-968.

A7. Devauchelle-Pensec V, Mariette X, Jousse-Jolin S, et al. Treatment of primary Sjögren syndrome with rituximab: a randomized trial. *Ann Intern Med.* 2014;160:233-242.

GENERAL REFERENCES

For the General References and other additional features, please visit Expert Consult at https://expertconsult.inkling.com.

INFLAMMATORY MYOPATHIES

STEVEN A. GREENBERG

OVERVIEW

The inflammatory myopathies are a heterogeneous group of acquired disorders in which the immune system is thought to play a major pathogenic role. Though some genetic disorders affecting muscle also have significant involvement of the immune system and are treated with immunosuppressive therapy as standard of care (e.g., treatment of Duchenne's muscular dystrophy with corticosteroids), these genetic disorders are not classified as inflammatory myopathies. The four major subtypes of inflammatory myopathy are: dermatomyositis (DM), polymyositis (PM), immune-mediated necrotizing myopathy (IMNM), and inclusion body myositis (IBM; also called sporadic inclusion body myositis [sIBM]). These disorders have distinct clinical and pathologic features and pathophysiologies (Table 269-1). Whereas DM and PM have been described in the medical literature for over 100 years, IMNM and IBM have only become defined as syndromes distinct from PM within the last few decades.

EPIDEMIOLOGY

The prevalence of DM has been estimated at 100[1] to 210 per million. The estimated prevalence of PM is confounded by frequent misdiagnosis of IBM and muscular dystrophies as PM. Traditionally, PM has been considered more prevalent (70 per million[2]), but comparative studies with attention to IBM have found a prevalence of PM of 35 per million, approximately half the prevalence of IBM of 70 per million. The prevalence of IMNM is unknown.

DM peaks in prevalence in childhood (7 to 15 years) and in midlife (30 to 50 years), whereas PM peaks in prevalence in midlife. IBM is rarely diagnosed before the age of 40 and is most common after the age of 50. DM and PM have female predominance; IBM has male predominance. Ethnicity and worldwide distribution influence the development of various inflammatory myopathies.

PATHOBIOLOGY

The pathophysiologies of various forms of inflammatory myopathy are poorly understood. These disorders do share in common injury to muscle by the immune system. Much of the theory of pathophysiology of these disorders comes from microscopic examination of muscle biopsies and the distinct pathologies of these disorders (Fig. 269-1).

The muscle pathology of DM involves loss of muscle blood vessels and injury to myofibers at the edges of muscle fascicles (i.e., perifascicular atrophy; see Fig. 269-1). The relationship of these two features to each other is uncertain but has been postulated to be due to a primary injury to muscle capillaries, followed by ischemic injury to myofibers. An alternative view is that a common factor injures both myofibers and capillaries.[3] Skin pathology shows features analogous to that of muscle, with an interface dermatitis consisting of injury to the basal layer of keratinocytes.

Much evidence points toward DM as mediated by the type 1 interferon cytokine family, consisting mainly of interferon (IFN)-α and IFN-β.[4,5] Numerous studies of DM skin and muscle samples show marked upregulation of type 1 IFN-inducible transcripts and proteins uniquely in DM among muscle diseases, and similarly to systemic lupus erythematosus among skin diseases. The presence of autoantibodies in some patients with DM, such as antibodies to the type 1 IFN-inducible protein MDA5, is of uncertain significance but seems likely due to an immune reaction to proteins that are not normally expressed at high levels or exposed to the immune system. The paraneoplastic associations of DM suggest that in such patients, an immune reaction against an underlying malignancy results in bystander injury to muscle and skin.

Because PM is a diverse group of disorders, the mechanisms involved are likely to be varied. Pathologically, there is an appearance of invasion of muscle fibers by adaptive immune system cells (T cells) that appears to be antigen driven, so that cytotoxic T cell–mediated autoimmunity directed against an unknown target has been a favored hypothesis. The antigens targeted by this process and the fundamental cause are unknown.

TABLE 269-1 CLASSIFICATION OF INFLAMMATORY MYOPATHIES

DISORDER	AGE RANGE	CLINICAL FEATURES	MUSCLE PATHOLOGY
Dermatomyositis	Juvenile and adult forms	Proximal weakness plus skin	Perimysial and perivascular inflammation, perifascicular atrophy
Polymyositis	Adult (rare in childhood)	Proximal weakness	Endomysial inflammation with invasion of non-necrotic muscle fibers
Immune-mediated necrotizing myopathy	Adult	Proximal weakness	Multifocal necrotic muscle fibers
Inclusion body myositis	Adult > 40 years old	Prominent quadriceps and finger flexor weakness; treatment refractory	Endomysial inflammation with invasion of non-necrotic muscle fibers plus rimmed vacuoles
Overlap syndromes	Adult	Myositis plus defined connective tissue disease	Nonspecific inflammation
Other (granulomatous myositis, eosinophilic myositis)	All ages	Proximal or distal weakness	Specific to type (e.g., granulomas present with granulomatous myositis)

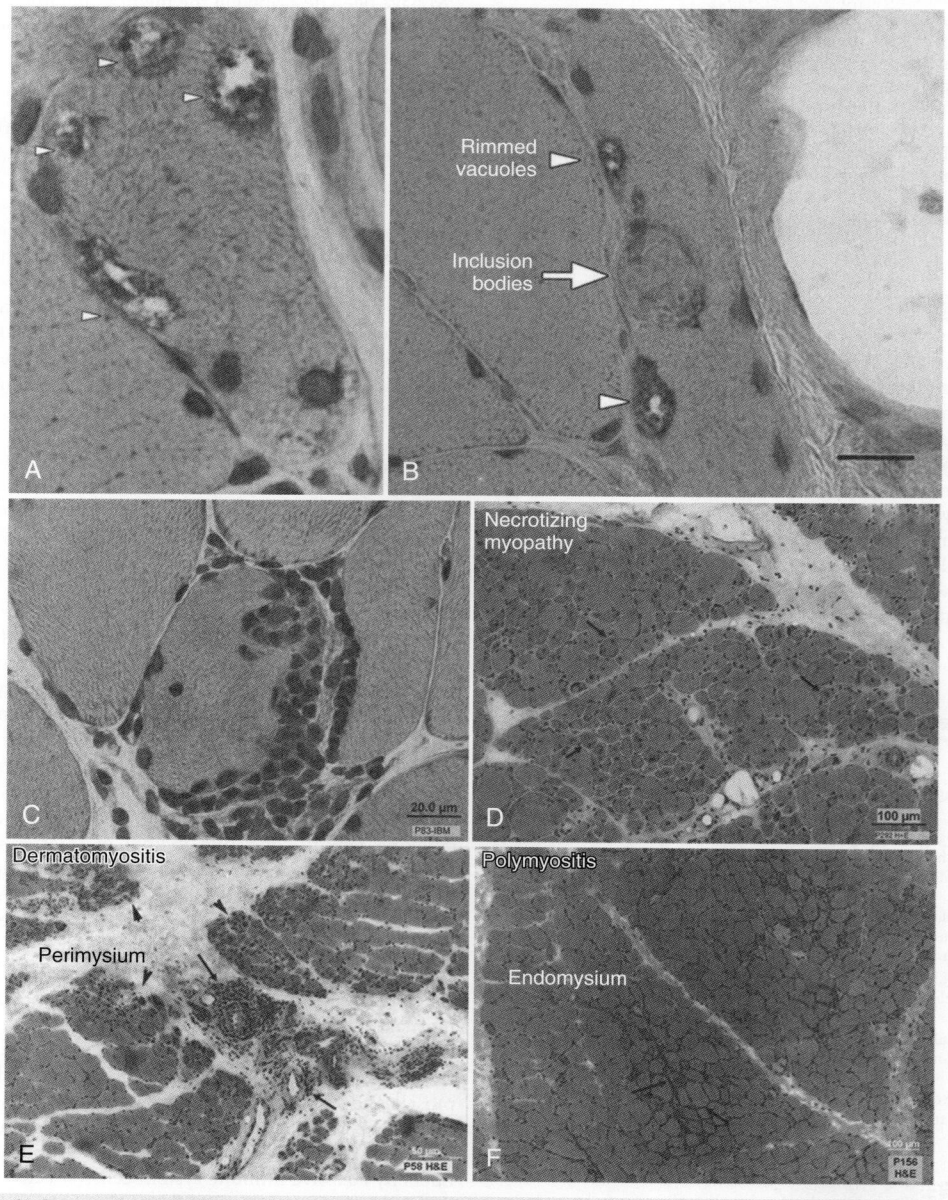

FIGURE 269-1. **Pathologies of inflammatory myopathies. A** and **B,** Rimmed vacuoles (*arrowheads*) of inclusion body myositis (IBM). **C,** Invasion of non-necrotic muscle fiber in IBM. **D,** Scattered necrotic and regenerating myofibers in immune-mediated necrotizing myopathy. **E,** Perivascular and perimysial inflammation (*arrows*), with perifascicular atrophy (*arrowheads*), in dermatomyositis. **F,** Endomysial inflammation in polymyositis. With permission from the Inclusion Body Myositis Foundation, Inc.

IMNM is also a poorly understood disorder.[6] It can also be paraneoplastic, suggesting cross-reactions by the immune system with the underlying malignancy and with muscle antigens. More commonly, IMNM occurs in association with treatment with statin drugs. The identification of autoantibodies against the target of statins, 3-hydroxy-3-methylglutaryl-coenzyme A reductase (HMGCR), in the majority of patients who develop IMNM in association with statin use suggests that the upregulation of HMGCR in muscle is directly toxic to muscle and triggers an immune reaction against it.

The pathogenesis of IBM is complex. Two dual pathologies have been noted: degeneration of myofibers and of myonuclei in particular, evident as formation of rimmed vacuoles (see Fig. 269-1A and B), and involvement of the immune system.[7] The accumulation of more than 75 different proteins into sarcoplasmic aggregates in a small percentage of IBM myofibers has been reported, and has given rise to a number of molecular toxicity hypotheses in which certain specific protein aggregates are theorized as injurious to myofibers.

The immune system involvement in IBM is notable in that whereas most other forms of inflammatory myopathy are generally responsive to immunomodulatory treatments, IBM is refractory to treatment. This is particularly remarkable in that IBM has the greatest evidence of all the inflammatory myopathies of a highly refined antigen-driven adaptive immune system involvement. Pathology shows very chronic and often marked but variable inflammatory infiltrates of T cells, myeloid dendritic cells, and plasma cells in muscle. Studies of the T-cell receptors have strongly suggested that T-cell autoimmunity is driven by one or more specific antigens, though the identity of any of these antigens is unknown.

Studies of a B-cell pathway in IBM have led to identification of an autoantibody that is highly specific to IBM among muscle diseases. Circulating autoantibodies against a 43-kD muscle protein were reported in 2011, and the identity of this 43-kD protein as cytoplasmic 5′ nucleotidase 1A (cN1A; NT5C1A) was reported in 2013.[8,9] cN1A is a nucleotidase that is most abundant in skeletal muscle and involved in the metabolism of nucleic acids. Serum anti-cN1A autoantibodies are present in 50 to 70% of patients with IBM, depending on which assays and what cutoffs are used, and highly specific to IBM (>90 to 95%) among muscle diseases. The role of blood testing for anti-cN1A autoantibodies in the diagnosis and management of patients with suspected IBM is currently being defined, potentially shortening the time to diagnosis, reducing the misdiagnosis rate, and avoiding more invasive muscle biopsy in some patients.

CLINICAL MANIFESTATIONS AND DIAGNOSIS

A diagnosis of inflammatory myopathy is considered when a patient presents with proximal or distal weakness without sensory symptoms, or in patients with the characteristic skin lesions of DM. Less frequently, asymptomatic elevated creatine kinase (CK) levels lead to a diagnosis of inflammatory myopathy. Most patients with DM, PM, or IMNM present with subacute proximal weakness of the arms and legs progressing over months, though these diseases may present acutely. Patients with IBM present later in life, usually symptomatic from slowly progressive weakness of knee extensors and finger flexors. More specific diagnostic considerations for these disorders are considered individually (Table 269-2). Most patients undergo muscle biopsy, or skin biopsy in the case of suspected DM, as part of the diagnostic evaluation.

Dermatomyositis

Patients with DM typically present with characteristic skin lesions or muscle weakness. Virtually pathognomonic skin features are a heliotrope rash, a violaceous periorbital macular erythema, sometimes with edema, and Gottron's papules, violaceous papules over dorsal metacarpophalangeal and interphalangeal joints of the hands (Fig. 269-2).[10] Periungual telangiectasias and thrombosed capillaries, poikiloderma over photoexposed areas such as the upper back ("shawl sign"), non-scarring alopecia, and subcutaneous calcification are other suggestive signs. Prominent pruritus is also a common feature of DM. Muscle weakness in DM is less specific, occurring in a pattern indistinguishable from many other muscle diseases.

Useful laboratory studies for the evaluation of suspected DM include serum CK (though CK can be normal or even below typical laboratory lower limits of normal in patients with highly active disease) and DM-associated autoantibody studies (e.g., anti-Jo-1, anti-Mi2, and anti-MDA5). Occasional patients have abnormal serum aldolase but normal serum CK. Skin biopsy showing a cell-poor interface dermatitis supports the diagnosis of DM. Muscle biopsy showing perimysial and perivascular inflammation also

TABLE 269-2	CLINICAL DIAGNOSTIC CRITERIA FOR INFLAMMATORY MYOPATHIES
DISORDER	**DIAGNOSIS**

Dermatomyositis	1. Diagnostic skin involvement (heliotrope rash, Gottron's papules) <u>OR</u> diagnostic muscle biopsy finding of perifascicular atrophy <u>OR</u>
	2. All of the following:
	  • Suggestive skin involvement
	  • Subacute or chronic proximal or distal weakness
	  • Muscle biopsy showing perimysial or perivascular inflammation without features suggesting another disorder (e.g., endomysial inflammation, rimmed vacuoles) <u>OR</u> skin biopsy showing interface dermatitis along with clinical exclusion of lupus erythematosus

Polymyositis	All of the following: 1. Subacute or chronic proximal weakness 2. Elevated serum creatine kinase (CK) 3. Muscle biopsy showing invasion of endomysial inflammation 4. Response to immunotherapy <u>OR</u> appropriate consideration and exclusion of limb-girdle muscular dystrophies and inclusion body myositis
Immune-mediated necrotizing myopathy	Both of the following: 1. Subacute or chronic proximal weakness 2. Muscle biopsy showing necrotizing myopathy, with scattered necrotic or regenerating myofibers and a lack of inflammation other than macrophage invasion of necrotic muscle fiber
Inclusion body myositis	All of the following: 1. Adult > 40 years old 2. Finger flexion or quadriceps weakness 3. Muscle biopsy showing endomysial inflammation <u>OR</u> the presence of serum anti-cN1A autoantibodies 4. Muscle biopsy showing rimmed vacuoles <u>OR</u> invasion of non-necrotic muscle fibers <u>OR</u> the presence of serum anti-cN1A autoantibodies

cNIA = cytoplasmic 5′ nucleotidase 1A.

supports a diagnosis of DM, whereas the presence of perifascicular atrophy in a muscle biopsy is pathognomonic for DM. Because DM is associated with malignancy, appropriate laboratory and radiologic studies should be performed to search for underlying malignancy in all newly diagnosed patients. The most common DM-associated malignancies tend to reflect the overall age and gender cancer rates within the individual patient's population (i.e., breast, lung, and colorectal cancer in Western countries; nasopharyngeal cancer in Asian populations). This observation supports the notion of DM as a paraneoplastic process that can develop in virtually any kind of cancer.

Research diagnostic criteria for DM have been defined.[11] Clinical diagnostic criteria are outlined in Table 269-2. The clinical features of muscle weakness in DM are entirely nonspecific, with no particular pattern indicative of DM rather than other muscle diseases. In practice, certain dermatologic clinical findings (heliotrope rash, Gottron's papules) or muscle biopsy findings (perifascicular atrophy) are considered nearly pathognomonic for DM.

Polymyositis

The diagnosis of PM is often problematic, with historically many patients with genetically defined limb-girdle muscular dystrophies and IBM being misdiagnosed as PM. The 1975 criteria for PM that are frequently cited allow for a diagnosis of "definite" PM without a muscle biopsy. Other research criteria require muscle biopsy. In clinical practice, the core criteria for the diagnosis of PM are subacute proximal weakness, elevated serum CK, and muscle biopsy showing endomysial inflammation without features suggestive of another diagnosis such as IBM (see Table 269-2). Patients with defined connective tissue disorders such as Sjögren's syndrome or mixed connective tissue disease have "overlap syndromes," often also classified as PM. Patients with IMNM have historically been classified as PM but are increasingly classified separately. Patients with IBM are frequently misdiagnosed as PM because of a lack of appreciation of characteristic IBM finger flexor weakness, and because muscle biopsies show endomysial inflammation. The presence of autoantibodies such as anti-Jo-1 argue more for PM than IBM, though these may be seen in DM as well.

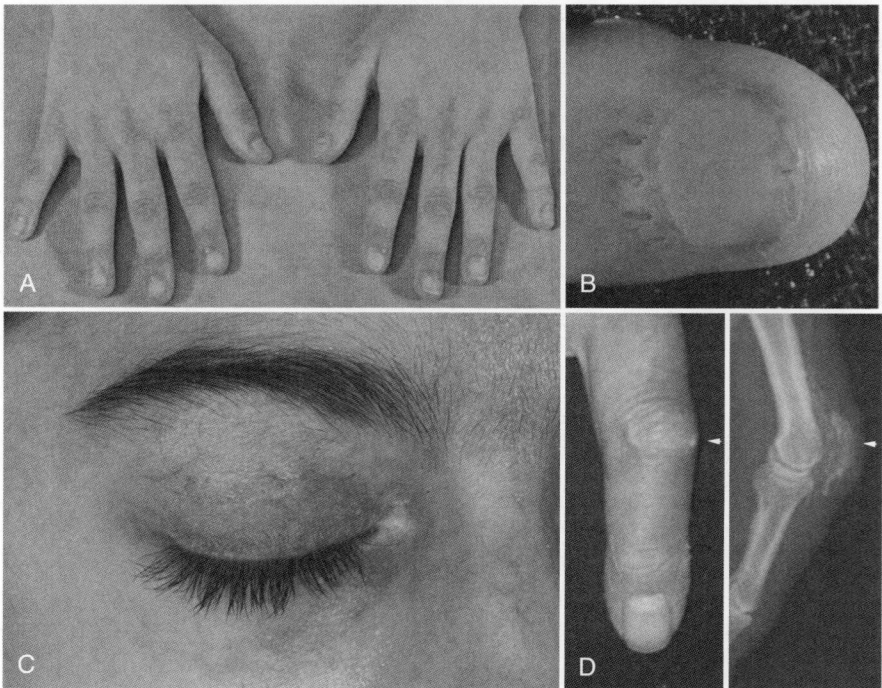

FIGURE 269-2. Clinical findings in dermatomyositis. **A,** Erythematous to violaceous raised papules overlying the metacarpal and interphalangeal joints, known as Gottron's papules. These are considered the hallmark finding in dermatomyositis. **B,** Cuticular overgrowth and periungual capillary changes, which include dilated and tortuous blood vessels with areas of atrophy, telangiectasia, vessel dropout, and bushy loop formation along the fingernail bed. **C,** Erythema and minimal edema involving the upper eyelids, with occasional telangiectasia, known as the heliotrope rash. **D,** Subcutaneous calcification erupting through skin (*arrowhead*), seen clinically and by x-ray.

Immune-Mediated Necrotizing Myopathy

IMNM has increasingly been separated from the PM category. Acute or subacute proximal weakness indistinguishable from that of PM or DM and an elevated CK are nonspecific, but muscle biopsy showing scattered necrotic or regenerating myofibers without inflammation other than macrophages invading these necrotic myofibers is typical of IMNM. The presence of anti-HMGCR (3-hydroxy-3-methylglutaryl-coenzyme A reductase) or anti-SRP (signal recognition particle) antibodies both suggest IMNM. IMNM, particularly when associated with anti-SRP antibodies, may be paraneoplastic, and laboratory and radiologic evaluation for malignancy should be considered.

Inclusion Body Myositis

IBM has a clinical presentation distinct from other inflammatory myopathies.[12] IBM weakness is always slowly progressive rather than the acute or subacute weakness more typically seen in other forms of inflammatory myopathies. Clinical diagnostic criteria are shown in Table 269-2. IBM has a high misdiagnosis rate, estimated at approximately 50% of patients. Symptoms of IBM rarely are present before the age of 40 years and most commonly occur after the age of 50. The distribution of weakness is usually in finger flexors or quadriceps rather than proximal arms (shoulder abduction) or proximal legs (hip flexion), more typical of PM or DM. IBM is a highly atrophying muscle disease, and loss of bulk in medial and lateral anterior thighs and ventral forearms is characteristic. Patients present with difficulty walking, buckling of knees, or weakness of grip. The diagnosis of IBM can be highly suspected in such patients of appropriate age and findings on examination of quadriceps atrophy and weakness of finger flexors, especially flexor digitorum profundi, responsible for flexion of distal fingertips. Examination of the strength in these distal fingertips, which needs to be done one finger at a time, is often the single most helpful approach to the diagnosis of IBM.

Serum CK is either normal or modestly elevated (typically < 5 times the upper limit of normal). A serum autoantibody, anti-cN1A (also called anti-NT5C1A), appears highly specific to IBM among muscle diseases and may be of diagnostic value. Most patients undergo muscle biopsy, with characteristic features being the presence of rimmed vacuoles seen on hematoxylin and eosin (H&E) and Gomori trichrome staining, along with endomysial inflammation or invasion of non-necrotic muscle fibers. Immunohistochemical stains detecting p62 or TDP-43 are of additional highly specific diagnostic value.

Generally, most patients with DM, PM, and IMNM respond to immunomodulatory therapies, whereas patients with IBM are almost universally refractory. A general approach to treatment is shown in Figure 269-3.

Treatment of Dermatomyositis and Polymyositis

Most patients with DM and PM are treated with and respond to corticosteroids.[13,14] Dosing is typically prednisone at 1 mg/kg/day orally until significant improvement occurs (typically 1 to 3 months), followed by gradual taper of 10 mg/day/month. Second-line agents include methotrexate, azathioprine, cyclosporine, and intravenous immunoglobulin. Second-line agents are used for two reasons: they may have a better side-effect profile than chronic higher doses of corticosteroids, and they may be necessary for patients whose responses are insufficient to corticosteroids alone. An important decision is whether to start second-line agents concurrently with initial corticosteroid treatment or wait and see how low a dose of corticosteroids offers satisfactory control, and then add agents only if the corticosteroid dose cannot be lowered sufficiently. Thus, in the former approach, prednisone 60 mg/day and methotrexate 7.5 mg PO weekly might be started concurrently, and the methotrexate dose increased weekly to 15 to 20 mg PO weekly. Once improvement is substantial, the dose of prednisone may be tapered over 3 to 6 months. Stability on methotrexate alone would then be followed by gradual reduction in its dose.

For patients with severe initial presentations, the combination of corticosteroids and periodic intravenous immunoglobulin (1 g/kg every 2 weeks) may offer a better chance for more rapid improvement.

Approximately seven randomized placebo controlled trials have been reported to date in DM or PM.[A1] These studies have almost always used the Bohan and Peter criteria for the diagnosis, which may result in inclusion of patients with limb-girdle muscular dystrophies and IBM misdiagnosed as having PM. The largest trial, rituximab in myositis (RIM), enrolling 200 subjects,[A2] used a trial design in which all subjects received active drug, but comparator groups were treated "early" or "late" (8 weeks later), and efficacy was based on time to improvement. This study found no significant differences between these early and late treatment groups' time to improvement, as defined by a specific definition of improvement (DOI) used in that study.

Treatment of Inclusion Body Myositis

A number of controlled and uncontrolled trials of IBM have been published. None of these demonstrated efficacies of the therapeutic

Suspected Inflammatory Myopathy

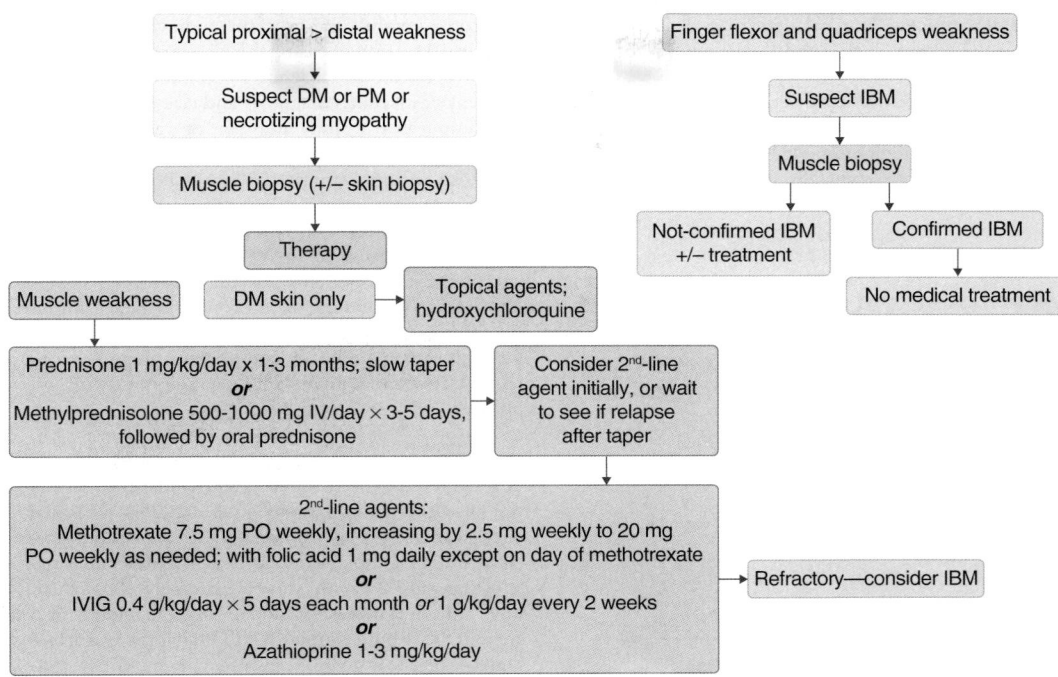

FIGURE 269-3. Approach to treatment of suspected inflammatory myopathy. DM = dermatomyositis; IBM = inclusion body myositis; IVIG = intravenous immunoglobulin; PM = polymyositis. With permission from the Inclusion Body Myositis Foundation, Inc.

interventions, which have included prednisone, intravenous immunoglobulin, methotrexate, antithymocyte globulin, oxandrolone, interferon-β, and alemtuzumab.[15] Current management of patients with IBM is supportive, involving avoidance of falls and the use of ankle supports and gait assistive devices. Tendon transfer to improve hand function has been used.

PROGNOSIS

Most patients with adult DM, PM, and statin-associated IMNM have a good prognosis but require long-standing immunomodulatory therapy. Many patients with juvenile DM may go into long-standing remission or cure with aggressive initial treatment. Patients with anti-SRP–associated IMNM may have severe and difficult-to-treat disease. Patients with IBM generally have a slowly progressive course, with one series showing a mean time to loss of ambulation of 12 years.

 Grade A References

A1. Gordon PA, Winer JB, Hoogendijk JE, et al. Immunosuppressant and immunomodulatory treatment for dermatomyositis and polymyositis. *Cochrane Database Syst Rev.* 2012;8:CD003643.
A2. Oddis CV, Reed AM, Aggarwal R, et al. Rituximab in the treatment of refractory adult and juvenile dermatomyositis and adult polymyositis: a randomized, placebo-phase trial. *Arthritis Rheum.* 2013;65:314-324.

GENERAL REFERENCES

For the General References and other additional features, please visit Expert Consult at https://expertconsult.inkling.com.

270
THE SYSTEMIC VASCULITIDES

JOHN H. STONE

DEFINITION

The vasculitides are a heterogeneous group of disorders linked by the common finding of destructive inflammation within blood vessel walls. The most current nomenclature scheme[1] identifies at least 27 different forms of primary vasculitis (Table 270-1). The major forms of vasculitis are discussed in this chapter.

CLASSIFICATION
Classification by Vessel Size

The etiology of most forms of vasculitis remains unknown, and major gaps exist in our understanding of the pathophysiologic processes. The most valid basis for classification of the vasculitides is the size of the predominant blood vessels involved. The vasculitides are categorized initially by whether the vessels affected are primarily large, medium, or small (Table 270-2). Large vessels are considered the aorta, its primary branches, and any vessel that is not located within an organ such as a muscle, kidney, nerve, or the skin. Medium-sized vessels, in contrast, consist of the main visceral arteries and their branches. (Thus, the renal artery is considered a large vessel, but its intrarenal branches—the interlobar and arcuate arteries—are medium-sized vessels). Finally, small vessels include smaller intraparenchymal arteries as well as arterioles, capillaries, and veins.

Medium-vessel vasculitis and even large-vessel vasculitis can also affect small arteries. However, Large-vessel vasculitis affects large arteries more often than medium or small-vessel vasculitis, medium-vessel vasculitis affects predominantly medium arteries, and small-vessel vasculitis affects predominantly small arteries and other small vessels.

Additional Considerations in Classification

Several considerations other than blood vessel size are relevant to the classification of vasculitis (see Table 270-2). These are (1) age, sex, and ethnic background of the patient; (2) tropism for particular organs; (3) presence or absence of granulomatous inflammation; (4) participation of immune complexes in the pathophysiologic process; and (5) detection of characteristic autoantibodies in the patients' serum, such as antineutrophil cytoplasmic antibodies (ANCAs).

Age, sex differences, and ethnic variation are discussed later in the section on Epidemiology. The organ tropisms of these disorders are illustrated by the following examples. Whereas immunoglobulin (Ig)A vasculitis (IgAV, also known as Henoch-Schönlein purpura) typically affects the skin, joints, kidneys, and gastrointestinal (GI) tract, granulomatosis with polyangiitis

(GPA; formerly Wegener granulomatosis) classically involves the upper airways, lungs, and kidneys. In contrast to both IgAV and GPA, Cogan syndrome involves the eyes, the audiovestibular apparatus of the inner ear, and (in 10 to 15% of cases) the large arteries.

The presence or absence of granulomatous inflammation is a crucial element of vasculitis diagnosis and classification. Granulomatous inflammation implicates a small number of vasculitides that bear this hallmark, including GPA, giant cell arteritis, Takayasu arteritis, and eosinophilic granulomatosis with polyangiitis (EGPA; Churg-Strauss syndrome).

Immune complexes are essential to the pathophysiologic mechanism of some forms of small- and medium-vessel vasculitis. Complexes of IgA1, for example, are found in IgAV. Immune complexes consisting of IgG, IgM, complement components, and the hepatitis C virion characterize most cases of mixed cryoglobulinemia. In contrast, "pauci-immune" types of small- and medium-vessel vasculitis, such as GPA and microscopic polyangiitis, have little immunoglobulin or complement deposition within diseased tissues. Many but not all patients with pauci-immune forms of vasculitis are ANCA positive.

EPIDEMIOLOGY

The epidemiologic features of individual forms of systemic vasculitis vary tremendously by geography (Table 270-3). This may reflect genetic influences, variation in environmental exposures, and other unknown disease risk factors. For example, whereas Behçet syndrome is rare in North Americans, affecting only 1 person in approximately 300,000, this condition is several hundred times more common among inhabitants of countries bordering the ancient Silk Route. Similarly, although Takayasu arteritis is rare in the United States—on the order of 3 new cases per million people per year—this disease is reportedly the most common cause of renal artery stenosis in India, where the incidence may be as high as 200 to 300 per million per year.

Age is an important consideration in the epidemiology of vasculitis. Eighty percent of patients with Kawasaki disease are younger than 5 years. In contrast, giant cell arteritis virtually never occurs in patients younger than 50 years, and the mean age of patients with this disease is 72. Age may also have an impact on disease severity and outcome. In IgAV, the overwhelming majority of cases in children (who represent 90% of all cases) have self-limited courses, resolving within several weeks. In adults, however, IgAV has a higher likelihood of chronicity and a poor renal outcome.

The distribution of sex varies across many forms of vasculitis. Buerger disease is the only form of vasculitis with a striking male predominance. The greater prevalence of smoking among males in most societies probably explains this predilection. In contrast, Takayasu arteritis has an overwhelming

TABLE 270-1 NAMES FOR VASCULITIDES ADOPTED BY THE 2012 INTERNATIONAL CHAPEL HILL CONSENSUS CONFERENCE ON THE NOMENCLATURE OF VASCULITIDES.[1]

LARGE-VESSEL VASCULITIS

Takayasu arteritis
Giant cell arteritis

MEDIUM-VESSEL VASCULITIS

Polyarteritis nodosa
Kawasaki disease
Buerger disease*

SMALL-VESSEL VASCULITIS

Antineutrophil cytoplasmic antibody (ANCA)-associated vasculitis
  Microscopic polyangiitis
  Granulomatosis with polyangiitis (formerly Wegener granulomatosis)
  Eosinophilic granulomatosis with polyangiitis (Churg-Strauss syndrome)
Immune complex small-vessel vasculitis
  Antiglomerular basement membrane disease
  Cryoglobulinemic vasculitis
  Immunoglobulin (Ig)A vasculitis (Henoch-Schönlein purpura)
  Hypocomplementemic urticarial vasculitis

VARIABLE-VESSEL VASCULITIS

Behçet syndrome
Cogan syndrome

SINGLE-ORGAN VASCULITIS

Cutaneous leukocytoclastic angiitis
Cutaneous arteritis
Primary central nervous system vasculitis
Isolated aortitis

VASCULITIS ASSOCIATED WITH SYSTEMIC DISEASE

Lupus vasculitis
Rheumatoid vasculitis
Sarcoid vasculitis
Others (e.g., IgG4-related aortitis)

VASCULITIS ASSOCIATED WITH PROBABLE ETIOLOGY

Hepatitis C virus–associated cryoglobulinemic vasculitis
Hepatitis B virus–associated vasculitis
Syphilis-associated aortitis
Drug-associated immune complex vasculitis
Drug-associated ANCA-associated vasculitis
Cancer-associated vasculitis
Others

*Buerger disease (thromboangiitis obliterans) is not always considered to be a primary form of vasculitis and was not included in this consensus statement on nomenclature.[1]

TABLE 270-2 CONSIDERATIONS IN THE CLASSIFICATION OF SYSTEMIC VASCULITIS

Size of predominant blood vessels affected
Epidemiologic features:
  Age
  Sex
  Ethnic background
Pattern of organ involvement
Pathologic features:
  Granulomatous inflammation
  Immune complex deposition vs. "pauci-immune" histopathology
Presence of ANCA in serum

ANCA = antineutrophil cytoplasmic antibody.

TABLE 270-3 EPIDEMIOLOGY OF SELECTED VASCULITIDES

DISEASE	UNITED STATES	ELSEWHERE	AGE, SEX, AND ETHNIC PREDISPOSITIONS
Giant cell arteritis	Incidence: 240/million (Olmsted County, MN)	220-270/million (Scandinavian countries)	Age > 50 yr, mean age 72 yr; females 3 : 1; northern European ancestry
Takayasu arteritis	Incidence: 3/million	200-300/million (India)	Age < 40 yr; females 9 : 1; Asian
Behçet syndrome	Prevalence: 3/million	3000/million (Turkey)	Silk Route countries
Polyarteritis nodosa	Incidence: 7/million	7/million (Spain)	Slight male predominance
Kawasaki disease	Incidence: 100/million*	900/million (Japan)	Children of Asian ancestry
Wegener granulomatosis	Incidence: 4/million	8.5/million (United Kingdom)	Whites ≫ blacks

*Among children younger than 5 years. From Gonzalez-Gay MA, Garica-Porrua C. Epidemiology of the vasculitides. *Rheum Clin North Am.* 2001;27:729-749.

tendency to occur in females (a 9 : 1 female-to-male ratio). The pauci-immune forms of vasculitis, such as GPA, EGPA, and microscopic polyangiitis, occur in males and females with approximately equal frequencies, but the phenotypic expression of these conditions may be affected by both age and sex.

The strongest link between any single gene and vasculitis is the association of HLA-B51 with Behçet syndrome. In Behçet syndrome, 80% of Asian patients have the HLA-B51 gene. The prevalence of HLA-B51 is significantly higher among patients with Behçet syndrome in Japan than among non-disease control subjects (55% versus < 15%). Among the sporadic cases of Behçet syndrome involving whites in the United States, however, HLA-B51 occurs in fewer than 15% of cases.

With the exception of Buerger disease and smoking, no definitive associations have been confirmed between disease and environmental or occupational exposures. Associations have been reported but not confirmed between exposures to silica and some types of pauci-immune vasculitis. Studies of potential associations between exposures of any type and vasculitis, however, are complicated frequently by difficulties in obtaining reliable measurements of the levels of the relevant exposure, the likelihood of recall bias among patients who are diagnosed with vasculitis, and the choice of appropriate control groups.

PATHOBIOLOGY

Table 270-4 illustrates the pathologic characteristics of selected forms of vasculitis. Specific pathologic features are discussed in the subsections on each disease. The type of inflammatory cell infiltrate in vasculitis is independent of the size of blood vessels involved. Mixed cell infiltrates in vasculitis are the rule rather than the exception, and histopathologic patterns of vasculitis may include leukocytoclasis (degranulation and destruction of neutrophils within blood vessel walls), granulomatous findings (with or without giant cells), lymphoplasmacytic infiltrates, varying degrees of eosinophilic infiltration, necrosis, and combinations of all these findings.

PATHOPHYSIOLOGY

Some pathophysiologic mechanisms are common to many different forms of vasculitis, regardless of the size of the predominant blood vessels involved. Immune complex deposition, for example, is present in several types of vasculitis that involve both medium-sized and small blood vessels. In this section, the general concepts related to the pathogenesis of large-vessel vasculitides are discussed separately from those of medium- and small-vessel vasculitides.

Large-Vessel Vasculitides

The pathologic process in large-vessel vasculitis appears to begin in the adventitia. In both Takayasu arteritis and giant cell arteritis, abundant numbers of activated T lymphocytes are found within inflamed arterial walls, centering on the adventitia. In Takayasu arteritis, most of these T cells appear to be of the $CD8^+$ subtype. Current evidence suggests that the cytotoxic functions of these cells, mediated by perforin and granzyme B, contribute to smooth muscle cell damage in this disease. $CD4^+$ T-cell responses in Takayasu arteritis have not been well defined.

In giant cell arteritis (Chapter 271), much evidence now suggests an antigen-driven disease, with the site of immunologic recognition events being the adventitia. $CD4^+$ T cells that secrete interferon (IFN)-γ appear to be recruited to the adventitia by a specific antigen(s), the identity of which remains unknown. Both the T cells that orchestrate the transmural inflammation and the inciting antigens are theorized to reach the adventitia through the vasa vasorum. Subsequently, T-cell signals from the adventitia stimulate macrophages and multinucleated giant cells to elaborate an array of downstream mediators, including metalloproteinases and platelet-derived growth factor. Interleukin (IL)-6, known to be a crucial cytokine in giant cell arteritis and probably Takayasu arteritis as well, is produced by macrophages residing in the blood vessel wall. The results of this inflammatory cascade are granulomatous inflammation, destruction of the internal elastic lamina, arterial wall hyperplasia, smooth muscle cell proliferation, intimal thickening, vascular occlusion, and in some cases, weakening of the vessel wall, leading to dilation and aneurysm formation.

Medium- and Small-Vessel Vasculitides

Several different pathophysiologic mechanisms are operative among the medium- and small-vessel vasculitides. In many cases, the mechanisms outlined in the following sections overlap.

Immune Complex–Mediated Vascular Injury

Immune complex–mediated tissue injury does not produce a single clinical syndrome but rather applies to many forms of vasculitis and overlaps with injuries caused by other immune mechanisms. Numerous variables influence immune complex–mediated injury, including the physical properties of the immune complexes (e.g., their size), the ability of the immune complexes to activate complement, the antigen-to-antibody ratio, and the hemodynamic features of specific vascular beds. Immune complexes participate in the pathophysiologic process of some forms of both medium- and small-vessel vasculitis, including polyarteritis nodosa, cryoglobulinemia, IgAV, cutaneous leukocytoclastic angiitis, and rheumatoid vasculitis.

Role of Antineutrophil Cytoplasmic Antibodies

ANCAs are directed against antigens that reside within the primary granules of neutrophils and monocytes. Two types of ANCA are relevant to vasculitis: (1) those directed against proteinase 3 (PR3), known as PR3-ANCA; and (2) those directed against myeloperoxidase (MPO), termed MPO-ANCA. ANCA interact with cytokines, neutrophils, monocytes, and other elements of the immune system to amplify ongoing inflammation in certain forms of vasculitis. A striking and still unexplained feature of ANCA-associated vasculitis (AAV) is that patients with primary forms of these conditions virtually never have antibodies to both PR3 and MPO. Despite the specificity of these antibodies, however, evidence for a primary role of ANCA in the etiology of human disease is still absent.

In GPA, abnormal cytokine regulation interacts with the production of ANCA to fuel the inflammatory response. T_H1 cytokines such as IFN-γ, IL-12, and tumor necrosis factor (TNF) appear to play important roles. Under the direction of IL-12, $CD4^+$ T cells from patients with GPA produce elevated levels of TNF, and peripheral blood mononuclear cells secrete increased amounts of IFN-γ. Serum levels of soluble receptors for TNF are elevated in patients with active GPA and normalize with the induction of remission. In vitro priming of activated neutrophils with TNF markedly

TABLE 270-4	PATHOLOGIC CHARACTERISTICS OF SELECTED FORMS OF VASCULITIS					
	TAKAYASU ARTERITIS	**POLYARTERITIS NODOSA**	**GRANULOMATOSIS WITH POLYANGIITIS (WEGENER GRANULOMATOSIS)**	**CHURG-STRAUSS SYNDROME**	**HENOCH-SCHÖNLEIN PURPURA**	**CUTANEOUS LEUKOCYTOCLASTIC ANGIITIS**
Vessels involved	Elastic (large) or muscle (medium-sized) arteries	Medium-sized and small muscle arteries	Small arteries and veins; sometimes medium-sized vessels	Small arteries and veins; sometimes medium-sized vessels	Capillaries, venules, and arterioles	Capillaries, venules, and arterioles
Organ involvement	Aorta, aortic arch and major branches, and pulmonary arteries	Skin, peripheral nerves, gastrointestinal tract, and other viscera	Upper respiratory tract, lungs, kidneys, skin, eyes	Upper respiratory tract, lungs, heart, peripheral nerves	Skin, joints, gastrointestinal tract, kidneys	Skin, joints
Type of vasculitis and inflammatory cells	Granulomatous with some giant cells; fibrosis in chronic stages	Necrotizing, with mixed cellular infiltrate	Necrotizing or granulomatous (or both); mixed cellular infiltrate plus occasional eosinophils	Necrotizing or granulomatous (or both); prominent eosinophils and other mixed infiltrate	Leukocytoclastic, with some lymphocytes and variable eosinophils; IgA deposits in affected tissues	Leukocytoclastic, with occasional eosinophils

enhances the ability of ANCA to stimulate neutrophil degranulation. Despite the strong rationale for anti-TNF strategies in GPA, however, a randomized trial of etanercept showed no efficacy in the maintenance of disease remissions.

B-cell depletion is a more effective approach to the treatment of AAV. The efficacy of this treatment strategy probably relates to the removal of several B-cell functions beyond their evolution into plasma cells and the production of ANCA. These other B-cell functions include cytokine production, antigen presentation, and B cell–T cell crosstalk.

Superantigen Model

The degree of immune activation in Kawasaki disease and the acute but generally self-limited nature of this illness imply a potential role for superantigens. Superantigens are proteins produced by microbial pathogens (e.g., *Staphylococcus aureus* or *Streptococcus* species) that are capable of stimulating large populations of T cells in a manner unrestricted by the class II major histocompatibility complex (MHC). Superantigens bind directly to conserved amino acid residues outside the antigen-binding groove on class II MHC molecules, thereby selectively stimulating T cells that express particular β-chain variable gene segments. Through the binding of this MHC-superantigen complex to its cognate T-cell receptors, as many as 20% of circulating lymphocytes may become activated, leading to a potentially enormous outpouring of cytokines. With regard to the etiology of Kawasaki disease, substantial attention has focused on toxic shock syndrome toxin 1, an exotoxin produced by *S. aureus*.[2] Superantigens have also been postulated to play roles in the susceptibility to disease flares in GPA. Nasal carriage of *S. aureus* and superantigens associated with these organisms has been linked to a greater likelihood of disease flares in some studies.

Anti–Endothelial Cell Antibodies

Anti–endothelial cell antibodies can induce endothelial cell injury and lysis through either complement-mediated cytotoxicity or antibody-dependent cellular cytotoxicity. Both of these mechanisms have been demonstrated to cause endothelial injury in in vitro assays employing sera from patients with systemic vasculitis. The ability of these antibodies to damage endothelial cells is an appealing argument for their potential role in forms of vasculitis in which the endothelium is the focus of the inflammation (as opposed to the more external vessel wall layers). However, the true relevance of anti–endothelial cell antibodies to human disease and their importance within the larger context of other disease mechanisms remain unclear.

CLINICAL MANIFESTATIONS

Large-Vessel Vasculitides
Takayasu Arteritis

Takayasu arteritis (Chapter 78) affects the aorta and its major branches. In contrast to atherosclerosis, which is characterized by focal irregular lesions, the lesions of Takayasu arteritis are long, smooth, tapered stenoses (E-Fig. 270-1). The most commonly involved arteries are the subclavian and innominate arteries. Takayasu arteritis has been termed "pulseless disease" because of its ability to obliterate peripheral pulses (particularly in the upper extremities). Exuberant collateral circulation develops over time in response to the gradual narrowing of major arteries, making the loss of digits or limbs from ischemia extremely rare. The pulmonary circulation is involved in approximately 50% of cases of Takayasu arteritis.

Patients with severe narrowing of the aortic arch vessels supplying the head may develop Takayasu retinopathy, a hypotensive retinopathy leading to neovascularization. In contrast, patients with prolonged hypertension associated with renal artery stenosis demonstrate the classic ocular features of hypertension: "copper wiring" and multiple retinal infarctions. This complication is particularly difficult to diagnose and dangerous because vascular narrowings of large arteries to the arms and legs can cause underestimations of the true central aortic pressure. Takayasu arteritis involvement of the ascending aorta may lead to aortic dilation, aortic regurgitation, aneurysm formation, and aortic rupture.

TREATMENT   Rx

The cornerstone of treatment of Takayasu arteritis is glucocorticoids. For patients with marked symptoms and signs of an inflammatory phase, prednisone (1 mg/kg/day) is usually effective in controlling the disease. This dose should be tapered within 8 to 12 weeks to less than 20 mg/day and ultimately to less than 10 mg/day as a maintenance dose. Emerging data support a role for IL-6 inhibition in patients with Takayasu arteritis whose prednisone doses cannot be tapered to reasonable levels. Patients have been treated with tocilizumab 8 mg/kg administered intravenously each month or with a corresponding subcutaneous preparation.

Giant Cell Arteritis

Giant cell arteritis is the other primary form of vasculitis that involves arteries far larger than vasculitides of any other category. This disease is discussed in detail elsewhere (Chapter 271).

Medium-Vessel Vasculitides
Polyarteritis Nodosa

Polyarteritis nodosa has a striking predilection for certain organs, particularly the skin, peripheral nerves, GI tract, and kidneys.[3] This disease usually begins with nonspecific symptoms such as malaise, fatigue, fever, myalgias, and arthralgias. Overt signs of vasculitis may not occur until weeks or months after onset of the first symptoms. Skin lesions of polyarteritis nodosa include livedo reticularis, subcutaneous nodules, ulcers, and digital gangrene. A majority of patients with polyarteritis nodosa (>80% in some series) have vasculitic neuropathy, typically in the pattern of a mononeuritis multiplex.

The classic GI manifestation of polyarteritis nodosa is "intestinal angina," the occurrence of postprandial abdominal pain. Polyarteritis nodosa can also affect individual GI tract organs such as the gallbladder or appendix, presenting as cholecystitis or appendicitis. The typical renal manifestation of polyarteritis nodosa is vasculitic involvement of the medium-sized intrarenal arteries, leading to renin-mediated hypertension and renal infarctions. Cardiac lesions, which usually remain subclinical, may lead to myocardial infarction or congestive heart failure. Polyarteritis nodosa usually spares the lungs.

The diagnosis of polyarteritis nodosa requires either a tissue biopsy or an angiogram that demonstrates microaneurysms (Fig. 270-1). Simultaneous nerve and muscle biopsies (e.g., sural nerve and gastrocnemius muscle) are of high yield if there is a clinical suspicion of vasculitic neuropathy. Symptoms suggestive of a neuropathy can be confirmed by electrodiagnostic studies that demonstrate a sensorimotor axonal neuropathy, often in a mononeuritis multiplex pattern. The pathologic changes in polyarteritis nodosa are limited to the arterial circulation, and the lesions are segmental, favoring the branch points of arteries. In gross pathologic specimens, aneurysmal bulges of the arterial wall may be visible. Histologic sections reveal infiltration and destruction of the blood vessel wall by inflammatory cells, accompanied by fibrinoid necrosis. Granulomatous inflammation is absent.

TREATMENT   Rx

Approximately half of patients with polyarteritis nodosa achieve remissions or cures with high doses of glucocorticoids alone. Cyclophosphamide (2 mg/kg/day, adjusted for renal dysfunction) is indicated for patients whose disease is refractory to glucocorticoids or who have serious involvement of major organs. In recent years, therapeutic regimens involving lamivudine or entecavir and plasma exchange have substantially improved the treatment of hepatitis B virus (HBV)-associated polyarteritis nodosa. Because of increasing use of the HBV vaccine, fewer than 10% of polyarteritis nodosa cases now are associated with HBV infections.

Kawasaki Disease

Kawasaki disease occurs exclusively in young children. Because of its striking mucocutaneous findings and lymphadenopathy, Kawasaki disease is also known as mucocutaneous lymph node syndrome. Features of Kawasaki disease include high fevers, cervical adenopathy, conjunctival congestion, buccal erythema, prominence of the tongue papillae ("strawberry tongue"), a polymorphous truncal rash, erythema of the palms and soles, and desquamation of skin from the fingertips occurring days to weeks into the illness.[4] In its acuity and severity, Kawasaki disease resembles toxic shock syndrome and scarlet fever, both of which are mediated by superantigens (see Pathophysiology).

In a small number of patients with Kawasaki disease, panvasculitis in the coronary vessels leads to acute cardiac complications. Coronary arteritis leads to narrowing of the vessel lumen by the migration of myointimal cells

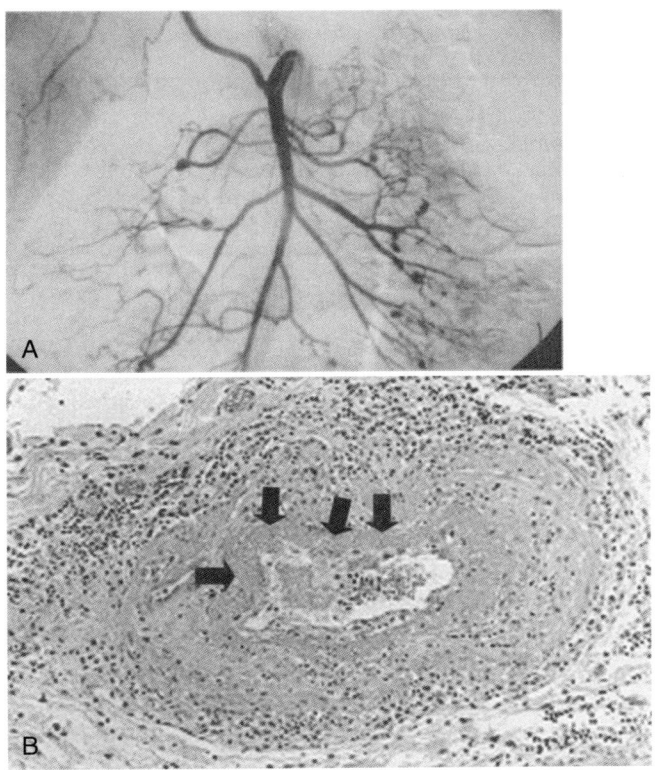

FIGURE 270-1. Vasculitis of medium-sized arteries in polyarteritis nodosa. A, Mesenteric angiogram showing numerous aneurysms in medium-sized arteries. B, Fibrinoid necrosis (*arrows*) in a jejunal artery from a patient who required surgical resection of necrotic bowel.

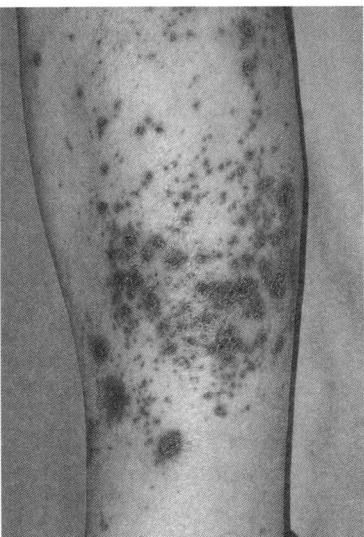

FIGURE 270-2. Cutaneous small-vessel vasculitis showing palpable purpuric lesions with necrosis and crusting.

TREATMENT $\quad$ Rx

Complete abstinence from tobacco is essential to the treatment of Buerger disease. Failure to stop smoking is associated with a dramatic increase in the risk of limb loss by amputation. No other therapeutic interventions, including glucocorticoids and anticoagulation, have dramatic effects on Buerger disease.

from the media through the fragmented internal elastic lamina. Direct complications include aneurysmal dilation and thrombosis of the coronary arteries, leading to myocardial infarction and possibly to death (in 1 to 2% of patients with Kawasaki disease during the acute illness). Late mortality from myocardial infarction may occur from the thrombosis of coronary artery aneurysms formed during the initial inflammatory stage. Such myocardial infarctions have been reported in middle-aged individuals who had febrile illnesses consistent with Kawasaki disease in childhood.

TREATMENT $\quad$ Rx

The recommended therapeutic regimen in Kawasaki disease is the combination of intravenous immune globulin (IVIG; 400 mg/kg/day on 4 consecutive days) and acetylsalicylic acid (100 mg/kg/day, lowered to 3 to 5 mg/kg/day after resolution of the fever). IVIG prevents the formation of coronary aneurysms in most cases. Glucocorticoids are reserved for salvage therapy in patients whose treatment with IVIG and acetylsalicylic acid has failed.[A1]

Buerger Disease

Buerger disease, also known as thromboangiitis obliterans (Chapter 80), is not always considered to be a primary form of vasculitis and was not included in the most recent consensus statement on nomenclature. Buerger disease has a remarkably strong yet poorly understood association with cigarette smoking and simply does not occur in the absence of exposure to tobacco. The vessels affected by Buerger disease are the distal medium-sized arteries and veins, particularly vessels at the levels of the ankles and wrists. The disease is characterized by thrombotic obliterations that begin distally and proceed proximally. Buerger disease tends to be segmental in nature, involving 5- to 10-cm lengths of blood vessels. Arterial obliteration leads to the development of collateral vessels with a "corkscrew" appearance on angiography. Vascular occlusion in Buerger disease often leads to the loss of digits and, if smoking persists, to loss of larger amounts of tissue (e.g., hands or feet). Despite the intense involvement of the extremities in Buerger disease, internal organ disease almost never occurs.

Small-Vessel Vasculitides
Antineutrophil Cytoplasmic Antibody–Associated Vasculitides
Granulomatosis with Polyangiitis

Classic GPA (formerly Wegener granulomatosis) involves the upper respiratory tract, lungs, and kidneys.[5] Distinctive features may also occur in the eyes, ears, and other organs. The three pathology hallmarks of GPA are (1) granulomatous inflammation in the upper or lower respiratory tract, (2) necrotizing vasculitis affecting arteries or veins, and (3) segmental glomerulonephritis associated with necrosis and thrombosis of capillary loops, with or without granulomatous lesions.

Approximately 90% of patients with GPA have nasal involvement, including crusting, bleeding, and obstruction. Cartilaginous inflammation may lead to nasal septal perforation and collapse of the nasal bridge ("saddle nose" deformity). Erosive sinus disease and subglottic stenosis (narrowing of the trachea just below the vocal cords) are highly characteristic of GPA.

Both conductive and sensorineural hearing loss can occur in GPA, though conductive lesions caused by middle ear disease are more common. Orbital masses ("pseudotumors" that develop behind the eye), scleritis, and peripheral ulcerative keratitis are the most dangerous ocular lesions. Episcleritis and conjunctivitis also occur. Anterior uveitis is rare. The clinical manifestations of GPA in the lung range from asymptomatic nodules to fulminant alveolar hemorrhage. The most common radiographic findings are pulmonary infiltrates, nodules, and cavitary lesions. Large-airway disease leading to bronchial narrowing is a challenging diagnosis to make because patients present with few symptoms until advanced disease is present.

The clinical presentation of renal disease in GPA is usually rapidly progressive glomerulonephritis: hematuria, red blood cell casts, and proteinuria (usually non-nephrotic). Without appropriate therapy, end-stage renal disease may ensue within weeks.

Sixty percent of patients with GPA have musculoskeletal symptoms during their disease course. The presenting complaint is frequently arthralgias or an oligoarthritis that is migratory in nature. Skin lesions in GPA include the full panoply of lesions associated with cutaneous vasculitis, including purpura (Fig. 270-2). Cutaneous nodules over the extensor surfaces of joints, particularly the elbow, may mimic rheumatoid nodules. These lesions are known as cutaneous extravascular necrotizing granulomata or Churg-Strauss lesions. Meningeal inflammation, presenting with headaches, cranial neuropathies, and a clinical picture compatible with chronic meningitis, is perhaps the most common central nervous system (CNS) manifestation of GPA. Mononeuritis multiplex may affect the peripheral nervous system.

GPA is the prototype of conditions associated with ANCA. Positive results of immunofluorescence tests for ANCA in either the cytoplasmic (C-ANCA) or perinuclear (P-ANCA) pattern should be confirmed by enzyme immunoassays for antibodies to either proteinase 3 (PR3) or myeloperoxidase (MPO). An ANCA-negative assay sample does not exclude GPA, because a substantial minority of patients (between 15 and 40% overall) lack these antibodies. Furthermore, ANCA titers do not correlate reliably with disease activity.

TREATMENT　Rx

Manifestations of GPA that constitute immediate threats either to the function of a vital organ or to the patient's life require treatment urgently. From the late 1960s until 2010, the combination of cyclophosphamide (2 mg/kg orally daily) and high doses of glucocorticoids (prednisone 1 mg/kg orally daily, tapered during 6 to 12 months) was the standard of care for GPA. Intermittent administration of cyclophosphamide by IV infusion is also effective in remission induction. However, a multicenter clinical trial that compared rituximab to cyclophosphamide in patients with either GPA or microscopic polyangiitis demonstrated that rituximab (375 mg/m² weekly times four) is at least as effective as the conventional regimen.[A2][A3] Rituximab appears to be more effective for AAV patients who present with disease flares. An alternative dosing regimen of rituximab, 1 g times two separated by 2 weeks, may also be effective. Limited forms of GPA may respond to the combination of methotrexate (up to 25 mg/week) and glucocorticoids, but rituximab is now often employed in this setting as well. Rituximab (e.g., 500 mg every 6 months) is more effective than azathioprine for maintaining remission in patients who demonstrate a tendency to flare.[A4]

Microscopic Polyangiitis

Microscopic polyangiitis is characterized by (1) nongranulomatous necrotizing vasculitis with few or no immune deposits, (2) involvement of small (and possibly medium-sized) blood vessels in the arterial or venous circulation, and (3) tropism for the kidneys and lungs. Many cases of small-vessel vasculitis once regarded as polyarteritis nodosa are now classified more properly as microscopic polyangiitis. In contrast to polyarteritis nodosa, an ANCA-negative disorder, 70% of microscopic polyangiitis patients are ANCA positive.[6] Thus, microscopic polyangiitis is considered to be a form of AAV. The ANCAs in microscopic polyangiitis are usually directed against myeloperoxidase, leading to a perinuclear pattern of staining on immunofluorescence testing (P-ANCA). Microscopic polyangiitis is not characterized by granulomatous inflammation, and upper respiratory tract symptoms, if present at all, are much milder than those associated with GPA.

TREATMENT　Rx

The approach to the treatment of microscopic polyangiitis is similar to the treatment of GPA. The combination of rituximab and glucocorticoids is the treatment regimen of choice for most patients with microscopic polyangiitis.

Eosinophilic Granulomatosis with Polyangiitis

EGPA is an eosinophil-rich form of granulomatous inflammation that involves the respiratory tract and other organs. The disease is associated with necrotizing vasculitis of small to medium-sized vessels. Two hallmarks of EGPA are asthma and eosinophilia. Several phases of EGPA are described:

- A prodromal phase characterized by the presence of allergic disease (typically asthma or allergic rhinitis), which may last months to many years
- An eosinophilia–tissue infiltration phase in which remarkably high peripheral eosinophilia may occur and tissue infiltration by eosinophils is observed in the lung, GI tract, and other tissues
- A vasculitic phase in which systemic necrotizing vasculitis afflicts a wide range of organs, ranging from the heart and lungs to peripheral nerves and skin

TREATMENT　Rx

Patients with mild disease may be treated with prednisone. Those with evidence of neurologic, cardiac, renal, or GI involvement should be treated with cyclophosphamide in addition to glucocorticoids. Although clinical remissions are obtained in more than 90% of patients with EGPA, disease recurrences are seen in 25%. In most cases, relapses are heralded by the return of eosinophilia. Approximately 50% of cases of EGPA are associated with

ANCA, usually directed against myeloperoxidase, but the percentage may be higher among untreated patients.

Immune Complex–Mediated Vasculitides

Anti–Glomerular Basement Membrane Disease

Anti–glomerular basement membrane (anti-GBM) disease is vasculitis affecting glomerular capillaries, pulmonary capillaries, or both, accompanied by the deposition of anti–basement membrane autoantibodies within basement membranes. Anti-GBM disease is discussed in detail elsewhere (Chapter 121).

Immunoglobulin A Vasculitis/Henoch-Schönlein Purpura

IgA vasculitis (IgAV) is characterized by non-thrombocytopenic purpura, arthritis, abdominal pain, and glomerulonephritis. The histopathologic findings are those of a leukocytoclastic vasculitis with IgA deposition. IgAV can develop at any age, but 80 to 90% of the cases occur in children. Although the cause is unknown, the disease's seasonal variation and the fact that two thirds of patients with IgAV experience antecedent acute upper respiratory illnesses suggest an infectious trigger. Medications such as antibiotics can also trigger IgAV, and environmental triggers are also likely. The diagnosis of IgAV can be confirmed only by demonstration of IgA deposition within and around blood vessel walls.

The classic IgAV patient presents with the acute onset of fever, palpable purpura on the lower extremities and buttocks, abdominal pain, arthritis, and hematuria. The clinician must be alert to the possibility of IgAV even when only parts of the syndrome are present. Most patients with IgAV, especially children, have a self-limited disease that lasts an average of 4 weeks.

TREATMENT　Rx

Glucocorticoids ameliorate the GI, joint, and skin symptoms in many cases, but some patients respond surprisingly poorly to conventional doses of glucocorticoids, even in doses on the order of 40 to 60 mg/day. Anecdotal evidence suggests that pulse glucocorticoids (e.g., methylprednisolone 500 to 1000 mg/day times three doses) may abort persistent bouts of IgAV. The efficacy of glucocorticoids in the glomerulonephritis associated with this condition is controversial. Uncontrolled studies suggest that methylprednisolone pulses (1 g/day for three doses), followed by oral prednisone combined with azathioprine or mycophenolate mofetil may be useful in severe glomerulonephritis associated with IgAV.

Hypocomplementemic Urticarial Vasculitis

At least three subtypes of urticarial vasculitis are known: (1) normocomplementemic, a form that is generally idiopathic and benign (which may be viewed as a manifestation of cutaneous leukocytoclastic angiitis); (2) hypocomplementemic, a form that is often associated with a systemic inflammatory disease; and (3) hypocomplementemic urticarial vasculitis syndrome (HUVS), a potentially severe condition usually associated with autoantibodies to the collagen-like region of C1q. Most patients with the hypocomplementemic subtype have an underlying systemic disorder, such as systemic lupus erythematosus (Chapter 266) or Sjögren syndrome (Chapter 268). Many HUVS patients have C1q "precipitins," IgG autoantibodies to the collagen-like region of C1q that trigger the classical pathway of complement activation. The role of anti-C1q antibodies in disease pathogenesis remains unclear.

The lesions of urticarial vasculitis must be distinguished from the far more common chronic idiopathic urticaria (Chapters 252 and 440). Unlike idiopathic urticaria, the lesions of urticarial vasculitis last more than 48 hours, often have a purpuric component (i.e., they do not blanch), and resolve with postinflammatory hyperpigmentation. In urticarial vasculitis, lesions associated with vasculitis are often accompanied by stinging or burning. Urticarial vasculitis affects the capillaries and postcapillary venules, showing leukocytoclastic vasculitis on light microscopy. Direct immunofluorescence studies reveal both immunoglobulin and complement deposition in or around blood vessels of the upper dermis or the dermoepidermal junction.

TREATMENT　Rx

Patients with urticarial vasculitis whose serum complement levels remain normal during attacks often have self-limited disease and require little therapy.

Other cases, especially HUVS, may cause life-threatening involvement of the lungs or other organs and require periods of intensive immunosuppression. Treatment decisions in HUVS must be individualized according to the patient's clinical status.

Cryoglobulinemia

Cryoglobulins are antibodies that precipitate from serum under conditions of cold and resolubilize on rewarming. Cryoglobulins are classified into types I, II, and III on the basis of whether monoclonality and rheumatoid factor activity (the ability to bind to the Fc portion of IgG) are present.[7] Type I cryoglobulins, which are monoclonal but lack rheumatoid factor activity, are associated with certain hematopoietic malignant neoplasms (e.g., multiple myeloma) and often lead to hyperviscosity rather than to vasculitis (Chapter 187). In contrast, type II and type III cryoglobulins may be associated with systemic vasculitis involving small (and often medium-sized) blood vessels. Vasculitis results from the deposition of cryoglobulin-containing immune complexes within blood vessel walls and the activation of complement.

Cryoglobulin types II and III are termed *mixed cryoglobulins* because they consist of complexes of both IgG and IgM antibodies. The IgM components in both type II and type III cryoglobulinemia possess rheumatoid factor activity (i.e., assays for rheumatoid factor are positive, indicating binding of the IgM antibody to the Fc portion of IgG). Whereas the IgM component in type II cryoglobulin is monoclonal, the IgM in type III cryoglobulin is polyclonal. Ninety percent of patients with vasculitis secondary to mixed cryoglobulins are hypocomplementemic, with C4 levels characteristically more depressed than C3. Infection with hepatitis C virus (HCV) accounts for at least 80% of the vasculitis cases associated with mixed cryoglobulins.[8]

TREATMENT Rx

Rapidly progressive sensorineural hearing loss requires early and requires aggressive therapy with high doses of systemic glucocorticoids. Some otolaryngologists also perform intratympanic injections of glucocorticoids. Cytotoxic agents can be considered for patients with suboptimal responses to glucocorticoids who still have salvageable hearing. Many Cogan syndrome patients become candidates for cochlear implants.

Variable-Vessel Vasculitides

The variable-vessel vasculitides have no predominant type of vessel involved but rather can affect vessels of any size (small, medium, and large) and any type (arteries, veins, and capillaries).

Cogan Syndrome

The combination of inflammatory eye disease and vestibuloauditory dysfunction is the sine qua non of Cogan syndrome.[9] In addition to inflammatory disease of the eyes and ears, up to 15% of patients with Cogan syndrome have vasculitis involving medium-sized to large blood vessels. Although the ocular manifestations vary, the classic presentation is the combination of interstitial keratitis and sensorineural hearing loss. Cogan syndrome may appear first in either the eyes or the ears. Although intervals as long as 1 to 2 years have been described between the start of disease in one organ and the appearance of disease in the other, the time between disease manifestations in these organs is usually only a matter of months. Patients usually present with photophobia and blurry vision, sometimes accompanied simultaneously by auditory or vestibular dysfunction. The vascular disease in Cogan syndrome resembles that of Takayasu arteritis.

TREATMENT Rx

The optimal therapy for most cases of cryoglobulinemic vasculitis is successful treatment of the underlying HCV infection. For cryoglobulinemic patients with relatively mild disease (e.g., frequent purpuric lesions, shallow cutaneous ulcers), short courses of prednisone followed by the institution of effective therapy for HCV may be sufficient. For patients with severe cutaneous ulcers, mononeuritis multiplex, glomerulonephritis, or other manifestations of severe disease, glucocorticoids, rituximab, and possibly a short course of plasma exchange may be indicated.

Behçet Syndrome

Behçet syndrome may affect small, medium, and large vessels in either the venous or the arterial circulation.[10] The most typical lesions in Behçet

syndrome are mucocutaneous, reflecting the involvement of small blood vessels. The triad of recurrent mouth ulcers, genital ulcers, and eye inflammation is the classic presentation. The criteria for diagnosis of the International Study Group for Behçet Syndrome consist of one required manifestation—recurrent oral ulceration—plus at least two of the following: recurrent genital ulceration, characteristic eye or skin lesions, or a pathergy reaction (see later). However, the spectrum of Behçet syndrome encompasses many manifestations not included in these criteria.

Large-vessel complications of Behçet syndrome may include aneurysms in the pulmonary and systemic arterial systems. Venous complications include thromboses of the deep venous system, vena cava, portohepatic vein, and cerebral sinus. Pathergy—the development of pustules at the sites of sterile needle pricks—is a distinctive feature in many patients with Behçet syndrome, particularly those of Turkish origin. The arthritis of Behçet syndrome is a nondeforming, oligoarticular, asymmetrical arthritis of large joints. GI lesions in Behçet syndrome typically consist of ulcerations of the distal ileum or cecum. Crohn disease, which can cause genital ulcers as well as GI tract disease, may be particularly difficult to distinguish from Behçet syndrome.

TREATMENT Rx

Low-dose glucocorticoids are effective for intransigent mucocutaneous disease and may have a better side-effect profile than other medications used for this purpose (e.g., thalidomide). Intermittent courses of glucocorticoids during periods of particular mucocutaneous disease activity may be sufficient for patients with mild disease.

Severe disease in any organ system almost always requires high doses of prednisone (e.g., 1 mg/kg/day). Azathioprine (2 mg/kg/day), cyclosporine (3 to 5 mg/kg/day in two divided doses), methotrexate (up to 25 mg/week), and interferon alpha (3 million to 5 million units three times a week) are appropriate therapies for many complications of Behçet's syndrome. TNF inhibition with infliximab (5 mg/kg IV every 4 to 6 weeks) or adalimumab (40 mg every other week) is the treatment of choice for patients with the most severe forms of uveitis or meningoencephalitis.

Selected Single-Organ Vasculitides

Single-organ vasculitis is defined as vasculitis within the vessels of any type or size of a single organ, in the absence of any features (e.g., ANCA) suggesting one of the systemic forms of vasculitis.

Cutaneous Leukocytoclastic Angiitis

Cutaneous leukocytoclastic angiitis has also been termed *hypersensitivity vasculitis*. Cutaneous leukocytoclastic angiitis is the preferred name because no hypersensitivity or allergy is evident in many cases. Histories of exposure to new medications or to infections may be elicited. An immune complex deposition is central to the pathophysiologic process. Although it is occasionally associated with synovitis, other signs of systemic involvement are absent.

The skin lesions in cutaneous leukocytoclastic angiitis occur in "crops," coinciding with some period of elapsed time following exposure to the inciting antigen. The usual time between the exposure and the onset of clinically evident vasculitis is 10 to 14 days. The lesions typically occur first in dependent regions, such as on the lower extremities or buttocks. The rash may be asymptomatic but is usually accompanied by burning or tingling sensations.

TREATMENT Rx

Keys to the management of cutaneous leukocytoclastic angiitis include (1) exclusion of any underlying form of vasculitis that may cause subclinical involvement of other organs and (2) removal of any agent (e.g., a medication) that may have triggered the vasculitis. For patients in whom a precipitant can be identified, removal of the offending agent usually leads to resolution of the vasculitis within days to weeks. The type, intensity, and duration of therapy for cutaneous leukocytoclastic angiitis are based on the degree of disease severity. Mild cases may be treated simply with leg elevation, H$_1$ antihistamines, or low-dose prednisone. For persistent disease not associated with cutaneous gangrene, colchicine, hydroxychloroquine, or dapsone may be tried. For severe cases, high doses of glucocorticoids are indicated to suppress inflammation quickly and prevent skin ulceration.

Vasculitis of the Central Nervous System

CNS vasculitis includes two major categories of disease, one of which is not a true vasculitis. These conditions are primary angiitis of the CNS (PACNS)

TABLE 270-5 PRIMARY ANGIITIS OF THE CENTRAL NERVOUS SYSTEM (PACNS) VERSUS REVERSIBLE CEREBRAL VASOCONSTRICTION SYNDROME (RCVS)

	PACNS	RCVS
Female-to-male ratio	1 : 1	2-3 : 1
Onset	Subacute (weeks to months)	Sudden (seconds to minutes)
Headache	Insidious, dull	Thunderclap
Typical lumbar puncture findings	Abnormal in 50-80%: lymphocytic pleocytosis; elevated protein	Normal
Typical MRI findings	Multifocal subacute infarctions	Normal Watershed infarcts in minority
Typical angiogram findings	Normal in up to 40% of cases. Abnormal angiographic features when present cannot be distinguished from RCVS	Multifocal stenoses/dilatations
Utility of brain biopsy	Reasonable sensitivity in appropriately selected patients Important for excluding disease mimickers	Little to no role Helpful if confusing clinical situation confounds differentiation from PACNS or PACNS mimickers

MRI = magnetic resonance imaging.

and reversible cerebral vasoconstriction syndrome (RCVS). The diagnosis and management of these two conditions differ dramatically. The clinical, radiologic, and pathologic characteristics of PACNS and RCVS are shown in Table 270-5.

Primary Angiitis of the Central Nervous System
PACNS[11] typically develops in a subacute fashion, with the evolution of multifocal strokes, encephalopathy, headache, and other clinical features over months. Headache is often the first symptom. As the condition progresses, most patients develop lethargy, confusion, and memory loss. Some patients develop multifocal strokes, seizures, evidence of increased intracranial pressure, or myelopathy. The results of routine laboratory tests (e.g., erythrocyte sedimentation rate) are often normal in PACNS. Lumbar puncture demonstrates abnormalities of the cerebrospinal fluid in approximately 80% of cases, usually a modest monocytosis and elevated protein. Lumbar punctures should be performed in all patients in whom the diagnosis of PACNS is considered seriously. Although the findings on lumbar puncture in PACNS patients are nonspecific, a normal lumbar puncture argues against PACNS, and the procedure frequently identifies important PACNS mimickers such as infection or malignancy.

Magnetic resonance imaging (MRI) is the critical imaging modality in PACNS. Because of the subacute nature of the disorder, MRI studies reveal multifocal CNS infarctions in most cases. Strokes, hemorrhagic lesions, and mass lesions typically occur in more than one vascular territory. A normal brain MRI argues strongly against the diagnosis of PACNS. Angiography is less helpful in the evaluation of patients with PACNS for two main reasons. First, the sizes of blood vessels involved in PACNS are often too small to be resolved adequately, even by conventional angiography. The false-negative rate of angiography in PACNS is on the order of 35%. Second, the "classic" string-of-beads abnormality on angiography, produced by segmental arterial narrowing alternating with dilations, is nonspecific and can be mimicked perfectly by a host of nonvasculitic conditions (the most common of which is RCVS). No angiographic pattern is pathognomonic for PACNS, and there is a significant tendency to overdiagnose "vasculitis" on angiographic grounds alone. A normal brain MRI in the setting of an abnormal angiogram suggests RCVS, not PACNS.

TREATMENT Rx

When employed in appropriately selected patients whose history and radiologic studies suggest PACNS, brain biopsy is associated with reasonable

positive and negative predictive values and frequently identifies important PACNS mimickers. Prednisone and cyclophosphamide are appropriate for treatment of patients who have abnormal findings on brain biopsy. Treatment courses of 6 to 12 months are recommended.

Reversible Cerebral Vasoconstriction Syndrome
Eighty percent of patients with RCVS[12] are women. RCVS is probably far more common than PACNS. Overtreatment of patients with RCVS who are misdiagnosed as having PACNS leads to substantial morbidity.

A careful history is the most important part of the evaluation. In contrast to the subacute course that typifies PACNS, RCVS usually begins in a more dramatic fashion with a "thunderclap" headache. Compared with PACNS, the neurologic signs are less severe in RCVS (e.g., encephalopathy is less common). RCVS frequently occurs in the setting of precipitants associated with vasospasm, such as in the postpartum setting or following the use of vasoactive agents such as nasal decongestants and recreational drugs.

The lumbar puncture is usually normal in RCVS, and brain MRI usually does not show multifocal CNS infarctions, with the exception of watershed infarctions mentioned earlier. The typical angiographic findings in RCVS—vascular narrowing and beading—are generally indistinguishable from those of PACNS and conditions that mimic PACNS. Multifocal vascular narrowing is particularly characteristic of RCVS. The most distinctive angiographic feature of RCVS is that the abnormalities are completely reversible, usually within 4 to 8 weeks. These abnormalities in RCVS are caused by vasospasm rather than true vasculitis. In the evaluation of patients with potential RCVS, a diagnostic strategy that can clinch the diagnosis is a follow-up angiogram 4 to 8 weeks after the first. Angiographic abnormalities due to RCVS will resolve in this interval.

TREATMENT Rx

Several approaches to the treatment of RCVS are reasonable. First, one may opt for watchful waiting. It is not clear that immunosuppression is either necessary or helpful. Moreover, attempts to treat vasospasm with calcium-channel blockers may lead to a vascular steal phenomenon, potentially causing harm. Second, because it is frequently difficult to do nothing for a patient with possibly serious CNS disease, calcium-channel blockers (e.g., nifedipine 30 mg three times daily) may be tried. Third, because of the frequent diagnostic uncertainty at the time of presentation, some clinicians opt to treat empirically with glucocorticoids (prednisone 1 mg/kg/day) for 1 month, followed by a taper over several weeks. Fourth, combinations of calcium-channel blockers and glucocorticoids are also reasonable, but cytotoxic therapy is not indicated in RCVS.

DIAGNOSIS
Differential Diagnosis
The major categories of diseases that can mimic vasculitis are displayed in Table 270-6. Certain features of a patient's case should raise the diagnostic suspicion for vasculitis. First, most cases of vasculitis do not begin suddenly but rather unfold subacutely during weeks or months. Second, pain is usually a prominent feature of vasculitis, resulting from arthritis or arthralgias, myalgias, headaches, neuropathy, testicular infarction, digital ischemia, sinusitis, otalgia, back pain (caused by aortic inflammation), postprandial abdominal pain (caused by mesenteric vasculitis), or other disease manifestations. Third, signs of inflammation such as fever, rash, weight loss, and elevated acute phase reactants are highly characteristic. Finally, multiorgan system involvement is the rule in vasculitis.

Ideally, the diagnosis of vasculitis is established through biopsy of an involved organ. Diagnoses based on angiography alone have many potential pitfalls, as discussed in the sections on PACNS and RCVS. Angiographic findings that are "consistent with vasculitis" must be interpreted in the proper context. A diverse array of other diseases, ranging from atherosclerosis to vasospasm to pheochromocytoma, may mimic the angiographic appearance of vasculitis. Systemic vasculitis can also be mimicked by two or more common medical problems or treatment complications occurring simultaneously in the same patient. Finally, high on the differential diagnosis of any individual form of vasculitis are other forms of vasculitis. For example, digital ischemia and splinter hemorrhages may be secondary to idiopathic polyarteritis nodosa. They may also be caused by polyarteritis nodosa associated with HBV infection, GPA, EGPA, microscopic polyangiitis, cryoglobulinemia, Buerger disease, or some other form of vasculitis. Because the

TABLE 270-6 MAJOR DISEASE CATEGORIES IN THE DIFFERENTIAL DIAGNOSIS OF VASCULITIDES
Other forms of vasculitis
Simultaneous occurrence of common medical problems in the same patient
Infections
Bacterial, viral, mycobacterial, fungal
Occlusive processes
Hypercoagulable states
Livedoid vasculopathy (atrophie blanche)
Atheroembolic disease
Malignant neoplasms
Lymphoma (including lymphomatoid granulomatosis)
Castleman disease
Amyloidosis
Paraproteinemias
Connective tissue disorders
Systemic lupus erythematosus, mixed connective tissue disease
Systemic sclerosis
Rheumatoid arthritis
Miscellaneous
Atrial myxoma
Calciphylaxis
Fibromuscular dysplasia
Neutrophilic dermatoses
Pyoderma gangrenosum
Sarcoidosis
Reversible cerebral vasoconstriction syndrome

appropriate interventions for these conditions vary widely, careful distinction among these potential etiologies is essential.

TREATMENT   Rx

The intensity of treatment in patients with vasculitis must be guided by the degree of disease activity. Specifically, the treatment of vasculitis should be predicated not only on abnormal laboratory test results but also on clear evidence of active disease. In addition, the intensity of treatment must be adapted to the type of vasculitis. Whereas giant cell arteritis responds to high doses of glucocorticoids in essentially all cases, for example, GPA nearly always requires an additional agent (rituximab, cyclophosphamide, or methotrexate) for disease control. In contrast, despite the dramatic fashion in which they sometimes present, most cases of IgA vasculitis and cutaneous leukocytoclastic angiitis require no immunosuppressive treatment at all.

Conventional therapies such as glucocorticoids, immunomodulating agents, and cytotoxic drugs induce remissions and control vasculitis in most cases. Moreover, in some cases—a variable percentage, depending on the type of vasculitis—the disease is curable. Unfortunately, the treatments of vasculitis have enormous potential for toxicity. Regular monitoring of patients' bone marrow, renal, and hepatic function is essential to avoid treatment-induced toxicity. Prophylaxis against opportunistic infections, particularly *Pneumocystis* pneumonia (Chapter 341), is an important part of many vasculitis treatment regimens. During the tapering of immunosuppressive medications, disease flares are common in many forms of vasculitis.

A common error is treating patients with high doses of immunosuppressive agents for too long. The most appropriate use of medications such as cyclophosphamide and glucocorticoids is to induce remission as quickly as possible with early, aggressive treatment regimens, and then to convert patients to safer treatments for the maintenance of remission. Rituximab is replacing cyclophosphamide as the drug of choice for some forms of vasculitis, particularly AAV. Patients with AAV who demonstrate a tendency to flare are often retreated with rituximab (500 mg or 1 g) every 4 to 6 months, at least until lengthy periods of disease control are established. Current treatment approaches to specific vasculitides are described under their "Clinical Manifestations."

PROGNOSIS

Assuming that the diagnosis is made before the patient has become catastrophically ill, the prognosis in systemic vasculitis is determined largely by the answers to four questions:

1. Was the diagnosis established before the occurrence of major irreversible organ damage?
2. Was aggressive (but appropriately dosed) treatment begun in a timely fashion?
3. Was there careful monitoring during treatment, and were specific steps taken to avoid drug-induced toxicity (e.g., opportunistic infection)?
4. Were the potentially toxic medications that induced remission stopped at an appropriate juncture and replaced with less dangerous medications (or was treatment stopped altogether)?

For most forms of vasculitis, the factors that determine long-term drug-free remissions remain poorly understood. The likelihood of achieving sustained remissions after discontinuation of all medications (or cures) varies according to the specific type of vasculitis.

FUTURE DIRECTIONS

Compelling laboratory and naturally occurring animal models of disease, combined with the known associations among HBV, HCV, and vasculitis in humans, suggest that additional links between infection and systemic vasculitis may be established in the future. Important strides have been made in the description of cytokine and chemokine pathways that are operative in vascular inflammation, but relevant anticytokine interventions remain to be defined for clinical therapies. B-cell depletion is emerging rapidly as the treatment of choice for some forms of severe vasculitis. IL-6 inhibition strategies are also likely to play important roles soon in the large-vessel vasculitides. Additional studies are required to define the full spectrum of clinical utility of these and other biologic agents.

Grade A References

A1. Newburger JW, Sleeper LA, McCrindle BW, et al. Randomized trial of pulsed corticosteroid therapy for primary treatment of Kawasaki disease. *N Engl J Med.* 2007;356:663-675.
A2. Stone JH, Merkel PA, Spiera R, et al. Rituximab versus cyclophosphamide for remission induction in ANCA-associated vasculitis. *N Engl J Med.* 2010;363:221-232.
A3. Specks U, Merkel PA, Seo P, et al. Efficacy of remission-induction regimens for ANCA-associated vasculitis. *N Engl J Med.* 2013;369:417-427.
A4. Guillevin L, Pagnoux C, Karras A, et al. Rituximab versus azathioprine for maintenance in ANCA-associated vasculitis. *N Engl J Med.* 2014;371:1771-1780.

GENERAL REFERENCES

For the General References and other additional features, please visit Expert Consult at https://expertconsult.inkling.com.

271

POLYMYALGIA RHEUMATICA AND TEMPORAL ARTERITIS

ROBERT F. SPIERA

DEFINITION

Polymyalgia rheumatica (PMR) and temporal arteritis, also called giant cell arteritis (GCA), are companion systemic inflammatory disorders of unknown etiology that represent a spectrum from severe proximal aches and pains and constitutional symptoms to an occlusive granulomatous vasculitis of medium and large vessels that can lead to permanent blindness or other organ and tissue damage. These disorders occur primarily in patients older than 50 years, in women more than in men; they are propagated by antigen-driven, cell-mediated (T_H1) immune mechanisms that may be associated with specific genetic markers and are highly responsive to corticosteroids.

EPIDEMIOLOGY

In the United States, the average annual incidence of PMR is 52.5 per 100,000 patients aged 50 years and older and increases with age. The prevalence is about 0.5 to 0.7%. Internationally, the frequency varies according to country, with the highest rates occurring in the Scandinavian countries.[1] The incidence and prevalence of GCA are approximately one third those of PMR.

PATHOBIOLOGY

The etiology of PMR and GCA is unknown, but both demonstrate familial aggregation and have a genetic association with human leukocyte antigen (HLA)-DR4 and a demonstrated sequence polymorphism encoded within the hypervariable region of the *HLA-DRβ1*04* gene.[2] Other genetic associations have been suggested, including polymorphisms that may be seen in increased frequency in patients with the disease. Disease in genetically predisposed patients may be triggered by environmental factors such as viruses or endogenous antigens such as elastin, and their inflammatory manifestations are directed by specific patterns of cell-mediated, T_H1-associated cytokines. The cytokine production by the mononuclear cells in the involved tissues appears to influence the clinical phenotype. Cytokine profiles characterized in temporal artery biopsy specimens obtained from patients with PMR and GCA differ. GCA tissue contains the T-lymphocyte products interferon-γ and interleukin (IL)-2 and the macrophage products IL-1β, IL-6, and transforming growth factor-β. In PMR vascular tissue, transcripts are found for transforming growth factor-β, IL-1, and IL-2 but not for interferon-γ.[3] Patients with GCA who present with fever of unknown origin and who do not have ischemic symptoms, such as visual loss, have low interferon-γ levels. Arteries that express high interferon-γ levels typically have multinucleated giant cells present; these cells remove debris and secrete cytokines that stimulate intimal hyperplasia and lead to angiogenesis. IL-17-producing T_H17 cells have also been found in involved vascular tissue and peripheral blood of patients with untreated GCA but disappear rapidly with institution of corticosteroid therapy, whereas T_H1 cells are more persistent, speaking to the possibility that more than one antigenic trigger may be involved.[4]

The adventitia is considered the immunologic center in the pathogenesis of GCA. Macrophages and T lymphocytes enter the vessel wall through the vasa vasorum with the aid of adhesion molecules and come into contact with an inciting antigen. Here, it is likely that clonal proliferation of CD4+ T cells is triggered by the presentation of unknown antigens by antigen-presenting cells. The activated CD4 cells produce interferon-γ that attracts macrophages to the arterial wall. Some of these macrophages fuse at the intima-media to form multinucleated giant cells. These cells produce vascular endothelial growth factor, which triggers neovascularization, both at the intima-media junction and at the level of the vasa vasorum, sprouting from the adventitia to the media. The subsequent immunologic events lead to a characteristic topography of mononuclear cells throughout the vessel wall. Products of the giant cells and macrophages at the intima-media junction include collagenase and nitric oxide, both of which probably contribute to tissue damage. The pathologic impact of cytokines leads not only to the characteristic medial damage but also to significant intimal hyperplasia that eventually, if it is not treated, may cause luminal narrowing and tissue ischemia.

In GCA, a transmural (involving all layers of the vessel) inflammatory infiltrate, comprising predominantly mononuclear cells and commonly with giant cells, is found in the superficial temporal arteries as well as in other large and medium-sized arteries. In elderly patients, fragmentation of the internal elastica is characteristic and helps differentiate this vascular lesion from that of atherosclerosis. Often, macrophages containing fragments of elastic tissue are found at the intima-media junction, the histologic center of the inflammatory process. As mentioned earlier, immunochemical techniques demonstrate differing patterns of cells and their proinflammatory and profibrotic products in the adventitia, media, and intima. Intimal proliferation may be prominent and lead to luminal narrowing. Fibrinoid necrosis, a common histologic feature in polyarteritis nodosa, is not seen in GCA.

In PMR, mononuclear cell inflammation can be found not only in the proximal joints, such as the shoulders, but also in the surrounding tendons, bursae, and soft tissues consistent with enthesitis. Although muscle pains may be present, no muscle inflammation is found.

CLINICAL MANIFESTATIONS

PMR and GCA are systemic inflammatory disorders that occur primarily in patients older than 50 years, in women more than in men (2:1), and in whites. PMR and GCA are particularly uncommon in African Americans. Shared characteristics of the two disorders include significant cytokine-driven constitutional symptoms, such as fever, fatigue, and weight loss, as well as a markedly elevated erythrocyte sedimentation rate (ESR), anemia, and thrombocytosis. The musculoskeletal hallmark of PMR is proximal, severe, and symmetrical morning and even day-long stiffness, soreness, and pain in the shoulder, neck, and pelvic girdles.[5] Fifty percent of patients with GCA share this characteristic proximal pain syndrome. Carpal tunnel syndrome and hand and knee synovitis may be seen in patients with PMR, but the overall presentation remains predominantly proximal, as opposed to rheumatoid arthritis, in which distal synovitis dominates. Whereas patients with PMR may appear to have proximal muscle weakness, this is invariably due to pain and not muscle inflammation (Table 271-1). Magnetic resonance imaging (MRI)[6] and ultrasound studies[7] in patients with PMR have

TABLE 271-1 GIANT CELL ARTERITIS: CLINICAL FEATURES
INFLAMMATORY
Polymyalgia rheumatica: constitutional symptoms
Fever
Weight loss
Fatigue
Laboratory abnormalities
Hematologic: anemia, thrombocytosis
Elevated sedimentation rate, C-reactive protein
ISCHEMIC
Ocular
Diplopia
Amaurosis fugax
Fixed vision loss
Complete blindness
Cranial symptoms
Headache
Jaw claudication
Scalp tenderness
Scalp or lingual necrosis (rare)
Cerebrovascular accidents
Large vessel disease
Leg or arm claudication
Diminished pulses, blood pressure asymmetry
Aortic aneurysms
LATE COMPLICATIONS
Aortic aneurysms
Thoracic aorta
Abdominal aorta
Corticosteroid complications
Osteoporosis
Fractures
Cataracts

confirmed the presence of inflammation of extra-articular synovial structures, in particular subacromial and subdeltoid bursae in the shoulders.

Specific signs and symptoms of GCA are best appreciated in their anatomic and physiologic contexts. GCA preferentially affects certain blood vessels, including the branches of the external carotid artery, the ophthalmic artery and particularly its posterior ciliary branches, and the large arteries that arise from the aortic arch and abdominal aorta. Headache and scalp pain are probably the most frequent symptoms, occurring in 50 to 75% of patients. Headache is often the first manifestation of GCA and is described as boring, severe, and constant, unresponsive to simple pain medications and persisting through the night. Classically, patients complain of persistent and prominent temporal headaches, but occipital pains can also occur. Ear, pinna, or parotid gland pain may occur secondary to involvement of the posterior auricular artery. Jaw claudication and pain due to masseter muscle ischemia on chewing occur in 50% of patients. Lingual and maxillary artery involvement can lead to jaw or tongue pain on chewing or talking. The superficial temporal artery may become tortuous, prominent, nodular, or tender, but these findings are not invariable, and an abnormal temporal artery may be found on biopsy in vessels that appear normal. It is important to note that a dry, nonproductive cough can be a feature of the disease because this often may direct the clinician away from considering GCA and more toward consideration of an infectious or neoplastic respiratory cause of the symptoms. Rarely, mononeuritis multiplex and/or sensorineural hearing loss can occur but should lead the clinician to consider other possible vasculitides such as antineutrophil cytoplasmic antibody (ANCA)-associated vasculitis or polyarteritis nodosa.

Fixed or intermittent symptoms related to vasculitic involvement of the ophthalmic arteries and its branches are the most dreaded in this illness and demand immediate therapeutic intervention. These symptoms are related to vascular narrowing due to both active inflammation and endothelial injury–mediated vasospasm. Decreased vision secondary to arteritis is the most common serious consequence of GCA, occurring in 20 to 50% of patients who present to ophthalmologists. It is the presenting symptom in 60% of patients with GCA who develop visual loss. A careful history of most patients who present with "sudden" visual loss reveals that preceding headache, constitutional symptoms, and PMR occurred in approximately 40% of patients. Even the evolution of the visual loss was often staggered, with amaurosis fugax in 10% and a partial field defect progressing to complete blindness over days. If GCA remains untreated, the second eye may become involved within

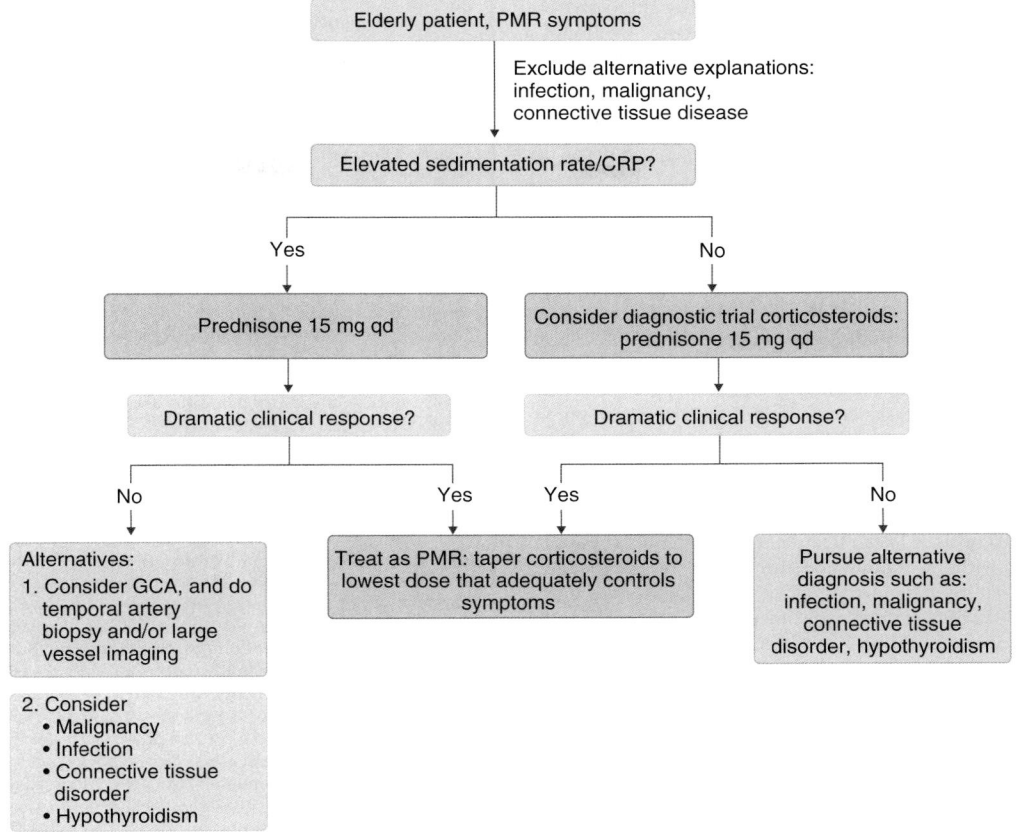

FIGURE 271-1. Diagnostic algorithm for polymyalgia rheumatica (PMR). CRP = C-reactive protein; GCA = giant cell arteritis.

1 to 2 weeks. The posterior ciliary arteries are the most frequently involved; thus, anterior ischemic optic neuropathy is the most common lesion, which can be easily defined by an ophthalmologist. Occlusion of the central retinal artery and its branches is uncommon; thus, exudates, hemorrhages, and frank vasculitis are infrequent. Five percent of patients with GCA may present with diplopia or ptosis, which may precede visual loss. The final visual abnormality can be a composite of many ischemic events occurring together in the optic nerve, the extraocular muscles, the chiasm, and the brain itself. Because GCA primarily involves arteries that contain elastica and the elastic lamina is lost as vessels pierce the dura, intracerebral lesions such as strokes are uncommon but not unheard of.

Large artery involvement most commonly presents as arm or leg claudication; rarer manifestations are stroke, subclavian steal syndrome, intestinal infarction, and symptomatic aortic aneurysm. Thus, a subclinical arteritis can exist and demands long-term monitoring. There is an emerging appreciation that some older patients classified as having GCA can present with large vessel disease resembling Takayasu's arteritis clinically, with a paucity of cranial ischemic symptoms but often the presence of PMR-like symptoms. Conversely, in patients presenting with typical GCA with cranial symptoms and a positive temporal artery biopsy, large vessel disease with aortic wall thickening is markedly more frequent than in matched controls without GCA, even early in the disease course. Steroid-treated PMR and GCA are self-limited illnesses lasting 1 to 2 years in most patients. However, a subgroup of patients with both disorders can have active inflammatory disease as manifested by persistent symptoms and blood test signs of active inflammation for 7 to 10 years. Of note is the fact that thoracic aneurysms with giant cells in the tissue can develop as long as 15 years after the diagnosis, successful treatment, and discontinuation of steroids. Indeed, the incidence of thoracic and aortic aneurysms is markedly higher in patients with prior history of presumably successfully treated GCA than in age-matched control subjects. Conversely, in studies of repaired aortic aneurysms, pathologic findings consistent with GCA have been found in approximately 2 to 4% of specimens from individuals without previously recognized or suspected arteritis. In most studies, survival rates for patients with PMR and GCA are similar to those of unaffected persons of the same age. However, one study did show that survival was decreased in a group of patients with GCA who had permanent visual loss and required more than 10 mg of prednisone per day at 6

months. This probably supports the experience that the morbidity and mortality are caused by steroid-related treatment complications in this high-risk, elderly group of patients possessing many comorbid conditions.

DIAGNOSIS

The diagnoses of PMR and GCA are based on clinical facts, with supporting but not diagnostic aid obtained from laboratory tests and temporal artery biopsy (Fig. 271-1).[8] No physician should await an abnormal finding on temporal artery biopsy or demand the presence of an elevated ESR before making the definitive diagnosis of GCA in the setting of a characteristic clinical picture. That said, the laboratory hallmark of PMR and GCA is an elevation in IL-6-stimulated acute phase reactants such as the ESR and C-reactive protein. The ESR is usually in excess of 50 mm/hour and may exceed 100 mm/hour. An ESR in the low 20s or 30s, however, does not exclude a diagnosis of PMR or GCA if other characteristic clinical features are present and especially if the patient is already taking steroids.

Normocytic, normochromic anemia and thrombocytosis occur in approximately 50% of patients with both disorders and are excellent guides to the state of inflammation. In both PMR and GCA, the frequency of rheumatoid factor, antinuclear antibody, ANCA, monoclonal proteins, and cryoglobulins is not higher than in age-matched control subjects, and complement is not reduced. Alkaline phosphatase activity may be elevated in one third of patients, primarily those with GCA. Although these tests are not indicated in PMR and GCA, muscle enzymes and electromyography are normal, and muscle biopsy shows type II fiber atrophy but no inflammation.

Superficial Temporal Artery Assessment

Temporal artery tenderness, nodularity, and diminished pulsation are typical findings on physical examination in a patient with GCA. Color duplex ultrasonography has been used as an adjunctive noninvasive diagnostic tool in GCA. A hypoechoic halo around the superficial temporal artery has been reported in 73% of patients with biopsy-proven GCA. The halo, representing edema in the arterial wall, was observed bilaterally in a significant subset of patients and disappeared in a mean of 16 days after the initiation of steroids in one study. The presence of the halo in this study had a sensitivity of 73% and was 100% specific for GCA. Other groups have been unable to replicate this experience, however, finding Doppler ultrasonography to be no more sensitive or specific than physical examination in patients thought to have the disease. Findings of stenosis or occlusion of temporal arteries by Doppler ultrasound have also been recognized as being modestly sensitive and specific for the diagnosis of GCA in some studies. Operator dependency remains a challenge to the more widespread use of this modality diagnostically. [^{18}F] Fluorodeoxyglucose–positron emission tomography may be helpful in identifying large vessel inflammation suggestive of GCA, but it is not helpful in assessing the temporal arteries themselves, given their relatively small size and high background uptake in that area. Conventional angiography is rarely used in the diagnosis of GCA. Some studies have suggested that MRI/magnetic resonance angiography (MRA) may be a helpful noninvasive diagnostic modality. Superficial cranial arteries can be visualized, and mural inflammatory changes and luminal narrowing can be identified. Large vessel involvement can also be assessed. Studies have suggested sensitivities and specificities of MRI/MRA similar to those of biopsy in the diagnosis of GCA. Nevertheless, temporal artery biopsy remains the diagnostic "gold standard" in GCA, and given the relatively easy accessibility of the artery and potentially significant morbidity of therapy in GCA, histologic confirmation is favored in most cases.

Although temporal artery biopsy continues to be an important diagnostic test for the presence of GCA, a few caveats must be stated. First, in a patient in whom the clinical diagnosis is likely, treatment with steroids should be instituted immediately without waiting for the biopsy results. Second, because of the skipped nature of the pathologic inflammatory lesions in the vessel wall, as many as 20 to 30% of biopsy specimens may be normal despite an overwhelming diagnostic likelihood of GCA. However, because the biopsy is helpful in confirming the diagnosis of GCA, in which high doses of steroids are used, the following guidelines are given. Patients with pure PMR and no GCA signs or symptoms do not need a biopsy. However, because 10% of these patients may develop such clinical manifestations of GCA within the next year, they should be told to report such symptoms immediately. When GCA is likely, an outpatient biopsy should be performed on the symptomatic side of the head, preferably including inflamed areas with tenderness or nodularity and incorporating 2 to 3 cm of vessel. Multiple sections should be requested because of the segmental nature of the disease process. Some rheumatologists routinely request bilateral biopsies, which may increase the likelihood of obtaining an abnormal finding by up to 5%, whereas others perform a contralateral biopsy if the first specimen is normal. Diagnostic biopsy findings continue to be present for as long as 2 to 4 weeks after the clinical diagnosis is made and steroid treatment instituted.[9]

Differential Diagnosis

The systemic nature of these disorders and the fact that they occur in elderly people demand careful diagnostic scrutiny to avoid missing a malignant neoplasm or major infection and possibly treating patients inappropriately with high-dose steroids. This is true in PMR because there is no diagnostic test and in GCA because the GCA biopsy finding may be normal in the face of active, vision-threatening vasculitis. Infections that must be considered and ruled out if clinically appropriate include tuberculosis, endocarditis, and hepatitis B and C. Malignant neoplasms such as lymphoma and multiple myeloma may mimic PMR, and an age-appropriate cancer evaluation is always indicated in this age group. Autoimmune disorders such as elderly-onset rheumatoid arthritis and systemic lupus erythematosus, as well as dermatomyositis and other types of vasculitis, must be considered in the differential diagnosis and sorted out by employing clinical information and serologic testing. There is support for the concept that elderly-onset rheumatoid arthritis is the same disorder as PMR with negative rheumatoid factor, a more proximal focus of joint inflammation, and a good response to low-dose prednisone. The distinction may be semantic because neither disorder tends to evolve into an erosive arthritis. A more protracted clinical course, however, is often seen in patients in whom distal synovitis is a prominent feature, and those patients are classified as having elderly-onset rheumatoid arthritis. PMR and GCA should always be thought of in the setting of a fever of unknown origin because symptoms and signs can be occult or the history incomplete.

TREATMENT Rx

Both PMR and GCA are highly responsive to corticosteroids, which are the preferred treatment choice.[10] This response is so characteristic that an immediate and dramatic improvement in PMR and GCA symptoms within 1 to 3 days after steroid institution supports the diagnosis. Conversely, a lack of rapid and significant improvement in signs, symptoms, and function within 5 to 7 days

should lead the clinician to suspect the initial impression and consider an alternative diagnosis (e.g., tumor or infection) or the presence of GCA in PMR patients that might require a higher steroid dose. Because the inflammatory burden of the two disorders is different, different doses of steroids are employed at the onset of treatment. Whereas PMR usually responds to 15 mg of prednisone daily, GCA usually requires 40 to 60 mg of prednisone per day in divided doses or higher doses if organ or tissue damage is present or threatened.[11] In GCA, if visual symptoms are present as a fixed loss or amaurosis fugax, the patient often should be treated with high-dose intravenous methylprednisolone with doses ranging from 40 mg every 8 hours to 1 g/day for 3 days, followed by high-dose oral steroids in divided doses.

Within 2 to 3 days after the institution of steroids, most symptoms of PMR or GCA clear rapidly, and patients describe a miraculous improvement. The steroid dose is then maintained for 2 to 3 weeks, during which the ESR, C-reactive protein, hemoglobin, and platelet counts normalize. Steroid taper is then instituted and guided by the clinical response. In PMR, taper is commonly by 1 mg every 7 to 10 days; in GCA, taper is by 5 to 10 mg every 7 to 10 days. In GCA, the use of alternate-day corticosteroid regimens to minimize steroid side effects is generally not recommended because randomized controlled trials have demonstrated higher rates of treatment failure with alternate-day dosing schedules. It is important that the taper be guided primarily by clinical findings (e.g., PMR stiffness, headache, fatigue) and that the level of ESR elevation be considered within that clinical context. One should never "chase the ESR" because the elderly patient would be subjected inappropriately to a dangerously high cumulative dose of steroids with their attendant side effects. An increased dose of prednisone should be based on a change in symptoms, not solely on an increase in the ESR. One possible exception is in a patient with a history of GCA and prior abrupt vision loss in one eye, in whom any further compromise of vision would be catastrophic. The effective dose demanded for a flare often can be as low as 5 to 10 mg of prednisone, and uncommonly up to 60 mg/day to control symptoms (e.g., visual abnormalities). A persistently elevated ESR (>50 mm/hour) without PMR or GCA symptoms should alert the physician to look for alternative causes, such as infection. Treatment is a careful balancing act between disease control and avoidance of steroid-related toxicity. The overall goal of the patient and the physician is to attain the best disease control with the lowest dose of steroids. In most patients, prednisone can be tapered safely in 1 to 2 years. However, other patients may need to take low doses of steroids for 2 years or more. The higher the initial dose and cumulative dose, the greater the likelihood that the patient will develop a major steroid side effect such as sepsis, osteoporosis, osteonecrosis, diabetes, emotional lability, or myopathy. Appropriate immunizations, osteoporosis regimens (calcium, vitamin D, and bisphosphonates), and metabolic monitoring are mandatory in all patients prescribed chronic steroid therapy.

The major feared outcome in GCA is ischemic complications of the disease, most often vision loss or, less frequently, cerebrovascular accident. Vision loss is usually irreversible, and although it is uncommon after the diagnosis is suspected and glucocorticoid therapy is instituted, it can occur early in the course of treatment. Aspirin is known to be protective against ischemic events in patients with atherosclerosis and has anti-inflammatory effects in inflamed blood vessels, including inhibition of interferon-γ. A recently reported cumulative meta-analysis of retrospective studies showed that antiplatelet or anticoagulant therapy has a marginal benefit when used together with corticosteroids in patients with established GCA.[12] Although this has not been demonstrated in prospective randomized controlled trials, in most patients, adjunctive therapy with low-dose aspirin should be considered unless there is a strong contraindication to its use.

Alternative immunosuppressive agents have been tested in both PMR and GCA patients in an attempt to "spare steroids" and to control the inflammatory state. Studies examining the efficacy of methotrexate in GCA have yielded mixed results, with the largest, most recent study showing no incremental benefit from combined therapy. One individual patient meta-analysis of three randomized placebo controlled trials suggested a modest benefit to methotrexate in GCA in terms of affording a steroid-sparing benefit and reducing likelihood of flares. Given the modest nature of the benefit demonstrated and the potential toxicities of methotrexate in this elderly population, methotrexate is not routinely incorporated as first-line therapy in GCA. In PMR, methotrexate has been shown in one study to afford a benefit in terms of steroid sparing and possibly reducing numbers of flares. The magnitude of the benefit appears modest, and no reduction in corticosteroid-related side effects was demonstrated. At present, methotrexate is not routinely used in the management of either disease, but in individual patients with refractory disease or excessive corticosteroid morbidities, addition of weekly rheumatoid arthritis–level doses of methotrexate (7.5 to 20 mg/week) or azathioprine (2 mg/kg/day) is employed in selected instances. There have been case series suggesting cyclophosphamide may be of value in patients with refractory disease and/or unacceptable corticosteroid toxicity, but adverse events were common, and it is rare to use this agent in GCA.

Randomized controlled trials of TNF inhibitors including infliximab and adalimumab in GCA have failed to demonstrate benefit in terms of preventing relapses or affording a steroid-sparing benefit.[13] Abatacept, a costimulatory molecule blocker, is presently being evaluated in large vessel vasculitis including GCA, in a large randomized trial, but those results are not yet available. Tocilizumab, an IL-6 inhibitor, has been of major interest in GCA and PMR because this cytokine seems pivotal in these disorders. Tocilizumab reliably reduces C-reactive protein and ESR, which in theory could be independent of a true beneficial effect on the underlying arteritis, but early controlled observations are encouraging.[14] This will be a challenge in assessing the true efficacy of Tocilizumab in GCA in the larger controlled clinical trials that are in progress.

FUTURE DIRECTIONS

Better understanding of the disease-causing roles of immunologically active cells and their cytokine products, along with genetics and correlations with clinical subsets, will lead to more focused treatment modalities and the avoidance of the need for long-term treatment with steroids. A recently published cohort study revealed that GCA is associated with increased risks for myocardial infarction, stroke, and peripheral vascular disease,[15] suggesting that greater attention should be paid to cardiovascular risk reduction in patients with this disease.

GENERAL REFERENCES

For the General References and other additional features, please visit Expert Consult at https://expertconsult.inkling.com.

272

INFECTIONS OF BURSAE, JOINTS, AND BONES

ERIC L. MATTESON AND DOUGLAS R. OSMON

INFECTION OF BURSAE
Septic Bursitis
DEFINITION

Bursae are the satellite structures that form to protect tissues from bony prominences. The superficial bursae, including the olecranon, prepatella, infrapatella, and bursae over the first metatarsophalangeal bunions, are more likely to become infected than are the deep bursae, such as the subacromial, trochanteric, and iliopsoas bursae.[1]

EPIDEMIOLOGY

Olecranon bursitis may occur in as many as 10 in 100,000 persons. The majority of cases occur in men, and antecedent trauma to the skin is frequent.

PATHOBIOLOGY

Septic bursitis of superficial bursae is most commonly due to direct inoculation through the overlying skin; less commonly, it is secondary to overlying cellulitis. Most cases of deep septic bursitis are due to contiguous spread from adjacent infected joints or hematogenous seeding.

Predisposing risk factors for septic bursitis include trauma to the skin, as may occur in plumbers, athletes, and patients with chronic obstructive pulmonary disease (COPD) who frequently lean on the elbows; prepatellar or infrapatellar septic bursitis occurs in housecleaners, gardeners, and carpet layers. At least one third of patients with septic bursitis have an underlying comorbid illness such as diabetes mellitus, rheumatoid arthritis, gout, COPD, or alcoholism.

CLINICAL MANIFESTATIONS

In immune-competent patients, septic bursitis often but not always presents with fever and erythema and warmth of the overlying skin; there may be swelling of the bursae. In contrast to those with septic arthritis, patients with septic bursitis of superficial bursae have intact range of motion of the joints, which may be limited only at the extremes of flexion. Pain on motion of the joint and restriction of joint range of motion are highly suggestive of septic arthritis. Acute phase reactants such as C-reactive protein, the sedimentation rate, and the white blood cell count (WBC) may be elevated

DIAGNOSIS

Radiography should be performed to look for a foreign body and to evaluate the surrounding bones. Aspiration of bursal fluid is helpful in the diagnosis of patients who have pain, erythema, and/or swelling of an affected area. However, given the risk for contaminating the bursa if the aspiration occurs through skin involved with cellulitis, many clinicians choose to aspirate a bursa only if empirical antimicrobial therapy has failed. Ultrasound or computed tomography (CT) guidance greatly enhances the successful aspiration of superficial bursae. Care must be taken not to violate the joint space when aspirating a bursa to avoid inoculating the joint space.

The leukocyte count of the bursal fluid is generally lower than that seen in septic arthritis, with a mean of 13,500 cells/mm³. Even in immune-competent hosts, cell counts can range from less than 1500 to greater than 100,000/mm³. A leukocyte count greater than 2000/mm³ has a sensitivity of 94% and a specificity of 79% for superficial (olecranon or prepatellar) bursitis. Bacterial culture and in vitro susceptibilities must be obtained; if additional fluid is available, a Gram stain may be obtained, although its sensitivity may be as low as 15%. The presence of crystals does not exclude the possibility of septic bursitis.

Staphylococcus aureus (Chapter 288) is the most common cause of septic bursitis, present in more than 80% of culture-proven cases, followed by β-hemolytic streptococci. Aerobic gram-negative bacilli, including *Escherichia coli*, *Campylobacter jejuni*, and *Pseudomonas* species, are rare causes of septic bursitis. Chronic bursitis may be associated with systemic infections due to *Brucella abortus*, atypical mycobacteria, or *Mycobacterium tuberculosis*, as well as fungi; the presence of these infections should raise the possibility of systemic infection.

Differential Diagnosis

In the immune-competent host, nonseptic bursitis (Chapter 263) may have a somewhat more indolent presentation than septic bursitis. The differential diagnosis includes gout, pseudogout, arthritis, and trauma with hemobursa. An overlying cellulitis may be confused with bursitis. Fever is usually not present in nonseptic bursitis due to mechanical or friction trauma.

TREATMENT [Rx]

Treatment of septic bursitis is guided by knowledge of the putative underlying organisms, in most cases, *S. aureus*. Because the Gram stain is positive in less than two thirds of patients and cultures may be delayed, empirical therapy is guided by the clinical presentation. Most patients can be treated as outpatients, but those who are immunocompromised may require hospitalization for intravenous antibiotic therapy. Initial ambulatory treatment in patients without comorbidities may consist of an oral antistaphylococcal penicillin or first-generation cephalosporin. If community-acquired methicillin-resistant *S. aureus* (MRSA) is suspected, co-trimoxazole or minocycline may be added to one of these agents. In patients who are allergic to penicillin, oral clindamycin or linezolid may be used. Patients who have severe inflammation, are septic, or are immunocompromised may require hospitalization for initiation of treatment with intravenous nafcillin, oxacillin, or cefazolin; if MRSA is suspected, intravenous vancomycin, daptomycin, or linezolid should be used. Guidelines on the treatment of MRSA have been published.[2] Vancomycin can also be used in patients who are allergic to penicillin.

The duration of antimicrobial therapy is guided by the clinical response and comorbid states. It should be continued until there is no longer bursal inflammation. This may require several weeks of intravenous or oral therapy and multiple aspirations. Failure of the septic bursitis to respond to initial antibiotic therapy mandates a second course of therapy; recurrence thereafter or inability to adequately drain the bursa with needle aspiration is an indication for surgical intervention.

PREVENTION

Because superficial septic bursitis is often associated with occasional or avocational activities involving kneeling or resting on the elbows, using protective padding may be helpful.

PROGNOSIS

The optimal duration of therapy is unknown, but prognosis of superficial bursitis is generally excellent. The presence of comorbid conditions, especially those associated with deep bursal infections, including septic arthritis, bacteremia, and osteomyelitis, is associated with more intractable and difficult disease.

INFECTION OF JOINTS
Septic Arthritis

DEFINITION

Septic arthritis refers to infection of a joint by a microorganism. It is associated with increased morbidity and mortality, as well as loss of articular integrity and function. Septic arthritis is usually caused by a bacterial infection.[3] Other microorganisms can cause infections with clinical characteristics that differ from those of bacterial infections; these are reviewed separately.

NONGONOCOCCAL SEPTIC ARTHRITIS

EPIDEMIOLOGY

The incidence of septic arthritis affecting native joints is about 5 to 8 in 100,000 patient years. Among patients presenting with an acutely swollen and painful joint, the prevalence of bacterial arthritis ranges widely, from less than 10% to as high as 27%, depending on the source population. Nongonococcal septic arthritis is the most common form of septic arthritis and is somewhat more common in men than in women.

PATHOBIOLOGY

More than 90% of cases of septic arthritis are due to staphylococci or streptococci (Table 272-1). Septic arthritis can result from direct inoculation (e.g., accidents, bites, surgery) or by extension from infected bone into an adjacent joint space. Approximately 75% of cases are due to hematogenous spread, particularly in patients with indwelling catheters and immunocompromised patients. Septic arthritis due to needle arthrocentesis (<1 in 10,000 procedures) or arthroscopy (4 cases per 1000 to 10,000 procedures) is very rare.

Bacteria causing septic arthritis produce an acute inflammatory reaction in the synovial membrane. Synovial hyperplasia and inflammatory cell immigration with the release of pro-inflammatory and cartilage-destroying cytokines and proteases result in damage to cartilage and bone. Bacterial toxins and DNA and superantigens, such as those seen in staphylococcal toxic shock syndrome, also contribute to cartilage and bone damage.

Risk factors for the development of septic arthritis include diabetes, alcoholism, cutaneous ulcers, intravenous drug use, prosthetic joints, rheumatoid arthritis, osteoarthritis, and low socioeconomic status, as well as advanced age, skin infection, indwelling intravenous catheters, cancer, and immunosuppressive therapies, including biologic response modifiers used in the management of autoimmune diseases such as rheumatoid arthritis and inflammatory bowel disease.

CLINICAL MANIFESTATIONS

Most patients with bacterial arthritis feel ill and have fever. Immunocompromised and elderly patients may not have a marked febrile response. Most cases (>80%) of septic arthritis are monoarticular; the knee is involved in more than 50% of cases. Polyarticular joint sepsis may be seen in immunocompromised patients and those with rheumatoid arthritis or systemic lupus erythematosus. Such patients frequently lack typical signs and symptoms of infection and may not appear to be particularly ill at presentation, but they may develop rapid cardiovascular decompensation. This is particularly true for patients who are taking glucocorticosteroids, other immunosuppressive agents, and biologic response modifiers, including tumor necrosis factor-α (TNF-α) inhibitors.

Patients with septic arthritis affecting nondiarthrodial joints, such as the acromioclavicular or sacroiliac joints, may have a history of intravenous drug use or may have intravenous catheters in place to treat other medical conditions. Infection of the symphysis pubis is associated with previous urinary tract surgery, pelvic malignancy, intravenous drug use, or vigorous weight-bearing physical activity, such as long-distance running, in female athletes.

A finding of microorganisms in the joint should lead to an appropriate history and physical examination to identify a source of hematogenous infection, such as cellulitis, pneumonia, or urinary tract infection. Staphylococci and β-hemolytic streptococci may enter directly through open wounds, whereas gram-negative infection may be associated with bowel or bladder disease.

DIAGNOSIS

Plain radiography should be performed to evaluate the surrounding bones and joint space and to provide a baseline for comparison after therapy is completed. Imaging modalities such as magnetic resonance imaging (MRI), CT, and plain radiography are useful to determine whether there is associated osteomyelitis and in cases of diagnostic uncertainty. Blood cultures are positive in up to 50% of patients with bacterial septic arthritis and should be obtained in all patients in whom this diagnosis is suspected.

TABLE 272-1 MICROORGANISMS RESPONSIBLE FOR ACUTE SEPTIC ARTHRITIS AND ACUTE AND CHRONIC OSTEOMYELITIS

SEPTIC ARTHRITIS		OSTEOMYELITIS: ACUTE AND CHRONIC	
MICROORGANISM	FREQUENCY (%)	MICROORGANISM	FREQUENCY (%)
Gram Positive	**60-90**	**Gram Positive**	**80-90**
Staphylococcus aureus	50-70	Staphylococcus aureus	60-80
Group A, B, C streptococci	15-30	Group A, B, C streptococci	10-20
Coagulase-negative staphylococci	6-20	Staphylococcus epidermidis	10-15
Streptococcus pneumoniae	1-3	Streptococcus pneumoniae	<1
Enterococcus sp	<1	Enterococcus sp	1-2
Corynebacterium sp	<1	Corynebacterium sp	1-2
Gram Negative	**5-25**	**Gram Negative**	**5-20**
Salmonella sp		Salmonella sp	
Pseudomonas aeruginosa		Enterobacter sp	
Escherichia coli		Pseudomonas aeruginosa	
Klebsiella pneumoniae		Brucella sp	
Enterobacter sp		Pasteurella multocida	
Kingella kingae		Bartonella henselae	
Haemophilus influenzae	<1-3*	Propionibacterium sp	
Anaerobes	**1-2**	**Anaerobes**	
Fusobacterium sp		Bacteroides sp	
Bacteroides fragilis			
Miscellaneous	**<5**	**Miscellaneous**	**5-7**
Mycoplasma		Mycobacterium sp	
Mycobacterium sp		Fungi (candidiasis, coccidioidomycosis, blastomycosis, histoplasmosis)	
Fungi			
Viruses			
Algae			

*Children.

Clinical Evaluation of Infections of Soft Tissues, Joints, and Bone

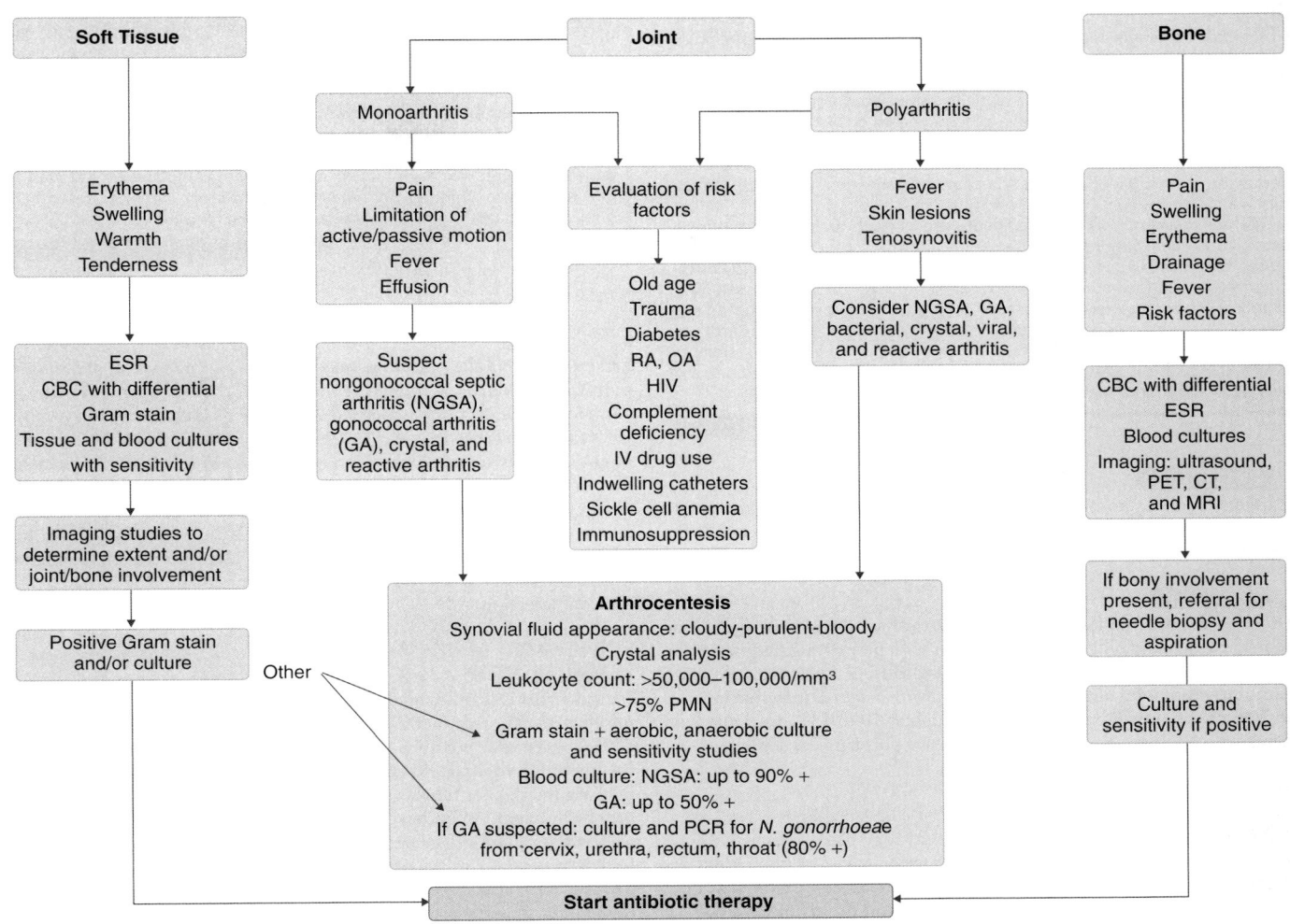

FIGURE 272-1. Clinical evaluation of infections of soft tissues, joints, and bone. CBC = complete blood count; CT = computed tomography; ESR = erythrocyte sedimentation rate; HIV = human immunodeficiency virus; IV = intravenous; MRI = magnetic resonance imaging; OA = osteoarthritis; PCR = polymerase chain reaction; PET = positron emission tomography; PMN = polymorphonuclear leukocyte; RA = rheumatoid arthritis.

If septic arthritis is suspected, synovial fluid arthrocentesis is indicated, and the fluid should be examined for bacterial culture and Gram stain; the latter is positive in only about 50% of patients. Specific cultures and stains for fungal and mycobacterial organisms should be done if there is a history of exposure or if antibacterial therapy has failed. Polymerase chain reaction (PCR) assays may be helpful for diagnosing less common joint infections such as *Borrelia,* but the value of PCR over standard culture for the diagnosis of staphylococcal or streptococcal joint infection has not yet been demonstrated. Other helpful examinations include leukocyte count and differential, as well as evaluation of the synovial fluid for the presence of crystals. The presence of gout or pseudogout crystals does not exclude the possibility of septic arthritis, particularly in patients whose WBC is above 50,000/mm³.

A frequent clinical scenario is the patient who is anticoagulated. Because of the rapidly destructive nature of septic arthritis and the often profound systemic consequences, anticoagulation is not a contraindication to arthrocentesis. The procedure may be assisted by ultrasound guidance, especially when only small amounts of joint fluid are present or when the joint is difficult to aspirate. CT-guided arthrocentesis is particularly useful for aspiration of deep joints such as the hips and nondiarthrodial joints.

The total WBC and differential in synovial fluid are helpful in distinguishing infected from noninfected joints in immunocompetent patients. A diagnosis of septic arthritis is present in 47% of patients with a synovial WBC greater than 50,000/mm³ and in 77% of patients with a WBC greater than 100,000/mm³. It is important to realize that a WBC less than 50,000/mm³, especially in immunocompromised patients, can be associated with septic

arthritis, so the absolute WBC in synovial fluid is not, by itself, a reliable way to confirm or exclude a diagnosis of septic arthritis.

Differential Diagnosis

Symptoms of septic arthritis, such as acute joint pain, swelling, and even fever, with an increase in acute phase reactants, can be caused by crystalline arthritis (Chapter 273), especially pseudogout and gout, as well as psoriatic arthritis and reactive arthritis (Chapter 265). In patients who have preexisting inflammatory joint disease, such as rheumatoid arthritis, septic arthritis may be suspected if there is a sudden onset of acute or subacute monoarticular or pauciarticular joint swelling when the disease is otherwise well controlled. The presence or absence of fever is not a reliable indicator of an infected joint (Fig. 272-1).

TREATMENT   **Rx**

As soon as the joint has been aspirated and, ideally, after blood cultures have been obtained, prompt treatment with antibiotics must be instituted. Removal of purulent material and, where appropriate, débridement are essential. The choice of empirical antimicrobial therapy is based on which organisms are thought to be the likely cause of the septic arthritis and on the results of Gram stain and culture. No advantage of one antibiotic regimen over another has been demonstrated. If the initial Gram stain of the synovial fluid reveals gram-positive cocci, vancomycin is recommended, given the increasing frequency of infection due to MRSA and the need to initiate effective antimicrobial therapy as soon as possible. Daptomycin and linezolid are alternative agents. If the initial Gram stain reveals gram-negative bacilli, an agent with broad coverage, including activity against *Pseudomonas aeruginosa*, is recommended. Such agents include ceftazidime, cefepime, imipenem, meropenem, piperacillin-tazobactam, and intravenous ciprofloxacin. If the Gram stain is negative, vancomycin alone in immunocompetent patients or in those unlikely to have gram-negative infection based on history and examination, or vancomycin plus one of the gram-negative antibacterials listed, is reasonable. Once culture and in vitro susceptibility results are available, therapy can be modified. The duration of antibacterial therapy usually ranges from 2 to 6 weeks. [A1]

The role of arthroscopic versus needle versus open drainage of the joint remains unsettled. Surgical management is appropriate for septic arthritis of the hip, for patients who fail to respond to serial needle aspiration and antibiotic therapy, and for patients who appear to be developing life-threatening complications such as necrotizing fasciitis. No studies have demonstrated the utility of lavage with or without synovectomy by arthroscopy versus arthrotomy or débridement. Patients should be mobilized as rapidly as possible to prevent joint contractures. In children, concomitant oral dexamethasone for 4 days can lead to more rapid symptomatic improvements. [A2]

PREVENTION

In patients requiring immunosuppression or glucocorticosteroid therapy to manage their underlying diseases, every effort should be made to use the lowest possible dose of these medications.

PROGNOSIS

Up to one third of patients with septic arthritis have a poor functional outcome, particularly older patients, patients with preexisting diseases of the joints such as osteoarthritis or rheumatoid arthritis, and patients with prosthetic joints. Poor joint outcome is associated with *S. aureus* infection in more than 50% of patients; mortality may be as high as 10 to 15%, particularly in patients who are immunocompromised or have polyarticular sepsis.

GONOCOCCAL SEPTIC ARTHRITIS

EPIDEMIOLOGY

Neisseria gonorrhoeae (Chapter 299) is a common cause of polyarthralgias and arthritis as well as oligoarticular arthritis and tenosynovitis in young, healthy patients. Disseminated gonococcal infection occurs in 0.5 to 3% of patients with gonorrhea (Chapter 299). Many of these patients have arthritis. Disseminated gonococcal infection and septic arthritis due to *N. gonorrhoeae* occur two to three times more often in women than in men. Most patients do not have a recent history of a symptomatic genital infection. The incidence of gonococcal arthritis is 133 cases per 100,000 population per year. Predisposing factors for disseminated gonococcal infection with arthritis include pregnancy, recent menstruation, complement deficiencies (C5, C6, C7, or C8), and systemic lupus erythematosus.

CLINICAL MANIFESTATIONS

Patients with gonococcal arthritis usually present with one of two clinical syndromes. The first is a purulent arthritis without skin lesions; the second is the triad of tenosynovitis, dermatitis, and polyarthralgias without purulent arthritis. The latter patients may have bacteremia and fever as well as maculopapular, vesicular, necrotic, pustular skin lesions anywhere on the integument. The arthritis is usually asymmetrical and may involve large or small joints, typically the elbows and knees or joints distal to these.

DIAGNOSIS

A high degree of clinical suspicion is required for diagnosis because many patients are asymptomatic for the primary infection. A thorough joint evaluation is important, as is an evaluation of soft tissues, particularly for tenosynovitis affecting the hands and feet. Cultures of blood, endocervix, and urethra are essential; cultures of the pharynx and rectum may be very helpful. *N. gonorrhoeae* is isolated in less than 30% of patients with the tenosynovitis-dermatitis syndrome and in about 50% of those with monoarthritis. PCR may be used to detect the gonococcal DNA in synovial fluid, skin lesions, urine, and throat samples, which are culture negative. Cultures should be submitted on Thayer-Martin media. Patients with suspected gonococcal arthritis should be screened for other coexisting sexually transmitted diseases (Chapter 285) such as syphilis, HIV, and chlamydia, as well as hepatitis B and C.

TREATMENT Rx

Ceftriaxone is given for 2 to 4 days, followed by oral therapy to complete a minimum of 7 days of therapy, although up to 14 days of therapy is recommended. There is emerging resistance to fluoroquinolones, and unless specific in vitro susceptibility testing is available, their use is not recommended. Patients should also be treated for concomitant chlamydia with the regimens recommended by the Centers for Disease Control and Prevention (CDC). Most patients respond well to outpatient therapy, with complete resolution of the infection. Given emerging antimicrobial resistance, the most recent CDC guidelines for treating *N. gonorrhoeae* should be reviewed.

Viral Arthritis

Patients with viral syndromes may have polyarthralgias or inflammatory polyarthritis, which can mimic rheumatoid arthritis (Chapter 264). The most common viral infections associated with arthritis include hepatitis A, B, and C; cytomegalovirus; parvovirus B19; rubella; measles; and HIV. Other forms of viral arthritis are caused by adenovirus, echovirus, Epstein-Barr virus, and herpes zoster in North America and Europe; chikungunya and o'nyong-nyong viruses, especially in Africa; and Ross River virus in Australia. Chikungunya virus, which can cause severe bone and joint pain, has spread to the Caribbean basin and mainland United States.[4] Arthritis related to viral infections is likely principally reactive in nature, rather than being caused by direct synovial infection.

Other Forms of Infectious Arthritis
FUNGAL ARTHRITIS

Fungal arthritis is unusual and most commonly occurs in immunocompromised patients. Treatment with high doses of immunosuppressants, anti-TNF agents, and possibly other biologic response modifiers used in the treatment of rheumatoid arthritis and other autoimmune diseases may increase the risk for fungal infections. The infections are often systemic and may be indolent. An understanding of the epidemiology of the organisms as well as the patient's risk factors, including occupational and avocational risk factors, is essential to the diagnosis. The most common fungi in the United States include *Blastomyces dermatitidis*, *Coccidioides immitis*, and *Histoplasma capsulatum*. *Sporothrix schenckii* fungal infections may be seen, especially in gardeners. More unusual infections occur in immunocompromised patients, including *Aspergillus*, *Candida*, *Cryptococcus*, and *Nocardia*. The reader is referred to the specific chapters regarding these organisms for up-to-date antimicrobial recommendations.

LYME ARTHRITIS

Lyme disease (Chapter 321) usually causes oligoarticular arthritis, most commonly affecting the knee. Antibiotic treatment, as outlined in Chapter 321, is effective. Polyarticular disease affecting the small joints has been associated with HLA-DR4, which is found in greater frequency in patients with rheumatoid arthritis.

MYCOPLASMA ARTHRITIS

Mycoplasma hominis (Chapter 317) causes an oligoarticular or monoarticular arthritis. Risk factors include an immunocompromised state and hypogammaglobulinemia. The treatment of choice is tetracyclines, usually doxycycline; alternatively, clindamycin or fluoroquinolones can be used.

TUBERCULOUS ARTHRITIS

Most cases of tuberculosis (TB; Chapter 324) in Canada, the United States, Western Europe, Australia, and New Zealand occur in immigrants. The arthritis is usually monoarticular or oligoarticular, affecting larger joints, and TB should be suspected in patients who have refractory monoarticular or pauciarticular arthritis thought to be secondary to another bacterial infection or to a systemic inflammatory disease such as rheumatoid arthritis. TB screening is mandatory for all patients before beginning treatment with immunosuppressive drugs or biologic response modifiers.

The diagnosis of TB may be delayed because of a lack of suspicion because patients may not have pulmonary disease. Atypical mycobacterial infection may occur in fishermen and immunocompromised patients. Appropriate treatment for septic arthritis due to TB is based on guidelines and in vitro susceptibility testing, but it often includes isoniazid, ethambutol, or rifampin and pyrazinamide as empirical therapy (Chapter 324). Atypical mycobacteria are often not susceptible to traditional antituberculous agents, and infectious disease consultation is recommended. Patients with a history of TB in whom anti-TNF therapies are being considered should be appropriately treated for TB before these drugs are started. Patients with a positive purified protein derivative (PPD) test or QuantIFERON assay for TB without a history of diagnosed tuberculosis should be treated prophylactically for several months before starting anti-TNF therapy. Clinical suspicion and culture of synovial fluid or synovial membrane obtained at biopsy are essential to the diagnosis.

SYPHILIS

Musculoskeletal involvement by syphilis (Chapter 319) is manifold in its manifestations and includes monoarticular or oligoarticular arthritis, polyarthralgias, tenosynovitis, sacroiliitis, spondylitis, chondritis, osteitis, and periostitis. Charcot's joints, osteitis, and chronic arthritis are typical of tertiary syphilis. Most patients with syphilis-related arthritis can be treated successfully. Arthritis may complicate congenital, secondary, and tertiary syphilis.

PROSTHETIC JOINT INFECTION

More than 1 million joint replacements (Chapter 276) are done each year in the United States, and this number continues to increase. Infection occurs in 0.3 to 1.7% of hip arthroplasties and 0.8 to 1.9% of knee arthroplasties, and the infection risk is two- to three-fold higher in patients with rheumatoid arthritis. Prosthetic joint infections are classified as (1) early infections, occurring within 3 months of joint replacement; (2) delayed infections, occurring 3 months to about 1 year after joint replacement; and (3) late infections, occurring more than 1 to 2 years after joint replacement.[5-7] Infections occurring within the first year are usually related to the implantation surgery itself, and late infections are usually due to hematogenous spread.

The development of a bacterial biofilm on the prosthetic joint is characteristic of prosthetic joint infection, increasing the susceptibility to infection in experimental animal models with as few as 100 colony-forming units. These biofilms are formed by bacterial glycocalyx, which increases the organisms' resistance to antimicrobial agents and likely accounts for the difficulty in obtaining viable organisms from the infected joint. More than half of all prosthetic joint infections of hips and knees are caused by staphylococci. Other organisms, including gram-negative bacilli, anaerobes, and *Candida* species, may also cause infection. In particular, *Propionibacterium* species are associated with infected shoulder arthroplasties. About 20% of cases are polymicrobial, and in 7%, cultures are negative.

Risk factors associated with the development of prosthetic joint infection include wound healing complications, prior superficial surgical site infection, prior infection of the joint, previous surgery on the joint, rheumatoid arthritis, advanced age, obesity, smoking, cancer, and diabetes mellitus. Other risk factors include simultaneous bilateral arthroplasty, prolonged operative time, requirement for blood transfusion, and infection occurring elsewhere in the body that can hematogenously seed the prosthesis.

Patients with early-onset infection may have classic symptoms and signs of septic arthritis, including joint pain, effusion, erythema, and fever. Patients with delayed infection may have only joint pain, with or without implant loosening, requiring a high degree of suspicion for the presence of infection.

The definitive diagnosis of prosthetic joint infection is based on the recovery of organisms from multiple specimens of synovial fluid and periprosthetic tissue, sonication of the prosthesis itself, acute inflammation suggestive of infection on pathologic examination of periprosthetic tissue obtained at surgery, or the presence of a sinus track communicating with the prosthesis, even in the absence of microorganisms.

An elevated sedimentation rate or C-reactive protein without another obvious cause, such as inflammatory arthritis or recent surgery, is very suggestive of infection in a patient with a painful, loose prosthesis. Plain radiographs may show loosening, new bone formation, and lucencies along the implant margin but are often nonspecific. Technetium-based scintigraphy combined with indium-labeled white blood cell scanning is suggestive of established infection but is often not performed owing to the expense. MRI and CT have low utility in diagnosing prosthetic joint infection.

Surgical treatment of prosthetic joint infection typically consists of débridement with retention of the prosthesis for acute infection, resection arthroplasty with or without staged reimplantation for chronic infection, or amputation in a few limited instances. Systemic antibiotic therapy in a patient with a prosthetic joint infection is pathogen directed and driven by the surgical therapy used to manage the infection. Following an attempt at salvage of

the prosthesis with 2 to 6 weeks of effective intravenous antibiotic therapy, chronic suppressive therapy with oral antimicrobial agents is often used. In rifampin-susceptible staphylococcal infections, its addition to a companion intravenous or oral antimicrobial is recommended to avoid the emergence of resistance, to treat biofilm organisms, and to improve the chance of salvaging the prosthesis. After resection arthroplasty, 4 to 6 weeks of pathogen-directed intravenous therapy is typical before an attempt at reimplantation several weeks later. The use of depot local antimicrobial therapy with antibiotic-impregnated polymethylmethacrylate spacers following resection arthroplasty is also very common. The reader is referred to recently released guidelines for more specific information on the diagnosis and management of prosthetic joint infection (Infectious Diseases Society of America guidelines).

PREVENTION

In addition to optimizing comorbidities such as diabetes mellitus and discontinuing tobacco use preoperatively, careful screening for infection, including asymptomatic urinary tract infection, is prudent when considering joint surgery. Perioperative antibiotic treatment with cephalosporin in patients undergoing prosthetic joint replacement reduces the risk for infection by approximately three-fold. Antimicrobial therapy should be given within 60 minutes of the initial incision, ideally before tourniquet application. Cefazolin or cefuroxime can be given to patients with normal renal function, and vancomycin can be used in patients who are allergic to penicillin.

Whether an antirheumatic agent should be stopped before joint replacement surgery is unclear. The usual practice is to hold drugs such as methotrexate, anti-TNF agents, and other biologics including abatacept and tocilizumab for one to four half-lives before and after surgery. No guidelines exist for tofacitinib or anakinra, but similar suggestions may be helpful. It may be prudent to wait at least 8 to 12 weeks after rituximab therapy for rheumatoid arthritis before performing elective joint replacement; it is unclear whether B-cell reconstitution plays a role in surgical infection risk. The impact of these strategies on reducing prosthetic joint infections is unknown.

OSTEOMYELITIS

DEFINITION

Osteomyelitis is a bacterial infection of bone that causes destruction and can occur through a variety of mechanisms.[8,9]

EPIDEMIOLOGY

Osteomyelitis of the bones of the foot in adult patients with diabetes, neuropathy, and arterial insufficiency is very common. Management of osteomyelitis in diabetic feet is discussed in updates for Chapter 229. Hematogenous seeding of the spine also occurs but less frequently. The incidence of osteomyelitis due to trauma and surgery is increasing.

PATHOBIOLOGY

Osteomyelitis can develop from (1) hematogenous seeding from a distant infection, (2) contiguous spread from nearby skin and joints, and (3) penetration of microorganisms into bone at the time of trauma or surgery. Unless there is trauma or the presence of a foreign body, bone is typically very resistant to infection. Organisms such as *S. aureus* cause disease more frequently because they colonize the skin in up to 30 to 40% of individuals, frequently cause cellulitis and bacteremia, and have the ability to bind to bone through the expression of receptors for fibronectin and collagen.

Hematogenous causes of osteomyelitis typically present in elderly people; it usually involves two or more vertebrae and their intervening disc spaces. Bacteria gain access to these structures through the arterial and venous systems (Batson's venous plexus). Bacteremia from any source can cause osteomyelitis of the spine, but cellulitis, urinary tract infection, and pneumonia are the most common sources.

Contiguous focus osteomyelitis is common in adults, typically occurring in elderly people. It results from the spread of infection from nearby skin, often in the feet of patients with diabetes, neuropathy, or vascular insufficiency, or in pelvic bones in patients with decubitus due to impaired sensation from spinal cord injury or disease. Alternatively, it can occur at the time of orthopedic surgery, from contamination at the time of an open fracture, or from a human or animal bite.

Acute osteomyelitis has a duration of less than 10 days, whereas chronic infection has a duration of more than 10 days. *S. aureus* is the most common cause of hematogenous and contiguous osteomyelitis in adults.

Osteomyelitis due to β-hemolytic streptococci and aerobic gram-negative bacilli is much less common, but it can occur if infections due to these organisms result in hematogenous seeding, if nosocomial contiguous osteomyelitis occurs due to surgical site infection, or if contamination occurs at the time of traumatic open fracture. Polymicrobial infection, including infection due to anaerobes, is very common in osteomyelitis of the bones of the feet associated with diabetes and vascular insufficiency. Coagulase-negative staphylococci can be pathogenic in patients with orthopedic implants.

CLINICAL MANIFESTATIONS

Localized pain over the affected bones is a hallmark of osteomyelitis. A sinus tract or swelling and erythema due to concomitant soft tissue infection or abscess may be present in osteomyelitis due to contiguous infection. Constitutional symptoms, including fever, are present in the minority of cases and more often in hematogenous osteomyelitis. If neurologic structures are involved, neurologic signs and symptoms may be present. Signs and symptoms due to a coexisting infection that has caused hematogenous osteomyelitis may be present as well. The differential diagnosis of osteomyelitis includes diseases that can cause acute and chronic bone pain in adults, including osteoarthritis, metastatic malignancy, fractures, and SAPHO (synovitis, acne, pustulosis, hyperostosis, and osteitis) syndrome, as well as postoperative pain and soft tissue infection without concomitant osteomyelitis.

DIAGNOSIS

The WBC is often elevated in hematogenous and acute osteomyelitis. Serum inflammatory markers such as the sedimentation rate and C-reactive protein are often abnormal, particularly in cases of hematogenous infection, but may be normal in chronic contiguous osteomyelitis. Blood cultures are positive in 25 to 50% of cases of hematogenous infection but are almost always negative in chronic osteomyelitis unless concomitant soft tissue infection is present. In the setting of chronic contiguous osteomyelitis, plain radiographs often show specific abnormalities; in vertebral osteomyelitis, they are often not helpful in confirming the diagnosis of infection.

The ability to percutaneously probe or palpate bone with a probe is a simple, effective diagnostic test in patients with diabetes mellitus and possible contiguous osteomyelitis of the feet. In one prospective study, the ability to palpate bone through a contiguous ulcer had a sensitivity of 66% and a specificity of 85% for osteomyelitis.

MRI is the most sensitive and diagnostic imaging technique to identify osteomyelitis, except when orthopedic implants are present. Gallium scans are more sensitive and specific than three-phase technetium (^{99m}Tc) bone scans or indium-labeled leukocyte scans for the diagnosis of vertebral osteomyelitis. Gallium scans are used when spinal hardware is present that degrades the magnetic resonance images and in cases of skull bone osteomyelitis due to malignant external otitis.

Multiple specimens of involved bone, contiguous soft tissue, and purulence should be sent for Gram stain, aerobic and anaerobic culture, and pathologic examination at the time of bone biopsy or surgical débridement. If the history, examination, or imaging is suggestive of atypical infection, culture for fungi and mycobacteria or other unusual organisms should be performed.

TREATMENT   Rx

There are no large randomized studies comparing antimicrobial therapy for osteomyelitis.[A2] Antimicrobials for specific pathogens based on in vitro susceptibility testing are recommended, and examples of antimicrobials used to treat common pathogens causing osteomyelitis and septic arthritis are shown in Table 272-2. Oral antibiotics can achieve adequate levels in bone, and oral and parenteral therapies may achieve similar cure rates in some cases.

The duration of antimicrobial therapy is almost always dictated by surgical therapy in chronic osteomyelitis. For example, if an amputation is performed, a short course of antimicrobial therapy may be required, whereas if an extensive débridement of chronic osteomyelitis is performed, prolonged intravenous antimicrobial therapy for 4 to 6 weeks is typically recommended. If the surgical therapy could lead to a worse outcome than no surgery, chronic oral antimicrobial suppression may be recommended. Acute hematogenous vertebral osteomyelitis in adults is typically treated with 6 weeks of intravenous antimicrobial therapy, without surgical intervention, after identification of the pathogen through percutaneous or open biopsy. Hyperbaric oxygen therapy for chronic osteomyelitis is controversial.

TABLE 272-2 ANTIMICROBIAL THERAPY FOR SELECTED MICROORGANISMS IN OSTEOMYELITIS OR SEPTIC ARTHRITIS IN ADULTS

MICROORGANISM	FIRST CHOICE*	ALTERNATIVE CHOICE
Methicillin/oxacillin/nafcillin-sensitive staphylococci	Nafcillin sodium or oxacillin sodium 1.5-2 g IV q4-6h for 4-6 wk or cefazolin 1-2 g IV q8h	Vancomycin 15 mg/kg IV q12h for 4-6 wk
Methicillin/oxacillin/nafcillin-resistant staphylococci (MRSA)	Vancomycin† 15 mg/kg IV q12h or daptomycin 6 mg/kg IV q24h	Linezolid 600 mg PO/IV q12h or levofloxacin† 500-750 mg PO/IV daily
Penicillin-sensitive streptococci	Aqueous penicillin G 20 × 10^6 U/24 hr IV either continuously or in 6 equally divided daily doses or ceftriaxone 1-2 g IV q24h or cefazolin 1-2 g IV q8h	Vancomycin 15 mg/kg IV q12h
Enterococci	Aqueous crystalline penicillin G 20 × 10^6 U/24 hr IV either continuously or in 6 equally divided daily doses or ampicillin sodium 12 g/24 hr IV either continuously or in 6 equally divided daily doses; the addition of gentamicin sulfate 1 mg/kg IV or IM q8h for 1-2 wk is optional	Vancomycin† 15 mg/kg IV q12h; the addition of gentamicin sulfate 1 mg/kg IV or IM q8h for 1-2 wk is optional
Enterobacteriaceae	Ceftriaxone 2 g IV q24h	Ciprofloxacin† 500-750 mg PO q12h
Pseudomonas aeruginosa	Cefepime 2 g IV q8-12h	Ciprofloxacin† 750 mg PO q12h or ceftazidime 2 g IV q8h

*Antimicrobial selection should be based on in vitro sensitivity data, as well as allergies, intolerances, and drug interactions in individual patients.
†Doses shown are based on normal renal and hepatic function and may need to be adjusted or serum levels monitored (vancomycin).
MRSA = methicillin-resistant *Staphylococcus aureus*.
Adapted from Berbari EF, Steckelberg JM, Osmon DR. Osteomyelitis. In: Mandell GL, Bennett JE, Dolin R, eds. *Mandell, Douglas, and Bennett's Principles and Practice of Infectious Diseases*, 7th ed. Philadelphia: Churchill Livingstone/Elsevier; 2010:1457-1467.

PREVENTION

Improving the control of diabetes and decreasing the incidence of peripheral vascular disease will reduce the incidence of diabetic foot bone infection. Optimal strategies to prevent surgical site infection after orthopedic procedures will prevent orthopedic implant infection after surgery and open fractures.

PROGNOSIS

The success of osteomyelitis management depends on the medical and surgical therapy employed and the ability to improve comorbidities such as arterial insufficiency. The ability of orthopedic surgeons to perform more extensive reconstructive surgery has allowed more extensive débridement and higher success rates, as well as restoration of function. Treatment failure can lead to relapse of infection or progression of infection to involve more of the affected bone. Long-standing osteomyelitis can be complicated by amyloidosis, squamous cell carcinoma of the skin in a chronic sinus tract, or primary bone malignancy.

Grade A References

A1. American Academy of Orthopedic Surgeons (AAOS). Advisory statement. Recommendations for the intravenous antibiotic prophylaxis in primary total joint arthroplasty. 2004. Retrieved October 6, 2014, from http://www.aaos.org/about/papers/advistmt/1027.asp.
A2. Conterno LO, da Silva Filho CR. Antibiotics for treating chronic osteomyelitis in adults. *Cochrane Database Syst Rev.* 2013;9:CD004439.

GENERAL REFERENCES

For the General References and other additional features, please visit Expert Consult at https://expertconsult.inkling.com.

273

CRYSTAL DEPOSITION DISEASES

N. LAWRENCE EDWARDS

The destructive potential of intrasynovial crystals has been recognized for more than a century. The mechanisms by which certain crystals induce inflammation and joint destruction have become much better clarified over the past several decades. The three most common crystal-induced arthropathies are caused by precipitation of monosodium urate monohydrate (MSU), calcium pyrophosphate dehydrate (CPPD), and basic calcium phosphate (BCP) and are termed *gout, CPPD arthropathy,* and *basic calcium arthropathy,* respectively.

At the turn of the 20th century, Wilhelm His and Max Freudweiler at the University of Leipzig proved that MSU crystals could induce inflammation when injected into normal joints. In 1961, Daniel McCarty and Joseph Hollander developed a way of identifying MSU crystals in synovial fluid using compensated polarized light microscopy. This technique also allowed for distinguishing MSU crystals from the other "phlogistic" crystals such as CPPD and BCP.

The role of calcium-containing crystals in cartilage pathology and joint disease was first suggested in serial radiographs by Zitnan and Sitaj that showed accretion of calcific deposits in articular cartilage leading to accelerated joint destruction. The nature and structure of CPPD crystals in inflamed synovial fluid was first described by McCarty and collaborators in 1962. This group also established the term *pseudogout* to describe this common crystalline arthropathy.

Basic calcium crystals are ultra-microscopic in size and are not detected by the compensated polarized microscopy used to identify MSU and CPPD crystals. Paul Dieppe and Ralph Schumacher independently identified these very small crystals in synovial fluid using electron microscopy in the mid-1970s. Like MSU and CPPD crystals, BCP crystals are biologically active and can accelerate atrophic changes in bone and cartilage. This chapter defines these separate crystalline arthropathies and describes their different pathogeneses and treatments.

GOUT AND HYPERURICEMIA

DEFINITION

Gout is an inflammatory arthritis of metabolic origin that is caused by crystallization of MSU crystals within joints. It is the most common inflammatory joint disease in men and in older women. Its incidence and prevalence are increasing worldwide. The metabolic derangement responsible for gout is the supersaturation of blood and body fluids with the urate ion to the point that crystal formation is possible. At physiologic pH and at normal body temperature, urate is considered to be supersaturated at concentrations of 6.8 mg/dL or greater. Therefore, from a biologic perspective, hyperuricemia is any serum urate level greater than 6.8 mg/dL in both men and women. Although hyperuricemia is a necessary prerequisite for developing gout, only 20% of all hyperuricemic subjects will ultimately develop gout.

The natural course of gout progresses from an intermittent monoarthritis or oligoarthritis in the lower extremities to a chronic, destructive, and debilitating polyarthritis involving almost any peripheral joint in the body. Also considered within the definition of gout is the spectrum of clinical conditions resulting from the deposition of MSU crystals in the subcutaneous tissues and kidney manifesting as tophaceous deposits, inflammatory cellulitis, urate nephropathy, and kidney stones.

EPIDEMIOLOGY

Hyperuricemia is very common in Western cultures, with prevalence as high as 15 to 20% being reported in some more recent population-based studies.[1] This rate of hyperuricemia is more than twice that observed just three decades earlier. A number of factors have been proposed to explain this dramatic rise. These include the overall increase in longevity; the increased prevalence of hypertension, metabolic syndrome, and obesity; the ubiquitous use of thiazide diuretics and low-dose aspirin; changes in dietary trends, including the greater use of high-fructose corn syrup as a sweetener; and finally, the increase in survival of patients end-stage renal disease and organ transplantation.

There is a direct correlation between the degree of serum urate elevation and the likelihood of developing gout. The reported annual incidence of gout in subjects with baseline serum urate levels greater than or equal to 9 mg/dL is 4.9%, compared with only 0.5% in people with serum urate levels of 7.0 to 8.9 mg/dL.

Epidemiologic surveys since the 1970s demonstrate a continuous increase in the prevalence of gout. According to the most recent National Health and Nutrition Examination Survey (NHANES 2007-2009), 8.3 million adults in the United States are followed by a health care provider for gout, a prevalence of 3.9%. Men continue to make up the majority of the gout population (73%). The prevalence of gout in women has been rising at a disproportionately higher rate.

PATHOBIOLOGY

Uric acid is the end product of purine metabolism in humans. In most mammals, purine catabolism is taken one step further through the enzyme uric acid oxidase or uricase, with the purine end product in these species being the very soluble allantoin. Humans and most other hominoids lost the ability to produce the enzyme uricase nearly 18 million years ago. As a result, uric acid accumulation is possible. Whether caused by overproduction of uric acid or its underexcretion by the kidneys, this accumulation leads to supersaturation of urate ion in blood and the precipitation of MSU crystals in synovial fluid, soft tissues, and organs. Urate is produced by the conversion of a very soluble molecule, hypoxanthine, to the less soluble xanthine, which, in turn, is converted to the very insoluble uric acid by progressive purine ring oxidations catalyzed by the enzyme xanthine oxidase. Xanthine oxidase is present in several organs, but most activity in the body is found in the liver and intestines. Because of its potential for causing disease, urate elimination is very important. The total daily accumulation of uric acid from de novo synthesis, nucleotide degradation, and dietary consumption is between 800 and 1200 mg/day and is balanced by renal excretion of approximately two thirds of the total amount and intestinal elimination by the remaining one third.

Simply put, hyperuricemia occurs when urate production is not balanced by renal excretion. In 90% of all gout patients, the cause of this imbalance is renal underexcretion. The remaining 10% of gout cases are caused by purine overproduction or a combination of overproduction and underexcretion. The nongenetic causes of hyperuricemia include other medical conditions, dietary components, and medications (Table 273-1). These factors may result in either overproduction or diminished renal clearance of uric acid. Similarly, the genetic causes of hyperuricemia (Table 273-2) may affect either production or elimination of uric acid.[2]

TABLE 273-1 NONGENETIC CAUSES OF HYPERURICEMIA

IMPAIRED URIC ACID EXCRETION

Clinical Conditions

Reduced glomerular filtration rate
Hypertension
Obesity
Systemic sclerosis
Lead nephropathy

Drugs

Diuretics
Ethanol
Low-dose salicylates (0.06-3.0 g/day)
Cyclosporine
Tacrolimus
Levodopa

EXCESSIVE URIC ACID PRODUCTION

Clinical Conditions

Myeloproliferative and lymphoproliferative neoplasms
Obesity
Psoriasis

Diet and Drugs

Alcoholic beverages (especially beer)
Red meat, organ meat, shellfish
High fructose corn syrup
Cytotoxic drugs
Nicotinic acid
Pancreatic extract

Renal Urate Underexcretion

Because uric acid is small and not protein bound, it is completely filtered by the glomerulus. In normal persons, approximately 8 to 10% of the filtered load is ultimately cleared in the urine. The various renal tubular transporters that are responsible for determining how much of the filtered uric acid is actually excreted are located in the proximal convoluted tubules and are referred to collectively as the *transportasome* (Fig. 273-1). Both reabsorption and secretion occur in this segment through the actions of several organic acid transporters (OATs), with the net effect being the reabsorption of nearly 90% of the uric acid filtered at the glomerulus. These OATs are also responsible for eliminating organic acids other than uric acid as well as many commonly used medications. The most important tubular transporter of uric acid is URAT1. This transporter swaps urate ions for other monocarboxylate organic ions in both directions across the luminal membrane of proximal tubular cells. This system can be driven to reabsorb more uric acid from the tubular lumen by raising tubular epithelial concentrations of lactate, pyruvate, or the ketoacids acetoacetate and β-hydroxybutyrate. Certain drugs, when present in the tubular lumen, can displace uric acid from the transporter, causing more uric acid to be lost in the urine. These compounds include probenecid, losartan, and high-dose aspirin and are considered uricosuric.

When renal clearance of uric acid is compared between normal adult men and gouty men, the gouty subjects excrete only 70% as much uric acid as normal individuals at any given serum urate concentration. In general, gouty subjects required a serum urate concentration to be 1.7 mg/dL higher to obtain the same level of excretion as seen in normal subjects.

Most genetic polymorphisms associated with gout in genome-wide association studies encode for the various components of the uric acid transportasome. Polymorphisms in the glucose transporter GLUT-9 (encoded by the *SLC2A9* gene) are statistically the most significant determinants of serum urate. ABCG2 is a multifunctional transporter that belongs to the adenosine triphosphate (ATP)-binding cassette family found in the proximal tubule of the kidney as well as in the small intestine and liver. Polymorphisms in the *ABCG2* gene have a larger effect on urate levels in men than in women. Polymorphisms in the gene encoding URAT1 may lead to either hypouricemia or hyperuricemia. A loss-of-function mutation results in familial renal hypouricemia. Other mutations have been detected that lead to hyperuricemia and gout in Mexican, Asian, and African American populations.

The serum urate variance explained by these common genetic variants is only about 6% of the total variance observed between gouty and nongouty subjects. Similar risk-stratifying techniques demonstrate that 67% of the variance is caused by nongenetic factors such as serum creatinine, ethanol consumption, and the components of the metabolic syndrome.

Urate Overproduction

In approximately 10% of gouty subjects, hyperuricemia is caused by uric acid overproduction rather than reduced renal excretion. In most of these people,

TABLE 273-2 GENETIC CAUSES OF HYPERURICEMIA	
SYNDROME	**PHENOTYPE**
INBORN ERRORS OF PURINE METABOLISM	
Hypoxanthine-guanine phosphoribosyl transferase deficiency	Neurologic dysfunction, renal stones, early-onset gout
Phosphoribosyl pyrophosphatase synthetase overactivity	Neurologic dysfunction, early-onset gout
EXCESSIVE CELL DEATH AND URATE GENERATION	
Glycogen storage disease I	Growth restriction, lactic acidosis, early-onset gout
Glycogen storage disease III	Early-onset gout
Glycogen storage disease V	Early-onset gout
Glycogen storage disease VII	Early-onset gout
Fructose-1-phosphate aldolase deficiency	Growth restriction, liver failure, early-onset gout
Myoadenylate deaminase deficiency	Myopathy, gout
Carnitine palmitoyltransferase II deficiency (late onset)	Rhabdomyolysis, gout
REDUCED RENAL EXCRETION OF URIC ACID	
Medullary cystic kidney disease	Renal dysfunction, early-onset gout
Familial juvenile hyperuricemic nephropathy	Renal dysfunction, early-onset gout
Uric acid transportasome mutations	
GLUT-9	Familial gout
ABCG2	Familial gout
URAT1	Familial gout

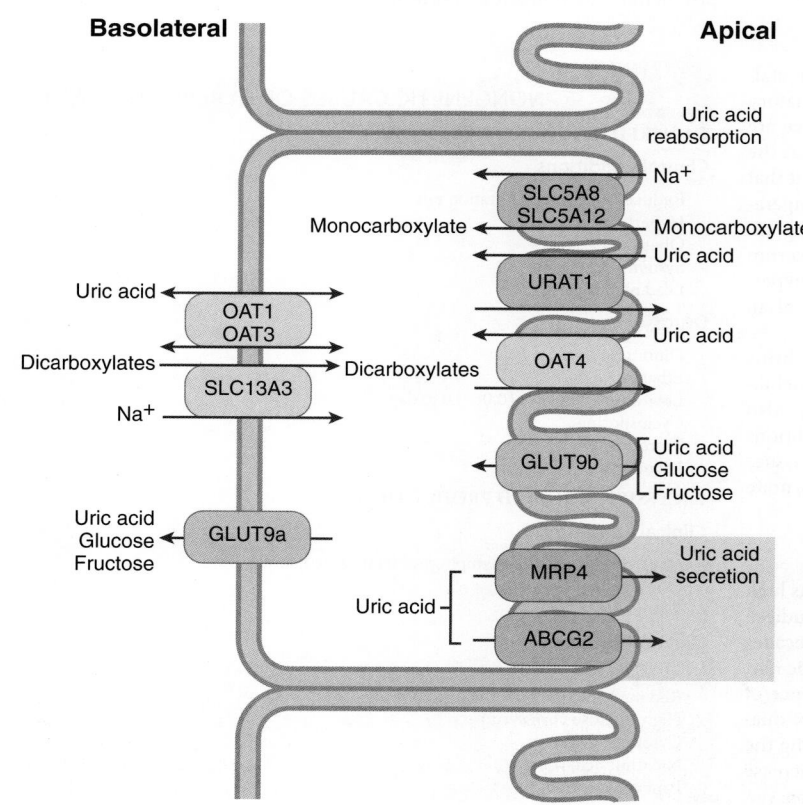

FIGURE 273-1. Renal transport of urate in proximal tubule of kidney. Serum urate reaches the tubule lumen by glomerular filtration and by secretion through the proximal tubular epithelium. Secretion of urate is facilitated in the luminal direction by MRP4, UAT, ABCG2, and NTP1, and at the basolateral membrane by OAT1 and OAT3. Reabsorption of urate from the tubular lumen is facilitated by URAT1, OAT4, OAT10, and the short isoform of GLUT (GLUT9b), and at the basolateral membrane by the long isoform (GLUT9a). ABCG2 = adenosine-triphosphate-binding cassette transporter; GLUT = glucose transporter; MRP = multidrug-resistance-related protein; NTP = sodium phosphate transport protein; OAT = organic acid transporters; URAT = uric acid transporter.

the hyperuricemia reflects accelerated cell turnover (e.g., lymphoproliferative and myeloproliferative diseases, psoriasis, chronic hemolytic states, polycythemia vera, and certain muscle glycogenoses) or other causes of enhanced purine nucleotide breakdown as seen with alcohol abuse or fructose ingestion. In addition to these secondary causes of urate overproduction, there are primary disease processes that are also responsible for urate overproduction. These are inborn errors of metabolism that result in increased de novo purine synthesis, as seen in PRPP synthetase overactivity or decreased purine salvage as seen in the complete and partial HPRT deficiencies (Lesch-Nyhan syndrome and Kelley-Seegmiller syndrome, respectively). Regardless of the cause, urate overproduction is determined by a 24-hour urine collection showing greater than 1000 mg of uric acid while eating a standard Western diet.

Pathogenesis of Monosodium Urate Monohydrate Crystals and Inflammation

MSU crystals in joints, soft tissues, and organs are the cause of pain and destruction in gout. Urate crystals will form only when physiologic conditions permit. In plasma, urate becomes insoluble at concentrations of 6.8 mg/dL (408 μmol/L) with a pH of 7.40 and normal body temperature. A reduction in pH or temperature will lower the solubility threshold even further. Not all people who are hyperuricemic will form crystals, however. There appears to be an additional requirement of a "nucleation factor" that is still poorly defined for gout and other local factors that either promote or inhibit further crystal growth.

MSU crystals form in joints and soft tissues of individuals long before they have any symptoms of gout. They deposit in small lattice structures called *microtophi* on the surface of cartilage and synovial lining. These microtophi slowly grow but are generally stable as long as the environment surrounding them does not change drastically with regard to pH, urate concentration, or temperature. At the time of the first and subsequent flares, something does change in the joint environment to cause these crystal lattice structures to break apart and shed a massive number of crystals into the joint space. These newly released and nonopsonized crystals activate receptors on synovial macrophages and are then phagocytized by monocytes and macrophages, leading to interaction with the NALP3 inflammasome. This results in the rapid production of interleukin-1 (IL-1), which is responsible for all the cardinal features of the severe inflammation associated with acute gout. The gout flare is self-limited probably as a result of a physical change in the MSU crystals after they have been repeatedly phagocytized and partially digested. A maturation of the resident monocytes in the inflamed joint also appears to help terminate the gouty flare. Even after the acute attack subsides, low-grade inflammation persists in the asymptomatic joint. It is this persistent, ongoing inflammatory process that will eventually lead to bony erosion, cartilage destruction, and synovial hypertrophy if the hyperuricemia is not treated and the MSU crystals dissolved.

CLINICAL MANIFESTATIONS
Classic Gout

The natural course of classic gout passes through three stages: asymptomatic hyperuricemia, acute intermittent gout, and chronic advanced gout.[3] The rate of progression from asymptomatic hyperuricemia to chronic advanced gout varies considerably from one person to another and is dependent on numerous factors, the most important being the degree of increase in serum urate levels.

Asymptomatic hyperuricemia[4] refers to a state in which serum urate exceeds the level of solubility (6.8 mg/dL), but symptoms of crystalline deposition have not occurred. Only 15 to 20% of all hyperuricemic people are prone to develop MSU crystals, and for this group, the period of asymptomatic hyperuricemia begins a stage of subclinical structural changes. In men, asymptomatic hyperuricemia frequently begins at puberty, whereas in women, it is usually delayed until menopause.

The initial episode of acute gout usually follows decades of asymptomatic hyperuricemia. In men, the first attack usually occurs between the fourth and sixth decades of life. In women, the age of onset is older and varies with several factors, most importantly the age of menopause. The classic acute gout attack is hallmarked by the rapid development of warmth, swelling, erythema, and exquisite pain in one or occasionally two joints. The characteristically severe pain evolves from its faintest twinge to its most intense level over an 8- to 12-hour period. Initial attacks are usually monoarticular and involve lower extremity joints. The most common joint involved is the first metatarsal phalangeal joint (termed *podagra*), followed by the ankle, midfoot, and knee (Fig. 273-2). After years of acute intermittent attacks, upper extremity joints, including the wrists, elbows, and small joints of the hands, can also become involved. Systemic symptoms of fever, chills, and malaise may accompany acute attacks, along with an intense erythema extending beyond the area of the involved joint. This may lead to confusion with a septic process.

Factors capable of provoking episodes of acute gout are those that cause fluctuations in serum urate levels, including trauma, surgery, starvation, overindulgence in certain high-purine foods, and the ingestion of any medication that raises or lowers serum urate.

The other characteristic of classic gout flares is the self-remitting nature. For the first several acute flares, the duration of the attack is 5 to 8 days. The resolution of symptoms is gradual but complete, even if no anti-inflammatory therapy is administered. The periods between the acute attacks are devoid of articular pain, although synovial fluid aspirates during this stage continue to show low-grade inflammation and the presence of MSU crystals.

Eventually, the untreated patient will progress to chronic polyarticular gout, also referred to as *advanced gout*. This stage usually develops after 10 or more years of acute intermittent gout and is evident when the pain-free intercritical periods have disappeared. Gouty flares can continue to occur against this constantly painful background. The intensity of the chronic pain is not nearly as severe as that experienced with the acute flares.

The subcutaneous tophus is the most characteristic lesion of advanced gout. The development of tophaceous deposits of MSU is a function of the duration and severity of hyperuricemia. Subcutaneous tophi may occur anywhere over the body but most commonly in the fingers, wrists, ears, knees, and olecranon bursa and at pressure points under the ulnar aspect of the forearm and Achilles tendon (Fig. 273-3). Gout at this stage can be confused with rheumatoid arthritis, especially if tophi are confused with rheumatoid nodules.

Atypical Gout Presentations

Approximately 5% of patients with gout exhibit the onset of symptoms before age 25 years. Early-onset gout represents a special subset of patients who generally have a genetic component (see Table 273-2), with a more

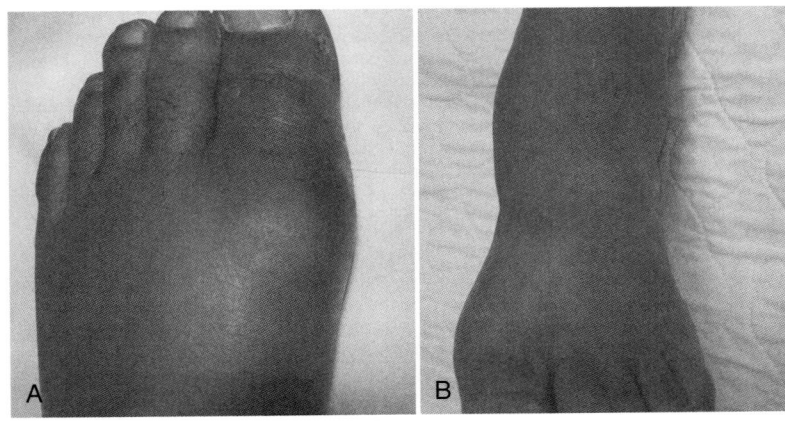

FIGURE 273-2. The intense inflammation of acute gouty arthritis. **A,** The marked swelling of the first metatarsophalangeal joint (podagra) is demonstrated. A dusky blue hue over an intense erythema is characteristic. **B,** Ankle swelling is shown with erythema extending beyond the area of the tibiotalar joint.

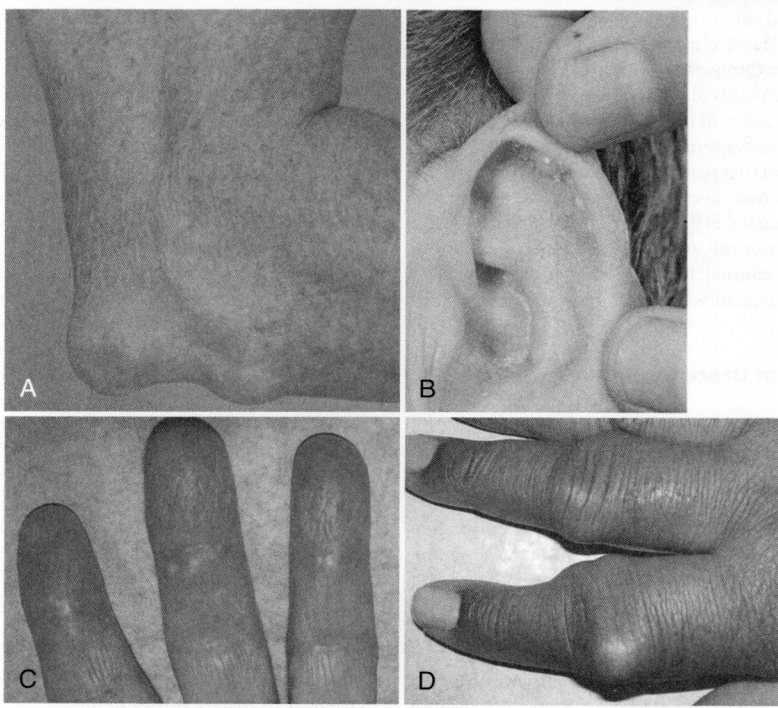

FIGURE 273-3. Characteristic locations of gouty tophi. **A,** At the elbow, tophi present as hard nodules along the ulnar ridge or as multiple nodules within the olecranon bursa. **B,** Ear tophi are uncommon but may be an easy source of crystal confirmation of gout when present. **C,** Small subcutaneous tophi can occur along the ventral creases of fingers. **D,** Tophi over the proximal interphalangeal or distal interphalangeal joints may be confused with Bouchard or Heberden nodes, respectively.

accelerated clinical course, requiring more aggressive antihyperuricemic therapy.

Gout develops in approximately 15% of heart transplant recipients who are taking cyclosporine to prevent allograft rejection. A slightly lower frequency of gout is seen in kidney and liver transplant recipients. Cyclosporine-induced gout has a marked shortening of the asymptomatic and acute intermittent stages, with a rapid appearance of tophi in 1 to 4 years.

In most large reviews, women account for no more than 5% of all gout subjects. This demographic is changing, with gout in older women becoming more common. Most women with gout are postmenopausal. Women who have premenopausal gout usually have renal insufficiency and hypertension and are taking thiazide diuretics, or they have a strong genetic predilection. Gout in older women may differ from classic gout in its propensity to occur in joints previously damaged by osteoarthritis such as the knees or the distal interphalangeal joints with Heberden nodes.

Saturnine gout is the term used to describe gout caused by chronic lead exposure. In the middle of the last century, this was most commonly observed in consumers of "moonshine" whiskey. Occupational exposure as seen in plumbers and environmental exposure from lead-based paints are other potential causes of this unusual form of gout.

DIAGNOSIS

Hyperuricemia is a critical risk factor for developing gout, but it is not a reliable diagnostic test because many people with elevated serum urate levels will never develop gout. Serum urate levels during an acute flare of gout are also unreliable because they may be suppressed by as much as 1.5 to 2.0 mg/dL from baseline values. The definitive diagnosis of gout is made by polarized compensated microscopy of a synovial fluid aspirate from the affected joint. The presence of intracellular needle-shaped crystals with strong negative birefringence is the diagnostic "gold standard." Similar microscopic results from a tophus aspirate or spontaneously draining fluid would also confirm the diagnosis of gout.

Synovial fluid confirmation is obtained in as few as 10% of patients said to have gout. The presumptive diagnosis of gout is based on a pattern of acute joint symptoms coupled with the patient's own medical history or a family history. The patient's medical history may reveal comorbidities frequently associated with gout or the use of medications associated with urate retention.

The characteristic clinical presentation is the rapid onset (over 8 to 12 hours) of severe pain in one or several lower extremity joints (especially the great toe, midfoot, and ankle). The presumptive diagnosis is given much greater credence if there have been similar previous attacks that spontaneously resolved to a symptom-free state.

Radiographic evaluation is not helpful in early attacks of gout except to rule out fracture. In advanced gout, affected joints may show punched-out periarticular erosions with classic overhanging edges. Ultrasonography can detect MSU crystals layered over articular cartilage in early disease and may be diagnostic. Magnetic resonance imaging is not part of a standard evaluation but will reveal soft tissue and intra-articular tophi long before they become clinically evident.

The differential diagnosis of acute gout includes bacterial infection, trauma, sarcoidosis, and CPPD arthropathy (pseudogout). Diseases occasionally confused with advanced gout include rheumatoid arthritis, reactive arthritis, and CPPD arthropathy.

TREATMENT AND PREVENTION   Rx

In 2012, the American College of Rheumatology (ACR) published its first guidelines on the management of gout.[5,6] Subsequent developments have been systematically reviewed.[7] There were several components of these guidelines that are applicable to all subjects with recurrent gouty flares. First, and foremost, is a heavy emphasis on patient education in order to obtain an optimal treatment outcome. Not only should patients be informed about dietary and other lifestyle changes that will lower their serum uric acid and lessen flares (Table 273-3), but they should also know that their disease is caused by an excessive burden of MSU crystals already present in their joints and soft tissues. This understanding of the disease process underlying gouty arthritis will help shift the focus from symptoms to "urate burden" as the real target of treatment.

Acute Gout

The treatment goal for acute gout flare is to relieve pain and terminate the flare as quickly as possible. Resting the painful joint and applying ice are generally helpful, but pharmacologic intervention is usually necessary to alter the excruciatingly painful course that may last for several days to more than a week. The therapeutic options include nonsteroidal anti-inflammatory drugs (NSAIDs),[A1] oral colchicine,[A2] and corticosteroids. NSAIDs are widely used but

TABLE 273-3 SPECIFIC AMERICAN COLLEGE OF RHEUMATOLOGY RECOMMENDATIONS ON LIFESTYLE AND DIET FOR GOUTY PATIENTS

Weight loss for obese patients	Avoid: Organ meats High fructose corn syrup–sweetened drinks Alcohol overuse
Healthy overall diet	Limit: Beef, pork, lamb, shellfish Beer
Exercise to achieve fitness	Encourage: Low-fat dairy
Smoking cessation	
Stay well hydrated	

may be inappropriate for patients with renal insufficiency or peptic ulcer disease. Oral colchicine administered as 1.2 mg (two tablets) at the time of flare onset followed in 1 hour by a third 0.6-mg tablet is the recommended dosing for the first 24 hours. This is followed by 7 to 10 days of once-daily or twice-daily colchicine depending on renal function. Corticosteroids can be administered orally, intramuscularly, or intra-articularly for acute gout symptoms and is a valuable option in patients with poor renal function or intolerance to colchicine. Issues critical to treatment success for a gouty flare are the early initiation of treatment, ensuring adequate dosing of anti-inflammatory therapy, and continuing the treatment until the flare has completely resolved (usually 6 to 10 days). During the acute flare, subjects already taking urate-lowering therapy (ULT) should continue the drug, whereas those not receiving this therapy should not be started.

Recurrent and Advanced Gout

The principal goal of treating gout is to lower the serum uric acid below its saturation point so that the process of crystallization will cease and the accumulated urate burden will be gradually diminished. The 2012 ACR guidelines recommend a target serum urate of less than 6 mg/dL in all subjects, with an even lower target (<5 mg/dL) for patients with advanced gout. ULT is recommended for all patients with two or more gouty flares per year, patients with advanced disease, and those with kidney stones. Allopurinol[A3] and febuxostat are both xanthine oxidase inhibitors and are considered first-line ULT. The ACR guidelines recommend that allopurinol starting dose be no greater than 100 mg/day. The dose is gradually escalated by 100 mg daily every 2 to 5 weeks, with serum urate monitoring until the target serum urate is achieved. The maximal U.S. Food and Drug Administration (FDA)-approved dose of allopurinol is 800 mg daily. In subjects with advanced chronic kidney disease, the initial dose should be reduced to 50 mg daily, with incremental dose escalations of 50 mg. Febuxostat is an alternative ULT and should be used in patients who have failed allopurinol treatment or have demonstrated sensitivity or intolerance to allopurinol.[8] The initial febuxostat dose of 40 mg daily can be increased to 80 mg daily after 2 weeks of therapy if the serum urate target is not achieved.

In patients with gout who have not attained the target serum urate despite maximal doses of either allopurinol or febuxostat, the uricosuric agent probenecid can be added to the xanthine oxidase inhibitor. Pegloticase is an intravenously administered monomethoxypoly (ethylene glycol)-conjugated recombinant uricase that dramatically lowers serum urate levels. It is approved by the FDA for the treatment of gout in patients for whom conventional therapy has been ineffective and who still have signs and symptoms of gout.

Before the initiation of any form of ULT, the patient should be placed on maintenance anti-inflammatory therapy. This is to prevent or minimize the anticipated increase in flare activity that is associated with starting ULT. Typically, this anti-inflammatory prophylaxis is in the form of colchicine once or twice daily or low-dose NSAIDs. Anti-inflammatory prophylaxis should be continued until the subject has been free of gout flares for 6 months or more.

CALCIUM PYROPHOSPHATE DIHYDRATE CRYSTAL DEPOSITION DISEASE

DEFINITIONS

The heterogeneous group of clinical conditions associated with CPPD crystals are collectively called *CPPD crystal deposition disease*. Within this spectrum is the common radiographic finding of chondrocalcinosis (CC) that is frequently asymptomatic. The acute synovitis associated with intra-articular CPPD crystals can closely mimic the findings of gout and is hence referred to as *pseudogout*. The more chronic changes associated with CPPD-induced

bone and cartilage destruction is referred to as *pyrophosphate arthropathy*. These conditions are further classified as familial (genetic), metabolic, and sporadic.

EPIDEMIOLOGY

The true prevalence of CPPD crystal deposition disease is unknown, but it is generally thought to be underdiagnosed because of its confusion with other forms of arthritis.[9] The prevalence of radiographically appearing chondrocalcinosis has been studied extensively and is clearly an age-related phenomenon. Chondrocalcinosis of the meniscal and articular cartilage of the knee is seen in 4% of people between the ages of 55 and 59 years; in 18% of those 80 to 84 years; and in approximately 27% of those older than 85 years.

PATHOBIOLOGY

Clinical CPPD disease is divided into three categories based on the etiology of altered inorganic pyrophosphate (PPi) metabolism. The categories are hereditary (familial), sporadic (idiopathic), and metabolic. All three types of CPPD disease are associated with extracellular PPi accumulation around chondrocytes, and extracellular PPi is necessary for the formation of CPPD crystals. Intracellular PPi is a common byproduct of many synthetic reactions, and if allowed to accumulate intracellularly, it impedes the further synthesis of proteins, nucleotides, and lipids. Therefore, there are multiple mechanisms for removing PPi from the cellular cytoplasm, including specific and nonspecific membrane transporters and both intracellular and extracellular (ecto-) pyrophosphate hydrolysis.

Hereditary forms of CPPD crystal deposition disease may be caused by increased transmembrane transport of chondrocyte intracellular PPi to its extracellular matrix by diminished activity of the protective pyrophosphate hydrolases, or because of altered influences of factors that lead to increased extracellular PPi, including transforming growth factor-β, bone morphogenic protein-2 and -4, ascorbic acid, and osteopontin. The best characterized of the hereditary causes is a gain of function mutation of the ANK anion transporter on the chondrocyte plasma membrane.

These types of mutations are rarely observed in the sporadic form of CPPD disease. Aging chondrocytes in culture produce considerably more PPi than do younger chondrocytes, although the exact mechanism for this is unclear.

The metabolic diseases that predispose to CPPD crystal deposition disease include hemochromatosis, hyperparathyroidism, hypomagnesemia (as in Gitelman syndrome), and hypophosphatasia. All of these metabolic conditions result in increased extracellular PPi or other alterations in the cartilage matrix that are permissive for CCPD crystal formation.

CLINICAL MANIFESTATIONS AND DIAGNOSIS

CPPD crystal deposition disease presents in a variety of fashions. It is frequently asymptomatic (lanthanic) and recognized only by the appearance of chondrocalcinosis on radiographs. The most common clinical manifestation accounting for approximately 60% of CPPD disease is a polyarticular, non-inflammatory arthritis affecting joints not typically involved in primary osteoarthritis, including the wrists, shoulders, and metacarpophalangeal joints (particularly the second and third metacarpophalangeals). This form of CPPD disease is called *pseudo-osteoarthritis* and may be associated with occasional inflammatory attacks. The acute monoarticular presentation is known as pseudogout. The pain and swelling of pseudogout can be similar to that seen in gout. The onset is usually not as abrupt as with gout, and the attacks tend to last longer—frequently months. Pseudogout occurs more often in the large joints than in small joints. CPPD crystal deposition disease can occasionally present as a chronic polyarticular inflammatory disease that may mimic rheumatoid arthritis or polymyalgia rheumatica.

CPPD disease is diagnosed by identifying chondrocalcinosis by radiography in a patient with a clinical history suggestive of the disease (Fig. 273-4). Definitive diagnosis is made by the finding of CPPD crystals by compensated polarized light microscopic examination of aspirated synovial fluid.[10]

PREVENTION AND TREATMENT   Rx

There are no specific therapies for CPPD crystal deposition disease.[11] In patients with metabolic disease–associated CPPD disease, treatment and control of the metabolic disease can afford some improvement in the arthritis, although this is not the case for phlebotomy-treated hereditary hemochromatosis. For both the acute and chronic forms of CPPD crystal deposition disease, therapy is directed at symptoms. NSAIDs are the mainstay of

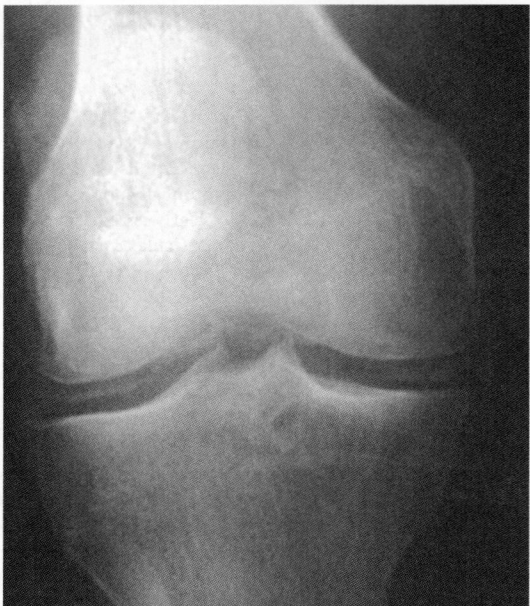

FIGURE 273-4. Calcium pyrophosphate dehydrate arthropathy of the knee. Radiographic evidence of chondrocalcinosis showing fibrocartilage calcification as thick, linear deposits parallel to and separate from subchondral bone.

treatment. Low-dose oral colchicine can be used in both acute and chronic settings. Intra-articular steroids have also been proved to be beneficial for symptomatic CPPD crystal deposition disease. The IL-1 inhibitor, anakinra, has been effectively used "off-label" for treating CPPD disease flares. On the other hand, intra-articular viscosupplementation (hyaluronic acid) may exacerbate joint symptoms.

APATITE (BASIC CALCIUM PHOSPHATE)-ASSOCIATED ARTHROPATHY

BCP crystals include several different crystal species. The most common of these is hydroxyapatite. The BCP crystals are unlike MSU or CPPD crystals in that they are not identifiable by polarized microscopy. These very tiny crystals are responsible for several important clinical conditions. Although BCP crystals are found in 50% of osteoarthritic synovial fluids, the incidence and prevalence of the individual apatite-associated clinical manifestations have not been established. This is especially true of the most severe and destructive apatite syndromes such as Milwaukee shoulder and tumoral calcinosis. The prevalence of the most common apatite-associated conditions, calcific periarthritis of the shoulder, was 3% in a large North American study.

PATHOBIOLOGY

Like MSU and CPPD crystals, BCP crystals exert their pro-inflammatory effects by being phagocytized by resident synoviocytes and influxing leukocytes. Unlike MSU and CPPD crystals, apatite crystals apparently do not act through the NALP3 inflammasome. Rather, BCP crystals are dissolved in the acidic phagosome and raise intracellular calcium levels and then activate the calcium-dependent signaling pathways. The synoviocytes are stimulated by these pathways to increase production of tumor necrosis factor-α and IL-6, and influxing neutrophils are stimulated to increase pro-inflammatory oxygen radicals. The fibroblasts in the joint lining and surrounding soft tissues are stimulated to increase production of many of the matrix metalloproteinases, such as collagenase 1, collagenase 3, and stromolysin 1.

CLINICAL MANIFESTATIONS OF BASIC CALCIUM PHOSPHATE DEPOSITION

The clinical manifestations of BCP deposition can be acute or chronic, and their cause can be idiopathic, hereditary, or secondary to other diseases that cause hypercalcemia (Table 273-4). BCP crystals can be found in 50% of synovial fluids from osteoarthritic knees. The presence of BCP crystals correlates with more severe radiographic changes secondary to more rapid dete-

TABLE 273-4	CLINICAL MANIFESTATIONS OF BASIC CALCIUM PHOSPHATE DEPOSITION DISEASE

Osteoarthritis and basic calcium phosphate deposition
Acute inflammatory arthritis
Acute calcific periarthritis
Chronic noninflammatory arthropathy
Diffuse idiopathic skeletal hyperostosis (DISH)
Tumoral calcinosis
Calcifications associated with hypercalcemic states
    Hyperparathyroidism
    Hypervitaminosis D
    Sarcoidosis
    Metastatic cancer
    Myeloma
    Leukemia

rioration in these osteoarthritic knees. Acute inflammatory arthritis associated with BCP deposition is similar in many ways to that of gout and pseudogout and has been referred to as *pseudo-pseudogout*. The patients tend to be younger and usually have evidence of soft tissue BCP deposition elsewhere in the body. Periarticular calcifications are often asymptomatic. However, BCP deposition can cause an acute and severe inflammation of the ligaments, tendons, and bursae surrounding a joint, termed *acute calcific periarthritis*. This frequently occurs around the shoulders and hips but can also occur in fingers, toes, wrists, and ankles.

The most destructive BCP-associated arthropathy is Milwaukee shoulder, which is characterized by large noninflammatory effusions containing BCP crystals with or without CPPD crystals. The process results in the destruction of the rotator cuff leading to marked instability and glenohumeral cartilage dissolution. This process can also affect knees. Like the acute calcific periarthritis discussed previously, Milwaukee shoulder is observed in women four times more frequently than in men.

Diffuse idiopathic skeletal hyperostosis (DISH) predominates in men and elderly people. The radiographic appearance of this condition is flowing ossifications along the anterolateral aspect of spinal vertebrae, especially in the thoracic spine. DISH is usually asymptomatic, but very large bridging osteophytes can cause pain; in the cervical spine, it can even result in dysphagia.

Idiopathic tumoral calcinosis is rare but most prevalent in young patients of African descent. These subjects have large irregular calcifying masses in the soft tissue surrounding the shoulders, hips, and elbows. Some cases show a familial occurrence and medical conditions associated with hyperphosphatemia.

Finally, metastatic calcifications can arise in any medical condition associated with hypercalcemia such as hyperparathyroidism, hypervitaminosis D, sarcoidosis, metastatic cancer, multiple myeloma, and leukemia.

TREATMENT AND PREVENTION   Rx

The treatment of most BCP-associated syndromes is conservative. In acute inflammatory arthritis and periarthritis, low-dose oral colchicine and NSAIDs are the mainstay of a symptomatic therapy. The persistent large effusion seen in Milwaukee shoulder should be serially aspirated to decrease intracapsular pressure. The added effectiveness of corticosteroid injections in this setting is unproved. The calcinosis associated with abnormal calcium and phosphate metabolism is best managed by treating the underlying metabolic process.

 Grade A References

A1. van Durme CM, Wechalekar MD, Buchbinder R, et al. Non-steroidal anti-inflammatory drugs for acute gout. *Cochrane Database Syst Rev.* 2014;9:CD010120.
A2. van Echteld I, Wechalekar MD, Schlesinger N, et al. Colchicine for acute gout. *Cochrane Database Syst Rev.* 2014;8:CD006190.
A3. Seth R, Kydd AS, Buchbinder R, et al. Allopurinol for chronic gout. *Cochrane Database Syst Rev.* 2014;10:CD006077.

GENERAL REFERENCES

For the General References and other additional features, please visit Expert Consult at https://expertconsult.inkling.com.

274

FIBROMYALGIA, CHRONIC FATIGUE SYNDROME, AND MYOFASCIAL PAIN

ROBERT M. BENNETT

Fibromyalgia (FM) and chronic fatigue syndrome (CFS) are multisymptomatic syndromes defined respectively by the core features of chronic widespread pain and chronic unexplained fatigue. Although there is a significant overlap in symptomatology between FM and CFS, they are generally considered to be separate disorders. Myofascial pain is a universal experience that is usually self-limited; when it becomes persistent, it may accentuate and perpetuate the experience of chronic fatigue and FM.

FIBROMYALGIA

EPIDEMIOLOGY

Chronic musculoskeletal pain is commonly encountered in the general population with an estimated prevalence of about 20%. It is subdivided into chronic regional pain, with a prevalence of about 25%, and chronic widespread pain, with a prevalence of about 10%.

FM is considered to be a subset of chronic widespread pain and has a prevalence of about 2% in women and 0.5% in men. There is a steady increase in FM with age, with about 12% of women in their 60s being affected. Chronic musculoskeletal pain is associated with a reduction in overall health status, and FM patients have more impairment than do patients with chronic widespread pain or chronic regional pain. The prevalence of FM in the medical setting is much greater, with about 20 to 30% of the rheumatology visits in the United States made for FM.

PATHOBIOLOGY

There is persuasive evidence that FM pain results from abnormal sensory processing within the central nervous system (Fig. 274-1).[1] This is commonly referred to as *central sensitization* and results from an amplification of peripheral sensory stimuli and a deficit of descending inhibitory control from the midbrain.[2] The magnification of peripheral sensory input is readily visualized as increased activity in somatosensory areas of the brain on magnetic resonance imaging (MRI) in FM subjects versus healthy controls. Central sensitization is the result of a persistent neuronal hyperexcitability that continues long after the original sensitizing input has waned. The pathophysiology of this phenomenon is based, in part, on temporal summation of neural impulses. This occurs when pain fibers (unmyelinated C) are repetitively stimulated at a rate greater than one impulse every 3 seconds. At a biochemical level, such stimulation results in depolarization of *N*-methyl-D-aspartate (NMDA) receptors, which causes transcriptional changes that affect pain processing. Thus, persistent pain input may eventually give rise to central sensitization in some individuals, probably based, in part, on a genetic predisposition.[3]

The frequent development of FM from focal pain states, such as in rheumatoid arthritis, post-traumatic injuries, and endometriosis, is thought to be a result of chronic nociceptive input stimulating central neuroplastic changes.

The descending pain system, originating in the periaqueductal gray nucleus of the midbrain and terminating in the dorsal horn, is important in modulating the transmission of nerve impulses to the brain. This inhibitory system is defective in FM patients. Activation of the nuclei in the midbrain involved in this system occurs in response to opioids, endorphins, emotions, and the placebo response. This modulation may upregulate or downregulate sensory processing, and in part, it underlies the influence of the psyche on the pain experience.

Understanding the biologic basis for central sensitization has provided an explanation for the common association of FM with other conditions such as irritable bowel syndrome, overactive bladder, multiple chemical hypersensitivity, and chronic daily headaches.

CLINICAL MANIFESTATIONS

FM patients always have the core symptom of widespread pain but also report a wide array of other symptoms (Table 274-1).[4]

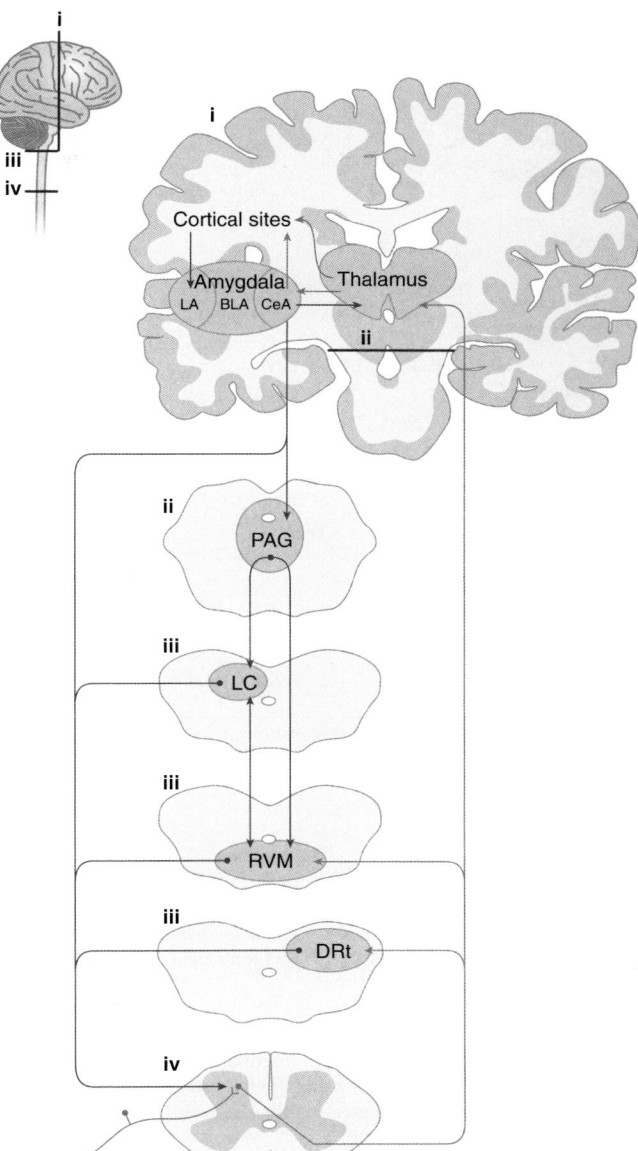

FIGURE 274-1. Neuroanatomy of pain pathways. Nociceptive inputs enter the spinal dorsal horn through primary afferent fibers that synapse onto transmission neurons. The projection fibers ascend through the contralateral spinothalamic tract. Ascending projections target the thalamus, and collateral projections also target mesencephalic nuclei, including the DRt, the RVM, and the midbrain PAG. Descending projections from the DRt are a critical component of the DNIC pathway. Rostral projections from the thalamus target areas that include cortical sites and the amygdala. The lateral capsular part of the CeA ("nociceptive amygdala") receives nociceptive inputs from the brain stem and spinal cord. Inputs from the thalamus and cortex enter through the lateral (LA) and basolateral (BLA) amygdala. The CeA sends outputs to cortical sites and the thalamus, in which cognitive and conscious perceptions of pain are integrated. Descending pain modulation is mediated through projections to the PAG, which also receives inputs from other sites, including the hypothalamus, and communicates with the RVM as well as other medullary nuclei that send descending projections to the spinal dorsal horn through the DLF. The noradrenergic locus coeruleus (LC) receives inputs from the PAG, communicates with the RVM, and sends descending noradrenergic inhibitory projections to the spinal cord. Antinociceptive and pronociceptive spinopetal projections from the RVM positively and negatively modulate nociceptive inputs and provide for an endogenous pain regulatory system. Ascending (red) and descending (blue) tracts are shown schematically. Areas labeled "i-iv" in the small diagram correspond with labeled details of the larger diagram. (From Ossipov MH, Dussor GO, Porreca F. Central modulation of pain. *J Clin Invest* 2010;120[11]:3779-3787.)

TABLE 274-1	SELF-REPORTED SYMPTOMS IN FIBROMYALGIA	
CURRENT SYMPTOM		**FREQUENCY (%)**
Low back pain		63
Recurrent headaches		47
Arthritis		46
Muscle spasm		46
Tingling		46
Balance problems		45
Irritable bowel syndrome		44
Numbness		44
Chronic fatigue		40
Bloating		40
Depression		40
Anxiety		38
Sinus problems		37
Tooth disorders		32
Restless legs		32
Tinnitus		30
Jaw pain		29
Bladder problems		26
Rashes		25

From Bennett RM, Jones J, Turk DC, et al. An internet survey of 2,596 people with fibromyalgia. *BMC Musculoskelet Disord.* 2007;8:27.

Pain

The core symptom of FM is chronic widespread pain and stiffness. Characteristically, the pain is described as a constant dull ache that is worsened by muscle overactivity. FM-related pain is usually perceived as arising from muscle; however, many patients also report joint pain but have no objective evidence of arthritis.

Fatigue

Easy fatigability from physical exertion, mental exertion, and psychological stressors is typical of FM. Patients with CFS have many similarities with FM patients; about 75% of patients meeting the diagnostic criteria for CFS also meet criteria for the diagnosis of FM.

Disordered Sleep

FM patients characteristically have nonrestorative sleep. Even if they sleep continuously for 8 to 10 hours, they awake feeling tired. Many exhibit an alpha-delta electroencephalographic pattern that would explain their never achieving the restorative stages of non–rapid eye movement sleep. A poor night's sleep is often followed by worsening of FM symptoms the next day. Restless legs syndrome and the associated periodic limb movement disorder occur in up to 60% of FM patients. A thorough evaluation for sleep disorders, such as sleep apnea, is warranted in all FM patients.

Cognitive Dysfunction

Cognitive dysfunction is a prominent complaint of many FM patients. They commonly describe difficulties with working memory, semantic memory, concentration, logical analysis, and motivation. It has been estimated that the working memory deficit in FM is comparable to 20 years of aging. Recent studies have documented that these neurocognitive deficits correlate with local brain morphology in the frontal lobe and anterior cingulate gyrus.

Psychological Distress

Having a chronic painful disorder for which there is currently no generally accepted cure often produces an existential crisis. Approximately 30% of FM patients have significant depression at any given time, and about 60% have a lifetime prevalence of depressive illness. Although psychiatric disorders are common in FM patients, they do not seem to be intrinsically related to the pathophysiology of FM; effective treatment of depression with a selective serotonin re-uptake inhibitor (SSRI) does not eliminate FM pain. FM

patients are at an increased risk for suicide and suicide ideation.[5] Fibromyalgia and depression show familial clustering, suggestive of an underlying genetic susceptibility.

Associated Problems

Fibromyalgia patients often have a spectrum of other pain disorders that share similar features, such as not having a well-defined etiology, having an association with mood disorders, and having no definitive cure. These accompanying disorders are often referred to as *central sensitivity syndromes* and include irritable bowel syndrome, overactive bladder syndrome, temporomandibular pain disorder, chronic pelvic pain, chronic daily headaches, and chemical hypersensitivity syndrome.

History
Initiation and Maintenance of Fibromyalgia

FM seldom emerges "out of the blue." Many patients relate an onset following an acute injury, repetitive workload, persistent stress, infections, and toxin exposure. It is not uncommon for a regional pain state to evolve into FM. FM is commonly found as an accompaniment of other painful disorders, such as rheumatoid arthritis, migraine, low back pain, systemic lupus erythematosus, Sjögren syndrome, inflammatory bowel disease, endometriosis, and osteoarthritis. There is increasing evidence that FM is a common occurrence in victims of post-traumatic stress disorder; for instance, both FM and CFS were common diagnoses after Operation Desert Storm in 1991. Childhood abuse and sexual trauma are often elicited during a careful and empathetic history.

DIAGNOSIS

The current "gold standard" for diagnosis of FM is based on the classification criteria of the American College of Rheumatology.[6] These criteria require persistent symptoms of at least 3 months' duration and widespread pain accompanied by tenderness at 11 or more of 18 tender point locations.

The following are the locations of the nine paired tender points:
Occiput: bilateral, at the suboccipital muscle insertions
Low cervical: bilateral, at the anterior aspects of the intertransverse spaces at C5-C7
Trapezius: bilateral, at the midpoint of the upper border
Supraspinatus: bilateral, at the origins, above the scapular spine near the medial border
Second rib: bilateral, at the second costochondral junctions just lateral to the junctions on the upper surfaces
Lateral epicondyle: bilateral, 2 cm distal to the epicondyles
Gluteal: bilateral, in the upper outer quadrants of the buttocks in the anterior fold of muscle
Greater trochanter: bilateral, posterior to the trochanteric prominence
Knee: bilateral, at the medial fat pad proximal to the joint line

Because the fibromyalgia tender point evaluation is seldom performed in clinical practice, more recent criteria have proscribed a diagnosis based on the combination of common symptoms and pain locations. Figure 274-2 is one example of such criteria that has an 80% diagnostic accuracy.

FM is not a diagnosis of exclusion; thus, laboratory tests and imaging studies play no role in establishing the diagnosis, although they are often indicated in the evaluation of concomitant peripheral pain generators and accompanying symptoms.

TREATMENT

Successful management of FM requires a thorough analysis in terms of the biopsychosocial model of disease. The major management issues that require attention are listed in Figure 274-3.[7]

Education

There is evidence that higher educational attainment is associated with a better prognosis in many chronic disorders, such as FM. Education has a positive effect through cognitive behavioral strategies, such as goal setting and reassessment of priorities. Educated patients are more likely to take an active role in self-management.

Pain

In considering the management of pain in FM, it is logical to focus on the major sites of pain processing, namely, peripheral pain generation and central pain pathways. There is no specific tissue pathology, at least in peripheral tissues, that is characteristic of FM. However, once the central nervous system

Pain location inventory (PLI):

Directions: For each of the following 28 sites, select those locations where you have experienced persistent pain during the past 7 days. The score will be between 0 and 28.

Neck	Left upper back	Right wrist	Left thigh
Right jaw	Right lower back	Left wrist	Right knee
Left jaw	Left lower back	Right hand	Left knee
Mid–upper back	Right shoulder	Left hand	Right ankle
Front of chest	Left shoulder	Right hip	Left ankle
Mid–lower back	Right arm	Left hip	Right foot
Right upper back	Left arm	Right thigh	Left foot

10–item Symptom Impact Questionnaire (SIQR):

Directions: For each of the following 10 questions, check the <u>one</u> box that best indicates the intensity of the following common symptoms over the last 7 days. Divide the total symptom score (0–100) by 2 (i.e., the range will be 0 to 50).

		0 1 2 3 4 5 6 7 8 9	
1.	*Pain*	No pain ☐☐☐☐☐☐☐☐☐☐	Unbearable pain
2.	*Energy*	Lots of energy ☐☐☐☐☐☐☐☐☐☐	No energy
3.	*Stiffness*	No stiffness ☐☐☐☐☐☐☐☐☐☐	Severe stiffness
4.	*Sleep*	Awoke rested ☐☐☐☐☐☐☐☐☐☐	Awoke very tired
5.	*Depression*	No depression ☐☐☐☐☐☐☐☐☐☐	Very depressed
6.	*Memory Problems*	Good memory ☐☐☐☐☐☐☐☐☐☐	Very poor memory
7.	*Anxiety*	Not anxious ☐☐☐☐☐☐☐☐☐☐	Very anxious
8.	*Tenderness to touch*	No tenderness ☐☐☐☐☐☐☐☐☐☐	Very tender
9.	*Balance problems*	No imbalance ☐☐☐☐☐☐☐☐☐☐	Severe imbalance
10.	*Sensitivity to loud noises, bright lights, odors and cold*	No sensitivity ☐☐☐☐☐☐☐☐☐☐	Extreme sensitivity

Criteria:

A patient fulfilling the following guidelines has a high likelihood of having FM:*

1. **The symptoms and pain locations have been persistent for at least the last 3 months**
2. **Pain location score is ≥ 17**
3. **SIQR symptom score is ≥ 21**

* • *Fibromyalgia patients have a continuum of symptoms; a diagnosis based on a strict numerical cutoff is subject to error.*
 • *The presence of another pain disorder or related symptoms does <u>not</u> rule out a diagnosis of fibromyalgia.*
 • *A careful clinical evaluation is always required in order to identify any condition that could <u>fully</u> account for the patient's symptoms and/or contribute to the severity of the symptoms.*

FIGURE 274-2. Alternative diagnostic criteria for fibromyalgia.[4] (From Bennett RM, Friend R, Marcus D, et al. Criteria for the diagnosis of fibromyalgia: validation of the modified 2010 preliminary American College of Rheumatology criteria and the development of alternative criteria. *Arthritis Care Res (Hoboken)*. 2014;66:1364-1373.)

is sensitized, not only are peripheral pain generators perceived as being more painful, but they also prolong and amplify the central neuroplastic changes. Thus, a critical first component of treating FM pain is to identify and effectively treat all peripheral pain generators, which commonly include peripheral arthritis, axial arthritis, spinal stenosis, myofascial trigger points, neuropathic pain, vascular headaches, visceral pain (e.g., irritable bowel syndrome, overactive bladder), postsurgical pain, and pelvic pain syndromes (e.g., endometriosis).

Management of central sensitization is typically initiated with heterocyclic antidepressant (HCA) medications such as amitriptyline, trazodone, cyclobenzaprine, or nortriptyline. (Chapter 397) There is evidence that antidepressant medications with both re-uptake inhibition of serotonin and norepinephrine (e.g., venlafaxine, duloxetine, milnacipran) are more effective in treating FM pain. Both duloxetine and milnacipran have U.S. Food and Drug Administration (FDA) approval for use in FM. Importantly, the mechanism of action of these drugs is independent of any antidepressant effect and results from upregulation of the descending pain system that originates in the brain stem and uses serotonin and norepinephrine as neurotransmitters at dorsal horn synapses. Anticonvulsant medications such as gabapentin, pregabalin, and topiramate are increasingly being used in FM and other chronic pain states; they inhibit the presynaptic release of glutamate and thus modulate the activation of NMDA receptors. Pregabalin has been beneficial in randomized trials[A1] and has FDA approval for use in FM. Sedative hypnotics such as zolpidem and zopiclone often help the nonrestorative sleep, but not pain. On the other hand, sodium oxybate, an FDA-approved drug for narcolepsy, has been shown to improve not only sleep but also pain, stiffness, and fatigue; it has not been approved for use in fibromyalgia.

Opioids are often used in the treatment of FM, but long-term trials are lacking. Opioids should not be the first choice for analgesia; however, they should not be withheld if less powerful analgesics have failed. Tramadol (both Ultram and Ultracet) has proved useful in reducing FM pain in two controlled trials. Tramadol is a weak opioid agonist that also inhibits the re-uptake of serotonin and norepinephrine at the level of the dorsal horn. It is metabolized by CYP2D6, as are many antidepressant medications. FM patients who are taking tramadol or any of several antidepressants that are eliminated by CYP2D6 are at risk for the development of a serotonin syndrome (Chapter 434). A careful review of concomitant medications is an important prerequisite in the prescription of any new medication, especially in difficult-to-treat patients who are often taking multiple medications.

Fatigue

A search for a treatable cause of fatigue is always indicated. Common treatable causes of chronic fatigue in FM patients are inappropriate dosing of medications, depression, aerobic deconditioning, primary sleep disorder (e.g., sleep apnea), non-restorative sleep, a coexisting inflammatory disorder, and neurally mediated hypotension. As in CFS, the underlying cause of *primary* fatigue in FM is not known. Sodium oxybate, methyl phenidate, and modafinil have provided worthwhile improvement in fatigue in some FM patients.

Sleep

Low-dose HCAs, particularly trazodone and cyclobenzaprine, are the mainstay of sleep pharmacotherapy in FM patients. Some patients cannot tolerate HCAs because of unacceptable levels of daytime drowsiness or weight gain.

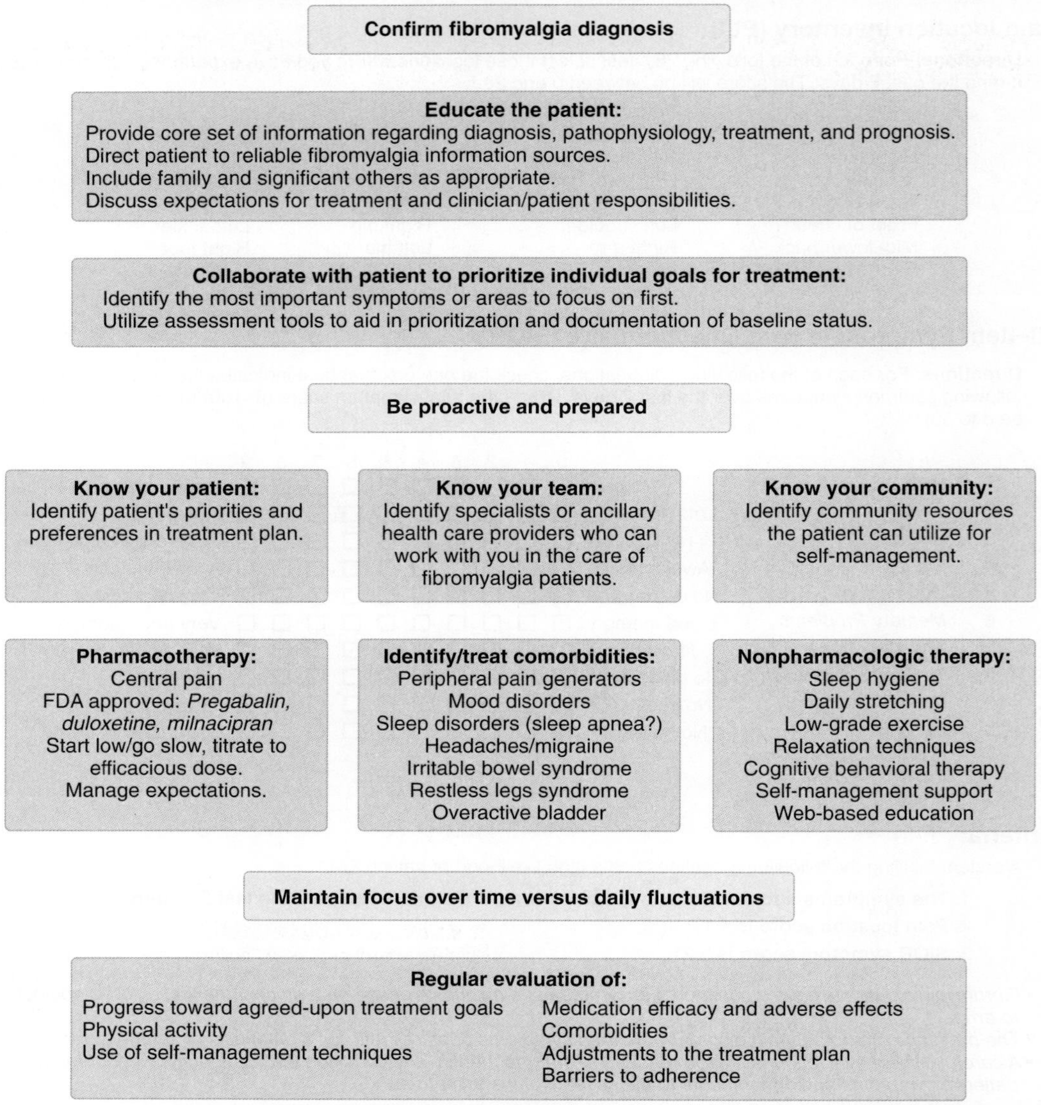

Confirm fibromyalgia diagnosis

Educate the patient:
Provide core set of information regarding diagnosis, pathophysiology, treatment, and prognosis.
Direct patient to reliable fibromyalgia information sources.
Include family and significant others as appropriate.
Discuss expectations for treatment and clinician/patient responsibilities.

Collaborate with patient to prioritize individual goals for treatment:
Identify the most important symptoms or areas to focus on first.
Utilize assessment tools to aid in prioritization and documentation of baseline status.

Be proactive and prepared

Know your patient:
Identify patient's priorities and preferences in treatment plan.

Know your team:
Identify specialists or ancillary health care providers who can work with you in the care of fibromyalgia patients.

Know your community:
Identify community resources the patient can utilize for self-management.

Pharmacotherapy:
Central pain
FDA approved: *Pregabalin, duloxetine, milnacipran*
Start low/go slow, titrate to efficacious dose.
Manage expectations.

Identify/treat comorbidities:
Peripheral pain generators
Mood disorders
Sleep disorders (sleep apnea?)
Headaches/migraine
Irritable bowel syndrome
Restless legs syndrome
Overactive bladder

Nonpharmacologic therapy:
Sleep hygiene
Daily stretching
Low-grade exercise
Relaxation techniques
Cognitive behavioral therapy
Self-management support
Web-based education

Maintain focus over time versus daily fluctuations

Regular evaluation of:

Progress toward agreed-upon treatment goals	Medication efficacy and adverse effects
Physical activity	Comorbidities
Use of self-management techniques	Adjustments to the treatment plan
	Barriers to adherence

FIGURE 274-3. Management algorithm for treatment of fibromyalgia. (Adapted from Arnold LM, Clauw DJ, Dunegan LJ, Turk DC. A framework for fibromyalgia management for primary care providers. *Mayo Clin Proc.* 2012;87[5]:488-496.)

In these patients, short-acting benzodiazepine-like medications such as zolpidem, zapelon, and eszopiclone may be beneficial. Sodium oxybate is proving to be a useful medication in improving the nonrestorative sleep of FM. About 25% of male and 15% of female FM patients have sleep apnea (Chapter 405), which usually requires treatment with continuous positive airway pressure or surgery. By far the most common sleep disorder in FM patients is restless legs syndrome or periodic limb movement disorder. Treatment is with dopamine agonists such as L-dopa/carbidopa, pramipexole, or ropinirole.

Psychological Distress
Stressors related to psychosocial/economic and health issues often develop in FM patients. Psychological intervention in terms of improving the internal locus of control and more effective problem solving is important in such patients. Cognitive-behavioral therapy is particularly well suited to effect these changes, although it does not affect pain.[A2] Although antidepressant medications are commonly used in the treatment of pain and disordered sleep in FM patients, the doses are often suboptimal for treating depressive illness.

Deconditioning
FM is invariably aggravated by excessive exertion. However, a carefully graded program of aerobic conditioning and stretching is a critical component of an effective FM treatment program. Daily stretching, progressive walking, and simple strength training have been shown to be an important component of FM treatment. In general, exercise needs to be incrementally added to the program *after* some control of pain, sleep, and depression has been achieved.

Endocrine Dysfunction
There is no good evidence that FM is primarily due to an endocrine disorder. However, common problems such as hypothyroidism and menopausal symptoms often aggravate pain and fatigue, and appropriate replacement therapy is frequently worth a trial. A subset of fibromyalgia patients have adult growth hormone deficiency and show a worthwhile response to growth hormone therapy.

PROGNOSIS

FM symptoms usually persist for many years. A 5-year longitudinal study of 1550 FM patients undergoing standard treatment by U.S. rheumatologists reported substantial improvement in 10%, moderate improvement in 15%, and a worsening of symptoms in 39%. The majority of patients continued with high levels of self-reported symptoms and distress, with about 25% having a trend toward improvement.[8] In general, recommended medications can be expected to effect a 30% improvement in about 30% of patients. Difficulty in accepting an FM diagnosis, hypervigilance, high levels of psychological distress, and poor social support are poor prognostic factors. The consequences of pain, fatigue, and cognitive dysfunction negatively influence the sustained performance of physical and mental tasks. Everyday activities

TABLE 274-2 SELF-REPORTED SYMPTOMS IN CHRONIC FATIGUE SYNDROME

SYMPTOM	FREQUENCY (%)
Non-refreshing sleep	97
Memory/concentration problems	94
Pain in two or more joints	90
Muscle pain	89
Muscle discomfort	87
Difficulty thinking	85
Sleep problems	85
Fatigue after exercise (>24 hr)	81
Migratory joint pain	76
Unexplained muscle weakness	75
Intolerance to exercise	72
Anxiety	71
Malaise after exertion (>24 hr)	69
Sweatiness/cold hands and feet	66
Light/noise sensitivity	66
Headaches	65
Intolerance to be on your feet	61
Difficulty in understanding things	58
Sore throat	57
Tender glands in the neck/armpits	57
Depression	56
Confusion or disorientation	55
Mild fever or chills	53
Migraine	28

From Nacul LC, Lacerda EM, Pheby D, et al. Prevalence of myalgic encephalomyelitis/chronic fatigue syndrome (ME/CFS) in three regions of England: a repeated cross-sectional study in primary care. *BMC Med.* 2011;9:91.

take longer for FM patients, who need more time to get started in the morning and often require extra rest periods during the day.

CHRONIC FATIGUE SYNDROME

CFS, also referred to as myalgic encephalomyelitis (ME), is a poorly understood disorder characterized by a subacute onset of disabling fatigue and other defining symptoms (Table 274-2).[9] There are no conclusive diagnostic tests or generally effective treatments.

EPIDEMIOLOGY

Fatigue is a common symptom; indeed, some 50% of individuals report "feeling fatigued" in population surveys. Fatigue is one of the most common problems reported to primary care doctors. In a series of 1000 consecutive patients seen in primary care, 8.5% reported debilitating fatigue lasting 6 months or longer without apparent cause; only 15% satisfied the clinical definition for CFS shown in Table 274-3. In many cases, fatigue is self-limited, or the causes are self-evident (e.g., insufficient rest, a medical illness, depression, or insomnia). On the other hand, well-documented CFS is relatively rare, with a frequency of 0.006 to 3.0% in various population surveys. CFS is diagnosed predominantly in women aged 30 to 55 years. They are typically highly functional before the onset of the illness.

PATHOBIOLOGY

The cause of CFS remains poorly defined. There are many reports linking CFS with chronic infections; most have not stood up to careful scrutiny. Although many CFS patients complain of nonrestorative sleep, polysomnographic studies have been inconclusive (Chapter 405). The similarity between CFS and early Addison disease has prompted numerous neuroendocrine studies. They have failed to show a clinically treatable endocrine deficiency. About 30% of CFS patients have abnormal results on tilt-table testing with evidence of autonomic dysfunction in terms of neurally mediated hypotension or postural orthostatic tachycardia syndrome. This may be of relevance

TABLE 274-3 1994 CFS INTERNATIONAL STUDY GROUP CRITERIA

A diagnosis of CFS requires the following features:
1. Persistent chronic fatigue (at least 6 months) or intermittent, unexplained chronic fatigue, which relapses, or with a definite start, and is not the result of recent exertions. The fatigue is not improved by rest and results in a significant reduction in the patient's previous level of activity.
2. Exclusion of other diseases that may cause chronic fatigue *plus* four of the following eight minor criteria that have been present concurrently for 6 months or longer, after the onset of fatigue:
   A. Recently impaired memory or concentration.
   B. Pain on swallowing
   C. Painful axillary or cervical lymph nodes
   D. Muscle pains
   E. Joint pain without swelling
   F. Headache with a new pattern or increased severity
   G. Sleep that does not improve after rest
   H. Postexertional discomfort lasting more than 24 hours

From Morris G, Maes M. Case definitions and diagnostic criteria for myalgic encephalomyelitis and chronic fatigue syndrome: from clinical-consensus to evidence-based case definitions. *Neuro Endocrinol Lett.* 2013;34(3):185-199.

in a subpopulation of patients, but treatment with fludrocortisone was of no benefit in one large placebo-controlled study. Many studies have suggested a low level of immune stimulation in CFS, the most common abnormalities being reduced natural killer cell function and increased numbers of cytotoxic T cells. However, these findings are not diagnostically useful, and clinical improvement has not been associated with any significant change in immune markers. Extensive psychological testing in CFS patients has failed to reveal a common psychiatric denominator. MRI studies[10] have reported significant reductions in gray-matter volume, which are consistent with the complaint of impaired memory; they also suggest subtle abnormalities in visual processing and discrepancies between intended actions and consequent movements.[11]

CLINICAL MANIFESTATIONS

The chief complaint is an abrupt onset of debilitating fatigue that causes significant impairment in daily activities, work ability, and social relationships. Typically, these patients report excellent health status just before the onset of fatigue, which is often preceded by a flulike prodrome. Symptoms suggestive of an infectious etiology include low-grade fever, night sweats, tender cervical lymph nodes, sore throat, myalgias, and headaches. As in FM, many CFS patients complain of generalized musculoskeletal pain, cognitive dysfunction, irritable bowel syndrome, temporomandibular pain disorders, nonrestorative sleep, and multiple chemical sensitivities (see Table 274-2).

DIAGNOSIS

There are several definitions of CFS; this has led to different clinical descriptions depending on the criteria used. The most widely used criteria are the 1994 CFS International Study Group Criteria.[12] Whereas the definition of FM contains no exclusionary criteria, the definition of CFS excludes patients with fatiguing medical disorders such as melancholic depression, psychotic disorders, substance abuse, and severe obesity (body mass index >40). Because CFS is not a diagnosis of exclusion, it is important to systematically evaluate the patient for treatable causes of fatigue.

TREATMENT Rx

Currently, there is no generally accepted pharmacologic intervention for patients with CFS. Antidepressants (HCAs and SSRIs) are of minimal benefit, although two studies have reported modest benefit with the use of monoamine oxidase inhibitors in patients with significant vegetative symptoms. Patients with presumed CFS should have a general medical work-up to exclude treatable causes of fatigue (e.g., sleep apnea, hypothyroidism, chronic infection, anemia, orthostatic hypotension). Patients with poorly defined chronic illnesses require affirmation that they have a real illness and that the clinician will provide them with ongoing empathetic care. Education is a critical component in managing CFS; acceptance of having a chronic disorder, avoidance of catastrophizing, and adoption of activity pacing are important facets of living with CFS[13]; such problems are often helped by cognitive behavioral therapy.[14] The mainstay of treatment is to engage the patient in a gently graded program of aerobic exercise.

PROGNOSIS

The prognosis for a full recovery varies between 0 and 37%; substantial improvement rates vary between 6 and 62%. Younger patients and those without a significant psychiatric overlay or catastrophizing have the best prognosis.

MYOFASCIAL PAIN

Pain arising from muscle is a universal human experience. In most instances, it is due to muscle *macrotrauma* (i.e., a muscle tear or sprain) or muscle *microtrauma* (i.e., injury at the sarcomere level resulting from repetitive muscle use or overexertion). After appropriate rest, the pain usually dissipates over a period of a few days to weeks. In some cases, a persistent pain focus develops that has the characteristics of a myofascial trigger point. This diagnosis should be considered if the patient complains of focal pain that is aggravated by muscle use or psychological stressors that cause increased muscle tension. Myofascial trigger points often play a role in poorly characterized focal pain syndromes such as low back pain, jaw pain, pelvic pain, and headache.[15]

A myofascial trigger point is a well-defined point of focal tenderness within a muscle (Fig. 274-4). Palpation usually reveals a ropelike induration referred to as a "taut band." In many instances, firm palpation of this area causes pain in a referred distribution that reproduces the patient's symptoms. Importantly, referred pain from a trigger point does not follow a nerve root distribution (i.e., it is not dermatomal). Trigger points frequently cause dysfunction in terms of a restriction in range of movement and weakness; the involved muscle or muscles often demonstrate easy fatigability (Table 274-4).

Electromyographic recordings from trigger points show spontaneous low-voltage activity resembling end-plate spike potentials. In normal muscle, depolarization of the motor end plate initiates the release of calcium ions from the sarcoplasmic reticulum, which in turn results in activation of the myosin-actin contractile elements ("contraction coupling"). It is thought that

the areas of electrical hyperexcitability in trigger points result from a non-physiologic focal contraction caused by an influx of calcium ions into the damaged sarcomeres. If this process is not "switched off," excessive utilization of adenosine triphosphate may result in a focal energy crisis in the injured muscle and thus perpetuate the problem. Functional MRI studies have confirmed the hyperalgesic features of myofascial trigger points in terms of increased activity of brain regions involved in processing stimulus intensity and negative affect. Microdialysis of trigger point foci have shown, compared with adjacent muscle, a more acidic pH and an increase of inflammatory cytokines, bradykinin, substance P, and calcitonin gene–related peptide.

Factors commonly cited as predisposing to trigger point formation include deconditioning, poor posture, repetitive mechanical stress, mechanical imbalance (e.g., leg length inequality), joint disorders, and nonrestorative sleep. The muscle pain experienced by FM patients is often the result of pain originating from myofascial trigger points and amplified by central sensitization.[16] It is hypothesized that myofascial pain is an important "peripheral pain generator" that may, in some FM patients, perpetuate and accentuate the process of central sensitization. The characteristic tender points used in FM diagnosis are in fact myofascial trigger points.

TREATMENT Rx

Management of myofascial trigger points is based on the following principles:

Postural and Ergonomic
An important issue in the effective management of myofascial pain syndromes is correction of predisposing factors (see earlier). These factors interfere with the ability of the muscle to fully recover and are the most common reason for treatment failure.

Stretching
Restoration of a muscle to its full stretch length breaks the link between the energy crisis and contraction of injured sarcomeres (see earlier). Commonly used stretching techniques include spray and stretch with ethyl chloride, acupressure, post-isometric relaxation, and deep stroking massage.

Strengthening
Muscles harboring trigger points usually become weak because of the inhibitory effects of pain. A program of slowly progressive strengthening is essential to restore full function and minimize the risk for recurrence and perpetuation of satellite trigger points.

Trigger Point Injections
Needling the myofascial trigger point with a "peppering technique" often provides a worthwhile and long-lasting benefit. Although dry needling is effective, the use of a local anesthetic (1% lidocaine or 1% procaine) helps confirm the accuracy of the injection and provides immediate relief. Validation of the accuracy of the injection is suggested by the patient's report that the pain is reproduced on entry of the needle into the trigger point; in superficial muscles a local twitch response may be observed, and this provides further evidence of an accurate injection.

Medications
Treatment of myofascial trigger points is mainly nonpharmacologic. Non-steroidal anti-inflammatory drugs and other analgesics often provide moderate symptomatic relief. As in FM, drugs that modulate pain at the central level are a useful adjunct in difficult-to-treat patients, especially if central sensitization is suspected.

FUTURE DIRECTIONS

Both FM and CFS represent a major challenge to modern medicine in understanding a constellation of common, often disabling symptoms that originate

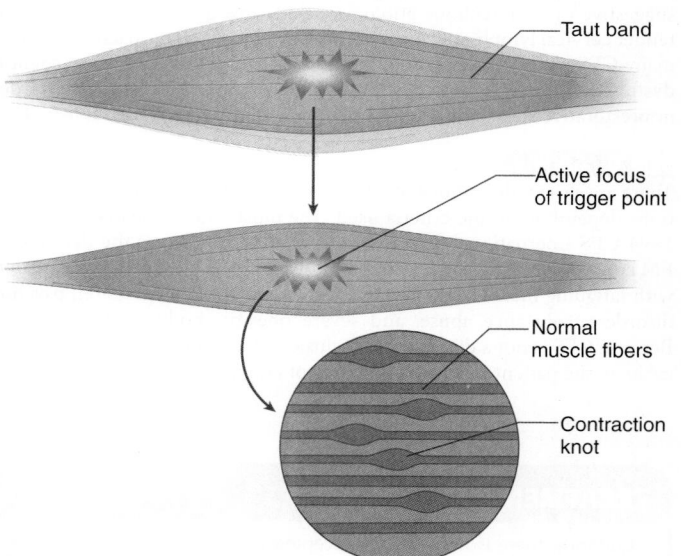

Trigger point complex

- Taut band
- Active focus of trigger point
- Normal muscle fibers
- Contraction knot

FIGURE 274-4. Schematic depiction of a myofascial trigger point. Depiction of a trigger point complex as seen in a longitudinal section of muscle. The top component represents a muscle with a taut band. The middle component represents a magnified view of the taut band containing an active trigger point focus. The lower component represents further magnification of the taut band and trigger point focus showing contraction knots (contracted sarcomere units). It is envisaged that these contraction knots are responsible for the nodularity of the taut band. Effective needling of myofascial trigger point requires piercing each contraction knot within the taut band. (From Bennett R. Myofascial pain syndromes and their evaluation. *Best Pract Res Clin Rheumatol.* 2007;21:427-445.)

TABLE 274-4	DIAGNOSTIC FEATURES OF A MYOFASCIAL TRIGGER POINT

- Focal point of tenderness on palpation of the muscle involved
- Reproduction of pain complaint by trigger-point palpation (about 3-kg pressure)
- Palpation reveals an induration of the adjacent muscle (the "taut band")
- Often pseudo-weakness of the muscle involved (no atrophy)
- Often referred pain on continued (at least 5 seconds' duration) pressure over trigger point

within the central nervous system but cannot be explained in terms of a classic psychological disorder. The central sensitization demonstrated in FM patients has provided important insight into the physiologic basis for the complaint of widespread pain, but no such breakthrough has occurred in the comprehensive understanding of fatigue in either FM or CFS. Current research suggests that both these conditions have a genetic predisposition that interacts with environmental insults such as infections, trauma, myofascial foci, and psychological stressors. In the next few years, epigenetic studies should start to unravel the complex interaction of environment and genes. Both these disorders are prime examples of the need to integrate the classic biomedical model of disease with psychosocial influences (i.e., the biopsychosocial model of disease).

Grade A References

A1. Moore A, Wiffen P, Kalso E. Antiepileptic drugs for neuropathic pain and fibromyalgia. *JAMA.* 2014;312:182-183.
A2. Bernardy K, Fuber N, Kollner V, et al. Efficacy of cognitive-behavioral therapies in fibromyalgia syndrome: a systematic review and metaanalysis of randomized controlled trials. *J Rheumatol.* 2010;37:1991-2005.

GENERAL REFERENCES

For the General References and other additional features, please visit Expert Consult at https://expertconsult.inkling.com.

275

SYSTEMIC DISEASES IN WHICH ARTHRITIS IS A FEATURE

STERLING G. WEST

Arthritis, arthralgias, and myalgias can be significant features of several systemic diseases and may be the presenting symptoms for some of these disorders (Table 275-1). Appropriate evaluation of these musculoskeletal symptoms, including selected laboratory tests and radiographs, can provide clues to the early diagnosis of these diseases. Synovial biopsies are rarely necessary but can be diagnostic. Brief descriptions of the arthritic manifestations of some of these systemic disorders follow; a more detailed discussion of each entity is found in the chapters devoted to these diseases. Because of the rarity of many of these diseases, evidence-based treatments with U.S. Food and Drug Administration–approved medications are lacking.

AUTOIMMUNE HEPATITIS

Patients with type I autoimmune hepatitis (Chapter 149) may present with a syndrome resembling systemic lupus erythematosus (SLE; Chapter 266). Patients with the early-onset subset are frequently young and female, with complaints of polyarthralgia and occasionally fever. Laboratory examination may show leukopenia, a positive antinuclear antibody (70 to 90%), elevated erythrocyte sedimentation rate, polyclonal gammopathy, and elevated liver-associated enzymes. Antibodies against double-stranded DNA are usually not seen, whereas antibodies against the smooth muscle antigen (F1 actin) support the diagnosis. Joint radiographs show soft tissue swelling without erosions or deformity. Joint pain resolves with corticosteroid therapy for the liver disease. Patients with autoimmune hepatitis have an increased risk for having a concurrent autoimmune disease.[1]

PRIMARY BILIARY CIRRHOSIS

Up to 50% of patients with primary biliary cirrhosis (Chapter 155) have other autoimmune disorders, including rheumatoid arthritis (RA), Sjögren's syndrome, limited scleroderma, and autoimmune thyroiditis.[2] In addition to antimitochondrial antibodies, rheumatoid factor, antinuclear antibodies, and anticentromere antibodies are often present. More than 10% of patients with primary biliary cirrhosis have a symmetrical or asymmetrical small joint inflammatory arthritis. Unlike RA, it can involve distal interphalangeal joints and is rarely erosive or deforming. Other musculoskeletal manifestations

TABLE 275-1 SYSTEMIC DISEASES ASSOCIATED WITH ARTHRITIS

DISEASE	TEST*
GASTROINTESTINAL DISEASES	
Autoimmune hepatitis	Liver-associated enzymes, *ASMA*
Primary biliary cirrhosis	Alkaline phosphatase, *antimitochondrial Ab*
Pancreatitis-arthritis syndrome	Lipase, amylase, *abdominal CT scan*
Whipple's disease	*Tissue biopsy, tissue immunohistochemical stain for Tropheryma whippelii, PCR for T. whippeli DNA*
Gluten-sensitive enteropathy	*Antitransglutaminase antibody, small bowel biopsy*
Inflammatory bowel disease	Stool guaiac, *colonoscopy*
Hepatitis B/hepatitis C	Liver-associated enzymes, *hepatitis serology, cryoglobulins*
Intestinal bypass arthritis	*Cryoglobulins*
HEMATOLOGIC DISORDERS	
Hemophilia	PTT, *factor VIII and IX levels*
Hemoglobinopathies	CBC, *hemoglobin electrophoresis*
Hypogammaglobulinemia	Low total protein, *SPEP, immunoglobulins*
Plasma cell dyscrasias	High total protein, *SPEP, UPEP, IEF*
ENDOCRINE DISORDERS	
Diabetes mellitus	Glucose, *hemoglobin A₁c*
Thyroid disorders	TSH, *thyroxine*
Parathyroid disorders	Calcium, phosphorus, *PTH*
Acromegaly	Radiographs, *growth hormone, IGF-1*
Hyperlipoproteinemia	Lipid panel
Paget's disease	Bone-specific alkaline phosphatase, radiographs, *bone scan*
MALIGNANT DISORDERS	
Hypertrophic osteoarthropathy	Radiographs (hands, wrists, chest)
Leukemia and lymphoma	CBC, LDH, *bone marrow/tissue biopsy*
Carcinomatous polyarthritis	*Cancer screen*
Palmar fasciitis and arthritis	CA-125, *pelvic CT scan, cancer screen*
OTHER DISEASES	
Hemochromatosis	Iron studies, radiographs, *HFE gene*
Multicentric reticulohistiocytosis	Radiographs, *skin/synovial biopsy*
Sarcoidosis	Chest radiograph, *ACE level, tissue biopsy*
IgG4-related disease	Serum IgG4 level, *histopathology of biopsy specimens including IgG4 immunostaining*
Alkaptonuria	Radiographs, *urine homogentisic acid level*
Fabry's disease	Angiokeratomas, *α-galactosidase A level or gene mutation*
Relapsing polychondritis	*Cartilage biopsy*
Cystic fibrosis	Chest radiograph, *sweat chloride, CFTR gene mutation*
Tenosynovial giant cell tumor: diffuse type (diffuse pigmented villonodular synovitis)	Synovial fluid analysis, *MRI, synovial biopsy*
Systemic infections	Cultures, serologies (RPR, HIV, EBV, parvovirus)

*Tests listed are common laboratory tests and radiographs that are frequently ordered; this information should provide a clue that a systemic disease is a possible cause of the patient's musculoskeletal symptoms. These tests, coupled with the history and physical examination, should be followed by more specific tests and biopsies (listed in italics) to confirm the diagnosis.
Ab = antibody; ACE = angiotensin-converting enzyme; ASMA = anti–smooth muscle antibody; CBC = complete blood cell count; CFTR = cystic fibrosis transmembrane conductance regulator; CT = computed tomography; EBV= Epstein Barr virus; HIV = human immunodeficiency virus; IEF = immunoelectrophoresis; IGF-1= insulin-like growth factor-1; IgG4 = immunoglobulin G4; LDH = lactate dehydrogenase; MRI = magnetic resonance imaging; PCR = polymerase chain reaction; PTH = parathyroid hormone; PTT = partial thromboplastin time; RPR = rapid plasmin reagin; SPEP = serum protein electrophoresis; TSH = thyroid-stimulating hormone; UPEP = urine protein electrophoresis.

include osteomalacia related to vitamin D deficiency, osteoporosis related to renal tubular acidosis, and hypertrophic osteoarthropathy associated with liver disease.

WHIPPLE'S DISEASE

An inflammatory arthritis occurs in 60 to 90% of patients with Whipple's disease (Chapter 140) and may precede other clinical manifestations by years.[3] The joint involvement is typically an intermittent, migratory oligoarthritis affecting large joints more than small joints or the spine, lasting from several hours to days. The synovial fluid is inflammatory, with a predominance of mononuclear cells. Subcutaneous nodules are occasionally seen, contributing to an erroneous diagnosis of rheumatic fever or RA. However, patients consistently test negative for rheumatoid factor and anti-nuclear antibodies. Synovial biopsies show rod-shaped bacilli on electron microscopy, which have been identified as *Tropheryma whipplei*. Diagnosis is suspected when duodenal, synovial, or lymph node biopsies show periodic acid–Schiff–positive macrophages. Infection is confirmed by demonstration of the organism in tissue by immunohistochemical staining with antisera specific for *T. whipplei*. Quantitative polymerase chain reaction to detect *T. whipplei* DNA is used as a confirmatory test performed on tissue and body fluids. Typically, the arthritis does not cause radiographic changes or defor-mities. Prolonged antibiotic therapy results in resolution of musculoskeletal as well as other symptoms of this disease. Relapses, especially neurologic, can occur in up to 35% of patients after cessation of antibiotic therapy.

GLUTEN-SENSITIVE ENTEROPATHY (CELIAC DISEASE)

An asymmetrical oligoarthritis or symmetrical polyarthritis occurs in up to 25% of adults with celiac disease (Chapter 140). It may precede the entero-pathic symptoms by months to years. Large joints such as knees and ankles, more than hips and shoulders, are most commonly involved. Axial involve-ment is reported. The arthritis does not cause deformities or radiographic changes and resolves with a gluten-free diet in 40 to 50% of cases. Another musculoskeletal manifestation is osteomalacia related to vitamin D malab-sorption, which may mimic diffuse fibromyalgia.

PANCREATITIS-ARTHRITIS SYNDROME

Pancreatic panniculitis is a systemic syndrome occurring in some patients with pancreatic acinar cell carcinoma and less commonly in patients with pancreatitis or hematologic malignancies. This syndrome is characterized by tender red nodules, usually on the extremities; these are frequently misdiag-nosed as erythema nodosum, but biopsy shows areas of lobular panniculitis with fat necrosis. Arthritis occurs in 60% of patients and usually involves the ankles and knees. Synovial fluid is typically noninflammatory and creamy in color. It contains multiple lipid droplets because of necrosis of fat in the synovial membrane. Other manifestations include osteolytic lesions (10%) from bone marrow fat necrosis, pleuropericarditis, fever, and eosinophilia. The prominent fat necrosis is due to the release of lipase, amylase, and trypsin from the diseased pancreas. Another musculoskeletal manifestation resulting from pancreatic disease is osteomalacia from vitamin D deficiency related to malabsorption.

HEMOPHILIA

Hemophilia A (factor VIII deficiency) and hemophilia B (factor IX defi-ciency) (Chapter 174) are associated with hemarthrosis.[4] Almost all patients with factor levels less than 1% of normal experience recurrent hemarthroses spontaneously or after minor trauma. Large joints (knees, elbows, ankles) are most commonly involved. Intramuscular hemorrhage can also occur. Recur-rent hemarthrosis can lead to proliferative synovitis and cartilage degrada-tion, resulting in both erosive and degenerative changes on radiographs. Physical examination shows bone enlargement, crepitus, atrophic muscles, and joint contractures. Treatment of acute monoarthritis consists of factor replacement to achieve a level of 30% or greater, given at the first sign of joint swelling. Patients with fever (temperature >38° C) or who fail to respond to factor replacement need joint aspiration to rule out septic arthritis, which occurs with an increased incidence in hemophilia. Chronic arthritis is treated with nonsteroidal anti-inflammatory drugs (NSAIDs), which do not inhibit platelet function; arthroscopic or radiation synovectomy for chronic synovi-tis; and total joint arthroplasty for end-stage joint disease. The regular pro-phylactic administration of factor replacement has reduced the risk for developing chronic arthropathy. Acute and chronic arthritis is less frequent and less severe in patients with hemophilia B compared with hemophilia A.

HEMOGLOBINOPATHIES

Patients with sickle cell anemia (Chapter 163) or the heterozygous states of sickle β-thalassemia and sickle–hemoglobin C disease frequently experience polyarthralgia. Local sickling of cells leads to obstruction of the microcircula-tion and to bone infarctions. Patients most commonly experience painful crises causing chest, back, and joint pain. A painful large joint arthritis (usually in the knees), often with noninflammatory synovial effusions, lasting days to 2 to 3 weeks can also occur. Infarcts in the metaphyses of bones are commonly found on joint radiographs. Vertebral bodies have a characteristic

"Lincoln log" appearance or a central cuplike indentation ("codfish verte-brae"). Femoral and humeral head osteonecrosis can occur in up to 33% of sickle cell anemia and sickle–hemoglobin C disease cases. Because of splenic autoinfarction, septic arthritis (*Staphylococcus aureus*) and osteomyelitis (50% caused by *Salmonella*) have been associated with sickle cell disease. In adults, gout has been reported, whereas in children younger than 2 years, an acute, painful, nonpitting swelling of the hands and feet (hand-foot syn-drome) associated with fever and leukocytosis may be the first manifestation of sickle cell anemia. Treatment includes intravenous hydration, oxygen, and analgesics. Hydroxyurea can reduce the frequency of painful crises. In patients with β-thalassemia major (Cooley's anemia; Chapter 162), significant expan-sion of bone marrow develops as a result of increased erythroid precursors, leading to osteoporosis and microfractures that affect primarily the lower extremities. Chelation therapy with deferiprone (to reduce iron overload from transfusions) can cause arthralgias in 20% of patients.

HYPOGAMMAGLOBULINEMIA

Patients with congenital X-linked hypogammaglobulinemia (Bruton's disease) or acquired common variable immunodeficiency (CVID; Chapter 250) can develop a nonerosive, noninfectious large joint oligoarthritis that responds to intravenous gamma globulin therapy. However, septic arthritis caused by common pathogens or *Mycoplasma* can also occur and must be rigorously excluded. In adults with acquired CVID, autoimmune conditions are also common (22%), including autoimmune cytopenias and pernicious anemia. Selective immunoglobulin A (IgA) deficiency (Chapter 250) is asso-ciated with various rheumatic manifestations, including positive autoanti-bodies, in the absence of clinical disease. Systemic autoimmune disorders, including SLE, juvenile idiopathic arthritis, and others, as well as organ-specific autoimmune disorders such as type 1 diabetes mellitus and myasthe-nia gravis, also occur in IgA-deficient individuals.

DIABETES MELLITUS

Diabetic stiff hand syndrome of limited joint mobility (diabetic cheiroar-thropathy) occurs in more than 30% of patients with long-standing, poorly controlled type 1 or type 2 diabetes mellitus (Chapter 229).[5] Patients present with the insidious development of flexion contractures and thickened skin of the fingers, which may be confused with scleroderma. These changes may be due to excess glycosylation of tendinous structures and accumulation of sugar alcohols, producing excess water content in the tissues and leading to increased stiffness. As a result of the inability to extend the fingers fully, the "prayer sign" is observed on physical examination. Unlike diabetic stiff hand syndrome, Dupuytren's contractures are due to a chronic thickening of the palmar aponeurosis, causing flexion deformities of the third and fourth digits. It is a frequent musculoskeletal complication, occurring in more than 20% of type 2 diabetic patients. A less common manifestation is Charcot's, or neu-ropathic, joints, occurring in less than 1% of all patients with long-standing diabetes. All patients have a diabetic peripheral neuropathy and typically present with painless swelling of the feet caused, most commonly, by destruc-tion of the tarsometatarsal joints. Deformities can occur with midtarsal col-lapse ("rocker bottom" feet), predisposing to ulceration and infection of the skin over desensate bony prominences. Radiographs are diagnostic, and treat-ment should include supportive footwear and protected weight bearing.

Unlike Charcot's joint, diabetic osteolysis and diabetic amyotrophy are unique to diabetes. The osteolysis is characterized by resorption of the distal metatarsal bone and proximal phalanges of the feet, giving radiographs a characteristic "licked candy" appearance. Pain is variable, and treatment is conservative because the process may terminate on its own. Diabetic amyot-rophy is a lumbar polyradiculopathy (L2 to L4) that arises with severe pain, dysesthesias, and rapid atrophy of the proximal muscles of one or both thighs. Carpal tunnel syndrome (25%), adhesive capsulitis of the shoulder (frozen shoulder), flexor tenosynovitis (trigger finger) of the hands, diffuse idio-pathic skeletal hyperostosis (type 2 diabetes), osteopenia (type 1 diabetes), diabetic muscle infarction (usually of the thigh), osteomyelitis of the foot, and septic joints are all musculoskeletal conditions that occur with increased frequency in diabetic patients. Aggressive control of blood glucose helps prevent some of these musculoskeletal complications.

THYROID DISORDERS

Musculoskeletal symptoms occur in 33% of patients with clinical hypothy-roidism (thyroid-stimulating hormone levels >20 μU/mL) (Chapter 226). Patients can present with carpal tunnel syndrome, Raynaud's phenomenon, or muscle aching and stiffness similar to fibromyalgia and polymyalgia rheumatica. Patients with severe hypothyroidism can experience a noninflammatory myopathy with proximal muscle weakness and elevated creatine kinase, which may be confused clinically with polymyositis. Similarly, myxedematous patients can develop a symmetrical arthropathy of the large joints, especially the knees, associated with noninflammatory synovial fluid with increased viscosity. The association of hypothyroidism with chondrocalcinosis is controversial, but clearly patients beginning thyroid replacement therapy can experience an acute attack of pseudogout. Patients with hyperthyroidism can develop proximal myopathy (70%), adhesive capsulitis of the shoulder (10%), osteoporosis, or thyroid acropathy. Thyroid acropathy occurs in less than 1% of patients with Graves' disease and consists of soft tissue swelling of the hands, digital clubbing, and periostitis, particularly involving the metacarpal and phalangeal bone shafts. Pain is usually mild, radiographs are characteristic, and there is no effective therapy. Patients with autoimmune thyroid disease have an increased prevalence of positive antinuclear antibodies and an increased association with systemic connective tissue diseases such as Sjögren's syndrome.

PARATHYROID DISORDERS

Primary hyperparathyroidism (Chapter 245) can develop with osteoporosis and fractures or with chondrocalcinosis and episodes of acute pseudogout.[5] In severe hyperparathyroidism, which is rare, vague myalgias and arthralgias resembling fibromyalgia; a reversible, painless, proximal myopathy with normal creatine kinase; and osteitis fibrosa cystica with bone pain can be seen. Osteitis fibrosa cystica occurs primarily in patients with secondary hyperparathyroidism associated with renal failure and has a characteristic radiographic appearance, with subperiosteal resorption on the radial side of the phalanges, small erosions in the hands and distal clavicles, and discrete lytic bone lesions (brown tumors). Ectopic calcifications, joint laxity, and tendon ruptures have been reported in patients with severe hyperparathyroidism. Hypoparathyroidism has also been associated with myopathy and ectopic calcifications. Patients with type Ia pseudohypoparathyroidism and pseudo-pseudohypoparathyroidism have a shortened fourth metacarpal bone bilaterally.

ACROMEGALY

Up to 75% of patients with acromegaly (Chapter 224) develop an atypical form of osteoarthritis. The knees, shoulders, hips, and lumbosacral and cervical spine are the most frequently symptomatic areas, although the hands reveal the most characteristic radiographic changes, with widened joint spaces due to cartilage hypertrophy. Carpal tunnel syndrome (50%), Raynaud's phenomenon (33%), and proximal muscle weakness with normal creatine kinase can also occur.

HYPERLIPOPROTEINEMIA

Type IIa familial hyperlipidemia (Chapter 206) is associated with tendinous and tuberous-osseous xanthomas as well as episodic Achilles tendinitis. An acute migratory, inflammatory arthritis persisting up to a month and resembling rheumatic fever occurs in up to 50% of patients. Predominantly large joints are affected. In addition, a self-limited, acute monoarticular or oligoarticular arthritis involving the knee or ankle can occur. Patients with type III familial hyperlipoproteinemia can develop tendon and bone xanthomas. Patients with human immunodeficiency virus (HIV) infection taking protease inhibitor drugs can develop dyslipidemia leading to tendon xanthomas. In all hyperlipidemias, gout must be excluded before ascribing the symptoms to hyperlipoproteinemia. Therapy with NSAIDs and treatment of the underlying lipid disorder should be pursued. Notably, some of the therapies used to treat hyperlipidemia can cause musculoskeletal symptoms, including hyperuricemia and gout from nicotinic acid and myalgias (with or without elevated creatine kinase) from statin therapy.

PAGET'S DISEASE

Paget's disease (Chapter 247) can cause bone pain and deformity. An elevated bone-specific alkaline phosphatase and characteristic radiographic changes can help make the diagnosis. Joint pain caused by secondary osteoarthritis in areas of bone involvement by Paget's disease most commonly occurs in the hips, knees, or vertebrae. Spinal stenosis from Paget's disease of the spine has been reported. Bisphosphonate therapy is highly effective.

HYPERTROPHIC OSTEOARTHROPATHY

Hypertrophic osteoarthropathy is a syndrome that includes clubbing of the fingers and toes, periostitis of long bones (distal tibia, femur, radius), and arthritis (Fig. 275-1). Hypertrophic osteoarthropathy is classified into primary (hereditary) and secondary forms. Between 80 and 90% of secondary hypertrophic osteoarthropathy is associated with intrathoracic neoplasms, especially non–small cell lung cancer.[6] Other causes include other neoplasms, chronic pulmonary infections, congenital heart disease, cirrhosis, HIV infection, medications (voriconazole), and inflammatory bowel disease. Patients with secondary hypertrophic osteoarthropathy can present with acute, severe, burning bone pain and a noninflammatory arthritis caused by periarticular periostitis. Pain is accentuated by dependency of the limbs. Pitting edema, warmth, and tenderness of the legs and forearms can be seen. Radiographs show diagnostic changes of periosteal elevation, new bone formation, or both along the distal ends of long bones. Therapy is symptomatic, and hypertrophic osteoarthropathy improves with successful treatment of the underlying primary disease. In resistant cases, treatment with intravenous bisphosphonate has been effective in modulating symptoms.

LEUKEMIA AND LYMPHOMA

Leukemia can arise as an asymmetrical or migratory polyarthritis, monoarthritis (rare), back pain (10%), or nocturnal bone pain. Articular manifestations occur in 14 to 50% of children and 4 to 16% of adults with acute leukemia and can precede the diagnosis by months. Joint pain is attributed to leukemic synovial infiltration and usually involves the ankle or knee, but it can be polyarticular, resembling juvenile or adult RA. The joint pain is disproportionately more severe than the clinical findings. Synovial effusions are uncommon, and evidence of leukemic cells in the synovial fluid is rare. Bone pain due to subperiosteal leukemic cell infiltration occurs in up to 50% of patients, with long bone pain (lower extremities) more common in children and back pain more common in adults. Radiographs are normal in 50%

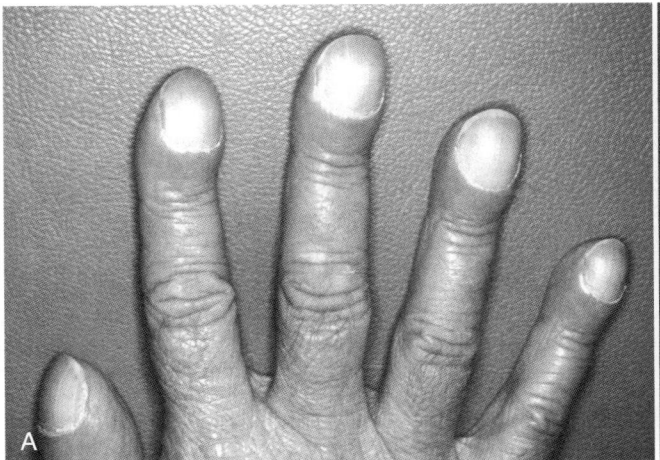
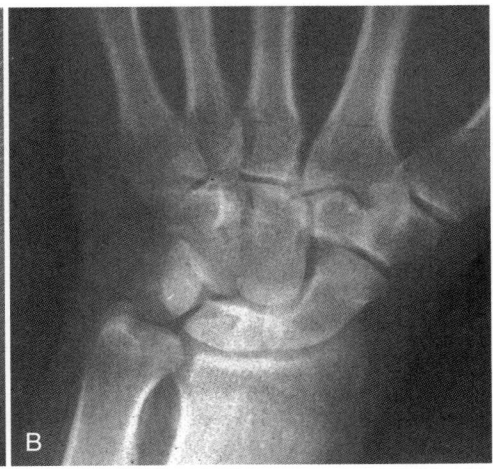

FIGURE 275-1. Hypertrophic osteoarthropathy. **A,** Severe clubbing of the nails. **B,** Radiograph demonstrating periosteal elevation of the distal radius and ulna.

of cases. The musculoskeletal symptoms are poorly responsive to NSAIDs but can resolve with successful therapy of the leukemia. Musculoskeletal symptoms occur in 25% of patients with non-Hodgkin's lymphoma. Nocturnal bone pain is the most common presenting musculoskeletal complaint. A seronegative monoarthritis or polyarthritis can occur and should be suspected in patients with severe constitutional symptoms or lymphadenopathy out of proportion to the degree of arthritis. Patients with angioimmunoblastic T-cell lymphoma (Chapter 185) may occasionally develop a chronic, nonerosive polyarthritis with erythroderma.

CARCINOMATOUS POLYARTHRITIS

Polyarthritis can rarely (<2%) be the presenting manifestation of an occult malignancy; it may precede the discovery of the malignancy by several months.[7] Breast, colon, lung, ovarian, and lymphoproliferative malignancies are the most commonly associated cancers. Clinical features suggesting carcinomatous polyarthritis include the explosive onset of a rheumatoid factor–negative, asymmetrical polyarthritis involving predominantly the lower extremities and sparing the hands and wrists in a patient older than 60 years. Polymyalgia rheumatica and RA must be excluded. Treatment of the underlying malignancy results in improvement of the arthritis.

PALMAR FASCIITIS AND ARTHRITIS SYNDROME

Ovarian carcinoma (Chapter 199) is the most common malignancy found in patients with palmar fasciitis and arthritis. This musculoskeletal manifestation can also be seen in patients with breast, gastric, or pancreatic cancer. Patients present with a severe, painful, symmetrical inflammatory polyarthritis and fasciitis causing contractures primarily of the hands and, less commonly, the feet. Patients may have vasomotor instability, causing diagnostic confusion with complex regional pain syndrome or RA. This syndrome portends a poor prognosis because it typically manifests after tumor metastasis. Response to treatment is poor, although clinical improvement can occur with successful eradication of the underlying tumor.

HEMOCHROMATOSIS

Joint involvement occurs in 40 to 75% of patients with hereditary hemochromatosis (Chapter 212) and may be the presenting symptom (Fig. 275-2).[8] The metacarpophalangeal (MCP) joints (especially the second and third MCP joints), wrists, knees, hips, shoulders, and ankles are most often involved in a symmetrical pattern. The arthropathy resembles osteoarthritis, with joint swelling resulting from bone enlargement, but it is distinguished clinically by the involvement of atypical joints, such as MCP joints, wrists, and ankles. Radiographs show joint space narrowing, subchondral cysts, sclerosis, and osteophytes that are hooklike at the MCP joints. Chondrocalcinosis is present in up to 50% of patients. It is typically asymptomatic, but in some patients it leads to attacks of acute inflammatory synovitis (pseudogout), which may result in the misdiagnosis of RA. The prevalence of overt arthritis increases with age, and it may be only minimally symptomatic when the disease arises in other organs. However, it is not uncommon for articular

pain to be the initial presenting complaint (33%). Consequently, all patients (especially male) presenting with premature osteoarthritis occurring in atypical joints, especially MCP joints and wrists, should be screened for hereditary hemochromatosis with iron studies. The mechanism whereby iron causes arthritis is unclear, but it may be related to hemosiderin deposits in the synovial membrane and chondrocytes activating degradative enzymes. Treatment is symptomatic with NSAIDs and, when severe, total joint arthroplasties. Phlebotomy for iron removal does not alter the course of the arthritis. Additional rheumatic manifestations in patients with hemochromatosis include osteoporosis related to hypogonadotropic hypogonadism, osteomalacia related to vitamin D deficiency when liver disease is severe, and an increased susceptibility to *Yersinia* septic arthritis.

MULTICENTRIC RETICULOHISTIOCYTOSIS

Multicentric reticulohistiocytosis (MRH) is a chronic, symmetrical, inflammatory polyarthritis most commonly affecting the hands and cervical spine.[9] It may resemble RA but can be differentiated by its prominent distal interphalangeal joint synovitis. Joint involvement remits and relapses initially, but in 50% of cases it worsens into a severely deforming arthritis mutilans. Firm, nonpruritic, reddish brown or yellow papulonodular lesions ("coral beads") that wax and wane occur around the nail beds and on the face, hands, ears, and other areas predominantly above the waist. The skin lesions have a diagnostic histology. In 50 to 66% of patients, these diagnostic nodules follow the onset of arthritis by months to years. Additional associations include xanthelasma (33%) and malignancies of various types (25%), which may precede or follow the onset of MRH. MRH usually remits spontaneously in 8 to 10 years but often leaves permanent cutaneous and joint damage. Treatment may include methotrexate or cytotoxic therapy if the arthritis is aggressive. Anti–tumor necrosis factor-α (anti-TNF-α) therapy is reportedly beneficial in resistant cases.

SARCOIDOSIS

Joint manifestations including arthritis, periarthritis, and arthralgias occur in 4 to 38% of patients with sarcoidosis (Chapter 95).[10] Rheumatic involvement is divided into acute and chronic types. The first consists of the triad of arthritis, erythema nodosum, and hilar adenopathy on chest radiographs (Löfgren's syndrome), which may be accompanied by fever. Arthritis arises most often in the knees and ankles, and periarticular pain can be severe. Treatment is with NSAIDs, colchicine, or both, and symptoms usually remit spontaneously over several weeks. The less common type of joint involvement in sarcoidosis consists of synovitis that accompanies the slower onset, more chronic, systemic form of sarcoidosis. Polyarthritis, oligoarthritis, or monoarthritis can affect the small or large joints; it is typically nondestructive but in some cases can be aggressive. Dactylitis resulting from sarcoid bone and soft tissue involvement can occur (Fig. 275-3). In contrast to the acute type, chronic sarcoid arthropathy is characterized by mildly inflammatory synovial fluid and histologic granulomas on synovial biopsy. Treatment consists of NSAIDs, low-dose corticosteroids, hydroxychloroquine, and methotrexate or azathioprine. In refractory cases, anti-TNF-α therapy has been successful. Other musculoskeletal manifestations of sarcoidosis include lytic or sclerotic bone lesions (3 to 13%) and symptomatic acute or chronic myopathy (3%). Notably, asymptomatic lesions involving bone and muscle are much more common on magnetic resonance imaging and tissue biopsies.

IMMUNOGLOBULIN G4–RELATED DISEASE

Patients with IgG4-related disease are typically men (70 to 75%) older than 50 years. Patients present with a variety of local and systemic manifestations, some of which can resemble several rheumatic diseases (Chapter 256).[11] For example, tumefactive lesions of the salivary glands can mimic Sjögren's syndrome. Destructive sinus and middle ear lesions or periorbital masses can suggest granulomatous polyangiitis (GPA) (formerly Wegener's granulomatosis). Furthermore, patients with IgG4-related disease frequently (40%) have allergic manifestations including chronic sinusitis and pulmonary symptoms, which may add to the diagnostic confusion with GPA. IgG4-related disease can also cause an inflammatory aortitis with aneurysm formation that can be mistaken for giant cell arteritis. A fibrosclerotic presentation in the abdomen can mimic retroperitoneal fibrosis. Other organs that can be involved include the pancreas, biliary tree, kidneys, lymph nodes, meninges, thyroid, breast, prostate, pericardium, and skin. Although up to 70% of patients will have an elevated serum IgG4 level, histopathologic analysis of biopsy specimens is the "gold standard" for diagnosis. The key pathologic features are a dense lymphoplasmacytic infiltrate organized in a storiform

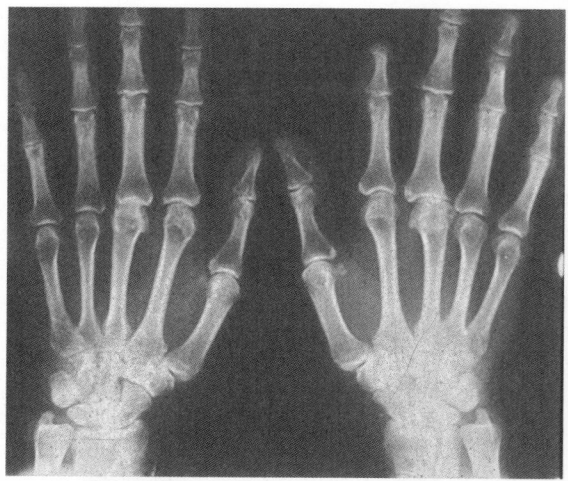

FIGURE 275-2. Hemochromatotic arthropathy. Radiograph demonstrating degenerative changes, with hooklike osteophytes of the second and third metacarpophalangeal joints bilaterally.

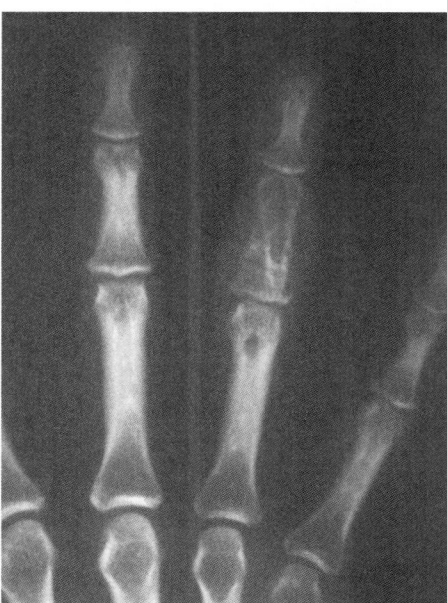

FIGURE 275-3. Sarcoid bone involvement. Punched-out lytic lesions of the middle phalanx, with soft tissue swelling.

pattern, obliterative phlebitis, and a mild or moderate eosinophilic infiltrate. The plasma cell infiltrate will show more than 30 IgG4-positive cells per high-power field and a ratio of IgG4 to IgG positive cells that is higher than 50%. Glucocorticoids are effective in most patients. Several medications (azathioprine, mycophenolate mofetil, methotrexate) have been used as steroid-sparing agents to maintain remission. For refractory disease, B-cell depletion therapy with rituximab is effective.

ALKAPTONURIA (OCHRONOSIS)

Although an inherited disorder, alkaptonuria is usually not diagnosed until the patient presents with progressive premature osteoarthritis as a young adult (before age 30 to 35 years). The spine is initially involved, followed by the knees, shoulders, and hips. Small peripheral joints are spared. Radiographs show multiple vacuum discs, disc space ossification, and osteoarthritic changes in the spine. Nonarticular features include bluish brown discoloration of ear pinna, sclera, and nasal cartilage. Deposition of ochronotic pigment onto collagen fibers causes the articular cartilage to become brittle and fragmented. The noninflammatory synovial fluid may show tiny shards of pigmented cartilage ("ground pepper"). The diagnosis of alkaptonuria is suspected when fresh urine turns dark brown or black on standing or with alkalinization. The diagnosis is confirmed by quantitative measurement of increased homogentisic acid in urine. A specific enzyme assay for homogentisic acid dioxygenase can also be performed. There is no effective therapy for alkaptonuria, although nitisinone is currently under investigation. The arthritis is treated symptomatically with analgesics.

FABRY'S DISEASE

Most patients with hereditary lysosomal storage diseases present and are diagnosed during childhood (Chapter 208). However, female heterozygotes and atypical variants of Fabry's disease may have a milder and later-onset phenotype. Fabry's disease is an X-linked lipid storage disease caused by a deficiency of lysosomal α-galactosidase A. Males with classic Fabry's disease usually develop neuromuscular symptoms in childhood, including painful crises with burning paresthesias of the distal extremities, often accompanied by fever. However, in female heterozygotes and males with low residual α-galactosidase A levels, disease manifestations may occur for the first time in adulthood. Neuromuscular manifestations can range from painful acroparesthesias to fibromyalgia. Progressive or isolated cardiac, cerebrovascular, and renal disease can develop later. Fabry's disease should be suspected in any patient with a paternal family history of early-onset renal failure. Patients should be examined for characteristic ocular stigmata (cornea verticillata) and dermal signs (angiokeratomas). The diagnosis is confirmed in males by determining α-galactosidase A activity in plasma or peripheral leukocytes. In

contrast, female carriers must be tested for one of the specific gene mutations. Early diagnosis is important because enzyme replacement therapy can prevent irreversible organ damage.

RELAPSING POLYCHONDRITIS

Relapsing polychondritis is an uncommon multisystem disorder characterized by recurrent episodes of inflammation of cartilaginous tissues.[12] Patients with relapsing polychondritis typically present with the sudden onset of pain and erythema involving the cartilage of the external ear, larynx, trachea, or nose. A nonerosive, seronegative polyarthritis or oligoarthritis affecting small, large, or parasternal joints (23 to 47%); ocular inflammation, including episcleritis or scleritis; and audiovestibular disturbances may also be presenting symptoms. The arthritis is typically acute, migratory, and episodic and resolves spontaneously over days to weeks. Rarely, it can become chronic. Tenosynovitis is also common. Relapsing polychondritis is presumably due to a cell-mediated and humoral immune response against cartilage components; biopsies showing acute and chronic inflammation destroying cartilage support the diagnosis. Late sequelae of relapsing polychondritis include deformity of the pinnae or nose, reduced vision or hearing, tracheal narrowing or collapse, and aortic insufficiency resulting from aortic ring dilation as well as other cardiovascular abnormalities. Patients with relapsing polychondritis frequently have associated coexisting diseases, such as systemic vasculitis, various connective tissue diseases (e.g., RA), myelodysplastic syndromes and other cancers, and thyroid disease. Treatment depends on the severity of the presentation and whether major organs are involved. Mild episodes of inflammation are treated with NSAIDs, colchicine, dapsone, and low-dose corticosteroids. Life-threatening or organ-threatening complications are treated with high-dose corticosteroids and immunosuppressive agents such as methotrexate or cyclophosphamide. Infliximab and tocilizumab have been anecdotally effective in treatment-resistant cases.

CYSTIC FIBROSIS

In up to 10% of patients with cystic fibrosis (Chapter 89), an episodic, nondestructive, inflammatory oligoarthritis develops, most commonly involving the fingers and lower extremity joints. This arthritis is thought to be due to immune complex deposition caused by chronic lung infections. Attacks last for a few days and may be associated with fever and painful nodular skin lesions and purpura. Other musculoskeletal manifestations include osteoporosis (30-75%) and osteomalacia related to malabsorption and, more rarely, hypertrophic osteoarthropathy (5%) and a small vessel vasculitis.

TENOSYNOVIAL GIANT CELL TUMOR: DIFFUSE TYPE

The diffuse type of tenosynovial giant cell tumor (TGCT) (also called diffuse pigmented villonodular synovitis) occurs most commonly in the third and fourth decades of life. It is characterized by the onset of unilateral pain and swelling of a joint, typically the knee (80%). Unusually, a tendon, bursa, or another joint can be involved. The synovial fluid is characteristically brown or hemorrhagic, and radiographs may show soft tissue swelling, osteolysis, subchondral cysts, and bone erosions. TGCT is a nonmalignant condition due to a translocation between chromosomes 1p13 and 2q35 in which the gene coding for colony-stimulating factor-1 (CSF-1) is fused to the collagen VI alpha-3 gene. Up to 15% of cells in the TGCT overexpress CSF-1. The remaining cells in the tumor are inflammatory cells recruited into the tumor because they contain the receptor for CSF-1. TGCT is best diagnosed by synovial biopsy. Microscopic examination reveals a characteristic histology, including marked synovial cell hyperplasia and subsynovial invasion by masses of polygonal cells, multinucleated giant cells, and lipid-filled macrophages. Hemosiderin deposits are between and within cells and have a characteristic appearance on magnetic resonance imaging, with nodular foci of decreased signal on both T1- and T2-weighted images. The treatment for pigmented villonodular synovitis is synovectomy with or without postoperative radiotherapy.[13]

FUTURE DIRECTIONS

With the advances being made in immunology and genetics, there will be an increased understanding of the pathogenesis of many of these diseases. Treatments such as immunomodulating biologic agents or cartilage-preserving therapies will be developed on the basis of new discoveries elucidating the etiology of these unusual disorders. Because of the rarity of many of these diseases, the establishment of registries and international databases detailing clinical characteristics and response to therapies would be a valuable resource.

GENERAL REFERENCES

For the General References and other additional features, please visit Expert Consult at https://expertconsult.inkling.com.

276

SURGICAL TREATMENT OF JOINT DISEASES

C. RONALD MACKENZIE AND EDWIN P. SU

Estimates of the prevalence of arthritis and other rheumatic diseases demonstrate the enormous impact that these conditions have on the U.S. populace and the health care system in general. More than 21% of U.S. adults (46 million people) currently report physician-diagnosed arthritis. Although the majority of this health burden arises as a consequence of osteoarthritis, the full span of the rheumatic diseases contributes to the impact of this class of conditions. Already the leading cause of disability in the nation, the number of people with arthritis and arthritis-attributable limitation in activity is anticipated to approach 67 million affected adults by the year 2030. Ultimately, surgical intervention is required in many of these individuals. Factors such as an increased patient awareness of the benefits of surgery, the desire for higher activity levels, and improvements in surgical techniques have, in concert with the increasing prevalence of chronic arthritis, fueled the growth in utilization of orthopedic surgery. In 2010, it was estimated that about 300,000 primary total hip replacements and about 650,000 primary total knee replacements were performed in the United States. By the year 2020, it is predicted that about 500,000 hip replacements and 1.5 million knee replacements will be performed each year.[1]

PATHOBIOLOGY

The pathobiology of joint arthritis leading to surgical intervention is essentially that of articular cartilage damage resulting in the loss of mechanical properties, accompanied by inflammation of the joint lining. With continued cartilage deterioration, stiffness and pain ensue. Without the protective layer of articular cartilage, the nociceptive and proprioceptive receptors in the periosteum are activated, leading to unremitting pain.

Osteoarthritis is the most common cause of end-stage arthritis (Chapter 262). Osteoarthritis may be primary, due to biochemical changes in the cartilage, or secondary to systemic disease affecting the cartilage, joint damage from preexisting inflammatory joint disease, or trauma. Mechanical overload and imbalances lead to further cartilage degradation. Important adaptive processes such as subchondral sclerosis and osteophyte formation occur in response to joint overload, and, if chronically present, cyst formation in the subarticular bone may also result. Over time, the osteophytes or bone spurs will lead to restricted range of motion (Fig. 276-1).

Inflammatory arthritis, by contrast, is a constellation of diseases involving the synovium. Included in this class of disorders are such important conditions as rheumatoid arthritis (Chapter 264), psoriatic arthritis, and the seronegative spondyloarthropathies (Chapter 265). On a pathologic level, all involve the release of inflammatory mediators in the adjacent synovium, leading secondarily to cartilage destruction. In contrast to osteoarthritis, there is no mechanical overload as a primary mechanism, and no bone sclerosis or osteophyte formation are seen. Rather, the inflammatory synovitis leads to characteristic loss of cartilage matrix, marginal bony erosions, and osteopenia (Fig. 276-2)

Trauma is another important cause of joint destruction. Post-traumatic arthritis is initiated by cartilage damage at the time of injury or by secondary mechanical imbalances that result from fractures of juxta-articular bone. Abnormal loading conditions will subsequently lead to a wear-and-tear form of cartilage damage.

Osteonecrosis is another entity that may lead to joint arthritis. In this process, the blood supply to the bone is compromised, leading to necrosis of the bone supporting the articular surface. The most commonly affected joints are the hip, shoulder, and knee. As the disease progresses, the necrotic bone may collapse, leading to the loss of articular integrity and progressive cartilage deterioration.

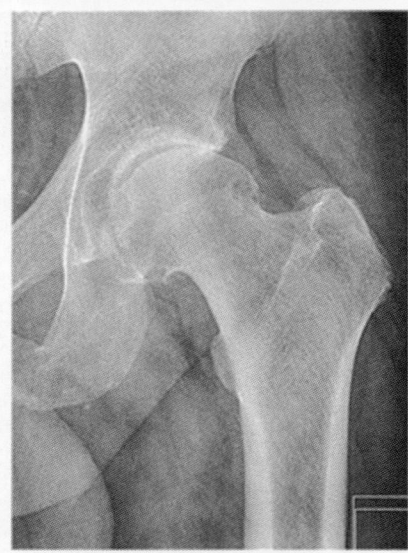

FIGURE 276-1. Radiograph of an osteoarthritic left hip. Note the asymmetrical joint space narrowing and subchondral sclerosis that are characteristic of a wear-and-tear pattern of joint deterioration.

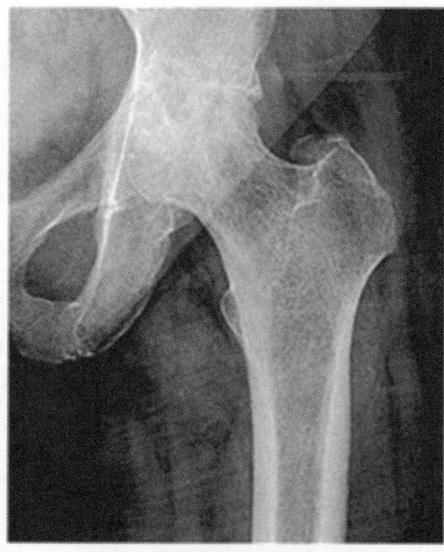

FIGURE 276-2. Radiograph of a left hip with end-stage inflammatory arthritis. Note the symmetrical pattern of cartilage loss and presence of osteopenia.

Other causes of arthritis that may lead to joint damage include metabolic disorders (chondrocalcinosis, gout), tumor (synovial chondromatosis), infections (post-septic), and bleeding disorders (hemophilia).

PREOPERATIVE CONSIDERATIONS

The indications for orthopedic surgery are refractory joint pain and disability. Ultimately, the patient and physicians need to agree that the possible benefits of surgery outweigh the risks (Chapter 431). The decision to proceed with surgery therefore reflects the outcome of a partnership among the patient, the orthopedic surgeon, and the patient's primary physician or rheumatologist (Chapter 430). Achieving the necessary decision-making balance may be complicated, especially given the increasing burden of comorbidity that accompanies the aging patient.

In the elective setting, joint replacement and spine surgery are the most common procedures under consideration. With the former, severe pain and functional limitation unrelieved by conservative treatment are the most common indications for surgical intervention. In the case of spinal surgery, severe radiculopathy, nerve dysfunction (e.g., acute foot drop), and myelopathy are additional considerations. In contrast to elective surgery, there are circumstances when a deliberative approach is not possible because of the development of more urgent, occasionally life-threatening clinical problems. Examples include hip fracture, acute myelopathy, or the patient with an infected native or prosthetic joint. Because the patient's general health is at risk in these settings, the medical-surgical team must stabilize the patient quickly in order to optimize the outcome. Owing to the coupling of medical advances with increasing financial and resource constraints, a dominant trend toward the performance of surgery in the ambulatory setting has emerged. Indeed the percentage of all surgical procedures performed on an outpatient basis in the United States rose from 20% in 1982 to 60% in 1995, a phenomenon particularly relevant to the arthroscopic techniques of orthopedic surgery. Among the benefits of these developments has been the opportunity to move the preoperative medical evaluation to the outpatient arena. This change in practice allows time for discourse with the other physicians involved in the patient's care, for supplementary consultation and investigation, and, when necessary, for the institution of therapy directed at optimizing the patient's medical status before the contemplated surgery. Approached in this manner, the preoperative evaluation becomes a focal point of communication among all members of the medical team, enhancing the collaborative nature of the consultative process and, ultimately, the patient's care.

Although the efficacy of preoperative assessment has not been definitively established, the aging and increasing complexity of modern-day surgical patients justifies this clinical practice. Although no consensus exists regarding what constitutes the optimal preoperative medical evaluation, a growing literature pertaining to perioperative medicine supports various core principles that underlie effective medical consultation in this clinical setting (Chapter 431).

● ANESTHESIA IN THE ORTHOPEDIC PATIENT

Given the protean clinical features that accompany chronic arthritis and the connective tissue diseases, a variety of issues, including airway considerations, the surgical site (joint region), the anticipated duration of surgery, and comorbidities are important determinants of the type of anesthesia to be employed, whether invasive monitoring will be necessary, and the length of time the patient will require intensive monitoring after surgery.

General anesthesia and regional anesthesia are commonly used in the orthopedic patient (Chapter 432). General anesthesia with endotracheal intubation may present a particular danger in patients with rheumatoid arthritis or ankylosing spondylitis. Patients with cervical spine instability or those with a rigid spine may require fiberoptic intubation. Regional anesthesia may involve local anesthesia or peripheral nerve block for minor procedures or epidural-spinal anesthesia for total joint arthroplasty.

Although the debate concerning the relative merits of regional versus general anesthesia remains unresolved, many procedures, particularly orthopedic surgery, are well suited for regional anesthetic techniques. Advantages of regional approaches include a reduction in blood loss, deep vein thrombosis and pulmonary embolism, adverse postoperative respiratory events, and death. Further postoperative pain, a significant problem for patients with a painful rheumatic disease, may be best managed with regional anesthesia. For example, peripheral nerve blocks using longer acting anesthetics and infusion methodologies are often employed because they provide excellent intraoperative anesthesia and postoperative pain relief.

A number of options exist for the control of postoperative pain, including the traditional intravenous and intramuscular routes of narcotic medications (systemic), the use of epidural analgesia, and the local infiltration of anesthetics into the surgical site.[A1] The direct administration of local mixtures of medications, including long-acting anesthetics and anti-inflammatory drugs, has become more popular because of the ease of use and excellent efficacy, particularly around the hip and knee joints. Patient-controlled analgesia (PCA) using an epidural route of administration is also an effective method of pain control after lower extremity surgery. Further, epidural PCA and local soft tissue injections facilitate postoperative physical therapy, which is important to the restoration of range of motion in patients undergoing orthopedic procedures. Both methods also reduce the systemic absorption of analgesics, thereby minimizing the problem of narcotic-induced respiratory depression. Parenterally administered nonsteroidal anti-inflammatory drugs (NSAIDs) are also useful and can be used to reduce narcotic requirements after major surgery. However, the common contraindications to NSAID therapy, such as peptic ulcer, renal, and ischemic heart disease, should be observed in the postoperative setting.

● SURGICAL MANAGEMENT

Surgical treatment of joint disease is focused primarily on the relief of pain; secondary objectives are improvement in joint motion, reduction in swelling,

return to function, and prevention of continued cartilage destruction. Realizing that surgical treatment has limitations and complications, the decision to move forward is one that must be individualized for each patient. Factors such as disease severity, the patient's desired activity level, and the anticipated longevity of the patient are all relevant to decision making. Typically, patients who are candidates for the surgical treatment of joint diseases have failed conservative measures (NSAIDs, physical therapy, intra-articular injections) and have daily pain that hinders their function and diminishes their quality of life.

● ORTHOPEDIC PROCEDURES
Osteotomy

In circumstances in which a structural abnormality around a joint has led to mechanical overload, an osteotomy (cutting bone) may be an option to correct alignment problems. The most common sites for osteotomy are the hip, to treat acetabular dysplasia, and the tibia, to realign the knee. In acetabular dysplasia, the hip socket is excessively shallow, leading to abnormal stresses on the articular cartilage and premature osteoarthritis. An acetabular osteotomy can be performed in patients in whom significant cartilage still remains. By rotating the pelvic bones, a deeper socket can be formed, reducing stresses on the cartilage and thereby slowing down the arthritic process. With tibial osteotomy, the knee joint can be realigned to direct forces away from the region of cartilage damage. Usually a varus (bow-legged) deformity indicates that the medial compartment of the knee is excessively worn and, as such, a tibial osteotomy realigns the joint in such a way to direct forces to the uninvolved, lateral compartment. Typically, osteotomy is considered an option for younger patients (<40 years); beyond this age, the loss of cartilage is generally such that more reproducible results would be attained with total joint arthroplasty.

Arthroscopy

Arthroscopic surgery is performed by inserting a camera and specialized instruments into a joint through small, puncture-type incisions. Arthroscopic surgery is effective in the treatment of intra-articular pathology such as meniscal tears of the knee, labral tears of the hip, cartilage flaps, small chondral defects, and loose bodies. However, after the articular cartilage is significantly damaged, arthroscopic débridement is usually ineffective in the absence of mechanical symptoms such as locking and clicking.[A2-A4] In some instances, underlying joint arthritis may lead to tears in the meniscus or labrum; if such a tear results in new mechanical symptoms, then arthroscopic surgery may be helpful in selected cases.

In the assessment of the hip, there has been an increased focus on the femoral head and neck architecture as a cause of osteoarthritis. In certain patients, the anatomy of the femoral head and neck may lead to impingement of the femoral neck upon the acetabular rim, typically in flexion and internal rotation. This condition, known as *femoroacetabular impingement*, results in the repetitive contact between the femoral neck and acetabular rim and is believed to result in labral tears, cartilage damage, and eventually arthritis.[2] Thus, there is currently much interest in reshaping the bones of the femur and acetabulum by so-called osteochondroplasty. This procedure is being performed as an open or arthroscopic procedure and provides good symptomatic relief in the short term. The long-term effects, specifically the impact on the future development of arthritis, have yet to be demonstrated for this procedure.

Synovectomy

Synovectomy refers to removal of the synovial lining of the joint, either through an open or an arthroscopic approach. In conditions such as rheumatoid arthritis, in which the disease process involves an actively inflamed synovium, it follows that debulking the pathologic tissue may reduce symptoms and slow the destruction of cartilage. In practice, synovectomy can be effective at relieving pain as long as there is remaining cartilage. However, the procedure is not predictable in terms of regaining joint motion. Further, after the cartilage is completely worn through, the joint deterioration is too advanced for synovectomy to be helpful. Therefore, synovectomy is generally performed in patients with rheumatoid arthritis (or other forms of inflammatory arthritis) who have active synovitis in the presence of relatively preserved articular cartilage. The most common joints that benefit from synovectomy are the knee and elbow. However, synovectomy should be considered as "buying time" because the synovium will reappear.

Arthrodesis

Arthrodesis, or fusion of a joint, achieves the goal of pain relief by creating a nonmobile joint. Rather than have the arthritic joint surfaces elicit pain with movement, a surgical fusion (arthrodesis) of the articulating bones creates a construct that can bear weight and is stable. This is achieved by removing the articular surfaces from the joint and immobilizing the bones such that they heal in a solid union. This procedure was formerly the treatment of choice for hip and knee arthritis in young, active laborers because of its durability and avoidance of implants with their propensity to wear. However, creating stiffness at one joint will increase stresses on the joints above and below the fused joint.

Hip fusion may be performed in young patients to treat the sequelae of slipped capital femoral epiphysis, Legg-Calvé-Perthes disease, post-septic arthritis, or osteonecrosis of the femoral head. Fusion surgery can achieve a painless, supportive joint that is capable of bearing heavy loads while avoiding artificial implants. However, the gait mechanics are altered, requiring more energy for ambulation. Further, the lack of motion at the hip increases stresses on the joints above and below the hip. Thus, the natural history of a hip fusion is the development of ipsilateral knee arthritis and low back pain after 20 to 25 years, necessitating much later the conversion of a fused hip to a hip replacement (fusion takedown). Although hip arthrodesis is still a viable option in the young arthritic patient, patients' desire for maintaining hip mobility in order to sit and drive has made this largely a treatment of the past.

Fusion of the knee joint is performed less commonly than hip fusion. In addition to the lack of motion that may make it difficult to sit or climb stairs, knee fusion cannot be successfully converted to total knee replacement. Thus, knee fusion is generally considered a salvage procedure, mainly employed in situations in which replacement is not possible (e.g., lack of muscle function or persistent infection).

Ankle fusion is still commonly performed as the treatment of choice of tibiotalar arthritis. Because the historical results of ankle replacement have not been durable, fusing the ankle is the best method of creating a pain-free joint. Furthermore, the ability of the knee and subtalar joints to compensate for a stiff ankle has made this procedure more tolerable.

Total Joint Arthroplasty

Joint arthroplasty refers to the re-creation of congruent joint surfaces, typically with artificial parts. In certain patients and in non-load-bearing joints such as the elbow, interpositional arthroplasty can be performed by placing a tissue graft between the arthritic surfaces. In the case of weight-bearing joints such as the hip and knee, however, metal and plastic materials produce the most durable results. In such circumstances, the articular surfaces are replaced by shaped materials designed to recreate the joint kinematics; thus, the procedures are commonly called total hip, knee, and shoulder replacements.

In general, after the articular cartilage is completely worn or destroyed on both sides of the joint, arthroplasty is the most predictable option to relieve pain. After total joint arthroplasty, it is advisable to reduce stresses on the joint to promote implant longevity. This includes weight loss and avoidance of impact activities; walking, cycling, and gliding type activities are permitted, but in general, running and jumping should not be performed. Because a total joint arthroplasty involves artificial, moving components, the replaced joints are subject to the same wear and tear as native joints. Thus, they have a finite lifespan that is dependent on a patient's weight and activity level and the implant materials. Subsequent revisions of joint replacements can be difficult and less durable; thus, it is wise to defer joint arthroplasty until there are no other options.

Total hip replacement was first developed in the 1950s in the United Kingdom using metal and plastic components attached to the bone with cement. The early results were so predictable and reproducible that the technique rapidly spread worldwide. The National Institutes of Health, in 1994, published a consensus statement that total hip replacement "is one of the most successful surgical procedures and provides immediate and substantial improvement in a patient's pain, mobility, and quality of life. Compared with treatments for other chronic debilitating diseases, total hip replacement is highly cost effective."

Total hip replacement is the treatment of choice for end-stage arthritis caused by any of the aforementioned pathobiologic processes. It involves the exposure of the joint, removal of the arthritic femoral head at the level of the femoral neck, and removal of enough acetabular bone to place a prosthetic socket. The femoral implant is inserted into the intramedullary canal and anchored with bone-ingrowth techniques or bone cement. The typical bearing materials for the hip joint are metal-on-polyethylene, ceramic-on-polyethylene, and ceramic-on-ceramic implants. These combinations of materials may be chosen based on the patient's age, activity level, and surgeon

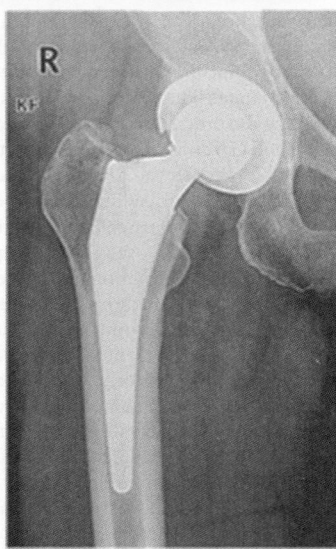

FIGURE 276-3. Radiograph of a total hip replacement consisting of uncemented acetabular and femoral components. The articulating materials are a metal ball and polyethylene liner.

preference (Fig. 276-3). Metal-on-metal total hip replacement, popular for a time period in early to mid-2000s, has now fallen out of favor because of findings of adverse local tissue reactions to the metal debris.

Using modern implant materials and surgical technique, the implant survival rates are 90 to 95% successful at 15 years; however, longevity will vary depending on patient factors such as weight and activity. There have been cases in which total hip replacement implants have lasted more than 30 years.

A major cause of failure of total hip replacement has been wearing of the implant materials coupled with the body's reaction to the particulate debris shed into the joint space over time. In the process of immunologic uptake of the debris, inflammatory cytokines are released, causing osteoclasts to resorb periprosthetic bone. The end result of this osteolytic process is that the implant attachments to bone may be compromised, causing loosening of the prosthesis and pain. The hope is that the current generation of implant materials will reduce the amount of particulate wear debris, thereby extending longevity further.

Total knee replacement was developed in the United States shortly after total hip replacement. The surgery involves the removal of the arthritic surfaces of the tibia and femur followed by their replacement with a metal femoral implant and a metal and/or polyethylene tibial component (Fig. 276-4). It is termed "total" knee replacement to distinguish it from a unicompartmental or "partial" knee replacement.

The recovery from total knee replacement is more difficult than after total hip replacement because of greater postoperative pain and the emphasis on regaining motion. Nonetheless, pain relief and function are usually excellent when recovery is complete. Current studies demonstrate modern implant survival to be 90 to 95% at 15 years, again depending on patient factors.

The long-term outcome after total hip or knee arthroplasty has improved steadily over recent decades. Despite more pre-surgical morbidity, rates are declining especially for cardiac disease, stroke, and pulmonary embolism.[3]

Although less commonly performed than hip and knee replacement, total shoulder replacement is an excellent pain-relieving procedure for glenohumeral arthritis. Developed from experience gained for total hip replacement and total knee replacement, total shoulder replacement uses a stemmed humeral implant with a metal ball and metal and/or polyethylene glenoid socket. Total shoulder replacement requires an extensive rehabilitation protocol to regain range of motion and strength; however, 1 year after surgery, 95% of patients have pain-free use of the shoulder.

Surgical Innovations in Joint Arthroplasty
Minimally Invasive Surgery

As in all surgical subspecialties, there has been a movement toward minimally invasive surgery. This may be a misnomer because the actual work done inside the joint has not changed. Some surgeons have suggested the terminology be changed to "smaller incision surgery" or "less invasive surgery." In any case, the idea is that the smallest incision possible be used to perform the operation, resulting in less tissue trauma. The interest in this type of surgery has resulted in improvements in instrument design and surgical training. Typically, a hip replacement, performed until recently using a 10-inch incision, can now be done through a 4- to 5-inch incision. Similarly, knee replacement incisions are about one half of their former length. Despite these surgical advances, even larger benefits have resulted from the increased attention to various nonsurgical modalities, all directed at more rapid surgical recovery. Examples include the increased use of peripheral nerve blocks and local tissue anesthetic infiltration, preemptive analgesia, and a more expeditious approach to rehabilitation. Such approaches have reduced the average hospital length of stay to 2 to 3 days after a total hip replacement and 3 to 4 days after a total knee replacement.

Improvements in Implant Technology

As the average age of patients undergoing hip and knee replacement decreases, while their activity levels increase, the number of revision surgeries is projected to grow. Therefore, much research is being performed to improve the longevity of implant materials.[4] The gold standard of arthroplasty is to use a cobalt-chrome (metal) implant against a polyethylene (plastic) surface. Unfortunately, the harder metal surface will eventually wear away the softer

plastic surface. Therefore, biomechanical engineers have developed a more resistant, "highly cross-linked" polyethylene that demonstrates greater wear resistance in laboratory simulators. Such highly cross-linked polyethylene has been in clinical use for about 10 years, and the early experience suggests significantly less wear compared with standard polyethylene.[5] Other materials such as ceramics and metals are also being used in an attempt to improve longevity. Nonetheless, to date, there is no consensus concerning the optimal weight-bearing surfaces.

Bone-preserving implants have also been developed in order to maintain more options when revision surgery becomes a necessity. Such procedures may require the removal of the implant and placement of a new prosthetic device; thus, with more bone available, surgical options are enhanced. One such bone-preserving implant is the hip-resurfacing device introduced in the United States in 2006. This is discussed more fully later.

Unicompartmental knee replacement is a bone-preserving implant for the knee. As suggested by its name, it involves replacing only one of the three knee compartments with a prosthetic device (Fig. 276-5). Therefore, candidates for unicompartmental knee replacement must have arthritis limited to a single compartment. Because the surgical trauma and dissection are significantly reduced compared with total knee replacement, patient recovery tends to be less painful and quicker. However, there remains a higher failure rate for unicompartmental knee replacement compared with total knee replacement because of the possibility for developing arthritic changes elsewhere in the joint.

Resurfacing Arthroplasty

Hip resurfacing is an alternative treatment to total hip replacement in the younger, active patient. The primary benefit is the preservation of proximal femoral bone in the event that future (revision) surgery is necessary. Rather than removing the femoral head and portion of the femoral neck as in total hip replacement, the bone is sculpted to accept a metal resurfacing cap (like a tooth), preserving an additional 4 to 5 centimeters of bone (Fig. 276-6). The acetabulum is prepared to accept a metal socket, creating a metal-on-metal joint. There are currently no alternatives to the metal-on-metal articulation of a hip-resurfacing implant; however, in contradistinction to metal-on-metal total hip replacements, there appear to be fewer issues arising from the materials in hip resurfacing.[A5] The likely explanation for this finding is that there are fewer pieces and junctions in a hip resurfacing compared with total hip replacement. The preservation of the proximal femoral bone raises an additional risk for failure (i.e., femoral neck fracture below the resurfacing implant), which is estimated to occur in 1% of cases. Although there are no defined age limits for hip resurfacing, the best candidates have been males younger than 55 years, likely because the bone quality in this demographic group is the strongest and most robust. In this age group, the 10-year results of hip resurfacing in Australia have demonstrated a 94% rate of survival (free of revision), which is superior to total hip replacement. However, concerns regarding longevity, a greater short-term failure rate than total hip

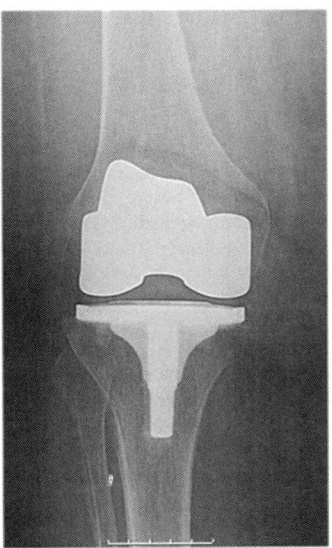

FIGURE 276-4. Radiograph of a total knee replacement. The components are metal, with a polyethylene insert between the tibial and femoral components.

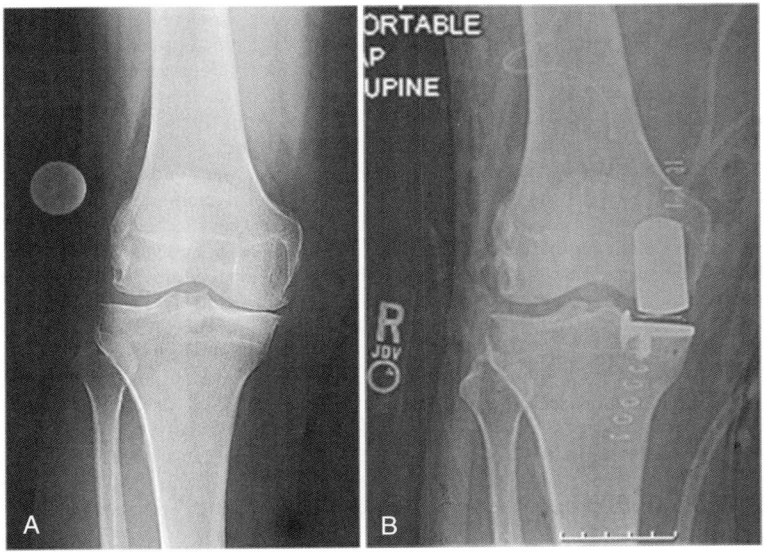

FIGURE 276-5. A, Radiograph of a knee with arthritis limited to the medial compartment. B, A medial unicompartmental knee replacement.

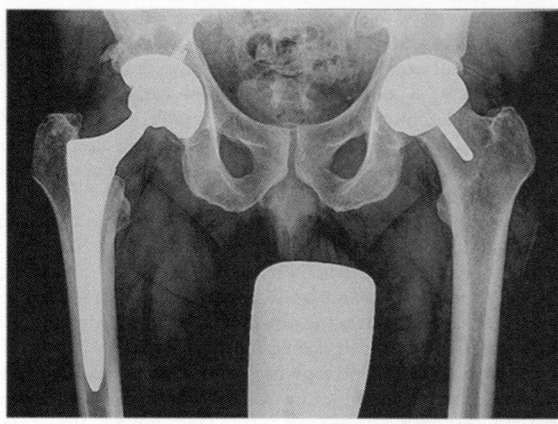

FIGURE 276-6. Radiograph of a patient with a right total hip replacement and a left hip resurfacing. The total hip replacement consists of a longer stem placed into the medullary canal of the femur. The hip resurfacing implant preserves the proximal femoral bone.

replacement, poorer results in women, and metal ion release have led to questions concerning the superiority of the procedure.

Computer Navigation

An orthopedic surgeon relies on visualization, instrument jigs, and experience in order to recreate the proper joint mechanics. Although the surgeon may know exactly how the artificial components are to be placed, it may be difficult to achieve perfect alignment in every operation. Computer navigation is a tool that can be used to aid in the reproducible positioning of implants. Although some errors are inherent in the precision of computer navigation, such techniques have reliably diminished outlier results. It has yet to be determined whether the longevity of hip and knee replacements inserted with the aid of computer navigation differ from those inserted by conventional approaches. For this reason, as well as the expense and time associated with its use, computer navigation is not universally practiced.

ORTHOPEDIC PROCEDURES ON OTHER JOINTS

Elbow, Ankle, and Wrist

The elbow, ankle, and wrist are less frequently replaced joints. With the exception of the rheumatoid wrist, these joints are less commonly afflicted by chronic arthritis. Further, the smaller bones making up these joints also translate to a diminished surface area for implant fixation, thus lowering the durability of the surgical procedures. Although total joint arthroplasty can be successful at relieving pain in the short term, 10-year results do not approach that of total hip or knee replacement. Synovectomy remains an effective surgical option in selected patients with inflammatory arthritis of the elbow, ankle, or wrist.

Spine

The spine consists of multiple levels of articulating bone, discs, and facets. Although not a "joint" in the typical sense of the word, various spinal segments may be differentially involved in chronic arthritis. Generally, the lumbar spine is the most affected, although a similar process can occur in the cervical spine; more than 95% of patients older than 50 years will demonstrate degenerative changes in the lumbar spine. With aging, the nucleus pulposus of the intervertebral disc loses water content and elasticity, resulting in disc space collapse and increased forces across the vertebral facets. As a consequence of the resultant increased pressure, bone spurs develop, leading to stenosis (narrowing) of the neural foramen. As a result of the degenerative process or *spondylosis*, patients may experience mechanical back pain with bending, extending, and twisting. Pain, numbness, or weakness radiating down the extremities in a radicular distribution can result from the neural foraminal stenosis.

Mechanical back pain is the most common affliction of the spine. Unfortunately, this constellation of back symptoms is not reproducibly relieved by surgical intervention. Physical therapy and use of proper back mechanics are the mainstay of treating mechanical back pain.

The advanced sequela of spinal arthritis is spinal stenosis, which can result in lower extremity pain and weakness. This disorder can reliably benefit from decompressive surgery with or without instrumented fusion. The spinal unit must be evaluated for stability in order to determine whether or not spinal fusion is necessary.

Newer surgical treatments such as lumbar disc replacement may be used in certain cases to treat spinal disorders. Whereas the gold standard, vertebral fusion, eliminates painful motion at degenerative disc levels, disc replacement attempts to preserve motion of the spinal unit. As in hip and knee arthrodesis, fusion of the spinal unit will increase forces at the levels above and below the fused segment; thus, further degeneration will often occur. Disc replacement surgery aims to eliminate the progression of arthritis at adjacent levels by retaining motion. Long-term studies comparing disc replacement and spinal fusion are not yet available.

MANAGEMENT ISSUES IN PATIENTS WITH ARTHRITIS UNDERGOING SURGERY

Prevention of Postoperative Infection

Efforts to prevent and detect any infectious processes before and after surgery are of utmost importance. The skin and urinary tract are sites of specific concern, and infection can be ruled out by a careful physical examination and routine preoperative urine culture. In addition, dental consultation may be appropriate in patients with poor oral hygiene and dentition.

Prophylactic antibiotic therapy for total joint arthroplasty patients should begin less than 2 hours before surgery and continue for 24 hours. A common protocol involves cefazolin (Ancef) 1 g every 8 hours (total of three doses) or, in penicillin allergic patients, vancomycin 1 g every 12 hours (total of two doses).

Peripheral Nerve Injuries

Peripheral nerve injuries arise more often after upper and lower extremity surgery because they generally result from excessive traction on the nerve or, alternatively, as a consequence of nerve compression resulting from prolonged positioning of the extremity during surgery or while in a cast. Early detection and intervention are critical to the outcome in these circumstances. Patients with chronic neurologic disorders, such as neuropathies in the setting of diabetes or spinal stenosis, are at increased risk for nerve injury.

Venous Thromboembolism

Prevention of venous thromboembolic phenomena after orthopedic surgery is the most thoroughly studied of potential postoperative complications, and pulmonary embolism remains an important cause of mortality. The orthopedic literature has concentrated on lower extremity arthroplasty, although a recent study suggests that similar approaches should also be considered after total shoulder arthroplasty, in which the risk for thromboembolism may be higher than generally appreciated.

After orthopedic surgery, a complicated balance exists between a possible life-threatening pulmonary embolus and the potential for postoperative bleeding. Numerous protocols have documented the effectiveness of prophylaxis, which should begin at the time of the procedure. Short intraoperative time reduces the risk for deep vein thrombosis, as does the type of anesthesia. Epidural anesthesia reduces the risk for proximal deep vein thrombosis following total hip replacement by two- to three-fold and also reduces the overall risk for deep vein thrombosis by at least 20%. Other intraoperative interventions, such as hypotensive anesthesia and intraoperative heparin administration, further reduce thrombogenesis. Mechanical methods also have proven efficacy at reducing risk for thromboembolism. These include compression methodologies such as stockings and various pneumatic devices, foot flexion-extension exercises, and early ambulation. These are safe, effective approaches that do not increase the risk for bleeding.

The mainstay of prevention is prophylactic anticoagulation, which should begin immediately after surgery. Regimes include aspirin, warfarin, low-molecular-weight heparin,[A6] and several new oral anticoagulants,[A7] often used in combination with various mechanical compression devices (Chapter 38). Continuing prophylaxis for 21 days rather than 7 days reduces risks of thromboembolism while increasing risks of minor bleeding.[6]

Fat Embolism Syndrome

Fat embolization, a well-described complication of skeletal trauma, may also occur after procedures involving instrumentation of the femoral medullary canal. Although the embolization of fat is believed to occur almost entirely in the setting of hip or femoral fractures, 1 to 3% of patients undergoing joint replacement surgery (particularly simultaneous bilateral procedures) develop fat embolism syndrome (FES).

The signs and symptoms of FES involve the respiratory, neurologic, and hematologic systems, as well as the skin.[7] Time of onset is variable, with hemodynamic instability developing almost immediately in some or insidiously over the first 2 to 3 postoperative days in others. In the latter, patients gradually become hypoxemic, may be hypotensive, and are often confused. Respiratory signs are the most common manifestation. Most patients develop mild to moderate hypoxemia or radiographic changes (mainly bilateral alveolar infiltrates), but only a minority will develop life-threatening adult respiratory distress syndrome. Neurologic manifestations range from mild drowsiness to acute confusional states or to severe obtundation and coma, all consequences of the hypoxemia and the direct effect of the embolization of fat on the brain. The skin eruption, which is rare in total joint arthroplasty patients, takes the form of a petechial rash involving the folds of the neck and axillae, as well as petechiae in the subconjunctiva and oral mucosa. Retinal edema and hemorrhage are also seen. Transient thrombocytopenia is common.

Although patients suspected to have developed FES need to be closely monitored, in most instances after total joint arthroplasty, the condition is relatively benign. Treatment is supportive and includes the administration of oxygen and the prevention of pulmonary hypertension (by fluid restriction and the use of diuretics and venodilators). Corticosteroids are not effective. In most patients, the condition resolves within 3 to 7 days, although in severe cases, the mortality rate has remained in the 5 to 15% range even with modern aggressive therapy.

Cervical Spine

In those rheumatoid arthritis patients who exhibit advanced destructive disease, cervical spine instability should be ruled out before surgery with flexion-extension films in patients with neck pain or crepitus on range-of-motion testing, radicular symptoms, or arm and/or leg weakness. Affected patients should wear a soft cervical collar to the operating room. When possible, epidural or spinal anesthesia should be employed.

Conversely, in patients with ankylosing spondylitis, the patient's rigid cervical spine may also present technical challenges for the anesthesiologist during intubation. Fiberoptic methods are often employed in this clinical setting.

Immunosuppressive and Anti-inflammatory Therapy

The potential contribution of corticosteroids, the disease-modifying antirheumatic drugs (DMARDs), and the newer biologic agents to the risk for postoperative infection and wound dehiscence are well recognized by clinicians, although the debate concerning how to manage these medications in the perioperative setting is not settled. The primary challenge in this context is to achieve an optimal balance between the maintenance of control of the underlying disease while minimizing the risk for postoperative wound infection and/or wound breakdown.

Methotrexate (MTX) is the most commonly used DMARD for the treatment of rheumatoid and other forms of inflammatory arthritis, so it is frequently seen in the perioperative setting. Given its importance in the maintenance of disease control, coupled with observations concerning the low rates of postoperative wound infection and dehiscence associated with its use, it appears safe, indeed desirable, to continue MTX throughout the perioperative period.

With respect to the biologic (anti–tumor necrosis factor) agents, recommendations have been formulated by international groups in which such

agents are discontinued for short periods of time before surgery, generally 2 to 4 weeks. Some favor the longer 4-week interval for agents with longer half-lives. There is virtually no information concerning postoperative infection and wound healing with the newer agents such as anakinra, rituximab, and abatacept. Recommendations similar to the other biologics must suffice until more data can be gathered.

The other important medication commonly encountered in the perioperative setting is corticosteroids. In addition to problems related to wound healing, there is the additional concern of postoperative adrenal insufficiency. Traditionally, steroids have been shown to increase the rate of wound infection and dehiscence in surgical patients, although data derived from the orthopedic setting per se remain scant. Similarly insecure is the published experience concerning postoperative adrenal insufficiency. In contrast to MTX and the biologic therapies, however, the question is not whether to stop corticosteroids before surgery because this is generally not feasible. Rather, management considerations pertain to how much and for how long steroid augmentation (stress doses) will be required. In this regard, a nuanced approach, premised on patient-specific considerations, is required. For the patient chronically managed with low doses of corticosteroid (i.e., prednisone ≤7.5 mg/day) or on any dosage for less than 3 weeks, stress dose steroid therapy is unnecessary, and maintenance of the patients' usual daily dosage should be sufficient. In contrast, for patients taking larger dosages (≥20 mg/day) for longer periods (>3 weeks) of time, it is prudent to assume secondary adrenal suppression exists, justifying the use of stress dose steroid therapy. For those taking intermediate dosages (i.e., 7.5 to 20 mg/day), decision making needs to be individualized. In addition to the dosage and duration of steroid therapy, other considerations, such as the presence of diabetes, the use of other immunosuppressive therapy, hypoalbuminemia, and poor nutritional status, as well as the magnitude of the surgical procedure, need to be taken into account.

Grade A References

A1. Yadeau JT, Goytizolo EA, Padgett DE, et al. Analgesia after total knee replacement: local infiltration versus epidural combined with a femoral nerve blockade: a prospective, randomised pragmatic trial. *Bone Joint J.* 2013;95-B(5):629-635.

A2. Moseley JB, O'Malley K, Petersen NJ, et al. A controlled trial of arthroscopic surgery for osteoarthritis of the knee. *N Engl J Med.* 2002;347:81-88.

A3. Kirkley A, Birmingham TB, Litchfield RB, et al. A randomized trial of arthroscopic surgery for osteoarthritis of the knee. *N Engl J Med.* 2008;359:1097-1107.

A4. Sihvonen R, Paavola M, Malmivaara A, et al. Arthroscopic partial meniscectomy versus sham surgery for a degenerative meniscal tear. *N Engl J Med.* 2013;369:2515-2524.

A5. Garbuz DS, Tanzer M, Greidanus NV, et al. The John Charnley Award: metal-on-metal hip resurfacing versus large-diameter head metal-on-metal total hip arthroplasty: a randomized clinical trial. *Clin Orthop Relat Res.* 2010;468:318-325.

A6. Sobieraj DM, Coleman CI, Tongbram V, et al. Comparative effectiveness of low-molecular-weight heparins versus other anticoagulants in major orthopedic surgery: a systematic review and meta-analysis. *Pharmacotherapy.* 2012;32:799-808.

A7. Adam SS, McDuffie JR, Lachiewicz PF, et al. Comparative effectiveness of new oral anticoagulants and standard thromboprophylaxis in patients having total hip or knee replacement: a systematic review. *Ann Intern Med.* 2013;159:275-284.

GENERAL REFERENCES

For the General References and other additional features, please visit Expert Consult at https://expertconsult.inkling.com.

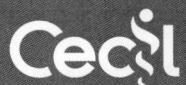

XXIII

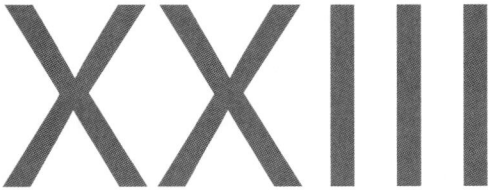

INFECTIOUS DISEASES

277

INTRODUCTION TO MICROBIAL DISEASE: HOST-PATHOGEN INTERACTIONS

W. MICHAEL SCHELD

Infectious diseases have profoundly influenced the course of human history. The "black death" (caused by *Yersinia pestis*) changed the social structure of medieval Europe, in the process eliminating approximately a third of the population. The outcomes of military campaigns have been altered by outbreaks of diseases such as dysentery and typhus. Examples include Napoleon's retreat from Russia, after typhus did more damage to his army than the opposition forces did; the decision by the French to sell the Louisiana Territory after French soldiers died from yellow fever in Cuba and the Gulf Coast; and the introduction of smallpox to the nonimmune population of the New World by Europeans, thus facilitating the "conquest" and the dawn of the colonial age. Malaria influenced the geographic and racial pattern and distribution of hemoglobins and erythrocyte antigens in Africa. The development of *Plasmodium falciparum* is inhibited by the presence of hemoglobin S, and Duffy blood group–negative erythrocytes are resistant to infection with *Plasmodium vivax*. Thus, populations with these erythrocyte factors are found in areas where malaria is common.

Infections are a major cause of morbidity and mortality in the world. Of the approximately 53 million deaths worldwide in 2009, at least a third were due to infectious diseases. In the United States, pneumonia is the fifth leading cause of death overall and the most common cause of death related to infection. Acquired immunodeficiency syndrome (AIDS) threatens to disrupt the social fabric in many countries of Africa and is severely distressing the health care system in the United States and other parts of the world. The year 2011 marked the 30th "anniversary" of the AIDS epidemic. Approximately 35.3 million people worldwide are currently infected with human immunodeficiency virus (HIV), and since 1981, approximately 36 million have died (≈600,000 in the United States alone). AIDS is now the leading cause of death in sub-Saharan Africa.

Infection can be defined as the multiplication of microbes (from viruses to multicellular parasites) in the tissues of the host. The host may or may not be symptomatic. For example, HIV infection may cause no overt signs or symptoms of illness for years. The definition of infection should also include the multiplication of microbes on the surface or in the lumen of the host that causes signs and symptoms of illness or disease. For example, toxin-producing strains of *Escherichia coli* may multiply in the gut and cause a diarrheal illness without invading tissues. Microbes can cause diseases without actually coming in contact with the host by virtue of toxin production. *Clostridium botulinum* may grow in certain improperly processed foods and produce a toxin that can be lethal on ingestion. A relatively trivial infection, such as that caused by *Clostridium tetani* in a small puncture wound, can cause devastating illness because of a toxin released from the organism growing in tissues. It has now become apparent that multiple virulence factors of microorganisms can be carried in tandem on so-called pathogenicity islands of the genome (the "virulome").

We live in a virtual sea of microorganisms, and all our body surfaces have indigenous bacterial flora. In fact, we are a "super organism" as our native flora outnumbers our own human cells by a ratio of 10 : 1. This normal flora actually protects us from infection. Reduction of gut colonization increases susceptibility to infection by pathogens such as *Salmonella enteritidis* serovar *typhimurium*. Bacteria that constitute the normal flora are thought to exert their protective effect by several mechanisms: (1) using nutrients and occupying an ecologic niche, thus competing with pathogens; (2) producing antibacterial substances that inhibit the growth of pathogens; and (3) inducing host immunity that is cross-reactive and effective against pathogens. These conclusions appear to be oversimplistic, however. For example, colonization of the gastrointestinal tract with *Bacteroides fragilis* expressing an immunodominant bacterial polysaccharide causes dendritic cell activation and induction of a T_H1-mediated response, leading to a splenic response characterized by normal numbers of $CD4^+$ T cells, lymphoid architecture, and systemic lymphocytic expansion. Thus, a single bacterial molecule in our gut is

necessary to make us "immunologically fit." Indeed, it has become apparent that a healthy, diverse microbiome is vital to proper immune system function. The timing of changes in the microbiome can also be of crucial importance. For example, pregnant mice fed antibacterials pass along their altered gut microbiome to their offspring. The neonates, in turn, display decreased total number and composition of gut microbes that is associated with decreased numbers of circulating and bone marrow neutrophils. This disordered neutrophil homeostasis leads to impaired host defense and increased susceptibility to *E. coli* K1 and *Klebsiella pneumoniae* sepsis, classic neonatal pathogens in humans.[1] Furthermore, because children are often prescribed multiple courses of antibacterials, one must wonder if these (often unnecessary) exposures later predispose them to epidemic disorders, such as asthma, autoimmunity, inflammatory bowel disease, and obesity.

Only a small proportion of microbial species can be considered primary or professional pathogens, and even among these species, a relatively small number of clones have been shown to cause disease. For example, epidemic meningococcal meningitis and meningococcemia are due to a small number of clones of *Neisseria meningitidis*, and the worldwide explosion of penicillin-resistant *Streptococcus pneumoniae* can be traced to a few clones originating in South Africa and Spain. This observation supports the concept that pathogenic organisms are highly adapted to the pathogenic state and have developed characteristics that enable them to be transmitted, to attach to surfaces, to invade tissue, to avoid host defenses, and thus to cause disease. In contrast, opportunistic pathogens cause disease principally in impaired hosts, and these organisms, which may be harmless members of normal flora in healthy persons, can act as virulent invaders in patients with severe defects in host defense mechanisms. Although opportunistic infection has traditionally been viewed as the exploitation of a weakened host through physiologic stress or immunocompromise (or both) by relatively "avirulent" pathogens, this is an oversimplification. For example, *Pseudomonas aeruginosa* recognizes host immune activation, specifically by binding interferon-γ to a cell surface protein OprF, which in turn, through a quorum-sensing signaling system, leads to the overexpression of virulence determinants such as PA-I (lecA) and pyocyanin. Thus, bacteria have developed a "contingency system" that recognizes immunologic perturbations in the host and counters this response by the expression of virulence factors.

Pathogenic organisms may be acquired by several routes. For example, direct contact has been implicated in the acquisition of staphylococcal disease. Airborne spread, usually by droplet nuclei, occurs in respiratory diseases such as influenza, in severe acute respiratory syndrome (SARS), and in the recently recognized Middle East respiratory syndrome (MERS). Contaminated water is the usual vehicle in *Giardia* infection and typhoid fever. Food-borne toxic illnesses may be caused by extracellular toxins produced by *Clostridium perfringens* and *Staphylococcus aureus*. Blood and blood products may be vectors for transmitting hepatitis B and C viruses as well as HIV. Sexual transmission is also important for these agents and for a variety of other pathogens, including *Treponema pallidum* (syphilis), *Neisseria gonorrhoeae* (gonorrhea), and *Chlamydia trachomatis* (nonspecific urethritis). The fetus may be infected in utero, and the infection may be devastating if the agent is rubella virus, cytomegalovirus, or parvovirus B19. Arthropod vectors may be important, as illustrated by mosquitoes for malaria and dengue, ticks for Lyme disease and ehrlichiosis, and lice for typhus.

Pathogens are able to cause disease because of a finely tuned array of adaptations, including the ability to attach to appropriate cells, often mediated by specialized structures such as the pili on gram-negative rods. Microbes such as *Shigella* species have the ability to invade cells and cause damage. Toxins may act at a distance or may intoxicate only infected cells. Pathogens have the ability to thwart host defenses by a variety of ingenious maneuvers. The antiphagocytic coat of the pneumococcus is an example. Organisms may change their surface antigen display at an astonishingly rapid rate to outmaneuver the host immune system. Examples include influenza virus and trypanosomes. Certain pathogens (e.g., *Toxoplasma gondii*) have the ability to inhibit the respiratory burst of phagocytes, and others (e.g., *Streptococcus pyogenes*) can destroy phagocytic cells that have engulfed them. The environment plays an important role in infection, both in transmission and in the host's ability to combat the invader. The humidity and temperature of air may affect the infectivity of airborne pathogens. The sanitary state of food and water, woefully lacking in many areas of the developing world, is an important factor in the acquisition of enteric pathogens, one of the major causes of mortality, morbidity, and disability, such as physical and mental developmental delay leading to poor performance in school. The malaria associated with the "bad air" of swamps is, in fact, due to the mosquitoes there, but the environmental association was appropriate. The nutritional status of the host is clearly a significant factor in certain infectious diseases. It is likely that micronutrient deficiency contributes to the invasion and multiplication of certain pathogens. A new concept is the possibility that infectious diseases cause malnutrition through a vicious circle of diarrhea leading to dehydration and poor oral intake, resulting in secondary diarrhea with a propensity for "stunting" and delaying intellectual development. Establishment of infection is a complicated interplay of factors involving the microbe, the host, and the environment.

Host reaction to infection may result in illness. For example, previous infection with *Campylobacter jejuni* is responsible for about 40% of cases of Guillain-Barré syndrome. The mechanism is thought to be the production of antibodies against *C. jejuni* lipopolysaccharides that cross-react with gangliosides in peripheral nerves. Similarly, much of the damage resulting from meningitis is due to the host's response to invading bacterial pathogens.

With some exceptions, infectious diseases are often treatable and curable. Thus, it is important to make an accurate etiologic diagnosis and to institute appropriate therapy promptly. In acute infections such as pneumonia, meningitis, or sepsis, rapid institution of therapy may be life-saving; thus, a presumptive etiologic diagnosis should be established before a definitive diagnosis. This presumptive diagnosis is based on the history, physical examination, epidemiology of illness in the community, and rapid techniques such as microscopic examination of appropriate gram-stained specimens or molecular techniques such as antigen detection or polymerase chain reaction. Antimicrobial therapy can then be instituted for the presumptive etiologic agents, but it must be reevaluated as more definitive diagnostic information becomes available.

The study as well as the understanding of infectious diseases is a dynamic process. A number of factors or themes of current interest contribute to this conclusion, including the following.

EMERGING INFECTIONS

The most obvious is AIDS, but recent examples with a major impact on the public health in the United States include community-associated methicillin-resistant *S. aureus*, a hypervirulent strain of *Clostridium difficile*, the 2009 H1N1 influenza, and multidrug-resistant gram-negative bacteria, such as carbapenamase-producing Enterobacteriaceae. More than 400 new, emerging infectious diseases have been described in the last 70 years; approximately 60% are zoonoses associated with geographic "hotspots." Their emergence is driven largely by ecologic, socioeconomic, and environmental factors.[2]

GENOMICS AND OTHER "OMICS"

The exact sequence of the genome of more than 2000 microbes relevant to humans has been determined. This new information, in concert with genomic information from multicellular organisms such as the *Anopheles* mosquito, offers significant promise for the development of new therapies and vaccines.[3] Careful analysis of the genomes of pathogens will continue to yield important information about the pathogenesis of infection. For example, genome sequencing of group A streptococci, collected over time with relevant robust clinical information, has detected the acquisition of new determinants (often by prophage) responsible for increased virulence and resulting in toxic shock syndrome, necrotizing fasciitis, or both, even within a single patient with sequential samples. Proteomics, transcriptomics, metabolomics, and virulomics have transformed research on infectious diseases and promise significant improvements in diagnostics and therapeutics in the future.

GENETIC FACTORS ALTERING SUSCEPTIBILITY TO INFECTION AND THE RESPONSE TO INFECTIOUS DISEASES

This field promises new and significant information relevant to the wide variety of responses to infectious diseases in humans. For example, an overvigorous response, with generation of tumor necrosis factor-α, may accentuate the development of cerebral complications in falciparum malaria. Analysis of single-nucleotide polymorphisms of the human genome will lead to an enhanced understanding of two fundamental issues in infectious diseases: why invasive, overt disease develops in only a small fraction of individuals colonized with a given microbe, and why infections are more severe in some people than in others. Variants in genes that encode molecules that mediate attachment, pathogen recognition, inflammatory cytokine response, and innate and adaptive immunity are being identified at an astonishing rate.

INNATE IMMUNITY

This is the most active field in the immunology of infectious diseases. The identification of pattern recognition receptors (e.g., Toll-like receptors and nucleotide oligomerization domain–like receptors) that recognize pathogen-associated molecular patterns, as well as endogenous substances reflecting tissue injury (e.g., alarmins), has revolutionized our understanding of the early host response to infection. Agonists or antagonists of Toll-like receptors have already entered clinical trials as adjuvant therapies or to improve the immunogenicity of vaccines. The other area that has exploded recently is the study of antimicrobial peptides (e.g., defensins, cathecidins, histatins, galectins) and their role in the early response to infectious disorders.

ANTIMICROBIAL RESISTANCE

The development of new antibacterial agents has slowed despite the burgeoning problem of antimicrobial resistance. This disconnect has been the focus of meetings among the pharmaceutical industry, the Infectious Diseases Society of America, the U.S. Food and Drug Administration, and internationally. Multiresistant pneumococci, vancomycin resistance in *S. aureus* and enterococci, and, perhaps most important, multidrug-resistant gram-negative bacilli are just a few examples. Some multidrug-resistant gram-negative bacilli are susceptible to only a few agents of "last resort," such as colistin or tigecycline; others are truly untreatable. Unfortunately, new agents active against these latter strains are years if not decades away from introduction.

THE ROLE OF INFECTIOUS AGENTS IN CHRONIC DISEASES

Many so-called idiopathic diseases may in fact have an infectious basis. Conditions for which there is some evidence (but not conclusive proof) of an infectious basis include diabetes, atherosclerosis, acute leukemia, collagen vascular diseases, and inflammatory bowel disease. Detection of "uncultivatable" microorganisms by newer techniques, such as 16S RNA analysis, may uncover agents responsible for "noninfectious" diseases or suggest a role in conditions that are considered infectious but in which the pathogen or pathogens are controversial (e.g., bacterial vaginosis). In addition, we know that hepatitis C virus, human papillomavirus, and *Helicobacter pylori* cause human cancers. Furthermore, changes in our own microbiome may lead to disease. Alterations in the gut microbiome are associated with obesity. Another recent example comes from experiments with mice lacking TLR5. These mice develop hyperphagia and hallmark features of the metabolic syndrome, including hyperlipidemia, hypertension, insulin resistance, and increased adiposity, associated with an altered gut microbiome. Further, transfer of this changed microbiota into germ-free wild-type mice induces most features of the metabolic syndrome in the recipients.[4] The explosion of new knowledge on the role of the human microbiome in health and disease has been so rapid and profound in the last decade that we thought a separate chapter on this subject was warranted (see Chapter 279).

GENERAL REFERENCES

For the General References and other additional features, please visit Expert Consult at https://expertconsult.inkling.com.

278

THE HUMAN MICROBIOME

ILSEUNG CHO AND MARTIN J. BLASER

Until recently, our understanding of the microbiota of humans (formerly called the normal flora) was handicapped by the limitations of traditional microbial cultivation. However, DNA-based analyses have expanded our horizons by generating enormous new data sets that can be mined for information about the composition and functional properties of our indigenous microbial communities (the human microbiome) and its collective genes (the metagenome). There has been great progress in characterizing the compositional range of the "normal" microbiome of healthy individuals.[1] Major clustering patterns at body sites such as the gastrointestinal tract provide new ways to classify individuals and, possibly, their disease risks. Substantial progress has been made in defining the overarching concepts that advance the field. However, the subject is vast, and the implications for human health and disease are wide-ranging. Although most focus has been on bacteria, inquiries aimed at eukaryotes, archaea, viruses, and retroviruses also are needed.

CHARACTERIZING THE MICROBIOME

Animals have had residential microbes for hundreds of millions of years, and comparisons of the phylogenies of animal hosts and their microbiota suggest the existence of specific selection based on co-adaptation. Cooperative interactions between microbes and their hosts typically involve microbial participation in host functions such as defense, metabolism, and reproduction. The composition of the microbiome varies by anatomic site (Fig. 278-1). The primary determinant of community composition is anatomic location, and individuals can be grouped according to the major types present at specific sites, such as the gastrointestinal tract. However, dietary changes can rapidly cause substantial changes in intestinal composition and function. Similarly, nasopharyngeal microbiota in young children varies seasonally, and vaginal microbiota may vary with menses. The aggregate microbiota of an individual appears to have a host-specific pattern, but large perturbations, such as antibiotic exposure or enteric infections, can lead to transient disequilibria or to the development of new stable states.

Among all mammals, the microbiota is extensively conserved at high taxonomic levels, but variation increases at progressively lower taxonomic levels. Consequently, most of the sequences obtained from the mouse gut represent genera that are not detected in humans. Furthermore, intraspecies variability

of the microbiota within the human population is also substantial. Indicator organisms such as *Helicobacter pylori* and *Streptococcus mutans* highlight some differences across the microbiota and metagenome among human ethnic groups; however, the extent of ethnic variation in overall metagenomic composition is unknown. The microbiomes of monozygotic twins are more closely related to one another than to those of unrelated individuals but not strikingly so, indicating important postnatal influences on composition.

The extensive lower-level taxonomic variation and large compositional differences observed even among highly related host organisms (e.g., mice and humans) are counterbalanced by the substantial conservation of metagenomic core functions (Fig. 278-2), reflecting the conservation of core bacterial properties involved in nucleic acid and protein synthesis and in metabolic and structural requirements. Of the more than 50 known phyla, most of the human microbiota is composed of fewer than 10 (and mostly six) phyla. Bacteria from other phyla, often of plant origin, that may be present in skin, nasopharyngeal, or gut samples are generally infrequent (<0.01% of the sequences) and probably represent transient carriage from food-borne and airborne exposures. The parallel needs of individual bacteria lead to competition for key substrates and to functional redundancy in the microbiota. Nevertheless, the enormous bacterial biomass also provides many unique or minimally redundant bacterial genes.

Resilience and Community Disturbance

Resilience, the ability to withstand disturbance, is a central concept in ecology. Whereas the microbiome of human adults appears highly resilient, the same may not be true for children. Because microbial population

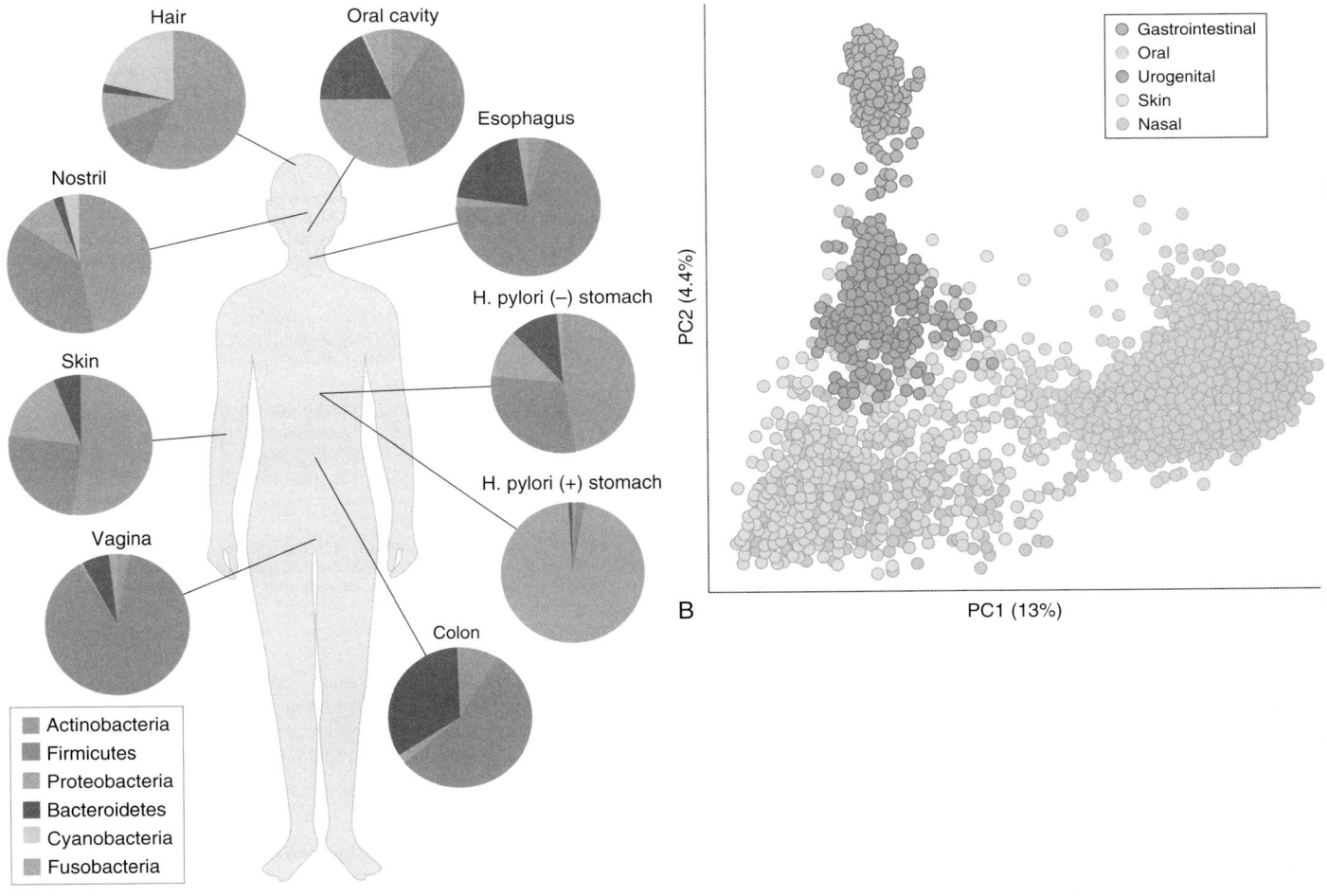

FIGURE 278-1. Compositional differences in the microbiome and metagenome by anatomic site. **A,** Substantial intersite microbiome variation. Higher level (e.g., phylum) taxonomic features display temporal (longitudinal) stability in individuals at specific anatomic sites. The figure indicates percentages of sequences at the taxonomic phylum level from selected references. Certain features, such as the presence or absence of *Helicobacter pylori*, are associated with alternative community composition states. (Modified from Cho I, Blaser MJ. The human microbiome: at the interface of health and disease. *Nat Rev Genet.* 2012;13:260-270.) **B,** Taxonomic variation and spatial relationships. Primary clustering, shown by principal coordinate analysis, is by anatomic site. Gastrointestinal, oral, urogenital, and skin populations separate, but samples from the nasal cavity bridge both the oral and skin populations. Site-specific differences as well as observed interpersonal conservation provide a framework to understand biologic and pathologic significance of particular microbiome compositions. (From Human Microbiome Project Consortium. Structure, function and diversity of the healthy human microbiome. *Nature.* 2012;486:207-214.)

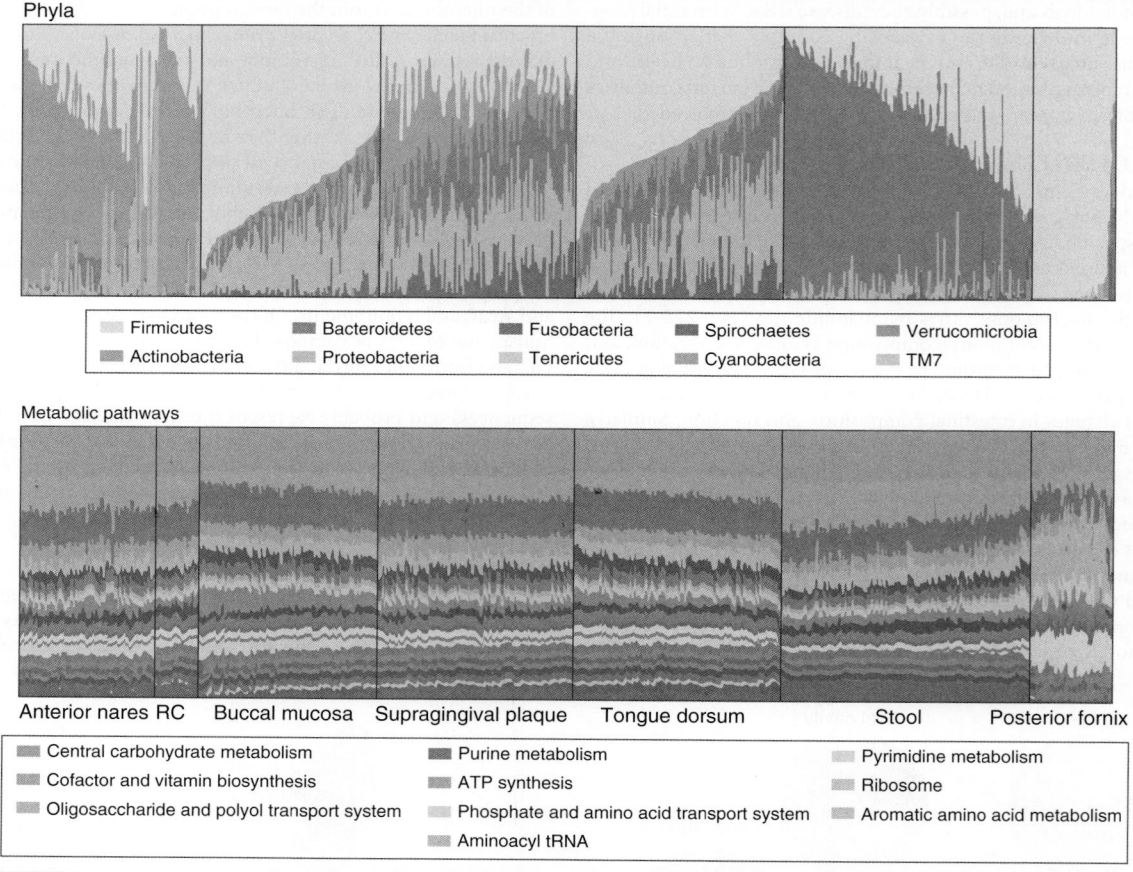

FIGURE 278-2. Variation and conservation in the microbiome and metagenomic functions of human anatomic sites. The phylogenetic composition of the microbiome at several anatomic sites shows substantial variation among individuals (*top panel*). Most but not all communities' membership consists of one or two dominant species (e.g., Firmicutes and Bacteroidetes in stool). However, the core metabolic functions of the microbial communities (*bottom panel*) are evenly distributed and highly conserved within a healthy population and across anatomic sites. Vertical bars represent microbiome samples of 242 individuals; colors represent relative abundance of microbial phyla or metabolic pathways in those samples. RC = retroauricular crease. (From Human Microbiome Project Consortium. Structure, function and diversity of the healthy human microbiome. *Nature.* 2012;486:207-214.)

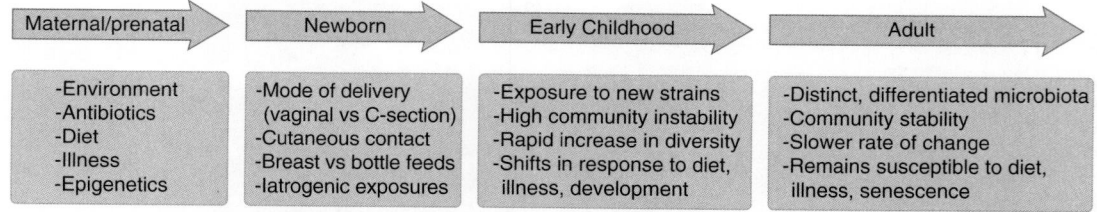

FIGURE 278-3. Factors and characteristics affecting acquisition and development of the microbiota from birth to adulthood. Numerous factors can affect the microbiome, beginning with prenatal exposures, such as to antibiotics, that can alter the composition of the maternal microbiome. Evidence exists that the mode of delivery can affect the initial composition of an infant's microbiome. The microbiome of young children is dynamic, but later in childhood (after 3 years of age), communities stabilize. At every stage of life, the microbiota are susceptible to external pressures, such as antibiotic exposure, diet, or disease.

structures appear more dynamic and developmental, resilience may be lower. An important natural experiment has been occurring during the past 70 years in which most of the world's population has been exposed to pharmacologic doses of antimicrobial agents. Such usage has been based on the implicit belief that the human microbiome is completely resilient and returns to the *status quo ante* after antibiotic-induced perturbation. These exposures also may cause medium- and long-term selection of resistant organisms and destabilization of the microbiome with new species compositions in the absence of further antibiotic exposure. Thus, despite the extensive resilience inherent in a complex ecosystem, there may be loss of recovery from continued perturbations, with important future implications for human health.

Extinctions

The human microbiome represents one or more complete ecosystems. Such communities may resist random perturbations, but if keystone species are lost, effects may cascade with secondary extinctions. High biodiversity diminishes this risk. In the short term, functional redundancy may mask extinction effects, but in the longer run, extinctions lead to loss of

contingency responses that can cause ecologic crashes. Considering the importance of guilds of bacteria exploiting parallel and sequential metabolic pathways and the extent of medical interventions that are perturbing them, these concepts are germane to the human metagenome.

● INFLUENCES ON THE MICROBIOTA DURING THE LIFE CYCLE

Differences in microbiota composition exist across body sites and between individuals.[2] However, changes are also evident across the human lifespan. Studies have answered important questions, such as whether temporal changes are life-stage specific and if they are predetermined by host genetic characteristics or environmental factors (Fig. 278-3).

Inheritance of Microbiota

The congruent phylogenies of mammals and their microbiota provide strong evidence for the inheritance of the microbiota. Increasing evidence supports maternal inheritance. Until the amniotic sac ruptures, a fetus has been considered to be essentially sterile. Immediately after vaginal delivery, microbial

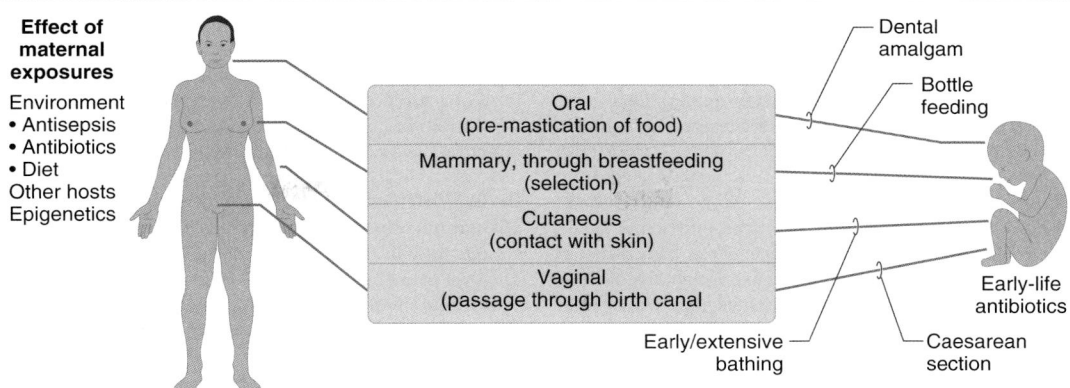

FIGURE 278-4. Factors affecting maternal exposures and vertical transmission of the microbiome between mother and child. Natural birth provides important opportunities for mother-to-child microbial transmission through a series of direct physical contacts. However, modern health practices can reduce flow of organisms and genes, thereby affecting the composition of the early infant microbiome. Many factors can affect early microbiomic development, including offspring genetics and epigenetics as well as dietary variation and environmental exposures. Organisms that have particular tissue or niche specificity explain conserved microbiome compositions at specific anatomic sites. (Modified from Cho I, Blaser MJ. The human microbiome: at the interface of health and disease. *Nat Rev Genet.* 2012;13:260-270.)

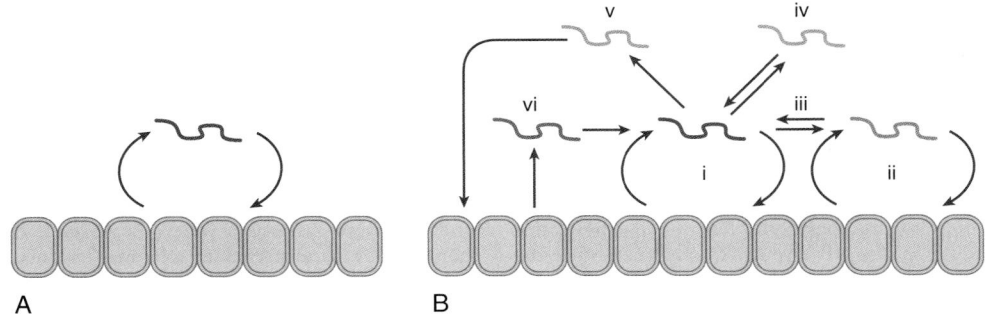

FIGURE 278-5. Equilibrium between co-evolved microbes and host cells. A, Single-organism equilibrium. In this model, there is a counter-regulatory interaction involving metabolic and physical signals between the microbe and host. B, Multiple organisms in equilibrium. This more complex model better approximates the interactions that occur in the human microbiome. Organisms may have individual equilibrium relationships (e.g., *i* and *ii*) with host cells. However, the interactions between these two microbes (*iii*) will affect their individual interactions. Similarly, another microbe (*iv*) may interact exclusively with an organism (*i*) but not with the host. Some interactions may be primarily unidirectional, as with a microbe (*v*) that is influenced by others and directly signals the host but does not receive direct host signals back. This may also proceed in the opposite direction as well (*vi*). (Modified from Plottel CS, Blaser MJ. Microbiome and malignancy. *Cell Host Microbe.* 2011;10:324-335.)

populations in the infant closely resemble those of the mother's vagina, with lactobacilli predominating. Because lactic acid–producing bacteria dominate both the vaginal canal and mother's milk, the initial bloom of lactobacilli cannot be considered accidental.

The multiple opportunities for the microbiota to be transferred from a mother to her baby may be disrupted by modern lifestyles.[3] Cesarean section instead of vaginal delivery is an obvious example of the potential impact of medical practice on microbiota composition, with substantial differences in founding populations that may persist for months. Such difference may alter infant immune responses, potentially leading to long-term consequences (Fig. 278-4).

Postnatal Influences on the Microbiota

Over a lifetime, each person develops a densely populated microbiome. The eruption of teeth is responsible for major successions in the oral microbiota, suggesting that succession may be a general property of human microbiome dynamics. Exposure (or not) to environmental microbes is another important but highly variable reservoir for the resident microbiota. Antibiotic use early in life produces major shifts in both microbiota characteristics and host developmental phenotypes, both on the farm and in experimental animals. Whether such precedents are applicable to human children is unknown but seems likely. If so, then both the timing of microbiome succession and the specific organisms present may affect metabolic, immunologic, and even cognitive development.

Microbiome Dynamics in Adults

Our knowledge of microbiome dynamics, especially age-related changes, during human adulthood is limited. We know that the postmenopause vaginal microbiota differs substantially from that during the reproductive period. Similarly, in the stomach, the age-related progressive development of gastric atrophy (enhanced by *H. pylori* presence) selects for gastric microbiota that are substantially different from the norm. Analogous changes may be

occurring in other body sites as senescence advances. In the gut, the ratio of Bacteroidetes to Firmicutes changes with age. The specific interactions that the microbiome has with human hosts are enormously complex (Fig. 278-5), and further studies will be needed to define the specific pathways that inform the maintenance of health or the pathogenesis of disease. These concepts are particularly relevant to oncogenesis, which is generally age related. In the multistep Nordling hypothesis of oncogenesis, four to six somatic cell mutations are needed for cancer development. Microbiota shifts may contribute to this multistep process. Residential microbes can contribute to host cell mutagenesis by inflammation, increased cell proliferation, and production of promutagenic metabolites (e.g., butyrate).

● DISEASE LINKS AND HEALTH IMPLICATIONS

How, then, does the microbiome affect human health? For many conditions, the challenge is to discover whether there is a causal link between microbiome variation and significant disease. Limitations in the definitions and stratification of clinical syndromes, including irritable bowel syndrome and nonulcer dyspepsia, reduce the potential of microbiome studies. Several examples of preliminary but promising observations follow.

Cutaneous Microbiome

The cutaneous microbiome could be involved in specific diseases, such as psoriasis, a chronic, idiopathic inflammatory condition. In some studies, Actinobacteria were significantly underrepresented in psoriatic lesions compared with unaffected skin both in psoriasis patients and in normal controls. Atopic dermatitis, another chronic inflammatory condition, has substantially increased in incidence in developed countries, suggesting a potential role for microbiome alterations. Classic atopic dermatitis occurs in areas, such as the antecubital and popliteal fossae, with similar microbial populations, suggesting a microbiome role. Similarly, *Propionibacterium acnes* has been implicated in the common dermatologic condition acne. Although *P. acnes* thrives in the cutaneous pilosebaceous units and secretes enzymes that cause local injury and inflammation, continuing investigations are identifying *P. acnes* strain differences as well as other microbes in acne development. In chronic skin ulcers, often secondary to venous stasis or diabetes, cutaneous microbiome shifts occur. For example, Pseudomonadaceae are increased in patients with chronic ulcers treated with antibiotics, and Streptococcaceae are increased in diabetic ulcers.

Gastric Microbiome
The discovery of *H. pylori* overturned the dogma that the stomach is sterile. In *H. pylori*–negative persons, gastric microbiota diversity is high. Most of the prominent gastric species also are abundant in the oropharynx, indicating that many constituents are swallowed from more proximal sites or that close relatives of the oral microbiota colonize more distally. In contrast, among *H. pylori*–positive persons, *H. pylori* often accounts for more than 90% of sequence reads from the gastric microbiota, reducing the overall diversity in this discrete niche. *H. pylori* is a classical amphibiont; the presence (or absence) of an *H. pylori*–dominated gastric microbiota is strongly associated with particular diseases with important age-related differences. Its presence increases risk for development of peptic ulcer disease, gastric mucosa-associated lymphoid tissue (MALT) tumors, and gastric adenocarcinoma, but its absence is associated with increased reflux esophagitis and childhood-onset asthma. These disease relationships illustrate our complex biologic interactions with our microbiota.

The Colonic Microbiota and Colorectal Cancer
Involvement of the colonic microbiota in the development of colorectal cancers has long been suspected.[4] Synthesis of short-chain fatty acids, in particular butyrate, may induce apoptosis, cell cycle arrest, and differentiation through Wnt signaling. Microbes may also be genotoxic to colonic epithelial cells, inducting polyploidy. The colonic microbiota also might promote colorectal cancer by eliciting host responses, for example, by stimulating exaggerated immune responses, potentially through T_H17 cells. Another link with colorectal cancer is suggested by antibiotic administration, altering the composition of the colonic microbiota, affecting expression of host genes involved in cell cycle regulation, and reducing epithelial proliferation. Early studies limited to identifying culture-dependent species, such as *Streptococcus bovis*, could not adequately assess anaerobic constituents. However, the anaerobic genus *Fusobacterium* has recently been associated with colorectal cancer, especially *Fusobacterium nucleatum*, a mucosally adherent, proinflammatory microbe first identified in the mouth. In colorectal cancer samples, *F. nucleatum* sequences were significantly enriched compared with control subjects, whereas both Bacteroidetes and Firmicutes were relatively depleted in those with *Fusobacterium*-rich malignant neoplasms. However, the causal direction of the association has not yet been ascertained. Finally, epigenetic phenomena, such as DNA hypermethylation, have been demonstrated to play an important role in the development of colorectal cancers through microsatellite instability and the sessile serrated adenoma pathway. It is possible that interactions with the microbiome may affect epigenetic pathways for colonic carcinogenesis.

The Colon Microbiota and Inflammatory Bowel Disease
The microbiome is essential for the activation of host immune responses.[5] For example, in mice, T_H17 cell differentiation in the lamina propria requires the presence of segmented filamentous bacteria, and polysaccharide A produced by *Bacteroides fragilis* mediates conversion of CD4$^+$ T cells into regulatory T cells. Accordingly, microbes are suspected to be involved in inflammatory bowel diseases (Chapter 141). Susceptibility to inflammatory bowel disease is associated with host polymorphisms in bacterial sensor genes such as nucleotide-binding oligomerization domain–containing protein 2 (*NOD2*; also known as *CARD15*) and toll-like receptor 4 (*TLR4*), and patients with inflammatory bowel disease sometimes improve after antibiotic treatment. Exposure to antibiotics in early childhood has been associated with significantly increased risk for Crohn's disease, suggesting that gut microbiome perturbations may enhance disease risk. Microbial diversity is significantly diminished in Crohn's disease, suggesting decreased gut microbiome resilience. Gut microbiome population structures of patients with ulcerative colitis or Crohn's disease are not normal and are clustered by disease. More recent investigations have implicated adherent-invasive *Escherichia coli* as a candidate pathogen in ileal Crohn's disease, given its ability to adhere to and invade epithelial cells and to replicate within macrophages. Specific bacteria among the Enterobacteriaceae may synergize with a disordered microbiome to increase the risk of ulcerative colitis. Among twins

discordant for ulcerative colitis, those affected had significantly reduced bacterial diversity but increased Actinobacteria and Proteobacteria. Patients with Crohn's disease have overrepresentation of *Enterococcus faecium* and several Proteobacteria compared with controls. The microbial patterns observed for the conditions described are preliminary, and their specificity and causal direction have not been established.[6]

The Gut Microbiota and Diseases of the Liver
The gut microbiota may be involved in hepatic conditions, including nonalcoholic fatty liver disease, alcoholic steatosis, and hepatocellular carcinoma. The liver is the first solid organ exposed to the metabolic products generated by the gut microbiome, including acetaldehyde, ammonia, and phenols. Compared with germ-free mice, the presence of a microbiome in conventional mice led to suppression of intestinal epithelium angiopoietin-related protein 4, which inhibits lipoprotein lipase, increasing downstream triglyceride accumulation in the hepatic parenchyma and adipocytes. Chronic ethanol exposure disturbs the gut microbiome, but roles for the microbiome in steatosis are unresolved. Particular murine colonic commensals (e.g., *Helicobacter hepaticus*) promote the development of hepatocellular carcinoma. Patients with cirrhosis have a substantially altered microbiome, including community-wide changes at multiple taxonomic levels, with enrichment of Proteobacteria and Fusobacteria (phyla) and of Enterobacteriaceae, Veillonellaceae, and Streptococcaceae (family). Although many observations suggest links between microbiome composition and liver disease, definitive associations in humans are lacking.

The Gut Microbiota and Obesity
Genetically obese (*ob/ob*) mice have decreased ratios of Bacteroidetes to Firmicutes compared with lean (*ob/+* and *+/+* wild-type) siblings. Transplantation of gut microbiota from the obese (*ob/ob*) to germ-free mice conferred an obese phenotype, which shows the transmissibility of metabolic phenotypes; the transferred microbiomes had increased capacity for energy harvest. Studies have shown that transplantation of human microbiota can achieve parallel effects. In humans, relative Bacteroidetes proportions increase with weight loss. In monozygotic and dizygotic twins, obesity has been associated with decreased Bacteroidetes and diminished bacterial diversity, with enrichment of genes related to lipid and carbohydrate metabolism. In early life, the administration of antibiotics or alterations in diet may select for altered microbiota compositions, contributing to development of obesity.[7] Antibiotic use in human infancy, before the age of 6 months, has been significantly associated with obesity development. In contrast, in another study, perinatal administration of a *Lactobacillus rhamnosus* GG–based probiotic decreased excessive weight gain during childhood. These preliminary studies provide support for the concept that the early-life microbiota is modifiable, with alterations affecting risk of childhood-onset obesity. Studies are ongoing in adults to determine specific characteristics of the microbiome that may predict the risk of adiposity-related comorbidities.[8] Interventions used to treat obesity, such as the Roux-en-Y gastric bypass, substantially alter the gut microbiome, which may contribute to the metabolic effects.

The Gut Microbiota and Rheumatoid Arthritis
Altered regulation of host responses secondary to dysbiosis within the gut lumen could affect distant anatomic sites. This may be a mechanism in rheumatoid arthritis, another chronic idiopathic inflammatory condition. In mice, the presence of segmented filamentous bacteria in the gut microbiome causes local expansion of T_H17 cells that then migrate to peripheral immune compartments and activate B cells into antibody-producing plasma cells. Antibody production leads to immune-mediated destruction of the joints that mirrors rheumatoid arthritis. Substantial alterations in the gut microbiota have been identified in patients in the early stages of rheumatoid arthritis, consistent with a pathogenic role.

The Effect of the Microbiota on the Brain and Behavior
Early work suggests potential links between the gut microbiome and specific neurologic processes and disorders. Germ-free mice showed an exaggerated hypothalamic-pituitary response to stress that diminished after conventionalization with fecal matter. Subsequent investigations showed that the microbiome could alter neurotransmitter levels, such as brain-derived neurotropic factor and serotonin.[9] The rising incidence of autism in developed societies has led investigators to question whether shifts in gut microbes may play a causative role in these neurodevelopmental disorders. However, causal associations are difficult to determine from existing studies because many affected

children have concomitant gastrointestinal symptoms and were repeatedly treated with antibiotics. Microbiome effects on multiple sclerosis and other neurologic diseases have been hypothesized.

CAUSE OR EFFECT?

Microbiome analysis in humans has been largely observational, associating disease phenotypes with particular microbiota constituents. But which is causal? Does factor A cause factor B, does factor B cause factor A, or does factor C cause both A and B? Bradford Hill developed criteria to address the questions, "In what circumstances can we pass from this observed association to a verdict of causation? Upon what basis should we proceed to do so?" The criteria include the strength of association; its consistency, specificity, temporality, and biologic plausibility; and whether biologic gradients are present, experimental support exists, and support can be extrapolated from known causal relationships. These criteria are applicable to understanding either environmental or genetic (including metagenomic) causal roles.

For understanding causation and pathogenesis, model organisms provide an important approach. Animal models approximate some human diseases (e.g., asthma, atherosclerosis), but others (e.g., psoriasis) are not well reproduced. For those diseases that can be studied in model organisms, microbiota roles can be explored. Standard models of inbred mice are limited by their uncontrolled microbiome diversity. Certain disease states are well studied in these models, such as the effects of segmented filamentous bacteria on T_H17 development or the susceptibility to type 1 diabetes in nonobese diabetic mice. The use of germ-free mice eliminates microbiome variability until the introduction of "test" microbiota but requires specialized facilities, limiting their widespread use. The recent availability of germ-free animals from commercial sources permits their conventionalization without requiring such facilities, permitting direct observation of microbiota effects.

PERSPECTIVES

To better understand the implications of microbiota and metagenome variation in human health and disease, improved informatics tools are needed. The multidimensionality of the human and microbial phenotypes and the dynamic, nonlinear interactions challenge simple linear solutions.

The inherent compositional complexity of the microbiome limits investigations of microbe-associated diseases by classical approaches, such as Koch's postulates. Instead of single organisms associated with disease, community characteristics (composition and metagenomic functionality) may be more relevant. The principles of host interaction with pathogens and commensals contain many parallel features, which can help tutor the new field, but the nature of the selection for commensalism is more complex and highly dynamic. The scale of the interface suggests that microbiome-host interactions have important bearings on disease susceptibility; microbial effects on host metabolism and immunity provide "proof-of-principle" for the broader phenomenon of disease susceptibility. Modifying disease risk by altering metabolic, immunologic, or developmental pathways is an obvious strategy. Study of the microbiome, leading to new understandings of complex traits, will ultimately lead to new preventives, diagnostics, and therapies.

GENERAL REFERENCES

For the General References and other additional features, please visit Expert Consult at https://expertconsult.inkling.com.

279

PRINCIPLES OF ANTI-INFECTIVE THERAPY

GEORGE M. ELIOPOULOS

Among the pharmaceutical agents used in the treatment of human disease, antimicrobial agents are distinctive because they target invading microorganisms rather than abnormal human cellular functions. As a result, to select an appropriate antimicrobial regimen, it is necessary to consider both the activity of the agent against the known or suspected pathogen and the effects that agent might have on the individual under treatment. Although the term *anti-infective agent* can be used more broadly to include substances that ameliorate infection by altering the virulence of the pathogen or modulating the host's response to infection, for purposes of this chapter, *anti-infective agent* and *antimicrobial agent* are used interchangeably to refer to drugs that inhibit the growth of microbial pathogens. This chapter focuses primarily on agents directed against bacterial pathogens, although many parallels can be drawn to the use of antimicrobial agents for the treatment of fungal, viral, or parasitic infections.

On the time scale of human history, the modern antibiotic era is short. Since the introduction of penicillin for general clinical use in the mid-1940s, the numerous antimicrobial agents developed for human use have saved countless lives and have led to amazing advances in cancer chemotherapy, organ transplantation, and implant surgery that have improved and extended the lives of many others. Unfortunately, over time, resistance to available antibiotics has become widespread among many common bacterial pathogens,[1] making the selection of appropriate antimicrobial regimens ever more challenging and threatening to thrust an unfortunate few into a situation resembling the pre-antibiotic era.

SELECTING ANTIMICROBIAL THERAPY TARGETING THE PATHOGEN

Empirical Antimicrobial Therapy

In most instances, selection of the initial antimicrobial therapy proceeds empirically, before a causative organism is identified or tested for susceptibility to antimicrobial agents. The clinician's first decision is whether a patient's symptoms are likely to represent infection. Fever may result from neoplastic, rheumatologic, or other noninfectious processes and does not necessarily imply the presence of infection. Noninfectious causes of fever, such as deep vein thrombophlebitis, drug reaction, and vasculitis, may pose just as great a risk to the patient as infection and must not be overlooked.

Additional symptoms, signs, and laboratory or radiographic data usually help define whether infection is likely and, if so, localize the organ systems involved. This information allows an initial prediction about the organisms likely to be involved. For example, if the initial data cause one to suspect a diagnosis of community-acquired pneumonia in a previously healthy person who does not have any unusual exposures, *Streptococcus pneumoniae* and atypical bacteria such as *Mycoplasma pneumoniae* or *Chlamydophila pneumoniae* would be prominent on the list of potential pathogens to be targeted in selecting antimicrobial therapy. Examination of a gram-stained slide of expectorated sputum may provide valuable information. The prominent appearance of gram-positive cocci in clusters, for example, would alert the clinician to the possible presence of *Staphylococcus aureus*, many isolates of which are now methicillin resistant, and thus lead the clinician to select treatment options to include targeting of these organisms.

Guidance regarding the probable pathogens for site-specific infections and the susceptibility of these organisms to antimicrobial agents is available from a number of sources.[2] In some cases, the susceptibility of suspected pathogens can be predicted with a high degree of certainty. For example, *Streptococcus pyogenes* remains uniformly susceptible to penicillin G. In other instances, resistance has emerged to antimicrobials previously considered to be highly active against a species. Resistance rates for a given organism may vary widely by region, by health care institution, or even by patient care area within a hospital. For this reason, access to periodically updated, cumulative antibiotic susceptibility profile data specific to an institution can be important. Typically presented in tabular form, these "antibiograms" show the percentage of recently isolated bacterial pathogens that proved "susceptible" to the antibiotics tested and can help guide the selection of appropriate empirical regimens at that practice site.

There is mounting evidence that selection of an appropriate regimen (i.e., one that contains an antimicrobial that can be expected to inhibit the causative pathogen at the site of infection) and the prompt initiation of that empirical treatment result in improved clinical outcomes in those with serious infections. Published guidelines for the treatment of community-acquired pneumonia (Chapter 97) advise administration of the first dose of appropriate antimicrobial therapy while the patient is still in the emergency department.

Whenever possible, samples of purulent exudates, blood, or other body fluids suspected to be infected should be obtained for culture before antimicrobial therapy is started. Identification and susceptibility testing of the microorganisms detected can be used to direct subsequent definitive treatment. At times, however, this principle must be overridden. For example, when bacterial meningitis is suspected, antibiotic therapy (often with adjunctive corticosteroids) must not be delayed when a lumbar puncture cannot be performed promptly to obtain material for culture. In such instances, blood samples taken for culture before the administration of antibiotics often reveal the causative organism, or the pathogen may grow from spinal fluid even if lumbar puncture is delayed.

Definitive Antimicrobial Therapy

Identification of the causative microorganism and determination of its susceptibility to available drugs are the basis for optimizing definitive antimicrobial regimens. Often, the antibiotics used for empirical therapy are appropriate for definitive therapy and can be continued. At other times, the results allow one to switch to a narrower spectrum, better tolerated, or less expensive antimicrobial.[3] In some instances, test results indicate the need to broaden the spectrum of an anti-infective regimen by adding or substituting agents active against pathogens inadequately targeted by the initial empirical regimen.

In almost all cases, it is desirable to test an infecting organism's susceptibility to antimicrobials that may be useful. To extend the example cited earlier, although it is not necessary to test the susceptibility of S. pyogenes to penicillin G, some isolates are resistant to macrolide antibiotics (e.g., erythromycin, azithromycin) and other drugs, so the testing of alternative agents might be useful for patients who are intolerant of β-lactam antibiotics. Even when the activity of certain antimicrobials can be predicted with great confidence, susceptibility testing is still useful. For example, surveillance studies examining hundreds of isolates have predicted that vancomycin or linezolid would inhibit virtually all S. aureus strains recovered from initial clinical specimens. Therefore, on statistical grounds, testing of these agents would not seem warranted; however, rare isolates resistant to these agents have now been encountered, and it is advantageous to detect such isolates for both therapeutic and epidemiologic purposes. For most bacterial pathogens, resistance to commonly used agents is sufficiently frequent that testing of antimicrobials being considered for definitive therapy is essential. Organisms of the family Enterobacteriaceae that are resistant to multiple antibiotics are isolated often enough, even among outpatients, that susceptibility to agents previously considered broadly active, including third-generation cephalosporins, fluoroquinolones, and aminoglycosides, is no longer ensured. Even more challenging problems of drug resistance are encountered among isolates of species such as Pseudomonas aeruginosa, Acinetobacter baumannii, and Stenotrophomonas maltophilia.

Susceptibility Testing

Several methods are available for determining the susceptibility of a bacterial isolate to antimicrobial agents being considered for therapy. Tests most frequently used in clinical microbiology laboratories today are variations of three methods: serial dilution, disc diffusion, and gradient diffusion. The minimal inhibitory concentration (MIC) represents the lowest concentration of an antimicrobial tested that inhibits growth of the microorganism in test media.

In the dilution method, the antimicrobial is diluted in broth or agar to span a range of (usually) two-fold decreasing concentrations, and the medium is then inoculated with a standardized number of organisms. After incubation for a specified period (usually 16 to 24 hours) at 35° to 37° C, the series of dilution tubes or microtiter wells (for broth dilution) or agar plates (for agar dilution) is examined for growth. The MIC is determined by direct inspection as the lowest concentration that prevents turbidity of the broth or colony formation on agar. Modifications of this method allow the automation of many steps in the process, permitting more efficient test performance in clinical laboratories.

In the disc diffusion method, paper discs impregnated with a standardized amount of the antimicrobial are placed on an agar plate, the surface of which has been seeded with the bacterium to be tested. During incubation, the antimicrobial diffuses from the disc into the surrounding agar and inhibits growth of the seeded organism. After a specified period of incubation, the zone of growth inhibition around the disc is measured. By this method, the MIC is not determined directly. Instead, relying on accumulated data correlating inhibition zones with MICs, the measured zone is used to predict the susceptibility of the organism to the drug tested.

The gradient diffusion method is similar to the disc diffusion method, except that instead of using a round paper disc impregnated with a single concentration of the antimicrobial, this test uses a strip impregnated with the antimicrobial applied in a concentration gradient along its length. The strip is laid on the surface of an agar plate that has been inoculated with a suspension of the organism to be tested, and the plate is then incubated. By visually inspecting where the zone of growth inhibition on the agar surface intersects the strip (which is marked at intervals corresponding to MIC equivalents), it is possible to determine the MIC value directly.

To perform susceptibility studies and to interpret the results, it is necessary to identify the organism to be tested. This knowledge allows the selection of appropriate methods and interpretive criteria to determine whether an organism is "susceptible," "intermediate," or "resistant" to an antimicrobial on the basis of measurement of the MIC or the inhibition zone diameter. To illustrate this point, consider that an enterococcus is determined to be susceptible to penicillin if the MIC is less than or equal to 8 µg/mL, whereas for viridans streptococci, the corresponding breakpoint for susceptibility to penicillin is the MIC of 0.12 µg/mL. Thus, knowledge that the MIC of penicillin against a gram-positive coccus growing in short chains is 2 µg/mL does not allow the determination of whether it is susceptible to penicillin unless the organism has been identified.

Additional tests are sometimes required to fully assess susceptibility to an antimicrobial. For oxacillin-susceptible S. aureus, a test for penicillinase production is performed to assess susceptibility to penicillin G. For erythromycin-resistant, clindamycin-susceptible S. aureus, the laboratory may perform a supplementary D-zone test or equivalent before reporting the clindamycin result. A positive D-zone test result (i.e., blunting of the inhibition zone around a clindamycin disc in proximity to an erythromycin disc) predicts the presence of erm genes. Their product, a ribosomal methylase, can confer resistance to clindamycin if it is expressed; however, clindamycin is a poor inducer of this resistance trait (in contrast to erythromycin, which is a good inducer). A positive test result thus implies the presence of inducible resistance traits. Mutants with constitutive production of methylase can be selected during treatment, resulting in the emergence of clindamycin resistance and an increased risk of clinical failure when this drug is used to treat serious staphylococcal infections caused by strains with the erm gene.

In principle, tests for the presence of resistance genes, their products, or both can be used in place of phenotypic resistance testing. Such methods have the potential to provide answers more rapidly than can be obtained with the usual susceptibility tests of growth inhibition, which generally require several hours of incubation. At present, these tests are not yet widely employed, with the exception of testing for methicillin resistance by detection of the mecA gene or its product, penicillin-binding protein 2a, or testing for rifampin resistance by detection of resistance mutations in Mycobacterium tuberculosis. Newer technologies, such as matrix-assisted laser desorption ionization–time of flight mass spectrometry, are being explored as a means of providing not only more rapid identification of organisms but also their predicted susceptibility to antimicrobial agents.[4]

Bactericidal Activity

In some circumstances, an antimicrobial regimen that kills pathogenic microorganisms would be preferable to an alternative regimen that only inhibits growth of the pathogen. Bactericidal activity is desirable in the treatment of endocarditis or meningitis; in these infections, bacteriostatic agents have generally performed poorly, possibly because of inadequate host responses to infection at these sites. Tests to measure the bactericidal activity of an antibiotic in vitro have been developed. Bactericidal activity is usually defined as a 99.9% reduction in the number of viable colony-forming units relative to the inoculum density at a specified incubation time, which is usually 20 to 24 hours.

Despite the theoretical benefit of determining the bactericidal activity of an antibiotic or drug regimen, these tests are rarely used clinically because of several factors, including (1) the labor-intensive nature of the tests, (2) the potential for discordant results due to the various methods and criteria for determining bactericidal activity, and (3) the imperfect correlation between bactericidal activity measured in vitro and clinical outcomes observed.

● SELECTING ANTIMICROBIAL THERAPY APPROPRIATE TO THE INFECTION AND PATIENT

Nature of the Infection

Determination that a pathogenic microorganism is susceptible to an antibiotic in vitro does not ensure that treatment with that drug will result in a successful clinical outcome. The antimicrobial must reach the site of infection in adequate concentration, which is generally assumed to be some multiple of the MIC, and it must demonstrate activity in the infection milieu. For some infections and antimicrobials, these requirements cannot easily be met.

A number of antimicrobials fail to penetrate into cerebrospinal fluid sufficiently well to permit their use for the treatment of bacterial meningitis in adults. First-generation cephalosporins or aminoglycosides given intravenously do not enter the subarachnoid space well enough to allow their use as primary agents for treatment of this disease. Aminoglycosides have been administered by intrathecal or intraventricular instillation when needed for the treatment of gram-negative meningitis, but the availability of newer β-lactams with broad activity, high potency, and reasonable cerebrospinal fluid penetration when administered intravenously has largely eliminated the need for direct instillation of antimicrobials.

In other situations, antimicrobials may penetrate to the site of infection, only to be inactivated by local factors. For example, daptomycin is inactivated by interaction with pulmonary surfactant, so this antibiotic is not indicated for the treatment of bronchopneumonia, even though it is highly active against *S. pneumoniae* isolates in vitro. Antibiotics can also be inactivated by cellular debris or macromolecules present within abscesses, and some exhibit reduced potency at the low pH and reduced oxygen tensions prevailing at these sites. Finally, high densities of microorganisms within abscesses may elaborate sufficiently high concentrations of β-lactamases to inactivate some relatively labile β-lactam antibiotics. All these factors provide a rationale for the drainage of large abscesses as an adjunct to antimicrobial therapy.

Bacterial infections associated with foreign bodies such as artificial joints, cardiac pacemakers, or prosthetic heart valves can be particularly difficult to eradicate without removal of the foreign material. The reasons are not completely understood, but they relate, at least in part, to the presence of biofilm, which is composed of bacteria embedded within extracellular material that is adherent to the foreign body. Bacteria recovered from biofilms are metabolically different from and less susceptible to antimicrobial agents than planktonic cells (i.e., those freely suspended in liquid medium) of the same organism. Rifampin is often added to antimicrobial regimens for the treatment of infections involving prosthetic material. This inhibitor of RNA polymerase rapidly penetrates into biofilms and demonstrates relatively similar activity against both biofilm-associated and planktonic cells of a susceptible organism. However, because resistance to rifampin emerges rapidly, it is not used as a single agent in these circumstances; rifampin must be combined with a second active drug to minimize the risk that resistance will emerge. Despite such approaches, many infections involving implanted devices prove refractory to antimicrobial therapy alone and require removal of the foreign material for eradication.

Host Factors

After consideration of the nature of the infection and the antimicrobials determined in vitro to be active against a bacterial isolate (or likely to be active against probable pathogens when an isolate is not yet available), the ultimate choice of an antimicrobial regimen must take into account a number of additional patient-specific factors, some examples of which are examined in the following paragraphs.

Allergies

It is imperative to obtain a history of previous allergic reactions to antimicrobial agents. Some reactions are by nature so severe and potentially life-threatening that one must avoid using the same agent or drugs within the same class for which cross-reactivity is likely to occur. Examples of such reactions include an immediate hypersensitivity reaction to penicillin (e.g., hives, lip swelling, laryngeal edema, circulatory collapse) and a mucocutaneous bullous eruption from a sulfonamide (e.g., Stevens-Johnson syndrome).

In cases in which the allergic reaction was mild, such as a faint, self-limited rash in a patient receiving penicillin, the clinician may elect to use a related antimicrobial, such as a cephalosporin, when the probability of cross-sensitivity and the risk for a severe adverse outcome if a reaction were to occur are both assessed to be low. In these instances, careful monitoring of the patient for adverse reactions is essential. Rarely, for patients with significant allergies to potentially life-saving antimicrobial agents for which no alternative exists, desensitization of the patient to the antimicrobial is attempted so that the agent can be used. For example, desensitization protocols are available for penicillin and for trimethoprim-sulfamethoxazole. Because of the risks involved, these procedures may need to be performed in intensive care unit settings.

Pregnancy

A number of antimicrobial agents have the potential to cause fetal harm if they are administered to a pregnant woman. For example, tetracyclines can cause tooth discoloration and hypoplasia of dental enamel and are thus avoided in pregnant women and young children. Streptomycin given during pregnancy can cross the placenta, and evidence of eighth nerve toxicity in the child has been reported. A few other antimicrobials are labeled by the Food and Drug Administration as pregnancy category D (evidence of human risk) or are contraindicated because of fetal harm (category X). Many more antimicrobials, however, are assigned to category C; for these drugs, the potential risk to the fetus is based on animal studies. In designing antimicrobial regimens, the possibility of pregnancy should be considered in any woman of childbearing age so that the risks of candidate agents can be individually reviewed and the safest possible therapy selected.

Many antibiotics used to treat lactating women can be found in breast milk. Thus, it may be necessary to suspend breast-feeding during treatment if exposure of the infant to the drug must be avoided.

Pregnant women may be particularly susceptible to certain antimicrobial-associated toxicities. Death resulting from hepatic failure has been described in pregnant women receiving large doses of tetracycline. Potentially life-threatening hepatic steatosis has been observed in patients treated with a combination of the antiretroviral agents didanosine plus stavudine; pregnant women may be especially vulnerable to this toxic effect.

Age

For reasons discussed earlier, tetracycline antibiotics are avoided in children during tooth development to prevent discoloration and enamel hypoplasia of the permanent teeth. Because fluoroquinolone antimicrobials produce erosion of cartilage and arthropathy in juvenile animals, they are avoided in children when alternative agents are available. Recently, limited pediatric indications were added for ciprofloxacin (for complicated urinary tract infection and pyelonephritis and after inhalational exposure to anthrax) and for levofloxacin (inhalational exposure to anthrax and for plague). Musculoskeletal complaints appear to be more frequent in children treated with ciprofloxacin than with nonfluoroquinolone antimicrobials.

Pediatric dosing regimens differ from those appropriate for adults. Some agents, such as linezolid, are eliminated much more rapidly in young children (excluding preterm neonates) than in older children and adults, so higher doses may be required. In premature infants and neonates, renal function has not yet reached full capacity, and elimination of some antimicrobials may be delayed. Similarly, hepatic clearance activity is not fully developed in the very young, which has led to cardiovascular collapse and fatalities from chloramphenicol treatment. Absorption of oral antimicrobials may also differ with age if their absorption is dependent on gastric pH. The gastric pH of young children is higher than that of adults, and achlorhydria resulting in higher gastric pH is more common in adults older than 60 years than in younger adults. Thus, in young children and older adults, the absorption of oral drugs that are unstable in acid, such as penicillin G, may be higher than that in younger adults. In contrast, antimicrobials such as ketoconazole require gastric acid for absorption and may be less bioavailable in persons with reduced gastric acid production.

A curious association between the appearance of a rash and the patient's age and sex was noted during development of the fluoroquinolone antimicrobial gemifloxacin. In clinical studies, rash was more common in young women than in men and older women, suggesting that there may be hormonal influences on the risk for development of a rash.

Renal and Hepatic Function

Renal excretion and hepatobiliary excretion are the major routes of elimination for antimicrobial agents. Relatively few antibacterial agents can be administered without dosage adjustments in patients with renal dysfunction. Included among these drugs are nafcillin, ceftriaxone, doxycycline, azithromycin, and linezolid. Although linezolid exposure is not significantly altered, microbiologically inactive metabolites of the compound do accumulate in end-stage renal disease; what, if any, effect this has is unknown.

A number of antimicrobial agents require major dosage adjustments in the presence of renal dysfunction. The dosing interval for ceftazidime, usually administered every 8 hours in patients with normal renal function, is extended to once every 24 to 48 hours in persons with creatinine clearance below 10 mL/minute. Vancomycin is also administered at substantially increased dosing intervals or at smaller doses as renal function declines. Because of the increased efficiency of newer hemodialysis membranes in removing vancomycin, dosages are usually based on measured serum drug concentrations, and dosing may be required after each dialysis session.

In some instances, clearance of the antimicrobial agent is not affected by renal dysfunction, but excipients may accumulate, with the potential for toxic effects. For example, clearance of the antifungal agent voriconazole is not dependent on renal function. However, its intravenous preparation contains the solubilizing agent sulfobutyl ether β-cyclodextrin, which does accumulate in the presence of renal insufficiency. The intravenous preparation should not be used in those with moderate to severe renal dysfunction, but the oral formulation, which does not contain β-cyclodextrin, can be administered. A number of other antimicrobials may accumulate in the presence of severe liver disease, with the possibility of an increased risk for adverse events. Antimicrobials requiring dose adjustments for various levels of hepatic insufficiency include metronidazole, chloramphenicol, tigecycline, caspofungin, and voriconazole. For ceftriaxone, dosage adjustments or careful monitoring may be required in patients with both hepatic and renal dysfunction.

Drug-Drug Interactions

One of the most important considerations in the selection of an appropriate antimicrobial regimen is to determine whether the drug or drugs will interact with other medications the patient is taking. Some drug-drug interactions can have severe or even fatal consequences. There are too many potential interactions to list comprehensively, but some examples are provided in this section. Fortunately, resources are now available that allow the clinician to check for potential drug-drug interactions when an antimicrobial agent is ordered.

A large number of antimicrobials are eliminated through cytochrome P-450 pathways. As a result, they may interfere with the elimination of other drugs cleared by these pathways, leading to their accumulation to potentially dangerous levels. Several macrolide antibacterials, some fluoroquinolones, and human immunodeficiency virus protease inhibitors are among the most likely antimicrobials to inhibit the clearance of other drugs. For example, use of the protease inhibitor darunavir/ritonavir is contraindicated with several drugs, including ergot derivatives, the neuroleptic drug pimozide, certain sedative-hypnotic agents, and others. Macrolides may result in increased levels of some 3-hydroxy-3-methylglutaryl coenzyme A reductase inhibitors, which can lead to rhabdomyolysis.

In contrast, administration of rifampin induces the cytochrome P-450 system and may enhance the clearance of other drugs, some of which have narrow therapeutic windows. This may result in a number of important effects, including reduced effectiveness of oral contraceptives and increased warfarin requirements to maintain desired levels of anticoagulation. It is important to consider these potential interactions not only when starting rifampin therapy but also when *stopping* treatment. When rifampin is stopped, unless the previously increased dose of warfarin is adjusted downward accordingly, excessive anticoagulation and possibly serious bleeding can occur.

A number of other drug interactions have been described. Linezolid has weak monoamine oxidase inhibitor activity. As such, it has the potential to enhance the hypertensive effect of adrenergic agonists and has been associated with the development of serotonin syndrome in patients taking serotonergic antidepressants. Patients with this syndrome can exhibit a number of signs and symptoms, including fever, tachycardia, tremulousness, agitation, confusion, and clonus, occasionally with fatal results. Serotonin syndrome (Chapter 434) has been described in patients taking linezolid together with drugs other than selective serotonin re-uptake inhibitors; in principle, it could occur when linezolid is combined with any of a large number of agents that increase serotonin concentrations in the central nervous system.

Other Host Factors

Several additional host factors may influence the choice of a suitable antimicrobial regimen. Some antimicrobials have the potential to induce hemolysis in persons with glucose-6-phosphate dehydrogenase deficiency (Chapter 161). Among the drugs that should be avoided in these individuals are primaquine, nitrofurantoin, and various sulfonamides.

Coexisting diseases should also be taken into account. Use of fluoroquinolones or linezolid has been associated with abnormalities in glucose homeostasis. Hyperkalemia has been observed in patients with renal insufficiency during treatment with trimethoprim-sulfamethoxazole because trimethoprim blocks the renal excretion of potassium in the distal tubule.

In some cases, the patient's occupation might play a role in the selection of a treatment regimen. Antibiotics that can cause transient (minocycline) or permanent (streptomycin) dizziness or unsteadiness may create hazardous situations in those whose occupations require excellent balance. Antimicrobial agents with the potential to cause photosensitivity, such as tetracyclines, fluoroquinolones, trimethoprim, and sulfonamides, may be problematic in persons with significant sun exposure during outdoor employment or other activities.

● ANTIMICROBIAL COMBINATIONS

It is common for hospitalized patients to receive more than one antimicrobial agent simultaneously. The rationale for using antimicrobials in combination is not always clearly defined, and there are a number of potential disadvantages to combination therapy. The basis for using combination therapy is considered in this section.

Reasons to Use Combination Antimicrobial Therapy

The clinical indications for using combination antimicrobial therapy can be divided into five categories. Two of these categories (empirical therapy and polymicrobial infections) relate to maximizing the likelihood that at least one agent in the combination will be active against known or suspected pathogens. The other three reasons (minimizing toxicity, preventing the emergence of resistance, and obtaining synergistic inhibition or killing) attempt to exploit the unique advantages of some combinations as compared with a component drug alone.

To Provide Broad Coverage during Empirical Therapy

A common reason for using more than one antimicrobial in hospitalized patients is to provide broad coverage against potential pathogens and to maximize the likelihood of delivering an active antimicrobial agent as quickly as possible to seriously ill patients. When the pathogen is unknown, the antimicrobial regimen often includes an agent broadly active against gram-positive bacteria, including methicillin-resistant S. aureus (MRSA), such as vancomycin, as well as an agent active against aerobic or facultative gram-negative bacteria. Selection of the latter is strongly influenced by local patterns of antimicrobial resistance specific to the institution and might include an extended-spectrum cephalosporin, an aminoglycoside, a fluoroquinolone, a β-lactam–β-lactamase inhibitor drug, or a carbapenem.[5] The last two choices also provide activity against gram-negative anaerobes. Alternatively, one could add an agent such as metronidazole to provide anaerobic activity. Because of the high frequency of antibiotic resistance in P. aeruginosa isolates, in settings in which that pathogen is encountered frequently, empirical use of two agents with antipseudomonal activity may be justified to maximize the likelihood that at least one of the agents will inhibit the organism.

Combination therapy is widely used in the initial treatment of hospitalized patients with community-acquired pneumonia. Commonly used regimens include a third-generation cephalosporin such as ceftriaxone with a macrolide or fluoroquinolone. This cephalosporin provides antimicrobial activity against S. pneumoniae, Haemophilus influenzae, Moraxella catarrhalis, and several other "typical" bacterial pathogens associated with community-acquired pneumonia, with the notable exception of MRSA. The macrolide azithromycin is commonly added to provide activity against "atypical" bacteria that cause pneumonia, including M. pneumoniae, C. pneumoniae, and Legionella species. One of the respiratory fluoroquinolones may also be added to attain coverage of the atypical organisms. Although fluoroquinolones approved for respiratory tract infections are likely to cover most or all of the organisms targeted by the cephalosporin, isolates of S. pneumoniae resistant to fluoroquinolones do exist, so guidelines recommend combination therapy in patients with severe pneumonia requiring hospitalization.

To Treat Documented Polymicrobial Infections

For many infections from which two or more pathogens are recovered, it is possible to provide adequate coverage with a single, broadly active antimicrobial agent. Switching to a single agent reduces the patient's exposure to potential antibiotic toxicities, is usually more convenient for nursing staff, and may be less expensive. For some patients, susceptibility profiles or allergies to broad-spectrum agents justify the use of antibiotic combinations for the treatment of polymicrobial infections.

To Attempt to Reduce Toxicity

It is theoretically possible to use two or more drugs of different classes with additive antimicrobial activities and independent toxicities, each at relatively low doses, to achieve sufficient potency while avoiding toxicity. However, there are no situations in which the approach of using submaximal doses of multiple agents is predictably effective in accomplishing this goal. This does not exclude the possibility that, in isolated instances, a successful response might be attained from additive effects when drugs with marginal activities are combined for treatment of infection due to multiply resistant organisms.

To Prevent the Emergence of Drug Resistance

The treatment of tuberculosis provides the paradigm for using combinations of drugs in an attempt to prevent the emergence of resistance to any one agent. The basis for this approach is that if resistance to two different agents occurs by independent mechanisms, the probability of resistance developing to both drugs is the product of the probability of resistance developing to each drug, which is likely to be very low, so resistance should not emerge. Similar reasoning has justified the use of combination regimens when rifampin is required for the treatment of nonmycobacterial infections. Rifampin is not used alone (with rare exceptions, such as brief courses for the eradication of meningococcal carriage) because resistance to this agent can emerge quickly. As mentioned earlier, rifampin is particularly useful in the treatment of infections related to foreign devices because of its activity against biofilm-associated bacteria. In such cases, it is combined with another active antimicrobial, such as vancomycin for coagulase-negative staphylococcal prosthetic valve endocarditis (usually with a brief course of gentamicin as well to reduce the bacterial inoculum further at the beginning of therapy) or a fluoroquinolone for orthopedic device–related infections.

It has been difficult to show unequivocally that combination therapy protects against the emergence of resistance to antimicrobial drugs in other situations, including infections caused by *P. aeruginosa* or *Enterobacter* species. There are two plausible explanations of why combinations do not prevent resistance predictably. First, there may be differential penetration of the two antimicrobials at an infected site or differences in activity at the site of infection. Thus, a more readily penetrating agent may be left relatively unprotected in a privileged site of infection. Second, for many commonly encountered bacteria, resistance mechanisms against unrelated antimicrobial classes may not be truly independent. Some bacterial efflux pumps recognize chemically unrelated substrates, so upregulation of pump activity may confer resistance to several classes of antimicrobials. In other instances, there may be coordinated upregulation of efflux mechanisms and downregulation of outer membrane protein channels (porins), again potentially conferring resistance simultaneously to two or more antimicrobial classes.

To Attain Synergism

Decades ago, the surprising benefits of using penicillin and streptomycin together for the treatment of enterococcal endocarditis were discovered empirically. Penicillin alone usually inhibits but does not kill enterococci, and failure rates were high when penicillin G was used alone to treat enterococcal endocarditis. Streptomycin has no significant activity against enterococci at clinically relevant concentrations. However, the combination results in bactericidal synergism in vitro and high cure rates in patients with enterococcal endocarditis. Detailed studies of this phenomenon demonstrated that in the presence of a cell wall–active antibiotic, uptake of the aminoglycoside into the bacterial cell increases substantially. Unfortunately, increasing rates of high-level resistance to streptomycin (MIC > 2000 µg/mL), gentamicin (MIC > 500 µg/mL), or both have nullified the benefit of such combinations against a substantial number of enterococcal isolates today. An example of bactericidal synergism between vancomycin and gentamicin against an *Enterococcus* isolate is illustrated in Figure 279-1A.

Combinations of cell wall–active agents plus aminoglycosides have been shown to achieve synergistic killing against a broad range of gram-positive and gram-negative bacteria when tested in vitro. Modest clinical benefits were shown when short courses of gentamicin were added to nafcillin for the treatment of *S. aureus* endocarditis, but at the cost of added nephrotoxicity. Against strains of viridans streptococci that are relatively insensitive to penicillin, the addition of an aminoglycoside for the first 2 weeks of a 4-week course of penicillin G is believed to result in a higher likelihood of cure.

Although it was once considered important in the treatment of gram-negative bacterial infections, especially in immunocompromised (e.g., neutropenic) patients, the clinical value of a synergistic combination of a cell wall–active agent and an aminoglycoside has been difficult to prove in recent experience. To a large extent, the introduction of agents with potent activity against gram-negative bacteria has diminished the perceived value of synergistic combinations. Nevertheless, there is some evidence that administration of two or more active drugs for empirical therapy may achieve a better outcome than is possible with a single active agent for *P. aeruginosa* infections, especially in neutropenic patients. The major value of combination therapy in this setting is to ensure that at least one active agent is administered

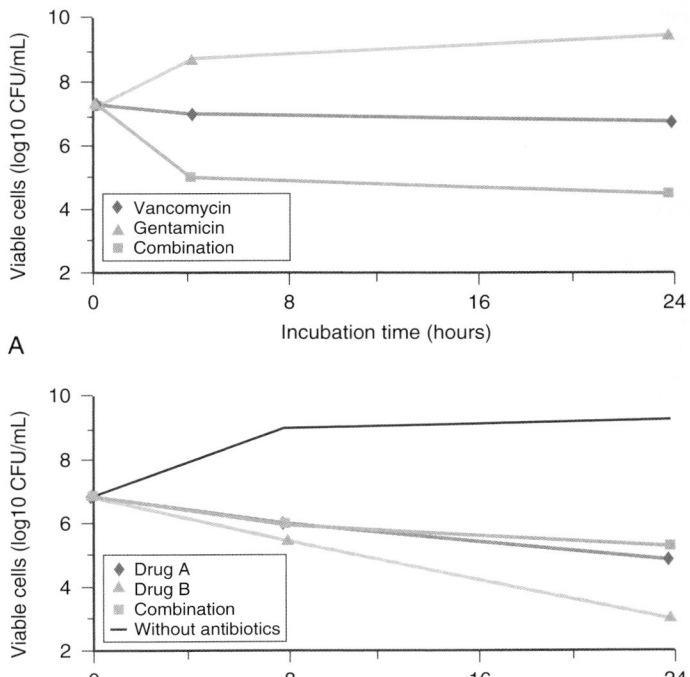

FIGURE 279-1. Bactericidal synergism and antagonism. **A,** Bactericidal synergism between vancomycin and gentamicin against an isolate of *Enterococcus* species. Killing by the combination of drugs is substantially greater than that by each agent alone. **B,** Antagonism of the bactericidal activity of drug B by the more slowly bactericidal drug A. Killing by the combination of drugs is less than that by drug B alone. Growth in the absence of antibiotics is also shown. CFU = colony-forming unit.

promptly. The combination of sulfamethoxazole and trimethoprim, agents that block sequential steps in folic acid synthesis, can also achieve bactericidal (or bacteriostatic) synergism against a number of important gram-positive and gram-negative pathogens. Quinupristin and dalfopristin are streptogramin antibiotics that display inhibitory activity against gram-positive organisms. Combining these two agents, as is done in the commercial formulation, results in bactericidal synergism against organisms susceptible to both.

β-Lactam–β-lactamase inhibitor antimicrobials represent another example of synergistic combinations. Five drugs in this category are currently marketed in the United States: amoxicillin-clavulanate, ampicillin-sulbactam, ticarcillin-clavulanate, piperacillin-tazobactam, and ceftolozane-tazobactam. The β-lactamase inhibitors themselves, clavulanic acid, sulbactam, and tazobactam, are devoid of significant antimicrobial activity, with rare exceptions. However, by inhibiting common β-lactamases that are sensitive to these agents, the inhibitors restore the activity of the hydrolyzable companion penicillins against many target pathogens elaborating these enzymes.

Antagonism

Antibiotic combinations can sometimes result in microbiologic antagonism, such that the combination may have *reduced* activity compared with the most active single agent of the treatment regimen. Time-kill curves illustrating in vitro antagonism are shown in Figure 279-1B. In this example, the more slowly bactericidal drug A antagonizes the killing effect of the intrinsically more bactericidal drug B. Antagonistic interactions against *S. aureus* between less bactericidal (linezolid) and more bactericidal (vancomycin) antimicrobials have also been demonstrated in vivo in experimental endocarditis. In vitro antagonism can be demonstrated when certain β-lactams are tested in combination against gram-negative bacteria with inducible β-lactamases. Here, exposure to one β-lactam can de-repress the synthesis of inducible β-lactamases, which then degrade the second antibiotic.

It is uncommon to encounter clinically apparent antagonism between antibiotics in the patient care setting, in part because offending combinations are not likely to be used in routine clinical care today. However, if unusual antimicrobial combinations are used, in desperation, against isolates exhibiting multiple drug resistance, it is possible that clinically relevant antagonism will be encountered more often in the future. Antagonism of bactericidal activities may also be difficult to detect in clinical practice because most common infections (with the exception of endocarditis and meningitis) do not unequivocally benefit from bactericidal therapy. As long as one agent maintains inhibitory activity, it is unlikely that failure resulting from antagonism will be observed.

CONSIDERATIONS IN ANTIMICROBIAL ADMINISTRATION

Route of Administration

In almost all instances, antimicrobial therapy for infections of mild to moderate severity that are treated in the outpatient setting can be undertaken with oral agents. There are notable exceptions, such as the use of intramuscular injections of benzathine penicillin for the treatment of syphilis or ceftriaxone for the treatment of otitis media or gonorrhea caused by strains resistant to oral agents.

Drugs such as levofloxacin and linezolid demonstrate virtually complete bioavailability when administered by the oral route in persons with normally functioning gastrointestinal tracts, and they can be used as an alternative to intravenous therapy in many patients with more serious infections. Even for these well-absorbed antimicrobials, however, treatment of seriously ill patients in the hospital is often initiated with intravenous formulations because of the uncertainty of gastrointestinal tract function under conditions of hemodynamic instability.

Antimicrobial therapy can be administered by other routes, including topical administration for the treatment of infected skin lesions (e.g., mupirocin or retapamulin ointments) and intravaginal administration for candidiasis (e.g., azole creams) or for bacterial vaginosis (e.g., metronidazole gel). Topical administration *onto* the eye is used to treat conjunctivitis or as adjunctive therapy for deeper infections; administration *into* the globe itself is a component of regimens for the treatment of endophthalmitis. Infections associated with peritoneal dialysis are frequently treated by intraperitoneal instillation of antimicrobials admixed with the dialysis solution. Rarely, direct administration into the thecal space or into the cerebral ventricles is necessary for the treatment of meningitis when the required antimicrobials do not achieve adequate concentrations in cerebrospinal fluid after systemic administration. For the treatment of *Clostridium difficile*–associated diarrhea, vancomycin reaches high concentrations in the intestine when it is given orally, but it is occasionally administered directly into the colon for the intraluminal treatment of severe infections.

The availability of protocols for the outpatient use of long venous catheters, whether inserted centrally or peripherally, has made it possible to administer antimicrobial agents that are not well absorbed orally. Thus, many patients who require long-term antibiotic treatment for infections such as endocarditis, osteomyelitis, neuroborreliosis, and other conditions can be treated as outpatients, often after an initial period of hospitalization for a full assessment of the infection, initiation of therapy, and stabilization of the medical condition. In addition to monitoring for adverse effects from the antibiotic itself, patients treated through indwelling intravenous devices require close observation for complications related to the catheter, such as thrombophlebitis, entry site infections, or line-related blood stream infections.

Pharmacodynamic Considerations

In recent years, the scientific basis for selection of a dosing regimen has extended well beyond empirical dosing strategies based primarily on the pharmacokinetic characteristics of antimicrobial agents. Pharmacodynamics relates the time course of antibiotic concentrations after dosing, the observed antimicrobial effects against likely pathogens, and the potential adverse effects of the agent.

Studies of the pharmacokinetic and pharmacodynamic properties of antimicrobial agents allow the prediction of their activities with various dosing regimens. For β-lactam antibiotics, the time during which the concentration of free drug (i.e., the non–protein-bound fraction) exceeds the MIC of the pathogen best relates to antimicrobial effectiveness in animal models. This provides the rationale for the frequent dosing schedules of β-lactams with short half-lives, such as penicillin G and the antistaphylococcal penicillins, and for the use of extended intravenous infusions when β-lactams are used to treat marginally susceptible organisms.

In contrast, the aminoglycosides and fluoroquinolones demonstrate concentration-dependent killing of bacteria. For these drugs, animal models show that the ratio of either peak concentration to MIC or the area under the 24-hour drug concentration curve to MIC better predicts effectiveness. With these agents, less frequent, higher dosing would be optimal (except perhaps when used with cell wall–active agents to achieve synergy). For the aminoglycosides, less frequent dosing may also allow more time for washout of the drug from the kidney, thus potentially minimizing the risk for nephrotoxicity.

For daptomycin, the adoption of once-daily dosing largely mitigated the muscle toxicity that had been seen with more frequent dosing and allowed the use of this agent for serious gram-positive infections.

MONITORING ANTIMICROBIAL CONCENTRATIONS

From a practical point of view, there are few situations in which assays to determine concentrations of antimicrobials in blood or body fluids are readily available. Commercial assays for the measurement of serum aminoglycoside concentrations are available and, because of these agents' great potential for toxicity, are used frequently. Commercial assays to measure vancomycin concentrations are also widely available. It may be prudent to monitor serum concentrations of vancomycin in patients with unstable renal function, those undergoing hemodialysis, patients at the extremes of body composition, or those with particularly serious infections in which high concentrations may be desirable. In some young adults, clearance of vancomycin may be so great that unexpectedly low concentrations result with the usual dosing regimens.

ADMINISTRATIVE ASPECTS OF ANTIMICROBIAL THERAPY

Formularies

In most practice settings today, the choice of antimicrobials is constrained in some way. For example, in hospitals and other facilities, institutional formularies may limit the choice of antimicrobial agents available, require special approval for the use of selected agents, or both. Such policies can, in principle, enhance efficiency by avoiding the need to stock and to dispense multiple agents with similar antimicrobial activities, minimize costs by allowing purchase of the most cost-effective alternatives, and potentially increase patient safety by encouraging clinical personnel to become familiar with a manageable number of agents. In the outpatient setting, it is common practice for health insurers to assign oral drugs to various tiers of coverage and copayment; as a result, there may be dramatic financial benefits or disincentives for the patient to receive specific agents. In both health care settings, the practitioner must be familiar with the options available to patients under these constraints.

Interchangeability

Although two drugs may have antimicrobial spectra that are so similar that only one need be included on a formulary, it is not always safe to assume that the activity of either agent can be predicted perfectly by susceptibility to the other. For example, for most bacterial species, the percentage of isolates susceptible to meropenem and imipenem are roughly comparable. However, there are differences in mechanisms of resistance to these two carbapenems, so it is possible that a specific strain will be susceptible to one but resistant to the other. For serious infections, even when two drugs are considered interchangeable, one should determine susceptibility to the specific antimicrobial that is to be used.

Impact on the Institutional Environment

In contrast to other medications, which almost always affect only the patient receiving them, antimicrobial use can have a significant impact on the institutional environment as well.[6] As a result, it is sometimes necessary or desirable to manage the use of antimicrobial agents on an administrative level to avoid selective pressure leading to the spread of antibiotic resistance. Within institutions, antimicrobial-resistant organisms not only threaten the patient treated with the antimicrobial but also can be transmitted to other vulnerable persons, including those who have not been exposed to the drug. These considerations have given rise to the movement to promote antimicrobial stewardship in health care environments.[7]

GENERAL REFERENCES

For the General References and other additional features, please visit Expert Consult at https://expertconsult.inkling.com.

280

APPROACH TO FEVER OR SUSPECTED INFECTION IN THE NORMAL HOST

JAMES E. LEGGETT

We are constantly exposed to microorganisms through our skin or mucous membranes. Most microorganisms are adapted to niches in the environment that make them avirulent to humans (Chapter 279). Pathogens in a normal host are relatively few, and most of the time, exposure results in only transient or stable colonization. Infection can be defined as invasion of a pathogen that triggers an immune response, whether the infection is asymptomatic or symptomatic. Manifestations of infection are protean and are due as much to our immune response as to the attributes of the particular pathogen.

The inflammatory response that accompanies infection is usually marked by fever. Fever is a tightly controlled elevation in body temperature above the normal range in response to a central nervous system change in the set point. Defining normal body temperature is somewhat problematic because it is dependent on both physiology and the method of measurement. Normal oral temperature in 99% of the population ranges from 36.0° to 37.7°C, with a circadian variation of 1°C or more between the morning nadir and the evening peak. Mean oral temperature in healthy adults is 36.8° ± 0.4°C, with women exhibiting slightly higher values than men (36.9° vs. 36.7°C). In menstruating women, the morning temperature may rise by 0.6°C with ovulation and remain higher until menses occur. Measured rectal temperatures are 0.4°C higher than oral and 0.8°C higher than aural (tympanic membrane) temperatures. However, considerable individual variability exists. Clinicians generally define significant fever as a temperature higher than 38.3°C (101.0°F). Despite historical claims, fever patterns are not especially helpful in establishing a specific diagnosis.

The majority of acute febrile illnesses lasting less than 2 weeks have an infectious cause. These infections occur predominantly where body surfaces interact with the environment, such as the upper and lower respiratory tracts, gastrointestinal and genitourinary systems, and skin. The majority of acute respiratory and gastrointestinal infections are viral in nature. As the duration of the febrile illness lengthens beyond 3 weeks, other inflammatory illnesses become more prominent in the differential diagnosis. Most chronic febrile illnesses are not caused by infection.

⬤ PATHOBIOLOGY OF INFECTION AND FEVER

Infection ensues only when a pathogen overcomes both nonspecific innate and specific adaptive humoral and cellular immune responses. The normal indigenous microflora, host physical barriers (e.g., skin, mucous membranes, cilia), and soluble factors (e.g., cytokines, complement) provide important barricades to pathogen invasion. Disruption of these barriers, which provide a first line of defense, permits the invasion of pathogens. The acute phase response triggered by such disruption provides direct antimicrobial activity and prompts the development of adaptive immunity mediated by lymphocytes and macrophages. This inflammatory response plays an important role in containing infection. Unfortunately, an exaggerated response may worsen the clinical condition. It is the neutrophil response that causes the damage seen in septic arthritis, and it is the unchecked immune response that precipitates the systemic inflammatory response syndrome.

Body temperature is regulated both physiologically and behaviorally. Basal metabolic processes, governed especially by thyroid hormones but also by catecholamines and growth hormone, are responsible for the normal resting body temperature. Thermogenesis may be increased up to 80% by hyperthyroidism and decreased as much as 50% by hypothyroidism. Moderate activity increases thermogenesis and results in a transiently increased temperature until heat-dissipating processes are engaged. Each 1°F increase in temperature results in a 7% increase in the basal metabolic rate. Vaporization from the lungs and skin accounts for a third of basal body heat loss and for as much as all heat loss at ambient dry temperatures above 36°C. The elderly have a decrease in basal metabolism as well as blunted responses to thermogenetic stimuli, but they have the same average core temperature as young people.

The hypothalamus contains temperature-sensitive neurons that have receptors for pro-inflammatory and anti-inflammatory cytokines, which are continuously balanced to maintain a homeothermic set point. When body temperature becomes elevated, cutaneous vasodilation and sweating occur, and people may reduce activity and seek a cooler environment. In contrast, low body temperature is increased by shivering, piloerection, cutaneous vasoconstriction, adding clothes, and seeking a warmer environment. In a febrile illness, symptoms may be due to the underlying disease or to the fever itself. Malaise is the rule, and many febrile patients experience myalgia secondary to the muscle contractions used to generate temperature elevation. Although it was once thought that the back and thigh pain related to rigors suggests bacteremia, any febrile stimulus can produce such symptoms. The chill associated with rigors may be related to the surface vasoconstriction that accompanies the increase in core temperature.

Fever is a complex physiologic process involving metabolic and immunologic responses (Fig. 280-1). Exogenous pyrogens cause fever largely mediated by endogenous pro-inflammatory pyrogenic cytokines produced by phagocytic leukocytes, including interleukin-1, interleukin-6, tumor necrosis factor-α, and interferon-γ. These cytokines stimulate the immune responses of T and B cells, macrophages, and polymorphonuclear leukocytes. They appear to act through a common mechanism involving the activation of Toll-like receptors and induction of prostaglandin synthesis. Feedback inhibitory responses are mediated by adrenocorticotropic hormone, arginine vasopressin, serotonin, dopamine, and other homeostatic mechanisms, thus emphasizing the orchestrated nature of fever production and response to infection. These thermoregulatory mechanisms rarely allow fevers to exceed 41°C (106°F). Temperatures exceeding 41°C are often due to a drug-induced imbalance in these mechanisms and may cause direct cellular damage.

Failure of fever to develop during severe bacterial infection has, in some studies, been associated with higher morbidity and mortality. Whether this is due to the absence of fever or to associated conditions, such as chronic renal failure or corticosteroid use, has not been determined. Favorable effects of fever on host-microbe interactions are suggested by inhibited multiplication of some pathogens (such as *Streptococcus pneumoniae* and *Treponema pallidum*), reduced proliferation of pathogens in the presence of

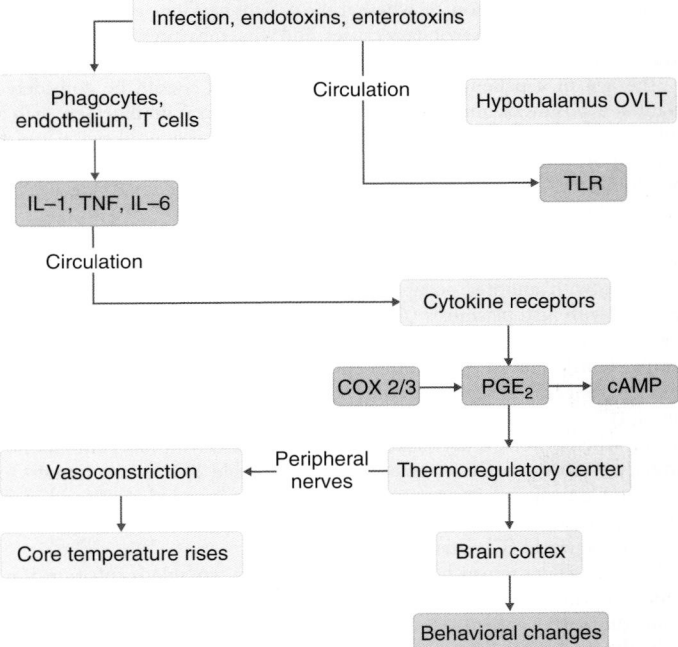

FIGURE 280-1. Pathways leading to the production of fever in bacterial infection, whether local or systemic. Bacteria release cell wall products such as peptidoglycans and endotoxin as well as enterotoxins, which bind to Toll-like receptors (TLRs) on phagocytes (neutrophils, macrophages) and endothelial cells. As a result, pyrogenic cytokines such as interleukin (IL)–1, IL-6, and tumor necrosis factor (TNF)–α are released into the circulation and bind to cytokine receptors in the hypothalamic organum vasculosum of lamina terminalis (OVLT). Bacterial products may also directly bind to TLRs on the OVLT. Activation of TLRs and cytokine receptors induces cyclooxygenase 2 (COX2), which leads to the production of prostaglandin E₂ (PGE₂) and elevates cyclic adenosine monophosphate (cAMP) in the brain. This, in turn, triggers neurons in the thermoregulatory center to raise the hypothalamic thermostatic set point. In addition, neuronal signals to the cortex prompt behavioral changes to conserve heat (e.g., posturing, adding clothing). The hypothalamus also triggers sympathetic peripheral efferent nerves that constrict peripheral blood vessels and conserve central heat until hypothalamic PGE₂ levels fall.

hypoferremia, augmented complement-mediated lysis, and increased neutrophil entry into inflammatory sites. Indeed, vertebrate endothermy restricts most fungi as potential pathogens in hosts with intact immune systems.

Temperature-pulse dissociation, in which there is relative bradycardia compared with the usual increase of 2.44 beats/minute per 1°F, has been described in typhoid fever, leptospirosis, rickettsiosis, dengue, legionellosis, and babesiosis, for unclear reasons.

No laboratory abnormalities accompany typical benign acute viral infections. Leukocytosis (Chapter 167) of various lineages is usually seen in other infections in immunocompetent adults. Neutrophilia is the norm in most acute infections, whatever the cause. The elderly, although not mounting a neutrophilic response, generally display bandemia during an acute bacterial infection. Neutropenia (Chapter 167) may be seen in rickettsial, severe viral, and overwhelming bacterial infections. Eosinophilia (Chapter 170) is typical of invasive helminthic and some protozoal infections. Lymphocytosis may accompany many viral and rickettsial infections and is common during convalescence from acute bacterial infection. Monocytosis may be seen in tuberculosis. Virtually all infections have an impact on the erythroid system, but given the long half-life of erythrocytes, usually only chronic infections or other inflammatory diseases result in anemia (Chapter 158). Few acute infections rapidly produce anemia. For instance, *Helicobacter pylori* may induce a bleeding ulcer, *Plasmodium falciparum* may directly lyse erythrocytes, overwhelming clostridial and other bacterial infections associated with disseminated intravascular coagulopathy may cause hemolytic anemia, and *Mycoplasma pneumoniae* may induce immunologically mediated hemolysis.

APPROACH TO FEBRILE ILLNESS IN OUTPATIENTS AND INPATIENTS

Infectious disease epidemiology depends on the interaction among pathogens, susceptible hosts, and environmental conditions allowing exposure. Most infections are transmitted horizontally between people by contact (e.g., hands, fomites), a common vehicle (e.g., food, water), air (e.g., tuberculosis), or vectors (e.g., mosquitoes). Evaluation of a patient with a known or possible infection should determine whether the condition might be due to a transmissible agent and its source, whether the patient has done any recent traveling, whether there are secondary causes, and what measures need to be taken to contact health department officials and to prevent additional infections.

The age of a patient influences which illnesses should be considered. Natural exposure or immunization generally limits certain illnesses, such as rubeola, rubella, and varicella. Waning of immunity may likewise lead to pertussis in young adults or reactivation of tuberculosis in the elderly. Other physiologic effects of aging, such as impaired bladder emptying, lead to increased rates of urinary tract infection in the elderly.

A patient's occupation and travel history should be noted. An abattoir worker is more likely to have been exposed to *Brucella* (Chapter 310) than is someone with another occupation. Indiana residents are more likely be infected with histoplasmosis (Chapter 332), whereas those from the Southwest desert may have coccidioidomycosis (Chapter 333), despite having a similar febrile illness. Many other illnesses are likewise directly related to specific geographic exposure, with varying incubation times before their onset (Chapter 286). Typhoid fever should be manifested within a few weeks, whereas amebic liver abscess might not cause symptoms until months after a traveler's return from an endemic area (Table 280-1). The Centers for Disease Control and Prevention website (http://www.cdc.gov) and many others provide more specific information about prevalent infections in all parts of the world (Chapter 286).

Many travelers return home with fever after a variable incubation time, generally with other symptoms and signs as well. The first consideration in evaluating such a patient is that an infection unrelated to travel is more likely to be the cause of the illness.[1] Once such routine infections have been ruled out, the differential diagnosis should include infections related to travel,[2] whether within a region of the United States (e.g., ehrlichiosis, Colorado tick fever, hantavirus) or abroad (e.g., visceral leishmaniasis, tick-borne encephalitis in Europe) (Chapter 286). For example, prompt evaluation of a patient who has traveled to a malaria-endemic area should be undertaken and blood tests performed to determine the presence of parasites.

The setting in which a febrile illness occurs influences both the diagnostic approach and the differential diagnosis. In the ambulatory arena, with a generally healthy febrile patient, the clinician should not necessarily pursue a diagnosis as aggressively as with a hospitalized or chronically ill patient. Empirical treatment of a presumed urinary tract infection is warranted in the outpatient setting, where the cost of a culture is often more than that of the antibiotic. However, the cost of a urine culture in a hospital setting is minimal

TABLE 280-1	SELECTED EXAMPLES OF FEVER ASSOCIATED WITH RECENT TRAVEL	
	INCUBATION PERIOD	
DISEASE	**<2-3 WEEKS**	**>3-4 WEEKS**
COMMON		
Dengue	+	
Dysentery	+	
Entamebic liver abscess		+
Enteric fever	+	
Malaria	+	+
Pulmonary tuberculosis		+
Viral hepatitis		+
LESS COMMON		
Ehrlichiosis	+	
Leptospirosis	+	
Schistosomiasis		+
Viral (hemorrhagic, encephalitic)	+	
Visceral leishmaniasis		+

in comparison to the daily cost of care, and accurate identification of the pathogen may speed hospital discharge. Likewise, the pathogens commonly causing febrile illness in health care facilities, including nursing homes, may differ from those seen in ambulatory settings. Most patients in the ambulatory setting have noncritical, self-limited infections.

Higher temperatures are usually due to invasive visceral disease, such as community-acquired pneumonia or pyelonephritis. Common viral respiratory infections and gastroenteritis as well as some cases of subacute bacterial endocarditis are accompanied by temperatures below 102°F. Moreover, many infections may not be associated with fever, such as Lyme disease, osteomyelitis, and most sexually transmitted diseases. The clinician must always keep in mind that certain infections, such as sexually transmitted diseases (Chapter 285) or herpes zoster, occur normally in immunocompetent hosts and may signal a higher risk for infection with human immunodeficiency virus (HIV) or an already established immunodeficiency.

Fever in Outpatients

In the ambulatory setting, an acutely febrile patient represents a common problem and only infrequently presents an enigmatic diagnostic challenge. In most instances, a febrile illness is accompanied by localizing symptoms and signs suggesting a specific diagnosis. For instance, leg erythema, pain, and fever in a patient with tinea pedis or a saphenous vein graft incision immediately suggests streptococcal cellulitis. Several diseases may masquerade as infectious cellulitis.[3] If the patient has had a gradual onset and does not appear toxic, only clinical observation and follow-up are required. If the patient appears toxic, with tachypnea and apprehension or confusion accompanying localized findings, clinically focused diagnostic studies should be performed immediately, and hospitalization should be considered. When a patient has fever and only nonspecific constitutional symptoms, it may be more difficult to address the problem in a single ambulatory clinic visit, requiring a balance between observation and investigation.

Fever in Inpatients

Fever and leukocytosis are probably the main clinical parameters for evaluating potential infections in hospitalized patients. However, about 10% of nosocomial bacteremias occur without fever, and health care–associated infections occur without fever in a substantial proportion of patients who are elderly or have significant comorbid conditions. Most cases of hospital-associated fever represent nosocomial infection, which typically involves the lower respiratory tract, urinary tract, or surgical wounds (Table 280-2). Some important causes of nosocomial fever may not exhibit easily discernible localizing symptoms or signs. Antibiotic-induced colitis secondary to *Clostridium difficile* (Chapter 296) is increasing in prevalence and may be characterized by little or no diarrhea. It is probably the most common cause of a leukemoid reaction in hospitalized patients. Other intra-abdominal processes involving the hepatobiliary system, bowel infarction, viscus perforation, or abscesses may have little in the way of localizing symptoms or signs.

Given the greater severity of illness and comorbid conditions in intensive care unit (ICU) patients, it is logical that fever and infection are more frequent in the ICU than elsewhere. Infection was recently found to be present in more than 80% of febrile ICU patients, although both infectious and noninfectious

TABLE 280-2   SELECTED CAUSES OF HOSPITAL-ASSOCIATED FEVER

COMMON	LESS COMMON
INFECTIOUS	**INFECTIOUS**
Clostridium difficile enterocolitis	Biliary tract disease
Pneumonia	Endometritis
Surgical wound	Intra-abdominal abscess
Urinary tract	Mediastinitis
Vascular catheter	Sinusitis
NONINFECTIOUS	**NONINFECTIOUS**
Drug-induced fever	Adrenal insufficiency
Hematoma	Gout
Immediate postoperative state	Myocardial infarction
Transfusion reaction	Organ infarction
Venous thromboembolism	Pancreatitis

TABLE 280-3   SELECTED INFECTIONS WITH FEVER AND RASH

ETIOLOGY	MACULES, PAPULES	VESICLES, BULLAE	PETECHIAE, PURPURA
BACTERIA			
Borrelia burgdorferi	+ (annular)		
Neisseria meningitidis			+
Rickettsia rickettsii	+		+
Treponema pallidum	+ (secondary)		
Vibrio vulnificus		+	
FUNGI AND MYCOBACTERIA			
Disseminated disease	+ (nodular)		
PROTOZOA			
Plasmodium falciparum			+
VIRUSES			
Enteroviruses	+	+	+
Epstein-Barr	+		+
Hemorrhagic fever			+
Herpes		+	
HIV	+		

TABLE 280-4   FEVER AND RASH INVOLVING THE PALMS AND SOLES

Erythema multiforme
Hand-foot-and-mouth disease
Neisseria infection
Rocky Mountain spotted fever
Streptobacillus moniliformis infection
Subacute bacterial endocarditis
Syphilis (secondary)
Toxic shock syndrome
Varicella-zoster infection

causes of fever may coexist. Indeed, ischemia or devitalization of tissue provokes an inflammatory response similar to that prompted by infection. About half of patients with acute myocardial infarction have a temperature between 38.0° and 38.5° C within 2 to 3 days of their infarction. Similarly, about half of patients with deep venous thrombosis and pulmonary embolism have a temperature in the same range, most commonly in the first 3 days after diagnosis. A third or more of patients with stroke demonstrate fever, which is also a common consequence of subarachnoid or intracerebral hemorrhage and subdural hematoma, especially within 72 hours of onset.[4] The fever in such cases may result from damage to the hypothalamus or pulmonary aspiration secondary to obtundation. Iatrogenic causes of fever should be considered. Fever and chills may be seen in up to a quarter of patients receiving platelet transfusions, although the frequency is much less with other blood products.

SYNDROMIC APPROACH

Fever and Rash

A syndromic approach is valuable to narrow the many possible causes of a suspected infection. Two approaches must be juxtaposed in this evaluation, and both are key in recognizing patterns. The clinician must be aware of (1) the differential diagnosis of the particular type of lesion observed and (2) the constellation of findings produced by individual pathogens. Because of the variety of possible manifestations and the often overlapping symptoms and signs, both elements are key in arriving at a probable diagnosis. Moreover, fever and associated findings, such as exanthem, lymphadenopathy, or jaundice, may be due to noninfectious systemic diseases as well as infectious ones. For instance, leukocytoclastic vasculitis and fever may be found in meningococcemia, Rocky Mountain spotted fever, and hepatitis C, but they are also seen in noninfectious inflammatory diseases. Likewise, fever and adenopathy may be due to lymphoma or to cat-scratch disease.

A recognizable exanthem may lead to the immediate recognition of a particular pathogen (Chapter 441), but often a larger differential diagnosis must be entertained. The clinician must recognize the type or types of skin lesions present, the distribution of the exanthem, and the chronologic progression with respect to the onset of fever and other symptoms (Table 280-3). Morphologic variations in skin lesions help in the differential diagnosis. Maculopapular exanthems are frequently seen in viral illness, hypersensitivity drug reactions, and immune complex–mediated diseases. Some of the most common viral causes include the many enteroviruses, but similar lesions may also be seen with hepatitis B and West Nile viruses. Erythema multiforme, a subset of maculopapular exanthem, can result from various viral infections or drug eruptions (Chapter 440). It may have a spectrum of disease that ranges from benign to the life-threatening Stevens-Johnson syndrome/toxic epidermal necrolysis complex. Herpes simplex virus is perhaps the most common cause of erythema multiforme. Although drugs, especially antibiotics, are the major precipitating factor in the Stevens-Johnson syndrome/toxic epidermal necrolysis complex, M. pneumoniae has been associated with it as well. Evolution of the cutaneous findings over time may give clues to the cause; for example, the initial blanching, erythematous, maculopapular lesions may later evolve into petechiae, as seen in meningococcemia, Rocky Mountain spotted fever, and dengue. Secondary syphilis may be manifested with a multitude of morphologic skin lesions. Sometimes, many different manifestations occur simultaneously in the same patient. Most vesiculobullous skin exanthems are immunologically mediated. The few infections associated with these eruptions include herpes simplex and varicella-zoster viruses and enteroviruses such as echovirus and coxsackievirus. The poxviruses, which can also cause such exanthems, are much rarer or are associated with bioterrorism. Pustules, or vesicles containing leukocytes, are usually associated with psoriasis or infections with *Pseudomonas*, *Staphylococcus*, or *Neisseria*. Bullous exanthems in the presence of sepsis suggest severe streptococcal cellulitis or necrotizing fasciitis, staphylococcal impetigo, or *Vibrio* infections.

Petechial and purpuric eruptions are due to the extravasation of red blood cells and should always lead to consideration of a potentially serious illness. Pathogens creating such lesions most commonly include *Neisseria meningitidis*, *Rickettsia*, and *Capnocytophaga canimorsus*, but these eruptions may be seen with a variety of other pathogens, including *Staphylococcus aureus*, group B streptococci, and other gram-negative bacilli. A petechial exanthem may also be seen with enteroviruses and viral hemorrhagic fevers. The most common causes of petechiae not attributable to infections include thrombocytopenia and vasculitis.

The presence of fever and rash involving the palms and soles allows considerable narrowing of the differential diagnosis (Table 280-4). In addition to the diffuse erythema associated with toxic shock syndrome, illnesses such as Rocky Mountain spotted fever, secondary syphilis, hand-foot-and-mouth disease, *Neisseria* infections, and rat-bite fever should be considered in patients with maculopapular exanthems involving these areas.

Nodular skin lesions may be either noninfectious, as seen in malignant disease or with certain drugs (e.g., sulfonamides), or infectious, as seen in a variety of inflammatory diseases. Atypical mycobacteria and disseminated fungi often produce skin nodules. The tender nodules of erythema nodosum usually occur in crops located pretibially, but they may be solitary or occur on other parts of the body. They do not typically suppurate, and they heal without scarring. Infectious agents are the most likely cause of erythema nodosum. Diffuse erythema may be seen with scarlet fever, toxic shock syndrome, Kawasaki disease, Stevens-Johnson syndrome, and toxic epidermal necrolysis, with desquamation occurring late in all these syndromes. Sweet's syndrome, a febrile neutrophilic dermatosis, represents a hypersensitivity reaction often preceded by an upper respiratory tract infection.

Fever and Musculoskeletal Complaints

Fever and localized tenderness, swelling, or erythema generally accompany septic arthritis and often accompany osteomyelitis (Chapter 272). Septic bacterial arthritis in adults usually is manifested acutely and involves a single large joint such as the knee, hip, or shoulder, unless the infection is directly inoculated by trauma or surgery. Septic oligoarthritis may be seen with endocarditis and rat-bite fever. Disseminated gonococcal disease is the usual cause of arthritis involving small joints of the wrist, ankle, and digits, often with tenosynovitis. Acute or subacute polyarthritis may be seen in several viral diseases, including parvovirus B19 and hepatitis B, and in Lyme disease, but it is more typical of immunologic disorders. Rheumatologic diseases generally have more subacute manifestations, with more symmetrical polyarthritis. Hematogenous osteomyelitis in adults frequently involves the vertebrae and is almost always initiated by discitis with symmetrical involvement of adjacent vertebrae (as opposed to malignant metastasis, which is asymmetrical and does not involve the disc).

Myositis secondary to clostridia, streptococci, *Aeromonas*, or mixed aerobic-anaerobic infections usually causes an acutely septic picture with painful, edematous involvement of the limb or torso. Pyomyositis frequently involves deep muscles such as the psoas or gluteus and is usually due to *S. aureus*. Diffuse myositis may be seen with leptospirosis or toxoplasmosis, and rhabdomyolysis occurs with a variety of viral infections and legionellosis.

Fever and Lymphadenopathy or Hepatosplenomegaly

Fever and lymphadenopathy may suggest a variety of illnesses, both infectious and noninfectious (Table 280-5). Lymphadenopathy (Chapter 168) may be regional or generalized. Local enlargement can occur with either a local infection or some systemic illnesses (e.g., posterior cervical lymphadenopathy with Epstein-Barr virus and other viral illnesses). Generalized lymphadenopathy usually suggests a systemic disorder, which may itself be either infectious or noninfectious. Although the combination of fever and lymphadenopathy secondary to infection is especially common during childhood, it is also frequently seen in adults. As in other syndromes, acute versus chronic adenopathy tilts the diagnosis toward different broad categories of illness. In chronic adenopathy, histopathologic evaluation of enlarged lymph nodes may point to a particular diagnosis. For instance, toxoplasmosis or cat-scratch disease can be easily differentiated from mycobacterial disease or sarcoidosis.

Fever and hepatosplenomegaly (Chapter 168) may provide an important clue to the cause of a febrile illness, which is typically either an infection or a malignant neoplasm arising from bone marrow or the reticuloendothelial system. Jaundice may also limit the differential diagnosis (Table 280-6).

Aside from the viral hepatitides and other diseases affecting primarily the liver, many pathogens producing sepsis can cause hyperbilirubinemia.

⬤ APPROACH TO FEVER OF UNKNOWN ORIGIN

The majority of febrile illnesses are short-lived, but fever may be prolonged for weeks or months as part of an infectious disease, inflammatory disorder, or occult neoplasm. When fever is caused by infection, the site is an area not easily controlled by host defenses, leading to the continued release of inflammatory cytokines. Likewise, macrophage and lymphocyte involvement in inflammatory disorders causes persistent cytokine production, as do certain neoplasms. Given this final common pathway, it is easy to understand why the majority of cases of classic fever of unknown origin (FUO), loosely defined as lasting longer than 3 weeks despite routine investigation, are found in these three broad categories.[5,6] Two other categories round out the bulk of FUO cases: miscellaneous illnesses and cases in which the fever remains undiagnosed (Table 280-7). The proportion of patients in each category varies by geographic locale, age, duration of fever, and immune status. As more effective methods of diagnosing viral and bacterial infections have become available, and with improved serologic studies to detect connective tissue disorders and better imaging techniques to detect occult malignant neoplasms, the proportion of patients with FUO in the miscellaneous and undiagnosed categories has increased to about a third of the total in developed countries. The longer a febrile illness persists without a diagnosis or appropriate therapy, the less likely it is to be due to an infection. In one study, only 6% of patients who had persistent FUO beyond 6 months were found to have infection. Most such cases resolve spontaneously, with a mortality rate of less than 3% at 5 years.

Bacterial species, particularly *Mycobacterium tuberculosis*, make up the largest category of infections that cause prolonged FUO. *M. tuberculosis* and other bacterial pathogens causing FUO have adapted to survive intracellularly or frequently change their surface antigens so that they are not readily eradicated by host defenses. Other infections causing FUO are localized in cryptic abscesses, especially intra-abdominally, or reside on heart valves, where the inflammatory response is blunted. Persistent viral infections constitute a small and shrinking subset of patients with FUO because modern techniques can more readily detect infection with Epstein-Barr virus, cytomegalovirus, and others. Among the pathogens likely to be characterized initially by fever alone, cytomegalovirus is the most common cause of mononucleosis in adults, and malaria is a common cause of fever in returning travelers.

Malignant disease may result in persistent fever due to the production of inflammatory cytokines, necrosis, or the presence of a complicating infection. The most common malignant neoplasms manifesting as FUO are lymphomas, leukemias, and solid tumors with metastases to the liver. Connective tissue disorders may lead to tissue inflammation, which produces fever as a prominent feature of the illness. In a recent series, adult Still's disease (Chapter 261) was the leading rheumatologic disorder manifesting as FUO. Temporal arteritis and polymyalgia rheumatica (Chapter 271) are seen almost exclusively in patients older than 50 years. Systemic lupus erythema-

TABLE 280-5	COMMON CAUSES OF FEVER AND LYMPHADENOPATHY	
REGIONAL		**GENERALIZED**
Cervical		Cytomegalovirus
Streptococci		Epstein-Barr virus
Tuberculosis		HIV
Viral upper respiratory tract infection		Lymphoma
		Sarcoidosis
Peripheral		Syphilis (secondary)
Bartonella henselae		Toxoplasmosis
Herpesviruses		Viral hepatitis
Lymphoma		
Metastatic cancer		
Sporotrichosis		
Streptococci		
Inguinal		
Chancroid		
Herpes		
Lymphogranuloma venereum		
Syphilis (primary)		

TABLE 280-6	COMMON INFECTIOUS CAUSES OF FEVER AND JAUNDICE
Bacterial sepsis	
Cholangitis	
Hepatic abscess	
Leptospirosis	
Malaria	
Viral hepatitis	
Yellow fever	

TABLE 280-7	FREQUENCY OF SELECTED CHRONIC FEBRILE ILLNESSES

INFECTION, 25-50%	MALIGNANT DISEASE, 20-30%	CONNECTIVE TISSUE DISEASE, 15-30%	MISCELLANEOUS, 10-20%	UNDIAGNOSED, 10-30%
Cytomegalovirus	Carcinomatosis	Polyarteritis nodosa	Drug-induced fever	
Endocarditis	Leukemia	Rheumatoid arthritis	Granulomatous hepatitis	
Intra-abdominal	Local tumor	Still's disease	Inflammatory bowel disease	
Mycoses	Lymphoma	Systemic lupus erythematosus	Pancreatitis	
Occult abscess		Temporal arteritis	Pulmonary embolism	
Tuberculosis				

tosus (Chapter 266) is an occasional cause of FUO, especially if it is manifested in an atypical fashion.

The miscellaneous category of FUO includes several disparate groups of diseases. Granulomatous diseases such as granulomatous hepatitis, Crohn's disease, or sarcoidosis may incite cellular immune responses that result in fever. Granulomatous hepatitis was present in up to 6% of National Institutes of Health cases with fever lasting longer than 6 months. Chronic pancreatitis may occasionally cause FUO, as may recurrent pulmonary embolism.

Drug-induced fever (Table 280-8) may be the only manifestation of an adverse drug event in up to 5% of cases of drug hypersensitivity. Recognition of drug-induced fever is important to avoid extra tests, additional therapy, and prolonged hospitalization.[7] The mechanisms by which drugs incite fever are not well understood in many cases. These events may result from hypersensitivity reactions, altered thermoregulatory homeostasis directly related to either drug administration or the drug's pharmacologic action, or idiosyncratic reactions. Hypersensitivity reactions are usually accompanied by an exanthem or enanthem and hepatic, renal, or pulmonary dysfunction in addition to fever. Antimicrobial agents appear to be the most common cause of drug-induced fever and are responsible for approximately a third of episodes in some studies. β-Lactams and sulfonamides account for most cases because they are among the most frequently administered antimicrobials. Anticonvulsants are also common causes of drug-induced fever secondary to hypersensitivity reactions. Altered thermoregulation is possible with a variety of drugs, including those with anticholinergic activity, such as phenothiazines and tricyclic antidepressants. Sympathomimetic agents, such as amphetamines and cocaine, may also cause fever. Drug administration itself may cause fever if the vehicle of the drug is contaminated with exogenous pyrogens or chemical phlebitis occurs. Some drugs appear to have intrinsic pyrogenic properties, such as amphotericin B and bleomycin. Others cause fever as a result of their pharmacologic activity, such as interferon alfa or interleukin-2. With antibiotics, drug-induced fever occurs with the rapid lysis of spirochetes or other bacteria, known as the Jarisch-Herxheimer reaction. Idiosyncratic drug-induced febrile reactions include malignant hyperthermia, neuroleptic malignant syndrome, and serotonin syndrome (Chapter 434). Drugs implicated in these reactions are inhaled anesthetic agents, central nervous system dopamine-depleting agents, and serotonin re-uptake inhibitors, among others. Drug-induced fever is usually a diagnosis of exclusion. The duration of drug exposure before the onset of fever, the clinical appearance of the patient, and the pattern of the fever are not particularly useful. Elimination of a single drug at a time, beginning with the one most likely to be implicated, is the usual means of identifying the causative agent. The fever abates once the drug has been eliminated from the body, usually within 3 to 4 days of discontinuing use of the drug.

Laboratory evaluation and diagnostic imaging studies should be chosen according to information derived from a detailed history and physical examination. These may initially include complete blood count and blood chemistry determinations, erythrocyte sedimentation rate or C-reactive protein, blood cultures, and antibody tests (antinuclear antibody, cytomegalovirus, Epstein-Barr virus, HIV) as well as a chest radiograph and computed tomography of the abdomen.[8] 18-Fluoro-2-deoxy-D-glucose positron emission tomography (FDG-PET) may also be useful in difficult cases.[9] Despite the

recent focus on "emerging" infectious diseases, the cause of FUO is still more likely to be a common pathogen presenting atypically.

INITIAL MANAGEMENT OF SUSPECTED INFECTION IN THE AMBULATORY SETTING

An acutely febrile patient in the ambulatory setting presents a common but often demanding diagnostic problem. In most cases, the history and physical examination reveal diagnostic clues and may guide decisions about additional studies or therapy. More difficult to diagnose is a fever that occurs without localizing symptoms or is accompanied only by nonspecific symptoms, such as malaise or anorexia. Fortunately, most such acute, undifferentiated febrile illnesses are benign and resolve spontaneously within 1 or 2 weeks without a specific diagnosis being made. In such cases, no further evaluation beyond the initial visit is warranted. If symptoms persist, the history and physical examination should be repeated, looking for previously unsought clues and new physical findings. Laboratory studies might be required.

In patients with an illness involving cough of less than 3 weeks' duration, the evaluation should focus on ruling out a serious disorder. Normal vital signs and normal findings on a chest examination effectively rule out most cases of pneumonia. Such cough illnesses are caused by viral pathogens in more than 90% of cases. Antibiotics are ineffective in such patients, and antimicrobial therapy does not prevent bacterial complications such as pneumonia. The presence of sputum and its characteristics are not helpful in distinguishing bacterial from viral infections. Adults with prolonged coughing lasting longer than 3 weeks or with recurrent episodes should be evaluated for reactive airway disease, gastroesophageal reflux, and other illnesses. Infections rarely causing prolonged cough include *Bordetella pertussis*, *M. pneumoniae*, and *Chlamydophila pneumoniae*. Clinicians in this case should obtain a chest radiograph; treat for exacerbation of chronic obstructive pulmonary disease (fever, leukocytosis, purulent sputum), if present; treat a confirmed bacterial infection; and direct therapy to a specific underlying cause or other causes.

Symptoms and signs of pharyngitis include fever, tonsillar exudates, tender anterior cervical lymph nodes, and absence of cough. If fewer than two of these criteria are present, the patient should be managed as though viral pharyngitis were the cause. With two or more of these criteria, one should consider obtaining a rapid streptococcal antigen test.[10] Because of the low incidence of streptococcal infection and acute rheumatic fever in adults, a negative rapid test result alone is sufficient to rule out infection with *Streptococcus pyogenes*. If the antigen test result is positive, the patient can be managed with a β-lactam antibiotic if not allergic. Ninety percent of cases of pharyngitis in adults are viral in origin. In a patient with symptoms of upper respiratory tract infection and a mucopurulent nasal discharge of less than 10 days' duration, purulent nasal secretions do not predict bacterial infection. Most cases of acute rhinosinusitis seen in the outpatient setting are caused by uncomplicated upper respiratory viral infection.[A1] If symptoms have been present for more than 10 days without improvement, or if there are specific symptoms of sinusitis of any duration (purulent nasal discharge lasting 3 to 4 days, unilateral facial pain and pressure, maxillary toothache, or worsening of symptoms after initial improvement), amoxicillin or another β-lactam should be considered, with other antimicrobial classes used in penicillin-allergic patients. Most clinical outcomes are not adversely affected by delayed antibiotics for upper respiratory infections.[A2]

Community-acquired pneumonia (Chapter 97) should be suspected in a patient with cough, sputum production, or dyspnea, especially if it is accompanied by fever and altered breath sounds. A chest radiograph should be performed to confirm the diagnosis. Determining where to care for the patient is the most important immediate decision. Outpatient care generally suffices for patients younger than 50 years with no cardiopulmonary disease; for patients with no comorbid conditions (including malignant disease, heart failure, diabetes, or hospitalization within the last year); and for patients with no physical examination findings, such as altered mental status, pulse of 125 beats/minute or greater, or respiratory rate of 30/minute or greater. Recent guidelines developed by the American Thoracic Society and the Infectious Diseases Society of America suggest a β-lactam, macrolide, or doxycycline. Fluoroquinolones should be used for outpatients only when the patient has failed to respond to first-line therapy, has a significant comorbidity, or has a known allergy to a first-line agent.

Skin and soft tissue infections are caused, for the most part, by streptococci; a minority are due to *S. aureus* and, rarely, other bacteria whose presence may be suggested by epidemiologic considerations (e.g., swimming in fresh water, where *Aeromonas* may be the pathogen). Pain may be present for

TABLE 280-8	SELECTED AGENTS ASSOCIATED WITH DRUG-INDUCED FEVER
COMMON	**LESS COMMON**
ANTIMICROBIAL	
Amphotericin B	Clindamycin
β-Lactams	Fluoroquinolones
Sulfonamides	Rifampin
CARDIOVASCULAR	
Procainamide	Diltiazem
Quinidine	Hydralazine
CENTRAL NERVOUS SYSTEM	
Carbamazepine	Haloperidol
Phenytoin	Serotonin re-uptake inhibitors
MISCELLANEOUS	
Bleomycin	Allopurinol
Interferon alfa	Cimetidine
Interleukin-2	Tacrolimus

12 hours or more before skin discoloration is noted. A furuncle or abscess formation should prompt consideration of *S. aureus* and, rarely, *Streptococcus anginosus* group. Incision and drainage may be sufficient for a skin abscess, although the rapidly expanding, virulent, community-acquired methicillin-resistant *S. aureus* phenotype may require antimicrobial therapy. Septic bursitis is nearly always due to *S. aureus*, and the infected bursa should be aspirated and drained, in addition to using antibiotics (Chapter 272).

Gastrointestinal infections may be due to ingested toxins, viruses, or, less commonly, bacteria, with or without associated toxin production. The appropriate approach depends on the epidemiologic setting, such as improper food storage, travel abroad, or contact with another ill person (Chapter 283). Symptoms of cystitis in a young, sexually active woman can be treated with empirical antibiotics, but when fever and flank pain are present and the patient is nauseated, consideration of a brief hospital admission or an initial intravenous dose of antibiotics may be necessary (Chapter 284). The possibility of pelvic inflammatory disease should also be entertained.

In the initial evaluation of a patient with a more chronic, persistent fever, a careful history and physical examination provide important diagnostic clues, directing further investigation. The initial goal is to characterize the illness accurately, in addition to eliciting important host and epidemiologic factors. A careful review of systems is necessary to understand the extent of involvement of various organ systems as well as to note previous medical conditions. The examination should be broader than for an acute febrile illness with localizing symptoms and signs. Laboratory tests may also play a more important role in guiding further investigation. Repeated evaluations are the norm rather than the exception in these cases.

Blindly initiating empirical therapy in febrile patients with no imminent risk of serious clinical harm or death should be discouraged because it may impede a timely diagnosis affording definitive care. Procalcitonin, which is a precursor of calcitonin, is an acute phase reactant that is more likely to be elevated with bacterial than with viral infections, and its use may reduce unnecessary antibiotics in some situations, such as patients with respiratory infections.[A3] However, procalcitonin distinguishes sepsis from nonseptic systemic inflammation poorly (71% sensitivity, 71% specificity, receiver operating characteristic curve 0.63),[11] and it appears to be less useful in such settings.[A4]

INITIAL MANAGEMENT OF SUSPECTED NOSOCOMIAL INFECTION

Determination of the nature of a febrile illness in a hospitalized patient must take into account the host, the setting, and the timing of recent trauma or type and duration of surgery, in addition to the general approach taken for ambulatory patients. A classic mnemonic—the six *w*'s—may help guide the evaluation: wind, water, wound, walk, wonder drug, and what we did. "Wind" refers to fever within the first 24 hours of surgery, when it is unusual to have an infection. A fever at this time is often thought to be related to the anesthetic agent, atelectasis, or surgical trauma. The only bacteria believed to cause significant infections within 24 hours of surgery are *S. pyogenes* and *Clostridium* species, both of which are unusual in the typical hospital patient. "Water" refers to a urinary tract infection occurring after the third day of urinary tract catheterization. Because nearly all nosocomial urinary tract infections occur in patients with indwelling urinary catheters or in those who have undergone urologic instrumentation, urinalysis or culture (or both) should be performed routinely only in febrile patients with such risk factors. There is a high prevalence of bacteriuria in patients who have been catheterized for 3 days or longer, and there is a relatively low incidence of true infection attributable to bacteriuria. "Wound" infections commonly occur about 5 to 7 days postoperatively, whether they are surface wounds or complications of dehiscence of gastrointestinal anastomoses. Some of the highest rates of skin and soft tissue infections in the National Nosocomial Infection Surveillance database are seen with gastrointestinal procedures. Toxin-producing *C. difficile* is the only significant nosocomial gastrointestinal infection seen in hospitalized patients, so a routine bacterial stool culture is not necessary. "Walk" refers to possible deep venous thrombosis or pulmonary embolism in someone who has not received appropriate prophylaxis or who is otherwise at risk for thrombosis. Fever induced by a "wonder drug" is typically seen after approximately 7 to 10 days of use if the patient does not already have an allergy to that medication, in which case it recurs immediately. An exception to this rule is sulfamethoxazole, for which approximately half of hypersensitivity reactions occur within 3 days of initiation. Finally, "what we did" alerts the clinician to the possibility of an iatrogenic infection, such as intravenous catheter–related bacteremia.

CONCLUSION

The initial management of patients with febrile illnesses requires three major considerations. First, is the illness more likely to be infectious or more likely to be related to some other process? Excessive antibiotic use when it is not warranted, such as for viral infections or collagen vascular disease, may cause an adverse reaction, in addition to contributing to the worldwide increase in antimicrobial resistance. However, an empirical antibiotic is appropriate in many cases of fever and localizing signs of bacterial infection. Second, the clinician must rapidly assess the severity of the illness and determine whether it is likely to cause significant organ damage or even death. In a febrile patient with signs of sepsis, the clinician must quickly decide which specific therapy is indicated because a delay in initiating antimicrobial therapy is correlated with increased morbidity and mortality.[12] Finally, the clinician needs to determine whether supportive care alone, including antipyretic therapy, is warranted.

The nearly universal prevalence of febrile adaptive responses to microbial challenge suggests that fever has a net benefit to the host. In addition to clinical studies correlating elevated core temperature and improved prognosis during infection, investigations of principal endogenous mediators have provided evidence of a protective effect of pyrogenic cytokines. Although the use of antipyretic medications is a long-established and widespread practice, the actual benefit of temperature reduction in febrile patients is uncertain. Antipyretic therapy does not protect against the recurrence of childhood febrile seizures, nor has its risk-benefit ratio been determined in patients with cardiopulmonary and other underlying disorders. In summary, fever is usually not harmful, and antipyretics may confuse the clinical picture by dampening it, although their anti-inflammatory effects are often beneficial.[A5]

Grade A References

A1. Lemiengre MB, van Driel ML, Merenstein D, et al. Antibiotics for clinically diagnosed acute rhinosinusitis in adults. *Cochrane Database Syst Rev.* 2012;10:CD006089.

A2. Little P, Moore M, Kelly J, et al. Delayed antibiotic prescribing strategies for respiratory tract infections in primary care: pragmatic, factorial, randomised controlled trial. *BMJ.* 2014;348:g1606.

A3. Long W, Li LJ, Huang GZ, et al. Procalcitonin guidance for reduction of antibiotic use in patients hospitalized with severe acute exacerbations of asthma: a randomized controlled study with 12-month follow-up. *Crit Care.* 2014;18:471.

A4. Shehabi Y, Sterba M, Garrett PM, et al. Procalcitonin algorithm in critically ill adults with undifferentiated infection or suspected sepsis. A randomized controlled trial. *Am J Respir Crit Care Med.* 2014;190:1102-1110.

A5. Jefferies S, Weatherall M, Young P, et al. The effect of antipyretic medications on mortality in critically ill patients with infection: a systematic review and meta-analysis. *Crit Care Resusc.* 2011;13:125-131.

GENERAL REFERENCES

For the General References and other additional features, please visit Expert Consult at https://expertconsult.inkling.com.

281

APPROACH TO FEVER AND SUSPECTED INFECTION IN THE COMPROMISED HOST

KIEREN A. MARR

DEFINITION

This chapter focuses on the approach to suspected infection and fever in compromised hosts.[1] Multiple conditions, including burns, critical illness, and inherited immunodeficiencies (to name only a few), can compromise the immune system and render a person at risk for different infections, but this chapter focuses primarily on hosts who have acquired defects in immune function secondary to medical therapies, or the "medically immunosuppressed." Examples include treatment of neoplastic diseases (particularly hematologic disorders such as leukemia and lymphoma), organ transplantation, and treatment of collagen vascular or autoimmune diseases. Management of people with the acquired immunodeficiency syndrome (AIDS) is discussed in Chapters 384 through 395, and a more thorough discussion of primary immunodeficiency is provided in Chapter 250.

TABLE 281-1 CONDITIONS, INTERVENTIONS, AND IMMUNE DEFECTS TYPICALLY ENCOUNTERED IN COMPROMISED HOSTS

UNDERLYING CONDITION	INTERVENTION	TYPE OF DEFECT
Treatment of neoplastic diseases (particularly hematologic malignant neoplasms)	Underlying disease (without intervention)	Defects in production of bone marrow cells associated with defects in cellular immunity and phagocytic function (e.g., cytopenias associated with bone marrow infiltration with malignant cells)
	Cytotoxic chemotherapies	Bone marrow suppression; defects in primary and secondary humoral and cellular immunity; breach in mucosal barriers (skin, gut); impairment in mucociliary clearance; defects in other organ function (e.g., kidney, liver)
Hematopoietic stem cell transplantation	Underlying disease, without intervention (e.g., hematologic malignant neoplasms)	Defects in primary and secondary humoral and cellular immunity; defects in phagocytic cell quantity and function
	Cytotoxic conditioning therapy (± total body irradiation)	Bone marrow suppression; defects in primary and secondary humoral and cellular immunity; breach in mucosal barriers; defects in organ function
	Stem cell manipulation (e.g., T-cell depletion)	Delay in cellular engraftment
	Prophylaxis and treatment of graft-versus-host disease (e.g., corticosteroids, calcineurin inhibitors, antimetabolites, TNF-α antagonists)	Defective function in phagocytic cells and dysfunction of primary and secondary humoral and cellular immunity
Solid organ transplantation	Underlying disease, without intervention (e.g., diabetes, end-stage liver disease)	Organ dysfunction and miscellaneous immune dysfunction
	Induction therapies (e.g., corticosteroids, antilymphocyte globulin, splenectomy, anti–interleukin-2 Ab, anti-CD52 Ab, calcineurin inhibitors	Depletion and impairment in primary and secondary cellular and humoral immunity
	Surgical intervention and altered anatomy	Breach in mucosal barriers; defects in organ function
	Acute and chronic rejection prophylaxis and treatment (e.g., corticosteroids, calcineurin inhibitors, antimetabolites and alkylating agents, plasmapheresis, antithymocyte globulin, monoclonal antibodies to B and T cells, anticytokine therapies, T-cell costimulation blockers)	Defective function in phagocytic cells, primary and secondary humoral and cellular immunity
Treatment of collagen vascular and autoimmune diseases	Anti-inflammatory and immunosuppressive agents (corticosteroids, nonsteroidal anti-inflammatory drugs, calcineurin inhibitors, sirolimus, mycophenolate mofetil)	Defective function in phagocytic cells, primary and secondary humoral and cellular immunity
	Antimetabolite and alkylating agents	Bone marrow suppression, defects in primary and secondary humoral and cellular immunity
	Biologic immune response modifiers (e.g., antithymocyte globulin, monoclonal antibodies to B and T cells, anticytokine therapies, T-cell costimulation blockers)	Defective function in primary and secondary humoral and cellular immunity

Ab = antibody; TNF = tumor necrosis factor.

APPROACH TO THE PATIENT

The approach to the immunosuppressed patient requires detailed knowledge of the type of immune defect and related risks. Table 281-1 outlines general defects in host responses with the types of conditions that characterize groups of medically immunosuppressed patients discussed in the context of this chapter (treatment of neoplastic diseases, hematopoietic stem cell and solid organ transplantation, and treatment of autoimmune and collagen vascular diseases). As the management of many of these conditions becomes more and more complex and dependent on biologic agents that affect immune responses at both broad and focused targets, knowledge of prior therapies received has become critically important in developing an informed approach to fever.

Patients with Malignant Disease

In patients with neoplastic diseases, particularly hematologic malignancies, the underlying condition plays a role in dictating infectious risks. For instance, the absolute number of phagocytic cells belonging to the polymorphonuclear leukocyte series may be reduced or the function of those cells impaired in the setting of specific malignancies (e.g., acute or chronic leukemias). In conditions such as acute leukemia, in which the cells are abnormal in morphology and function and only a small proportion of normally functioning cells circulate, risks for bacterial infections are enhanced, even in the absence of administered cytotoxic therapies. In certain conditions, such as in the setting of chronic lymphocytic leukemia, there may be quantitative defects in humoral factors that are critical in host defense, such as circulating immunoglobulin G and immunoglobulin M antibodies, secretory immunoglobulin A antibodies, and components of the complement cascade that can directly lyse some bacteria. Another component of the population of phagocytic cells includes circulating monocytes and tissue macrophages and the fixed mononuclear cells of the reticuloendothelial system. These cells collaborate with helper T cells in defense against pathogens that can survive intracellularly, such as mycobacteria, fungi, and some viruses and parasites. The spectrum of infectious risks is further enhanced and prolonged after treatment with cytotoxic drugs. These therapies affect other organ functions that are critical to defense, especially the integrity of the gastrointestinal tract mucosal barrier and airway innate clearance mechanisms, posing additional susceptibilities to bacterial and fungal pathogens. In this manner, the neoplastic disorder itself and the specific therapies used to treat it combine to define both acute and chronic risks for infection.

Transplant Recipients

Hematopoietic stem cell transplantation (HSCT) (Chapter 178) posits additional risks to the patient as a result of the agents used for conditioning therapy in preparation for the stem cell transplantation, variable rate and magnitude of cellular engraftment, and, in recipients of allogeneic HSCT, administration of additional agents to modulate risks for and treatment of graft-versus-host disease (GVHD). Thus, risks for specific infections can be roughly divided on a time scale relative to engraftment. Organ dysfunction, loss of natural barriers (skin and gut), and neutropenia dictate enhanced early risks for bacteria and fungi that inhabit the gastrointestinal tract; impaired humoral and secondary immunity enhance late risks for infections caused by viruses, fungi, and encapsulated bacteria, especially in people treated aggressively for GVHD.

Immunodeficiency in solid organ transplant recipients (Chapter 49) is largely related to the acute initiation and chronic maintenance requirements of therapies to suppress T- and B-cell function to minimize the impact of allosensitization and to decrease risks for early and late graft rejection. Therapies have evolved over time, with increased use of targeted biologic therapies, but in general, risks are largely related to those associated with acute and chronic cellular and humoral dysfunction. The type and amount of therapy differ according to immunologic risk of recipients. Additional variables modulating overall risks for infection include the altered anatomy, surgical intervention, and potential of infection transmitted from the graft itself (i.e., donor derived).

Transplant recipients have increased risks both for acute infection and for reactivation of latent infections after initiation of immunosuppression. Hence, pretransplantation evaluation should be focused on detection of latent herpes viruses (e.g., cytomegalovirus [CMV]) and other pathogens (e.g., *Mycobacterium tuberculosis*) that can be transferred or reactivated with transplantation and immunosuppression.

Two important concepts regarding immunosuppression that have emerged from the field of transplantation include observations of the immunomodulatory effects of viral reactivation and infection and the "net state of immunosuppression."[2] It was long ago noted that viral infections (both reactivation and disease) enhance risks for other infections. This has been particularly well documented for CMV (Chapter 376), which is recognized as a risk for other infections in recipients of both hematopoietic stem cell and solid organ transplant grafts. Overall risks for infection are related to epidemiologic exposures and the net state of immunosuppression, dictated by multiple host, donor, and medical variables. This net state is variable in both quantity and changes in character over time, largely influenced by therapies to prevent rejection or GVHD, and other complications, such as viral reactivation. This concept, which originated from an understanding of solid organ transplantation, can perhaps be applied to the care of all immunosuppressed patients.

Patients Treated for Autoimmune Disease

Table 281-1 also outlines the types of immunosuppressive therapies frequently administered to patients for the control of connective tissue diseases and autoimmune conditions. This is detailed here to emphasize that this group of patients is growing in importance in both hospitalized and outpatient populations, with increased use of biologic immune response modifiers (Chapters 35 and 36) enhancing risks for both reactivation of latent infection (e.g., *M. tuberculosis* and *Histoplasma capsulatum*) and severe manifestations of acute infection. Infectious risks should be considered in balancing need for these therapies, designing preventive regimens, and creating differential diagnoses of suspected infection.

● FEVER IN THE COMPROMISED HOST

The onset of fever in a compromised patient can be an ominous development, and depending on the nature and magnitude of the impaired host defenses, a febrile response can herald the onset of a life-threatening systemic infection. A diagnostic approach should be derived by careful consideration of the patient's signs and symptoms of infection, immunosuppression, and whether the patient is at heightened risk for reactivation of latent infection. Because infection can progress rapidly, empirical antimicrobial therapy may be indicated even before an infection is definitively diagnosed. In this situation, empirical antimicrobial therapy may be indicated even before an infection is definitively diagnosed. Here, the common scenario of fever in the neutropenic host is discussed in depth.

Fever during Neutropenia: Diagnostic Considerations

If fever occurs in the setting of chemotherapy-induced neutropenia, the risk for bacterial infection increases proportionally with the decline in neutrophil count, especially with prolonged durations of significant neutropenia. Early pivotal studies documented that infection rates increase with neutrophil levels lower than 1000 cells/mm^3, progressively increasing as counts decline to less than 100 cells/mm^3. The duration of significant neutropenia is also an important determinant of the type of infection most likely to occur, with the risk for bacterial and fungal infections increasing with each successive week in which leukocyte counts are less than 500 cells/mm^3. In these studies, neutropenia and lymphopenia played significant roles in influencing infection rates in the setting of acute leukemia; however, neutropenia alone was more important than lymphopenia alone. These studies marked some of the earliest efforts that laid the foundation for our current approach to treatment of fever during neutropenia.

Historically, the most common causes of fever during neutropenia were gram-negative bacteria arising from the gastrointestinal tract. These observations drove establishment of empirical and prophylactic antibiotic practices designed to prevent and to treat unrecognized infection caused by the most common predicted pathogens. In the 1990s, concurrent with increased use of prophylactic and empirical antibiotics, especially quinolones and extended-spectrum β-lactams, reported rates of gram-negative bacteremias declined, with proportional increases in the numbers of bacteremias caused by gram-positive organisms. Why the change in epidemiology occurred is a matter of debate, but it is likely multifactorial; in addition to increased use of effective preventive antibacterials, there may be a role played by increased use of

TABLE 281-2	APPROACH TO FEVER DURING CHEMOTHERAPY-INDUCED NEUTROPENIA

PAST AND CURRENT CLINICAL CONSIDERATIONS

What is the type and duration of immunologic deficiency?
Does the patient have any organ dysfunction that would predispose to particular infection?
Does the patient have any unique environmental or epidemiologic exposures?
What are the patient's prior infections and colonizing organisms?
What are the current and recently administered antimicrobial agents?
Are there any specific presenting signs or symptoms that suggest a particular type of infection or syndrome?

indwelling intravascular devices, positing higher risks for gram-positive bacteremias. It has also been recognized that fever that persists despite administration of broad-spectrum antibacterial therapy may herald the onset or presence of undiagnosed invasive fungal infections.

The importance of mucositis in driving inflammation and leading to development of bacterial or fungal infection through mucosal barrier injury cannot be overemphasized in patients administered cytotoxic therapies. Studies have shown that mucositis can produce inflammation adequate to drive development of fever. It is also likely that some people develop fever by transient seeding of the blood stream with colonizing bacterial or fungal pathogens. Some of these infections may be caused by organisms that are less well adapted to growth with standard microbiologic methods. These concepts support liberal use of empirical antimicrobials in the febrile neutropenic setting, with the focus on administration of a compound that is active against the most likely pathogens, considering the patients' epidemiologic exposures and colonizing organisms, especially in the gastrointestinal tract.

Table 281-2 lists multiple questions and considerations that the clinician should entertain when approaching fever in the neutropenic patient. The differential diagnosis of fever in the setting of chemotherapy-induced neutropenia is influenced by local and hospital exposure and the type of preventive antibiotics administered to the patient, which serve to alter microbial epidemiology within the gastrointestinal tract (see Table 281-2). Importantly, the type and the duration of immunodeficiency can alter overall risks, with "latent" infections presenting at development of first fever. Specific organ dysfunction, such as underlying pulmonary disease or renal impairment, can predispose to unique infectious syndromes (see later). Epidemiologic exposures should be thoroughly solicited; for instance, diagnostic evaluation should consider whether the patient previously or currently resides in areas endemic for *M. tuberculosis* or other infections that become latent. Current and previously administered antimicrobial drugs both affect risks for specific infections and can alter host microbial epidemiology. With this in mind, it is useful to have some information on colonizing organisms that may display complex resistance profiles, such as vancomycin-resistant enterococci and bacteria that express extended-spectrum β-lactamases or other resistance determinants (carbapenemases). Knowledge of recent colonization with these organisms should tailor initial antibiotic management, especially in patients who present severely ill.

One early consideration in treatment of fever during neutropenia is whether the patient requires hospitalization for therapy.[3] Risk assessment is an integral part of early evaluation to determine whether outpatient therapy is feasible. Two risk assessment systems have been developed, with the Multinational Association of Supportive Care in Cancer score validated to serve as a useful predictor of outcome, potentially assisting in identifying patients who can be treated with oral antibiotics and close monitoring rather than with inpatient therapy. Although the score is useful as a general guide to risk stratification, other variables that are important to consider in making risk assessment are underlying disease (e.g., lymphoma vs. leukemia), past and anticipated duration of neutropenia, symptoms and signs of infection foci, other comorbidities, and, perhaps most important, whether the patient has access to immediate and reliable medical attention if discharged from the medical facility. Recent guidelines suggest that febrile neutropenic patients can be managed as outpatients, provided the risk index is low enough and empirical antibacterial therapy is administered within an hour of triage, with close monitoring for stability to ensure safety in outpatient management.🅐

The onset of fever should trigger a prompt and thorough bedside evaluation of the patient. Beginning with examination of the head and neck, there should be a specific examination for evidence of central nervous system (CNS) infection as well as a general evaluation of mental status. The oropharynx must be examined for evidence of pharyngitis and focal tenderness. Sinus membranes should be evaluated for the presence of erythema or necrosis. Complete examination of the heart, lung fields, and abdomen is critical, with attention to the potential presence of new murmurs, pneumonia, and intra-abdominal tenderness. The perirectal area and the entire integument should be examined. Intravenous catheter exit sites and tunnels should be carefully examined, and blood should be drawn through all catheter channels for culture. Because catheter exit sites and tunnels can be infected in neutropenic patients without showing early signs of inflammation and erythema and with classic signs of infection presenting only after recovery of neutrophils, examination should be performed daily and with close scrutiny for evolving localized infection that may necessitate catheter removal.

Laboratory studies should be undertaken, with emphasis placed on procedures that can yield prompt results, such as Gram stain of body fluids, exudates, or aspirates. Routine blood work should include a complete blood count with differential, serum creatinine concentration, and screening liver function studies. A chest radiograph should be part of the initial evaluation, as should routine urinalysis. Because routine radiographs are insensitive for detection of small nodular lesions, especially those caused by filamentous fungi, computed tomography (CT) should be performed in evaluating persistent fever, especially in the presence of airway symptoms. No biomarker has yet to be proved reliable in discriminating between severe infection or other causes of fever during neutropenia, although studies have focused attention on the utility of lipopolysaccharide-binding protein, interleukins 6 and 8, procalcitonin, and C-reactive protein, to name only a few.

Although fever is the hallmark of infection, it is not specific for the presence of an infectious process. The development of fever may be a result of multiple causes, including medications, reaction to blood components, Sweet's syndrome, and GVHD. The fundamental principle is that infection should be suspected as the most likely cause of fever in a compromised host, and therapy should be applied empirically, even as diagnostic tests are being

performed. Multiple episodes of fever during prolonged hospitalization and neutropenia are not uncommon; each episode requires comprehensive assessment. After a documented infection, it should not be assumed that a subsequent episode of fever is caused by the same recrudescent pathogen; the law of diagnostic parsimony tends to be less reliable in immunosuppressed patients.

Fever during Neutropenia: Management

Progression of infection can occur rapidly in neutropenic hosts. Very high mortality rates associated with bacteremia, especially that caused by gram-negative bacteria, triggered the introduction of routine empirical therapies (i.e., treatment of fever before diagnosis of infection). There are now many options for initial antibiotic therapy; choice should be tailored according to patient and institutional variables, as outlined in Table 281-1 and Figure 281-1. The first therapeutic distinction is whether a patient is at high risk, warranting inpatient management and intravenous antibiotic therapy, or low risk, potentially treated with oral regimens as an outpatient.[A2] In low-risk patients, the combination of a fluoroquinolone such as ciprofloxacin with amoxicillin-clavulanate has been shown to be effective. In high-risk patients, admission for treatment and prompt administration of a broad-spectrum antibiotic regimen is necessary. An international guideline panel of the Surviving Sepsis Campaign recommends starting antibiotics as soon as possible, preferably within an hour of recognition of fever during neutropenia. Although these recommendations were not specifically developed for this population, recent outcomes studies suggest that delays in administering antibiotics may be associated with prolonged hospital stays.[4]

Early studies demonstrated that the combination of an antipseudomonal β-lactam and an aminoglycoside is effective, but a recent meta-analysis showed that monotherapy with one of the new broad-spectrum β-lactams is associated with better outcomes compared to the combination therapy.[A3] Extended-spectrum agents, such as third- and fourth-generation cephalosporins and

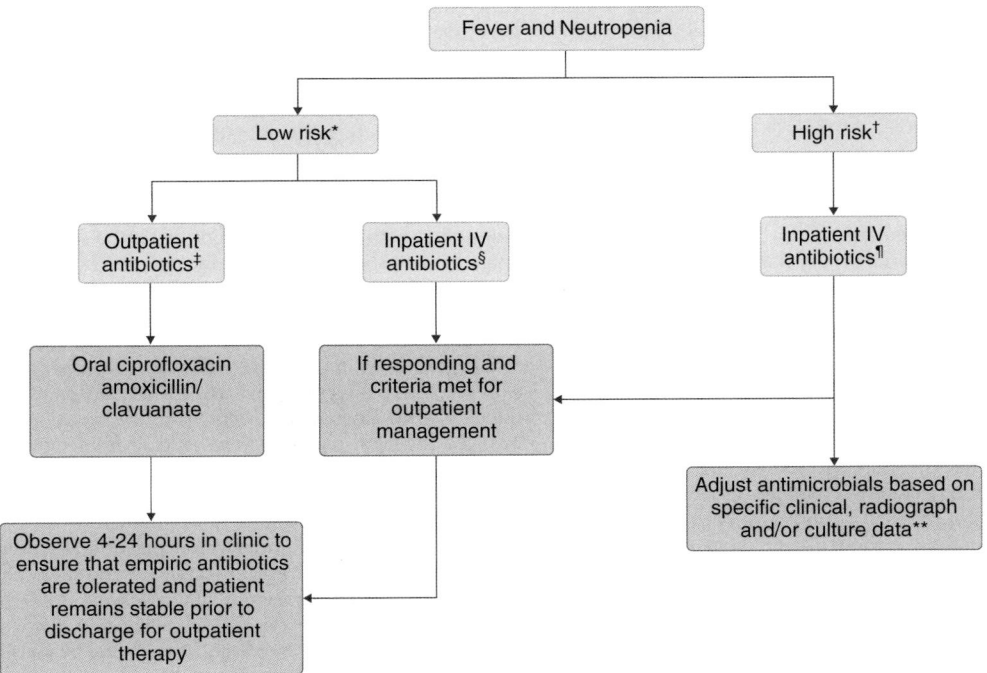

* Low Risk = anticipated neutropenia ≤7 days and clinically stable and no medical comorbidities.
† High Risk = anticipated neutropenia >7 days, or clinically unstable, or any medical comorbidities.
‡ If able to tolerate and absorb; caregiver, access, and transportation are available; patient and physician decide.
§ If there is documented infection requiring IV antibiotics; there is gastrointestinal intolerance; patient and physician decide.
¶ Empiric antibiotic monotherapy with any of the following: Piperacillin/tazobactam, or Carbapenem, or Ceftazidime, or Cefepime.
** For example: vancomycin and linezolid for cellulitis or pneumonia; add aminoglycoside and switch to carbapenem for pneumonia or gram negative bacteremia; metronidazole for abdominal symptoms of suspected C. difficile infection.

FIGURE 281-1. Initial management of fever (≥38.3°C) and neutropenia (≤0.5 × 10⁹ cells/mL). Limited data to support recommendation. (Modified from Freifeld AG, Bow EJ, Sepkowitz KA, et al. Clinical practice guideline for the use of antimicrobial agents in neutropenic patients with cancer: 2010 update by the Infectious Diseases Society of America. *Clin Infect Dis.* 2011;52:e56-e93.)

carbapenems, were then shown to be effective options administered as monotherapy. Meta-analyses have now shown that the routine use of an aminoglycoside in combination may result in more toxicities and no better outcomes.

One major decision point in early therapy involves when to initiate vancomycin in high-risk patients. Advocates point to the risk for gram-positive infections that may carry a higher morbidity in neutropenic patients, including those caused by *Staphylococcus aureus* and viridans streptococci. However, because initiation of vancomycin with fever does not affect outcomes except in the case of treating breakthrough viridans streptococcal infection, in a setting where toxicities may offset benefits, most guidelines do not support its administration except in the case of documented or suspected catheter-related infection, colonization with penicillin- and cephalosporin-resistant pneumococci or methicillin-resistant *S. aureus*, positive blood cultures for gram-positive bacteria, or hemodynamic instability.[A4]

The median time to defervescence is shorter (2 days) in low-risk patients and longer (5 to 7 days) in high-risk patients. Clinical response to the first few days of therapy is a critical determinant of the course of extended antimicrobial therapy. Therapy should be tailored to the diagnostic findings. If patients are stable yet still febrile during a period of prolonged and severe neutropenia, clinical judgment must be used in deciding whether to maintain the initial regimen or to switch to an alternative regimen. If patients become afebrile after 3 to 5 days of antibacterial treatment but cultures are negative, some authorities recommend continuing the broad-spectrum intravenous coverage until recovery of the neutrophil count. This, however, may not be practical for patients with leukemia in blast crisis or refractory aplastic anemia, in whom periods of aplasia lasting weeks or more are common. Others believe that a switch to oral treatment is justifiable (e.g., a fluoroquinolone possibly paired with a β-lactam) if the patient becomes afebrile and appears to be clinically stable. If the patient remains afebrile, there is rapid improvement in the underlying condition, such as with recovery of the circulating neutrophil count to higher than 500 cells/mm^3, and no focus of infection is identified, discontinuation of treatment is an option. If the neutrophil count recovers to above 500 cells/mm^3 and fever persists, clinical judgment must be used to define needs for antimicrobial therapy while a search for the cause of the fever is continued. If the patient was initially treated with vancomycin and no confirmatory cultures supporting continued vancomycin use are obtained after 3 days (e.g., no coagulase-negative staphylococci from blood or methicillin-resistant *S. aureus*), intravenous vancomycin therapy should be discontinued.

Clinical deterioration should trigger consideration of infections resistant to the empirical regimen. Classic examples include breakthrough streptococcal bacteremia in patients not receiving vancomycin; vancomycin-resistant enterococci; breakthrough extended-spectrum β-lactamase–producing gram-negative bacteria in patients taking single-agent β-lactams; *Stenotrophomonas* species infections occurring in the setting of carbapenem monotherapy; and infections with multidrug-resistant pathogens, such as *Acinetobacter* species and organisms that produce carbapenemases.

There are many causes of persistent fever, both noninfectious and infectious. Noninfectious causes include hematomas, drug reactions, transfusion reactions, pulmonary emboli, splenic infarcts, and the underlying malignant disease. The possibility of infection caused by nonbacterial pathogens, such as fungi (especially *Candida* and *Aspergillus* species), should prompt evaluation and consideration of antifungal empirical therapies in the setting of fever that persists more than 4 to 7 days. Many drugs have been evaluated and shown to be effective in this setting, including azole drugs, echinocandins, and polyenes.[A5] Choice should be tailored to current antifungal prophylaxis, diagnostic findings, suspicion of *Candida* versus *Aspergillus* infection, and organ function. Current efforts are focused on developing reliable screening methods to negate the need for potentially toxic antifungals and to derive "preemptive" strategies for guiding use.

There are no hard and fast rules for duration of therapies; the simplest recommendation is to treat documented pathogens until the signs and symptoms of infection subside. On the other hand, persistently compromised hosts may remain febrile for weeks without identification of the cause. For a patient with persistent fever in whom no pathogen is identified, the duration of therapy must be based on integration of clinical data and the best estimate of the direction of the host's status. As mentioned previously, therapy can be discontinued in stable, afebrile patients, assuming that the absolute neutrophil count exceeds 500 cells/mm^3. Clearly, if broad-spectrum antibacterial therapy is to be discontinued, the patient must be monitored carefully thereafter. For patients whose neutrophil counts remain at levels less than 500 cells/mm^3, particularly the subset with severe profound neutropenia of less than 100 cells/mm^3, it is prudent to continue empirical antibacterial and antifungal therapy, with reappraisal of all diagnostic measures. The decision to stop therapy at whatever arbitrary interval may be justified if the patient's condition is stable.

The use of granulocyte colony-stimulating factors for the prevention of febrile neutropenia is discussed in Chapter 167. For the management of established fever in neutropenic patients, evidence-based guidelines have been published by the American Society of Clinical Oncology and by the Infectious Diseases Society of America. The National Comprehensive Cancer Network and the German Society for Haematology and Medical Oncology have likewise published recommendations for the use of myeloid growth factors in the oncology setting. [5,6] The guidelines generally agree, and they support the use of colony-stimulating factors in similar circumstances that indicate high risk for infection-associated complications and poor clinical outcomes, such as in patients with anticipated long and profound durations of neutropenia, age older than 65 years, uncontrolled primary disease, pneumonia, hemodynamic compromise, and invasive fungal infections.

The remainder of this chapter discusses diagnosis and evaluation of specific syndromes that are common in individuals who are immunocompromised because of multiple conditions, including transplantation. Table 281-3 summarizes some of the most common infectious and noninfectious syndromes that involve the skin, lungs, gastrointestinal tract, and nervous system, as discussed next.

● CUTANEOUS SYNDROMES

Cutaneous abnormalities can provide a clue to bacteremia, and aspiration and culture of suspicious lesions can be as valuable as a blood culture. Ascending streptococcal or staphylococcal cellulitis can occur in both immunocompromised and non-compromised patients. Metastatic abscesses are a well-recognized part of the *S. aureus* bacteremia syndrome. Necrotizing vasculitis is classically associated with *Pseudomonas aeruginosa* infections; its cutaneous lesion of ecthyma gangrenosum is an erythematous, indurated target or "bull's-eye" lesion with an area of central necrosis that can appear in crops (Fig. 281-2). However, other gram-negative endotoxin-producing bacteria have been associated with similar cutaneous lesions.

In the neutropenic host, disseminated fungal infections may be initially recognized by characteristic cutaneous lesions. Disseminated candidiasis in neutropenic patients can be manifested with diffuse maculopapular, erythematous, and sometimes tender lesions. The appearance of cutaneous lesions typically changes in character with engraftment of neutrophils (Fig. 281-3). Disseminated infections caused by filamentous organisms such as *Aspergillus* species cause similar lesions, but usually fewer in number and more often with some component of central necrosis. Other filamentous fungi, namely, those with which infection is characterized by a high fungal burden, such as *Fusarium* species, typically cause more skin lesions in multiple stages of evolution, ranging from papules to larger erythematous lesions with central necrosis. Multiple filamentous fungi such as *Aspergillus* species and Zygomycetes can also cause primary cutaneous lesions, especially with a breech in skin integrity associated with catheter sites, trauma, and surgery. Infection with *Cryptococcus neoformans* can be accompanied by cutaneous involvement, with manifestations ranging from molluscum-like lesions to primary cutaneous cellulitis, which may be especially common in solid organ transplant recipients. Cutaneous lesions are an opportunity to establish diagnosis through aspiration, biopsy, and culture.

Morbilliform eruptions or maculopapular exanthems are frequent in neutropenic patients and transplant recipients, and they can be caused by drug reactions, GVHD, and numerous viral infections. Primary infection and reactivation with herpes viruses such as CMV and Epstein-Barr virus can be accompanied by rashes, and diagnostics should be considered in the appropriate context. Human herpesvirus 6, the primary cause of roseola infantum in childhood, leads to latency and can cause disease in immunocompromised hosts both by reactivation and by primary infection. Disease can be accompanied by fever, rash, myelosuppression, and involvement of other organ systems (e.g., CNS). In immunocompromised patients, adenovirus can be both primarily acquired, usually through the respiratory tract, and reactivated; it causes fever, rash, and potentially disease involving multiple organ systems (lungs, gastrointestinal tract, kidneys, liver, CNS). In HSCT recipients, the constellation of fever, rash, diarrhea, and hepatitis may be confused for severe GVHD. Parvovirus B19 infection can be severe in immunocompromised hosts and associated with fever, rash, and manifestations of hemophagocytosis, although there are other infectious causes of hemophagocytic syndromes as well (Chapter 169). The characteristic vesicular rashes of

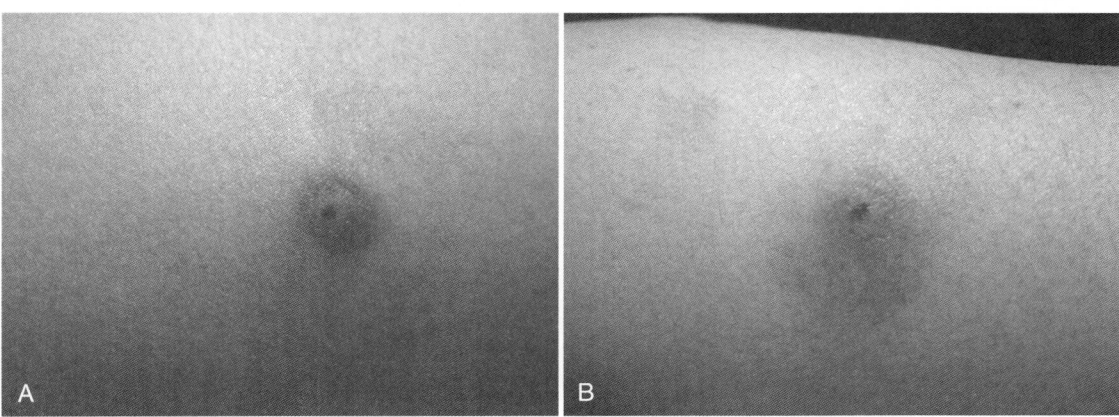

FIGURE 281-2. **Ecthyma gangrenosum.** A 28-year-old woman with fever and neutropenia while receiving chemotherapy for acute leukemia developed several tender edematous papules on her thighs. A, Central crust and surrounding erythema are shown. B, The papules became necrotic during 1 to 2 days, with the formation of black, well-demarcated eschar. Cultures from blood and the necrotic eschar grew *Pseudomonas aeruginosa*. (© DermAtlas; http://www.DermAtlas.org.)

TABLE 281-3 COMMON INFECTIOUS AND NONINFECTIOUS SYNDROMES IN IMMUNOCOMPROMISED HOSTS

PRIMARY ORGAN SYSTEM	BACTERIA	FUNGI	VIRUSES	NONINFECTIOUS
Cutaneous	Disseminated gram-positive and gram-negative bacteria, e.g., *Staphylococcus aureus* *Pseudomonas aeruginosa* *Mycobacterium* spp *Nocardia* spp	*Candida* spp. Filamentous fungi, e.g., *Aspergillus* spp Zygomycetes *Fusarium* spp *Scedosporium* spp *Cryptococcus* spp	Herpes simplex Varicella-zoster CMV HHV-6 Adenovirus Parvovirus B19	Drug eruptions GVHD Sweet's syndrome
Sinopulmonary	Gram-positive and gram-negative causes of sinusitis and pneumonia *S. aureus* *Streptococcus pneumoniae* *P. aeruginosa* *Haemophilus influenzae* Anaerobes Legionella *Nocardia* spp *Mycobacterium* spp	Filamentous fungi, e.g., *Aspergillus* spp Zygomycetes *Fusarium* spp *Scedosporium* spp *Cryptococcus* spp Endemic fungi, e.g., *Histoplasma capsulatum* *Coccidioides immitis* *Blastomyces dermatitidis* *Pneumocystis jiroveci*	Respiratory viruses, e.g., RSV Parainfluenza Influenza Adenovirus Reactivation herpes viruses, e.g., VZV	Drug-related pulmonary toxicities Pneumonitis (sirolimus) Diffuse alveolar damage Bronchiolitis obliterans syndromes
Gastrointestinal	Bacterial enterocolitis ("typhlitis") Mixed gram-positive, gram-negative *Clostridium difficile* colitis Enteric diarrheal pathogens *Salmonella* spp *Shigella* spp *Escherichia coli* *Campylobacter* spp	*Candida* spp.	CMV EBV-PTLD Adenovirus Coxsackievirus Rotavirus Norovirus	Drug-related toxicities, e.g., MMF
Neurologic	Gram-positive and gram-negative bacteria *Listeria* spp Pneumococcus Meningococcus *Mycobacterium tuberculosis*	Filamentous fungi *Cryptococcus* spp	Herpes viruses HSV HHV-6 VZV JC virus West Nile virus Miscellaneous viral encephalitides	Drug-related toxicities, e.g., carbapenem-related seizures PRES

CMV, cytomegalovirus; EBV-PTLD = Epstein-Barr virus–post-transplantation lymphoproliferative disorder; GVHD = graft-versus-host disease; HHV-6 = human herpes virus 6; HSV = herpes simplex virus; MMF = mycophenolate mofetil; PRES = posterior reversible encephalopathy syndrome; RSV = respiratory syncytial virus; VZV = varicella-zoster virus.

varicella reactivation are frequent in stem cell and solid organ transplant recipients with chronic T-cell deficiencies, especially in the absence of antiviral prophylaxis; an important therapeutic consideration is to recognize and aggressively treat disease that involves viscera because disseminated disease is associated with high mortality rates. Antivirals administered as prophylaxis in high-risk HSCT and solid organ transplant recipients can decrease both early morbidity and late mortality associated with herpes simplex virus (HSV), varicella-zoster virus (VZV), and CMV disease, although drug-related toxicities need to be measured in risk-benefit calculations.

There are numerous noninfectious causes of rashes and lesions that are common in immunocompromised individuals. Drug-induced hypersensitivity syndromes can be both mild and severe, potentially associated with life-threatening toxic epidermal necrolysis. As in other populations,

antimicrobial agents are frequently implicated as causative agents. GVHD, especially during the acute phase, frequently is manifested as suspected infection, with fever, nonspecific rashes, and frequently disease involving the gastrointestinal tract (diarrhea, hepatitis).

Sweet's syndrome, or acute febrile neutrophilic dermatosis, is characterized by skin lesions with neutrophilic infiltration in the dermis (see Fig. 440-22). This presents a diagnostic dilemma in neutropenic patients and has been described in the setting of impending neutrophil recovery or treatment with granulocyte colony-stimulating factor. It is also associated with numerous drugs and can appear as a paraneoplastic phenomenon. Biopsy with appropriate microbial stains and culture is essential to distinguish these lesions from infectious causes of ecthyma gangrenosum and other disseminated infections, such as those caused by fungi.

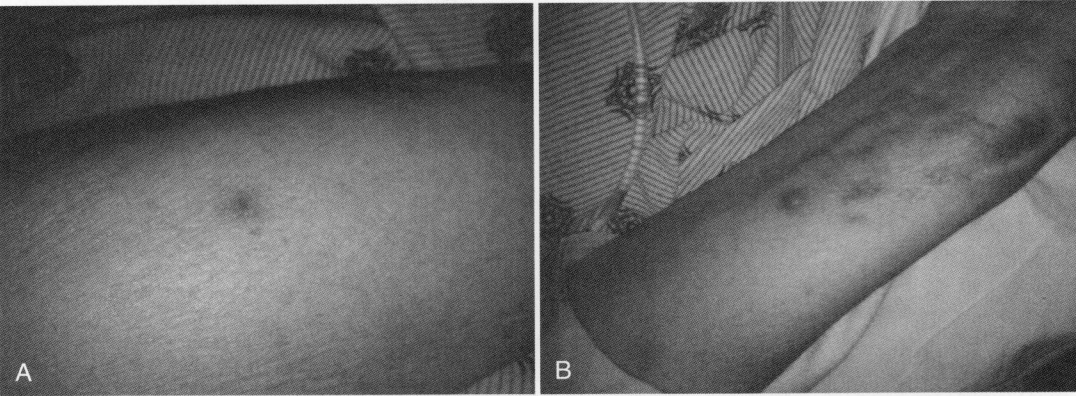

FIGURE 281-3. Disseminated candidiasis. A 60-year-old woman with fever during neutropenia that developed after receipt of therapy for acute leukemia developed tender papular lesions on her extremities, trunk, and back. **A,** Blood cultures returned positive for *Candida tropicalis*. **B,** After resolution of neutropenia, lesions developed a more pustular appearance.

RESPIRATORY SYNDROMES

The lungs are a challenging site in evaluating fever in a compromised patient because detection of abnormalities is easy but obtaining lung secretions or infected tissues can be difficult. Pneumonia should be suspected in a patient who has respiratory symptoms as manifested by cough, shortness of breath, chest pain, and hypoxia. In the early stages of pneumonitis, routine chest radiographs may be normal, whereas more expensive imaging procedures such as CT can reveal pulmonary infiltrates or abscesses. Both community-acquired pathogens such as pneumococci and *Haemophilus influenzae* can cause lobar or diffuse pneumonia. Gram-negative bacilli can cause pneumonia of a necrotizing type in severely neutropenic patients. All patients who are receiving ventilator support are at risk for secondary gram-negative bacillary pneumonia or staphylococcal pneumonia. Clusters of outbreaks of *Legionella pneumophila* infection have occurred in immunocompromised patients maintained in dialysis, transplant, or intensive care units; these outbreaks reflect institutional environmental contamination.

Opportunistic fungi have been increasingly recognized as causes of lung infection in compromised neutropenic patients and transplant recipients. A travel history is essential in a compromised patient who has evidence of lung disease; epidemic mycoses such as blastomycosis, coccidioidomycosis, and histoplasmosis may be manifested as acute pneumonia after recent exposure (although more typically, initial exposure in a normal host leads to containment in an initial focus of fungal lung disease). After immune suppression, the primary focus can be the source of reactivated disease. *Candida* species, in contrast, are uncommon primary lung pathogens. Although *Candida* species commonly colonize indwelling vascular and urinary catheters, candidal pneumonia is unusual in the absence of systemic candidiasis. Systemic candidiasis usually originates from the gastrointestinal tract if it is not secondary to vascular catheter infection, but *Candida* lung nodules can occur after systemic infection, especially with high fungal burden. Although traditionally associated with an "interstitial pattern" of lung infiltration, *Pneumocystis* species pneumonia can be manifested as local consolidation or pulmonary nodules, exhibiting granulomatous inflammation on pathologic examination. Filamentous fungi, which include *Aspergillus*, Zygomycetes, and less frequently diagnosed *Fusarium* species and *Scedosporium* species, are difficult to treat. These infections may be accompanied by chest pain and occasionally hemoptysis. From an initial focus, *Aspergillus* infection can spread through the pulmonary vasculature, which sets the stage for localized hemorrhage, creating a halo sign on CT scan, and infarction and necrosis, which progress to cavitary lesions. Non-neutropenic hosts frequently also develop less specific radiographic findings, such as bronchopneumonia. These organisms can also cause primary airway disease, presenting with features typical of tracheobronchitis, with or without findings apparent on CT scan. This infection is particularly well described in lung transplant recipients, who may also have involvement of the bronchial anastomosis.

Attention has recently been drawn to the high risks for severe pulmonary infection caused by reactivation of *M. tuberculosis* in people who are treated with biologic immune response modifiers (Chapter 36) in the setting of autoimmune or other inflammatory diseases, such as with rheumatoid arthritis, psoriasis, and inflammatory bowel diseases. High risks are particularly well described in the setting of treatment with tumor necrosis factor antagonists, justifying enhanced vigilance, including routine screening for prior infection, and consideration of preventive chemotherapy.[7] These patients are also at increased risk for invasive fungal infections, including reactivation of endemic infections such as histoplasmosis, warranting enhanced screening and high suspicion for disease.

Viral infections that involve the lung are difficult to diagnose in immunocompromised patients. A particularly common concern is reactivation pneumonitis caused by members of the herpesvirus family, especially CMV, which occurs most frequently in the setting of chronic T-cell depression associated with transplantation. Respiratory viruses, which infect immunocompromised hosts with the same frequency as in the general population, cause lower tract disease and pneumonitis more frequently in hosts with suppressed cellular immunity. Essentially any respiratory virus can cause upper and lower tract disease, depending on geographic and seasonal epidemiology; most frequently recognized are respiratory syncytial virus, parainfluenza viruses, influenza viruses, and adenoviruses. Patients who have defects in cellular immunity typically exhibit higher viral loads and prolonged shedding, presenting considerations with regard to enhanced therapy, emergence of antiviral resistance, and infection control. The transplant population has served as a sentinel population in recognizing multiple emerging viral pathogens, including human metapneumovirus, bocavirus, and the KI and WU polyomaviruses.

There are numerous recognized noninfectious causes of pulmonary infiltrates in immunosuppressed hosts. These include early complications of chemotherapy administration, such as diffuse alveolar damage and hemorrhage, and late complications of GVHD and organ rejection (e.g., bronchiolitis obliterans syndromes). Certain drugs that are frequently administered in these populations of patients can cause direct lung toxicity; one classic example is the proliferation signal inhibitor sirolimus.

GASTROINTESTINAL SYNDROMES

There are multiple causes of diarrhea in a compromised host, including conventional enteric pathogens such as *Salmonella* (Chapter 308), *Shigella* (Chapter 309), and *Campylobacter* (Chapter 303). More recently, attention has been drawn to the frequency of noroviruses as an important cause of chronic gastroenteritis in immunocompromised patients, in whom diagnoses have been classically elusive and misapplied to noninfectious syndromes (e.g., GVHD), and outcomes can be poor.[8] In patients who have been in the hospital and have been receiving multiple courses of antibiotic treatment, *Clostridium difficile* (Chapter 296) is a common occurrence, and colitis can be both severe and persistent in immunosuppressed hosts. Two acid-fast staining parasites are *Isospora belli* and *Cryptosporidium* species, and they are associated with predisposing impairments in cell-mediated immunity. More recently recognized are the microsporidians. *Giardia lamblia* is classically associated with hypogammaglobulinemia. Individuals who have received long courses of chemotherapy, radiation, and antibiotics commonly experience *Candida* mucosal overgrowth in the mouth and esophagus. HSV and CMV can cause symptoms identical to those of *Candida* esophagitis. In severely neutropenic patients, anaerobic streptococci and gram-negative pathogens such as *P. aeruginosa* can cause severe mucositis and pharyngitis. In cancer patients, these organisms take advantage of the cytotoxic effects of chemotherapy, which promotes sloughing of mucosal surfaces and subsequently predisposes to infection.

Neutropenic patients may develop enterocolitis that can be of mixed anaerobic and aerobic bacterial origin. Neutropenic enterocolitis, also known as typhlitis or *ileocecal syndrome*, results from chemotherapeutic damage to the intestinal mucosa in the setting of neutropenia. Presentation usually includes fever, abdominal pain, nausea, vomiting, and diarrhea. Because neutropenic enterocolitis can rapidly progress to intestinal perforation, sepsis, and multi-system organ failure, prompt diagnosis and aggressive medical or surgical intervention are required.

CMV colitis can be focal or diffuse; in some solid organ transplant recipients, disease can be present without demonstration of a positive blood polymerase chain reaction for CMV, so endoscopy is required for diagnosis. Because the differential diagnosis of colitis and diarrhea is broad and includes multiple infections, focal Epstein-Barr virus–associated post-transplantation lymphoproliferative disorder, GVHD, and drug-induced toxicity such as that caused by mycophenolate mofetil, these patients should be evaluated with endoscopy to reach definitive diagnosis.

NEUROLOGIC SYNDROMES

Both gram-positive and gram-negative bacteria (including anaerobes) can cause brain abscess or meningitis. *Listeria monocytogenes* is a common cause of meningitis in a compromised host. This pathogen is a gram-positive pleomorphic bacillus that may be difficult to identify on routine Gram stain of cerebrospinal fluid. Encapsulated bacteria such as pneumococci and staphylococci can cause metastatic CNS disease and meningitis. In patients with impaired cell-mediated immunity, *C. neoformans* is also a leading cause of CNS infection. Other fungal pathogens, such as *Aspergillus* and other molds, can invade the CNS, both by direct sinus invasion and by hematogenous spread. Focal brain lesions and meningoencephalitis in individuals who have chronic deficiency in cellular immunity can be caused by reactivation or acute severe infection by typically latent organisms such as *Toxoplasma gondii*, *M. tuberculosis*, and *H. capsulatum*. Reactivated or quiescent CNS syphilis should also be considered in patients with severe immunologic impairment.

There are numerous viral causes of meningoencephalitis. Similar to other populations, one needs to consider enteroviruses, measles, and neurotropic herpesviruses (HSV-1, CMV, VZV). Human herpesvirus 6 is a common cause of encephalitis and post-transplantation acute limbic encephalitis in transplant recipients, characterized by seizures, anterograde amnesia, and neuroimaging abnormalities involving the temporal lobes. Progressive multifocal leukoencephalopathy caused by JC polyomavirus occurs in patients with chronic CD4 deficiency, such as with human immunodeficiency virus (HIV) type 1 infection. Studies have emphasized that transplant recipients are at increased risk for meningoencephalitis caused by West Nile virus compared with the general population. Anyone presenting early after transplantation should be considered at risk for potentially severe infections acquired from the donor; West Nile virus, rabies, HIV, HSV, and multiple other viruses have been documented to be transmitted through organ donation.

There are multiple noninfectious causes of neurologic symptoms, which include drug toxicities and immunologic disorders, such as paraneoplastic syndromes and Guillain-Barré syndrome. Particularly relevant in the transplant recipient, patients with autoimmune diseases, and recipients of high doses of cancer chemotherapy is the *posterior reversible encephalopathy syndrome*. The classic presentation of the posterior reversible encephalopathy syndrome encompasses a sudden onset of severe "thunderclap" headache, seizures, confusion, and visual disturbance, accompanied by a CT or magnetic resonance imaging pattern of predominantly posterior cerebral edema and angiographic evidence of reversible vasoconstriction. It may be caused by endothelial injury, vasospasm, or edema associated with drugs such as calcineurin inhibitors (cyclosporine, tacrolimus).

CONCLUSION

Infections are a major cause of mortality in immunocompromised hosts. The approach to fever and suspected infection requires knowledge of specific risks inherent to the type and duration of immunodeficiency, diagnostic diligence, and tailored therapeutics designed to avoid rapid progression and poor outcomes.

Grade A References

A1. Flowers CR, Seidenfeld J, Bow EJ, et al. Antimicrobial prophylaxis and outpatient management of fever and neutropenia in adults treated for malignancy: American Society of Clinical Oncology clinical practice guideline. *J Clin Oncol.* 2013;31:794-810.

A2. Vidal L, Ben Dor I, Paul M, et al. Oral versus intravenous antibiotic treatment for febrile neutropenia in cancer patients. *Cochrane Database Syst Rev.* 2013;10:CD003992.

A3. Paul M, Lador A, Grozinsky-Glasberg S, et al. Beta lactam antibiotic monotherapy versus beta lactam-aminoglycoside antibiotic combination therapy for sepsis. *Cochrane Database Syst Rev.* 2014;1:CD003344.

A4. Averbuch D, Orasch C, Cordonnier C, et al. European guidelines for empirical antibacterial therapy for febrile neutropenic patients in the era of growing resistance: summary of the 2011 4th European Conference on Infections in Leukemia. *Haematologica.* 2013;98:1826-1835.

A5. Goldberg E, Gafter-Gvili A, Robenshtok E, et al. Empirical antifungal therapy for patients with neutropenia and persistent fever: systematic review and meta-analysis. *Eur J Cancer.* 2008;44:2192-2203.

A6. Yahav D, Gafter-Gvili A, Muchtar E, et al. Antiviral prophylaxis in haematological patients: systematic review and meta-analysis. *Eur J Cancer.* 2009;45:3131-3148.

GENERAL REFERENCES

For the General References and other additional features, please visit Expert Consult at https://expertconsult.inkling.com.

282

PREVENTION AND CONTROL OF HEALTH CARE–ASSOCIATED INFECTIONS

DAVID P. CALFEE

THE BURDEN OF HEALTH CARE–ASSOCIATED INFECTIONS

The Centers for Disease Control and Prevention (CDC) defines health care–associated infections (HAIs) as infections that patients acquire during the course of receiving health care treatment for other conditions. *Nosocomial infection* is a term that refers specifically to an HAI that develops in association with hospital care. The development of infection during the course of health care is not, however, limited to the acute care hospital setting. Thus, *health care–associated infection* is the preferred term in referring to the broader spectrum of infections that develop during the course of health care, wherever that care may be provided, including acute care hospitals, long-term care facilities, rehabilitation facilities, dialysis facilities, and even the patient's home during the receipt of home care services.

The most extensive data regarding the incidence of and outcomes associated with HAIs come from the acute care hospital setting. On the basis of data reported by U.S. hospitals to the CDC in 2002, it has been estimated that 1.7 million HAIs occur in U.S. hospital patients each year, with almost 99,000 associated deaths (Table 282-1). A point prevalence survey conducted in 2010 in 183 U.S. hospitals that the prevalence of HAI was 4%.[1] Previous European studies have estimated that 4.1 million HAIs occur in European acute care hospitals each year. Thus, approximately one of every 14 to 20 patients admitted to U.S. and European hospitals develops an HAI, making HAI one of the most common complications associated with the receipt of health care. Moreover, these data indicate that HAIs are one of the top 10 causes of death in the United States. Whereas many of these HAI-associated deaths occur among patients who are already severely ill and who have a high likelihood of death due to their underlying disease, a substantial proportion of HAI-related deaths occur among persons who were otherwise expected to survive their hospitalization. In a single-center study, 31% of unexpected in-hospital deaths were determined to be possibly or probably related to an HAI. In addition to an increased risk of death, patients who develop HAI suffer a number of other adverse outcomes, including prolonged hospital stays, additional medical interventions and antibiotic treatment, discomfort, and loss of function and income. It has been estimated that these HAIs cost U.S. hospitals between $28.4 billion and $45 billion each year.[2] These statistics are particularly concerning when they are considered with the knowledge that many of these infections are preventable. In fact, a systematic review found that 55 to 70% of four of the most common types of HAIs are preventable through the use of currently available, evidence-based preventive strategies (see Table 282-1).

Although the majority of HAI statistics come from acute care hospitals, there are data to demonstrate that HAIs are significant problems in other health care settings as well. Point prevalence surveys conducted in European and the U.S. Veterans Affairs system long-term care facilities found that the prevalence of HAI among long-term care facility residents ranged from 2.4 to 5.2%. The overall burden of HAI among long-term care facility residents has been estimated to be 1.64 to 3.83 million infections per year in the United States and at least 2.6 million infections per year in Europe. Vascular access–related infections are the most common HAIs among patients requiring

TABLE 282-1 ESTIMATES OF THE BURDEN, COSTS, AND PREVENTABILITY OF HEALTH CARE–ASSOCIATED INFECTIONS IN U.S. HOSPITALS

TYPE OF INFECTION	NUMBER OF INFECTIONS PER YEAR[a]	AVERAGE ATTRIBUTABLE COST* PER INFECTION[b]	NUMBER OF DEATHS (CASE-FATALITY RATE)[a]	PROPORTION PREVENTABLE[c]
Urinary tract infection	561,667	$749-$1007	13,088 (2.3%)	65-70%
Catheter-associated urinary tract infection	449,334			
Surgical site infection	290,485	$11,087-$34,670	8205 (2.8%)	55%
Pneumonia	250,205	$14,806-$28,508	35,967 (14.4%)	55%
Ventilator-associated pneumonia	52,543			
Blood stream infection	248,678	$6461-$29,156	30,665 (12.3%)	65-70%
Central line–associated blood stream infection	92,011			
Other	386,090	$5682-$9124	11,062 (2.9%)	
C. difficile infection	178,000			

*In 2007 U.S. dollars.
[a]Klevens RM, Edwards JR, Richards CL, Jr., et al. Estimating health care-associated infections and deaths in U.S. hospitals, 2002. *Public Health Rep.* 2007;122:160-166.
[b]Scott RD. The direct medical costs of healthcare-associated infections in U.S. hospitals and the benefits of prevention. Centers for Disease Control and Prevention; 2009. Available at: http://www.cdc.gov/hai/pdfs/hai/scott_costpaper.pdf. Accessed January 25, 2015.
[c]Umscheid CA, Mitchell MD, Doshi JA, et al. Estimating the proportion of healthcare-associated infections that are reasonably preventable and the related mortality and costs. *Infect Control Hosp Epidemiol.* 2011;32:101-114.

chronic hemodialysis for end-stage renal disease, with approximately 37,000 catheter-related blood stream infections occurring in U.S. end-stage renal disease patients each year. The magnitude of HAIs related to care provided in other settings, such as ambulatory surgery and endoscopy centers, has not been as thoroughly studied, but such infections have been well described.

Pathogenesis

HAIs can be caused by organisms that are a part of the patient's normal flora (i.e., endogenous infection) or by pathogens acquired during exposure to health care (i.e., exogenous infection) through the contaminated hands of health care workers, the environment, contaminated medical equipment, other patients, or visitors. A variety of factors can contribute to the development of an HAI, and in many cases, HAIs are multifactorial in nature. These factors can be related to the pathogen, the host, the specific health care interventions that a patient receives, the setting in which health care is received, and the methods by which these interventions are made. HAI prevention strategies focus on eliminating, reducing, or modifying one or more of these risk factors.

Pathogen-Related Factors

A variety of pathogen-related factors contribute to the ability of an organism to cause infection. These factors include the organism's normal reservoir, mode of transmission (e.g., direct or indirect contact transmission, respiratory droplets, airborne particles), ability to survive on inanimate objects and surfaces, ability to produce biofilm, virulence factors, and resistance to antimicrobial agents and, for some organisms (e.g., *Clostridium difficile*), disinfectants.

Host-Related Factors

Many host-specific factors are associated with an inherent increased risk of one or more types of infection, regardless of the receipt of health care; however, when a patient with one or more of these risk factors enters the health care system, these factors contribute to an increased risk of HAI. Such risk factors include age (with neonates and older adults having an increased risk of infection because of incomplete development or senescence of the immune system, respectively), obesity, smoking, severity of illness, and certain medical conditions (e.g., burns, end-stage liver or renal disease, poorly controlled diabetes, some cancers, congenital or acquired immune deficiency). These factors reflect suppression of the immune system or breaches of other normal host defense mechanisms. Whereas many of these factors are not amenable to intervention or cannot be effectively modified in the short term, interventions that address remediable risk factors (e.g., obesity, smoking, poorly controlled diabetes mellitus) have the potential to reduce the risk of HAI during future episodes of health care.

Health Care–Related Factors

Health care–related HAI risk factors are those resulting from interventions that are intended to treat or otherwise provide benefit for a patient's existing medical conditions but that also introduce an increase in the risk of infection. These factors may disrupt normal host defenses or alter the patient's normal microbiologic flora. Health care–related risk factors include the use of invasive devices (e.g., central venous catheters, urinary catheters, endotracheal tubes), surgical procedures, exposure to antibiotics, receipt of immunosuppressive medications, and prolonged hospitalization. Because each of these interventions poses at least some degree of increased risk of infection, the risk-to-benefit ratio of each intervention must frequently be reassessed so that patients are not exposed to unnecessary risk. For example, central venous catheters and indwelling urinary catheters are major risk factors for primary blood stream infection and urinary tract infection, respectively. In a patient who has a true medical need for one of these devices, the benefits of the catheter exceed the risk of infection. However, once the patient recovers from the condition that necessitated the catheter, the risks associated with the device then outweigh the benefits.

Exposure to antibiotics is a well-established risk factor for colonization and infection with multidrug-resistant organisms (MDROs) and development of *C. difficile* infection (CDI) through a mechanism known as antibiotic selection pressure. Antimicrobial use is common in acute care hospitals and other health care settings, such as long-term care and dialysis facilities and ambulatory care practices. A 2009 point prevalence survey of hospitals in 25 European countries found that 29% of hospitalized patients receive one or more antimicrobials during their hospital stay. Among 70 academic hospitals in the United States, 49.6 to 76% of hospitalized adults received at least one dose of an antibacterial drug, and mean total antimicrobial use was 839 days of therapy (range, 594 to 1109) per 1000 patient-days in 2009. Even more important, studies have shown that a large proportion of antimicrobial use is inappropriate. Inappropriate antimicrobial use includes administration of antimicrobial regimens that are broader in spectrum or longer in duration than necessary, use of antibiotics that do not provide activity against the causative pathogen, treatment for test results that do not reflect the presence of infection (e.g., specimen contamination, asymptomatic colonization), use of antibacterial agents for treatment of conditions that are not due to bacterial infection (e.g., viral respiratory tract infections), and prescription of inappropriate doses of an antibiotic. Other studies have found that approximately 30% of antimicrobial use in acute care hospitals is inappropriate. Similar proportions of inappropriate antimicrobial use have been reported among long-term care facility residents and chronic hemodialysis patients. Misuse and overuse of antimicrobial agents in the outpatient setting are also well-recognized problems in the United States and other countries, including many countries where antimicrobials can be obtained without a prescription. This inappropriate use of antimicrobial agents introduces unnecessary risk for the development of complications of antibiotic therapy, including CDI, MDRO infection, and toxicity, and represents an important target for intervention.

Health Care Delivery–Related Factors

This group of risk factors includes those that are introduced as a result of the way in which health care is delivered. These risk factors do not offer any potential benefit to patients but rather are associated only with risk. Health care delivery–associated risk factors include, among other things, failure to perform hand hygiene when indicated or to use aseptic or sterile technique during invasive procedures, unsafe injection practices (e.g., entering

TABLE 282-2 RATES OF ANTIMICROBIAL RESISTANCE AMONG PATHOGENIC ISOLATES FROM HEALTH CARE–ASSOCIATED INFECTIONS

		PROPORTION OF ISOLATES RESISTANT TO ANTIBIOTIC		
ORGANISM	ANTIBIOTIC CLASS	United States (2009-2010)[a]	ICUs in 36 Developing Countries (2004-2009)[b]	ICUs in 13 European Countries (2007)[c]
Staphylococcus aureus	Anti-staphylococcal penicillins (e.g., oxacillin, methicillin)	44-59%	71-84%	34.5%
Klebsiella species	Extended-spectrum cephalosporins	13-29%	72-76%	22%
	Carbapenems	8-13%	7-8%	2%
Pseudomonas aeruginosa	Carbapenems	11-30%	36-47%	38%
Enterococcus faecium	Glycopeptides (vancomycin)	62-83%	NR	2.7%
Acinetobacter baumannii	Carbapenems	37-74%	52-66%	73%
Escherichia coli	Extended-spectrum cephalosporins	11-19%	50-68%	11.7%
	Carbapenems	2-3%	4-6%	1.2%
	Fluoroquinolones	25-42%	32-55%	32%

ICUs, intensive care units; NR, not reported.

[a]Sievert DM, Ricks P, Edwards JR, et al. Antimicrobial-resistant pathogens associated with healthcare-associated infections: summary of data reported to the National Healthcare Safety Network at the Centers for Disease Control and Prevention, 2009-2010. *Infect Control Hosp Epidemiol.* 2013;34:1-14.

[b]Rosenthal VD, Bijie H, Maki DG, et al. International Nosocomial Infection Control Consortium (INICC) report, data summary of 36 countries, for 2004-2009. *Am J Infect Control.* 2012;40:396-407.

[c]European Centre for Disease Prevention and Control. Surveillance of healthcare-associated infections in Europe, 2007. Stockholm: ECDC; 2012. Available at: http://ecdc.europa.eu/en/publications/Publications/120215_SUR_HAI_2007.pdf.

a multidose vial with a used needle), and failure to adequately clean and disinfect or to sterilize the patient environment and medical equipment and instruments. These risks are all potentially modifiable and are thus important targets for HAI prevention initiatives. Antibiotic use, which has already been discussed as a patient-specific health care–related risk factor, can also be considered a health care delivery–related risk factor. Unlike with other types of drugs, use and misuse of antibiotics in one patient or population can introduce risks among the larger population through changes in microbial ecology (i.e., selection and increased prevalence of antimicrobial-resistant pathogens).

Many of these health care delivery–related factors are the result of poor adherence to recommended, evidence-based infection prevention practices. Despite recognition that poor hand hygiene practice is a leading cause of pathogen transmission, the existence of major national and international guidelines, and initiatives to improve hand hygiene practices among health care workers, compliance with recommended hand hygiene practices among health care personnel remains unacceptably low. In the United States, average rates of health care worker compliance with recommended hand hygiene practices have been reported to be less than 50%, with some individual studies reporting rates as low as 20% in some intensive care units (ICUs). Similarly, unsafe injection practices continue to be identified as the cause of health care–related transmission of blood-borne pathogens, such as hepatitis B and C viruses.

In recent years, there has been an increasing recognition of the role of environmental contamination in the transmission of health care–associated pathogens. Environmental contamination with these organisms is common, and many of these organisms can persist in the health care environment for prolonged periods. For example, environmental contamination with *C. difficile* has been detected in 100% of hospital rooms occupied by patients with CDI, whereas methicillin-resistant *Staphylococus aureus* (MRSA) has been detected on environmental surfaces in approximately 70% of hospital rooms housing patients infected and colonized with MRSA. Some but not all studies have identified similarly high rates of environmental contamination with multidrug-resistant gram-negative pathogens. This contamination can result in patient-to-patient transmission through transient contamination of health care workers' hands and equipment or by direct contact of the patient with the contaminated environment. Studies have shown that admission to a hospital room in which the prior occupant was colonized or infected with one of several MDROs is a significant risk factor for acquisition of that organism. Environmental contamination is, however, a potentially modifiable risk factor for HAI. Cleaning and disinfection of the environment and portable medical equipment that is shared among patients is often suboptimal. For example, one multicenter study conducted in 36 acute care hospitals in the United States found that at baseline, only 48% of high-risk environmental surfaces were cleaned during routine cleaning after discharge of the patient. Improvement in cleaning practices and other interventions to reduce the microbiologic burden in the health care environment has been shown to reduce the microbiologic burden of organisms in the environment and has been associated with a reduction in the risk of acquisition of MDROs and CDI. In

addition to cleaning and disinfection of environmental surfaces and disinfection or sterilization of shared medical equipment, environmental infection control interventions are important for preventing patients from acquiring pathogens due to exposure to water (e.g., *Legionella* species) and air (e.g., environmental fungi) within the health care setting.

Pathogens in Health Care–Associated Infections

The organisms most commonly identified in device- and procedure-associated infections (i.e., central line–associated blood stream infection, catheter-associated urinary tract infection, ventilator-associated pneumonia, and surgical site infection) vary somewhat among the different types and sites of infection. Overall, eight pathogen groups accounted for more than 80% of pathogens identified in device- and procedure-related infections reported to the CDC through the National Healthcare Safety Network in 2009 and 2010.[3] These pathogen groups and the proportion of reported pathogens that they represented include *Staphylococcus aureus* (16%), *Enterococcus* species (14%), *Escherichia coli* (12%), coagulase-negative staphylococci (11%), *Candida* species (9%), *Klebsiella* species (8.0%), *Pseudomonas aeruginosa* (8%), and *Enterobacter* species (5%). Whereas many of these pathogens represent patients' endogenous flora, further discussion of several of the organisms that may be acquired during exposure to health care is warranted.

Multidrug-Resistant Organisms

An increasingly concerning problem is the emergence of acquired antimicrobial resistance among many of the bacterial pathogens that are common causes of HAIs (Table 282-2). MDROs represent a significant health threat because infections caused by many of these MDROs have been associated with worse outcomes than those caused by antimicrobial-susceptible strains of the same organism, including excess length of hospital stay, increased health care costs, and higher mortality, with mortality rates approaching 50% in some studies. Possible explanations for the observed increased rate of adverse outcomes associated with MDRO infections include the presence of more severe underlying disease, delays in initiating effective therapy, and the use of more toxic or less effective therapy for treatment of the infection. Regardless of their cause, the poor outcomes associated with MDRO infections highlight the critical need for effective preventive measures and development of new antibiotics with activity against these MDROs, particularly multidrug-resistant gram-negative bacilli (MDR-GNB).

Organisms can develop resistance to antimicrobial agents to which they were previously susceptible through a variety of mechanisms, including induction, genetic mutation, and acquisition of new genetic material (e.g., conjugation with cell-to-cell transfer of genetic material by plasmids or transposons). In the health care setting, however, patient-to-patient transmission of MDROs is more common than de novo development of resistance in a previously susceptible organism within the patient's existing flora. Identified risk factors for acquisition of MDROs include exposure to antibiotics, frequent or prolonged exposure to health care facilities (e.g., hospitals, nursing homes), poor infection control practices among health care workers, environmental contamination with MDROs, and prevalence of MDROs among other patients within a health care facility.

Among the pathogens reported to the CDC between 2009 and 2010 as causes of device-associated infections and surgical site infections, approximately 20% had antimicrobial susceptibility profiles that met the CDC's definition of multidrug resistance (see Table 282-2). Of note, 62 to 83% of *Enterococcus faecium* isolates were vancomycin resistant (VRE), and 44 to 59% of *S. aureus* isolates were resistant to methicillin (MRSA). These multidrug-resistant gram-positive pathogens have been recognized as significant health care–associated pathogens for several decades. More recently, the emergence of multidrug resistance among several gram-negative pathogens has been identified as a growing global health threat among persons receiving health care. For example, 65% of *Acinetobacter baumannii* isolates reported to the CDC in 2009 and 2010 demonstrated acquired resistance to at least one drug in three or more antibiotic classes. Such multidrug resistance definitions were also met by 15% of *Klebsiella* isolates and 14% of *P. aeruginosa* isolates. Antimicrobial resistance is an important problem in many regions of the world. For example, International Nosocomial Infection Control Consortium data from 36 developing countries in Asia, Africa, Europe, and Latin America collected between 2004 and 2009 demonstrated methicillin resistance in 84% of *S. aureus* isolates and extended-spectrum cephalosporin resistance in 76.3% of *Klebsiella pneumoniae* isolates and 66.7% of *E. coli* isolates.[4] The lack of use of a standardized definition of multidrug resistance limits direct comparisons of resistance data from different populations. Standardized definitions for multidrug resistant, extensively drug resistant, and pandrug resistant have recently been proposed.[5] Adoption of these or other standardized definitions is needed to allow a more thorough understanding of the global burden of antimicrobial resistance among health care–associated pathogens.

One example of the emergence and rapid dissemination of MDR-GNB is carbapenem-resistant Enterobacteriaceae (CRE), particularly *K. pneumoniae* (Chapter 305). Carbapenem resistance among these organisms was rare in the United States before the year 2000, at which time less than 1% of *K. pneumoniae* isolates reported to the CDC demonstrated such resistance. By 2009-2010, 8 to 13% of *K. pneumoniae* isolates from hospital-associated infections were resistant to carbapenems. In the United States, carbapenem resistance among the Enterobacteriaceae is most commonly due to the production of *K. pneumoniae* carbapenemase (KPC), a class A serine β-lactamase enzyme that hydrolyzes all β-lactam antibiotics. The KPC enzyme, which was first described in 2001, is encoded by the *bla*$_{KPC}$ gene carried on a transmissible plasmid that also carries additional genes that confer resistance to several other classes of antimicrobial agents. Thus, in addition to carbapenem resistance, these organisms demonstrate resistance to other β-lactam antibiotics and to several other classes of antibiotics. Other mechanisms of carbapenem resistance among the Enterobacteriaceae, including other carbapenemases such as New Delhi metallo-β-lactamase-1 (NDM-1), OXA, VIM, and IMP, contribute to the growing threat of CRE around the world.

Asymptomatic carriage of MDROs is relatively common among persons with health care exposures. In fact, patients with clinically apparent MDRO infections represent a relatively small proportion of the total burden of these pathogens. Reported rates of MRSA carriage have ranged from 4.6 to 13.6% among hospital patients, 2 to 22% among U.S. ambulatory dialysis patients, and 10 to 100% among residents of long-term care facilities. The prevalence of VRE carriage among hospital patients and ambulatory dialysis patients has been reported to range from 6.3 to 67% and 0 to 16%, respectively. It is more difficult to describe the prevalence of MDR-GNB carriage because of use of different definitions of multidrug resistance and the inclusion of multiple and different organisms (e.g., *P. aeruginosa, A. baumannii, K. pneumoniae*) among reported studies. Studies that have included a variety of MDR-GNB have reported carriage rates of 19 to 32% in ICU patients and hospital patients with diarrhea, 25% among residents of long-term care facilities, and 16% among chronic hemodialysis patients. Studies that have focused specifically on carbapenem-resistant Enterobacteriaceae have demonstrated prevalence rates ranging from 2 to 5.4% among high-risk hospital patients in the United States and 2 to 49% among post–acute care facility patients in Israel. These asymptomatic carriers play an important role in the epidemiology of MDRO infections. First, they are at substantial risk of subsequent infection with the colonizing organism, with up to one third of carriers of MRSA, VRE, and MDR-GNB developing symptomatic infection within 12 months. Second, asymptomatic MDRO carriers can contribute to MDRO transmission within the health care system through contamination of their surrounding environment and of health care workers' hands, clothing, and medical equipment. In fact, several studies have demonstrated that the risk of acquiring an MDRO, such as MRSA, VRE, and MDR-GNB, during hospitalization is related to the

prevalence, or colonization pressure, of that MDRO among other patients. Finally, admission to a hospital room in which the prior patient was colonized or infected with the MRSA, VRE, or MDR-GNB has been associated with an increased risk of acquisition of those organisms.

There are, however, some encouraging data related to the incidence of some MDROs, particularly MRSA. In the United States, the incidence of hospital-onset invasive MRSA infections decreased 9.4% per year between 2005 and 2008.[6] During a similar period (2005 to 2011), the incidence of invasive MRSA infections among dialysis patients, a group with a rate of invasive MRSA infection that is approximately 100 times greater than that of the general population, was also observed to have significantly decreased in the United States, with annual decreases of 6.7% for health care–associated community-onset cases and 10.5% for hospital-onset cases.[7] These changes occurred despite the emergence of community-associated MRSA as a significant cause of skin and soft tissue infections among persons without typical health care–associated risk factors and the introduction of community-associated MRSA as a health care–acquired pathogen. In England, a 56% reduction in the number of cases of MRSA bacteremia reported through a mandatory reporting system was observed between 2004 and 2008. The specific cause of these observed decreases in MRSA HAIs is uncertain and may be the result of improvements in basic infection control practices, introduction of specific MRSA prevention practices, or other changes in the epidemiology of this pathogen.

Clostridium Difficile

C. difficile, the etiologic agent of pseudomembranous colitis, is the most common cause of health care–associated infectious diarrhea (Chapter 296). Although community-associated CDI occurs, most cases are associated with receipt of health care. Analysis of CDC data from 2010 found that 94% of cases of CDI were associated with health care exposure but that 75% of cases had their onset outside of the hospital (e.g., in the community or in long-term care facilities). Clinical manifestations of CDI range from asymptomatic carriage to mild diarrhea to life-threatening colitis, toxic megacolon, and sepsis. The overall mortality associated with CDI has been reported to range from 2 to 6%, with substantially higher mortality among patients who develop toxic megacolon and other severe manifestations of the disease. Compared with patients without CDI, hospital patients who develop CDI experience an extended duration of hospitalization of 2.8 to 6.4 days, and approximately 15 to 30% of these patients will experience at least one recurrence of the disease, typically within 1 to 2 months of the initial episode. Persons who experience one recurrence have a 50 to 60% chance of additional recurrences. U.S. data from 2009 indicate that 4.8% and 12.8% of hospital patients with CDI are readmitted to the hospital with a principal diagnosis or any diagnosis of CDI, respectively, within 30 days and that by 90 days, rates of hospital readmission increase to 6.8% and 17.2%, respectively. Estimates of CDI-attributable hospital costs range from $5682 to $9124 per case (in 2007 U.S. dollars), amounting to a total cost of $1 billion to $4.8 billion per year.

C. difficile has become one of the most common health care–associated pathogens, and several studies have suggested that more HAIs are now due to *C. difficile* than to MRSA. The incidence of CDI among hospitalized patients in the United States more than doubled between 2000 and 2009. Reported rates of hospital-onset CDI in the United States and Europe are 7.4 and 4.1 per 10,000 patient-days, respectively. In addition to an increased incidence of CDI, the rate of *C. difficile*–related death increased more than four-fold in the United States during the past decade, causing approximately 14,000 deaths per year. The observed increases in the incidence of and mortality associated with CDI were temporally associated with the emergence and dissemination of the 027/NAP1/BI strain of *C. difficile*, which has been associated with greater mortality and higher rates of recurrence than other circulating strains. Initially identified in North America, this epidemic strain has now disseminated globally. Data from England show a 50% reduction in CDI between the fourth quarter of 2009 and the first quarter of 2013 after the introduction of a national CDI surveillance and prevention program. In the United States, however, *C. difficile* remains a challenge, and reductions like those reported in the United Kingdom have not been observed. In fact, between 2008 and 2012, *C. difficile* hospitalizations increased by 11.2%, and from 2010 to 2012, the incidence of hospital-onset CDI increased by 28%.

The problem of *C. difficile* extends beyond the acute care hospital setting. For instance, data from Ohio indicate that 62% of CDI cases in 2006 occurred in nursing homes. Another study conducted in Montgomery County, New York, found that 52% of cases of CDI in long-term care facility residents developed within 4 weeks of discharge from an acute care hospitalization.[8] Data from the CDC's Emerging Infections Program showed that 20% of hospital-onset CDI occurred among persons with recent (i.e., <12 weeks) residence in a nursing home and that 67% of nursing home–onset CDI cases occurred among residents who had been recently discharged from an acute care hospital. These latter findings demonstrate the complex epidemiology of CDI.

The development of CDI is a two-step process that first requires acquisition of *C. difficile* through fecal-oral transmission and then the presence or introduction of factors that allow progression to symptomatic disease. Although some healthy individuals without health care exposure are intestinal carriers of *C. difficile*, acquisition of the organism during contact with the health care system plays a critical role in the epidemiology of CDI. Transmission in the health care setting can occur as the result of exposure to organisms on health care workers' hands, environmental surfaces, or medical equipment. Hand contamination of health care workers is common after contact with the skin or environment of persons with CDI. For example, a prospective study of 30 CDI patients found that hand contamination occurred in 50% of health care workers after contact with patients' skin and in 50% of health care workers after contact with the patient's immediate environment, particularly the bed rails.[9] In the absence of effective hand hygiene practices, contaminated health care workers may transmit the organism to other patients. Contamination of the environment and medical equipment with *C. difficile* is also common. Testing performed in hospital rooms has identified *C. difficile* on environmental surfaces in up to 100% of rooms housing patients with active CDI and in as many as 33% of non-CDI patient rooms. Commonly contaminated surfaces include bed rails, bedside tables, telephones, call buttons, and blood pressure cuffs. *C. difficile* spores are resistant to killing by many common hospital disinfectants and can persist in the environment for long times, further contributing to the risk of exposure to a contaminated environment. Patients who are admitted to a hospital room in which the previous occupant had CDI have been found to be at greater risk for development of CDI than patients admitted to hospital rooms in which the previous occupant did not have CDI. The risk for development of CDI has also been demonstrated to be directly related to the prevalence, or colonization pressure, of *C. difficile* among other patients in a health care facility. This likely reflects an increased risk of exposure to the organism through contaminated hands of health care workers, environment, or medical equipment as the number of persons with CDI increases.

Once *C. difficile* has been ingested, several factors are known to be associated with development of symptomatic CDI. The major risk factor is receipt of antibiotics. Such exposures disrupt the normal intestinal flora and allow *C. difficile* to multiply to larger numbers and to produce toxins that result in disease. Although exposure to any antimicrobial agent may increase the risk for development of CDI, clindamycin, third-generation cephalosporins, penicillins, and fluoroquinolones may present the highest risk. Other factors that have been associated with an increased risk for development of CDI include receipt of cytotoxic chemotherapeutic agents and gastric acid suppressive medications such as proton pump inhibitors, failure to develop an antibody response to *C. difficile*, and older age (i.e., age older than 64 years).

Viruses
Respiratory Viruses
Common respiratory viruses, such as influenza, can be transmitted in the health care setting by health care workers, visitors, and patients, resulting in health care–acquired disease. Higher rates of morbidity and mortality have been observed among those who acquire infection during hospitalization, probably due to the presence of significant underlying medical illness. Despite several studies that have associated higher influenza immunization rates of health care workers with lower rates of nosocomial influenza transmission, the uptake of influenza vaccination among health care workers remains relatively low. This has led many public health agencies and professional societies to call for mandatory influenza vaccination policies for all eligible health care workers. The health care–associated transmission of newly emerged respiratory viruses, such as the severe acute respiratory syndrome coronavirus (SARS-CoV) in 2003, pandemic influenza in 2009, and the Middle East respiratory syndrome coronavirus (MERS-CoV) in 2013, highlights the importance of syndromic surveillance to allow rapid identification of patients with potentially communicable diseases and implementation of appropriate infection control precautions.

Blood-borne Viruses
Although routine screening of the blood supply for the blood-borne pathogens (BBPs) hepatitis B virus, hepatitis C virus, and human immunodeficiency virus has dramatically decreased the incidence of health care–associated

BBP infections, transmission of these pathogens within health care settings continues to occur. Most health care–associated BBP transmission that occurs now is due to failure to adhere to recommended basic infection control practices. Unsafe injection practices (e.g., reuse of syringes, contamination of multidose vials, improper use and disinfection of blood glucose monitoring devices that are used for multiple patients) and inadequate cleaning, disinfection, and sterilization of medical equipment and the health care environment (e.g., dialysis facilities) have been identified in several recent outbreaks of patient-to-patient transmission of BBPs. Between 2001 and 2011, an estimated 130,198 patients from 17 U.S. states were notified of possible health care–associated exposures to BBPs as the result of 35 reported unsafe injection practice events.[10] A large proportion of documented health care–associated hepatitis B virus and hepatitis C virus transmission events has occurred in outpatient settings and long-term care facilities, highlighting the importance of infection prevention programs throughout the entire health care system. Transmission of BBPs from health care worker to patient is uncommon but can occur, typically in the setting of "exposure-prone" invasive procedures. Guidelines are available to assist health care workers and health care facilities in minimizing the risk posed to patients by a BBP-infected health care worker while allowing most such health care workers to remain involved in patient care activities.

Fungi
Candida albicans and other *Candida* species accounted for approximately 9.5% of all pathogens reported to the CDC between 2009 and 2010 as causes of device-associated infections and surgical site infections, placing them among the most common pathogens implicated in HAIs. *Candida* species were particularly common causes of catheter-associated urinary tract infection and catheter-associated blood stream infection, accounting for 12.7% and 14.6% of pathogens reported among these types of infection, respectively. Exposure to environmental fungi, such as *Aspergillus* species, in the health care setting can result in HAI, particularly in immunocompromised hosts. Such exposure and resulting infection are most commonly associated with inadequate environmental control measures during construction, demolition, or water damage within the health care facility. A recent multistate outbreak of invasive fungal infections in the United States, mostly due to *Exserohilum rostratum*, associated with contaminated methylprednisolone injections demonstrates that contaminated medications and other medical products are additional potential sources of exposure to fungal pathogens during health care.

Device-Associated Infections
Central Line–Associated Blood Stream Infections
Central line–associated blood stream infections (CLABSIs) are blood stream infections that occur in patients with a central venous catheter and in whom there is no other identified source of the infection. Development of CLABSI has been associated with longer hospital stays, increased risk of death, and greater hospital costs than those observed among otherwise similar patients who do not develop CLABSI (see Table 282-1). Rates of morbidity and mortality, however, vary substantially, depending on the causative pathogen and characteristics of the patient in whom the infection occurs. The CLABSI definition was developed for epidemiologic surveillance purposes rather than for medical decision making for individual patients. It differs in definition from that of a catheter-related blood stream infection, a term that may be used for research or clinical purposes, in which more specific testing, such as catheter segment cultures, quantitative blood cultures, or differential time to positivity of paired blood cultures, is done to definitively determine that the catheter is the true source of a blood stream infection. Although CLABSIs are often thought of as a complication that occurs among ICU patients, the use of central venous catheters in non-ICU hospital wards has expanded substantially during the past few decades. Thus, the incidence of and the overall burden of CLABSI in some non-ICU wards now often exceeds that in ICUs. CLABSIs are also important problems among nonhospitalized persons with central venous catheters, such as persons receiving chronic total parenteral nutrition, chemotherapy, or dialysis in the outpatient or home care setting. In 2008, for example, approximately 37,000 CLABSIs occurred among outpatient hemodialysis patients in the United States.

Blood stream infections due to central venous catheters are largely the result of contamination or colonization of the external surface or the intraluminal surface of the catheter. This contamination can occur either during catheter insertion or after insertion, related to a number of aspects of catheter use and care. Research has identified a number of effective strategies to reduce the risk of catheter contamination during insertion and throughout the time that the catheter remains in situ. This research has led to the development of evidence-based guidelines for prevention of vascular catheter–related infections. A review of the scientific literature concluded that 65 to 70% of CLABSIs are preventable with the use of currently available strategies and technologies.[11] The "central line bundle" refers to a small number of evidence-based practices that, when used together, can reduce the risk of CLABSI even more than would be expected when the components are introduced individually. The central line bundle includes hand hygiene, maximal barrier precautions during insertion (i.e., use of sterile gown and gloves and a surgical cap and mask by the operator and covering the patient with a sterile, full-body drape), chlorhexidine skin antisepsis, optimal insertion site selection (i.e., avoidance of the femoral site in adult patients), and daily review of catheter necessity with immediate removal of catheters that are no longer necessary. Other interventions that have been associated with reductions in CLABSI rates include the use of antimicrobial or antiseptic catheters, covering of the insertion site with a sterile gauze or semipermeable transparent dressing, cleansing of the catheter insertion site with an antiseptic such as chlorhexidine, use of aseptic technique to access and to manipulate the catheter, scrubbing of the catheter hub with a disinfectant before accessing the catheter lumen for administration of medications or other products or for aspiration of blood, use of antimicrobial- or antiseptic-coated catheters, and use of chlorhexidine rather than regular soap and water for daily bathing of ICU patients.

Widespread adoption of the central line bundle and other CLABSI prevention strategies has been associated with a substantial reduction in the incidence of CLABSI in U.S. hospitals. Data from the CDC demonstrate a 58% decrease in the incidence of CLABSI in ICUs between 2001 and 2009. More recent data from the CDC's National Healthcare Safety Network show a further 41% reduction in CLABSI in U.S. acute care hospitals between 2008 and 2011, with reductions noted in both ICU and non-ICU settings. In these most recent data, the incidence of CLABSI ranged from 0.9 to 3.7 per 1000 catheter-days in ICUs. The highest rate was observed in burn units.[12] Most other types of ICUs had rates ranging from 1.0 to 1.6 per 1000 catheter-days. In non-ICU wards, the highest CLABSI rates were reported from hematopoietic stem cell units and hematology-oncology wards.

Catheter-Associated Urinary Tract Infections

A catheter-associated urinary tract infection (CAUTI) is a urinary tract infection that develops in a patient who has or who recently had an indwelling urinary catheter. Similar to the pathogenesis of catheter-related blood stream infections, CAUTIs develop by the introduction of pathogens into the bladder as a result of contamination and colonization of the internal or external surface of the catheter. Among patients with indwelling urinary catheters, the incidence of bacteriuria is 3 to 8% per day, and 10 to 25% of those with bacteriuria will subsequently develop symptoms consistent with a urinary tract infection. Compared with the mortality and costs associated with many other HAIs, those associated with individual CAUTI events are substantially lower (see Table 282-1). CAUTI, however, occurs 5 to 10 times more frequently than CLABSI and ventilator-associated pneumonia, and thus the total burden of suffering and expense due to CAUTI is substantial. It has been estimated that 65 to 70% of CAUTIs that occur in acute care hospitals are preventable. Data reported to the CDC's National Healthcare Safety Network in 2011 show that the mean incidence of CAUTI in U.S. ICUs ranged from 1.2 to 4.5 per 1000 catheter-days, with substantial variation between different types of ICUs. In non-ICU inpatient wards, the mean rate ranged from 0.2 to 3.2, with the highest rates being observed on rehabilitation units. These data demonstrate a small but statistically significant 7% reduction in CAUTI between 2009 and 2011. The large reductions observed among many published studies of CAUTI prevention initiatives compared with the relatively small overall reduction observed in U.S. hospitals suggest that substantial opportunities remain for additional CAUTI prevention.

A number of basic practices, such as aseptic technique during insertion, maintenance of proper cleanliness and hygiene, securement of the catheter to avoid piston-like movement of the catheter within the urethra, and maintenance of a closed system with unobstructed flow of urine from the bladder into the collection system, are recommended to reduce the risk of CAUTI. Several studies have demonstrated that indwelling urethral catheters are often inserted for inappropriate reasons and that many catheters that were initially inserted for an appropriate indication remain in place even after the initial indication for catheterization has resolved. This may be due in part to lack of familiarity with appropriate indications for catheter insertion or with options that exist regarding alternatives to the use of indwelling urethral catheters. Additional studies have found that physicians are often unaware that their patient has a urinary catheter. Thus, perhaps the greatest opportunity for

CAUTI prevention is avoidance of unnecessary catheter insertion and prompt removal of catheters that are no longer necessary. Development of protocols that explicitly define appropriate indications for insertion of urinary catheters, introduction of interventions that remind clinicians to reassess the appropriateness of a patient's urinary catheter, and nurse-driven protocols that allow nurses to remove unnecessary urinary catheters have been associated with reduced catheter use and lower rates of CAUTI.

Ventilator-Associated Pneumonia

In hospitalized patients, mechanical ventilation is one of the most common risk factors for the development of pneumonia. Mechanical ventilation and the interventions required to provide mechanical ventilation (e.g., endotracheal intubation, sedation) increase the risk of pulmonary infection through a variety of mechanisms, including an increased risk of aspiration of oropharyngeal and gastrointestinal secretions and impairment of the cough reflex. From both a clinical and epidemiologic standpoint, ventilator-associated pneumonia (VAP) is a difficult diagnosis to establish with certainty because of the subjective nature of many of the variables considered (e.g., chest radiograph findings, changes in the characteristics of respiratory tract secretions), alternative explanations for clinical and radiographic abnormalities (e.g., acute respiratory distress syndrome, atelectasis), and difficulty in determining whether the results of respiratory tract cultures represent true infection or colonization of the airway.

In 2011, the incidence of VAP in U.S. hospital ICUs ranged from 0.2 to 3.2 per 1000 ventilator-days, with the highest rates observed in trauma and burn units.[12] These infections are associated with mortality rates and health care costs that are among the highest observed among all HAIs (see Table 282-1). Studies suggest that at least 55% of VAP cases are preventable. As with other device-associated infections, avoiding the use of the device is the most effective means of preventing infection. For preventing VAP and other complications of mechanical ventilation, the use of noninvasive methods of ventilation, daily sedation interruption and assessment of readiness to be weaned, and early mobilization can eliminate or at least reduce the duration of mechanical ventilation. For patients who do require mechanical ventilation, the following are routinely recommended for VAP prevention: proper cleaning, disinfection, sterilization, use, and maintenance of respiratory equipment; elevation of the head of the bed (unless it is medically contraindicated); and routine oral hygiene care, typically with an antiseptic such as chlorhexidine. In some randomized, controlled trials, selective oropharyngeal or digestive decontamination has been associated with a significant reduction in VAP, but this approach has not yet been widely adopted as a standard of care in the United States, at least in part because of concerns that this intervention may lead to selection of antimicrobial-resistant organisms.

Other Device-Related Infections

With the advances that have occurred in medical technology in recent years, there have been substantial improvements in the capabilities of existing medical devices and the development of new implantable devices to treat and to manage a variety of medical conditions, particularly of the cardiovascular and nervous systems. These devices include cardiovascular implantable electronic devices such as pacemakers and implantable cardioverter-defibrillators, ventricular assist devices, deep brain stimulators, and intrathecal pumps. The potential benefits that these devices may offer to patients come with at least some degree of risk of device-related infection.

Surgical Site Infections

Surgical site infections (SSIs) are infections that develop at the site of an operative procedure. Although only a relatively small proportion of patients who undergo surgery subsequently develop SSI and the overall mortality rate associated with SSI is relatively low, the absolute number of SSIs that occur and the overall cost and burden of morbidity and mortality associated with SSI are large because of the volume of surgical procedures performed each year (see Table 282-1). A number of factors contribute to the risk of SSI: the specific site and type of surgical procedure; duration of the procedure; tissue hypoxia at the surgical site; wound contamination with endogenous or exogenous organisms; surgical technique; perioperative infection prevention practices; environmental controls related to temperature, humidity, and air purity within the operating room; and the patient's underlying medical conditions, smoking status, and other factors that may increase the inherent risk of infection. Although some of these factors are not amenable to corrective intervention, many of them are, and a number of interventions have been proved to reduce the risk of SSI. In fact, through routine application of evidence-based preventive measures, it has been estimated that 55% of SSIs could be prevented. The use of sterile technique, preoperative skin preparation with an antiseptic agent, administration of antimicrobial prophylaxis within 60 minutes before the surgical incision, and perioperative glucose control are practices that have been demonstrated to reduce the risk of infection associated with a wide variety of surgical procedures. There is also evidence that at least in some types of surgeries, maintenance of normothermia and the use of supplemental oxygen (e.g., 80% fraction of inspired oxygen) in the perioperative period may reduce the risk of SSI. Although substantial opportunities for improvement remain, a report from the CDC's National Healthcare Safety Network that compares SSI data from 2008 and 2011 shows during that 4-year period a statistically significant 17% reduction in the incidence of SSI occurring in association with several common surgical procedures.[13]

HEALTH CARE–ASSOCIATED INFECTION PREVENTION STRATEGIES

As noted in the preceding paragraphs, many HAIs are preventable. This has been recognized since at least as early as the mid-1800s, when Semmelweiss demonstrated a dramatic reduction in sepsis-related deaths among maternity ward patients after an intervention to improve hand hygiene among health care workers. The degree to which HAIs are preventable was more clearly quantified in a multicenter study conducted in the 1970s. In that study, it was found that 32% of HAIs could be prevented through establishment of an effective infection control program. More recent estimates that take into account newer research and the technology that has been developed during the following three decades suggest that at least 55 to 70% of some of the most common HAIs can be prevented. Scientific research and clinical experience have led to the publication of evidence-based guidelines for the prevention of HAIs.[14]

Strategies to prevent HAI are designed to interrupt one or more of the factors associated with pathogen transmission or the development of infection due to endogenous or exogenous organisms. HAI prevention strategies are sometimes described by one of two categorization schemes that classify the intervention on the basis of either the applicability of the intervention for the prevention of a variety of HAIs or the priority an intervention should be given with regard to the overall HAI prevention program within a health care facility. The first categorization scheme classifies interventions as either "horizontal" or "vertical" infection prevention strategies. Horizontal prevention strategies are those that have the potential to prevent a wide variety of HAIs or to prevent transmission of a variety of pathogens. Vertical strategies, on the other hand, are those that target a specific pathogen. Examples of horizontal prevention strategies include hand hygiene, education of health care workers, environmental cleaning and disinfection, antimicrobial stewardship, and use of aseptic technique for invasive procedures. Vertical or pathogen-specific prevention strategies include the use of transmission-based precautions that are applied to patients known or suspected to be colonized or infected with a specific pathogen to prevent transmission of that pathogen. Preventing its transmission could involve interrupting its normal routes of transmission (e.g., contact, droplet, airborne), active surveillance testing for the pathogen (e.g., MRSA) to detect asymptomatic carriers who may serve as unrecognized reservoirs for its transmission, targeted decolonization therapy for persons identified as carriers of the pathogen of interest (e.g., MRSA), and vaccination programs (e.g., health care worker influenza vaccination campaigns).

The second categorization scheme classifies interventions as either basic or advanced (or special) preventive practices. Basic practices are those that should routinely be implemented in all health care facilities. Basic practices for acute care hospitals include most of the horizontal approaches described before as well as a few vertical approaches, such as transmission-based precautions. Special or advanced interventions are additional interventions that a facility may implement when basic practices fail to adequately control or prevent HAIs or transmission of one or more specific pathogens within the facility. This approach is consistent with recommendations and guidelines from the CDC and several professional societies that promote a tiered approach to the implementation of various HAI prevention strategies. The selection of specific strategies to be implemented within a specific health care facility should be based on an assessment of risk, local data and epidemiology, scientific evidence and guidelines, regulatory and accreditation requirements, and facility-specific cost-benefit calculations. Many of the prevention strategies that have been proven effective for prevention of device-associated infections and SSIs have already been discussed. Several additional preventive strategies are discussed in more detail here.

Antimicrobial Stewardship

Antimicrobial stewardship refers to interventions designed to improve the appropriateness of antimicrobial use by promoting the selection of an optimal antimicrobial regimen (i.e., the most appropriate drug, dose, duration, and route of administration) for a specific patient. The goals of an antimicrobial stewardship program are to optimize clinical outcomes (e.g., cure of infection related to antimicrobial use, minimize toxicity and other adverse events) and to limit the antimicrobial selection pressure that drives the emergence of antimicrobial-resistant strains. Multidisciplinary antimicrobial stewardship programs have been associated with several desirable outcomes, including significant reductions in antimicrobial use, reduced rates of antimicrobial resistance among health care–associated pathogens, reduced incidence of adverse outcomes associated with antibiotic use (e.g., toxicity, *C. difficile* infection), and significant reductions in hospital antimicrobial-associated costs. Thus, antimicrobial stewardship can be considered a horizontal infection prevention strategy.

A variety of approaches have been used by successful antimicrobial stewardship programs, and guidelines describing these strategies have been published. One of the most commonly used and most effective strategies includes formulary restriction and requirement of preauthorization before prescribing of certain antibiotics (e.g., antibiotics that are broad in their antimicrobial spectrum, are associated with significant toxicity, or are expensive). A second approach that has been considered to be a core strategy for antimicrobial stewardship activities is prospective audit of the appropriateness of prescribed antimicrobial therapy with provision of feedback to the prescribing clinician if opportunities for further optimization of therapy are available (e.g., narrowing or broadening spectrum of therapy, discontinuing antimicrobial therapy, or altering drug dose or dosing interval on the basis of available clinical data). Additional approaches that have been included in successful antimicrobial stewardship programs include education, development of guidelines and clinical pathways, computer-assisted decision support, and protocols to optimize conversion from the parenteral to the oral route of administration when appropriate.

Despite a substantial amount of data indicating that antimicrobial stewardship activities are an effective means of reducing inappropriate antimicrobial use and the clinical and financial consequences of excessive antimicrobial use, many acute care hospitals do not yet have formal antimicrobial stewardship programs in place, and many of those that do are not adequately resourced to reach their full potential. In addition to the standard challenges associated with implementation of interventions that require a change in human behavior and clinical practice, antimicrobial stewardship programs must also address the complex and constantly changing problems and issues associated with antimicrobial resistance. Antimicrobial stewardship programs are most commonly found in academic hospitals and large community hospitals, but there is a recognized need for development of such programs in smaller community hospitals, long-term care facilities, dialysis facilities, and outpatient practices.

Decolonization Therapy

Decolonization refers to the administration or application of antimicrobial or antiseptic agents to a person to eliminate or to reduce the burden of carriage of one or more pathogens. Perhaps most commonly recognized as a vertical measure that has been used in some MRSA control programs, decolonization therapy has also been used as a horizontal preventive measure. For example, selective oropharyngeal or digestive decontamination has been used for prevention of VAP and SSI after colorectal surgery. More recently, topical decolonization has been studied as a horizontal intervention for prevention of a variety of HAIs and prevention of transmission of a variety of pathogens. Several quasi-experimental, before-after studies have associated the use of chlorhexidine, compared with nonantimicrobial soap, for daily bathing of patients with significant reductions in rates of blood stream infections, including CLABSI, acquisition of MDROs, blood culture contamination, and contamination of the environment and health care workers. Thus far, two higher quality studies of daily chlorhexidine bathing have been completed and published. A multicenter, cluster-randomized trial conducted in eight adult ICUs and one bone marrow transplant unit in the United States found that daily bathing with chlorhexidine, compared with nonmedicated soap, was associated with a 23% reduction in the combined outcome of MRSA and VRE acquisition.[A3] A similar study in pediatric ICUs showed a significant reduction in the incidence of bacteremia in the per-protocol analysis, although the difference observed in the intention-to-treat analysis did not reach statistical significance.[A2] A third cluster-randomized trial conducted in 74 adult ICUs in the United States found that providing all ICU patients with decolonization therapy that consisted of intranasal application of mupirocin for 5 days and daily chlorhexidine bathing significantly reduced the MRSA-positive clinical cultures attributable to the ICU by 37% and was associated with a lower incidence of all-cause blood stream infections compared with the use of active surveillance and contact precautions for MRSA-colonized patients without decolonization therapy.[A3] Selective decontamination of the digestive tract reduces ICU-acquired bacteremia even more than does selective oropharyngeal decontamination, but it also increases carriage of aminoglycoside-resistant gram-negative bacteria.[A4] Most of the data supporting the use of universal decolonization come from studies conducted in ICUs, and the role of this intervention in preventing infection and pathogen transmission in other settings is not well established.

Active Surveillance Testing

Active surveillance testing is a vertical intervention that identifies asymptomatic carriers of a pathogen of interest (e.g., MRSA, VRE, MDR-GNB) with the intention to introduce additional interventions for identified carriers to prevent infection in the carrier or transmission to others. The interventions that may be applied to the identified carriers include transmission-based precautions (e.g., contact precautions), decolonization therapy (mostly applicable to *S. aureus*), and altered antimicrobial therapy (e.g., surgical antimicrobial prophylaxis). The role of active surveillance has long been the subject of debate and investigation. It is commonly used in outbreak control efforts in conjunction with other interventions. In the non-outbreak setting, there are numerous reports of use of active surveillance as part of a comprehensive program to reduce transmission of or infection with MDROs in individual hospitals, large hospital systems, and health care facilities within specific geographic regions, such as a number of northern European countries. A cluster-randomized trial conducted in U.S. ICUs found that there was not a significant difference in the incidence of colonization or infection with MRSA and VRE in ICUs that performed active surveillance testing with introduction of contact precautions for patients found to be carriers of MRSA or VRE compared with ICUs that did not conduct active surveillance testing.[A5] However, there was a delay in reporting the results of surveillance testing that was longer than would be anticipated in normal clinical practice, which may limit the ability to generalize the study findings to all settings. A comparative effectiveness review of MRSA screening strategies concluded that the strength of evidence for universal screening to prevent MRSA HAIs was low and that there was insufficient evidence to assess other outcomes associated with universal screening or to assess the comparative effectiveness of other MRSA screening strategies (e.g., targeted screening).[15]

As previously mentioned in the discussion of decolonization therapy, a more recently published cluster-randomized trial found that providing universal decolonization to all ICU patients without the use of active surveillance testing was associated with a significantly greater reduction in MRSA clinical cultures attributable to the ICU than was active surveillance testing with isolation of MRSA-positive patients. Although data from these recent, cluster-randomized trials of active surveillance testing and the emergence of data supporting the use of horizontal measures such as universal decolonization therapy have contributed substantial new data regarding the control of multidrug-resistant gram-positive pathogens (e.g., MRSA and VRE) in the ICU in non-outbreak situations, additional study of these interventions in other settings and for other pathogens, such as MDR-GNB, is needed.

Interfacility and Regional Collaboration

Given the frequency with which patients are shared among hospitals and other health care settings within geographic regions and the evidence of interfacility patient transfer as a risk factor of introduction of MDROs and *C. difficile* into a health care facility, implementation of comprehensive prevention programs in all facilities within a region may be more effective in preventing HAIs and MDRO transmission than implementation of the same interventions in a single health care institution. The establishment of regional infection prevention initiatives offers several potential benefits, including the ability to more effectively address the complex epidemiology of HAIs that involve multiple health care facilities (e.g., MDRO acquisition, transmission, and infection) than single-institution interventions and opportunities for collaboration and sharing of information, experiences, and resources. A number of successful regional and national initiatives for the prevention of HAI, including CLABSI, dialysis-related blood stream infections, MRSA, VRE, CRE, and *C. difficile*, have been described.

 Grade A References

A1. Climo MW, Yokoe DS, Warren DK, et al. Effect of daily chlorhexidine bathing on hospital-acquired infection. *N Engl J Med.* 2013;368:533-542.
A2. Milstone AM, Elward A, Song X, et al. Daily chlorhexidine bathing to reduce bacteraemia in critically ill children: a multicentre, cluster-randomised, crossover trial. *Lancet.* 2013;381:1099-1106.
A3. Huang SS, Septimus E, Kleinman K, et al. Targeted versus universal decolonization to prevent ICU infection. *N Engl J Med.* 2013;368:2255-2265.
A4. Oostdijk EA, Kesecioglu J, Schultz MJ, et al. Effects of decontamination of the oropharynx and intestinal tract on antibiotic resistance in ICUs: a randomized clinical trial. *JAMA.* 2014;312:1429-1437.
A5. Huskins W, Huckabee C, O'Grady N, et al. Intervention to reduce transmission of resistant bacteria in intensive care. *N Engl J Med.* 2011;364:1407-1418.

GENERAL REFERENCES

For the General References and other additional features, please visit Expert Consult at https://expertconsult.inkling.com.

283

APPROACH TO THE PATIENT WITH SUSPECTED ENTERIC INFECTION

HERBERT L. DUPONT

EPIDEMIOLOGY

Enteric infections are second only to respiratory tract infections as common infectious medical problems. In certain populations, enteric infections are hyperendemic: poorly nourished infants living in developing tropical countries showing excessive rates of mortality; infants in certain daycare centers; unhygienic residents of custodial institutions for the mentally retarded; immunosuppressed persons; and visitors from industrialized areas to developing regions with traveler's diarrhea.

ETIOLOGY

In approaching a patient with an enteric infection, epidemiologic (Table 283-1) and clinical features (Table 283-2) are used to identify the type of etiologic agent responsible for illness and to develop a plan for evaluation (Table 283-3) and management (Table 283-4).

Recent travel (Chapter 286) to mountainous regions or recreational lakes of North America should raise the suspicion of infection caused by *Giardia* species.[1] When diarrhea occurs during or after travel to a developing tropical region, a bacterial enteropathogen should be suspected.[2] The leading causes of traveler's diarrhea worldwide are the diarrheogenic *Escherichia coli*[3]: enterotoxigenic *E. coli* (ETEC) and enteroaggregative *E. coli* (EAEC). The invasive bacteria (*Shigella*, *Salmonella*, and *Campylobacter* species) cause diarrhea among travelers to all regions but are more common in Asia. Infection with *Cyclospora* species should be suspected when persistent or recurrent diarrhea follows travel to Nepal, Haiti, or Peru or other regions of the developing world (travel-related infections are discussed in detail in Chapter 286).

A specific food or water vehicle cannot be suspected unless multiple cases of illness with a common exposure occur. All too frequently, persons assume that food consumed during their last meal before an illness onset is responsible for the symptoms. The highly variable incubation period for diarrheal disease, which may be as short as 2 hours after eating a food, for preformed toxins, to a week or even longer for microbial enteropathogens, makes the determination of a specific food or beverage in a single case of illness impossible. When an outbreak of diarrhea results in multiple cases, a category of etiology (preformed toxin versus enteric infection) can be determined by calculating the incubation period after looking at timing of the common exposure and the time of first symptoms. Short incubation periods are characteristic of food poisoning associated with enterotoxins (2 to 7 hours for cases caused by *Staphylococcus aureus*, 2 to 4 hours for *Bacillus cereus* enterotoxin food poisoning). Longer incubation periods (usually 12 to 72 hours or longer) are associated with most cases of intestinal infection.

The clinical expression of diarrheal illness will give clues to the etiologic agent involved in disease (see Table 283-2). In the patient with diarrhea who is receiving or recently has completed a course of an antimicrobial drug, a proton pump inhibitor, or an anticancer drug, particularly with recent or current hospitalization, *Clostridium difficile* infection (Chapter 296) should be suspected. An increasing number of cases of *C. difficile* diarrhea are occurring in the community. When a person has close contact with an infant or infants attending a daycare center, a number of low-dose pathogens found in this setting (e.g., *Giardia*, *Cryptosporidium*, or *Shigella* species or viral pathogens, particularly norovirus) should be suspected. Some homosexuals may show high rates of enteric infection acquired through fecal-oral contamination, often associated with infection by multiple pathogens or through the practice of unprotected receptive anal intercourse leading to proctitis due to sexually transmitted organisms. When persons experience advanced acquired immunodeficiency syndrome (AIDS) or other forms of severe immunodeficiency associated with metastatic malignant disease or chronic use of immunosuppressive drugs, depressed intestinal immunity may lead to enteric infection with a variety of parasitic, bacterial, or viral pathogens (see Table 283-1) (Chapter 281). Infants with malnutrition may develop persistent diarrhea and substantial long-term morbidity due to protozoal parasites, including *Giardia* and *Cryptosporidium*.

Enteric infection syndromes may be divided into at least five groups on the basis of the clinical presentation: (1) febrile systemic disease (enteric fever); (2) acute watery diarrhea (secretory diarrhea); (3) recurrent vomiting as the primary manifestation of enteric disease (gastroenteritis); (4) passage of many small-volume stools containing blood and mucus (dysentery); and (5) diarrhea lasting 2 weeks or longer (persistent diarrhea). Table 283-2 lists the major syndromes along with the expected cause.[4]

Noroviruses (Chapter 380) have become the major cause of food-borne gastroenteritis and the most commonly identified cause of waterborne enteric disease.[5] They have been identified as causes of persistent diarrhea in immunocompromised patients, especially in those undergoing hematopoietic stem cell transplantation. *Campylobacter* species (Chapter 303) is a commonly reported bacterial enteropathogen in industrialized countries and is the most important definable cause of Guillain-Barré syndrome (Chapter 420), often resulting in severe disease requiring assisted ventilation, intensive care unit confinement, and permanent neurologic sequelae. *E. coli* O157:H7 and other Shiga toxin–producing *E. coli* (STEC) (Chapter 304) are important causes of food-borne and waterborne colitis complicated by hemolytic-uremic syndrome in children and occasionally in elderly people.

The most commonly detected pathogens in endemic diarrhea in the United States in one study were noroviruses (26%), rotavirus (18%), and *Salmonella* species (5.3%). EAEC strains are being shown to be important causes of pediatric diarrhea in the United States as diagnostic methods improve.[6] In May and June of 2011, there was a large outbreak of diarrhea and hemolytic-uremic syndrome reported from Germany and France due to an *E. coli* O104:H4 strain of EAEC that had picked up the STEC phage controlling production of Shiga toxin. In the future, with improved diagnostic tools, we are likely to see more of these hybrid superpathogens with multiple virulence properties.

DIAGNOSIS
Laboratory Findings
Laboratory tests (Fig. 283-1; see Table 283-3) can be useful and are of particular value in the more severely ill patients, when subjects are forced by their illness to alter activities or are totally disabled and confined to bed or when many patients are afflicted during an outbreak. In each of these situations, the laboratory may help establish cause and allow development of a proper plan of treatment (see Table 283-3). Useful laboratory tests include procedures looking for fecal inflammatory markers, such as microscopic detection of fecal leukocytes or the more sensitive, commercially available test, fecal lactoferrin or calprotein. These tests are particularly helpful to suggest the presence of the invasive bacterial pathogens *Shigella*, *Salmonella*, and *Campylobacter* species or the noninvasive but inflammatory *C. difficile*. Stool culture is performed in more severe cases of sporadic diarrhea and in disease outbreaks

TABLE 283-1 EPIDEMIOLOGIC FEATURES IMPORTANT IN DETERMINING POTENTIAL CAUSE OF ENTERIC INFECTION IN A PERSON OR PERSONS WITH DIARRHEA

EPIDEMIOLOGIC FEATURE	ETIOLOGIC AGENT TO SUSPECT
Travel to mountainous areas of North America	*Giardia* spp
Travel to Russia (especially St. Petersburg)	*Cryptosporidium*, *Giardia* spp
Travel to Nepal	*Cyclospora* spp
Travel to the developing tropical/semitropical world from an industrialized region	Enterotoxigenic *Escherichia coli*, enteroaggregative *E. coli*; *Shigella*, *Campylobacter*, *Salmonella* spp; other bacterial causes; *Giardia*, *Cyclospora*, *Cryptosporidium* spp and noroviruses
Presence of associated cases (an outbreak)	Use incubation period and clinical features to determine probable cause
Antibiotic, chemotherapy, or proton pump inhibitor use in the past 2 months, particularly with a history of recent or current hospitalization	*Clostridium difficile*
Contact with daycare centers	Any enteropathogen, often the low-dose organisms: *Giardia*, *Cryptosporidium*, *Shigella* spp or viral pathogens
Homosexual person practicing unprotected sex	Any organism spread by fecal-oral route; in those with proctitis, suspect *Neisseria gonorrhoeae*, *Chlamydia trachomatis*, herpes simplex, or *Treponema pallidum*
Immunosuppressed person	Any agent, especially *Cryptosporidium*, *Cyclospora*, *Isospora*, *Shigella*, and *Salmonella* spp; *C. jejuni*, *C. difficile*, *Mycobacterium avium-intracellulare*, microsporidia, herpes simplex virus, and cytomegalovirus
Recent or current cruise ship travel	Norovirus, less frequently enterotoxigenic *E. coli*

TABLE 283-2 CLINICAL FEATURES OF ENTERIC INFECTION

CLINICAL SYNDROME	ETIOLOGIC AGENTS SUSPECTED	SPECIAL CONSIDERATIONS
Sustained fever, often with systemic toxicity (enteric or typhoid fever)	*Salmonella typhi*, nontyphoid *Salmonella* spp, *Campylobacter* spp, *Shigella* spp, *Yersinia enterocolitica*	Stool and blood cultures; empirical antibiotics generally indicated
Acute watery (secretory) diarrhea	Any agent. Consider *Vibrio cholerae* (if water losses are major), enterotoxigenic or enteroaggregative *Escherichia coli*, *Shigella* spp, *Salmonella* spp, *Campylobacter jejuni*, viral or parasitic protozoal pathogen	Fluid and electrolyte therapy crucial for recovery in dehydration
Recurrent vomiting (gastroenteritis)	Viral agents (rotavirus or noroviruses) or preformed toxin (*Staphylococcus aureus* or *Bacillus cereus*)	In case of an outbreak, incubation period suggests the etiology
Bloody diarrhea (dysentery)	*Shigella* spp, *C. jejuni*, *Salmonella* spp, Shiga toxin–producing *E. coli* (e.g., O157:H7 or other serotype) or invasive *E. coli*, *Aeromonas hydrophila*, noncholera *Vibrio* spp, *Yersinia enterocolitica*, *Entamoeba histolytica*, or inflammatory bowel disease	Stool culture and occasionally parasite examination important to determining cause; hemolytic-uremic syndrome may complicate diarrheal disease caused by Shiga toxin–producing *E. coli* or rarely *Shigella dysenteriae*
Diarrhea lasting ≥2 weeks (persistent diarrhea)	*Giardia* spp and other protozoal parasites, bacterial overgrowth, bacterial diarrhea, lactase deficiency, Brainerd diarrhea, postinfectious irritable bowel syndrome (PI-IBS), unmasked inflammatory bowel disease (IBD), or celiac sprue	Stool culture and parasite examination indicated; empirical anti-*Giardia* therapy may be useful; remove milk from diet; prior raw milk or untreated (well or surface) water consumption or international travel may predispose to Brainerd diarrhea; with illness lasting >30 days, consider Brainerd diarrhea, PI-IBS, celiac disease, or IBD

TABLE 283-3 LABORATORY TESTS AND PROCEDURES USEFUL IN THE DIAGNOSIS OF INFECTIOUS DIARRHEA

SPECIFIC TEST OR PROCEDURE	WHEN INDICATED	CLINICAL SIGNIFICANCE
Fecal leukocyte test	For moderate to severe cases	When present, indicates diffuse colonic inflammation, often due to *Shigella*, *Salmonella*, *Campylobacter* spp, Shiga toxin–producing *Escherichia coli*, or *Clostridium difficile*
Fecal lactoferrin	For moderate to severe cases to help identify inflammatory forms of enteric infection, to use in health care–associated diarrhea to help determine whether *C. difficile* toxin test should be performed	More sensitive test than fecal leukocytes and will pick up the same pathogens as fecal leukocytes but also pathogens associated with less striking degrees of inflammation (enteroaggregative *E. coli* and *C. difficile*)
C. difficile toxins A and B	Diarrhea associated with use of antibiotics, chemotherapy, or proton pump inhibitors, especially associated with current or recent hospitalization	Most sensitive tests are culture and tissue culture assay. Polymerase chain reaction is sensitive but lacks specificity. Most specific tests are enzyme immunoassay for toxins A and B; a two-step procedure can be used: sensitive but nonspecific *C. difficile* glutamate dehydrogenase antigen test followed by toxin assay
Stool culture for *Shigella*, *Salmonella*, *Campylobacter* spp, and Shiga toxin–producing *E. coli* (O157:H7 and others)	Moderate to severe diarrhea and when stools are positive for inflammatory markers or contain gross blood and mucus (dysentery)	The four mucosa-inflammatory bacteria are the only bacteria routinely sought by most laboratories.
Specialized stool culture for *Vibrio* spp	For cases of profuse watery diarrhea in cholera-endemic areas and outbreaks of seafood-associated diarrhea or dysentery	Cholera cases may need aggressive fluid therapy. Non-cholera vibrios can cause dysentery.
Parasite examination: (1) enzyme immunoassay for *Giardia* spp, *Cryptosporidium* spp, or *Entamoeba histolytica*; (2) acid-fast stain for *Cyclospora* or *Cryptosporidium* spp or *Isospora*; or (3) trichome stain and microscopic examination	In any patient with persistent diarrhea and when diarrhea follows visits to mountainous or recreational lakes in North America, Nepal, Haiti, Peru, or Russia (particularly St. Petersburg)	If microscopic evaluation is performed, experience of the laboratory personnel is important. The commercially available enzyme immunoassay tests are sensitive.
Esophagogastroduodenoscopy and flexible sigmoidoscopy	Persistent diarrhea in patients without evidence of cause of illness	Identified cause of diarrhea is treated; without diagnosis, subjects may be treated symptomatically.

TABLE 283-4 THERAPY FOR AND PREVENTION OF INFECTIOUS DIARRHEA

THERAPEUTIC OPTION	INDICATION	PHARMACOLOGIC AGENT
Oral fluid and electrolyte therapy	For infants, elderly patients, and anyone with profuse watery diarrhea	Soups, soft drinks, and saltine crackers are sufficient; formal oral replacement therapy may be needed with dehydrating forms of diarrhea
Diet	In all forms of diarrhea to facilitate enterocyte renewal and recovery	Soups and broth, saltine crackers, steamed vegetables, baked or broiled meats
Nonspecific therapy	For temporary (≤48 hours) control of diarrhea in older children and adults without evidence of severe diarrhea caused by an invasive or inflammatory bacterial or parasitic pathogen	Loperamide is the most effective symptomatic treatment and will decrease number of stools passed by 60%; bismuth subsalicylate is much less effective and will reduce number of stools by 40%; the antisecretory agent crofelemer is of value in HIV-associated diarrhea
Empirical antibacterial drugs	Enteric fever with toxicity. Febrile dysenteric diarrhea. Traveler's diarrhea	Fluoroquinolones for 7-10 days. Azithromycin is recommended when fever or dysentery complicates illness. Rifaximin for 3 days, fluoroquinolone for 1-3 days, or azithromycin 1000 mg in single dose
Specific antibacterial therapy	Shigellosis, campylobacteriosis, cholera	See Chapters 302, 303, and 309
Antiparasitic drugs	Giardiasis, amebiasis, cryptosporidiosis, cyclosporiasis	See Chapters 350, 351, and 353
Prophylaxis in traveler's diarrhea	Persons traveling to developing areas on tight schedules, those with history of prior traveler's diarrhea, persons with unstable underlying medical disorders, and those interested in prophylaxis	Rifaximin, 200 mg twice daily with meals, while in a high-risk region

and is carried out with blood culture in a patient with fever and systemic toxicity. Other indications for stool culture are presence of dysentery (passage of grossly bloody stools) and when fecal inflammatory markers are found. In dysenteric diarrhea, particularly in the presence of an outbreak, the laboratory should also be instructed to look for *E. coli* O157:H7 and other Shiga toxin–producing *E. coli*. Parasite examination is indicated by diarrhea and persistent (≥14 days) illness; a recent trip to Nepal, Haiti, Peru, or Russia; evidence that the subject practices oral-anal sex or unprotected receptive anal intercourse; or associated immunosuppression. Other tests are indicated in special situations, including stool culture for *Vibrio cholerae* in a patient with severe watery diarrhea with excessive fluid losses in a cholera-endemic area and culture for *Mycobacterium avium* complex, herpes simplex virus, and cytomegalovirus in those with immunosuppression. For patients with persistent diarrhea without etiologic diagnosis when routine tests are employed, endoscopy (esophagogastroduodenoscopy and flexible sigmoidoscopy or colonoscopy) may be indicated in attempting to determine the nature and cause of illness.

The broad range of conventional diagnostic approaches currently available to identify enteropathogens associated with infectious diarrhea will be increasingly supplemented by or replaced with new molecular methods, including real-time polymerase chain reaction, quantitation of pathogen load, and next-generation sequencing.[7]

TREATMENT   Rx

Treatment of diarrhea should be tailored to the clinical syndrome. Oral rehydration therapy with fluids and electrolytes is used to treat acute watery diarrhea and gastroenteritis and all forms of enteric infection, especially when complicated with any degree of dehydration. Oral rehydration therapy is particularly important in infants; it can be life-saving in developing countries for infants with severe diarrhea. Patients with diarrhea should be fed easily digestible foods to facilitate enterocyte renewal and to speed up disease recovery.

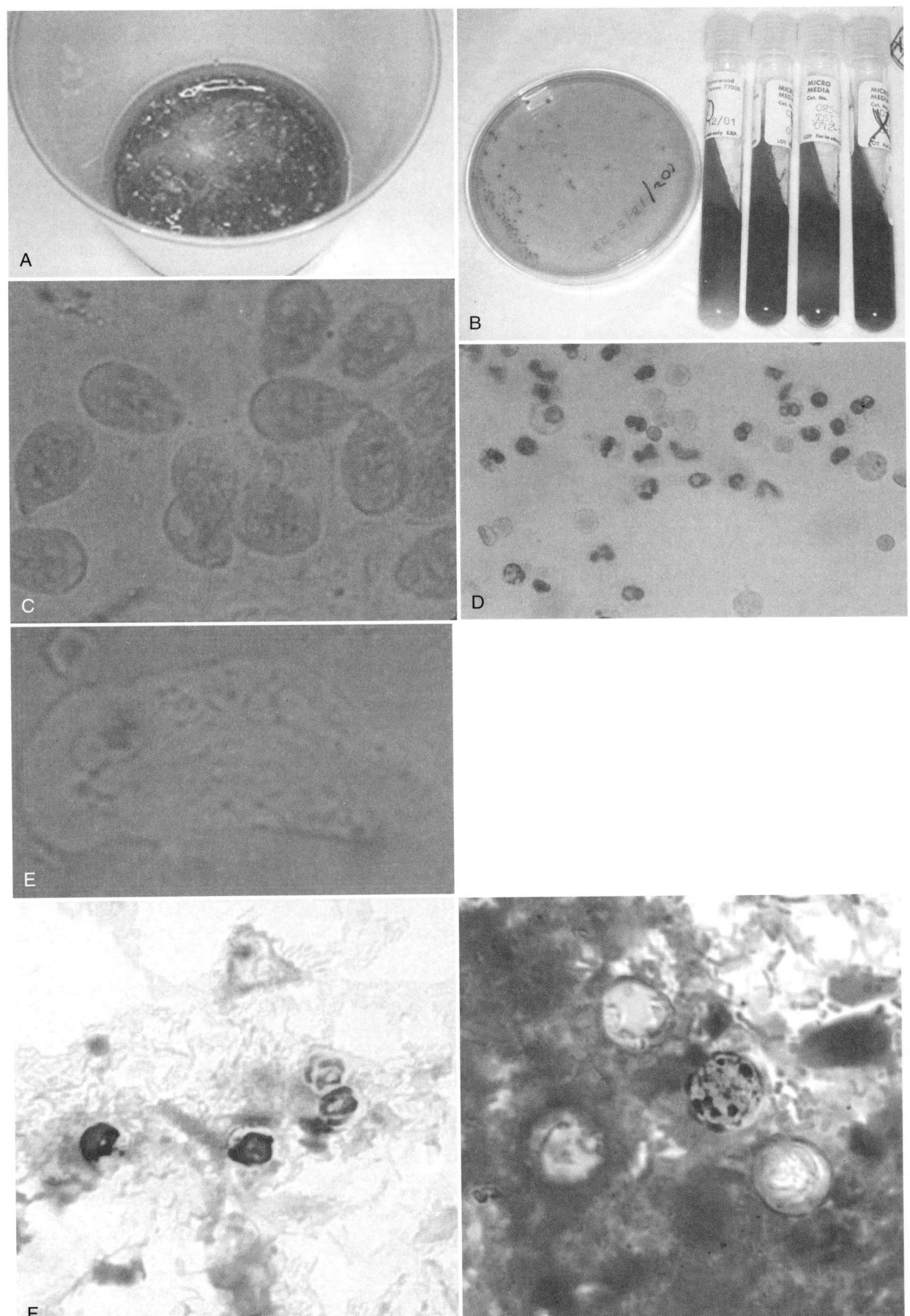

FIGURE 283-1. Laboratory tests to diagnose causes of diarrhea. **A,** Dysenteric stool. **B,** Stool culture and biochemical tests confirm *Salmonella*. **C,** *Giardia* trophozoites. **D,** Many leukocytes in diffuse colonic inflammation. **E,** *Entamoeba histolytica* trophozoite with ingested red blood cells. **F,** Oocysts of *Cryptosporidium* (*left*) and *Cyclospora* (*right*). (From the CDC Public Health Information Library. http://phil.cdc.gov/phil/home.asp: images 7829 and 7827.)

TABLE 283-5 NONINFECTIOUS CAUSES OF DIARRHEA

Running	Small bowel bacterial overgrowth
Fecal impaction	Systemic mastocytosis and eosinophilic
Drugs and laxatives	gastroenteritis
Enteral feeding	Tropical sprue
Irradiation	Celiac sprue
Pancreatic insufficiency	Dermatitis herpetiformis
Intestinal lymphangiectasia	Whipple's disease
Foods (especially dietetic)	Thyrotoxicosis
Cirrhosis and biliary obstruction	Adrenal insufficiency
Diabetic diarrhea	Factitious
Alcoholism	Inflammatory bowel disease
Collagenous colitis	Food allergy
VIPoma	Carcinoid
Ischemic bowel disease	Villous adenoma
Irritable bowel syndrome	Stress with autonomic stimulation

In afebrile, nondysenteric diarrhea, symptomatic drugs may allow older children and adults with illness to return earlier to school or work. Loperamide is the most active drug for improvement of symptoms. Bismuth subsalicylate can reduce diarrhea and is mildly effective in reducing nausea and vomiting associated with viral gastroenteritis.

For enteric fever, febrile dysenteric disease, and moderate to severe cases of traveler's diarrhea, empirical antimicrobial therapy is indicated (see Table 283-4).[8] For outbreaks of dysenteric diarrhea, particularly in children in whom fever is not significant, antibacterial and antimotility drugs should be initially withheld while the etiology of the outbreak is being established to prevent patients infected by STEC strains from being predisposed to hemolytic-uremic syndrome. For bacterial and parasitic pathogen-specific diarrhea, antimicrobial therapy is often advised (see other chapters in the text for specific treatments). Because of the importance of diarrhea when persons travel from industrialized regions to developing countries, prophylaxis with the orally administered, poorly absorbed rifaximin can be employed for some groups (see Table 283-4), with expected protection rates exceeding 70%.

In sporadic cases of acute or persistent diarrhea, infectious agents are not always responsible. Table 283-5 offers a partial list of the noninfectious causes of diarrhea that should be considered.

GENERAL REFERENCES

For the General References and other additional features, please visit Expert Consult at https://expertconsult.inkling.com.

284

APPROACH TO THE PATIENT WITH URINARY TRACT INFECTION

LINDSAY E. NICOLLE AND S. RAGNAR NORRBY

DEFINITIONS

Urinary tract infection (UTI) is bacterial or fungal infection of the normally sterile urine. The clinical presentation varies from asymptomatic bacteriuria, when the urine culture is positive but there are no symptoms, to cystitis (bladder or lower tract infection), pyelonephritis (renal or upper tract infection), and urosepsis (systemic inflammatory response syndrome or septic shock from a urinary source). Urethritis caused by *Chlamydia trachomatis, Ureaplasma urealyticum* (Chapter 285), or *Neisseria gonorrhoeae* (Chapter 299) and prostatitis (Chapter 129) and renal tuberculosis (Chapter 324) are addressed elsewhere in this text.

Uncomplicated UTI occurs in women with a normal genitourinary tract. Most episodes are manifested as cystitis; acute nonobstructive pyelonephritis also occurs in these women, at a lower frequency. Complicated UTI occurs in patients with functional or structural abnormalities of the urinary tract. Complicating factors are host factors facilitating the establishment and persistence of bacteriuria or infection (Table 284-1). Uncomplicated UTI occurs rarely in young men. Men presenting with UTI should be assumed to have

TABLE 284-1 HOST FACTORS ASSOCIATED WITH COMPLICATED URINARY TRACT INFECTION

	EXAMPLES
Obstruction	Urethral or ureteric strictures, tumor
	Diverticula
	Pelvicalyceal junction obstruction
	Prostate enlargement
	Urolithiasis
	Extrinsic compression
Functional	Neurogenic bladder
	Vesicoureteral reflux
	Anatomic defects
	Pregnancy
	Turbulent urethral urine flow
	Cystocele
Urologic interventions	Indwelling or suprapubic catheters
	Endourologic surgery
	Ureteric stents
	Nephrostomy tubes
	Cystoscopy
	Neobladders
Metabolic or congenital diseases	Urethral valves
	Polycystic kidneys
	Nephrocalcinosis
	Medullary sponge kidney
Immunologic abnormalities	Renal transplantation

complicated infection until it is proved otherwise. Recurrent infection is considered a reinfection when it is caused by a new bacterial strain and relapse when the same strain that caused preceding infections is isolated. It is clinically important to classify UTIs by site of infection, presence or absence of symptoms, tendency to recur, and presence or absence of complicating factors.

EPIDEMIOLOGY

UTI is the most common bacterial infection. It is somewhat more common in boys than in girls in the newborn period because of the higher frequency of urethral malformations in boys. Later in childhood, symptomatic UTIs and asymptomatic bacteriuria are more common in girls. More than half of all healthy women experience at least one symptomatic UTI in their lifetime, and each year, 2 to 10% of women experience at least one episode. UTI is uncommon in men with a normal genitourinary tract but increases after the age of 65 years, primarily attributable to prostate hypertrophy and prostatitis. The frequency of infection in patients with complicated infection varies by the abnormality promoting infection. For instance, patients with spinal cord injury and neurogenic bladder have continuing high rates of infection, but patients with abnormalities that can be corrected will no longer be at risk of infection. UTI is also one of the most common hospital-acquired infections; about 80% of these are a consequence of the use of an indwelling bladder catheter.

Asymptomatic bacteriuria is common. The prevalence increases from 1 to 2% of schoolgirls to 3 to 5% of sexually active premenopausal women, 10 to 20% of healthy postmenopausal women, and 40 to 50% of elderly women in nursing homes. It is infrequent in men until older ages, with 5 to 10% of elderly men in the community and 35 to 40% in nursing homes having bacteriuria. Some patients with genitourinary complications also have a very high prevalence. For instance, 50% of spinal cord–injured patients with a neurogenic bladder and without an indwelling catheter and 100% of patients with chronic indwelling urethral catheters have bacteriuria.

PATHOBIOLOGY

Acute uncomplicated UTI follows ascension into the bladder or kidney of uropathogenic organisms in the normal gut flora that have colonized the vagina and periurethral mucosa. The ability of these organisms, usually *Escherichia coli*, to colonize and to persist within the urinary tract is dependent on an array of virulence factors that include adhesins, toxins, and iron-scavenging proteins. Organism virulence is a major determinant of whether infection is asymptomatic or symptomatic or is manifested as cystitis or pyelonephritis. All strains causing uncomplicated infection express the FimH adhesin, but this adhesin is not specific for UTI. *E. coli* isolated from uncomplicated pyelonephritis are characterized by the presence of the P fimbria adhesin Gal(α1-4) Galβ disaccharide globoside, which initiates mucosal inflammation. Adherence of organisms in the bladder or kidney activates the innate immune response leading to release of cytokines, particularly interleukin-6 and interleukin-8, and mobilizes leukocytes. This results in pyuria and local or systemic symptoms, including fever in patients with pyelonephritis.

The occurrence of acute uncomplicated UTI in healthy premenopausal women is determined by both genetic and behavioral factors. A genetic predisposition is supported by observations that a history of prior UTI is consistently one of the strongest associations with recurrent uncomplicated UTI, and women who experience these infections report a higher proportion of first-degree female relatives with recurrent UTI than do those without infection. One established genetic association is being a nonsecretor of the ABH blood group antigen. There is more avid binding of uropathogenic organisms to the vaginal epithelium in nonsecretors. Genetic polymorphisms affecting the innate immune response have been correlated with increased frequency of infection as well as with specific presentations.[1] The strongest behavioral factors associated with uncomplicated UTI are sexual intercourse and spermicide use. For sexually active premenopausal women, 75 to 90% of episodes are attributed to intercourse. The normal lactobacillus flora of the vagina maintains an acid environment that prevents colonization by potential uropathogens, and spermicide suppresses these organisms. Use of the birth control pill or condoms, postcoital voiding, type of underwear used, personal hygiene after voiding or defecating, and taking a bath rather than a shower are not associated with an increased risk for recurrent episodes of UTI, despite popular perceptions. Behavioral risk factors are similar for women for all clinical presentations—asymptomatic bacteriuria, cystitis, or pyelonephritis. Sexual intercourse is not a major contributor to UTI in postmenopausal women. The most important determinants of infection in these women are having a history of UTI at a younger age and nonsecretory status.

The risk of complicated UTI is determined by the underlying abnormality. Genitourinary abnormalities facilitate infection through increased entry of organisms into the bladder, such as intermittent catheterization or urologic procedures, and persistence of organisms within the urinary tract because of incomplete voiding or in biofilm on urologic devices. The determinants that promote symptomatic rather than asymptomatic infection are not well characterized. However, obstruction and mucosal trauma with bleeding are well-recognized antecedents for bacteremia and sepsis in patients with preexisting bacteriuria. Although it is generally accepted that patients with diabetes have an increased incidence of UTI, this correlates with long-term complications of diabetes, such as neurogenic bladder, rather than with diabetes.[2] Patients with poorly controlled diabetes, however, are at risk for more severe manifestations of infection.

Acquisition of bacteriuria in individuals with indwelling urinary devices, including indwelling catheters, stents, and nephrostomy tubes, is primarily attributable to biofilm development along the device.[3] Biofilm is composed of an extracellular polysaccharide material produced by the organisms that incorporates urine components including Tamm-Horsfall protein and magnesium or calcium ions. After insertion of the device, a conditioning layer composed of proteins and other host components immediately coats the device. Organisms adhere to this conditioning layer and initiate biofilm formation. Colonization usually begins at the urethral orifice or in the drainage bag, and the biofilm then ascends the catheter. Organisms growing in the biofilm persist in an environment relatively protected from antibiotics or host defenses. For patients with an indwelling catheter, the acquisition of bacteriuria occurs at a rate of 3 to 7% per day. The initial episode that follows indwelling catheter insertion is usually with a single organism, but polymicrobial flora is the norm in mature biofilms on chronic indwelling devices. *Proteus mirabilis* is a particularly important organism for biofilm formation on chronic devices. These strains may produce copious biofilm, and urease production creates an alkaline environment leading to precipitation of calcium and magnesium ions. This creates a "crystalline biofilm" that is similar to the material causing infection stones and may cause catheter obstruction. About 80% of episodes of urinary catheter obstruction are attributed to *P. mirabilis*.

ETIOLOGY

Table 284-2 summarizes the most common infecting organisms. In all types of UTI, *E. coli* is the dominant bacterial species, causing up to 85% of all symptomatic UTIs in women with community-acquired infections.[4] The second most common species causing uncomplicated cystitis is *Staphylococcus saprophyticus*, which is isolated more frequently in later summer and early fall. In patients with recurrent complicated UTI, species such as *Enterococcus faecalis*, *Enterococcus faecium*, *Klebsiella* species, *Proteus* species, *Providencia stuartii*, and *Morganella morganii* become more common. Patients with very frequent recurrences or with bladder catheters, particularly those in hospitals and nursing homes where antimicrobials are frequently used,

TABLE 284-2	MICROBIAL ETIOLOGY OF URINARY TRACT INFECTIONS
ORGANISMS	**CLINICAL CHARACTERISTICS**
GRAM-NEGATIVE BACTERIA	
Escherichia coli	Typical
Klebsiella pneumoniae	Often reinfection
Enterobacter spp	Often reinfection or health care–associated infection*
Proteus spp	May indicate calculi; frequent with devices
Providencia stuartii	Often reinfection or health care–associated infection*
Morganella morganii	Often reinfection or health care–associated infection*
Serratia marcescens	Often health care–associated infection*
Acinetobacter baumannii	Often health care–associated infection*
Burkholderia spp	Often health care–associated infection*
Pseudomonas aeruginosa	Often health care–associated infection*
Stenotrophomonas maltophilia	Often health care–associated infection*
GRAM-POSITIVE BACTERIA	
Staphylococcus saprophyticus	Most common during late summer and fall
Staphylococcus aureus	May indicate focus outside the genitourinary tract
Enterococcus spp	Often reinfection
Other gram-positive bacteria	In most cases contaminants or colonizers
FUNGI	
Candida spp	May indicate focus outside the genitourinary tract

*Includes hospital and nursing home care.

may have *Pseudomonas aeruginosa*, *Acinetobacter baumannii*, *Serratia marcescens*, and *Stenotrophomonas maltophilia* isolated. In such patients, *E. coli* accounts for less than 50% of infections. Urolithiasis attributed to infection stones is associated with urease-producing organisms; the alkaline urine created facilitates struvite formation.[5] Patients with frequent recurrent complicated UTI, including those with chronic indwelling catheters, often acquire organisms of increased antimicrobial resistance because of repeated exposure to antimicrobials. In health care facilities, the catheterized urinary tract is the most common site of isolation of multiply drug–resistant gram-negative organisms, including extended-spectrum β-lactamase–producing and carbapenemase-producing Enterobacteriaceae. *Candida* sp is the most common fungal UTI. Patients with *Candida* infection are characterized by the presence of diabetes or of an indwelling urinary catheter and broad-spectrum antimicrobial exposure.[6]

CLINICAL MANIFESTATIONS

Typical symptoms of cystitis, pyelonephritis, and urosepsis are listed in Table 284-3. The onset of cystitis is rapid, and symptoms usually develop during less than 24 hours. Clinically, the lack of vaginal discharge differentiates cystitis from urethritis caused by chlamydia, ureaplasma, or gonococci. Women who experience recurrent episodes of acute uncomplicated UTI are more than 90% reliable for self-diagnosis.

Pyelonephritis may also have a rapid onset and may or may not be associated with cystitis symptoms. Bacteremia occurs in 10 to 30% of patients but does not have prognostic significance. The typical flank pain and tenderness, resulting from inflammation and edema of the renal parenchyma, may be masked by the intake of analgesic drugs such as acetaminophen, which may also reduce the fever. An important differential diagnosis is renal calculus. This may have a similar location of pain but does not cause fever unless it is complicated by infection.

Complicated UTI is manifested across a clinical spectrum from minimal voiding abnormalities to symptoms consistent with cystitis, pyelonephritis, or severe sepsis. Urosepsis is a life-threatening condition, usually associated with bacteremia.[7] Obstruction or trauma to the mucosa from an indwelling catheter or with urologic surgery may precipitate bacteremia. Patients who present with urosepsis invariably have complicated UTI rather than nonobstructive pyelonephritis.

TABLE 284-3 CLINICAL SYMPTOMS OF URINARY TRACT INFECTIONS

TYPE OF URINARY TRACT INFECTION	TYPICAL SIGNS OR SYMPTOMS
Cystitis	Frequency Dysuria Urgency Stranguria (difficulty in micturition) Suprapubic pain Hematuria or cloudy urine
Pyelonephritis	Costovertebral angle pain or tenderness Fever Chills Cystitis symptoms (may be absent)
Urosepsis	Fever Chills, rigors Sepsis syndrome

TABLE 284-4 INTERPRETATION OF THE QUANTITATIVE URINE CULTURE

	QUANTITATIVE BACTERIAL COUNT
Asymptomatic bacteriuria	$\geq 10^5$ CFU/mL (two consecutive specimens for women)
Acute uncomplicated cystitis	$\geq 10^2$ CFU/mL of *Escherichia coli* or *Staphylococcus saprophyticus*
Acute uncomplicated pyelonephritis	$\geq 10^4$ CFU/mL (95% have $\geq 10^5$ CFU/mL)
Complicated urinary tract infection	$\geq 10^5$ CFU/mL (lower counts may occur with diuresis)
Intermittent or in and out catheter collection	$\geq 10^2$ CFU/mL
Suprapubic or percutaneous aspiration	Any organisms isolated

TABLE 284-5 DECISION PROCESS FOR DIAGNOSIS AND TREATMENT OF UPPER (PYELONEPHRITIS) VERSUS LOWER (CYSTITIS) URINARY TRACT INFECTIONS

	CYSTITIS	PYELONEPHRITIS
SIGNS AND SYMPTOMS		
Fever	No	Yes
Dysuria	Yes	May be present
Frequency	Yes	May be present
Flank pain	No	Yes
DIAGNOSIS		
Pyuria	Yes	Yes
Nitrite test result	Normally positive	Normally positive
Bacteriuria	Yes	Yes
C-reactive protein	Normal	Increased
Blood cultures	Negative	Positive in $\approx$10-30%
TREATMENT		
First line	Short-term oral therapy (Table 284-6)	Oral: fluoroquinolone for 7 days Parenteral: cephalosporin, fluoroquinolone, or aminoglycoside for 7-14 days (Table 284-7)
Second line	Fluoroquinolone for 3 days or cephalosporin for 7 days	Injectable cephalosporin until afebrile, followed by oral step-down for total of 2 weeks
Pregnant women	Nitrofurantoin or cephalosporin for 5-7 days	Injectable cephalosporin until afebrile, followed by oral cephalosporin for 14 days

DIAGNOSIS

Laboratory Findings

The hallmark of UTI diagnosis is demonstration of bacteriuria in a urine sample that has been incubated in the bladder for at least 2 hours to allow the growth of bacteria. A pretherapy urine culture specimen should be obtained for all patients presenting with pyelonephritis, urosepsis, or complicated UTI or when the diagnosis is uncertain. It is not generally recommended for acute uncomplicated cystitis because the clinical presentation is characteristic, and use of empirical short-course therapy means symptoms are often resolved by the time the culture is available. The urine specimen must be collected in a manner that will limit contamination. The usual collection method is a mid-stream urine sample. All specimens should be taken promptly to the laboratory to prevent growth during transportation. Urine specimens for culture must be collected before institution of antimicrobial therapy as the urine is rapidly sterilized after initiation of systemic antimicrobials.

Interpretation of the quantitative urine culture varies with the clinical presentation and collection method (Table 284-4). *Significant bacteriuria* is usually 10^5 CFU/mL or more, where one colony-forming unit (CFU) is one or more bacterial cells forming a colony when growing on an agar plate. In women with symptoms of uncomplicated cystitis, 10^2 CFU/mL or more in midstream urine of *E. coli* or *S. saprophyticus* is consistent with infection. Other gram-positive organisms at any quantitative count should be interpreted as contaminants.[8]

Pyuria is present in most patients with symptomatic UTI or asymptomatic bacteriuria. Many other abnormalities are, however, associated with pyuria, and the presence of pyuria does not diagnose infection or differentiate symptomatic from asymptomatic infection. The absence of pyuria has a high negative predictive value to exclude UTI for most patients. However, the absence of pyuria in a urine specimen from a woman with symptoms compatible with cystitis is not an indication to withhold empirical antimicrobial therapy.

For screening of bacteriuria, identification of nitrite in the urine may be useful. Gram-negative bacteria, with the exception of *P. aeruginosa*, will metabolize nitrate to nitrite, which can be demonstrated by a color reaction on a dipstick. Gram-positive bacteria and fungi do not metabolize nitrate. The technique is rapid (<1 minute) and inexpensive. It has a high degree of speci-

ficity but is insensitive because it does not detect infections caused by gram-positive organisms.

Blood culture specimens should be obtained in all patients with suspected urosepsis. Patients with acute pyelonephritis, but not those with acute cystitis, have increased serum levels of C-reactive protein.

Imaging

Early imaging should be performed in any patient with urosepsis to identify abnormalities that require immediate source control. The optimal imaging modality is an infused computed tomography scan. Magnetic resonance imaging may not identify gas in tissues or small stones. Ultrasound may provide a rapid examination to exclude significant obstruction. Investigations would also be indicated for patients with delayed response or failure to respond to appropriate antimicrobial therapy or if there is early relapse of pyelonephritis after completion of therapy. The optimal management of complicated urinary infection requires characterization of underlying abnormalities and correction of these, whenever possible. Selected patients may require studies for diagnosis of vesicoureteral reflux or to characterize differential renal function.

Differential Diagnosis

Clinical manifestations will usually differentiate acute cystitis and acute pyelonephritis (Table 284-5). New-onset frequency, dysuria, and urgency without accompanying vaginal discharge or pain have a positive predictive value of 90% for acute cystitis. The differential diagnosis for women presenting with acute irritative lower tract symptoms includes sexually transmitted infections, vulvovaginal candidiasis, and noninfectious causes such as interstitial nephritis. Some patients who present with only lower tract symptoms may have renal infection, referred to as occult pyelonephritis. Patients with appendicitis and cholecystitis can present with flank pain similar to right-sided pyelonephritis, and pelvic inflammatory disease may be misdiagnosed as urinary infection.

TREATMENT   Rx

Symptomatic UTIs should be treated with antimicrobials to decrease the duration of symptoms and, for pyelonephritis, to limit damage to renal tissue. Antimicrobials selected for treatment should be excreted renally, so

TABLE 284-6 ANTIMICROBIALS USED TO TREAT CYSTITIS

ANTIMICROBIAL	DOSE* AND DURATION
FIRST-LINE THERAPY	
Trimethoprim	100-150 mg q12h for 3 days
Trimethoprim-sulfamethoxazole	80/400 mg q12h for 3 days or 320/1600 mg single dose
Nitrofurantoin	50 mg q8h for 5-7 days
Nitrofurantoin macrocrystals	100 mg bid for 5 days
Fosfomycin trometamol	3 g single dose
Pivmecillinam	400 mg bid for 3-5 days
OTHER	
Amoxicillin-clavulanate	500 mg (amoxicillin dose) q8h for 7 days
Amoxicillin	500 mg tid for 7 days
Cefpodoxime proxetil	100 mg bid for 3 days
Cefuroxime axetil	500 mg bid for 7 days
Cefixime	400 mg/day for 7 days
Ceftibuten	400 mg/day for 5-7 days
Norfloxacin	400 mg q12h for 7 days
Ciprofloxacin	250 mg q12h for 7 days (500 mg qd extended release)
Levofloxacin	250-500 mg/day for 7 days
Doxycycline	100 mg bid for 7 days

*Doses given are for adults with normal renal function. The need to reduce dosages because of renal impairment related to infection in the kidneys, other renal diseases, or advanced age should always be considered.

TABLE 284-7 ANTIMICROBIALS USED TO TREAT PYELONEPHRITIS

ROUTE OF ADMINISTRATION AND ANTIMICROBIAL	DOSE* AND DURATION
PARENTERAL	
First-Line Therapy	
Gentamicin	4.5 mg/kg/day × 10-14 days
Tobramycin	4.5 mg/kg/day × 10-14 days
Ciprofloxacin	400 mg q12h × 7 days
Levofloxacin	750 mg/day × 5 days
Cefotaxime	1 g q8h × 10-14 days
Ceftriaxone	1-2 g qd × 10-14 days
Other	
Ceftazidime	1 g q12h × 10-14 days
Ertapenem	1g qd × 10-14 days
Meropenem	500 mg q6h × 10-14 days
Piperacillin-tazobactam	3-375 g q6h × 10-14 days
Doripenem	500 mg q8h × 10-14 days
Amikacin	15 mg/kg/day × 10-14 days
Trimethoprim-sulfamethoxazole	160/800 mg q12h × 14 days
ORAL	
First-Line Therapy	
Ciprofloxacin	500 mg q12h × 7 days
Levofloxacin	250-500 mg/day × 5-7 days
Other	
Amoxicillin-clavulanate	500 mg (amoxicillin dose) q8h × 14 days
Cefuroxime axetil	500 mg q12h × 14 days
Cefixime	400 mg/day × 14 days
Ceftibuten	400 mg/day × 14 days
Cefepime	2 g q12h × 14 days

*Doses given are for adults with normal renal function. The need to reduce dosages because of renal impairment should always be considered.

high antimicrobial concentrations are achieved in the renal parenchyma and urine.

Cystitis

Table 284-6 lists recommended choices for the antimicrobial treatment of cystitis.[9] The shortest effective treatment duration for the antimicrobial should be used. Trimethoprim, trimethoprim-sulfamethoxazole, fosfomycin, pivmecillinam, and nitrofurantoin are recommended first-line treatments[A1] because they are effective with relatively short courses, and because there is limited impact on normal flora, resistance emergence is not a concern. Trimethoprim or trimethoprim-sulfamethoxazole should be selected for initial empirical therapy only if the local prevalence of resistance to these agents in community-acquired E. coli infections is less than 20%. Fluoroquinolones are not recommended for first-line therapy as widespread use may lead to the emergence of resistance. β-Lactam antimicrobials are about 10% less effective than the first-line agents.[A2] Patients with recurrent cystitis can be effectively managed with a strategy of early self-treatment. Early empirical treatment usually leads to prompt improvement of symptoms. Nitrofurantoin and oral cephalosporins are preferred therapy for pregnant women as these are safe for the fetus.[A3]

Pyelonephritis

For antimicrobial treatment of pyelonephritis, the initial decision is whether parenteral treatment is needed or whether oral treatment alone will suffice. Table 284-7 lists antimicrobials suitable for the treatment of pyelonephritis. After initial treatment with a parenteral drug, a transition to oral treatment is normally possible at 24 to 48 hours if the patient has clinically improved. The recommended treatment time is 7 to 14 days.[A4]

Complicated Urinary Infection

The antimicrobial regimen selected for treatment of complicated UTI is individualized on the basis of the site of infection, severity of the manifestations, new or presumed infecting organism and susceptibility, tolerance of the patient, and nature of the underlying abnormalities.[10] When symptoms are mild, it is preferable to delay initiation of antimicrobial therapy until results of urine culture are available to allow optimal antimicrobial selection. Empirical antimicrobial therapy should be initiated when severe symptoms are present. Oral or parenteral therapy is selected on the basis of the presentation and the likelihood of resistant organisms. Previous urine culture results from the patient and recent history of antimicrobial exposure are helpful to assess the likelihood of resistant organisms. Nitrofurantoin may be used for episodes of bladder infection but is not effective for renal infection and is contraindicated in individuals with renal failure. The empirical therapy selected should be reassessed after 48 to 72 hours, by which time the urine culture result should be available and the response to initial therapy can be assessed. If the organism

isolated from a pretherapy urine culture specimen is resistant to the empirical antimicrobial therapy initiated, the antimicrobial regimen should be modified to an agent to which the organism is susceptible, irrespective of the clinical response.[11] Antibiotic prophylaxis at the time of catheter removal can reduce the risk of subsequent symptomatic infection.[A5]

Asymptomatic Bacteriuria

Asymptomatic bacteriuria should be treated only in pregnant women[12] or when antimicrobials are given as perioperative prophylaxis before a urologic procedure with trauma to the genitourinary mucosa. For all other populations, including elderly women,[13] treatment of asymptomatic bacteriuria has not been associated with improved outcomes but is uniformly followed by reinfection with organisms of increasing antimicrobial resistance. For some populations, evidence suggests that asymptomatic bacteriuria may protect subjects from symptomatic UTI. Bacteriuria in patients with indwelling catheters should not be treated unless the patient has symptoms attributed to urinary infection. Administration of antimicrobials to catheterized patients with asymptomatic bacteriuria inevitably results in reinfection with more resistant organisms.

Urosepsis

The principles of management of urosepsis are similar to those for patients with severe sepsis from any site. Parenteral empirical antimicrobial treatment and supportive care should be initiated promptly. The antimicrobial selected should provide broad-spectrum coverage for potential uropathogens, including resistant bacteria. Antimicrobial therapy is reassessed when urine and blood culture results become available and the specific infecting organism and susceptibilities are identified.

Funguria

Funguria in catheterized patients should be treated only when there is a symptomatic UTI. Symptomatic infection is treated with fluconazole 400 mg

TABLE 284-8	PROPHYLACTIC REGIMENS TO PREVENT RECURRENT URINARY TRACT INFECTION IN WOMEN	
PREFERRED		**OTHER**
Long-term low dose		
Nitrofurantoin 50 mg od or 100 mg qd		Cephalexin 250-500 mg qd*
Trimethoprim-sulfamethoxazole, 40/200 mg qd or every other day		Norfloxacin 200 mg qd
		Ciprofloxacin 125 mg qd
Postcoital (single dose)		
Nitrofurantoin 50 or 100 mg*		Cephalexin 250 mg*
Trimethoprim-sulfamethoxazole 40/200 mg		Ciprofloxacin 125 mg
Trimethoprim 100 mg		Norfloxacin 200 mg

*Suitable for use in pregnancy.

once daily for 1 day, followed by 200 mg once daily for 7 to 14 days. If *Candida* sp resistant to fluconazole is isolated, amphotericin B deoxycholate is the recommended alternative therapy as other antifungals have limited renal excretion.

Follow-up

Patients do not require follow-up urine cultures unless symptomatic infection persists or recurs. When there is early (<30 days) symptomatic recurrence, the infecting organism should be re-evaluated to ensure that it was susceptible to the antimicrobial given.

PREVENTION

Premenopausal women with recurrent acute uncomplicated UTI should avoid spermicide use. For women with frequent recurrent acute uncomplicated UTI (more than two in 6 months or three in 12 months) presenting as either cystitis or pyelonephritis, prophylactic antimicrobial therapy is effective. This may be given as long-term low-dose prophylaxis or as postintercourse prophylaxis. Suggested regimens for prophylactic antimicrobial therapy are provided in Table 284-8. The use of cranberry tablets or juice does not reliably decrease the frequency of recurrent infection,[A6] and probiotics are not effective. For postmenopausal women, use of topical vaginal estrogens may decrease the frequency of infection.[A7] The use of systemic estrogen, however, is associated with an increased frequency of UTI. Prophylactic antimicrobial therapy is more effective than topical vaginal estrogen in these women.

Pregnant women should be screened for asymptomatic bacteriuria early in the pregnancy, usually at 12 or 16 weeks. If bacteriuria is present, these women should be treated and have subsequent follow-up culture specimens obtained monthly. If either asymptomatic or symptomatic recurrent infection occurs, prophylactic antimicrobial therapy with either cephalexin or nitrofurantoin should be continued through the duration of the pregnancy to decrease the risk for development of pyelonephritis in later pregnancy.

Prophylactic antimicrobial therapy has not been shown to be effective for patients with complicated UTI, including those with spinal cord injury or with chronic indwelling catheters. In these patients, the abnormality leading to impaired voiding means that bacteriuria is unavoidable, and antimicrobial therapy simply promotes bacteriuria with increasingly resistant organisms.

Infection control programs of health care facilities should include practices to prevent catheter-acquired UTI. Evidence-based guidelines provide clear recommendations for program components, including ongoing surveillance.[14] The most important intervention is to avoid the use of an indwelling catheter wherever possible and, when there are clear indications for catheter use, to limit the duration to as short a time as possible. The ultimate solution to the problem of catheter-acquired UTI, however, will require development of biofilm-resistant materials.[15]

PROGNOSIS

The prognosis of uncomplicated cystitis and pyelonephritis is good. Women with acute uncomplicated cystitis who do not receive antimicrobial therapy will usually have resolution of symptoms by 1 to 2 weeks, and about half will be culture negative by 6 weeks. Women with even very frequent recurrent acute uncomplicated UTI[16] experience no long-term adverse outcomes, such as renal impairment or hypertension. A small proportion of women with severe presentations of acute nonobstructive pyelonephritis develop renal

scars, but these are not associated with impaired renal function. Patients with frequent recurrent complicated UTI may experience substantial morbidity with recurrent infections, but poor long-term medical outcomes are usually determined by the underlying abnormality rather than by infection. Patients with urosepsis have a fatality rate of about 10%. Factors increasing the risk of death are advanced age and significant underlying diseases as well as inadequate initial antimicrobial treatment.

Grade A References

A1. Grigoryan L, Trautner BW, Gupta K. Diagnosis and management of urinary tract infections in the outpatient setting: a review. *JAMA.* 2014;312:1677-1684.
A2. Hooton TM, Roberts PL, Stapleton AE. Cefpodoxime vs ciprofloxacin for short course treatment of acute uncomplicated cystitis. *JAMA.* 2012;307:583-589.
A3. Vazquez JC, Abalos E. Treatments for symptomatic urinary tract infections during pregnancy. *Cochrane Database Syst Rev.* 2011;1:CD002256.
A4. Sandberg T, Skoog G, Hermansson AB, et al. Ciprofloxacin for 7 days versus 14 days in women with acute pyelonephritis: a randomised, open-label and double-blind, placebo-controlled, non-inferiority trial. *Lancet.* 2012;380:484-490.
A5. Marschall J, Carpenter CR, Fowler S, et al. Antibiotic prophylaxis for urinary tract infections after removal of urinary catheter: meta-analysis. *BMJ.* 2013;346:f3147.
A6. Jepson R, Craig J, Williams G. Cranberry products and prevention of urinary tract infections. *JAMA.* 2013;310:1395-1396.
A7. Beerepoot MA, Geerlings SE, van Haarst EP, et al. Nonantibiotic prophylaxis for recurrent urinary tract infections: a systematic review and meta-analysis of randomized controlled trials. *J Urol.* 2013;190:1981-1989.

GENERAL REFERENCES

For the General References and other additional features, please visit Expert Consult at https://expertconsult.inkling.com.

285

APPROACH TO THE PATIENT WITH A SEXUALLY TRANSMITTED INFECTION

HEIDI SWYGARD AND MYRON S. COHEN

SEXUALLY TRANSMITTED INFECTIONS

DEFINITION

Sexually transmitted infections (STIs) include a wide variety of organisms that are transmitted through intimate contact involving skin or mucosal surfaces of the oropharynx, vagina, penis, and rectum. STIs can generally be divided into five broad categories (syndromes): urethritis, genital ulcers, epithelial cell disorders, female vaginal discharge, and ectoparasites (Table 285-1).

ETIOLOGY

The interaction between the host and the STI pathogen plays a critical role, and characteristic tissue changes offer exceptionally strong clues about etiology. Several STI pathogens cause local inflammation only (*Neisseria gonorrhoeae, Chlamydia trachomatis, Trichomonas vaginalis*), with the potential for local tissue invasion (*N. gonorrhoeae, C. trachomatis*) or systemic dissemination (*N. gonorrhoeae*). Some STI pathogens cause tissue ulceration (*Treponema pallidum, Haemophilus ducreyi*, herpes simplex viruses 1 and 2). Human papillomaviruses (HPVs) cause epithelial cell changes and predispose to neoplasm. Several STI pathogens (human immunodeficiency virus [HIV], hepatitis B and C viruses, cytomegalovirus) routinely use the genital tract for access without causing any local changes.

EPIDEMIOLOGY

STIs are among the most common infections worldwide, and most are never reported. Each year there are almost 10 million new STIs reported among persons aged 15 to 24 years in the United States alone; many infections are subclinical and may escape detection, suggesting that these numbers are an underestimate. Of great concern, STIs are generally transmissible whether they are symptomatic or asymptomatic.

TABLE 285-1	SYNDROMES OF SEXUALLY TRANSMITTED DISEASES
SYNDROME	**ORGANISM**
URETHRITIS	
Gonococcal	*Neisseria gonorrhoeae*
Nongonococcal	*Chlamydia trachomatis*
	Trichomonas vaginalis
	Mycoplasma genitalium
	Ureaplasma urealyticum
	Herpes simplex (primary infection)
GENITAL ULCERS	
Syphilis	*Treponema pallidum*
Genital herpes	Herpes simplex
Chancroid	*Haemophilus ducreyi*
EPITHELIAL CELL INFECTIONS	
Genital warts	Human papillomavirus
Molluscum	Molluscum contagiosum
Cervical neoplasia	Human papillomavirus types 16 and 18
FEMALE GENITAL DISCHARGE	
Cervicitis	*Neisseria gonorrhoeae*
	Chlamydia trachomatis
	Trichomonas vaginalis
	Herpes simplex
Pelvic inflammatory disease	*Neisseria gonorrhoeae*
	Chlamydia trachomatis
Vaginitis	*Trichomonas vaginalis*
	Candida albicans
Bacterial vaginosis	*Gardnerella vaginalis*, anaerobes
ECTOPARASITES	
Pubic lice	*Phthirus pubis*
Scabies	*Sarcoptes scabiei*

Chlamydia, gonorrhea, and syphilis are reportable to the U.S. Centers for Disease Control and Prevention. The incidence of primary and secondary syphilis declined in the 1990s, but since 2000, rates have been increasing among men (8.2 cases per 100,000 in 2011, a 3.8% increase compared with 2010) and men aged 20 to 29 years (23.4 cases per 100,000). Rates declined 9.1% in women (from 1.1 cases per 100,000 to 1.0 case per 100,000). Men who have sex with men accounted for 72% of all cases of primary and secondary syphilis reported in 2011. Following a nadir of 98.1 cases per 100,000 in 2009 (since reporting for gonorrhea began), gonorrhea rates increased slightly (104.2 cases per 100,000 in 2011). Rates are highest among the 15- to 24-year age group for both sexes.

For other STIs, seroprevalence and national surveys provide data that suggest a high burden of viral STIs. From the 2005 to 2008 National Health and Nutrition Examination Survey (NHANES), herpes simplex virus 2 (HSV-2) was shown to affect 16.2% of the survey sample for those aged 14 to 49 years; of 20- to 49-year-old participants seropositive for HSV-2, only 18.9% had been previously diagnosed. Data from NHANES collected between 2001 and 2004 show an overall prevalence of 3.1% for women, with the highest percentage among African American women (13.3%).

The spread of STIs depends on the organism and the host, the length of time an infected person remains contagious, and the number of people exposed. These parameters have been reduced to the following formula:

$$R_o = B \times D \times C$$

where R_o is the basic reproductive rate of an infection, or the mean number of secondary cases a typical single infected person will cause in a population; B is the efficiency of transmission; D is the duration of infectiousness; and C is the number of sexual partners.

PATHOBIOLOGY

The STI pathogens depend entirely on human-human transmission, although *T. vaginalis* may have some inanimate sources. The efficiency of transmission reflects the infectiousness of the index case (which depends on the concentration and phenotype of the organism in the genital tract) and the susceptibility of the sexual partner (which reflects the resistance of the host, whether

it is hereditary, acquired, or innate). Because immunity to STIs is rare, reinfections are common, and vaccine development has been difficult; the only STI vaccines available target hepatitis B and HPV.

STIs produce syndromes precisely because each pathogen has a proclivity for one or more tissues and (when symptomatic) can evoke a predictable inflammatory response. For example, gonococci that infect the male urethra generally produce an intense neutrophil response that leads to a purulent discharge and pain with urination, whereas *C. trachomatis* is less likely to produce such a response in the same tissue and is more likely to produce a mild, watery discharge or no symptoms at all.

STIs serve as markers for sexual risk-taking behavior, so coinfections are common. The detection of an STI should lead to a variety of other (seemingly unrelated) tests. STI pathogens move together: gonorrhea and chlamydia cause urethritis; genital ulcers greatly increase the probability of HIV acquisition.

DIAGNOSIS AND TREATMENT

Syndromic Strategies

For a variety of common STI syndromes, treatment of the index case (based on signs and symptoms) is empirical, as is treatment of sexual partners. This approach reflects the facts that the diagnostic accuracy of some tests is imperfect, coinfection demands concomitant therapy that overrides the search for individual pathogens, and patients who are not treated immediately may not return for therapy. Genital ulcer disease and urethral discharge have high sensitivity and specificity compared with laboratory diagnosis, and empirical therapy is so successful that follow-up care ("proof of cure") is usually unnecessary. However, the vaginal discharge syndrome is far less sensitive or specific in terms of true STI diagnosis.[1] In a study of South African women, almost 90% with a laboratory-confirmed STI diagnosis had no clinical symptoms and would therefore not have been treated.[2]

The syndromic approach is particularly critical in resource-constrained countries or in areas of the United States where laboratory tests are not available or their cost is prohibitive. In the United States, concomitant microbiologic diagnosis is preferred because it (1) confirms the choice of empirical therapy or redirects subsequent care; (2) permits the detection and monitoring of resistance to treatment; and (3) enables specific diagnoses to be reported to public health authorities, which is required by state law for many STIs. However, even when laboratory tests are ordered, the most appropriate agents should be provided empirically at the point of care to resolve infection and to reduce onward transmission.

Relationship of STIs to HIV Infection

Diagnosis of an STI demonstrates increased sexual risk-taking behavior and inconsistent condom use and serves as a marker for potential HIV infection. Any patient undergoing evaluation or treatment for an STI should be tested for HIV infection. Early diagnosis of HIV infection has major personal and public health benefits.

Nevertheless, STIs also contribute to HIV acquisition and hamper efforts at optimal prevention of HIV transmission. Genital ulcers increase HIV replication in the infected person. Genital ulcers disrupt the epithelium and allow the entry of HIV; inflammation caused by ulceration recruits macrophages and lymphocytes, increasing the number of target cells for HIV.

SYNDROMES

Urethritis

Urethritis is characterized by some combination of urethral discharge and dysuria, but prostatitis can cause similar complaints. Urethritis is caused by a limited group of pathogens (see Table 285-1) that may be difficult to visualize microscopically or to grow in culture. Accordingly, empirical therapy is provided to treat a spectrum of potentially causative organisms.

Urethritis is diagnosed when one or more of the following are demonstrated: (1) mucopurulent or purulent urethral discharge, (2) Gram stain of urethral secretions demonstrating five or more leukocytes per oil immersion microscopic field, (3) positive leukocyte esterase test result on first-void urine, or (4) microscopic examination of first-void urine demonstrating 10 or more leukocytes per high-power field. If no discharge can be expressed from the urethral meatus, a calcium alginate swab can be inserted 5 mm into the urethra; the material collected is transferred to a slide by rolling the swab along the glass.

A Gram stain of urethral discharge is a simple and rapid diagnostic test to document both urethritis and gonococcal infection (Chapter 299),

TABLE 285-2 SYNDROMIC TREATMENT OF URETHRITIS

GONOCOCCAL*

Recommended

Ceftriaxone 250 mg injected intramuscularly once, *and*
Azithromycin 1 g orally (single dose)

NONGONOCOCCAL

Recommended

Azithromycin 1 g orally (single dose), *or*
Doxycycline 100 mg orally twice daily for 7 days

Alternative

Erythromycin base 500 mg orally four times daily for 7 days, *or*
Erythromycin ethylsuccinate 800 mg orally four times daily for 7 days, *or*
Ofloxacin 300 mg orally twice daily for 7 days, *or*
Levofloxacin 500 mg orally once a day for 7 days

*Uncomplicated anorectal and genital disease.

characterized by the detection of leukocytes containing intracellular gram-negative diplococci. Confirmation of gonococcal urethritis does not rule out concomitant infection with *Chlamydia* or *Mycoplasma*. As culture and Gram stain have become less popular or less available, nucleic acid amplification tests that are highly sensitive and specific for the detection of organisms have been used routinely. Nucleic acid amplification tests for gonorrhea, *Chlamydia*, and *Trichomonas* can be applied to first-void urine samples (the meatus is intentionally not cleaned so that the urine is contaminated with these organisms) or urethral swab material. Specific diagnosis may enhance the management of sexual partners, and the results from such tests should be reported to the health department. However, in practice, patients and (in most cases) sexual partners must be treated before the results of these tests are available.

Treatment for urethritis should be initiated as soon as possible after the clinical diagnosis and should be directly observed if feasible (Table 285-2). *N. gonorrhoeae* (Chapter 299) has become resistant to many antimicrobials, including quinolones and oral cephalosporins, which are no longer recommended. Thus, the choice of optimal therapies is limited. Dual therapy with azithromycin and ceftriaxone increases the cure rate of uncomplicated urogenital, anorectal, and pharyngeal gonorrhea. [A1][A2] Azithromycin can also be expected to cure most cases of nongonococcal urethritis (NGU), including those caused by *Mycoplasma genitalium*, an increasingly recognized cause of NGU. Some studies suggest that doxycycline is more effective than azithromycin for NGU, but a longer course of treatment dependent on the patient's adherence must also be considered. Currently, there is no commercially available diagnostic test for *M. genitalium*, which complicates the treatment question. In some settings in which *M. genitalium* is a consideration, persistent or recurrent NGU should be treated with moxifloxacin for 7 to 10 days.[3] *T. vaginalis*, which is susceptible to metronidazole or tinidazole, also causes urethritis and should be considered in the face of NGU treatment failure.

Women with urethritis present with some combination of dysuria and pyuria, which must be differentiated from bacterial cystitis. Because treatment for urinary tract pathogens may also resolve sexually transmitted urethritis, the clinician treating a presumed bladder infection should consider an STI as well.

Genital Ulcers

In the United States, HSV-1 and HSV-2 (Chapter 374) and *T. pallidum* are responsible for virtually all the ulcers encountered, and HSV-1 and HSV-2 are by far the most common cause.

LYMPHOGRANULOMA VENEREUM

Lymphogranuloma venereum, caused by a serovar of *C. trachomatis* (Chapter 318), is characterized by local lymph node suppuration, ulceration and subsequent fibrosis, fistula formation, and distal edema. Lymphogranuloma venereum has increasingly been emerging as a concern in HIV-infected men who have sex with men, particularly in Europe.

GENITAL HERPES

Genital herpes usually develops after an incubation period of less than 21 days and arises as clustered vesicles on an erythematous base. The vesicles become pustular and then rupture to form shallow, painful ulcers, which may coalesce. The ulcers heal by crusting over, and the process is usually

completed 2 to 3 weeks after the initial lesions. Recurrences proceed through the same stages but generally last only about 5 to 7 days. The first (incident) episode of HSV-2 infection may be accompanied by systemic signs and symptoms including fever and headache, the latter reflecting the spread of HSV to the central nervous system. HSV-2 is the putative cause of Mollaret's recurrent meningitis. It may appear after a primary genital infection or as reactivation. It may also occur in the absence of genital lesions or a known diagnosis of HSV-2 infection.

About 20% of infected individuals manifest the classic genital presentation, 60% have mild and atypical signs and symptoms, and at least 20% are completely asymptomatic. Individuals who have acquired HSV-2 shed the virus approximately 3 to 4% of the time (even while asymptomatic), posing an ongoing risk to sexual partners.

SYPHILIS

The ulcerative lesion of syphilis (Chapter 319)—the chancre—is indurated and painless, and in many cases it escapes detection. Dark-field examination of scrapings suspended in saline from a genital ulcer may reveal motile spirochetes, and this finding is diagnostic. Secondary syphilis results when the spirochetes spread systemically, leading to a characteristic rash, alopecia, oral mucous patches, or condyloma latum. These skin manifestations should prompt testing for syphilis. The serologic screening test of choice for syphilis is based on the formation of antibodies to cardiolipin, a constituent of the spirochetal cell wall (e.g., rapid plasma reagin test, Venereal Disease Research Laboratory [VDRL] test, toluidine red unheated serum test [TRUST]). Confirmatory testing requires the search for an antitreponemal antibody (e.g., microhemagglutination assay–*T. pallidum*, fluorescent treponema antibody test). The anticardiolipin test provides a titer that must be used to monitor the response to treatment.

Some larger commercial laboratories have reversed the order of testing, using an antitreponemal test followed by an anticardiolipin test, which allows automation and may be cost-effective in areas of low endemicity. This represents a change in testing and interpretation and must be done with caution[4] because such an approach cannot immediately separate old, treated infections from new infections (Fig. 285-1).

Later stages of syphilis may be identified only serologically or on pathologic specimens. Late latent syphilis and syphilis of unknown duration are managed similarly. Neurosyphilis can occur at any stage of infection and should be suspected in any patient with a positive serologic test result who also has findings suggestive of nervous system involvement, including ocular and vestibular symptoms.

Worldwide, syphilis infection has been detected in a substantial number of people with recognized or unrecognized HIV infection, especially men who have sex with men. Accordingly, the diagnosis of syphilis requires HIV testing.

CHANCROID

Chancroid (Chapter 301), infection with *H. ducreyi*, produces painful, ragged ulcers and tender inguinal lymphadenopathy, which may be fluctuant. Unlike the lesions of HSV infection, these genital ulcers are likely to vary in size.

Epithelial Cell Infections

HUMAN PAPILLOMAVIRUS

Sexually transmitted HPV infection (Chapter 373) is generally transient and asymptomatic, but some patients develop visible genital warts. These warts are painless, soft, moist, pink or flesh-colored swellings that vary in shape and can be raised or flat, single or multiple, small or large, and sometimes cauliflower shaped. Warts occur in the vulva, vagina, and anus; on the cervix; and on the penis, scrotum, groin, or thigh. Genital warts are diagnosed by visual inspection. Treatment is primarily with topical agents but is generally not curative.

Two oncogenic HPV genotypes (16 and 18) are responsible for at least 85% of all cervical neoplasia, and HPV types 6 and 11 are responsible for most cases of genital warts. HPV vaccines are available that target these genotypes. Papanicolaou smears are recommended for sexually active women beginning at the age of 21 years, regardless of risk factor or age at coitarche; HPV testing, however, is not recommended for women younger than 30 years. Frequency of rescreening is influenced by age, previous screening results, and HPV results. An increasing incidence of oral HPV is associated with head and neck squamous cell carcinomas, with more than 70% of U.S. cases demonstrating detectable HPV. Male gender, smoking, and HIV-positive status are significantly associated with prevalent oral HPV.[5]

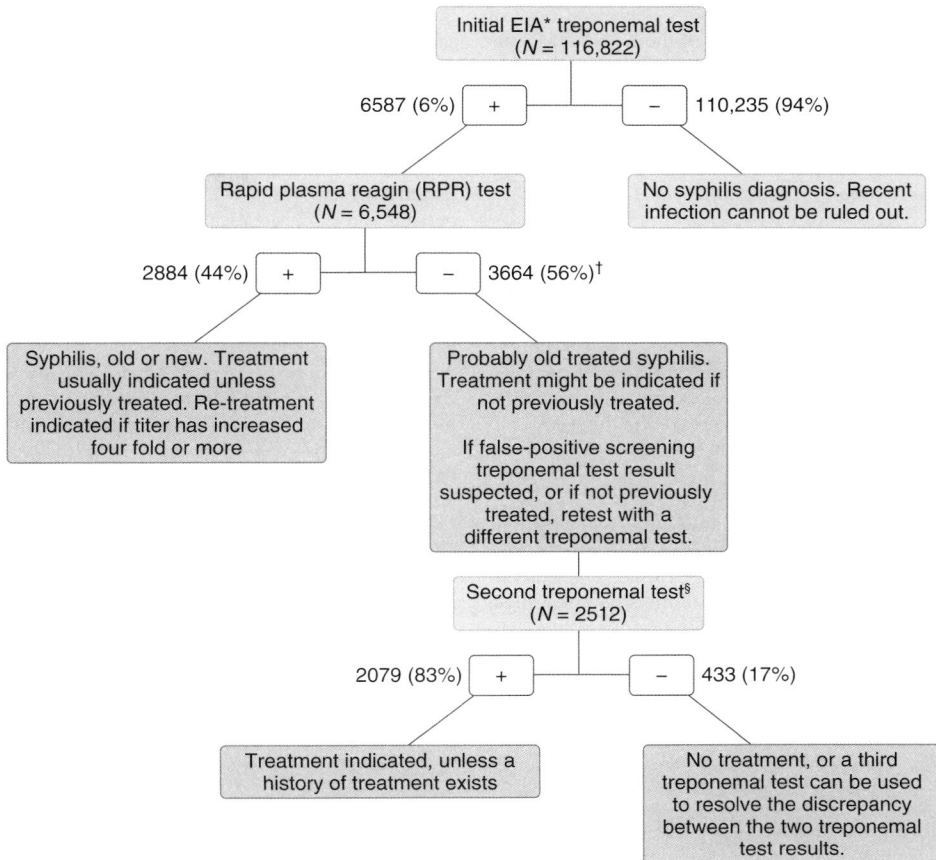

FIGURE 285-1. Syphilis testing algorithms using treponemal tests for initial screening and recommendations from the Centers for Disease Control and Prevention, 2008. *Enzyme immunoassay. †Reactive with EIA treponemal test but nonreactive with RPR test. §Using *Treponema pallidum* particle agglutination or fluorescent treponemal antibody tests. (Redrawn from the Centers for Disease Control and Prevention. Syphilis testing algorithms using treponemal tests for initial screening—four laboratories, New York City, 2005-2006. *MMWR Morb Mortal Wkly Rep.* 2008;57:872-875.)

Two HPV vaccines are currently approved by the Food and Drug Administration for use in males and females: a quadrivalent vaccine (protecting against HPV types 6, 11, 16, and 18), and a bivalent vaccine (protecting against HPV types 16 and 18). The quadrivalent vaccine protects against anal precancers and may influence future vaccine recommendations.

Female Genital Discharge

Infections of the female genitourinary tract produce several syndromes with overlapping symptoms (dysuria, vaginal discharge, vulvar irritation), the cause of which can usually be established with a careful history, examination, and laboratory tests. The initial approach depends on the primary anatomic site of infection—urinary tract, endocervix, or vagina. The columnar epithelium of the endocervix is susceptible to infection with *N. gonorrhoeae*, *C. trachomatis*, and *T. vaginalis*, and the vagina is susceptible to infection with *Candida albicans*, *T. vaginalis*, and the syndrome of bacterial vaginosis. The cervix may appear completely normal in women with cervical infection, but mucopurulence at the cervical os or mucosal friability suggests infection. Vaginitis is associated with a visible discharge, and the characteristics of the vaginal fluid offer diagnostic clues.

Female genital discharge is a condition in which syndromic management strategies generally lack sensitivity and specificity. In women with vaginal discharge, microscopic examination of a wet mount preparation may enhance the effectiveness of syndromic treatment, but interpretation of results is difficult and cannot exclude infection with several pathogens concurrently.

BACTERIAL VAGINOSIS

Bacterial vaginosis (BV) is the most common cause of vaginal discharge in the United States. Women with BV are often minimally symptomatic but may note mild vaginal discharge and vaginal odor (which is often increased after coitus). The normal vaginal flora contains hydrogen peroxide–producing lactobacilli such as *Lactobacillus crispatus* and *Lactobacillus jensenii*, which

probably help "defend" the vagina against a number of pathogens (an example of innate immunity). *Lactobacillus acidophilus* is rarely found in the normal vagina, which explains the failure of yogurt to serve as a remedy or a preventive. BV begins with the unexplained disappearance of the normal vaginal flora and its replacement with *Gardnerella vaginalis* and many species of anaerobic bacteria. The precise mechanism causing this shift in vaginal flora is poorly understood. Most recently, previously unrecognized anaerobic bacterial species (BV-associated bacteria) have been described as potentially causative. In a study of 220 women with BV, the vaginal milieu demonstrated great species diversity. African American women without BV at the time of sampling had higher numbers of BV-associated bacteria, which could contribute to an increased risk of BV.[6]

The discharge of BV is homogeneous and may contain bubbles. Vaginal pH is elevated above the normal 4.0 to 4.5. Adding 10% potassium hydroxide to the vaginal discharge on the microscope slide or to the discharge present in the extracted speculum elicits an amine-like, fishy odor, yielding a positive "whiff" test result because of the elaboration of amines from the anaerobic flora. Examination of vaginal material as a wet mount reveals the absence of bacilli and their replacement with clumps of coccobacilli. Some vaginal epithelial cells are coated with coccobacilli, which may obscure their edges (clue cells) or the normally clear appearance of the cytoplasm. Relatively few polymorphonuclear leukocytes are observed; large numbers of leukocytes in the wet mount of a woman with BV suggest a coincident infection, possibly trichomoniasis or bacterial cervicitis.

BV is not necessarily a benign change in flora. It is associated with an increased rate of upper tract infection (endometritis, salpingitis) and, on occasion, with complications of pregnancy, including premature rupture of the membranes and preterm delivery. However, treatment of asymptomatic women with BV who are not at high risk for preterm delivery appears to confer no benefit. Women with BV may have increased risk for the acquisition of HIV. Treatment is generally directed against the anaerobic flora and consists of metronidazole or clindamycin for 7 days. A single oral dose of metronidazole is not recommended for BV because of the high failure rate. The BV relapse rate is about 30%, and treatment of male sexual partners offers no benefit.

CANDIDIASIS

Vulvovaginal candidiasis (Chapter 338) is common and is seen most frequently in women taking antibiotics or using oral contraceptives when endogenous Candida species outgrow normal bacterial flora. Women usually complain of vulvar itching and discomfort and may or may not notice an accompanying discharge. The vagina generally maintains normal numbers of lactobacilli, so the vaginal pH is usually normal, which is helpful in discriminating between candidiasis and other vaginal infections. The labia and vaginal walls may be erythematous. Although classically described as "curdy," the discharge of candidiasis is frequently loose and is difficult to distinguish from other discharges. Vaginal material may be treated with 10% potassium hydroxide to destroy other cellular elements and to make the fungi easier to observe. Wet mount, however, has a sensitivity of only about 50%, and a woman with a classic clinical presentation should be treated even if fungal elements are not observed.

A wide range of topical antifungal medications are available (many without a prescription), and all these drugs are approximately equally effective, although the cure rate with some single-dose topical treatments appears to be lower than that with longer regimens. Fluconazole administered as a single oral dose of 150 mg is highly effective. Infection with yeasts other than C. albicans may require longer therapy. Recurrent vulvovaginal candidiasis is a problem for many women, and optimal management has not been defined. Recurrent infection should lead the clinician to consider underlying diabetes mellitus or HIV infection. Treatment of sexual partners of women with candidiasis confers no benefit.

TRICHOMONIASIS

Women with T. vaginalis infection complain of a purulent discharge and vulvar irritation. The vaginal walls are red, and the vagina may contain excessive yellow or green discharge displaying large bubbles. The ectocervix may also be inflamed or have punctate microhemorrhages, causing the pathognomonic "strawberry cervix" (colpitis macularis). Vaginal pH is elevated, but the whiff test result is generally negative. Wet mount reveals large numbers of polymorphonuclear leukocytes as well as motile protozoa about the same size as the leukocytes, with visible flagella; motile organisms may be recognized in about two thirds of cases. Therapy for trichomoniasis requires metronidazole or tinidazole, but resistant organisms are encountered with increasing frequency.

CERVICITIS

The diagnosis of cervicitis is suggested by tenderness on bimanual examination, visible inspection revealing inflammation, or discharge. The specific diagnosis can be made only by detecting microorganisms from the cervix. N. gonorrhoeae and C. trachomatis have tropism for cervical tissue, whereas other pathogens (including HIV) can apparently infect the vaginal tissues as well.

PELVIC INFLAMMATORY DISEASE

Each year, more than 800,000 women develop pelvic inflammatory disease (PID) in the United States. The majority of PID cases involve N. gonorrhoeae, C. trachomatis, and Mycoplasma (especially M. genitalium); however, one third of PID cases are due to other anaerobic and aerobic bacteria that ascend from the cervix into the uterine cavity, producing endometritis, and then extend to the fallopian tubes, causing salpingitis. Treatment should include therapy directed at anaerobes.[A3] Chlamydial salpingitis may be mild, and patients may not seek medical attention. Some intrauterine devices have been associated with an increased risk of salpingitis, and some data suggest that vaginal douching is a predisposing factor.

Adnexal tenderness on bimanual examination leads to the clinical diagnosis of salpingitis. Cervical tenderness, fever, leukocytosis, and an elevated sedimentation rate are sometimes observed. The clinical diagnosis is confirmed laparoscopically in only about 70% of cases, suggesting considerable error in diagnosis. Vaginal ultrasonography or computed tomography is often helpful in defining the cause of pelvic pain syndromes. Pregnant women with evidence of salpingitis should be hospitalized. Other indications for hospitalization include nonresponse to or intolerance of an oral regimen, presence of a tubo-ovarian abscess, and inability to rule out a surgical emergency, such as appendicitis.[7] Infertility complicates approximately 15% of initial attacks of salpingitis and about 75% of women who suffer three or more attacks.

Ectopic pregnancy, infertility, and tubo-ovarian abscess are complications of salpingitis.

● PREVENTION

STIs are preventable. The Centers for Disease Control and Prevention recommends five strategies as the foundation for an effective prevention program: (1) education and counseling of persons at risk to motivate the adoption of safer sexual behavior; (2) identification of asymptomatic infected persons and symptomatic persons unlikely to seek diagnostic and treatment services; (3) rapid and effective diagnosis and treatment of infected persons; (4) evaluation, treatment, and counseling of exposed sexual partners; and (5) preexposure vaccination of persons at risk for vaccine-preventable STIs.

Behavioral Interventions

Abstaining from sexual intercourse or being in a long-term, mutually monogamous relationship with an uninfected partner is the most reliable way to prevent STIs. Abstinence should be recommended during treatment for an STI and for anyone who wants to avoid STIs and unintended pregnancy. Both partners should be tested for STIs, including HIV infection, before initiating sexual intercourse.

Counseling is essential for people with STIs. Interactive counseling, video presentations, peer groups, and other formats that emphasize correct condom use have reduced the incidence of subsequent infections among STI clinic patients and adolescents. Randomized controlled trials demonstrate that structured risk reduction counseling can reduce the incidence of infections by 25 to 40% among some STI clinic populations.[A4] HIV testing is preceded by a counseling session, but there is little evidence of a preventive benefit from this communication.

Barrier Methods

When used consistently and correctly, male latex condoms are effective in preventing the sexual transmission of HIV infection and can reduce the risk of other STIs (gonorrhea, chlamydia, and trichomoniasis). However, because condoms do not cover all exposed areas, they are likely to be more effective in preventing infections transmitted by fluids from mucosal surfaces (e.g., gonorrhea, chlamydia, trichomoniasis, HIV infection) than in preventing those transmitted by skin-to-skin contact (e.g., HSV, HPV, syphilis, chancroid). Male condom failure usually results from inconsistent or incorrect use rather than from condom breakage. Non-latex condoms (those made of polyurethane or other synthetic material) can be used by persons with latex allergy. There is less information available on the effect of female condoms on the incidence of STIs. Although cervical caps and diaphragms cover the cervix, there is little evidence that they can prevent STIs or HIV infection.

Male Circumcision

Male circumcision reduces mucosal tissue susceptible to HIV and STI pathogens. Circumcision of adult men reduces the acquisition of HIV by more than 70% for up to 5 years after circumcision.[A5] Circumcision also appears to reduce the acquisition of other viral STI pathogens, including HSV-2 and HPV.

Partner Services

The detection of an STI demands consideration of the infected person's sexual partners, who may have undetected and serious disease. In addition, in the absence of partner treatment, reinfection of the index case can be expected. The probability that a sexual partner is also infected reflects the efficiency of transmission of the STI pathogen, as described earlier. For example, most men with gonococcal urethritis infect their partners, whereas only about half of patients with HIV infection have infected their partners at the time of outreach; partners who differ in terms of STI or HIV infection status are referred to as discordant.

Sexual partners can be notified directly by the infected person or by health care workers, sometimes through proactive contact tracing. In general, dependence on the infected person is a less reliable way to get partners treated. However, in many states it is legal to pursue expedited care by providing the infected patient with the appropriate treatment for his or her partners. Expedited partner care appears to work well for the treatment of gonorrhea and chlamydia infections.[A6]

Preexposure Interventions

Preexposure vaccination is the most effective method for preventing the transmission of certain STIs. For example, because hepatitis B virus is frequently transmitted sexually, hepatitis B vaccination is recommended for all unvaccinated persons being evaluated for an STI. In addition, hepatitis A vaccine is recommended for men who have sex with men and for drug users (both injection and noninjection). Vaccines for HPV are now available for both females and males (Chapter 373). The HPV vaccines now have more than 5 years of follow-up and demonstrate continued high rates of protection in women. HPV vaccination for males may reduce acquisition of genital warts and is protective against anal precancerous lesions, leading to a "permissive" vaccine recommendation for boys aged 9 to 26 years from the Advisory Committee on Immunization Practices.

Several studies have evaluated the effectiveness of antiretroviral agents for HIV preexposure prophylaxis. Results have indicated HIV prevention but only in the setting of high-level (>85%) medication adherence. Furthermore, because the only currently Food and Drug Administration–approved antiretroviral for HIV prevention is also a drug combination used for therapy, regular HIV screening is necessary to prevent the development of resistance should the patient become infected.[8] Topical HIV prevention by vaginal microbicides has been only partially successful, in large part because of poor adherence. Long-acting injectable drugs, vaginal rings, and coformulated options (i.e., contraceptive and antiretroviral agents) are under evaluation.

Postexposure Prophylaxis
After consensual or nonconsensual sexual exposure, a variety of STIs can be prevented with empirical antibiotics. Prevention of HIV infection appears to require several antiretroviral agents that must be used in combination for 28 days.

Contraception
All methods of birth control can influence the acquisition and outcome of an STI. In addition, pregnancy itself (in the absence of effective birth control) affects STI acquisition and the health of the pregnancy and the neonate. Accordingly, STI management demands consideration of the reproductive health of both partners as well as family planning issues. A systematic review suggested that there was no increased risk of HIV infection in oral contraceptive users; however, the data for injectable hormonal contraceptives were more difficult to interpret.[9] Women using injectable hormonal birth control should be cautioned about consistent condom use for STI prevention until these relationships are better clarified.

● TOWARD A COMPREHENSIVE MANAGEMENT STRATEGY
Although most STIs are self-limited and readily treated, the comprehensive and proper management of the patient with an STI requires considerable skill.[10] First, the correct syndrome must be recognized, and a decision about specific diagnostic tests must be made. Second, empirical therapy must be provided and must be sufficiently broad to promise cure or reduced duration of illness. Third, the clinician is obligated to search for other STIs of public health or personal significance. Fourth, the clinician must deal with the patient's sexual partners, through either referral or expedited partner therapy. Fifth, the patient needs counseling and adjunctive preventive measures, where appropriate. Such measures might include vaccination for hepatitis B or HPV or antibiotics to prevent another STI, such as incubating syphilis or HIV infection.

Grade A References

A1. Centers for Disease Control and Prevention (CDC). Update to CDC's sexually transmitted diseases treatment guidelines, 2010: oral cephalosporins no longer a recommended treatment for gonococcal infections. *MMWR Morb Mortal Wkly Rep.* 2012;61:590-594.
A2. Creighton S. Gonorrhoea. *Clin Evid (Online).* 2014;2014.
A3. Ross JD. Pelvic inflammatory disease. *Clin Evid (Online).* 2013;2013.
A4. Westhoff CL, Jones HE. Guiahi M. Do new guidelines and technology make the routine pelvic examination obsolete? *J Womens Health (Larchmt).* 2011;20:5-10.
A5. Gray R, Kigozi G, Kong X, et al. The effectiveness of male circumcision for HIV prevention and effects on risk behaviors in a posttrial follow-up study. *AIDS.* 2012;26:609-615.
A6. Ferreira A, Young T, Mathews C, et al. Strategies for partner notification for sexually transmitted infections, including HIV. *Cochrane Database Syst Rev.* 2013;10:CD002843.

GENERAL REFERENCES
For the General References and other additional features, please visit Expert Consult at https://expertconsult.inkling.com.

286

APPROACH TO THE PATIENT BEFORE AND AFTER TRAVEL

DAVID O. FREEDMAN

Prevention strategies and medical interventions for the traveler need to be individualized according to a risk assessment that considers both the itinerary and factors that are dependent on the prospective traveler. A structured approach to patient interaction (Table 286-1) is the most efficient way to cover the necessary educational and preventive interventions. As many of these measures will be initiated only much later at the traveler's destination, clearly printed instructions in lay language are advisable. The worldwide epidemiology of travel-related diseases is constantly changing. Special needs travelers, such as those who are immunocompromised, are pregnant, or have significant underlying disease, should be referred to a specialized travel medicine clinic.

Globally, approximately 100 million people travel from industrialized to developing countries each year. Several recent analyses have provided much needed new data on the profiles of travel-related illness determined by destination of travel.[1] Depending on destination, 22 to 64% of travelers report some illness; most of these problems are mild, self-limited illnesses, such as diarrhea, respiratory infections, and skin disorders. Infectious diseases account for up to 10% of the morbidity during travel but only 1% of the deaths, with malaria being the most common disease.

● IMMUNIZATION
The choice of vaccines for an individual traveler is based on risk of exposure to vaccine-preventable diseases on the chosen itinerary, the severity of disease if it is acquired, and any risks presented by the vaccine itself. Travelers differ in their tolerance of risk. For the vaccine-preventable diseases, the monthly incidence for nonimmune travelers to developing countries is most significant for symptomatic hepatitis A at 0.03% per month overall; the risk of symptomatic hepatitis B is most significant for long-stay travelers at 0.25% per month. Enteric fever (typhoid and paratyphoid) has a risk of 0.03% per month on the Indian subcontinent and is 10 times lower in Africa and parts of Latin America. Risk of yellow fever may be as high as 0.1% per month of travel to an area with current epidemic transmission, but the risk varies greatly between destinations encompassed by the endemic area map. The risk of meningococcal meningitis, rabies, cholera, polio, measles, varicella, and Japanese encephalitis in travelers is not known but is thought to be small (<0.0001%).

Table 286-2 provides data on dosing, administration, need for boosters, and possible accelerated regimens for vaccines administered in the travel medicine setting. Details on vaccine composition, mechanism of action, use for routine adult and childhood primary vaccination, and adverse reactions can be found in Chapter 18. The following discussion focuses on indications for vaccines in the context of travel.

Verification and Update of Routine Immunizations
Because of the increased prevalence of many infections in the developing world, routine adult immunizations need to be current.[2] If no adult doses of tetanus/diphtheria/acellular pertussis (Tdap) have ever been given, a dose of Tdap should be given regardless of the time elapsed since the last tetanus/diphtheria vaccination. Persons born in the United States before 1957 or born anytime in the developing world are considered immune to measles. Other adult travelers should have received at least two doses of live measles–containing vaccine during their life unless a history of measles infection can be documented. Unvaccinated persons who have the accepted routine indications for influenza or pneumococcal vaccines (Chapter 18) should receive these during the pretravel consultation. Two doses of varicella vaccine spaced by at least 4 weeks should be considered for adult travelers without evidence of varicella immunity. Adults born before 1980 in the United States are considered immune.

Vaccines to Consider for All Developing World Travelers
A number of additional vaccines should be administered depending on the travel destinations.[3]

Hepatitis A
Hepatitis A vaccine is indicated for every nonimmune traveler to countries or areas with moderate to high risk of infection, which includes essentially

TABLE 286-1	THE PRETRAVEL CONSULTATION WITH A TRAVELER TO THE DEVELOPING WORLD—A STRUCTURED APPROACH

PERFORM RISK ASSESSMENT

The following must always be ascertained initially to determine appropriate preventive medical recommendations. Preprinted medical record forms may be used to record these.

Exact itinerary, including regions within each country to be visited
Dates of travel to assess risk of seasonal diseases
Age
Past vaccination history
Underlying illnesses
Current medications
Pregnancy status
Allergies
Purpose of trip
Risk exposures—blood, body fluids, adventure or extensive outdoor exposures
Urban versus rural travel
Type of accommodations
Level of aversion to risk
Financial limitations that may necessitate prioritization of interventions

ADMINISTER IMMUNIZATIONS

Administer routine vaccinations that are not up to date.
Administer indicated travel vaccines.
Provide to patient legally mandated Vaccine Information Statements from the Centers for Disease Control and Prevention (http://www.cdc.gov/vaccines/pubs/vis/).
Provide printed checklist to patient listing vaccines administered.
Record in the clinic record vaccines administered, lot number, and date.
Document vaccines offered to but declined by patient as well as nonrecommended vaccines administered at the patient's request.

PROVIDE MALARIA PREVENTION (IF INDICATED)

Determine whether malaria risk exists for the destination country. If yes:
Does the patient's itinerary within that country put him or her at risk? If yes:
Recommend malaria chemoprophylaxis. Several equally effective drugs of choice may be indicated. Ascertain which is best suited to the individual patient and itinerary.
Educate on personal protection against arthropods.

EDUCATE ON TRAVELER'S DIARRHEA

Recommend food and water precautions.
Prescribe and educate on standby therapy with a quinolone antibiotic or azithromycin and advise on use of loperamide and oral hydration if needed.

TEACH ESSENTIAL PREVENTIVE BEHAVIORS

Most travel-related health problems, including vaccine-preventable diseases, can be avoided through simple behaviors initiated by the traveler.
Educate on appropriate strategies in the following categories (some topics are not applicable to all destinations): blood-borne and sexually transmitted diseases, safety and crime avoidance, injury prevention, swimming safety, rabies, skin/wound care, tuberculosis, packing for healthy travel, obtaining health care abroad.

DISCUSS OTHER APPLICABLE HEATH ISSUES

Advise and prescribe for altitude illness, motion sickness, or jet leg.
Discuss prevention of specific travel-related infections that are of some risk to the traveler and have a possible preventive strategy not included in strategies above.
Discuss any minimal-risk conditions (e.g., hemorrhagic fevers) that are a frequent cause of patient anxiety.

everyone traveling outside the United States, Canada, Japan, Australia, New Zealand, Scandinavian countries, and developed countries in Europe. A single dose of hepatitis A vaccine given any time before travel provides adequate protection. Persons with a history of hepatitis or who previously lived in an endemic country for a prolonged period may benefit from prevaccination serum antibody testing.

Hepatitis B

Pretravel hepatitis B vaccination is indicated for all nonvaccinated travelers with standard indications, such as health care workers, and all longer-stay travelers who will be visiting or residing in high- or moderate-risk areas. Transmission by routes such as sexual contact, blood transfusions, contaminated medical equipment, body piercing, tattooing, acupuncture, and sharing of cooking and bathroom facilities is difficult to control or to predict in the context of travel. Vaccination is usually advocated for short-term travelers, especially younger travelers and those anticipating close contact with local populations, even if they have no specific risk factors. Adventure travelers

(accident prone), backpackers, and those with underlying medical conditions are more likely to require contact with the medical system. Accelerated and hyperaccelerated schedules (see Table 286-2) are used widely in practice and are approved in many countries. These are helpful in administering all three primary doses necessary for high assurance of protection in the frequent circumstance in which the traveler is leaving in a very short time and is at risk of hepatitis B exposure.

Combination Hepatitis A and Hepatitis B Vaccine

The combined hepatitis A and hepatitis B vaccine provides convenience for travelers with an overlap of indications for use of the individual vaccines. A less well known accelerated 3-week schedule (see Table 286-2) is approved by the Food and Drug Administration.

Typhoid

Typhoid vaccine is indicated for all travelers to the Indian subcontinent and considered for those traveling to other endemic areas under all but the most deluxe and protected of conditions. Risk increases with trip duration, lodging and eating with local residents, and extent of travel off the usual tourist itineraries. Current typhoid vaccines do not protect against *Salmonella paratyphi*, which is emerging in many areas.[4] Adherence to the oral vaccine regimen may be as low as 70%.

Influenza

Influenza is transmitted year-round in the tropics. Increasing data show that influenza may be the most common vaccine-preventable illness in travelers. An increased risk of influenza has been reported among cruise ship passengers. All travelers to destinations with current influenza virus circulation, not just those with the usual risk factors, should strongly consider influenza vaccination.[5]

Vaccines for Certain Destinations
Yellow Fever

The primary indication for yellow fever vaccination is to prevent infection in individuals at risk. A map of risk areas can be found at www.cdc.gov/travel. However, yellow fever is currently the only vaccine that falls under the International Health Regulations that may necessitate vaccination purely for regulatory reasons. A number of African countries and one in South America (French Guiana) require proof of yellow fever vaccination from all arriving travelers. Other countries, both within and outside the risk zone, have submitted more complex requirements to the World Health Organization. Current country-by-country yellow fever entry requirements are at www.who.int/ith/chapters/en/index.html. A Centers for Disease Control and Prevention–designated yellow fever vaccination center should be consulted for detailed requirements. Neither yellow fever vaccine nor any other vaccine is currently required for readmission to the United States. In general, all healthy adult travelers to areas with a risk of yellow fever transmission should be vaccinated. The true duration of immunity from yellow fever vaccination is probably much longer than the stated 10 years and may exceed 30 years.[6]

Meningococcus

Meningococcal vaccine is recommended for travelers to Africa's sub-Saharan "meningitis belt" during the dry season from December through June, especially if prolonged contact with the local populace is likely. Out-of-season epidemics have occurred in Ethiopia, Somalia, and Tanzania, indicating possible changes in epidemiologic trends perhaps due to climate changes. Muslims undertaking Hajj and Umrah pilgrimages in Saudi Arabia are at a higher risk of meningococcal disease, and proof of vaccination with quadrivalent vaccine within the past 3 years is required to obtain pilgrimage visas.

Rabies

A preexposure rabies series is indicated for long-stay travel to endemic areas of Latin America, Asia, or Africa where the rabies threat is constant and where access to adequate postexposure rabies immune globulin and vaccine is likely to be limited. For short-term travel, risk groups for whom immunization should be considered include adventure travelers, bikers, hikers, cave explorers, and business travelers who travel for short but frequent trips and plan to go running outdoors on these trips.

Japanese Encephalitis

Japanese encephalitis is endemic to many rural farming areas of Southeast Asia and the Indian subcontinent. Sporadic cases with severe sequelae

TABLE 286-2 TRAVEL-RELATED VACCINES OF ADULTS

DISEASE	VACCINE	PRIMARY COURSE	ROUTE	FURTHER BOOSTERS
VACCINES TO CONSIDER FOR ALL DEVELOPING WORLD TRAVELERS				
Hepatitis A	Killed virus	0, 6-18 months	IM	None
Hepatitis B	Recombinant viral antigen	0, 1, 6 months	IM	None
		A: 0, 1, 2 weeks and 12 months	IM	None
		A: 0, 1, 3 weeks and 12 months*	IM	None
Hepatitis A/B	Combination of monovalent preparations	0, 1, 6 months	IM	None
		A: 0, 1, 3 weeks and 12 months	IM	None
Typhoid	Capsular Vi polysaccharide	Single dose	IM	2-3 years
	Live attenuated Ty21a bacteria	0, 2, 4, 6 days	Oral	5 years
Influenza	Inactivated viral	Single dose	IM	Annual
	Live attenuated virus	Single dose (<50 years of age only)	Nasal	Annual
Varicella	Live attenuated virus	0, 4-8 weeks	SC	None
VACCINES FOR CERTAIN DESTINATIONS				
Yellow fever	Live attenuated 17D virus	Single dose	SC	10 years
Meningococcus	Quadrivalent conjugated polysaccharide (A, C, Y, W135)	Single dose	IM	5 years
Rabies	Inactivated viral cell culture	0, 7, 21-28 days	IM†	None routinely but two doses after each exposure
Japanese encephalitis (Vero cell)	Inactivated viral	0, 28 days	IM	1 year if at continued risk; no data on subsequent doses
Polio‡	Inactivated viral	Single dose if adequate childhood series	SC; IM acceptable	None
Cholera§	Killed bacteria + recombinant B toxin subunit‖	0, 1 week	Oral	2 years for cholera; 3 months for ETEC

*Regimen not approved by the U.S. Food and Drug Administration for monovalent hepatitis B vaccine but approved for combination hepatitis A/B vaccine containing the same quantity of hepatitis B antigen.
†Intradermal rabies preexposure vaccine is no longer produced, and the intramuscular 1.0-mL vials are not licensed for intradermal use in a 0.1-mL dose.
‡Oral polio vaccine is no longer produced in the United States.
§Not available in the United States but available in Canada and most European countries. No cholera vaccine of any kind is currently available in the United States.
‖Also licensed in some countries for traveler's diarrhea due to enterotoxigenic *Escherichia coli*.
A = accelerated regimen to be used for imminent departures; ETEC = enterotoxigenic *E. coli*; IM = intramuscular; SC = subcutaneous.

continue to occur in travelers.[7] In temperate regions, the transmission season is from April through November. In tropical or subtropical regions of Oceania and Southeast Asia, transmission may occur year-round. Vaccination is recommended for (1) long-stay travel to an endemic rural area; (2) expatriation to anywhere in an endemic country; (3) short-term travel to endemic rural areas with extensive unprotected outdoor exposure, such as with adventure travel; and (4) short-term travel in the face of a current local epidemic.

Polio

Because of eradication efforts, poliomyelitis remains in only a few countries, but complete control remains elusive. Adults traveling to countries that are currently polio endemic (updated information at www.polioeradication.org) and who have previously completed a primary vaccine series should receive a one-time single dose of inactivated polio vaccine as a booster if the last dose or booster dose was administered at least 10 years previously.

Cholera

Cholera vaccination is no longer required by any country, and the risk to typical travelers is insignificant.[8] However, medical and aid workers staying for short periods in disaster areas or refugee camps may consider cholera vaccine. A highly effective oral killed whole cell–B subunit vaccine is available widely outside the United States.

Sequence of Travel-Related Vaccines

All currently indicated immunizations can and should be given at the same time and in any combination (Chapter 18). If two live viral antigens are not administered on the same day, they must be spaced by a month. However, yellow fever vaccine can be given at any interval with respect to single-antigen measles vaccine. Minimum intervals between vaccine doses must be respected, although 4 days or fewer before the next interval are acceptable. Regimens that involve 1-week intervals (rabies, Japanese encephalitis, accelerated hepatitis) are exceptions. There is not a maximum interval between doses of a primary vaccine series; interrupted series (except oral typhoid and rabies) need not be restarted but can be resumed beginning with the dose that is overdue.

● MALARIA CHEMOPROPHYLAXIS

An average of 1500 imported cases of malaria are reported annually in the United States. Estimates of risk in travelers not taking chemoprophylaxis vary widely by destination but range from 3.4% per month in West Africa to one tenth that on the Indian subcontinent and a further 10-fold reduction in South America. The majority of cases of imported malaria in the United States and Europe occur in noncitizen immigrants visiting friends and relatives abroad.

Resources describing current country-specific malaria microepidemiology should be accessible immediately to those prescribing malaria prophylaxis. Dosing and pharmaceutical properties of antimalarial drugs are described in Chapter 345. In the limited number of countries where it is still effective, chloroquine, 500 mg salt (300 mg base) per week beginning the week before the first exposure to malaria and continuing for 4 weeks after the last exposure, is still the drug of choice. However, atovaquone/proguanil may still be used by short-stay travelers who prefer the shorter duration of that regimen.

For all other areas of the world, three drugs are equally effective, and the choice depends on both traveler and itinerary factors. Atovaquone/proguanil (250/100 mg) is a well-tolerated, once-a-day drug that should be started 1 day before arrival in the malarious area (may not coincide with first overseas destination) and continued for 7 days after the last exposure. The short period of postexposure use makes it convenient for the many travelers on typical 1- to 3-week itineraries. High cost and daily dosing make it difficult to use for extended periods. Weekly mefloquine (250 mg) is given 2 and preferably 3 weeks before the first exposure to malaria and continued for 4 weeks thereafter. Weekly dosing and a long track record of efficacy make this drug the most effective for long-stay travelers. If contraindications to mefloquine exist for long-stay travelers, daily doxycycline (100 mg) beginning 1 day before exposure can be used; unlike atovaquone/proguanil, it must be continued for 4 weeks after exposure. Approximately 5% of individuals who take either mefloquine or doxycycline discontinue therapy because of side effects. Chemoprophylaxis may be started well before departure (3 to 4 weeks for mefloquine) in those concerned about possible intolerance to any drug.

Travelers should be reminded in writing to continue antimalarial drugs for the appropriate period after the last possible exposure, that malaria can still occur despite chemoprophylaxis, and that a malaria smear or malaria rapid diagnostic test is mandatory for any febrile illness occurring within 3 months after travel. Prevention of malaria in travelers residing in malarious areas for 6 months or more presents complex problems that have been reviewed elsewhere.

● DENGUE

An estimated 100 million cases of dengue fever and 250,000 cases of dengue hemorrhagic fever occur annually (Chapter 381). The past 20 years have seen a dramatic geographic expansion of epidemic dengue fever and dengue hemorrhagic fever. Dengue accounts for up to 2% of all illness in returned travelers, and dengue is the most common systemic febrile illness in returned travelers from every region except sub-Saharan Africa, where malaria still predominates. Several dengue vaccine candidates are in advanced clinical trials. Dengue fever is transmitted by day-biting *Aedes* mosquitoes, reinforcing the need to instruct travelers to the tropics in the need for both day and night use of repellents.

● TRAVELER'S DIARRHEA

The most frequent cause of traveler's diarrhea is enterotoxigenic *Escherichia coli* and in some locations enteroaggregative *E. coli*. *Salmonella*, *Shigella*, and *Campylobacter* each account for about 5 to 15%, and in Asia noncholera vibrios are significant.[9] Protozoa account for less than 5%. In adults, norovirus and rotavirus are increasingly detected. The mean duration of traveler's diarrhea, even if it is untreated, is 4 days.

All travelers to the developing world should be thoroughly educated in self-therapy for diarrheal disease and carry the appropriate agents while traveling.[10] Eighty percent of patients respond to a regimen of loperamide and an antibiotic within 24 hours. A single dose of a self-administered quinolone is usually sufficient, but patients should be instructed to complete 3 days of therapy with 500 mg of levofloxacin daily or 500 mg of ciprofloxacin twice daily should the traveler's diarrhea not resolve within 24 hours. Because of a significant increase in quinolone-resistant *Campylobacter* in Southeast Asia, India, and Nepal, travelers to those destinations should self-treat with azithromycin, 500 mg/day for 3 days or a single dose of 1000 mg.

Most guidelines do not recommend prophylaxis for the typical traveler because of potential adverse drug effects while away from medical care and because effective rapid-onset therapy is available for diarrhea should it occur. Exceptions include travelers with advanced human immunodeficiency virus (HIV) infection, those who have an underlying chronic medical problem that makes them more prone to adverse consequences from diarrhea, and travelers on a vital mission for a short period (less than 1 week) who cannot tolerate even a day of disability. Antibiotic prophylaxis should be carried out with a quinolone once per day or with rifaximin twice per day[A1]; prophylaxis should be used only for trips of 2 weeks or less.

● PREVENTIVE BEHAVIORS

Most travel-related health problems, including many infectious diseases, can be significantly reduced through appropriate behavior by the traveler.

Mosquito Protection

Antimalarial chemoprophylactic drugs are less than 100% effective. Protection against arthropods will help prevent dengue, leishmaniasis, filariasis, and a number of important arboviral diseases. Travelers should be instructed to clothe themselves to reduce as much exposed skin as practicable and to apply a repellent containing DEET (concentration of 30% to 35%) to all exposed, nonsensitive areas of the body every 4 to 6 hours.[11] More frequent application is required for agents containing lower concentrations of DEET. Travelers should sleep under a permethrin-impregnated bed net in malarious areas unless they are in a sealed air-conditioned environment. Although anopheline mosquitoes are night biters, *Aedes* spp and culicine mosquitoes are usually day biters, so vigilance at all times of day is necessary.

Food and Water Precautions

Travelers to developing countries should be diligent in washing their hands frequently; avoiding food from dubious eating places, markets, and roadside vendors; avoiding buffets where there are no food covers or fly controls; avoiding high-risk food such as shellfish, reef fish (ciguatera risk), undercooked meats and poultry, dairy products, unpeeled fruits, cold sauces, and salads; avoiding both tap water and drinks or ice made from tap water; and using sealed bottled water or chemically treated, filtered, or boiled water for drinking and brushing their teeth.

Sex

Education on the incidence of HIV infection and sexually transmitted diseases among professional sex workers abroad, on the use of condoms, and on the failure rate of condoms (3 to 5% breakage/slippage) should be given regardless of the apparent circumstances of the traveler. Unprotected sex even with fellow travelers is considered high risk.[12] Travel is a disinhibiting experience in itself, and alcohol consumption tends to increase during travel.

Blood-borne Pathogens

Blood, blood products, syringes, and contaminated medical or dental instruments are a risk following accidents or trauma. Travelers should consider carrying an infusion set, needles, and a suture kit for high-risk areas. If possible, they should defer medical treatment and travel to a facility where safety can be ensured. Tattooing, acupuncture, and body piercing carry similar risks. Health care workers and others at risk in areas of high HIV prevalence without sophisticated medical infrastructure may consider carrying a 1- to 2-week supply of Truvada (200 mg of emtricitabine plus 300 mg of tenofovir), 1 tablet per day, plus raltegravir 400 mg, 1 tablet twice a day to begin immediate twice-daily postexposure prophylaxis, with the understanding that this is only an initial measure to allow time for travel to an adequate medical facility able to provide sophisticated testing and counseling.

Protection Against Skin Diseases

Infected mosquito bites are common. Practicing good hand hygiene in dirty environments and covering open wounds are preventive measures that all travelers should take. Scabies and lice infestations can be prevented by carrying out good personal hygiene. In Africa, all clothes dried outdoors should be ironed to avoid cutaneous myiasis due to the tumbu fly. Hats and sunscreen are mandatory in the tropics. Sunscreen should always be applied to skin before, and not after, an application of DEET.

Swimming and Water Exposure

Travelers should be instructed to avoid recreational (swimming, rafting, wading) or other exposure to fresh water in areas that are endemic for schistosomiasis. Hikers, bikers, and adventure travelers should consider prophylaxis with 200 mg of doxycycline once per week because of the significant risk of leptospirosis that exists in fresh water throughout the developing world. Walking barefoot in tropical areas predisposes to hookworm, *Strongyloides* infection, cutaneous larva migrans, and tungiasis.

Prevention of Tuberculosis

A predeparture baseline tuberculin skin test with annual retesting is indicated for long-stay travelers to developing countries. Aggressive treatment of skin test converters will prevent cases of active tuberculosis later. Travelers should avoid crowded public transportation or crowded public places and distance themselves immediately from anyone with a chronic or heavy cough. Expatriates should screen domestic help for tuberculosis.

● NONINFECTIOUS TRAVEL PROBLEMS
Traveler's Thrombosis and Jet Lag

A causal relationship between travel-related immobility and deep venous thrombosis or pulmonary embolism in otherwise healthy travelers has become established. Risk of pulmonary embolus is essentially absent on flights lasting less than 6 hours. Those with clear, known risk factors are at highest risk. All travelers should avoid dehydration, avoid alcohol, and exercise the legs regularly in flight. Of many recommendations for prevention, only the use of graded 15 to 30 mm Hg compression stockings for those at higher risk is supported in trials,[A2] although prophylactic subcutaneous low-molecular-weight heparin just before departure and again 24 hours later for those with thrombophilia or previous thrombotic events is often used in practice. Aspirin therapy is of no proven benefit in this setting.

Jet lag (Chapter 405) occurs after crossing three or more time zones, and zolpidem (5 mg) taken for a few nights at bedtime at the destination is generally effective.

Altitude Illness

Whether ascending by car or airplane, acute mountain sickness occurs in at least 25% of people who ascend rapidly to 2500 m or more and in most people who go quickly to 3000 m or more. Gradual ascent during days is rarely practiced by modern travelers. For prevention of altitude illness, acetazolamide, 125 mg twice a day beginning the morning of the day before ascent and continuing through the day after ascent, is effective.[A3][A4] If symptoms of mountain sickness, such as nausea, vomiting, anorexia, light-headedness, fatigue, or insomnia, persist beyond the day after ascent, travelers may continue to take one tablet each evening.[13] Other medications such as dexamethasone also can be used (Chapter 94). Severe complications, such as pulmonary or cerebral edema, occur uncommonly above 3500 m and are best treated by oxygen and immediate descent. Those traveling above 3500 m for longer than a brief transit of a few hours should consult an expert.

POST-TRAVEL CARE

The approach to the patient requires knowledge of world geography, the epidemiology of disease patterns in 230 or so countries, and the clinical presentation of a wide spectrum of disorders. Most illnesses are mild, most are self-limited, and many are noninfectious. Based on 43,000 ill-returned travelers seen by the GeoSentinel Surveillance Network, specific travel destinations are associated with the probability of the diagnosis of certain diseases. Diagnostic approaches and empirical therapies can be guided by these destination-specific differences. Important region-specific disease occurrence data indicate that (1) febrile illness is most important from Africa and Southeast Asia; (2) malaria is one of the top three diagnoses from every region, yet during the past decade, dengue has become the most common febrile illness from every region outside of sub-Saharan Africa;[14] (3) in sub-Saharan Africa, rickettsial disease is second only to malaria as a cause of fever; (4) respiratory disease is most important in Southeast Asia and sub-Saharan Africa; and (5) acute diarrhea is disproportionately from South Central Asia.

Fever in a traveler who has recently returned from the tropics is a potential emergency and must be evaluated immediately so that antimalarial or other definitive treatment can be initiated rapidly if it is indicated. Persistent gastrointestinal symptoms in a returning traveler require prompt evaluation and treatment.[15] Certain long-term travelers should be evaluated by a travel or tropical medicine specialist when they return to be screened for conditions that may be asymptomatic, such as schistosomiasis or strongyloidiasis.

Travelers who become ill during or any time up to several months after a foreign trip will frequently associate that illness with a possible travel-specific etiology. This may be the case, but often it is not. Routine things are common, and common things are common whether they are actually acquired during travel or at some time after the trip.

Grade A References

A1. Zanger P, Nurjadi D, Gabor J, et al. Effectiveness of rifaximin in prevention of diarrhoea in individuals travelling to south and southeast Asia: a randomized, double-blind, placebo-controlled, phase 3 trial. *Lancet Infect Dis.* 2013;13:946-954.

A2. Kahn SR, Lim W, Dunn AS, et al. Prevention of VTE in nonsurgical patients: Antithrombotic Therapy and Prevention of Thrombosis, 9th ed: American College of Chest Physicians Evidence-Based Clinical Practice Guidelines. *Chest.* 2012;141:e195S-e226S.

A3. Low EV, Avery AJ, Gupta V, et al. Identifying the lowest effective dose of acetazolamide for the prophylaxis of acute mountain sickness: systematic review and meta-analysis. *BMJ.* 2012;345:e6779.

A4. Ritchie ND, Baggott AV, Andrew Todd WT. Acetazolamide for the prevention of acute mountain sickness—a systematic review and meta-analysis. *J Travel Med.* 2012;19:298-307.

GENERAL REFERENCES

For the General References and other additional features, please visit Expert Consult at https://expertconsult.inkling.com.

287

ANTIBACTERIAL CHEMOTHERAPY

GEORGE L. DRUSANO

Antibiotics have been classified as "miracle drugs" since their introduction and have transformed our expectations regarding the outcome of infection. More recently, they have been the backbone of modern interventional medicine. Barriers not meant to be breached have been. Catheters have been inserted into veins and arteries, the bladder, and the tracheal tree. These interventions support the seriously ill patient, but they also give bacteria access to normally sterile areas. Therapies for cancer and immune-mediated disease often leave patients severely immunosuppressed. Bacterial infections

in such patients are serious and, when untreated or treated late, frequently result in death. Antibacterial agents allow critical life-saving support for such patients.

What is clear is that the overuse and poor use of antibiotics have allowed many pathogens to develop resistance to drugs. Multiresistant *Staphylococcus aureus* has become a plague both in the hospital and, of late, in the community. Extended-spectrum β-lactamases and *Klebsiella pneumoniae* carbapenemase enzymes have mediated resistance to many of our most potent and broad-spectrum β-lactam agents, including the carbapenems. Consequently, it is important to understand the principles of antibacterial chemotherapy to obtain the best clinical outcomes for our patients but also, in a broader sense, to lower the probability of the emergence of resistance and to maintain the potency of the drugs we currently have in our therapeutic armamentarium.[1,2]

CHOICE OF ANTIBIOTIC, ANTIBIOTIC DOSE, AND SCHEDULE TO OPTIMIZE CLINICAL OUTCOME

As in all of clinical medicine, a well-done history and physical examination are central to proper decision making and to the achievement of optimal therapeutic outcomes in patients with infections. Key to choosing the correct drug, dose, and schedule is recognition that an infection exists. The next step is to document where the infection exists and then to identify the dominant organisms present at each site of infection. The next step is to determine whether there are any risk factors that might predict the presence of drug-resistant pathogens.

As an example, we know that community-acquired pneumonia is caused by certain traditional pathogens. *Streptococcus pneumoniae, Haemophilus influenzae,* and perhaps *Moraxella catarrhalis* are the "classic" bacterial pathogens associated with this entity. "Atypical" pathogens such as *Legionella* species, *Mycoplasma pneumoniae,* and *Chlamydophila pneumoniae* may also be seen. In contrast, intra-abdominal infections are dominated by *Escherichia coli* and other Enterobacteriaceae and anaerobic organisms such as *Bacteroides* species. Consequently, it is important to understand the dominant pathogens present at different infection sites so that the best drug or combination of drugs can be chosen to treat the infection.

Knowing the source of infection is also critical because drugs penetrate differently into different spaces.[3] Classically, penetration is poorer into spaces where there are tight junctions, such as the central nervous system, the eye, and the prostate. In general, the penetration of many classes of antibacterial agents is good into complicated skin and skin structure infection sites. What is often not appreciated is the divergent penetrations of different agents and even agents within the same class into the lung to treat bacterial pneumonia. For instance, the penetration by macrolide antibiotics into skin infection sites is modest, but their penetration into the lung is good, with penetration ratios (area under the concentration-time curve [AUC] in epithelial lining fluid/AUC in plasma) ranging from 4 to 20. The penetration of β-lactam drugs can range from 15 to 100%, but there is no set of variables (at least to date) that explains such a range of penetrations. Table 287-1 presents a partial list of

TABLE 287-1	PRIMARY INFECTION SITES AND THE DOMINANT BACTERIAL SPECIES PRESENT	
SITE	**BACTERIA**
Complicated skin or skin structure infection	*Staphylococcus aureus* and *Streptococcus* spp
Diabetic foot ulcer	Organisms above plus Enterobacteriaceae
Intra-abdominal infections	*Escherichia coli* and other Enterobacteriaceae plus anaerobes
Community-acquired bacterial pneumonia	*Streptococcus pneumoniae, Haemophilus influenzae, Moraxella catarrhalis,* "atypical" pathogens
Hospital-acquired pneumonia	*S. aureus, Klebsiella pneumoniae, Enterobacter* spp, *Pseudomonas aeruginosa, Acinetobacter* spp
Meningitis	*S. pneumoniae, H. influenzae* (nontypable), meningococci; in hospital settings, *S. aureus* and gram-negatives may be seen
Urinary tract infections	Enterobacteriaceae, particularly in sexually active women; multiresistant gram-negatives in patients with complicated urinary tract infections or those instrumented; enterococci, particularly in elderly men
Prostatitis	Enterobacteriaceae, enterococci, atypical pathogens

infection sites and their dominant pathogens. The point is not to have an encyclopedic knowledge of infection sites or of pathogens but to appreciate that different infection sites require different drugs to provide adequate coverage for the most likely pathogens present.

It is also important to understand other factors that increase the probability that a resistant organism is present at the primary infection site. An example is a patient who has recently taken antibiotics before acquiring the present infection. Other examples are the acquisition of an infection in the hospital or in an extended care facility and in a patient who is immunosuppressed. In such patients, the choice of antimicrobial agents must be carefully considered to cover more resistant pathogens.

● CULTURE AND GRAM STAIN

Once the site of infection has been definitively identified or the most likely source of infection has been determined, it is critical to obtain culture specimens from that site as well as to obtain blood culture samples. Coordination with the microbiology laboratory is key to make sure that culture specimens are handled appropriately. Also of great importance is the performance and interpretation of a Gram stain on the specimen. This can be straightforward if the specimen is from a normally sterile space, or it may require considerable skill in interpretation if the specimen is from an area where mixed flora is normally present, such as sputum.

Although it is not possible to make a definitive diagnosis on the basis of the cellular morphology of the organism, it is possible to combine information on the morphology, the organism's gram positivity or negativity, the infection site, and the most likely pathogens to make an initial antimicrobial choice with the highest probability of producing effective chemotherapy. The initial antibiotic chosen to cover organisms present at the primary infection site has a significant influence on the outcome of therapy. Initial choices should err on the side of caution. When definitive cultures are available, the chemotherapy can be "streamlined" to provide the most effective and least toxic antimicrobial for the patient. As the seriousness of the infection increases, providing the correct initial coverage becomes more important with regard to the ultimate outcome.

● SUSCEPTIBILITY

Because infections occur at a specific place, it is important to have an understanding of the antimicrobial susceptibility patterns in one's particular hospital. Most frequently, the microbiology susceptibility patterns are different in the culture specimens taken from patients on the general wards as opposed to those in intensive care units (ICUs) because the former are generally (but not always) infected with pathogens derived from the community setting. In severely infected patients, particularly those whose infections were acquired in the ICU, it is critical to know the susceptibility patterns for these pathogens, which are likely to be multiply resistant to different classes of agents.

After the definitive culture, the identified pathogen must be examined in an antimicrobial susceptibility test. This can be automated, in which case the information returned is the minimal inhibitory concentration (MIC), or it can be reported from a disc diffusion test, where the results are typically reported as S (susceptible), I (intermediate), or R (resistant). The MIC is often misunderstood as the concentration of drug that prevents the pathogen from growing, but it is actually the concentration of drug that allows a tube (or well) containing the pathogen to remain clear by visual examination after 18 to 24 hours. If one starts with an organism concentration of 1 to 5×10^5 colony-forming units (CFUs)/mL, this criterion can actually allow almost a $1 \log_{10}$ (CFU/mL) increase in bacterial count over this time frame and still be read as the MIC. With all its limitations, the MIC provides critical information about drug choice. For several infections, such as meningitis, endocarditis, and perhaps bacteremia, knowing the minimal bactericidal concentration (defined as the concentration required for kill of 99.9% of organisms during 18 to 24 hours) is valuable. In these cases, it is important to obtain multi-log killing of the organism to ensure a high probability of a good clinical outcome. For meningitis and endocarditis, there is also the confounding problem of penetration of the drug to the primary infection site. In other circumstances (e.g., ventilator-associated pneumonia) in which bacterial burdens are high, optimizing the probability of cure requires highly bactericidal therapy.

● DETERMINING THE "CORRECT" DRUG DOSE

The correct drug dose is the one that produces a high likelihood of achieving a good clinical response with a low probability of causing a concentration-driven adverse event. Another consideration is that the optimal dose should

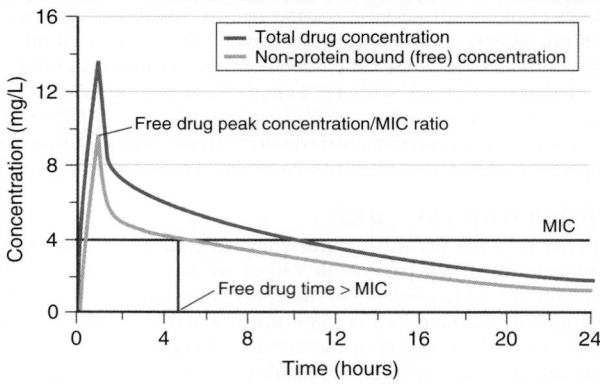

FIGURE 287-1. Three measures of drug exposure are important to the measure of potency, or the minimal inhibitory concentration (MIC). These measures are free drug peak concentration/MIC ratio, free drug time greater than MIC, and free drug area under the curve (AUC)/MIC ratio.

have a high probability of suppressing the emergence of resistant mutants. To be confident that a drug dose has a high likelihood of producing a good clinical outcome requires an understanding of the relationship between the measure of drug exposure and infection outcome, that is, pharmacodynamics (Chapter 29).

When we administer a drug either intravenously or orally, the drug concentration starts low, increases to a maximal value, then declines over time until another dose of the drug is given (in a multidose regimen). This drug concentration–time profile should be seen relative to a measure of drug potency against the pathogen in question: the MIC (or minimal bactericidal concentration). It is also critical to note that protein binding is important because in almost all cases, it is the free or non–protein bound drug that kills the causative pathogen. So understanding the pharmacodynamics of a drug or class of agents first requires knowledge of the concentration-time profile, protein binding, and MIC (Fig. 287-1). For drugs that kill organisms much faster as their concentrations rise (e.g., fluoroquinolones, aminoglycosides), the free drug AUC/MIC ratio is most closely linked to drug effect. For other drugs (e.g., penicillins, carbapenems, cephalosporins, monobactams), the rate of organism kill rises with concentration and plateaus quickly, in which case the free drug time greater than MIC is most closely linked to drug effect. On occasion, the free drug peak concentration/MIC ratio is linked to drug effect. This is seen when there is a rapid and frequent emergence of resistance and the peak concentration helps suppress the amplification of resistant mutant subpopulations.

These measures of drug exposure need to be linked to drug effect. There are a number of ways to do this, but two are most common. In the first and most valuable way, patients are studied during the course of a clinical trial. Multiple plasma samples are taken for documentation of the drug's pharmacokinetics and corrected for protein binding. The MIC of the infecting pathogen is determined for the drug being administered, and the three measures of drug exposure cited earlier are calculated. The outcome of the patient is then determined (usually success or failure, but in some instances, time to success or failure serves as the outcome measure). If the outcome is success or failure, the appropriate measure of drug exposure is linked to the outcome through logistic regression analysis. By creating such a relationship, we can directly estimate the probability of a patient's having a successful outcome if a certain measure of drug exposure is achieved. For example, if a patient receiving a drug that is a concentration-dependent killing agent achieves a free drug AUC/MIC ratio of 88, the logistic regression relationship allows the calculation that the probability of a good outcome is a specific number (perhaps 91%). During the past 10 years, we have been able to generate such relationships for a great number of drugs and across drug classes. The most common relationships are for the fluoroquinolone antimicrobials, but examples can be found for the aminoglycosides, oxazolidinones, β-lactams, and glycylcyclines, among others.

The second way to link exposure to antibacterial effect is through preclinical animal models of infection. Here, the end point is most often microbiologic, although survivorship models have been employed. We observe the drug concentration–time profile in the animals and at the end of the experiment determine the number of organisms left after therapy at the infection site (the baseline number of organisms having been previously determined).

We can then link the measure of drug exposure (as earlier) to the number of bacterial cells killed by a specific regimen. It is most often the case that drugs are administered to the animals in a "dose fractionation" fashion. For example, 400 mg/kg/day regimen of a β-lactam may be administered as the whole dose daily, half the dose every 12 hours, or one quarter of the dose every 6 hours. In this way, we can determine whether free drug peak concentration/ MIC ratio, free drug AUC/MIC ratio, or free drug time greater than MIC is the best measure of drug exposure for the class of drug being studied.

How does knowing the relationship between drug exposure and microbiologic effect in an animal infection model help in treating patients? On the basis of experience with different drugs and drug classes, it has become possible to link a drug's microbiologic effect in an animal model to clinical outcome.[4] For instance, in the therapy of complicated skin and skin structure infections, a drug exposure in the animal model that stops organisms from growing for 24 hours or reduces their number by approximately 1 $\log_{10}$ (CFU/g) is adequate to generate a high probability of a good clinical outcome. This has been documented for oxazolidinones and glycylcyclines. For severe community-acquired pneumonia or for hospital-acquired pneumonia, a greater cell kill—generally 2 $\log_{10}$ (CFU/g) or greater—is required for a high likelihood of a good clinical outcome.

When we have clinical data with a logistic regression function, it is possible to identify an exposure target that is associated with a specific probability of a good outcome (e.g., a free drug AUC/MIC ratio of 88 generates a 91% probability of a good outcome). In the case of the animal model, it is possible to identify a target drug exposure that will achieve a certain microbiologic effect associated with a good clinical outcome (the logic is one step removed). In both cases, we have a target drug exposure, and this is used to identify the "correct" dose.

When the same dose of a drug is administered to a number of patients, no two concentration-time curves will be identical. Indeed, it is not unusual to have a 10-fold range in measures of drug exposure (e.g., peak concentration, trough concentration, AUC). When these are transformed by incorporating MIC values, ranges of 100- to 1000-fold are commonly encountered. As part of the drug development process, the pharmacokinetics of new agents are now identified in a large number of patients with the infection of interest. As part of this process, the interpatient variability in important pharmacokinetic parameters (e.g., drug clearance = 10 ± 4 L/hour) is determined. This information is then used with a tool called Monte Carlo simulation to ask and answer a key question: If I give this specific drug dose to a large number of patients and I recognize that the MIC values I am likely to encounter will range (for example) between 0.06 and 8 mg/L, how many patients will achieve the desired measure of drug exposure to give them a high likelihood of a good clinical outcome? This can be calculated directly from the data indicated earlier plus the MIC distribution for the drug and the type of infection one wishes to treat. Indeed, many of the dosage recommendations for new drugs are calculated in this manner and validated in large phase III clinical trials. It provides the clinician with a degree of confidence that the recommended doses are likely to work if the infecting pathogen is still susceptible to the drug.

⬤ EMERGENCE OF RESISTANCE

If the drug is properly chosen, the organism should have a high probability of being susceptible to it. However, during the course of therapy, the organism has many mechanisms available to make it less susceptible (the MIC increases) to the drug being used. This leads to less effect than was originally envisioned, which results in a lower probability of cure.

When are organisms likely to become resistant? There are many determinants, but five factors account for the majority of cases of resistance emerging during therapy. The first is the mutational frequency of the organism being treated. Because mistakes are made by the organism during replication, mutations occur in the genome at a specific rate, which is organism dependent. For antibiotic resistance, the mutational frequency rate is generally around $1/10^8$ to $1/10^6$. There are organisms, however—referred to as hypermutators—that have mutations in other places in the genome (often mutS) that alter their DNA replication error-checking mechanisms. These organisms' mutational frequencies are generally 10- to 100-fold higher than those of organisms without these other mutations.

The second factor is related to the bacterial burden. The higher the bacterial burden, the more likely it is that a preexistent mutant is already extant in the bacterial population. Antibiotic pressure then provides this mutant with a selective advantage, and it amplifies in the population while its more susceptible cousins are killed by the antibiotic. As the bacterial burden increases and ultimately surpasses the inverse of the mutational frequency to resistance, it becomes more and more likely that a resistant mutant exists in the population. For instance, if the mutational frequency to resistance is $1/10^7$ (1 resistant organism per a population of 10^7) and the patient has a bacterial infection in which the total bacterial burden is 10^9 organisms, it is highly likely that a resistant organism is present in the population a priori. A calculation of the actual probability can be performed by a Poisson distribution, the bacterial burden, and the mutational frequency to resistance. Consequently, infections in which the bacterial burden is high are more likely to generate resistance during therapy. For example, in clinical trials of ventilator-associated pneumonia, single-agent β-lactam drugs or fluoroquinolones allowed the emergence of resistance during therapy 33 to 50% of the time.

The third issue is drug penetration. There are circumstances (e.g., empyema) in which the bacterial burden is high but the drug's penetration to the infection site is reduced. In this case, the emergence of resistance is more likely. In contrast, poor penetration with relatively low bacterial burdens (e.g., meningitis) generally does not result in a high probability of the emergence of resistance.

The fourth issue has to do with error-prone replication in bacterial pathogens. When resistance occurs relatively late in therapy and the bacterial burden is modest, error-prone replication is often to blame. Antibiotics differ greatly with respect to their ability to induce the bacterial isolate to perform error-prone replication. Perhaps the best example is the fluoroquinolone antimicrobials because these drugs strike at the heart of DNA replication. The organism senses the attack of the antibiotic, and a whole cascade of events takes place, the most important of which is the induction of error-prone polymerases (e.g., pol V). These polymerases markedly increase the error rate in DNA replication. Most of these errors are lethal to the organism and therefore unhelpful to it. However, because this is a totally random process, by chance, a mutation can occur in a spot that provides protection from the onslaught of the antibiotic (e.g., a mutation in the DNA gyrase when the patient is receiving a fluoroquinolone). We perceive this as the organism's having a selective replication advantage (emergence of resistance), and we see an increase in the MIC of the mutant organism relative to the baseline organism.

The fifth factor has to do with mechanisms other than antibacterial target site mutations that allow the organisms to survive in the face of appropriate antibiotic chemotherapy. One extremely common mechanism seen in the majority of both gram-positive and gram-negative organisms is the upregulation of efflux pumps. These pumps are indiscriminate in their ability to pump molecules; they can eject multiple classes of antibacterials from the organism as well as natural substances that can harm it, such as metal ions. These pumps keep drug concentrations at their target sites much lower than they would be in the absence of the pumps. The pumps can be induced and then downregulated once the threat has passed, or occasionally, the organism can pick up a mutation in the part of the genome where expression of the pump is regulated, so the pump is always expressed (constitutive expression).

A similar process is seen with the production of β-lactamases. Often, these enzymes are situated on plasmids and are produced all the time. Sometimes, as with the efflux pumps, they sense the attack by the β-lactam, and their production is markedly increased (the phenomenon of induction, seen with ampC-type enzymes, which generally reside on the chromosome). Sometimes, also like the pumps, the organisms pick up a mutation in the part of the genome that regulates production of the β-lactamase. This is referred to as stable de-repression, and the enzyme is made all the time. The enzyme hydrolyzes its substrate (the β-lactam drug), thus preventing the binding to the target sites, the β-lactam–binding proteins.

Finally, in gram-negative organisms, the drug must cross the diffusional barrier of the outer membrane before binding to β-lactam–binding proteins (if the drug is a β-lactam) in the periplasm of the organism, or it must cross the inner membrane if its target site is actually inside the organism. For many agents, particularly those that are water soluble, a large percentage of their influx is due to passage through porin proteins. These proteins are water-filled channels that pass through the entirety of the outer membrane of gram-negative bacteria. Part of their function is to provide access to nutrients for the organism and allow the easy diffusion of waste products. These channels are also used to obtain passage by water-soluble antibacterial agents. The organism has the ability to downregulate these channels, either temporarily or permanently (by mutation). An example is *Pseudomonas aeruginosa*, in which downregulation of the porin channel oprD markedly diminishes the penetration of carbapenem antibiotics (β-lactam agents), with a resultant two- to eight-fold rise in MIC. With all these mechanisms that can be brought to bear, it is no surprise that poor dosing and prolonged courses of therapy often lead to the emergence of resistance.

These mechanisms also interact. In the case of fluoroquinolone antimicrobials, where error-prone replication almost always occurs under pressure, the upregulation of efflux pumps relieves some of the antibiotic pressure, allowing the organisms to undergo more rounds of replication per unit of time, giving the error-prone replication mechanism more time to find a mutation that is not lethal and provides protection against the drug at the primary target site.

SUPPRESSING THE EMERGENCE OF RESISTANCE

Suppressing the emergence of resistance is an end point that is different from achieving a good clinical or microbiologic outcome. The antimicrobial exposure (free drug peak concentration/MIC ratio, free drug AUC/MIC ratio, or free drug time greater than MIC) necessary to suppress resistance is always at least as high as that required to attain maximal killing of bacterial cells, and in many instances, it is substantially higher.

Recently, it has been shown experimentally that it is possible to identify doses and schedules of drugs that suppress the emergence of resistance as well as provide optimal killing of bacterial cells. Unfortunately, many of the exposures necessary to achieve such an outcome are high enough to result in increased drug toxicity. Nevertheless, as new agents are developed, it will become important to identify resistance-suppressive exposures and to ascertain whether they are too toxic to be used clinically, as a way of retaining the potency of the antibacterial therapeutic armamentarium.

The other way to help suppress the emergence of resistance is to employ combination chemotherapy. Combination therapy has major advantages, but there are significant disadvantages as well. Among the advantages are that combination therapy can improve the spectrum of coverage in the setting of empirical treatment as well as help suppress the emergence of resistance. This is best seen in the treatment of *Mycobacterium tuberculosis*, although there is growing evidence that this may also be true for difficult-to-treat pathogens such as *P. aeruginosa* and *Acinetobacter* species. Combination therapy can be effective against some pathogens in serious infections for which a single agent would not be adequate. Enterococcal endocarditis is the classic example; ampicillin or vancomycin is generally static and not up to the task of curing this disease, and the second agent (an aminoglycoside, streptomycin, or gentamicin) is somewhat resistant when it is used alone (MIC values <500 mg/L). Yet the combination produces excellent bacterial kill in the endocarditic vegetation, with a high probability of cure if the patient can tolerate the combination for the requisite time. Some authors have discussed reducing drug doses in combination as a way of ameliorating toxicity, but this theoretical advantage is difficult to demonstrate convincingly in the clinical setting.

The disadvantages of combination therapy are also well known. At full doses of each, there may be added toxicity, and there are certainly greater costs associated with combinations. Finally, combinations of agents may interact antagonistically instead of either additively or synergistically. For example, the combination of tetracycline and penicillin is somewhat antagonistic and caused a number of failures in the treatment of pneumococcal meningitis in the 1950s. However, there are circumstances in which weak antagonism is tolerable. It has been shown that isoniazid plus rifampin, part of the standard therapy for *M. tuberculosis*, is somewhat antagonistic with respect to cell killing, but the combination provides superb protection against the emergence of resistance. Consequently, in discussing drug interactions (synergy, additivity, antagonism), it is important to be specific about the end point to which one is referring.

MECHANISM OF ACTION

The search for new antimicrobials begins with the principle that the target that affects pathogens must not be in the human genome or must be sufficiently different that the agent in question does not cause appreciable human toxicity. β-Lactam antibiotics are a good example; the inhibition of peptidoglycan synthesis has no effect on humans because this target is simply not present. An example of differing susceptibility to inhibition because of poor sequence homology between bacteria and humans can be seen in the inhibitors of the bacterial ribosome. The bacterial ribosome is much smaller than that in humans and has differing affinities for such drugs as aminoglycosides, tetracyclines, macrolides, and clindamycin. Consequently, such agents are an important part of the therapeutic armamentarium and cause only minor adverse effects related to their primary mode of action. In some cases,

so-called off-target toxicity may take place. Again, an example is the β-lactams; a major toxicity is accelerated allergic reaction, even though the target for the agents is not present in humans. Table 287-2 lists the sites of action and the effects of many antimicrobial agents.

Often, antimicrobials are thought of as either *bacteriostatic* or *bactericidal*, for which there are standard definitions. An agent that causes a 1000-fold decline (3 $\log_{10}$ [CFU/mL] decrease) in an in vitro test system during 18 to 24 hours is defined as being bactericidal. Any agent that causes a smaller decline is defined as bacteriostatic. It is clear that these definitions are arbitrary; however, there is a clinical connection. In some circumstances, such as meningitis and endocarditis, it is critical to kill every last organism with the combination of drugs employed and the immune system. Obviously, the more organisms the antimicrobial kills, the easier this is to accomplish. In other circumstances, such as multilobar pneumonia, it is critical to kill as many of the organisms as possible so as not to overwhelm the body's immunologic defenses. For these reasons, clinicians generally prefer bactericidal to bacteriostatic agents.

MECHANISMS OF RESISTANCE

Earlier, how to suppress the emergence of resistance was examined. Here, the mechanisms by which organisms can become less susceptible to antimicrobial agents are examined. As stated earlier, in most cases, resistance is caused by an alteration in the target site; by an enzyme that alters the drug, resulting in a lack of activity; by the drug's being pumped out of the organism; or, in the case of gram-negative pathogens, by the loss or downregulation of a transmembrane porin protein. These mechanisms, along with error-prone replication, can interact to cause large increases in the MIC. For example, a gram-negative pathogen that acquired a mutation in its gyrase enzyme would generally have only a four-fold increase in its MIC value for a fluoroquinolone antimicrobial; however, if this isolate also had an efflux pump upregulated, the MIC could change 8- to 16-fold. Table 287-3 shows the mechanisms of resistance for multiple drug classes as well as the most common organisms in which these mechanisms are seen.

EFFECTS OF PHARMACOKINETIC CHANGES

Whereas antimicrobial pharmacodynamics is the study of the effect of a drug on an infecting organism, pharmacokinetics is the study of the effect of the body's processes on the drug concentration–time profile and the drug's ability to penetrate to the infection site (or the toxicity site). As such, it is a prime determinant of whether a drug will be able to kill or to inhibit the offending pathogen and, because many toxicities are concentration related, whether a serious drug-related toxicity will occur.

Earlier, the algorithm for identifying appropriate drug doses and schedules was outlined. Table 287-4 shows recommended doses and schedules of important antimicrobial agents as well as their protein-binding ability and whether alterations in renal or hepatic function generate major changes in the concentration-time profile. As in all chemotherapy, the aim is to generate a concentration-time profile in the plasma to generate a concentration-time profile at the infection site that allows the drug to inhibit or to kill the pathogen without causing toxicity.

Although there is almost always a guide to the concentration-time profile that results in an appropriate antimicrobial effect, it is more difficult to identify a linkage between drug exposure and the occurrence of toxicity. Data in this regard are available for the aminoglycosides, including a considerable amount of information on the association between drug concentrations and the likelihood of nephrotoxicity, and for daptomycin, for which a link between exposure and the likelihood of creatine kinase elevation has been elucidated.

For aminoglycosides, the relationships between drug exposure and the likelihood of a good clinical outcome and between drug exposure and the likelihood of nephrotoxicity have been determined. These are in the form of logistic regression functions, so the actual probability of both outcomes can be calculated. The one difference is that for the relationship with good outcome, the MIC value is part of the evaluation, whereas it does not figure in the toxicity relationship. Nevertheless, it is possible to derive appropriate information by making the outcome relationship MIC specific. Figure 287-2 illustrates the effect and toxicity relationships for aminoglycosides at three different MIC values. As shown, it is relatively easy to achieve a high probability of good clinical outcomes with aminoglycosides when the MIC is 0.25 mg/L, but it is virtually impossible to do so when the MIC rises to a value of 1.0 mg/L. The evaluation in the figure is based on twice-daily dosing; daily aminoglycoside dosing markedly improves this circumstance. Also,

TABLE 287-2 MECHANISMS OF ACTION OF ANTIMICROBIAL AGENTS

AGENT	SITE OF ACTION	EFFECT	BACTERICIDAL	BACTERIOSTATIC
β-Lactams (penicillins, cephalosporins, carbapenems, aztreonam)	Cell wall: penicillin-binding proteins	Inhibit cross-linking of peptidoglycan (transpeptidation), impair cell wall synthesis	+	Occasionally (enterococci)
Vancomycin, teicoplanin, dalbavancin, telavancin	Cell wall: terminal D-alanyl-D-alanine of pentapeptide peptidoglycan precursor	Inhibit polymerization of disaccharide precursors to peptidoglycan (transglycosylation), impair cell wall synthesis	+	Occasionally (enterococci)
Daptomycin	Cell membrane	Rapid depolarization of membrane potential	+	Occasionally (enterococci)
Aminoglycosides	Protein synthesis: 30S ribosome subunit	Inhibit peptide elongation, cause misreading of genetic code, inhibit protein synthesis	+	
Tetracyclines, glycylcyclines	Protein synthesis: 30S ribosome subunit	Inhibit binding of transfer RNA, inhibit protein synthesis	Occasionally	+
Chloramphenicol	Protein synthesis: 30S ribosome subunit	Blocks attachment of aminoacyl transfer RNA, inhibits protein synthesis	Occasionally	+
Macrolides, azalides, ketolides	Protein synthesis: 50S ribosome subunit	Block transfer of amino acids to peptide chain, inhibit protein synthesis	Occasionally	+
Clindamycin	Protein synthesis: 50S ribosome subunit	Blocks transfer of amino acids to peptide chain, inhibits protein synthesis	Occasionally	+
Quinupristin-dalfopristin	Protein synthesis: 50S ribosome subunit	Block extrusion of peptide chains, inhibit protein synthesis	+	+ (with quinupristin resistance)
Linezolid	Protein synthesis: 50S ribosome subunit	Blocks formation of 70S initiation complex, inhibits protein synthesis	Occasionally	+
Rifampin	Nucleic acid synthesis: β-subunit of DNA-dependent RNA polymerase	Inhibits RNA synthesis	+	
Metronidazole	Nucleic acid synthesis	Damages nucleic acids, inhibits DNA synthesis	+	
Quinolones	Nucleic acid synthesis: DNA gyrase, topoisomerase IV	Impair supercoiling of DNA, prevent decatenation of DNA molecules after replication, inhibit DNA synthesis	+	
Sulfonamides	Folic acid synthesis: dihydropteroate synthetase	Competitive inhibition of synthesis of dihydrofolate from p-aminobenzoic acid, pteroate, and glutamic acid	Occasionally (when used with trimethoprim)	+
Trimethoprim	Folic acid synthesis: dihydrofolate reductase	Inhibits reduction of dihydrofolate to tetrahydrofolic acid	Occasionally (when used with sulfonamide)	+

these relationships permit one to calculate the probabilities of effect and toxicity when, for example, aminoglycoside AUC is increased owing to renal dysfunction because these agents are largely eliminated renally.

When no toxicity relationship is available, there is still a target for good clinical effect. Achievement of this target should be paramount, and alterations for renal or hepatic impairment should strive to maintain the high likelihood of effect seen in patients with a relatively normal clearance function. One can change the dose or schedule of a drug to decrease its accumulation in the presence of renal or hepatic impairment (depending on the drug) and then recalculate the impact on the likelihood of attaining a good clinical outcome. One can also calculate the amount of accumulation with the proposed dose reduction or extension of the dosing interval. For the increase in exposure (relative to that in normally clearing patients), there is no clear guidance, but one can accept a certain maximal amount of accumulation as long as the proposed dose adjustment maintains a high likelihood of a good outcome. The acceptability of the increased drug exposure after dosage adjustment is usually based on a combination of preclinical toxicology and the largest exposures seen in phase I and phase II clinical trials. However, the overarching issue is that the proposed dose or schedule alteration maintains a high probability of a good clinical outcome.

DRUG CLASSES AND THEIR PROPERTIES

During the past 70 years, a large number of different classes of antimicrobial agents have been developed. These classes differ in their mechanisms of action, mechanisms of emergence of resistance, and whether they kill substantial numbers of organisms or only shut off bacterial growth. The following sections examine some of the properties of the major classes of antimicrobial agents in use today.

β-Lactam Agents

This class of drugs is arguably the most important group of antimicrobials. With chemical modification, they have an exceptionally broad spectrum of activity and, in general, an excellent safety profile. The major toxicity is related to allergic reactions to a degradation product of the drug. There are a number of different types of β-lactams, including the penicillins, the cephalosporins, the monobactams, and the carbapenems.

These agents bind to their targets, the β-lactam–binding proteins (sometimes referred to as penicillin-binding proteins). These binding proteins have an active site serine, and the drug forms a covalent bond with this site through the carbonyl of the β-lactam ring. Sometimes, the binding has direct effects on the organism's shape. For example, in gram-negative organisms, binding to penicillin-binding protein (PBP)–2 causes the organism to assume a spherical shape, whereas binding to PBP-3 causes the formation of long chains of organisms. In general, high-affinity binding to PBP-1 leads to the rapid death of the organism, sometimes accompanied by lysis. The classic response of S. pneumoniae to penicillin G is rapid lysis of the organism. Binding to PBP-1 (1a or 1b) leads to activation of N-acetylmuramic acid amidase, which destroys the bacterial cell wall, resulting in lysis.

The most common way for pathogens to protect themselves from β-lactams is by elaborating β-lactamases.[5] The genes for these enzymes may be on plasmids or other bits of transmissible DNA, or they may reside on the bacterial chromosome. Some drugs, such as the carbapenems, are resistant to hydrolysis by many enzymes (but certainly not all of them, especially the metallo-β-lactamases and K. pneumoniae carbapenemase-type β-lactamases). One of the ways developed to protect these drugs is to add a second agent, the β-lactamase inhibitor. Examples include potassium clavulanate,

TABLE 287-3 MECHANISMS OF ANTIMICROBIAL RESISTANCE

ANTIBACTERIAL AGENT	MECHANISM	REPRESENTATIVE ORGANISM
β-Lactams (penicillins, cephalosporins, carbapenems, aztreonam)	Altered target (penicillin-binding proteins)	Methicillin-resistant *Staphylococcus aureus* (MRSA), penicillin-resistant *Streptococcus pneumoniae*, *Enterococcus faecium*
	Reduced permeability	*Enterobacter* spp, *Pseudomonas aeruginosa*, *Acinetobacter* spp
	Enhanced efflux	*P. aeruginosa*, *Acinetobacter* spp
	β-Lactamases	*S. aureus*, Enterobacteriaceae (includes ESBLs), *Haemophilus influenzae*, *Moraxella catarrhalis*, *Neisseria gonorrhoeae*, *Enterococcus faecalis*, *P. aeruginosa*, *Acinetobacter* spp
Aminoglycosides	Inactivating enzymes (acetylation, adenylation, phosphorylation)	*S. aureus*, enterococci, *P. aeruginosa*, Enterobacteriaceae
	Reduced permeability	Enterobacteriaceae, *P. aeruginosa*, enterococci
	Enhanced efflux	*P. aeruginosa*
	Decreased ribosomal binding	*S. aureus*, *E. faecalis*, mycobacteria (streptomycin), gram-negative pathogens (aminoglycoside ribosomal methylase)
Chloramphenicol	Enhanced efflux	*H. influenzae*
	Reduced permeability	Enterobacteriaceae
	Inactivating enzyme (acetylation)	*S. aureus*, *S. pneumoniae*, enterococci
Daptomycin	Altered target	*S. aureus*
Glycylcyclines	Enhanced efflux	Enterobacteriaceae, especially *Proteus*
Macrolides, clindamycin, ketolide, quinupristin	Altered target (methylation of ribosomal RNA)	*S. aureus*, *S. pneumoniae* (not ketolide), streptococci, *Bacteroides fragilis*
	Enhanced efflux (not clindamycin or ketolide)	*S. pneumoniae*, streptococci
	Reduced permeability	Enterobacteriaceae
	Inactivating enzymes	*Escherichia coli*, *Klebsiella pneumoniae*, *S. aureus*
Linezolid	Altered target	Enterococci, *S. aureus*
Quinolones	Altered target (DNA gyrase, topoisomerase IV)	Enterobacteriaceae, *P. aeruginosa*
	Reduced permeability	Enterobacteriaceae, *P. aeruginosa*
	Enhanced efflux	*E. coli*, *P. aeruginosa*
Tetracyclines	Altered target (ribosome)	*N. gonorrhoeae*, streptococci
	Enhanced efflux	*E. coli*, *S. pneumoniae*
	Reduced permeability	Enterobacteriaceae
	Drug inactivation	*B. fragilis*
Rifampin	Altered target (β-subunit of polymerase)	*E. coli*, *S. aureus*, *Mycobacterium tuberculosis*
Sulfonamides, trimethoprim	Altered target (dihydropteroate synthetase or dihydrofolate reductase)	Enterobacteriaceae, *M. catarrhalis*
	Enhanced *p*-aminobenzoic acid production	*S. aureus*, *N. gonorrhoeae*
	Reduced permeability	*P. aeruginosa*, Enterobacteriaceae
Vancomycin	Altered target (peptidoglycan precursor binding site)	*E. faecium*, *E. faecalis*, *S. aureus*

ESBLs = extended-spectrum β-lactamases.

sulbactam, tazobactam, and, most recently, NXL-104 (an experimental drug now referred to as avibactam). These agents inhibit different types of β-lactamases, with NXL-104 being the only one able to inhibit the ampC-type enzymes carried by *P. aeruginosa*, *Enterobacter* species, *Citrobacter* species, *Serratia marcescens*, and indole-positive *Protea* (SPICE organisms).

All β-lactams are relatively non–concentration dependent in their kill rate, and free drug time greater than MIC is the important factor for increased organism killing. The classes differ somewhat, with carbapenems requiring approximately 40% free drug time greater than MIC for near-maximal cell killing. For penicillins, this percentage is approximately 50%, and for cephalosporins and monobactams, it is 60 to 70%. When these agents need to penetrate to a site of infection, such as epithelial lining fluid or central nervous system, the targets may change somewhat.

Aminoglycosides

These important agents were discovered in the late 1940s for the treatment of *M. tuberculosis* (streptomycin). Screening of natural products identified a number of different aminoglycosides, such as kanamycin, neomycin, gentamicin (actually a combination of three congeners), and tobramycin. Other semisynthetic agents, such as amikacin, netilmicin, and arbekacin (among others), have been discovered and used for therapy in the United States and elsewhere.

Nephrotoxicity and middle ear toxicity (hearing loss or loss of balance) are the defining dose-limiting toxicities of aminoglycosides and resulted in

their going out of favor in the 1990s and early in the first decade of the 21st century. It has now been recognized that most (but not all) of the nephrotoxic potential can be ameliorated by intermittent dosing of these drugs (usually once daily). Even with daily therapy, however, prolonged use can still result in nephrotoxicity or ototoxicity.

The recent rise in resistance, particularly among gram-negative isolates, and new resistance mechanisms mediating resistance to even our best β-lactam agents have resulted in renewed interest in existing aminoglycosides and a search for new ones that are more resistant to inactivation by the aminoglycoside-modifying enzymes.[6]

These drugs are concentration dependent in terms of their kill rate and are rapid killers. Hence, the AUC/MIC ratio (or, as sometimes reported, peak concentration/MIC ratio) is the factor most closely associated with bacterial cell killing. Therefore, large doses administered daily to patients with normal renal function would be expected to optimize bacterial cell killing while minimizing the probability of inducing an aminoglycoside-related toxic event.

The older aminoglycosides (streptomycin and gentamicin) have the best profile for synergizing with drugs active against gram-positive streptococci (particularly enterococci). Tobramycin generally has the most potent activity against *P. aeruginosa* (depending on the aminoglycoside-modifying enzymes present in a specific locale), and less resistance is generally seen with amikacin (again, depending on the locale). Streptomycin and amikacin, because of the number of amino groups carried, are usually about four-fold less potent

TABLE 287-4 DOSAGE REGIMENS OF ANTIBACTERIALS, PHARMACOKINETICS, AND DOSE ADJUSTMENT IN PATIENTS WITH RENAL OR HEPATIC FAILURE

CLASS/AGENT	DOSE* FOR SYSTEMIC INFECTION	ORAL FORMULATION	PEAK SERUM CONCENTRATION (μg/mL)	PROTEIN BINDING (%)	NORMAL SERUM HALF-LIFE (hr)	HEPATIC FAILURE	RENAL FAILURE	SERUM LEVELS AFFECTED BY DIALYSIS
AMINOGLYCOSIDES								
Amikacin	5-6.7 mg/kg q8h or 15-20 mg/kg q24h	—	35	0	2-3	No	Major	Yes (H, P)
Gentamicin	1.7 mg/kg q8h or 5 mg/kg q24h	—	7	0	2-3	No	Major	Yes (H, P)
Netilmicin	1.7 mg/kg q8h or 5 mg/kg q24h	—	7	0	2-3	No	Major	Yes (H, P)
Tobramycin	1.7 mg/kg q8h or 5 mg/kg q24h	—	7	0	2-3	No	Major	Yes (H, P)
ANTITUBERCULOUS AGENTS								
Ethambutol	15 mg/kg q24h (PO)	Yes	2	10	3.3	No	Major	Yes (H, P)
Isoniazid	5 mg/kg q24h or 300 mg q24h (PO)	Yes	4.5	10	3	Yes	Major	Yes (H, P)
Pyrazinamide	10 mg/kg q8h (PO)	Yes	12	10	10	Yes	Yes	Yes (H)
Rifampin	10 mg/kg or 600 mg q24h (PO)	Yes	7	81-89	3	Yes	Minor	No (H)
CARBAPENEMS								
Doripenem	0.5-1.0 g q8h	—	23	<10	1	No	Yes	Yes (H)
Ertapenem	1 g q24h	—	155	95	4-5	Unknown	Yes	Yes (H)
Imipenem	0.5-1 g q6-8h	—	40	15	1	No	Avoid in severe renal dysfunction	Yes (H)
Meropenem	0.5-2 g q8h	—	50	<10	1	No	Yes	Yes (H)
FIRST-GENERATION CEPHALOSPORINS								
Cefadroxil	1000 mg q12h (PO)	Yes	16	20	1.5	No	Yes	Yes (H)
Cefazolin	0.5-2 g q8h	—	180	80	2	No	Major	Yes (H) No (P)
Cephalexin	250-500 mg q6h (PO)	Yes	18	15	1	No	Yes	Yes (H, P)
Cephradine	500-1000 mg q6-12h	Yes†	140	10	103	No	Yes	Yes (H, P)
SECOND-GENERATION CEPHALOSPORINS								
Cefaclor	250-500 mg q8h (PO)	Yes†	10	25	0.8	No	Yes	Yes (H)
Cefoxitin	1-2 g q6-8h	—	220	70	0.8	No	Yes	Yes (H) No (P)
Cefprozil	250-500 mg q12h (PO)	Yes	10	35	1.4	No	Yes	Yes (H)
Cefuroxime	750-1500 mg q8h	—	100	50	1.5	No	Yes	Yes (H, P)
Cefuroxime axetil	250-500 mg q12h (PO)	Yes	9	50	1.5	No	Yes	Yes (H, P)

TABLE 287-4 DOSAGE REGIMENS OF ANTIBACTERIALS, PHARMACOKINETICS, AND DOSE ADJUSTMENT IN PATIENTS WITH RENAL OR HEPATIC FAILURE—cont'd

CLASS/AGENT	DOSE* FOR SYSTEMIC INFECTION	ORAL FORMULATION	PEAK SERUM CONCENTRATION (μg/mL)	PROTEIN BINDING (%)	NORMAL SERUM HALF-LIFE (hr)	HEPATIC FAILURE	RENAL FAILURE	SERUM LEVELS AFFECTED BY DIALYSIS
THIRD-GENERATION CEPHALOSPORINS								
Cefdinir	300 mg q12h (PO)	Yes	2	65	1.7	Unknown	Minor	Yes (H)
Cefditoren pivoxil	400 mg q12h (PO)	Yes	4	88	1.6	No	Yes	Yes (H)
Cefixime	400 mg q24h (PO)	Yes	3-5	67	3	No	Yes	No (H, P)
Cefotaxime	1-2 g q6-8h	—	200	50	1.5	Minor	Minor	Yes (H), No (P)
Cefpodoxime proxetil	200-400 mg q12h (PO)	Yes	3	25	2.5	No	Yes	Yes (H)
Ceftazidime	1-2 g q8h	—	160	60	2	No	Major	Yes (H, P)
Ceftibuten	400 mg q24h (PO)	Yes	15	65	2.5	Unknown	Yes	Yes (H)
Ceftizoxime	1-2 g q6-8h	—	130	30	1.3	No	Major	Yes (H), No (P)
Ceftriaxone	1-2 g q12-24h	—	250	90-95	8	No	No	No (H)
FOURTH-GENERATION CEPHALOSPORINS								
Cefepime	1-2 g q8h	—	193	20	2	No	Major	Yes (H, P)
Ceftaroline	600 mg q8-12h	—	21.3	20	2.6	No	Major	Yes (H)
PENICILLINS								
Amoxicillin	500 mg q8h (PO)	Yes	10	20	1	No	Yes	Yes (H), No (P)
Amoxicillin–clavulanic acid#	875/125 mg q8-12h	Yes	2.7	25	1.3	Unknown	Moderate	Yes (H, P)
Ampicillin	1 g q6h	Yes+	200	20	1	No	Yes	Yes (H), No (P)
Cloxacillin	500 mg q6h (PO)	Yes+	9	95	0.5	No	No	No (H, P)
Dicloxacillin	500 mg q6h (PO)	Yes+	18	97	0.5	No	No	No (H, P)
Nafcillin	1-2 g q4-6h	—	160	90	0.5	Yes	No	No (H, P)
Oxacillin	1-2 g q4-6h	—	200	90	0.5	Yes	No	No (H, P)
Penicillin G	3-4 million units q4-6h	Yes+	60	60	0.5	No	Yes	Yes (H), No (P)
Penicillin V	500 mg q6h (PO)	Yes	5	80	1	No	No	Yes (H), No (P)
Piperacillin/tazobactam	3.375-4.5 g q6-8h	—	240	50	1	Minor	Minor	Yes (H)
Ticarcillin/clavulanate	3.1 g q4-8h	—	220	50	1	Minor	Major	Yes (H, P)
MONOBACTAMS								
Aztreonam	1-2 g q8h	—	250	60	2	No	Major	Yes (H, P)
QUINOLONES								
Ciprofloxacin	400 mg q8-q12h / 500-750 mg q12h (PO)	Yes+	2-3	30	4	No	Minor	No (H, P)
Levofloxacin	250-750 mg q24h (IV or PO)	Yes	6-9	30	7	No	Yes	No (H, P)
Moxifloxacin	400 mg q24h (IV or PO)	Yes	4-5	50	10	No-minor	No	No (H, P)

TETRACYCLINES, GLYCYLCYCLINES

Drug	Dose							
Doxycycline	100 mg q12-24h (PO) after 200-mg loading dose	Yes	1.5-2.1	93	15-20	Avoid	No	No (H, P)
Minocycline	100 mg q12-24h (PO) after 200-mg loading dose	Yes	2.2	75	15	No	Avoid	No (H, P)
Tetracycline	500 mg q6h (PO)	Yes†	4	50	7	Avoid	Avoid	No (H, P)
Tigecycline	100 mg, then 50 mg q12h	—	0.6-0.9	70	37-38	Minor	No	No (H, P)

SULFONAMIDES

Drug	Dose							
Sulfadiazine	15 mg/kg q6h	Yes	30	50	3	Avoid	Avoid	Unknown
Sulfamethoxazole	0.5-1 g q6-8h (PO)	Yes	100	50	9	Avoid	Major	Yes (H) No (P)
Trimethoprim (with sulfamethoxazole)	3-5 mg/kg q6-8h (based on trimethoprim component)	Yes	3-9	60	10	No	Avoid	Yes (H) No (P)

MACROLIDES, LINCOSAMIDES, KETOLIDES

Drug	Dose							
Azithromycin	500 mg first dose, followed by 250 mg q24h or 500 mg ×3 days (PO) Single-dose therapy of 1-2 g for STIs	Yes†	0.4	25	12-50	Unknown	No	No (H, P)
Clarithromycin	500 mg q12h (PO)	Yes	2-3	70	7	No	Minor	Yes (H) No (P)
Clindamycin	0.3-0.9 g q8h	Yes	15	90	2.5	Minor	No	No (H, P)
Erythromycin	500 mg q6h (PO)	Yes†	1.8	70	2	Minor	No	No (H, P)
Telithromycin	800 mg q24h (PO)	Yes	2	65	10	No	No	No (H)

OTHER AGENTS

Drug	Dose							
Chloramphenicol	0.25-1 g q6h Oral administration produces higher blood concentrations than IV administration.	Yes	8-14	60	1.5	Minor	No	Yes (H) No (P)
Daptomycin	4-6 mg/kg q24h	—	58-100	90	8-9	No	Minor	No (P) Minor (H)
Linezolid	600 mg q12h	Yes	18	30	5	No–minor	No	Yes (H)
Metronidazole	500 mg q6h (anaerobes) 250 mg q8h (trichomoniasis) 750 mg q8h (amebiasis) (IV or PO)	Yes	25	20	8	Yes	No	Yes (H) No (P)
Nitrofurantoin	100 mg q6h (PO)	Yes	Nil	60	0.3	No	Avoid	Yes (H) No (P)
Quinupristin-dalfopristin (30:70)	7.5 mg/kg q8-12h	—	3.2/8§	90/30	3/1§	Minor	No	No (P)
Spectinomycin	2 g/24hr	—	100	0	2	No	Avoid	Unknown
Vancomycin	15 mg/kg q12h	Yes¶	35	50	6	No	Major	No (H, P)

Dose in milligrams per kilogram body weight at hour intervals and/or oral dose in milligrams in patients with normal renal function; all doses are parenteral unless specified PO.

†Significant decrease or delay in absorption when administered with food.

‡Refers to information for clavulanic acid.

§Includes parent compound and active metabolites.

¶Oral vancomycin is not absorbed; it is used for intraluminal therapy only.

H = hemodialysis; P = peritoneal dialysis; STI = sexually transmitted infection.

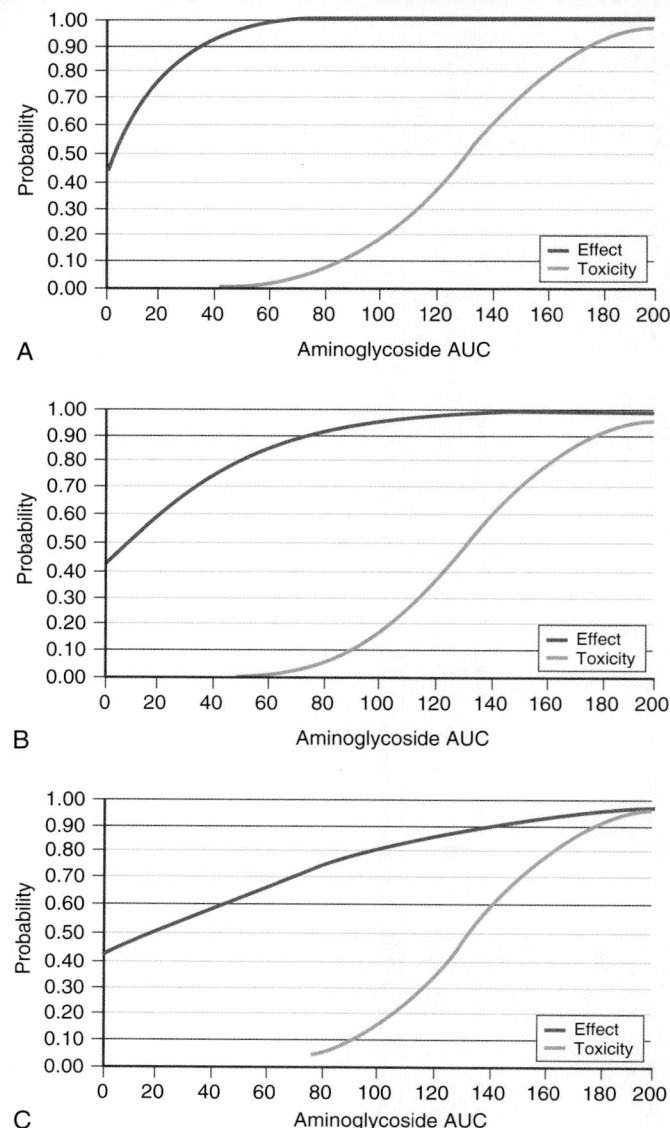

FIGURE 287-2. Probability of clinical effect versus nephrotoxicity as a function of aminoglycoside area under the curve (AUC). **A,** Minimal inhibitory concentration (MIC) = 0.25 mg/L. **B,** MIC = 0.5 mg/L. **C,** MIC = 1.0 mg/L.

than gentamicin or tobramycin. Consequently, their dosages are approximately three- to four-fold higher.

These agents should be thought of as components of combination regimens for seriously ill patients, particularly those thought to be infected by gram-negative organisms, in the empirical therapy setting.

Quinolones

These agents are completely synthetic and do not exist in nature. They are inhibitors (depending on the drug and the organism) of topoisomerases II and IV. This means that they strike at the heart of DNA replication, making them rapidly bactericidal. The use of a fluorine substitution markedly enhanced the microbiologic activity of these drugs, so they became useful for both community-acquired infections (especially urinary tract infections and pneumonia) and hospital-acquired gram-negative infections.

These drugs penetrate well into most spaces, with substantial concentrations inside cells. This makes them active against obligate intracellular pathogens such as *Chlamydophila*, *Legionella*, and *Mycoplasma*. They also penetrate well into spaces with tight junctions (prostate, eye, central nervous system) and into epithelial lining fluid.

Typically, the toxicities associated with these drugs are "off target." A number of these drugs were either withdrawn from the marketplace or given black box warnings by health authorities because of the infrequent

occurrence of torsades de pointes (Chapter 65) or other serious and life-threatening toxicities, such as eosinophilic hepatitis.

These agents are concentration-dependent bacterial killers, indicating that the free drug AUC/MIC ratio is best associated with a regimen's ability to kill bacterial cells. Of interest, particularly for a drug that is completely synthetic, there are a number of resistance mechanisms that allow bacterial escape from drug pressure. The combination of efflux pump overexpression and error-prone replication, resulting in target site mutants as well as serious underdosing for some of the earlier drugs in the class, has resulted in the emergence of considerable resistance, particularly among gram-negative isolates and in the ICU setting.[7]

Macrolides, Tetracyclines, Ketolides, Clindamycin, and Linezolid

These agents bind to different places in the bacterial ribosome, making them inhibitors of protein synthesis and, for the most part, drugs with limited bactericidal activity. An exception may be their activity against *S. pneumoniae*.

Macrolides (particularly clarithromycin and azithromycin) are most useful for community-acquired respiratory tract infections, for two reasons. First, their spectrum is well suited to the classic and atypical pathogens encountered in these patients. Second, they concentrate well in the epithelial lining fluid, with an accumulation that ranges from 6-fold to almost 20-fold that in plasma. This accumulation also partially explains why these agents have fared much better in the respiratory tract setting than in the skin and skin structure setting. Telithromycin, a ketolide, retains activity against many (but not all) macrolide-resistant isolates.

The macrolides and telithromycin are free drug AUC/MIC ratio–driven drugs with respect to bacterial activity, but for different reasons. Telithromycin is somewhat concentration dependent with regard to its microbiologic activity, whereas classic macrolides are not. Telithromycin is more like aminoglycosides or quinolones in terms of the association between exposure indices and bacterial effect. Classic macrolides, especially azithromycin, induce a long persistent or post-antibiotic effect and are *not* concentration dependent in their bacterial effect. This post-antibiotic effect suppresses bacterial regrowth after the drug concentration declines below the MIC until the next dose of drug is administered. In this way, we perceive the linkage to be driven by the free drug AUC/MIC ratio, but with a mechanism different from that of agents whose bacterial kill rate is concentration dependent.

Most of the toxicities seen here are off target and gastrointestinal. However, there is also some elongation of the QT interval (Chapter 54).

Tetracyclines have an exceptionally broad spectrum of activity, including both gram-positive and gram-negative pathogens, and are active against atypical pathogens. The latest incarnation of a tetracycline-type agent (tigecycline, a glycylcycline) has good activity against methicillin-resistant *S. aureus* (MRSA) as well. Tigecycline differs from previous tetracyclines (e.g., doxycycline, minocycline) in that its structure prevents many efflux pumps from removing the drug from the bacteria and also provides a degree of ribosomal protection.

The lincosamide antibiotic clindamycin has a spectrum that covers most clinically significant anaerobes, including many in the *Bacteroides* group (although some resistance is being seen). It is thus a useful agent for infections in which anaerobes play a prominent role, such as lung abscesses and intra-abdominal infections. In many areas of the country, it retains activity against MRSA, but this should be verified with a D-test (inducible macrolide-lincosamide-streptogramin resistance) in the microbiology laboratory. It also has good activity against many streptococci. Because it is a protein synthesis inhibitor, it may provide improved results when the staphylococcal or streptococcal isolate elaborates a great deal of toxin.

Again, most toxicity is off target, with gastrointestinal symptoms being most frequent. Antibiotic-associated diarrhea and the more serious *Clostridium difficile* colitis can occur.

Linezolid is a member of the oxazolidinone class of antibiotics and is a protein synthesis inhibitor. It is distinguished by having excellent gram-positive activity and robust activity against MRSA. It has been used in skin and skin structure infections and has been evaluated in MRSA nosocomial pneumonia. Linezolid penetrates well into skin as well as into the epithelial lining fluid, which is the reason for its evaluation in hospital-acquired MRSA against vancomycin. It is also distinguished by having an oral formulation that is highly bioavailable.

The free drug AUC/MIC ratio is the pharmacodynamic index most associated with cell killing for linezolid. Its toxicity is reflected by dropping counts of bone marrow–derived cells, particularly platelets, seen most frequently

TABLE 287-5 DIVERSE EFFECTS OF ANTIMICROBIAL AGENTS

AGENT	GENERAL	SKIN	GI TRACT	BLOOD CELLS	KIDNEY	NERVOUS SYSTEM	OTHER
Penicillins	Hypersensitivity, anaphylaxis, serum sickness	Rash, urticaria, erythema multiforme	Diarrhea (ampicillin, amoxicillin-clavulanate), hepatitis (oxacillin)	Coombs-positive hemolytic anemia, impaired platelet function (ticarcillin), leukopenia, thrombocytopenia	Nephritis (methicillin), hypokalemia (carboxy- and ureido-penicillins)	Seizures, twitching (high doses, renal failure)	Inactivates aminoglycosides when admixed; possible with concurrent therapy in renal failure
Cephalosporins	Serum sickness (cefaclor), hypersensitivity, anaphylaxis (rare)	Rash, urticaria	Diarrhea, hepatic dysfunction, precipitates in bile (ceftriaxone), mild increase in LFTs	Neutropenia, increased prothrombin time, bleeding (due to MTT side chain), positive Coombs test	Enhances aminoglycoside toxicity, acute renal failure (rare), interstitial nephritis		Disulfiram-like reaction with alcohol use (MTT side chain)
Carbapenems	Hypersensitivity	Rash, urticaria, erythema multiforme	Vomiting with rapid infusion (imipenem), abnormal LFTs	Bone marrow suppression, positive Coombs test	Renal dysfunction	Seizures, myoclonus	
Aminoglycosides	Fever	Rash			Reversible renal failure	Irreversible vestibular toxicity and/or auditory damage, muscle blockade (with anesthetics and myasthenia gravis)	
Vancomycin	Allergy, fever	Rash		Leukopenia, thrombocytopenia	Nephrotoxic	Decreased hearing, neuropathy	Histamine release with flushing and hypotension (infusion <1 hr, antihistamines can prevent)
Quinolones	Headache, allergy, anaphylaxis (rare)	Rash (gemifloxacin), urticaria, photosensitivity (lomefloxacin)	GI distress, abnormal LFTs			Dizziness, insomnia, nervousness, tremors, visual changes, seizures	Tendon rupture arthropathy in young animals
Sulfonamides	Hypersensitivity, anaphylaxis, serum sickness, fever	Rash, Stevens-Johnson syndrome, photosensitivity	Hepatitis	Hemolysis (G6PD deficiency), agranulocytosis, marrow suppression	Crystalluria	Neuropathy	Vasculitis
Trimethoprim ± sulfamethoxazole	Fever	Rash, erythema multiforme, Stevens-Johnson syndrome, TEN	Hepatitis, pancreatitis	Marrow suppression	Hyperkalemia, acute renal failure		
Chloramphenicol	Fever		GI discomfort	Marrow suppression (dose related), aplastic anemia		Optic neuritis, neuropathy	Circulatory collapse (gray baby syndrome in neonates)
Tetracyclines	Hypersensitivity	Photosensitization (doxycycline)	GI discomfort, hepatotoxicity in azotemia or pregnancy		Antianabolic aggravation of azotemia (except doxycycline)	Vertigo (minocycline)	Deposition in bone (dysplasia) and teeth (staining)
Macrolides	Fever	Rash	GI discomfort			Reversible decreased hearing	Phlebitis (IV erythromycin), metallic taste (clarithromycin)
Clindamycin	Fever	Rash	Diarrhea, pseudomembranous colitis				
Metronidazole	Headache, hypersensitivity		Nausea, metallic taste, pancreatitis	Leukopenia		Peripheral neuropathy, ataxia	Mutagenic, carcinogenic in rodents, disulfiram-like reaction with alcohol

GI = gastrointestinal; G6PD = glucose-6-phosphate dehydrogenase; LFT = liver function test; MTT = methylthiotetrazole; TEN = toxic epidermal necrolysis.

with prolonged use. Resistance occurs rarely and is seen with enterococci more frequently than with *S. aureus*. There are five or six gene copies of the target site. As more and more copies become mutated through homologous recombination, the MIC increases almost linearly. Because these mutated targets have some biofitness cost, there is a slow reversion to wild-type targets when therapy is discontinued. If all copies become mutated, however, they cannot revert to wild type. The early detection of MIC changes should lead to the consideration of changing or stopping therapy.

Vancomycin, Quinupristin-Dalfopristin, and Daptomycin

Although structured differently, these agents (along with linezolid) are distinguished by having reliable activity against MRSA.

Vancomycin acts at the cell wall and is bactericidal. The free drug AUC/MIC ratio is the driver of antimicrobial effect. Vancomycin has activity against many gram-positive pathogens and has lately become distinguished for its activity against *C. difficile* when it is administered orally. As with most drugs, wide use has caused the emergence of vancomycin resistance in both enterococci and *S. aureus* (although the latter is rare).

Although vancomycin has a reputation for being a somewhat slow killer, no new agent has significantly outperformed it, at least in trials of skin and skin structure infections. MIC creep has been documented. Although many *S. aureus* isolates were once susceptible with MIC values of 0.25 and 0.5 mg/L, these are now in the distinct minority; 1.0 mg/L represents the modal value, with a few isolates having values of 2.0 mg/L. The higher MICs make these isolates more difficult to treat reliably with standard dosing (1 g IV every 12 hours). Also, it has recently become clear that higher vancomycin doses are associated with a significantly higher risk of nephrotoxicity, even when the agent is administered alone. In addition to nephrotoxicity, vancomycin causes histamine release ("red man syndrome") when it is administered too quickly intravenously. Infusion times of approximately 1 hour are recommended for standard doses.

Quinupristin-dalfopristin is a combination of streptogramin A and streptogramin B antibiotics. Although each is bacteriostatic, the combination can produce some cell killing because the two drugs are synergistic. The synergy is lost, however, with the emergence of resistance to either drug. Further, the amount of bacterial cell killing is modest because of the drugs' rapid half-lives and the imposition of a 12-hour dosing interval. This combination product has activity against resistant enterococci as well as MRSA. Its toxicity includes relatively severe muscle pain in some patients. It is also phlebitogenic and has to be administered with a central venous catheter, limiting its utility.

Daptomycin is a lipopeptide antibiotic discovered in the 1980s and resurrected in the 1990s with a greater understanding of the relationship between exposure and effect versus exposure and toxicity. It was discovered that the antibacterial effect against MRSA was driven by the free drug AUC/MIC ratio. Muscle effects were seen early in its development that limited therapy. Trough concentrations of daptomycin drive this toxicity and can be ameliorated by once-daily dosing (thus minimizing trough concentrations).

This agent has been licensed for skin and skin structure infections and, of note, for complicated *S. aureus* bacteremia and right-sided endocarditis. It also has activity against enterococci. The drug is bound up in epithelial lining fluid by surfactant, excluding its use in the therapy for pneumonia.

Daptomycin may cause muscle toxicity, which is rare, but this may be preceded by the harbinger of an elevated creatine kinase level. The muscle damage is driven by daptomycin trough concentrations, generally above a concentration of about 25 mg/L. Monitoring of creatine kinase concentration is useful in the management of patients receiving daptomycin therapy.

TOXICITIES

All antimicrobials have toxicities. The most common observed toxicities for many antimicrobial agents are presented in Table 287-5.

DURATION OF THERAPY

Relatively little is known about the optimal duration of therapy. Some work has been done to define certain circumstances in which short courses of chemotherapy are effective. For instance, gonorrhea is highly likely to be cured by a single dose of drug (ceftriaxone, cefixime, fluoroquinolones), as long as the organism is susceptible to the drug given.

For trimethoprim-sulfamethoxazole and fluoroquinolones, controlled trials have shown that 3 days of therapy is adequate for uncomplicated urinary tract infections. For β-lactam antimicrobials, a somewhat longer duration is required.

In community-acquired pneumonia, controlled trials with fluoroquinolones have demonstrated optimal results with 5 days of therapy, most likely because of concentration-dependent killing. For bacterial sinusitis, direct sampling from the infected sinus has demonstrated that bacterial pathogens were eradicated by day 3 of therapy or earlier, particularly for *S. pneumoniae* infections.

In ventilator-associated pneumonia, a double-blind comparison of 8 versus 15 days of therapy demonstrated that, with a single exception, clinical outcomes were just as good, there was less emergence of resistance, fewer antibiotics were administered, and there was less toxicity in the group receiving 8 days of therapy. The single exception was when a nonfermenting gram-negative rod was recovered (*P. aeruginosa* or *Acinetobacter* species). In this circumstance, there were significantly more relapses with 8-day versus 15-day treatment, but clinical outcomes were no different.

In some infections, the organisms are slow growing and require more time for control. Both endocarditis and osteomyelitis are examples. Therapy durations of 4 to 6 weeks and occasionally longer may be required for cure in this circumstance.

Finally, one of the longest durations of therapy is seen in the treatment of tuberculosis. In this case, some organisms are in the "non-replicative persister" (NRP) state, indicating that they are not growing or metabolically active. When recovered, they are still fully susceptible to the antimicrobials being used, but while in the NRP state, they cannot be readily killed with current chemotherapy (phenotypic, not genotypic resistance). Therapy durations of 6 months for wild-type organisms and 18 to 24 months for multidrug-resistant tuberculosis are required because of the need to use suboptimal regimens. Indeed, it is a major research goal to find drugs that will readily kill organisms in the NRP state and thus substantially shorten the therapeutic course for *M. tuberculosis*.

FAILURE OF ANTIMICROBIAL THERAPY

Antimicrobial therapy occasionally fails, with failure defined as the persistence of signs and symptoms of infection or the persistence of fever. When one is confronted with failure after what was thought to be adequate antimicrobial therapy, it should set off a sequence of investigations: Did resistance emerge, or did superinfection occur? Is there an obstructed hollow viscus (e.g., urinary or gastrointestinal tract)? Is there an undrained abscess or infected collection (e.g., empyema)? Is there an infected foreign body (e.g., intravenous catheter or prosthesis), or is there devitalized tissue (e.g., sequestrum in osteomyelitis)? Is the fever (if present) attributable to a drug being administered? Thoughtful re-examination should sort out the cause in many instances.

GENERAL REFERENCES

For the General References and other additional features, please visit Expert Consult at https://expertconsult.inkling.com.

288

STAPHYLOCOCCAL INFECTIONS

HENRY F. CHAMBERS

DEFINITION

Staphylococci are well adapted as both commensals and pathogens. Coagulase-negative species constitute a significant proportion of the normal human cutaneous microbiome. *Staphylococcus aureus*, a coagulase-positive species, is present in nasopharyngeal flora in a third of individuals, most of whom will not become infected. As a pathogen, *S. aureus* is one of the most common causes of bacterial infections, which range in severity from relatively trivial skin infections to lethal invasive disease. Coagulase-negative species are intrinsically less virulent and less invasive than *S. aureus* but are responsible for one in four health care–associated infections, frequently involving an indwelling medical device. Prevalence of antibiotic-resistant strains of staphylococci has a profound impact on therapy.

The genus *Staphylococcus* consists of more than 30 distinct species. These organisms have coevolved as normal flora of mammals and birds. They are gram-positive spherical cells (i.e., cocci) 0.5 to 1.5 μm in diameter that divide in multiple planes to form clusters resembling grapes (*staphylo*- is derived from the Greek word for "bunch of grapes") when viewed under the microscope. Staphylococci are nonmotile, nonsporulating, hardy organisms that are resistant to desiccation, extremes of pH, and high salt concentrations and are capable of growth under aerobic or anaerobic conditions. Staphylococci produce catalase, an enzyme that degrades hydrogen peroxide into water and oxygen, which definitively distinguishes them biochemically from streptococci and enterococci. The coagulase test is the basis for differentiating *S. aureus* from the numerous other nonpathogenic, coagulase-negative species. Coagulase is a secreted cell surface protein that, in the presence of a prothrombin-like plasma protein, converts fibrinogen to fibrin, forming a clot. *S. aureus* produces a variety of other species-specific surface proteins (e.g., protein A) that differentiate it from other species.

The staphylococcal chromosome is circular. Approximately 75% of the genes constitute a core genome common to all staphylococcal species. The remaining 25% contains species-defining elements and mobile genetic elements acquired by horizontal gene transfer. The *S. aureus* genome is abundant in genes encoding toxins, superantigens, and adhesins, whereas coagulase-negative species contain few adhesin and no toxin or superantigen genes. Genetically, *S. aureus* is sufficiently uniform to classify it as a single species; greater diversity among coagulase-negative species merits their classification as distinct species.

STAPHYLOCOCCUS AUREUS

EPIDEMIOLOGY

S. aureus is maintained in the human population primarily through asymptomatic colonization of the anterior nares, mucous membranes, and other moist areas of the body as well as of the groin, perineum, and perianal area in healthy children and adults. Infants become colonized by strains from their mothers within weeks of birth. Carriage rates are higher in children than in adults. Higher than average *S. aureus* carriage rates are associated with atopic dermatitis, eczema, chronic skin ulcers, and other acute and chronic skin conditions; insulin-dependent diabetes; dialysis; human immunodeficiency virus infection; and recreational injection drug use. Carriers have a several-fold higher risk for development of a subsequent *S. aureus* infection compared with noncarriers. The principal mode of transmission of *S. aureus* is direct contact with an infected individual or an asymptomatic carrier, probably through transient hand carriage. *S. aureus* may also contaminate environmental surfaces, where it can persist for days. The role of environmental contamination in transmission is not well defined, but it may be important if heavily contaminated surfaces or materials are contacted. Droplet and aerosol transmission of *S. aureus* plays little if any role.

S. aureus is responsible for millions of infections in the United States each year, most of which are community-acquired skin infections. Approximately 5 to 10% of *S. aureus* infections are invasive and are often associated with bacteremia. *S. aureus* also causes hundreds of thousands of health care–associated infections each year, 50 to 60% of which are caused by methicillin-resistant *S. aureus* (MRSA). Before the mid-1990s, MRSA strains were almost exclusively hospital or health care associated, but they have now become prevalent in the community. Community-associated MRSA strains are distinct from classic health care–associated MRSA strains in several ways.

PATHOBIOLOGY

Virulence Factors

S. aureus is highly adapted to humans through millions of years of coevolution with hominids. Well above 50 virulence factors, including adhesins, toxins, enzymes, surface-bound proteins, and capsule polysaccharides, may be produced. Genes encoding virulence factors may be located on the chromosome either as part of the core genome or within mobile genetic elements (or their remnants), including bacteriophages, pathogenicity islands, and cassettes, or on plasmids. Alpha-toxin, Panton-Valentine leukocidin, and phenol-soluble modulins, all of which provoke potentially deleterious host inflammatory response and cause host cell lysis, appear to be important virulence factors mediating disease severity, especially in community MRSA strains.[1] Protein A, a B-cell superantigen that promiscuously triggers B-cell proliferation and supraclonal expansion and apoptosis, interferes with host antibody-mediated adaptive immunity.[2]

Virulence factors serve to promote binding to host tissues; to evade, circumvent, or disrupt host immune responses; and to facilitate cell injury and tissue invasion. Variability in both the presence of virulence determinants and their expression among strains allows extreme diversity among clinical isolates and the remarkable adaptability and versatility of *S. aureus* as a pathogen. An extensive network of two component response systems, DNA-binding proteins and regulatory RNAs, controls the expression of virulence (and other) factors in response to environmental conditions. Principal among these is the accessory gene regulator *agr*, a two-component quorum sensing and global gene regulator that controls the expression of numerous surface and secreted proteins. Mutations in *agr* have been associated with reduced susceptibility to vancomycin and loss of virulence.

Biofilm formation occurs in the presence of foreign material, such as vascular catheters or implanted devices. Biofilm is a complex network of extracellular polysaccharides, DNA, and protein in which bacterial cells become embedded, rendering them inaccessible to clearance by host defense mechanisms. Organisms within biofilms tend to be metabolically inactive and tolerant to killing by antimicrobial agents.

Mechanisms of Disease

Pathogenesis of *S. aureus* disease occurs by two mechanisms: tissue invasion, which may be local or systemic; and toxin mediated. The characteristic lesion of tissue invasion is the abscess, a focal collection of pus (liquefied and necrotic host tissue, blood, inflammatory cells, DNA, and cellular debris) and bacterial cells surrounded by an ill-defined layer of edematous and inflamed tissue infiltrated by acute and chronic inflammatory cells.

Host defenses against *S. aureus* infection primarily consist of an intact, normal skin barrier and the innate immune system. Conditions in which these defenses are impaired are associated with increased risk of *S. aureus* infection. Among these conditions are injection drug use, presence of vascular access devices, burns, chronic skin diseases, use of systemic steroids, traumatic wounds, minor skin abrasions or trauma, surgical procedures, insulin-dependent and non–insulin-dependent diabetes, peritoneal dialysis, hemodialysis, subcutaneous and intramuscular injections, acupuncture, prosthetic implants, and congenital or acquired neutrophil disorders (e.g., chronic granulomatous disease, Job's syndrome). If the cutaneous barrier is breached, the next line of defense is the innate immune system. Neutrophils recruited to the site of infection ingest and kill staphylococci. Staphylococci elaborate numerous virulence factors specifically designed to thwart each step of the host response. If large numbers of organisms are present, the host response is overwhelmed, infection is not contained, and dissemination occurs. Endothelial cell injury and invasion can also occur. Intracellular organisms and small colony variants within phagocytes and endothelial cells may play a role in relapse and persistent bacteremia. High tissue burdens of organisms and bacteremia are usually but not always accompanied by fever, tachycardia, and other signs of the systemic inflammatory response syndrome, including frank septic shock.

The three toxin-mediated syndromes, which can occur in the absence of invasive disease, are staphylococcal food poisoning, staphylococcal toxic shock syndrome, and staphylococcal scalded skin syndrome. Staphylococcal food poisoning is caused by the ingestion of a preformed heat-stable enterotoxin. The emetogenic activity of enterotoxin is mediated by the intestinal release of 5-hydroxytryptamine and the stimulation of receptors present on afferent vagal neurons. Toxic shock syndrome is caused by a specific toxin, TSST-1, or other staphylococcal enterotoxins acting as superantigens that bind to major histocompatibility complex class II molecules of antigen-presenting cells and T-cell receptors, stimulating the massive release of cytokines from T cells and resulting in septic shock and death. Staphylococcal scalded skin syndrome and bullous impetigo are caused by either of two exfoliative toxins, A or B. These toxins are serine proteases that specifically cleave desmoglein 1, a desmosomal protein that anchors the overlying superficial epidermis to the stratum granulosum.

CLINICAL MANIFESTATIONS

Skin and Soft Tissue Infections

Skin and soft tissue infections are by far the most common infections caused by *S. aureus*; millions of cases occur annually in the United States (Chapter 441). Community MRSA strains have been associated with a 50% increase in the rates of skin and soft tissue infections in the United States. This heterogeneous group of skin diseases includes impetigo, folliculitis, furuncle, abscess, erysipelas and cellulitis, mastitis (cellulitis of the breast), necrotizing fasciitis, and wound infections.

Impetigo, folliculitis, and furuncle are superficial infections; fever and other systemic signs of infection are not present. Impetigo is a focal infection of the epidermis that occurs most commonly in children (Fig. 441-1). The typical lesion, which may be multiple or in clusters, is about 1 cm in diameter, with erythema surrounding a bulla or bullae (caused by the production of exfoliative toxin) containing cloudy fluid or with a crusty or scabbed-over appearance. Gram stain of the fluid or drainage from the lesion shows the organism. Folliculitis is a superficial infection with tender, erythematous, maculopapular or pustular lesions centered around hair follicles. Both impetigo and folliculitis readily respond to local measures, such as application of soap and water, topical antibiotics, or antiseptics; systemic antimicrobial therapy may be indicated for extensive or refractory infections.

A furuncle is simply a boil, an erythematous, suppurative infection measuring 1 to 2 cm that extends through the dermis into the subcutaneous tissue (Fig. 441-2). It may drain spontaneously with application of hot compresses or can be surgically drained with simple incision and drainage. Antimicrobial therapy is not needed. The distinction between a furuncle and an abscess is somewhat arbitrary. Abscesses tend to be larger and deeper and may be associated with systemic signs of infection and bacteremia. Furuncles may extend to fascia or deeper tissues and coalesce into carbuncles, a more severe form of infection that may be accompanied by bacteremia. Large abscesses and carbuncles, particularly in the presence of fever and the systemic inflammatory response syndrome, require surgical drainage and systemic antimicrobial therapy.

Erysipelas (Fig. 441-4) and cellulitis, which are similar in appearance, are painful, warm, indurated, erythematous, nonlocalized infections that may be accompanied by lymphangitis. Cellulitis extends into the dermis and subcutaneous fat; erysipelas is more superficial. Surrounding cellulitis is often associated with an obvious cutaneous abscess, but it may also overlie a deeper abscess, in which case the primary therapy is surgical drainage. Cellulitis without an associated abscess should be treated with systemic antimicrobial therapy. Cellulitis due to streptococci (Chapter 290) cannot reliably be distinguished from that caused by S. aureus owing to their similar appearance. The presence of an associated purulent lesion suggests staphylococcal infection.

Necrotizing fasciitis is an infection of the deep layers of skin and subcutaneous tissues, extending to muscle and along fascial planes. It is associated with systemic toxicity, leukocytosis, and severe pain often out of proportion to the physical findings. The overlying skin may appear to be uninvolved, belying the serious nature of this infection, which requires immediate surgical intervention for débridement of involved tissue. Necrotizing fasciitis, which is more typically caused by group A streptococci (Chapter 290) or occurs as a mixed infection, has been associated with community MRSA infection.

Pyomyositis (also termed tropical myositis) is an infection of the skeletal muscle; S. aureus is the most common cause. The patient presents with fever, pain, and swelling and induration that can be felt on deep palpation. The overlying skin and soft tissue may appear normal. There is often a history of trauma to the infected area. Although it can occur in otherwise normal children and adults, acquired immunodeficiency syndrome and other immunocompromising conditions are predisposing factors. This infection is thought to occur as a consequence of metastatic seeding from a subclinical bacteremia, and blood cultures may not be positive at the time of diagnosis. The diagnosis is established by culture of pus collected by needle aspirate. Surgical or percutaneous drainage should be performed, and systemic antimicrobial therapy is indicated.

S. aureus causes 30% of surgical site infections overall in the United States, and approximately 50% of those follow neurosurgical or orthopedic procedures. These infections occur at the site of incision, typically after the second or third postoperative day. Signs and symptoms are fever accompanied by erythema, edema, induration, drainage, pain, and tenderness at the surgical site. Superficial infections respond to removal of stitches, débridement of devitalized tissue, opening of the wound to allow drainage, and a short course of antimicrobial therapy. Deeper infections may require more extensive débridement and longer courses of therapy (4 to 6 weeks), particularly if bone or a prosthetic device is involved. Removal of infected prosthetic material or a foreign body greatly increases the chance of cure.

Bacteremia

Bacteremia, the presence of bacteria in the blood stream, exemplifies the pathogenicity of S. aureus. It is present in approximately 75% of cases of invasive, deep tissue infections. The most common sources of bacteremia are skin and soft tissue infections, central venous catheters and other intravascu-

lar devices, bone and joint infections, pneumonia, and endocarditis. Bacteremia can emanate from any source, which may not be obvious in 25% of cases. Invasion of the blood stream allows the organism to disseminate widely throughout the body, establishing multiple metastatic sites of infection and thereby perpetuating bacteremia. Fever is usually but not always present. Sepsis syndrome and septic shock are common, and death occurs in 10 to 20% of cases. Patients with occult S. aureus bacteremia have high rates of organ failure, septic shock, and intensive care unit (ICU) admissions, prolonged ICU stays, and high mortality.[3]

The presence of bacteremia dictates the approach to the diagnosis, management, and therapy of S. aureus infection. When blood cultures are positive, even if the primary source is known, there is always the possibility of endocarditis or other secondary foci of infection. Echocardiography has been generally recommended in cases of S. aureus bacteremia to look for valvular vegetations or other signs of endocarditis, although its role is evolving.[4] If it is available, transesophageal echocardiography is preferable to transthoracic echocardiography because it has better sensitivity. An echocardiogram should be obtained in cases of complicated bacteremia, defined by the presence of any one of the following: positive blood cultures for 3 days or more, presence of an intracardiac device (e.g., pacemaker, prosthetic valve), presence of a secondary or metastatic focus of infection, relapse or recurrence of S. aureus bacteremia, or clinically suspected endocarditis.

Source control is the cornerstone of management and therapy. Both primary and secondary foci of infection should be identified and eliminated whenever possible because these may lead to treatment failure or relapse once therapy is discontinued. Computed tomography or magnetic resonance imaging should be considered if signs and symptoms point to deep tissue abscesses or osteomyelitis. Follow-up blood cultures should be obtained to document clearance. Persistent bacteremia is suggestive of endovascular infection, and failure to clear blood cultures after 3 to 4 days of appropriate therapy is a strong predictor of complicated bacteremia, necessitating a longer course of therapy. Antimicrobial therapy should always be administered. A shorter duration of therapy (i.e., 14 days) is appropriate for uncomplicated bacteremia (Table 288-1). Longer courses of 4 to 6 weeks are recommended for the treatment of endocarditis or bacteremia complicated by slow resolution or the presence of metastatic infection.

Endocarditis

S. aureus is the leading cause of both native valve and prosthetic valve endocarditis (Chapter 76), accounting for approximately 30% or more of all cases. Most are community-acquired infections, often occurring as a complication of injection drug use. The number of health care–associated infections has been increasing in recent years.[5] Risk factors are diabetes mellitus, hemodialysis, and presence of a prosthetic valve. The presentation is that of an acute febrile illness with high fever developing during a few days. The patient may appear toxic and septic. The intracardiac source of infection may not be evident at first because a pathologic murmur may not be evident when the patient first presents. A quarter or more of patients have an associated infection of bone, joint, or skin and soft tissue. The aortic and mitral valves are most commonly involved in native valve infection except in injection drug users (discussed later). Systemic embolization to the brain, kidneys, spleen, gut, or other large vessels is clinically evident in about one third of cases. Peripheral manifestations, including Roth's spots, Osler's nodes, Janeway's lesions, and petechiae, occur with a similar frequency. Morbidity and mortality are high, in part due to the occurrence of this infection in older patients,

TABLE 288-1	CRITERIA FOR DIAGNOSIS OF UNCOMPLICATED *STAPHYLOCOCCUS AUREUS* BACTEREMIA*

Resolution of fever and systemic signs of infection by day 3 of therapy
Sterile blood cultures within 2 or 3 days of initiation of antimicrobial therapy
Presence of an identifiable and easily removable focus of infection
Prompt removal of the primary focus of infection
No echocardiographic or clinical signs of endocarditis
No osteomyelitis
No hematogenous secondary foci of infection
No preexisting valve abnormalities predisposing to endocarditis (e.g., prosthetic valve, rheumatic heart disease, bicuspid aortic valve)
No implanted prosthetic device (e.g., prosthetic hip)

*Uncomplicated S. aureus bacteremia can be treated with a shorter course of antibiotics (see text).

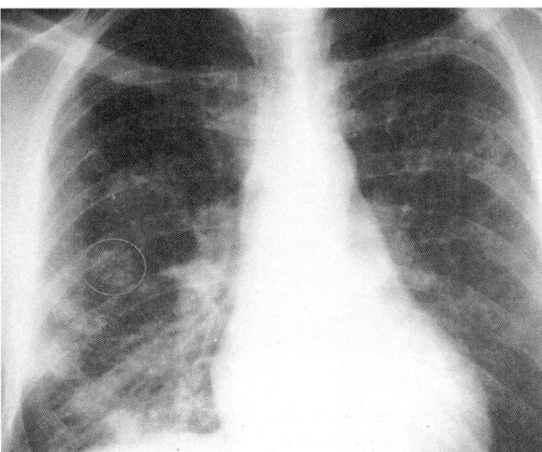

FIGURE 288-1. Chest radiograph shows multiple nodular pulmonary lesions, suggestive of septic embolization, in a patient with tricuspid valve *S. aureus* endocarditis. The *red circle* shows a lesion with signs of cavitation.

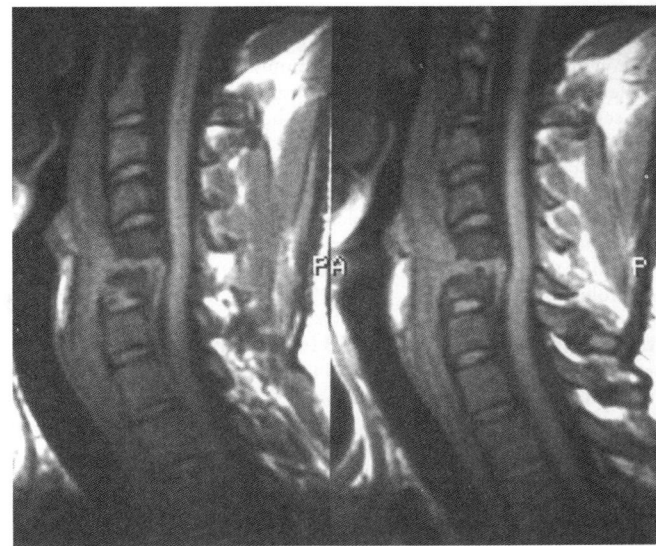

FIGURE 288-2. Noncontrast, non–fat-saturated, T1-weighted, sagittal sequence shows discitis, osteomyelitis, prevertebral and epidural abscess, and cord compression in a patient with *S. aureus* infection of the cervical spine.

many of whom have medical comorbidities. Strokes occur in approximately 20% of patients, and congestive heart failure occurs in 40 to 50%. Twenty-five percent to 30% of patients do not survive the initial hospitalization.

Native valve endocarditis in injection drug users involves the tricuspid valve in approximately three quarters of cases. Patients typically have fever, cough, hemoptysis, and pleuritic chest pain as a consequence of hematogenous seeding of the lung and septic emboli from the valve. The chest radiograph may show pulmonary infiltrates, signs of consolidation or pleural effusion, or multiple, often peripheral nodular pulmonary infiltrates with cavitation, hallmark features of septic embolization (Fig. 288-1). Patients tend to be young and otherwise healthy, so mortality is relatively low, 5% or less. Injection drug users can also have aortic valve or mitral valve endocarditis, in which case the presentation is similar to that described earlier. Conversely, patients who are not injection drug users may have tricuspid valve endocarditis with pulmonary findings.

S. aureus prosthetic valve endocarditis is associated with a 40% or higher in-hospital mortality. Although prosthetic valve endocarditis can be managed medically in some cases, outcomes tend to be worse, and surgery and valve reimplantation are usually required to cure the infection or to manage its complications.[6]

Pericarditis

S. aureus is the most common cause of purulent pericarditis in children and following cardiac surgery in adults. It may occur by contamination at the time of surgery; by bacteremic seeding from another site of infection; as a complication of endocarditis, paravalvular abscess, or myocardial abscess; or by direct extension of infection from pneumonia, lung abscess, or empyema. The presentation is that of acute pericarditis (Chapter 77), with fever and severe chest pain, tachycardia, and hemodynamic instability. The clinical course may be extremely rapid, terminating in septic shock or cardiac tamponade. Immediate drainage of the infected pericardial space and administration of systemic antimicrobial therapy are indicated. Needle pericardiocentesis is useful for confirming the diagnosis and providing temporary decompression of the pericardial space, but definitive therapy requires surgical or continuous tube drainage.

Osteomyelitis

S. aureus is the most common cause of osteomyelitis, both acute and chronic (Chapter 272). The primary mode of infection is hematogenous seeding. Up to a quarter of cases of bacteremia are complicated by osteomyelitis, and concurrent bacteremia is present in 50% or more of osteomyelitis cases. Acute osteomyelitis—defined as an initial episode with a clinical course of days to weeks, but not months—is manifested with fever and pain at the site of infection. Long bones are more commonly infected in children, whereas vertebrae are more commonly infected in adults.[7] Adults can also have long bone osteomyelitis, usually from a contiguous focus of infection or at a site of fracture or prior trauma. Vertebral osteomyelitis is frequently accompanied by paravertebral or epidural abscess (Fig. 288-2). Back pain accompanied by

signs of cord compression, such as radicular pain, sensory loss, lower extremity weakness, urinary retention, and bowel or bladder incontinence, is an emergency. Magnetic resonance imaging should be performed as soon as possible to define the location and extent of infection, and neurosurgical consultation should be obtained in anticipation of surgical decompression and drainage.

Septic Arthritis

S. aureus is the most common cause of septic arthritis (Chapter 272), usually as a consequence of bacteremic seeding, trauma, or a surgical procedure. Risk factors include diabetes, recent joint surgery or joint prosthesis (Chapter 276), and rheumatoid arthritis (Chapter 264). Cardinal features are joint pain, history of joint swelling, and fever. The diagnosis is established by analysis of synovial fluid, in which the white blood cell count typically exceeds 25,000/mm^3, with 90% neutrophils. Blood cultures are positive in 30 to 50% of cases, organisms are seen on Gram stain of synovial fluid in about 50% of cases, and synovial fluid culture is almost always positive. Hip, knee, ankle, and wrist are most commonly affected. *S. aureus* also has a predilection for infecting the sternoclavicular, sacroiliac, and symphysis pubis joints. Multiple joints are involved in 5% of cases. Both antimicrobial therapy and drainage of the infected joint (by repeated needle aspiration, by arthrotomy, or arthroscopically) are required to prevent destructive arthritis.

Central Nervous System Infections

S. aureus is an uncommon cause of community-acquired central nervous system infections, such as bacterial meningitis, primary brain abscess, or subdural empyema. These infections are often associated with endocarditis or a contiguous focus of infection, such as cavernous sinus thrombosis. Mortality of these infections is as high as 30 to 50%. *S. aureus* is an important cause of nosocomial meningitis after head trauma, craniotomy, or implantation of intraventricular or extraventricular catheters.

Pulmonary Infections

S. aureus is an uncommon cause of community-acquired pneumonia (Chapter 97), accounting for 1 to 5% of cases. It is typically a severe, often fatal, fulminant necrotizing pneumonia accompanied by evidence of cavitation on chest radiographs. Production of Panton-Valentine leukocidin has been associated with severe pneumonia. Community-acquired staphylococcal pneumonia should be considered, and coverage for MRSA strains should be included in the empirical regimen, in two clinical settings: severe pneumonia requiring admission to an ICU and pneumonia in a patient with influenza.

Hospital-acquired and ventilator-associated pneumonias often are caused by *S. aureus* and MRSA in particular. Mortality can be as high as 40 to 50%, reflecting the virulence of the organism and the comorbid conditions that contribute to poor outcomes. The diagnosis is readily established by examination of a Gram stain and culture of sputum, tracheal aspirate, or lavage fluid (obtained to avoid oropharyngeal contamination), which typically shows organisms and numerous neutrophils. The culture is less specific than the Gram stain because it can be positive in colonized patients, but it is highly sensitive. Coverage for *S. aureus* can be discontinued if the organism is not isolated in culture.

Lung abscess and pleural empyema, infections most commonly caused by oral anaerobic bacteria, are occasionally caused by *S. aureus*. The clinical course may be subacute or even indolent. Empyema occurs as a complication of prior chest tube placement, surgery, trauma, staphylococcal pneumonia, or tricuspid valve endocarditis. These infections are treated with drainage and antimicrobial therapy.

Orthopedic Device–Associated Infections

Prosthetic joint and implant-associated infections occurring within the first 12 weeks of surgery are most commonly caused by *S. aureus*. *S. aureus* is second only to coagulase-negative staphylococci as a cause of later infections. The presentation may be acute, with joint pain, evidence of arthritis, fever, and systemic signs of infection. Alternatively, the infection may run a more chronic course, with pain and loosening of the prosthesis but little or no fever. Formation of biofilm makes treatment of these infections a challenge. Intraoperative inspection, débridement, and hardware retention may be appropriate for infections of less than 3 weeks in duration or occurring within the first month of implantation.[8] Otherwise, débridement and removal of the prosthesis or implant in conjunction with antimicrobial therapy offer the best chance of cure. This can be accomplished either as a one-stage procedure, in which the infected prosthesis or implant is removed and immediately replaced, or as a two-stage procedure, in which the device is removed and replaced after completion of a 4- to 6-week course of antimicrobial therapy.

Genitourinary Infections

Genitourinary infections arise by hematogenous dissemination or as an ascending infection, usually as a result of instrumentation, urinary catheterization, or surgery. These infections include cystitis, pyelonephritis, microabscess, perinephric abscess, prostatitis, and prostatic abscess. *S. aureus* can also be a contaminant introduced during the collection of urine from a patient with asymptomatic vaginal or perineal colonization. Contamination should be suspected if the urine colony counts are low, repeated urine cultures are negative, pyuria is absent, and there are no signs or symptoms of urinary tract infection. If contamination seems unlikely and there is no well-documented history of an event that could lead to ascending infection, hematogenous dissemination should be suspected. Blood culture samples should be obtained to determine whether there is ongoing bacteremia and appropriate imaging studies performed to identify a deep focus of infection and the presence of renal and perinephric abscesses.

Toxin-Mediated Diseases

These diseases are caused by the ingestion of preformed toxin or the elaboration of toxin by *S. aureus* from a site of colonization or infection. Staphylococcal food poisoning is a gastroenteritis caused by the ingestion of a preformed enterotoxin produced in food contaminated with *S. aureus* from an infected or colonized food handler. When contaminated food is kept at room temperature for several hours, organisms replicate and produce a heat-stable toxin that is not inactivated by cooking or digestive enzymes. Nausea, vomiting, abdominal pain, and diarrhea occur within 2 to 6 hours of eating the contaminated food. There is no fever, and the illness is self-limited, generally lasting about a day. Antibiotics have no role in therapy, which consists of fluid replacement to prevent dehydration. Infants, small children, and the elderly are more severely affected and may require intravenous fluids.

Toxic shock syndrome is caused by colonization or infection with a strain that elaborates a specific toxin, TSST-1, or certain staphylococcal enterotoxins. TSST-1 is responsible for 100% of menstrual cases due to its ability to cross the vaginal mucosa and to achieve systemic concentrations. TSST-1 and the staphylococcal enterotoxins SEA, SEB, and SEC are responsible for nonmenstrual toxic shock syndrome, which is characteristically associated with an identifiable focus of infection, usually of the skin. The diagnosis is clinical, defined by fever, erythroderma, hypotension, involvement of three or more organ systems (renal, hematologic, hepatic, pulmonary, gastrointestinal, muscle, central nervous system, mucous membranes), and desquamation, especially of the palms and soles, 1 to 2 weeks after the onset of illness. Bacteremia is present in only 5% of cases. The case fatality rate is about 5%. Treatment consists of systemic antimicrobial therapy, removal of the source

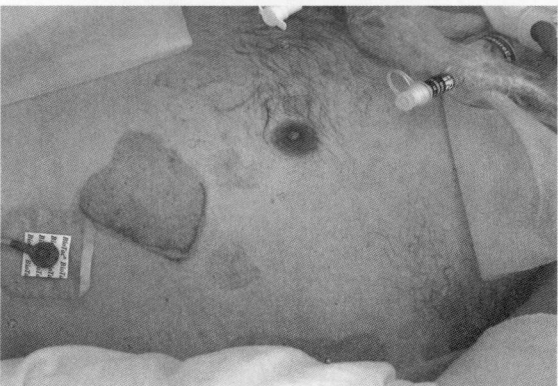

FIGURE 288-3. Scalded skin–type lesions with multiple ruptured bullae and desquamation in a patient with aortic valve endocarditis caused by an exfoliative toxin–producing strain of *S. aureus*.

of toxin production, and treatment of septic shock. Streptococcal toxic shock syndrome is discussed in Chapter 290.

Colonization or infection with an *S. aureus* strain that produces exfoliative toxin A or B may cause staphylococcal scalded skin syndrome, a disease primarily of infants but occasionally seen in adults (Fig. 288-3), and bullous impetigo, a pustular skin lesion. The appearance is that of a scald, burn, or blister. The differential diagnosis of staphylococcal scalded skin syndrome includes drug reaction (Chapter 440), toxic epidermal necrolysis (Chapter 439), Kawasaki disease (Chapter 439), and pemphigus foliaceus (Chapter 439).

DIAGNOSIS

S. aureus infection is diagnosed by isolating the organism in culture specimens of blood, tissue, or pus. Non–culture-based methods, such as nucleic acid amplification tests, are becoming available, but their utility is still being defined.[9] Culture remains the "gold standard." Gram stain is useful for making a presumptive diagnosis of staphylococcal infection and should be performed whenever possible to look for gram-positive cocci in tetrads or clusters in pus, bone or tissue samples, respiratory secretions, or body fluids such as cerebrospinal fluid, pleural or pericardial fluid, synovial fluid, or urine. Failure to isolate the organism in culture is strong evidence against *S. aureus* infection unless a patient is being actively treated with an antibiotic; even then, infected sites may remain culture positive for several days. The specificity of isolating *S. aureus* from blood or other sterile body sites is essentially 100%. Because of nasopharyngeal colonization in some uninfected individuals, isolation of *S. aureus* from culture of a respiratory specimen lacks specificity; however, if Gram stain also shows gram-positive cocci in tetrads and clusters and many neutrophils, this is suggestive of *S. aureus* pneumonia.

Susceptibility Testing

Susceptibility testing should be performed for clinically significant isolates to guide antimicrobial therapy. The critical determination is whether the isolate is methicillin resistant (i.e., resistant to β-lactam antibiotics). Resistance to macrolides and fluoroquinolones is common, and these drugs should not be used to treat suspected staphylococcal infection without confirmation of in vitro susceptibility. Clindamycin is usually active, although macrolide-resistant strains that produce a ribosomal methylase, inducibly or constitutively, are cross-resistant. Tetracyclines and trimethoprim-sulfamethoxazole are active against 80 to 90% of strains. Resistance to vancomycin, daptomycin, telavancin, or linezolid, although rare, may occur, particularly when there has been prior exposure to the drug, making susceptibility testing important for these antibiotics.

TREATMENT

The two principles of therapy for *S. aureus* infections are (1) source control by elimination of focal infection and infected foreign material whenever feasible and (2) administration of systemic antimicrobial therapy. For boils and cutaneous abscesses, incision and drainage may be all that is required. Antimicrobial therapy is indicated if the infection is not amenable to removal (e.g., cellulitis, pneumonia), drainage is impossible or inadequate, systemic signs and symptoms of infection are present, or there is invasive disease (i.e., metastatic sites of infection; involvement of deep tissues, vital organs, sterile sites) and in all cases of bacteremia. An undrained focus of infection or retention of an infected foreign body is the most common reason for unsatisfactory clinical response, treatment failure, or relapse.

The most important consideration in selecting an antibiotic is susceptibility of the *S. aureus* isolate to β-lactams. A penicillinase-resistant penicillin, such as nafcillin (1 to 2 g every 4 to 6 hours IV, depending on the severity of the infection), oxacillin, or flucloxacillin, or a cephalosporin (e.g., cefazolin 1 to 2 g every 8 hours IV) is the agent of choice for the treatment of methicillin-susceptible *S. aureus* (MSSA) infections; no other antibiotic is as safe or as effective as a β-lactam. An orally administered β-lactam (e.g., dicloxacillin 500 mg four times daily or cephalexin 500 mg four times daily) is appropriate for most cutaneous infections; a parenteral agent is recommended, at least initially, for invasive infections. Only if the patient is allergic or has a serious reaction is an agent other than a β-lactam preferred for the treatment of infection caused by an MSSA strain.

Methicillin-resistant strains are cross-resistant to all currently available β-lactams, except for ceftaroline (dose of 600 mg IV every 12 hours), which is indicated for treatment of skin and skin structure infections caused by methicillin-resistant strains. Otherwise, a β-lactam should not be used for treatment of infection known or suspected to be caused by a methicillin-resistant strain. The prevalence of methicillin resistance in *S. aureus* isolates from hospital-acquired and health care–associated infections in the United States and in many European countries is 25 to 50% or higher. MRSA also causes a substantial proportion of community-onset infections in individuals lacking other risk factors, especially in the United States. Trimethoprim-sulfamethoxazole (one or two 80/160-mg tablets twice a day), clindamycin (300 mg three times a day), and doxycycline or minocycline (100 mg twice a day) are active in vitro against most community-acquired MSSA and MRSA strains and are effective when administered orally for the treatment of skin and soft tissue infections in outpatients. Fluoroquinolones should not be used because most methicillin-resistant strains are also fluoroquinolone resistant.

For invasive infections, vancomycin is still a drug of choice.[10] It must be administered intravenously; doses of 30 to 60 mg/kg/day, adjusted on the basis of creatinine clearance, are recommended to achieve trough serum concentrations of 15 to 20 µg/mL for patients with bacteremia, endocarditis, or other serious infections. Treatment failures are not uncommon with bacteremia or endocarditis. Patients can remain persistently bacteremic (≥3 days or longer) or relapse, even when the strain is susceptible (minimal inhibitory concentration [MIC] ≤2 µg/mL) in vitro. Other than the presence of an undrained focus of infection, the reasons for this are unclear. Possible explanations include vancomycin's slowly bactericidal activity; tolerance, in which the isolate is inhibited at low concentrations but not killed; or so-called heteroresistance, in which a small fraction of the population of organisms has a higher MIC. Vancomycin MIC of 2 µg/mL has been associated with treatment failure in some retrospective studies but not in others.[11-13] Strains with intermediate susceptibility to vancomycin (MICs of 4 or 8 µg/mL), which account for 1 to 3% of MRSA isolates, should be considered resistant because this is highly predictive of vancomycin treatment failure. Vancomycin-resistant strains (MIC >8 µg/mL), which express the *vanA* gene, are rare. Alternatives to vancomycin include quinupristin-dalfopristin (7.5 mg/kg every 8 to 12 hours, rarely used because of poor tolerability and limited efficacy data), linezolid (600 mg every 12 hours, Food and Drug Administration [FDA] approved for pneumonia and skin and soft tissue infection), daptomycin (FDA-approved doses of 4 mg/kg once daily for complicated skin and soft tissue infections and 6 mg/kg once daily for bacteremia), telavancin (10 mg/kg once daily, approved for skin and soft tissue infection and pneumonia when alternative treatments are not suitable), and ceftaroline (skin and soft tissue infection). These alternative agents have been shown to be noninferior to vancomycin in high-quality, randomized controlled trials, and none has demonstrated superiority.[A1-A4]

Some authorities recommend higher doses of daptomycin (e.g., 10 mg/kg/day) for treatment of bacteremia or endocarditis, particularly when the infection has failed to respond to vancomycin. Daptomycin should not be used to treat primary staphylococcal pneumonia because it is inactivated by pulmonary surfactant, although it is indicated for treatment of hematogenous pneumonia, as occurs in tricuspid valve endocarditis or septic pulmonary embolization.

The role of combination therapy is ill defined. Aminoglycoside combination regimens have not been shown to improve outcomes, but there are good data demonstrating increased toxicity and adverse events with aminoglycoside combinations. Aminoglycoside combinations should not be used routinely, and if used at all, they should be reserved for patients who have failed to respond to first-line therapy. Rifampin combination therapy is recommended for the treatment of osteomyelitis, device-related bone infection[A5] and prosthetic joint infection, or prosthetic valve endocarditis, particularly those that caused by methicillin-resistant strains of staphylococci. Rifampin (300 to 450 mg twice daily) must always be administered in combination with a second active agent because resistance emerges rapidly during therapy.

PREVENTION

The emergence of community MRSA and the large burden of hospital-acquired and health care–associated staphylococcal infections have stimulated renewed interest in prevention strategies. The organisms that cause these infections are usually resident flora (either *S. aureus* or coagulase-negative staphylococci), or they are acquired by direct contact with a contaminated source, such as a wound or dressing, the skin or hands of an asymptomatically colonized individual, or a contaminated health care provider. The most effective strategy is adherence to principles of basic infection control, the key component of which is hand hygiene, whether it is handwashing or use of an alcohol-based hand rub. This disrupts transmission of organisms by the hands of care providers, a well-documented source of bacterial contamination. Barrier precautions (gloves and gowns) are important for minimizing contact with infected wounds, contaminated secretions, and dressings. Isolation precautions and screening for asymptomatic carriage are more controversial and less well documented in terms of their efficacy. For patients undergoing surgical procedures, surgical hand and surgical site antisepsis, aseptic surgical technique, and antimicrobial prophylaxis are important preventive measures.

Another potentially effective means of preventing infection is screening and decolonization of *S. aureus* carriers. Studies to determine whether screening, decolonization, and isolation actually prevent MRSA infection have had mixed results. In the ICU setting, universal decolonization with 2% chlorhexidine bath cloths and 2% intranasal mupirocin ointment was found to be more effective than targeted screening and decolonization in reducing MRSA rates.[A6] This approach has yet to be widely adopted, and one concern is emergence of resistant strains.

Decolonization may be considered in two other settings: prevention of recurrent infection in individuals who have had several prior episodes and prevention of surgical site infections. The best-studied regimens are topically applied mupirocin nasal ointment (0.5 g twice daily in each nostril for 5 days), with or without bathing with chlorhexidine soap, and orally administered rifampin (600 mg in one or two divided doses) in combination with another active agent (e.g., a fluoroquinolone if the isolate is susceptible, trimethoprim-sulfamethoxazole, doxycycline). In a randomized, double-blind, placebo-controlled, multicenter trial, the number of surgical site *S. aureus* infections acquired in the hospital was reduced by the rapid screening of nasal carriers by a real-time polymerase chain reaction assay and the decolonization of carriers with mupirocin nasal ointment and chlorhexidine soap.[A7] Several antistaphylococcal vaccine candidates are currently in phase I and phase II clinical trials; the availability of an effective vaccine would be an important tool in preventing staphylococcal infections.

PROGNOSIS

Prognosis of *S. aureus* infections and outcomes depend on the site of infection, adequacy of source control, presence of comorbidities (e.g., diabetes; immunosuppression; underlying cardiac, renal, or liver disease), presence of bacteremia, presence of secondary foci of infection, presence of severe sepsis or septic shock, antibiotic effectiveness, and duration of therapy for complicated disease. Methicillin resistance is a risk factor for poorer outcome largely because of its health care association, and thus occurrence in a population that is elderly and in which comorbid medical illnesses are prevalent, and possibly because less effective antibiotics (non–β-lactams) are used to treat these infections. Historically, untreated *S. aureus* bacteremia was lethal in 85% or more of cases. Antibacterial therapy, 4 to 6 weeks or longer for complicated bacteremia or infections of deep tissues, and recognition of the importance of source control have dramatically improved outcome. Mortality remains high, in the range of 20 to 40%, in patients with severe sepsis, septic shock, or endocarditis.

COAGULASE-NEGATIVE STAPHYLOCOCCI

More than 30 different species of coagulase-negative staphylococci have been identified, and about half of these colonize humans. *Staphylococcus epidermidis* is the species that most commonly causes infection. Coagulase-negative staphylococci infrequently cause infection unless there is a foreign body in place, and although bacteremia occurs, metastatic seeding of secondary sites of infection is distinctly uncommon. Coagulase-negative staphylococci are typically resistant to methicillin and multiple other antibiotics, and they are an important reservoir of drug resistance elements that are horizontally transferrable to *S. aureus*. They are the most common cause of health care–associated infections overall in the United States (Chapter 282); they account for one third of central line–associated blood stream infections; and they are the second most common cause of surgical site infections, particularly when a prosthetic device or other foreign material has been implanted. Infections are often indolent, causing little in the way of fever or systemic signs of infection, but they may also be acute and life-threatening, as in the case of prosthetic valve endocarditis. Coagulase-negative staphylococci are proficient biofilm producers; consequently, débridement and removal of the infected prosthetic device or foreign body are paramount. Prosthetic joint infections occurring more than 1 month after device implantation are best managed with removal of the prosthesis and reimplantation in a one-stage or two-stage procedure. Antimicrobial therapy for these infections is similar to that for *S. aureus*, except that hematogenous seeding rarely occurs, so attention is focused primarily on source control.

Coagulase-negative staphylococci, because they are normal skin flora, are the most common blood culture contaminant. In approximately 75% of cases, when the blood culture is positive for coagulase-negative staphylococci, this reflects contamination rather than infection. Sorting out whether a positive culture represents contamination or true infection can be a challenge. A single positive blood culture or blood cultures in which more than one strain is present are likely to be due to contamination. Time to blood culture positivity, quantitative blood cultures, and the presence of multiple positive cultures can be useful in determining whether a positive blood culture represents true infection. Isolation of coagulase-negative staphylococci from the blood of a patient with a prosthetic valve, intravenous pacemaker, or vascular graft can be especially problematic because these patients are at high risk for true infection. Unless the patient is hemodynamically unstable or otherwise seriously ill, it is advisable to withhold antibiotics until additional culture specimens are obtained to document the presence of true bacteremia. Isolation of coagulase-negative staphylococci from culture specimens of deep tissue, bone, prosthetic devices, or other normally sterile sites, especially if multiple cultures are positive, strongly suggests true infection.

Staphylococcus lugdunensis, in contrast to other coagulase-negative staphylococci, is pathogenic and causes infections in the absence of a foreign body and in otherwise normal hosts that clinically resemble *S. aureus* infections. These include prosthetic valve and native valve endocarditis, bacteremia, skin and soft tissue infection, septic arthritis, prosthetic joint infection, and osteomyelitis. It lacks free coagulase, but some strains produce a membrane-bound form that can lead to its misclassification as *S. aureus*. *S. lugdunensis* lacks protein A and is positive for ornithine decarboxylase and pyrrolidonyl arylamidase, differentiating it from *S. aureus*. *S. lugdunensis* is susceptible to most antibiotics, including penicillin (approximately 75% of isolates), and resistance to nafcillin and oxacillin is rare. The management of these infections is similar to that of *S. aureus* infections.

Grade A References

A1. Wang Y, Zou Y, Xie J, et al. Linezolid versus vancomycin for the treatment of suspected methicillin-resistant Staphylococcus aureus nosocomial pneumonia: a systematic review employing meta-analysis. *Eur J Clin Pharmacol.* 2015;71:107-115.
A2. Fowler VG Jr, Boucher HW, Corey GR, et al. Daptomycin versus standard therapy for bacteremia and endocarditis caused by Staphylococcus aureus. *N Engl J Med.* 2006;355:653-665.
A3. Corey GR, Wilcox MH, Talbot GH, et al. CANVAS 1 investigators. CANVAS 1: the first Phase III, randomized, double-blind study evaluating ceftaroline fosamil for the treatment of patients with complicated skin and skin structure infections. *J Antimicrob Chemother.* 2010;65(suppl 4): iv41-iv51.
A4. Rubinstein E, Lalani T, Corey GR, et al. ATTAIN Study Group. Telavancin versus vancomycin for hospital-acquired pneumonia due to gram-positive pathogens. *Clin Infect Dis.* 2011;52:31-40.
A5. Zimmerli W, Widmer AF, Blatter M, et al. Role of rifampin for treatment of orthopedic implant-related staphylococcal infections: a randomized controlled trial. Foreign-Body Infection (FBI) Study Group. *JAMA.* 1998;279:1537-1541.
A6. Huang SS, Septimus E, Kleinman K, et al. CDC Prevention Epicenters Program; AHRQ DECIDE Network and Healthcare-Associated Infections Program. Targeted versus universal decolonization to prevent ICU infection. *N Engl J Med.* 2013;368:2255-2265.
A7. Bode LG, Kluytmans JA, Wertheim HF, et al. Preventing surgical-site infections in nasal carriers of Staphylococcus aureus. *N Engl J Med.* 2010;362:9-17.

GENERAL REFERENCES

For the General References and other additional features, please visit Expert Consult at https://expertconsult.inkling.com.

289

STREPTOCOCCUS PNEUMONIAE INFECTIONS

LIONEL A. MANDELL

DEFINITION

The term *pneumococcal pneumonia* refers to infection of the pulmonary parenchyma and its associated structures by *Streptococcus pneumoniae*. There are an estimated 5 million cases annually worldwide, and community-acquired pneumonia (CAP) of all etiologies is the commonest cause of death from infection in the United States and Europe.[1]

The Pathogen

S. pneumoniae is a gram-positive coccus that typically grows in pairs or short chains. Careful examination of the diplococcal form reveals slightly tapered ends that give rise to its lancet-shaped appearance. It is a facultative anaerobe that grows best on blood agar plates in a 5% carbon dioxide ambient environment. The colonies are typically surrounded by a greenish zone of hemolysis resulting from degradation of hemoglobin by a pneumococcal toxin. The organism can be distinguished from other streptococci by its susceptibility to ethyl hydrocupreine (Optochin) and bile solubility.

The surface of the pneumococcus consists of a capsule and a cell wall. The capsule, which helps prevent phagocytosis, is composed of polysaccharides that define at least 92 different pneumococcal serotypes. The cell wall is a dynamic structure composed of more than a dozen distinct glycopeptides.

EPIDEMIOLOGY

The pneumococcus is one of the most common causes of CAP and can cause hospital-acquired and health care–associated pneumonia as well.[2] The false impression that *S. pneumoniae* is uncommon has arisen because at least one third of patients with CAP are unable to produce sputum and, even if they do, often provide an inadequate sample. Moreover, if the patient has recently taken just one dose of a drug to which the pneumococcus is susceptible, it may not be possible to isolate the organism.

The ecologic niche of the pneumococcus is the nasopharynx, and up to 80% of infants and 20% of healthy adults may be colonized. Colonizing and invasive strains of pneumococci have developed adaptive mechanisms allowing them to escape host responses. Simultaneous colonization with more than one capsular type has been reported. The horizontal transfer of genes that can occur can expand the gene pool of the colonizing pneumococci, thereby enhancing their adaptive abilities and virulence properties. Asymptomatic colonization is an immunizing experience because homologous anticapsular antibodies may be demonstrated in individuals after colonization with a specific serotype.

A particular serotype may colonize the nasopharynx for varying periods, but the average duration in infants is 7 weeks. Carriage rates are highest during the late fall, winter, and early spring. Although each of the 92 serotypes is potentially pathogenic, the most frequently encountered are types 3, 4, 6, 7, 9, 12, 14, 18, 19, and 23.

Person-to-person transmission results from close interpersonal contact. Although pneumococcal pneumonia is typically a sporadic illness, epidemics can occur in crowded settings such as daycare centers, barracks, nursing homes, and prisons.

The incidence of pneumococcal pneumonia is about 18 per 100,000 people per year. For persons 5 years or younger and 75 years or older, rates are about 23 and 35.8 per 100,000 people, respectively. For pneumococcal bacteremia, the incidence is about 7.5 per 100,000 people per year and increases with age; the case-fatality rate is 21%.

Risk factors for pneumococcal pneumonia include dementia, seizure disorders, heart failure, cerebrovascular disease, chronic obstructive pulmonary disease (COPD), human immunodeficiency virus (HIV) infection, previous viral respiratory illness, alcoholism, malnutrition, diabetes, cirrhosis, and renal insufficiency.

Certain ethnic groups such as Native Americans, particularly Alaskan natives, and Australian Aboriginals, appear to be particularly susceptible to invasive pneumococcal infection. Any individual who has a defect in immunoglobulin G (IgG) synthesis (Chapter 250) or phagocyte function (Chapter 169) or who has undergone splenectomy is also at increased risk for invasive pneumococcal infection.

PATHOBIOLOGY

Pneumonia is the result of a breakdown in the interplay between colonizer and host as well as pneumococcal virulence factors that can influence both colonization and invasion. In pneumococcal pneumonia, the microorganism first colonizes the nasopharynx. Aspiration of small amounts of oropharyngeal contents occurs in deep sleep, even in normal individuals, but if the oropharyngeal material includes pneumococcal serotypes associated with invasive infection and if normal clearance mechanisms fail, the colonizers may become pathogens. Whether or not a particular pneumococcus results in active infection is related to a number of virulence factors that allow it to avoid or mitigate host defenses and to attack host cells. These include capsular polysaccharides, which allow avoidance of opsonophagocytosis; exoglycosidases, which enable access to cell receptors and choline-binding proteins; and divalent metal-ion binding lipoproteins, which can act as adhesins. Autolysins can cause lysis of host cells and pneumolysin, and choline-binding proteins may enable the pathogen to gain access to the vascular system, potentially resulting in bacteremia and metastatic infection.[3] The risk for infection is increased by any process or condition that exposes the host to the pathogen, that allows oropharyngeal secretions to bypass upper airway defenses, or that interferes with the host's ability to ingest and kill the pneumococci (Table 289-1).

It appears that aspirated pneumococci adhere to type II cells in the alveolus if they are not cleared by normal defense mechanisms. Attachment to resting cells is mediated by two classes of glycoconjugates, but local inflammatory mediators upregulate host cell receptors, such as those for platelet-activating factor (PAF), and provide a site of attachment for the bacteria. This interaction between PAF receptor and pathogen appears to be an important step in internalization of the bacteria by means of an endocytic vacuole and may promote invasion. Expression of pili by certain pneumococcal strains facilitates binding to epithelial cells and results in a more vigorous tumor necrosis factor (TNF)–dependent inflammatory response, which can cause further tissue damage.

In the lung, the pneumococci are able to activate complement and stimulate the cytokine response. Initially, the alveoli fill with fluid exudate (Fig. 289-1), which allows the infection to spread to adjacent uninfected alveoli. In healthy lungs, polymorphonuclear leukocytes (PMNs) constitute less than 1% to 2% of alveolar cells and normally reside in the interstitial areas of the lung and in adjacent capillaries. Recruitment of PMNs into alveoli depends on the generation of chemoattractants necessary for the directed migration of neutrophils.

Ultimately, the signs and symptoms of disease are both attributable to the pathogens themselves and to the body's response to them. The bacterial cytotoxin pneumolysin and various pneumococcal cell wall components are able to induce a variety of effects that initiate and then enhance the inflammatory response, thereby resulting in the various signs and symptoms of pneumonia.

The effects of pneumococcal infection are ultimately manifested as changes in lung mechanics secondary to reductions in lung volumes and lung compliance, as well as gas exchange problems resulting from intrapulmonary shunting and subsequent arterial hypoxemia. If severe enough, death may ensue.

Antibiotic Resistance

The phenotypic expression of antibiotic resistance corresponds to genetic alterations resulting from horizontal acquisition of foreign genetic information or from mutations in the microbial genome. The impact of antibiotic resistance as documented in vitro is not as straightforward as one might imagine, and there is not a direct relationship between resistance and clinical outcomes.

With *S. pneumoniae*, resistance may be acquired by direct DNA incorporation and remodeling from closely related oral commensal bacteria by the process of natural transformation. Pneumococcal resistance to β-lactams such as penicillin is solely attributable to the presence of low-affinity penicillin-binding proteins (PBPs). Increasing the concentration of the β-lactams can usually overcome such resistance. Revision of the break points for resistance in nonmeningeal isolates has resulted in a lower prevalence of penicillin resistance than was previously reported.[4] The PBPs themselves are *trans* and carboxypeptidase enzymes that are involved in bacterial cell wall synthesis and represent the primary sites of action for β-lactam drugs.

Resistance to macrolides, in contrast, can occur through multiple mechanisms, including target site modification or an efflux pump. Target site modification is caused by a ribosomal methylase encoded by the *ermB* gene. A change in 23S recombinant RNA mediated by this gene can result in resistance to macrolides, lincosamides, and streptogramin B–type antibiotics (MLS_B phenotype). The efflux mechanism is encoded by the *mefA* gene, which results in an M phenotype. The former is typically associated with high-level resistance with minimal inhibitory concentrations (MICs) of 64 μg/mL or higher, but the latter is usually associated with low-level resistance with MICs of 1 to 32 μg/mL. These two mechanisms account for approximately 45% and 55%, respectively, of resistant isolates. Clonal dissemination is important in the spread of macrolide resistance. Some pneumococcal isolates have been found with both the *erm* and *mef* genes, but the significance of such a finding is unknown.

Resistance to fluoroquinolones may be mediated by changes in one or both target sites (topoisomerase II and IV) of the pneumococcus, which usually result from mutations in the *gyrA* and *parC* genes, respectively. Low-level resistance may result from changes in one site, but high-level resistance can result when dual mutations occur. An efflux pump may have a role as well. Also of concern is the fact that the incidence of multidrug-resistant isolates is increasing.

TABLE 289-1	PREDISPOSING FACTORS FOR PNEUMOCOCCAL PNEUMONIA

INCREASED EXPOSURE TO *STREPTOCOCCUS PNEUMONIAE*

Prisons
Military barracks
Daycare centers
Shelters for the homeless

DECREASED HOST DEFENSES

Complement deficiency
Antibody deficiency
Functional or anatomic asplenia
Decreased numbers or function of phagocytes

SPECIFIC DISEASE ENTITIES

Multiple myeloma
Lymphoma
Chronic lymphocytic leukemia
Human immunodeficiency virus infection

RESPIRATORY AND PULMONARY PROBLEMS

Chronic obstructive pulmonary disease
Smoker
Allergies
Previous viral infection

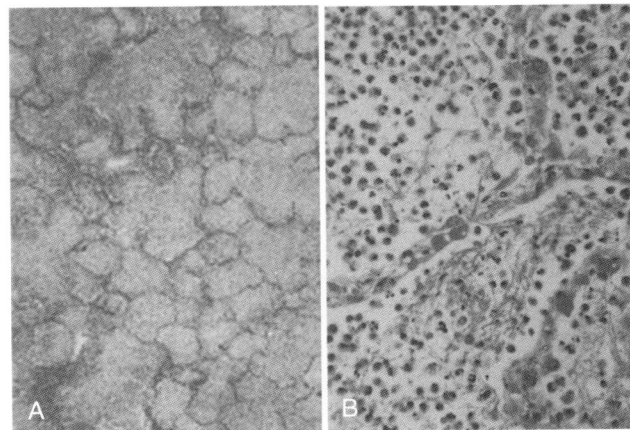

FIGURE 289-1. Pneumonia. **A,** Low-power magnification (×100) of hematoxylin and eosin (H&E) stain of tissue section from the left lower lobe of the lung. Note the intact alveolar walls and alveoli filled with edema and thick cellular exudates. **B,** Higher magnification (× 500) H&E stain of the same section shown in A. Note the heavy infiltrate of polymorphonuclear cells and the intact alveolar walls.

CLINICAL MANIFESTATIONS

The clinical features of pneumococcal pneumonia depend on factors such as whether the patient is immunocompetent or immunosuppressed, the severity of illness, and whether the patient has taken antibiotics. Temperatures can vary from 101° F to higher than 103° F (38° to 39.5° C), can be accompanied by chills and rigors, and are usually associated with a tachycardic response. A cough, typically productive of purulent and occasionally blood-tinged sputum, is often present, and as many as 46% of patients report chest pain. About 20% have gastrointestinal symptoms such as nausea, vomiting, or diarrhea. In elderly people, symptoms and signs may be more subtle; for example, older patients may have predominantly confusion.

On examination, the patient is often listless and may be cyanotic. The respiratory rate is increased; if pleuritic pain is marked, the patient may be splinting the affected side. Whereas dullness to percussion over a lung segment suggests consolidation, a flat percussion note is typically associated with a pleural effusion. Breath sounds may be "distant" if there is an overlying effusion, but they are bronchial in nature if the underlying lung is consolidated. Rales may be noted. If the patient has pleurisy without much pleural fluid, a friction rub may be heard.

No radiographic appearance is characteristic of pneumococcal pneumonia (Chapter 97). Typically, however, involvement is limited to one or more segments within a single lobe. Involvement is unilateral approximately 80% of the time, and the presence of cavitation or lung abscess is uncommon. Among patients with pneumococcal pneumonia, necrotizing changes in the lungs were seen in 6.6% of cases in a large series but were often overlooked on initial readings of chest radiographs or computed tomography (CT) scans. Forty-five percent of patients have an associated pleural effusion, but only 15% have an effusion of sufficient size to warrant drainage (>10 mm on lateral decubitus views). Purulent pericarditis can also be seen (Chapter 77).

Patients with lobar consolidation are more likely to be bacteremic, but there are no consistently significant differences in the radiologic manifestations of bacteremic and nonbacteremic pneumococcal pneumonia. Bacteremic pneumococcal pneumonia may seed distant sites and cause meningitis (Chapter 412), endocarditis (Chapter 76), or septic arthritis (Chapter 272).

With sepsis, sepsis syndrome, or septic shock (Chapter 108), the patient may be hypotensive, and the findings of organ failure vary depending on the target organ(s) involved. For example, oliguria, anuria, and acidosis suggest renal failure; myocardial impairment suggests heart failure; and jaundice is consistent with hepatic failure. Systemic activation of coagulation together with consumption of clotting proteins can result in simultaneous clotting and bleeding (Chapter 175). In some cases, peripheral gangrene and purpura fulminans may be seen.

DIAGNOSIS

Despite extensive testing, a specific etiologic agent is not found in 50% or more of patients with CAP. The history, physical examination, chest radiograph, sputum Gram stain, and blood and sputum cultures are insensitive and lack specificity, but more invasive methods (e.g., endotracheal aspirate, bronchoscopy techniques, pleural fluid aspiration, and lung biopsy) require special expertise and are infrequently indicated. As a general rule, routine diagnostic tests to identify a pathogen are optional for outpatients with CAP, but more extensive testing is recommended for hospitalized patients (Table 289-2).[5]

Ultimately, the diagnosis should be based on suggestive clinical features and a chest radiograph with or without corroborating microbiologic data. Because *S. pneumoniae* is the most common etiologic agent of CAP, virtually any recommended treatment regimen must provide adequate coverage for it,

TABLE 289-2	INDICATIONS FOR MORE EXTENSIVE DIAGNOSTIC TESTING IN COMMUNITY-ACQUIRED PNEUMONIA

Intensive care unit admission for community-acquired pneumonia
Failure of outpatient treatment
Radiographic appearance of cavities on initial evaluation
Infection resulting in neutropenia
Alcohol abuse
Chronic severe liver disease
Severe chronic obstructive lung disease
Asplenia (anatomic or functional)
Recent travel (within 2 weeks)
Positive rapid *Legionella* spp. or pneumococcal urinary antigen test result
Pleural effusion

so documentation of its presence has little or no effect on ultimate clinical outcomes. From the point of view of epidemiology and antimicrobial susceptibility, however, documentation of a pathogen is desirable.

The sputum Gram stain is a relatively simple and inexpensive procedure to document the presence of certain pathogens. The adequacy of the specimen is based on the relative number of neutrophils and squamous epithelial cells (SECs). There should be at least 25 neutrophils and fewer than 10 SECs per low-power field (×100 magnification). The sensitivity of sputum Gram stain for *S. pneumoniae* is 55%, but the specificity is higher than 80%. Unfortunately, approximately 30% of patients overall are unable to produce an appropriate sputum sample. In elderly patients, this figure reaches almost 70%. Overall, only 28% at best of sputum samples are of good quality. Sputum cultures are neither sensitive nor specific, particularly when dealing with relatively fastidious pathogens such as *S. pneumoniae*.

Blood cultures are positive in only 5% to 14% of patients with CAP. If patients have taken a previous dose of antibiotic, culture results are even less useful. As a result, sputum Gram stain, sputum culture, and blood cultures are generally recommended only in patients with selected clinical indications (see Table 289-2). In patients with severe CAP, an expectorated sputum sample should be replaced by an endotracheal aspirate sample if the patient is intubated.

Pneumococcus can also be detected by polymerase chain reaction (PCR), but this is not done routinely and there currently is no evidence that such testing will change clinical outcomes.[A1] Nevertheless, an increased pneumococcal bacterial load demonstrated by real-time PCR is associated with an increased risk for septic shock, need for mechanical ventilation, and death, suggesting that such a test may be of help in identifying patients suitable for care in the intensive care unit.[6] Pneumococcal capsular polysaccharide can be detected in urine, and this may occasionally be helpful for diagnosis after antibiotic therapy has been started. The overall sensitivity of the pneumococcal urinary antigen test is less than 80% but can reach 90% or higher in patients with pneumococcal bacteremia and those with high-risk pneumonia. The specificity in adult patients with CAP can exceed 95%. Detection of antibody to pneumococcal polysaccharide is not useful.

Newer methods which may help in the diagnosis of pneumococcal pneumonia include real-time polymerase chain reaction (RT-PCR) to detect pneumococcal DNA in blood and the use of host biomarkers such as C-reactive protein (CRP) and procalcitonin (PCT).[7] These are acute phase reactants which increase in the presence of an inflammatory response, particularly to bacterial pathogens. CRP may help to identify worsening disease, and PCT may help in determining the need for antibacterial therapy.

PREVENTION

Two types of pneumococcal vaccines are available, each with its own particular advantages and disadvantages.[8]

Polysaccharide Vaccine

A polysaccharide vaccine contains 25 μg of each of the 23 capsular polysaccharides that account for 90% of invasive infections (Chapter 18). Polysaccharide vaccines stimulate B-cell responses, thereby resulting in type-specific antibody production that enhances ingestion and killing of the pathogens by phagocytes. The antigens, however, are T-cell independent and therefore do not result in long-lasting immunity. Two types of polysaccharide vaccine have been available, Pneumovax (Merck) and Pnu-Imune (Lederle).

The effectiveness of the pneumococcal polysaccharide vaccine ranges from 56% to 81%. Data suggest that it is effective in preventing both pneumococcal and all-cause pneumonia.[A2] A randomized trial demonstrated that the immunogenicity of the 23-valent polysaccharide vaccine is comparable to that of the 7-valent pneumococcal conjugate vaccine (see later) in frail, hospitalized, elderly patients.[A3] It is not effective in immunocompromised patients, such as those with sickle cell disease, chronic renal failure, immunoglobulin deficiency, Hodgkin's disease, non-Hodgkin's lymphoma, leukemia, and multiple myeloma.. The vaccine is recommended for (1) persons 65 years or older; (2) persons 2 to 64 years old with chronic illnesses such as cardiovascular disease, chronic pulmonary disease (not asthma), diabetes mellitus, alcoholism, chronic liver disease, or cerebrospinal fluid leaks; (3) persons 2 to 64 years old with functional or anatomic asplenia; and (4) persons 2 to 64 years old living in special environments or social settings (Alaskan natives, certain Native American populations, residents of long-term care facilities).

Although the effectiveness of the vaccine is less in these subgroups, the following immunocompromised patients 2 years or older should also be immunized: (1) persons with HIV infection, leukemia, lymphoma, or Hodgkin's disease and (2) those with multiple myeloma, generalized malignancy, chronic renal failure, nephrotic syndrome, or organ or bone marrow transplants and individuals being treated with immunosuppressive chemotherapy, including steroids.

The lack of an anamnestic response with polysaccharide vaccines means that antibody levels decrease over time, and revaccination is required. Although the exact timing is unclear, most experts suggest revaccination at 5 years. For immunocompetent persons 65 years or older, a second dose is suggested if the patient was given the first vaccine 5 years earlier at an age younger than 65 years. For persons 2 to 64 years of age with asplenia, a single revaccination is suggested 5 years after the initial dose if the patient is older than 10 years. However, if the patient is younger than 10 years, revaccination should be given 3 years after the first dose. For immunocompromised patients, revaccination should be given 5 years after the first dose if the patient is older than 10 years and 3 years after the first dose if the patient is younger than 10 years.

Conjugated Vaccine

This vaccine contains capsular polysaccharide from 13 of the most frequent pneumococcal pathogens affecting children linked to an immunogenic protein, thereby producing T cell–dependent antigens, which results in long-term immunologic memory. A heptavalent vaccine was effective in reducing the risk of pneumonia in young children. Use of a 7-valent vaccine resulted in an overall decrease in the prevalence of antimicrobial resistant pneumococci and in the incidence of invasive pneumococcal disease in both children and adults and with replacement with nonvaccine serotypes such as 19A and 35B. As a result, in 2010, the U.S. Food and Drug Administration licensed a new 13-valent pneumococcal conjugate vaccine to replace the 7-valent vaccine. Overall data demonstrate a superior antibody response in adults vaccinated with the 13-valent pneumococcal conjugate vaccine compared with the pneumococcal polysaccharide vaccine, whether or not they were previously vaccinated with the latter.[9] This vaccine is recommended for children, elderly adults, and younger immunocompromised patients.[10]

TREATMENT Rx

A number of prediction rules have been developed to help determine the appropriate site of care. This step, together with optimal antimicrobial therapy and supportive measures, can help to maximize chances for a satisfactory outcome.[11]

Empirical therapy is usually used for CAP. If pneumococcal infection can be documented, however, antibiotic therapy can be targeted against this specific pathogen.

Treatment Regimens
Directed Therapy Against Known *S. pneumoniae*

S. pneumoniae can be treated with a number of antimicrobials, including various β-lactams, macrolides, and selected fluoroquinolones (Table 289-3). Resistance has been described for virtually all of these agents, and the prevalence of resistant serotypes has risen since the introduction of the 13-valent conjugate vaccine.[12] For nonmeningeal infections such as pneumonia, susceptibility is now defined by a penicillin MIC of 2 µg/mL or less, intermediate as an MIC of 4 µg/mL, and resistant as an MIC of more than 8 µg/mL. Multidrug-resistant pathogens, which are resistant to three or more antimicrobial agents with different mechanisms of action, have been seen in a number of countries. Risk factors for drug-resistant pneumococcal infection include recent antimicrobial therapy, age younger than 2 years or older than 65 years, attendance at a daycare center, recent hospitalization, and HIV infection.

If a good-quality Gram stain of sputum reveals sheets of PMNs with lancet-shaped gram-positive diplococci as the only organism, if the patient has no risk factors for infection with resistant *S. pneumoniae*, and if the patient is not living in an area endemic for penicillin-resistant *S. pneumoniae*, it is reasonable to initiate parenteral treatment with penicillin G, 2.4 million U/day. For outpatients, oral therapy is usually given in the form of amoxicillin, 500 mg three times daily. For infection with *S. pneumoniae* with penicillin MICs of up to 1 µg/mL, penicillin is still an appropriate agent. For strains with penicillin MICs of 2 to 4 µg/mL, data regarding efficacy are conflicting, and higher doses may be better. If the patient is allergic to penicillin, a macrolide such as azithromycin (500 mg on day 1; then 250 mg/day) or clarithromycin (500 mg twice daily) may be used. Monotherapy with a macrolide should not be used in areas where there is a high prevalence of macrolide-resistant pneumococci.

Five days is the minimal recommended duration of treatment of CAP that is not complicated, severe, or associated with bacteremia.

For patients who are hospitalized because of CAP, higher doses of parenteral antibiotics are generally used, including penicillin in the range of 12 million U (2-3 million every 4 hours) or ampicillin, 4 g/day (1 g every 6 hours). Third-generation cephalosporins such as ceftriaxone (1-2 g every 24 hours) and cefotaxime (1-2 g every 8 hours) are other alternatives.

TABLE 289-3 ANTIMICROBIAL DOSES AND FREQUENCY OF ADMINISTRATION

ANTIMICROBIAL	DOSE AND ROUTE	FREQUENCY
MACROLIDES		
Azithromycin	500 mg × 1; then 250 mg PO	q24h
Clarithromycin	500 mg PO	q12h
Erythromycin	500 mg PO	q6h
TETRACYCLINE		
Doxycycline	100 mg PO	q12h
FLUOROQUINOLONES		
Moxifloxacin	400 mg PO or IV	q24h
Gemifloxacin	320 mg PO	q24h
Levofloxacin	750 mg PO or IV	q24h
β-LACTAMS		
Amoxicillin	1 g PO	q8h
Amoxicillin–clavulanate	2 g PO	q12h
Ampicillin–sulbactam	2 g IV	q6h
Cefepime	1-2 g	q12h
Cefixime	400 mg PO	q12h
Cefotaxime	1-2 g IV	q8h
Ceftriaxone	1-2 g IV	q24h
Cefpodoxime	100-200 mg	q12h
Cefuroxime	500 mg PO	q12h
Ertapenem	1 g IV	q24h
Imipenem	500 mg IV	q6h
Meropenem	1 g IV	q8h
Piperacillin–tazobactam	3.375 g IV	q6h
MISCELLANEOUS		
Linezolid	600 mg PO or IV	q12h
Vancomycin	0.75-1 g IV	q12h

IV = intravenous; PO = oral; q = every. Five days is the minimal recommended duration of treatment of community-acquired pneumonia that is not complicated, severe, or associated bacteremia.

The patient can be switched to an oral regimen when cough and shortness of breath are improving, the white blood cell count is normalizing, and oral intake and gastrointestinal tract absorption are adequate. Febrile patients are frequently treated outside the hospital, so absence of a fever is not a prerequisite for switching to an oral regimen.

Some studies have suggested that initial combination antimicrobial treatment of bacteremic pneumococcal pneumonia that includes a macrolide is associated with lower mortality rates possibly because of an immunomodulatory effect of the macrolides.

Empirical Treatment

This is discussed in the chapter dealing with CAP (Chapter 97). The body of evidence supporting the positive effects of guidelines on outcomes in CAP patients is compelling, particularly for those ill enough to require hospitalization.[13]

PROGNOSIS

In an otherwise well, relatively young patient with no comorbid conditions and with mild to moderate infection, the elevated temperature and white blood cell count usually resolve by days 2 to 4 and 4, respectively. The patient looks and feels better within a few days, but it is important to keep in mind that even in patients younger than 50 years, only 60% of cases will have resolved radiologically by 1 month. In patients older than 50 years or those with more severe infection or COPD, only 25% may clear radiographically by 1 month.

A patient who fails to respond or deteriorates after initial treatment must be carefully reassessed with a detailed review of the history and treatment course plus appropriate radiographic studies and cultures.[14] If the diagnosis is incorrect, other infectious causes of pneumonia, such as *Haemophilus influenzae* (Chapter 300) or the atypical agents (Chapter 97), must be considered. Noninfectious illnesses must also be considered; these include heart failure (Chapter 58), pulmonary embolism (Chapter 98), pulmonary neoplasm (Chapter 191), radiation injury (Chapter 20), drug reaction (Chapter 254), and inflammatory lung disease, to name a few. If the original diagnosis was correct, metastatic infection, lung abscess (Chapter 90) or empyema, and unsuspected drug resistance must be considered. Drug factors such as errors in selection, dose, or route of administration are possible explanations, especially in patients who receive oral medication.

There also appears to be an increased risk of cardiovascular events after certain respiratory infections, including pneumococcal pneumonia. This may be attributable to an enhanced inflammatory state and its effects on coronary arteries.[15]

Grade A References

A1. Nicholson KG, Abrams KR, Batham S, et al. Randomised controlled trial and health economic evaluation of the impact of diagnostic testing for influenza, respiratory syncytial virus and Streptococcus pneumoniae infection on the management of acute admissions in the elderly and high-risk 18- to 64-year-olds. *Health Technol Assess.* 2014;18:1-274.
A2. Maruyama T, Taguchi O, Niederman MS, et al. Efficacy of 23-valent pneumococcal vaccine in preventing pneumonia and improving survival in nursing home residents: double blind, randomized and placebo control trial. *BMJ.* 2010;340:c1004.
A3. Macintyre CR, Ridda I, Gao Z, et al. A randomized clinical trial of the immunogenicity of the 7-valent pneumococcal conjugate vaccine compared to 23-valent polysaccharide vaccine in frail, hospitalized elderly. *PLoS ONE.* 2014;9:e94578.

GENERAL REFERENCES

For the General References and other additional features, please visit Expert Consult at https://expertconsult.inkling.com.

290

NONPNEUMOCOCCAL STREPTOCOCCAL INFECTIONS AND RHEUMATIC FEVER

DONALD E. LOW

THE PATHOGENS

The *Streptococcus* genus contains a number of species that inhabit a broad range of hosts, including humans and domesticated animals, where they often colonize as part of the normal flora and cause infection. They are gram-positive cocci that grow in chains. The two most useful methods of classifying streptococci are by the type of hemolytic reaction displayed on blood agar on which they are grown and the serologic reactivity of the cell wall polysaccharide antigens as originally described by Rebecca Lancefield (Table 290-1). On blood agar plates, streptococci may cause complete (β), incomplete (α), or no (γ) hemolysis. Hemolytic streptococci from humans can be classified into Lancefield groups A, B, C, F, G, and L on the basis of carbohydrate antigens of the cell wall and can be subdivided into large- and small-colony (<0.5 mm in diameter) formers. The β-hemolytic group A and group B streptococci (GBS) are considered the major pathogenic β-hemolytic streptococci. The β-hemolytic large-colony–forming species, *Streptococcus dysgalactiae* subspecies *equisimilis*, may possess Lancefield group A, C, G, or L antigens. The small-colony–forming β-hemolytic strains with Lancefield group A, C, F, or G or no group antigens belong to the *anginosus* (or previously termed *Streptococcus milleri*) group. Members of the *anginosus* group (*Streptococcus anginosus*, *Streptococcus constellatus*, and *Streptococcus intermedius*) are considered part of the viridans group streptococci (VGS), most of which display α-hemolytic or nonhemolytic reactions.

STREPTOCOCCUS PYOGENES (GROUP A STREPTOCOCCUS)

The most clinically significant of the streptococcal human pathogens are *Streptococcus pyogenes* (also referred to as group A streptococci [GAS]), which contain the Lancefield group A antigen on their cell surface. GAS causes primarily infections of the upper respiratory tract and the skin. It is also responsible for a toxic shock–like syndrome; necrotizing fasciitis; and delayed nonsuppurative sequelae, including acute rheumatic fever and poststreptococcal glomerulonephritis. The major virulence factor of the organism is the M protein. This protein, a stable dimer, is anchored to the cell membrane and traverses and penetrates the cell wall. Whereas the proximal portion of the molecule is highly conserved among GAS, the distal portions contain type-specific epitopes localized on the tips that protrude from the cell surface. This variation in the distal region of the M proteins provides the basis of widely used epidemiologic typing schemes that use serologic methods (M type) or nucleotide sequence analysis of the M protein gene (*emm* type). There are more than 150 distinct *emm* and *emm*-like genes recognized. Epidemiologic studies have revealed that certain disease manifestations are commonly associated with particular M types, such as M1 and M3 types, which are associated with the most severe invasive manifestations such as toxic shock syndrome and necrotizing fasciitis. Humans are the natural host, and there is no animal or environmental reservoir. The throat and skin of the human host are the principal reservoirs for GAS. GAS is transmitted primarily person to person by either contact or droplet transmission.

EPIDEMIOLOGY

All GAS infections have the highest incidence in children younger than 10 years. The asymptomatic prevalence is also higher (15%-20%) in children than in adults. Age is not the only factor; crowded conditions in temperate climates during the winter months are also associated with epidemics of pharyngitis in school children as well as in military recruits. The peak incidence for streptococcal pharyngitis and impetigo varies with season and locale. In many temperate regions of the world, the incidence of pharyngitis peaks in winter; impetigo, although less common, peaks during the summer months. In contrast, for many tropical host populations, impetigo is hyperendemic year round, but throat infection, whether pharyngitis or asymptomatic carriage, ranges from very low to moderate levels.

CLINICAL MANIFESTATIONS

Respiratory Tract Infections
Pharyngitis

Group A streptococci are a major cause of pharyngitis and remains the only agent of this syndrome requiring etiologic diagnosis and treatment. The burden and economic costs of GAS pharyngitis are great. It has been estimated that in the United States alone, more than 7 million cases of acute pharyngitis are diagnosed by pediatricians annually. *S. pyogenes* is the cause in only 15% to 30% of them, but antibiotics are prescribed in 55% to 75% of the cases. Although a major consequence of GAS pharyngitis, acute rheumatic fever (see later), is much less common now than in the past, it is still a considerable problem in the developing world. The World Health Organization (WHO) estimates that there are about half a million cases of acute rheumatic fever worldwide annually. On clinical grounds, streptococcal pharyngitis (Fig. 290-1) is strongly suggested by the presence of fever, tonsillar exudate, tender enlarged anterior cervical lymph nodes, and absence of cough.

Because these findings are nonspecific and are also commonly found in cases of viral origin, however, even experienced physicians may accurately diagnose streptococcal pharyngitis based on the clinical findings alone in no more than 75% of the cases. Treatment of suspected GAS pharyngitis at the time of initial clinical evaluation has only a modest effect on relieving acute symptoms and perhaps on preventing suppurative complications. However, antibacterial treatment may be delayed for several days and still achieve the goal of preventing rheumatic fever and spread of disease. Prospective studies to compare the impact of various pharyngitis management strategies on clinically relevant outcomes have been recommended. A particular focus of recent guidelines has been to reduce overall use of antibiotics for treatment of pharyngitis in both children and adults in order to limit antibiotic resistance (Table 290-2).

TABLE 290-1	IDENTIFICATION OF THE β-HEMOLYTIC STREPTOCOCCI		
SPECIES	**LANCEFIELD GROUP**	**COLONY SIZE**	**ORIGIN**
S. pyogenes	A	Large	Human
S. agalactiae	B	Large	Human, bovine
S. dysgalactiae subsp. *equisimilis*	A, C, G, L	Large	Human, animals
S. equi subsp. *zooepidemicus*	C	Large	Animals, human
S. canis	G	Large	Dog, human
S. anginosus (group)*	A, C, G, F, none	Small	Human

*Group carbohydrate antigen.

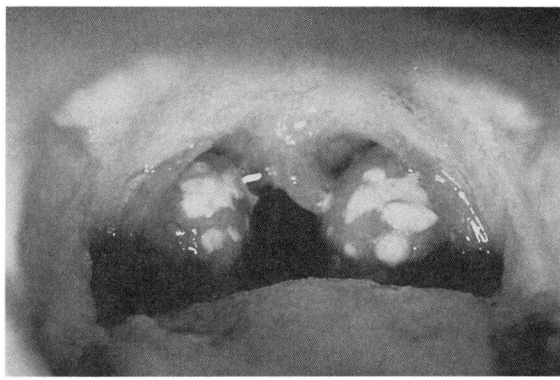

FIGURE 290-1. Acute streptococcal pharyngitis. Pus is present in the tonsillar crypts, and some palatal petechiae are seen. (From Forbes CD, Jackson WF. *Color Atlas and Text of Clinical Medicine*. 3rd ed. London: Mosby; 2003).

TABLE 290-2	SCORE FOR USE IN BOTH CHILDREN AND ADULTS WITH SORE THROAT TO ESTIMATE PROBABILITY OF POSITIVE CULTURE AND GUIDE MANAGEMENT APPROACH			
DIAGNOSTIC CRITERIA		*MANAGEMENT*		
FINDINGS	**POINTS**	**SCORE**	**RISK FOR STREPTOCOCCAL INFECTION (%)**	**RECOMMENDATION**
Temperature >38°C	+1	≤0	1-2.5	No culture or antibiotics
Absence of cough	+1	1	5-10	
Swollen, tender anterior cervical nodes	+1	2	11-17	Culture: antibiotics only if culture positive
Tonsillar swelling or exudate	+1	3	18-35	
Age		≥4		Antibiotics
3-14 yr	+1			
>44 yr	−1			

Adapted from McIsaac WJ, Kellner JD, Aufricht P, et al. Empirical validation of guidelines for the management of pharyngitis in children and adults. *JAMA.* 2004;291:1587-1595.

Throat culture is the conventional method for establishing the diagnosis of GAS pharyngitis. In an untreated patient with GAS pharyngitis, results of a properly obtained throat culture (by vigorous swabbing of both tonsils and posterior pharynx) are almost always positive; however, a positive throat culture may reflect chronic colonization by GAS, and the acute illness may be caused by another agent. Quantitation of GAS from the throat swab culture cannot be used to differentiate carriage from infection because sparse growth may be associated with true infection. A negative throat culture result permits the physician to withhold antibiotic therapy from most patients with sore throats.

Many GAS antigen detection tests are available commercially. These tests vary in method. Most of these tests have a high degree of specificity, but their sensitivity in clinical practice can be unacceptably low. Therefore, treatment is indicated for patients with acute pharyngitis who have a positive rapid antigen detection test result.

Otitis Media and Rhinosinusitis

During the past several decades, a number of studies have reported isolation of GAS from 2% to 5% of cultures of middle ear fluid specimens obtained from children with acute otitis media. Thus, in contrast to the very striking role of GAS as the major bacterial agent of acute pharyngitis, GAS has been fairly consistently the fourth most predominant pathogen causing pediatric acute otitis media, after *Streptococcus pneumoniae, Haemophilus influenzae,*

and *Moraxella catarrhalis.* GAS acute otitis media is associated with increased risk for development of mastoiditis. Although the risk is small (<1%), it is much greater than with acute otitis media caused by *S. pneumoniae, H. influenzae,* or *M. catarrhalis.* GAS is the etiologic agent of acute bacterial rhinosinusitis in 2% to 7% of cases.

Pneumonia

The occurrence of pneumonia has increased with the resurgence of invasive GAS disease during the past several decades, with 10% of patients with invasive GAS disease presenting with pneumonia. Small outbreaks of GAS pneumonia have been described in chronic care facilities and within families, as well as sporadic cases occurring in the community. GAS pneumonia now occurs with a frequency similar to that of other well-recognized causes, such as *Staphylococcus aureus* or *Klebsiella pneumoniae.* A Canadian population-based surveillance program of invasive GAS disease confirmed that GAS pneumonia is a severe illness of sudden onset frequently associated with local and systemic complications, particularly empyema (19%), toxic shock (32%), and death (38%).

Skin and Soft Tissue Infections
Scarlet Fever

Scarlet fever is a diffuse erythematous eruption that generally occurs in association with pharyngitis, most commonly in children 5 to 15 years of age. The development of the scarlet fever rash requires prior exposure to *S. pyogenes* and occurs as a result of delayed-type skin reactivity to pyrogenic exotoxin (erythrogenic toxin, usually types A, B, or C) produced by the organism. The rash of scarlet fever is a diffuse erythema that blanches with pressure, with numerous small (1-2 mm) papular elevations, giving a sandpaper quality to the skin. It usually starts on the head and neck and is accompanied by circumoral pallor and a strawberry tongue. Subsequently, the rash expands rapidly to cover the trunk followed by the extremities and then ultimately desquamates; the palms and soles are usually spared. The rash is most marked in the skinfolds of the inguinal, axillary, antecubital, and abdominal areas and about pressure points. It often exhibits a linear petechial character in the antecubital fossae and axillary folds, known as Pastia's lines.

Erysipelas

Erysipelas is an acute, superficial, non-necrotizing dermal or hypodermal infection that is mainly caused by streptococci. The definitive diagnosis is based on clinical findings that usually include a sharply demarcated shiny erythematosus plaque associated with pain, swelling, and fever (see Fig. 441-1). Erysipelas affects predominantly adult patients in the sixth or seventh decade of life and is located on the lower limb in more than 80% of cases. A female predominance exists, except in young patients. Risk factors include disruption of the cutaneous barrier (leg ulcer, wound, fissured toe-web intertrigo, and pressure ulcer), lymphedema, chronic edema, or local surgical operations (lymph node dissection, saphenectomy). Toe-web intertrigo appears to be a major portal of entry whether or not due to dermatophytes. Erysipelas is less commonly caused by group B, C, or G streptococci and rarely by staphylococci. Bulla formation is considered as a relatively severe but frequent local complication of the disease. Although most cases of erysipelas are caused by β-hemolytic streptococci, many other bacteria can produce non-necrotizing cellulitis, which can often occur in particular circumstances, such as *Pasteurella multocida* after cat or dog bites, *Aeromonas hydrophila* after immersion in fresh water, *Vibrio* spp. after saltwater exposure, or *H. influenzae* in periorbital cellulitis in children. Recurrence is the main complication of erysipelas; it occurs in about 20% of cases. Measures to reduce recurrences of erysipelas include treatment of any predisposing factor, such as toe-web intertrigo or wound, and reducing any underlying edema. If frequent infections occur despite such measures, prophylactic antibiotics may be warranted.

Impetigo

Impetigo is a highly contagious infection of the superficial epidermis that most often affects children 2 to 5 years of age (see Fig. 441-1), although it can occur in any age group. Impetigo is classified as bullous or nonbullous impetigo; the latter is the most common form. Bullous impetigo simply means that the skin eruption is characterized by bullae (blisters). The infection usually heals without scarring, even without treatment. *S. aureus* is the most important causative organism, especially in bullous impetigo. GAS causes fewer cases, either alone or in combination with *S. aureus,* and is more often found in nonbullous impetigo. The diagnosis usually is made clinically and can be confirmed by Gram stain and culture, although this is not usually necessary. Culture may be useful to identify patients with nephritogenic strains of GAS during outbreaks of poststreptococcal glomerulonephritis. Impetigo usually is transmitted through direct contact. Patients can further spread the infection to themselves or others after excoriating an infected area. Infections often spread rapidly through schools and daycare centers.

The Cochrane Collaboration reviewed interventions for impetigo. There was little evidence found for the use of disinfecting measures, such as chlorhexidine. There was good evidence that topical mupirocin and topical fusidic acid are equally or more effective than oral antibiotics for people with limited disease.[A1] Fusidic acid and mupirocin were of similar efficacy. It was found to be unclear whether oral antibiotics are superior to topical antibiotics for people with extensive impetigo.

Cellulitis

Bacterial cellulitis refers to a diffuse, spreading skin infection. Associated regional lymphadenopathy and lymphatic streaking are variable, and local complications (abscesses, necrosis) are more frequent than in erysipelas. Petechiae and ecchymoses with frequent bullae may develop in inflamed skin, resulting in hemorrhagic cellulitis. *Cellulitis* usually refers to a more deeply situated skin infection than erysipelas. However, the distinction between these entities is not clear-cut, and the two conditions share the typical clinical features, including sudden onset, usually with a high fever, and the tendency to recur. GAS has been considered the main causative agent of cellulitis, although groups B, C, and G streptococcus and *S. aureus* can also be a cause.

The predominant infection site for cellulitis is on the lower extremities. Lymphedema and disruption of the cutaneous barrier, which serves as a site of entry for the pathogens, are risk factors for infections. About 20% to 30% of patients have a recurrence during a 3-year follow-up period. Blood cultures are positive for β-hemolytic streptococci in fewer than 5% of cases.

Invasive Group A Streptococcus Disease

Invasive disease is defined as the isolation of GAS from an otherwise sterile site. GAS is capable of producing a variety of bacterial exotoxins, including a family of toxins known as superantigens (SAg). Severe invasive GAS disease includes streptococcal toxic shock syndrome and necrotizing fasciitis. *S. anginosus* plays a significant role as a reservoir of antimicrobial resistance genes, transferring different resistance traits to more pathogenic organisms such as *S. pneumoniae* and *S. pyogenes*. Both manifestations are associated with high morbidity and mortality.

Toxic Shock Syndrome

Streptococcal *toxic shock syndrome* is defined as hypotension accompanied by multiple organ failure, indicated by two of the following signs: renal impairment, coagulopathy, liver involvement, acute respiratory distress syndrome, a generalized rash, and soft tissue necrosis. In contrast to the other major form of toxic shock syndrome that is caused by toxin-producing *S. aureus* (Chapter 288), in which blood cultures are positive in fewer than 5% of cases, most (60%) patients with streptococcal toxic shock syndrome have positive blood cultures. In the late 1980s, patients with severe GAS infections were characterized and reported. Most patients were younger than 50 years old and otherwise healthy. All had invasive GAS infections characterized by signs that included shock; multiorgan system involvement; and rapidly progressive, destructive soft tissue infection (necrotizing fasciitis). The case-fatality rate was 30% even though most patients received appropriate antimicrobial therapy. M-types 1 and 3 were the most common type, and 80% of the isolates produced pyrogenic exotoxin A.

A focus of infection in staphylococcal toxic shock syndrome, if present at all, tends to be superficial, a complication of surgical wounds or burns or a foreign body (e.g., tampons). Streptococcal toxic shock syndrome can originate from an unknown focus or from a deep-seated soft tissue infection (e.g., necrotizing fasciitis, myositis, and cellulitis). Mortality rates are much higher with streptococcal than staphylococcal toxic shock, reported at up to 80% when associated with myositis.[1]

Necrotizing Fasciitis

Necrotizing fasciitis is defined by infection of the subcutaneous tissue and fascia that often results in necrosis with relative sparing of the underlying muscle. Histopathology demonstrates both necrosis of superficial fascia and polymorphonuclear infiltrates as well as edema of the reticular dermis, subcutaneous fat, and superficial fascia. GAS organisms in this disorder secrete proteases that disrupt host tissue and exotoxins that can cause local tissue

injury or systemic manifestations as the result of an excessive and inappropriate inflammatory response, leading to a life-threatening infection.

In the early stages of necrotizing fasciitis caused by GAS, the clinical findings can be nondescript, with as many as one third of patients initially being given a diagnosis other than necrotizing fasciitis. The only feature that might alert the clinician is a complaint of pain out of proportion to that expected on examination, even for patients who report previous trauma to the area. Necrotizing fasciitis has been found to occur more frequently during the winter months and in older men. More then half of patients give a history of an antecedent skin lesion or injury at the site of infection. In adults, most cases occur in persons with at least one chronic underlying illness, and in children, the most frequent underlying illness is an infection caused by varicella-zoster virus (Chapter 375). The most common primary site of infection is the lower extremity followed by the upper extremity, trunk, and groin or perineum.

Streptococcal exotoxins, which are superantigens, have been recognized as central mediators of the systemic effects associated with severe GAS infections.[2] Superantigens interact with antigen-presenting cells and T cells to induce T-cell proliferation and massive cytokine production, which leads to fever, rash, capillary leak, and subsequent hypotension, the major symptoms of severe GAS disease (Fig. 290-2). Twelve distinct superantigens produced by GAS have been identified, and many GAS strains harbor genes encoding four to six different superantigens. The magnitude of the inflammatory response is determined by the patient's human leukocyte antigen class II type. Another important risk factor for invasive GAS infections is lack of opsonic anti-M1 protein and neutralizing antisuperantigen antibodies.

Treatment of either streptococcal toxic shock or necrotizing fasciitis has not been critically studied because of the low incidence of disease and difficulty in patient recruitment for clinical trials. The dogma for the management GAS necrotizing fasciitis is that when necrotizing fasciitis is suspected, early surgical debridement is warranted. Despite the lack of clinical or scientific evidence to support this approach, it is widely endorsed in standard textbooks and treatment guidelines. The published studies are all based on retrospective chart review of patients with necrotizing fasciitis from multiple etiologies, including mixed aerobic and anaerobic organisms.

The finding that lack of protective antibodies against streptococcal M protein and superantigens correlates with risk for developing invasive streptococcal diseases, highlights the importance of antibodies in protection against these infections and suggests that intravenous immunoglobulin (IVIG) might be a potential adjunctive therapy. IVIG exhibits high polyspecificity generated by antibodies pooled from several thousands of donors and has been shown to contain broad-spectrum antibodies against streptococcal superantigens and M proteins. In addition, IVIG has a general anti-inflammatory effect that is largely attributable to Fc receptor–mediated mechanisms. The documentation of clinical efficacy of IVIG includes several case reports and two observational cohort studies, one case-control study, and one multicenter placebo-controlled trial.

Nonsuppurative Sequelae of Streptococcal Infections
Acute Rheumatic Fever

Acute rheumatic fever is a delayed, nonsuppurative sequela of a pharyngeal infection with the GAS. After the initial pharyngitis, a latent period of 2 to 3 weeks occurs before the first signs or symptoms of acute rheumatic fever appear. The disease presents with various manifestations that may include arthritis, carditis, chorea, subcutaneous nodules, and erythema marginatum. In developing areas of the world, acute rheumatic fever and rheumatic heart disease are estimated to affect nearly 20 million people and are the leading causes of cardiovascular death during the first five decades of life. The story is much different in developed countries. In the latter half of the 20th century, rheumatic fever receded as an important health problem in almost all wealthy countries. Today, most physicians in these countries are unlikely ever to see a case of acute rheumatic fever. Most of the reduction is attributable to improved living conditions, which have resulted in less overcrowding and better hygiene, with consequent reductions in transmission of group A streptococci. In other words, rheumatic fever is now a disease of poverty.

Worldwide, at least 350,000 deaths are attributable to rheumatic fever or rheumatic heart disease each year; most occur in developing countries and among indigenous groups.[3] The observation in some studies that only a few M serotypes (types 3, 5, 6, 14, 18, 19, 24, and 29) were implicated in outbreaks of rheumatic fever suggested a particular "rheumatogenic" potential of certain strains of GAS. The decrease in the incidence of acute rheumatic fever in developed countries with the replacement of rheumatogenic types by

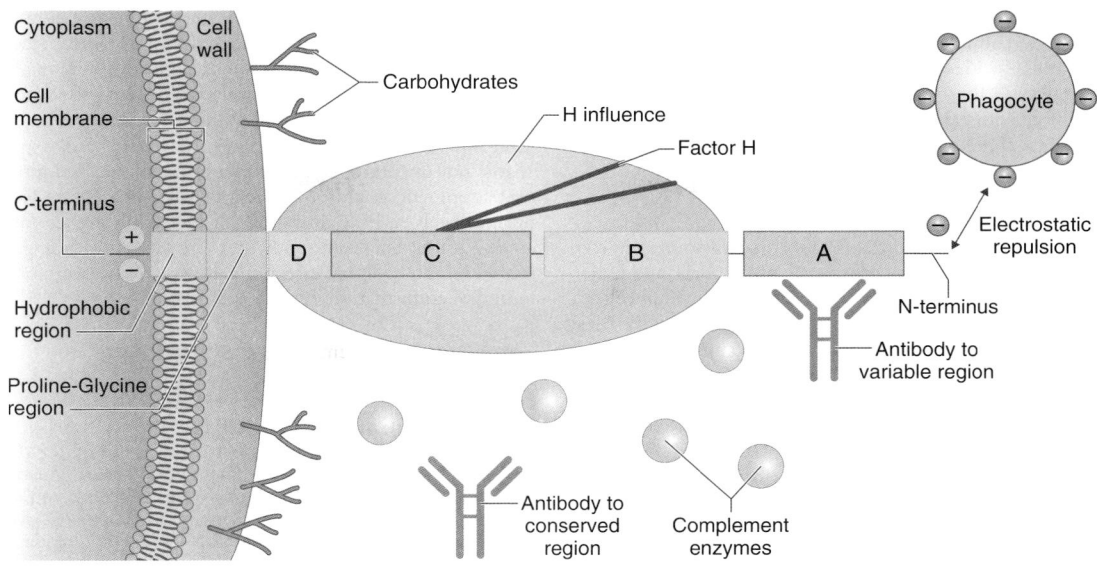

FIGURE 290-2. Thwarting the immune system is the primary job of the M protein. Negative charges at the N-terminus may repel phagocytic white blood cells. By binding with factor H—a regulatory protein produced by the human host—the M protein protects its most conserved regions from antibodies and complement enzymes. Only antibodies against the antigenically shifting hypervariable region can clear an established streptococcal infection from the host's body. (Reprinted from Fischetti VA. Streptococcal M protein. *Sci Am.* 1991;264(6):58-65; with permission from Mr. Tomoyuki Narashima from Tane+1 LLC for reproduction of illustration).

nonrheumatogenic types is not solely responsible for the decrease in acute rheumatic fever, and the issue of potential rheumatogenic strains remains unresolved. A streptococcal strain capable of causing a well-documented pharyngitis almost always is potentially capable of causing rheumatic fever. The lack of specific rheumatogenic strains also can explains the relatively high risk for recurrent disease with new streptococcal infections, in contrast to poststreptococcal glomerulonephritis, in which only a few "nephritogenic" strains appear to be capable of inducing the disease (e.g., type 12 with pharyngitis and type 49 with impetigo), and recurrent disease is uncommon.

Modified Jones criteria were first published in 1944 to be able to define persons with acute rheumatic fever. They have been periodically revised by the American Heart Association in collaboration with other groups.[4] According to revised Jones criteria, the diagnosis of rheumatic fever can be made when two of the major criteria or one major criterion plus two minor criteria are present along with evidence of streptococcal infection. Exceptions are chorea and indolent carditis, each of which by itself can indicate rheumatic fever. Major criteria include the following:

1. Migratory polyarthritis: a temporary migrating inflammation of the large joints, usually starting in the legs and migrating upward
2. Carditis: inflammation of the heart muscle, which can manifest as congestive heart failure, pericarditis with a rub, or a new heart murmur
3. Subcutaneous nodules: painless, firm collections of collagen fibers over bones or tendons, commonly appearing on the back of the wrist, the outside elbow, and the front of the knees
4. Erythema marginatum: a long-lasting rash that begins on the trunk or arms as macules and spreads outward to form a snakelike ring while clearing in the middle. This rash never starts on the face, and it is made worse with heat.
5. Sydenham's chorea (St. Vitus' dance): a characteristic series of rapid movements of the face and arms without purpose, generally occurring late in the disease

Minor criteria include the following:

1. Fever
2. Arthralgia: joint pain without swelling
3. Raised erythrocyte sedimentation rate (ESR) or C-reactive protein (CRP)
4. Leukocytosis
5. Electrocardiogram showing features of heart block, such as a prolonged PR interval
6. Supporting evidence of streptococcal infection: elevated or rising antistreptolysin O titer or anti-DNAse B
7. Previous episode of rheumatic fever or inactive heart disease

The pathogenic mechanisms that lead to the development of acute rheumatic fever remain incompletely understood. Clearly, streptococcal pharyn-

geal infection is required, and genetic susceptibility may be present. On the other hand, evidence is sparse that toxins produced by the streptococcus are important. Molecular mimicry is thought to play an important role in the initiation of the tissue injury. As a result of molecular mimicry, antibodies directed against GAS antigens cross-react with host antigens. In addition to the role of antibody, observations suggest a role for cellular immunity in molecular mimicry.

Primary prevention of acute rheumatic fever is accomplished by proper identification and adequate antibiotic treatment of GAS tonsillopharyngitis.[5,6] The diagnosis of GAS pharyngitis is best accomplished by combining clinical judgment with diagnostic test results, the criterion standard of which is the throat culture. Penicillin (either oral penicillin V or injectable benzathine penicillin) is the treatment of choice because it is cost effective, has a narrow spectrum of activity, and has long-standing proven efficacy. In addition, GAS resistant to penicillin has not been documented. For penicillin-allergic individuals, acceptable alternatives include a narrow-spectrum oral cephalosporin, oral clindamycin, or various oral macrolides. An individual who has had an attack of rheumatic fever is at very high risk of developing recurrences after subsequent GAS pharyngitis and needs continuous antimicrobial prophylaxis to prevent such recurrences (secondary prevention). The recommended duration of prophylaxis depends on the number of previous attacks, the time elapsed since the last attack, the risk for exposure to GAS infections, the age of the patient, and the presence or absence of cardiac involvement. Penicillin is again the agent of choice for secondary prophylaxis, but sulfadiazine or a macrolide is an acceptable alternative in penicillin-allergic individuals.

Poststreptococcal Reactive Arthritis

The term *poststreptococcal reactive arthritis* (PSRA) was first used to describe patients with arthritis after documented GAS infection but who failed to meet the Jones criteria for the diagnosis of acute rheumatic fever. Since then, the differentiation of PSRA from acute rheumatic fever has remained unsettled.[7] Compared with acute rheumatic fever, the arthritis of PSRA is more likely to occur within 10 days after infection, be symmetrical and nonmigratory, last longer than 3 weeks, and be poorly responsive to aspirin or other nonsteroidal anti-inflammatory drugs (NSAIDs). Periarticular findings, such as tenosynovitis, have not been considered to be part of the clinical spectrum of acute rheumatic fever but have been described with PSRA. However, some studies have reported that an additive and prolonged pattern of arthritis, as well as aspirin unresponsivity, may be seen in 19% to 36% of patients with acute rheumatic fever. Some have suggested that patients with higher ESR and CRP, a shorter duration of joint symptoms after NSAID therapy, and without relapse when NSAIDs were stopped were diagnosed as having acute rheumatic fever rather than PSRA. Although all patients with PSRA have serologic evidence of a recent GAS infection, no more than half of these patients who have a throat culture performed have GAS isolated. Because a small proportion of patients with PSRA have been reported to develop subsequent valvular heart disease, these patients should be observed carefully for several months for clinical evidence of carditis. If valvular disease is detected, the patient should be classified as having had acute rheumatic fever and should continue to receive secondary prophylaxis.

Poststreptococcal Glomerulonephritis

Acute poststreptococcal glomerulonephritis (PSGN) is a disease characterized by the sudden appearance of edema, hematuria, proteinuria, and hypertension (Chapter 121).[8] It is now known to follow infection by nephrogenic strains of GAS, which are M types 1, 2, 4, 12, 18, 25, 49, 55, 57, and 60. These may cause skin or throat infections, but specific M types, such as 49, 55, 57, and 60, are most commonly associated with skin infections. In addition, nontypeable GAS is frequently isolated from the skin or throats of patients with glomerulonephritis, representing presumably unclassified nephritogenic strains. The overall risk of developing acute PSGN after infection by these nephritogenic strains is about 15%. The risk for nephritis may also be related to the M type and the site of infection. The risk of developing nephritis infection by M type 49 is 5% if it is present in the throat. This risk increases to 25% if infection by the same organism is present in the skin. The time lapse between infection and onset of PSGN symptoms is typically 1 to 3 weeks after a throat infection and 3 to 6 weeks after a skin infection.

The pathogenic mechanism of PSGN remains largely unknown (Chapter 121). Diffuse glomerular hypercellularity, C3 and immunoglobulin G (IgG) deposition, and proteinuria and hematuria are cardinal features. However, it can occur without all of these signs present concurrently. For a reliable diagnosis of PSGN, clear evidence that a streptococcal infection preceded the glomerulonephritis is required. However, streptococcal infection has often cleared by the time the patient appears in the clinic because the symptoms generally arise 1 to 3 weeks after the patient was infected. Acute PSGN most often follows upper respiratory tract GAS infections in colder climates and skin infections in warmer climates. Occasionally, it may also be seen after group C or G streptococcal infections. A high incidence of PSGN is noted in other parts of the world, especially in areas with tropical climates where skin infections are common. Epidemic episodes tend to occur in highly populated areas where poor hygiene, malnutrition, anemia, and parasites are common, and episodes are separated by periods of 5 to 7 years in certain communities. Epidemics occur also in the Western world, especially in closed communities. Acute PSGN affects all age groups but most commonly children and young adults. Males are affected more often than females, often in the ratio of 2 : 1. Acute PSGN rarely strikes the same individual twice. Thus, it appears likely that protective immunity is acquired as a result of an infection with a nephritogenic strain.

Although penicillin treatment of the antecedent streptococcal infections is highly efficacious in preventing acute rheumatic fever, it does not appear to be the case in PSGN. Studies carried out during epidemics of nephritis found that prior antibiotics had little, if any, effect in preventing PSGN. Penicillin is, nevertheless, effective in epidemiologic attempts to eradicate nephritogenic strains by treatment of acute glomerulonephritis patients and their colonized family contacts. Because recurrent episodes of acute glomerulonephritis are so rare, continuous antibiotic prophylaxis, such as is used in the secondary prevention of rheumatic fever, is unnecessary.

The ultimate prognosis in persons with acute glomerulonephritis depends largely on the severity of the initial insult. In an extremely small proportion of patients, the initial injury is so severe that either persistent renal failure or progression to renal failure occurs. However, in most patients, histologic regression of the disease is the rule, and the ultimate prognosis is good.

DIAGNOSIS

Streptococcal Antibody Tests

Ant streptococcal antibody titers reflect past and not present immunologic events and therefore cannot be used to determine whether an individual with pharyngitis and GAS in the pharynx is truly infected or merely a streptococcal carrier. When present, elevated or rising antistreptococcal antibody titers provide reliable confirmation of a recent GAS infection and are of value in identifying a preceding GAS infection in a patient suspected of having rheumatic fever. The most commonly used and commercially available antibody assays are antistreptolysin O and anti-DNAse B. These tests are valuable in patients who have possible nonsuppurative complications of GAS infections (acute rheumatic fever or acute glomerulonephritis). The antistreptolysin O

test is usually obtained first, and if the result is not elevated, an anti-DNAse B test may be performed. Antistreptolysin O titers begin to rise approximately 1 week and peak 3 to 6 weeks after the infection. Anti-DNAse B titers begin to rise 1 to 2 weeks and peak 6 to 8 weeks after the infection. Elevated titers for both tests may persist for several months after even uncomplicated GAS infections.

It is not uncommon for laboratory personnel and physicians to misinterpret streptococcal antibody titers because of a failure to appreciate that the normal levels of these antibodies are higher among school-aged children than among adults. Single antibody titers are often misleading. Sequential samples more accurately define infection, allowing correlation of titer increases with temporal confirmation of GAS acquisition.

TREATMENT   Rx

Antimicrobial Susceptibility

Penicillin and the cephalosporins continue to be the drugs of first choice for the treatment of most GAS infections.[A2] The continued susceptibility of *S. pyogenes* to β-lactams is remarkable, especially compared with the emergence of resistance to β-lactams among pneumococci and VGS over the past decade. A limited ability to acquire foreign DNA and a physiologic fitness cost associated with β-lactam resistance are possible explanations for this organism's continued susceptibility to penicillin. The macrolides are the second-line drug of choice and are used in penicillin-hypersensitive patients. Clindamycin is also the drug of choice for chronic, recurrent pharyngitis. However, resistance has emerged in this organism. Elevated rates of macrolide resistance (>25%) among GAS reported in Korea, Taiwan, Spain, and Italy are causes of concern. Limited surveillance data suggest that the overall rate of macrolide-resistant GAS in North America is 3% to 9%. There are two primary mechanisms of macrolide resistance in GAS: efflux (encoded by *mefA*) and target modification caused by ribosomal methylation (encoded by *ermB* or *ermA*). Isolates with the *mefA* gene have a pattern of resistance known as the M phenotype: they are macrolide resistant but clindamycin susceptible. GAS isolates with the *ermB* gene are usually resistant to macrolides and clindamycin. Isolates with the *ermA* gene typically have an inducible phenotype that requires exposure to a macrolide inducer before clindamycin resistance becomes evident. There are rare reports of L4 ribosomal protein and 23S recombinant RNA mutations in macrolide-resistant GAS isolates.

Fluoroquinolones are a useful therapeutic alternative for the treatment of skin and soft tissue infections in adults. Although strains of GAS nonsusceptible to the fluoroquinolones have been reported, they are rare. The mechanisms of decreased susceptibility to the fluoroquinolones among *Streptococcus* spp. are mainly mediated by point mutations in the quinolone resistance–determining region of the bacterial topoisomerase II enzymes, namely, DNA gyrase and topoisomerase IV. DNA gyrase and topoisomerase IV enzymes are homologs, with each enzyme consisting of a tetramer with two subunits (two *gyrA* and two *gyrB* molecules in DNA gyrase, two *parC* and two *parE* molecules in topoisomerase IV). *S. pyogenes* isolates that are resistant or have reduced susceptibility to fluoroquinolones have been reported, but isolates with a high level of resistance have been detected very infrequently.

Tetracycline resistance in GAS is quite common. In gram-positive organisms, resistance to tetracycline is typically conferred by ribosome protection genes, such as *tet*(M) and *tet*(O). Tetracycline resistance is usually acquired by GAS through horizontal gene transfer. A global sample of GAS revealed 80 or more separate acquisitions of tetracycline resistance. Of 244 clones, 38% and 25% displayed resistance to tetracycline and erythromycin, respectively; a relatively high proportion (15%) were resistant to both classes of drugs. *tet*(M) displayed a highly significant association with *erm*(B). Trimethoprim–sulfamethoxazole is not active against GAS and therefore should not be used as monotherapy for infections potentially caused by GAS.

STREPTOCOCCUS AGALACTIAE (GROUP B STREPTOCOCCUS)

EPIDEMIOLOGY

Group B streptococci, also known as *Streptococcus agalactiae*, was once considered a pathogen of only domestic animals, causing mastitis in cows. Although asymptomatic vaginal carriage of GBS was described in 1935, the first report of GBS sepsis in a neonate was not reported until 1964. Since the 1970s, GBS is recognized as one of the most common causes of neonatal infectious morbidity and mortality in developed countries. GBS causes significant maternal and perinatal morbidity, asymptomatic bacteriuria in pregnancy, and urinary tract and other infections in the adult nonpregnant population. The virulence of *S. agalactiae* is related to the polysaccharide toxin it produces. Immunity is mediated by antibodies to the capsular polysaccharide and is serotype specific. Several serotypes are known, including Ia, Ib, Ic, II, III, IV, V, VI, VII, and VIII.

CLINICAL MANIFESTATIONS
Neonatal Group B Streptococcus Disease

Group B streptococci colonizes the vaginal and gastrointestinal (GI) tracts in healthy women, with carriage rates ranging from 15% to 45%. Neonates can acquire the organism vertically in utero or during delivery from the maternal genital tract. Although the transmission rate from mothers colonized with *S. agalactiae* to neonates delivered vaginally is approximately 50%, only 1% to 2% of colonized neonates go on to develop invasive GBS disease. Neonatal GBS disease is divided into early and late disease. Early GBS neonatal sepsis often presents within 24 hours of delivery but can become apparent up to 7 days postpartum. Pneumonia with bacteremia is common, but meningitis is less likely. Late GBS neonatal sepsis is defined as infection that presents between 1 week postpartum and age 3 months. Late disease commonly involves GBS serotype III, typically characterized by bacteremia and meningitis.

PREVENTION

The current approach to the prevention of early-onset GBS infection in pregnancy is to provide intrapartum antimicrobial prophylaxis in women at term with culture evidence of recent vaginal or rectal GBS infection.[A3] Women without a known GBS status delivering before 37 weeks' gestation with premature rupture of the membranes or intrapartum fever are also candidates for intrapartum antimicrobial prophylaxis. Penicillin or ampicillin is the initial approach. Clindamycin and macrolides are standard in individuals with penicillin allergy, but GBS infections are no longer always sensitive to these two drugs. Despite these recommendations, there is lack of evidence from well-designed and well-conducted trials to recommend intrapartum antibiotic prophylaxis to reduce neonatal early-onset GBS disease.

Invasive Group B Streptococcus Disease

S. agalactiae infection is extremely rare in healthy adults and is almost always associated with underlying abnormalities. Bacteremia with an unknown source accounts for approximately 25% of all cases of invasive GBS disease. Diabetes mellitus and malignancy are the most common underlying diseases associated with infection. Urinary tract infections are a common manifestation of GBS disease and are observed in both pregnant and nonpregnant adults. Other presentations of GBS infection include pneumonia, skin and soft tissue infections, septic arthritis, osteomyelitis, meningitis, peritonitis, and endo-ophthalmitis.

Invasive GBS disease is a major cause of illness and death in older adults and is even more frequent among long-term care facility residents, possibly because of concurrent conditions such as advanced age, diabetes, cirrhosis, and stroke, which are known risk factors for GBS infection.[9] Case-fatality rates are about 13% for persons 65 years and older. An increased prevalence of serogroup V has been reported in adult populations. Serotype V has been associated with higher rates of antimicrobial drug resistance.

> ## TREATMENT   Rx
>
> Although β-lactams remain the preferred therapy for GBS infections, strains with elevated penicillin minimal inhibitory concentrations have been reported but are rare.

STREPTOCOCCUS DYSGALACTIAE SUBSPECIES EQUISIMILIS (HUMAN GROUP C AND G STREPTOCOCCI)

EPIDEMIOLOGY

Non–group A or B β-hemolytic streptococci that are frequently normal inhabitants of the oropharynx, skin, and GI and genitourinary (GU) tracts are also capable of causing significant disease. These include groups C, G, F, and L, of which the most common are groups G and C (see Table 290-1). Large-colony-forming human groups C and G streptococci are currently clas-

sified as *Streptococcus dysgalactiae* subspecies *equisimilis* (SDSE). Infections caused by SDSE are transmitted person to person; an animal reservoir for these strains has not been reported. Zoonotic group C or G streptococcal infections are comparatively rare and are mostly caused by other streptococcal species after animal contact or are associated with the consumption of unpasteurized dairy food products. Nonhuman large-colony-forming β-hemolytic group G streptococci usually belong to *Streptococcus canis*, an animal pathogen that has been found only rarely in humans.

CLINICAL MANIFESTATIONS

A population-based study carried out in North America demonstrated a substantial morbidity and mortality associated with infections caused by SDSE, comparable to that caused by invasive GAS infection during the same study period. Both SDSE and GAS affected similar adult populations, tended to be community acquired, and affected primarily persons with underlying medical conditions. The mortality rate was similar to that (8%-21%) reported in other studies. Whereas SDSE primarily presented as skin and soft tissue infection in older patients, individuals with invasive *S. anginosus* group infections were more likely to be younger patients with intra-abdominal infections; these were typically polymicrobial and represented sequelae of perforated appendicitis and associated peritonitis. This finding is supported by the fact that *S. anginosus* group isolates have been recovered from 20% to 40% of healthy appendices.

Pharyngitis is a classic presentation in adult patients, and SDSE has clearly been responsible for epidemic outbreaks of pharyngitis in children. The etiologic role of SDSE in pharyngitis is supported by reports on acute poststreptococcal glomerulonephritis and, more recently, on acute rheumatic fever after SDSE isolation from the upper respiratory tract.

In a 1-year study of 90 patients presenting with 98 disease episodes of acute bacterial cellulitis in Finland, SDSE instead of GAS was strikingly the most common finding. Some patients and household members also carried SDSE in the pharynx; it was not detected in the control participant. Whereas SDSE was isolated either from skin lesions or blood from 22% of patients, GAS was isolated from 7% of patients.

> ## TREATMENT   Rx
>
> The non–group A or B β-hemolytic streptococci are typically susceptible to penicillins and cephalosporins, although α-hemolytic VGS have shown increasing resistance to penicillin and other β-lactams. In contrast, the resistance to erythromycin and tetracycline among SDSE is similar to rates found in GAS.

VIRIDANS GROUP STREPTOCOCCI
Streptococcus anginosus Group (Streptococcus milleri Group)

The *S. anginosus* group includes three distinct species and more subspecies. *S. anginosus*, *S. constellatus*, and *S. intermedius* have all been collectively known as either *S. anginosus* or *S. milleri*. Members of the *S. anginosus* group are nonmotile, facultative anaerobes that demonstrate variable hemolysis patterns (α, β, or γ) on sheep blood agar. Colonies are typically small (colony < 0.5 mm). A caramel or butterscotch smell is useful for identifying the *S. anginosus* group when present but is not a sufficiently sensitive screening test. There are β-hemolytic strains of each of the three species, and the strains may possess one of four different Lancefield group antigens (group A, C, F, or G) or no group antigen. Non--hemolytic varieties of each of the three species are grouped into the general classification of viridans streptococci.

The organisms, although normal flora of the human oral cavity and GI tract, have the ability to cause abscesses and systemic infections, unlike *S. pyogenes* and *S. agalactiae*. The *S. anginosus* group should be considered true pathogens when isolated from humans. *S. anginosus* often presents as part of a polymicrobial infection in patients with oral, head and neck, and abdominal infections. Copathogens in such infections may include other bacteria such as *Eikenella corrodens* and *Fusobacterium nucleatum*. This group is less commonly the cause of endocarditis than other viridans streptococci. Whereas *S. intermedius* has an apparent tropism for the brain and liver, *S. anginosus* and *S. constellatus* have been isolated from a wider range of sites and infections.

Thoracic infections caused by *S. anginosus* group are largely pleural. They are polymicrobial in one third of cases and in most patients are associated with major surgery or surgical procedures of the respiratory or digestive tract. The empyema frequently requires thoracotomy for complete resolution. In the chest, infections tend to cause loculated empyemas that are not conducive to tube thoracostomy drainage or to antibiotic treatment. About 75% of infections of the chest require surgical intervention. The optimal method and timing of intervention for thoracic empyema remains debated, likely because of the presentation of pleural space disease in one of three stages: exudative effusions, fibrinopurulent collections, and organized loculations. In the fibrinopurulent stage, the lung can be thoracoscopically dissected off the chest wall without much difficulty.

Members of the *S. anginosus* group are largely susceptible to β-lactam agents. Minimal inhibitory concentrations (MICs) to penicillin G are usually 0.125 mcg/mL or less. Some strains with penicillin G MICs between 0.25 and 2 mcg/mL have been reported; rare strains have penicillin MIC 4 mcg/mL or greater. Penicillin-intermediate or -resistant strains have altered penicillin-binding proteins; these are more likely to be *S. anginosus* or *S. intermedius* than *S. constellatus*. Vancomycin is an appropriate alternative agent for penicillin-allergic patients. A parental third-generation cephalosporin is recommended for brain abscesses and bacteremia caused by members of the *S. anginosus* group.

Fluoroquinolone MICs among *S. anginosus* group members are high but in the susceptible range (0.5-1.0 mcg/mL); resistance tends to develop easily, and therefore fluoroquinolones are not appropriate first-line antimicrobial agents. Macrolide resistance appears to be emerging among the *S. anginosus* group. Most strains of the *S. anginosus* group are resistant to aminoglycosides. Sulfonamides have no activity against *S. anginosus* group isolates.

S. anginosus plays a significant role as a reservoir of antimicrobial resistance genes, transferring different resistance traits to more pathogenic organisms such as *S. pneumoniae* and *S. pyogenes*.

Other Viridans Group Streptococci

There are now at least 30 recognized species of VGS, including those discussed earlier. Although often found as commensals whose pathogenic abilities appear to be much more subtle than those of the pyogenic streptococci, they may also participate in various infections such as subacute bacterial endocarditis; catheter-related and neutropenia-related bloodstream infections; and purulent abdominal, hepatobiliary, brain, and dental infections. Antimicrobial resistance is substantial in the viridans streptococci as a group. Penicillin resistance is from 30% to 50% in strains isolated from patients in North America. *S. mitis* and *S. oralis* are the most common strains found in blood cultures of cancer patients and are commonly resistant to β-lactam antimicrobials. *S. sanguinis*, *S. oralis*, and *S. gordonii*, in descending order, are the most common strains isolated from cultures of blood of endocarditis patients.

⬤ ZOONOTIC STREPTROCOCCI
Streptococcus suis

S. suis is a pathogen in pigs that can cause severe infection in humans.[10] *S. suis* was first reported by veterinarians in 1954 after outbreaks of meningitis, septicemia, and purulent arthritis occurred among piglets. Fourteen years later, the first human *S. suis* cases were diagnosed in Denmark, and subsequently, other cases were reported in more than 30 countries, including Canada, the United States, Japan, Vietnam, and Thailand. It can be clinically manifested with meningitis, arthritis, and sepsis. *S. suis* is the name assigned to streptococci that were formally called Lancefield groups R, S, and T. Of the 35 known serotypes, the most frequent serotype identified from humans has been serotype 2 (group R). Human *S. suis* infections are most often reported from countries where pig rearing is common. The relatively high mean patient age (47-55 years) and almost complete absence of children in case series, as well as the high male-to-female patient ratio (3.5 : 1 to 6.5 : 1), support the notion that infection with *S. suis* is generally an occupational disease. The annual risk of developing *S. suis* meningitis among abattoir workers and pig breeders has been estimated to be 3 cases per 100,000 population; the risk is lower for butchers, at 1.2 cases per 100,000 population in developed countries. The incubation period of *S. suis* is from hours to 14 days (median, 2.2 days). A very short incubation time is consistent with direct entry of *S. suis* into the blood through skin wounds. Patients have generally been healthy before infection with *S. suis,* although predisposing factors, such as splenectomy, diabetes mellitus, alcoholism, malignancy, and structural

heart diseases, have been reported. An outbreak in China was associated with an overall case-fatality rate of 18%, but this reached 63% among patients with severe sepsis and septic shock.

Data from Vietnam show that *S. suis* is susceptible to penicillin, ceftriaxone, and vancomycin. Resistance was seen to tetracycline (83%), erythromycin (20%), and chloramphenicol (3%). In a European study, 384 *S. suis* strains from diseased pigs were susceptible to penicillin, but resistance was detected to gentamicin (1.0%), trimethoprim–sulfamethoxazole, (6.0%), and tetracycline (75%). There may be a role for the use of dexamethasone as an adjunctive treatment to reduce mortality and improve the outcome of bacterial meningitis caused by infection with *S. suis*. In a randomized, double-blind, placebo-controlled clinical trial in Vietnam, dexamethasone (0.4 mg/kg twice daily for 4 days) resulted in a significant reduction in the risk for death at 1 month and in the risk for death and disability at 6 months in patients with confirmed bacterial meningitis; *S. suis* accounted for 25% of pathogens.

Currently, a human vaccine is not available, but simple preventive measures, such as wearing gloves during processing pig meat or slaughtering, handwashing after handling raw pork meat, and thorough cooking of pork, should prevent most cases. Travelers should be aware that dietary habits in some countries may pose a risk for infectious diseases, including *S. suis* infection.

Streptococcus canis

S. canis is an organism that was described in 1986 as having the Lancefield group G antigen and was isolated from animals, most frequently dogs. Extensive phenotypic testing of isolates from dogs was described in 1994, and the isolation of *S. canis* from a human with sepsis was reported in 1997. Despite its name, *S. canis* has also been isolated from animals other than dogs, including cats, harbor porpoises, cows, mice, rats, and rabbits. In healthy dogs, *S. canis* is found as commensal flora of the skin, oropharynx, GU tract, and anus. Rare cases of *S. canis* infection in humans have been reported in the literature. Resistance to erythromycin and tetracycline is common. In the clinical laboratory, group G streptococci are not usually identified to the species level. In addition, laboratory tests have only recently been able to identify *S. canis* accurately. Thus, the true incidence of *S. canis* infection is unknown.

Streptococcus bovis Group

Members of the *Streptococcus bovis* group have long been regarded as opportunistic pathogens in humans, causing up to 11% to 14% of all endocarditis cases and 24% of streptococcal endocarditis. *S. bovis* group isolates from human infections are divided into three biotypes, designated biotypes I, II/1, and II/2. Most *S. bovis* group endocarditis isolates belong to biotype I, for which a reclassification as *Streptococcus gallolyticus* subspecies *gallolyticus* has been proposed. The human intestinal tract is a major natural reservoir of *S. bovis* group strains with a reported carriage rate of about 10%. There is a strong association between the presence of malignant or premalignant lesions in the GI tracts of patients and isolation of *S. bovis* as a causative agent of bacteremia or endocarditis.

Streptococcus iniae

S. iniae is a β-hemolytic streptococcus without a group antigen. It is a major fish pathogen in many regions of the world. These bacteria are also zoonotic, with infections in humans associated with the handling and preparation of infected fish. The first human infections were reported in 1996. Most cases of human *S. iniae* infections have been in persons of Asian descent, who are elderly and commonly have underlying conditions such as diabetes mellitus, chronic rheumatic heart disease, cirrhosis, or other conditions.

Carrier fish have been implicated in fish-to-fish transmission of *S. iniae*, and these carriers may be responsible for human infection because fish with overt signs of disease are unmarketable. Soft tissue injuries that occur during the preparation of fresh fish from wet markets usually result in bacteremic cellulitis of the hand followed by one or more of the following conditions: endocarditis, meningitis, arthritis, sepsis, pneumonia, osteomyelitis, and toxic shock. *S. iniae* is susceptible to penicillin and other antimicrobials. The expression of a suite of virulence factors, many of them similar to those found in GAS, is responsible for successful entry, propagation, and evasion of immune defenses of the host by this bacterium. Underreporting of human cases is likely because identification of *S. iniae* is based on biochemical testing of isolates with commercial kits; the use of kits is associated with problems because *S. iniae* is not listed in commercial or clinical databases, and many atypical strains are assigned low matches.

Grade A References

A1. Koning S, van der Sande R, Verhagen AP, et al. Interventions for impetigo. *Cochrane Database Syst Rev.* 2012;1:CD003261.
A2. Van Driel ML, De Sutter AL, Keber N, et al. Different antibiotic treatments for group A streptococcal pharyngitis. *Cochrane Database Syst Rev.* 2013;4:CD004406.
A3. Ohlsson A, Shah VS. Intrapartum antibiotics for known maternal Group B streptococcal colonization. *Cochrane Database Syst Rev.* 2014;6:CD007467.

GENERAL REFERENCES

For the General References and other additional features, please visit Expert Consult at https://expertconsult.inkling.com.

291

ENTEROCOCCAL INFECTIONS

TRISH M. PERL

DEFINITION

Enterococci, formerly called group D streptococci, are endogenous human gut flora that had been considered pathogens with low virulence in the past. However, more recently, they have emerged as increasingly important health care–associated pathogens. This emergence is primarily because of their inherent resistance to commonly used antimicrobials, acquisition of high-level resistance to vancomycin and aminoglycosides, persistence in the environment, and transmission from patient to patient by way of the contaminated hands of health care workers. Hence, the emergence of vancomycin-resistant enterococci (VRE) has limited therapeutic options in confirmed enterococcal infections and in empirical therapy for infections in severely ill hospitalized patients and it represents a challenge for infection control in the health care setting. This chapter reviews the most important clinical manifestations of enterococci and their diagnosis and the importance of infection prevention.

The Pathogen

Members of the genus *Enterococcus* were long classified within group D of the genus *Streptococcus*. However, in the past 30 years, they have been reclassified based on new molecular and genetic analyses. Enterococci are catalase-negative gram-positive cocci that can appear singly or in pairs or short chains. They are facultative anaerobes that grow optimally at 35° to 37° C and are usually α-hemolytic or nonhemolytic on sheep blood agar. Enterococci can grow in broth containing 6.5% NaCl and hydrolyze esculin in the presence of 40% bile salts (bile-esculin medium) that can distinguish them from most streptococci. *Enterococcus faecalis*, the most common cause of enterococcal infections in humans, is the causative agent for 80% to 90% of the enterococcal infections followed by *Enterococcus faecium*, which is found in 5% to 10% of the infections. *Enterococcus casseliflavus*, *Enterococcus gallinarum*, and *Enterococcus raffinosus* are less frequently associated with infections, but clusters of infections have been reported. Other species isolated from different sources in humans include *Enterococcus avium*, *Enterococcus caccae*, *Enterococcus cecorum*, *Enterococcus dispar*, *Enterococcus durans*, *Enterococcus gilvus*, *Enterococcus italicus*, *Enterococcus hirae*, *Enterococcus malodoratus*, *Enterococcus mundtii*, *Enterococcus pallens*, *Enterococcus pseudoavium*, and *Enterococcus sanguinicola*.

EPIDEMIOLOGY

Enterococci are part of the normal human gut flora, and infections in both hospitalized and nonhospitalized patients can arise from either an endogenous or exogenous source. The proportion of infections caused by enterococci in hospitalized patients has been increasing over the past several decades. Overall, urinary tract infections (UTIs) are the most common clinical condition caused by enterococci. Based on data reported to the Centers for Disease Control and Prevention (CDC), enterococcal species are now the second most common isolates for any health care–associated infection and prominent causes of catheter-associated bloodstream, UTIs, and surgical site infections, causing approximately 15% of these infections in North America. Enterococci are the second most common cause of catheter-associated UTIs

and cause both complicated and uncomplicated UTIs. They are also the second most common cause of central line–associated blood stream infections and are involved in approximately 5% to 15% of all cases of infective endocarditis. They are also the third most frequent pathogen recovered in surgical site infections. Outside of the United States, these organisms are less common but increasingly important causes of infections.

In the 1970s, *E. faecalis* accounted for up to 95% of isolates and was associated with the introduction of third-generation cephalosporins. Increasingly, hospitalized patients, if they are colonized or infected with an *Enterococcus* species, tend to have a strain resistant to vancomycin and sometimes ampicillin (i.e., VRE).[1] *E. faecium* is the most common strain to acquire vancomycin resistance. VRE was first reported in Europe in 1986. Since the mid-, the proportion of enterococcal strains resistant to vancomycin, primarily *E. faecium,* has risen steadily. According to the CDC's National Healthcare Safety Network (NHSN), 62% to 82.6% of *E. faecium* isolates and 6.2% to 9.5% of *E. faecalis* isolates were resistant to vancomycin in 2009 to 2010.[2] Also, according to a recent report by the CDC on antimicrobial resistance in the United States, 66,000 *Enterococcus* health care–associated infections are reported yearly, and 20,000 of them are caused by VRE. There are two major genotypes for acquired vancomycin resistance, VanA and VanB. The genes encoding the VanA phenotype result in high-level resistance to vancomycin and teicoplanin and are carried on a transposon usually found on a plasmid that is transferable to other gram-positive cocci, including *Staphylococcus aureus*. VanA is mostly found in *E. faecium* and, less frequently, in *E. faecalis*. VanB is associated with variable resistance to vancomycin, but isolates are usually susceptible to teicoplanin. VanB is usually recovered from *E. casseliflavus* and *E. gallinarum*. Importantly, these genetic elements have been integrated into the genome of *S. aureus* that is resistant to vancomycin. The vancomycin-resistant *S. aureus* (VRSA) acquired a vancomycin resistance gene (*VanA*) from a VRE isolate that colonized a patient coinfected with methicillin-resistant *S. aureus*.

The epidemiology of VRE differs between Europe and North America. In Europe, VRE is often detected in farm animals, likely because of the use of the antibiotic avoparcin in animal feeds until it was banned in 1997. The proportion of VRE among enterococcal clinical isolates in hospitalized Europeans has been historically lower than in the United States; however, these rates are increasing. In the United States, avoparcin was never used in animal feeds, and therefore VRE is not usually found in farm animals or healthy humans. In contrast, the proportion of enterococcal isolates resistant to vancomycin is higher in U.S. hospitals than European hospitals. The proportion of enterococcal isolates from hospitalized European patients that are highly resistant to vancomycin varies by geographic region from less than 1% to up to 35%.

Most VRE infections are associated with health care and result from an exogenous source, meaning transmission from the environment, another patient, or on the hands of a health care worker. Nearly all infections are preceded by a period of colonization, primarily in the gastrointestinal (GI) tract. A study of hospitalized patients found that the most sensitive predictor of VRE colonization was previous admission to an acute care hospital in the past year. Importantly, after being colonized with VRE, patients may harbor the strain in their GI tract for years. Similarly, a study among hemodialysis patients demonstrated that the primary risk factor for VRE colonization was hospitalization in the prior year. Although many colonized patients do not develop infections, they are still able to contaminate the environment and shed and transmit bacteria to other hospitalized patients. The organism has a predilection to contaminate the hospital environment and equipment and has been associated with outbreaks.

Apart from preexisting GI colonization, risk factors for enterococcal infections, particularly VRE infections, include severe underlying conditions such as renal failure, previous solid organ or bone marrow transplantation, solid and hematologic malignancy, diabetes mellitus, and neutropenia. Other factors associated with infection include prior surgical or GI procedures, presence of a vascular or urinary indwelling catheter, hospital factors such as location in the intensive care unit (ICU) or oncology ward, proximity to colonized patients, prolonged length of hospitalization, and recent antimicrobial exposure.

Numerous epidemiologic investigations have revealed that most classes of antimicrobials have been associated with VRE infections. In particular, vancomycin, cephalosporins, and drugs with anaerobic organism coverage use have been linked to VRE acquisition. However, measuring the attributable impact of a particular antibiotic on VRE acquisition is difficult. Increasingly, an association between VRE colonization and *Clostridium difficile* infection is reported in high-risk patients such as those with hematologic malignancies.

PATHOBIOLOGY

Enterococci are commensal organisms that colonize the human GI tract and female genital tract. Although they are not as intrinsically virulent as other gram-positive pathogens, under certain conditions, the commensal relationship is disrupted, and serious infections occur. Several adhesion factors have been identified, including aggregation substance, which allow binding to epithelial surfaces and enhance the ability for colonization. The ability to adhere to heart valves and urinary tract epithelium enables enterococci to cause endocarditis and UTIs. Enterococci are also known to secrete potential virulence factors. These include cytolysin–hemolysin, which is a bacterial toxin that is produced in a higher proportion of infecting strains compared with stool-colonizing strains. Infecting strains also possess the ability of intestinal translocation, although the exact mechanisms of this process have yet to be determined. In addition, some cell surface determinants that are encoded may mediate adherence to host tissues that may be important in this organism's role in endocarditis. To this point, little is known about the host defense mechanisms in enterococcal infections. In addition, the exact role of capsular polysaccharides in colonization or infection is unknown. Strains have been shown to survive within phagocytic cells, yet it is unclear whether this represents successful host defense or evasion by the enterococci. The intrinsic resistance to multiple antimicrobials that enterococci possess, along with their ability to acquire new resistance mechanisms through mutation or acquisition of new genes, enhances their ability to survive and multiply in the many hospitalized patients treated with broad-spectrum antimicrobials.

CLINICAL MANIFESTATIONS

No specific clinical manifestations can help distinguish enterococcal infections from infections caused by other bacteria. Enterococci are not thought to cause lower respiratory tract infections or ventilator-associated pneumonia and, if found in these settings, likely represent colonization and not infection. Enterococci act as opportunistic pathogens in severely ill and compromised patients. They are known to cause UTIs, intra-abdominal abscesses, wound infection, bacteremia (including catheter-associated blood stream infections), and endocarditis.

Urinary Tract Infections

Urinary tract infections are the most frequent type of infection caused by enterococci.[3] Most infections are nosocomial in origin and include uncomplicated cystitis, pyelonephritis, prostatitis, and perinephric abscess. These infections are typically secondary to urinary catheterization or instrumentation. In contrast to nosocomial UTI, enterococci cause fewer than 5% of uncomplicated cystitis or pyelonephritis cases in otherwise healthy nonhospitalized women. Patients with diabetes mellitus appear to be at increased risk for enterococcal UTI. Bacteremia is only infrequently associated with enterococcal UTI.

Bacteremia

Importantly, enterococci can cause infection or contaminate cultured blood via contaminated catheter hubs and contaminated skin. Determining a true bacteremia versus a blood culture that is not clinically significant can be a challenge. Given this backdrop, the incidence of bacteremia caused by enterococci continues to increase. Specific risk factors include prolonged hospitalization, preexisting urethral catheters or intravascular lines, recent surgery, malignancy, neutropenia, and biliary pathology. Secondary bacteremia without endocarditis usually arises from the urinary tract, hepatobiliary tract, or soft tissue infection. Bacteremia secondary to an intra-abdominal source carries a high mortality rate. Risk factors for VRE bacteremia parallel those mentioned previously but additionally include severe preexisting comorbid conditions, including hematologic malignancy, human immunodeficiency virus (HIV) infection, chronic renal insufficiency, and liver transplantation. Prior exposure to broad-spectrum antimicrobials, including those with antianaerobic activity such as clindamycin or metronidazole, and exposure to multiple and prolonged antimicrobial therapy are consistent risk factors. Enterococcal bacteremia is frequently polymicrobial, and the clinical picture is often influenced by whether it is isolated alone or with other bacteria. When enterococci are isolated alone, the course is typically indolent, and frequently fever is the only sign. In contrast, polymicrobial bacteremia is more severe, often presenting with shock or disseminated intravascular coagulation. VRE bacteremia is associated with higher mortality rates than bacteremia caused by vancomycin-susceptible strains, and early treatment with an appropriate antibiotic within the first 48 hours of presentation has been associated with improved outcomes.

Endocarditis

Enterococci, particularly E. faecalis, are an increasingly frequent cause of endocarditis even though most enterococcal bacteremias are not complicated by endocarditis. The disease occurs most frequently in older patients, with a male predominance. Most cases appear to arise in the community. Patients with preexisting valvular heart disease, including prosthetic valves, are at highest risk, yet many patients lack underlying heart disease. Enterococci more commonly cause left-sided endocarditis primarily affecting the mitral valve. Clinically, these patients present with symptoms that closely resemble a subacute bacterial endocarditis caused by viridans streptococci. Many patients have symptoms for weeks or months before seeking medical care.

Intra-abdominal Infections

In intra-abdominal infections, enterococci are often detected as part of a polymicrobial process.[4] These infections typically arise from a hepatobiliary source, including postoperative infection in liver transplantation, and are complicated by secondary bacteremia.

Skin and Soft Tissue Infections

Enterococci rarely cause cellulitis or other soft tissue infections alone but are often isolated in mixed surgical site infections, diabetic foot infections, and decubitus ulcers along with other gram-negative bacilli, gram-positive cocci, and anaerobic bacteria. Their clinical significance in these situations has not been adequately determined. Enterococci are not thought to be primary pathogens in chronic osteomyelitis. When they are identified, it is thought they may solely represent superinfection, and thus adequate therapy may not require antibiotics directed at enterococcal eradication.

DIAGNOSIS

The diagnosis of an *Enterococcus* infection is made by isolating the organism through culture of a sterile site, such as blood or urine. Recently, molecular techniques have been developed to identify *Enterococcus* more quickly. The diagnosis and differential diagnosis of specific conditions are the same as discussed for UTIs (Chapter 284) and endocarditis (Chapter 76).

TREATMENT   Rx

Therapy for enterococcal infections is complicated by the fact that strains exhibit inherent resistance to many commonly used antibiotics, including cephalosporins.[5] In addition, enterococci can acquire resistance to a wide range of antibiotic classes, including aminoglycosides (high-level resistance), β-lactams, fluoroquinolones, and vancomycin. Thus, effective directed therapy for any severe enterococcal infection requires susceptibility testing by experienced microbiology laboratories, with therapy adjusted based on the results. Optimal therapy for most infections includes intravenous ampicillin, penicillin, or vancomycin. Given the resistance or tolerance to cell wall–targeting antibiotics, including penicillins and vancomycin, standard therapy with these antibiotics, except in UTIs, should include the addition of a synergistic aminoglycoside (i.e., gentamicin or streptomycin), as long as high-level resistance is not detected. This strategy of two-drug therapy has been associated with improved outcomes. This is particularly important in the setting of suspected endocarditis. Even when enterococcus appears susceptible to trimethoprim–sulfamethoxazole in vitro, it should not be used in therapy because clinical failures have been reported secondary to the ability of enterococci to use exogenous folate. Similarly, E. faecalis is intrinsically resistant to quinupristin–dalfopristin, which therefore should not be used in therapy for infections caused by this species. Recently, there has been increasing isolation of E. faecium strains with intrinsic resistance to penicillins. Still, most E. faecalis strains remain susceptible to ampicillin and the related piperacillin, in contrast to most E. faecium strains, which are resistant to ampicillin.

If the VRE strains are known to be susceptible, potential therapy in these infections includes linezolid, tigecycline, and daptomycin. Linezolid is commonly the drug of choice,[A1] although its use is associated with bone marrow suppression, including thrombocytopenia, and has only bacteriostatic activity against the enterococci. Linezolid, when used in combination with selective serotonin reuptake inhibitors, can be associated with serotonin syndrome (Chapter 434). Although daptomycin is not approved by the U.S. Food and Drug Administration (FDA) to treat VRE, it treats skin and soft tissue infections and bacteremia.[6] Tigecycline is FDA approved to treat complicated skin and soft tissue infections and complicated intra-abdominal infections caused by vancomycin-susceptible isolates of E. faecalis, but a recent black box warning by the FDA limits its use. Nitrofurantoin remains an option for VRE UTIs. Given the complexity of enterococcal infections, an infectious disease consult should be considered for therapeutic guidance.

Urinary Tract Infections

A single agent can usually be used to treat enterococcal UTIs, including ampicillin, amoxicillin, penicillin, quinolones, fosfomycin, or vancomycin. Vancomycin is typically reserved for penicillin-allergic patients or if the strain has high-level penicillin resistance. β-Lactam–β-lactamase inhibitor combinations are usually reserved for polymicrobial infections. Nitrofurantoin is also occasionally used because most strains remain susceptible. Fosfomycin is also indicated for UTIs caused by susceptible *E. faecalis.*

Bacteremia without Endocarditis

Many cases of enterococcal bacteremia are transient or self-limited, yet antibiotic therapy with penicillin or ampicillin has been shown to improve outcomes. Unlike in endocarditis therapy, it is not known whether patients benefit from combination therapy (penicillin or ampicillin or vancomycin plus an aminoglycoside), except perhaps when an indwelling intravascular catheter is present. In the setting of an indwelling intravascular catheter, especially for VRE, removal of the catheter is indicated. If the bacteremia is secondary to another site such as an intraabdominal abscess, drainage of the source is critical to cure.

Endocarditis

Combination therapy (intravenous penicillin, ampicillin, or vancomycin plus an aminoglycoside) is the standard therapy for enterococcal endocarditis. Various combinations have been tried with varying success depending on the species and susceptibilities of the organisms. Doses and durations are found in Chapter 76, but in general, consultation with infectious diseases experts is indicated. Importantly, the aminoglycoside is used to provide synergistic killing of the organism. The duration of therapy is typically 4 to 6 weeks with longer therapy given to patients who had prolonged symptoms before seeking therapy, prosthetic valve infection, or relapsed after initial treatment. If the causative enterococcal strain is highly resistant to both gentamicin and streptomycin, then alternative agents and durations must be explored, and surgery to excise infected valves should be considered. Optimal therapy of VRE strains that are resistant to ampicillin is not known but includes combination therapy under the guidance of an infectious diseases consultant. Several newly approved agents, including linezolid, and daptomycin could be considered if the strain is found to be susceptible. VRE endocarditis may require early surgery because outcomes with antibiotic therapy alone can be poor. Careful microbiologic and clinical assessment of all patients with enterococcal endocarditis and VRE in particular is helpful in deciding when surgery is necessary. If repeated blood cultures grow for more than 7 days after the initiation of medical therapy or other signs of uncontrolled infection (persistent fever or leukocytosis) are present, surgical repair of the valve or valve replacement should be considered early in the treatment course if there are no absolute contraindications for surgery.

Of note, linezolid resistance is increasingly reported even in patients without previous exposure to the antibiotic. Daptomycin resistance is also reported in both *E. faecalis* and *E. faecium* after prolonged courses of therapy.

Optimal infection prevention for VRE, similar to many multidrug-resistant bacteria, includes proper use and compliance with hand hygiene, use of contact precautions, proper management and timely removal of urinary and vascular catheters, reduction of antibiotic selective pressure through antimicrobial stewardship, and environmental cleaning of equipment and patient rooms. The latter is particularly important for VRE. A study in a U.S. hospital's medical ICU found that the number of patients already colonized with VRE in a defined geographic area ("colonization pressure") was the most significant variable in predicting new acquisition of VRE. Hence, decontamination of patients' skin, called source control, may broadly control transmission of resistant pathogens and reduce device-related infections such as central venous catheter–associated blood stream infections. Source control using daily bathing of patients with chlorhexidine gluconate-saturated cloths has been associated with reduced VRE contamination of patients' skin and health care workers' hands. A multicenter cluster randomized, cross-over clinical study in ICUs found daily bathing with chlorhexidine gluconate (CHG) solution reduced VRE acquisition by 25% and decreased the risk for VRE bacteremia in known VRE-colonized patients,[A2] although a subsequent trial has cast doubt on the efficacy of such an approach.[7]

The methods for VRE-specific prevention are directed at preventing incident colonization in high-risk hospitalized patients. Nearly all enterococcal infections, including VRE infections, are preceded by GI colonization, and although most colonized patients do not develop infections, they are still able to shed and transmit bacteria to other hospitalized patients. At least with VRE, a colonization-to-infection ratio of 10 : 1 has been reported, suggesting for every one clinical infection in an ICU, there may be 10 colonized patients lurking undetected in the unit. Thus, the unrecognized colonized patients represent the target population for infection prevention and control efforts such as active surveillance. Active surveillance programs use rectal or perirectal surveillance swabs to detect previously unrecognized, colonized patients and isolate them to prevent further transmission. Currently, surveillance cultures are recommended at the time of hospital admission for patients at high risk for carriage of VRE, and colonized patients or infected patients should be placed in isolation using contact precautions. Contact precautions typically entail private rooms, dedicated equipment such as stethoscopes, and gloves and gowns for all patient contact, although in a recent randomized trial in medical and surgical ICUs, the use of gloves and gowns for all patient contact compared with usual care did not result in a difference in the acquisition of VRE (or methicillin-resistant *S. aureus*).[A3] Implicit in this is the continued use of standard precautions that requires cleaning and disinfection of equipment that is used in patient rooms. Many hospitals do use active surveillance in the ICU and other wards with a high prevalence of VRE, although the overall adoption of this strategy has been hindered by the perceived high costs of surveillance programs and lack of available randomized control trial data.

Enterococcal bacteremia is associated with prolonged hospitalization and added costs compared with similar patients without enterococcal bacteremia. Still, apart from enterococcal endocarditis, the attributable mortality of enterococcal infections is difficult to quantify owing to its predilection to infect patients with preexisting comorbid conditions and high levels of illness severity. In certain patient populations, including those with liver and bone marrow transplants, studies have suggested increased morbidity, length of stay, and mortality associated with vancomycin resistance. Furthermore, a recent meta-analysis reported that the odds of dying from a vancomycin-resistant enterococcal blood stream infection were 2.5 times higher than dying from an infection caused by a susceptible enterococcus. The unadjusted mortality in susceptible enterococcal bacteremia was 20%. It is unclear why resistance is associated with higher mortality, although it is thought that delayed adequate empirical therapy may play a role. These studies should be interpreted cautiously because the clinical impact of resistance in enterococci was assessed before the availability of newer antimicrobials with activity against VRE.

Grade A References

A1. Chuang YC, Wang JT, Lin HY, et al. Daptomycin versus linezolid for treatment of vancomycin-resistant enterococcal bacteremia: systematic review and meta-analysis. *BMC Infect Dis.* 2014; 14:687.
A2. Climo MW, Yokoe DS, Warren DK, et al. Effect of daily bathing with chlorhexidine on hospital acquired infection. *N Engl J Med.* 2013;368:533-542.
A3. Harris AD, Pineles L, Belton B, et al. Universal glove and gown use and acquisition of antibiotic-resistant bacteria in the ICU: a randomized trial. *JAMA.* 2013;310:1571-1580.

GENERAL REFERENCES

For the General References and other additional features, please visit Expert Consult at https://expertconsult.inkling.com.

292

DIPHTHERIA AND OTHER *CORYNEBACTERIUM* INFECTIONS

ROLAND W. SUTTER

DEFINITION

Diphtheria is an acute infectious disease caused by toxigenic *Corynebacterium diphtheriae,* a gram-positive bacillus. The hallmark of the disease is the presence of a thick, firmly adherent pseudomembrane at the site of infection. The organism primarily infects the mucosa of the nose, pharynx, tonsils, or larynx (respiratory diphtheria). Rarely, other mucosal sites may be infected (e.g., conjunctiva, genitals, or ear). In developing countries, a variety of indolent skin lesions (cutaneous diphtheria) are common. Absorption of toxin can result in severe complications such as life-threatening myocarditis or polyneuritis.

The Pathogen

C. diphtheriae is a member of a group of aerobic, nonmotile, unencapsulated, nonsporulating, pleomorphic gram-positive bacilli.[1] Its name comes from the Greek *korynee* (meaning "club"), which describes the shape of the organism on stained smears with one end usually being wider, and *diphtheria* (meaning "leather hide"), for the characteristic adherent membrane.[2] The genus *Corynebacterium* is characterized by bacilli that line up in parallel groups and bend when dividing to create "Chinese character" arrangements. Both nontoxigenic and toxigenic *C. diphtheria* strains exist. Toxigenicity is conferred when a nontoxigenic organism is infected with a β-phage carrying the gene for the toxin (*tox*). *C. diphtheriae* has four biotypes—*gravis, mitis, intermedius,* and *belfanti*—that are distinguished by colonial morphology and varying biochemical and hemolytic reactions. Strains may be distinguished for epidemiologic purposes by molecular techniques. Diphtheria toxin-producing strains of *Corynebacterium ulcerans* can produce classic respiratory diphtheria-like disease, including distal toxic complications.

EPIDEMIOLOGY

Humans are the only natural reservoir of *C. diphtheriae,* although the organism has occasionally been isolated from a variety of domestic and other animals, including horses. Spread occurs in close-contact settings through respiratory droplets or by direct contact with respiratory secretions or skin lesions. The organism may survive for weeks and possibly months on environmental surfaces and in dust, and fomite transmission can occur. The majority of nasopharyngeal *C. diphtheriae* infections may abort or result in asymptomatic carriage, with clinical disease developing in only about one in seven individuals. However, asymptomatic carriers are important in maintaining transmission.

In the prevaccine era, respiratory disease dominated in temperate climates, with a fall and winter peak in incidence. Most individuals acquired natural immunity by the midteen years. Cutaneous disease is more common in tropical countries, but the contribution of cutaneous diphtheria in inducing or maintaining diphtheria immunity in tropical countries is unknown. Over the past 3 decades, outbreaks of cutaneous diphtheria have occurred in the United States and Europe, typically in homeless and alcoholic inner-city adults.

Diphtheria immunization protects against disease but does not prevent carriage. Vaccination with diphtheria toxoid (formalin-treated toxin) was introduced in the 1920s. Immunization of children in an era when the majority of older individuals had natural immunity resulted in a dramatic drop in the incidence of diphtheria and an even more rapid decline in the proportion of toxigenic strains isolated, presumably because the selective advantage of the *tox* gene—promotion of greater replication and spread of the organism—is lost in an immune host. In the postvaccine era, the respiratory diphtheria has virtually been eliminated from developed countries with excellent childhood vaccination coverage.[3] In the United States, reported cases fell from 147,991 in 1920, to 15,536 in 1940, to a total of 55 cases from 1980 to 2012. The absence of reported diphtheria cases in the United States in recent years, however, does not indicate that circulation of toxigenic *C. diphtheriae* has ceased. Investigations in a Northern Plains Indian community in North Dakota and First Nations communities in Ontario, Canada, suggested that *C. diphtheriae* strains might have circulated independently for more than 2 decades in these communities despite the absence of reported respiratory diphtheria cases.

In the absence of natural environmental boosting, vaccine-induced immunity wanes with increasing age and duration since a previous vaccination dose. There is a growing cohort of individuals with no natural diphtheria immunity. Serosurveys indicate that 20% to 60% of adults in industrialized countries have diphtheria antitoxin levels below minimal protective levels. A level of 0.01 IU/mL from an in vitro neutralization assay, the "gold standard" test, is considered the lower limit of protection. Long-term protection against diphtheria requires a level of greater than 0.1 IU/mL. As long as a high proportion of the population remains susceptible, the danger of reintroduction or reemergence of toxigenic strains exists.

Large outbreaks of diphtheria have occurred in the vaccine era. In the 1990s, there was a major resurgence of diphtheria in several countries of the

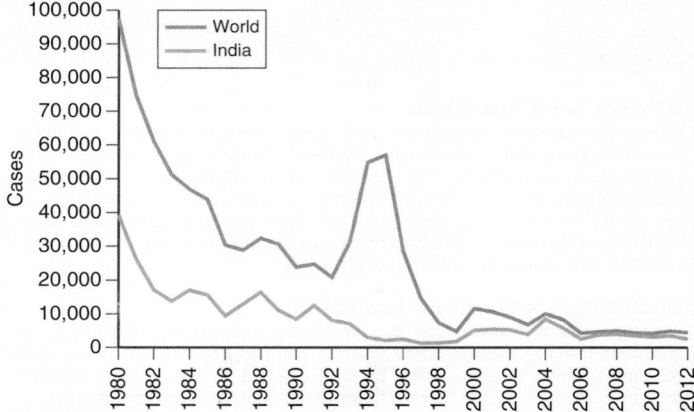

FIGURE 292-1. Reported diphtheria cases, worldwide, 1980 to 2012. (Data from the World Health Organization.)

former Soviet Union. In Russia, the number of reported cases rose from 593 in 1989 to 39,582 in 1994, with more than two thirds of cases occurring in adults. Large-scale campaigns of mass administration of diphtheria toxoid to virtually the entire population in the affected new independent states of the former Soviet Union have since led to significant decreases in the incidence of diphtheria, from a peak of 50,449 cases in 1995, to 7197 cases in 1997, to preresurgence levels by the late 1990s (Fig. 292-1). A large outbreak occurred in Indonesia from 2010 to 2012 and in Thailand in 2012.[4] Low vaccination coverage, and non- or inadequate vaccination have been the underlying causes. In general, outbreaks of diphtheria may occur in a suceptible population caused by clonal spread of the organism or transfer of the bacteriophage to nontoxigenic strains of *C. diphtheriae.* Although the reported diphtheria cases have declined globally in the past decade, some countries (e.g., India) continue to have endemic foci.

PATHOBIOLOGY

In classic respiratory diphtheria, *C. diphtheriae* colonizes the mucosal surface of the nasopharynx or larynx and multiplies locally without blood stream invasion.[5] The symptoms and signs of diphtheria are attributable to toxin production. Diphtheria toxin is an extremely potent inhibitor of protein synthesis, and the estimated human lethal dose is 0.1 mg/kg. Released toxin causes local tissue necrosis with the formation of a tough pseudomembrane composed of a mixture of fibrin, dead cells, and bacteria that is firmly adherent to the underling submucosal tissue. The membrane usually begins on the tonsils, on the posterior pharynx, or in the nose. In more severe cases, it progressively extends over the pharyngeal wall, fauces, and soft palate and into the larynx and may result in respiratory obstruction. Toxin entering the blood stream causes tissue damage at distant sites, particularly the heart (myocarditis), nerves (demyelination), and kidney (tubular necrosis). The extent of toxin absorption varies with the site of infection, being much less from the skin or nose than from the pharynx. Nontoxigenic strains may cause mild local respiratory disease and rarely a membrane.

CLINICAL MANIFESTATIONS
Respiratory Diphtheria

Infection limited to the anterior nares (nasal diphtheria) is manifested as a chronic serosanguineous or seropurulent discharge without fever or significant toxicity. A whitish membrane may be observed on the septum. The faucial (pharyngeal) form is most common. After an incubation period of 1 to 7 days, the illness begins with a sore throat, malaise, and mild to moderate fever. Initially, there is mild pharyngeal erythema, usually followed by progressive formation of a whitish tonsillar exudate, which over a period of 24 to 48 hours consolidates into a firmly adherent grayish membrane that bleeds on attempted removal. In more severe cases, the patient appears toxic, and the membrane is more extensive. Cervical lymphadenopathy and soft tissue edema may occur and result in the typical bull neck appearance and stridor. Laryngeal involvement (laryngeal diphtheria), which may develop on its own or as a result of membrane extension from the nasopharynx, is manifested as hoarseness, stridor, and dyspnea. The following clinical classification has been proposed by the World Health Organization: (1) catarrhal form (erythema of pharynx, no membrane), (2) follicular form (patches of exudate, no pharynx or tonsillar involvement), (3) spreading form (membranes covering the tonsils and the posterior pharynx), and (4) combined form (more than one anatomical site involved, e.g., throat and skin). The more severe clinical manifestations are associated with increasing toxin absorption levels.

The likelihood of toxic complications depends primarily on the interval between disease onset and administration of antitoxin. The severity of disease at initial evaluation closely predicts the likelihood of a severe clinical course, complications, and death. Myocarditis typically occurs in the first or second week after the onset of respiratory symptoms and develops either suddenly or insidiously with signs of low cardiac output and congestive failure. Conduction disturbances, which may occur without other signs of myocarditis, include ST-T wave abnormalities, arrhythmias, and heart block. Neurologic impairment is manifested as cranial nerve palsies and peripheral neuritis.[6] Palatal or pharyngeal paralysis (or both) occurs during the acute phase; peripheral neuritis, symmetrical and predominantly motor, occurs 2 to 12 weeks after onset of the disease. Motor deficit may range from minor proximal weakness to complete paralysis. Complete recovery is the rule. In fulminant, sometimes called "hypertoxic," diphtheria, toxic circulatory collapse with hemorrhagic features occurs.

Cutaneous Diphtheria

Cutaneous diphtheria lesions are classically indolent, deep, punched-out ulcers that may have a grayish-white membrane. However, the lesions may be indistinguishable from impetigo, or *C. diphtheriae* may infect chronic dermatoses such as stasis dermatitis. Coinfection with *Streptococcus pyogenes*, *Staphylococcus aureus*, or both occurs frequently. Toxic complications of only cutaneous diphtheria are rare.

DIAGNOSIS

A high index of suspicion is required. Specimens for culture should be taken from beneath the membrane, from the nasopharynx, and from any suspicious skin lesions. Because special media are required, the laboratory should be alerted to the concern about diphtheria. *C. diphtheriae* is best isolated on selective media that inhibit the growth of other nasopharyngeal organisms; one containing potassium tellurite is generally used. Based on colonial morphology and Gram stain appearance, a presumptive diagnosis may be possible within 18 to 24 hours. Culture results may be negative if the patient previously received antibiotics. Toxigenicity testing should be performed on all *C. diphtheriae* isolates. Because both nontoxigenic and toxigenic strains may be isolated from the same patient, more than one colony should be tested. Traditional testing methods include guinea pig inoculation and the modified Elek test, in which the isolate and appropriate controls are streaked on a culture plate in which a filter strip soaked with antitoxin has been embedded; toxin production is confirmed by an immunoprecipitation line in the agar. Identification of the diphtheria tox gene allowed the development of rapid and accurate polymerase chain reaction–based methods for identification of toxigenic strains.

Differential Diagnosis

The differential diagnosis includes streptococcal and viral tonsillopharyngitis, infectious mononucleosis, Vincent's angina, candidiasis, and acute epiglottitis. A history of travel to a region with endemic diphtheria or a history of contact with a recent immigrant from such an area increases the suspicion of diphtheria, as does a pre-antitoxin treatment serum antitoxin level of less than 0.01 IU/mL.

TREATMENT Rx

The decision to initiate therapy should be based on clinical grounds because delayed treatment, especially delays in antitoxin administration, is associated with worse outcomes. The goals of treatment are to neutralize the toxin rapidly, eliminate the infecting organism, provide supportive care, and prevent further transmission (Table 292-1). The mainstay of therapy is equine diphtheria antitoxin. Because only unbound toxin can be neutralized, treatment should commence as soon as the diagnosis is suspected, and each day of delay in administration increases the likelihood of a fatal outcome. A single dose ranging in quantity from 20,000 units for localized tonsillar diphtheria up to 100,000 units is given for extensive disease with severe toxicity. Antitoxin may be administered intramuscularly or intravenously; particularly for more severe cases, the intravenous route is preferred. Tests for sensitivity to antitoxin should be performed according to package insert instructions before administering it and desensitization carried out if necessary. Antibiotic therapy, by

TABLE 292-1	GOALS AND PROPOSED INTERVENTIONS FOR THE MANAGEMENT OF SUSPECTED DIPHTHERIA CASES
GOALS	**PROPOSED INTERVENTIONS**
Neutralize toxin as soon as possible to reduce severe complications, including death.	After a presumptive diagnosis of diphtheria, immediately obtain and administer antitoxin, initiate antimicrobial treatment, and arrange for appropriate supportive care.
Prevent further spread of *Corynebacterium diphtheriae* to close contacts, including hospital staff.	Isolate the patient; strictly observe respiratory barrier procedures. Notify the health department. Review the vaccination status of the family and other close contacts and initiate postexposure prophylaxis.
Confirm the diagnosis.	Collect appropriate specimens for culture (alert the laboratory to ensure that it can prepare specific culture media).
Induce long-term protection against *C. diphtheriae* in case and close contacts.	Complete the primary series with diphtheria toxoid as needed.

eliminating the organism, halts toxin production, limits local infection, and prevents transmission. Parenteral penicillin (4-6 million U/day) and erythromycin (40 mg/kg/day in four divided doses; maximum of 2 g/day, usually orally if the patient can swallow) are the drugs of choice. General supportive care includes ensuring a secure airway (with tracheotomy, if necessary), electrocardiographic monitoring for evidence of myocarditis, treating heart failure and arrhythmias, and preventing secondary complications of neurologic impairment such as aspiration pneumonia. The patient should be in strict isolation until follow-up culture results are negative. Convalescing patients should receive diphtheria toxoid.

The local health department must be notified. Close contacts should have cultures performed and be administered prophylactic antibiotics and brought up to date with an age-appropriate diphtheria toxoid-containing vaccination. A positive culture result in a contact may confirm the diagnosis if the patient is culture negative. All contacts without full primary immunization and a booster within the preceding 5 years should receive diphtheria toxoid.

The availability and access to diphtheria antitoxin has become problematic in recent years. Currently, very few manufacturers exist. In the United States, because manufacturers discontinued diphtheria antitoxin production in 1997, no licensed product is available. However, diphtheria antitoxin for therapeutic purposes can be obtained from the Centers for Disease Control and Prevention (CDC; 770-488-7100), which distributes a Brazilian-produced antitoxin (Instituto Butantan, Sao Paulo, Brazil) under an Investigational New Drug protocol.

PREVENTION

Immunization with diphtheria toxoid is the only effective means of primary prevention. The primary series is four doses of diphtheria toxoid (given with tetanus toxoid and pertussis vaccine) at 2, 4, 6, and 15 to 18 months; a preschool booster dose is given at 4 to 6 years of age. Thereafter, boosters should be given as part of the adolescent immunization visit (i.e., between 11 and 13 years of age) followed by doses administered every 10 years.

For additional protection against pertussis during adolescence, the CDC recommends the routine use of tetanus toxoid, reduced diphtheria toxoid, and acellular pertussis vaccine, adsorbed (Tdap), in adolescents 11 to 18 years of age in place of tetanus and diphtheria toxoid (Td) vaccines. Similarly, for adults who have never received a dose of Tdap, the CDC recommends routine use of a single dose of Tdap for adults older than 19 years of age to replace the next booster dose of Td (Chapter 18), although a second dose five years later may be needed to protect against diphtheria.[7]

Genetically altered, fully immunogenic mutants of diphtheria toxin have been created (e.g., CRM197) CRM197 is used as a protein carrier in several polysaccharide–protein conjugate vaccines. However, the role of CRM197 in contributing to or maintaining immunity has not been evaluated.

PROGNOSIS

Diphtheria, at the beginning of the 21st century, remains a serious disease associated with a high case-fatality rate. In the United States, the diphtheria

TABLE 292-2   CORYNEBACTERIA AND RELATED ORGANISMS ASSOCIATED WITH HUMAN DISEASE

SITE OF INFECTION	PATHOGEN	CLINICAL SYNDROME	COMMENTS
Respiratory tract	Corynebacterium diphtheriae Corynebacterium ulcerans Corynebacterium pseudodiphtheriticum Arcanobacterium haemolyticum	Classic diphtheria Diphtheria Pharyngitis Rarely, pneumonia in patients with advanced AIDS Pharyngitis, tonsillar abscess, rash	Zoonotic infection; may produce diphtheria toxin Clinically indistinguishable from streptococcal pharyngitis
Skin and soft tissue	Corynebacterium pseudotuberculosis Corynebacterium minutissimum Corynebacterium kroppenstedtii	Granulomatous lymphadenitis Erythrasma Granulomatous breast abscess	Zoonotic infection, especially in sheep; occupational risk for veterinarians and butchers
Genitourinary tract	Corynebacterium glucuronolyticum Corynebacterium urealyticum Corynebacterium riegelli	UTIs in men; chronic prostatitis Chronic and recurrent UTIs Encrusted cystitis	More common in elderly, chronically ill, and immunosuppressed patients and in those with indwelling catheters
Health care–associated infections	Corynebacterium jeikeium and less commonly many others, including Corynebacterium amycolatum, Corynebacterium striatum, and Corynebacterium urealyticum	Catheter- and device-associated infections Postprocedure wound and soft tissue infections Prosthetic valve joint infections Nosocomial pneumonia CSF shunt infections	C. jeikeium is the most common corynebacterial pathogen in hospitals and causes severe infections in immunosuppressed patients and those with indwelling devices

CSF = cerebrospinal fluid; UTI = urinary tract infection.

case-fatality rate has remained virtually unchanged (between 5% and 10%) over recent decades.

OTHER *CORYNEBACTERIUM* SPECIES

Corynebacteria other than *C. diphtheriae* are ubiquitous in the environment and are among the normal flora colonizing humans and animals. The pathogenic potential of many of these organisms was not appreciated in the past, but many are now known to be associated with specific and often serious infectious diseases, especially in immunosuppressed, chronically ill, and hospitalized patients (Table 292-2). In general, these organisms remain susceptible to vancomycin, but resistance to other classes of antimicrobials is common and varies among species.

GENERAL REFERENCES

For the General References and other additional features, please visit Expert Consult at https://expertconsult.inkling.com.

293

LISTERIOSIS

BENNETT LORBER

DEFINITION

Listeriosis is a food-borne infection caused by the gram-positive rod *Listeria monocytogenes*. Most patients have impaired cell-mediated immunity and are seen with life-threatening bacteremia or meningitis. However, a self-limited, febrile gastroenteritis in healthy persons also occurs.

The Pathogen

Widely distributed in nature, *L. monocytogenes* may be found in soil, on vegetation, and in the stool of healthy mammals, including humans. It causes disease in animals, especially herd animals, and in humans. The organism has been isolated from many foods, including raw vegetables, raw milk, fish, poultry, and meat. Unlike most food-borne pathogens, *L. monocytogenes* can grow at refrigerator temperatures.

EPIDEMIOLOGY

Non-perinatal listeriosis is almost always the result of food-borne infection.[1,2] Listeriosis is a relatively rare food-borne illness (≈1% of U.S. cases) but is associated with a case-fatality rate of 16 to 20% (second only to *Vibrio vulnificus* at 35 to 39%) and causes approximately 19 to 28% of all food-borne disease–related deaths.[3] Outbreaks have been documented in association with coleslaw, milk, soft cheeses, pâté, ready-to-eat pork products, deli counter meats, hot dogs, smoked fish, butter, sprouts, taco or nacho salads, and cantaloupes. In 2011, *L. monocytogenes*–contaminated cantaloupes were responsible for the deadliest food-borne disease outbreak in U.S. history, with 28 states reporting illness in 146 persons and death in 30 (21% mortality).[4]

Listeriosis was made a nationally reportable disease in 2000. The Centers for Disease Control and Prevention has established PulseNet (http://www.cdc.gov/pulsenet/), a network of public health and food regulatory laboratories that use pulsed-field gel electrophoresis to subtype food-borne pathogens to detect promptly disease clusters that may have a common source. Presently, the annual incidence of listeriosis is 3 cases per million population, and it accounts for 1800 cases per year and about 400 deaths. Neonates and adults older than 60 years have the highest infection rates. Pregnant women represent 20% of all affected individuals[5]; other adults at increased risk for invasive listeriosis (bacteremia, meningitis) include those with hematologic malignant disease, advanced acquired immunodeficiency syndrome (AIDS), a solid organ transplant, or iron overload and anyone treated with corticosteroids or an anti–tumor necrosis factor agent. However, as many as a fourth of all cases of invasive listeriosis occur in apparently healthy persons, particularly those older than 60 years.

PATHOBIOLOGY

L. monocytogenes enters the human body through the intestine, most often after the ingestion of contaminated food.[6] The bacterium induces its own uptake by gastrointestinal cells and macrophages. Mother-to-child transmission occurs transplacentally or through an infected birth canal. Within the host cell, the bacterium is enclosed in a phagolysosome, but through the production of an exotoxin called listeriolysin O, it destroys the phagolysosome membrane and gains access to the cytoplasm. All pathogenic strains of *L. monocytogenes* produce listeriolysin O, the major virulence factor. Listeriae actively divide in the cytoplasm, migrate to the periphery of the cell by polymerization of host cell actin, and then push out the cell membrane to form pseudopods, which are taken up by adjacent host cells. The bacteria move from cell to cell in this fashion and repeat their life cycle without exposure to antibodies or complement.

After invasion through the gastrointestinal tract, listeriae may disseminate hematogenously to any body site but show a particular tropism for the central nervous system (CNS). Less commonly, listeriae may spread intra-axonally through cranial nerves to reach the CNS; this mode of CNS invasion may result in rhombencephalitis (brain stem infection).

Immunity to listerial infection is handled chiefly through the cell-mediated arm of the immune system. Persons who have had splenectomy or have abnormalities solely of humoral immunity or leukocytes are not at increased risk for infection.

CLINICAL MANIFESTATIONS

The incubation period for invasive listeriosis (time from ingestion of contaminated food to illness) averages about 30 days. Invasive listeriosis in an immunocompromised adult is most often manifested as bacteremia without an obvious focus. In such cases, patients have nonspecific complaints, such as fever, malaise, myalgia, and back pain. Bacteremia is the form of invasive listeriosis that complicates pregnancy; CNS infection is extremely rare in the absence of other risk factors. Listeriosis during pregnancy may lead to spontaneous abortion or neonatal sepsis, but early antimicrobial therapy may result in the birth of a healthy child.[7] Endocarditis with *L. monocytogenes* can occur on both native and prosthetic valves and carries a high rate of septic complications. Endocarditis, but not bacteremia per se, may be a clue to underlying colon cancer; colonoscopy should be considered in all cases of listerial endocarditis.

Persons in whom *L. monocytogenes* bacteremia develops may progress to CNS infection, most commonly manifested as meningitis. *Listeria* has a predilection for infecting brain tissue as well as the meninges, and unlike other common bacterial causes of meningitis, it not infrequently causes encephalitis or brain abscess. Brain abscess as a result of infection by *L. monocytogenes* exhibits unusual features compared with other bacteria: listerial brain abscess coexists with bacteremia in nearly all cases and with meningitis in a fourth; in addition, abscesses are often subcortical.

L. monocytogenes is the most common cause of bacterial meningitis in patients with lymphomas, organ transplant recipients, and patients treated with corticosteroids for any reason. Affected persons usually have the classic acute symptoms of meningitis, but the presentation is subacute (>24 hours) in 60% of cases. Nuchal rigidity is absent in 20%. Focal neurologic findings, including ataxia, tremors, myoclonus, and seizures, may be seen, consistent with the tropism of *Listeria* for brain parenchyma. Gram stain of cerebrospinal fluid (CSF) reveals small gram-positive rods in only about one third of cases. The glucose content in CSF is normal in more than 60% of cases; mononuclear cells predominate in 30%.

Listerial rhombencephalitis[8] is an unusual form of listerial encephalitis that involves the brain stem and, unlike other listerial CNS infections, usually occurs in healthy adults. The typical clinical picture is one of a biphasic illness with a prodrome of fever, headache, nausea, and vomiting lasting about 4 days, followed by the abrupt onset of asymmetrical cranial nerve deficits, cerebellar signs, and hemiparesis or hemisensory deficits or both. Respiratory failure develops in about 40% of patients. Nuchal rigidity is present in about half, and CSF findings are only mildly abnormal, with a positive CSF culture in about 40%. Almost two thirds of patients are bacteremic. Magnetic resonance imaging is superior to computed tomography for demonstrating rhombencephalitis. Mortality is high, and serious sequelae are common in survivors.

Localized infection may occur after hematogenous seeding (e.g., liver abscess, septic arthritis) or, rarely, after direct inoculation (e.g., papulopustular rash, conjunctivitis). Osteoarticular listeriosis[9] primarily involves prosthetic joints, occurs in immunocompromised patients, and requires implant removal for cure.

Well-documented reports of food-borne outbreaks have demonstrated that ingestion of *L. monocytogenes* in a sufficiently large inoculum can result in a self-limited illness consisting of fever, chills, diarrhea, abdominal cramps, and sometimes nausea and vomiting. Symptoms follow exposure by 1 to 2 days and last for about 2 days.

DIAGNOSIS

Differential Diagnosis

Clinical situations in which a diagnosis of listeriosis should be considered include the following:
- neonatal sepsis or meningitis;
- meningitis or parenchymal brain infection in patients with subacute presentations, hematologic malignant neoplasms, AIDS, organ transplantation, corticosteroid immunosuppression, treatment with anti–tumor necrosis factor agents, or age older than 50 years;
- simultaneous infection of the meninges and brain parenchyma;
- subcortical brain abscess;
- fever during pregnancy;
- blood, CSF, or other normally sterile specimen reported to have "diphtheroids" on Gram stain or culture; and
- food-borne outbreak of febrile gastroenteritis when routine cultures fail to identify a pathogen.

The differential diagnosis of listerial CNS infection includes the more common causes of bacterial meningitis and brain abscess; indolent listerial meningitis or rhombencephalitis may mimic CNS tuberculosis.

Laboratory Findings

The diagnosis of listeriosis is made by routine bacterial culture of specimens from usually sterile sites, such as blood or CSF. The laboratory must exercise caution because *L. monocytogenes* may be mistaken for diphtheroids, streptococci, or enterococci. Specific stool culture is recommended only when routine stool cultures are negative in the setting of an outbreak of gastroenteritis; many people have enteric colonization with *L. monocytogenes* without invasive disease. The laboratory must be advised that listerial infection is suspected because the organism is unlikely to be identified with routine stool culture media.

Serologic testing (antibody to listeriolysin O) is not useful for invasive disease but may be helpful in the retrospective identification of food-borne outbreaks of febrile gastroenteritis when routine cultures are negative. Real-time polymerase chain reaction analysis of CSF for the *hly* gene, which encodes listeriolysin O, has been useful in diagnosing CNS listeriosis, including cases in which routine bacterial cultures were negative, but this test is not yet commercially available.[10]

PREVENTION

Guidelines for preventing listeriosis are similar to those for preventing other food-borne illnesses. In general, one should thoroughly cook raw food from animal sources; wash raw vegetables thoroughly before eating; keep uncooked meats separate from vegetables and from cooked and ready-to-eat foods; avoid raw (unpasteurized) milk or foods made from raw milk; and wash hands, knives, and cutting boards after each handling of uncooked foods.

People at high risk for listeriosis (those immunocompromised by illness or medications, pregnant women, and the elderly) may choose to avoid soft cheeses such as feta, Brie, Camembert, blue veined, and Mexican-style cheese such as queso fresco. Hard cheeses, processed cheeses, cream cheese, cottage cheese, and yogurt are safe. Leftover foods or ready-to-eat foods such as hot dogs should be cooked until steaming hot. It is best to avoid foods from delicatessen counters, such as prepared salads, meats, and cheeses, or at least to reheat cold cuts thoroughly until they are steaming hot before eating.

Listeriosis is effectively prevented by trimethoprim-sulfamethoxazole given as *Pneumocystis* prophylaxis to organ transplant recipients, those receiving corticosteroid immunosuppression, or individuals infected with human immunodeficiency virus. Second episodes of neonatal listerial infection are virtually unheard of, and intrapartum antibiotics are not recommended for women with a history of perinatal listeriosis.

Except for transmission from infected mother to fetus, human-to-human transmission of listeriosis does not occur; patients do not need to be isolated.

TREATMENT ℞

Recommendations for the treatment of infection with *L. monocytogenes* derive from in vitro data, animal models, and clinical experience with small numbers of patients; no controlled trials have been performed to prove the efficacy of one drug over another. Many antimicrobials show in vitro activity against *L. monocytogenes*. Clinical utility is more relevant than in vitro susceptibility test results because cephalosporins and other drugs to which the bacterium appears to be susceptible are inadequate to treat infection.

Twenty percent of cases of bacterial meningitis in those older than 50 years are due to *L. monocytogenes*. Therefore, empirical therapy for bacterial meningitis in all adults older than 50 years should include either ampicillin or trimethoprim-sulfamethoxazole, especially in the absence of associated pneumonia, otitis, sinusitis, or endocarditis, which would suggest a cause other than *L. monocytogenes*. Cephalosporins, commonly used for the treatment of bacterial meningitis, should not be used alone when *Listeria* is a diagnostic consideration.

Ampicillin is generally considered the drug of choice for treating confirmed cases of listeriosis. In cases of meningitis and endocarditis and in patients with severely impaired T-cell function, many authorities recommend the addition of gentamicin to ampicillin for synergy on the basis of in vitro testing and animal models. For meningitis, therapy should be continued for at least 3 weeks; bacteremic patients without CNS involvement may be treated for 2 weeks. Endocarditis and brain abscess should be treated for at least 6 weeks. Meningitis doses should be used to treat all cases of invasive listeriosis, even in the absence of CNS or CSF abnormalities.

In patients with penicillin hypersensitivity, trimethoprim-sulfamethoxazole is the preferred agent. It is bactericidal and appears to be as effective as the combination of ampicillin and gentamicin. Drugs that should be avoided because of treatment failure and relapse include cephalosporins, chloramphenicol, tetracycline, vancomycin, and erythromycin.

Corticosteroids appear to be important adjunctive agents in treating the most common forms of bacterial meningitis. Their role in the treatment of listerial CNS infection is unknown.

Iron is a virulence factor for *L. monocytogenes*, and clinically, iron overload states are risk factors for listerial infection. Therefore, in patients with listeriosis and iron deficiency, it may be prudent to withhold iron replacement until antimicrobial therapy is complete.

PROGNOSIS

Listeria meningitis carries a mortality of about 25%,[11] and mortality is higher in those with underlying malignant disease. Mortality from brain abscess and endocarditis is about 50%; survivors of brain abscess commonly have significant neurologic residua.

GENERAL REFERENCES

For the General References and other additional features, please visit Expert Consult at https://expertconsult.inkling.com.

294

ANTHRAX

DANIEL R. LUCEY AND LEV M. GRINBERG

DEFINITION

Anthrax is caused by *Bacillus anthracis*, a spore-forming, gram-positive rod that is aerobic or facultatively anaerobic. Its name derives from a Greek word for "coal," in reference to the black color of the eschar that forms in cutaneous anthrax. Although it is primarily a disease of animals (zoonosis), anthrax was developed as a biowarfare weapon by several nations in the 20th century and used for bioterrorism in the United States in 2001 when spores were mailed in letters.

The Pathogen

The bacterium is a large (1 to 1.5 by 3 to 5 μm), gram-positive rod. It has a ground-glass appearance of growth on sheep blood agar, with 2- to 5-mm, nonhemolytic, tenacious ("beaten egg white") colonies within 24 hours of culture; oval, central to subterminal spores; and a capsule that can be visualized by India ink staining.

EPIDEMIOLOGY

Human infection with *B. anthracis* is often linked to a zoonotic source, such as cattle, sheep, goats, water buffalo, and other animals. Meat, bones, hides, and hair have been reported to transmit infection. Spores can persist in soil for many years. Spores infect animals or humans, then germinate into the vegetative form of *B. anthracis* and cause disease. The World Health Organization provides an online global epidemiology database for anthrax along with guidelines for management of the disease in animals, humans, and the environment.

A systematic review of the worldwide medical literature found that between 1900 and 2005, at least 82 patients with inhalational anthrax were reported in clinical detail.[1] These 82 cases included 18 patients from the United States with naturally acquired, animal-related disease in the 20th century and 11 patients with inhalational anthrax due to the bioterrorism-related events of 2001. The dozens of patients with inhalational anthrax from the 1979 outbreak in Sverdlovsk that was linked to an accidental release of spores downwind from a military facility, however, were not included in these 82 cases because of unavailability of their clinical records. Only the autopsy records from 1979 were preserved by the pathologists (Abramova and Grinberg),

and these were published first in Russian in 1993 and then in English for the 41 cases confirmed by histopathology or microbiology.[2,3]

Between 2006 and 2013, an additional five patients with naturally acquired inhalational anthrax were diagnosed, three in the United Kingdom and two in the United States. In 2009, the first human case in the United States of culture-confirmed gastrointestinal anthrax was diagnosed.[4] At least three of these six sporadic cases, including the gastrointestinal case, were linked to exposure to spores contaminating drums made from animal hides. The source of exposure was uncertain for the others. More typically, gastrointestinal anthrax is linked to consumption of meat from infected animals.

Importantly, *B. anthracis* is not transmitted from person to person through the air. Moreover, only one quarter of the 41 autopsy-confirmed inhalational cases in 1979 had any evidence of pneumonia, specifically an acute hemorrhagic pneumonia. All had the characteristic hemorrhagic mediastinal adenopathy, edema, and pleural effusions caused by the primary inhalation of spores. Infection by reaerosolization was suspected in a small number of these patients in 1979.

In support of this reaerosolization hypothesis, a detailed review of the experimental literature found evidence that spores from *Bacillus* species could reaerosolize under outdoor conditions.[5] Moreover, a study of the spores in a contaminated U.S. Senate Office concluded that spores used in a terrorist incident reaerosolized under common office activities.

The most common form of anthrax is the cutaneous form. Direct contact with infected animals or contaminated animal products is the usual mode of transmission. One of the lessons from the 2001 bioterrorist attacks in the United States, however, is that spores in the mailed letters caused cutaneous anthrax in 11 persons, none of whom had inhalational anthrax. Of note, therefore, unexplained cutaneous anthrax cases could be an early clue to an intentional release of spores, especially given that the shortest part of the incubation period in humans for cutaneous anthrax (1 to 12 days) is less than that for laboratory-documented inhalational anthrax (4 to 43 days).

In 2009-2010, at least 80 confirmed or probable cases of anthrax occurred in persons who injected heroin in Europe, primarily in the United Kingdom.[6] In 2012-2013, at least another 14 cases occurred, again in the United Kingdom[7] but also in Denmark, France, and Germany. A new term, *injection anthrax*, was applied to this novel route of infection and distinct clinical syndrome that involved severe soft tissue infection at the site of the injection and sometimes systemic disease. The single strain of *B. anthracis* in these outbreaks most closely matched that reported from a goat in Turkey, suggesting that heroin originating in Afghanistan or Pakistan and smuggled overland in an animal skin may have been the source of these spores in Europe.

PATHOBIOLOGY

Major virulence factors of *B. anthracis* include its two binary toxins, edema toxin and lethal toxin, and also its antiphagocytic poly-D-glutamic acid capsule. Edema toxin consists of edema factor bound to a third anthrax toxin component, protective antigen. Similarly, lethal toxin consists of lethal factor bound to protective antigen. These three toxin components, edema factor, lethal factor, and protective antigen, are encoded on one plasmid (pX-01). The antiphagocytic capsule is encoded on a second plasmid (pX-02). Both plasmids are necessary to cause disease.

The pathogenesis of anthrax has been attributed primarily to its two binary toxins. However, more recently, key roles for both nontoxin and toxin components have been implicated in the pathogenesis of the characteristic cardiac and endovascular abnormalities,[8] bleeding, and shock. Nontoxin components include the peptidoglycan part of the bacterial cell wall and nontoxin metalloproteinases. Moreover, inhibition of both innate and adaptive immune responses occurs by the activities of both toxins and the antiphagocytic capsule.

Similarly, the sepsis model has been proposed to explain the high lethality of inhalational anthrax, rather than the toxin model.[9] In this sepsis model, the primary role of anthrax toxin is to inhibit the immune response against the vegetative form of the bacteria, thus allowing the typically high levels of bacteremia to develop and subsequent shock, multiorgan failure, and death to occur.

Lethal toxin[10] is a metalloproteinase and inhibitor of the mitogen-activated protein kinase intracellular signal transduction pathway. It contributes to the coagulation disorder, hemolysis, and hemorrhage seen with inhalational anthrax. Whether lethal toxin contributed to the vasculitis lesions reported in the 1979 outbreak in Sverdlovsk is uncertain. Edema toxin contributes to the typical "gelatinous" fluid in the mediastinum and abdomen as well as the marked edema seen in both cutaneous anthrax and injection anthrax. The mechanism is attributed to excessive production of cyclic adenosine mono-phosphate from adenosine triphosphate, by edema toxin acting as an adenyl-ate cyclase enzyme. The result is water and calcium dysregulation with marked edema.

CLINICAL MANIFESTATIONS

Major clinical manifestations of anthrax infection—inhalational, cutaneous, gastrointestinal, injection, and meningeal—are related to the routes through which *B. anthracis* can enter the body: inhalation, contact, ingestion, or injec-tion (e.g., by contaminated heroin).[11]

Inhalational anthrax[12] almost always causes hemorrhagic mediastinitis, gelatinous edema, and mediastinal adenopathy, resulting in mediastinal wid-ening, as well as pleural effusions due to blockage and reversal of normal lymphatic flow and drainage within the mediastinum. These pleural effusions can be large, bloody, and recurring unless repeatedly drained by thoracentesis or chest tube. Such effusions were found to contribute to respiratory failure in the 1979 outbreak in Sverdlovsk, in part due to compression of lung paren-chyma and impaired gas exchange. During the outbreak, the pleural fluid was drained by thoracentesis, rather than by chest tube, and antibiotics were injected into the pleural space. Nevertheless, nearly every patient with inha-lational anthrax who underwent autopsy in this outbreak was found to have large (average, 1776 mL) pleural effusions. Although it was not known in 1979 or in 2001, these pleural effusions can serve as a reservoir for toxin. Pleural fluid toxin levels were not tested until the two U.S. patients in 2006 and 2011. High levels of lethal factor were reported.

Radiography demonstrated pulmonary infiltrates in 7 of the 11 patients in 2001 in the United States as well as in both U.S. patients in 2006 and 2011. Thus, although inhalational anthrax has been stated by some not to cause pneumonia, these radiologic findings serve to emphasize the important diag-nostic point for clinicians that not only mediastinal widening and pleural effusions but also pulmonary infiltrates are often seen. Moreover, in the 1979 outbreak in Sverdlovsk, one quarter of the 41 autopsy-confirmed cases had a hemorrhagic pneumonia. Thus, pulmonary infiltrates on radiologic imaging, whether or not interpreted as pneumonia, do not rule out the diagnosis of inhalational anthrax.

In 2005, a new three-part clinical staging system for inhalational anthrax (Table 294-1) was published, adding an intermediate progressive stage based on clinical, microbiologic, and radiologic information acquired from the 11 patients in 2001. Previously, these patients would have been included in the late stage, for whom death was considered almost certain. Importantly, all six of the patients who survived the anthrax attacks in 2001 had rapid therapy initiated, including pleural drainage, during this intermediate progressive stage. This three-part symptomatic clinical staging system is cited at www .cidrap.umn.edu/idsa/bt/anthrax/biofacts/anthraxfactsheet.html.

Although in 2001 none of the five patients in the late fulminant stage survived, the two U.S. patients in 2006 and 2011 both survived even though they required mechanical ventilation, placing them in the late fulminant stage. One additional treatment they received was anthrax antitoxin, which was not available in 2001.

The shortest incubation period that has been *documented* microbiologically or histopathologically is 4 days. The range is 4 to 43 days. Although shorter incubation periods may have occurred, none have been documented in the English literature by these laboratory criteria.

Cutaneous anthrax accounts for about 95% of patients with anthrax. The incubation period ranges from 1 to 12 days. Like the three clinical stages of symptomatic inhalational anthrax, three stages of cutaneous anthrax can be delineated: (1) an initial pruritic papule progressing to (2) a central vesicular or bullous lesion with surrounding nonpitting edema and finally (3) a necrotic and hemorrhagic central lesion that evolves into the classic painless eschar with surrounding edema. Resolution can take up to 2 months. This three-stage progression can occur even if appropriate antibiotics are given. During the anthrax letter attacks of 2001, some of the cutaneous lesions were initially considered to be due to brown recluse spider bites. These lesions are usually painful, unlike the painless lesions of anthrax.

In contrast to cutaneous anthrax, injection anthrax[13] described from Europe in persons injecting spore-contaminated heroin does not typically develop a black crusted eschar, can be painful, and can present with severe gastrointestinal or central nervous system manifestations that can rapidly lead to death. The 2011 official report from Health Protection Scotland on outbreaks of this novel form of anthrax advises physicians to suspect injection anthrax in heroin users who demonstrate any of three presentations: (1) severe soft tissue infection including necrotizing fasciitis and cellulitis/

TABLE 294-1	CLINICAL STAGING SYSTEM FOR INHALATIONAL ANTHRAX

I. EARLY PRODROMAL STAGE

Nonspecific illness sometimes described as "flulike" and including any of the following: fever, cough, headache, chills, nausea, chest pain, or abdominal pain. Laboratory tests and radiographs are nondiagnostic. The prognosis for cure is good with appropriate therapy, but the diagnosis is difficult to confirm acutely in this stage.

II. INTERMEDIATE PROGRESSIVE STAGE

Any of the following findings are defining inclusion criteria for this stage:
1. Positive blood cultures (typically positive in <24 hours)
2. Mediastinal adenopathy
3. Pleural effusions: bloody, often large, require drainage, and may recur

Findings in this stage may include high fever, dyspnea, confusion or syncope, or increasing nausea and vomiting. Exclusion criteria for this stage include the following:
1. Meningitis
2. Respiratory failure requiring intubation and mechanical ventilation or
3. Shock

Importantly, patients in the intermediate progressive stage can still be cured with appropriate antibiotics and drainage of pleural effusions by repeated thoracentesis or preferably chest tube to keep the pleural space dry in order to reduce the adverse mechanical effect on respiration by large-volume effusions and to remove potentially toxin-producing *Bacillus anthracis* from the pleural space.

III. LATE FULMINANT STAGE

Inclusion criteria include any one of the following findings:
1. Meningitis
2. Respiratory failure requiring intubation and mechanical ventilation
3. Shock: end-organ hypoperfusion

Findings in this stage may also include any of those from previous stages, so there are no exclusion criteria. The probability of survival is lowest in this stage. Novel therapeutics that safely and effectively neutralize anthrax toxin may be needed to increase survival.

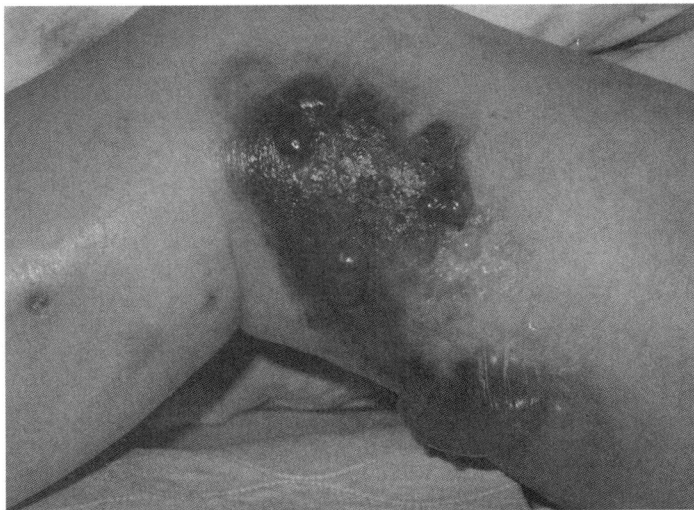

FIGURE 294-1. An example of the lesions due to injection anthrax.

abscess, especially if marked edema is present (Fig. 294-1); (2) signs of sepsis even if no soft tissue infection is evident; and (3) meningitis or subarachnoid hemorrhage/intracranial bleed.

Gastrointestinal anthrax is divided into an oropharyngeal form and an intestinal form. The oropharyngeal form has painful cervical adenopathy and an incubation period between 2 hours and 6 days. The oral lesions can ulcer-ate. They also can progress to cause a white pseudomembrane with dysphagia and hoarseness. The intestinal form has been described to have three clinical phases, much like the three-part progressive clinical stages of inhalational anthrax and cutaneous anthrax: (1) a prodromal phase with fever, malaise, and sometimes syncope; followed by (2) a progressive phase with abdominal pain, nausea, vomiting, abdominal distention, ascites, and severe weakness; and finally (3) a fulminant phase with rapidly increasing abdominal girth and expanding ascites, paroxysmal abdominal pain, and shock. Of note, the U.S. patient with gastrointestinal anthrax in 2010 who survived had more than 50 liters of ascitic fluid drained as part of her therapy along with antibiotics and anthrax antitoxin.

Anthrax meningoencephalitis can occur in association with any of the other forms of anthrax, inhalation, cutaneous, gastrointestinal, or injection, and rarely without a known portal of entry. Cerebral edema, parenchymal brain hemorrhage, vasculitis, and subarachnoid hemorrhage can occur. The cerebrospinal fluid is often bloody with anthrax meningitis. At autopsy, the extensive bleeding gives a characteristic macroscopic appearance termed the cardinal's cap. This form of anthrax remains fatal in more than 95% of cases.

DIAGNOSIS

If anthrax is suspected, blood should be obtained immediately before any antibiotics are given, primarily for microbiologic culture and possibly for newer assays for anthrax toxins whenever available. Notably, blood cultures from patients with inhalational anthrax will grow the large, gram-positive rods within 24 hours. Given such high levels of bacteremia, it is surprising that even one dose of an effective antibiotic has been reported to turn blood cultures negative, hence the need to draw blood culture samples before antibiotics are given. Toxin assays could still be positive after initial antibiotics, but these assays are still investigational at this time. Nasal cultures should not be performed as a routine clinical diagnostic test for individual patients because a negative result does not rule out inhalation of spores. Nasal cultures could be epidemiologically useful, however, as part of an investigation to help estimate the perimeter of exposure to spores.

In the microbiology laboratory, if the initial culture is suggestive of *B. anthracis*, three tests can be performed with a biosafety cabinet. These are assays for motility (nonmotile), catalase (positive), and hemolysis (negative). If these characteristics are found, identification is still not proved until a sample is sent to a reference laboratory where polymerase chain reaction analysis can identify *B. anthracis* and gamma-phage lysis of the encapsulated bacteria can provide confirmation. One or more antibody tests also are available, although results are unlikely to be positive during the earliest part of the disease. In contrast, a number of investigational anthrax toxin tests (e.g., for lethal factor, edema factor, or protective antigen) are being developed that should have positive results early in the disease, even if antibiotics have been given, and may also have prognostic value. At the time of this writing, these assays are available in the United States only through the Centers for Disease Control and Prevention (CDC).

A noncontrast computed tomography scan of the chest can be a valuable adjunctive diagnostic tool for inhalational anthrax. It is more sensitive than a chest radiograph for demonstrating the characteristic hyperattenuating mediastinal adenopathy causing the mediastinal widening and pleural effusions. The hyperattenuation is consistent with bleeding into lymph nodes and thus helps differentiate inhalational anthrax from tularemia, histoplasmosis, tuberculosis, sarcoidosis, and most other causes of mediastinal or hilar adenopathy.

Anthrax meningitis is typically neutrophilic and bloody. Very large gram-positive rods in the cerebrospinal fluid distinguish anthrax meningitis from other causes of gram-positive meningitis, such as the smaller *Listeria monocytogenes*. In the February 2014 *Emerging Infectious Diseases* online journal, the CDC published its first formal updated guidelines on anthrax since 2001, including diagnostic tests, prophylaxis, treatment, and monitoring.[14] New diagnostic recommendations include a lumbar puncture at admission unless it is contraindicated because new treatment recommendations will be based in part on whether meningitis has been excluded.

TREATMENT   Rx

Treatment of symptomatic anthrax includes antibiotics and, in the case of inhalational anthrax, pleural fluid drainage. In addition, in December 2012, the Food and Drug Administration (FDA) licensed the first anthrax antitoxin for treatment of inhalational anthrax. The CDC recommendations for prevention and treatment were updated in 2014, and the reader is referred to their webpage for complete details.[14]

Treatment with three intravenous antibiotics is recommended in the 2014 CDC recommendations if meningitis is possible or confirmed. These include a bactericidal fluoroquinolone (ciprofloxacin is the preferred drug), a bacteri-

cidal β-lactam (meropenem is the preferred drug), and a protein synthesis inhibitor (linezolid is the preferred drug). If meningitis is excluded, a bactericidal drug (ciprofloxacin is preferred) and a protein synthesis inhibitor (either clindamycin or linezolid) is preferred.

A total 60-day course of antibiotic therapy, of at least 2 weeks intravenously with more than one drug followed by the remainder with one oral drug, is recommended for inhalational anthrax because of concern that spores may germinate into vegetative bacteria if therapy is stopped sooner.

An essential treatment modality for inhalational anthrax is pleural drainage. The CDC 2014 guidelines state: "Drainage of pleural fluid and ascites is believed to improve survival by reducing the toxin level and by decreasing mechanical lung compression. These data support the need for early and aggressive drainage of any clinically or radiographically apparent pleural effusions; chest tube drainage is recommended over thoracentesis because many effusions will require prolonged drainage. Thoracotomy or video-assisted thoracic surgery might be required to remove gelatinous or loculated effusions."

As of 2014, there are two types of anthrax toxin antibodies in the Strategic National Stockpile. One is polyclonal, called intravenous anthrax immune globulin, and is derived from the plasma of persons who have received the anthrax vaccine. It is still investigational, and the investigational new drug protocol is held by the CDC in Atlanta. Intravenous anthrax immune globulin has been given as adjunctive therapy to several patients, including three in the United States in 2006, 2009, and 2011 as well as several patients in the United Kingdom. The other antitoxin is a humanized monoclonal antibody called raxibacumab that was licensed by the FDA in December 2012 for treatment of inhalational anthrax in both adults and children.[15] It has not been given to any patients with anthrax as of February 2015 but was licensed by the FDA on the basis of efficacy in animal models of inhalational anthrax plus human safety data in healthy volunteers. It does not cross the blood-brain[16] barrier. It is given intravenously during 2 hours and 15 minutes, after a single dose of the antihistamine diphenhydramine.

PREVENTION

Clinical anthrax can be prevented by preexposure vaccination or by postexposure prophylaxis with antibiotics. Moreover, in December 2012, the monoclonal antibody antitoxin (raxibacumab) was licensed by the FDA for postexposure prophylaxis in both adults and children "when alternative therapies are not available or not appropriate."

The current FDA-licensed anthrax vaccine (as of 1970) contains protective antigen as the vaccine antigen and alum as an adjuvant.[17] It requires five injections during an 18-month period when it is given before exposure. In contrast, postexposure prophylaxis, which is an off-label use of this same vaccine and thus needs an investigational new drug or emergency use authorization protocol, requires only three injections given during a 1-month period. This vaccine is in limited supply and is dedicated primarily for use by the military; however, it is available to civilian populations through at least one commercial travel clinic.

Antibiotics that are approved by the FDA for postexposure prophylaxis include ciprofloxacin, doxycycline, and procaine penicillin G as well as levofloxacin. Either doxycycline or ciprofloxacin is recommended as the preferred drug by the CDC for initial prophylaxis when the antibiotic susceptibility of an anthrax strain is unknown. During pregnancy, however, ciprofloxacin is preferred to doxycycline according to 2014 CDC guidelines. The CDC website on anthrax (at http://www.bt.cdc.gov/agent/anthrax) has detailed recommendations regarding the choice of antibiotics, doses, and durations for both prevention and treatment of anthrax.

Prevention of anthrax due to bioterrorism remains a national priority. A suspicion of clinical anthrax or exposure to spores warrants immediate involvement of law enforcement authorities because of the possibility of a criminal act. Evolving approaches for detecting and responding to any future bioterrorism attacks with anthrax include the BioWatch system to detect aerosolized threats and the Autonomous Detection System in postal facilities. The Cities Readiness Initiative was initially described on the CDC website in June 2004 as a program for multiple U.S. cities to help prepare for large-scale public health emergencies, including bioterrorism attacks (e.g., with aerosolized anthrax or another organism). Large volumes of medical supplies, including but not limited to antibiotics, can be delivered rapidly from the Strategic National Stockpile to one or more cities followed by local distribution. The 2012 Institute of Medicine report titled *Prepositioning Antibiotics for Anthrax* discusses the Strategic National Stockpile, Cities Readiness Initiative, BioWatch, and antibiotic issues including defining multidrug-resistant and extremely drug-resistant strains.

PROGNOSIS

The inhalational anthrax of all six patients who survived the attacks of 2001 was diagnosed during the intermediate progressive stage, and prompt therapy prevented progression beyond this stage. The 45% case-fatality rate in 2001 was much improved over the 88% rate seen in the United States from 1900 to 1976. Survival is more likely in patients who undergo pleural drainage, receive multidrug antibiotic regimens, do not require intubation or tracheotomy, and do not progress to anthrax meningoencephalitis. Of note, two patients with inhalational anthrax in the United States (in 2006 and 2011) with respiratory failure requiring mechanical ventilation have survived. Whether the addition of antitoxin to their intensive care, multiple antibiotics, and pleural drainage played a causal role in their survival is uncertain. Their survival emphasizes, however, that even patients in the late fulminant stage can sometimes survive.

The mortality from cutaneous anthrax is approximately 20% if it is untreated, particularly in patients in whom upper airway compression develops from a lesion on the neck or in whom secondary bacteremic anthrax meningitis develops. Anthrax meningitis remains fatal in more than 95% of victims, and thus better therapies are needed. The FDA licensure of the first anthrax antitoxin for both children and adults, as therapy and also as postexposure prophylaxis when alternative therapies are not available or not appropriate, may improve clinical outcome in systemic forms of anthrax. An antitoxin is still needed, however, that can treat anthrax meningitis.

FUTURE DIRECTIONS

A rapid test is still needed for the diagnosis of infection with *B. anthracis* in the early prodromal stage of the illness or in later clinical stages if the patient received antibiotics before blood culture samples were obtained. Such a test is likely to be based on a toxin or a toxin component. Ideally, it should be available at the point of care.

Anthrax toxin inhibitors, in conjunction with antibiotics, could be particularly useful in treating patients who have progressed into the systemic stages of anthrax as a result of inhalational, gastrointestinal, or injection anthrax causing serious soft tissue infection. In addition, antitoxin could be useful in the setting of infection with an engineered form of multidrug-resistant or extremely drug-resistant anthrax. New anthrax vaccines are still being tested. A shorter series of primary and booster doses for the only licensed vaccine was reported in December 2013. Criteria have been established for approval by the FDA of this vaccine specifically in the setting of postexposure prophylaxis. Meeting these criteria and obtaining licensure of the vaccine for postexposure prophylaxis will be a major advance.

GENERAL REFERENCES

For the General References and other additional features, please visit Expert Consult at https://expertconsult.inkling.com.

295

ERYSIPELOTHRIX INFECTIONS

ANNETTE C. REBOLI

DEFINITION

Erysipelothrix rhusiopathiae causes three well-defined patterns of human infection: (1) erysipeloid, a cellulitis of the fingers and hands (also known as whale finger or pork finger), which is the most common manifestation of infection with *E. rhusiopathiae*; (2) a diffuse cutaneous form; and (3) a bacteremic form, with or without cutaneous involvement, usually complicated by endocarditis.

The Pathogen

E. rhusiopathiae is a thin, pleomorphic, nonsporulating, microaerophilic gram-positive rod. It may be confused with other gram-positive bacillary organisms, particularly *Listeria monocytogenes* (Chapter 293) and *Corynebacterium* species (Chapter 292). It can be differentiated from *L. monocytogenes*

by its lack of motility, lack of catalase and coagulase production, and resistance to neomycin. Most strains of *E. rhusiopathiae* produce hydrogen sulfide on triple sugar iron agar slants, a feature that distinguishes *E. rhusiopathiae* from *L. monocytogenes* and from corynebacteria. Because α-hemolysis may be seen after 48 hours of incubation of *E. rhusiopathiae*, confusion with streptococci may also occur. The term *erysipeloid* refers to cutaneous infection by *E. rhusiopathiae* and should not be confused with erysipelas (see Fig. 441-4), which is a superficial cellulitis caused by streptococci or staphylococci.

EPIDEMIOLOGY

E. rhusiopathiae is found worldwide as a commensal or as a pathogen in a variety of wild and domestic animals, including swine, sheep, cattle, horses, dogs, cats, rodents, chickens, ducks, turkeys, penguins, and parrots, as well as in flies, ticks, mites, and lice. The greatest commercial impact of *E. rhusiopathiae* infection is due to disease in swine, but infection of sheep and poultry is also important economically. Environmental surfaces in contact with infected animals or their products are potential sources of *E. rhusiopathiae*. It can persist for prolonged periods in contaminated soil. *E. rhusiopathiae* is killed within 15 minutes by heating to 55° C and by several commercially available home disinfectants.

The incidence of cutaneous infection in humans seems to be decreasing because of technologic advances in animal industries. Infection is usually the result of contact with infected animals or their products. Persons at greatest risk for infection include fishers, fishmongers, farmers, butchers, slaughterhouse workers, and veterinarians.[1] The organism gains entry through cuts and abrasions on the skin. The seasonal incidence of erysipeloid parallels that of swine erysipeloid and is highest in the summer and early fall. The rare instances of systemic infection that do not have an occupational link tend to occur in immunocompromised hosts, suggesting that oropharyngeal or gastrointestinal colonization with the organism may occur. Chronic alcoholism has been acknowledged as a common underlying condition. Erysipeloid and erysipeloid with bacteremia have been reported rarely after cat and dog bites, suggesting that *E. rhusiopathiae* may be part of the oral flora of these animals.

PATHOBIOLOGY

The virulence of *E. rhusiopathiae* is associated, at least in part, with resistance to phagocytosis by polymorphonuclear leukocytes. This antiphagocytic ability results from the organism's possession of a capsule. In the absence of specific antibodies, *E. rhusiopathiae* evades phagocytosis, but even if it is phagocytosed, it is able to replicate intracellularly in these cells. Other virulence factors include enzymes (neuraminidase and hyaluronidase) and surface proteins.

CLINICAL MANIFESTATIONS

Because of the mode of acquisition (contact with infected animals or their products, with organisms inoculating abrasions on the skin), lesions are usually confined to the fingers and hands (Fig. 295-1). A well-defined, slightly elevated, violaceous lesion accompanied by a very painful, throbbing, burning, or itching sensation develops within 2 to 7 days of traumatic dermal inoculation. The infected area is swollen. Vesicles may be present, but suppuration is absent. The lesion spreads slowly to other fingers but rarely involves the fingertips or the skin above the wrist. As the lesion spreads peripherally, the central area clears.[2] Systemic signs and symptoms are rare. There may be sterile arthritis of an adjacent joint. Regional lymphadenopathy or lymphadenitis occurs in about 20% of cases, and low-grade fever develops in approximately 10%. Lesions usually resolve within 3 weeks without treatment. Relapse occurs in 1% of cases.

The diffuse cutaneous form is rare. The cutaneous lesion progresses proximally from the site of inoculation or appears at remote areas. Patients often have fever and arthralgias, but blood cultures are generally negative.

Systemic infection with *Erysipelothrix* is uncommon. More than 90 cases of bacteremia have been reported; most of the patients had endocarditis. Although cases of prosthetic valve endocarditis have been reported, most cases have involved native valves. In 60% of cases, infection developed on apparently normal heart valves. One third of patients had an antecedent or concurrent skin lesion of erysipeloid. The clinical manifestations of endocarditis secondary to *E. rhusiopathiae* and other microorganisms are similar. *E. rhusiopathiae* endocarditis correlates highly with occupation, exhibits a tropism for the aortic valve, affects more males than females, and is associated with high mortality.[3] The high mortality may reflect a delay in appropriate therapy because of the empirical use of vancomycin, which is not an effective treatment of *E. rhusiopathiae*. Cases of *E. rhusiopathiae* endocarditis have been

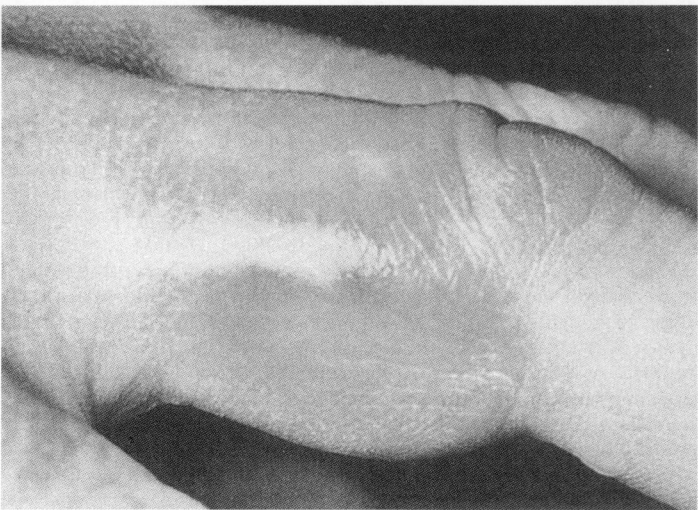

FIGURE 295-1. Erysipeloid with its characteristic purple, nonpurulent swelling of the finger. Also known as whale finger or pork finger, this form of cellulitis caused by *Erysipelothrix rhusiopathiae* should not be confused with streptococcal or staphylococcal erysipelas (see Fig. 441-4). (From Farrar WE, Wood MJ, Innes JUA, Tubbs H. *Infectious Diseases: Text and Color Atlas.* 2nd ed. New York: Gower Medical Publishing; 1992.)

complicated by paravalvular and myocardial abscess formation, cerebral emboli, congestive heart failure, valve perforation, and acute renal failure. *E. rhusiopathiae* bacteremia without endocarditis occurs more frequently than was previously believed. Bacteremia is occurring with increased frequency in immunocompromised patients, whereas endocarditis usually occurs in immunocompetent patients. Focal infections, including brain abscess, meningitis, endophthalmitis, osteomyelitis, septic arthritis, epidural and paravertebral abscesses, liver abscess, necrotizing fasciitis, intra-abdominal abscess, and peritonitis, have been reported. Some of these infections were complications of bacteremia. Septic arthritis has occurred in native joints, in prosthetic joints, and after arthroscopic surgery.[4] Peritonitis has complicated peritoneal dialysis.

DIAGNOSIS

E. rhusiopathiae grows on routine laboratory media. Because *E. rhusiopathiae* is located only in deeper parts of the skin in cases of erysipeloid, biopsy of the entire thickness of the dermis from the edge of the lesion yields maximal recovery of the organism. Definitive diagnosis by skin biopsy is rarely necessary because of the classic clinical presentation and the rapid response to therapy. Routine blood culture techniques are adequate for growth and isolation of the organism in suspected cases of bacteremia or endocarditis. Various selective media have been used to improve the isolation of *E. rhusiopathiae* from contaminated specimens. Molecular techniques, such as polymerase chain reaction with primers specific for *E. rhusiopathiae*, have been developed and improve the efficiency of detection and identification.[5]

TREATMENT Rx

Most isolates of *E. rhusiopathiae* are susceptible to penicillin, cephalosporins, imipenem, clindamycin, ciprofloxacin, ofloxacin, and daptomycin. Some resistance has been observed with erythromycin, tetracycline, and chloramphenicol. *E. rhusiopathiae* is resistant to vancomycin, aminoglycosides, trimethoprim-sulfamethoxazole, and sulfonamides. Penicillin G is the treatment of choice. Uncomplicated cutaneous lesions generally respond well to a 5- to 7-day course of oral penicillin. Treatment hastens healing, although relapse may still occur. Bacteremia should be treated with intravenous penicillin; cases of endocarditis should be treated with 12 million to 20 million units of penicillin G daily or ceftriaxone 1 g daily for 4 to 6 weeks. Two weeks of intravenous therapy followed by 2 weeks of oral therapy has been successful. The use of quinolones or daptomycin may be considered for *Erysipelothrix* infections when the patient is allergic to β-lactams. Oral linezolid was used to complete therapy in a case of bacteremia complicated by endophthalmitis. Valve replacement may be necessary in patients with endocarditis. Infected prosthetic devices should be removed.

PREVENTION

Proper cleaning and disinfection of work surfaces and attention to hygienic work practices, including the use of gloves and hand hygiene, reduce the risk for infection. Vaccines are available for commercial use in animals only.

GENERAL REFERENCES

For the General References and other additional features, please visit Expert Consult at https://expertconsult.inkling.com.

296

CLOSTRIDIAL INFECTIONS

DALE N. GERDING AND STUART JOHNSON

Clostridial infections are characterized by disease produced by toxins. They include tetanus and botulism, both caused by neurotoxins, and clostridial myonecrosis or gas gangrene, caused by the toxins of *Clostridium perfringens* as well as those of other clostridial species. Although these clostridial infections remain important clinically, their frequency has declined markedly with the advent of vaccines and better public health measures. Several previously little known species of clostridia that produce very large clostridial cytotoxins (LCCs) varying in size from 250 to 308 kD have become increasingly prominent. They include, in particular, *Clostridium difficile*, which is responsible for one of the most common health care–associated infections and for increasing mortality among elderly patients. Another LCC-producing organism, *Clostridium sordellii*, has caused devastating infections in young women in association with pregnancy and medical abortion, in injection drug users, and in patients with traumatic wounds. *Clostridium novyi* type A is a third LCC organism that has also caused severe infections in injection drug users.

CLOSTRIDIUM DIFFICILE INFECTION

DEFINITION AND PATHOGEN

C. difficile infection (CDI) is a gastrointestinal infection characterized by diarrhea (three or more loose or unformed stools in ≤24 hours) and a positive test result for *C. difficile* toxin A or toxin B in stool, evidence of a toxin-producing strain of *C. difficile* in stool, or evidence of pseudomembranous colitis on direct visualization of the colon. *C. difficile* is a spore-forming, anaerobic, gram-positive organism that survives well in water, soil, and animals and has a worldwide distribution.

EPIDEMIOLOGY

CDI occurs most frequently in health care settings, particularly in long-term care facilities and acute care hospitals, and is most frequent and lethal among the elderly, especially those older than 75 years. Rates in U.S. hospitals have nearly tripled in the decade since 2000, and it is now estimated that there are 500,000 to 750,000 CDIs each year. A specific strain of *C. difficile*—identified as the restriction endonuclease group BI, pulsed-field gel type NAP1, polymerase chain reaction ribotype 027 (BI/NAP1/027) strain—is thought to be responsible for much of the epidemic that has extended to Canada and Europe. Rates of community-onset CDI have also increased during the past decade, in association with the rising rates in hospitals and nursing homes.[1] However, 94% of community-onset cases in this population-based study were associated with receiving some kind of recent health care, including outpatient visits, recently discharged patients, and nursing home residents. It is unlikely that community-associated cases (with no health care exposure) account for more than 10 to 15% of all CDIs. Risk factors for CDI include antimicrobial use, advanced age, and stay in an acute or chronic care facility. Hospitals are considered a particularly high-risk environment because patients are elderly, antibiotic use is frequent, the environment is contaminated with *C. difficile* spores (which are difficult to eradicate), asymptomatic patients carry *C. difficile* in their stools, and health care workers carry *C. difficile* on their hands if they do not practice good hand hygiene. In about 2 to 3% of healthy adults, *C. difficile* can be cultured from their stools, but the frequency in asymptomatic hospitalized patients increases with the duration of hospitalization and may reach 20% or more. Exposure to nearly all antimicrobials has been associated with subsequent CDI, but those with the highest risk are clindamycin, the cephalosporins, and the fluoroquinolones. CDI is rare in children and young adults, despite their frequent exposure to antimicrobials. However, children younger than 1 year are commonly colonized with *C. difficile* but remain asymptomatic, an observation that remains largely unexplained.

PATHOBIOLOGY

CDI risk appears to be minimal in the absence of antimicrobial therapy. When antimicrobials are administered, they have the unintended consequence of disrupting the normal protective bowel microbiota, which may persist for days to weeks after the antimicrobial is stopped. If *C. difficile* is ingested during this time, the spores germinate in the gut, and the vegetative form of the organism multiplies and begins to make toxins. At this point, whether the patient will develop diarrhea is dictated by the status of his or her immunity to the toxins, which is best correlated with serum immunoglobulin G antibodies directed at toxin A and toxin B of *C. difficile*. Those with good antibody responses will be asymptomatic but will remain colonized with *C. difficile*, whereas those with little or no antibody response will develop diarrhea and CDI. Toxin A is primarily an enterotoxin, and toxin B is a cytotoxin. Both act by glucosylation that disrupts the cell cytoskeleton, resulting in colonic epithelial cell rounding, fluid leakage, and cell death. In the presence of pseudomembranous colitis, the colon appears to be covered in yellow to white pseudomembranes that vary in size from punctate to completely confluent and covering the entire colon in advanced cases. On histologic evaluation, the colon demonstrates a marked neutrophil infiltration throughout the colon wall, with mucosal necrosis and volcano-like lesions from which the pseudomembrane is seen to "erupt." The pseudomembrane is composed of proteinaceous material and cellular debris.

CLINICAL MANIFESTATIONS

Clinical symptoms of CDI range from asymptomatic carriage to severe and sometimes life-threatening pseudomembranous colitis complicated by major fluid losses and systemic complications. With mild CDI, patients may simply have "nuisance diarrhea" that resolves when the implicated drug is discontinued. Others with more severe CDI have substantial fluid and protein losses combined with fever, cramps, hypoalbuminemia, leukocytosis, and hypotension. Leukocytosis is common (occurring in up to 50% of patients) and is a marker of severe CDI when it exceeds 15,000/mm^3. Extremely high levels (>50,000/mm^3) are an indication of fulminant and potentially fatal illness. Other factors that may be indicative of severe or late-stage disease include toxic megacolon, high fever, renal failure, hypotension, and a lactic acidosis greater than 5.0 mmol/L.

DIAGNOSIS

The diagnosis should be suspected in any patient who has otherwise unexplained diarrhea (three or more loose or unformed stools in ≤24 hours) in association with recent or concurrent antibiotic use. Only about 10 to 20% of patients in this category actually have CDI, but this is the group of patients that should be tested. The standard test to establish the diagnosis is to detect toxins A and B in stool or to detect a toxin-producing strain of *C. difficile* in stool. Tests that detect only toxin A are not acceptable because about 1 to 3% of strains that cause CDI produce toxin B but not toxin A. The most common laboratory method has been an enzyme immunoassay, but its sensitivity is only 50 to 80%. Repeated testing does not improve the diagnostic accuracy because enzyme immunoassays also have specificity deficiencies that increase the rate of false-positive test results with repeated testing. Polymerase chain reaction tests for *C. difficile* in stool are widely available commercially and markedly improve test sensitivity to 90 to 95% (compared with the "gold standard" of culture for a toxigenic strain). The polymerase chain reaction tests are more expensive, but their use by clinical laboratories is increasing rapidly. They increase the sensitivity of CDI diagnosis, but some studies have shown that a positive test result for stool toxin should also be present to confirm the diagnosis.[2] The standard cell cytotoxin assay is little used but more sensitive than enzyme immunoassay, but it has the disadvantages of a 24- to 48-hour turnaround and the requirement for tissue culture facilities. Stool culture for *C. difficile*, which is the most sensitive test available, is likewise slow and requires confirmation of toxin production by the organism before reporting. Testing of stools for glutamate dehydrogenase, or "common antigen," can be used as a rapid screening test, but it is only about 50% specific and requires confirmation with a toxin test, which can increase the turnaround time for reporting positive results. CDI can also be diagnosed by observing pseudomembranous colitis directly through sigmoidoscopy or colonoscopy or at surgery. When a negative test result does not confirm the diagnosis in a patient whose clinical symptoms are highly suggestive of CDI, empirical treatment of CDI should be given rather than repeating the test. The cause of infectious diarrhea in an adult patient with an onset longer than 48 hours after hospital admission is almost always CDI because other infectious enteric pathogens (with the exception of norovirus) are extremely rare in the hospital setting. Also common in the differential diagnosis are noninfectious causes of diarrhea, such as antibiotic or other drug-associated diarrhea, ischemic colitis, and idiopathic inflammatory bowel disease. For patients with antibiotic-associated diarrhea and no evidence of colitis, the cause of diarrhea with a negative *C. difficile* toxin assay is usually not defined.

PREVENTION

Two major prevention strategies are employed. The first is traditional infection control, in which barriers to transmission (gowns, gloves, isolation, hand hygiene, environmental cleaning) are used to prevent the spores of *C. difficile* from reaching the patient. The second strategy is to reduce the likelihood of infection if the patient does encounter *C. difficile* while in the hospital. The most efficacious strategy, also known as antimicrobial stewardship, is to avoid or to minimize exposure to antimicrobials, especially those with a high CDI risk, such as clindamycin, cephalosporins, and fluoroquinolones. Interventions to restrict exposure to clindamycin and to cephalosporins have been highly effective in interrupting outbreaks of CDI in hospitals.[3]

TREATMENT   Rx

Treatment of CDI begins with discontinuation of the implicated antibiotic, supportive care, and avoidance of antiperistaltic agents. Mildly ill patients may recover with these simple conservative measures, but most require specific treatment. Continuation of the offending antibiotics while CDI is being treated with vancomycin and other agents results in lower cure rates and higher CDI recurrence rates in patients. Metronidazole, at a dose of 500 mg orally three times a day for 10 to 14 days, has been the recommended treatment for patients with mild CDI because it is much less expensive and it avoids some of the concern about vancomycin-resistant enterococcus colonization. However, a large randomized prospective trial of vancomycin versus metronidazole has placed the recommendation into question as it showed vancomycin to be statistically superior to metronidazole for all patients with CDI (P = .02).[A1] Patients with severe CDI (variously defined as a white blood cell count >15,000 or a creatinine increase to >1.5-fold above baseline) should be treated with vancomycin 125 mg orally four times a day for 10 days.[4] Vancomycin can be substituted for metronidazole if there is a delayed response in patients with mild illness. A newer option is fidaxomicin (200 mg orally twice daily), a narrow-spectrum macrocycle that is as efficacious as vancomycin and reduces recurrent infection.[A2][A3] The anticipated response to these drugs is rapid defervescence, with gradual normalization of bowel habits. Mean time to resolution of diarrhea is about 3 days; if symptoms have not resolved by day 5 or day 6 of treatment, a change in therapy should be considered. However, there are no data to support the use of more than one drug at a time to treat CDI. Failure to respond often means that either the disease has progressed too far or another condition is causing the symptoms. For patients with severe complicated or fulminant CDI, medical management includes vancomycin at a higher dose (500 mg four times a day) orally or by nasogastric tube; if ileus is present, metronidazole (500 mg IV every 8 hours) is added, with vancomycin also administered by enema. If symptoms progress with this therapy, colectomy may be life-saving and should be performed before the white blood cell count reaches 50,000/mm^3 or lactate concentration reaches 5.0 mmol/L. A colon-sparing loop ileostomy procedure followed by infusion of polyethylene glycol and vancomycin has demonstrated reduced mortality compared with historic colectomy controls and may be a preferred procedure to colectomy.[5]

Other antibiotic options include oral fusidic acid, teicoplanin, nitazoxanide, rifaximin, and bacitracin, but most of these drugs have been evaluated in only a small number of patients, and none (like metronidazole) has Food and Drug Administration approval for the treatment of CDI. There is no convincing evidence that toxin-binding agents, such as cholestyramine and probiotics, are useful in treating CDI. About 20 to 25% of patients treated with either vancomycin or metronidazole have a recurrence of symptoms when treatment is stopped because of the persistence of *C. difficile* spores or acquisition of a new strain. Treatment with vancomycin, fidaxomicin, or metronidazole is recommended, depending on the severity of the recurrence. Patients with multiple recurrences of CDI are extremely difficult to treat and may benefit from consultation with an infectious disease specialist or gastroenterologist. Observational data and one prospective randomized controlled trial suggest that fecal microbiota transplantation might be an effective treatment for recurrent *C. difficile* infection.[A4]

The majority (≈80%) of patients respond to simple withdrawal of the implicated antibiotic combined with a single course of metronidazole, vancomycin, or fidaxomicin. Some patients with fulminant disease eventually require colectomy. The attributable mortality rate is as high as 7% in large series, and the majority of lethal cases occur in patients older than 65 years. Patients with multiple recurrences require repeated courses of antibiotics, usually vancomycin with tapering and pulse-dose regimens that may need to be continued for weeks to months, or may require resorting to fecal microbiota transplantation.

NECROTIZING CLOSTRIDIAL TISSUE INFECTION
Clostridium sordellii
DEFINITION AND PATHOGEN

C. sordellii is another clostridial species that produces LCCs, and it has become more common as a cause of septic shock and necrotizing fasciitis in association with trauma, childbirth, medical abortion, and injection drug use. C. sordellii antitoxin cross-neutralizes the cytotoxic effect of C. difficile toxins, indicating the similarity of these LCCs.

EPIDEMIOLOGY

The organism is commonly found in soil and in the intestines of animals and occasionally humans worldwide. Soil contamination of wounds is the usual suspected route of infection. Infections have been described after traumatic wounds, childbirth, medical abortion, and intramuscular or subcutaneous injection drug use.

PATHOBIOLOGY

C. sordellii produces up to seven identified toxins; of these, hemorrhagic toxin (TcsH) and lethal toxin (TcsL), which are both LCCs and analogous to TcdA and TcdB of C. difficile, are considered major virulence factors. TcsL has been shown to be essential for virulence.[6] The toxins produce local necrosis, progressive edema, and shock that results in high mortality. The toxins are glucosyltransferases that glucosylate the Rho, Rac, or Ras proteins, causing impaired cytoskeletal organization and massive capillary leakage, leading to the progressive edematous state.

CLINICAL MANIFESTATIONS

Initial symptoms are nonspecific and include nausea, lethargy, dizziness, and tenderness at the infection site. Tachycardia and hypotension follow within hours. Laboratory tests show a marked leukocytosis or leukemoid reaction. Hypotension and tachycardia are refractory to treatment. Edema secondary to capillary leakage is prominent, resulting in hemoconcentration but little or no fever. Peritoneal and pleural effusions are common. White blood cell elevations greater than $75,000/mm^3$ are associated with a fatal outcome.

Infection Associated with Childbirth and Medical Abortion
This is a rare infection in which patients present 4 to 7 days after the administration of oral mifepristone and vaginal misoprostol for medical abortion with nausea, vomiting, weakness, abdominal pain, hypotension, and tachycardia but little or no fever and, often remarkably, a lack of findings on pelvic examination. The presentation is similar to toxic shock syndrome. There is rapid progression to vascular collapse and cardiac arrest. Leukocytosis is dramatic, with white blood cell counts near $100,000/mm^3$ in most patients. After delivery, the presentation is similar, but localized swelling and discoloration of the labia and perineum may be evident if the episiotomy site is infected. All patients to date have died.

Infection Associated with Injection Drug Use
Black tar heroin (a dark, gummy, less refined and cheaper form of heroin) has been associated with necrotizing fasciitis at the subcutaneous or intramuscular injection site, presumably a result of the contaminants mixed with the heroin. Patients present with 2 to 7 days of symptoms of necrotizing fasciitis of the upper or lower extremity where they injected heroin, in some cases accompanied by hypotension. Aggressive surgical débridement is required at the infection site, together with fluids and pressors. Cultures of débrided tissue reveal multiple organisms in addition to C. sordellii. Mortality in these patients is 50%.

DIAGNOSIS

Diagnosis is difficult because of the lack of specific symptoms, but it is usually made by identifying the likely source of infection and isolating C. sordellii from the infection site or blood cultures. Polymerase chain reaction analysis for C. sordellii in infected tissues may be required to make the diagnosis when cultures are negative. Other bacteria are also commonly found at the infection site. Computed tomography or magnetic resonance imaging may be helpful in identifying localized infections, which can then be excised or drained surgically, providing material for microbiologic diagnosis.

PREVENTION

C. sordellii infections are very rare, and the exact mechanism of infection, especially after medical abortion, is not known. However, careful attention to wound cleansing, avoidance of injecting drugs into skin or muscle, and good hygiene during childbirth are likely to help prevent C. sordellii infection.

TREATMENT Rx

Definitive treatment information is lacking. The infection progresses so rapidly that therapeutic interventions are rarely successful. Surgery to remove necrotic sites of infection and administration of intravenous fluids and pressors to treat hypotension and tachycardia are supportive. Antibiotic susceptibility suggests that β-lactams, clindamycin, tetracyclines, and chloramphenicol are active, but no clinical treatment efficacy data are available. Theoretically, use of an antibiotic such as clindamycin to suppress toxin synthesis could be a useful adjunct to treatment. At present, there is no antitoxin available.

PROGNOSIS

Infections after childbirth or medical abortion have been uniformly fatal. Mortality in injection drug users or patients after trauma or surgery is about 50%.

Clostridium novyi Infection in Injecting Drug Users

C. novyi α-toxin causes an LCC-producing disease in humans. C. novyi has long been recognized as a cause of fatal toxemia in animals with contaminated wounds. An extended outbreak of human infections occurred in Scotland, Ireland, and elsewhere in the United Kingdom in 2000 to 2009 among persons injecting heroin extravascularly (skin or muscle popping).[7] A localized necrotizing infection with painful edema, sepsis, and significant mortality was recognized. The findings include soft tissue inflammation, edema and necrosis at the injection sites, circulatory collapse, marked leukocytosis, and pleural effusions. Treatment usually involves débridement and antibiotic administration (gentamicin, flucloxacillin, penicillin, metronidazole, and clindamycin were used during this outbreak because infections are typically polymicrobial in origin).

Clostridial Myonecrosis (Gas Gangrene)
DEFINITION

Clostridial myonecrosis, or gas gangrene, can be caused by several Clostridium species, most commonly C. perfringens after trauma or tissue injury and Clostridium septicum after dissemination from a colonic source.[8]

EPIDEMIOLOGY

Gas gangrene has historically been a complication of battlefield injuries and of trauma in noncombat settings. The estimated number of cases in the United States is about 1000 per year. Traumatic injuries account for about 50% of cases, with vehicular accidents accounting for the majority; the remaining cases develop in patients after crush injuries, industrial accidents, gunshot wounds, and burns. Minor injuries such as puncture wounds, intramuscular injections, simple lacerations, and subcutaneous injections with epinephrine may occasionally precipitate clostridial myonecrosis. Postoperative complications account for about 30% of cases and are most frequently associated with surgery on the appendix, biliary tract, or intestine. Approximately 20% are "spontaneous" or nontraumatic and are invariably associated with an occult colonic malignant neoplasm.

PATHOBIOLOGY

Clostridia are widely distributed in nature and can be cultured from nearly all soil samples, from environmental sites in the hospital, and from the human intestine. A critical factor is a physiologic state of the wound with conditions that support germination and toxin production by toxigenic clostridia. Particularly critical are a low oxidation-reduction potential, hypoxia, appropriate substrates, and calcium ions. The probability of infection is substantially increased by devitalized muscle and the presence of foreign material such as soil. C. perfringens elaborates at least 12 recognized toxins, most importantly α-toxin and θ-toxin of C. perfringens type A. Although the interaction is complex, good evidence supports a central role for α-toxin, a phospholipase C, and θ-toxin or perfringolysin O, a cholesterol-dependent cytolysin, in the extensive cell death and disruption of microvascular perfusion that are characteristic of clostridial myonecrosis. The vascular perfusion changes are likely mediated by toxin-induced platelet aggregation and leukocyte margination. The α-toxin of C. septicum, a pore-forming cytolysin unrelated to α-toxin of C. perfringens, also causes cell death and microvascular perfusion changes.

CLINICAL MANIFESTATIONS

Initial symptoms of traumatic myonecrosis usually occur 1 to 4 days after the precipitating event, although the range is 8 hours to 3 weeks. The initial symptom is pain that is often sudden and severe at the site of surgery or trauma. The involved skin has intense edema and is initially pale before progressing to a bronze or magenta color, followed by the formation of bullae. The bullae contain fluid that may be clear or hemorrhagic. The discharge has an odor that is described as "foul-sweet."

Circulatory collapse and hypotension unresponsive to fluid challenge are common and may reflect the effect of α-toxin, which suppresses cardiac contractility. About 15% of patients have bacteremia that is usually complicated by rapid hemolysis with a dramatic drop in the hematocrit, which may even decrease to 0%. Common complications include jaundice, hypotension, hepatic failure, and renal failure. The renal failure is often due to hemoglobulinuria and myoglobulinuria, but it may also be due to acute tubular necrosis from hypotension. Despite the severity of the illness, the patient's mental status is usually remarkably good until very late in the disease. Surgical intervention shows necrotic muscle that does not contract with stimulation. Deeper dissection reveals beefy red necrotic muscle that becomes black and extremely friable in the late stages.

Uterine gas gangrene, which was once common after septic abortions, is now rare but may complicate normal delivery, amniocentesis, cesarean section, or abortion. The onset is usually sudden, with fever, tachycardia, hypotension, renal failure, and jaundice. Radiography may show gas in the uterine wall. The urine is often "port wine" in color as a result of hemoglobulinuria, and there is often jaundice because of massive intravascular hemolysis. The usual causes are C. perfringens and C. sordellii.

Spontaneous myonecrosis occurs in the absence of trauma and is usually caused by C. septicum. One distinctive association is with colon cancer and neutropenic enterocolitis, which represent portals of entry for hematogenous seeding of C. septicum. This infection is also seen with acute leukemia and is most common with chemotherapy for solid tumors and after stem cell transplantation. The usual portals of entry are the terminal ileum, cecum, and ascending colon, hence the term *typhlitis*. The usual manifestation is a necrotizing infection in an extremity or in the abdominal wall, accompanied by hypotension and renal failure. Examination shows spreading crepitations with rapid clinical deterioration during a period of hours, and imaging reveals gas.

DIAGNOSIS

The diagnosis of gas gangrene is usually based on a constellation of characteristic clinical features, including myonecrosis, shock, and renal failure. The patient typically complains of severe pain. Early recognition is important because early institution of treatment may strongly influence the prognosis. The diagnosis is established by examination of skin and muscle, which shows putrid discharge, characteristic bullae, and crepitations. Gram stain demonstrates abundant gram-positive bacilli and no inflammatory cells. Histopathologic examination of the lesion shows myonecrosis without polymorphonuclear leukocytes, a finding that is remarkably different from most soft tissue infections, which do not feature necrosis and have abundant inflammatory cells. Gas is present in the tissue and may be detected by physical examination, radiography, or other imaging methods.

PREVENTION

The basic principle of prevention is adequate management of traumatic wounds—establishing adequate drainage, removing foreign bodies, draining hematomas, and ensuring good hemostasis.

TREATMENT   Rx

The most important facet of treatment is prompt surgical débridement. Many cases require extensive, often mutilating surgery. Penicillin and clindamycin are recommended but are rarely adequate without radical surgery, except in patients with neutropenic enterocolitis, who can often be managed with antibiotics. The rationale for penicillin combined with clindamycin is that some strains of clostridia are resistant to clindamycin, but clindamycin is probably the superior drug for reducing toxin formation. Other antibiotics that are generally effective include metronidazole and chloramphenicol. The use of hyperbaric oxygen is controversial, in part because the therapeutic trials have been either of poor quality or not convincing.

PROGNOSIS

Factors associated with a poor prognosis include advanced age, location on the trunk, association with severe underlying disease, leukopenia, renal failure, hemolysis, and shock. The best results are seen in young patients with involvement of a single extremity. Management plays an important role, particularly the use of early and aggressive surgery as well as antibiotics. The overall mortality rate of patients with traumatic gas gangrene in tertiary centers is about 25%.

NEUROTOXIC CLOSTRIDIAL INFECTIONS
Botulism
DEFINITION

Botulism is a severe neuroparalytic disease characterized by a descending flaccid motor neuron paralysis. It is caused by botulinum toxin produced by *Clostridium botulinum*.

The Pathogen

C. botulinum is a gram-positive, spore-forming obligate anaerobe that is widely distributed in nature and is frequently found in soil, marine environments, and agricultural products. Each strain produces one of seven toxins designated by the letters A to G. A new botulism toxin designated H, the first new neurotoxin identified in more than 40 years, was recently isolated from a patient with infant botulism.[9] Botulinum toxin may also be produced by the related clostridial species *Clostridium baratii* and *Clostridium butyricum*. All these neurotoxins produce the same syndrome; the usual causes of disease in humans are types A, B, and E, with rare cases caused by type F.

EPIDEMIOLOGY

Botulism in humans is generally one of three types: food-borne botulism, infant botulism, or wound botulism. Rarely, botulism may be acquired as a result of iatrogenic misadventures with botulinum toxin, which is a potential bioterrorism agent if it is inhaled or ingested.

Food-borne botulism is the most common form of botulism in the world but is a distant second to infant botulism in the United States. Nevertheless, 20 cases from ingestion of prison-made alcohol (pruno) and the first eight cases in more than 30 years from ingestion of a commercially canned product (hot dog chili sauce) have occurred recently.[10,11] Foods most frequently implicated are home-canned vegetables or fermented foods, and most cases are sporadic single cases occasionally involving two or three people. Commercially preserved and restaurant-prepared foods are also rare causes of food-borne botulism. Type A toxin is predominant in the United States. Alaska has the highest rate of any state, with approximately 35% of all cases; 80% of events and cases in Alaska are caused by type E and are most often associated with fermentation methods used to prepare fish and marine mammals by native Alaskans.[12] Meat and meat products are frequently implicated in Europe, where the predominant toxin is type B. In China, the most frequent vehicle is a vegetable product, and type A predominates.

Infant botulism is the most frequently recognized form in the United States and is the most recently discovered type of botulism, first described in 1976. It is caused by production of botulinum toxin in the intestine after presumed spore ingestion and colonization in 2- to 36-week-old infants. Honey has been identified as the source of C. botulinum spores, but in most cases the source is never identified. Nearly all cases are caused by type A or type B toxin. The symptoms usually begin with constipation followed by poor feeding, weak cry, lethargy, and generalized weakness characterized as the "floppy baby syndrome" because of loss of head control. This form of botulism is rare in adults, occurring most often in patients with anatomic or functional abnormalities of the intestines.

Wound botulism, first described in 1943, is the least frequent form of the disease and is usually caused by either type A or type B toxin. Sporadic cases in traumatic wounds contaminated by soil are rarely reported. Outbreaks have been described in black tar heroin users in the western United States, particularly if they inject the drug intramuscularly or subcutaneously (skin popping). These drug users also develop other clostridial infections, including necrotizing fasciitis caused by *C. sordellii* and *C. novyi* and tetanus caused by *Clostridium tetani*.

Inhalation or ingestion of botulinum toxin is considered one of the top six bioweapon agents in terms of probability of use. The presumed method would be contamination of the food supply, water supply, or commercial beverages or aerosolization in a highly populated area to cause inhalational botulism. It is estimated that a point-source aerosol release of the toxin could incapacitate or kill 10% of people within a 0.5-km radius.

Iatrogenic botulism results from the misuse of botulinum toxin for cosmetic or therapeutic purposes. Cosmetic treatment doses are far too low to cause systemic disease, but the use of unlicensed products with high concentrations of botulinum toxin can cause systemic symptoms. Higher doses used for the management of muscle movement disorders have caused occasional cases with systemic botulism-like symptoms.

PATHOBIOLOGY

Pathologic findings are due to absorption of toxins from the intestine (ingested preformed toxin in foods or in situ production in the intestine in infants), inhalation (aerosol from bioterrorism), absorption from cutaneous infection sources (wounds), or iatrogenic injection. The toxin is disseminated by the systemic circulation and causes flaccid paralysis by binding presynaptic motor neuron terminals and blocking acetylcholine transmission across the neuromuscular junction. The estimated lethal doses of purified botulinum toxin A for a 70-kg human are 0.09 to 0.15 μg when given intravenously, 0.8 to 0.9 μg when inhaled, and 70 μg when given orally.

CLINICAL MANIFESTATIONS

In contrast to Guillain-Barré syndrome (Chapter 420), which is an ascending paralysis, botulism is characterized by generalized weakness and a descending paralysis. Symptoms are due to absorption of botulinum toxin from the gut, the lung, or a wound. Clinical symptoms consist of highly distinctive and usually symmetrical cranial nerve palsies, followed by a symmetrical descending flaccid paralysis. Prominently involved cranial nerves III, IV, and VI cause blurred vision and diplopia; involvement of cranial nerve VII causes the characteristic expressionless facies and dysphagia; and involvement of cranial nerve IX causes dysarthria. Thus, the initial symptoms include the "four d's"—diplopia, dysarthria, dysphagia, and dysphonia—although the last is rarely reported, and blurred vision is reported more commonly than diplopia. These findings are followed by a descending upper extremity paralysis and respiratory paralysis. Neurologic examination shows bilateral cranial nerve VI paresis, ptosis, dilated pupils with a sluggish reaction, and diminished gag reflex, followed by descending involvement of motor neurons. Deep tendon reflexes are diminished or absent. Mentation remains clear, vital signs are normal, and the neurologic findings are symmetrical. The most common cause of death is respiratory failure. The tempo of the disease and the extent of paralysis in the absence of treatment are highly variable. The symptoms may be restricted to a few cranial nerves, or there may be complete paralysis of all voluntary muscles. Progression may occur during a period of hours or days. The timing and extent of neurologic deficits depend on the size of the botulinum toxin inoculum.

DIAGNOSIS

Botulism should be suspected in patients with an acute flaccid paralysis involving the cranial nerves, particularly in the presence of bilateral cranial nerve VI dysfunction, associated neurologic findings, and a 10-hour to 5-day history of consuming suspect food, such as preserved or home-canned foods. Nausea, vomiting, abdominal pain, and diarrhea are common early in the illness, with constipation present when paralysis develops. The finding of two or more cases that are epidemiologically linked is virtually diagnostic of food-borne botulism because other causes of paralysis are rare and sporadic. In the absence of a history of suspect food ingestion, potentially infected wounds should be sought, including injection sites in users of black tar heroin. With bioterrorism, the epidemiology may reflect a common source exposure, such

as a local water supply or an aerosolized toxin, but it could also be widely distributed with a contaminated food source, such as the milk supply.

Laboratory tests for suspected food-borne botulism include analysis of serum, stool, gastric contents, or food for botulinum toxin and culture of stool and suspect food or wounds for *C. botulinum*. Toxin assay specimens should be collected before treatment with antitoxin. With wound botulism, recovery of *C. botulinum* from wound cultures or detection of toxin in serum is diagnostic. The toxin assays are generally available only at public health laboratories. The standard is a mouse bioassay for detection and quantification of toxin. Toxin type is determined by type-specific antibody neutralization. In general, adult patients with clinical evidence of food-borne botulism have detectable toxin in sera in a third of cases and detectable toxin in stool in a third of cases, but the organism is recovered from stool in about 60%.

The differential diagnosis includes myasthenia gravis, Guillain-Barré syndrome, tick paralysis, cerebrovascular accident, trichinosis, Eaton-Lambert syndrome, hypocalcemia, hypermagnesemia, organophosphate poisoning, atropine poisoning, and paralytic poisoning by shellfish or puffer fish. Electromyography using repetitive stimulation at 2 to 50/second may be helpful in distinguishing causes of flaccid paralysis. Electromyography patterns with slow and rapid supramaximal stimulation show similar responses in botulism and Eaton-Lambert syndrome. Findings on cerebrospinal fluid analysis and cranial imaging are normal in botulism.

PREVENTION

The disease can be prevented by destroying spores in the original food source, inhibiting germination, or destroying preformed toxin.

TREATMENT Rx

Clinicians who suspect botulism should immediately seek clinical consultation, notify public health authorities, and administer antitoxin. The agency to contact in the United States is the state health department, which will contact the Centers for Disease Control and Prevention (CDC) if needed. Additional emergency consultation is available from the CDC botulism duty officer through the CDC Emergency Operations Center (telephone: 770-488-7100); similar public health agencies should be contacted in other countries. Treatment consists of supportive care and passive neutralization with equine botulinum antitoxin.

The standard treatment of adults since 2010 in the United States is heptavalent botulinum antitoxin (HBAT) through a CDC-sponsored Food and Drug Administration investigational new drug protocol.[13] HBAT contains equine-derived antibody to the seven known botulinum toxin types (A to G) with the following nominal potency values: 7500 U anti-A; 5500 U anti-B; 5000 U anti-C; 1000 U anti-D; 8500 U anti-E; 5000 U anti-F; and 1000 U anti-G. BabyBIG (botulism immune globulin) is a human-derived treatment of infant botulism types A and B and is available for infant botulism through the California Infant Botulism Treatment and Prevention Program. The antitoxin should be given as early as possible and should not be delayed while awaiting microbiologic results. This treatment does not reverse paralysis or neutralize toxin already bound to nerve endings, but it does neutralize unbound toxin in the circulation to prevent progression. The HBAT antitoxin is derived from horses, and as a result, hypersensitivity reactions may occur.

Respiratory failure is a major risk, and patients must be monitored carefully with liberal criteria for ventilatory support. The requirement for mechanical ventilation varies from about 20% in adults with food-borne disease to 60% in patients with infant botulism. Other forms of supportive care include enteral or parenteral feeding and positioning in the reverse Trendelenburg position.

Toxin can be removed from the gastrointestinal tract by gastric lavage, cathartics, and enemas early in the course. Antibiotic treatment is unnecessary, except for wound botulism.

PROGNOSIS

The case-fatality rate for untreated food-borne botulism was once 60 to 70% but is currently 3 to 5% with treatment. Infant botulism in the United States now has a mortality rate of less than 1%; the use of human antitoxin has reduced the median duration of hospitalization from 6 to 3 weeks. Patients who survive any form of botulism generally have a complete recovery.

Tetanus

DEFINITION

Tetanus is a neurologic syndrome characterized by generalized rigidity and convulsive spasm of skeletal muscles caused by a neurotoxin elaborated at the site of injury by *Clostridium tetani*.

The Pathogen

C. tetani is an anaerobic, gram-positive, slender, motile bacillus. When it sporulates, the terminal spore gives the organism a characteristic "drumstick" or "tennis racket" shape. The vegetative form produces tetanospasmin, a protein neurotoxin with a molecular mass of approximately 151 kD, including a heavy chain (100 kD) that binds neuronal cells and a light chain that blocks the release of neurotransmitters.

EPIDEMIOLOGY

C. tetani can be found in 2 to 23% of soil samples, with the highest yield in manure-treated soil. The organism can also be found in stool from a variety of domestic and farm animals and poultry. Tetanus is most common in warm climates and in highly cultivated rural areas. The greatest problem occurs in resource-limited countries because of high numbers of unimmunized mothers and unhygienic practices. The estimated annual toll from neonatal tetanus in developing countries is greater than 257,000, mostly secondary to inadequate passive immunity caused by absence of immunity in the mother. In the United States, an average of 29 cases of tetanus were reported annually from 2001 to 2008 with a mortality of 13.2%, and almost all occurred in unimmunized or inadequately immunized persons.[14] In the U.S., patients 65 years of age and older constituted 31% of patients and had the highest mortality at 31%.

PATHOBIOLOGY

Tetanospasmin, also known as tetanus neurotoxin or TeNT, ranks with botulinum toxin as one of the most potent known microbial toxins; 2.5 ng/kg is a lethal human dose. Clinical tetanus usually results from entry of the organism into a wound and low oxygen conditions that allow spore germination and survival of the vegetative organism to produce toxin. Entry is usually through a traumatic or surgical wound, drug injection site, burn, skin ulcer, or infected umbilical cord. Tetanospasmin binds the peripheral nerve terminals and is then carried intra-axonally within membrane-bound vesicles to spinal neurons at a transport rate of approximately 75 to 250 mm/day. The light chain passes to the presynaptic terminals, where it blocks the release of neurotransmitters in inhibitory afferent motor neurons. Loss of the inhibitory influence results in sustained muscle contraction. Binding of the toxin is irreversible, so recovery requires the generation of new axon terminals.

CLINICAL MANIFESTATIONS

Forms of tetanus include generalized, local, cephalic, and neonatal. Generalized tetanus, which is the most common form, accounts for 80 to 90% of reported cases in the United States. The usual incubation period is 3 to 21 days (mean, 8 days), depending largely on the distance between the site of injury and the central nervous system. A short incubation period is associated with more severe symptoms. Generalized tetanus is characterized by a persistent tonic spasm with brief exacerbations. The neck and jaw are almost always involved. Trismus (lockjaw) is the initial complaint in 75% of cases, so the patient is often initially seen by a dentist or oral surgeon. Other early features include irritability, restlessness, diaphoresis, and dysphagia with hydrophobia and drooling. Persistent spasm of the back musculature may cause opisthotonos. These early manifestations reflect involvement of the paraspinous muscles. With progression, all muscles contract, with stronger muscles overtaking weaker muscles. Noise or tactile stimuli may precipitate spasms and generalized convulsions. Involvement of the autonomic nervous system may result in severe arrhythmias, blood pressure oscillation, profound diaphoresis, hyperthermia, rhabdomyolysis, laryngeal spasm, and urinary retention. In most cases, the patient remains lucid and afebrile. The condition may continue for 3 to 4 weeks, despite antitoxin therapy, because of the time required for intra-axonal toxin transport. Complications include fractures from sustained contractions, pulmonary emboli, bacterial infections, and dehydration.

Local tetanus, in which the patient has persistent muscle contractions in the extremity involving a contaminated wound, is rare and shows considerable variation in severity. In mild cases, a patient may simply have spasms of the involved extremity; in more severe cases, local painful spasms progress to generalized tetanus. This relatively unusual form of tetanus has an excellent prognosis, with only about 1% mortality.

Cephalic tetanus is also rare and generally follows a head injury or occurs with *C. tetani* infection of the middle ear. Clinical symptoms consist of isolated or combined dysfunction of the cranial motor nerves, most frequently cranial nerve VII. This dysfunction may remain localized or progress to generalized tetanus. The incubation period is only 1 or 2 days, and the prognosis for survival is usually poor.

Neonatal tetanus is generalized tetanus resulting from *C. tetani* infection in neonates. It occurs primarily in underdeveloped countries, where it accounts for up to half of all neonatal deaths.

DIAGNOSIS

The diagnosis of tetanus is usually based on clinical observations. The putative agent, *C. tetani*, is recovered from wound culture only about 30% of the time. Results of cerebrospinal fluid analysis are entirely normal. Diagnostic testing is usually not necessary except in cases lacking an identified portal of entry. The differential diagnosis depends on the dominant clinical features and includes dystonic reactions as a result of neuroleptic toxicity, seizure disorders, hypocalcemic or alkalotic tetany, alcohol withdrawal, and strychnine poisoning. Strychnine also antagonizes glycine, and strychnine poisoning is the only condition that truly mimics tetanus. Strychnine levels in blood and urine establish the diagnosis. Dystonic reactions may resemble tetanus and are distinguished by rapid response to anticholinergic agents.

PREVENTION

Immunization with tetanus toxoid is virtually 100% effective, so nearly all cases of tetanus occur in unimmunized or inadequately immunized individuals. The Advisory Committee on Immunization Practices has recommended diphtheria and tetanus toxoids and acellular pertussis vaccine (DTaP) for active immunization of infants and children at 2 months, 4 months, 6 months, 15 to 18 months, and 4 to 6 years of age. Protective levels of serum antitoxin in persons who complete the primary series persist for at least 10 years. Td (tetanus and diphtheria toxoids adsorbed for adult use) is recommended every 10 years, but this recommendation has been modified because of concerns about waning adult pertussis antibody protection; as a result, the Advisory Committee on Immunization Practices recommends that all adults aged 19 years and older who have not yet received a dose of Tdap (tetanus toxoid, reduced diphtheria toxoid, and acellular pertussis) should receive a single dose regardless of the interval since last Td.[15] The recommended primary immunization series for unimmunized persons older than 7 years is Td at time 0, 4 to 8 weeks, and 6 to 12 months after the second dose, and then every 10 years. Nearly all states now require DTaP immunization for school enrollment. Immunization of childbearing women with Tdap confers protection to their infants through transplacental maternal antibody and is recommended during the third trimester of each pregnancy for optimal fetal passive antibody protection.[16]

Prevention of tetanus after injury (Table 296-1) requires appropriate wound management, assurance of adequate immunity, and consideration of antibiotic prophylaxis. The aim of surgery is to eliminate necrotic tissue, purulent collections, and foreign bodies that promote the environmental conditions necessary for spore germination. Passive immunization with tetanus immune globulin (TIG) is recommended only for "tetanus-prone"

TABLE 296-1 GUIDE TO TETANUS PROPHYLAXIS IN ROUTINE WOUND MANAGEMENT				
HISTORY OF ADSORBED TETANUS TOXOID (NO. OF DOSES)	**CLEAN MINOR WOUNDS**		**ALL OTHER WOUNDS***	
	Tdap or Td[†]	*TIG*[‡]	*Tdap or Td*[†]	*TIG*[‡]
<3 or unknown	Yes	No	Yes	Yes
≥3	No[§]	No	No[¶]	No

*Such as (but not limited to) wounds contaminated with dirt, feces, soil, and saliva; puncture wounds; avulsions; and wounds resulting from missiles, crushing, burns, and frostbite.
[†]For children younger than 7 years, DTaP (pediatric diphtheria–tetanus toxoid plus acellular pertussis vaccine) is recommended; if pertussis vaccine is contraindicated, DT (pediatric diphtheria–tetanus toxoid) is given. For persons aged 7 to 9 years or 65 years or older, Td (adult tetanus–diphtheria toxoid) is recommended. For persons 10 to 64 years, Tdap (adult tetanus–diphtheria toxoid plus acellular pertussis vaccine) is preferred to Td if the patient has never received Tdap and has no contraindication to pertussis vaccine. For persons 7 years and older, if Tdap is not available or not indicated because of age, Td is preferred to TT (tetanus toxoid alone). Note that pediatric formulations (DT and DTaP) contain an amount of tetanus toxoid similar to that of adult Td, but they contain three to four times as much diphtheria toxoid. DTaP and Tdap vaccines do not contain thimerosal as a preservative.
[‡]TIG is human tetanus immune globulin. Equine tetanus antitoxin should be used when TIG is not available.
[§]Yes, if more than 10 years since the last dose.
[¶]Yes, if more than 5 years since the last dose.

wounds in patients with an inadequate or unknown primary immunization status. The determination of whether a wound is tetanus prone depends on the interval between injury and treatment, the degree of contamination, the extent of devitalized tissue or foreign bodies at the site of injury, and the depth of injury. Antimicrobial agents, such as penicillin and metronidazole, may be given to inhibit replication of the vegetative forms of *C. tetani*, but immunization and wound cleansing are considered more important.

TREATMENT   Rx

Patients with tetanus require intensive care with particular attention to respiratory support, treatment with benzodiazepines, autonomic nervous system support, passive and active immunization, surgical débridement, and antibiotics directed against *C. tetani*.[17] There may be clinical progression for 2 to 4 weeks, despite antitoxin treatment, because of the time required to complete the transport of toxin. The severity of disease may be reduced by partial immunity; as a result, some patients have mild disease with minimal mortality, whereas others have mortality rates as high as 60% despite expert care.

Supportive Care

It is most important to assess airway function. Many patients require endotracheal intubation with benzodiazepine sedation and neuromuscular blockade; a tracheostomy should be placed if the endotracheal tube causes spasms. A feeding tube is usually required for nutritional support.

Control of Muscle Spasms

Benzodiazepines have become the mainstay of therapy to control spasms and to provide sedation. The most extensively studied is diazepam given in 5-mg increments; lorazepam and midazolam are equally effective. Patients with tetanus may have high tolerance for the sedative effects of these drugs and may require exceptionally high doses. When tetanus symptoms resolve, the drugs must be tapered during at least 2 weeks to prevent withdrawal reactions. If control of spasms cannot be achieved by benzodiazepines, long-term neuromuscular blockade is performed with vecuronium (6 to 8 mg/hour).

Passive Immunization

Human TIG should be given as soon as possible to neutralize toxin that has not entered neurons. The usual dose is 500 IU intramuscularly. Higher doses or intrathecal administration does not appear to be more effective. An alternative to TIG is pooled intravenous immune globulin. Equine TIG is equally effective, but the rate of allergic reactions is high because of the equine source; this preparation should not be used if human TIG is available.

Active Immunization

The standard three-dose schedule of immunization with tetanus toxoid should be given at an injection site separate from that used for immune globulin.

Antibiotic Therapy

C. tetani is susceptible in vitro to penicillins, cephalosporins, imipenem, macrolides, metronidazole, and tetracyclines. Clinical studies favor the use of metronidazole, which should be given in an intravenous dose of 2 g/day for 7 to 10 days.

Autonomic Nervous System Dysfunction

This complication generally reflects excessive catecholamine release and is usually treated with labetalol (0.25 to 1.0 mg/minute) for blood pressure control. Hypotension may require norepinephrine infusion. Bradycardia may require a pacemaker.

Surgery

Any wounds should be appropriately débrided.

PROGNOSIS

The overall mortality rate for generalized tetanus is 20 to 25%, even in modern medical facilities with extensive resources. Patients with moderate or severe generalized tetanus generally require treatment for 3 to 6 weeks. The highest mortality rates are at the extremes of age. The most frequent cause of death is pneumonia, but many patients have no obvious findings at autopsy, suggesting that death was directly due to the neurotoxin. Patients who recover usually recover completely.

OTHER CLOSTRIDIAL INFECTIONS

Clostridium perfringens Type C Enteritis

C. perfringens type C enteritis, also called enteritis necroticans, is a necrotizing disease involving the proximal small intestine caused by β-toxin–producing strains of *C. perfringens*. Enteritis necroticans occurs as sporadic cases or in outbreaks, most often in underdeveloped countries, most notably in Papua New Guinea in the 1960s and 1970s, where it was called pigbel because of its association with pork feasts by aboriginal people in the highlands. Outbreaks have also been reported among Khmer refugees in Thailand in the 1980s and in Sri Lanka in 2007. Enteritis necroticans also occurs rarely in isolated cases in the developed world, particularly among patients with diabetes mellitus.

PATHOBIOLOGY

Experimental and clinical evidence supports infection with *C. perfringens* type C and β-toxin as the causative agent of and key virulence factor in enteritis necroticans. The organism has been identified at the site of necrotic lesions, the disease can be reproduced in guinea pigs, isogenic β-toxin gene null mutants are avirulent, and vaccination with a toxoid preparation of β-toxin is protective. β-Toxin production is rapidly upregulated in the presence of Caco-2 enterocytes, and the toxin localizes to the endothelium in humans and piglets infected with *C. perfringens* type C.[18] These findings may explain key histopathologic hallmarks of this disease, that is, deep small intestinal necrosis with vascular necrosis and hemorrhage in the lamina propria.

CLINICAL MANIFESTATIONS

In Papua New Guinea, affected patients usually develop severe abdominal pain 12 hours to several days after a ritual pork feast (or, presumably, other infected food). Vomiting and bloody diarrhea are frequently associated findings. The abdomen becomes distended, and thickened bowel loops are sometimes appreciated on palpation. Disease severity and whether the patient experiences spontaneous recovery or bowel perforation and death depend on the extent of intestinal involvement.

DIAGNOSIS

Recognition of the clinical syndrome is critical to making the diagnosis. Culture to identify specific β-toxin–producing strains of *C. perfringens* remains a research tool and is not helpful in the management of patients. Plain radiographs of the abdomen may show dilated small bowel loops and ileus.

PREVENTION

An effective toxoid vaccine was available and used in Papua New Guinea (where the disease is endemic) as well as in the Khmer refugee camp outbreak in 1986. Vaccination was discontinued in the mid-1990s, and the vaccine is no longer available. A 2002 survey of Papua New Guinea children in the highlands suggested that pigbel was responsible for 9 to 16% of acute abdominal cases and clustered in three close geographic regions.

TREATMENT   Rx

Treatment is primarily supportive, including nasogastric suction and intravenous hydration. Surgical resection of the infected bowel is often required for those who do not initially respond to supportive measures. Antibiotics (penicillin, chloramphenicol, metronidazole) are almost always given empirically, but their role has not been defined. Prognosis depends on the extent of disease and the availability of surgery for those with more extensive intestinal involvement.

Clostridium perfringens Type A Diarrhea

C. perfringens type A is a well-recognized cause of food poisoning due to the ingestion of food, usually meat, heavily contaminated with enterotoxin-producing *C. perfringens* after storage at inappropriate temperatures. Enterotoxin production is associated with sporulation of ingested vegetative bacteria in the small intestine. The incubation period is 7 to 15 hours after ingestion, and the most prominent symptoms are diarrhea and abdominal pain. The syndrome is usually mild and self-limited.

In contrast to food poisoning due to *C. perfringens* type A, a more severe and protracted infectious diarrhea syndrome due to this organism has been recognized among hospitalized or institutionalized patients. These patients often have a history of prior or concomitant antibiotic use, and an enzyme immunoassay for *C. perfringens* enterotoxin is commercially available for investigative use. Metronidazole treatment is recommended for those with protracted diarrhea. As with CDI, diarrhea may recur after successful treatment.

Despite the self-limited nature of most food-associated diarrheal syndromes, *C. perfringens* type A has also been responsible for outbreaks of fatal illness in institutionalized mentally ill patients. A recent outbreak in a state psychiatric hospital linked to improperly prepared chicken was notable for three deaths (7% case-fatality rate) in patients taking antimotility agents and in whom necrotizing colitis was found at autopsy.[19]

Grade A References

A1. Johnson S, Louie TJ, Gerding DN, et al. Vancomycin, metronidazole, or tolevamer for *Clostridium difficile* infection: results from two multinational, randomized, controlled trials. *Clin Infect Dis.* 2014;59:345-354.

A2. Louie TJ, Miller MA, Mullane KM, et al. Fidaxomicin versus vancomycin for *Clostridium difficile* infection. *N Engl J Med.* 2011;364:422-431.

A3. Cornely OA, Nathwani D, Ivanescu C, et al. Clinical efficacy of fidaxomicin compared with vancomycin and metronidazole in Clostridium difficile infections: a meta-analysis and indirect treatment comparison. *J Antimicrob Chemother.* 2014;69:2892-2900.

A4. van Nood E, Vrieze A, Nieuwdorp M, et al. Duodenal infusion of donor feces for recurrent *Clostridium difficile. N Engl J Med.* 2013;368:407-415.

GENERAL REFERENCES

For the General References and other additional features, please visit Expert Consult at https://expertconsult.inkling.com.

297

DISEASES CAUSED BY NON–SPORE-FORMING ANAEROBIC BACTERIA

ITZHAK BROOK

DEFINITION

Anaerobic bacteria are the predominant members of the indigenous, normal human flora, including the skin and the oral, gastrointestinal, and vaginal mucosa (Fig. 297-1; Table 297-1). However, the types of predominant anaerobes are different at each location.

The Pathogens

Advances in taxonomics have led to reclassification of many anaerobic species. The genus *Bacteroides* is used only for species of the *Bacteroides fragilis* group. The "oral" *Bacteroides* and "pigmented" *Bacteroides* species have been reclassified as *Prevotella* (saccharolytic, pigmented species), *Porphyromonas* (asaccharolytic species), and other genera. Capnophilic organisms (which require an elevated concentration of carbon dioxide for growth), sometimes referred to as microaerophiles, are not true anaerobes and are often more related to *Campylobacter, Capnocytophaga*, and other genera. In addition, many new genera and several new species have been created to accommodate pathogens such as *Bilophila wadsworthia, Sutterella wadsworthensis, Centipeda periodontii*, and *Anaerobiospirillum thomasii. Fusobacterium nucleatum* is the predominant *Fusobacterium* species isolated from clinical specimens.

EPIDEMIOLOGY

Anaerobes are opportunistic pathogens that can cause serious infections, generally in synergistic infections in combination with aerobic bacteria. Because the microbiology of these infections is often complex and culture results may be delayed, awareness of the normal bacterial flora at the site of infection is an indispensable guide for selection and institution of empirical antimicrobial therapy.

TABLE 297-1	LOCATION OF VARIOUS GROUPS OF ANAEROBES AS NORMAL MICROFLORA IN HUMANS		
LOCATION	**NO. OF ORGANISMS PER GRAM**		**PREDOMINANT ANAEROBIC BACTERIA**
	Aerobes	*Anaerobes*	
Skin	—	—	*Propionibacterium acnes* Peptostreptococcus spp
Mouth/upper respiratory tract (in saliva)	10^8-10^9	10^9-10^{11}	Pigmented *Prevotella* and *Porphyromonas* spp *Fusobacterium* spp *Peptostreptococcus* spp *Actinomyces* spp
Gastrointestinal tract (in fecal material)			
Upper	10^2-10^5	10^3-10^7	*Bacteroides fragilis* group *Clostridium* spp
Lower	10^5-10^9	10^{10}-10^{12}	*Peptostreptococcus* spp *Bifidobacterium* spp *Eubacterium* spp
Female genital tract (in vaginal secretions)	10^8	10^9	*Peptostreptococcus* spp *Prevotella bivia* *Prevotella disiens*

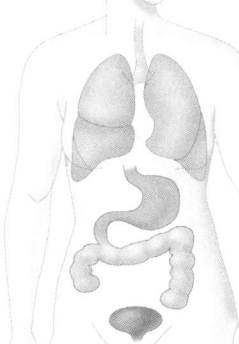

Skin
Propionibacterium acnes
Gram-positive cocci

Oral cavity and upper respiratory passages
Prevotella melaninogenica
Prevotella oralis
Other *Prevotella* sp
Porphyromonas sp
Fusobacterium nucleatum
Anaerobic cocci—peptostreptococci, *Veillonella*, microaerophilic streptococci
Actinomyces

Female genital tract
Prevotella melaninogenica
Other *Prevotella*
Other *Bacteroides*
Peptostreptococcus
Clostridium
Porphyromonas

Colon
Bacteroides fragilis group
Anaerobic cocci—peptostreptococci, *Veillonella*
Clostridium
Eubacterium
Bifidobacterium

FIGURE 297-1. Anaerobes as the predominant normal microflora of the human body by general anatomic location. (Modified from Finegold SM, Sutter VL. *Diagnosis and Management of Anaerobic Infections.* Kalamazoo, MI: Upjohn; 1976. Copyright by Dr. Finegold.)

TABLE 297-2   POTENTIAL VIRULENCE FACTORS IN VARIOUS ANAEROBES

FACTOR	SPECIES
ADHESION	
Capsule	*Bacteroides fragilis* group, *Prevotella melaninogenica*
Pili/fimbriae	*B. fragilis* group
	Porphyromonas gingivalis
Hemagglutinin	*P. gingivalis*
Lectin	*Fusobacterium nucleatum*
INVASION/TISSUE DAMAGE	
Proteases	*Fusobacterium necrophorum*
	Bacteroides spp
	Porphyromonas spp
Hemolysins	Many species
Endotoxin	*B. fragilis*
Fibrinolysin	*B. fragilis* group
	Porphyromonas spp
Heparinase	*B. fragilis* group
	Porphyromonas spp
Neuraminidase	*B. fragilis* group
	Porphyromonas spp
ANTIPHAGOCYTIC	
Capsule	*B. fragilis* group
	P. gingivalis
Lipopolysaccharide	*B. fragilis* group
	F. necrophorum, P. gingivalis
Metabolic products	Most anaerobes
TOXINS	
Endotoxin	*B. fragilis*
	F. necrophorum
Enterotoxin	*B. fragilis*

Modified from Duerden BI. Virulence factors in anaerobes. *Clin Infect Dis.* 1994;18(Suppl 4):253.

PATHOBIOLOGY

Anaerobic bacteria range from those that cannot survive even a brief exposure to oxygen to those that can survive even in the presence of atmospheric oxygen (e.g., *B. fragilis*). Most anaerobes require an environment with a low oxidation-reduction potential (E_h gradient), which can be achieved in association with low pH, tissue destruction, byproducts from aerobic bacterial metabolism, or low oxygen content. Although they are not true anaerobes, some organisms, such as microaerophilic streptococci and other capnophilic or difficult-to-cultivate bacteria, are sometimes lumped together with anaerobes because of their fastidious nature. Some genera, such as *Lactobacillus* and *Actinomyces*, include both aerobic and anaerobic species.

Anaerobic bacteria possess a variety of virulence factors that are species specific (Table 297-2).

CLINICAL MANIFESTATIONS

Bacteremia

Transient anaerobic bacteremia occurs in about 85% of patients immediately after dental cleaning or manipulation. It is estimated that more than 200 cases of endocarditis from anaerobes are reported annually in the United States, usually in association with anatomic abnormalities or damaged cardiac valves (Chapter 76). Most anaerobic bacteremias are intermittent and associated with serious intra-abdominal or female genital tract, skin, and soft tissue infections, often proximal to the gastrointestinal tract. Which organisms are involved depends on their portal of entry and the underlying disease. The most common isolates are the *B. fragilis* group (60 to 75% of isolates). About 5 to 15% of bacteremias are caused by anaerobes, and they are the sole isolates in two thirds of these. Mortality associated with *B. fragilis* group bacteremia is 15 to 30%. Bacteremia with the *B. fragilis* group generally originates from a gastrointestinal source; with pigmented *Prevotella*, *Porphyromonas*, and *Fusobacterium* spp, from oropharyngeal and pulmonary sources; with *Fusobacterium* spp, from the female genital tract; and with *Propionibacterium acnes*, from foreign body sources. Bacteremia with peptostreptococci is associated with all sources but especially with the oropharyngeal, pulmonary, and female genital tracts.

Central Nervous System Infections

Anaerobes can cause brain abscess, subdural empyema, epidural abscess, and meningitis. The main source of brain abscess is an adjacent, generally chronic infection in the ears, mastoids, sinuses, oropharynx, teeth, or lungs. Rarely, bacteremia of another origin or endocarditis can cause such infection.

Meningitis caused by anaerobes is uncommon and can follow respiratory or dental infection or develop as a complication of a cerebrospinal fluid shunt. The isolates usually isolated from brain abscesses that complicate respiratory and dental infections include *Prevotella*, *Porphyromonas*, *Bacteroides*, *Fusobacterium*, and *Peptostreptococcus* spp. Microaerophilic and other streptococci are also often isolated. *Propionibacterium acnes* is common in shunt infections.

Head and Neck

Dental infections (Chapter 425) associated with a variety of oral anaerobes include periodontal disease, gingivitis, pulpitis, acute necrotizing ulcerative gingivitis, localized juvenile periodontitis, adult periodontitis, pericoronitis, endodontitis, periapical and dental abscesses, and postextraction infection.[1] Peritonsillar, retropharyngeal, and parapharyngeal abscesses (Chapter 429) are deep-seated, potentially life-threatening infections that may spread into the various potential spaces of the neck or mediastinum and cause jugular vein thrombosis. Oral anaerobes can be recovered in more than 50% of such cases, usually mixed with aerobes. Other regional infections include cervicofacial actinomycosis (Chapter 329), Ludwig's angina, *Fusobacterium necrophorum* sepsis with metastatic infection (Lemierre's syndrome), suppurative sialoadenitis (including parotitis), neck space infections, thyroiditis and chronic sinusitis (Chapter 426), otitis media (Chapter 426), and mastoiditis. Management involves surgical drainage and appropriate antimicrobial therapy.

Pleuropulmonary

Anaerobes predominate in oral and upper respiratory tract normal flora, and most aspiration pneumonias are due to this flora (Chapter 97).[2] Aspiration can result from altered consciousness, dysphagia, or mechanical devices such as intubation equipment. Poor oral hygiene is associated with an increased anaerobic bacterial burden, and the presence of aerobes or necrotic tissue lowers the pH, which facilitates the growth of anaerobes. Anaerobes are involved in 90% of community-acquired aspiration pneumonia and in about a third of nosocomial aspiration pneumonia, empyema, lung abscess, and pneumonia associated with tracheostomy. If the anaerobic component of aspiration pneumonia is not treated, the anaerobes can cause a lung abscess. Management requires good pulmonary toilet and antimicrobial therapy.

Intra-abdominal

Because anaerobes outnumber aerobes by 1000 to 1 in the large intestine, they play a major role in almost all intra-abdominal infections. Most visceral abscesses (e.g., hepatic; Chapter 151), chronic cholecystitis (Chapter 155), perforated and gangrenous appendicitis (Chapter 142), postoperative wound infections and abscesses, diverticulitis (Chapter 142), and any infection associated with fecal contamination of the abdominal cavity involve both aerobes and anaerobes. *B. fragilis* group members predominate because they are encapsulated, resist phagocytosis, are often resistant to many antimicrobials, and promote abscess formation. They may also be associated with concomitant bacteremia and sepsis. Randomized controlled trials have found that prophylactic antibiotics covering both anaerobic and aerobic bacteria administered orally and/or intravenously prior to elective colorectal surgery reduce the risk of surgical wound infection by as much as 75%. **A1**

Obstetric-Gynecologic

A variety of obstetric-gynecologic infections involve anaerobes. These are polymicrobial and include bacterial vaginosis; soft tissue perineal, vulvar, and Bartholin gland abscesses; endometritis; pyometra; salpingitis; tubo-ovarian abscesses; adnexal abscess; pelvic inflammatory disease, which may include pelvic cellulitis and abscess; chorioamnionitis; vaginal cuff cellulitis; septic pelvic thrombophlebitis; intrauterine contraceptive device–associated infection; septic abortion; and postsurgical obstetric and gynecologic infections. Bacterial vaginosis has been associated with preterm labor or delivery, chorioamnionitis, low birthweight, postpartum endometritis, and postabortal pelvic inflammatory disease. Bacterial vaginosis can increase the risk for infection with human immunodeficiency virus type 1 and the development of other sexually transmitted diseases (Chapter 285).

Skin and Soft Tissue

Cutaneous infections include infected ulcers, cellulitis (including synergistic necrotizing cellulitis), pyoderma, paronychia, hidradenitis suppurativa, and a variety of secondarily infected sites. Such sites include secondarily infected gastrostomy or tracheostomy site wounds, subcutaneous sebaceous or inclusion cysts, eczema, psoriasis, poison ivy, atopic dermatitis, eczema herpeticum, scabies or kerion, and postsurgical wounds.

Subcutaneous infections include abscesses, decubitus ulcers, infected diabetic (vascular or trophic) ulcers, human and animal bite wounds, anaerobic cellulitis and gas gangrene, bacterial synergistic gangrene, Fournier's gangrene, infected pilonidal cyst or sinus, and burn wounds. Anaerobic soft tissue infections that occur deeper are necrotizing fasciitis, necrotizing synergistic cellulitis, and gas gangrene. These infections can involve the fascia and can induce myositis and myonecrosis.

Cultures frequently yield isolates that are members of the normal flora of the region of the infection. In addition to oral and skin flora, human bite infections often contain *Eikenella* species, and animal bites harbor *Pasteurella multocida*.

The infections are generally polymicrobial, and some (e.g., decubitus ulcers, diabetic foot ulcers) are often complicated by osteomyelitis or bacteremia. Deep tissue infections, such as necrotizing cellulitis, fasciitis, and myositis, often involve *Clostridium* species, *Streptococcus pyogenes*, or a polymicrobial aerobic and anaerobic flora. They are often associated with gas in the tissues and putrid-like pus with a gray, thin quality and have a high rate of bacteremia and mortality. Management of deep-seated soft tissue infection includes surgical débridement, drainage, and vigorous surgical management.

Osteomyelitis and Septic Arthritis

Anaerobes can be involved in osteomyelitis of the long bones after trauma and fracture, osteomyelitis related to peripheral vascular disease, decubitus ulcers, and osteomyelitis of the cranial and facial bones. Most of these infections are polymicrobial.

Cranial and facial bone osteomyelitis is generally caused by spread from a contiguous soft tissue source or from sinus, ear, or dental infection. Intestinal anaerobes originating from decubitus ulcers are involved in pelvic osteomyelitis. Osteomyelitis of long bones and septic arthritis are generally caused by hematogenous spread, trauma, or the presence of a prosthetic device.

The most commonly recovered anaerobes are peptostreptococci and *P. acnes* (often in prosthetic joint infection), *B. fragilis* group and fusobacteria (often of hematogenous origin), and clostridia (associated with trauma).

DIAGNOSIS

Anaerobic infections should be suspected in a number of specific clinical scenarios (Table 297-3). An appropriately collected microbiologic specimen (Table 297-4) is critical for accurate diagnosis.

TREATMENT   Rx

General principles of treatment (Table 297-5) include appropriate antimicrobial therapy coupled with prompt drainage, decompression of closed space infections, relief of obstructions, and surgical débridement.[3,4] The various clinically important anaerobes can be characterized by reasonably predictable antimicrobial susceptibility patterns (Table 297-6). However, some anaerobes have become resistant to antimicrobials, and many can develop resistance during therapy.[5] Reliable culture and sensitivity results should ultimately guide therapy. The efficacy of hyperbaric oxygen is unproved, but its use in conjunction with other therapeutic measures is not contraindicated.

In choosing antimicrobials for the treatment of mixed infections, their aerobic and anaerobic antibacterial spectra and their availability in oral or parenteral form should be considered. Some antimicrobials have a limited range of activity.[6] For example, metronidazole is active only against anaerobes and therefore cannot be administered as a single agent for the treatment of mixed infections. Others (i.e., carbapenems, a penicillin plus a β-lactamase inhibitor) have wide spectra of activity against aerobes and anaerobes.

Aside from susceptibility patterns, other factors influencing the choice of antimicrobial therapy include the pharmacologic characteristics of the various drugs, their toxicity, their effect on normal flora, and their bactericidal activity. Although identification of the infecting organisms and their antimicrobial susceptibility may be needed for selection of optimal therapy, the clinical setting and Gram stain preparation of the specimen may suggest the types of anaerobes present in the infection and the nature of the infectious process.

Even though the length of therapy for anaerobic infections is generally longer than that for aerobic and facultative infections, the length of treatment must be individualized, depending on the response. In some cases, treatment may require 6 to 8 weeks, but therapy may be shortened with proper surgical drainage. An anti–gram-negative enteric agent is generally added to treat Enterobacteriaceae in managing intra-abdominal infections.

The available parenteral antimicrobials for most infections are metronidazole, chloramphenicol, clindamycin, cefoxitin, a penicillin (i.e., ticarcillin, ampicillin, piperacillin) and a β-lactamase inhibitor (i.e., clavulanic acid, sulbactam, tazobactam), a carbapenem (i.e., imipenem, meropenem, doripenem, ertapenem), and tigecycline.

An agent effective against gram-negative enteric bacilli (e.g., an aminoglycoside, fluoroquinolone) or an antipseudomonal cephalosporin (e.g., cefepime) is generally added to metronidazole and, occasionally, cefoxitin in treatment of intra-abdominal infections. Penicillin can be added to metronidazole for the treatment of intracranial, pulmonary, or dental infections to cover microaerophilic streptococci and *Actinomyces* species. Penicillin is added to clindamycin to supplement its coverage against *Peptostreptococcus* species and other gram-positive anaerobic organisms. For *Chlamydia* and

TABLE 297-4 SPECIMEN ACCEPTABILITY FOR ANAEROBIC CULTURE

SPECIMENS THAT SHOULD NOT BE CULTURED FOR ANAEROBES

Feces or rectal swabs
Throat or nasopharyngeal swabs
Sputum or bronchoscopic specimens
Routine or catheterized urine
Vaginal or cervical swabs
Material from superficial wounds or abscesses not collected properly to exclude surface contamination
Material from abdominal wounds obviously contaminated with feces, such as an open fistula

SPECIMENS APPROPRIATE FOR ANAEROBIC CULTURE

All normally sterile body fluids other than urine, such as blood, pleural fluid, and joint fluid
Urine obtained by suprapubic bladder aspiration
Percutaneous transtracheal aspiration, direct lung puncture, or double-lumen catheter bronchial brushing and bronchoalveolar lavage (both cultured quantitatively)
Culdocentesis fluid obtained after decontamination of the vagina
Material obtained from closed abscesses
Material obtained from sinus tracks or draining wounds

TABLE 297-3 CLINICAL INDICATORS OF ANAEROBIC INFECTION

Infection adjacent to a mucosal surface
Foul-smelling discharge
Necrotic gangrenous tissue and abscess formation
Free gas or crepitus in tissue
Bacteremia or endocarditis with no growth on aerobic blood cultures
Infection related to the use of antibiotics effective against aerobes only (e.g., trimethoprim-sulfamethoxazole, aminoglycosides, older quinolones)
Infection related to tumors or other destructive processes
Infected thrombophlebitis
Infection after bites
Black discoloration of exudates containing *Prevotella melaninogenica*, which may fluoresce under ultraviolet light
"Sulfur granules" in discharges caused by actinomycosis
Clinical finding of gas gangrene or necrotizing fasciitis
Clinical condition predisposing to anaerobic infection (e.g., after maternal amnionitis, fistulous tracks, bites, dental infection, bowel perforation)

TABLE 297-5 GENERAL PRINCIPLES OF THERAPY FOR ANAEROBIC INFECTIONS

Decompression of closed spaces
Débridement
Drainage
Relief of obstructions
Irrigation
Provision of adequate circulation when possible
Removal of foreign bodies
Antimicrobials
Activity against most likely pathogen or pathogens: location dependent, minimal effect on normal flora
Absorption, appropriate route of administration (intravenous, oral)
Penetration into site of infection
Dosage appropriate for local tissue levels, body mass of patient, renal and liver function
Duration appropriate for condition
Susceptibility testing of isolate to guide specific therapy

TABLE 297-6 ANTIMICROBIAL SUSCEPTIBILITY PATTERNS FOR ANAEROBIC BACTERIA*

BACTERIA	PENICILLIN	β-LACTAMASE[†]	CEFOXITIN	CEFOTETAN	CARBAPENEMS, TIGECYCLINE	MOXIFLOXACIN	CLINDAMYCIN	METRONIDAZOLE
Bacteroides fragilis	−	+	+	+	+	+	V	+
Bacteroides thetaiotaomicron	−	+	V	V	+	V	V	+
B. fragilis group, other	−	+	V	V	+	+	V	+
Prevotella spp	V	+	+	+	+	+	+	+
Fusobacterium nucleatum	V	+	+	+	+	V	+	+
Fusobacterium necrophorum	+	+	+	+	+	V	+	+
Porphyromonas spp	+	+	+	+	+	+	+	+
Peptostreptococcus	+	+	+	+	+	+	+	V
Propionibacterium acnes	+	+	+	+	+	+	+	−
Veillonella	+	+	+	+	+	+	+	+
Actinomyces	+	+	+	+	+	+	+	−

*Based on a variety of in vitro susceptibility studies from different laboratories and using different techniques.
[†]β-Lactamase inhibitor–β-lactam combination (e.g., ticarcillin-clavulanate, ampicillin-sulbactam, piperacillin-tazobactam).
+ = Susceptible; − = resistant; V = variable.

Mycoplasma species, doxycycline is added to most regimens in treatment of pelvic infections. Oral therapy is often substituted for parenteral therapy. The agents available for oral therapy are clindamycin, amoxicillin and clavulanate, and metronidazole.

Grade A Reference

A1. Nelson RL, Gladman E, Barbateskovic M. Antimicrobial prophylaxis for colorectal surgery. *Cochrane Database Syst Rev.* 2014;5:CD001181.

GENERAL REFERENCES

For the General References and other additional features, please visit Expert Consult at https://expertconsult.inkling.com.

298

NEISSERIA MENINGITIDIS INFECTIONS

DAVID S. STEPHENS

DEFINITION

Neisseria meningitidis (the meningococcus) is the cause of epidemic bacterial meningitis, fulminant sepsis (meningococcemia), milder bacteremia, and, less commonly, focal infections (such as pneumonia, septic arthritis, purulent pericarditis, and conjunctivitis).[1-3]

The Pathogen

N. meningitidis is an aerobic, diplococcal gram-negative β-proteobacterium and a member of the family Neisseriaceae, which also includes *Neisseria gonorrhoeae* (Chapter 299), another important human pathogen. The meningococcus is a commensal of the human upper respiratory tract, but it can also cause local and devastating invasive human disease. Human mucosal surfaces, most commonly the nasopharynx, are the only known reservoir. There are 12 confirmed serogroups of *N. meningitidis*, based on different capsular polysaccharide structures, but only 6 serogroups (A, B, C, W, X, and Y) cause almost all invasive meningococcal disease (Fig. 298-1). Highly pathogenic meningococci are also distinguished by genetically defined clonal complexes that can emerge and spread worldwide.[4] Dissecting the basis of meningococcal disease has provided important scientific lessons for bacterial emergence and

pathogenesis, antibiotic resistance mechanisms, innate and adaptive human immune responses, and vaccine development.

EPIDEMIOLOGY

For at least 200 years, *N. meningitidis* has inflicted rapid death, disability, and fear on disparate human populations. Beginning with the initial descriptions of outbreaks in Geneva in 1805 and New Bedford, Massachusetts, in 1806, the meningococcus has caused endemic disease, case clusters, epidemics and pandemics of meningitis and septicemia, and less commonly pneumonia. An estimated 500,000 cases occur worldwide each year. The greatest burden of disease occurs in Africa and in parts of Asia, where endemic rates of disease have been 3 to 10 per 100,000 population. In sub-Saharan Africa, seasonal increases in disease and cyclic pandemics occurred every 8 to 10 years since 1905. During epidemics and cyclic pandemics, the incidence can climb to 1 per 1000 population for weeks before the frequency of disease declines in the immediate outbreak area. For example, until the introduction in 2010 of a new meningococcal conjugate vaccine for serogroup A, the dry seasons in Burkina Faso, located in the sub-Saharan meningitis belt, were accompanied by more than 5000 cases of meningitis per week (>680/100,000 population), an almost yearly occurrence in the country. Meningococcal epidemics in developing countries have been catastrophic and contribute to a cycle of poverty and hence the disorganization of social structures.

Meningococcal disease remains endemic, with focal outbreaks/clusters, in the United States, Canada, Europe, Japan, Australia, and other industrialized countries, with a lower overall incidence now at 0.1 to 2 per 100,000 population. The introduction and widespread use of new meningococcal conjugate vaccines in North America, Australia, and Europe have helped to lower the incidence,[5,6] but slow declines in industrialized countries began before new vaccine introductions. Endemic disease and outbreaks also occur in China, eastern Europe, Russia, South America, India, and Southeast Asia. Before and during World War II, large epidemic outbreaks (mainly due to serogroup A) affected the United States, Europe, Japan, and Australia; after the war, these outbreaks disappeared, for reasons that are not understood. Meningococcal disease has the highest incidence in children younger than 4 years and in adolescents, but in endemic settings, half of all cases occur in adults.

PATHOBIOLOGY

N. meningitidis is transmitted among humans through close contact by large respiratory droplets. Colonization of the upper respiratory mucosal surfaces (e.g., nasopharynx) by *N. meningitidis* is the first step in establishment of a human carrier state and invasive meningococcal disease. Acquisition of meningococci through contact with respiratory secretions or saliva can be transient, lead to colonization (carriage), or result in invasive disease. The inoculum size needed for transmission is unknown. Meningococcal disease usually occurs within 1 to 14 days of acquisition. Meningococci can be found in the urogenital tract and rectum and may be transmitted sexually.

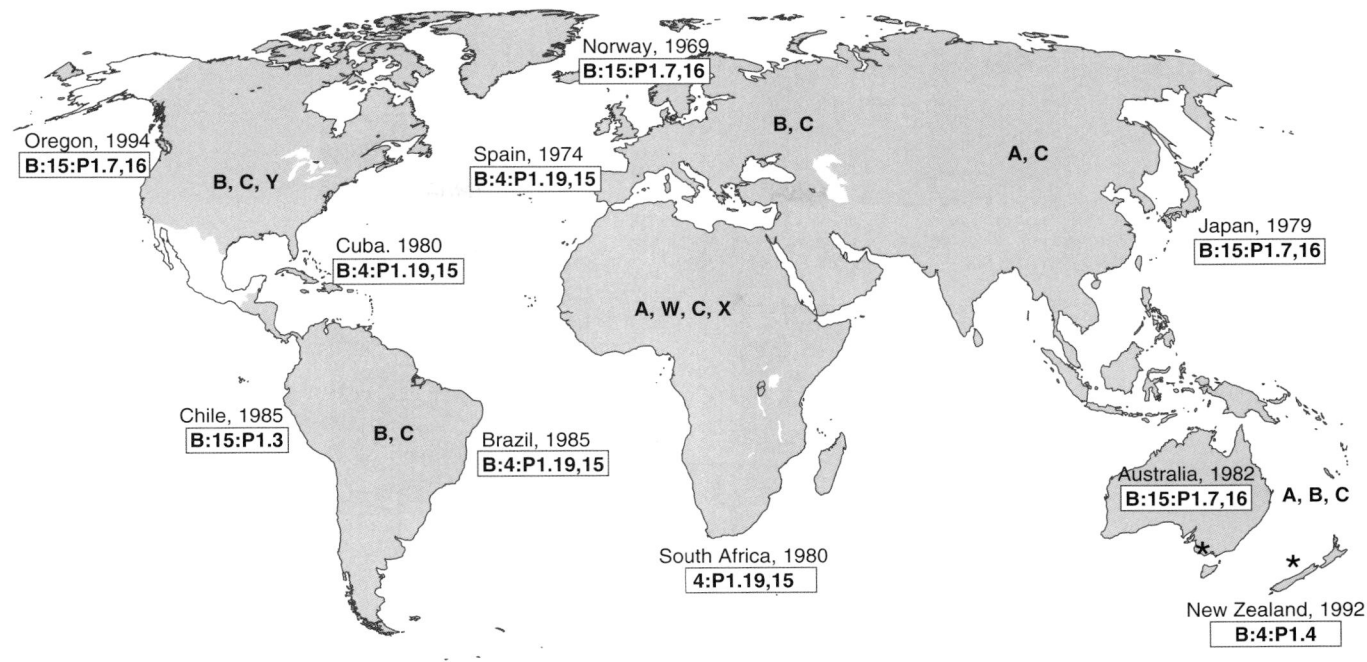

*Group B by serotype, modified from Caugant, APMIS 1998; 106:505-525

FIGURE 298-1. **Epidemiology of meningococcal disease** (major serogroups causing disease by region and serogroup B epidemics). (Modified from Stephens DS, Greenwood B, Brandtzaeg P. Epidemic meningitis, meningococcemia and *Neisseria meningitidis*. Lancet. 2007;369:2196-2210.)

Initial contact of meningococci with mucosal epithelial cells is mediated by type IV pili. These structures provide mobility ("twitching motility") to penetrate mucus and are the initial adhesins for human epithelial cells. Meningococci proceed to proliferate on the surface of human nonciliated epithelial cells, forming small microcolonies at the site of attachment; they can disseminate from colonies by post-translational glycan modifications of pili and migrate to adjacent cells by the pili-mediated motility.[7,8] Meningococci can also spread from the nasopharynx to adjacent epithelial surfaces and can infrequently cause local infections, including pneumonia, sinusitis, and otitis media. Other less common local infections include conjunctivitis, urethritis, and proctitis. Close adherence of meningococci to the host epithelial cells results in the formation of epithelial cell cortical plaques and leads to the recruitment of factors ultimately responsible for the formation and extension of host epithelial cell pseudopodia that can surround the meningococcus. Intimate meningococcal association with the epithelial cell is mediated by the bacterial opacity proteins Opa and Opc with CD66/carcinoembryonic antigen–related cell adhesion molecules and integrins, respectively, on the surface of the cell. However, other meningococcal epithelial cell mediators include the meningococcal adhesin NadA and meningococcal lipo-oligosaccharide. The formation of epithelial cell membrane protrusions and pseudopodia stems from the organization of specific molecular complexes involving the linkers ezrin and moesin along with the clustering of several membrane-integral proteins, including CD44, intracellular adhesion molecule 1, and cortical actin polymerization.[9] These events can lead to internalization of *N. meningitidis* in epithelial cells (Fig. 298-2). Intracellular meningococci reside within a membranous vacuole and are capable of translocating through the epithelial layers within 18 to 40 hours. Meningococci are capable of intracellular replication (in part because of the protective capsule), can survive under microaerophilic conditions, use lactate as a carbon source, and have the capacity to acquire iron through specialized transport systems.

Meningococci cross mucosal surfaces, enter the blood stream, and, in some individuals, produce systemic infections. Damage to the mucosal surface by coinfection, drying (e.g., very low humidity), or smoke exposure may increase this risk of meningococcal invasion. Similar molecular interactions noted for meningococci and epithelial cells also occur with endothelial cells, and meningococci can translocate across the blood-meninges barrier, possibly at the choroid plexus or by opening of intercellular junctions, and proliferate in the subarachnoid space, resulting in meningitis. In the vasculature and cerebrospinal fluid (CSF), high levels of multiplying bacteria lead to an intense inflammatory response, with pronounced increases in concentrations of tumor necrosis factor-α, interleukins (1β, 6, 8, and 10), different chemokines, and other inflammatory mediators.[10]

Resistance to complement-mediated lysis or phagocytosis is due to the expression of the capsule, lipo-oligosaccharide, and several surface-exposed proteins (factor H–binding protein, NspA, Opc, NalP). Meningococcal endotoxin released in blebs plays a major role in the inflammatory events of meningococcemia and meningococcal meningitis. Meningococcal lipid A is responsible for much of the biologic activity and toxicity of meningococcal endotoxin. The toll-like receptor 4 (TLR4) is critical to the innate immune response to bacterial endotoxins, and meningococcal endotoxin is no exception. Activation of TLR4 by endotoxin requires association with the accessory protein MD-2, an *N*-glycosylated 19- to 27-kD protein expressed in both a soluble and a membrane-bound form. Binding of endotoxin to MD-2 in association with TLR4 leads to dimerization or oligomerization of two or more TLR4s, subsequent cellular activation, and cytokine and chemokine release.

In contrast to invasive disease, an asymptomatic *N. meningitidis* carrier state is found in up to 8 to 25% of healthy individuals. Meningococcal carriage is affected by age, intimate personal contact, crowding (e.g., bars, dormitories), and vaccination or chemoprophylaxis interventions in the community. Variable carriage rates have been reported, even during epidemics. Meningococcal carriage is a dynamic process, is less common in young children (<3% and *Neisseria lactamica* predominates) than in older children and adolescents (7 to 37%), and increases in closed populations (e.g., military recruits, hajj pilgrims). Rates as high as 36 to 71% have been reported in military recruits. Damage to the upper respiratory tract by coinfections (e.g., mycoplasma, influenza, other respiratory viral infections), smoking, very low humidity, drying of mucosal surfaces, and trauma induced by dust predisposes to both meningococcal carriage and meningococcal disease. Meningococcal carriage has also been linked to status as a secretor of glycoprotein ABO blood group antigens, which are water soluble, and to ethnic background. In a large U.K. study, social behavior (e.g., attendance at pubs or clubs, intimate kissing, cigarette smoking or exposure to passive smoke) was highly associated with the risk of meningococcal carriage. Carriage can be transient or last for days, weeks, or months and is an immunizing event leading to protective immunity (e.g., serum bactericidal activity against the meningococcus).

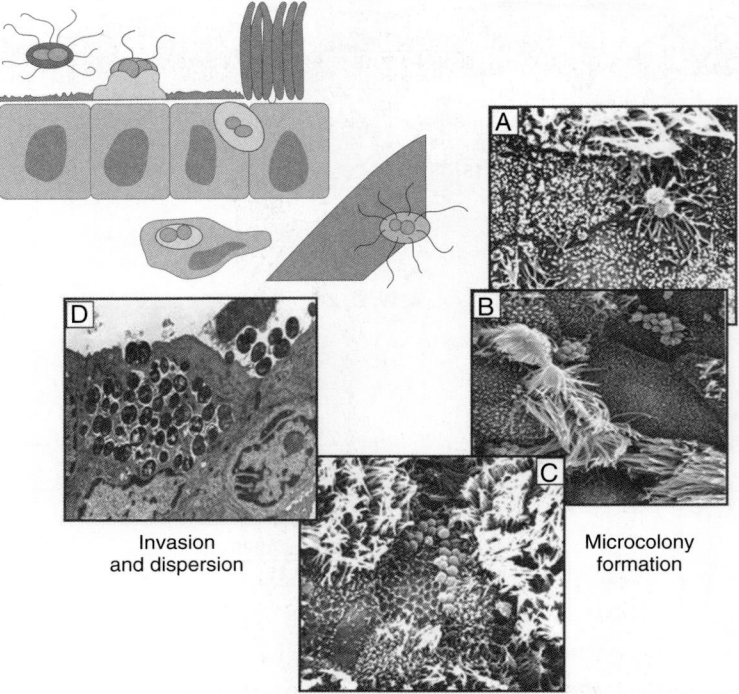

FIGURE 298-2. Steps in initiation of meningococcal colonization and invasion at the human nasopharynx. **A,** Adhesion and introduction of cell microvilli. **B,** Microcolony formation. **C,** Cortical plaque formation and close adherence. **D,** Human epithelial cell invasion. (Modified from Stephens DS. Biology and pathogenesis of the evolutionarily successful, obligate human bacterium *Neisseria meningitidis. Vaccine.* 2009;27S:B71-B77.)

The absence of protective bactericidal antibodies is the most important predisposing factor for systemic meningococcal disease, but complement deficiencies, genetic polymorphisms, and other host cofactors can contribute to meningococcal disease and disease severity. Disappearance of protective maternal antibodies increases the risk in older infants and young children. Congenital and acquired antibody deficiencies also increase risk. Opsonization and phagocytic function do contribute to meningococcal host defense mechanisms, as shown by disease reduction after polysaccharide vaccination in individuals with complement deficiencies. Rapidly progressive, fatal meningococcemia can arise in patients without properdin, and there is a marked risk of recurrent meningococcal infections in those with defects in the terminal complement pathway (C5-C9) and C3 deficiency.[11]

Polymorphisms in genes coding for the Fcγ-receptor II (CD32), Fcγ-receptor III (CD16), mannose-binding lectin, TLR4, and β_2-adrenoceptor gene have been associated with increased risk. Mannose-binding lectin is a plasma opsonin that initiates complement activation; specific polymorphisms in the gene are identified more frequently in children with meningococcal disease than in controls in some studies. Plasminogen activator inhibitor 1 concentrations appear to affect the severity and mortality of meningococcal sepsis, suggesting that impaired fibrinolysis is an important factor in its pathophysiology. Meningococcal disease is occasionally linked to immunosuppressive disorders, such as nephrotic syndrome, congenital or acquired hypogammaglobulinemia, splenectomy, and human immunodeficiency virus (HIV) infection/AIDS (about a 10-fold increased risk for sporadic disease). However, there has been no documented increase in epidemic outbreaks of meningococcal disease in countries with very high rates of HIV infection.

Meningococci can multiply rapidly in the vascular compartment, with an estimated doubling time of 30 to 45 minutes in some patients, or in the CSF.[12] The release of high levels of inflammatory mediators such as meningococcal endotoxin in the circulation or CSF triggers an exaggerated release of chemokines, cytokines, bradykinin, and nitric oxide. Vascular dilation, hypovolemia, capillary leak, and pronounced reduction in myocardial function are the result. At a later stage, substantial complement activation contributes to the altered endothelial barrier function and relaxation of the smooth muscles in the vessel wall through the generation of high levels of anaphylatoxins (C3a and C5a). The capillary leak syndrome results in an increased flux of albumin and water across the altered capillary wall to the extravascular space. A patient with fulminant meningococcemia accumulates a large amount of fluid in the extravascular tissue. Circulatory collapse and multiorgan dysfunction are the primary causes of death due to meningococcemia. In meningitis, morbidity and death are due predominantly to cerebral edema.

Unraveling the pathogenic mechanisms of this devastating, evolutionarily successful obligate human pathogen has significance for the understanding of human sepsis as well as for prevention through vaccines directed at mucosal pathogens.

CLINICAL MANIFESTATIONS

The meningococcus causes meningitis (37 to 50% of cases), septicemia (meningococcemia, 10 to 18% of cases), or both in 7 to 12% of cases. The presentations are less commonly a mild bacteremia or pneumonia (10% of cases) and much less commonly (<5% of cases) septic arthritis, pericarditis, chronic bacteremia, or conjunctivitis . Very rarely, meningococci can cause urethritis or proctitis. In endemic and epidemic disease outbreaks, hemorrhagic skin lesions (petechiae, purpura; Fig. 298-3) are present in 28 to 77% of patients with invasive meningococcal disease on admission, but these lesions may be absent or difficult to see in patients with dark skin. Hemorrhagic lesions sometimes occur on mucous membranes and sclera, but they are especially prevalent on the limbs. Petechiae of meningococcemia are usually larger and bluer than the pinpoint petechiae caused by thrombocytopenia, leukocytoclastic vasculitis induced by other infections or drugs, or vomiting or coughing. A nonblanching macular rash can also be a manifestation of meningococcal bacteremia. Evolving ecchymoses and purpura (diameter >10 mm) are noted mainly in patients with meningococcemia and disseminated intravascular coagulation (Chapter 175), but they may not appear until 12 hours into the illness. In addition to vasculitis, other conditions in the differential diagnosis of meningococcemia include Rocky Mountain spotted fever and enteroviral infections.

Meningitis is the most common clinical presentation of invasive meningococcal disease.[13] Headache, fever, and rash with meningismus and altered mental status are the characteristic features; however, the rash may be absent, and the presentation can resemble pneumococcal or bacterial meningitis of other causes, viral meningitis, or early-stage encephalitis. Bacteremic meningococcal pneumonia has been linked most often to serogroup Y and is more common in adolescents and adults, especially older adults (approximately one third of cases occur in those older than 65 years). Isolated septic pericarditis or septic arthritis can also be a presentation, and an autoimmune- or antibody-mediated polyarthritis can be seen in the recovery phase following invasive meningococcal disease. Chronic meningococcemia can be

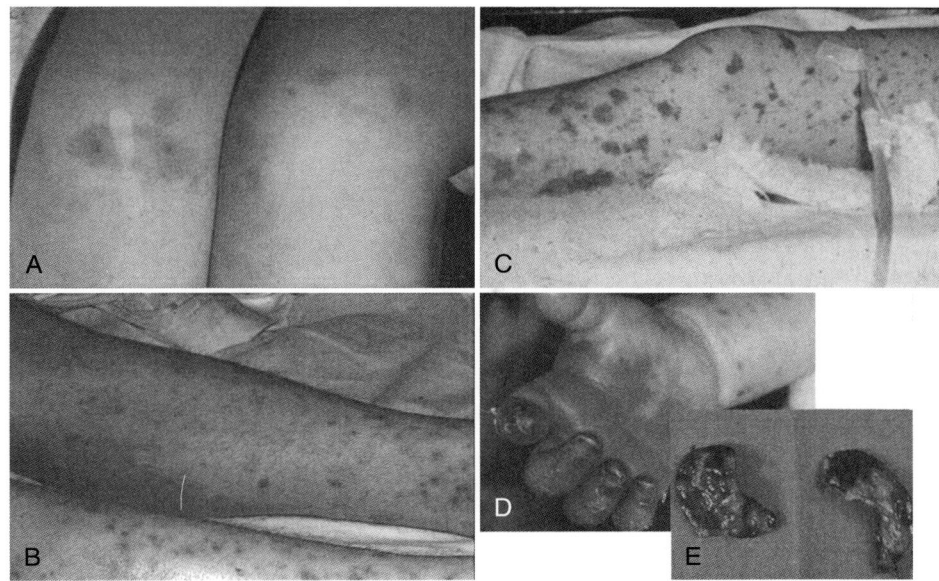

FIGURE 298-3. Clinical manifestations of meningococcal disease. **A** and **B,** Macular and petechial rashes of meningococcal bacteremia. **C,** Fulminant meningococcal sepsis with ecchymoses. **D,** Digital necrosis of meningococcemia sepsis. **E,** Hemorrhagic adrenals in fulminant meningococcal sepsis. (Modified from Stephens DS, Greenwood B, Brandtzaeg P. Epidemic meningitis, meningococcemia and *Neisseria meningitidis. Lancet.* 2007;369:2196-2210.)

manifested with low-grade fever and a polyarticular arthritis that can be confused with rheumatoid arthritis.

DIAGNOSIS

The clinical diagnosis of meningococcal meningitis relies on the recognition of fever, rash, meningeal signs, and altered mental status. The early clinical diagnosis of meningococcemia is a challenge because a rash, meningeal signs, and high fever may not be present. The course can be fulminant (<24 hours), and the early stages of disease can mimic viral infections such as those caused by enterovirus or influenza. Thus, it can be difficult to identify and to treat the disease quickly. General symptoms of sepsis (nausea and vomiting, drowsiness, irritability, leg pains, cold hands and feet, abnormal skin color) are present. However, these symptoms (in contrast to fever and rash) are not likely to be specific markers. Parents and relatives should be instructed to undress and inspect a febrile child, adolescent, or adult for a rash, and physicians and other health care providers should be alert to the concerns of parents or relatives about the abrupt or rapid deterioration of a patient.

The definitive diagnosis of invasive meningococcal disease is based on bacteriologic isolation or antigen or DNA identification of *N. meningitidis* in a usually sterile body fluid, such as blood, CSF, synovial fluid, pleural fluid, urine, or pericardial fluid. Blood and CSF are the most fruitful sources of positive cultures and for DNA identification by the polymerase chain reaction (PCR), but urine and skin lesions can also yield results in systemic meningococcal disease. The diagnosis of meningococcal meningitis is confirmed by CSF pleocytosis and Gram stain showing gram-negative diplococci (often inside neutrophils) and CSF culture, latex agglutination detecting meningococcal capsular polysaccharide in CSF, or PCR identifying *N. meningitidis* in CSF.

PCR is increasingly used for the diagnosis of meningococcal disease, including serogrouping and multilocus sequence typing, and has the potential to detect antibiotic resistance determinants. PCR techniques include real-time PCR of CSF, blood, and other sterile sites. Urine is a less sensitive fluid for PCR. An increasing number of patients are now diagnosed by PCR without culture, especially if they have received empiric prehospital antibiotic treatment.[14] The sensitivity of PCR for the diagnosis of meningococcal meningitis is more than 90 to 95%; in contrast, the sensitivity of CSF or blood culture is less than 65%.

TREATMENT   Rx

Early recognition and antibiotic administration (Table 298-1) are critical for effective treatment because effective antibiotics immediately stop the growth of *N. meningitidis*. Ceftriaxone, cefotaxime, and penicillin are effective

TABLE 298-1	ANTIBIOTIC TREATMENT OF MENINGOCOCCAL MENINGITIS AND MENINGOCOCCEMIA	
DRUG	**AGE GROUP**	**DOSAGE**
Ceftriaxone*	Children > 3 months Adults	50 mg/kg IV q12h 1-2 g IV q12h
Cefotaxime	Adults	50-75 mg/kg q6-8h; maximum dose, 12 g/day
Penicillin G	Adults	50,000 U/kg IV q4h; up to 4 million U q4h
Meropenem	Adults	2 g IV q8h, 6 g/day
If penicillin and cephalosporin allergic, chloramphenicol	Adults	25 mg/kg IV q6h, up to 1 g q6h

*Because of concerns in neonates from calcium/ceftriaxone precipitates and displacement of bilirubin from albumin by ceftriaxone, babies younger than 3 months should be started on cefotaxime 50 mg/kg q6-8h.

antibiotics, as are meropenem and chloramphenicol.[15] Meningococci in CSF are killed within 3 to 4 hours after intravenous treatment with an adequate dose of a third-generation cephalosporin or penicillin, and concentrations of endotoxin in plasma fall by 50% within 2 hours. The concentrations of key cytokines and chemokines fall in parallel. Antibiotic treatment does not induce a large release of meningococcal endotoxin or lead to an increased inflammatory response.

Prehospital antibiotic treatment is advocated if the disease is suspected. One goal is to reduce the case-fatality rate for patients with fulminant meningococcal sepsis or meningitis with rapidly increasing concentrations of meningococci and inflammatory mediators in the circulation or CSF. If antibiotic treatment is initiated before admission, ceftriaxone or another effective antibiotic can be injected intravenously or intramuscularly. During epidemics in developing countries, a single injection of ceftriaxone or long-acting chloramphenicol may be sufficient for patients with meningitis,[A1] and this simple treatment has saved many thousands of lives. The sensitivity of meningococci to penicillin is decreasing worldwide because of a reduced affinity for penicillin-binding protein 2, although high-level penicillin resistance remains rare in most countries. Fluoroquinolone resistance of meningococcal isolates, although rare, has also emerged. Ceftriaxone and cefotaxime can achieve CSF concentrations 45- to 8750-fold higher than the minimal inhibitory concentrations for meningococci. First-generation cephalosporins should not be used.

Patients with suspected bacterial meningitis of unknown cause are often given ceftriaxone or cefotaxime, often combined with vancomycin, until the causative agent has been identified. When *N. meningitidis* is identified, antibiotic treatment can be continued with a third-generation cephalosporin or possibly benzylpenicillin alone. Meropenem is also active clinically in the treatment of meningococcal meningitis, or chloramphenicol is a choice in penicillin- and cephalosporin-allergic patients. Traditionally, patients with meningococcal meningitis were treated for 7 days or longer, but 3 or 4 days of intravenous treatment can provide a cure without relapse.

Recognition of the different pathophysiologic processes associated with meningococcal meningitis (which causes death and morbidity predominantly by cerebral edema) and meningococcal septic shock (which causes death and morbidity predominantly through hypovolemia, capillary leak, myocardial dysfunction, and multiorgan failure) has led to improved management strategies for these two different forms of disease. Early and aggressive management of shock through the use of volume expansion, intensive care monitoring, and inotropic support can reduce fatality rates of meningococcal sepsis from higher than 30% to 5 to 10%. In meningococcemia with hypotension, the primary goal is to increase the circulating blood volume by aggressive fluid treatment. Both colloids and crystalloids (saline 0.9%) can be used without a demonstrated difference in effectiveness. Adults are given saline starting with 1 L infused intravenously during 15 to 20 minutes, followed by several liters at a reduced rate. Some patients require two to three times their own blood volume during the first 24 hours. The total fluid volume needed per 24 hours is determined by response to treatment—tissue perfusion, blood pressure, urine output, and evidence of intravascular volume overload. The volume treatment may be combined with a vasopressor such as dopamine, norepinephrine, epinephrine, or dobutamine. Fluid treatment may be complicated in patients with reduced renal function. They may need dialysis or hemofiltration to compensate for renal failure and to reduce the substantial edema that accumulates.

Patients with meningitis or mild meningococcemia should be given the normal daily fluid requirement, supplemented with the volume lost before admission unless there is evidence of the syndrome of inappropriate antidiuretic hormone. Excessive volume treatment in patients with meningitis can induce fatal brain edema and herniation. Management of raised intracranial pressure (hyperosmolar solutions, diuretics, mechanical ventilation), seizures, and hyponatremia is indicated.

Anticoagulant treatment of patients with meningococcemia and disseminated intravascular coagulation has not been documented to improve outcome. A phase III study of recombinant activated protein C in children with sepsis of all causes, including meningococcemia, was stopped because no benefit was noted, and recombinant activated protein C has been withdrawn from the market. Administration of activated protein C is associated with an increased risk of cerebral hemorrhage. The use of recombinant human tissue plasminogen activator does not appear to be beneficial. Randomized controlled clinical trials using hyperimmune serum, antibodies, or recombinant bactericidal or permeability-increasing protein (designed to inactivate *N. meningitidis* endotoxin) have not demonstrated a beneficial effect on survival. Blockade of other specific inflammatory mediators has not been adequately tested in meningococcal septic shock.

Patients with fulminant meningococcal septicemia can develop adrenal hemorrhage (Waterhouse-Friderichsen syndrome). The corticotropin concentration is higher, the cortisol concentration is lower, and the corticotropin-to-cortisol ratio is higher in patients with fatal meningococcal shock than in survivors. Adults with septic shock and indications of inadequate adrenal function are given low doses of steroids. Although the benefit has not been documented, many intensive care specialists use stress replacement doses of hydrocortisone in children with shock caused by *N. meningitidis*.

Plasmapheresis, blood exchange, and extracorporeal membrane oxygenation have been used in patients with meningococcemia; however, no controlled trials to assess the results have been done. Plasmapheresis and blood exchange appear to have little additive effect on the endogenous clearance of endotoxin and cytokines from the circulation. Extracorporeal membrane oxygenation has been used in several centers, with better results in children with acute pulmonary failure than in those with refractory septic shock. The use of insulin to control mild hyperglycemia in critically ill adults has not shown benefits (Chapter 108).

Pharmacologic doses of dexamethasone have been shown to reduce morbidity in pneumococcal and *Haemophilus influenzae* type b meningitis. The use of dexamethasone to reduce death caused by brain edema or to prevent sequelae such as deafness in patients with meningococcal meningitis remains unproved on the basis of large randomized controlled trials, but trends toward reductions in hearing loss, mortality, and arthritis after meningococcal disease are reported. Many now recommend that dexamethasone (10 mg every 6 hours for the first 4 days and in children at a dose of 0.15 mg/kg every 6 hours for 4 days beginning before or with the first dose of antibiotics) be given early in suspected or confirmed bacterial meningitis.[A2] Glycerol has been used to reduce intracranial pressure in bacterial meningitis, but its value is not proven. Other major life-threatening complications necessitating therapy include adult respiratory distress syndrome, neurologic sequelae ranging from coma to diabetes insipidus, pneumonia that is not necessarily meningococcal but may be secondary to aspiration during the obtunded state, and pericarditis.

Immune complex–mediated complications, such as arthritis, cutaneous vasculitis, iritis, episcleritis, pleuritis, and pericarditis, can first appear several days to 2 to 3 weeks after onset of illness, when the patient is otherwise improving. These complications, which can be multiple, are due to the deposition of antigen-antibody complexes composed of meningococcal capsular polysaccharide or other antigens, meningococcal-specific immunoglobulins, and C3 and complicate 6 to 15% of meningococcal meningitis or septicemia. Treatment is with aspirin or nonsteroidal anti-inflammatory drugs, and resolution is complete, usually within 14 days from the onset and usually without residual sequelae.

PREVENTION

Chemoprophylaxis to eliminate meningococcal carriage is recommended for close contacts of patients to prevent further transmission and disease (Table 298-2). The occurrence of meningococcal disease in household contacts is approximately 100-fold higher than in the general population. Secondary cases usually occur within 1 to 14 days of the primary case. Chemoprophylaxis can be helpful to control localized outbreaks, but it is generally not recommended for the control of large epidemics (see the later discussion of vaccines). Rifampin, ceftriaxone, azithromycin, and quinolones (but not penicillin) have the ability to eradicate meningococci in the nasopharynx. A majority of meningococcal isolates are now resistant to sulfonamides; resistance to rifampin can develop rapidly, and quinolone resistance in meningococci is reported.

Prevention through vaccination is the best option for the long-term control of meningococcal disease.[16] Capsular polysaccharide vaccines to decrease serogroup A, C, Y, and W-135 meningococcal disease were introduced in the 1970s and 1980s. These vaccines were safe, with mild local adverse events, and effective (>85%) in children older than 2 years and adults but less immunogenic in younger children; immunity to the polysaccharide vaccines was limited to 3 to 5 years of protection, and immunologic hyporesponsiveness was induced by repeated doses of the polysaccharide. Also, meningococcal polysaccharide vaccines do not induce immunologic memory and have little or no effect on nasopharyngeal carriage. Although these vaccines were used extensively to control disease in military populations and in epidemics in the African meningitis belt, in the latter they were often deployed too late in the course of an outbreak. There was no evidence that widespread use of polysaccharide vaccines reduced the frequency of epidemics in Africa.

A major advance in the past 15 years has been the development and now widespread use of meningococcal polysaccharide-protein conjugate vaccines and their introduction first into the United Kingdom and then other parts of Europe, Canada, Australia, the United States, and, more recently, the African meningitis belt. These vaccines are safe and immunogenic in young children, induce immunologic memory, and can decrease nasopharyngeal carriage of meningococci.[A3] In the United Kingdom, the introduction of the serogroup C conjugate meningococcal vaccine in 2000 to all children and young adults greatly reduced the rate of serogroup C disease (90% vaccine effectiveness at 3 years for patients aged 11 to 18 years). A major protective effect of the C conjugate vaccine is mediated through herd immunity.[17] Rates of serogroup C carriage and disease in nonvaccinated individuals were reduced by more than 50% through herd immunity. Polysaccharide-protein conjugate meningococcal vaccines containing serogroups A, C, Y, and W-135 were introduced for adolescents in the United States in 2005 and subsequently extended to children aged 2 months to 10 years at increased risk for meningococcal disease. In addition to routine use in older children and adolescents (first dose at the age of 11 or 12 years with booster at 16 years), populations that should benefit from the new conjugate vaccines are college freshmen, military recruits, patients with immunoglobulin or complement deficiencies (inherited or chronic deficiencies such as C3, properdin, factor D, or late complement components), patients with anatomic or functional asplenia, microbiologists who are routinely exposed to isolates of *N. meningitidis*, adults with HIV type 1 infections, and people who travel to or reside in countries where *N. meningitidis* is epidemic. An important example of a new approach to meningococcal conjugate vaccine development is the Meningitis Vaccine Program, a partnership between PATH, the World Health Organization, and the Global Alliance for Vaccines and Immunization for the development of a group A meningococcal conjugate vaccine for Africa, designated MenAfriVac, at less than $0.50 a dose.[18] Because of the huge impact of herd immunity of the serogroup C conjugate vaccines in the United Kingdom, MenAfriVac was introduced as a mass vaccination strategy for those 1 to 29 years old. The MenAfriVac vaccination campaign began in Burkina Faso in December 2010 and has been extended to Mali, Chad, Niger, Nigeria, Benin, Ghana, Senegal, Cameroon, Sudan, and other regions of the African meningitis belt. More than 100 million doses have been administered. Initial results

TABLE 298-2 CHEMOPROPHYLAXIS AGAINST MENINGOCOCCAL INFECTION

DRUG	AGE GROUP	DOSAGE	DURATION AND ROUTE OF ADMINISTRATION*	CONSIDERATIONS
Rifampin	Children <1 month	5 mg/kg q12h	2 days	
	Children >1 month	10 mg/kg q12h (maximum, 600 mg)	2 days	
	Adults	600 mg q12h	2 days	Rifampin can interfere with efficacy of oral contraceptives and some seizure prevention and anticoagulant medications; may stain soft contact lenses Not recommended for pregnant women
Ceftriaxone	Children <15 years	125 mg	Single IM dose	
	Children >15 years and adults	250 mg	Single IM dose	Ceftriaxone is recommended for prophylaxis in pregnant women.
Ciprofloxacin	Adults	500 mg	Single dose	Not recommended routinely for persons <18 years of age, but use in infants and children (20 mg/kg) may be justified after careful assessment of the risks and benefits Not recommended for pregnant or lactating women Cases of ciprofloxacin resistance have been reported, and use for prophylaxis should be based on local sensitivity of the meningococcus to the drug.
Azithromycin		10 mg/kg (maximum, 500 mg)	Single dose	Equivalent to rifampin for eradication of meningococci from nasopharynx, but data are limited

ANTIBIOTIC CHEMOPROPHYLAXIS FOR HOUSEHOLD OR INTIMATE CONTACTS:

- Household contacts and persons sharing the same living quarters, particularly young children
- Daycare center, nursery school, or child care contacts; frequent playmates of young children
- Close social contacts that were exposed to oral secretions in the week before onset, such as by kissing and sharing of eating and drinking utensils or toothbrushes
- For airline travel lasting more than 8 hours, passengers who are seated directly next to an infected person should receive prophylaxis.
- Routine prophylaxis is not recommended for health care professionals unless they have had intimate exposure to respiratory secretions.
- As the risk of secondary cases is highest during the first few days after exposure, chemoprophylaxis should be initiated as soon as possible, ideally <24 hours after identification of the index patient.
- If more than 14 days have passed since the last contact with the index patient, chemoprophylaxis is not likely to be of benefit.
- Pharyngeal cultures are not helpful in determining the need for chemoprophylaxis and may unnecessarily delay the use of effective chemoprophylaxis.
- Chemoprophylaxis has also been recommended for patients given penicillin or chloramphenicol for treatment because pharyngeal carriage may not be eliminated with these antibiotics and the patient could remain colonized with a virulent strain.
- Ceftriaxone is recommended for pregnant women.
- May want to avoid ciprofloxacin or azithromycin in individuals at risk of QT-prolongation.

Recommended groups for chemoprophylaxis based on exposure to the case in the week before onset of illness.
*Administered orally unless otherwise stated.

show the virtual elimination of serogroup A meningococcal disease in the countries vaccinated in the first 2 years after the mass campaigns.

The development of vaccines for serogroup B *N. meningitidis* has also shown progress. Serogroup B can cause prolonged outbreaks during many years, such as those seen in the past two decades in the Pacific Northwest (Oregon, parts of Washington), Brazil, Norway, and New Zealand. The serogroup B capsule has an identical structure to polysialic structures expressed in fetal neural tissue and does not induce a protective bactericidal immunoglobulin G response. Thus, strategies have been focused on noncapsular antigens, such as outer membrane proteins containing vesicles (OMV) or conserved protein antigens. The diversity of major outer membrane structures in meningococci has limited OMV approaches, but this approach has been successful in controlling serogroup B epidemics that are strain specific (e.g., in New Zealand). New serogroup B vaccines based on semiconserved surface protein antigens identified by "reverse vaccinology" are the most advanced candidates and are obtaining licensure. One of these, 4CMenB or Bexosero,[A4] recently approved in Europe, contains three semiconserved surface protein antigens—a member of the factor H–binding protein family, neisserial adhesin A (NadA), and neisserial heparin-binding antigen—and a meningococcal serogroup B PorA-containing OMV preparation previously used to control the serogroup B clonal outbreak in New Zealand. Alum is the adjuvant. A second serogroup B vaccine is based on two members of the factor H–binding protein family and was recently licensed in the United States.[19] Initial evaluation of the immunogenicity and safety of these vaccines appears promising. The prevention of serogroup B disease appears to be a significant step closer with these new vaccines.

PROGNOSIS

Historically, the mortality of untreated systemic meningococcal disease was 70 to 90%. Despite highly effective antibiotics and aggressive supportive care, the mortality of invasive meningococcal disease remains at about 10%. The failure to recognize disease early, the very rapid development of disease (especially meningococcemia), and the time to administration of antibiotics remain the most significant challenges. The chance of surviving shock is

directly correlated to plasma concentrations of endotoxin, and half the nonsurviving patients with shock die within the first 12 hours of hospital admission.

Long-term sequelae and morbidity after invasive meningococcal disease are significant.[20] Neurologic impairment occurs in 7 to 10% with meningococcal meningitis, with palsies of the sixth, seventh, and eighth cranial nerves and hemiparesis and quadriparesis. Unilateral or bilateral sensorineural hearing loss occurs in 2 to 9% of cases, which is profound in 2% of affected individuals and necessitates cochlear implantation in 0.4%. Neurodevelopmental impairment, including behavioral and psychological problems, learning difficulties, memory deficits, executive function problems, decreased academic performance, spasticity, seizures, and focal neurologic signs, is seen in approximately 10%. Visual difficulties, seizures, and motor deficits are reported in 2 to 3%, with multiple neurologic disabilities occurring in 1 to 2% of affected individuals. Survivors of meningococcal sepsis in childhood have, in 5 to 20% as young adults, long-term behavioral and emotional problems, decreased intellectual functioning, and illness-related physical or social consequences.

Scarring of the skin, secondary to necrotic purpura, may vary from unnoticeable to requiring skin grafting. Multiple areas may be involved; the lower limbs are most frequently affected, followed by the arms, chest, and face. Amputations, of the digits or limbs, are frequently multiple; these result from necrosis of the skin, muscle, and bone of the affected parts (Fig. 298-3D) and, depending on the site and extent, may require prostheses to improve function or appearance. Bone growth disturbances, stump overgrowth, scar contractures, and soft tissue and bone infections may complicate amputations. Limb length discrepancies, which may result from the growth plate infarction, often necessitate further surgical intervention. Following acute renal failure at presentation, renal function recovers in the majority of individuals; however, evidence of renal dysfunction may persist for more than 4 years in both children and adults, with the risk being higher in those who required renal replacement therapy.

Meningococcal disease and its complications, often occurring rapidly in otherwise healthy individuals, also produce significant family, community, health care, and public health impact. The emotional toll on individuals who survive and on the families of those with meningococcal disease in intensive care units, of those who survive with complications, and of those who die is considerable and a global phenomenon. In communities, meningococcal disease may also create considerable fear and anxiety. Post-traumatic stress disorder occurs at a higher frequency in both patients and families, often months after the illness. In one study, post-traumatic stress disorder occurred in 15% of children, in half of the mothers, and in 19% of fathers at 3 months. Meningococcal disease and its complications also result in substantial hospital and long-term health care costs. Furthermore, delay in the diagnosis of meningococcal sepsis and meningitis and septicemia is a common reason for litigation.

If parents and health care professionals recognize the importance of fever and headache with a nonblanching rash and seek treatment early, morbidity and mortality can be reduced with prehospital antibiotic treatment, rapid transportation to medical facilities, and stabilization in an intensive care unit. Prevention of meningococcal disease with new vaccines and vaccine strategies remains the major worldwide goal.

Grade A References

A1. Nathan N, Borel T, Djibo A, et al. Ceftriaxone as effective as long-acting chloramphenicol in short-course treatment of meningococcal meningitis during epidemics: a randomised non-inferiority study. *Lancet.* 2005;366:308-313.

A2. Brouwer MC, McIntyre P, Prasad K, et al. Corticosteroids for acute bacterial meningitis. *Cochrane Database Syst Rev.* 2013;6:CD004405.

A3. Cohn AC, MacNeil JR, Clark TA, Centers for Disease Control and Prevention (CDC), et al. Prevention and control of meningococcal disease: recommendations of the Advisory Committee on Immunization Practices (ACIP). *MMWR Recomm Rep.* 2013;62(RR-2):1-28.

A4. Read RC, Baxter D, Chadwick DR, et al. Effect of a quadrivalent meningococcal ACWY glycoconjugate or a serogroup B meningococcal vaccine on meningococcal carriage: an observer-blind, phase 3 randomised clinical trial. *Lancet.* 2014;384:2123-2131.

GENERAL REFERENCES

For the General References and other additional features, please visit Expert Consult at https://expertconsult.inkling.com.

299

NEISSERIA GONORRHOEAE INFECTIONS

MATTHEW R. GOLDEN AND H. HUNTER HANDSFIELD

DEFINITION

Neisseria gonorrhoeae is a sexually transmitted organism that infects primarily the columnar epithelia of mucosal surfaces and causes urethritis in men and endocervicitis and urethritis in women. Other sites of primary infection include the rectum, pharynx, and conjunctiva, and vulvovaginitis can occur in prepubertal girls. The most common complication of gonococcal infection is pelvic inflammatory disease, which can lead to infertility, ectopic pregnancy, and chronic pelvic pain. Other much less common complications include epididymitis, posterior urethritis, urethral stricture, Bartholin's gland abscess, and perihepatitis. Bacteremia may occur, with the production of characteristic cutaneous lesions, arthritis, and, rarely, endocarditis or meningitis. Neonatal conjunctivitis (ophthalmia neonatorum) was formerly a common cause of blindness. Gonococcal infections are also thought to increase the risk of human immunodeficiency virus (HIV) transmission from persons dually infected with HIV and *N. gonorrhoeae* and to increase the risk of HIV acquisition among persons with gonorrhea who are exposed to HIV.

The Pathogen

The gonococcal envelope is similar in its basic structure to that of other gram-negative bacteria and is composed of an inner cytoplasmic membrane, a middle peptidoglycan cell wall, and an outer membrane. The outer membrane contains several surface components that play a central role in the organism's interaction with the host and its pathogenicity. Pili, hairlike projections also referred to as fimbriae, are composed of several different protein subunits and, along with other outer membrane adhesins (i.e., opacity-related

proteins), facilitate attachment and invasion of host cells. Gonococci vary the composition of these proteins and surface lipo-oligosaccharides over time, allowing the organism to elude host defenses. This phase variation has also been a barrier to successful vaccine development.

EPIDEMIOLOGY

Gonorrhea is the second most commonly reported infectious disease in the United States, with 334,826 cases reported to the Centers for Disease Control and Prevention (CDC) in 2012.[1] The incidence of gonorrhea in the United States in 2012 was 107.5 per 100,000 population, although this number, which is based on cases reported to U.S. health departments, is undoubtedly an underestimate. The overall incidence of gonorrhea in the United States has been relatively stable for more than a decade, and current rates are more than 70% lower than the incidence observed in the mid-1970s. The prevalence of gonorrhea varies widely, depending on the population tested. The National Longitudinal Study of Adolescent Health (Add Health) tested a representative sample of U.S. 18- to 26-year-olds in 2001 and 2002 and found that 0.43% were infected, with wide variations geographically and among population groups. This prevalence estimate is almost identical to one derived from the National Health and Nutrition Examination Survey of 1998 to 2008, another population-based survey.[2] Among women aged 15 to 24 years tested for gonorrhea in family planning clinics in 48 U.S. states and territories in 2011, the median prevalence of gonorrhea was 0.7%, but it varied from 0 to 3.5%. By comparison, the prevalence of chlamydial infection in the Add Health study was 4.19%, and among 15- to 24-year-old females tested in U.S. family planning clinics in 2011, it was 8.3% (range, 3.8 to 15.9%).

Like virtually all other sexually transmitted infections (STIs; Chapter 285), gonorrhea rates vary widely with age, geographic location, sexual orientation, and race or ethnicity. In the United States, the rate of reported infection is highest among 15- to 24-year-olds, and rates in the South are more than twice those observed in the West and Northeast. However, the most glaring disparities are observed in comparing rates of infection among different racial and ethnic groups and in comparing heterosexuals to men who have sex with men (MSM).

Rates of reported gonorrhea among U.S. African Americans are almost 15 times higher than those among non-Hispanic whites, and rates among American Indians/Alaska Natives and Hispanics are 4 and 1.9 times higher, respectively, than those among non-Hispanic whites. Variations in reporting probably account for some of these observed differences because low socioeconomic status is associated with receiving care in public health clinics and other venues where there is more complete reporting than in the private health care sector. However, the marked disparity in reported rates is also apparent in population-based studies, clearly establishing that the different rates of infection in different racial and ethnic groups are not simply a result of reporting bias. The reasons for this profound disparity are certainly multifactorial and are not entirely clear. Different racial groups in the United States vary little in terms of their number of sex partners, so this cannot explain the different rates of STIs. Although inadequate access to medical care is likely to play a role in the racial disparities in STI rates, profound racial and ethnic disparities are also observed in the United Kingdom and the Netherlands, nations with nationalized health care systems in which access to care should be more uniform than it is in the United States. Research has highlighted the importance of concurrency (i.e., partnerships that overlap in time) and patterns of sexual mixing based on age, race, and level of sexual activity as critical determinants of a population's risk of STI. These factors are thought to be shaped by social factors (e.g., poverty, incarceration, joblessness, racism) that play a central role in defining the epidemiology of all STIs worldwide.

Gonorrhea also disproportionately affects gay and bisexual men and other MSM. Numerous cities in the United States, western Europe, and Australia have reported increases in the rate and number of gonorrhea cases among MSM since the mid-1990s. For example, in King County, Washington State, in 2012 the estimated incidence of reported gonorrhea in MSM was more than 2114 cases per 100,000, compared with 40 and 41 per 100,000 heterosexual men and women, respectively.

Gonorrhea is highly transmissible. Although it is not precisely defined, the risk of transmission from a man to a woman during a single episode of unprotected vaginal intercourse is thought to be 50 to 70%, and the risk of transmission from a woman to a man is 20%. The transmission risks associated with anal sex, fellatio, or cunnilingus are not well defined, but anal intercourse is probably a relatively efficient mode of transmission, and receipt of fellatio is likely to be an important source of gonococcal infections in at least some populations (e.g., MSM). Gonococci die rapidly on drying, and with the exception of occasional acquisition by laboratory personnel working with the organism, nonsexual transmission does not occur in adults. Perinatal transmission causing neonatal ophthalmitis or pharyngeal infection is now rare.

PATHOBIOLOGY

After attachment to host epithelial cells, gonococci are endocytosed into the cell in a process thought to be facilitated by Por (or protein 1). Gonococci then replicate within the host cell and are released into the subepithelial space.

Typical urethral infections result in prominent inflammation, probably as a result of the release of toxic lipo-oligosaccharide and peptidoglycan fragments as well as the release of chemotactic factors that attract neutrophilic leukocytes. The reasons that some gonococcal strains selectively cause asymptomatic genital infection are poorly understood, but this propensity may be related to differences in the organism's ability to bind complement-regulatory proteins that downregulate the production of chemotactic peptides. In particular, gonococcal strains that express PorB1A appear to bind factor H and complement-binding protein and have an increased propensity for causing disseminated gonococcal infections.

Although the gonococcus is not highly mutable, many gonococci possess conjugative plasmids and are consequently able to efficiently transfer other, nontransferable plasmids, such as those conferring resistance to penicillin and tetracycline. Gonococci are also capable of efficiently transferring naked DNA (transformation). These characteristics are important in the organism's ability to develop resistance to antimicrobials. For example, recent evidence suggests that the gonococci with diminished susceptibility to oral cephalosporins possess genetic resistance mutations acquired from commensal *Neisseria* species commonly found in the oropharynx.[3,4]

CLINICAL MANIFESTATIONS

Gonococcal infections can result in a number of specific clinical syndromes, each of which has its own manifestations, differential diagnosis, and recommended evaluation. The major clinical manifestations of gonococcal infection are discussed separately later. Gonococcal ophthalmia, now a rare complication, can result from direct contact or by autoinoculation in individuals with anogenital gonorrhea and is manifested as an acute, purulent conjunctivitis that can result in corneal ulceration if it is not treated promptly.

DIAGNOSIS
Microscopy

Microscopy of a Gram-stained smear is positive when polymorphonuclear neutrophils are observed to contain intracellular gram-negative diplococci of typical morphology (Fig. 299-1). Gram-stained urethral smears are 90 to 98% sensitive in the diagnosis of symptomatic gonococcal urethritis in men and have a specificity greater than 95%. However, Gram stain is only approximately 50% sensitive for cervical or rectal infection and for asymptomatic urethral gonorrhea. Although Gram stain is often considered highly specific

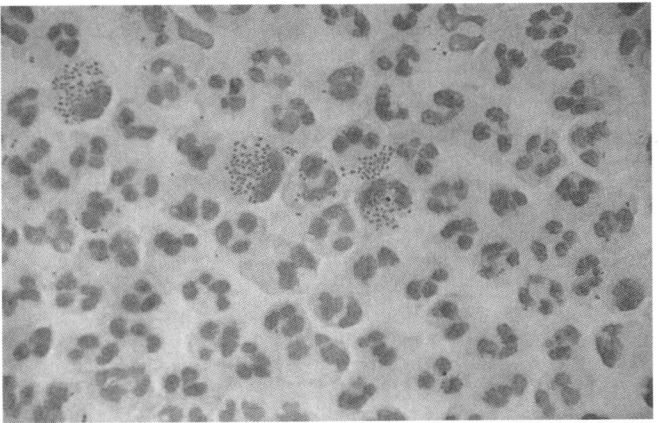

FIGURE 299-1. Gram stain in an acute case of gonococcal urethritis. This slide is used to demonstrate the nonrandom distribution of gonococci among polymorphonuclear neutrophils. Note that there are both intracellular and extracellular bacteria in the field of view.

for such infections, the actual performance varies with the skill and experience of the examiner, and rectal and cervical smears are unreliable in many clinical settings. Smears are both insensitive and nonspecific for pharyngeal gonococcal infection and are not recommended.

Culture

Isolation of *N. gonorrhoeae* by culture, generally with antibiotic-containing selective media, is the historic mainstay of the diagnosis of gonorrhea. Despite the proliferation of molecular diagnostic methods, culture retains important roles in surveillance for antimicrobial resistance and selected clinical settings. Ideally, growth media should be inoculated directly and placed promptly into a humid atmosphere with increased carbon dioxide, such as a candle extinction jar. However, standard transport systems (e.g., Culturette) are acceptable if specimens are kept moist, are not refrigerated, and are processed within 6 hours. In testing of specimens not likely to be colonized by competing flora (e.g., synovial fluid), nonselective chocolate agar should be used.

Nucleic Acid Amplification Tests

In most settings in the United States, nucleic acid amplification tests (NAATs) have now supplanted culture as the dominant laboratory test used to diagnose gonorrhea.[5] NAATs approved by the Food and Drug Administration include polymerase chain reaction, transcription-mediated amplification (TMA), and DNA strand displacement (SDA). The advantages of NAATs include a slight increase in sensitivity over culture, the ability to test urine specimens and self-obtained vaginal swabs, and the fact that most NAATs are now marketed as combination assays that allow simultaneous testing for *N. gonorrhoeae* and *Chlamydia trachomatis*. The disadvantages of NAATs include the inability to perform antimicrobial susceptibility testing and the poor or inadequately defined positive predictive value of some NAATs when they are used to test low-prevalence populations. Because the prevalence of *N. gonorrhoeae* in family planning clinics in many parts of the United States and other nations is now well below 1%, the risk of false-positive screening results may be high, and reliable results depend on the use of assays with exquisite specificity. Existing evidence suggests that TMA has a high positive predictive value even in very low-prevalence settings; the positive predictive value of SDA and the current-generation Roche polymerase chain reaction is not well defined.

Although NAATs have been approved by the Food and Drug Administration only for the testing of genital tract and urine specimens, increasing evidence suggests that at least some NAATs (e.g., TMA, SDA) are substantially more sensitive than culture in detecting *N. gonorrhoeae* in pharyngeal and rectal specimens and that these NAATs are sufficiently specific to screen high-risk populations for rectal and pharyngeal gonorrhea. Given the decreasing availability of gonococcal culture, the poor sensitivity of culture on non–genital tract specimens, and the high prevalence of asymptomatic rectal and pharyngeal infections in some populations (particularly MSM), clinicians caring for patients at high risk for nongenital gonococcal infections should be able to use NAATs. Recent studies suggest that self-obtained rectal and pharyngeal specimens yield accurate results and are acceptable to MSM.

CLINICAL SYNDROMES
Urogenital Gonorrhea in Males
CLINICAL MANIFESTATIONS AND DIAGNOSIS

Gonococcal urethritis in men is typically characterized by a purulent urethral discharge and dysuria. The usual incubation period is 2 to 6 days. A small minority of men who acquire urethral infection—generally estimated at 1 to 10%, and varying between specific strains of *N. gonorrhoeae*—remain asymptomatic.

Physical examination typically reveals purulent urethral exudate (Fig. 299-2); this is usually readily apparent, but compression of the urethra is sometimes required to express the exudate. Erythema of the meatus is sometimes present. Nongonococcal urethritis (Chapter 285) is typically characterized by less copious and less purulent discharge.

The diagnosis of gonococcal urethritis is usually suspected clinically, confirmed preliminarily by a Gram-stained smear showing leukocytes with intracellular gram-negative diplococci (see Fig. 299-1), and made definitively when *N. gonorrhoeae* is identified by culture or NAAT. Despite the usual clinical differences between gonococcal urethritis and nongonococcal urethritis, substantial overlap exists, and microbiologic diagnosis should be routine even in clinically typical cases.

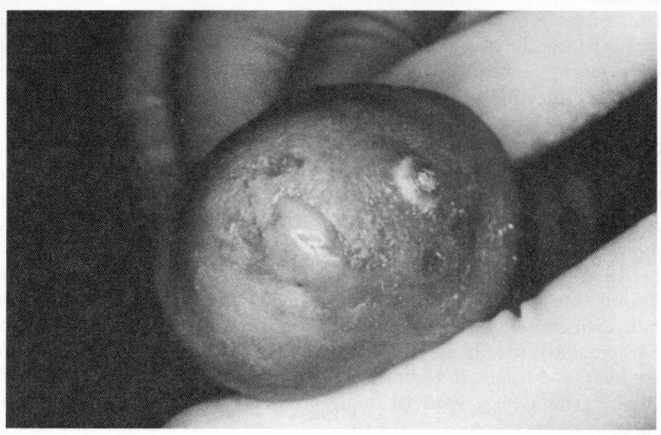

FIGURE 299-2. Male patient with a purulent penile discharge from gonorrhea and an overlying penile pyodermal lesion. Pyoderma involves the formation of a purulent skin lesion, which in this case is located on the glans penis.

PROGNOSIS

With prompt treatment, urethral gonorrhea seldom results in significant long-term morbidity. Acute epididymitis complicates gonococcal urethritis in less than 1% of cases. Patients with epididymitis usually present with unilateral testicular pain and swelling, sometimes with fever. Posterior urethritis or prostatitis, typically manifested as pelvic or perineal pain and urinary retention, was once fairly common but is now rare. Urethral stricture, another formerly common complication, is now very rare. Gonorrhea is associated with an elevated risk of HIV infection, both directly and as an epidemiologic risk factor. Diagnosis of gonorrhea should alert clinicians to counsel such patients about sexual risks, test them for HIV infection, and encourage patients to seek frequent follow-up testing for HIV infection and other STIs.

Lower Genital Tract Gonorrhea in Females

CLINICAL MANIFESTATIONS, DIAGNOSIS, AND PROGNOSIS

The primary site of infection in women is the endocervical canal. The proportion of infected women who develop symptoms is not precisely known, but probably about 50% of incident infections are symptomatic. In any case, asymptomatic infections accumulate in populations, whereas many or most symptomatically infected women present for diagnosis and treatment. Therefore, most prevalent infections among women are asymptomatic or are associated with mild symptoms not perceived by patients as abnormal or important. Gonorrhea is sometimes associated with an abnormal vaginal discharge, but other lower genital tract infections, such as bacterial vaginosis, trichomonas vaginitis, and candidal vaginitis, are much more common causes of this symptom. Lower genital tract gonorrhea in women can be associated with abnormal vaginal bleeding, which typically is manifested as metrorrhagia, scant intermenstrual bleeding, or postcoital spotting. *N. gonorrhoeae* sometimes causes dysuria and can be isolated from the urethra in up to 80% of women with gonorrhea. However, the urethra is rarely the only infected site, except in women who have had hysterectomies. In a minority of women, physical examination is notable for a purulent or mucopurulent cervical discharge, cervical edema, or easily induced cervical bleeding, signs of mucopurulent cervicitis. In uncomplicated infections, purulent exudate can sometimes be expressed from a Bartholin's gland duct, near the vaginal introitus laterally, or from Skene's glands, adjacent to the urethral meatus.

Microbiologic diagnosis usually rests on identifying *N. gonorrhoeae* in cervical secretions by NAAT or culture. Gram-stained smears are insensitive and seldom used.

The most important common complication of lower genital tract gonorrhea in women is pelvic inflammatory disease (see later). Rarer complications include Bartholin's gland abscess, which is manifested as a tender introital mass and may involve superinfection with facultative and anaerobic bacteria.

Pelvic Inflammatory Disease

CLINICAL MANIFESTATIONS

Pelvic inflammatory disease (PID) refers to an infection of the lower female genital tract and can involve the uterus (endometritis), fallopian tubes (salpingitis), and ovaries (oophoritis) as well as neighboring pelvic structures.[6] An estimated 10 to 40% of women with endocervical gonococcal infections develop PID, and gonorrhea is thought to be the cause of approximately 5 to 30% of all diagnosed cases of PID in the United States. However, this proportion varies with overall rates of gonorrhea and other causes of PID in the population, such as chlamydial infection.

Low abdominal pain is the dominant symptom of PID. Pain is variable in intensity and is often mild; it is usually bilateral, typically present for days to weeks before clinical presentation, and can be exacerbated by coitus. Symptoms often coincide with the onset or cessation of menses. Approximately one third of women have abnormal vaginal bleeding. Fever, chills, anorexia, vaginal discharge, urethritis, and proctitis occur, but they are neither sensitive nor specific in identifying women with PID. There is little if any difference in the severity of symptoms and signs of PID associated with *N. gonorrhoeae*, *C. trachomatis*, or neither of these pathogens.

The physical examination is typically notable for diffuse abdominal tenderness that is greatest in the lower quadrants and for tenderness of the pelvic organs on bimanual examination, with or without manipulation of the cervix. Most women have signs of cervicitis or bacterial vaginosis. Fever is present in a minority of cases. Abdominal or adnexal signs are occasionally unilateral, and this finding can cause confusion with appendicitis (Chapter 142), ectopic pregnancy, and other conditions. Right upper quadrant abdominal tenderness due to perihepatitis (Fitz-Hugh–Curtis syndrome) is sometimes present, which can mimic acute cholecystitis or viral hepatitis. Perihepatitis sometimes occurs in the absence of other abdominal or pelvic findings typical of PID, especially when it is caused by *C. trachomatis*. Severe PID may be accompanied by signs of generalized peritonitis.

DIAGNOSIS

The clinical diagnosis of PID is imprecise. Published studies, which have used somewhat variable criteria in populations with different prevalences of the syndrome, have reported positive predictive values of 65 to 90% compared with the "gold standard" of laparoscopically defined PID. Although nonspecific, the presence of neutrophils on a saline wet mount of vaginal secretions was 91% sensitive for endometritis in one study. The absence of white blood cells on a wet mount of vaginal secretions, particularly if mucopurulent cervicitis is also absent, should prompt the consideration of alternative diagnoses. The differential diagnosis of PID includes ectopic pregnancy; appendicitis; rupture, bleeding, or torsion of an ovarian cyst; endometriosis; urinary tract infection or pyelonephritis; renal or ureteral stones; inflammatory bowel disease; and, rarely, viral hepatitis or cholecystitis.

Because of the potential seriousness of the infection and the relative simplicity, low cost, and low toxicity of treatment, clinical diagnostic criteria emphasize sensitivity at the cost of specificity. Clinicians therefore should maintain a low threshold for tentative diagnosis and presumptive treatment of PID. The CDC recommends that all sexually active women with pelvic or lower abdominal pain and uterine, adnexal, or cervical motion tenderness be treated for possible PID if no other cause of their symptoms and signs is readily apparent. Furthermore, screening of asymptomatic sexually active young women with NAATs is recommended by the U.S. Preventive Services Task Force.[7] Factors such as fever, an elevated erythrocyte sedimentation rate or C-reactive protein level, and concurrent bacterial vaginosis or mucopurulent cervicitis further support the clinical diagnosis, but these are frequently absent. Definitive diagnosis requires histologic evidence of endometritis on endometrial biopsy; transvaginal ultrasound or other diagnostic imaging showing thickened or fluid-filled fallopian tubes or tubo-ovarian abscess; or laparoscopy demonstrating purulent tubal exudate, erythema, or edema.

PROGNOSIS

Fallopian tube scarring secondary to PID often results in tubal factor infertility (TFI), ectopic pregnancy, and chronic pelvic pain. Previous gonococcal and chlamydial infections are among the most common antecedents of these complications. Each episode of PID, whether due to *N. gonorrhoeae*, *C. trachomatis*, or neither of these organisms, significantly increases the risk for recurrent salpingitis.

The natural history of clinically apparent PID is well defined. In what is probably the best single study on the subject, TFI occurred in 8% of women after a single episode of laparoscopically proved PID, in 20% after two such episodes, and in 40% after three or more episodes. The first pregnancy after an episode of PID was ectopic in almost 8% of women, and like TFI, the risk of ectopic pregnancy increased with each successive episode of the syndrome. Chronic pelvic pain, sometimes disabling in its severity, occurs in almost 20% of women after one or more episodes of PID. Importantly, these outcomes were best studied in women with clinically apparent PID, and the pertinent studies were undertaken at a time when clinical recognition and treatment were likely delayed. Many women suffer clinically mild or silent

PID. The risk of sequelae associated with silent PID is not well defined, but more clinically severe PID is associated with a higher risk of sequelae. Most women with TFI deny a history of PID, and it seems likely that silent PID, particularly silent PID associated with *C. trachomatis*, is responsible for most cases of STI-related reproductive tract sequelae. For example, *C. trachomatis* seropositivity is strongly associated with TFI, independent of clinical or historical evidence of PID.

Rectal Infection
CLINICAL MANIFESTATIONS

Gonococcal infection of the rectum is common in women and in MSM. In women, infection is acquired either through perineal contamination with cervicovaginal secretions or by anal intercourse; the latter is the exclusive route of infection in MSM. In women with cervical gonorrhea and in MSM with gonorrhea at any anatomic site, about 40% have rectal infection. More than 80% of rectal infections are subclinical, but symptomatic proctitis sometimes is manifested as varying combinations of anal pruritus, mucopurulent discharge (often characterized by the patient as mucus-coated feces), pain, tenesmus, and bleeding. Symptomatic proctitis seems to be more common in MSM than in women with rectal gonorrhea, which suggests that the size of the infecting inoculum or trauma from anal intercourse may influence the clinical manifestations. Among MSM, rectal gonorrhea is a potent epidemiologic risk marker for the acquisition of HIV and may be a direct risk factor because anorectal inflammation enhances susceptibility to HIV infection.

DIAGNOSIS

Diagnosis of rectal gonorrhea depends on the identification of *N. gonorrhoeae*, usually by NAAT. The Gram-stained smear is insensitive and nonspecific. The differential diagnosis of symptomatic proctitis includes other traditional STIs (herpes, syphilis, and chlamydial infection, including lymphogranuloma venereum; Chapter 318) as well as ulcerative colitis, Crohn's colitis, anal fissure, rectal lacerations, and proctocolitis caused by *Shigella*, *Campylobacter*, *Yersinia enterocolitica*, and other enteric pathogens. Recent studies using NAAT among STI clinic patients suggest that approximately 5% of tested MSM and 1% of tested women have rectal infections without concurrent genital tract infections. Although less than 20% of women with gonorrhea have extragenital infections, more than half of MSM with gonorrhea have only extragenital infections, highlighting the importance of routine screening of MSM, but not women, for rectal gonorrhea.

Pharyngeal Infection
CLINICAL MANIFESTATIONS

Pharyngeal gonococcal infection results from orogenital exposure. It is more efficiently acquired by fellatio than by cunnilingus and is typically found in 3 to 7% of heterosexual men, 10 to 30% of women, and 10 to 30% of MSM with genital tract gonorrhea. Asymptomatic infection is the rule, although rare cases may exhibit exudative pharyngitis and cervical lymphadenopathy. Isolated pharyngeal infection is common is MSM and may also be common in at least some populations of heterosexuals. Complications are infrequent, and most infections eventually resolve spontaneously or in response to therapy for genital or rectal infection. Although the modest morbidity associated with pharyngeal infections probably does not justify extensive screening efforts, the oropharynx may be an important reservoir for infection in some populations, particularly MSM. The oropharynx is also a site of gene exchange between *N. gonorrhoeae* and commensal Neisseriaceae, and pharyngeal infections are thought to play a critical role in fostering the emergence of antimicrobial-resistant gonococci. Failure to identify and to eradicate pharyngeal infections probably helps sustain high levels of gonococcal transmission and may foster the spread of antibiotic-resistant gonococci. Accordingly, current guidelines suggest that MSM at risk for STIs be tested periodically for pharyngeal gonorrhea.

Gonorrhea in Children

Gonococcal conjunctivitis may develop in infants born to mothers with gonorrhea, a condition termed ophthalmia neonatorum. Formerly a common cause of blindness, gonococcal ophthalmia is now rare in industrialized countries because of both improved control of gonorrhea and routine use of neonatal ocular prophylaxis with topical antibiotics or 1% silver nitrate. Neonates may also acquire pharyngeal or rectal infection and, rarely, gonococcal pneumonia or sepsis. Beyond the neonatal period, purulent vaginitis is the most common manifestation of gonorrhea or chlamydial infection in girls, and rectal or pharyngeal infection is the most common manifestation in prepubertal boys. Most cases are acquired through sexual abuse, but occasional cases in young children may be acquired from fomites or by nonsexual personal exposure in crowded conditions, especially in tropical climates.

Disseminated Gonococcal Infection
CLINICAL MANIFESTATIONS

Disseminated gonococcal infection (DGI) usually is manifested with various combinations of polyarticular tenosynovitis, dermatitis secondary to focal septic embolization, and septic arthritis. Studies undertaken in the 1960s and 1970s estimated that DGI occurred in 1 to 3% of adults with gonorrhea, but the risk depends on characteristics of the particular strains of *N. gonorrhoeae* circulating in the population. Today, DGI probably occurs in well under 1% of gonococcal infections in most geographic areas. Women may be somewhat more susceptible to DGI than men, and the onset often coincides with menstruation. Severity varies from a mild illness with slight joint discomfort, a few skin lesions, and little or no fever to a fulminant illness with overt polyarthritis, innumerable skin lesions, high fever, and prostration. Most persons with DGI have no symptoms of genital gonorrhea, probably because some strains of *N. gonorrhoeae* that are prone to disseminate are also associated with subclinical mucosal infections. The absence of clinical symptoms and signs of mucosal infection in these strains is probably due to their ability to bind complement downregulatory molecules, thereby diminishing the local inflammatory response.

The presentation of DGI can be divided into the clinical syndromes of tenosynovitis-dermatitis and monarticular or oligoarticular arthritis, although these presentations sometimes overlap. Tenosynovitis-dermatitis is thought to predominate early in the course of dissemination, and approximately 70% of DGI cases in published series present with this syndrome. These patients usually suffer migratory polyarthralgias without purulent arthritis. There is often tendon inflammation affecting the wrists, fingers, ankles, or toes. Skin lesions are typically painless, are few in number (5 to 30), affect predominantly the extremities, and are pustular or vesiculopustular (Fig. 299-3), although petechiae, hemorrhagic macules, papules, bullae, and nodules rarely occur (see Fig. 441-5). Axial skeletal involvement is uncommon, a feature that can help differentiate DGI from reactive arthritis (Chapter 265). The tenosynovitis-dermatitis syndrome often subsides spontaneously, or it may evolve during a period of several days into an overt septic arthritis with purulent synovial fluid, usually involving only one or two joints. Approximately 25 to 50% of persons with DGI present initially with purulent monarticular or oligoarticular arthritis, often without apparent sequential evolution from arthritis-dermatitis syndrome. This form of DGI typically affects the knee, ankle, elbow, or wrist, but any joint may be involved.

DIAGNOSIS

Sexually active young persons with arthritis, tenosynovitis, or papulopustular skin lesions should be tested for *N. gonorrhoeae* at all potentially exposed anatomic sites. The diagnosis of DGI is secure when gonococci are identified by culture or NAAT in the blood, a skin lesion, or synovial fluid, but it is often made presumptively when genital, rectal, or pharyngeal gonorrhea is present in a patient with a compatible clinical syndrome that responds promptly to antibiotics.

Blood, synovial fluid, and mucosal tract cultures are positive in approximately 4 to 35%, 10 to 34%, and 80% of patients, respectively. However, the yield from culture varies with the clinical presentation. The performance of NAAT versus culture of blood, synovial fluid, or skin lesions has not been studied in patients with DGI. Patients with tenosynovitis-dermatitis more frequently have bacteremia, whereas patients with septic gonococcal arthritis are seldom bacteremic, and close to 50% have positive synovial fluid cultures; it is reasonable to suspect that the yield might be higher with NAAT. Because bacteremia is intermittent, clinicians should obtain more than one set of blood cultures to maximize the likelihood of isolating the organism. Similarly, NAAT or culture specimens should be obtained from all potentially exposed anatomic sites (genital tract, pharynx, rectum). Cultures of skin lesions are generally negative despite demonstrable gonococci by fluorescent antibody, but NAAT results may be positive in persons with negative blood and mucosal site cultures. The peripheral blood leukocyte count is generally elevated but may be normal. The synovial fluid leukocyte count is usually 20,000 to 60,000/mm^3, with higher numbers of white blood cells seen in persons with clinically apparent arthritis than in those with tenosynovitis-dermatitis. Liver function tests often show elevations in aminotransferase levels, suggestive of mild hepatitis.

The differential diagnosis of DGI includes reactive arthritis (Chapter 265), meningococcemia (Chapter 298), other kinds of septic arthritis (Chapter 272), rheumatoid arthritis (Chapter 264), systemic lupus erythematosus

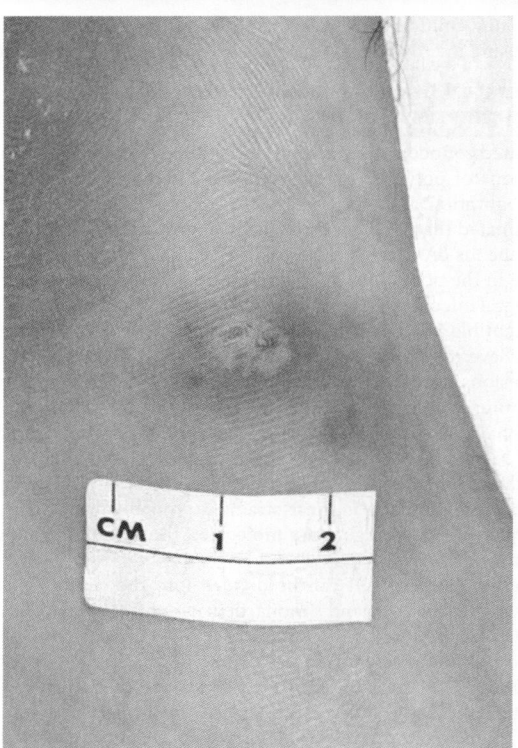

FIGURE 299-3. Cutaneous gonococcal lesion secondary to disseminated *Neisseria gonorrhoeae* infection. Although gonorrhea is a sexually transmitted disease, if it remains untreated, the *N. gonorrhoeae* bacteria responsible for the infection can disseminate throughout the body and form lesions in extragenital locations (also see Fig. 441-5). (From Handsfield HH. *Color Atlas and Synopsis of Sexually Transmitted Diseases.* 3rd ed. New York: McGraw-Hill; 2011.)

(Chapter 266), acute HIV infection (Chapter 385), syphilis (Chapter 319), and other rheumatologic conditions and infectious diseases. Reactive arthritis, often triggered by sexually acquired chlamydial infection, is the principal consideration in young adults. The skin lesions of the two conditions, when present, are generally distinct and often pathognomonic for one syndrome or the other. In addition, conjunctivitis and involvement of the axial skeleton (e.g., sacroiliitis) are common in reactive arthritis and infrequent in DGI.

PROGNOSIS

Many cases of arthritis-dermatitis syndrome resolve spontaneously; with prompt treatment, few patients suffer sequelae of DGI, but untreated septic arthritis can lead to contiguous osteomyelitis or joint destruction. Endocarditis, meningitis, and myocarditis are occasionally seen, with or without a typical DGI syndrome. Gonococcal endocarditis usually involves the aortic valve and often progresses rapidly, leading to valve destruction and heart failure.

PREVENTION

Control of gonorrhea depends on prompt diagnosis and effective treatment of infected persons, screening of sexually active women and MSM in settings where gonorrhea is prevalent, treatment of patients' partners, rescreening of persons with a recent history of gonorrhea, and efforts to promote safer sexual behaviors (e.g., condom use, abstinence, fewer partners). Sexually active MSM outside of mutually monogamous relationships, including HIV-infected men, are at high risk for gonorrhea and should be tested at least annually for rectal and pharyngeal gonococcal infection as well as for chlamydial infection, syphilis, and HIV infection. The value of screening of asymptomatic men for urethral infection (by NAAT of urine) is uncertain; the yield is low in most settings. Gonococcal screening criteria for woman are not well defined. However, because most NAATs for *C. trachomatis* also test for *N. gonorrhoeae*, most chlamydia screening includes gonorrhea testing.

Public education and personal counseling of persons with gonorrhea or at risk of contracting it should emphasize the effectiveness of mutual monogamy and condoms for vaginal or anal sex for new or casual partnerships. Every patient with gonorrhea should be counseled about the risks for HIV infection

and should be tested for HIV, *C. trachomatis*, and syphilis. Because accurate epidemiologic data are essential to generate and to maintain resources for the prevention and control of STIs, all cases of gonorrhea, chlamydial infection, syphilis, and HIV infection should be promptly reported to the health department in accordance with local laws. Ultimate control of gonorrhea may require immunization, but no effective vaccine is on the horizon, despite intensive research for more than four decades.

TREATMENT   Rx

Antimicrobial Susceptibility

Gonococci with chromosomal or plasmid-borne mutations that confer relative or absolute resistance to the penicillins, tetracyclines, and sulfonamides are prevalent worldwide, and none of these drugs is acceptable as empirical therapy anywhere in the world. The prevalence of β-lactamase (penicillinase) plasmids, which confer absolute resistance to penicillin, ampicillin, and amoxicillin, varies from about 10% of gonococci in the United States and western Europe to almost 50% in some developing countries. Approximately 27% of gonococcal infections in MSM and 9% of infections in heterosexuals are caused by organisms that are resistant to ciprofloxacin and other fluoroquinolones. Resistant gonococci are still more prevalent in Europe (up to 50% in some countries). Fluoroquinolone-resistant gonococci are prevalent worldwide, and fluoroquinolones are no longer suitable for routine use unless recent local data demonstrate low levels of resistance. Approximately 5% of gonococcal isolates in the United Kingdom are no longer susceptible to azithromycin, and azithromycin-resistant *N. gonorrhoeae* has been identified in the western United States, although such strains were rare as recently as 2012.

Gonococcal resistance to cephalosporins is now a major public health concern. Strains with relative resistance to oral cephalosporins (e.g., cefixime, heretofore a mainstay of gonorrhea treatment) are common in Japan, and in 2011 almost 8% of gonococcal isolates in Europe and 1.4% of isolates in the United States had reduced susceptibility to cefixime. In the United States, organisms with diminished susceptibility to oral cephalosporins are more common on the West Coast than in other parts of the country and more common among MSM than among heterosexuals.[8] Diminished susceptibility to ceftriaxone remains very rare, although isolated cases of multidrug-resistant gonorrhea—organisms that are resistant to ceftriaxone therapy—have been identified in Japan and Europe. Although recent data suggest that the proportion of gonococcal infections caused by organisms with diminished susceptibility to oral third-generation cephalosporins is now declining, ongoing surveillance for cephalosporin resistance remains a high priority, and decisions on how to treat gonorrhea need to incorporate strategies for diminishing the development of population-level antimicrobial resistance. Clinicians who treat patients for gonorrhea and other STIs should keep abreast of regional trends in resistance and be alert to modified therapeutic recommendations.[9]

Principles of Treatment

Because of the need to curtail transmission, therapy is usually based on clinical or epidemiologic suspicion before the diagnosis is confirmed microbiologically.[10] Clinicians should presumptively treat all patients evaluated as contacts to persons with known gonococcal infections, all women with PID or mucopurulent cervicitis, and, if Gram staining cannot be performed, all men presenting with a clinical syndrome of urethritis. (Men with urethritis and no evidence of gonorrhea on Gram stain should be treated for nongonococcal urethritis.) Diagnosis by NAAT precludes antimicrobial resistance testing, and even when *N. gonorrhoeae* is isolated by culture, susceptibility testing is rarely performed routinely. Accordingly, treatment of uncomplicated gonorrhea is dictated by national or local patterns of antimicrobial susceptibility, without knowledge of susceptibility in individual patients. However, susceptibility testing should be used to guide the treatment of gonococcal septic arthritis, endocarditis, or other serious complications and may increasingly become routine even in genitourinary infections.[11]

Dual treatment of uncomplicated gonorrhea, typically with both a cephalosporin and either azithromycin or doxycycline, has long been recommended to cover the possibility of simultaneous chlamydial infection, typically present in 5 to 10% of MSM, 15 to 25% of heterosexual men, and 35 to 50% of women with gonorrhea in North America. In addition, dual therapy using antibiotics with differing mechanisms of action may reduce selection pressure for antimicrobial resistance in *N. gonorrhoeae*, so that dual therapy is now recommended routinely even when chlamydial infection is unlikely or has been excluded by negative testing.

Treatment Regimens

Ceftriaxone 250 mg intramuscularly plus azithromycin 1 g orally is the preferred treatment regimen for uncomplicated gonorrhea (Table 299-1).[12] This regimen is highly effective against pharyngeal gonorrhea, which may be relatively resistant to oral therapies, and is designed to diminish the spread of cephalosporin-resistant *N. gonorrhoeae* as well as to cover simultaneous chlamydial infection.[A1] Cefixime 400 mg orally (with azithromycin 1.0 g orally)

TABLE 299-1	ANTIBIOTIC REGIMENS FOR THE TREATMENT OF GONORRHEA IN THE UNITED STATES*

UNCOMPLICATED GONORRHEA OF THE URETHRA, CERVIX, OR RECTUM

Preferred

Ceftriaxone 250 mg IM single dose *plus* azithromycin 1 g PO

Alternatives

Cefixime 400 mg PO single dose *plus* azithromycin 1 g PO

or

Azithromycin 2 g PO single dose

plus gentamicin 240 mg IM single dose *or* gemifloxacin 320 mg PO as a single dose

INFECTION OF THE PHARYNX

Ceftriaxone 250 mg IM single dose *plus* azithromycin 1 g PO as a single dose

CONJUNCTIVITIS (NOT OPHTHALMIA NEONATORUM)

Ceftriaxone 1 g IM single dose *plus* azithromycin 1 g PO as a single dose

DISSEMINATED GONOCOCCAL INFECTION

Preferred

Ceftriaxone 1 g IM or IV q24h[†]

or

Ceftizoxime 1 g IV q8h

plus

Azithromycin 1 g PO as a single dose

Alternative

Cefotaxime 1 g IV q8h

*Treatment of gonorrhea in adults should always include treatment of sex partners and advice to abstain from sex for 7 days.

[†]Treat with intravenous therapy until the patient has been clinically improved for 24 to 48 hours. Then switch to cefixime 400 mg orally twice a day to complete a 7-day course.

remains appropriate when ceftriaxone therapy is not feasible (e.g., if a patient declines injection) or in expedited (unobserved) treatment of patients' sex partners. Clinicians should be mindful that ensuring that all patients and partners are treated is more important than always using intramuscular ceftriaxone. Persons with severe β-lactam allergies should receive azithromycin 2 g orally once, *plus* either a single dose of gentamicin 240 mg IM *or* a single dose of gemifloxacin 320 mg orally.[A2]

Women with acute PID should be treated with antibiotics active against *N. gonorrhoeae* and *C. trachomatis*.[13] The role of anaerobic bacteria in PID is uncertain, although it is not known whether anaerobic treatment is required for PID. Most women can be treated as outpatients, but the following factors should prompt hospital admission: possible surgical cause of symptoms (e.g., appendicitis), pregnancy, failure to respond to oral therapy within 72 hours of initiation, inability to tolerate or to adhere to oral therapy, severe symptoms, and tubo-ovarian abscess. The suggested outpatient regimen is ceftriaxone 250 mg IM plus doxycycline 100 mg PO twice daily for 14 days or cefoxitin 2 g IM plus probenecid 1 g PO as a single dose and doxycycline 100 mg twice daily for 14 days. Either regimen can be given with or without metronidazole (500 mg twice daily) for 14 days. For hospitalized patients or others who require parenteral therapy, the CDC recommends intravenous cefotetan or cefoxitin plus oral doxycycline or parenteral therapy with clindamycin plus gentamicin. Intravenous ampicillin-sulbactam plus oral doxycycline can also be used. Parenteral therapy is continued until improvement is observed, after which oral therapy is prescribed to complete 14 days' total treatment.

Most persons with DGI should be hospitalized and treated with a parenteral third-generation cephalosporin such as ceftriaxone, cefotaxime, or ceftizoxime. Joint irrigation or drainage appears to be unnecessary for septic arthritis, although repeated aspiration of synovial fluid may speed clinical improvement. Oral treatment (e.g., cefixime, cefpodoxime, or a fluoroquinolone) can usually be substituted after improvement begins and then continued to complete 7 days' therapy. More prolonged parenteral treatment and higher doses are indicated for the treatment of gonococcal meningitis or endocarditis, although modern data are lacking. Gonococcal epididymitis, bartholinitis, and other localized complications should generally be treated for 7 to 14 days with drugs active against both *N. gonorrhoeae* and *C. trachomatis*. Gonococcal conjunctivitis in adults can be managed with a single dose of ceftriaxone, 1 g IM, with optional saline lavage. The diagnosis of all forms of complicated gonococcal infection should be confirmed by culture with determination of antimicrobial susceptibility, which can guide completion of treatment after initial empirical therapy.

Management of Sex Partners

Failure to ensure treatment of patients' sex partners contributes to the continued transmission of gonorrhea and other bacterial STIs and often results in reinfection of the index case. For gonorrhea and chlamydial infection, all partners in the preceding 2 months should be treated; if the patient has not had sex in the preceding 2 months, the most recent partner should be treated. Very few U.S. health departments routinely make an effort to ensure that sex partners receive treatment, and the responsibility to ensure partner treatment lies jointly with the patient and the diagnosing clinician. Optimally, the partners of persons with gonorrhea should undergo diagnostic testing for gonorrhea, chlamydial infection, syphilis, and HIV infection. However, clinicians should not wait to obtain the results of diagnostic testing before treating a potentially exposed sex partner; all partners of infected persons should be treated when they initially present for evaluation.

In most settings, approximately 50% of potentially exposed sex partners go untreated, risking ongoing transmission and reinfection of the original patient. In an effort to address this problem, the CDC and several state health departments recommend that clinicians offer heterosexual patients with gonorrhea or chlamydial infection medication to give to their sex partners. This practice, termed patient-delivered partner therapy (PDPT)—sometimes termed expedited partner therapy—is supported by three randomized controlled trials showing that treating sex partners without requiring attendance for care in person decreases the risk of reinfection and increases the proportion of partners treated.[A3] PDPT requires single-dose treatment, typically with cefixime plus azithromycin for gonorrhea or azithromycin alone for the partners of patients with chlamydial infection. PDPT currently is legal in most states of the United States and is likely to become permissible in other states, and clinicians should offer PDPT as an option for most heterosexual patients with gonorrhea or chlamydial infection. The CDC website maintains up-to-date information on the legality of PDPT in U.S. states and territories (http://www.cdc.gov/STD/ept/legal/default.htm). In addition to direct delivery of drugs to the patient for PDPT, it is often feasible to write or to telephone a prescription to a cooperating pharmacy. However PDPT is implemented, when practical, clinicians should provide written information about the medication and STI prevention as well as advice to seek clinical care in addition to taking the drugs provided. Examples of forms that can be dispensed with PDPT can be found at the following websites: http://www.doh.wa.gov/YouandYourFamily/IllnessandDisease/SexuallyTransmittedDisease/ExpeditedPartnerTherapy; http://www.cdph.ca.gov/HealthInfo/discond/Pages/SexuallyTransmittedDiseases.aspx. PDPT is not recommended for MSM with gonorrhea or chlamydial infection owing to potentially high rates of syphilis and HIV infection; the partners of such patients should be evaluated and treated in person.

Follow-up

The recommended treatment regimens cure 96 to 100% of uncomplicated cases of genital or rectal gonorrhea caused by susceptible strains and at least 90% of pharyngeal infections. Retesting of infected patients to document eradication of *N. gonorrhoeae* ("test of cure") is not recommended except in pregnant women, when adherence to therapy is in doubt, or when atypical treatment regimens are employed. When test of cure is indicated, culture can be performed a week after treatment is completed, but retesting by NAAT should be delayed at least 3 weeks after treatment to reduce the possibility of detecting persistent gonococcal DNA despite the eradication of viable organisms.

Although test of cure is generally not advised, all persons diagnosed with gonorrhea should be rescreened 3 to 4 months after treatment. In prospective studies, 10 to 20% of both men and women with gonorrhea or chlamydial infection are infected when they are retested 3 to 4 months later. The likelihood of recurrent or persistent gonococcal infection appears to be reduced by up to 70% when partners are managed with PDPT. Rescreening can be done with urine or self-obtained vaginal swab testing by NAAT and does not require a second visit with a clinician.

Grade A References

A1. Creighton S. Gonorrhoea. *Clin Evid (Online)*. 2014;2014.

A2. Kirkcaldy RD, Weinstock HS, Moore PC, et al. The efficacy and safety of gentamicin plus azithromycin and gemifloxacin plus azithromycin as treatment of uncomplicated gonorrhea. *Clin Infect Dis.* 2014;59:1083-1091.

A3. Ferreira A, Young T, Mathews C, et al. Strategies for partner notification for sexually transmitted infections, including HIV. *Cochrane Database Syst Rev.* 2013;10:CD002843.

GENERAL REFERENCES

For the General References and other additional features, please visit Expert Consult at https://expertconsult.inkling.com.

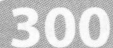

HAEMOPHILUS AND *MORAXELLA* INFECTIONS

MICHAEL S. SIMBERKOFF

● *HAEMOPHILUS* INFECTIONS

DEFINITION

The name *Haemophilus* is derived from the Greek nouns *haima*, meaning "blood," and *philos*, meaning "lover." *Haemophilus* species colonize the respiratory tract; cause infections of the respiratory tract, skin, or mucous membranes of humans; and from these sites can invade and cause bacteremia, meningitis, epiglottitis, endocarditis, septic arthritis, or cellulitis (Table 300-1).

The Pathogen

Haemophilus species are small, nonmotile, aerobic or facultative anaerobic, pleomorphic, gram-negative bacilli. The prototype of this genus, *Haemophilus influenzae*, was originally recovered from patients with influenza by Pfeiffer in 1893, and it was considered the cause of that disease for many years. Primary isolation of *Haemophilus* species is best accomplished on chocolate agar medium in a carbon dioxide–enriched atmosphere.

EPIDEMIOLOGY

The precise prevalence and incidence of *H. influenzae* infections are unknown.[1] This organism can be detected in the nasopharynx of both children and adults. Before the introduction of an effective vaccine, between 3 and 5% of infants harbored *H. influenzae* type b in their nasopharynx. Children who have been immunized against *H. influenzae* type b are far less likely to be colonized and infected with this organism. However, the risk for infection in nonimmune household contacts of a patient with invasive *H. influenzae* disease is approximately 600-fold greater than the risk in the age-adjusted general population. Nontypeable *H. influenzae* can be detected in the nasopharyngeal cultures of more than 70% of young children, but infection occurs in only a small proportion of colonized individuals.

H. influenzae type b was the most common cause of meningitis in young children before effective vaccines were introduced in the 1980s. Vaccination has had a dramatic impact on the incidence of infection in this group. In a population-based study in Atlanta during the 18-month period from December 1, 1988, through May 31, 1990, invasive *H. influenzae* disease occurred in only 5.6 per 100,000 children and 1.7 per 100,000 adults. Forty of the 47 strains associated with invasive disease from adult patients in this study were serotyped. Twenty of these isolates (50%) were *H. influenzae* type b, 19 (47.5%) were nontypeable, and 1 (2.5%) was type f. A more recent study covering the period from 1989 to 2008 from the Centers for Disease Control and Prevention's Active Bacterial Core surveillance system showed that the

overall incidence of invasive *H. influenzae* infections fell from 4.39 cases per 100,000 population in 1989 (shortly after introduction of the *H. influenzae* type b conjugate vaccine in the United States) to 1.55 cases per 100,000 in 2008, and the percentage of invasive infections caused by *H. influenzae* type b fell from 87 to 3%, whereas the percentage caused by nontypeable *H. influenzae* strains increased from 16.8 to 68.4%.[2]

Patients with human immunodeficiency virus (HIV) infection are at increased risk for *H. influenzae* infection. Rates of invasive *H. influenzae* infection in men aged 20 to 49 years with HIV infection and acquired immunodeficiency syndrome (AIDS) were 14.6 and 79.2 per 100,000, respectively. The majority of these infections were caused by nontypeable *H. influenzae* strains, although in a second study, 10 of 15 bacteremic *H. influenzae* type b infections observed in adults occurred in patients at risk for HIV infection, and AIDS was documented in seven of these patients.

Other factors also increase the risk for *H. influenzae* infection, including immunoglobulin deficiencies, sickle cell disease, splenectomy, malignant disease, pregnancy, cerebrospinal fluid (CSF) leaks, head trauma, alcoholism, chronic obstructive pulmonary disease (COPD), and race. Eskimo, Navajo, and Apache children have *H. influenzae* type b infection rates that are significantly greater than those in comparable non-native populations. In addition, daycare attendance, crowding, the presence of siblings, prior hospitalizations, and previous otitis media have been shown to increase the risk for *H. influenzae* type b disease in young children, whereas breast-feeding decreases this risk.

PATHOBIOLOGY

H. influenzae consists of encapsulated (typeable) and nonencapsulated (nontypeable) forms. The encapsulated forms are responsible for most of the invasive infections in children and acute epiglottitis in both children and adults, whereas the nonencapsulated forms cause respiratory mucosal infections, conjunctivitis, female genital tract infections, and invasive disease in adults. The capsules of *H. influenzae* consist of polysaccharide antigens. Six capsular serotypes (a through f) exist and are important virulence factors that inhibit opsonization, clearance, and intracellular killing of the organisms. *H. influenzae* type b, formerly the most common cause of meningitis in infancy and childhood worldwide, contains a pentose capsular polysaccharide consisting of polyribosyl ribitol phosphate (PRP). Other serotypes contain hexose polysaccharides. *H. influenzae* type b is more virulent than the other serotypes, probably because it is highly resistant to clearance once bacteremia has been initiated. Since the introduction of *H. influenzae* serotype b conjugate vaccines in the 1990s, most infections are now caused by non-b serotypes, and *H. influenzae* serotype a has emerged as a cause of serious morbidity and mortality.[3] Recent findings suggest that *H. influenzae* strains have the capacity to induce variations in their surface oligosaccharides when serially passed in the presence of human antibody and complement. It has been hypothesized that this may contribute to the organism's capacity to colonize and to survive in nares of patients before causing respiratory tract infections including otitis, sinusitis, epiglottitis, bronchitis, and pneumonia.

Fimbriae are important virulence factors that enhance the adherence of *H. influenzae* to mucosal surfaces. Both typeable and nontypeable *H. influenzae* isolates contain fimbriae. The lipo-oligosaccharides of *H. influenzae* also contribute to their virulence. Lipo-oligosaccharides appear to play a crucial role in facilitating the survival of *H. influenzae* on mucosal surfaces within the nasopharynx and in initiating invasive disease (blood stream invasion) from these sites.[4]

Outer membrane proteins also serve as virulence factors in *H. influenzae* disease. At least 15 different *H. influenzae* outer membrane proteins have been identified. One of these (P2, 39 to 40 kD) functions as a porin, and others are associated with iron binding. Successful scavenging of iron within the human host is crucial for multiplication of *H. influenzae*.

Antibodies have been recognized for decades as an important part of host defenses against *H. influenzae* diseases. The classic studies of Fothergill and Wright in 1933 demonstrated that most cases of *H. influenzae* meningitis occur in young children after they lose passively acquired maternal antibodies and before active humoral immunity to the organism develops. These protective antibodies function primarily to opsonize and to facilitate the clearance of *H. influenzae* rather than to kill virulent organisms directly.

Complement is also an essential component of host defenses against some *H. influenzae* diseases. Children with congenital deficiencies of C2, C3, and factor I have an increased incidence of *H. influenzae* infections. Patients who lack a functional spleen (e.g., those with sickle cell disease) or who have undergone splenectomy also are at risk for the development of overwhelming infection with *H. influenzae* type b.

TABLE 300-1	SITES OF COLONIZATION AND INFECTIONS BY *HAEMOPHILUS INFLUENZAE*	
SPECIES	**NORMAL FLORA**	**ASSOCIATED DISEASES**
H. influenzae	Nasopharynx Upper respiratory tract	Meningitis Epiglottitis Sinusitis Otitis Pneumonia Cellulitis Arthritis Osteomyelitis Obstetric infections Endocarditis
H. influenzae, biogroup *aegyptius*		Purulent conjunctivitis Brazilian purpuric fever

CLINICAL MANIFESTATIONS

Meningitis

H. influenzae meningitis commonly occurs in children younger than 5 years and in adults with a history of skull trauma or CSF leaks. *H. influenzae* type b strains cause most of these cases. A review of 493 episodes of acute bacterial meningitis in adults at the Massachusetts General Hospital during the 27-year period from 1962 through 1988 showed that 19 cases (4%) were due to *H. influenzae*.

H. influenzae meningitis is clinically indistinguishable from other forms of acute bacterial meningitis. Most patients with *H. influenzae* meningitis have CSF white blood cell counts greater than 1000/mm^3 and hypoglycorrhachia. CSF Gram stain shows pleomorphic gram-negative bacilli in 60 to 70% of untreated cases. In some patients, however, the bipolar staining may result in a mistaken diagnosis of pneumococcal meningitis. Thus, Gram stain is neither sensitive nor specific for diagnosis of *H. influenzae* meningitis.

A diagnosis of *H. influenzae* type b meningitis can be rapidly and reliably established by detecting PRP capsular antigens in CSF. The diagnosis can be established in most cases even when antibiotics have been given before CSF is obtained. Other serotypes (most commonly type f) can also cause meningitis in adults. Therefore, serologic tests for type b antigen in CSF cannot be relied on to rule out *H. influenzae* meningitis in all cases.

Epiglottitis

H. influenzae type b is the most common cause of acute epiglottitis in both children and adults. Epiglottitis is a life-threatening infection in children that usually occurs in those younger than 5 years. The symptoms are fever, drooling, dysphagia, and respiratory distress or stridor, which appear during the course of hours. In adults, fever, sore throat, dysphagia, and odynophagia occur. Cervical tenderness and lymphadenopathy can be found at all ages. Laryngoscopy demonstrates a swollen, cherry-red epiglottis. However, this procedure should be avoided or undertaken only by experts because it may precipitate acute airway obstruction and thus make emergency tracheotomy necessary. A lateral radiograph of the neck more safely confirms the diagnosis of acute epiglottitis. The patient must be maintained in an upright position during this procedure, however, to avoid additional compromise of the airway. The cause is usually established by blood culture. Cultures of the pharynx and other mucosal surfaces are less useful because *H. influenzae* may be part of the normal flora. One review suggests that although vaccination has effectively reduced the incidence of this disease in children, it may be increasing in adults.

Pneumonia

H. influenzae is a common cause of pneumonia in both children and adults. These organisms can also cause nosocomial infections, including ventilator-associated pneumonia. The clinical features of *H. influenzae* pneumonia include fever, cough, and signs and radiographic findings of lobar consolidation.[5] Parapneumonic effusions or empyema occur commonly in patients with *H. influenzae* pneumonia. Gram-negative bacilli in sputum suggest the diagnosis, but isolation of *H. influenzae* from sputum culture alone is inadequate to prove a cause because of the high frequency with which this organism colonizes the respiratory tract. A diagnosis can be established by isolating *H. influenzae* from either blood or pleural fluid. Most isolates are nontypeable.

Tracheobronchitis

Tracheobronchitis is a condition characterized by fever, cough, and purulent sputum that occurs in the absence of radiographic infiltrates suggestive of pneumonia.[6] It frequently develops in patients with known chronic lung disease. Blood cultures are rarely positive. A combination of pleomorphic gram-negative bacilli predominating in purulent sputum, antibody titers to *H. influenzae* that rise after infection, and a response, at least transiently, to treatment of *H. influenzae* infection strongly suggests this diagnosis.

Sinusitis

H. influenzae and *Streptococcus pneumoniae* are the most frequent bacterial isolates from antral punctures or surgical specimens of patients with acute purulent sinusitis. Most *H. influenzae* isolates are nontypeable. Although patients may respond initially to treatment directed against *H. influenzae*, the response is transient if the sinus obstruction is not relieved. *H. influenzae* is not an important pathogen in patients with chronic sinusitis.

Otitis Media

H. influenzae is the most frequent cause of otitis media in young children. Approximately 90% of the *H. influenzae* isolates obtained by tympanocentesis are nontypeable; *H. influenzae* type b causes most of the remaining 10% of cases. Patients with otitis media may have ear pain or exhibit irritability. Drainage can be present. An inflamed, opaque, bulging, or perforated tympanic membrane is usually demonstrated. The cause can be proved by Gram stain and culture of purulent fluid obtained by tympanocentesis. Otitis caused by *H. influenzae* type b may occur in association with bacteremia and meningitis.

Cellulitis

H. influenzae type b is the cause of 5 to 15% of cases of cellulitis in young children. Most of the infections occur on the face or neck. *H. influenzae* cellulitis is often described as causing a distinctive blue or violaceous discoloration of the skin. However, the fever, erythema, and tenderness observed may not be distinguishable from those attributable to other causes. The diagnosis is established by culture of blood or tissue aspirates from the involved area, or both.

Bacteremia without a Primary Focus of Infection

H. influenzae causes primary bacteremia in both children and adults. In infants or children, occult meningitis or epiglottitis can be present. Rigorous clinical and laboratory evaluation is essential to avoid missing a diagnosis of life-threatening focal infection in these patients. In adults, primary *H. influenzae* bacteremia often occurs in those with underlying diseases, such as lymphoma, leukemia, or alcoholism.

Obstetric and Gynecologic Infection

Pregnancy is associated with a significant risk for *H. influenzae* infection. In the Atlanta study, 7 of 47 adult *H. influenzae* invasive infections occurred in pregnant women. Nontypeable *H. influenzae* is also an important cause of tubo-ovarian abscess and salpingitis in women. A recent study of women in England and Wales showed that pregnancy was associated with an increased risk of invasive, mostly unencapsulated *H. influenzae* infection and that these infections were associated with poor pregnancy outcomes, including fetal loss and extremely premature births or stillbirths.[7]

Pericarditis

H. influenzae type b is an important cause of primary bacterial pericarditis in children. It rarely causes this infection in adults; however, pericarditis can occur in association with pneumonia, probably as a result of contiguous spread of the infection.

Endocarditis

H. influenzae is an unusual cause of endocarditis in view of the frequency with which invasive disease occurs. Most infections occur in patients with preexisting valvular heart disease. Because of its slow initial growth in blood culture media, diagnosis of this infection may be delayed or missed. Patients with *H. influenzae* endocarditis are at high risk for arterial embolic phenomena.

Septic Arthritis

H. influenzae type b is a common cause of septic arthritis in young children; it is rare in adults. *H. influenzae* type b arthritis is clinically indistinguishable from other causes of pyogenic arthritis.

Purulent Conjunctivitis and Brazilian Purpuric Fever

H. influenzae, biogroup *aegyptius* (Koch-Weeks bacillus), causes epidemic purulent conjunctivitis in children. This disease commonly occurs in hot climates or in the summer season.

The infection is characterized by conjunctival erythema, edema, mucopurulent exudate, and varying discomfort in the eyes. An unusually virulent clone of *H. influenzae*, biogroup *aegyptius*, causes an invasive infection called Brazilian purpuric fever, which is characterized by petechial or purpuric skin lesions and vascular collapse; it occurs days to weeks after an initial episode of conjunctivitis in infants and children younger than 10 years.

TREATMENT

Third-generation cephalosporins are considered the treatment of choice for serious *H. influenzae* infections, such as meningitis or epiglottitis. Treatment with ceftriaxone (adult dose, 1 to 2 g intravenously every 12 hours) or cefotaxime (adult dose, 2 g intravenously every 6 hours) should be started in patients with proven or suspected *H. influenzae* infection, and it should be continued at least until full susceptibility data are available.

Ampicillin was effective treatment of all *H. influenzae* infections until the mid-1970s. Since the first reports of ampicillin-resistant *H. influenzae* isolates in 1972, however, the prevalence of resistance has increased dramatically. Most resistance is due to a plasmid-mediated, R-factor enzyme (tumor endothelial marker 1) β-lactamase, which can be detected rapidly in the laboratory. A small number of isolates, however, have altered penicillin-binding proteins that have decreased binding affinity to penicillin and other β-lactam antibiotics. As a consequence, the isolates may be resistant to some cephalosporins, such as cefaclor, cefamandole, and cefuroxime, in addition to ampicillin. Therefore, patients with proven or suspected *H. influenzae* infections should not be treated with ampicillin or second-generation cephalosporins until susceptibility to these antibiotics has been proved. Chloramphenicol resistance also occurs in *H. influenzae*; an inactivating enzyme, chloramphenicol acetyltransferase, causes resistance. A small number of *H. influenzae* isolates are resistant to both ampicillin and chloramphenicol.

Oral antibiotics are commonly used to treat tracheobronchitis in patients with COPD and otitis media in children, in whom *H. influenzae* isolates are common. Because of resistance, ampicillin and amoxicillin cannot be recommended for the more serious of these infections unless the susceptibility of isolates is known. Most *H. influenzae* isolates are susceptible to amoxicillin-clavulanate. They are also susceptible to azithromycin and clarithromycin, the newer macrolide antibiotics. Fluoroquinolones, such as ciprofloxacin, ofloxacin, levofloxacin, and gatifloxacin, are active against these organisms. Trimethoprim-sulfamethoxazole is also effective for most isolates.

PREVENTION

The first *H. influenzae* type b vaccines were licensed for use in the United States in 1985. They contained purified PRP antigens. However, postlicensing studies of PRP vaccines in the United States showed variable efficacy. The PRP vaccines elicit a type 2, thymus-independent B-cell response, generate few (if any) memory B cells, and fail to stimulate a response in neonates and infants.

Protein-conjugated PRP vaccines were developed to overcome the problem of lack of immune response in the most susceptible infants and some young children. Several are now licensed for use in infants.[8] At present, protein-conjugated PRP vaccines are recommended for use in all infants older than 2 months but not earlier than 6 weeks of age. Studies have shown that protein-conjugated vaccines are effective in diverse populations, including adults with COPD.

Antibiotic prophylaxis should be used for the nonimmunized household or daycare contacts of patients with invasive *H. influenzae* type b disease. Rifampin is the treatment of choice. It should be given in a dosage of 10 mg/kg once daily for 4 days to neonates younger than 1 month, 20 mg/kg (up to a maximum of 600 mg) once daily for 4 days to older children, and 600 mg/day for 4 days to adults.

Other *Haemophilus* Species

Haemophilus parainfluenzae can be found as part of the normal flora of the mouth and pharynx (Table 300-1). It is a rare cause of meningitis in children and an even rarer cause of meningitis in adults. It may cause dental infections or dental abscesses. Cases of brain abscess, epidural abscess, liver abscess, osteomyelitis, pneumonia, empyema, epiglottitis, peritonitis, septic arthritis, and bacteremia have been reported to be caused by this organism. *H. parainfluenzae* also causes subacute endocarditis, often in young adults. *Haemophilus* species are responsible for approximately 1% of cases of infective endocarditis in non–drug-abusing patients. *H. parainfluenzae*, *Haemophilus aphrophilus*, and *Haemophilus paraphrophilus* are the species most frequently recovered from these patients. *H. parainfluenzae* forms bulky vegetations on heart valves. Arterial embolization is common in patients with *H. parainfluenzae* endocarditis. Most isolates are sensitive to ampicillin, but some produce β-lactamases.

⬤ *MORAXELLA* INFECTIONS

DEFINITION

Moraxella species are associated with a variety of infections, the most common of which is exacerbation of chronic bronchitis by *Moraxella catarrhalis*.[9]

The Pathogen

Moraxella organisms are small, gram-negative bacteria that grow well on blood or chocolate agar. They are catalase and oxidase positive. These small diplococci are morphologically difficult to distinguish from *Neisseria*. Some *Moraxella* species are gram-negative bacilli. *M. catarrhalis* is the most important pathogen of this genus (Table 300-2).

PATHOBIOLOGY

The organism is isolated exclusively from humans and is found predominantly in the respiratory tract. *M. catarrhalis* adheres to mucosal cells with the aid of pili. Infection is believed to result from contiguous spread of the organism from sites of colonization, possibly as a result of the introduction of new, more virulent strains to which the host lacks immunity. *M. catarrhalis* possesses multiple virulence factors that can be carried through biologically active outer membrane vesicles to contribute to the pathobiology of otitis media.[10]

M. catarrhalis can often be found in respiratory secretions together with *H. influenzae*. Although the mechanism for coexistence of these pathogens is not known, evidence suggests that the outer membrane vesicles of *M. catarrhalis* inactivate complement, thus enhancing survival of *H. influenzae*.

CLINICAL MANIFESTATIONS

M. catarrhalis is associated with exacerbations of chronic bronchitis. Studies indicate that this organism can be isolated from 0.2 to 8.1% of the sputum aspirates of patients with this disease. It is the third most common pathogen isolated from these patients behind *S. pneumoniae* and *H. influenzae*.

M. catarrhalis can cause pneumonia, particularly in elderly patients with COPD and other underlying conditions such as diabetes mellitus. Sir William Osler is believed to have died as a result of *M. catarrhalis* pneumonia. Cases of bacteremic pneumonia have been reported. In addition, *M. catarrhalis* can cause nosocomial pneumonia with evidence of patient-to-patient spread of the organism.

M. catarrhalis is a common cause of otitis media in young children. Microbiologic studies indicate that this organism is present in approximately 15% of the aspirates from such patients. The organism also causes sinusitis and is a rare cause of bacteremia in children and adults.

Serious infections with other *Moraxella* species are uncommon. However, these organisms are associated with chronic conjunctivitis. Furthermore, case reports have documented the rare occurrence of invasive infections, including bacteremia, endocarditis, arthritis, pericarditis, and meningitis. Meningitis may occur in patients with complement deficiency.

TREATMENT   Rx

Oral antibiotics are sufficient for the treatment of most *M. catarrhalis* infections. Inducible β-lactamases are present in many isolates. Therefore, treatment with a β-lactamase–stable antibiotic such as amoxicillin-clavulanate (usual adult dose, 500 mg every 12 hours), a cephalosporin (e.g., cefaclor, usual adult dose, 500 mg every 8 hours), or a non–β-lactam antibiotic such as trimethoprim-sulfamethoxazole (usual adult dose, 1 double-strength tablet every 12 hours) should be initiated pending susceptibility test results.

TABLE 300-2   SITES OF COLONIZATION AND INFECTION BY *MORAXELLA* SPECIES

SPECIES	NORMAL FLORA	ASSOCIATED DISEASES
M. catarrhalis	Oral cavity and upper respiratory tract	Chronic bronchitis exacerbation Otitis media Pneumonia Sinusitis Bacteremia, endocarditis Arthritis, osteomyelitis, epiglottitis (all extremely rare)
M. lacunata	Upper respiratory tract	Chronic conjunctivitis
Other *Moraxella*	Upper respiratory tract	Rare cases of bacteremia, endocarditis, arthritis, meningitis

301

CHANCROID

STANLEY M. SPINOLA

DEFINITION

Chancroid is a sexually transmitted disease characterized by painful genital ulcers and inguinal lymphadenitis. Chancroid is caused by *Haemophilus ducreyi*, a gram-negative coccobacillus that is not a true *Haemophilus* species. Within the Pasteurellaceae, *H. ducreyi* is grouped in a distinct lineage with *Mannheimia haemolytica* and *Actinobacillus pleuropneumoniae*. *H. ducreyi* is likely to have diverged from these animal respiratory pathogens to occupy its niche in the human genital epithelium.

EPIDEMIOLOGY

Chancroid is endemic in resource-poor regions of Africa and Asia and facilitates the transmission of human immunodeficiency virus (HIV-1). In the 1990s, the World Health Organization estimated the annual global prevalence of chancroid to be 4 million to 6 million cases. Because of the widespread use of syndromic management, which consists of treatment for syphilis and chancroid without diagnostic testing, the prevalence of chancroid has dramatically declined in endemic areas. Chancroid can be maintained only in networks with high sex partner change rates; female sex workers play an important role in its epidemiology. Targeted treatment of infected sex workers leads to eradication of the disease in endemic areas. Despite these successes, reports of chancroid persist from many countries. Such reports imply a reservoir of untreated sex workers. Urban outbreaks of chancroid associated with sex work occurred in the United States in the 1980s and 1990s. Owing to contact tracing and treatment efforts, the number of domestic cases of chancroid has decreased steadily, with a 65-year low of eight cases in 2013; such sporadic cases are likely to be imported after contact with infected persons in endemic areas.

The male-to-female ratio of chancroid is 3 : 1. The excess number of male cases is usually attributed to the infection of multiple partners by sex workers. However, human inoculation experiments indicate that men are twice as susceptible as women for development of pustules, suggesting that male gender is a risk factor for disease progression.[1]

PATHOBIOLOGY

Much of what is known about the pathogenesis of *H. ducreyi* is derived from experiments in which bacteria are inoculated into the skin of the upper arm of human volunteers. Puncture wounds are required to initiate infection, and the estimated infectious dose is as low as one bacterium. Papules develop within 24 hours and either spontaneously resolve or evolve into pustules in 2 to 5 days. Neutrophils and macrophages surround the organism and form an abscess that erodes the epidermis. Below the abscess, there is a collar of macrophages and regulatory T cells and a dermal infiltrate of macrophages, CD4 and CD8 T cells, natural killer (NK) cells, and dendritic cells. This histopathology resembles a suppurative granuloma and is identical to that of natural ulcers. In both experimental and natural infection, *H. ducreyi* associates with neutrophils and macrophages, which fail to ingest the organism. Mutant versus parent trials have revealed bacterial components that are required for infection; several are involved with adherence and resistance to serum killing and phagocytosis. In addition to gender, the human model has shown that there are host effects on disease progression. Differential host susceptibility is associated with distinct dendritic cell responses to the organism, which may shape T-cell and NK-cell responses that influence the ability of phagocytes to ingest the organism.

CLINICAL MANIFESTATIONS

H. ducreyi enters the skin through breaks in the epithelium that occur during intercourse.[2] Papules form within hours to days and evolve into pustules in 2

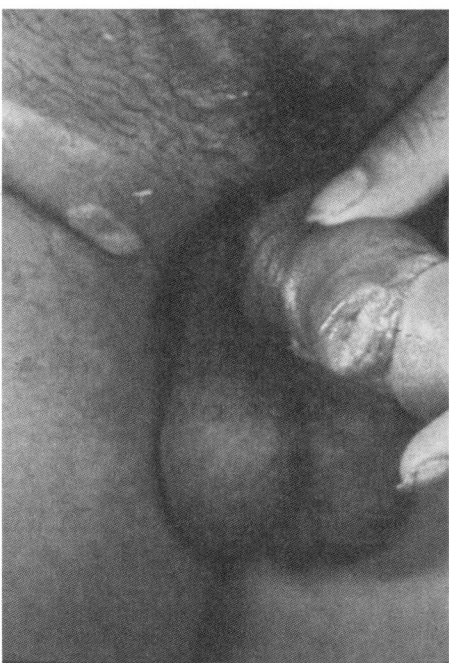

FIGURE 301-1. Typical chancroidal ulcer and lymphadenitis in a man. (From Herpes-Coldsores.com. http://www.herpes-coldsores.com/std/chancroid_pictures.htm.)

to 3 days. After a few days to 2 weeks, the pustules ulcerate. Patients typically develop one to four painful ulcers (Fig. 301-1) but do not seek treatment until they have had ulcerative symptoms for 1 to 3 weeks. By this time, 10 to 40% have suppurative inguinal lymphadenopathy or buboes (see Fig. 301-1).

Natural ulcers are classically very painful and nonindurated, with ragged edges. The ulcer may be covered by a yellow or gray necrotic exudate and bleeds when scraped. However, this presentation occurs in a minority of patients; chancroid is frequently indistinguishable from syphilis and genital herpes. Lesions in men are usually on the foreskin, coronal sulcus, or penile shaft. Lesions in women are usually on the labia; but women may have internal vaginal and cervical ulcers that are painless. Lesions also occur on the thighs and buttocks or at distant sites; extragenital lesions are thought to be due to autoinoculation. Untreated, chancroid persists for months and causes giant ulcers, erosion of the infected area, or fibrosis, leading to phimosis in men.

In the western Pacific, *H. ducreyi* causes a chronic limb ulceration syndrome that is not sexually transmitted and occurs primarily in children.[3] Close contact with family members with ulcers is implicated in these cases. In a cohort study done in yaws-endemic villages in Papua New Guinea, the prevalence of this syndrome is 3.2 cases per 100 persons. *H. ducreyi, Treponema pallidum* subspecies *pertenue*, and dual infections accounted for 58%, 26%, and 16% of the ulcers, respectively. The overall prevalence of *H. ducreyi* infection in children aged 5 to 15 years is an astoundingly high 7%. Similar data are emerging from other yaws-endemic areas.[4]

DIAGNOSIS

Diagnosis requires either a positive culture or a polymerase chain reaction (PCR) test. In research settings, PCR has a resolved sensitivity of 95 to 98% and a specificity of 99% for *H. ducreyi*. In comparison, the sensitivity for culture is approximately 75%, but clinical diagnosis is neither sensitive (range, 50 to 75%) nor specific (range, 50 to 75%). Unfortunately, PCR-based tests are not commercially available.[5] Most sexually transmitted disease clinics do not routinely test patients for chancroid, and the diagnosis is typically made by the exclusion of genital herpes and syphilis. If patients with genital ulcers and lymphadenitis or treatment failure for primary syphilis appear in a community, public health authorities should be notified so that specific diagnostic testing can be initiated.

The differential diagnosis includes syphilis, genital herpes, lymphogranuloma venereum, and granuloma inguinale. Mixed infections with herpes simplex virus or syphilis are common, occurring in approximately 17% of chancroid cases diagnosed by PCR. Patients with suspected chancroid should be tested for genital herpes and have serologic tests for syphilis and HIV-1 and a dark-field examination.

TREATMENT Rx

Because of syndromic management, little is known about the current prevalence of antibiotic resistance in *H. ducreyi*, but most clinical isolates have had plasmid-mediated resistance to ampicillin, tetracyclines, and sulfonamides. The only reliable treatment regimens are macrolides, quinolones, and third-generation cephalosporins; there have been isolated reports of erythromycin and ciprofloxacin resistance. Owing to the propensity of *H. ducreyi* to acquire plasmids, the fact that some Enterobacteriaceae harbor plasmids that encode extended-spectrum β-lactamases and quinolone resistance is a concern. Current treatment recommendations include single-dose azithromycin 1 g orally or ceftriaxone 250 mg intramuscularly, ciprofloxacin 500 mg orally twice a day for 3 days, and erythromycin base 500 mg orally three times a day for 7 days.[6]

Repeated aspiration of buboes may be required to effect a cure. In a randomized study comparing repeated aspiration versus incision and drainage, incision and drainage was considered preferable. However, incision and drainage may cause excessive scarring, especially in persons of African descent, and should be avoided according to some experts.

Initial reports of coinfection with HIV infection and chancroid suggest that such individuals have a greater number of ulcers that do not heal as readily after antibiotic treatment compared with patients infected with *H. ducreyi* alone and that single-dose regimens may not be effective in this setting. Antibiotic treatment failure is also associated with lack of circumcision. If close follow-up cannot be ensured, most experts recommend multidose regimens in HIV seropositives.

PROGNOSIS

Clinical cure correlates with a reduction in pain and purulence and re-epithelialization of the ulcer within 7 days. Patients who do not show improvement within 7 days should be regarded as treatment failures and given an alternative agent. Even if *H. ducreyi* is eradicated, ulcers may persist if genital herpes or syphilis is present and not treated. Most ulcers heal in 2 weeks; large ulcers may take 4 weeks to heal.

PREVENTION

Circumcision protects against chancroid in men. Condoms are likely to be protective. Although several antigens that may afford protection in animal models have been identified, there is no vaccine. Contacts of patients with chancroid should be treated with an approved regimen.

GENERAL REFERENCES

For the General References and other additional features, please visit Expert Consult at https://expertconsult.inkling.com.

302

CHOLERA AND OTHER *VIBRIO* INFECTIONS

EDUARDO GOTUZZO AND CARLOS SEAS

CHOLERA

DEFINITION

Cholera is a feared epidemic diarrheal disease caused by *Vibrio cholerae* serogroup O1 and, since 1992, by the new serogroup O139. The disease is characterized by acute watery diarrhea. In its more severe form, a person may be severely dehydrated and in hypovolemic shock; the patient may die in a matter of a few hours after contracting the infection if treatment is not provided. Cholera is endemic today in Africa and Asia, and cases are also reported from Latin America, North America, and Europe. Seven pandemics have been registered in history since 1816; the most recent has lasted more than five decades since its recognition in Indonesia in 1961.

The Pathogen

V. cholerae is a curved gram-negative bacillus that belongs to the family Vibrionaceae and shares common characteristics with the family Enterobacteriaceae. *V. cholerae* O1 can be classified into three serotypes according to the presence of somatic antigens and into two biotypes, classic and El Tor, according to specific phenotypic characteristics. There is no evidence of different clinical spectra among the three serotypes of *V. cholerae*. The classic biotype, responsible for the first six pandemics of cholera, causes an approximately equal number of symptomatic and asymptomatic cases, whereas the El Tor biotype causes more asymptomatic infections. The classic biotype is confined to the south of Bangladesh, and the El Tor biotype is responsible for the current pandemic. The O139 serogroup is composed of a variety of genetically diverse strains, both toxigenic and nontoxigenic; it is genetically closer to El Tor *V. cholerae*.

EPIDEMIOLOGY

Cholera has both a predisposition to cause epidemics with pandemic potential and an ability to remain endemic in all affected areas. People of all ages are at risk to contract the infection in epidemic settings, whereas children older than 2 years are mainly affected in endemic areas. *V. cholerae* lives in riverine, brackish, and estuarine ecosystems, where both O1 and non-O1 strains coexist, with non-O1 and nontoxigenic O1 strains predominating over toxigenic O1 strains. In its natural environment, *V. cholerae* lives attached to algae or to crustacean shells and copepods, with which it coexists in a symbiotic manner. Several conditions, such as temperature, salinity, and availability of nutrients, determine the survival of *V. cholerae*; when these conditions are adverse, vibrios survive in a viable but nonculturable state. More recent data suggest that cholera phages modulate the abundance of *V. cholerae* in the environment and determine the beginning and end of epidemics. Phages may also play a role in the emergence of new *V. cholerae* serogroups by transferring genetic material to nontoxigenic strains.

From its aquatic environment, *V. cholerae* is introduced to humans through contamination of water sources and food. Once humans are infected, very high attack rates may take place, particularly in previously naïve populations.[1] Acquisition of the disease by drinking contaminated water from rivers, ponds, lakes, and even tube well sources has been documented. Drinking unboiled water, introducing hands into containers used to store drinking water, drinking beverages from street vendors, drinking beverages to which contaminated ice has been added, and drinking water outside the home are risk factors; these factors contributed to the acquisition of cholera during the large Peruvian epidemic of 1991. Drinking boiled water, acidic beverages, and carbonated water and using narrow-necked vessels for storing water are protective measures. Epidemics of cholera associated with the ingestion of leftover rice, raw fish, cooked crabs, seafood, raw oysters, and fresh vegetables and fruits have been documented. Person-to-person transmission is less likely to occur because a large inoculum is necessary to transmit disease. High transmission rates (approximately 50%) are reported among household contacts of patients with cholera in endemic areas.[1]

Epidemics of cholera tend to occur during the hot season. Factors affecting climate change and climate variability have an impact on the incidence of cholera. The El Niño–southern oscillation (ENSO), a periodic phenomenon representative of global climate variability, affects the transmission of cholera and vector-borne diseases. ENSO causes the warming of normally cool waters in the Pacific coastline of Peru, thereby promoting phytoplankton bloom, zooplankton bloom, and *V. cholerae* proliferation.

Some host factors are important in the transmission of cholera. The chronic gastritis associated with *Helicobacter pylori* predisposes to cholera by inducing hypochlorhydria, which reduces the ability of the stomach to contain the infection. An unexplained predisposition to severe disease in persons with the O blood group has been observed in Asia and more recently in Latin America. Thus, complex associations among climatic, seasonal, bacterial, and human factors affect cholera transmission. Although for the most part developing countries are affected by cholera, several developed countries, such as the United States, Canada, and Australia, have reported indigenous and imported cases.[2] The most recent epidemic occurred in Haiti in 2010. During the first 2 years of the epidemic, 604,634 cases were reported; the cumulative case-fatality rate was 1.2%.[3] Figure 302-1 shows the distribution of cholera in the world from 1990 to 2011.[4]

Number of cholera cases per continent

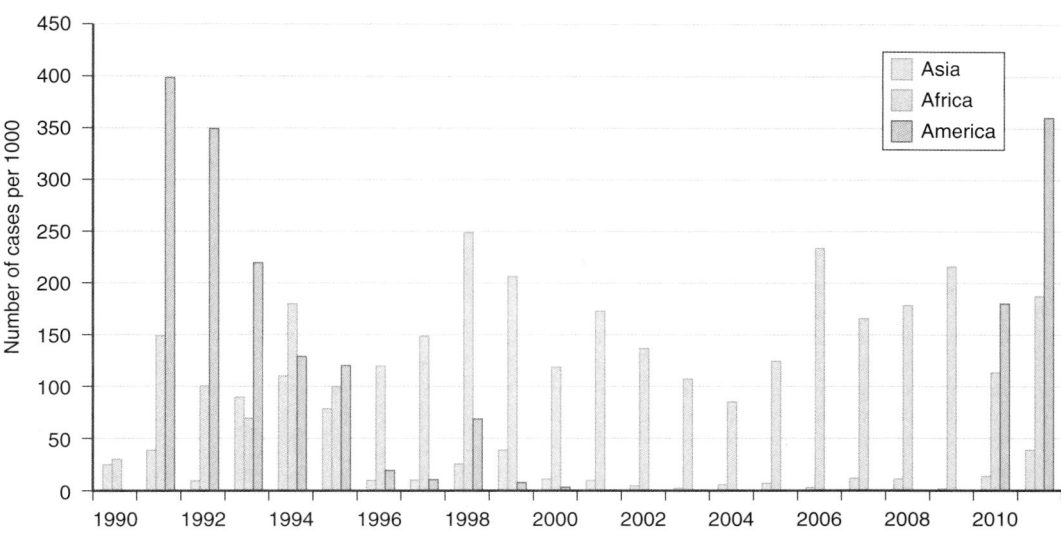

FIGURE 302-1. World distribution of cholera from 1990 to 2011 based on reports to the World Health Organization. (Reprinted with permission from the World Health Organization. Cholera, 2011. *Wkly Epidemiol Rec.* 2012;87:289-304.)

TABLE 302-1 ELECTROLYTE COMPOSITION OF CHOLERA STOOLS AND SOLUTIONS RECOMMENDED FOR TREATMENT

	Na$^+$	Cl$^-$	K$^+$	HCO$_3^-$	GLUCOSE	OSMOLARITY
Stools of adults with severe cholera	130	100	20	44		
Intravenous lactated Ringer solution	130	109	4	28*	0	271
Intravenous normal saline	154	154	0	0	0	308
Standard oral rehydration solution promoted by the WHO	90	80	20	10†	111	311
Reduced-osmolarity oral rehydration solution promoted by the WHO	75	65	20	10†	75	245
Rice-based oral rehydration solution	90	80	20	10†		270

*Lactated Ringer solution contains citrate instead of bicarbonate.
†Bicarbonate is replaced by trisodium citrate.
Glucose concentration is in mg/dL, electrolyte concentrations are in mEq/L, and osmolarity is in mOsm/L. WHO = Word Health Organization.
Modified with permission from Seas C, DuPont HL, Valdez LM, et al. Practical guidelines for the treatment of cholera. *Drugs.* 1996;51:966-973.

PATHOBIOLOGY

V. cholerae O1 and O139 cause clinical disease by secreting an enterotoxin that promotes the secretion of fluids and electrolytes by the small intestine. The infectious dose of bacteria varies with the vehicle. When water is the vehicle, more bacteria are needed to cause disease (10^3 to 10^6), but when the vehicle is food, lower amounts are needed (10^2 to 10^4). The incubation period varies from 12 to 72 hours; the median is 1.4 days.[5] Cholera toxin (CTX) has two subunits, a pentamer B subunit and a monomer A subunit. The B subunit allows binding of the toxin to a specific receptor, a ganglioside (GM$_1$) located on the surface of cells lining the mucosa along the intestine of humans and certain suckling mammals. The active, or A, subunit has two components, A1 and A2, linked by a disulfide bond. Activation of adenylate cyclase by the A1 component results in an increase in cyclic adenosine monophosphate in intestinal epithelial cells, which blocks the absorption of sodium and chloride by microvilli and promotes the secretion of chloride and water by crypt cells. These events lead to the production of watery diarrhea with electrolyte concentrations similar to those of plasma, as shown in Table 302-1. A few other toxins have been isolated from pathogenic *V. cholerae*, but their roles in genesis of the disease are less clear.

The genetic material of El Tor *V. cholerae* O1 is included in two circular chromosomes, the larger containing 3 megabases and the smaller containing 1.07 megabases. The main virulence genes are *ctxA* and *ctxB*, which encode CTX subunits A and B, respectively, and *tcpA*, which codes for toxin coregulated pilus. Regulation of expression of these genes is complex. Recent data suggest that vibrios are able to upregulate the expression of CTX in response to intestinal fluid components as well as in the presence of certain environmental factors. Genes unique to El Niño–southern oscillation (ENSO) *V. cholerae* may encode specific features that allow this biotype to better survive in the environment as well as to be more infectious to humans.

CLINICAL MANIFESTATIONS

Cholera is characterized by watery diarrhea and dehydration, which ranges from mild to severe and life-threatening. Patients with mild dehydration cannot be differentiated from those infected by other enteric pathogens causing watery diarrhea. In contrast, patients with severe dehydration secondary to cholera are easy to identify in that their stools have the appearance of rice water and no other clinical illness produces such severe dehydration as quickly (in a matter of a few hours) as cholera. Onset of the disease is abrupt and characterized by watery diarrhea, vomiting, generalized cramps, and oliguria. Physical examination shows a feeble pulse, fever is rarely present, patients look anxious and restless, the eyes are very sunken, mucous membranes are dry, the skin has lost its elasticity and when pinched retracts very slowly, the voice is almost nonaudible, and intestinal sounds are prominent. Although watery diarrhea is the hallmark of cholera, some patients do not have diarrhea but instead have abdominal distention and ileus, a relatively rare type of cholera called cholera sicca.

Laboratory findings in patients with severe dehydration consist of an increase in hematocrit, urine specific gravity, and total serum protein; azotemia; metabolic acidosis with a high anion gap; normal or low serum potassium levels; and normal or slightly low sodium and chloride levels. The calcium and magnesium content in plasma is high as a result of hemoconcentration. Leukocytosis is observed in patients with severe cholera. Hyperglycemia, caused by high concentrations of epinephrine, glucagon, and cortisol stimulated by hypovolemia, is more commonly seen than hypoglycemia. Acute renal failure is the most severe complication of cholera. Incidence rates of 10.6 cases per 1000 were reported in Peru during the first months of the

1991 epidemic. Patients with acute renal failure almost always have a history of improper rehydration. Cholera in pregnant women carries a poor prognosis. Pregnant women have more severe clinical illness, especially when the disease is acquired at the end of the pregnancy. Fetal loss occurs in as many as 50% of these pregnancies. Cholera in the elderly also carries a poor prognosis because of an increase in complications, particularly acute renal failure, severe metabolic acidosis, and pulmonary edema.

DIAGNOSIS

Chaotic movement under dark-field microscopy and a high number of bacteria in a stool sample from patients with diarrhea are characteristic of *V. cholerae* infection. Specific antisera against the serotype block the movement of vibrios and allow confirmation of the diagnosis. Under epidemic conditions, observing bacteria with a darting movement in a stool sample from a patient with suspected infection under dark-field microscopy is adequate to make the diagnosis. Definitive confirmation requires isolation of the bacterium in culture. Specific medium is needed to isolate *V. cholerae* from stool. Higher sensitivity and specificity have been reported with DNA amplification by polymerase chain reaction for detection of vibrios in stool and environmental samples.

TREATMENT   Rx

The objectives of therapy are to restore the fluid losses caused by diarrhea and vomiting, to correct the metabolic acidosis, to restore potassium deficits, and to replace continuous fluid losses.[6] Treatment of patients with milder forms of dehydration is easy, but treatment of patients with severe dehydration requires experience and proper training. The intravenous route should be restricted to patients with some dehydration who do not tolerate the oral route, those who purge more than 10 to 20 mL/kg/hour, and all patients with severe dehydration. Rehydration should be accomplished in two phases: the rehydration phase and the maintenance phase. The purpose of the rehydration phase is to restore normal intravascular volume, and it should last no longer than 4 hours. Intravenous fluids should be infused at a total volume of 100 mL/kg during the rehydration phase in severely dehydrated patients. Lactated Ringer solution is preferred, but other solutions may be used as well (see Table 302-1). All signs of dehydration should have disappeared and the patient should pass urine at a rate of 0.5 mL/kg/hour or greater after the rehydration phase is finished. The maintenance phase follows immediately. During this phase, the objective is to maintain normal hydration status by replacement of ongoing losses. The oral route is preferred during this phase, and the use of oral rehydration solutions is highly recommended. Oral rehydration therapy uses the principle of common transportation of solutes, electrolytes, and water by the intestine not affected by cholera toxin. People with diarrhea can undergo successful rehydration with simple solutions containing glucose and electrolytes. The World Health Organization recommends an oral rehydration solution with reduced osmolarity (245 mOsm/L) to treat all diarrheal diseases. This solution contains lower sodium than the standard oral rehydration solution promoted since 1975 (75 vs. 90 mEq/L). No more symptomatic hyponatremia is observed with the reduced-osmolarity solution than with the standard solution. The addition of L-histidine to rice-based oral rehydration solutions has been shown to reduce the volume and duration of diarrhea and the unscheduled use of intravenous therapy in adult cholera patients.[A1] Patients without severe dehydration who tolerate the oral route can be rehydrated with oral rehydration solutions exclusively and discharged promptly from the health center. Recommendations for treatment of cholera patients are shown in Table 302-2. Treatment of cholera caused by *V. cholerae* O139 is the same as described earlier.

Antimicrobial agents are not life-saving and always need to be accompanied by fluid therapy.[7] Effective antibiotics in patients with severe dehydration decrease the duration of diarrhea and the volume of stool by nearly half.[A2] Oral tetracycline and doxycycline are the agents of choice in areas of the globe where sensitive strains predominate. A single dose of doxycycline (300 mg) is the preferred regimen. Pregnant women can be treated with erythromycin or furazolidone. Because of the emergence of resistance to tetracyclines and other antimicrobials in many endemic areas, the quinolones and, more recently, azithromycin have been tested in clinical trials. A single-dose regimen of azithromycin (20 mg/kg) showed clinical and bacteriologic results that were comparable to a 3-day regimen with erythromycin in children and comparable to a single-dose regimen of ciprofloxacin (1 g) in adults.[A3] The addition of oral zinc (30 mg/day) to an erythromycin regimen in children reduced the duration of diarrhea by 12%, with an additional 11% reduction in the volume of diarrhea in comparison to placebo.[A4] Antimotility agents such as loperamide or diphenoxylate, adsorbents, analgesics, and antiemetics are not recommended. Antisecretory drugs, including racecadotril, an enkephalinase inhibitor, are not useful in patients with severe cholera. Chemoprophylaxis of household contacts of cholera cases is not routinely recommended.

PREVENTION

Access to potable water and ensuring proper management of excreta to avoid contamination of other water sources are important measures to reduce transmission of cholera. Alternative ways to prevent cholera transmission are necessary in developing countries. Water can be made safer to drink by boiling, adding chlorine, or filtering it with cloth made of cotton. An inability to implement these measures to curtail cholera transmission has prompted a search for vaccines. An ideal vaccine against cholera should elicit a fast and long-lasting immune response with minimal side effects. Parenteral vaccines are no longer recommended. Two oral vaccines, the two-dose regimen of the inactivated vaccine WC-BS (whole cell plus B subunit) and a single dose of the live attenuated CVD 103-HgR vaccine, have been tested extensively in epidemic settings and in field trials in endemic areas. Although the WC-BS vaccine showed good short-term protective efficacy (85% at 6 months), the results at 3 and 5 years were less impressive (60%), particularly in children. A large effectiveness study in Mozambique confirmed the high short-term protection against cholera (80%) by this vaccine, especially against severe dehydration (90%). In Guinea, oral vaccine was 87% protective.[8] In addition, reanalysis of data on this vaccine in field trials and in Zanzibar has shown that it may also confer herd protection in the unvaccinated population.[9] Cost-effectiveness of interventions like this require prices of the oral vaccine below 1.3 USD.[10] A large field trial of the live attenuated vaccine showed no protective efficacy. Indications for use of the currently available cholera vaccines include travel to endemic areas and situations in which high attack rates of cholera are expected, such as after environmental disasters, in refugee camps, and in urban slums in highly endemic areas. Preemptive and reactive vaccination approaches should be thoroughly evaluated in epidemic settings.[11] New oral vaccines, including both killed and live *Vibrio*, are being evaluated in endemic areas, with promising preliminary reports.

PROGNOSIS

Patients with severe cholera left untreated or improperly treated carry a poor prognosis, with mortality rates higher than 50%. However, case-fatality rates during epidemics may be reduced to values below 1% even in disaster situations, provided adequate access to health care centers and proper management of patients can be ensured. In contrast, figures higher than 10% have been reported in epidemic settings when patients had no access to health care or received improper treatment.

OTHER *VIBRIO* INFECTIONS

Noncholera vibrios have worldwide distribution and coexist in environments in which *V. cholerae* lives. They cause a spectrum of clinical syndromes, including acute diarrhea, soft tissue infections, and sepsis, especially in immunocompromised hosts. In the United States, 7700 cases of *Vibrio* infections

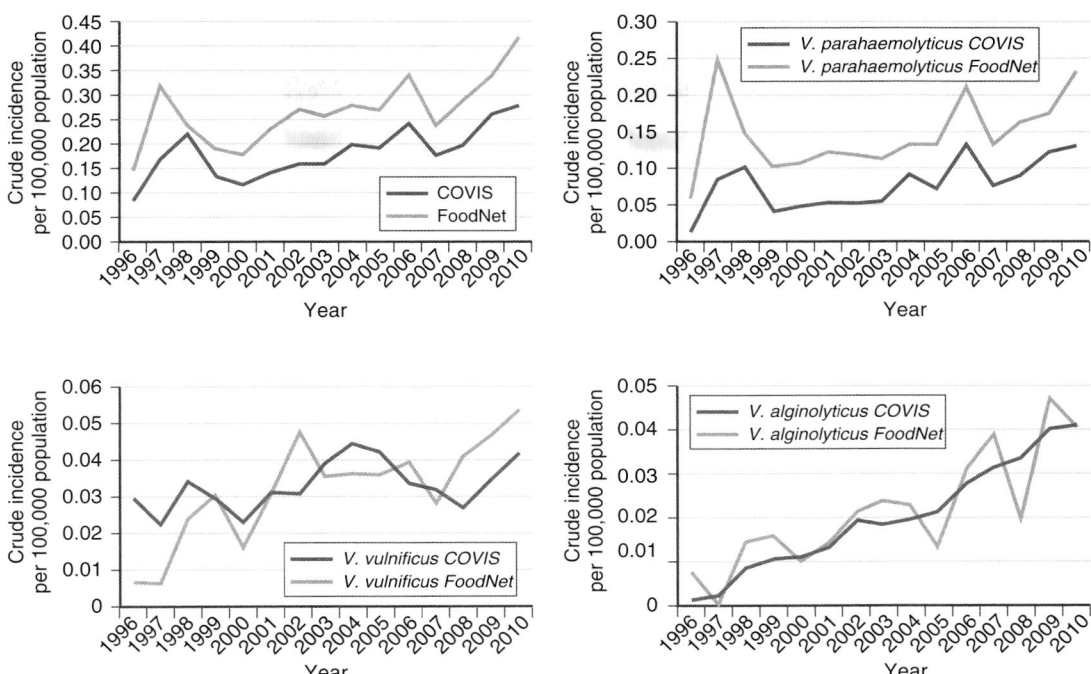

FIGURE 302-2. Crude incidence rates per 100,000 population of noncholera *Vibrio* infections based on two U.S. surveillance reports from 1996 to 2010. COVIS = Cholera and Other *Vibrio* Illness Surveillance; FoodNet = Foodborne Diseases Active Surveillance Network. (Redrawn from Newton A, Kendall M, Vugia DJ, et al. Increasing rates of vibrosis in the United States, 1996-2010: review of surveillance data from 2 systems. *Clin Infect Dis.* 2012;54[Suppl 5]:S391-S395.)

were reported by two surveillance networks covering the period from 1996 to 2010.[12] The incidence of *Vibrio* infection increased during the study period; *Vibrio parahaemolyticus* predominated (44.9% of isolates) but was associated with a low case-fatality rate of 0.7%. In contrast, *Vibrio vulnificus* accounted for 18.8% of the isolates but was associated with a case-fatality rate of 31.9%. *Vibrio* illnesses in the United States are seasonal and peak during the summer (Fig. 302-2). The incubation period for noncholeragenic *Vibrio* infection is usually 12 to 72 hours but can be as long as 1 week.

Nontoxigenic *V. cholerae* causes gastroenteritis, but unlike toxigenic *V. cholerae* O1 or O139, nontoxigenic *V. cholerae* does not cause epidemics. Illness ranges in severity from mild diarrhea to severe watery diarrhea. Fever and bloody diarrhea are unusual, but immunocompromised persons and those with liver disease can experience more severe illness, including fever, chills, and septic shock.

V. parahaemolyticus lives in marine environments and is a source of intestinal illness associated with the ingestion of contaminated shellfish. Certain serovars have shown pandemic spread (O3:K6 and O4:K68). It is not well known how this *Vibrio* causes infection in humans, but the clinical illness may mimic cholera, although most cases are milder and self-limited forms of acute watery diarrhea. Acute dysentery is reported rarely.

In the United States, *V. parahaemolyticus* and *V. vulnificus* as well as other noncholeragenic vibrios caused skin and soft tissue infections in victims and responders affected by the Gulf Coast hurricane disasters in fall 2005. *V. parahaemolyticus* wound infections are generally less severe than those caused by *V. vulnificus*.[13] However, in persons with liver disease or those who are immunocompromised, fatal infections can occur.

V. vulnificus is associated with wound infections in persons in contact with contaminated water as well as with primary sepsis in immunocompromised hosts. Wound infections follow trauma and are characterized by rapid progression of skin and soft tissue involvement, with necrosis and bulla formation occurring in more severe cases. Fever, chills, and sepsis syndrome may ensue rapidly. Primary sepsis with bacteremia and metastatic lesions on the skin, characterized by disseminated erythematous lesions that may evolve to necrotic lesions, is a distinctive clinical manifestation in patients with chronic liver illnesses, alcoholics, and patients with blood disorders such as thalassemia. A history of seafood ingestion, usually oysters, is typical. Patients are acutely ill with high fever and need to be managed aggressively with fluid resuscitation, surgical débridement, general supportive care, and antibiotic coverage. An intravenous combination of cefotaxime, 2 g four times a day, plus doxycycline, 100 mg two times a day, is recommended. This combina-

tion is synergistic in vitro. Alternative antimicrobials are ceftazidime and ciprofloxacin.

Grade A References

A1. Rabbani GH, Sack DA, Ahmed S, et al. Antidiarrheal effects of L-histidine supplemented rice-based oral rehydration solution in the treatment of male adults with severe cholera in Bangladesh: a double-blind, randomized trial. *J Infect Dis.* 2005;191:1507-1514.

A2. Leibovici-Weissman Y, Neuberger A, Bitterman R, et al. Antimicrobial drugs for treating cholera. *Cochrane Database Syst Rev.* 2014;6:CD008625.

A3. Saha D, Karim MM, Khan WA, et al. Single-dose azithromycin for the treatment of cholera in adults. *N Engl J Med.* 2006;354:2452-2462.

A4. Roy SK, Hossain MJ, Khatun W, et al. Zinc supplementation in children with cholera in Bangladesh: randomised controlled trial. *BMJ.* 2008;336:266-268.

GENERAL REFERENCES

For the General References and other additional features, please visit Expert Consult at https://expertconsult.inkling.com.

303

CAMPYLOBACTER INFECTIONS

BAN MISHU ALLOS

DEFINITION

Campylobacter jejuni is one of the most commonly recognized bacterial causes of diarrhea in developed and developing nations. More than 95% of campylobacters isolated in developed countries are *C. jejuni* or *Campylobacter coli.* However, other *Campylobacter* species are also associated with human disease.

The Pathogen

Campylobacters are motile, curved, gram-negative rods that are found in domestic and wild animals—especially poultry—all over the world. *C. jejuni* is microaerophilic, requires 3 to 15% oxygen for growth, and is oxidase and catalase positive. It grows best at 42° C; however, other *Campylobacter* species that may also be pathogenic grow best at 37° C. The whole genome sequences for multiple *Campylobacter* species have been determined.

EPIDEMIOLOGY

C. jejuni infections are endemic in young children in developing nations,[1] where they may be isolated in up to 20% of children younger than 5 years with diarrhea. In developed nations, *Campylobacter* infections are among the most common bacterial causes of diarrhea in children and adults. The incidence of *C. jejuni* infection in the United States fell by more than 30% from 21.7 per 100,000 population in 1998 to 12.7 in 2008, but by 2012 the incidence had increased again to its highest level since 2000. The actual burden of disease caused by *Campylobacter* is probably much higher because even active surveillance systems substantially underreport the true incidence of infection. Epidemiologic studies have estimated that more than 2 million people in the United States are infected with *C. jejuni* each year. For reasons that are not clear, the incidence is highest in western states, such as California and Hawaii. Similarly high rates of infection are observed in Europe. In the United States, Europe, and Australia, *C. jejuni* infections show a substantial peak in warmer months. Such seasonality is not observed in tropical developing countries, perhaps because of the absence of extreme temperature variations.

The incidence of *Campylobacter* infections is highest in early childhood, an epidemiologic feature common to many food-borne bacterial pathogens. However, in the United States and other industrialized countries, the incidence of *Campylobacter* infections peaks again in early adulthood. The incidence of infection is also higher in men, a gender difference most pronounced in young adults.

Most human *C. jejuni* infections occur sporadically, with only a tiny fraction occurring as part of outbreaks. The dominant source of sporadic infections in both developed and developing countries is consumption or handling of poultry. Other sources of transmission in developed nations include foreign travel, contact with pets and other animals, contaminated drinking water, and consumption of unpasteurized milk.[2] Cross-contamination within a kitchen (e.g., use of the same utensils or cutting boards to prepare uncooked chicken and to chop fruit) has led to a variety of foods being implicated as sources of human *C. jejuni* infection. In contrast to sporadic infections, the most common source of *C. jejuni* outbreaks is unpasteurized milk; large waterborne outbreaks occasionally occur. Transmission of *C. jejuni* infection from ill food handlers is uncommon. Even in households in which an individual has culture-proven *C. jejuni* gastroenteritis, secondary transmission to other family members is unusual.

PATHOBIOLOGY

Persons become infected with *C. jejuni* as a result of orally ingesting the organism, usually in food or water. Factors that affect whether *Campylobacter* infection leads to illness include the dose of bacteria ingested, the virulence of the organism, and the specific immunity of the host to the ingested organism.[3] The minimum number of bacteria needed to cause illness varies between people, but it may be quite low; because *C. jejuni* is susceptible to gastric acidity, ingestion of very few organisms may cause illness if gastric pH is elevated as a result of illness or medication. The median incubation period is 2 to 4 days, although it may range from 1 to 7 days.

In early infection, *C. jejuni* multiplies in the bile-rich upper intestines; subsequently, tissue injury is seen in the jejunum, ileum, and colon. Gross inspection of the bowel shows a diffuse, bloody, edematous enteritis. Microscopic examination shows an inflammatory infiltrate consisting of neutrophils, mononuclear cells, and eosinophils in the lamina propria. The mucosal epithelium is ulcerated, and crypt abscesses may be seen. The pathologic appearance is nonspecific and may mimic ulcerative colitis or Crohn's disease.

Invasion of the epithelium by *C. jejuni* appears to be central to its pathogenesis, and many factors influence how *C. jejuni* adheres to and invades intestinal tissues. A superficial conserved antigen, PEB1, appears to be a major adhesin and is a target of the immune response to *C. jejuni* infection. Other factors contributing to the invasiveness and pathogenicity of *C. jejuni* that may be encoded by a virulence plasmid include type IV secretion systems and mechanisms that disrupt microtubules in host cells. The presence of the plasmid pVir in clinical isolates is significantly associated with bloody stools. *C. jejuni* also may invade in an actin- and microtubule-independent manner. Glycolipids and glycoproteins on the surface of *C. jejuni* are important in the organism's survival in the intestinal lumen and in pathogenesis because they

have an impact on cell-to-cell interactions as well as on the host's immune response to infection. The bacteria's flagella facilitate its ability to colonize the gastrointestinal tract by promoting the organism's motility and chemotaxis. *C. jejuni* may produce extracellular toxins, but their role in pathogenesis has not been confirmed, with the possible exception of the cytoskeletal distending toxin (cdt), which may facilitate intracellular activities that lead to apoptosis.

Regardless of the organism's virulence, host factors are pivotal in affecting the clinical outcome of infection. In healthy volunteers fed a fixed dose of a single *C. jejuni* strain, a spectrum of illnesses develops. Patients infected with *C. jejuni* excrete the organism in feces for 2 to 3 weeks. In developing nations, where the level of immunity to *C. jejuni* is higher because of recurrent exposure, the period of convalescent excretion of *C. jejuni* is shorter.

After recovery from *Campylobacter* infection, at least short-term immunity develops. The decreasing illness-to-infection ratio with age seen in developing nations also suggests that individuals are acquiring immunity. Specific immunoglobulin A, G, and M antibodies in serum and immunoglobulin A antibodies in intestinal secretions develop in patients infected with *C. jejuni*. Patients with congenital or acquired hypogammaglobulinemia are at risk for severe or recurrent *C. jejuni* infections. Because the incidence of *C. jejuni* infection is markedly higher in persons infected with human immunodeficiency virus (HIV), cell-mediated immunity might also play a role in preventing and terminating infection.

CLINICAL MANIFESTATIONS

The clinical consequences of *Campylobacter* infection range from complete absence of symptoms to fulminant sepsis and death. In most cases, however, illnesses are brief and do not require hospitalization. In developed nations, detection of *C. jejuni* in the stool of asymptomatic persons is rare. However, in developing nations, where infections are endemic and recurrent infections occur frequently, asymptomatic infections are more common. In both developing and developed nations, persons infected with *C. jejuni* typically contract a diarrheal illness that resolves within a week. The case-fatality rate associated with this infection is low, about 0.05 death per 1000 infections, and is not surprisingly highest among the elderly and persons with comorbid conditions.

The gastroenteritis that is caused by infection with *C. jejuni* is clinically indistinguishable from that caused by other bacterial enteric pathogens, such as *Salmonella* (Chapter 308), *Shigella* (Chapter 309), or *Escherichia coli* O157:H7 (Chapter 304). The most common symptoms are diarrhea, malaise, fever, and abdominal pain (Table 303-1). Most patients with *C. jejuni* gastroenteritis experience at least 1 day with 10 or more stools; the diarrhea may be loose, watery, or bloody. Nausea is reported by some patients, but vomiting is less common. More than half the patients describe subjective fever. The abdominal cramping may be severe and is sometimes the predominant symptom. Although in most patients the symptoms resolve within 7 days, symptoms may persist in 10 to 20% of patients, and another 5 to 10% may experience a relapse.

Almost regardless of the nature of the symptoms, fecal leukocytes are found in 75% of infected patients; gross or occult blood is seen in 50%. Peripheral white blood cell counts may be elevated, but liver function test results, the hematocrit, and serum electrolyte values are usually normal.

TABLE 303-1	CLINICAL FEATURES OF *CAMPYLOBACTER* ENTERITIS DERIVED FROM OUTBREAKS IN WHICH MORE THAN 50 PATIENTS WERE INFECTED	
SYMPTOM	**MEDIAN FREQUENCY (%)**	**RANGE (%)**
Fever	50	6-75
Diarrhea	84	52-100
Headache	41	6-69
Abdominal pain	79	56-99
Myalgia	42	28-59
Vomiting	15	1-42
Blood in feces	15	0.5-32

Modified from Blaser MJ, Engberg J. Clinical aspects of *Campylobacter jejuni* and *Campylobacter coli* infections. In: Nachamkin I, Szymanski CM, Blaser MJ, eds. *Campylobacter.* 3rd ed. Washington, DC: ASM Press; 2008:99-121.

Sigmoidoscopic examination reveals diffuse colonic inflammation, which is nonspecific.

Local complications of *C. jejuni* gastroenteritis are rare. In its most severe form, infection may lead to massive gastrointestinal hemorrhage or toxic megacolon. Infection of the biliary tract may result in obstructive hepatitis, cholecystitis (Chapter 155), or pancreatitis (Chapter 144). Other reported local complications include peritonitis (Chapter 142), splenic rupture, and exacerbations of inflammatory colitis. Bacteremia is detected in 1.5 per 1000 intestinal infections, with higher rates in persons who are immunocompromised or elderly, but transient bacteremia may be more common because blood cultures are infrequently obtained in patients with diarrhea and the bacteria are killed rapidly by normal human serum. Other extraintestinal complications, such as meningitis, endocarditis, osteomyelitis, and purulent arthritis, are rare.

Guillain-Barré syndrome (Chapter 420), which is a postinfectious complication of *C. jejuni* infection, occurs about once in every 2000 infections; between 30 and 50% of all cases may be triggered by a preceding *C. jejuni* infection.[4] Because the onset of neurologic symptoms occurs about 1 to 3 weeks after the onset of gastrointestinal symptoms, cross-reactivity between antibodies formed against the lipopolysaccharide and capsule of *C. jejuni* and proteins in peripheral nerve myelin or other glycolipids in peripheral nerves is probably the cause. Certain *C. jejuni* serotypes (O type 19, O type 41) are overrepresented in patients in whom Guillain-Barré syndrome develops after culture-documented *C. jejuni* infection. Other postinfectious complications of *C. jejuni* infection include reactive arthritis (seen mostly in persons with HLA-B27 histocompatibility antigens), uveitis, hemolytic-uremic syndrome, erythema nodosum, encephalitis, carditis, hemolytic anemia, and chronic gastrointestinal consequences such as irritable bowel syndrome, inflammatory bowel disease, and celiac disease.[5]

DIAGNOSIS

The diagnosis of *C. jejuni* infection should be considered in any patient with an acute febrile diarrheal illness. The diagnosis is established by culturing the organism from stool or tissue. Primary isolation of *Campylobacter* species from blood may take up to 14 days.

The presence of curved gram-negative rods on a Gram stain of stool is specific but only 50 to 75% sensitive for detecting *C. jejuni*. Examination of fecal specimens by dark-field microscopy is useful if it is done within 2 hours of passage; the characteristic darting motility of *Campylobacter* provides a presumptive diagnosis. Serum serologic studies of stool are currently available only as research tools. Use of polymerase chain reaction techniques for direct detection of organisms has been successful in research studies but has not yet been applied to the general clinical setting.

Differential Diagnosis

In patients with acute colitis and bloody diarrhea, especially those whose symptoms last longer than 1 week, *Campylobacter* enteritis may be mistaken for ulcerative colitis or Crohn's disease (Chapter 141). In such cases, it is critical to exclude infectious colitis before starting immunosuppressive therapy. In patients with severe abdominal pain, appendicitis may be suspected and unnecessary appendectomy may result (Chapter 142).

PREVENTION

Because the most common source of transmission of *C. jejuni* infection to humans in developed countries is by consumption and handling of poultry, interrupting this route of infection will probably have the greatest effect on reducing the burden of disease caused by *Campylobacter*. The nearly universal colonization of poultry flocks with *C. jejuni* makes eradication of the organism in chickens unlikely, but improvements in slaughtering plants appear to be reducing the level of contamination of products reaching humans. For the consumer, careful food preparation methods are critical; chicken must be cooked thoroughly. To avoid cross-contamination in the kitchen, cutting boards, knives, and other utensils used to prepare raw chicken should be washed with hot soapy water before being used to prepare foods eaten uncooked, such as fruits and vegetables. Person-to-person transmission of *Campylobacter* is not common; nevertheless, all persons with diarrhea, especially those who handle food, should wash their hands after using the bathroom. Travelers and campers should be cautioned against drinking untreated water. Many outbreaks of *C. jejuni* infection might also be avoided if persons abstain from drinking unpasteurized milk. Antibiotic prophylaxis for travelers is not advised. An effective anti-*Campylobacter* vaccine has not yet been developed.

TREATMENT   Rx

As is true for most patients with infectious or noninfectious diarrhea, the most important principle of treatment of *Campylobacter* gastroenteritis is restoration of proper hydration and electrolyte balance, typically with oral fluids. On occasion, intravenous fluids are needed, especially in elderly patients or young children. Most *C. jejuni* infections are self-limited and resolve without specific antibiotic treatment. Furthermore, treatment with antibiotics shortens the duration of illness by less than 48 hours.[A1] Prompt antimicrobial therapy is indicated for patients with high fever (>38.5° C), prolonged illness (>1 week), bloody stools, or worsening symptoms and for those who have relapsed. Antimicrobial treatment is also warranted in the elderly, infants, pregnant women, and persons who are immunocompromised, including those infected with HIV.

For many decades, the antibiotic of choice for the treatment of *C. jejuni* gastroenteritis has been erythromycin (500 mg twice daily for 5 days). A single 1-g dose of azithromycin is at least as effective,[A2] but it and clarithromycin are considerably more expensive. One concern with erythromycin, which is primarily metabolized by CYP3A4, is the risk of sudden cardiac death. The risk is increased five-fold when erythromycin is given with medications that inhibit CYP3A4. In patients taking one or more of these medications, azithromycin may be substituted for erythromycin.

Fluoroquinolones, carbapenems, aminoglycosides, and clindamycin may also be effective, but resistance to quinolones is now common in many parts of the world.[6] In general, rates of resistance to ampicillin, amoxicillin, and cephalosporins are too high for them to be useful in the treatment of *C. jejuni* infections.

Critically ill or septic persons with *Campylobacter* infection may benefit from carbapenems or aminoglycosides, agents to which campylobacters are exquisitely susceptible, with resistance rates consistently less than 1%. In contrast, persons with persistent or relapsing infection, especially those who are immunocompromised, may require prolonged use (sometimes months) of antibiotics. In the absence of continuing sepsis, oral agents may be used.

OTHER *CAMPYLOBACTER* SPECIES

Campylobacter fetus may cause systemic and diarrheal illnesses in compromised hosts and diarrheal illnesses in normal hosts.[7] Most *C. fetus* strains, unlike *C. jejuni*, are not susceptible to the lethal effect of normal human serum because they possess a protein capsule (S layer). In immunocompromised persons, *C. fetus* can cause extraintestinal illnesses such as bacteremia, vascular infections, and meningitis. *C. fetus* infection may also cause perinatal infection and fetal loss. Prolonged treatment with erythromycin plus either imipenem, meropenem, an aminoglycoside, or a third-generation cephalosporin is indicated for serious *C. fetus* infections.

Campylobacter upsaliensis may cause acute or chronic diarrhea in healthy or immunocompromised persons. The organism is frequently isolated from dogs with diarrhea, which could be a source for transmission to humans. Some *C. upsaliensis* strains are resistant to erythromycin, but most are susceptible to fluoroquinolones, doxycycline, third-generation cephalosporins, and amoxicillin-clavulanate.

Campylobacter hyointestinalis was first recognized as a cause of proliferative enteritis in swine; *Campylobacter lari* is most often cultured from gulls and other birds. Both organisms have now been identified as rare causes of watery diarrhea and abdominal cramping in immunocompetent children and adults. Most infected patients do not require antimicrobial therapy; all isolates studied in vitro have been susceptible to erythromycin.

Campylobacter concisus, long believed to be part of the microbiota of healthy persons, is now considered a possible cause of human gastrointestinal illness. An increasing body of evidence also has linked *C. concisus* infection with childhood Crohn's disease.

Helicobacter cinaedi and *Helicobacter fennelliae*, once called *Campylobacter*-like organisms, are causes of proctocolitis or enterocolitis and have also been reported to cause bacteremia in immunocompromised patients. The organisms are frequently resistant to erythromycin; fluoroquinolones are considered the treatment of choice in patients who require antimicrobial therapy. The organisms are also susceptible to third-generation cephalosporins, aminoglycosides, and carbapenems.

Other *Campylobacter* or related species that have been associated with human illness include *Campylobacter mucosalis*, *Campylobacter doylei*, *Campylobacter curvus*, *Campylobacter insulaenigrae*, *Campylobacter rectus*, *Campylobacter helveticus*, *Arcobacter butzleri*, and *Arcobacter cryaerophila*. Illnesses include diarrhea and localized infections, presumably as a result of transient bacteremia from intestinal sources. Recently identified *Campylobacter* species that may be clinically relevant include *Campylobacter ureolyticus*, *Campylobacter troglodytis*, *Campylobacter lari* subspecies *concheus*, and *Campylobacter peloridis*. New pathogenic species of *Campylobacter* are being identified with some regularity.

PROGNOSIS

Even in critically ill patients, 1 week of therapy is generally sufficient to eradicate infection. *Campylobacter* infections in HIV-positive patients may be more severe, persist, recur, and be antibiotic resistant. More severe and extraintestinal illness is also more likely to occur in patients with acquired or congenital hypogammaglobulinemia. Most *C. jejuni* gastrointestinal infections in pregnant women are mild and self-limited, with no severe consequences for the mother or baby. However, if bacteremia develops in the mother, placental infection and fetal death may ensue. Infection during the third trimester can also cause neonatal sepsis and death if the woman is excreting *Campylobacter* in her stool at the time of delivery.

Grade A References

A1. Ternhag A, Asikainen T, Giesecke J, et al. A meta-analysis on the effects of antibiotic treatment on duration of symptoms caused by infection with *Campylobacter* species. *Clin Infect Dis.* 2007;44: 696-700.

A2. Vukelic D, Trkulja V, Salkovic-Petrisic M. Single oral dose of azithromycin versus 5 days of oral erythromycin or no antibiotic in treatment of Campylobacter enterocolitis in children: a prospective randomized assessor-blind study. *J Pediatr Gastroenterol Nutr.* 2010;50:404-410.

GENERAL REFERENCES

For the General References and other additional features, please visit Expert Consult at https://expertconsult.inkling.com.

304

ESCHERICHIA COLI ENTERIC INFECTIONS

THEODORE S. STEINER

DEFINITION

Bacteria belonging to the species *Escherichia coli* are a normal component of the intestinal microbiota (Chapter 279). The majority of *E. coli* are harmless commensals, but specific isolates have acquired pathogenicity genes that enable them to cause diseases, including urinary tract infections, bacteremia, meningitis, and diarrheal illness. One particular challenge to the clinician and microbiology laboratory is how to distinguish these pathogenic *E. coli* from harmless commensal strains to better guide diagnosis and treatment.

Enteric infections caused by *E. coli* may involve the small intestine, colon, or both, depending on the organism's genetic codes for virulence traits. These virulence traits include a variety of toxins, adherence factors, and secreted mediators that work together to perturb host intestinal physiology. Specific combinations of these factors produce six major pathotypes of diarrheogenic *E. coli*: enterotoxigenic (ETEC), enteroinvasive (EIEC), enterohemorrhagic (EHEC), enteropathogenic (EPEC), enteroaggregative (EAEC), and diffusely adherent (DAEC). In addition, these pathotypes can overlap; for example, some strains can express Shiga-like toxins that are characteristic of EHEC without the usual associated adherence factors; these are collectively known as shigatoxigenic *E. coli* (STEC). Taken together, diarrheogenic *E. coli* not only constitute the major category of bacterial enteric pathogens but also provide important scientific models for the many ways in which enteric pathogens can cause disease.

The Pathogen

E. coli is a small catalase-positive, oxidase-negative, gram-negative bacillus in the family Enterobacteriaceae. It characteristically reduces nitrates, ferments glucose and usually lactose, and is either motile (with peritrichate flagella) or nonmotile. It exhibits a positive methyl red reaction and negative reactions with Voges-Proskauer, urease, phenylalanine deaminase, and citrate agents. *E. coli* is the predominant member of the Gammaproteobacteria in the intestinal tract of humans and other mammals, although it is greatly outnumbered by members of other bacterial phyla, which largely consist of strict anaerobes.

As with other gram-negative organisms, the lipopolysaccharide cell wall of *E. coli* contains immunostimulatory lipid A attached to a core oligosaccharide chain. Most *E. coli* have immunogenic carbohydrate chains known as O antigens attached to this core glycolipid to produce 173 O serogroups. There are also at least 56 distinct flagellar (H) antigens based on variable domains of the flagellin gene. Some 80 variably heat-labile capsular (K) antigens have also been described. These O, H, and K antigen combinations have allowed serotyping of thousands of different strains, which historically was the simplest way to distinguish them. Whereas serotypes are sometimes useful in identifying specific pathotypes of *E. coli*, there are numerous adherence, enterotoxic, cytotoxic, and invasiveness factors that may be gained or lost by a particular serotype because they are characteristically encoded on transmissible genetic elements such as plasmids or bacteriophages. It is these factors that convey disease pathotype because they allow colonization and perturbation of host intestinal physiology. Indeed, molecular analysis available during the past decade has shown that commensal and pathogenic *E. coli* cluster into phylogenetic groups that are often independent of O:H serotype. Nevertheless, relatively few O serogroups tend to predominate in the normal human colon (O groups 1, 2, 4, 6, 7, 8, 18, 25, 45, 75, and 81), whereas others (Table 304-1) tend to be associated with specific virulence traits and thus different types of pathogenesis in the intestine.

Well-established mechanisms of *E. coli* pathogenesis include secretion of enterotoxins (ETEC), *Shigella*-like tissue invasion (EIEC), and epithelial necrosis as a result of Shiga-like toxins (SLTs SLT-1/2 or Stx1/Stx2) causing food-borne hemorrhagic colitis (EHEC and STEC) (see Table 304-1). By comparison, the classically recognized EPEC serotypes are neither enterotoxigenic nor invasive but rather attach and efface the epithelium. Still other types of "enteroadherent" *E. coli* exhibit aggregating (EAEC) or diffuse adherence (DAEC) traits, and EAEC in particular is associated with prolonged diarrhea in children in tropical developing areas, in patients infected with human immunodeficiency virus (HIV), and in acute diarrhea in outbreak settings and travelers from developed areas.

EPIDEMIOLOGY

Part of the challenge in studying the epidemiology of enteric *E. coli* infections is that, with the exception of EHEC/STEC strains, they are not identified in routine microbiology procedures in most clinical laboratories. In addition, the diagnostic methodologies have evolved, making it difficult to compare older and more recent studies. Nevertheless, several clear epidemiologic patterns have been revealed. In addition, specific single-nucleotide polymorphisms in the lactoferrin, osteoprotegerin, CD14, and interleukin-8 genes are associated with traveler's diarrhea caused by ETEC, EAEC, or both.[1]

Enteric *E. coli* infections are acquired by the fecal-oral route, although the fecal sources and infectivity differ among the pathotypes. It is believed that a human reservoir is required for most recognized types of EPEC and ETEC, although domestic dogs and cats can also harbor human pathogenic strains.[2] Different ETEC strains can also be important veterinary pathogens, especially in calves and piglets, but the attachment and virulence traits of animal strains are different from those of strains that infect humans. The infectious dose of ETEC in volunteers is 10^6 to 10^{10} organisms, meaning that it usually requires multiplication in contaminated food or water vehicles for its transmission, rather than spreading directly from person to person. Heavy contamination with ETEC has been documented in foods prepared in homes and restaurants and by street vendors as well as in drinking water in many tropical areas. Contaminated water and food probably represent the major sources of their acquisition, primarily in warm or wet seasons.

As with most diarrheal illnesses, the highest age-specific attack rates of ETEC are found in young children, especially at the time of weaning, when ETEC accounts for anywhere from 3% to 39% (average, 13%) of acute diarrheal illnesses, depending on the population studied. Like immunologically inexperienced young children, a traveler visiting tropical areas has a 30 to 50% chance of acquiring traveler's diarrhea (Chapters 283 and 286) during a 2- to 3-week stay unless untreated water or ice and uncooked foods such as salads are strictly avoided. The most commonly recognized pathogen associated with traveler's diarrhea in most tropical areas of the world is ETEC that produces the heat-stable toxin STa, the heat-labile toxin LT, or both. A close second to ETEC as a cause of traveler's diarrhea is EAEC, now reported in 19 to 33% of affected travelers to India or Mexico.

Typical EPEC strains have been recognized primarily in poor urban areas, especially among hospitalized infants in their first year of life, with apparent

TABLE 304-1 DIFFERENT TYPES OF ENTERIC *ESCHERICHIA COLI* INFECTIONS

TYPE	MECHANISM	PREDOMINANT O SEROGROUPS	GENETIC CODE	DETECTION	CLINICAL SYNDROMES
ENTEROTOXIGENIC *E. COLI* (ETEC)					
Heat-labile toxin (LT)	Activates intestinal adenylate cyclase	6, 8, 11, 15, 20, 25, 27, 63, 80, 85, 139	Plasmid	Gene probe, PCR for LT	Watery diarrhea, traveler's diarrhea
Heat-stable toxin (STa: STh or STp)	Activates intestinal guanylate cyclase	12, 78, 115, 148, 149, 153, 155, 166, 167	Plasmid (transposon)	EIA, suckling mice, 6-hour ileal loop assay, gene probes, PCR	Watery diarrhea, traveler's diarrhea
ENTEROINVASIVE *E. COLI* (EIEC)					
	Cell invasion and spread	11, 28ac, 29, 124, 136, 144, 147, 152, 164, 167	Plasmid (140 MIa, pWR110)	Sereny test, gene probe, PCR for *ipaH*	Inflammatory dysentery
SHIGATOXIGENIC *E. COLI* (STEC)					
Enterohemorrhagic (EHEC)	Shiga-like toxins (SLTs/Stxs) and attaching/effacing ability	26, 39, 113, 121, 128, 139, 145, 157, occ 55, 111	SLT phages and adhesin plasmids; type III secretion system	EIA or PCR for SLT, serotype, cell adhesion with pedestal formation; Vero cell cytotoxicity; sorbitol agar; PCR for *eae*	Afebrile, bloody diarrhea; HUS in some cases
Non-EHEC STEC	SLTs only without attaching/ effacing	26, 111, 103, 121, 45, 104, 145	SLT phage; may possess other virulence traits (e.g., O104:H4 EAEC)	SLT EIA or PCR; negative for *eae*	Hemorrhagic colitis, HUS, or benign watery diarrhea
ENTEROADHERENT *E. COLI*					
Typical enteropathogenic (EPEC)	Attach, then efface the mucosa	55, 86, 111, 114, 119, 127, 142	Bundle-forming pili on plasmid and chromosomal LEE	Serotype, focal HEp2/HeLa cell adhesion, pedestal formation, gene probe or PCR *eae*	Infantile diarrhea in developing areas
Atypical enteropathogenic (EPEC)	Attaching and effacing but different microcolony formation	26, 55, 86, 111, 119, 125, 128	Possess the LEE but not bundle-forming pili	Gene probe or PCR for LEE; cell adherence (variable)	Infantile and animal diarrhea in developed areas
Enteroaggregative (EAEC)	Colonize in aggregates; toxins (EAST, Pet), biofilm formation	3, 15, 44, 51, 77, 78, 91	Plasmid (AA); chromosome (Pic/ ShET and type VI secretion)	HEp2 cell adherence; AA probe; PCR for *aggR* or other virulence genes; biofilm formation	Endemic persistent diarrhea, acute traveler's diarrhea, sporadic acute diarrhea
Diffusely adherent (DAEC)	Colonize (F 1845 afimbriate adhesin)	86, 75, 15	Chromosomal/plasmid	HEp2 cell adherence; DA gene probe/PCR	Persistent diarrhea in children >18 months old

AA = aggregative adherence; DA = diffuse adherence; EIA = enzyme immunoassay; HUS = hemolytic-uremic syndrome; LEE = locus of enterocyte effacement; PCR = polymerase chain reaction.

cross-infection in hospital nurseries. Although sporadic cases still occur, nosocomial outbreaks of EPEC diarrhea during the summer appear to have become less common and less severe in industrialized countries in the past few decades. "Atypical" EPEC strains lacking certain virulence factors have tended to predominate in developed areas but can be found in developing areas as well.[3]

EHEC frequently colonizes commercial livestock but does not infect them. EHEC (O157:H7 and others) infections were first attributed to eating undercooked hamburgers, but subsequent large outbreaks have been associated with contamination of unpasteurized apple juice, spinach, seed sprouts, and other vegetable items. Approximately 600 people were infected in a large outbreak caused by contamination of the domestic water supply in Walkerton, Ontario, in 2000. More recently, a 2011 outbreak of shigatoxigenic EAEC strain O104:H4 (ST/EAEC) associated with fenugreek sprouts sickened almost 4000 people in Europe.[4] In addition, the low infectious dose of EHEC O157:H7 means that person-to-person spread can occur, leading to secondary cases. Secondary cases of ST/EAEC O104:H4 may also have occurred but appear to be very rare. EHEC and STEC infections are especially alarming because of the risk of hemolytic-uremic syndrome (HUS) (Chapter 172). HUS can be fatal despite antimicrobial therapy, which in some instances may actually induce SLT production from bacteriophage carried within the organism and hence is generally not recommended. Patients who recover from HUS may also suffer chronic kidney injury as a result.

The natural reservoir of EAEC is not known, but outbreaks have been traced to contaminated food, and live organisms can be found in drinking water, table salsa, and other consumable items in endemic tropical areas. Volunteer studies demonstrated that a high infectious dose is required for acquisition of EAEC, suggesting that direct person-to-person spread may be difficult. In addition to its role in traveler's diarrhea, EAEC is an important cause of both acute diarrhea and persistent diarrhea and malnutrition, especially in children in tropical areas and in patients with HIV/AIDS. It was also shown in several studies to be a major cause of sporadic diarrhea in the United States and the United Kingdom.

Limited data on EIEC suggest that infectious doses are relatively high, but as with ETEC infections, adequate numbers of organisms have readily been spread in food with high attack rates in outbreak situations. This distinguishes EIEC epidemiologically from *Shigella*, which is easily spread person to person as well as in contaminated food and water.

DAEC remains the least well understood pathotype and has not consistently been found more often in diarrheal cases than in controls. Nevertheless, some studies have shown a clear association with acute diarrhea in developing areas, particularly in children 1 to 4 years of age. Part of the difficulty is the heterogeneity of strains, some of which express different types of adhesins and different groups of virulence traits, leading to inconsistent pathogenicity.

PATHOBIOLOGY

The pathogenesis of enteric *E. coli* infection begins with ingestion of the organism in contaminated food or water or rarely direct person-to-person spread, in the case of EHEC. It then faces the normal gastric acid barrier. Both ETEC and EIEC appear to be sensitive to gastric acid; neutralization of gastric acid reduces the infectious dose by 100- to 1000-fold. Hypochlorhydria increased the risk of EPEC diarrhea in a volunteer study. Whereas EHEC expresses acid tolerance factors that may facilitate its survival in the stomach, hypochlorhydria was shown to be a risk factor for HUS in one study.

After ingestion and passage through the stomach, enteric *E. coli* colonize the involved part of the intestinal tract using specialized adhesins and the coordinated expression of virulence traits. This can lead to toxin production, intracellular invasion, or other disruptions of host cell physiology. These virulence traits may be shared among different enteric *E. coli* as well as related enteric pathogens, and it is their combination that leads to the characteristic pathogenic and clinical features of infection. The incubation period between ingestion and symptom development varies from pathogen to pathogen. For example, it averaged 14 hours for EAEC and 2 days for ETEC in volunteer studies; epidemiologic studies found an average incubation period of 3 to 4 days for EHEC O157:H7 but 8 days for ST/EAEC O104:H4.

ETEC colonizes the upper portion of the small bowel using fimbriate or fibrillar surface proteins known as colonization factor antigens. The colonization factor antigens bind the organism to cell surface receptors on enterocytes. Whereas this colonization itself can lead to mild inflammatory changes in the epithelium, the majority of ETEC illness is due to its enterotoxins. LT, with a molecular weight of about 86,000, has a binding and active subunit and, like the closely related choleratoxin, binds to a monosialoganglioside (GM$_1$) receptor. Also like choleratoxin (Chapter 302), the active subunit is an enzyme that ADP-ribosylates the regulatory subunit of adenylate cyclase, leading to constitutive production of cyclic adenosine monophosphate. The consequently increased chloride secretion and reduced sodium absorption combine to cause net isotonic electrolyte loss that can be as great as 1 liter/hour. Other human ETEC strains produce heat-stable toxin (STa), which is a much smaller molecule than LT (18 to 19 amino acids) and activates intestinal particulate guanylate cyclase. Like cyclic adenosine monophosphate, the cyclic guanosine monophosphate thus formed also causes net secretion. The roles of other enterotoxins, such as LTII, EAST, EIET, and others seen in ETEC, EAEC, and EIEC, respectively, are unclear at present. Both the colonization traits and production of enterotoxin are encoded on transmissible plasmids. Besides the complications of dehydration, the only significant pathologic change with ETEC is depletion of mucus from intestinal goblet cells.

EIEC, like the closely related *Shigella*, can invade and multiply in epithelial cells, cause experimental conjunctivitis in guinea pigs (known as the Sereny test), and produce inflammatory colitis and dysenteric or bloody diarrhea. As seen with shigellosis, a striking inflammatory response occurs, with numerous polymorphonuclear leukocytes in stool. The colon shows patchy, acute inflammation in the mucosa and submucosa with focal denuding of the surface epithelium, usually without deeper invasion or systemic spread. Although epithelial cell invasiveness in both EIEC and *Shigella* appears to be encoded on a large 120- to 140-Md plasmid, several chromosomal determinants, including the O antigen, are crucial for full invasive virulence.

Typical EPEC strains are well-established causes of infantile diarrhea. They express both plasmid-encoded localized adherence to epithelial cells (through specialized bundle-forming pili) and chromosomally mediated attachment and effacement of microvilli. The latter is characterized by the formation of cellular pedestals that hold the bacteria intimately to the cell surface. These changes in the host epithelia are mediated through protein effectors injected directly into host cells by a specialized type III secretion system encoded on the chromosomal locus of enterocyte effacement. These secreted effectors cause cellular changes that lead to villous atrophy, mucosal thinning, inflammation in the lamina propria, and variable crypt cell hyperplasia. These morphologic changes are associated with a reduction in mucosal brush border enzymes and may contribute to the impaired absorptive function and diarrhea.[5] Atypical EPEC strains are generally defined as those expressing the locus of enterocyte effacement but not the bundle-forming pili; they maintain the ability to attach/efface and cause disease.

EHEC, most notably serotype O157:H7 but also serogroups O26, O39, and others, cause type III secretion-dependent intimate adherence and microvillous effacement like EPEC, but they also produce SLTs that are responsible for the characteristic colonic mucosal disruption and hemorrhage as well as the complication of HUS. These toxins bind to the Gb3 surface ganglioside, leading to internalization and enzymatic inactivation of ribosomes, halting protein synthesis. Gb3 is highly expressed on vascular endothelial cells in the colon, kidney, and brain, which may explain the predilection for HUS to affect these organs. Organisms that produce SLTs without intimate adherence and pedestal formation are known as STEC or VTEC (Shiga-toxigenic or verotoxigenic *E. coli*), and often they lack the other virulence traits necessary for colonization and disease production. A notable exception was the ST/EAEC O104:H4 that caused the 2011 European outbreak; this strain was essentially an EAEC that also expressed SLT. The terms EHEC, STEC, and VTEC were often used interchangeably in the older literature, until the important role of the attaching/effacing ability of true EHEC strains like O157:H7 was understood.

EAEC is defined by a characteristic aggregative adherence pattern to cells and the substrata associated with biofilm formation. This adherence requires a large plasmid known as the AA plasmid, which encodes specialized aggregative adherence fimbriae and other virulence genes, including a serine protease autotransporter toxin known as Pet and an antiaggregative protein called dispersin. Chromosomal virulence traits include a mucinase, Pic, and a second enterotoxin, ShET, as well as type VI secretion systems. Limited studies on human infections with EAEC suggest that the organisms do not intimately adhere or invade but reside within a biofilm at the epithelial surface, where secreted factors contribute to a damaging host inflammatory response.

The fundamental pathogenesis of DAEC is still an area of active investigation but appears to depend on direct interactions between specialized adhesins (Afa/Dr) and host membrane proteins such as CD55 (decay-accelerating factor) or carcinoembryonic antigen. Many DAEC strains are closely related to uropathogenic *E. coli* with similar virulence traits. Some also express other virulence factors, including the serine protease autotransporter toxin SAT and a type III secretion system.

Host risk factors for diarrheogenic *E. coli* infection differ among the various bacterial pathotypes but in general include age, recent antibiotic use, and loss of gastric acid.

CLINICAL MANIFESTATIONS

The clinical manifestations of enteric *E. coli* infections differ among the pathotypes. ETEC infections generally produce watery diarrhea, particularly in young children and travelers to tropical or developing areas. Diarrhea may range from mild to severe and cholera-like; it may be life-threatening, especially in small children and elderly individuals, who are particularly prone to dehydration, undernutrition, and electrolyte imbalance (especially hypokalemia and acidosis). Other characteristic symptoms include malaise, abdominal cramping, anorexia, and occasionally nausea, vomiting, or low-grade fever. The illness is generally self-limited to 1 to 5 days and rarely extends beyond 10 to 14 days. Infections with ETEC that produce both ST and LT or ST alone may be more severe than those caused by ETEC that produce only LT. The persistence of impaired mucosal absorptive capacity for 1 to 3 weeks may further compound the cycle of malnutrition that complicates diarrheal illnesses in children in developing, tropical areas.

Infection with EIEC is characterized by inflammatory colitis, often with abdominal pain, high fever, tenesmus, and bloody or dysenteric diarrhea, essentially like that seen with *Shigella*. The incubation period is usually 1 to 3 days, with the duration generally self-limited to 7 to 10 days.

Outbreaks of EPEC infection in newborn nurseries have ranged from mild transient diarrhea to severe and rapidly fatal diarrheal illnesses, especially in premature or otherwise compromised infants. The more severe illnesses appear to have been more common in industrialized countries before 1950. However, more recent outbreaks and sporadic cases are well documented.

Hemorrhagic colitis associated with EHEC classically begins with watery diarrhea that quickly turns grossly bloody, with a conspicuous absence of fever or inflammatory exudate in stool but with significant abdominal pain. Although this diarrheal illness is self-limited, potentially fatal HUS or thrombotic thrombocytopenic purpura subsequently develops in a significant number of children and older adults (Chapter 172). Outbreaks of hemorrhagic colitis secondary to EHEC in nursing homes or other institutions may be common and severe. The incubation period in two outbreaks has been 3 to 4 days (range, 1 to 7 days), and the illness is characteristically self-limited to 5 to 12 days (mean, 7.8 days). The clinical manifestations in the ST/EAEC O104:H4 outbreak were similar, although rates of HUS were significantly higher (more than 20%) and women were disproportionately affected.[6]

EAEC has been associated with persistent diarrhea and malnutrition in children in developing areas, in HIV/AIDS patients, and in travelers who experience diarrhea (especially those genetically predisposed to greater inflammatory responses). No characteristic clinical features of EAEC have been consistently identified, although some outbreaks were associated with bloody diarrhea and several studies suggest that elevated inflammatory markers in stool are fairly common. DAEC has also been associated with diarrhea with no particular identifying features in children older than 18 months.

DIAGNOSIS

With the exception of EHEC, definitive etiologic diagnosis of *E. coli* diarrhea requires documentation of a specific virulence trait or serotype, which requires specialized immunologic tests, tissue culture, animal bioassay, and molecular testing[7] that are usually available only in research and reference laboratories. Other than for EHEC, such tests are rarely cost-effective or clinically indicated, except in outbreak or research situations. Fortunately, a probable diagnosis can often be suspected by the clinical and epidemiologic setting.

EHEC O157:H7 can be identified with reasonable accuracy by culture on sorbitol-MacConkey agar to identify nonfermenting colonies. However, it has long been recommended that any stool sample with visible blood should also be tested specifically for SLTs by enzyme-linked immunosorbent assay, polymerase chain reaction, or other molecular methods, which can identify non-O157 serotypes and rare sorbitol-fermenting O157 strains.[8] Many experts recommend that all stools submitted for culture be tested in this way. In hemorrhagic colitis due to EHEC, sigmoidoscopy, which is rarely indicated, generally reveals only moderately hyperemic mucosa, and barium enema or CT scan may show a thumbprint pattern of segmental or diffuse colonic wall thickening. Some patients have superficial ulceration with mild neutrophil infiltration in the edematous submucosa. These changes are not pathognomonic.

Differential Diagnosis

Numerous other causes of diarrhea must be considered, depending on the clinical circumstances (Chapters 140 and 283). For example, self-limited, noninflammatory diarrhea in tropical, developing areas is most likely due to ETEC, EAEC, rotaviruses (young children), or noroviruses (older children and adults) (Chapter 380). Noninflammatory diarrhea in older children or adults in temperate areas is more likely to be due to noroviruses (Chapter 380). *Vibrio* infections (Chapter 302) are common in areas endemic for cholera or in any coastal area where inadequately cooked seafood may be eaten. If noninflammatory diarrhea persists beyond a week, especially with weight loss, other possibilities include *Giardia lamblia* (Chapter 351), *Cryptosporidium* (Chapter 350), *Cyclospora* (Chapter 353), and microsporidial infection (Chapter 353). In outbreaks of food poisoning, *Staphylococcus aureus* (Chapter 288), *Clostridium perfringens* (Chapter 296), and *Bacillus cereus* should be considered.

Inflammatory colitis with high fever and tenesmus as well as leukocytes, mucus, and blood in the stool may well be due to EIEC but should prompt a stool culture for more common invasive pathogens, such as *Campylobacter jejuni* (Chapter 303), *Shigella* (Chapter 309), *Salmonella* (Chapter 308), *Yersinia enterocolitica* (Chapter 312), or noncholera *Vibrio* (Chapter 302). Any patient with diarrhea and a history of recent antibiotic use, gastrointestinal surgery, or parturition should be screened for toxigenic *Clostridium difficile* (Chapter 296). EHEC should be strongly considered in any case of bloody diarrhea, particularly in the absence of fever; it is recommended that laboratories now routinely screen for this pathogen in all stool cultures, and they should automatically screen any grossly bloody samples. Ischemic colitis and cytomegalovirus colitis can mimic EHEC but should occur only in people at risk (vascular disease and immune compromise or inflammatory bowel disease, respectively)

TREATMENT Rx

As with all diarrheal illnesses, the primary treatment for most *E. coli* diarrhea is replacement and maintenance of water and electrolytes, usually with a simple oral rehydration solution that uses the intact, sodium-coupled glucose or amino acid absorption (or both) to replace the fluid losses.[9] Oral rehydration solution should be given ad libitum with free water, and in breast-fed infants, continued breast-feeding and early refeeding can compensate for the nutritional losses without an adverse effect on diarrhea output.[A1] Zinc supplementation is also recommended for diarrhea in children older than 6 months in developing areas where zinc deficiency is common as it significantly reduces diarrhea volume.[A2] The enkephalinase inhibitor racecadotril, which is available in Europe but not currently in North America, also reduces diarrheal volume in children with acute gastroenteritis and is as effective as loperamide in adults but less likely to cause constipation. Certain probiotic preparations have been shown in small studies to improve symptoms when they are added to oral rehydration solution in children with infectious diarrhea[A3] but are not yet universally recommended. Antimotility agents reduce the frequency of diarrheal stools but should not be used when fever or bloody diarrhea is present as they can increase the risk of mortality due to toxic megacolon or HUS. Bismuth subsalicylate may reduce symptoms in traveler's diarrhea but should be used with caution to avoid toxic doses of salicylate.[10]

Because most *E. coli* diarrhea is self-limited, the role of antimicrobial agents is debated and remains of secondary importance to rehydration. One situation in which treatment is generally favored is traveler's diarrhea (Chapter 286) because strong clinical studies have shown a benefit of antibiotics in reducing the duration of symptoms.[A4][A5] Unfortunately, rising antimicrobial resistance has narrowed the options for empirical therapy; currently, azithromycin, a fluoroquinolone, or rifaximin is recommended, with trimethoprim-sulfamethoxazole a somewhat less reliable alternative.[11] Antimicrobials are not recommended in EHEC infection because of the possibility of increasing the risk of HUS and a lack of evidence of efficacy.

PREVENTION

Prevention of most *E. coli* enteric infections is ultimately related to basic economic development, adequate sanitary facilities, and sufficient availability of safe water. In the interim, especially in areas where adequate water supplies and sanitary facilities are not available, measures such as exclusive breast-feeding for at least 6 to 12 months and hand hygiene reduce the likelihood of acquiring *E. coli* enteric infections. Simple, portable water filters to reduce bacterial contamination are also in development.

Travelers to developing or tropical areas should avoid drinking untreated or unboiled water or ice and eating uncooked fruits or vegetables that may have been washed with highly contaminated water. Although a number of antimicrobial agents are effective during short periods when taken prophylactically, their effectiveness is ultimately limited by rapidly emerging resistance to antimicrobial drugs as well as by the potential side effects of their indiscriminate, widespread use. For example, tetracycline resistance among ETEC is now common, and resistance to trimethoprim-sulfamethoxazole and fluoroquinolones is quickly emerging around the world. This, combined with the rapid effect of empirical antibiotics at the onset of diarrhea symptoms, has diminished enthusiasm for prophylactic antibiotics. Bismuth subsalicylate is modestly effective at preventing traveler's diarrhea, although with side effects. Another option is the killed *Vibrio cholerae*/cholera toxin B subunit vaccine (Dukoral), which provides transient, partial protection against ETEC in travelers and hence may somewhat reduce the incidence of traveler's diarrhea, although strong evidence is lacking.

Sporadic EHEC infections may be reduced by adequately cooking beef, especially hamburger, and by careful handwashing and other hygienic measures in daycare centers and nursing homes. Unfortunately, large outbreaks due to contaminated produce continue to occur and are frequently associated with items meant to be eaten raw (such as sprouts). A vaccine composed from type III secreted effectors of EHEC to reduce colonization of livestock (Econiche) is on the market but has not yet entered widespread use.

PROGNOSIS

The greatest concern with enteric *E. coli* infections in developed areas is EHEC/STEC-associated HUS, which develops in 3 to 7% of sporadic cases up to as high as 20% in outbreaks. Whereas most patients with HUS recover, they frequently require intensive medical care (including temporary hemodialysis), and as many as 30% of survivors have renal sequelae such as proteinuria, hypertension, reduced glomerular filtration rate, or, more rarely, dialysis dependence.[12]

On a global scale, the greatest impact of diarrheogenic *E. coli* is in children in poor, developing areas, who are prone to death from dehydration from these otherwise self-limited infections. Moreover, children who survive repeated episodes of infectious diarrhea (due to *E. coli* and other pathogens) may experience permanent deficits in growth and even cognitive development, the full impact of which remains unknown.[13]

Grade A References

A1. Gregorio GV, Dans LF, Silvestre MA. Early versus delayed refeeding for children with acute diarrhea. *Cochrane Database Syst Rev.* 2011;7:CD007296.

A2. Lazzerini M, Ronfani L. Oral zinc for treating diarrhoea in children. *Cochrane Database Syst Rev.* 2013;1:CD005436.

A3. Francavilla R, Lionetti E, Castellaneta S, et al. Randomised clinical trial: *Lactobacillus reuteri* DSM 17938 vs. placebo in children with acute diarrhoea—a double-blind study. *Aliment Pharmacol Ther.* 2012;36:363-369.

A4. Taylor DN, Bourgeois AL, Ericsson CD, et al. A randomized, double-blind, multicenter study of rifaximin compared with placebo and with ciprofloxacin in the treatment of travelers' diarrhea. *Am J Trop Med Hyg.* 2006;74:1060-1066.

A5. Tribble DR, Sanders JW, Pang LW, et al. Traveler's diarrhea in Thailand: randomized, double-blind trial comparing single-dose and 3-day azithromycin-based regimens with a 3-day levofloxacin regimen. *Clin Infect Dis.* 2007;44:338-346.

GENERAL REFERENCES

For the General References and other additional features, please visit Expert Consult at https://expertconsult.inkling.com.

305

INFECTIONS DUE TO OTHER MEMBERS OF THE ENTEROBACTERIACEAE, INCLUDING MANAGEMENT OF MULTIDRUG-RESISTANT STRAINS

DAVID L. PATERSON

DEFINITION

The Enterobacteriaceae are a family of gram-negative bacilli that are responsible for a broad range of infections in humans and in animals. They may be motile or nonmotile, depending on the species. They are aerobic or facultatively anaerobic in growth and have a predilection for inhabiting the gastrointestinal tract. Only extra-gastrointestinal manifestations of disease are discussed in this chapter. Enteric infections caused by *Escherichia coli* are discussed in Chapter 304.

From a microbiologic perspective, the members of the Enterobacteriaceae ferment sugars. They grow on a variety of solid media and are usually readily identified by clinical microbiology laboratories. A number of subtleties arise in detection of antibiotic resistance mechanisms by laboratories, however, sometimes leading to issues in reporting of antibiotic susceptibilities. A worldwide trend is the development of multidrug resistance in all gram-negative bacilli, including the Enterobacteriaceae. Particular emphasis is placed in this chapter on treatment and prevention of these multidrug-resistant strains.

Medically important members of the Enterobacteriaceae are listed in Table 305-1. Infections due to *Salmonella*, *Shigella*, and *Yersinia* are discussed in Chapters 308, 309, and 312, respectively.

EPIDEMIOLOGY

The Enterobacteriaceae are among the most common pathogens to infect humans worldwide. They are responsible for community-acquired, hospital-acquired, and health care–associated infections. Examples of the last category include infections acquired in nursing homes and those associated with outpatient management of cancers or hematologic malignant disease. As resident components of the flora of the gastrointestinal tract, isolates of Enterobacteriaceae may represent examples of colonization rather than true infection. This may apply to isolates from rectal swabs, urine, or respiratory secretions. In many hospitals, multidrug-resistant Enterobacteriaceae have become endemic, leading to substantial problems in the management of serious infections.[1]

E. coli is the most common cause of urinary tract infections (UTIs), accounting for more than 80% of isolates from urine in most clinical situations. Any of the remaining members of the Enterobacteriaceae can cause this infection; *Klebsiella* spp and *Proteus mirabilis* are among other common

TABLE 305-1 SELECTED MEDICALLY IMPORTANT MEMBERS OF THE FAMILY ENTEROBACTERIACEAE

GENUS	SOME IMPORTANT SPECIES
Enterobacter	*E. cloacae*
Escherichia	*E. coli*
Klebsiella	*K. pneumoniae, K. oxytoca*
Morganella	*M. morganii*
Plesiomonas	*P. shigelloides*
Proteus	*P. mirabilis, P. vulgaris*
Providencia	*P. stuartii*
Salmonella	*S. enterica*
Serratia	*S. marcescens*
Shigella	*S. sonnei*
Yersinia	*Y. pestis, Y. enterocolitica*

causes of UTI. *Providencia stuartii* is notable as a cause of UTI among chronically catheterized patients. The Enterobacteriaceae can cause uncomplicated UTI in healthy women as well as acute pyelonephritis and UTI complicating renal tract abnormalities or catheterization. The Enterobacteriaceae may colonize the urine or be found in contaminated, improperly collected samples.

Antibiotic-resistant, uropathogenic *E. coli* may spread clonally. In other words, *E. coli* isolates from multiple different people with UTI may be identical or closely related at a genetic level. Trimethoprim-sulfamethoxazole–resistant *E. coli* is notable for its spread in a clonal fashion in the United States (e.g., "clonal group A" and *E. coli* O15:K52:H1). A widely spread *E. coli* clone, defined by multilocus sequence typing as sequence type 131 (ST131), has been found to be associated with ciprofloxacin resistance and production of extended-spectrum β-lactamases (ESBLs).[2,3] This clone is typically associated with community-acquired UTI. It has been detected in every inhabited continent.

Given the niche of most Enterobacteriaceae in the gastrointestinal tract, it is not surprising that these bacteria are prominent as causes of peritonitis. *E. coli* ranks most common as a cause of both spontaneous bacterial peritonitis (occurring in cirrhotic patients) and bacterial peritonitis arising from visceral perforation. Pyogenic liver abscess and intra-abdominal abscess may also be due to *E. coli*. Other members of the Enterobacteriaceae may also cause these intra-abdominal infections, especially in patients with "tertiary" peritonitis occurring after prior surgery for intra-abdominal disease.

The Enterobacteriaceae may also be the causative pathogens of pneumonia. They are more frequently the cause of hospital- and health care–associated pneumonia than community-acquired pneumonia. *Klebsiella pneumoniae* was once renowned as a cause of community-acquired pneumonia in alcoholics but has declined in significance during the last few decades. One exception is the finding of community-acquired pneumonia, liver abscess, or meningitis in Asia due to highly mucoid strains of *K. pneumoniae*.[4] Hospital-acquired pneumonia due to the Enterobacteriaceae may be ventilator associated. The Enterobacteriaceae rank most common as causes of ventilator-associated pneumonia after *Staphylococcus aureus*, *Pseudomonas aeruginosa*, and *Acinetobacter baumannii*. The Enterobacteriaceae may also cause hospital-acquired pneumonia in non–mechanically ventilated patients, such as those with neurologic impairment from head injury or cerebrovascular accident.

Outbreaks of antibiotic-resistant *K. pneumoniae* infection in hospitals have been prominent for more than three decades. In the hospital setting, *K. pneumoniae* is usually the cause of peritonitis, pneumonia, or complicated UTI. Blood stream infection arising from these sites of infection, from vascular catheters, or in association with neutropenia may also occur. In the 1970s, outbreaks due to gentamicin-resistant strains occurred. In the 1980s and 1990s, hospital outbreaks of ESBL-producing *K. pneumoniae* became commonplace. Finally, in the last decade, *K. pneumoniae* carbapenemase (KPC)–producing *K. pneumoniae* became a substantial infection control issue. The KPC-producing organisms are discussed in detail in a subsequent section of this chapter.

PATHOBIOLOGY

The virulence factors associated with *E. coli* causing enteric infections are discussed in detail in Chapter 304. At least 40 different virulence genes have been described in *E. coli* causing extraintestinal infections. Among the virulence properties of these strains is the renowned ability of *E. coli* to adhere to uroepithelial cells. The ST131 *E. coli* clone is typically highly virulent. It belongs to "phylogenetic group" B2, which is known for extraintestinal pathogenic infections. In an evaluation of the ST131 clone, numerous extraintestinal virulence genes were found. Enterobacteriaceae other than *E. coli* also possess a number of virulence mechanisms, but it is beyond the scope of this chapter to describe these in detail.

Many Enterobacteriaceae are now multidrug resistant. Resistance of the Enterobacteriaceae to aminoglycosides is usually mediated by production of aminoglycoside-modifying enzymes. However, 16S ribosomal RNA methylation is a more recently described mechanism that results in resistance to gentamicin, tobramycin, and amikacin. Resistance of the Enterobacteriaceae to fluoroquinolones is a growing problem. In most areas, more than 20% of *E. coli* strains are resistant to fluoroquinolones. Resistance is usually mediated by mutations at target sites and is associated with the ST131 strain. Mechanisms such as efflux pump overexpression and expression of the plasmid-mediated *qnr* genes may also play a role in quinolone resistance. The mechanisms of resistance of the Enterobacteriaceae to β-lactam antibiotics are worthy of detailed description (Table 305-2).

TABLE 305-2	ANTIBIOTIC RESISTANCE ISSUES IN THE ENTEROBACTERIACEAE	
ORGANISM	**β-LACTAMASE**	**COMMENTS**
NARROW-SPECTRUM β-LACTAMASES		
Escherichia coli	TEM-1	Present in at least 40% of strains globally
Klebsiella pneumoniae	SHV-1	Universally found
EXTENDED-SPECTRUM β-LACTAMASES		
E. coli	CTX-M-15	International clone ST131
K. pneumoniae	SHV, TEM, CTX-M	Hospital outbreaks
AmpC β-LACTAMASES		
Enterobacter cloacae	AmpC	Universally found
E. coli	AmpC	Occasional plasmid-mediated strains
CARBAPENEMASES		
K. pneumoniae	KPC	Endemic in many parts of the United States
K. pneumoniae	NDM	Hospital outbreaks in India

Narrow-Spectrum β-Lactamases

Ampicillin was introduced into clinical practice in the early 1960s. Enterobacteriaceae, with genes encoding β-lactamases inherent to their chromosome, were found to be intrinsically resistant to this antibiotic. Examples of these include the production of the SHV-1 β-lactamase by *K. pneumoniae* and the AmpC β-lactamase by *Enterobacter cloacae*. Other Enterobacteriaceae (e.g., *E. coli*, *Proteus mirabilis*, or *Salmonella*) lacked substantial production of chromosomally encoded β-lactamase. However, within months of the release of ampicillin, a plasmid-mediated β-lactamase leading to resistance of *E. coli* to the antibiotic was discovered. This β-lactamase was coined the TEM β-lactamase, in honor of the patient (Temoneira) from whom the TEM β-lactamase–producing *E. coli* was first isolated. Plasmids encoding resistance to ampicillin have now become widespread, with at least 40% of *E. coli* in most parts of the world now being TEM β-lactamase producers.

Extended-Spectrum β-Lactamases

Third-generation cephalosporins (such as ceftriaxone) were active against Enterobacteriaceae producing narrow-spectrum β-lactamases. However, mutant genes encoding β-lactamases capable of inactivating third-generation cephalosporins were discovered in the 1980s. The genes encoding these β-lactamases were identical to TEM or SHV, except for point mutations that led to an altered amino acid sequence. The subsequent structural change led to an ability to hydrolyze and thus to inactivate third-generation cephalosporins. In view of the extended spectrum of antibiotic-hydrolyzing abilities compared with the parent TEM and SHV enzymes, these β-lactamases were coined extended-spectrum β-lactamases (ESBLs). In addition to the TEM and SHV types of ESBLs, many new types of ESBLs have now been described, most notably the CTX-M type.

Frequently, the ST131 *E. coli* clone produces a CTX-M type of ESBL (especially CTX-M-15). Although ESBLs are typically susceptible to β-lactamase inhibitors (e.g., clavulanic acid), many ST131 *E. coli* isolates produce an additional β-lactamase (OXA-1) that confers resistance to β-lactamase inhibitors. The antibiotic resistance phenotype of the ST131-positive *E. coli* is that the organisms are typically resistant to ceftriaxone, cefotaxime, fluoroquinolones, trimethoprim, trimethoprim-sulfamethoxazole, penicillin–β-lactamase inhibitor combinations, and tetracyclines. Resistance to aminoglycosides is variable. The clone confers multidrug resistance by the presence of multiple antibiotic resistance genes. These are usually encoded on plasmids.

AmpC β-Lactamases

A number of genera within the Enterobacteriaceae have a chromosomally encoded β-lactamase capable of producing resistance to all penicillins and all cephalosporins except cefepime. In addition, these β-lactamases are not inhibited by β-lactamase inhibitors, such as clavulanic acid or tazobactam. These β-lactamases are known as AmpC β-lactamases. They are not derived from narrower-spectrum parent β-lactamases, so it is not correct to call these extended-spectrum β-lactamases. These AmpC β-lactamases may be overproduced in the presence of certain antibiotics (i.e., the genes encoding the AmpC β-lactamases are "inducible"). *Enterobacter* spp, *Citrobacter freundii*, *Serratia marcescens*, and *Morganella morganii* have inducible, chromosomally

encoded AmpC β-lactamases. The genes encoding these β-lactamases have now been found on plasmids in *E. coli*, *Salmonella*, and other gram-negative bacteria.

KPC, NDM, and Other Carbapenemases

In 2001, a novel carbapenem-hydrolyzing β-lactamase from a carbapenem-resistant strain of *K. pneumoniae* was first described. This enzyme was described as the *K. pneumoniae* carbapenemase (KPC). KPC-producing organisms are typically resistant to penicillins, cephalosporins, and carbapenems and are not inhibited by clavulanic acid or other commonly used β-lactamase inhibitors, such as sulbactam and tazobactam. KPC production has been documented in *E. coli* and in many genera of the Enterobacteriaceae, such as *Enterobacter*, *Citrobacter*, *Proteus*, and *Salmonella*.

The epicenter of KPC-producing *K. pneumoniae* has been New York City. By 2004, approximately one quarter of *K. pneumoniae* isolates in a surveillance study in Brooklyn, New York, were KPC producing. The Centers for Disease Control and Prevention now reports KPC-producing organisms in numerous cities across the United States. International spread of KPC-producing organisms has been well described, with outbreaks in Israel, Italy, and Greece being particularly problematic. Parts of China and South America have also reported endemic KPC-producing organisms.[5]

Another carbapenem-hydrolyzing β-lactamase, the New Delhi metallo-β-lactamase (NDM), has emerged in the last decade as a major cause of carbapenem resistance. As its name suggests, its epicenter is the Indian subcontinent. However, it has also been found to be endemic in some hospitals in the Balkan states as well as causing outbreaks in North America and Europe. Many outbreaks of NDM-producing organisms have been associated with interhospital transfers from hospitals in the Indian subcontinent.[6] Worryingly, NDM-producing organisms have been found in drinking water in India[7] and in food-producing animals in China.[8]

Other carbapenem-hydrolyzing β-lactamases include the OXA-48 type, which is found in North Africa, the Middle East, and India and has since spread to other parts of the world, as well as a variety of metallo-β-lactamases (such as of the IMP and VIM types). These enzymes have in common the ability to render Enterobacteriaceae resistant to carbapenems and other β-lactam antibiotics.

CLINICAL MANIFESTATIONS

The clinical manifestations of UTI, peritonitis, pneumonia, and blood stream infection due to the Enterobacteriaceae are described in other chapters.

DIAGNOSIS

Infection with the Enterobacteriaceae is readily diagnosed in clinical microbiology laboratories after collection of appropriate specimens. Examination of the Gram stain enables a rapid differentiation of gram-negative bacilli from other pathogens. However, it is frequently difficult on clinical grounds and by Gram stain results to differentiate infection with the Enterobacteriaceae from other gram-negative bacilli, such as *Pseudomonas aeruginosa*.

Once a member of the Enterobacteriaceae has been identified, it is important to ensure that appropriate antibiotic susceptibility testing has been performed. In some instances, specialized tests need to be performed by the clinical microbiology laboratory to detect ESBL or carbapenemase production. Molecular epidemiologic assessment may need to be undertaken to determine if an isolate belongs to an outbreak strain.

TREATMENT Rx

Treatment depends on the site of infection and the extent of antibiotic resistance. Empirical antibiotic choices for orally administered therapy for UTI due to *E. coli* and the other Enterobacteriaceae may include fluoroquinolones, trimethoprim-sulfamethoxazole, amoxicillin-clavulanate, and nitrofurantoin. *P. mirabilis* is resistant to nitrofurantoin. Empirical parenteral choices may include third-generation cephalosporins, penicillin–β-lactamase inhibitor combinations, aminoglycosides, fluoroquinolones, and carbapenems.

The advent of antibiotic resistance in the Enterobacteriaceae has the potential to have a huge impact on treatment of common infections. UTI is a pertinent example. Orally administered choices such as fluoroquinolones, trimethoprim-sulfamethoxazole, and amoxicillin-clavulanate are typically inactive in the ST131 *E. coli* strain. There may be a need to now admit some patients for parenteral antibiotics because of this antibiotic resistance. Worse still, some patients with hospital-acquired infection may need "last-line" antibiotics like colistin or polymyxin B. Specific details of treatment choices for antibiotic-resistant Enterobacteriaceae are given in Table 305-3.

TABLE 305-3 TREATMENT OPTIONS FOR MULTIPLY RESISTANT ENTEROBACTERIACEAE

ESBL PRODUCERS

Carbapenems (first choice, serious infections)
Piperacillin-tazobactam, cefepime (second choice, serious infections)
Nitrofurantoin, fosfomycin (first choice, UTI)
Ciprofloxacin, amoxicillin-clavulanate (second choice, UTI)

KPC OR NDM PRODUCERS

Colistin, polymyxin B, tigecycline, meropenem (as part of a combination)

ESBL = extended-spectrum β-lactamases; KPC = *K. pneumoniae* carbapenemase; NDM = New Delhi metallo-β-lactamase; UTI = urinary tract infection.

Treatment of ESBL-Producing Organisms

In vitro, the carbapenems (including imipenem, meropenem, doripenem, and ertapenem) have the most potent activity against ESBL-producing organisms. This is not surprising because these antibiotics are not inactivated by ESBLs. Carbapenems should be regarded as the drugs of choice for serious infections with ESBL-producing organisms on the basis of extensive positive clinical experience. No randomized trials have been completed comparing carbapenems with other antibiotic classes against ESBL producers. Although a substantial proportion of ESBL-producing organisms will be resistant to piperacillin-tazobactam, observational studies have shown a similar mortality from carbapenem-treated blood stream infections due to ESBL-producing compared with β-lactam/β-lactamase inhibitor–treated infections.[9] There is no evidence that combination therapy involving a carbapenem is superior to use of a carbapenem alone for ESBL producers.

Thus, meropenem or piperacillin-tazobactam is the treatment of choice for serious infections due to ESBL producers. The ability to use ertapenem once daily makes it potentially useful in serious infections with ESBL producers in nursing home residents or patients continuing parenteral therapy out of the hospital. UTIs may be treated with orally administered fosfomycin, nitrofurantoin, or amoxicillin-clavulanate if susceptible.

Treatment of Carbapenem-Resistant Organisms

Treatment of carbapenem-resistant organisms (e.g., due to KPC or NDM production) is difficult because they may lack susceptibility to all β-lactam antibiotics (including penicillins, cephalosporins, aztreonam, and carbapenems), fluoroquinolones, and aminoglycosides. Carbapenemase-producing organisms may sometimes appear susceptible to carbapenems such as meropenem and imipenem (although they are almost always recognized as resistant to ertapenem), but these antibiotics should not be relied on as monotherapy.

No randomized controlled trials have yet been performed evaluating different antibiotic options for carbapenemase producers. On the basis of observational studies, combination therapy appears to be superior to single-drug therapy. Combinations of a polymyxin, tigecycline, and meropenem have met with the greatest success.[10-12] Meropenem has been used in these combinations despite a lack of in vitro susceptibility.

A variety of new antibiotics with activity against ESBL producers and some carbapenemase producers are undergoing evaluation. These include the combination of ceftazidime and a novel β-lactamase inhibitor called avibactam and a new aminoglycoside, plazomicin. These appear to have significant activity against KPC producers. Unfortunately, avibactam does not inhibit NDM or other metallo-β-lactamases. Furthermore, plazomicin is not active against NDM producers because most exhibit aminoglycoside resistance by way of 16S ribosomal RNA methylation.

atic colonization with ESBL-, KPC-, or NDM-producing organisms without signs of overt infection. These patients represent an important reservoir of organisms. In some hospital wards with ongoing issues with ESBL, KPC, or NDM producers, more than 30% of patients have gastrointestinal tract colonization with these organisms at any one time. These patients should be nursed with use of contact precautions. Hand carriage by health care workers is usually eliminated by hand hygiene with alcohol-based agents. Compliance with contact isolation precautions and hand hygiene needs to be high to maximize the effectiveness of these interventions.

Changes in antibiotic policy may play a role in controlling outbreaks of ESBL, KPC, or NDM producers, but this concept remains controversial. In one reported outbreak of ESBL producers, no effort was made to change infection control procedures. Instead, at this hospital, ceftazidime use decreased and piperacillin-tazobactam was introduced into the formulary. This coincided with curtailment of the outbreak. In another institution, cephalosporins as an entire class were removed to exact control over endemic ESBL producers. The difficulty with this approach is that replacement of one antibiotic class with another may result in replacement of one antibiotic resistance issue with another. No study has demonstrated that removal of carbapenems from a hospital formulary leads to elimination of KPC or NDM producers. Because these organisms are resistant to multiple antibiotic classes, classes as diverse as β-lactam/β-lactamase inhibitor combinations and fluoroquinolones have been more commonly received than carbapenems before colonization or infection with KPC producers. Prudent use of all antibiotic classes with an emphasis on reducing duration of antibiotic use may be more useful than individual antibiotic class restriction.

PROGNOSIS

The prognosis of infection with the Enterobacteriaceae depends on multiple factors, such as site of infection, presence of underlying diseases, and adequacy of empirical antibiotic therapy. At one extreme, inadequate orally administered antibiotic therapy for uncomplicated UTI due to an ESBL producer may have no impact on mortality, although it may have an impact on duration of symptoms and need for parenteral therapy for treatment failure. At the other extreme, patients in an intensive care unit with serious infections due to KPC or NDM producers may have an in-hospital mortality rate exceeding 70%. This may compare with in-hospital mortality rates of 20 to 30% in comparable patients without infection due to a KPC or NDM producer.

GENERAL REFERENCES

For the General References and other additional features, please visit Expert Consult at https://expertconsult.inkling.com.

306

PSEUDOMONAS AND RELATED GRAM-NEGATIVE BACILLARY INFECTIONS

MATTHEW E. FALAGAS AND PETROS I. RAFAILIDIS

PREVENTION

Prevention of hospital-acquired outbreaks of ESBL, KPC, or NDM producers rests on a number of basic infection control principles. First, if a focus of infection exists in the hospital environment, it should be removed. Examples have included contamination of ultrasonography coupling gel and bronchoscopes. Outbreaks have been dramatically curtailed when these sources of contamination have been properly cleaned or removed from the hospital environment.

Present evidence suggests that transient carriage on the hands of health care workers is the most important means of transfer of ESBL-, KPC-, or NDM-producing Enterobacteriaceae from patient to patient. The hands of health care workers are presumably colonized by contact with the skin of patients with skin colonization of the organism or by contact with a contaminated environment around the patient. Many patients may have asympto-

DEFINITION

Infections due to *Pseudomonas* spp are caused by members of the family Pseudomonadaceae. The Pseudomonadaceae is a group of gram-negative rods, including *Pseudomonas aeruginosa*, the most frequently recovered human pathogen in the family. Other *Pseudomonas* spp include *Pseudomonas putida, Pseudomonas alcaligenes, Pseudomonas fluorescens, Pseudomonas luteola, Pseudomonas mendocina, Pseudomonas oryzihabitans, Pseudomonas pseudoalcaligenes, Pseudomonas stutzeri, Pseudomonas chlororaphis, Pseudomonas delafieldii, Pseudomonas kingii, Pseudomonas pertucinogena,* and *Pseudomonas* CDC group 1.

Related gram-negative bacillary infections include infections due to *Stenotrophomonas maltophilia* (formerly known as *Pseudomonas maltophilia* and *Xanthomonas maltophilia*) and members of the genus *Burkholderia* (*Burkholderia pseudomallei, Burkholderia mallei,* and *Burkholderia cepacia* complex).

The Pathogens

Pseudomonas aeruginosa is a gram-negative, lactose nonfermenting, straight or slightly curved rod with a length ranging from 1.5 to 7 μm and a width of 0.5 to 1.0 μm. It is catalase positive, oxidase positive, and motile with one or more polar flagella. Most species oxidize glucose and reduce nitrate to nitrite or nitrogen gas. It has the ability to grow at 42° C. This pathogen is admirably armed on its exterior: a polysaccharide capsule along with lipopolysaccharides, pili, and flagella. Furthermore, the interior arsenal includes toxins such as exotoxin A, pyocyanin (blue or blue-green pigment), pyorubin (red or red-brown pigment), pyomelanin (black pigment), and pyoverdin (yellow-green pigment). *P. aeruginosa* is notorious for its ability to acquire resistance genes and to spread by horizontal transfer.

Stenotrophomonas maltophilia is a gram-negative nonfermenting bacillus motile by polar flagella. It is also catalase positive; the majority of strains are oxidase negative, but some strains are oxidase positive. *Burkholderia cepacia* and *Burkholderia pseudomallei* are also motile gram-negative lactose nonfermenting bacteria. In contrast, *Burkholderia mallei* is nonmotile.

EPIDEMIOLOGY

P. aeruginosa is one of the most common pathogens in health care–associated infections. Ventilator-associated pneumonia, bacteremia associated with central venous catheters or secondary to infections present elsewhere in the body, urinary tract infections, and surgical site infections are the main types of infections associated with *P. aeruginosa* in the hospital setting. Data from the National Healthcare Safety Network at the Centers for Disease Control and Prevention indicate that during 2009 to 2010, *P. aeruginosa* was responsible for 8% of a total of 69,475 health care–associated infections and was the sixth most frequent culprit among 81,139 pathogens.[1] Approximately 2% of these strains are resistant to carbapenems, a powerful antibiotic against them. This organism is able to survive in environments that have only minimal nutritional components. *P. aeruginosa* can colonize moist surfaces of the axilla, ear, and perineum. It is also isolated from other moist, inanimate environments within the hospital, including water in sinks and drains, mechanical ventilation equipment, dialysis equipment, toilets, showers, hydrotherapy pools, mops, water for flowers, and even cleaning solutions.

Strains of *P. aeruginosa* resistant to multiple classes of antibiotics, including quinolones and β-lactams, are a major cause of morbidity and mortality worldwide. During a relatively short time, a multidrug-resistant *P. aeruginosa* strain spread through neighboring countries.[2] The use of broad-spectrum antibiotics is certainly a risk factor for the development of multidrug-resistant *P. aeruginosa*, as are deficiencies in infection control implementation.

A range of hosts are particularly prone to infections by this pathogen: patients with neutropenia, patients with burns, cystic fibrosis (CF) patients, cancer patients, transplant recipients, diabetics, and patients with AIDS. Patients with compromised immunity due to treatment or by the disease, either humoral (hypogammaglobulinemia) or cellular (steroid treatment), as well as patients with foreign bodies (e.g., vascular grafts, orthopedic implants) are also more vulnerable to *P. aeruginosa* infections.

Community-acquired *P. aeruginosa* infection is related to exposure to water by the use of hot tubs, whirlpools, swimming pools, spas, and other types of baths as well as to the use of contact lenses, particularly the extended-wear variety. Puncture wounds including those through tennis shoes can give rise to *P. aeruginosa* infection. *P. aeruginosa* endophthalmitis after eye trauma can result in visual compromise, and *P. aeruginosa* endocarditis is frequently found in intravenous injection drug users. In addition, there is the possibility for drug-resistant *P. aeruginosa* in the community, and this risk has to be taken into account in prescribing antibiotic therapy.

S. maltophilia, once thought to be of limited virulence, is a significant emerging pathogen.[3] It is an environmental gram-negative, multidrug-resistant organism that mainly causes pneumonia and acute exacerbation of chronic obstructive pulmonary disease. Bacteremia, urinary tract infection, skin and soft tissue infections including cellulitis, osteomyelitis, endocarditis, and meningitis are among the infections caused by *S. maltophilia*.

Once isolated in the geographic setting of Southeast Asia and Australia with an incidence of approximately 50/100,000 in the general population, infections due to *B. pseudomallei* are of special interest because they are reported now more frequently also from the Indian subcontinent.[4] Fortunately, infection due to *B. mallei* is rare in humans.

Burkholderia cepacia belongs to the *Burkholderia cepacia* complex, which includes also *Burkholderia ambifaria*, *Burkholderia anthina*, *Burkholderia arboris*, *Burkholderia cenocepacia*, *Burkholderia contaminans*, *Burkholderia*

diffusa, *Burkholderia dolosa*, *Burkholderia latens*, *Burkholderia lata*, *Burkholderia metallica*, *Burkholderia multivorans*, *Burkholderia pyrrocinia*, *Burkholderia seminalis*, *Burkholderia. stabilis*, *Burkholderia ubonensis*, and *Burkholderia vietnamiensis*. *B. cepacia* was previously reported under the name of *Pseudomonas cepacia*. *B. cepacia* infects mainly patients with CF and chronic granulomatous disease. However, there are many reports of *B. cepacia* infections in hospitalized patients without CF. Patients with central venous catheters, manipulation of the urogenital tract (catheterization, instrument insertion, and biopsy), burns, and wounds (surgical and other) may develop infection due to *B. cepacia*.

PATHOBIOLOGY

Pathogenesis and Pathophysiology

Innate immunity, primarily through inflammatory cytokine production and phagocytic clearance by neutrophils and macrophages, is the key to endogenous control of *P. aeruginosa* infection.[5] Patients with neutropenia and also patients in whom there are defects of recruitment and activation of polymorphonuclear neutrophils, such as those with CF, are susceptible to *P. aeruginosa* infections. This happens because the lipopolysaccharide of *P. aeruginosa* binds to the CF transmembrane conductance regulator (CFTR), which is a channel involved in chloride movement across the cell. When there is normal CFTR, release of interleukin-1 and signaling through the interleukin-1 receptor and adaptor molecule MyD88 occur. Furthermore, CFTR lipid rafts are formed and NF-κB is translocated, followed by transcription of NF-κB–dependent genes and the production of interleukin-6, interleukin-8, and intercellular adhesion molecule 1. After that follows the recruitment of polymorphonuclear neutrophils to infected tissue and the induction of apoptosis and resolution of infection. In the absence of MyD88, however, lethal pneumonia and sepsis can be induced by fewer than 60 bacterial cells applied to the noses of mice. Patients with CF have a defective CFTR and thus cannot mount a normal defensive response to *P. aeruginosa*. The major challenge has been to correlate the genetic defect leading to the synthesis of either no CFTR protein or dysfunctional CFTR to the pathogenesis of *P. aeruginosa* infection.

Other host factors that predispose to *Pseudomonas* infections are burns and wounds, especially necrotic tissue, and AIDS/HIV infection. In addition, loss of mucosal function of the tracheobronchial tree of mechanically ventilated patients and patients with cancer and disruption of the normal bacterial flora in the gastrointestinal tract are ideal settings for the growth of *P. aeruginosa*.

Bacterial Factors in Pathogenesis

P. aeruginosa is one of the ESKAPE (*Enterococcus faecium*, *Staphylococcus aureus*, *Klebsiella pneumoniae*, *Acinetobacter baumannii*, *Pseudomonas aeruginosa*, and *Enterobacter* species) group of bacteria that the Infectious Diseases Society of America has specifically addressed as a cause of concern. It survives in aquatic as well as in soil environments. Its armamentarium is vast and adaptable to the challenges faced, and its intraspecies but also interspecies communication in the microbial kingdom is noteworthy. Several factors including flagella, pili, exopolysaccharides, phospholipases, proteases, endotoxins, secreted toxins (types I, II, II, IV, and VI), exotoxins, and iron-binding proteins are involved in pathogenesis. Defensive weapons of *Pseudomonas* are the production of high levels of an extracellular mucoid polysaccharide called alginate, which is the main constituent of the glycocalyx allowing growth in a biofilm. Furthermore, the expression of O side chains on the bacterium's lipopolysaccharide prevents lysis by complement. Aggressive mediators to kill immune cells and to invade and degrade tissues are the toxins and enzymes produced by the bacterium. Exotoxin A, an adenosine diphosphate–ribosylating toxin, has activity similar to that of diphtheria. The production of this cellular toxin is affected by iron levels. *P. aeruginosa* uses pyoverdin and pyochelin, typical siderophore systems, to acquire iron.

P. aeruginosa can induce hemolysis by PlcHR, a hemolytic phospholipase C. A nonhemolytic phospholipase C, PlcN, is also made by *P. aeruginosa* strains. *P. aeruginosa* type III secretion systems allow direct injection of bacterial toxins into eukaryotic cells and disrupt cellular trafficking by inhibiting the actin cytoskeleton and by affecting protein synthesis. For *P. aeruginosa*, clinical isolates expressing type III toxins are isolated significantly more frequently from patients who have poor clinical outcomes. Four major effector proteins are known: ExoS, ExoT, ExoU, and ExoY. More than these factors, the ability of *Pseudomonas* to communicate with other members of its microbial community through quorum sensing leads to the formation of biofilms, a daunting obstacle in attempting to eradicate the pathogen. Quorum sensing systems of *Pseudomonas* are lasR1, rhlR1, and *Pseudomonas* quinolone system. These systems have a complex interaction with other factors in the context of regulation of gene transcription and production of virulence factors.

Both intrinsic (mutation-driven) and transferable (such as β-lactamase production) mechanisms confer *Pseudomonas* resistance to antibiotics, including carbapenems. Transferable resistance to aminoglycosides entails modification of aminoglycosides through phosphoryltransferases, acetyltransferases, nucleotidyltransferases, or ribosomal methyltransferases (RmtA, RmtB, RmtC, RmtD, and ArmA). Chromosomally encoded resistance involves the following:

- AmpC cephalosporinase overproduction or derepression;
- porin OprD, which facilitates diffusion of basic amino acids and carbapenems;
- class D oxacillinase (OXA-50); and
- efflux-mediated resistance through efflux pumps of the RND (resistance-nodulation-division) family, such as the MexXY, which among others affects fluoroquinolones, β-lactams, and aminoglycosides; MexAB-OprM and MexCD-OprJ, which among others affect fluoroquinolones and β-lactams; and MexEF-OprN (F), MexGHI-opmD (F), MexVW (F), and MexPQ-OpmE, which among others affect fluoroquinolones.

Chromosomally mediated resistance also is related to mutations in the quinolone resistance-determining region of gyrase A and the topoisomerase IV gene parC, which hamper the attack of fluoroquinolones on the bacterium. Aminoglycoside-inactivating enzymes are related to the *P. aeruginosa* chromosome and involve 3-*N*-aminoglycoside acetyltransferases [AAC(6)-I, AAC(6)-II, AAC(3)-I, AAC(3)-II, AAC(3)-III, AAC(3)-IV] or nucleotidyltransferases ANT(2)-I and ANT(4)-II and phosphotransferase APH(3)-VI. Impermeability resistance to aminoglycosides is also chromosomally mediated.

The production of such powerful enzymes as the metallo-β-lactamase (such as VIM-1, VIM-2, VIM-4, and IMP-29) is capable of destroying the carbapenem antibiotics, which are important for the treatment of patients with multidrug-resistant gram-negative bacteria. Furthermore, as reported in a study from French intensive care units,[6] additional intrinsic mechanisms may be present concurrently, such as the complete loss of porin OprD as a consequence of mutations or gene disruption by insertion sequences. Downregulation of OprD may be coupled with overexpression of efflux pumps (MexXY, MexEF-PprN, CzcCBA).

Pathology

The pathologic spectrum of *P. aeruginosa* infections depends on the site afflicted. Hemorrhage and necrosis may be present in severe *Pseudomonas* infections, such as in pneumonia and endocarditis. Notably, as regards the skin in the case of ecthyma gangrenosum, bacteria invade the arteries and veins of the skin, but there is little accompanying inflammation. This is reflected in the small quantity, if any, of pus present in these skin lesions. The pathology of *B. pseudomallei* infection is in sharp contrast, with intense inflammation leading to abscess formation and necrosis in the affected organs, as in the skin, liver, spleen, or lungs.

CLINICAL MANIFESTATIONS

A constellation of manifestations are included in the clinical spectrum of *P. aeruginosa* infections. There are no symptoms or signs to effectively discriminate *P. aeruginosa* infection from infections by other pathogens. Even ecthyma gangrenosum, which was once thought to represent a unique effect of *P. aeruginosa* infection, can be caused by other bacteria, such as *S. aureus* or *Citrobacter freundii*.

Febrile Neutropenia

P. aeruginosa infections during febrile neutropenia (Chapters 167 and 281) have a cardinal role. It is the organism against which empirical coverage must always be included. This principle remains unaltered in the span of time. The importance of *P. aeruginosa* infection in neutropenic patients has not diminished, and the antimicrobial resistance of the bacterium has evolved to a painstaking therapeutic challenge. Mortality is high if infection is not appropriately treated by empirical therapy. The classic clinical syndromes in febrile neutropenic patients are bacteremia, pneumonia, and soft tissue infection, mainly manifested as ecthyma gangrenosum.

Bacteremia

Bacteremia due to *P. aeruginosa* remains one of the most difficult challenges a physician may face. It is usually caused by primary infection at different sites, such as pneumonia, urinary tract infection, complicated intra-abdominal

tract infection (peritonitis, abscess), and endocarditis. Manifestations can include those of sepsis and septic shock, that is, fever, tachycardia, tachypnea, hypotension, and mental status changes ranging from confusion to coma (Chapter 108). Multiorgan failure with adult respiratory distress syndrome and acute renal failure along with coagulation defects (disseminated intravascular coagulation) may occur. In the ventilated patient, an increased index of suspicion for *P. aeruginosa* must be present in case of clinical deterioration.

Eye Infections

Keratitis is among the most frequent type of disease seen, and it is associated with contact lens wear, especially extended-wear lenses. However, any form of trauma may predispose to keratitis by direct inoculation into tissue, including surgery and burns. *P. aeruginosa* keratitis is a medical emergency because of the speed with which it can progress and lead to loss of vision. Pain and redness of the eye are cardinal manifestations of keratitis. The entire cornea is opacified, and sometimes perforation occurs.

Endophthalmitis is another fulminant *P. aeruginosa* eye infection that may result from penetrating injuries, surgery, perforation of a corneal ulcer, or seeding from bacteremia. Severe pain, chemosis, decreased visual acuity or even loss of vision, anterior uveitis, vitreous involvement, and panophthalmitis are manifestations of endophthalmitis.

Other rarer eye infections include orbital cellulitis in neutropenic patients and gangrene necrosis of the eyelids, both of which are metastatic foci of bacteremia.

Ear Infections

Acute otitis externa presenting with otalgia (ear pain) is commonly seen in children and results from infection of moist, macerated skin of the external ear canal. The source of the organism is likely to be hot tubs or swimming pools (swimmer's ear), particularly if they are not sufficiently chlorinated. The natural history is usually resolution without sequelae, but chronic drainage occurs in some patients. Chronic suppurative otitis media has been associated with *P. aeruginosa*. The main clinical manifestation is drainage of fluid. Cultures are usually polymicrobial, including *P. aeruginosa*. In a third of patients, it is found in isolation.

One of the most dramatic clinical manifestations of *Pseudomonas* infections is malignant otitis externa. The diagnosis is made easily as long as there is a high index of suspicion, which should be the case in diabetics and patients with AIDS. Although literally a misnomer (as this is not a cancerous process), the fulminant evolution to death if it is not diagnosed and treated appropriately justifies this nomenclature. It usually afflicts the diabetic patient and is manifested with pain in the ear accompanied by fever (not always), drainage, and nerve palsies that may even be bilateral. Traction of the pinna will elicit pain in the majority of patients. Most commonly, cranial nerves VI to XII (in various combinations) may be involved, and thus hoarseness and dysphagia accompanying facial paralysis may be evident. Mental status may be affected (obtundation, coma) and signifies intracranial spread of the infection. A characteristic of the disease is the presence of granulation tissue at the junction of bone and cartilage in the meatus, in contrast with the generally intact tympanic membrane. Culture specimens should be taken from the external auditory canal. Computed tomography or magnetic resonance imaging findings include temporomandibular joint destruction, infratemporal fossa or nasopharyngeal soft tissue involvement, and evidence of meningitis or empyema.

Ventilator-Associated Pneumonia and Health Care–Associated Pneumonia

The respiratory tract is among the most frequent sites of infection due to *P. aeruginosa*. This organism is a well-established and frequent cause of ventilator-associated pneumonia (VAP) and health care–associated pneumonia.[7] Identification of the bacterium as a culprit can be based on culture of endotracheal tube aspirates as well as bronchoalveolar lavage fluid in the corresponding clinical setting. Ventilator-associated tracheobronchitis is usually far from innocuous, and treatment is needed to avoid progression to the more severe VAP. Obviously, for the ventilated patient, the liberation of the patient from the mechanical ventilation when feasible is a key management issue. Even when only colonization of the tracheobronchial tree is thought to be present, a watchful and vigilant eye by the clinician has to be in place as the pathogen is notorious.

Pseudomonas necrotizing pneumonia is not uncommon, and its significance is reflected by the fact that the currently suggested 8 days of antimicrobial treatment for most microbial causes of VAP does not apply to VAP related to *P. aeruginosa*. The duration of treatment of VAP due to nonfermentative, gram-negative bacteria (such as *P. aeruginosa* and *A. baumannii*) has been proposed by the American Thoracic Society to be 14 days. Pneumonia due to *P. aeruginosa* can also be community acquired.

Chronic Respiratory Tract Infections

P. aeruginosa is responsible for chronic infections of the airways associated mainly with CF and chronic obstructive pulmonary disease. A description and management of *P. aeruginosa* infection in patients with CF can be found in Chapter 89. Patients with advanced chronic obstructive pulmonary disease may become infected by *P. aeruginosa* and present with an exacerbation.

Another chronic infection of the respiratory tract associated with *P. aeruginosa* is diffuse panbronchiolitis. Diffuse panbronchiolitis affects mainly Asian populations. Nevertheless, forms of this disease have also been reported in white, Hispanic, and African American patients. Criteria have been established for diagnosis of this disease[8]:

1. persistent cough, sputum and exertional dyspnea;
2. history of chronic paranasal sinusitis;
3. bilateral diffuse small nodular shadows on a plain chest radiograph or centrilobular micronodules on chest computed tomography images;
4. coarse crackles;
5. FEV_1/FVC <70% and PaO_2 <80 mm Hg; and
6. titer of cold hemagglutinin >64.

Criteria for definite diagnosis are a compilation of criteria 1 to 3 plus two criteria from criteria 4 to 6. *P. aeruginosa* is isolated in advanced stages of the disease. It shows similarities to CF in terms of respiratory tract involvement, but it is characterized by the lack of affliction of other systems (pancreas, genital tract). Furthermore, the amount of sputum produced is usually at least 50 to 100 mL/day, and the genetic background is different, with associations to HLA-Bw52 and HLA-A11 reported.

Bone and Joint Infections

P. aeruginosa is not a frequent cause of bone or joint infections (Chapter 272) in patients without foreign bodies. Such infections result from bacteremia, direct inoculation into bone, or spread from contiguous infection. Bacteremia secondary to either injection of contaminated illicit drugs or infective endocarditis in the population of intravenous drug users has been well documented to cause vertebral osteomyelitis and septic arthritis of the sternoclavicular joint. The clinical manifestations of vertebral *P. aeruginosa* osteomyelitis are more indolent than those of staphylococcal osteomyelitis. The duration of symptoms in the addict population with vertebral osteomyelitis is generally prolonged, ranging from weeks to months. Tenderness of the affected region has to be elicited, and there may be a decreased range of motion. Low-grade fever is more likely to be encountered than the high fever associated more classically with staphylococcal osteomyelitis. Sternoclavicular and sacroiliac septic arthritis from *P. aeruginosa* is seen almost exclusively in intravenous drug users. It may occur with or without endocarditis, but a primary site of infection is often not found. Its causative role seems to lag behind *S. aureus* in the affliction of the sternoclavicular joint. *P. aeruginosa* is also a cause of bone infections when medical material is present, such as that used in orthopedic surgery or neurosurgery.

Pseudomonas osteomyelitis of the foot most frequently follows puncture wounds through sneakers. The bacterium has been found between the rubber sole layers of sneakers in many cases. Most of these cases are reported in children, but it is also seen in adults. The main manifestation is pain in the foot, and there may be superficial cellulitis around the puncture wound and tenderness on deep palpation of the wound. Also, a group of patients that seems prone to *Pseudomonas* infections are those with Charcot's arthropathy. Prolonged hospital stay and more surgical operations are associated with *P. aeruginosa* secondary bone infection in patients with Charcot's arthropathy. *P. aeruginosa* also has the potential to affect the diabetic foot, especially when there is high local prevalence of the bacterium, warm climate, and frequent exposure to water.

Central Nervous System Infections

Involvement of the central nervous system is almost always secondary to a surgical procedure or penetrating head trauma and is rare after bacteremia. The entities seen most often are postoperative or post-traumatic meningitis, subdural empyema, and epidural infections resulting from initial contamination of access areas. Brain abscess secondary to embolic disease from endocarditis may be seen. Extension of the infection in necrotizing malignant otitis to the brain heralds an ominous clinical course. The cerebrospinal fluid profile of *P. aeruginosa* meningitis is that of pyogenic meningitis. Brain abscess

and epidural and subdural empyema generally require surgical drainage in addition to antibiotics.

Urinary Tract Infections

P. aeruginosa urinary tract infections usually occur as a complication of the presence of a foreign body, such as a catheter or stent in the urinary tract or an obstruction (mainly stone or malignant neoplasm) of the urinary system, or after instrumentation or surgery in the urinary tract. Notwithstanding the relationship between obstructive lesions and *P. aeruginosa* urinary tract infections, there have been descriptions of *P. aeruginosa* urinary tract infections in outpatient children and adults without relevant foreign bodies, stones, or other causes of evident obstruction. *P. aeruginosa* urinary tract infection frequently is associated with bacteremia.

Skin and Soft Tissue Infections, Including Burns

P. aeruginosa causes ecthyma gangrenosum in neutropenic patients. These are small, round lesions that occur either isolated or as aggregates. There is no skin site immune to their presence. More commonly, the limbs and the perineum are affected. The mouth may be involved as well. There is an evolution from vesicles to nodules that become hemorrhagic and necrotic and eventually ulcerate. Thus they best fit in the vesiculonodular type of skin lesion description. Secondary infection of chronic skin ulcers or burns can also occur. Maceration of normal skin, such as from soaking in a hot tub, can lead to superficial infection. Folliculitis and other papular or vesicular lesions have also been attributed to *P. aeruginosa*. Other types of skin and soft tissue involvement are cellulitis, abscesses, and myositis.

Burn wound infections by *P. aeruginosa* constitute one of the most significant problems caused by this organism. A distinct clinical picture of sepsis, in which high colony counts of *P. aeruginosa* exceed 10^5 organisms per gram of tissue, is the defining feature. Patients generally exhibit the progressive formation of a black necrotic eschar, with or without bacteremia. *P. aeruginosa* remains a major pathogen in settings in which burn patients have high rates of infection. The diagnosis may be made by culture of blood or by the pathognomonic clinical picture of an expanding burn lesion caused by infection with *P. aeruginosa*.

Endovascular Infections

P. aeruginosa may cause endovascular infections, including infective endocarditis, mainly of native valves but also of prosthetic ones. In intravenous drug users, the source is generally contaminated material, needles, or other paraphernalia; in this population, *P. aeruginosa* may even lead to outbreaks of endocarditis. The manifestations of *P. aeruginosa* endocarditis resemble those of other forms of acute endocarditis in addicts except that it appears to be more indolent than *S. aureus* endocarditis. *P. aeruginosa* endocarditis occurs also in non–intravenous injection drug users.

Gastrointestinal Infections

P. aeruginosa is a pathogen involved in complicated intra-abdominal infections,[9] usually as part of a polymicrobial infection. It is recovered in cases of secondary peritonitis, tertiary peritonitis, peritonitis associated with continuous ambulatory peritoneal dialysis, and intra-abdominal abscesses. Gastrointestinal infections due to *P. aeruginosa* include necrotizing enterocolitis in children and typhlitis in neutropenic patients (neutropenic enterocolitis).

Uncommon *P. aeruginosa* Infections

P. aeruginosa can cause a number of infrequently seen syndromes: noma neonatorum, a necrotizing mucosal and perianal infection of newborns; toe web infections; the "green nail syndrome" caused by *P. aeruginosa* paronychia as a result of diffusion of pyocyanin into the nail bed; and *Pseudomonas* hot-foot syndrome, which is manifested with tender plantar nodules. Shanghai fever is a sporadic community-acquired disease of previously healthy infants that is manifested as a necrotizing enteritis with fever and diarrhea and may lead to bowel perforation, seizures, and ecthyma gangrenosum. Laboratory parameters include leukopenia, thrombocytopenia, high C-reactive protein levels, coagulopathy, and hypoalbuminemia. The mortality is approximately 15%.

Infection due to *Pseudomonas* spp Other than *P. aeruginosa*

Infection due to other *Pseudomonas* spp may occur. *P. fluorescens* may lead to bacteremia associated with central venous catheters or transfusion-related bacteremia. Notably, a multistate outbreak due to contaminated heparinized saline flush occurred in the United States. Reports of *P. stutzeri* infections include peritonitis, meningitis, endocarditis, pneumonia, bacteremia, and endophthalmitis. *P. putida* has been reported as a causative pathogen in bacteremia, pneumonia, cholecystitis, cholangitis, and skin and soft tissue infections.

DIAGNOSIS

Diagnosis rests on the culture of the pathogen from various human biologic samples or fluids pertinent to the clinical presentation. Newer methods, including multiplex polymerase chain reaction tests, which are based on the detection of the bacterial DNA, have received clearance from the Food and Drug Administration (FDA) for use in clinical practice. They are especially of value in the setting of the intensive care unit, where speed is important in decreasing the mortality associated with delay in treatment of sepsis. Serology is not helpful in the diagnosis of *P. aeruginosa* infections. Pulsed-field gel electrophoresis, restriction fragment length polymorphism, multilocus sequence typing, and random amplified polymorphic DNA polymerase chain reaction are used mainly for epidemiologic purposes.

The differential diagnosis lies between *P. aeruginosa* and pathogens that can lead to the same spectrum of diseases, especially in the hospital environment. External otitis, infection after a nail injury, or infection after immersion in water can provide some important clues that narrow the differential diagnosis spectrum in their respective settings. Nevertheless, diagnostic considerations have to include other pathogens as well. For example, fungal otitis has to be included in the differential diagnosis of external otitis as well as of other causes of earache.

In addition, the specific population of patients (e.g., neutropenic patients, patients with burns and wounds, CF patients, patients who have medically inserted equipment or foreign bodies) should be considered to have a high pretest probability of having a *P. aeruginosa* infection. Other types of infection in the hospital environment necessitate coverage for *Pseudomonas* until microbiologic data are available either from cultures or from molecular tests detecting the bacterium's DNA. A de-escalation protocol can then be performed to narrow the antibiotic spectrum.

At times, clinical acumen has to differentiate frank infection due to *P. aeruginosa* from colonization mainly on the basis of local symptoms and signs (pain, erythema, necrosis, exudate, edema, loss of function, dysuric symptoms, productive cough) or systemic symptoms and signs (fever, hypotension, tachycardia, dyspnea, hypoxia, rash, organ failure, radiologic change of previous imaging) of infection.

TREATMENT   Rx

Treatment of *P. aeruginosa* Bacteremia

Guidelines from the Surviving Sepsis Campaign for patients with severe infections associated with respiratory failure and septic shock suggest combination therapy with an extended-spectrum β-lactam and either an aminoglycoside or a fluoroquinolone for *P. aeruginosa* bacteremia. Empirical combination therapy should not be administered for more than 3 to 5 days. De-escalation to the most appropriate single-agent therapy should be performed as soon as the susceptibility profile is known.[10] This recommendation is based on the higher possibility that at least one of the antibiotics used will have activity against the potentially multidrug-resistant pathogen. This recommendation is not based on better synergistic effect between the two antibiotics. Indeed, evidence-based data from meta-analyses suggest that a combination may not provide an advantage in terms of clinical outcomes, such as cure of the infection, or less emergence of resistance. Furthermore, a combination of a β-lactam and an aminoglycoside carries a higher rate of nephrotoxicity. There is therefore currently a trend that a β-lactam/β-lactamase inhibitor (piperacillin-tazobactam) or an antipseudomonal carbapenem (meropenem or imipenem-cilastatin) may be used alone as monotherapy without compromising patient outcomes. Nevertheless, monotherapy with an aminoglycoside is not suggested as it is associated with poor clinical outcomes. Local in vitro antimicrobial susceptibility data regarding the level of resistance of local clinical isolates of *P. aeruginosa* to various antibiotics have to be taken into consideration.[11]

Removal of an infected vascular catheter or another infected foreign device (urinary catheter, implant) may be needed to control device-related infection due to *P. aeruginosa*. Source control of an infection nidus (drainage of an abscess or empyema, excision of necrotic tissue) is also of paramount significance.

Depending on the antibiotic susceptibility of *P. aeruginosa* isolates routinely found in a specific setting, one of the following regimens would be appropriate for *P. aeruginosa* bacteremia, provided renal function as assessed by creatinine clearance is relatively normal (>50 to 60 mL/minute): intravenous piperacillin-tazobactam, 3.375 to 4.5 g every 6 to 8 hours; ceftazidime, 2 g

every 8 hours; cefepime, 2 g every 8 to 12 hours; meropenem, 1 to 2 g every 8 hours; imipenem, 0.5 to 1 g every 6 hours; doripenem, 0.5 g (1-hour infusion) every 8 hours; or aztreonam, 1.5 to 2 g every 6 to 8 hours (aztreonam has been used mainly for patients with β-lactam allergy). The addition of an aminoglycoside to the other regimens depends on the level of resistance to β-lactam antibiotics seen at any given institution. If administration of a second drug is indicated, amikacin 15 mg/kg every 24 hours may be added to the β-lactam antibiotic therapy. Addition of ciprofloxacin 400 mg every 8 to 12 hours IV (instead of an aminoglycoside) has been suggested to fare equally well.

Antibiotics that have to be considered on a compassionate basis if resistance to carbapenems with antipseudomonal spectrum is encountered include colistimethate sodium (polymyxin E or colistin parenteral form)[12] and polymyxin B. Two forms of colistin are commercially available: colistin sulfate and colistimethate sodium (also called colistin methanesulfonate, pentasodium colistimethanesulfate, and colistin sulfonyl methate). Colistimethate sodium is less potent than colistin sulfate. Specifically, activity as assessed biologically is 20,500 IU/mg for colistin sulfate and approximately 12,500 IU/mg for colistimethate sodium. Colistimethate sodium is produced by the reaction of colistin with formaldehyde and sodium bisulfite. Colistin sulfate is administered orally (tablets or syrup) in bowel decontamination regimens and topically as a powder for the treatment of bacterial skin infections. Colistimethate sodium is available in parenteral formulations. The term *colistin* throughout this chapter refers to the formulation of colistimethate sodium, except if otherwise specified.

The suggested dosage of intravenous colistin for adult patients with normal renal function is different for manufacturers in the United States and the United Kingdom. Specifically, recommended dosage in the United States is 2.5 to 5 mg/kg/day of colistin base activity (75,000 to 150,000 IU/kg), divided into two to four equal doses (1 mg of colistin base activity, ≈30,000 IU; 1 mg of colistimethate sodium activity, ≈12,500 IU). In the United Kingdom, the suggested dosage is 4 to 6 mg/kg/day of colistimethate sodium activity (50,000 to 75,000 IU/kg) in three divided doses for adults and children with body weight of 60 kg or less and 80 to 160 mg of colistimethate sodium activity (1 to 2 million IU) every 8 hours for body weight of more than 60 kg. However, we and others have treated patients with higher daily doses of intravenous colistin, up to 720 mg/day (9 million IU) in three divided doses. For serum creatinine level of 1.3 to 1.5 mg/dL, 1.6 to 2.5 mg/dL, or 2.6 mg/dL and higher, the dosage of intravenous colistin recommended by the manufacturers is 160 mg (2 million IU) every 12 hours, 24 hours, or 36 hours, respectively. During hemodialysis, the recommended dose is 80 mg (1 million IU) after each hemodialysis session. However, further studies are needed to better clarify the appropriate dosing regimens of colistin, especially for patients with renal dysfunction or failure. In a small study, on the basis of pharmacokinetic and pharmacodynamic data, a loading dose of intravenous 9 million IU of colistimethate sodium followed by 4.5 million IU every 12 hours was used successfully.[13] When dosing colistin, clinicians should be aware of the existing differences in dosage recommendations based on the specific formulation of colistin used. Lately, the parenteral formulation of fosfomycin sodium has been used in various European countries in combination with other antibiotics with an antipseudomonal spectrum.[14]

Another important consideration is the prolonged intravenous infusion of the antibiotics to exploit the pharmacodynamic properties of β-lactams in the treatment of *P. aeruginosa* and other infections. β-Lactam antibiotics have time-dependent antimicrobial activity, and thus their concentration in blood achieved by their prolonged intravenous administration is above the minimum inhibitory concentration for longer periods (proportion of the time between doses above minimum inhibitory concentration). There are data, mainly from nonrandomized studies and a relevant meta-analysis, that support the fact that a prolonged infusion of piperacillin-tazobactam during 4 hours may provide a survival benefit.[15] Meropenem is usually infused in a relatively short infusion of 30 minutes; an extended meropenem infusion is one that extends to 3 hours. Doripenem should not be used in pneumonia according to an FDA warning based on a study comparing it with imipenem-cilastatin.

Despite the introduction of new broad-spectrum antibiotics in the antibiotic arsenal, one should remember that ertapenem, ceftaroline, and tigecycline do not possess antipseudomonal activity.

Treatment of Pneumonia

The principles of treatment that apply to bacteremia are also the basis for treatment of pneumonia. Patients with nosocomial pneumonia may have *P. aeruginosa* isolates resistant to many antibiotics, a problem that appears to be becoming progressively worse. Provided renal and liver function is normal, the following recommendations have been made by the American Thoracic Society and the Infectious Diseases Society of America: IV ceftazidime, 2 g every 8 hours; cefepime, 1 to 2 g every 8 to 12 hours; imipenem, 500 mg every 6 hours or 1 g every 8 hours; meropenem, 1 g every 8 hours; or piperacillin-tazobactam, 4.5 g every 6 hours plus an aminoglycoside (amikacin 15 to 20 mg/kg once daily, with a trough level of less than 4 to 5 µg/mL for amikacin).

Aminoglycosides are not optimally active in the lungs at concentrations used for intravenous administration. The administration of aerosolized aminoglycoside may provide adequate drug levels in the tracheobronchial tree.

Tobramycin (300 mg inhaled daily) and inhaled aztreonam lysine (75 mg three times daily for 28 days) have shown safety and efficacy for CF patients and have FDA approval only in patients with CF. Another antibiotic that has been used in different parts of the world on a compassionate basis is the inhaled form of colistin. The effectiveness and safety of inhaled colistin in patients with CF have led to a revival of the use of the medication also in patients with *P. aeruginosa* infection in the critical care setting. Inhaled colistin does not have FDA approval.

Treatment of Other Infections

Standard therapy to treat meningitis due to *P. aeruginosa* includes ceftazidime or cefepime. Alternative therapies are aztreonam, ciprofloxacin, and meropenem; the addition of aminoglycosides to these alternatives should be considered as well. The duration of treatment extends to 3 weeks or 2 weeks after the first sterile cerebrospinal fluid culture. No antimicrobial agent has been approved by the FDA for intraventricular use, and the specific recommendations are not well defined. The daily intraventricular dose is 1 to 8 mg for gentamicin, 5 to 20 mg for tobramycin, 5 to 50 mg (usually 30 mg) for amikacin, 5 mg for polymyxin B, and 10 mg for colistin. The removal of all components of the infected shunt, in combination with appropriate antimicrobial therapy, appears to be the most effective treatment for cerebrospinal fluid shunt infections. The ventriculitis of the shunt infection appears to clear more rapidly with the drainage catheter still in place, and the presence of the catheter allows continued treatment of the hydrocephalus until the infection has cleared. Reshunting (placement of a new shunt) necessitates 10 to 14 days of sterile cerebrospinal fluid culture.

Formulations of aminoglycosides or fluoroquinolones for topical use are recommended for the treatment of keratitis. In cases in which involvement is extensive, ceftazidime or gentamicin may be given by subconjunctival injection. Therapy for endophthalmitis includes both systemic antibiotics at high doses to achieve better concentrations in the eye and intravitreal antibiotics. Ceftazidime has been the most frequently used antibiotic for this entity. Aminoglycosides are also injected subconjunctivally and by intraocular routes and sometimes given intravenously. Adjunctive surgery is generally performed to remove infected vitreous.

Management of otitis externa involves also the use of topical antibiotic agents (otic solutions). Protection of the ear from additional moisture and avoidance of further mechanical injury by scratching are also important. Aminoglycoside-containing otic solutions (neomycin plus polymyxin B and hydrocortisone) and quinolone-containing otic solutions (ciprofloxacin 0.2% or ofloxacin 0.3%) are the most frequently used. Gentle removal of debris and cleaning with a mixture of acetic acid, alcohol, and distilled water may also help. Chronically draining ears may require more intensive topical therapy.

Treatment of malignant external otitis involves débridement of the ear canal, including any necrotic tissue cartilage and adjacent bone, rather than extensive bone débridement or facial nerve decompression. Furthermore, treatment with ciprofloxacin or an antipseudomonal β-lactam (cephalosporin such as ceftazidime or cefepime, carbapenem, or monobactam) is necessary for a period of 6 to 8 weeks.

The majority of *P. aeruginosa* urinary tract infections are complicated. Urinary catheters, stents, or stones should be removed if possible to prevent relapse. In general, 7 to 10 days of antibiotic treatment will suffice, with up to 2 weeks for severe pyelonephritis. Quinolones (ciprofloxacin, levofloxacin) have the pharmacodynamic advantage of excellent concentrations in the urinary tract. Antipseudomonal β-lactam/β-lactamase inhibitors and carbapenems (doripenem is approved for the treatment of complicated and uncomplicated urinary tract infections and intra-abdominal infections) are equally acceptable, given their normally high levels of urinary excretion.

Management of *P. aeruginosa*–infected burn wounds is both surgical and medical. Extensive débridement of colonized eschar or necrotic tissue is required in addition to antibiotic treatment. Medical treatment follows the principles detailed in the bacteremia treatment section.

For treatment of chronic osteomyelitis due to *Pseudomonas*, ciprofloxacin has been used extensively. Experts infer that oral treatment is acceptable as an alternative to parenteral treatment.[16] Of note, an increased dosage of orally administered ciprofloxacin (750 mg twice a day) is used in the majority of the relevant studies. There are relatively few data regarding the appropriate duration of treatment. A duration of 6 to 12 weeks is most commonly reported.

Infections Caused by Organisms at One Time Classified as Pseudomonads

Most of these infections are due to members of the genus *Burkholderia*, including *B. cenocepacia*, a complex of about 10 related species previously referred to as genomovars that are phenotypically similar but distinguished primarily by nucleic acid sequences, as well as *B. mallei* and *B. pseudomallei*, causes of glanders and melioidosis, respectively.

S. maltophilia causes a variety of organ afflictions. It is manifested as pneumonia, acute exacerbation of chronic obstructive pulmonary disease, bacteremia, soft tissue and skin infection, cellulitis, myositis, osteomyelitis, catheter-related bacteremia or septicemia, meningitis, endophthalmitis, keratitis, scleritis, dacryocystitis, endocarditis, urinary tract infection, and biliary sepsis. One notices the commonalities with the clinical manifestations of *P.*

aeruginosa as well as the commonalities regarding the sources of infection. Whereas it has been regarded as a rare pathogen in the past, this is far from the truth. Indeed, it is the 11th most frequently cultured microorganism in a U.S. multiple hospital study covering 1993 to 2004 (4.3% of 74,934 gram-negative bacilli). Furthermore, the prevalence of *S. maltophilia* in patients with CF has increased in a relevant study from 6% to 12.7% from 1995 to 2008. Selective media (vancomycin–imipenem–amphotericin B, gram-negative selective agar, BTB, and SM2i) have been developed to ease detection of *S. maltophilia*, especially because the pathogen is frequently co-cultured in samples of polymicrobial infections. Polymerase chain reaction amplification of 16 rRNA in blood has also been used. The bacterium is usually susceptible to trimethoprim-sulfamethoxazole, which is regarded as the first-choice antibiotic.[17] However, resistant strains are emerging. Other antibiotics that have been effective against *S. maltophilia* isolates include ciprofloxacin, ceftazidime, and ticarcillin-clavulanate; sometimes these are used in combination with trimethoprim-sulfamethoxazole. Inherent resistance to carbapenems is a notable characteristic of this bacterium.

Melioidosis is an infection due to *B. pseudomallei* and occurs mainly in Southeast Asia and Australia. A notable current addition to these geographic regions is the Indian subcontinent and Sri Lanka. One should also be aware of potential niduses in the Americas (Mexico and the northern part of South America) and Africa (Madagascar). Risk factors for acquisition of melioidosis include renal failure, diabetes mellitus, heavy alcohol consumption, chronic respiratory disease, thalassemia, glucocorticoid therapy, and cancer. It can also afflict immunocompetent travelers to the regions mentioned. Interestingly, there is a seasonal association with the rainy season in more than three quarter of cases. Clinical manifestations vary from asymptomatic infection to localized skin infection, pneumonia, and fulminant sepsis due to bacteremia. The formation of abscesses is a usual feature of the disease. Other manifestations include septic arthritis, osteomyelitis, prostatitis, neurologic manifestations such as brain stem encephalitis associated with cranial nerve palsies or myelitis with peripheral motor weakness, and kidney and spleen involvement. Suppurative parotitis, even bilateral in 10%, is a feature present in patients with melioidosis in Thailand and Cambodia. Parotitis afflicts mainly children. The bacterium may remain dormant and then reactivate. The portal of entry includes the respiratory system, the skin, and the gastrointestinal system. Indeed, recurrence of melioidosis is due to reactivation in approximately three quarters of cases. There is a need for prolonged treatment of the bacterium that entails a 2- to 4-week regimen of intravenous antibiotic administration: ceftazidime, 2 g every 8 hours; meropenem, 1 g every 8 hours; or imipenem, 1 g every 8 hours.[18] An extended course of oral eradication with trimethoprim-sulfamethoxazole for 3 to 6 months is necessary after initial intravenous antibiotics.[A1] In the case of allergy or adverse events, amoxicillin-clavulanate and doxycycline have been proposed as alternatives to trimethoprim-sulfamethoxazole. Of note, *B. pseudomallei* is a bioterrorism factor B, and thus appropriate infection control and notification of authorities are mandatory.

Glanders is an equine infection due to *B. mallei*. Humans acquire the disease from contact with horses or more rarely donkeys or mules in an occupational setting. It mainly is manifested with tracheobronchitis, pneumonia, skin lesions, or lymphadenopathy. The disease has been eradicated in many countries. Nevertheless, cases can occur especially in association with an occupational risk in veterinarians, veterinary students, farriers (hoof care workers), flayers (hide workers), transport workers, soldiers, slaughterhouse personnel, farmers, and horse fanciers. *B. mallei* remains a significant cause of zoonosis, and therefore appropriate veterinary surveillance is necessary, especially because *B. mallei* is also a significant bioterrorism agent (class B). Treatment of glanders in humans is based on limited data. The approach to treatment is similar to that used for melioidosis, with intravenous meropenem, imipenem, or ceftazidime initially and then oral trimethoprim-sulfamethoxazole for 3 to 12 months.

B. cepacia is a bacterial pathogen that is a plant and human pathogen. Its classification has evolved, as has its name. It was previously known as *Pseudomonas cepacia* and then *Xanthomonas cepacia*. *B. cepacia* belongs to the *B. cepacia* complex and is a pathogen mainly of patients with CF and chronic granulomatous disease. Relatively recent reports have implicated *B. cepacia* in infections of the lung, blood, and other sites in immunocompromised patients and even in immunocompetent patients and children in the hospital environment due to outbreaks. Aerosolized medications, chlorhexidine solutions, napkins, and prefabricated clothes along with horizontal transmission have led to significant morbidity and mortality. Patients with CF typically present initially with asymptomatic carriage. Nevertheless, progressive decline of lung function is associated with *B. cepacia*. The most dramatic presentation of the lung ailment is the cepacia syndrome, a fulminant lung infection often accompanied by bacteremia. Other types of infection include meningitis, pericarditis, endocarditis, cholangitis, peritonitis, and abscesses in the abdomen, perineum, or scrotum.

PREVENTION

Primary prevention of *Pseudomonas* infections applies to preventing pollution of water by *Pseudomonas*. This applies to both the public environment and the hospital environment. Outbreaks have been linked to aquatic environments such as whirlpools, swimming pools, and spas. Thus, control of growth of this organism in the recreational environment by proper antibacterial treatment of water is essential, comparable to the control practiced in hospitals. Contamination of various equipment and devices (i.e., breast implants, ocular implants, and sinus irrigation devices) must be avoided. Handwashing cannot be emphasized enough in the prevention of infections due to *P. aeruginosa*, *S. maltophilia*, and *B. cepacia*. Hospital point-of-use water filtration has also been employed in the battle against *P. aeruginosa* and *S. maltophilia* infections. Barrier nursing practices may decrease horizontal transmission, especially in the critical care environment. Isolation of patients infected with extensively drug-resistant and pandrug-resistant *P. aeruginosa* and strict infection control measures (dedicated personnel and equipment, use of gowns and gloves) may be needed to avoid intrahospital spread. The most important measure is the washing of hands. Nevertheless, even antiseptic solutions may be contaminated by *P. aeruginosa*, *S. maltophilia*, and *B. cepacia*. Factors that shorten hospital length of stay and decrease the use of antibiotics are likely to decrease the incidence of these infections.

PROGNOSIS

P. aeruginosa infections carry a high mortality, even with treatment. Mortality rates of 26 to 36% have been reported. Differences also exist between appropriately and inappropriately treated *P. aeruginosa* infections, with mortality rates even double when inappropriate antibiotics are used. Furthermore, *P. aeruginosa* infections are associated with increased length of hospitalization and medical costs. Loss of vision is the grave outcome of ophthalmic infection. Antibiotic resistance associated with *P. aeruginosa* will most likely continue to pose an enormous burden on human lives and financial resources in years to come.

S. maltophilia infections are associated with attributable mortality of up to about 37% if they are not appropriately treated. Melioidosis is associated with a 14% mortality rate in Australia and up to 40% in countries in Southeast Asia when it is treated. Fortunately, reports of glanders are rare in humans. Mortality of glanders with treatment is about 40 to 50%. *B. cepacia* has a predilection for CF patients and often signals impaired overall prognosis in these patients. Furthermore, *B. cepacia* seems to adversely affect transplantation. Indeed, in patients presenting with the cepacia syndrome, survival is unusual. Furthermore, many transplant centers do not support transplantation when *B. cepacia* is present because of the grave prognosis associated with the infection in the post-transplantation period.

 Grade A Reference

A1. Chetchotisakd P, Chierakul W, Chaowagul W, et al. Trimethoprim-sulfamethoxazole versus trimethoprim-sulfamethoxazole plus doxycycline as oral eradicative treatment for melioidosis (MERTH): a multicentre, double-blind, non-inferiority, randomised controlled trial. *Lancet.* 2014;383:807-814.

GENERAL REFERENCES

For the General References and other additional features, please visit Expert Consult at https://expertconsult.inkling.com.

307

DISEASES CAUSED BY *ACINETOBACTER* AND *STENOTROPHOMONAS* SPECIES

KEITH S. KAYE AND ROBERT A. BONOMO

ACINETOBACTER SPECIES

DEFINITION
The Pathogen
Acinetobacter species are gram-negative aerobic bacteria that are coccobacillary in shape and are generally described as aerobic, non–lactose-fermenting,

nonfastidious, nonmotile, catalase positive, and oxidase negative. Unique among microbial pathogens, the appearance of *Acinetobacter* species visualized with a Gram stain is highly dependent on the life cycle. In the early growth phases, *Acinetobacter* species appear rod shaped. In the stationary phase, they acquire a coccobacillary *Acinetobacter* spp. morphology.

In the context of this chapter, *Acinetobacter* species refers specifically to *Acinetobacter baumannii* and *Acinetobacter baumannii-calcoaceticus* complex.

EPIDEMIOLOGY

Acinetobacter species can colonize all body surfaces and cause infection in almost any organ system. Consequently, there are a number of common clinical syndromes associated with infection by *Acinetobacter*. The most common infections are respiratory (pneumonia), blood stream (bacteremia), urinary tract, wound, skin and soft tissue, and burn infections; osteomyelitis secondary to trauma; and meningitis.[1,2] In general, infection is observed only in critically ill, immunocompromised, or injured hosts. Recently, infections by *Acinetobacter* spp. are being described in patients without significant medical problems from the community setting.

During the past several years, *Acinetobacter* spp emerged in the United States from a pathogen that was primarily found in intensive care units (ICUs) to one that can affect patients in non-ICU wards, patients in long-term care settings, and military personnel with combat injuries acquired in the Middle East.[3] Overall, there are few distinguishing features of *Acinetobacter* infection except for skin manifestations. The frequency of *Acinetobacter* infections is often greater in the summer than in other seasons.

CLINICAL MANIFESTATIONS
Pneumonia
Because of colonization of the oropharynx and tracheostomy tubes in patients on ventilators, the upper respiratory tract is the most common site for infection by *Acinetobacter* species. The two distinct syndromes associated with respiratory tract infection due to *Acinetobacter* are community-acquired pneumonia (CAP) and healthcare-associated pneumonia (HCAP). In tropical regions of China, Asia, Australia, and the South Pacific, CAP due to *Acinetobacter* species is increasingly recognized. In some locations, the incidence can exceed 15%. Reports have highlighted the emergence of *Acinetobacter* as a common cause of CAP in western China.[4] In Saudi Arabia, *Acinetobacter* is the most common pathogen associated with late-onset and recurrent ventilator-associated pneumonia (VAP) in one adult ICU.[5]

The common comorbid conditions predisposing to CAP due to *Acinetobacter* species are mainly chronic obstructive pulmonary disease (emphysema), renal disease, diabetes mellitus, and alcoholism. CAP due to *Acinetobacter* species appears to be associated with a high incidence of bacteremia, acute respiratory distress syndrome, sepsis, and death (mortality rates ≥50%). The reasons for these fulminant presentations are still unknown. Rarely, CAP due to *Acinetobacter* species can be manifested with consolidation and multiple lung abscesses.

More frequently, *Acinetobacter* species are a cause of HCAP, often manifested as VAP. In the United States, *Acinetobacter* species are the third leading cause of VAP. HCAP due to *Acinetobacter* largely resembles the clinical spectrum of gram-negative pneumonias (bilateral infiltrates, pleural effusion, cavitations, hypoxemia, and bacteremia). Most cases are described in patients on ventilators. The main factors associated with HCAP due to *Acinetobacter* species are mechanical ventilation, previous antibiotic exposure, ICU stay, surgery, and underlying pulmonary disease. The major challenge complicating nosocomial pneumonia due to *Acinetobacter* species is the frequent recovery of MDR and sometimes XDR strains. When isolates are MDR or XDR, the options for treatment are limited, and complications quickly arise. HCAP due to MDR *Acinetobacter* has been associated with excess lengths of stay and mortality, although some studies have reported similar outcomes compared with control patients matched by severity of illness and duration of ICU stay.

Bacteremia
Blood stream infection due to *Acinetobacter* species is often a consequence of infection of intravenous catheters (i.e., central line–associated blood stream infection or CLABSI) or is secondary to HCAP due to *Acinetobacter*. *Acinetobacter* is the ninth most common cause of CLABSI among U.S. hospitals reporting to the Centers for Disease Control and Prevention. Less commonly, wound infections can cause bacteremia. In most series,

mortality associated with blood stream infection ranges from approximately 15 to 50%.

Urinary Tract Infection

Urinary tract infections are most commonly caused by enteric gram-negative bacilli; only rarely are these infections caused by *Acinetobacter* species. The indwelling bladder catheter has been implicated as the major risk factor for urinary tract infection (cystitis and pyelonephritis) due to *Acinetobacter* species.

Wound, Burn, and Skin and Soft Tissue Infections

In many clinical series to date, traumatic or postoperative wounds, burns, and skin and soft tissue infections (SSTIs) are the most common causes of *Acinetobacter* infections. Most likely, the combination of antibiotic use, colonization, and compromised or devitalized tissues is responsible. The spectrum of infection can extend from cellulitis to necrotizing fasciitis.

As a result of the outbreak of *A. baumannii* among military personnel in Iraq and Afghanistan, reports of severe wound infections and SSTIs caused by this pathogen are increasing in frequency. Necrotizing SSTI associated with *A. baumannii* occurs in hosts with underlying comorbidities (e.g., trauma, cirrhosis) and is often accompanied by bacteremia. *Acinetobacter* infection has become increasingly common among patients residing in burn units, sometimes resulting in unit-wide outbreaks. Multiple drug resistance and the presence of copathogens frequently complicate treatment. Most cases require surgical débridement and lead to substantial mortality. In addition, the use of central venous catheters and total parenteral nutrition is more common among patients with SSTIs. *Acinetobacter* species–associated SSTIs can be manifested with a peau d'orange appearance, with overlying tiny vesicles (Fig. 307-1), and, when untreated, can progress to necrotizing infection with bullae (hemorrhagic and nonhemorrhagic).

Osteomyelitis

The conflicts in Iraq and Afghanistan highlighted the first cases of osteomyelitis due to *Acinetobacter* species. Before this time, rare cases of osteomyelitis occurring in soldiers were reported during the Korean and Vietnam wars. Most of the initial reports from the Middle East described "contiguous focus" osteomyelitis. These patients had open fractures or exposed bone, with gross findings of infection: purulence, necrotic tissue, or environmental contamination with exposed bone; temperature higher than 38° C; leukocyte count greater than 12,000/μL; and *Acinetobacter* species identified from culture of deep wound tissue obtained intraoperatively. Frequently, these infections require multiple surgical débridements of necrotic bone.

Meningitis

Acinetobacter meningitis is occasionally found in the post-neurosurgical setting, with mortality exceeding 15 to 30%. Infection often involves intraventricular catheters. Although *Acinetobacter* is an uncommon cause of meningitis from the community, the frequency is almost 4% in cases of hospital-acquired meningitis and almost 11% among patients with meningitis involving an indwelling intraventricular catheter. Treatment is problematic because some cephalosporins do not achieve high enough levels in cerebrospinal fluid to be effective and because of the increasing incidence of MDR and XDR *Acinetobacter* (see later).

DIAGNOSIS

There are now more than 30 different species in the genus *Acinetobacter*, and their classification and identification remain problematic for clinicians (to date, 38 species are known; 27 are named and 11 are unnamed genospecies).[6] Automated and biochemical systems are sometimes inaccurate for the identification of *Acinetobacter* species. The introduction of matrix-assisted laser desorption/ionization time-of-flight into the clinical laboratory may facilitate better diagnosis.[7]

TREATMENT Rx

An increasing number of strains of *Acinetobacter* species are resistant to all antibiotics, and these strains are often responsible for outbreaks in large hospitals. These multidrug-resistant (MDR) or extremely drug-resistant (XDR) strains are often resistant to three or more classes of antibiotics. Among the resistance genes found in *Acinetobacter* species are a large collection of genes encoding β-lactamases, aminoglycoside-modifying enzymes, and many efflux

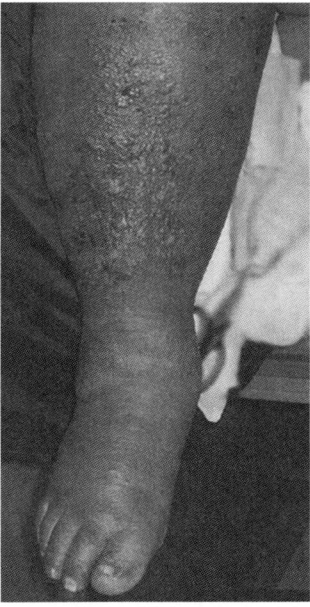

FIGURE 307-1. Cellulitis caused by *Acinetobacter baumannii*. There is characteristic edematous peau d'orange erythema, with associated vesicles that may coalesce to form nonhemorrhagic bullae. (From Guerrero DM, Perez F, Conger NG, et al. *Acinetobacter baumannii*–associated skin and soft tissue infections: recognizing a broadening spectrum of disease. *Surg Infect [Larchmt]*. 2010;11:49-57.)

pumps. Even more concerning is the emergence of XDR strains of Acinetobacter that are resistant to carbapenems and ampicillin-sulbactam, leaving few treatment options.[8] Unfortunately, resistance to "last-line" agents, such as the cationic antimicrobial peptides colistin (polymyxin E) and its close relative polymyxin B, also occurs. Regrettably, colistin resistance is becoming more common as clinicians are forced to use this agent more frequently. In hospital environments, Acinetobacter species can withstand drying (desiccation) and may even be transmitted by aerosol/respiratory droplet. Combined with drug resistance, these characteristics create a formidable infection control challenge.

Increasing resistance to a variety of antimicrobial agents complicates the treatment of Acinetobacter species infections. In general, infections due to more resistant strains of Acinetobacter are associated with less favorable outcomes than are infections due to more susceptible strains. These worse outcomes are likely due in part to limited treatment options as well as delays in the time to implementation of effective antimicrobial therapy for patients with infections due to MDR and XDR Acinetobacter strains.

The treatment doses that follow all assume normal renal function; doses need to be adjusted on the basis of the degree of renal insufficiency. When it is susceptible, Acinetobacter is typically treated with sulbactam (in the formulation of ampicillin-sulbactam in the United States, 3 g IV every 6 hours); the carbapenems imipenem (500 to 1000 mg IV every 6 hours) or meropenem (500 to 1000 mg IV every 8 hours); or broad-spectrum cephalosporins.[9] Based on ampicillin component, aminoglycosides are an option for treatment of urinary tract infection. One must be cautious: susceptibility to imipenem does not always translate to susceptibility to meropenem, and susceptibility to ceftazidime does not always indicate that cefepime can be used. In addition, there are data suggesting that doripenem may be the carbapenem with the most in vitro activity.

Treatment of infection with XDR Acinetobacter is challenging.[10] Tigecycline (100 mg loading dose, then 50 mg IV every 12 hours) and minocycline (200 mg IV or PO initially, followed by 100 mg IV or PO every 12 hours) have good in vitro activity against many strains of XDR Acinetobacter. Some experts recommend higher maintenance dosages of tigecycline (100 mg IV every 12 hours) and minocycline (200 mg IV or PO every 12 hours). These agents are appropriate for treatment of SSTI, but because of poor serum concentrations and lack of clinical experience in the treatment of MDR and XDR Acinetobacter, monotherapy with these should be avoided for invasive infections such as bacteremia and pneumonia. Sometimes, there is no choice but to use tigecycline as it might be the only available agent with in vitro activity against infecting Acinetobacter strains.

Invasive infections, such as bacteremia, pneumonia, and deep wound infections, are often treated with a polymyxin antimicrobial, either colistimethate sodium (CMS, often referred to as colistin) or polymyxin B. If CMS is used, a loading dose of 5 mg/kg colistin base activity, with a maximum dose of

300 mg, should be administered, followed by daily administration of 5 mg/kg colistin base activity per day in divided doses every 8 hours. If polymyxin B is used, a loading dose of 2.5 mg/kg × 1 should be administered intravenously, followed by a dose of 1.5 to 2.5 mg/kg/day by continuous IV infusion or in divided doses every 12 hours infused during a period of 60 minutes.[11]

Clinicians often treat invasive infections due to XDR *Acinetobacter* with combination therapy, although there is a lack of prospective controlled data demonstrating the superiority of combination therapy. Agents often combined with the polymyxins include rifampin (10 mg/kg/day, not to exceed 600 mg), imipenem or meropenem, sulbactam (ampicillin-sulbactam), tigecycline or minocycline, and aminoglycosides. At the time of this writing, data obtained from clinical trials conducted in Italy suggest that rifampin may not add measurable benefit to the treatment of MDR or XDR *Acinetobacter* despite the in vitro efficacy of the combination.[A1] In addition, the benefit of aerosolized colistin has not yet been established. Interest is rising in the use of the combination of colistin and tigecycline or fosfomycin, but further studies are needed.

The major adverse effect of polymyxin therapy is nephrotoxicity.[12] Current advances have improved our understanding of the pharmacokinetics, pharmacodynamics, and dosing of the polymyxins, but this is still an emerging and changing field. There is promising interest in the use of antioxidants (e.g., ascorbic acid) to prevent nephrotoxicity, but these studies are still preliminary.

In cases of meningitis due to *Acinetobacter* species, treatment should be intravenous meropenem (2000 mg every 8 hours) plus the intraventricular administration of an aminoglycoside (gentamicin or amikacin, depending on susceptibilities). Intraventricular gentamicin is administered at a dose of 4 mg once daily every 1 to 3 days until clinical and microbiologic improvement occurs. Amikacin can be used in place of gentamicin at the dose of 30 mg once a day, if required. For cases of meningitis due to XDR *Acinetobacter*, intravenous CMS or polymyxin B should be supplemented with intraventricular or intrathecal administration of CMS 10 mg/day, colistin base activity, or polymyxin B 5 to 10 mg/day for the initial 3 days of therapy and then every other day.

PREVENTION

Infection prevention practices, including hand hygiene, use of contact precautions, maintenance of environmental cleanliness, and implementation of antimicrobial stewardship, can help prevent spread of *Acinetobacter* in the hospital. During outbreaks, cohorting of patients and use of dedicated staff to care for cohorted patients might be necessary to control spread. Removal of indwelling devices from patients, including vascular catheters and endotracheal tubes, can help prevent colonization and infection with *Acinetobacter*.

PROGNOSIS

Invasive infection due to *Acinetobacter* has been associated with crude mortality rates in excess of 50% and increases in duration of ICU stay of 6 days and duration of total hospital stay of more than 14 days. With appropriate early empiric therapy, however, the mortality rate for community-acquired infection can be as low as 11%.[13] By comparison, infections due to strains of MDR and XDR *Acinetobacter* are associated with increases in mortality and durations of hospitalization compared with more susceptible *Acinetobacter* strains.[14]

STENOTROPHOMONAS MALTOPHILIA

DEFINITION

Stenotrophomonas maltophilia has attracted significant attention because it is often MDR due to intrinsic and acquired factors. *S. maltophilia* contributes significantly to morbidity, but usually not mortality, in immunocompromised patients.

The Pathogen

S. maltophilia are gram-negative bacteria that need methionine for growth and, like *Pseudomonas aeruginosa* and *Acinetobacter* species, are non–lactose fermenters. *S. maltophilia* possess flagella that are multitrichous (more than one flagellum arising from the pole) and are distinguished from *P. aeruginosa* as oxidase negative. Colonies of *S. maltophilia* may appear pale yellow or lavender-green on blood agar plates. The organism emits a mild ammonia-like odor that is used for preliminary identification.[15]

S. maltophilia can colonize inanimate surfaces in the hospital, including catheters, intravenous fluid, water supplies, and hospital equipment. This pathogen may also survive in hospital-grade disinfectant. Other health

TABLE 307-1	RISK FACTORS FOR INFECTION BY *STENOTROPHOMONAS MALTOPHILIA*

Prolonged hospitalization or intensive care unit stay
Intravascular catheters
Indwelling devices
Mechanical ventilation or tracheostomy
Neutropenia or cytotoxic chemotherapy
Solid organ transplantation
Immunocompromised state
Mucositis
Malignant disease
Chronic lung disease (especially cystic fibrosis and chronic obstructive pulmonary disease)
HIV infection
Hemodialysis
Antibiotic exposure (especially to carbapenems, extended-spectrum cephalosporins, and fluoroquinolones)
Exposure to other patients with *S. maltophilia*

care–associated sources of *S. maltophilia* include contaminated intravenous fluids, hospital water and ice supplies, nebulizers, dialysis machines, ventilator circuits, thermometers, blood gas analyzers, intra-abdominal balloon pumps, and central venous or arterial pressure monitors.

EPIDEMIOLOGY

Despite its harboring many resistance genes, little is known about the virulence of *S. maltophilia*. Nevertheless, a number of risk factors are associated with infection by *S. maltophilia* (Table 307-1).[16] Although *S. maltophilia* is regarded as primarily a nosocomial pathogen (it is the third most common nonfermenting gram-negative bacillus health care–associated pathogen), community-acquired infection can occur. *S. maltophilia* infection primarily affects patients who are immunocompromised (including patients with hematologic malignant neoplasms[17] and patients who underwent solid organ transplantation), patients cared for in ICUs who are mechanically ventilated, hemodialysis patients with intravascular catheters, neonates, and patients with cystic fibrosis. Colonization or infection with *S. maltophilia* among patients with cystic fibrosis (Chapter 89) has been associated with reduction in lung function.[18]

CLINICAL MANIFESTATIONS

Respiratory Tract

The respiratory tract is the most common site of isolation of *S. maltophilia* in the hospital. Surveillance programs reveal a rate of recovery of *S. maltophilia* from hospitalized patients with pneumonia of more than 3% in the United States. Nosocomial pneumonia due to *S. maltophilia* is often associated with significant pulmonary disease such as emphysema, bronchiectasis, lung transplantation, or endobronchial obstruction. In addition, many of these patients are on mechanical ventilators, have tracheostomy tubes in place, or are receiving broad-spectrum antibiotics. Among mechanically ventilated patients, it can be challenging to differentiate colonization due to *S. maltophilia* from infection. CAP due to *S. maltophilia* has been reported but is very rare.

The incidence of respiratory tract infection due to *S. maltophilia* in patients with cystic fibrosis (Chapter 89) is increasingly being reported. There may be clear links with resistance to antipseudomonal antibiotics (tobramycin, imipenem, ceftazidime) used to treat these patients. The presence of chronic *S. maltophilia* infection has been associated with increases in cystic fibrosis exacerbations, hospitalizations, need for lung transplantation, and mortality. It remains unclear whether *S. maltophilia* has a causative association with poor outcomes or is merely a marker for severe underlying disease.

Blood Stream Infection and Endocarditis

Bacteremia may be secondary to a respiratory, urinary, or gastrointestinal source but is most commonly due to infection of an indwelling intravascular device. In many cases, except for those involving intravenous catheters, the portal of entry is not apparent. Immunocompromised patients with indwelling intravascular catheters, including those with hematologic malignant disease, are at particularly high risk for CLABSI due to *S. maltophilia*. In cases of CLABSI due to *S. maltophilia*, removal of the infected catheter is an important component of management. On occasion, an environmental reservoir or contaminated vascular access device is linked to the presence of bacteremia. Intravenous drug users are at especially high risk for

TABLE 307-2	MECHANISMS OF RESISTANCE IN *STENOTROPHOMONAS MALTOPHILIA*
DRUG	**MECHANISM OF RESISTANCE**
β-Lactams, including imipenem	L1 and L2 β-lactamases Outer membrane permeability/efflux
Aminoglycosides	Aminoglycoside-modifying enzymes, transport

contaminating prosthetic valves with S. *maltophilia*. In the case of endocarditis, favorable outcomes are reported with antimicrobial therapy, but surgery may also be required.

Urinary Tract Infection

Although *S. maltophilia* is frequently recovered from urine specimens in patients with indwelling urinary catheters, the role of this organism as a pathogen in this setting is unclear.

Meningitis

Cases of central nervous system infection due to *S. maltophilia* are reported rarely. These are often associated with central nervous system devices or antecedent neurosurgery.

Skin and Soft Tissue Infection

S. maltophilia can be isolated from postoperative wounds, but its role as a pathogen in this setting is unclear. In contrast, *S. maltophilia* can cause burn wound sepsis, manifested as a syndrome very similar to ecthyma gangrenosum (Chapter 441) in immunocompromised oncology patients.

TREATMENT　　　　　　　　　　　　　Rx

As a pathogen that is an increasingly important cause of nosocomial infections, *S. maltophilia* exhibits intrinsic resistance to many antibiotics. The complexity of resistance genes and mechanisms is summarized in Table 307-2. Resistance to imipenem, piperacillin-tazobactam, ceftazidime, and aminoglycosides is common. Despite significant resistance to many agents, trimethoprim-sulfamethoxazole remains the drug of choice (10 to 15 mg/kg/day IV, based on the trimethoprim component).[19] Treatment duration is uncertain, but it is usually 14 days or longer. In addition, in vitro studies indicate that ticarcillin-clavulanate (3.1 g every 6 hours), minocycline (200 mg followed by 100 mg every 12 hours, not to exceed 400 mg in 24 hours), some of the fluoroquinolones, and tigecycline may be useful agents. Polymyxin-based regimens may serve as alternatives in the face of resistance to trimethoprim-sulfamethoxazole (see earlier for details regarding polymyxin treatment). New regimens attempting to combine tigecycline and colistin for invasive *S. maltophilia* infections appear promising. Aztreonam is effective against strains exhibiting resistance to β-lactams by metallo-β-lactamases.

PROGNOSIS

Among patients with VAP or bacteremia due to *S. maltophilia*, crude mortality rates in the range of 60% have been reported. The attributable mortality of invasive *S. maltophilia* infection has been reported to be between 12 and 37.5%,[20] but patients who receive early appropriate antibiotic therapy appear to do better.[21]

PREVENTION

Standard infection control practices including hand hygiene and thorough environmental cleaning can help prevent spread of *Stenotrophomonas* in the hospital. In outbreak settings, contact precautions and possibly cohorting of patients have been used to control spread.

Grade A Reference

A1. Durante-Mangoni E, Signoriello G, Andini R, et al. Colistin and rifampicin compared with colistin alone for the treatment of serious infections due to extensively drug-resistant *Acinetobacter baumannii*: a multicenter, randomized clinical trial. *Clin Infect Dis.* 2013;57:349-358.

GENERAL REFERENCES

For the General References and other additional features, please visit Expert Consult at https://expertconsult.inkling.com.

308

SALMONELLA INFECTIONS (INCLUDING ENTERIC FEVER)

JOHN A. CRUMP

DEFINITION

A member of the family Enterobacteriaceae, *Salmonella enterica* subspecies *enterica* includes more than 2500 serovars (also called serotypes) found in humans and other warm-blooded animals. These serovars may be associated with human asymptomatic intestinal carriage, intestinal infection, and invasive disease with extraintestinal infection. Each serovar designation follows the species name (e.g., *Salmonella enterica* subspecies *enterica* serovar Typhimurium) and is frequently abbreviated as simply *Salmonella* followed by the serovar name (e.g., *Salmonella* Typhimurium).

The Pathogen

Salmonellae are gram-negative, non–spore-forming bacilli. They are differentiated from other Enterobacteriaceae by biochemical tests. They ferment glucose, maltose, and mannitol but typically not lactose or sucrose. They reduce nitrates and do not produce cytochrome oxidase. Almost all salmonellae produce acid and gas with fermentation. Most *Salmonella* serovars cannot be distinguished by biochemical reactions. However, *Salmonella* Typhi may be preliminarily identified by its production of only trace amounts of hydrogen sulfide and diminished biochemical activity compared with other serovars.

Salmonellae can be differentiated into more than 2500 serovars by their somatic (O) antigens, which are composed of lipopolysaccharides and are part of the cell wall, and by their flagellar (H) and capsular (Vi) antigens. *Salmonella* serogroups were traditionally designated by letters based on O antigens (e.g., A, B, C1, C2). More recently, the growing number of serogroups has made it necessary to move to a numeric designation. During the transition, the traditional letter-based serogroup may be retained in brackets after the numeric designation (e.g., O:2 [A], O:4 [B], O:6,7 [C1], O:8 [C2]). Some of the important serovars and their serogroups are Typhi (group O:9 [D1]), Choleraesuis (group O:7 [C1]), Typhimurium (group O:4 [B]), and Enteritidis (group O:9 [D1]). *Salmonella* Enteritidis and Typhimurium are the most common nontyphoidal serovars causing human disease.

EPIDEMIOLOGY

Salmonella Typhi, *Salmonella* Paratyphi A, *Salmonella* Paratyphi B, *Salmonella* Paratyphi C, and *Salmonella* Sendai are either solely or almost exclusively pathogens of humans; they cause primarily enteric fever rather than diarrhea, and transmission between humans is usually through water or food. As a result of modern sewage and water treatment facilities and improved food safety practices, typhoid fever and paratyphoid fever have become rare in developed countries but remain a problem in countries that lack adequate sanitation and a safe water supply. There are usually fewer than 500 cases of typhoid fever each year in the United States, mainly acquired abroad[1]; in contrast, an estimated 26.9 million cases occurred globally in 2010.[2]

Other serovars of *Salmonella* (described here as nontyphoidal *Salmonella*) have reservoirs in warm-blooded animals and cause human foodborne illness after the consumption of contaminated meat or animal products, contamination of produce or water by animal feces or animal products, or contact with animals and their environments. Some nontyphoidal *Salmonella* serovars appear frequently in particular animal species, and human illness is often associated with exposure to these animals and their products. For example, *Salmonella* Enteritidis has a reservoir in chickens, and infection is often linked to the consumption of undercooked eggs and poultry products or exposure to live chicks. Such a relationship is less clear for some other nontyphoidal serovars (e.g., *Salmonella* Typhimurium). Foodborne nontyphoidal *Salmonella* was estimated to be associated with approximately 1.0 million domestically acquired illnesses and 378 deaths in the United States in 2006.[3] A disproportionate number of infections occur in July through October, probably related to warm weather. *Salmonella* infections are most common among infants and children younger than 5 years. Worldwide, nontyphoidal

Salmonella was estimated to cause 93.8 million diarrheal illnesses, 80.3 million food-borne illnesses, and 155,000 deaths in 2005.[4]

Antimicrobial Resistance

Salmonellae have become increasingly resistant to antimicrobial agents, usually by acquiring resistance transfer factors (e.g., plasmid mediated). It is thought that antimicrobial resistance in the human-restricted salmonellae (e.g., *Salmonella* Typhi) is driven primarily by antimicrobial use in humans, whereas antimicrobial resistance among the nontyphoidal salmonellae (e.g., *Salmonella* Typhimurium) is associated with the use of antimicrobial agents in farm animals. Among *Salmonella* Typhi isolated in the United States during 1999 to 2006, 13% were resistant to the traditional first-line antimicrobials ampicillin, chloramphenicol, and trimethoprim-sulfamethoxazole, and 38% showed decreased fluoroquinolone susceptibility. Resistance to extended-spectrum cephalosporins is rare in *Salmonella* Typhi and *Salmonella* Paratyphi. Among nontyphoidal *Salmonella* isolated from humans in the United States, resistance to three or more antimicrobial classes is common but declining, whereas resistance to ceftriaxone and nonsusceptibility to ciprofloxacin are uncommon but increasing.[5] Susceptibility breakpoints and interpretive criteria were established for azithromycin in 2015 in response to reports of *Salmonella* with elevated azithromycin minimum inhibitory concentrations.

PATHOBIOLOGY
Etiology

Salmonellae are transmitted by the ingestion of fecally contaminated food or water; contact with animals, their environments, and other fomites; and, rarely, close contact with infected persons (e.g., oral-anal intercourse). The ultimate sources of contamination are humans or animals that are acutely ill or are asymptomatic carriers.

Contaminated Animal Products

Salmonella infection in humans usually occurs from ingestion of contaminated animal food products, most often eggs, poultry, and meat. *Salmonella* Choleraesuis is associated with pig products, *Salmonella* Dublin with cattle and unpasteurized milk from cattle, and *Salmonella* Enteritidis with poultry and poultry products, including eggs. Fecal material on poultry and other animal carcasses can spread at slaughterhouses, such as when many poultry carcasses are placed in the same hot-water tank to remove feathers. *Salmonella* contaminating carcasses can multiply to high levels if meat or other animal products are not refrigerated. Human illness may result if such animal products are inadequately cooked or if utensils or other uncooked foods are cross-contaminated during preparation. A wide range of foods can be contaminated with animal or human feces, from production on the farm through consumption in the home. Reports of produce-associated *Salmonella* outbreaks, due to contamination by animal or human feces during production, are increasing.[6] *Salmonella* outbreaks have occurred from contaminated cheese, ice cream, vegetables, fruit, juice, and alfalfa sprouts.

Contaminated Food and Water
Contamination by Pets

Salmonella infections may be acquired after contamination of food or water with the feces of pet turtles, chicks, ducks, birds, dogs, cats, and many other species.

Contamination by Humans

Salmonella infection can also be acquired by eating food or by drinking water contaminated by human carriers who have not adequately washed their hands. Infection has been spread by the fecal-oral route among children, by contaminated enema and fiberoptic instruments, by diagnostic and therapeutic preparations made from animal or insect products (e.g., pancreatic extract, carmine dye), and from intentional or unintentional contamination of restaurant salad bars. Outbreaks of salmonellosis may occur in institutionalized patients, who are probably more prone to the development of *Salmonella* infections for three reasons. First, within institutionalized populations, there is an increased prevalence of underlying diseases that decrease host defense mechanisms against salmonellae, such as disorders of gastric acidity and intestinal motility; second, the use of antimicrobial agents modifies the normal, protective intestinal flora; and third, institutional food prepared in bulk may be more likely to be contaminated than are individually prepared meals. Outbreaks in nurseries and among the elderly in nursing homes are associated with the highest case-fatality ratios (>5%).

Contact with Animals and Their Environments

Both healthy and sick animals may harbor and shed *Salmonella*. Transmission of *Salmonella* from animals and their environment to humans occurs primarily by the fecal-oral route. Animal hides and saliva often harbor fecal organisms, and transmission can occur when persons pet, touch, feed, or are licked by animals. Transmission has also been associated with contaminated animal bedding, flooring, barriers, other environmental surfaces, and clothing and shoes. Contact with calves, turtles and other reptiles, rodents, and young poultry and their environments has been associated with *Salmonella* outbreaks. Humans may also become infected when animals come into contact with their food or water. Infections can be prevented by education, supervision of animal contact, provision and promotion of handwashing facilities, and separation of food handling and consumption from animal areas.[7]

Contact with Infected Persons

Close contact with persons shedding *Salmonella* is an occasional source of infection. Transmission has been documented among persons handling feces (e.g., parents changing the diapers of an infected infant) and is associated with certain sexual practices (e.g., oral-anal intercourse).

Pathophysiology

After the ingestion of organisms, the likelihood for development of infection, as well as the severity of infection, is related to the dose, the virulence of the *Salmonella* strain, and the status of host defense mechanisms. Usually at least 10^2 to 10^3 bacteria are required to produce clinical infection in a normal host. Higher inocula are associated with increased disease severity, whereas smaller inocula are more likely to result in transient intestinal carriage. Gastric acid serves as a host defense mechanism by killing many of the ingested organisms, and intestinal motility is probably another host defense mechanism. In the absence of or with a decrease in gastric acidity (e.g., in infants and the elderly; after gastrectomy, vagotomy, or gastroenterostomy; or with the use of drugs that reduce gastric acidity) and with decreased intestinal motility (e.g., the use of antimotility drugs), much smaller inocula can produce infection, and the infection tends to be more severe.

Administration of antimicrobial agents before the ingestion of salmonellae can markedly reduce the size of the inoculum needed to produce infection, presumably by reducing the concentration of protective bowel flora.

Although any *Salmonella* serovar can produce any of the *Salmonella* syndromes (transient asymptomatic carrier state, enterocolitis, enteric fever, bacteremia, and chronic carrier state), each serovar tends to be associated with certain syndromes much more frequently than with others. For example, *Salmonella* Anatum usually causes asymptomatic intestinal infection, whereas *Salmonella* Typhimurium generally causes enterocolitis. *Salmonella* Choleraesuis is more likely to produce bacteremia (often with metastatic infection) than asymptomatic infection or enterocolitis, and some serovars such as *Salmonella* Typhi and *Salmonella* Paratyphi are most likely to cause enteric fever as well as the chronic carrier state. Fortunately, most *Salmonella* serovars are of relatively low pathogenicity for humans. Therefore, although food products are commonly contaminated, large outbreaks tend to involve the more virulent serovars.

To produce infection, invasion must occur across the mucosa of the intestine. When the organisms reach the lamina propria, an influx of polymorphonuclear leukocytes serves as a host defense mechanism to prevent invasion of the lymphatics. Certain serovars seem to have a greater ability than others to invade the lymphatics and subsequently to produce bacteremia (e.g., *Salmonella* Choleraesuis and *Salmonella* Dublin, which commonly produce bacteremia after intestinal infection). Both the small intestine and the colon are involved in the inflammatory process.

In the case of *Salmonella* Typhi and other causes of enteric fever, salmonellae invade the mononuclear phagocytes in Peyer's patches in the ileum and mesenteric lymph nodes. Some intracellular salmonellae form a nonreplicating population of "persisters" that could provide a reservoir for relapsing infection; intracellular persistence is determined by conditions in the vacuolar environment of the infected cells.[8] Others multiply intracellularly and are carried through the lymphatic system and blood stream to the liver, spleen, bone marrow, and other parts of the reticuloendothelial system. Once in the reticuloendothelial system, they multiply intracellularly in mononuclear phagocytes and produce the systemic manifestations of enteric fever. The onset of fever is associated with bacteremia and the release of cytokines (e.g., tumor necrosis factor and interleukins) from mononuclear phagocytes.

Ulcerations over Peyer patches are responsible for the intestinal manifestations of enteric fever, such as pain, perforation, and bleeding.

In *Salmonella* enterocolitis, the organisms remain localized in the intestinal mucosa, and diarrhea results from the inflammation produced by polymorphonuclear leukocytes. In addition, watery diarrhea may occur, apparently the result of the secretion of water and electrolytes by small intestinal epithelial cells in response to an enterotoxin secreted by some of the *Salmonella* strains or in response to tissue mediators of inflammation.

Patients with diseases that impair host defense mechanisms seem to have an increased frequency of severe *Salmonella* infection. A striking association has been recognized between diseases producing hemolysis and *Salmonella* bacteremia. Specifically, *Salmonella* bacteremia is common in patients with sickle cell disorders, malaria, and bartonellosis. In fact, because of the frequency of *Salmonella* bacteremia in sickle cell diseases and the underlying bone disease in these patients to which salmonellae localize, these organisms are the most common cause of osteomyelitis in patients with sickle cell disorders (Chapter 163). Prolonged *Salmonella* bacteremia may occur in patients with hepatosplenic schistosomiasis, possibly related to localization on and in the intravascular schistosomes. Patients with lymphoma and leukemia are also more prone to the development of *Salmonella* bacteremia. A markedly increased frequency and severity of *Salmonella* infections in general have been observed in patients with human immunodeficiency virus (HIV) infection, particularly those with CD4+ T-lymphocyte counts less than 200 cells/mm^3. Prolonged and recurrent, refractory *Salmonella* bacteremia is common among these patients. Other risk factors that increase the frequency and severity of *Salmonella* infection are extremes of age, immunocompromised states (e.g., from immunosuppressive agents), malnutrition, and probably diabetes. Nontyphoidal *Salmonella* serovars are a leading cause of community-acquired blood stream infection in sub-Saharan Africa, where children younger than 3 years and HIV-infected adults carry most of the burden of invasive disease.[9]

CLINICAL MANIFESTATIONS

Asymptomatic Intestinal Carrier State

The asymptomatic intestinal carrier state may result from inapparent infection (which is the most common form of *Salmonella* infection), or it may follow clinical disease (in which case the patient becomes a convalescent carrier). The carrier state is usually self-limited to several weeks to months, with the prevalence of positive stool cultures rapidly decreasing over time. By 1 year, far less than 1% of carriers still have positive stools. The main exception is *Salmonella* Typhi; about 3% of those infected excrete the organism for life. Women and older men are most likely to become chronic carriers of *Salmonella* Typhi, related to the presence of biliary tract disease, especially calculi. A patient who has had salmonellae in stool for 1 year (chronic carrier) is likely to become a lifelong carrier; the reservoir is in the biliary tree, usually in calculi in the gallbladder. Patients with *Schistosoma haematobium* infection are predisposed to become chronic urinary carriers of salmonellae.

Enterocolitis

After an incubation period of usually 12 to 48 hours, the illness starts suddenly with crampy abdominal pain and diarrhea. Nausea and vomiting may occur but are usually not prominent or persistent. The diarrhea may be watery and of large or small volume. Stools may contain mucus and are occasionally bloody. Polymorphonuclear leukocytes are present in the stool. Diarrhea may be mild or severe, with up to 20 to 30 stools a day. Fever is present in most patients, and the temperature may reach 40° C (104° F) or higher. The abdomen is tender to palpation. Transient bacteremia may occur and is most commonly seen in infants, the elderly, and patients with impaired host defense mechanisms.

Symptoms generally improve during a period of days, with fever lasting no more than 2 to 3 days and diarrhea lasting no more than 5 to 7 days. However, these symptoms occasionally persist for up to 14 days. More severe disease is seen with malnutrition, inflammatory bowel disease, and HIV infection. Reactive arthritis may follow enterocolitis in up to 7% of cases, especially among those with the HLA-B27 phenotype.

Enteric Fever

Enteric fever is produced by *Salmonella* Typhi (typhoid fever), *Salmonella* Paratyphi A, B, and C (paratyphoid fever), and occasionally other serovars. Sometimes it immediately follows classic enterocolitis caused by the same organism. The syndrome is characterized by prolonged, sustained fever and

may be associated with relative bradycardia, splenomegaly, rose spots, and leukopenia. In Africa, the common symptoms of invasive nontyphoidal *Salmonella* disease, which is seen predominantly in patients with HIV infection, malaria, and malnutrition, are fever, hepatosplenomegaly, and respiratory symptoms; features of enterocolitis are often absent.[10]

Therapy aborts the course of the disease. The following is a description of untreated illness. After an incubation period of 5 to 21 days (generally 7 to 14 days), fever and malaise develop, often associated with cough. A small proportion of patients may have diarrhea during the incubation period. The fever tends to rise in a stepwise fashion during the first few days to a week and then becomes sustained, usually at 39.4° to 40.0° C (103° to 104° F) or higher. Relative bradycardia is seen in up to half of patients. Apathy, confusion, delirium, and even psychosis may occur. Abdominal distention, pain, and tenderness may occur in the first week and may be associated with diarrhea or constipation; these symptoms are generally more pronounced during the second week of fever. Most patients have abdominal tenderness during the course of the illness.

In about 30% of patients, rose spots develop on the abdomen or chest (or both) toward the end of the first week or during the second week of fever. These faint, salmon-colored maculopapular lesions are subtle and may be difficult to see, particularly in dark-skinned patients. Salmonellae can be cultured from punch biopsies of these lesions. Hepatosplenomegaly occurs in about half of patients. Leukopenia and neutropenia are seen in about 20%. Abnormal liver function test results are common.

After 2 weeks of illness, the severe complications of intestinal hemorrhage and perforation related to necrosis of Peyer patches may be observed in about 5% of patients. These perforations may require surgical as well as medical therapy and can occur even in a patient treated with antimicrobials. Intestinal perforation is the leading cause of death from enteric fever.

The illness usually resolves by the end of the fourth week in an untreated patient. Relapse may occur in untreated as well as in treated patients, but the illness is milder than the original episode.

Rarely, some of the following complications may occur: pancreatitis, cholecystitis, infective endocarditis, meningitis, pneumonia, hepatic or splenic abscess, orchitis, or focal infection at virtually any site.

Bacteremia

Patients with *Salmonella* bacteremia usually complain of fever and chills lasting days to weeks. Gastrointestinal symptoms are unusual, but in some patients *Salmonella* bacteremia follows classic enterocolitis. Other symptoms are nonspecific, such as malaise, anorexia, and weight loss. Metastatic infection of bones, joints, aneurysms (particularly of the abdominal aorta), meninges (mainly in infants), pericardium, pleural space, lungs, heart valves, cysts, uterine myomas, malignant neoplasms, and other sites is common, and symptoms may be related to the site of metastatic infection. Stool cultures are often negative for salmonellae, but blood cultures are positive.

Although any *Salmonella* serovar can produce bacteremia, *Salmonella* Dublin, *Salmonella* Choleraesuis, *Salmonella* Heidelberg, *Salmonella* Oranienburg, *Salmonella* Panama, and *Salmonella* Sandiego are associated with increased likelihood of bacteremia.

Salmonella bacteremia occurs with increased frequency in infants, the elderly, and patients with diseases associated with hemolysis (e.g., sickle cell diseases, malaria, bartonellosis), HIV infection, lymphoma, leukemia, disseminated histoplasmosis, and perhaps systemic lupus erythematosus. Localization to bone is common in patients with sickle cell diseases (Chapter 163).

Prolonged *Salmonella* bacteremia lasting for months may occur in patients with hepatosplenic schistosomiasis. In patients with HIV infection, recurrent, relapsing *Salmonella* bacteremia may develop, which may be difficult to cure with antimicrobial agents.

DIAGNOSIS

Although *Salmonella* enterocolitis is an invasive disease, the differential diagnosis includes all causes of acute diarrhea, including invasive bacteria such as *Campylobacter jejuni*, *Shigella* species, invasive *Escherichia coli*, *Yersinia enterocolitica*, and *Vibrio parahaemolyticus*; toxigenic bacteria such as *Vibrio cholerae*, enterotoxigenic *E. coli*, enterohemorrhagic *E. coli* (e.g., *E. coli* O157:H7), *Staphylococcus aureus*, *Bacillus cereus*, *Clostridium perfringens*, and *Clostridium difficile*; viruses; and protozoa such as *Entamoeba histolytica*, *Giardia intestinalis*, and *Cryptosporidium* species. The invasive bacterial causes of diarrhea, enterohemorrhagic *E. coli* and *C. difficile* infection, are also associated with polymorphonuclear leukocytes in stool, whereas bacterial toxigenic causes (other than *C. difficile* and enterohemorrhagic *E. coli*), viruses, and protozoa generally are not. The bacterial toxigenic causes of diarrhea other than *C. difficile* and enterohemorrhagic *E. coli* do not produce fever.

Stool culture is definitive for the diagnosis of *Salmonella* enterocolitis, but by the time the results of stool culture are available, most patients are recovering. A stained smear of the stool usually demonstrates polymorphonuclear leukocytes. Serologic studies are of little clinical value in *Salmonella* enterocolitis, but they may be of use in epidemiologic studies.

The differential diagnosis of *Salmonella* bacteremia includes virtually all acute infectious and noninfectious causes of fever, including bacteremia caused by other organisms. The diagnosis is proved by isolation of the microorganism from blood or from another normally sterile site.

The differential diagnosis of enteric fever is broad and depends in part on the area of the world where the infection was acquired. All causes of sustained fever are in the differential diagnosis, including infective endocarditis, disseminated tuberculosis, brucellosis, tularemia, *Mycoplasma pneumoniae* infection, rickettsial infections, Q fever, and viral infections such as infectious mononucleosis. Depending on the site of acquisition, diseases such as malaria, amebic abscesses of the liver, and visceral leishmaniasis also enter into the differential diagnosis.

The diagnosis of enteric fever is best proved by isolation of the microorganism from blood, stool, or bone marrow.[11] During the first week of illness, blood cultures are positive in about 90% of patients, but culture positivity decreases in the next 2 weeks to less than 50% during the third week of illness. Stool cultures are usually negative during the first week but are generally positive by the third week. Bone marrow cultures give the highest yield, with up to 95% being positive; they should be considered in suspected cases with negative blood cultures. Bone marrow cultures may be positive even after several days of antimicrobial treatment, when blood cultures have become negative. Urine cultures and cultures of punch biopsies of rose spots may also be positive. The string test to obtain samples of bile from the duodenum has also yielded positive cultures.

The peripheral leukocyte count is usually normal, but leukopenia, which occurs in about 20% of cases, may be suggestive of enteric fever. Fecal leukocytes are generally present.

The Widal and other serologic tests that detect serum antibodies against *Salmonella* Typhi are limited by shortcomings of both sensitivity and specificity and rarely provide useful information to guide management of the patient. Polymerase chain reaction and other molecular techniques lack sensitivity for diagnosis from blood and other specimens, but they have been used to determine the *Salmonella* serovar of bacterial isolates.

TREATMENT   Rx

Enterocolitis

The primary approach to the treatment of *Salmonella* enterocolitis is fluid and electrolyte replacement. Drugs with antiperistaltic effects, such as loperamide or diphenoxylate with atropine, can relieve cramps, but they should be used sparingly because they can prolong the diarrhea.

Salmonella enterocolitis is self-limited, and antimicrobial therapy is usually not indicated, except perhaps in groups of patients at high risk for invasive disease. Antimicrobial therapy reportedly has little effect on the clinical course, and in some studies, it has prolonged the duration of *Salmonella* excretion in stool. In addition, most patients are improving by the time salmonellae or other bacterial pathogens are isolated from stool.

The fluoroquinolones are active against virtually all bacterial pathogens that cause diarrhea (including salmonellae), except for *C. difficile* and many *Campylobacter* organisms. Thus, it is reasonable to use fluoroquinolones for patients with suspected or known *Salmonella* enterocolitis who are severely ill and suspected of being bacteremic. The threshold for antimicrobial treatment is also decreased in those at increased risk for severe illness (e.g., infants, the elderly, patients with sickle cell disease, immunosuppressed individuals). As an example, in adults, ciprofloxacin, 500 mg every 12 hours orally or 400 mg every 12 hours intravenously for 3 to 5 days, or until defervescence, has been widely used. An extended-spectrum cephalosporin such as ceftriaxone is an alternative. In the presence of gross bloody diarrhea, antimicrobial therapy should be withheld until the possibility of *E. coli* O157:H7 infection has been eliminated because antimicrobial therapy may increase the frequency of hemolytic-uremic syndrome.

Other agents, such as amoxicillin and trimethoprim-sulfamethoxazole, have also been widely used in severely ill adults. However, many strains of *Salmonella* are now resistant to these agents.

Enteric Fever

Resistance to the traditional first-line antimicrobial agents (ampicillin, chloramphenicol, trimethoprim-sulfamethoxazole) has emerged worldwide among the salmonellae causing enteric fever. Consequently, alternative antimicrobial agents are now preferred.

The fluoroquinolones have become the agents of choice for the treatment of enteric fever, for several reasons.[A1] They can be administered orally and have high bioavailability, they concentrate in bile and the bowel, and they often retain activity against multidrug-resistant strains of *Salmonella* Typhi and other causes of enteric fever. Most important, the fluoroquinolones have proved to be effective in the treatment of enteric fever, even with short courses (e.g., 3 to 7 days). The proportion of patients cured exceeds 95%, and relapse and chronic fecal carriage after therapy are uncommon. Ciprofloxacin (500 mg orally twice a day) for 7 to 14 days has been the fluoroquinolone of choice for enteric fever. If a patient cannot tolerate oral therapy, the fluoroquinolones can be administered intravenously. Reduced susceptibility and resistance to fluoroquinolones are increasingly reported in *Salmonella* Typhi and *Salmonella* Paratyphi strains both in the United States and elsewhere and are associated with treatment failure. If decreased fluoroquinolone susceptibility or resistance is suspected or demonstrated, alternative agents include extended-spectrum cephalosporins (e.g., intravenous ceftriaxone) and azithromycin.

Extended-spectrum cephalosporins such as ceftriaxone are reliable agents for the treatment of enteric fever. Ceftriaxone dosed at 1 to 2 g every 12 to 24 hours for adults and 75 mg/kg/day for children, given intravenously or intramuscularly for 10 to 14 days, results in cure of 95% of patients. Resistance to ceftriaxone has been described in clinical strains of *Salmonella* Typhi, but this occurs rarely.

If the *Salmonella* isolate is shown to be susceptible by antimicrobial susceptibility testing, ampicillin, chloramphenicol, or trimethoprim-sulfamethoxazole may be considered. The ampicillin dose is 25 mg/kg intravenously every 6 hours. The use of chloramphenicol should be weighed against the risk of bone marrow toxicity. The chloramphenicol dose is 50 mg/kg/day orally, divided into four doses. Chloramphenicol can be given intravenously at the same dose if oral therapy is not possible. Trimethoprim-sulfamethoxazole (4/20 mg/kg intravenously or orally every 12 hours) is given for 10 to 14 days.

Azithromycin (10 mg/kg/day orally for 7 days) is effective in the treatment of patients with uncomplicated typhoid fever caused by multidrug-resistant strains.[A2] The oral route of administration makes it a particularly attractive choice in settings where multidrug resistance is common and intravenous extended-spectrum cephalosporins are impractical, unavailable, or too expensive.

Patients often require supportive care with intravenous saline, correction of electrolyte and acid-base disturbances, and, in the setting of intestinal bleeding, blood transfusion. If perforation is suspected, abdominal imaging should be performed to evaluate for free air. If perforation seems likely, laparotomy should be performed as soon as possible to repair the perforation. In the setting of perforation, antimicrobial therapy should be broadened to cover bowel flora.

Steroid therapy is beneficial in some patients with severe enteric fever and coma, delirium, or shock. Dexamethasone is administered at doses of 3 mg/kg initially, followed by 1 mg/kg every 6 hours for 48 hours. Steroids can mask the signs and symptoms of abdominal perforation and should not be continued for more than 48 hours. Salicylates should be avoided.

Relapses of typhoid fever may be treated with the same antimicrobial regimen as the initial attack.

Bacteremia

The agents of choice to treat *Salmonella* bacteremia are the fluoroquinolones, such as ciprofloxacin, and the extended-spectrum cephalosporins, such as ceftriaxone. Typical doses are ciprofloxacin 400 mg every 12 hours intravenously and ceftriaxone 1 to 2 g every 12 to 24 hours intravenously. When the salmonellae are known to be susceptible, ampicillin 1 to 2 g intravenously every 4 to 6 hours or trimethoprim-sulfamethoxazole 8 mg/kg/day (of the trimethoprim component) intravenously can be used. Chloramphenicol is another option. Antimicrobial susceptibility testing is necessary because of the emergence of infections resistant to the fluoroquinolones or extended-spectrum cephalosporins.

In cases of sustained bacteremia, the possibility of endovascular infection should be investigated. For transient bacteremia or bacteremia without localization, therapy is continued for 7 to 14 days. With localization to bone, aneurysms, heart valves, and various other sites, antimicrobial therapy should be given for much longer periods (e.g., 6 weeks). Surgical drainage, removal of foreign bodies, or resection of an aneurysm is often necessary to cure localized infection. The possibility of schistosomiasis should be considered and treated, when present, in patients with sustained *Salmonella* bacteremia (Chapter 355). Patients with HIV infection tend to experience repeated relapses after treatment courses for *Salmonella* bacteremia. In this group, initial treatment with ciprofloxacin for 2 weeks or longer is recommended. Long-term suppressive therapy has been suggested for those experiencing frequent relapses.[12]

Carriers

Chronic carriers (i.e., >1 year) of salmonellae other than *Salmonella* Typhi are rare. Stools of convalescent carriers spontaneously become negative during a period of weeks to months, and no therapy should be given. The rare chronic carrier of *Salmonella* serovars other than Typhi (usually infected with *Salmonella* Paratyphi A, B, or C) may be treated with a fluoroquinolone, amoxicillin, or trimethoprim-sulfamethoxazole in the doses listed later for 4 to 6 weeks. Patients who experience relapse usually have gallbladder disease (most often calculi) and will not be cured with antimicrobial therapy alone. Cholecystectomy plus antimicrobial therapy may cure these patients, but it is doubtful that the carrier state is a sufficient indication for cholecystectomy.

Chronic fecal carriers of *Salmonella* Typhi can be treated with ciprofloxacin (500 to 750 mg twice daily) for 6 weeks or with amoxicillin at doses of 6 g/day in three or four divided doses plus probenecid 2 g/day in divided doses for 6 weeks. Trimethoprim-sulfamethoxazole (160/800 mg twice daily) plus rifampicin (300 mg twice daily) for 6 weeks may be considered as an alternative regimen. Patients with persistent urinary carriage and *S. haematobium* infection should be treated with praziquantel before eradication of *Salmonella* Typhi is attempted. For patients with persistent carriage and anatomic abnormalities (e.g., gallstones), cholecystectomy combined with antimicrobial therapy is often necessary. For patients with persistent carriage despite adequate antimicrobial therapy and without an identifiable anatomic abnormality, chronic suppressive therapy may be considered. Chronic carriers who do not prepare food and who practice adequate personal hygiene usually do not constitute a public health hazard. Therefore, after the institution of appropriate personal hygienic precautions, and in the absence of evidence of a chronic carrier infecting others, cholecystectomy is probably not indicated to eradicate the carrier state.

PREVENTION

Salmonella infection is best prevented by protecting the water supply, preventing fecal contamination during food production, cooking and refrigerating foods, pasteurizing milk and milk products, and handwashing before preparing foods. Travelers should judiciously avoid consuming untreated water (including ice), raw vegetables, and fruits. Food should be cooked or peeled, and drinks should be boiled, carbonated, or commercially bottled. The widespread presence of salmonellae in the animal kingdom means that reducing the risk for *Salmonella* infections requires a multifaceted approach.

There is no vaccine for *Salmonella* infection other than that for *Salmonella* Typhi. Travelers should be vaccinated before going to areas that are endemic for typhoid fever.[13] Two vaccines are available in the United States. One is the typhoid Vi capsular polysaccharide vaccine, which is administered as a single intramuscular injection, with booster doses given every 2 years if needed. This vaccine provides a degree of herd protection against typhoid fever when it is used at the population level. The other licensed typhoid fever vaccine is the oral live attenuated Ty21a vaccine. Revaccination is necessary every 5 years, if indicated. Ty21a vaccine should not be used in immunocompromised persons or those receiving antimicrobials. Both these vaccines confer greater than 75% protective efficacy. Efforts are under way to develop typhoid vaccines that are effective in young children.

Vaccines afford only partial immunity to typhoid fever. Persons who have been vaccinated should still restrict their diets to avoid potentially contaminated food and fluids. When cases of imported typhoid are identified in the United States, the local health department should be informed and will monitor stool cultures. Typhoid fever acquired in the United States is typically investigated by the public health department to identify potential sources and chronic carriers.

PROGNOSIS

Mortality in patients with *Salmonella* enterocolitis is rare; infants and the elderly are at greatest risk, with death occurring as a result of dehydration and electrolyte imbalance. Mortality from *Salmonella* bacteremia is not uncommon and is most likely to occur in the very young, the very old, the malnourished, and the immunocompromised.

Before the advent of antimicrobial therapy, typhoid fever had a case-fatality ratio of 15 to 20%. This has been reduced to less than 1% in industrialized countries. However, the case-fatality ratio remains high in some developing countries. The case-fatality ratio of invasive nontyphoidal *Salmonella* in Africa is approximately 20%. In treated patients, the temperature usually returns to normal after 3 to 5 days of therapy, but this may take longer in patients treated with extended-spectrum cephalosporins than in those treated with fluoroquinolones and in those infected with isolates with decreased fluoroquinolone susceptibility who are treated with ciprofloxacin.

In the era before antimicrobial therapy, 5 to 10% of patients who recovered from typhoid fever had relapses. Relapses continued to occur in 10 to 15%

of patients treated with chloramphenicol, ampicillin, and trimethoprim-sulfamethoxazole, but this seemed to be much less frequent (<5%) among those treated with ceftriaxone and fluoroquinolones. Intestinal bleeding or perforation occurs in about 5% of patients. With perforation, case-fatality ratios of 10 to 30% have been reported. Up to 3% of patients recovering from *Salmonella* Typhi infection become chronic fecal carriers.

Grade A References

A1. Effa EE, Lassi ZS, Critchley JA, et al. Fluoroquinolones for treating typhoid and paratyphoid fever (enteric fever). *Cochrane Database Syst Rev.* 2011;10:CD004530.
A2. Effa EE, Bukirwa H. Azithromycin for treating uncomplicated typhoid and paratyphoid fever (enteric fever). *Cochrane Database Syst Rev.* 2008;4:CD006083.

GENERAL REFERENCES

For the General References and other additional features, please visit Expert Consult at https://expertconsult.inkling.com.

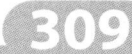

SHIGELLOSIS

GERALD T. KEUSCH

DEFINITION

Shigellosis is an acute infection of the large bowel due to bacteria of the genus *Shigella*, characterized by mucosal inflammation and fever. Clinical disease ranges from watery diarrhea to bloody diarrhea or dysentery, a syndrome consisting of multiple small-volume bloody stools per day, abdominal cramping, and tenesmus, a painful straining with the urge to defecate.

The Pathogen

The etiologic agents of shigellosis are gram-negative bacilli of the family Enterobacteriaceae, tribe Escherichieae, and genus *Shigella*. The organism is so closely related to *Escherichia coli* (Chapter 304) that if it were discovered today, *Shigella* would be classified as distinct serotypes of *E. coli*. Indeed, a number of *E. coli* serotypes causing *Shigella*-like illness and possessing conserved virulence factors are now well described.

EPIDEMIOLOGY

In the United States, the incidence of microbiologically confirmed cases has been steadily trending down during the past four decades on the basis of data compiled from voluntary reporting by state health departments to the Centers for Disease Control and Prevention (CDC) (Fig. 309-1). In 2011, the latest year for which data are available, 7062 cases were identified, corresponding to an all-time low incidence rate of 2.3 per 100,000.[1] However, this is not uniform across the country. For example, the incidence rate of *Shigella sonnei* infection, which accounts for more than 75% of all isolates reported to the CDC, was considerably higher in the seven southern states from Alabama across to Arizona. In addition, the incidence rate was nearly 11 per 100,000 in children 0 to 4 years old and more than 8 per 100,000 in children 5 to 9 years old, reflecting the fact that about one third of cases occur in these age groups.[2] Pediatric shigellosis in the United States is commonly associated with daycare centers, where hygiene is difficult to maintain. However, most cases of acute shigellosis are never reported because they are mild or not part of an outbreak and therefore never microbiologically investigated. For this reason, the CDC estimates that around 450,000 cases of *Shigella* infection occur each year in the United States, primarily self-limited watery diarrheas. The small inoculum, from just 10 to 10,000 organisms, documented to cause infection and illness in experimental human infections explains why shigellosis is so readily transmitted from person to person from the stool of an infected person to a susceptible individual, often by the hands and direct skin contact or indirectly through objects (fomites) previously handled by the infected person. It also explains why one case in a family is associated with transmission to 20 to 40% of household members, although children are much more likely to develop clinical illness than are adults, who may be immune as a

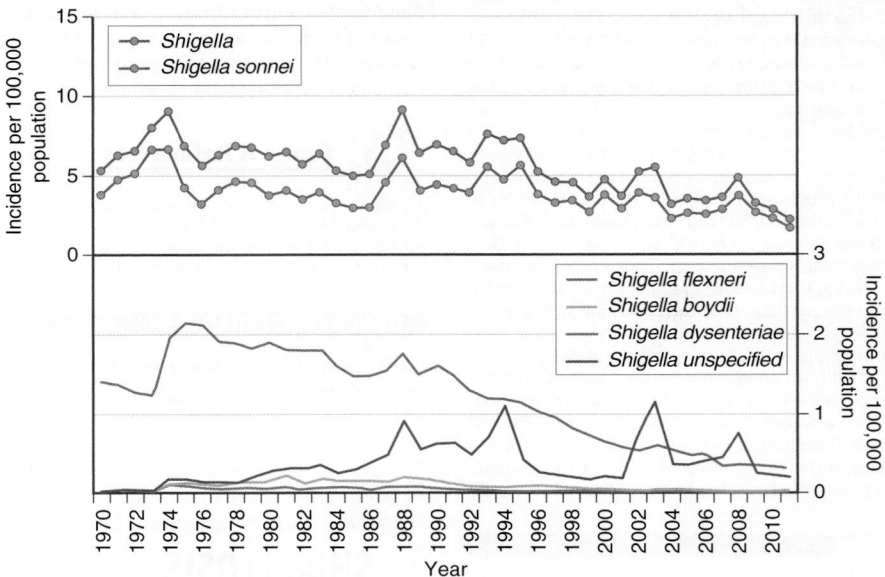

Incidence Rate of Laboratory-Confirmed *Shigella* Infection Reported to CDC (All Species), United States, 1970-2011

FIGURE 309-1. Incidence rate of laboratory-confirmed *Shigella* infection reported to the Centers for Disease Control and Prevention (all species), United States, 1970-2011. *Top panel,* The incidence rates of infection with *Shigella* (all species) and *Shigella sonnei*. Since 1970, the incidence rate of infection with *Shigella* (all species) has been driven by the incidence of infection with *Shigella sonnei*. *Bottom panel,* The incidence rate of infection with all *Shigella* species other than *Shigella sonnei,* including infections with an unspecified species. The incidence rate of infection with *Shigella flexneri* has been decreasing since the 1980s. Since the mid-1980s, the incidence rate of *Shigella* infection in which the species is not indentified has fluctuated, likely representing, at least to some extent, outbreak situations in which public health laboratories did not characterize all outbreak-associated *Shigella* isolates to the species level. *Shigella boydii* and *Shigella dysenteriae* infections are rare in the United States.

result of prior contact with the organism.[3] Asymptomatic carriage of *Shigella* is typically limited to a few weeks; but because an etiologic diagnosis of *S. sonnei* is rarely made, except in common-source outbreaks most likely to be investigated by public health officials, convalescent carriers often return to their normal activities while still able to transmit infection. This may account, in part, for the predilection for outbreaks in daycare centers.

Fecal contamination of food or water is another route for transmission. In settings where there are no facilities for sanitary disposal of feces, flies can serve to transfer the organism to food or water. In the United States, food-borne shigellosis results in multiperson or multistate outbreaks.[4] In 2012, the CDC Foodborne Diseases Active Surveillance Network (FoodNet) identified *Shigella* in 2128 individuals, the third leading cause, of whom 23% were hospitalized and two died. The overall incidence rate was 4.5 per 100,000 at risk in the sentinel populations, but it was four times higher in children 0 to 9 years old. These events are generally related to an infected food handler and continually seem to involve new vehicles, such as recent outbreaks traced to fresh salsa or guacamole prepared in restaurants. Multicountry outbreaks of *S. sonnei* due to contaminated fresh foods shipped from Africa or Southeast Asia demonstrate how globalization of the food supply can also globalize infection with particular strains of *Shigella*. This has important implications for the importation of antibiotic-resistant strains from areas of the world where the prevalence is particularly high. In the United States, contamination of swimming pools or bathing areas, usually by young children harboring the organism who defecate in the water, can result in common-source outbreaks. Because of the small infectious inoculum, outbreaks readily occur during complex humanitarian emergencies such as floods, landslides, earthquakes, or the gathering of refugees of conflict into crowded camps with limited sanitary facilities.

Shigella dysenteriae type 1 and *Shigella flexneri* generally cause more severe illness, resulting in bloody diarrhea or dysentery, whereas *S. sonnei* and *Shigella boydii* are typically mild infections causing self-limited watery diarrhea.[5] For still unknown reasons, *S. sonnei* is most common in high-income countries; most *Shigella* infections in developing countries are due to *S. flexneri* strains,[6] with *S. dysenteriae* type 1 periodically causing outbreaks that may last several years. *S. boydii* is present primarily in the Indian subcontinent and clinically resembles *S. sonnei*. Wherever there is severe underlying childhood malnutrition, however, any *Shigella* infection can be lethal.

In the United States, the incidence peaks in summer and fall. Females are more often infected than are males in the age range of 5 to 29 years, whereas

males predominate in the 30- to 49-year age group, possibly related to anal-oral sex among men who have sex with men. Among the latter, *S. flexneri* is more common than *S. sonnei*, the reverse ratio observed in the general population. Thus, the median age of individuals with *S. sonnei* infection is 6 years, in contrast to a median age of 26 years in those harboring *S. flexneri*. In developing countries, seasonal peaks occur in the rainy season, when organisms from open defecation can be washed into the water used for drinking, or in the dry season, when water for personal hygiene is scarce. In contrast to the low case-fatality rate for *Shigella* in the United States (approximately 50/100,000 infected in the FoodNet survey), the rate in developing countries may be as high as 100-fold greater, despite the continuing decline in global diarrhea mortality during the past three decades. However, it is difficult to determine how many of the currently estimated 700,000 annual global diarrheal disease deaths are due to *Shigella* because bloody diarrhea or dysentery is not separately reported and cultures are not routinely performed, but it is likely to be a substantial proportion.[7] A careful microbiologic study of moderate to severe diarrhea in nearly 10,000 patients 0 to 5 years of age in seven sites in Africa and South Asia revealed *Shigella* as the fourth leading cause in the age group younger than 1 year, the second leading cause in the age group 1 to 2 years, and the leading cause in the age group 3 to 5 years.[8]

PATHOBIOLOGY

When *Shigella* exit an infected host in feces, they are resistant to acid pH. This facilitates their ability to survive gastric acid when ingested and accounts in large part for the small inoculum required. Once past the stomach, the organisms turn off genes governing acid resistance and turn on genes that allow them to invade the host's colon. *Shigella* initially gain entry into M cells overlying lymphoid Peyer's patches; they are then transcytosed to the lamina propria, where they are ingested by macrophages and induce inflammatory cytokines, leading to macrophage death and the recruitment and migration of polymorphonuclear leukocytes through the mucosa.[9] This forces open the tight junctions between epithelial cells and allows many more organisms from the lumen to gain access to the basolateral membrane of colonic epithelial cells, where they induce the host cells to ingest them by a mechanism resembling phagocytosis. *Shigella* then lyse the phagocytic vesicle to enter the cytoplasm and multiply; although they are nonmotile, they use their capacity to cross-link actin in the cytoplasm to propel themselves to the host cell membrane. There, by the induced phagocytosis-like mechanism, they pass laterally from one epithelial cell to another. The inflammation and death of contiguously invaded host epithelial cells result in mucosal ulcerations and further exudation of blood and leukocytes into the colonic lumen and ultimately in stool. At the same time, regulatory pathways are engaged to transmit alarm signals that activate the innate immune system in bystander cells to confine the invading organisms to the localized area of involvement. Mucosal inflammation and ulceration are the characteristic pathologic changes caused by *Shigella*. The difference between infection by one species and that by another is the severity of the process, which is proportional to the severity of the illness they cause.

The attributes of virulence are present in a large virulence plasmid present in all *Shigella* and in enteroinvasive *E. coli* serotypes capable of causing a similar clinical illness. The virulence plasmid encodes the proteins for a type III secretion system that is capable of transferring microbial effector proteins into the host cell; these proteins regulate the cytoskeleton of the host cell to ingest the organism. Once inside the epithelial cell, shigellae are sequestered from host immune responses. Whereas the short-term gain for the organism is microbial multiplication and excretion in feces, the same mechanisms subsequently act to eliminate the organisms. For example, at later stages of infection, neutrophils play a major role in disease resolution by killing the bacteria and degrading some *Shigella* virulence proteins. *S. dysenteriae* type 1 also produces a chromosomally encoded toxin, Shiga toxin, that inhibits protein synthesis and directly causes cell death. It is one important reason that infection due to this species is so severe.

Structurally and antigenically similar toxins are produced by certain *E. coli*, notably serotype O157:H7, responsible for cases of hemorrhagic colitis (Chapter 304). All Shiga toxin–producing organisms are known causes of hemolytic-uremic syndrome (HUS; Chapter 172), a potentially lethal complication due to the toxin's effects on vascular endothelium within the kidneys.

CLINICAL MANIFESTATIONS

Infections due to *S. sonnei* or *S. boydii* typically are manifested after an incubation period of 1 to 3 days with fever and mild to moderate watery diarrhea (Table 309-1). They do not cause serious dehydration and generally resolve without treatment in 3 to 5 days. However, if the stool is examined under the microscope, white and red blood cells are found, indicative of the underlying inflammation of the mucosa. When the inflammation is more severe, as with *S. flexneri*, the watery diarrhea turns bloody and may progress to dysentery, with its characteristic small-volume bloody mucoid stool passed many (10 to >40) times per day, abdominal cramps, and tenesmus. The most severe infections are due to *S. dysenteriae* type 1 and progress rapidly from watery to bloody diarrhea and frequently to frank dysentery.

The variety of consequences and complications of *S. flexneri* and *S. dysenteriae* type 1 contributes to their importance as causes of death in children in developing countries. Bacteremia with the infecting strain or other enteric flora occurs in up to 10% of cases of severe dysentery due to *S. dysenteriae* type 1 and in some patients with *S. flexneri* infection. Intense mucosal inflammation can result in toxic megacolon, associated in many patients with leukemoid reactions and HUS. Colonic perforation and pancolitis are rare complications that may require surgical intervention. In resource-limited settings, where colostomy management may be difficult to ensure, conservative management with fluids and antibiotics or limited surgery to oversew perforations is the prudent choice; however, mortality may still be as high as 50%. In young children, in whom mesenteric support for the rectosigmoid colon is not fully developed, the intense proctitis that results in straining to pass stool may cause rectal prolapse. A rapid rise in temperature can lead to a seizure in this age group and is distinguishable from typical febrile seizures by the older age of the child and the rarity of multiple seizures. However, patients may become obtunded or even comatose, usually with *S. dysenteriae* type 1 or *S. flexneri* infections. This is often associated with hypoglycemia, due to poor food intake and inadequate gluconeogenesis, or hyponatremia, secondary to inappropriate secretion of antidiuretic hormone. Anorexia may be intense and prolonged. Combined with ongoing catabolism of host muscle protein associated with excessive pro-inflammatory cytokine production and protein-losing enteropathy due to colitis, this always results in some degree of protein-energy malnutrition (Chapter 215). Even with adequate protein-containing and energy-dense diets after infection, replacement of nutrient stores may take as long as four times the duration of the clinical illness. This is more of a problem in developing countries where the diet is poor and full nutritional recovery may not be possible before the next infection occurs, causing further nutritional deterioration. Because of its prolonged metabolic effects, shigellosis is often the precipitating cause of severe and often fatal protein-energy malnutrition or kwashiorkor. *S. flexneri* infection is also associated with reactive arthritis and other autoimmune inflammatory manifestations, such as tendinitis, conjunctivitis, uveitis, urethritis, or erythema nodosum, a constellation of findings commonly termed Reiter's syndrome (Chapter 265). This occurs primarily in individuals positive for HLA-B27 antigen and may be a consequence of molecular mimicry.

Routine laboratory studies document leukocytosis with many immature "band" forms, especially in patients with bloody diarrhea or dysentery. In as many as 20% of hospitalized patients with *S. dysenteriae* type 1 infection and 1 to 2% with *S. flexneri* infection, this may progress to a leukemoid reaction with thrombocytopenia and microangiopathic hemolytic anemia. HUS (Chapter 172) occurs in approximately 8% of patients with *S. dysenteriae* type 1 infection, usually preceded by a leukemoid reaction, and results in some degree of acute renal failure that might progress and require dialysis.

DIAGNOSIS

Shigellosis presenting with watery diarrhea is clinically indistinguishable from the many other causes of watery diarrhea, except for the frequency of fever in *Shigella*, unless the stool is examined microscopically to demonstrate the presence of red and white blood cells or infection is confirmed microbiologically. Bloody diarrhea or dysentery in patients in the developed world is most commonly due to a Shiga toxin–producing *E. coli* (STEC), such as serotype O157:H7, or *S. flexneri* and less often *Campylobacter jejuni*, nontyphoidal *Salmonella* species, or rarely *Yersinia enterocolitica* or *Entamoeba histolytica*. In patients who have recently received antibiotics, bloody diarrhea is often the consequence of *Clostridium difficile* (Chapter 296). In developing countries, *Shigella* (*S. flexneri* or *S. dysenteriae* type 1) is the most common cause of bloody diarrhea or frank dysentery. Although more sophisticated and more sensitive methods of diagnosis are available, such as quantitative

TABLE 309-1 CLINICAL SYNDROMES AND COMPLICATIONS OF SHIGELLOSIS

STAGE	TIME OF APPEARANCE AFTER ONSET OF ILLNESS	SYMPTOMS AND SIGNS	PATHOLOGY AND PATHOGENESIS
Prodrome	Earliest findings	Fever, chills, myalgias, anorexia	None or early colitis
Watery diarrhea	0-3 days	Fever, abdominal cramps, loose stools	Colitis with fecal leukocytes and erythrocytes
Bloody diarrhea	1-3 days	Frequent stools containing blood and mucus, abdominal cramps and tenderness, fever, anorexia	Colitis with fecal leukocytes and erythrocytes
Dysentery	1-5 days	Frequent small-volume stools consisting of blood, mucus, and pus; severe abdominal cramps; tenesmus	More extensive colitis with crypt abscesses and mucosal ulcerations
Acute complications	3-7 days	Seizures, obtundation, bacteremia, colonic obstruction, mucosal perforation, peritonitis	Severe colitis, terminal ileitis
Additional acute complications due to infection with *Shigella dysenteriae* type 1	3-7 days	Toxic megacolon, leukemoid reaction, hemolytic-uremic syndrome	Severe colitis, expression of Stx toxin
Postinfectious syndromes	1-3 weeks	Reactive arthritis, with or without urethritis and conjunctivitis	Autoimmune inflammatory response, most common in individuals expressing HLA-B27 antigen

polymerase chain reaction (which may double the positivity rate), the standard method remains microbiologic culture. For a genus capable of causing such severe illness, *Shigella* species are remarkably fragile outside the intestine and will rapidly die unless samples (preferentially stool and not rectal swabs) are processed rapidly, ideally at the bedside. Using more than one selective culture medium (e.g., MacConkey and xylose-lysine-deoxycholate or *Salmonella*-*Shigella* agar) and obtaining multiple culture specimens will increase the yield. Initially, laboratory screening is based on the failure of *Shigella* species to ferment lactose. Subculture of lactose-negative colonies to differential media such as triple sugar–iron confirms this property and reveals the ability to ferment glucose anaerobically, whereas the lack of motility or production of hydrogen sulfide distinguishes *Shigella* from *Salmonella* species. Specific diagnosis can then be made by standard serologic methods for *Shigella* O antigens. In the case of mild watery diarrhea due to *S. sonnei*, the patient is often recovered by the time the laboratory results are available, so they are of little use in guiding treatment. Culture yields are maximized when patients with bloody diarrhea or dysentery are studied. Typically in the United States, it is only these patients who are likely to be cultured, and the results are valuable for selection of empirical treatment and for epidemiologic purposes when antibiotic sensitivity is also determined to track the emergence of antibiotic resistance.

TREATMENT Rx

Because of the typically mild nature of *S. sonnei* infection in well-nourished children, cultures are not performed, the diagnosis remains unproven, and no specific treatment is given or required. Although it might be sensible from a public health perspective to eliminate convalescent carriers with antibiotics to prevent subsequent transmission (e.g., in the setting of daycare centers), it cannot be justified because of the predilection for *Shigella* to acquire antibiotic resistance, resulting in the loss of valuable therapeutics to treat more severe illness. Hence, antibiotics should be reserved for such episodes, even in outbreak settings. Some authorities have suggested that culture-positive patients—particularly food handlers, caretakers in daycare or clinical care settings, teachers or other school employees, and the immunocompromised—should be kept at home until three consecutive stool cultures are negative; however, the question of who pays means this recommendation is unlikely to be followed in most instances.

In the case of bloody diarrhea or dysentery, antibiotics are the mainstay of treatment. This is particularly problematic in developing countries, where many of the inexpensive, safe, and useful oral drugs, such as ampicillin and trimethoprim-sulfamethoxazole, have become ineffective because of drug resistance. Presently, a fluoroquinolone, such as ciprofloxacin, or azithromycin is reliable in most patients, but these drugs are expensive (particularly azithromycin), and resistance in some isolates has been documented, especially in clusters of men who have sex with men with *S. sonnei* infection. Parenteral ceftriaxone has been useful in severe or drug-resistant illness. However, intravenous treatment requires hospitalization and monitoring and seriously increases the cost of treatment in both developed and developing countries. Isolates of *S. sonnei* expressing the CTX-M type of β-lactamase that confers resistance to all β-lactam antibiotics except cephamycins and carbapenems are increasingly being identified in Asia and elsewhere.

In severe shigellosis, the prompt initiation of effective antibiotic treatment shortens the duration of illness and achieves a more rapid improvement in symptoms such as fever, cramps, and tenesmus.[A1] Evidence from Bangladesh in patients with *S. dysenteriae* type 1 infection also demonstrates that prompt treatment reduces the frequency of HUS and presumably other complications due to colonic inflammation, such as megacolon, perforation, and rectal prolapse. In the United States and other developed countries where *S. dysenteriae* type 1 is not present, HUS is almost exclusively associated with STEC. The toxin genes in these *E. coli* are present on plasmids, in contrast to the chromosomal location of the *stx* gene in *S. dysenteriae* type 1, and are actually upregulated by commonly used antibiotics. Hence, most experts recommend that antibiotic treatment be withheld in patients with STEC infections; but if it is necessary, a drug should be selected that does not have this effect, such as azithromycin, rifaximin, or intravenous meropenem.

Given the known epidemiology of antibiotic resistance among *Shigella* species, empirical therapy for adults with bloody diarrhea or dysentery can be initiated with ciprofloxacin 500 mg orally twice daily for 3 to 5 days.[10] There is increasing evidence that shorter courses are sufficient, even for known or suspected *S. dysenteriae* type 1 infections, but given its severity, many experts would still recommend a full 5-day course. A still reliable oral alternative is azithromycin, with an initial dose of 500 mg followed by 250 mg/day for an additional 4 days, although the identification of *S. sonnei* with reduced susceptibility to azithromycin during an outbreak in Los Angeles in 2012 is of concern. Depending on the epidemiology of resistance in specific geographic areas,

ampicillin (500 mg orally four times daily for 3 days) or trimethoprim-sulfamethoxazole (160/800 mg combination twice daily for 3 days) may still be effective. Doses for young children are ciprofloxacin 10 mg/kg twice daily for 3 days; azithromycin 10 mg/kg on day 1, followed by 5 mg/kg for 4 days more; ampicillin 25 mg/kg four times daily for 5 days; and a pediatric syrup of trimethoprim-sulfamethoxazole containing 4/20 mg, respectively, twice daily for 5 days. β-Lactam antibiotics, such as amoxicillin and oral cephalosporins, are not recommended because initial studies have shown that they are less effective in vivo than predicted by in vitro drug sensitivity studies. This may be due to efficient absorption, leaving insufficient amounts in the intestinal lumen. Pivamdinocillin (mecillinam; marketed as Coactin) is effective but is not available in the United States. Nonabsorbable antimicrobial agents are not recommended because optimal treatment requires therapeutic levels of the drugs in both the lumen and the mucosal compartments.

In more severe infections, complications such as hypoglycemia or hyponatremia can be managed with appropriate glucose or saline given intravenously, but patients must be monitored by trained clinical staff. Colitis with toxic megacolon and intestinal perforation represent difficult problems, especially in resource-poor settings where these complications are most likely to occur. In such settings, conservative medical or surgical management is best, even if it is not optimal. Renal failure due to HUS can generally be managed conservatively or with peritoneal dialysis, if it is available. Seizures are usually self-limited, and other neurologic complications respond to fluid and electrolyte management and correction of hypoglycemia and hyponatremia. Reactive arthritis is a greater problem as it is an autoimmune response that occurs primarily in genetically susceptible individuals positive for HLA-B27 antigen. In addition to effective antibiotic treatment to eliminate the causative organism, chronic arthritis may ensue, requiring nonsteroidal anti-inflammatory agents, steroids, or inflammatory cytokine inhibitors. In the susceptible host, infection-induced reactive arthritis can result in troublesome destructive joint disease that requires ongoing medical management. Some evidence suggests that antimotility agents are contraindicated in shigellosis, particularly in cases of bloody diarrhea or dysentery in young children, because these drugs may slow peristalsis and prolong contact between the organisms and the mucosa, thereby increasing microbial invasion, pathologic changes, and severity, including toxic megacolon.

Because of the prolonged anorexia and catabolic responses in shigellosis, attention to nutritional rehabilitation, especially in malnourished children in developing countries, is an important component of early and continuing management.

PREVENTION

Personal hygiene (in particular handwashing after handling the diapers of infected children and before food preparation), the sanitary disposal of feces, and protection of food and water sources from microbial contamination are essential to limit the spread of shigellosis. Preventing spread in daycare settings is a particular problem because it is so difficult to stop young children from constantly exploring their world, picking up bacteria on their hands, and bringing their potentially contaminated fingers or fomites to their mouths. In such settings, it is particularly important for the adult caretakers to observe good personal hygiene and to supervise children in handwashing. Soap and water are sufficient, but hand sanitizers do work and may be more convenient. In environments where soap is unavailable, water used with sand or ash for scrubbing is helpful. Keeping infected children away from daycare until their stool is negative, if indeed it was cultured, or separating recently ill children from the susceptible has been recommended but is not easy to accomplish. Household hygiene in the setting of an index case, including frequent handwashing, caution in the disposal of soiled diapers or underwear, regularly wiping down the area where these are collected with a disinfectant such as Lysol, and precautions in food preparation, can help limit intrahousehold spread.

Vaccines, particularly for the more virulent species, would be useful. However, despite much effort, a safe and effective vaccine has not been developed or approved for general use. It is doubtful whether a vaccine for *S. sonnei* infection would be recommended for children in a developed country such as the United States, even if it is safe and effective, because the illness is so mild and self-limited and because other vaccines are more important to administer in the context of an increasingly antivaccine public. Once it is available, it could be useful for travelers or among military who are deployed to high-risk locations. In contrast, effective and safe vaccines for *S. flexneri* or *S. dysenteriae* type 1 would be extremely useful in developing countries, where shigellosis accounts for a significant portion of the annual mortality due to diarrheal diseases.[11,12] Our current understanding of immunity in shigellosis indicates that serotype-specific immunity is most important; however, whether this is best conveyed by antibody (and, if so, immunoglobulin G or A) or by cell-mediated mechanisms remains uncertain. Vaccine development has focused on attenuated live oral vaccines; unfortunately, vaccines most effective in inducing immunity have also been the most reactogenic, causing fever and often diarrhea in recipients. Recent efforts employ killed whole cells, O antigen–protein conjugates, and subunit candidates. Unless common protective antigens are identified, the most likely vaccine strategy will be based on a combination of serotype-specific antigens from the most common *S. flexneri* strains and *S. dysenteriae* type 1. We are a long way from having an approved vaccine for shigellosis.

PROGNOSIS

S. sonnei infection and most cases of *S. boydii* infection are mild and self-limited, with no sequelae. Infection with *S. flexneri* or *S. dysenteriae* responds to proper treatment with antibiotics. When treatment is not effective, either a drug-resistant strain or another etiologic agent should be suspected. In some instances, severe shigellosis with pancolitis has been misdiagnosed as inflammatory bowel disease. This can be a disaster if the patient is treated with steroids. Whereas early and effective treatment of *S. dysenteriae* type 1 reduces the risk of complications such as HUS and probably megacolon and bowel perforation, about 25% of those with HUS will have some permanent renal impairment, and a small percentage may progress to end-stage renal failure. Because of the autoimmune nature of reactive arthritis, usually associated with *S. flexneri*, early treatment might not prevent its occurrence but could mitigate its severity. Infection with one serotype of *Shigella* generally provides durable immunity to reinfection with the same strain but leaves the individual susceptible to other antigenically distinct strains and serotypes.

 Grade A Reference

A1. Christopher PRH, David KV, John SM, et al. Antibiotic therapy for *Shigella* dysentery. *Cochrane Database Syst Rev.* 2010;8:CD006784.

GENERAL REFERENCES

For the General References and other additional features, please visit Expert Consult at https://expertconsult.inkling.com.

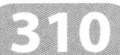

BRUCELLOSIS

EDSEL MAURICE T. SALVANA AND ROBERT A. SALATA

DEFINITION

Brucellosis is a zoonotic disease with protean manifestations caused by bacteria of the genus *Brucella*. Human infection is acquired via ingestion or inhalation of bacteria in contaminated material. Although occupational exposure is a common risk factor for infection, the vast majority of disease occurs through ingestion of unpasteurized dairy products. Despite continuing efforts to control its spread, brucellosis remains a significant health and economic burden in many countries.

The Pathogen

Brucellae are slow-growing, small, aerobic, nonmotile, nonencapsulated, non–spore-forming, gram-negative coccobacilli. *Brucella abortus* (from cattle), *Brucella suis* (from pigs), *Brucella melitensis* (from sheep, goats and camels), and *Brucella canis* (from dogs) are the species that most commonly infect humans. Genome sequencing shows a high degree of homology among strains despite disparate preferred hosts.[1]

EPIDEMIOLOGY

Etiology

Virulence traditionally varies among the four major species of *Brucella*, although this concept has been recently challenged. Because of its pathogenicity and ability to remain viable in storage for long periods, *Brucella* spp.

are potential agents for bioterrorism. *B. abortus* is usually associated with mild to moderate sporadic disease. *B. suis* and *B. melitensis* infections are associated with suppurative or disabling complications and can have a prolonged course. Infection with *B. canis* has an insidious onset, relapses frequently, and has a chronic but relatively mild course. Two marine species, *Brucella pinnipediae* and *Brucella cetaceae*, related to seals and cetaceans, respectively, can cause mild infection in humans. *Brucella microti*, with a high potential for pathogenicity, has been isolated from the common vole, red fox, and soil, but no instances of human infection have been reported. Other newly described *Brucella* species with known or potential human pathogenicity include *Brucella inopinata* (one human case of breast implant infection), *Brucella ovis* (sheep infection; no human cases reported), and *Brucella neotomae* (rodent infection; no human cases reported). BO2, a proposed future species closely related to *B. ovis*, has caused one human case of chronic destructive pneumonia.[1,2]

Incidence and Prevalence

More than 500,000 cases of brucellosis are reported yearly to the World Health Organization (WHO) from 100 countries. *B. melitensis* infection accounts for the majority of cases, distributed primarily in the Mediterranean region (particularly Spain and Greece), Latin America, the Arabian Gulf, and the Indian subcontinent. *B. abortus* infection occurs worldwide but has been effectively eradicated in several European countries, Japan, and Israel. Whereas *B. suis* occurs mainly in the Midwestern United States, South America, and Southeast Asia, *B. canis* infection is most common in North America, South America, Japan, and central Europe. Identification of the infecting *Brucella* species helps determine the likely source of infection.[3]

In animals, brucellosis is a chronic infection that can persist throughout life. Because of effective control programs in animals, the incidence of human brucellosis has decreased dramatically in the United States, from more than 6000 cases in 1947 to fewer than 200 cases each year since 1980. States reporting the greatest number of cases include Texas, California, Virginia, and Florida. In North America, brucellosis occurs mainly in the spring and summer, is more common in men, and is usually related to occupational exposure.

Brucella infection in the United States occurs mostly through direct contact with animals or animal secretions in high-risk groups, including slaughterhouse workers, farmers, dairy workers, veterinarians, and travelers returning from endemic areas. Laboratory workers handling infected animals or *Brucella* cultures are also at risk. More than half of the reported cases are associated with the meat-processing industry, particularly the "kill areas," where infection is spread through abraded or lacerated skin; the conjunctiva, possibly by aerosolization; and, rarely, by ingestion of infected tissue. Many cases of *B. abortus* infection in veterinarians have resulted accidentally from exposure to the strain 19 vaccine used to immunize cattle. In the southern United States, 20% of feral swine are positive for *B. suis*, and human infections in hunters have been reported. *B. melitensis* infection, transmitted through the ingestion of goat's milk cheese, has been seen in U.S. travelers to and immigrants from Mexico. Brucellosis contracted abroad may not become symptomatic until the patient returns to the United States. Although persons with human immunodeficiency virus (HIV) infection are generally at higher risk for intracellular pathogens, the clinical manifestations of brucellosis in HIV-infected and noninfected individuals are similar in the few cases of coinfection that have been reported. Human-to-human transmission is rare, but there have been increasing reports of sexually transmitted brucellosis.[4]

Brucellosis in pregnancy has been associated with spontaneous abortions, congenital abnormalities, and neonatal infections. Childhood brucellosis also occurs, mostly in school-aged children, but accounts for only 3% to 10% of all reported cases worldwide. It is more common in endemic areas, where it may account for 20% to 25% of cases, and is often a mild, self-limited process.[5]

PATHOBIOLOGY
Pathogenesis

After penetrating the epithelial cells of human skin, conjunctiva, pharynx, intestine, or lung, *Brucella* organisms in naive individuals induce a delayed inflammatory response (up to 48 hours) with polymorphonuclear leukocyte infiltration at the infection site. *Brucella* organisms are then ingested by dendritic cells, neutrophils and tissue macrophages, and these subsequently spread to regional lymph nodes. If host defenses within the lymph nodes are overwhelmed, bacteremia follows. The usual incubation period from infection to bacteremia is 2 to 4 weeks. Bacteremia is accompanied by phagocytosis of free *Brucella* organisms by macrophages, and localization of the disease primarily to the spleen, liver, and bone marrow, with the formation of small, noncaseating granulomas, which can serve as persistent sources of infection.

As an intracellular organism, *Brucella* spp. have to avoid detection by the immune system on entry and must be able to survive a hostile intracellular environment. *Brucella* organisms avoid initial detection by the host through multiple mechanisms. Its cell wall lipopolysaccharide (smooth LPS) differs significantly from regular bacterial LPS in two important ways: it has very little effect on Toll-like receptor type 4 (TLR4) activation, and it is resistant to complement activation. In addition, *Brucella* organisms deploy a protein that interferes with TLR signaling. Upon successful entry into the host, *Brucella* organisms in phagosomes are able to survive acidification and lysosome fusion through the induction of specific virulence factors such as the VirB type IV secretion system (T4SS). To replicate, *Brucella* organisms intercept traffic between the endoplasmic reticulum and the Golgi apparatus. They also seem to inhibit apoptosis of the infected cell, thereby maintaining a persistent presence protected from the immune system.[2]

Immunity

Humoral factors play an important role in host defense against *Brucella* spp. Even in the absence of specific agglutinating antibody, normal human serum is bactericidal for *Brucella* organisms; *B. abortus* is more susceptible to serum lysis than is *B. melitensis*. The intracellular location of *Brucella* spp. within macrophages enables it to escape the lethal effects of serum to a certain extent. Specific serum agglutinating antibody has opsonic activity but does not correlate with the development of protective immunity.

A role for mononuclear phagocytes and cell-mediated immunity in brucellosis has been demonstrated. Prior infection with *Listeria monocytogenes* or *Mycobacterium tuberculosis,* both of which stimulate cell-mediated immune mechanisms, is protective against *Brucella* infection in animals. Skin testing with *Brucella* proteins elicits a typical delayed hypersensitivity response in infected individuals. Macrophages, activated with T helper 1 (T_H1)–type cytokines (including interferon-γ, tumor necrosis factor-α, interleukin-1, interleukin-12), kill *Brucella*. Studies have shown that despite high levels of T_H1 cytokine production, deficient effector phagocytic activity persists. Later in the course of infection, there is evidence of an unexpected inhibitory effect from neutrophils. Animal models have demonstrated more efficient killing of *Brucella* organisms in the absence of polymorphonuclear cells, which somehow dampen the immune response to this pathogen.[6]

CLINICAL MANIFESTATIONS

Clinically, human brucellosis can be divided into subclinical illness, acute or subacute disease, localized disease, relapsing infection, and chronic disease (Table 310-1).[7]

Subclinical Illness

Asymptomatic or clinically unrecognized human brucellosis often occurs in high-risk groups, including slaughterhouse workers, farmers, and veterinarians. The diagnosis is usually made through serologic means. More than 50% of abattoir workers and up to 33% of veterinarians have high anti-*Brucella* antibody titers but no history of recognized clinical infection. Children in endemic areas frequently have subclinical illness.

Acute and Subacute Disease

After an incubation period of several weeks or months, acute brucellosis may occur as a mild, transient illness (*B. abortus* or *B. canis*) or as an explosive, toxic illness with the potential for multiple complications (*B. melitensis*). Approximately 50% of patients have an abrupt onset over days, but the remainder have an insidious onset over weeks. Symptoms in brucellosis are protean and nonspecific. More than 90% of patients experience malaise, chills, sweats, fatigue, and weakness. More than 50% of patients have myalgias, anorexia, and weight loss. Fewer patients complain of arthralgias, cough, testicular pain, dysuria, ocular pain, or blurring of vision. Few localizing physical signs are apparent. Fever, with temperatures often greater than 39.4° C (103° F), occurs in 95% of patients. An undulating or intermittent fever pattern is not unusual. A pulse–temperature deficit (i.e., relative bradycardia) may occur. Splenomegaly is present in 10% to 15% of cases, and lymphadenopathy occurs in about 14% of patients. Axillary, cervical, and supraclavicular lymphadenopathy are most frequent and may be related to hand wounds or oropharyngeal routes of infection. Hepatomegaly is less frequent. Other laboratory findings in acute or subacute disease may include mild anemia; lymphopenia; or neutropenia (especially with bacteremia); lymphocytosis; thrombocytopenia; or, in rare cases, pancytopenia. The majority of infected individuals recover completely without sequelae if diagnosed early with prompt initiation of therapy.[8]

Localized Disease and Complications

Brucella organisms can localize to almost any organ but usually target the bones, joints, central nervous system, heart, lung, spleen, testis, liver, gallbladder, kidney, prostate, pancreas, and skin. Disease may occur at multiple sites. Complications with local manifestations most often appear in association with chronic illness, although complications may also occur with acute disease caused by *B. melitensis* or *B. suis*. In the United States, localized disease is most frequently related to *B. suis*. Osteoarticular complications account for 10% to 80% of localized disease in most reported series. Whereas sacroiliitis is the most common manifestation in young persons, spondylitis is more frequently encountered in elderly adults. Vertebral osteomyelitis, particularly in the lumbar area, is also a well-recognized complication and can be associated with paravertebral, epidural, and psoas abscesses.

Relapsing Infection

Up to 10% of patients with brucellosis relapse after antimicrobial therapy. The intracellular location of *Brucella* organisms predisposes to recurrence because the organisms are relatively protected from host defense mechanisms, and antimicrobial agents may be unable to penetrate efficiently enough to kill all the bacteria. Acquired resistance to antibiotics is another factor that can lead to treatment failure. Relapses usually occur 3 to 6 months after completion of therapy but may be seen up to 2 years after initial treatment. Relapsing

TABLE 310-1	CLINICAL CLASSIFICATION OF HUMAN BRUCELLOSIS			
CLASSIFICATION	**DURATION OF SYMPTOMS BEFORE DIAGNOSIS**	**MAJOR SYMPTOMS AND SIGNS**	**DIAGNOSIS**	**COMMENTS**
Subclinical	—	Asymptomatic	Positive (low-titer) serology, negative cultures	Occurs in abattoir workers, farmers, and veterinarians
Acute and subacute	Up to 2-3 mo and 3 mo-1 yr, respectively	Malaise, chills, sweats, fatigue, headache, anorexia, arthralgias, fever, splenomegaly, lymphadenopathy, hepatomegaly	Positive serology, positive blood or bone marrow cultures	Presentation can be mild, self-limited (*B. abortus*) or fulminant with severe complications (*B. melitensis*)
Localized	Occurs with acute or chronic untreated disease	Related to involved organs	Positive serology, positive cultures in specific tissues	Bone or joint, genitourinary, hepatosplenic involvement most common
Relapsing	2-3 mo after initial episode	Same as acute illness but may have higher fever and more fatigue, weakness, chills, and sweats	Positive serology, positive cultures	May be extremely difficult to distinguish relapse from reinfection
Chronic	>1 yr	Nonspecific presentation, but neuropsychiatric symptoms and low-grade fever most common	Low titer or negative serology, negative cultures	Most controversial classification; localized disease may be associated

infection is difficult to distinguish from reinfection in high-risk groups with continued exposure. Relapses are associated with inappropriate or insufficient antimicrobial therapy, growth on blood cultures during the initial presentation, and an acute onset of disease.

Chronic Disease

Disease with a duration of more than 1 year is referred to as *chronic brucellosis.* A majority of patients classified as having chronic brucellosis really have persistent disease caused by inadequate treatment of the initial episode, or they have focal disease in bone, liver, or spleen. About 20% of patients diagnosed with chronic brucellosis complain of persistent fatigue, malaise, and depression; in many respects, this condition resembles chronic fatigue syndrome. These symptoms are frequently not associated with clinical, microbiologic, or serologic evidence of active infection and may represent a preexisting psychoneurosis.

DIAGNOSIS

Culture

Many common illnesses mimic the clinical presentation of brucellosis, and a thorough history is essential, including occupation, travel to endemic areas, avocations, and ingestion of at-risk food and beverages. The most conclusive means of establishing the diagnosis of brucellosis is the recovery of the organism from a culture from normally sterile body fluid or tissue. Sensitivity of cultures have ranged from 15% to 90%, depending on the methods used and the specimen type. In cases of suspected brucellosis, the microbiology laboratory should be asked to extend the length of incubation because it may take more than 5 days for *Brucella* organisms to grow. Handling of *Brucella* cultures is potentially hazardous to laboratory personnel.

In acute brucellosis, blood cultures are positive in 10% to 30% of cases, but this may be as high as 85% with *B. melitensis*. The sensitivity of blood cultures decreases with increasing duration of illness. With *B. melitensis* infection, bone marrow cultures are more sensitive than blood cultures. With localized brucellosis (e.g., lymph nodes, spleen, liver, skeletal system), cultures of purulent material or tissues usually yield *Brucella* organisms. Culture of cerebrospinal fluid turns positive in 45% of patients with meningitis. Antibodies against *Brucella* may be demonstrated in cerebrospinal fluid by enzymelinked immunosorbent assay (ELISA).

Standard Tube Agglutination

In the absence of microbiologic confirmation, a presumptive diagnosis can be made by history and serology. The most frequently used test is the standard tube agglutination (STA) test, measuring antibody titers against *B. abortus* antigen. A fourfold or greater rise in titer over 2 weeks is considered significant. A presumptive case is one in which the agglutination titer is positive (1:160 in endemic areas; 1:80 in nonendemic areas) in single or serial specimens, with symptoms consistent with brucellosis. By 3 weeks of illness, more than 97% of patients demonstrate serologic evidence of infection. This test detects antibodies to *B. abortus, B. suis,* and *B. melitensis* but not to *B. canis.* Serologic confirmation of *B. canis* infection requires *B. canis* or *B. ovis* antigen. After adequate antibiotic treatment, significant STA titers can persist for up to 2 years in 5% to 7% of cases. Because of this, STA titers are not useful in

differentiating relapsing infection from other febrile illnesses in patients with a history of past *Brucella* infections. Individuals with subclinical infection may demonstrate significant STA titers. In chronic localized brucellosis, STA titers may appear absent or low owing to a prozone phenomenon. This prozone effect appears to be related to the presence of immunoglobulin G or immunoglobulin A blocking antibodies; it can be eliminated if dilutions are carried out to at least 1:1280. False-positive STA titers related to immunologic cross-reactivity have been associated with *Brucella* skin testing, cholera vaccination, or infection with *Vibrio cholerae, Francisella tularensis,* or *Yersinia enterocolitica.*

Other Tests

Newer generation antibody tests, including ELISA, are more sensitive and specific than STA and are being used more widely. Preliminary studies using polymerase chain reaction of blood and other fluids or tissues offers rapid and highly accurate diagnosis of brucellosis.[9] Sequencing of specific gene products can identify the organism up to the species level. However, protocols still need to be standardized on a wider scale, and access to expertise and adequate laboratory facilities remains a significant limiting factor.

TREATMENT   Rx

Effective treatment of *Brucella* infection requires antibiotics that can penetrate the intracellular compartment, have little or no toxicity even with prolonged use for preventing relapse, and are bactericidal for adequate treatment of central nervous system infection and endocarditis. There remains considerable debate over which antibiotic regimen is best. In adults, the combination of oral doxycycline at 100 mg orally twice a day for 6 weeks plus intramuscular gentamicin at 5 mg/kg for 5 to 7 days is equally effective as traditional therapy using doxycycline for 6 weeks plus streptomycin 1 g intramuscularly for 14 days.[A1] The WHO recommends doxycycline plus rifampin 15 mg/kg orally for 6 weeks. This regimen is less effective for cases of spondylitis, which may require up to 3 months of treatment with any of the above regimens. Monotherapy with fluoroquinolones has been disappointing, and if these agents are used, they should always be combined with another active agent. Recent in vitro studies have demonstrated significant activity and synergy of tigecycline with gentamicin and rifampin; these observations must be supported in clinical trials. A prospective, non-randomized trial of triple combination doxycycline, streptomycin, and rifampicin versus the standard double combination doxycycline plus streptomycin showed a significantly higher rate of undetectable Brucella DNA on follow-up.[10] Recommendations are summarized in Table 310-2.

PREVENTION

The control of human brucellosis is directly related to prevention programs in domestic animals and the avoidance of unpasteurized milk and milk products. In slaughterhouses, important means of prevention include careful wound dressing, the use of protective glasses and clothing, the prohibition of raw meat ingestion, and the use of previously infected (immune) individuals in high-risk areas. Work is ongoing to find an effective vaccine for humans. Postexposure antimicrobial prophylaxis is controversial.

TABLE 310-2	TREATMENT FOR BRUCELLOSIS	
	TREATMENT	**COMMENTS**
Acute, with no endocarditis or CNS involvement	Doxycycline (200 mg/day) plus rifampin (15 mg/kg/day) for 6 wk *Or* Tetracycline (2 g/day) for 6 wk plus streptomycin (1 g/day) or gentamicin (5 mg/kg/day) for 1 wk	Treatment of choice by WHO; widely used; low rate of relapse; IMG administration of streptomycin may be difficult
Alternative agents: chloramphenicol, fluoroquinolones, TMP-SMX, imipenem	Combination therapy still preferred; fluoroquinolones plus rifampin is an alternative	
In children	TMP-SMX plus rifampin	
CNS	Doxycycline plus rifampin and TMP-SMX	Third-generation cephalosporin can be substituted if susceptible in vitro
Localized	Surgically drain abscesses plus antimicrobial therapy for ≥6 wk	
Brucella endocarditis	Bactericidal drugs; early valve replacement may be necessary	Possible aortic valve destruction and/or major arterial emboli

CNS, Central nervous system; *IM,* intramuscular; *TMP-SMX,* trimethoprim–sulfamethoxazole; *WHO,* World Health Organization.

PROGNOSIS

Brucellosis treated appropriately within the first month of symptom onset is curable. Acute brucellosis often produces severe weakness and fatigue, and patients are frequently unable to work for up to 2 months. Immunity to reinfection follows initial *Brucella* infection in the majority of individuals. With early antimicrobial therapy, cases of chronic brucellosis or localized disease and complications are rare. Of the patients who die of brucellosis, 84% have endocarditis involving a previously abnormal aortic valve, often associated with severe congestive heart failure. A recent retrospective review showed a much higher risk of death with medical treatment alone compared with a combined medical and surgical approach for *Brucella* endocarditis, although this needs to be confirmed in prospective trials.[11]

Grade A Reference

A1. Roushan MR, Amiri MJ, Janmohammadi N, et al. Comparison of the efficacy of gentamicin for 5 days plus doxycycline for 8 weeks versus streptomycin for 2 weeks plus doxycycline for 45 days in the treatment of human brucellosis: a randomized clinical trial. *J Antimicrob Chemother*. 2010;65: 1028-1035.

GENERAL REFERENCES

For the General References and other additional features, please visit Expert Consult at https://expertconsult.inkling.com.

311

TULAREMIA AND OTHER *FRANCISELLA* INFECTIONS

WILLIAM SCHAFFNER

DEFINITION

Tularemia is an infectious zoonosis caused by *Francisella tularensis*, a small aerobic, pleomorphic, gram-negative bacillus. Many animal species harbor the organism, most prominently rabbits, squirrels, and muskrats. Humans acquire the infection through various means, including direct contact with infected animal tissues, ingestion of contaminated water or meat, the bite of an infected tick or deer fly, or breathing an aerosol of bacteria.[1,2] Although *F. tularensis* is highly infectious and is a well-recognized risk to laboratory personnel manipulating culture plates of the organism, it is a paradox that the illness is not communicable from person to person. Edward Francis established that deer flies can transmit the infection from animals to humans and provided detailed descriptions of its clinical manifestations. Colloquially, the disease is often referred to as *rabbit fever* or *deer fly fever*.

The Pathogen

The organism occurs in two major subspecies (biovars). *F. tularensis* biovar *tularensis* (type A) is more virulent in animals and humans, has distinctive biochemical reactions (it produces acid from glycerol and has citrulline ureidase activity), and is the common North American biovar. In contrast, *F. tularensis* biovar *holarctica* (type B) is less virulent and occurs commonly in Europe and Asia. Type B is most frequently isolated from rodent species, including muskrats (*Ondatra zibethicus*), mice (*Mus musculus*), beavers (*Castor canadensis*), voles (*Microtus* spp.), and water voles (*Arvicola terrestris*), and has been associated with an outbreak of infection in wild-caught prairie dogs. Specific virulence factors for *F. tularensis* have not been identified.

EPIDEMIOLOGY

Tularemia has been reported in the United States, Canada, Mexico, Japan, and Europe (particularly Scandinavia). It has not been reported in the United Kingdom or the Southern Hemisphere. In the United States, reported cases diminished during the second half of the 20th century from a high of 2291 cases in 1939 to the approximately 125 cases reported annually at present. Tularemia has occurred in all the continental states, but four states account

for 56% of reported cases: Arkansas, Missouri, Oklahoma, and South Dakota. The island of Martha's Vineyard off the coast of Massachusetts is also a focus of tularemia.

In the United States, tularemia is usually acquired from tick bites or from contact with infected animals, especially rabbits. Tick-associated cases now constitute the majority and occur during the summer. The most common vectors in the United States are the wood tick (*Dermacentor andersoni*), the dog tick (*Dermacentor variabilis*), and the Lone Star tick (*Amblyomma americanum*). A smaller peak of autumn and winter cases is a consequence of rabbit hunters skinning and eviscerating their game. Public health education materials aimed at decreasing the hazards of handling wild animals have contributed to the reduction of tularemia in hunters. Mosquitoes are the common vectors in northern Europe. Occasional individuals acquire infection from the bite of an infected animal or, more likely, from the bite of an animal whose mouth was contaminated from recently eating a diseased animal. The latter likely explains most instances of cat-bite tularemia.

Males experience a higher incidence of disease than females in all age groups, probably as a consequence of their greater exposure to the outdoors and animal-related activities and less use of protective measures against tick bites. Persons in all age groups are affected, with children 5 to 14 years of age and older adults most prominently represented. In the United States, American Indians and Alaska natives experience the highest annual incidence (0.5 per 100,000); whites have a lower risk (0.04 per 100,000), and African Americans and Asians/Pacific Islanders have the lowest occurrence of tularemia (≤0.01 per 100,000).

Although tularemia is usually a sporadic infection, outbreaks of disease have been traced to laboratory exposure, contaminated groundwater, muskrat handling, lawn mowing, and brush cutting. In the latter two cases, primary pneumonic tularemia apparently occurred when the affected individuals created an environmental aerosol by mowing grass and cutting brush that had been contaminated with *F. tularensis* excreted in the urine and feces of infected rodents. The organism can survive in water, mud, and straw for weeks to months.

Interest in tularemia has been enhanced because of its potential use as a bioterrorism agent.[3] Its high infectivity (as few as 10 organisms have induced pneumonic disease), its ease of dissemination, and the difficulty of rapidly diagnosing acute illness are characteristics that merit its inclusion among threat agents. Thus, tularemia must be reported immediately to local public health authorities. Unusual patterns of disease will be investigated for both conventional and bioterrorist sources.

PATHOBIOLOGY

F. tularensis can infect humans through several portals of entry, including the skin, mucous membranes, and gastrointestinal and respiratory tracts. It requires intracellular residence and can multiply within macrophages and other cells. After inoculation into the skin and subcutaneous tissue, local bacterial multiplication occurs and evokes a suppurative necrotic reaction characterized by an initial polymorphonuclear response followed by an influx of macrophages and lymphocytes. These suppurative lesions evolve into granulomas. Bacteremia can occur both early and late during this process. The infection can disseminate to the lymph nodes, liver, spleen, lungs, and pleura. Viable *F. tularensis* can persist in tissues for long periods, contributing to the tendency to relapse after treatment.

CLINICAL MANIFESTATIONS

Classically, the clinical manifestations of tularemia have been separated into six categories: ulceroglandular, glandular, oculoglandular, typhoidal, oropharyngeal, and pneumonic. Although this classification has historic roots, it should not be used rigidly because many patients have features of several types. The course of illness is determined by the portal of entry, the degree of systemic involvement, and the dose and virulence of the infecting strain of *F. tularensis*.[4]

The general features of tularemia are similar regardless of the portal of entry. After exposure, the usual incubation period is 3 to 5 days (range, 1-21 days). The disease begins abruptly with the onset of fever (≥101° F), chills, malaise, and headache. Myalgia, vomiting, sore throat, and abdominal pain can also occur. Almost half the patients have a pulse rate that is substantially slower than would be anticipated based on the degree of fever (pulse–temperature dissociation). The fever may abate somewhat after 1 to 3 days, only to recur and continue along with other symptoms for 2 to 3 weeks. Untreated, weight loss, easy fatigue, and lymphadenopathy may persist for weeks longer.

Ulceroglandular Disease

Ulceroglandular disease is the form of infection most readily recognized by physicians. Along with fever and other constitutional symptoms, the patient calls attention to tender, swollen lymph nodes that drain an inoculation site. The nodes are usually axillary or inguinal, and a local lesion appears concurrently or 1 or 2 days before or after the lymphadenopathy. The lesions at the site of inoculation begin as small, red, tender, or painful papules that progress to pustules and then undergo necrosis to produce an ulcer with sharp, somewhat elevated edges and a flat base that becomes black. Untreated, the ulcers heal over a period of weeks and leave scars. Tick-induced infections produce lesions on the trunk, about the waist, and in the perineum, along with the expected local adenopathy. Children typically have occipital and cervical adenopathy from tick bites on the neck and in the hair. Animal exposure often produces lesions on the hands and forearms. Lesions may be multiple. Because the organisms evoke a localized granulomatous response, frank lymphangitis does not occur in uncomplicated tularemia, but an occasional patient manifests a chain of nodules in "sporotrichoid" fashion along the lymphatic drainage.

Patients with such apparently "localized" disease often have symptoms and findings indicating a more widespread infection. Sore throat with or without an erythematous pharynx occurs, as well as chest radiographic findings of patchy infiltrates in the lower lobes, pleural effusions, and hilar adenopathy.

Glandular and Typhoidal Disease

Glandular disease is essentially the same clinical syndrome as ulceroglandular disease but without the local lesion. Thus, the patient has fever, constitutional symptoms, and lymphadenopathy. The local lesion may have been on a part of the body where it was not seen, or it may have been small and already healed by the time the patient sought medical care. Glandular disease accounts for only 3% to 20% of cases. Typhoidal disease does not show evidence of lymphadenopathy and is essentially characterized by fever of unknown cause. These illnesses evade diagnosis unless the physician specifically considers the possibility of tularemia and inquires about tick or animal exposure. Occasionally, the diagnosis is made fortuitously when a positive blood culture is reported.

Oculoglandular Disease

Oculoglandular disease is rare (<5% of cases) and occurs when the conjunctival sac is the portal of entry via an aerosol, splash, or contaminated fingers. It is almost always unilateral and can have a dramatic manifestation with inflamed, swollen eyelids, chemosis, and painful conjunctivitis. The palpebral conjunctiva often shows small yellow nodules and ulcers, counterparts to the skin lesions of ulceroglandular disease. The affected regional lymph nodes are those of the head and neck.

Oropharyngeal Disease

Oropharyngeal disease is also uncommon in the United States and occurs when the mucous membranes of the mouth and pharynx are the portal of entry. Contaminated water or food (inadequately cooked game meat) is the source. Painful exudative pharyngitis and tonsillitis, pharyngeal ulcers, and swollen retropharyngeal and cervical lymph nodes are seen.[5]

Pneumonic Disease

Although pneumonia may be one aspect of the other tularemic syndromes, *pneumonic tularemia* refers to an illness that manifests as a distinctive pneumonia.[6] It accounts for about 10% of reported cases and occurs from inhalational exposure. This is the form of the disease that would result from bioterrorism. In addition to fever and malaise, patients may have a dry cough, substernal discomfort, pleural pain, dyspnea, and sore throat. These pulmonary symptoms may not be very prominent in the context of the systemic illness. Hemoptysis is unlikely. The results of physical examination reflect the extent and distribution of the pneumonic process, which may range from barely evident to frank consolidation with pleural effusion. Radiographic findings range from modest peribronchial infiltrates early in the illness to distinctive bronchopneumonia with effusion. Hilar adenopathy is present in more than one third of cases. Sputum examination is not helpful. Pleural effusions generally contain more than 1000 lymphocytes/mm^3. Gram stain results are negative, and pleural biopsies occasionally contain granuloma, thus inviting confusion with tuberculosis. Without a suggestive history of tick or animal exposure, patients with tularemic pneumonia may be thought to have poorly responding community-acquired pneumonia. Fluoroquinolone

antibiotics are commonly used as empirical therapy in this circumstance to treat some patients with undiagnosed tularemia pneumonia.

DIAGNOSIS

The diagnosis of tularemia usually involves serologic testing with tube agglutination or microagglutination techniques. Antibody concentrations do not reach diagnostic levels until after the 11th day of illness. A single acute titer of 1 : 160 is considered presumptive; a confirmed diagnosis requires a fourfold rise in titer between acute and convalescent specimens. Titers of both immunoglobulin M and immunoglobulin G antibodies may remain elevated for many years after the illness.

Differential Diagnosis

The differential diagnosis of patients with tularemia is substantial. The local lesions can be confused with cat-scratch disease, brown recluse spider bites, *Mycobacterium marinum* infection, herpes simplex infection (Chapter 374), and even syphilis (Chapter 319) and chancroid (Chapter 301) when the lesions are in the perineum or on the penis. Pneumonic tularemia resembles common community-acquired pneumonia (Chapter 97), as well as less common infections such as psittacosis, legionellosis, and Q fever. The glandular and typhoidal forms can resemble typhoid fever (Chapter 308), brucellosis (Chapter 310), ehrlichiosis, and other illnesses accompanied by nonspecific fevers.

Routine laboratory studies do not provide specific results. Leukocyte counts may be within normal limits or elevated; thrombocytopenia, elevated liver enzymes, and sterile pyuria occur with some frequency. *F. tularensis* may be isolated from blood cultures and tissue specimens when media containing cysteine are used. Laboratory personnel should be notified when tularemia is suspected so that appropriate media can be used and to ensure that safeguards are in place to protect against the production of hazardous aerosols.

TREATMENT Rx

Because tularemia is a relatively uncommon disease, therapeutic recommendations are based on a combination of in vitro studies and accumulated clinical experience. The preferred antimicrobials are streptomycin and gentamicin; either one is given for 10 days. Streptomycin is given at a dose of 1 g intramuscularly twice daily. Gentamicin may be more readily available and is administered at a dose of 5 mg/kg intramuscularly or intravenously once daily. Both chloramphenicol and the tetracyclines have been used in the past to treat tularemia; however, use of both these bacteriostatic agents has resulted in higher rates of relapse than treatment with streptomycin or gentamicin. Because chloramphenicol may produce bone marrow toxicity, it is rarely used today. Doxycycline is administered at a dose of 100 mg intravenously twice daily for 14 days. In recent years, ciprofloxacin has been used successfully in a growing number of patients; the dosage is 750 mg intravenously twice daily for 10 days. Both of these drugs can be switched to oral administration of the same doses as soon as tolerated by the patient. There is a need to develop new therapeutic strategies to improve the management of patients with tularemia.[7,8]

PREVENTION

Prevention of tularemia entails minimizing exposure to ticks and avoiding direct exposure to wild animals. Tick protection includes clothing that extends to the wrists and ankles, regular inspection for attached ticks, and the use of insect repellents containing diethyltoluamide (DEET). Gloves should be worn when skinning and dressing game animals, especially rabbits, and all wild rabbit and other game meats should be cooked thoroughly.

A live, attenuated vaccine has been used in the past to provide some protection to researchers working with *F. tularensis*. The vaccine is not available commercially.

PROGNOSIS

Before treatment became available, acute tularemia often lasted as long as 1 month followed by several months of debility. The mortality rate approached 10%. When appropriately diagnosed and treated, the mortality rate from tularemia is now 1% or less.

GENERAL REFERENCES

For the General References and other additional features, please visit Expert Consult at https://expertconsult.inkling.com.

312

PLAGUE AND OTHER *YERSINIA* INFECTIONS

KENNETH L. GAGE AND PAUL S. MEAD

The genus *Yersinia* currently contains at least 18 species, only three of which are known to be significant human pathogens (*Yersinia pestis, Yersinia enterocolitica,* and *Yersinia pseudotuberculosis*). The remaining species are normally considered nonpathogenic and are most frequently isolated from environmental specimens, including fish, water, and fecal samples. Although these minor yersiniae have been identified primarily from environmental samples, they are occasionally recovered from patient samples, suggesting a possible role as human pathogens.

● *YERSINIA PESTIS*

DEFINITION

Plague is a highly fatal flea-borne disease that is best known as the cause of the Black Death of the Middle Ages.[1] Its etiologic agent, *Y. pestis,* is a gram-negative coccobacillus belonging to the family Enterobacteriaceae.

The Pathogen

Y. pestis is microaerophilic, gram negative, nonmotile, and nonsporulating; it can exist as a facultative intracellular pathogen and exhibits bipolar staining with Wayson, Giemsa, and Wright stains (Fig. 312-1). It is fragile outside its hosts or vectors but can be grown within 24 to 48 hours on a variety of bacteriologic media at temperatures ranging from 4° to 40° C. *Y. pestis* lacks a true capsule but has a carbohydrate-protein envelope comprised of the *capsular* or *fraction 1 antigen*. Production of this antigen occurs only at temperatures above 33° C. Wild-type strains typically bear three plasmids with sizes of approximately 100 to 110 kilobases (kb), 70 to 75 kb, and 9.5 kb (19 kb if present as a dimer), respectively. Although only one serotype is thought to exist, strains can be classified into biotypes. The three classic biotypes (*antiqua, mediaevalis,* and *orientalis*) differ in their ability to ferment glycerol and reduce nitrates. All three biotypes occur in Asia, which is generally accepted as the continent where plague originated. Two biotypes exist in Africa (*antiqua* and *orientalis*), but only the *orientalis* biotype occurs in the Americas. Although these three biotypes have historical and biogeographic significance, all are highly virulent and appear to cause virtually identical signs and symptoms in humans. Recently, a fourth biotype (*microtus* or *pestoides*), which is purportedly nonpathogenic for humans, was reported from east-central Asia.[2] More modern typing methods, including ribotyping, multiple-locus variable-number tandem repeat assays, and single-nucleotide polymorphism analysis, are proving useful for molecular epidemiology

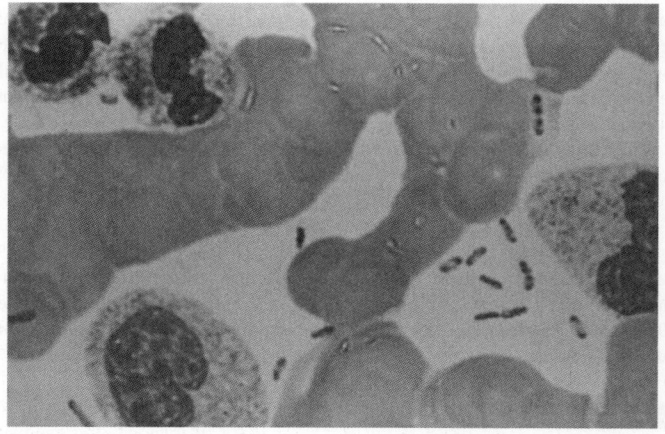

FIGURE 312-1. Wayson-stained blood smear from a fatal case of human septicemic plague (Centers for Disease Control and Prevention).

studies, identification of probable environmental sources of human infection, and phylogenetic analyses.

EPIDEMIOLOGY

Y. pestis is maintained in nature through transmission cycles involving certain rodent species and their fleas, which act as vectors. Although other mammals often become infected with *Y. pestis* and occasionally succumb to plague, the only nonrodent species reported to be important hosts for infecting vector fleas and perhaps contributing to the maintenance of plague in some natural foci are certain species of rabbits and hares, the steppe pika of central Asia, and the house shrew of southeastern Asia and Madagascar. Rodent-consuming carnivores and raptors might play indirect roles in spreading plague by transporting infected rodent fleas from one area to another.

Foci of *Y. pestis* infection occur in rodent populations in many regions of Africa, Asia, and the Americas, although only about 2000 to 5000 human cases were reported each year to the World Health Organization (WHO) in the period 1987 to 2009. In the 1960s and 1970s, the majority of human cases occurred in Southeast Asia, which was the site of civil wars and political unrest. However, beginning in the 1980s, this situation began to change, and most cases now occur in Africa, especially the Congo,[3] and nearby Madagascar.[4] According to the most recently released WHO statistics for 2004 to 2009, 96.6% of the world's cases occurred in the Democratic Republic of Congo, Madagascar, Uganda, and other countries in Africa (Fig. 312-2). Asian countries reported only 1.6% of the total cases, and another 1.8% were reported from five countries in the Americas, including the Brazil, Bolivia, Ecuador, Peru, and the United States. Since 1970, evidence of *Y. pestis* infection has been identified in animals or their fleas in 17 western states, and human cases have been identified in 13 of these states (Fig. 312-3). Most of these cases have occurred in three southwestern states (New Mexico, Arizona and Colorado) and California.

Humans most frequently acquire plague as a result of being bitten by infectious fleas (Fig. 312-4). On a worldwide basis, the risk of flea bite exposure is highest in poverty-stricken areas that are situated near natural plague foci and have large infestations of commensal rats (*Rattus* spp.) heavily infested with fleas, particularly the oriental rat flea (*Xenopsylla cheopis*). *X. cheopis* readily feeds on humans and is an efficient vector of *Y. pestis* to people as well as to rats. Persons are most likely to be bitten by infectious *X. cheopis* when plague epizootics cause massive mortality among susceptible rats, forcing these fleas to seek new hosts. Currently, certain regions of central and southern Africa (including Madagascar), southeastern Asia and India, and a few areas in South America remain at relatively high risk for rat-associated plague outbreaks. The spread of rat-associated plague from one region to another, perhaps by the natural movement of rats or their transport along with trade goods, poses a threat of epidemics in large rat-infested cities, as demonstrated by the repeated spread of plague from the central highlands of Madagascar to the port city of Majunga, where the disease has caused multiple outbreaks in the past 2 decades. The appearance of bubonic cases acquired via flea bite in large cities also greatly increases the possibility that secondary pneumonic plague with hemoptysis will develop in untreated bubonic cases and that the infection will spread to others through inhalation of infectious respiratory droplets expelled by coughing pneumonic plague patients. Such spread will result in cases of primary pneumonic plague, a form of the disease that is often fatal and can spread rapidly from person to person under appropriate circumstances. The persons most at risk for acquiring plague through respiratory droplet spread are those who fail to take appropriate respiratory precautions and come into close contact (≤2 m) with coughing pneumonic plague patients experiencing hemoptysis. Human-to-human spread of primary pneumonic plague has not been reported in the United States since 1924, when an outbreak occurred in Los Angeles, California. The few cases of naturally acquired primary pneumonic plague that have occurred in this country since that time, and for which likely sources of exposure were identified, have involved pet owners or veterinary staff handling cats with signs of plague pneumonia, pharyngitis, or oral abscesses. Although rare in the United States, primary pneumonic plague still poses a threat in developing countries, with outbreaks occurring in the past 20 years in India, Ecuador, Madagascar, the Democratic Republic of Congo, and Uganda. It should be noted, however, that the spread of pneumonic plague depends on many factors, and relatively simple control measures can quickly and effectively stop the respiratory droplet spread of pneumonic plague.[5]

At present, rat-associated plague poses little risk to persons in the United States, with most cases resulting from exposure to the bites of infectious wild rodent fleas (79% in one case series), although a significant number (19%)

Reported* Plague Cases by Country, 2000-2009

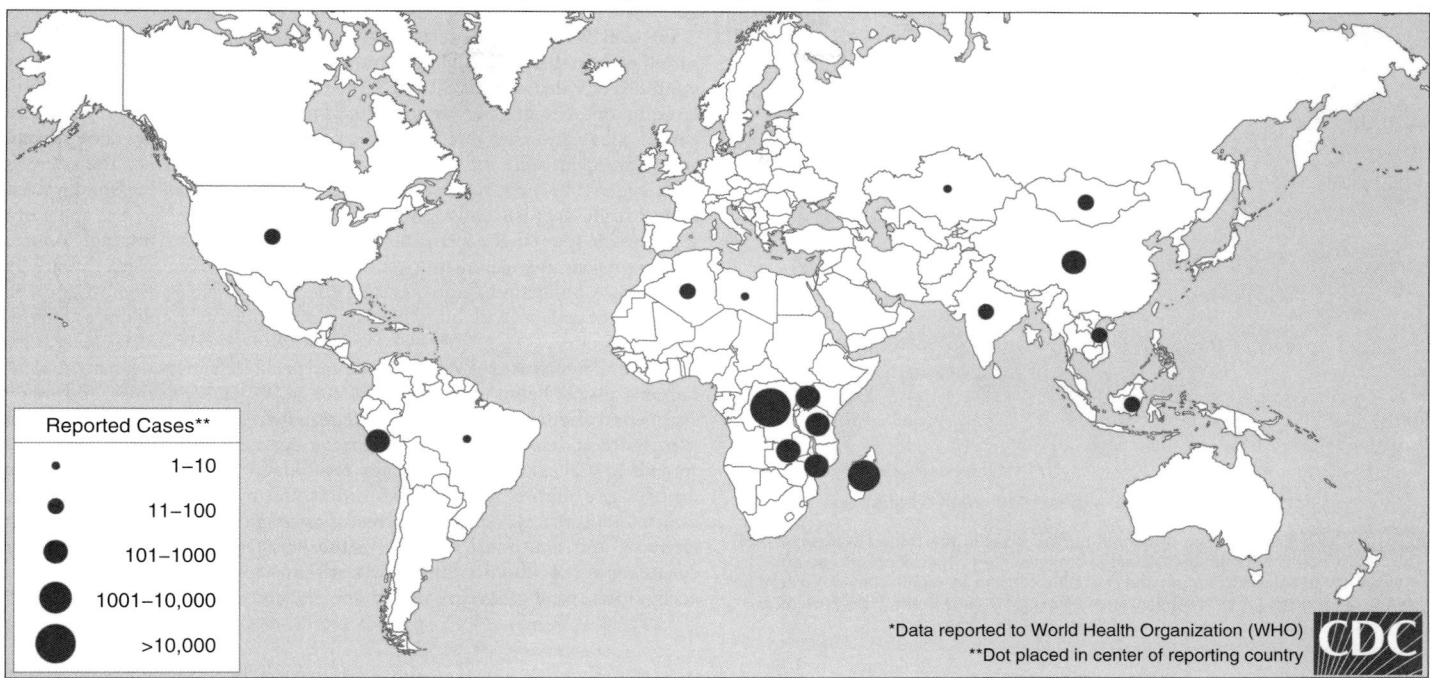

Reported Cases**

· 1–10

● 11–100

● 101–1000

● 1001–10,000

● >10,000

*Data reported to World Health Organization (WHO)
**Dot placed in center of reporting country

CDC

FIGURE 312-2. Worldwide distribution of plague in humans, 2000 to 2009. (Data compiled from the World Health Organization, Centers for Disease Control and Prevention, and other sources.)

were exposed while handling *Y. pestis*–infected animals, including rabbits, domestic cats, wild rodents, and wild carnivores. These direct-contact exposures occurred primarily in persons who had been bitten or scratched by infected cats or had skinned infectious rabbits or rodents for meat or certain wild carnivores for their fur. The risk of exposure to infectious wild rodent fleas or animals is typically greatest when epizootics cause high mortality rates in certain rodent species in the western United States, particularly ground squirrels, prairie dogs, wood rats, and chipmunks. Epizootics appear to progress most rapidly during late spring to early fall, when human cases also peak, probably because this is the period of greatest flea vector activity. Most cases arising from flea bite occur when persons are exposed to fleas as a result of close contact with dead hosts that are flea infested or with the nests or burrows of infected hosts. Evidence also exists that allowing dogs from plague-endemic areas to sleep in their owners' beds increases plague risk for these persons, presumably because these animals carry infectious fleas into beds. The few human cases reported during the winter months are typically acquired through direct contact with infected animals, and affected individuals have a history of hunting or trapping wild animals or handling domestic cats. The exposure sites for most U.S. cases are peridomestic environments, with smaller numbers of exposures occurring during recreational activities such as hunting or camping.[6] Occupational exposure has also rarely occurred among veterinary staff, biologists, and trappers. Rarely, primary pneumonic plague has been acquired in the United States through the inhalation of infectious materials (2% of cases) by means of close face-to-face contact with *Y. pestis*–infected cats that had oral lesions or signs of plague pneumonia, including cough.

Recently, concern has been raised that plague could be used as an agent of bioterrorism (Chapter 21). In most projected scenarios, bioterrorists would spread plague in an aerosol form, potentially resulting in numerous primary pneumonic cases, a high mortality rate, and widespread panic, especially if the *Y. pestis* strains released had been engineered to be resistant to antimicrobial agents commonly used to treat plague.

PATHOBIOLOGY

Y. pestis possesses a variety of virulence factors that promote its initial invasion of the host, evasion of the host's immune system, survival in lymph nodes, and the development of a fulminant bacteremia that can lead to fatal gram-negative sepsis and the spread of the pathogen to other organs.[7] Few bacteria rival the pathogenicity of *Y. pestis* for humans. *Y. pestis* usually enters the body at the site of a flea bite or perhaps as a result of contact between abraded or cut skin and blood or other body fluids from a *Y. pestis*–infected animal. On entering the body, plague bacteria come under attack by host phagocytes and other host defenses. Although many of the invading *Y. pestis* are killed by arriving polymorphonuclear leukocytes, some enter into and survive in mononuclear cells, where they are carried via the lymphatics to regional lymph nodes. The ability to escape from the host's innate immune defenses and disseminate to regional lymph nodes depends in part on a protease (Pla) encoded on the 9.5 kb plasmid that helps degrade fibrin clots and promote the production of excess plasmin, which can affect inflammatory exudates, break down extracellular proteins and basement membranes, and reduce levels of chemoattractants, possibly because of the inhibition of interleukin-8 production at the site of initial infection. Another virulence factor, YopM, is one of many *Yersinia* outer proteins (Yops), encoded by genes on the midsized (70-75 kb) plasmid of *Y. pestis*. Although most other Yops are degraded by the Pla protease, YopM is resistant to its activity and probably aids in the dissemination of *Y. pestis* by competing with platelets for thrombin, a factor that not only reduces clotting but also inhibits the activation of platelets, thereby lowering local inflammatory responses and promoting the dissemination of *Y. pestis* to regional lymph nodes. Initial invasion and dispersal to regional lymph nodes also depend on the ability of *Y. pestis* to survive for at least brief periods in host phagocytes. Survival in such environments is promoted by other Yops that work in concert with a type III secretory apparatus to deliver into host phagocytes those Yops that act as intracellular effectors. These effector Yops disturb the cytoskeletal dynamics of phagocytic cells and block their production of proinflammatory cytokines. Affected phagocytes are rendered incapable of killing the invading *Y. pestis*, thereby allowing this bacterium to survive extracellularly in lymphoid tissues. Survival of *Y. pestis* in mammalian hosts also depends on its ability to acquire sufficient quantities of iron for growth. The most important means of iron uptake in *Y. pestis* is a siderophore (yersiniabactin) system that can effectively compete with host iron-binding molecules for this essential nutrient. Although the ability of *Y. pestis* to resist host phagocytic killing and survive intracellularly in phagocytes is thought to be particularly important during the early stages of infection, plague bacteria also express a glycoprotein capsular antigen (caf1 or fraction 1 antigen) that confers resistance to phagocytosis. Expression of caf1 is temperature dependent, being repressed at the

Reported cases of human plague—United States, 1970–2012

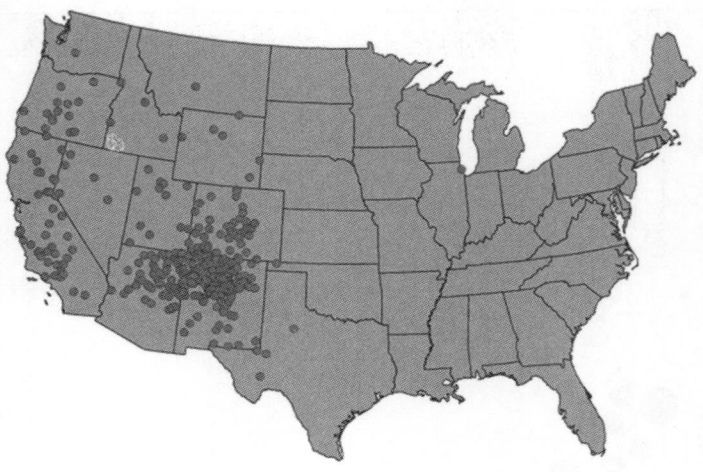

1 dot placed in county of exposure for each plague case

FIGURE 312-3. **Distribution of human plague cases in the United States, 1970 to 2012. Case points were randomly placed within counties where exposures occurred to indicate the general distribution and clustering of cases by region. One dot placed in county of exposure for each plague case (Centers for Disease Control and Prevention).**

cooler temperatures found in the flea vector and upregulated at mammalian host body temperatures.

Infected lymph nodes, termed *buboes*, can appear edematous and congested early in the course of illness but exhibit little evidence of inflammatory infiltrates or vascular injury. These buboes represent the most obvious manifestation of the lymphatic system's efforts to arrest the spread of *Y. pestis*, and within a few days after infection, they contain massive numbers of *Y. pestis* and heavy neutrophil infiltrates, which cause them to swell to the size of a hen's egg and become surrounded by serous fluid. As the illness progresses, hemorrhagic necrosis and vascular damage in the node become apparent; some nodes spontaneously rupture, and abscesses appear. Although *Y. pestis* can be present in small quantities in blood samples taken relatively early in the course of infection, large quantities of plague bacteria usually appear in the blood of patients with bubonic plague only after the lymph node defenses are overwhelmed.

As the bacteria escape from the node and proliferate in blood, patients with bubonic plague begin to exhibit evidence of plague septicemia (secondary septicemic plague). Patients with inadequately treated septicemic plague can experience widespread and overwhelming destruction of tissues as *Y. pestis* spreads to various organs, eventually resulting in their failure. Patients who die of plague often experience diffuse interstitial myocarditis, cardiac dilation, diffuse hemorrhagic splenic necrosis, renal glomeruli containing fibrin thrombi, and multifocal necrosis in the liver. Disseminated intravascular coagulation can lead to thrombosis within capillaries, vascular necrosis, ecchymoses, acral gangrene, and cutaneous, mucosal, and serosal petechiae

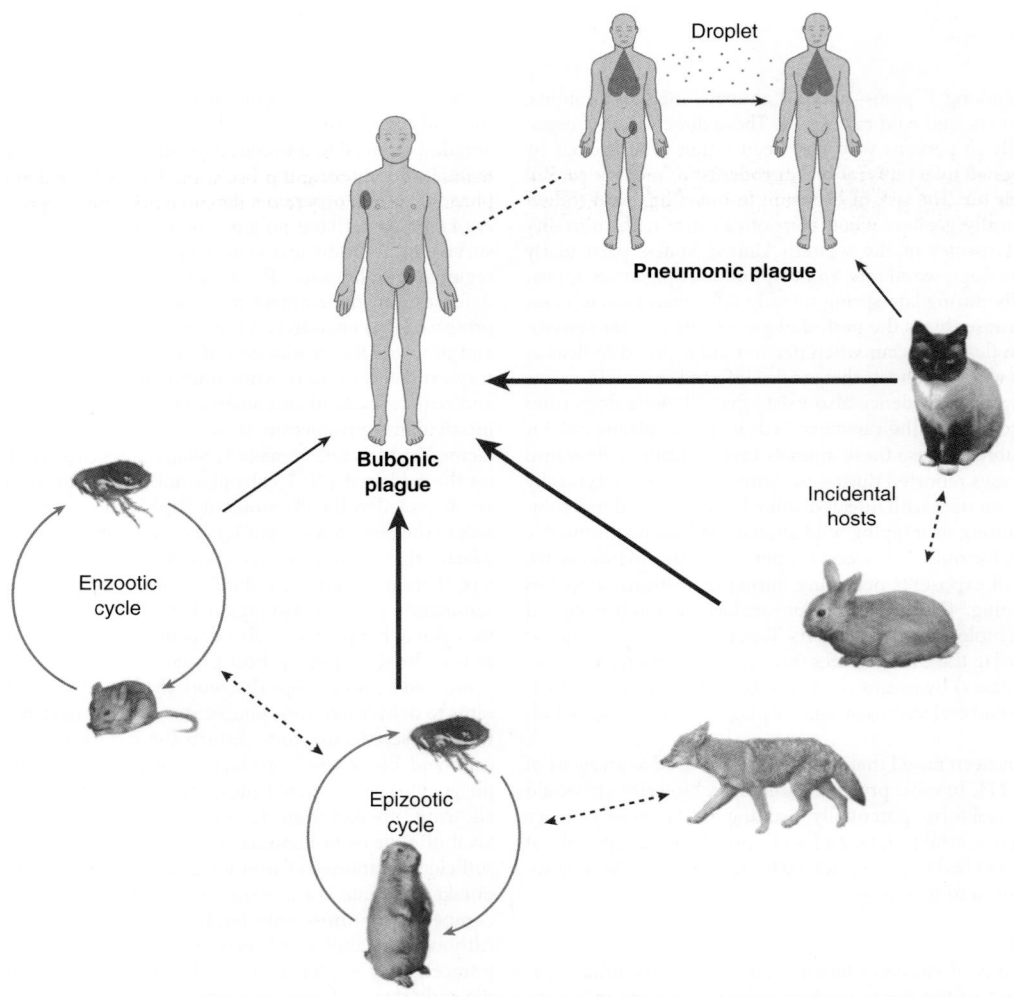

FIGURE 312-4. **Ecology and transmission of plague.** *Red circles* indicate zoonotic cycles. Common routes of transmission to humans indicated by *wide solid arrows* and uncommon routes by thin *arrows* (Centers for Disease Control and Prevention).

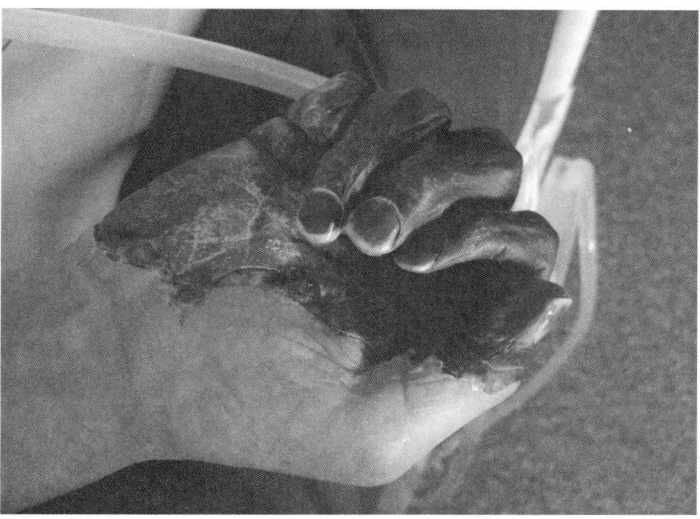

FIGURE 312-5. Hand of a patient with plague displaying acral gangrene, a manifestation that may have given rise to the term "black death" (Centers for Disease Control and Prevention).

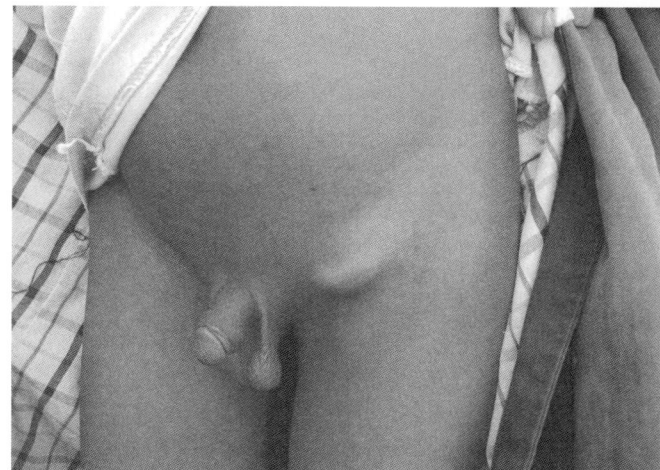

FIGURE 312-7. Young Malagasy boy with a bubo. (Courtesy Brook Yockey, Centers for Disease Control and Prevention.)

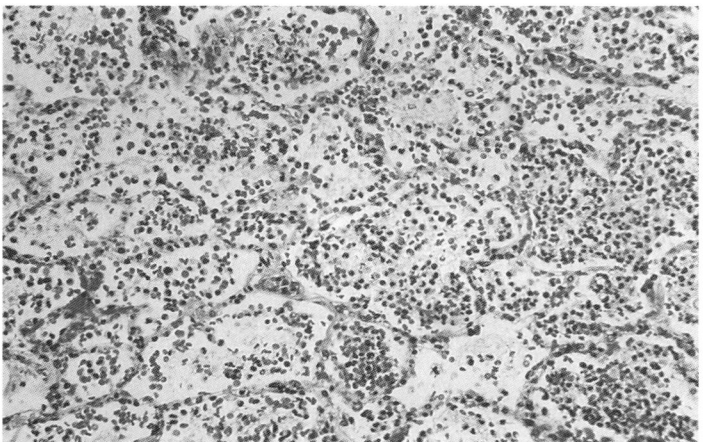

FIGURE 312-6. Photomicrograph of lung tissue from fatal case of primary pneumonic plague and septicemic plague. Note filling of alveolar spaces with inflammatory cells and debris (Centers for Disease Control and Prevention).

(Fig. 312-5). In a small proportion of cases, septicemia occurs in the absence of buboes or other signs of localized infection, a condition referred to as *primary septicemic plague*. Septicemic plague can also occur secondary to primary pneumonic plague.

Rarely, plague can be acquired through the inhalation of infectious respiratory droplets or other materials. Patients with primary pneumonic plague typically experience a rapidly progressing lung infection that is initially lobular, then lobar, and finally multilobar, with large numbers of *Y. pestis* being present in the alveoli and pulmonary secretions of affected sites (Fig. 312-6). Pneumonic plague can also occur secondary to bubonic or primary septicemic plague. In these instances, *Y. pestis* invades the lungs in a diffuse manner, with most bacilli appearing in interstitial spaces. The most common pathologic findings are edema, diffuse pulmonary congestion, limited neutrophilic infiltration, and hemorrhagic necrosis. Cavitation and liquefaction necrosis can also occur and result in scarring of the lungs, particularly at sites of consolidation.

CLINICAL MANIFESTATIONS

The three most commonly observed forms of plague (in order of decreasing occurrence) are bubonic, septicemic, and pneumonic. Unusual manifestations of plague include meningitis and pharyngitis. In rare instances, *Y. pestis* has been inoculated through the conjunctiva, resulting in oculoglandular plague. The incubation periods are 2 to 6 days for bubonic plague and 1 to 3 days for primary pneumonic plague.

The characteristic swollen and tender lymph nodes (buboes) of bubonic plague usually appear in the node or nodes located closest to the site of initial infection (Fig. 312-7). Most cases of bubonic plague in the United States are thought to be acquired from flea bites on the legs, as indicated by the appearance of inguinal or femoral lymph node involvement on the side where the flea bite occurred. Axillary buboes are also common, often indicating the handling of an infected animal or other flea-infested object. Cervical buboes are much less common in the United States than in many developing countries, perhaps because persons in the latter are more likely to sleep on dirt floors in flea-infested huts, thus increasing their chances of being bitten about the head and neck by infectious fleas. Rarely, a skin lesion appears at the site of an infectious flea bite or other source of inoculation.

Symptoms of bubonic plague include fever, chills, myalgia, arthralgia, headache, malaise, and prostration. Untreated patients with bubonic plague become increasingly toxic, remain febrile, and experience tachycardia, agitation, confusion, delirium, and convulsions.

Septicemic plague manifests as a rapidly progressive, overwhelming endotoxemia. Patients often complain of gastrointestinal (GI) symptoms, including nausea, vomiting, diarrhea, and abdominal plain. Disseminated intravascular coagulation can also occur with the appearance of petechiae, ecchymoses, bleeding, and ischemia in the tips of the extremities. Later-stage septicemic patients are likely to experience refractory hypotension, renal shutdown, obtundation, and other signs of shock. Patients with late-stage septicemic plague can also exhibit acute respiratory distress syndrome (Chapter 104), which has occasionally been confused with hantaviral pulmonary syndrome (Chapter 381) in the American Southwest. Because septicemic plague is likely to be fulminant and fatal, favorable outcomes depend on rapid diagnosis and prompt treatment with appropriate antimicrobials.

Pneumonic plague can be accompanied by fever, cough, chest discomfort that becomes increasingly painful, tachycardia, dyspnea, bacteria-laden sputum, chills, headache, achiness, weakness, and dizziness. As the illness progresses, patients may experience increasing respiratory distress, hemoptysis, cardiopulmonary insufficiency, and circulatory collapse. In the early stages of illness, patients with primary pneumonic plague may have signs of localized pulmonary involvement, beginning in a single lung and rapidly progressing to segmental consolidation and later bronchopneumonia, with death ensuing in as little as 1 to 3 days after the onset of symptoms. Localized infection is unlikely to be observed in the lungs of patients with secondary pneumonic plague because the lung tissues are infected initially through circulatory spread, which results in a diffuse interstitial pneumonitis. The appearance of sputum also differs in primary versus secondary pneumonic plague, being watery or mucoid, frothy, and perhaps tinged with blood in primary pneumonic cases but scanter, thicker, and more tenacious in secondary pneumonic cases.

DIAGNOSIS

Plague fatalities are typically related to delay in seeking treatment or misdiagnosis. The differential diagnosis of plague in its various clinical forms includes staphylococcal (Chapter 288) or streptococcal adenitis (Chapter 290) or pneumonia (Chapter 97); cat-scratch disease (Chapter 315); tularemia (Chapter 311); chancroid (Chapter 301); acute filarial lymphadenitis (Chapter 358); mycobacterial infection (Chapter 325); septicemia caused by other bacteria; meningococcemia; bacterial endocarditis; mycoplasmal pneumonia and other community-acquired pneumonias; legionnaires' disease (Chapter 314); Q fever; influenza pneumonitis (Chapter 364); hantaviral pulmonary syndrome (Chapter 381); viral pneumonia caused by respiratory syncytial virus (Chapter 362), cytomegalovirus (Chapter 376) or other viruses; and strangulated inguinal hernia.

Laboratory confirmation relies on bacterial culture accompanied by specific bacteriophage lysis tests or detection of a fourfold rise in antibody titer to the *Y. pestis* F1 capsular antigen over a period of 2 to 4 weeks. Although the procedures for confirming the laboratory diagnosis of *Y. pestis* infection are relatively simple, delays can occur because the relevant expertise and reagents are often limited to a few public health or reference laboratories. Because cases of plague can rapidly progress to a life-threatening illness and because culture of *Y. pestis* on bacteriologic media may require 48 hours or longer before colonies become visible, it is essential that patients suspected of having plague receive appropriate antimicrobial therapy immediately after samples have been taken. Direct fluorescent antibody assays can be used to identify *Y. pestis* bacteria in bubo aspirates, sputum samples, and tracheal washes; this procedure requires about 1 hour and provides strong presumptive evidence of infection. A presumptive diagnosis can also be obtained rapidly by detecting *Y. pestis* DNA in polymerase chain reaction (PCR) assays or *Y. pestis*–specific antigens in immunologic assays, but these tests are not widely available. Recently, rapid immunochromatographic tests have been developed that can detect plague antigen or antibodies. The potential advantages of these tests are that they require few laboratory resources, can be done in field settings, and yield results in less than 1 hour. One such test designed to detect *Y. pestis* antigens in patient samples has been used in some developing countries to diagnose plague, but these assays are still being evaluated and are not widely available. Preferred laboratory samples include blood, serum, bubo aspirates, tracheal washes, and swabs of skin lesions or pharyngeal mucosa. Cerebrospinal fluid can also be collected from patients in whom plague meningitis is suspected.

PREVENTION

No commercially available plague vaccine exists in the United States. Newer recombinant vaccines designed to stimulate immune responses to the F1 and V antigens of *Y. pestis* are undergoing clinical trials and have yielded promising results, but they are unlikely to be available in the near future.

Human plague risk can be reduced through the implementation of effective surveillance programs to rapidly identify human cases and threatening epizootics and allow effective intervention measures to be implemented. When appropriate, affected areas can be treated with insecticides to reduce the risk for flea bite exposure. Measures also should be taken to reduce the amount of food and shelter available to rodents. In rare instances, rodenticides can be used to reduce host numbers, but their use is not recommended before the implementation of effective flea control measures. Persons living in or visiting areas endemic for plague should avoid sick and dead animals and use insect repellents to reduce the risk for infectious flea bites. Dogs and cats should be prevented from roaming freely in rodent-infested areas, and these animals should be treated with flea control agents that safely and effectively kill fleas. Although most dogs appear to be somewhat resistant to plague, cats are highly susceptible, often experience severe illness, and can serve as sources of infection for their owners or veterinary staff. Cats that roam outside in endemic areas and suddenly become seriously ill should be taken to a veterinarian for evaluation.

Persons with pneumonic plague should be held in respiratory isolation for at least 48 hours after the initiation of appropriate antimicrobial therapy, and persons caring for such patients should follow respiratory droplet precautions (masks, gloves, gowns, and eye protection). Although human-to-human transmission has not been reported in the United States for many decades, rare cases of primary pneumonic plague have occurred after face-to-face contact with infected cats that had oral lesions or symptoms of pneumonic plague. Veterinary staff from plague-enzootic areas should take appropriate precautions (masks, gloves, gowns, eye protection) when handling sick cats with illnesses suggestive of plague.

Prophylactic antimicrobial therapy is generally recommended for persons with possible plague exposure only in relatively high-risk situations, such as after close contact with patients with pneumonic plague, handling of *Y.*

pestis–infected animals, or being bitten by rodent fleas in an area with a recent history of epizootic activity. The most recently recommended prophylactic antimicrobials are doxycycline and ciprofloxacin (Table 312-1).

TREATMENT   Rx

The most commonly recommended agent for treating plague is streptomycin (see Table 312-1), but a randomized trial in Tanzania concluded that gentamicin and doxycycline are effective for treating plague in adults and children and cause few adverse responses.[A1] A review of human cases treated in New Mexico also strongly suggests that gentamicin is effective and can be substituted for streptomycin. Tetracyclines are effective for treating uncomplicated cases of bubonic plague, and chloramphenicol is believed to be effective, particularly for plague meningitis. Although antimicrobial resistance is not believed to be a problem in the United States, strains resistant to tetracyclines and other agents have been described occasionally, and resistance to streptomycin and chloramphenicol may also occur. Recently, the Food and Drug Administration approved levofloxacin (Levaquin) to treat patients with plague under the agency's Animal Efficacy Rule, which allows evidence from animal studies, in this case those involving nonhuman primates, to be used to demonstrate the efficacy of a proposed treatment when it is not possible to conduct adequate trials in humans.

PROGNOSIS

Patients with uncomplicated bubonic plague respond quickly to appropriate antimicrobial therapy and typically defervesce, with relief from most other systemic manifestations within 2 to 5 days. Large buboes can remain swollen, however, for more than 1 week and may require incision and drainage if necrotic. In rare instances, ischemic necrosis in septicemic cases has resulted in the amputation of digits.

ENTEROPATHOGENIC YERSINIAE

DEFINITION

Y. enterocolitica and *Y. pseudotuberculosis* differ significantly from *Y. pestis* in that they are enteropathogenic, rarely cause death, and are spread via the fecal–oral route. Similar to *Y. pestis,* both of these bacteria are gram-negative members of the family Enterobacteriaceae.

The Pathogens

Y. enterocolitica is genetically quite distinct from *Y. pseudotuberculosis* and *Y. pestis;* the plague bacterium is thought to have arisen as a recent clone of *Y. pseudotuberculosis,* and the chromosomal DNA of these two species is extremely similar but markedly different from that of *Y. enterocolitica.*[8] All three species, however, share an approximately 70-kb plasmid that encodes for various proteins (Yops) that are key virulence factors. Unlike *Y. pestis,* the enteropathogenic yersiniae are urease positive and motile at temperatures lower than 30° C. *Y. pseudotuberculosis* is rhamnose positive, thereby distinguishing it from the closely related *Y. pestis* and the more distantly related *Y. enterocolitica.* The enteropathogenic yersiniae are genetically more diverse than the more recently evolved plague bacterium. *Y. enterocolitica* contains six biogroups, five of which are known to be pathogenic for humans, and nearly 60 serogroups; *Y. pseudotuberculosis* has been classified into six distinct serogroups (O groups 1-6).

EPIDEMIOLOGY

Enteropathogenic yersiniae are transmitted via the fecal–oral route, and successful infection of the host requires large doses of bacteria (median infective dose of 10^8 to 10^9 bacteria). Typical sources of infection include the consumption of contaminated foods such as dairy products, inadequately cooked pork, and certain vegetables. Both *Y. enterocolitica* and *Y. pseudotuberculosis* can survive and proliferate slowly at refrigerator temperatures. Although far less common, person-to-person transmission has been reported, as has transmission via blood transfusion. Pigs, rodents, rabbits, sheep, goats, cattle, horses, dogs, cats, and sometimes birds serve as reservoirs for these yersiniae. Most hosts act as asymptomatic carriers, but a few human cases have been associated with handling sick animals. Symptomatic patients shed large amounts of yersiniae for as long as 2 to 3 weeks. Untreated, infected persons can become carriers and shed for 2 to 3 months.

Yersiniosis is a reportable disease in many countries. Most cases result from *Y. enterocolitica* infection, and this agent reportedly accounts for 1% to

TABLE 312-1 RECOMMENDATIONS FOR THE TREATMENT OF PATIENTS WITH PNEUMONIC PLAGUE IN CONTAINED AND MASS CASUALTY SETTINGS AND FOR POSTEXPOSURE PROPHYLAXIS*

PATIENT CATEGORY	RECOMMENDED THERAPY
CONTAINED CASUALTY SETTING	
Adults	Preferred choices: Streptomycin 1 g IM twice daily Gentamicin 5 mg/kg IM or IV once daily or 2 mg/kg loading dose followed by 1.7 mg/kg IM or IV 3 times daily Alternative choices: Doxycycline 100 mg IV twice daily or 200 mg IV once daily Ciprofloxacin 400 mg IV twice daily[†] Chloramphenicol 25 mg/kg IV 4 times daily[‡]
Children[§]	Preferred choices: Streptomycin 15 mg/kg IM twice daily (maximum daily dose, 2 g) Gentamicin 2.5 mg/kg IM or IV 3 times daily[‖] Alternative choices: Doxycycline: if ≥45 kg, give adult dosage; if <45 kg, give 2.2 mg/kg IV twice daily (maximum, 200 mg/day) Ciprofloxacin 15 mg/kg IV twice daily[†] Chloramphenicol 25 mg/kg IV 4 times daily[‡]
Pregnant women[§]	Preferred choice: Gentamicin 5 mg/kg IM or IV once daily or 2 mg/kg loading dose followed by 1.7 mg/kg IM or IV 3 times daily[‖] Alternative choices: Doxycycline 100 mg IV twice daily or 200 mg IV once daily Ciprofloxacin 400 mg IV twice daily[†]
MASS CASUALTY SETTING AND POSTEXPOSURE PROPHYLAXIS	
Adults	Preferred choices: Doxycycline 100 mg PO twice daily[††] Ciprofloxacin 500 mg PO twice daily[†] Alternative choices: Chloramphenicol 25 mg/kg PO 4 times daily[‡‡]
Children[§]	Preferred choices: Doxycycline[††]: if ≥45 kg, give adult dosage; if <45 kg, give 2.2 mg/kg PO twice daily Ciprofloxacin 20 mg/kg PO twice daily Alternative choice: Chloramphenicol 25 mg/kg PO 4 times daily[‡‡]
Pregnant women[§]	Preferred choices: Doxycycline 100 mg PO twice daily[††] Ciprofloxacin 500 mg PO twice daily Alternative choice: Chloramphenicol 25 mg/kg PO 4 times daily[‡‡]

*These are consensus recommendations of the Working Group on Civilian Biodefense and are not necessarily approved by the U.S. Food and Drug Administration. In general, one antimicrobial agent should be selected, and therapy should be continued for 10 days. Oral therapy should be substituted when the patient's condition improves. Although animal and limited human studies support their use, gentamicin and ciprofloxacin are not currently approved by the U.S. Food and Drug Administration (FDA) for treatment of plague in humans. The related drugs, streptomycin and levofloxacin, are FDA approved for treatment of plague.

[†]Other fluoroquinolones can be substituted at doses appropriate for age. The ciprofloxacin dosage should not exceed 1 g/day in children.

[‡]The concentration should be maintained between 5 and 20 μg/mL. Concentrations >25 μg/mL can cause reversible bone marrow suppression.

[§]In children, the ciprofloxacin dose should not exceed 1 g/day, and the chloramphenicol dose should not exceed 4 g/day. Children younger than 2 years should not receive chloramphenicol.

[‖]Aminoglycoside dosages must be adjusted based on renal function. Evidence suggests that gentamicin 5 mg/kg intravenously or intramuscularly once daily would be efficacious in children, although this is not yet widely accepted in clinical practice. Neonates up to 1 week of age and premature infants should receive gentamicin 2.5 mg/kg intravenously twice daily.

[¶]In neonates, a gentamicin loading dose of 4 mg/kg should be given initially.

**The duration of treatment of plague in a mass casualty setting is 10 days. The duration of postexposure prophylaxis to prevent plague infection is 7 days.

[††]Tetracycline can be substituted for doxycycline.

[‡‡]Children younger than 2 years should not receive chloramphenicol. An oral formulation is available only outside the United States.

IM, Intramuscular; IV, intravenous; PO, oral.

Adapted from Inglesby TV, Dennis DT, Henderson DA, et al. Plague as a biological weapon: medical and public health management. Working Group on Civilian Biodefense. *JAMA.* 2000;283:2281-2290.

3% of all cases of acute enteritis in some areas. From 1996 to 2009, the overall annual incidence in the United States was about 0.5 cases per 100,000 persons, with higher rates among children and African Americans.[9] The incidence has decreased over the past decade, especially among African American children younger than 5 years of age. Nevertheless, rates remain markedly higher among African American and Asian American children, at 3.5 and 5.1 cases per 100,000, respectively. In the past, high rates among African American populations were associated with the home preparation of chitterlings made from contaminated pork intestines. Exposure of contaminated pork products was also considered a likely source of infection for Asian Americans.

Y. enterocolitica serotypes O:3, O:8, O:9, and O:5,27 have been associated with human disease. Serotype O:3 (biotype 4) predominates in most countries and is found most commonly in swine. Serotype O:9 (biotype 2) has been isolated from sheep, cows, and goats. These last two serotypes are the most common causes of human infection worldwide but are considered less pathogenic than strains of the O:8 (biotype 1B) serotype, which are associated with the most severe outbreaks. Although serotype O:8 infections appear to be decreasing in incidence in the United States, they are becoming increasingly important in Japan, Italy, and France. In Europe, most cases involve serotype O:3 infections, although a few are associated with serotypes O:9 and O:5,27. Biotype 1A appears to be nonpathogenic, and biotype 5 has been isolated only from hares. Strains pathogenic in humans are esculin, salicin, and pyrazinamidase negative.

Y. pseudotuberculosis has been isolated from rodents, cattle, sheep, cats, dogs, and birds.[10] It occurs worldwide but human infections are most commonly reported in northern Europe and in Asia, including Japan. O group 1, 2, and 3 strains are associated with human disease, with most cases being attributed to O:1 or O:2 strains. Infected animals serve as chronic carriers and sources for the infection of water and foods such as meat, dairy products, and stored vegetables. Some cases have been associated with the handling of kittens and puppies. Recent outbreaks of *Y. pseudotuberculosis* in Finland were traced to eating iceberg lettuce and carrots (serotypes O:3 and O:1, respectively). A large Canadian outbreak was associated with milk that had been pasteurized but nevertheless became contaminated. Outbreaks in the former Soviet Union have been associated with the consumption of root vegetables that were stored underground for winter consumption and presumably became contaminated with rodent excreta containing *Y. pseudotuberculosis*.

PATHOBIOLOGY

Y. enterocolitica possesses numerous virulence factors responsible for its persistence in the GI tract and ability to cause disease in susceptible hosts. Upon reaching the ileum, *Y. enterocolitica* adheres to the mucosa, where intracellular infections in Peyer's patches, mucosal cells, and macrophages can occur. Invasion of the ileal mucosa is favored by the presence of invasin, an outer membrane protein, and a 17-kD surface factor (Ail). An inflammatory response causes abdominal pain and diarrhea, as well as ulcerative ileitis, mesenteric adenitis, and necrosis within Peyer's patches. If the regional defenses are breached, the bacteria can disseminate and cause sepsis and hepatic and splenic abscesses. Polyarthritis can also occur later in the course of illness, particularly in human leukocyte antigen (HLA)-B27–positive individuals.

Similar to *Y. pestis*, the enteropathogenic yersiniae attack host lymphoid tissues. Invasion of these tissues and resistance against host defenses depend on the possession of the approximately 70-kb plasmid that is shared by each of the three pathogenic yersiniae and bears genes encoding for various Yops and the so-called V antigen. The products of this plasmid work in concert to inhibit phagocytosis and reduce inflammation, thereby suppressing the host immune response and favoring persistence of these microbes.

When *Y. enterocolitica* and *Y. pseudotuberculosis* become established in the lymph nodes, they can resist phagocytosis, which allows them to replicate extracellularly and form aggregates in the nodes. The ability to acquire host iron can be a significant factor contributing to the virulence of *Y. enterocolitica* strains. O:8 serotypes, which are virulent for mice, have the *irp2* (iron repressible 2) gene that encodes for a pair of high-molecular-weight outer membrane proteins, but the mouse avirulent O:3 and O:9 serotypes lack *irp2*. O:3 and O:9 serotypes typically remain confined to the guts of their hosts, except when iron overload is present or patients are being treated with an iron chelator.

Patients with reactive arthritis (Chapter 265) are more likely to have fewer GI symptoms, lower T-cell proliferative responses to *Yersinia* antigens, lower initial immunoglobulin (Ig) M responses, higher and more persistent IgG and IgA responses, and increased levels of IgA with a secretory component. *Yersinia*-specific antibody responses are also more likely to persist in patients with reactive arthritis than in those with uncomplicated GI disease. *Yersinia* antigens thought to contribute to reactive arthritis include Yops and released proteins, which stimulate host CD4 cells, and heat shock protein 60, which has been hypothesized to work in conjunction with other antigens to modulate the host immune response. Evidence exists that hosts can maintain chronic *Y. enterocolitica* infections for years after the initial infection, a factor that may induce the inflammation associated with reactive arthritis (Chapter 265).

CLINICAL MANIFESTATIONS

After an incubation period of about 3 to 7 days, a gastroenteritis typically develops that can be difficult to distinguish from *Salmonella* (Chapter 308) or *Campylobacter* (Chapter 303) gastroenteritis. The most common clinical syndromes associated with *Y. enterocolitica* infection are acute enteritis with fever, diarrhea, vomiting, right lower quadrant pain suggestive of appendicitis (Chapter 142), erythema nodosum, and reactive arthritis. Other common symptoms include associated pharyngitis, rash, joint pain, and headache. Stool examination reveals leukocytes or erythrocytes, and one fourth of patients experience bloody diarrhea.

Y. pseudotuberculosis infections most commonly manifest as enterocolitis, pharyngitis, and pseudoappendicitis.

Whereas enterocolitis is most likely to occur in young children, older children more frequently experience acute terminal ileitis, mesenteric adenitis, and systemic disease. Pseudoappendicitis has been reported in patients with mesenteric lymphadenitis. Sepsis is uncommon and is most likely to occur in persons with underlying conditions such as diabetes mellitus, cirrhosis, immunosuppression, older age, and hemochromatosis. Splenic abscesses, meningitis, or endocarditis can develop in septic patients, and the mortality rate can approach 50%. Erythema nodosum is identified in about one third of all patients and in 10% of adults.

DIAGNOSIS

Yersiniosis should be suspected in patients with abdominal pain and fever, especially if they live in high-incidence areas. The diagnosis is best accomplished by isolation of the bacterium from stool, blood, or other appropriate samples.[11] Recovery of *Y. enterocolitica* and *Y. pseudotuberculosis* from clinical and environmental samples can be greatly complicated by the presence of other bacteria that are likely to predominate. The preferred selective agar for isolation from stool specimens is CIN (cefsulodin–irgasan–novobiocin) agar prepared with relatively low cefsulodin concentrations. Isolation of yersiniae is also helped by culture at 25° to 30° C, which results in better growth than when cultures are kept at 35° C and favors growth of the more cold-tolerant yersiniae over other bacteria that require higher temperatures. After being obtained, isolates can be confirmed as enteropathogenic *Yersinia* by biochemical tests. Biotyping and serotyping, which are often available only in research or reference laboratories, can provide useful epidemiologic information. Isolation difficulties and the reported low sensitivity (about 10^3 to 10^6 colony-forming units per gram of sample) of current isolation techniques have led some to suggest that PCR or other DNA-based methods are likely to result in the more rapid and sensitive detection of these bacteria.[12]

Tube or microagglutination tests can identify antibodies to the pathogenic *Y. enterocolitica* serogroups O:3, O:9, O:5,27, and O:8, but cross-reactivity can be a problem, particularly between *Y. enterocolitica* O:9 and *Brucella* spp. PCR for O genotyping of *Y. pseudotuberculosis* could eventually replace traditional serotyping methods. Immunologically mediated *Yersinia* illnesses, including reactive arthritis, are associated with the production of IgA antibodies that can be detected by enzyme-linked immunosorbent assay (ELISA) or immunoblotting. IgG antibodies can persist for many years, but persistence of IgA antibodies for more than a few months could indicate a chronic *Yersinia* infection.

PREVENTION

Prevention depends on measures intended to protect persons from contact with contaminated environments, foods, and wastes. These include using proper sewage disposal methods, protecting water supplies from contamination with human or animal wastes, following appropriate procedures for animal husbandry and slaughtering, thoroughly cooking meats (especially pork), avoiding long-term storage of meats at temperatures higher than 39° F, and consuming only pasteurized milk. Individuals should thoroughly wash their hands after handling potentially contaminated pork or other foods. Persons with diarrhea should not work in food-handling areas, care for young

children, or work with patients, and hospital staff should follow enteric precautions. Vaccines are not available.

TREATMENT   Rx

Antibiotics do not improve the course of uncomplicated enterocolitis or mesenteric adenitis, and the use of antimicrobial therapy is not generally recommended for intestinal forms of the disease. Such therapy is, however, recommended for immunocompromised patients, patients with septicemia, and those with systemic disease or extraintestinal foci of infection. It should be noted that in vitro susceptibility does not necessarily indicate efficacy in vivo.

Broad-spectrum cephalosporins, sometimes accompanied by aminoglycosides, have resulted in successful outcomes in patients with extraintestinal forms of yersiniosis, including septicemia. Ciprofloxacin, cefotaxime, and ceftriaxone are considered the most effective agents for treating *Y. enterocolitica* serogroup O:3 infection. In addition, *Y. enterocolitica* serogroup O:3 and O:9 isolates possess chromosomally determined β-lactamases that can confer resistance to ampicillin, carbenicillin, and cephalothin. Although serogroup O:8 strains, which produce type A β-lactamase, show resistance to the latter two agents, they are susceptible to ampicillin. It has yet to be determined whether antimicrobial therapy is useful for treating immunologically mediated forms of yersinial illness, including reactive arthritis.

PROGNOSIS

Cases of *Y. enterocolitica* enteritis are generally mild and self-limited after a 2- to 3-week course of illness. Sequelae most commonly include reactive arthritis and erythema nodosum.[13] Glomerulonephritis and myocarditis have also been reported, particularly with serogroup O:3, biotype 4, phage type 8 infections. Other sequelae can include endocarditis, pericarditis, and osteitis. *Y. enterocolitica*–induced reactive arthritis, which can appear 1 to 3 weeks after infection, is oligoarticular, asymmetrical, and peripheral; it occurs most frequently in the lower limbs and eventually resolves over a period of a few weeks to months. HLA-B27–positive patients are more likely to experience severe and prolonged arthritis.

Y. pseudotuberculosis infections are also generally mild and self-limited. Reported complications include erythema nodosum, iritis, reactive arthritis, and nephritis. Although infection of the bloodstream by *Y. pseudotuberculosis* is rare, one review of 72 such cases reported that 26 (36%) were fatal.

Grade A Reference

A1. Mwengee W, Butler T, Mgema S, et al. Treatment of plague with gentamicin or doxycycline in a randomized trial in Tanzania. *Clin Infect Dis.* 2006;42:614-621.

GENERAL REFERENCES

For the General References and other additional features, please visit Expert Consult at https://expertconsult.inkling.com.

313

WHOOPING COUGH AND OTHER *BORDETELLA* INFECTIONS

ERIK L. HEWLETT

DEFINITION

Pertussis (whooping cough), an acute respiratory illness with a potentially protracted clinical course, is caused by infection with *Bordetella pertussis* or related members of the genus, especially *Bordetella parapertussis*. The infection is highly contagious and can have both endemic and epidemic features in a population, but there are no known chronic carriers of the organism. Pertussis is currently a serious public health problem worldwide, with reported U.S. cases in 2012 the highest in more than 50 years.[1,2] The greatest risks of morbidity and mortality are in infants, but increases in incidence in recent years include adolescents and adults and are highest in the cohort of children who have only ever received acellular pertussis vaccines.[3,4]

The Pathogens

There are now eight species in the genus *Bordetella*, but *B. pertussis*, *B. parapertussis*, and *B. bronchiseptica* (primarily a veterinary pathogen) are most likely to cause respiratory infections in humans. Recently identified species such as *B. holmesii* and *B. trematum* have been associated with bacteremia, meningitis, and wound infections, and *B. holmesii* has been isolated concurrently with *B. pertussis* in an outbreak of respiratory illnesses.[5] The *Bordetellae* are gram-negative, coccobacilli, and particularly fastidious and small relative to other gram-negative organisms. *B. pertussis* was first isolated by Bordet and Gengou in 1906, and a medium used for culture (Bordet-Gengou agar) still bears their names.

EPIDEMIOLOGY

In the prevaccine era (before the mid-1950s), pertussis was primarily a childhood illness; as a result, the disease received little attention in adult medicine. The extensive use of whole-cell pertussis vaccines in the United States and other parts of the world resulted in a marked reduction of pertussis. In addition, however, the vaccine elicited a change in the age-specific incidence of disease, with the majority of cases subsequently occurring in infants too young to be vaccinated and in adolescents and adults, who become susceptible because of waning immunity after childhood vaccination.[6,7] In recent years, this shift has been particularly notable, with 48,277 cases of pertussis reported in the United States in 2012, approximately 50% of those occurring in patients 7 to 19 years old. In fact, seroepidemiologic data suggest that 25% of adolescents and adults with a cough lasting more than 1 week have pertussis. The disease is endemic in the United States, but epidemics also occur every 3 to 4 years.

B. pertussis is highly contagious and the presumption that transmission can occur by aerosol droplet has recently been documented for the first time in nonhuman primate studies. There is no classic "carrier" state such as that recognized for other infectious organisms. In recent studies, however, nonhuman primates (baboons) immunized with acellular pertussis vaccine and challenged directly with *B. pertussis* were without clinical signs of disease but were able to transmit *B pertussis* to susceptible cage mates.[8] Dissemination in a community is often caused by symptomatic (or now perhaps asymptomatic) adolescents, who spread the organism during school attendance and social events. Health care personnel are also important sources of transmission, and health care–associated outbreaks can affect both vulnerable patients and their care providers.

PATHOBIOLOGY

Although *B. pertussis* and related organisms produce a number of interesting toxins, and pertussis has been described as a "toxin-mediated" disease, there is no clear pathophysiologic link between the known virulence factors and clinical manifestations of disease.[9] The infection is localized to the respiratory tract, where organisms adhere to the ciliated surface of epithelial cells. Mucous secretion is prominent, especially during later stages of the illness. Intracellular *B. pertussis* organisms have been demonstrated both *in vitro* and in samples collected from patients, but it is not an obligate intracellular organism, and the significance of these observations remains unknown.

Toxins and adhesins are important both for their potential role in the pathogenesis of disease and for their use as antigens in acellular pertussis vaccines. Filamentous hemagglutinin (FHA), pertactin (PRN), and fimbriae are adhesins that are components of some acellular vaccines, and all currently available vaccines include chemically inactivated pertussis toxin (PT). In addition to their adhesin function, FHA, PRN, and fimbriae have been shown to modulate the functions of host immune-effector cells. PT is a member of the family of adenosine diphosphate–ribosylating toxins that includes cholera toxin and diphtheria toxin, and its intracellular targets consists of several guanosine triphosphate–binding proteins such as $G_{i\alpha}$. Although PT causes lymphocytosis and enhances insulin secretion, its target cell or cells and its contribution to the clinical manifestations of pertussis are still a mystery. *Bordetellae* also possess adenylate cyclase (AC) toxin, a bacterial AC that enters host cells to produce supraphysiologic levels of cyclic adenosine monophosphate (cAMP). AC toxin acts against phagocytic cells, such as polymorphonuclear leukocytes and alveolar macrophages, whose antibacterial functions are inhibited by the increased cAMP. Additional "toxins,"

including the tracheal cytotoxin, tracheal colonization factor, and heat-labile or dermonecrotic toxin, have been identified by virtue of their activities in vitro or in animals. The relationship of these toxins to disease also remains ill defined.

CLINICAL MANIFESTATIONS

Although the classic paroxysmal cough of pertussis is striking and unforgettable, not all patients experience this characteristic symptom. Infants may have apnea as their only manifestation of pertussis; in others, the characteristic cough develops subsequently. Existing clinical case definitions of pertussis are decades old and based largely on presentations in infants and children. Because of the increasing incidence in adolescents and adults, who may manifest distinct symptoms and signs, the Global Pertussis Initiative has developed an algorithm based on different age groups in order to encourage expanded use of laboratory testing in suspected cases.[10]

Incubation Period

After exposure of an individual to active pertussis (typically by way of aerosol from an infected patient who is coughing), the onset of symptoms is not experienced until 1 to almost 3 weeks later. This relatively long incubation period makes it difficult to track transmission and increases the time necessary for intervention and implementation of control measures.

Catarrhal Phase

Importantly, the symptoms that reflect onset of the catarrhal phase (rhinorrhea, increased lacrimation, conjunctival injection, and sometimes low-grade fever) are nonspecific and are not suggestive of pertussis, except in the setting of an ongoing hospital or community outbreak. This phase, which can last from a few days to as long as 1 week, is often associated with a nonproductive cough.

Paroxysmal Phase

A patient's transition to the paroxysmal phase and initiation of the typical cough can suggest the diagnosis of pertussis. This striking cough consists of a series of uncontrollable expirations followed by gasping inhalation, which, depending on the airway anatomy, can result in the characteristic "whooping" sound. The whoop is more frequent in children than in adults. It is common for each episode of coughing to be associated with cyanosis and end with gagging and vomiting, which in infants can result in dehydration and malnutrition. The paroxysmal stage can last up to 4 weeks, and the development of fever or worsening pulmonary function during this time suggests the possibility of secondary pneumonia. Eighty percent or more of adolescents and adults with pertussis have paroxysmal cough, but the frequency of whoop and posttussive vomiting in this population is quite variable. In addition, during the paroxysmal stage, adults experience symptoms, such as a scratchy throat, other pharyngeal symptoms, and episodes of sweating, which are not described in children.

Convalescent Phase

A reduction in the frequency and severity of coughing attacks marks the transition to the convalescent phase, which can last weeks to months. It is often during this time that adults present to the health care system with "chronic cough" and may be evaluated for conditions such as asthma, tuberculosis, other chronic lung diseases, malignancies, and gastroesophageal reflux. After the coughing spells have ended, patients may experience a return of the paroxysmal cough in conjunction with unrelated upper respiratory illnesses or stimuli or irritants; this phenomenon is often incorrectly interpreted as a recurrence of pertussis. Eighty percent of adults with pertussis have an illness of at least 3 weeks' duration, and 27% are still coughing after 90 days.

Complications

In infants and children younger than 5 years, hospitalization is common; 5% to 10% have pneumonia, nearly 1% of infants experience seizures, and encephalopathy is seen in 0.1%. Pertussis in infants and small children can be associated with pulmonary hypertension, now known to result from the elevated white blood cell (WBC) count, which can exceed 100,000/mm³ in a naïve host. In one study, this phenomenon occurred in fewer than 15% of cases but was present in 75% of patients who died.[11] Adolescents and adults have these same complications with a lower frequency, but adults can experience other problems associated with underlying medical conditions. For example, there are anecdotal reports of cough syncope, herniated

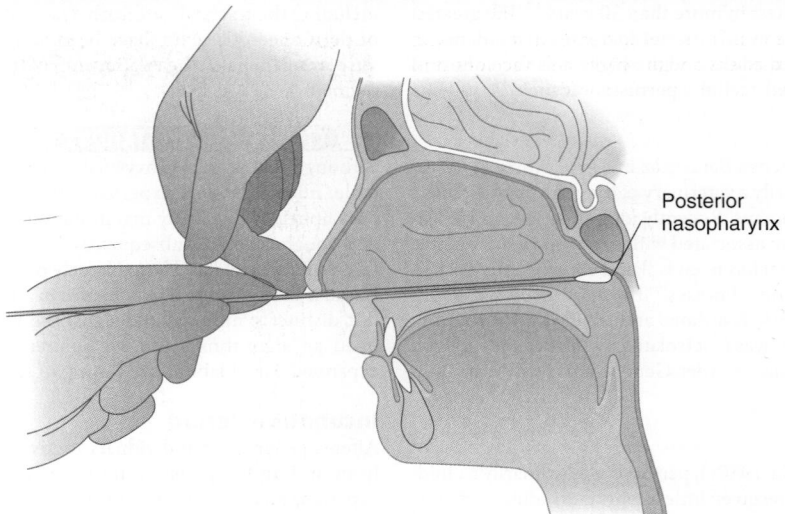

Posterior
nasopharynx

FIGURE 313-1. Technique for obtaining a nasopharyngeal specimen for the isolation of *Bordetella pertussis.* Dacron or calcium alginate swabs are recommended to obtain culture specimens. Dacron swabs are appropriate if polymerase chain reaction testing will be performed. (Redrawn from Cornia PB, Lipsky BA, Saint S, Gonzales R. Clinical problem solving: nothing to cough at. *N Engl J Med.* 2007;357:1432-1437.)

intervertebral disc, sudden-onset hearing loss, angina episodes, and carotid artery dissection.

DIAGNOSIS

Several methods can be used to detect *B. pertussis,* its products, and the host response to them, but each has its limitations. Culture of a nasopharyngeal swab or aspirate (Fig. 313-1) is the "gold standard" (specificity approaching 100% in symptomatic patients), but even with the use of specialized transport medium and processing in a careful, interested laboratory, recovery rates are often less than 50% and are completely dependent on the duration of illness and whether antimicrobial treatment was initiated before specimen collection. Polymerase chain reaction (PCR)–based diagnostic tests of nasopharyngeal swabs or aspirates are much more sensitive than culture, and results can remain positive for several days after the initiation of antimicrobial treatment. In addition, appropriately designed PCR assays can identify and distinguish among *B. pertussis, B. parapertussis,* and *B. bronchiseptica* and detect insertion sequence elements suggestive of other *Bordetella* species.[12] However, several apparent "outbreaks" of pertussis have later been found to represent false-positive PCR results. Detection of serum antibodies to products of *B. pertussis* can be used to identify patients during infection, but care must be taken to distinguish an acute response from residual antibodies elicited by prior immunization.

In view of the limited resources and equipment available for the diagnosis of pertussis, the World Health Organization has established a clinical case definition, which is 21 or more days of paroxysmal coughing with laboratory confirmation or epidemiologic linkage. Although this definition is often used for clinical trials, it is now clear that its application can result in cases of lesser severity or shorter duration being missed.

TREATMENT   Rx

Supportive Therapy
Because infants and young children have the highest risk for complications and death, supportive therapy is often the most important component of their medical care. Close observation (preferably in the hospital) is essential to ensure adequate feeding, oxygenation, and hydration to minimize complications in this age group. None of the pharmacologic interventions tested for the amelioration of cough and other symptoms is effective in pertussis.[A1] Leukophoresis has been used to reduce the WBC count and thus ameliorate pulmonary hypertension in infants and young children, but there is no agreement as to whether this approach affects mortality rates.

Antimicrobial Agents
There are two reasons to use antimicrobials in a patient with pertussis: (1) to eliminate the causative organism and reduce transmission and (2) to limit the course of illness in the treated patient. Because individuals can remain culture positive and can potentially transmit *B. pertussis* for several weeks after

onset of symptoms, it is appropriate to treat patients who are seen within that time frame. Antimicrobials do not provide symptomatic relief or affect the course of the illness in the later stages of the infection, but they can do so when treatment is started within the first few days of symptoms. Although macrolide resistance is not a significant problem, it has been reported.

The recommendation of the Centers for Disease Control and Prevention for the treatment of pertussis in adults is azithromycin (500 mg on day 1 followed by 250 mg/day on days 2-5), clarithromycin (1 g/day in two divided doses for 7 days), erythromycin (2 g/day in four divided doses for 14 days), or trimethoprim–sulfamethoxazole (trimethoprim 320 mg/day, sulfamethoxazole 1600 mg/day, in two divided doses for 14 days). It has now been shown that treatment with erythromycin for 7 days is as effective as treatment for 14 days.[A2][A3] The newer macrolides (azithromycin and clarithromycin) are better tolerated but more expensive.

PREVENTION

Chemoprophylaxis

Chemoprophylaxis with the aforementioned antimicrobial agents is an important mechanism for controlling outbreaks in hospitals or in the community. This approach is effective when initiated before the onset of symptoms and is recommended for individuals exposed within the preceding 3 weeks; high-risk persons with underlying health problems, particularly infants; or those who might have occupational or other contact with susceptible hosts.

Immunization

A killed, whole-cell vaccine was introduced in the late 1940s. Use of that product had a dramatic effect on the incidence of pertussis, with the number of reported cases in the United States falling from more than 200,000 annually to less than 2000 in 1980. In the 1970s and 1980s, recognition of the adverse events associated with the whole-cell product and public concern about the extent of those reactions led to the development of the purified acellular pertussis vaccines that are in use today.[13]

Current pediatric acellular pertussis vaccines (DTaP), which contain one or more purified protein antigens (all contain PT and other combinations of FHA, pertactin, and fimbriae types 2 and 3), are administered to infants and children up to the age of 6 years and cause significantly fewer adverse reactions than the whole-cell vaccines. In recognition of the significant incidence of pertussis in adolescents and adults and their role in transmitting the disease to infants and small children, Tdap (tetanus, diphtheria and pertussis) vaccines, which contain reduced quantities of the pertussis components, are now licensed for administration to these age groups. Their use is recommended to boost immunity in adolescents and adults who completed the recommended childhood vaccination series. Importantly, this adult booster immunization is now recommended for women during each pregnancy to prevent acquisition of *B. pertussis* and transmission to their neonates.

The increasing incidence of pertussis, including in immunized populations, appears to be attributable to a markedly reduced duration of protection relative to that anticipated from experience with whole-cell vaccines and prior infection. There is, however, an increasing number of *B. pertussis* isolates that do not express pertactin.[14] In addition, there is increasing prevalence of strains harboring the *ptxP*3 allele, which is associated with increased production of PT and with alterations in expression of other virulence factors.[15,16]

In consideration of the adverse events and negative publicity associated with the whole-cell vaccines and the poor efficacy of the current acellular vaccines, there is active development of a live, attenuated pertussis vaccine, which would be administered intranasally.[17]

PROGNOSIS

Most patients will eventually clear *B. pertussis* even without antimicrobial treatment, but in most cases, the illness lasts weeks to months. Antimicrobials are of limited effectiveness in altering the course of the illness unless they are started before the paroxysmal phase. The introduction of booster doses of vaccines for adolescents and adults has not, however, resulted in the control of pertussis in well-immunized populations as had been anticipated. The next steps to address this serious public health problem are still being debated. Of major concern is the recent demonstration that baboons immunized with acellular pertussis vaccine can become infected and transmit *B. pertussis* in the absence of symptoms.

Grade A References

A1. Wang K, Bettiol S, Thompson MJ, et al. Symptomatic treatment of the cough in whooping cough. *Cochrane Database Syst Rev.* 2012;9:CD003257.
A2. Centers for Disease Control and Prevention. Recommended antimicrobial agents for the treatment and post-exposure prophylaxis of pertussis: 2005 CDC guidelines. *MMWR Recomm Rep.* 2005; 54(RR–14):1-16.
A3. Altunaiji SM, Kukuruzovic RH, Curtis NC, et al. Antibiotics for whooping cough (pertussis) [review]. *Cochrane Database Syst Rev.* 2007;3:CD004404.

GENERAL REFERENCES

For the General References and other additional features, please visit Expert Consult at https://expertconsult.inkling.com.

314

LEGIONELLA INFECTIONS

THOMAS J. MARRIE

DEFINITION

Legionellosis is the term for infection due to bacteria in the *Legionella* genus, of which there are two main manifestations—pneumonia (legionnaires' disease) and Pontiac fever (named after Pontiac, Michigan, where it was first recognized). Pontiac fever is usually a mild febrile illness presumed to be a reaction to lipopolysaccharide of *Legionella* species.

The 58th annual convention of the American Legion was held at a hotel in Philadelphia from July 21 to July 24, 1976. Subsequently, 182 of the delegates became ill (hence the name legionnaires' disease), and 146 were hospitalized at 87 institutions across the United States. Most had radiographic evidence of pneumonia, and 29 (16%) died. Within about 6 months of the outbreak, a new microorganism, *Legionella pneumophila*, was isolated from the pulmonary tissue of some of those who had died in the Philadelphia outbreak. In retrospect, the organism had first been isolated in 1943.

The Pathogen

Legionellae are small, gram-negative, aerobic, non–spore-forming bacilli that measure 0.3 to 0.9 μm wide by 2 to 20 μm long (Fig. 314-1A to D). These organisms require special media for growth, and many laboratories are unable to isolate legionellae; thus, when laboratory expertise is uncertain, a negative culture is meaningless. They usually do not stain with Gram stain. In tissue specimens, Dieterle or Warthin-Starry stain is used to visualize these organisms. *Legionella micdadei* retains the modified acid-fast stain and can appear as acid-fast bacilli in clinical specimens. Legionellae are aquatic organisms

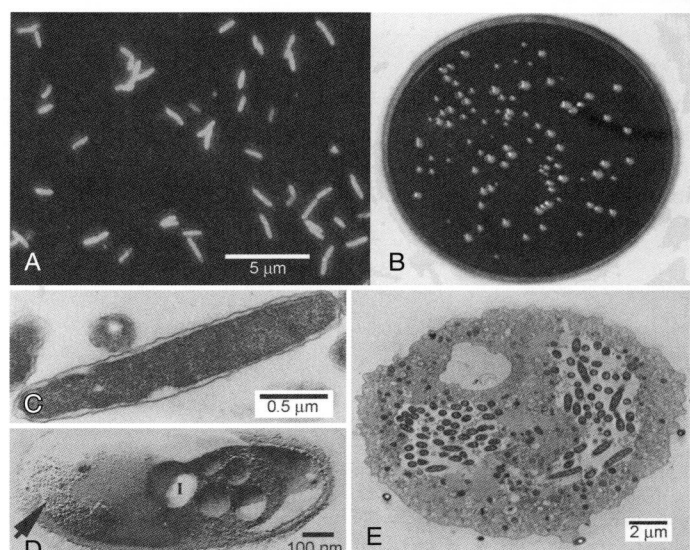

FIGURE 314-1. **A,** Direct fluorescent antibody stain of *Legionella pneumophila*. **B,** Colonies of *L. pneumophila* growing on a BCYE plate. **C,** Thin section of replicative form of *L. pneumophila*. **D,** Freeze-fracture replica of the mature infectious form obtained after growth in ameba. The latter shows prominent cytoplasmic inclusions (I) and a polar distribution of membrane proteins (*arrow*). **E,** Electron micrograph of *L. pneumophila* growing within *Acanthamoeba castellani*. (A Courtesy Dr. Paul Hoffman, University of Virginia. B courtesy Dr. Sharon Berk, Tennessee Technical University. C to E courtesy Drs. Rafel Garduno and Gary Faulkner, Dalhousie University.)

that thrive in both natural and man-made waterways and distribution systems, especially hot-water pipes, water heaters (electrical more so than gas heaters), cooling towers, and water fountains. In these systems, they are found in biofilms that help confer resistance to biocides and chlorine. They are also found in moist soil and mud. They can survive in these environments for long periods and can tolerate temperatures of 0° to 68° C and a pH range of 5 to 8.5. In their natural environments, they are intracellular parasites of protozoa, such as the freshwater ameba *Acanthamoeba* and *Hartmannella* species (Fig. 314-1E). Indeed, legionellae can live in at least 20 species of ameba, two species of ciliated protozoa, and one species of slime mold. Free-living legionellae in biofilms are inactivated within a few weeks, whereas those residing in amebae survive for 6 months or more. Humans are accidental hosts who become infected by inhaling *Legionella* bacteria or amebae laden with these bacteria. Genomes of four different strains of *L. pneumophila* have been sequenced, and they range in size from 3.3 to 3.5 Mb. Legionellae have many eukaryotic-like proteins, which may help the intracellular growth of these organisms in human macrophages by mimicking host proteins. *Legionella* species have type I, II, IV, and V secretion systems, which allow the efficient and rapid delivery of molecules into the phagocytic host cell.

The number of new *Legionella* species continues to grow; there are now at least 56 *Legionella* species and 73 serogroups or more, including 15 serogroups of *L. pneumophila*. A variety of typing systems can be used to further refine the isolates so that individual strains can be identified, a factor that is important for determining the source of an outbreak or understanding the difference between environmental and clinical isolates. It is noteworthy that *L. pneumophila* and all its serotypes cause disease in humans (with serotype 1 predominant), whereas only about 50% of the remaining species of *Legionella* cause such disease.[1]

Legionella longbeachae was first isolated in 1980 from a patient with pneumonia in Long Beach, California. In Australia, New Zealand, and Japan, reported cases of *L. longbeachae* infection occur as often as cases of *L. pneumophila* infection. This organism is rarely isolated from aquatic environments. The primary environmental reservoir remains unknown, but the major source of human infection is considered to be commercial potting mixes and other decomposing material, such as bark and sawdust. The *L. longbeachae* genome encodes for a range of proteins that might assist in the degradation of plant material. These enzyme systems are not present in *L. pneumophila*.

EPIDEMIOLOGY

The incubation period for legionnaires' disease (LD) is most commonly cited as 2 to 10 days, with extremes of 1 to 28 days. Person-to-person transmission

TABLE 314-1 RISK FACTORS FOR LEGIONNAIRES' DISEASE

RISK FACTOR	APPROXIMATE INCREASED RISK (-FOLD) OVER PERSONS WITHOUT THIS RISK FACTOR
HOST FACTORS	
Renal failure requiring dialysis	20
Corticosteroid therapy	5-10
Hairy cell leukemia	20
Lung or hematologic malignant neoplasm	7-20
Cytotoxic chemotherapy	5
>3 Alcoholic drinks/day	3-4
Cigarette smoking	2-10
Age older than 50 years	2
Diabetes mellitus	2
Solid organ transplantation (immunosuppression)	2
Anti–tumor necrosis factor treatment	16-21
Chronic heart or lung disease	>1
Splenectomy (non-*pneumophila* strains only)	—
ENVIRONMENTAL FACTORS	
Travel	2
Recent plumbing work in home or at work	2
Hospitalization	—
Exposure to contaminated water sources—cooling towers, hot tubs, decorative fountains	—
Exposure to potting soil (Australia) for *Legionella longbeachae*	—

does not occur. Legionellosis is found worldwide, predominantly in developed countries owing to the frequent use of cooling towers and complex plumbing systems. Underdiagnosis may be a feature in developing countries because of the laboratory facilities required. In recent years, there has been an increase in *Legionella* cases in Japan from 56 cases in 1999 to 804 cases in 2011, reaching a rate of 1.15 per 100,000 population; in Europe, the rate in 2010 was 1.25 cases per 100,000, and in the United States, the rate increased from 0.39 to 1.15 per 100,000. From 1990 to 2005, 23,076 cases of LD were reported in the United States. Only 1.7% of these cases occurred in children, whereas 63% occurred in those aged 45 to 64 years. Males accounted for 61% of cases, and rates were highest in the eastern United States, where most cases occur in the summer or fall. More recent U.S. data show an annual increase of 217% in the number of cases from 2000 to 2009, with the highest rates in the Mid-Atlantic states at 2.60 per 100,000. Twenty-four percent were travel related, and 81% of these cases involved domestic travel; noteworthy is that 5% involved cruise ship travel. The overall case-fatality rate was 8%. Eastern Canada also has higher rates of LD than the rest of that country. The epidemiology of LD in Europe is not dissimilar to that of the United States. The countries with rates of more than 2 per 100,000 were France, Denmark, Spain, Netherlands, and Italy. Twenty percent were travel associated, and the overall case-fatality rate was 11%.

There is an association between increased rainfall and cases of LD. The connection may be aerosolization of *Legionella* from rain puddles on roads. In one study, 33 (47.8%) of puddle water samples were positive for *Legionella*, yielding 325 isolates. Among the 14 sequence types of the clinical isolates, 4 were present in puddle water isolates.

The most common risk factors for the acquisition of LD are listed in Table 314-1. *Legionella* species account for 1 to 5% of community-acquired pneumonia requiring admission to a hospital. In some areas, *Legionella* accounts for about the same percentage of pneumonia treated on an ambulatory basis. *Legionella* infections can be sporadic or occur in outbreaks.[2] Outbreaks have been associated with exposure to a variety of aerosol-producing devices, including showers, a grocery store mist machine, cooling towers, whirlpool spas, decorative fountains, and evaporative condensers. Other water sources implicated in transmission of LD include water on trains, birthing pools, dental units, asphalt paving machines, and windscreen wiper fluid without added screen wash. LD can be acquired up to 10 to 11 km away from contaminated cooling towers. Aspiration of contaminated potable water by immunosuppressed patients is another mechanism by which *Legionella* is acquired. From 1985 to 2007, 14 of 2946 (0.5%) solid organ transplant

recipients developed LD at one center in Barcelona; 5 (36%) were nosocomially acquired.

Exposure to contaminated potting soil is a risk factor for *L. longbeachae* infection in Australia and New Zealand.

Pontiac fever occurs predominantly in outbreaks with very high attack rates. *L. pneumophila*, *L. micdadei*, and *L. anisa* have been implicated in outbreaks of Pontiac fever. Among residents of nursing homes, Pontiac fever has been associated with *L. pneumophila* concentrations of greater than 10^4 colony-forming units/L in shower water. Those receiving corticosteroid therapy have a six-fold higher risk for development of Pontiac fever.

PATHOBIOLOGY

After being inhaled, legionellae are phagocytosed in the lungs by alveolar macrophages.[3] Only virulent strains of *Legionella* are capable of initiating organism-directed endocytosis when attachment to the alveolar macrophage through E-cadherin and β1 integrin receptors occurs. Legionellae abrogate phagosome-lysosome fusion and replicate in an endosome surrounded by the endoplasmic reticulum. Once it is intracellular, the bacteria-laden endosome recruits small vesicles, mitochondria, and ribosomes, and within 4 to 6 hours it becomes enveloped by the endoplasmic reticulum, thereby establishing the replicative endosome. After a latent period of about 12 hours, the bacteria start dividing. During this latent period, there is synthesis of up to 35 proteins and repression of 32 proteins. Iron must be available in the phagosome for growth. Growth continues in the macrophages for approximately 24 hours, at which time the macrophage disintegrates by apoptosis and the bacteria are released. The released bacteria are often phagocytosed by other macrophages, dendritic cells, and epithelial cells, perpetuating the infection. Cell-mediated immunity is necessary for recovery from *Legionella* infection. Production of type 1 interferons has a protective effect by promoting the activation of macrophages. Activated macrophages limit the intracellular replication of legionellae by downregulating the expression of their transferrin receptors and limiting the availability of iron to the bacteria. Toll-like receptors 2, 4, 5, and 9 are activated during infection with *L. pneumophila*. Interleukins 1α, 1β, 4, 6, 12, and 18 are detected during *Legionella* infection. Vaccination of guinea pigs with the purified major outer membrane protein OmpS protects against an LD_{100} lethal challenge, whereas immunization with purified heat shock protein 60 provides little protection. Polymorphonuclear leukocytes are present in abundance in the infected lung, but their role in clearing the infection is unclear. Bacteria can spread beyond the lung and cause metastatic infection. However, many extrapulmonary effects of LD, such as cerebellar ataxia and confusion, are not due to metastatic infection; they are presumably due to as yet unidentified toxins. The infected lung is consolidated, and there is usually no parenchymal damage once recovery occurs. Abscess formation and bronchiolitis obliterans or fibrosing alveolitis are occasionally seen.

The pathogenesis of Pontiac fever is unclear. The onset of illness occurs within 12 to 36 hours after the inhalation of, presumably, endotoxin. This period is too short for bacterial multiplication to cause the symptoms.

CLINICAL MANIFESTATIONS

Most of our knowledge of the clinical features of LD comes from studying patients who have been hospitalized with this illness, that is, those with the most severe manifestations. Fever (often high), malaise, and cough are present in most patients. Chills occur in about 75%, and dyspnea in just more than half the patients. Other features include myalgias, headache, chest pain, and diarrhea. The cough is nonproductive in 50% of patients; others have scant sputum production that is usually mucoid, rarely purulent, and very rarely bloody. There are no clinical features that distinguish individual patients with LD from those with pneumonia caused by other pathogens.[4-6] However, when patients with LD are compared with those with community-acquired pneumonia due to other agents, the patients with LD are more likely to have myalgias, headache, diarrhea, and a higher mean oral temperature at the time of presentation. They also present to the hospital sooner after the onset of symptoms, 4.7 days versus 7.7 days. When patients with LD were compared with patients with bacteremic pneumococcal pneumonia, the following features were associated with *Legionella* pneumonia: male sex (odds ratio [OR], 4.6), heavy drinking of alcohol (OR, 4.8), previous β-lactam therapy (OR, 19.9), axillary temperature higher than 39° C (OR, 10.3), myalgias (OR, 8.5), and gastrointestinal symptoms (OR, 3.5). Pleuritic chest pain and purulent sputum were less likely to be present. In a young, otherwise healthy person with rapidly progressive pneumonia (especially if the progression occurs in the setting of β-lactam therapy), LD should be strongly suspected. Mental confusion is common, and on occasion, the presentation is dominated by extrapulmonary manifestations such as reactive arthritis, cerebellar ataxia, seizures, myoclonus, or encephalitis. Rarely, extrapulmonary infection, such as prosthetic valve endocarditis, sinusitis, dialysis shunt infection, or abscess formation, occurs.

Physical findings include fever, tachypnea, relative bradycardia, and initially only a few crackles on chest examination. Later, the findings of pulmonary consolidation are not uncommon. Abdominal examination is usually unremarkable. Rash as a manifestation of LD is very rare. Progression of the illness is not uncommon, even after the institution of antibiotic therapy. This is more likely in immunocompromised patients, who may require up to a week to respond to therapy. About half the patients with LD who require hospitalization have a complicated course.

Pontiac fever has an incubation period of about 36 hours. Fever, severe myalgia, headache, and extreme fatigue are the dominant manifestations. The illness is of short duration, lasting, on average, 3 days.

DIAGNOSIS

It is most important to have a high index of clinical suspicion that a patient might have LD. Routine laboratory test results are nonspecifically abnormal. Leukocytosis is common; leukopenia, thrombocytopenia, and disseminated intravascular coagulation also occur. Other laboratory abnormalities may include hyponatremia (in about half the patients, sometimes severe), hypophosphatemia (also common, occurring early and resolving within a few days of the initiation of treatment), mild liver function test abnormalities (except for alkaline phosphatase, which is occasionally very elevated), elevated creatine kinase (occasionally with rhabdomyolysis), microscopic hematuria, and mild proteinuria. High procalcitonin levels exceeding 1.5 are associated with a higher rate of admission to intensive care units and death. Combinations of findings may be suggestive of LD. These include high temperature, absence of sputum production, high lactate levels, increased C-reactive protein level, and low platelet counts.

There are a number of specific tests for the diagnosis of LD. Tests to detect *L. pneumophila* SG 1 antigen in urine are available commercially.[7] These are easy to use, but there is a false-negative rate of up to 26%. The sensitivity of the urinary antigen test in a review of published data was 0.74 (0.68 to 0.81), and the specificity was 0.991 (0.984 to 0.997). Rarely, the urinary antigen test result can remain positive for up to 1 year. Use of this test has allowed early diagnosis of LD because of the very short time required to do the test. This may be a factor in the lower mortality rates from LD compared with historic rates. Sputum culture has a low sensitivity but is 100% specific. It should be performed on all patients suspected of having LD. Serologic tests are not useful in the immediate management of a patient because of the long time (6 to 12 weeks) required to seroconvert; however, they do have a role in the work-up of outbreaks of LD. False-negative and false-positive serologic results do occur. A four-fold or greater increase in antibody titer between the acute and convalescent phase serum samples is diagnostic. A former criterion of a high stable antibody titer of 1:256 or higher is no longer considered diagnostic. Polymerase chain reaction can be used to amplify *Legionella* DNA in sputum, bronchoalveolar lavage fluid, pleural fluid, pulmonary tissue, or serum. Polymerase chain reaction can detect 1 fg of *Legionella* DNA, equivalent to one microorganism. These tests have not yet gained widespread use clinically. *Legionella* can be isolated from the blood with special media or by subculturing onto BCYE (buffered charcoal–yeast extract) agar plates, but this is not used in practice.

A chest radiograph is necessary to establish a diagnosis of pneumonia. About half the patients with LD have unilateral pulmonary involvement. The lower lobes are involved most commonly. About one third of patients have a pleural effusion. Dense opacification is common, but interstitial and nodular opacities also occur. Cavitation is uncommon; 70% of the 79 patients reported to date with lung abscess due to *Legionella* were receiving corticosteroids. Figures 314-2 to 314-5 illustrate some of the radiographic findings in LD.

The diagnosis of Pontiac fever is based on demonstration of *Legionella* in water to which the patient was exposed, seroconversion to *Legionella*, and a compatible clinical course.

Differential Diagnosis

LD should be considered in any patient with pneumonia who is admitted to the hospital, especially those who require treatment in an intensive care unit. If *Legionella* is present in a hospital's water supply, LD should be considered in all patients with nosocomial pneumonia.

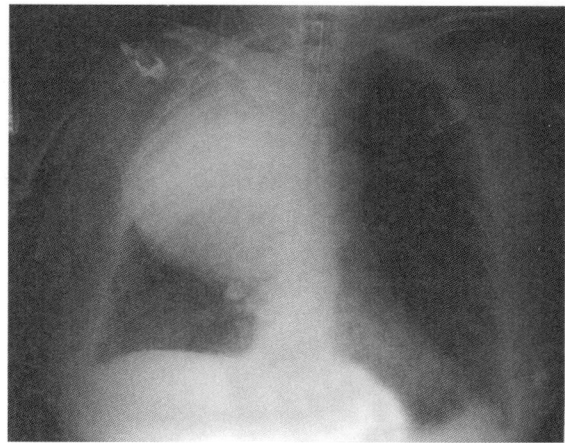

FIGURE 314-2. Posteroanterior chest radiograph of a patient with community-acquired pneumonia due to *Legionella pneumophila*. Note the dense consolidation of the right upper lobe, with bulging of the fissure. Such dense consolidation is a common radiographic appearance of legionnaires' disease.

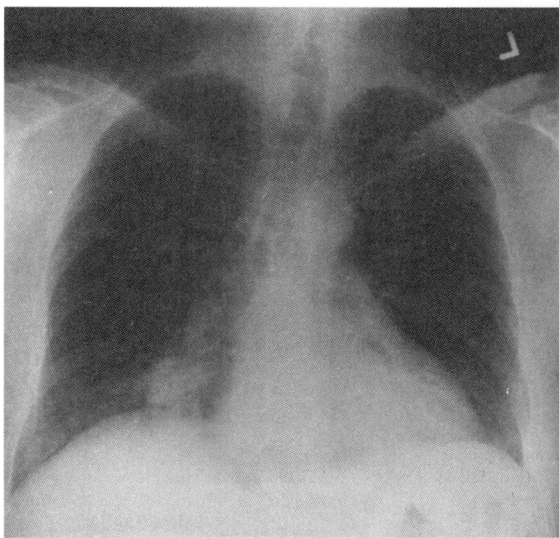

FIGURE 314-3. Posteroanterior chest radiograph of a patient with community-acquired legionnaires' disease (*L. pneumophila*) manifesting as a right lower lobe nodular opacity.

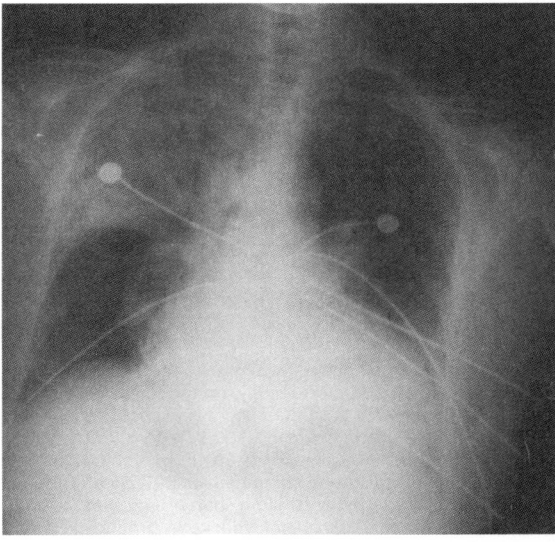

FIGURE 314-4. Posteroanterior chest radiograph of a patient with community-acquired *Legionella feeleii* pneumonia. There is patchy consolidation of the right upper lobe.

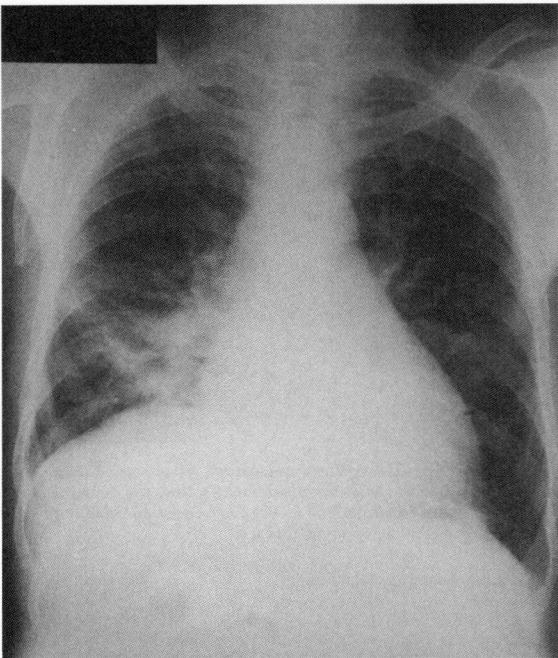

FIGURE 314-5. Posteroanterior chest radiograph of a patient with community-acquired pneumonia due to *Legionella pneumophila*. There is patchy consolidation at the right base, with subsegmental atelectasis and elevation of the right hemidiaphragm.

TABLE 314-2 TREATMENT FOR LEGIONNAIRES' DISEASE

SEVERITY OF *LEGIONELLA* PNEUMONIA	DRUG	DOSAGE
Mild pneumonia in a nonimmunocompromised person treated at home	Azithromycin	500 mg once daily for 5 days
	Clarithromycin	500 mg bid for 10 days
	Doxycycline	200 mg loading dose, then 100 mg bid for 10 days
	Levofloxacin	500 mg once daily for 10 days
	Moxifloxacin	400 mg once daily for 10 days
Pneumonia requiring hospitalization or pneumonia in an immunocompromised person	Levofloxacin	750 mg once daily (IV initially) for 10-14 days*
	Azithromycin	500 mg once daily for 10 days*
	Moxifloxacin	400 mg once daily for 10 days*
	Ciprofloxacin	400 mg q8h IV for 14 days*
	Erythromycin	1000 mg IV qid for 3 days; then 500 mg qid for a total of 21 days
	plus	
	Rifampin	600 mg bid for 5 days

*Increase duration of treatment to 21 days for immunocompromised persons.

TREATMENT   Rx

If the diagnosis of LD is known, levofloxacin and moxifloxacin are first-choice agents (Table 314-2). Unfortunately, no randomized controlled trials have studied the therapy for LD. Data from a prospective, nonrandomized study indicate that levofloxacin is superior to macrolides for the treatment of severe LD. In this study carried out in Murcia, Spain, 3.4% of the patients receiving levofloxacin had complications, compared with 27.2% of those receiving macrolides; the levofloxacin patients had a shorter length of stay, 5.5 versus 11.3 days. The addition of rifampin to levofloxacin produced no additional benefit. In one clinical trial, 20 of 21 patients with LD were cured when treated with azithromycin. In another study, the authors selected 139 cases of *L. pneumophila* pneumonia in a prospective series of 1934 consecutive cases of community-acquired pneumonia. The overall mortality rate was 5%. Eighty patients received initial therapy with a macrolide, and 40 received levofloxacin. Those who received levofloxacin had a faster time to defervescence (2 vs. 4.5 days) and to clinical stability (3 vs. 5 days) and a shorter median length of stay (8 vs. 10 days); there were no significant differences in complications or mortality. In a review of data from six clinical trials, 75 patients with *Legionella* infection were treated with levofloxacin, and 90% of these infections had resolved clinically at the post-therapy visit 2 to 14 days after the termination of treatment. The authors concluded that treatment with levofloxacin 500 mg/day for 7 to 14 days or 750 mg/day for 5 days was effective. In a study of 33 patients admitted to an intensive care unit with LD, fluoroquinolone administration within 8 hours of arrival was associated with decreased mortality. There are no good data on the duration of treatment of LD. The consensus is that 7 to 10 days of treatment with azithromycin or a quinolone is sufficient. However, longer treatment is required if there is lung abscess, empyema, or endocarditis. In immunosuppressed patients, therapy should last for 21 days.

A meta-analysis of 24 trials involving 5015 patients with pneumonia showed that for patients with LD, there was a significant benefit when empirical therapy for pneumonia included agents active against *Legionella*. All patients who are severely ill with pneumonia should receive empirical therapy that treats *Legionella* as well as other pathogens. This is in line with the pneumonia guidelines issued by the American Thoracic Society and the Infectious Diseases Society of America.

Rifampin is frequently added to the treatment regimen of patients who are seriously ill with LD. There are no data suggesting synergy when this antibiotic is used in combination with antibiotics other than a macrolide. When it is used in this context, patients have a longer length of stay and higher bilirubin levels.

PROGNOSIS

In one study, the case-fatality rate from LD fell from 35% in 1993 to 5.6% in 2004. Such a decline in mortality was substantiated in a 15-year study of 217 cases of LD requiring admission to the hospital from Barcelona, Spain. The mortality decreased over time from 9% in 1995 to 2007 to 4% in 2007 to 2010.

In general, the fatality rate is higher in sporadic cases than in outbreak cases, and it is higher in nosocomial cases compared with community-acquired cases. The highest fatality rate is seen in nosocomial LD, for which it is still about 30%. Earlier diagnosis by the urinary antigen test and more effective antibiotic therapy account for much of the reduction in mortality. Factors associated with mortality are older age, immunosuppression, and severity of pneumonia.

Cases of LD should be reported to local health officials. An investigation is often required to determine the source of the *Legionella*.

GENERAL REFERENCES

For the General References and other additional features, please visit Expert Consult at https://expertconsult.inkling.com.

315

BARTONELLA INFECTIONS

JEAN-MARC ROLAIN AND DIDIER RAOULT

DEFINITION

Bartonella species belong to the alpha-2 subgroup of Proteobacteria and are closely related to the genera *Brucella*, *Agrobacterium*, and *Rhizobium*. Since 1993, the genus *Bartonella* has been reorganized by addition of the genera *Rochalimaea* and *Grahamella* to the family Bartonellaceae. More than 30 known *Bartonella* species have been isolated from both animals and humans.[1] These bacteria are considered emerging pathogens that are associated with zoonosis and human infections. Among them, 14 validated species have been implicated in human diseases: *B. henselae*, *B. quintana*, *B. bacilliformis*, *B. elizabethae*, *B. clarridgeiae*, *B. vinsonii* subsp. *arupensis*, *B. vinsonii* subsp. *berkhoffii*, *B. alsatica*, *B. tamiae*, *B. grahamii*, *B. washoensis*, *B. rochalimae*, *B.*

TABLE 315-1 *BARTONELLA* SPECIES CAUSING HUMAN DISEASE

BARTONELLA SPECIES	FIRST CULTIVATION		YEAR OF DESCRIPTION	RESERVOIR HOST/VECTOR	HUMAN DISEASE
	Mammal	*Country*			
B. alsatica	Wild rabbit (*Oryctolagus cuniculus*)	France	1999	Rabbit	Endocarditis, lymphadenopathy
"*Candidatus* B. ancashi"		Peru	2013		Verruga peruana
B. bacilliformis	Human		1909	Human/sandfly	Carrión's disease, Oroya fever, verruga peruana
B. clarridgeiae	Cat		1996	Cat/cat flea	Cat-scratch disease
B. elizabethae	Endocarditis patient	United States	1993	Rat	Endocarditis, neuroretinitis
B. grahamii	Woodland mammal (*Clethrionomys glareolus*)	United Kingdom	1995	Rat, insectivore	Neuroretinitis
B. henselae	Cat		1990	Cat/cat flea	Cat-scratch disease, endocarditis, bacillary angiomatosis, bacillary peliosis, Parinaud oculoglandular syndrome, neuroretinitis, osteomyelitis, arthropathy, bacteremia with fever
B. koehlerae	Domestic cat	United States	1999	Cat	Endocarditis
B. mayotimonensis	Endocarditis patient	United States	2009	Unknown	Endocarditis
B. quintana	Human		1920	Human/body louse	Trench fever, endocarditis, bacillary angiomatosis
B. rochalimae	Human	United States	2007		Bacteremia, fever, splenomegaly
B. tamiae	Human	Thailand	2008		Febrile illness
B. vinsonii arupensis	Cattle rancher	United States	1999	Dog, rodent/ticks	Bacteremia with fever
B. washoensis			2000	Ground squirrel	Myocarditis

koehlerae, and "*Candidatus* B. ancashi" (Table 315-1). The other *Bartonella* species have been isolated only from the blood of animals, including rodents, felids, canids, dolphins, and ruminants. The route of transmission of *Bartonella* species in mammals and humans is by fleas, ticks, mites, and lice (see Table 315-1).

Bartonella infections are emerging infectious diseases that lead to a wide spectrum of either acute or chronic diseases. The status of the host immune response plays an important role in the development of the different manifestations. Four different clinical syndromes may occur with *Bartonella* infections: (1) infection of red blood cells and erythrophagocytosis, (2) granulomatous disease controlled by the immune response, (3) blood culture–negative endocarditis and bacteremia, and (4) vasculoproliferative diseases. A single *Bartonella* species can cause either acute or chronic infections and either vasculoproliferative or suppurative manifestations, but with different pathogenetic mechanisms that mainly depend on the patient's immune status. For example, *B. quintana* is responsible for trench fever as well as for endocarditis, bacteremia in the homeless population, and vasculoproliferative diseases, whereas *B. bacilliformis* is the agent of Carrión's disease, which corresponds to either an acute intraerythrocytic bacteremic disease (Oroya fever) or a chronic vasculoproliferative disease (verruga peruana). Infection of red blood cells has been well established for *B. bacilliformis* (Oroya fever) and *B. quintana* (trench fever and bacteremia in the homeless), whereas *B. henselae* and *B. koehlerae* have been seen in erythrocytes of infected cats. *B. henselae* can cause granulomatous disease, that is, cat-scratch disease (CSD), which affects lymph nodes, but can also be responsible for other clinical manifestations or complications, such as endocarditis. Vasculoproliferative diseases include bacillary angiomatosis caused by *B. henselae* and *B. quintana*, peliosis hepatis caused by *B. henselae*, and verruga peruana caused by *B. bacilliformis*. The immune status of the host plays a critical role in the development of these different forms of the disease. *B. henselae* usually causes CSD (a self-limited disease) in immunocompetent hosts, whereas it is responsible for bacillary angiomatosis in immunocompromised patients. In patients with a previous valvulopathy, any *Bartonella* infection may lead to endocarditis.

The Pathogen

Bartonella species are small, gram-negative, fastidious, pleomorphic coccobacilli or slightly curved rods (0.5 by 1 to 2 μm). Because of the slow growth of these bacteria and the lack of reproducible biochemical methods for their identification, they are usually identified by molecular methods. Matrix-assisted laser desorption/ionization time-of-flight mass spectrometry has emerged as a new technique for species identification and is an accurate and reproducible method for the rapid and inexpensive identification of

Bartonella species. The bacteria can grow on enriched blood-containing media with a 5% carbon dioxide atmosphere after 5 to 15 days to up to 45 days on primary culture. The optimal growth temperature ranges from 28° C for *B. bacilliformis* to 35° to 37° C for the other species. *Bartonella* species can also be cocultured with endothelial cells. *Bartonella* species are either flagellated or nonflagellated cells. *B. bacilliformis* uses flagella for binding and deforming into the surface of erythrocytes. Bacteria can either persist in the blood stream of the host as intraerythrocytic parasites or colonize human endothelial cells.

EPIDEMIOLOGY

Almost all *Bartonella* species are vector-borne bacteria (see Table 315-1). Some are limited geographically, such as *B. bacilliformis*, which is found only in the Andes Mountains in South America at high altitudes, where its principal vector, *Lutzomyia verrucarum*, is distributed; others have a worldwide distribution, such as *B. henselae* and *B. quintana*. Each *Bartonella* species is highly adapted to its mammalian reservoir, in which bacteria usually cause a long-lasting intraerythrocytic bacteremia that may be asymptomatic. Humans are the hosts and reservoirs for *B. bacilliformis* and *B. quintana*. *B. quintana* is transmitted by the human body louse by inoculation of arthropod feces through broken skin (Chapter 359). Cats represent the main reservoir hosts for *B. henselae* infection; this pathogen is the agent of CSD in humans, caused by cat bites or scratches. *B. henselae* infection is transmitted from cat to cat by the cat flea. Cat fleas may also be infected by *B. quintana*. The role of dogs as reservoir hosts has been documented for several species, including *B. vinsonii* subsp. *arupensis*, *B. vinsonii* subsp. *berkhoffii*, and *B. henselae*. Wild rabbits are the reservoir hosts for *B. alsatica*, which is an agent of endocarditis and lymphadenopathy[2] in humans in close contact with rabbits. For other *Bartonella* species known to cause diseases in humans (see Table 315-1), their pathogenic role and mode of transmission are not fully understood.

INFECTION OF RED BLOOD CELLS: OROYA FEVER AND TRENCH FEVER

PATHOBIOLOGY

In Oroya fever, *B. bacilliformis* invades up to 80% of erythrocytes and produces their massive lysis, which results in severe hemolytic anemia, the major symptom of the disease.[3] Similarly, trench fever is characterized by an intracellular erythrocyte parasitism by *B. quintana*, with the percentage of infected red blood cells ranging from 0.001 to 0.005% (Fig. 315-1). Bacteria can also be seen extracellularly and in erythroblasts. This intracellular erythrocyte parasitism can presumably preserve the pathogens for efficient transmission by body lice, protect *B. quintana* from the host immune response, and contribute to decreased antimicrobial efficacy.[4] During bacteremia in the homeless, *B. quintana* can also be seen in red blood cells.

CLINICAL MANIFESTATIONS

The main clinical manifestations of infection by *Bartonella* species are summarized in Table 315-2.[5]

Oroya fever is the acute or hemolytic phase of Carrión's disease, caused by *B. bacilliformis*; it usually develops 3 to 12 weeks after inoculation. Oroya fever results from the massive invasion of erythrocytes by *B. bacilliformis*, and without antibiotic treatment, it causes death in up to 85% of infected humans by hemolysis or when complicated by opportunistic infections such as salmonellosis. The onset is usually abrupt, with high fever, chills, headache, and anorexia. Patients have intense myalgias and arthralgias, abdominal pain, and jaundice. Complications are frequent, including meningoencephalitis, dyspnea, delirium, and superinfection leading to death. Asymptomatic persistent bacteremia may serve as the reservoir of the organism.

Trench fever is transmitted by lice (Chapter 359) and is the clinical manifestation of *B. quintana*. Trench fever affected more than 1 million people during World War I; more recently, *B. quintana* has been recognized in immunocompromised hosts, homeless people, and chronic alcoholics.[6] Clinical manifestations of trench fever may range from asymptomatic infection to severe, life-threatening illness. After an incubation period of 2 to 3 weeks, there is a sudden onset of fever that lasts 1 to 3 days associated with headache, shin pain, and dizziness. Although fatal cases have not been reported, the disease may persist for 4 to 6 weeks and result in prolonged disability. Relapses may occur years later, and in some cases there may be bacteremia with no clinical signs.

● CAT-SCRATCH DISEASE

PATHOBIOLOGY

Little is known about the pathogenesis of the long-lasting lymphadenopathy in CSD. Immunopathogenesis is assumed to play an important role in CSD

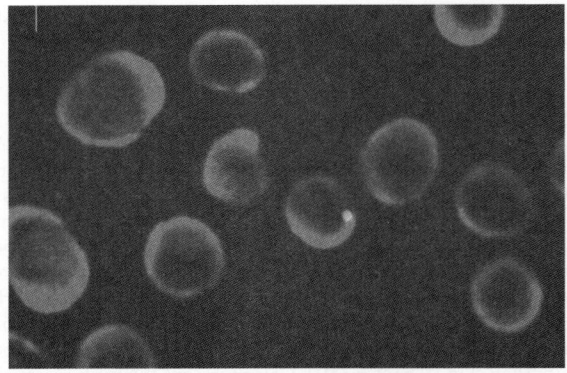

FIGURE 315-1. Section of human red blood cell infected with *Bartonella quintana* as viewed by confocal microscopy.

because bacteria have only rarely been isolated from affected lymph nodes. Thus, the disease is usually controlled by the host immune response, and there are few or no viable bacteria when lymph node biopsy specimens are analyzed; they are necrotic by pathologic examination.

CLINICAL MANIFESTATIONS

Typical CSD is the most common manifestation of infection with *B. henselae* and usually is manifested as a self-limited regional lymphadenitis.[7] Transmission from cat to human occurs directly by a cat scratch or cat bite or possibly by a cat flea or tick bite. A typical papule or pustule may be seen 3 to 10 days after the scratch or bite at the site of inoculation and may last for 1 to 3 weeks. The subsequent lymphadenopathy is localized mainly to the axillary, cervical, or submaxillary nodes that drain the area where the cat scratch occurred. The enlarged lymph node is often painful and tender. Lymphadenopathy sometimes lasts for months, and in a few cases it can persist for as long as 1 to 2 years. In some cases, the lymph node may suppurate if it is not drained. Most patients are not febrile during the course of typical CSD. Systemic or severe disease may occur in about 5 to 14% of patients, with most of them suffering severe systemic symptoms due to disseminated infection. *B. alsatica* has been reported as a cause of lymphadenitis in a woman scratched on the finger while butchering a wild rabbit. After exposure to *B. henselae*, patients may develop bacteremia with or without clinical signs of typical CSD, and in patients with valvular lesions, this may result in infective endocarditis. Thus, CSD represents the primary infection of *B. henselae*, and endocarditis may follow in patients with heart valve lesions.

Approximately 10% of patients with CSD have atypical clinical manifestations, including prolonged fever (>2 weeks), malaise, neuroretinitis, encephalitis, erythema nodosum, hepatitis, fatigue, weight loss, and splenomegaly. A recent clinical study showed that musculoskeletal manifestations (myalgia, arthritis, arthralgia, tendinitis, osteomyelitis, neuralgia) were present in more than 10% of patients with CSD, demonstrating that these clinical manifestations are not as rare as might be expected from the cases reported in the past. In this series of 913 patients, myalgia and arthropathy were the most common manifestations, with an incidence of 5.8% and 5.5%, respectively. Moreover, these manifestations occurred primarily in adults whose ages ranged from 20 to 59 years. Myalgia had a mean duration of 4 weeks and was often severe. Arthropathy had a mean duration of 5.5 weeks, was more common in female patients older than 20 years, affected large and medium joints (half of those involved being weight-bearing joints), and was associated with symmetrical erythema nodosum early in the course of CSD. These musculoskeletal manifestations are often severe and may evolve into chronic forms that persist for more than a year. Tendinitis, neuralgia, and osteomyelitis are less common, with incidences lower than 1%.

Ocular and Neurologic Manifestations

Parinaud oculoglandular syndrome is a self-limited conjunctivitis associated with preauricular lymphadenopathy. Other atypical manifestations include neurologic syndromes (meningoencephalitis, meningitis, neuroretinitis). Encephalopathy may occur in 2 to 4% of CSD patients, mainly adolescents and adults. Patients usually have persistent headaches with or without fever and may develop seizures. Acute neurologic disorders range from self-limited nuchal rigidity to pupillary dilation or aphasia and hemiplegia; they may last

TABLE 315-2 CLINICAL MANIFESTATIONS ASSOCIATED WITH *BARTONELLA* SPECIES					
CLINICAL MANIFESTATION	***B. BACILLIFORMIS***	***B. QUINTANA***	***B. HENSELAE***	***B. ALSATICA***	**OTHERS**
Intraerythrocytic bacteremia	+	+			
Chronic bacteremia	+	+	+		+
Infective endocarditis		+	+	+	+
Verruga peruana	+				
Bacillary angiomatosis		+	+		
Peliosis hepatis			+		
Lymphadenopathy		+	+ (CSD)	+	+
SENLAT with skin lesion			+		
Meningoencephalitis			+		
Uveitis-retinitis		+	+		+

CSD = cat-scratch disease; SENLAT = scalp eschar and neck lymphadenopathy.

for several weeks to months. Neuroretinitis has been associated with CSD in patients experiencing a sudden unilateral loss of visual acuity.[8] The most common picture remains papilledema associated with macular exudates causing stellar retinitis. A few reports have now established that *B. henselae* can be responsible for uveitis, along with *B. grahamii* and *B. quintana*. Patients present with either nongranulomatous or granulomatous uveitis.

Finally, tick-borne *B. henselae* infection has been described, including scalp eschar and neck lymphadenopathy after tick bites in three patients during the colder months in France. *B. henselae* was detected by molecular tools both in skin biopsy specimens (cervical and occipital) and in a *Dermacentor marginatus* tick removed from the scalp of one patient. All three patients had asthenia, but none had alopecia.

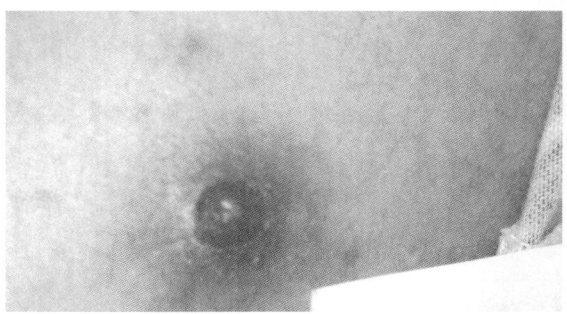

FIGURE 315-2. Skin lesion of bacillary angiomatosis.

ENDOCARDITIS

PATHOBIOLOGY

B. quintana, B. henselae, B. alsatica, B. vinsonii subsp. *berkhoffii, B. elizabethae*, and "*Candidatus* Bartonella mayotimonensis" have been associated with blood culture–negative endocarditis, whereas *B. vinsonii* subsp. *arupensis* has been detected in a patient with fever and bacteremia; *B. washoensis* has been identified in one patient with myocarditis; *B. rochalimae* was reported in a patient with fever, bacteremia, and splenomegaly; and *B. tamiae* has been isolated in a patient with a febrile illness. Patients with endocarditis usually have preexisting heart valve disease that promotes the development of infective endocarditis and, in some cases, a definite risk factor for infection specifically with *Bartonella*. Endocarditis caused by *Bartonella* species exhibits slight inflammation, with a few inflammatory mononuclear cells and small vegetations; the bacteria are seen extracellularly in dense immunopositive clusters that are mainly included in vegetations and in neutrophil and macrophage cytoplasm.

CLINICAL MANIFESTATIONS

The most commonly identified agents of *Bartonella* endocarditis are *B. quintana*, followed by *B. henselae* and other *Bartonella* species.[9] Patients appear to have chronic, blood culture–negative endocarditis, usually with fever (90%). Echocardiography reveals vegetations (in 90%) that should be removed by surgery in the majority of patients. Infections with *B. henselae* are epidemiologically linked to close contact with cats or cat fleas and previous valvular heart disease, whereas *B. quintana* endocarditis is frequently described in homeless and alcoholic patients with body lice infection and can be observed in patients without previous valve lesions. The onset is usually subacute, with some patients being afebrile at the time of admission. About half the patients have embolic phenomena. Interestingly, there is a north (Europe) to south (North Africa) gradient for the proportion of *Bartonella* endocarditis in humans; thus *Bartonella* is apparently a common cause of endocarditis in North Africa. Sporadic cases of endocarditis have also been associated with *B. koehlerae, B. vinsonii* subsp. *berkhoffii, B. vinsonii* subsp. *arupensis, B. elizabethae, B. alsatica*, and "*Candidatus* Bartonella mayotimonensis."

VASCULOPROLIFERATIVE DISEASE: VERRUGA PERUANA, BACILLARY ANGIOMATOSIS, AND PELIOSIS HEPATIS

PATHOBIOLOGY

Bartonella species have the ability to cause vasculoproliferative lesions through a process of pathologic angiogenesis resulting in the formation of new capillaries from preexisting ones. These typical vasoproliferations can be expressed as skin lesions called bacillary angiomatosis, which are caused by *B. quintana* and *B. henselae*[10]; there is also a cystic form in the liver and spleen called peliosis hepatis, which is caused only by *B. henselae*.[11] Skin lesions are similar to those reported for verruga peruana, the chronic form of Carrión's disease. Bacillary angiomatosis is a neovascular proliferation that has been reported most commonly in AIDS patients and involves the skin (Fig. 315-2) and lymph nodes; it occurs less frequently in patients with other causes of immunosuppression and only exceptionally in immunocompetent patients. In bacillary angiomatosis, lesions comprise proliferating endothelial cells, bacteria, and mixed infiltrates of macrophages/monocytes and polymorphonuclear neutrophils, leading to chronic inflammation. Bacteria are clustered as aggregates both surrounding and within endothelial cells, indicating that the vascular endothelium represents a target tissue for intracellular and extracellular colonization in vivo. On histologic evaluation, bacillary angiomatosis

is a lobular proliferation of small blood vessels containing endothelial cells and bacteria, usually seen in clusters when stained with Warthin-Starry. As in bacillary angiomatosis, lesions of verruga peruana are characterized by lobular proliferations and atypical endothelial cells forming both relatively solid sheets and small, well-formed vessels with patent lumens. Lesions are typically infiltrated, indicating a chronic inflammatory process.

CLINICAL MANIFESTATIONS

As already noted, bacillary angiomatosis is seen most often in AIDS patients. Cutaneous lesions often arise in crops and can be subcutaneous or dermal nodules with red or purple papules millimeters to centimeters in diameter. When cutaneous lesions are absent, the diagnosis is often difficult and delayed because signs of visceral involvement are usually nonspecific. The potentially systemic nature of bacillary angiomatosis is reflected by the involvement of brain, bone, lymph node, bone marrow, skeletal muscle, conjunctiva, and mucosal surfaces of the gastrointestinal and respiratory tracts. Peliosis hepatis affects solid internal organs, primarily the liver, with reticuloendothelial elements; in the liver, it is defined as a vascular proliferation of sinusoidal hepatic capillaries resulting in blood-filled spaces. The spleen, abdominal lymph nodes, and bone marrow may also be involved.

Following acute Oroya fever, patients usually develop angioproliferative cutaneous tumors called verruga peruana after a latent period ranging from weeks to months. The infection is characterized by benign cutaneous vascular lesions typically consisting of round papules that are frequently pruritic and bleeding. The infection is accompanied by malaise and arthralgias. Skin lesions may change over time from miliary to nodular subcutaneous lesions to large mulaire lesions. These large lesions are often engorged with blood and prone to ulceration and bleeding. This eruptive phase clinically resembles Kaposi's sarcoma or bacillary angiomatosis. However, it has a low morbidity, and there are no reports of mortality.

DIAGNOSIS OF *BARTONELLA* INFECTION

Methods used for the diagnosis of *Bartonella* infection include serology, microscopy, culture, molecular amplification of *Bartonella* species genes, direct immunofluorescence, and immunohistochemistry. The usefulness of these techniques may vary according to the disease involved (Table 315-3).

Serologic Tests

Serology remains the most widely used method for the diagnosis of CSD and *Bartonella* endocarditis because culture and isolation are difficult and time-consuming, and molecular methods are not available in all laboratories. There are currently two classic serologic methods for the diagnosis of *Bartonella* infections: enzyme-linked immunosorbent assay and immunofluorescence assay. By immunofluorescence assay, an immunoglobulin G titer of 1 : 64 or greater should be considered positive for CSD, whereas patients with endocarditis usually have higher antibody titers (≥1 : 800). In homeless patients, bacteremia has been associated with serologic tests that were positive for *B. quintana*. However, reported sensitivities of immunofluorescence assay vary considerably, from nearly 100% to less than 30%, depending on the nature of the antigens used and the selected patients. Moreover, owing to cross-reactive antibodies between *Bartonella* species, the diagnosis of *Bartonella* infection at the species level is usually not possible. More sophisticated methods should be used, especially Western blot with cross-adsorption analysis. Western blot is also useful for the differential diagnosis of endocarditis

TABLE 315-3 LABORATORY METHODS FOR THE DIAGNOSIS OF *BARTONELLA* INFECTIONS

CLINICAL MANIFESTATION	SEROLOGY	CULTURE	MOLECULAR METHODS	IMMUNOHISTOCHEMISTRY (WARTHIN-STARRY STAIN)	MICROSCOPY FOR INTRAERYTHROCYTIC ORGANISM (GIEMSA OR IF)
Oroya fever	−	+	+	−	+++
Verruga peruana	−	−	+	+	−
Trench fever	+/−	+	+	−	+
Chronic bacteremia	+/−	+++	+	−	−
Infective endocarditis	+++	+++	+++	+++	−
Bacillary angiomatosis	+/−	++	+++	+++	−
Peliosis hepatis	+/−	++	+++	+++	−
Cat-scratch disease	+	−	+++	+/−	+/−
SENLAT with skin lesion	+	+	+++	+	−
Meningoencephalitis	++	−	++	−	−
Uveitis-retinitis	++	−	++	+	−

IF = immunofluorescence; SENLAT = scalp eschar and neck lymphadenopathy.

because the profile obtained for endocarditis is specific compared with that for CSD or chronic bacteremia.

Microscopy, Immunofluorescence, and Immunohistochemistry

The diagnosis of Oroya fever is based on examination of a peripheral blood smear stained by Giemsa; the percentage of infected red blood cells is sufficiently high so that bacteria are visible. Similarly, *B. quintana* can be seen within red blood cells with use of specific monoclonal antibody by immunofluorescence and confocal microscopy (see Fig. 315-1). Microscopic examination after Warthin-Starry silver staining or immunohistochemistry of a cardiac valve or skin biopsy specimen is also useful for the detection of *Bartonella* organisms in patients with endocarditis and bacillary angiomatosis.

Culture

Bartonella species can be recovered from the blood of bacteremic patients as well as from cardiac valves, skin and liver biopsy specimens, and, rarely, lymph nodes. Bacteria can be isolated directly from these specimens after plating onto blood agar solid media, blood culture in broth, and cocultivation in endothelial cells. Cultures are usually positive after 2 weeks of incubation, but up to 45 days may be necessary for primary isolation.

Molecular Detection Methods

Direct detection and final identification of *Bartonella* species from blood and tissue specimens, including lymph node, cardiac valve, skin, and liver, can be achieved by polymerase chain reaction amplification and sequencing of various housekeeping genes. Real-time polymerase chain reaction with TaqMan probes has been added to the panel of molecular techniques for the specific detection of *Bartonella* at the species level from lymph nodes in CSD, directly from cardiac valves in patients with endocarditis, and in patients with bacillary angiomatosis or peliosis hepatis.

Differential Diagnosis

The differential diagnosis of bacillary angiomatosis is Kaposi's sarcoma, but visualization of bacteria in the tissue specimen can help distinguish between these two entities. Trench fever may be confused mainly with typhus group rickettsiosis, relapsing fever, and malaria. CSD may be confused with tularemia, pyogenic lymphadenitis, mycobacterial infection, and neoplasia.

TREATMENT Rx

Trench Fever

Before the advent of antibiotics, acetylsalicylic acid was the most effective drug for the pain caused by trench fever. However, a randomized clinical trial in homeless persons with episodes of bacteremia demonstrated that the combination of gentamicin and doxycycline is more effective in stopping bacteremia compared with no treatment or the use of β-lactams or doxycycline alone.

Because the intraerythrocytic presence of *B. quintana* decreases antimicrobial efficacy, the duration of treatment is critical in trench fever. Patients with *B. quintana* bacteremia should be treated with gentamicin (3 mg/kg body weight/day IV for 14 days), in combination with doxycycline (200 mg/day PO) for 28 days.

Oroya Fever and Verruga Peruana

In Oroya fever, treatment with penicillin, streptomycin, fluoroquinolones, tetracycline, or erythromycin produces rapid defervescence and disappearance of the organisms from the blood, usually within 24 hours. As an alternative treatment, chloramphenicol can be used alone or in combination with a β-lactam. Treatment with chloramphenicol may also have the advantage of covering commonly associated *Salmonella* species. Patients with Oroya fever should be treated with chloramphenicol (500 mg PO four times a day) for 14 days in combination with another antibiotic (especially a β-lactam compound). Streptomycin (15 to 20 mg/kg/day for 10 days) was the traditional treatment for verruga peruana. However, its use is problematic, especially in children, and rifampin has become the drug of choice for the treatment of eruptive-phase bartonellosis. Failures of rifampin treatment have been reported in verruga peruana. Finally, ciprofloxacin (500 mg PO twice daily for 7 to 10 days) has been used successfully for the treatment of multiple eruptive-phase lesions in adults and has been proposed as an appropriate alternative. Doxycycline in association with gentamicin may be used to treat the eruptive phase of Carrión's disease.

Cat-Scratch Disease

Typical CSD is a self-limited illness that resolves within 2 to 6 months and usually does not respond to therapy because the bacteria within necrotic lymph nodes are not alive. In cases of long-lasting lymphadenopathy, patients should be reassured that it is benign and will probably subside spontaneously within 2 to 4 months. Management consists of analgesics for pain and prudent follow-up.[12] However, azithromycin (500 mg PO on day 1 and 250 mg PO on days 2 to 5 as single daily doses) is an alternative for patients with large, bulky lymphadenopathy.[13] If lymphadenopathy does not resolve, lymph nodes can be removed surgically. For atypical presentations of CSD, there are no data regarding the benefit of specific antimicrobial therapy for immunocompetent patients. For neuroretinitis, the combination of doxycycline (100 mg PO or IV twice daily) with rifampin (300 mg PO twice daily) seems to promote disease resolution, to improve visual acuity, to reduce optic disc edema, and to decrease disease duration.

Endocarditis

Patients with *Bartonella* endocarditis have a higher death rate and undergo valvular surgery more frequently than patients with endocarditis caused by other pathogens. Patients with suspected (but culture-negative) *Bartonella* endocarditis or proved *B. quintana* endocarditis should be treated with oral doxycycline 100 mg twice a day for 6 weeks in combination with gentamicin 3 mg/kg/day in one intravenous daily dose for 14 days.[14] The American Heart Association consensus on treating infective endocarditis is ceftriaxone plus gentamicin, with or without doxycycline, when *Bartonella* is suspected, and doxycycline plus gentamicin when *Bartonella* endocarditis is confirmed. However, there is direct evidence that patients receiving an aminoglycoside are more likely to fully recover, and those treated with aminoglycosides for at least 14 days are more likely to survive than those receiving a shorter duration of therapy. In the absence of any prospective study for the treatment of *Bartonella* endocarditis, the same regimen as for *B. henselae* and *B. quintana* should be used for endocarditis when another *Bartonella* species has been identified as the causative agent.

Bacillary Angiomatosis and Peliosis Hepatis

Without appropriate therapy, infection spreads systemically and can involve virtually any organ, and the outcome is sometimes fatal. Thus, antibiotic treatment is warranted in all cases of *Bartonella*-associated vasculoproliferative disease. On the basis of empirical clinical reports, erythromycin remains the treatment of choice and has been used successfully to treat many patients with bacillary angiomatosis. The response to treatment in bacillary angiomatosis can be dramatic in immunocompromised patients, with resolution of palpable subcutaneous lesions within hours. Erythromycin also has an antiangiogenic effect on microvascular endothelial cells that could explain this quick disappearance of lesions. Erythromycin (500 mg four times daily) for 3 months is first-line therapy. Doxycycline (100 mg PO or IV twice daily) is currently proposed as an appropriate alternative. In patients with serious infections, erythromycin or doxycycline can be used in combination with rifampin (300 mg PO twice daily). The duration of therapy is critical. We recommend that treatment be given for at least 3 months for bacillary angiomatosis and 4 months for peliosis hepatis. Peliosis hepatis responds slowly, and hepatic lesions continue to improve after several months of treatment, whereas cutaneous bacillary angiomatosis demonstrates improvement after 4 to 7 days of treatment and resolves after about 1 month of treatment. Relapses of peliosis hepatis and bacillary angiomatosis lesions after antibiotic treatment have been reported frequently, especially in immunocompromised patients with a shorter duration of therapy. Patients who relapse after the recommended treatment should probably be re-treated for 4 to 6 months with erythromycin (500 mg PO four times daily) or doxycycline (100 mg PO twice daily), and those with repeated relapses should receive antibiotic therapy as long as they are immunocompromised.

PREVENTION

Because arthropods play an important role in the transmission of feline *Bartonella* species to humans, rigorous arthropod control (Chapter 359) should be recommended by health care workers, particularly when advising immunocompromised individuals on the risks related to pet ownership. Cat fleas live on both cats and dogs and are best controlled by fumigating areas where these animals live.

PROGNOSIS

Mortality in those with Oroya fever was as high as 50% before the antibiotic era but is now limited by the use of antibiotics. Trench fever should be treated with antibiotics to avoid more severe disease, especially in patients with valvulopathy who are at risk for development of endocarditis. CSD usually resolves spontaneously without any treatment in immunocompetent patients. In the case of complications or in immunocompromised patients, antibiotic therapy should be given, and patients usually respond well to treatment. Finally, for vasculoproliferative diseases, antibiotics are usually effective if they are given for a long time, but cutaneous lesions in verruga peruana may benefit from surgery.

GENERAL REFERENCES

For the General References and other additional features, please visit Expert Consult at https://expertconsult.inkling.com.

316

GRANULOMA INGUINALE (DONOVANOSIS)

EDWARD W. HOOK III

DEFINITION

Granuloma inguinale, also known as donovanosis, is a slowly progressive ulcerative disease that involves principally the skin and subcutaneous tissues of the genital, inguinal, and anal regions.

The Pathogen

The causative organism is *Klebsiella granulomatis* (formerly *Calymmatobacterium granulomatis*), a facultative intracellular parasite. The organism is challenging to cultivate but can sometimes be grown in yolk sacs, and successful cell culture has been reported from South Africa and Australia. Successful culture, in turn, has permitted the development of polymerase chain reaction assays, currently for research purposes.

EPIDEMIOLOGY

The organism is primarily transmitted sexually, but it can probably be transmitted by nonsexual contact as well. Transmission efficiency is relatively low, and multiple sexual contacts with an infected partner seem to be necessary for the transmission of infection. The disease is rarely encountered in the United States. Although still relatively rare, it is more common in other areas of the world, including India, Papua New Guinea, the Caribbean, southern Africa, and parts of Australia, and it may be becoming less common even in these areas.

CLINICAL MANIFESTATIONS

After an incubation period of up to 50 days, the initial lesion usually appears as a subcutaneous nodule that erodes through the surface and develops into a beefy, elevated granulomatous lesion (Fig. 316-1).[1,2] The lesion is painless but tends to bleed easily, and it is not associated with systemic symptoms. Lesion exudate is often described as foul smelling. Secondary bacterial infection may cause a necrotic, painful, ulcerative lesion that may be rapidly destructive. A cicatricial form may also occur, with a depigmented elevated area of keloid-like scar containing scattered islands of granulomatous tissue. About 90% of lesions occur on the genitals and are commonly associated with pseudobuboes; these swellings usually are not due to involvement of the inguinal lymph nodes but rather are due to granulomatous involvement of subcutaneous tissue. Metastatic infection of bones or viscera is occasionally seen. Clinical experience suggests that secondary carcinomas may be a rare complication of granuloma inguinale.

DIAGNOSIS

The diagnosis is made by demonstrating intracellular Donovan's bodies in histiocytes or other mononuclear cells from lesion scrapings or biopsy samples. Wright stain and Giemsa stain of fresh impression smears or unfixed biopsy specimens usually demonstrate the bacilli relatively easily, although multiple biopsies may be necessary in chronic cases. Histologic examination of biopsy specimens shows plasma cells with some infiltration by polymorphonuclear leukocytes but no giant cells. In infected lesions, *K. granulomatis* is found primarily in histiocytes or other mononuclear cells. Cell culture and polymerase chain reaction methods are currently primarily research tools. No serologic test is clinically available.

Differential Diagnosis

The differential diagnosis includes squamous cell carcinoma, chancroid (Chapter 301), lymphogranuloma venereum (Chapter 318), syphilis

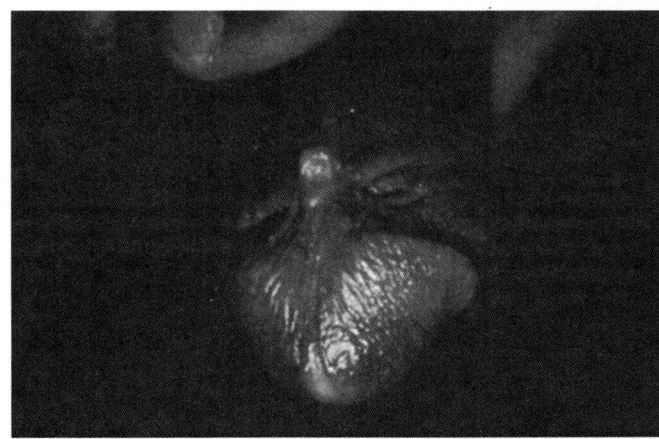

FIGURE 316-1. Typical primary lesion of granuloma inguinale. (Reproduced with permission from Herpes-Coldsores.com. http://www.herpes-coldsores.com/std/lymphogranuloma-pictures.htm.)

(Chapter 319), and other ulcerative granulomatous diseases.[3] In the absence of therapy, patients may not present until lesions have been present for months, long after the lesions of syphilis and other ulcerative sexually transmitted diseases have resolved. Chancroid is usually differentiated by its irregular undermined borders, which are not seen in typical cases of granuloma inguinale. Dark-field examination and serologic tests should help distinguish syphilis. Biopsy of lesions may be necessary to distinguish granuloma inguinale from certain tumors.

TREATMENT   Rx

There are no recent clinical trials of therapy for granuloma inguinale. Recommended treatment consists of azithromycin administered either as 1.0 g weekly or 500 mg daily or doxycycline 100 mg twice daily.[4] One double-strength trimethoprim-sulfamethoxazole tablet twice daily or erythromycin base 500 mg four times daily is recommended as alternative therapy. An aminoglycoside (e.g., gentamicin 1 mg/kg intravenously every 8 hours) may be added if these regimens do not result in clinical improvement within a few days. Treatment should be administered for at least 3 weeks and until lesions are completely healed. Patients should be monitored for at least several weeks after treatment is discontinued because of the possibility of relapse. Although the risk of communicability appears to be low, sexual contacts should also be examined; at present, treatment of contacts is not indicated in the absence of clinically evident disease.

GENERAL REFERENCES

For the General References and other additional features, please visit Expert Consult at https://expertconsult.inkling.com.

317

MYCOPLASMA INFECTIONS

STEPHEN G. BAUM

DEFINITION

Mycoplasma organisms of the class Mollicutes are ubiquitous as pathogens and colonizing agents in the plant, animal, and insect kingdoms. They represent the smallest known free-living forms, but because they have fastidious growth requirements, they are difficult to culture. However, the presence of several species of *Mycoplasma* as commensals in animals and on human oral and genital mucosa frequently resulted in contamination of cell cultures. Such contamination led to the false implication of mycoplasmas as causative agents in many human diseases, both trivial and life-threatening. Of the human diseases proved to be due to mycoplasmas, pneumonia caused by *Mycoplasma pneumoniae* is by far the most clinically important. This infection constitutes a significant proportion of cases previously classified as atypical pneumonia, a nonspecific term for patchy pneumonias that generally do not respond to β-lactam antibiotics and have etiologic agents that are not easily cultured or visible on Gram stain. The term *atypical pneumonia* persists despite our increasing ability to identify specific etiologic agents, such as viruses, *Legionella*, and *Chlamydophila*. Other proven *Mycoplasma* infections include those in the urogenital tract caused by *Ureaplasma* species, *Mycoplasma hominis*, and *Mycoplasma genitalium*; wound infections caused by *M. hominis*; and overwhelming systemic infection in immunocompromised patients caused by *Mycoplasma fermentans* (*incognitus* strain).

The Pathogen

Mycoplasmas are short rods (10×200 nm) that have no cell wall and are bounded by a sterol-containing membrane; thus, they are unaffected by cell wall–inhibiting antimicrobials such as β-lactams. In tissue culture, mycoplasmas are intracellular; but in vivo, infection is primarily extracellular and affects epithelial cells and their organelles, such as cilia. Attachment to respiratory epithelium is by way of terminal adhesin proteins in specialized tip organelles.

EPIDEMIOLOGY

M. pneumoniae infection is spread person to person by respiratory droplets produced by coughing. Relatively close association with the index case appears to be required. The disease is usually introduced into families by a young child; in some studies, most of the infected adults were the parents of young children. As opposed to most viral respiratory infections, which are manifested 1 to 3 days after infection, *Mycoplasma* has an incubation period of 2 to 3 weeks. Therefore, a careful history showing several weeks between cases within a family may be an important clue to the mycoplasmal etiology. Organisms can be cultured from the sputum of infected individuals for weeks to months after clinically efficacious treatment.

Most cases of *Mycoplasma* respiratory infection occur singly or as family outbreaks. However, in closed populations, such as military recruit camps and boarding schools, *Mycoplasma* can cause mini-epidemics and may be responsible for 25 to 75% of cases of pneumonia in such settings. Serologically based epidemiologic studies have documented the high incidence of *Mycoplasma* respiratory infection throughout the world. In the United States, it is estimated that each year at least one case of *Mycoplasma* pneumonia occurs for every 1000 persons, or more than 2 million cases annually. The incidence of *Mycoplasma* nonpneumonic respiratory infection may be 10 to 20 times greater. The highest attack rates are in individuals 5 to 20 years old, but *M. pneumoniae* infection can occur at any age and may cause particularly severe disease in neonates.

As opposed to viral respiratory infections that peak in winter in temperate climates, a few studies have reported a peak incidence of *M. pneumoniae* outbreaks in the fall. Most surveys, however, show little or no seasonal predominance in sporadic cases. There is an age-related relationship of upper versus lower respiratory tract infection caused by *M. pneumoniae*. In children younger than 3 years, primarily upper respiratory tract infection develops, whereas in those 5 to 20 years old, bronchitis and pneumonia tend to occur. In older adults, pneumonia predominates.

The prevalence and incidence of clinical urogenital disease caused by *Ureaplasma urealyticum*, *Ureaplasma parvum*, *M. hominis*, and *M. genitalium* are much less well documented (Table 317-1). These organisms are rarely cultured outside the realm of clinical studies, and they exist as clinically inapparent commensals of the genitourinary tract. Diseases attributed to *Ureaplasma* species include urinary tract infection with and without calculus formation. The organism has been implicated as a cause of low birthweight in neonates. *M. hominis* is a common genitourinary and oral commensal as well and has been documented as a cause of endometritis and postpartum fever.

M. hominis has also caused sternal wound infection after cardiothoracic surgery and has been implicated in arthritis in immunocompromised patients. *Mycoplasma salivarium* may be involved in periodontal disease, and *M. genitalium* is implicated in some cases of nongonococcal urethritis and vaginitis.

TABLE 317-1   SITES AND INFECTIONS RELATED TO HUMAN MYCOPLASMAS

SUBGROUP	SITES OF ISOLATION	DISEASES	OCCURRENCE
M. hominis	GU tract (F > M)	Cervicitis, vaginitis, ?prostatitis	Common
	Conjunctivae (neonate)	Conjunctivitis	
	Blood (peripartum)	Peripartum sepsis	
	Surgical wounds, joints	Sternotomy infection, arthritis	
M. orale	Oropharynx	?	Common
M. pneumoniae	Respiratory tract	URI, pneumonia	Common
M. salivarium	Oropharynx, gingiva	?Periodontal disease	Common
M. fermentans	GU tract, blood, tissues	Multisystem disease in AIDS	Uncommon
M. genitalium	GU tract	Urethritis, cervicitis, PID	Uncommon
Ureaplasma spp	GU tract	Urethritis, upper GU infection	Common

AIDS = acquired immunodeficiency syndrome; F = female; GU = genitourinary; M = male; PID = pelvic inflammatory disease; URI = upper respiratory tract infection.

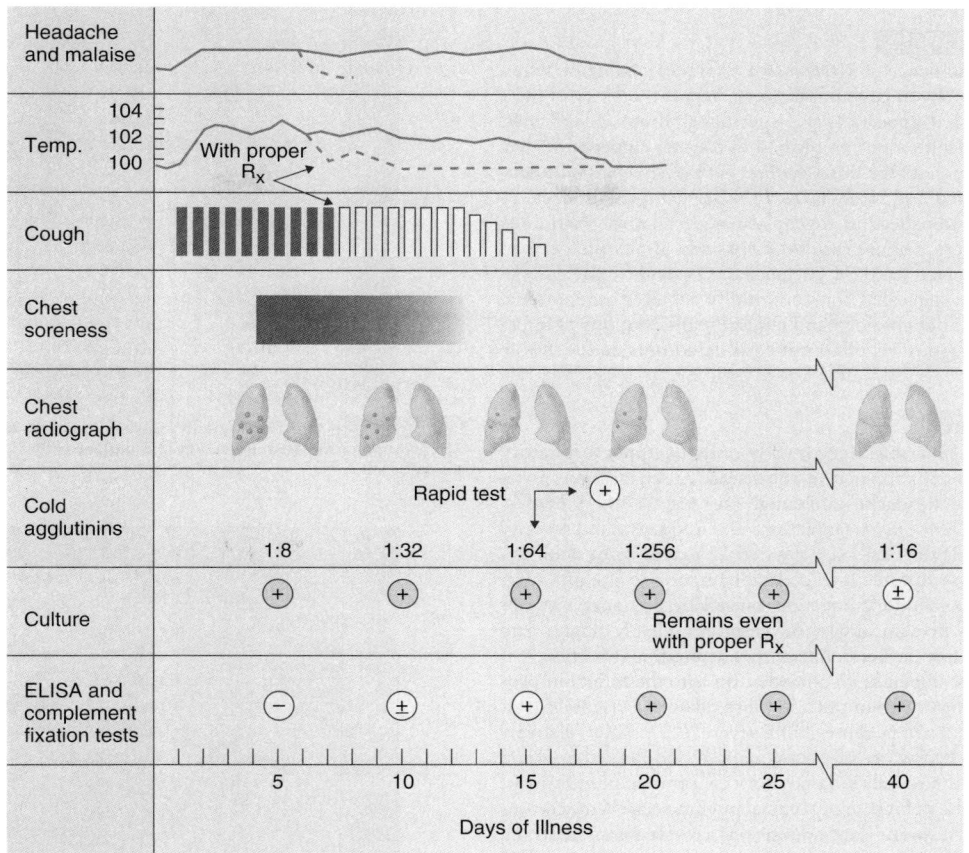

FIGURE 317-1. Major clinical and laboratory manifestations of mycoplasmal pneumonia. ELISA = enzyme-linked immunosorbent assay. (Modified from Baum SG. Mycoplasmal infections. In: Wyngaarden JB, Smith LH Jr, eds. *Cecil Textbook of Medicine*.17th ed. Philadelphia: Saunders; 1985:1506.)

M. fermentans, incognitus strain, was identified about four decades ago as an infectious agent in immunocompromised patients, in whom it causes overwhelming multisystem involvement.

PATHOBIOLOGY

Because of the low fatality of most *Mycoplasma* infections, there is little human pathologic material. Inoculation onto animal tracheal organ cultures is followed by ciliary damage and desquamation of surface epithelium. This latter effect is probably responsible for the hacking cough in *Mycoplasma* respiratory infection.

Several characteristics of *M. pneumoniae* probably play a direct role in the respiratory pathogenicity of this organism. The first is the affinity of *M. pneumoniae* for respiratory epithelial cells. Attachment appears to be between a terminal organelle at one end of the filamentous organism and a sialated glycoprotein (I-FI) on the surface of both respiratory epithelium and erythrocytes that acts as a receptor. *M. pneumoniae* attaches to ciliated epithelial cells at the base of cilia and appears to produce most of its physiologic and cytolytic changes while remaining extracellular. Hydrogen peroxide produced by *M. pneumoniae* (the only human mycoplasma to do so) may be responsible for some in vivo cell damage, as it is for the hemolysis seen when the organisms are grown on blood agar plates. *Mycoplasma* infection activates T and B cells and induces many pro-inflammatory and anti-inflammatory cytokines and chemokines that may play a role in inflammation-related cell destruction. Strain-specific elaboration of biofilms probably plays a role in protecting the organism from host immune cells and may decrease antimicrobial penetration.

In the course of *M. pneumoniae* infection, some patients produce cold agglutinins. These oligoclonal M-type immunoglobulins (IgM) cross-react with I antigens, one of the blood group antigens common to almost all mature human erythrocytes, and high titers may cause hemolysis (presumably as a result of complement-activated, Coombs-positive erythrocyte destruction) and lead to some of the complications described in the Clinical Manifestations section. Like other IgM antibodies, the *Mycoplasma*-induced cold

agglutinins (Chapter 160) develop early in the disease (7 to 10 days) and are often present by the time the patient seeks medical attention. The titer of these agglutinins peaks at 2 to 3 weeks, and they persist for 2 to 3 months (Fig. 317-1).

Several theories about the factors triggering the formation of cold agglutinins in *Mycoplasma* pneumonia have been proposed. One is that the organism alters the I antigen such that it becomes antigenic to the patient. The hydrogen peroxide elaborated by *M. pneumoniae* could be responsible for this alteration. One study indicated that the I antigen in a sialated state may serve as a receptor for *M. pneumoniae* and that the cold agglutinins are directed at the modified receptor. Other studies indicate that the cold agglutinins are directed at mycoplasmal substructures themselves and merely cross-react with the I antigen (altered or native) on red cells. Given their apparent target, these antibodies could either contribute to cytolysis and exacerbate infection or interfere with cell-to-cell spread by blocking or disrupting the cell receptor for the mycoplasma. High titers of cold agglutinins have also been associated with hemolysis, presumably as a result of the activation of complement-mediated erythrocyte destruction (Chapter 160). Although clinically significant hemolysis is uncommon, subclinical levels of red cell destruction are common.

Sickle cell disease, sickle-related hemoglobinopathies, and hypogammaglobulinemia predispose to increased severity and mortality. Therefore, some of the available pathologic data may be influenced by the pathophysiologic mechanisms of these underlying conditions. Deaths have occurred in patients with diffuse pneumonia, acute respiratory distress syndrome, thromboembolism, and disseminated intravascular coagulation.

In nonfatal cases in which lung biopsy was performed, the inflammatory process involved primarily the trachea, bronchioles, and peribronchial tissue. The lumen of the respiratory tree was filled with a purulent exudate rich in polymorphonuclear leukocytes. The lining of the bronchial and bronchiolar walls showed metaplastic cells, and the walls themselves were infiltrated with monocytic elements, especially plasma cells. There was widening of the peribronchial septa and hyperplasia of type II pneumocytes.

CLINICAL MANIFESTATIONS

In view of the very high incidence of *Mycoplasma* respiratory infection when it is studied epidemiologically in large populations, versus the rarity of individual sporadic diagnoses, it appears that a specific, laboratory-confirmed diagnosis of this entity is seldom accomplished in routine clinical practice. There are probably four reasons for this. The first is that *Mycoplasma* pneumonia is usually self-limited and rarely fatal. This fact dampens the zeal to establish the cause of infection. Second, mycoplasmas are relatively fastidious and slow growing; therefore, culture results, if obtained at all, often return after the patient has recovered. Third, *M. pneumoniae* responds to the empirical antimicrobial therapy suggested for community-acquired pneumonia. Finally, knowledge of the epidemiology and clinical manifestations of infection is deficient, so the diagnosis is often not considered outside the classic age group.

Respiratory Infection

The majority of *M. pneumoniae* infections involve only the upper respiratory tract. After a 2- to 3-week incubation period, the disease has an insidious onset consisting of fever, malaise, headache, and cough (see Fig. 317-1). Cough is the clinical hallmark of *M. pneumoniae* infection. The frequency and severity of the cough increase during the next 1 to 2 days, and it may become debilitating. The gradual onset of symptoms is in contradistinction to the often fulminant manifestation of respiratory infection caused by influenza virus or adenovirus. Unfortunately, no clinical signs or symptoms reliably differentiate *M. pneumoniae* infections from other community-acquired pneumonias.[1]

In 5 to 10% of patients, depending somewhat on age, the infection progresses to tracheobronchitis or pneumonia. In these cases, the original manifestations persist, and the cough becomes more severe. It is usually relatively nonproductive but may yield white or occasionally blood-flecked sputum. Gram staining of this sputum reveals inflammatory cells but no predominant bacterial species (part of the definition of atypical pneumonia). With continued cough, parasternal chest soreness may develop as a result of muscle strain, but true pleuritic pain is unusual. Fever is usually at the level of 101° to 102° F and may be associated with chilly sensations. As opposed to pneumonia caused by *Streptococcus pneumoniae* (Chapter 289), that caused by *M. pneumoniae* rarely produces true shaking chills. In comparison to influenza, which can also be manifested as an atypical pneumonia syndrome, myalgias and gastrointestinal complaints of nausea and vomiting are unusual. Diarrhea, sometimes a concomitant of adenoviral or *Legionella* pneumonia, is uncommon in *Mycoplasma* infection.

On physical examination, the patient does not appear to be terribly ill. In fact, this disease is the paradigm of the term *walking pneumonia*. The pharynx may be injected and erythematous, usually without the marked cervical adenopathy seen with group A streptococcal pharyngitis. *M. pneumoniae* is not a common cause of isolated pharyngitis in the pediatric or adult population. Much has been made of the finding of bullous myringitis in this disease. Although this abnormality was present in about 20% of volunteers with experimentally induced *M. pneumoniae* infection, true bullous myringitis in naturally occurring *Mycoplasma* disease is rare. In a study involving children, otitis was rarely associated with isolation of *Mycoplasma* and, on the contrary, was often associated with bacterial and viral upper respiratory tract pathogens. Thus, the absence of myringitis, bullous or otherwise, should not dissuade one from a diagnosis of *Mycoplasma* pneumonia.

Examination of the chest in patients with *Mycoplasma* pneumonia is often unrevealing, even in those with severe, productive cough. There may be no auscultative or percussive findings, or only minimal rales (crackles) may be present. The disparity between physical findings and radiographic evidence of pneumonia in this condition may be the greatest of any of the atypical pneumonia syndromes (Fig. 317-2). Although wheezing can occur in this disease, in one study of asthmatic patients, the presence of wheezing had a negative correlation with isolation of *M. pneumoniae* compared with isolation of viral respiratory pathogens such as respiratory syncytial virus (Chapter 362). *M. pneumoniae* does not seem to be a common pathogen in patients with preexisting chronic obstructive lung disease, either. Bacterial superinfection after *M. pneumoniae* respiratory infection is rare. The radiographic finding of interstitial or patchy alveolar pneumonia does not allow differentiation from any of the other causes of the atypical pneumonia syndrome.

Pleural effusion (usually small) occurs in 5 to 20% of patients with *M. pneumoniae* pneumonia. This low incidence of pleural inflammation is consistent with the rarity of pleuritic pain. If effusion is present, thoracentesis reveals serous fluid that is exudative, with minimal inflammatory reaction.

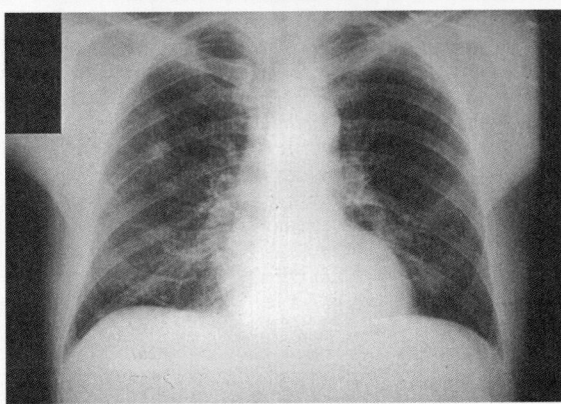

FIGURE 317-2. Chest radiograph showing moderate interstitial pneumonia due to *Mycoplasma pneumoniae* infection in a patient with a paucity of findings on chest auscultation.

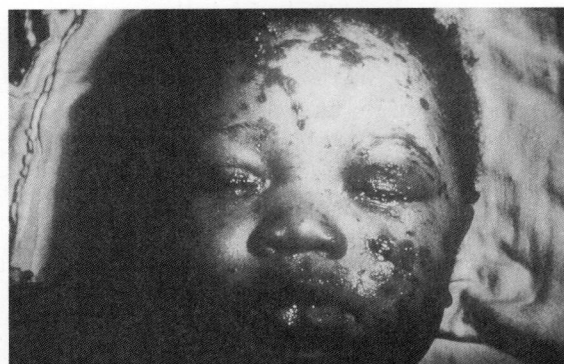

FIGURE 317-3. Stevens-Johnson syndrome in a child with *Mycoplasma* pneumonia. (From Baum SG. *Mycoplasma pneumoniae* and atypical pneumonia. In: Mandell GL, Bennett JE, Dolin R, eds. *Mandell, Douglas, and Bennett's Principles and Practice of Infectious Diseases.* 6th ed. Philadelphia: Churchill Livingstone; 2005:2274.)

The cell differential count in the fluid is variable, and bloody effusions are rare. It is unusual to isolate *M. pneumoniae* from effusions when they do occur, but several reports of such isolation exist. Although the pneumonia is generally mild and self-limited, fulminant, severe, and lethal cases have been reported in normal young adults and may be underdiagnosed.

Extrapulmonary Involvement

Abnormalities in almost every organ system have been described as examples of the extrapulmonary manifestations of *M. pneumoniae* infection. The frequency of these extrapulmonary manifestations varies greatly from one report to another, and they are much less common when viewed as part of a prospective epidemiologic study rather than as the sum of isolated case reports. The conclusion appears to be that the high prevalence of *Mycoplasma* infection predisposes to the reporting of many concurrent but perhaps unrelated events as though they were part of the mycoplasmal disease. Several clinical syndromes have been reported with sufficient frequency to provide some support for a causal relationship.

Dermatologic Involvement

A wide variety of transient dermatologic conditions have been reported in conjunction with *Mycoplasma* pneumonia, including macular, morbilliform, and papulovesicular eruptions as well as erythema nodosum and urticaria. Again, the variety and high incidence of these rashes in the absence of *Mycoplasma* infection make it difficult to define the relationships, if any, among these occurrences. Furthermore, the role of concurrent antibiotic therapy in the development of exanthems during *M. pneumoniae* infection is unknown. One skin condition that occurs often enough in concert with *M. pneumoniae* infection to provide some basis for relatedness is erythema multiforme majus, or Stevens-Johnson syndrome (Fig. 317-3). This rash has been reported in up to 7% of patients with *Mycoplasma* pneumonia and consists of erythematous vesicles, plaques, and bullae involving the skin, with particular localization at mucocutaneous junctions. The conjunctivae as well as organs of the gastrointestinal and genitourinary tracts and the joints may also be involved. Stevens-Johnson syndrome has been associated with isolated cases of many other infections, including some that can be manifested as atypical pneumonia syndrome, such as legionnaires' pneumonia, adenovirus respiratory-conjunctivitis syndrome, and influenza B infection. However, the association with *M. pneumoniae* infection is by far the most common. Stevens-Johnson syndrome tends to occur in younger patients with *Mycoplasma* pneumonia and has a definite male preponderance (2 : 1 to 4 : 1).

The pathogenesis of Stevens-Johnson syndrome is unclear. It has long been supposed that immunity plays a major role, but several reports have noted the culture of *M. pneumoniae* from the lesions. The relationship to the level of cold agglutinins in this disease is variable. It has been suggested that the development of Stevens-Johnson syndrome may be the result of augmented sensitivity to antibiotics in the presence of *M. pneumoniae* infection, but erythema multiforme majus develops in some patients in the absence of previous or concurrent antibiotic therapy. Most patients clear the lesions in 1 to 2 weeks without scarring unless impetiginization supervenes.

A debilitating form of *M. pneumoniae*–associated mucositis without skin involvement has been described as an atypical Stevens-Johnson syndrome, but it is now increasingly recognized as a separate entity, termed *M. pneumoniae*–associated mucositis.[2]

Raynaud's syndrome (Chapter 80), a transient, reversible vasospasm of the digits that develops on exposure to cold, is not technically a dermatologic syndrome; however, it is manifested in the skin. This phenomenon occurs in many people, usually women, without any association with infection. It has been reported in patients with acute *Mycoplasma* pneumonia, regardless of whether they exhibited the syndrome before infection. Although the pathophysiologic mechanism of this condition in *M. pneumoniae* infection is unclear, it may be related to the in vivo action of cold agglutinins (see Diagnosis, later). Other vascular complications reported in *M. pneumoniae* infection include internal carotid artery occlusion and cerebral infarction.

Cardiac Complications

Cardiac abnormalities are among the most commonly reported extrapulmonary manifestations of *M. pneumoniae* infection. Signs and symptoms suggesting involvement of the heart are arrhythmia, congestive failure, chest pain, and electrocardiographic abnormalities, particularly conduction defects. Although cardiac abnormalities have been reported in as many as 10% of cases of *M. pneumoniae* infection, other reports indicate a much lower prevalence. Cardiac complications are more common with increasing age. They prolong the illness but rarely lead to death. The mechanism of heart damage is unknown, but *M. pneumoniae* has been isolated from the pericardial fluid of at least one patient.

Neurologic Complications

Neurologic complications are said to occur in about 0.1% of *Mycoplasma* infections, but proof of the cause of central nervous system involvement is somewhat tenuous. Central nervous system involvement is most common in children, with encephalitis the most common and perhaps the most devastating.[3] Aseptic meningitis and meningoencephalitis, transverse myelitis, brain stem dysfunction, Guillain-Barré syndrome, cerebral ataxia, and peripheral neuropathy have all been reported. Cerebrospinal fluid findings in these cases are variable, but the cellular response is usually minimal, with slightly elevated protein level and normal to slightly depressed glucose concentration. Most often, the diagnosis of *Mycoplasma*-related central nervous system involvement is based on the exclusion of other causes, the presence of an antecedent or intercurrent respiratory illness, and a rise in antibody titer to *M. pneumoniae* in serum. On occasion, *Mycoplasma*-specific antibodies have been demonstrated in cerebrospinal fluid, but these titers have paralleled serum antibody titers. Neurologic complications are usually reversible; however, mortality in patients with central nervous system involvement is higher than in those without such involvement. Although *M. pneumoniae* has been isolated from a few of these patients, polymerase chain reaction (PCR) failed to detect *M. pneumoniae* DNA in the cerebrospinal fluid of 11 patients deemed to have *M. pneumoniae*–related central nervous system disease on serologic grounds. Therefore, immune mechanisms of neural damage have been suggested. Some mycoplasmas elaborate a neurotoxin, but this has not been described for *M. pneumoniae*.

Musculoskeletal, Renal, and Hematopoietic Complications

Polyarthralgias are common in *Mycoplasma* pneumonia, but monarticular or migratory arthritis is rare. Immune mechanisms have been postulated, but

there have been a few reports of the isolation of *M. pneumoniae* from joint fluid. Several of the cases of frank arthritis were reported in patients with hypogammaglobulinemia. Nonhuman mycoplasmas probably cause arthropathy in several animal species, and *M. hominis* has been associated with human arthritis. Rhabdomyolysis has also been increasingly reported and may be associated with very high muscle enzyme, interleukin-18, and tumor necrosis factor-α levels.[4]

Renal complications associated with immune complex deposition and high-titer cold agglutinins have been reported. There are several case reports of *M. pneumoniae*–associated aplastic anemia.

Conditions Leading to Increased Susceptibility

Several reports have emphasized the unusual severity of *M. pneumoniae* infection in patients with sickle cell disease or sickle-related hemoglobinopathies (Chapter 163). Large pleural effusions and marked respiratory distress may develop in these patients. Functional asplenia and its attendant opsonization deficiencies may contribute to overwhelming infection with *M. pneumoniae*, as they do with *S. pneumoniae* infection. Some patients with sickle cell disease and *M. pneumoniae* infection in whom extremely high cold agglutinin titers develop may experience digital necrosis, as they do with *S. pneumoniae* infection. A hypothesis about the pathogenesis is provided in the discussion on cold agglutinins in the Diagnosis section. Children with immunodeficiency syndromes have been the subjects of case reports of *M. pneumoniae* infection. Because *Mycoplasma* infections are so common in normal children, the contribution of immunodeficiency is unclear. *M. pneumoniae* is not a very common opportunistic agent in patients with acquired immunodeficiency syndrome (AIDS), but *M. fermentans* (*incognitus* strain) has been identified in these patients. Unusually severe but nonlethal *M. pneumoniae* infection has also been reported in children with Down syndrome.

⬤ DIAGNOSIS

The diagnosis of *Mycoplasma* pneumonia is made primarily on clinical grounds. The organism can be grown in cell-free media, but most hospital diagnostic laboratories are not prepared to culture mycoplasmas. Because of this, there is considerable interest in developing rapid diagnostic tests with high sensitivity and specificity. These assays fall into three categories: detection of *M. pneumoniae*–specific immunoglobulins in serum and detection of *M. pneumoniae*–specific antigens or nucleotide sequences directly in clinical specimens. Diagnostically, the most useful *M. pneumoniae*–specific immunoglobulin to detect is IgM because it is most likely to indicate recent infection. Enzyme-linked immunoassays have been developed to detect IgM and IgG directed against *M. pneumoniae*. When used in patients with positive assays for complement-fixing antibodies, the enzyme immunoassay had a specificity of more than 99% and a sensitivity of 98%. Specificity was retained but sensitivity dropped to only 46% when IgG alone was the target. Variations on this theme detect IgM antibodies directed at specific *M. pneumoniae* antigens. The tests are simple to perform and have high sensitivity and specificity, but because all these tests are designed to detect IgM antibody, results may be negative early in the course of infection (<7 to 10 days). Therefore, they do not provide the desired confirmation early enough to guide initial therapy.

Detection of *M. pneumoniae* antigens directly in sputum specimens has been accomplished with the use of an antigen capture, indirect enzyme immunoassay. The specificity of the assay was high, the reagents reacting only with *M. pneumoniae* and *M. genitalium*. Sensitivity was also relatively high (91%) when the assay was used on sputum and nasopharyngeal aspirates from patients who were shown by culture or serologically to have *M. pneumoniae* infection.

The high sensitivity and specificity of real-time PCR performed on sputum, nasopharyngeal aspirate, or throat swab material suggest that this test could serve as a specific and rapid diagnostic method. Detection of *M. pneumoniae*–specific nucleotide sequences directly in clinical material has been accomplished with the use of tests developed locally or by large reference laboratories. These tests, which can be completed in a few hours, detect either *M. pneumoniae* DNA (PCR) or ribosomal RNA (reverse transcriptase nucleic acid amplification).[5] Compared with PCR as the "gold standard" of proven infection, very few of the available antibody assays have acceptable sensitivity and specificity. Although the nucleic acid probe assays show excellent specificity, they fail to detect infection in some antibody-positive patients, and their sensitivity varies considerably, depending on the source of the specimen tested: highest for sputum, but lower for nasopharyngeal aspirate or throat swab material. This latter point is important in evaluating comparative studies, many of which use different specimen sources for their assays.[6]

In the course of *M. pneumoniae* infection, several classes of antibody are produced. Some of these fulfill the desired role of antibody production—neutralization of the agent—and others appear to be autoantibodies. The latter include agglutinins to lung, brain, cardiolipins, and smooth muscle. These best studied of these autoagglutinins are the cold isohemagglutinins. These agglutinins were found to be capable of clumping erythrocytes at 4° C. Agglutination was reversible by warming the serum-erythrocyte mixture to 37° C and, unlike hemagglutination by myxoviruses and paramyxoviruses, was repeatable with the same sample, indicating that receptor-destroying enzyme (neuraminidase) plays no role in the dissociation at 37° C.

The cold agglutinin phenomenon, when positive, occurs early, but it is neither sensitive nor specific. Other diseases that can give rise to cold agglutinins are mononucleosis caused by Epstein-Barr virus (anti-i), cytomegalovirus infection (anti-I), some other viral diseases, and lymphoma. A titer of 1 : 32 or greater is highly suggestive of infection with *M. pneumoniae*.

When this test is performed in a laboratory, the results will not be available for at least a day and in some cases a week, but a rapid version can be done at the bedside. In this test, 1 mL of the patient's blood is drawn into a tube containing anticoagulant. The type of tube used to collect specimens for prothrombin determination is preferred. Before cooling, examination shows a smooth coating of the tube by red cells. The blood is cooled to 4° C by placing it on liquid ice or in a standard refrigerator. After several minutes, the tube is examined for the presence of macroscopic erythrocyte agglutination. The tube is then rewarmed to 37° C in an incubator or by exposure to body heat and reexamined. The agglutination should dissociate at 37° C, and the appearance should be as it was before cooling. This temperature-associated agglutination and dissociation can be repeated many times on the same sample. A positive result in the bedside test correlates with a laboratory titer of 1 : 64 or greater and is therefore less sensitive than the laboratory test. It can be accomplished in minutes, however, and if positive, it is highly suggestive of *Mycoplasma*-related cold agglutination. The presence of cold agglutinins can also artifactually give rise to macrocytic indices secondary to in vitro clumping of erythrocytes, as measured by the Coulter counter method. In this case, the red cell distribution width would be high, indicative of heterogeneity in measured red cell size.

Finally, PCR should become the gold standard for diagnosis because of its high sensitivity and specificity and the rapidity with which results can be obtained. A multiplex assay kit for this test has been approved for rapid diagnosis of *M. pneumoniae* infection. However, the test may not be available in many medical centers. Widespread availability of real-time definitive diagnostic assays will enhance the ability to apply organism-specific treatment.[7]

TREATMENT   Rx

Despite the number and variety of tests for the diagnosis of *M. pneumoniae* infection, most cases are encountered in the ambulatory setting, and the institution of antimicrobial therapy is empirical and based on clinical recognition of the syndrome.

Antimicrobial therapy is not necessary for mycoplasmal upper respiratory tract infection, and the mycoplasmal cause of this syndrome most often goes undiagnosed. The pneumonia caused by *Mycoplasma* is self-limited and not life-threatening in most cases. However, treatment with effective antimicrobials may shorten the duration of illness[8] and, by reducing cough and the number of organisms per unit volume of sputum, may reduce the spread of infection to contacts. Because *Mycoplasma* pneumonia is sporadic, most of the studies of antimicrobial efficacy are directed not at this single agent but rather at the treatment of community-acquired pneumonia, of which *Mycoplasma* makes up a variable percentage. Retrospective analysis of specific causes then allows microbe-specific efficacy.

As would be predicted by the lack of a cell wall, all mycoplasmas, including *M. pneumoniae*, are unaffected by β-lactam antibiotics such as the penicillins and cephalosporins. Aminoglycosides are effective in vitro but have not been evaluated for efficacy in vivo. The mainstays of treatment of *M. pneumoniae* respiratory tract infection are macrolides and tetracyclines. Use of either drug class significantly shortens the duration of illness. The radiographic findings may take a week or longer to resolve, even with appropriate therapy (see Fig. 317-1), and organisms may continue to be cultured from sputum for several weeks after a complete course of clinically effective treatment. This may be a result of the fact that although *M. pneumoniae* causes respiratory disease as an extracellular parasite, it has the capacity to reside intracellularly as well, thus making it difficult to eradicate the organism in vivo as opposed to cell cultures. The effect of therapy on extrapulmonary manifestations is unknown. *M. hominis* is not sensitive to erythromycin.

Although the tetracyclines are very active against *M. pneumoniae*, their use is precluded in young children because of adverse effects on developing teeth and bones. Erythromycin is poorly tolerated by many people because of its gastrointestinal side effects, including nausea, vomiting, abdominal pain, and diarrhea. Erythromycin also raises theophylline levels, a consideration in the few asthmatic patients who may still be taking this drug.

Because of the adverse effects of erythromycin and tetracycline, there is considerable interest in the antimycoplasmal efficacy of other agents. Doxycycline is somewhat better tolerated than tetracycline and can be administered in two daily doses rather than three. In vitro, doxycycline is as effective as tetracycline against *M. pneumoniae*, but it is contraindicated in young children.

Several other classes of antimicrobials have significant in vitro and in vivo activity against *M. pneumoniae* and other *Mycoplasma* species, including the fluoroquinolones,[A1] broad-spectrum macrolides (azithromycin, clarithromycin), and members of the macrolide-lincomycin-streptogramin-ketolide (MLSK) class of antimicrobials. There are no good data on the optimal duration of therapy needed to minimize carriage and relapse with these agents.

The macrolides are more active in vitro than the tetracyclines are. Fluoroquinolones have adequate activity for the treatment of these infections. They are more active than the tetracyclines but are at least 100 times less active than the macrolides. The streptogramins are also less active than the macrolides but more active than the tetracyclines. There is a significant cost differential in the use of these drugs. The newer macrolides and quinolones are 50 to 60 times more expensive than the tetracyclines and 6 to 10 times more costly than erythromycin.

During the past decade, there have been increasing reports, first from Asia and later spreading to other areas including the United States,[9] describing decreasing susceptibility of *M. pneumoniae* isolates to the macrolides. By 2012, one study from China reported 95% macrolide resistance. Taking all this into account, recommended therapy includes doxycycline 100 mg every 12 hours in older children and adults,[10] or azithromycin 500 mg on day 1 and then 250 mg every 24 hours. Young children should be given erythromycin (10 mg/kg every 6 hours) or an extended-spectrum macrolide (10 to 12 mg/kg on day 1, followed by 5 mg/kg/day).[A2] The usual duration of therapy is 14 days; shorter courses may lead to relapse. The addition of corticosteroids (e.g., prednisolone 1 mg/kg twice daily for three days then tapered over one week) has been reported to shorten the duration of symptoms in patients with severe or refractory infections,[A3][A4] especially when the serum lactate dehydrogenase level is above about 300 IU/L.[11] *M. hominis* is not sensitive to macrolides, but it is sensitive to the other antimicrobials recommended for *M. pneumoniae* infection. Azithromycin (1-g single dose) achieves a significantly higher cure rate for *Mycoplasma genitalium*–associated urethritis than does multidose doxycycline.

PREVENTION

Outbreaks of *M. pneumoniae* respiratory infection among military recruits led to interest in producing a vaccine to protect against this organism. The resulting vaccines induced specific antibody responses, but protection was limited to no more than 50% of vaccine recipients. Live vaccines using attenuated wild-type and temperature-sensitive mutant mycoplasmas have proved no more effective. In one study, volunteers who received vaccine but did not mount an antibody response had more severe disease when rechallenged with wild-type *Mycoplasma* than did nonvaccinated personnel.

Although *M. pneumoniae* is perhaps the leading cause of atypical pneumonia syndrome in closed populations, the enthusiasm for developing a vaccine for this disease has waned. New technology involving DNA expression library immunization has proved successful in animal studies with nonhuman mycoplasmas, and these methods may breathe new life into *M. pneumoniae* vaccine development.

Secondary Prevention

Prophylactic antibiotic use in family members exposed to *Mycoplasma* decreases clinical disease in these patients, but seroconversion is not prevented. One study showed that azithromycin prophylaxis, given as a 500-mg loading dose and 250 mg/day on days 2 through 5, significantly reduced the secondary attack rate of *M. pneumoniae* infection in a long-term care facility.

Grade A References

A1. Bradley JS, Arguedas A, Blumer JL, et al. Comparative study of levofloxacin in the treatment of children with community-acquired pneumonia. *Pediatr Infect Dis J.* 2007;26:868-878.

A2. Mulholland S, Gavranich JB, Gillies MB, et al. Antibiotics for community-acquired lower respiratory tract infections secondary to *Mycoplasma pneumoniae* in children. *Cochrane Database Syst Rev.* 2012;9:CD004875.

A3. Huang L, Gao X, Chen M. Early treatment with corticosteroids in patients with *Mycoplasma pneu-moniae* pneumonia: a randomized clinical trial. *J Trop Pediatr.* 2014;60:338-342.
A4. Luo Z, Luo J, Liu E, et al. Effects of prednisolone on refractory *Mycoplasma pneumoniae* pneumonia in children. *Pediatr Pulmonol.* 2014;49:377-380.

GENERAL REFERENCES

For the General References and other additional features, please visit Expert Consult at https://expertconsult.inkling.com.

318

DISEASES CAUSED BY CHLAMYDIAE

WILLIAM M. GEISLER

DEFINITION

Chlamydiae are obligate intracellular bacteria that cause a variety of human and animal diseases and much morbidity. Chlamydiae were originally classified taxonomically into one genus, *Chlamydia*. On the basis of sequence analysis of 16S rRNA genes, it had been proposed that chlamydial taxonomy be revised to contain two genera: *Chlamydia* and *Chlamydophila*. However, on the basis of additional data on chlamydia genome sequences and meetings within the *Chlamydia* scientific community, it has been agreed that the family Chlamydiaceae will contain a single genus, *Chlamydia*. Within the family are now nine recognized species: *C. trachomatis, C. pneumoniae, C. psittaci, C. pecorum, C. muridarum, C. felis, C. abortus, C. suis,* and *C. caviae. C. trachomatis* is classified into a trachoma biovar and lymphogranuloma venereum (LGV) biovar. This chapter is limited to human diseases caused by chlamydiae.

The Pathogen

Chlamydiae have a gram-negative cell wall structure consisting of an outer membrane that contains lipopolysaccharide and an inner cytoplasmic membrane. The outer membrane contains a single 40-kD major outer membrane protein, OmpA (also known as MOMP), and two cysteine-rich minor outer membrane–associated proteins (OmcA and OmcB); through intermolecular and intramolecular disulfide bonding, these proteins form a complex that provides structural rigidity.

Chlamydiae grow only within intracellular membrane-bound vacuoles, termed inclusions,[1] that seclude the organism from extracellular and cytoplasmic environments. They share a distinct biphasic developmental cycle (Fig. 318-1) that includes an extracellular, metabolically inactive, infectious form (an elementary body) and an intracellular replicative form (a reticulate body). In vitro studies have shown that chlamydiae may enter a persistent state under certain conditions (penicillin treatment,[2] challenge with certain cytokines, restriction of select nutrients) in which they have reduced metabolic activity and may be more refractory to antibiotic treatment; whether this occurs in vivo is unclear. Chlamydiae are unable to synthesize adenosine triphosphate and therefore depend on the host cell for nutrients to meet their energy requirements.

Additional knowledge of chlamydial cell biology emerged after several chlamydial genomes were sequenced. Polymorphic outer membrane proteins were identified, but their role in pathogenesis is unclear. Chlamydiae were also found to express proteins that localize to the cytoplasmic surface of the inclusion membrane (e.g., Inc A). *C. trachomatis* was demonstrated to have type III secretion genes, which may encode a secretion apparatus providing a means for protein transport. Chlamydiae have small genomes (*C. trachomatis* contains 894 protein-coding genes, and *C. pneumoniae* contains 1052 genes). Most strains of *C. trachomatis* and some strains of *C. psittaci* contain a 7-kilobase cryptic plasmid.

PATHOBIOLOGY

Macrophages are the principal host cells for *C. psittaci* and *C. trachomatis* LGV biovar, whereas the principal host cells for *C. trachomatis* trachoma biovar and *C. pneumoniae* strains are columnar epithelial cells at mucosal sites. Host cell tropism correlates with the type of inflammation elicited by chlamydiae. The LGV biovar and *C. psittaci* produce granulomatous inflammation, characteristic of delayed hypersensitivity reactions. The trachoma biovar produces neutrophilic exudate during acute infection and submucosal mononuclear infiltration with lymphoid follicle formation during later stages of infection.

Chlamydiae elicit both humoral and cellular immune responses. Infection can persist or recur even after an adaptive immune response develops, suggesting that the organism has evolved strategies for immune evasion. Persistent or recurrent infections can elicit inflammatory cellular immune responses that cause tissue injury.

CHLAMYDIAL DISEASES

Table 318-1 summarizes the diseases caused by chlamydiae in humans and the associated clinical and laboratory characteristics.

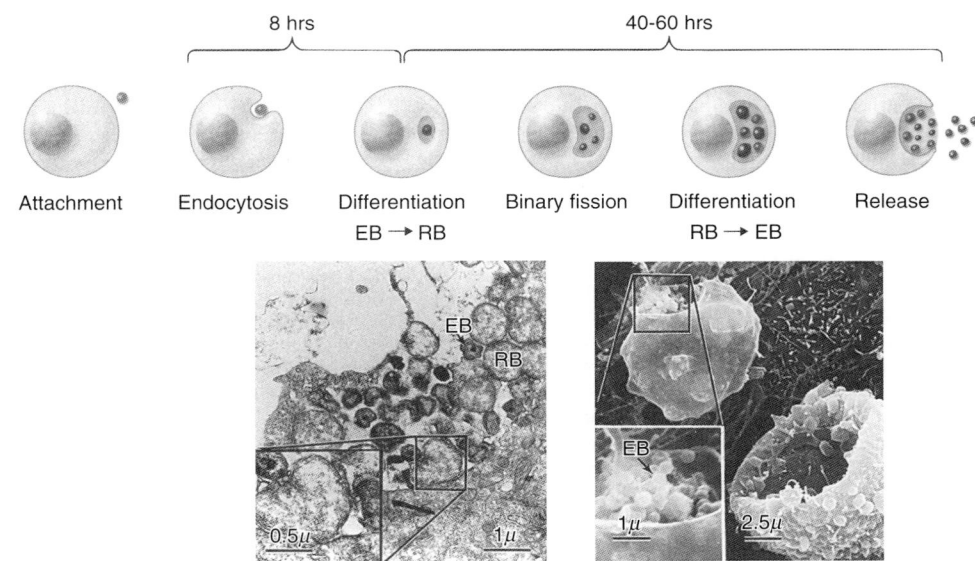

FIGURE 318-1. **Developmental cycle of chlamydiae.** The *top panel* shows the developmental cycle common to all chlamydiae. The *red circles* represent elementary bodies (EBs), and the *blue circles* represent reticulate bodies (RBs). Chlamydiae infect eukaryotic cells through multiple attachment mechanisms. After attachment, EBs enter the cell within a membrane-bound vacuole that remains unfused with lysosomes. EBs reorganize into RBs and asynchronously replicate 8 to 12 times, with a doubling time of 2 to 3 hours. At the conclusion of the growth cycle, RBs differentiate back to EBs, and each inclusion yields 100 to 1000 new infectious EBs. The *bottom left panel,* a transmission electron micrograph taken 40 hours after infection, shows the large RBs and the smaller EBs, which have a condensed nucleoid structure within their cytoplasm. The *bottom right panel,* a scanning electron micrograph taken 60 hours after infection, shows a membrane-bound vacuole containing many EBs exiting from an infected HeLa cell.

TABLE 318-1   MAJOR DISEASES CAUSED BY CHLAMYDIAE IN HUMANS AND ASSOCIATED CLINICAL AND LABORATORY FEATURES

SPECIES	SEROVAR	DISEASE	TRANSMISSION ROUTE	DIAGNOSIS	PREVENTION
C. trachomatis	A–C	Trachoma	Fomites, eye-seeking flies	Clinical criteria or culture/NAAT	SAFE strategy
	D–K	Urethritis, cervicitis, proctitis, epididymitis, PID	Sexual contact	NAAT	Abstinence or monogamy, education, condoms, partner treatment
	D–K	Inclusion conjunctivitis, infant pneumonia	Perinatal contact	Culture, DFA, NAAT, or serology (for pneumonia)	Prenatal chlamydia screening: treat infected mothers
	L1–L3	Lymphogranuloma venereum	Sexual contact	Serology or culture/NAAT plus OmpA typing	Abstinence or monogamy, education, condoms, partner treatment
C. pneumoniae	One	Upper respiratory infections, atypical pneumonia, asthma exacerbations	Respiratory droplet	Serology or culture/PCR	None
C. psittaci	Multiple	Psittacosis, atypical pneumonia, febrile illness	Aerosolized bird secretions, dust	Serology	Quarantine and chlortetracycline for imported birds, avoidance or precautions for at-risk subjects

DFA = direct fluorescent antibody test; NAAT = nucleic acid amplification test; PCR = polymerase chain reaction; PID = pelvic inflammatory disease; SAFE = World Health Organization's recommended strategy: acronym for surgery (for trichiasis), antimicrobials (periodic community-wide treatment), facial cleanliness, and environmental improvement.

Chlamydia trachomatis

C. trachomatis infection is a common bacterial infection in humans and accounts for significant morbidity worldwide. *C. trachomatis* isolates have been differentiated into 18 major serovars (i.e., OmpA types) based on variations in OmpA that are identified on antigen cross-reactivity in the microimmunofluorescence test. The major diseases caused by *C. trachomatis* are trachoma, caused by serovars A, B, Ba, and C; sexually and perinatally transmitted diseases, caused by serovars D through K (and, rarely, serovars B and Ba); and sexually transmitted LGV, caused by serovars L1, L2, L2a, and L3. Sequencing of the *ompA* gene has led to the recognition of more OmpA variants, including L2b. Multilocus sequencing typing is a newer tool that has been used to further discriminate between *C. trachomatis* strains of the same OmpA genotype. Trachoma and LGV are endemic in developing areas of the world (although LGV outbreaks have also occurred in populations of men who have sex with men in developed countries), whereas sexually and perinatally transmitted non-LGV chlamydial infections occur worldwide.

TRACHOMA

EPIDEMIOLOGY

Trachoma is a chronic follicular conjunctivitis. The overall incidence is unknown, but it has been estimated by the World Health Organization (WHO) that 21.4 million people have active trachoma.[3] Trachoma is endemic in more than 50 countries and is especially common in poor areas of sub-Saharan Africa, where the disease prevalence in children may exceed 40%. According to the Trachoma Atlas provided by the International Coalition for Trachoma Control, there are an estimated 110 million people living in endemic areas and another 210 million living in suspected endemic areas. Trachoma is a major public health problem because scarring from trachoma causes blindness, affecting 7.2 million people by WHO estimates. Trachoma is the most common preventable cause of blindness worldwide. Active trachoma often occurs in the first few years of life. The inflammation from recurrent or persistent trachoma can lead to conjunctival scarring, which can ultimately cause corneal damage and blindness later in life. The *C. trachomatis* serovars that produce trachoma are spread by direct contact with fingers or fomites (e.g., washcloths, handkerchiefs) contaminated with eye discharge from an infected person or by eye-seeking flies. Because of this mode of transmission, trachoma often clusters in households. Risk factors for trachoma include poor facial hygiene, limited access to water, poor sanitation, and proximity to other infected persons or to a heavy density of eye-seeking flies.

CLINICAL MANIFESTATIONS

There are two stages of trachoma disease, and they can overlap. Initially, trachoma begins as an inflammatory follicular conjunctivitis (i.e., active trachoma). On eversion of the upper eyelid, white to pale yellow lymphoid follicles can be visualized on the superior tarsal conjunctival surface, and papillae may be noted between follicles. Minimal watery or mucoid ocular discharge may also be seen. In more severe active trachoma, the conjunctiva

can be thickened and edematous. Subsequently, conjunctival inflammation can progress to cause scarring of the upper tarsal conjunctiva (the cicatricial stage of disease). Scarring deforms the eyelid and can lead to an inward turning of the eyelashes, which can result in corneal abrasion (trichiasis). Over time, trichiasis causes corneal edema, ulceration, vascularization (pannus), scarring, and opacification. The corneal damage leads to decreased vision or blindness, occurring mostly in young adults and middle-aged persons. Viral conjunctivitis (e.g., adenovirus) is manifested in a clinical fashion similar to active trachoma, but it is self-limited and usually resolves within a week. Trachoma can be complicated by superinfection with other bacterial pathogens (e.g., *Haemophilus influenzae*), which should be considered when purulent ocular discharge or significant inflammation of the bulbar conjunctiva is present.

DIAGNOSIS

Because the majority of trachoma cases occur in developing countries without access to laboratory testing or the necessary resources, trachoma is often diagnosed clinically on the basis of findings of active trachoma (follicles on the upper tarsal conjunctiva or pronounced inflammatory thickening of the tarsal conjunctiva) or cicatricial disease. When laboratories are available, detection of *C. trachomatis* provides definitive evidence of active trachoma and may identify infection in subjects with minimal clinical evidence of active trachoma. Isolation of the organism in cell culture is one means to detect *C. trachomatis*, but the test's sensitivity is less than 50% and the methods are labor-intensive. Nonculture tests have higher sensitivities in active trachoma. For instance, nucleic acid amplification tests (NAATs) are the most sensitive diagnostic tests, but they are not widely available in many trachoma-endemic areas. It is uncommon for adults with late scarring to have *C. trachomatis* detected by any of these assays.

TREATMENT

Active trachoma can be treated with a tetracycline eye ointment twice daily for 6 weeks or oral macrolide therapy. The latter is preferred in part because extraocular sites such as the nasopharynx may be infected in young children. Single-dose oral azithromycin (20 mg/kg; maximum of 1 g) is as effective as tetracycline ointment and is more advantageous in terms of compliance and side effect profile; tetracycline application can irritate the ocular surface.

Surgical intervention is the only effective management for trichiasis. Eyelid rotation surgery prevents the eyelashes from abrading the cornea, preventing blindness and other nonvisual symptoms. Trichiasis recurrence after surgery is a major concern, and recurrence rates are highly variable across studies. Other concerns include accessibility to surgery and the patient's acceptance.

PREVENTION

The WHO is committed to eliminating blinding trachoma by 2020 and recommends that all countries with endemic trachoma adopt the SAFE strategy: surgery (for trichiasis), antimicrobials (periodic community-wide treatment), facial cleanliness, and environmental improvement. Mass treatment of a community with single-dose oral azithromycin is safe and has dramatically reduced the prevalence of infection for up to 1 year after treatment, without an increase in antimicrobial resistance; it has also been shown to reduce mortality in children.[A1] Annual azithromycin treatment is recommended for trachoma-endemic areas. Reintroduction of trachoma after mass treatment has been demonstrated, which may be due in part to decreased herd immunity. Repeated mass treatment (every few months) provides herd protection to the entire community.[A2]

Mass antibiotic treatment as the sole intervention for eliminating trachoma is unlikely to be successful if other factors that facilitate transmission are not addressed. Face washing and good hygiene help reduce the risk of transmission through contact with fingers and flies. Although the promotion of facial cleanliness through educational campaigns may be one of the most important interventions, sustaining such behavioral changes can be challenging. Achieving better environmental conditions through measures that reduce household and community fly density and improve waste management and access to clean water can also limit transmission. Improvement in socioeconomic conditions in a community correlates with a decline in trachoma prevalence.

SEXUALLY AND PERINATALLY TRANSMITTED CHLAMYDIAL INFECTIONS

EPIDEMIOLOGY

Chlamydia is the most prevalent bacterial sexually transmitted infection in the United States. Currently, more than 1.4 million infections are reported to the Centers for Disease Control and Prevention (CDC) annually.[4] The number of reported cases is increasing each year; this may reflect increased chlamydia screening efforts rather than a true increase in infection burden, but this remains unclear. Taking into account underreporting and under-screening, it is estimated that more than 2.8 million new chlamydial infections occur annually in the United States. Higher chlamydia prevalence rates have been associated with younger age (sexually active adolescents and young adults), select minority ethnic groups (especially African Americans), and new or multiple sexual partners.[5] Chlamydia prevalence is higher in women than in men; it is unclear whether this is due to higher screening rates in women or whether women may be more susceptible to infection acquisition or persistence. Chlamydia prevalence is highest in the southeastern United States. The estimated total cost attributable to chlamydial disease in the United States exceeds $2.4 billion annually. From a global perspective, WHO estimated from 2005 data that there were approximately 98 million adults with chlamydia. In addition to the adverse effects on the reproductive health of women, chlamydia has a substantial impact on perinatal outcomes and facilitates the transmission of human immunodeficiency virus (HIV).

CLINICAL MANIFESTATIONS
Urethritis

C. trachomatis is the most common cause of nongonococcal urethritis in men,[6] being responsible for 20 to 55% of cases. Although the majority of men with chlamydial urethritis are asymptomatic, studies in high-prevalence venues (e.g., sexually transmitted disease clinics) have reported that 40 to 60% of men with chlamydial urethritis are symptomatic. The most frequent symptoms are urethral discomfort (itching or pain) with urination and urethral discharge. On examination, a mild to moderate amount of clear or cloudy/mucoid (rarely purulent) urethral discharge may be visualized (Fig. 318-2A). Urethral discharge sometimes becomes apparent only after stripping the urethra from the base of the penis to the glans; this should be considered in men reporting urethral symptoms but without urethral discharge on initial inspection. Gram stain from a urethral swab specimen demonstrates

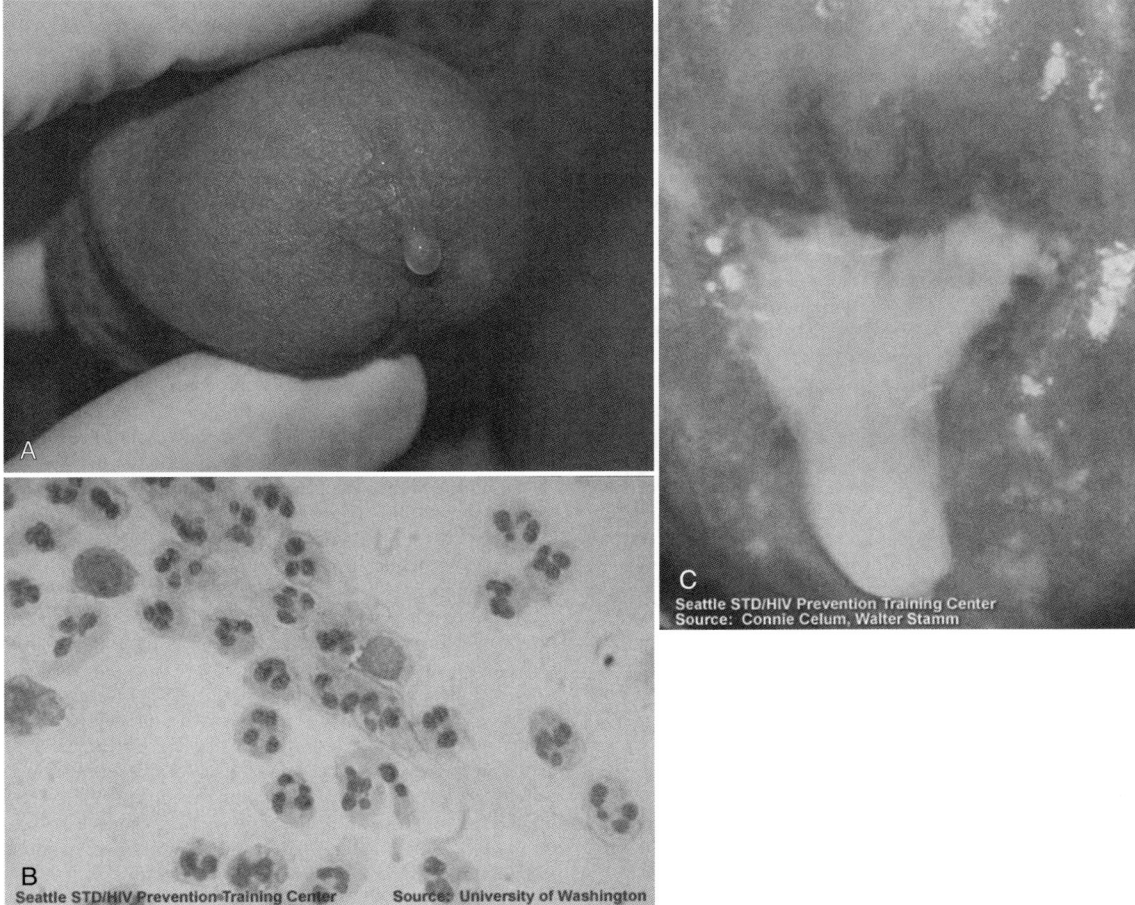

FIGURE 318-2. Clinical manifestations of genital *Chlamydia trachomatis* infection. **A,** Cloudy urethral discharge of urethritis. **B,** Urethral specimen Gram stain revealing nongonococcal urethritis findings: five or more polymorphonuclear cells per oil field (1000×) and the absence of intracellular gram-negative diplococci. **C,** Purulent endocervical discharge of mucopurulent cervicitis. (A courtesy James Sizemore, MD. **B** and **C** from *Practitioner's Handbook for the Management of Sexually Transmitted Disease.* http://depts.washington.edu/handbook. Accessed March 18, 2015.)

five or more polymorphonuclear leukocytes (PMNs) per oil field (1000×) in the majority of chlamydial infections (Fig. 318-2B). Chlamydial organisms cannot be visualized on Gram stain. Up to 20% of men with chlamydial urethritis have fewer than five PMNs per oil field on urethral Gram stain, reflecting the fact that minimal inflammation may be elicited in some cases of chlamydial urethritis. Urethral inflammation can also be detected by a positive urinary leukocyte esterase test result on unspun first-void urine.

C. trachomatis urethritis also occurs in women, who may be asymptomatic or present with an acute urethral syndrome characterized by dysuria, urinary frequency, and pyuria. This acute urethral syndrome mimics a urinary tract infection, and chlamydia should be suspected in women with pyuria but negative urine nitrite or negative urine culture, especially in sexually active adolescents and young adults; many urinary tract infection treatments are not effective against chlamydia. Mild urethral discharge may be seen. Pelvic examination should be performed in women with suspected chlamydia urethritis to search for other clinical findings of chlamydia (e.g., cervicitis).

Epididymitis
Chlamydia can spread from the urethra to the epididymis, causing epididymitis in up to 1 percent of infected men. Symptoms include testicular pain and scrotal erythema and swelling that are typically unilateral. On examination, there is palpable swelling and tenderness of the epididymis; accompanying findings may include testicular tenderness, scrotal erythema and swelling, urethral discharge, or hydrocele. In men younger than 35 years, *C. trachomatis* is the principal cause of epididymitis, whereas in men older than 35 years, complicated urinary tract infection with uropathogens is a more common cause, especially in those with prostate disorders. Up to 15% of epididymitis cases are complicated by chronic pain that is usually idiopathic and often unresponsive to antibiotics. Other complications include decreased fertility and, rarely, testicular abscess.

Cervicitis
C. trachomatis is the most common cause of cervicitis, being responsible for up to 50% of cases. The majority of women with endocervical chlamydial infection are asymptomatic. Symptoms, when present, are often mild and nonspecific for chlamydia and include the following: vaginal discharge, intermenstrual vaginal bleeding, dysuria, and pain during intercourse (dyspareunia). Approximately 10% of women with asymptomatic cervical chlamydial infection have mucopurulent cervicitis detected on pelvic examination (Fig. 318-2C); this is characterized by a purulent or cloudy endocervical discharge visible in the endocervical canal or on the tip of an endocervical swab. A similar proportion may have endocervical bleeding that is easily induced with passage of a swab through the cervical os. Nonspecific findings may include vaginal discharge and edematous ectopy (a darker red area of columnar epithelium visible on the face of the cervix). Gram stain of an endocervical sample usually shows more than 10 PMNs per oil field. A vaginal wet mount often shows more than 5 to 10 PMNs per 400× field.

Pelvic Inflammatory Disease
Chlamydia can spread from the cervix to the endometrium (causing endometritis), fallopian tubes (causing salpingitis), and peritoneum (causing peritonitis or perihepatitis). These upper genital tract infections are collectively referred to as pelvic inflammatory disease (PID). Estimates of the proportion of cervical chlamydial infections that progress to PID vary greatly but are most commonly around 10 to 20%. The majority of PID cases are subclinical or silent. PID symptoms include pelvic or lower abdominal pain (especially during menses or the first 2 weeks of the menstrual cycle) and nausea. Fever is less common. Examination findings include cervical motion tenderness and tenderness of the uterus or adnexa. Although most cases of chlamydial PID are due to the natural progression of infection, they may also occur post partum or after pregnancy termination. The long-term consequences of PID include infertility, ectopic pregnancy, and chronic pelvic pain.

Complications during Pregnancy
There is some evidence that genital chlamydial infection during pregnancy can lead to adverse outcomes, including preterm labor, low birthweight, miscarriage, and stillbirth.

Reactive Arthritis
Reactive arthritis, characterized by the classic triad of trigger infection (e.g., chlamydia), conjunctivitis, and arthritis, can complicate chlamydial infection (Chapter 265). There is a male predominance in reactive arthritis cases triggered by chlamydia, and it has been estimated that reactive arthritis occurs in about 1% of men presenting with chlamydial urethritis.

Proctitis
Proctitis caused by non-LGV *C. trachomatis* OmpA types is usually asymptomatic. Subjects with acute symptomatic proctitis may report rectal pain or bleeding, tenesmus, pruritus, rectal discharge, or diarrhea. Anoscopy or sigmoidoscopy may reveal friable mucosa and a mucoid or mucopurulent discharge. A rectal swab Gram stain often reveals many PMNs per oil field.

Conjunctivitis
An acute follicular conjunctivitis may rarely occur in adolescents or adults with genital chlamydial infection. The presumed mode of acquisition is autoinoculation with infected genital secretions. The typical clinical presentation is subacute or chronic infection characterized by unilateral conjunctival redness, mucoid or mucopurulent ocular discharge, a foreign body sensation, and preauricular adenopathy.

Oropharyngeal Infection
C. trachomatis has been detected in the oropharynx of sexually active subjects and is asymptomatic in most instances. Recent evidence suggests that *C. trachomatis* can be transmitted from oropharyngeal sites to the genital tract, providing rationale for treatment of oropharyngeal chlamydia. However, because oropharyngeal chlamydia prevalence is very low in most populations and the clinical significance of *C. trachomatis* detected in the oropharynx is unclear, routine oropharyngeal chlamydia screening is not recommended.

Infant Inclusion Conjunctivitis and Pneumonia
Because the prevalence of chlamydia in pregnant adolescents and young adults in the United States can be high (>5%), the morbidity associated with perinatally transmitted chlamydia is considerable. Neonates exposed to *C. trachomatis* during passage through the birth canal may develop inclusion conjunctivitis (≈20 to 40%) or pneumonia (≈10 to 20%). The conjunctivitis, termed inclusion conjunctivitis because the cytoplasmic chlamydia inclusion bodies demonstrated in neonatal conjunctival scrapings are the same as those seen in genital scrapings from adults with genital chlamydia, usually develops 5 to 12 days after birth but may occur as long as 4 to 6 weeks after birth. Clinical manifestations include conjunctival injection and thickening, a clear or mucopurulent ocular discharge, and eyelid swelling. Chlamydia pneumonia in infants usually occurs subacutely between 1 and 3 months of age. Characteristic clinical features include a repetitive staccato cough and absence of fever. Other clinical findings may include tachypnea, crackles on auscultation of the lungs, nasal discharge, and eosinophilia. Chest radiographs may reveal bilateral diffuse infiltrates.

Lymphogranuloma Venereum
LGV is a sexually transmitted infection caused by *C. trachomatis* LGV OmpA types. In contrast to infection with non-LGV strains, LGV is a more invasive systemic infection that involves lymphoid tissue (causing lymphadenitis) and can be ulcerative. LGV is endemic in Africa, India, Southeast Asia, South America, and the Caribbean. LGV had been uncommon in the United States, with fewer than 100 cases reported annually. However, in 2003, an LGV outbreak was reported in the Netherlands, and since then, the LGV epidemic has continued to spread throughout Europe and to North America and Australia. LGV outbreaks are primarily occurring in men who have sex with men with high-risk sexual behaviors (most are HIV infected) who are presenting with proctitis and are infected with LGV OmpA variant L2b.[7]

The clinical manifestations of LGV differ in early versus later stages of infection. In the early stage (3 to 30 days after acquisition) of genital LGV, a primary skin lesion or lesions may develop on the genital mucosa or adjacent skin in the form of a papule, ulcer, or herpetiform lesion. The lesion is usually asymptomatic and goes unnoticed, but it may be erosive; it heals quickly without scarring. Early genital LGV may also be manifested as a nonspecific inflammatory syndrome (e.g., urethritis and cervicitis), similar to infection with non-LGV strains. Genital LGV can progress to an inguinal syndrome 2 to 4 weeks later, characterized by painful, erythematous inguinal lymphadenopathy (buboes; see Fig. 312-3) and systemic manifestations including fever, headache, arthralgias, myalgias, and leukocytosis. The buboes are commonly unilateral, and about one third spontaneously rupture and drain pus, which can be complicated by fistulas or sinus tracks; unruptured buboes usually heal. In later stages, genital tract fibrosis can lead to complications such as infertility, elephantiasis, strictures, fistulas, and subcutaneous sclerosis.

LGV may also be manifested as an anogenital syndrome with invasive proctitis. Symptoms include fever, tenesmus, anal pruritus, and a rectal discharge that may be mucoid or, less commonly, mucopurulent or bloody. Up to 20 to 30% of patients are asymptomatic. The rectal mucosa is friable, with multiple superficial ulcerations, and biopsy may reveal submucosal granulomas and crypt abscesses; these clinical and histopathologic findings resemble Crohn's disease (Chapter 141). Late complications include rectal strictures, anal fistulas, and lymphorrhoids (perianal growths of lymphatic tissue).

Natural History

The natural history of untreated genital *C. trachomatis* infection has not been fully elucidated, in part because ethical considerations limit such research. Outcomes of untreated genital chlamydia include spontaneous resolution (i.e., immune-mediated clearance) and persisting infection; the latter may be subclinical or may progress to clinical manifestations (e.g., urethritis, cervicitis), which can remain uncomplicated or lead to a complication (e.g., PID). On the basis of limited evidence in subjects with chlamydia detected initially by a screening test who returned within weeks to months for treatment and were retested, anywhere from 10 to 40% of infections resolve spontaneously before treatment.[8] Some patients with persisting infection develop clinical manifestations before returning for treatment, including a small proportion of females (up to 4%) who develop symptomatic PID. Other sparse data in females suggest that up to 50% of genital chlamydial infections resolve after a year, but a small percentage (<10%) could persist for several years. There is recent evidence to suggest that chlamydia resolution before treatment may lower the short-term risk for reinfection.[9] An improved understanding of the natural history of chlamydia could have an impact on screening and treatment recommendations.

DIAGNOSIS

C. trachomatis infections are difficult to diagnose clinically because the majority are asymptomatic, and even when symptoms or signs are present, they are nonspecific. Therefore, a definitive diagnosis relies on detecting the organism. Laboratory diagnosis confirms the clinical diagnosis in those with clinical manifestations and detects infection in asymptomatic individuals (i.e., screening). The CDC recommends annual chlamydia screening for sexually active women aged 25 years and younger as well as for older women with risk factors (e.g., new or multiple sexual partners). Select studies have demonstrated that chlamydia screening reduces the prevalence of chlamydia in women and the rate of PID. Surveillance data from the United States, England, and British Columbia during the last decade have demonstrated a steady decline in PID rates. Universal chlamydia screening in men is not recommended; selective chlamydia testing is appropriate in venues with high prevalences (e.g., sexually transmitted disease clinics, correctional facilities), for high-risk men, or for symptomatic men.

The reference standard for the detection of *C. trachomatis* has been isolation of the organism in cell culture. Development of nonculture tests was important because culture is technically demanding, expensive, and not widely available. Earlier nonculture tests included enzyme immunoassay, direct fluorescent antibody, and nucleic acid hybridization. These tests were less expensive and less technically demanding than culture but had lower sensitivities (lower limit of detection $\geq 10^3$ elementary bodies) and therefore detected fewer infections. These earlier tests have been replaced in most laboratories by NAATs, which are now the recommended diagnostic tests for chlamydia.[10] NAATs have the highest sensitivity (detecting a small number of elementary bodies) and can be performed on genital swabs and on noninvasively collected specimens (first-void urine or self-collected vaginal swabs) with similar accuracy. The CDC's recommended specimens for screening with NAATs are first-void urine in males and vaginal swabs in females. NAATs have not been cleared by the Food and Drug Administration for use with rectal, oropharyngeal, or conjunctival swab specimens; however, some laboratories have validated the assays to meet Clinical Laboratory Improvement Amendments (CLIA) requirements.

The role of serology in diagnosis of *C. trachomatis* infection is limited primarily to two indications: (1) infant pneumonia syndrome, the diagnosis of which is suggested by a *C. trachomatis* immunoglobulin M (IgM) antibody titer of 1 : 32 or greater with the microimmunofluorescence (MIF) assay; and (2) LGV, the diagnosis of which is suggested by a complement fixation (CF) antibody titer greater than 1 : 64 or MIF antibody titer greater than 1 : 256 in the appropriate clinical context. MIF has a higher specificity than CF. LGV can be more definitively diagnosed by demonstrating an LGV OmpA type on *C. trachomatis* DNA from infected material.

TREATMENT   Rx

C. trachomatis is susceptible to tetracyclines, macrolides, and select quinolones (ofloxacin and levofloxacin, but not ciprofloxacin). The CDC's recommended treatment for uncomplicated chlamydia is either doxycycline 100 mg orally twice daily for 7 days or azithromycin 1 g orally in a single dose.[11] A meta-analysis of genital chlamydia treatment trials that used primarily chlamydia culture revealed that these regimens are equally efficacious, with cure rates around 97 to 98%. A subsequent study in women using the more sensitive NAAT suggested that the cure rate in genital chlamydia may be slightly lower (≈92%).[12] Recent retrospective studies have raised concern about the efficacy of azithromycin for rectal chlamydia; however, these studies had limitations, and prospective clinical trials comparing azithromycin versus doxycycline regimens for rectal chlamydia are needed. Treatment compliance is higher with azithromycin. Alternative treatment regimens include erythromycin base 500 mg orally four times a day for 7 days, ofloxacin 300 mg orally twice daily for 7 days, and levofloxacin 500 mg orally once a day for 7 days. Azithromycin is the recommended treatment for chlamydia-infected pregnant women. *C. trachomatis* epididymitis and PID should be treated with doxycycline for 10 and 14 days, respectively. Treatment of these syndromes is usually empirical before test results are available; therefore, ceftriaxone 250 mg intramuscularly in a single dose is added to doxycycline to cover gonorrhea. LGV should be treated with doxycycline for 3 weeks; some experts recommend azithromycin 1 g orally weekly for 3 weeks as an alternative.[13] Infant chlamydial infections are treated with erythromycin base 50 mg/kg/day orally divided into four daily doses for 14 days; data on other macrolides are limited, but a shorter treatment course with azithromycin 20 mg/kg/day orally may be effective.

A test of cure (approximately 3 weeks after completion of chlamydia treatment) is recommended only for pregnant women. Sexual partners (including current partners and those with contact in the preceding 60 days) and parents of chlamydia-infected infants should be evaluated and treated empirically. Expedited partner therapy, whereby chlamydia-infected patients are offered medication or a prescription to give to their sexual partners, or clinicians provide medication to contacts without an examination, may reduce the risk for recurrent chlamydia.[14] Patients and their partners should remain abstinent until treatment is completed.

PREVENTION

Education and the provision of condoms are preventive measures that should accompany chlamydia treatment. Recurrent chlamydia occurs in approximately 10 to 20% of chlamydia-infected subjects within a few months of treatment; therefore, repeated chlamydia testing is recommended approximately 3 months after treatment. Routine screening may reduce the risk of pelvic inflammatory disease in sexually active young women.[15]

Chlamydia pneumoniae

In 1986, a new chlamydial pathogen that caused acute respiratory tract infections was identified and designated *Chlamydia* strain TWAR. It was initially thought to be a novel *C. psittaci* strain but was later recognized as the species *C. pneumoniae*. Pneumonia and upper respiratory tract infections (bronchitis, pharyngitis, laryngitis, and sinusitis) are the most frequently identified diseases caused by *C. pneumoniae*.[16] However, *C. pneumoniae* may also contribute to exacerbations of chronic bronchitis and asthma. There is evidence suggesting that *C. pneumoniae* may contribute to atherosclerosis, although large *C. pneumoniae* treatment trials have not demonstrated benefit in preventing adverse cardiovascular events. Select central nervous system disorders (e.g., Alzheimer's disease, multiple sclerosis) have been linked to *C. pneumoniae*, but a causal relationship has not been established.

EPIDEMIOLOGY

The majority of adults in the United States and other developed countries are seropositive for *C. pneumoniae*, up to 80% in some populations. Seroconversion often occurs during childhood or adolescence and may be subclinical. Studies incorporating culture or polymerase chain reaction (PCR) suggest that infection is not uncommon in children younger than 5 years. *C. pneumoniae* causes an atypical pneumonia syndrome, with an estimated annual incidence of 1 case per 1000 population; epidemiologic studies suggest a 4-year cycle of increased pneumonia incidence. Up to 10% of community-acquired pneumonias are attributed to *C. pneumoniae*, and coinfection with other respiratory pathogens such as *Streptococcus pneumoniae* and *Mycoplasma pneumoniae* is not uncommon. The organism is believed to be acquired through the inhalation of infected respiratory droplets from persons with disease and possibly asymptomatic carriers. This mode of transmission can facilitate the spread of infection among household members and can cause epidemics in enclosed populations, such as persons in military barracks, nursing homes, and schools.

CLINICAL MANIFESTATIONS

Most *C. pneumoniae* infections occur in children, who often have mild clinical manifestations or are asymptomatic. Clinical manifestations are more evident in adults, especially the elderly, who have the highest incidence of *C. pneumoniae* pneumonia. *C. pneumoniae* causes an atypical pneumonia that is usually of mild to moderate severity. The incubation period may be several weeks, and the disease onset is gradual. A nonproductive cough is usually present and is often preceded or accompanied by nasal congestion, sore throat, and hoarseness. Headache may occur in up to half of patients. Fever and dyspnea occur less commonly. On examination, localized pulmonary crackles or rhonchi are often heard. Chest radiography shows pneumonitis, most often evident as a single subsegmental lower lobe infiltrate. The leukocyte count is usually normal. *C. pneumoniae* may also be manifested as isolated bronchitis, sinusitis, laryngitis, or nonexudative pharyngitis. The clinical course of these upper respiratory tract infections may be protracted for several weeks.

DIAGNOSIS

C. pneumoniae infection is usually diagnosed by serology or direct detection of the organism in respiratory specimens by cell culture or other nonculture methods. Serology is the test used in most clinical settings, with the MIF assay considered the reference standard for serodiagnosis. Acute infection is suggested by a four-fold rise in IgG from paired sera or a single high IgM (>1:16) or IgG (>1:512) titer. However, serology is limited by its specificity, reproducibility, and clinical correlation. *C. pneumoniae* can be isolated in cell culture, but culture is technically challenging and time-consuming. Antigen detection with use of fluorescent monoclonal antibodies has a lower sensitivity than culture and is also technically challenging. *C. pneumoniae* PCR is more sensitive than culture, and real-time PCR appears to have advantages over conventional PCR. Although there are still issues involving the standardization of PCR methods for *C. pneumoniae* detection, PCR is promising and will likely become the test of choice.

TREATMENT Rx

C. pneumoniae is susceptible to tetracyclines, macrolides, and fluoroquinolones. Treatment trials using culture have demonstrated that select macrolide and fluoroquinolone regimens eradicate *C. pneumoniae* in approximately 70 to 85% of subjects with pneumonia. The clinical response to treatment may be slow, and some patients may need re-treatment. The suggested treatment duration for most regimens is typically 10 to 14 days, except that shorter courses may be effective for azithromycin (10 mg/kg on day 1, followed by 5 mg/kg during the next 4 days; up to 1.5 g orally during 5 days). Chronic *C. pneumoniae* infections may require even longer courses of treatment (e.g., 6 weeks), and macrolides are suggested in this setting. Protective immunity after *C. pneumoniae* infection may not occur, and therefore reinfection is common.

Chlamydia psittaci
EPIDEMIOLOGY

C. psittaci naturally infects a variety of mammals and birds. *C. psittaci* strains appear to be host specific, and most human infections are linked to contact with an infected bird. *C. psittaci* infection in humans is termed psittacosis, in part because exposure to psittacine birds (parrots, parakeets, and budgerigars) is commonly implicated in infections. However, because human cases have been linked to exposure to finches, pigeons, pheasants, ducks, turkeys, chickens, seagulls, and other birds, ornithosis may be a more appropriate term. Psittacosis disease in birds ranges from an asymptomatic carriage state to a mild symptomatic illness manifested by ruffled feathers, anorexia, shivering, dyspnea, diarrhea, or depression. Infected birds shed *C. psittaci* in urine, feces, or secretions from their beaks or eyes. Their feathers and surrounding

environment become contaminated. Transmission to humans is primarily by inhalation of aerosolized bird secretions or dust. Infected birds may shed the organism for months. Person-to-person transmission rarely occurs.

Human psittacosis is a rare infection, due in part to antibiotic-laced bird feed and a mandated quarantine for imported birds. The number of cases of psittacosis in the United States has been stable for the past 10 years, with fewer than 50 confirmed cases reported annually; a larger number of cases are reported but not confirmed.

CLINICAL MANIFESTATIONS

Psittacosis initially involves the lungs and then spreads to the reticuloendothelial system. The clinical spectrum of infection ranges from asymptomatic to fulminant, and clinical manifestations may resemble several other nonspecific febrile systemic illnesses, including Q fever, typhoid fever, and legionnaires' disease.[17] After an incubation period of 5 to 14 days, some patients may present with a nonspecific virus-like illness or a mononucleosis-like syndrome. The presentation most suggestive of psittacosis is an acute febrile atypical pneumonia.[18] Patients initially have an abrupt onset of shaking chills and a fever as high as 40.5° C. Temperature-pulse dissociation (i.e., elevated temperature with a normal pulse) may occur. Constitutional symptoms, including headache, myalgias, and arthralgias, are prominent. A cough, usually nonproductive, appears early in the illness and may accompany chest pain, which is usually nonpleuritic. Auscultation may be normal or reveal bilateral crackles. Chest radiograph findings are usually more dramatic than lung examination findings; the most common finding is single lower lobe consolidation, but multiple localized bronchopneumonic patches, diffuse ground-glass changes, and a miliary pattern have been described. Small pleural effusions may be seen. In contrast to *C. pneumoniae* pneumonia, psittacosis is more severe, with high fever and absent or minimal upper respiratory complaints.

Extrapulmonary findings frequently occur in psittacosis. Splenomegaly is common. A faint erythematous, blanching, maculopapular rash (Horder's spots), resembling the rose spots of typhoid fever, can occur, as can erythema nodosum. Signs of hepatitis, endocarditis (culture negative), pericarditis, myocarditis, meningoencephalitis, hemolytic anemia, or disseminated intravascular coagulation may be noted. *C. psittaci* infection has also been associated with nongastrointestinal extranodal marginal zone lymphomas of mucosa-associated lymphoid tissue, including ocular and central nervous system sites.

DIAGNOSIS

Psittacosis should be suspected in patients with a febrile illness (especially atypical pneumonia) who report exposure to sick or imported birds or who have regular exposure to birds, including bird owners, pet shop workers, veterinarians, zookeepers, and poultry processing plant workers. The diagnosis can be made with serology or by isolating the organism in cell culture. *C. psittaci* is a biocontainment level 3 agent because of its stability in the environment and aerosol transmission. Because laboratory-acquired *C. psittaci* infections are well documented, culture is discouraged and serology is preferred. If culture is attempted, laboratory staff should be notified in advance so that appropriate precautions can be taken. A serologic diagnosis of psittacosis is made by demonstrating (1) a four-fold or greater rise in CF or MIF antibody against *C. psittaci* to a titer of at least 1:32 from acute to convalescent sera collected at least 2 weeks apart (3 to 6 weeks is recommended) or (2) an IgM titer of 1:16 or greater against *C. psittaci* by MIF.

TREATMENT Rx

Untreated psittacosis can be fatal, but mortality is rare with prompt antimicrobial treatment. Because of the delay in laboratory diagnosis of psittacosis, empirical therapy should be provided on the basis of clinical suspicion. *C. psittaci* susceptibility has been demonstrated to tetracyclines, macrolides, and some of the newer fluoroquinolones. The recommended treatment regimen, based on clinical experience, is either tetracycline 500 mg four times a day or doxycycline 100 mg twice a day for 10 to 21 days. Further studies on the clinical efficacy of azithromycin and newer fluoroquinolones are needed. The initial treatment response can be dramatic, with defervescence and marked clinical improvement within 24 to 48 hours. Full recovery may take several weeks, and relapse or reinfection can occur. Endocarditis treatment includes prolonged antibiotic therapy and consideration of valve replacement.

It is possible to culture *T. pallidum*, but sustained in vitro cultivation is not yet possible, and yields are very low. Culture is of limited use in research and of no use in clinical practice. All isolates studied have been susceptible to penicillin and are antigenically similar. The only known natural hosts for *T. pallidum* are humans and certain monkeys and higher apes.

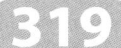

EPIDEMIOLOGY

With the exception of congenital syphilis, syphilis is acquired almost exclusively by intimate contact with the infectious lesions of primary or secondary syphilis (e.g., chancres, mucous patches, condylomata lata). Disease is usually acquired through sexual intercourse, including anogenital and orogenital intercourse. Health care workers are sometimes infected during the unsuspecting examination of patients with infectious lesions. Infection by contact with fomites is extremely uncommon. Before the advent of modern blood banking techniques, syphilis was occasionally transmitted through the transfusion of blood from persons with *T. pallidum* bacteremia, and occasional parenteral transmission still occurs as a result of the sharing of contaminated needles.

Syphilis is most common in large cities and in young, sexually active individuals. The highest rate is found in men between the ages of 20 and 29 years. In 2012, 67% of the 3142 U.S. counties reported no cases of primary or secondary syphilis, and just 28 locales accounted for about 50% of all reported infections.[3] The disease is most prevalent in the Southeast and California.

Syphilis spares no class, race, or group but is more prevalent among persons living on the margins of society. U.S. syphilis rates are about six-fold greater in African Americans than in non-Hispanic whites. In 2012, more than 75% of reported early syphilis occurred in men who acknowledged sex with other men. Increased numbers of different partners and perhaps indiscriminate choice of partners increase the risk of acquiring sexually transmitted disease (Chapter 285). A traditional cornerstone of syphilis control has been the epidemiologic investigation and treatment of sexual contacts of patients with primary or secondary lesions and patients with early latent disease. Patients with primary and secondary syphilis name, on average, nearly three different sexual contacts within the previous 90 days. As syphilis has become associated with drug use and anonymous sex, epidemiologic investigations have become less efficacious.

The incidence of syphilis has generally declined worldwide for more than 100 years, with the exception of periods of war or social upheaval. With the introduction of penicillin, there was a rapid decline in primary and secondary syphilis, to approximately 4 cases per 100,000 people in 1957. This decline was followed by reductions in federal expenditures for syphilis control, which resulted in resurgence of infectious primary and secondary syphilis in the United States; peaks of more than 12 cases per 100,000 people were attained several times from 1965 through the mid-1990s. Because many cases of syphilis are not reported, the true incidence may be much higher.

During the past 40 years, syphilis epidemics have occurred serially in at least three U.S. population subgroups. In the 1970s and 1980s, men who had sex with other men accounted for a disproportionate number of the total cases of infectious syphilis. Similar trends occurred in other countries. Then, after a period of decline, U.S. syphilis rates nearly doubled from 1986 to 1990, with 50,578 cases reported in 1990 in an epidemic disproportionately affecting multiracial heterosexual men and women and occurring contemporaneously with an epidemic of crack cocaine use. After 1990, syphilis rates again declined; in 2001, there were 6103 cases of primary and secondary syphilis reported, one of the lowest numbers since 1959. The epidemic of the late 1980s probably contributed to the spread of human immunodeficiency virus (HIV) infection (see Syphilis-HIV Interactions) and to dramatic increases in the rate of congenital syphilis. Since 2001, syphilis rates have again begun to increase in men, and now especially men infected with HIV.

In 2013, the rate of reported primary and secondary syphilis in the United States was 5.3 cases per 100,000 population, more than double the lowest-ever rate of 2.1 in 2000. During 2005 to 2013, primary and secondary syphilis rates increased among men of all ages, races, and ethnicities across all regions. Recent years have shown an accelerated increase occurring among men who have sex with men. Among women, rates increased during 2005 to 2008 and decreased during 2009 to 2013.[4]

Patients with clinically evident late syphilis, particularly those with cardiovascular or gummatous syphilis, are becoming less common, perhaps as a result of the effectiveness of penicillin therapy for early syphilis. However, surveys indicate that there are still significant numbers of patients with untreated neurologic syphilis, especially in older age groups.

PREVENTION

Epidemic psittacosis is preventable by a 30-day period of quarantine for all imported psittacine birds and their treatment with feed containing chlortetracycline. The U.S. Department of Agriculture recommends extending treatment for an additional 15 days after quarantine. Prevention of epidemic and endemic psittacosis also relies on avoidance of or protection from exposure to dust or body secretions from birds or their living areas as well as avoidance of the handling of sick birds. Environmental sanitation is another important preventive measure, considering the organism's resistance to drying.

Grade A References

A1. Porco TC, Gebre T, Ayele B, et al. Effect of mass distribution of azithromycin for trachoma control on overall mortality in Ethiopian children: a randomized trial. *JAMA.* 2009;302:962-968.
A2. House JI, Ayele B, Porco TC, et al. Assessment of herd protection against trachoma due to repeated mass antibiotic distributions: a cluster-randomised trial. *Lancet.* 2009;373:1111-1118.

GENERAL REFERENCES

For the General References and other additional features, please visit Expert Consult at https://expertconsult.inkling.com.

319

SYPHILIS
EDWARD W. HOOK III

DEFINITION

Syphilis, which is a chronic infectious disease caused by the bacterium *Treponema pallidum* subspecies *pallidum*, is usually acquired by sexual contact with another infected individual. Syphilis is remarkable among infectious diseases for its large variety of clinical manifestations. If untreated, it progresses through primary, secondary, and tertiary stages. The early stages (i.e., primary and secondary), when lesions are present, are infectious. Spontaneous healing of early lesions occurs, followed by a long latent period. In about 30% of untreated patients, late disease of the heart, central nervous system (CNS), or other organs may develop years after the initial infection. Although the disease is less common now than previously, it remains a challenge to clinicians because of its protean manifestations, and it is of interest to biologists because of the prolonged, tenuous balance between the host and the invading spirochete.[1,2]

The Pathogen

The causative agent of syphilis, *T. pallidum* subspecies *pallidum*, is closely related to other pathogenic spirochetes (Chapter 320), including those causing yaws (*T. pallidum* subspecies *pertenue*) and pinta (*Treponema carateum*). *T. pallidum* is a thin, helical bacterium approximately 0.15 μm wide and 6 to 15 μm long. The organism has 6 to 14 spirals and is tapered on either end. It is too thin to be seen by ordinary Gram stain microscopy but can be visualized in wet mounts by dark-field microscopy or in fixed specimens by silver stain or fluorescent antibody methods.

Unlike most bacteria, which have protein-rich outer membranes, the *T. pallidum* outer membrane appears to be composed of predominantly phospholipids, with few surface-exposed proteins. It has been hypothesized that because of this structure, syphilis can progress despite the brisk antibody response to non–surface-exposed internal antigens, which is the basis for serologic tests for the diagnosis and management of syphilis. Between the outer membrane and the peptidoglycan cell wall are six axial fibrils; three are attached at each end, and they overlap in the center of the organism. They are structurally and biochemically similar to flagella and are in part responsible for the organism's motility.

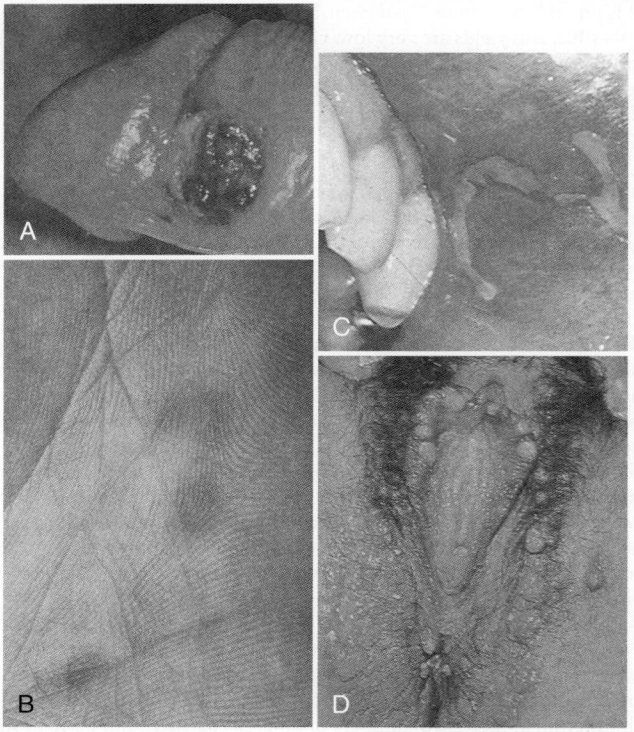

FIGURE 319-1. Syphilis lesions. A, Chancre in primary syphilis. B, Palmar lesions of a coppery color in secondary syphilis. C, Mucous patch in secondary syphilis. D, Condylomata lata in secondary syphilis. (A, C, and D from Forbes CD, Jackson WF. *Color Atlas and Text of Clinical Medicine.* 3rd ed. London: Mosby; 2003. B from Habif TP, Cambell JI, Quitadamo MJ, et al. *Skin Disease: Diagnosis and Treatment.* St. Louis: Mosby; 2001.)

Natural Course of Untreated Syphilis

The incubation period from the time of exposure to development of the primary lesion averages approximately 21 days (range, 10 to 90 days). Initially, a painless papule develops at the site of inoculation and soon breaks down to form a clean-based ulcer—the chancre—with raised, indurated margins (Fig. 319-1A). The chancre persists for 2 to 6 weeks and then heals spontaneously. Several weeks later, a secondary stage characterized by low-grade fever, headache, malaise, generalized lymphadenopathy, and a mucocutaneous rash typically develops. There may be involvement of visceral organs. The secondary eruption may occur while the primary chancre is still healing or up to several months after disappearance of the chancre. Secondary lesions also heal spontaneously within 2 to 6 weeks, and the infection then becomes latent. In more than 20% of patients with untreated latent syphilis, relapsing lesions later develop, similar to those of the secondary stage; rarely, the relapse takes the form of recurrence of the primary chancre. In the era before antibiotics, late, destructive tertiary lesions involving the eyes, the CNS, the heart, and other organs, including the skin, eventually developed in about a third of untreated patients. These lesions may occur a few years to as long as 25 years after infection.

The incidence of late complications of untreated syphilis is currently unknown, but it seems to be less than that seen previously. Cases of gumma are now so rare as to be reportable.

PATHOBIOLOGY

T. pallidum may penetrate through normal mucosal membranes and minor abrasions on epithelial surfaces. The first lesions appear at the site of direct, primary inoculation. The minimal number of treponemes needed to establish infection is not known but may be as low as one. Multiplication of organisms is slow, with a division time in rabbits of approximately 33 hours. The slow growth of treponemes in humans probably accounts in part for the protracted nature of the illness, the relatively long incubation period, and the need for relatively long duration of therapy.

Syphilis is a systemic disease from the onset. Treponemes are capable of specific attachment to host cells, but it is not known whether attachment

results in damage to the host cells. Most treponemes are found in the intercellular spaces, but they are occasionally seen within phagocytic cells. However, there is no evidence of prolonged intracellular survival of treponemes. *T. pallidum* is not known to produce toxins.

The primary pathologic lesion of syphilis is a focal endarteritis with an increase in adventitial cells, endothelial proliferation, and the presence of an inflammatory cuff around affected vessels. Lymphocytes, plasma cells, and monocytes predominate in the inflammatory lesion, and polymorphonuclear cells are seen in some cases. The vessel lumen is frequently obliterated. With healing, there is considerable fibrosis. Treponemes may be seen in most early lesions of syphilis and in some of the late lesions, such as the meningoencephalitis of general paresis.

Granulomatous reaction is common in secondary and late syphilis. The granulomas are histologically nonspecific, and cases of syphilis have been incorrectly diagnosed as sarcoidosis or other granulomatous diseases. Human inoculation studies suggest that the pathogenesis of the gumma, which is a granulomatous lesion, involves hypersensitivity to small numbers of virulent treponemes introduced into a previously sensitized host.

Intracutaneous inoculation of partially purified antigens of *T. pallidum* into patients with syphilis in various stages has shown that delayed cellular hypersensitivity develops only late in secondary syphilis but is uniformly present in latent syphilis. There may be temporary hyporesponsiveness of lymphocytes to treponemal antigens in patients with primary and secondary syphilis. It is possible that the waxing and waning of lesions in early syphilis depend on the balance between the development of effective cellular immunity and the suppression of thymus-derived lymphocyte function.

The host responds to infection by producing numerous antibodies; in some instances, circulating immune complexes may be formed as well. For example, nephrotic syndrome has occasionally been recognized in secondary syphilis, and renal biopsy specimens from such patients have shown membranous glomerulonephritis characterized by focal subepithelial basement membrane deposits containing immunoglobulin G, C3, and treponemal antibody.

CLINICAL MANIFESTATIONS

Primary Syphilis

The typical lesion of primary syphilis, the chancre, is a painless, clean-based, indurated ulcer (Fig. 319-1A). The chancre starts as a papule, but then superficial erosion results in ulceration. The borders of the ulcer are raised, firm, and indurated. On occasion, secondary infections change the appearance and cause a painful lesion. Most chancres are single, but multiple ulcers are sometimes seen, particularly when skinfolds are apposed (i.e., kissing chancres). An untreated chancre heals in several weeks and leaves a faint scar. The chancre is usually associated with regional adenopathy, which may be unilateral or bilateral. The regional nodes are movable, discrete, and rubbery. If the chancre occurs in the cervix or the rectum, the affected regional iliac nodes are not palpable.

Chancres can occur at any site of potential inoculation by direct contact, with most occurring in anogenital locations. Chancres may also be seen in the pharynx, on the tongue, around the lips, on the fingers, on the nipples, and in other diverse areas. The morphology depends in part on the area of the body where they occur and on the host's immune response. Chancres in previously infected individuals may be small and remain papular. Chancres of the finger may appear more erosive and can be quite painful. Chancres of the anal canal may be missed in men who have sex with men unless a careful examination is undertaken.

Secondary Syphilis

Between 4 and 8 weeks after the appearance of the primary chancre, signs and symptoms of secondary syphilis typically develop. Symptoms may include malaise, fever, headache, sore throat, and other systemic complaints. Most patients have generalized lymphadenopathy, including involvement of the epitrochlear nodes. Approximately 30% of patients have evidence of a healing chancre, although many patients (including a disproportionate number of women and of men who have sex with men) give no history of a primary lesion.

At least 80% of patients with secondary syphilis have cutaneous or mucocutaneous lesions at some point in their illness. The diagnosis is frequently first suspected on the basis of the cutaneous eruption. The rash is often minimally symptomatic, and many patients with late syphilis do not recall primary or secondary lesions. The rashes are varied in appearance but have certain characteristic features. The lesions are usually widespread, are symmetrical in distribution, and are frequently pink, coppery, or dusky red (particularly the earliest macular lesions). They are generally nonpruritic, although occasional exceptions have been reported, and they are rarely vesicular or bullous in adults. They are indurated, except for the very earliest macular lesions, and frequently have a superficial scale (i.e., papulosquamous lesions). The lesions tend to be polymorphic and rounded, and on healing, they may leave residual pigmentation or depigmentation. They may be faint and difficult to visualize, particularly on dark-skinned individuals.

The earliest pink macular lesions are typically seen on the trunk, with later spread to the rest of the body. The face is often spared, except around the mouth. Subsequently, a papular rash appears that is usually generalized but is marked on the palms and soles (Fig. 327-1B). These rashes are often associated with a superficial scale and may be hyperpigmented. When the rash occurs on the face, it may be pustular and resemble acne vulgaris. On occasion, the scale may be so great that it resembles psoriasis. Ulceration may occur and produce lesions resembling ecthyma. In malnourished or debilitated patients, extensive and destructive ulcerative lesions with a heaped-up crust may occur, the so-called rupial lesions. Lesions around the hair follicles may result in patchy alopecia of the beard or scalp.

Ringed or annular lesions may occur, especially around the face and particularly on dark-skinned individuals. A lesion at the angle of the mouth or the corner of the nose may have a central linear erosion, the so-called split papule.

The palate and pharynx may be inflamed. In approximately 30% of secondary syphilis patients, so-called mucous patches (Fig. 319-1C) develop; these slightly raised, oval areas are covered by a grayish white membrane that, when raised, reveals a pink base that does not bleed. These lesions may be seen on the genitalia, in the mouth, or on the tongue.

In warm, moist areas such as the perineum, large, pale, flat-topped papules may coalesce to form condylomata lata (Fig. 319-1D). Papules may also be seen in the axilla and rarely occur in a generalized form. These papules are not to be confused with the common venereal warts (i.e., condylomata acuminata), which are small, often multiple, and more sharply raised than condylomata lata. Like mucous patches, condylomata lata are highly infectious.

Other manifestations of secondary syphilis include hepatitis, which has been reported in up to 10% of patients in some series. Jaundice is rare, but an elevated alkaline phosphatase level is common. Liver biopsy reveals small areas of focal necrosis and mononuclear infiltrate or periportal vasculitis. Spirochetes can often be visualized with silver stains. Periostitis with widespread lytic lesions of bone has been reported occasionally; bone scanning appears to be a sensitive test for early syphilitic osteitis. An immune complex type of nephropathy with transient nephrotic syndrome has been documented rarely. There may be iritis or an anterior uveitis. Between 10 and 30% of patients have pleocytosis in cerebrospinal fluid (CSF), but symptomatic meningitis is seen in less than 1% of patients. Symptomatic gastritis may occur.

Relapsing Syphilis

After resolution of the primary or secondary skin lesions, 20 to 30% of patients experience cutaneous recurrences. Recurrent lesions may be fewer or more firmly indurated than the initial lesions. Like the typical lesions of primary or secondary syphilis, they are infectious for exposed sexual partners.

Latent Syphilis

By definition, latent syphilis is the stage at which there are no clinical signs of syphilis and the CSF is normal. Latency, which begins when the first attack of secondary syphilis has passed and may last for a lifetime, is usually detected by reactive serologic tests for syphilis (see Diagnosis). Congenital syphilis must also be excluded before the diagnosis of latent syphilis can be made. Patients may or may not have a clinical history of earlier primary or secondary syphilis manifestations.

Latency has been divided into two stages: early and late. Most infectious relapses occur in the first year, and epidemiologic evidence shows that the most infectious period is during the first year of infection. Early latency is therefore defined as the first year after resolution of the primary or secondary lesions or as a newly reactive serologic test response for syphilis in an otherwise asymptomatic individual who has had a negative serologic test result within the preceding year. Late latent syphilis, or, more accurately, latent

TABLE 319-1	NEWLY DIAGNOSED TERTIARY SYPHILIS IN 105 PATIENTS IN DENMARK, 1961-1970
TYPE OF TERTIARY SYPHILIS	**NO. OBSERVED***
Neurosyphilis	72
Asymptomatic	45
Tabes dorsalis	11
General paresis	13
Meningovascular	1
Optic atrophy	2
Cardiovascular syphilis	44
Aortic insufficiency	16
Aortic aneurysm	13
Uncomplicated aortitis[†]	15
Late benign syphilis (gumma)	4

*Some patients had more than one form of late syphilis.
[†]Autopsy diagnoses only.

syphilis of unknown duration, is ordinarily not infectious, except for pregnant women, who can transmit infection to the fetus despite long-standing infection.

Late Syphilis

Late syphilis (Table 319-1) is usually slowly progressive, although certain neurologic syndromes may have a sudden onset because of endarteritis and CNS thrombosis. Late syphilis is not infectious through sexual contact. Any organ of the body may be involved, but three main types of disease can be distinguished: late benign (gummatous), cardiovascular, and neurosyphilis.

Late Benign Syphilis

In the penicillin era, gummas are rare. They typically develop 1 to 10 years after initial infection and may involve any part of the body. Although gummas may be destructive, they respond rapidly to treatment and are therefore relatively benign. On histologic evaluation, the gumma is a granuloma.

Gummas may be solitary or multiple and most often come to medical attention as space-occupying lesions. They are usually asymmetrical and are often grouped. Gummas may start as a superficial nodule or as a deeper lesion that breaks down to form punched-out ulcers. They are ordinarily indolent, slowly progressive, and indurated on palpation. Cutaneous gummas may resemble other chronic granulomatous ulcerative lesions caused by tuberculosis, sarcoidosis, leprosy, and other deep fungal infections. Precise histologic diagnosis may not be possible. However, syphilitic gummas are the only such lesions to heal dramatically with penicillin therapy.

Gummas may also involve deep visceral organs, particularly the respiratory tract, gastrointestinal tract, and bones. In addition, they may involve the larynx or the pulmonary parenchyma. Gummas of the stomach may masquerade as carcinoma of the stomach or lymphoma. Gummas of the liver were once the most common form of visceral syphilis and often manifested as hepatosplenomegaly and anemia and occasionally as fever and jaundice. Skeletal gummas typically produce lesions in the long bones, skull, and clavicle; a characteristic symptom is nocturnal pain. Radiologic abnormalities, when present, include periostitis and lytic or sclerotic, destructive osteitis.

Cardiovascular Syphilis

The primary cardiovascular complications of syphilis are aortic insufficiency (Chapter 75) and aortic aneurysm (Chapter 78), usually of the ascending aorta. Less commonly, other large arteries may be affected, and involvement of the coronary ostia rarely results in coronary insufficiency. All these complications are caused by obliterative endarteritis of the vasa vasorum, with resultant damage to the intima and media of the great vessels. This damage results in dilation of the ascending aorta, but the valve cusps remain normal. An aneurysm occasionally is manifested as a pulsating mass bulging through the anterior chest wall. Syphilitic aortitis[5] may also involve the descending aorta proximal to the renal arteries.

Cardiovascular syphilis usually begins within 5 to 10 years of the initial infection but may not be manifested clinically until 20 to 30 years later. Cardiovascular syphilis does not occur after congenital infection, a phenomenon that remains unexplained.

Asymptomatic aortitis is best diagnosed by visualizing linear calcifications in the wall of the ascending aorta by radiography. The signs of syphilitic aortic insufficiency are the same as for aortic insufficiency of other causes. In aortic insufficiency resulting from dilation of the aortic ring, the decrescendo murmur is often loudest along the right sternal margin. Syphilitic aneurysms may be fusiform but are more typically saccular and do not lead to aortic dissection. Between 10 and 20% of patients with cardiovascular syphilis have coexistent neurosyphilis.

Neurosyphilis

CNS involvement occurs throughout the natural history of syphilis. Neurosyphilis[6] can be divided into five groups: asymptomatic, syphilitic meningitis, meningovascular syphilis, tabes dorsalis, and general paresis. Asymptomatic neurosyphilis can occur at any time, whereas syphilitic meningitis is most common during the secondary stage of infection. Meningovascular syphilis, tabes dorsalis, and general paresis are typically manifestations of late syphilis. The divisions are not absolute, and overlap between syndromes is typical. Current cases of neurosyphilis are likely to be variants of the classic syndromes, possibly as a result of the use of antimicrobial agents for other diseases.

Syphilitic Meningitis

Acute to subacute aseptic meningitis can occur at any time after the primary stage, but it usually occurs within the first year of infection. It frequently involves the base of the brain and may result in unilateral or bilateral cranial nerve palsies. Mild aseptic meningitis may be relatively common in patients with early syphilis, but severe disease occurs in only about 1.5% of untreated patients. Syphilitic meningitis typically resolves without treatment.

Meningovascular Syphilis

Some patients have sufficient endarteritis and perivascular inflammation to result in cerebrovascular thrombosis and infarction, generally 5 to 10 years after the initial infection. However, case reports suggest that in syphilis patients with coexistent HIV infection, meningovascular syphilis may be manifested earlier or may be a manifestation of treatment failure. Patients frequently have associated aseptic meningitis. Most cerebrovascular accidents are not caused by syphilitic arteritis, even in patients with a reactive serologic test result for syphilis. However, syphilis should be considered a potential cause in relatively young patients with a history of syphilis and without other risk factors for cerebrovascular accidents.

Tabes Dorsalis

Tabes dorsalis, which appears to be far less common than in the prepenicillin era, is a slowly progressive, degenerative disease that involves the posterior columns and posterior roots of the spinal cord and results in progressive loss of peripheral reflexes, impairment of vibration and position sense, and progressive ataxia. Sensory changes may lead to chronic destructive changes in the large joints of the affected limbs in advanced cases (i.e., Charcot's joints). Incontinence of the bladder and impotence are common. Sudden and severely painful crises of uncertain origin are a characteristic part of the syndrome. Severe, sharp abdominal pain may lead to exploratory surgery.

Optic atrophy is seen in 20% of cases. In 90% of patients, the pupils are bilaterally small and fail to constrict further in response to light, but they do respond normally to accommodation (i.e., Argyll Robertson pupils).

The onset of tabes dorsalis is usually first noticed 20 to 30 years after the initial infection. Its cause is unclear, and spirochetes cannot be demonstrated in the posterior column or dorsal root.

General Paresis

This form of neurosyphilis is a chronic meningoencephalitis resulting in the gradual and progressive loss of cortical function. It typically occurs 10 to 20 years after the initial infection. On pathologic examination, there is a perivascular and meningeal chronic inflammatory reaction, with thickening of the meninges, granular ependymitis, degeneration of the cortical parenchyma, and abundant spirochetes in tissues.

In its early stages, general paresis results in nonspecific symptoms of early dementia, such as irritability, fatigability, headaches, forgetfulness, and personality changes. Later, there is impaired memory, defective judgment, lack of insight, confusion, and often depression or marked elation. Patients may be delusional, and seizures sometimes occur. There may also be loss of other cortical functions, including paralysis or aphasia.

Physical signs are primarily those of the altered mental status. Cranial nerve palsies are uncommon, and optic atrophy is rare. The complete Argyll Robertson pupil is also uncommon, but irregular or otherwise abnormal pupils are not infrequent. Peripheral reflexes are often somewhat increased.

Syphilis-HIV Interactions

Syphilis, like other genital ulcer diseases, is associated with a three- to five-fold increased risk for acquisition of HIV infection. Presumably, genital ulcers act as portals of entry through which HIV may more readily infect exposed individuals. As a result, HIV serologic testing 3 months after a diagnosis of syphilis is recommended for all patients. Conversely, in individuals with HIV infection who acquire syphilis, the natural history of the infection may be modified. HIV-infected syphilis patients are somewhat more likely than non–HIV-infected patients to present initially with secondary syphilis. HIV-infected secondary syphilis patients are also more likely than HIV-negative secondary syphilis patients to have coexistent chancres, suggesting that the healing of chancres is delayed or the appearance of secondary manifestations is accelerated in the presence of HIV coinfection.

Congenital Syphilis

Congenital syphilis results from the transplacental, hematogenous spread of syphilis from the mother to the fetus. In 2012, 322 cases of congenital syphilis were reported in the United States. A serologic test for syphilis should be performed in all expectant mothers at the beginning of pregnancy and should be repeated near the end of pregnancy in women living in areas where syphilis is relatively common.[7]

The risk for fetal infection is greatest in the early stages of untreated maternal syphilis and declines slowly thereafter, but the untreated mother can infect her fetus during at least the first 5 years of her infection. Adequate treatment of the mother before the 16th week of pregnancy usually prevents clinical illness in the neonate. Later treatment may not prevent late sequelae of the disease in the child. Untreated maternal infection may result in stillbirth, neonatal death, prematurity, or syndromes of early or late congenital syphilis in surviving infants.

Manifestations of early congenital syphilis are often seen in the perinatal period but may not develop until the infant has been discharged from the hospital. The disease resembles secondary syphilis in adults, except that the rash may be vesicular or bullous. The child often has rhinitis, hepatosplenomegaly, hemolytic anemia, jaundice, and pseudoparalysis (i.e., immobility of one or more extremities) as a result of painful osteochondritis.

Late congenital syphilis is defined as congenital syphilis diagnosed more than 2 years after birth. The disease may remain latent, with no manifestations of late damage. Cardiovascular alterations have not been observed in patients with congenital syphilis. Neurologic manifestations are common and may include eighth cranial nerve deafness and interstitial keratitis. Periostitis may result in prominent frontal bones of the skull, depression of the bridge of the nose (saddle nose), poor development of the maxilla, and anterior bowing of the tibia (saber shins). There may be late-onset arthritis of the knees (Clutton's joints). The permanent dentition may show characteristic abnormalities known as Hutchinson's teeth; the upper central incisors are widely spaced, centrally notched, and tapered in the manner of a screwdriver. The molars may show multiple poorly developed cusps (mulberry molars).

DIAGNOSIS

Dark-Field Examination

The most definitive means of syphilis diagnosis is finding typical spirochetes in lesions of early acquired or congenital syphilis. Dark-field examination is often positive in cases of primary syphilis and in patients with the moist mucosal lesions of secondary and congenital syphilis. The result may occasionally be positive for aspirates of lymph nodes in secondary syphilis. False-negative results may occur in primary syphilis because of the application of soaps, antiseptics, or other compounds toxic to *T. pallidum* to the lesions. A single negative result is therefore insufficient to exclude syphilis. For high-risk individuals (e.g., drug users, homosexually active men), it is appropriate to treat presumptively on the basis of suspicious lesions after performing serologic tests. Confusion may also arise because of the presence of spirochetes that are morphologically indistinguishable from *T. pallidum* organisms in the mouth, particularly around the gingival margins. Living *T. pallidum* organisms demonstrate gradual motion to and fro, rotational movement around the long axis, and rather sudden 90-degree flexing near the center of the organism. Because most physicians do not have the proper equipment and are not familiar with dark-field microscopy techniques, public health authorities can be called for assistance. *T. pallidum* may also be demonstrated in biopsy or pathologic specimens by fluorescent antibody stains or by silver stains.

Serologic Tests

Two basic types of serologic tests (Table 319-2) are widely used to diagnose infection with *T. pallidum*: (1) nontreponemal tests that detect antibodies reactive with diphosphatidylglycerol (cardiolipin), which is a normal component of many tissues; and (2) tests that detect antibodies to specific treponemal antigens.

Nontreponemal Tests

The standard tests to detect anticardiolipin antibody are the rapid plasma reagin (RPR) and Venereal Disease Research Laboratory (VDRL) tests, which are slide flocculation tests. The RPR and VDRL are readily quantified, so they are the tests of choice for monitoring patients' responses to treatment. The relative proportion of patients with a false-positive RPR result depends on the prevalence of syphilis in the community; the lower the prevalence of syphilis, the higher the proportion of reactive RPR test results from nonsyphilitic causes.

The RPR test result begins to turn positive less than 1 week after onset of the chancre; thus, a nonreactive RPR test result does not exclude primary syphilis, particularly if the lesion is less than 1 week old. The RPR test result is positive in 99% of patients with secondary syphilis (Table 319-3). Patients with advanced HIV infection may have negative test results, and some patients have such high titers of antibody that they are in antibody excess; dilution of their serum paradoxically results in conversion of a negative test result to a positive one, the so-called prozone reaction. RPR reactivity tends to diminish in later stages of syphilis, and only about 70% of patients with cardiovascular syphilis or late neurosyphilis have positive RPR test results.

The *quantitative titer* of the RPR or VDRL test is somewhat useful in diagnosis and is quite useful for monitoring of the therapeutic response. Most patients with secondary syphilis have titers of at least 1 : 16. Most patients with false-positive RPR test results have titers of less than 1 : 8. No single titer is diagnostic by itself. Significant rises (four-fold or greater) in paired sera, however, strongly indicate acute syphilis.

Treponemal Tests

Several types of treponemal tests are widely used. Recently, treponemal enzyme immunoassays (EIAs) using cloned treponemal antigens for treponemal antibody detection have become available from several manufacturers

TABLE 319-2	SEROLOGIC TESTS FOR SYPHILIS	
TYPE	**USE**
NONTREPONEMAL (ANTICARDIOLIPIN) ANTIBODIES	
VDRL (slide flocculation)	Screening, quantitation of response to treatment
RPR (circle card) (agglutination)	Screening, quantitation of response to treatment
SPECIFIC TREPONEMAL ANTIBODIES	
FTA-ABS (immunofluorescence with absorbed serum)	Confirmatory, diagnostic; not for routine screening
TP-PA (microhemagglutination)	Similar to FTA-ABS but can be quantified and automated
EIA	Confirmatory and increasingly used for screening; automated

EIA = enzyme immunoassay; FTA-ABS = fluorescent treponemal antibody absorption test; RPR = rapid plasma regain test; TP-PA = *Treponema pallidum* particle agglutination; VDRL = Venereal Disease Research Laboratory.

TABLE 319-3	FREQUENCY OF POSITIVE SEROLOGIC TEST RESULTS IN UNTREATED SYPHILIS		
STAGE	**VDRL (%)**	**FTA-ABS (%)**	**TP-PA (%)**
Primary	70	85	50-60
Secondary	99	100	100
Latent or late	70	98	98

FTA-ABS = fluorescent treponemal antibody absorption test; TP-PA = *Treponema pallidum* particle agglutination; VDRL = Venereal Disease Research Laboratory.

and have gained favor because of their low cost and ease of use. In addition to EIA tests, agglutination of particles to which *T. pallidum* antigens have been fixed is the basis of the widely used *T. pallidum* particle agglutination (TP-PA) test. The fluorescent treponemal antibody absorption (FTA-ABS) test has been widely used as well and is reported in terms of relative brilliance of fluorescence, from borderline to 4 plus; most laboratories report only test results with 2 plus or greater reactivity as positive. For patients lacking historical or clinical evidence of syphilis but with a reactive FTA-ABS test result, the test should be repeated. Use of another treponemal test may be helpful in problem cases. The TP-PA test is slightly less sensitive than the RPR or FTA-ABS test in primary syphilis. Its sensitivity and specificity are otherwise nearly identical to those of the FTA-ABS test.

Because EIA serologic tests permit the screening of large numbers of sera and have performance characteristics (sensitivity, specificity, predictive values) similar to those of other treponemal tests, they have been increasingly used recently for syphilis screening.[8,9] Persons with reactive treponemal antigen EIAs should be tested with a quantitative nontreponemal test, such as the RPR or VDRL test, for confirmation and to permit the use of that test to evaluate the subsequent response to therapy. It is not unusual for patients to have a reactive EIA test result for syphilis and a nonreactive RPR or VDRL test result. A substantial proportion of these EIA-only positive test results are falsely positive or are detecting long-standing, often previously treated syphilis, but occasionally they may detect very recent infection before RPR or VDRL test results become positive.

When nontreponemal tests such as the RPR and VDRL are used for screening, treponemal tests are used to confirm that persons with reactive nontreponemal test results have antibodies to *T. pallidum*. Results of treponemal tests are not reliably quantified. They are sensitive and have a high degree of specificity, in that only approximately 1% of normal individuals have reactive treponemal test results. They are reactive in 85% of patients with primary syphilis, 99% with secondary syphilis, and at least 95% with late syphilis. They may therefore be the only test with a positive result in patients with cardiovascular or neurologic syphilis. For patients with late syphilis, treponemal test results often remain reactive for life, despite adequate therapy.

Differential Diagnosis

The differential diagnosis of a genital ulcer (Chapter 285) includes genital herpes (Chapter 374), chancroid (Chapter 301), lymphogranuloma venereum (Chapter 318), and a number of other ulcerative processes. Classically, herpetic ulcers are multiple, painful, superficial, and, if seen early, vesicular. However, atypical manifestations may be indistinguishable from a syphilitic chancre. Genital herpes is much more common than syphilis and is now the most common cause of a "typical chancre" in North America. Syphilitic chancres may also be coinfected with herpes simplex virus in about 15% of cases. The ulcers of chancroid are usually painful, often multiple, and frequently exudative and nonindurated. Lymphogranuloma venereum may produce a small, papular lesion associated with regional adenopathy. Other conditions that must be distinguished include granuloma inguinale (Chapter 316), drug eruptions, carcinoma, superficial fungal infections (Chapter 438), traumatic lesions, and lichen planus (Chapter 438). In most cases, the final distinction is based on dark-field examination, which is positive only in syphilis, and on serologic test results.

The differential diagnosis of the skin lesions of secondary syphilis includes pityriasis rosea (Chapter 438), which can be differentiated by the occurrence of lesions along lines of skin cleavage and frequently by the presence of a herald patch. Drug eruptions, acute febrile exanthems, psoriasis, lichen planus, scabies, and other diseases must also be considered in some cases. A mucous patch may superficially resemble oral candidiasis (i.e., thrush). Infectious mononucleosis (Chapter 377) may appear similar to secondary syphilis, with sore throat, generalized adenopathy, hepatitis, and a generalized rash. Hepatitis (Chapter 148) may also cause confusion.

False-Positive Serologic Test Results for Syphilis

The RPR or VDRL test result is reactive in patients with other treponemal diseases, such as pinta, yaws, and endemic syphilis (Chapter 320). These test results may also be falsely reactive in persons who do not have treponemal infections based on a negative clinical history or negative results of serum treponemal tests.[10]

The origins of false-positive results are better studied for nontreponemal tests than for treponemal tests. Acute (<6 months) false-positive RPR test results occur with low frequency in patients with atypical pneumonia, malaria, and other bacterial or viral infections, and they may occur after smallpox or other vaccinations as well. Chronic false-positive RPR test results (persisting >6 months) are relatively common in patients with autoimmune disorders such as systemic lupus erythematosus (Chapter 266), parenteral drug users, HIV-infected patients, patients with leprosy, and the aged. Between 8 and 20% of patients with systemic lupus erythematosus have false-positive RPR test results. Chronic false-positive RPR test results in female patients 20 years or younger indicate a significant risk for the future development of systemic lupus erythematosus, thyroiditis, or other autoimmune disorders. As many as a third of parenteral drug users have false-positive RPR test results. More than 1% of persons 70 years old and 10% of those older than 80 years also have low-titer, false-positive RPR test results. In most cases of false-positive RPR test results, the titer is less than 1 : 8, although a few patients with lymphoma and other diseases have very high-titer, false-positive results.

There is also an increased incidence of false-positive treponemal test results in other chronic inflammatory diseases associated with hyperglobulinemia, including rheumatoid arthritis and biliary cirrhosis. On occasion, reproducible positive FTA-ABS results are obtained in patients with no clinical or historical evidence of syphilis and no evidence of diseases typically associated with false-positive FTA-ABS results. If the diagnosis is in doubt and if the patient is not allergic to penicillin, it is often prudent to treat for possible syphilis.

Neurosyphilis

Asymptomatic neurosyphilis is diagnosed when there are CSF abnormalities, such as lymphocytic pleocytosis, protein elevation, or a reactive VDRL test result, in a syphilis patient in the absence of signs and symptoms of neurologic disease. Unlike serologic tests, the VDRL and RPR tests do not perform equally for CSF, and only the VDRL is recommended. Although numerous other processes can cause CSF pleocytosis or protein elevations, false-positive CSF VDRL test results are rare in the absence of a traumatic tap. If the CSF is normal 2 years or longer after the initial infection, a positive CSF finding is not likely to develop later. Routine lumbar punctures to examine CSF are not indicated in early syphilis unless the patient is known to have HIV infection. Lumbar puncture in HIV-infected persons with early syphilis is the subject of controversy. Although a nonreactive CSF FTA-ABS result may be useful to rule out the diagnosis, no diagnosis of neurosyphilis should be based solely on the CSF FTA-ABS test.

In syphilitic meningitis, the CSF shows a lymphocytic pleocytosis, with increased protein and usually normal glucose concentrations. The CSF VDRL test is nearly always reactive. Rarely, the CSF glucose concentration is decreased. Without treatment, syphilitic meningitis generally resolves, similar to the course of other manifestations of early syphilis. This syndrome can mimic tuberculous or fungal meningitis or nonpurulent meningitis of various causes.

In tabes dorsalis, the VDRL test for serum is nonreactive in as many as 30 to 40% of patients, and 10 to 20% of patients (even before the advent of penicillin) have normal CSF VDRL results. The FTA-ABS test for serum is nearly always reactive. In general paresis, the CSF is nearly always abnormal, with lymphocytic pleocytosis and an increased total protein concentration. The VDRL test is usually reactive for CSF and serum.

Congenital Syphilis

Because many infants with congenital syphilis may be clinically normal at birth but develop serious, symptomatic disease some weeks later, it is important to determine whether a newborn with a reactive serologic test result for syphilis has passively transferred maternal antibody or is actively infected. If the mother has been adequately treated for syphilis during pregnancy and the infant is clinically normal at birth, one option is to monitor the infant carefully by serial examinations and RPR titers. If the reactive RPR result for the infant is caused by passively transferred maternal antibody, the titer will fall markedly in the first 2 months of life; a rising titer indicates active disease and the need for treatment. However, the risk of improper follow-up of RPR-positive but clinically normal neonates makes the immediate empirical administration of effective therapy an attractive alternative.

TREATMENT Rx

T. pallidum is inhibited by less than 0.01 µg/mL of penicillin G. Because treponemes divide slowly and penicillin acts only on dividing cells, it is necessary to maintain serum levels of penicillin for many days (Table 319-4).

Early Infectious Syphilis

Early syphilis (<1 year) can be treated with a single injection of 2.4 million units of benzathine penicillin G, which provides low but effective serum levels for about 2 weeks and cures approximately 95% of patients.[11] It is not necessary to examine CSF at this stage because penicillin prevents the later development of neurosyphilis.[12]

Individuals with other sexually transmitted diseases may have been exposed to syphilis at the time they became infected. Treatment with a single dose of β-lactam antibiotics (penicillins, cephalosporins), which provide relatively high serum levels for a brief period, is ineffective in established early syphilis but is curative if the disease is still in the incubating stage. The ceftriaxone regimen used for gonorrhea (Chapter 299) is probably curative for incubating syphilis, but careful follow-up is indicated if there is reason to suspect exposure to syphilis in a patient treated for gonorrhea with ceftriaxone. Single-dose therapy with 2.0 g of azithromycin administered orally was as effective as benzathine penicillin therapy in several studies of early syphilis,[A1] but treatment failures have been reported in persons with coexistent HIV infection. Currently, azithromycin should not be used for the treatment of early syphilis unless close follow-up can be ensured.

For patients allergic to penicillin, 100 mg of doxycycline orally twice daily for 14 days is recommended. Particularly careful follow-up is necessary for patients treated with drugs other than penicillin because they may not be fully compliant with these prolonged courses of oral therapy and these regimens have been less fully evaluated clinically. Ceftriaxone, given in doses of 500 mg to 1.0 g intramuscularly daily for 10 days, may be effective but has been studied only in small numbers of patients with syphilis. Quinolone antibiotics have essentially no effect on syphilis.

Syphilis of More than 1 Year in Duration

Prolonged therapy with intramuscular injections of 2.4 million units of benzathine penicillin G weekly for 3 weeks is recommended for the treatment of late latent syphilis and latent syphilis of unknown duration. Limited evidence suggests that treatment of latent syphilis with a total dose of 7.2 million units of benzathine penicillin during a 3-week period is curative, even if the patient has asymptomatic neurosyphilis. However, because of the possible lack of efficacy of benzathine penicillin G in some patients with CNS syphilis, CSF examination should be considered in those with latent syphilis to exclude asymptomatic neurosyphilis, particularly in HIV-positive patients, in whom the prevalence of asymptomatic neurosyphilis is higher. Alternatively, a lumbar puncture can be performed at the conclusion of the follow-up period (2 years); if the CSF is normal, the patient can be reassured that neurosyphilis will not develop.

Larger doses of penicillin are recommended for persons with proven neurosyphilis (see Table 319-4). General paresis responds well to penicillin therapy if it is administered early, although progressive neurologic decline may develop later in as many as a third of treated patients. Carbamazepine in doses of 400 to 800 mg/day reportedly treats the lightning pains of tabes dorsalis effectively. Published studies show that a total of 6.0 to 9.0 million units of penicillin G results in a satisfactory clinical response in approximately 90% of patients with neurosyphilis who do not have HIV infection. There are anecdotal reports of increased treatment failures in patients with concomitant HIV infection, and there is considerable rationale to treat these patients with intravenous penicillin G (20 million units/day for at least 10 days). Therapy for neurosyphilis can result in increased CSF pleocytosis for 7 to 10 days after treatment is started and may transiently convert a normal CSF to abnormal.

Although there is no evidence that therapy with antimicrobial drugs is clinically beneficial in patients with cardiovascular syphilis, treatment is recommended to prevent further progression of disease and because approximately 15% of patients with cardiovascular syphilis have associated neurosyphilis. If patients are allergic to penicillin, it is mandatory that the CSF be examined before therapy is undertaken; if the CSF is abnormal, desensitization to penicillin is generally recommended. With a normal CSF, tetracycline (500 mg orally four times a day) or doxycycline (100 mg orally two times a day) taken for 4 weeks is probably effective.

Syphilis in Pregnancy

Because of the risk to the fetus, evaluation and treatment of a pregnant RPR-positive patient must be rapid, particularly for those patients first seen in the later stages of pregnancy. If a confirmatory treponemal test result is positive and the patient has not been treated, penicillin should be administered in doses appropriate for early or late syphilis, as outlined earlier. For penicillin-allergic patients, penicillin desensitization is preferred; patients should not be treated with tetracycline or erythromycin because of toxicity (tetracycline) or lack of efficacy (erythromycin). For patients who are RPR positive but treponemal test negative and have no clinical signs of syphilis, treatment may be withheld; a quantitative RPR test and another treponemal test should be repeated in 4 weeks. If the treponemal titer has risen four-fold or more, or if clinical signs of syphilis have developed, the patient should be treated. If, after repeated examination, the diagnosis remains equivocal, the patient should be

TABLE 319-4   PENICILLIN TREATMENT FOR SYPHILIS AS RECOMMENDED BY THE U.S. PUBLIC HEALTH SERVICE

INDICATIONS FOR SYPHILIS THERAPY*	DOSAGE AND ADMINISTRATION†	
	Benzathine Penicillin G	*Aqueous Benzylpenicillin G or Procaine Penicillin G*
Primary, secondary, and early latent syphilis (<1 year); epidemiologic treatment	Total of 2.4 million units; single IM dose of two injections of 1.2 million units in one session	Total of 4.8 million units IM in doses of 600,000 units/day for 8 consecutive days
Late latent (>1 year) or when CSF was not examined in "latency"; cardiovascular syphilis, late benign (cutaneous, osseous, visceral gumma)	Total of 7.2 million units IM in doses of 2.4 million units at 7-day intervals during a 21-day period	Total of 9 million units IM in doses of 600,000 units/day during a 15-day period
Symptomatic or asymptomatic neurosyphilis	2-4 million units aqueous (crystalline) penicillin G IV q4h for at least 10 days	2-4 million units procaine penicillin IM daily and probenecid 500 mg orally four times daily, for 10-14 days
Congenital		
Infants	CSF normal: total of 50,000 units/kg IM in a single or divided dose at one session	CSF abnormal: total of 50,000 units/kg/day IM for 10 consecutive days‡
Older children	CSF normal: same as for early congenital syphilis, up to 2.4 million units	CSF abnormal: 200,000-300,000 units/kg/day aqueous crystalline penicillin IV for 10-14 days

*In *pregnancy*, treatment depends on the stage of syphilis.
†Individual doses can be divided for injection in each buttock to minimize discomfort.
‡For aqueous penicillin, give in two divided intravenous doses per day; for procaine penicillin, give as one daily dose intramuscularly.
CSF = cerebrospinal fluid.

treated to prevent possible disease in the neonate. After treatment, a quantitative RPR titer should be monitored monthly; if it rises four-fold, the patient should be treated a second time.

Congenital Syphilis

Proper treatment of the mother usually prevents active congenital syphilis in the neonate. However, infected infants may be clinically normal at birth, and the infant may be seronegative if the mother's infection was acquired late in pregnancy. The infant should be treated at birth if the mother has received no treatment or inadequate treatment or has been treated with drugs other than penicillin, if the mother has not yet responded to possibly effective therapy, or if the infant cannot be carefully monitored for several months after birth. The infant's CSF should be examined before treatment. If the CSF is normal, the child can be treated with a single intramuscular injection of 50,000 units/kg (up to 2.4 million units) of benzathine penicillin G. If the CSF is abnormal, the infant should be treated with 50,000 units/kg of aqueous penicillin G given intramuscularly or intravenously twice daily for a minimum of 10 days. Alternatively, a single daily intramuscular injection of 50,000 units/kg of procaine penicillin may be given for 10 days. Antimicrobial agents other than penicillin are not recommended for treatment of congenital syphilis.

Jarisch-Herxheimer Reactions

Up to 60% of patients with early syphilis and a significant proportion of patients with later stages of syphilis experience a transient febrile reaction after therapy for syphilis. The pathogenesis is unclear, but it may be caused by the liberation of antigens from spirochetes.

This reaction usually occurs in the first few hours after therapy, peaks at 6 to 8 hours, and disappears within 12 to 24 hours of therapy. On occasion, Jarisch-Herxheimer reactions are mistaken for allergic reactions to syphilis therapy. Temperature elevation is usually low grade, and there is often associated myalgia, headache, and malaise. The skin lesions of secondary syphilis are frequently exacerbated during the Jarisch-Herxheimer reaction, and cutaneous lesions that were not visible may become visible. The reaction is generally of no clinical significance and in most cases can be treated with salicylates. Corticosteroids have been used to prevent adverse effects of the Jarisch-Herxheimer reaction, but there is no evidence that they are clinically beneficial (other than reducing fever) or necessary. Institution of treatment with small doses of penicillin does not prevent the reaction.

PREVENTION

All patients with syphilis should be reported to public health authorities. In the absence of an effective vaccine, control of syphilis depends on finding and treating persons with infectious lesions of primary and secondary syphilis before they can transmit the disease as well as finding and treating individuals with incubating syphilis before infectious lesions develop. All patients with early syphilis (primary, secondary, or early latent) should be carefully interviewed by qualified persons to determine the nature of their recent sexual contacts. Approximately 16% of the named recent contacts of patients with early syphilis are found to have active, untreated syphilis on examination, and a similar proportion of individuals named as suspects or associates also have active syphilis.

Treatment of the sexual contacts of patients with early syphilis with 2.4 million units of benzathine penicillin G intramuscularly is recommended even if the contacts are clinically and serologically normal on examination. This is because syphilis eventually develops in 30% of clinically normal contacts who are untreated. In general, preventive treatment is given to all sexual contacts in the past 90 days, although nearly all cases of syphilis in contacts develop within 60 days of exposure.

PROGNOSIS

Follow-up Examinations

All HIV-seronegative patients with early or congenital syphilis should return for quantitative VDRL titers and clinical examination 6 and 12 months after treatment. For HIV-positive patients, serologic tests should be repeated at 1, 2, 3, 6, 9, and 12 months. Patients with late latent syphilis should also be examined 24 months after therapy.

In about 80 to 85% of patients with early (i.e., primary, secondary, or early latent) syphilis, quantitative RPR titers decline two or more dilutions (fourfold) by 6 and 12 months after therapy. In serofast patients, prolonged reactive RPR test results are associated with older age, lower initial RPR titers, prolonged infection, or more advanced stage (primary < secondary < early latent) infection.[13] Re-treatment of patients with serofast RPR results at 6 months leads to serologic response to syphilis in a minority of patients.[14] Chronic, low-titer RPR reactivity after therapy is much more common in cases of late syphilis and should not be viewed with alarm. Treponemal test results may remain positive for years despite adequate therapy. A four-fold or greater rise in RPR titer after therapy is sufficient evidence for repeated treatment. Patients with treated early syphilis are susceptible to reinfection, and many clinical and serologic relapses after therapy are probably reinfections. As such, they represent failures of proper epidemiologic case finding and preventive therapy for the patient's sexual contacts.

Patients with neurosyphilis should be monitored with serologic tests for at least 3 years and with repeated CSF examinations at 6-month intervals. CSF pleocytosis is the first abnormality to disappear, but cell counts may not be normal for 1 to 2 years. Elevated CSF protein levels fall even more slowly, followed by a change in the positive CSF VDRL test result, which may take years to become negative. It is not known whether high-dose intravenous penicillin therapy accelerates the return of CSF to normal. Rising CSF cell counts, protein level, and CSF VDRL titer obtained at follow-up are an indication for repeated treatment.

Antibiotic therapy should ultimately cure essentially all patients with early or secondary syphilis, although treatment failures may occur in patients with concomitant HIV infection. In tabes dorsalis, penicillin usually arrests progression but does not reverse the symptoms. Meningovascular syphilis generally responds well, except for residual damage resulting from ischemic infarcts.

Grade A Reference

A1. Bai ZG, Wang B, Yang K, et al. Azithromycin versus penicillin G benzathine for early syphilis. *Cochrane Database Syst Rev.* 2012;6:CD007270.

GENERAL REFERENCES

For the General References and other additional features, please visit Expert Consult at https://expertconsult.inkling.com.

320

NONSYPHILITIC TREPONEMATOSES

EDWARD W. HOOK III

DEFINITION

The nonsyphilitic treponematoses—yaws, endemic syphilis (previously known as bejel), and pinta—are the spirochetal diseases caused by *Treponema pallidum* subspecies (yaws and endemic syphilis) or by the closely related organism *Treponema carateum* (pinta). Like syphilis, the nonsyphilitic treponematoses are usually transmitted through direct contact with an infectious cutaneous or mucosal lesion. The natural history of the nonsyphilitic treponematoses also has a number of similarities to that of syphilis (Chapter 319).

The Pathogen

Yaws is caused by *T. pallidum* subspecies *pertenue*, endemic syphilis is caused by *T. pallidum* subspecies *endemicum*, and pinta is caused by *T. carateum*. The *T. pallidum* subspecies causing nonsyphilitic treponematoses are closely related to *T. pallidum* subspecies *pallidum*, which causes venereal syphilis; there is a high degree (more than 99%) of DNA homology, and they share unique pathogen-restricted antigens.[1] Analyses of recently described genetic sequence variations among *T. pallidum* subspecies promise the eventual clarification of pathophysiologic differences among the subspecies as well as answers to the age-old question of the origins of syphilis. Like *T. pallidum*, these treponemes are spirochetal bacteria with helical structures and measure about 0.2 μm in diameter and 10 μm in length. They are visible by dark-field microscopy but cannot be cultivated for prolonged periods in vitro.

EPIDEMIOLOGY

Worldwide, the nonsyphilitic treponematoses are rare. However, rates are increasing (particularly for yaws) in some regions where previous World Health Organization (WHO)–coordinated control programs had dramatically reduced disease prevalence. Yaws is prevalent in moist, humid regions, including rural areas of tropical Africa, the Americas, Southeast Asia, and Oceania. The highest incidence occurs in children between 2 and 5 years of age. Endemic syphilis occurs in more arid climates, including Africa, eastern Mediterranean countries, the Arabian peninsula, central Asia, and Australia. Pinta occurs in rural areas of tropical Central and South America and affects mostly older children and adolescents. Humans are the only known carriers of the nonsyphilitic treponematoses, although *T. pallidum* strains associated with genital lesions have recently been described in African baboons, potentially providing a clue to the origin of human treponemal infections, including syphilis.[2] The spirochete enters the skin only after it is broken, such as by a scratch or an insect bite. Transmission is believed to occur by contact of the skin directly or by indirect contamination through hands or fomites; it is facilitated by conditions of poor personal hygiene and crowding.

PATHOBIOLOGY

Primary nodular or ulcerative lesions typically develop at sites of inoculation after an incubation period of several weeks. Untreated primary lesions serve as a source for local spread through scratching or for hematogenous dissemination, which gives rise to a secondary stage of infection characterized by the development of widespread manifestations involving the skin, lymph nodes, and bone or cartilage. Without therapy, the primary and secondary manifestations of infection resolve, and the infection becomes latent, detectable only with serologic testing; however, periodic recurrent secondary manifestations may occur for several years. A proportion of persons with long-standing untreated infection are at risk for late sequelae, which may include bone deformity, destruction of nasal cartilage, or chronic skin changes. Unlike syphilis, the nonsyphilitic treponematoses are primarily diseases of children, are not transmitted across the placenta, and do not invade the central nervous system to cause clinical disease.

CLINICAL MANIFESTATIONS

Yaws,[3] the most common nonsyphilitic treponematosis, produces a skin papule at the inoculation site after an incubation period of 3 to 4 weeks. The most common sites are the legs and buttocks. The papule enlarges, ulcerates, and forms a serous crust from which treponemes can be recovered. Regional lymphadenitis may accompany the papule, which heals spontaneously within 6 months. A generalized secondary rash occurs before or after the initial lesion heals; this rash is also papular and is often covered with brown crusts. Relapsing crops of lesions can occur. Papillomas may result, and the plantar surfaces of the feet are involved with hyperkeratotic lesions. Periostitis of the long bones leads to tenderness, and fever may be present. Relapsing lesions of early yaws may occur during a period of several years and result in chronic ulcerations and destructive gummatous lesions affecting the skin and bones.

Endemic syphilis produces patches on the mucous membranes of the oral cavity and pharynx and can cause split papules at the mucocutaneous junction of the oral angles. Anal, genital, and other intertriginous skin areas can be affected by lesions that resemble secondary syphilis. Regional lymphadenitis is common, and generalized rashes are rare. Healing of these early lesions is followed by latency, manifested as seropositivity, or by late lesions that resemble gummatous tertiary syphilis (Chapter 319). Lesions include nodular skin ulcers, bone deformities, and ulcerative lesions that can perforate the palate.

Pinta starts similarly as a cutaneous papule with regional lymphadenitis, followed by a generalized maculopapular eruption. One to 3 years after healing of the initial lesion, large hyperpigmented brown or blue macules develop; they subsequently lose their pigment and become white. The time required for lesions to pass through these stages varies, so the same patient may have coexisting areas of increased pigment and loss of pigment.

DIAGNOSIS

The clinical differentiation of the nonsyphilitic treponematoses from one another and from syphilis may be challenging, requiring the integration of epidemiologic features, clinical findings, and supportive but not diagnostic laboratory test results. The skin lesions of the endemic treponematoses may resemble other cutaneous processes, including impetigo (Chapter 439), scabies, cutaneous fungal infections (Chapter 438), and other diseases. By dark-field microscopy, the causative spirochetes from early skin lesions can be observed directly; however, dark-field microscopy is rarely available in settings where nonsyphilitic treponematoses are seen. There is no specific test for any of the nonsyphilitic treponematoses, but serologic tests for syphilis detect cross-reacting antibodies in these diseases. The rapid plasma reagin (RPR) test, the Venereal Disease Research Laboratory (VDRL) test, and the fluorescent treponemal antibody absorption (FTA-ABS) test as well as other specific treponemal tests give positive results if serum is obtained at least 2 weeks after the lesions initially appear.

PREVENTION

The prevalence of these diseases was reduced dramatically in the 1950s by mass penicillin treatment campaigns. The WHO campaign treated about 53 million cases of yaws and 350,000 cases of pinta in the 1950s, with good results. These campaigns, however, were not adequate to eradicate the disease, and in recent years, the prevalence of yaws has increased, with foci of infection now reported in sub-Saharan Africa, several Pacific islands including Indonesia, and the Amazon region of South America. Current estimates are that as many as 2.5 million persons are infected worldwide, 75% of whom are younger than 15 years. Whereas penicillin is effective for both treatment and prevention of infection, requirements for cold chain transport, parenteral administration, and allergies sometimes compromise the utility of the drug.

Recent studies demonstrating the efficacy of single-dose oral azithromycin have expanded practical intervention strategies and led to renewed emphasis on yaws eradication by the WHO with targeted mass therapy.[4]

TREATMENT AND PROGNOSIS   Rx

Single-dose, long-acting benzathine penicillin G, 1.2 million units intramuscularly, has been the preferred treatment in patients with early lesions. For patients with late manifestations, this therapy should be repeated twice at approximately 7-day intervals. The early lesions heal rapidly, and most seropositive cases convert to seronegative status. Late destructive lesions take longer to show improvement. A randomized trial demonstrated oral azithromycin, 30 mg/kg up to a maximal dose of 2.0 g, to be as effective as penicillin for yaws therapy, providing the first readily administered, single-dose alternative to penicillin for treatment and prevention of nonsyphilitic treponematoses.[A1]

Grade A Reference

A1. Mitja O, Hays R, Ipai A, et al. Single-dose azithromycin versus benzathine benzylpenicillin for treatment of yaws in children in Papua New Guinea: an open-label, non-inferiority, randomized trial. *Lancet.* 2012;379:342-347.

GENERAL REFERENCES

For the General References and other additional features, please visit Expert Consult at https://expertconsult.inkling.com.

321

LYME DISEASE

GARY P. WORMSER

DEFINITION

Lyme disease (also known as Lyme borreliosis) is a zoonotic infection that is transmitted by certain *Ixodes* tick species and caused by a group of related spirochetes referred to formally as *Borrelia burgdorferi* sensu lato, or more simply as Lyme borrelia.[1] Lyme disease was first described in 1977 after an investigation of a cluster of cases of arthritis among children living in the area of Lyme, Connecticut. With more than 25,000 cases reported annually, it is the most common vector-borne infection in the United States; Lyme disease is also an infection of public health importance in both Europe and Asia. The most common clinical manifestation is a characteristic skin lesion called erythema migrans. This lesion is a result of inflammation associated with the centrifugal spread of the spirochete within the skin from the site where the tick deposited the microorganism. The spirochete may also spread hematogenously to other skin locations, resulting in secondary erythema migrans skin lesions, or to non-skin sites, such as the joints, nervous system, or heart, leading to a variety of extracutaneous clinical manifestations.[2]

The Pathogen

In the United States, the only species of Lyme borrelia known to cause human infection is *B. burgdorferi* (also referred to as *B. burgdorferi* sensu stricto). Although *B. burgdorferi* also causes Lyme disease in Europe, collectively other species of Lyme borrelia that can be distinguished genotypically account for the majority of infections there, especially *Borrelia afzelii* and *Borrelia garinii*. The fact that at least six species of Lyme borrelia may cause infection in Europe has created serodiagnostic challenges and accounts for a wider variety of possible clinical manifestations there than in the United States (see later). *B. garinii* appears to be the most neurotropic and *B. burgdorferi* the most arthritogenic among the species of Lyme borrelia.

Lyme borrelia are motile, microaerophilic, spirochetal bacteria with 3 to 10 loose coils arranged in a helical shape. The cells are 10 to 30 μm in length and 0.2 to 0.5 μm in width and contain at least seven periplasmic flagella that are responsible for the organism's motility. Borrelia are too thin to be seen by Gram stain, but live organisms can be visualized by dark-field or phase contrast microscopy. In tissues, they can be recognized by light microscopy after application of silver stains or by fluorescent microscopic methods. *B. burgdorferi* was the first spirochete for which the complete genome was sequenced. Genetic studies suggest the nearly complete absence of biosynthetic pathways, making the microorganism dependent on its environment for nutritional requirements.[3] Lyme borrelia can be grown in vitro in a highly enriched culture medium.

EPIDEMIOLOGY

In the United States, more than 95% of cases of Lyme disease are concentrated in just 14 states: 12 eastern states and two in the North Central region. The states with the largest number of cases are Pennsylvania, Massachusetts, New York, New Jersey, and Connecticut. *Ixodes scapularis* (also known as the deer tick or black-legged tick) is the tick vector in these states. *Ixodes pacificus* is the vector for cases that occur in the Northwest region. Lyme disease also occurs in limited areas of Canada. Cases of Lyme disease occur throughout the temperate regions of Europe and are especially common in Scandinavia and countries of central Europe such as Slovenia, Austria, and Germany. *Ixodes ricinus* transmits the infection in Europe, and *Ixodes persulcatus* is the vector in the Asian region of Russia, China, and Japan.

The principal reservoirs for Lyme borrelia (i.e., source of infection for ticks) in the United States and Eurasia are small mammals such as mice and certain species of birds. Deer play an essential role in the life cycle of the *I. scapularis* tick species but are not a competent reservoir for *B. burgdorferi*.

Although Lyme borrelia exist in enzootic cycles in the southern United States, cases of Lyme disease arising indigenously have not been well documented in states south of Virginia. A skin lesion that resembles erythema migrans does occur in the southern United States, however, but it is associated with the bite of the *Amblyomma americanum* tick, a tick species that is not a competent vector for *B. burgdorferi*. This condition is of unknown etiology and is referred to as southern tick-associated rash illness (STARI).

The likelihood of acquiring Lyme disease is directly related to exposure to environments in which infected ticks are present. Of the three feeding stages in the life cycle of *I. scapularis*, the second or nymphal stage is the most important epidemiologically for transmission of infection to humans. The first or larval stage is uninfected and cannot transmit this infection. Although the third stage (i.e., the adult stage of the tick) is more likely to be infected with *B. burgdorferi* than the nymphal stage is, it is less important in transmission to humans because this stage is present in smaller numbers in the environment and because there is less human activity outdoors during the time periods in the spring and fall when this stage is seeking a blood meal. In addition, adult ticks are larger and their bites cause more skin irritation than bites of nymphal ticks do, thereby increasing the likelihood that they will be noticed and detached by a person who has been bitten. If they are not removed, *Ixodes* ticks will usually feed for at least 3 days (Fig. 321-1). Transmission of *B. burgdorferi* by *I. scapularis* or *I. pacificus* ticks is typically delayed for more than 36 hours from the start of the blood meal, providing the opportunity to prevent infection simply by finding and removing the tick.[4] Transmission of *B. afzelii* by the European tick *I. ricinus* is considerably faster, however, often occurring within the first 24 hours of feeding.

Most cases of erythema migrans in the United States occur during June through August. There is a bimodal age distribution, with the highest incidences in children 5 to 9 years old and in adults 45 to 54 years of age, but individuals of all ages are at risk. The reported incidence of Lyme disease in the United States is rising, partially as a result of expansion of the deer population and the spread of infected *I. scapularis* ticks to new geographic areas.

Extracutaneous manifestations are somewhat less likely than erythema migrans to occur during June to August because the time from the tick bite until the onset of these manifestations is longer. Because adult *I. scapularis* ticks may become active on warm days during the winter, cases of erythema migrans may occasionally occur even in the colder months.

PATHOBIOLOGY

B. burgdorferi resides in the midgut of the *Ixodes* tick through attachment of its outer surface protein A (OspA) to the cells lining this site. With the onset

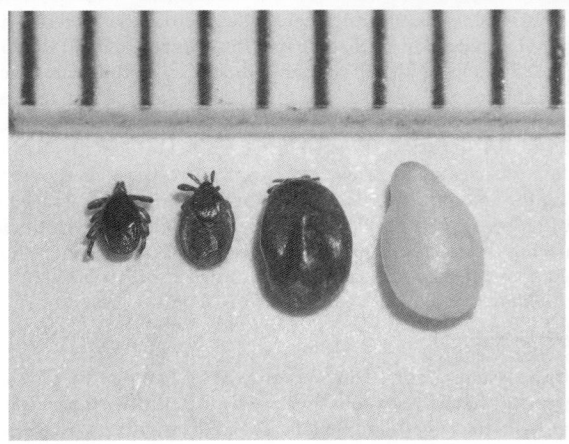

FIGURE 321-1. From left to right is an unfed nymphal stage *Ixodes scapularis* tick, a nymphal stage *I. scapularis* tick after about 48 hours of feeding, a nymphal stage *I. scapularis* tick after about 126 hours of feeding, and a sesame seed. The distance between the ruler marks is 1 mm. (Courtesy Kam Truhn of Fordham University.)

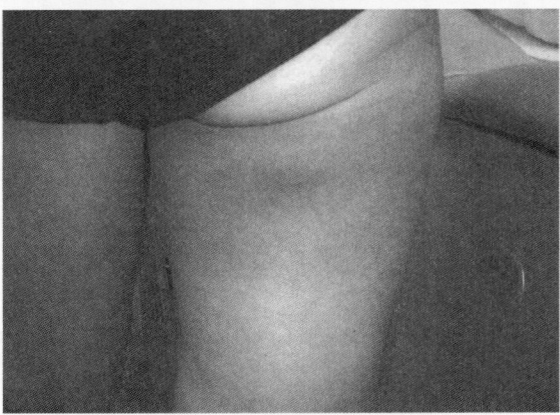

FIGURE 321-2. Erythema migrans skin lesion on the posterior aspect of the right thigh.

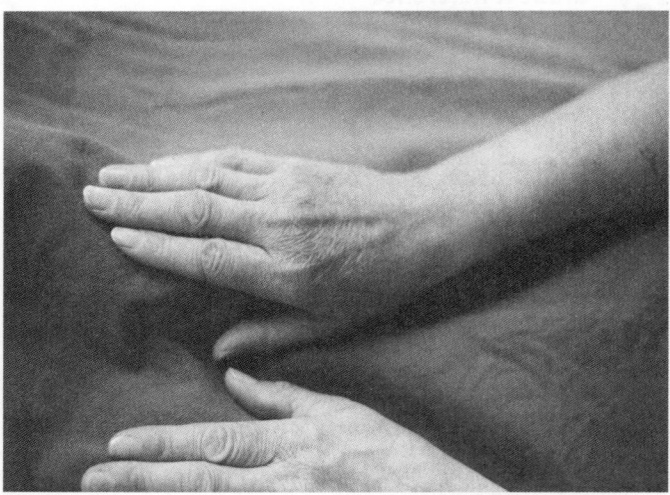

FIGURE 321-3. Acrodermatitis chronica atrophicans. This late cutaneous manifestation of Lyme borreliosis is characterized by slowly expanding red violaceous lesions that typically involve the dorsal surfaces of acral sites and do not heel spontaneously. The lesions are initially inflammatory and later on more and more atrophic. (Courtesy Dr. Franc Strle.)

of the blood meal, because of changes in temperature, pH, and probably other factors, the spirochete increases in number and undergoes a sequence of phenotypic changes including downregulation of OspA expression and upregulation of another outer surface protein, OspC.[5] This set of events releases the spirochete from the midgut and permits migration to the salivary gland. At that site, OspC binds to a salivary protein, Salp15, that is induced during the blood meal in borrelia-infected ticks; this protects the spirochete from antibody-mediated killing and aids in transmission to a vertebrate host. *Ixodes* tick saliva also contains other components with anti-inflammatory and immunomodulatory actions that serve to promote infection with Lyme borrelia and other tick-transmitted pathogens. Expression of OspC by the spirochete in the mammalian host is essential for infection to be established because in some manner this protein protects the microorganism from immediate elimination by the innate immune system.

The spirochete is deposited by the tick into the skin rather than directly into the blood stream. Hematogenous dissemination seems to be an important mechanism responsible for spread of the spirochete to other sites. Alternatively, spread of the spirochete to other sites might occur through tissue planes. The likelihood of entry into the blood stream is affected by the strain of Lyme borrelia causing the infection.[6] Unlike patients who are bacteremic with more conventional pathogens, patients with spirochetemia rarely appear "septic." In one study, only 5% of 93 spirochetemic patients were febrile when the blood culture specimen was obtained, and almost none was found to have leukocytosis. The lack of fever and other clinical signs of sepsis may be due to the absence of lipopolysaccharide within the borrelial cell wall.

Infection of humans or animals elicits innate and adaptive immune responses resulting in both macrophage and antibody-mediated killing of the spirochete. The inflammatory response in tissue typically shows an infiltration of lymphocytes, macrophages, and plasma cells, although granulocytes predominate in synovial fluid samples of Lyme arthritis patients. The potential for persistence of infection despite a robust humoral and cellular immunologic response is, however, typical of infection with Lyme borrelia, as it is with *Treponema pallidum* infection. The virulence factors responsible for persistence of infection include the spirochete's ability to downregulate expression of certain immunogenic surface-exposed proteins, including OspC, and to alter rapidly and continually by recombination the antigenic properties of a surface lipoprotein known as variable major protein–like sequence expressed (VlsE). In addition, the ability of the spirochete to bind avidly to various components of the extracellular matrix may also contribute to persistence.

All of the objective clinical manifestations of Lyme disease are thought to be due to an inflammatory response to live spirochetes or to their undegraded antigens. Obliterative endarteritis has been seen histologically in synovial tissue, but its importance in pathogenesis is unclear. Lyme borrelia are not known to produce toxins. In humans, the only role so far established for host genetic factors is in the development of antibiotic-refractory Lyme arthritis, which is seen most often in patients with certain HLA DR alleles, some of which coincide with those associated with rheumatoid arthritis.

CLINICAL MANIFESTATIONS

The clinical manifestations are often categorized as follows:
- Early localized infection, typically manifested by a single erythema migrans (Fig. 321-2) skin lesion, with or without viral infection–like symptoms, but without objective extracutaneous manifestations
- Early disseminated infection, usually manifested by multiple erythema migrans skin lesions or by an objective manifestation of early neurologic Lyme disease or Lyme carditis
- Late disease, usually manifested by arthritis but may also include certain rare neurologic manifestations or the skin condition known as acrodermatitis chronica atrophicans (Fig. 321-3)

Children and adults have similar clinical manifestations. The expected frequency of the various clinical presentations is well illustrated by a study of 313 cases of Lyme disease diagnosed in Wurzburg, Germany, during a 12-month period. In this series, erythema migrans by itself was seen in 89% of cases, early neurologic manifestations in 3%, cardiac manifestations in less than 1%, borrelial lymphocytoma in 2%, arthritis in 5%, and acrodermatitis chronica atrophicans in 1%. None of the patients had late neurologic Lyme disease. A similar distribution of cases has been seen in recent case series in the United States, except for the absence of borrelial lymphocytoma and acrodermatitis chronica atrophicans. In earlier studies in the United States from the 1980s, there was a much higher proportion of patients who had neurologic, cardiac, or joint manifestations. This may have been due to a bias of ascertainment in the older studies or to improved recognition and

TABLE 321-1	CLINICAL SYMPTOMS AND SIGNS PRESENT IN AT LEAST 20% OF PATIENTS WITH ERYTHEMA MIGRANS	
CHARACTERISTIC	**UNITED STATES (95% CI)**	
Viral infection-like	65% (52-76%)	
Fatigue	47% (37-58%)	
Headache	36% (27-46%)	
Myalgias	35% (26-45%)	
Arthralgias	35% (25-46%)	
Fever	33% (23-43%)	
Stiff neck	31% (21-43%)	
Lymphadenopathy	22% (13-33%)	
Dysesthesia	20% (12-32%)	
	EUROPE (95% CI)	
Viral infection-like	37% (27-49%)	
Dysesthesia	35% (25-47%)	
Headache	20% (14-29%)	

CI = confidence interval.
Modified from Tibbles CD, Edlow JA. Does this patient have erythema migrans? *JAMA.* 2007;297:2617-2627.

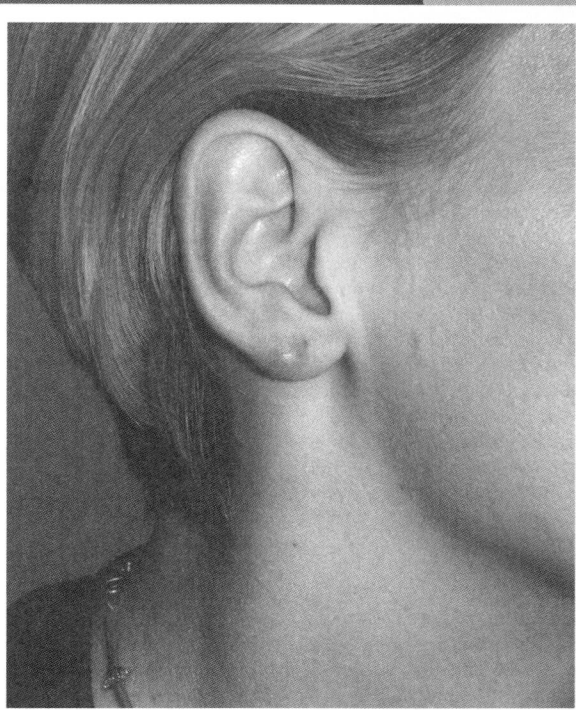

FIGURE 321-4. Borrelial lymphocytoma. A rare cutaneous manifestation of Lyme disease that is seen predominantly outside the United States, it is manifested as a solitary bluish red swelling most commonly on the earlobe of children and the breast in adults. (Courtesy Dr. Franc Strle.)

treatment of patients with erythema migrans more recently, thereby preventing the development of extracutaneous complications because they occur later.

Early Localized Infection
Single Erythema Migrans Skin Lesion
Erythema migrans is by far the most common clinical manifestation of Lyme disease. Although the appearance of the skin lesion is often distinctive (see Fig. 321-2), it is not pathognomonic for Lyme disease. Erythema migrans appears 7 to 14 days (range, 3 to 30 days) after tick detachment and is characterized by an expanding, flat to slightly raised, erythematous skin lesion (usually ≥5 cm in diameter) that is round or oval. The bite mark from the preceding tick bite can sometimes be identified at or near the center of the lesion and is called a punctum. Approximately 80% of patients in the United States with erythema migrans have just a single skin lesion. Nonspecific viral infection–like symptoms or signs, such as malaise, neck pain, headache, fatigue, migratory arthralgias, or chills and fever, may be present (Table 321-1) but are more common in patients infected with *B. burgdorferi* or *B. garinii* compared with *B. afzelii.* Prominent respiratory or gastrointestinal symptoms are highly atypical for Lyme disease. An acute febrile illness in the absence of a skin lesion or other objective clinical manifestation has been attributed to early Lyme disease, but the possibility of misdiagnosis is greater in this situation because of the potential for false-positive serologic test results.

Erythema migrans skin lesions can vary in appearance. Some (especially lesions of short duration) are nearly uniform in color, whereas others may show central clearing or a target-like appearance. About 5% have a vesicular-pustular center. Erythema migrans on the lower extremities may sometimes be purpuric. Erythema migrans lesions may be scaly when they are long-standing and fading or after topical corticosteroid creams have been applied. The most common locations include the thigh, back, shoulder, and calf. Lesions are often asymptomatic but can be mildly painful or pruritic, and tender regional lymphadenopathy may be present. The majority of U.S. patients with erythema migrans, as for all other clinical manifestations, do not recall a preceding tick bite.

Certain signs and symptoms that have been described in small numbers of patients with erythema migrans in early case series, such as hepatomegaly, splenomegaly, sore throat, conjunctivitis, or testicular swelling, may have been coincidental findings. There has been no microbiologic confirmation of borrelia infection at these sites.

Borrelial Lymphocytoma
Borrelial lymphocytoma is a rare cutaneous manifestation of Lyme disease that almost never occurs in the United States. It often is manifested at or near

a preceding tick bite as a solitary bluish red swelling with a diameter of up to a few centimeters. The most common locations are the earlobe in children and the breast in adults (Fig. 321-4). Histologic examination shows a dense polyclonal infiltration of the cutis and subcutis by predominantly B lymphocytes, frequently with germinal center formation. Histologic evaluation may be necessary to exclude malignant disease for patients with suspected borrelial lymphocytoma at a location other than the earlobe.

Early Disseminated Infection
Multiple Erythema Migrans Skin Lesions
In the United States, approximately 20% of patients with erythema migrans have multiple skin lesions at the time of presentation. Secondary erythema migrans skin lesions can be smaller than 5 cm, do not have a punctum, and are usually not tender or pruritic. They arise from hematogenous dissemination to the skin rather than from additional tick bites.

Early Neurologic Lyme Disease
Within weeks to several months after infection, patients may develop neurologic manifestations, the most common of which are cranial neuropathy (particularly peripheral seventh nerve palsy that may be bilateral), lymphocytic meningitis, and sensory (often painful) radiculopathy.[7] Less common manifestations, among others, include mononeuritis multiplex (multifocal involvement of anatomically unrelated nerves) and brachial or lumbosacral plexopathies. A pseudotumor cerebri–like picture has been reported occasionally in children. The presence of a concomitant erythema migrans lesion or the patient's recollection of a recent lesion consistent with erythema migrans may be helpful diagnostically. Studies suggest that approximately 90% of children with Lyme meningitis in the United States have at least one of the following three findings: concomitant erythema migrans, cranial nerve palsy, or papilledema.

Cardiac Lyme Disease
Weeks to months after infection, patients may develop cardiac manifestations of Lyme disease, most often fluctuating degrees of atrioventricular heart block or other manifestations of a myopericarditis, which may cause the patient to complain of lightheadedness, palpitations, dyspnea, chest pain, or syncope. Heart block is typically at or above the atrioventricular node.

Erythema migrans is often but not invariably present concurrently. Valvular dysfunction is not known to occur, and chronic cardiomyopathy has been reported only rarely in Europe.

Late Lyme Disease
Lyme Arthritis
If patients with erythema migrans in the United States are not treated with antibiotics, approximately 60% will develop a monarticular or oligoarticular arthritis at a mean time of 6 months after disease onset (range, 4 days to as long as 2 years). In untreated patients, Lyme arthritis is characterized by intermittent attacks of synovitis that last for a few weeks to several months. One or two joints are involved at a time. Primarily large joints are affected,[8] but there may be involvement of the temporomandibular joint, small joints, and periarticular sites. The most commonly involved joint is the knee. Baker's cysts may form and rupture. Joint swelling is often pronounced, but pain is usually relatively modest. Particularly in children, there may be concomitant fever, but adults are often minimally symptomatic aside from the arthritis.

In about 10% of adult patients with Lyme arthritis in the United States, involvement of a large joint (almost always the knee) may persist despite appropriate antibiotic treatment. Erosion of cartilage or bone may develop in such cases.

Late Neurologic Lyme Disease
After months to years of infection, late neurologic manifestations may develop. These include encephalomyelitis, peripheral neuropathy, and encephalopathy. Because most patients with Lyme disease are now diagnosed and treated early in the course of infection, these more indolent forms of neurologic Lyme disease are rare.

In untreated patients, encephalomyelitis has been monophasic and slowly progressive, mainly involving white matter. It is the most severe neurologic manifestation and, although infrequent, is probably more common in Europe than in the United States. Cerebrospinal fluid (CSF) examination typically shows a lymphocytic pleocytosis, a moderately elevated protein level, and a normal glucose level, with evidence of intrathecal production of antibody to borrelia. Magnetic resonance imaging of the affected part of the brain or spinal cord can demonstrate areas of inflammation, typically with increased signal on T2 and fluid attenuation inversion recovery imaging and enhancement after administration of contrast material.

In the United States, peripheral neuropathy typically is manifested as a mild, diffuse "stocking-glove" process. Patients typically complain of intermittent limb paresthesias and sometimes radicular pain. The most common abnormality on neurologic examination is reduced vibratory sensation of the distal lower extremities. Electrophysiologic studies show a patchy axonal neuropathy. Nerve biopsy shows axonal loss and small perivascular collections of lymphocytes without spirochetes. CSF findings are often normal without evidence of intrathecal antibody production.

Encephalopathy is an imprecisely defined clinical entity characterized by mild abnormalities of memory or other cognitive functions that are demonstrable on either a careful mental status examination or on formal neuropsychological testing. CSF examination findings may be completely normal or may show intrathecal antibody production, mild CSF protein elevation, or a mild pleocytosis. Cranial imaging studies may occasionally demonstrate focal areas of presumed parenchymal inflammation, but findings are most often normal.

Acrodermatitis Chronica Atrophicans
Acrodermatitis chronica atrophicans is a late skin manifestation of Lyme disease that is most commonly seen in women older than 40 years.[9] This skin lesion develops insidiously several years after initial infection, usually on the extensor surfaces of the hands and feet. Early lesions are characterized by a slight bluish red discoloration and doughy swelling. Histologic examination shows lymphocytes and plasma cells in the skin and sometimes in the subcutis, with or without atrophy. Initially unilateral, the lesion may later become bilateral. Over time, there is resolution of the edema with development of skin atrophy. Nodules may develop over bone prominences. About two thirds of patients have an associated peripheral neuropathy of the affected extremity, manifested primarily as local sensory loss.

Although presumably any of the species of Lyme borrelia may cause acrodermatitis chronica atrophicans, by far the most common etiologic agent is *B. afzelii*.[1] Therefore, this manifestation is rarely seen in the United States.

General Laboratory Testing
White blood cell count, hemoglobin and hematocrit levels, and platelet count are usually normal in Lyme disease, unless coinfection with *Anaplasma phagocytophilum*, *Babesia microti*, or a tick-borne encephalitis virus is present (see later). Lymphopenia, however, may be found in the absence of a recognized coinfection.[10] In patients with erythema migrans, mild abnormalities of liver function tests (particularly elevations of aspartate and alanine aminotransferase levels) can be seen in approximately 35% of patients. The erythrocyte sedimentation rate may be modestly elevated in all stages of Lyme disease, but values greater than 80 mm/hour are distinctly uncommon.

CSF examination in Lyme meningitis typically shows a pleocytosis with more than 90% lymphocytes, a modestly elevated protein level, and a normal glucose level. Synovial fluid examination in Lyme arthritis typically shows approximately 25,000 white cells/mm^3 (range, 500 to 110,000/mm^3) with a polymorphonuclear predominance.

Serologic Testing
Erythema migrans skin lesions may go unnoticed by the patient because of the absence of prominent local symptoms and occurrence on parts of the body that are difficult for the patient to visualize. Therefore, a complete skin examination should be performed for any patient thought to have early localized or disseminated Lyme disease. Erythema migrans is the only clinical manifestation sufficiently distinctive to allow a clinical diagnosis in the absence of a supporting laboratory test. Erythema migrans is diagnosed on the basis of recognition of the characteristic appearance of the skin lesion in persons who live in or have recently traveled to areas endemic for Lyme disease. Because of the short duration of infection at this stage, serologic assays for antibodies to Lyme borrelia are infrequently positive and thus should be obtained only in atypical cases, then in conjunction with convalescent-phase serologic testing 2 to 4 weeks after the acute sample is obtained (Table 321-2).

For non–erythema migrans presentations of Lyme disease, the mainstay of laboratory diagnosis is two-tier serologic testing in which the first tier test is usually a sensitive enzyme-linked immunosorbent assay (EIA). If the EIA result is positive or equivocal, separate IgM and IgG immunoblots are performed on the original serum sample. If symptoms have persisted for at least 4 weeks, then specifically the IgG immunoblot should be positive for the results to be interpreted as evidence of seropositivity. Untreated patients who remain seronegative for 6 to 8 weeks are unlikely to have Lyme disease, and other possible diagnoses should be pursued.

Omitting the first-tier EIA or interpreting the immunoblot with alternative criteria that are not evidence based will potentially decrease the specificity of testing and is not recommended. False-positive results on the IgM immunoblot may be due to cross-reactive antibodies that arise from polyclonal B-cell

TABLE 321-2	DIAGNOSIS OF LYME DISEASE	
DIAGNOSTIC MODALITY	**APPLICATION**	**COMMENT**
Visual inspection	Erythema migrans	Usually seronegative at time of presentation
Two-tier serology with a positive IgM and/or IgG immunoblot	Lyme carditis	Look for concomitant erythema migrans
	Early neurologic Lyme disease	Look for concomitant erythema migrans; intrathecal antibody may be detectable before serum antibody in Europe; PCR sometimes positive in CSF
	Borrelial lymphocytoma	Biopsy may be needed to exclude malignant neoplasm
Two-tier serology with a positive IgG immunoblot	Lyme arthritis	PCR often positive in synovial fluid
	Late neurologic Lyme disease	Intrathecal antibody positivity expected in Lyme encephalomyelitis
	Acrodermatitis chronica atrophicans	

CSF = cerebrospinal fluid; Ig = immunoglobulin; PCR = polymerase chain reaction.

stimulation. Probably the most common cause of false-positive results, however, is the overreading of nonspecific weak bands.[11] Background rates of seropositivity, which may exceed 4% in highly endemic areas of the United States with even higher rates than this in Europe, may also confound the interpretation of seroreactivity. Therefore, a positive serologic test result does not mean that the patient necessarily has active Lyme disease. The positive predictive value is most informative when the pretest probability based on the clinical features is at least 20%. Serologic testing is not indicated in routine follow-up of patients after treatment as either IgM or IgG borrelial antibodies may persist for many years in successfully treated patients.

Testing for borrelial antibody that is produced locally in the central nervous system (i.e., intrathecal antibody) may be helpful in the diagnosis of neurologic Lyme disease and has been reported to precede detection of serum antibody in a minority of European patients. Positive test results for intrathecal antibody may persist, however, for long periods after successful antibiotic treatment.

Other Diagnostic Modalities

Culture for Lyme borrelia is not routinely done or available to diagnose Lyme disease. It is unnecessary for patients with erythema migrans and too insensitive for patients with extracutaneous manifestations of Lyme disease. In contrast, polymerase chain reaction (PCR) for detection of borrelial DNA is positive on synovial fluid specimens in up to approximately 80% of untreated patients with Lyme arthritis, and a positive result lends support for this diagnosis in a patient who is IgG seropositive. The sensitivity of PCR in CSF tends to be much lower, however, and was only approximately 5% in a study of children from the United States with early neurologic Lyme disease. A negative PCR result on either type of fluid does not exclude Lyme disease.

Differential Diagnosis
Erythema Migrans

Tick-bite hypersensitivity reactions can be mistaken for erythema migrans, but these reactions occur within 48 hours of a tick bite, are usually pruritic, and tend to wane within a few days. In contrast, erythema migrans skin lesions in untreated patients will last for a median time of approximately 4 weeks in the United States and even longer in Europe. Bacterial cellulitis rarely occurs at the most frequent skin sites for erythema migrans and would not be expected to demonstrate central clearing or a target-like appearance. Erythema migrans, unlike erythema multiforme, does not involve the mucous membranes, palms, or soles. Southern tick-associated rash illness (STARI) is the most likely diagnosis in patients with erythema migrans–like skin lesions who were bitten by an *A. americanum* tick or developed this lesion in the southern United States (see under Pathobiology). Other considerations in the differential diagnosis of erythema migrans that usually can be readily distinguished include tinea (often pruritic with a thin, raised, scaly border), nummular eczema (symmetrical pruritic lesions with a tendency to scale and crust), granuloma annulare (acral location, especially on the dorsum of hands and feet, relatively fixed in size and <5 cm in diameter), contact dermatitis (pruritic with streaking along the area of contact and a vesicular component), urticaria (raised, pruritic, and usually <5 cm in diameter), fixed drug eruption (usually on genitals, hands, feet, or face and fixed in size), pityriasis rosea (multiple, moderately pruritic lesions with peripheral scale and relatively fixed in size), and spider bite (often very painful and necrotic with a central eschar).

Extracutaneous Lyme Disease

Included in the differential diagnosis of early neurologic Lyme disease is Bell's palsy. Even in highly endemic areas of the United States, other causes of seventh nerve palsy outnumber Lyme disease by a margin of 3 : 1. Viral meningitis and mechanical radiculopathy can also potentially be confused with manifestations of early neurologic Lyme disease. Viral or other causes of myopericarditis may resemble cardiac Lyme disease. Many causes of synovitis might be considered in the differential diagnosis of Lyme arthritis, but the pattern of joint involvement, such as symmetrical small joint involvement in rheumatoid arthritis, is often distinctly different from that found in Lyme arthritis. Lyme encephalomyelitis may occasionally be confused clinically with a first episode of relapsing-remitting multiple sclerosis or primary progressive multiple sclerosis. Testing for borrelial antibody in serum (and CSF for the last condition) usually suffices to differentiate these conditions from Lyme disease.

TREATMENT Rx

In vitro studies have shown that Lyme borrelia are highly susceptible to tetracyclines, most penicillins, and many second- and third-generation cephalosporins. *B. burgdorferi* is resistant to certain fluoroquinolones, rifampin, and first-generation cephalosporins. Whether macrolides are active in vitro depends on the borrelial strain tested and the assay technique used. Although most manifestations of Lyme disease will resolve spontaneously without treatment, antibiotic therapy may hasten resolution and prevent progression.

Oral antibiotic therapy is used to treat patients with erythema migrans (Table 321-3). Doxycycline, amoxicillin, and cefuroxime axetil are each highly effective and are the preferred agents for this indication. Macrolides such as azithromycin are somewhat less effective than other oral antibiotics and consequently are not recommended as first-line therapy.

Doxycycline alone among the first-line agents is effective against *A. phagocytophilum* coinfection and is the only agent for which a prospective clinical trial has demonstrated that just 10 days of treatment is effective.[A1] Doxycycline, however, may cause photosensitivity, which is a concern because early Lyme disease occurs most commonly during the summer months; in addition, this drug is relatively contraindicated in children younger than 8 years and in women who are pregnant or breast-feeding. When erythema migrans cannot be reliably distinguished from community-acquired bacterial cellulitis, either cefuroxime axetil or amoxicillin–clavulanate potassium (Augmentin) is preferred because these antimicrobials are generally effective against both types of infection.

Within 24 hours of initiation of antimicrobial therapy, up to 15% of patients treated for erythema migrans will experience a Jarisch-Herxheimer–like reaction characterized by an increase in the size or intensity of erythema in the skin lesion and more intense viral infection–like systemic symptoms. Fever, if present, should resolve within 48 hours and the skin lesion itself within 7 to 14 days. Other symptoms, such as fatigue or arthralgia, tend to improve but not invariably to resolve within this time frame, lasting for more than 3 months in one quarter of patients. Extending the initial course of treatment does not cause faster relief of symptoms. Oral antibiotic therapy is also used as first-line treatment for the other cutaneous manifestations of Lyme disease discussed elsewhere in this chapter and as initial treatment of patients with Lyme arthritis.

The preferred parenteral agent for Lyme disease is ceftriaxone because it is highly active against Lyme borrelia in vitro, crosses the blood-brain barrier well, and has a long serum half-life, allowing the convenience of once-daily administration. Alternative choices for parenterally administered antibiotics are cefotaxime and intravenous penicillin. Parenteral antibiotic therapy is recommended to treat patients with late neurologic Lyme disease and those with cardiac Lyme disease who are admitted to the hospital for monitoring (see Table 321-3). Parenteral antibiotics are often given to patients with Lyme arthritis who have failed to respond to one or more courses of oral antibiotic treatment.

TABLE 321-3 RECOMMENDED THERAPY FOR ADULT PATIENTS WITH LYME DISEASE*

THERAPY	MANIFESTATION	DURATION
Doxycycline 100 mg PO bid *or*	Erythema migrans	14 days
	Borrelial lymphocytoma	14 days
Amoxicillin 500 mg PO tid *or*	Acrodermatitis chronica atrophicans	21 days
	Lyme arthritis	28 days
Cefuroxime axetil 500 mg PO bid	Lyme carditis—mild	14 days
	Cranial neuropathy	14 days[†]
Doxycycline 100 mg PO bid	Lyme meningitis or radiculopathy in Europe and possibly in the United States	14 days
Ceftriaxone 2 g IV daily	Lyme arthritis that failed to respond to oral therapy	14-28 days
	Late neurologic Lyme disease	14-28 days
	Lyme carditis requiring hospitalization	14 days
	Lyme meningitis or radiculopathy in the United States	14 days
Azithromycin 500 mg PO daily	Erythema migrans in a patient intolerant of doxycycline and β-lactam antibiotics	6-10 days

*Regardless of the clinical manifestations of Lyme disease, complete response to treatment may be delayed beyond the treatment duration. Relapse may occur with any of these regimens; patients with objective signs of relapse may need another course of treatment.

[†]Although any one of first-line oral antibiotics appears to be effective in patients with cranial neuropathy, there is only limited experience in patients with a cranial neuropathy other than seventh nerve palsy or with agents other than doxycycline.

Modified from Wormser GP, Dattwyler RJ, Shapiro ED, et al. The clinical assessment, treatment, and prevention of Lyme disease, human granulocytic anaplasmosis, and babesiosis: clinical practice guidelines by the Infectious Diseases Society of America. *Clin Infect Dis.* 2006;43:1089-1134.

In the United States, parenteral therapy has been the preferred management strategy for early neurologic Lyme disease, especially for meningitis and radiculitis, with oral therapy reserved for patients with uncomplicated seventh nerve palsy. Studies conducted in Europe, however, have provided convincing evidence that oral doxycycline is just as effective as ceftriaxone for any of the primary manifestations of early neurologic Lyme disease.[A2] Although the same may be true in the United States, studies are lacking. Other oral antibiotics, such as amoxicillin, have been used successfully to treat patients with uncomplicated seventh nerve palsy, but published data on efficacy are much more limited for these agents. Available data indicate that seventh nerve palsy will resolve, with or without antibiotic treatment, and that the rate of recovery is not accelerated by antibiotics. Therefore, the primary reason to treat such patients is to prevent the subsequent development of later complications, particularly Lyme arthritis.

The presence of either papilledema or sixth cranial nerve palsy may indicate the presence of increased intracranial pressure in patients with neurologic Lyme disease. The elevated pressure will typically fall in response to antibiotic therapy, but other measures conventionally used to lower pressure may need to be considered in individual cases.

Symptomatic patients with cardiac Lyme disease and those with high-grade first-degree atrioventricular heart block (PR interval of ≥300 msec) and second- or third-degree block should be hospitalized and closely monitored. Temporary cardiac pacing may be required. In treated patients, complete heart block generally resolves within 1 week, and lesser conduction disturbances resolve within 6 weeks.

Lyme arthritis typically responds to antibiotic treatment. Patients whose arthritis is improved but not resolved after an initial course of oral therapy may be re-treated with a second course of oral antibiotics, with parenteral antibiotic therapy reserved for those without any significant clinical response. Approximately 10% of adult patients in the United States, however, do not respond clinically to antibiotic therapy and are said to have antibiotic-refractory Lyme arthritis; this condition has been defined as persistent synovitis for at least 2 months after completion of a course of intravenous ceftriaxone (or 1 month after completion of two 4-week courses of an oral antibiotic) in conjunction with negative PCR test results on synovial fluid and on synovial tissue if it is available. Because these patients are no longer believed to be actively infected, they are customarily treated with nonsteroidal anti-inflammatory agents, intra-articular injections of corticosteroids, or disease-modifying antirheumatic drugs. Arthroscopic synovectomy has also been used successfully for patients with this condition.

Pregnant patients with Lyme disease are generally treated similarly to non-pregnant patients except that doxycycline should be avoided because of the potential for adverse effects to both the fetus and the mother. No published data convincingly support a congenital Lyme disease syndrome.

Post–Lyme Disease Symptoms and Syndrome

The outcome of treatment in most patients with erythema migrans is excellent. Studies show, however, that when questioned at 6 months or more after treatment of erythema migrans, approximately 5 to 15% of patients will report purely subjective symptoms such as fatigue or musculoskeletal pains. These subjective symptoms are typically mild and may wax and wane in intensity. Patients who have them are referred to as having post–Lyme disease symptoms or syndrome, depending on the symptom duration and severity. The cause of these symptoms is currently unknown. Carefully done microbiologic evaluations in the United States have failed to find evidence of either persistent B. burgdorferi infection or a coinfection with a second Ixodes-transmitted pathogen. Furthermore, re-treatment has provided either no measurable benefit or a benefit so modest or ambiguous that it was outweighed by the risks associated with the antibiotic therapy.[A3] Therefore, symptomatic treatment is recommended for such patients. In addition, a prospective study conducted in Europe that for the first time also incorporated a "healthy control" group has challenged the notion that such a syndrome even exists. In this study, the frequency of unexplained subjective symptoms in the Lyme disease group was no higher than that in the control group by 6 months into follow-up.[12]

Chronic Lyme Disease

The term *chronic Lyme disease* is poorly defined but widely used. In Europe, the term has been used to refer to the objective manifestations that most authorities prefer to call late Lyme disease. Others have used the term to refer to patients with post–Lyme disease subjective complaints. Most often, chronic Lyme disease is used as a diagnosis for patients with persistent pain, neurocognitive complaints, or fatigue, without objective clinical or serologic evidence of past or present B. burgdorferi infection. In this usage, the term is a misnomer and has become the latest in a series of postulated syndromes that attempt to attribute "medically unexplained symptoms" to particular infections.[13]

Coinfections

Ixodes ticks may be coinfected with and transmit Lyme borrelia along with other pathogens, such as *A. phagocytophilum*, *B. microti* (the primary cause of babesiosis), and a tick-borne encephalitis virus. The likelihood of coinfection is dependent on the particular species of *Ixodes* tick and on the geographic area. Thus, bites from *I. scapularis* ticks in certain areas may lead to the development of Lyme disease, human granulocytic anaplasmosis, or babesiosis as a single infection or less frequently as a coinfection. In addition, this tick species can potentially transmit the deer tick virus subtype of the Powassan virus, an *Ehrlichia* species referred to as the *Ehrlichia muris*-like agent, and *Borrelia miyamotoi*.[14-16] In Europe, the most common coinfection is Lyme disease with tick-borne encephalitis virus infection.

Coinfection should be considered in patients from geographic areas endemic for these pathogens who present with more severe initial symptoms than are commonly observed with Lyme disease alone. In this situation, coinfection should be considered especially in those who have high-grade fever for more than 48 hours despite antibiotic therapy appropriate for Lyme disease; those who develop recurrent fever; and those who have unexplained leukopenia, thrombocytopenia, or anemia. Coinfection might also be considered in the situation in which there has been resolution of the erythema migrans skin lesion but either no improvement or worsening of the viral infection–like symptoms.

Reinfection

Patients treated for early Lyme disease do not appear to develop an immunologic response that is adequate to protect against reinfection with a different strain of *B. burgdorferi*.[17] Therefore patients with erythema migrans may become reinfected at a different skin site if they get a bite from another infected tick.[18] Reinfection has been well documented only in patients who were treated for early infection (nearly always erythema migrans) and not after late manifestations of Lyme disease, such as Lyme arthritis. Clinical manifestations of reinfection appear to be similar to those of the primary infection.

PREVENTION

Lyme disease can be prevented by avoiding tick-infested environments and by covering bare skin and using tick repellents on skin and clothing when in such environments. The tick density around individual residences can be reduced by removing leaf litter, placing wood chips where lawns abut forests, applying acaricides to property, and constructing fences to keep out deer. Bathing within 2 hours of tick exposure has been shown to decrease the risk of Lyme disease. Daily inspections of the entire skin surface (including scalp) to remove attached ticks is recommended because of the grace period between the time of tick attachment and transmission of *B. burgdorferi*. Removal is accomplished by grasping the tick as close to its mouth parts as possible with a forceps (or tweezers) and then gently pulling it out. Clinical studies have demonstrated that without any other intervention, more than 96% of patients who find and remove an attached *I. scapularis* tick will remain free of Lyme disease, even in highly endemic geographic regions. If the tick is not found or removed, the probability of infection approaches the infection rate in the regional tick population (typically >20% of nymphal stage *I. scapularis* ticks are infected in highly endemic areas of the Northeast and Midwest United States).

Evidence shows that doxycycline chemoprophylaxis can further reduce the chance for development of Lyme disease after removal of an *I. scapularis* tick. A single 200-mg dose of doxycycline is about 90% effective in preventing erythema migrans at the tick bite site.[A4] Use of a single dose of doxycycline within 72 hours of tick removal should be considered for persons in highly endemic areas who are known to have been bitten by a nymphal or adult *I. scapularis* tick that was estimated to have been attached for at least 36 hours. Given the uncertain efficacy of a short course of amoxicillin in this situation, observation rather than chemoprophylaxis has been recommended for individuals for whom doxycycline is contraindicated. No vaccine is currently available to prevent Lyme disease in humans.

Grade A References

A1. Wormser GP, Ramanathan R, Nowakowski J, et al. Duration of antibiotic therapy for early Lyme disease. A randomized, double-blind, placebo-controlled trial. *Ann Intern Med*. 2003;138:697-704.

A2. Ljostad U, Skogvoll E, Eikeland R, et al. Oral doxycycline versus intravenous ceftriaxone for European Lyme neuroborreliosis: a multicentre, non-inferiority, double-blind, randomised trial. *Lancet Neurol*. 2008;7:690-695.

A3. Klempner MS, Hu LT, Evans J, et al. Two controlled trials of antibiotic treatment in patients with persistent symptoms and a history of Lyme disease. *N Engl J Med*. 2001;345:85-92.

A4. Warshafsky S, Lee DH, Francois LK, et al. Efficacy of antibiotic prophylaxis for the prevention of Lyme disease: an updated systematic review and meta-analysis. *J Antimicrob Chemother*. 2010;65:1137-1144.

GENERAL REFERENCES

For the General References and other additional features, please visit Expert Consult at https://expertconsult.inkling.com.

322

RELAPSING FEVER AND OTHER *BORRELIA* INFECTIONS

WILLIAM A. PETRI, JR.

DEFINITION

Relapsing fever is a spirochetal infection with bacteria of the genus *Borrelia*. There are two modes of transmission: epidemic louse-borne and endemic tick-borne relapsing fever. Disease is characterized by recurrent bouts of fever and spirochetemia separated by short fever-free periods.

The Pathogen

Members of the genus *Borrelia* are motile spirochetes that measure 0.5 μm in diameter and 5 to 40 μm in length. They are aerophilic and require long-chain fatty acids for growth. Louse-borne relapsing fever is caused by *Borrelia recurrentis*. Tick-borne relapsing fever organisms are named after their tick vector and include the closely related species *Borrelia duttonii* (Old World); *Borrelia hermsii*, *Borrelia turicatae*, and *Borrelia parkeri* (North America); and *Borrelia miyamotoi* (Old and New World).[1]

EPIDEMIOLOGY

Louse-borne epidemic relapsing fever is caused by *B. recurrentis* and is carried from person to person by the human body louse (*Pediculus humanus*). There is no animal reservoir. The spirochete lives in the louse hemolymph; infection is transmitted to humans when the louse is crushed on human skin and infective spirochetes penetrate the skin or mucous membranes. Epidemics have occurred during famines and at wartime when breakdown in sanitation favors the transmission of body lice. Louse-borne disease remains endemic in central and east Africa (Ethiopia, Somalia, Chad, and the Sudan) and in the South American Andes (Bolivia and Peru).

Tick-borne endemic relapsing fever occurs throughout the world and is transmitted to humans by *Ornithodoros* soft ticks. The ticks become infected by feeding on wild rodents (including mice, rats, squirrels, and chipmunks), which serve as natural reservoirs for the organisms. In the United States, relapsing fever is limited to humid mountainous areas of the West at altitudes of 1500 to 8000 feet, where the tick vector *Ornithodoros hermsii* resides in forests of ponderosa pine and Douglas fir trees. A key diagnostic clue has been a history of sleeping in rodent-infested rustic cabins in western U.S. national parks.[2] In Tanzania, where house infestation with *Ornithodoros* tick vectors can be very high, relapsing fever was identified in 11% of children seen at a clinic with fever. In the northeastern U.S., the prevalence of antibodies to *Borrelia miyamotoi* is nearly 50%, as high as for *Borrelia burgdorferi* (Chapter 321).[3]

PATHOBIOLOGY

Borrelia infection begins in the skin at the site of the louse or tick bite and is followed by rapid dissemination of the spirochetes through the blood stream. Spirochetes are visible on Wright-stained peripheral blood smears during the initial febrile episode and during each febrile relapse in most patients. The spirochete burden in blood positively correlates with symptom severity. Clearance of spirochetes from blood is associated with the production of serotype-specific immune sera; anti-*Borrelia* antibodies have been shown in animal models to be the major mechanism of immune clearance of infection.

Relapses are associated with cyclic antigenic variation in the variable major proteins (VMPs), which are the abundant outer membrane proteins of the spirochete that carry the serotype-specific epitopes. Antigenic variation is the consequence of recombination events that occur between VMP genes at silent and expression sites on linear plasmids. A single *B. hermsii* bacterium may produce as many as 40 distinct serotypes. Because spirochetes undergo one or several antigenic phases during infection, no specific or standard procedure has been developed for routine serodiagnosis of relapsing fever.

CLINICAL MANIFESTATIONS

An abrupt onset of fever (temperature > 39° C in most patients), headache, myalgia, and shaking chills characterizes the onset of illness. Cough, nausea and vomiting, and fatigue are less frequent complaints. Signs include fever, tachycardia, lethargy or confusion, conjunctival injection, and epistaxis. Hepatosplenomegaly, jaundice, and often a truncal petechial rash are common signs in louse-borne relapsing fever. Neurologic findings may occur,[4] including meningitis, meningoencephalitis, and facial palsy, although these entities are more common with tick-borne relapsing fever. Untreated louse-borne disease lasts 6 days, and relapses occur once after an afebrile period of 9 days. The initial illness of tick-borne relapsing fever lasts about 4 days without antibiotic treatment, with an average of two relapses (each after an average 10-day afebrile period) before the diagnosis is made.

Relapsing fever in pregnancy can cause placental damage and intrauterine growth retardation and results in miscarriage in a third of patients. Neonatal infection by both the tick- and louse-borne forms is accompanied by jaundice, hepatosplenomegaly, and often sepsis and hemorrhage. Fever and hepatosplenomegaly are also common signs in children. It has been also recognized in immunocompromised patients.[5]

DIAGNOSIS

The diagnosis should be considered in patients with fever who are returning from a stay in cabins in the mountainous and high-elevation areas of the western United States. Only a few patients will remember tick exposure, because *O. hermsii* is a night feeder, has a painless bite, and remains attached for only 15 minutes. Internationally, relapsing fever can occur sporadically wherever dwellings are infected with *Ornithodoros* ticks, as well as in epidemics with louse-borne disease.

Because the number of organisms in blood is extremely high, the diagnosis is most often made by direct visualization of the organism in a blood smear (Fig. 322-1), although the diagnosis can also be made with polymerase chain reaction and serodiagnostic tests. Spirochetes can be demonstrated in peripheral blood smears taken during febrile episodes in 70% of patients. Additional sensitivity may be gained by examination of a buffy coat preparation of peripheral blood. Because of their characteristic locomotion, spirochetes can be readily detected by direct visualization of thick blood films under low-power microscopy. Culture of the organism requires a special medium and is not practical in a clinical laboratory setting. The white blood cell count is generally normal, but platelet counts of less than 50,000/mm³ occur in up to 90% of cases of louse-borne disease. Prothrombin and activated partial thromboplastin times are often prolonged. In louse-borne disease, elevations in liver function test results (serum transaminases and bilirubin) and blood urea nitrogen are common. Urinalysis may reveal proteinuria and microscopic hematuria. Examination of cerebrospinal fluid may show a lymphocytic pleocytosis, and spirochetes may be directly visualized.

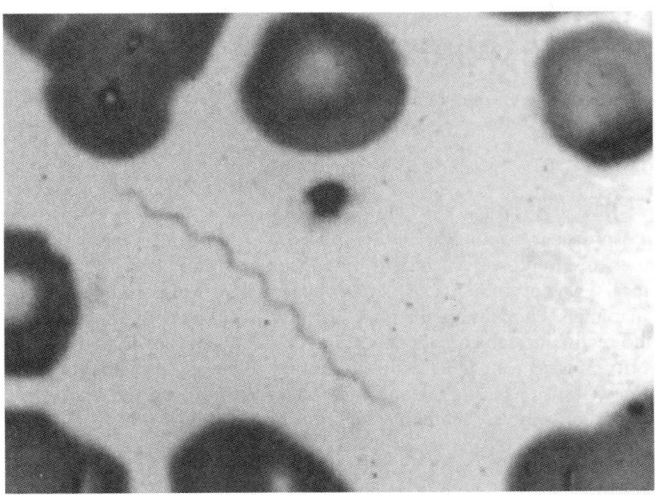

FIGURE 322-1. A single spirochete is seen in a Wright-stained thin blood smear from a patient with relapsing fever.

TREATMENT Rx

Borrelia is generally quite sensitive to antibiotics, which has led to recommendations for single-dose treatments. Although this may be sufficient, especially for louse-borne disease, recent reports suggest that silent residual infections occur and may best be addressed by longer treatments. For tick-borne relapsing infection, treatment should extend for 7 days to reduce the risk for persistent infection. Tetracycline, doxycycline, and erythromycin are all effective antibiotics. Erythromycin should be used in pregnant women and children younger than 7 years (in whom tetracyclines can stain the permanent teeth). Penicillin treatment has been reported to clear the spirochetemia more slowly than tetracycline does.

The Jarisch-Herxheimer reaction (typically characterized by a rise in body temperature of 1°C, rigors, a rise in blood pressure followed by a fall, and transient leukopenia) occurs 2 to 3 hours after treatment in many patients with louse-borne disease, less commonly in tick-borne disease, and should be anticipated and managed supportively. Death as a result of shock from the Jarisch-Herxheimer reaction occurs rarely. The Jarisch-Herxheimer reaction has been associated with accelerated phagocytosis of spirochetes by neutrophils and transient elevations in tumor necrosis factor (TNF)-α, interleukin (IL)-6, IL-8, and IL-10. In small numbers of patients with louse-borne relapsing fever, anti–TNF-α antibodies have been effective in prevention.

PREVENTION

Prevention of louse-borne relapsing fever hinges on improving hygienic conditions, delousing affected areas, and antibiotic treatment of patients and close contacts. Tick-borne relapsing fever can be prevented by reducing the risk of contact with rodents and ticks, including repair of structural flaws in cabins and other residences so rodents cannot nest in or around them, as well as spraying infested indoor environments. Tick-bite screening and prophylactic treatment with doxycycline in highly endemic areas has been reported to be a practical, safe, and effective policy in preventing tick-borne relapsing fever.[6]

PROGNOSIS

Epidemics of louse-borne relapsing fever have been reported, with mortality rates approaching 40%; as much as 5% of the mortality is related to Jarisch-Herxheimer reactions with treatment. Mortality from tick-borne disease is less than 5%. Autopsies of patients with louse-borne disease have documented intracranial hemorrhage, brain edema, bronchopneumonia, hepatic necrosis, and splenic infarcts.

GENERAL REFERENCES

For the General References and other additional features, please visit Expert Consult at https://expertconsult.inkling.com.

323

LEPTOSPIROSIS

ATIS MUEHLENBACHS AND SHERIF R. ZAKI

DEFINITION

Leptospirosis is a zoonotic disease caused by pathogenic *Leptospira* species spirochetes. Leptospirosis is distributed worldwide and is most prevalent in tropical developing countries. Leptospires frequently infect wild and domestic mammals. Humans are infected directly by contact with infected animals or indirectly through contact with urine-contaminated soil or water. Disease severity ranges from mild and self-limiting to severe with life-threatening manifestations including massive pulmonary hemorrhage and Weil's disease (the triad of jaundice, acute renal failure, and bleeding).

The Pathogen

Leptospires are thin, coiled, highly motile spirochetes measuring 6 to 20 microns in length. They are obligate aerobes that can survive for several weeks in the environment. *Leptospira* is currently genetically classified into nine pathogenic species (*L. interrogans, L. kirschneri, L. borgpetersenii, L. santarosai, L. noguchii, L. weilii, L. alexanderi, L. alstoni, L. kmetyi*) and those of intermediate pathogenesis (*L. inadai, L. broomii, L. fainei, L. wolffii, L. licerasiae*). Pathogenic leptospires are further classified into over 25 serogroups and 250 serovars that differ by geographic range and host specificity, which is useful information for outbreak and other epidemiologic investigations.

EPIDEMIOLOGY

Over 350,000 cases of leptospirosis are estimated to occur each year and are generally underreported. In the United States, around 100 to 200 leptospirosis cases are identified each year, with most occurring in Hawaii and Puerto Rico; the incidence is likely higher.[1] The majority of infections are mild and self-limiting, but case fatality in reported cases may be as high as 10%. In endemic areas, up to 20 to 30% of acute undifferentiated fever cases may be due to leptospirosis,[2] and seroprevalence can range from 5 to 15%. The major groups at risk are slum dwellers, subsistence farmers, and animal workers, owing to exposure to rodent, domestic, and wild animal reservoirs. In both tropical and temperate climates, the urban poor are an underrecognized population at risk.[3] Fresh water exposure is a risk factor, particularly during heavy rainfall and natural disasters, in addition to exposure during travel, extreme outdoor sports activities, and military operations. Humans are considered accidental hosts; rare human-to-human transmission by transplacental infection and breast-feeding has been reported.

PATHOBIOLOGY

Leptospires can directly penetrate abraded skin and mucous membranes and spread hematogenously to target organs. The classic illness is biphasic, with the first phase characterized by leptospiremia and the second phase with organism clearance by agglutinating antibodies and an associated host response that can be immunopathogenic.[4,5] Leptospires can persist for a period of time in target organs. In asymptomatic reservoir animals, leptospires can reach massive densities within the renal tubules, resulting in continued urinary excretion.

Pathologic findings (Fig. 323-1) may include pulmonary hemorrhage, diffuse alveolar damage, mild to marked hepatocellular dissociation, mild portal hepatitis, lymphohistiocytic interstitial nephritis, renal tubular necrosis, and mild renal glomerular mesangial hyperplasia. Hemorrhage in other organs, multifocal myocarditis, myositis, and hemophagocytosis may also be present. By immunohistochemistry or silver stains (Fig. 323-2), leptospires can be seen within the renal interstitium, hepatic parenchyma, and within the walls of small, medium, and large pulmonary blood vessels.

Leptospire tissue penetration may be mediated by a burrowing motion and secreted enzymes including collagenase and sphingomyelinase. Leptospiral proteins interact directly with host extracellular matrix components such as collagen, fibronectin, and laminins. Leptospires are resistant to the alternative pathway of complement-mediated lysis and can bind inhibitory complement factor H. Leptospiral lipopolysaccharides and lipopeptides have low endotoxic potency but can activate innate immune response through toll-like receptor (TLR)-2 signaling and are thought to generate a cytokine response. Immunity is considered to be primarily humoral and serotype specific. Circulating immune complexes may contribute to renal damage and endothelial dysfunction. An expansion of γδ T cells occurs during infection. Leptospires may also directly activate plasminogen to plasmin, the main enzyme of the fibrinolytic system, which could promote hemorrhage.[6]

Genomic studies of pathogenic intermediate and saprophytic *Leptospira* species have revealed a relatively large genome that contains genes involved in environmental survival, chemotaxis, and motility that may be involved in pathogenesis.[7] Little is known about host genetic risk factors, although the HLA-DQ6 allele has been associated with increased susceptibility to infection.

CLINICAL MANIFESTATIONS

The incubation period is typically 7 to 12 days (range, 2 to 30 days). During the early phase of illness (first 3 to 7 days), the majority of patients present with high fever (38° to 40° C) and myalgia. Cough, nausea and vomiting, diarrhea, headache, photophobia, and rash may be seen. Conjunctival suffusion is a characteristic finding (Fig. 323-3), but it is only seen in a third of patients near the end of early-phase illness. Myalgia may be pronounced and most frequently involves the calves and lumbar musculature, with creatine phosphokinase elevation. Severe cervical and abdominal myalgia may mimic nuchal rigidity or an acute abdomen, respectively. Rash occurs in 10 to 20% of patients and may be urticarial, maculopapular, or purpuric in a typically

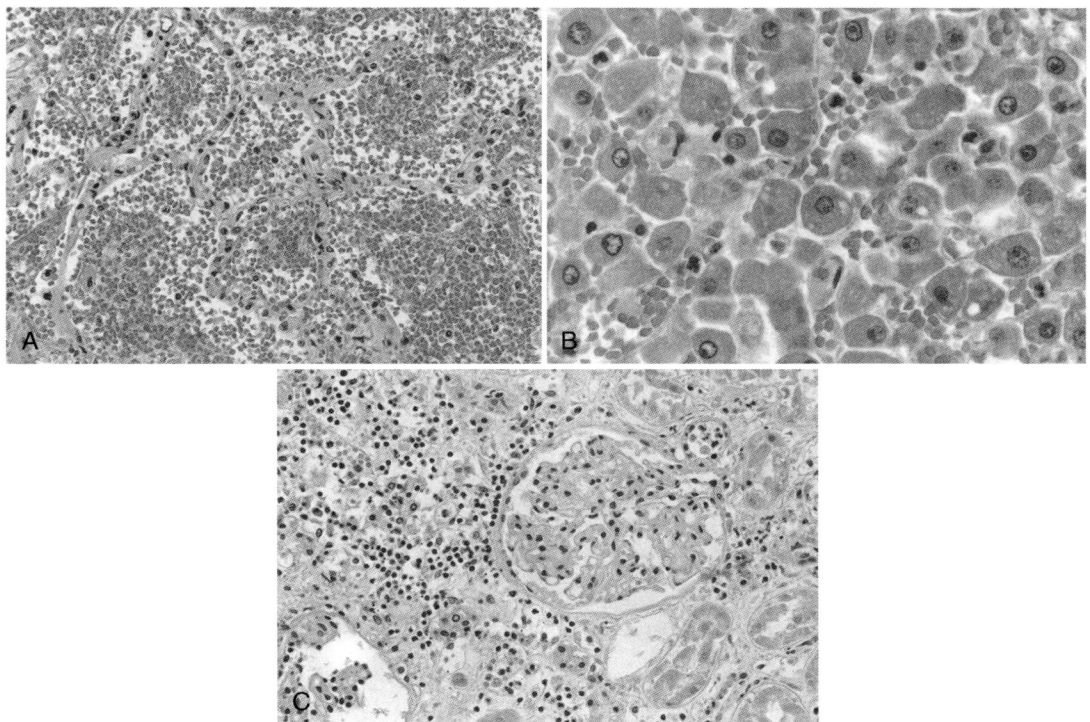

FIGURE 323-1. Pathologic features of severe leptospirosis. A, Pulmonary hemorrhage. B, Hepatocellular dissociation. C, Interstitial nephritis.

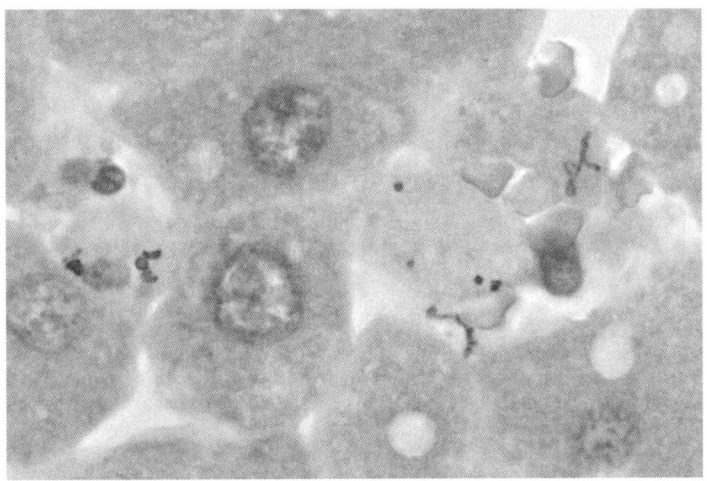

FIGURE 323-2. Immunostaining of *Leptospira* in liver. Note the coiled nature of the spirochetes. Granular antigen staining is also seen.

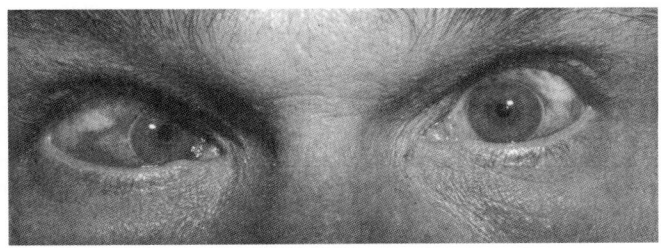

FIGURE 323-3. Conjunctival suffusion in a patient with severe leptospirosis. Conjunctival suffusion is a characteristic sign of leptospirosis and best seen along the right upper palpebral border above the subconjunctival hemorrhage. (Courtesy Antonio Seguro and Paulo Marotto, Hospital Emílio Ribas and Universidade de São Paulo.)

pretibial and truncal distribution. Hepatosplenomegaly and lymphadenopathy may also be present. Resolution of symptoms coincides with the presence of agglutinating immunoglobulin (Ig)M antibodies and reduction in leptospiremia. As a classic biphasic disease, fever may recur 3 to 4 days after remission. In this later immune phase, severe headache is often present and can be associated with photophobia, meningeal signs, and cerebrospinal fluid (CSF) pleocytosis.

Severe disease may occur progressively at initial presentation or during late-phase leptospirosis and result in 10 to 50% mortality. Life-threatening manifestations are renal failure, hypotension, hemorrhage, and respiratory failure. Jaundice occurs in 5 to 10% of patients, and serum bilirubin levels can be elevated up to 40 to 80 mg/dL, with only moderate and minor elevations in transaminase and alkaline phosphatase levels, respectively. Leptospirosis may present as acute cholecystitis. Long-term hepatic sequelae are typically not seen. Renal findings are typically of nonoliguric hypokalemic renal insufficiency and impaired tubular sodium reabsorption. Volume loss may result in oliguric renal insufficiency and acute tubular necrosis, and renal failure occurs in about half of severe cases. Common urinalysis findings are proteinuria, white blood cells, hematuria, and hyaline and granular casts.

Pulmonary findings may include cough, dyspnea, and hemoptysis. Leptospirosis-associated pulmonary hemorrhage and acute respiratory distress syndrome is now recognized as a common clinical presentation. Radiographic findings may show a patchy alveolar infiltrate to large areas of consolidation due to hemorrhage.[8] Cardiac conduction abnormalities can be seen and tend to be nonspecific in mild disease. First-degree atrioventricular block and features of pericarditis are the most common findings in severe disease. Arrhythmias including ventricular fibrillation may also occur.

Thrombocytopenia is frequent and does not appear to be due to platelet consumption, but disseminated intravascular coagulopathy can occur. Prothrombin and partial thromboplastin times are typically normal or only mildly elevated. Petechiae, conjunctival hemorrhage, and purpura can be seen in addition to the more severe hemorrhagic manifestations.

Aseptic meningitis is the most frequent neurologic manifestation. CSF findings include pleocytosis with neutrophil predominance in early disease, followed by lymphocyte predominance in later disease. Glucose is generally normal, and CSF pressure may be elevated. Less common are intracerebral hemorrhage, encephalitis, myelitis, and peripheral neuropathy. Ocular leptospirosis, including chronic uveitis, is thought to be primarily caused by an immunopathogenic mechanism and occurs late in the disease process.

DIAGNOSIS

Few clinical signs differentiate early stage leptospirosis, and severe leptospirosis may be recognized in the form of Weil's disease. Reference tests require specialized laboratories, and there is a need for point-of-care testing in tropical areas. Culture and serologic assays may provide false negatives.[9-11]

Culture of the organism requires specialized media (Ellinghausen-McCullough-Johnson-Harris (EMJH) or Fletcher media, with often more than 4 weeks needed with observation under darkfield microscopy. Cultures generally have low sensitivity, with the best yield obtained from peripheral blood during days 1 through 4 of the acute illness; urine may be positive for up to day 10. Direct darkfield microscopy of clinical specimens can also be attempted but has low sensitivity and specificity.

The gold standard serologic test is the microagglutination test (MAT), available at the Centers for Disease Control and Prevention. MAT is considered positive if there is a four-fold rise in titer between acute and convalescent sera. This assay requires cultured *Leptospira*; it provides serotype data and has a very high specificity but lower sensitivity. U.S. Food and Drug Administration–approved IgM enzyme-linked immunosorbent assay (ELISA) and indirect hemagglutination assays are also available. Multiple lateral flow rapid diagnostic "dipstick" tests are manufactured and used in other countries; however, their performance may not be well characterized. Diagnostic polymerase chain reaction (PCR) assays are being investigated and hold promise for diagnostic accuracy.[12,13] Organisms within tissues can be detected by Warthin-Starry silver stain or immunohistochemistry. In the United States, leptospirosis is a nationally notifiable disease.

DIFFERENTIAL DIAGNOSIS

As previously discussed, few clinical or laboratory findings differentiate leptospirosis from other causes of acute fever. Differential diagnosis depends on other diseases in the geographic area, most frequently malaria, dengue, typhoid fever, and rickettsial diseases including scrub typhus. Other diseases in the differential include influenza, acute viral hepatitis, yellow fever, bacterial and viral meningitis, bacterial sepsis, and hantavirus infection. A high index of suspicion is needed in endemic areas. Useful diagnostic clues are conjunctival suffusion, muscle tenderness, and pulmonary bleeding. High serum bilirubin in the presence of relatively mild transaminitis would argue against viral hepatitis and favor leptospirosis. Hypokalemia, elevated creatinine, elevated creatine phosphokinase, and thrombocytopenia are nonspecific but may also suggest leptospirosis.

TREATMENT   Rx

The World Health Organization guidelines and widespread clinical practice are to treat patients early with antibiotics for leptospirosis. Penicillin, doxycycline, or a cephalosporin appear to be equally efficacious, and doxycycline has the advantage of also treating rickettsial infections. Of note, a recent meta-analysis of seven randomized trials over the past 30 years concluded there is insufficient "grade A" evidence to recommend for or against the use of antibiotics to treat leptospirosis[A1]; antibiotic therapy may decrease the duration of clinical illness by 2 to 4 days; however, in severely ill patients, penicillin may be associated with a higher rate of dialysis. Additional randomized controlled trials are needed.

Treatment regimens for mild leptospirosis include doxycycline (100 mg PO bid), ampicillin (500 mg PO q6h), amoxicillin (500 mg orally [PO] q8h), or azithromycin (1 g followed by 500 mg daily for 2 days); and for severe disease, intravenous (IV) penicillin (1.5 million units q6h), ceftriaxone (1 g daily), cefotaxime (1 g q6h), or doxycycline (100 mg IV q12h). Treatment duration is typically 7 days. The Jarisch-Herxheimer reaction, a febrile inflammatory reaction that occurs with initiation of treatment and results from clearance of the organism from the circulation (Chapter 319), can occur shortly after antimicrobial therapy is started,[14] so patients require monitoring at initiation of antibiotics.

Prompt triage of high-risk patients and aggressive supportive care are essential. Hypotension should be treated, and volume repletion is useful in limiting renal damage. Patients with nonoliguric hypokalemic renal insufficiency may be treated by volume and potassium repletion. Prompt dialysis is indicated for oliguric renal insufficiency, either by continuous hemofiltration or by peritoneal dialysis. Serial electrocardiograms are helpful to monitor for arrhythmia. Aggressive therapy may be needed to treat hemorrhage and respiratory failure.

PREVENTION

Preventive measures include sanitation to prevent population exposure to contaminated water, and limiting water contamination by animal reservoirs

such as dogs, pigs, and cattle. Vaccination is available for domestic and livestock animals. Rodent control is important.[15] Workers with occupational exposure to animals or contaminated water or soil are encouraged to use protective equipment such as gloves and boots. Travelers to endemic areas should be counseled on fresh water exposure. A vaccine is not available for human use within the United States. Vaccine trials have been performed in Cuba, Russia and China, however vaccine safety and efficacy are uncertain.

Prophylaxis with doxycycline (200 mg PO weekly) is widely used for persons with exposure to contaminated water or at high risk for leptospirosis. Prophylaxis may work better in reducing risk of clinical disease for short-term travelers with high risk, rather than residents in an endemic area. Of interest, a recent meta-analysis concluded that there is insufficient grade A evidence to recommend for or against the use of antibiotic prophylaxis[A2]; additional randomized controlled trials are needed.

PROGNOSIS

The majority of infections are self-limiting, but there may be 10% case fatality among patients who seek medical attention. Severe leptospirosis is associated with a 10 to 50% risk of death. Death is more frequent during infection if there is renal failure, altered mental status, older age, oliguria, pulmonary hemorrhage, or respiratory insufficiency. Ocular disease, including chronic uveitis, may result in severe visual impairment.

 Grade A References

A1. Brett-Major DM, Coldren R. Antibiotics for leptospirosis. *Cochrane Database Syst Rev.* 2012;2:CD008264.
A2. Brett-Major DM, Lipnick RJ. Antibiotic prophylaxis for leptospirosis. *Cochrane Database Syst Rev.* 2009;3:CD007342.

GENERAL REFERENCES

For the General References and other additional features, please visit Expert Consult at https://expertconsult.inkling.com.

324

TUBERCULOSIS

JERROLD J. ELLNER

DEFINITION

Tuberculosis (TB) is a chronic granulomatous disease with a unique latent stage usually caused by the acid-fast bacillus (AFB) *Mycobacterium tuberculosis* (Mtb). The most common site of disease is the lung; frequent extrapulmonary sites are the lymph nodes, pleura, bones, and joints. TB is spread from person to person by inhalation of infectious droplet nuclei aerosolized by patients with pulmonary TB (PTB). TB is a major cause of morbidity and mortality worldwide, with over 95% of cases and 99% of deaths occurring in resource-limited settings. The human immunodeficiency virus (HIV) pandemic led to a resurgence of TB and promoted explosive nosocomial outbreaks of multiple-drug resistant TB. The result was increased attention to TB as a global public health emergency and increased funding for TB control and research. The problems posed for TB control are compounded by increasing drug-resistant disease that is expensive to treat and may be refractory to available drugs.

The Pathogen

TB is caused by infection with one of the three members of the Mtb complex: Mtb, *Mycobacterium africanum*, or *Mycobacterium bovis*. The causative organism is a slender, non-motile, non–spore-forming, non–toxin-producing bacillus that may be beaded and is approximately 2 to 4 μm in length. It is a slow-growing (doubling time of 18 to 24 hours) facultative aerobe that can persist intracellularly for prolonged periods. The organism is identified in clinical specimens as an acid-fast bacillus (AFB). Mtb can be stained with carbol fuchsin by either alkalinization (Kinyoun) or heat (Ziehl-Neelsen) methods. The waxy coat of Mtb, composed of mycolic acid and other complex

TABLE 324-1 RISK FACTORS FOR TUBERCULOSIS

RISK FACTOR	INCREASED RISK OF RECENT INFECTION*	INCREASED RISK OF PROGRESSION FROM INFECTION TO DISEASE	TST CUT POINT
Household contact of PTB	X		>5 mm
Solid organ transplant recipients, immunosuppressive treatment (TNF inhibitors, prednisone > 15 mg/day for > 1 month), fibrotic lesions on chest radiograph consistent with prior TB		X	>5 mm
HIV infection	X	X	>5 mm
Foreign-born, injecting drug users, TST-positive children, adolescents, young adults	X		>10 mm
Residents or workers in hospitals, homeless shelters, correctional facilities, nursing homes, residences for the HIV-infected	X		>10 mm
Underweight (>15%), silicosis, diabetes mellitus (particularly insulin-dependent or poorly controlled), renal failure, hemodialysis, gastrectomy, jejuno-ileal bypass, carcinoma of the head and neck, lung cancer, lymphoma, leukemia		X	>10 mm
None			>15 mm

*Recent infection per se increases risk of progressing from infection to disease (12.9 cases per 1000 person-years in the first year compared to 1.6 per 1000 person-years in the subsequent 7 years).
HIV = human immunodeficiency virus; PTB = pulmonary TB; TNF = tumor necrosis factor; TST = tuberculin skin test.

lipopolysaccharides, precludes decolorization of the stain with a mixture of acid and alcohol.

DNA sequencing of Mtb and genetic manipulations have promoted basic understanding of the metabolism and virulence of the organism, its immunodominant antigens, and capacity to survive adverse conditions and persist intracellularly. Clinical isolates of Mtb differ in their virulence in experimental models, potential for transmission in humans, and interaction with the host (immunopathology, induction of host cytokines, delayed-type hypersensitivity [DTH]). For example, the hypervirulent Beijing strain family overexpresses a phenolic glycolipid that inhibits innate immunity and may thereby contribute to its pathogenicity.

There are six main phylogeographic lineages of Mtb, each associated with a specific human population. The families differ in geographic distribution and in some cases the potential for transmission and pathogenesis. Strain typing is particularly useful in outbreak investigations and can be performed by several techniques, restriction fragment length polymorphism (RFLP) of the insertional element IS 6110 or spoligotyping. The finding that multiple cases of TB are caused by the same strain and constitute a "cluster" suggests that they are epidemiologically linked. Whole-genomic sequencing has emerged as a more powerful tool to establish transmission even in the absence of epidemiologic links.

TB caused by *M. africanum* is clinically identical to that caused by Mtb. *M. bovis* has greater than 95% DNA homology with Mtb and causes disease in humans, cattle, deer, badgers, and other animals. The main route of transmission of Mtb is person to person through respiratory aerosols generated by coughing. Bacilli in small droplet nuclei (1 to 5 μm in diameter) remain suspended in air for long periods and once inhaled can reach the airways, where only 1 to 5 organisms are sufficient to cause infection. Laryngeal involvement renders the patient highly infectious. Direct cutaneous inoculation ("prosector's wart") does occur. *M. bovis* can be transmitted by the gastrointestinal route, usually through ingestion of contaminated milk.

EPIDEMIOLOGY

In 2012, there were an estimated 8.6 million new cases of TB (13% in HIV-infected persons) and 1.3 million deaths as a result of TB.[1] Fifty-eight percent of cases of TB occurred in Asia and 25% in Africa. The largest number of cases was in India (26% of all cases) and China (12%). Worldwide, TB occurs more commonly in males than females, but 210,000 women died of TB; the prevalence of disease peaks in young adults, with major economic consequence. Globally, both TB incidence (declining 2% per year) and case-fatality rates have been falling.

HIV infection has a profound effect on the epidemiology of TB, promoting and accelerating progression from infection to active TB and both reactivation and reinfection disease. Some 80% of HIV-infected TB cases are in sub-Saharan Africa, resulting in TB case rates as high as 1% in South Africa and Swaziland.

In the United States in 2013, the incidence of TB was 3.0 per 100,000, with 9588 new cases reported (6.8% were HIV-infected, 5.7% homeless, and 3.8% incarcerated).[2] The incidence rate in foreign-born individuals was 13-fold higher than in those born in the United States and foreign-born individuals

accounted for 64% of new cases. Rates were 26-fold higher in non-Hispanic Asians than non-Hispanic whites. The age-specific prevalence of TB in the United States is skewed toward older adults, presumably representing reactivation disease in the foreign born and U.S. born that were infected when TB was more common.

Country of origin is a large determinant of both the risk of latent TB infection (LTBI) and of disease. In a low-prevalence setting such as the United States, the prevalence of LTBI (defined as a positive tuberculin skin test [TST] or interferon-γ release assay [IGRA] and no active disease) is approximately 4%. Those infected are at markedly increased risk of disease compared to uninfected, a risk that is further increased by medical comorbidities and other factors shown in Table 324-1. The risk is not homogeneous within groups affected, for example, by extent of immunosuppression in HIV or duration, severity, and control of diabetes. Smoking and alcoholism also confer an increased risk for TB, although smaller than the conditions listed.

TB caused by drug-resistant organisms is a particular and emerging threat to public health.[3] Multidrug-resistant (MDR) TB (resistant to isoniazid [INH] and rifampin [RIF]) and extensively drug-resistant (XDR) TB (MDR plus resistance to fluoroquinolones [FQs] and a second-line injectable (kanamycin, amikacin, or capreomycin) are much more difficult and expensive to treat and in some cases may be incurable. There are 450,000 incident cases of MDR TB each year, with an increasing prevalence because most are untreated, and 170,000 deaths. About 5 to 10% of these new cases of MDR TB are XDR. Twenty-seven countries account for 85% of the cases of MDR TB, with most occurring in India, China, and the Russian Federation. Eighty-six U.S. cases of MDR TB and two cases of XDR TB were reported in 2012. Most cases of MDR TB are not treated, which results in increasing transmission and prevalence.

PATHOBIOLOGY

Typically, the chain of transmission of TB begins with an infectious case of pulmonary TB (PTB) (Fig. 324-1). Infectiousness of a patient is determined by sputum smear status (3 to 4+ AFB), cough strength and frequency, the presence of cavitary lung disease, and the characteristics of the physical space shared with the source (ventilation and air recirculation). However, not all strongly AFB smear–positive patients with PTB are equally infectious, and there may be high transmitters, owing to host or bacterial factors or both. Recent studies, in fact, show that only about 50-60% of strongly sputum smear–positive persons with PTB generate aerosols that contain viable organisms.[4]

In both low- and high-prevalence countries, exposure/infection usually occurs in the household. In this setting, where exposure may be intense and protracted, 50 to 75% of contacts become infected. The higher numbers result from studies in which repeated testing identifies all TST convertors. In outbreaks occurring in residential shelters, hospitals, and prisons, Mtb infection or disease has been documented after brief exposure. Important variables that may explain differences in transmission include virulence of the organism, innate immunity, and susceptibility of the exposed populations (e.g., HIV infected). Human genetic factors such as polymorphisms in expression or regulation of toll-like receptors (TLR), pattern recognition

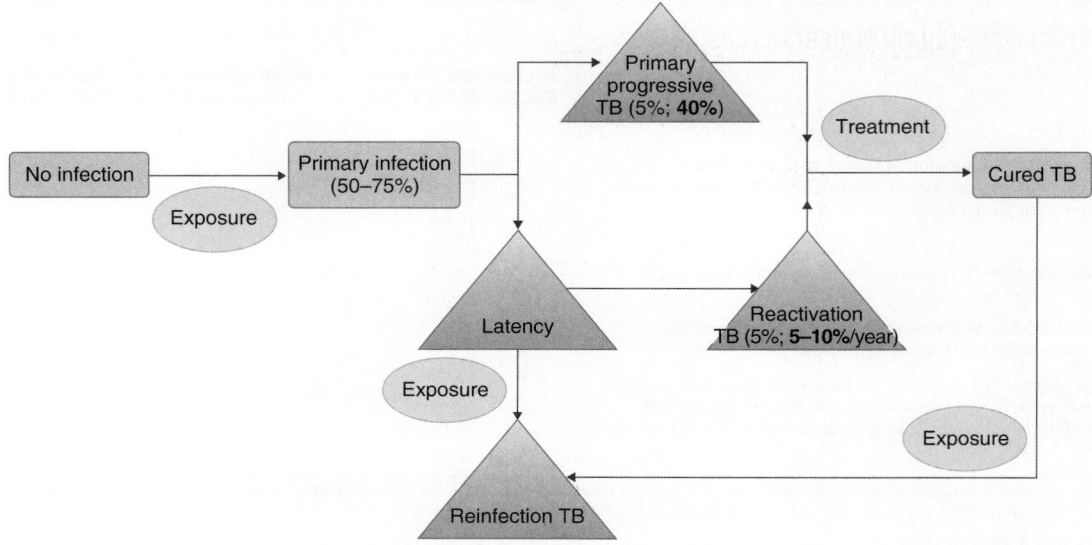

FIGURE 324-1. Natural History of TB. The proportion of individuals affected are shown in parentheses. Bolded figures are for HIV infection with severe immunosuppression. A number of medical risk factors besides HIV promote progression from *Mycobacterium tuberculosis* infection to disease (see Table 324-1).

receptors important to innate immunity, may modulate risk of infection and expression of infection (TST) as well as risk and expression of disease. Predisposition to disease is seen with defects in interferon (IFN)-γ and interleukin (IL)-12 receptors, consistent with their role in immunity. Polymorphisms that modify inflammation (e.g., by affecting leukotriene A₄ hydrolase) also may affect disease manifestations and response to therapy.

Two models of the natural history of TB are shown in Figures 324-1 and 324-2. There is increasing evidence that that the natural history represents a continuum rather than distinct entities of latent and active TB.[5] Diagnostic biomarkers that stratify risk of progression from LTBI to active TB would be of enormous value for targeting public health interventions.

The lung is the site of most cases of reactivation TB. The hallmark of the pathology is granuloma formation with caseation necrosis and multinucleated Langerhans giant cells. The caseous material found in necrotic cavities contains AFB. Mtb multiplies exuberantly in the liquid caseum. Immunologically, expectorated sputum contains cytokines and both upregulators and downregulators of the immune and inflammatory response, the downregulation being dominant. Bronchoalveolar lavage shows a lymphocytic alveolitis, with an influx of immature macrophages representing monocytes attracted from blood.[6] In sum, there is an active but downregulated immune response concomitant with bacterial replication. As a consequence of the inflammation, extensive apoptosis occurs and may lead to the deletion of Mtb-responsive T cells, which may play a role in the requirement for a long duration of therapy and in the susceptibility to reinfection TB. In HIV-infected persons with advanced immunosuppression, granulomas may be poorly formed or absent. Lung tissue is infiltrated with foamy epithelioid cells, which are macrophages laden with AFBs. Caseation may or may not be present, but there is extensive inflammation and necrosis.

Extrapulmonary TB can involve any organ. Persistence of organisms in areas that are relatively well oxygenated may explain the more frequent sites of reactivation, such as the apices of the lung, cortices of the kidney, and vertebral bodies.

Several forms of extrapulmonary TB have a shared pathogenesis: discharge of a contiguous tuberculous focus into a serosal cavity, a brisk inflammatory reaction based on preexisting delayed-type hypersensitivity (DTH), fever, frequently negative smears of exudative fluid for AFBs, and sometimes a transiently negative TST. The focus that discharges may be a long-standing focus or one seeded during recent dissemination associated with primary infection. This basic scenario also occurs in pleural TB, TB pericarditis, TB meningitis (the parameningeal focus is called a "Rich focus"), TB peritonitis, and TB arthritis.

Pleural TB represents an in situ DTH reaction with activation of T_H1 helper T cells, abundant cytokines, including IFN-γ and tumor necrosis factor (TNF)-α, and apoptosis. In non–HIV-infected individuals, organisms are sparse, which may be why self-cure of pleural TB can take place. However, in the absence of chemotherapy for TB, there is a high risk for TB recurrence, usually as PTB on the side contralateral to the effusion.

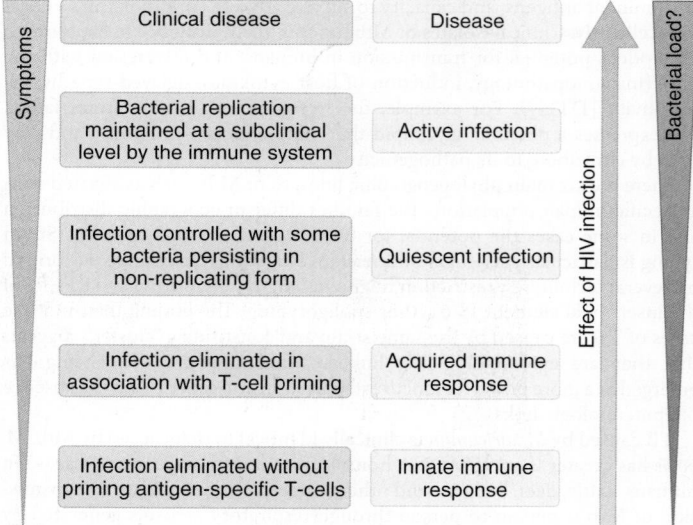

FIGURE 324-2. Tuberculosis infection as a spectrum. The outcome of infection by *Mycobacterium tuberculosis* is generally represented as a bimodal distribution between active tuberculosis (TB) and latent TB on the basis of the presence or absence of clinical symptoms. It is proposed that latent TB is usefully represented as part of a spectrum of responses to infection. One consequence of this model is that there may be a subpopulation within the group that is currently defined as having latent TB that should be preferentially targeted for preventive therapy. A second consequence is that efforts to develop drugs for effective treatment of latent TB would overlap the search for drugs that shorten treatment times for active TB. (From Barry CE 3rd, Boshoff HI, Dartois V, et al. The spectrum of latent tuberculosis. Rethinking the biology and intervention strategies. *Nat Rev Microbiol.* 2009;7:845-855, Figure 1.)

In addition to reactivation of a latent focus, reinfection with Mtb may occur and progress to disease. Reinfection is more likely if the host is immunosuppressed or there is repeated or intense exposure. Treated cases of PTB also are predisposed to reinfection disease as discussed earlier. LTBI is over 70% protective against reinfection TB.

CLINICAL MANIFESTATIONS
Primary Tuberculosis
Most cases of primary TB are unrecognized clinically except for conversion of the TST. There may be fever, shortness of breath, nonproductive cough, and rarely erythema nodosum. Crepitations and focal wheezes may be present. Chest radiographs show small patchy opacities in the mid-lung fields, often with unilateral hilar lymphadenopathy. Upper or middle lobe collapse may also be seen as a result of bronchial compression by enlarged nodes or transient pleural effusion. Recent studies with positron emission

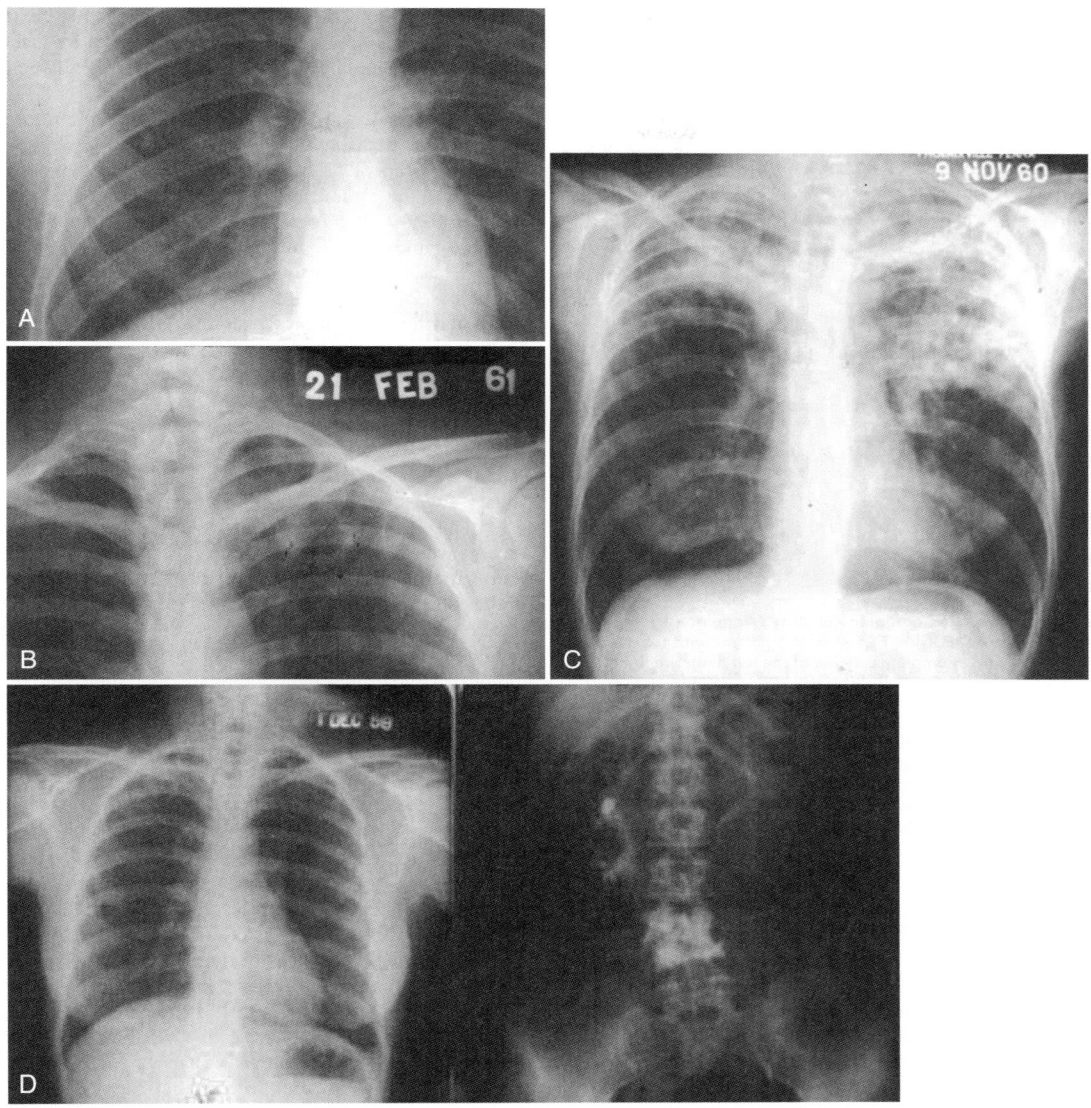

FIGURE 324-3. A, Ghon complex. B, Moderately advanced pulmonary tuberculosis (TB). C, Far advanced pulmonary TB. D, Pulmonary (*left*) and extrapulmonary (*right*) TB. (Radiographs courtesy Thomas M. Daniel, MD.)

tomographic computed tomography (PET-CT) scan show that most household contacts of infectious TB cases with a positive TST have mediastinal adenopathy that resolves with INH preventive therapy. HIV-infected persons with LTBI studied with this modality may show parenchymal uptake consistent with subclinical disease. In most individuals (immunosuppression being the exception), the manifestations of primary TB resolve without treatment, concurrent with the development of an adaptive immune response. During the subsequent period of clinical latency, evidence of the primary infection may be found as a small calcified parenchymal scar in the mid-lung fields (Ghon complex), sometimes associated with similar findings in the draining hilar nodes (Ranke complex) (Fig. 324-3A). A small scar caused by an arrested lesion in the apices of the lung is called a Simon focus.

Progressive Primary Tuberculosis

Failure to develop adaptive immunity is most common in young children, the elderly, and the immunocompromised. Progressive primary TB manifested as TB meningitis may develop in this setting. Primary infection also may progress to PTB within the first 1 to 2 years. In this case, PTB usually is upper lobe and cavitary, distant from the site of primary infection. Recent data indicate that in high-prevalence areas, most PTB cases represent progressive primary disease. Clinically, it is not possible to distinguish between progressive primary and "post-primary" or reactivation TB.

Reactivation Tuberculosis

The terms *reactivation TB* and *post-primary TB* are used interchangeably to connote that primary TB is followed by a variable period of at least 2 years

of clinical latency, after which TB develops in the setting of existing DTH/adaptive immunity, which contributes importantly to the pathogenesis and clinical manifestations.

PTB is the most common form of reactivation TB. Typical clinical findings in PTB consist of the insidious onset of a productive cough, night sweats, anorexia, and weight loss. Fever is present in approximately half of those affected. Patients may be asymptomatic and the diagnosis suggested by a chest radiograph obtained for other reasons (subclinical TB). The sputum may be purulent, blood streaked, or frankly bloody. Pleuritic chest pain may occur when there is subpleural inflammation. Dyspnea is not a hallmark of PTB, in part because thrombosis of vessels limits the perfusion of inflamed areas, so hypoxemia is not a prominent clinical feature. Physical examination may show dullness to percussion, low-pitched amphoric (hollow-sounding) breath sounds, and occasionally crepitations that may be post-tussive. Chest radiographs often reveal more disease than suggested by physical examination (see Fig. 324-3B and C). Typically (>95% of cases), lesions are found in the apical and posterior segments of the upper lobes and the superior (dorsal) segment of the lower lobe. There is a progression from patchy opacities and consolidation to cavitation reflective of caseation and liquefaction. Advanced imaging with PET-CT shows a heterogeneity in metabolic activity of different lesions within the same patient (Fig. 324-4), which may be associated with variable response to treatment. Rupture and discharge into bronchi and intrabronchial spread may lead to disease in multiple areas, including the other lung (so-called TB bronchopneumonia). There may be involvement of the larynx and middle ear. Early cavities are thin walled and evolve into characteristic chronic thick-walled cavities. Ten percent of all cavities have an

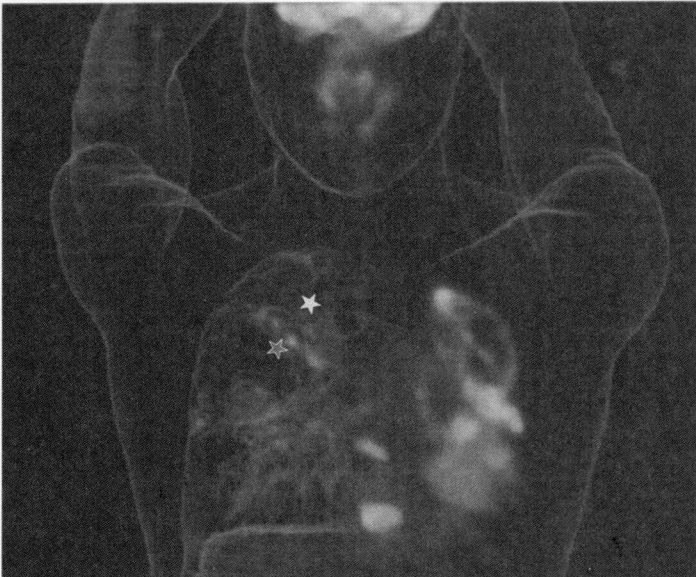

FIGURE 324-4. Positron emission tomographic computed tomography (PET-CT) imaging. An ¹⁸F-fluorodeoxyglucose (FDG) PET-CT scan of a patient with tuberculosis with extensive bilateral disease and a complete collapse of the left lung. The right lung also shows extensive disease throughout and illustrates the variability of FDG-PET uptake among lesions within even a single infected patient. The yellow star illustrates one lesion that fails to take up FDG that lies immediately adjacent to a string of three lesions that take up label avidly (*red star*). These different types of lesions respond to chemotherapy with different kinetics, indicating that they represent distinct bacterial subpopulations in different microenvironments. (From Barry CE 3rd, Boshoff HI, Dartois V, et al. The spectrum of latent tuberculosis. Rethinking the biology and intervention strategies. *Nat Rev Microbiol.* 2009;7:845-855, Figure 2.)

air-fluid level. There may be an associated pleural effusion or rarely, with rupture of cavities into the air space, pyopneumothorax. If the disease is minimal, it may best be seen on apical lordotic chest radiographs or on CT. Rarely, chest radiographs are normal, and the accompanying symptoms and positive sputum smears may be the result of endobronchial lesions or rupture of a tuberculous node into bronchi. Healing, fibrosis, and contraction obliterate small cavities, although large cavities may persist and even become the eventual nidus for an aspergilloma or a "scar" carcinoma.

In immunocompromised persons, the opacities may be located in the mid- and lower lung fields and be manifested as poorly resolving lobar or segmental pneumonitis, atelectasis, nodules, and cavities. Early in the course of HIV infection when the CD4⁺ count exceeds 200/μL, PTB may be typical in its manifestation. At lower CD4⁺ counts, mid- and lower lung abnormalities are more common. At a CD4⁺ count below 100/μL, the findings may be quite atypical, with prominent hilar and mediastinal adenopathy, pleural disease, interstitial or miliary opacities, or any combination of these manifestations. This picture resembles primary TB and, in fact, may represent progressive primary TB or reinfection disease. Chest radiographs are normal in up to 20% of persons with culture-confirmed TB, sometimes in the presence of a smear that contains AFB. In this CD4 strata, disseminated and extrapulmonary TB are the rule, with or without concurrent PTB.

Reinfection Tuberculosis

Reinfection TB is clinically indistinguishable from other forms and an important pathogenetic mechanism in high transmission settings. A shift in the drug susceptibility profile, a documented change in the DNA fingerprint or sequence, or occurrence in an outbreak setting may be the only evidence supporting the diagnosis of reinfection TB. Reinfection TB typically affects those with preexisting LTBI or following treatment of PTB.

Extrapulmonary Tuberculosis

Approximately 20% of cases of TB in non–HIV-infected populations are extrapulmonary (see Fig. 324-3D). In areas endemic for TB, extrapulmonary TB often occurs concurrently with PTB and is more common in children and young adults, in whom it represents progressive primary infection. By contrast, in low-prevalence areas, isolated extra-pulmonary TB is more common, and there is a shift to the elderly that represents reactivation TB. HIV infection is associated with a higher frequency of extrapulmonary disease, including the more serious forms, disseminated TB and TB meningitis.

Pleural Tuberculosis

Pleural TB occurs by direct extension when a subpleural caseous focus discharges into the pleural space or through hematogenous seeding. There may be concurrent PTB. Its peak occurrence is 3 to 6 months after primary infection. The typical manifestation is abrupt onset of fever, pleuritic chest pain, and cough. Occasionally there is an insidious presentation consisting of fever, weight loss, and malaise. If the pleural effusion is large enough, shortness of breath may be seen. Physical examination shows dullness to percussion and decreased breath sounds. Above the area of dullness there may be true egophony. Chest radiographs typically show unilateral pleural effusion, more frequently in the right hemithorax. Bilateral disease occurs in 10% of cases. Pleural effusions may be medium-sized, large, or, uncommonly, massive.

Miliary Tuberculosis

Miliary TB usually has an insidious manifestation consisting of fever, weight loss, night sweats, and little in the way of localizing symptoms or signs. There may be concurrent TB meningitis with associated symptoms. Physical examination may show choroidal tubercles (raised white-yellow plaques on funduscopic examination, present in 15% of cases), lymphadenopathy, and hepatomegaly. Chest radiographs may show multiple bilateral small opacities termed *miliary infiltrates* because of their resemblance to millet seeds. The findings on initial chest radiographs are often subtle and may be clear-cut only in retrospect after 3 months of follow-up. Performance of CT or high-resolution CT is useful because of its increased sensitivity (Fig. 324-5). A variant of miliary TB is disseminated are active TB, as may occur in HIV-infected patients or those treated with TNF inhibitors. In this entity, chest radiographic findings may be even more minimal. In the HIV-infected individual with advanced immunodeficiency, blood cultures are positive for Mtb in 20 to 40% of patients and may be the only manifestation of TB.

Tuberculous Meningitis

TB meningitis is usually characterized by less than 2 weeks of fever, headache, and meningismus. There may be depressed levels of consciousness, diplopia, and (rarely) hemiparesis. Physical examination shows a stiff neck and occasionally cranial neuropathy (VI, III, IV, VII in order of frequency) and long-tract signs. Chest radiographs may be consistent with PTB or miliary TB. CT of the head may show contrast enhancement over the basilar meninges, hypodense areas consistent with infarcts, hydrocephalus, and sometimes focal inflammatory lesions (tuberculomas). CT angiography may show entrapment of vessels or vasculitis.

Tuberculous Lymphadenitis

Lymphadenitis may be the sole manifestation of TB or, more frequently, particularly in the HIV infected, may accompany PTB. Patients with isolated lymph node disease may be afebrile. The supraclavicular and posterior cervical lymph nodes are most frequently involved. This is in contrast to scrofula caused by atypical mycobacteria or *M. bovis* and often seen in children, in whom submandibular and high anterior cervical adenopathy predominates. The lymphadenitis is not usually painful, and aspiration of the lymph node with the finding of AFB is an excellent approach to establish the diagnosis.

Tuberculous Pericarditis

The usual manifestation of TB pericarditis is chronic but may occasionally be subacute with fever, night sweats, chest pain, shortness of breath, pedal edema, and other signs of right heart failure. Physical examination shows signs of pericardial disease, right-sided heart failure, and tamponade (in ≈ 10%). Pericardial aspiration and biopsy are the diagnostic procedures of choice. When tamponade is present, a pericardial window can be both diagnostic and therapeutic.

Tuberculous Peritonitis

TB peritonitis may be accompanied by abdominal pain and fever, at times mimicking an acute abdomen. Alternatively, there may be an insidious manifestation consisting of abdominal pain, swelling, night sweats, and weight loss. The clinical syndrome is caused by discharge of tuberculous lymph nodes into the peritoneal space. Exudative ascites is usually present unless TB is superimposed on preexisting transudative ascites, as in alcoholic liver

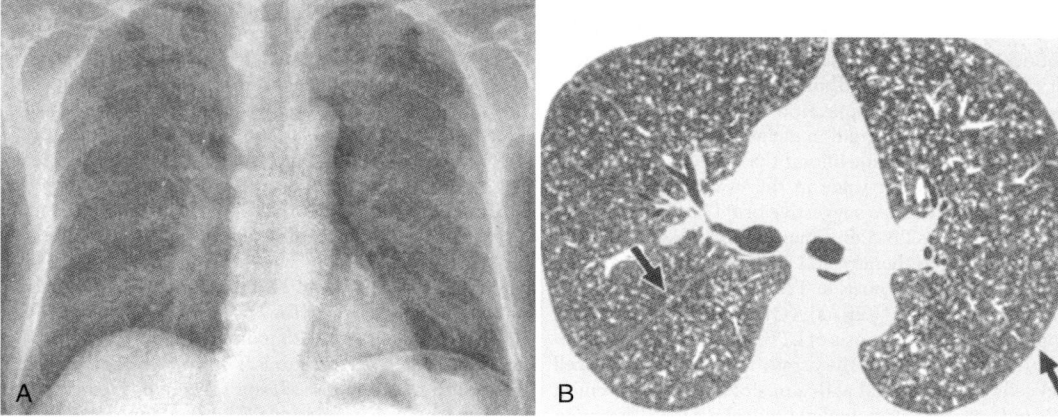

FIGURE 324-5. Miliary tuberculosis in a 70-year-old man. **A,** Posteroanterior chest radiograph shows evenly distributed, discrete, uniformly millet-sized nodular opacities in both lungs. **B,** High-resolution computed tomography (1.0-mm section thickness) at the level of the right upper lobar bronchus shows uniformly sized small nodules randomly distributed throughout both lungs. Note the subpleural and subfissural nodules *(arrows)*. (From Jeong YJ, Lee KS. Pulmonary tuberculosis: up-to-date imaging and management. *AJR Am J Roentgenol.* 2008;191:834-844.)

disease. On physical examination, the abdomen has been described as "doughy," because matted loops of bowel may be palpable. A variant of this syndrome is perhaps best termed *abdominal TB*. In this case, the abdominal pain is subacute, the associated findings on physical examination less striking, and ascites less prominent or absent. The best method for diagnosis when ascites is present is laparoscopically guided peritoneal biopsy. In areas endemic for TB and HIV, the finding of intra-abdominal lymphadenopathy on abdominal ultrasound or CT is often used to support the diagnosis of abdominal TB.

Gastrointestinal Tuberculosis

Patients with gastrointestinal TB have fever, abdominal pain, diarrhea, and gastrointestinal bleeding or obstruction. Roentgenograms of the small bowel and abdominal CT show involvement of the terminal ileum, similar to Crohn's disease. The diagnosis is made on clinical suspicion in areas endemic for TB and HIV or by the finding of TB elsewhere. Occasionally, intraluminal biopsy of the terminal ileum or other involved sites is used to establish the diagnosis.

Renal Tuberculosis

There may be few symptoms and signs associated with renal TB, although occasionally dysuria, hematuria, and flank pain are present. The diagnosis is often suggested by the finding of sterile pyuria or hematuria as initial abnormalities that trigger evaluation. Physical examination is usually unremarkable. CT shows renal cortical scarring, occasionally with mass or cavitary lesions, papillary necrosis with calyceal and ureteral dilation, or "beading" of the ureter because of ureteral strictures.

Vertebral Osteomyelitis

The initial site of disease is the subchondral region of the anterior portion of the vertebral body. The lower thoracic and lumbar vertebrae are involved most commonly. The disc space is initially spared but becomes involved late with spread to adjacent vertebrae. Paravertebral "cold abscesses" may dissect through tissue planes. Patients have back and sometimes radicular pain. Occasionally and more often with cervical disease, there may be weakness of the legs and incontinence of stool and urine. Physical examination may show a gibbus deformity caused by anterior compression fractures or paraparesis. Radiographs of the spine, as well as CT and magnetic resonance imaging, may show abnormalities in adjacent vertebrae, with anterior compression (see Fig. 324-3D). Cold abscesses may be appreciated as well.

Other Forms of Extrapulmonary Tuberculosis

TB of the bone or joints may be manifested subacutely as a combination of synovitis and osteomyelitis. The joints involved may have sustained previous trauma. TB of the female genital tract may result in pelvic pain, menorrhagia, vaginal discharge, or infertility. Males may have an epididymal mass, sometimes seen in patients with miliary TB. TB can cause granulomatous uveitis.

DIAGNOSIS

Infection with *Mycobacterium Tuberculosis*

The diagnosis of latent TB infection (LTBI) is one of exclusion, based on the finding of delayed-type hypersensitivity (DTH) and the absence of active TB. The tuberculin skin test (TST) has been used widely, and there is strong epidemiologic evidence supporting its interpretation. Tuberculin purified protein derivative (PPD) derived from autoclaved culture filtrates of Mtb is used to elicit DTH. The response elicited by PPD is nonspecific because of broad cross-reactivity among tuberculous and nontuberculous mycobacteria and other organisms as well. The TST is performed by injecting 5 tuberculin units of PPD in 0.1 mL intradermally. The reaction is assessed as induration after 48 to 72 hours. Problems with the TST are legion. It is the only bioassay used in clinical medicine, and there is no quality control of the application or reading of the TST. The sensitivity of the TST is less in immunosuppressed patients, such as those with HIV infection, and also less in the presence of active TB. The TST may revert to negative over time, and it may be boosted by the application of PPD. On repeat testing the result is a "pseudoconversion" that does not represent new infection with Mtb. The greatest limitation of the TST is its nonspecificity. There has been uncertainty in its interpretation, particularly in the setting of previous vaccination with *M. bovis* bacille Calmette-Guérin (BCG). In fact, BCG administered once at birth has little effect on the TST beyond the first year. By 10 years of age, only 1% of positive TSTs can be ascribed to previous BCG administration.

The TST remains of value in the diagnosis of LTBI in at-risk individuals who are candidates for treatment (preventive therapy). Interpretation of the TST is based on a "sliding scale" that takes into account an individual's a priori risk for Mtb infection and, if infected, the risk for progressing to disease (see Table 324-1). Changing the cut point for positives, in effect, modifies the sensitivity and specificity of the TST. Routine testing is not recommended for low-risk populations; however, testing may be performed because of employment. Certain populations should undergo annual testing, including staff or individuals living or working in congregate settings (incarcerated, homeless, HIV-infected, correctional facility staff), injection drug users, and others at risk because of sociodemographic factors. For individuals who will undergo an annual TST, a true baseline should be established by two-step skin testing. After the initial negative TST, the test is repeated in 1 to 3 weeks (there is no need to repeat the test if the first TST is positive). An increased reaction size on the second TST is known as "boosting" and may be due to previous infection with non-tuberculous mycobacteria or Mtb or vaccination with BCG. TST conversion from negative to positive is the best indicator of intervening new infection with Mtb and is defined as an increase in reaction size of 6 mm or greater from less than 10 mm to 10 mm or greater. It also may be of value to perform a two-step TST on individuals older than 60 years and therefore at risk for TST reversion.

In HIV infection, the TST may be negative before administration of antiretroviral therapy (ART) and convert to positive with treatment. For this reason, it is recommended that the TST be repeated in TST-negative

HIV-infected persons once their CD4$^+$ count reaches 200/μL and annually thereafter.

The sensitivity of the TST is decreased in individuals with active TB, more so in certain forms of extrapulmonary TB. Though insensitive for the diagnosis of active TB, the TST has another application in low-prevalence areas. If the differential diagnosis of a clinical condition includes TB, establishment of previous Mtb infection increases the likelihood that the clinical findings represent TB. The TST is of particular value in the evaluation of smear-negative patients with pulmonary disease suggestive of PTB and in patients suspected of having extrapulmonary TB. Confirmatory findings such as positive culture or histology, response to therapy, and lack of an alternative diagnosis are necessary to establish the diagnosis of TB.

Interferon gamma releasing assays (IGRAs) (QuantiFERON-TB Gold test) have also been approved for the diagnosis of LTBI, and the CDC considers them interchangeable with the TST.[7] The assays represent in vitro cell culture in which blood cells are stimulated with a mix of antigens present in Mtb but not in BCG and most nontuberculous mycobacteria. The main advantage of IGRAs is specificity. The antigens used to stimulate cells are present in Mtb but not BCG. IGRAs also require only a single patient visit. The disadvantages of IGRAs are expense, technical requirements, and controversy over test sensitivity in certain situations such as HIV infection and in household contacts of patients with PTB. Another issue has been instability of the result in individuals undergoing annual testing with IGRAs close to the cut point. The main indication for performing an IGRA, therefore, is to diagnose LTBI in a person who received BCG vaccination beyond the first year of life. There are several other situations in which IGRAs may be useful, for example, confirmation of a positive TST.

Because treatment of LTBI is effective in TST-positive HIV-infected persons, and the risk for progression of infection is inordinately high in such individuals, it is important to perform tests with high negative predictive value. Therefore, both a TST and IGRA should be performed in HIV-infected persons and others at high risk of progression from Mtb infection to disease or of a poor outcome. If either TST or IGRA is positive, the individual is a candidate for treatment of LTBI. Recent studies indicate that IGRAs may be less sensitive than TST in household contacts recently infected with Mtb, a particularly high-risk group.[8] This may be due to delayed conversion of IGRAs relative to TST. Mathematical modeling suggests IGRAs should replace TST in immunocompromised and perhaps all individuals, and that despite their increased cost, they are cost-effective in the United States. Unfortunately, modeling currently is based on data that are quite variable between studies. A fourth-generation test, Quantiferon-Gold Plus will undergo evaluation shortly and may show improved and stable accuracy.

In high TB–prevalence areas, the World Health Organization (WHO) recommends preventive therapy for all HIV-infected persons because of the difficulty in implementing a TST program that would identify those that will achieve the greatest benefit of INH preventive therapy.

Active Tuberculosis

In countries with a high TB burden, the diagnosis of TB is often based on clinical symptoms and sputum microscopy. Clinical diagnosis without the benefit of culture confirmation or radiography is the norm in endemic countries where access to diagnostics is limited. The diagnosis is also made on clinical grounds alone when smears are negative and suspicion for TB is high. Cultures, if available, require several weeks to months, and the decision to begin therapy must be made promptly. Clinical diagnosis is particularly important in HIV-infected persons because of the risk for rapid progression of the TB if left untreated, the more frequent occurrence of AFB smear–negative PTB, and in those with forms of TB that are "paucibacillary" (pediatric, meningeal, miliary, abdominal, pleural, pericardial), in which bacteria are few and AFB smears typically negative. The diagnosis of miliary, abdominal, pleural, and pericardial TB may be confirmed by the finding of AFBs in biopsied tissue or by culture. In the absence of bacteriologic confirmation, either because cultures are negative or because they are unavailable, the final diagnosis often relies on response to therapy or establishment of an alternative diagnosis. It should be noted that the empirical approach, taken of necessity in resource-limited settings, leads to overdiagnosis and overtreatment of TB, which expends TB program resources and delays treatment of other infections. It is therefore preferable to attempt to establish a definite diagnosis based on demonstration of Mtb by smears, cultures, or nucleic acid amplification tests of infected secretions or tissue specimens.

Sputum microscopy is the standard approach to the diagnosis of PTB. A smear requires 1000 to 10,000 bacilli/mL to be read as positive. Both hot and cold carbol fuchsin methods (Ziehl-Neelsen and Kinyoun) are used

extensively. The use of fluorochrome stains such as auramine-rhodamine allows more rapid screening of sputum smears and improves sensitivity by about 10%. Three specimens, preferably early morning samples, should be examined to establish the diagnosis. Yield is higher in the presence of cavitary lung disease. Approximately half of individuals with PTB are AFB sputum smear negative, and this proportion is higher in the HIV infected. The quantity of AFBs present in the sputum smear is a rough measure of the infectiousness of patients with PTB, and it is a convenient way to monitor response to treatment. On this basis, additional roles have evolved for the sputum smear as a tool to monitor the potential for transmission and response to therapy.

HIV-infected persons with PTB carry a particular risk for transmission to health care workers and have been documented as sources of nosocomial outbreaks. Therefore, in the United States, in areas of high prevalence of TB, HIV-infected persons with pulmonary symptoms may be placed into respiratory isolation until infectious TB can be reasonably excluded by three negative sputum smears for AFB on specimens separated by at least 8 hours.

The diagnosis of pediatric TB has always been problematic. Children do not produce sputum readily, and TB is often noncavitary, extrapulmonary, or both. Sputum samples may not be readily obtained from infants and children. Options in this case include sputum induction and gastric aspiration. The sensitivity of AFB smears of gastric aspirates and induced sputum is 25 to 30%. Therefore, the diagnosis often is based on clinical and epidemiologic features as well as response to therapy.

Bronchoscopy with bronchoalveolar lavage or transbronchial biopsy is another option for the diagnosis of TB and is useful in all severely ill individuals and the immunocompromised, in whom the diagnosis of TB or an alternative infection must be made quickly if treatment is to have an impact on patient outcome.

AFB smears should be performed on normally sterile fluid obtained from all patients suspected of having TB. The yield of smears from pleural fluid, pericardial fluid, ascitic fluid, and cerebrospinal fluid (CSF) is low in patients with TB but may be higher in those with HIV coinfection, particularly if immunodeficiency is advanced. In TB meningitis, CSF may clot spontaneously, and AFB stains of the clot have increased yield. Rapid diagnosis of some forms of extrapulmonary TB may be made by biopsy of tissue (pleural, pericardial, peritoneal, synovial, terminal ileum); the presence of granulomas, particularly if necrotizing, virtually confirms the diagnosis. Necrotizing granulomas are seen in TB and fungal diseases (particularly histoplasmosis, blastomycosis, coccidioidomycosis, and sporotrichosis). AFBs may also be seen in tissue histology, and Mtb cultured from the specimen.

The diagnosis of miliary TB can be suggested by CT of the chest and confirmed by transbronchial lung biopsy (highest yield), as well as biopsy of the liver, bone marrow, or abnormal lymph nodes. If TB meningitis is suspected and the patient is immunosuppressed, it is particularly important to exclude cryptococcal meningitis by performing a cryptococcal polysaccharide antigen test, as well as an India ink preparation on CSF sediment.

The diagnosis of TB from specimens of normally sterile fluid can be difficult and is increased by culturing relatively large volumes. In addition, the yield of biopsy and culture of tissue (pleura, pericardium) is additive. There are particular diagnostic features for various forms of extrapulmonary TB. In TB meningitis, the initial CSF examination may show neutrophil predominance, but this evolves into a lymphocytic meningitis (100 to 500 cells/μL) with high protein and depressed glucose. TB of the pleura, pericardium, and peritoneum is associated with an exudative effusion, often with a lymphocyte predominance. Low glucose may be found in 20% of TB effusions but limits the differential diagnosis considerably. For example, malignancy, empyema, and rheumatoid arthritis are the other causes of pleural effusion with low glucose. Pericardial fluid in patients with TB pericarditis may be bloody. Eosinophilic meningitis and chylous pleural effusions or ascites may also be seen in TB.

Currently, the gold standard for the diagnosis of TB is culture on solid (Löwenstein-Jensen) or in liquid (BACTEC MGIT 960 system) media. The mycobacteria growth indicator tube (MGIT) system, which has replaced BACTEC, is non-radiometric and based on oxygen quenching in the presence of replicating mycobacteria. When compared with solid media, culture with liquid media is more sensitive and growth is more rapid (1 to 3 weeks vs. 3 to 8 weeks for solid media). Once an isolate is available, drug susceptibility testing should be performed to guide therapy. This takes an additional 2 to 4 weeks on solid media, although isoniazid (INH) and rifampicin (RIF) susceptibility results are available in several days when the molecular line probe assay (described later) is used. Liquid medium can be inoculated with smear-positive specimens for direct drug susceptibility testing, which also accelerates the process. Once mycobacterial growth occurs, speciation is possible within hours with commercially available DNA probes. Nuclear acid amplification tests are approved and commercially available for use in TB diagnostics. Their sensitivity is somewhat higher than that of AFB smears, and their specificity is excellent. Expense precludes routine use of such tests, however.

The Xpert MTB-RIF has transformed TB diagnosis globally, although there is limited uptake in the United States because of delays in approval. Through in situ DNA amplification reaction, this test allows a specific diagnosis of TB and determination of susceptibility to rifampicin within 90 minutes.[9] After minimal processing, sputum is added to a cartridge. Gene amplification is done with primers based on the *rpoB* gene, which encodes the target of RIF, and resistance-conferring mutations are detected. This method is capable of establishing the diagnosis of TB in 97% of patients with PTB, including 98% of AFB sputum smear–positive and 73% of smear-negative individuals, thus rivaling the sensitivity of solid culture. It does not require molecular expertise by the technician and is not subject to amplicon (DNA) contamination, because it is a closed system. The uptake of GenXpert has been remarkable. The government of South Africa is replacing sputum smear analysis with GenXpert for the diagnosis of TB. The government of Brazil is developing a similar policy. In Uganda, there will be a single reference laboratory for culture and drug susceptibility testing (DST). GenXpert will be available regionally and used mainly for the diagnosis of smear-negative cases. GenXpert is priced differently for low-income countries, but cost still may be prohibitive in some settings. The test allows more rapid diagnosis and initiation of treatment but may not affect the outcome of treatment depending on a site's effectiveness in treating smear-negative patients.[10]

There are other candidate nucleic acid amplification tests (NAATs) about to undergo evaluation that are less expensive than GenXpert and may be truly point of care. Diagnostics for pediatric and extrapulmonary TB more sensitive than NAATs are likely to be based on host responses. As regards host-based diagnostics, there are promising data based on transcriptomics, proteomics, and metabolomics.

TB in the HIV-infected patient poses particular diagnostic issues because of increased likelihood of smear-negative PTB, and in advanced HIV, atypical presentation and extrapulmonary disease.

The HIV-infected TB suspect poses unique difficulties in diagnosis. Recent data indicate that a dipstick to detect lipoarabinomannan, the major cell wall glycolipid of Mtb, has a sensitivity of 60% when $CD4^+$ cell count is below 100 cells/μL.[11] This would be the first point-of-care test.

The development of new diagnostics also targets rapid determination of drug susceptibility. The Xpert MTB-RIF test described earlier is promising in this regard. The commercially available molecular line probe assay (Hain Genotype MTBDR plus) has been approved in Europe and is recommended by the WHO. This assay is based on probing for mutations in the targets of INH and RIF. The assay requires the technician be trained in molecular methods, and results require several days. This assay also is useful for rapidly establishing drug susceptibility once cultures are positive.

TREATMENT   Rx

Comprehensive reviews of TB treatment have been published and provide complete information on drugs for TB, monitoring of therapy, management of adverse events, and treatment of pregnant women, children, and other special populations:

- http://www.cdc.gov/mmwr/preview/mmwrhtml/rr5211a1.htm (treatment)
- http://www.cdc.gov/mmwr/preview/mmwrhtml/rr5804a1.htm (treatment and prevention in HIV-infected persons)

Treatment of TB is both a clinical and a public health issue. The goals are to cure the patient and minimize transmission. For that reason, the treating physician has the obligation to ensure that treatment is completed with good adherence to medications. Because of the declining number of TB cases in the United States, with subsequent decline in expertise in TB management, treatment is more likely to occur in a public health clinic than in the private sector. The cornerstone of TB treatment is multidrug therapy. This is necessary because Mtb undergoes spontaneous mutation to drug resistance at a frequency such that most patients with cavitary lung disease—and therefore patients with a high burden of organisms—are likely to harbor resistant mutants.

For the treatment of TB caused by drug-susceptible organisms, there is an intensive phase of therapy for the first 2 months aimed at the rapidly dividing and metabolizing organisms and usually resulting in sterilization of sputum in those with PTB. This is followed by a 4- to 6-month continuation phase that kills the slowly metabolizing persisting organisms. The five first-line anti-TB drugs, INH, RIF, ethambutol (EMB), pyrazinamide (PZA), and streptomycin (SM), form the foundation of chemotherapy for TB. The precepts of therapy have

been largely defined by controlled clinical trials. Standard short-course therapy for PTB requires a 2-month intensive phase of four drugs (INH, RIF, EMB, and PZA), followed by a 4-month continuation phase with INH and RIF.

The use of intermittent dosing regimens increases the feasibility of directly observed therapy (DOT) but is controversial. Intermittent regimens may be slightly less effective than daily 5/7 regimens (5 weekdays observed, 2 weekend days self-administered). For patients with extensive cavitary disease and the severely immunosuppressed, daily therapy should be administered throughout the entire course. For HIV-infected persons with TB who are not severely immunosuppressed, treatment should be daily during the intensive phase and at least three times weekly during the continuation phase. Non–HIV-infected persons without extensive cavitary disease can be treated with intermittent regimens throughout. Originally, EMB was perceived to be a "place holder" should the isolate prove to be resistant to INH, and the recommendation was to eliminate its use once drug susceptibility test results were available. There is recent evidence that EMB may be important because of its synergistic or additive activity with other first-line drugs, thereby providing an argument against its premature discontinuation before a full 2 months of therapy has been received.

The problem of nonadherence has led to the directive to provide DOT. The addition of PZA to the intensive phase allows for the so-called short-course chemotherapy; if PZA is not tolerated, comparable outcomes can be obtained with 9 months of INH-RIF. Treatment of drug-susceptible TB with this standard regimen can be expected to cure approximately 90 to 95% of cases. Routine monitoring of liver function test results is not recommended unless there is preexisting liver disease. Patients should return to the clinic promptly with any signs of drug toxicity, particularly those of early hepatotoxicity (nausea, malaise, anorexia, upper abdominal discomfort). Visits should be scheduled monthly and include clinical assessment and sputum examinations. For those with PTB, sputum cultures are continued until two consecutive cultures are negative. In uncomplicated PTB, defervescence is expected within 2 weeks, and there should be weight gain and diminution of cough and chest pain. About 20% of patients with cavitary PTB remain sputum culture positive after 2 months of therapy. A positive sputum culture at 3 months or failure to improve on chest radiographs suggests nonadherence with therapy, drug-resistant TB, or an alternative or complicating diagnosis. Positive sputum culture at 4 months is defined as treatment failure.

Extrapulmonary TB is usually associated with a smaller bacterial burden than is the case with PTB and can be treated with standard short-course regimens of 6 to 9 months' duration. However, because of the serious ramifications of treatment failure, more prolonged treatment of at least 9 to 12 months is recommended for miliary, meningeal, and skeletal TB. Adjunctive surgical débridement and stabilization may be necessary for skeletal TB. Adjunctive corticosteroids are indicated for TB pericarditis and severe pleurisy, as well as extensive PTB with clinical toxicity or respiratory failure. In TB meningitis, dexamethasone improves survival but has not had an impact on the proportion surviving with severe neurologic sequelae. Ventricular shunting may be necessary to relieve hydrocephalus.

HIV-TB coinfection creates additional management issues. Fortunately, the response to treatment of TB is comparable to that in HIV-uninfected individuals, except for higher early mortality. Intermittent regimens have a tendency to lead to RIF resistance; therefore, daily administration of drugs is recommended in the intensive phase, and drugs should be administered no less than three times weekly in the continuation phase. In resource-limited settings, the administration of cotrimoxazole prophylaxis is associated with improved survival. Integration of the treatment of TB and HIV rather than sequential treatment of first TB and then HIV is associated with a 56% reduction in mortality. The results of three randomized controlled trials support the current Department of Health and Human Services and Infectious Diseases Society of America guideline to start ART 2 weeks after initiation of TB treatment if $CD4^+$ count is below 50 cells/μL.[A1][A2] Early initiation of ART does incur a risk for paradoxical reaction, a form of immune reconstitution inflammatory syndrome (IRIS) (Chapter 395). TB-IRIS is more likely to occur when the $CD4^+$ count is low, the viral load is high, and the interval between starting TB drugs and ART is short.[12] Immune reconstitution is associated with inflammation and transient exacerbation of disease mimicking progression of TB. There may, for example, be fever, lymphadenitis, and pleural or worsening parenchymal disease, including consolidation and new or progressing nodular opacities on chest radiographs. In about one third of dually infected patients, IRIS will develop within the first 2 months of treatment and often within the first 2 to 3 weeks of starting ART. TB-IRIS usually is not an important cause of mortality. A controlled trial has shown that corticosteroid therapy limits morbidity,[A3] although it is not useful for treating tuberculous pericarditis.[A4] More problematic is IRIS associated with respiratory failure or neurologic involvement. Initiation of ART in HIV-infected persons may also be associated with "unmasking TB," which occurs within 3 months. This may be due to a missed diagnosis of TB in screening, the development of inflammation at sites of mycobacterial replication in tissue, or progression of latent infection consequent to ART. Unmasking TB is common in countries endemic for TB (5 to 10% in Uganda, for example, but about 25% in South Africa) and associated with morbidity, mortality, and risk for nosocomial transmission.

In general, TB does not affect the response of HIV to ART. A major issue, however, is the interactions between rifamycins that induce CYP3A hepatic microsomal enzymes and protease inhibitors and some non-nucleoside reverse transcriptase inhibitors (NRTIs). Because of its potency, simplicity, and proven clinical efficacy, efavirenz 600 mg with two NRTIs, along with rifampin-based TB regimens, is the preferred strategy for co-treatment of HIV and TB. Rifabutin is off-patent and increasingly available as a less potent inducer of cytochrome enzymes, but its own pharmacokinetics can be affected by certain ARTs. Rifampin is the preferred rifamycin for efavirenz containing regimens, whereas rifabutin should be used at a does of 150 mg daily with a boosted protease inhibitor. Guidelines for other drug combinations for managing adverse events were updated June 2013 and are available at http://www.cdc.gov/tb/TB_HIV_Drugs/default.htm.[13]

Management of TB-HIV coinfection may be complicated for the clinician. For example, a new fever may be due to drug reaction, TB-IRIS, drug resistance, or a complicating opportunistic infection.

Drug-resistant TB is more difficult to cure than drug-susceptible TB and in some instances may be incurable. DOT is particularly important to prevent acquisition of additional drug resistance. Selection and monitoring of treatment for drug-resistant TB should be the responsibility of those experienced with the unique drug regimens and issues involved. General issues concerning the management of drug-resistant TB are listed in Table 324-2. A major problem, however, is the lack of information on drug susceptibility at the time of initiation of treatment. In resource-limited settings, drug susceptibility testing may not be available at all. Drug resistance is more likely in retreatment cases, so standardized retreatment regimens are administered. The risk for drug resistance is greater if the initial regimen was not administered in a DOT program. For patients who relapse, did not receive DOT, were not treated with a RIF-containing regimen, were known or presumed to have irregular treatment, or have severe disease, an expanded regimen should be started. An example would be INH, RIF, and PZA plus an injectable (streptomycin if not previously used) and a fluoroquinolone, with or without an additional oral agent (ethionamide, para-aminosalicylic acid [PAS], or cycloserine). Ideally, the retreatment regimen should contain at least three drugs to which the isolate is likely to be susceptible. In resource-poor environments, streptomycin alone is often added to INH, RIF, EMB, and PZA. Although most retreatment cases remain drug susceptible, about 25% do not respond adequately to the standard regimen.[14] This approach is clearly inadequate for MDR or XDR TB. Ideally, drug susceptibility testing should be performed for all patients being retreated to ensure success of treatment and prevent acquisition of additional resistance.

Monoresistance to INH or streptomycin has little effect on the outcome of TB treatment. INH-resistant TB can be treated with RIF, PZA, and EMB for 6 months. Ofloxacin may be added for extensive or refractory disease. RIF-resistant TB can be treated with 12 to 18 months of INH, EMB, ofloxacin, and PZA (plus an injectable for the first 2 months if there is extensive disease). Acquisition of additional drug resistance is more likely if the initial isolate was resistant to one drug (6%) or more than one drug (14%) versus being pansusceptible (0.8%).

MDR TB represents a problem of a different order of magnitude. Not only is cure difficult and extremely expensive, but unrecognized MDR TB can also lead to nosocomial outbreaks and rapid and high rates of fatality in the HIV infected.

There is no substitute for performing drug susceptibility testing that includes all first-line and available second-line drugs. MDR TB is not a homogeneous entity. Frequently, the first diagnosis of MDR TB occurs in the setting of residual susceptibility to most other drugs. However, after repeated treatments, the isolate usually acquires additional drug resistance and, regardless of whether it fulfills the definition, is essentially XDR.

The cornerstone of treatment of MDR TB is administration of at least four drugs to which the isolate is susceptible (see Table 324-2). Typically, the regimen will include first-line drugs with retained activity, a fluoroquinolone (FQ), an injectable (amikacin, kanamycin, or capreomycin), and a second-line drug if disease is extensive (ethionamide, cycloserine, PAS). The duration of treatment is set at 12 to 18 months (12 to 15 months after sterilization of sputum). Residual susceptibility to FQ treatment and capreomycin has been shown to be a determinant of treatment outcome. Surgical resection is a consideration if the disease is localized, sputum remains culture positive, medical therapy is not tolerated, or massive hemoptysis is present. A recent review of published case series and cohort studies showed that surgical resection is beneficial in the adjunctive treatment of drug-resistant TB; however, the results might not be applicable in all settings, and well-designed studies are needed. Cure rates of 60 to 80% can be expected if therapy is targeted to drug susceptibility test results and MDR organisms remain sensitive to enough chemotherapeutic drugs that a reasonable regimen can be established. The U.S. Food and Drug Administration (FDA) recently approved both bedaquiline and delamanid for the treatment of MDR TB.[A5,15] Bedaquiline, a diarylquinoline, targets mycobacterial ATP synthase, and delamanid, a nitrodihydroimidazooxazole inhibits Mtb mycolic acid synthesis. Both accelerate sterilization of sputum when added to regimens for treatment of MDR TB. It is recommended that bedaquiline be added to three drugs active against the isolate. These are the first new classes of TB treatment drugs to be approved by the FDA in 40 years. They should revolutionize management of MDR TB. Spectinamides, a new class of semisynthetic anti-TB agents, have been shown to overcome the efflux pump that is upregulated in MDR strains.[16]

The definition of XDR TB requires that an organism be MDR with additional resistance to an FQ plus at least one of three injectables (amikacin, kanamycin, capreomycin). The outcome of treatment of XDR TB has been variable. The best reported results have been obtained in Peru, with a comprehensive approach that included therapeutic regimens that were tailored according to drug susceptibility testing. Effective regimens included cycloserine, capreomycin, and PAS. Moxifloxacin may be active even if the isolate is resistant to first-generation FQs. Adjunctive surgery should be considered. A recent study indicates that linezolid has remarkable activity against XDR TB,[A6] and other oxazolidinones are in development for TB treatment.

The emergence of drug resistance has emphasized the need for new drugs and new drug regimens. A drug regimen that shortens the course of TB would lessen the emergence of drug resistance, because adherence would increase and DOT would be simplified. Once MDR TB develops, particularly in the setting of XDR TB, new drugs are necessary to improve efficacy and shorten treatment.

There are promising developments with existing classes of drugs, as well with as new classes about to enter or already in clinical trials. Rifapentine, a rifamycin with a longer half-life than RIF, shows remarkable enhancement of sterilization of sputum at 2 months. Moxifloxacin has increased activity against Mtb, although data of its efficacy in 4-month regimens have been disappointing to date. PA-824 and delamanid are nitroimidazole derivatives that are active against slowly replicating bacilli. Also in development are SQ-109 (ethylenediamine), an ethambutol derivative, and sutezolid (an oxazolidinone more active than linezolid).

TABLE 324-2	PRINCIPLES OF MANAGEMENT OF TUBERCULOSIS CAUSED BY DRUG-RESISTANT ORGANISMS

- Do not add a single drug to a failing regimen.
- When starting or modifying therapy, add three previously unused drugs (one an injectable) to which there is susceptibility.
- In MDR TB where there is resistance to first-line drugs, in addition to INH and RIF, treat with 4-6 drugs.
- Patients with MDR TB have highest priority for DOT, because treatment failure may mean XDR TB.
- Intermittent therapy should not be used (except for injectables after 2-3 mo).
- Do not use drugs to which the Mtb isolate is resistant. Low-level INH resistance may be the exception.
- There is cross-resistance among rifamycins but not between streptomycin and other aminoglycosides.
- There may be susceptibility to moxifloxacin but resistance to other fluoroquinolones.
- Drug susceptibility testing for PZA is complex technically and not performed in most laboratories. Monoresistance to PZA suggests *Mycobacterium bovis*.
- Always consult with an expert. There is predisposition to acquisition of additional drug resistance that will decrease the chances of cure.

DOT = directly observed therapy; INH = isoniazid; MDR TB = multidrug-resistant tuberculosis; Mtb = *Mycobacterium tuberculosis*; PZA = pyrazinamide; RIF = rifampin; XDR TB = extensively drug-resistant tuberculosis.

PREVENTION

The issues surrounding prevention are presented in a comprehensive statement published in 2000 (http://www.cdc.gov/mmwr/preview/mmwrhtml/rr4906a1.htm), and prevention in HIV-infected persons is presented at the website http://www.cdc.gov/mmwr/preview/mmwrhtml/rr5804a1.htm.

The approach taken in a low-prevalence setting such as the United States is to target tuberculin skin testing to those at high risk for recent Mtb infection and to those with comorbid conditions that predispose to progression from infection to disease. In either category, a positive TST becomes an indication for treatment of LTBI. The cut point of TST is adjusted according to risk of MTB infection and risk of progressing from infection to disease (see Table 324-1).

LTBI can be treated with rifampicin for 3 to 4 months, INH for 6 to 12 months, or the combination for 3 to 4 months,[17] thereby decreasing the lifetime risk for development of TB by approximately 75 to 90%, depending on the level of adherence to treatment. Pyridoxine should be administered to prevent INH-induced peripheral neuropathy. Monitoring of liver function is indicated in older individuals (the risk for hepatotoxicity increases beyond the age of 35 years) and in those with significant alcohol intake or underlying liver disease (or both). INH should be discontinued if symptoms develop (see Treatment) or hepatic transaminase levels rise to more than three to five times the upper limit of normal. Rifapentine plus INH once weekly for 3 months (12 doses) is as effective as 9 months of INH alone in preventing active TB in patients with latent infection.[A7] Administration of this regimen should be directly observed. In HIV-infected persons, treatment of LTBI confers short-term efficacy (≈1 year), but this may be extended if ART is administered. Treatment for 3 years confers an additional benefit that is most marked in the TST positives. Unfortunately, treatment of LTBI has not been applied broadly. This is in part due to the concern that if screening is inadequate, patients with active TB will be treated with a single drug and thereby acquire drug resistance. The available data do not support this concern. In a recently reported cluster-randomized study, a trial of mass screening and INH preventive therapy for TB control among gold mine workers in South Africa (where TB is epidemic) had no significant effect on TB control despite the successful use of INH in preventing TB during treatment.[A8] In a low-resource setting in the HIV infected, the absence of current fever, weight loss, or night sweats has a negative predictive value of 97%, may obviate the need for chest radiography if it is not routinely available, and identifies a group that should be treated with INH preventive treatment regardless of TST status. Although INH preventive therapy is the preferred regimen, there is renewed interest in the possibility that rifamycin-containing regimens may confer more sustained protection. There are no data on how to treat LTBI caused by a known or probably drug-resistant isolate. PZA plus EMB or ofloxacin has been used after known exposure to MDR TB that is susceptible to the combination, but gastrointestinal intolerance is very common. Studies of linezolid are planned in this population.

Secondary preventive therapy after completion of TB treatment is indicated in HIV-infected persons in the setting of intense exposure to Mtb. Data demonstrating efficacy of secondary prevention largely result from studies of adults in Congo and gold miners in South Africa.

A randomized controlled trial has now demonstrated that in HIV-positive patients, early initiation of ART as compared with delayed treatment (where there was a decline in CD4 counts or AIDS-related illness had already occurred) led to a significant decrease in the development of TB.[A9]

Tracing of household contacts is a critical element of TB programs. The household is a major site of TB transmission, particularly in an area of low endemicity, so treatment of TST converters is an important strategy for elimination of TB. It is essential that transmission be limited in hospitals and other settings in which infectious PTB patients may comingle with susceptible hosts. The risk of transmission to health care workers should be ascertained annually by skin testing. The finding of excessive risk for new TB infection should lead to focused measures for reducing transmission. All TB suspects should be placed in respiratory isolation in negative-pressure rooms with at least six air exchanges per hour and high-efficiency particulate air (HEPA) filtration or ultraviolet irradiation. N-95 personnel respirator devices that are fit-tested are necessary for individuals entering areas with a known high risk for exposure.

BCG vaccine is widely used and relatively safe except in the setting of immunosuppression. Unfortunately, efficacy has been variable by age and by latitude. A meta-analysis indicated an overall efficacy of 50%. It is approximately 80% effective in preventing the severe forms of TB in childhood, miliary TB, and TB meningitis. However, its failure to prevent adult TB, particularly at low latitudes that include the most endemic areas, means that BCG vaccine does not have an impact on the public health problem of TB. The development of a more effective protective vaccine has been hampered by the absence of good animal models and the lack of correlates of protective immunity in humans. The issue is further compounded by the natural history of TB such that large, lengthy, and expensive trials may be needed to establish protective efficacy. Nonetheless, several vaccine candidates have been developed and their potential efficacy supported by preclinical studies in animal models. Two of the 12 currently in clinical trials are MVA85A, a recombinant modified vaccinia virus expressing the 85A antigen, a major secretory product of Mtb, and Mtb72f, a combination of two immunogenic antigens, Mtb 32a and Mtb 39a, in two adjuvants, ASO2a and ASO1B. A recent trial of the MVA85A vaccine in infants to boost the BCG response failed to show efficacy.

PROGNOSIS

In the pre-chemotherapeutic era, minimal PTB stabilized in about 50% of cases. Pleural TB also self-cured, with a risk for reactivation as noted previously. With treatment, the prognosis of patients with TB depends on the extent of PTB, the sites of extrapulmonary TB, drug susceptibility of the isolate, and the presence of HIV infection and other comorbid conditions. With extensive PTB, respiratory failure may supervene with a poor prognosis. There is also increased risk for serious, sometimes lethal, hemoptysis and pneumothorax. Miliary TB is associated with a high case-fatality rate, in part related to delays in diagnosis. TB meningitis is associated with serious neurologic residua, as well as high mortality. MDR TB and XDR TB are accompanied by high rates of treatment failure, morbidity, and mortality. TB in HIV-infected persons is associated with high early mortality that is poorly characterized. In the absence of ART, there is increased risk for other opportunistic infections and progression of HIV disease. The addition of ART, however, results in the morbidities associated with the concurrent administration of TB and HIV medications and with TB-IRIS. Long-term outcomes of patients with XDR TB were recently reported from South Africa. Their outcomes were poor irrespective of HIV status, and because of the scarcity of long-stay or palliative care facilities, substantial numbers of patients with XDR TB who had failed treatment and had positive sputum cultures were being discharged to likely transmit disease into the wider community.[18]

Grade A References

A1. Havlir DV, Kendall MA, Ive P, et al. Timing of antiviral therapy for HIV-1 and tuberculosis. *N Engl J Med.* 2011;365:1482-1491.
A2. Blanc F-X, Sok T, Laureillard D, et al. Earlier vs later start of antiviral therapy in HIV-infected adults with tuberculosis. *N Engl J Med.* 2011;365:1471-1481.
A3. Meintges G, Wildkinson RJ, Morroni C, et al. Randomized placebo-controlled trial of prednisone for paradoxical tuberculosis-associated immune reconstitution syndrome. *AIDS.* 2010;24:2381-2390.
A4. Mayosi BM, Ntsekhe M, Bosch J, et al. Prednisolone and *Mycobacterium indicus pranii* in tuberculous pericarditis. *N Engl J Med.* 2014;371:1121-1130.
A5. Diacon AH, Pym A, Grobusch M, et al. The diaryquinoline TMC 207 for multidrug resistant tuberculosis. *N Engl J Med.* 2009;360:2397-2405.
A6. Lee M, Lee J, Carroll MW, et al. Linezolid for treatment of chronic extensively drug resistant tuberculosis. *N Engl J Med.* 2012;367:1508-1518.
A7. Sterling TR, Villarino ME, Borisov AS, et al. Three months of rifapentine and isoniazid for latent tuberculosis infection. *N Engl J Med.* 2011;365:2155-2166.
A8. Churchyard GJ, Fielding KL, Lewis JJ, et al. A trial of mass isoniazid preventive therapy for tuberculosis control. *N Engl J Med.* 2014;370:301-310.
A9. Grinsztejn B, Hosseinipour MC, Ribaudo HJ, et al. Effects of early versus delayed initiation of antiretroviral treatment on clinical outcomes of HIV-1 infection: results from the phase 3 HPTN 052 randomised controlled trial. *Lancet Infect Dis.* 2014;14:281-290.

GENERAL REFERENCES

For the General References and other additional features, please visit Expert Consult at https://expertconsult.inkling.com.

325

THE NONTUBERCULOUS MYCOBACTERIA

STEVEN M. HOLLAND

DEFINITION

Nontuberculous mycobacteria generally include the growing number of mycobacteria other than *Mycobacterium tuberculosis* and its close relatives (Chapter 324) and *Mycobacterium leprae* (Chapter 326). Other names that have been used include *atypical mycobacteria, mycobacteria other than tuberculosis,* and *environmental mycobacteria.* The number of nontuberculous mycobacteria is growing rapidly as a result of the advent of DNA sequence typing for determining criteria for speciation. Accordingly, the number of species of nontuberculous mycobacteria has increased to almost 170 and will continue to increase for the near future.

The Pathogens

Identification of any mycobacterium requires that the appropriate tests be thought of ahead of time and be performed, because routine microbiological testing does not identify mycobacteria. Nontuberculous mycobacteria are typically first detected on acid-fast smears of sputum or other body fluids. When levels of organisms are high, mycobacteria may be seen on Gram stain

TABLE 325-1	COMMON NONTUBERCULOUS MYCOBACTERIA
ORGANISM	**DISEASE**
RAPIDLY GROWING NONTUBERCULOUS MYCOBACTERIA	
M. abscessus	Lung, disseminated, lymph node
M. chelonae	Skin
M. fortuitum	Line infections, lung
M. smegmatis	Almost never associated with disease
SLOWLY GROWING NONTUBERCULOUS MYCOBACTERIA	
M. avium complex	Lung, disseminated, lymph node
M. kansasii	Lung
M. marinum	Skin, tendons (fish tank granuloma)
M. xenopi	Lung
M. simiae	Lung
M. szulgai	Lung
M. malmoense	Lung
M. scrofulaceum	Lymph node
M. haemophilum	Disseminated, skin
M. genavense	Disseminated
M. ulcerans	Skin (Buruli ulcer; toxin producing)
M. neoarum	Disseminated
M. celatum	Disseminated
M. gordonae	Almost never causes disease
M. terrae complex	Disseminated

M = *Mycobacterium*.

as gram-positive beaded rods, but this finding is unreliable. The first step in identification is to request the appropriate smear (acid-fast or fluorochrome) and culture. Nontuberculous mycobacteria are broadly differentiated into rapidly growing (<7 days) and slowly growing (>7 days) forms. *M. tuberculosis*, by contrast, typically takes 2 or more weeks to grow. Formation of pigment in light (photochromogens) or dark (scotochromogens) and lack of pigment (nonchromogens) have also been used to help categorize nontuberculous mycobacteria. Current diagnostics use biochemical, nucleic acid, or cell wall composition on high-performance liquid chromatography for speciation (Table 325-1). For purposes of diagnosis, prognosis, and therapy, identification of nontuberculous mycobacteria should be taken to the species level.

EPIDEMIOLOGY

As a group, the nontuberculous mycobacteria are ubiquitous in soil and water and are often found in certain animals, but they rarely cause disease in humans. There are very few instances of human-to-human transmission of nontuberculous mycobacteria. However, *Mycobacterium massiliense* has caused outbreaks of infection in cystic fibrosis centers. Because these infections are not reported to health agencies and their identification is sometimes problematic, reliable data on incidence and prevalence are lacking. In the United States, however, isolates of nontuberculous mycobacteria have exceeded those for *M. tuberculosis* for many years. In patients with cystic fibrosis (Chapter 89), for example, rates of clinical nontuberculous mycobacterial infection range up to 40%, but even more patients harbor the organism. Differentiating active disease from commensal harboring of the organism remains problematic. Other patient groups, such as those with bronchiectasis, also have elevated rates of nontuberculous mycobacterial infection, but the rates are undefined.[1] The bulk of nontuberculous mycobacterial disease in North America is due to *Mycobacterium kansasii*, *Mycobacterium avium* complex (MAC), and *Mycobacterium abscessus*.

PATHOBIOLOGY

Because exposure is essentially universal and disease is rare, normal host defenses against nontuberculous mycobacteria must be highly effective. Therefore, otherwise healthy individuals in whom disease develops must have specific susceptibility factors that permit these infections to become established, multiply, and cause disease.

With the advent of human immunodeficiency virus (HIV) infection, CD4+ T lymphocytes were identified as key effectors against nontuberculous mycobacteria. Much of the genetic basis of susceptibility to disseminated nontuberculous mycobacterial infection outside HIV infection has been found to be due to specific mutations in the interferon (IFN)-γ/interleukin

(IL)-12 synthesis and response pathways. However, only about 70% of disseminated cases unassociated with HIV infection have a genetic diagnosis, and genetic causes of predisposition to nontuberculous mycobacterial lung disease are still very few.

Mycobacteria are typically phagocytosed by macrophages, which respond with the production of IL-12, a heterodimer composed of p35 and p40 moieties that together constitute IL-12p70 (Fig. 325-1). IL-12 activates T lymphocytes and natural killer (NK) cells through binding to its receptor (composed of IL-12Rβ1 and IL-12Rβ2/IL-23R) and results in phosphorylation of STAT4 (signal transducer and activator of transcription 4). IL-12 stimulation leads to production and secretion of IFN-γ, which activates neutrophils and macrophages to produce reactive oxidants and increase major histocompatibility complex display and Fc receptors. IFN-γ signals through its receptor (composed of IFN-γR1 and IFN-γR2), thereby leading to phosphorylation of STAT1, which in turn regulates IFN-γ–responsive genes such as those for the production of IL-12 and tumor necrosis factor (TNF)-α. Therefore, the positive feedback loop between IFN-γ and IL-12/IL-23 is pivotal in the immune response to mycobacteria and other intracellular infections (most importantly *Salmonella*, *Histoplasma*, *Coccidioides*). The advent of potent TNF-α inhibitors such as infliximab, adalimumab, certolizumab, etanercept, and golimumab (Chapter 36) has provided the ability to neutralize this critical cytokine, which has occasionally resulted in mycobacterial and fungal infections.

CLINICAL MANIFESTATIONS

Disseminated Disease

Disseminated nontuberculous mycobacterial disease secondary to MAC used to occur commonly in the setting of advanced acquired immunodeficiency syndrome (AIDS) but is now uncommon in North America because of MAC prophylaxis and improved treatment of HIV infection. The portal of entry was the bowel, with spread to bone marrow and the blood stream. Rapidly growing mycobacteria such as *Mycobacterium fortuitum* sometimes infect deep indwelling lines. The severe disseminated infection seen with immune defects is typically associated with malaise, fever, and weight loss, and it is often accompanied by organomegaly and lymphadenopathy. Disseminated (two or more organ) involvement in a child without an underlying iatrogenic cause should always prompt an investigation of the IFN-γ/IL-12 pathway.[2] Nontuberculous mycobacterial osteomyelitis is especially common with dominant negative mutations in IFN-γR1. A male with conical or peg teeth or an abnormal hair pattern and disseminated nontuberculous mycobacterial infection should be evaluated for defects in the pathway that activates nuclear factor (NF)κB. Some patients with disseminated rapidly growing infections (predominantly *M. abscessus*) have high-titer autoantibodies to IFN-γ.

Pulmonary Disease

Lung disease caused by nontuberculous mycobacteria is by far the most common form of the infection in North America. Predisposing factors include underlying lung disease, such as bronchiectasis (Chapter 90), pneumoconiosis (Chapter 93), chronic obstructive pulmonary disease (Chapter 88), primary ciliary dyskinesia, and cystic fibrosis.[3] The manifestations of *M. kansasii* infection can be very similar to those of tuberculosis (Chapter 324) and consist of hemoptysis, chest pain, and cavitary lung disease. MAC infection most commonly occurs in women in their sixth or seventh decade who have had months to years of nagging intermittent cough and fatigue, with or without sputum production or chest pain. Bronchiectasis and nontuberculous mycobacterial infection often coexist and progress in tandem, thus making causality difficult to determine. When compared with male smokers with upper lobe cavitary disease, who tend to carry the very same single strain of MAC indefinitely, nonsmoking females with nodular bronchiectasis tend to have several strains simultaneously and change them over the course of their disease process. Patients with pulmonary alveolar proteinosis (Chapter 91) are prone to pulmonary nontuberculous mycobacterial and *Nocardia* infections, likely reflecting their association with anti-GM-CSF autoantibodies and impaired alveolar macrophage function. Esophageal motility disorders such as achalasia (Chapter 138) have been associated with pulmonary disease, especially that caused by rapidly growing nontuberculous mycobacteria such as *M. abscessus*. It is important to note that lung disease rarely disseminates, illustrating that the defects leading to isolated pulmonary involvement are specific to the respiratory epithelium, whereas those defects leading to disseminated disease affect immune cells.

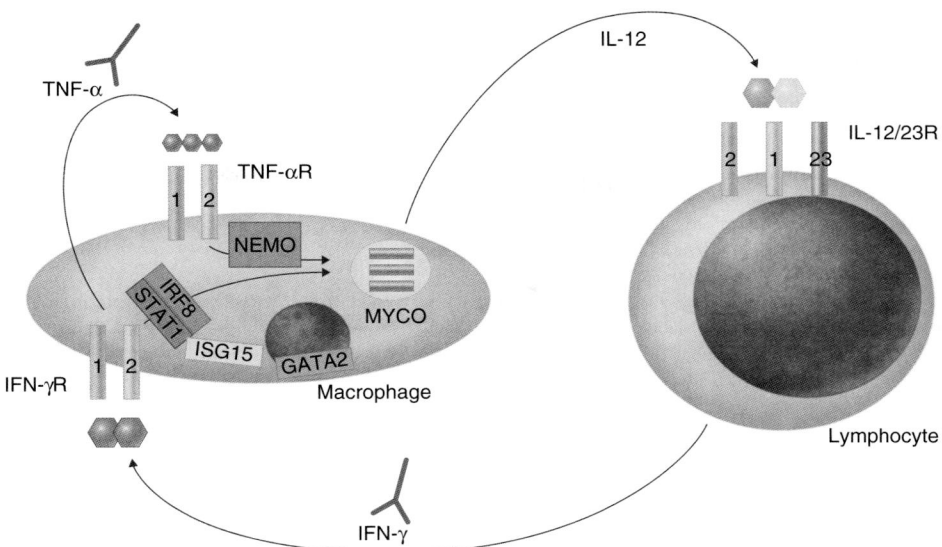

FIGURE 325-1. Schematization of the critical cytokine interactions between infected macrophages and T and natural killer lymphocytes. Organisms (MYCO) infect macrophages, which release heterodimeric interleukin (IL)-12. This acts on the IL-12/23 receptor complex and leads to the production of homodimeric interferon (IFN)-γ. IFN-γ acts on its receptor to stimulate the production of tumor necrosis factor (TNF)-α and kill intracellular organisms such as mycobacteria, salmonellae, and some fungi. Homotrimeric TNF-α acts on its own receptor and also contributes to killing of intracellular organisms. Both IFN-γ and TNF-α lead to upregulation of IL-12. TNF-α–blocking antibodies work either by blocking the ligand (infliximab, adalimumab, certolizumab) or by providing soluble receptor (etanercept). Mutations in both chains of IFN-γR, IL-12p40, and IL-12Rβ1, IL-12Rβ2 and signal elements for IFN-γR and TNF-αR have been identified through their predisposition to mycobacterial infections. IRF8 = interferon regulatory factor 8; ISG = interferon stimulated gene; NEMO = nuclear factor kappa-B essential modulator; STAT1 = signed transducer and activator of transcription 1.

Therefore, evaluation of isolated lung disease should focus on respiratory tract causes.[4]

Cervical Lymph Nodes

Isolated cervical lymphadenopathy, most frequently caused by MAC, is the most common form of nontuberculous mycobacterial infection in young children in North America. The organism is generally MAC, but other nontuberculous mycobacteria can also cause disease. The cervical swelling is often firm and relatively painless with a paucity of systemic signs. Because the differential diagnosis of painless adenopathy includes malignancy, many of these infections are incidentally diagnosed at biopsy. Local fistulas usually resolve completely with resection or antibiotic therapy or both.

Skin and Soft Tissue Disease

Mycobacterium marinum causes skin infections, usually papules or ulcers, associated with water exposure and is known as "fish tank granuloma." Numerous outbreaks of skin infections caused by rapidly growing mycobacteria (especially *M. abscessus*, *M. fortuitum*, and *Mycobacterium chelonae*) have been due to skin contamination from instruments used for surgical procedures (especially cosmetic surgery), injections, and other procedures.[5] These infections are typically accompanied by painful, erythematous, draining subcutaneous nodules, usually without associated fever or systemic symptoms.

DIAGNOSIS

With the continued decline in cases of tuberculosis, nontuberculous mycobacteria are now the most common mycobacteria isolated from humans in North America. The conventional tuberculin skin test (purified protein derivative [PPD]) evokes a cell-mediated response to secreted mycobacterial antigens. Unfortunately, the PPD test does not differentiate well between nontuberculous mycobacterial and tuberculosis infection, although large PPD reactions (>15 mm) more commonly signify tuberculosis. With the progressive decline in active tuberculosis in the United States, nontuberculous mycobacteria are likely to account for significant proportions of PPD reactivity. Newer IFN-γ release assays (IGRAs) incubate blood with relatively tuberculosis-specific recombinant proteins and elicit T-cell secretion of IFN-γ, thereby helping to clarify whether PPD reactivity is due to tuberculosis.

Isolation of nontuberculous mycobacteria from blood specimens is clear evidence of disease. However, because the slow-growing nontuberculous mycobacteria typically do not grow well in routine blood culture media, the diagnosis must be suspected. Isolation of nontuberculous mycobacteria from a biopsy specimen is strong evidence of infection, but cases of laboratory

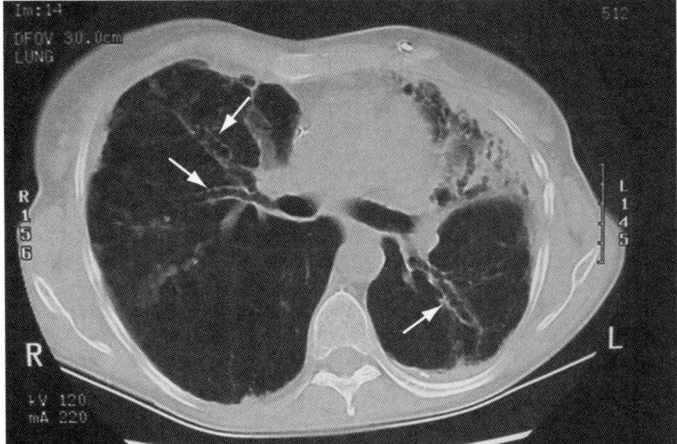

FIGURE 325-2. Chest computed tomography in a patient with severe pulmonary *Mycobacterium abscessus* infection. Arrows indicate bronchiectasis. Note the extensive left upper lobe destruction and diffuse pleural reaction. In addition, the left lung is smaller than the right as a result of extensive loss of lung parenchyma.

contamination do occur. Identification of organisms on stained sections of biopsy material confirms the authenticity of the culture. Some unusual nontuberculous mycobacteria require lower incubation temperatures or special additives for growth (e.g., *Mycobacterium hemophilum*).

The radiographic appearance of nontuberculous mycobacterial disease in the lung ranges from normal to nodules, bronchiectasis, air space disease, and extensive cavity formation, similar to that seen in tuberculosis (Fig. 325-2). Isolation of nontuberculous mycobacteria from respiratory samples presents special problems in both sensitivity and specificity. *Mycobacterium gordonae* is often recovered from respiratory samples and is almost never thought to be a real pathogen. Many patients, especially those with bronchiectasis, will occasionally have nontuberculous mycobacteria recovered from sputum culture without such mycobacteria being seen on smear. Specific criteria for definitive diagnosis of nontuberculous mycobacterial lung disease exist for MAC, *M. abscessus*, and *M. kansasii*, but they are probably good guidelines for other nontuberculous mycobacteria as well. A positive diagnosis requires that two of three sputum samples grow nontuberculous mycobacteria, regardless of smear findings; a positive bronchoscopic alveolar sample, regardless of smear findings; or a biopsy specimen of pulmonary parenchyma with granulomatous inflammation or mycobacteria found on section and nontuberculous mycobacteria on culture.

Once isolated, identification of nontuberculous mycobacteria is important because it will determine the broad class of antimycobacterial therapy to be used. Many laboratories now use DNA probes to identify MAC, *M. gordonae*, and *M. kansasii*.[6] Drug susceptibility testing is of limited and largely unproven value, although clarithromycin susceptibility testing for MAC and rifampin susceptibility testing for *M. kansasii* are indicated. Initial isolates of MAC that have not been exposed to macrolides are almost always susceptible to macrolides. Any nontuberculous mycobacteria that have resisted a course of antimicrobials should probably be tested for antibiotic susceptibility as well.

PREVENTION

Prophylaxis of MAC disease in patients infected with HIV is started when the CD4+ T-lymphocyte count is less than 50 cells/μL. Azithromycin 1200 mg weekly, clarithromycin 1000 mg daily, and rifabutin 300 mg daily are effective.

TREATMENT   Rx

It is rarely an emergency to initiate treatment of nontuberculous mycobacterial infections, which are relatively slow-growing chronic infections that evolve over a period of weeks to years, not hours to days. Therefore, empirical therapy is not usually needed, and identification of the species is advisable before starting complex, often poorly tolerated and potentially toxic, regimens. Similar to the case with tuberculosis, single-drug therapy is almost always associated with the emergence of antimicrobial resistance and is strongly discouraged.

MAC infection frequently requires complex multidrug therapy, the foundation of which is a macrolide (clarithromycin or azithromycin), ethambutol, and a rifamycin (rifampin or rifabutin). For disseminated nontuberculous mycobacterial disease in HIV-infected patients, the use of rifamycins poses special problems of drug interactions with protease inhibitors. For pulmonary MAC disease, three-times-weekly administration of drugs has been used successfully. The duration of therapy is prolonged, generally for 12 months after culture conversion and typically for a total of at least 18 months. Other drugs with activity against MAC include aminoglycosides, fluoroquinolones, and clofazimine.

M. kansasii lung disease is similar to tuberculosis in many ways and is also effectively treated with isoniazid (300 mg/day), rifampin (600 mg/day), and ethambutol (15 mg/kg/day). Treatment should continue until cultures have been negative for at least 1 year. Other drugs with very high activity against *M. kansasii* include clarithromycin, fluoroquinolones, and aminoglycosides.

Rapidly growing mycobacteria pose special therapeutic problems. Extrapulmonary disease in an immunocompetent host is usually due to inoculation (e.g., surgery, injection, trauma) or line infection and is often treated successfully with a macrolide and another drug (based on in vitro susceptibility), along with removal of the offending focus. By comparison, pulmonary disease, especially that caused by *M. abscessus*, is extremely difficult to eradicate, although repeated courses of treatment are usually effective in reducing the infectious burden and symptoms. Therapy generally includes a macrolide along with an intravenous agent such as amikacin, a carbapenem, cefoxitin, or tigecycline.[7] Other oral agents used according to in vitro susceptibility testing and tolerance include fluoroquinolones, doxycycline, and linezolid. Inhaled amikacin may be an option for treatment-refractory pulmonary infections.[8]

Treatment of the other nontuberculous mycobacteria is less well defined, but macrolides and aminoglycosides are usually effective, with other agents added as indicated. Expert consultation is strongly encouraged for difficult or unusual nontuberculous mycobacterial infections.

PROGNOSIS

The effect of nontuberculous mycobacterial infection on longevity is closely tied to the underlying condition (e.g., IFN-γ/IL-12 pathway defect, cystic fibrosis). With no or inadequate treatment, symptoms are intrusive, and the infections can lead to fatal complications, including overwhelming infection or severe lung destruction.

GENERAL REFERENCES

For the General References and other additional features, please visit Expert Consult at https://expertconsult.inkling.com.

326

LEPROSY (HANSEN DISEASE)

JOEL D. ERNST

DEFINITION

Leprosy (Hansen disease) is a chronic infection caused by *Mycobacterium leprae*, an acid-fast slowly growing bacterium that cannot yet be cultured in vitro. Leprosy is found worldwide, although three countries of high prevalence (India, Brazil, and Indonesia) currently account for more than 80% of reported cases.[1] The primary manifestations of infection with *M. leprae* occur in the skin and peripheral nerves. The skin lesions of leprosy are classically hypopigmented, hypoesthetic or anesthetic, and nonpruritic. Peripheral nerves can be damaged by direct infection with *M. leprae* or by the immune response to the infection; the result is loss of sensation and motor function. Additional morbidity is due to the peripheral nerve dysfunction, including painless traumatic and burn injuries, secondary bacterial infections, and muscle atrophy and contractures. Leprosy per se is not a cause of death, but the debility associated with leprosy contributes to the severity of poverty and the likelihood of death from malnutrition or other infections. Despite the low transmissibility of *M. leprae* and the ability of multiple-drug therapy to cure leprosy, it remains a stigmatized disease that can pose a challenge to diagnosis and therapy.

The Pathogen

M. leprae is an acid-fast bacillus that contains a mycolic acid–rich cell wall and a single membrane. Despite nearly 150 years of effort, *M. leprae* remains uncultivatible in vitro. For biochemical and structural characterization, *M. leprae* can be grown in large quantities in nine-banded armadillos (*Dasypus novemcinctus*), and inoculation of the footpads of athymic mice allows semiquantitation of viable bacilli.

The genome of *M. leprae* consists of 3,268,203 base pairs (bp), compared with the *Mycobacterium tuberculosis* genome of 4,411,529 bp, and the number of expressed genes of *M. leprae* is approximately 60% fewer than that of *M. tuberculosis*. Because *M. leprae* and *M. tuberculosis* probably evolved from a common mycobacterial ancestor, *M. leprae* appears to have lost approximately 2000 genes since this divergence, leaving it dependent on specialized ecologic niches for its survival. Among the genes lacking in *M. leprae* are those of the *mbt* complex, whose products are involved in bacterial acquisition of iron. *M. leprae* also lacks many of the genes for lipid biosynthesis and modification that are characteristic of *M. tuberculosis*. The genome sequence has also allowed a directed approach to identification of 16 strains of *M. leprae* from geographically diverse sources. Genome sequence analyses have revealed that leprosy was introduced to the United States from Europe,[2] and also facilitated discovery that armadillos in the southeastern United States have the same unique strain as the U.S.-born leprosy patients have in the same region, suggesting that armadillos may be a reservoir for the pathogen in that region.

EPIDEMIOLOGY

Leprosy is found worldwide, although endemic leprosy is absent from northern Europe, where it was present in epidemic form as recently as the 19th century. The global prevalence of leprosy is about 180,000 known cases, and the current incidence is about 220,000. By definition of the World Health Organization (WHO) Strategic Plan for the Elimination of Leprosy, a newly diagnosed patient who has been treated with multidrug therapy is removed from the prevalence registry, which explains the lower prevalence than incidence of this chronic infection. Since initiation of the WHO Strategic Plan (whose goal is to eliminate leprosy as a public health problem, i.e., a prevalence of < 1 in 10,000 in all regions), an estimated 14 million people have been cured of leprosy.

The success of multidrug therapy notwithstanding, leprosy remains a public health problem in Brazil, Indonesia, Philippines, Democratic Republic of Congo, India, Madagascar, Mozambique, Nepal, and the United Republic of Tanzania. India and Brazil currently have the largest number of cases. Although domestic transmission of leprosy is extremely rare in the United States, 82 cases of leprosy were diagnosed in 2011, including cases in immigrants from India, Brazil, the Philippines, the Dominican Republic, and Mexico. Because leprosy is not highly transmissible, it is not considered a disease of travelers other than immigrants.

Inability to culture *M. leprae* in vitro has been a major hindrance to understanding the modes of transmission and reservoirs of the organism. Observational studies reveal a low frequency of leprosy in casual travelers or temporary residents of high-incidence regions, thus indicating that *M. leprae* is not highly transmissible. Even in areas of high incidence, clusters of leprosy are rare outside families or others with prolonged close contact. It is believed that transmission of *M. leprae* commonly occurs through the respiratory route, because nasal secretions of people with lepromatous leprosy may contain 10^7 viable bacilli per milliliter. In addition, transmission of *M. leprae* is thought to occur through contact with contaminated soil, although soil has not been found to be a reservoir for the bacilli.

PATHOBIOLOGY

Immunology

There is an inverse correlation between the number of lymphocytes and the number of acid-fast bacteria present in skin lesions. Tuberculoid lesions have abundant lymphocytes, well-formed granulomas, and few bacteria (hence this form of leprosy is also termed *paucibacillary*). In contrast, lepromatous lesions have very few lymphocytes, poorly organized or no granulomas, and large numbers of bacteria (also termed *multibacillary leprosy*). Between these polar extremes are intermediate forms that represent a continuum of the histopathologic and bacteriologic findings, termed *borderline tuberculoid, borderline,* and *borderline lepromatous* (Fig. 326-1). In addition to correlating with the number of bacteria in individual lesions, the polar forms of leprosy correlate with the total number of skin lesions in an individual patient: tuberculoid leprosy exhibits few (<five) lesions, whereas lepromatous leprosy is characterized by multiple lesions (≥five, up to hundreds).

Leprosy provides a paradigm for the effect of the cellular immune response to a bacterial pathogen on the clinical manifestations of the infection.[3] Individuals in whom a T helper 1 (T_H1) immune response (characterized by antigen-specific T cells that produce interferon [IFN]-γ, lymphotoxin [LTA], or interleukin [IL]-2 and no IL-4 or IL-5) develops to *M. leprae* exhibit few skin lesions and few bacteria within the lesions (paucibacillary leprosy). In contrast, persons in whom a T_H2 immune response develops (T cells that produce little IFN-γ, lymphotoxin, or IL-2, but produce IL-4, IL-5, and IL-13) have larger numbers of skin lesions and large numbers of bacteria within lesions (multibacillary leprosy). The roles of other T-cell subsets, such as T_H17 or T-regulatory cells, remain to be defined in leprosy. The primary determinant of the differential immune response to *M. leprae* is incompletely understood, although substantial evidence indicates that host genetic polymorphisms contribute to the likelihood of paucibacillary versus multibacillary leprosy.

Pathogenesis of Nerve Damage

Peripheral nerve damage, the most important consequence of infection with *M. leprae*, occurs in all forms of leprosy and underlies the complications of the infection. *M. leprae* invades Schwann cells, the glial cells of peripheral nerves. Schwann cells form a functional unit with peripheral nerve axons and are surrounded by laminin-2, a neural-specific extracellular matrix protein. The G domain of laminin-2 can bind simultaneously to *M. leprae* and to the Schwann cell laminin receptor α-dystroglycan, which promotes binding of *M. leprae* to Schwann cells by use of laminin-2 as a bridging molecule. Laminin-2 interacts with two distinct molecules on the surface of *M. leprae*, a 21-kD protein and phenolic glycolipid-1 (PGL-1); either can mediate internalization by Schwann cells. Once *M. leprae* is bound and internalized by Schwann cells, it can cause direct demyelination of peripheral nerves in the absence of an immune response, apparently by signaling through ErbB2 and Erk1/2. *M. leprae*–mediated demyelination occurs without early cell death or toxicity, although Schwann cells and neurons can die by apoptosis after infection. In addition, dead *M. leprae* or PGL-1 shed from live or dying *M. leprae* can mediate peripheral nerve demyelination and may contribute to the ongoing nerve damage that can follow initiation of chemotherapy. In addition to PGL-1–mediated demyelination, an *M. leprae* 19-kD lipoprotein can mediate Schwann cell apoptosis in vitro, and apoptotic Schwann cells can be found in human leprosy lesions. These mechanisms may be responsible for the nerve damage in multibacillary leprosy.

In addition to direct damage to peripheral nerves by *M. leprae*, the immune response in leprosy also contributes to nerve damage, especially in paucibacillary (tuberculoid) leprosy, in which the bacteria or PGL-1 or both are present in insufficient quantity to cause widespread nerve damage, and in reversal reactions, in which inflammation is particularly prominent.[4] Several distinct immunologic mechanisms probably contribute to the nerve damage in leprosy. Pro-inflammatory cytokines such as tumor necrosis factor (TNF)-α, IL-1β, and IFN-γ are especially prominent in lesions during reversal reactions, when irreversible nerve damage can occur. Because these molecules can contribute to inflammatory tissue damage and can induce apoptosis of Schwann cells in vitro, it is likely these mediators play an active role in nerve damage. Reversal reactions are also characterized by an increase in the number of CD4+ T lymphocytes in lesions, and at least some of these CD4+ cells exhibit a cytotoxic phenotype and kill *M. leprae*–infected Schwann cells through antigen- and major histocompatibility complex class II–dependent secretion of cytotoxic granule contents. Whether these mechanisms of nerve damage occur in chronic tuberculoid leprosy is not established, but similar cytokines and T lymphocytes are found in tuberculoid lesions.

Genetics

Cases of leprosy cluster in families, partly because of shared environments and similar exposure but also probably because of genetic determinants of susceptibility. Genetic loci whose allelic variants are related to altered susceptibility to infection with *M. leprae* include *PARK2*, *NRAMP1*, *TNF*, *TLR1*, *FCN2*, *LTA*, *NOD2*, *RIPK2*, *IL23R*, and *RAB32*. Parkin, the product of *PARK2*, is an E3 ubiquitin ligase that promotes autophagy and killing of intracellular bacteria, including mycobacteria. *NRAMP1*, *NOD2*, *RIPK2*, and *TNF* are expressed by macrophages, and quantitative or temporal differences in their expression may account for differences in innate susceptibility to infection. TLR1 and ficolin-2 are pattern recognition molecules that recognize bacterial lipopeptides and polysaccharides, respectively, whereas NOD2 and its downstream kinase RIPK2 are involved in responses to bacterial peptidoglycan. The overlap in susceptibility genes for leprosy and for Crohn's disease suggests one or more shared mechanisms of pathogenesis.[5] Genes with polymorphisms associated with a predisposition to distinct clinical forms of leprosy (i.e., lepromatous vs. tuberculoid) include HLA-DRB1*1501 and HLA-DRB1*1502, *NRAMP1*, *TNF*, *IL-10*, and *TAP2*.

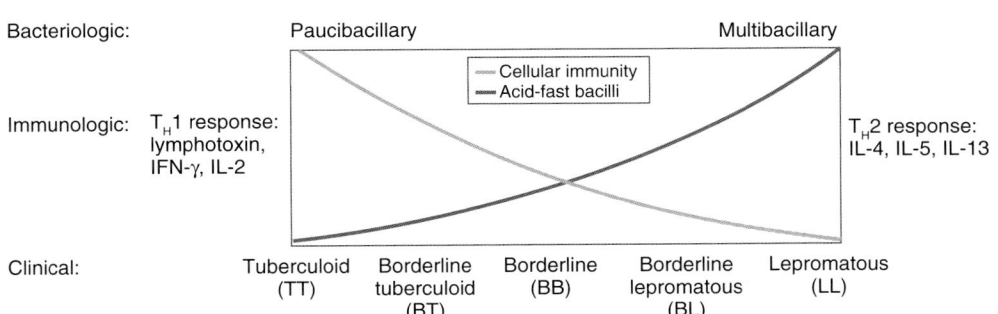

Bacteriologic, immunologic, and clinical spectrum of leprosy. Tuberculoid (paucibacillary) leprosy is characterized by a T_H1 immune response and few or no detectable bacilli in biopsy specimens of skin lesions or smears of skin slits. At the opposite pole of the spectrum, lepromatous (multibacillary) leprosy is accompanied by a T_H2 immune response, numerous skin lesions, and numerous acid-fast bacilli on skin biopsy specimens or smears. The intermediate forms can be classified according to their resemblance to tuberculoid or lepromatous leprosy. IFN = interferon; IL = interleukin.

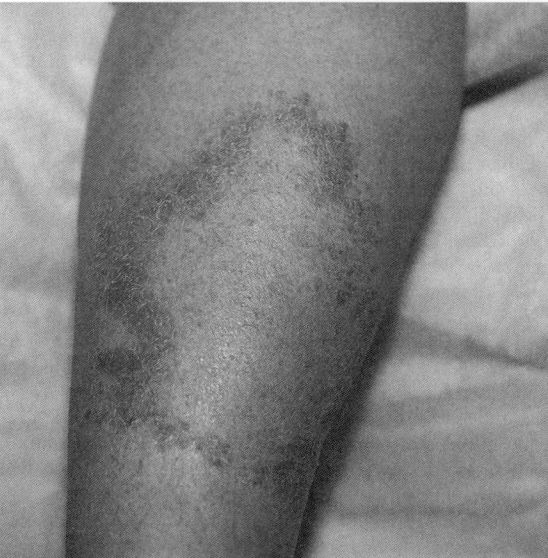

FIGURE 326-2. Tuberculoid leprosy. A single large lesion with irregular, raised, erythematous borders and a depressed, hypopigmented center is shown. (From Hansen's disease [leprosy]. In: James WD, Berger TG, Elston DM, eds. *Andrews' Diseases of the Skin.* 10th ed. Philadelphia: Elsevier; 2006.)

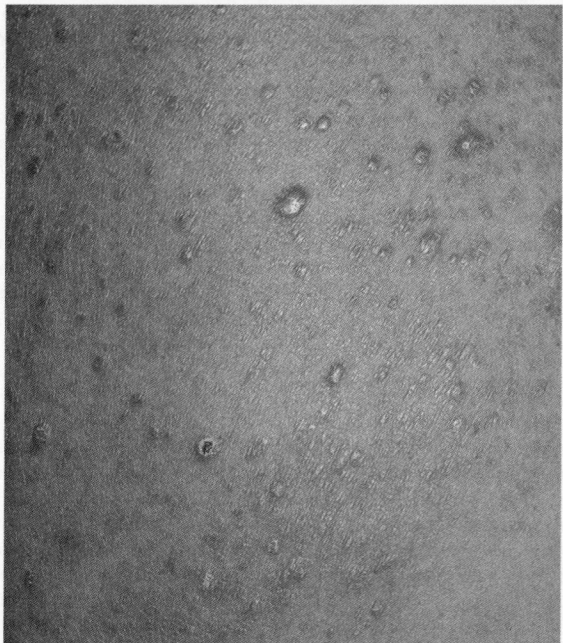

FIGURE 326-3. Lepromatous leprosy. Numerous papules and nodules are apparent. Lepromatous macules have ill-defined borders, with normal sensation usually maintained. (From Hansen's disease [leprosy]. In: James WD, Berger TG, Elston DM, eds. *Andrews' Diseases of the Skin.* 10th ed. Philadelphia: Elsevier; 2006.)

CLINICAL MANIFESTATIONS

The most common manifestations of leprosy involve the skin and peripheral nerves and are determined by the polarity of the disease: paucibacillary (tuberculoid) or multibacillary (lepromatous). The onset of leprosy is usually insidious. Depending on the form of leprosy, numbness may be an initial complaint or finding, and skin lesions may become apparent only months or years later. The classification of leprosy as tuberculoid, lepromatous, or one of the borderline forms is based on the combination of clinical examination, the number of bacteria seen on skin slit smears or skin biopsy specimens, and the histologic appearance. Because the nature of the potential complications and the specific course of chemotherapy are determined by the form of leprosy, accurate diagnosis and classification are essential.

Tuberculoid Leprosy

Tuberculoid leprosy is characterized by the presence of fewer than five skin lesions, which are typically hypopigmented or erythematous macules with raised erythematous borders and an atrophic center (Fig. 326-2). The skin lesions in tuberculoid leprosy are usually hypoesthetic or anesthetic; when multiple lesions are present, their distribution is asymmetrical. The skin lesions may be large and are most commonly found on the face, trunk, or extremities; however, they are not found in the axillae, groin, perineum, or on the scalp, presumably because of the preference of *M. leprae* for lower temperatures.

Local peripheral nerve involvement is common in tuberculoid leprosy and is asymmetrical. In addition to hypoesthesia or anesthesia of the skin lesions, nerve involvement in tuberculoid leprosy is manifested as enlargement or tenderness (or both) of the peripheral nerves that serve the region of the skin lesions. Superficial nerves such as the ulnar, superficial peroneal, or greater auricular nerves may be visibly enlarged, depending on the location of the skin lesions. Functional complications of nerve involvement, such as muscle atrophy and contractures, may be present at the time of diagnosis of tuberculoid leprosy. Tuberculoid leprosy is a stable form; it does not convert to borderline or lepromatous forms.

Lepromatous Leprosy

Lepromatous leprosy is characterized by multiple skin lesions that are smaller than those observed in tuberculoid leprosy (Fig. 326-3). Although the sites of skin lesions are similar to those of tuberculoid leprosy, the multiple lesions of lepromatous leprosy are often symmetrically distributed. Lepromatous macules may have poorly defined borders and no loss of sensation; local nerve enlargement is not characteristic. In addition to macules, lepromatous skin lesions may be nodules or plaques, or they may diffusely infiltrate the skin, especially on the face (which may cause loss of eyebrows and "leonine facies").

Nerve involvement in lepromatous leprosy is characteristically symmetrical and exhibits a stocking-glove distribution unrelated to the location of skin lesions. Peripheral nerve involvement may initially be manifested as loss of temperature sensation, followed by loss of light touch, pain, and deep pressure sense. In addition, dysesthesia is common. Motor complications, including muscle weakness and atrophy of the muscles of the hands, feet, and face, develop in the absence of effective antileprosy chemotherapy. Involvement of the facial nerve may result in corneal exposure, ulceration, and blindness. Persons with lepromatous leprosy may also have prominent rhinorrhea as a result of nasal mucosal involvement, and they may shed large numbers of *M. leprae* in their nasal secretions—one of the major sources of bacilli for transmission to other individuals. Like tuberculoid leprosy, lepromatous leprosy is stable; conversion to other forms does not occur.

Borderline Forms of Leprosy

Borderline tuberculoid leprosy is characterized by skin lesions similar to those of tuberculoid leprosy, but they are more numerous and may be accompanied by satellite lesions around large lesions. In borderline leprosy, skin lesions are numerous but remain asymmetrical. The lesions are usually plaques rather than macules and exhibit satellite lesions. Nerve involvement in borderline leprosy is manifested as thickening or tenderness of local nerves, but the skin lesions retain sensation. Borderline lepromatous leprosy is characterized by numerous symmetrical small macules, papules, plaques, and nodules but not the diffuse skin infiltration found in full-blown lepromatous leprosy. Unlike tuberculoid and lepromatous leprosy, the borderline forms are unstable and progress to the lepromatous form over time unless effective treatment is provided. Reactional states, including both reversal reactions and downgrading reactions, occur in those with borderline forms of leprosy.

Reactional States

Individuals with leprosy who may otherwise avoid care may exhibit acute reactional symptoms and signs. Physicians in developed countries may encounter patients with reactional states in acute care settings.[6]

Type 1 reactions, which are mediated by cellular immune responses to *M. leprae* antigens in skin lesions and nerves, occur in borderline tuberculoid, borderline, and borderline lepromatous leprosy. Type 1 reactions are frequently accompanied by worsening of peripheral nerve manifestations and may result in permanent nerve damage; they should be considered medical emergencies. Reversal reactions, which are type 1 reactions that occur after initiation of therapy for leprosy or for human immunodeficiency virus (HIV) infection, are associated with enhanced T_H1 immune responses that develop in patients with a large burden of *M. leprae*; they are most severe in those with borderline lepromatous leprosy. Downgrading reactions occur in association with the transition of borderline disease toward the lepromatous form. Although the immune mechanisms that underlie reversal reactions and downgrading reactions are believed to be distinct, their clinical manifestations are indistinguishable. Type 1 reactions may have an acute or insidious onset, and they are characterized by inflammation of preexisting skin and nerve lesions. Skin lesions, which become erythematous and edematous, may also become tender and thereby resemble cellulitis, but type 1 reactions are not accompanied by fever or other systemic symptoms or signs. Increased expression of TNF has been found in lesions during type 1 reactions and may contribute to the clinical and functional consequences. Moreover, type 1 reactions have been reported when TNF antagonist therapy has been withdrawn after diagnosis of borderline lepromatous leprosy. Recent transcriptomic analyses have also implicated the complement system in the pathogenesis of type 1 and type 2 leprosy reactions.[7]

Type 2 reactions, also known as erythema nodosum leprosum (ENL), occur in persons with borderline lepromatous and lepromatous leprosy; they may be mediated by immune complexes rather than cellular immune responses. Type 2 reactions, which occur most often after initiation of antileprosy chemotherapy or during pregnancy, are generally accompanied by fever and arthralgias. Additional signs of systemic inflammatory disease may appear, including hepatosplenomegaly, lymphadenopathy, arthritis, nephritis, keratitis, and iritis. The skin lesions of ENL resemble those of classic erythema nodosum (Chapter 440), with widely distributed erythematous dermal and subcutaneous nodules whose location is unrelated to the leprosy lesions. Biopsy of ENL lesions shows leukocytoclastic vasculitis.

Leprosy and Human Immunodeficiency Virus
CD4$^+$ T-cell–mediated immunity is essential for control of *M. leprae*, and the extent of T_H1 immunity determines whether an individual will have tuberculoid or lepromatous leprosy. However, coinfection with HIV and depletion of CD4$^+$ T lymphocytes does not affect the rate of progression of leprosy, nor does it cause conversion of tuberculoid leprosy to the lepromatous form. In contrast, type 1 reversal reactions may accompany immune reconstitution subsequent to initiation of effective antiretroviral therapy for HIV infection (Chapter 395). The manifestations of these reversal reactions are similar to those observed in patients who are not infected with HIV.

DIAGNOSIS

The diagnosis of leprosy should be considered in any patient with skin and peripheral nerve manifestations, especially those who have lived in countries where leprosy is endemic. Although leprosy is a chronic infection, its acute complications require prompt diagnosis and therapy to prevent irreversible peripheral nerve damage. It is also important to classify a patient's disease as tuberculoid, lepromatous, or one of the specific borderline forms, because correct classification is necessary for selecting optimal therapy and anticipating potential reactional states. Because *M. leprae* cannot be cultured in vitro and there is currently no reliable serologic test or other diagnostic biomarker for leprosy, diagnosis and classification of leprosy depend on the combination of clinical examination, histopathologic evaluation, and acid-fast staining of skin slit or biopsy specimens.

Clinical Examination
Examination of an individual with possible or confirmed leprosy must include evaluation and documentation of the number, location, and characteristics of skin lesions. In addition to descriptions of the skin lesions, accurate classification of leprosy depends on whether the lesions are distributed symmetrically and whether they are hypoesthetic or anesthetic. The examination must also include a search for (1) enlarged and tender peripheral nerves, (2) the presence of sensory deficits (especially temperature sensation and pain) and skin ulcerations, and (3) the nature and distribution of motor deficits, muscle atrophy, and contractures. Because some medications used for the treatment of leprosy are contraindicated in pregnancy, women of childbearing age should be evaluated for pregnancy.

Skin Smears and Biopsies
In developing countries, classification of multibacillary or paucibacillary leprosy is made by the combination of clinical examination findings and bacterial counts as determined on acid-fast–stained smears made from skin slits of lesions and skin from cool areas of the body, such as the earlobes. In developed countries, skin biopsies are usually performed instead of skin slits. Skin specimens should be obtained from the active borders of lesions and should include subcutaneous tissue. On hematoxylin-eosin staining, tuberculoid leprosy is characterized by granulomas with giant cells, aggregates of epithelioid macrophages that are neither vacuolated nor foamy, and lymphocytes at the periphery. Although granulomas may be found in other skin diseases, selective destruction of nerve trunks and perineural fibrosis are specific features of leprosy. Acid-fast stains (preferably done with the Fite procedure) show rare or undetectable bacilli in tuberculoid leprosy. Lesions of lepromatous leprosy show poorly organized granulomas without giant cells or lymphocytes; macrophages are foamy and lipid laden. Acid-fast staining of lepromatous leprosy lesions reveals abundant bacilli that usually appear in large clumps ("globi"). The borderline forms of leprosy exhibit less well-organized granulomas with fewer giant cells and lymphocytes but more foamy macrophages and acid-fast bacilli as the spectrum varies from borderline tuberculoid to borderline lepromatous.

Specialized immunohistochemistry stains, such as for CD4$^+$ T lymphocytes or cytokine expression, are useful in research studies but are not currently used for the diagnosis or classification of leprosy. Polymerase chain reaction amplification of *M. leprae* genomic DNA from skin slits or skin biopsy specimens has not yet contributed to enhanced sensitivity or specificity of diagnosis or classification.

Diagnosis of Reactional States
The diagnosis of type 1 reactions is based on clinical findings in a patient with borderline tuberculoid, borderline, or borderline lepromatous leprosy and acute inflammation of preexisting skin lesions, with or without worsening of nerve lesions. Type 1 reactions are not accompanied by systemic findings such as fever or arthritis. At highest risk for type 1 reactions are patients who have recently initiated antileprosy chemotherapy, although type 1 reactions can occur spontaneously. Diagnosis of a type 2 reaction (ENL) is also based on clinical findings of new erythematous subcutaneous or dermal nodules in a patient with borderline lepromatous or lepromatous leprosy. There are currently no diagnostic tests or biomarkers for ENL, and skin biopsy will not distinguish ENL from classic erythema nodosum.

TREATMENT   Rx

Agents to Treat Leprosy
The first-line antimicrobial agents for leprosy are dapsone and rifampin. Clofazimine, minocycline, certain fluoroquinolones, and clarithromycin are also useful in specific contexts, including drug intolerance or resistance.

Dapsone is inexpensive and well tolerated, has a long serum half-life ($\approx$28 hours), and is safe for use during pregnancy. Glucose-6-phosphate dehydrogenase (G6PD)-deficient individuals (Chapter 161) are susceptible to dapsone-induced methemoglobinemia and hemolysis, and all patients should be screened for G6PD deficiency before starting dapsone. Patients with mild G6PD deficiency (the African type, caused by mutations that lead to instability of the enzyme) can begin dapsone at 25 mg/day but require close monitoring for hemolytic anemia. Dapsone can also cause bone marrow suppression and profound neutropenia. Other rare adverse effects of dapsone include hepatitis, cholestatic jaundice, and a hypersensitivity syndrome that usually occurs within 4 to 6 weeks of initiation of dapsone and is characterized by exfoliative dermatitis, generalized lymphadenopathy, fever, and hepatosplenomegaly. A recent study in China found that the presence of the HLA class I allele B*13:01 confers a seven-fold higher risk of the dapsone hypersensitivity syndrome, strongly implicating CD8$^+$ T cells in its pathogenesis.[8]

Rifampin, the most bactericidal drug against *M. leprae*, is well absorbed after oral administration and has a serum half-life of approximately 3 hours. Rifampin should never be used as monotherapy because resistance can develop with single point mutations in its target, RNA polymerase II. Because rifampin is bactericidal and rapid release of components from dead bacteria can have pro-inflammatory effects, some experts withhold rifampin during reversal reactions. Adverse effects of rifampin include maculopapular rash, hepatotoxicity, an influenza-like syndrome (most frequent with intermittent therapy), and orange discoloration of tears, urine, saliva, and sweat. Thrombocytopenia occurs occasionally but is not usually severe. Rifampin also induces metabolism and decreases serum concentrations of other drugs, including antiretroviral protease inhibitors and non-nucleoside reverse transcriptase inhibitors, methadone, and oral contraceptives. Rifampin decreases serum concentrations of dapsone, but this effect is not clinically significant with a dapsone dose of 100 mg/day.

Clofazimine is a lipophilic dye that is bacteriostatic against *M. leprae*. It has a very long ($\approx$70 days) half-life and appears to have anti-inflammatory activity as well as direct bacteriostatic activity. Because of its anti-inflammatory activity, clofazimine is useful in the treatment of type 1 reactional states. Clofazimine is generally well tolerated; its major side effect is discoloration of the skin, which occurs in nearly all clofazimine-treated patients. The skin discoloration can range from reddish tan to bluish black and can be blotchy, but it is reversible within 6 to 12 months of discontinuation of the drug. In chronic reactional patients maintained with high doses of clofazimine (200 to 300 mg/day), enteropathy with crampy abdominal pain, mild nausea, or diarrhea (or both) and even bowel obstruction can develop.

Regimens to Treat Leprosy

Chemotherapy for leprosy involves the use of multiple drugs to optimize the rate of cure and prevent emergence of drug resistance.[9] The regimen currently recommended in the United States for paucibacillary (tuberculoid and borderline tuberculoid) leprosy in adults consists of dapsone, 100 mg, and rifampin, 600 mg, both given daily for 12 months. The U.S. recommended regimen for multibacillary leprosy in adults is dapsone, 100 mg, plus rifampin, 600 mg, and clofazimine, 50 mg, each given daily for 24 months (available at http://www.hrsa.gov/hansensdisease/diagnosis/recommendedtreatment .html). Clofazimine is currently not commercially available, but it can be obtained in the United States through the National Hansen's Disease Program (1-800-642-2477). In resource-limited countries where the burden of leprosy is highest, the WHO regimen for paucibacillary leprosy is dapsone, 100 mg daily, plus rifampin, 600 mg once a month, for 6 months. The WHO regimen for adults for multibacillary leprosy (which differs from the U.S. recommendation) is dapsone, 100 mg daily, plus rifampin, 600 mg once a month, plus clofazimine, 50 mg daily, each given for 12 months, plus an additional dose of clofazimine, 300 mg once a month (available at http://www.who.int/lep/mdt/ regimens/en/index.html). The monthly doses of rifampin and clofazimine should be administered under supervision. Alternative agents for patients with drug intolerance or drug resistance include clarithromycin (may be substituted for any of the first-line drugs), minocycline (may be substituted for dapsone or clofazimine), and ofloxacin (may be substituted for clofazimine).

Response to Therapy

Response to effective therapy for leprosy is seen clinically as flattening and resolution of the papules, nodules, or plaques, with or without improvement in nerve function. Clinical improvement may begin within the first months of therapy, but resolution of skin lesions is often delayed as long as 1 to 2 years after completion of therapy. Quantitation of the bacillary load to assess response to treatment is cumbersome, semiquantitative, and not recommended.

Patients who have been adequately treated may experience worsening of nerve and skin symptoms, perhaps because of a late reversal reaction or relapsed leprosy. If skin specimens do not reveal acid-fast organisms, a therapeutic trial of corticosteroids, which will ameliorate the symptoms of reversal reactions but not those of relapsed leprosy, can help make the distinction and assist in choosing subsequent therapy. Patients who experience relapse after treatment of paucibacillary disease should be treated for multibacillary disease, because the most likely cause of relapse is previous multibacillary disease that was misclassified. Patients with multibacillary disease who relapse should be retreated with a regimen containing dapsone and rifampin with the addition of at least two drugs that were not used in the initial treatment regimen, unless susceptibility testing is available and confirms that the organisms remain susceptible to dapsone and rifampin. The choices among additional drugs include minocycline, ofloxacin or moxifloxacin, and clarithromycin. Relapsed multibacillary patients may benefit from lifelong maintenance therapy after completing 2 years of a salvage regimen. Because susceptibility testing cannot be performed with in vitro assays, an alternative approach to determination of susceptibility by detecting mutations in the targets of dapsone and rifampin (*folP1* and *rpoB*, respectively) is beginning to be widely used and is commercially available. The mouse footpad assay has been used, but it is becoming less available.

Treatment of Reactional States

Type 1 reactions may develop before, during, or years after completion of antileprosy chemotherapy.[10] Type 1 reactions that involve worsening of nerve symptoms are medical emergencies because permanent nerve damage can occur. Type 1 reactions usually respond at a daily dose of prednisone of 60 to 80 mg, which can be tapered slowly once symptoms are controlled. Type 1 reactions can also respond to high-dose clofazimine (200 to 300 mg/day), although reactions with worsening nerve symptoms should be treated initially with prednisone. Patients who have type 1 reactions that occur before or during antileprosy chemotherapy and whose reactions include nerve involvement should have rifampin withheld until the worsened nerve symptoms resolve, because release of pro-inflammatory components from dying bacteria may contribute to inflammation and nerve damage. Dapsone and clofazimine should be continued during treatment of type 1 reactions.

The treatment of choice for severe type 2 reactions (ENL) is thalidomide, except in pregnant or potentially pregnant women. Thalidomide requires that

patients and the prescribing physician be enrolled in the System for Thalidomide Education and Prescribing Safety (STEPS) program to avoid the drug's teratogenic effects. The mechanism of action of thalidomide is incompletely understood but is likely to include inhibition of TNF. The dose of thalidomide for ENL varies, depending on the severity of the reaction. In patients with ENL and high fever, frank arthritis, and large subcutaneous plaques, up to 100 mg four times daily may be required to achieve a clinical response. Once a clinical response is achieved, the dose of thalidomide may be tapered to a maintenance dose of 50 to 100 mg given once daily at night (because thalidomide is sedating). For milder cases of ENL, 50 to 100 mg per night may be sufficient to achieve and maintain control. ENL in women of childbearing age and thalidomide-unresponsive cases may respond to corticosteroids. Methotrexate may be efficacious in otherwise treatment-resistant ENL, but methotrexate has been assigned by the U.S. Food and Drug Administration to pregnancy category X (teratogenic risks "clearly outweigh" potential benefits) and is also contraindicated in nursing mothers. Antileprosy chemotherapy, including rifampin, should be continued in patients with ENL.

Other Therapy

Nerve damage in leprosy, which can result in muscle atrophy, contractures, and autoamputation, is the major cause of debility. Supportive care, reconstructive surgery, physical and occupational therapy, and rehabilitation can be extremely valuable in allowing patients to achieve and maintain optimal function.

PREVENTION

There is currently no effective specific vaccine for leprosy, but several trials have observed a partial protective effect of bacille Calmette-Guérin vaccination.[11] It is likely that improved understanding of transmission of *M. leprae* will be generated by the use of DNA-based strain typing, so better preventive measures are likely to become available in the near future.

PROGNOSIS

Multidrug chemotherapy cures a high proportion of people with paucibacillary and multibacillary leprosy. The currently recommended regimens provide high rates of response, with relapse rates of approximately 0.1% per year in paucibacillary cases and up to 5% per year in multibacillary cases. Some cases of paucibacillary leprosy may enter remission or even self-cure, but all cases of multibacillary leprosy are progressive. Because of its efficacy and low toxicity and to minimize long-term morbidity, multidrug chemotherapy should be used in all persons in whom leprosy is diagnosed.

GENERAL REFERENCES

For the General References and other additional features, please visit Expert Consult at https://expertconsult.inkling.com.

327

RICKETTSIAL INFECTIONS

DIDIER RAOULT

DEFINITION

Rickettsioses are emerging infectious diseases. Because of better diagnostic tools and changes in tick exposure, many new rickettsial diseases have been described in the past 20 years. Three families of diseases are grouped under this name: (1) rickettsioses, (2) ehrlichioses and anaplasmoses, and (3) Q fever.

The Pathogens

The agents of rickettsial diseases (formerly grouped in the order Rickettsiales) are small gram-negative bacteria that grow within eukaryotic cells. They have never been grown in axenic media thus far and for culture require living hosts such as cell cultures, embryonated eggs, or susceptible animals. With the exception of *Rickettsia prowazekii*, the agent of epidemic typhus, these

TABLE 327-1 GENETIC CLASSIFICATION OF RICKETTSIALES

	GENUS	GROUP	SPECIES	SUBSPECIES	FIRST YEAR OF ISOLATION OR DISCOVERY
Rickettsiae	Rickettsia	Typhus	R. prowazekii		1916
			R. typhi		1920
		Spotted fever	R. conorii	conorii	1932
				israeli	1974
				caspia	1991
				indica	2001
			R. rickettsii		1919
			R. sibirica	sibirica	1946
				mongolotimonae	1996
			R. slovaca		1997
			R. honei		1991
			R. japonica		1992
			R. parkeri		2003
			R. massiliae		2006
			R. monacencis		2007
			R. heilongjiangensis		1998
			R. aeschlimannii		2001
			R. helvetica		2000
			R. australis		1950
			R. felis		2001
			R. akari		1946
			R. raoultii		2008
	Orientia	Scrub typhus	O. tsutsugamushi		1920
Ehrlichiae	Ehrlichia		E. chaffeensis		1991
			E. ewingii		1999
			E. canis		1996
	Anaplasma		A. phagocytophilum		1992
	Neorickettsia		N. sennetsu		1957
	Wolbachia		W. pipientis		2001
Coxiellae	Coxiella		C. burnetii		1931

bacteria infect humans incidentally and are mainly animal pathogens. On the basis of molecular phylogeny, the bacteria causing rickettsial diseases have been reclassified into three phyla (Table 327-1).

Because of their difficult growth in vitro, the main diagnostic tool for rickettsioses is serology. Serologic evaluation is frequently hampered by late positivity and cross-reactivity. The development of direct staining in blood smears or skin biopsy samples, as well as polymerase chain reaction (PCR) amplification of DNA in blood samples or biopsy specimens, has considerably helped identification at the species level and led to the description of emerging pathogens.[1]

● RICKETTSIOSES (DISEASES CAUSED BY *RICKETTSIA* SPECIES AND *ORIENTIA TSUTSUGAMUSHI*)

DEFINITION

Rickettsia species are small gram-negative bacteria that multiply free in the cytoplasm of their host cells. The target cells in humans are endothelial cells or monocytes, and vasculitis is the most prominent clinical manifestation. These bacteria invade cells by phagocytosis and escape the phagosome vacuole.[2]

The genome of *Rickettsia* is small, between 1.1 and 1.6 Mb; some have plasmids and potential for conjugation. These bacteria have a family of outer membrane proteins of the surface cell antigen family, including rOmpA (lacking in typhus group) and rOmpB. These proteins are major antigens that help identify the rickettsial species, and their encoding genes are used for amplification and sequencing for diagnostic or taxonomic purposes. Among

rickettsiae, two subgroups, the typhus group and the spotted fever group, were identified on the basis of growth conditions and antigenicity. A specific group antigen determined to be lipopolysaccharide has been identified. The optimal growth temperature is 37° C for the typhus group and 32° to 35° C for the spotted fever group. The complete genome sequencing of *R. prowazekii* (from the typhus group) showed that it is mainly a subset of *Rickettsia conorii* (a member of the spotted fever group).

Tick-Borne Rickettsioses
ROCKY MOUNTAIN SPOTTED FEVER

EPIDEMIOLOGY

Rocky Mountain spotted fever (RMSF), the most severe of the rickettsioses, is caused by *Rickettsia rickettsii* (Table 327-2).[3] It is the major tick-transmitted rickettsiosis (Chapter 359) recognized in America, with *Rickettsia africae* in the West Indies, *Rickettsia parkeri* in the southern states of the United States,[4] and perhaps *Rickettsia amblyommii*. It was described first in the 19th century in the western United States. RMSF is prevalent in at least 44 U.S. states (Fig. 327-1) and in Central and South America (Argentina, Brazil, Colombia, Costa Rica, Mexico, and Panama).[5]

Rickettsia is transmitted transovarially to tick progeny from one generation to the next. The infecting ticks are mainly *Dermacentor andersoni* (a wood tick) in the western United States; *Dermacentor variabilis* (the American dog tick) in the East, the Midwest, and the South; and *Rhipicephalus sanguineus* in Arizona. In Central and South America, *Amblyomma cajennense* is the major vector. Humans are infected through infected saliva after a tick bite. The duration of attachment is critical in any tick-borne rickettsiosis, and transmission is unlikely when the tick feeds for less than 20 hours. The tick

TABLE 327-2 RICKETTSIAL DISEASES IN HUMAN BEINGS

DISEASE	ORGANISM	ARTHROPOD HOST	GEOGRAPHIC AREA	RASH	ESCHAR TACHE NOIRE	REGIONAL LYMPH NODE	HIGH FEVER	FATALITY RATE
TICK-TRANSMITTED SPOTTED FEVERS								
Rocky Mountain spotted fever	R. rickettsii	Dermacentor andersoni Dermacentor variabilis Rhipicephalus sanguineus Amblyomma cajennense	America (North, Central, and South)	Yes, may be purpuric	Very rare	No	Yes	High
Mediterranean spotted fever, Astrakhan fever, Israeli spotted fever	R. conorii	Rhipicephalus sanguineus	Mediterranean, India, Caspian Sea, Africa	Yes, papular; may be purpuric	Yes	No	Yes	Moderate
African tick bite fever	R. africae	Amblyomma hebraeum Amblyomma variegatum	Sub-Saharan Africa, West Indies	Yes, half of cases may be vesicular	Yes (frequently multiple)	Yes	No	Low
Queensland tick typhus	R. australis	Ixodes holocyclus	Eastern Australia	Yes, may be vesicular	Yes	?	Yes	Moderate
Siberian tick typhus	R. sibirica	Dermacentor nuttallii	Siberia, China, Mongolia	Yes	Yes	No	Yes	Low
Scalp eschar, neck lymphadenopathy after tick bite (SENLAT)	R. slovaca or R. raoultii	Dermacentor marginatus Dermacentor reticulatus	Europe, Pakistan	Very rare	Yes, may be erythematous	Yes (painful)	No	Low
Lymphangitis-associated rickettsiosis (LAR)	R. sibirica mongolotimonae	Hyalomma asiaticum	Mongolia, Africa, Europe	Yes	Yes	Yes	Yes	Low
Unnamed	R. aeschlimannii	Hyalomma sp.	Mediterranean, Africa	Yes	Yes	Yes	Yes	Unknown
Flinders Island spotted fever	R. honei	Ixodes granulosus	Flinders Island, eastern Australia	Yes	Yes	Yes	Yes	Low
Japanese spotted fever	R. japonica	Ixodes ricinus	Japan, Korea (China?)	Yes	Yes	No	Yes	Low
Unnamed	R. parkeri	Amblyomma maculatum	America	Yes	Yes	No	Yes	
Unnamed	R. helvetica	Ixodes ricinus	Europe, Asia	No	Yes	No	No	
	R. massiliae	Rhipicephalus sanguineus	Europe, United States	Yes	Yes	No	Yes	Unknown
	R. monacensis	Ixodes ricinus	Europe	Yes	Yes	No	Yes	Unknown
FLEA-TRANSMITTED DISEASES								
Murine typhus	R. typhi	Xenopsylla cheopis Ctenocephalides felis (mosquitoes)	Worldwide	Yes	No	No	Yes	Low
Flea-borne spotted fever	R. felis	Ctenocephalides felis	Worldwide	Sometimes	Sometimes	Unknown	Yes	Unknown
LOUSE-TRANSMITTED DISEASE								
Epidemic typhus	R. prowazekii	Pediculus humanus corporis Amblyomma ticks (?)	Worldwide	Yes	No	No	Yes	High
American sylvatic typhus	R. prowazekii	Flying squirrel ectoparasites	United States	Yes	No	No	Yes	Low
Brill-Zinsser disease (relapse of epidemic typhus)	R. prowazekii		Worldwide	Yes, could lack	No	No	No	Low
MITE-TRANSMITTED DISEASE								
Rickettsialpox	R. akari	Liponyssoides sanguineus	Worldwide	Yes, vesicular	Yes	Yes	Yes	Low
Scrub typhus	Orientia tsutsugamushi	Leptotrombidium sp. (chiggers)	Central and eastern Asia, Australia	Yes	Yes	Yes	Yes	High, may relapse

bite is painless and frequently unnoticed. Rarely, an eschar at the site of the tick bite is observed in RMSF. The epidemiology of RMSF undergoes largely unexplained yearly variations. This temporal repartition is determined by tick activity and human encounter. More than 500 cases occur each year, and more than 90% are reported from April to September. The disease is more prevalent in children younger than 10 years. A recent increase has been reported, but the current diagnostic tools do not allow discrimination between RMSF and other rickettsioses.

CLINICAL MANIFESTATIONS

Two to 14 days after the tick bite, fever and headaches appear. The fever is high (temperature > 102° F) and associated with nonspecific symptoms

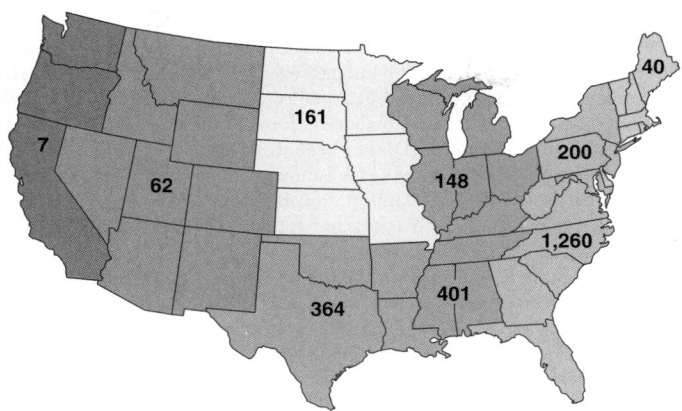

FIGURE 327-1. Number of reported cases of Rocky Mountain spotted fever by region, 1994 to 1998.

including malaise, myalgias, nausea, vomiting, anorexia, and diarrhea. At this stage, RMSF is not frequently diagnosed, but during the "tick season," patients with high fever who live in or have a history of travel to an endemic location and possibly a history of tick bite should be considered as possibly having RMSF.

The most characteristic feature is a rash. However, the classic triad of fever, headache, and rash is present in only 44% of confirmed cases. Rash is found in 14% of cases on the first day of disease and in less than 50% in the first 3 days. The rash is macular; it appears first on the ankles and wrists and then generalizes. Spots are 1 to 5 mm in diameter and can evolve from pink to purpuric. A rash can appear later or even not at all; Rocky Mountain "spotless" fever represented 34% of cases in a series from the Centers for Disease Control and Prevention (CDC). Involvement of the palms and soles theoretically differentiates the typhus diseases (in which it is absent) from the spotted fevers.

Untreated patients worsen progressively. The disease is associated in various degrees with general manifestations related to vascular inflammation and increased vascular permeability and with multiple organ involvement that can lead to multiple organ dysfunction syndrome (MODS). In severe forms, patients suffer from edema, hypovolemia, hypoalbuminemia, and hypotension leading to shock. In very severe cases, necrosis and gangrene of the extremities occur. In some instances, noncardiogenic pulmonary edema develops; pulmonary involvement leading to respiratory distress can cause death. Renal failure can result either from hypovolemia and shock and be reversible or from acute tubular necrosis and require hemodialysis. The usual neurologic symptoms are confusion, lethargy, and stupor. In severe cases, delirium, coma, and seizures are observed. Cerebrospinal fluid (CSF) sampling exhibits meningitis in a third of cases; in general, a few monocyte cells (10 to 100) are observed, along with increased protein but normal glucose levels. Heart involvement can cause arrhythmia. Liver involvement is manifested as an increase in transaminases in a third of patients and jaundice in 8%. Jaundice can also reflect hemolysis. Intestinal tract involvement is manifested as abdominal pain, diarrhea, vomiting, and severe bleeding (upper gastrointestinal hemorrhage can cause death). Ocular involvement consists of conjunctivitis and retinal abnormalities, including hemorrhages, papilledema, and arterial occlusion.

The blood cell count shows a normal number of white blood cells but often immature myeloid cells. Thrombocytopenia is observed in 30 to 50% of cases and may be marked in severe cases. Anemia develops in 30% of patients. Coagulopathy with decreases in clotting factors (including fibrinogen) and prolonged coagulation times may contribute to bleeding; serum albumin may be low and proteins of the acute phase response increased (C-reactive protein, ferritin, fibrinogen). Hyponatremia and hypocalcemia may be noted and correlate with severity, as with an increase in creatinine. Increased concentrations of serum enzymes such as aminotransferases (aspartate [AST] and alanine [ALT] aminotransferase), lactate dehydrogenase (LDH), and creatine kinase usually reflect the severity of organ involvement—including the lung, heart, and liver—and multifocal rhabdomyolysis.

DIAGNOSIS

The diagnosis of RMSF should be based on clinical and epidemiologic findings and lead to early use of doxycycline. The most important clue is

unexplained fever in a patient with a history of tick exposure in an endemic area. When a rash is present, RMSF should be suspected and the patient treated accordingly unless another cause is demonstrated. The differential diagnosis includes other rickettsioses (e.g., those caused by *R. parkeri* in southeastern states), meningococcemia, enterovirus infections, typhoid, leptospirosis, ehrlichiosis, gonococcemia, toxic shock syndrome, syphilis, rubella, measles, and the Kawasaki syndrome. Drug hypersensitivity, especially after antimicrobial use for febrile illness, is sometimes confused with RMSF.

The main diagnostic test relies on serology, and treatment should never be delayed to obtain diagnostic confirmation. Criteria for laboratory confirmation include a four-fold or greater change in antibody titer determined by serology (measured by immunofluorescence assay [IFA], complement fixation, or latex agglutination) and direct detection of the bacterium by demonstration of specific antigens by immunodetection, genomic amplification by PCR, or culture. A biopsy specimen of a skin lesion is the best sample for this purpose. Culture of *Rickettsia* takes 3 to 7 days and is restricted to specialized laboratories. It is performed on cell lines such as Vero, L929, or HEL cells. Immunodetection by IFA or immunohistochemistry is sensitive and specific. It can be performed with frozen or fixed and paraffin-embedded material and allows retrospective diagnosis. PCR amplification and identification give promising results in rickettsioses in general but have not been properly evaluated for diagnosis of RMSF. Skin biopsy and direct detection in removed ticks yield the best results because blood contains inhibitors and only few copies of rickettsial DNA.

Two serum samples should be tested (early and convalescent). The early serum is usually negative because patients seroconvert between the 7th and 15th days. IFA is highly sensitive and specific. A cutoff value of 1 : 64 for total immunoglobulin and 1 : 32 for IgM antibodies is required for diagnosis. The latex agglutination cutoff is 1 : 64 or 1 : 128. Cross-reactive antibodies have been reported with infections caused by other rickettsioses, *Ehrlichia, Bartonella, Legionella,* and *Proteus.* False-positives, including IgM, may be observed when rheumatoid factor is present in serum and in patients with viral infection generating nonspecific B-lymphocyte proliferation (cytomegalovirus, Epstein-Barr virus). Complement fixation (which lacks sensitivity) and the Weil-Felix test (using antibodies that cross-react with *Proteus* strains) should not be used.

TREATMENT

The prognosis for patients with RMSF depends on the timing of antimicrobial treatment. Doxycycline saves patients with RMSF. The recommended dose is 100 mg twice daily, and treatment should be continued for at least 3 days after the fever resolves. Oral treatment is effective, but in patients with gastric intolerance or coma, the intravenous route is advised. Several antimicrobials are effective in vitro against *R. rickettsii*, including fluoroquinolones, rifampin, and new macrolide antimicrobials (but not erythromycin), but lack of clinical experience precludes their use for RMSF. β-Lactam antimicrobials, aminoglycosides, and cotrimoxazole are not effective.

Severely ill patients should be treated in intensive care units and fluid administration carefully monitored. Mechanical ventilation is used in case of respiratory distress, hemodialysis in patients with renal insufficiency, and antiseizure drugs in patients with seizures. Anemia and coagulation abnormalities may also be corrected. For patients with gangrene of the extremities, amputation may be necessary. Glucocorticoids have not proved useful.

PREVENTION

Prevention is based on avoidance of tick bites (Chapter 359) by use of repellents, protective garments, or both. To discourage tick attachment, repellents containing permethrin can be sprayed on boots and clothing and will last for several days. Repellents containing DEET (*N,N*-diethyl-*m*-toluamide) can be applied to the skin but will last only a few hours before reapplication is necessary. It is also useful to check for ticks after exposure. Careful examination of the scalp, groin, and axillae is recommended. The tick can be removed by forceps, and the skin should be disinfected (Fig. 327-2).

PROGNOSIS

The evolution of RMSF depends strongly on the timing of diagnosis and antimicrobial treatment. The current fatality rate is 2.4% on the basis of a 4-year national survey in the United States (27 deaths were attributable to RMSF during this period). This rate is currently declining, but this may result from reporting of confounding rickettsial diseases. No significant difference in outcome was observed between blacks and whites, but the case-fatality rate was highest in individuals older than 70 years (9%). Patients with glucose-6-phosphate dehydrogenase (G6PD) deficiency are more susceptible to severe infection. Treatment with chloramphenicol has been associated with a poorer outcome than treatment with doxycycline. Recovery from RMSF is usually complete, but neurologic sequelae can remain, and amputation of extremities may be necessary after gangrene.[6]

OTHER TICK-BORNE RICKETTSIOSES

EPIDEMIOLOGY

Like other tick-transmitted diseases (Chapter 359), rickettsioses have a limited geographic distribution that is determined mainly by the tick vector ecology (Fig. 327-3). *R. parkeri* has recently been identified in the United States and South America. *R. conorii* is found in Europe around the Mediterranean and Caspian seas (*caspia* subspecies); *Rickettsia slovaca*, *Rickettsia raoultii*, and possibly *Rickettsia helvetica* in western and central Europe; and *Rickettsia sibirica mongolotimonae* in France and Greece. Elsewhere, a number of specific agents of rickettsial disease have been identified (see Table 327-2).

CLINICAL MANIFESTATIONS

R. conorii comprises different but closely related subspecies. Many names are given to the infection caused by *R. conorii*: Mediterranean spotted fever (MSF), boutonneuse fever, Marseilles fever, Kenya tick typhus (caused by the subspecies *R. conorii conorii*), Astrakhan fever (caused by *R. conorii caspia*), Israeli spotted fever (caused by *R. conorii israeli*), and Indian tick

typhus (caused by *R. conorii indica*). *R. conorii* is closely related to *R. rickettsii*, with which it shares many common antigens that generate cross-reactive antibodies. MSF resembles RMSF but has several distinct characteristics. The spontaneous evolution is milder, but a fatality rate of 1.5 to 2.5% in hospitalized patients is still observed. A malignant form of the disease that includes purpuric rash, shock, and MODS has been described in alcoholic, diabetic, human immunodeficiency virus (HIV)-infected, and elderly or debilitated patients. The typical clinical manifestation is that of a patient with fever, a rash, and a tache noire (i.e., a black eschar at the site of the tick bite). A tache noire is found in 50 to 80% of cases. Multiple lesions do not occur because the dog tick vector, *R. sanguineus*, seldom bites humans. The rash is frequently clearly papular, which led to one of the names of the disease, boutonneuse fever. Israeli tick bite fever and Astrakhan fever appear to be milder than typical MSF, and tache noire is usually lacking.

R. africae, which causes African tick bite fever, may be responsible for most of the rickettsioses worldwide. It is extremely common in travelers visiting southern Africa. It is transmitted by African ticks, *Amblyomma hebraeum* and *Amblyomma africanum*. These ticks are often infected; as many as 60% can harbor *R. africae*. They usually feed on ungulates but attack human beings in groups and cause a high prevalence of infection in rural Africa (60% of tested patients exhibit antibodies) and in travelers. The tick attacks typically generate clusters of cases in Safari tourists. The disease differs from MSF in that it is much milder, fever is frequently absent, a rash is observed in only half the patients, and the rash may be vesicular (which has never been reported in confirmed MSF). Moreover, several taches noires are frequently observed. They are prevalently found on the lower limbs and often associated with draining lymphadenopathy in the groin.

Japanese spotted fever (caused by *Rickettsia japonica*) and Siberian tick typhus (caused by *R. sibirica*) resemble MSF. Infections caused by *R. sibirica mongolitimonae* resemble MSF but in some cases exhibit specific clinical features, including a tache noire, groin lymphadenopathy, and lymphangitis joining these two lesions. The disease has recently been named lymphangitis-associated rickettsiosis. *Rickettsia australis* (Queensland tick typhus) and *Rickettsia honei* (Flinders Island spotted fever) cause diseases resembling MSF, but their rash can be vesicular.

R. slovaca and *R. raoultii* cause a disease apparently common in Europe named scalp eschar and neck lymphadenopathy transmitted by ticks (Hungary, Germany, France, Spain). Its tick vectors, *Dermacentor marginatus* and *Dermacentor reticulatus*, preferentially bite in cold months and bite the scalp because they prefer hairy prey. In contrast to other tick-borne rickettsioses, the disease is more prevalent in children and women. It is rarely exanthematic; the typical clinical picture consists of an erythematous skin lesion at

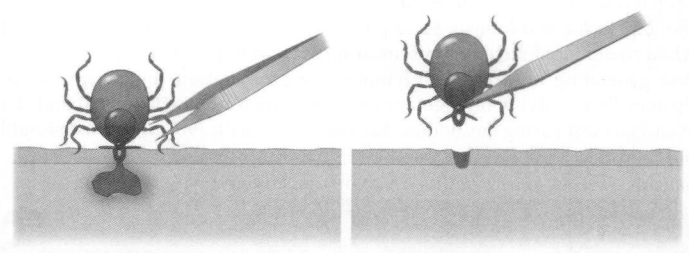

FIGURE 327-2. Tick removal technique.

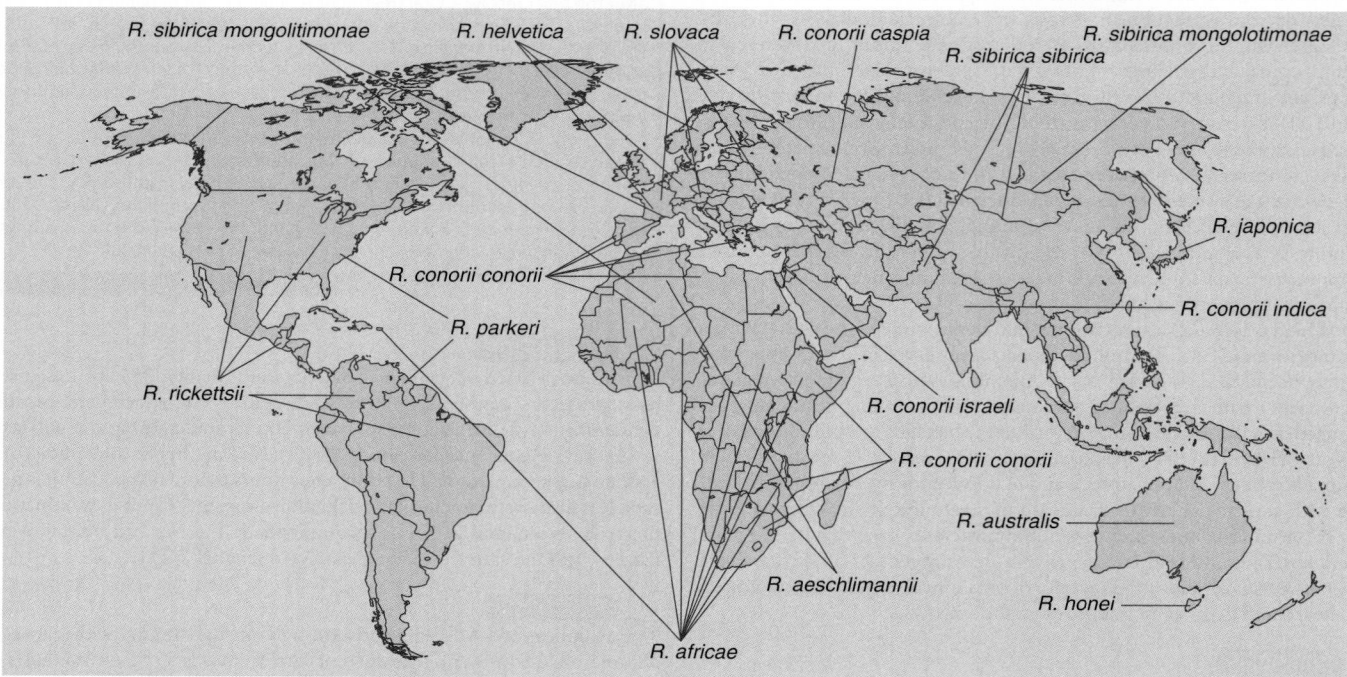

FIGURE 327-3. Geographic distribution of tick-borne rickettsioses.

the site of the tick bite on the scalp that ranges from 2 to 8 cm in diameter, and a draining neck lymphadenopathy that may be painful. Rarely, patients may exhibit fever and a rash. Deep postinfectious asthenia and residual alopecia at the site of the tick bite can be observed. The occurrence of this rickettsiosis without rash may stimulate research on other new rickettsial diseases with only localized manifestations.

DIAGNOSIS

The diagnosis of other tick-borne rickettsioses is similar to that of RMSF, mainly by serology (IFA; see earlier). An exception is *R. slovaca* infection, in which the serologic response is weak, possibly because of its lack of general infection; in this case, PCR of a skin lesion sample by a swab or a lymph node aspirate is the best solution. In *R. africae* infection, the serologic response occurs later than in RMSF and MSF, and late serum samples are therefore recommended.

TREATMENT Rx

Doxycycline (100 mg twice daily for adults or 4.4 mg/kg body weight per day in two divided doses for children under 45.4 kg [100 lb]) is the drug of choice for treatment. A single day of therapy usually suffices, but in adults with more severe disease, it should be administered until the patient is afebrile for 24 hours. In pregnant women, josamycin, a macrolide antimicrobial, has proved efficient at a dose of 3 g daily for 7 days for MSF; quinolones and newer macrolide antimicrobials give results comparable to those of doxycycline but with longer regimens.

Flea-Transmitted Diseases

Fleas (Chapter 359) can harbor two rickettsial species: *Rickettsia typhi*, the agent of murine typhus, and *Rickettsia felis*, the agent of flea-borne spotted fever. Both rickettsiae can be transmitted transovarially in the flea. Vectors are *Xenopsylla cheopis* and *Pulex irritans* but also *Ctenocephalides felis*, a cat flea. Rats, cats, opossums, and dogs can propagate infected fleas. These reservoirs and vectors are distributed worldwide, and thus these diseases have a global distribution. Fleas can be infected by both species at the same time.

MURINE TYPHUS

DEFINITION

Fleas are usually infected by *R. typhi* when feeding on apparently healthy rats that have blood-borne infection. Humans and other mammals are infected through autoinoculation by scratching a fleabite that is contaminated with feces from an infected flea. Murine typhus, because of its cycle, is more prevalent in hot and humid areas when rats proliferate.

EPIDEMIOLOGY

In the United States, 50 to 100 cases are reported yearly, mainly in southern California and southern Texas. In California, a transmission cycle involving opossums and cat fleas has been demonstrated. Murine typhus is extremely common in Southeast Asia and North Africa and is a common cause of fever in travelers.

CLINICAL MANIFESTATIONS

On the basis of studies of infected volunteers, the incubation period is generally 8 to 16 days. The disease begins with abrupt fever, nausea, vomiting, myalgias, arthralgias, and headache. A rash is observed in 40 to 50% of patients about 6 days after the onset.[7] It is detected even less frequently in patients with dark skin. The rash begins as pink maculae that can evolve to be maculopapular. It is often discrete, starting in the axilla; it generalizes to the trunk but does not usually involve the face, palms, and soles. In severe cases, it can become purpuric. The most frequently involved organ is the lung. A third of patients have a cough, and in a fourth, a nonspecific interstitial pneumonia develops that is sometimes associated with a pleural effusion. In severe forms, respiratory failure occurs. In patients with severe disease, neurologic symptoms range from confusion and stupor to coma and seizures. Cerebral hemorrhages may occur. Gastrointestinal involvement can be manifested as vomiting, abdominal pain, jaundice, and in severe cases, hematemesis.

The white blood cell count initially shows leukopenia and then leukocytosis. Thrombocytopenia can be noted as well as anemia, specifically when hemolysis is observed (frequently in patients with G6PD deficiency). A moderate increase in serum liver enzymes is common. In patients with severe disease, hyponatremia and hypoalbuminemia are observed.

DIAGNOSIS

The diagnosis of murine typhus is based mainly on serology (IFA), with titers similar to those of RMSF. On serologic evaluation, *R. typhi* cross-reacts with *R. prowazekii*; it can be differentiated either by comparing titers (two dilutions or more if IgG and IgM titers are discriminative) or by cross-adsorption. In this technique, the serum is absorbed with either antigen and then retested, and the causative agent is that removing antibodies to both bacteria. Skin biopsies and blood samples for culture and PCR may be valuable.

TREATMENT Rx

Treatment is the same as that for RMSF.

PROGNOSIS

The prognosis is usually favorable, but 10% of patients require intensive care and 1% die. Older patients and those with G6PD deficiency (Chapter 161) or chronic debilitating conditions are at higher risk.

FLEA-BORNE SPOTTED FEVER CAUSED BY *RICKETTSIA FELIS*

R. felis is mainly transmitted transovarially. Its genome comprises one or two plasmids, one being apparently conjugative. This is a new, incompletely defined disease. The bacterium is found in fleas in the Americas, Asia, Europe, Africa, and New Zealand. Isolated cases have been reported from Texas, Mexico, Brazil, France, and Germany. Reported cases all exhibited fever, a rash in six of seven cases, and inoculation eschar in some cases. The diagnosis can be based on serologic evaluation using specific *R. felis* antigen or PCR of blood or skin biopsy samples. Treatment has not been established, but the bacterium is highly susceptible to doxycycline and resistant to erythromycin. *R. felis* has been found at very high prevalence in the blood of febrile sub-Saharan Africans and is suspected to be transmitted by mosquitoes.

Louse and Mite Infections
EPIDEMIC LOUSE-BORNE TYPHUS

EPIDEMIOLOGY

The human body louse (Chapter 359) lives in clothes and multiplies rapidly when cold weather and lack of hygiene allow it to. The body louse transmits three bacterial diseases: (1) trench fever (caused by *Bartonella quintana*), (2) relapsing fever (caused by *Borrelia recurrentis*), and (3) exanthematic typhus (caused by *R. prowazekii*). The name *typhus* is derived from the Greek *tuphos*, which describes the neurologic condition associated with this disease and with typhoid. The body louse is prevalent during war, in poor countries, and in the homeless population of rich countries, including the United States and Europe. A 100,000-person outbreak of typhus was reported during the civil war in Burundi in 1997, and cases were reported in Russia, Peru, the United States, Algeria, and France in the 1990s. Louse-transmitted diseases killed more people than weapons did during central and eastern European wars in the 19th and 20th centuries.

The epidemiology of *R. prowazekii* is mainly related to humans as reservoirs and lice as vectors. In the United States, the eastern flying squirrel (*Glaucomys volans volans*) is also a reservoir, and its fleas, lice, and mites can be infected.

R. prowazekii has also been found in *Amblyomma* ticks, but their role is not known. The louse is infected when feeding on blood, which it does five times a day. *R. prowazekii* multiplies in the gut of the louse and is released in feces; after a few days, it destroys intestinal epithelium, which causes bright red blood to spread from the gut (typhus was also named the red louse disease). The patient is usually contaminated by infected feces (in which *R. prowazekii* survives for weeks), through aerosols, or by skin autoinoculation after scratching. Patients who recover from typhus may harbor the bacterium in a dormant form and suffer relapses under stressful conditions years later; this relapsing form is called Brill-Zinsser disease. During the relapse, a bacteremia occurs that may allow the start of a new outbreak if lice bite the patient.

CLINICAL MANIFESTATIONS

Typhus begins abruptly with fever, headaches, and myalgias, which may have led to the crouched posture termed *sutama* in the largest recent outbreak in Burundi. Cough and neurologic signs (stupor, confusion, or coma) are common. A rash is observed in 20 to 80% of patients, depending on the population studied; it is probably commonly underobserved on dark skin. It generally starts in the axilla and then spreads. The rash is usually macular but can be papular or purpuric in severe cases. In some cases, diarrhea and jaundice are reported. Splenomegaly is infrequently found. In severe cases, shock occurs and the fatality rate is 20 to 30%. Leukopenia, thrombocytopenia, and anemia as well as an increase in serum hepatic enzymes may be noted.

Sylvatic typhus in the United States is caused by an *R. prowazekii* variant and is a milder disease. The most prominent clinical features are neurologic. Few cases have been described, and nearly all occurred in areas where the eastern flying squirrel is found, east of the Mississippi.

Brill-Zinsser disease is difficult to diagnose because rash is rare and recent exposure to lice can be lacking. Interviewing the patient may reveal prior exposure to lice, associated or not with a diagnosis of typhus in previous years. The disease is mild and the prognosis is good.

DIAGNOSIS

The diagnosis of typhus should be considered when grouped cases of high fever with confusion are observed in patients exposed to lice. The most common diagnostic error is to attribute the findings to typhoid, which can have fatal consequences because the antimicrobials typically prescribed for that condition (β-lactams, cotrimoxazole, and quinolones) are ineffective treatment of typhus. In tropical countries, typhus is frequently confused with malaria, hemorrhagic fever, and dengue. In persons with lice, it can be confused with trench fever and relapsing fever, but treatment for both can be prescribed.

The diagnosis of typhus should be clinical because the fatality rate is high and the treatment safe and efficient. Any outbreak of unexplained fever in unhygienic environments may suggest typhus, including outbreaks during civil wars (such as in Algeria, Rwanda, and Burundi), during social collapses (such as in Russia and Ukraine), in jails (such as in Rwanda and Burundi), and in chronically poor and cold countries. The diagnosis is based mainly on serology, in which there is cross-reaction with *R. typhi* (see earlier). When the investigation is performed under difficult field conditions, a drop of blood applied on filter paper and sent to a reference laboratory is valuable for serologic testing. Culture and PCR are helpful and can be performed with a skin biopsy sample or blood. Lice are good diagnostic tools because they can be tested even when dry and can be sent in closed containers without specific temperature conditions.

TREATMENT Rx

Treatment of typhus is extremely simple, cheap, and effective; 200 mg of doxycycline orally in two divided doses is life-saving. Comatose patients should be treated parenterally. In allergic patients, chloramphenicol is the only known alternative, prescribed at a dose of 2 g/day for 10 days. There is no current vaccination, and the fight against lice is the major prevention strategy. Because lice are fragile, changing and boiling clothes are efficient. When this is not possible, insecticides (primarily permethrin) or ivermectin orally should be used.

SCRUB TYPHUS (*ORIENTIA TSUTSUGAMUSHI*)

EPIDEMIOLOGY

Scrub typhus is transmitted by the bite of trombiculid mite (Chapter 359) larvae infected by *O. tsutsugamushi*. These mites, also named chiggers, are vertically infected through their mother. Scrub typhus distribution is limited to a triangle extending between northern Japan, eastern Australia, and eastern Russia and includes the Far East, China, and the Indian subcontinent. All together, 1 billion people may be exposed. Seasonality is determined by the emergence of larvae. It is one of the three most common causes of prolonged fever in rural Asia; in temperate zones, it occurs mainly in autumn and to a lesser extent in spring. *O. tsutsugamushi* species have a wide heterogenicity that may allow the definition of several species, but a single species is currently recognized with many serotypes.

CLINICAL MANIFESTATIONS

The disease occurs in patients exposed to rural or urban foci of scrub typhus after a delay of 10 or more days. The onset is usually sudden and includes fever, headache, and myalgias. Attentive examination may reveal an inoculation eschar at the site of the mite bite and tender draining lymph nodes. Generalized lymphadenopathy and rash may be observed. The symptoms vary according to organ involvement. Neuromeningeal symptoms are relatively common. Severe forms can be manifested as septic shock. Abortion commonly occurs in pregnant women.

Leukopenia, thrombocytopenia, and increased levels of hepatic enzymes can occur. Evolution depends on the hosts and strains, and the fatality rate ranges from 0 to 30%. Scrub typhus is not more severe in HIV-infected patients, and surprisingly, HIV suppressive factors appear to be produced during infection. Relapses may occur in this disease.

DIAGNOSIS

Diagnosis may be difficult. Because the clinical features are frequently not specific, epidemiologic factors are critical.[8] A diagnosis of infectious mononucleosis has erroneously been made in patients with scrub typhus. The bacterium can be detected by culture (in cells or mice) or by PCR in blood and biopsy specimens. The serologic technique first used was agglutination of *Proteus mirabilis* serotype OXK in the Weil-Felix reaction. This test lacks sensitivity and specificity and should be replaced by IFA or enzyme-linked immunosorbent assay tests using the three or four major serotypes.

TREATMENT Rx

Chloramphenicol was the mainstay of treatment for many years, but now doxycycline is recommended. Single-day treatment with doxycycline is followed by relapses, and even repeated treatment for 2 days at a 7-day interval does not prevent all relapses. Hence, the currently recommended regimen is doxycycline, 100 mg orally twice a day for 7 days. Cases resistant to doxycycline have been reported, and rifampin (600 mg orally daily) is a reasonable alternative. Quinolones should be avoided. Prophylaxis is based on the use of repellents.

RICKETTSIALPOX (*RICKETTSIA AKARI*)

EPIDEMIOLOGY

Rickettsialpox was first described by a general practitioner in 1946 in New York City, where it is still prevalent. *R. akari*, the causal agent, is transmitted by the bite of the mouse mite (*Liponyssoides sanguineus*). Its prevalence is probably underestimated; an active search revealed 13 cases in a New York hospital in the 1980s. Cases have been reported in Arizona, Utah, and Ohio. After the terrorist attacks of 9/11/01, cases of black skin eschars were investigated as possible anthrax in New York but were in fact rickettsialpox. High seroprevalence was reported among intravenous drug users in Baltimore. Cases have also been reported from Russia, Ukraine, Slovenia, and Korea.

CLINICAL MANIFESTATIONS

Ten days after the mite bite, the beginning of the illness is marked by fever, headache, and myalgia. Careful examination reveals an inoculation eschar and a draining lymphadenopathy that could be mistaken for cutaneous anthrax. Two to 6 days later, a rash appears and comprises 5 to 40 macular then papular and vesicular spots. This aspect led to the name of the disease. It is frequently mistaken for chickenpox. The disease is usually mild.

DIAGNOSIS

The diagnosis can be made by serologic testing with IFA. Specific antigens react with high titer, but antibodies to other *Rickettsia* may be detected. The diagnosis may also be made on skin specimens by culture, immunodetection, or PCR.

TREATMENT Rx

Doxycycline is highly effective in these patients. Prevention is based on the control of mice.

EHRLICHIOSES AND ANAPLASMOSES

DEFINITION

The index case of modern ehrlichiosis was reported in the United States in 1987.[9] The patient died of fever, presumably acquired after a tick bite in Arkansas, despite receiving chloramphenicol. The patient had several initially confusing diagnostic features; on blood smears, morulae in polymorphonuclear (PMN) cells were seen, and antibodies to *Ehrlichia canis*, a pathogen of dogs but not humans, were detected. He was then thought to have *Ehrlichia chaffeensis*, but this bacterium infects monocytes, not PMN cells. A diagnosis of *Anaplasma phagocytophilum* infection (or human granulocytic ehrlichiosis [HGE]) was considered, but the tick vector of this disease is absent in Arkansas. The most likely diagnosis is currently believed to be infection with *Ehrlichia ewingii*, an agent transmitted by *Amblyomma americanum* that is prevalent in Arkansas, infects PMN cells, and cross-reacts with *E. canis*, although it typically affects immunocompromised hosts. This case illustrates the progress in knowledge on ehrlichioses and how difficult it is to conclude the etiology of an atypical infection definitively on the basis of serology alone.

All *Ehrlichia* pathogenic for humans—except *E. ewingii*—can be cultured.[10] The ehrlichiae have been reclassified into four genera, mainly on the basis of 16S ribosomal RNA–derived phylogenetic analysis. Two are the tick-associated genera *Ehrlichia* and *Anaplasma* (*A. phagocytophilum*, or the HGE agent that was formerly named *Ehrlichia phagocytophila*). One is a helminth-associated genus, *Neorickettsia*, including *Neorickettsia sennetsu* (formerly *Rickettsia sennetsu*, then *Ehrlichia sennetsu*). The fourth is *Wolbachia pipientis*, a bacterium associated with arthropods (insects, crustaceans, and acarids) and helminth worms (mainly filaria). These organisms elicit cross-reactive antibodies.

Ehrlichiae multiply exclusively in vacuoles of their eukaryotic cell host, where they form clusters known as morulae. The vacuoles are derived from phagosomes and help the organism escape bactericidal lysosomal fusion. In humans, ehrlichiae are associated with monocytes (*E. chaffeensis*, *E. canis*, *N. sennetsu*) or PMN cells (*A. phagocytophilum*, *E. ewingii*).

Ehrlichioses can be acquired through tick bites, by ingestion of nematodes through contaminated water or animals (fish, snails), or as a consequence of filariasis.

American Human Monocytic Ehrlichiosis (*Ehrlichia chaffeensis*)

EPIDEMIOLOGY

Human monocytic ehrlichiosis (HME) is caused by *E. chaffeensis*. This organism has been isolated or identified by PCR mainly in the United States in the southeastern, south central, and mid-Atlantic states and California (Table 327-3). In the United States, *A. americanum* (Lone Star tick) is the vector (Chapter 359), and the white-tailed deer is the main mammalian reservoir. Immature ticks are infected by blood while feeding on persistently bacteremic reservoirs. *E. chaffeensis* is transmitted transstadially (remaining with the same vector from one life stage to the next) in the tick and infects its next host (deer or human) during its next blood meal. The disease epidemiology reflects the tick habitat and activity, with most cases being contracted in the southern United States, in rural areas, and from April to September. In highly endemic areas, the incidence can reach 100 cases per 100,000 inhabitants. The severity is age dependent, which may explain the lower incidence reported in children. Males are more often affected than females, with a sex ratio of 4:1.

CLINICAL MANIFESTATIONS

The incubation lasts for 7 to 10 days after an identified tick exposure in 80% of cases. Patients have fever, headache, malaise, nausea, and anorexia. Untreated patients worsen and may require intensive care. Gastrointestinal tract involvement consisting of nausea, vomiting, diarrhea, and abdominal pain is common. Central nervous system infection is manifested in many forms from confusion to coma. A rash is observed in a third of cases and lymphadenopathy in a fourth. In severe forms, sepsis syndrome and multiple organ dysfunction syndrome may occur.

The white blood cell count typically shows leukopenia, caused by both lymphopenia and neutropenia. Thrombocytopenia is also frequently found; anemia may appear later. Coagulopathy may be observed in severe forms. Increases in serum enzymes, including AST, ALT, and LDH, may reflect organ involvement, as does an elevated serum creatinine. CSF examination in patients with neurologic symptoms reveals pleocytosis and increased protein levels. Cells may be monocytic or PMN. The prognosis depends on early antimicrobial treatment, but the fatality rate is still high at 2.5%. In persons coinfected with HIV, it may be most severe; in one series, 6 of 13 patients died.

DIAGNOSIS

The diagnosis of HME should be considered in patients with a history of tick exposure and unexplained fever. HME resembles RMSF, but rash is less frequent. Later in the disease, it can be misdiagnosed as anything that causes severe sepsis.

Leukopenia associated with thrombocytopenia and an increase in liver enzyme levels may establish the etiology. Careful examination of blood and CSF smears may help identify typical morulae. Treatment should be started in any suspected case. The diagnosis can be confirmed by culture in specialized laboratories using a canine cell line, DH82. However, PCR is more practical; confirmatory PCR using a second target gene is useful. Most cases are currently diagnosed serologically by a four-fold or greater increase in antibody titer or by seroconversion. The reference technique is IFA. A single titer of 25 is indicative of the diagnosis. There are cross-reactive antibodies among *Ehrlichia* species and with *A. phagocytophilum*. Western blotting may be valuable to distinguish among these bacteria.

TREATMENT ℞

Doxycycline (100 mg twice daily for adults) is the drug of choice for patients with ehrlichiosis. The optimal duration of therapy has not been established, but current regimens recommend continuation of treatment for at least 3 days after the fever subsides and until evidence of clinical improvement, for a minimum total course of 5 to 7 days. Severe or complicated disease may require longer treatment courses. Because tetracyclines are contraindicated in pregnancy, rifampin has been used successfully in a limited number of pregnant women with documented HME.

Human Granulocytic Ehrlichiosis (*Anaplasma phagocytophilum*)

EPIDEMIOLOGY

The first human case of *A. phagocytophilum* infection was recognized in 1990. The disease is found in America, Asia, and Europe (Fig. 327-4). It is transmitted by *Ixodes scapularis* (eastern North America), *Ixodes pacificus* (western North America), *Ixodes ricinus* (Europe), and *Ixodes persulcatus* (Asia), the vectors of Lyme disease (Chapter 321), and its epidemiology is similar. Coinfection with the two diseases may occur. The temporal distribution of the disease parallels that of nymph tick activity, with two peaks in spring and autumn. Ticks are born free of *Ehrlichia* and are infected while feeding on bacteremic small mammals. Deer play a major role as hosts of adult ticks and reservoirs. In highly endemic areas, the incidence can reach 50 per 100,000

TABLE 327-3 EHRLICHIOSES AND ANAPLASMOSES

DISEASE	AGENT	VECTOR	GEOGRAPHIC REPARTITION
American monocytic ehrlichiosis	*Ehrlichia chaffeensis*	*Amblyomma americanum*	South central, southeastern, mid-Atlantic coastal states
Human granulocytic ehrlichiosis	*Anaplasma phagocytophilum*	*Ixodes ricinus*	Europe, China
		Ixodes scapularis	Northeast, upper Midwest, northern California
E. ewingii	*Ehrlichia ewingii*	*Amblyomma americanum*	South central, southeastern, mid-Atlantic coastal states
Japanese monocytic ehrlichiosis	*Neorickettsia sennetsu*	Helminth of the gray mullet?	Japan
E. canis	*Ehrlichia canis*	*Rhipicephalus sanguineus*	Venezuela

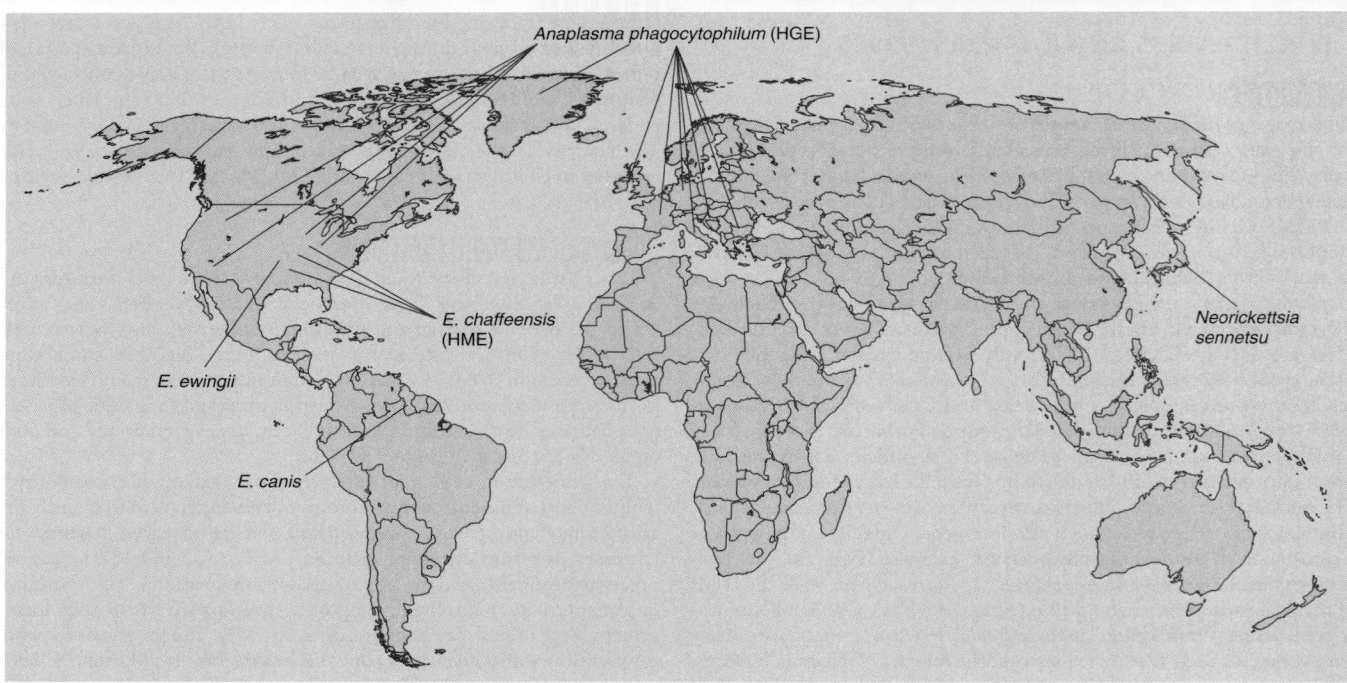

FIGURE 327-4. Geographic distribution of ehrlichioses. HGE = human granulocytic ehrlichiosis; HME = human monocytic ehrlichiosis.

inhabitants per year. The mean age of diagnosed patients is high, and males are more frequently infected than females, with a sex ratio of 3 : 1.

CLINICAL MANIFESTATIONS

The incubation time is usually between 7 and 10 days, and 80% of patients report a history of tick exposure. Many infections may be asymptomatic or too mild to require a diagnostic procedure. The disease frequently begins abruptly, with fever, headache, malaise, and myalgias that may be particularly severe. Rash is found in less than 10% of cases. Visceral involvement may be observed and includes digestive symptoms such as nausea, vomiting, and diarrhea. Neurologic symptoms may include confusion, meningitis, and meningoencephalitis.

The evolution of the disease is favorable in most cases, even without specific therapy, but the disease may evolve to septic shock in some individuals. Patients with underlying diseases are more at risk of dying. Most deaths are the consequence of *Anaplasma*-induced immunosuppression, and patients may experience invasive aspergillosis, candidiasis, cryptococcosis, or herpes esophagitis.

DIAGNOSIS

Laboratory findings consist of the association of thrombocytopenia and leukopenia (lymphopenia or neutropenia). An increase in serum transaminases is also frequent. The diagnosis can be made by careful examination of blood smears for morulae within PMN cells (Fig. 327-5). Culture from blood is possible in appropriate cells (HL-60), and PCR is useful as for HME. Most cases are diagnosed by serologic testing with IFA, which is comparable to that in HME (see earlier).

TREATMENT   Rx

Treatment is also similar to that of HME except that *A. phagocytophilum* is susceptible to fluoroquinolones in vitro, but these drugs have not been tested in patients.

Ehrlichia ewingii

Canine granulocytic ehrlichiosis, reported in the United States in 1972, is caused by *E. ewingii*. This bacterium was characterized by amplification and sequencing of the 16S ribosomal RNA gene. The vector of *E. ewingii* is *A.*

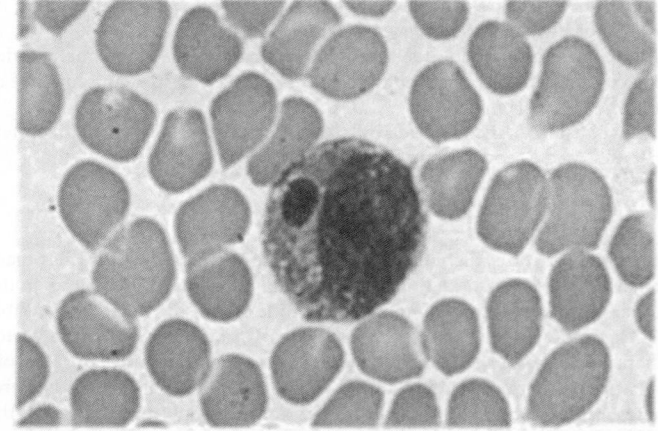

FIGURE 327-5. Peripheral blood leukocyte (monocyte) containing ehrlichial morula in a patient with human monocytic ehrlichiosis. (Courtesy Centers for Disease Control and Prevention. http://www.cdc.gov/ehrlichiosis/symptoms.)

americanum (Chapter 359), which also transmits *E. chaffeensis*. Among 60 cases of ehrlichiosis in Missouri in 1999, four were caused by *E. ewingii*; four other cases have been reported since by the CDC. The disease was prevalent in immunocompromised hosts (seven of eight) coinfected with HIV or receiving immunosuppressive drugs. Patients who report tick exposure are noted to have fever, thrombocytopenia, leukopenia, and various symptoms, including meningitis. Morulae may be seen on blood smears in PMN cells. The evolution in reported cases was good; patients responded dramatically to doxycycline. Patients have antibodies to *E. chaffeensis*, and PCR has been shown to be useful when it is applied to blood samples. This diagnosis should be considered when ehrlichiosis is suspected in immunocompromised patients exposed to *A. americanum* ticks.

Ehrlichia canis

Canine monocytic ehrlichiosis was reported first in Algeria in the 1930s. It is caused by *E. canis* and transmitted by the dog tick *R. sanguineus* (Chapter 359). This tick is found worldwide and is prevalent in temperate and hot areas. In 1996, a single case of infection was reported in an asymptomatic man from Venezuela who owned an infected dog. Recently, cases have been reported in patients in South America.

A New *Ehrlichia* in Wisconsin

In four patients from Wisconsin, a new *Ehrlichia* species closely related to *E. muris* was cultured and identified[11] as *Ixodes scapularis* ticks. All patients had fever, malaise, headache and lymphopenia, and some also had thrombocytopenia and elevated transaminases.

Candidatus Neoehrlichia mikurensis

Candidatus Neoehrlichia mikurensis, transmitted by Ixodes ticks, has been reported based on PCR on the blood of febrile immunocompromised European patients and in China.

Wolbachia Species

Wolbachia bacteria are endosymbionts of arthropods and nematodes. They were known to be present in filarial worms, but it was later shown that they may play a role in human disease. These bacteria manipulate the fertility of their host. Eradication of *Wolbachia* in filariae may lead to infertility and stop the microfilariae from spreading. This effect was demonstrated by field treatment with doxycycline in patients with onchocerciasis. The patients improved when treated with this drug, which is effective on *Wolbachia* and subsequently on the worm's fertility but not on the worm itself. In 2001, it was shown that the adverse reactions observed after treatment of lymphatic filariasis may be caused by the release of *Wolbachia* from destroyed worms. Some authors suggested that eradicating *Wolbachia* before the anthelmintic prescription would avoid these reactions. For some reason, *Loa loa* (Chapter 358) do not harbor *Wolbachia*, and the genome of *Wolbachia* integrated in the *Brugia malayi* genome makes it inaccessible to therapy.

Q FEVER

DEFINITION

Q fever is a worldwide zoonosis caused by *Coxiella burnetii*. The name Q fever is derived from "query" to emphasize the surprising aspect of the disease first described in Queensland, Australia, in 1935 by Derrick. The infection in humans is variable in its severity, clinical expression, and natural course (i.e., acute or chronic). It is considered by the CDC to be a potential agent of bioterrorism. Ungulates and pets are the major sources of human infection.[12]

The Pathogen

C. burnetii is a gram-negative bacterium that naturally infects its host's monocytes. It multiplies in an acidic vacuole. Strains are heterogeneous genetically and antigenically and are associated with acute infections of variable severity. *C. burnetii* in vitro generates a deleted avirulent mutant also named phase II. This mutant exhibits diagnostic antigens that are useful because they are more reactive during acute infection.

C. burnetii is incompletely eliminated after acute infection. In immunocompromised hosts and patients with cardiac valve lesions, *C. burnetii* continues to multiply despite high levels of antibodies and causes chronic infection. Control of the disease in acute Q fever is associated with formation of a granuloma.

EPIDEMIOLOGY

C. burnetii infects a wide range of animals, including mammals, birds, and ticks. Ungulates and pets (cats and dogs) are the most common source of the disease. Mammals are infected through aerosols and may shed *Coxiella* in feces, urine, milk, and birth products. Humans are usually infected by aerosols or less frequently by exposure to milk products. Interhuman infections through sexual intercourse, during delivery, or by blood transfusion have been reported. *Coxiella* survives in the environment and can be spread far by the wind. In the past few years, major outbreaks were related to sheep and goats. The disease is partly seasonal and related to lambing time. The current geographic repartition is largely unknown. Males have more severe disease but are not more often exposed to Q fever, and middle-aged people are more frequently affected and hospitalized. The number of reported cases recently increased dramatically in Europe and Asia. Many American soldiers were infected during the war in Iraq. A giant outbreak was observed more recently in the Netherlands.

CLINICAL MANIFESTATIONS

After contamination by *C. burnetii*, 60% of patients seroconvert without apparent disease, 38% experience a self-limited disease, and only 2% require

TABLE 327-4	SITUATIONS THAT SHOULD PROMPT SEROLOGIC TESTING FOR Q FEVER

ACUTE Q FEVER (PHASE II ANTIGEN AND IgG ≥ 200 AND IgM ≥ 50)

Fever in a patient in contact with ungulates
Unexplained prolonged fever (>7 days)
Granulomatous hepatitis
Fever and thrombocytopenia
Meningoencephalitis
Myocarditis
Erythema nodosum
Fever during pregnancy
Fever in a patient in contact with a parturient pet
Unexplained atypical pneumonia
Fever and an increase in transaminases (2-5 times the normal level)
Aseptic meningitis
Guillain-Barré syndrome
Pericarditis
Spontaneous abortion

CHRONIC Q FEVER (PHASE I ANTIGEN AND IgG ≥ 800 AND IgA ≥ 100)

Blood culture–negative endocarditis
Patient with a valvulopathy and unexplained
    Fever
    Weight loss
    Fatigue
    Increased erythrocyte sedimentation rate
    Increased transaminases
    Thrombocytopenia
Patient with unusually rapid degradation of a prosthetic valve
Fever in a patient with a vascular aneurysm or prosthesis
Aseptic osteomyelitis
Chronic pericarditis
Multiple spontaneous abortions

diagnostic evaluation. Months to years after the primary infection, a chronic infection associated with an immunocompromised situation, a cardiac valve lesion, or a vascular prosthesis or aneurysm develops in 0.2 to 0.5% of patients.

Patients with diagnosed acute infection may have a variety of symptoms (Table 327-4). Isolated prolonged fever was observed in 14% of more than 1000 patients. Pneumonia was found in 37% and was the only symptom in 17%. This percentage may vary according to the place of study and reach 90% of diagnosed cases. Some cases may be associated with respiratory distress. Hepatitis is found in 60% of patients and is the sole manifestation in 40%. The association of fever and a moderate increase in transaminases is an important clue. Some hepatitides, specifically in middle-aged men, are associated with an inflammatory syndrome and autoantibodies and may be resistant to antimicrobial treatment. Liver biopsy, when it is performed, exhibits granulomas that may be typified by a lipid vacuole and surrounded by a fibrinoid ring in the form of a doughnut. Less frequently (1.5% of cases), patients exhibit a rash. Patients can have specific neurologic manifestations such as meningitis, encephalitis, meningoencephalitis, or peripheral neuropathy. In 1 to 2% of cases, patients have cardiovascular manifestations such as pericarditis or, more rarely, myocarditis.

Evolution is usually favorable even without treatment, except in special hosts. In pregnant women, symptomatic or not, Q fever compromises the pregnancy. When infected during the first trimester, the patient usually aborts spontaneously. When the patient is infected later, the disease can result in fetal death or prematurity, or the outcome may be normal. Chronic uterine infection may develop in half the patients infected during pregnancy, and they may later experience multiple spontaneous abortions. From 30 to 50% of patients with heart valve or vascular lesions may experience chronic endocarditis within 2 years. This evolution is not prevented by regular treatment.

Patients with Q fever endocarditis have a chronic infection with low-grade fever, progressive degradation of valve function, and progressive heart failure. Fever is intermittent, and vegetations are frequently absent on echocardiography. Endocarditis is therefore not frequently considered in the initial differential diagnosis. If it is not diagnosed, the disease progressively worsens, and emboli (mainly cerebral) as well as renal insufficiency, splenomegaly, and hepatomegaly may be observed. Digital clubbing may also be seen. The main clue to the diagnosis in a patient with a valvulopathy is unexplained sickness (unexplained fatigue, weight loss, fever), a biological abnormality (leukopenia, increased erythrocyte sedimentation rate, thrombocytopenia, increase in hepatic enzymes), or rapid degradation of a prosthetic valve. Chronic osteomyelitis, hepatitis, and infection of an aneurysm and vascular prosthesis have been reported.

Leukopenia may be observed; thrombocytopenia is frequent, as are increases in hepatic enzymes. Circulating anticoagulant associated with antiphospholipid antibodies may be observed, as may anti–smooth muscle antibodies. During endocarditis, antinuclear antibodies, microhematuria, and rheumatoid factor are frequently found.

DIAGNOSIS

The diagnosis is based mainly on serology (see Table 327-4). Direct detection by culture and PCR or immunochemistry in valve, liver, or blood samples is also useful, but serologic evaluation by IFA is the best method. Two antigens (phase I and phase II) can be tested. Acute Q fever is diagnosed when seroconversion or a four-fold increase is obtained with phase II antigen. A single serum test exhibiting IgG antibodies of 200 or greater and IgM of 50 or greater against phase II is also diagnostic. During chronic Q fever, antibodies are at higher titer and directed against both phase I and phase II. IgG against phase I at a titer of 800 or 1600 is diagnostic of chronic infection, as is IgA at 100 or greater. Serology is useful for follow-up of patients with acute Q fever and underlying disease and those with treated chronic Q fever.

TREATMENT Rx

Treatment is easy during acute Q fever. Doxycycline is the most efficient antimicrobial and should be prescribed for 2 weeks. Some patients with hepatitis do not respond well because of an excessive immune response. They rapidly improve with a short course of glucocorticoids. In pregnant women, cotrimoxazole during the entire pregnancy may decrease the chance of an unfavorable outcome. As for endocarditis, bactericidal treatment is necessary. In vitro, antimicrobial efficacy is impaired by the low pH of the vacuoles in which *C. burnetii* resides. Hydroxychloroquine increases the pH of these vacuoles and restores the bactericidal effect of doxycycline. In patients with endocarditis, the recommended treatment is a combination of doxycycline (200 mg daily) and hydroxychloroquine (600 mg/day, then adjusted to reach a 1-mg/mL plasma concentration). This regimen is prescribed for 18 to 36 months according to serologic results. We recently observed that a more rapid favorable outcome was obtained with doxycycline serum levels higher than 5 μg/mL. Some strains may be resistant to doxycycline, and new macrolides may be an alternative. The major problem with this treatment is photosensitivity; sun exposure should be avoided. An alternative treatment is a combination of doxycycline and ofloxacin for 3 years or more.

PREVENTION

Prevention is based on veterinary control in animals. A vaccine is currently available in Australia.

GENERAL REFERENCES

For the General References and other additional features, please visit Expert Consult at https://expertconsult.inkling.com.

328

ZOONOSES

STUART LEVIN AND KAMALJIT SINGH

DEFINITION

Zoonoses are classically defined as infections or diseases naturally transmitted between humans and vertebrate animals. There are approximately 1400 human pathogens, of which about 800 species are zoonotic. Zoonoses may be bacterial, viral, fungal, parasitic, or due to unconventional agents such as prions.[1] Of the approximate 400 emerging or reemerging pathogens in the past 70 years, 60% are known to be zoonotic, with a disproportionate number of the new zoonoses being caused by RNA viruses. Arthropod-transmitted diseases are prototypic zoonoses, but whereas infections such as West Nile fever, *Schistosoma japonicum*, *Trypanosoma rhodesiense*, and *Plasmodium knowlesi* malaria are zoonoses, other related diseases such as *Schistosoma mansoni*, *Trypanosoma gambiense*, and *Plasmodium vivax* malaria are not zoonoses, because these pathogens are transferred from human to human and do not depend on vertebrate reservoirs. Human infestations with ectoparasites are likewise not considered to be zoonoses.

We have little ability to predict how an emerging zoonotic pathogen will act. Most zoonotic pathogens like rabies enter a human and cause disease; however, in these cases, humans are dead-end hosts and are unlikely to transmit the disease to others. Less commonly, pathogens such as human immunodeficiency virus (HIV) or recombinant swine H1N1 (pH1N1/2009) enter the human population with great difficulty but are then successfully transmitted from human to human to cause global epidemics. The recent emphasis on emerging infections that are predominantly zoonoses and the potential for new pandemics markedly enhance the need for human medicine to be integrated with veterinary medicine and veterinary research. This is the concept of One Health, which calls for enhanced collaboration between physicians, veterinarians, and environmental health professionals for the optimal health of all species on the planet.[2,3]

EPIDEMIOLOGY

During the course of evolution, humans have sought the company of vertebrates for many reasons, including their companionship as pets. In the United States, fewer than 60% of households have pets; a surprising 56% of dog owners sleep with their dog next to them, whereas among cat owners, 75% sleep with their pets.[4] The over 100 million dogs and cats in the United States facilitate the transmission of more than 250 different infectious species and cause more than 1 million bite injuries each year. Other pets include birds, fish, and reptiles (particularly common are small pet turtles that can transmit salmonellosis). Another popular trend is the keeping of exotic animals as pets, many of which are important reservoirs of a variety of viral and bacterial human pathogens.

Almost all arthropod-transmitted infectious agents acquired from vertebrates in the United States are due to either ticks or mosquitoes. Ticks are the more common villain,[5] and Lyme disease is the most frequent arthropod-transmitted infectious disease in the United States (Chapter 321). At least five tick-borne pathogens are known to be transmitted by *Ixodes scapularis* (the principal tick vector for Lyme disease): *Borrelia burgdorferi*, *Anaplasma phagocytophilum* (an agent for anaplasmosis, previously known as human granulocytic ehrlichiosis), *Babesia microti* (an agent of human babesiosis), *Borrelia miyamotoi* (an agent of relapsing fever), and the Powassan encephalitis virus. Two or more of these pathogens can be transmitted by a single tick bite, resulting in 30 different permutations of mixed infections. In addition, two geographically distinct species of *Borrelia* (Chapter 322) cause relapsing fevers in the United States, with *Borrelia hermsii* described in the mountain states west of the Mississippi River and *Borrelia turicatae* in the southwest plains states. Threats from mosquito bites include almost all the vector-borne encephalitides, such as St. Louis encephalitis and West Nile virus (Chapter 383).

The recognition of novel zoonoses such as Hendra and Nipah (henipaviruses) and the SARS (severe acute respiratory syndrome) coronavirus has intensified research in wildlife reservoirs especially among the more than 1000 species of Chiroptera or bats. Bats have been known as the origin of a number of "old" viruses such as yellow fever virus (Chapter 381) and Japanese encephalitis virus but are now also recognized as the source of a succession of highly pathogenic emerging zoonoses, including Ebola, Marburg, and MERS (Middle East respiratory syndrome) coronavirus. (Dromedary camels have also been identified as hosts for MERS.) Another area of great interest is in the highly pathogenic avian influenza viruses (HPAIV) that spread from wild birds and ducks to chickens and humans, such as A/H5N1, with over 640 cases and 380 deaths since 2003, and other avian viruses, such as A/H7N9, with 132 laboratory-confirmed cases and 38 fatalities since March 2013. Emerging swine zoonoses include the 2009 novel swine-origin A/H1N1 virus that began in February 2009 in Veracruz, Mexico. Other novel swine influenza virus infections (e.g., vH3N2) have been documented in fairgoers and pigs in agricultural fairs in the United States since 2007.[6] In addition, living in close contact with swine, a common husbandry practice in Asia, has been associated with an emerging rapidly fatal meningitis due to *Streptococcus suis*.

The risk of contracting a zoonosis is increased by direct animal contact in meat handlers, poachers, hunters, exotic animal smugglers, and international travelers; by exposure to and inhalation of infectious air particles; by insect

TABLE 328-1 NEWER ZOONOSES IN THE UNITED STATES (EMERGING INFECTIONS)

DISEASE*	INFECTIOUS AGENT	CLINICAL FINDINGS	VECTOR/ACQUISITION
Ehrlichiosis, monocytic	*Ehrlichia chaffeensis* (Chapter 327)	Fever, myalgia, leukopenia; monocyte inclusions not often seen; maculopapular rash in a minority	*Amblyomma* (Lone Star) tick bite
Human granulocytic anaplasmosis (HGA)	*Anaplasma phagocytophilium* (Chapter 327)	Fever, myalgia, leukopenia; granulocyte inclusions often seen on blood smear	*Ixodes* (deer) tick bite
"Flu syndrome"	*Ehrlichia ewingii* (Chapter 327)	Immunocompromised host—fever, myalgia	*Amblyomma*
STARI (Southern tick-associated rash illness)	Unknown	Lyme disease–like illness	*Amblyomma*
Relapsing fever	*Borrelia hermsii* & *Borrelia turicatae* (Chapter 322)	Fever, headaches, myalgias	*Ornithodorus* ticks
Cat-scratch disease	*Bartonella* spp. (there are 8 identified zoonotic *Bartonella* spp.) (Chapter 315)	Cervical lymphadenopathy in normal hosts and cutaneous and hepatic angiomatosis in AIDS patients	Cat scratch or bite
Hemorrhagic diarrhea	Enterohemorrhagic *Escherichia coli* O157:H7 (other Shiga toxin–producing strains) (Chapter 304)	Rectal bleeding, dysentery, hemolytic-uremic syndrome	Contaminated undercooked meat
Hantavirus pulmonary syndrome	*Hantavirus*—Sin Nombre (Chapter 381)	Noncardiac pulmonary edema, elevated hematocrit	Fomites of wild rodents
Cryptosporidium diarrhea	*Cryptosporidium parvum* (Chapter 350)	Prolonged watery diarrhea	Contaminated water—cattle and sheep
Paragonimiasis	*Paragonimus kellicotti* (Chapter 356)	Diarrhea, cough, pleuritic chest pain, hemoptysis	Freshwater crayfish
Dysentery	*Campylobacter jejuni* (Chapter 303)	Dysentery, reactive arthritis, Guillain-Barré syndrome	Contaminated chicken
Pyogenic skin ulcer	*Capnocytophaga canimorsus* (Chapter 280)	Sepsis, skin infection	Dog bites
West Nile fever encephalitis	West Nile virus (Chapters 382 and 383)	Encephalitis, myelitis, Guillain-Barré syndrome, West Nile fever	Mosquito bite, birds
SARS	Coronavirus (Chapter 366)	Severe lower respiratory tract infection	Horseshoe bats
Cutaneous leishmaniasis	*Leishmania mexicana* (Chapter 348)	Skin nodules and ulcers	Wood rat

*See table of contents and index to locate a more detailed discussion of each disease.
AIDS = acquired immunodeficiency syndrome; SARS = severe acute respiratory syndrome.

bites, contact with previously infected human blood products, contact with and ingestion of infectious agents transmitted by animal-contaminated water; by insufficiently cooked meat, eggs, dairy products, and fish; and by acts of bioterrorism. Patrons of petting zoos, pet owners, farmers, hunters, laboratory researchers, cave explorers, hikers, and veterinarians, among others, are at higher risk for a zoonosis than the general population is. Infectious agents transmitted by these routes from animal sources essentially include members of all microbial classes: viruses and prions, bacteria and rickettsia, fungi, helminths, and protozoa. Immunocompromised hosts, such as splenectomized individuals, transplant recipients, patients with acquired immunodeficiency syndrome (AIDS), patients on chemotherapeutic agents (including biologics used in rheumatology and oncology), and pregnant women and their fetuses, are at higher risk for clinical disease when exposed to these various infectious agents. Chagas disease, a protozoal infection, is a zoonosis in South America but is not endemic to the United States (with only seven Autochthonous cases described since 1955); however, immigration from Latin America has led to "globalization" of this disease, with an estimated 300,000 persons with *Trypanosoma cruzi* infection in the United States and the potential for transmission of the infection through blood, birth, or organ donations. *Leishmania donovani* is almost always a small-animal reservoir zoonosis, but in India, it has become established in the human population, with female sandflies as the vector for human-to-human transmission.

As the world shrinks, warms, flattens, and remains in conflict, new infectious diseases seem inevitable, and previously rare ones are seen in unexpected places (Table 328-1) because of global warming, human intrusion into previously underexplored or never explored sites, world travel, deforestation, and the increasing threat of biological terrorism or warfare. Tens of thousands of years ago, human communities consisted of small groups of people living in vastly disparate regions that posed a very low risk for global epidemics. Increasing urbanization, intermingling of humans and domestic animals, and lack of adequate sanitation threaten to dramatically increase the incidence and severity of epidemic infectious diseases.

CLINICAL MANIFESTATIONS

Zoonoses can manifest as a variety of clinical syndromes, including respiratory disease (Table 328-2), central nervous system disease (Table 328-3), and rash or skin lesions (Table 328-4). Other zoonotic clinical syndromes

may present as sepsis, polyarthritis, jaundice, acute renal failure, endocarditis, or diarrhea (Table 328-5).

Emerging zoonotic infectious diseases include Nipah virus and Hendra virus encephalitis, *Hantavirus* pneumonia and *Hantavirus* fever with renal failure, the SARS and MERS coronaviruses, West Nile encephalitis (which spread coast to coast in the United States in 3 years and is now apparently a permanent resident), monkeypox (an outbreak of which in the upper Midwest was caused by pet prairie dogs housed next to an imported Gambian rat infected with the virus), *Leishmania mexicana* in Texas, and at least 8 to 10 newly identified tick-borne rickettsial spotted fevers worldwide, including the flea-borne *Rickettsia felis* in California and tick-borne *Rickettsia parkeri* in the Gulf Coast states. Avian H5N1 and A/H7N9, pH1N1/2009 (swine) influenza, SARS and MERS coronaviruses, and West Nile fever have recently exposed the fragility of our world village. Nevertheless, exotic zoonoses remain a less frequent cause of fever in travelers than the well-known ordinary gastrointestinal and pulmonary pathogens.

DIAGNOSIS

Non–animal-associated environment- or travel-related infectious diseases can be confused with zoonoses. The vast majority of clinical diseases caused by *Legionella pneumophila*, *Entamoeba histolytica*, *Giardia lamblia*, *Burkholderia pseudomallei*, *Chromobacterium violaceum*, *Aeromonas hydrophila*, and airborne fungi such as *Blastomyces dermatitidis*, *Coccidioides immitis*, and *Histoplasma capsulatum* are acquired through environmental exposure and are only rarely related to animal hosts. *Sporothrix schenckii*, almost always an environmentally acquired pathogen stemming from vegetation-related injuries, has also been transmitted from cats with draining cutaneous ulcers to owners and animal handlers. Histoplasmosis has been acquired by explorers (spelunkers) in caves contaminated by bat guano.

Unfortunately, some descriptive disease titles can be misleading to clinicians and interfere with reaching the correct diagnosis. The transmission of tick-borne Rocky Mountain spotted fever actually occurs much more commonly in the southeastern United States than in the Rocky Mountains and has even occurred in the middle of New York City. In turn, the geographic range of Southern tick-associated rash illness (STARI), a Lyme disease–like infection transmitted by the Lone Star tick, *Amblyomma americanum*, has expanded to areas where *Ixodes scapularis* transmission of *B. burgdorferi*

TABLE 328-2   RESPIRATORY TRACT ZOONOSES

DISEASE*	MICROORGANISM†	CLINICAL FINDINGS	RESERVOIR AND/OR VECTOR
Psittacosis‡	*Chlamydophila psittaci* (Chapter 318)	Pneumonia, often severe	Aerosols from parrots, ducks, turkeys
Q fever	*Coxiella burnetii* (Chapter 327)	Pneumonia, hepatitis, myocarditis	Airborne from soil contaminated by sheep, goats, and cats, particularly if parturient
Tularemia	*Francisella tularensis* (Chapter 311)	Cutaneous ulcer and regional node, pneumonia and hilar node, pleural effusion	Rabbit contact (winter) and tick/fly bites
Plague	*Yersinia pestis* (Chapter 312)	Inguinal nodes, bubonic plague (basilar pneumonia develops in 10%), hilar node enlargement	Fleas from prairie dogs, rock squirrels, rats
Hantavirus cardiopulmonary syndrome	Hantavirus (Chapter 381)	Upper respiratory to lower respiratory to adult respiratory distress syndrome (ARDS) to death	Deer mouse fomites: urine, feces, saliva
Rhodococcus pneumonia	*Rhodococcus equi*	Pneumonia often cavitates in those with AIDS and in other immunosuppressed patients.	Horse manure, soil
Mycoplasma arginini pneumonia	*Mycoplasma arginini* (Chapter 317)	Pneumonia, sepsis, neutropenia	Sheep, goats
Foot-and-mouth disease	Aphthovirus	Nonspecific upper respiratory tract infection, oral vesicles	Cloven-footed mammals
Whooping cough	*Bordetella bronchiseptica* (Chapter 313)	Pneumonia, bronchitis, whooping cough	Dogs
Histoplasmosis	*Histoplasma capsulatum* (Chapter 332)	Pneumonia or fever of unknown origin	Bats
Anthrax	*Bacillus anthracis* (Chapter 294)	Mediastinal widening with CT scan; pneumonia often absent	Herbivore mammals
Glanders	*Burkholderia mallei* (Chapter 306)	Pneumonia, erosive tracheobronchitis	Horses, mules

*See table of contents and index to locate a more detailed discussion of each disease.
†Because of the fastidious nature of some organisms, the rapid development of diagnostic tools, and the risk some agents pose to laboratory workers, a clinical microbiologist should be consulted if these agents are considered in a patient's differential diagnosis.
‡Occurs in more than 1000 animal species.
AIDS = acquired immunodeficiency syndrome; CT = computed tomography.

TABLE 328-3   CENTRAL NERVOUS SYSTEM ZOONOSES

DISEASE*	ORGANISM	CLINICAL FINDINGS	ACQUISITION
Listeriosis	*Listeria monocytogenes* (Chapter 293)	Purulent meningitis during pregnancy, in patients > 65 yr, in neonates, and immunosuppressed	Unpasteurized cheese and other dairy products; cattle, goats
Leptospirosis	*Leptospira interrogans* (Chapter 323)	Aseptic meningitis, hepatorenal syndrome	Asymptomatic dogs, cattle; common water source
Herpes B encephalitis	Cercopithecine herpesvirus (herpes B virus) (Chapter 414)	Diffuse progressive encephalitis	Macaca monkey bites or scratches
Lyme disease	*Borrelia burgdorferi* (Chapters 321 and 322)	Lymphocytic meningitis, motor-sensory neuropathy, facial palsy	Tick bite
Lymphocytic choriomeningitis	Lymphocytic choriomeningitis virus (Chapter 412)	Lymphocytic meningitis, occasionally with pneumonia	Inhalation of mouse secretions: urine, feces, saliva
Mosquito-borne encephalitis (U.S.)	Eastern, Western equine, St. Louis, California encephalitis; West Nile virus (Chapter 383)	Diffuse encephalitis least severe; California encephalitis most severe; Eastern equine encephalitis, myelitis, meningitis	Mosquito-borne from horses, birds
Rabies encephalitis	Rabies virus (Chapter 414)	Encephalitis; almost always fatal	Bites from dogs, skunks, bats, raccoons, foxes
Toxoplasmosis	*Toxoplasma gondii* (Chapter 349)	Multiple brain masses in AIDS patients	Cat feces or ingestion of undercooked lamb or pork
Cerebral cysticercosis	*Taenia solium* (Chapter 354)	Epilepsy, CNS cysts, eosinophilic meningitis, hydrocephalus	Fecal-oral; contamination of food with pork tapeworm eggs
New-variant Creutzfeldt-Jakob disease	Prion (proteinaceous infectious particle) (Chapter 415)	Dementia, ataxia, myoclonus	Beef from cattle fed scraps from contaminated sheep carcasses
Nipah virus (Chapter 414)	Paramyxovirus	Acute encephalitis, death	Pig contact, fruit bats
Hendra virus	Paramyxovirus	Pneumonitis, encephalitis	Horses, fruit bats

*See table of contents and index to locate a more detailed discussion of each disease.
AIDS = acquired immunodeficiency syndrome; CNS = central nervous system.

occurs, resulting in misdiagnosis as Lyme borreliosis. Urban New York City continues to be a major source of rickettsialpox, where it was first described 60 years ago.[7] Vegetarians and other strict non–pork-eating persons have been seriously infected with the pig tapeworm *Taenia solium* as a result of fecal contamination of food from infected human food handlers. Recent outbreaks of food-borne zoonotic disease with Shiga toxin–producing *Escherichia coli*–infected brussels sprouts in Germany and *Listeria*-infected cantaloupes in the United States in 2011 highlight the difficulties in identifying the original source of the disease outbreak. The separation of an infection from the source of transmission, or a lack of knowledge, often blurs the diagnosis of a zoonoses. For example, unexpected outbreaks of leptospirosis among triathlon athletes exposed to water bodies that are contaminated by animal urine may not be recognized by physicians in a nonendemic setting. Emerging parasitic zoonosis such as the lung fluke, *Paragonimus kellicotti* (acquired by ingestion of contaminated crayfish from the Mississippi River basin), although unknown to most physicians and microbiologists, is well recognized by veterinarians in North America.

Until recently, human influenza A was not well recognized as a zoonosis; however, interspecies spread and mixing of swine, avian, and human influenza viruses can occur in unique geographic areas such as southern China or Mexico (pH1N1/2009), where dense concentrations of ducks, pigs, and people cohabit. Viral incubation of the three influenza species in the pig, with

TABLE 328-4 ZOONOSES CAUSING RASH OR SKIN NODULE, ULCER

DISEASE*	MICROORGANISM†	CLINICAL FINDINGS	RESERVOIR AND/OR VECTOR
Ehrlichiosis (monocytic)	Ehrlichia chaffeensis (Chapter 327)	Macular rash (seen in < half of patients) with a central distribution; prevalent in south-central United States	Tick bite
Leptospirosis	Leptospira interrogans (Chapter 323)	Central macular rash in 20%; occasional enanthem, conjunctival suffusion, hepatorenal syndrome	Urine-contaminated water; dogs, cattle
Lyme disease	Borrelia burgdorferi (Chapters 321 and 322)	Erythema migrans; 20% have multiple lesions	Mouse reservoir—tick bite
Rocky Mountain spotted fever	Rickettsia rickettsii (Chapter 327)	Acral or peripheral distribution of maculopapular to hemorrhagic rash to gangrenous lesions—no eschar	Tick bite
Typhus (epidemic)	Rickettsia prowazekii (Chapter 327)	Macular rash with a central distribution (can be hemorrhagic)	Flying squirrel fleas or fomites
Spotted fever	Rickettsia parkeri (Chapter 327)	Eschar, fever, headache, generalized rash involving palms and soles	Amblyomma maculatum
Cat-scratch disease	Bartonella spp. (Chapter 315)	Bacillary angiomatosis, peliosis hepatis in HIV patients, cervical adenopathy, subacute bacterial endocarditis, fever of unknown origin	Cat scratch or bite
Tularemia	Francisella tularensis (Chapter 311)	Ulcer and node, typhoidal syndrome, pneumonia	Rabbit contact and tick bite
Anthrax	Bacillus anthracis (Chapter 294)	Painless, edematous, nonpurulent ulcer that becomes black and necrotic over days; mediastinitis	Herbivore animal products, including animal hides
Rickettsialpox (spotted fever Rickettsia)	Rickettsia akari, Rickettsia conorii, Rickettsia africae (8 others found on all continents) (Chapter 327)	Fever, rash, eschar (multiple), tache noire (R. africae, often multiple)	House mouse mite
Monkeypox	Orthopoxvirus (Chapter 372)	Multiple maculopustular lesions with lymphadenopathy	Prairie dog (U.S.), African rodents
Erysipeloid	Erysipelothrix rhusiopathiae (Chapter 295)	Red, tender, swollen finger; subacute bacterial endocarditis	Skin pricked while cleaning fish, domestic meat animals

*See table of contents and index to locate a more detailed discussion of each disease.
†Because of the fastidious nature of some organisms, the rapid development of diagnostic tools, and the risk some agents pose to laboratory workers, a clinical microbiologist should be consulted if these agents are considered in a patient's differential diagnosis.

TABLE 328-5 OTHER ZOONOTIC CLINICAL SYNDROMES

DISEASE*	ORGANISM
Sepsis syndrome	Streptococcus suis, Capnocytophaga canimorsus, Yersinia enterocolitica, Pasteurella multocida, Rickettsia rickettsii, Streptobacillus moniliformus, Rickettsia conorii, Leptospira icterohaemorrhagiae
Polyarthritis	Streptobacillus moniliformus, Borrelia burgdorferi, Spirillum minus, Brucella spp., alpha virus—six groups (Ross River, Sindbis, Mayaro, chikungunya, o'nyong-nyong, igbo-ora)
Jaundice	Coxiella burnetii, Leptospira icterohaemorrhagiae, yellow fever (sylvatic), hepatitis E, echinococcosis, Fasciola hepatica
Renal failure (acute)	Leptospira, Hantavirus, Rickettsia rickettsii, Rickettsia conorii, Escherichia coli O157
Endocarditis	Bartonella, Coxiella burnetii, Erysipelothrix rhusiopathiae, Brucella, Streptococcus suis, Listeria monocytogenes, Chlamydia psittaci
Diarrhea	Salmonella, Campylobacter jejuni, Shiga toxin–positive E. coli, Giardia intestinalis, cryptosporidia, Yersinia pseudotuberculosis, Yersinia enterocolitica

*See table of contents and index to locate a more detailed discussion of each disease.

Despite the large number of zoonoses described, clinicians evaluating an individual patient usually need to consider only a limited number of historical details to arrive at an appropriate differential diagnosis:

1. A history of direct contact with animals or animal products, animal bites, arthropod exposure, and food ingestion may offer clues to the correct cause.
2. All hobbies such as hunting and pet exposures (including contact with other owners' pets) should be elicited. Ownership of exotic pets or reptiles is often denied.
3. The patient's travel history must be considered because a number of zoonoses are still quite limited in geographic distribution.
4. Occupational and recreational high-risk activities such as cave exploration must be ascertained.
5. The patient's clinical manifestations (course and organ involvement) are used to focus on the most likely cause (see Tables 328-2 through 328-5).
6. Though neither specific nor sensitive, the inoculation nodule (eschar, tache noire, chancre, necrotic ulcer), with or without fever, rash, or local lymphadenopathy, is the only general clue from the physical examination that might alert the physician to a zoonosis when the history does not.
7. Significant unilateral hilar adenopathy in the presence of acute pneumonia can be a clue to anthrax, plague, or tularemia.

TREATMENT Rx

The approach to treatment of the various zoonoses is presented in their respective chapters.

PREVENTION

Guidelines have been published to help prevent nosocomial transmission of zoonotic diseases. Preventive measures to decrease infection in compromised hosts include the routine immunization of pets, neutering of pets, use of caution when handling pet fomites, rigorous handwashing practices, and avoidance of ingesting undercooked meat, fish, shellfish, and eggs.

Isolation is recommended for anthrax, Andes Hantavirus disease, herpes B, monkeypox, Q fever, rabies, plague, SARS and MERS coronavirus (Chapter 366), influenza, and the hemorrhagic fever illnesses (Chapter 381)

a reassortment of antigens and subsequent spread of virulent "new" influenza strains to humans, can lead to massive influenza pandemics that in sheer numbers (billions) surpass any past epidemics of smallpox or plague.[8] Initially, HIV-1 and HIV-2 were transmitted as simian immunodeficiency viruses from chimpanzees and mangabey primates, respectively, to humans. As with influenza, the subsequent 60 million (and counting) cases of HIV no longer require an animal reservoir for continuing transmission. Because these pandemics of AIDS and influenza now spread from human to human without the help of the initiating animal host, the World Health Organization no longer considers them zoonoses.

Leprosy, an illness of biblical notoriety transmitted from human to human, is endemic in at least three animal species, including the armadillo. This animal has rarely been implicated in the transmission of leprosy to humans in the United States.

TABLE 328-6 HIGHLY FATAL ZOONOSES

DISEASE*	FATALITY RATE (%)
Creutzfeldt-Jakob disease (new variant)	100
Rabies	100
Anthrax, inhalational	80-90
Herpes simiae	50-75[†]
Ebola virus	70
Eastern equine encephalitis	50-70
Hantavirus pulmonary syndrome (U.S.)	60[†]
H5N1 influenza	60
Yellow fever (sylvatic)	20-50[§]
Lassa fever	15-25[§]
Plague	50-80[†]
Rocky Mountain spotted fever	20-60[†]
East African sleeping sickness	20-30[†]
Anthrax, cutaneous	20[†]
Tularemia, pneumonic	30-60[†]
Tularemia, cutaneous	2-10
Visceral leishmaniasis	5-25[†]
Louse-borne relapsing fever	5-40[†]

*See table of contents and index to locate a more detailed discussion of each disease.
[†]If untreated.
[‡]Case mortality of hospitalized patients.
[§]If jaundiced.

caused by Argentine, Bolivian, Crimean-Congo, Ebola, Lassa, and Marburg viruses.

PROGNOSIS

The prognosis of zoonoses varies widely, but a number of these diseases have very high case-fatality rates (Table 328-6).

GENERAL REFERENCES

For the General References and other additional features, please visit Expert Consult at https://expertconsult.inkling.com.

329

ACTINOMYCOSIS

ITZHAK BROOK

DEFINITION

Actinomycosis is an uncommon, subacute to chronic bacterial infection that induces both suppurative and granulomatous inflammation. Localized swelling with suppuration, abscess formation, tissue fibrosis, and draining sinuses characterize this disease. The infection spreads contiguously and often forms draining sinuses that extrude characteristic but not pathognomonic "sulfur granules." Infections of the oral and cervicofacial regions are the most common, but any site in the body can be infected, including the thoracic region, abdominopelvic region, and central nervous system (CNS). Musculoskeletal or disseminated disease is rare but does occur.

The Pathogen

Actinomycetes of the genera *Actinomyces, Propionibacterium,* and *Bifidobacterium* act as the principal pathogens. However, 98 to 99% of actinomycoses are caused by non–spore-forming anaerobic or microaerophilic bacterial species of the genus *Actinomyces,* family Actinomycetaceae, order

Actinomycetales.[1] Of the 30 *Actinomyces* spp, 8 may cause disease in humans: the strictly anaerobic *A. israelii, A. gerencseriae* (formerly known as *A. israelii* serotype II), *A. odontolyticus, A. naeslundii, A. meyeri, A. viscosus, A. pyogenes,* and *A. georgiae. A. israelii* is the most common species causing human disease. *Propionibacterium propionicum* (formerly known as *Arachnia propionica*) and *Bifidobacterium dentium* (formerly known as *Actinomyces eriksonii*) also are associated with clinically indistinguishable infection. The organisms are filamentous, branching, gram-positive, pleomorphic, non–spore-forming, non–acid-fast anaerobic or microaerophilic bacilli. *Actinomyces* organisms are fastidious bacteria that require enriched culture media; 6 to 10% ambient CO_2 may aid in their growth, which takes up to 2 to 3 weeks in culture. Most actinomycotic infections are polymicrobial and involve other aerobic and anaerobic bacteria. The most common co-isolates depend on the infection site and are *Actinobacillus actinomycetemcomitans, Aggregatibacter aphrophilus, Eikenella corrodens, Bacteroides, Fusobacterium, Capnocytophaga,* aerobic and anaerobic streptococci, *Staphylococcus,* and Enterobacteriaceae.

EPIDEMIOLOGY

Actinomyces spp are members of the endogenous mucous membrane flora in the oral cavity, lower gastrointestinal tract, bronchi, and female genital tract. No external environmental reservoir, such as soil or straw, has been documented, nor has person-to-person transmission of pathogenic *Actinomyces* spp been demonstrated. Although infection can occur in all age groups, it is rarely seen in children or patients older than 60 years. Most cases are encountered in individuals in the middle decades of life. A male-to-female infection ratio of 3:1 is reported in most series. The explanation for this ratio is the higher prevalence of poor oral hygiene and oral trauma in men. The annual reported incidence in the United States is fewer than 100 cases. However, because of the fastidious nature of the organism, many cases are undiagnosed and the true incidence is probably much higher.

PATHOBIOLOGY

Actinomyces spp are agents of low pathogenicity and require mucosal barrier disruption to cause disease.[2] Actinomycosis usually occurs in immunocompetent persons but may afflict those with diminished host defenses. Risk factors include steroids, bisphosphonates, leukemia with chemotherapy, human immunodeficiency virus (HIV), alcoholism, lung and renal transplant receipt, and local tissue damage caused by trauma, recent surgery, or irradiation. Oral and cervicofacial diseases are commonly associated with dental caries and extractions, gingivitis and gingival trauma, infection in erupting secondary teeth, chronic tonsillitis, otitis or mastoiditis, diabetes mellitus, immunosuppression, immunodeficiency, malnutrition, and neoplastic disease. Pulmonary infections generally arise after aspiration of oropharyngeal or gastrointestinal secretions and has been reported in patients with underlying lung disorders, such as emphysema, chronic bronchitis, and bronchiectasis. Gastrointestinal infection frequently follows loss of mucosal integrity, such as with surgery, trauma, foreign bodies, perforated appendix or diverticulitis, neoplasia, foreign bodies, and emergency colonic surgery. Extended use (>2 years) of intrauterine contraceptive devices (IUDs) increases risk for the development of actinomycosis of the female genital tract.

Other bacterial species that are frequently copathogens with *Actinomyces* spp may assist in the spread of infection by inhibiting host defenses and reducing local oxygen tension. Once the organism is established locally, it may spread progressively to surrounding tissues. The infection tends to spread without regard for anatomic barriers, including fascial planes and lymphatic channels. The end result is a chronic, indurated, suppurative infection (usually with draining sinuses and fibrosis, especially in pelvic and abdominal infection). The fibrotic walls of the mass before suppuration are "wooden" in nature and may be confused with a neoplasm. Hematogenous spread can be fulminant but is rare.

Actinomyces spp grow in microscopic or macroscopic clusters of tangled filaments surrounded by neutrophils. Plasma cells and multinucleated giant cells are often observed with lesions, as are large macrophages with foamy cytoplasm around purulent centers. When visible, these clusters are pale yellow and exude through sinus tracks; they are called sulfur granules (originally called drusen). These granules (1 to 2 mm in diameter) are made of aggregates of organisms and contain calcium phosphate. A central purulent loculation surrounds the granules. Their centers have a basophilic staining property, with eosinophilic rays terminating in pear-shaped "clubs." One to six granules can be present per loculation, and up to 50 loculations can be present in a lesion. Multicenter giant cells can be seen as well.

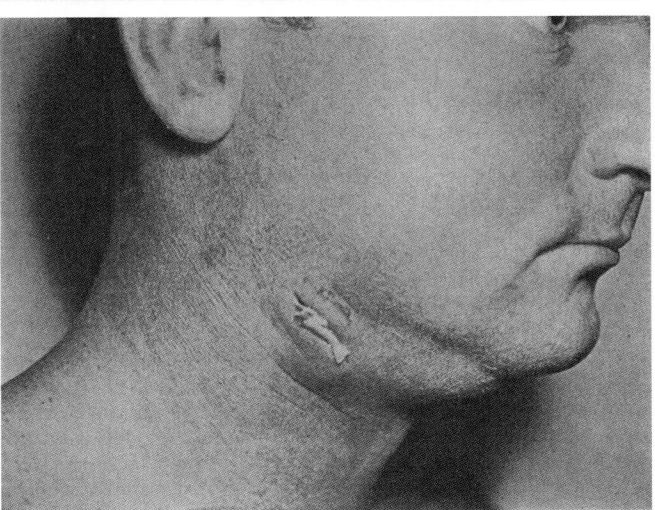

FIGURE 329-1. Actinomycosis of the jaw, observed at Letterman General Hospital, San Francisco, Calif., in a sergeant who had punctured the floor of his mouth while picking his teeth. (Courtesy Office of Medical History, Office of the Surgeon General, U.S. Army.)

CLINICAL MANIFESTATIONS

Cervicofacial

Cervicofacial infection is the most common manifestation of actinomycosis (Fig. 329-1).[3] It is generally odontogenic and evolves as a chronic or subacute painless or painful soft tissue slowly progressive, nontender swelling or mass involving the submandibular or paramandibular region. However, the submental and retromandibular spaces, temporomandibular joint, cheek, chin, and upper jaw can be involved. The swelling may have a ligneous consistency caused by tissue fibrosis. Depending on the composition of the concomitant synergistic flora, the onset of actinomycosis may be acute, subacute, or chronic. When *Staphylococcus aureus* or β-hemolytic streptococci are involved, an acute painful abscess or a phlegmatous cellulitis may be the initial manifestation. Pain and trismus can be disproportionate to the degree of inflammation apparent. The chronic form of the disease is the most common form and is characterized by painless infiltration and bluish or reddish induration that generally progresses to form multiple abscesses and draining sinus tracts discharging pus that may contain sulfur granules in up to 25% of instances. Periapical infection, trismus, dyspnea, dysphagia, fever, pain, and leukocytosis may be present. The infection can extend to the carotid artery, tongue, sinuses, ears, mastoid, orbit, salivary glands, pharynx, masseter muscle, thyroid, larynx, trachea, or thorax. Bone (most commonly the mandible) may be invaded from the adjacent soft tissue and results in periostitis or osteomyelitis. Cervical spine or cranial bone infection may lead to subdural empyema and invasion of the CNS. The differential diagnosis includes tuberculosis (scrofula), fungal infections, nocardiosis, suppurative infections by other organisms, and neoplasms.

Thoracic

Thoracic actinomycosis is an indolent, slowly progressive process involving the pulmonary parenchyma and pleural space.[4,5] This form accounts for 15 to 30% of actinomycosis cases and is caused by aspiration of infective material from the oropharynx, as well as rarely after esophageal perforation, by extension into the mediastinum from the neck, by spread from an abdominal site, or by hematogenous spread to the lung. Infection can spread from a pneumonic focus across lung fissures to involve the pleura and the chest wall, with eventual fistula formation and drainage containing sulfur granules (Fig. 329-2). The mediastinum, pericardium, and myocardium also rarely can be affected. Granules are seldom present in sputum. The incidence of this complication, as well as the destruction of thoracic vertebrae and adjacent ribs, has declined in the antimicrobial era.

The complaints of patients with thoracic actinomycosis are nonspecific. The most common are chest pain, productive cough, dyspnea, weight loss, and fever. Anemia, mild leukocytosis, and elevated sedimentation rate are relatively common. There is often a history of underlying lung disease, and patients are rarely initially seen in an early stage of infection. The pulmonary lesion is either a mass lesion or pneumonitis and may resemble tuberculosis,

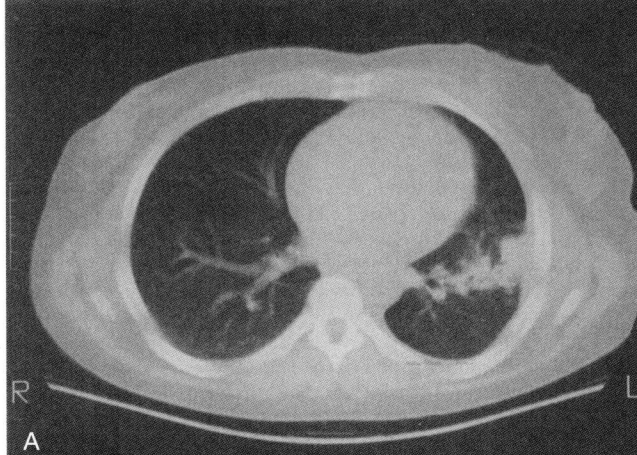
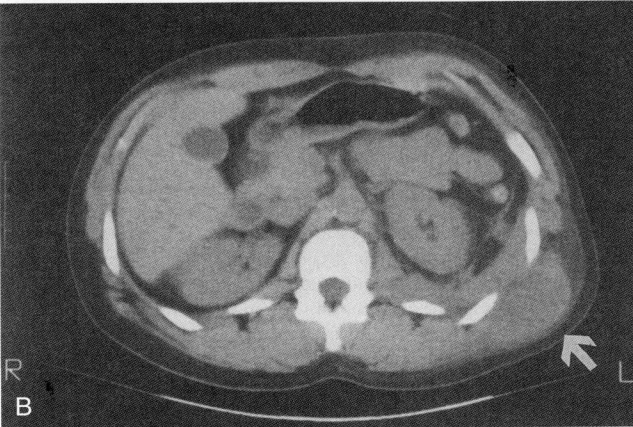

FIGURE 329-2. Thoracic computed tomography scan of a 43-year-old woman with pulmonary actinomycosis. A, There is consolidation of the lung with pleural thickening adjacent to the parenchymal disease. B, Abscess extended into the left breast and inferiorly to the costophrenic sulcus, to the retroperitoneum, and into the lateral abdominal wall (*arrow*).

especially when cavity formation occurs, or blastomycosis, which may destroy ribs posteriorly but rarely forms sinuses.[6] Nocardiosis, bronchogenic carcinoma, cryptococcosis, aspiration pneumonia, pulmonary infection, and lymphoma also can mimic thoracic actinomycosis. Pleural thickening, effusion, or emphysema is common.

Abdominal

Abdominal actinomycosis makes up approximately 20% of actinomycosis.[7] It is a chronic, localized inflammatory process that can occur weeks, months, or years after the integrity of the gastrointestinal mucosa is breached by surgery or trauma. Extension from the thorax or pelvis or through hematogenous dissemination also can occur. The ileocecal region is involved most frequently (usually after a perforated appendix) with the formation of a mass lesion. The infection extends slowly to contiguous organs, especially the liver, and may involve retroperitoneal tissues, the spine, or the abdominal wall. Hepatic, renal, or splenic dissemination is an uncommon complication. Persistent draining sinuses may form, and those involving the perianal region can simulate Crohn's disease (Chapter 141) or tuberculosis. The extensive fibrosis of actinomycotic lesions, recognized by the examiner as a mass, often suggests tumor. A frequent finding on computed tomography (CT) is an infiltrative mass with dense inhomogeneous contrast medium enhancement. Constitutional symptoms and signs are nonspecific, the most common being fever, diarrhea or constipation, weight loss, nausea, vomiting, pain, and sensation of a mass.

Pelvic

Pelvic infection is observed in patients with prolonged use of IUDs and also may occur from extension of intestinal infection, commonly from indolent ileocecal disease.[8] Manifestations may range from a chronic vaginal discharge to pelvic inflammatory disease with tubo-ovarian abscesses or pseudomalignant masses. Patients generally have abnormal vaginal bleeding or discharge, abdominal or pelvic pain, menorrhagia, fever, and weight loss.

Endometritis is the earlier form of the infection, followed by tubo-ovarian abscesses. Extension to the uterus, bladder, rectal area, abdominal wall, peritoneum, pelvic bones, thorax, and systemic circulation also can occur.

Central Nervous System

Infections of the CNS are very rare and generally manifest as single or multiple encapsulated brain abscesses that appear as ring-enhancing lesions with a thick wall that may be irregular or nodular on contrast-enhanced CT scans. There are no features that readily distinguish actinomycosis from other causes of brain abscesses. Rarely, solid nodular or mass lesions termed *actinomycetomas* or *actinomycotic granulomas* are found. Headache and focal neurologic signs are the most common finding. Most actinomycotic infections of the CNS are seeded hematogenously from a distant primary site, but direct extension of cervicofacial disease also occurs. Sinus formation is not a characteristic of CNS disease. The rare meningitis caused by *Actinomyces* is chronic and basilar in location, and the cerebrospinal fluid pleocytosis is usually lymphocytic. Thus, it may be misdiagnosed as tuberculous meningitis. Extension to the cranial epidural or subdural space and spinal epidural space also can occur from adjacent foci.

DIAGNOSIS

Appropriate microbiologic and pathologic studies are essential for diagnosis. A high index of suspicion should be communicated to the microbiology laboratory, along with material from draining sinuses, from deep-needle aspiration, or from biopsy specimens. CT or ultrasound needle aspiration can be used to obtain a biopsy specimen. It is important to avoid contamination of the specimen by normal flora and administration of antimicrobial therapy before a specimen is obtained. Anaerobic culture is required, and no selective media are available to restrict overgrowth of the slow-growing *Actinomyces* by associated microflora. The presence, in pus or tissue specimens, of non–acid-fast, gram-positive organisms with filamentous branching is suggestive of the diagnosis. The characteristic morphologic features of sulfur granules within are helpful. In tissue sections stained with hematoxylin-eosin, sulfur granules are round or oval basophilic masses with a radiating arrangement of eosinophilic terminal clubs. However, *Actinomyces* spp are infrequently visible in sections stained with hematoxylin-eosin; visualization is facilitated by special stains such as Gomori methenamine silver, *p*-aminosalicylic acid, McCallen-Goodpasture, and Brown-Brenn. Multiple biopsy sections from different tissue levels are recommended to improve the histopathologic diagnosis. The granules must be distinguished from similar structures that are sometimes produced in infections caused by *Nocardia, Monosporium, Cephalosporium, Staphylococcus* (botryomycosis), and others. *Actinomyces* and *Arachnia* can generally be differentiated from other gram-positive anaerobes by means of their growth rate (slow), by catalase production (negative, except for *A. viscosus*), and by gas-liquid chromatographic detection of the acetic, lactic, and succinic acids produced in peptone-yeast-glucose broth. Specific staining with fluorescent-conjugated monoclonal antibody testing can be used, but this method is not readily available to clinical microbiology laboratories.

Imaging methods such as conventional radiography, CT, and magnetic resonance imaging do not provide a specific diagnosis but allow more accurate definition of the dimensions and extension of the infection.

TREATMENT · Rx

Prolonged antimicrobial therapy (i.e., 6 to 12 months) has typically been recommended for patients with all clinical forms of actinomycosis to prevent disease recrudescence. However, individualization of courses of therapy is recommended because the duration of treatment depends on the initial burden of disease, the site of infection, and the clinical and radiologic response. Adequate drainage is indicated if abscesses are present.

Penicillin G is the drug of choice for treatment of an infection caused by any of the *Actinomyces*. It is given in high dosage during a prolonged period because the infection has a tendency to recur. Most deep-seated infections can be expected to respond to intravenous penicillin G, 18 to 24 million units/day given for 2 to 6 weeks, followed by an oral phenoxypenicillin in a dosage of 2 to 4 g/day. A few additional weeks of oral penicillin therapy may suffice for uncomplicated cervicofacial disease; complicated cases and extensive pulmonary[9] or abdominal disease may require treatment for 12 to 18 months. Little evidence exists of acquired resistance to penicillin G by *Actinomyces*

during prolonged therapy. The combination of a penicillin (i.e., amoxicillin, piperacillin) and a β-lactamase inhibitor (i.e., clavulanate, tazobactam) offers the advantage of coverage against penicillin-resistant aerobic and anaerobic copathogens. Alternative first-line antibiotics include amoxicillin, tetracycline, erythromycin, and clindamycin. Ceftriaxone, imipenem, and fluoroquinolones have also been used successfully. Metronidazole, aminoglycosides, oxacillin, and cephalexin are not effective. In vitro antimicrobial susceptibility testing of *Actinomyces* is difficult, and the results may not be predictive of antimicrobial effects in vivo.

The need to use combination antimicrobial therapy to eradicate microorganisms that are isolated in association with *Actinomyces* has not been established. However, because many of these organisms are known pathogens, treatment is usually appropriate, especially with lower abdominal infections. Surgical removal of infected tissue also may be necessary in some cases, especially if extensive necrotic tissue or fistulas are present, if malignant disease cannot be excluded, and if large abscesses cannot be drained by percutaneous aspiration. When well-defined IUD-related symptoms and Papanicolaou smears demonstrate *Actinomyces* by specific fluorescence-labeled antibody, the IUD should be removed. Antimicrobial administration for a 2-week period may be indicated. More serious infections require prolonged therapy.

PROGNOSIS

The availability of antimicrobial treatment has greatly improved the prognosis for all forms of actinomycosis. At present, cure rates are high and neither deformity nor death is common.

GENERAL REFERENCES

For the General References and other additional features, please visit Expert Consult at https://expertconsult.inkling.com.

330

NOCARDIOSIS

FREDERICK S. SOUTHWICK

DEFINITION

Nocardiosis refers to infections caused by *Nocardia* spp. *Nocardia* most commonly causes pneumonia but also can infect the central nervous system (CNS) and the skin. Less commonly, this organism can disseminate throughout the body. These infections usually occur in patients with defective immunity.

Etiology

Nocardia spp are thin, aerobic, gram-positive bacilli that form branching filaments. The bacteria stain irregularly and appear beaded on Gram stain. The speciation of *Nocardia* has been problematic. The original classification was based on the ability to use specific nutrients and decompose substrates such as adenine, casein, urea, gelatin, and xanthine. However, gene sequencing and DNA-DNA hybridization have now defined the true taxonomy. The species called *N. asteroides* was previously reported to be the most common cause of human disease. However, the majority of these bacteria were misidentified by today's standards. The number of species causing human disease is large and includes *N. abscessus, N. brevicatena/paucivorans* complex, *N. nova* complex, *N. transvalensis* complex, *N. farcinica, N. cyriacigeorgica, N. otitidis-caviarum, N. veterana, N. brasiliensis,* and *N. pseudobrasiliensis.*

EPIDEMIOLOGY

Nocardia spp are ubiquitous and primarily originate in soil. Despite being found throughout the environment, they rarely cause symptomatic infection in humans. Because nocardiosis is not a reportable disease, the frequency of this disease is unknown. The annual incidence has been estimated to be 0.4 in 100,000. The risk for symptomatic *Nocardia* infection is greatly increased (estimated to be 140 to 340 times greater) in individuals who are immunocompromised, including patients who are receiving immunosuppressive agents following bone marrow or solid organ transplant, and patients with acquired immunodeficiency syndrome (AIDS). Corticosteroids are the most frequent immunosuppressant associated with nocardiosis[1]; however, cases also have been reported in patients receiving anti–tumor necrosis factor-α antibody (infliximab) as well as other immunosuppressants. It is important to keep in mind that trimethoprim-sulfamethoxazole prophylaxis does not always protect against *Nocardia*. Other risk groups include patients with cancer, Cushing's disease, chronic granulomatous disease, and dysgammaglobulinemia. Patients with chronic pulmonary disorders, particularly alveolar proteinosis, are also more susceptible to this infection. In approximately one third of patients with nocardiosis, no predisposing condition can be identified.

PATHOBIOLOGY

Most *Nocardia* spp gain entry to the host via the respiratory tract or less commonly by skin inoculation. Invading bacteria elicit a neutrophil response that inhibits but does not kill the organism. The bacteria are phagocytosed by neutrophils and macrophages and become enclosed in a membrane-bound phagolysosome. In this closed environment neutrophils and macrophages are able to kill many species of bacteria by synthesizing superoxide and hydrogen peroxide. However, *Nocardia* are able to survive in this hostile environment by producing superoxide dismutase, an enzyme that inactivates these toxic oxygen byproducts. In addition, *Nocardia* spp produce a mycolic acid called cord factor that inhibits the fusion of lysosomes with the phagolysosomal compartment, preventing toxic proteases and other antibacterial products from reaching the intracellular bacteria. Cell wall extractable lipids impair phagocytosis and also inhibit bacterial killing.[2] In addition to neutrophils and macrophages, cell-mediated[3] and humoral immunity also play roles in protecting the host against *Nocardia* invasion, explaining the wide range of immunocompromised patients that are at increased risk for contracting nocardiosis.

CLINICAL MANIFESTATIONS

Nocardiosis has no pathognomonic characteristics, and delays in diagnosis are common. Failure of a pulmonary or skin infection to respond to conventional antibiotic therapy should raise the possibility of a *Nocardia* spp infection. Nocardiosis always should be considered in the immunocompromised patient.

Pulmonary Nocardiosis

Approximately two thirds of patients with nocardiosis present with pulmonary infection.[4,5] Pulmonary disease is usually subacute in onset, mimicking a fungal or mycobacterial infection, and is most commonly misdiagnosed as tuberculosis. The most common complaints are a persistent cough producing purulent sputum, fever, anorexia, and weight loss. Less commonly, patients may report pleuritic chest pain and dyspnea. Hemoptysis is rare but can develop in patients with large cavitary lesions. Acute onset of pneumonia has occasionally been reported in the immunocompromised host.

Central Nervous System Infection

Approximately 5% of patients with a *Nocardia* infection have CNS involvement.[6] Multilocular brain abscess is the most common CNS manifestation[7] and is usually the consequence of transient bacterial dissemination from the lung. Lesions can occur in any region of the brain, and symptoms depend on location. Headache is the usual initial complaint and frequently localized to the site of the abscess. Patients also may present with neurologic deficits and seizures. The combined findings of a lung nodule on chest x-ray and a ring-enhancing CNS lesion are often mistaken for metastatic lung carcinoma. Other diagnoses that should be considered when the immunocompromised host presents with both a lung and CNS focus are disseminated aspergillosis and toxoplasmosis. Meningitis is a less common CNS manifestation and is often associated with brain abscess (40% of meningitis cases). The CSF cell count usually reveals neutrophils and the CSF culture may be positive, particularly if the culture is held for a prolonged period.

Cutaneous Infection

Skin infection is usually caused by *N. brasiliensis* and typically follows a break in the skin that is contaminated by soil. Cutaneous disease has been reported in association with trauma, a postoperative wound, insect bites, thorn bush scratches, or even a cat scratch. Initially a pustule or a moderately erythematous, nonfluctuant nodule develops at the site of inoculation. Erythema can

extend along the lymphatic system and is associated with tender lymphadenopathy.[8] This form of cutaneous infection has been termed *lymphocutaneous* or *sporotrichoid* disease. Similar skin manifestations are seen with other etiologies, including cat scratch disease, tularemia, *Mycobacterium marinum,* and sporotrichosis. In the immunocompromised host, disseminated infection may be manifest by multiple erythematous raised nodules and is an ominous finding. In tropical regions of South and Central America *Nocardia* spp can cause ulcerations and large tumor-like lesions called *mycetomas* that are usually found on the lower legs.

DIAGNOSIS

Radiology

In pulmonary disease, chest x-ray findings are variable, with pulmonary nodules or mass lesions being seen most often (Fig. 330-1). Less frequently, consolidation, cavitary lesions with air-fluid levels, interstitial infiltrates, and pleural effusions are found. Chest CT often demonstrates areas of low attenuation within consolidations, multiple nodules, and chest wall extension of the infection. Patients with AIDS are more likely to have multiple pulmonary nodules, cavitary lesions, and upper lobe infiltrates. In some patients the infiltrate may resolve, particularly in patients with normal immune function. However, the patient may present with brain abscess several months later as a consequence of transient dissemination. In CNS infection CT or magnetic resonance imaging with contrast usually demonstrates one or more ring-enhancing lesions (Fig. 330-2). *Nocardia* brain abscess is more commonly multiloculated; otherwise the radiologic findings are similar to those in other

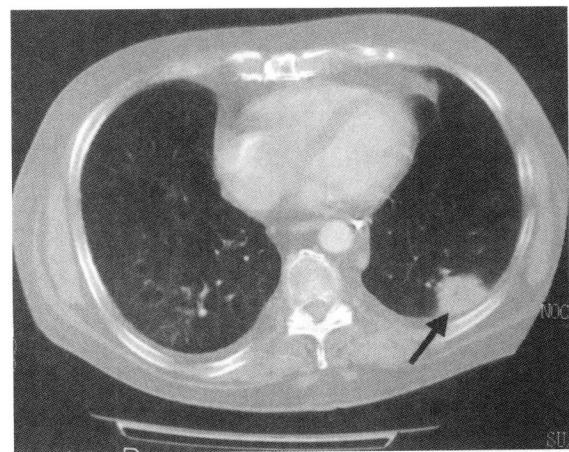

FIGURE 330-1. Chest computed tomography showing a peripheral nodular lung lesion (*arrow*) caused by *Nocardia* infection.

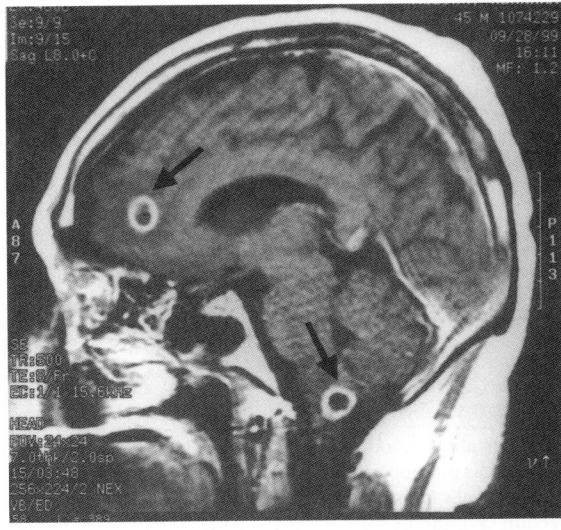

FIGURE 330-2. Multiple, gadolinium-enhanced brain lesions (*arrows*) caused by *Nocardia* infection.

bacterial causes of brain abscess. Positron emission tomography is not helpful in differentiating *Nocardia* brain abscess from tumor; both demonstrate increased uptake.

Histopathology

Invasive procedures are generally required for specific diagnosis. For pulmonary infection, bronchoscopy with transbronchial biopsy or skinny needle biopsy is recommended. CT-guided needle aspirate is the diagnostic procedure of choice for brain abscess. Histopathologic examination usually reveals an acute inflammatory response with a predominance of neutrophils. Micronodular abscesses with minimal capsular formation are usually found. Gram stain or Brown-Brenn stains reveal gram-positive, beaded, branching forms. The morphology is identical to that of *Actinomyces*; however, the high lipid content of its cell wall often renders *Nocardia* modified acid-fast positive, whereas *Actinomyces* spp are modified acid-fast negative. However, acid fastness may be variable when staining *Nocardia* colonies from cultures and is unreliable for direct clinical samples.

Culture

Isolation of the organism on culture provides a definitive diagnosis from needle aspirate samples of brain abscess, and a presumptive diagnosis when grown from respiratory and cutaneous samples. *Nocardia* grows best under aerobic conditions with 5 to 10% carbon dioxide. Because the organism grows slowly on blood agar, taking 3 to 5 days to form colonies, other organisms can overgrow. When *Nocardia* is suspected the clinical laboratory should be notified to allow the use of selective media and prolonged incubation. 16S ribosomal RNA gene sequencing allows rapid speciation of isolates. Antibiotic susceptibility testing always should be performed to guide the choice of therapy.

TREATMENT   Rx

Because of the rarity of nocardiosis, no prospective treatment trials have been performed, and all recommendations are based on retrospective studies and in vitro sensitivity testing. Sulfonamides remain the treatment of choice for pulmonary and cutaneous disease. Trimethoprim-sulfamethoxazole given orally at a dose of 160/800 mg (one double strength) three times daily is the most commonly used adult regimen. When patients with disseminated and/or CNS *Nocardia* are treated with sulfonamides alone, survival has been less than 50%. One of the most common species to cause disseminated diseases, *N. farcinica*, is also one of the most common *Nocardia* spp to be resistant to sulfonamides. In these more serious conditions combination therapy is generally recommended, the exact regimen being guided by antibiotic susceptibility testing. One recommended empirical regimen is trimethoprim-sulfamethoxazole 15 mg/kg/day IV of the trimethoprim component divided into 2 to 4 doses, amikacin (7.5 mg/kg every 12 hours), and either ceftriaxone (2 g twice daily) or imipenem (500 mg four times daily). In a retrospective study, patients failing trimethoprim-sulfamethoxazole responded to imipenem with or without amikacin.[9] Linezolid (600 mg twice daily) has been used successfully in a small number of CNS infections. However, prolonged therapy with this agent can lead to bone marrow toxicity and warrants weekly monitoring of the peripheral cell counts.[10] The newer fluoroquinolone moxifloxacin (400 mg/day PO) has been shown to have activity against several strains of *Nocardia,* including *N. farcinica* and *N. brasiliensis,* and this agent may prove useful in patients who cannot tolerate sulfonamides; however, relapse has been reported. Minocycline (100 mg PO twice daily) and amoxicillin-clavulanate (875/125 mg PO twice daily) are other potentially effective alternative treatments for *Nocardia.* Because of the intracellular nature of *Nocardia* and the slow rates of bacterial growth, antibiotic treatment for 6 to 12 months in the immunocompromised host and 4 to 6 months in the normal host is usually required to prevent relapse.

In addition to antibiotics for patients with brain abscess or subcutaneous abscesses, surgical drainage is required for cure.

PROGNOSIS

The overall mortality for nocardiosis is approximately 25%. In otherwise healthy individuals pulmonary nocardiosis has a better prognosis (15% mortality). The survival rate is worse in patients with bacteremia, patients with acute infection (symptoms for < 3 weeks), patients receiving corticosteroids or cytotoxic agents, patients with disseminated disease involving two or more noncontiguous organs, and patients with meningitis.

GENERAL REFERENCES

For the General References and other additional features, please visit Expert Consult at https://expertconsult.inkling.com.

331

SYSTEMIC ANTIFUNGAL AGENTS

DAVID A. STEVENS

Methods for in vitro susceptibility testing are available as standardized tools. A variety of assays are available for therapeutic drug monitoring of serum and other body fluids. As more common mutations inducing resistance are uncovered,[1] it becomes possible to develop molecular screening methods that can detect the resistance genes in clinical isolates, in advance of susceptibility test results.[2]

AMPHOTERICIN B–BASED PREPARATIONS

Mechanism of Action

Amphotericin B is a lipophilic molecule that exerts its antifungal effect by insertion into the fungal cytoplasmic membrane. Amphotericin B causes membrane permeability to increase. Loss of intracellular molecules impairs fungal viability. The onset of action is rapid. Amphotericin B also has effects on oxidation that may enhance antifungal activity and in vivo may activate endothelial cells.

Spectrum of Activity and Mechanisms of Resistance

Amphotericin B is active against most fungi, and its spectrum of activity is not influenced by the choice of formulation. When resistance occurs, it is generally attributed to reductions in ergosterol biosynthesis and the synthesis of alternative sterols that lessen the ability of amphotericin B to interact with the fungal membrane; oxidant scavengers also may be produced. Primary resistance is common for *Scedosporium* and *Trichosporon* spp. Among the *Candida* spp, primary resistance is noted at meaningful frequencies most often for *Candida lusitaniae*. Development of resistance in isolates of normally susceptible species is uncommon. In some studies, the principal pharmacodynamic driver of in vivo response has been the ratio of the peak serum concentration to the minimal inhibitory concentration (MIC).

Available Formulations

There are four commercially available amphotericin B formulations: amphotericin B deoxycholate (ABD) and three lipid-associated formulations—amphotericin B colloidal dispersion (ABCD), amphotericin B lipid complex, and liposomal amphotericin B. All formulations must be infused in 5% dextrose with no electrolytes added. Infusion bottles need not be protected from light. In attempts to produce less expensive lipid-associated formulations, some have advocated mixing ABD with a parenteral fat emulsion. Although less nephrotoxicity has been observed in adults given this preparation at a dose of 1 mg/kg/day compared with infusions of ABD in 5% dextrose, no advantage was found in children. Serum amphotericin B concentrations were also lower with the fat emulsion, raising the possibility that amphotericin B was simply aggregating in the fat emulsion, but the cloudiness could not be perceived in the milky-looking lipid. Use of such preparations should be reserved for investigational settings.

Amphotericin B Deoxycholate
Formulation

ABD for intravenous use is a colloidal suspension. If a filter with a 0.22-μm pore diameter is placed in the infusion line, considerable drug is removed by the filter. The addition of electrolyte aggregates the colloids, so the solution becomes cloudy; this is to be avoided. ABD is available from several generic manufacturers, and significant differences in the formulations have been reported, which may account in part for the intersubject variation in toxicities observed.

Pharmacology

Most of the drug leaves the circulation promptly, with only a small percentage being excreted in urine or bile. Amphotericin B is stored in the liver and other organs; the drug appears to re-enter the circulation slowly. Blood levels are not influenced by hepatic or renal failure. Hemodialysis does not alter blood levels, except in an occasional patient with lipemic plasma who may be losing drug owing to its adherence to the dialysis membrane. Concentrations of amphotericin B in fluid from inflamed areas, such as pleura, peritoneum, joint, vitreous humor, and aqueous humor, are roughly two thirds of the nadir serum level. Amphotericin B penetrates poorly into either normal or inflamed meninges, saliva, bronchial secretions, brain, pancreas, muscle, bone, vitreous humor, and normal amniotic fluid. Urine concentrations are similar to serum concentrations. Peak serum concentrations with conventional intravenous doses are roughly 0.5 to 2 μg/mL; these concentrations fall rapidly and then slowly approach a plateau of roughly 0.2 to 0.5 μg/mL. The initial half-life is approximately 24 hours; the β-phase half-life is roughly 15 days. Serum concentrations can be detected for at least 7 weeks after the end of therapy, presumably reflecting release from cell membranes. The drug also has complex immunomodulatory properties that are potentially of clinical significance.

Nephrotoxicity

ABD causes a dose-dependent decrease in the glomerular filtration rate. The direct vasoconstrictive effect of amphotericin B on afferent renal arterioles results in reduced glomerular and renal tubular blood flow. Other effects on the kidney include potassium, magnesium, and bicarbonate wasting and decreased erythropoietin production. Loss of renal function is due to the destruction of renal tubular cells, disruption of tubular basement membrane, and loss of functioning nephron units. Saline loading, such as the infusion of 1 L saline before ABD, has been associated with reduced nephrotoxicity in some studies. Potassium wasting often requires supplemental oral or intravenous potassium. Renal tubular acidosis from bicarbonate wasting rarely requires base replacement, but other drugs and diseases that promote acidosis may act synergistically.

Azotemia caused by amphotericin B is often worse in patients taking other nephrotoxic drugs. Hypotension, intravascular volume depletion, and other preexisting renal disease all magnify the management problems associated with amphotericin B–induced azotemia. These toxicities are lessened by use of the lipid-associated formulations of amphotericin B.

Early in the course of therapy with ABD, azotemia may increase rapidly; it often improves a little and then stabilizes after several days. Adults with no other renal disease have an average serum creatinine level of 2 to 3 mg/dL at therapeutic doses, and therapy should not be withheld unless azotemia exceeds this level. Attempting to give ABD to an adult without causing azotemia usually leads to inadequate therapy.

Other Chronic Toxicity

Nausea, anorexia, and vomiting are common. Phlebitis occurs if peripheral vein catheters are used. Normocytic normochromic anemia occurs gradually. The hematocrit rarely falls below 20 to 25% unless other causes of anemia are present. Rarely, thrombocytopenia, modest leukopenia, arrhythmias, coagulopathy, hemorrhagic enteritis, tinnitus, vertigo, encephalopathy, seizures, hemolysis, or dysesthesia of the soles of the feet may be observed. Amphotericin B remains the first choice parenteral agent in pregnancy despite its potential toxicities.[3]

Acute Reactions

Approximately 30 to 45 minutes after beginning the first few ABD infusions, chills, fever, and tachypnea may occur, peak in 15 to 30 minutes, and then slowly abate over 2 to 4 hours. A patient with underlying cardiac or pulmonary disease may have hypoxemia. These reactions are less common in young children or in patients receiving corticosteroids. Subsequent infusions of the same dose cause progressively milder reactions. Premedication with acetaminophen or the addition of hydrocortisone 25 to 50 mg to the infusion solution can diminish the reaction. Meperidine given early in a chill shortens the rigors but may induce nausea or emesis. Concern about this kind of reaction in an unstable patient has led some physicians to use a test dose of 1 mg given over a 15-minute period to assess the subsequent reaction over 1 hour before deciding whether to administer a full therapeutic dose. Patients with rapidly progressive mycoses should receive a full therapeutic dose within 24 hours. These reactions should not be mistaken for anaphylaxis or considered a contraindication to further amphotericin B. True allergic reactions are extremely rare.

Administration

ABD is infused over a 2- to 4-hour interval. Infusions 1 hour in duration generally appear to be safe for persons who have tolerated slower infusions. Rapid infusion in patients with severely compromised renal function may lead to acute, marked hyperkalemia and ventricular fibrillation.

Patients receiving a stable daily dose can be changed to a double dose on alternate days to reduce the frequency of infusion-associated toxicity, particularly anorexia, and to make outpatient therapy more convenient. Doses above 1.5 mg/kg are generally not given on this schedule because the toxicity of such infusions is not well described. Continuous infusion of amphotericin B with doses up to 2 mg/kg/24 hours is another approach (based on limited data) to reducing toxicity, but this is not consistent with the observation that the principal pharmacodynamic driver of efficacy for amphotericin B is peak drug concentration.[4]

Dosage

Daily ABD doses of 0.3 mg/kg often suffice for esophageal candidiasis. A dose of 0.5 mg/kg is appropriate for blastomycosis, disseminated histoplasmosis, and extracutaneous sporotrichosis. Patients with cryptococcal meningitis are generally given doses of 0.6 to 0.8 mg/kg; those with coccidioidomycosis may require doses of 1 mg/kg. Patients with mucormycosis or invasive aspergillosis are given daily doses of 1 to 1.5 mg/kg until improvement is clearly present. Doses of 0.5 to 1 mg/kg are often used in neutropenic patients receiving empirical amphotericin B. Local instillation of amphotericin B into cerebrospinal fluid (CSF), joints, or pleura is rarely indicated. One exception is coccidioidal meningitis, which may be treated with intrathecal ABD because it may produce superior results to systemic azole therapy, particularly in the long term, although with far greater toxicity. Intraocular administration for fungal endophthalmitis is occasionally used; doses of 10 μg appear to avoid retinal toxicity. Corneal baths with 1 mg/mL in sterile water are useful for fungal keratitis but are irritating.

Lipid-Associated Formulations of Amphotericin B
Pharmacology and Toxicity

The three lipid-associated formulations have quite different pharmacokinetic patterns. When compared on the basis of equal dosages (milligram/kilogram), the lipid-associated formulations produce tissue amphotericin B concentrations that range from 90% lower to 500% higher than those seen with ABD, with the most consistent relative reduction seen in the kidney. The lipid-associated formulations are typically given at doses that are 3- to 12-fold higher than those used for ABD. All three formulations generally require higher doses in experimental animals to achieve the same therapeutic effect as ABD.

These higher but equipotent doses are notably better tolerated than ABD, with reductions in both the frequency and the severity of acute infusion-related reactions and chronic nephrotoxicity. An exception is ABCD, which generally induces acute infusion-related reactions similar to those for ABD.

Randomized clinical trials comparing ABD as therapy for a defined mycosis are limited to demonstrations that liposomal amphotericin B has a similar efficacy for cryptococcal meningitis and a greater efficacy for histoplasmosis. Randomized comparisons with ABD in persistently neutropenic and febrile cancer patients consistently demonstrate a better tolerability profile, but few data on differential antifungal effect. The aggregate open-label data on efficacy rates for the lipid-associated formulations are similar to those for ABD. Although the lipid-associated formulations are notably more costly than ABD, the purchase cost of the compound must be balanced against the morbidity of ABD-related nephrotoxicity and the financial costs of monitoring, treating, and managing it.

● FLUCYTOSINE
Formulation and Pharmacology

Flucytosine (5-fluorocytosine) is the fluorine analogue of a normal body constituent, cytosine. Flucytosine is marketed as 250- and 500-mg capsules. Absorption from the gastrointestinal tract is rapid and complete, and approximately 90% is excreted unchanged in the urine. CSF concentrations are approximately 74% of simultaneous serum concentrations; the drug also penetrates well into aqueous humor, joints, bronchial secretions, peritoneal fluid, brain, bile, and bone, and it is readily cleared by hemodialysis and peritoneal dialysis.

The half-life of the drug in the serum of patients with normal renal function is 3 to 5 hours and is longer in newborns. Abnormal hepatic function has no influence, but decreased renal function prolongs the half-life.

Mechanisms of Action and Resistance

Isolates of *Candida* spp are usually susceptible, as are most isolates of *Cryptococcus neoformans*. Flucytosine is often active against isolates of *Aspergillus* spp and against the melanin-pigmented molds that cause chromoblastomycosis. The mechanism of antifungal action appears to be deamination to 5-fluorouracil and then conversion through several steps to 5-fluorodeoxyuridylic acid monophosphate, a noncompetitive inhibitor of thymidylate synthetase, which interferes with DNA synthesis, or conversion to 5-fluouridine triphosphate, which is incorporated into RNA and causes aberrant transcription. In some studies, the principal pharmacodynamic driver of response was the proportion of time the blood level exceeded the minimum inhibitory concentration (MIC). Resistance may be due to loss of the cytosine permease that permits flucytosine to cross the fungal cell membrane or loss of any of the enzymes that lead to its conversion into forms that interfere with DNA or RNA synthesis.

Administration and Dosage

Flucytosine is administered orally, 100 to 150 mg/kg/day, in four divided doses. As an approximation, the total daily dose should be reduced to 75 mg/kg with a creatinine clearance of 26 to 50 mL/minute and to 37 mg/kg when the creatinine clearance is 13 to 25 mL/minute. Ideally, the blood level should be measured in azotemic patients 2 hours after the last dose and immediately before the next dose. These values should range between 10 and 100 μg/mL. Patients requiring hemodialysis can be given a single post-dialysis dose of 37.5 mg/kg. Further doses are adjusted by blood level.

Flucytosine given alone to patients with normal renal, hematologic, and gastrointestinal function is infrequently associated with adverse effects, including rash, diarrhea, and hepatic dysfunction. In the presence of azotemia (such as that caused by concomitant amphotericin B), leukopenia, thrombocytopenia, and enterocolitis may appear. These complications seem to be far more frequent among patients whose flucytosine blood levels attain, and especially if they exceed, 100 to 125 μg/mL. Patients receiving flucytosine whose renal function is changing should have their serum flucytosine concentrations determined twice weekly, and the leukocyte count, platelet count, alkaline phosphatase, and aminotransferase levels should be measured at a similar frequency. Patients in whom loose stools or dull abdominal pain suddenly develops or who have laboratory evidence consistent with flucytosine toxicity should have their flucytosine blood levels determined, and consideration should be given to withholding the drug until the situation is clarified. Patients with bone marrow and gastrointestinal toxicity from flucytosine often tolerate the drug at a reduced dosage. Uncommonly, vomiting, bowel perforation, confusion, hallucinations, headache, sedation, and euphoria have been reported. Flucytosine is contraindicated in pregnancy.

Conversion of flucytosine to 5-fluorouracil within the human body occurs to a sufficient degree to possibly account for the drug's toxicity to bone marrow and the gastrointestinal tract. It is likely that the drug is secreted into the gut, where flucytosine becomes deaminated by intestinal bacteria and is reabsorbed as 5-fluorouracil.

Flucytosine has a beneficial effect in patients with cryptococcosis, candidiasis, and chromoblastomycosis. It is not the drug of choice for any infection, however, because its clinical efficacy in the first two mycoses is inferior to that of amphotericin B, primary drug resistance is not uncommon in *Candida* infection, and secondary drug resistance is common in cryptococcosis and chromoblastomycosis.

Flucytosine and amphotericin B are at least additive in their effects. Flucytosine permits a lower dose of amphotericin B to be used to achieve the same therapeutic effect, and amphotericin B prevents the emergence of secondary drug resistance. These advantages have been confirmed in large multicenter studies of cryptococcal meningitis, and a more rapid antifungal effect has been shown.

Flucytosine therapy is more difficult to manage in patients with diminished bone marrow reserve. Intravenous flucytosine is no longer available in the United States, but it is used at the same dosage as the capsule formulation.

Flucytosine resistance has occurred, albeit uncommonly, during combination therapy. Use of combination therapy in such patients incurs the risk for

toxicity without evidence that flucytosine adds to the therapeutic effect. An MIC of 20 μg/mL or less is considered susceptible.

● AZOLE ANTIFUNGAL AGENTS

Mechanism of Action

The azole ring confers antifungal activity on a variety of synthetic organic compounds. *N*-substitution of imidazoles has created a family of drugs called *triazoles* that have the same mechanism of action as imidazoles, a similar or broader spectrum of activity, and less effect on human sterol synthesis. Both imidazoles and triazoles inhibit C-14α demethylation of lanosterol in fungi; this leads to reduced concentrations of ergosterol, which is essential for a normal fungal cytoplasmic membrane. In some studies, the principal pharmacodynamic driver for response to the triazole antifungal agents has been the ratio of total drug exposure (area under the curve) to the MIC. Because of their interaction with the cytochrome P-450 (CYP) system and, in some cases, the P-glycoprotein pumps, the azoles as a class have a large number of drug-drug interactions, only some of which are covered here. In any patient in whom azole therapy is contemplated, package inserts for the drug should be consulted to determine which of the patient's other medications could result in a significant drug-drug interaction.

Newer triazoles have properties that make them preferable to ketoconazole. These include not only less hormonal inhibition but also better distribution into body fluids, both parenteral and oral formulations, less hepatotoxicity, and a broader spectrum. Some have fewer drug interactions. Resistance to azoles in previously susceptible species is emerging. Resistance mechanisms include increased drug efflux and altered or increased C-14α demethylase. It has been speculated that some of the common mutations in this demethylase in *Aspergillus* isolates from certain geographic areas, resulting in resistance, may have arisen owing to the widespread agricultural use of azole fungicides. All agents in this class have the potential for embryotoxicity and teratogenicity and should be avoided during pregnancy, particularly the first trimester.

Ketoconazole

Formulations and Pharmacology

Ketoconazole is available in tablet form. It is metabolized in the liver and excreted as inactive drug in bile and, to a small extent, urine. The drug is not removed significantly by hemodialysis or peritoneal dialysis. Decreased renal or hepatic function does not alter plasma drug levels. The initial half-life is approximately 2 hours, with a β-phase half-life of approximately 9 hours commencing 8 to 12 hours after ingestion.

Oral absorption of ketoconazole differs among individuals. Serious gastrointestinal disease may lead to low blood levels. Inhibitors of gastric acid secretion should not be given to patients taking ketoconazole because blood levels of the latter drug are drastically reduced. The drinking of citrus fruit juices or cola beverages with ketoconazole improves absorption in hypochlorhydric patients. Patients who need antacids should take them 1 to 2 hours after ketoconazole. Low concentrations are found in vaginal secretions, saliva, and breast milk, but penetration into inflamed joints is better.

Uses

The main advantage of ketoconazole is its lower cost compared with the cost of triazoles. Although at a dose of 400 mg/day the drug is effective in many mycoses, usage has been supplanted by the triazoles, but least so in cutaneous mycoses. Therapy is continued for 6 to 12 months or longer, if the response is slow, to prevent relapse. Improvement may not be evident for weeks to months. Although the dose can be advanced to 600 or 800 mg/day in patients who are not responding to therapy, there is more evidence of increased toxicity than increased efficacy. Aspergillosis does not respond to ketoconazole; additionally, the subsequent use of amphotericin B may be antagonized.

Adverse Effects

The most frequent toxic effects are anorexia, nausea, and vomiting. Dividing doses greater than 400 mg/day is not recommended because hormonal suppression is prolonged. Ketoconazole causes a dose-dependent depression in the serum testosterone-stimulated and adrenocorticotropic hormone–stimulated cortisol response. The effect of doses of 800 to 1200 mg/day is profound enough to have prompted trials in the treatment of Cushing's syndrome and prostate cancer. Hypertension is seen in a few of these high-dose patients, associated with increased levels of mineralocorticoid precursors.

Gynecomastia, oligospermia, and menstrual irregularities may be seen during prolonged therapy. Allergic rash and pruritus have been noted.

Perhaps the most serious complication is hepatitis. Fortunately, this complication is estimated to occur in only 1 in 15,000 exposed individuals. A slight, asymptomatic elevation of transaminase levels occurs in 5 to 15% and is generally transient. Ketoconazole-associated hepatitis begins as anorexia, malaise, nausea, and vomiting. Eighty percent of cases occur within the first 3 months. Progression can be swift. If hepatotoxicity is suspected, serum transaminase and alkaline phosphatase levels should be measured. Some authorities have recommended that liver function be measured periodically. This procedure does not protect a patient who has a rapid onset of hepatitis in the interval between tests, but it does require that all patients with abnormalities be contacted to inquire about symptoms and to arrange for repeat testing.

Itraconazole
Formulations and Pharmacology
Itraconazole (Sporanox) is marketed as a capsule and as an oral suspension in cyclodextrin (an oligosaccharide ring). The ring entraps the hydrophobic, water-insoluble drug, thus making it soluble; it is then released either at the lipid membrane of the enterocyte after oral administration or directly into tissues after intravenous administration. The solution can be delivered through a nasogastric tube in intubated patients, and it makes the dosing of infants and small children more convenient. Oral absorption of the capsule is significantly enhanced by food, whereas absorption of the solution is best on an empty stomach. Coadministration of a cola beverage with itraconazole capsules increases absorption. Peak levels with either preparation are achieved 4 to 6 hours after a dose. Steady state is achieved only after 13 to 15 days, at which time the β-elimination half-life is approximately 19 to 22 hours. Absorption of the capsule is markedly depressed in bone marrow transplant recipients, probably because of hypochlorhydria, mucositis, and graft-versus-host intestinal changes, and in patients with acquired immunodeficiency syndrome (AIDS) because of enteritis, but this problem can be alleviated by using the solution.

For deep mycoses, an initial itraconazole dose of 200 mg three times daily is recommended for the first 3 days to quickly achieve high serum and tissue levels. Hydroxyitraconazole, a metabolite of itraconazole, appears in the blood in amounts roughly twice that of the parent drug; it has antifungal activity and pharmacokinetics similar to those of the parent compound.

Bioassays of itraconazole yield much higher concentrations than measurement by high-pressure liquid chromatography; the difference depends on the susceptibility of the bioassay organism to hydroxyitraconazole. Concentrations of itraconazole in tissue, pus, and bronchial secretions are generally higher than those in plasma. Ocular levels are low. Saliva concentrations persist for 8 hours after administration of the solution and may be beneficial in treating oral disease or eradicating oral colonization. The drug is metabolized in the liver and excreted in feces as metabolites. Of the liquid administered, less than 0.5% of the cyclodextrin is absorbed. No significant amount of bioactive itraconazole appears in urine. Plasma concentrations do not increase in patients with renal insufficiency or decrease with hemodialysis. The half-life is prolonged in those with cirrhosis.

Adverse Effects
The most common adverse effect is dose-related nausea and abdominal discomfort, but symptoms rarely necessitate stopping therapy. Dividing the dose and administering the drug twice daily can improve tolerance and raise blood levels. Hypokalemia and edema may occur at doses of 400 mg/day or higher. Allergic rash is seen occasionally. Itraconazole is rarely hepatotoxic. Diarrhea, nausea, and other gastrointestinal complaints are more frequent with the solution. A negative inotropic effect is rarely seen.

Drug Interactions
Blood levels are reduced by about half in patients taking drugs that decrease gastric acidity. Some of the most notable drug interactions are rifampin, rifabutin, isoniazid, phenytoin, carbamazepine, and phenobarbital, which decrease itraconazole blood levels. Itraconazole decreases rifampin blood levels and increases blood levels of some antihistamines, potentially causing polymorphic ventricular tachycardia (torsades de pointes), as well as increasing levels of warfarin, benzodiazepines, hepatic hydroxymethylglutaryl–coenzyme A (HMG-CoA) reductase cholesterol-lowering agents, dihydropyridine calcium-channel blockers, digoxin, quinidine, cyclosporine, tacrolimus, methylprednisolone, human immunodeficiency virus (HIV)

protease inhibitors (ritonavir, indinavir), and vinca alkaloids (vincristine, vinblastine).

Uses
Itraconazole is useful for the treatment of invasive aspergillosis, allergic bronchopulmonary aspergillosis, blastomycosis, histoplasmosis, meningeal and nonmeningeal coccidioidomycosis, paracoccidioidomycosis, sporotrichosis, phaeohyphomycosis, mucosal candidiasis, ringworm (including onychomycosis), and tinea versicolor. Itraconazole is also useful for the prevention of relapse of disseminated histoplasmosis in patients with AIDS. Itraconazole may be useful for prophylaxis against fungal infections during neutropenia and as empirical therapy for febrile episodes in neutropenia.

Fluconazole
Formulations and Pharmacology
Fluconazole is currently available in oral and vaginal tablets, as a powder for oral suspension, and as an intravenous formulation. Fluconazole is well absorbed from the gastrointestinal tract. Of the oral dose, 60 to 75% appears unchanged in the urine. Oral absorption is not decreased in patients with AIDS or patients taking H_2-blocking agents. Fluconazole penetrates into the brain, saliva, sputum, and urine.

The half-life in patients with normal renal function is 27 to 34 hours; it increases to 59 and 98 hours in groups with creatinine clearances of 35 and 14 mL/minute, respectively. The normal dose should be reduced to 50% when the creatinine clearance is reduced to 50 mL/minute and to 25% when the creatinine clearance is below 20 mL/minute. A loading dose of twice the daily dose is recommended. Patients receiving hemodialysis should have one daily dose after each session.

Drug Interactions
Among other drug interactions, fluconazole can cause significant increases in the blood level of phenytoin, glipizide, glyburide, tolbutamide, warfarin, rifabutin, cisapride, quinidine, or cyclosporine. Rifampin lowers fluconazole blood levels by approximately one fourth.

Adverse Effects
Adverse effects are uncommon. Even with chronic therapy, including doses exceeding 400 mg/day, headache, hair loss, and anorexia were the most common symptoms; 10% of patients had rises in aspartate aminotransferase levels. Alopecia is reversible, in some cases, even when the drug is continued at lower doses. Neurotoxicity has been described after heroic doses of 2000 mg/day. Rarely, anaphylaxis after the first dose or Stevens-Johnson syndrome has been observed.

Indications
Candidiasis
Provided the infection is not caused by fluconazole-resistant *Candida*, fluconazole is effective for the treatment of oropharyngeal and esophageal candidiasis. A single dose of 150 mg is approximately as effective as topical treatment of vulvovaginal candidiasis. Patients with candidemia who are not neutropenic or otherwise seriously immunosuppressed respond as well to intravenous fluconazole therapy as to amphotericin B. A study comparing fluconazole with a combination of fluconazole plus amphotericin as initial therapy of candidemia found that the combination might produce more rapid clearance of the pathogen from the blood stream. In a few patients with *Candida* endocarditis, long-term fluconazole therapy has been used to prevent relapse after amphotericin B therapy. For immunosuppressed patients and for rapidly progressing or severely ill patients with deep-seated candidiasis, amphotericin B or an echinocandin is preferred.

Cryptococcal Meningitis
Clinical trials in AIDS have engendered the conventional practice of therapy with amphotericin B or amphotericin B plus flucytosine for at least the first 2 weeks. Therapy can then be changed to fluconazole 400 mg/day for 2 months if the patient is clinically stable. The propensity of patients with AIDS to relapse has led to maintenance therapy with fluconazole 200 mg/day, at least until antiretroviral therapy causes CD4 counts to approach normal. Itraconazole capsules are inferior to fluconazole for maintenance therapy. Relapse because of fluconazole resistance is rare. Fluconazole is effective for the eradication of genitourinary foci. For patients without AIDS, fluconazole is useful for those who have completed a course of amphotericin B and seem to be at high risk for relapse.

Other Mycoses

Fluconazole is useful for coccidioidal meningitis and disseminated nonmeningeal coccidioidomycosis, but a direct comparison with itraconazole found a trend favoring itraconazole owing to its superior efficacy for skeletal infections. The two drugs were similarly efficacious for soft tissue and pulmonary infections. Cutaneous sporotrichosis, ringworm, histoplasmosis, and blastomycosis may respond to fluconazole, but the results are inferior to those with itraconazole.

Prophylaxis in Neutropenic Patients

Fluconazole decreases the incidence of death from deep-seated candidiasis in bone marrow transplant recipients. In a long-term follow-up of one study, bone marrow transplant recipients who received at least 75 days of fluconazole prophylaxis also had improved survival. Use of this drug for prophylaxis may result in shifts to less susceptible species in patient flora.

Prophylaxis in Patients with Acquired Immunodeficiency Syndrome

Fluconazole has reduced the incidence of oral and vulvovaginal candidiasis and cryptococcosis in patients with advanced HIV infection, but it has negligible effects on other mycoses. Cost, lack of effect on survival, and the possibility of azole resistance have led the advisory committee of the Infectious Diseases Society of America to recommend against routine fluconazole prophylaxis in patients with AIDS.

Voriconazole
Formulations and Pharmacology

Voriconazole is marketed as a tablet and as a solution in sulfobutyl ether β-cyclodextrin for intravenous administration. Voriconazole is cleared by hepatic metabolism, with less than 2% of the dose excreted unchanged in the urine. Voriconazole exhibits nonlinear pharmacokinetics owing to saturation of the clearance pathways at higher doses. The principal enzyme involved in clearance is hepatic CYP2C19. This enzyme has significant genetic polymorphisms that affect the metabolism of this drug. Despite these differences in metabolism, the achieved plasma levels overlap, and an initial dose adjustment based on genotype or racial group is not necessary. Different studies have suggested that favorable outcomes correlate with serum concentrations greater than 1 to 2 μg/mL, and neurologic/psychiatric, hepatic or cardiac side effects occur with levels greater than 5 μg/mL, so therapeutic drug monitoring is recommended, with dose adjustments as necessary.

Standard loading doses followed by maintenance doses that are 50% of normal are recommended for individuals with mild-to-moderate hepatic cirrhosis. Dosage adjustments are not required for renal dysfunction, and voriconazole is not significantly cleared by hemodialysis. Because of nephrotoxicity from the cyclodextrin, the intravenous formulation should not be used in patients with a creatinine clearance less than 50 mL/minute.

Drug Interactions

Voriconazole has many drug interactions. Rifampin, carbamazepine, long-acting barbiturates, glucocorticoids, and ritonavir induce the hepatic enzymes responsible for the clearance of voriconazole and thereby reduce voriconazole levels. Sirolimus levels are increased dramatically. Reduction in the clearance of pimozide, quinidine, and some antihistamines may be sufficient to place the patient at risk for QTc prolongation. Reduction in the clearance of ergot alkaloids could lead to chronic ergot poisoning. Cyclosporine, tacrolimus, warfarin, oral coumarins, lipid-lowering statin agents, benzodiazepines, calcium-channel blockers, sulfonylureas, methadone, and vinca alkaloids can be coadministered, but the dosages of these drugs may need to be reduced, and clinical or laboratory monitoring is suggested. Voriconazole significantly reduces the rate of clearance of omeprazole. Voriconazole with rifabutin, phenytoin, or efavirenz results in lower voriconazole levels and elevated levels of the other drug. Other interactions are possible, and any cytochrome P450 (CYP 450) inhibitors, blockers, or inducers could have an interaction with voriconazole.

Adverse Effects

The most frequently reported adverse event is a transient, reversible visual disturbance beginning approximately 30 minutes after a dose. Patients should be advised to avoid activities that require keen visual acuity while experiencing visual changes. Hallucinations and confusion also have been reported, associated with higher blood levels. Liver enzyme abnormalities appear to correlate with higher blood levels. Photosensitivity can be severe and has been associated with skin cancers in rare instances. Prolongation of the QT interval and tachyarrhythmias have been noted in patients with proarrhythmic risk factors, such as electrolyte abnormalities. Periostitis has been noted after prolonged therapy, apparently related to the fluoride atoms in the molecule. Leukoencephalopathy has been rarely reported.

Indications
Aspergillosis

Voriconazole was licensed for the treatment of invasive aspergillosis[5] on the basis of a randomized, unblinded comparative trial in which patients were randomized to receive initial therapy with either voriconazole or amphotericin B. Following the initial randomization, patients could be switched to other licensed therapies, as dictated by clinical events. After 12 weeks, 53% of the patients randomized to voriconazole, but only 32% of those randomized to amphotericin B, had a successful outcome.

Other Mycoses

Voriconazole is also licensed for the treatment of invasive fusariosis and scedosporiosis, based on high response rates for these diseases. Infections by *Scedosporium apiospermum* complex may respond, but *Scedosporium prolificans* infections are commonly resistant. The drug is efficacious in esophageal candidiasis, invasive candidiasis, and refractory candidiasis. Although the drug has appeal for use in prophylaxis, there has been concern about breakthrough zygomycoses with long-term use.

Posaconazole
Formulations and Pharmacology

Posaconazole has been available as an oral suspension, and a tablet form has been introduced. Absorption of the suspension is usually maximized by dividing the daily dose into four administrations and enhanced by taking the suspension with or after fatty food. Some commercial dietary supplements have the same effect as fatty meals and are better tolerated. The half-life is 20 to 35 hours. Clearance is primarily by fecal excretion, with only 13% excreted via renal clearance. Hepatic metabolism via uridine diphosphate glucuronidation plays only a small role in clearance, and CYP-mediated oxidation does not occur. The drug is concentrated in phagocytes. The dose is 800 mg/day for treatment of deep-seated mycoses, although 600 mg has been used successfully for prophylaxis, and 100 to 200 mg has been used for mucosal candidiasis. At steady state, 800 mg/day produces a peak concentration (C_{max}) of 4.2 μg/mL. Blood levels appear to be rather unpredictable, and outcomes in the treatment of aspergillosis correlate with levels. Therapeutic drug monitoring is advisable, and levels greater than 0.7 μg/mL have correlated with efficacy in prophylaxis. Dosage adjustment is not needed for hepatic or renal failure or hemodialysis. The dosing for the 100-mg oral tablet is 300 mg twice daily as a first day loading dose, then 300 mg/day. Blood concentrations after administration of the tablets exceed those after optimal dosing of the solution and appear negligibly affected by food or by medications that affect gastric pH or motility. Side effects of the tablets reported include somnolence, diarrhea, and flatulence. An intravenous formulation of posaconazole was introduced in early 2014.

Drug Interactions

Although posaconazole has fewer interactions than itraconazole and voriconazole, there are many significant ones, including increased levels of calcium-channel blockers, cyclosporine, sirolimus, tacrolimus, quinidine, atazanavir, amiodarone, cisapride, corticosteroids, digoxin, benzodiazepines, and drugs for erectile dysfunction. Posaconazole levels are reduced by cimetidine, efavirenz, metoclopramide, rifampin, and, in some studies, with diarrhea and proton pump inhibitors. Posaconazole with phenytoin, carbamazepine, or rifabutin result in lower posaconazole levels and elevated levels of the other drug.

Adverse Effects

The paucity of side effects is similar to that of fluconazole. Gastrointestinal symptoms, headache, and acneiform rashes of the face are occasionally seen. Electrolyte abnormalities should be rectified before therapy to avoid arrhythmias.

Indications

Posaconazole appears to possess a very broad spectrum of activity against molds, including many zygomycetes, a unique property among azoles, and the least cross-reactivity among the azoles to mutations in the ergosterol synthesis pathway that cause resistance to other azoles. The main interest in the drug has been as prophylaxis and for salvage therapy of refractory mycoses. Efficacy in preventing opportunistic mycoses has been shown in the patients at highest risk, transplant patients with graft-versus-host disease, and those with hematologic malignancies and neutropenia. Impressive results in salvage have been demonstrated in aspergillosis and coccidioidomycosis. Superficial candidiasis is also responsive.

ECHINOCANDIN ANTIFUNGAL AGENTS

General Features

The echinocandin antifungal agents act by inhibiting the synthesis of 1,3-β-D-glucan in the fungal cell wall. In studies, the principal pharmacodynamic driver of in vivo response has been the ratio of the peak concentration to the MIC. There are now three licensed echinocandins: caspofungin, micafungin, and anidulafungin. These agents are similar to one another, having very few drug interactions, an admirably low adverse event rate, and essentially identical antifungal spectra. Of the three drugs, caspofungin has the broadest array of approved indications and the most clinical data. Micafungin has the most detailed data on its use in neonates and children. Anidulafungin appears to have somewhat fewer drug-drug interactions. All are cyclic lipopeptides that must be given intravenously.

They are fungicidal against all *Candida* spp, including isolates resistant to other agents. Reduced activity against isolates of *Candida parapsilosis* and *Candida guilliermondii* and a paradoxical effect whereby high concentrations that permit growth in vitro have been noted in a minority of *Candida* isolates and do not appear to be clinically relevant. Resistance, while uncommon, is increasingly noted, and instances of resistance development on therapy have been described. All are active against *Aspergillus* spp, but activity is limited to growing and dividing hyphal elements. Their activity against other fungi is variable.

Caspofungin

Formulations and Pharmacology

Caspofungin is marketed for intravenous infusion. The clearance of caspofungin is through a combination of spontaneous chemical degradation, hydrolysis, and *N*-acetylation. Dose adjustments are not required for impaired renal function or hemodialysis. The clearance of caspofungin is modestly reduced in subjects with moderate hepatic insufficiency, and a reduction of the usual daily dose is recommended. Penetration into infected tissues appears to be good.

Drug Interactions

Caspofungin has few meaningful drug interactions. Cyclosporine coadministration increases caspofungin exposure and has been associated with increased hepatic transaminase levels, so concomitant use requires caution. Caspofungin reduces tacrolimus exposure by approximately 20%, and dosage adjustments may be required. Rifampin reduces caspofungin blood levels by approximately 30%, so the daily dosage of caspofungin should be increased from 50 to 70 mg if these drugs are co-administered. Likewise, limited data on other inducers of drug clearance (efavirenz, nevirapine, phenytoin, dexamethasone, carbamazepine) suggest that reduced caspofungin levels are possible and that increasing the daily dose to 70 mg should be considered.

Adverse Effects

Overall, the adverse reactions with caspofungin have been infrequent and minor. Symptoms possibly related to histamine release during rapid infusion have been reported.

Indications

Caspofungin is indicated for the treatment of invasive candidiasis and esophageal candidiasis. Caspofungin is also indicated for invasive aspergillosis in patients who are refractory to or intolerant of other therapies. With its activity against these two major opportunistic pathogens, the use of caspofungin for empirical therapy in high-risk situations is logical and is supported by clinical trials.

Micafungin

Micafungin has an in vitro spectrum and properties similar to those of caspofungin. It is similarly cidal for *Candida* spp and noncidal in vitro for *Aspergillus*.

Formulations and Pharmacology

The drug is light sensitive. After an intravenous infusion, the terminal half-life is approximately 15 hours. The recommended dose is 100 mg/day. Once daily dosing produces steady state in 3 days. Metabolism appears to be mostly through fecal excretion; less than 1% is excreted in the urine. The drug appears to penetrate particularly well into the lungs, liver, kidneys, and gastric mucosa. No adjustment for hepatic or renal insufficiency is needed.

Drug Interactions

Micafungin has fewer drug interactions than caspofungin. There is no interaction with cyclosporine or rifampin.

Adverse Effects

Micafungin has an excellent safety profile. Histamine release, manifested most prominently by erythema over the body, can be avoided by slow infusion. Phlebitis has been reported.

Indications

Efficacy is good in invasive candidiasis, similar to that of amphotericin or caspofungin. In clinical dose-finding studies against *Candida* esophagitis, doses of 75 to 150 mg/day were particularly effective. A trial of prophylaxis in neutropenic patients with hematopoietic stem cell transplant showed efficacy at 50 mg/day. Limited experience suggests comparable activity to caspofungin against aspergillosis.

Anidulafungin

Formulations and Pharmacology

Anidulafungin is slowly degraded by the chemical opening of its ring structure. A 100-mg dose produces a C_{max} (peak concentration achieved) of 8.6 μg/mL at a time of peak concentration (T_{max}) of 6 to 7 hours. The half-life is 30 to 50 hours. Steady state is achieved in 3 to 10 days. Dose adjustments are not required for renal or hepatic insufficiency.

Drug Interactions

Anidulafungin has no meaningful CYP enzyme interactions. It is not an inducer, inhibitor, or substrate and has no interaction with drugs cleared by these pathways or drugs that induce these pathways. The lack of metabolism suggests this would be the best echinocandin to use in the presence of liver failure.

Adverse Effects

Histamine-mediated symptoms (e.g., rash, urticaria, flushing, pruritus, dyspnea, hypotension) have been noted on occasion, but they are infrequent when the rate of infusion does not exceed 1.1 mg/minute. Other adverse reactions to anidulafungin have generally been infrequent and minor (diarrhea, hypokalemia, elevated liver function tests, neutropenia, nausea, headache, dermatitis).

Indications

Anidulafungin is indicated for the treatment of invasive candidiasis and esophageal candidiasis. Randomized trials indicate that anidulafungin is at least as efficacious as fluconazole. Inefficacy against *C. parapsilosis* may be of greatest concern with this echinocandin.

OTHER AGENTS

Combinations of antifungal agents are increasingly being used in an effort to improve the very poor response rates in some diseases and to combine drugs with different mechanisms of action. Although synergy in vitro may be relatively easy to demonstrate, there are few examples of synergy in animal model studies. In patients, the costs are high and the side effects are likely to be increased. The clinical advantages of the amphotericin-flucytosine combination in cryptococcosis have yet to be documented definitively in other situations.

Immunomodulators, particularly cytokines, hold promise, but insufficient clinical data exist to determine where and how these drugs might be used.[4] Granulocyte-macrophage colony-stimulating factor was shown to be effective in one trial when given prophylactically during induction therapy of patients with leukemia who are high risk.

Therapy of the various forms of tinea and of onychomycosis with systemic agents is discussed in Chapter 438. Although *Pneumocystis jiroveci* (formerly

Pneumocystis carinii) is now classified among the fungi, the drugs used to treat it are principally those used to treat parasitic infections (Chapter 344).

GENERAL REFERENCES

For the General References and other additional features, please visit Expert Consult at https://expertconsult.inkling.com.

332

HISTOPLASMOSIS

CAROL A. KAUFFMAN

DEFINITION

Histoplasmosis is the most common endemic mycosis in the United States. Most infections are self-limited, but the organism has the ability to cause acute and chronic pulmonary infections and disseminated infection.[1,2]

The Pathogen

Histoplasma capsulatum var *capsulatum* is a thermally dimorphic fungus. In the environment and at temperatures lower than 35° C, it exists as a mold that produces conidia. It produces both tuberculate macroconidia, which are helpful for identification purposes in the laboratory, and microconidia, which are the infectious form. In tissues and at 35 to 37° C, *H. capsulatum* transforms into tiny 2- to 4-μm oval yeasts that reproduce by budding and parasitize macrophages. African histoplasmosis is caused by a different subspecies, *H. capsulatum* var *duboisii,* and has different disease manifestations, particularly involvement of skin, subcutaneous tissues, lymph nodes, and bone, and only rarely the lungs and other internal organs.

EPIDEMIOLOGY

Histoplasmosis, though found worldwide, is primarily a disease of North and Central America. *H. capsulatum* is endemic in the Mississippi and Ohio River valleys, with extension into the St. Lawrence basin; microfoci exist in discrete isolated areas in several eastern states. Soil, caves, and abandoned buildings containing high concentrations of bird or bat guano support luxuriant growth of the organism. Every year, hundreds of thousands of individuals who live in areas endemic for *H. capsulatum* are infected. Most cases are sporadic and the exact source of exposure is unknown. Point source outbreaks that have included as few as 4 persons and as many as 100,000 have been well described in association with disruption of soil; cleaning attics, bridges, or barns; renovating or tearing down old structures laden with guano; and spelunking.[3]

PATHOBIOLOGY

After inhalation of microconidia into the alveoli, a localized pulmonary infection ensues. Neutrophils and macrophages phagocytize the organism, now in the yeast phase; the organism is able to survive and travels within macrophages to the hilar and mediastinal lymph nodes and throughout the reticuloendothelial system by hematogenous dissemination. Such dissemination probably occurs in most persons who are infected and in normal hosts is associated with no symptoms. After several weeks, T cells specifically sensitized by *H. capsulatum* antigens activate macrophages, which are then able to kill the intracellular fungi. Histoplasmosis is a classic example of the pivotal importance of the cell-mediated immune system in containing intracellular pathogens.

The extent of disease is determined by both the number of conidia inhaled and the immune response of the host. A small inoculum can cause severe pulmonary infection or progress to acute symptomatic disseminated histoplasmosis in immunosuppressed patients. Conversely, severe life-threatening pulmonary infection may develop in a healthy individual if a large number of conidia are inhaled, as might occur during the demolition of old buildings or while spelunking in a heavily infested cave.

Reinfection can occur in persons who previously had histoplasmosis but is uncommon and almost always occurs in the setting of heavy exposure. Reactivation of latent infection takes place in patients who have deficient cell-mediated immunity, as evidenced by the occurrence of histoplasmosis in immunosuppressed persons who grew up in the endemic area but have not been back in that area for years.

CLINICAL MANIFESTATIONS

Acute Pulmonary Histoplasmosis

Infection is asymptomatic in most people infected with *H. capsulatum.* Those who do have symptomatic pulmonary infection usually have a self-limited illness that begins several weeks after exposure and is characterized by fever, chills, fatigue, nonproductive cough, anterior chest discomfort, and myalgias. A patchy lobar or multilobar nodular infiltrate is noted on chest radiographs.

The differential diagnosis of acute pulmonary histoplasmosis includes pneumonia from *Blastomyces dermatitidis, Mycoplasma pneumoniae, Legionella* sp, and *Chlamydia pneumoniae.* When enlarged hilar or mediastinal lymph nodes are present, histoplasmosis should be strongly considered. The most difficult to differentiate is acute pulmonary blastomycosis (Chapter 334) because the endemic areas overlap, a comparable history of outdoor activities is often obtained, and radiographs show similar findings.

In patients who have experienced heavy exposure to *H. capsulatum* and in those who are immunosuppressed, acute pulmonary histoplasmosis can be life-threatening. High spiking fevers, chills, prostration, dyspnea, and cough are prominent.[4] Chest radiographs show diffuse reticulonodular pulmonary infiltrates, and acute respiratory distress syndrome (ARDS) can occur.

Chronic Pulmonary Histoplasmosis

Chronic cavitary pulmonary histoplasmosis is a progressive, often fatal form of histoplasmosis that develops almost exclusively in older patients who have chronic obstructive pulmonary disease.[5] Symptoms include fever, fatigue, anorexia, weight loss, cough productive of purulent sputum, and hemoptysis. On chest radiography the usual findings are unilateral or bilateral upper lobe infiltrates with multiple cavities and extensive fibrosis in the lower lobes. Chronic pulmonary histoplasmosis mimics tuberculosis, other fungal pneumonias (especially blastomycosis and sporotrichosis), and nontuberculous mycobacterial infections with regard to symptoms, signs, and radiographic findings.

Complications of Pulmonary Histoplasmosis

The mediastinal and hilar lymph nodes frequently calcify as the infection resolves; years later they can erode into bronchi and cause hemoptysis and expectoration of broncholiths. Granulomatous mediastinitis is an uncommon syndrome characterized by continuing inflammation and necrosis in the mediastinal lymph nodes. The enlarged nodes are readily apparent on chest radiographs, and computed tomography (CT) shows central necrosis and, in some cases, impingement on adjacent structures, including the esophagus, airways, and blood vessels. Although the symptoms usually resolve without treatment, obstructive syndromes can be severe and the nodes can persist for years.

Fibrosing mediastinitis[6] is a rare complication of histoplasmosis in which the host responds to the infection with an inappropriate excessive fibrotic response. Obstruction of the airways, superior vena cava, or pulmonary arteries and veins can occur with resultant progressive right heart failure and respiratory insufficiency. Bilateral obstruction of the pulmonary vasculature is less common than unilateral involvement and carries a worse prognosis. Mediastinal widening is seen on chest radiographs, and CT and angiography define the extent of invasion and obstruction of mediastinal structures.

Pericarditis is a manifestation of a local inflammatory reaction to adjacent histoplasmosis. Patients respond promptly to anti-inflammatory medications without antifungal therapy. Hemodynamic compromise, though unusual, requires drainage of pericardial fluid; only rarely has progression to constrictive pericarditis been documented.

Disseminated Histoplasmosis

Symptomatic disseminated histoplasmosis occurs mostly in immunosuppressed patients. Patients with acquired immunodeficiency syndrome (AIDS) and CD4+ counts lower than 150/μL, infants, and those who have a hematologic malignancy, have received an organ transplant, or are taking corticosteroids or tumor necrosis factor antagonists are at greatest risk for acute disseminated histoplasmosis.[7] Symptoms and signs include chills, fever, anorexia, weight loss, hypotension, dyspnea, hepatosplenomegaly, and skin and mucous membrane lesions. Pancytopenia, diffuse pulmonary infiltrates on chest radiography and CT, findings of disseminated intravascular coagulation, and acute respiratory failure are common. This syndrome is indistinguishable from sepsis of any bacterial or viral cause. In patients with acquired immunodeficiency syndrome (AIDS), the differential diagnosis includes cytomegalovirus, disseminated *Mycobacterium avium* complex infection, and tuberculosis.

Chronic progressive disseminated histoplasmosis is a fatal form of histoplasmosis that occurs mostly in middle-aged to elderly men who have no known immunosuppressive illness. The illness is characterized by fever, night sweats, weight loss, anorexia, and fatigue. Patients appear chronically ill, hepatosplenomegaly and mucocutaneous ulcerations are common, and adrenal insufficiency can develop. An increased erythrocyte sedimentation rate, elevated alkaline phosphatase, pancytopenia, and diffuse reticulonodular infiltrates on chest radiography and CT are typical. Patients with this form of histoplasmosis often have fever of unknown origin. Miliary tuberculosis, lymphoma, and sarcoidosis must be excluded.

Involvement of almost every organ system has been reported with disseminated infection. Adrenal insufficiency must be sought in any patient who has unexplained hypotension, hyponatremia, and hyperkalemia. Abdominal CT shows markedly enlarged adrenal glands. Central nervous system involvement manifests as either meningitis or focal lesions seen on magnetic resonance imaging and is more common in patients with AIDS. Skin lesions, also more common in patients with AIDS, can be papular, pustular, or ulcerated. *Histoplasma* endocarditis is a rare form of disseminated infection.[8]

DIAGNOSIS

The definitive diagnostic test for histoplasmosis is growth of the organism in culture. Unfortunately, *H. capsulatum* may take as long as 6 weeks to grow in vitro. Tissue samples, bronchoalveolar lavage fluid, sputum, and blood are appropriate for culture. For patients who have evidence of dissemination, blood cultures are best performed with the lysis-centrifugation (Isolator tube) system; bone marrow and liver biopsy material often yield *H. capsulatum* in the setting of dissemination. If pulmonary histoplasmosis is a diagnostic consideration, the laboratory should be informed so that a special medium that decreases the growth of commensal fungi can be used for the culture of pulmonary samples. As soon as growth of a mold has been detected, highly specific DNA probes for *H. capsulatum* allow rapid identification of the organism.

If the patient is acutely ill, tissue biopsy should be performed to search for the distinctive 2- to 4-μm oval yeasts with single buds, which allows a tentative diagnosis to be made as quickly as possible. Routine tissue stains do not show the tiny yeasts; biopsy material must be stained with methenamine silver or periodic acid–Schiff stains. In patients with disseminated disease, bone marrow, liver, skin, and mucocutaneous lesions usually reveal many organisms. The organisms also can be seen within neutrophils in peripheral blood smears from patients with acute disseminated infection. In patients with chronic pulmonary histoplasmosis or granulomatous mediastinitis, biopsy of the lung or lymph nodes may reveal the organism.

Serology plays an important role in the diagnosis of some forms of histoplasmosis. Complement fixation assays that use two different antigens—mycelial and yeast—and immunodiffusion tests are available. Serology is helpful in diagnosing acute pulmonary histoplasmosis when a four-fold rise in complement fixation titer, a complement fixation titer higher than 1:32, or the appearance of an M precipitin band by immunodiffusion assay is found. These tests also are useful in patients with chronic forms of pulmonary or disseminated histoplasmosis, but they are rarely helpful in immunosuppressed patients, who often cannot mount an antibody response. Because serologic tests are not definitive in patients with mediastinal lymphadenopathy, the results always should be confirmed by tissue biopsy. An enzyme immunoassay for *H. capsulatum* polysaccharide antigen in urine and serum is extremely helpful in patients with disseminated infection and in those with acute pulmonary histoplasmosis.[9] Almost 75% of patients who have experienced heavy exposure and demonstrate diffuse pulmonary infiltrates and more than 90% of patients who have disseminated histoplasmosis will have a positive urinary antigen test. However, the assay is not useful for patients who have chronic cavitary histoplasmosis, granulomatous mediastinitis, or fibrosing mediastinitis. False-positive reactions have been noted commonly with blastomycosis, paracoccidioidomycosis, and penicilliosis and occasionally with acute coccidioidomycosis. Antigen levels usually become undetectable with successful therapy. Polymerase chain reaction has been used for diagnosis in some cases, but the assays are not standardized.

TREATMENT   Rx

Guidelines for the treatment of histoplasmosis have been published by the Infectious Diseases Society of America (IDSA).[10] Itraconazole is the drug of choice for mild-to-moderate histoplasmosis, and lipid formulations of amphotericin B should be used as initial therapy for severe, life-threatening infections. Fluconazole is less active and should be considered a second-line agent. There is less experience using voriconazole or posaconazole, although both appear to be effective therapy. The echinocandins are not effective for histoplasmosis.

For all patients who are treated with itraconazole, serum levels should be determined when a steady state has been reached after 2 weeks of therapy to ensure adequate absorption. Serum concentrations should be greater than 1 μg/mL.

Pulmonary Histoplasmosis

Treatment is not usually given for acute pulmonary histoplasmosis; many times the diagnosis is not made until after the symptoms have resolved. However, if the patient remains symptomatic after 4 weeks, therapy with itraconazole, 200 mg once or twice daily for 6 to 12 weeks, should be given. All patients who have severe pulmonary histoplasmosis and all immunosuppressed patients should be treated with an antifungal agent. Lipid formulation amphotericin B, 3 to 5 mg/kg/day, is recommended for several weeks until a response is noted, at which time therapy can be changed to oral itraconazole, 200 mg three times daily for 3 days and then 200 mg twice daily. A short course of methylprednisolone is recommended in the IDSA guidelines for patients in whom respiratory distress develops in association with acute pulmonary histoplasmosis.

Antifungal therapy should be given to all patients with chronic pulmonary histoplasmosis. Itraconazole, 200 mg twice daily for 12 to 24 months, is recommended. A trial of itraconazole for 6 to 12 weeks is often given to patients with symptomatic granulomatous mediastinitis, although there are no data proving such therapy to be effective. Surgical resection of nodes causing obstructive symptoms may be beneficial. Antifungal therapy offers no benefit for patients with fibrosing mediastinitis. Surgery is not indicated and carries a high operative mortality rate. Intravascular stents have been used successfully in patients who have vascular obstruction.

Disseminated Histoplasmosis

All patients with symptomatic disseminated histoplasmosis should receive antifungal therapy. Patients who have only mild-to-moderate symptoms with acute disseminated disease and most patients with chronic progressive disseminated histoplasmosis can be treated with itraconazole, 200 mg twice daily after a loading dose of 200 mg three times daily for 3 days. A total of 12 months of therapy is generally adequate, but for those with chronic progressive disease, the duration of treatment may need to be longer.

Patients who have moderately severe to severe disseminated histoplasmosis should be treated with liposomal amphotericin B, 3 mg/kg/day. Therapy can be changed to itraconazole after the patient has responded to therapy, generally in a few weeks. Therapy should continue for a total of 12 months. For those who are immunosuppressed, therapy with itraconazole, 200 mg/day, should continue until the immunosuppression resolves. For patients with AIDS, suppressive therapy can be safely stopped in those who have had a year of therapy, are receiving antiretroviral therapy, and have CD4+ counts greater than 150 cells/μL.[11]

Prevention of histoplasmosis is difficult because exposure can occur without the person's knowledge in highly endemic areas. Persons who are immunosuppressed should be advised to avoid demolition areas, spelunking, and cleaning of farm buildings or attics. A randomized, blinded, placebo-controlled trial in patients with AIDS found that itraconazole, 200 mg/day, was effective in preventing infection. Recommendations are to use prophylaxis only for patients whose CD4+ counts are lower than 150/μL and who live in a highly endemic area with a rate of histoplasmosis that is greater than 10 cases per 100 patient years. There are no recommendations for prophylaxis for other immunosuppressed patients.

PROGNOSIS

Acute pulmonary histoplasmosis is usually a self-limited disease. Patients who require treatment generally respond promptly to antifungal agents. However, the response of patients with chronic cavitary pulmonary histoplasmosis is often poor, primarily because of their severe underlying pulmonary disease. Mediastinal fibrosis has a poor prognosis, but intravascular stenting has led to improvement in many patients. Patients with disseminated histoplasmosis, even those with advanced AIDS, usually respond promptly to antifungal therapy; most deaths in immunosuppressed patients occur when the diagnosis is delayed. Older patients with chronic progressive disseminated histoplasmosis have a slower, but usually complete response to therapy.

GENERAL REFERENCES

For the General References and other additional features, please visit Expert Consult at https://expertconsult.inkling.com.

333

COCCIDIOIDOMYCOSIS

JOHN N. GALGIANI

DEFINITION

Coccidioidomycosis is a systemic fungal infection caused by *Coccidioides* spp endemic to some arid regions of the Western Hemisphere (Table 333-1).

The Pathogen

Coccidioides immitis and *C. posadasii* are dimorphic fungi classified as Ascomycetes by ribosomal gene homology. In their vegetative state, mycelia with true septations mature to produce arthroconidia, single cells approximately 2 to 5 μm in diameter. After infection, an arthroconidium enlarges to a spherule up to 75 μm in diameter and undergoes internal septation to produce scores of endospores. When the spherules rupture, packets of endospores are released and produce more spherules in infected tissue or revert to mycelia if removed from the body.

EPIDEMIOLOGY

Coccidioides organisms can be recovered from the soil of the low deserts of Arizona; the Central Valley of California; parts of other states, including New Mexico and Texas; and parts of Central and South America.[1] Isolated pockets of endemnicity have been found unexpectedly elsewhere such as in Washington State.[2] Endemic regions follow the climatologic Sonoran life zone, which is characterized by modest rainfall, mild winters, and low humidity. However, even in the most highly endemic areas, fungal colonies are sparse and occupy only a tiny fraction of the total acreage. Mycelia bloom beneath the surface during periods of rain, and arthroconidia develop as the earth dries.[3] Rates of infection are highest during dry months, occasionally accentuated when soil is disturbed by windstorms or construction equipment. Exposure to contaminated bales of cotton or other fomites can rarely result in infection beyond the endemic regions. Person-to-person transmission of pulmonary infection has not been reported, and isolation precautions are unnecessary, even in acute care areas. As of 2013, *Coccidioides* spp are no longer listed and controlled by the Centers for Disease Control and Prevention as select agents.

Incidence and Prevalence

In general, the annual risk for infection within the most strongly endemic areas is 3%, resulting in approximately 150,000 new infections per year. Reported clinical illness following infection is increasing. For example, from 1998 to 2011, reported infections increased more than eight-fold.[4] With unusually intense exposure, such as at archaeology sites or during military maneuvers within endemic regions, infections can develop in the majority of persons exposed for only a matter of days. Arizona and California contribute 66% and 31%, respectively, of all U.S. infections.

PATHOBIOLOGY

Inhaling even a single arthroconidium to the level of the terminal bronchiole initiates virtually all coccidioidal infections. Fungal proliferation engenders both granulomatous inflammation, which is associated with intact spherules, and acute inflammation, including eosinophils, which is associated with spherule rupture and proliferation. Focal pneumonia is often associated with ipsilateral hilar adenopathy; less frequently, infection enlarges the paratracheal, supraclavicular, and cervical nodes. Lesions occurring elsewhere are the result of hematogenous dissemination, and most become apparent within 2 years of the initial infection. Although progressive dissemination occurs in less than 1% of infections, as many as 8% of persons with self-limited infection manifest asymptomatic chorioretinal scars, suggesting that subclinical hematogenous spread may be frequent. Within weeks after infection, durable T-cell immunity normally arrests fungal proliferation, which allows the inflammation to resolve and prevents reinfection in the future. However, control of the infection occurs without sterilizing lesions, and reactivation of the dormant infection is possible even many years later in patients whose cell-mediated immunity becomes deficient.

CLINICAL MANIFESTATIONS

Two thirds of infections are asymptomatic and are detected only by finding dermal hypersensitivity to coccidioidal antigens. Those who become ill usually experience pulmonary syndromes that eventually are self-limited. However, some patients develop complications or progressive forms of infection that display a broad variety of manifestations and pose difficult management problems.

Primary Pulmonary Infections

Symptoms develop within 5 to 21 days after exposure. For residents of or recent visitors to southern Arizona, coccidioidomycosis accounts for approximately one third of cases of community-acquired pneumonia.[5] Fever, weight loss, fatigue, dry cough, and pleuritic chest pain are common but nonspecific complaints. Arthralgia of multiple joints without significant effusion is also frequent and is referred to as "desert rheumatism." Occasionally, skin manifestations develop, including a short-lived nonpruritic maculopapular rash, erythema multiforme, or erythema nodosum. These arthritic and dermatologic manifestations are mediated by circulating immune complexes or other immunologic phenomena rather than by fungal dissemination and resolve without tissue destruction. Radiographs of the chest may not detect any abnormalities or may demonstrate pulmonary infiltrates that are either segmental or lobar. Hilar adenopathy is often a distinctive finding and may suggest lymphoma by its appearance. Peripneumonic pleural effusions may occur and generally resolve without intervention, although cultures of pleural biopsies usually yield *Coccidioides* spp. Eosinophilia may be a prominent finding in differential leukocyte counts of peripheral blood, and the erythrocyte sedimentation rate is generally elevated. Symptoms frequently persist for many weeks before improvement is clearly under way, and the illness, especially lassitude, may persist for months.[6]

The primary pulmonary process produces a variety of sequelae. The most frequent is the development of a pulmonary nodule (Fig. 333-1), typically measuring 1 to 4 cm and lying within 5 cm of the hilum. Despite their harmless nature, coccidioidal nodules may cause concern because of their similarity to a malignant mass (Chapters 84 and 191). Positron emission tomography scans are typically positive. For these reasons, management usually requires percutaneous needle aspiration or resection. Another consequence of pulmonary coccidioidomycosis is cavitation of the infiltrate, which occurs in approximately 5% of cases of pneumonia.[7] Most cavities are solitary and thin walled and reside in an upper lobe, close to the pleura. Occasionally, they produce pain, hemoptysis, or adjacent infiltrates. Cavities may acquire mycetomas from either *Coccidioides* spp or some other colonizing mold. Infrequently, a cavity ruptures and forms a pyopneumothorax. Half of the time,

TABLE 333-1	COCCIDIOIDOMYCOSIS: CLINICAL CHARACTERISTICS AND TREATMENT	
CHARACTERISTIC	**DESCRIPTION**
Causative fungi	*Coccidioides immitis* and *Coccidioides posadasii*
Primary geographic distribution	Lower Sonoran deserts of the Western Hemisphere, including parts of Arizona, California, and New Mexico; western Texas; parts of Central and South America
Primary route of acquisition	Respiratory (inhalation of arthroconidia)
Principal site of disease	Lungs most common; spread to skin, bones, meninges, and other viscera uncommon but serious
Opportunistic infection in compromised hosts	Diffuse pneumonia and widespread infections common in patients with T-lymphocyte defects or during high-dose corticosteroid therapy
Drug of choice for most patients	No antifungal is required for uncomplicated pneumonia; fluconazole or itraconazole for progressive forms of infection
Alternative therapy	Amphotericin B (especially with diffuse pneumonia or rapidly progressive infections), voriconazole, posaconazole

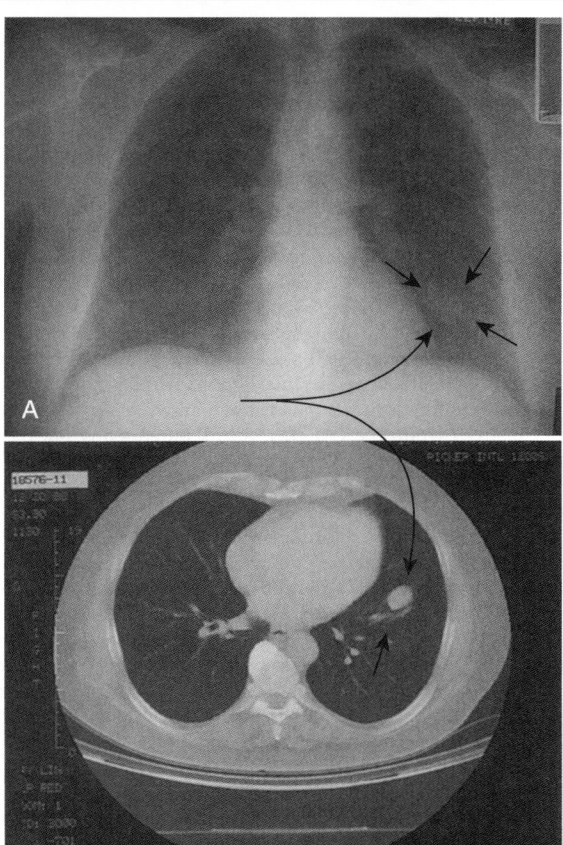

FIGURE 333-1. Coccidioidomycosis. A, Benign nodule secondary to coccidioidomycosis (*arrows*). B, Computed tomography scan of the nodule shown in A (*arrows*).

this is the first symptom of coccidioidal infection and typically occurs in otherwise healthy young men. An air-fluid level in the pleural space, detectable by roentgenography, often helps differentiate this problem from a spontaneous pneumothorax. Prompt surgical resection of the cavity is the preferred treatment of this complication. The least common pulmonary complication is persistent fibrocavitary infection that progresses to involvement of both lungs. Rarely, a mutation of the *STAT1* gene results in chronic progressive noncavitary pulmonary destruction.[8]

Extrapulmonary Dissemination

Coccidioidomycosis in patients with deficiencies in cellular immunity, such as solid organ recipients, those with acquired immunodeficiency syndrome (AIDS) or lymphoma, and women during their third trimester of pregnancy, usually results in dissemination beyond the lungs. Mutations of the genes for γ-interferon or the interleukin-12 receptor also predispose persons to dissemination.[9] However, disseminated infection occurs in some patients who have no underlying disease and do not manifest heightened susceptibility to other infections. Disseminated infection is more likely in men than in women and in persons of certain ancestry such as Africans, Filipinos, or Native Americans compared to Caucasians. The most common locations for disseminated lesions are the skin (cutaneous papules or subcutaneous abscesses); joints (especially the knee); bones, including the vertebrae; and basilar meninges.[10] Such infections may produce one or many lesions and are frequently subacute or chronic in their manifestation. In broadly immunosuppressed patients, coccidioidal infections may be more fulminant, with fungemia detectable in blood cultures and the development of diffuse reticulonodular embolic pulmonary infiltrates. Although the kidneys and the urinary bladder are rarely involved, *Coccidioides* may be recovered from concentrated specimens of urine, usually because of focal dissemination to the prostate. In contrast to histoplasmosis, the gastrointestinal tract is rarely involved in coccidioidomycosis.

DIAGNOSIS

The diagnosis is definitively established by recovering *Coccidioides* spp from clinical specimens. On direct examination of respiratory specimens or tissue,

spherules appear as large structures with refractile walls and internal organization; they are also seen on hematoxylin-eosin, silver, or periodic acid–Schiff stains of histologic preparations. Gram stain does not detect spherules. In culture, mycelial growth is often evident within the first week of incubation, and DNA probing with commercially available kits allows rapid genus identification. Recovery of *Coccidioides* spp from patients with only scant respiratory secretions associated with the initial pneumonia and from the cerebrospinal fluid of patients with meningitis may be difficult.

A presumptive diagnosis of coccidioidal infection is often based on the detection of specific antibodies in serum. Within the first weeks of the initial infection, a precipitin-type antibody is detected, usually by immunodiffusion techniques. Later, complement fixation–type antibodies generally appear. However, these tests may be falsely negative as often as half the time during the first weeks of illness.[11] When reported quantitatively, concentrations of complement fixation antibodies are usually highest in the most extensive infections and decrease in patients whose infections are controlled. An important means of diagnosing coccidioidal meningitis is the detection of complement fixation antibodies in cerebrospinal fluid, along with other abnormalities such as leukocytosis, elevated protein concentration, or low glucose concentration. Newer enzyme immunoassay commercial kits are also available, are generally more sensitive than the older serologic tests, but occasionally produce falsely positive results. Coccidioidal antigens are sometimes found in the urine or serum of patients with widespread infection. A *Coccidioides* genus–specific, quantitative, real-time polymerase chain reaction assay has been developed for the early diagnosis of coccidioidomycosis.[12] In 2014, a coccidioidal skin test became clinically available and, if positive, indicates past infection.

TREATMENT Rx

The role of antifungal therapy for primary uncomplicated infections is unsettled because clinical trials have not been performed to determine whether treatment either shortens the course of symptoms or diminishes the chance of complications.[13,14] However, the value of treatment is clear for patients with progressive illness.[15] Because many coccidioidal infections are chronic, initial treatment often consists of oral azole antifungal agents, such as fluconazole and itraconazole. Responses to these two drugs are similar, but itraconazole is preferred in patients with skeletal infections. Doses of these azoles are 400 mg/day or higher, and treatment is usually continued for a year or more. Satisfactory responses are obtained in approximately two thirds of patients. Fluconazole is effective therapy for coccidioidal meningitis and has greatly reduced the number of patients treated with intrathecal amphotericin B. Unfortunately, cessation of azole therapy is often followed by a recurrence of symptoms, especially in those with coccidioidal meningitis. Therefore, many patients need protracted or even lifelong therapy to control disease activity. The limited evidence available for the newer azole antifungals (voriconazole, posaconazole) indicates that they are also effective in some patients and are sometimes useful for refractory infections. Amphotericin B remains a rational choice when treatment with azole antifungals has failed. Daily doses range from 0.4 to 1 mg/kg for the original deoxycholate formulation and up to 5 mg/kg per day for newer lipid formulations. Occasionally, in a patient with rapid disease progression, amphotericin B may produce a more rapid therapeutic response and is therefore the preferred initial therapy. In addition to antifungal agents, surgical removal of necrotic tissue may be essential to control the progressive damage from specific lesions.

PROGNOSIS

After resolution of the initial infection, most patients maintain lifelong immunity, and infections after re-exposure are rare. However, cessation of symptoms is frequently accomplished without eradicating *Coccidioides* completely, and recurrence of the original infection many years after the original episode is a well-recognized risk for intercurrent profound immunosuppression. Re-treating patients with rheumatic disease with biologic response modifiers and/or disease-modifying antirheumatic drugs after coccidioidomycosis appears to be safe in some patients.[16] For patients in whom the initial infection cannot be resolved, the disease typically follows a protracted course. Although infection is more often debilitating than fatal, fulminant respiratory failure can occur, and, if untreated, coccidioidal meningitis is nearly always fatal within 2 years.

GENERAL REFERENCES

For the General References and other additional features, please visit Expert Consult at https://expertconsult.inkling.com.

334

BLASTOMYCOSIS

CAROL A. KAUFFMAN

DEFINITION

Blastomycosis (North American blastomycosis) is an endemic mycosis that primarily causes infection of the lungs and skin and, less commonly, infection of the osteoarticular and genitourinary systems.[1]

The Pathogen

Blastomyces dermatitidis is a thermally dimorphic fungus. In the environment in the mold phase, the organism produces conidia, which when aerosolized and inhaled cause infection. At 37°C on culture media and in tissues, the organism is a yeast that is 5 to 20 μm in diameter, has a thick refractile cell wall, and produces single broad-based buds (Fig. 334-1)

EPIDEMIOLOGY

B. dermatitidis exists in many diverse geographic areas worldwide, but most cases of blastomycosis are reported from the south central and north central regions of the United States[2] and the Canadian provinces surrounding the Great Lakes. The natural niche of *B. dermatitidis* is thought to be soil and decaying vegetation, especially in areas associated with rivers and lakes. Although most cases occur sporadically, several well-described outbreaks have occurred in association with activities along waterways. The largest community outbreak was reported in 2009 and 2010 in Wisconsin, with geographic and ethnic clustering likely related to multifocal environmental sources.[3] The typical patient in whom blastomycosis develops is a middle-aged man who has an outdoor occupation or hobby. The association of blastomycosis developing in both hunters and their dogs is well known in endemic areas.

PATHOBIOLOGY

After the inhalation of conidia, *B. dermatitidis* transforms into the yeast phase and causes pulmonary infection. Although many patients manifest only pulmonary symptoms, others have cutaneous lesions in the absence of other organ involvement or have disseminated infection. It is likely that most patients have asymptomatic hematogenous dissemination after the initial pulmonary infection. Thus, cutaneous lesions should be viewed as a manifestation of hematogenous spread of the organism. Except in rare instances, blastomycosis is not acquired by inoculation. Cellular immunity involving T lymphocytes and macrophages is an important component of the host response to infection with *B. dermatitidis,* but neutrophils also play a role. Most patients with blastomycosis are healthy hosts. Patients who are immunosuppressed are more likely to have severe disease. Infection in an immunosuppressed host can occur after new exposure to *B. dermatitidis* or from reactivation of a latent focus of infection acquired years earlier.[4]

CLINICAL MANIFESTATIONS

Pulmonary

Most patients with acute pulmonary blastomycosis are asymptomatic or are thought to have community-acquired pneumonia. Patients with acute pneumonia have fever, malaise, a nonproductive cough, and a pulmonary infiltrate that shows lobar or multilobar patchy or nodular infiltrates on chest radiographs. Development of skin lesions is a strong clue for blastomycosis. Chronic pulmonary blastomycosis must be differentiated from tuberculosis, other fungal infections, and lung cancer.[5] Fever, night sweats, weight loss, fatigue, cough, sputum production, hemoptysis, and dyspnea are commonly noted. On chest radiograph the lesions are cavitary, nodular, fibrotic, or mass-like in appearance. Hilar and mediastinal lymphadenopathy and pleural effusions are not commonly seen. Overwhelming pulmonary disease with acute respiratory distress syndrome (ARDS) occurs infrequently but has a high mortality rate. Whether this is due to inhalation of a large number of conidia or to an exuberant host response is not known. Given improvement in some patients with corticosteroids, the latter may be important.

Disseminated Infection

Cutaneous lesions are the most common manifestation of disseminated blastomycosis. The lesions are usually well-circumscribed, painless papules, nodules, or plaques that become verrucous and develop multiple punctate draining areas in the center. Some patients have predominantly ulcerative lesions. Cutaneous lesions, sometimes single but more often multiple, are most common on the face and extremities but can appear anywhere. The skin lesions of blastomycosis clinically mimic those associated with nontuberculous mycobacteria, other fungal infections, pyoderma gangrenosum, and bromide use. An uncommon manifestation, seen more often in immunocompromised patients, is the appearance of hundreds of pustular lesions that readily reveal the organism when aspirated.

Another manifestation of disseminated blastomycosis is osteoarticular involvement. Osteomyelitis can be associated with contiguous skin lesions or can appear at sites distant from cutaneous lesions. It is helpful to obtain a bone scan in all patients with disseminated blastomycosis because of the propensity of the organism to infect bone. Genitourinary involvement may be asymptomatic or be associated with signs of prostatism and the presence of a nodule on digital examination. Infrequently occurring findings include laryngeal and oropharyngeal nodules; ocular lesions; central nervous system (CNS) involvement, either meningitis or intracerebral mass lesions; and dissemination to the liver, spleen, and lymph nodes.

DIAGNOSIS

The definitive diagnostic test for blastomycosis is growth of the organism from an aspirate, tissue biopsy specimen, sputum, or body fluid. Urine obtained before and after prostatic massage should be sent for fungal culture in those with disseminated blastomycosis. The mold phase takes several weeks to grow at room temperature. Once growth has occurred, the organism can be rapidly identified as *B. dermatitidis* with a highly specific and sensitive DNA probe. Histopathologic examination of cutaneous or pulmonary lesions, cytologic examination of sputum, bronchoalveolar lavage fluid, or other tissue fluids, and calcofluor fluorescent staining of sputum or purulent material from pustular lesions should be performed to look for the distinctive large, thick-walled yeast with a single broad-based bud. Identification of characteristic organisms allows a tentative diagnosis of blastomycosis and initiation of antifungal therapy before culture results are known. An enzyme immunoassay for *B. dermatitidis* cell wall antigens can be performed on urine and serum and is a useful rapid diagnostic test in patients who have severe pulmonary or disseminated blastomycosis.[6] Because *B. dermatitidis* and *H. capsulatum* share many cell wall antigens, this assay is often positive in patients with histoplasmosis, as well as in those with blastomycosis. Antibody tests for blastomycosis are neither sensitive nor specific. Polymerase chain reaction on tissue samples has proved useful if histopathology and culture are not diagnostic.[7]

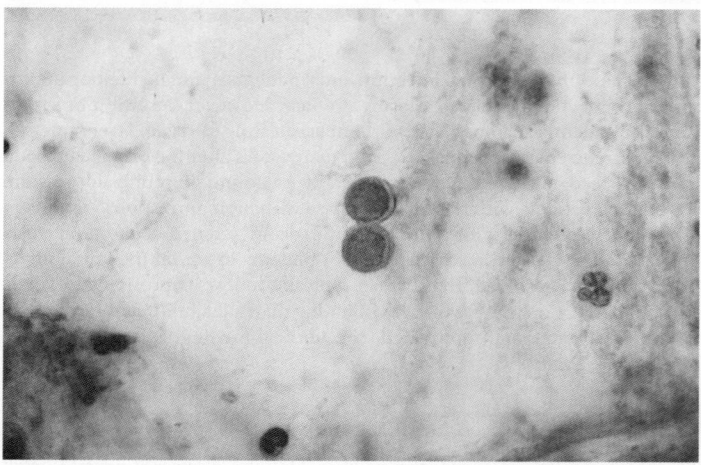

FIGURE 334-1. Papanicolaou stain of sputum showing a thick-walled yeast with broad-based budding typical of Blastomyces dermatitidis.

TREATMENT   Rx

Guidelines for the treatment of blastomycosis have been published by the Infectious Diseases Society of America (IDSA),[8] and the American Thoracic Society.[9] With the exception of patients who have acute pulmonary blastomycosis that has totally resolved before the diagnosis is established, all patients with blastomycosis should be treated with an antifungal agent. Patients who have mild-to-moderate pulmonary or disseminated blastomycosis should be treated with itraconazole, 200 mg once or twice daily. The length of treatment is 6 to 12 months to achieve mycologic cure and prevent relapse. Fluconazole is not as effective as itraconazole. However, if the patient is unable to take itraconazole, fluconazole can be used, but the dosage should be 400 to 800 mg/day for 6 to 12 months. Voriconazole is increasingly reported to be effective in patients unable to tolerate itraconazole. Successful use of posaconazole has been reported in only a few patients. The echinocandins are not active against *B. dermatitidis* and should not be used.

Patients who have severe pulmonary or disseminated blastomycosis, all patients with CNS infection,[10] and most immunosuppressed patients should be treated initially with a lipid formulation of amphotericin B. The dosage is 3 to 5 mg/kg daily, except for CNS infection, for which 5 mg/kg daily should be used. After clinical improvement has occurred, usually within several weeks, therapy can be changed to itraconazole, 200 mg twice daily for a total of at least 12 months of therapy. For all patients who are treated with itraconazole, serum levels should be determined when steady state has been reached after 2 weeks of therapy to ensure adequate absorption. Serum concentrations should be greater than 1 µg/mL. Corticosteroids have been helpful as adjunctive therapy for patients with ARDS associated with blastomycosis, but this practice remains controversial.

PROGNOSIS

The prognosis for patients with pulmonary or disseminated blastomycosis treated with itraconazole is excellent; more than 90% are cured.[11] If relapse does occur, a second course of itraconazole is usually successful. Most reported deaths occur in patients with overwhelming pneumonia and ARDS.

GENERAL REFERENCES

For the General References and other additional features, please visit Expert Consult at https://expertconsult.inkling.com.

335

PARACOCCIDIOIDOMYCOSIS

CAROL A. KAUFFMAN

DEFINITION

Paracoccidioidomycosis (South American blastomycosis) is a subacute to chronic mycosis that is endemic in Central and South America. The disease is characterized primarily by pulmonary, mucous membrane, and cutaneous lesions, but disseminated disease also occurs.[1]

The Pathogen

Paracoccidioides brasiliensis is a thermally dimorphic fungus. In the environment and at temperatures below 35° C, the organism is a mold that produces conidia, the infectious form. In tissues and at 37° C in vitro, the organism assumes the yeast form with multiple narrow-based daughter cells attached to the mother cell.

EPIDEMIOLOGY

P. brasiliensis exists only in humid areas of Central and South America. More than 80% of cases are from Brazil. The presumed ecologic niche is in soil, but the exact conditions that favor growth of the organism have not been elucidated. The disease is most prevalent in middle-aged to elderly men from rural areas. The reason for the sexual imbalance (male-to-female ratio of 13 : 1 in many reports, but as high as 70 : 1 in one report from Colombia) is possibly related to the inhibitory effects of estrogens on transition from the mold to the yeast phase of the organism,[2] rather than solely environmental exposure. Although the disease classically develops later in life, it is likely that initial exposure occurs many years earlier. Cases seen in areas outside Central and South America have all been linked to previous residence in the endemic area.

PATHOBIOLOGY

Paracoccidioidomycosis develops after the inhalation of aerosolized conidia encountered in the environment. Once in the alveoli, the mycelial phase converts to the yeast phase. The infection may remain localized to the lungs, although it is likely that asymptomatic hematogenous dissemination occurs during most infections. In most patients, manifestations of disease do not develop at the time of the initial infection. The primary host defense mechanism against *P. brasiliensis* appears to be cell-mediated immunity, but neutrophils also play a role in host defense. The histopathologic picture includes both neutrophilic and granulomatous responses. There have been increasing reports of paracoccidioidomycosis in patients infected with human immunodeficiency virus (HIV)[3] and in other immunosuppressed patients; in these patients there is widespread dissemination, and histopathologic examination shows poorly formed granulomas. Reactivation of latent infection acquired years earlier is the presumed pathogenesis of most cases of the chronic adult form of paracoccidioidomycosis and cases that appear years after the patient has left the endemic area.

CLINICAL MANIFESTATIONS

Acute-Subacute (Juvenile) Paracoccidioidomycosis

The acute-subacute form of paracoccidioidomycosis occurs in less than 10% of patients. It is a disease of the reticuloendothelial system with widespread dissemination to the liver, spleen, lymph nodes, and bone marrow. Patients younger than 30 years typically have this form of paracoccidioidomycosis; however, older adults, especially those who are immunosuppressed, also can manifest this type of rapidly progressive disease. In patients with HIV infection, rapid progression occurs with multiple cutaneous lesions, lymphadenopathy, hepatosplenomegaly, and severe pulmonary involvement with hypoxemia.

Chronic (Adult) Paracoccidioidomycosis

Chronic paracoccidioidomycosis is slowly progressive over many years and is the form seen in more than 90% of patients. Most patients with this type of paracoccidioidomycosis are older men. Pulmonary involvement is prominent and clinically mimics tuberculosis and other chronic fungal pneumonias.[4] Radiographically, nodular, interstitial, or cavitary lesions are seen but differ from those of tuberculosis and histoplasmosis in that the infiltrates tend to be in the middle and lower lung fields rather than the apices. Many patients with the adult form of paracoccidioidomycosis also have ulcerative or nodular mucous membrane lesions, primarily in the anterior nares, the oral cavity, and the larynx; these are slowly destructive and can lead to dysphonia and stenosis of the airway. Cutaneous lesions, particularly on the face, are also common and may be papular, nodular, ulcerative, or plaquelike. The mucocutaneous lesions must be differentiated from mucocutaneous leishmaniasis and squamous cell carcinoma. Adrenal involvement has been reported in more than 90% of cases at autopsy, but adrenal insufficiency is only noted in about half.

DIAGNOSIS

Definitive diagnosis of paracoccidioidomycosis is established by growth of *P. brasiliensis* in culture. The organism may take as long as 4 weeks to grow. For seriously ill patients, direct examination of body fluids, sputum, or purulent material treated with potassium hydroxide or calcofluor fluorescent stain or histopathologic examination of tissue biopsy samples can provide a presumptive diagnosis while awaiting culture results. The characteristic appearance of *P. brasiliensis* consists of thick-walled yeast cells that have multiple small, circumferentially attached, narrow-based budding daughter yeast cells—a distinctive morphologic picture likened to a ship's steering wheel.

A variety of immunodiffusion assays, enzyme immunoassays, and complement fixation assays are available in endemic areas, but sensitivity and specificity vary greatly. The immunodiffusion assay appears to be most useful.[5] An assay for circulating cell wall antigens of *P. brasiliensis* has also been developed in endemic areas, but its role has not been established.

TREATMENT

The drug of choice for the treatment of paracoccidioidomycosis is itraconazole (200 mg/day for 6 to 12 months). Ketoconazole at a dosage of 200 to 400 mg daily for 1 year is effective and certainly less expensive than itraconazole, but the incidence of side effects is greater and relapses occur more frequently than with itraconazole. Fluconazole is less effective and should not be used unless no other agent is available. Voriconazole has been shown to be as effective as itraconazole in a randomized open-label pilot study, and there are scattered reports of the successful use of posaconazole as salvage therapy. Sulfonamides have been used for years to treat paracoccidioidomycosis and are clearly the most inexpensive form of treatment. However, relapse rates are higher than with the azoles. Amphotericin B is effective but rarely required, except in immunosuppressed patients with life-threatening disseminated disease. Most HIV-infected patients with paracoccidioidomycosis have been treated with amphotericin B as initial therapy, followed by lifelong suppressive therapy with either itraconazole or trimethoprim-sulfamethoxazole. Adjunctive corticosteroids have been used in a few patients with severe infection and appeared to be useful, but this remains controversial.[6]

PROGNOSIS

Patients with paracoccidioidomycosis have an excellent response to antifungal therapy, with overall relapse rates of about 5% with itraconazole therapy.[7] Although HIV-infected patients respond less well. Patients who have extensive pulmonary involvement at the time of diagnosis are at high risk for progressive fibrosis despite antifungal therapy.

GENERAL REFERENCES

For the General References and other additional features, please visit Expert Consult at https://expertconsult.inkling.com.

336
CRYPTOCOCCOSIS
CAROL A. KAUFFMAN

DEFINITION

Cryptococcosis occurs most often in persons who are immunosuppressed, especially those infected with human immunodeficiency virus (HIV). Meningitis is the most common clinical manifestation, but pulmonary and other organ involvement occur as well.

The Pathogen

Among the approximately 40 species of *Cryptococcus*, *Cryptococcus neoformans* and, much less often, *Cryptococcus gattii* are the predominant pathogens in humans.[1] In the environment, *Cryptococcus* species exist as yeasts that have minimal capsules and are easily aerosolized and inhaled. In tissues, *C. neoformans* and *C. gattii* are enveloped by a large polysaccharide capsule that is a major virulence factor. *C. neoformans* is found in the soil and grows well in avian droppings that have high nitrogen content. *C. gattii* is more restricted geographically and has been described mostly in Australia and Southeast Asia, where the ecological niche is the eucalyptus tree. However, the epidemiology of *C. gattii* is evolving with its emergence in the past decade in the Pacific Northwest and now in other areas of North America; the ecologic niche has not been definitively established in these areas. Most of this chapter focuses on *C. neoformans*, which is more common and which has been studied extensively.

EPIDEMIOLOGY

Before the widespread availability of antiretroviral therapy (ART), cryptococcosis occurred in 5 to 10% of patients with acquired immunodeficiency syndrome (AIDS), and almost always in those with fewer than 50 CD4 cells/μL. Cryptococcosis is less commonly seen now in Europe and North America but is extremely common in Africa, where it is estimated that the prevalence among HIV-infected patients is as high as 30%.

In the non-AIDS population, cryptococcosis is a frequent opportunistic infection in patients who have received a solid organ transplant,[2] have been treated with corticosteroids, or have diabetes mellitus, renal failure, cirrhosis, or chronic pulmonary disease. For some patients, the only risk factor appears to be older age. In every reported series, separate from those dealing only with HIV infection, approximately 20% of patients have no known underlying illness. *C. gattii* most often causes illness in normal hosts.[3]

PATHOBIOLOGY

The organism is inhaled from the environment and causes pulmonary infection initially. The primary host defense at this stage is complement-dependent macrophage and neutrophil phagocytosis and killing. Natural killer cells also have the ability to kill the organism. Ultimately, however, T-cell immunity is the most important host determinant in limiting the replication of *C. neoformans*. In most normal hosts, the infection remains localized to the lungs and does not cause symptomatic infection. It is likely that a few organisms exist as walled-off subpleural granulomas in many who have had pulmonary infection. If the host becomes immunosuppressed, the organism can then reactivate and disseminate to other sites. *C. neoformans* is clearly neurotropic, and the primary disease manifestation is meningoencephalitis. However, dissemination to many organs is likely, especially in those with deficient T-cell immunity.

Virulence factors for *C. neoformans* include the capsule, which requires opsonization for efficient phagocytosis, and the production of melanin, which has been shown to occur in vivo and enables the organism to resist intracellular killing. Both of these factors may help explain the virulence of the organism once it has reached the central nervous system (CNS). Antibody and complement levels are low in the brain, and thus phagocytosis of the organism is minimal. Brain tissue provides high concentrations of substrates, such as catecholamines, for the phenol oxidase enzyme systems of *C. neoformans* that produce melanin, thereby aiding survival of the organism.

CLINICAL MANIFESTATIONS

Central Nervous System Infection

The most common manifestation of cryptococcosis is CNS infection.[4] The typical picture is subacute to chronic meningoencephalitis. Patients usually have increasingly severe headaches over a period of several weeks. Other symptoms and signs include nuchal rigidity, lethargy, personality changes, confusion, visual abnormalities (photophobia, diplopia, decreased visual acuity, papilledema, extraocular nerve palsies), and nausea and vomiting. Less commonly, hearing loss, ataxia, and seizures occur. Fever is present in only approximately half the patients. Elderly persons with cryptococcal meningitis may have just dementia, without other neurologic findings. AIDS patients often have subtle CNS symptoms but usually have fever and other constitutional symptoms and rapidly manifest signs of dissemination.

Pulmonary Infection

In non-HIV-infected patients, the most common underlying risk factor for pulmonary cryptococcal infection is chronic obstructive pulmonary disease, followed by corticosteroid use and receipt of a solid organ transplant. *C. neoformans* may merely be an airway colonizer in some patients; in others, symptomatic infection, manifested by fever, cough, and dyspnea, requires treatment with an antifungal agent. The typical lesion noted with pulmonary cryptococcosis is a pleural-based nodular lesion. However, patchy pneumonitis, multiple nodular lesions, cavitary lesions, masslike lesions, and diffuse pulmonary infiltrates have all been noted with pulmonary cryptococcosis. Patients with advanced HIV infection are likely to have diffuse infiltrates that can progress rapidly to acute respiratory insufficiency. All immunosuppressed patients who have pulmonary cryptococcosis and all patients with any CNS symptoms should undergo lumbar puncture to be certain that meningitis is not present. Whether normal hosts with isolated pulmonary cryptococcosis and negative serum antigen tests require lumbar puncture remains controversial.

Involvement of Other Organs

C. neoformans has been reported to infect most organs during the course of disseminated infection, especially in AIDS patients. Skin lesions are a prominent clue to dissemination. Papules that resemble molluscum contagiosum or an acneiform rash, nodules, ulcers, plaques, draining sinuses, and cellulitis have all been reported. Focal involvement can occur in the prostate and other organs of the genitourinary tract, in osteoarticular structures, in the breast, and in the eye, larynx, and other head and neck structures. The prostate, in particular, has been noted as a sanctuary from which persisting organisms can later disseminate.

DIAGNOSIS

The diagnosis of cryptococcosis is established when the yeast is grown in culture. Appropriate specimens for culture include cerebrospinal fluid (CSF), blood, sputum, material from skin lesions, and other body fluids or tissues that appear to be infected. The organism grows in several days on most standard agar media. Most automated blood culture systems allow rapid growth of *C. neoformans*. Visualization of the capsule and performance of a few simple tests differentiate *C. neoformans* from other yeasts. Tissue biopsy shows the 5- to 10-μm yeast surrounded by the capsule. Definitive diagnosis of cryptococcosis can be made by mucicarmine staining, which selectively stains the polysaccharide capsule a deep rose color. In CSF or other body fluids, an India ink preparation allows visualization of the budding yeast cells surrounded by the large capsule, but this test is not currently done by many laboratories.

The latex agglutination assay for cryptococcal polysaccharide antigen (CRAG) is a highly sensitive and specific diagnostic test.[5] CRAG is positive in CSF in almost 100% and in serum in about 75% of patients who have meningitis. In AIDS patients, serum CRAG is almost always positive and is an excellent screening tool, and in these patients, titers in both CSF and serum are exceptionally high because of the enormous burden of organisms. In non-AIDS patients who have pulmonary cryptococcosis, the CRAG assay is positive in only 25 to 50% of cases. False-positive results with the CRAG assay are uncommon but have been reported in patients with *Trichosporon asahii* infections because of cross-reacting antigens shared by both fungi.

A newer technique, lateral flow analysis (LFA) to detect cryptococcal polysaccharide antigen has been developed as a dipstick assay, similar to that of pregnancy tests, that can be performed in serum or urine at the point of care by clinicians caring for the patient. This technique appears to be as sensitive and specific as the classic CRAG test.

The CSF of patients with cryptococcal meningitis typically has an increased number of white blood cells (but rarely >500/μL), a predominance of lymphocytes (although neutrophils are sometimes prominent early in the course), elevated protein, and decreased glucose. AIDS patients most often have normal or only mildly abnormal findings as a result of their markedly defective immune response. Despite normal CSF findings with regard to cells, protein, and glucose, every AIDS patient with a headache must have a CRAG or LFA test and culture performed on CSF. It is extremely important that an opening pressure be obtained when lumbar puncture is performed. Especially in AIDS patients, extremely high intracranial pressure (>350 mm H_2O) has been associated with poor outcomes and must be aggressively lowered.

All patients with cryptococcal meningitis should undergo computed tomography or magnetic resonance imaging of the brain to look for mass lesions and to assess ventricular size. Obstructive hydrocephalus is uncommon but requires a shunting procedure to decrease the pressure. More commonly, the increased intracranial pressure with cryptococcal infection is associated with normal-sized ventricles and is due to blockage at the arachnoid villi or increased brain edema (or both), perhaps related to the osmotic effect of the polysaccharide capsule. Different methods for reducing pressure are used in this situation.

TREATMENT   Rx

Guidelines for the treatment of cryptococcal infection have been published by the Infectious Diseases Society of America (IDSA).

Central Nervous System Infection

Early multicenter randomized trials in non-AIDS patients showed superiority of the combination of amphotericin B and flucytosine for 6 weeks over amphotericin B alone for 10 weeks. Subsequent randomized trials in the azole era have been performed only in the AIDS population. They have confirmed the benefit of flucytosine added to amphotericin B for induction therapy and have shown that initial therapy with fluconazole alone or with amphotericin B alone is not as effective as therapy with amphotericin B and flucytosine. The combination of amphotericin B and flucytosine has been shown to be the most rapidly fungicidal regimen, and increasing number of reports have documented that rapid fungicidal activity that clears the organism from the CSF is associated with improved outcomes. Regimens using amphotericin B with fluconazole or flucytosine with fluconazole[A1] are less effective but reasonable alternatives when the preferred regimen of amphotericin B plus flucytosine is not available.

Current recommendations for AIDS patients are to give induction therapy with intravenous amphotericin B deoxycholate, 0.7 to 1 mg/kg daily, combined with oral flucytosine, 100 mg/kg daily given in four divided doses for at least 2 weeks, followed by consolidation therapy with oral fluconazole, 400 mg daily for a minimum of 8 weeks, and then suppressive therapy with fluconazole, 200 mg daily. Lipid formulations of amphotericin B at daily dosages of 3 to 5 mg/kg daily are increasingly used because they are less nephrotoxic; however, they are often not available in developing countries. Induction therapy with amphotericin B (1 mg/kg per day for 4 weeks) plus flucytosine (100 mg/kg per day for 2 weeks) is associated with improved survival among HIV-positive patients with cryptococcal meningitis compared with either amphotericin B alone or amphotericin B plus fluconazole (400 mg twice daily for 2 weeks).

For patients who have undergone 12 months of antifungal therapy, who have CD4+ counts higher than 100/μL, and whose HIV viral load is undetectable on antiretroviral therapy, the suppressive therapy can be stopped. Suppressive therapy with fluconazole for transplant recipients is recommended for 6 to 12 months. The IDSA guideline recommendations[6] for non-HIV-infected, non–transplant recipients are to treat with amphotericin B deoxycholate, 0.7 to 1.0 mg/kg daily, plus flucytosine, 100 mg/kg daily, in four divided doses for at least 4 weeks for induction therapy, followed by consolidation therapy with fluconazole, 400 mg daily for 8 weeks, and suppressive therapy with fluconazole, 200 mg daily for 6 to 12 months. Again, many physicians use lipid formulations of amphotericin B, 3 to 5 mg/kg daily, in this population, many of whom are older and have underlying medical illnesses.

Only one treatment trial used voriconazole in combination with amphotericin B, and there are just a few case reports on the use of voriconazole and posaconazole for salvage treatment of cryptococcal meningitis. These are reasonable alternatives if no other azoles can be used. The echinocandins are not active against *C. neoformans* and should not be used.

A significant observation from the AIDS treatment trials was the role of increased intracranial pressure as a cause of early death from cryptococcal meningitis. An aggressive approach to the diagnosis and treatment of increased intracranial pressure in both AIDS and non-AIDS patients is mandatory and should include daily lumbar puncture or placement of a temporary lumbar drain or ventriculostomy until the opening pressure remains lower than 190 mm H_2O. Treatment with corticosteroids, acetazolamide, or mannitol has not proved efficacious in this setting.

Another issue that has emerged is the development of immune reconstitution inflammatory syndrome (IRIS), which can occur in patients with AIDS who are receiving effective antiretroviral therapy (ART) that increases the CD4 count (Chapter 395). Symptoms of meningitis reappear and are due to the inflammatory response and not to a relapse of disease. In a recently reported trial, HIV-positive patients with cryptococcal meningitis who had not previously received ART were randomized to initiate either earlier ART (1 to 2 weeks after meningitis diagnosis) or deferred ART (5 weeks after diagnosis), with all patients treated for cryptococcal meningitis with amphotericin B (0.7 to 1.0 mg/kg/day) plus fluconazole (800 mg per day) for 14 days, followed by fluconazole consolidation therapy. Although the incidence of recognized cryptococcal IRIS did not differ significantly between the earlier and deferred ART groups, deferring ART for 5 weeks after diagnosis was associated with significantly improved survival, especially among patients with a paucity of CSF white cells.[A3] IRIS can also occur in transplant recipients in whom immunosuppressive therapy is decreased rapidly. Generally, no specific therapy is needed for mild IRIS, but sometimes corticosteroids are needed if increased intracranial pressure occurs.

Pulmonary and Other Nonmeningeal Infections

Treatment of nonmeningeal cryptococcosis depends on the severity of the infection. Many patients with isolated pulmonary or other focal infections are not severely ill, and oral fluconazole, 400 mg daily for 6 to 12 months, is recommended. For patients who are severely ill, therapy is the same as noted earlier for CNS infection.

PROGNOSIS

The outcome for both AIDS and non-AIDS patients with cryptococcal meningitis has improved markedly in the developed world. However, in Africa the mortality from cryptococcal meningitis in AIDS patients approaches 100% in some areas because of lack of access to specific therapy. Dementia, which usually occurs in older patients, hearing loss, and visual loss may not be reversed even though mycologic cure is achieved. Fluconazole, 200 mg three times per week, is safe and effective as primary prophylaxis against cryptococcal disease in cryptococcal antigen-negative, HIV-infected adults with CD4 counts lower than 200 cells/μL, both before and during early antiretroviral treatment.[A4]

 Grade A References

A1. Nussbaum JC, Jackson A, Namarika D, et al. Combination flucytosine and high-dose fluconazole compared with fluconazole monotherapy for the treatment of cryptococcal meningitis: a randomized trial in Malawi. *Clin Infect Dis.* 2010;50:338-344.

A2. Day JN, Chau TT, Wolbers M, et al. Combination antifungal theory for cryptococcal meningitis. *N Engl J Med.* 2013;368:1291-1302.

A3. Boulware DR, Meya DB, Muzoora C, et al. Timing of antiretroviral therapy after diagnosis of cryptococcal meningitis. *N Engl J Med.* 2014;370:2487-2498.

A4. Parkes-Ratanshi R, Wakeham K, Levin J, et al. Primary prophylaxis of cryptococcal disease with fluconazole in HIV-positive Ugandan adults: a double-blind randomised, placebo-controlled trial. *Lancet Infect Dis.* 2011;11:933-941.

GENERAL REFERENCES

For the General References and other additional features, please visit Expert Consult at https://expertconsult.inkling.com.

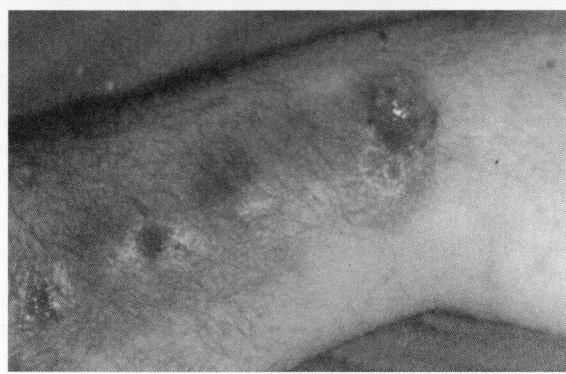

FIGURE 337-1. Lymphocutaneous sporotrichosis. The lesion at the inoculation site has ulcerated. (From Watanakunakorn C.: Photoquiz. *Clin Infect Dis.* 1996;22:765.)

337

SPOROTRICHOSIS

CAROL A. KAUFFMAN

DEFINITION

Sporotrichosis is a subacute or chronic infection that is usually localized to cutaneous and lymphocutaneous structures, but pulmonary, osteoarticular, and disseminated infection can occur in patients who have certain underlying diseases.

The Pathogen

Sporothrix schenckii is a thermally dimorphic fungus. In the environment at temperatures lower than 35° to 37° C, the organism is a mold and produces conidia, the infectious form. In tissues and at 35° to 37° C, *S. schenckii* transforms into the yeast phase; the yeasts are 4 to 6 μm in diameter; are cigar shaped, round, or oval; and reproduce by budding.

EPIDEMIOLOGY

S. schenckii is found worldwide in climates ranging from temperate to tropical.[1] The organism exists in a variety of environmental niches, including soil, sphagnum moss, hay, decaying wood, and other vegetation. Infection is seen almost entirely in persons whose vocation, avocation, or living condition brings them into contact with the organism in the environment. Landscaping activities, gardening, farming, and motor vehicle collisions have been associated with sporotrichosis. Inhalation of *S. schenckii* conidia occurs less commonly and results in pulmonary and, rarely, disseminated sporotrichosis. Most cases of sporotrichosis are sporadic, but outbreaks have been described. An extensive outbreak extending over many years in Rio de Janeiro and occurring mostly in children and women has been traced to infected domestic cats.

PATHOBIOLOGY

Infection is almost always acquired by inoculation of conidia and remains localized to the immediate and contiguous cutaneous, subcutaneous, and lymphatic structures. Some strains of *S. schenckii* grow poorly at temperatures higher than 35° C; these strains usually cause fixed cutaneous lesions without lymphatic spread. The typical host response to infection with *S. schenckii* is a mixed neutrophilic and granulomatous reaction. Antibody is not protective; cell-mediated immunity is important in containing the infection. In individuals who have underlying illnesses, including alcoholism, diabetes mellitus, and chronic obstructive pulmonary disease, *S. schenckii* is more likely to involve osteoarticular structures and the lungs. Widespread dissemination develops in persons infected with human immunodeficiency virus (HIV) but is a distinctly unusual event in normal hosts.[2]

CLINICAL MANIFESTATIONS

Lymphocutaneous

Days to weeks after inoculation of *S. schenckii* conidia, a papular lesion develops at the inoculation site; the lesion becomes nodular and often ulcerates (Fig. 337-1). Drainage is not grossly purulent, and the lesion is not terribly painful. Similar lesions occur along the lymphatic distribution proximal to the primary lesion. Verrucous or ulcerative fixed cutaneous lesions do not exhibit lymphatic extension. The differential diagnosis of lymphocutaneous sporotrichosis includes *Nocardia* infections (Chapter 330), particularly *Nocardia brasiliensis*; atypical mycobacterial infections (Chapter 325), especially *Mycobacterium marinum*; *Leishmania brasiliensis* infections (Chapter 348); and tularemia (Chapter 311).

Visceral and Osteoarticular

Pulmonary sporotrichosis[3] occurs most often in middle-aged men who have chronic pulmonary disease and abuse alcohol. Fever, night sweats, weight loss, fatigue, dyspnea, cough, purulent sputum, and hemoptysis are common. Chest radiographs show unilateral or bilateral upper lobe cavities with variable amounts of fibrosis and nodular lesions. The disease mimics reactivation tuberculosis in many aspects. Osteoarticular sporotrichosis is found most often in middle-aged men and occurs more frequently in alcoholics. Infection may involve one or multiple joints; the joints most commonly affected are the knee, elbow, wrist, and ankle. Isolated bursitis, tenosynovitis, and nerve entrapment syndromes have been reported. Osteoarticular infection can follow local inoculation, but in most patients this occurs secondary to hematogenous spread. Isolated case reports document sporotrichosis involving the pericardium, eye, perirectal tissues, larynx, breast, epididymis, spleen, liver, bone marrow, lymph nodes, and meninges. Disseminated sporotrichosis, manifested as widespread ulcerative cutaneous lesions with or without visceral involvement, is uncommon; most cases have been reported in patients with advanced HIV infection.

DIAGNOSIS

Growth of *S. schenckii* from culture of material aspirated from a lesion, a tissue biopsy specimen, sputum, or body fluid is the most effective method of establishing the diagnosis of sporotrichosis. Growth of the mold phase of the organism is usually evident within a few days. Histopathologic examination of biopsy material shows a mixed granulomatous and pyogenic process; however, the organisms are often present in small numbers and are frequently not visualized. Serology is not useful in the diagnosis of sporotrichosis. Polymerase chain reaction testing has been used to confirm the diagnosis[4] but must be obtained at a fungal reference laboratory.

TREATMENT   Rx

Because sporotrichosis is usually a localized subacute to chronic infection, oral antifungal agents are preferred; amphotericin B is reserved for severe visceral infections. Guidelines for the management of sporotrichosis have been published by the Infectious Diseases Society of America.[5] Itraconazole is the drug of choice for lymphocutaneous sporotrichosis.[6] The usual dosage is 200 mg daily, and treatment should continue for several weeks after all lesions have disappeared, generally for a total of 3 to 6 months. Saturated solution of potassium iodide (SSKI) has been used to treat sporotrichosis for almost a century. The initial dose is 5 to 10 drops three times daily in water or juice, with the dose increasing over a period of several weeks to a maximum of 40 to 50 drops three times daily. SSKI has many side effects, including salivary gland swelling, metallic taste, rash, and fever; the only advantage is that it is inexpensive. Fluconazole is less effective than itraconazole but for occasional patients can be used at a dosage of 400 to 800 mg daily. Voriconazole is not active against *S. schenckii*, and there is minimal experience using posaconazole. Terbinafine appears to be effective for sporotrichosis at a dosage of 500 mg twice daily. Local hyperthermia, induced by a variety of different warming devices or baths, has been shown to be effective in some patients with fixed cutaneous lesions.

Osteoarticular and pulmonary sporotrichosis are usually treated with itraconazole, 200 mg twice daily for 1 to 2 years. Other azoles are less effective, and SSKI is ineffective. In a seriously ill patient with pulmonary sporotrichosis, a lipid formulation of amphotericin B at a dosage of 3 to 5 mg/kg daily should be used as initial therapy. After the patient has shown improvement, therapy can be changed to itraconazole. A lipid formulation of amphotericin B, at a dosage of 3 to 5 mg/kg daily, is the drug of choice for disseminated sporotrichosis. Therapy can be changed to itraconazole, 200 mg twice daily, once the patient has stabilized. Patients with HIV infection and disseminated sporotrichosis should remain on lifelong maintenance therapy with itraconazole, 200 mg daily.

For all patients who are treated with itraconazole, serum levels should be determined when steady state has been reached after 2 weeks of therapy to ensure adequate absorption. Serum concentrations should be greater than 1 µg/mL.

PROGNOSIS

The prognosis for patients with cutaneous and lymphocutaneous sporotrichosis is excellent. Almost all patients are cured with one course of therapy; relapses occur in only a small proportion of patients. Extracutaneous forms of sporotrichosis do not respond well to therapy, partly because of delays in diagnosis and partly because of the underlying diseases that are frequently found in those who have extracutaneous sporotrichosis. The outcome of disseminated sporotrichosis in patients with HIV infection has improved in recent years with effective antiretroviral therapy.

GENERAL REFERENCES

For the General References and other additional features, please visit Expert Consult at https://expertconsult.inkling.com.

338

CANDIDIASIS

CAROL A. KAUFFMAN

DEFINITION

Candidiasis encompasses a wide variety of clinical syndromes caused by yeasts of the genus *Candida*. Of the species that cause infection in humans, *Candida albicans* is the most common; *Candida glabrata*, *Candida parapsilosis*, and *Candida tropicalis* are responsible for most of the remaining infections. Organisms such as *Candida krusei*, *Candida lusitaniae*, and *Candida guilliermondii* are less common causes of infection.

The Pathogen

Candida species are 2- to 6-µm yeastlike organisms that reproduce by budding. Most species, with the exception of *C. glabrata*, form pseudohyphae (elongated buds that remain attached to the mother cell) and hyphae in tissues.

Candida species cause a wide spectrum of diseases ranging in severity from localized mucous membrane infection to life-threatening disseminated disease. The major determinant of the severity of infection is the host's immune response. Local infections are often related to overgrowth of *Candida* as a result of changes in the normal microbiota. Invasive infections that remain within an organ system, such as urinary tract infections, usually occur because of local anatomic abnormalities. In an immunosuppressed host, especially a patient with neutropenia, widespread visceral dissemination is common.

EPIDEMIOLOGY

Candida species reside normally in the gastrointestinal and genitourinary tracts and on the skin. As colonizers, *Candida* species do not cause infection unless there is a defect in host defense mechanisms or unless exogenous factors, such as antibiotic use, have upset the ecology of the normal microbiota. *C. albicans* is the species most commonly found colonizing humans; *C. glabrata* is the second most common species, and *C. tropicalis*, *C. parapsilosis*, and others are found less often. The species of *Candida* colonizing and infecting patients has changed in recent decades in that *C. glabrata*, a species that is increasingly resistant to fluconazole, has become a prominent pathogen in many hospitals.

Though uncommon, acquisition of *Candida* from environmental sources has been noted. The *Candida* species most often associated with transmission from contaminated fluids or devices, especially central intravenous catheters, has been *C. parapsilosis*.

Candidiasis is the most common opportunistic fungal infection as a result of both the organisms' ubiquity and the increasing number of patients with risk factors for infection with these organisms.[1] The classic immunosuppressed host at risk for serious *Candida* infections is a neutropenic patient with a hematologic malignancy who has received cytotoxic agents and corticosteroids. Increasingly, however, candidiasis is seen in patients in intensive care units (ICUs). Risk factors for the development of serious *Candida* infections in ICU patients include the use of broad-spectrum antimicrobials, indwelling central venous catheters, previous surgical procedures, renal failure, parenteral nutrition, and high Acute Physiology and Chronic Health Evaluation (APACHE) score. Certain ICU populations, especially very-low-birthweight neonates and burn victims, are at even higher risk for *Candida* infection than is the typical ICU patient.

The primary manifestation of *Candida* infection in patients with HIV/AIDS is mucocutaneous infection, primarily oropharyngeal candidiasis. The development of mucosal *Candida* infection is related to deficient T-cell immunity as reflected by a low CD4 lymphocyte count. With appropriate antiretroviral therapy, oropharyngeal candidiasis has become an uncommon opportunistic infection.

PATHOBIOLOGY

The usual mode of infection with *Candida* is egress from its normal niche into the bloodstream or other tissues; the source is usually the gastrointestinal tract, but the skin and genitourinary tract are other sources. The primary host defense in response to this event is phagocytosis and killing by neutrophils, monocytes, and macrophages. C-C chemokine receptor 2 (CCR2)-expressing inflammatory monocytes and their tissue-resident derivatives play an essential antifungal role, particularly in the first 48 hours after *Candida* infection.[2] Phagocytosis is enhanced in the presence of specific anti-*Candida* antibody and complement. Several different mechanisms are operative within neutrophils and macrophages that allow the killing of yeasts. Thus, patients who are leukopenic, especially those with chemotherapy-induced disruption of the gut mucosa, are at great risk for invasion with *Candida* species. Once *Candida* gains access to the bloodstream, widespread hematogenous dissemination is the rule. Biopsy of involved organs shows multiple microabscesses composed of neutrophils (in a host who has these cells), budding yeasts, and often pseudohyphae or hyphae. Over time, the lesions show a mixed neutrophilic and granulomatous response.

T-cell immunity is an important host defense against infection with *Candida* at mucosal surfaces. In contrast to those with neutropenia, patients with deficient T-cell immunity are at risk for persistent and recurrent mucocutaneous candidiasis, but invasive infection rarely develops.

CLINICAL MANIFESTATIONS

Mucocutaneous Candidiasis

Oropharyngeal Candidiasis

Local mucous membrane and cutaneous lesions are the most common forms of *Candida* infection. Oropharyngeal candidiasis, or *thrush* (Chapter 425), can be due to either local factors or T-cell dysfunction. Local factors include the use of broad-spectrum antimicrobials or inhaled corticosteroids, xerostomia, and radiation treatment of the head and neck. Denture stomatitis occurs frequently in persons who wear full upper dentures, especially those who do not remove their dentures at night.

Thrush secondary to T-cell dysfunction is most commonly seen in patients with HIV infection (Chapter 390) and is the most frequent opportunistic infection noted in patients with AIDS. The appearance of thrush in a

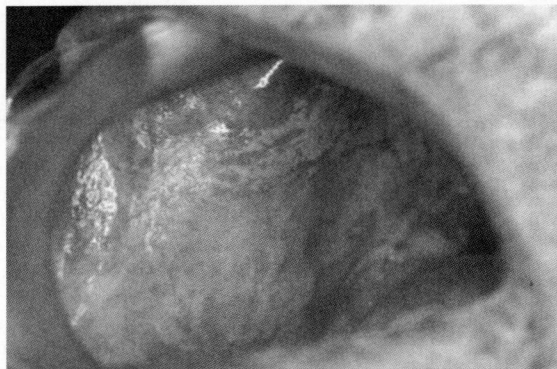

FIGURE 338-1. Thrush.

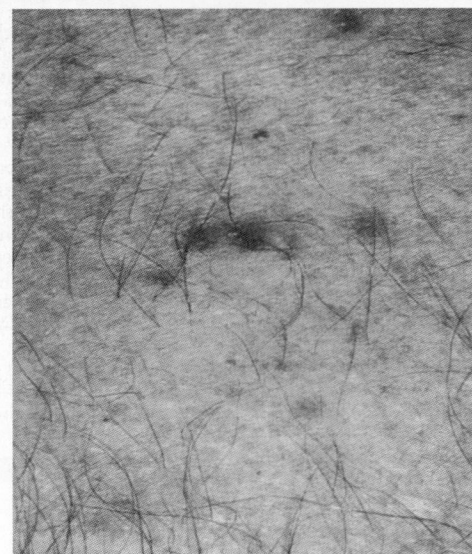

FIGURE 338-2. Skin lesions in invasive candidiasis.

previously healthy individual with no known risk factors should immediately raise suspicion of HIV infection.

Thrush manifests with white plaques on the buccal mucosa, palate, oropharynx, or tongue (Fig. 338-1). Scraping the lesions with a tongue depressor reveals an erythematous, nonulcerated mucosa under the plaques. Denture stomatitis almost always manifests as a painful erythematous palate without plaques. Angular cheilitis, or perlàche, which is the presence of painful cracks at the corners of the mouth, can occur with or without thrush.

Esophagitis

Esophagitis may accompany oropharyngeal candidiasis or may occur independently of lesions in the oropharynx (Chapter 138). The development of *Candida* esophagitis is almost always related to immune dysfunction and not simply to local factors. *Candida* esophagitis occurs in AIDS patients with low CD4 counts, patients with leukemia, and others taking immunosuppressive agents. The classic symptom of *Candida* esophagitis is odynophagia localized to a discrete substernal area. The differential diagnosis includes ulcerations due to herpes simplex or cytomegalovirus and, in AIDS patients, idiopathic ulcers.

Vulvovaginitis

Candida vulvovaginitis is a common infection in women of childbearing age and is the most frequent mucocutaneous manifestation of *Candida* infection.[3] Risk factors include conditions associated with increased estrogen levels, such as the use of oral contraceptives and pregnancy, diabetes mellitus, therapy with corticosteroids or broad-spectrum antimicrobials, and HIV infection. Symptoms include vaginal discomfort, discharge, and vulvar pruritus. The discharge is usually curdlike, but it can also be thin and watery. The labia are erythematous and swollen, and the vaginal walls show erythema and white plaques. Although most women have only a few episodes throughout their lives, a minority have frequent recurrences; in most of these patients, no discrete risk factor is found, and the cause is presumed to be local immune dysregulation.

Cutaneous Candidiasis

Candida infection of the skin (Chapter 441) occurs mostly in the intertriginous areas or under a large pannus or pendulous breasts. The lesions are erythematous, pruritic, and frequently pustular; have a distinct border; and are almost always associated with smaller satellite lesions, which helps distinguish candidiasis from tinea cruris or corporis. *Candida* onychomycosis results in thickened, opaque, and onycholytic nails. *Candida* can also cause paronychia, especially in those whose occupation involves frequent immersion of the hands in water.

Chronic Mucocutaneous Candidiasis

This uncommon syndrome usually begins in childhood and is characterized by recalcitrant and relapsing thrush, vaginitis, onychomycosis, and hyperkeratotic skin lesions on the face, scalp, and hands. Autosomal dominant chronic mucocutaneous candidiasis is associated with mutations in the CC domain of *STAT1* leading to defective T_H1 and T_H17 responses.[4] Some patients have associated autoimmune endocrinopathies, including hypoparathyroidism, hypothyroidism, and hypoadrenalism (autoimmune polyendocrinopathy-candidiasis-ectodermal dystrophy [APECED], which is

caused by a loss-of-function mutation of the autoimmune regulator gene, *AIRE*, and in these patients autoantibodies against interleukin-17 (IL-17) and IL-22 are found.[5] (See Autoimmune Polyglandular Syndrome Type 1 in Chapter 231.)

Disseminated Infections
Candidemia

The most common manifestation of disseminated *Candida* infection is candidemia. However, candidemia merely implies the presence of *Candida* in blood; it does not define the extent of visceral involvement. *Candida* obtained from a blood culture should never be considered a contaminant and should always prompt a search for the probable source and the extent of infection. Risk factors for candidemia include broad-spectrum antimicrobial therapy, central intravenous catheters, parenteral nutrition, renal failure, surgical procedures involving the gastrointestinal tract, neutropenia, and corticosteroid therapy. The attributable mortality from candidemia approaches 40%; overall mortality is higher in elderly patients and neonates.

Although candidemia is the most obvious manifestation of serious infection with *Candida* species, septic shock can occur, along with invasion of multiple viscera, in the absence of positive blood cultures.[6] The clinical picture of invasive candidiasis is indistinguishable from that of bacterial infection. The characteristic histologic picture consists of multiple microabscesses in many organs. The eyes, kidneys, liver, spleen, and brain are the most commonly involved sites, but virtually all organs can be involved. Clinical clues to the diagnosis of invasive candidiasis include the appearance of skin and retinal lesions. The nonpainful, nonpruritic skin lesions are papular to pustular and surrounded by a zone of erythema (Fig. 338-2). The eye lesions appear as distinctive white exudates in the retina (Fig. 338-3); with extension into the vitreous body, the retina becomes obscured.

Endocarditis

Candida endocarditis is an uncommon and often fatal complication of candidemia. It occurs most often in intravenous drug users, patients who have prosthetic cardiac valves, and those with central venous catheters in place. Blood cultures are usually persistently positive, and echocardiography reveals large vegetations that can readily embolize to major vessels.

Chronic Disseminated (Hepatosplenic) Candidiasis

This syndrome almost always occurs in leukemic patients who have had an episode of neutropenia. After the neutrophil count returns to normal, fevers that are often quite high, right upper quadrant tenderness, and nausea develop. The alkaline phosphatase level is generally elevated, and distinctive punched-out lesions are seen in the liver, spleen, and sometimes the kidneys on computed tomography (Fig. 338-4). Biopsy of these lesions shows microabscesses that contain budding yeasts.

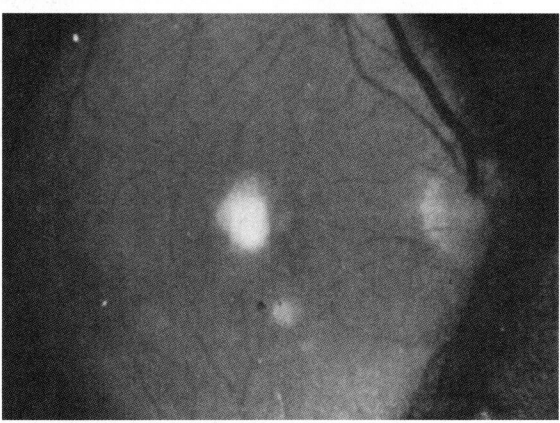

FIGURE 338-3. Retinal involvement.

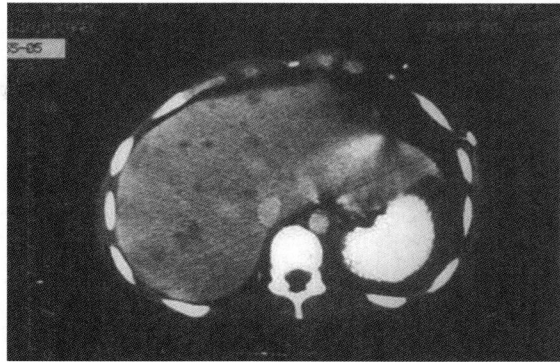

FIGURE 338-4. Computed tomography scan of a patient with chronic disseminated candidiasis (hepatosplenic candidiasis). Note the distinctive punched-out lesions in the liver.

Focal Invasive Infections

These forms of candidiasis result from local inoculation, contiguous spread, or hematogenous spread. Hematogenous spread, which often goes undetected, is probably the most common pathogenetic mechanism.

Urinary Tract Infections

Candiduria is a frequent finding in hospitalized patients and is related to factors such as diabetes mellitus, broad-spectrum antimicrobial treatment, indwelling urinary devices, and genitourinary tract structural abnormalities. Most patients with candiduria have only bladder colonization and not infection. Urinary tract infection with *Candida* species can arise by two mechanisms. Patients with candidemia can develop multiple microabscesses secondary to hematogenous spread to the kidneys. Other patients, who have the risk factors noted earlier, can develop cystitis or ascending infection with pyelonephritis. Patients with cystitis or pyelonephritis have symptoms indistinguishable from those of bacterial infections. A fungus ball composed of fungal hyphae can develop at any level of the collecting system and lead to obstruction, with subsequent infection.

Osteoarticular Infections

Osteoarticular infections arise secondary to hematogenous seeding or exogenous inoculation during intra-articular injection, a surgical procedure, or trauma. Vertebral osteomyelitis is the most common manifestation of osteoarticular candidiasis. The symptoms of back pain and fever may occur many weeks after an episode of fungemia.

Endophthalmitis

Exogenous endophthalmitis occurs secondary to trauma or ophthalmic surgery. Most often, the procedure involved is cataract extraction, with or without lens implantation, and the most common infecting species is *C. parapsilosis*. Primary infection occurs in the anterior chamber, but ultimately the posterior chamber is also involved. Endogenous *Candida* endophthalmitis results from hematogenous seeding of the choroid and retina and is one of the most serious complications of candidemia. Characteristic white lesions are visible in the retina, and with progression of the infection, vitritis occurs; the risk for loss of vision is quite high.

Peritonitis

Candida peritonitis can follow bowel surgery or perforation. Symptoms are the same as those noted in bacterial peritonitis. Usually, this type of infection is polymicrobial, and abscess formation is common. In patients maintained on continuous ambulatory peritoneal dialysis, *Candida* peritonitis generally develops as a late infection after previous episodes of bacterial peritonitis. A cloudy dialysate, abdominal pain, and fever are typically noted.

Meningitis

Acute *Candida* meningitis occurs as part of disseminated infection, especially in low-birthweight neonates. Chronic meningitis, an uncommon manifestation of candidiasis, resembles cryptococcal or tuberculous meningitis with regard to symptoms and cerebrospinal fluid findings.

DIAGNOSIS

The diagnosis of mucocutaneous candidiasis is often made clinically. Culture is rarely indicated. Confirmation can be sought by scraping the lesions and performing either a potassium hydroxide preparation or a Gram stain to look for budding yeasts (Chapter 436). In cases in which the disease is recurrent or unresponsive to standard therapy, lesions should be cultured to establish whether a more resistant species, such as *C. glabrata* or *C. krusei*, is the causative agent. In the event of suspected esophagitis, endoscopy shows plaque-like lesions or ulcerations, and biopsy shows mucosal invasion with budding yeasts and pseudohyphae.

The diagnosis of invasive candidiasis is more difficult. Evidence of dissemination is usually sought by culturing blood or other sterile body sites. The automated blood culture systems used by most hospitals are as sensitive as the lysis-centrifugation system for growing *Candida* from blood. However, no system is sensitive enough for clinicians to rely on blood cultures to establish the diagnosis of invasive candidiasis in all cases or to rule out candidiasis as a diagnostic possibility. In addition, 1 to 4 days is required for growth to occur; in a desperately ill patient, this delay is problematic.

The tips of intravenous catheters that have been removed should be sent for culture. However, no studies have evaluated the number of yeasts that is indicative of infection, and many physicians accept the growth of any yeast as affirming infection that requires treatment. Many focal forms of candidiasis are indistinguishable from bacterial infection, and biopsy should be performed for histopathologic and culture studies.

In a seriously ill patient suspected of having candidiasis, the development of pustular skin lesions or typical retinal lesions can be helpful. Budding yeasts typical of *Candida* species should be sought by smearing material from a pustule on a slide and staining it with Gram stain or by performing a biopsy of a lesion and staining the tissue section with a silver stain. All patients who are candidemic or suspected of having disseminated *Candida* infection should undergo a dilated ophthalmologic examination, preferably by an ophthalmologist, to look for typical retinal lesions.

Imaging studies are invaluable for certain forms of candidiasis, especially chronic disseminated candidiasis, and they can be of major help in defining the extent of infection in other types of *Candida* infection, such as osteoarticular and urinary tract infections and endocarditis.

There are increasing reports of using an assay for β-D-glucan, a cell wall component of fungi, or polymerase chain reaction (PCR) as diagnostic aids for invasive candidiasis.[7,8] The β-D-glucan assay is commercially available; sensitivity and specificity vary depending on the patient populations studied and further studies need to be performed to establish its role in diagnosis. PCR is not standardized, but some studies show that it is more sensitive than β-D-glucan and it may prove useful for earlier diagnosis.

TREATMENT   Rx

Guidelines for treatment of the various forms of candidiasis have been published by the Infectious Diseases Society of America (IDSA).[9] Mucocutaneous disease is obviously treated in a much different fashion than disseminated life-threatening infection. Because diagnostic tests are not sensitive, empirical therapy is indicated in some circumstances, and for patients at the highest risk for *Candida* infection, antifungal prophylaxis can decrease that risk.

Mucocutaneous Infections

Most mucocutaneous infections should initially be treated with local creams, solutions, troches, or suspensions.[10] For thrush, clotrimazole troches (10 mg four or five times daily) are preferred to nystatin suspension (commonly given as "swish and swallow" four times daily). Patients with AIDS may not respond to local therapy, especially when their CD4 counts are low; in this situation, oral fluconazole 100 to 200 mg daily is given. For vaginitis, a variety of creams and vaginal tablets (miconazole, clotrimazole, and others) are effective, but many women prefer to take a single 150-mg fluconazole tablet orally. Recurrent vaginitis is a more complicated therapeutic issue and often requires chronic suppressive therapy with fluconazole. Esophagitis should always be treated with a systemically absorbed agent; the usual treatment is fluconazole 200 mg/day for 14 days.

In patients with advanced AIDS and low CD4 counts, who are often taking fluconazole to prevent recurrent candidiasis, fluconazole-refractory disease may develop. For these patients, increasing the dosage of fluconazole or switching to itraconazole suspension 200 mg daily, voriconazole 200 mg twice daily, or posaconazole suspension 400 mg daily should be effective. If oral tablets and solutions are no longer effective, intravenous amphotericin B, caspofungin, anidulafungin, and micafungin are alternative agents that can be used. Patients with the syndrome of chronic mucocutaneous candidiasis require lifelong suppressive therapy with oral azole agents.

Candidemia and Invasive Candidiasis

All patients with candidemia should be treated with an antifungal agent, including patients who have only one blood culture that yields *Candida* and those with a vascular catheter tip that yields *Candida*. The rationale for this recommendation is related to the high rate of metastatic foci in major organs associated with hematogenously disseminated candidiasis. Randomized controlled trials have shown the effectiveness of the following antifungal agents for the treatment of candidemia: fluconazole 400 or 800 mg/day; the three echinocandins—caspofungin 50 mg/day, anidulafungin 100 mg/day, and micafungin 100 mg/day; voriconazole 3 mg/kg twice daily; amphotericin B 0.7 mg/kg/day; and a lipid formulation of amphotericin B 3 to 5 mg/kg/day. The IDSA guidelines recommend fluconazole for patients who are not severely ill and have not had recent azole exposure and an echinocandin for severely ill patients and those who have had recent azole exposure. Patients who have stabilized clinically and are found to have an isolate, such as *C. albicans*, that is likely to be susceptible to fluconazole can be transitioned to fluconazole from an echinocandin. Voriconazole is recommended for step-down therapy rather than initial therapy, and amphotericin B formulations are used infrequently, except for patients who are neutropenic and for neonates.

All vascular catheters should be removed because removal has been shown to help clear *Candida* from blood more quickly. Repeated blood cultures should be obtained to ascertain that the fungemia has resolved, and treatment should continue for 2 weeks after the date of the first negative blood culture. An individual patient-level quantitative review of seven randomized trials for the treatment of invasive candidiasis found an overall mortality in the entire data set of 31.4%.[11] Significant predictors of mortality included increasing age; use of immunosuppressive therapy; and infection with *C. tropicalis*. Improved survival and clinical success was found with the use of an echinocandin and the removal of central venous catheters.

Because diagnostic tests are not sensitive, seriously ill patients who could have invasive candidiasis may need to be treated before culture confirmation. This approach is used frequently in neutropenic patients and is increasingly used in the ICU setting.[12] Liposomal amphotericin B, caspofungin, and voriconazole have been shown to be effective for empirical use in neutropenic patients. A placebo-controlled, randomized trial of fluconazole empirical therapy in ICU patients failed to show a benefit; however, there were acknowledged problems with the chosen end point, and the rate of candidemia was too low to allow a proper evaluation of empirical therapy.[A1] The IDSA guidelines recommend that empirical therapy be reserved for febrile, critically ill patients who have risk factors for invasive candidiasis. The agents recommended are either fluconazole or an echinocandin, with the caveats noted earlier for treating patients with documented candidemia. Compelling data for early treatment come from a study of 224 candidemic patients who had septic shock. Mortality rates as high as 98% were found in patients in whom there was a delay beyond 24 hours of the onset of shock in initiating antifungal therapy and in effecting source control, defined as draining abscesses and removing central venous catheters.

Endocarditis should be treated with a lipid formulation of amphotericin B, with or without flucytosine. Echinocandins are an acceptable alternative. Infected valves should be replaced. In a few patients for whom valve replacement was not an option, lifelong suppression with fluconazole appeared to be effective.

Chronic disseminated candidiasis generally requires months of therapy for cure. Most patients begin therapy with a lipid formulation of amphotericin B and are then switched to fluconazole and treated until the lesions disappear on computed tomography scanning.

Focal Invasive Infections

Treatment of focal infections depends on the organ system involved. Perhaps the simplest to treat are urinary tract infections. Most patients with candiduria are not infected but merely colonized; removing the selective pressure of antimicrobials and indwelling catheters eliminates candiduria in many of these patients. For those who have infection, oral fluconazole at a dosage of 200 mg/day for 2 weeks is recommended. Bladder irrigation with amphotericin B should not be used because it eradicates only bladder colonization, requires that a catheter be placed in the bladder, and is associated with a high recurrence rate. None of the newer antifungal agents has a role in the treatment of urinary tract infections.

Osteoarticular infections require months of therapy; a lipid formulation of amphotericin B or an echinocandin can be given initially, followed by long-term therapy with an azole. Peritonitis associated with chronic ambulatory peritoneal dialysis can be treated with amphotericin B, fluconazole, or an echinocandin, depending on the species of *Candida* causing infection. Intraperitoneal administration of amphotericin B can be extremely irritating and should not be attempted. The dialysis catheter should be removed. Meningitis should be treated initially with a lipid formulation of amphotericin B and flucytosine; patients with more chronic disease can be switched to fluconazole for a longer duration of therapy.

Treatment of *Candida* eye infections varies with the extent of ocular involvement.[13] Lesions discovered early at the stage of choroidal or retinal involvement perhaps can be treated effectively with systemic antifungal agents (amphotericin B, an echinocandin, fluconazole, or voriconazole) alone. Many experts prefer to use an agent, such as voriconazole or fluconazole, that achieves higher concentrations in the eye. Lesions extending into the vitreous require more aggressive therapy. The best results have been obtained with pars plana vitrectomy, injection of amphotericin B or voriconazole into the vitreous; and a systemic antifungal agent such as fluconazole or voriconazole. Management must be individualized and performed in concert with an ophthalmologist experienced in the treatment of this infection. Treatment of endophthalmitis associated with an intraocular lens implant requires removal of the implant, vitrectomy, and local amphotericin B injections, as well as therapy with fluconazole or voriconazole.

PREVENTION

For certain populations at the highest risk for invasive fungal infection, prophylactic antifungal agents can prevent infection. The populations for whom prophylaxis is recommended include stem cell transplant recipients, patients with acute leukemia who are undergoing induction chemotherapy, high-risk liver transplant recipients, and pancreas and small bowel transplant recipients; in these groups, a variety of different agents are effective. In the ICU population, prophylaxis with fluconazole can be effective, but it is recommended only in units that have a high rate of invasive candidiasis, and only in those patients at the highest risk for infection. In a placebo-controlled trial of caspofungin as antifungal prophylaxis in adults who were in the ICU for at least 3 days, were ventilated, received antibiotics, had a central line, and had at least one additional risk factor, caspofungin was safe and tended to reduce the incidence of invasive candidiasis when used for prophylaxis, but the difference was not statistically different.[A2] Restricting the use of prophylaxis is essential to prevent the widespread use of azoles, with subsequent selection of resistant species.

PROGNOSIS

The prognosis for patients with mucocutaneous infections is excellent. The prognosis for focal invasive infections depends on the organ involved and the patient's immune status. For example, whereas pyelonephritis may respond well to antifungal therapy, endocarditis and meningitis are more difficult to treat and have poor outcomes. Invasive candidiasis has a high mortality rate. Early treatment with an effective antifungal agent is extremely important for a favorable outcome.

Grade A References

A1. Schuster MG, Edwards JE Jr, Sobel JD, et al. Empirical fluconazole versus placebo for intensive care unit patients: a randomized trial. *Ann Intern Med.* 2008;149:83-90.

A2. Ostrosky-Zeichner L, Shoham S, Vasquez J, et al. MSG-01: a randomized, double-blind, placebo-controlled trial of caspofungin prophylaxis followed by preemptive therapy for invasive candidiasis in high-risk adults in the critical care setting. *Clin Infect Dis.* 2014;58:1219-1226.

GENERAL REFERENCES

For the General References and other additional features, please visit Expert Consult at https://expertconsult.inkling.com.

339

ASPERGILLOSIS

THOMAS J. WALSH

DEFINITION

Aspergillosis is defined as an infection with one or more of the species of the genus *Aspergillus.* Sporelike structures called *conidia* are aerosolized from the mold form of the organism growing in the environment. When conidia reach tissue, they germinate to form invasive filaments called *hyphae.*

The Pathogens

The most common species infecting humans are *Aspergillus fumigatus, Aspergillus flatus, Aspergillus terreus,* and *Aspergillus niger.* The species are usually identified in culture by characteristic microscopic features of hyphae and the structures producing conidia. When some species are not readily identifiable, they may be reported by the clinical laboratory as "*Aspergillus* species or *Aspergillus* sp." Molecular methods are increasingly used for identification. *Aspergillus fumigatus* may be reported as "*A. fumigatus* species complex." Some species within *A. fumigatus* complex may be particularly drug resistant. *Aspergillus terreus* is resistant to amphotericin B. Aspergilli within tissue appear as dichotomously branched (Y-shaped) septate hyphae. *Scedosporium* and *Fusarium* species also may produce septate hyphae in tissue. The presence of septa and dichotomous branching differentiates *Aspergillus* species from the Mucorales, which are the causative organisms of mucormycosis (Chapter 340).

EPIDEMIOLOGY

Aspergillus species. are ubiquitous organisms in the external environment, including soil, decaying matter, and air in temperatures as high as 40 to 50° C.[1] Aspergilli are easily isolated from houses, particularly from basements, crawl spaces, bedding, humidifiers, ventilation ducts, potted plants, dust, condiments (e.g., pepper), and marijuana samples. Aspergilli cause abortion in cattle and are important pathogens of marine organisms, insects, and domesticated and wild birds. Aflatoxin, which is one of the most potent carcinogens known, is produced by strains of *Aspergillus flavus* at ambient temperature on stored grain, spices, and nuts. Foodborne ingestion of preformed aflatoxin may cause hepatic necrosis or hepatocellular carcinoma (Chapter 196) in animals and humans.

Aspergillus species may be acquired from airborne conidia in inpatient and outpatient settings. Nosocomial aspergillosis is associated with building renovation, new construction, unfiltered air, contaminated ventilation systems, and fireproofing materials.[2] Hospital water, which may become aerosolized during activities such as showering, is a newly described potential source of aspergilli. As human pathogens, *Aspergillus* species may cause acute invasive disease, chronic infection, or allergic symptoms. A classification of aspergillosis is presented in Table 339-1.

Acute invasive aspergillosis develops in immunocompromised patient populations, particularly those with hematologic malignancies, hematopoietic stem cell transplantation (HSCT), severe aplastic anemia, primary immunodeficiencies, and solid organ transplantation, especially of heart, lung, and liver.[1] Genetic deficiency of the soluble pattern-recognition receptor called PTX3 (long pentraxin 3) caused by homozygous haplotype (h2/h2) in the *PTX3* gene of donor cells has been found to lead to impaired neutrophil antifungal capacity and increased risk for invasive aspergillosis in recipients of HSCT.[3] Persistent neutropenia, corticosteroids, other immunosuppressive agents, graft versus host disease (GVHD), and cytomegalovirus (CMV) disease are the most frequently observed clinical risk factors. The

TABLE 339-1 CLASSIFICATION OF ASPERGILLOSIS

CATEGORY	SPECIFIC FORMS OF ASPERGILLOSIS

Acute invasive aspergillosis	Invasive pulmonary aspergillosis
	  Empyema
	  Tracheobronchial infection
	Extrapulmonary aspergillosis
	  Acute sinusitis
	  Focal rhinitis
	  Cerebral, cerebellar, or brain stem infarction
	  Endophthalmitis
	  Osteomyelitis
	  Epidural abscess
	  Cardiac aspergillosis
	    Myocarditis
	    Endocarditis
	    Pericarditis
	  Gastrointestinal aspergillosis
	  Renal infection
	  Cutaneous lesions (nodules, ulcers)
	Disseminated aspergillosis

Chronic aspergillosis	Aspergilloma Chronic necrotizing pulmonary aspergillosis Chronic cavitary pulmonary aspergillosis *Aspergillus* otomycosis
Allergic forms of aspergillosis	Allergic bronchopulmonary aspergillosis Extrinsic allergic alveolitis Allergic *Aspergillus* sinusitis

mortality of acute invasive aspergillosis varies from as much as 100% with central nervous system (CNS) infection to approximately 65% with pulmonary infection in HSCT recipients. Early recognition of clinical manifestations followed by initiation of antifungal therapy may improve the ominous prognosis of acute invasive aspergillosis.

CLINICAL MANIFESTATIONS

Invasive Aspergillosis

The classic clinical manifestations of *invasive pulmonary aspergillosis* (IPA) in immunocompromised hosts are fever and focal pulmonary infiltrates, nodules, or wedge-shaped densities resembling infarcts (see Table 339-1).[4] Cough, pleuritic pain, and hemoptysis also may be present. Focal pulmonary infiltrates may progress to a cavity on recovery from neutropenia. Pulmonary infiltrates may also present as bronchopneumonia in an immunosuppressed patient. The pulmonary pathology in all these entities is that of hemorrhagic infarction caused by the organism's capacity to invade blood vessel walls (angioinvasion). These processes lead to formation of a necrotic center surrounded by a ring of hemorrhage and edema, which correlates with a "halo sign" surrounding the nodular density. Concomitant pleural effusion may develop and represent *Aspergillus* empyema. Tracheobronchial aspergillosis in immunocompromised patients presents as ulcerative, pseudomembranous, or plaquelike large airway disease that may presage pulmonary parenchymal invasion.

Acute Aspergillus sinusitis may occur concomitantly or independently of IPA. Although symptoms may include fever, localized pressure, and pain, they may be absent in severely immunocompromised patients. Eschar may be observed by speculum examination or endoscopy on the nasal septum and turbinates. Acute *Aspergillus* sinusitis of the ethmoid and sphenoid sinuses may progress to cavernous sinus thrombosis with symptoms referable to cranial nerves III, IV, $V_{1,2}$, and VI. *Aspergillus flavus* has a high propensity for causing acute sinus infection.

The tissue targets of *extrapulmonary* and *disseminated aspergillosis* most commonly include the CNS, where abscesses and infarcts are characteristic.[5] Patients with CNS aspergillosis present with focal paresis, cranial nerve deficits, and seizures. The glucose level in cerebrospinal fluid (CSF) is usually normal, and cultures of CSF are negative. Other extrapulmonary manifestations include endophthalmitis, myocardial infarction, gastrointestinal disease, renal infarction, cutaneous lesions, and Budd-Chiari syndrome. Esophageal ulcers and mesenteric thrombosis may produce gastrointestinal bleeding. Renal infection may present as flank pain and hematuria.

Aspergillus endocarditis usually begins as an isolated infection in intravenous drug users or after cardiac valvular surgery.[6] *Aspergillus* endocarditis most commonly presents as major arterial emboli. Blood cultures, which are

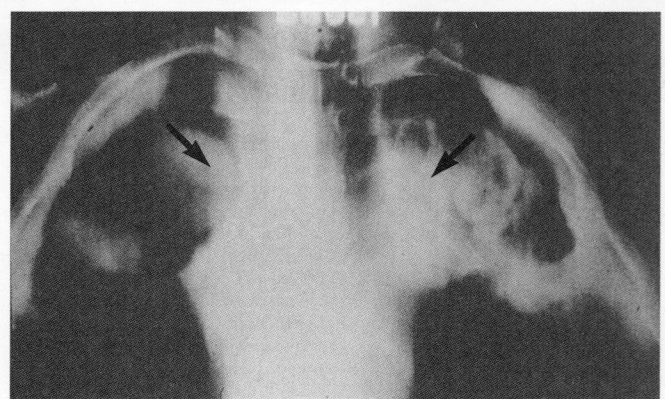

FIGURE 339-1. Tomogram of pulmonary aspergillomas (arrows).

seldom positive, may be delayed in growth by as much as 14 to 21 days. Diagnosis is difficult, and despite valve replacement with antifungal therapy, mortality approaches 100%. *Aspergillus pericarditis* may arise from contiguous pulmonary lesions or through transmural infection from endocardial infection.

Locally invasive aspergillosis usually develops in immunocompromised patients as cutaneous ulcers, focal rhinitis, osteomyelitis, and septic arthritis.[7] Cutaneous ulcers have been associated with use of contaminated adhesive tape and arm boards. Blood-borne infection in illicit intravenous drug users may present as foci of dissemination in brain, lung, kidney, and bone. Keratitis, endophthalmitis, and infection of burn wounds may develop from traumatic inoculation in otherwise immunocompetent patients.

Chronic Pulmonary Aspergillosis

Aspergilloma appears on chest radiograph as a ball in a cavity. The fungus ball consists of matted hyphae and debris in a preformed cavity from previous pulmonary tuberculosis, histoplasmosis, or fibrocystic sarcoidosis (Fig. 339-1). Symptomatic patients present with cough, hemoptysis, dyspnea, weight loss, fatigue, chest pain, or fever. Sputum culture is typically positive for *Aspergillus* species, particularly *Aspergillus niger*. Pleural aspergillosis may complicate surgical resection of aspergilloma or develop spontaneously as a bronchopleural fistula or concomitantly with tuberculosis.

As a stage in the repair process of infarcted lung tissue in neutropenic patients, one or more apparent "aspergillomas" may develop in consolidated lesions during recovery from neutropenia. These apparent aspergillomas do not develop in preexisting cavities and create an "air-crescent sign," or Monod sign, during their formation.

Chronic necrotizing pulmonary aspergillosis (CNPA) and *chronic cavitary pulmonary aspergillosis* (CCPA) occur in patients with underlying chronic lung disease, chronic immunosuppression, such as that due to prolonged use of systemic corticosteroids, or both. CNPA characteristically causes a slowly progressive inflammatory destruction of lung tissue superimposed on chronic lung disease. Clinical manifestations of worsening pulmonary function, cough, and dyspnea in CNPA may be indistinguishable from concomitant primary chronic respiratory disease.

CCPA is defined as the presence of multiple *Aspergillus*-related cavities, which may or may not contain an aspergilloma. Patients with CCPA may have genetically mediated deficits in innate host defenses. Occurring in association with symptoms of cough, hemoptysis, and dyspnea, the progressive cavities of CCPA tend to coalesce with the loss of functional lung tissue.

Aspergillus otomycosis is a chronic infection that usually involves the external auditory canal with symptoms of pain, pruritus, hypoacusis, and otic discharge in patients with impaired mucocutaneous immunity, such as those with chronic eczema, hypogammaglobulinemia, diabetes mellitus, or HIV infection and those receiving corticosteroids. *Aspergillus* may involve the middle ear and extend into the mastoid sinus if the tympanic membrane has been perforated.

Allergic Forms of Aspergillosis

Allergic bronchopulmonary aspergillosis (ABPA) develops most frequently in patients with a history of chronic asthma or cystic fibrosis.[8,9] Occurring in genetically susceptible patients exposed to specific *Aspergillus* antigens,

ABPA is characterized by episodic airway obstruction, fever, eosinophilia, positive sputum cultures, mucous plugs containing hyphae, the presence of grossly visible brown flecks in sputum (hyphae), transient infiltrates and parallel "tramline" or ring markings on chest radiographs, proximal bronchiectasis, upper lobe contraction, and elevated levels of total immunoglobulins G and E (IgG and IgE). Eosinophilia may be present in blood, sputum, and lung tissue. Mucous plugs contribute to development of pulmonary infiltrates, atelectasis, and peribronchial inflammation. The parallel or ring markings are caused by thickened ectatic bronchi, whereas the upper lobe changes are due to progressive apical fibrosis. Pulmonary infiltrates in ABPA may be nonsegmental and transient in association with eosinophilia and asthma; alternatively, they may be segmental and associated with bronchial obstruction by mucous plugs, wherein asthma and eosinophilia may be absent.

Extrinsic allergic alveolitis is an unusual allergic form of *Aspergillus* lung disease that has been most frequently associated with *Aspergillus clavatus* in malt workers. A hypersensitivity pneumonitis with dyspnea and fever develops approximately 4 hours after exposure. Diffuse reticulonodular interstitial infiltrates may be present at the time of symptoms. Patients have IgG precipitins and cell-mediated immune reactions against *Aspergillus* antigens. Granulomas are present in lung tissue. In comparison to ABPA, eosinophilia is not a feature of *Aspergillus* extrinsic allergic alveolitis.

Allergic Aspergillus sinusitis (AAS) is a noninvasive form of sinus disease that typically presents in patients with asthma, nasal polyps, sinus opacification, and eosinophilia. Sinus aspirate yields mucinous material containing eosinophils, Charcot-Leyden crystals, and hyphal elements. AAS and ABPA may coexist in some patients. Advanced forms of AAS may present with proptosis and optic neuropathy, necessitating prompt surgical intervention.

DIAGNOSIS

Invasive Aspergillosis

Diagnosis of IPA and disseminated aspergillosis is difficult. None of the aforementioned clinical manifestations are diagnostic for invasive aspergillosis. Advances in computed tomography (CT) have revealed characteristic features of nodules, halo signs, wedge-shaped infiltrates, and air-crescent signs during IPA in immunocompromised patients (Fig. 339-2). However, infections caused by *Fusarium* species, *Scedosporium* species, the Mucorales, as well as *Pseudomonas aeruginosa* may be radiologically indistinguishable from IPA. Microbiologic confirmation, where possible, is important to differentiate aspergillosis from other filamentous fungal infections. Bronchoalveolar lavage (BAL), percutaneous needle aspiration, video-assisted thoracoscopic (VATS) biopsy, and if necessary, open lung biopsy are standard procedures for establishing a microbiologic diagnosis of invasive aspergillosis. Specimens obtained from these procedures may demonstrate dichotomously branching septate hyphae by direct microscopy or grow *Aspergillus* species in culture. Each of these procedures is associated with false-negative results, as well as with complications. Conversely, the presence of *Aspergillus* by direct examination or culture in an immunocompromised host with pulmonary nodules or well-circumscribed infiltrates carries a high probability for diagnosis of invasive aspergillosis.

Galactomannan, which is a heteropolysaccharide of the *Aspergillus* cell wall, is a useful biomarker that is released into the circulation and alveolar spaces during IPA.[10] Detection of galactomannan by enzyme immunoassay (EIA) in serum or BAL above certain thresholds is strong microbiologic evidence for a diagnosis of invasive aspergillosis in immunocompromised patients with characteristic clinical manifestations. Nonetheless, false-positive results have been reported in patients who have received piperacillin-tazobactam or amoxicillin-clavulanate, in cases in which Plasmalyte was used for BAL, and in other deeply invasive mycoses such as blastomycosis and histoplasmosis. Serum galactomannan may be falsely negative in patients receiving antifungal prophylaxis or empirical therapy.

$(1{\to}3)\text{-}\beta\text{-D-glucan}$ is another *Aspergillus* cell wall polysaccharide that is detected in serum during invasive disease. The sensitivity of the *Limulus* spectrophotometric assay for detection of $(1{\to}3)\text{-}\beta\text{-D-glucan}$ in patients with invasive aspergillosis appears to be comparable to that of the galactomannan EIA. However, because $(1{\to}3)\text{-}\beta\text{-D-glucan}$ also is present in the cell wall of other medically important fungi, including *Candida* species, the specificity of $(1{\to}3)\text{-}\beta\text{-D-glucan}$ for *Aspergillus* species is less than that of galactomannan.

Although molecular diagnostic tools, such as quantitative polymerase chain reaction (PCR), for diagnosis of invasive aspergillosis are promising, they also remain investigational for this infection. Ultimately, the combined use of improved diagnostic imaging, microscopy, culture methodology, cell

Neutropenia

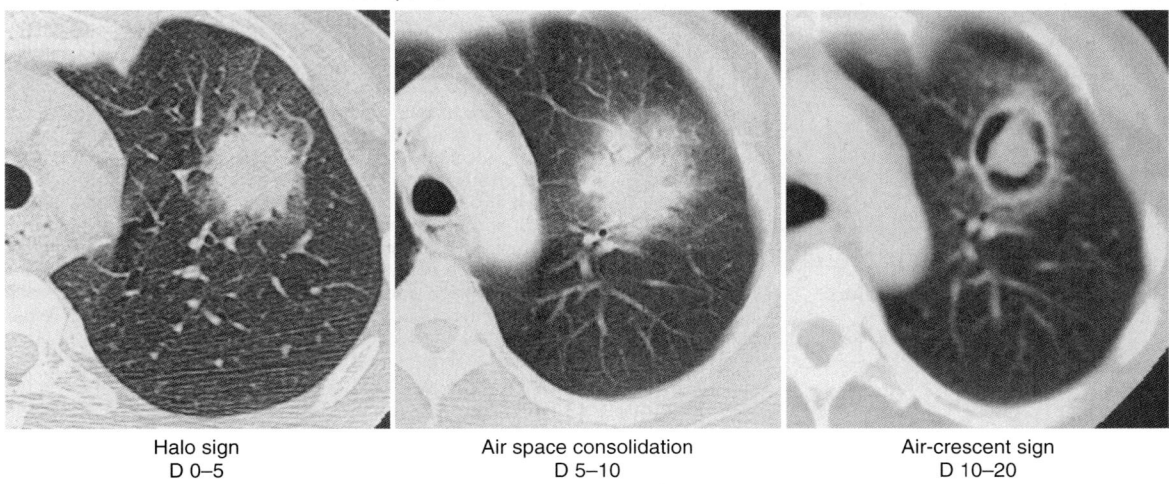

| Halo sign | Air space consolidation | Air-crescent sign |
| D 0–5 | D 5–10 | D 10–20 |

FIGURE 339-2. Evolution of radiography of invasive aspergillosis in an immunocompromised host. D = days after the lesion is first noted.

wall biomarkers, and possibly PCR in conjunction with careful bedside assessment of risk factors and clinical manifestations will improve the diagnosis of invasive aspergillosis and early initiation of therapy.

Diagnosis of locally invasive extrapulmonary aspergillosis causing mucocutaneous lesions, osteomyelitis, and septic arthritis is best accomplished with biopsy, direct microscopy, and culture. A diagnosis of *Aspergillus* keratitis is established by careful culture of corneal lesions by an ophthalmologist.

Allergic Forms of Aspergillosis

Diagnosis of ABPA is based on the presence of a combination of clinical, biologic, and radiologic, criteria (Fig. 339-3). The consensus criteria for establishing a diagnosis of ABPA differ depending on the presence of cystic fibrosis. For patients with ABPA without the presence of cystic fibrosis (Chapter 89), criteria for ABPA include asthma, an immediate cutaneous reaction to *A. fumigatus* antigen, total serum IgE concentration higher than 1000 ng/mL, elevated *A. fumigatus*–specific serum IgE levels, precipitating serum antibodies to *A. fumigatus*, central bronchiectasis, peripheral blood eosinophilia, and characteristic pulmonary infiltrates. The latter two features (eosinophilia and pulmonary infiltrates) are considered nonessential because they only may be present during an acute phase of ABPA.

Among patients with cystic fibrosis, distinguishing between ABPA and an episode of clinical deterioration with colonization by *Aspergillus* species is challenging. The current criteria of the Cystic Fibrosis Foundation help to define ABPA in that setting: clinical deterioration (coughing, wheezing, increased sputum production, exercise intolerance, and decrease in pulmonary function); immediate hypersensitivity to *A. fumigatus* (positive skin test or IgE response); total serum IgE concentration higher than 1000 kUI/L; precipitating antibodies to *A. fumigatus*; abnormal chest radiograph (infiltrate, mucous plugs, or unexplained changes compared with previous chest radiograph).

A biphasic skin test response may assist in the diagnosis. A scratch test with *Aspergillus* antigens produces an immediate wheal-and-flare reaction that is mediated by IgE and blocked by antihistamines but not by corticosteroids. An intracutaneous test with the antigens produces a later (6 to 8 hours) reaction that is mediated by IgG and complement and blocked by corticosteroids.

An occupational history of exposure is critical to the diagnosis of *extrinsic allergic alveolitis*. A typical history of recurrent episodes developing within 24 hours after inhalation of conidial antigens in an agricultural environment in conjunction with a negative scratch test, a positive intradermal test, and granulomas with immunoglobulins and complement in tissue is diagnostically consistent with *Aspergillus* extrinsic allergic alveolitis.

Recurrent sinusitis in a patient with asthma, nasal polyps, eosinophilia, sinus opacification, and a sinus aspirate yielding mucinous material containing eosinophils, Charcot-Leyden crystals, and hyphal elements establishes a diagnosis of AAS.

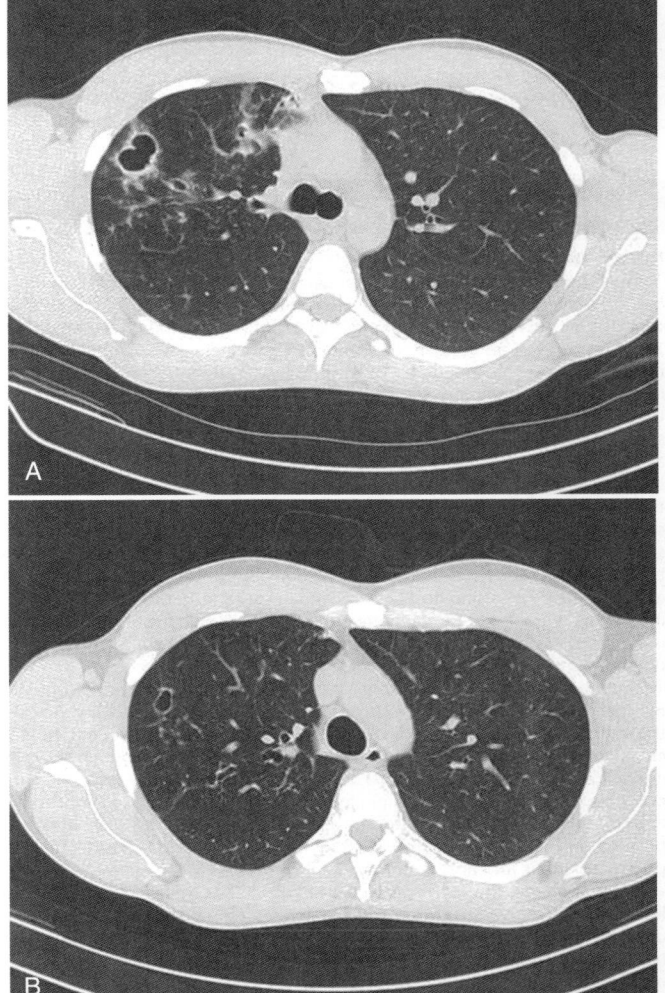

FIGURE 339-3. Allergic bronchopulmonary aspergillosis in a patient with a long history of asthma. **(A)** is a thin slice CT image showing bronchiectasis with cystic changes in the right upper lobe. This patient had an underlying history of asthma and a markedly elevated IgE level and other findings consistent with allergic bronchopulmonary aspergillosis. **(B)** is the same patient after treatment with systemic steroids; the cystic bronchiectasis has markedly improved. (Courtesy of Anne E. O'Donnell, MD.)

TABLE 339-2 ANTIFUNGAL THERAPY OF INVASIVE ASPERGILLOSIS*

FIRST-LINE TREATMENT IN ADULTS[†]

Drug of choice:	
Voriconazole	IV therapy: 6 mg/kg q12h for two doses, then 4 mg/kg q12h
	Oral therapy: 300 mg or 4mg/kg bid
Alternate (see text for conditions):	
Liposomal amphotericin B	3-5 mg/kg IV daily

SECOND-LINE OR SALVAGE TREATMENT IN ADULTS[†]

Amphotericin B lipid complex *or*	5 mg/kg IV daily
Caspofungin *or*	70 mg IV daily for first dose, then 50 mg IV daily
Posaconazole *or*	200 mg PO qid or 400 mg PO bid
Itraconazole	400 mg PO (capsules) daily (in either one or two doses); or 2.5 mg/kg PO (solution) bid

*Refer to package insert for dosage modification of antifungal agents in liver disease or renal impairment.

[†]Duration of antifungal therapy depends on therapeutic response of documented lesions, burden of disease, host immunocompetence, and type of aspergillosis (e.g., acute invasive vs. chronic, vs. allergic). Guidelines of Infectious Diseases Society of America recommend at least 6 to 12 weeks for invasive pulmonary aspergillosis. Patients who are immunosuppressed continue treatment throughout the period of immunosuppression and until resolution of lesions. In patients with previously diagnosed invasive aspergillosis, antifungal therapy should be continued or reinitiated during subsequent periods of immunosuppression (e.g., chemotherapy, stem cell transplantation, graft vs. host disease) to prevent recrudescence

(see Walsh TJ, Anaissie EJ, Denning DW, et al. Treatment of aspergillosis: clinical practice guidelines of the Infectious Diseases Society of America (IDSA). *Clin Infect Dis.* 2008: 46:327-360.)

TREATMENT   Rx

Invasive Aspergillosis

The foundation of treatment of invasive aspergillosis consists of (1) antifungal medical therapy (Table 339-2), (2) reversal of immunosuppression and, where appropriate, (3) surgical resection of infected lesions (see Table 339-2).[11,12] Dosages of antifungal agents are listed in Table 339-2. Voriconazole is recommended in most patients for the primary treatment of invasive aspergillosis, including pulmonary, disseminated, and extrapulmonary isolated infection. This recommendation is based on the randomized controlled trial showing that voriconazole is superior to deoxycholate amphotericin B (D-AmB) as primary treatment for invasive aspergillosis. However, not all patients are candidates to receive voriconazole. This includes patients with substantially elevated hepatic transaminases, hepatic dysfunction, and a history of hypersensitivity to or intolerance of voriconazole. Such patients should receive liposomal amphotericin B (L-AmB) as primary therapy. This recommendation is based on the randomized trial that demonstrated comparable efficacy of approximately 70% using dosages of 3 mg/kg/day and 10 mg/kg/day of LAmB in patients who had predominantly hematologic malignancies.[A1] L-AmB also is indicated as primary therapy for patients in whom there is a suspicion for or documentation of concurrent mucormycosis.

Second-line or salvage antifungal therapy is indicated in patients who are intolerant of or whose infection is unresponsive to primary therapy. Among the antifungal agents used in this setting are a lipid formulation of amphotericin B, posaconazole, itraconazole, or an echinocandin (caspofungin is the only agent licensed for this indication). For patients who are already receiving voriconazole, a change of class to a lipid formulation, addition of an echinocandin, and use of another azole are alternative possibilities. Such decisions are complicated and warrant infectious diseases consultation with consideration of pharmacokinetic and host factors.

Antifungal therapy for invasive aspergillosis should be continued until lesions have resolved, cultures and biomarkers are negative, and reversible underlying predispositions have abated. Reinstating therapy in patients who have previously responded should be considered if immunosuppression is reinstituted or if neutropenia recurs.

Preliminary reports of a randomized multicenter study demonstrate that a new antifungal triazole known as isavuconazole is as effective but better tolerated than voriconazole in the primary treatment of invasive aspergillosis.

Reversal of immunosuppression is a critical factor in the successful management of invasive aspergillosis. Recovery from neutropenia and decreasing the daily dosage or discontinuation of corticosteroids, where feasible, are two of the most important forms of improving host response. Depending on the protocol used, granulocyte transfusions may stabilize *Aspergillus* lesions until

recovery from neutropenia. Granulocyte colony-stimulating factor (G-CSF) and granulocyte-macrophage colony-stimulating factor (GM-CSF) may accelerate recovery from neutropenia. The role of GM-CSF, G-CSF, or interferon-γ in immunocompromised non-neutropenic patients with invasive aspergillosis remains to be further defined.

Surgical management of infected lesions is an important adjunctive component of primary therapy for several forms of invasive aspergillosis: endocarditis, pericarditis, osteomyelitis, epidural abscess, infected vascular catheters and prosthetic devices, and skin and soft tissue infection. Surgical management also is important for several conditions of invasive pulmonary aspergillosis: recurrent hemoptysis from a single cavitary lesion, invasion of a pulmonary lesion into the chest wall, and pulmonary lesions contiguous with great vessels or the pericardium. *Aspergillus* empyema requires closed chest tube drainage and possibly débridement of the infected pleural cavity. Débridement of sinus aspergillosis, particularly when the ethmoid and frontal sinuses are infected, may prevent extension into the orbit or into the cavernous sinus. Surgical resection of selected lesions of the CNS may be indicated for establishing a diagnosis, reducing increased intracranial pressure, and/or protecting critical neural centers. Location of CNS lesions and neurologic sequelae after resection are critical factors in neurosurgical management of aspergillosis.

Local infusion of antifungal agents, particularly intravitreal therapy for endophthalmitis, provides high concentrations to compartments that may not be reached by systemic therapy. Topical irrigation with voriconazole, amphotericin B, or if available, pimaricin is an important adjunct to management of *Aspergillus* keratitis.

Chronic Aspergillosis

Medical therapy has limited benefit in treatment of aspergilloma; however, some patients may benefit from extended use of an antifungal triazole. Lifelong commitment to an antifungal triazole should be balanced against the natural history of approximately 10% of aspergillomas resolving spontaneously. By comparison, medical therapy with itraconazole or voriconazole is the standard of treatment for CCPA. Patients with CCPA typically achieve improvement of symptoms and stabilization or improvement of radiologic changes. Patients with CNPA also receive an antifungal triazole; however, assessment of response is more difficult because of the underlying chronic lung disease. The role of surgical resection in patients with solitary aspergilloma or CCPA is limited because of development of bronchopleural fistula, *Aspergillus* infection of the pleural space, and potentially further worsening of already compromised pulmonary function. However, surgical resection may have a more important role in treating patients with recurrent and severe hemoptysis, for which the benefits of removing the cavity usually outweigh the known risks. Bronchial artery embolization and transthoracic direct intracavitary instillation of antifungal agents for aspergilloma have only transient benefits but substantial risk.

Topical irrigating solutions of boric acid, acetic acid, or an antifungal azole cream may be effective in treating *Aspergillus* otomycosis. Voriconazole, posaconazole, or itraconazole may be necessary for refractory cases or perforated tympanic membranes.

Allergic Forms of Aspergillosis

ABPA is treated with a combination of corticosteroids and itraconazole. This recommendation is based on two double-blind, randomized, placebo-controlled trials for treatment of ABPA. These studies demonstrated that itraconazole (200 mg twice daily orally for 16 weeks) resulted in significant amelioration of disease, as evidenced by improvement in exercise tolerance and pulmonary function, reduction in corticosteroid dose, increased interval between corticosteroid courses, as well as decreased eosinophilic inflammatory parameters and IgE concentration. Although corticosteroid therapy is the mainstay of treatment of ABPA, chronic administration of corticosteroids causes severe immunosuppression and multisystem metabolic abnormalities. Addition of itraconazole reduces organism burden, attenuates antigenic stimulus for destructive bronchial inflammation, and provides a corticosteroid-sparing effect. Intermittent use of corticosteroids or substantially raising the dose in patients receiving chronic therapy can produce rapid resolution of marked symptomatic episodes or deteriorating forced expiratory volume in 1 second (FEV$_1$).

Extrinsic allergic alveolitis is best managed by removing patients from the allergic environment. An accurate occupational history is critical to this intervention.

AAS is treated by endoscopic drainage to relieve obstruction by tenacious mucin. Itraconazole, nasal corticosteroids, and systemic corticosteroids, alone or in combination, may be beneficial in some patients with AAS. Caution is warranted with chronic use of systemic or nasal corticosteroids. Itraconazole may have a corticosteroid sparing effect.

Combination Antifungal Therapy

Combinations of polyenes, triazoles, and echinocandins are being explored. The aggregate of well-conducted in vitro, in vivo, and clinical observational studies support the additive or synergistic interaction of a triazole and echinocandin in primary treatment of invasive pulmonary aspergillosis. In a randomized trial designed to study combination therapy for invasive aspergillosis, patients with hematologic malignancies and/or allogeneic HSCT were randomized at study entry to receive initial treatment with a combination of voriconazole and anidulafungin or voriconazole monotherapy.[A2] Combination therapy was associated with reduced all-cause mortality at 6 weeks compared with voriconazole monotherapy, but this difference did not reach statistical superiority. In patients with probable invasive aspergillosis, combination therapy was associated with a significant survival benefit.

GENERAL REFERENCES

For the General References and other additional features, please visit Expert Consult at https://expertconsult.inkling.com.

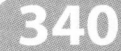

MUCORMYCOSIS

D.P. KONTOYIANNIS

PREVENTION

Several strategies may be used for prevention of invasive aspergillosis in immunocompromised patients: primary prophylaxis, empirical therapy, and secondary prophylaxis. Posaconazole is licensed for prophylaxis of invasive aspergillosis in patients with hematologic malignancies and in HSCT recipients.[A3] This recommendation in hematologic malignancies is based on a randomized clinical trial in patients undergoing chemotherapy for acute myelogenous leukemia or myelodysplasia. Posaconazole significantly prevented invasive fungal infections more effectively than did either fluconazole or itraconazole and improved overall survival. There were, however, more adverse events with posaconazole. Voriconazole also is used for this indication but with less evidence.[A4] A multicenter, randomized, double-blind trial comparing fluconazole versus voriconazole in HSCT recipients for the prevention of mycoses found nonsignificant trends of fewer *Aspergillus* infections with voriconazole. The study also demonstrated that in the context of intensive monitoring and structured empirical antifungal therapy, 6-month fungal-free survival did not differ in allogeneic HSCT recipients given prophylactic fluconazole or voriconazole. Empirical antifungal therapy provides early treatment for persistently febrile immunocompromised patients and systemic prophylaxis for high-risk hosts with or without pulmonary infiltrates. Liposomal amphotericin B (D-AmB), caspofungin, and voriconazole have been used for this strategy. Secondary prophylaxis of invasive aspergillosis with voriconazole is used for patients with a history of previous aspergillosis who are scheduled for a subsequent cycle of immunosuppression that may increase the risk for recurrence.

Reduction of exposure to airborne conidia, such as by HEPA filtration of hospital air, avoiding activities that increase conidial aerosols (room maintenance, dust exposures, and contaminated materials (e.g., potted plants), as well as providing clean water distribution systems, may reduce acquisition of *Aspergillus* by immunosuppressed or neutropenic patients.

For patients with allergic forms of aspergillosis, use of corticosteroids and itraconazole, alone or in combination, may prevent debilitating exacerbations. The toxicity of chronic administration of prednisone warrants strategies for intermittent administration of prednisone or corticosteroid-sparing use of itraconazole.

PROGNOSIS

Untreated invasive aspergillosis is associated with severe morbidity and high mortality in immunocompromised patients. Prognosis is improved by both early initiation of antifungal therapy, reversal of immunosuppression, and successful treatment of the underlying primary disease. For patients with chronic aspergillosis, multidisciplinary specialized supportive care may improve outcome and quality of life.

Grade A References

A1. Cornely OA, Maertens J, Bresnik M, et al. Liposomal amphotericin B as initial therapy for invasive mold infection: a randomized trial comparing a high-loading dose regimen with standard dosing (AmBiLoad trial). *Clin Infect Dis.* 2007;44:1289-1297.
A2. Marr KA, Schlamm HT, Herbrecht R, et al. Combination antifungal therapy for invasive aspergillosis: a randomized trial. *Ann Intern Med.* 2015;162:81-89.
A3. Cornely OA, Maertens J, Winston DJ, et al. Posaconazole compared with fluconazole or itraconazole prophylaxis in high-risk neutropenic patients receiving chemotherapy. *N Engl J Med.* 2007;356:348-359.
A4. Wingard JR, Carter SL, Walsh TJ, et al. Randomized, double blind trial of fluconazole vs. voriconazole for the prevention of invasive fungal disease after allogeneic hematopoietic cell transplantation. *Blood.* 2010;116:5111-5118.

DEFINITION

Mucormycosis is the accurate unifying term used to describe infections caused by fungi belonging to the order Mucorales. Zygomycosis, an alternative term used to describe these life-threatening infections, has become less accurate based on a recent taxonomic reclassification (using molecular methods) that abolished Zygomycetes as a class (and placed the order Mucorales in the subphylum Mucormycotina).[1] Mucorales typically cause aggressive, acute-onset, frequently fatal angioinvasive infections, especially in immunosuppressed hosts.

EPIDEMIOLOGY

Mucorales fungi are distributed worldwide and found in decaying organic substrates. The true incidence of mucormycosis is not known and probably is underestimated because of difficulties in antemortem diagnosis. The relative frequency of Mucorales families causing infection differs. In a recent review of more than 900 reported cases, the most common microbiologically confirmed infecting species were *Rhizopus* (47%), *Mucor* (18%), *Cunninghamella bertholletiae* (7%), *Apophysomyces elegans* (5%), *Absidia* (5%), *Saksenaea* (5%), and *Rhizomucor pusillus* (4%). Some Mucorales causing infection have specific geographic and host associations. For example, the thermophilic Mucorales *Saksenaea vasiformis elegans* have specific geographic distributions, as recently shown in victims of combat-related injuries from Afghanistan who developed necrotizing soft tissue infections.[2] Also, major natural disasters have been associated with rapidly progressing necrotizing soft tissue infections by infrequently isolated species, such as those caused by *Apophysomyces elegans* in the Joplin tornado victims in 2011.[3]

The classic risk factors for mucormycosis include hematologic malignancy, hematopoietic stem cell or solid organ transplantation, poorly controlled diabetes mellitus, chronic acidemia, prematurity, profound chronic debilitation, trauma, burns, and very rarely intravenous drug use.[4] Nosocomial cutaneous infections can develop at surgical wound and intravenous catheter insertion sites. Finally, breakthrough mucormycosis has been increasingly observed in patients with leukemia and in recipients of hematopoietic stem cell transplants receiving *Aspergillus*-active drugs such as voriconazole (which has no anti-Mucorales activity). This association has been a topic of debate.

PATHOBIOLOGY

Mucorales species are saprophytic, rapidly growing fungi. Angioinvasive growth results in infarction and necrosis of surrounding tissue, which is the hallmark of mucormycosis. The major modes of transmission are inhalation, ingestion, and cutaneous inoculation, with inhalation of spores from environmental sources being the most common. Cutaneous or percutaneous transmission occurs with traumatic disruption of skin barriers, and it is the most important mode of transmission in immunocompetent hosts. Gastrointestinal acquisition, while less common, has occurred in patients with repeated ingestion of spores during severe malnutrition, non-nutritional substances (pica), contaminated herbal/homeopathic products, or allopurinol tablets.

Host immunity in healthy hosts prevents germination of fungal spores unless the inoculum is heavy.[5] To establish invasive infection, spores must overcome both innate and adaptive immune responses to germinate into hyphae. Defects in phagocytic activity caused by insufficient numbers (i.e., neutropenia) and functional defects caused by glucocorticoids, hyperglycemia, and/or acidosis allow unimpeded proliferation of fungi because of the absence of coordinated, effective host responses. Unsurprisingly, mucormycosis is often disseminated in severely immunosuppressed patients, with high mortality rates. However, lymphopenia may not be as critical in patients with acquired immunodeficiency syndrome.

Free iron is an essential component of the pathogenesis of mucormycosis, as suggested by the predisposition of patients with iron overload and ketoacidosis to such infections. These patients often receive the iron chelator deferoxamine. Both iron overload and use of deferoxamine (which is also used to treat aluminum overload in dialysis recipients) are risk factors for angioinvasive mucormycosis. *Rhizopus oryzae* can utilize deferoxamine as a xenosiderophore to form a ferrioxamine complex and to obtain more iron for use. Reassuringly, the newer iron chelators agents (e.g., deferasirox) are not associated with increased risk for mucormycosis; on the contrary, in preclinical models, deferasirox has exhibited direct fungicidal effects against Mucorales via iron starvation.

Historically, poorly controlled diabetes mellitus (types 1 and 2) has been a major predisposing factor, reported in 36 to 88% of all cases of mucormycosis. In particular, diabetic patients with ketoacidosis are susceptible to mucormycosis. Normal human serum cannot support the growth of *R. oryzae*, whereas serum in diabetic patients can do so. Acidosis disrupts the normal inhibitory activity of serum by attenuating the ability of transferrin to bind iron from the fungus. In addition, quantitative and qualitative neutrophil and phagocytic cell dysfunction occurs in diabetic patients with ketoacidosis and may play a role in the pathogenesis.

CLINICAL MANIFESTATIONS

The clinical presentation of mucormycosis depends on the host's underlying immune and medical condition. Hence, pulmonary mucormycosis is most common in neutropenic or corticosteroid-treated patients (e.g., hematopoietic stem cell and solid organ transplant recipients). In contrast, rhino-orbital or rhinocerebral mucormycosis is the characteristic presentation in patients with diabetic ketoacidosis. Finally, cutaneous mucormycosis in both immunocompetent and immunocompromised hosts is typically seen following local trauma or burns resulting in breakdown of skin integrity and/or subcutaneous tissue injuries. Infectious syndromes associated with Mucorales are grouped based on clinical presentation into one of six categories: (1) rhinocerebral, (2) pulmonary, (3) cutaneous, (4) gastrointestinal, (5) disseminated, and (6) unusual presentations, as follows:

Rhinocerebral Mucormycosis

Rhinocerebral mucormycosis describes an infection originating in the paranasal sinuses after inhalation of Mucorales spores and extending to the orbit (sino-orbital) or brain (rhinocerebral), particularly in patients with diabetic ketoacidosis or those with profound neutropenia.[6] Rhinocerebral mucormycosis is the most common manifestation. Early signs and symptoms of sinus invasion may be indistinguishable from common causes of sinusitis. Common symptoms include sinus pain, congestion, headache, mouth pain, otologic symptoms, and hypo-osmia/anosmia. Involved tissues become red and then violaceous and, finally, black with thrombosis, and tissue necrosis. Necrotic eschar of the nasal cavity and turbinates, facial lesions, and exophytic or necrotic lesions of the hard palate are signs of extensive, rapidly progressing infection. A painful black eschar on the palate or nasal mucosa is a classic diagnostic but late sign. Absence of this finding does not rule out rhinocerebral infection, as necrotic nasal or palate lesions occur in only 50% of patients within 3 days of onset of infection. Extension into the periorbital region is not uncommon at presentation. Signs and symptoms of periorbital and orbital involvement include periorbital swelling, preseptal and/or orbital cellulitis, proptosis, chemosis, blurred vision or rapidly progressing external ophthalmoplegia, diplopia, eyelid gangrene, retinal detachment, and endophthalmitis. Also, patients with extensive rhino-orbital or rhinocerebral disease may present with trigeminal or other cranial nerve palsy, which is consistent with frequent histologic findings of perineural invasion. Infection can rapidly progress through the cavernous sinuses into the central nervous system, resulting in cavernous sinus and internal carotid artery thrombosis. A bloody nasal discharge may be the only sign indicating that the infection has invaded through the nasal turbinates and into the brain. Patients with advanced infection may have cranial neuropathies and/or altered consciousness; bone destruction; retinal artery, internal carotid artery, cavernous, and less often, sagittal sinus, thrombosis; frontal lobe necrosis; epidural and subdural abscesses; and/or basilar artery aneurysm.

Plain films and cerebrospinal fluid findings lack sensitivity in diagnosing rhinocerebral mucormycosis. Computed tomography (CT) and magnetic resonance imaging (MRI) are more useful for revealing soft tissue involvement around the nerve sheaths and bone destruction. CT frequently shows mucosal thickening, air-fluid levels, and bony erosion. Orbital thickening may be detected earlier by using MRI. CT and MRI scans of the orbits may be unremarkable during the initial stages of mucormycosis, highlighting the importance of serial radiographic imaging in monitoring disease progression. Extraorbital muscle thickening is often the first sign of orbital involvement and should prompt empirical antifungal therapy followed by surgical exploration or biopsy.

Accurate diagnosis and prompt medical and surgical intervention are critical because of the rapid progression of the infection. Definitive diagnosis of necrotic lesions using biopsy and rapid histologic assessment of frozen sections should be performed as soon as possible because it directly impacts outcome. In a review of 929 documented mucormycosis cases, the mortality rate was as follows: 62% in rhinocerebral mucormycosis, 24% in sino-orbital involvement, and 16% in isolated sinus disease. Isolated sinusitis is curable by following timely surgical intervention and systemic antifungal therapy.

Pulmonary Mucormycosis

The clinical manifestations of pulmonary mucormycosis are indistinguishable from those of invasive pulmonary aspergillosis. Patients may present with fever refractory to broad-spectrum antibiotics, nonproductive cough, and progressive dyspnea. Less commonly, pleuritic chest pain, hemoptysis, and pleural effusion are seen. If the major pulmonary blood vessels are invaded by fungal hyphae, massive, potentially fatal hemoptysis can occur. Pulmonary mucormycosis can progress and invade adjacent organs via traverse tissue planes, including the diaphragm, chest wall, and pleura (Fig. 340-1). Clues for distinguishing pulmonary mucormycosis from invasive pulmonary aspergillosis include the presence of pansinusitis, a history of prophylaxis with antifungals against *Aspergillus* but not Mucorales (e.g., voriconazole, echinocandins), and possibly continual absence of detectable *Aspergillus galactomannan* antigen in serum. In rare circumstances, pulmonary mucormycosis can present as an endobronchial or tracheal lesion with a less fulminant course, especially in diabetics. Endobronchial mucormycosis may cause airway obstruction or erosion of major pulmonary blood vessels and fatal hemoptysis. In more immunocompetent hosts, pulmonary mucormycosis may present with more atypical, slowly progressing forms. Like *Aspergillus* species, Mucorales can form mycetomas in preexisting lung cavities and cause slowly necrotizing pneumonia and hypersensitivity syndromes. Investigators have also implicated *Rhizopus* species in allergic alveolitis among farm workers or sawmill workers (wood-trimmer's disease).

Because the first-line antifungal typically used for aspergillosis is voriconazole, which lacks activity against Mucorales, failure to achieve a timely diagnosis of pulmonary mucormycosis and delayed antifungal therapy (e.g., amphotericin B) rapidly worsens outcome.

Skin and Soft Tissue Mucormycosis

Cutaneous mucormycosis typically occurs in victims of severe skin or muscular injury. It starts as erythema and a skin induration at a puncture site and progresses to necrosis with a black eschar. Cutaneous infections can quickly extend into the deep fascia and muscle layers. Necrotizing fasciitis is rare and has a poor prognosis. Neutropenic patients in particular are susceptible to lymphatic and blood vessel invasion, infarction, and necrosis with eventual dissemination. Interestingly, the skin appears to be a less common site of secondary involvement with disseminated mucormycosis than of infections by other hyaline molds such as *Fusarium* or *Scedosporium* species. Even so, skin lesions in patients with suspected mucormycosis should raise concerns about disseminated disease and prompt, careful clinical work-up. Because the differential diagnosis of necrotic skin lesions is broad, especially in neutropenic patients, biopsy specimens should be obtained from the center of the lesion down to the subcutaneous fat. Excision and wide débridement of cutaneous lesions, coupled with systemic antifungal therapy and, on occasion, hyperbaric oxygen therapy, can further reduce mortality rates.

Gastrointestinal Mucormycosis

Primary gastrointestinal mucormycosis is rare and can present as necrotizing enterocolitis and involve any part of the alimentary system with mortality rates of more than 85%. It occurs primarily in malnourished patients and premature infants, in which the stomach is the most commonly affected site, followed by the colon and ileum. The liver, spleen, and pancreas also can be involved. Physicians have described liver abscesses following ingestion of herbal products contaminated by *Mucor indicus*. Fungi can invade the bowel wall and blood vessels, resulting in bowel perforation, peritonitis, and massive gastrointestinal hemorrhage. In neutropenic patients, seeding of the gastrointestinal tract is likely more common than previously thought because 75% of gastrointestinal mucormycoses are diagnosed postmortem. Symptoms and

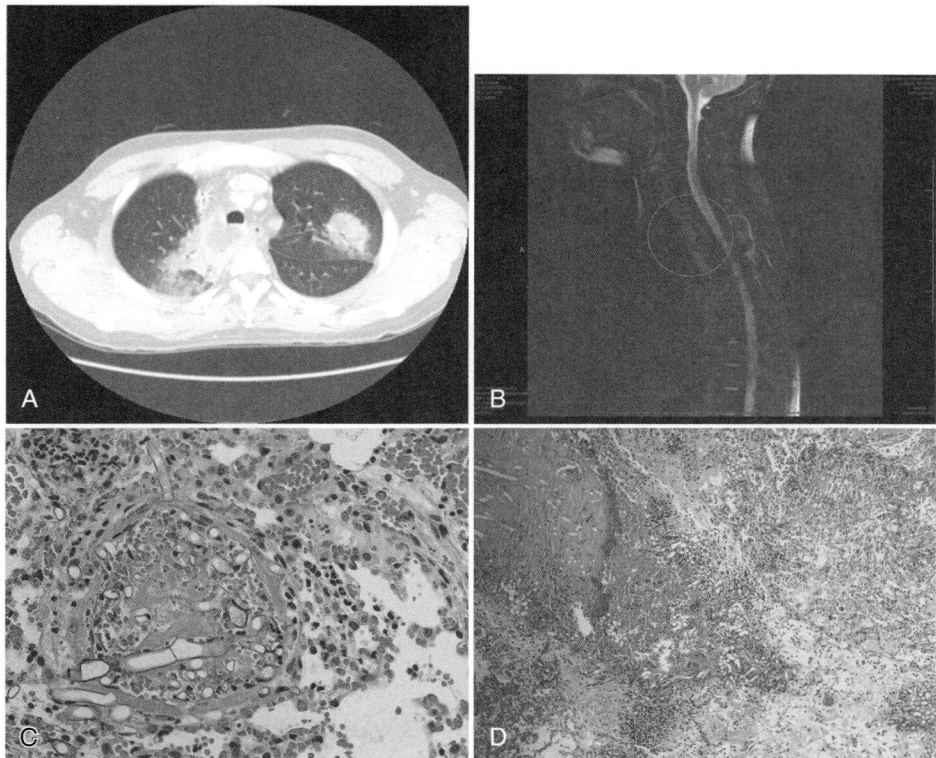

FIGURE 340-1. Extensive, progressive pulmonary mucormycosis in a patient with active leukemia and neutropenia. Characteristic extension of the infection across tissue planes to trachea (producing a fistula) and mediastinum (A) and adjacent spine (B) are shown. The histopathologic characteristics of profound necrosis and hemorrhage and pauciseptate, broad-based, ribbon-like Mucorales are also shown (C and D). Culture of a tissue biopsy specimen remained negative. The patient died 3 weeks after diagnosis, despite aggressive use of a high-dose lipid formulation of amphotericin B (AMB) and adjunct immune therapy.

signs of gastrointestinal mucormycosis include fever, abdominal distention, nausea, vomiting, abdominal pain, diarrhea, melena, hematemesis, hematochezia, and masslike appendiceal and ileal lesions.

Disseminated Mucormycosis

Disseminated mucormycosis is rarely apparent antemortem. Severely immunosuppressed patients (e.g., those with prolonged and profound neutropenia, allogeneic stem cell transplant recipients with severe graft-versus-host disease) and patients receiving deferoxamine are at the highest risk. Symptoms vary depending on the site of dissemination and degree of vascular infarction of the affected organs. The most common organ as source of dissemination is the lung, and the most common site of spread is the brain. Diagnosis of disseminated mucormycosis is challenging and requires a high level of suspicion because the infection may present as an unexpected acute vascular event. Biopsy of suspected sites is critical because of the low yield of blood cultures and suboptimal recovery of the fungus from respiratory specimens. Without appropriate timely treatment, virtually all patients with disseminated mucormycosis die.

Rare Clinical Presentations of Mucormycosis

Mucormycosis has protean manifestations that involve any organ. Authors have reported isolated cases of tracheal, mediastinum, bone, heart, kidney, otitis externa, and corneal involvement. More recently, there have been reports of renal mucormycosis in patients with intravenous drug abuse and/ or those receiving corticosteroids. Cerebral mucormycosis often presenting as brain abscess involving the basal ganglia, and in conjunction with infective endocarditis, has been typically observed in patients using illicit intravenous drugs. Reports of peritonitis in patients undergoing continuous ambulatory peritoneal dialysis have been rare. In all cases of device-related mucormycosis, prompt removal of the device and several weeks of systemic antifungal therapy are essential for resolution of the infection.

___DIAGNOSIS___

The clinical signs and symptoms of mucormycosis are nonspecific. Therefore, a high level of suspicion in susceptible patient populations is of paramount importance.[7] Biopsy analysis and culture from sterile sites remain critical.

Tissue swabs and cultures of sputum, sinus secretions, and bronchoalveolar lavage fluid are usually nondiagnostic. For example, fungal contamination of clinical specimens occurs because the small size of sporangiospores (approximately 6 μm in width) allows easy dispersion via the airborne route. Particles of this size may remain airborne even with very slight movements in air and contaminate clinical samples. Therefore, growth in culture may not represent clinically significant invasive mucormycosis. However, the value of Mucorales-positive cultures (especially repetitive cultures) as an important indication of infection in immunocompromised patients is quite high. The site of infection has a major impact on the likelihood of histopathologic diagnosis. With their ease of accessibility, sinuses are the major site of definite infection.

Histopathology

A variety of stains, including hematoxylin and eosin, Grocott-Gomori methenamine-silver nitrate, and periodic acid–Schiff, reveal characteristic hyphal elements in tissue. Histopathologic examination of infected tissue typically shows characteristic broad (3 to 25 μm in diameter), thin-walled, primarily aseptate hyphae; focal bulbous dilation; and nondichotomous irregular branching at occasional right angles accompanying tissue necrosis and fungal angioinvasion (see Fig. 340-1). Perineural invasion is found in 90% of tissues containing nerves. The inflammatory responses to mucormycosis can range from neutrophilic, granulomatous, and/or pyogranulomatous to minimal inflammation with hemorrhage. Also, fungal hyphae can be examined directly using a potassium hydroxide preparation of a tissue specimen or bronchial alveolar lavage fluid. Although contamination is always a possibility, discovery of fungal elements in a specimen obtained from an immunocompromised host is considered significant. Treatment with fluorescent stains such as Calcofluor White and Blankofluor may enhance detection of hyphal elements during microscopic examination. Improved staining procedures may be important when the number of organisms is small or the amount of tissue is limited.

Culture

Mucorales fungi characteristically produce large, ribbon-like hyphae with irregular diameters and only occasionally septa, resulting in characterization of these organisms primarily as aseptate fungi. Identification can be

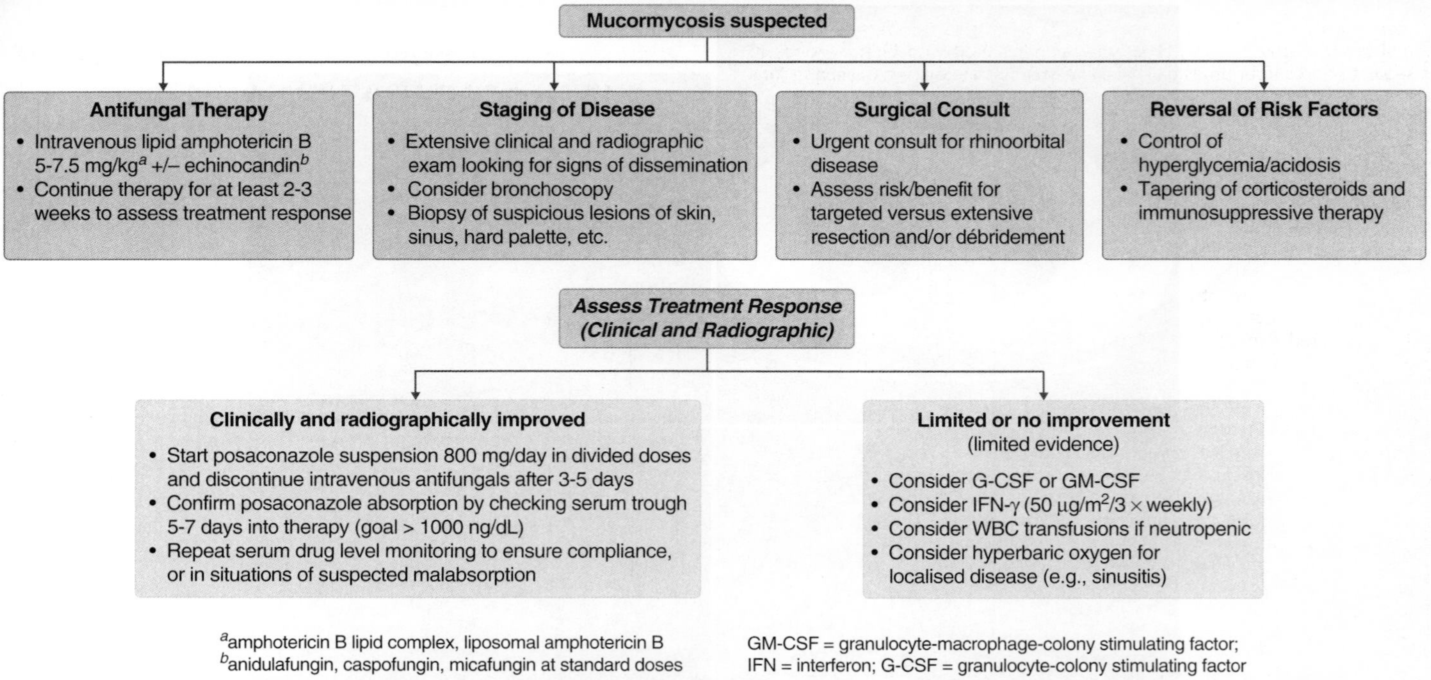

FIGURE 340-2. Diagram of the management approach to patients with suspected mucormycosis.

confirmed by observing the characteristic saclike fruiting structures (sporangia), which produce internally spherical yellow or brown spores (sporangiospores). Spores range from 3 to 11 µm in diameter and are easily aerosolized. Blood cultures are rarely positive for these pathogens despite their angioinvasive nature. Paradoxically, even when fungal hyphae are seen in histopathologic analysis, fungal cultures may not be positive because of the friability of nonseptated hyphae, making them more susceptible to damage during tissue manipulation. However, collection of several proper clinical specimens is important. Recovery of Mucorales from tissue can be improved by mincing (not homogenizing) tissue specimens and using culture techniques that simulate in vivo fungal growth, including incubation at 35° to 37°C under relatively semianaerobic conditions.

Morphologic identification of Mucorales requires their cultivation to examine reproductive fruiting structures. Most of these fungi grow rapidly on most fungal media (e.g., Sabouraud dextrose agar) when incubated at 25° to 30° C. These fungi are sensitive to the protein inhibitor cycloheximide, and addition of this agent to fungal media may not ensure optimal recovery. Morphologic features alone, especially when assessed by individuals with expertise in fungal identification, can provide a high level of accuracy comparable to that of molecular methods.

Data on the antifungal susceptibility of Mucorales species. are limited, and minimal inhibitory concentration (MIC) testing is rarely available outside research or research laboratories. The MIC end points for these rapidly growing fungi are inconsistent, not standardized, and at times difficult to interpret. Because interpretive MIC break points for Mucorales have yet to be defined, the correlation between clinical responses and MIC values is uncertain. Mucorales are resistant to many antifungals, including flucytosine, ketoconazole, fluconazole, voriconazole, and the echinocandins. Also, they have variable susceptibility to itraconazole. Amphotericin B (AMB) and posaconazole, a new triazole, are the most active agents in vitro, although their activities differ among different Mucorales families. The activity of antifungal combinations against these fungi has yet to be proved in vivo.

The importance of early differentiation of Mucorales from more common opportunistic molds such as *Aspergillus* species has generated considerable interest in development of culture- or histopathology-independent diagnostic tests such as detection of specific antigens or nucleic acids using polymerase chain reaction or in situ hybridization techniques. Molecular techniques for detecting Mucorales are few, not widely available, and investigational. This is an important unmet need for the management of mucormycosis.

TREATMENT Rx

Approach to the management of suspected mucormycosis and assessment of treatment response are shown in Figure 340-2. Successful treatment of mucormycosis relies on a multifaceted strategy that includes (1) aggressive attempts at diagnosis and rapid initiation of effective antifungal therapy and (2) extensive surgical débridement, and (3) rapid control of underlying medical conditions.[8]

Again, early diagnosis is critical to the outcome. Small focal lesions can be surgically resected before they progress to involve critical structures or distal organs. Patients often have indolent clinical presentations until extensive invasion or dissemination of the infection occurs.[9]

Antifungal Therapy

Delayed administration of systemic antifungal therapy increases the probability of patient death. Most of the knowledge about the activity of currently used antifungals comes from small case series, anecdotes, and animal models of infection. Therefore, the optimal treatment approach is uncertain.[10] Most of the clinical experience has been with AMB. Previously, the recommended antifungal therapy for mucormycosis included AMB deoxycholate at the maximum tolerated dosage, usually 1.0 to 1.5 mg/kg/day. The nephrotoxic and systemic toxic effects of regular AMB led to the development of the lipid formulations of AMB (liposomal AMB, AMB lipid complex, AMB colloidal dispersion). These agents are less nephrotoxic than regular AMB and can be given at higher doses (e.g., 5 to 10 mg/kg per day). Lipid formulations of AMB are now considered the drugs of choice for mucormycosis. Furthermore, use of percutaneous or aerosolized AMB in conjunction with concomitant systemic therapy has been successful in selected patients with pulmonary mucormycosis. Topical therapy with AMB as well as other polyenes (natamycin) may be effective against primary cutaneous and ocular mucormycosis. Treatment of mucormycosis with AMB-based combinations has been successful in small retrospective case series. In particular, a benefit has been suggested for echinocandin-liposomal AMB combination in 41 diabetic patients with rhino-orbital mucormycosis compared with the ones who received amphotericin B lipid complex (ABLC) or liposomal AMB alone. This benefit was most pronounced in patients with cerebral involvement.

Although azoles traditionally have been inactive against Mucorales, the new broad-spectrum triazole posaconazole demonstrated promising activity. Among open-label studies and retrospective surveys evaluating posaconazole suspension as salvage therapy (800 mg/day) in patients with refractory mucormycosis, the agent showed a response rate approaching 70%. Furthermore, posaconazole has been well tolerated. Determining whether posaconazole alone or combined with a lipid formulation of AMB or other agent (e.g., deferasirox) is of value requires further study. Posaconazole has limitations because absorption of the oral suspension is suboptimal in patients with mucositis, severe diarrhea, acid suppression therapy, or poor oral intake. Absorption of oral posaconazole is maximized when administered with high-fat foods in separate doses (four times daily). Finally, steady-state plasma concentrations of posaconazole are not reached until around 1 week of therapy. The new formula of posaconazole (posaconazole tablets 300 mg/daily) has not been studied adequately in mucormycosis.

The duration of antifungal therapy should be determined on an individual basis. Near normalization of radiographic imaging, negative follow-up biopsy specimens, and cultures from the affected site, as well as recovery from immunosuppression, are important indicators for stopping antifungal therapy.

Surgery

Surgical débridement of cutaneous lesions is crucial and must be done without delay because of the aggressively invasive nature of mucormycosis. A coordinated effort among all subspecialties involved (surgery, infectious diseases, head and neck, ophthalmology, pathology, clinical microbiology, and plastic surgery) is crucial, and the internist can play a vital role coordinating it.

Repeated removal of necrotic tissue or aggressive surgical measures such as enucleation of the eye may be required for control of the infection. Decisions regarding the extent of débridement are often made at the bedside. A CT or MRI scan before surgery and intraoperative frozen section analysis help determine the extent of tissue and tissue margin involvement. Low platelet counts, as may be seen in patients with underlying hematologic malignancies, must be corrected with transfusions before surgical intervention. Unfortunately, bleeding problems can limit surgical options. Surgery in conjunction with systemic antifungal therapy has been shown to significantly improve survival rates.

Management of Comorbidity and Adjunct Treatments

Adjunct measures have been proposed to improve host immunity, tissue viability, and impeding fungal proliferation. Rapid correction of underlying conditions, such as control of hyperglycemia, reversal of ketoacidosis, rapid tapering of glucocorticoid therapy, and discontinuation of deferoxamine-based treatment, can influence outcomes. Hyperbaric oxygen is a beneficial adjunct therapy for mucormycosis, particularly in diabetic patients with rhinocerebral disease. Specifically, the increased oxygen pressure achieved seems to improve neutrophil activity and oxidative killing by polyene antifungals. Also, high concentrations of oxygen can inhibit growth of the organism in vitro and improve the rate of wound healing by increasing the release of tissue growth factors. However, this treatment has not been studied vigorously to determine efficacy and cannot be routinely recommended. Investigators have proposed several immune augmentation strategies as adjunct therapy, including administration of cytokines (e.g., granulocyte colony-stimulating factor [G-CSF], interferon). In refractory neutropenic patients, granulocyte transfusion may be beneficial until granulocyte recovery. These adjunct measures, although promising, are yet to be studied sufficiently. Finally, the new iron chelator deferasirox has been considered as an adjunct antifungal agent based on preclinical studies and very limited human experience with patients with refractory mucormycosis. Results of the small randomized, double-blinded DEFEAT Mucor trial were published in 2012.[A1] Twenty patients with proven or probable mucormycosis were randomized to treatment with liposomal amphotericin B plus deferasirox (20 mg/kg per day for 14 days) or liposomal amphotericin B plus placebo. Although reported adverse events were similar between the two study groups, significantly higher mortality rates were found in patients randomized to receive deferasirox at 30 (45% vs. 11%) and 90 days (82% vs. 22%, P = .01). However, patients in the deferasirox arm were more likely than patients in the placebo arm to have active malignancy, neutropenia, and/or corticosteroid therapy, and less likely to have received additional antifungals, making the results of this pilot trial less conclusive. Nevertheless, currently available data do not support a role for initial deferasirox therapy for mucormycosis. Further knowledge of the unique virulence attributes of Mucorales based on genomic analysis might aid the development on novel therapeutic targets.

Grade A Reference

A1. Spellberg B, Ibrahim AS, Chin-Hong PV, et al. The Deferasirox-AmBisome Therapy for Mucormycosis (DEFEAT Mucor) study: a randomized, double-blinded, placebo-controlled trial. *J Antimicrob Chemother*. 2012;67:715-722.

GENERAL REFERENCES

For the General References and other additional features, please visit Expert Consult at https://expertconsult.inkling.com.

341

PNEUMOCYSTIS PNEUMONIA

JOSEPH A. KOVACS

DEFINITION

Pneumocystis jirovecii is a fungus that causes pneumonia almost exclusively in immunodeficient patients. In the 1950s, it was recognized as the cause of an epidemic interstitial plasma cell pneumonia that occurred primarily in premature and malnourished infants. During the 1960s and 1970s, *Pneumocystis* pneumonia (PCP) was seen with increasing frequency in immunodeficient patients, especially those receiving immunosuppressive chemotherapy. In the early 1980s, an epidemic of PCP in previously healthy adults heralded the onset of the HIV/AIDS epidemic; in the United States and in many other parts of the world, PCP has been the most common life-threatening opportunistic infection in this population. Although the frequency of PCP decreased in HIV-infected patients first in association with the widespread use of anti-*Pneumocystis* prophylaxis and later with the introduction of effective combination antiretroviral therapy for HIV/AIDS, it continues to be seen with regularity in HIV-infected and other immunodeficient patients.[1] Over the past decade, there has been a marked increase in outbreaks of PCP among renal transplant recipients, especially in Europe and Australia.

The Pathogen

Pneumocystis, which was long thought to be a protozoan, has now been definitively classified as an ascomycete fungus, based primarily on molecular studies demonstrating that a large number of genes have a high level of homology to other fungi rather than to protozoa. Molecular as well as antigenic studies have further demonstrated that the genus *Pneumocystis* includes a group of closely related organisms that are unique species, each of which can infect only a single host species. This has led to the application of species names to the group of organisms previously called *Pneumocystis carinii*. *P. carinii* is reserved for a species that infects rats (there is also a second species, *P. wakefieldiae*, that can infect rats). The organism infecting humans has been renamed *P. jirovecii*, in honor of Otto Jirovec, one of the investigators who recognized that this organism is the causative agent of interstitial plasma cell pneumonia. Despite the name change, the acronym PCP (for *Pneumocystis* pneumonia) continues to be used to designate the disease in humans.

Pneumocystis species show a strict host specificity: attempts to transmit, for example, rat or human *Pneumocystis* to mice have been unsuccessful. Molecular evolutionary studies suggest that *Pneumocystis* species coevolved with their hosts, with rat and mouse *Pneumocystis* diverging an estimated 33 million years ago, similar to the time rat and mouse species diverged.

Studies of *Pneumocystis* have been substantially hampered by an inability to grow any species in culture for a sustained period. Thus, the life cycle of *Pneumocystis* is unknown, although putative life cycles based on morphologic studies have been proposed; there is accumulating evidence supporting a sexual phase in the life cycle. There are two easily recognized forms of the organism: trophic forms ($\approx$2 to 6 μm in diameter) and cysts (also called asci; $\approx$6 to 8 μm in diameter), which can contain up to eight intracystic bodies (ascospores); additional intermediate forms are also seen. Trophic forms, which have an amorphous shape, are estimated to outnumber cysts, which are spherical, by approximately 10 : 1 in an infected lung. β-1,3-Glucan is found in the cyst form only, where it contributes to the rigidity of the cell wall. The estimated genome size is approximately 8 million base pairs.[2] The most abundant surface protein of *Pneumocystis*, the major surface glycoprotein, is found on both cysts and trophic forms and is encoded by a multicopy gene family, only one of which is apparently expressed in a given organism; this provides *Pneumocystis* with the potential for antigenic variability. Although, to date, only a single *Pneumocystis* species has been found that infects humans, molecular typing techniques have demonstrated a high level of diversity among human *Pneumocystis* isolates.

EPIDEMIOLOGY

Pneumocystis has a worldwide distribution. Serologic studies show a high prevalence of anti-*Pneumocystis* antibodies in all populations studied to date.

In America and Europe, serologic studies have demonstrated that most humans develop antibodies to *Pneumocystis* by an early age, suggesting that this is a ubiquitous organism. In support of this, an autopsy study in infants younger than 1 year with no major underlying medical problems identified *Pneumocystis* infection in lung tissue by polymerase chain reaction (PCR) in 100% of cases.

Animal studies have demonstrated that *Pneumocystis* is transmitted by the respiratory route. Human infection appears to be transmitted in the same manner. There is no evidence that water or fomites play a role in transmission. A small number of animal studies and very limited human data suggest that transmission can occur transplacentally, although the clinical relevance is unknown.

Given the strict host specificity of *Pneumocystis*, the source of organisms infecting humans is presumably other humans, by either direct or indirect exposure; *Pneumocystis* is not a zoonosis. PCR-based studies have identified *Pneumocystis* DNA in air sampled in close proximity to patients with PCP, and outbreaks, especially in renal transplant patients, have been linked to a single strain of *Pneumocystis*, both of which suggest that patients with PCP can transmit it to other susceptible patients.[3] Because clinically apparent PCP is rare, and given the high penetration of infection into healthy human populations at a young age, *Pneumocystis* infection is also likely acquired from apparently healthy humans, in whom subclinical infection (either asymptomatic or minimally symptomatic) must be quite common to allow such rapid and broad dissemination. The high frequency of detection in infants suggests an important role in transmission.

Although infection with *Pneumocystis* is widespread, in immunocompetent hosts, it does not appear to cause significant disease. Clinically significant PCP occurs exclusively in patients with severe levels of immunodeficiency that are usually associated with a high risk for other opportunistic pathogens. Populations at risk include those with congenital immunodeficiencies (Chapter 250), especially severe combined immunodeficiency (SCID) and hyper–immunoglobulin M (IgM) syndrome; patients with HIV infection (Chapter 384) and human T-lymphotropic virus-1–associated lymphoma (Chapter 378); patients receiving chemotherapy for the treatment of malignancies, especially lymphoma; transplant patients receiving immunosuppressive therapy; and patients being treated with prolonged courses of immunosuppressive drugs (Chapter 35), especially corticosteroids, for inflammatory diseases such as Wegener's granulomatosis or systemic lupus erythematosus. Biologic agents such as rituximab and those targeting tumor necrosis factor-α (TNF-α) are also associated with an increased, though low, absolute risk for PCP (e.g. 0.18 to 0.4% in patients receiving anti-TNF-α agents in Japan).[4] Among patients with HIV infection, the best predictor of the risk for developing PCP is the CD4 count: patients with CD4 counts less than 200 cells/mm^3, and especially those with CD4 counts less than 100 cells/mm^3, are at greatest risk. Patients with a prior history of PCP and those with unexplained fever, weight loss, or thrush are also at increased risk. Among other patient populations, laboratory parameters are not as useful in quantifying risk, although non-HIV patients with CD4 counts less than 200

cells/mm^3 may be at increased risk. Additional information on risk is provided in the section on prophylaxis.

For many years, development of PCP was thought to result from a reactivation of latent infection by organisms that remained viable following infection at an early age, similar to tuberculosis. However, recent molecular epidemiologic studies based on the detection of mutations in the dihydropteroate synthase (DHPS) gene of *Pneumocystis*, as well as genotyping of isolates from outbreaks of PCP primarily in renal transplant patients, have provided compelling evidence that the infecting strain is often recently acquired. Molecular studies have further documented that in the majority of non-outbreak cases of PCP, more than one strain can be identified in respiratory samples. In patients who develop recurrent PCP, this recurrence can be due to relapse, especially for early recurrences, or to reinfection with a novel strain. Recurrent PCP occurs almost exclusively in HIV-infected patients, in whom the risk was greater than 50% early in the AIDS epidemic, before the availability of highly active antiretroviral therapy (HAART) and the broad use of anti-*Pneumocystis* prevention.

PATHOBIOLOGY

Animal studies have provided important insights into the pathogenesis of *Pneumocystis* infection. Exposure for as little as 1 day to a *Pneumocystis*-infected animal results in transmission of infection. In healthy animals, an adaptive immune response develops by approximately 5 to 6 weeks, which leads to control and clearance before the organism burden produces symptoms. CD4 cells are critical to this control, although other populations, including B cells and macrophages, also play important roles. CD8 cells can contribute to the associated inflammation. In immunodeficient animal models, inability to control *Pneumocystis* replication leads to severe pneumonia by 2 to 3 months. Limited human data suggest a similar time course. Host inflammatory responses appear to play a critical role in the development of pulmonary symptoms. This may account for the development of symptoms of PCP in patients in whom corticosteroids are being tapered, as well as the exacerbation of hypoxia that develops approximately 4 days after the initiation of anti-*Pneumocystis* therapy (in the absence of concomitant corticosteroid therapy).

The lung pathology in patients with PCP is characteristic. Staining with hematoxylin and eosin demonstrates an acellular, foamy, eosinophilic, intraalveolar exudate associated with mild interstitial inflammation (Fig. 341-1). With disease progression, hyaline membrane formation and interstitial as well as intraluminal fibrosis develop. Although methenamine silver stain highlights cysts scattered throughout the eosinophilic exudate, based on Giemsa staining of thin sections as well as electron micrographs, this exudate is composed almost entirely of *Pneumocystis* organisms. Atypical pathology, including noncaseating granulomas and intrapulmonary cystic changes, can also be seen.

As noted earlier, patients with certain congenital immunodeficiencies, especially SCID patients, who have global T- and B-cell defects, and hyper-IgM syndrome patients, whose primary defect is in CD40-CD40L signaling,

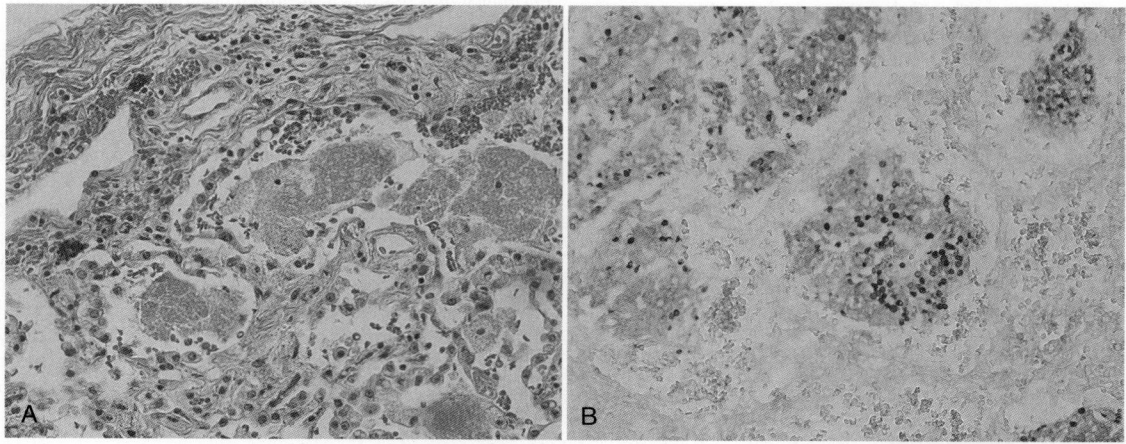

FIGURE 341-1. Histopathology of the lung of a patient who died from *Pneumocystis* pneumonia (PCP). **A,** The hematoxylin and eosin–stained section shows the characteristic acellular, eosinophilic, intra-alveolar exudate that is typical of PCP. **B,** Methenamine silver staining of lung tissue from the same patient demonstrates black-staining cysts scattered throughout the intra-alveolar exudates.

are at increased risk for developing PCP. Among HIV-infected patients, polymorphisms in the FcγRIIa gene and in the chemokine receptor gene for CCRL2 were each associated with an increased risk for developing PCP in single studies.[5]

CLINICAL MANIFESTATIONS

In nonimmunosuppressed humans, no well-defined clinical syndrome is associated with *Pneumocystis* infection. *Pneumocystis* has been identified in infants by PCR and may be associated with a mild respiratory syndrome, but a postulated association with sudden infant death syndrome has not been supported by data from well-controlled studies. *Pneumocystis* has been detected by PCR in pulmonary samples from patients with chronic obstructive pulmonary disease (COPD), but what role, if any, it plays in the development or progression of COPD (Chapter 88) remains to be elucidated.[6]

Pneumonia is the primary clinical manifestation of *Pneumocystis* infection in immunosuppressed patients. PCP typically presents with a fever, nonproductive cough, and shortness of breath that initially occurs only on exertion but, without therapy, inevitably progresses to dyspnea at rest. Only one or two of these symptoms may be present initially. Development of symptoms may be insidious, over the course of a few weeks, as is common in patients with HIV infection; a more rapid onset, over the course of only a few days, is more common in non-AIDS patients. Purulent sputum production is unusual, and chills and chest pain occur in a minority of patients. Patients with HIV infection may present with other manifestations of immunodeficiency, including weight loss and thrush.

In non-AIDS patients, corticosteroids are a common risk factor.[7] Clinical manifestations may develop as corticosteroids are being tapered, which presumably represents the unmasking of an inflammatory response to the infection as immunosuppression is decreased.

Rarely, extrapulmonary disease can involve the skin, eye (choroiditis), central nervous system, bone marrow, thyroid, spleen, liver, gastrointestinal tract, lymph node, or multiple organs in disseminated disease. Extrapulmonary disease can occur with or without concurrent pneumonia. Use of aerosol pentamidine for prophylaxis has been associated with an increased risk for extrapulmonary disease in HIV-infected patients, but even in that circumstance, it remains extremely rare. Symptoms are related to the specific site involved and may be nonspecific; diagnosis is often made at autopsy.

DIAGNOSIS

Given the nonspecific symptoms, especially early in the disease process, clinicians must have a high index of suspicion for PCP even in patients not known to be immunosuppressed; many patients with HIV infection are unaware of their status until they present with an opportunistic infection. Knowledge of the most recent CD4 count is helpful in assessing HIV-infected patients because PCP is rare in those whose CD4 counts are above 200 cells/mm³.

Physical examination and routine laboratory tests are usually not helpful in making the diagnosis because many pulmonary processes, both infectious and noninfectious, can present in a similar manner. Moreover, even though patients may be tachypneic and appear to be in respiratory distress, those presenting early in the disease course may have an entirely normal lung examination. Lymphopenia is common but is a manifestation of the underlying disease rather than PCP. Lactate dehydrogenase levels may be elevated but have poor specificity.

The initial evaluation should include a chest radiograph and assessment of arterial oxygenation, either by blood gas measurement or by pulse oximetry. The chest radiograph typically shows perihilar or diffuse bilateral interstitial infiltrates that progress to a diffuse alveolar pattern (Fig. 341-2). However, PCP has been associated with unilateral disease, focal disease, consolidation, nodules, cavities, pneumothorax, and, rarely, pleural effusions. In up to 30% of patients with HIV infection, the chest radiograph appears normal; in this situation, a computed tomography (CT) scan of the chest, especially high-resolution CT, is invariably abnormal, usually showing a patchy or diffuse ground-glass pattern (see Fig. 341-2).[8]

Arterial oxygenation at rest is often abnormal, although in 30% or more of cases, it is within normal limits. Exercise testing induces desaturation and an increase in the alveolar-arterial oxygen (A-a O₂) gradient in the majority of patients with PCP, even those with normal oxygenation at rest or a normal chest radiograph. An abnormal resting diffusing capacity is also common. However, although many of these tests have a high sensitivity for PCP, their specificity is poor because other respiratory processes show similar abnormalities.

Serologic tests are not helpful in diagnosing PCP. Although antibody titers against recombinant *Pneumocystis* proteins such as major surface glycoprotein may be increased in patients with PCP, such tests have not shown utility for diagnosis in individual patients. Although serum and bronchoalveolar lavage (BAL) β-D-glucan levels are elevated in many patients, this again is a nonspecific test because other fungal infections can also lead to elevations, and conditions unrelated to fungal infection can lead to false-positive results. To date, there are inadequate data from well-conducted prospective trials to support routine use of this assay for definitive diagnosis of PCP.

Because *Pneumocystis* cannot be cultured, a definitive diagnosis of PCP requires detection of the organism in a pulmonary sample. This can be accomplished by any number of colorimetric or immunologic stains or by molecular techniques. Until the development of anti-*Pneumocystis* monoclonal antibodies in the 1980s, colorimetric stains were routinely used, and they continue to be used at many centers owing to cost considerations. Such stains include Gomori methenamine silver, toluidine blue O, Gram-Weigert, and cresyl echt violet, which stain the cyst wall of *Pneumocystis*, as well as Giemsa-type stains, including Diff-Quik, which can stain both trophic forms, the more abundant form of the organism, and intracystic bodies within cysts, but not the cyst wall. *Pneumocystis* can also be detected by Calcofluor white, Papanicolaou, periodic acid–Schiff, and, rarely, Gram stain. None of the colorimetric stains is specific for *Pneumocystis*. Cyst wall stains such as Gomori methenamine silver and toluidine blue O can stain other fungi, and Giemsa-type stains also stain background cells and cellular debris. The latter requires substantial expertise for correct interpretation.

Immunofluorescent assays using anti-*Pneumocystis* monoclonal antibodies provide a number of advantages over colorimetric stains. They are specific for *Pneumocystis* and do not show cross-reactivity with other organisms, including fungi; they can be performed and interpreted rapidly; and they have increased sensitivity, especially when examining induced sputum samples (Fig. 341-3).

Molecular techniques, primarily PCR-based assays, have been extensively evaluated for diagnosing PCP. PCR assays are 10- to 100-fold more sensitive than stains for the detection of *Pneumocystis*; this may allow for diagnosis using samples such as oral washes, which have a lower organism burden than induced sputum or BAL.[9] This increased sensitivity, however, is associated with decreased specificity because it allows the detection of organisms in patients ultimately shown not to have PCP.[10] The latter situation presumably reflects colonization or subclinical infection that does not require specific anti-*Pneumocystis* therapy. PCR-based assays are currently not broadly used because of limited availability, lack of standardization among laboratories, and the lack of a commercial product with U.S. Food and Drug Administration approval.

As detection methods for *Pneumocystis* improved, there was a parallel improvement in sample acquisition. Before the AIDS epidemic, open lung biopsy was required for diagnosis. During the 1980s, bronchoscopy, initially with brushings and biopsy, and subsequently with BAL, was shown to have a greater than 90% sensitivity for diagnosing PCP; BAL continues to be the primary diagnostic modality at many centers today. Although expectorated sputum has a low diagnostic yield, induced sputum, especially when combined with immunofluorescent staining, can have a sensitivity approaching 90%, although in many centers the diagnostic yield is much lower, likely due in part to variability in the methods used for induction and processing. Ideally, sputum induction should be the first step in diagnosis, followed by bronchoscopy with BAL (Fig. 341-4). Bronchoscopic or open lung biopsy is only rarely needed to make the diagnosis.

The differential diagnosis of pulmonary infiltrates in immunosuppressed patients is very broad and includes infections such as adenovirus, cytomegalovirus, tuberculosis, cryptococcosis, histoplasmosis, aspergillosis, and toxoplasmosis, as well as noninfectious processes such as tumor, congestive heart failure, pulmonary emboli, radiation- and chemotherapy-induced pneumonitis, and, especially in HIV-infected patients, nonspecific interstitial pneumonitis and Kaposi's sarcoma.

TREATMENT   Rx

Specific anti-*Pneumocystis* therapy should be initiated promptly when the diagnosis is suspected in a potentially susceptible patient. Dosing regimens with documented efficacy are listed in Table 341-1. Although there are no controlled studies defining the optimal duration of therapy, HIV-infected patients should be treated for 21 days and non-HIV patients for at least 14

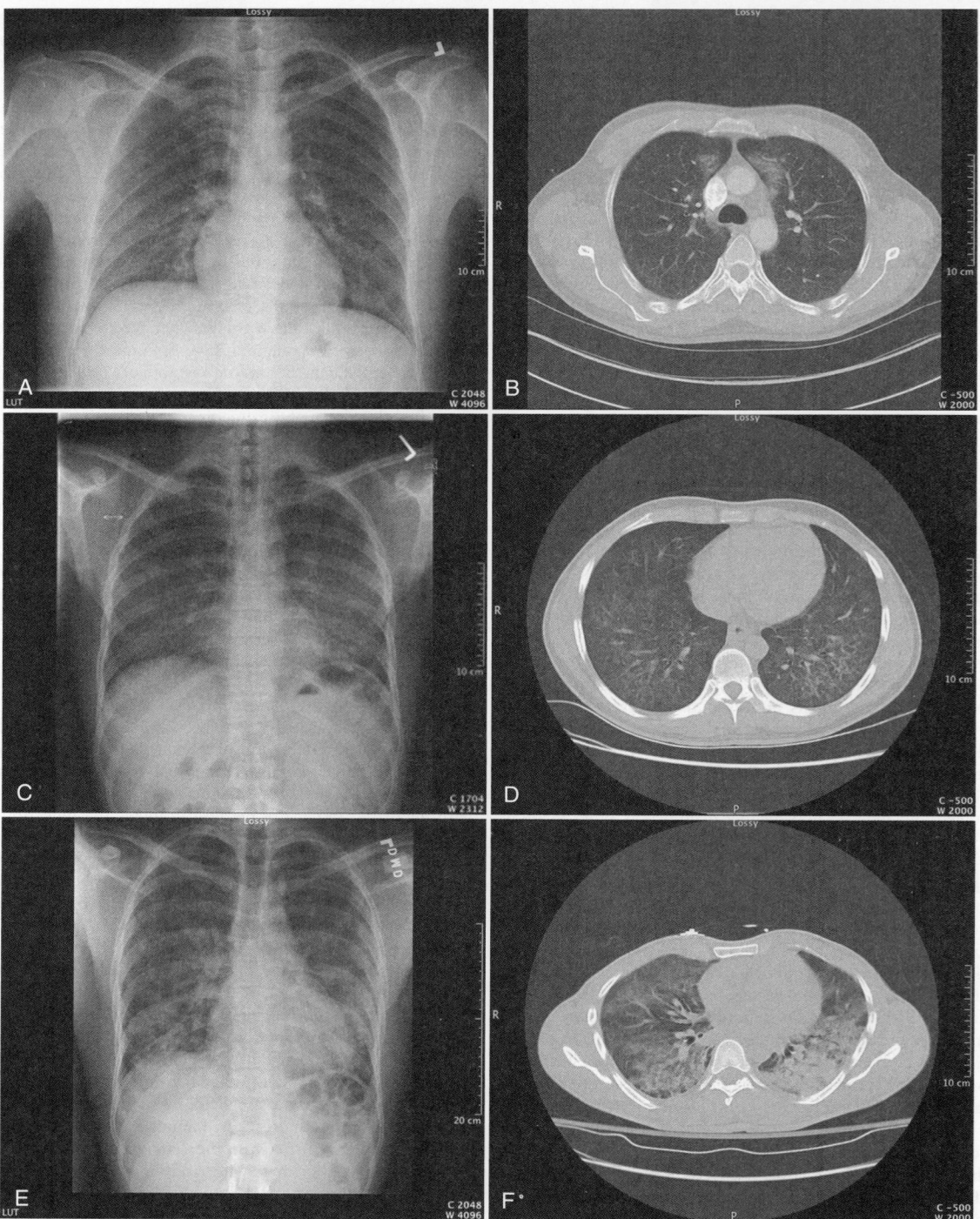

FIGURE 341-2. Chest radiographs (**A, C, E**) and corresponding computed tomography (CT) scans (**B, D, F**) from three HIV patients diagnosed with laboratory-confirmed *Pneumocystis* pneumonia. Patient 1 presented with no symptoms; had minimal abnormalities on an incidental chest radiograph (**A**), suggesting an interstitial process; and had focal infiltrates on CT (**B**). Patient 2 presented with fever and weight loss but no shortness of breath. Pulse oximetry demonstrated 99% saturation at rest, with a decrease to 89% with exercise. Chest radiograph (**C**) showed bilateral lower lobe infiltrates, and CT (**D**) showed bilateral lower lobe interstitial infiltrates with patches of ground-glass attenuation. Patient 3 presented with a 2-week history of fever, night sweats, shortness of breath, and weakness. His PaO$_2$ at diagnosis was 67 mm Hg, and his A-a O$_2$ gradient was 53 mm Hg. Chest radiograph (**E**) showed bilateral mid and lower lung field infiltrates, and CT (**F**) showed bilateral infiltrates with lower lung consolidation.

days.[11,12] For HIV-infected patients with moderate to severe disease (PaO$_2$ <70 mm Hg or A-a O$_2$ gradient >35 mm Hg), concomitant corticosteroid therapy should be administered. In contrast, the use of corticosteroids in non-HIV patients is not well defined, as discussed later. The diagnosis should be definitively confirmed by sputum induction or bronchoscopy as soon as possible; however, delaying such confirmation for a few days after the initiation of therapy will not decrease the diagnostic yield because organisms can be detected in clinical samples for more than 3 weeks after the initiation of therapy. Empirical therapy in the absence of a confirmed diagnosis runs the risk of delaying appropriate therapy for another infection, giving inappropriate

therapy with known toxicities, and performing a definitive procedure such as bronchoscopy when the patient is failing therapy and consequently has more severe pulmonary compromise.

The treatment of choice for PCP or extrapulmonary disease, regardless of severity, is trimethoprim-sulfamethoxazole, which combines inhibitors of two enzymes in the folate synthetic pathway of *Pneumocystis*: sulfamethoxazole, an inhibitor of DHPS, and trimethoprim, an inhibitor of dihydrofolate reductase (DHFR). Trimethoprim-sulfamethoxazole is available in both oral and intravenous formulations. Oral therapy should be reserved for patients with mild to moderate disease in whom poor absorption is not a concern.

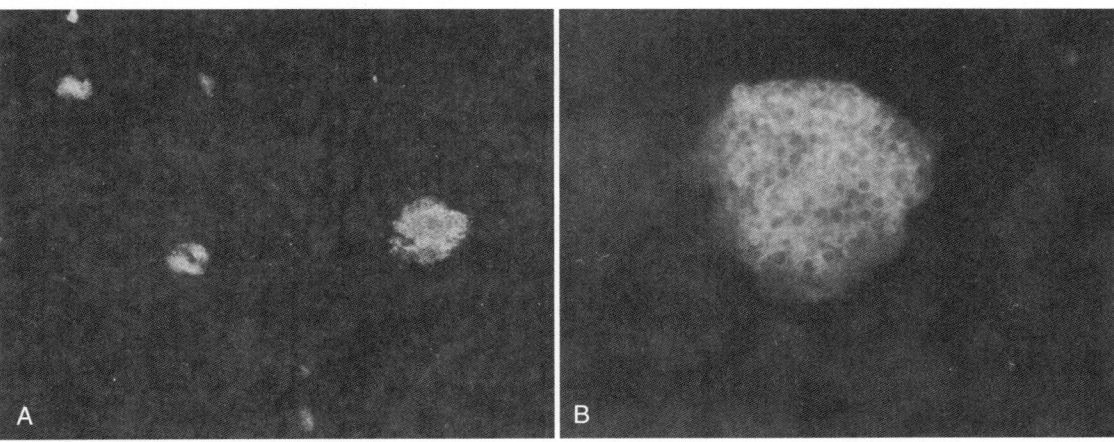

FIGURE 341-3. Immunofluorescent detection of *Pneumocystis* using a direct fluorescent antibody test to examine an induced sputum sample. **A,** Low power (100× original) allows visualization of multiple clusters of organisms staining bright green. **B,** Under high power (400× original), individual organisms can be seen within a single cluster.

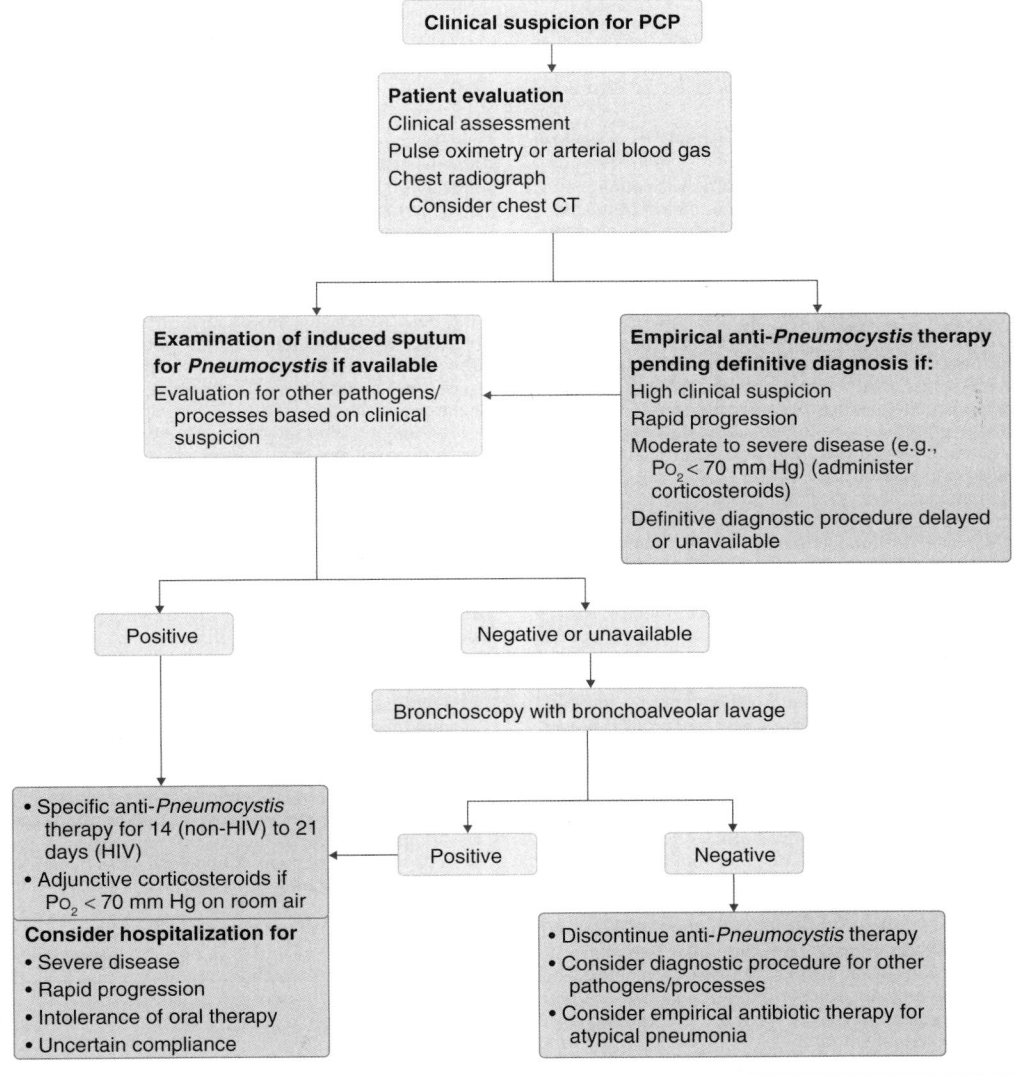

FIGURE 341-4. Algorithm for the evaluation of patients with suspected *Pneumocystis* pneumonia (PCP). CT = computed tomography; HIV = human immunodeficiency virus.

TABLE 341-1 DRUG REGIMENS FOR TREATMENT OF *PNEUMOCYSTIS PNEUMONIA* (PCP)

INDICATION	REGIMEN PREFERENCE	DRUG	ROUTE	DOSE	COMMENTS
Mild PCP: PaO$_2$ ≥70 mm Hg or (A-a) O$_2$ gradient ≤35 mm Hg	Preferred	Trimethoprim-Sulfamethoxazole (TMP-SMX)	PO	2 double-strength (160 TMP+800 SMX) tablets TID	
	Alternative	Trimethoprim plus Dapsone	PO PO	5 mg/kg TID (15 mg/kg/d) 100 mg QD	If possible test for G6PD deficiency before use
	Alternative	Clindamycin plus Primaquine	PO PO	450 mg QID or 600 mg TID 30 mg (base) QD	If possible test for G6PD deficiency before use
	Alternative	Atovaquone	PO	750 mg BID with food	
Moderate to severe PCP: PaO$_2$ <70 mm Hg or (A-a) O$_2$ gradient >35 mm Hg; moderate PCP ((A-a) O$_2$ gradient 35 to 45 mm Hg); can be treated with an oral regimen	Preferred	Trimethoprim-Sulfamethoxazole (TMP-SMX)	IV	5 mg/kg Q8H TMP and 25 mg/kg Q8H SMX (15 mg/kg/d TMP and 75 mg/kg/d SMX)	May switch to oral therapy following clinical improvement
	Alternative	Pentamidine	IV	3-4 mg/kg QD	Infuse over >60 minutes
	Alternative	Clindamycin plus	IV	600 mg Q6H or 900 mg Q8H	May switch to oral therapy following clinical improvement
		Primaquine	PO	30 mg (base) QD	No parenteral formulation is available
Adjunctive therapy for moderate to severe PCP: PaO$_2$ <70 mm Hg or (A-a) O$_2$ gradient >35 mm Hg	Preferred	Prednisone	PO	40 mg BID, days 1-5; 40 mg QD, days 6-10; 20 mg QD days 11-21	Begin as early as possible and within 72 hours; efficacy if started later has not been demonstrated
	Preferred	Methylprednisolone	IV	30 mg BID, days 1-5; 30 mg QD, days 6-10; 15 mg QD days 11-21	Use if parenteral therapy is necessary

Note: HIV-infected patients should receive 21 days of therapy; non-HIV patients should receive at least 14 days of therapy.

Outpatient therapy should be reserved for patients with mild to moderate disease who will reliably return for follow-up.

The efficacy of trimethoprim-sulfamethoxazole for both the treatment and the prevention of PCP was first demonstrated in a pediatric cancer population in the 1970s; it has been the first-line therapy since then, when the only alternative was pentamidine. The high incidence of PCP during the early years of the AIDS epidemic led to the identification of a number of new agents with anti-*Pneumocystis* activity, and these were extensively evaluated in randomized controlled trials, primarily in HIV-infected patients. In patients with mild to moderate disease (A-a O$_2$ gradient <45 mm Hg), trimethoprim-sulfamethoxazole has superior efficacy compared with atovaquone and similar efficacy compared with trimethoprim-dapsone and clindamycin-primaquine. In patients with moderate to severe disease (A-a O$_2$ gradient >30 mm Hg), it showed superior efficacy to trimetrexate, a potent inhibitor of *Pneumocystis* DHFR that is approved for the treatment of PCP but is no longer commercially available. In smaller, lower power studies, trimethoprim-sulfamethoxazole and pentamidine showed similar efficacy.

The major toxicities associated with trimethoprim-sulfamethoxazole include fever, rash, neutropenia, thrombocytopenia, nausea, vomiting, and transaminase elevations. Hyperkalemia and crystalluria have also been reported, and hyponatremia is seen primarily in association with intravenous administration. Toxicities usually appear after the first week of therapy. Toxicities are much more common in HIV-infected patients, occurring in about 50 to 60%; 15 to 35% of these patients discontinue therapy because of the adverse events. Although folinic acid can decrease the toxicities associated with some DHFR inhibitors such as pyrimethamine, it should not be administered with trimethoprim-sulfamethoxazole; in one placebo-controlled trial, it did not decrease side effects but was associated with an increased risk for therapeutic failure and death.

Alternative regimens for patients with mild to moderate disease include trimethoprim-dapsone, clindamycin-primaquine, and atovaquone. Like sulfamethoxazole, dapsone is an inhibitor of *Pneumocystis* DHPS. Adverse reactions to trimethoprim-dapsone include rash, fever, nausea and vomiting, transaminase elevations, methemoglobinemia, anemia, and mild hyperkalemia. Approximately 20 to 30% of patients with adverse reactions to trimethoprim-sulfamethoxazole experience adverse reactions to trimethoprim-dapsone. Toxicities associated with clindamycin-primaquine include fever, rash, diarrhea, anemia, neutropenia, transaminase elevations, and methemoglobinemia. For both dapsone and primaquine and, to a lesser extent, sulfamethoxazole, glucose-6-phosphate dehydrogenase deficiency (Chapter 161) can increase the risk for hemolytic anemia and methemoglobinemia. In a randomized trial comparing trimethoprim-sulfamethoxazole, trimethoprim-dapsone, and clindamycin-primaquine in 181 HIV-infected patients with mild to moderate disease, response rates and toxicities were similar among the three arms, with an overall therapeutic failure rate of 9% by day 21 and a dose-limiting toxicity rate of 31%. Serious transaminase elevations were more common in the trimethoprim-sulfamethoxazole group, and serious hematologic toxicities were more common in the clindamycin-primaquine group.

Atovaquone is a hydroxynaphthoquinone with activity against *Toxoplasma* and malaria as well as *Pneumocystis*. Atovaquone (tablet formulation) was less effective than trimethoprim-sulfamethoxazole in a randomized trial in HIV-infected patients with mild to moderate disease and showed a trend toward lesser efficacy compared with pentamidine in another study. Low serum atovaquone levels and preexisting diarrhea were associated with therapeutic failure. The current formulation is a suspension that has approximately 50% greater bioavailability than the tablet formulation, which may result in improved responses. Atovaquone should be taken with food because this increases its bioavailability, and it should be avoided in patients with potentially decreased gastrointestinal absorption (e.g., diarrhea). Toxicities of atovaquone include rash, fever, transaminase elevations, nausea, vomiting, diarrhea, neutropenia, and anemia.

Therapeutic alternatives to trimethoprim-sulfamethoxazole for patients with disease requiring parenteral therapy are limited to clindamycin-primaquine (but only clindamycin is available for intravenous administration) and pentamidine. Caspofungin and other echinocandins, which are β-1,3-glucan synthase inhibitors, cannot be recommended because there have been no clinical trials documenting their efficacy; β-1,3-glucan is present in the cyst but not in the trophic form of the organism.

Pentamidine was the first drug demonstrated to have anti-*Pneumocystis* activity. Available data suggest that trimethoprim-sulfamethoxazole and pentamidine have similar efficacy; trimethoprim-sulfamethoxazole is the preferred regimen because the toxicities associated with pentamidine are more frequent and potentially more severe. Intravenous pentamidine was originally associated with severe hypotension, but a slow (>1 hour) infusion is usually well tolerated. Intramuscular administration is associated with a high frequency of sterile abscesses at the injection site. Toxicities associated with pentamidine, which occur in about 50 to 60% of patients and frequently result in discontinuation of the drug, include nephrotoxicity, hypoglycemia, hyperglycemia, fever, neutropenia, thrombocytopenia, hypotension, hyperkalemia, transaminase elevations, and pancreatitis. Hypoglycemia may be life-threatening and may precede the development of hyperglycemia; hyperglycemia may be irreversible. Torsades de pointes (Chapter 65) has also rarely been reported.

Adjunctive Corticosteroid Therapy

Initiation of specific anti-*Pneumocystis* therapy is associated with deterioration in oxygenation after approximately 3 to 4 days; this likely results from a host inflammatory response to organisms damaged by therapy. Randomized controlled trials have demonstrated that the early addition of corticosteroids to specific anti-*Pneumocystis* therapy in HIV-infected patients can prevent this deterioration and improve survival, without a significant increase in opportunistic complications other than localized herpes simplex infection. In the largest such study, corticosteroid therapy was associated with a 50% decrease in respiratory failure and mortality; this benefit was limited to patients with moderate to severe disease. For HIV-infected patients, corticosteroids and specific anti-*Pneumocystis* therapy should be started at the same time; the addition of corticosteroids after 72 hours has shown no benefit, although it is reasonable to add them if patients exhibit deterioration after this time. Although the optimal regimen has not been defined by controlled trials, the tapering regimen from the largest study is most commonly used (see Table 341-1).

The optimal utilization of corticosteroids in non-HIV patients who are often receiving them as part of the treatment regimens for their underlying disease is less clear because data from randomized controlled trials are not available; dosing may need to be individualized to balance the immunosuppressive effects that potentially contributed to the development of PCP against the anti-inflammatory effects that may ameliorate life-threatening pulmonary dysfunction. One retrospective analysis of 31 patients suggested that increasing corticosteroids to a prednisone equivalent of 60 mg/day or more was associated with clinical benefit. It is reasonable to administer corticosteroids to non-HIV patients with moderate or severe disease if they were not receiving corticosteroids, using the same regimen as for HIV-infected patients; for patients already taking corticosteroids at lower doses, the dosage can be increased to those levels.[13]

Initiation of Antiretroviral Therapy

Given that many patients with HIV infection who are diagnosed with PCP are not receiving antiretroviral therapy, an important issue is how soon to start HAART after a diagnosis of PCP. Retrospective and prospective studies have suggested that, in general, it is safe to initiate HAART while patients are being treated for PCP, and early HAART may be associated with an improved outcome. In a randomized 282-patient trial that examined early versus late initiation of HAART in patients with acute opportunistic infections, 63% of whom had PCP, the early initiation arm (HAART started a median of 12 days after starting therapy for the opportunistic infection) had a decreased rate of AIDS progression or death. Similar findings for tuberculosis in developing countries have emphasized the benefit of early initiation of HAART.

Major concerns about initiating HAART include the risk for adverse drug reactions, which may be confused with adverse reactions to anti-PCP therapy; the risk for overlapping toxicities, which may complicate management; and the risk for immune reconstitution. There are several reports describing apparent immune reconstitution inflammatory syndrome (Chapter 395), which can be life-threatening, in patients who started HAART soon after being diagnosed with PCP. Thus, many clinicians initiate HAART during or immediately after completion of anti-Pneumocystis therapy, assuming the patient has shown clinical improvement, is able to tolerate oral medications, and accepts the commitment to lifelong therapy. However, the parameters for such an approach are difficult to define precisely. Patients who start HAART early should be closely monitored for a recurrence of symptoms that may represent immune reconstitution.

Treatment Failure

The optimal approach to the management of patients who are failing therapy has not been well defined. In patients with progressive respiratory deterioration, it is critical that the diagnosis of PCP be confirmed rather than presumptive and that other concurrent processes (e.g., other infections, congestive heart failure, pulmonary emboli) have been ruled out; bronchoscopy should be considered to facilitate these determinations. Parenteral therapy should be used to eliminate absorption concerns, and corticosteroid medications should be added if this has not already been done. Because patients who will ultimately respond can show clinical deterioration at 3 to 4 days, as noted earlier, it is reasonable to wait 5 to 8 days before considering a change in drug therapy.

Only trimethoprim-sulfamethoxazole and pentamidine are available in parenteral formulations. Parenteral clindamycin is available, but primaquine is available only as a tablet. No randomized trials have examined the relative efficacy of these agents in patients who are failing therapy. For patients who have not received trimethoprim-sulfamethoxazole, this should be the first choice as an alternative agent, assuming the patient did not have a life-threatening adverse reaction previously. Rapid desensitization (similar to penicillin desensitization), ideally in consultation with an allergy specialist, can be considered in patients with prior adverse reactions; however, patients with a history of Stevens-Johnson syndrome or toxic epidermal necrolysis should not be rechallenged. Although retrospective cohort studies and meta-analyses have found that clindamycin-primaquine is superior to pentamidine in patients failing a first-line regimen, there are potential biases in such analyses (e.g., severity of illness or ability to take oral medications may have affected the choice of salvage regimen). There are no data to recommend switching to an alternative agent rather than adding an alternative agent (if toxicity is not an issue); both approaches have been used.

Resistance

Although Pneumocystis cannot be cultured, molecular studies have identified mutations in genes that are the targets of anti-Pneumocystis therapy, and these mutations appear to represent the development of resistance by Pneumocystis to these agents. The best-characterized mutations have been identified in the DHPS gene of Pneumocystis, which is the target of sulfamethoxazole and dapsone. Two mutations at the active site of this enzyme, which can occur

either individually or together, have been identified with greater frequency in patients receiving trimethoprim-sulfamethoxazole or dapsone for prophylaxis; in vitro studies suggest that these mutations confer resistance. The clinical relevance of these mutations remains uncertain; some studies have found worse outcomes in patients with these mutations, but others have found no such association.[14] Most patients in whom these mutations were identified retrospectively were successfully treated with sulfa-containing drugs. In contrast to DHPS, there are very limited reports suggesting that the DHFR gene of Pneumocystis, which is the target of trimethoprim and pyrimethamine, has developed potential drug-resistant mutations.

Atovaquone presumably binds to the mitochondrial bc_1 complex of Pneumocystis and thus inhibits electron transport. Multiple mutations have been identified in the cytochrome B gene of Pneumocystis, which presumably represent resistance in patients receiving atovaquone for prophylaxis; these mutations have not, however, been associated with clinical outcome.

Because the presence of these mutations has not been definitively associated with worsening prognosis, clinical decisions should not be based on their identification. Methods for identifying these mutations are not readily available, and their detection should remain a research tool until their clinical relevance can be better defined.

PREVENTION

Although Pneumocystis is transmitted by the airborne route, exposure to the organism appears to be ubiquitous in humans, suggesting that avoidance of exposure may be difficult. In animal models, it takes 2 to 3 months following exposure to develop a heavy infection. If the pattern of growth were similar in humans, clinical symptoms would develop only months after exposure to a source that is likely unknown. Currently, respiratory isolation of patients with active PCP is not required, although it is reasonable to avoid having a susceptible patient share a room with a PCP patient. Recent outbreaks in renal transplant patients strongly suggest a common source of infection; a better understanding of the patterns of transmission in these settings may lead to improved guidelines for preventing the spread of infection. It is noteworthy that in these outbreaks, broad institution of anti-Pneumocystis prophylaxis was the intervention that terminated the outbreaks.

A major advance in the management of patients at risk for the development of PCP was the demonstration that trimethoprim-sulfamethoxazole was highly effective in preventing the disease in a susceptible pediatric population. Subsequent studies, primarily in HIV-infected patients, demonstrated that additional drug regimens were also effective. This has led to the broad use of anti-Pneumocystis prophylaxis in a wide range of susceptible populations.

Two important issues in administering prophylaxis are identifying populations at risk and defining the period of risk during which prophylaxis should be provided. AIDS patients are at especially high risk; before the use of prophylaxis or HAART, the lifetime incidence of PCP in this population was estimated at 60 to 80%. The most recent CD4 count is a validated surrogate marker for HIV-infected patients: patients with CD4 counts below 200 cells/mm^3 are at substantially increased risk for developing PCP, and prophylaxis is recommended for this group.[15] Although 10 to 15% of patients who develop PCP have higher CD4 counts, the incidence is very low in this population, given the large number of patients who fall in this category. Patients with CD4 counts greater than 200 cells/mm^3 but a CD4 percentage of less than 14% or a history of an AIDS-defining illness are also candidates for prophylaxis. For pediatric patients with HIV infection, in whom the normal CD4 count changes with age, guidelines are based on age. Prophylaxis is recommended for children older than 6 years with CD4 counts below 200 cells/mm^3 or 15%, for children between 1 and 5 years old with CD4 counts below 500 cells/mm^3 or 15%, and for all children younger than 12 months.[16]

Before the availability of HAART, when patients with HIV infection initiated prophylaxis, they were committed to continuing it for life because immunologic decline was irreversible. With HAART, however, control of HIV replication leads to an increase in the CD4 count, which is associated with a concomitant decrease in the risk for developing PCP. Multiple studies have shown that when the CD4 count has been above 200 cells/mm^3 for at least 3 months (ideally in the setting of controlled HIV replication), prophylaxis can be safely discontinued because the risk for developing PCP is no greater than in patients whose CD4 counts never fell below 200 cells/mm^3. In most of these studies, the median CD4 count was greater than 300 cells/mm^3, and HIV viral loads were below detection limits in the majority of patients. Recent uncontrolled studies have suggested that prophylaxis can also be safely discontinued in patients with CD4 counts between 100 and

200 cells/mm^3 who have virologically suppressed HIV, but specific criteria for discontinuation (e.g., duration of viral suppression) were not defined in these studies.[17]

Among non-HIV-infected patients, the CD4 count is not routinely measured, and it has not been shown to have the same predictive value for the development of PCP as in HIV-infected patients; however, CD4 counts below 200 cells/mm^3 do appear to increase their susceptibility. Recommendations for PCP prophylaxis in these populations are based on clinical parameters, including empirical identification of periods of risk and estimation of levels of immunosuppression. Very broad prophylaxis has not been implemented because of the side effects associated with these regimens; for example, there is concern that trimethoprim-sulfamethoxazole might cause bone marrow suppression that would interfere with engraftment or cause nephrotoxicity that would damage a transplanted kidney.

Risk factors for non-HIV-infected patients include underlying disease, older age, use of immunosuppressive drugs, radiation therapy, graft-versus-host disease, and concomitant cytomegalovirus infection (Chapter 376). Patients with malignancies, especially hematologic malignancies, but increasingly solid tumors as well, are at risk for PCP primarily owing to the therapies they receive; the incidence can range from 1 to 43% in the absence of prophylaxis and is highly dependent on the intensity and duration of immunosuppression. In the absence of prophylaxis, the risk for developing PCP in transplant patients, whether hematopoietic stem cell or solid organ transplants, is reportedly about 5 to 15%, although lung and heart-lung transplant patients appear to have a higher incidence (up to 43%). Among patients with collagen vascular disease, the reported risk is less than 2% without prophylaxis, although patients with Wegener's granulomatosis (Chapter 270) reportedly have a risk up to 12%, presumably because of the use of more immunosuppressive treatment regimens.[18] In patients with inflammatory bowel disease, the incidence in one large retrospective cohort study, was about 1% per year, with a greater risk for Crohn's disease compared with ulcerative colitis.[19] The current risk for developing PCP in non-HIV populations is difficult to quantify because of the widespread use of prophylaxis and because immunosuppressive regimens are evolving.

To facilitate the management of prophylaxis in at-risk populations, a number of guidelines have been developed by expert panels that have made recommendations based on the strength of the available data. HIV guidelines have already been summarized. For allogeneic stem cell transplant recipients, prophylaxis is recommended from the time of engraftment to at least 6 months after transplantation, and longer for patients who continue receiving immunosuppressive therapy or who have chronic graft-versus-host disease. For autologous stem cell transplant recipients, who have a lower risk for PCP, prophylaxis for 3 to 6 months should be considered if the degree of immunosuppression is substantial owing to underlying disease or therapy (e.g., patients with leukemia or lymphoma receiving intensive conditioning or immunosuppressive therapy).

For solid organ transplant patients, prophylaxis has not been universally adopted; it has been used primarily in centers with a known incidence greater than 3%. Guidelines recommend the administration of prophylaxis for 3 to 12 months in renal transplant patients and for longer periods, up to lifelong, in heart, lung, liver, and intestine transplant recipients. As noted earlier, a number of outbreaks of PCP have recently been reported in renal transplant centers, and many of those patients developed disease more than 1 year after transplantation. Risk factors identified in case-control studies have included older age, recent or concurrent cytomegalovirus infection, and treatment for rejection. Specific immunosuppressive drugs, such as mycophenolate mofetil and cyclosporine, have not been consistently implicated.

For patients with inflammatory bowel disease (Chapter 141), who appear to be at increased risk as newer immunosuppressive agents are used, data are limited; however, consensus-based guidelines recommend prophylaxis for patients receiving triple immunomodulators that include either a calcineurin inhibitor or an anti-TNF agent. No consensus was reached for less intensive regimens. For patients with connective tissue disorders or vasculitis, there are currently no consensus guidelines.

Corticosteroid therapy (Chapter 35) is a well-described risk factor in non-HIV-infected patients, with approximately 90% of patients receiving such therapy before developing PCP in some studies. Higher dose and longer duration increase the risk. Not all patients who receive corticosteroids are at risk, however; for instance, asthmatic patients receiving corticosteroid therapy are at low risk. Although there are no consensus guidelines on the use of prophylaxis for patients receiving corticosteroids, one reasonable approach is to provide prophylaxis to patients with an underlying immunosuppressive or inflammatory disease who receive at least 20 mg of prednisone or equivalent for longer than 1 month. Other immunosuppressive agents (Chapter 35), such as calcineurin inhibitors, sirolimus, TNF antagonists, and rituximab, also appear to increase the risk for developing PCP, primarily in the patient populations noted earlier. Based on the manufacturer's recommendations, patients receiving temozolomide plus radiotherapy for glioblastoma multiforme should receive anti-*Pneumocystis* prophylaxis.

Trimethoprim-sulfamethoxazole is the first-line agent for prophylaxis in all populations (Table 341-2). [A2] Alternatives include dapsone alone or combined with pyrimethamine plus leucovorin, atovaquone, and aerosol pentamidine administered by the Respirgard II nebulizer. In a randomized trial of 843 HIV-infected patients comparing trimethoprim-sulfamethoxazole with dapsone and aerosol pentamidine, no significant differences were seen on an intent-to-treat basis, but the lowest failure rates were seen while patients were receiving trimethoprim-sulfamethoxazole. Conversely, trimethoprim-sulfamethoxazole was superior to aerosol pentamidine in another randomized study. In other large randomized trials in HIV-infected patients, the following regimens showed similar efficacy: atovaquone suspension and dapsone, atovaquone suspension and aerosol pentamidine, and dapsone-pyrimethamine and aerosol pentamidine. No randomized trials of these regimens have been conducted in non-HIV-infected populations, but clinical experience suggests that they are effective in these populations as well. Patients receiving pyrimethamine plus sulfadiazine plus leucovorin for treatment of toxoplasmosis do not require additional anti-*Pneumocystis* prophylaxis as this regimen also prevents PCP.

Although the combination of sulfadoxine and pyrimethamine is also efficacious, it is contraindicated in patients with sulfonamide allergies. Moreover, because Stevens-Johnson syndrome and other potentially life-threatening cutaneous reactions are more common with this combination than with trimethoprim-sulfamethoxazole, and because its long half-life results in slow

TABLE 341-2 DRUG REGIMENS FOR PREVENTION OF *PNEUMOCYSTIS PNEUMONIA* (PCP)

INDICATION	DRUG	ROUTE	DOSE	COMMENTS
Preferred	Trimethoprim-Sulfamethoxazole (TMP-SMX)	PO	1 double-strength tablet (160 mg TMP+800 mg SMX) or one single-strength tablet (80 mg TMP+400 mg SMX) QD	Also active in preventing toxoplasmosis
Alternative	Trimethoprim-Sulfamethoxazole (TMP-SMX)	PO	1 double-strength tablet (160 mg TMP+800 mg SMX) 3 times weekly	Also active in preventing toxoplasmosis
Alternative	Dapsone	PO	100 mg QD or 50 mg BID	Test for G6PD deficiency before use
Alternative	Dapsone plus	PO	50 mg QD	Also active in preventing toxoplasmosis
	Pyrimethamine plus	PO	50 mg once weekly	
	Leucovorin	PO	25 mg once weekly	Should be administered with pyrimethamine to minimize toxicity
Alternative	Atovaquone	PO	1,500 mg QD with food	Likely active in preventing toxoplasmosis
Alternative	Pentamidine	Aerosol	300 mg via the Respirgard II nebulizer once monthly	Not active in preventing toxoplasmosis

Note: Patients receiving pyrimethamine-sulfadiazine and atovaquone therapy for toxoplasmosis do not appear to need additional prophylaxis for PCP; patients receiving clindamycin-pyrimethamine therapy for toxoplasmosis will need additional prophylaxis for PCP. GGPD = glucose-6-phosphate dehydrogenase.

clearance after the drug is discontinued, sulfadoxine plus pyrimethamine should probably not be used in sulfa-tolerant patients if trimethoprim-sulfamethoxazole is available.

HIV-infected patients with a prior history of a mild sulfa allergy (e.g., mild rash, excluding those with prior Stevens-Johnson syndrome or toxic epidermal necrolysis) can often be safely rechallenged with trimethoprim-sulfamethoxazole. Randomized trials have demonstrated that dose escalation over a 6- to 13-day period is associated with better tolerance than direct rechallenge with full-dose trimethoprim-sulfamethoxazole, and that up to 75% of patients can continue to receive trimethoprim-sulfamethoxazole for at least 6 months.

PROGNOSIS

Mortality for untreated PCP approaches 100%. With therapy, the survival rate for HIV-infected patients with confirmed PCP is now as high as 95%, but a poorer survival rate of 75% has been reported in patients without HIV infection.[20] Risk factors for death in HIV-infected patients include more severe hypoxia, older age, recurrent episodes of PCP, low hemoglobin, and the presence of comorbid conditions. Although mortality for patients admitted to an intensive care unit is high, survival for HIV-infected patients has improved in recent years, now approaching 75%.[21]

Grade A References

A1. Briel M, Bucher HC, Boscacci R, et al. Adjunctive corticosteroids for *Pneumocystis jiroveci* pneumonia in patients with HIV-infection. *Cochrane Database Syst Rev.* 2006;3:CD006150.
A2. Stern A, Green H, Paul M, et al. Prophylaxis for Pneumocystis pneumonia (PCP) in non-HIV immunocompromised patients. *Cochrane Database Syst Rev.* 2014;10:CD005590.

GENERAL REFERENCES

For the General References and other additional features, please visit Expert Consult at https://expertconsult.inkling.com.

342

MYCETOMA

D. P. KONTOYIANNIS

DEFINITION

Mycetoma (a tumor produced by fungi) was first described in 1842 in the Madura district of India, hence the terms "Madura foot," "maduromycosis," and "maduromycetoma." However, there is evidence of its existence from as far back as the Byzantine era and ancient India.

Mycetoma is a chronic, slowly progressive infection that starts in the subcutaneous tissue and spreads across tissue planes to contiguous structures. The disease has diverse etiology; also, the offending organism is inoculated into the subcutaneous tissues by trauma typically associated with soil contamination. The hallmarks of mycetoma are the presence of "grains" that consist of colonies of the infectious organism and chronically draining sinus tracts. There is some confusion in the literature, however, because the term pulmonary mycetoma is used inappropriately to describe fungus balls typically caused by *Aspergillus* species that colonize a preexisting lung cavity; the term *aspergilloma* is more appropriate for this entity, the pathogenesis of which is distinctly different from that of true mycetoma.

The Pathogen

Two groups of soil-inhabiting pathogens, each of which accounts for approximately 50% of the cases, cause mycetoma: (1) the filamentous aerobic actinomycetes, hence the term actinomycetoma, and (2) a wide range of saprophytic soil and woody plant fungi, hence the term eumycetoma. Eumycetoma accounts for approximately 50% of cases of mycetoma.[1,2]

A variety of *Nocardia* species (e.g., *Nocardia brasiliensis*, *Nocardia asteroides*), *Actinomadura* species (e.g., *Actinomadura pelletierii*, *Actinomadura madurae*), and *Streptomyces* species (e.g., *Streptomyces somaliensis*) have been reported to cause actinomycetoma. Even more numerous are the agents that

cause eumycetoma, such as *Madurella* species (e.g., *Madurella mycetomatis* causes 70% of all cases of eumycetoma,), which are probably the most prevalent mycetoma-causative fungal species worldwide. Other eumycetoma include *Fusarium* species, *Acremonium* species, *Pseudallescheria boydii, Exophiala* species, and *Curvularia* species. There is controversy about whether the various dermatophytes and *Aspergillus* species can cause mycetoma. Eumycetoma is often further characterized on the basis of the color of the grains; specifically, white- to yellow-grain mycetomas (white piedra) are typically caused by hyalohyphomycetes (e.g., *P. boydii, Fusarium* species, *Acremonium* species), and black-grain eumycetomas (black piedra) are caused by *Madurella* species and other less common fungi. However, the geographic distribution of the fungi that cause black grain eumycetoma is variable.

EPIDEMIOLOGY

Although mycetoma has a global distribution, it occurs primarily in the tropical and, to a lesser extent, the temperate zones. More specifically, the infection is quite prevalent in India, Mexico, Central America, South America, the Middle East, and especially sub-Saharan Africa (the "mycetoma belt"); Sudan has a particularly high burden of mycetoma. Indigenously acquired mycetoma is sporadic in North America and Europe. However, the globalization of tourism and the increase in immigration from countries of high endemicity of mycetoma to the western countries necessitates awareness of this entity, even in the developed word.

The relative frequency of actinomycetoma and eumycetoma differs among geographic areas. Hence, eumycetoma is more common in India and Africa, and actinomycetoma is more common in Central and South America. Furthermore, the causative agents of mycetoma differ in their geographic distribution. For example, *Scedosporium apiospermum* (*P. boydii*) is the most common agent of mycetoma in North America, and *Actinomadura* and *Nocardia* species are predominant in Central and South America. Finally, *Luidia senegalensis* and *M. mycetomatis* are predominant in sub-Saharan Africa and India (Fig. 342-1). The recent development of molecular typing procedures such as polymerase chain reaction restriction fragment length polymorphism holds promise in expanding our knowledge on the environmental sources and the pathogenesis of some agents of eumycetoma such as *M. mycetomatis*.

PATHOGENESIS

Local trauma (e.g., wood splinters) introduces a mycetoma-causative organism into the skin and subcutaneous tissues and initiates a chain of events that leads to chronic, suppurative granulomatous inflammation, tumefaction, formation of multiple fistulous tracts and sinuses, deep abscesses, fibrosis and scar formation, and extension to adjacent connective tissue across the lines of least resistance (fascia) and ultimately to bones, muscles, nerves, and tendon sheaths, leading to gross anatomic distortion of the affected site. In addition, a chronic suppurative granuloma featuring reactive fibrosis and grains (sclerotia), which is a matrix consisting of vegetative aggregates of the etiologic agents and host-derived inflammatory response, is characteristic of mycetoma in histologic sections. This infection is not contagious, however. Even though the genetics and immunopathogenesis of mycetoma are not well defined, it appears that there are differences in host susceptibility because some affected persons have impaired or delayed hypersensitivity reactions or polymorphisms in genes encoding for chemokines (e.g., CCL50) and cytokines (e.g., IL-10).[3] However, mycetoma does not appear to be more common in immunocompromised hosts. The lack of appropriate animal models that simulate the macroscopic features of subcutaneous human infection limits our understanding of the pathogenesis of mycetoma.

CLINICAL MANIFESTATIONS

The clinical manifestations and natural history of mycetoma are variable and, to some degree, related to the pathogenic agent involved.[4] For example, the progression of eumycetoma tends to be slower than that of actinomycetoma. In addition, eumycetoma lesions tend to be more confined and have less inflammation and fewer granulomas and fistulas but more fibrosis compared with actinomycetoma lesions. Furthermore, male mycetoma patients predominate (5 : 1 over female patients), and the disease is typically seen in rural areas and in persons susceptible to local trauma and contamination from soil (e.g., thorns). Hence, farmers, gardeners, woodcutters, herders, and people who work outside while barefoot are more susceptible to this infection. Not surprisingly, the foot is the most common site involved in mycetoma (Fig. 342-2), but any other part of the body, such as the hands, thighs, torso, and back of the head, may become involved. Location is typically solitary. Painless

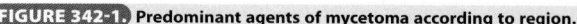

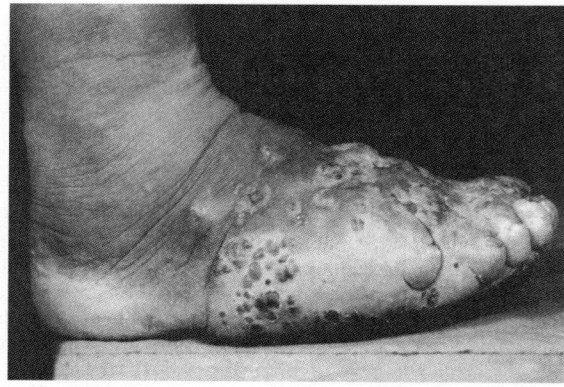

FIGURE 342-1. Predominant agents of mycetoma according to region.

United States
Pseudallescheria boydii
(Scedosporium apiospermum)

Middle East/East Africa
Madurella mycetomatis
Streptomyces somaliensis

India
Nocardia spp
Madurella grisea

West Africa
Leptoshaeria senegalensis

Central and South America
Madurella grisea
Nocardia spp

FIGURE 342-2. **Madura foot.** A 40-year-old farmer from rural Venezuela with a 10-year history of foot edema and slowly progressive deformity following an injury caused by being struck by a hammer presented with chronic crusted plaques, multiple confluent tender abscesses with fistulization, and release of black grains. The range of motion of the patient's ankle and foot joints was limited, but the joints were not painful. A deep skin biopsy with hematoxylin and eosin staining, periodic acid–Schiff staining, foot radiography, sampling of black grain smears, and a mycology culture were performed. The foot radiograph showed osteofibrosis, destruction of articular surfaces, osteoporosis, and ankylosis, and *Madurella* species grew in the culture. (Courtesy Dr. M. Mendoza, Instituto De Biomedicina, Laboratorio de Micología, San José Caracas, Venezuela.)

nodular and/or papular swelling is the most common early manifestation of mycetoma, which is followed by a slow evolution to painless, fixed woody induration. This infection typically runs a chronic, relentless course, sometimes spanning several decades. It is characterized by recurring, vicious cycles of suppuration, draining sinuses, bacterial superinfection, and scar formation. Old sinuses may close up, but new ones may occur, and satellite lesions may be seen. Constitutional symptoms are surprisingly rare. In particular, the presence of fever indicates bacterial superinfection. Bone involvement mimicking clinically chronic osteomyelitis with osteolytic cavitary bone lesions, periosteal reaction or sclerosis (seen with radiography, computed tomography [CT], or magnetic resonance imaging [MRI] studies), osteoporosis, and reactive periosteal bone formation may occur; such involvement can be substantial. However, pathologic fractures are rare. In addition, because nerves are relatively spared from involvement, neuropathic manifestations are uncommon. Inexorable limb deformity and misuse because of destruction of

deeper tissues may be seen in chronic, refractory, and advanced cases. Finally, because mycetoma does not spread hematogenously, visceral dissemination is not seen. However, because lymphatic spread may occur (typical incidence of 1 to 3% but more common with actinomycetoma and especially after surgery), regional lymphadenitis may develop.

DIAGNOSIS

Mycetoma, especially in its advanced forms, has a rather characteristic presentation. The classic triad of painless soft tissue swelling, draining sinus tracts, and extrusion of grains facilitates diagnosis with a high degree of accuracy, especially in endemic areas. For instance, the macroscopic and microscopic appearance of grains in pus-filled draining sinuses frequently allows presumptive diagnosis of the offending pathogen. However, basing the diagnosis on the presence of grains in tissue may be difficult because these grains might be composed of dead organisms. Furthermore, grains may be contaminated by surface bacteria or fungi. Therefore, a deep-tissue biopsy specimen is ideal for staining with hematoxylin and eosin, and appropriate selective bacterial (e.g., Löwenstein-Jensen culture medium) and fungal (e.g., blood agar and modified Sabouraud dextrose agar with antibiotics) cultures and stains (Gram stain, modified Ziehl-Neelsen stain, Gomori methenamine silver, periodic acid–Schiff stain) are preferable for primary detection. Alternatively, aspiration of grains from unopened sinus tracts might provide material for culture.

The culture should be maintained for several weeks because some of the causative agents of mycetoma (e.g., *Nocardia* and *Streptomyces* species) are slowly growing and can take 4 to 6 weeks to grow. Histopathology differentiates eumycetoma from actinomycetoma; however, the multitude of fungi causing eumycetoma necessitates culture identification because agents of eumycetoma might respond differently to antifungal agents. Similarly, cross-reactivity, lack of standardization, and the multitude of agents causing eumycetoma limit the practical value of serology. Finally, there are no studies correlating in vitro susceptibility testing with outcome in either actinomycetoma or eumycetoma.

Differential Diagnosis

The specific manifestations of mycetoma are sometimes confused with other entities.[5] For example, early lesions could be confused with soft tissue neoplasms or foreign body granulomas. In addition, mycetoma without fistulas must occasionally be distinguished from chronic cutaneous fungal infections such as sporotrichosis (mycetomatous lymphatic sporotrichosis) and dermatophytic mycetoma. The latter infection, which is typically seen in Africans and sometimes called pseudomycetoma, is a painless granulomatous induration of the skin and subcutaneous tissues caused by ringworm that may be associated with grains consisting of fungi. However, unlike mycetoma, dermatophytic mycetoma is confined to the skin and subcutaneous tissue and does not spread to fasciae or bone. Similarly, chronic severe botryomycosis (typically caused by gram-positive cocci) with purulent exudates, grains, and draining sinus tracts may be confused with mycetoma; however, the presence of visceral dissemination supports a diagnosis of (severe) botryomycosis. Actinomycosis (Chapter 329), which is caused by endogenous microaerophilic actinomycetes (part of normal mucosa flora), also has a propensity for grains and formation of draining sinus tracts, but unlike mycetoma, its location (e.g., neck, chest, pelvis) is rather characteristic. In addition, differentiation between mycetomas with bone involvement and chronic osteomyelitis or osseous tumors may be difficult. Ultrasonography has been used to reliably differentiate mycetoma from either tumor or osteomyelitis. The dot-in-circles sign seen at MRI (tiny hypodense foci, believed to be grains, within high-hyperintensity spherical lesions, believed to be granulomas scattered by areas of fibrosis) might provide an early and specific diagnostic clue for mycetoma, Finally, in cases of mycetoma without draining sinus tracts, benign or malignant skin tumors, chronic granulomatous lesions (e.g., thorn granuloma, cutaneous tuberculosis), chromomycosis, and verrucous leishmaniasis are diagnoses that should be excluded. Unfortunately, delays of specific diagnosis by many months or even years is not uncommon, even in areas of high endemicity.

TREATMENT Rx

Therapy for mycetoma should be individualized.[6] Optimal management has not been well defined, however, because the literature consists of rather heterogeneous and uncontrolled small studies. There is no "gold standard" approach for therapy, and no single agent is effective against all causative agents of mycetoma. Hence, successful treatment necessitates a reliable diagnosis, differentiation between actinomycetoma and eumycetoma, assessment of the extent of the lesion, and identification of the causative agent. Specifically, the degree of tissue invasion, especially bone involvement (as determined by radiology studies), site affected, and specific etiologic diagnosis determine the type and intensity of therapy. Recent studies indicate that MRI and CT (more sensitive especially for mycetoma involving bone) are especially useful in "staging" the disease.

In general, considering the refractoriness of eumycetoma to medical therapy, surgery plays a more prominent role.[7] In contrast, considering the satisfactory response of actinomycetoma to medical therapy (success rate of up to 90%) and recognized risk for lymphatic spread following surgery, chronic antibiotic administration is the mainstay of actinomycetoma management.

For actinomycetoma, treatment consists primarily of chronic antibiotic therapy (for at least 9 to 12 months) in conjunction with limited debulking surgery in selected cases; combination therapy designed for potential synergy is preferred. A variety of drugs (trimethoprim-sulfamethoxazole, tetracyclines, dapsone, streptomycin) have been used in different sequences and combinations according to the specific cause of actinomycetoma (e.g., trimethoprim-sulfamethoxazole with or without dapsone for Nocardia species, streptomycin with dapsone for A. madurae). Parenteral streptomycin is usually reserved for cases that do not respond to oral therapy. Responses to these drugs tend to occur slowly (within at least 1 month). Also, relapse is not uncommon, and multiple cycles of therapy may be needed for chronically recurrent disease. Side effects and compliance issues after prolonged administration of antibiotics are common problems.

For eumycetoma, however, medical therapy has produced mixed results. The best results were obtained with prolonged (9 to 12 months) use of oral imidazoles (e.g., ketoconazole 200 to 400 mg/day or itraconazole 200 to 400 mg/day). The experience using newer triazoles (e.g., voriconazole or posaconazole) or the allylamine terbinafine (with or without concomitant itraconazole), although encouraging, is not as extensive, however.[8] Posaconazole or voriconazole might prove to be especially useful for treatment of eumycetoma due to S. apiospermum (P. boydii), a fungus that is not susceptible to either ketoconazole or itraconazole. Also, intravenous amphotericin B and its lipid formulations have been used for refractory cases with rather disappointing results. This is not surprising because most eumycetoma-causative agents (e.g., P. boydii) are resistant to amphotericin B in vitro.

The need for and extent of surgery for mycetoma depend on the etiologic agent and, more important, extent of the lesion. Early wide-margin surgery for early localized lesions is curative. Although it is potentially curative, major disfiguring or mutilating surgery (e.g., amputation) is reserved for very advanced or refractory cases. Furthermore, primary reliance on surgery could result in recurrence or even spreading of the disease of incomplete excision.

The prognosis for mycetoma depends on the site and degree of tissue involvement (e.g., worse with involvement of the back because of poor healing or in the presence of bone destruction) and, more important, the timeliness of the diagnosis and monitoring of recurrence and extension to other tissues, especially bone. CT and MRI are important modalities for early detection of bone involvement.

Finally, since mycetoma represents a significant, yet frequently ignored, socioeconomic burden for tropical and subtropical countries,[1] every effort for its prevention should be made. There is vaccine for that entity, and education of persons at risk in endemic areas is crucial (e.g., avoidance of walking barefoot). Finally, prompt recognition for early curative chemotherapy and/or surgery could lead to a better outcome of this difficult-to-manage, chronic infection.

GENERAL REFERENCES

For the General References and other additional features, please visit Expert Consult at https://expertconsult.inkling.com.

343

DEMATIACEOUS FUNGAL INFECTIONS

PETER G. PAPPAS

DEFINITION

Dematiaceous fungi represent a large group of fungal organisms characterized by the presence of abundant melanin in the cell wall, which gives rise to a brown-black coloration on artificial culture media and which can be seen on histopathologic specimens. A related term, *phaeohyphomycosis*, refers broadly to infection by these pigmented fungi. The two terms are often used interchangeably, but when dematiaceous fungi are reviewed, three distinct clinical conditions are encountered: eumycetoma (e.g., Madura foot), chromomycosis (also known as chromoblastomycosis), and phaeohyphomycosis. Eumycetoma are covered in Chapter 342. This chapter focuses on the latter two entities.

The Pathogens

More than 100 dematiaceous fungi have been identified as causes of colonization or disease in humans. The most common organisms and their related conditions are listed in Table 343-1. The taxonomy of the dematiaceous fungi is somewhat confusing because these agents belong to different classes, including Hyphomycetes, Ascomycetes, Basidiomycetes, Coelomycetes, and Zygomycetes. The most common agents of phaeohyphomycosis include species in the following genera: *Bipolaris, Curvularia, Exophiala, Cladosporium, Cladophialophora, Alternaria, Exserohilum, Ochroconis, Wangiella, Phialophora, Scedosporium, Phaeoacromonium,* and *Chaetomium.* These agents are ubiquitous saprophytes of soil and decaying matter, and some are important plant pathogens. In tissue, these organisms exist as yeastlike cells, septated hyphae, or a combination of yeast and hyphae. Many have a histologic appearance similar to *Aspergillus* and *Fusarium* species, but they can be easily distinguished on the basis of positive melanin staining with the Fontana-Masson procedure.

Chromomycosis (formerly known as chromoblastomycosis) is a chronic skin and subcutaneous infection that is observed most frequently in the tropics. Virtually all cases of chromomycosis are caused by three species: *Fonsecaea pedrosoi, Cladosproium carrionii,* and *Phialophora verrucosa.* The distinctive histologic appearance is characterized by the presence of thick-walled, dark brown bodies known as *sclerotic cells* or *copper pennies,* which represent individual organisms and may be seen in clusters or as single cells. The etiologic fungi causing chromomycosis are indistinguishable on histologic examination of tissue.

EPIDEMIOLOGY AND PATHOBIOLOGY

The agents of chromomycosis and phaeohyphomycosis are found worldwide. Although there is no unique endemic area for most of these infections, some

TABLE 343-1   DEMATIACEOUS FUNGI AND ASSOCIATED DISEASES

CLINICAL CONDITION	COMMON ETIOLOGIC AGENTS
Chromomycosis	*Fonsecaea pedrosoi* *Cladophialophora carrionii* *Phialophora verrucosa*
Cutaneous or subcutaneous disease	*Exophiala jeanselmei* *Wangiella dermatitidis* *Phialophora* spp *Bipolaris* spp *Alternaria* spp
Sinusitis	*Bipolaris* spp *Curvularia* spp *Exserohilum* spp *Alternaria* spp
Central nervous system	*Cladophialophora bantiana* *Ochroconis gallopavum* *Rhinocladiella mackenziei* *Chaetomium altrobrunnium*
Healthcare-associated	*Exserohilum rostratum* *Exophilia* spp
Disseminated	*Wangiella dermatitidis* *Exophiala jeanselmei* *Bipolaris* spp *Ochroconis gallopavum* *Phialophora* spp *Scedosporium prolificans*

observations are relevant. Allergic fungal sinusitis associated with dematiaceous fungi appears to be more common in the southern United States. Chronic infections of the lower extremities are more commonly seen in men and in tropical areas. Chromomycosis is more prevalent in rural populations in the tropics and is hyperendemic in certain geographic areas such as Madagascar, Brazil, and other Latin American countries, where most infections are caused by *Fonsecaea pedrosoi* and *Cladosporium carrionii*.[1]

Most cutaneous infections occur as a result of minor skin trauma and direct inoculation of the organism. Other risk factors include intravenous drug abuse, chronic sinusitis, freshwater immersion, and chronic corticosteroid therapy.

In the developed world, phaeohyphomycosis is an important emerging fungal infection, particularly among immunocompromised patients such as solid organ and hematopoietic stem cell transplant recipients, patients with prolonged neutropenia, and other chronically immunocompromised individuals. Phaeohyphomycosis is reported in HIV-infected patients but is far less common than other opportunistic fungi. Extracutaneous invasive disease occurs in otherwise normal patients but is much less common.

The recent U.S. epidemic of fungal meningitis, epidural abscess, sacroiliitis, vertebral osteomyelitis, discitis, and peripheral arthritis caused by *Exserohilum rostratum* following injection of contaminated methylprednisolone acetate from a single compounding pharmacy is a striking example of the risk for dematiaceous fungal infections following invasive procedures in the health care setting.[2-4] In this epidemic, more than 750 persons with injection associated infection were identified, of whom almost 10% died as a direct result of the infection. Previous reports of infection due to *Exophiala* species following contaminated steroid injections, infected breast implants, other prosthetic materials, and, rarely, contaminated intravascular catheters and intravenous fluids further underscore the importance of these pathogens as potential health care–associated infections.

CLINICAL MANIFESTATIONS

Chromomycosis is manifested as a cutaneous or subcutaneous lesion that may range in size from a small papule to a large confluent plaque involving a major portion of an extremity. Single or multiple lesions may be seen, and ulceration may occur. Lesions may remain unchanged in size and consistency for months or years, although most tend to progress in the absence of specific therapy. Chronic lesions may become dry and crusted with a raised border, which may be smooth or irregular. Multiple lesions can coalesce to form

larger plaques in which central scarring may develop. Occasionally, lesions assume a verrucous, warty appearance. The differential diagnosis includes other fungal infections such as blastomycosis, coccidioidomycosis, sporotrichosis, histoplasmosis, and paracoccidioidomycosis. Nocardiosis and cutaneous mycobacteriosis can also mimic the lesions of chromomycosis. Cutaneous lesions usually remain confined to one anatomic site, although nodular lymphangitis and autoinoculation resulting in multifocal cutaneous disease may occur. Common complications include local disfigurement due to scarring and extensive tissue involvement. Disseminated disease involving visceral organs may occur, but this is rare.

Phaeohyphomycosis is associated with several well-described clinical syndromes. *Superficial* infection is characterized by tinea nigra and black piedra. Tinea nigra is a darkening of the skin caused by growth of *Phaeoannellomyces werneckii* in the stratum corneum. Black piedra is associated with the development of focal thickening on the hair shaft and results from colonization of the shaft by *Piedraia hortae*. *Cutaneous* phaeohyphomycosis involves deeper skin structures and results in dermatomycosis and onychomycosis; this is frequently due to agents such as *Scytalidium* and *Phyllosticta* species.

Subcutaneous phaeohyphomycosis is relatively common and may be confused with chromomycosis. Patients have discrete subcutaneous nodules or cysts that result from direct inoculation or penetrating trauma. The most common organisms are *Exophiala jeanselmei*, *Wangiella dermatitidis*, and *Phialophora* species. *Mycotic keratitis* as a result of infection with *Curvularia*, *Exophiala*, and *Exserohilum* species may occur after corneal trauma or surgery.

Foreign body–related infections are seen in patients undergoing chronic ambulatory peritoneal dialysis in whom fungal peritonitis develops, in patients with indwelling intravenous catheters, and rarely in other devices such as breast implants.

Fungal sinusitis is commonly associated with dematiaceous fungi and can be manifested as allergic fungal sinusitis, a fungus ball (eumycetoma) in a sinus cavity, and invasive fungal sinusitis associated with extension into bone, soft tissue, and the central nervous system.[5] This latter manifestation is indistinguishable from rhinocerebral zygomycosis or invasive *Aspergillus* sinusitis. *Bipolaris*, *Curvularia*, and *Alternaria* species are the most common organisms causing invasive fungal sinusitis.

Systemic phaeohyphomycosis may result from direct extension from a colonized area or dissemination from a distant source. Most patients with systemic disease have significant underlying immunosuppression, and the organisms have a proclivity for involvement of the brain, lungs, endocardium, and other visceral organs. Among patients with primary central nervous system disease, *Cladophialophora bantiana*, *Ochroconis gallopavum*, *Rhinocladiella mackenziei*, and *Chaetomium altrobrunnium* are the most common etiologic agents, and the majority of these are otherwise healthy patients with no known underlying immunodeficiency. Among immunocompromised patients, *Ochroconis gallopavum*, *Bipolaris* species, and *Exophiala* species are seen more commonly.

A unique form of systemic phaeohyphomycosis has been seen recently in the fungal meningitis epidemic due to *Exserohilum rostratum* from contaminated methylprednisolone acetate injections as mentioned earlier. Patients with the meningeal form of this infection presented with symptoms ranging from local symptoms due to epidural abscess to devastating complications such as severe meningitis and basilar infarctions. Persons with extraneural involvement included those with focal sacroiliitis and peripheral joint arthritis.[6]

DIAGNOSIS

The diagnosis of phaeohyphomycosis is suggested by direct examination of a clinical specimen with a 10% potassium hydroxide preparation or special stains to demonstrate pigmentation in the cell walls of these organisms. For patients with chromomycosis, the finding of sclerotic cells or copper pennies on skin biopsy is characteristic, and special stains are usually unnecessary. For patients with other forms of phaeohyphomycosis, the Fontana-Masson stain is useful in distinguishing organisms with significant melanin content. Culture remains the "gold standard" by which a specific etiologic diagnosis is established, and the identity of the organism is largely based on colony and microscopic morphology. A polymerase chain reaction–based diagnostic assay for *Exserohilum rostratum* was developed in the context of the fungal meningitis outbreak, and it has served as a reliable marker of infection in patients who were exposed to contaminated steroid injections.[7] Serologic studies and molecular diagnostics for other organisms are not generally available.

TREATMENT

For chromomycosis, surgical excision of a cutaneous or subcutaneous lesion is often curative, although antifungal therapy is usually given in conjunction with surgery.[8] There are limited clinical studies and no large randomized trials that have assessed the efficacy of antifungal therapy for this condition. Historically, 5-flucytosine (5-FC, 150 mg/kg/day) has been advocated for the oral treatment of chromomycosis based on moderate in vitro activity and clinical experience. Because of limited availability, the need for prolonged therapy, and the necessity of monitoring serum levels, 5-FC is uncommonly used for this purpose. The triazoles, including itraconazole (200 mg orally twice daily), voriconazole (200 mg twice daily), and posaconazole (300 mg daily), demonstrate the best in vitro activity, although clinical studies with these agents are very limited. Terbinafine (500 mg orally twice daily) has also been used successfully for the treatment of chromomycosis and is an effective alternative to azole therapy.

Amphotericin B has modest in vitro activity against most of the dematiaceous fungi and is most often reserved for patients with life-threatening or disseminated disease. Among the triazoles, posaconazole offers the most potential in the clinical setting based on scattered reports from patients with central nervous system infection, but comparative clinical data are not available because of the relative rarity of these infections. Most patients with epidemic *Exserohilum rostratum* infections have been treated with voriconazole (intravenous, then oral) with or without a lipid formulation of amphotericin B for severe central nervous system involvement, and anecdotal reports suggest that this approach has been generally successful. The length of antifungal therapy for any of the systemic dematiaceous fungal infections is unclear but should probably be continued for at least 6 months or until 1 month after resolution of all signs and symptoms of disease.

GENERAL REFERENCES

For the General References and other additional features, please visit Expert Consult at https://expertconsult.inkling.com.

344

ANTIPARASITIC THERAPY

RICHARD D. PEARSON

International travel, widespread immigration, and a growing number of persons with compromised immunity due to HIV/AIDS, organ transplants, corticosteroids and other conditions have resulted in increased attention to parasitic diseases worldwide. A number of drugs are available to treat them, but physicians practicing in industrialized countries often are not familiar with their use. The focus of this chapter is on their therapeutic indications, pharmacology, and major side effects. Generalizations emerge that help in organizing an otherwise vast amount of information.

In considering the chemotherapy of parasitic diseases, it is helpful to classify infections into those caused by helminths, multicellular worms with complex internal structures, and protozoa, single-celled organisms that multiply by cell division. Helminths are further divided into nematodes, or roundworms, which can be grouped into those that live in the gastrointestinal tract and those found elsewhere in the body, and platyhelminths, or flat worms, which are subdivided into cestodes, or tapeworms, and trematodes, or flukes.

The protozoa can be grouped into those that reside under anaerobic conditions in the gastrointestinal tract or vagina and those that live aerobically in the body. The most prevalent systemic protozoan infections are attributable to members of the Apicomplexa, which cause malaria, babesiosis, and toxoplasmosis, and the Kinetoplastida, which are responsible for Chagas disease, human African trypanosomiasis (sleeping sickness), and leishmaniasis.

The Centers for Disease Control and Prevention (CDC) provide detailed information about the diagnosis and treatment of parasitic diseases through their website (www.cdc.gov). An excellent compilation of therapeutic recommendations is available in tabular form in *The Medical Letter on Drugs and Therapeutics*, "Drugs for Parasitic Infections" (available at www.medicalletter.org). Many antiparasitic drugs are commercially available in the United States, whereas others can only be obtained from the manufacturer, special pharmacies, or the CDC Drug Service. Some are available through investigational new drug protocols. Several drugs that are used for the treatment of parasitic diseases are also active against common bacterial or fungal pathogens. They are discussed elsewhere (Chapters 287 and 331).

● TREATMENT OF HELMINTHS
Intestinal Roundworms (Nematodes)

Soil-transmitted intestinal roundworms (Chapter 357) are among the world's most prevalent parasites, and there are good therapeutic options for them. *Ascaris lumbricoides*, the hookworms *Ancylostoma duodenale* and *Necator americanus*, and *Trichuris trichiura* each infect on the order of 1 billion people worldwide. Many residents of impoverished areas harbor more than one soil-transmitted pathogen.

Albendazole has a broad spectrum of activity against intestinal roundworms. It is active against *A. lumbricoides*, the hookworms, and *T. trichiura*. Administered as a single 400-mg dose, it has been used successfully in mass treatment programs for children living in high prevalence areas. However, reinfection is common, and treatment is often repeated at 3- to 4-month intervals. The CDC recommends presumptive treatment of refugees from endemic regions with a single dose of albendazole (600 mg), administered overseas before departure for the United States. It has been highly effective and well tolerated in refugees from Africa and Southeast Asia.[1] Daily doses of albendazole for 3 days are recommended for persons with heavy *T. trichiura* infection. Twice-daily doses of albendazole, 600 mg for 7 days, are used as an alternative to ivermectin for the treatment of *Strongyloides stercoralis* infection. Failures can occur with either drug, and they are often used together for longer periods to treat those with disseminated hyperinfection. Albendazole is effective against pinworms in a single dose that is repeated in 2 weeks. It can be used for cutaneous larva migrans, which is caused by migrating stages of *Ancylostoma braziliense* and other intestinal helminths of animals. It is the drug of choice for trichinosis, and it is an alternative for the treatment of *Trichostrongylus* species and *Capillaria philippinensis*.

Mebendazole, administered twice daily at a dosage of 100 mg orally for 3 days, has a similar spectrum of activity as albendazole against *A. lumbricoides*, hookworms, and *T. trichiura*. In this regimen, it is more effective than a single dose of albendazole and is considered the treatment of choice for *T. trichiura*. A single 500-mg dose of mebendazole has been used in mass treatment programs. Mebendazole is effective in treating pinworm when given at 100 mg orally in one dose followed by a second dose after 2 weeks. It is an alternative to albendazole for the treatment of trichinosis. Mebendazole is poorly absorbed and not effective against *S. stercoralis*.

Pyrantel pamoate is a relatively safe, poorly absorbed, over-the-counter drug with activity against *A. lumbricoides*, hookworms, and pinworms, but it is not effective against *T. trichiura* or *S. stercoralis*. When used for pinworms, it is administered as an oral suspension at a dose of 11 mg/kg (to a maximum of 1 g), which is repeated after 2 weeks. The combination of ***oxantel pamoate***, 20 mg/kg, and ***albendazole***, 400 mg, taken on consecutive days, has been recently found to result in higher cure and egg-reduction rates for *T. trichiura* infection then the rates with standard therapy.[A1]

Ivermectin at an oral dose of 200 μg/kg daily for 2 days is considered the treatment of choice for *S. stercoralis*.[2] It is also effective against cutaneous larva migrans and *A. lumbricoides*, but not hookworms. It is considered an alternative to mebendazole for the treatment of *T. trichiura*. Albendazole, mebendazole, pyrantel pamoate, and ivermectin replaced a number of older anthelmintics that were more toxic, such as piperazine and thiabendazole, or less effective.

Systemic Roundworms (Nematodes)

Diethylcarbamazine is the drug of choice for lymphatic filarial infections (Chapter 358) caused by *Wuchereria bancrofti*, *Brugia malayi*, and *Brugia timori*, as well as for tropical pulmonary eosinophilia. It promotes the host's killing of microfilariae of these species and also damages or kills the adult worms. Inflammatory side effects are common and due in part to the release of lipopolysaccharide from endosymbiotic *Wolbachia* bacteria within dying filaria. *Wolbachia* are necessary for filarial development and are a potential drug target. Long-term therapy with doxycycline has been shown to result in their elimination and has been used for therapy. Diethylcarbamazine is also used for *Loa loa* infections in persons with acceptably low microfilaremia (<8000/mL). Encephalopathy may result from treatment of those with higher levels. In that case, apheresis or treatment with albendazole is used first to reduce the number of microfilaria. Diethylcarbamazine can also be used prophylactically for *L. loa*. Ivermectin has activity against the microfilariae of *W. bancrofti*, *Brugia* species, and *L. loa*, but it does not kill adult worms and is not recommended for treatment of these organisms.

Ivermectin is the treatment of choice for onchocerciasis.[A2] It is administered as a single dose of 150 µg/kg. It does not kill adult *Onchocerca volvulus*, but it decreases ova production and reduces microfilariae in the skin and eyes. Retreatment is usually necessary at 6- to 12-month intervals until the patient is free of symptoms. Profits from the use of ivermectin for treatment of the dog heartworm *Dirofilaria immitis* have permitted the manufacturer to provide the drug free to persons with onchocerciasis in developing areas. Diethylcarbamazine should not be used for onchocerciasis. It kills the microfilariae of *O. volvulus* rapidly, but the release of parasite and *Wolbachia* antigens can result in severe ocular and systemic inflammatory responses. The latter is known as the Mazzotti reaction. Ivermectin is associated with less rapid killing of microfilariae and less severe reactions.

Tapeworms (Cestodes)

Praziquantel has a broad spectrum of activity against tapeworms (Chapter 354) and flukes. It is the drug of choice for adult tapeworms in the human intestinal tract. It is effective against *Taenia solium* (pork tapeworm), *Taenia saginata* (beef), *Diphyllobothrium latum* (fish), and *Hymenolepis nana* (dwarf tapeworm) when administered as a single dose. Niclosamide, which is not absorbed, is an effective alternative for the treatment of *T. saginata* and *D. latum*. It also kills adult *T. solium*, but disintegration of the worm and release of viable ova into the intestinal lumen raise the theoretical possibility of autoinfection. In the case of *H. nana*, a dose of nitazoxanide, 500 mg twice daily for 3 days, provides an alternative to praziquantel. It also has activity against *T. saginata* and potentially other tapeworm species.

Neurocysticercosis caused by the larval or tissue phase of *T. solium* is a major cause of seizures and other central nervous system (CNS) abnormalities in residents of and immigrants from endemic areas in Latin America and elsewhere. Symptoms can result from the physical presence of cysticerci, but the inflammation elicited by the release of antigens from dying cysticerci is often more important. Both albendazole and praziquantel are capable of killing cysticerci in the brain; albendazole is the drug of choice for pharmacokinetic reasons. Their use depends on the clinical syndrome. Corticosteroids are administered concurrently—and sometimes alone—to reduce the inflammatory response and the increase in intracranial pressure associated with it. Albendazole is administered for 15 to 30 days at 400 mg twice a day. Praziquantel is administered at 100 mg/kg in three divided doses the first day and then at 50 mg/kg in three divided doses for 29 days. The concurrent use of corticosteroids increases the serum level of albendazole but decreases that of praziquantel. Neither albendazole nor praziquantel should be used in persons with cysticerci in the eye or spinal cord because the release of antigens can trigger a locally destructive inflammatory reaction.

Surgery or PAIR (percutaneous aspiration, injection of chemicals, and reaspiration) is the preferred approach for *Echinococcus granulosus* cysts. Albendazole is used for inoperable *E. granulosus* and *Echinococcus multilocularis* disease and in persons in whom medical treatment is preferred for other reasons. Administered at a dose of 400 mg twice daily for adults, generally for 1 to 6 months, albendazole may cure one third of uncomplicated *Echinococcus granulosus* liver cysts. Albendazole is also administered before ultrasound-guided PAIR or surgery to prevent seeding of the peritoneum should the cyst's contents spill. Potentially fatal bone marrow suppression and hepatitis are concerns in persons receiving high-dose, prolonged albendazole therapy.

Flukes (Trematodes)

Praziquantel is the drug of choice for the treatment of all forms of schistosomiasis (Chapter 355), as well as intestinal, lung, and liver flukes (Chapter 356), with the exception of the liver fluke *Fasciola hepatica*. For schistosomiasis, two or three doses are given in 1 day depending on the species. The flukes are treated with three doses on 1 or 2 days, depending on the species. Oxamniquine is an alternative for *Schistosoma mansoni*, but it is more toxic and less effective. Higher doses of oxamniquine are recommended for *S. mansoni* infections acquired in areas of Egypt or equatorial Africa where the parasite is less susceptible. Either praziquantel or albendazole can be used to treat the liver fluke *Clonorchis sinensis*. *F. hepatica* responds to the veterinary agent triclabendazole. Bithionol, which is more toxic, and nitazoxanide are alternatives.

Drugs Used for Helminthic Infections

Albendazole is poorly soluble in water, but it is well absorbed when administered with a fatty meal. It undergoes rapid first-pass metabolism in the liver to albendazole sulfoxide, which has excellent anthelmintic activity. The serum half-life of albendazole sulfoxide is 8 to 9 hours. Elimination of albendazole sulfoxide and other metabolites is achieved primarily through the kidney. Albendazole binds to tubulin in susceptible parasites, inhibits microtubule assembly, and decreases glucose absorption. It does not affect human tubulin. It also inhibits fumarate reductase in helminths. Concurrent administration of dexamethasone, which is frequently given to prevent cerebral edema in persons with neurocysticercosis, increases serum levels by approximately 50%. The cerebrospinal fluid (CSF) concentration of albendazole is approximately 40% of that in serum.

Albendazole is generally well tolerated when given as a single dose for the treatment of intestinal nematode infections, although gastrointestinal discomfort may develop or patients may experience migration of adult *A. lumbricoides* from the nose or mouth or see them in their stools. Albendazole at higher doses and for longer duration is also used for persons with neurocysticercosis. Corticosteroids are administered concurrently to reduce intracranial inflammation and resulting increased pressure. Albendazole is contraindicated in those with cysticerci in the eye or spinal cord. High-dose, prolonged therapy with albendazole, such as that recommended for echinococcal disease, can be complicated by alopecia, hepatitis, or bone marrow suppression, which is not always reversible after discontinuation of the drug. Albendazole is embryotoxic in animals and contraindicated during pregnancy.

Mebendazole is only slightly soluble in water and is relatively poorly absorbed from the gastrointestinal tract. This is advantageous for the treatment of intestinal parasites but limits its effectiveness against tissue-dwelling helminths. Absorbed drug is metabolized in the liver and excreted in urine. Mebendazole selectively binds to helminthic tubulin, blocks its assembly into microtubules, and inhibits glucose uptake, thereby leading to depletion of glycogen stores and ultimately death of the parasite. It is relatively well tolerated in the doses used to treat intestinal helminths. Transient abdominal pain and diarrhea occur in a small number of recipients. Mebendazole is contraindicated during pregnancy.

Ivermectin is a macrocyclic lactone produced by *Streptomyces avermitilis*. It has a broad spectrum of activity against helminths and arthropods, including *Sarcoptes scabiei*, the cause of scabies. It is well absorbed after oral administration. Ivermectin is highly protein bound, has a serum half-life of 12 hours, and accumulates in adipose tissue and the liver. It is subject to enterohepatic recirculation and ultimately eliminated in stool. Ivermectin activates the opening of gated chloride channels in susceptible helminths and arthropods. The result is an influx of chloride ions and paralysis of the pharyngeal pumping mechanism of helminths. Ivermectin is generally well tolerated in humans, although inflammatory reactions can result in response to antigens released from dying parasites.

Diethylcarbamazine, a piperazine derivative, is well absorbed orally and has a half-life of 8 hours. The parent drug and its metabolites are excreted through the kidney. Although the mechanism of action is uncertain, the piperazine moiety may result in paralysis of sensitive helminths. Diethylcarbamazine also alters the surface membranes of susceptible microfilariae, thereby resulting in destruction by the host's immune system. Side effects include those caused by the drug and those that result from release of the parasite antigens and lipopolysaccharide from filaria-harbored, endosymbiotic *Wolbachia*. Adverse effects include nausea, vomiting, anorexia, headache, malaise, weakness, arthralgias, and rarely, acute psychotic reactions. In patients with lymphatic filariasis, localized swelling or nodules may develop along the lymphatics during treatment, or transient lymphedema or hydrocele formation may occur.

Praziquantel is well absorbed after oral administration. It undergoes extensive first-pass metabolism, and the metabolites, which are inactive, are excreted in urine. Praziquantel is approximately 80% protein bound, with a serum half-life of 4 to 6 hours. It is rapidly taken up by susceptible cestodes and trematodes. In the case of schistosomes, praziquantel damages the tegument, which results in intense vacuolation and increased permeability to calcium. Adult schistosomes are paralyzed and translocated to the liver through the portal circulation. Sequestered antigens are exposed on their surface, permitting binding of antibodies and phagocytes and resulting in immune destruction. Praziquantel is an alternative to albendazole for the treatment of neurocysticercosis. The concurrent administration of corticosteroids, which are necessary to decrease inflammation and edema in the brain, reduces the serum concentration of praziquantel. The concentration in CSF is approximately 15 to 20% that of serum.

Praziquantel is frequently associated with mild, transient side effects, including headaches, lassitude, dizziness, nausea, vomiting, and abdominal discomfort, but they are seldom severe enough to interrupt therapy. Untoward reactions attributed to release of parasite antigens have been reported in patients treated for schistosomiasis and pulmonary paragonimiasis. Increased intracranial pressure resulting from release of cysticercal antigens is a potentially life-threatening consequence in patients receiving praziquantel for neurocysticercosis. Corticosteroids should be administered concurrently. Praziquantel is contraindicated in persons with cysticerci in the eye or spinal cord.

● TREATMENT OF PROTOZOAL DISEASES

Intestinal and Vaginal Protozoa

Several major luminal pathogens, including *Entamoeba histolytica* (Chapter 352), *Giardia lamblia* (Chapter 351), and *Trichomonas vaginalis* (Chapter 353), live in anaerobic conditions in the intestine or vagina and are susceptible to metronidazole and tinidazole. The latter has favorable pharmacodynamics and is generally better tolerated. Because neither metronidazole nor tinidazole reliably eradicates cysts of *E. histolytica*, either paromomycin or iodoquinol, which are active in the lumen of the bowel, is administered as well. Either one of these drugs or diloxanide furoate can be used alone to treat persons with asymptomatic cyst excretion.

Giardiasis can also be treated with nitazoxanide. It is well tolerated, and an oral formulation is available for children. Nitazoxanide is the only drug available for the treatment of cryptosporidiosis (Chapter 350). It is effective in immunocompetent persons, but not in those with AIDS. Trimethoprim-sulfamethoxazole, which inhibits successive steps in the folic acid pathway, is the drug of choice for *Cystoisospora* (*Isospora*) *belli* and *Cyclospora cayetanensis*. Ciprofloxacin, a fluoroquinolone antibiotic, is an alternative. Tetracycline is the treatment of choice for *Balantidium coli*; metronidazole and iodoquinol are alternatives. Finally, albendazole is effective in the treatment of intestinal and disseminated microsporidiosis caused by *Encephalitozoon* (*Septata*) *intestinalis* and for some other microsporidial species that cause disease in persons with AIDS.

Metronidazole, a nitroimidazole, is rapidly absorbed after oral administration and has a half-life of 8 hours. More than half of each dose is metabolized in the liver. The metabolites and remaining parent drug are excreted in urine. Metronidazole is activated by reduction of its 5-nitro group through a sequence of intermediate steps involving microbial electron transport proteins of low redox potential. It is concentrated in susceptible anaerobic organisms and serves as an electron sink. Nausea, vomiting, diarrhea, and a metallic taste are often associated with the use of metronidazole. They are less common with the lower doses recommended for the treatment of giardiasis than with the higher doses used for amebiasis. Other untoward effects include headache, dizziness, vertigo, and numbness. Potentially severe disulfiram-like reactions occur in patients who ingest alcohol while taking metronidazole.

Tinidazole, another 5-nitroimidazole, has a similar mechanism of action and spectrum of activity as metronidazole but more favorable pharmacodynamics, and it is generally better tolerated. It has been used widely around the world for the treatment of giardiasis, intestinal amebiasis, and trichomoniasis. In comparison with metronidazole, it has a longer half-life, a shorter and less complicated dosing regimen, and fewer gastrointestinal side effects. It, too, can cause severe disulfiram-like reactions after alcohol ingestion.

Nitazoxanide, a 5-nitrothiazole salicylamide derivative, has a broad spectrum of activity against protozoa and helminths. It is formulated as a liquid for use in children. Nitazoxanide is well absorbed orally and hydrolyzed to its active metabolite tizoxanide, which undergoes conjugation to tizoxanide glucuronide. The parent compound is not detectable in serum. Maximum concentrations of the metabolites are observed in 1 to 4 hours. They are excreted in urine and bile. Tizoxanide is highly protein bound. Although its antiparasitic mechanism of action is uncertain, tizoxanide inhibits pyruvate : ferredoxin oxidoreductase–dependent electron transport reactions essential for the metabolism of susceptible anaerobic organisms. It is very well tolerated in children and adults.

Malaria: Prophylaxis and Treatment

As discussed in this section, a number of drugs are available for the prophylaxis and treatment of malaria. Most act against *Plasmodium* stages within erythrocytes. Only primaquine kills *Plasmodium vivax* and *Plasmodium ovale* hypnozoites in the liver. The antimalarial drug of choice depends on the geographic site visited and the *Plasmodium* species encountered (Chapter 345). Antimicrobial resistance is now widespread among *Plasmodium falciparum* isolates and well documented in *P. vivax* from some regions. Country-specific recommendations for prophylaxis and treatment are provided by the CDC at www.cdc.gov/travel/ and in "CDC Health Information for International Travel 2014."[3,4] Major additions to the therapeutic armamentarium in the United States include the fixed drug combination of artemether and lumefantrine (Coartem), which is used for the oral treatment of acute malaria acquired in areas with chloroquine-resistant *P. falciparum*, and artesunate for intravenous administration in those with severe malaria who cannot take oral medications and for whom quinidine is contraindicated or not available. Artesunate can be obtained from the CDC on an emergency basis as an investigational new drug.

Atovaquone plus **proguanil** (adult tablets contain 250 mg of atovaquone and 100 mg of proguanil) is used for prophylaxis and treatment of chloroquine-resistant and sensitive malaria. Atovaquone is a highly lipophilic compound with low aqueous solubility. Administration with food enhances its absorption two-fold. Plasma concentrations do not increase proportionally with dose. Atovaquone is highly protein bound with a half-life exceeding 60 hours. It undergoes extensive enterohepatic cycling and is eventually excreted unchanged in feces. Atovaquone selectively inhibits electron transport in the mitochondria of susceptible *Plasmodium* species at the level of the cytochrome bc_1 complex, which results in collapse of mitochondrial membrane potential. It also affects pyrimidine biosynthesis, which is obligatorily coupled to electron transport in *Plasmodium*. Resistance develops rapidly when atovaquone is used alone to treat malaria. Atovaquone is generally well tolerated but can cause nausea, vomiting, diarrhea, rash, and pruritus.

Proguanil is absorbed slowly after oral administration. Its serum level falls to zero within 24 hours, so it must be administered daily. Its triazine metabolite, cycloguanil, inhibits dihydrofolate reductase in susceptible *Plasmodium* species. Resistance is well documented when proguanil is used alone. Proguanil also acts synergistically with atovaquone to collapse mitochondrial membrane potential in susceptible *Plasmodium* species.

The combination of atovaquone and proguanil is considered the best tolerated of the options for prevention of chloroquine-resistant malaria. It is begun 1 to 2 days before departure and continued during the time of exposure and for 7 days thereafter. Higher doses are administered over a period of 3 days to treat acute, uncomplicated malaria. Potential side effects include abdominal pain, nausea, vomiting, diarrhea, headache, pruritus, and rash. Asymptomatic, transient elevations in liver enzymes have been observed with treatment doses.

Doxycycline 100 mg taken daily by adults provides effective prophylaxis against all *Plasmodium* species. It is begun 1 to 2 days before departure and continued during the time of exposure and for 4 weeks after leaving the malaria-endemic area. Doxycycline or tetracycline is also often administered with quinine for the treatment of acute chloroquine-resistant malaria, but neither drug acts rapidly enough to be used alone for treatment. Doxycycline is generally well tolerated, although it can cause gastrointestinal symptoms and "pill" esophagitis. To avoid the latter, it should be taken with a full glass of water, and the recipient should remain upright for an hour or more after ingestion. Other potential side effects include photosensitivity dermatitis, *Candida albicans* vaginitis, and antibiotic-associated colitis. Finally, doxycycline and tetracycline should not be used in children younger than 8 years or in women who are pregnant or breastfeeding.

Mefloquine, a quinoline methanol compound derived from quinine, was once used widely for the prophylaxis and occasionally treatment of chloroquine-resistant *P. falciparum* malaria. Mefloquine is available for oral administration only. Slowly and incompletely absorbed, it is 99% protein bound. It has a variable half-life ranging from 6 to 23 days with a mean of approximately 14 days. It is metabolized and excreted slowly through bile and feces.

Concern about neuropsychiatric and other toxicities and the availability of better-tolerated alternatives have limited its use in recent years. It is associated with nausea, dizziness, vivid dreams, fatigue, and lassitude. Less common but of greater concern are anxiety, depression, acute psychosis, and seizures. Mefloquine is contraindicated in persons with a history of epilepsy or psychiatric disorders. It now carries a U.S. Food and Drug Administration (FDA) black-box warning. It also depresses atrioventricular conduction and should not be used in persons taking β-blockers for cardiac indications.

Although not approved for use during pregnancy or in children weighing less than 15 kg, mefloquine has been used in situations in which its potential benefits were judged to outweigh the risks.

Chloroquine, a 4-aminoquinoline, has a bitter taste but is well absorbed from the gastrointestinal tract. Its half-life, which varies among persons, averages 4 days, thus permitting once-weekly administration for prophylaxis. Chloroquine is concentrated in the hemoglobin-containing digestive vesicles of asexual intraerythrocytic parasites. It inhibits the parasite's heme polymerase that incorporates ferriprotoporphyrin type IX complexes, which are potentially toxic to the parasite, into insoluble, nontoxic, crystalline hemozoin. Chloroquine-resistant strains of *P. falciparum* actively transport chloroquine out of the intraparasitic compartment. Although this action can be blocked by calcium-channel inhibitors in vitro, chloroquine resistance has not been effectively reversed in humans. Hydroxychloroquine (Plaquenil), which is used for rheumatologic diseases, is also effective against chloroquine-sensitive *Plasmodium* species.

Chloroquine is generally well tolerated when used at the doses recommended for the prophylaxis and treatment of malaria. Side effects include headache, nausea, vomiting, blurred vision, dizziness, and fatigue. Some Africans and African Americans experience pruritus, which responds to antihistamines. Rare side effects include depigmentation of hair, exacerbation of psoriasis, blood dyscrasias, seizures, neuropsychiatric effects, and reactions in persons with porphyria. Retinal damage has occurred in persons receiving chloroquine at high doses for the treatment of rheumatologic disorders, but it has not been documented as a problem in those taking it weekly over a period of many years for malaria prophylaxis. Cardiopulmonary collapse and death have occurred after accidental overdose and in adults attempting suicide. As little as 5 g of chloroquine can be fatal unless treatment is initiated with mechanical respiration, medications to control seizures, and blood pressure support.

Primaquine, an 8-aminoquinoline, eradicates the hepatic hypnozoite stage of *P. vivax* and *P. ovale* and is used as a 14-day course at the end of treatment or prophylaxis to prevent late relapses in persons who are or may be infected with these *Plasmodium* species. It is also an alternative for daily prophylaxis for *Plasmodium vivax* and other species. In that case, it is begun 1 or 2 days before exposure and continued during and for 7 days after the traveler leaves the endemic area.

Primaquine is well absorbed orally and rapidly converted to carboxyprimaquine, which has a half-life of approximately 7 days. It is generally well tolerated, although some recipients experience abdominal cramps, epigastric distress, and nausea. The major concern is hemolysis in persons with glucose-6-phosphate dehydrogenase (G6PD) deficiency (Chapter 161). The G6PD status of the recipient should be determined before it is administered. Rarely, primaquine causes neutropenia, methemoglobinemia, hypertension, or arrhythmias. Primaquine is contraindicated during pregnancy and in breastfeeding mothers because life-threatening hemolysis may occur if the fetus or baby is deficient in G6PD. Travelers should be warned not to give the drug to fellow travelers who have not been screened for G6PD deficiency.

Quinine sulfate, a cinchona alkaloid, is the oldest of the antimalarials. It has a very bitter taste. It is rapidly absorbed after oral administration and has a half-life of 16 to 18 hours in persons with malaria. Quinine has the poorest therapeutic-to-toxicity ratio of any antimalarial drug. The side effects, known collectively as cinchonism, include tinnitus, decreased hearing, headache, nausea, vomiting, dysphoria, and visual disturbances. They are dose related and reversible. Quinine has also been associated with severe hypoglycemia in persons with heavy *P. falciparum* infection as a result of the utilization of glucose by the parasites and release of insulin from the pancreas. Hypoglycemia can be prevented or treated by the intravenous administration of glucose. Rare complications with quinine include massive hemolysis in patients with heavy *P. falciparum* infection resulting in hemoglobinuria and renal failure (blackwater fever), cutaneous hypersensitivity reactions, agranulocytosis, and hepatitis. Quinine can cause respiratory paralysis in persons with myasthenia gravis. It stimulates uterine contractions and can produce abortions, but it has saved the lives of many pregnant women with *P. falciparum* malaria. Quinine dihydrochloride given intravenously can cause myocardial depression, peripheral vascular collapse, respiratory depression, and potentially death.

Quinidine gluconate, the stereoisomer of quinine, is recommended for the intravenous treatment of patients with severe malaria and in those who cannot take antimalarials orally. Quinidine gluconate was once widely used for the treatment of ventricular ectopy, but it has been replaced by newer antiarrhythmic agents, which has decreased its availability in many

hospitals. Side effects include prolongation of the QT interval, arrhythmias, and hypotension, particularly if it is infused too rapidly. Persons receiving intravenous quinidine should be monitored in an intensive care setting, and therapy should be switched to an oral antimalarial medication as soon as possible.

Artemether,[5] **artesunate,**[6] and other artemisinins are sesquiterpene lactone derivatives of the wormwood plant *Artemisia annua*, from which qinghaosu, the Chinese herbal medication for fever, is derived. They are endoperoxide-containing compounds. In the presence of intraparasitic iron, they are converted into free radicals and other intermediates that alkylate specific malarial proteins and act rapidly to kill intraerythrocytic parasites. The artemisinins have been used widely around the world for the treatment of acute malaria caused by chloroquine-resistant *P. falciparum*, as well as other *Plasmodium* species. They are usually administered with a second antimalarial drug that has a different mechanism of action and longer half-life to prevent the development of resistance. The route of administration with artemisinins varies; some are well absorbed orally, whereas others are administered intravenously, intramuscularly, or by suppository. Their short half-lives preclude their use for prophylaxis. Side effects in humans are common but seldom result in discontinuation of the drug. Neurologic toxicity and cerebellar dysfunction have been observed in dogs receiving chronic, high-dose therapy.

Artemether plus lumefantrine (Coartem), a fixed drug combination, is available in the United States and has been widely used around the world to treat chloroquine-resistant malaria. It should be taken with food, but grapefruit juice should be avoided. Common adverse reactions in adults are headache, anorexia, dizziness, asthenia, arthralgia, and myalgia. The most common in children are fever, cough, vomiting, anorexia, and headache. They do not usually require discontinuation of therapy. Of greater concern, artemether-lumefantrine can result in prolongation of the QT interval and is contraindicated in persons with abnormal QT. It also inhibits CYP206 and can hereby reduce the metabolism of other medications that prolong the QT interval. It can also decrease the effectiveness of birth control pills. Care must be taken in reviewing the recipient's medication list for potential interactions before artemether-lumefantrine is prescribed.

Artesunate is available from the CDC as an investigational new drug for the intravenous treatment of severe malaria in persons who cannot take quinidine gluconate, in those who have failed quinidine, or when it is not available (contact the CDC Malaria Hot Line for information). Artesunate is rapidly hydrolyzed to dihydroartemisinin, which is responsible for the antimalarial effect. Studies in malaria endemic regions suggest that parenteral artesunate has a higher success rate and lower adverse event rate than quinidine. In addition to the side effects with Coartem described previously, artesunate has been associated with delayed hemolysis approximately 2 weeks after completion of therapy.

Toxoplasmosis, Babesiosis, and Amoebic Encephalitis

Toxoplasma gondii (Chapter 349) and *Babesia* species (Chapter 353) are other important pathogens of the phylum Apicomplexa. Pyrimethamine and sulfadiazine are recommended for the treatment of toxoplasmosis. They inhibit sequential steps in the folic acid metabolic pathway. Pyrimethamine preferentially inhibits dihydrofolate reductase in susceptible parasites. It is well absorbed orally. The major side effect is macrocytic anemia, which can be prevented by the concurrent administration of leucovorin. Sulfonamides reduce the activity of dihydropteroate synthetase and the binding of *p*-aminobenzoic acid to it. In ocular toxoplasmosis with macular involvement, corticosteroids are used along with anti-*Toxoplasma* therapy to minimize the local inflammatory response. Clindamycin plus pyrimethamine and atovaquone plus pyrimethamine are therapeutic options in sulfonamide-intolerant patients. Persons with AIDS, $CD4^+$ counts less than $100/mm^3$, and serologic evidence of *T. gondii* infection should receive prophylaxis with one of the following regimens: daily trimethoprim-sulfamethoxazole, pyrimethamine plus dapsone, pyrimethamine plus atovaquone, or atovaquone alone. Spiramycin, a macrolide, is used for the treatment of toxoplasmosis during pregnancy. Two therapeutic regimens are available for babesiosis. The greatest experience has been with the combination of clindamycin plus quinine, but side effects are common. Atovaquone plus azithromycin is effective and better tolerated (Chapter 353). Finally, the addition of miltefosine, an antileishmanial drug (see later), to multidrug regimens has improved the outcome of persons with encephalitis due to the free-living *Acanthamoeba* and *Balamuthia*. It is now recommended as part of regimens to treat them as well as *Naegleria* infections. It is available from the CDC for these infections.

CHAGAS' DISEASE, AFRICAN TRYPANOSOMIASIS, AND LEISHMANIASIS

The *Leishmania* species that cause cutaneous, mucosal, and visceral leishmaniasis; *Trypanosoma cruzi*, the etiology of Chagas' disease; and *Trypanosoma brucei rhodesiense* and *Trypanosoma brucei gambiense*, which are responsible for human African trypanosomiasis (sleeping sickness); pose difficult therapeutic challenges.

Nifurtimox and benznidazole orally are the only drugs available to treat *T. cruzi* (Chapter 347).[7] Benznidazole has been used widely in endemic areas in Latin America and nifurtimox in the United States. They lower mortality and shorten the duration of acute Chagas' disease. Treatment is also recommended for persons with recent infection as well as asymptomatic children and adults through middle age with indeterminate-stage *T. cruzi* infection. The percentage of those who are parasitologically cured by treatment has been debated. Neither benznidazole nor nifurtimox can reverse the manifestations of chronic Chagas' disease after they have developed. Side effects are common with both drugs and increase in frequency and severity with age. Benznidazole is associated with allergic dermatitis, peripheral neuropathy, insomnia, and gastrointestinal symptoms, including anorexia and weight loss. Nifurtimox causes anorexia, nausea, vomiting, weight loss, headache, dizziness or vertigo, paresthesias, weakness, and polyneuropathy.

Suramin, pentamidine, eflornithine, and melarsoprol are used for the treatment of human African trypanosomiasis (Chapter 346). Suramin is recommended for the hemolymphatic stage of *T. brucei rhodesiense* infection, and melarsoprol is used in those with CNS involvement. Both drugs are associated with potentially severe side effects. Eflornithine, which is much better tolerated, is effective against both the hemolymphatic and CNS stages of *T. brucei gambiense* infection. It does not have activity against *T. brucei rhodesiense*. Unfortunately, eflornithine is costly and not available in many endemic areas, and supplies are limited. When eflornithine is not available, pentamidine, which has substantial untoward effects, is used for the hemolymphatic stage of *T. brucei gambiense* infection, with suramin being used as an alternative. Melarsoprol is used for CNS disease.

Liposomal amphotericin B (AmBisome) and miltefosine are the only drugs approved by the FDA for treatment of visceral leishmaniasis (Chapter 348) in the United States. Amphotericin B deoxycholate is also effective. Liposomes deliver amphotericin to macrophages and are theoretically attractive because leishmania reside within them. Liposomal amphotericin B is also better tolerated than amphotericin B. Other lipid-associated amphotericin B preparations appear to be effective, but they have been less extensively studied and are not FDA approved for this indication.

For many years, two pentavalent antimony drugs, stibogluconate sodium and meglumine antimoniate, were used to treat visceral leishmaniasis, but resistance is now common among *Leishmania donovani* isolates in India, and therapeutic failures occur in other areas. In addition, pentavalent antimonials require parenteral administration. Side effects increase with age and include gastrointestinal complaints, pancreatitis, myalgias, headache, malaise, elevated liver enzyme levels, and occasionally, bone marrow suppression. Nonspecific ST-T wave changes are common. Sudden death has been reported in persons receiving more than the recommended dose.

Miltefosine,[8] an alkylphospholipid and phosphocholine analogue, that was initially developed as an antineoplastic drug, has proved effective for the treatment of antimony-resistant visceral leishmaniasis in the Indian subcontinent and for cutaneous leishmaniasis in a number of other geographic locations. A major advantage is oral administration. The pharmacokinetics are characterized by a long elimination half-life and extensive drug accumulation. The mechanism of action is uncertain, but it induces apoptosis-like changes in the parasite and has immune modulatory effects in the host. Side effects are frequent but typically are mild to moderate. Dose-dependent gastrointestinal toxicity can result in nausea, vomiting, and diarrhea. They tend to decrease with continued administration of the drug. Elevations in liver enzymes and creatinine are common but usually transient. Miltefosine is embryotoxic and is thus contraindicated during pregnancy. Contraceptive cover is mandatory in females of childbearing years during and for 4 months after therapy. Although miltefosine has proved effective in the treatment of visceral leishmaniasis on the Indian subcontinent, relapses have been reported in 10 to 20% of cases and are even more frequent in persons coinfected with HIV/AIDS. Resistance has also been reported.

Treatment of cutaneous leishmaniasis depends on the size, number, complexity, and location of the skin lesions, their cosmetic impact, the infecting *Leishmania* species, and its propensity to cause mucosal disease. Simple lesions acquired in Europe, Africa, and Asia where mucosal dissemination is rare are often treated topically, or if they are spontaneously healing, followed without therapy. Lesion-directed treatment options include cryotherapy; heat therapy, which requires a specialized delivery system; or intralesional injection of pentostam, which is not available in the United States. Topical therapy with direct application of paromomycin is another option. An ointment containing 15% paromomycin and 12% methylbenzethonium chloride in white paraffin developed in Israel has been the most widely used. Recent results with a U.S. Army formulation of topical paromomycin appear very promising.[9]

Parenteral or oral antileishmanial therapy is used for persons with complicated cutaneous disease and those who are or may be infected with a New World *Leishmania* species potentially associated with mucosal leishmaniasis. Stibogluconate sodium and meglumine antimoniate have been used widely over the years, but toxicity and the requirement for parenteral administration are problematic. Miltefosine has also been used in the treatment of cutaneous and mucosal leishmaniasis. The efficacy has varied with the *Leishmania* species and geographic location. The imidazole antifungals vary in their activity against different *Leishmania* species. Recent clinical experience in Brazil suggests that higher doses of fluconazole are more effective than the 200-mg/day dose used in earlier trials. Liposomal amphotericin B and amphotericin B deoxycholate are effective but more toxic and expensive parenteral alternatives.

Mucosal leishmaniasis is less responsive than cutaneous leishmaniasis to treatment, and relapses are common. Therapeutic options include stibogluconate sodium, meglumine antimoniate, liposomal amphotericin B, amphotericin B deoxycholate, and miltefosine.

Grade A References

A1. Speich B, Ame SM, Ali SM, et al. Ozantel pamote-albendazole for *Trichuris trichiura* infection. *N Engl J Med*. 2014;370:610-620.
A2. Basanez MG, Pion SD, Boakes E, et al. Effect of single-dose ivermectin on *Onchocerca volvulus*: a systematic review and meta-analysis. *Lancet Infect Dis*. 2008;8:310-322.

GENERAL REFERENCES

For the General References and other additional features, please visit Expert Consult at https://expertconsult.inkling.com.

345

MALARIA

PHILIP J. ROSENTHAL AND MOSES R. KAMYA

DEFINITION

Malaria is caused by infection with protozoan parasites of the genus *Plasmodium*, all of which are transmitted by bites of infected anopheline mosquitoes.[1] Malaria is typically characterized by an acute febrile illness, with parasites infecting large numbers of erythrocytes, and classically entails recurrent episodes of fever and chills. It was first described thousands of years ago and is named on the basis of the belief that it was caused by the bad air of the marshes surrounding Rome. Malaria is common, causing hundreds of millions of illnesses each year throughout most of the tropics. Severe disease can occur, primarily with *Plasmodium falciparum* infection, with the acute development of serious organ dysfunction or when chronic and repeated infection leads to severe anemia. *P. falciparum* malaria kills an estimated 660,000 people each year, mostly children in sub-Saharan Africa.

The Pathogen

P. falciparum is responsible for most episodes of severe malaria. It is endemic in most malarious areas and is by far the predominant species in Africa. *Plasmodium vivax* is about as common as *P. falciparum*, except in Africa, but causes severe disease much less commonly. However, studies suggest that severe illness associated with *P. vivax* infection is more common than had previously been appreciated.[2] *Plasmodium ovale* and *Plasmodium malariae* are much less common causes of disease and generally do not cause severe illness. A fifth parasite causing human infections is *Plasmodium knowlesi*, a parasite of macaque monkeys that is a fairly common zoonosis in parts of Southeast Asia and has been responsible for malarial illnesses, including severe disease, in individuals exposed to macaque-biting vectors in forested areas.

EPIDEMIOLOGY
Malaria in Endemic Countries

Malaria is the most important parasitic disease of humans, causing hundreds of millions of illnesses and hundreds of thousands of deaths each year. The disease is endemic in most of the tropics, including many parts of South and Central America, Africa, the Middle East, the Indian subcontinent, Southeast Asia, and Oceania. Transmission, morbidity, and mortality are greatest in Africa, where infection with *P. falciparum* predominates. In most other endemic areas, disease caused by both *P. falciparum* and *P. vivax* is common. In highly endemic areas, the group at greatest risk is young children, who experience most episodes of disease and the most deaths. A second high-risk group is pregnant women, with high risks of maternal and fetal morbidity from *P. falciparum* malaria, including many deaths secondary to low birthweight. In highly endemic areas, in addition to extensive mortality, malaria exerts a massive toll through adverse effects on child development; contributions to school and work absenteeism; and, overall, billions of dollars in lost income among the poorest citizens of the poorest countries of the world. In areas of developing countries with lower levels of malaria transmission, malaria can be epidemic, with intermittent increases in transmission that cause major morbidity in relatively nonimmune populations.

Malaria in Travelers

Malaria is also common in travelers of any age from nonendemic areas to the tropics and may be manifested in those who have returned to nonendemic areas up to many months after travel. Indeed, malaria is the most common documented cause of febrile illness in travelers returning from the tropics to developed countries. Malaria is also rarely transmitted in areas considered nonendemic, including the United States, when imported parasites are transmitted by local anopheline mosquitoes, by blood products, or through congenital spread of infection.

Malaria Transmission

Malaria is transmitted by multiple species of mosquitoes of the genus *Anopheles,* which vary in geographic distribution, ecologic preferences, and susceptibility to mosquito control measures. Anopheline mosquitoes bite at night, so personal mosquito control measures focus on avoidance of mosquito bites overnight. Levels of malaria transmission in endemic areas vary greatly, from areas where residents experience only rare infectious bites to regions of Africa where individuals may receive hundreds of infectious bites each year.

Recent Changes in the Epidemiology of Malaria

A major effort to eradicate malaria after World War II led to elimination of the disease in many areas, including the United States and Europe, but eventually failed to control the disease in most of the tropics. During the ensuing decades, improvements in malaria control were few, and malarial morbidity worsened in many areas, driven by the loss of enthusiasm for vector control; increasing resistance of mosquitoes to insecticides; and, in particular, resistance of parasites to commonly used antimalarial drugs. More than 50 years later, a new large effort to control and eventually to eradicate malaria has been initiated.[3] Key control measures include indoor residual spraying of insecticides, distribution of insecticide-impregnated bed nets, prompt provision of effective drugs to those with malaria, and targeted administration of drugs to prevent infection in high-risk groups. Recent efforts have led to documented decreases in levels of malarial morbidity and mortality in some areas, notably parts of Africa,[4] Asia, and Oceania with relatively low levels of transmission intensity. It is of great interest to learn whether recent advances due to intensified control efforts can bring significant improvements to those parts of the world most affected with malaria, in particular, highly endemic regions of Africa and Asia.

Malaria and Human Immunodeficiency Virus Infection

Malaria does not differ as markedly between those with human immunodeficiency virus (HIV) infection and others as is the case with typical opportunistic infections. However, several interactions between malaria and HIV infection have been established. First, HIV infection appears to disrupt the

acquired immune response to malaria and thereby increases the incidence and severity of malaria. Second, acute malaria elevates HIV viral load and so may increase the risk of HIV transmission. Third, HIV infection may be associated with reduced efficacy of antimalarial treatment, especially in the setting of severe immune suppression. Fourth, therapies for each infection may have an impact on the other, leading to unanticipated effects on drug efficacy or toxicity. Fifth, routine interventions for HIV infection may affect the incidence of malaria; notably, daily trimethoprim–sulfamethoxazole, a routine regimen in HIV-infected patients, offers partial protection against malaria. Because both HIV infection and malaria are common in many areas, in particular sub-Saharan Africa, even modest associations are important. Thus, malaria coinfection in HIV-infected individuals may be an important factor in promoting the spread of HIV infection in Africa. However, increasing implementation of insecticide treated bed nets, prophylaxis against opportunistic infections with trimethoprim–sulfamethoxazole, and antiretroviral therapy will likely substantially lessen malaria risk in HIV-infected patients, such that the risk in those receiving optimal management will not be substantially greater than that in the general population.

PATHOBIOLOGY
Parasite Life Cycle

Malaria is transmitted by the bite of infected female anopheline mosquitoes. During feeding, mosquitoes inject sporozoites, which circulate to the liver and infect hepatocytes, causing asymptomatic liver infection (Fig. 345-1). Merozoites are subsequently released from the liver, and they rapidly infect

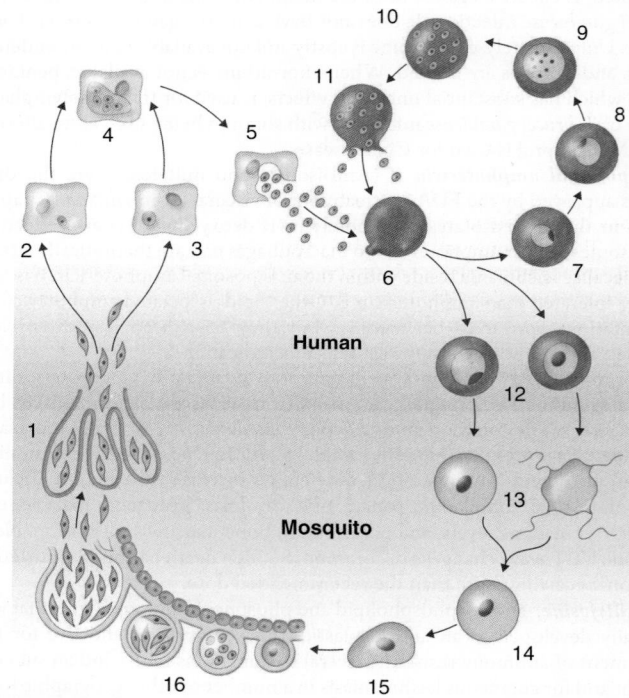

FIGURE 345-1. Life cycle of the malaria parasite. The *upper* and *lower halves* of the diagram indicate the human and anopheline mosquito parts of the cycle, respectively. Sporozoites from the salivary gland of a female *Anopheles* mosquito are injected under the skin (1). They then travel through the blood stream to the liver (2) and mature within hepatocytes to become tissue schizonts (4). Up to 30,000 parasites are then released into the blood stream as merozoites (5) and produce symptomatic infection as they invade and destroy red blood cells. However, in *Plasmodium vivax* and *Plasmodium ovale* infection, some parasites remain dormant in the liver as hypnozoites (3), which can later develop to tissue schizonts and merozoites, leading to relapse. Within the blood stream, merozoites (5) invade erythrocytes (6) and mature to the ring (7, 8), trophozoite (9), and schizont (10) asexual stages. Mature schizonts lyse their host erythrocytes and release the next generation of merozoites (11), which invade previously uninfected cells. Some erythrocytic parasites differentiate to sexual forms (male and female gametocytes) (12). When taken up by a mosquito, the gametocytes mature to male and female gametes (13), fuse to form zygotes (14), and then develop into ookinetes that invade the gut of the mosquito (15) and develop into oocysts (16). Mature oocysts produce sporozoites, which migrate to the salivary gland of the mosquito (1) to allow another human infection. (From Krogstad DJ: Blood and tissue protozoa. In: Schaechter M, Medoff G, Eisenstein BI, eds. *Mechanisms of Microbial Diseases.* 2nd ed. Baltimore: Williams & Wilkins; 1993:600.)

erythrocytes[5] to begin the asexual erythrocytic stage of infection that is responsible for human disease. Multiple rounds of erythrocytic development, with production of merozoites that invade additional erythrocytes, lead to large numbers of circulating parasites and clinical illness. Each erythrocytic cycle lasts approximately 24 hours for *P. knowlesi*; 48 hours for *P. falciparum, P. vivax,* and *P. ovale;* and 72 hours for *P. malariae.* Some erythrocytic parasites also develop into sexual gametocytes, which are taken up by mosquitoes. In the mosquito, gametocytes mature to gametes, and after fusion of male and female gametes to produce zygotes, parasites develop into ookinetes, oocysts, and then salivary gland sporozoites that are infectious for humans, allowing completion of the life cycle and infection of others. *P. vivax* and *P. ovale* also cause a chronic liver infection, in which hypnozoites persist in hepatocytes in a dormant state not eradicated by most therapies for acute disease and subsequently can progress to erythrocytic infection and a relapse of clinical illness.

Pathogenic Features of Malaria Parasites

The most common clinical feature of malaria is fever. Fever coincides with rupture of large numbers of schizont-infected erythrocytes at the completion of the erythrocytic cycle and with high circulating levels of tumor necrosis factor-α (TNF-α). Severe falciparum malaria is associated with very high levels of TNF-α and other inflammatory cytokines, but the specific roles of cytokines in pathogenesis are not well understood. *P. falciparum* infects erythrocytes of all ages, so it is capable of routinely causing high parasitemias, with infection of more than 1% of erythrocytes and more than 10^5 infected erythrocytes per microliter of blood. Non–*P. falciparum* parasites infect smaller numbers of erythrocytes, limiting the extent of infection and morbidity. Non–*P. falciparum* parasites are more likely to cause highly synchronous infections, leading if untreated to regular cycles of fever every 48 (*P. vivax* and *P. ovale*) or 72 (*P. malariae*) hours, often with minimal symptoms between fever episodes.

The contribution of parasite virulence determinants to the severity of malaria is poorly understood. A key biologic feature of *P. falciparum* infection is the ability of parasites to mediate the adherence of infected erythrocytes to a number of ligands on endothelial cells. By this mechanism, erythrocytes infected with the more mature stages of erythrocytic parasites do not circulate but rather adhere within small blood vessels in the brain and other organs. This phenomenon, termed cytoadherence, allows parasites to avoid passing through the spleen, where abnormal erythrocytes would be cleared. Cytoadherence is also likely to play a major role in mediating severe manifestations of *P. falciparum* malaria, with local inflammatory changes mediated by large numbers of adherent parasites leading to organ dysfunction. In particular, *P. falciparum* malaria can progress to cerebral malaria, including coma; noncardiogenic pulmonary edema, including severe respiratory compromise; and renal failure, severe anemia, acidosis, hypoglycemia, and other syndromes of organ dysfunction. Pregnancy selects for a subset of *P. falciparum* strains that specifically bind to ligands in the placenta. Pregnant women in endemic areas, in particular those in their first pregnancy who lack antibodies specific for placenta-binding parasites, are at high risk of morbidity, including anemia, from high parasite loads in the placenta and of poor fetal outcomes, including intrauterine growth retardation, spontaneous abortion, and low birthweight.

A common cause of death from *P. falciparum* malaria, in particular in children in endemic areas, is severe anemia. Anemia is caused by destruction of infected and uninfected erythrocytes, decreased hematopoiesis, and bleeding. In many endemic areas, most asymptomatic young children are infected with *P. falciparum,* with chronic infection contributing to chronic anemia. Other factors contributing to anemia are nutritional deficits and intestinal roundworm infections. With frequent malarial infections and chronic anemia, children are ill equipped to manage acute worsening of the anemia caused by acute malarial illness. With limited access to health care, children often present for medical care late in the course of illness if at all, and many deaths result.

P. falciparum parasites use antigenic variation to evade the host immune response. The principal protein that mediates the cytoadherence of infected erythrocytes to endothelial cells, *P. falciparum* erythrocyte membrane protein-1 (PfEMP-1), is transported to the erythrocyte surface and is a target of host immune responses that limit infection. The PfEMP-1 family comprises about 60 proteins, but only one PfEMP-1 variant is expressed on the surface of infected erythrocytes at a time. During the course of an infection, parasites frequently vary the expression of PfEMP-1s to stymie host responses. This factor and the high variability in sequence of many PfEMP-1

molecules present a broad repertoire of antigens and probably help explain the slow acquisition of protective antimalarial immunity. Antigenic variation and other aspects of immunologic diversity are poorly understood for non–*P. falciparum* malaria parasites, but each species appears capable of repeated infections.

Plasmodial parasites other than *P. falciparum* do not cause cytoadherence of infected erythrocytes, infect lower numbers of erythrocytes, and are much less commonly responsible for complicated and severe disease. However, recent reports suggest that *P. vivax* can cause severe disease, in particular respiratory compromise, more commonly than has previously been appreciated. *P. vivax* is also particularly prone to cause splenic rupture, although this complication can be seen with all malarial species. *P. malariae* most commonly causes a mild febrile illness, but chronic or repeated infection has been associated with an immune complex–mediated glomerulonephritis (Chapter 121) with nephrotic syndrome (Chapter 121). Recent reports indicate that *P. knowlesi* can cause severe illness, including deaths. The short (24-hour) erythrocytic cycle of *P. knowlesi,* which allows more rapid replication of these parasites compared with others, may partly explain the propensity of this zoonotic parasite to cause severe illness.

Host Immunity and Genetics

The nature of human immune responses to malaria remains poorly characterized, but protective responses require multiple infections and apparently humoral and cell-mediated responses. Where *P. falciparum* malaria is common, disease occurs primarily in children. After some protection during the first few months of life, probably because of protective effects of maternal antiplasmodial antibodies and fetal hemoglobin, young children are infected frequently, experience repeated febrile malaria illnesses, and are at high risk of severe disease. With repeated episodes of malaria, children develop partial immunity. Immunity develops gradually, with some protection against severe malaria after only a few infections, increasing protection against symptomatic illness in children, and eventually strong protection against infection. Thus, in highly endemic areas, young children experience frequent episodes of malaria, especially at about age 6 months to 5 years; older children are frequently infected but uncommonly symptomatic; and adults experience identifiable malarial parasitemia only uncommonly. However, antimalarial immunity is not complete; malaria can occur in individuals of any age. In addition, immunity requires boosting by repeated infections, so adults are at increased risk of disease if they return to a highly endemic site after an extended stay in a nonendemic area.

A number of human genetic polymorphisms offer protection against malaria.[6] The best characterized is sickle hemoglobin (Chapter 163). Hemoglobin S heterozygotes are partially protected against severe *P. falciparum* malaria, leading to a balanced polymorphism in which the survival advantage of the polymorphism allows persistence of sickle cell disease in homozygotes. Other erythrocyte polymorphisms that also are likely to offer protection against malaria include hemoglobin C and E, thalassemias (Chapter 162), glucose-6-phosphate dehydrogenase deficiency (Chapter 161), and ovalocytosis (Chapter 161). The Duffy antigen, an erythrocyte chemokine receptor of uncertain function, is the principal receptor on human erythrocytes for attachment and subsequent invasion of *P. vivax.* Most Africans lack the erythrocyte Duffy antigen, explaining the nearly complete absence of *P. vivax* malaria in most of Africa.

CLINICAL MANIFESTATIONS
Uncomplicated Malaria

Most malarial episodes, even with *P. falciparum* infection, are uncomplicated. The incubation period after an infectious bite is usually 10 to 14 days for *P. falciparum* and about 2 weeks for other species, but this can be much longer, especially in non–*P. falciparum* malaria and in individuals with prior immunity. The hallmark of malaria is fever, often with a nonspecific influenza-like prodrome including headache and fatigue followed by a classic malarial paroxysm including chills, high fever, and then sweats. Patients may be remarkably well between febrile episodes. Fevers are typically irregular early in the illness but without therapy may become regular, with 48-hour (*P. vivax* and *P. ovale*) or 72-hour (*P. malariae*) cycles, especially with non–*P. falciparum* disease. Headache, malaise, myalgias, arthralgias, rigors, confusion, cough, chest pain, abdominal pain, anorexia, nausea, vomiting, and diarrhea are common. Seizures are often simple febrile convulsions, especially in young children, but they also may represent evidence of severe neurologic disease. Physical findings may be absent or include signs of anemia, jaundice, splenomegaly, and mild hepatomegaly. Rash and lymphadenopathy are not typical in malaria and thus are suggestive of another cause of fever. Laboratory studies commonly show anemia, thrombocytopenia, and liver and renal function abnormalities.

Severe *P. falciparum* Malaria

Severe malaria can be defined as presentation with signs of severe illness or organ dysfunction (including prostration, impaired consciousness, convulsions, respiratory distress, shock, acidosis, severe anemia, excessive bleeding, hypoglycemia, jaundice, hemoglobinuria, and renal impairment) or a high parasite load (generally peripheral parasitemia >5% or >200,000 parasites/μL). Cerebral malaria, the most common severe complication in children, is generally defined as altered consciousness in the setting of *P. falciparum* malaria. Seizures are common, and deep coma, abnormal posturing, focal neurologic findings, and abnormal respiratory patterns can be seen. The mortality rate is 15% to 25%, with about 10% with persistence of neurologic sequelae, but many patients do remarkably well with appropriate therapy.

Severe anemia is a common presentation, particularly in young children. Transfusions are avoided when possible but play a key role in management of those with severe compromise. Respiratory failure is caused by noncardiogenic pulmonary edema and is more common in adults than in children. Mechanical ventilation can be life saving, if available. Acute renal failure is also more common in adults and generally due to hypoperfusion and acute tubular necrosis; hemofiltration and hemodialysis are valuable, if available. Blackwater fever, including intravascular hemolysis and hemoglobinuria, has an uncertain etiology but can be caused by quinine. Hepatic dysfunction, including jaundice, can be seen; jaundice may also be caused by hemolysis. Splenic enlargement is common, and splenic rupture can be seen. Hypoglycemia is common because of glucose consumption by parasites, increased demand, impaired gluconeogenesis, and quinine-induced insulin secretion; blood glucose levels should be observed closely, with glucose replacement as needed. Metabolic acidosis caused by lactic acidosis and other factors is common; the value of specific therapies for acidosis or aggressive fluid resuscitation is uncertain. Electrolyte derangements can be seen. Coagulopathy, caused by consumption of clotting factors, and marked thrombocytopenia, caused by increased platelet turnover, can lead to significant bleeding. Bacterial infection and sepsis can coexist with malaria; presumptive use of antibiotics is warranted when signs of sepsis are seen.

Complications of Non–*P. falciparum* Malaria

The large majority of infections with non–*P. falciparum* parasites are uncomplicated both in endemic areas and in nonimmune travelers. Nonetheless, *P. vivax* infection is common in many areas, and studies from a number of sites in Asia and Oceania have shown that it makes up about a quarter of children hospitalized with severe malaria, with a mortality rate of about 1%. Important features of severe *P. vivax* malaria include severe anemia and respiratory distress. All malarias, but in particular *P. vivax* infection, can be complicated by splenic rupture. Chronic malaria infections can be complicated by hyperreactive malarial splenomegaly, with massive splenomegaly and findings of hypersplenism. Chronic infections can also lead to the nephrotic syndrome, particularly with *P. malariae* infection.

DIAGNOSIS

Clinical Features

In individuals with febrile illness and malaria risk, it is essential to make a diagnosis promptly and important to distinguish the different species that infect humans because management differs according to the infecting species. Malaria is the most common cause of febrile illness in many areas, and with limited diagnostic capabilities, it is frequently diagnosed based only on presentation with a febrile illness. However, formal diagnosis is preferred. In travelers returning from endemic areas with fever, historical details can aid in the diagnosis. Malaria is most likely in individuals who failed to use measures to prevent infection and in travelers to the most highly endemic areas, such as rural sub-Saharan Africa. *P. falciparum* malaria generally has a fairly short incubation period in nonimmune individuals, so it presents within 1 to 2 months of return in more than 90% of travelers. Infection with the other malarial species can present a number of months and uncommonly more than 1 year after exposure.

Blood Smears

The standard means of diagnosis in malaria-endemic areas is by thick blood smear. In this procedure, 1 drop of blood is allowed to dry on a slide, erythrocytes are lysed, and parasites are then stained with Giemsa. Parasites are easily identified by trained microscopists, and parasite density can be estimated on the basis of counts relative to those of leukocytes. However, thick blood smears do not allow identification of erythrocyte morphology, which is helpful in species diagnosis, and are difficult for those with limited training. Giemsa-stained thin blood smears offer an improved means of characterizing parasite morphology, but the process is much less efficient than for thick smears. Thus, thick smears are the standard means of diagnosis in highly endemic areas, and thin smears are preferred where malaria is uncommon and where laboratory personnel have ample time to examine multiple microscopic fields. It is important to distinguish infecting species of malaria parasites. In *P. falciparum* infection, generally only ring-form asexual parasites are seen. Trophozoites of *P. vivax* and *P. ovale* are present in enlarged (and ovoid in the case of *P. ovale*) erythrocytes that contain inclusions known as Schüffner's dots. Intraerythrocytic *P. malariae* and *P. knowlesi* trophozoites are often elongate in shape. Sexual stage gametocytes (which have a characteristic oblong shape in *P. falciparum*) are also seen on blood smears; most treatments do not eradicate gametocytes, so persistence of these forms for a few weeks is not a sign of treatment failure.

Antigen Detection

An important new means of malaria diagnosis is antigen detection. Multiple simple tests are now available, incorporating colorimetric detection of one or two antigens in an assay that requires limited training and only a few minutes.[7] The most used assays in Africa use histidine-rich protein-2, a protein that is abundant and long-lived but expressed only by *P. falciparum*. Other assays identify plasmodial lactate dehydrogenase and aldolase, which are produced by all human malarial species. Some tests use two antigens to separately identify *P. falciparum* and all-species plasmodial infection. Rapid diagnostic tests have recently become a standard component of many malaria control programs. One test is approved in the United States. However, with many different tests available around the world, standardization is not optimal, and the specific role of rapid antigen tests for the diagnosis of malaria in different epidemiologic settings is not yet established.

Other Diagnostic Tests

Serologic tests are available to identify prior malaria infection, but responses develop slowly and persist for an extended period, so these tests have limited clinical value unless it is helpful to diagnose the cause of a febrile illness retrospectively in an individual without prior history of malaria. Malaria parasites can be identified readily with polymerase chain reaction (PCR) using primers encoding genus- and species-specific sequences. These tests are convenient for research purposes because they can be conducted on DNA extracted from blood spotted onto filter paper in field settings. PCR is more sensitive than other diagnostic modalities. It is not practical for routine diagnosis because of the time required to complete an assay, the uncertain significance of a positive test result in endemic areas where low-level parasitemia may be common and clinically insignificant, and the cost and logistical requirements of the procedure in developing countries.

TREATMENT   Rx

The treatment of falciparum malaria has been challenged by drug resistance for many years[8,9] and has changed dramatically recently, with recommendations for artemisinin-based combination therapy (ACT) in nearly all countries endemic for *P. falciparum* malaria (Table 345-1). Non–*P. falciparum* malaria is still generally treated with chloroquine, although chloroquine resistance is increasing in *P. vivax*; resistant vivax malaria can be treated with other drugs that are standard to treat falciparum malaria.

Chloroquine and Other Aminoquinolines

Chloroquine has been widely used to treat malaria for more than 60 years. It remains the treatment of choice for non–*P. falciparum* malaria and *P. falciparum* malaria in the few areas where resistance has not been seen (primarily Central America and the Caribbean) and is generally rapidly effective and well tolerated. For *P. vivax* and *P. ovale* infections, primaquine must also be given to eradicate dormant liver forms and thereby prevent subsequent relapse. Chloroquine remains effective as weekly chemoprophylaxis to prevent malaria in areas without resistance. Amodiaquine and piperaquine probably share mechanisms of action with chloroquine, but they are routinely active against chloroquine-resistant parasites because of increased potency compared with chloroquine and some differences in mechanisms of resistance. Monotherapy with either drug is discouraged, but each is now a component of a leading ACT (Table 345-2). Amodiaquine is somewhat less well tolerated than other

TABLE 345-1 TREATMENT OF MALARIA*

CHLOROQUINE-RESISTANT *PLASMODIUM FALCIPARUM*, RESISTANT *PLASMODIUM VIVAX*, OR SPECIES UNIDENTIFIED

UNCOMPLICATED DISEASE

Coartem (artemether 20 mg, lumefantrine 120 mg)	4 tablets orally twice daily for 3 days
or	
Malarone (atovaquone 250 mg, proguanil 100 mg)	4 tablets daily for 3 days
or	
Quinine	650 mg quinine sulfate 3 times daily for 3-7 days
plus	
Doxycycline	100 mg twice daily for 7 days
or plus	
Clindamycin	600 mg twice daily for 7 days
or	
Mefloquine	750 mg followed by 500 mg in 6-8 hours; can also be given as a single 1250-mg dose, although this is less well tolerated than the divided dose

COMPLICATED *P. FALCIPARUM* MALARIA OR UNABLE TO TOLERATE ORAL MEDICATIONS†

IV artesunate‡	2.4 mg/kg every 12 hr on day 1; then daily for 2 additional days
or	
IV quinidine gluconate§	10 mg/kg over 1 to 2 hr; then 0.02 mg/kg/min *or* 15 mg/kg over 4 hr; then 7.5 mg/kg over 4 hr every 8 hr
or	
IV quinine dihydrochloride§,‖	20 mg/kg over 4 hr; then 10 mg/kg every 8 hr
or	
IM artemether‖	3.2 mg/kg IM; then 1.6 mg/kg/day

CHLOROQUINE-SUSCEPTIBLE *P. FALCIPARUM* AND OTHER SPECIES

Chloroquine phosphate	1 g, followed by 500 mg at 6, 24, and 48 hr *or* 1 g at 0 and 24 hr; then 0.5 g at 48 hr
plus (for *P. vivax* and *P. ovale* only)	
Primaquine¶	30-mg base (52.6 mg primaquine phosphate) daily for 14 days

*Dosages refer to salts unless indicated and are for adults. For pediatric dosing and full Centers for Disease Control and Prevention (CDC) recommendations, see http://www.cdc.gov/malaria/pdf/treatmenttable.pdf.
†IV regimens should be given until the patient can tolerate oral agents and then followed by a course of oral therapy (doxycycline, clindamycin, or full treatment courses of other drugs, as listed) when patients can tolerate this.
‡Available in the United States on an investigational basis through the CDC.
§Cardiac monitoring should be in place during IV administration of quinidine or quinine.
‖Not available in the United States.
¶Use primaquine only after demonstrating normal levels of glucose-6-phosphate dehydrogenase.
IM, Intramuscular; *IV*, intravenous.

TABLE 345-2 RECOMMENDATIONS FOR THE TREATMENT OF *PLASMODIUM FALCIPARUM* MALARIA IN DEVELOPING COUNTRIES*

REGIMEN	NOTES
Artemether–lumefantrine (Coartem, Riamet)	First-line therapy in many countries; FDA approved
Artesunate–amodiaquine (ASAQ)	First-line therapy in many African countries; efficacy limited by resistance to amodiaquine in many areas
Artesunate–mefloquine	Standard therapy in parts of Southeast Asia
Artesunate–sulfadoxine–pyrimethamine	Efficacy low compared with other regimens in most areas
Dihydroartemisinin–piperaquine	Newer regimen; highly effective in studies in Asia and Africa

*Recommendations modified from World Health Organization. *Guidelines for the Treatment of Malaria.* Geneva: World Health Organization; 2010.
FDA, Food and Drug Administration.

Tolerability of chemoprophylactic and especially treatment doses of mefloquine is often limited by neurologic and gastrointestinal (GI) toxicity. Halofantrine is an effective drug; however, its use is limited by uncommon but dangerous cardiac rhythm disturbances. Lumefantrine is a related drug that does not share this toxicity and offers effective therapy in combination with artemether as Coartem.

Quinine and Quinidine

Quinine has been used to treat malaria for hundreds of years. It offers rapid action against all species, with limited known resistance except in Southeast Asia, where failures against *P. falciparum* malaria are fairly common. Quinine can be used to treat uncomplicated malaria, but GI and other nonspecific toxicities lead to difficulty in tolerating a full 7-day treatment course. This problem is circumvented by combining a 3-day course of quinine with other agents. For severe disease, intravenous (IV) quinine or, in the United States, IV quinidine has been standard therapy for many years; therapy should be accompanied by cardiac monitoring because of cardiac toxicities of the drugs.

Primaquine

Primaquine is the only available drug to eradicate dormant liver forms of *P. vivax* and *P. ovale* that are not cleared by other drugs and can lead to relapses after therapy with chloroquine and other agents. Primaquine is also an alternative agent for chemoprophylaxis against *P. falciparum* and other species. Primaquine use is limited principally by hemolysis or methemoglobinemia (Chapter 158) in individuals with deficiency in glucose-6-phosphate dehydrogenase (Chapter 161). Testing for deficiency should be performed before use of the drug.

Inhibitors of Folate Metabolism

Inhibitors of two parasite enzymes involved in folate metabolism, dihydrofolate reductase and dihydropteroate synthase, are used in fixed-dose combination regimens for the treatment and prevention of malaria. For treatment, sulfadoxine–pyrimethamine (Fansidar) was heavily used to treat uncomplicated *P. falciparum* malaria, but resistance has increased markedly in most endemic areas. The dihydrofolate reductase inhibitor proguanil is combined with atovaquone in Malarone (see later). For chemoprophylaxis, sulfadoxine–pyrimethamine is no longer recommended because of drug resistance and rare life-threatening dermatologic toxicities. However, less frequent dosing in intermittent preventive therapy regimens has been well tolerated and has decreased malaria in high-risk African groups, particularly pregnant women and young children. Seasonal malaria chemoprevention with monthly combined sulfadoxine–pyrimethamine and amodiaquine during the transmission season is now recommended for malaria control in areas of Africa with highly seasonal transmission and limited drug resistance. Daily trimethoprim-sulfamethoxazole, a common prophylactic to prevent opportunistic infections in individuals with HIV infection, has offered some protection against malaria in Africa.

Artemisinins

Artemisinin, the active component of an herbal medicine from China, and a number of its analogues offer rapid elimination of circulating malaria parasites and activity against gametocytes to limit disease transmission. The drugs are all short-acting, leading to frequent recrudescences of infection after short-course monotherapy. For this reason and to limit selection of resistance, artemisinins are now used in combination with longer acting drugs to treat malaria in 3-day regimens. A number of these combinations have become the standard therapies for *P. falciparum* malaria in most endemic

aminoquinolines. It is generally safe with short-term use but can cause rare serious toxicities, including hepatic and bone marrow toxicity, especially with chronic use, and so it is not recommended for chemoprophylaxis. Piperaquine was well tolerated during extensive use in China a few decades ago; although resistance was reportedly common in China, it does not appear to be a problem at present.

Mefloquine, Halofantrine, and Lumefantrine

Mefloquine offers effective therapy and chemoprophylaxis for most chloroquine-resistant strains of *P. falciparum* and for other species. Resistance to mefloquine is uncommon but has been seen in parts of Southeast Asia. Mefloquine is now used to treat *P. falciparum* malaria in combination with artesunate and is one of three drugs recommended for chemoprophylaxis against *P. falciparum* by the Centers for Disease Control and Prevention (CDC).

countries (see Table 345-2). Leading regimens are fixed-dose combinations of artemether–lumefantrine, artesunate–amodiaquine, artesunate–mefloquine, and dihydroartemisinin–piperaquine, and artesunate–pyronaridine will soon be available.[A1-A10] In some settings rank orders of efficacy are seen for leading ACTs, typically with optimal efficacy for artemether–lumefantrine or dihydroartemisinin–piperaquine, although results have varied based on study details and geography. Of these, artemether–lumefantrine is most widely advocated, is now approved in the United States, and includes a partner drug that has never been available as monotherapy, but it requires twice-daily therapy. The other regimens offer once-daily therapy but have potential problems with resistance to partner drugs. Resistance to artemisinins is a recent concern, with evidence for prolonged times to parasite clearance in Southeast Asia suggestive of diminished drug responsiveness of *P. falciparum*.[9-11] Artemisinins also have an increasing role for the treatment of severe malaria. IV artesunate has been shown to be superior to quinine for the treatment of severe malaria in a mostly adult population in Asia[A11] and in African children,[A12] notably with survival advantages over quinine in both populations. For settings with limited infrastructure, intramuscular artemether and intrarectal artesunate have also shown good efficacy. IV artesunate should now be considered the first-line therapy for severe malaria in the United States, where it is available from the CDC. Artemisinins are generally very well tolerated, with minimal toxicity.

Atovaquone–Proguanil (Malarone)

This fixed-dose combination of a dihydrofolate reductase inhibitor and atovaquone, which has a unique antimalarial mechanism, has excellent efficacy against most *P. falciparum* infections. It is approved for both treatment and chemoprophylaxis of *P. falciparum* malaria and other species in the United States, where it is now widely used for both indications. Malarone offers excellent efficacy with minimal toxicity. Adverse effects may include GI symptoms, elevations in liver enzymes, headache, and rash. Widespread use in developing countries is limited by high cost and concerns about resistance because resistance to each component drug is readily selected.

Antibiotics

A number of antibacterials are slow-acting antimalarials. Tetracyclines and clindamycin should not be used alone to treat malaria but are combined with quinine to allow a shorter duration of therapy with that drug. In addition, doxycycline is effective in chemoprophylaxis of most *P. falciparum* malaria and is recommended for this purpose by the CDC, in particular for travelers to regions of Southeast Asia with high-level resistance to other drugs. Macrolides also have antimalarial activity and are currently under study for use against malaria.

Treatment of Severe Malaria

Severe malaria is a medical emergency and requires parenteral therapy. With appropriate prompt therapy and supportive care, rapid recoveries may be seen even in very ill individuals. As noted before, standard therapy for severe malaria has been IV quinine or quinidine, with continuous cardiac monitoring if possible. However, as noted above, IV artesunate showed superior efficacy and decreased toxicity. Although it is not yet available in all endemic areas, it has become the worldwide standard to treat severe malaria. In the United States, IV quinidine is not available in all hospitals and IV artesunate must be obtained from the CDC; initial treatment should be with whichever drug is most rapidly available. Appropriate care of severe malaria includes close nursing care; maintenance of fluids, electrolytes, and glucose; respiratory and hemodynamic support; and consideration of blood transfusions, anticonvulsants, antibiotics for bacterial infections, and hemodialysis or hemofiltration. Aggressive fluid resuscitation, blood transfusion for moderate anemia, exchange transfusion, and specific treatment of acidosis are of uncertain value. After the acute illness, parenteral quinine, quinidine, or artesunate should be followed with oral longer acting drugs, typically a full course of an oral ACT, Malarone, mefloquine, or quinine plus doxycycline or clindamycin.

PREVENTION

Recent years have been marked by a dramatic increase in interest and investment in the control of malaria. Key malaria control interventions in malaria-endemic regions are control of mosquito vectors by indoor residual spraying of insecticides; personal protection against mosquito bites with insecticide-impregnated bed nets; routine use of artemisinin-based combination therapies, which offer prompt control of malaria infections and activity against gametocytes to limit transmission to mosquitoes; and selected use of intermittent preventive therapies to decrease malarial incidence in high-risk groups. No vaccine to prevent malaria is yet available, but extensive research on potential vaccines is under way. RTS,S, which is based on an immunogenic sporozoite antigen, is the most advanced vaccine candidate. Recent clinical

TABLE 345-3	CHEMOPROPHYLAXIS OF MALARIA*
AREAS WITH CHLOROQUINE-RESISTANT *PLASMODIUM FALCIPARUM*	
Malarone	1 tablet (250 mg artesunate/100 mg proguanil) daily
Mefloquine	250 mg weekly
Doxycycline	100 mg daily
Primaquine[†]	30 mg daily during exposure (chemoprophylaxis) or 30 mg daily for 14 days (terminal prophylaxis against *P. vivax* and *P. ovale*)
AREAS WITHOUT CHLOROQUINE-RESISTANT *P. FALCIPARUM*	
Chloroquine phosphate	500 mg weekly

*Recommendations may change on the basis of drug resistance patterns. For additional details and pediatric dosing, see Centers for Disease Control and Prevention guidelines (http://www.cdc.gov). Begin 1 to 2 weeks before travel for mefloquine and 2 days before for doxycycline, Malarone, and primaquine; continue for 4 weeks after leaving the endemic area (1 week for Malarone; 2 weeks for primaquine). All doses refer to salts unless indicated.
[†]Use primaquine only after demonstrating normal levels of glucose-6-phosphate dehydrogenase.

trials have consistently shown protection in children immunized with RTS,S, with protection against malaria of about 30% to 60% in the year after immunization, but lower levels of protection in very young children, in areas of highest malaria exposure, and when assessed over longer periods of time after immunization.[A13-A15]

Preventive Measures for Travelers to Malaria-Endemic Regions

It is important for nonimmune travelers (Chapter 286) to endemic areas to be protected against potentially lethal malaria. Travelers should decrease exposure to night-biting anopheline mosquitoes by use of insecticide repellants and sleeping in rooms that are screened or equipped with insecticide-impregnated bed nets. Standard advice for travelers to endemic areas is also to use low doses of preventive drugs chosen on the basis of the resistance profile of the particular region. Chloroquine is still recommended for malaria-endemic regions of Central America and the Caribbean. For nearly all other areas, the CDC recommends use of daily Malarone, weekly mefloquine, or daily doxycycline; details of dosing vary, but it is important to continue therapy after return from travel to eliminate parasites as they emerge from the liver (Table 345-3). For areas with high risk of *P. vivax* malaria, some authorities recommend a full treatment course of primaquine after travel to eliminate dormant liver stages. For all chemoprophylaxis, it is important to appreciate that no mosquito avoidance methods or drug regimens are fully protective, so consideration of malaria as a cause of fever in returned travelers is essential (Chapter 286).

PROGNOSIS

Patients with malaria caused by *P. vivax*, *P. ovale*, or *P. malariae* generally respond well to chloroquine and make an uneventful recovery. Chloroquine-resistance is increasing with *P. vivax* from many areas; failures of initial treatment are usually not dangerous but should be followed by treatment with another regimen, such as an ACT, Malarone, or mefloquine. Patients with *P. falciparum* malaria also generally respond well to prompt therapy as long as the disease is not overly advanced at presentation. The mortality rate in those with uncomplicated *P. falciparum* malaria is about 0.1%. Key contributing factors to most deaths from *P. falciparum* malaria are probably a delay between the appearance of symptoms and presentation for definitive therapy and the use of suboptimal therapies. Presentation with high-level parasitemia (>200,000 parasites/μL or >5% parasitemia) or signs of severe malaria are predictive of a poor outcome. However, with aggressive support, even individuals with severe disease can often experience complete recoveries.

Grade A References

A1. Mutabingwa TK, Anthony D, Heller A, et al. Amodiaquine alone, amodiaquine+sulfadoxine-pyrimethamine, amodiaquine+artesunate, and artemether-lumefantrine for outpatient treatment of malaria in Tanzanian children: a four-arm randomised effectiveness trial. *Lancet.* 2005;365: 1474-1480.
A2. Smithuis F, Kyaw MK, Phe O, et al. Efficacy and effectiveness of dihydroartemisinin-piperaquine versus artesunate-mefloquine in falciparum malaria: an open-label randomised comparison. *Lancet.* 2006;367:2075-2085.
A3. Yeka A, Lameyre V, Afizi K, et al. Efficacy and Safety of Fixed-Dose Artesunate-Amodiaquine vs. Artemether-Lumefantrine for Repeated Treatment of Uncomplicated Malaria in Ugandan Children. *PLoS ONE.* 2014;9:e113311.

A4. Gogtay N, Kannan S, Thatte UM, et al. Artemisinin-based combination therapy for treating uncomplicated Plasmodium vivax malaria. *Cochrane Database Syst Rev.* 2013;10:CD008492.

A5. Zongo I, Dorsey G, Rouamba N, et al. Randomized comparison of amodiaquine plus sulfadoxine-pyrimethamine, artemether-lumefantrine, and dihydroartemisinin-piperaquine for the treatment of uncomplicated *Plasmodium falciparum* malaria in Burkina Faso. *Clin Infect Dis.* 2007;45: 1453-1461.

A6. Esu E, Effa EE, Opie ON, et al. Artemether for severe malaria. *Cochrane Database Syst Rev.* 2014;9:CD010678.

A7. Tshefu AK, Gaye O, Kayentao K, et al. Efficacy and safety of a fixed-dose oral combination of pyronaridine-artesunate compared with artemether-lumefantrine in children and adults with uncomplicated Plasmodium falciparum malaria: a randomised non-inferiority trial. *Lancet.* 2010; 375:1457-1467.

A8. Four Artemisinin-Based Combinations (4ABC) Study Group. A head-to-head comparison of four artemisinin-based combinations for treating uncomplicated malaria in African children: a randomized trial. *PLoS Med.* 2011;8:e1001119.

A9. Zani B, Gathu M, Donegan S, et al. Dihydroartemisinin-piperquine for treating uncomplicated Plasmodium falciparum malaria. *Cochrane Database Syst Rev.* 2014;1:CD010927.

A10. Bukirwa H, Unnikrishnan B, Kramer CV, et al. Artesunate plus pyronaridine for treating uncomplicated Plasmodium falciparum malaria. *Cochrane Database Syst Rev.* 2014;3:CD006404.

A11. Dondorp A, Nosten F, Stepniewska K, et al. Artesunate versus quinine for treatment of severe falciparum malaria: a randomised trial. *Lancet.* 2005;366:717-725.

A12. Dondorp AM, Fanello CI, Hendriksen IC, et al. Artesunate versus quinine in the treatment of severe falciparum malaria in African children (AQUAMAT): an open-label, randomised trial. *Lancet.* 2010;376:1647-1657.

A13. Agnandji ST, Lell B, Soulanoudjingar SS, et al. First results of phase 3 trial of RTS,S/AS01 malaria vaccine in African children. *N Engl J Med.* 2011;365:1863-1875.

A14. Agnandji ST, Lell B, Fernandes JF, et al. A phase 3 trial of RTS,S/AS01 malaria vaccine in African infants. *N Engl J Med.* 2012;367:2284-2295.

A15. Olotu A, Fegan G, Wambua J, et al. Four-year efficacy of RTS,S/AS01E and its interaction with malaria exposure. *N Engl J Med.* 2013;368:1111-1120.

GENERAL REFERENCES

For the General References and other additional features, please visit Expert Consult at https://expertconsult.inkling.com.

346

AFRICAN SLEEPING SICKNESS

WILLIAM A. PETRI, JR.

DEFINITION

Human African trypanosomiasis (HAT), commonly known as sleeping sickness, is a vector-borne parasitic disease transmitted to humans and animals by the bite of the tsetse fly (genus *Glossina*). Infection is caused by protozoa of the genus *Trypanosoma* and species *brucei*. In humans, there are two forms of illness caused by two distinct subspecies that are morphologically identical but differ in their geographic range and clinical presentations. *Trypanosoma brucei gambiense* is typically found in west and central Africa and *Trypanosoma brucei rhodesiense* in east Africa. *T. b. gambiense* has a more chronic course, and *T. b. rhodesiense* causes a rapid disease course; both have late stages marked by meningoencephalitis, resulting in coma and death if untreated. There is a third subspecies, *Trypanosoma brucei brucei*, known to cause chronic infection called nagana in cattle; however, humans are not susceptible to this organism.

The Pathogen

As an extracellular microbe, the parasite must evade immune clearance to establish a persistent infection. The surface of the blood stream form of the trypanosome is covered by a dense, homogeneous coat of variant surface glycoproteins (VSGs), which are immunodominant. Each individual trypanosome expresses only one VSG at a time but possesses more than 1000 different silent copies of the VSG gene, and switching to a new VSG occurs at a frequency of about 1×10^{-6} parasites. Hence, the trypanosomes expressing a given VSG will eventually be cleared by the host antibody response, but any individual trypanosome that has switched to a new VSG will evade immune clearance, resulting in a new peak of parasitemia. Recombination between VSG alleles ensures a virtually limitless repertoire of new VSGs; therefore, antibody-mediated parasite eradication is impossible.

EPIDEMIOLOGY

Human African trypanosomiasis is relatively less of a problem now than it has been in the prior century, partly because of cyclic epidemics in the past as well as recent increases in public health efforts for control. However, it remains a looming threat to an estimated 60 million people living in tsetse fly–inhabited areas among 36 countries of sub-Saharan Africa and causes significant morbidity, accounting for 1.5 million disability-adjusted life years in Africa as a whole.

The causative organism was first identified during the latter half of the 19th century, roughly corresponding to the first of three epidemics occurring during the past century. The first epidemic occurred in the Congo basin and Uganda between 1896 and 1906, driven in part by various natural disasters that decimated populations of livestock and regional droughts as well as changes in population distribution influenced by colonialism. The second epidemic occurred in numerous endemic countries in the 1920s; control was achieved after major efforts to systematically screen and treat individuals followed by extensive vector control programs, including bush clearing and insecticide spraying. These acts were nearly successful in halting transmission by the 1960s; however, the independence of many African nations around this time hindered the sustainability of prevention and control programs. The incidence began to rise by the 1970s and surged a decade later, leading to the third epidemic of the 20th century. However, in the past 15 years, increased access to at-risk populations for diagnosis and treatment has led to a 68% reduction in the incidence of reported cases.

Despite increased surveillance efforts during the past 15 years, there are still at-risk areas that lack active monitoring programs, and many people are thought to die of HAT without an accurate diagnosis. The World Health Organization reported an annual incidence of 12,000 cases in 2007, a dramatic decrease from the estimated incidence of 300,000 cases a decade earlier. It is estimated that 300,000 to 500,000 people are infected, contributing to approximately 100,000 deaths each year. More than 90% of reported cases are due to *T. b. gambiense*, the majority being from the Democratic Republic of the Congo.

The geographic distribution includes areas where the vector, parasite, reservoir hosts, and human hosts cohabit (Fig. 346-1). In general, these include focal areas on the African continent within 15 degrees North and 15 degrees South latitude, with a predilection for rural areas. Humans at greatest risk for infection are those who rely on animal husbandry, agriculture, fishing, and hunting for their livelihoods. Often, disease is concentrated among foci of rural areas, having significant socioeconomic impact on affected villages. With a few exceptions, this infection is never found in urban areas. There have

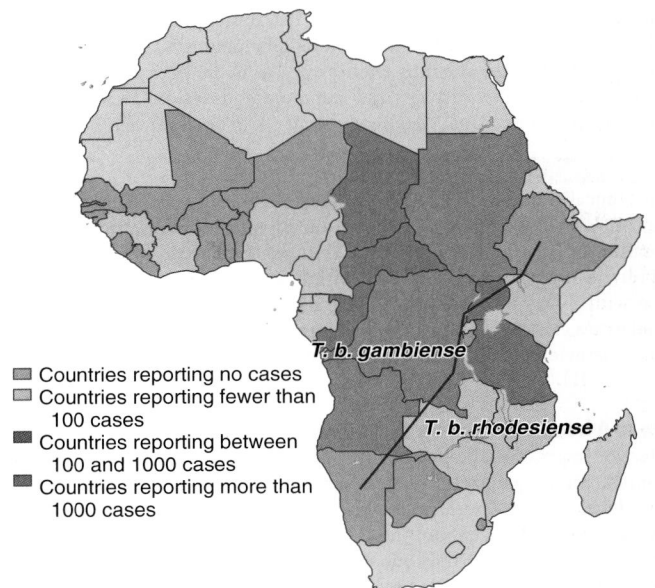

FIGURE 346-1. Map of human African trypanosomiasis (HAT). These 36 sub-Saharan African countries are considered endemic for HAT. *Shaded areas* represent the reported incidence from 1997 to 2006. The *black line* roughly represents the dividing line for the two parasites, although some overlap may already occur.

Legend:
- Countries reporting no cases
- Countries reporting fewer than 100 cases
- Countries reporting between 100 and 1000 cases
- Countries reporting more than 1000 cases

T. b. gambiense
T. b. rhodesiense

been fewer than 50 cases reported annually outside of Africa, usually the result of travel by North Americans or Europeans to African game reserves.[1]

T. b. gambiense is transmitted by tsetse flies from the *Glossina palpalis* group, the annotated genome sequence of which was recently reported. Teste flies are typically found along riverbanks among wooded areas in the more tropical regions of central and West Africa. The reservoir hosts for *T. b. gambiense* and the focus of public health campaigns are mainly humans. Because of this, *T. b. gambiense* is not generally considered a zoonotic disease; the role of the animal reservoir for this organism remains undetermined, although natural infections have been reported in domestic animals such as dogs, sheep, cattle, and pigs.

T. b. rhodesiense is transmitted by tsetse flies belonging to the *Glossina morsitans* group,[2] which are commonly found among woodland and savannah areas of east and central Africa. *T. b. rhodesiense* is a zoonotic disease with numerous wild and domestic species of animals acting as reservoirs. With this infection, the animal reservoir serves an important role in the cycle, sustaining parasite transmission and human infections. Domestic species, especially cattle, have the potential to drive outbreaks and, not surprisingly, have served as the focus of successful prevention campaigns.

PATHOBIOLOGY

After the bite of a tsetse fly carrying metacyclic trypomastigotes, a local reaction (chancre) may form at the inoculation site. This symptom is seen with *T. b. rhodesiense* infection and is more frequently observed in travelers but is rarely seen with *T. b. gambiense* infection. Parasites subsequently disseminate into the blood and lymphatic systems in what is considered stage I of the disease. Spread of the parasites into the central nervous system (CNS) defines stage II of the disease, which is invariably fatal if untreated. The parasite appears to remain extracellular throughout the course of infection.

Peaks and waves of parasitemia occur during stage I disease and result in the classic symptom of intermittent fever. These bouts of fever correspond to a type 1 inflammatory response (Chapter 48), in which classically activated macrophages produce high levels of tumor necrosis factor (TNF) and nitric oxide. This helps in the control of parasitemia but also contributes to tissue damage. Type 2 inflammatory responses with high interleukin-10 production may subsequently occur, which limit TNF and nitric oxide production after initial parasitemia has been controlled. Antibody responses are directed to VSGs and other trypanosome antigens (e.g., antigens from lysed parasites), but autoantibodies are also produced. Generalized febrile episodes are observed together with lymphadenopathy and myocardial and pericardial inflammation. Cardiac involvement is typically more severe with *T. b. rhodesiense* infection. Anemia, thrombocytopenia, disseminated intravascular coagulation, and renal disease may also be observed.

In stage II of the disease, parasites cross the blood-brain barrier and invade the CNS. Acute meningoencephalitis develops, with a variety of inflammatory cells infiltrating the brain, including macrophages, lymphocytes, plasma cells, Mott cells, and morular cells. These inflammatory cells are found in the meninges, which become thickened, as well as in the perivascular spaces and neuropil. Edema, hemorrhage, and granulomatous lesions are often present; thrombosis and neuronal degeneration may also be observed.

CLINICAL MANIFESTATIONS

The clinical manifestations of HAT differ on the basis of the infecting organism.[3] *T. b. gambiense* is more of a chronic disease, with an estimated average duration of 3 years; infection with *T. b. rhodesiense* progresses much more rapidly, leading to coma and death within weeks to months. However, infection with *T. b. gambiense* has been known to cause a rapid decline. Other similarities exist, including an early hemolymphatic stage (stage I) and a late stage characterized by prominent CNS disease including meningoencephalitis (stage II).[4,5]

West African Sleeping Sickness

Infection starts after the bite of a fly infected with *T. b. gambiense*. At the site of inoculation, a painful, indurated, and erythematous trypanosomal chancre may develop 1 to 2 weeks after the bite and resolves spontaneously after several weeks. On occasion, the chancre may ulcerate. However, these features are rarely seen at the time of clinical presentation and sometimes are not known to have occurred on history; thus, many develop disseminated disease without awareness of a localized infection.

The hemolymphatic stage, when parasites disseminate throughout the body, may not be manifested clinically until weeks or months after the initial bite. Typical symptoms include intermittent spiking fevers, occasionally

accompanied by headaches and malaise. These features may persist for weeks or months because of the cyclic nature of parasitemia and antibody production against the various antigens sequentially expressed by the parasite.

Lymphadenopathy (Chapter 168) is a common finding in West African sleeping sickness. Whereas regional lymphadenopathy may develop after the initial bite, generalized lymphadenopathy around the head and neck is often found as chronic illness develops. Enlargement of nodes in the posterior cervical triangle, commonly known as Winterbottom's sign, is the classic finding, but other cervical and supraclavicular nodes may also be involved. Affected nodes are discrete, movable, rubbery nodes that are nontender to palpation; over time, they may become more indurated because of fibrosis.

Other symptoms reported include pruritus, occasionally accompanied by rash, arthralgias, and periarticular swelling as well as by transient edema of the extremities and face. Less common symptoms include features consistent with neuroendocrine dysfunction, including loss of libido and impotence, amenorrhea and infertility, alopecia, and gynecomastia. Signs of disease include hepatomegaly and splenomegaly; cardiac dysfunction, including tachycardia; electrocardiographic abnormalities such as prolonged QTc intervals and repolarization changes; and, less commonly, pericarditis or myocarditis. Hemolytic anemia and derangements in liver function test results may occur.

Months or even years after the initial infection, stage II disease develops and is characterized by headaches, daytime somnolence, and neuropsychiatric features. Behavioral changes, including irritability, confusion, inability to concentrate, and lassitude, are among the first signs of CNS disease; psychosis has also been described. Neurologic findings are numerous and include a variety of motor and sensory disturbances, including extrapyramidal features, dysesthesias, and visual impairment. These symptoms have given the infection its common name of sleeping sickness and are manifested by daytime somnolence and nocturnal irritability. Late-stage disease is marked by cerebral edema and meningoencephalitis. Progressively, a loss of neurologic function can lead to paralysis, and many may succumb to aspiration pneumonias or malnutrition; otherwise, coma leads to death in the absence of treatment.

East African Sleeping Sickness

Compared with Gambian sleeping sickness, East African sleeping sickness is more rapidly progressive. The infective bite is more frequently associated with the development of a chancre, although some studies report this in only 20% of patients. An incubation period lasting days to weeks is needed before symptoms are demonstrated. Initial symptoms include severe intermittent fevers that may resemble those found with malaria. Lymphadenopathy is not as common with this infecting organism; Winterbottom's sign is typically absent. Skin changes are more prominent, and rashes in the early stage of infection are particularly common in expatriates with the infection. In addition, cardiac manifestations are more commonly and clinically relevant; tachycardia, arrhythmias, myocarditis, and congestive heart failure have been documented and may be severe enough to cause death before the development of severe CNS disease. CNS disease mirrors that of West African sleeping sickness, but the onset occurs earlier, and the rate of deterioration is more rapid. Hematologic abnormalities include anemia, thrombocytopenia, and disseminated intravascular coagulation. Death may ensue after weeks or months without treatment.

DIAGNOSIS

Epidemiologic clues and clinical findings may together suggest the diagnosis of HAT, but definitive diagnosis relies on demonstration of the parasite. In the early stage of disease, light microscopy and Giemsa stain may be used to visualize the highly motile parasites directly from fresh specimens of fluid expressed from chancres or lymph node aspirates. Peripheral blood smears, including Giemsa-stained thick and thin smears and bone marrow aspirates, have been successful. Blood smears have increased sensitivity when they are performed during stage I disease, when parasitemia is high (Fig. 346-2); the threshold for visualization of parasites by thick smear is approximately 5000 parasites/mL. Performance is superior with *T. b. rhodesiense* infection, given the higher parasite load. If the initial smear analysis is negative, subsequent examinations should be pursued. Concentration techniques, including buffy coat examination, should be used when technically feasible. Culture of any of these fluids may yield higher sensitivity than smear preparations.

Cerebrospinal fluid (CSF) must also be analyzed to determine the most appropriate treatment. Abnormalities in CSF analysis often start with increased cell counts and progress to include an elevated opening pressure and total protein levels with an increased polyclonal IgM. Stage II disease is defined by the presence of more than 5 white blood cells/µL, the presence of trypanosomes, or an elevated total protein count (>370 mg/L) in the CSF. Newer diagnostic methods, including polymerase chain reaction analysis of CSF and a latex-agglutination test for CSF IgM, hold promise but require validation to determine outcomes after treatment of patients with positive test results.

Allocation of resources to this neglected tropical disease in recent years has allowed slow but exciting progress in the field of HAT diagnostics. The genomes of *T. brucei* species have been mapped, and molecular assays have been developed that can distinguish among species of HAT with a single polymerase chain reaction test. Novel uses of mass spectrometry have been developed that use proteomic signature analysis to identify specific fingerprints of HAT with the host.

In contrast to these highly technical and expensive methods, other tests suitable for the field are being validated, including the dot-ELISA test, which would be able to provide information on stage of disease. Serology tests are also available for diagnosis of *T. b. gambiense* infection. The card agglutination test for trypanosomiasis with *T. b. gambiense* (CATT) is commonly used by screening programs; the sensitivity ranges from 87% to 98%, depending on the population under study, and the specificity may be as high as 95%. No serology tests are available for *T. b. rhodesiense* infection. Rapid diagnostic tests for infection with *T. b. gambiense* include HAT Sero-Strop (which uses a dipstick method) and the HAT Sero + K SeT test (which uses a lateral flow device) for testing blood or plasma, respectively, with results available in 15 minutes at an estimated price of $2.50 each.[6]

parenteral administration for 1 week; however, studies are ongoing to determine the efficacy of shortening therapy to three doses.

Suramin is also used for stage I disease with *T. b. rhodesiense*. This medication is complex to mix and to administer. The drug must be administered in a slow intravenous infusion periodically during 3 weeks. Although anaphylaxis is rare (approximately one in 20,000 patients), a test dose is recommended before full treatment is initiated. A number of side effects require close monitoring, the most important being nephrotoxicity. Urinalysis is recommended before each dose, and the drug should be discontinued if proteinuria persists and casts are seen in the urine sediment.

Melarsoprol is a highly effective but impressively toxic drug used for stage II disease with either organism. The side effects are numerous, but the most important is the life-threatening encephalopathy that may develop from the arsenic (highly fatal) or as an inflammatory reaction. Concomitant steroid use is helpful in reducing the risk of encephalopathy and death without compromising the efficacy of melarsoprol. Gradual increase in the first round of treatment between 2 and 3.6 mg/kg in divided doses three times daily during 3 days has also been shown to reduce the risks of encephalopathy. Melarsoprol has been replaced by eflornithine for *T. b. gambiense* infection but remains the only agent available for the treatment of stage II *T. b. rhodesiense* infection.

Developed more than 20 years ago, eflornithine is the newest agent and drug of choice for treatment of stage II disease with *T. b. gambiense*. Unfortunately, it is not effective as monotherapy for *T. b. rhodesiense* because of reduced susceptibility of this organism to the drug. Eflornithine requires frequent intravenous administration, and up to 40% of patients may report some adverse effects. The drug is much more tolerable than its predecessor melarsoprol and is associated with a comparatively reduced mortality rate.

TREATMENT   Rx

There are very few drugs for treatment of HAT, and those that are commonly used are quite toxic (Table 346-1).[7] Treatment depends on the infecting organism and the stage of disease. For stage I disease with *T. b. gambiense* infection, pentamidine is the drug of choice. The standard regimen consists of daily

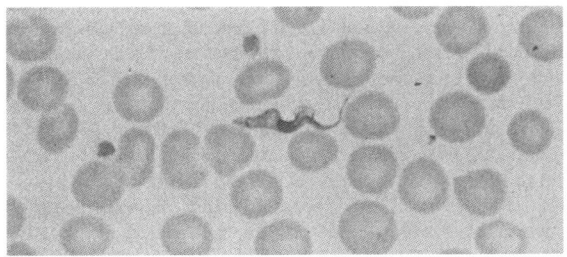

FIGURE 346-2. *Trypanosoma rhodesiense* in peripheral blood. It has a nucleus, posterior kinetoplast, undulating membrane, and flagellum (×1500).

PREVENTION

To date, there is no vaccine against HAT. The mainstays of prevention include active case finding with early treatment and vector control. Given the nature of each infection, active case surveillance is more suitable for infection with *T. b. gambiense*, but vector control is more effective for prevention of infection with *T. b. rhodesiense*. The goal of active case finding is to identify infected individuals who may still be in the asymptomatic stage or early stage. This approach, which is more suited for disease from *T. b. gambiense*, typically consists of a screening examination for lymphadenopathy followed by a CATT test. If results are positive for both, the patient should undergo further evaluation with lymph node aspirate and blood testing. If trypanosomes are found, the patient should be treated. Vector control measures include tsetse fly traps and insecticide-impregnated screens; the traps are easily maintained by locals, but the screens require regular retreatment and thus are more labor intensive and costly to maintain. Mass spraying, once a successful method until the 1960s, is no longer practiced. However, if an epidemic does occur, ground or aerial spraying combined with disruption of the animal reservoir's habitat may be the most effective method of achieving rapid vector control.

Travelers to endemic areas should be aware of this disease and should use basic protective measures. Protective clothing of at least medium weight should be worn; neutral colors are most effective because flies are attracted

DRUG	CLASS	STAGE	ROUTE	ADULT DOSE	ADVERSE EFFECTS
TABLE 346-1	**DRUGS USED TO TREAT HUMAN AFRICAN TRYPANOSOMIASIS**				
TRYPANOSOMA BRUCEI GAMBIENSE					
Pentamidine	Aromatic diamidine	I	IM or IV	4 mg/kg daily for 7 days	Pain, GI symptoms, hypoglycemia or hyperglycemia, electrolyte abnormalities, leukopenia, thrombocytopenia
Eflornithine	Ornithine carboxylase inhibitor	II	IV	100 mg/kg every 6 hr for 14 days	GI symptoms, bone marrow toxicity, seizures
Melarsoprol (alternative option)	Trivalent arsenical	II	IV	2.2 mg/kg daily for 10 days (maximum daily dose, 180 mg)	Encephalopathic syndromes, peripheral neuropathy, paralysis, cardiac dysrhythmias, GI symptoms, rash, pruritus, thrombophlebitis
TRYPANOSOMA BRUCEI RHODESIENSE					
Suramin	Polysulfonated naphthylamine derivative of urea	I	IV	1 g IV on days 1, 3, 7, 14, and 21 (after test dose of 100-200 mg)	Anaphylaxis, nephrotoxicity, fever, rash, pruritus, arthralgias, reversible peripheral neuropathy, and bone marrow toxicity
Melarsoprol	Trivalent arsenical	II	IV	1.2 mg/kg every 8 hr for 3 consecutive days each week for 3 weeks (maximum daily dose, 180 mg)	Encephalopathic syndromes, peripheral neuropathy, paralysis, cardiac dysrhythmias, GI symptoms, rash, pruritus, thrombophlebitis

GI, Gastrointestinal; IM, intramuscular; IV, intravenous.

to bright and dark colors. Tsetse flies are attracted to moving vehicles but rest in the shade or bushes. Although use of insect repellant is prudent for other vector-borne illnesses that may be endemic in these areas, it has not been proven to substantially reduce the risk of tsetse fly bites. There is no recommended chemoprophylaxis for travelers.

GENERAL REFERENCES

For the General References and other additional features, please visit Expert Consult at https://expertconsult.inkling.com.

347

CHAGAS DISEASE

LOUIS V. KIRCHHOFF

DEFINITION

Chagas disease, or American trypanosomiasis, is caused by the protozoan parasite *Trypanosoma cruzi*. The terms *Chagas disease, American trypanosomiasis,* and *T. cruzi infection* are synonyms.

The Pathogen

Several dozen species are included in the genus *Trypanosoma*, but only the African trypanosome *Trypanosoma brucei* (subspecies *T. b. gambiense* [West African] and *T. b. rhodesiense* [East African]) (Chapter 346) and the American trypanosome *T. cruzi* cause disease in humans. Many species of triatomine insects, also called kissing bugs, act as vectors for *T. cruzi*, and many species of wild and domestic mammals, as well as humans, are involved in the complex life cycle of this fascinating organism. The vectors become infected by ingesting blood from mammals that have parasites in their blood stream. The parasites then multiply in the gut of the insects and are ultimately discharged in the feces of the vector. Transmission to a new mammalian host occurs when parasite-laden vector feces contact vulnerable surfaces such as the mucosae of the mouth or nose, the conjunctivae, or breaks in the skin. When in contact with tissues of the new host, the contaminating parasites enter local cells and multiply intracellularly, and as parasitized cells rupture, are released into the lymphatics and blood stream. The circulating organisms enter new cells at distant sites and in this manner maintain an endless process of asynchronous multiplication. The life cycle is completed as parasites are swept up in blood meals taken by vectors. In addition to vector-borne transmission, *T. cruzi* can be transmitted by blood or organs donated by infected persons, from mother to unborn child, by the ingestion of contaminated food or drink,[1] and in laboratory accidents.

EPIDEMIOLOGY
Epizootiology of *T. cruzi*

The triatomine vectors that transmit *T. cruzi* are found in the Americas from southern Argentina through the southern half of the United States. The parasite has been isolated from more than 100 species of domestic and wild mammals, which for the most part probably become infected when they eat infected vectors. Armadillos, wood rats, raccoons, and opossums are typical wild mammalian reservoirs, and these and other species that harbor *T. cruzi* can be found in large numbers in the southern and western parts of the United States.

Typically, humans acquire *T. cruzi* infection when they live in houses in enzootic areas where the sylvatic cycle of transmission is active. The process begins when vector species adaptable to living in human dwellings take up residence in niches in the primitive wood, mud, and stone houses that are typical in many regions of Latin America. These vectors become domiciliary and they then take blood meals, mostly at night, from the humans who occupy the dwellings that they have invaded, as well as from domestic animals that sleep there, particularly dogs. Thus, Chagas disease is primarily a public health problem among poor people who live in rural areas.

Epidemiology of Chagas Disease in Latin America

Chagas disease is a zoonosis that is endemic in Mexico and all countries of Central and South America. None of the Caribbean islands are endemic. In 2006, the Pan American Health Organization estimated that 8 million people are chronically infected with *T. cruzi* and that up to 12,000 deaths result from Chagas disease annually.[2] Since 1991 a major international vector control program in the southern cone countries of South America (Chile, Argentina, Paraguay, Brazil, Bolivia, and Uruguay) has achieved a marked reduction in transmission of *T. cruzi* through housing improvement, education of people at risk for acquiring the infection, and spraying of residual insecticides. Substantial reductions in prevalence rates in school-aged children and in blood donors constitute clear evidence of the success of the program. Uruguay, Chile, and Brazil were certified as being free of vector transmission in 1997, 1999, and 2006, respectively. Marked reduction in transmission has been achieved in Argentina as well. Similar programs have been initiated in Central America and the Andean countries. In parallel with the vector control programs, donor screening has been implemented throughout almost the entire endemic range, and with the notable exception of Mexico, transmission of *T. cruzi* by transfusion has largely been eliminated.

Epidemiology of Chagas Disease in the United States

As noted, the sylvatic cycle of *T. cruzi* exists in much of the southern and western regions of the United States, but only six cases of autochthonous transmission have been reported: three in Texas and one each in Tennessee, Louisiana, and California. Moreover, the nationwide blood donor screening that started in January 2007, in which more than 50 million units have been tested, has uncovered only 17 *T. cruzi*–infected donors, who appear to have acquired the infection autochthonously.[3] In the past 30 years, only about 15 laboratory-acquired and imported cases of acute Chagas disease have been reported to the Centers for Disease Control and Prevention (CDC). Only one of the latter infections occurred in a tourist returning to the United States, but three such instances have been reported in Europe as well as one in Canada. Thus, acute Chagas disease is extremely rare in the United States.

Census data indicate that including illegal and legal immigrants, 23 million persons born in countries endemic for Chagas disease currently live in the United States. Roughly 17 million of these individuals are from Mexico, where the overall prevalence of *T. cruzi* infection is thought to range from 0.5% to 1.0%. Moreover, more than half of the non-Mexican immigrants have come from Central America, a region where the prevalence of *T. cruzi* infection is relatively high. A recent estimate puts the number of *T. cruzi*–infected persons currently living in the United States at 300,000. Several studies done before blood donor screening began in 2007 identified *T. cruzi*–infected persons in the donor pool, and nine instances of transmission by transfusion in the United States and Canada were described. Since screening began in 2007, more than 50 million units have been screened, and nearly 3000 *T. cruzi*–infected donors have been identified and permanently deferred from donation. The confirmed rate of *T. cruzi* infection in donors is about 1 in 13,300.[4] With the goal of reducing the enormous cost of universal screening ($100 to $200 million per year), a selective screening protocol based on previous negative test results has been implemented.

The transplantation in the United States of organs from three persons with undiagnosed chronic *T. cruzi* infection resulted in acute Chagas disease in five recipients, one of whom died of the infection. To date, only one instance of congenital transmission of *T. cruzi* here has been reported. A reasonable estimate of the number of babies born in the United States each year with congenital Chagas disease puts it in the range of 63,000. The fact that most babies with congenital Chagas disease are asymptomatic[5] and the low level of knowledge about Chagas disease among caregivers likely underlie the dearth of reported cases.

PATHOBIOLOGY

In acute Chagas disease, an inflammatory lesion, called a chagoma, may appear at the site of entry of the parasites. Local histologic changes include intracellular parasitism of muscle and other subcutaneous tissues, lymphocytic infiltration, interstitial edema, and hyperplasia of lymph nodes that drain the area. As the parasites spread systemically through the lymphatics and blood stream, muscles, including the myocardium, are the most heavily parasitized tissues, but the organisms can invade essentially any tissue. Myocarditis may develop in association with focal areas of infected cardiomyocytes, inflammation, and necrosis. The characteristic pseudocysts seen in sections of *T. cruzi*–infected tissues are actually host cells filled with multiplying forms of the parasite (Fig. 347-1). In some patients, parasites can be seen in cerebrospinal fluid (CSF).

In persons with chronic Chagas disease, the heart is the organ most commonly affected. Hearts obtained at autopsy from patients who died of Chagas cardiomyopathy usually have a global appearance reflecting biventricular enlargement and thinning of ventricular walls (Fig. 347-2). Mural thrombi are frequently present, and an apical aneurysm of the left ventricle is typical in patients with advanced disease. At the cellular level, the process that underlies these gross pathologic abnormalities is a chronic inflammation with mononuclear cell infiltration, diffuse interstitial fibrosis, and atrophy of myocardial cells. The chronic inflammation affects the conduction system as well and causes a variety of rhythm disturbances, including atrial bradyarrhythmias and fibrillation; premature ventricular contractions; bundle branch blocks, often of the right bundle; ventricular tachycardia; and third-degree atrioventricular block. Parasites are rarely seen in diseased tissues by conventional histologic methods, but several studies using polymerase chain reaction (PCR) assays found a correlation between the intensity of inflammation and the presence of parasites. Evidence accumulated to date implicates the persistence of parasites and the resulting chronic inflammation in affected tissues—rather than autoimmune mechanisms—as the basis for the pathogenesis in patients with chronic *T. cruzi* infection.

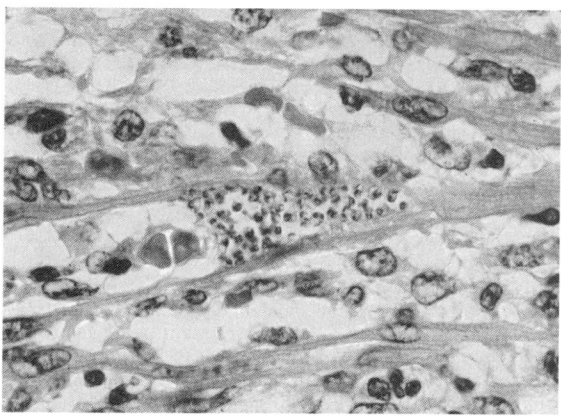

FIGURE 347-1. *Trypanosoma cruzi* in cardiac muscle of a child who died of acute Chagas myocarditis. An infected myocyte containing several dozen *T. cruzi* amastigotes is in the center of the field (hematoxylin-eosin staining, ×900).

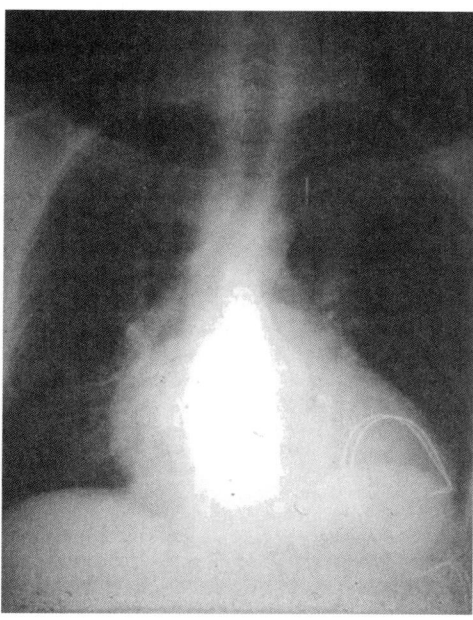

FIGURE 347-2. Chest radiograph of a patient from Bolivia with chronic *Trypanosoma cruzi* infection, rhythm disturbances, and cardiomyopathy. Pacemaker wires can be seen in the area of the left ventricle.

The dilation and hypertrophy observed on gross examination of the esophagus or colon of a patient with chronic Chagas disease of the digestive tract (megadisease) is striking. Focal inflammatory lesions with lymphocytic infiltration are seen on microscopic examination of affected tissues. In addition, the number of neurons in the myenteric plexus is reduced, and periganglion and intraganglion fibrosis with Schwann cell proliferation and lymphocytosis is present. In most patients, the clinical consequences of this parasympathetic denervation are limited to the esophagus or colon (or to both), but the ureters, biliary tree, and other hollow viscera can be affected as well.

CLINICAL MANIFESTATIONS

Acute Chagas Disease

Acute Chagas disease is usually an illness of children but can occur at any age.[6] Symptoms are typically mild and nonspecific. When the parasite has entered through a break in the skin or the site of a vector's puncture, as noted, a chagoma may appear with local lymphadenopathy. The Romaña sign, the classic finding in acute Chagas disease, consists of painless edema of the palpebrae and periocular tissues and may appear when the conjunctiva is the portal of entry. These initial local signs can be followed by fever, malaise, anorexia, and edema of the face and lower extremities. Generalized lymphadenopathy and hepatosplenomegaly may also be present. Severe myocarditis may develop as well, and most deaths are caused by the resulting congestive heart failure. Meningoencephalitis is a rare complication. In untreated patients the acute illness resolves spontaneously over a period of 6 to 8 weeks as the patient enters the indeterminate phase of Chagas disease, which is characterized by subpatent parasitemia, absence of associated signs and symptoms, and easily detectable antibodies to *T. cruzi*.

Chronic Chagas Cardiopathy

In only 10% to 30% of persons chronically infected with *T. cruzi* does clinically manifested disease develop. It most often involves rhythm disturbances or cardiomyopathy.[7,8] Symptoms of cardiac Chagas disease can develop insidiously over years and often decades after the initial infection. Clinical findings reflect the rhythm disturbances, congestive heart failure, and thromboembolism that characterize the illness. Dizziness, syncope, and even seizures can result from a wide variety of arrhythmias. The cardiomyopathy often leads to biventricular failure, and right-sided heart failure can predominate in patients with advanced disease. A validated risk score assessment tool has been developed to gauge prognosis. Chronic Chagas disease is an independent risk factor for stroke.

Chronic Gastrointestinal Chagas Disease (Megadisease)

The esophagus and colon are the segments of the gastrointestinal (GI) tract most commonly affected in persons with chronic *T. cruzi* infection. In patients with megaesophagus, the symptoms are similar to those of idiopathic achalasia (Chapter 138) and may include cough, dysphagia, odynophagia, and regurgitation. Hypersalivation and consequent salivary gland hypertrophy develop in some patients with advanced esophageal dysfunction. Aspiration can occur, especially during sleep, and in untreated patients, repeated episodes of aspiration pneumonitis are common. Weight loss and even cachexia in patients with severe megaesophagus can combine with pneumonitis to cause death. Patients with chagasic megacolon have intermittent abdominal pain and chronic constipation and in advanced cases can go for several weeks between bowel movements. Rarely, acute obstruction, occasionally with volvulus, can lead to perforation, sepsis, and death.

IMMUNOSUPPRESSION AND TRANSPLANTATION IN PATIENTS INFECTED WITH *T. CRUZI*

When persons with chronic carriage of *T. cruzi* become immunosuppressed, reactivation of the infection can occur, sometimes with an intensity that is atypical of acute Chagas disease in immunocompetent persons.[9] The overall incidence of reactivation in immunosuppressed persons who harbor the parasite chronically is not known. Reactivation after renal transplantation has been reported, and in rare instances central nervous system abscesses and skin lesions were involved. The consensus view is that Chagas disease should not be a contraindication to kidney transplantation. In *T. cruzi*-infected patients who do undergo the procedure, periodic monitoring for signs and symptoms of acute Chagas disease should nonetheless be carried out, including careful neurologic evaluation, and parasitologic testing should be performed when acute illnesses occur postoperatively.

Reactivation of *T. cruzi* infection can also occur in persons coinfected with the parasite and human immunodeficiency virus (HIV). Dozens of such patients have been described. It is striking that in many of these patients *T. cruzi* brain abscesses developed, which do not occur in immunocompetent patients with chronic Chagas disease. It has been shown that HIV viral loads increase in the context of reactivated acute Chagas disease. Calculations based on the overlapping epidemiologies of HIV and *T. cruzi* infections in the endemic countries suggest that the incidence of reactivation of the latter in coinfected persons is low.

DIAGNOSIS

Acute Chagas Disease

The first step in considering the diagnosis of acute Chagas disease is establishing that a person is at risk for *T. cruzi* infection. Risk factors include recent residence or blood transfusion in an endemic area, birth to a mother with geographic- or transfusion-associated risk in the case of a newborn, or a laboratory accident involving the parasite. Definitive diagnosis of acute Chagas disease can be made only by detecting parasites. Serologic assays for *T. cruzi*–specific IgM are not accurate enough to justify their use. In immunocompetent persons suspected of having acute Chagas disease, the most productive approach is examination of wet preparations of anticoagulated blood or buffy coat for the highly motile blood stream parasites. They can be seen in Giemsa-stained smears as well. In infected immunocompromised patients, moreover, parasites can sometimes be found in other specimens such as lymph node aspirates, biopsy specimens of skin lesions, bone marrow, endomyocardial tissue, CSF, and pericardial fluid.

When these direct methods fail to detect organisms in an at-risk person, samples should be tested with a PCR assay (see later).[10] PCR assays have been shown to be more sensitive than the direct methods described earlier for detecting *T. cruzi*. Another method is to culture blood or other samples in specialized liquid medium, but the usefulness of this approach is limited by low sensitivity (50%-70% for hemoculture) and by the fact that cultures take a minimum of 2 weeks before turning positive. In newborns whose blood is negative both by direct examination and in a PCR assay right after birth, serologic evaluation for *T. cruzi*–specific IgG should be performed 6 to 9 months later, by which time maternal antibodies will have disappeared.

Chronic Chagas Disease

Chronic *T. cruzi* infection is usually diagnosed by detecting IgG antibodies that specifically bind to parasite antigens, and in almost all instances isolation of the organism is not necessary. More than 30 serologic assays for diagnosing Chagas disease are currently available commercially in endemic countries, where they are used widely for testing clinical specimens and screening blood donors. Even though these tests usually have good sensitivity and reasonable specificity, false-positive reactions do occur, typically with specimens from people who have other infectious diseases or autoimmune conditions. The World Health Organization has recommended that testing be done with two assays based on different formats. In the United States, the Ortho *T. cruzi* ELISA Test System (Ortho-Clinical Diagnostics, Raritan, NJ) and the Abbott Prism Chagas Assay (Abbott Laboratories, Abbott Park, IL) are used to screen donated blood. The Abbott ESA Chagas and the Chagas RIPA[11] are used for confirmatory testing of donor samples that are positive in the screening tests.

Since the publication in 1989 of two reports describing the use of PCR tests to detect *T. cruzi*, well over 100 articles dealing with this approach have appeared. In human studies, the sensitivity of the PCR assays ranged from 44.7% to 100%, with most being higher than 90%. It is generally accepted that the level of sensitivity of these assays is not high enough to justify their use for confirmatory testing of serologically positive donor samples. In contrast, PCR assays may be useful in persons who have borderline serologic results, in patients suspected of having congenital or acute Chagas disease in whom parasites are not detected microscopically, and in infected patients who have received specific treatment. In all such persons, because of the sensitivity issue, only positive PCR results can be taken as being truly indicative of infection status.

TREATMENT   Rx

Antiparasitic Drugs (also see Chapter 344)

The two drugs currently available for treating Chagas disease are unsatisfactory, and the need for a parasitologically curative drug regimen is the most important current challenge in Chagas disease research.[12] Nifurtimox (Lampit, Bayer 2502, Leverkusen, Germany) is a nitrofuran derivative that has been used for more than 3 decades. Nifurtimox reduces symptoms and decreases mortality rates in patients with acute Chagas disease, approximately 70% of whom are cured parasitologically. Nifurtimox also can cure a substantial portion of children in the indeterminate phase, but unfortunately, cure rates may be less than 10% in adults with long-standing chronic *T. cruzi* infection.

Disadvantages of nifurtimox include its long course of treatment and occasionally bothersome side effects, including GI complaints such as anorexia, nausea, vomiting, weight loss, and abdominal pain. Patients taking the drug may also have neurologic symptoms such as insomnia, restlessness, paresthesias, twitching, polyneuritis, and even seizures.[13] For adults, the recommended oral dosage is 8 to 10 mg/kg body weight per day. For adolescents, the dose is 12.5 to 15 mg/kg/day, and for children 1 to 10 years of age, it is 15 to 20 mg/kg/day. The drug should be given each day in four divided doses, and treatment should be continued for 90 to 120 days. In the United States, nifurtimox can only be obtained from the CDC Drug Service (404-639-3670).

The second drug for treating *T. cruzi* infection is the nitroimidazole derivative benznidazole (Rochagan, Radinil, Roche 7-1051; LAFEPE, Pernambuco, Brazil). Cure rates are similar or perhaps a bit higher than those achieved with nifurtimox. A cure rate higher than 90% in babies with congenital infection has been observed with benznidazole. Side effects can include rash, peripheral neuropathy, and granulocytopenia.[14] Benznidazole is considered the drug of choice by most Latin American experts. The recommended oral dosage of benznidazole is 5 to 10 mg/kg body weight per day for children and 5 mg/kg body weight per day for adults, in both cases for 60 days.

There is broad agreement among experts that treatment is indicated in all patients with acute or congenital infections, as well as in chronically infected children up to 18 years old. This recommendation is supported by several studies showing that a majority of such patients can be cured parasitologically. By extension, it would be reasonable to treat anyone 18 years or older known to have acquired *T. cruzi* infection within the past 17 years. There is also broad agreement that persons with advanced symptomatic *T. cruzi* infection should not be given specific treatment. The remaining question, then, is whether adults with long-standing indeterminate-phase infections, who by far constitute the largest group of *T. cruzi*–infected persons, should be treated. This is a thorny question because the burden of taking a full course of either drug can be substantial and because parasitologic cure rates are so low. Importantly, there is no clear evidence from randomized controlled trials that therapy with either drug delays the onset of symptoms or the progression of pathology or reduces mortality rates in adults with chronic *T. cruzi* infection. In 2006, a panel of experts convened at the CDC recommended that adults 19 to 50 years old in the indeterminate phase or with mild symptoms be offered treatment. A large randomized trial (the BENEFIT multicenter trial) designed to assess the clinical and parasitologic efficacy of benznidazole in patients with Chagas disease 18 to 75 years old without advanced disease is being conducted in Colombia, Bolivia, Brazil, and Argentina. Initial findings will be available in 2015. A recently reported randomized trial comparing benznidazole (150 mg twice daily) with posaconazole, which had shown trypanocidal activity in mouse models, given at two doses (400 mg twice daily or 100 mg twice daily) all for 60 days for chronic Chagas disease showed that benznidazole had a significantly smaller percentage of treatment failures than did either treatment dose of posaconazole.[A1] A recently reported study from Argentina showed that treatment with either benznidazole or nifurtimox before pregnancy can reduce the probability of subsequent congenital transmission of the parasite.[15]

Management of Symptomatic Chagas Disease

An algorithm for the evaluation of persons with newly diagnosed Chagas disease has been developed (Fig. 347-3). *T. cruzi*–infected patients in whom symptomatic cardiac or GI disease develops should be referred to appropriate subspecialists. Beyond the possible use of nifurtimox or benznidazole, treatment of acute and chronic Chagas disease is symptomatic. In patients with symptomatic chronic Chagas cardiac disease, treatment should be directed at managing symptoms with the anticoagulants and cardiotropic drugs used in patients with cardiomyopathy of other causes. Pacemakers are useful in patients with ominous arrhythmias. The usefulness of implantable cardioverter-defibrillators in patients with Chagas heart disease has not been established and needs further investigation in prospective randomized trials.

Heart transplantation (Chapter 82) is an option in patients with end-stage Chagas cardiac disease, and more than 150 such patients have undergone the procedure in Brazil and the United States.[16] As is the case with other *T. cruzi*–infected patients who are immunosuppressed, reactivation is a risk but it is manageable. The usefulness and side effects of long-term prophylaxis for reactivation with either benznidazole or nifurtimox in *T. cruzi*–infected patients after heart transplantation have not been evaluated. The long-term survival of Chagas patients with heart transplants appears to be longer than that in patients undergoing cardiac transplantation for other reasons, probably because the lesions of *T. cruzi*–associated pathology affect mostly the heart.

Chagas megaesophagus should be treated as normally done for idiopathic achalasia (Chapter 138), which usually responds to balloon dilation of the lower esophageal sphincter when symptoms are mild. Surgical treatment may

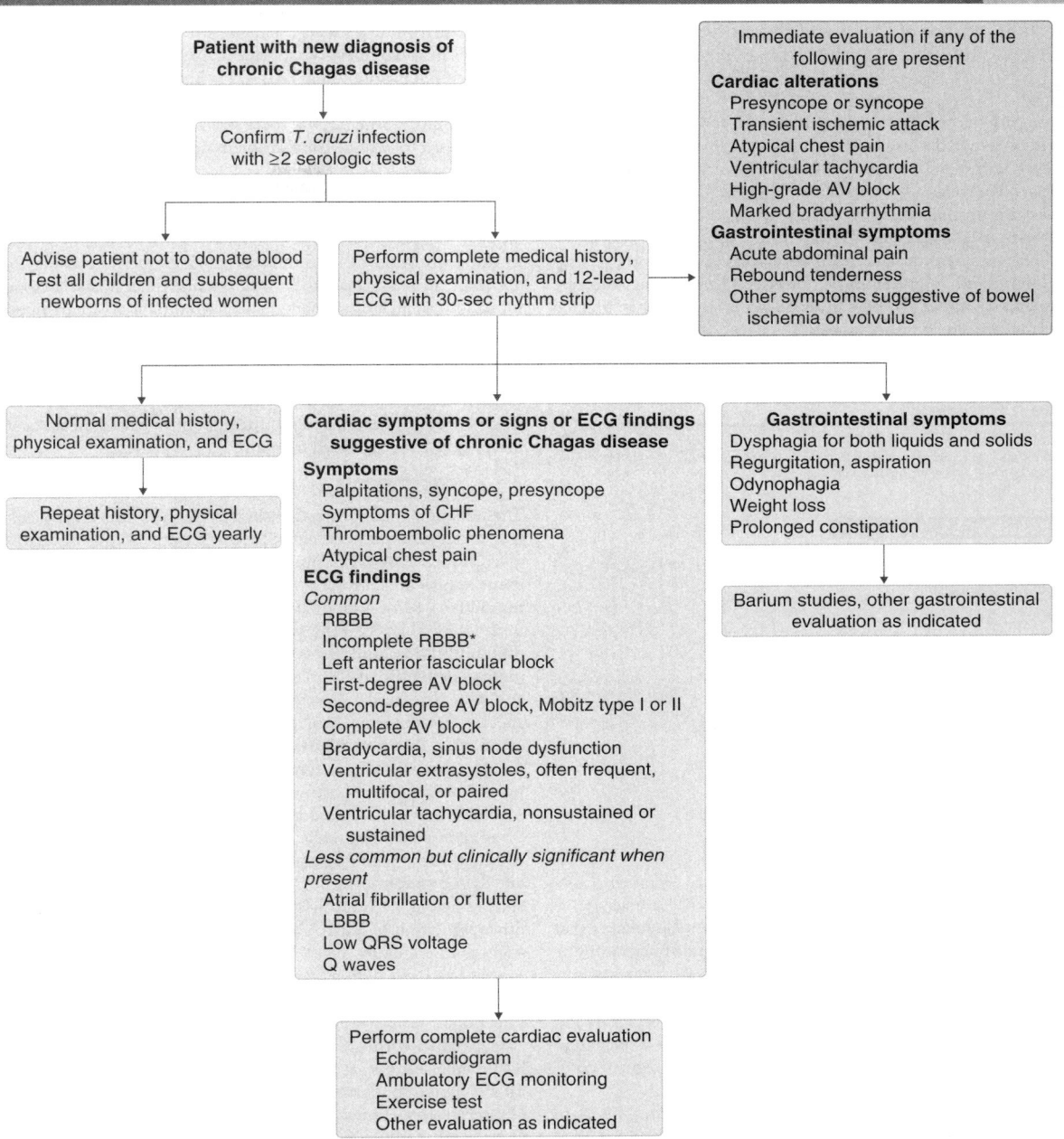

FIGURE 347-3. Algorithm for baseline evaluation of a patient with newly diagnosed chronic *Trypanosoma cruzi* infection. *AV,* Atrioventricular; *CHF,* congestive heart failure; *ECG,* electrocardiogram; *LBBB,* left bundle branch block; *RBBB,* right bundle branch block. (From Bern C, Montgomery SP, Herwaldt BL, et al. Evaluation and treatment of Chagas disease in the United States: a systematic review. *JAMA.* 2007;298:2171-2181.)

be required in patients who do not respond to repeated attempts at balloon dilation. Laparoscopic myotomy is being used with increasing frequency to treat Chagas megaesophagus, as is the case with achalasia.

Chagas megacolon in its early stage can be treated with a high-fiber diet and occasional laxatives or enemas. Fecal impaction requiring manual disimpaction can occur, and toxic megacolon requires surgery. In patients with advanced megacolon, volvulus (Chapter 142) can develop when an enlarged and lengthened sigmoid colon twists and folds on itself; volvulus causes a constellation of symptoms and in many cases requires immediate surgery. Even if the symptoms associated with volvulus are resolved without operative intervention, however, surgical treatment is usually ultimately necessary because the volvulus tends to recur. Several surgical procedures are used to treat advanced Chagas megacolon, all of which include resection of the sigmoid and removal of part of the rectum.

PREVENTION

Reducing human contact with triatomine vectors through education of at-risk persons, housing improvement, and spraying of residual insecticides in endemic countries has resulted in reduction or elimination of vector transmission of *T. cruzi* in a major part of the endemic range, and progress in this regard is expected to continue. Serologic screening of donated blood has essentially eliminated transfusion-related transmission of the parasite in most endemic areas. Outbreaks of acute Chagas disease through oral transmission can be avoided by the implementation of better food safety standards. Drug treatment of *T. cruzi*–infected women before pregnancy reduces the likelihood of congenital transmission. No protocols have been defined and validated for preventing reactivation of *T. cruzi* infection in chronically infected persons who are immunosuppressed iatrogenically or by HIV. A treatment regimen that reliably results in parasitologic cure is needed to prevent the onset or progression of chronic symptomatic Chagas disease.

PROGNOSIS

The prognosis for patients with acute Chagas disease is generally excellent because most acutely infected persons have only mild symptoms that resolve spontaneously, even without specific treatment. The occasional patient who has symptomatic acute Chagas myocarditis should generally do well if treated early. In persons with chronic *T. cruzi* infection, the lifetime risk for the development of related cardiac or GI dysfunction is only 10% to 30%.[17] A validated risk score assessment tool has been developed to gauge prognosis.[18] It has not been determined in randomized controlled trials whether this rate of progression to clinical disease or overall mortality is significantly affected by treatment with nifurtimox or benznidazole.

Visit *expertconsult.com* for the e-expanded chapter.

Grade A Reference

A1. Molina I, Gomez I, Prat J, et al. Randomized trial of posaconazole and benznidazole for chronic Chagas' disease. *N Eng J Med.* 2014;370:1899-1908.

GENERAL REFERENCES

For the General References and other additional features, please visit Expert Consult at https://expertconsult.inkling.com.

348

LEISHMANIASIS

SIMON L. CROFT AND PIERRE A. BUFFET

DEFINITION

Leishmaniasis is caused by protozoan parasites of the genus *Leishmania* that are generally transmitted between mammalian hosts by female phlebotomine sandflies. The disease in humans has a number of clinical manifestations ranging in severity from self-curing, limited cutaneous lesions to disseminated, potentially fatal visceral disease. The parasite exists in the sandfly gut as an extracellular flagellated form, the promastigote, and as an intracellular form, the amastigote, that survives and multiplies in a phagolysosomal compartment of macrophages in the mammalian host.

This disease complex is caused by 17 species of *Leishmania*, which are widely distributed in Europe, Asia, Africa, and South and Central America, with limited foci in Southeast Asia.[1] The characteristics of the main *Leishmania* species are summarized in Table 348-1. There are an estimated 1.5 to 2.0 million new cases each year, with up to 70,000 deaths, although this is probably an underestimate as leishmaniasis is not a reportable disease in many of the 101 countries and territories in which it is known to occur. Many *Leishmania* infections are either asymptomatic or misdiagnosed.

Because leishmaniasis is a disease complex, clinical aspects are considered under separate sections for visceral leishmaniasis (VL) and cutaneous leishmaniasis (CL).

EPIDEMIOLOGY

Infection is established in the mammalian host following a bite of the female sandfly belonging to either *Phlebotomus* spp in Europe, Asia, and Africa or *Lutzomyia* spp in the Americas. Different species of sandfly are associated with transmission of different *Leishmania* species. Most species that cause CL have a zoonotic (acquired from another mammal) transmission cycle, with the exception of *Leishmania tropica*, which is sometimes anthroponotic (transmitted between human beings). VL is either normally anthroponotic (in the case of *Leishmania donovani*) or zoonotic (in the case of *Leishmania infantum*). The predominant mammalian hosts (the reservoirs) are associated with different *Leishmania* species in diverse ecosystems (Fig. 348-1).

VL is caused by either *L. donovani* or *L. infantum* (which is identical to *Leishmania chagasi* in South America). These species have different geo-graphic distributions, with the highest incidence found in the poorest communities in six countries (Bangladesh, Nepal, India, Sudan, Ethiopia, Brazil), and infection is potentially fatal if it is untreated. An estimated 1 in 5 to 1 in 50 infections are asymptomatic, depending on the parasite species and host immunity. Since 2005, there has been a regional program to eliminate VL (aiming to reduce annual incidence to <1 per 10,000) in the Indian subcontinent.[2]

CL, which undergoes self-cure in more than 90% of patients within 3 to 18 months, is widely distributed, but its prevalence is difficult to estimate because of underreporting. Prevalence is associated with age, possibly related to the acquisition of immunity and risk factors, including the presence of domestic animals, rodents, or other mammalian hosts.[3] Ecologic conditions for sandflies, including shaded and humid habitats in crevices and mammal burrows, have been identified. The disease also must be considered in travelers returning from endemic areas.[4]

Urbanization, deforestation, and migration have resulted in changing patterns of disease, with transmission occurring in peridomestic cycles.[5] Other forms of transmission, such as through intravenous needles shared by drug users, have been reported in Spain.

PATHOBIOLOGY

The infection is initially established in the skin after the inoculation of infective metacyclic promastigotes by the sandfly. These infective forms have a glycoprotein coat (a lipophosphoglycan) that enables them to resist complement and to attach to and invade host cells. Peptides in sandfly saliva (e.g., maxadilan) cause vasodilation and erythema and help establish infection in the dermal layer of the skin. Early responses to infection involve neutrophil infiltration and invasion of resident macrophages. Progress of the disease depends on the parasite species and host responses. For both VL and CL, disease progression depends on the maintenance of a parasite-specific immunosuppressive state. Host cell macrophages are in a deactivated state, but cure follows when macrophages become activated and kill the parasites, which are sensitive to nitric oxide and oxygen radicals, in the phagolysosomal compartment. Resolution of disease, after the activation of macrophages, is mediated by a T-helper cell T_H1 response after interaction of antigen-presenting cells (e.g., dendritic cells) with $CD4^+$ and $CD8^+$ T cells and subsequent secretion of pro-inflammatory cytokines (e.g., interleukin 2, interferon-γ, tumor necrosis factor-α). However, in clinical forms such as active VL or diffuse CL, a T_H2 cell response predominates whereby downregulation of macrophage activity follows the production of cytokines such as interleukins 4, 10, and 13 and transforming growth factor-β. This profile has been defined in experimental models, mainly inbred mice, and ongoing clinical studies support the notion of a similar profile in human infection.

In patients with VL, the absence of a T cell–specific immune response to leishmanial antigens is associated with uncontrolled progression of infection. This is linked to elevated levels of interleukin 10 and decreased production of interferon-γ. Genetic susceptibility to *L. donovani* in Sudan has been associated with a solute carrier family (formerly NRAMP1) that regulates macrophage activation and with a polymorphism in the interleukin 4 gene. In localized simple CL, patients show a T_H1-type response and a delayed-type hypersensitivity (DTH) response. DTH is frequently measured by a Montenegro skin test, which can also be used in epidemiologic prevalence studies. Chronic infections show a T_H2-type response, most predominantly in patients with diffuse CL, in whom there is complete anergy to leishmania antigen and no DTH response. Patients with mucosal leishmaniasis (ML) have both T_H1 and T_H2 cell responses and a strong DTH response. Post–kala-azar dermal leishmaniasis (PKDL), a rare sequela to cure from VL, is poorly understood. The roles of $CD4^+$ and $CD25^+$ T cells appear to be different in Indian and Sudanese forms of PKDL.[6]

VISCERAL LEISHMANIASIS

CLINICAL MANIFESTATIONS

The onset of VL, often referred to as kala-azar when it is caused by *L. donovani*, occurs weeks to months after the initial infection. Clinical signs and symptoms do not distinguish VL from hyperreactive malarial splenomegaly or other infectious or hematologic conditions. Anemia, leukopenia, thrombocytopenia, systemic inflammation, or polyclonal hypergammaglobulinemia, either isolated or combined, suggests but does not confirm the diagnosis. Parasitologic tests are therefore indispensable before a therapeutic decision is made.[7]

TABLE 348-1 CHARACTERISTICS OF THE MAIN *LEISHMANIA* SPECIES

LEISHMANIA SPP	LEISHMANIA SUBGENUS	DISTRIBUTION: OLD WORLD	DISTRIBUTION: NEW WORLD	PRIMARY FORM	SECONDARY FORMS	ANTHROPONOTIC: AREAS OF TRANSMISSION	ZOONOTIC: RESERVOIR	ALTERNATIVE NAME
L. donovani	Leishmania	Indian subcontinent E. Africa		VL	PKDL CL, ML OIVL	Indian subcontinent E. Africa		Kala-azar
L. infantum (L. chagasi)	Leishmania	Europe Asia	S. & C. America	VL	CL, ML OIVL		Canid	
L. major	Leishmania	Asia N. & E. Africa Europe		CL			Rodent	
L. tropica	Leishmania	Asia Europe		CL	Recidivans	Syria Afghanistan	Rodent	Aleppo boil
L. aethiopica	Leishmania	Ethiopia		CL	DCL		Hyrax	
L. mexicana	Leishmania		C. America	CL			Rodent	Chiclero's ulcer
L. amazonensis	Leishmania	C. & S. America		CL	DCL		Rodent	
L. braziliensis	Viannia	S. America		CL ML	DissCL Lymph		Rodent, marsupial	ML-espundia
L. panamensis	Viannia	C. & S. America		CL	ML Lymph		Edentate rodent	Ulcera de bejuco
L. guyanensis	Viannia	S. America		CL	ML Lymph		Rodent, edentates	Pian bois
L. peruviana	Viannia	S. America		CL			Canids	Uta
L. siamensis		Southeast Asia		CL VL				

CL = cutaneous leishmaniasis; DCL = diffuse cutaneous leishmaniasis; DissCL = disseminated cutaneous leishmaniasis; Lymph = nodular lymphangitis; ML = mucosal leishmaniasis; OIVL = opportunistic infection with VL in HIV-infected patients; PKDL = post–kala-azar dermal leishmaniasis; VL = visceral leishmaniasis.

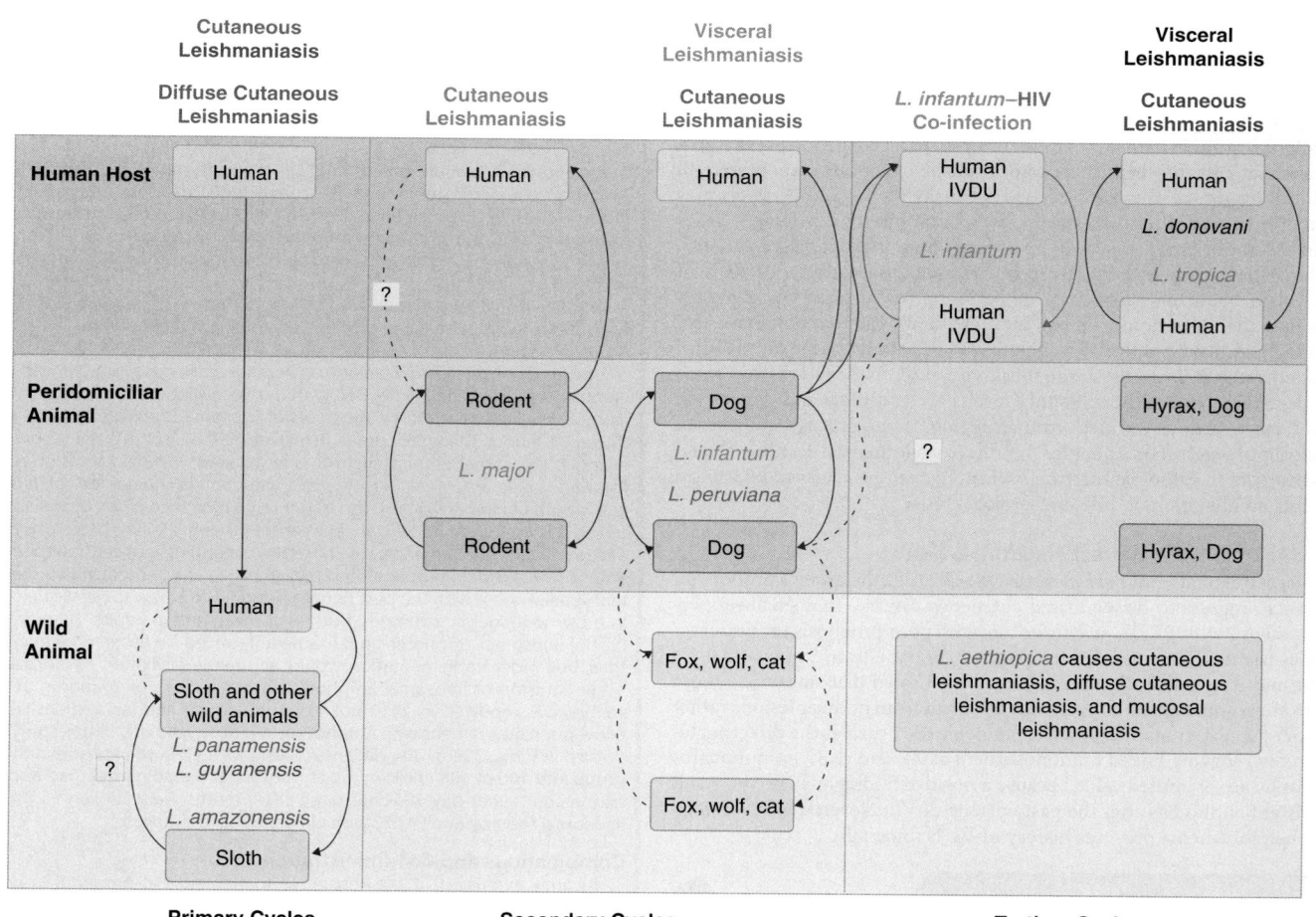

FIGURE 348-1. Old World and New World zoonotic and anthroponotic life cycles of the main species of *Leishmania*. Leishmaniasis is often referred to as a disease complex because different forms of disease can be caused by the same parasite species and similar forms of disease can be caused by different parasite species. IVDU = intravenous drug use.

DIAGNOSIS

Parasitology

Microscopic visualization of amastigotes in samples from the lymph nodes, bone marrow, liver, spleen, or other organs was usually the first step. Because spleen aspiration causes life-threatening complications in approximately 0.1% of patients, it should be performed only in trained facilities and only if other, lower-risk methods cannot be used. It is still used in the field because of the higher cost, logistic constraints, and lower sensitivity of bone marrow aspiration. Polymerase chain reaction (PCR) is more sensitive than microscopic examination and has become the first-line test in several referral hospitals and research centers.[8] Quantitative PCR with validated thresholds allows accurate diagnosis with venous blood samples, thereby avoiding bone marrow aspiration.

Serology

Serologic tests based on indirect fluorescent antibody, enzyme-linked immunosorbent assay, or Western blot display high performance but require equipment that is poorly adapted to field settings. The field-friendly direct agglutination test and immunochromatography (dipstick) with the rK39 antigen have high diagnostic accuracy and can be used in peripheral health centers.[9] Whatever the serologic test used, specific antibodies remain detectable for several years after cure or asymptomatic infection.

Antigen Detection Tests

A latex agglutination test that detects a heat-stable, low-molecular-weight carbohydrate antigen in the urine of patients with VL showed good specificity but low to moderate sensitivity in East Africa and the Indian subcontinent. Further optimization is required.

Complex Manifestations of Visceral Leishmaniasis

VISCERAL LEISHMANIASIS–HUMAN IMMUNODEFICIENCY VIRUS COINFECTION

Although the clinical manifestations in VL patients infected with human immunodeficiency virus (HIV) without severe immunosuppression are similar to those in immunocompetent patients, atypical clinical features can be found in patients with low CD4+ T-cell counts (<200/μL). In the latter group, physicians may order investigations for VL even in the absence of classic signs (e.g., lack of splenomegaly). A substantial proportion of HIV-VL–coinfected patients may have other opportunistic infections that complicate the clinical diagnosis. The parasitic load is usually higher and parasites may be found in tissues other than spleen, liver, bone marrow, or lymph nodes (e.g., in the gut or lung), especially in severely immunosuppressed patients. Therefore, the sensitivity of microscopic examination, culture, or PCR of blood (plain blood or buffy coat) or bone marrow aspirates is generally higher than that in immunocompetent VL patients. Limited data have also shown high sensitivity of the latex agglutination test in the urine of HIV-VL–coinfected patients. In contrast, the sensitivity of serologic tests is decreased in coinfected patients, although study results are equivocal and depend on several factors, such as the test's format, region of endemicity, and level of immunosuppression. For example, the direct agglutination test has shown high sensitivity in Ethiopia. Increased sensitivity can be achieved by using a sequential combination of different serologic tests.

POST–KALA-AZAR DERMAL LEISHMANIASIS (PKDL)

After successful treatment of visceral disease due to *L. donovani*, a proportion of patients progress to disseminated cutaneous disease. In a small proportion of patients with PKDL, uveitis occurs with poor prognosis for preservation of eyesight. This is reported in up to 20% of patients in Sudan and 0.5% in India and Bangladesh. Studies in India have shown that smears are more likely to show amastigotes if specimens are taken from nodular lesions rather than from papular or macular lesions. Serologic tests such as the direct agglutination test, enzyme-linked immunosorbent assay, and rK39 immunochromatography are of limited value because a positive finding may be the result of persistent antibodies after the past episode of VL. Nevertheless, serology can be helpful when a previous history of VL is uncertain.

TREATMENT Rx

General Principles

The therapeutic management of patients with VL requires renutrition; broad-spectrum antibiotics if bacterial superinfection is suspected; transfu-

sion in case of severe anemia; and proper hydration, especially when amphotericin B is used as the specific antileishmanial treatment.

The clinical response to antileishmanial agents depends on the clinical form and the infecting species or even the subspecies (zymodeme). Many antileishmanial agents are toxic, expensive, or difficult to administer in field conditions. No single satisfactory option for treating most of the clinical forms or species has been validated. Although therapeutic decisions and follow-up have become relatively simple for the treatment of VL in nonendemic and some endemic countries based on the powerful, well-tolerated agent liposomal amphotericin B,[10] more complexity persists for the treatment of VL in East Africa and in endemic countries where liposomal amphotericin B is not available.[11] The treatment decision for CL or ML often requires expert advice.[12]

Visceral Leishmaniasis in Immunocompetent Patients

Single-Agent Therapies

Pentamidine is efficient in treating VL only when high doses (more than seven injections of 4 mg/kg) are used. These are toxic, and pentamidine is no longer used for the treatment of VL. Lower doses (fewer than four injections of 4 mg/kg) induce much less severe adverse events and are still used for the secondary prophylaxis of VL in HIV-infected patients (fortnightly to monthly injections) and in those with CL caused by *Leishmania guyanensis* or *Leishmania panamensis* (one to three injections).

Pentavalent antimonials (sodium stibogluconate, meglumine antimoniate) are still prescribed as first-intention drugs in many areas. In the Indian subcontinent (mainly in northern Bihar), *L. donovani* is resistant to pentavalent antimonials.[13] Their efficacy has decreased from 90% to less than 40% during the past 40 years. In other VL foci, failure rates of initial treatment do not exceed 10% as long as the dosage is respected (20 mg of pentavalent antimony per kilogram per day for 28 days). In an endemic country, mortality in treated patients may exceed 10%, with toxicity positively correlating with age. Pentavalent antimonials are contraindicated in patients with heart, kidney, or liver disease or advanced age and in pregnant women. Generic formulations have generally but not constantly demonstrated activity and tolerance identical to those of sodium stibogluconate.

Miltefosine is an alkyl phosphocholine. The oral form (2.5 mg/kg/day for 28 days) is effective for VL in India. In Ethiopian patients with VL (28% with HIV infection), there was significantly higher mortality with sodium stibogluconate (generic) than with miltefosine (9.7% vs. 2.1%) despite the lower parasitologic efficacy of miltefosine (92.1% vs. 99.3%). Miltefosine is contraindicated in pregnant women or those who may become pregnant. Because of persistent levels of the drug, contraceptive measures must be observed for 3 months after therapy. Compared with a decade ago, substantial increase in the failure rate of oral miltefosine has been noted in the treatment of visceral leishmaniases in India and Nepal since 2012.

Paromomycin (aminosidine sulfate) (15 mg/kg in sulfate form equivalent to 11 mg of base per kilogram intramuscularly for 21 days) is highly effective in India, where it was registered in 2006. In East Africa, its efficacy is significantly lower. Similar to the situation with miltefosine, the longevity of the product would probably be better preserved in combination than as a single-agent therapy.

Amphotericin B (cumulative dose of 7 to 15 mg/kg) cures more than 98% of patients in India, whereas treatment of visceral infection with *L. infantum/chagasi* requires at least 14 mg/kg.

Liposomal amphotericin B achieves very high cure rates in India with lower cumulative doses than are needed with the deoxycholate formulation. In preliminary studies in East Africa, the doses of liposomal amphotericin B required to cure VL (about 30 mg/kg cumulatively) are markedly higher than those used in India. Liposomal amphotericin B is associated with less infusion-related fever and chills, less renal toxicity, and a reduction in the number of infusions and length of hospitalization. The better renal tolerance of liposomal amphotericin B is especially beneficial in patients with renal failure or a kidney graft and in those with an increase in serum creatinine concentration during amphotericin B deoxycholate therapy. Liposomal amphotericin B is the antileishmanial agent with the best benefit-risk ratio. It is now the first-line option in most nonendemic countries, both in children and in adults. The very high cost of liposomal amphotericin B has been reduced for use in endemic countries, but wider implementation would be greatly facilitated by donation. A single infusion of liposomal amphotericin B at a dose of 10 mg/kg of body weight was reported in 2010 not to be inferior to and less expensive than conventional treatment with amphotericin B deoxycholate. In this study, conducted in India, 304 of 304 patients (100%) with VL in the liposomal therapy group and 106 of 108 (98%) in the conventional therapy group had apparent cure responses at day 30. Cure rates at 6 months were similar: 95.7% with liposomal therapy and 96.3% with conventional therapy.

Combinations and Coadministration

To limit extension of the resistance to pentavalent antimonials and to prevent the emergence of resistance to paromomycin or miltefosine, shorter courses of therapy are being investigated. Because only miltefosine may be administered orally, this approach is based at least partly on products administered parenterally. As high cure rates have been reported, the combination of antimony and paromomycin is approved for use in East Africa but still requires many injections. Combinations of amphotericin with oral miltefosine (sequential) and of intramuscular paromomycin with miltefosine can achieve cure rates of up to 98% with 7- to 10-day courses of therapy. A single infusion of liposomal amphotericin B followed by oral miltefosine has been highly effective in India, but confirmation studies are required here and elsewhere.

Visceral Leishmaniasis in Immunodeficient Patients
Leishmania infantum–HIV Coinfection

As with other major opportunistic infections during HIV infection, treatment may be subdivided into initial course and secondary prophylaxis. With initial treatment, the efficacy of meglumine antimoniate and that of amphotericin B are similar. The severe adverse effects of antimony derivatives are more common in this context. Doses of liposomal amphotericin B administered to immunodeficient patients are higher (30 to 40 mg/kg in cumulative dose) than those administered to immunocompetent patients. When therapeutic immunosuppression may not be reduced or optimization of highly active antiretroviral therapy is not possible, secondary prophylaxis is often proposed. Amphotericin B lipid complex moderately reduces the frequency of recurrences. Discontinuous administration of liposomal amphotericin B is generally used, but a progressive reduction in its efficacy has been reported, although apparently not associated with decreased parasitic sensitivity in vitro. Miltefosine is another option, especially if the reduction in parasitic load is backed up by quantitative PCR with a validated threshold (low residual load probably being associated with a lower risk for resistance). Administration of pentamidine once or twice a month is another potentially interesting option because drug levels persist for weeks or months after a single administration. Pancreatic tolerance should be monitored closely.

Leishmania donovani–HIV Coinfection

Patients should benefit from effective antiretroviral treatment. The experience with L. infantum–HIV coinfection is in part transposable. The potential risk for the emergence of resistance to antileishmanial agents is still more significant in this context because L. donovani (but not L. infantum) can be transmitted from human to human. Important clinical research is ongoing in East Africa.

CUTANEOUS LEISHMANIASIS

CLINICAL MANIFESTATIONS

Although the signs and symptoms of CL vary considerably (Fig. 348-2)—from pure nodular lesions to developing ulceration through dry crusty lesions and squamous plaques—there are some fairly constant features. First, firm infiltration is almost constant (the exception being the initial macule of PKDL). Second, the evolution is subacute, which is a useful criterion in practice. A lesion reaching its maximum size in less than a week is most likely not due to CL. Finally, except in patients with numerous satellite papulopustules, the lesion or lesions are sharply defined. Colonization of the CL ulceration with bacteria may give the lesion a purulent appearance, whereas patent superinfection adds an erythematous ring distinctly overflowing the infiltrated edge of the ulceration and making a usually cold and painless lesion feel hot and painful. Several dermatologic conditions, such as staphylococcal or streptococcal infection, mycobacterial ulcer, leprosy, fungal infection, cancer, sarcoidosis, and tropical ulcer, can mimic CL or ML lesions (see Fig. 348-2). Because treatment is costly and potentially toxic, diagnostic confirmation is necessary.

DIAGNOSIS
Parasitology

Scraping, fine-needle aspiration, or biopsy of lesions provides appropriate samples in which amastigotes can be identified (Fig. 348-3). Scraping should be performed at both the center and edges of the lesion with a curved scalpel blade. Local anesthesia considerably reduces patients' discomfort and increases sensitivity. Use of an epinephrine-containing local anesthetic (contraindicated for lesions on extremities) or pinching of the lesion between the thumb and finger until blanching appears helps obtain a bloodless scraping, thus optimizing microscopic examination. The 2- to 4-mm skin fragment obtained by punch biopsy provides abundant material, which facilitates the search for scarce parasites and for an alternative diagnosis by culture (e.g., mycobacteria, fungi) as well as by histopathologic examination. Culture of a biopsy sample requires homogenization in saline or culture medium under sterile conditions.

The material obtained by any of these methods can be used for microscopic examination, culture, and PCR. Microscopic examination of Giemsa-stained material is the most widely available method. Culture of the parasite

in specific media (such as fetal calf serum–supplemented Schneider's or Novy-Nicolle-McNeal media) allows identification, characterization, and storage of the isolate. Detection of parasitic nucleic acids by molecular diagnosis (mainly PCR) increases sensitivity and allows identification of the Leishmania species (see Table 348-1). This is particularly useful in regions (e.g., New World) where several Leishmania species—with various clinical outcomes and responses to treatment—coexist. Both culture and molecular-based diagnosis require substantial laboratory infrastructure and technical expertise.

Serology

Serologic diagnosis is of limited use for CL because of low sensitivity and variable specificity. The leishmanin (or Montenegro) skin test (LST) evaluates the cell-mediated response against Leishmania spp. The LST requires culture and preferentially fixation of local species of Leishmania and therefore lacks standardization. The production of commercial formulations of the LST lacks sustainability. Like serologic tests, the LST does not distinguish between past and present infections.

Complex Manifestations of Cutaneous Leishmaniasis
MUCOSAL LEISHMANIASIS

A proportion of CL infections (about 1 to 10% in Brazil, Bolivia, and Peru) caused by Leishmania braziliensis or L. guyanensis progress to a metastatic infection of the mucosa of the oral or nasal cavity or larynx, often 1 to 5 years after healing of the initial simple cutaneous lesion. An immunopathologic response results in extensive destruction of local tissue. Allergic rhinitis, paracoccidioidomycosis or other deep mycosis, cancrum oris, leprosy, and sarcoidosis may mimic the lesions of ML. Positive serology (e.g., indirect fluorescent antibody, enzyme-linked immunosorbent assay) or LST indicates possible ML. Parasites are scarce in mucosal lesions. Therefore, a search for parasites in mucosal samples—obtained by scraping or biopsy—by microscopic examination or by culture lacks sensitivity. PCR has proved to be the most sensitive approach to confirm ML.

DIFFUSE CUTANEOUS LEISHMANIASIS

Patients with diffuse CL have an anergic response to Leishmania antigens, and nonulcerative nodules, loaded with parasites, disseminate from the initial site of infection to multiple sites on the patient's body. There is no self-cure, and treatment is difficult. This form of the disease is found in South America and East Africa, often associated with Leishmania amazonensis and Leishmania aethiopica infection.

RECIDIVANS CUTANEOUS LEISHMANIASIS

Recidivans CL is characterized by the development of lesions containing granulomatous tissue. The lesions often take many years to heal and may arise years after healing of a simple localized lesion. New ulcers and papules may form over the edge of the old scar. Infections are normally associated with L. tropica infection and are difficult to treat.

TREATMENT ℞

The clinical consequences of CL are dermatologic; concomitant visceral impairment is exceptional. The intensity of the discomfort, related to one or several oozing or unsightly lesions, and the impact of atrophic, hypopigmented or hyperpigmented scars depend on the lesions' topography. In the New World, mucosal impairment may affect up to 1 to 15% of patients (higher in Bolivia). The risk for metastasis (initially nasal and then affecting the entire otorhinolaryngeal zone) has strongly influenced therapeutic decisions. Systemic treatment of any New World CL has been recommended, but recent data indicate that a different strategy should probably be considered.[14] Inadequate surgical excision and pentavalent antimonials or systemic pentamidine administered in excessive doses or without sufficient follow-up may paradoxically be a major risk for patients with CL. Analysis of the number and size of the lesions and their topography, the clinical signs of spread (cutaneous, mucous, or lymphatic), and the predictable cosmetic or functional impact helps in estimating the benefit-risk ratio.[15]

Oral therapy with relatively nontoxic drugs (ketoconazole, fluconazole, itraconazole, miltefosine) would be the simplest option, and oral miltefosine monotherapy has been successful in Brazil.[A2] Local therapy with intralesional injections of pentavalent antimonials (with or without cryotherapy), photodynamic therapy, and thermotherapy are therefore attractive options to avoid potentially toxic, expensive, or impractical systemic schedules. However, implementation of these methods is hampered by logistic constraints and requires skilled health care providers. An efficient topical ointment would

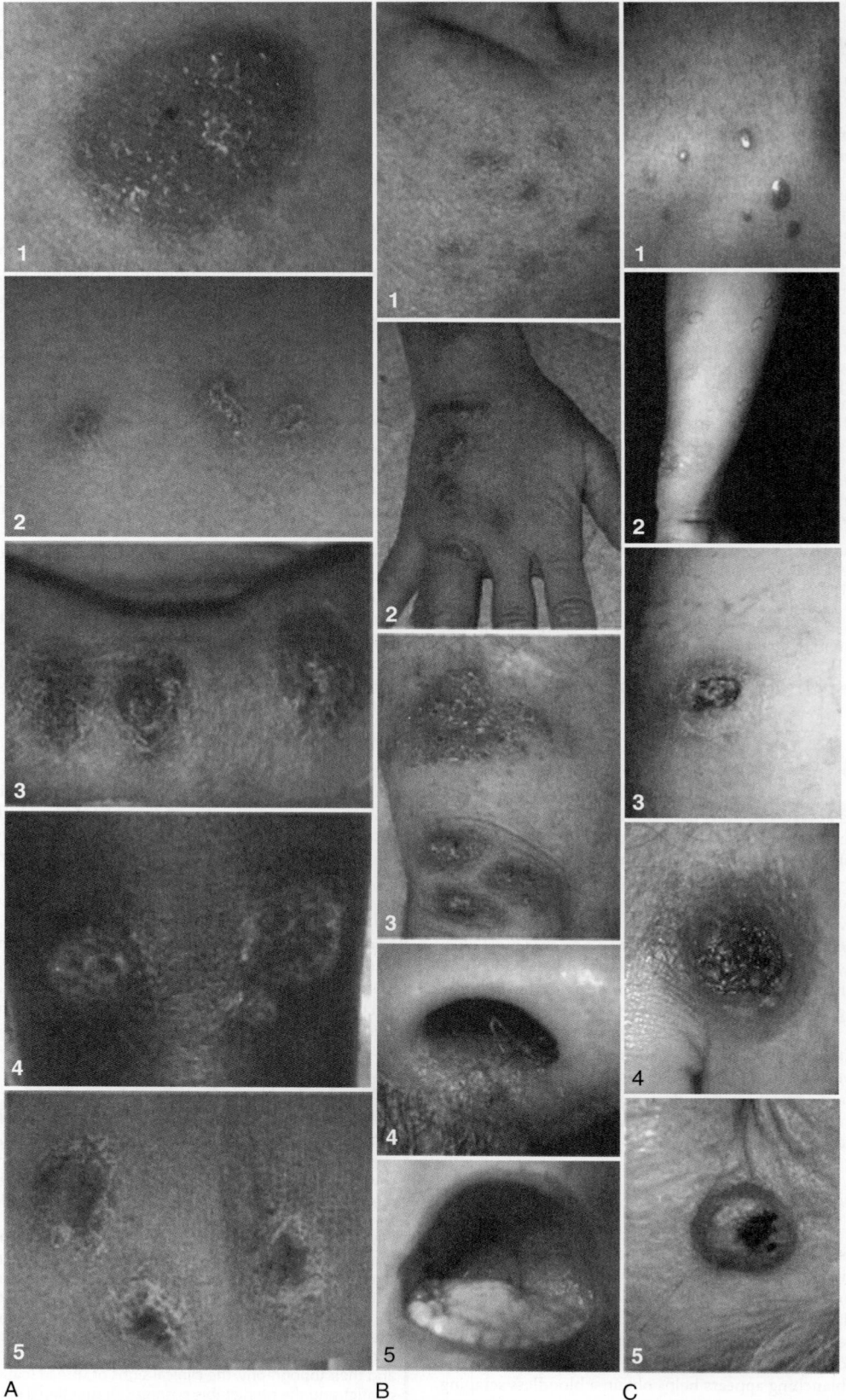

FIGURE 348-2. Clinical features of cutaneous leishmaniasis (CL). **A,** Typical forms of CL. **A1,** Papular-nodular lesion. **A2,** Squamous lesion. **A3,** Crusty lesion. **A4,** Ulcerated lesion. **A5,** Superinfected lesion. **B,** Atypical forms of CL and mucosal leishmaniasis. **B1,** Multiple papules on the face (*L. infantum*, Balearic Islands). **B2,** Nodular lymphangitis (*L. braziliensis*, Brazil). **B3,** Multiple lesions with numerous peripheral papules (*L. major*, Tunisia). **B4,** Initial spread to the nasal mucosa (anterior septum, *L. braziliensis*, Bolivia). **B5,** Infiltration and ulceration of the tonsils (*L. infantum*, France). **C,** Clinical manifestations that are not CL. **C1,** Multiple papules (late secondary syphilis) (Chapter 319). **C2,** Nodular lymphangitis (sporotrichosis) (Chapter 337). **C3,** Single crusty ulceration (*Mycobacterium ulcerans* infection) (Chapter 325). **C4,** Ulcerated acute *Staphylococcus aureus* infection (Chapter 288). **C5,** Ulcerated nodule keratoacanthoma (Chapter 203).

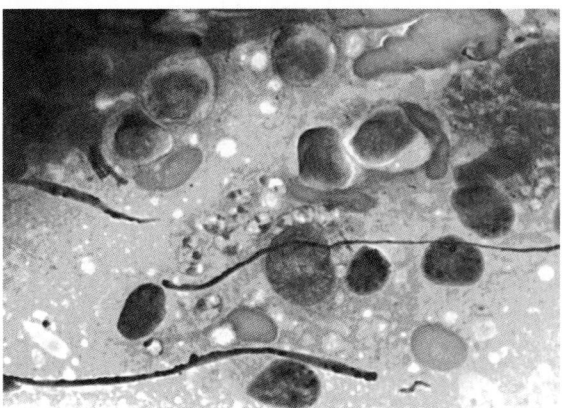

FIGURE 348-3. Amastigotes of *Leishmania major* in scrapings from a skin ulcer.

resolve most of these issues, but no efficient formulation is widely available. Several formulations of topical paromomycin have been tested with variable results. Recently, an ointment containing paromomycin and gentamicin has shown efficacy with acceptable local tolerance in patients with CL caused by *L. major* and *L. panamensis*.[A3][A4]

PREVENTION

There are no modern vaccines for human disease and no prophylactic drug regimens. Leishmanization, or inoculation of people with live virulent parasites to cause a local limited lesion and provide protection, was used for CL (e.g., in Iran) but is not recommended by the World Health Organization. Sandflies are sensitive to most insecticides, and transmission has been controlled with malaria eradication campaigns and residual spraying in houses. Insecticide-impregnated bed nets and dog collars (to prevent transmission of zoonotic CL) have been investigated. The high incidence of vertical and venereal transmission in dogs may cause elimination programs to fail in *L. infantum* foci.

PROGNOSIS

Most untreated patients with established disease ultimately die of the disease. VL has an excellent prognosis with less than a 2% death rate in patients treated soon enough with liposomal amphotericin B. Mortality increases when bleeding (mainly from the digestive tract or lung) or secondary bacterial infection occurs, usually after prolonged untreated evolution or unresponsiveness of VL to first-line agents. Post-therapeutic relapse is frequent in HIV-coinfected patients with low initial or persistently low CD4+ counts. In immunosuppressed patients, VL is rarely the direct cause of death but may give rise to complex therapeutic situations. A proportion of *L. donovani*–infected patients experience PKDL weeks to years after the initial episode, which may rarely lead to severe ocular involvement. CL caused by *L. braziliensis* may metastasize to the nose and other mucous membranes with variable frequency in different areas. CL caused by *L. tropica* often relapses (recidivans CL). A small proportion of patients infected with *L. amazonensis* and *L. aethiopica* experience diffuse CL. Even when treated, most CL lesions leave disfiguring, hypotrophic, hypopigmented, or hyperpigmented scars.

Grade A References

A1. Sundar S, Chakravarty J, Agarwal D, et al. Single-dose liposomal amphotericin B for visceral leishmaniasis in India. *N Engl J Med.* 2010;362:504-512.

A2. Chrusciak-Talhari A, Dietze R, Chrusciak Talhari C, et al. Randomized controlled clinical trial to access efficacy and safety of miltefosine in the treatment of cutaneous leishmaniasis Caused by *Leishmania (Viannia) guyanensis* in Manaus, Brazil. *Am J Trop Med Hyg.* 2011;84:255-260.

A3. Ben Salah A, Ben Messaoud N, Guedri E, et al. Topical paromomycin with or without gentamicin for cutaneous leishmaniasis. *N Engl J Med.* 2013;368:524-532.

A4. Sosa N, Capitan Z, Nieto J, et al. Randomized, double-blinded, phase 2 trial of WR 279,396 (paromomycin and gentamicin) for cutaneous leishmaniasis in Panama. *Am J Trop Med Hyg.* 2013;89:557-563.

GENERAL REFERENCES

For the General References and other additional features, please visit Expert Consult at https://expertconsult.inkling.com.

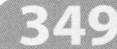

TOXOPLASMOSIS

JOSE G. MONTOYA

DEFINITION

The ubiquitous parasite *Toxoplasma gondii* is the etiologic agent of toxoplasmosis. The term *toxoplasmosis* is reserved for the disease process in which clinical manifestations are present, whereas *Toxoplasma infection* best describes the asymptomatic presence of the parasite. Toxoplasmosis may result in significant morbidity and mortality of the fetus, newborn, and immunocompromised patient. However, *T. gondii* can also be responsible for chorioretinitis, lymphadenopathy, pneumonia, brain abscesses, myositis, myocarditis, and hepatitis in immunocompetent patients.

A more aggressive form of congenital and adult toxoplasmosis appears to occur in certain geographic locales in Latin America, where pneumonia, fever of unknown origin, brain abscesses, and death have been reported in HIV-negative and otherwise immunocompetent individuals. Recent epidemiologic studies have established the role of novel risk factors for the acquisition of the acute infection, including the ingestion of untreated water, oysters, mussels, or clams.

The Pathogen

T. gondii is an intracellular parasite with a high capacity for host cell invasion due to a motile invasive form (tachyzoite or trophozoite) characterized by an evolutionarily unique apical complex and a mechanism of actin-based motility.

T. gondii maintains a highly clonal population structure in North America and Europe that consists of three main lineages: types I, II, and III. This relatively low genetic diversity comes as a surprise, given the fact that the parasite has the capacity to infect any warm-blooded animal. It has a sexual life cycle that takes place in the small intestine of cats. In Europe, type II strains predominate and are most commonly associated with human toxoplasmosis, both in congenital infections and in immunocompromised patients. In North America, types II and I appear to be equally common. In Latin America, type I strains are common, but *Toxoplasma* strains appear to be genetically more diverse, with many different genotypes described mainly in Brazil and French Guiana. These atypical Latin American strains, initially called exotic strains, belong to several haplogroups that are endemic to Latin America and have been found to be associated with more severe clinical manifestations; physicians need to entertain the diagnosis of toxoplasmosis in their patients presenting with pneumonia, fever of unknown origin, brain abscesses, lymphadenopathy, or chorioretinitis who are from or were traveling in these endemic areas.

In nature, the parasite exists in several forms, including the tachyzoite (Fig. 349-1A), the oocyst that contains sporozoites (Fig. 349-1B), the tissue cyst that contains bradyzoites (Fig. 349-1C), and the sexual forms (macrogametes and microgametes). The tachyzoite is the rapidly proliferating form of the parasite responsible for the clinical manifestations of toxoplasmosis observed in the setting of the acute infection or reactivation of a latent infection. The tissue cyst is the slower metabolic form of the parasite responsible for chronic infection and for its transmission through meat consumption in humans and animals. Tissue cysts persist in tissues for the life of the host and cannot be eradicated by drugs. Tissue cysts vary in shape and size from younger ones that contain only a few bradyzoites to older tissue cysts that may contain several thousand bradyzoites and may reach more than 100 μm in size. The central nervous system (CNS), eye, and skeletal, smooth, and heart muscles appear to be the most common sites of tissue cyst formation (i.e., latent infection). Oocysts are primarily responsible for the worldwide and large-scale spread of the parasite among different populations of other animals and humans. Domestic and feral animals belonging to the Felidae family shed

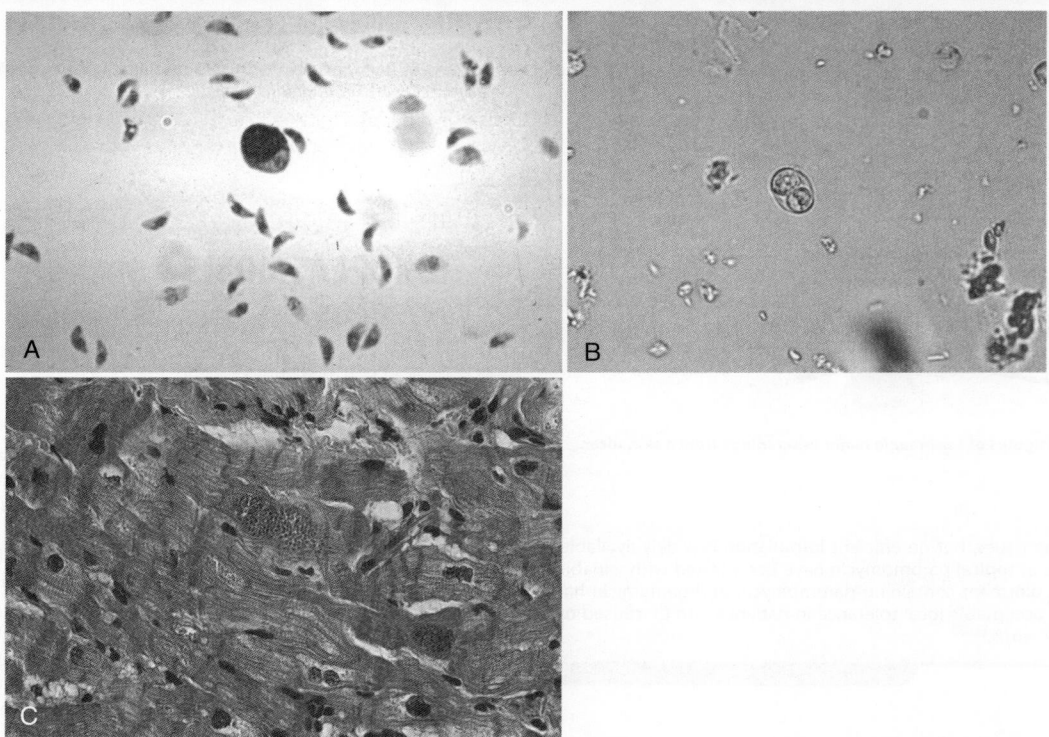

FIGURE 349-1. *Toxoplasma gondii* **exists in nature primarily in three forms. A,** Tachyzoites are bow or banana shaped, measure 2 to 3 μm wide and 5 to 7 μm long, and can be stained with Wright-Giemsa stain. **B,** Oocysts isolated from cat's feces are subspherical to spherical and measure 10 × 12 μm in diameter. **C,** Tissue cyst observed in human myocardial tissue stained with hematoxylin and eosin. Tissue cysts vary in shape and size and may reach more than 100 μm.

oocysts after they ingest any of the infectious forms of the parasite: tachyzoites, tissue cysts, and oocysts. As many as 10 million oocysts may be shed in the feces of an infected animal in a single day for periods varying from 7 to 20 days. Oocysts may remain viable for as long as 18 months in moist soil; this results in an environmental reservoir from which incidental hosts may be infected.

EPIDEMIOLOGY

The prevalence of *T. gondii* infection varies significantly according to geographic locale and the socioeconomic status of the population. It can be as low as 7% in England and as high as 80% in the Central African Republic. Seroprevalence increases with age because of increasing length of exposure with age, and it is inversely associated with socioeconomic status because of the strong influence of hygienic and alimentary habits in the transmission of the parasite. The overall age-adjusted seroprevalence of *T. gondii* infection in the United States has been recently reported at 11%, but it may be higher in certain geographic areas or socioeconomic groups. The seroprevalence of the parasite has declined during the past 30 years in the United States[1] and several other countries but appears to be stable or increasing in certain geographic locales, such as in the tropics (e.g., Latin America).

Humans and non-felid animals are incidental hosts and become infected primarily by the ingestion of infected meat containing tissue cysts or of contaminated food, water, or soil material containing oocysts. They can also become infected during gestation by vertical transmission of the parasite from the mother to her offspring. In addition, humans can become infected through organ transplantation and, more rarely, in the setting of laboratory accidents. Ingestion of raw or undercooked meat contaminated with tissue cysts is probably one of the major routes of transmission in humans. Ingestion of untreated water, food, or soil contaminated with oocysts is another significant route of infection with the parasite. Untreated water has been found to be the source of large epidemics of toxoplasmosis in Canada and Brazil.

The main risk factors for *T. gondii* infection in the United States include eating raw ground beef; eating rare lamb; eating locally produced cured, dried, or smoked meat; working with meat; drinking unpasteurized goat's milk; having three or more kittens. In this study, eating raw oysters, clams, or mussels was also identified as a novel risk factor. Untreated water as a potential vehicle for the transmission of *T. gondii* has been established in several large epidemiologic studies and was found to have a trend toward increased risk for acute infection in the United States.

In up to 50% of individuals acutely infected with *T. gondii*, it is not possible to identify the presence of a known risk factor for their acute infection. Thus, attempting to establish whether a patient is at risk for toxoplasmosis solely on the basis of the epidemiologic history is a futile task. Patients may have been infected with *T. gondii* even if they have not owned or been in contact with cats, have not eaten undercooked meat or shellfish, and have not ingested untreated water.

The seroprevalence of *T. gondii* infection in immunocompromised patients reflects the seroprevalence of the particular population from which they come. Latent *T. gondii* infection can reactivate in these patients, particularly in those with the acquired immunodeficiency syndrome (AIDS) and in hematopoietic stem cell transplant (HSCT, including bone marrow transplant) and liver transplant patients. In these patients, it is important to establish whether they have been infected with the parasite before severe immunosuppression ensues or their transplant procedure because serologic testing in severe immunosuppression or after transplantation may be unreliable. Approximately 30% of AIDS patients who are infected with *T. gondii* will develop toxoplasmosis by reactivation of their chronic infection if their CD4 count falls below 200 cells/μL and they are not taking anti-*Toxoplasma* primary prophylaxis. The advent of highly active antiretroviral therapy, in addition to the use of primary anti-*Toxoplasma* prophylaxis, has clearly contributed to the decline in the incidence of toxoplasmosis in AIDS patients. Among HSCT (including bone marrow transplant) patients, those recipients who are *Toxoplasma* seropositive before transplantation, receive an allogeneic graft, and develop graft-versus-host disease have the highest risk of reactivation.

For solid organ transplants, the highest risk for toxoplasmosis is observed when an allograft from a *Toxoplasma*-seropositive donor (D⁺) is transplanted into a seronegative recipient (R⁻). In D⁺/R⁻ patients, there is a 25% risk for development of potentially life-threatening toxoplasmosis if effective anti-*Toxoplasma* prophylaxis is not instituted. It is highly advised that the *Toxoplasma* serologic status of the donor and the recipient be established before transplantation. Serologic test results are less reliable in the post-transplantation period, and they may significantly vary without any clinical relevance.

Transmission of *T. gondii* to the fetus can occur during pregnancy when a woman acquires her primary infection during gestation. The incidence of seroconversion for pregnant women in the United States has been estimated at 0.27%. The overall rate of transmission of the parasite (prevalence of congenital toxoplasmosis) in seroconverting women has been estimated between 50 and 60% before spiramycin was instituted as an attempt to decrease vertical transmission and 25 to 30% thereafter. The transmission rate increases with the gestational age at which maternal infection is acquired. In women who have been treated for toxoplasmosis during gestation, it can be as low as 4.5% during the first trimester, 31.7% during the second trimester, and as high as 63% during the third trimester. The likelihood of severe disease is inversely proportional to the gestational age at which maternal infection was acquired. Although objective data are lacking on the prevalence of congenital toxoplasmosis in the United States, it has been estimated that among the approximately 4.2 million live births per year, congenital *T. gondii* infection occurs in 500 to 5000 newborns. The global annual incidence of congenital toxoplasmosis has been estimated to be 190,100 cases. This is equivalent to a burden of 1.2 million disability-adjusted life years. Particularly high burdens are seen in South America and in some Middle Eastern and low-income countries.[2]

Congenital transmission in women who were infected before conception has only rarely been reported in immunosuppressed patients, in those who were acutely infected shortly before conception (i.e., within 3 months of conception), and in those who have been reinfected with a more virulent strain.

PATHOBIOLOGY

Pathogenesis

After oral infection with tissue cysts (e.g., contaminated meat) or oocysts (e.g., contaminated soil, water, or food), the wall of both infectious forms is disrupted by the digestive juices of the gastrointestinal tract. Bradyzoites (from cysts) and sporozoites (from oocysts) are released and converted to the tachyzoite form. Tachyzoites have the capacity to infect contiguous cells or distant tissues by hematogenous or lymphatic spread. Tachyzoites appear to actively and rapidly migrate across epithelial cells and may traffic to distant sites while they are extracellular (acute infection).[3] Their histologic hallmark is necrosis surrounded by inflammation.

In immunocompetent individuals, the immune system controls the proliferation of the tachyzoite and induces its conversion to bradyzoites, facilitating the final formation of tissue cysts (chronic infection). Tissue cysts persist for the life of the host, and *T. gondii* can be isolated from tissues of individuals who have died from causes other than toxoplasmosis.

It appears that the activation of well-orchestrated immune responses is required for the successful resistance against *T. gondii*. Innate, humoral, and cellular immune responses likely to be involved in preventing the uncontrolled proliferation of tachyzoites include activation of the monocyte-macrophage system, dendritic cells, natural killer cells, and $\alpha\beta$ and $\gamma\delta$ T cells; *T. gondii*–specific and cytotoxic CD4$^+$ and CD8$^+$ T cells; and interferon-γ, interleukin 12, tumor necrosis factor–α, interleukin 10 and other cytokines, transforming growth factor-β, costimulatory molecules (e.g., CD28, CD40 ligand), and, to some degree, immunoglobulins. Recent studies have shown that innate type 1 immune responses that involve interferon-γ–producing natural killer cells and neutrophils, rather than interferon-γ–producing T cells, predetermine host resistance to *T. gondii*.[4]

In immunocompromised patients previously infected with *T. gondii*, decreased T cell–mediated or severe impairment in B cell–mediated immune responses can facilitate the reactivation of their infection (i.e., conversion of bradyzoites in their tissue cysts into rapidly proliferating tachyzoites). Toxoplasmosis in this setting is 100% lethal if untreated.

Pathology

Most of the data on the pathology of toxoplasmosis come from studies of congenitally infected babies and immunosuppressed patients. CNS lesions of patients with toxoplasmosis are characterized by significant necrosis and surrounding inflammation. In congenitally infected cases, necrotic areas may calcify and lead to typical radiographic findings suggestive but not diagnostic of toxoplasmosis. Hydrocephalus may result from obstruction of the aqueduct of Sylvius or foramen of Monro. Tachyzoites and tissue cysts may be visualized near necrotic foci, near or in glial nodules, in perivascular regions, and in cerebral tissue uninvolved by inflammatory changes.

Formation of multiple brain abscesses is relatively common in patients with AIDS. In the areas around the abscesses, edema, vasculitis, hemorrhage,

and cerebral infarction secondary to vascular involvement may also be present. Important associated features in toxoplasmic encephalitis are arteritis, perivascular cuffing, and astrocytosis. A "diffuse form" of toxoplasmic encephalitis has been described with histopathologic findings of widespread microglial nodules without abscess formation in the gray matter of the cerebrum, cerebellum, and brain stem.

Pulmonary involvement by *T. gondii* in the immunodeficient patient can lead to interstitial pneumonitis, necrotizing pneumonitis, consolidation, pleural effusion or empyema, or all of these. Chorioretinitis in AIDS patients is characterized by segmental panophthalmitis and areas of coagulative necrosis associated with tissue cysts and tachyzoites.

Toxoplasmic lymphadenitis in immunocompetent individuals may result in patterns of findings that are often diagnostic of the disease: a reactive follicular hyperplasia; irregular clusters of epithelioid histiocytes encroaching on and blurring the margins of the germinal centers; and focal distention of sinuses with monocytoid cells.

CLINICAL MANIFESTATIONS

Toxoplasmosis should be entertained in the differential diagnosis of several clinical syndromes in immunocompetent, unborn, newborn, infant, pediatric, adult, and immunocompromised patients (Table 349-1). Symptoms result from the primary infection or reactivation of the parasite due to T cell–mediated or severe B cell–mediated immunodeficiency. Primary infection can be asymptomatic in a significant number of individuals, and conventional risk factors for the acute infection may not be present in a particular patient. Thus, the possibility of acute toxoplasmosis or *T. gondii* infection should not be ruled out because of the absence of epidemiologic risk factors (e.g., exposure to cats or undercooked meat) or symptoms in a given patient. For this reason, if the goal is to detect each case of primary *T. gondii* infection in a population of patients (e.g., pregnant women), only systematic and universal screening methods can achieve such an objective; testing of only symptomatic patients or those with conventional epidemiologic risk factors will miss a significant number of acute cases.

Severity of toxoplasmosis due to primary infection or reactivation in a given patient or population may be influenced by the infecting strain (e.g., type I strain), size of the inoculum, infectious form (e.g., oocyst vs. cyst), or genetics of the host (e.g., presence of HLA-DQ3). During the past decade, it has become clear that patients infected in certain geographic locales (e.g., South America) have more aggressive clinical presentations, including a more severe primary infection and disease due to reactivation. These observations need to be kept in mind on seeing ill travelers returning from the endemic areas or patients who were born in these areas and in whom toxoplasmosis by reactivation has been included in their differential diagnosis.

Lymphadenopathy due to toxoplasmosis may be completely asymptomatic or be accompanied by other symptoms, such as fever (temperature as high as 104° F), headache, general malaise, and fatigue. It can be localized or generalized. A solitary, occipital, and painlessly enlarged lymph node can be the sole manifestation of toxoplasmosis in a child, pregnant woman, or adult. However, more generalized cervical, axillary, and abdominal lymphadenopathy has also been reported. Lymph nodes are usually 1 to 3 cm in size, nonsuppurative, and nontender on palpation. They usually regress within 12 weeks, but a mild relapse of the lymphadenopathy has been observed between months 3 and 6. Recurrence of toxoplasmic lymphadenopathy beyond the sixth month is extremely rare.

Ocular disease due to *T. gondii* can be asymptomatic or symptomatic and can be the result of congenital or postnatally acquired infection. In both settings (congenitally and postnatally acquired), toxoplasmic chorioretinitis can be discovered at the time of the diagnosis of the infection or as a reactivation of the subsequent latent infection months to years later.[5] Up to 17% of patients acutely infected with the parasite in Brazil and in a Canadian outbreak of toxoplasmosis presented with concurrent symptomatic toxoplasmic chorioretinitis at the time their acute infection was diagnosed. Similar cases have been described in Europe and the United States. *T. gondii* strain type appears to be a contributing factor determining severity and recurrence of ocular toxoplasmosis.[6] Symptomatic ocular disease primarily consists of a retinochoroiditis that can result in blurred vision, eye pain, decreased visual acuity, floaters, scotoma, photophobia, or epiphora. The morphology of the retinal lesions on funduscopic examination is thought to be characteristic of toxoplasmosis. An active whitish infiltrate is usually attached to the darkly pigmented border of an older scar (Fig. 349-2). However, retinal lesions tend to be less typical in older or immunocompromised patients.

TABLE 349-1	CLINICAL MANIFESTATIONS OF TOXOPLASMOSIS IN HUMANS
CLINICAL CATEGORIES	**CLINICAL MANIFESTATIONS AND SYNDROMES**
Primary infection	
Immunocompetent individuals and pregnant women	Most patients are asymptomatic. However, in ≈10% of patients, the following symptoms or syndromes, alone or in various combinations, have been reported: fever, lymphadenopathy, headache, myalgias, arthralgias, sore throat, stiff neck, nausea, abdominal pain, anorexia, rash, confusion, earache, eye pain, general malaise, fatigue. Chorioretinitis resulting in blurred vision, eye pain, decreased visual acuity, floaters, scotoma, photophobia, or epiphora Hepatitis; myositis; myocarditis Disseminated disease, pneumonia, brain abscesses, and even death have been observed in immunocompetent individuals infected with atypical strains of *T. gondii* (e.g. in Latin America).
Congenital toxoplasmosis	
Fetus	Ultrasound study can be normal or reveal hydrocephalus, brain or hepatic calcifications, splenomegaly, ascites, pericarditis. Fetal death can also result from overwhelming infection.
Newborn	Newborn can be entirely normal, have a nonspecific illness, or have abnormal findings on physical examination including chorioretinitis, strabismus, blindness, seizures, encephalitis, abnormal cephalic perimeter (microcephaly or hydrocephalus), psychomotor or mental retardation, hepatosplenomegaly, pneumonitis, diarrhea, hypothermia, jaundice, petechiae, rash. Intracranial calcifications can be present in brain imaging studies. Newborns can also die as a result of overwhelming infection.
Children and adults	Children can continue to suffer the chronic sequelae of the congenital disease. However, children may be born apparently normal and become symptomatic for the first time during childhood, adolescence, or adulthood, primarily in the form of reactivation of congenitally acquired chorioretinitis.
Chronic infection	Asymptomatic. However, some investigators have proposed a role of chronic infection in individuals with schizophrenia, bipolar disease, and behavioral issues including a higher incidence of motor vehicle accidents. Chorioretinitis can occur as a reactivation of congenital or postnatally acquired disease in otherwise immunocompetent individuals.
Reactivation of chronic infection in immunocompromised patients	Multiple brain abscesses, diffuse encephalitis, seizures, chorioretinitis, fever of unknown origin, pneumonia, myocarditis, hepatosplenomegaly, lymphadenopathy, rash

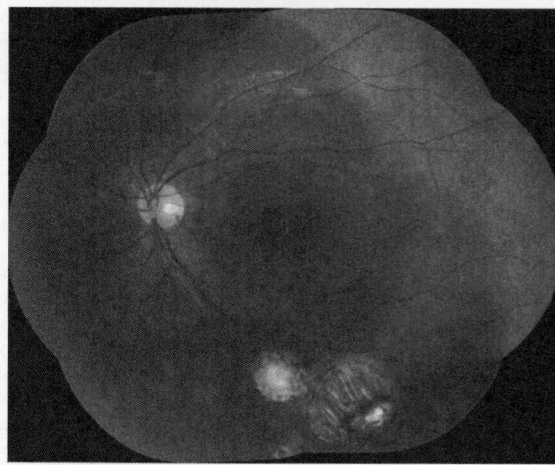

FIGURE 349-2. The morphology of the retinal lesions on funduscopic examination believed to be characteristic of toxoplasmic retinochoroiditis. An active whitish infiltrate is usually attached to the darkly pigmented border of an older scar.

Other less common but well-documented syndromes have been associated with the acute infection, including hepatitis, myositis, myocarditis, and skin lesions. More aggressive disease, including pneumonia, brain abscesses, and death, has been observed in immunocompetent patients in Latin America.

Primary infection can be observed in solid transplant patients when an allograft from a seropositive donor is transplanted into a seronegative recipient (D+/R−). Disseminated and localized toxoplasmosis has been reported in this setting, including myocarditis, pneumonia, fever of unknown origin, and encephalitis.

Congenital disease can be asymptomatic in the fetus, newborn, child, or adult. However, most of the infected offspring will eventually develop signs and symptoms of toxoplasmosis (see Table 349-1). The classic triad of chorioretinitis, hydrocephalus (Fig. 349-3A and B), and brain calcifications is highly suggestive of toxoplasmosis and is primarily seen in babies whose

mothers have not been treated against the parasite during gestation. Eye examination by an experienced pediatric ophthalmologist may reveal active or inactive toxoplasmic chorioretinitis. New lesions have been reported in up to 30% of congenitally infected children observed up until 11 years of age when their mothers have been treated but in up to 70% when their mothers have not.

Chronic infection is believed to be asymptomatic. However, several investigators have recently suggested the possibility that chronic infection may play a role in the predisposition of infected individuals to have a higher frequency of traffic accidents, mental illness (e.g. schizophrenia, bipolar disease), and behavioral abnormalities.

Reactivation of the chronic infection is usually observed in patients with significant impairment of T cell–mediated immunity or severe impairment of B cell–mediated immunity. Toxoplasmosis by reactivation can cause brain abscesses, diffuse encephalitis, seizures, chorioretinitis, fever of unknown origin, pneumonia, myocarditis, hepatosplenomegaly, lymphadenopathy, and rash. Although multiple brain abscesses (Fig. 349-3C) are commonly described in patients with toxoplasmic encephalitis, diffuse encephalitis without space-occupying lesions by magnetic resonance imaging has been reported with a very high mortality. Fever with pneumonia can be the sole manifestation of toxoplasmosis in immunocompromised patients, including HSCT and solid organ transplant recipients. Toxoplasmic pneumonitis can be manifested with cough, dyspnea, hypoxia, and diffuse bilateral or localized infiltrates. Most patients with pneumonia have been reported to have bilateral ground-glass opacities that can be confused with *Pneumocystis* pneumonia or viral etiologies. Fever alone has frequently been described in patients with allogeneic HSCT and liver transplant patients. Reactivation in heart tissue causing congestive heart failure, arrhythmias, and pericarditis has been described.

DIAGNOSIS

Laboratory methods for the diagnosis of *T. gondii* infection and toxoplasmosis include serologic tests, polymerase chain reaction (PCR), microscopy examination of tissue and body fluids, and attempts to isolate the parasite (Table 349-2).

The first step is to establish whether the patient has never been infected with *Toxoplasma* or has an acute or latent *T. gondii* infection; this can be accomplished by serologic testing. Serologic tests can establish whether a patient has never been infected or is acutely or chronically infected regardless of the presence or absence of symptoms. Available serologic tools include methods to detect *T. gondii*–specific IgG-, IgM-, IgA-, IgE-, and IgG-based avidity and differential agglutination (AC/HS).

With the use of commercial kits for the detection of IgG and IgM, most hospital-based or commercial laboratories can reliably diagnose the absence of *T. gondii* infection (negative IgG/negative IgM) and the presence of chronic infection (positive IgG/negative IgM). However, the diagnosis of acute infection is more challenging. A positive IgM test result is observed during the acute infection, but it may remain positive for months to years in

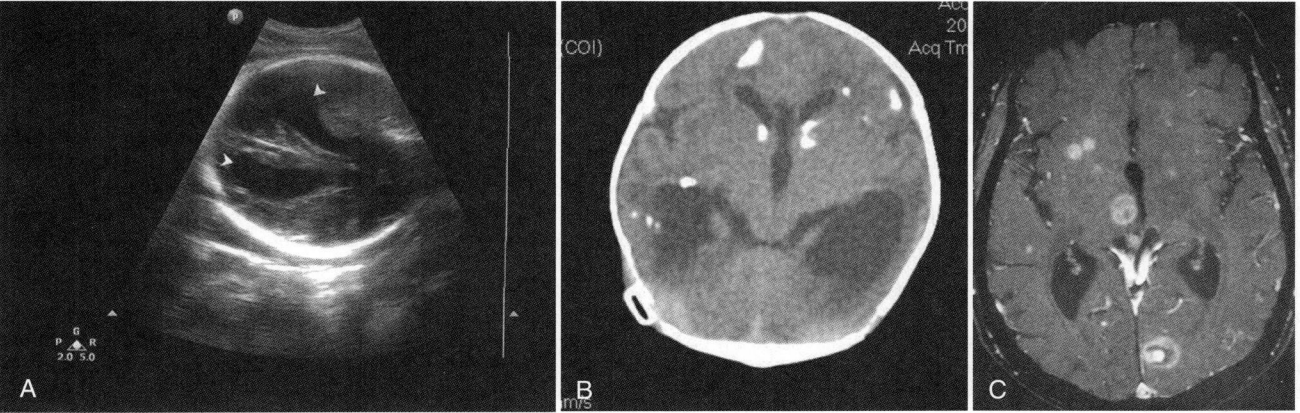

FIGURE 349-3. Radiologic manifestations of central nervous system toxoplasmosis. **A,** Fetal ultrasound of a fetus congenitally infected with *T. gondii* in the United States reveals hydrocephalus. **B,** Computed tomography scan of the brain of a newborn congenitally infected with *T. gondii* in the United States reveals hydrocephalus and calcifications. **C,** Magnetic resonance image of the brain of an AIDS patient revealing multiple ring-enhancing brain lesions.

TABLE 349-2 LABORATORY METHODS FOR THE DIAGNOSIS OF *T. GONDII* INFECTION AND TOXOPLASMOSIS* IN HUMANS

METHOD	CLINICAL INTERPRETATION
Serologic tests	
IgG	A positive test result establishes that the patient has been infected with *T. gondii*. However, a negative test result can be seen in patients infected within 4 weeks before serum sampling or in patients unable to produce IgG (e.g., immunocompromised hosts).
IgM	A positive test result suggests but is not necessarily diagnostic of an acute infection.
	Sera with positive IgM test results should be sent to a reference laboratory for confirmatory testing that includes a more specific IgM assay and additional tests, including avidity, acetone (AC)–fixed versus formalin (HS)–fixed (AC/HS) differential agglutination test of tachyzoites, and IgA and IgE.[†] Positive IgM test results can be seen in chronically infected patients because of persistence of the IgM response or false-positive results observed in certain commercial kits.
Confirmatory testing for positive IgM test results	IgG avidity test; differential agglutination (AC/HS); IgA, IgE performed at a reference laboratory.[†] At PAMF, a high IgG avidity test result[‡] or a nonacute AC/HS test result indicates that the patient has been infected for more than 4 months (avidity) or 12 months (AC/HS).
Polymerase chain reaction (PCR)	B1 and AF487550 genes are the most commonly used targets for amplification.
	PCR test can be performed in any body fluid, including amniotic fluid, peripheral blood, cerebrospinal fluid, bronchoalveolar lavage fluid, vitreous fluid, aqueous humor, peritoneal fluid, pleural fluid, ascitic fluid, and urine. PCR can also be performed in any tissue.
	A positive test result in any body fluid establishes that the patient has either acute or reactivated toxoplasmosis. However, a positive PCR test result in tissue is more difficult to interpret because it does not differentiate symptomatic toxoplasmosis from a latent infection.
	Although DNA extraction is more cumbersome, it can be attempted in paraffin-embedded tissue.
Direct visualization of the parasite	Identification of tachyzoites in any body fluid or tissue is diagnostic of toxoplasmosis due to acute infection or reactivation of a chronic infection. Tachyzoites can be identified by hematoxylin and eosin or cytologic studies but are better visualized with Wright-Giemsa and immunoperoxidase stains.
	Identification of cysts by hematoxylin and eosin or immunoperoxidase stains confirms the presence of *T. gondii* in the host but does not necessarily establish that the patient has toxoplasmosis.
	However, a strong inflammatory response surrounding the cysts is highly suggestive of toxoplasmosis, possibly explaining the patient's symptoms.
Attempts to isolate the parasite	A positive isolation study in any body fluid establishes the diagnosis of toxoplasmosis.
	Isolation of *T. gondii* in cell cultures or peritoneal cavity of mice can be attempted at reference laboratories. These studies can be important in trying to establish a correlation between the genetics of the parasite and its clinical manifestations.
Histology of the lymph node	Classic histologic triad is considered diagnostic: follicular hyperplasia, epithelioid histiocytes impinging on the margins of the germinal centers, and monocytoid cells focally distending sinus walls.

T. gondii infection = asymptomatic presence of the parasite. Toxoplasmosis = active symptoms and signs are present.
[†]For example, Palo Alto Medical Foundation Toxoplasma Serology Laboratory (PAMF-TSL), Palo Alto, Calif; *www.pamf.org/serology*; 650-853-4828; *toxolab@pamf.org*.
[‡]The window of exclusion for acute infection varies for different avidity kits (usually between 3 and 5 months).

certain individuals without any apparent clinical relevance. In addition, commercial IgM kits have been designed to be extremely sensitive so that an acute infection will be rarely missed; as a consequence, their specificity is somewhat sacrificed. Of patients who are found to be IgM positive at hospital-based or commercial laboratories, 60% are found to be chronically infected when their serum is tested at the national reference laboratory for the study and diagnosis of toxoplasmosis in the United States (Palo Alto Medical Foundation Toxoplasma Serology Laboratory [PAMF-TSL], Palo Alto, Calif; www.pamf.org/serology; 650-853-4828; toxolab@pamf.org). At PAMF-TSL, a battery of confirmatory tests (avidity, differential agglutination, IgA, IgE) are performed in addition to the "gold standard" dye test for IgG and the "double" sandwich capture enzyme-linked immunosorbent assay for IgM for confirmatory testing of positive IgM test results obtained at hospital-based or commercial laboratories. These tests are used in various combina-

tions, depending on the clinical scenario of each patient and the questions of the treating physician. For an appropriate interpretation of the serologic test results obtained at PAMF-TSL, it is also crucial to have relevant clinical information available for the medical consultants (for instance, low positive IgG and positive IgM test results with a high IgG avidity test result will mean no risk of congenital toxoplasmosis for a 16-week pregnant woman, but the same results can be highly supportive of the diagnosis of toxoplasmic encephalitis for an AIDS patient with multiple brain lesions). At PAMF-TSL, three interpretations can be given to final serologic test results: (1) acute, results are consistent with a recently acquired infection; (2) chronic, consistent with an infection acquired in the distant past; and (3) equivocal, cannot exclude a recently acquired infection; an earlier or subsequent sample is required to attempt to establish whether the infection is acute or chronic. For serologic test results consistent with an acute infection, an attempt is made by the medical consultants at PAMF-TSL to establish the approximate date that the infection was acquired.

The definitive diagnosis of toxoplasmosis (due to primary infection or reactivation of a chronic infection) requires the identification of tachyzoites in tissues or body fluids or the amplification of parasite DNA in any body fluid (see Table 349-2). Tachyzoites can be visualized in histologic sections stained with hematoxylin and eosin or in cytologic preparations without any specific staining, but they are better visualized with Wright-Giemsa (see Fig. 349-1A) and *T. gondii*–specific immunoperoxidase stains. Real-time PCR has become a useful method for the diagnosis of toxoplasmosis in the cerebrospinal fluid (CSF), and it is the diagnostic tool of choice for toxoplasmic encephalitis in immunocompromised patients (in CSF, assuming the lumbar puncture is deemed safe and feasible) and for the prenatal diagnosis of congenital toxoplasmosis (in amniotic fluid). Isolation of the parasite in any body fluid is also diagnostic of toxoplasmosis and can be attempted at reference laboratories. The diagnosis of toxoplasmosis can be indirectly supported by the use of serologic tools, demonstration of cysts in tissues (see Fig. 349-1C) surrounded by an inflammatory response, and attempts to isolate the parasite (see Table 349-2); in cases of toxoplasmic lymphadenitis, histologic features can be diagnostic.

Immunocompetent Patients, Pregnant Women, and Patients with Lymphadenopathy

The first diagnostic goal in these patients is to establish whether they have ever been infected with *T. gondii*. If *T. gondii*–specific IgG and IgM test results are negative, the possibility that the patient's symptoms are due to the parasite can be ruled out. During pregnancy, these results confirm that the mother has not been exposed to *T. gondii* but that she is at risk, if exposed, to acquire the primary infection during pregnancy and therefore can potentially transmit *T. gondii* to her offspring.[7] In attempting to determine whether the patient is infected with *T. gondii*, it is important to perform both IgG and IgM tests because during the first 4 weeks of the acute infection, the IgG can still be negative while the IgM will be positive. In these cases, seroconversion can be diagnosed by having a new positive IgG test result in a subsequent serum sample. In rare instances, infected patients may be IgG negative because of their incapacity to produce IgG.

If the patient is found to be IgG positive, the next goal is to determine whether the patient is having an acute infection or has been chronically infected (e.g., >6 months). If the IgG titer is low (e.g., a dye test at PAMF-TSL ≤512) and the IgM test result is negative, the patient has essentially been infected for more than 6 months. With these results, a patient whose symptoms or lymphadenopathy had a date of onset within 6 months of serum sampling will be considered unlikely to have toxoplasmosis. For a pregnant woman whose serum was obtained within 6 months of gestation, these results will mean that her infection was acquired before conception and that the risk for congenital toxoplasmosis is essentially zero.

If the patient is found to have a positive IgM test result confirmed to be indicative of a recently acquired infection at a reference laboratory and the onset of symptoms or lymphadenopathy falls within the time predicted by the serologic test results for the acquisition of *T. gondii*, the patient will be diagnosed as having acute toxoplasmosis. For a pregnant woman, if the predicted time for when the infection was acquired falls within her gestational age, she will be diagnosed with toxoplasmosis during pregnancy and at risk for transmitting the parasite to her baby.

In patients with lymphadenopathy, the histologic examination of the lymph node tissue obtained by excisional biopsy can be diagnostic or pathognomonic of toxoplasmic lymphadenitis (see earlier under Pathology).

Prenatal and Postnatal Diagnosis of Congenital Toxoplasmosis

Once the diagnosis of acute toxoplasmosis or *T. gondii* infection has been confirmed or is highly suspected in the mother, the next step is to attempt to establish whether her offspring has been infected. Consultation with reference centers for the study and diagnosis of congenital toxoplasmosis is highly recommended.

Ultrasound abnormalities can be consistent with or suggestive of congenital toxoplasmosis (see Fig. 349-3A), but they are not diagnostic. The method of choice for the prenatal diagnosis of congenital toxoplasmosis is a PCR in amniotic fluid obtained at 18 weeks of gestation. Attempts to diagnose congenital toxoplasmosis from amniotic fluid obtained before 18 weeks of gestation should be avoided because the studies reported to date have included only pregnant women whose gestational age was 18 weeks or more.

In addition, false-negative results have been reported in women whose amniocentesis was performed before 18 weeks of gestation. The overall sensitivity of the amniotic fluid PCR has been reported between 64 and 92% and is highly dependent of the gestational age at which the mother acquired the infection.

In the newborn, congenital toxoplasmosis can be confirmed by positive *T. gondii*–specific serologic test results or PCR.[8] Samples for serology should be obtained in the peripheral blood of the baby. Cord blood should be avoided because of the high rate of maternal blood contamination. However, there is still a small degree of maternal blood contamination in newborn blood obtained by peripheral venipuncture, during the first 5 days of life for IgM antibodies and the first 10 days of life for IgA antibodies. A positive IgM immunosorbent agglutination assay (after 5 days of life) or IgA enzyme-linked immunosorbent assay (after 10 days) is diagnostic of congenital disease. Congenitally infected babies can be positive for both; positive for either one, but negative for the other test; or negative for both. A positive *T. gondii*–specific IgM in CSF is diagnostic of congenital disease, but testing of the CSF by PCR rather than for IgM is strongly recommended because of the higher sensitivity of the PCR test. The diagnosis can also be made by a positive PCR in peripheral blood, CSF, or urine. The CSF of infected infants may exhibit very high levels of protein (e.g., 1000 mg/dL). Cellular response in CSF is characterized by lymphocytosis, and eosinophilia may be present. Brain imaging studies may reveal calcifications or hydrocephalus; computed tomography scan is superior to ultrasound examination in the detection of these CNS abnormalities (see Fig. 349-3B).

Ocular Disease

Serologic and PCR testing can be helpful in the diagnosis of toxoplasmic chorioretinitis. An IgG-negative/IgM-negative patient is unlikely to have ocular disease due to toxoplasmosis. However, patients should be tested at reference laboratories (e.g., PAMF-TSL) because their *T. gondii*–specific IgG can be present but at very low levels such that only a gold standard method like the dye test can detect it. In patients with eye lesions typical of toxoplasmic chorioretinitis (see Fig. 349-2), a positive IgG test result at a relatively low titer (e.g., a dye test at PAMF-TSL ≤512) and a negative IgM test result are diagnostic of ocular disease due to the parasite reactivation. If the serologic test reveals a positive IgM result and confirmatory testing at PAMF-TSL establishes the diagnosis of an acute infection in patients 1 year of age or older, the eye disease is most likely the result of eye involvement in the setting of a recent and postnatally acquired infection.

In patients with atypically appearing lesions or in whom the response to anti-*Toxoplasma* drugs is atypical or absent, a *T. gondii*–specific immune load (aqueous humor) or PCR in ocular fluids (vitreous fluid is preferable to aqueous humor because of probable higher sensitivity, but it is riskier to obtain) should be considered.

Immunocompromised Patients

It appears that acute infection rarely occurs in immunocompromised patients. However, life-threatening disease can occur when the patient's latent infection is reactivated by AIDS, HSCT, liver transplantation, or other diseases characterized by severe T-cell deficiency.

Toxoplasmosis can also develop when *T. gondii* is transmitted from a seropositive donor to a seronegative recipient through an infected allograft (e.g., heart, liver, kidney).[9] Therefore, to establish the risk for toxoplasmosis and to have a high index of suspicion when patients develop illnesses suggestive of toxoplasmosis, all immunocompromised patients should be tested for *T. gondii*–specific IgG as soon as they have been diagnosed with the underlying disease or it has been established that they will be subsequently immunosuppressed. In addition, serologic testing may not be reliable when immunosuppression is advanced or severe. Post-transplantation serologic test results for IgG antibodies may remain positive or may rise, decrease, or even become negative. Thus, pretransplantation *Toxoplasma* serologic studies are critical for interpretation of subsequent test results and clinical evaluation. Solid organ donors should also be tested for *T. gondii*–specific IgG as their allograft has the potential to transmit the parasite to the transplanted patient (e.g., heart, heart-lung, kidney, kidney-pancreas, liver, liver-pancreas). Toxoplasmosis in solid organ transplant recipients causes substantial morbidity, including disseminated disease, and mortality.

In AIDS patients suspected of having toxoplasmic encephalitis with the presence of multiple brain-occupying and ring-enhancing lesions (see Fig. 349-3C), a CD4 count below 200 cells/μL, and a positive *T. gondii*–specific IgG, the response to anti–*Toxoplasma*-specific treatment is considered an additional "diagnostic" indicator of toxoplasmic encephalitis. In these patients, invasive diagnostic tests (e.g., lumbar puncture, brain biopsy) are considered unnecessary unless they do not respond to treatment within a 7- to 10-day period. This diagnostic paradigm should not be applied to other populations of immunosuppressed patients (e.g., transplant patients) because their differential diagnosis often includes other pathogens, such as invasive mold infections. In those patients, examination of the CSF by PCR or brain biopsy should be attempted at the outset of the illness.

The definitive diagnosis of toxoplasmosis in immunosuppressed patients relies on PCR, direct visualization of the parasite, and attempts for isolation of the organism (see Table 349-2). PCR testing in body fluids is the diagnostic method of choice for immunosuppressed patients at risk for toxoplasmosis who develop unexplained fever (e.g., in whole blood), pneumonia (e.g., in bronchoalveolar lavage fluid), brain lesions (e.g., in CSF), or other compatible syndromes. Theoretically, PCR can be performed in any body fluid or tissue, and laboratories have validated its use in most fluids and some tissues. Attempts to identify the tachyzoite or tissue cyst in tissues by microscopy can be enhanced with the use of the *T. gondii*–specific immunoperoxidase stain. CSF examination by PCR or brain biopsy should be initially considered in AIDS patients who have a low likelihood of having toxoplasmic encephalitis, such as those who have a single lesion by magnetic resonance imaging examination, have tested seronegative for *T. gondii* infection, have a CD4 count of more than 200 cells/μL, or who are not responding to an appropriate anti-*Toxoplasma* regimen.

TREATMENT Rx

Principles of antiparasitic therapy are discussed in Chapter 344. Treatment of toxoplasmosis is indicated for immunocompetent patients with acute infection in the setting of ongoing fever, myocarditis, myositis, hepatitis, pneumonia, brain lesions or skin lesions, and lymphadenopathy accompanied by severe or persisting symptoms. Treatment is indicated as well for patients with active chorioretinitis due to primary infection or reactivation of a latent infection (Table 349-3).[10] In immunocompetent patients, treatment is prescribed for 3 to 4 weeks or until symptoms have subsided, whichever is longer. For toxoplasmic lymphadenitis, trimethoprim-sulfamethoxazole (TMP-SMZ) (8 mg TMP/40 mg SMZ per kilogram per day divided into two doses for 1 month) increased the cure rate to 65% compared with a 13% resolution rate with placebo.[A1] Treatment is also often recommended for all pregnant women suspected of having or diagnosed with primary infection during gestation (Table 349-4) in an attempt to prevent transmission of the parasite to the fetus (spiramycin) or, if congenital infection has occurred, to start treatment of the fetus in utero (pyrimethamine, sulfadiazine, and folinic acid). During pregnancy, treatment regimens are prescribed for the duration of the gestation. There was a worldwide controversy about the efficacy of spiramycin to decrease the incidence of congenital toxoplasmosis and of pyrimethamine, sulfadiazine, and folinic acid to decrease the frequency of clinical signs in infected offspring. Although no definitive studies ever disproved their efficacy, several epidemiologic studies erroneously concluded that there was no evidence of benefit. However, since 2006, several studies have reported a strong association between prenatal treatment of women infected during gestation (with spiramycin or pyrimethamine, sulfadiazine, and folinic acid) and decreases in the incidence of congenital toxoplasmosis and frequency of clinical signs in infected offspring. Spiramycin is recommended for pregnant women who have been definitively diagnosed to have or are highly suspected of having an acute infection during pregnancy and acquired before 18 weeks of gestation. Spiramycin should be given throughout pregnancy unless fetal infection is suspected or documented. Fetal infection should be investigated with amniotic fluid PCR at 18 weeks of gestation to see whether *Toxoplasma* DNA is amplified and with monthly follow-up ultrasound examinations. Therapy with pyrimethamine, sulfadiazine, and folinic acid is recommended for pregnant women who have been definitively diagnosed to have or are highly suspected of having an acute infection during pregnancy and acquired after 18 weeks of gestation, whose amniotic fluid PCR is positive for the presence of *Toxoplasma* DNA, or whose follow-up ultrasound examinations are suggestive of congenital toxoplasmosis in the setting of acute *Toxoplasma* infection during gestation. In addition, newborns and infants diagnosed with or suspected of having congenital toxoplasmosis should also be treated during their first year of life (see Table 349-4).

Treatment at higher doses is urgently indicated for all immunocompromised patients with toxoplasmosis due to reactivation of their latent infection or primary infection acquired by natural exposure to the parasite or by solid organ transplantation (see Table 349-3). If untreated, toxoplasmosis in these patients has a very high rate of morbidity and mortality.

TABLE 349-3	TREATMENT REGIMENS FOR PATIENTS WITH ACUTE OR PRIMARY TOXOPLASMOSIS AND IMMUNOCOMPROMISED PATIENTS WITH TOXOPLASMOSIS DUE TO REACTIVATION*	
	IMMUNOCOMPETENT PATIENTS WITH ACUTE INFECTION†	**IMMUNOCOMPROMISED PATIENTS**
Pyrimethamine (PO) *plus*	50 mg every 12 hr for 2 days, followed by 25 to 50 mg daily	200 mg loading dose, followed by 50 mg/day (<60 kg) to 75 mg/day (>60 kg)
Folinic acid‡	10-20 mg daily (during and 1 week after therapy with pyrimethamine)	10-20 mg daily (up to 50 mg/day)
	plus either sulfadiazine or clindamycin or atovaquone as follows:	*plus either sulfadiazine or clindamycin or atovaquone as follows:*
Sulfadiazine (PO)	75 mg/kg (first dose), followed by 50 mg/kg every 12 hr (maximum 4 g/day)	1000 mg (<60 kg) to 1500 mg (>60 kg) every 6 hr
or		
Clindamycin (PO or IV)	300 mg every 6 hr	600 mg every 6 hr (up to 1200 mg every 6 hr)
or		
Atovaquone (PO)	1500 mg orally twice daily	1500 mg orally twice daily
Trimethoprim-sulfamethoxazole (PO or IV)	10 mg/kg/day (trimethoprim component) in two or three doses	10 mg/kg/day (trimethoprim component) in two or three doses (doses as high as 15-20 mg/kg/day have been used)
Pyrimethamine and folinic acid *plus*	Same doses as above	Same doses as above
Clarithromycin (PO) *or*	500 mg every 12 hr	500 mg every 12 hr
Dapsone (PO) *or*	100 mg/day	100 mg/day
Azithromycin (PO)	900 to 1200 mg/day	900 to 1200 mg/day

After the successful use of a combination regimen during the acute or primary therapy phase, the same agents at half-dose are usually used for maintenance or secondary prophylaxis.
*Preferred regimens: pyrimethamine, sulfadiazine, and folinic acid or trimethoprim-sulfamethoxazole. Assistance is available for the diagnosis and management of patients with toxoplasmosis at the Palo Alto Medical Foundation Toxoplasma Serology Laboratory (PAMF-TSL), Palo Alto, Calif; www.pamf.org/serology; 650-853-4828; toxolab@pamf.org.
†Particularly in the setting of myocarditis, myositis, hepatitis, pneumonia, brain or skin lesions, and lymphadenopathy accompanied by severe or persisting symptoms. Also indicated for those with active ocular disease due to primary infection or reactivation.
‡Folinic acid = leucovorin; folic acid must not be used as a substitute for folinic acid.

PREVENTION
Primary Infection

Because approximately 50% of patients may inadvertently become infected with the parasite without having a recognized risk factor for acute infection, only systematic serologic testing can establish whether a patient has been exposed to *T. gondii*. Thus, each pregnant woman and immunocompromised patient should be screened for *T. gondii*–specific IgG and IgM regardless of their epidemiologic history. Seronegative pregnant women and immunocompromised individuals should be counseled on how to maximize their prevention efforts to avoid infection with *T. gondii*. In addition, seronegative pregnant women should be tested serially during gestation in an attempt to diagnose seroconversion at the earliest time possible. In some countries, such as France, seronegative pregnant women are mandated by law to be tested every month for *T. gondii*–specific IgG and IgM. Women who seroconvert are offered spiramycin (if infected before 18 weeks of gestation) or pyrimethamine, sulfadiazine, and folinic acid (if infected after 18 weeks). Mothers whose amniotic fluid is found to be positive by PCR or those in whom fetal ultrasound study is highly suggestive of congenital toxoplasmosis are offered pyrimethamine, sulfadiazine, and folinic acid. Although infection often occurs in the absence of known risk factors for the acute infection, educational interventions to avoid exposure to the parasite have been shown to be effective in decreasing the incidence of seroconversion during gestation.

The majority of epidemiologic studies worldwide have recognized contaminated and undercooked meat as one of the main risk factors for the

TABLE 349-4 TREATMENT REGIMENS FOR PREGNANT WOMEN WHO HAVE LIKELY ACQUIRED *T. GONDII* INFECTION DURING GESTATION AND INFANTS SUSPECTED OF HAVING OR CONFIRMED TO HAVE CONGENITAL TOXOPLASMOSIS

	DURING PREGNANCY	IN CONGENITAL DISEASE
Spiramycin (oral)	Recommended for pregnant women suspected of having or confirmed to have acquired the infection during gestation and before 18 weeks of gestation. Spiramycin should be administered until delivery in those with negative amniotic fluid PCR test results and normal follow-up ultrasound studies or low suspicion of fetal infection. Spiramycin is not teratogenic, and it is available in the United States only through the Investigational New Drug (IND) process at the Food and Drug Administration (301-796-1600). Prior medical consultation is required.* Dosage: 1 g (3 million units) every 8 hr (for a total of 3 g or 9 million units per day)	Not recommended during pregnancy if the fetus has been documented to be or suspected to have been infected. In the setting of fetal infection, pyrimethamine, sulfadiazine, and folinic acid should be instituted (see below)
Pyrimethamine (oral) plus sulfadiazine (oral) plus folinic acid† (oral)	Recommended for women ≥18 weeks of gestation in whom it is suspected or confirmed that the acute infection has been acquired at or after 18 weeks of gestation or who have a positive amniotic fluid PCR test result or an abnormal ultrasound study suggestive of congenital toxoplasmosis. Pyrimethamine is teratogenic and should not be used during pregnancy before week 18 (in some centers in Europe, it is used as early as week 14). Sulfadiazine should not be used alone. Dosages: Pyrimethamine: 50 mg every 12 hr for 2 days followed by 50 mg daily Sulfadiazine: 75 mg/kg (first dose) followed by 50 mg/kg every 12 hr (maximum 4 g/day) Folinic acid† (leucovorin): 10-20 mg daily (during and for 1 week after pyrimethamine therapy)	**Infant** (treatment regimen is usually recommended for 1 year): Pyrimethamine: 1 mg/kg every 12 hr for 2 days; followed by 1 mg/kg/day for 2 or 6 months; followed by 1 mg/kg/day every Monday, Wednesday, Friday Sulfadiazine: 50 mg/kg every 12 hr Folinic acid† (leucovorin): 10 mg three times weekly Prednisone (if CSF protein ≥1 g/dL or severe chorioretinitis): 0.5 mg/kg every 12 hr (until CSF protein <1 g/dL or resolution of severe chorioretinitis) **Older children with active disease** (usually 1-2 weeks beyond resolution of clinical manifestations): Pyrimethamine: 1 mg/kg every 12 hr (maximum 50 mg) for 2 days followed by 1 mg/kg/day (maximum 25 mg) Sulfadiazine: 75 mg/kg (first dose) followed by 50 mg/kg every 12 hr Folinic acid† (leucovorin): 10-20 mg three times weekly Prednisone (severe chorioretinitis): 1 mg/kg/day, divided bid, maximum 40 mg/day, rapid taper

*Palo Alto Medical Foundation Toxoplasma Serology Laboratory (PAMF-TSL), Palo Alto, Calif; *www.pamf.org/serology*; 650-853-4828; *toxolab@pamf.org*; or U.S. (Chicago) National Collaborative Treatment Trial Study (NCCTS), 773-834-4152.
†Folic acid should not be used as a substitute for folinic acid.
CSF = cerebrospinal fluid; PCR = polymerase chain reaction.

transmission of the parasite. This appears to be the case in Europe, North America, and Latin America. Tissue cysts in meat are rendered nonviable by γ-irradiation (0.4 kGy), heating throughout to 67° C, or freezing to −20° C for 48 hours and then thawing. Cured, dried, or smoked meat has been associated with the acute infection and should not be considered *Toxoplasma* free. Soil exposure and soil-related activities have been reported to play a more prominent role in transmission in certain geographic areas, such as Latin America.

In seronegative recipients of a solid organ from a seropositive donor, TMP-SMZ for at least 6 months or pyrimethamine for at least 6 weeks has been reported to be effective in the prevention of primary infection in the newly immunosuppressed patient.

Reactivation of Latent Infection in Immunocompromised Patients and Those with Ocular Disease

Drugs used to prevent reactivation of the latent infection in immunosuppressed hosts include TMP-SMZ (e.g., single strength or 80 mg TMP and 400 mg SMZ, 1 tablet per day) and atovaquone (1500 mg/day). Dapsone-pyrimethamine and sulfadoxine-pyrimethamine have been also reported to be effective, but their use appears to be limited because of potential hematologic toxicity.

Prophylaxis against reactivation of latent infection has been successful in AIDS patients dually infected with HIV and *T. gondii* (*Toxoplasma* IgG seropositive) and whose CD4+ T-cell counts are below 200 cells/μL. For prophylactic purposes, TMP-SMZ should probably not be used below a minimum dose of 160 mg TMP/800 mg SMZ orally twice a day on a thrice-weekly regimen or 80 mg TMP/400 mg SMZ once a day. In AIDS patients, 100 mg of dapsone plus 50 mg of pyrimethamine orally twice weekly or atovaquone (1500 mg/day) has also been effective in preventing toxoplasmic encephalitis. Findings in these studies have been extrapolated to non-AIDS immunosuppressed patients because of the absence of data in this population of patients.

Toxoplasma-seropositive recipients of an allogeneic HSCT (Chapter 178) who develop graft-versus-host disease represent a unique challenge. Reactivation of toxoplasmosis can be manifested by a nonspecific illness (e.g., fever or pneumonia) and be life-threatening. The disease is often not recognized.

Atovaquone prophylaxis has been proposed as an alternative regimen in these patients, given the potential bone marrow toxicity of TMP-SMZ. Some investigators have proposed a preemptive strategy in which *Toxoplasma*-seropositive patients who receive an allogeneic HSCT are monitored on a routine basis (e.g., weekly for the first 100 days) with *T. gondii* PCR. Those found positive would receive preemptive prophylaxis with TMP-SMZ or atovaquone.

Discontinuation of prophylaxis against toxoplasmic encephalitis has proved safe in AIDS patients receiving highly active antiretroviral therapy who demonstrate an increase in their CD4+ T-cell counts to at least 200 cells/μL and whose viral load has been undetectable for at least 6 months.

In patients with ocular toxoplasmosis who experience frequent relapses (e.g., more than two episodes per year), 80 mg TMP/400 mg SMZ daily for at least 1 year has been shown to be effective in the prevention of their recurrences.[A2]

PROGNOSIS

The primary infection has a wide spectrum of manifestations in humans, from asymptomatic in most individuals to pneumonia or life-threatening disease if it is acquired in certain areas of the world. Primary infection can also be fatal in the fetus and in immunocompromised individuals. Early diagnosis and treatment can make a significant difference in the prognosis of these patients.

It is not clear at this time whether chronic infection in immunocompetent individuals is clinically irrelevant. Several investigators have proposed that latent infection with the parasite may play a significant role in mental illness (e.g., schizophrenia) or in the propensity of the infected individual to incur motor vehicle accidents. Immunocompetent patients can reactivate chronic infection in their retina, and the prognosis is influenced by the proximity of the lesions to the macula, involvement of one or both eyes, and number of relapses. It is believed that treatment can slow the progression of these lesions and expedite their healing.

Reactivation of latent infection in immunosuppressed individuals with significant defects in their T cell–mediated or B cell–mediated immunity, if untreated, is 100% fatal. Even when treated in an intensive care unit, disseminated toxoplasmosis in immunocompromised patients has a mortality rate of about 80%.[11]

Grade A References

A1. Alavi SM, Alavi L. Treatment of toxoplasmic lymphadenitis with co-trimoxazole: double-blind, randomized clinical trial. *Int J Infect Dis*. 2010;3:e67-e69.
A2. Felix JP, Lira RP, Zacchia RS, et al. Trimethoprim-sulfamethoxazole versus placebo to reduce the risk of recurrences of *Toxoplasma gondii* retinochoroiditis: randomized controlled clinical trial. *Am J Ophthalmol*. 2014;157:762-766.e1.

GENERAL REFERENCES

For the General References and other additional features, please visit Expert Consult at https://expertconsult.inkling.com.

350

CRYPTOSPORIDIOSIS

ALDO A. M. LIMA AND RICHARD L. GUERRANT

DEFINITION

Cryptosporidiosis is the clinical disease in humans and animals caused by protozoal parasites of the genus *Cryptosporidium* (Apicomplexa). *Cryptosporidium* spp are recognized as major waterborne parasites worldwide, and 14 species of 30 to date have been documented to infect humans. Two named species, *C. hominis* and *C. pestis*, are considered of major public health significance. Four (*C. cuniculus, C. meleagridis, C. viatorum,* and *C. felis*) and eight (*C. parvum, C. fayeri, C. canis, C. suis, C. ubiquitum, C. scrofarum, C. muris,* and *C. andersoni*) of 14 named species are considered of moderate and minor public health significance, respectively. There are nine species of 30 that are shared between humans and cattle.

The Pathogen

The family Cryptosporidiidae has a hidden sporocyst and undergoes monoxenous completion of its cycle in one host, where it can cause predominantly intestinal, cloacal, and gastric infections.

EPIDEMIOLOGY

The life cycle begins with ingestion of *Cryptosporidium* oocysts (2 to 5 μm) by the vertebrate host, with subsequent excystation within the lumen of the small intestine to release four sporozoites (Fig. 350-1). The sporozoites attach to and enter the host's epithelial cells to form intracellular but extracytoplasmic parasitophorous vacuoles, where they develop into trophozoites and subsequently type 1 meronts (schizonts). By asexual nuclear division, they multiply and release six to eight type 1 merozoites that invade neighboring host cells and develop into type 2 meronts, or trophozoites, to complete the asexual reproductive cycle. Type 2 meronts undergo two nuclear divisions and release four type 2 merozoites that can infect the host's cells and further develop into male (microgamont) or female (macrogamete) forms. Microgametes released from the microgamont can penetrate the macrogametes to form zygotes. Approximately 20% of the zygotes develop into thin-walled autoinfective oocysts; some 80% become thick-walled oocysts, which are excreted in stool.

Cryptosporidium oocysts have at least five characteristics that make this organism a common problem and that help define the potential risk for person-to-person spread and for waterborne and food-borne disease outbreaks. First, *Cryptosporidium* oocysts are resistant to many chemical disinfectants, such as chlorine. Second, the organism is highly infectious, with the median *C. parvum* infectious dose being 132 or fewer oocysts. Third, the size of the oocysts, 2 to 5 μm, allows them to pass through many conventional filters. Fourth, the monoxenous life cycle allows infectious oocysts to be excreted in large numbers in feces, which can easily spread. Fifth, the organism is associated with geographic, seasonal, and socioeconomic differences in the distribution of *Cryptosporidium* spp.

Cryptosporidiosis is seasonal and related to precipitation and temperature fluctuations worldwide.[1] Excystation of *C. parvum* increases in water temperatures up to 46° C (natural sunlight for 12 hours). Two waterborne outbreaks brought cryptosporidiosis to public health attention. In January 1989, an increased number of cases of cryptosporidiosis were reported in Swindon

and Oxfordshire, United Kingdom, with a peak reached in March. Mapping of the addresses of early cases showed associations with water supplies. In late February, the water authority detected *Cryptosporidium* oocysts in samples from the water that supplied the affected areas and in the treated water. Contamination of the raw Thames River water used at three water treatment plants was found, with evidence of pollution by farm effluent. This outbreak resulted in 516 cases and thus ignited public interest and led to an official inquiry. The second outbreak occurred in early spring 1993 in Milwaukee, Wisconsin, and was the largest documented outbreak of waterborne disease ever in the United States, with an estimated 403,000 people having acute watery diarrhea and potentially 112 deaths. Findings from this outbreak indicated that *Cryptosporidium* oocysts passed through the filtration system of one of the city's water treatment plants. Again, this suggested that the water quality standards and detection methods for *Cryptosporidium* were inadequate. Swimming pool contamination, especially of bigger pools, pools with more heterogeneous mixing such as municipal pools, and pools catering to young children (wading pools), is associated with more cases.[2] Food-borne outbreaks have also been reported in association with contaminated apple cider, unpasteurized milk, chicken salad, vegetables, raw produce, and shellfish.[3]

The prevalence of cryptosporidiosis varies by geographic region, with the highest rates seen in developing countries. Most cases of cryptosporidiosis occur in young children, thus suggesting that the host's immune response plays a role in susceptibility. Furthermore, cryptosporidiosis in individuals infected with human immunodeficiency virus (HIV) and in those with acquired immunodeficiency syndrome (AIDS) is persistent and occasionally life-threatening and may involve infections of the hepatobiliary and respiratory tracts in addition to the entire gastrointestinal tract. Only effective antiretroviral therapy with restoration of immune function controls this devastating disease. The prevalence of cryptosporidiosis in patients with AIDS varies from 31% in those with $CD4^+$ cell counts equal or higher than 200/μL to 38% in those with $CD4^+$ cell counts lower than 100/μL.

PATHOBIOLOGY

Cryptosporidium oocysts and sporozoites interact with host cells, including the processes of excystation, gliding motility, attachment, invasion, parasitophorous vacuole formation, intracellular maintenance, and host cell damage.[4] Oocysts of *Cryptosporidium* spp use their cysteine and serine proteases and aminopeptidase for excystation in the upper part of the small bowel and release infective sporozoites that invade the mucosal epithelium and occasionally Peyer's patch M cells, often extending to the terminal ileum and colon. The sporozoites secrete proteins from the apical organelles for locomotion and attachment. In immunocompromised patients, the organisms can be found throughout the gut, biliary tract, pancreas, and respiratory tract. As noted earlier, trophozoites undergo asexual reproduction by merogony to form type 1 and then type 2 meronts. Sporozoites and merozoites are internalized by similar invasion machinery and actin reorganization. Two classes of proteins, mucin-like glycoproteins and thrombospondin-related adhesive proteins, mediate adhesion of the parasite. The parasite uses proteases for the proteolytic processing of surface and apical complex proteins for invasion and for egress from the host cells. Entry into the host's cell occurs within 30 seconds and is dependent on the parasite's actinomyosin cytoskeleton to enter host-derived bimembrane parasitophorous vacuoles in a unique intracellular but extracytoplasmic niche.[5] Dense polymerized actin forms at the base fusion of the host-parasite bimembranes. Invasion of cells of the host leads to displacement of the microvillous border, villous atrophy, blunting and crypt cell hyperplasia, and marked infiltration by lymphocytes, plasma cells, and some neutrophils into the lamina propria, with apoptosis of infected cells and significant alteration in intestinal permeability, as measured by mannitol and lactulose markers. This noninvasive functional test shows both reduced absorptive area and disrupted barrier function, which is even more severe in patients with HIV/AIDS. Upregulation of nuclear factor κB and the pro-inflammatory cascade causes secretory and mildly inflammatory diarrhea. Pro-inflammatory cytokines and potential biomarkers, such as tumor necrosis factor-α, interleukins 1β and 8, and lactoferrin, are significantly increased in murine and human infections. Interleukins 1β and 8 both upregulate cyclooxygenase 2, which results in prostaglandin synthesis in the epithelial cells and production of substance P by the inflammatory cells; these products together decrease net sodium absorption and increase net chloride secretion, which causes the secretory diarrhea often seen with this infection.

Both innate and adaptive immune responses are associated with immunity to cryptosporidiosis. Two chemokines, CXCL-10 and perhaps CXCL-8, are initially implicated in the attraction of pro-inflammatory cells. Activation of

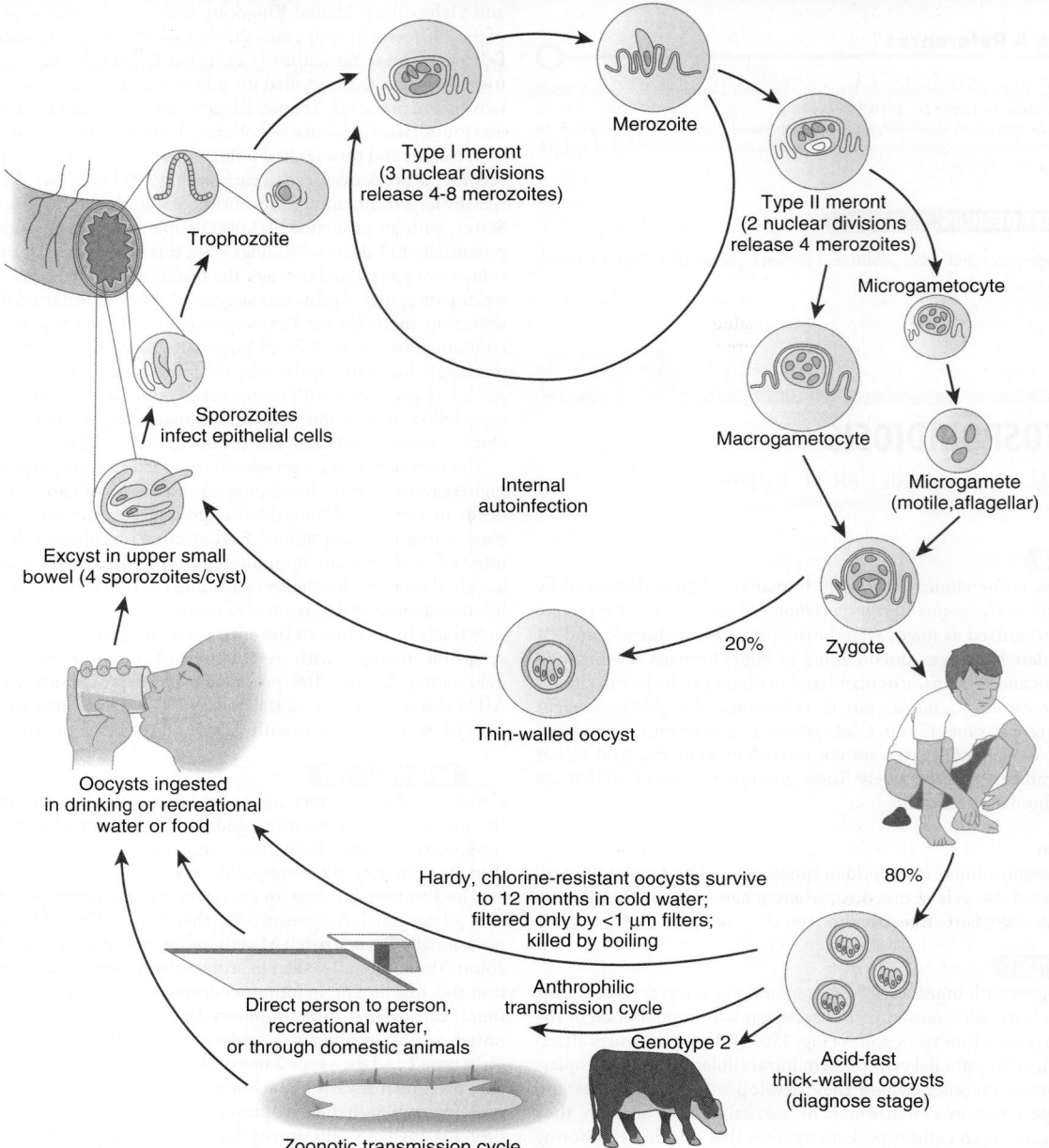

FIGURE 350-1. Life cycle of *Cryptosporidium* spp. (Redrawn with permission from Kosek M, Alcantara C, Lima AAM, et al. Cryptosporidiosis: an update. *Lancet Infect Dis.* 2001;1:262-269.)

the immune system involves early stimulation by interleukin 15, which may be important for initial clearance of the parasite. CD4⁺ T cells and interferon-γ play important roles in the eventual immune defense against this infection, probably more so than B cells or CD8⁺ cells.

CLINICAL MANIFESTATIONS

Cryptosporidiosis is a cosmopolitan, self-limited infection in immunocompetent hosts that affects all age groups and both sexes. In developing countries, the disease occurs most frequently in children younger than 5 years because of high rates of fecal-oral exposure and the development of partial immunity in older children and adults. In developed countries, the disease occurs at all ages, and most cases are associated with small waterborne outbreaks, frequently with contamination of recreational water. Patients from developed countries are more often adults. The incubation period is approximately 1 week, with a range of 1 to 30 days.[6] The diarrhea can have a sudden onset, frequently with voluminous watery stools, abdominal pain, nausea or vomiting, bloating, malaise, fatigue, weight loss, and occasional fever. In young children at risk in developing countries, it may have a long-term impact on physical activity, school performance, and development of cognitive function. Rarely, respiratory infection and cough have been reported. In normal hosts, the disease usually lasts 1 to 3 weeks but sometimes for more than a

month. Oocyst shedding typically lasts 1 to 2 weeks but can occur for up to 2 months. Patients with T-cell immune deficiency, such as those with hematologic malignant neoplasms (particularly children), primary T-cell deficiencies (severe combined immunodeficiency and CD40 ligand deficiency), and HIV/AIDS, are at high risk for the development of more severe disease and have an increased risk for death.

Immunocompetent Host

Data on the natural history of cryptosporidiosis in immunocompetent hosts have been obtained mostly from developed countries, and such data are derived from waterborne outbreaks, patients seeking medical assistance, travelers, animal workers, children in daycare, and their contacts. Most patients in outbreaks and travelers are adults and usually have diarrhea with a median duration of 14 days and a range of 1 to 100 days. The duration and severity of diarrhea appear to be similar for *C. parvum* and *C. hominis* infections. Recurrence of diarrhea is common and occurs in 30 to 41% of patients. Reports from the United Kingdom describe abdominal pain (96%), vomiting (65%), fever (59%), and bloody diarrhea (11%). The clinical manifestations in 285 people surveyed with a confirmed laboratory diagnosis of *Cryptosporidium* infection in the massive outbreak in Milwaukee showed a median duration of 9 days (range, 1 to 55 days), with watery diarrhea in 93%, abdominal cramps in 84%, fever in 57%, and vomiting in 48%. Patients may continue to shed oocysts for seven months despite being asymptomatic.[7]

Childhood Cryptosporidiosis in Developing Countries

In developing countries, cryptosporidiosis is associated with prolonged (7 to 13 days) or persistent (≥14 days) diarrhea, increased overall burden of diarrhea, risk for malnutrition, and infant mortality. A nested case-control study from a cohort of children in Brazil has shown that children younger than 1 year with cryptosporidiosis have subsequent increased diarrheal burdens and growth shortfalls. These findings have been extended in a shantytown in Peru, where cryptosporidiosis has been associated with growth faltering and stunting. This was also true for children with asymptomatic infections, which are even more common in endemic areas. The long-term impact of childhood diarrhea and cryptosporidiosis has also been evaluated in a cohort study in Brazil, in which it was shown that children with more diarrhea morbidity or cryptosporidiosis early in life (0 to 2 years) have reduced fitness and impaired cognitive function at 6 to 9 years of age. Several studies have now shown that oocysts are shed longer and the number of oocysts is higher with *C. hominis* than with *C. parvum* infection. In Brazil, a birth cohort study demonstrated that children with *C. hominis* infection have higher fecal lactoferrin and delayed growth in comparison to those with *C. parvum* infections. Diarrhea, nausea, vomiting, and general malaise are more frequently associated with *C. hominis* infection. Subtype family analysis of *C. hominis* (Ia, Ib, Id, and Ie) has indicated that Ib is more commonly associated with nausea, vomiting, and general malaise.

Immunocompromised Hosts

Low CD4[+] lymphocyte counts in HIV-infected patients are associated with severe cryptosporidial diarrhea. For example, patients with CD4[+] counts higher than $180/mm^3$ usually have transient or self-limited disease, whereas those with CD4[+] counts lower than $50/mm^3$ often have severe disease with more than 2 L of stool per day. The introduction of highly active antiretroviral therapy (HAART) heralded reduced rates of cryptosporidiosis in patients with HIV/AIDS. HAART may also directly inhibit sporozoite development and invasion in the host's cells. Patients with other immune disorders, such as T-cell immune deficiency (severe combined immunodeficiency and CD40 ligand deficiency) or hematologic malignant neoplasms, particularly children, are at higher risk for more severe, prolonged, or extensive disease, with infection occasionally extending to the gallbladder, the pancreatic duct, and even the bronchial tree. Several complications in these patients have been described, including pancreatitis, cholecystitis, sclerosing cholangitis, papillitis, and terminal bile duct stenosis with subsequent biliary cirrhosis.

DIAGNOSIS

The clinical manifestations and physical examination findings in patients with cryptosporidiosis are not unique, and the differential diagnosis should include other causes of infectious gastroenteritis, such as *Giardia*, *Cyclospora*, *Isospora*, microsporidia, *Escherichia coli* pathotypes (enteropathogenic [EPEC], enteroaggregative [EAEC], diffusely adherent [DAEC], enterohemorrhagic [EHEC], enteroinvasive [EIEC], and enterotoxigenic [ETEC]), *Campylobacter*, *Salmonella*, *Shigella*, rotavirus, norovirus, and others. Definitive diagnosis of *Cryptosporidium* enteric infection is made by stool examination. Up to three fecal samples with fixation and concentration before permanent staining or polymerase chain reaction analysis[8,9] may increase detection rates. Oocysts are stained with the acid-fast stain, modified Ziehl-Nielsen stain, fluorescence staining with auramine-phenol, or immunofluorescent stains. Acid-fast staining requires around 500,000 oocysts per gram for detection in formed stools, whereas immunofluorescence is at least 10 times more sensitive, and commercially available enzyme-linked immunoassays have a sensitivity and specificity approaching 100% for *Cryptosporidium*. Polymerase chain reaction testing can detect as few as 50 to 500 oocysts per milliliter of liquid stool and can be used to differentiate or even to quantify *Cryptosporidium* species and genotypes.

TREATMENT Rx

Nitazoxanide has emerged as the only promising candidate for treatment of cryptosporidiosis. It is licensed in the United States for treatment of cryptosporidiosis in nonimmunodeficient children and adults and has reportedly reduced the duration of diarrhea and oocyst shedding in several double-blind, placebo-controlled clinical trials. A clinical trial in Egypt in adults (500 mg twice daily for 3 days) and children (200 mg for 4- to 11-year-olds and 100 mg for 1- to 3-year-olds, twice daily for 3 days) with cryptosporidiosis showed that 80% exhibited resolution of diarrhea versus 41% of the placebo group.[A1] A second clinical trial of a 3-day course of treatment showed resolution of symptoms at 4 days in 96% of the patients receiving nitazoxanide tablets (500 mg twice daily for 3 days) versus only 41% of those receiving placebo tablets.[A2]

Prevention and treatment of cryptosporidiosis in immunocompromised patients have been reviewed; there has been no evidence of a reduction in the duration or frequency of diarrhea with nitazoxanide. However, nitazoxanide has resulted in significantly greater oocyst clearance than has placebo in all children.[A3] In patients with HIV/AIDS, HAART has emerged as the most important therapy to prevent and to reduce the severity and frequency of cryptosporidiosis. Oral rehydration therapy or intravenous fluid replacement for more severe disease is key to preventing dehydration and risk for immediate death.

PREVENTION

Prevention of person-to-person spread should be achieved with personal hygiene guidelines such as frequent handwashing after using or cleaning the toilet, changing diapers, and caring for a person with diarrhea. It is recommended that people with cryptosporidiosis be excluded from the workplace setting until 48 hours after the last diarrheal episode. Handwashing facilities should be available and used at farms to facilitate personal hygiene. Because most outbreaks of cryptosporidiosis are linked to oocysts in source water, routine survey of treated water for this parasite is key to preventing major spread of this disease. Optimization of multibarrier approaches, including chemical treatment and water filtration and treatment systems, is highly recommended. Ultraviolet irradiation and ozone are effective in inactivating *Cryptosporidium* and *Giardia* cysts in water and may prove useful in controlling the transmission of waterborne protozoa.

Grade A References

A1. Rossignol JF, Ayoub A, Ayers MS. Treatment of diarrhea caused by Cryptosporidium parvum: a prospective randomized, double-blind, placebo-controlled study of nitazoxanide. *J Infect Dis.* 2001;184:103-106.

A2. Rossignol JF, Kabil SM, Younis AM, et al. Effect of nitazoxanide in diarrhea and enteritis caused by Cryptosporidium species. *Clin Gastroenterol Hepatol.* 2006;4:320-324.

A3. Abubakar I, Aliyu SH, Arumugam C, et al. Treatment of cryptosporidiosis in immunocompromised individuals: systemic review and meta-analysis. *Br J Clin Pharmacol.* 2007;63:387-393.

GENERAL REFERENCES

For the General References and other additional features, please visit Expert Consult at https://expertconsult.inkling.com.

351

GIARDIASIS

THEODORE E. NASH AND DAVID R. HILL

DEFINITION

Giardia lamblia (*Giardia duodenalis*, *Giardia intestinalis*) is a ubiquitous, small intestinal protozoan parasite of humans and other mammals. It is the most common parasitic infection of the gastrointestinal tract in the United States as well as worldwide and is responsible for outbreaks of diarrhea and sporadic endemic disease.[1,2]

The Pathogen

Giardia has a simple life cycle. The trophozoite, which is 9 to 21 μm long, 5 to 15 μm wide, and 2 to 4 μm thick (Fig. 351-1), resides in the small intestine and is responsible for manifestations of disease. It has four pairs of flagella, two nuclei, and a ventral sucking disc by which it may adhere to intestinal epithelial cells. The dorsal surface is pear shaped and bilaterally symmetrical, with the two highly characteristic nuclei best visualized after staining. In the lower small intestine, the trophozoite develops into an environmentally resistant cyst. Detection of soluble cyst wall proteins in the feces forms the basis of many stool antigen assays.

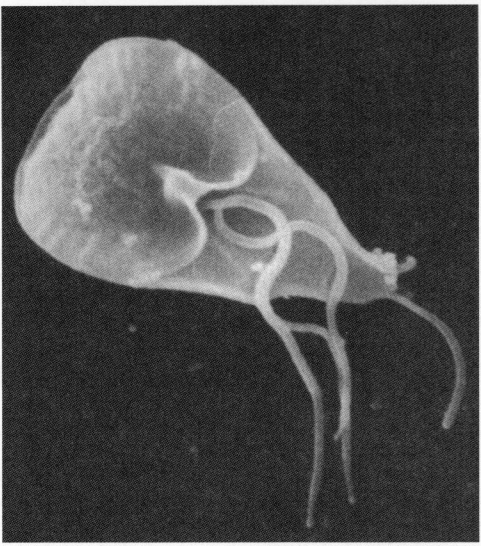

FIGURE 351-1. *Giardia lamblia.* This scanning electron micrograph reveals some of the external ultrastructural details displayed by a flagellated *G. lamblia* protozoan parasite.

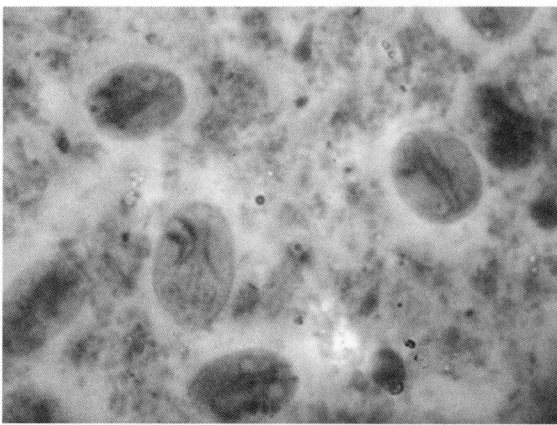

FIGURE 351-2. Iron hematoxylin stain of *Giardia lamblia* cysts from stool.

Excreted cysts are mature and infectious. They are oval and about 8 to 12 μm in length and 7 to 10 μm in width (Fig. 351-2). After ingestion and exposure to acid and proteases in the stomach and intestines, they excyst in the small intestine, yielding two trophozoites from each cyst, which quickly divide again. In vitro trophozoites double in number every 6 hours for the fastest growing isolates.

A number of morphologically identical but genetically distinct *Giardia* infect humans and animals that are now divided into eight assemblages. Humans and some animals are infected with either assemblage A or B. These two assemblages are genetically and biologically diverse and appear to be two separate species.[3]

Giardia is well adapted to its existence as a parasite. It has two equal functioning nuclei and lacks mitochondria and peroxisomes. It has a simplified metabolism and is dependent on the host for nutrients such as purines, pyrimidines, cysteine, and cholesterol. The WB isolate, assemblage A, has a compact genome (11.7 Mb) with unusually short promoters. The parasite's rigid cytoskeleton is composed of unique families of structural proteins and carbohydrates.

Giardia is the only bowel-dwelling parasite that undergoes antigenic variation. Only one of a family of about 250 variant-specific proteins (VSPs) is expressed on the surface of the trophozoite at a time.[4] Both immune and biologic selection of trophozoites that express specific VSPs occurs in humans and animals with giardiasis. Expressed VSPs must be compatible with the host's intestinal environment and are probably not recognized by the host's immune system because antibodies to VSPs are inhibitory or cytotoxic. Whereas all VSPs are transcribed, all but one of the transcripts are eliminated by RNA interference–based mechanisms, resulting in expression of a single VSP surface protein.[5] Exactly how selection and switching occur is unclear.

EPIDEMIOLOGY

Giardia is among the most common parasitic infections of humans; it is highly infectious, and cysts are frequently excreted in large numbers (as high as 10^7 cysts per gram of feces), especially in young children. Cysts can survive for months in cold water, are relatively resistant to chlorination, but are intolerant of desiccation and heat in comparison to the relatively resistant ova of cryptosporidia and helminths. Experimentally, between 10 and 100 cysts is sufficient to establish infection 100% of the time. Consequently, ingestion of water or food that contains small levels of contamination can result in infection. Approximately 20,000 infections are reported annually in the United States, but because of underreporting, actual infections are estimated at more than 100,000 cases per year.

Infections are most common in young children and are more frequent in summer and fall months. Giardiasis is acquired after ingestion of contaminated water or food or through person-to-person contact. In past decades, large outbreaks in high-income countries such as the United States occurred after ingestion of contaminated drinking water obtained from surface sources such as reservoirs, lakes, and mountain streams. However, with improved water treatment measures, ingestion of contaminated recreational water from pools or lakes is now a more common source of outbreaks. Backpackers who ingest untreated surface water remain at risk of infection.

Although outbreaks from contaminated food or infected food handlers are well described, they are not often documented. Worldwide, person-to-person transmission may be the most frequent mode of infection and is the primary way children are infected in daycare centers, where infection can be common. Person-to-person spread occurs among family members with infected children and following sexual practices that lead to fecal-oral contact.[6] In low-income, highly endemic regions, almost all children are infected by 2 to 3 years of age. Although partial immunity can develop in previously exposed adults, reinfection of children after treatment is common in highly endemic regions. Longer-term travel, particularly to south Asia, increases the risk of giardiasis. For the returned traveler with persistent diarrhea, giardiasis should be ruled out.

The understanding of immunity in humans is based mostly on animal models that have limited applicability to human infection and disease. In addition, some of the findings are conflicting. In the classic human experimental infections reported by Rendtorff and colleagues in the 1950s, self-cure occurred in about 84% of the persons. In a more recent experimental human challenge study, in which the infecting parasite was well characterized and the inoculum known, rechallenge with the same isolate after treatment resulted in brief, asymptomatic infections in two persons, suggesting development of partial immunity. Humans with hypogammaglobulinemia are susceptible to *Giardia* and have more severe disease that is resistant to treatment. Studies in animals support a major role of intestinal antibodies (particularly IgA) in protective immunity and an essential role of T-cell immunity in the control of *G. lamblia* infection.

Giardia infections are neither more severe nor more common in most other immunosuppressed states and in persons with selective IgA deficiency. Even though most human immunodeficiency virus–infected patients respond to usual treatment, a subset develop recurrent or repeated infections that are difficult to treat.

PATHOBIOLOGY

Giardia infections involve complex interactions between host and parasite. The two assemblages (A and B) that infect humans are composed of genetically distinguishable isolates, which may vary in infectivity, antigenicity, and virulence. In addition, human hosts vary in susceptibility to infection and disease and in the response or tolerance to infection. Pathogenic mechanisms need to explain the varied clinical manifestations as well as the contrasting situation in which there are high rates of infection and disease seen in waterborne outbreaks of giardiasis in regions where infections are sporadic, like in the United States, compared with the large number of asymptomatic infections in children in low-income regions. In addition, infection with *Giardia* can lead to malabsorption, weight loss, and nutritional deficiencies in some settings and little effect on nutritional parameters in other settings.

Giardia is strictly an intraluminal parasite that adheres to the epithelium by way of an adhesive or sucking disc. Invasion of the epithelium either does not occur or is rare. The number of trophozoites in the intestine can be so large that adherent organisms cover much of the epithelial surface. This could disrupt the epithelial brush border and contribute to disaccharidase deficiency seen in some patients. A number of studies demonstrate direct epithelial cell barrier dysfunction in vitro and in vivo in humans. Exactly how this occurs is not known. There is no evidence of production of a classic enterotoxin, although it is possible that secreted or surface proteins may be injurious to cells. Of patients with persistent giardiasis after treatment, nearly half exhibited inflammation on small bowel biopsy specimens, supporting the view that chronic inflammatory responses contribute to disease at least in this subset.

CLINICAL MANIFESTATIONS

The clinical manifestations, course, and duration of *Giardia* infections are variable. Infections may be self-limited or persistent, asymptomatic or symptomatic. In general, patients are not as sick as those with bacterial diarrheas. Acute disease manifestations occur commonly in travelers and in outbreaks and are characterized by diarrhea, nausea, anorexia, dehydration, flatulence, eructation, foul-smelling stools, distention, abdominal cramping, and weight loss. Malabsorption is more commonly seen in chronic infection. Fever and vomiting are uncommon. Blood, mucus, and polymorphonuclear cells in the stool, which are not usual features of small bowel infections, should suggest an alternative or additional diagnosis. Dehydration, although uncommon, may be severe and require hospitalization; hospitalization for giardiasis has occurred in the United States with a frequency similar to that for shigellosis. On occasion, nausea and vomiting will predominate and suggest other causes.

In experimental infections using inoculated cysts, presence of cysts in the stool occurred 6 to 15 days (mean, 9 days) after inoculation. In more recent experimental infections, *Giardia* antigen was detected 1 day before cyst excretion. In one well-documented food-borne outbreak, 74% became ill, with an incubation period of 2 to 19 days and peak symptoms at 5 to 6 days. Symptoms continued for a median of 18 days.

Acute symptoms can resolve, wax and wane, or settle into a chronic phase, which can be prolonged and last weeks to months. Long-lasting symptoms should indicate a search for the parasite. Lactose deficiency is common and can persist for some weeks after treatment, and it needs to be distinguished in symptomatic patients from relapse or reinfection. In extreme cases, malabsorption and weight loss are severe and mimic sprue. Infants and children are particularly susceptible to infection and disease, which can result in growth failure that is reversed on successful treatment.

A typical scenario is a mildly to moderately ill person who complains of an increased number of urgent loose stools, with flatus, cramping, anorexia, and weight loss. There may be periods when the person feels better only to relapse and become noticeably worse. After days to several weeks, the individual will seek medical help. Similar to other causes of infectious diarrhea, symptoms can continue after successful treatment and evolve into irritable bowel syndrome (Chapter 136).[7] Uncommonly, *Giardia* is found in biliary and pancreatic ducts and can cause cholecystitis and pancreatitis. Extraintestinal manifestations and long-term consequences are usually uncommon, but a series of sporadic cases documented them in a third of the patients.[8] The manifestations can include rash, reactive arthritis, eye complaints, and cognitive deficiencies.[9]

Disease and symptoms caused by *Giardia* in children in low-income regions are variably present despite almost universal infection by the age of 3 years and frequent reinfection with prevalence rates that are commonly above 20%. Although there are convincing studies showing detrimental growth and nutritional effects in some populations, other studies show little or no effects. An analysis of published studies indicated that persistent diarrhea as a result of infection with *Giardia* is a cause of malnutrition.[10] The reasons for these disparate results may be due to differences in the populations, such as prior exposures, maternal factors, nutritional status, and diet, or variability in the organism, including the genetics of the isolate (e.g., assemblage type) and properties of the expressed VSP. In contrast, *Giardia*-naïve visitors frequently develop symptomatic giardiasis while visiting or working in highly endemic regions, in contrast to a mostly asymptomatic population, suggesting that the endemic population has developed an accommodation to the disease. Some studies suggest giardiasis protects against other acute diarrhea episodes.[11]

DIAGNOSIS

The diagnosis of giardiasis is based on detection of cysts, trophozoites, or, more recently, parasite-specific antigens in fecal samples. Polymerase chain reaction has been largely experimental but is being increasingly used in field and laboratory settings. Polymerase chain reaction is sensitive and specific and can determine the infecting assemblages.[12] Because excretion of cysts may be variable or in low concentrations, a single examination for ova and parasites is only 50 to 80% sensitive, and two or three examinations may be necessary. Stool antigen tests are standard in most laboratories and are highly sensitive (>90%), specific (close to 100%), and relatively inexpensive and do not require a trained microscopist. Examination of small intestine biopsy specimens or intestinal contents for trophozoites was the previous "gold standard" for diagnosis but is now uncommonly needed to establish or to confirm the diagnosis. In low-intensity infections, all testing methods can be falsely negative and require repeated testing.

The laboratory findings are nonspecific. The white blood cell count and liver function test results are usually normal. Electrolyte disturbances can be present if diarrhea and vomiting are severe. White blood cells, lactoferrin, blood, and mucus are not found in the stool. Immunoglobulin levels are usually normal but abnormally low or absent in susceptible hypogammaglobulinemic individuals.

TREATMENT   Rx

Details of antiparasitic therapy in general are provided in Chapter 344. Tinidazole (Tindamax), a Food and Drug Administration (FDA)–approved nitroimidazole drug similar to metronidazole (Flagyl), has been the treatment of choice[A1][A2]; other nitroimidazoles (e.g., ornidazole and secnidazole) that are not approved in the United States are also effective. Tinidazole is given as a single dose, and compared with metronidazole, it has fewer side effects and greater efficacy. In adults, the dose is 2 g orally; in children, the dose is 50 mg/kg as a single dose with a maximum of 2 g. Metronidazole has been used to treat giardiasis for decades but has never been approved by the FDA for this indication; it requires multiple dosing at 250 mg orally three times a day for 5 to 7 days for adults and 15 mg/kg/day in three divided doses for 5 to 7 days for children. Gastrointestinal side effects of metronidazole are relatively common, and alcohol should not be taken concomitantly because of the possibility of a disulfiram reaction with both drugs. A meta-analysis indicated that albendazole (400 mg/day for 5 days), not presently approved by the FDA for treatment of giardiasis, has efficacy similar to that of metronidazole and fewer side effects.[A3] However, many studies test for efficacy shortly after therapy is stopped, so recurrent infection cannot be adequately determined, and there is only limited experience with albendazole. Nitazoxanide is a drug with broad activity against protozoa, helminths, and bacteria and is FDA approved for the treatment of giardiasis. It is given at a dose of 100 mg orally every 12 hours for 3 days for children aged 12 months to 3 years, 200 mg orally every 12 hours for 3 days for children 4 to 11 years of age, and 500 mg orally every 12 hours for 3 days for persons older than 12 years. Because it is available in a liquid suspension as well as in a 500-mg tablet, it may be easier to give to young children. It should be given with food. Most of the side effects are gastrointestinal symptoms and headache.

Paromomycin, a nonabsorbable aminoglycoside, has activity against *Giardia* and has been used in pregnant women to avoid the theoretical fetal adverse events of nitroimidazoles, particularly during the first trimester. It is given to adults at 500 mg three times a day for 5 to 10 days and to children at 25 to 35 mg/kg/day orally in three divided doses for 5 to 10 days. Quinacrine and furazolidone (FDA approved but not usually available) are also active against *Giardia* but should be reserved for use in particular situations.

Patients usually experience relief of symptoms on treatment. Failure of treatment is frequently heralded by a return of symptoms days to weeks after cessation of therapy and requires either re-treatment with an alternative class of drug or an increased dosing of the initial therapy. Clinically resistant cases usually respond to combination treatment; quinacrine and metronidazole have been most effective, with metronidazole plus albendazole also showing efficacy.[13]

PREVENTION

Infection is prevented by scrupulous personal hygiene, proper disposal of sewage, removal or killing of cysts from water supplies, and preventing contamination of food and water. Cysts are relatively labile and are susceptible to heating and filtration with small water volume filters of 0.2 to 1 μm. Heating (bringing water to a boil) is preferred because other pathogens found in feces are also inactivated. Cysts are not reliably susceptible to chlorination because the concentrations of chlorine, water temperatures, turbidity, and pH present when treating commercial water supplies are suboptimal. Four drops of 5.25% bleach to 1 liter for 1 hour at room temperature is sufficient for killing. At lower temperatures, inactivation may not be complete.

Grade A References

A1. Escobedo AA, Alvarez G, Gonzalez ME, et al. The treatment of giardiasis in children: single-dose tinidazole compared with 3 days of nitazoxanide. *Ann Trop Med Parasitol.* 2008;102:199-207.
A2. Pasupulet V, Escobedo AA, Despande A, et al. Efficacy of 5-nitroimidazoles for the treatment of giardiasis: a systematic review of randomized controlled trials. *PLoS Negl Trop Dis.* 2014;8:e2733.
A3. Solaymani-Mohammadi S, Genkinger JM, Loffredo CA, et al. A meta-analysis of the effectiveness of albendazole compared with metronidazole as treatments for infections with *Giardia duodenalis.* *PLoS Negl Trop Dis.* 2010;4:e682.

GENERAL REFERENCES

For the General References and other additional features, please visit Expert Consult at https://expertconsult.inkling.com.

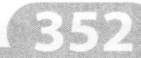

AMEBIASIS

WILLIAM A. PETRI, JR. AND ALDO A.M. LIMA

DEFINITION

Amebiasis is due to infection with the enteric protozoan parasite *Entamoeba histolytica*. Amebiasis can cause asymptomatic colonization, diarrhea, dysentery, and colitis as well as spread extraintestinally to cause liver and rarely brain abscess (Fig. 352-1).

The Pathogen

E. histolytica has a low infectious dose (<100 organisms), is resistant to chlorine, and is environmentally stable. These properties make it a threat to food and water supplies, as the 1998 municipal water outbreak of amebic liver abscess in Tbilisi, Georgia, demonstrated. Its tissue-destructive properties are the reason for the parasite's being named *histolytica*.

EPIDEMIOLOGY

Most *E. histolytica* infections occur in the developing world, including the Indian subcontinent, Southeast Asia, sub-Saharan Africa, and Central and South America, as a result of fecal-oral transmission. A national serologic survey in Mexico demonstrated antibody to *E. histolytica* in 8.4% of the population. In an urban slum of Fortaleza, Brazil, 25% of the population tested carried antibody to *E. histolytica*, and the prevalence in children 6 to 14 years of age was 40%. In Dhaka, Bangladesh, where diarrheal diseases are the leading cause of childhood death, the annual incidence of *E. histolytica* infection in a cohort of preschool children was 40%. The annual incidence of amebic liver abscess was 21 cases per 100,000 inhabitants in Hue City, Vietnam. The best current estimate by the World Health Organization is that *E. histolytica* infection results in 34 to 50 million symptomatic cases each year worldwide and as many as 100,000 deaths.

In the United States, amebiasis is the third most common parasitic infection after giardiasis and cryptosporidiosis (1.2 cases/100,000 U.S. population). Most cases in industrialized countries occur in travelers to and immigrants from endemic regions as well as in institutionalized individuals. In returning travelers, diarrhea is the predominant reason for a patient to visit a physician, and amebiasis is the second most common cause of diarrhea in returning travelers. Previously reported high rates of *E. histolytica* infection in homosexual men in the United States actually reflect a high prevalence of *Entamoeba dispar* infection in this population. In contrast, in Asia, amebiasis is more frequently an initial symptom of human immunodeficiency virus (HIV) infection and acquired immunodeficiency syndrome because of the common risk for acquisition of both HIV infection and amebiasis through the sexual practices of men who have sex with men. The typical patient with an amebic liver abscess in the United States is a 20- to 40-year-old Hispanic male immigrant. Several groups are at increased risk for severe amebiasis, including the very young or old, malnourished persons, pregnant women, and patients treated with corticosteroids.

PATHOBIOLOGY

Killing of host cells is required for invasion of the intestine by the parasite. The process of host cell destruction has been experimentally separated into sequential steps of adherence, contact-dependent cytotoxicity, followed finally by phagocytosis of the host cell corpse. The initial contact of parasite to host is mediated by the parasite's galactose and *N*-acetyl-D-galactosamine (Gal/GalNAc)–specific lectin, which binds to carbohydrate determinants on the host's intestinal epithelium. Human cells die by apoptosis induced by *E. histolytica*, a process that requires attachment of the Gal/GalNAc lectin to a host cell's receptor, as well as the parasite's acid intracellular vesicles, which may serve as delivery vehicles for an amebic pore-forming protein. *E. histolytica* initiates apoptosis in host cells by directly activating the host cell's distal apoptotic machinery; caspase 3 is activated within minutes of *E. histolytica* adherence, a caspase 3 inhibitor blocks *E. histolytica* killing, and caspase 3–deficient or bcl-2–overexpressing mice are resistant to amebic infection. Recognition and ingestion of the apoptotic host cell's corpse are required for colonic infection by the parasite, and multiple ligands and receptors are involved, including the Gal/GalNAc lectin, a phosphatidylserine receptor, serine-rich *E. histolytica* protein, and collectins. After ingestion of the corpse of the host cell, additional parasitic factors participate in invasion into the intestinal mucosa. For example, *E. histolytica* encodes at least 44 cysteine proteinase genes that have been implicated in degradation of colonic mucin glycoproteins; digestion of extracellular matrix, hemoglobin, and villin; and inactivation of interleukin-18 (IL-18).

The innate immune response to amebic infection includes activation of the alternative complement pathway, with C3a and C5a recruiting neutrophils to the site of infection but with amebae resisting killing by the membrane attack complex through the Gal/GalNAc lectin. In the murine model of intestinal amebiasis, innate resistance is conferred by nonhematopoietic cells, thus suggesting importance of the epithelial production of cytokines such as tumor necrosis factor-α (TNF-α), IL-1α, IL-6, IL-8, growth-related oncogene-α (GROα), and granulocyte-macrophage colony-stimulating factor. Neutrophils are the earliest innate cellular immune response (within 1 to 2 days) for both intestinal and hepatic amebiasis. Depletion of neutrophils with anti–Gr-1 neutralizing antibody in a murine model results in exacerbated amebic hepatic and intestinal disease. Macrophages and T lymphocytes are also recruited by day 3 of an infection. Macrophages acquire amebicidal activity after in vitro stimulation with interferon-γ (IFN-γ), TNF-α, or colony-stimulating factor 1. Natural killer cells may be important in part as a source of IFN-γ, as well as infiltrating mast cells for their ability to contribute to the innate immune response by the production of IL-6 and TNF-α.

The acquired immune response reflects the opposing roles of IL-4 and IFN-γ in persistence and clearance of amebic infection, respectively. Inbred mice of the CBA strain are susceptible to intestinal amebiasis and develop a rapid T_H2 phenotypic immune response, and this response is deleterious insofar as inhibition of IL-4 can convert the response to a healing IFN-γ response. Effective acquired immunity in humans is associated with both a systemic IFN-γ and a mucosal IgA response directed at the Gal/GalNAc lectin. Children with mucosal IgA against the Gal/GalNAc lectin were found to have 86% fewer new *E. histolytica* infections in the following year. Similarly, the risk for amebiasis was 50% lower in children who were in the 50th percentile and above for the production of IFN-γ by peripheral blood mononuclear cells stimulated with soluble amebic antigen. In contrast, there is an association between higher TNF-α production and *E. histolytica* diarrhea,[1] thus indicating that there is a fine line between a pro-inflammatory cellular immune response that is protective and one that is disease enhancing.

CLINICAL MANIFESTATIONS

Asymptomatic Intraluminal Amebiasis

The asymptomatic cyst-passing carrier state is the most common type of amebic infection. All *Entamoeba moshkovskii* and *E. dispar* infections and as many as 80% of *E. histolytica* infections are asymptomatic. Asymptomatically infected individuals represent a risk to the community because they are a source of new infections and a risk to themselves because 1 in 10 to 20 colonized individuals progress to symptomatic infection. The host has a bearing on whether infection is asymptomatic in that children heterozygous for the HLA class II DQB1*0601/DRB1*1501 haplotype have been found to be protected from symptomatic infection with amebiasis. In addition, certain genotypes of *E. histolytica* appear to be associated with the propensity for colonization as opposed to invasion.

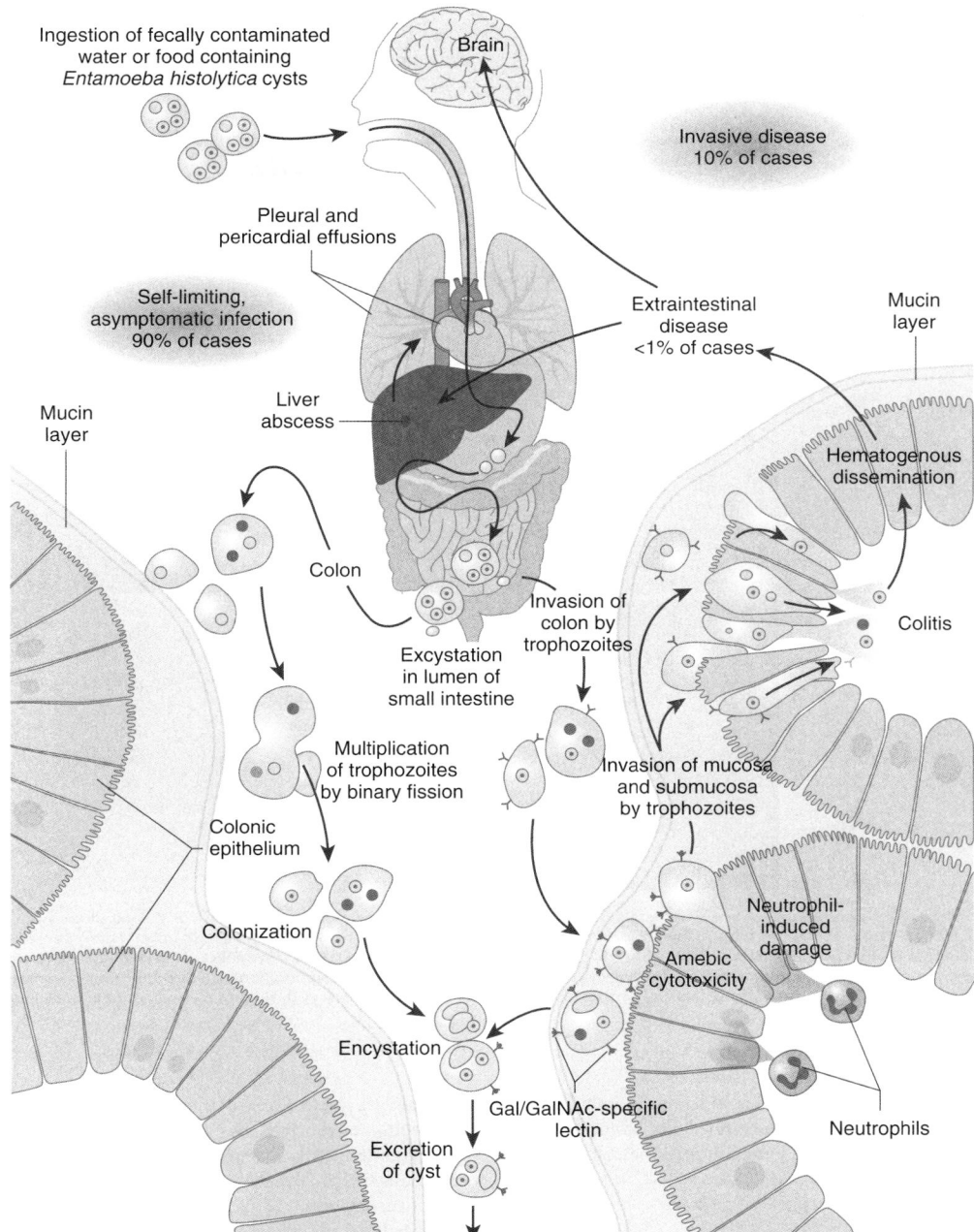

FIGURE 352-1. Life cycle of *Entamoeba histolytica*. Infection is normally initiated by the ingestion of fecally contaminated water or food containing *E. histolytica* cysts. The infective cyst form of the parasite survives passage through the stomach and small intestine. Excystation occurs in the bowel lumen, where motile and potentially invasive trophozoites are formed. In most infections, the trophozoites aggregate in the intestinal mucin layer and form new cysts, which results in a self-limited and asymptomatic infection. In some cases, however, adherence to and lysis of the colonic epithelium, mediated by the galactose and *N*-acetyl-D-galactosamine (Gal/GalNAc)–specific lectin, initiates invasion of the colon by trophozoites. Neutrophils responding to the invasion contribute to cellular protection at the site of invasion. Once the intestinal epithelium is invaded, extraintestinal spread to the peritoneum, liver, and other sites may follow. Factors controlling invasion, as opposed to encystation, probably include parasitic "quorum sensing" signaled by the Gal/GalNAc-specific lectin, interactions of amebae with the bacterial flora of the intestine, and innate and acquired immune responses of the host. (Redrawn with permission from Haque R, Huston CD, Hughes M, et al. Current concepts: amebiasis. *N Engl J Med.* 2003;348:1565-1573.)

Amebic Diarrhea

Amebic diarrhea without dysentery is the most common amebic disease. It is defined as diarrhea in an *E. histolytica*–infected individual. There is no requirement for the presence of mucus or visible or microscopic blood in stool for the diagnosis of amebic diarrhea. In one community-based study of a cohort of preschool children in Bangladesh, the annual incidence of amebic infection, diarrhea, and dysentery was 45%, 9%, and 3%, respectively. The mean duration of amebic diarrhea was 3 days in one study. It causes approximately 2% of cases of diarrhea severe enough to warrant hospital evaluation in developing countries such as Bangladesh.

Amebic Dysentery or Colitis

Diarrhea with mucus or visible or microscopic blood in a patient with *E. histolytica* infection is the definition of amebic dysentery or colitis. Approximately 15 to 33% of patients with *E. histolytica* diarrhea also have amebic dysentery. The onset of symptoms is typically gradual during a period of 3 or 4 weeks after infection, with abdominal tenderness and increasingly severe diarrhea being the primary complaints. Patients with bacterial causes of dysentery usually have only 1 or 2 days of symptoms. Surprisingly, fever is present in only a minority of patients with amebic colitis. In young children, intussusception, perforation, peritonitis, or necrotizing colitis may develop

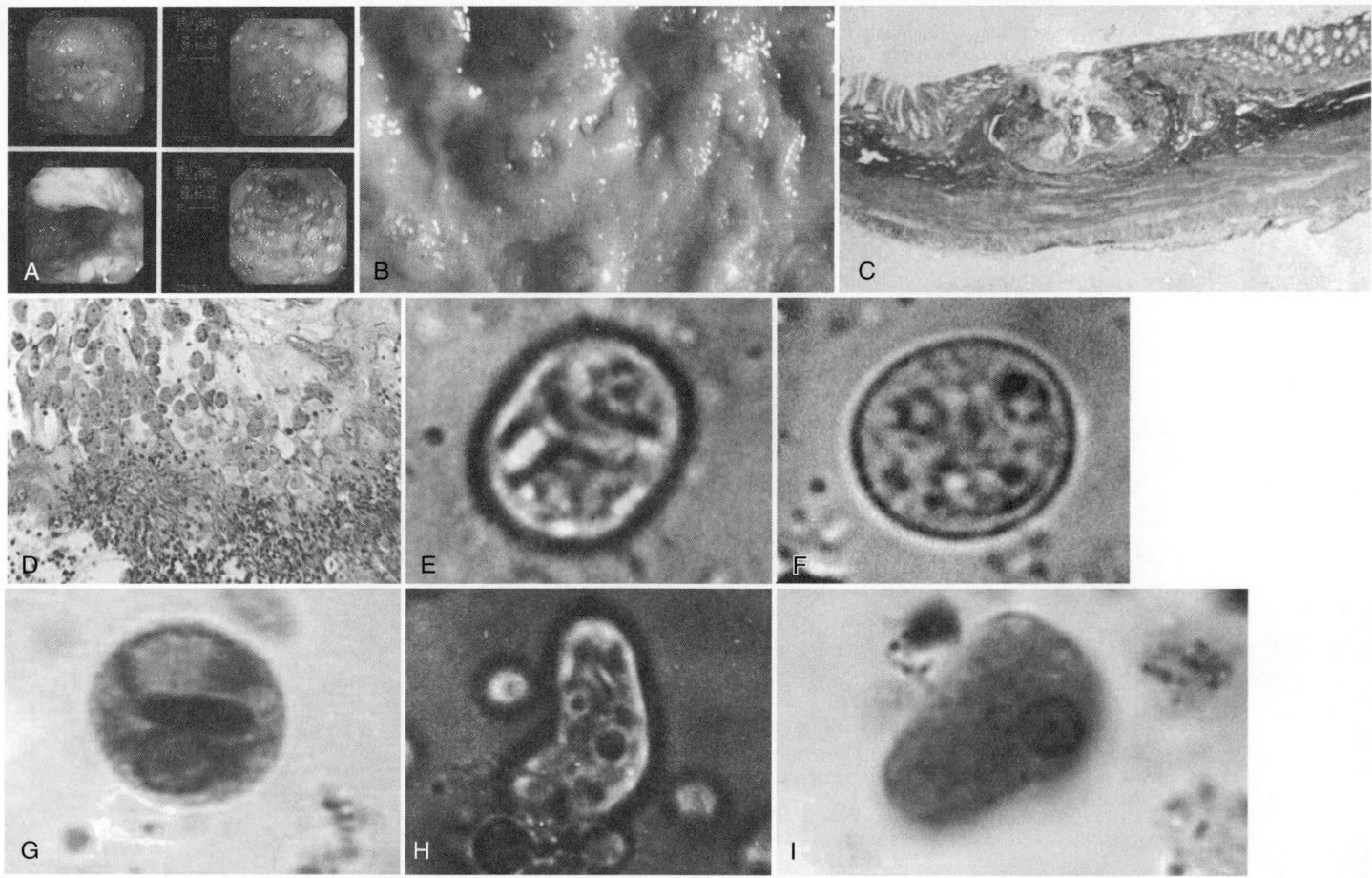

FIGURE 352-2. Endoscopic and pathologic features of intestinal amebiasis. **A,** Colonoscopic appearance of intestinal amebiasis. **B,** Colonic ulcers averaging 1 to 2 mm in diameter on gross pathologic examination. **C,** Cross section of a flask-shaped colonic ulcer (hematoxylin-eosin stain, magnification ×20). **D,** Inflammatory response to intestinal invasion by *Entamoeba histolytica* (hematoxylin-eosin stain, magnification ×100). **E** and **F,** *E. histolytica* cysts in a saline preparation (magnification ×1000). **G,** Iodine-stained cyst from stool (magnification ×1000). **H,** *E. histolytica* trophozoite with an ingested erythrocyte in a saline preparation from stool (magnification ×1000). **I,** Trophozoite from stool stained with trichrome (magnification ×1000). (B-D from the slide collection of the late Dr. Harrison Juniper.) (From Haque R, Huston CD, Hughes M, et al. Current concepts: amebiasis. *N Engl J Med.* 2003;348:1565-1573.)

rapidly (Fig. 352-2). Unusual manifestations of amebic colitis include toxic megacolon (0.5% of cases, usually requiring surgical intervention) and ameboma (granulation tissue in the colonic lumen mimicking colon cancer in appearance).[2]

Amebic Liver Abscess

Amebic liver abscess is 10 times as common in men as in women and is unusual in children. The typical patient with an amebic liver abscess in the United States is an immigrant from an endemic area, a man aged 20 to 40 years with fever, right upper quadrant pain, leukocytosis, abnormal serum transaminase and alkaline phosphatase levels, and a defect seen on hepatic imaging studies.[3] Most patients have 2 to 4 weeks of prior fever, cough, and abdominal pain in the right upper quadrant or epigastrium. Involvement of the diaphragmatic surface of the liver may lead to right-sided pleural pain or referred shoulder pain and an elevated right hemidiaphragm seen on chest radiography (Fig. 352-3). Hepatomegaly with point tenderness over the liver, below the ribs, or in the intercostal spaces is a typical finding.

If a space-filling defect in the liver is observed, the differential diagnosis includes (1) amebiasis (most common in men with a history of travel to or residence in a developing country), (2) pyogenic or bacterial abscess (particularly suspected in women, patients with cholecystitis, the elderly, individuals with diabetes, and patients with jaundice), (3) echinococcal abscess (which would be an incidental finding because echinococcal abscess should not cause pain or fever), and (4) cancer. Most patients with amebic liver abscess will have detectable circulating antigen in serum as well as serum antiamebic antibodies.

In children, abdominal pain is reported infrequently with amebic liver abscess. More commonly, high fever, abdominal distention, irritability, and

tachypnea are noted. Some of these children are admitted to the hospital with fever of unknown origin. Hepatomegaly occurs frequently, but elicitation of hepatic tenderness is not well documented. In one report, four of five children younger than 5 years died of amebic liver abscess because the diagnosis was not suspected.

Unusual extraintestinal manifestations of amebiasis include direct extension of the liver abscess to the pleura or pericardium and brain abscess. Death usually results from rupture of the liver abscess into the peritoneum, thorax, or pericardium, but it may also be caused by extensive hepatic damage and liver failure.

Other Extraintestinal Infections

Thoracic amebiasis is the most common type of extra-abdominal amebiasis after liver abscess and occurs in about 10% of patients with amebic liver abscess. It develops by direct extension from the liver. Pericardial amebiasis is the next most common form of extraintestinal involvement and may result from rupture of a liver abscess in the left lobe of the liver into the pericardium or from extension of the right-sided pleural amebiasis. Cerebral amebic abscesses have been found in about 0.5 to 5% of patients with amebic liver abscess. In one series of 18 patients with proven cerebral amebiasis, findings on the initial neurologic examination were normal in 13. Other foci of infection are rare, but amebic rectovesical fistula formation and involvement of the pharynx, heart, aorta, and scapula have been reported. Cutaneous infection may arise from trophozoites emerging from the rectum.

DIAGNOSIS

Diagnosis of amebiasis is best accomplished by the combination of serology and identification of the parasite in feces or at extraintestinal sites of invasion

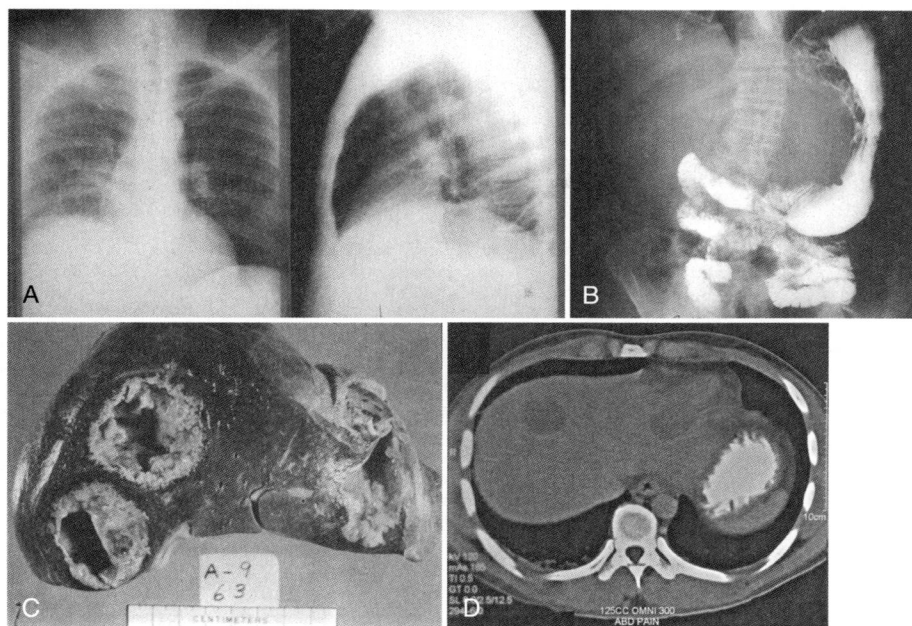

FIGURE 352-3. Radiographic and pathologic features of extraintestinal amebiasis. **A,** Left posteroanterior and right lateral chest radiographs in a patient with amebic liver abscess. The findings include an elevated right hemidiaphragm and evidence of atelectasis. **B,** Luminal narrowing revealed by barium enema examination in a patient with an ameboma. **C,** Two abscesses in the right lobe and one abscess in the left lobe of a patient with amebic liver abscess. **D,** Abdominal computed tomography showing one abscess in the right lobe and one abscess in the left lobe in a patient with amebic liver abscess. (From Haque R, Huston CD, Hughes M, et al. Current concepts: amebiasis. *N Engl J Med.* 2003;348:1565-1573.)

TABLE 352-1 SENSITIVITY OF TESTS FOR DIAGNOSIS OF AMEBIASIS

TEST	COLITIS	LIVER ABSCESS
Microscopy: stool	25-60%	10-40%
Stool antigen detection	80%	≈40%
Serum antigen detection	65%	>95%
Microscopy: abscess fluid	N/A	≤20%
Real-time PCR	>95%	>95%
Serologic testing (indirect hemagglutination)		
Acute	70%	70-80%
Convalescent	>90%	>90%

N/A = not available; PCR = polymerase chain reaction.
Modified from Haque R, Huston CD, Hughes M, et al. Current concepts: amebiasis. *N Engl J Med.* 2003;348:1565-1573.

(such as pus obtained by fine needle aspiration of a liver abscess).[4] Examination of stool for ova and parasites should *not* be used to diagnose amebiasis (Table 352-1). The most sensitive diagnostic approach is the combined use of *E. histolytica*–specific antigen detection or polymerase chain reaction plus serology.

TREATMENT   Rx
(also see Chapter 344)

Therapy for invasive infection differs from that for noninvasive infection, which may be treated with paromomycin (Table 352-2). Invasive infections require treatment with nitroimidazoles, particularly metronidazole, tinidazole, secnidazole, or ornidazole. For amebic colitis, tinidazole reduces treatment failure rates and adverse effects compared with metronidazole.[A1] In the rare case of fulminant amebic colitis, it is prudent to add broad-spectrum antibiotics to treat intestinal bacteria that may spill into the peritoneum. Parasites persist in up to half of the patients who are treated with a nitroimidazole, so treatment should be followed with paromomycin or the second-line agent

TABLE 352-2 DRUG THERAPY FOR TREATMENT OF AMEBIASIS

DRUG	ADULT DOSAGE	SIDE EFFECTS
AMEBIC LIVER ABSCESS		
Metronidazole	750 mg PO tid × 10 days	Primarily GI side effects: anorexia, nausea, vomiting, diarrhea, abdominal discomfort, or unpleasant metallic taste Disulfiram-like intolerance reaction to alcoholic beverages Neurotoxicity, including seizures, peripheral neuropathy, dizziness, confusion, irritability
or		
Tinidazole	2 g PO once daily × 5 days	Primarily GI side effects and disulfiram-like intolerance reaction to alcoholic beverages as for metronidazole
Followed by a luminal agent		
Paromomycin	30 mg/kg/day PO in 3 divided doses per day × 5-10 days	Primarily GI side effects: diarrhea, GI upset
or		
Diloxanide furoate	500 mg PO tid × 10 days	Primarily GI side effects: flatulence, nausea, vomiting Pruritus, urticaria
AMEBIC COLITIS		
Metronidazole	750 mg PO tid × 5-10 days	Same as for amebic liver abscess
Plus a luminal agent (same as for amebic liver abscess)		
ASYMPTOMATIC INTESTINAL COLONIZATION		
Treatment with a luminal agent as for amebic liver abscess		

GI = gastrointestinal.
Modified from Haque R, Huston CD, Hughes M, et al. Current concepts: amebiasis. *N Engl J Med.* 2003;348:1565-1573.

TABLE 352-3　FREE-LIVING AMEBAE

ORGANISM	DISEASE	EPIDEMIOLOGY	DIAGNOSIS	CLINICAL COURSE	THERAPY
Naegleria fowleri	Primary amebic encephalitis	Warm freshwater exposure	CSF wet mount for ameba, PCR	Death within 1-2 weeks of onset	Amphotericin B
Acanthamoeba spp	Keratitis	Corneal trauma, usually from contact lens	Corneal scraping for amebae and cysts	Subacute	Polyhexamethylene biguanide, chlorhexidine, propamidine, hexamidine
Acanthamoeba spp	Granulomatous amebic encephalitis	Immunodeficient (organ transplants, HIV/AIDS)	Biopsy of brain or skin abscess—IFA or PCR	Subacute	Combination therapy with pentamidine, an azole (fluconazole or itraconazole), flucytosine, and sulfadiazine
Balamuthia mandrillaris	Granulomatous amebic encephalitis	Immunodeficient but also immunocompetent	Biopsy of brain	Subacute	Combination therapy with flucytosine, pentamidine, fluconazole, and sulfadiazine plus either azithromycin or clarithromycin
Sappinia	Amebic encephalitis	Single patient was not immunodeficient			Azithromycin, pentamidine, itraconazole, flucytosine

AIDS = acquired immunodeficiency syndrome; CSF = cerebrospinal fluid; HIV = human immunodeficiency virus; IFA = indirect fluorescent antibody; PCR = polymerase chain reaction.
Modified from Visvesvara GS, Moura H, Schuster FL. Pathogenic and opportunistic free-living amoebae: *Acanthamoeba* spp, *Balamuthia mandrillaris*, *Naegleria fowleri*, and *Sappinia diploidea*. *FEMS Immunol Med Microbiol.* 2007;50:1-26.

diloxanide furoate to cure luminal infection. High-throughput drug screening has identified auranofin, a Food and Drug Administration–approved drug used for treatment of rheumatoid arthritis, as a potentially active agent against *E. histolytica*. Drainage of a liver abscess should be considered in patients who do not show a clinical response to drug therapy within 5 to 7 days or in those with a high risk for rupture of the abscess, as defined by a cavity with a diameter of greater than 5 cm or by the presence of lesions in the left lobe. Percutaneous needle aspiration or catheter drainage is the procedure of choice for drainage of a liver abscess. Surgical intervention is occasionally required for drainage of a liver abscess, acute abdomen, gastrointestinal bleeding, or toxic megacolon.

PREVENTION

The feasibility of prevention by vaccination with the parasite's Gal/GalNAc lectin is supported by substantial data from human, animal model, and in vitro studies.[5] This vaccine is in the late stages of preclinical development for the prevention of amebiasis in infants and children in the developing world. Provision of sanitation and clean water and safe sexual practices to prevent fecal-oral transmission are of great importance but not universally effective because of the low infectious dose and chlorine resistance of the cyst.

PROGNOSIS

Therapy for amebiasis is highly effective. Drug resistance is not reported.

● FREE-LIVING AMEBAE

Rare infections of the central nervous system can be seen with infection by free-living amebae of the genera *Naegleria*, *Balamuthia*, *Acanthamoeba*, and *Sappinia*. *Naegleria fowleri* is the agent of primary amebic meningoencephalitis, which occurs in previously healthy children and young adults who have swum in fresh water 2 to 5 days before the onset of meningoencephalitis. Cerebrospinal fluid has a polymorphonuclear predominance, and motile amebae can be seen in a wet mount of cerebrospinal fluid. The disease is relentlessly progressive to death in most patients. In one case of successful treatment, a combination of intrathecal and intravenous amphotericin B and miconazole and oral rifampin was used. *Acanthamoeba* can cause keratitis[6] in individuals with corneal injuries (usually from contact lens use) as well as granulomatous amebic encephalitis in the immunocompromised. Granulomatous amebic encephalitis can also be caused by *Balamuthia* and *Sappinia*; it is usually associated with focal neurologic findings and has a subacute course (Table 352-3).

Grade A Reference

A1. Gonzales ML, Dans LF, Martinez EG. Antiamoebic drugs for treating amoebic colitis. *Cochrane Database Syst Rev.* 2009;2:CD006085.

GENERAL REFERENCES

For the General References and other additional features, please visit Expert Consult at https://expertconsult.inkling.com.

353

BABESIOSIS AND OTHER PROTOZOAN DISEASES

SAM R. TELFORD III AND PETER J. KRAUSE

● BABESIOSIS

Babesiosis is a tick-borne malaria-like disease caused by sporozoan parasites of the genus *Babesia*.

EPIDEMIOLOGY

Three worldwide epidemiologic patterns are apparent. The first involves the rodent-maintained *Babesia microti*, which is a species complex distributed across the Holarctic. On average, more than 1000 cases of *B. microti* babesiosis have been reported from the northeastern United States and upper Midwestern states from 2011 through 2013, the first 3 years that human babesiosis has been designated as a notifiable infectious disease by the Centers for Disease Control and Prevention (CDC). By comparison, about 30,000 Lyme disease cases are reported each year in the United States. The vector for *B. microti* is the same as that for Lyme disease (Chapter 321), the deer tick, *Ixodes dammini*, also known as northern populations of *I. scapularis*. Indeed, concurrent babesiosis and Lyme disease is common. Immune-intact as well as immunocompromised individuals are at risk. Within the last decade, *B. microti* has been increasingly reported in an expanded distribution from the original foci in coastal New England and the Upper Midwest, and it is now possible that babesiosis cases may be found wherever Lyme disease is intensely zoonotic. In addition, cases of *B. microti* or *B. microti*–like babesiosis have been reported from Australia, China, Germany, Japan, and Taiwan; the vectors have not been definitively identified.[1] The second pattern is represented by fewer than 50 cases of babesiosis due to *Babesia divergens*, *B. divergens*–like, or closely related species (e.g., *Babesia venatorum* or EU1) that have been reported from Europe. Almost all have been in splenectomized patients residing in sites where European castor bean ticks (*Ixodes ricinus*) and deer are common.[2] A few cases have been described in the United States and the Canary Islands. The third pattern of babesiosis involves sporadic cases due to diverse *Babesia* spp. These include a *Babesia duncani* (WA-1) and CA-type parasites of the western United States; a *B. divergens*–like species (MO-1); a *Babesia motasi*–like infection (KO-1) in Korea; and unidentified

Babesia spp from Colombia, Egypt, India, Mexico, and South Africa. There are at least 100 described *Babesia* spp from mammals and birds, and these hemoparasites are common animal infections on all continents. With few exceptions, *Babesia* spp are transmitted by ixodid ticks. Thus, wherever humans are intensely exposed to hard-bodied ticks, babesiosis should be part of a differential diagnosis for a patient presenting with fever and hematologic abnormalities.

Although the known zoonotic tick vectors (*I. dammini, I. ricinus*) have marked seasonal periods of activity (May to August) and the majority of reported cases are acquired during these times, babesiosis may be diagnosed at any time of the year. More than 150 cases of transfusion-acquired babesiosis due to *B. microti* and three due to *B. duncani* have been reported. The actual number of cases is thought to be much greater. *B. microti* is currently the most commonly reported transfusion-transmitted pathogen in the United States, and the number of such cases is increasing, including those ending in death.[3] Cases occur throughout the year, and about 10% of cases occur in nonendemic areas because *Babesia*-infected blood is exported to nonendemic areas or persons become infected in endemic areas and subsequently donate blood in nonendemic areas. A few cases of transplacentally transmitted babesiosis have been reported.

PATHOBIOLOGY

The pathophysiology of *Babesia* infection is directly related to the development of parasitemia. Peripheral blood parasitemias of 70% or greater have been reported, although most cases sustain parasitemias on the order of 0.5 to 5%. In hamsters infected by inoculation of a human-derived *B. microti* strain, intravascular hemolysis develops as the parasitemia rises and results in profound anemia. The hematocrit may fall to less than 20%. During this acute phase of disease, there is extramedullary hematopoiesis and hyperplasia of the splenic red pulp. Livers of infected hamsters contain hypertrophied Kupffer cells, many with ingested parasitized erythrocytes but little hemoglobin breakdown products. The proximal convoluted tubules of the kidneys contain abundant hemosiderin, an observation consistent with the occurrence of marked intravascular hemolysis.

Excessive production of pro-inflammatory cytokines seems to best explain the most common clinical manifestations, which include fever, sweats, chills, headache, myalgia, nausea, vomiting, diarrhea, and pallor. Administration of recombinant tumor necrosis factor (TNF) to human volunteers induces most of the symptoms of babesiosis and malaria. Such findings are not seen when erythrocyte lysis is due to noninfectious causes, which suggests that the release of merozoites serves as a trigger for the pro-inflammatory cascade. Elevated serum concentrations of TNF as well as of interferon-γ, interleukins 2 and 6, E-selectin, vascular cell adhesion molecule 1, and intracellular cell adhesion molecule 1 are detected during the acute phase of human *B. microti* infection and return to baseline within 3 months after resolution of infection.

Severe illness caused by infection with *Babesia* includes a complex array of metabolic abnormalities and organ dysfunction. Pulmonary disease is the most common complication in people experiencing severe *Babesia* infection, with up to 20% of patients suffering from noncardiogenic pulmonary edema. Pro-inflammatory cytokines appear to mediate the pulmonary complications of *Babesia* infection, at least in part. TNF and interferon-γ mRNA are upregulated in the lungs of *B. duncani*–infected mice, whereas TNF-knockout mice are less likely to die of fulminating *B. duncani* infection than are those with an intact TNF response. It is also likely that lung and other end-organ disease is mediated, at least in part, by vascular stasis, which has been described in the lungs of hamsters and mice infected with *B. duncani*.

CLINICAL MANIFESTATIONS

About a quarter of *B. microti* infections in adults and half of those in children are subclinical. This estimate is derived from an epidemiologic study that determined the frequency of people who seroconverted during the course of the summer transmission season but reported no illness, coupled with a careful accounting of symptomatic cases. Most people experience a mild to moderate illness lasting about a week. There is a gradual onset of malaise, anorexia, fatigue, fever (temperature as high as 40°C), sweats, and myalgia. Nausea, vomiting, headache, shaking chills, emotional lability, depression, hemoglobinuria, and hyperesthesia also have been reported. Findings on physical examination consist of fever, pallor, splenomegaly, and hepatomegaly. Laboratory abnormalities include anemia, thrombocytopenia, and leukopenia. Parasitemia generally ranges from barely detectable on blood smear to 5% in previously healthy people but may reach 85% in asplenic and other immunocompromised patients. Lactate dehydrogenase, bilirubin, and

transaminase levels may be elevated in more severe cases. Persistent relapsing illness may occur in highly immunocompromised people who fail to clear the infection for months or more than a year despite multiple courses of antibiotics. The case-fatality rate for *B. microti* babesiosis has been estimated to be 6 to 9% in hospitalized patients but may be as high as 20% in immunocompromised hosts, including those who acquire the infection through blood transfusion. Severe babesiosis usually occurs only in people with asplenia, malignant disease, coinfection with human immunodeficiency virus (HIV), immunosuppressive treatment, or age younger than 2 months or older than 50 years.

Cases of babesiosis caused by species other than *B. microti* tend to be severe, at least in part because they are primarily reported in immunocompromised patients. Virtually all European patients experiencing *B. divergens* infection have been splenectomized, and about a third of the patients died. In these patients, there was an acute onset of illness with hemoglobinuria, a persistent nonperiodic high fever (temperature of 40° to 41°C), shaking chills, intense sweats, headaches, and myalgia as well as lumbar and abdominal pain. Vomiting and diarrhea may occur. Pulmonary, renal, or liver failure may develop rapidly. In fatal cases, patients become comatose with multiorgan failure. *B. duncani, B. venatorum*, and *B. divergens*–like infections also have often been reported in immunocompromised hosts with a similarly severe course of illness.

DIAGNOSIS

The diagnosis of babesiosis is based on epidemiologic and clinical findings and confirmed by laboratory testing. Given clinical findings consistent with babesiosis, the diagnosis may be confirmed by examination of a Giemsa-stained thin blood smear for the presence of parasites within erythrocytes. In an immunocompromised patient, parasitemias are likely to exceed one infected cell per oil immersion field and thus are quickly detected. For *B. microti* babesiosis (Fig. 353-1), examination of a slide for 10 minutes or as many fields as needed to tally 200 leukocytes (that are not infected but serve as a marker for effort) and repeated smears performed twice a day may be required. Standard Romanowsky stains (Giemsa, Wright) with malaria protocols are optimal. Artifactual inclusions are limited mainly to stain precipitates (which can be determined by their presence in the plasma spaces between cells), Howell-Jolly or Heinz bodies (Chapter 157), or platelets superimposed on erythrocytes, which always have a light colored halo when visualized this way. *Babesia* spp have clearly defined chromatin with a lighter-colored cytoplasm (Fig. 353-2A). They may be mistaken for early malarial trophozoites. Neither malarial nor babesial rings have hemozoin (malarial pigment), so this is not a good feature to distinguish between the two. Paired piriform parasites, arranged in a *v*, are suggestive of *B. divergens* or *B. divergens*–like infection (Fig. 353-2B). Rings of all sizes may be seen in all species. Multiple parasites may frequently be seen in single erythrocytes, as well as clumps of extracellular parasites. Tetrad forms (Fig. 353-2C) and Maltese cross forms (Fig. 353-2D) are diagnostic but are rarely seen in *B. microti* babesiosis. They seem to be more common with *B. duncani* or CA-type infections.

Polymerase chain reaction (PCR) assays are an important adjunct to blood smears. PCR is usually more sensitive than blood smears in cases in which parasitemias are sparse. Real-time PCR assays performed in-house would

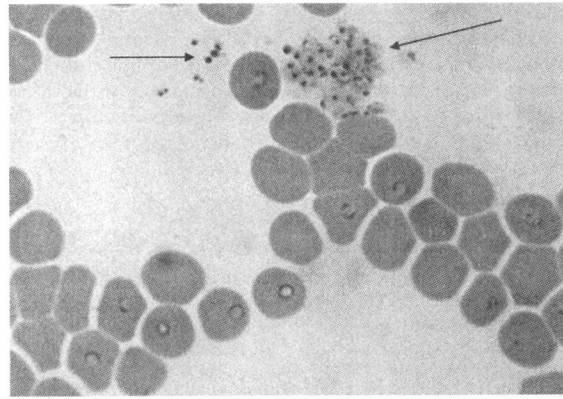

FIGURE 353-1. *Babesia microti.* Human infection, Nantucket Island. Predominance of ring forms with a cluster of extraerythrocytic parasites (*arrow*) free in the plasma.

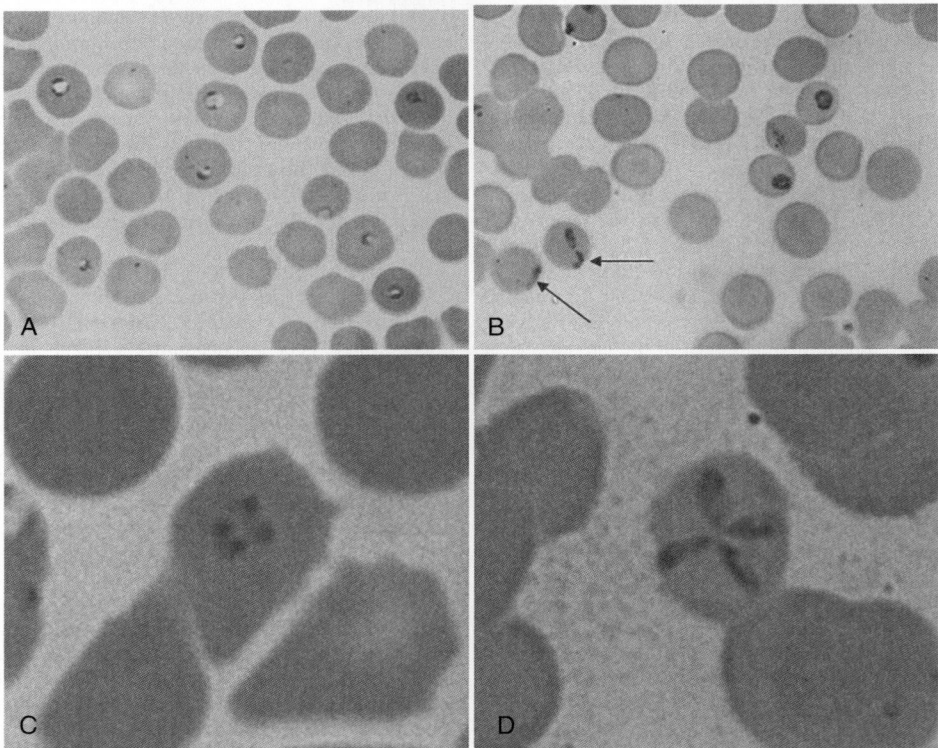

FIGURE 353-2. Diagnosis of *Babesia* infection. **A,** Typical thin-film field demonstrating ring forms of *B. microti* with vacuole or "whitish" cytoplasm demarcated by a dark-staining, defined chromatin. **B,** *B. Divergens*–like (MO-1) with robust rings; accolé form and paired piriform parasites are marked by *arrows*. **C,** Tetrad forms of *B. microti*. **D,** MO-1, classic Maltese cross. (Microscope slide from human case of MO-1 kindly provided by Dr. J. F. Beattie, Department of Pathology, The Medical Center, Bowling Green, Ky).

provide confirmation nearly as quickly as microscopy with the added advantage of increased sensitivity.[4] As with many molecular diagnostic assays, use of PCR for babesia (either conventional or real-time quantitative) is limited by false positives, validation of experimental assays, and insurance reimbursement. PCR sequencing, performed by collaborating research laboratories, is extremely valuable in retrospectively identifying the species of *Babesia* when the identity is not clear.

Serologic testing is useful for confirming *B. microti* infection. The indirect immunofluorescence test, using antigen from infected hamster red cells, is sensitive and specific and is currently the serologic method of choice. Analysis of paired acute and convalescent serum samples is most useful for a confirmation of *B. microti* infection. The presence of parasite-specific IgM may indicate that the patient has an acute infection even in the absence of readily demonstrable parasitemia. Serology is not generally useful for *B. divergens* babesiosis, given its fulminant natural history. Because parasitemia occurs before an antibody response and the doubling time of *B. divergens* can be as short as 8 hours, treatment needs to be initiated immediately on the basis of clinical suspicion and initial laboratory results.

The known vectors for human babesiosis are ticks that also transmit the agents of Lyme disease, human granulocytic anaplasmosis, *Borrelia miyamotoi* infection, *Ehrlichia muris*–like infection, and tick-borne encephalitis virus. Thus, coinfections should be considered in all patients with babesiosis. Acute illness in patients coinfected with Lyme disease and babesiosis is more severe and more persistent than in patients experiencing Lyme disease alone.

TREATMENT   Rx

Therapy for mild to moderate *B. microti* cases should consist of the combination of atovaquone (750 mg orally twice daily for 7 to 10 days) and azithromycin (500 to 1000 mg initial dose followed by 250 mg orally daily for 7 to 10 days; for immunocompromised hosts, 600 to 1000 mg orally daily for 7 to 10 days). A prospective randomized trial demonstrated that patients treated with atovaquone and azithromycin cleared parasitemia as effectively as did those receiving clindamycin and quinine and with fewer side effects. For severe

babesiosis, a 7- to 10-day course of the combination of clindamycin (either 300 to 600 mg every 6 hours intravenously or 600 mg orally every 8 hours) and quinine (650 mg orally every 8 hours) should be used. The pediatric regimen is clindamycin, 7 to 10 mg/kg given every 6 to 8 hours (maximum of 600 mg/dose) and quinine 8 mg/kg given every 8 hours orally (maximum of 650 mg per dose).

Treatment may occasionally fail in high-risk patients or in those who must discontinue quinine because of side effects, such as severe tinnitus and gastrointestinal distress. Multiple courses of treatment for a prolonged duration may be required to clear parasitemia in immunocompromised patients; combination therapy should be used that may include two or more of the following antimicrobials: artemisinin, atovaquone, azithromycin, clindamycin, doxycycline, atovaquone-proguanil (Malarone), pentamidine, quinine, and trimethoprim-sulfamethoxazole. Once an effective combination is identified, it should be continued for at least 6 weeks and 2 weeks beyond the time when *Babesia* can no longer be visualized on blood smear or blood samples become PCR negative.

Exchange transfusion should be considered in severely ill patients with parasitemias in excess of 10%, evidence of severe hemolysis, or organ compromise. In particularly severe babesiosis cases, partial or complete blood exchange transfusion (1 to 3 blood volumes) should be undertaken, in addition to treatment with clindamycin and quinine.

PREVENTION

Prevention depends on reducing the risk for tick bites. Immunocompromised individuals should be especially careful to use personal protection and may even consider avoiding highly endemic sites such as coastal New England and Long Island during May through July, when risk is the greatest.[5] Use of repellants such as DEET or application of permethrin to clothing will greatly reduce tick attachment. Such products should be applied to shoes, socks, and trouser cuffs. Wearing light-colored long pants and tucking the cuffs into socks will also help prevent ticks from gaining access to attachment sites. Daily examination for attached ticks should be performed; the best way to do this is to feel for new bumps on a soapy body in the shower. Any attached ticks should be promptly removed by simple traction, which is best accomplished with the use of tweezers. As with the agent of Lyme disease, ticks must be attached at least 36 to 48 hours before a sufficient inoculum of *Babesia* sporozoites is delivered. Community-level prevention should focus on public education about the risks of tick-borne infection, reducing habitat for ticks (brush removal and landscaping around yards), or reducing the reproductive hosts for the tick. Deer reduction will reduce the abundance of the deer tick vector for *B. microti* babesiosis. Currently, screening of blood donations for *Babesia* spp consists only of targeted questions about a history of previous *Babesia* infection, but laboratory screening methods are being developed.

PROGNOSIS

Death may occur in patients with severe babesiosis, but other long-term sequelae have not been reported for patients who have been adequately treated. In most patients who complete a full treatment regimen, *B. microti* DNA becomes undetectable by PCR within 3 months. Infection does not imply protective immunity based on laboratory rodent models, although subsequent infections are limited in duration and intensity. Recrudescent infections have been reported, mainly in immunocompromised individuals.

● MISCELLANEOUS ENTERIC PROTOZOA

The gastrointestinal and urogenital tracts may contain representatives of the four major groupings of protozoa (amebae, sporozoa, flagellates, and ciliates). Diarrhea and other lower gastrointestinal signs and symptoms may be caused by diverse protozoa. Specific clinical diagnosis is not possible; expert clinical parasitology support is required to determine whether an agent that has been detected in a stool sample is a pathogenic species.[6] Identification is necessary because treatment options differ by the agent. With the exception of *Trichomonas vaginalis* infection (sexually transmitted), all of the enteric protozoa are acquired by the ingestion of food or materials contaminated by human feces; a small subset may have extraintestinal manifestations. Given a shared mode of transmission (fecal-oral), demonstrating the presence of any one of these protozoa within a stool sample from a patient is justification for an intensified search for those that are recognized as clinically significant pathogens (*Entamoeba histolytica, Giardia lamblia/intestinalis, Cyclospora cayetanensis, Cystoisospora belli,* and *Cryptosporidium parvum/hominis*). Other protozoa, many of which morphologically resemble true pathogens, are commonly detected within stools of patients with lower gastrointestinal disturbances, but support for their role as etiologic agents is weak.

Cryptosporidiosis (Chapter 350), giardiasis (Chapter 351), and amebiasis (Chapter 352) are discussed in separate chapters. Trichomoniasis and coccidian enteritis are discussed here because they are relatively common infections.

Trichomoniasis

EPIDEMIOLOGY

Trichomonas vaginalis is among the most prevalent of all pathogenic protozoa and is one of the most common sexually transmitted infections in the United States and likely worldwide.[7] As many as 30% of female college students and 40% of pregnant Nigerian women were found to be infected. The highest incidence of infection occurs in women with multiple sexual partners and those with other sexually transmitted diseases (Chapter 285). *T. vaginalis* can also be passed from infected mothers to their newborn daughters, but it is seldom symptomatic in girls before menarche. The parasite is able to survive for some time in moist environments, and nonvenereal transmission, although uncommon, can occur. Trichomoniasis, like other sexually transmitted diseases, may increase the likelihood of transmission of HIV.

PATHOBIOLOGY

T. vaginalis, known colloquially as a flagellate, is classified in the phylum Metamonada and class Parabasalia along with another human pathogen, *Dientamoeba fragilis* (previously thought to be an ameba). The 10- to 15-μm-long trophozoites multiply by longitudinal binary fission on the epithelial surface of the vagina or urethra as well as in vaginal or urethral secretions and are thereby transmitted by sexual intercourse. No cyst form is known, and the trophozoites are easily killed by drying.

The parabasalids are a phylogenetic sister group to the class Eopharingia, which includes *Giardia* spp. The parabasalids lack mitochondria and are anaerobic; they all have a unique cellular organelle, the hydrogenosome, which is a relic of the mitochondrion and serves as the site of anaerobic pyruvate metabolism. A hemolysin is produced and may cause epithelial damage.

CLINICAL MANIFESTATIONS

Trichomoniasis is one of three common causes of vaginitis or vaginosis (along with bacterial vaginosis and vulvovaginal candidiasis). It is characterized by a thin gray to yellowish green frothy discharge; vulvovaginal erythema; ectocervical erythema or "strawberry cervix," observable mainly by colposcopy; pH higher than 4.5; increased presence of polymorphonuclear leukocytes; and a positive result of the whiff test, in which a foul fishy odor is intensified on addition of potassium hydroxide. The incubation period for trichomoniasis is 5 to 28 days. In addition to a frothy discharge, vaginitis can be accompanied by vulvovaginal irritation, dyspareunia, abdominal pain, and dysuria. Symptoms may worsen during menstruation. Population-based studies indicate that as many as half of *T. vaginalis* infections in women and the majority in men are asymptomatic. *T. vaginalis* can frequently be isolated from the male partners of infected women and can produce symptomatic urethritis. Urethral discharge is generally scant in these cases. Rarely, *T. vaginalis* is associated with epididymitis, superficial penile ulcerations that are usually located under the prepuce, or prostatitis.

DIAGNOSIS

The CDC guidelines (http://www.cdc.gov/std/treatment/2010/vaginal-discharge.htm#a2) state that all women with a sexually transmitted infection should be specifically tested for evidence of *T. vaginalis* infection, and HIV-positive women should be tested annually. In women, vaginal and urethral secretions should be examined. *T. vaginalis* is seen in wet mounts of vaginal secretions in approximately 60% of infected women, thus confirming the diagnosis. Live *T. vaginalis* have a twitching or tumbling motion in wet mounts, and polymorphonuclear leukocytes are usually present. Direct immunofluorescent antibody staining is more sensitive than wet mounts but technically more difficult. Culture is an even more sensitive method of diagnosis; commercial kits for culture are available, but the results are not available for 3 to 7 days. *T. vaginalis* is occasionally identified in Papanicolaou-stained smears; Giemsa stain may also be used (Fig. 353-3). For men, a wet mount of material from a platinum loop scraping of the anterior urethra reveals the organism in approximately half the cases. Prostatic massage before collection of urine for *Trichomonas* culture is a more sensitive diagnostic approach. *T. vaginalis* is not found in the gastrointestinal tract, and the presence of trichomonads in wet fecal mounts or stained fixed fecal smears (iron hematoxylin or trichrome) most likely represents the commensal *Pentatrichomonas* (formerly *Trichomonas*) *hominis*. Serology has limited clinical use because of issues of sensitivity and specificity and because evidence of exposure does not imply current disease. New modes of testing are becoming available and will eventually supplant microscopy. One Food and Drug Administration (FDA)–approved (and CLIA waived) point-of-care antigen assay (OSOM Trichomonas Rapid Test; Sekisui Diagnostics, Framingham, Mass) has

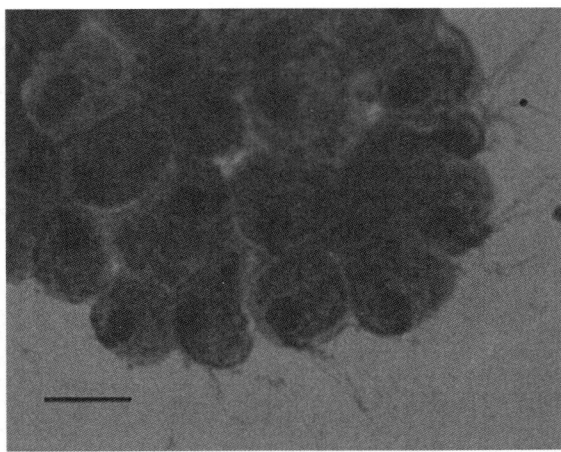

FIGURE 353-3. *Trichomonas vaginalis,* **Giemsa-stained smear of cultivated trophozoites.** (Bright-field microscopy, ×630. Scale bar is 15 μm.)

greater sensitivity and specificity in comparison with microscopy. The FDA has also cleared a single PCR-based assay (APTIMA *Trichomonas vaginalis* Assay; Hologic GenProbe, San Diego, Calif) with excellent sensitivity and specificity, but the assay requires specimens (swab samples) fixed in a proprietary solution.

TREATMENT
(also see Chapter 344) **Rx**

Tinidazole, a single 2-g oral dose in adults, or metronidazole, either as a single 2-g oral dose or 500 mg twice daily for 7 days, is the treatment of choice. Tinidazole is the better tolerated of the two. Single-dose therapy (metronidazole or tinidazole) ensures compliance of the patient but can produce nausea and a metallic taste, particularly with metronidazole. Both tinidazole and metronidazole have a disulfiram-like effect, and patients who consume alcohol within 24 hours of metronidazole or 72 hours of tinidazole may experience severe nausea, vomiting, and flushing. The use of tinidazole and metronidazole is relatively contraindicated during pregnancy, given the lack of well-controlled studies. Treatment failures with metronidazole are uncommon but well documented. HIV-positive women should be treated for 7 days with 500 mg of metronidazole because of frequent recrudescence with the single-dose therapy. Some instances of treatment failure in immune-intact women result from reinfection, others from poor compliance, but some are caused by metronidazole-resistant parasites. A repeated course of metronidazole (2 g orally daily for 5 days) may be tried. If patients remain refractory to appropriate treatment, metronidazole sensitivity can be tested by the CDC (available at www.dpd.cdc.gov/dpdx/HTML/DiagnosticProcedures.htm).

PREVENTION

Condoms (male or female) reduce risk of acquiring trichomoniasis. Sexual partners should be treated concurrently to prevent reinfection because nearly 20% of male partners are coinfected.

PROGNOSIS

Rare complications include pelvic inflammatory disease. Infection during gestation may lead to fetal growth retardation. There is no natural or acquired immunity, so reinfection may be common.

Coccidian Enteritis

EPIDEMIOLOGY

The coccidia, with 43 genera and more than 1700 recognized species, are well-known veterinary pathogens.[8] At least two of the coccidia, *Cyclospora cayetanensis* (an eimeriid) and *Cystoisospora belli* (a sarcocystid), are causative agents of enteritis in humans. Despite their ubiquity (nearly 100 species have been described), *Sarcocystis* spp have been rare causes of enteritis in humans and an even less common cause of myositis, although *Sarcocystis nesbitti*

caused a disease comprising fever, myalgia, headache, and myositis in 89 college students who had traveled to Malaysia.[9] *C. cayetanensis* may have both an animal and human reservoir, but *C. belli* is thought to be an anthroponosis. Cyclosporiasis is a cause of gastroenteritis in tropical and subtropical areas, with Peru, Mexico, Haiti, Caribbean countries, and Nepal commonly reporting such cases. Since 1990, at least 11 food-borne outbreaks affecting approximately 3600 persons have been documented in the United States and Canada among persons who have eaten contaminated raspberries, fresh basil, snow peas, or mesclun. Cyclosporiasis is not uncommonly diagnosed in international travelers, and large outbreaks have been reported from cruise ships.[10]

PATHOBIOLOGY

Oocysts are passed in feces and must sporulate for at least a day (*C. belli*) or 5 to 11 days (*C. cayetanensis*) before attaining infectivity. Sporozoites are liberated in the small bowel, penetrating enterocytes (for *C. cayetanensis*, mainly in the jejunum). *C. cayetanensis* appears to have a complicated developmental cycle with at least two merogonic cycles in the bowel, leading to the formation of gametes. The gametes fuse within the enterocyte cytoplasm, and an oocyst wall is deposited around the zygote. The sexual cycle begins about a week after infection, with oocysts sloughing into the bowel lumen and subsequently out of the body through feces. Biopsy specimens from infected patients demonstrate mononuclear and eosinophilic infiltrates in the lamina propria as well as alterations to the morphology of villi. Humans appear to be intermediate hosts for *S. nesbitti*, with sporozoites liberated in the small bowel, entering the vasculature, and forming cysts in muscle.

CLINICAL MANIFESTATIONS

After an incubation period of approximately 1 week, either organism produces watery diarrhea, nausea, vomiting, abdominal pain, myalgias, anorexia, and fatigue. Illness is usually self-limited, but symptoms can be prolonged (10 to 12 weeks) and associated with steatorrhea, flatulence, and substantial weight loss in persons who are immunocompromised, especially those with AIDS. Infections may also be asymptomatic. With *S. nesbitti*, fever and prominent myalgias are the dominant presentation.

DIAGNOSIS

The diagnosis is confirmed by identifying coccidia in stool samples stained with modified acid-fast or modified safranin preparations or by phase contrast microscopy or bright-field microscopy (using iodine as a contrast medium) of wet mounts (Fig. 353-4). *C. cayetanensis* and *C. belli* may be sensitively detected by fluorescent microscopy of wet mounts. PCR is specific and can be sensitive, depending on the mode of DNA extraction, but there are no FDA-approved assays available; PCR support may be requested from the CDC through state public health departments. *S. nesbitti* appears to undergo an aberrant asexual cycle only within humans and may not produce oocysts to be liberated into the bowel; therefore, diagnosis has required muscle biopsy and demonstration of sarcocysts by histology or detection of the agent's DNA by PCR.

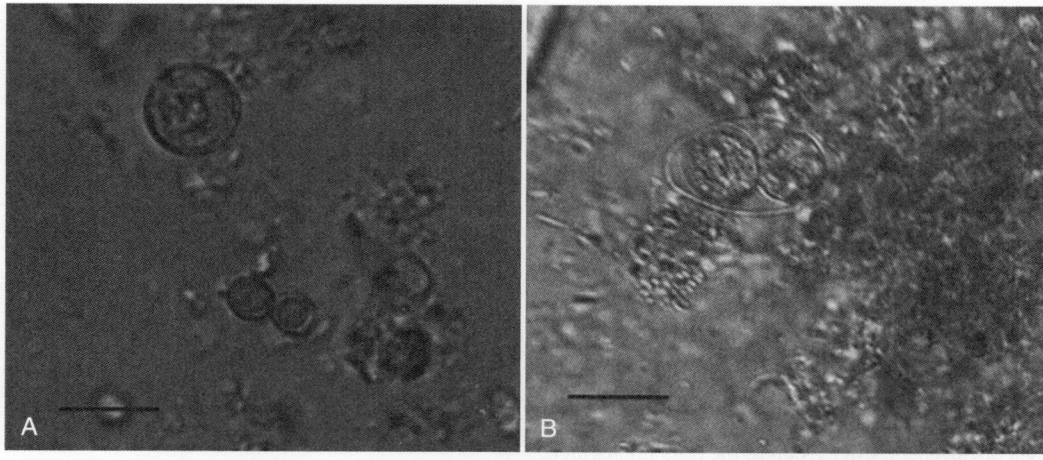

FIGURE 353-4. Diagnosis of coccidian enteritis. **A,** *Cyclospora cayetanensis,* seen on formalin-fixed human feces, unsporulated. (Bright-field microscopy, ×1000 with green contrast filter. Scale bar is 10 μm.) Note the doublet of yeast cells in lower right of the photomicrograph. **B,** *Cystoisospora belli,* seen on formalin-fixed human feces, partially sporulated. (Bright-field microscopy, ×400. Scale bar is 15 μm.)

TABLE 353-1 OTHER ENTERIC PROTOZOA

ORGANISM	EPIDEMIOLOGY	MANIFESTATIONS	THERAPY*
Balantidium coli	Primarily an infection of animals, especially pigs, but also affects humans	Asymptomatic or mild and self-resolving; occasionally more severe with abdominal pain, blood, and mucus in stool	Tetracycline (500 mg qid for 10 days) Alternative: metronidazole (750 mg tid for 5 days) or iodoquinol (650 mg tid for 20 days)
Blastocystis hominis	Probably worldwide, including North America; often found concomitantly with *Giardia lamblia*	Pathogenicity is debated	The need for treatment is debated, but symptomatic improvement has been reported with metronidazole (750 mg tid for 10 days), or trimethoprim-sulfamethoxazole (160 mg TMP/800 mg SMX bid for 7 days)
Dientamoeba fragilis	Worldwide distribution; frequently found concomitantly with the pinworm *Enterobius*	Often asymptomatic; diarrhea reported	Paromomycin (25-35 mg/kg body weight per day in 3 doses for 7 days), tetracycline (500 mg qid for 10 days), metronidazole (500-750 mg tid for 10 days), or iodoquinol (650 mg tid for 20 days)
Microsporidia[†] (*Enterocytozoon bieneusi* and *Encephalitozoon intestinalis*)	Apparent worldwide distribution	AIDS patients with persistent diarrhea and wasting; self-limited cases in immunocompetent persons	Oral fumagillin (20 mg tid) has been effective for *E. bieneusi*, but it has been associated with thrombocytopenia. Albendazole (400 mg bid) has been effective for *E. intestinalis.* Treatment with HAART may lead to clinical response in HIV-infected patients with microsporidial diarrhea.
Sarcocystis species	Common pathogens of animals; rare in humans; acquired by ingesting contaminated beef or pork	Often asymptomatic; nausea, vomiting, abdominal pain, and diarrhea may occur; eosinophilic necrotizing enteritis has been reported	No specific therapy

*Based on CDC recommendations, www.cdc.gov/parasites/az/index.html. Accessed March 9, 2015. The dosages and durations are for adults.
[†]Associated with persistent, severe diarrhea in persons with AIDS.
AIDS = acquired immunodeficiency syndrome; HAART = highly active antiretroviral therapy; HIV = human immunodeficiency virus.

TREATMENT   Rx

Rehydration is important, as it is for any severe diarrheal disease. Both infections may respond to treatment with 160 mg trimethoprim and 800 mg sulfamethoxazole taken twice daily for 7 to 10 days. HIV-infected patients may require a longer course of therapy. The widespread use of trimethoprim-sulfamethoxazole (Bactrim) prophylaxis for *Pneumocystis* has reduced the incidence of coccidial diarrhea in patients with HIV infection. No specific treatment has been recommended for sarcocystosis.

PREVENTION

At the community level, preventing the contamination of water and food (mainly vegetables and fruits) by animal or human feces reduces the risk of transmission. Washing vegetables and fruits in water will reduce the potential inoculum but does not eliminate all risk. Sarcocystosis may be prevented by ensuring that meat is well cooked.

PROGNOSIS

Reactive arthritis, Guillain-Barré syndrome, Reiter's syndrome, cholecystitis, and cholangitis have been reported as complications of either coccidian enteritis, mainly in patients with AIDS. Otherwise, treatment appears to eradicate the organism. Whether reinfection may occur is not known. Reports of extraintestinal development of *C. belli* and *C. cayetanensis* suggest the possibility of reinvasion of the bowel with ensuing recrudescence of signs and symptoms.

Other Enteric Protozoans

A number of other protozoa transmitted by fecal-oral contamination have been associated with enteric disease (Table 353-1). Some reside in the lumen of the bowel, and others invade and multiply within enterocytes. Enteric protozoa should be considered in the differential diagnosis of patients with persistent diarrhea and abdominal symptoms, particularly those with a history of recent international travel. A clinical diagnosis is rarely possible; laboratory tests, mainly for ova and parasites in stools, establish the diagnosis. Expert microscopists are required because these parasites may be confused with fecal debris. Pathogenic protozoa must also be differentiated from commensals such as *Entamoeba coli, Endolimax nana, Iodamoeba bütschlii, Pentatrichomonas hominis,* and *Chilomastix mesnili.* Therapy includes administration

of the appropriate antiprotozoal drug and rehydration, as listed in Table 353-1[11] (also see Chapter 344).

GENERAL REFERENCES

For the General References and other additional features, please visit Expert Consult at https://expertconsult.inkling.com.

354

CESTODES

A. CLINTON WHITE AND ENRICO BRUNETTI

DEFINITION
The Pathogens

Cestode parasites are members of the animal kingdom, subphylum Cestoda. The organisms are characterized by several life cycle stages, which typically develop in distinct hosts. The adult stage is the tapeworm, which is acquired by ingestion of uncooked tissues harboring larval forms. After ingestion, the larvae excyst and the scolex attaches to the intestines. Segments, termed *proglottids*, develop at the base of the scolex and are displaced from the scolex by new proglottids to form a chain or tapeworm. The host in which the tapeworm develops is termed the *definitive host.* The proglottids contain male and female sexual organs and produce large numbers of ova. The proglottids or their ova are shed in stools. Humans are the definitive hosts for a number of different tapeworms, including the *Taenia* species, *Diphyllobothrium* species, and *Hymenolepis nana.* Humans can also be an accidental host for the dog and cat tapeworms of the genus *Dipylidium* (Table 354-1).

The intermediate hosts harbor the larval form of the parasite. Infection follows ingestion of the ova. Under the influence of gastric and intestinal fluids, the ova hatch, releasing the invasive larvae (oncospheres), which migrate to tissues, forming tissue forms. The forms in tissue vary between

TABLE 354-1 COMMON HUMAN TAPEWORM INFECTIONS

ORGANISM	INTERMEDIATE HOST	COMMON NAME	CLINICAL PRESENTATION	TREATMENT
Diphyllobothrium spp	Fish	Fish tapeworm	Passing segments, pernicious anemia	Praziquantel, niclosamide
Hymenolepis nana	Humans	Dwarf tapeworm	Asymptomatic, diarrhea	Praziquantel, niclosamide
Taenia saginata	Cattle	Beef tapeworm	Asymptomatic, passing segments	Praziquantel, niclosamide
Taenia asiatica	Pigs	Asian tapeworm	Asymptomatic, passing worms	Praziquantel, niclosamide
Taenia solium	Pigs	Pork tapeworm	Asymptomatic, passing segments	Praziquantel, niclosamide
Dipylidium caninum	Fleas	Dog tapeworm	Passing segments	Praziquantel, niclosamide

TABLE 354-2 HUMAN LARVAL CESTODE INFECTIONS

ORGANISM	COMMON NAME	ORGANS INVOLVED
Taenia solium	Cysticercosis	Brain, spinal fluid, eye, muscle
Echinococcus granulosus group	Cystic hydatid disease	Liver, lung, other
Echinococcus multilocularis	Alveolar hydatid disease	Liver
Taenia multiceps, Taenia spp	Coenurosis	Brain, eyes
Spirometra species	Sparganosis	Subcutaneous tissue, viscera

TABLE 354-3 THERAPY FOR INTESTINAL TAPEWORM INFECTIONS

	PRAZIQUANTEL	NICLOSAMIDE	NITAZOXANIDE
Dosage			
Adults	5-10 mg/kg for all age groups (25 mg/kg for *Hymenolepis nana*)	2 g (4 tablets)	500 mg
Children >34 kg		1.5 g (3 tablets)	200 mg
Children 11-34 kg		1 g (2 tablets)	100 mg
Administration	Taken as a single dose	Taken as a single dose; tablets must be chewed and swallowed	Taken twice a day for 3 days
Side effects	Mild but frequent, including dizziness, myalgias, nausea, vomiting, diarrhea, abdominal pain	Nausea, vomiting, abdominal pain, diarrhea, drowsiness, dizziness, headache, pruritus	
Pregnancy		No known mutagenic effects; considered safe if indicated	

organisms and may include the cysticercus (a bladder containing a single invaginated scolex), the coenurus (a bladder with multiple scolices), the hydatid (a cystic structure with a germinal layer, which forms numerous protoscolices), or the plerocercoid (a solid form seen in *Spirometra* species). Humans can harbor the intermediate forms of *Taenia solium* (cysticercosis), *Echinococcus granulosus* group (cystic hydatid disease), *Echinococcus multilocularis* (alveolar hydatid disease), and rarely other organisms (Table 354-2). Humans can serve as both the definitive host and an intermediate host for two species, *T. solium* and *H. nana*. In the case of *T. solium*, humans are the obligate host for the tapeworm stage (pork tapeworm) but can also harbor the cystic form (cysticercosis). In the case of *H. nana*, both stages typically develop in a single person, with the cysticercoid form in the intestinal wall and the tapeworm in the lumen.

⬤ INTESTINAL TAPEWORM INFECTIONS
Diphyllobothrium Species (Fish Tapeworm)

Diphyllobothrium tapeworms are large segmented parasites that are acquired by ingestion of undercooked or pickled freshwater fish dishes (sushi, sashimi, ceviche, carpaccio, gefilte fish). The tapeworms develop within a few weeks and can live for more than 10 years.

EPIDEMIOLOGY AND PATHOBIOLOGY

Diphyllobothrium species are found worldwide, including foci in Europe, North and South America, and Asia. Perhaps 20 million people are thought to be infected worldwide. Major foci include Russia, Japan, and South America. Disease was formerly highly endemic in Scandinavia, where it is now rarely diagnosed.

In most cases, infection has little impact on the host. However, one species, *Diphyllobothrium latum*, contains vitamin B$_{12}$ receptors on the surface of the tapeworm, which can out-compete the host, leading to vitamin B$_{12}$ deficiency (Chapter 164). This manifestation has been described only in Scandinavia.

CLINICAL MANIFESTATIONS AND DIAGNOSIS

In most of those infected, *Diphyllobothrium* species produce few or no symptoms. Some may complain of gastrointestinal symptoms (abdominal discomfort, nausea, weight loss). The main clinical manifestation is the observation of proglottids being passed in stool. Pernicious anemia with symptoms of anemia or peripheral neuropathy may develop with *D. latum* infection. The diagnosis depends on observation of the characteristic operculated eggs in stool.

TREATMENT AND PREVENTION   **Rx**

A single oral dose of praziquantel (5 to 10 mg/kg) is usually adequate for therapy (Table 354-3). Niclosamide can be used as an alternative (2 g [adults] or 50 mg/kg [children] in a single dose chewed and swallowed), but it is not available in the United States. Parasites in fish can be killed by cooking (>56°C, >5 minutes) or freezing (−20°C, 24 hours). Infected fish may also be identified by inspection.

Hymenolepis nana

Hymenolepis nana is the human dwarf tapeworm. *Hymenolepis diminuta*, a rat tapeworm, can also cause human infection.

EPIDEMIOLOGY AND PATHOBIOLOGY

H. nana is widely prevalent worldwide, with estimates of 50 to 75 million people infected. Infection follows ingestion of ova. The larvae are released, invade, and develop into cysticercoid forms in the intestinal villi. After a few days, the cysticercoids mature, invade the lumen, and are transformed into a scolex, forming small tapeworms (up to 5 cm long), which begin producing eggs within 2 to 3 weeks. Autoinfection either in the intestines or by the fecal-oral route can lead to heavy infection.

CLINICAL MANIFESTATIONS AND DIAGNOSIS

Most infections are asymptomatic. However, some children may be infected by hundreds or thousands of worms, which can cause abdominal pain, loose stools, diarrhea, and malabsorption. Diagnosis depends on observation of the characteristic eggs in stool. More than one specimen may be required.

Praziquantel (15 to 25 mg/kg as a single oral dose) is usually effective in treating *H. nana* infection,[1] but it may need to be repeated in heavy infection (see Table 354-3). Nitazoxanide (100 mg by mouth twice daily for 3 days for children 1 to 3 years of age, 200 mg by mouth twice daily for 3 days for children 4 to 11 years of age, and 500 mg by mouth twice daily for 3 days for older children) is a reasonable alternative therapy; efficacy is about 75 to 82%. Niclosamide can be used as an alternative. Transmission is by the fecal-oral route and could be prevented by improved hygiene. Mass chemotherapy has been used to control infection in some populations.

Dipylidium caninum

Dipylidium caninum is a common tapeworm of dogs and cats. Dogs are infected by ingestion of fleas, which carry the cysticercoid form in their body cavities. The tapeworms can also develop in children who have ingested the fleas. It is widespread worldwide, but human infections are unusual.

CLINICAL MANIFESTATIONS AND DIAGNOSIS

Infection may be asymptomatic. In some cases, the motile proglottids may be noted in stool. The proglottids are similar in size and shape to rice grains. Diagnosis depends on identification of the ova in stool or identification of the proglottids.

TREATMENT AND PREVENTION Rx

There are no controlled trials of treatment for *Dipylidium* infection, but infection is likely to respond to regimens used for other tapeworms (see Table 354-3). The main measure for prevention is treatment of pets for fleas and tapeworms.

Taenia saginata

Taeniasis refers to infection with the tapeworm form of one of three *Taenia* species. *Taenia solium* and *Taenia asiatica* are acquired from ingestion of undercooked pork. *Taenia saginata*, called the beef tapeworm, is a common intestinal infection worldwide. Cattle are the intermediate hosts, harboring the tissue cysticerci in their muscle. Humans are the obligate definitive host, harboring the tapeworm form.

EPIDEMIOLOGY AND PATHOBIOLOGY

T. saginata is common worldwide in areas where cattle are raised and human fecal material contaminates the pastures. Approximately 45 to 60 million people are thought to be infected. It is found on most continents. Very high rates (>20% of the population) have been noted in east Africa, Bali, and Tibet. It is likewise endemic in the Middle East, the Americas, and Europe. *T. saginata* is also common in other parts of Asia, but many of the epidemiologic studies did not differentiate *T. saginata* from *T. asiatica*.

T. saginata tapeworms are acquired by ingestion of undercooked beef. The scolex attaches to the intestinal wall, and proglottids form at the base of the scolex. The proglottids gradually enlarge as they are displaced from the scolex by newer proglottids. The chain of proglottids can reach a length of up to 30 feet. The terminal proglottids are shed periodically in the stool. Terminal proglottids are typically off-white, 2 to 3 cm long, 0.5 to 1 cm wide, and 1 to 2 mm thick.

CLINICAL MANIFESTATIONS AND DIAGNOSIS

Mild symptoms (e.g., nausea, abdominal discomfort, anorexia, and pruritus) may be noted. The motile proglottids may cause discomfort as they exit the anus or may be noted in stool.

Ova may be noted in stool. The ova are 40 μm in diameter, surrounded by brown radial striations, and the embryos have six hooks. However, the ova of the three *Taenia* species are morphologically indistinguishable. The proglottids can be distinguished from those of *T. solium* by counting the number of uterine branches (≥14 branches suggests *T. saginata*). However, the proglottids of *T. saginata* cannot be readily distinguished from *T. asiatica*.

TREATMENT, PREVENTION, AND PROGNOSIS Rx

Taeniasis can be treated with praziquantel in a single dose (see Table 354-3). Single doses of niclosamide are also effective. Nitazoxanide has also been used for *T. saginata*. Taeniasis can be prevented by inspection of beef. Also, cooking to 56°C for 5 minutes or freezing at −20°C for 7 to 10 days destroys the infective larvae. Only minor symptoms are noted and are eventually self-limited with or without treatment.

Taenia asiatica

T. asiatica is a cause of taeniasis in Asia, termed *Asian taeniasis*. Infection is acquired by ingestion of undercooked pork. Pigs are infected by ingestion of the ova from tapeworm carriers. *T. asiatica* has been widely described in China, Taiwan, Korea, Indonesia, and Southeast Asia. The clinical manifestations, diagnosis, treatment, and prevention of *T. asiatica* infection are similar to those noted for *T. saginata* infection.

Taenia solium

T. solium, also known as the pork tapeworm, can cause both tapeworm infection and larval infection termed *cysticercosis*. *T. solium* tapeworm infections are caused by ingestion of infected undercooked pork. The scolex evaginates and attaches to the intestines, forming proglottids. The proglottids gradually mature as they are separated from the scolex by new proglottids. The adult worms are often 10 to 20 feet long. Within the mature proglottids, thousands of microscopic ova develop. The ova are either excreted into the stool or shed with the proglottids. By contrast, ingestion of the ova results in development of larval infection, termed cysticercosis (see later). Thus, the tapeworm carrier poses risk of self-infection as well as infection to other people.

EPIDEMIOLOGY AND PATHOBIOLOGY

T. solium is common worldwide in areas where pigs are raised and where pigs have access to human fecal material. Only a few million people are thought to harbor the tapeworm form. Pork tapeworm infection is highly endemic in Latin America, sub-Saharan Africa, south Asia, and Southeast Asia.

T. solium tapeworms are acquired by ingestion of undercooked pork. The scolex attaches to the intestinal wall and proglottids form at the base of the scolex. The proglottids gradually enlarge as they are displaced from the scolex by newer proglottids. The terminal proglottids are shed periodically in the stool. Terminal proglottids are typically off-white, 2 cm long, 0.5 to 1 cm wide, and 1 to 2 mm thick.

CLINICAL MANIFESTATIONS AND DIAGNOSIS

Mild symptoms (e.g., nausea, abdominal discomfort, anorexia, and pruritus) may be noted. The proglottids may be noted in stool. Diagnosis is made by the finding of ova in stool. The ova are 40 μm in diameter, surrounded by brown radial striations, and embryos have six hooks and are morphologically indistinguishable from the other *Taenia* species. The proglottids can be distinguished from those of *T. saginata* and *T. asiatica* by counting the number of uterine branches (<14 branches suggests *T. solium*).

TREATMENT AND PREVENTION Rx

Taeniasis can be treated with praziquantel in a single dose. Single doses of niclosamide are also effective. Taeniasis can be prevented by inspection of pork. Also, cooking to 56°C for 5 minutes or freezing at −20°C for 7 to 10 days destroys the infective larvae. Current control measures include mass chemotherapy for entire populations with praziquantel. Comprehensive control programs include mass chemotherapy to eliminate tapeworm carriers, treatment of porcine cysticercosis with drugs such as oxfendazole, and improved hygiene to limit access of pigs to human fecal material.

● TISSUE CESTODE (CYST) INFECTION
Taenia solium (Cysticercosis)

DEFINITION

T. solium is the cause of human larval infection termed cysticercosis. The normal hosts for the larval (cysticercus) forms are pigs. When ingested by pigs, the ova hatch, releasing the invasive larvae (termed *oncospheres*), which invade the intestines, migrate to tissues (especially muscle), and mature into cysticercus forms within the tissues. The cysticercus consists of a thin translucent bladder containing an invaginated scolex, which is poised to form a tapeworm after being ingested by a human host. The ova are also infectious to people, including the tapeworm carrier. The sticky ova attach to the hands of the tapeworm carrier and are transmitted by the oral route to the carrier or close contacts. After ingestion, the ova can migrate to tissues and form cysts (cysticercosis). The presence of cysticerci in the central nervous system is termed *neurocysticercosis*.[2] Neurocysticercosis includes cysticerci in the brain parenchyma (parenchymal neurocysticercosis) and cysticerci in the ventricles, subarachnoid space, spine, and eye (extraparenchymal neurocysticercosis).

EPIDEMIOLOGY

Cysticercosis is found in all regions of the world where pigs are raised with access to human fecal material. Some estimate that 60 million people are infected with *T. solium* cysticerci. However, exact data on incidence and prevalence are available from only a limited number of studies because of the requirement for neuroimaging studies to make a diagnosis. In the 19th century, infection was highly endemic in Europe. However, with improving standards of living, local transmission is now limited to a few rural areas in southern and eastern Europe. Cysticercosis is widespread in rural areas of Latin America. High prevalence rates have been documented in parts of Mexico, Guatemala, Honduras, Ecuador, Peru, Brazil, and Bolivia. In endemic villages, more than 10% of the population may have abnormalities on neuroimaging studies consistent with neurocysticercosis. Studies have highlighted the importance of cysticercosis in sub-Saharan Africa. Cysticercosis is widespread in India, Nepal, Southeast Asia, and parts of China. In India, neurocysticercosis most commonly is manifested with single enhancing lesions, which are the main lesion associated with seizure disorders in that country. In the United States, approximately 2000 cases are diagnosed each year. Most cases are in immigrants from pig-raising villages in Mexico and Latin America. However, there are also imported cases from Asia and a few locally acquired infections.

PATHOBIOLOGY

For cysticercosis, the pathogenesis and pathophysiology vary with the location of the cysticerci and the host inflammatory response. Cysticerci in the brain parenchyma initially suppress the host inflammatory response. After a silent period, estimated to be several years, the cysticerci lose the ability to suppress the host inflammatory response, leading to parenchymal inflammation, which typically is manifested by seizures. The cysticerci induce a granulomatous response, which gradually degrades the parasites. In some cases, the lesions resolve. However, in others, degradation leads to formation of calcified granulomas. These calcified lesions may intermittently become inflamed (as evidenced by edema or contrast enhancement on magnetic resonance imaging [MRI] scan) and may cause recurrent seizures during a period of years. In some cases, cysticerci develop within the ventricles of the brain and can mechanically cause obstructive hydrocephalus. Cysticerci in the subarachnoid space may cause a chronic arachnoiditis, which can be manifested by vasculitis and stroke, communicating hydrocephalus, basilar meningitis, and, in some cases, mass effect. Cysticerci can also develop in the spine (manifested as radiculitis), eye, subcutaneous tissue, and muscle.

CLINICAL MANIFESTATIONS

The clinical manifestations vary with the location of the cysticerci and the associated host response (Fig. 354-1).[3,4] Neurocysticercosis can lead to a spectrum of cognitive abnormalities, ranging from impairment in a single domain, to cognitive impairment, and occasionally to dementia. All forms of disease may be associated with headaches. In general, parenchymal cysticerci are associated with seizures,[5] whereas ventricular and subarachnoid cysticercosis are associated with hydrocephalus.

Single Enhancing Lesion

A single enhancing lesion is the most common manifestation of cysticercosis in India and the United States. Patients typically present with seizures, which can be focal or focal with secondary generalization. Many will have a single seizure or a few seizures during the period when the cysticercus is degenerating, but the duration of seizures is eventually self-limited in most cases. However, a few go on to develop calcified lesions, which are a risk factor for recurrent seizures.

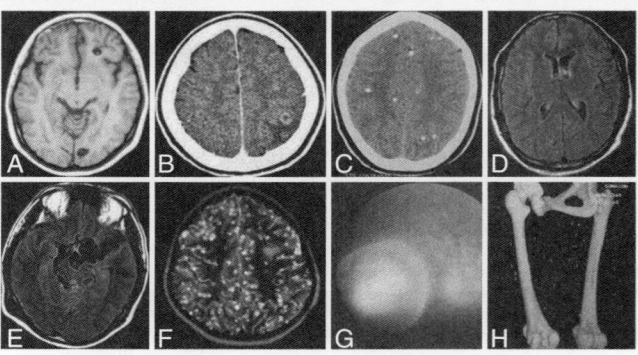

FIGURE 354-1. Human neurocysticercosis can be classified on the basis of neuroimaging studies. **A,** Multiple cystic lesions. **B,** Single enhancing lesion. **C,** Multiple calcifications. **D,** Intraventricular cysticerci. **E,** Subarachnoid cysticerci. **F,** Diffuse infection with cerebral edema, termed cysticercal encephalitis. **G,** Ocular cysticerci. **H,** Diffuse muscle calcifications. (Reprinted from Garcia HH, Del Brutto OH. Neurocysticercosis: updated concepts about an old disease. *Lancet Neurol.* 2005;4:653-661.)

Multiple Parenchymal Cysticerci

In patients with multiple lesions, the main presentation is with seizures, associated with parenchymal inflammation. In contrast to those with single lesions, seizures are more likely to recur.

Calcified Lesions

Many patients do not present until after they have calcified lesions. Patients with calcified lesions may develop recurrent seizures during a period of years.

Ventricular Cysticerci

The cysticerci typically are manifested by obstructive hydrocephalus. The patient may present with headache, nausea and vomiting, dizziness, altered mental status, or papilledema with altered vision. This is a medical emergency and can be fatal if it is not treated.

Subarachnoid Cysticerci

Cysticerci in the basilar cisterns are often accompanied by cysticerci in other locations, including parenchymal cysticerci or calcifications, ventricular cysticerci, and spinal or ocular cysticerci; patients may present with disease attributable to cysticerci at these sites. Cysticerci in the basilar cisterns are particularly prone to cause arachnoiditis. Manifestations of arachnoiditis may include vascular involvement (large- or small-vessel strokes), meningeal signs, or communicating hydrocephalus (headaches, nausea, vomiting, dizziness, and altered mental status).

DIAGNOSIS

The major clinical manifestations of neurocysticercosis (e.g., seizures and hydrocephalus) are not specific, and it is difficult to identify the parasites. The main tools used to diagnose neurocysticercosis are neuroimaging studies. Computed tomography (CT) scans are sensitive for identification of parenchymal calcifications, which appear as 2- to 5-mm nodules. CT may also reveal parenchymal cysticerci or obstructive hydrocephalus. MRI scans are more sensitive for identification of the cysticerci, especially in the subarachnoid space and ventricles. Three-dimensional fast imaging employing steady-state acquisition (FIESTA) sequences are particularly effective for ventricular cysticerci. The cysticerci are typically round, 1 to 2 cm in diameter. The cyst fluid is usually isodense with spinal fluid. In uninflamed cysticerci, the walls may not be visible. However, most cases demonstrate enhancement of the cyst walls or surrounding tissues and associated edema. In some cases, the scolex may be visible as a 1- to 2-mm solid nodule, cylinder, or spiral on the side of the cystic lesions. Serologic tests are useful to confirm the diagnosis. Assays using crude antigen, including enzyme-linked immunosorbent assay, are associated with poor sensitivity and specificity and are not reliable. An immunoblot assay using semipurified membrane glycoproteins is highly specific for the diagnosis. The sensitivity is excellent in cases with extraparenchymal or multiple parenchymal cysticerci. However, the sensitivity is poor in those with single enhancing lesions or just calcifications. Antigen detection assays are sensitive and more specific for viable cases and are increasingly available in the United States.

TREATMENT Rx

Treatment varies with the clinical manifestations and form of infection. Seizures should be treated with antiepileptic drugs (Chapter 403). Phenytoin and carbamazepine are typically used and can control the seizures. Newer antiepileptic drugs may be more effective. There are no viable parasites in those with just calcified lesions, so the main measure is to control symptoms (e.g., antiepileptic drugs for those with seizures). In patients presenting with hydrocephalus, surgery to reestablish cerebrospinal fluid flow is the critical initial step in management. The role of antiparasitic drugs (Chapter 344) varies with the form of infection. Randomized controlled trials have demonstrated more rapid resolution of parenchymal cystic lesions in those treated with corticosteroids and albendazole (15 mg/kg/day in two daily doses) compared with those treated with placebo.[A1] Praziquantel (50 to 100 mg/kg/day in three daily doses) can be used as an alternative. There are emerging data on the use of the two drugs in combination, which may have greater cysticidal activity.[A2] A number of clinical trials in subjects with single enhancing lesions have demonstrated a slightly more rapid radiologic resolution and fewer seizures in those treated with steroids or antiparasitic drugs.[A3] However, the benefits of even high-dose steroids are not dramatic.[A4] For patients with cysticerci in the ventricles, management usually involves removal of the cysticerci, which can be best achieved by neuroendoscopy.[6] However, the main alternative approach is placement of a ventriculoperitoneal shunt. Chronic steroids or antiparasitic drugs may decrease the rate of shunt failure, which usually results from clogging of the shunts by the cysticerci or proteinaceous debris. There are no controlled trials on the management of subarachnoid cysticercosis. However, expert opinion supports treatment of subarachnoid cysticercosis with prolonged courses of antiparasitic drugs (e.g., albendazole for months), higher doses of albendazole, or combinations of albendazole and praziquantel. Chronic anti-inflammatory medications (e.g., prednisone 1 mg/kg/day, or 24 mg/day of dexamethasone) are also critically important. Patients who will be treated with chronic steroids should be screened for *Mycobacterium tuberculosis* and *Strongyloides* infections before initiation of steroid therapy. Methotrexate is increasingly recommended as a steroid-sparing agent. Patients with hydrocephalus should be treated by cerebrospinal fluid diversion (e.g., ventriculoperitoneal shunting). Before treatment with antiparasitic drugs, patients should undergo a funduscopic examination. Intraocular parasites may develop brisk inflammatory responses after treatment with antiparasitic drugs. Because this inflammation could lead to blindness, most authorities recommend extraction of the parasites before antiparasitic therapy. However, there are also reports of treatment of intraocular parasites with antiparasitic drugs.

PROGNOSIS

The prognosis varies significantly between the different forms of neurocysticercosis. Parenchymal enhancing lesions and parenchymal cystic lesions will eventually resolve, but this may take months to years. Patients who have or develop calcifications are at lifelong risk for recurrent seizures. Patients with ventricular or subarachnoid disease are at high risk for morbidity and mortality. However, a recent case series noted no deaths with optimal management.

Cystic Hydatid Disease (*Echinococcus granulosus* group)

DEFINITION

Cystic echinococcosis (CE), also called cystic hydatidosis, is caused by the larval stage of cestodes of the *Echinococcus granulosus* complex. All of these parasites were initially thought to be a single species, *E. granulosus*. However, molecular studies demonstrate that *E. granulosus* comprises a number of different species and genotypes. In humans, the clinical manifestations range from asymptomatic infection to severe, potentially fatal disease.

Echinococcal cysts consist of a periparasitic host tissue (pericyst or adventitia), which encompasses the larval endocyst, and the endocyst itself. The endocyst has an outer, acellular laminated layer and an inner, or germinative, layer that gives rise to brood capsules and protoscolices. The cyst is filled with clear fluid, numerous brood capsules, and protoscolices. Some cysts may also harbor daughter cysts of variable size. The protoscolices convert to tapeworms in the canine definitive hosts but can also form new cysts when released in mammalian tissues.

EPIDEMIOLOGY

E. granulosus species occur on all continents and in circumpolar, temperate, subtropical, and tropical zones. The highest prevalence of the parasite is found in parts of Eurasia, Africa, Australia, and South America. Within the endemic zones, the prevalence of the parasites varies from sporadic to high, but only a few countries can be regarded as being free of *E. granulosus*.

It is difficult to determine the true incidence of CE because of the slow rate of growth and variable clinical presentation. Most epidemiologic reports are based on hospital- and surgery-based surveys that greatly underestimate the actual rates of infection, especially in low socioeconomic groups with limited access to diagnosis and treatment.

Since the mid-1980s, however, mass community-based surveys using portable ultrasound scanners have been conducted in many remote, rural areas of the world. The sensitivity and specificity of ultrasound have been shown to be superior to those of serology in prevalence surveys. These studies showed the real burden of disease, uncovering population infection rates of up to 6.6%.

E. granulosus exists as a complex of species and strains that differ in a variety of criteria that may have an impact on the epidemiology, pathology, and control of CE. To date, 10 distinct genotypes (G1 to G10) have been identified. Some distinct species have been identified (*Echinococcus equinus*, *Echinococcus ortleppi*). The great majority of *E. granulosus* isolates from human patients thus far have been of the sheep genotype (G1).

CLINICAL MANIFESTATIONS

The presentation of human CE is protean.[6] Patients seek medical attention when a large cyst has some mechanical effect on organ function or rupture of a cyst causes acute hypersensitivity reactions. The cyst is often diagnosed incidentally during ultrasound examination, chest radiography, or body scanning performed for other clinical reasons. The liver is the most frequent location of echinococcal cysts, representing approximately 70% of cases.[7,8] The lungs are the second most common location. However, CE can occasionally occur in virtually any other organ.

Common symptoms are upper abdominal discomfort and pain, poor appetite, and a mass in the abdomen. Physical findings are hepatomegaly, a palpable mass on the surface of the liver or other organs, and abdominal distention. Other manifestations include jaundice, colic-like pains, portal hypertension, ascites, and compression of the inferior vena cava. If cysts in the lung rupture into the bronchi, symptoms may include intense cough, a salty taste in the mouth, or vomiting of hydatid material and cystic membranes. Patients may present with a chest mass, chest pain, chronic cough, pneumothorax, eosinophilic pneumonitis, pleural effusion, parasitic lung embolism, hemoptysis, or biliptysis. Cysts in the heart can cause a cardiac mass, pericardial effusion, and embolism. Cysts in the breast must be differentiated from neoplasms. Cysts located in the spine and in the brain can cause serious neurologic symptoms, including paralysis and seizures.

DIAGNOSIS

The diagnosis of CE is based on imaging methods and on serology, but serology has only a confirmatory role. Routine laboratory tests are nonspecific. Cyst rupture into the biliary tree may cause elevation of alkaline phosphatase, sometimes in association with hyperamylasemia and eosinophilia (up to 60%). Unless the cyst has ruptured, eosinophilia is low grade or absent.

Imaging

Modern imaging tools (ultrasound, CT, and, to a lesser extent, MRI) are central to the diagnosis and clinical management of CE. Ultrasound is the procedure of choice for diagnosis of asymptomatic CE. Ultrasound is also useful for longitudinal studies, such as monitoring the response of cysts to treatment and recording cyst growth rate. In 2003, the World Health Organization (WHO) Informal Working Group on Echinococcosis proposed a standardized ultrasound classification (Fig. 354-2). This classification defines six cyst stages that are assigned to three clinical groups. The active group comprises developing cysts, which may be unilocular (CE1) or multivesicular with daughter cysts (class CE2) and are usually found to be viable. The transitional group (class CE3) contains cysts that are usually starting to degenerate. There are two types of CE3: the "water lily sign" for floating membranes, which is now known as subclass CE3a; and predominantly solid cysts with daughter cysts, or subclass CE3b. This subdivision is based on their different response to percutaneous treatment (see later) and albendazole, which is generally good for CE3a and poor for CE3b. A study using nuclear magnetic resonance spectroscopy has found that CE3a and CE3b may have different metabolic characteristics. The inactive group (classes CE4 and CE5) exhibits involution and signs of solidification of cyst content with increasing degrees of calcification and is nearly always found to be nonviable.

CT scanning has the advantage of inspecting any organ, detecting smaller cysts located outside the liver, locating cysts precisely, and sometimes differentiating parasitic from nonparasitic cysts. MRI may have some advantages

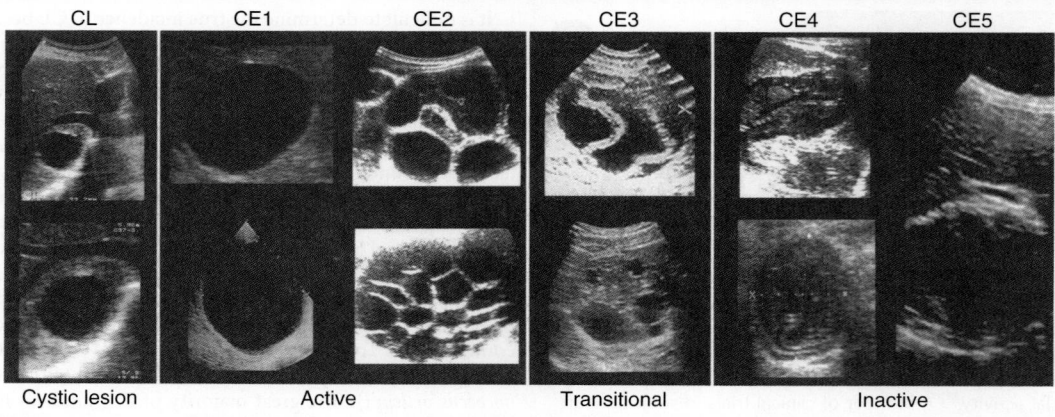

CL   CE1   CE2   CE3   CE4   CE5

Cystic lesion   Active   Transitional   Inactive

FIGURE 354-2. WHO Informal Working Group on Echinococcosis standardized ultrasound classification of cystic echinococcosis. CL lesions are cystic lesions lacking a distinct wall and may have other diagnoses. CE1 lesions are cystic lesions with a visible wall that may demonstrate protoscolices ("hydatid sand"). CE2 lesions include internal septation. CE3 lesions may be detached from the wall (CE3a, top row) or have daughter cysts with internal thickening (CE3b, bottom row). CE4 lesions are heterogeneous lesions with degeneration. CE5 lesions show thick calcification.

over CT scanning in the evaluation of postsurgical residual lesions, recurrences, and selected extrahepatic infections, such as cardiac infections. Furthermore, a study has shown that MRI reproduces the ultrasound-defined features of CE better than CT does. If ultrasound cannot be performed because of cyst location or patient-specific reasons, MRI with heavily T2-weighted series is preferable to CT. Plain radiographs are used for cysts in the lungs, bone, and muscle and for detection of calcified cysts.

Serology
Serologic tests are useful for confirmation of presumptive imaging diagnoses. However, many tests are available, and they are not standardized. Their sensitivity varies with the location of the cysts. Hepatic cysts are more likely to elicit an immune response than are pulmonary, brain, or splenic cysts. Serologic test results are usually positive when the endocyst is detached (CE3a) and in active (CE2) and transitional (CE3b) stages. Serologic test results are generally negative in patients with inactive cysts (CE4 and CE5). Titers tend to slowly decrease when a cyst becomes inactive (CE4, CE5) and after radical surgery. Titers may remain positive after conservative surgery in which the antigen source (the germinal layer) is not completely removed. Antibody titers usually increase immediately after medical or percutaneous treatments because of the mobilization of the antigen following disruption of cyst integrity.[9]

Other Diagnostic Procedures
Fine-needle aspiration of the cyst performed under ultrasonographic guidance, with a transhepatic approach, under anthelmintic coverage, is useful for differentiation of CE, malignant neoplasms, abscesses, and nonparasitic cysts. The procedure must be carried out in the presence of an anesthesiologist ready to manage the rare but possible anaphylactic reaction.

TREATMENT   Rx

The appropriate treatment depends on factors of the individual patient, the characteristics of the cyst, the therapeutic resources available, and the physician's preference. There are few randomized clinical trials evaluating treatment options, so a low level of evidence supports one therapeutic modality over another.

Surgery
Surgery has long been the only option in the treatment of CE. However, in the past two decades, medical treatment, percutaneous procedures, and a "watch and wait" approach have been successfully introduced and replaced surgery as the treatment of choice in selected cases. Surgery remains the main therapy in complicated cysts (i.e., those with rupture, biliary fistula, compression of vital structures, superinfection, or hemorrhage), cysts at high risk of rupture, or large cysts with many daughter vesicles that are not suitable for percutaneous treatments. Surgery can be performed as an open procedure, with either radical or conservative techniques, or laparoscopically, but there are controversies as to the safest and most effective technique and in which cases it should be applied. In all cases, perioperative albendazole prophylaxis, from 1 week before surgery until 4 weeks postoperatively, is recommended as

a cautionary measure to minimize the risk of fluid spillage and consequent secondary echinococcosis from seeding of protoscolices in the abdominal cavity. Some authorities treat with praziquantel as well.

Percutaneous Treatments
Percutaneous techniques provide an alternative to surgery and benzimidazole derivatives. These treatment modalities aim either to destroy the germinal layer with scolicidal agents or to evacuate the entire endocyst. The most popular method aimed at destroying the germinal layer is PAIR (puncture, aspiration, injection of a scolicidal agent, and reaspiration). Many modified catheterization techniques are used to evacuate the endocyst and are generally reserved for cysts that are difficult to drain or tend to relapse after PAIR, such as multivesiculated cysts or cysts with predominantly solid content and daughter cysts. A growing number of articles have reported its safety in treating abdominal, especially liver, echinococcal cysts. In a study on 5943 percutaneous punctures of echinococcal cysts, lethal anaphylaxis occurred in 0.03% of procedures, whereas reversible allergic reactions complicated 1.7% of procedures. Prophylactic administration of albendazole for at least 30 days after puncture is a cautionary measure that should always accompany PAIR. PAIR is generally successful at inducing permanent solidification in CE1 and CE3a cysts. A few reports with long-term follow-up indicate that multivesicular cysts (i.e., CE2 and CE3b) tend to relapse repeatedly after PAIR.

Chemotherapy
Albendazole (Chapter 344) is the antiparasitic drug of choice for CE. It is administered orally at a dosage of 10 to 15 mg/kg/day; administration should be continuous without treatment interruptions. However, the optimal dosage and optimal duration of treatment with albendazole have not been formally assessed, and data from the small clinical trials generally fail to take into account the cyst's characteristics. A recent systematic review on the effect of albendazole showed that the efficacy of the drug may have been overstated in previous retrospective, nonrandomized studies. Albendazole induces solidification in small and medium-sized CE1 and CE3a cysts, whereas it has generally little effect on giant (diameter > 10 cm) CE1 and CE3a cysts. It has no effect on most cases of CE2 and CE3b cysts.

Adverse effects of benzimidazoles (Chapter 344) include hepatotoxicity, leukopenia, thrombocytopenia, and alopecia. Increases in aminotransferases may be due to drug-related efficacy or real drug-related toxicity. Whereas teratogenic risks are theoretical, it is nonetheless good practice to avoid use during pregnancy when possible and to delay treatment until after delivery unless it is absolutely necessary.

Watch and Wait
Inactive liver cysts that are free of complications, such as compression on neighboring organs, are increasingly monitored without being treated.[10] Prospective studies need to be carried out to confirm the safety of this option.

Follow-up
Follow-up is crucial to evaluate the efficacy of treatment. Long-term follow-up, generally more than 5 years, is required to evaluate local recurrences, which have been reported up to 10 years after apparently successful treatment. When the combination of imaging and serology is inconclusive, fine-needle aspiration should be performed to ascertain the viability of the cyst contents.

355

Alveolar Hydatid Disease (*Echinococcus multilocularis*)

Alveolar hydatid disease is caused by the tissue forms of *Echinococcus multilocularis*. In tissues, typically the liver, *E. multilocularis* grows as a budding mass rather than as a large cystic lesion. The tissues resemble lung tissues, hence the name "alveolar." The normal definitive hosts are canines, including wolves and foxes. The normal intermediate hosts are rodents. Humans are accidentally infected by contact with soil containing the ova.

EPIDEMIOLOGY

E. multilocularis is endemic in arctic and alpine areas of the Northern Hemisphere. It is highly endemic in western China, Tibet, and central Asia. In recent years, *E. multilocularis* has emerged as an important problem in Alpine areas of central Europe and adjacent forested areas.

CLINICAL MANIFESTATIONS AND DIAGNOSIS

Human *E. multilocularis* infection almost invariably involves the liver, in which it is manifested as a tumor-like mass that gradually expands during decades. The main symptoms are liver discomfort and swelling. Diagnosis is by demonstration of a characteristic mass on imaging studies, with the etiology confirmed by serologic tests.[11]

TREATMENT AND PROGNOSIS Rx

Surgery remains the mainstay of treatment of *E. multilocularis*. When feasible, all infected tissues should be removed. Apparently curative therapy should be followed by a 2-year course of albendazole to decrease the risk of relapse. In some cases, resection is feasible only when it is accompanied by liver transplantation. In cases that are not amenable to surgical resection, prolonged courses of albendazole can suppress growth of the lesion. After treatment with benzimidazoles, mortality is similar to that of the age- and sex-matched general population.

Other Larval Cestode Infections

Sparganosis is caused by infection with the larval (plerocercoid) stage of *Spirometra mansonoides*. Infection is acquired by ingestion or application of infected meat (frogs, birds, fish) or exposure of skin to infected flesh (e.g., poultices of infected tissues). After infection, plerocercoids develop in the tissues, typically presenting as subcutaneous or central nervous system nodules or occasionally larva migrans symptoms. Treatment usually involves removal of the nodule.

Coenurosis is a rare larval cestode infection caused by human infection with the larval stage of the dog tapeworms *Taenia multiceps* and *Taenia serialis*. In the tissue, the larva forms a cystic lesion containing multiple scolices (the coenurus). The cystic lesion is usually single and most frequently identified in brain, eye, or soft tissues. Treatment usually involves removal.

Echinococcus oligarthrus and *Echinococcus vogeli* have been associated with polycystic hydatid disease in northern South America. *Taenia crassiceps* has been identified in the eye and in tissues of compromised hosts. *Hymenolepis*-like organisms have also been identified in tissues of AIDS patients.

Grade A References

A1. Baird A, Wiebe S, Zunt JR, et al. Evidence-based guideline: treatment of parenchymal neurocysticercosis: report of the Guideline Development Subcommittee of the American Academy of Neurology. *Neurology.* 2013;80:1424-1429.
A2. Garcia HH, Gonzales I, Lescano AG, et al. Efficacy of combined antiparasitic therapy with praziquantel and albendazole for neurocysticercosis: a double-blind, randomised controlled trial. *Lancet Infect Dis.* 2014;14:687-695.
A3. Otte WM, Singla M, Sander JW, et al. Drug therapy for solitary cysticercus granuloma: a systematic review and meta-analysis. *Neurology.* 2013;80:152-162.
A4. Garcia HH, Gonzales I, Lescano AG, et al. Enhanced steroid dosing reduces seizures during antiparasitic treatment for cysticercosis and early after. *Epilepsia.* 2014;55:1452-1459.

GENERAL REFERENCES

For the General References and other additional features, please visit Expert Consult at https://expertconsult.inkling.com.

SCHISTOSOMIASIS (BILHARZIASIS)

EDGAR M. CARVALHO AND ALDO A. M. LIMA

DEFINITION

Schistosomiasis, which is caused by trematodes of the genus *Schistosoma*, is one of the most important parasitic diseases of humans and is a global public health problem in the developing world.[1] *S. mansoni, S. haematobium, S. japonicum, S. intercalatum,* and *S. mekongi* are the five major species of *Schistosoma* affecting humans. Other *Schistosoma* species that occasionally infect humans include *S. bovis, S. mattheei,* and some avian schistosomes.

EPIDEMIOLOGY

Schistosomiasis occurs mainly in tropical and subtropical areas, especially in poor communities without access to safe drinking water and adequate sanitation.[2] It is estimated that 200 million people are infected by the helminth and 600 to 799 million are at risk of infection.[3] *S. mansoni* is found in 55 countries, mainly in Africa, the Middle East, the Caribbean, Brazil, Venezuela, and Suriname. *S. haematobium* is endemic in 53 countries in the Middle East and most of the African continent. *S. japonicum* is endemic in China, Indonesia, and the Philippines. *S. intercalatum* has been reported from 10 countries in Africa. *S. mekongi* is found in Cambodia and Laos.

The endemicity of schistosomiasis depends on the urban disposal of urine (*S. haematobium*) and feces (*S. mansoni, S. japonicum, S. intercalatum, S. mekongi*), the presence of suitable snail hosts, and human exposure to cercariae.[4] The freshwater snail intermediate hosts are *Biomphalaria* sp in Africa and *Biomphalaria glabrata (Australorbis)* and *Tropicarbis* in South America and the West Indies. In some cases, the endemicity of schistosomiasis may be maintained by animal reservoirs. Such is the case with *S. japonicum*, which infects dogs and cows. Rodents, monkeys, and baboons have been found infected in nature, but the role of these animals as reservoirs does not seem to be epidemiologically important.

Etiology and Life Cycle

The schistosomes are digenetic parasitic trematodes (Fig. 355-1). Although they are morphologically distinct, the species of *Schistosoma* that infect humans share some common characteristics. The large male (0.6 to 2.2 cm × 2 to 4 mm) has a ventral gynecophoric canal, in which the female (1.2 to 2.6 cm × 1 to 2 mm) is held during copulation. The sequencing of the *S. mansoni* genome has been determined.

Adult worms live in the mesenteric veins (*S. mansoni, S. japonicum, S. mekongi,* and *S. intercalatum*) or in the venous plexus around the lower ends of the ureters and the urinary bladder (*S. haematobium*). In these sites, they start their sexual reproduction by releasing eggs. Once deposited in the host, eggs can stay in the mesenteric vein, be trapped in the intestines, escape to the

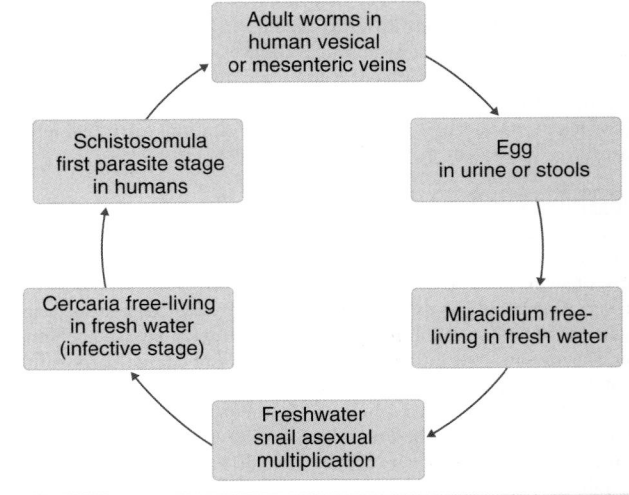

FIGURE 355-1. Schistosome life cycle.

intestinal lumen, and migrate by portal blood to the liver (*S. mansoni*, *S. japonicum*). Eggs of *S. haematobium* can be trapped in the intestines and bladder, escape to the intestinal or bladder lumen, and be trapped in the female genital tract. After being excreted with feces or urine into fresh water, the eggs hatch and release ciliated motile miracidia that penetrate into the snail intermediate host. Following asexual multiplication in the snail, the development of cercariae, the infective forms for humans, takes 4 to 7 weeks. After leaving the snails, the cercariae can survive in fresh water for almost 72 hours. When penetration of the skin in the human host occurs, the cercariae lose their tails and change into schistosomula. Schistosomula migrate to the lungs and in about 6 weeks mature into adult worms, after which they descend to their final habitat. Viable eggs can be seen in excretions (i.e., stool or urine) 5 to 9 weeks after cercarial penetration. The lifespan of the worms ranges from 5 to 10 years.

PATHOBIOLOGY

The pathogenesis of acute human schistosomiasis is mainly related to egg deposition and liberation of antigens of adult worms and eggs. A strong inflammatory response characterized by high levels of pro-inflammatory cytokines, such as interleukins 1 and 6 and tumor necrosis factor-α, and by circulating immune complexes participates in the pathogenesis of the acute phase of the disease.

In chronic schistosomiasis, tissue injury is mediated by egg-induced granulomas and the subsequent appearance of fibrosis. Because the habitat of *S. mansoni*, *S. japonicum*, *S. mekongi*, and *S. intercalatum* worms is the mesenteric blood vessels, the intestines are involved primarily, and egg embolism results in secondary involvement of the liver. Host genetics, immunologic response, and parasite load measured by egg count in the stool are associated with a greater chance of liver fibrosis resulting in hepatosplenomegaly. Polymorphisms within the interferon-γ receptor 1 (*IFNGR1*) gene may be related to severe hepatic disease caused by *S. mansoni* infection. There is also evidence that increased levels of interleukin 5 and tumor necrosis factor-α are associated with fibrosis.[5] The granuloma is mainly composed of macrophages, eosinophils, fibroblasts, and collagen deposition. The size of these granulomas and the resulting fibrosis lead to most of the chronic fibro-obstructive lesions in schistosomiasis. In the liver, the granulomas result in perisinusoidal obstruction of portal blood flow, portal hypertension, splenomegaly, esophageal varices, and portosystemic collateral circulation. Liver cell perfusion is consequently preserved, and liver function test results remain normal well into the course of the disease. In *S. haematobium* infection, eggs and granuloma formation are predominantly found in the ureters, bladder, and genital tract.

In schistosome-infected persons, the intensity of infection increases during the first two decades of life as children accumulate worms, with infection intensity declining thereafter. In the *S. haematobium*–infected population, IgE increases progressively with age, and IgE antibodies directed against adult worm antigens are associated with subsequent low intensities of reinfection. Alternatively, in subjects who are highly exposed to contaminated water but have negative stool examination results, there is evidence of higher interferon-γ production in response to *S. mansoni* antigens.[6] The existence of a major codominant gene, called *SM1*, which controls the intensity of infection by *S. mansoni*, has been demonstrated. *S. mansoni* infection levels are controlled by a locus that maps to chromosome 5q31-q33, which is close to a locus regulating IgE levels, indicating that genetic factors are probably critical to susceptibility and resistance to schistosome infection.

Because modulation of the immune response is a characteristic of chronic schistosomiasis, *S. mansoni* infection attenuates the clinical manifestations of autoimmune and inflammatory diseases, but it may also impair the immunologic response to vaccines and change manifestations of other infectious diseases.

CLINICAL MANIFESTATIONS

Clinical manifestations of schistosomiasis are divided into schistosome dermatitis, acute schistosomiasis, and chronic schistosomiasis. Schistosome dermatitis, or swimmer's itch, is an uncommon manifestation seen mainly when avian cercariae penetrate the skin and are destroyed. Schistosome dermatitis is a sensitization phenomenon occurring in previously exposed persons. The cercariae evoke an acute inflammatory response with edema, early infiltration of neutrophils and lymphocytes, and later invasion of eosinophils. A pruritic papular rash occurs within 24 hours after the penetration of cercariae and reaches maximal intensity in 2 to 3 days.

Acute schistosomiasis occurs usually 20 to 50 days after primary exposure. Although it is asymptomatic in endemic areas, acute schistosomiasis is becoming a frequent and major clinical problem in nonimmune individuals from urban regions who are exposed for the first time to a heavy infectious

dose in an endemic area. The clinical syndrome (i.e., fever, chills, liver and spleen enlargement, and marked eosinophilia) originally described for *S. japonicum* infection, and still common for this species, is increasingly being diagnosed in Brazil in individuals with *S. mansoni* infection. Malaise, diarrhea, weight loss, cough, dyspnea, chest pain, restrictive respiratory insufficiency, and pericarditis are important findings in this phase. High levels of circulating immune complexes correlate with respiratory manifestations, and tumor necrosis factor-α levels correlate with the presence of abdominal pain, diarrhea, and weight loss. Abdominal ultrasound may show hepatosplenomegaly. Acute disease is not observed in individuals living in endemic areas of schistosomiasis because of the down-modulation of the immune response by antigens or idiotypes transferred from mother to child.

In chronic schistosomiasis, abdominal pain, irregular bowel movements, and blood in the stool are the main symptoms of intestinal involvement. Colonic polyposis may occur, especially in Egypt. Hepatosplenic involvement is the most important cause of morbidity with *S. mansoni* and *S. japonicum* infection. Patients may remain asymptomatic until the manifestation of hepatic fibrosis and portal hypertension develops. Hepatic fibrosis is caused by a granulomatous reaction to *Schistosoma* eggs that have been carried to the liver. Hematemesis from bleeding esophageal or gastric varices may occur. In such cases, anemia and decreasing levels of serum albumin are observed. Some patients have severe hepatosplenic disease with decompensated liver disease. Jaundice, ascites, and liver failure are then observed. Concomitant infection by *Salmonella* species, and less extensively by other gram-negative bacteria, with *S. mansoni* or *S. haematobium* leads to a picture of prolonged fever, hepatosplenomegaly, and mild leukocytosis with eosinophilia. Glomerulonephritis, infantilism, and hypersplenism are other complications associated with hepatosplenic schistosomiasis. The detection of pulmonary hypertension is increasing with the use of more advanced diagnostic technology. Pulmonary hypertension, which used to be exclusively linked to the hepatosplenic form of the disease, has been documented in patients without liver fibrosis.[7] In hospitalized adult patients with *S. japonicum* infection, cerebral schistosomiasis occurs in 1.7 to 4.3%.[8] It may occur as early as 6 weeks after infection, and the most common sign is focal jacksonian epilepsy. Signs and symptoms of generalized encephalitis may occasionally be found. In *S. mansoni* infection, neurologic involvement is rare and mainly characterized by transverse myelitis, which occurs mainly in patients without liver fibrosis and hepatosplenomegaly.[9]

In *S. haematobium* infection, the main organ system involved is the urogenital tract. The acute granulomatous response to parasite eggs in the early stages causes urinary tract disease, such as urethral ulceration and bladder polyposis. In chronic disease, usually in older patients, granulomas at the lower end of the ureters obstruct urinary flow and may cause hydroureter and hydronephrosis. Bladder fibrosis and calcification are also seen in this phase. Up to 70% of infected individuals have hematuria, dysuria, or urinary frequency. Urine examination reveals proteinuria and hematuria. Radiologic findings include hydronephrosis; hydroureter; ureteral strictures, dilation, or distortion; ureteral calcifications; ureterolithiasis; calcified bladder; polyps; reduction in bladder capacity; irregular contraction of the bladder wall; or a dilated bladder because of bladder neck fibrosis. An increased incidence of squamous cell carcinoma of the bladder has been reported in endemic areas of *S. haematobium* infection.[10] *S. haematobium* eggs have occasionally been found in the lungs, with subsequent focal pulmonary arteritis and pulmonary hypertension. Genital schistosomiasis has been documented in up to 75% of women in *S. haematobium*–endemic areas[11] and has also been documented in girls.[12] Spontaneous bleeding, burning sensation in the genitals, dyspareunia, itching, tumors due to granulomas, and infertility are the more common complaints. The association of genital schistosomiasis and HIV infection has been recognized. Monocytes and CD4$^+$ T cells as well as high expression of chemokine receptors CCR5 and CXCR4 documented in schistosomiasis may facilitate binding of the virus after penetration through an ulcerated friable epithelium.

DIAGNOSIS

A definitive diagnosis of schistosomiasis can be made only by finding schistosome eggs in feces, urine, or a biopsy specimen, usually from the rectum (Table 355-1). However, a steep decrease of sensitivity is found in low-endemicity areas. A history of contact with contaminated water and appropriate clinical manifestations are important steps in establishing the diagnosis. Because schistosome eggs may be few, concentration by sedimentation should be performed. All eggs from feces, urine, or tissues should be examined under high power to determine their viability by visualizing the activity of cilia of the excretory flame cells of the enclosed miracidium. Dead eggs

TABLE 355-1   DIAGNOSIS OF SCHISTOSOMIASIS

SCHISTOSOME	EGGS	DIAGNOSIS
S. haematobium	Mainly found in urine but may be found in stools or rectal biopsy specimens Eggs: 143 × 50 µm; spindle shaped: rounded anterior, conical posterior, tapering to a terminal delicate spine	Obtain urine sample at midday (when eggs are excreted); more than one sample may be needed Examine urine directly or by filtering 10 mL of urine through a Nuclepore membrane Rectal biopsy in suspected cases with normal urine Serologic testing to diagnose early or light infection
S. mansoni	Eggs: 155 × 66 µm; oval with lateral, long spine	Examine stool for eggs Use the Kato-Katz thick smear method for quantification purposes Rectal biopsy or serologic testing to diagnose stool-negative cases, particularly in lightly infected patients
S. japonicum	Found in stool Eggs: 89 × 67 µm; oval or rounded with a lateral, short, sometimes curved spine	Examine stool for eggs Kato-Katz thick smear (for quantitative assessment) Rectal biopsy for those with light infections, especially with less common manifestations (i.e., cerebral schistosomiasis)
S. mekongi	Found in stool Eggs: 60 × 32 µm; smaller than eggs of S. japonicum	Examine stool for eggs
S. intercalatum	Found in stool Eggs: 180 × 65 µm; terminal spine	Examine stool for eggs

may persist for a long time after successful therapy or natural death of the worms. Because the intensity of infection is associated with morbidity, quantitative techniques such as the Kato-Katz thick smear method are recommended for *S. mansoni* and *S. japonicum*. Rectal biopsy may be used for those with light infection. Ultrasonography allows determination of the degree of liver fibrosis. *S. mekongi* and *S. intercalatum* infection is diagnosed by examination of the stool for eggs.

Urine examination for *S. haematobium* eggs can be performed by direct or concentration methods. Samples should be obtained at midday, when excretion of eggs is maximal. Rectal biopsy may be performed in patients with negative urine results. Schistosome real-time polymerase chain reaction is sensitive and specific in urine and stool.[13] After *S. haematobium* infection is diagnosed, assessment of urinary tract disease by ultrasonography is recommended. Because of an increased incidence of carcinoma of the bladder, cancer surveillance should be performed in patients with *S. haematobium* infection.

Serologic tests may help the diagnosis of acute infection because the symptoms are not specific and the finding of eggs in stool may reflect chronic infection.

Quantification of circulating antigens in serum and urine is an alternative for the diagnosis of schistosome infection. However, the sensitivity of the method decreases in patients with light infection (<100 eggs per gram of feces). This test has also been used to monitor the efficacy of antischistosome chemotherapy. A significant decrease in antigen levels or negativity of the test is observed as early as 10 days after therapy.

TREATMENT   Rx

Chemotherapy is by far the major method used for prophylaxis, control, and cure of schistosomiasis. Several compounds are in use: metrifonate, oxamniquine, praziquantel, and artemisin derivatives (artesunate and artemether).[14] Praziquantel, a pyrazinoisoquinoline derivative, is the drug of choice for the treatment of schistosomiasis for four reasons: high efficacy against all schistosome species and against cestodes, lack of serious short-term and long-term side effects, administration as a single oral dose, and competitive cost. Recent reviews confirm that a single dose of praziquantel (40 mg/kg) is an effective treatment for *S. mansoni* infection.[A1][A2] Doses lower than 40 mg/kg may be less effective, with no additional benefit for higher doses. Oxamniquine (40 mg/

kg) is also effective, and on the basis of current limited evidence, it is uncertain which intervention is more effective. A meta-analysis study also confirmed that artemisinin derivatives, unlike oxamniquine, used in combination with praziquantel increased the cure rates in schistosomiasis treatment, but artemisinin derivatives or oxamniquine alone did not.[A3]

The standard recommended treatment consists of a single dose of praziquantel, 40 mg/kg, for *S. mansoni, S. haematobium,* and *S. intercalatum* infection. In *S. japonicum* infection, a total dose of 60 mg/kg is recommended, split into two or three doses in a single day. Although no significant difference was found in the overall cure rates between single-dose (40 mg/kg) and double treatment (40 mg/kg with 2-week interval) regimens of praziquantel for *S. haematobium,* the effect of double treatment resulted in significant reduction in infection intensity and microhematuria, which may have an impact in reducing morbidity.[A4] *S. mekongi* may require two treatments at 60 mg/kg body weight. With these dosages of praziquantel, recorded cure rates are 75 to 85% for *S. haematobium,* 63 to 85% for *S. mansoni,* 80 to 90% for *S. japonicum,* 89% for *S. intercalatum,* and 60 to 80% for double infections with *S. mansoni* and *S. haematobium.* A decrease in the efficacy of praziquantel has been observed in patients coinfected with human T-cell leukemia virus type 1.

Praziquantel is well tolerated and effective in patients of all ages and for different clinical forms of schistosomiasis, including advanced hepatosplenic cases (*S. mansoni*), cerebral schistosomiasis (*S. japonicum*), and neurologic syndromes (*S. mansoni* and *S. haematobium*), possibly in association with corticosteroids.[15] However, praziquantel has a poor prophylactic effect, which reduces its efficacy in areas of high transmission. There have been several reports of persistent schistosome egg shedding after treatment, thus posing a concern about the emergence of drug resistance.[16] A systematic review and meta-analysis show that either artesunate or artemether has a confirmed prophylactic effect across different trials performed in China. Further studies will be necessary to examine the combination of antischistosome chemotherapy for *S. haematobium* infection in which repeated standard treatment fails to clear the infection.

The most common adverse events observed with praziquantel or oxamniquine are related to the gastrointestinal tract: abdominal pain or discomfort, nausea, vomiting, anorexia, and diarrhea. These symptoms can be observed in up to 50% of patients but are usually well tolerated. Other side effects are related to the central nervous system (e.g., headache, dizziness, drowsiness) and the skin (e.g., pruritus, eruptions) or may be nonspecific (e.g., fever, fatigue). In general, the cumulative experience from a large number of studies allows the conclusion that praziquantel is an extremely well tolerated drug that requires minimal medical supervision and is therefore particularly suitable for mass chemotherapy programs. Although a reduction in the intensity of infection and morbidity has been documented after mass chemotherapy, to control the disease, provision of clean water, use of molluscicides, implementation of adequate sanitation, and improvement of socioeconomic conditions should also be undertaken.

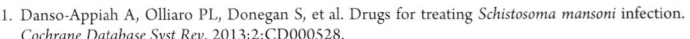

Grade A References

A1. Danso-Appiah A, Olliaro PL, Donegan S, et al. Drugs for treating *Schistosoma mansoni* infection. *Cochrane Database Syst Rev.* 2013;2:CD000528.

A2. Kramer CV, Zhang F, Sinclair D, et al. Drugs for treating urinary schistosomiasis. *Cochrane Database Syst Rev.* 2014;8:CD000053.

A3. Pérez del Villar L, Burguillo FJ, López-Abán J, et al. Systematic review and meta-analysis of artemisinin based therapies for the treatment and prevention of schistosomiasis. *PLoS ONE.* 2012;7:e45867.

A4. Sacko M, Magnussen P, Traore M, et al. The effect of single dose versus two doses of praziquantel on Schistosoma haematobium infection and pathology among school-aged children in Mali. *Parasitology.* 2009;136:1851-1857.

GENERAL REFERENCES

For the General References and other additional features, please visit Expert Consult at https://expertconsult.inkling.com.

356

LIVER, INTESTINAL, AND LUNG FLUKE INFECTIONS

EDUARDO GOTUZZO

Flukes belong to the phylum Platyhelminthes and class Trematoda. The major flukes of medical importance, other than *Schistosoma*, are discussed in this chapter; they belong to the families Fasciolidae, Opisthorchiidae,

TABLE 356-1 CLINICAL MANIFESTATIONS, DIAGNOSIS, AND TREATMENT OF LIVER, INTESTINAL, AND LUNG FLUKE INFECTIONS IN HUMANS

FLUKE, NUMBER OF PEOPLE INFECTED, AND GEOGRAPHIC DISTRIBUTION	CLINICAL MANIFESTATIONS ACUTE AND CHRONIC PHASES	DIAGNOSIS*	TREATMENT[†]
LIVER FLUKES			
Fasciola spp 17 million Cosmopolitan	Acute [‡]Hepatomegaly, eosinophilia, fever, abdominal pain, metastatic-like lesions on liver CT Chronic [§]Biliary obstruction, gallstones, fibrosis, cholangitis	Stools are negative Serology (Fas2 ELISA) Eggs in stool Fas2 ELISA	TCZ
Opisthorchis spp 11.2 million Asia	[‡]Fever, malaise, arthralgia, lymphadenopathy, and rash [§]Jaundice, cholangitis, cholangiocarcinoma	Serology Eggs in stool	PZQ
Clonorchis spp 35 million Asia Eastern Europe	[‡]Fever, rash, malaise, and RUQ discomfort [§]Choledocholithiasis, cholangitis, cholecystitis, liver abscess, and possible cholangiocarcinoma	Serology Eggs in stool	PZQ
INTESTINAL FLUKES			
Fasciolopsis buski and others[¶] 50 million Asia and North Africa	Small bowel inflammation, ulceration, mucus secretion, protein-losing enteropathy, malabsorption	Eggs in stool	PZQ
LUNG FLUKE			
Paragonimus spp 22 million Asia, Americas, Africa	[‡]Abdominal pain, pleuritic pain, cough, eosinophilia [§]Hemoptysis, cough, chronic pleural effusions, pulmonary cysts, abscess	Serology Eggs in sputum or stool	PZQ or TCZ

*For egg morphology and size, refer to text in the Diagnosis section.
[†]For drug regimens, refer to text in the Treatment section.
[‡]Acute.
[§]Chronic. For chronic infection, a sedimentation technique is preferred (suggested technique: rapid sedimentation technique or Kato-Katz technique).
[¶]Diagnosis and treatment also apply for other intestinal flukes.
CT = computed tomography; ELISA = enzyme-linked immunosorbent assay; PZQ = praziquantel; RUQ = right upper quadrant; TCZ = triclabendazole.

Heterophyidae, Echinostomatidae, and Troglotrematidae. With the exception of schistosomes, all flat worms of clinical significance are hermaphroditic. Blood flukes, or schistosomes, are discussed in Chapter 355. The epidemiology, clinical manifestations, diagnosis, and treatment are summarized in Table 356-1.

LIVER FLUKES
Fascioliasis

Fascioliasis is a zoonosis caused by *Fasciola hepatica* (adult: 30 by 13 mm) or *Fasciola gigantica* (adult: 75 by 20 mm). The most common natural hosts are sheep, cattle, and goats.

EPIDEMIOLOGY

The infection is distributed globally. The highlands of Peru, Bolivia, Ecuador, Egypt, and Vietnam are the most affected regions in the world. Prevalence rates higher than 60% have been reported in Peru and Bolivia. Estimates of the number of people infected in some countries are 830,000 in Egypt, 742,000 in Peru, 360,000 in Bolivia, 37,000 in Yemen, 20,000 in Ecuador, and 10,000 in Iran. It has been estimated that between 2.4 and 17 million people are infected worldwide.[1]

PATHOBIOLOGY

The life cycle begins when the parasite's eggs in stool are deposited in water; miracidia appear, develop, and hatch in 9 to 14 days and invade many species of freshwater snails (*Lymnaea* spp), in which they multiply as sporozoites, rediae, and cercariae during a period of 4 to 7 weeks. They then leave as free-swimming cercaria that subsequently attach to watercress, water lettuce, alfalfa, mint, parsley, or khat. The main source of infection is consumption of raw vegetables or water contaminated with metacercariae. Women have a higher incidence of the disease, with more severe infections and complications than seen in men.

CLINICAL MANIFESTATIONS

After consumption of contaminated vegetables, the larvae excyst in the duodenum and then migrate through the bowel wall to the liver through the peritoneal cavity. In 4 weeks, they reach the liver, penetrate Glisson's capsule,

and cause inflammation and pain. An acute diarrhea of 2 to 5 days' duration may occur before liver invasion. During their migration through the liver, the ongoing inflammatory process is accompanied by fever, pain, and hypereosinophilia. In a few cases, intense hemorrhage manifested as subcapsular liver hematoma may develop. Computed tomography (CT), magnetic resonance imaging, or ultrasonography can detect these initial lesions. Furthermore, migration of the parasite leaves a trail or track that can be observed in histologic sections or by imaging (CT). The flukes sometimes die and leave cavities filled with necrotic debris that are eventually replaced by scar tissue and then become calcified. After 3 to 5 months of migration in the liver, the juvenile larvae finally reach the bile ducts. During this invasive, migratory, or acute phase the clinical manifestations are prolonged fever, hepatomegaly, abdominal pain, and eosinophilia. Multiple hypodense lesions are seen on CT, similar to metastases, but they change in position, attenuation, and shape in time because the parasites are still migrating. Acute fascioliasis is clinically similar to acute cholecystitis but with the addition of significant eosinophilia. It can occur in travelers with acute subcapsular hematoma or "metastatic-like lesions" seen on CT of the liver. Hyperbilirubinemia is notably absent in this phase. Other manifestations are anorexia, weight loss, nausea, vomiting, cough, diarrhea, urticaria, lymphadenopathy, and arthralgias. Occasionally, the juvenile larvae reach other ectopic or extrahepatic locations, such as subcutaneous tissue, the pancreas, the eye, the brain,[2] and the stomach wall, among others. In endemic areas, the acute phase manifestations can be superimposed on chronic infection.

Arrival of the parasite in the bile ducts marks the beginning of the chronic phase. Mature flukes consume hepatocytes and duct epithelium and reside for years in the hepatic and common bile ducts and sometimes in the gallbladder. In this chronic phase, the liver contains large dilated, thick-walled, and calcareous bile ducts with yellowish-brown bile. The bile ducts have a thickened hyperplastic wall with marked fibrosis. Symptoms usually reflect biliary obstruction with colicky pain in the right upper quadrant and epigastric area. Eosinophilia is absent in half of the chronic cases. Bacterial superinfection of these cysts and consequent cholangitis can develop. Other complications are hemobilia and liver fibrosis. Alkaline phosphatase is commonly elevated because of biliary obstruction, which sometimes requires surgical intervention. On imaging, the initial lesions may be often confused with hepatic metastases. Other findings on CT are hepatomegaly, tracklike hypodense lesions in subcapsular locations, multiple hypodense nodular areas (abscess-like lesions), or low-density, serpiginous, tortuous, tunnel-like branching lesions ranging from 2 to 10 mm. CT also can show subcapsular hematoma, enhancement of Glisson's capsule, necrotic granuloma, and cystic calcifications. After maturation, the adult flukes start laying eggs, which are passed from the sphincter of Oddi to the intestines and evacuated to the environment along with stool. Adult parasites can live in the bile ducts for up to 13 years. In endemic populations, chronic infection has been reported as mildly symptomatic, whereas in travelers or temporary residents, it has been reported to cause biliary obstruction, with adult parasites being seen on endoscopic retrograde cholangiopancreatography (ERCP).

In summary, the typical clinical presentation of acute fascioliasis must be differentiated from cholecystitis; "liver metastasis" with fever and hypereosinophilia should raise the possibility of this infection; and in children and adolescents, systemic toxocariasis will be the differential diagnosis

Clonorchiasis and Opisthorchiasis

Clonorchiasis is the disease caused by *Clonorchis sinensis,* also called the Chinese or oriental liver fluke (adult: 10 to 25 mm by 3 to 5 mm). Opisthorchiasis is caused by *Opisthorchis viverrini* (adult: 5 mm to 10 mm by 1 mm to 2 mm) and *Opisthorchis felineus* (adult: 7 to 12 mm by 2 to 3 mm). The most common natural hosts are dogs, cats, pigs, and some small wild mammals.

EPIDEMIOLOGY

The global estimate of the number of people infected is 46.2 million: 35 million with *C. sinensis* (15 million in China), 10 million with *O. viverrini* (8 million in Thailand), and 1.2 million with *O. felineus.* There are 601 million and 79.8 million people at risk for infection with *Clonorchis* and *Opisthorchis,* respectively. Both infections are endemic in the Far East, Southeast Asia, and Eastern Europe. *C. sinensis* is endemic in northeast China, southern Korea, Japan, Taiwan, northern Vietnam, and the far eastern part of Russia, whereas *O. viverrini* is endemic in Laos, Thailand, Vietnam, and Cambodia. *O. felineus* infection is prevalent in Russia, Ukraine, and Kazakhstan.

PATHOBIOLOGY

The life cycle starts when the adult worm deposits fully developed eggs, which are then passed to the environment through feces. They hatch in water and the miracidia infect their first intermediate host, a freshwater snail (*Bithynia* spp or *Parafossarulus* spp), where they transform into sporocysts, rediae, and cercariae. Cercariae are released from the snail and then penetrate freshwater fish, which are the second intermediate host (*Cyclocheilichthys* spp, *Puntius* spp, *Hampala dispar*); the cercariae encyst as metacercariae in the muscles or under the scales. In general, the infection is acquired by eating raw or uncooked cyprinoid fish products in rural areas or dishes such as koi-pla, a salad made with raw fish. The metacercariae pass through the stomach and reach the small intestine unharmed. Then, through the ampulla of Vater, they reach the bile ducts, where they mature into adult worms within 4 weeks and deposit yellow, operculated eggs. The parasites may live for up to 45 years in a human host.

CLINICAL MANIFESTATIONS

Clonorchiasis as an acute infection caused by *C. sinensis* is usually asymptomatic, but some patients may have fever, rash, malaise, and right upper quadrant abdominal discomfort.[3] Chronic infections may be manifested as recurrent pyogenic cholangitis, cholecystitis, obstructive jaundice, hepatomegaly, cholecystitis, multiple hepatic tumors, cholelithiasis, or pancreatitis. In chronic carriers with a high load of parasites, cholangiocarcinoma may develop, especially in Thailand.

Opisthorchiasis as an acute infection caused by *O. viverrini* can cause right upper quadrant abdominal pain, flatulence, fatigue, and a hot sensation over the abdomen. In the chronic phase, mild hepatomegaly occurs, mainly in more heavily infected patients (egg counts >10,000/g). Jaundice and splenomegaly are not observed. Intrahepatic duct stones and recurrent suppurative cholangitis are common manifestations of opisthorchiasis. Whenever jaundice and ascending cholangitis are detected, fluke-related cholangiocarcinoma should be suspected.[4]

In opisthorchiasis caused by *O. felineus,* infestation usually follows the consumption of raw, slightly salted, and frozen fish ("stroganina"), and acute symptoms occur 2 to 4 weeks later, including high-grade fever, nausea, vomiting, abdominal pain, malaise, arthralgias, lymphadenopathy, and rash. Peripheral eosinophilia is a common finding, especially during the initial 2 to 6 weeks of the infection, together with raised liver enzyme levels. In chronic

infection, the eosinophilia is usually milder. Patients may have suppurative cholangitis and liver abscesses because of biliary obstruction. Ultrasonography or CT demonstrates the pathologic changes in the liver, including intrahepatic duct dilation and periductal changes.

The pathologic and clinical consequences of these flukes are related to the intensity and duration of cumulative infestations. In general, they cause inflammation around the biliary tree, severe hyperplasia of epithelial cells, metaplasia of mucin-producing cells in the mucosa, and progressive periductal fibrosis. There are clear associations between *O. viverrini* infection and cholangiocarcinoma.[5] Several *N*-nitroso compounds and their precursors occur at low levels in fermented food, such as preserved mud fish paste (*pla ra*), a condiment that is a ubiquitous component of the cuisine of northeastern Thailand and Laos.

● INTESTINAL FLUKES

The most common human intestinal trematode is *Fasciolopsis buski* (adult: 20 to 75 mm by 8 to 20 mm). It is found mainly in the central and southeast parts of Asia. *F. buski* is a common parasite in pigs. Others are *Heterophyes* (adult: 1 to 2 mm in length), *Metagonimus yokogawai* (adult: 1 to 2.5 mm by 0.4 to 0.75 mm), and *Echinostoma* spp (adult: 6.5 by 1 to 2 mm).

EPIDEMIOLOGY

More than 50 species of intestinal trematodes from the Far East, Middle East, and North Africa have been reported to cause human infection. *H. heterophyes* also can be found in the Nile delta region of Egypt. An estimated 40 to 50 million people are infected with one or several species of intestinal flukes. Their life cycles are similar. The adult worm, attached to the intestinal wall of humans, produces eggs that are passed in feces. The eggs reach water, and miracidia develop and penetrate the first intermediate host—snails. During the course of 6 to 7 weeks inside the host snails, they develop into sporocysts, rediae, and cercariae. The cercariae leave the snails to encyst in the second intermediate host, which can be freshwater snails, fish, tadpoles, or vegetables. Humans are infected by the ingestion of raw stems, leaves (especially bamboo shoots), watercress, or water chestnuts with encysted metacercariae. In the human duodenum, the metacercariae attach to the walls and become adult worms in approximately 3 months.

PATHOBIOLOGY AND CLINICAL MANIFESTATIONS

Despite the fact that the majority of intestinal fluke infections are asymptomatic, they may cause inflammation, ulceration, and mucus secretion at the site of attachment, particularly in the duodenum and jejunum. In fact, gastrointestinal hemorrhage, perforation, and abscesses have been observed. The differential diagnoses include typhoid fever, intestinal tuberculosis, and amebiasis. In these endemic cases, ulcerative colitis and other inflammatory diseases of the bowel are uncommon. In heavy infection, intestinal obstruction, protein-losing enteropathy, malabsorption, impaired vitamin B_{12} absorption, hypoalbuminemia, and anasarca have been reported. The adult worm causes traumatic, toxic, and obstructive damage to the intestinal mucosa. Some cases have been diagnosed by direct visualization of the adult parasite via esophagogastroduodenoscopy.

● PULMONARY FLUKES

Paragonimiasis is a zoonosis caused by *Paragonimus* spp (adult size: 10 by 5 mm).[6] Reservoir hosts include felids, canids, viverrids, mustelids, some rodents, and pigs. At least 10 species of *Paragonimus* are known to cause human disease; of these, *Paragonimus westermani* is the most common.

EPIDEMIOLOGY

An estimated 22 million people are infected worldwide with *Paragonimus* spp, and 293 million are at risk. Human paragonimiasis is distributed mainly in Southeast Asia, Japan, Korea, China, and the Philippines, where *P. westermani* is the main species. In other areas of low endemicity, other species have been reported, such as *Paragonimus mexicanus* in Latin America, *Paragonimus kellicotti* in North America, *Paragonimus heterotremus* in India, and *Paragonimus africanus,* and *Paragonimus uterobilateralis* in West Africa.

PATHOBIOLOGY

The life cycle starts when the eggs are excreted unembryonated in sputum, or alternatively they can be swallowed and passed in stool. In the external environment the eggs become embryonated, and miracidia hatch, seek the first intermediate host, a snail (families Pleuroceridae and Thiaridae), and penetrate its soft tissues. Within the snail, asexual reproduction occurs for several weeks, with transformation into sporocysts, rediae, and cercariae; the last emerge from the snail and invade the second intermediate host, a crustacean such as a crab or crayfish, where they encyst and become metacercariae. This is the infective stage for the mammalian host. Human infection occurs by eating inadequately cooked or pickled crab or crayfish that harbor metacercariae of the parasite. The metacercariae excyst in the duodenum, penetrate the intestinal wall, and migrate through the peritoneal cavity toward the lungs. During migration through the peritoneum and diaphragm, the inflammatory process causes abdominal pain and dry cough. When invading the lungs, they become encapsulated and develop into adults. Infections may persist for 20 years in humans.

CLINICAL MANIFESTATIONS

Paragonimiasis typically results from the consumption of raw or improperly cooked crustaceans, especially crabs. Recently in the United States, some autochthonous cases have been reported in the Midwest in people who consumed raw crayfish while camping during the summer.[7] Most of the infected people are asymptomatic and have subclinical disease. During the first month of infection, abdominal pain may represent the juvenile larvae migrating through the abdominal cavity before reaching the lungs. Irritation of the diaphragm or pleura may cause dry cough. Fever, chest pain, fatigue, and urticaria may follow, as well as eosinophilia. Pleural effusions may be seen at this stage, with significant eosinophilia noted on analysis of pleural fluid, which can be the first clue to the diagnosis. In fact, pleural manifestations predominate early in the disease process, whereas lesions of the pulmonary parenchyma predominate later in the course of disease. Moreover, pneumothorax and mild eosinophilia may occur only 1 month after the initiation of infection. The migrating worms may cause bronchiectasis, interstitial pneumonitis, transient hemorrhage, or bronchopneumonia. Again, pulmonary lesions and eosinophilia raise the possibility of paragonimiasis. Cough and recurrent hemoptysis are common clinical findings in this phase. The chronic stage occurs when the worms are paired in a cyst in the pulmonary parenchyma. Eggs are produced 6 weeks after infection, and if there is communication with the bronchial tree, eggs may be seen in a sputum sample under microscopy, or they can be swallowed and passed with stool. The rusty discoloration of sputum is caused by the presence of the tan- to brown-pigmented *Paragonimus* eggs; the sputa of these patients have been classically described as resembling "iron filings." Charcot-Leyden crystals can be seen.

Peripheral blood eosinophilia and elevated total serum IgE levels are observed in approximately 80% of patients. Common findings on CT are pleural effusion, hydropneumothorax, pulmonary nodules or consolidation of air spaces, and cysts. The most common ectopic form is cerebral paragonimiasis, which is manifested as eosinophilic meningitis or meningoencephalitis, brain tumor, or just residual calcifications from a past infection.

DIAGNOSIS AND TREATMENT OF LIVER, INTESTINAL, AND LUNG FLUKE INFECTIONS

DIAGNOSIS

In general, transmission of food-borne trematodiases is restricted geographically and distribution is one of the most important factors in suspecting this diagnosis. In the appropriate clinical setting, laboratory and imaging data can add information to narrow the differential diagnosis. Acute fluke infections require a high level of suspicion. Serologic tests, direct visualization of the migrating larvae, or empirical therapy with a significant clinical response (including reduction of eosinophilia) are major criteria to confirm the diagnosis. In the chronic phase, the diagnosis is usually made by visualization of the eggs in stool or, in the case of *Paragonimus*, in sputum. A sedimentation technique must be performed on a series of at least three stool specimens from alternate days or even weeks. Some of the sedimentation or concentration parasitologic techniques used for these infections include the Lumbreras rapid sedimentation technique, the Kato-Katz technique, and the ether-formalin concentration technique. Immunodiagnostics is an excellent tool, particularly for patients who do not have demonstrable eggs in clinical specimens.

If acute fascioliasis is strongly suspected, serology would be the next step. Cathepsin L1–based antibody enzyme-linked immunosorbent assay (ELISA) has a sensitivity of 92% and a specificity of 84%. If negative, the diagnosis is unlikely. If serology is not available, CT of the liver can visualize the characteristic tracklike lesions. However, because the parasitic lesions are very similar to metastases, liver biopsy may be necessary. If serology or CT is not available, a trial of triclabendazole with clinical (including eosinophilia)

resolution is the major criterion for diagnosis. In chronic fascioliasis, the Lumbreras rapid sedimentation technique is the method of choice to detect the eggs in stool. At least three stool examinations are preferred. If negative, serology can be helpful. Ultrasonography and CT have low sensitivity in this phase. ERCP usually finds the adult parasites in the bile duct when performed for other reasons. Nonetheless, ERCP can be useful to eliminate the adult parasites causing biliary obstruction.

In opisthorchiasis, serology or stool examinations can be performed to approach the diagnosis. The Ov-CP-1–based enzyme-linked immunosorbent assay (ELISA) has a sensitivity of 95% and a specificity of 96%. For *C. sinensis*, ELISA has a sensitivity between 81.3 and 96% and a specificity between 92.6 and 96.2%. For detection of eggs and to measure the intensity of infection, the Kato-Katz technique is preferred. Intestinal fluke eggs can be detected by performing a sedimentation stool technique, preferably in consecutive stool samples.

For paragonimiasis, an immunoblot assay performed with a crude antigen extract of *P. westermani* has been in use at the Centers for Disease Control and Prevention; the sensitivity of the test is 96%, and its specificity is 99%. This would be the ideal first step to confirm the diagnosis. In the acute phase, the precise location of the migrating larva is unknown and a biopsy may not necessarily target the parasite. When serologic findings are negative (or not available), a trial of praziquantel or triclabendazole with a positive clinical response in 48 to 72 hours is a major criterion for diagnosis. In the chronic phase, several sputum samples have to be examined by a sedimentation technique to increase sensitivity. Stool examinations are complementary because the eggs can be swallowed by the host and then passed through stool. If a pulmonary cyst contains adult parasites with eggs but they do not have communication to the main bronchi, serologic examination is indicated to confirm the diagnosis. If not available, biopsy is warranted.

Under the light microscope, the morphologic characteristics and size of the eggs may be sufficient to identify the specific fluke. For *Fasciola*, the egg is large, ellipsoid, and oval, with an indistinct operculum and thin shell. The *F. hepatica* egg measures 120 to 150 μm by 63 to 90 μm, the *F. gigantica* egg measures 160 to 190 μm by 70 to 90 μm, and the *F. buski* egg measures 130 to 159 μm by 78 to 98 μm. *Opisthorchis* eggs are elongated with an operculum on the anterior end and a pointed terminal "knob" on the posterior end (26 to 30 μm by 11 to 15 μm). *C. sinensis* eggs (27 to 35 μm by 11 to 20 μm) are small, ovoid, or elongated, with broad rounded posterior ends, a convex operculum resting on "shoulders," and a small "knob" on the posterior ends. *H. heterophyes* and *M. yokogawai* eggs are similar in size, 26 to 30 μm by 15 to 17 μm. *Echinostoma* eggs are brownish, operculated, and measure 83 to 116 μm by 58 to 69 μm. *Paragonimus* eggs measure 68 to 118 μm by 39 to 67 μm, are reddish-brown and ovoid or elongated, and have a thick shell; the operculum is slightly flattened and fits into the shoulder area of the shell, and the posterior end is thickened. The egg is often asymmetrical, with one side slightly flattened.

TREATMENT   Rx

The general principles and details of antiparasitic therapy are provided in Chapter 344. For fascioliasis, 10 mg/kg of triclabendazole once or twice has a cure rate higher than 90%, and it is the treatment of choice.[A1] Cure is achieved if stool examinations remain negative for at least 3 months. Serology usually can take more than a year to resolve. In treatment of the chronic phase, the dead parasites can occasionally cause biliary obstruction, which may need surgical consultation. In case of failure, some experts recommend double doses of triclabendazole for 2 days. Recently, in Mexico, nitazoxanide has appeared promising, but more experience is needed. For *O. viverrini*, a single dose of praziquantel (40 to 50 mg/kg) has a cure rate of 91 to 97%. For clonorchiasis, the recommended dose of praziquantel is 25 mg/kg three times for 1 day (total dose of 75 mg/kg), which has a cure rate of 83 to 85%. Tribendimidine has been found to be comparably effective as praziquantel in the treatment of *C. sinesis* infection with fewer adverse events in an open-label trial in 74 patients.[A2] For intestinal flukes, praziquantel, 25 mg/kg by mouth three times daily for 1 day, is recommended. For paragonimiasis, praziquantel, 25 mg/kg by mouth three times daily for 3 days, or triclabendazole, 10 mg/kg by mouth once or twice, is highly effective. For ectopic cases, surgery may be necessary. In follow-up, negative stool examinations in the ensuing weeks can confirm cure. However, because the rate of reinfection is high in individuals from endemic areas, a suddenly positive stool examination is highly suggestive of a new infection rather than failure to respond to treatment.

PREVENTION

Prevention of infection with these flukes depends on several factors, including recognizing their geographic distribution and avoiding the consumption of raw vegetables, fish, crayfish, or contaminated water in endemic areas. Proper medical advice must be given to individuals traveling or planning to reside in endemic areas, not only to prevent fluke infection but also to inform them about the risk for coinfection with other parasites. Control of these flukes in animals is impractical because of wild animal reservoirs. However, control of human infections is challenging because it involves changing long-established cultural, dietary, and sanitary habits. Massive chemotherapy in highly endemic populations may reduce the infection in humans and in selected animals.

Grade A References

A1. Hien TT, Truong NT, Minh NH, et al. A randomized controlled pilot study of artesunate versus triclabendazole for human fascioliasis in central Vietnam. *Am J Trop Med Hyg.* 2008;78:388-392.
A2. Qian MB, Yap B, Yang YC, et al. Efficacy and safety of tribendimidine against *Clonorchis sinesis. Clin Infect Dis.* 2013;56:e76-e82.

GENERAL REFERENCES

For the General References and other additional features, please visit Expert Consult at https://expertconsult.inkling.com.

357

INTESTINAL NEMATODE INFECTIONS

DAVID J. DIEMERT

DEFINITION

Nematodes are nonsegmented roundworms belonging to the phylum Nematoda. Most species are free-living in soil or water, but a few parasitize humans. Nematode infections are highly prevalent and affect millions worldwide. They are complex multicellular organisms with specialized organs that include a protective outer coating or cuticle, a complete and functional gastrointestinal tract, and muscular, nervous, and reproductive systems.

Nematodes of medical importance can be divided into those that primarily affect the gastrointestinal tract, where adult worms become established and cause disease, and those that affect other tissues and organ systems. The former group is covered in this chapter and includes the roundworm *Ascaris lumbricoides,* the hookworms *Ancylostoma duodenale* and *Necator americanus,* the pinworm *Enterobius vermicularis,* the whipworm *Trichuris trichiura,* and the threadworm *Strongyloides stercoralis.* Zoonotic intestinal nematodes such as *Trichostrongylus* and *Anisakis* also occasionally infect and cause disease in the gastrointestinal tract of humans. Nematodes that invade and cause disease primarily in tissues outside the gastrointestinal tract include those that cause lymphatic filariasis (*Wuchereria bancrofti, Brugia malayi,* and *Brugia timori*), *Onchocerca volvulus, Loa,* the guinea worm *Dracunculus medinensis,* as well as *Trichinella* and *Angiostrongylus* spp (Chapter 358).

Nematodes that infect humans measure from several millimeters to more than a meter in length and often survive for months to years within their host. With the exception of *S. stercoralis* and *Capillaria philippinensis,* adult worms cannot complete their life cycle within a human host. Instead, sexually mature adult worms mate and produce eggs or larvae that must have at least one stage of development outside the host, either in the environment or in an intermediate host.

Nematode infections are rarely fatal; they more commonly result in chronic morbidity such as iron deficiency anemia caused by hookworm or blindness due to onchocerciasis. For most nematodes, the severity of the clinical manifestations of infection is proportional to the number of worms harbored by a given host; although light infections with only a few worms are usually asymptomatic, pathologic features appear with heavier worm burdens.

Nematode infections are prevalent in the temperate and tropical regions of Africa, Asia, and Latin America. They are transmitted by the oral ingestion of embryonated eggs or by penetration of infective larvae through the skin, either by direct contact with contaminated soil or by arthropod vectors. Nematode infections are most common in areas with poor sanitation, where the environment is contaminated by human waste, and in climates that support survival of the insect vector, if one is involved in the life cycle.

In endemic areas most individuals harbor low numbers of worms and a minority have relatively high worm burdens and contribute disproportionally to both transmission and morbidity.

ASCARIASIS

The Pathogen

A. lumbricoides, colloquially known as *roundworm,* is acquired by oral ingestion of embryonated eggs. In the stomach, the egg's protective outer shell is dissolved by gastric acid, releasing larvae into the small intestine, where they penetrate the intestinal wall and enter the portal circulation. The larvae migrate to the liver and then the pulmonary vasculature, where they break into the alveolar spaces, ascend the bronchial tree, and are swallowed to re-enter the small intestine, developing there into adult worms approximately 9 to 11 weeks after egg ingestion. Adult worms (Fig. 357-1) range in length between 15 and 50 cm and survive in the host for approximately 18 months.[1] Female adult *Ascaris* worms produce approximately 240,000 eggs per day, which are expelled in feces. Fertilized eggs embryonate in warm, moist, shady soil, after which they are infectious (Fig. 357-2). Eggs can survive up to 15 years in the environment, being extremely hardy and resistant to extreme temperatures and desiccation.

EPIDEMIOLOGY

A. lumbricoides is the most prevalent nematode infection worldwide, with approximately a billion people chronically infected.[2] Infection is common in sub-Saharan Africa, south and Southeast Asia, and Latin America, especially in rural areas of high population density with inadequate sanitation or treatment of sewage and where untreated human feces are used as fertilizer.

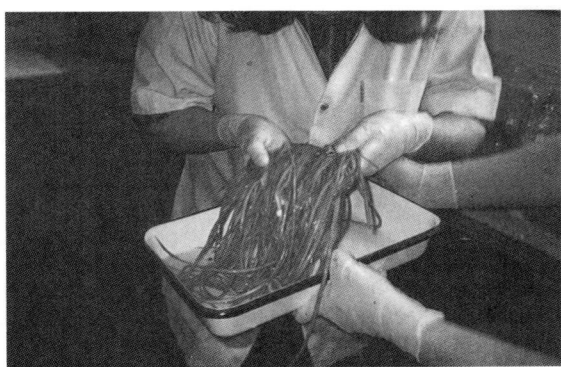

FIGURE 357-1. Mass of adult *Ascaris lumbricoides* worms recovered from a child after the administration of mebendazole. (Reproduced with permission from Dickson Despommier.)

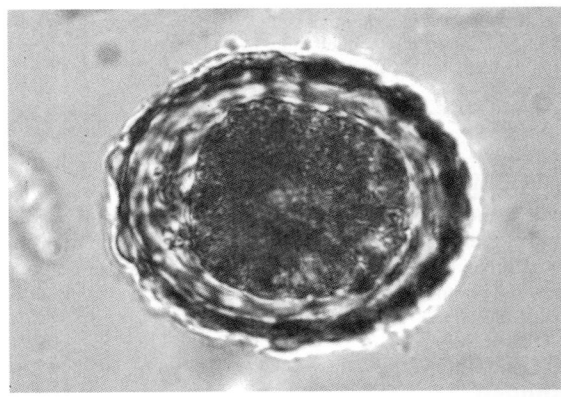

FIGURE 357-2. Fertilized, unembryonated egg of *Ascaris lumbricoides.* (Reproduced with permission from Dickson Despommier.)

Climate is an important determinant of disease in that warm temperature and adequate moisture are required for embryonation of eggs in soil. In endemic areas, the prevalence and intensity of infection with *A. lumbricoides* increase dramatically during the first 2 to 3 years of life; it remains high between the ages of 4 and 15 years and then declines during adulthood.[3]

CLINICAL MANIFESTATIONS

Infection with *A. lumbricoides* is usually asymptomatic. Clinical manifestations are associated with heavy worm burdens and can be classified into those resulting from larval migration through the lungs and those due to parasitism of the gastrointestinal tract by adult worms.

When migrating through the lungs, *A. lumbricoides* larvae can induce an intense reaction that is due to both the physical disruption that their migration causes and a dramatic inflammatory hypersensitivity response to secreted antigens. This phenomenon is more common in areas in which transmission is seasonal, such as on the Arabian Peninsula, where outbreaks of pneumonitis typically follow the rainy season because of resumption of transmission. Symptoms may last for 2 to 3 weeks and include the sudden onset of wheezing, dyspnea, paroxysmal nonproductive cough, and high fever. Respiratory symptoms may coincide with or be preceded by urticarial rash, angioedema, abdominal pain, and vomiting. These symptoms usually resolve spontaneously.

With moderate or heavy infections, signs and symptoms can result from obstruction caused by a mass of worms in the small intestine or migration of worms to the biliary tree, pancreatic duct, or appendix. Intestinal obstruction is more common in young children because of their smaller lumen size and is characterized by colicky abdominal pain and vomiting that may progress to signs of intestinal perforation. Hepatobiliary and pancreatic ascariasis is more common in adults, presumably because their biliary tree is large enough to accommodate a migrating worm. Chronic intestinal infection also can manifest as abdominal pain and distention, diarrhea, and nausea. More insidious effects, especially in children, include decreased protein and fat absorption, development of vitamin A and C deficiencies, and lactose intolerance, which together lead to stunted growth and impaired cognitive development.

DIAGNOSIS

The diagnosis of ascariasis is usually made by microscopic examination of a sample of feces for characteristic thick-shelled eggs.[4] Pulmonary ascariasis cannot be diagnosed on the basis of identification of ova in feces because adult worms have not yet matured and begun producing eggs; instead, larvae, as well as eosinophils or Charcot-Leyden crystals (formed from the breakdown of eosinophils), may be visualized on microscopic examination of sputum. Pulmonary disease is also usually marked by peripheral eosinophilia and transient infiltrates on chest radiographs. The diagnosis of intestinal or biliary obstruction caused by *A. lumbricoides* relies increasingly on radiologic evaluation with ultrasound or endoscopic retrograde cholangiopancreatography (ERCP).

TREATMENT Rx

Intestinal ascariasis is usually treated with a single oral dose of albendazole (Table 357-1).[A1] Alternatives include mebendazole, ivermectin, or pyrantel pamoate. No specific treatment is recommended for symptoms of pulmonary ascariasis because the condition is self-limited. In severe cases of biliary obstruction, including cholangitis, ERCP with or without resection of the ampulla of Vater is highly successful and may reduce the need for surgical intervention.

PREVENTION

The definitive means of preventing *Ascaris* infection is improvement of hygiene and proper disposal of human waste. In endemic communities where this is not feasible, control efforts center on regular (at least annual) mass administration of an anthelmintic medication such as albendazole or mebendazole.[5]

⬤ HOOKWORM

The Pathogen

Hookworm infection in humans is due almost exclusively to two species: *N. americanus* and *A. duodenale*. Humans may also be incidentally infected by

TABLE 357-1 TREATMENT OF INTESTINAL NEMATODES

NEMATODE	TREATMENT
Ascaris lumbricoides	Albendazole, 400 mg once. Alternatives: Mebendazole, 100 mg bid for 3 days; ivermectin 150-200 μg/kg once, or pyrantel pamoate, 11 mg/kg for 3 days with the maximum daily dose not to exceed 1 g
Hookworm (*Necator americanus* and *Ancylostoma duodenale*)	Albendazole, 400 mg/day for 3 days. Alternatives: Mebendazole, 100 mg bid for 3 days, or pyrantel pamoate, 11 mg/kg for 3 days with the maximum daily dose not to exceed 1 g
Trichuris trichiura	Mebendazole, 100 mg bid, or albendazole, 400 mg/day, for 3 days; or oxantel pamoate, 20 mg/kg, plus albendazole, 400 mg, administered daily for 2 days*
Enterobius vermicularis	Pyrantel pamoate, 11 mg/kg once, with a second dose 2 wk later; maximum dose of 1 g. Alternatives: Mebendazole, 100 mg once, or albendazole, 400 mg once, repeated in 2 wk
Strongyloides stercoralis	Uncomplicated infection: Ivermectin, 200 μg/kg/day for 2 days.† Alternative: Albendazole, 400 mg/day for 7 days
Trichostrongylus spp	Pyrantel pamoate, 11 mg/kg once; maximum dose of 1 g. Alternatives: Albendazole, 400 mg once, or mebendazole, 100 mg bid for 3 days
Capillaria philippinensis	Albendazole, 400 mg/day for 10 days. Alternative: Mebendazole, 200 mg bid for 20 days

*Oxantel pamoate is not approved by the U.S. Food and Drug Administration for this use at the time of this writing.
†Treatment may need to be extended in immunocompromised patients with disseminated disease.

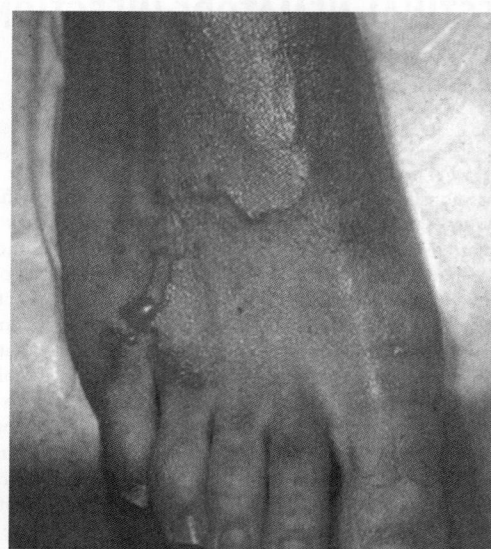

FIGURE 357-3. Typical lesion of cutaneous larva migrans. An erythematous, serpiginous track caused by intradermal migration of a dog (*Ancylostoma caninum*) or cat (*Ancylostoma braziliense*) hookworm larva is apparent. (Reproduced with permission from Gregory L. Zalar.)

the zoonotic hookworms *Ancylostoma caninum*, *Ancylostoma braziliensis*, *Bunostomum phlebotomum*, and *Uncinaria stenocephala*, which can cause self-limited dermatologic lesions known as cutaneous larva migrans (Fig. 357-3). Additionally, *Ancylostoma ceylanicum*, normally a hookworm infecting cats, has been reported to cause intestinal hookworm disease in humans, especially in Asia, whereas *A. caninum* has been implicated as a cause of eosinophilic enteritis in Australia.

Infection occurs when exposed skin comes in contact with infective filariform larvae in contaminated soil or grass. Larvae penetrate the skin, enter the afferent circulation, and migrate to the pulmonary vasculature, where they break into the alveolar spaces, ascend the bronchial tree to the trachea, and are swallowed into the gastrointestinal tract. Larvae undergo two molts to mature into adult worms approximately 5 to 9 weeks after skin penetration.

Adult hookworms reside in the lumen of the upper part of the small intestine, where they attach to the mucosa by means of cutting teeth (*A. duodenale*) or a rounded cutting plate (*N. americanus*). After mating in the host intestinal tract, a female adult worm produces thousands of eggs per day, which then exit the body in feces; *A. duodenale* female worms lay approximately 28,000 eggs daily, whereas the output from *N. americanus* worms is considerably less, averaging around 10,000 a day. Hookworm eggs hatch in warm, moist soil and release larvae that can infect another host. Humans are the only major definitive host for these two parasites, and there are no intermediate or reservoir hosts. *A. duodenale* survives on average for 1 year in the human intestine, whereas *N. americanus* lives for 3 to 5 years.

EPIDEMIOLOGY

More than 500 million people are infected with hookworms worldwide. *N. americanus* is the most widespread hookworm, whereas *A. duodenale* is more geographically restricted in distribution. The highest prevalence of infection occurs in rural areas of tropical and less developed countries, where environmental and socioeconomic conditions favor transmission. Climate is an important determinant of hookworm transmission, with adequate moisture and warm temperature being essential for larval development in soil. An equally important determinant of infection is poverty and inadequate sanitation and supply of clean water. In endemic areas, prevalence increases with age in young children and reaches a plateau by approximately 10 years of age, whereas the intensity of infection rises at a slower rate during childhood, reaches a plateau by around 20 years, and then increases again in the elderly. Whether such age dependency reflects differences in exposure, acquired immunity, or a combination of both is controversial.

Although cutaneous larva migrans is found throughout the tropics, in the United States it is diagnosed primarily in tourists who have recently returned from a vacation to a tropical beach destination, especially in the Caribbean, Brazil, Mexico, and Southeast Asia. Occasionally, autochthonous cases (originating where found) have been reported in the United States, usually from southeastern coastal states such as Florida and South Carolina. Most commonly, cutaneous larva migrans occurs when exposed skin comes in contact with the larval stages of the dog or cat hookworms *A. caninum* or *A. braziliense*, respectively, present in moist soil or sand (especially on beaches) contaminated with animal feces. Other animal hookworms such as *U. stenocephala* and *B. phlebotomum* are less common causes.

PATHOBIOLOGY

The major pathology of hookworm infection is due to the associated gastrointestinal blood loss and the resulting iron deficiency anemia. Hookworms attach to the intestinal mucosa and secrete enzymes that enable them to invade submucosal tissues and ingest villous tissue and blood. Hemoglobinases within the hookworm's digestive canal enable degradation of human hemoglobin for use as an essential nutrient source. The amount of blood loss is directly related to the total worm burden. *A. duodenale* causes more blood loss than *N. americanus*; each *N. americanus* worm results in a daily blood loss of 0.03 to 0.1 mL, and the corresponding figure for *A. duodenale* is between 0.15 and 0.26 mL.

CLINICAL MANIFESTATIONS

The clinical features of hookworm infection can be separated into acute manifestations associated with larval migration through the skin and other tissues and acute and chronic manifestations resulting from parasitism of the gastrointestinal tract by adult worms. Repeated skin exposure to hookworm larvae can result in a hypersensitivity reaction known as "ground itch," a pruritic erythematous and papular rash that appears most commonly on the hands and feet. In contrast, when zoonotic hookworm larvae penetrate the skin to produce cutaneous larva migrans, most commonly on the feet, thighs, and buttocks, they are unable to complete their life cycle in the human host and eventually die after causing a typical clinical syndrome of intensely pruritic, erythematous serpiginous tracks (see Fig. 357-3). Tracks appear after an incubation period of a few days, can be single or multiple, and advance by millimeters to a few centimeters each day. Vesiculobullous or papular lesions may develop along the tracks, as can secondary bacterial infection as a result of scratching. Untreated, lesions usually heal spontaneously within weeks to months following death of the larvae in the skin.

Migration of hookworm larvae through the lungs may induce mild and transient pulmonary symptoms consisting of dry cough, sore throat, wheezing, and low-grade fever. Acute symptomatic disease may uncommonly result from the oral ingestion of *A. duodenale* larvae, referred to as the Wakana syndrome, which is characterized by nausea, vomiting, pharyngeal irritation, cough, dyspnea, and hoarseness.

Abdominal symptoms and signs caused by hookworm infection are rare. Instead, the manifestations of hookworm disease occur when intestinal blood loss exceeds the nutritional reserves of the host and results in iron deficiency anemia. Usually only moderate- and high-intensity (≥2000 eggs per gram of feces) hookworm infections produce clinical disease, which resembles that of iron deficiency anemia secondary to other causes (Chapter 159). In addition, the protein losses associated with heavy hookworm infection can result in hypoproteinemia and anasarca. As iron deficiency anemia develops and worsens, an infected individual may have weakness, palpitations, fainting, dizziness, dyspnea, lassitude, and headache. Uncommonly, there may be constipation or diarrhea with occult blood in the stool or frank melena, especially in children; there also may be an urge to eat soil (pica). Overwhelming hookworm infection may cause listlessness, coma, and even death, especially in infants. Because children and women of reproductive age have reduced iron reserves, they are at particular risk for symptomatic disease. Severe iron deficiency anemia caused by hookworm during pregnancy can result in adverse consequences for the mother, her unborn fetus (miscarriage, intrauterine growth restriction), and the neonate (anemia, failure to thrive). In children, the anemia and protein malnutrition associated with chronic intestinal parasitism cause long-term impairments in physical and cognitive development.

DIAGNOSIS

The diagnosis of hookworm infection is made by microscopic identification of characteristic eggs in the stool. The eggs of *N. americanus* and *A. duodenale* cannot be distinguished because both are colorless and have a single thin hyaline shell with blunted ends; they range in size from 55 to 75 μm by 36 to 40 μm. Egg concentration techniques, such as the formalin–ethyl acetate sedimentation method, can be used to detect even light infections, although a direct wet mount examination is adequate for detecting moderate-to-heavy infections. In addition, eosinophilia is a common finding in chronic infection and also during larval migration through the lungs.

TREATMENT   Rx

Three daily oral doses of albendazole, 400 mg, is the recommended treatment for intestinal hookworm infection (see Table 357-1).[A2] Less effective alternatives include mebendazole, pyrantel pamoate, and single-dose albendazole. For cutaneous larva migrans, although the disease is self-limited and will resolve spontaneously within weeks to a few months, treatment with a single dose of ivermectin will lead to more rapid resolution of symptoms and skin manifestations. Albendazole is an alternative treatment of cutaneous larva migrans.

PREVENTION

The ideal method for preventing hookworm infection is improvement in hygiene and proper disposal of human waste. Until this occurs, in endemic communities control of disease consists of regular (at least annual) mass administration of an anthelmintic medication such as albendazole or mebendazole. For cutaneous larva migrans, tourists should be advised to wear shoes or sandals when walking to and on beaches and to avoid beaches frequented by stray cats and dogs.

● TRICHURIASIS

The Pathogen

Infection with *T. trichiura*, also known as *whipworm*, does not have a tissue migratory phase like *A. lumbricoides* and hookworm, and its entire life cycle in the host is limited to the gastrointestinal tract. After embryonated eggs are ingested orally, larvae are released into the small intestine, where they undergo a series of molts before being carried passively to the transverse and descending colon. The narrow anterior end of adult worms embeds in the columnar epithelium, with the posterior portion protruding into the lumen, thereby allowing eggs to be released into feces, which are then passed into the environment, where they must embryonate in warm, moist soil to complete the life cycle. Adult worms can measure up to 50 mm in length and survive in the host for approximately 1.5 to 2 years. The period between ingestion of eggs and detection of eggs in feces is approximately 90 days.

Like the other soil-transmitted helminths, trichuriasis is most common in poor, mostly rural areas of the tropics and subtropics where disposal of human waste is inadequate. The estimated prevalence worldwide is 800 million. Children are more frequently infected than adults and more likely to have higher worm burdens. Humans are the only host.

CLINICAL MANIFESTATIONS

Most *T. trichiura* infections are asymptomatic. Disease is mostly seen in children because the majority of heavy infections (>10,000 eggs per gram of feces) occur in this age group. Heavy infections can be accompanied by acute dysentery or chronic colitis resembling inflammatory bowel disease and result in abdominal pain and diarrhea. Chronic mucosal inflammation and edema of the colon and rectum can lead to protracted tenesmus that results in rectal prolapse. Chronic *Trichuris* colitis also can lead to malnutrition, impaired growth, and anemia.

DIAGNOSIS

Infection is diagnosed by microscopic identification of the typical barrel-shaped eggs with bipolar plugs in direct or concentrated smears of fecal specimens.

TREATMENT   Rx

Although *T. trichiura* responds less effectively than *A. lumbricoides* or hookworm to treatment with albendazole or mebendazole, a 3-day course of one of these two benzimidazole drugs has been the recommended therapy, as listed in Table 357-1. The addition of ivermectin (200 μg/kg) to either drug increases the response rate significantly.[A3] More recently, the combination of oxantel pamoate, 20 mg/kg, plus albendazole, 400 mg, administered daily for 2 days, was found to result in higher cure and egg-reduction rates for *T. trichiura* infection then the rates with standard therapy.[A4] (Oxanetel is not approved for this by the U.S. Food and Drug Administration at the time of this writing.)

PREVENTION

As for *A. lumbricoides* and hookworm, control of trichuriasis in endemic areas centers on regular mass anthelminthic drug administration, primarily to school-age children, although single doses of albendazole or mebendazole are poorly effective for this intestinal nematode.

● ENTEROBIASIS
The Pathogen

E. vermicularis, or pinworm, is transmitted by the fecal-oral route. Embryonated eggs on fingernails, bedding, or clothing are ingested and hatch in the upper small intestine, where they develop into adults before taking residence in the large intestine. Adult worms measuring between 2 and 5 mm live freely in the lumen of the colon, where they mate. Gravid female worms migrate nightly out of the rectum and deposit large numbers of eggs (11,000 per worm) on the perianal and perineal skin, where they rapidly embryonate within 6 hours of being deposited. If they are still on the skin, infective larvae are released that can migrate back through the anus into the rectum (retroinfection); alternatively, autoinfection occurs when eggs are transferred to the mouth via scratching the perianal skin on which eggs have been deposited, commonly in children. In infected females, larvae may also migrate into the genital tract and establish an ectopic infection.

EPIDEMIOLOGY

E. vermicularis is found worldwide and is the most prevalent nematode infection in temperate climes. Transmission is especially frequent in primary schools and daycare centers, where children are in close contact. Up to a quarter of all children worldwide are estimated to be infected with pinworm.

CLINICAL MANIFESTATIONS

Although most pinworm infections are asymptomatic, perianal pruritus is the most common symptom and is caused by an allergic response to worm proteins. The pruritus can be intense and result in chronic sleep deprivation. Rarely, adult *E. vermicularis* may precipitate appendicitis. When hatched larvae migrate into the female genital tract, vulvovaginitis, salpingitis, or peritonitis may develop.

DIAGNOSIS

Pinworm infection is diagnosed by identifying eggs by examination under a microscope on a piece of cellophane tape applied to the perianal region immediately after waking and before bathing. Characteristic *E. vermicularis* eggs are oval and slightly flattened on one side. It is unusual to find eggs in feces or adult worms in the perianal area. Repeated examination may be necessary.

TREATMENT   Rx

Pinworm infection is treated with a single dose of pyrantel pamoate, mebendazole, or albendazole, which must be repeated 2 weeks later because the drugs do not kill eggs or developing larvae (see Table 357-1). Given the high rate of transmission, all household members and individuals in close contact with the patient (e.g., other children attending the same daycare center) should be treated as well. Bedding and underclothes should be thoroughly laundered in hot water followed by a hot dryer to kill the eggs.

● STRONGYLOIDIASIS
The Pathogen

S. stercoralis, or threadworm, is endemic in warm climates worldwide, including parts of the United States.[6] Infection occurs when exposed skin comes in contact with free-living filariform larvae in soil contaminated with human feces. After penetrating the skin, larvae enter the afferent circulation and travel to the pulmonary vasculature, where they rupture into the alveolar spaces, ascend the bronchial tree to the pharynx, and are swallowed into the gastrointestinal tract. Further development into adult worms occurs in the upper small intestine, where parasites live embedded in the mucosa. Unlike most nematodes, *S. stercoralis* reproduces by parthenogenesis, with no apparent parasitic male worm present in human infection. Female worms begin laying eggs within 25 to 30 days after infection. The embryonated eggs hatch rapidly in the lumen of the small intestine and release noninfectious rhabditiform larvae that migrate to the colon and are excreted in feces. Alternatively, larvae may directly penetrate the colonic mucosa or perianal skin after migrating out of the anus and enter the circulation directly, a mechanism known as *autoinfection*. This phenomenon can lead to maintenance of parasitism in the host for decades.

Infectious filariform larvae develop in the soil by direct transformation from rhabditiform larvae or indirectly from eggs produced by free-living adult worms that have developed from rhabditiform larvae in warm, moist, sandy soil.

A less common type of strongyloidiasis, called *swollen belly syndrome*, has been attributed to infection with *Strongyloides fuelleborni* in infants living in sub-Saharan Africa and Papua New Guinea.

EPIDEMIOLOGY

S. stercoralis infection is endemic in the tropical and subtropical regions of sub-Saharan Africa, Asia, Latin America, and areas of eastern and southern Europe, with a worldwide prevalence of between 30 and 100 million. In the United States, infection is diagnosed most frequently in immigrants, commonly from Southeast Asia, although strongyloidiasis is still endemic in parts of rural Appalachia. *S. stercoralis* also be transmitted sexually through oral-anal contact, most often among men who have sex with men. Cases of transmission through solid organ transplantation have also been reported.

PATHOBIOLOGY

In immunologically competent individuals, infection is usually asymptomatic or is associated with mild gastrointestinal symptoms. The main complications of infection, however, occur in individuals with cell-mediated immunodeficiency such as those chronically taking corticosteroids, renal transplant recipients, patients with Hodgkin disease and other lymphomas, leukemic patients, and those infected with human T-cell lymphotropic virus type 1.[7] In these individuals, the autoinfection cycle of the *S. stercoralis* life cycle can become amplified and lead to a hyperinfection syndrome with a large increase in the total worm load in the infected person. Hyperinfection can lead to life-threatening dissemination of larvae and adult worms to aberrant sites such as the brain, pancreas, and kidneys. For unknown reasons, advanced acquired immunodeficiency syndrome has not been associated with hyperinfection syndrome or with disseminated strongyloidiasis. Disseminated strongyloidiasis is frequently accompanied by bacterial sepsis, probably as a result of translocation of enteric organisms carried by migrating larvae.

CLINICAL MANIFESTATIONS

Most *S. stercoralis* infections, especially in immunocompetent hosts, are asymptomatic or are associated with only mild gastrointestinal manifestations such as abdominal pain, bloating, and watery diarrhea. Gastrointestinal bleeding, manifested by hematochezia or melena, occurs in less than 20% of those infected. Rare causes of morbidity include small bowel obstruction, paralytic ileus, and a malabsorption syndrome (especially in children).[8]

During the migratory phase of larvae through the lungs, symptoms are rare in immunocompetent patients, although there may be peripheral eosinophilia. However, pulmonary signs and symptoms in immunocompromised persons with hyperinfection syndrome can be severe and resemble those of acute respiratory distress syndrome with dyspnea, productive cough, and hemoptysis accompanied by fever, tachypnea, and hypoxemia.

Migration of filariform larvae from the anus can lead to a dermatologic manifestation known as larva currens, which is characterized by serpiginous erythematous maculopapular tracks that migrate by 5 to 15 cm/hour, primarily on the skin of the buttocks, upper aspect of the thighs, and lower part of the abdomen.

Autoinfection leading to exceptionally high worm loads (i.e., hyperinfection) and disseminated strongyloidiasis can occur in persons with deficient cell-mediated immunity. Because asymptomatic infection with *S. stercoralis* may persist for decades after initial infection, it is important to remember that a change in immune status associated with conditions such as the administration of immunosuppressive drugs following solid organ transplantation may result in hyperinfection syndrome even though the infection was previously asymptomatic. Massive increases in the number of *Strongyloides* larvae because of hyperinfection can present as acute enteritis with severe diarrhea and ulcerative disease of the small and large intestine. During disseminated infection, larvae and sometimes adult worms penetrate the intestinal mucosa, migrate to aberrant sites, including the central nervous system, and result in metastatic abscesses and gram-negative meningitis due to enteric bacteria being carried by the migrating parasites. Less common complications of disseminated disease include glomerulonephritis and minimal-change nephrotic syndrome, acute respiratory distress syndrome, and alveolar hemorrhage. Mortality from hyperinfection and disseminated disease can be high, although early diagnosis and prompt initiation of treatment are associated with improved outcomes.

Infants with swollen belly syndrome caused by *S. fuelleborni* are often seen acutely with abdominal ascites that is not accompanied by diarrhea or fever. The ascites is due to gastrointestinal protein loss; it can be significant enough to cause respiratory impairment and is associated with a high rate of mortality.

DIAGNOSIS

Definitive diagnosis of *S. stercoralis* infection relies on microscopic identification of larvae in feces or other fluids (such as sputum) or tissues. Detection of filariform larvae in feces implies active autoinfection. Intestinal strongyloidiasis can be diagnosed by identification of larvae in direct smears of freshly passed stool, although the sensitivity of examining a single fecal sample is as low as 30%. Sensitivity can be increased by examining multiple fecal specimens, by using concentration techniques, and by plating feces on an agar plate and inspecting for tracks of colonies created by bacteria being dragged by migrating larvae.

Hyperinfection syndrome and disseminated strongyloidiasis can be diagnosed by detection of filariform larvae in duodenal fluid obtained by endoscopy, in sputum, or in bronchoalveolar lavage specimens. Larvae have also been recovered from cerebrospinal fluid, urine, peritoneal washings, skin, and the brains of immunocompromised persons.

Fluctuating eosinophilia is common with uncomplicated intestinal strongyloidiasis, especially during the pulmonary migration phase of initial infection. However, eosinophilia may be absent in patients with hyperinfection and dissemination. In fact, those with hyperinfection and eosinophilia appear to have a better prognosis than do those without eosinophilia.

Serologic diagnosis using an enzyme-linked immunosorbent assay (ELISA) that detects antibodies to filariform larval antigens is very sensitive, even in immunocompromised hosts with disseminated strongyloidiasis, although false positives may occur in cases of coinfection with other nematodes, particularly filaria. Specificity is improved by using the newer luciferase immunoprecipitation systems (LIPS) assays that incorporate *Strongyloides*-specific recombinant antigens. LIPS assays have the additional advantage of rapid reversion to seronegativity following treatment compared to the slow decline in ELISA titers.[9]

TREATMENT   Rx

Uncomplicated intestinal strongyloidiasis can be treated effectively with ivermectin (200 µg/kg body weight daily for 2 days), with cure rates in excess of 90%.[A5] Albendazole is an alternative treatment (see Table 357-1). Decreases in serologic antibody titer and eosinophilia indicate a treatment response in the absence of continued exposure. After 6 months, ELISA titers should decrease significantly whereas LIPS assays should revert to negative.

In immunocompromised patients with hyperinfection or disseminated disease, daily treatment should be extended. Some experts recommend continuing treatment until 2 weeks after fecal examinations have become negative (i.e., for one autoinfection cycle). For severely ill patients who are unable to tolerate oral therapy, parenteral veterinary and enema ivermectin preparations have been used. Combination therapy with ivermectin and albendazole may also be used to treat disseminated strongyloidiasis, but data on whether this improves prognosis over monotherapy are lacking.

PREVENTION

In endemic areas, the risk for infection can be reduced by minimizing skin contact with contaminated soil, although elimination of this infection will occur only with improvements in sanitation and treatment of human waste. To prevent hyperinfection in individuals already infected, diagnosis should be attempted before the onset of immunosuppression if possible, such as before organ transplantation or cancer chemotherapy. Anyone who has resided in or traveled to an endemic area should undergo screening for asymptomatic infection, preferably by serologic tests or, if not possible, by microscopic examination of at least three fecal samples for the presence of larvae. Patients with positive screening test results should be treated empirically with ivermectin. Individuals with negative screening test results but unexplained eosinophilia and a history of exposure should also be considered for empirical treatment. In those undergoing hematopoietic stem cell transplantation, documentation of cure with at least three consecutive negative fecal examinations or a negative LIPS assays is recommended before proceeding with transplantation.

● UNCOMMON INTESTINAL NEMATODIASES

Humans may serve as accidental hosts for several nematodes that ordinarily parasitize the intestines of other mammals.

Trichostrongylus

Human infection with several different species of the genus *Trichostrongylus* has been reported in Iran, the Far East, and Australia. Humans are incidentally infected when larvae are ingested with leafy vegetables that have been contaminated with soil containing the feces of herbivorous animals. *Trichostrongylus* worms are similar to hookworms in their morphology, appearance of their eggs on fecal examination, and the pathology that they induce. Heavy infections may be accompanied by diarrhea and anemia. Drugs recommended for treatment are pyrantel pamoate, albendazole, or mebendazole (see Table 357-1).

Anisakiasis

Anisakiasis results from ingestion of the larvae of nematodes that normally infect sea mammals such as dolphins, whales, and seals. Larvae of the genera *Anisakis*, *Phocanema*, and *Pseudoterranova* infect the flesh of a number of saltwater fish species as intermediate hosts. Consumption of raw or undercooked fish, often in the form of sushi or sashimi, results in release of the infective larvae into the stomach, followed by invasion of the stomach or duodenal wall, which causes upper abdominal pain that can be intense. Anisakid worms cannot further develop in humans and die within a few days; an eosinophilic granulomatous reaction may result that mimics a gastric tumor. Diagnosis and treatment are accomplished by endoscopic removal of the parasite. Infection is prevented by cooking or freezing seafood before consumption. Of note, salting, smoking, and marinating fish do not kill anisakid larvae.

Capillaria philippinensis

C. philippinensis can cause a serious intestinal infection that has been reported primarily in the Philippines and Thailand, although it has also been observed in Japan, Taiwan, Korea, and Egypt. Adult worms resemble those of *Trichinella spiralis*, although biologically they mimic *S. stercoralis* in that they have an autoinfectious cycle of reproduction in which larvae can develop into adult worms without having to leave the host. Even though the life cycle is not completely known, this nematode probably parasitizes waterfowl that feed on fish and crustaceans, which serve as intermediate hosts. Humans become infected by eating raw or undercooked infected shrimp or fish. Adult worms travel to the mucosal crypts of the small intestine, where they deposit living larvae, sometimes resulting in overwhelming infection. Clinical disease consists of severe diarrhea associated with anorexia, vomiting, and weight loss. Mortality rates as high as 10% have been reported, with death resulting from severe malabsorption and protein-losing enteropathy. Diagnosis depends on finding eggs or larvae in feces. The treatment of choice is albendazole or mebendazole (see Table 357-1).

Other Intestinal Nematode Infections

Several nematodes that normally parasitize the intestine of nonhuman primates very rarely infect the human gastrointestinal tract. *Oesophagostomum bifurcum* infections have been reported from Africa, Asia, and South America and result from the oral ingestion of infective larvae. Adult worms can result in the formation of nodules in the intestinal wall that may be manifested as abdominal masses. Finally, infection with *Ternidens diminutus* has been reported to result in colonic ulcerations and nodular lesions in people living in southern Africa.

Grade A References

A1. Keiser J, Utzinger J. Efficacy of current drugs against soil-transmitted helminth infections: systematic review and meta-analysis. *JAMA.* 2008;299:1937-1948.
A2. Steinmann P, Utzinger J, Du ZW, et al. Efficacy of single-dose and triple-dose albendazole and mebendazole against soil-transmitted helminths and *Taenia* spp.: a randomized controlled trial. *PLoS ONE.* 2011;6:e25003.
A3. Knopp S, Mohammed KA, Speich B, et al. Albendazole and mebendazole administered alone or in combination with ivermectin against *Trichuris trichiura:* a randomized controlled trial. *Clin Infect Dis.* 2010;51:1420-1428.
A4. Speich B, Ame SM, Ali SM, et al. Oxantel pamoate-albendazole for *Trichuris trichiura* infection. *N Engl J Med.* 2014;370:610-620.
A5. Supputtamongkol Y, Premasathian N, Bhumimuang K, et al. Efficacy and safety of single and double doses of ivermectin versus 7-day high dose albendazole for chronic strongyloidiasis. *PLoS Negl Trop Dis.* 2011;5:e1044.

GENERAL REFERENCES

For the General References and other additional features, please visit Expert Consult at https://expertconsult.inkling.com.

358
TISSUE NEMATODE INFECTIONS

DAVID J. DIEMERT

The tissue nematodes can be broadly divided into those for which humans serve as the principal host (the filariases) and those that usually infect animals but can incidentally infect humans. Several zoonotic nematodes, such as *Toxocara, Trichinella,* and *Angiostrongylus,* can infect humans through accidental oral ingestion of helminth eggs or larvae but are unable to complete their life cycle in the host. Clinical manifestations are primarily due to the aberrant migration of larvae through various tissues.

TOXOCARIASIS

DEFINITION

Accidental ingestion of embryonated eggs of the dog roundworm *Toxocara canis,* or less frequently of the cat ascarid *Toxocara cati,* can lead to the clinical syndromes of visceral larva migrans and ocular larva migrans.[1] Symptoms are caused by the migration of larvae through the body, invading organs to cause serious disease and even death.

EPIDEMIOLOGY

Toxocara infections in animals are ubiquitous in their distribution throughout the world and are more common in younger animals than in adults. In humans, children are most frequently infected, probably due to exposure to soil contaminated with dog or cat feces when playing in sandboxes or playgrounds. Visceral larva migrans occurs most commonly in children younger than 5 years of age, whereas ocular larva migrans typically affects older children between the ages of 5 and 10 years.

PATHOBIOLOGY

The life cycle of *Toxocara* in the animal host resembles that of *Ascaris lumbricoides* in humans; larvae penetrate the intestinal wall after being released into the lumen from ingested eggs, migrate through the vasculature to the lungs, enter into the alveolar space, and ascend the bronchial tree until they are swallowed back into the gastrointestinal tract, where they develop into adult worms that can produce eggs. However, when embryonated *Toxocara* eggs are ingested by humans, the released larvae migrate throughout the body (most commonly to the lungs, the liver, the central nervous system [CNS], and occasionally the eyes) but cannot develop into adult worms. Ultimately, the larvae die, inducing significant immediate-type and delayed-type hypersensitivity reactions that result in eosinophilic granuloma formation. Visceral larva migrans and ocular larva migrans seem to be mutually exclusive, suggesting that different *Toxocara* strains may have different tissue tropisms. Alternatively, visceral larva migrans may result from repeated infections whereas ocular larva migrans may be a manifestation of infection in children who have not been previously sensitized.

CLINICAL MANIFESTATIONS

Most *Toxocara* infections in humans are asymptomatic. Visceral larva migrans is characterized by low-grade fever, pulmonary symptoms including cough and wheeze,[2] and less frequently hepatosplenomegaly accompanied by right upper quadrant pain. Symptoms appear gradually and resolve over 4 to 8 weeks. Myocarditis, nephritis, and CNS disease are less common. CNS involvement can result in seizures, encephalopathy, neuropsychiatric symptoms, or eosinophilic meningoencephalitis. A more subtle syndrome referred to as *covert toxocariasis* has been described that may result from less dramatic migration of larvae through organs. For example, *T. canis* has been suggested as an environmental risk factor for asthma in inner-city populations.

Ocular larva migrans typically manifests as unilateral visual impairment that is sometimes accompanied by strabismus.[3] The degree of vision loss depends on the particular ocular structure involved, and permanent blindness can occur. Ocular larva migrans involving the retina can be difficult to distinguish from other causes of focal intraretinal lesions, such as retinoblastoma or tuberculosis.

DIAGNOSIS

Toxocariasis can be presumed on the basis of a compatible clinical presentation and history of exposure to dogs or cats. Eosinophilia and hypergammaglobulinemia are often present. Serologic diagnosis by an enzyme-linked immunosorbent assay (ELISA) that employs antigens secreted by second-stage larvae to measure anti-*Toxocara* antibodies may be informative. Although establishment of sensitivity and specificity is difficult because of the inability to make a definitive parasitologic diagnosis, it is estimated that when a titer cutoff of 1 : 32 is used, the sensitivity of the ELISA is 78% for visceral larva migrans but lower for ocular larva migrans; specificity for both syndromes is greater than 90%. Biopsy of tissues to document the presence of larvae is not recommended because of low sensitivity.

Computed tomography and fluorescein angiography may be helpful in the diagnosis of ocular larva migrans, especially to differentiate it from retinoblastoma and other causes of intraocular space-occupying lesions. Anti-*Toxocara* antibodies can be detected in aqueous and vitreous humor fluid, and elevated levels relative to serum are suggestive of ocular larva migrans.

TREATMENT   Rx

Albendazole (400 mg twice daily for 5 days) is the treatment of choice for toxocariasis (Table 358-1). Mebendazole is not recommended because of its poor oral bioavailability. In patients with severe pulmonary, cardiac, or neurologic involvement, corticosteroids may reduce the severity and duration of symptoms. Ocular larva migrans is treated by vitrectomy, corticosteroids, or albendazole. See also Chapter 344.

TABLE 358-1	TREATMENT OF TISSUE NEMATODE INFECTIONS
NEMATODE INFECTION	**TREATMENT**
Toxocariasis	Albendazole, 400 mg twice daily for 5 days
Trichinellosis	Albendazole, 400 mg twice daily for 8-14 days*
Angiostrongyliasis	Treatment with albendazole or mebendazole is controversial but may relieve symptoms.
Gnathostomiasis	Albendazole, 400 mg daily for 3 wk Alternative: Ivermectin, 200 µg/kg/day for 2 days ± Surgical removal
Lymphatic filariasis	Diethylcarbamazine, 6 mg/kg/day divided in three doses for 12 days[†] Alternative: Doxycycline, 100-200 mg/day for 4-8 wk
Onchocerciasis	Ivermectin, 150 µg/kg once, repeated every 6-12 mo until resolution of symptoms
Loiasis	Diethylcarbamazine, 9 mg/kg/day divided in three doses for 21 days[†,‡]
Mansonella perstans	Doxycycline, 200 mg/day for 6 wk
Mansonella ozzardi	Ivermectin, 200 µg/kg once
Mansonella streptocerca	Diethylcarbamazine, 6 mg/kg/day divided in three doses for 12 days Alternative: Ivermectin, 150 µg/kg once
Dracunculiasis	Extraction of the adult worm

*Treatment is effective only if it is initiated during the intestinal phase of infection.
[†]Start at a dose of 50 mg on the first day, 50 mg three times daily on the second, 100 mg three times daily on the third, and then 6 mg/kg/day on day 4 onward.
[‡]Repeated treatment after 6 mo is often necessary if symptoms and eosinophilia persist.

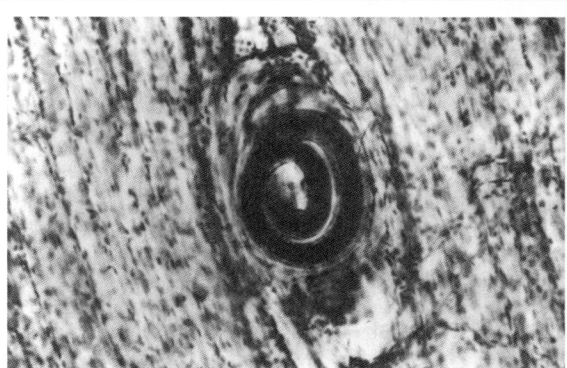

FIGURE 358-1. Nurse cell in muscle tissue containing a larva of *Trichinella spiralis*. (Courtesy Dr. I. Kagan, Centers for Disease Control and Prevention, Atlanta, GA.)

PREVENTION

Visceral larva migrans and ocular larva migrans may be prevented by periodic anthelminthic treatment of dogs and cats, proper disposal of pet feces, covering sandboxes, washing hands after playing with dogs or cats, and keeping children from playing in areas where pets have defecated.

BAYLISASCARIASIS

Baylisascariasis is a rare zoonosis caused by infection with the ascarid *Baylisascaris procyonis*, which is primarily a nematode parasite of raccoons and other small carnivores. In North America, infection is most commonly associated with contact with raccoons or environments contaminated with their feces and occurs predominantly in infants and young children who ingest the embryonated eggs while playing with soil. Clinically, disease is manifested as neural larva migrans because of the larval invasion of the CNS after release from ingested eggs in the gastrointestinal tract. Characteristic findings include fever and altered mental status accompanied by focal neurologic deficits and seizures; examination of the cerebrospinal fluid (CSF) reveals eosinophilic meningitis. *B. procyonis* also has been associated with ocular larva migrans, usually in otherwise healthy adults. Infection can be fatal or result in significant permanent neurologic or visual impairment. Once neural larva migrans is present, response to treatment with anthelmintics is poor, although corticosteroids may be helpful. Successful use of photocoagulation in ocular larva migrans has been reported. Prophylactic albendazole (25 mg/kg/day for 20 days) started within days of an exposure may prevent clinical disease.

TRICHINELLOSIS

DEFINITION

Trichinella infects a range of mammalian hosts, with the domestic pig serving as the most important reservoir worldwide. Humans are infected through eating raw or undercooked pork or other meats of domestic or wild animals that are contaminated with larvae that are encysted in muscle tissue. Although larvae develop into adults in the human intestinal tract, mate, and produce offspring larvae, clinical disease is characterized not so much by the intestinal infection as by the newborn larvae that penetrate the intestinal wall and disseminate throughout the body.

EPIDEMIOLOGY

Several different species of *Trichinella* can cause disease in humans, although *Trichinella spiralis* is the most important. *T. spiralis* is enzootic throughout the world in omnivorous and carnivorous wild animals, including bears, boars, and rats. *Trichinella nativa* affects predominantly carnivores (e.g., walruses, polar bears, and seals) living in the Arctic and subarctic regions of North America, Europe, and Asia. *Trichinella* is introduced into domestic animal populations, usually pigs or horses, by giving them unprocessed feed containing meat scraps of infected animals, most commonly rats. Because of regulations banning this practice in the United States, Canada, and the European Union, human infection by consumption of undercooked or smoked pork products or beef contaminated with the encysted larvae has been virtually eliminated, although it still occurs throughout the rest of the world. Instead, ingestion of poorly cooked wild game, especially bear or boar meat, is now the most common source of infection in these places. An important source of infection with *T. nativa* in Alaskan and Canadian Arctic native populations is eating of uncooked walrus meat.

PATHOBIOLOGY

Trichinellosis results from ingestion of striated muscle containing encysted infective larvae.[4] Larvae are released from muscle tissue by digestive enzymes in the stomach and then migrate to the upper two thirds of the small intestine, where they rapidly develop into sexually mature adult worms after only 2 days. Adults live embedded in the columnar epithelium, where they grow to a length of 3 mm (females) or 1.5 mm (males). Females begin producing newborn larvae within 5 days of mating. Adult worms remain viable for an additional 3 to 5 weeks, after which acquired immunity develops that leads to their expulsion from the host.

Newborn larvae possess a sword-like stylet in their oral cavity that permits them to penetrate the lamina propria and enter the lymphatic and blood vessels of the host, allowing them to migrate throughout the body. Larvae enter all types of cells, where they usually die, with the exception of striated skeletal and cardiac muscle cells. Unique among nematodes, mature *Trichinella* larvae have an intracellular phase, developing and transforming muscle cells into "nurse cells" that support larval growth and development (Fig. 358-1). In nurse cells, *Trichinella* larvae can survive for decades. Although nurse cells do not result in any disease in most mammals, they can induce an eosinophilic granulomatous reaction in humans that may result in significant tissue damage and dysfunction.

CLINICAL MANIFESTATIONS

Clinical disease in humans can be divided into an initial intestinal phase followed by a systemic or muscle phase. The initial phase of infection that occurs within days after ingestion of larvae may be associated with mild diarrhea, abdominal pain, and vomiting. This phase is self-limited and usually resolves spontaneously within 10 days.

The systemic dissemination of *Trichinella* larvae can result in myocardial, pulmonary, and focal neurologic manifestations,[5] although usually only in the most heavily infected persons. This systemic phase of infection usually begins 2 to 3 weeks after ingestion of infective larvae and may persist for several weeks. Clinical manifestations typically include fever, periorbital or facial edema, a diffuse inflammatory myositis (Chapter 421) that is characterized by myalgias and muscle tenderness, and petechial hemorrhages most easily observed in the subungual skin and conjunctivae. Larval invasion of the myocardium can lead to myocarditis (Chapter 60) that may result in heart failure or arrhythmias.

As with most nematodes, the severity of symptoms is related to the total worm burden. Because adult worms are incapable of reproducing within the host, the number of encysted larvae ingested is the most important determinant of the number of larvae that invade muscle and other tissues.

DIAGNOSIS

A diagnosis of trichinellosis should be suspected in individuals with a compatible clinical presentation, a history of eating raw or undercooked meat, eosinophilia, and increased muscle enzymes such as creatine kinase and lactate dehydrogenase. Definitive diagnosis depends on visualization of nurse cells in a muscle biopsy specimen or detection of *Trichinella*-specific DNA by the polymerase chain reaction (PCR) technique, although this tool is not widely available. Findings on muscle biopsy may be normal even in heavily infected patients because of sampling error. Detection of anti-*Trichinella* antibodies can be very useful in making a diagnosis; ELISA is the most commonly used method. Antibodies can be detected as early as 12 days after initial infection.

TREATMENT Rx

If patients present during the intestinal phase of infection, albendazole is recommended at a dosage of 400 mg twice daily for 8 to 14 days to kill the adult worms and thus prevent release of more newborn larvae (see Table 358-1). Although it is not known if albendazole is effective against newborn larvae, administration of this drug during the systemic phase of infection could potentially worsen symptoms by exacerbating the host inflammatory response to dying larvae. Treatment of severe systemic disease, including myocarditis and neurologic disease, should be directed toward reducing inflammation, most commonly with corticosteroids, although albendazole also should be given in such cases because corticosteroids may delay expulsion of adult worms from the intestine, thus increasing the number of newborn larvae that may be released. Symptomatic treatment with antipyretics and analgesics also should be considered. See also Chapter 344.

PREVENTION

Trichinella infection is prevented by thoroughly cooking meat products to kill the encysted larvae. Freezing meat solid at −20° C for at least 3 days will kill *T. spiralis* but not all other species of *Trichinella*. Of note, curing and smoking techniques do not reliably kill this nematode.

ANGIOSTRONGYLIASIS

DEFINITION

Angiostrongylus cantonensis and *Angiostrongylus costaricensis* are nematodes that normally infect rodents, primarily rats.[6] The adult worms of *A. cantonensis*, or rat lungworm, inhabit the pulmonary arteries of rodents; larvae are produced that migrate to the pharynx, are swallowed, and then are passed in the feces. Mollusks such as snails, slugs, and prawns serve as intermediate hosts until they are ingested by definitive hosts. Released larvae migrate to the brain, where they develop into immature adult worms before traveling to the pulmonary vasculature to become sexually mature adults. Humans are incidentally infected after eating poorly cooked or raw intermediate mollusk hosts; larvae can migrate to the CNS but cannot develop further. Fresh vegetables also may serve as a vehicle of human infection if they are contaminated with parts of mollusks containing infective larvae. As opposed to *A. cantonensis*, the larvae of *A. costaricensis* can develop into sexually mature adult worms in the local lymphatics and mesenteric arterioles of humans and release eggs and larvae into the intestinal tissue, causing an intense eosinophilic granulomatous reaction.

EPIDEMIOLOGY

Human infections with *A. cantonensis* occur mainly in Southeast Asia and the South Pacific and less frequently in Brazil, the Caribbean, and recently, in the United States in Louisiana. Abdominal angiostrongyliasis due to *A. costaricensis* has been reported mainly in Latin America, mostly in young children.

CLINICAL MANIFESTATIONS

In human cases of *A. cantonensis* infection, ingested larvae penetrate the intestinal wall and migrate to the brain, the meninges, and less commonly the spinal cord and eye. Fever, severe headache, meningismus, nausea, vomiting,

seizures, and focal neurologic deficits may develop. *A. costaricensis* infection can mimic appendicitis with right-sided abdominal pain, vomiting, and fever. Less frequently, gastrointestinal bleeding may occur.

DIAGNOSIS

Diagnosis of *A. cantonensis* infection is based on a history of ingestion of potentially contaminated food, the presence of peripheral eosinophilia, and detection of eosinophils and rarely larvae in the CSF.[7] In neither CNS nor intestinal angiostrongyliasis are larvae or eggs found in the feces, although both may be seen in tissue specimens for *A. costaricensis*. Serology is not commercially available.

TREATMENT AND PREVENTION   Rx

Most patients infected with either species of *Angiostrongylus* recover completely after approximately 2 weeks. The use of anthelmintics (Chapter 344) is controversial, with only a few reports of benefit with albendazole or mebendazole, usually administered in combination with analgesics and corticosteroids to relieve symptoms. Serial lumbar punctures to remove CSF can relieve symptoms of raised intracranial pressure caused by infection with *A. cantonensis*. Proper cooking of food and washing of vegetables can prevent this infection.

GNATHOSTOMIASIS

Gnathostoma spinigerum is an intestinal nematode of dogs and cats; intermediate hosts include tiny crustaceans (copepods), amphibians, freshwater fish, and birds.[8] Accidental human infection occurs throughout the Far East, Thailand, and Latin America, particularly Mexico, on eating of raw or undercooked invertebrate hosts harboring larvae. Larvae are released in the intestine and subsequently migrate through the body but are unable to reach sexual maturity in humans. The most common clinical presentation is migrating painful and pruritic subcutaneous swellings. Eosinophilic meningitis and ocular larva migrans also may occur, with potentially devastating results, including paralysis, subarachnoid hemorrhage, and permanent visual loss. Peripheral eosinophilia, often marked, is usually present; with meningitis, eosinophils are also present in the CSF. Although serologic testing is not available in the United States, laboratories in Thailand and Mexico can perform it. Treatment of cutaneous disease with either a 3-week course of albendazole or a 2-day course of ivermectin (200 μg/kg/day) is recommended (see Table 358-1); for neurologic or ocular involvement, anthelminthics are not advised because they may worsen manifestations. Gnathostomiasis may be prevented by thoroughly cooking fish.

FILARIASES

DEFINITION

The filariases are a group of arthropod-borne nematode infections that are endemic mostly in tropical areas of the world. Instead of residing in the intestine, mature adult filarial worms live in the lymphatics or in connective tissue (Table 358-2). Eight filarial species infect humans: *Wuchereria bancrofti*, *Brugia malayi*, *Onchocerca volvulus*, *Brugia timori*, *Loa loa*, *Mansonella streptocerca*, *Mansonella perstans*, and *Mansonella ozzardi*. The first three are the most common filariases worldwide. Although not usually fatal, these infections can result in significant disability and disfigurement, such as irreversible limb lymphedema (*W. bancrofti* and *B. malayi*) or blindness (*O. volvulus*). Most of the filariases require prolonged exposure for disease to manifest and are therefore uncommon in short-term travelers to endemic areas. The one exception is loiasis, which can occur in returned travelers and expatriates who have spent extended periods in endemic regions.

For all of the filarial nematodes, infection begins with the bite of an infected arthropod vector that deposits infective larvae called *microfilariae* into the skin or blood. Over several months, microfilariae mature into adult worms capable of mating to produce microfilariae that can be ingested by another arthropod vector to complete the life cycle. Adult worms can survive for 5 to 17 years in the human host; microfilariae live for between 5 months and 5 years. For most of the filarial nematodes except *B. malayi* and *M. perstans*, humans are the only definitive host.

Clinical manifestations of infection are varied and are caused by either adult worms or migrating microfilariae. Severity of disease is in most cases

TABLE 358-2 FILARIAL PARASITES OF HUMANS

SPECIES	DISTRIBUTION	VECTOR	MICROFILARIAE		
			PRIMARY LOCATION	PERIODICITY	PRESENCE OF SHEATH
Wuchereria bancrofti	Tropics worldwide	Mosquitoes	Blood	Nocturnal, subperiodic	+
Brugia malayi	India, Southeast Asia	Mosquitoes	Blood	Nocturnal, subperiodic	+
Brugia timori	Indonesia	Mosquitoes	Blood	Nocturnal	+
Onchocerca volvulus	Africa, Central and South America	*Simulium* black flies	Skin, eye	None or minimal	−
Loa loa	West and Central Africa	*Chrysops* flies	Blood	Diurnal	+
Mansonella perstans	Africa, South America, Caribbean	Midges	Blood	None	−
Mansonella ozzardi	Central and South America, Caribbean	Midges, *Simulium* black flies	Blood	None	−
Mansonella streptocerca	West and Central Africa	Midges	Skin	None	−

proportional to the worm burden harbored by an individual, with relatively light infections commonly being asymptomatic. For several of the filariases, the host inflammatory response to infection becomes apparent only on the death of the adult worm or microfilariae. This may be triggered by exposure to filarial antigens that were previously hidden from the immune system or by release of bacterial endosymbionts of the genus *Wolbachia* that live inside several of the filariae. *Wolbachia* are of the order Rickettsiales and are found in the hypodermis of adult worms and in oocysts, embryos, and microfilariae; they play a critical role in worm viability and fertility.[9]

Diagnosis of filarial infections usually depends on the microscopic examination of either blood or skin specimens for characteristic microfilariae (see Table 358-2). Microfilariae of the different filarial species measure between 170 and 320 μm in length and can be distinguished on the basis of the tissue source of the specimen, the presence or absence of a sheath, and the arrangement of nuclei in the tail. For some filarial species, microfilariae are present in the blood only during certain periods of the day to coincide with biting habits of the arthropod vector, which must be taken into account in timing blood sampling for diagnosis based on microscopy. Serology is not useful in endemic areas because a positive result does not distinguish between previous and current infection, and there is considerable antigenic cross-reactivity between the filariae and other nematodes. Detection of antifilarial antibodies may, however, be useful in returned long-term travelers or expatriates who are not originally from endemic areas.

Diethylcarbamazine (DEC), ivermectin, and albendazole are the principal antifilarial drugs, although they have varying efficacies against the different filarial species (see Table 358-1). DEC is macrofilaricidal (active against the adult worm) for *W. bancrofti*, *Brugia* spp, and *L. loa*, although prolonged or repeated courses are required for this effect. More commonly, the goal is to suppress microfilaria production by adult female worms, which can be achieved by single doses of antifilarial drugs administered alone or in combination annually or biannually. In some cases, reduction of microfilariae in the blood or skin can ameliorate symptoms or prevent progression of disease and interrupt transmission. Furthermore, targeting the *Wolbachia* endosymbionts of some filarial species with extended courses of antibiotics such as doxycycline can be macrofilaricidal.

Lymphatic Filariasis
DEFINITION
The three etiologic agents of lymphatic filariasis, *W. bancrofti*, *B. malayi*, and *B. timori*, are transmitted to humans through the bite of an infected mosquito.[10] Microfilariae deposited at the bite wound subsequently migrate through the subcutaneous tissue to the lymphatic system, where adult worms develop after approximately 4 to 12 months. The worms reside coiled in lymph nodes and may extend into afferent lymph vessels and surrounding subcutaneous tissue. The lymphatics of the lower and upper extremities and male genitalia are most commonly affected. After mating, females, which measure between 4 and 10 cm in length, twice the length of males, release more than 10,000 microfilariae per day that migrate into the blood stream until ingestion by mosquito intermediate hosts taking a blood meal. In most endemic areas, microfilariae are present in the peripheral blood only at night, when mosquito vectors are most likely to bite. Adult filariae live between 5 and 8 years within the host, although infections lasting for decades have been reported.

EPIDEMIOLOGY
An estimated 120 million people are affected by lymphatic filariasis worldwide; most cases are caused by *W. bancrofti*, and only approximately 10 to 20 million are due to *B. malayi*. *B. timori* is of minor importance, being restricted to southeastern Indonesia. *W. bancrofti* is widely distributed in the tropics, especially in Southeast Asia, the Indian subcontinent, Africa, South America, the Caribbean, and the South Pacific. The major vectors of bancroftian filariasis are *Culex* mosquitoes in urban areas, anopheline mosquitoes in rural areas of Africa, and *Aedes* species in the Pacific.

Humans are the only definitive host for *W. bancrofti*. *B. malayi*, however, can be zoonotic, with both monkey and feline species serving as reservoir hosts and transmission to humans by *Mansonia* mosquitoes. Brugian filariasis is found primarily in India, Malaysia, and other areas in Southeast Asia.

PATHOBIOLOGY
The pathologic process of filarial infections is primarily due to obstruction of lymphatic circulation resulting from damage induced by adult worms, specifically a local inflammatory lymphangitis with components of the innate and adaptive immune response that lead to hypertrophy of the vessel walls.[11] This inflammatory response can be triggered by release of antigens from dead or dying worms, although evidence suggests that it also is induced by living worms and *Wolbachia* antigens that are excreted or secreted into the surrounding milieu. Inflammatory damage is also exacerbated by secondary bacterial and fungal infections.

The initial inflammatory response leads to endothelial and connective tissue proliferation and vessel dilation, which impairs normal lymphatic function and results in lymphedema that is initially reversible. However, worm death results in a granulomatous reaction to released worm and *Wolbachia* antigens. The infiltration of giant cells, plasma cells, eosinophils, and neutrophils can completely occlude the lumen of the lymphatic vessel. Over time, progressive fibrosis and obstruction of lymph flow result in irreversible edema.[12] Although recanalization and collateralization of lymph vessels may occur, lymphatic function remains compromised.

CLINICAL MANIFESTATIONS
The clinical manifestations of lymphatic filariasis cover a wide spectrum from asymptomatic infection to severe chronic lymphatic obstruction accompanied by lymphedema and enlargement of the affected limb or body part (referred to as *elephantiasis*). Other common clinical outcomes include acute episodic lymphadenitis (also called *filarial fever*) and tropical pulmonary eosinophilia. Most infected individuals living in endemic regions are clinically asymptomatic, although microfilariae can be observed in their blood. Despite the absence of a significant inflammatory response, these individuals may nevertheless exhibit dilation of the affected lymphatics on ultrasound, which precedes the onset of clinically apparent disease.

For unknown reasons, newly exposed individuals may develop acute inflammatory reactions that can rapidly progress to chronic or irreversible changes compared with those born in endemic areas. Severe episodes of lymphadenitis, often with genital involvement, may lead to the relatively rapid development of lymphedema and elephantiasis within a year of arrival. Findings usually resolve quickly if the individual is promptly removed from the endemic area. Microfilariae are usually not detected in these patients.

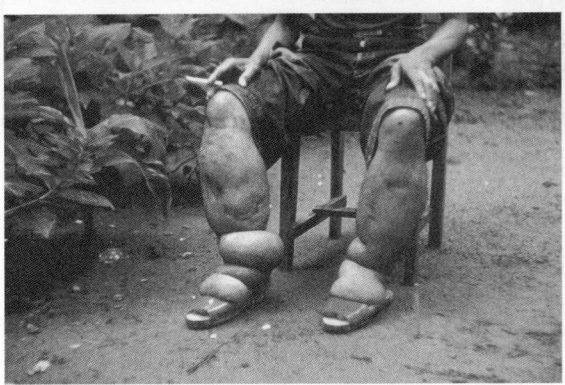

FIGURE 358-2. Elephantiasis, or chronic lymphedema due to infection with *Wuchereria bancrofti*. (Courtesy Centers for Disease Control and Prevention, Atlanta, GA.)

ACUTE LYMPHADENITIS

Acute episodes of retrograde lymphadenitis occur most commonly in adolescents in endemic areas, often in response to dying adult worms. Painful, erythematous enlargement of an affected lymph node, most commonly inguinal, precedes the onset of lymphangitis and is accompanied by fever and chills. Episodes usually last for approximately a week, frequently recur, and can be incapacitating. Defervescence is abrupt and associated with desquamation of the overlying skin. In men, inguinal lymphadenitis can be complicated by epididymitis and orchitis. Patients with filarial fevers may be microfilaremic but often are not.

ELEPHANTIASIS

Repeated episodes of lymphadenitis eventually lead to dilation of the lymphatic vessels, resulting in chronic lymphedema over the course of months to years (Fig. 358-2). The extremities, breasts, and genitalia are most commonly affected, although with *B. malayi* infection, usually only the lower parts of the legs are involved. The edema is initially pitting, but the subcutaneous tissue eventually loses its elasticity, resulting in woody edema with thickening of subcutaneous tissue and hyperkeratosis. Secondary bacterial or fungal infection contributes significantly to the chronic pathologic process of elephantiasis.

In bancroftian filariasis, development of hydrocele is a common manifestation of chronic filariasis in men and sometimes can become massive and debilitating; lymphedema of the vulva is less commonly seen in women. Involvement of the retroperitoneal lymphatics can lead to their rupture to produce intermittent chyluria or chylocele.

TROPICAL PULMONARY EOSINOPHILIA

Tropical pulmonary eosinophilia develops in a small minority of individuals with filarial infections. The syndrome is most commonly seen in young men living in southern India, although it also occurs in Pakistan, Sri Lanka, Southeast Asia, and Brazil. Characteristic clinical findings include nocturnal paroxysmal cough, wheeze, and low-grade fever that are accompanied by weight loss and prominent peripheral eosinophilia. Levels of both total IgE and antifilarial antibodies are typically high. Chest radiographs may show diffuse interstitial infiltrates or mottled opacities in the middle and lower lung fields. Without treatment, chronic restrictive lung disease may develop.

DIAGNOSIS

Definitive diagnosis usually relies on microscopic examination of a Giemsa-stained blood smear for microfilariae. Although thick blood smears are relatively insensitive except in cases of high microfilaremia, concentration or filtering techniques can increase diagnostic yield. Characteristic microfilariae are 250 to 320 μm in length. Collection of blood should be timed according to the known periodicity of the microfilariae.

A rapid immunochromatographic card test is available for *W. bancrofti* (there is no equivalent test for *Brugia* infections), and has the advantage of not requiring nocturnal collection of blood because it detects circulating antigen of the adult worm and not microfilariae. PCR methods also have been developed to detect filarial antigens in blood, although these are not widely available. Serologic detection of antifilarial antibodies is of limited value

because of extensive antigenic cross-reactivity with other nematodes. Furthermore, actively infected individuals cannot be distinguished from those previously infected, and those merely exposed but not infected also may have positive serologic test results.

Ultrasound examination of the lymphatic vessels of the spermatic cord of men can be used to visualize the "filarial dance sign," which is pathognomonic for a nest of filarial parasites.

Individuals with elephantiasis may be amicrofilaremic. Diagnosis therefore depends on a compatible clinical history and physical examination in the context of the appropriate epidemiology, and it may be supported by a positive antigen test or, in men, by a suggestive scrotal ultrasonogram. It should be distinguished from podoconiosis, a tropical lymphedema that results from long-term barefoot exposure to red-clay soil derived from volcanic rock and that may be a T-cell–mediated inflammatory disease.

TREATMENT   Rx

Management of lymphatic filariasis differs according to whether the aim is disease control or curative treatment of an individual patient. In endemic areas, annual mass drug administration with a combination of two antifilarial drugs can reduce transmission by decreasing the number of microfilariae in the blood available to biting mosquitoes. These programs use different combinations of single-dose DEC, ivermectin, and albendazole, administered at least once a year. DEC is administered with albendazole except in areas where onchocerciasis or loiasis is also found, in which case ivermectin plus albendazole is used.

It is recommended that all individuals with active infection by a lymphatic filarial parasite, whether symptomatic or asymptomatic, be treated with an antifilarial medication (see Table 358-1). The treatment of choice is DEC (6 mg/kg/day in three divided doses for 12 days). In the United States, DEC is available only through the Centers for Disease Control and Prevention (CDC) drug service (http://www.cdc.gov/laboratory/drugservice/formulary.html). For patients with high levels of microfilariae in the blood, treatment can be started at a low dose of 50 mg daily and scaled up during the first 3 days to reduce side effects of treatment such as fever, headache, dizziness, nausea, vomiting, rash, myalgias, and arthralgias. These normally resolve after a few days of treatment and can be treated with antipyretics, antihistamines, and, if symptoms are severe, corticosteroids.

DEC is both microfilaricidal and partially macrofilaricidal. In individuals who will not be returning to endemic areas, repeated treatments with DEC are often attempted to kill the adult worms instead of just reducing the levels of microfilariae in the blood. Typically, courses of DEC are repeated every 6 to 12 months. Although the adult worm burden is reduced in most treated individuals, all parasites are eliminated in less than a quarter. In men with dancing live adult worms visible by ultrasound in the scrotal lymphatics, serial studies may be performed to monitor the effects of therapy.

Unfortunately, lymphedema due to lymphatic filariasis usually is not reversible with DEC treatment, except in the very early stages. Nevertheless, several management modalities can be employed to limit the chronic sequelae of lymphatic filariasis. Critical among these is the prevention of secondary bacterial and fungal infection through meticulous hygiene and prompt treatment of suspected infections with antimicrobials. Limb elevation, physiotherapy, and use of elastic stockings may slow the worsening of lymphedema. Surgery is usually not indicated except for cases of hydrocele.

Interestingly, treatment directed against the *Wolbachia* endosymbiont has been shown to be effective in killing adult *W. bancrofti* and *Brugia* worms. Doxycycline, 100 or 200 mg daily for 4 to 8 weeks, reduces female worm fertility, with a resulting suppression of microfilaremia for up to a year, and reduces the number of live adult worms.[A1] Given the duration of treatment, these regimens are not ideal for disease control programs in endemic countries.

DEC is highly effective in the treatment of tropical pulmonary eosinophilia. Treatment with 6 mg/kg/day for 14 to 21 days results in resolution of symptoms within a week, although relapse may occur even after an interval of years. See also Chapter 344.

PREVENTION

Annual mass treatment with single doses of two antifilarial drugs can significantly reduce the prevalence of infection within a community.[13] In some areas, DEC-fortified table salt has been used to reduce the levels of microfilaremia in affected communities to interrupt the transmission cycle. Vector control through use of insecticide-treated bed nets and residual indoor spraying of insecticides appears to be effective.[14]

Onchocerciasis

DEFINITION

Onchocerciasis, or river blindness, caused by the nematode *O. volvulus,* is transmitted to humans by *Simulium* black flies. Infective microfilariae develop into male and female adult worms over several months and live for 9 to 14 years coiled within subcutaneous fibrous nodules (onchocercomas). Adult females measure between 20 and 70 cm in length and remain confined to the nodules; males are only 3 to 5 cm long and freely migrate through the subcutaneous tissues between nodules to inseminate females. Mature female worms produce up to 1500 microfilariae per day, which leave the nodule to migrate primarily through the skin and ocular tissues.[13] Microfilariae live within the host for 12 to 18 months.

EPIDEMIOLOGY

Onchocerciasis is endemic in equatorial Africa, with small foci in four Latin American countries (Guatemala, southern Mexico, Venezuela, and Brazil) and in Yemen. More than 37 million people are estimated to be infected, 500,000 of whom have significant visual impairment and 270,000 of whom are blind.[15] More than 99% of cases occur in sub-Saharan Africa, with Nigeria being the most highly endemic country. Because *Simulium* black flies require fast-flowing, well-oxygenated water for egg laying and reproduction, onchocerciasis is concentrated around streams and rivers, often in the most fertile farming areas. In communities bordering such waterways in endemic areas, up to 50% of the population can be affected.

Blindness caused by *O. volvulus* results in significant morbidity, long-term disability, and reduced economic productivity. In addition, onchocerciasis has been associated with a reduced life expectancy of at least 10 years compared with that of uninfected individuals in the same area, an effect that appears to be independent of the blindness that develops.

PATHOBIOLOGY

The pathologic changes of onchocerciasis are primarily due to an inflammatory reaction elicited by microfilariae, mostly in the skin, eyes, and lymph nodes. Adult worms contained in nodules are relatively isolated from the host immune response. Tissue damage results from a cell-mediated immune response to dying microfilariae, which becomes more pronounced as infection persists. The degree of tissue damage is directly related to the intensity of infection and magnitude of the host response. Sclerosing keratitis, the major cause of blindness, is caused by an inflammatory reaction to dying intraocular microfilariae that appears to be dependent on T helper cell type 2 (T_H2) cytokines. With time, neovascularization and scarring of the cornea lead to corneal opacification and eventual blindness. In the skin, similar immune responses result in pruritus and angioedema. Ongoing low-grade inflammation in the skin eventually leads to loss of elasticity and atrophy. Chronic inflammatory changes and fibrosis are also seen in lymph nodes.

Like the nematodes responsible for lymphatic filariasis, *O. volvulus* adult worms contain endosymbiotic *Wolbachia* bacteria that are obligatory for the development, survival, and fertility of these worms. Pro-inflammatory *Wolbachia* proteins released by dying microfilariae may be responsible for a significant amount of the immunopathology associated with onchocerciasis. For example, *Wolbachia* antigens have been shown to interact with the innate immune system through a toll-like receptor 2–mediated mechanism (Chapter 45).

CLINICAL MANIFESTATIONS

Onchodermatitis

Onchocerciasis commonly manifests with a diffuse papular dermatitis that is intensely pruritic. In heavily infected individuals in endemic areas, the pruritus is intractable, leading to scratching and excoriation to the point of bleeding and even suicide. Hypersensitivity reactions, scabies, insect bites, and atopic or contact dermatitis should be considered in the differential diagnosis of the acute papular dermatitis seen with onchocerciasis. The skin of affected areas becomes edematous and thickened, losing its elasticity and taking on an orange-peel texture. A lichenified dermatitis (referred to as *sowda*) may occur; it consists of an intensely pruritic eruption limited to one extremity, usually a leg, with hyperpigmented papules and plaques accompanied by edema of the entire limb. Over time, the skin will atrophy and fine wrinkles appear, especially over the buttocks. Pruritus is uncommon at this point. Areas of depigmentation may occur most commonly over the shins, a phenomenon called *leopard skin.*

Subcutaneous Nodules

Subcutaneous onchocercomas containing adult worms are most often palpable over bony prominences. In Africa, the nodules are most commonly found over the hips and lower limbs; in Latin America, they are often located on the head and upper part of the body. Nodules usually measure between 0.5 and 3 cm in diameter and are freely mobile. In lightly infected individuals, such as expatriates, nodules are usually not detectable.

Ocular Lesions

Initial ocular involvement is characterized by conjunctivitis, excess tearing, and photophobia in response to dying microfilariae. At this time, the corneal disease consists of a punctate keratitis or snowflake corneal opacities. Over 20 to 30 years, this leads to sclerosing keratitis, neovascularization, and corneal opacification. The anterior chamber of the eye also may be involved, with iritis, iridocyclitis, and secondary glaucoma. Posterior ocular disease can manifest as chorioretinitis, optic neuritis, and optic atrophy.

Lymphadenopathy

Lymphadenopathy is frequently found in the inguinal and femoral areas in Africa and in the head and neck in Latin America. Advanced disease in the inguinal region can result in the so-called hanging groin, with elongated atrophic skin containing nontender and fibrotic lymph nodes.

DIAGNOSIS

Definitive diagnosis has traditionally been made by observing unsheathed motile microfilariae measuring 200 to 300 μm in length that are released from superficial skin snips. To take a skin snip, a thin piece of skin overlying a bone prominence that has been tented up with a needle is sliced with a scalpel blade, or a corneal-scleral punch instrument is used to obtain a small piece of skin without drawing blood. Avoidance of blood contamination is critical so as to avoid confusion with blood-borne microfilariae in cases patients are coinfected with other filariases. Typically, six snips are taken, one from over each scapula, iliac crest, and lateral aspect of each calf, and then incubated with warm physiologic saline and examined microscopically for motile microfilariae after at least 30 minutes of incubation, although longer periods of up to 24 hours may be necessary. Newer techniques include PCR amplification of filarial DNA directly from skin snips that are far more sensitive than direct visualization. With ocular disease, free microfilariae may be visible by slit lamp examination in the anterior chamber or aqueous humor.

Subcutaneous nodules can be sampled or examined by ultrasound to demonstrate the presence of adult worms. Serologic tests are usually positive for antifilarial antibodies but are not specific because of extensive antigenic cross-reactivity with other nematodes. Eosinophilia is a common but inconsistent finding.

In the past, the Mazzotti test was used to diagnose onchocerciasis. In this test, a challenge dose of DEC was administered to patients suspected of having onchocerciasis; with *O. volvulus* infection, an intense pruritic skin reaction would develop within hours. However, in patients with high-intensity infections, the Mazzotti reaction could be severe and even worsen ocular disease, resulting in permanent visual loss. Therefore, this test is no longer recommended, although some instead suggest the application of a small amount of cream that contains DEC to the skin to provoke a localized Mazzotti reaction.

TREATMENT   Rx

Ivermectin is the treatment of choice for onchocerciasis (see Table 358-1).[16] Administration of a single dose of ivermectin (150 μg/kg) is effective in ameliorating ocular and dermatologic disease by destroying microfilariae and suppressing their release from female worms. Because ivermectin is not active against the encapsulated adult worms, treatment must be repeated every 6 to 12 months, probably for at least 10 years in those without further exposure. For unknown reasons, pruritus in lightly infected expatriates may require more aggressive and frequent treatment for the first 2 years. Within 24 hours of treatment with ivermectin, fever and pruritus may occur in reaction to the dying microfilariae or released *Wolbachia* antigens, especially in those with high pretreatment levels of microfilariae. Use of ivermectin in areas where *L. loa* (see later) is co-endemic should be undertaken with caution because treatment may precipitate severe reactions including encephalopathy in those with high levels of microfilaremia. DEC should never be used for treatment of onchocerciasis because of frequent unacceptable reactions to dying microfilariae ranging from urticaria and angioedema to hypotension and death. Although the drug suramin (available from the CDC drug service) is active against adult *O. volvulus* worms, because of its excessive toxicity and potentially life-threatening effects, it is used only in rare situations. Surgical removal of palpable nodules has been successful in resolving the infection in some areas, notably in Central America.

Doxycycline, 200 mg/day administered for 4 to 6 weeks, followed by single-dose ivermectin, has been shown to deplete *Wolbachia* endosymbionts from adult worms and to suppress *O. volvulus* embryogenesis and production of microfilariae for up to 18 months.[A2] Some experts now recommend this regimen for patients with onchocerciasis who have left an endemic area and will not be re-exposed. See also Chapter 344.

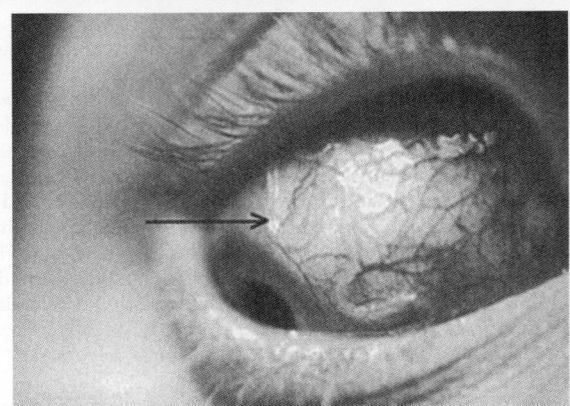

FIGURE 358-3. Adult *Loa loa* worm migrating across the eye (*arrow*).

PREVENTION

Regular mass administration of ivermectin to affected communities forms the core of the global eradication strategy for onchocerciasis.[17] Implementation of this program has been made easier because the drug is donated by the manufacturer. In addition to benefiting infected individuals, mass drug administration reduces the microfilariae available to vectors and thus interrupts the transmission cycle. For travelers to endemic areas, use of insect repellent may be beneficial.

Loiasis

DEFINITION

Loiasis is caused by infection with the filarial nematode *Loa*, otherwise known as the African eye worm. *L. loa* are transmitted by flies of the genus *Chrysops* during a blood meal. Adult worms develop during a period of 1 to 4 years and live for up to 17 years.[18] They migrate freely in the subcutaneous tissue, including the subconjunctiva or sclera of the eye. Adult females measure between 40 and 70 mm in length; males are shorter, measuring between 25 and 35 mm. After mating, females release microfilariae into the blood. *L. loa* microfilariae exhibit a diurnal periodicity coinciding with the feeding habits of *Chrysops,* with microfilaremia peaking around noon.

EPIDEMIOLOGY

Loiasis is endemic in the rain forest regions of central and western Africa. Although accurate numbers are not available, loiasis appears to be most prevalent in Gabon, Cameroon, the Democratic Republic of the Congo, Nigeria, and the Central African Republic. Loiasis requires a shorter period of exposure than other filarial infections and can be seen in returning travelers or expatriates who have spent extended periods in Africa.

PATHOBIOLOGY

Neither adult *L. loa* worms nor microfilariae have any direct pathologic effects. In a subset of infected individuals, a hypersensitivity response, termed a *Calabar swelling*, develops to secretions from adult worms or released microfilariae, resulting in recurrent localized angioedema that often precedes the migrating worm. These patients have very high serum levels of immunoglobulin E (IgE) antibodies and eosinophilia. This reaction is more commonly observed in visitors to endemic areas rather than in native residents. Unlike other filariae, *L. loa* does not contain *Wolbachia* endosymbionts.

CLINICAL MANIFESTATIONS

Most individuals with loiasis are asymptomatic despite being microfilaremic. Clinical manifestations of infection are more common in long-term visitors to endemic areas than in people native to the regions. Recurrent Calabar swellings are the most common finding in these individuals, who are not usually microfilaremic. They are nonerythematous swellings measuring 5 to 20 cm in diameter that typically occur on the extremities and the face and last for a few days. The onset is often preceded by pruritus and pain. On occasion, adult worms may migrate across the subconjunctiva or sclera of the eye in both groups of patients, causing severe pain and inflammation (Fig. 358-3). Rare complications of infection include nephropathy and encephalitis, which usually develop in those with high levels of microfilariae after receiving DEC or ivermectin treatment for other filarial infections. Endomyocardial fibrosis resulting from eosinophilic infiltration of the myocardium has been reported in association with loiasis.

DIAGNOSIS

Definitive diagnosis depends on microscopic examination of a Giemsa-stained blood film for characteristic sheathed microfilariae. Blood should be collected between 10 AM and 2 PM because of the diurnal periodicity of the microfilariae. Because individuals who are not native to endemic areas usually are not microfilaremic, diagnosis relies on a compatible history, clinical findings, peripheral eosinophilia, and elevated antifilarial antibody levels. Adult worms sometimes can be surgically removed while migrating across the eye or through subcutaneous tissues. Calabar swellings must be distinguished from onchocercomas and other causes of angioedema.

TREATMENT   Rx

DEC (9 mg/kg/day for 21 days) is active against both adult *L. loa* worms and microfilariae (see Table 358-1). Treatment usually is increased from a dose of 50 mg/day on the first day to the full dose on the fourth day to minimize the likelihood of treatment-associated complications, the most serious of which are glomerulonephritis and potentially fatal encephalopathy. Treatment-associated complications are more common with high pretreatment microfilarial levels and result from host allergic reactions to dying microfilariae. Antihistamines and corticosteroids may be employed to reduce allergic side effects. Alternatively, apheresis can be used to remove circulating microfilariae before initiation of DEC in these individuals. Albendazole, which is microfilaricidal but has no activity against adult worms, also has been used to reduce microfilaria levels before treatment with DEC. Repeated courses of DEC may be necessary in approximately half of patients before clinical manifestations completely resolve. Persistent or increasing eosinophilia or levels of antifilarial antibodies 6 months after treatment also should prompt re-evaluation for repeated treatment. Adult worms in the eye may be surgically removed.

Ivermectin is microfilaricidal but has no macrofilaricidal effect and may cause toxic encephalopathy in individuals with high microfilaria levels. In areas where onchocerciasis is co-endemic, this infection should be ruled out before the initiation of DEC for loiasis to prevent toxicity from dying *O. volvulus* microfilariae. See also Chapter 344.

PREVENTION

Weekly chemoprophylaxis with DEC administered as a 300-mg dose is effective in preventing loiasis in long-term residents of endemic areas.

Less Common Filarial Infections

MANSONELLA PERSTANS

M. perstans infection occurs throughout central Africa, in northeastern South America, and in parts of the Caribbean. Microfilariae are transmitted by *Culicoides* midges and develop into adult worms that live in serous body cavities, such as the pleural, pericardial, and peritoneal spaces, as well as in mesenteric and retroperitoneal tissues. Most infections are asymptomatic, although painless conjunctival nodules with eyelid edema have been reported. Transient angioedema and Calabar-like swellings, fever, headache, arthralgias, and neurologic manifestations also may occur. Microfilariae do not exhibit periodicity and can be observed on stained blood films. Eosinophilia is common.

M. perstans harbor *Wolbachia* endosymbionts, and treatment with doxycycline, 200 mg/day for 6 weeks, has been shown to be highly effective in suppressing microfilaremia for up to 3 years, suggesting that the treatment is macrofilaricidal.[A3]

MANSONELLA OZZARDI

Infections with *M. ozzardi* occur in Central and South America and parts of the Caribbean, especially Haiti. Vectors include *Simulium* black flies and midges. Adult worms locate to the peritoneal and thoracic cavities or the lymphatics; microfilariae circulate in the blood without periodicity. Infection usually results in asymptomatic eosinophilia, although arthritis and allergic symptoms such as urticaria and lymphadenopathy may occur. Administration of ivermectin as a single dose of 200 μg/kg has been reported to provide long-term suppression of microfilaremia and improvement of symptoms. Neither DEC nor the benzimidazoles are effective.

MANSONELLA STREPTOCERCA

M. streptocerca is endemic in the tropical forest zone of western and central Africa and is transmitted by biting midges. Similar to *O. volvulus,* adult worms live in the subcutaneous tissues, as do microfilariae. In contrast to onchocerciasis, however, microfilariae do not invade the eye. Infection is usually asymptomatic, although a pruritic dermatitis with depigmentation similar to onchodermatitis can affect the trunk and upper extremities. Associated axillary or inguinal adenopathy is common. Microfilariae have characteristic hooked tails and can be visualized in skin snips. In areas where onchocerciasis is co-endemic, skin specimens must be stained to differentiate *M. streptocerca* from *O. volvulus.* DEC is microfilaricidal and macrofilaricidal and is given as 6 mg/kg/day for 12 days. Ivermectin is effective against microfilariae but not adult worms.

ZOONOTIC FILARIAL INFECTIONS

A rare accidental filarial infection of humans with the dog heartworm *Dirofilaria immitis* occurs worldwide. Transmitted by mosquitoes, *D. immitis* microfilariae cannot reach maturity in humans but embolize to the lung after dying in the right ventricle. Most infections are asymptomatic, but some people experience cough, chest pain, and hemoptysis consistent with lung infarction. Chest radiographs demonstrate typical coin lesions that may be mistaken for carcinoma. Other animal filariae, including *Dirofilaria repens* of dogs and *Dirofilaria tenuis* of raccoons, can infect humans and result in subcutaneous nodules that may be migratory. Eosinophilia and antifilarial antibodies are not usually present in zoonotic filarial infections. Surgical removal of lesions is both diagnostic and curative.

⬤ DRACUNCULIASIS

Dracunculiasis is a disfiguring disease caused by the nematode *Dracunculus medinensis,* also known as the Guinea worm. Although previously found in India, Pakistan, and Latin America, it is now endemic in only five countries in sub-Saharan Africa (South Sudan, Sudan, Chad, Mali, and Ethiopia) because of concerted efforts at eradication. As of 2014, fewer than 200 cases are thought to exist, with the largest concentration being in South Sudan. Transmission to humans occurs through ingestion of tiny crustacean intermediate hosts called *copepods* that harbor infective larvae. Released larvae penetrate the intestinal wall and migrate to the subcutaneous tissues, where they develop into adult worms. After approximately a year, female worms induce vesicular skin lesions, usually on the lower extremities, that eventually ulcerate. On direct contact with fresh water, the female worm releases thousands of motile larvae that can then complete the transmission cycle by infecting copepods in the water. Adult worms can measure up to a meter in length. Fever and allergic symptoms, including wheezing and urticaria, may precede rupture of the blister or occur with attempts to extract the worm. Secondary bacterial infection of the skin lesions is frequent. Although not usually fatal, dracunculiasis can result in significant disability.

Traditionally, emerging worms are extracted by slowly winding a few centimeters of the parasite on a stick each day, taking care not to break it. Surgical removal can be attempted but may exacerbate allergic symptoms. There is no effective chemotherapy for this infection. Prevention efforts have been highly successful in breaking the transmission cycle and have led to eradication of the parasite from many countries. Strategies include filtering of drinking water through finely woven cloth, education of infected individuals not to enter fresh water, treatment of water sources with larvicides, and provision of safe drinking water from wells.

Grade A References

A1. Taylor MJ, Makunde WH, McGarry HF, et al. Macrofilaricidal activity after doxycycline treatment of *Wuchereria bancrofti*: a double-blind, randomised placebo-controlled trial. *Lancet.* 2005;365: 2116-2121.
A2. Hoerauf A, Specht S, Büttner M, et al. *Wolbachia* endobacteria depletion by doxycycline as antifilarial therapy has macrofilaricidal activity in onchocerciasis: a randomized placebo-controlled study. *Med Microbiol Immunol.* 2008;197:295-311.
A3. Coulibaly YI, Dembele B, Diallo AA, et al. A randomized trial of doxycycline for *Mansonella perstans* infection. *N Engl J Med.* 2009;361:1448-1458.

GENERAL REFERENCES

For the General References and other additional features, please visit Expert Consult at https://expertconsult.inkling.com.

359

ARTHROPODS AND LEECHES

DIRK M. ELSTON

⬤ ARTHROPODS

The Pathogens

Arthropods act as disease vectors and cause human injury by means of the direct toxic effects of their venom or via an immune response to their antigens (Tables 359-1 to 359-4). Immediate reactions to stings may be related to histamine, serotonin, formic acid, or kinins contained within the venom. Delayed reactions to bites and stings generally represent a host response to proteinaceous allergens contained within venom or saliva.[1]

Whereas many diseases are spread by a single vector, others have multiple potential vectors. For example, tularemia is commonly acquired from ticks or handling of infected carcasses but also may be spread by deerflies and horseflies. Rickettsiae are spread by both ticks and fleas. It is important to note that the vector may influence manifestations of the disease. For example, *Bartonella* transmitted by a flea may produce bacillary angiomatosis, whereas the same organism transmitted by a louse is much more likely to manifest as endocarditis. Disease manifestations also may reflect the underlying immune status of the host, previous sensitization, or associated comorbidities. For example, hypersensitivity reactions to insect stings are more common in those with an atopic diathesis and anaphylaxis may be a manifestation of underlying mastocytosis. Exaggerated bite reactions (Fig. 359-1) may be a manifestation of an underlying lymphoproliferative disease.

TABLE 359-1 MEDICALLY IMPORTANT ARTHROPODS

Arachnida
    Acari—mites, ticks
    Araneida—spiders
    Scorpionida

Pentastomida—tongue worms
Chilopoda—centipedes
Diplopoda—millipedes

Crustacea
    Copepoda—*Cyclops, Diaptomus*
    Decapoda—shrimp, lobster, crayfish, crab

Insecta
    Anoplura—lice
    Coleoptera—beetles
    Diptera—mosquitoes, black flies, midges, horse flies, deer flies, greenheads, tsetse
    flies, stable flies, sand flies, houseflies, bluebottle flies

Hemiptera—bed bugs, reduviids
Hymenoptera—ants, bees, wasps
Lepidoptera—moths, caterpillars
Siphonaptera—fleas

TABLE 359-2   ARTHROPOD VECTORS

DISEASE	VECTOR
African trypanosomiasis	Tsetse flies
American trypanosomiasis	Triatome bugs
Arboviridae	*Culex* mosquitoes
Babesiosis	*Ixodes scapularis* (deer tick)
Bartonellosis	Fleas, lice, sandflies
Dengue	*Aedes* mosquitoes
Endemic typhus	*Ctenocephalides felis* and *Xenopsylla cheopis* (fleas)
Filariasis	Anopheline and *Aedes* mosquitoes
Human anaplasmosis	*Ixodes scapularis*
Human monocytic ehrlichiosis	*Amblyomma americanum* (lone star tick)
Leishmaniasis	Sandflies
Lyme disease	*Ixodes scapularis*
Malaria	Anopheline mosquitoes
Onchocerciasis	*Simulum* flies
Plague	*Xenopsylla cheopis* and *Pulex irritans* (human flea)
Rickettsial pox	*Liponyssoides sanguineus* (house mouse mite)
Rocky Mountain spotted fever	*Dermacentor variabilis* (dog tick) *Dermacentor andersoni* (wood tick) *Amblyomma americanum*
Tick paralysis	*Dermacentor andersoni* *Dermacentor variabilis*
Tick-borne relapsing fever	*Ornithodoros* genus (soft tick)
Trypanosomiasis	*Tsetse* fly, hemipterids
Tularemia	*Amblyomma americanum* *Dermacentor andersoni* *Dermacentor variabilis* *Chrysops* deer flies Horseflies
Tyhpus	*Pediculus humanus* (lice)
Typhus, endemic	Fleas
Typhus, scrub	Chigger mites
Viral encephalitis	*Aedes* mosquitoes
West Nile fever	*Culex* mosquitoes
Yellow fever	*Aedes* mosquitoes

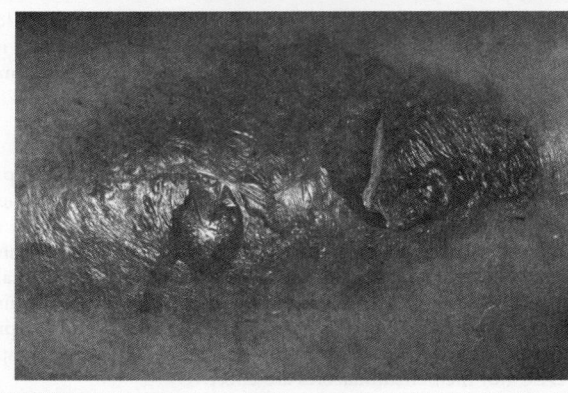

FIGURE 359-1. Exaggerated arthropod bite response in a patient with chronic lymphocytic leukemia.

TABLE 359-3   MEDICALLY IMPORTANT MITES

FAMILY	
Acaridae	Commonly found in grain, flour, and other foods
Cheyletidae	Walking dandruff in dogs, cats, and rabbits
Demodicidae	Human hair follicle mites
Dermanyssidae	Bird and rodent mites
Glycyphagidae	Associated with food, animals, and leaf litter
Hemoganasidae	Straw mites
Psoroptidae	Scab mites
Pyemotidae	Grain and straw mites
Sarcoptidae	Scabies mites
Trombiculidae	Chigger or harvest mites

TABLE 359-4   CAUSES OF DIRECT TOXIC INJURY BY ARTHROPODS AND LEECHES

ORGANISM	TYPE OF INJURY	DISTRIBUTION AND POPULATION AFFECTED
Australian funnel web spiders (*Hadronyche* and *Atrax*)	Neurotoxin producing tingling around the mouth, muscle twitching, nausea, vomiting, profuse sweating, coma, myocardial injury	Australians
Blister beetles	Bullous reactions	Widely distributed, but more common in hot climates
Brazilian wandering spider (*Phoneutria* spiders)	Neurotoxin resulting in paralysis	Brazilians
Brown *Loxosceles* spiders	Dermonecrotic reactions	Contact through attics and woodpiles
Centipedes	Neurotoxin that may produce pain, paresthesia, erythema, edema, and profuse bleeding. Rarely, coronary ischemia, rhabdomyolysis, proteinuria, and renal failure.	Most toxic species in Asia
Hymenopterids	Anaphylactic reactions	Wide distribution
Leeches	Bleeding	Fresh water exposure
Lepidopterids *Lonomia* caterpillars	Rash, ophthalmia nodosa, keratoconjunctivitis Fatal bleeding diathesis	Wide distribution Brazil
Millipedes	Chemical burns	Most toxic species in Australia and Africa
Pacific funnel web spider (*Tegenaria agrestis*)	Dermonecrotic reactions	Basements in the Pacific Northwest
Scorpions *Centruroides sculpturatus* Buthid scorpions	Mild systemic symptoms, sometimes severe in children Severe cardiac toxicity	Southwestern United States Asia, Africa, and Latin America
Tarantulas	Contact urticaria and ophthalmia nodosa	Hot climates
Widow spiders (*Latrodectus*)	Neurotoxin mimicking acute abdomen	Contact through outhouses and woodpiles

INFECTION BY ARACHNIDA

SCABIES

DEFINITION

Human scabies is caused by the mite *Sarcoptes scabiei* variant *hominis,* an obligate human pathogen, belonging to the class Arachnida, subclass Acari, order Astigmata, and family Sarcoptidae. Animal mange or scabies is caused by related *Sarcoptes* or *Psoroptes* mites. These zoonotic mites can produce transient symptoms in exposed humans, but are rarely capable of producing sustained infestation. *Sarcoptes scabiei* variant *hominis* is round to oval with a small anterior portion, dorsal spines, and hairlike projections on the rudimentary legs.

PATHOBIOLOGY

After mating on the skin surface, the female mite begins to burrow and lay eggs at a rate of 1 to 3 per day. The eggs mature and hatch over 3 to 4 days. The larvae pass through protonymph and tritonymph stages before molting into adults. The entire life cycle ranges between 30 and 60 days. All stages of the mite are capable of penetrating the stratum corneum via secretion of enzymes. In immunosuppressed individuals, mite populations may reach staggering proportions within thick, white, highly infectious crusts.

In immunocompetent patients, scabies mites induce a strong host response characterized by a superficial and deep perivascular inflammatory infiltrate composed of lymphocytes, histiocytes, and eosinophils. There is marked production of interleukin-6 (IL-6) resulting in proliferation of keratinocytes, activation of Th1 CD4+ cells causing production of IL-2, and activation of Th2 CD4+ cells causing production of IL-4. Disease manifestations relate to the complex balance of the immune response.

CLINICAL MANIFESTATIONS

In immunocompetent adults, the eruption manifests with severe pruritus with nocturnal exacerbation and a symmetrical erythematous, papulovesicular eruption. Pruritus can be present on both affected and unaffected skin. There is a predilection for involvement of the interdigital web spaces, wrists (Fig. 359-2), anterior axillary folds, periumbilical skin, the areolae in females, and the penis and scrotum in males. In the pediatric population, head, neck, face, palms, and soles are commonly involved. Nodular scabies is a clinical variant accounting for 7% of all cases. Those affected present with intensely pruritic red-brown nodules 2 to 20 mm in size on the genitalia, buttocks, groin, and axillary region. These nodules do not contain mites but represent hypersensitivity to mite products. Crusted scabies manifests in immunosuppressed individuals as silver to white crusts involving any portion of the body, but with a predilection for the hands and ears. In elderly patients, the manifestations may be quite subtle with mild pruritus and prurigo-like papules on the trunk and extremities. In patients with human T-lymphotropic virus type I infection, scabies often manifests with linear, psoriasiform, hyperkeratotic lesions on the dorsal hands and feet. Crusted scabies can result in sepsis, with a 5-year mortality rate of up to 50%.

The most pathognomonic findings are the presence of burrows and genital nodules. The burrow is a short serpiginous gray to white keratotic line measuring 1 to 4 mm in length. They are most common on the hands and feet, particularly on the finger web spaces, the thenar and hypothenar eminences, and the wrists. Genital nodules may involve the glans, scrotum, or labia majora. A history of itch in other family members or sexual partners is highly suggestive of the diagnosis.

DIAGNOSIS

The diagnosis is established by identification of the female mite, ova, or feces in a scraping from a burrow (Fig. 359-3). Definitive diagnosis relies on direct visualization of mites, eggs, or mite pellets under microscopy. Additional diagnostic methods include the burrow ink test, video-dermoscopy, and polymerase chain reaction (PCR) and enzyme-linked immunosorbent assay (ELISA) for mite product or specific immunoglobulin E (IgE).

TREATMENT Rx

Commonly employed topical agents include permethrin 5% and precipitated sulfur 2 to 10% in petrolatum. Topical agents used worldwide include benzyl benzoate 10 to 25%, monosulfiram 5 to 25%, malathion 0.5%, and esdepallethrin 0.63%. The topical agent crotamiton 10% has relatively weak antiscabetic activity but has antipruritic as well as antibacterial actions. An alternative to topical therapy is the use of oral ivermectin, 200 to 400 µg/kg given as a single dose, then repeated in 10 days.[2]

Proper application of any topical must include the umbilicus, genitalia, under the nails, and the skin up to the edge of all body orifices. Fomites are important in the spread of crusted scabies, with hospital linens being of particular concern. Caregivers involved in bathing or lifting, sexual partners, and family members are at high risk for infection and should be treated at the same time as the patient regardless of symptomatology. Clothes and bed linens should be machine washed at 60°C followed by heated drying.

OTHER MITES

Mites are ubiquitous in the environment and are a frequent cause of dermatitis. The most common medically important mites are listed in Table 359-3.

The majority of mites are free-living, but thousands of species are obligate parasites of animals or plants. Like ticks, mites mature through various life stages. Typically, there is a single six-legged larval stage, followed by several nymphal stages and an adult stage. Both nymphs and adults typically have eight legs. Although most mites lay eggs, the spiny rat mite (*Laelaps echidninus*) is viviparous, and the straw itch mite (*Pyemotes tritici*) protects its young internally throughout their life cycle until they emerge as sexually mature adults. Manifestations of mite infestations are protean and include papular, vesicular, urticarial, and morbilliform eruptions. Chigger mites most often affect the lower legs, the edges of underwear, and the genitalia. Summer penile syndrome is a manifestation of chigger mite infestation. It presents with tender to itchy papules of the glans and scrotum and may mimic scabies infestation. Chigger (Trombiculid) mites in Asia are vectors for scrub typhus,

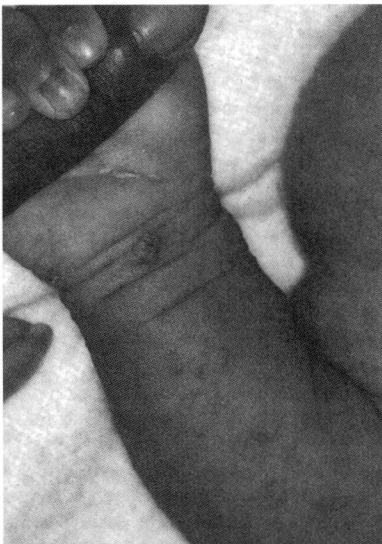

FIGURE 359-2. Scabies infestation in children commonly manifests with burrows (shown here between the thenar and hypothenar eminences), papulovesicles, and crusts involving the wrists and flexures.

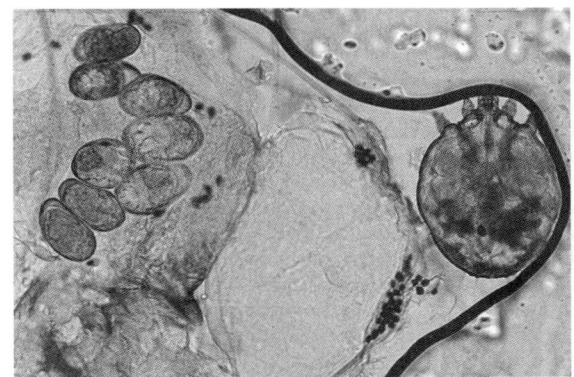

FIGURE 359-3. Scabies preparation demonstrating an adult mite, ova, and feces.

whereas house mouse mites in New York City transmit rickettsial pox. In endemic areas, the presence of an eschar in a patient with acute febrile illness has a high diagnostic value for rickettsial infection.

Most mite-induced rashes represent a "bite and run" injury and can be treated with topical corticosteroids or camphor and menthol lotion for symptomatic relief.

TICKS

Ticks are important disease vectors, and *Dermacentor* ticks can cause fatal tick paralysis in children. It is caused by a neurotoxin secreted by the salivary glands of an engorged female tick. Tick paralysis manifests as the development of unsteady gait, followed by progressive, ascending flaccid paralysis. As the tick attaches to the scalp, often behind the ear, it frequently goes unnoticed, and death occurs in over 10% of affected children due to respiratory failure. Nodular lesions are commonly pseudolymphomatous histologically.

Rickettsial illnesses typically manifest with fever and a headache, and treatment with a tetracycline should never be withheld because of the absence of a rash. Any delay in the initiation of antibiotic therapy may prove fatal, and empirical treatment should never be delayed until confirmatory tests are available. Doxycycline is generally recommended in both adults and children.

Rickettsial diseases, including Rocky Mountain spotted fever, continue to emerge in much of the world, especially in South America. Most of these agents produce milder syndromes similar to Rocky Mountain spotted fever.

Exclusion of animal hosts from recreational areas is key to control of tick-borne illness.[3] Oral agents, including avermectin-laced feed corn can be used to kill ticks that feed on deer. Removal of leaf debris leads to a reduction in tick numbers via dehydration of adults and ova. Permethrin, a pyrethroid insecticide with neurotoxic activity, is widely marketed as a topical acaricide to be applied to clothing. It is stable through several wash cycles. Some North African *Hyalomma* ticks have demonstrated high-level resistance, and permethrin may produce a pheromone-like attachment response in these ticks. Resistance in North American ticks can be esterase-based or related to sodium channel gene mutations, and permethrin resistance has been linked to outbreaks of bovine babesiosis and anaplasmosis.

A veterinarian should be consulted concerning control of ticks in pets and livestock.

Antibiotic prophylaxis after tick bites is rarely justified; it is indicated mostly in highly endemic areas where the ticks are heavily engorged. When signs and symptoms appear, a 10-day course of antibiotic is typically sufficient. A controlled trial comparing 10 days of oral doxycycline (with or without intravenous ceftriaxone) with 20 days of oral doxycycline for the treatment of early Lyme disease found a similar response rate in all three treatment groups.

SPIDERS

Toxic spiders are found worldwide.[4] The most feared include the funnel web spiders of Australia and *Phoneutria* wandering spiders in Brazil, which can be fatal. In North America, brown recluse spiders can produce a severe dermonecrotic reaction, but it should be noted that most spider bites result only in a mild local cutaneous reaction.

Black and brown widow spiders have a worldwide distribution. *Latrodectus mactans* is the most widely distributed black widow spider in North America. *Latrodectus curacaviensis* is common in South America and *Latrodectus tredecimguttatus* in Europe. Both black (*Latrodectus indistinctus*) and brown (*Latrodectus geometricus*) widow spiders are found in Africa and Madagascar, whereas Australia and New Zealand have red-black spiders (*L. mactans hasselti*).

Widow spiders are commonly encountered in woodpiles, and bites are typically defensive, frequently involving the hand after the spider has been disturbed. Latrotoxins act by increasing intracellular calcium concentrations, depolarizing neurons, and stimulating uncontrolled release of neurotransmitters, particularly norepinephrine and acetylcholine. Divalent cation-dependent tetramers of α-latrotoxin produce membrane pores in mammalian cells. Only the females have the ability to deliver venom and can be identified by the red hourglass pattern and shiny, black abdomen. Bites cause an envenomation syndrome comprising localized pain, diaphoresis, hypertension, weakness, muscle cramping, and severe pain in areas such as the abdomen and back. The syndrome may mimic an acute surgical abdomen. Both benzodiazepines and intravenous calcium gluconate have been used to treat associated tetany, but antivenin produces more rapid relief and is indicated for unresponsive tetany and priapism. Purified F(ab)2

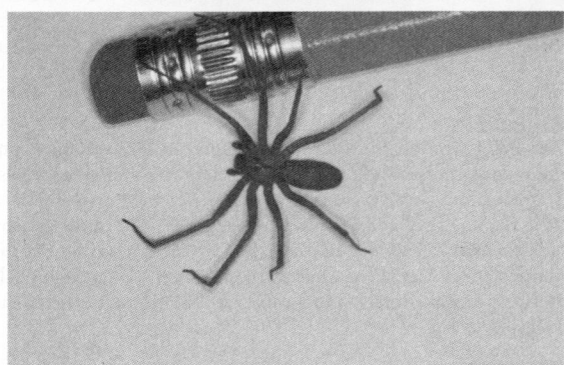

FIGURE 359-4. Brown recluse spiders are characterized by a dorsal violin case pattern.

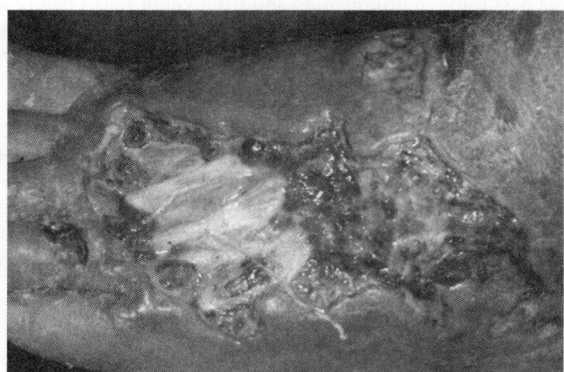

FIGURE 359-5. Dermonecrotic reactions from brown recluse spiders can be severe, but most are mild conditions. Furuncles or pyoderma gangrenosum are common misdiagnoses in patients who actually have brown recluse spider bites. (Courtesy Larry Becker, MD.)

fragment antivenin is now available and associated with a low risk for adverse reactions.

Brown *Loxosceles* spiders are found throughout the world, with the most famous being the brown recluse spider, *Loxosceles recluse* (Fig. 359-4).[5] The resulting necrosis can be severe (Fig. 359-5), but most bites do not result in skin necrosis, and those of related spiders, including *Loxosceles rufescens*, *Loxosceles deserta*, and *Loxosceles arizonica*, are even milder. Brown recluse spiders are endemic to southeastern and midwestern United States. They are quite shy and bites are very uncommon; however, envenomation can cause severe dermatonecrosis and hemolytic anemia. Most skin reactions diagnosed as "brown recluse bites" represent furuncles or pyoderma gangrenosum. The diagnosis can be confirmed by an enzyme immunoassay, glycophorin A measurement, or a passive hemagglutination inhibition test.

Sphingomyelinase D is the major toxin in brown recluse venom, and hyaluronidase allows the eschars to spread in a gravity-dependent fashion. Systemic reactions include disseminated intravascular coagulation and Coombs'-positive hemolytic anemia, but these reactions are rare as well. Most bites can be treated supportively with rest, ice, and elevation. Intradermal injection of polyclonal anti-*Loxosceles* Fab fragments or antivenin may reduce the ultimate size of the necrotic area, but these agents are not readily available. Studies with dapsone, colchicine, hyperbaric oxygen, and prednisone have generally been disappointing. Dapsone produces hemolysis, especially in individuals who have inherited G6PD deficiency (Chapter 161). Based on limited animal data and anecdotal human data, intralesional triamcinolone appears to be appropriate for patients with rapidly expanding areas of necrosis. The complement inhibitor eculizumab has demonstrated the ability to prevent venom-induced hemolysis in vitro.

Hadronyche and *Atrax* funnel-web spiders are endemic to a region in eastern Australia. Their venom contains small peptide neurotoxins, including the δ-atracotoxins that slow tetrodotoxin-sensitive voltage-gated sodium channel inactivation. Catecholaminergic and cholinergic excess can result in bradycardia or tachycardia, hypertension, shock, hypersalivation, and diaphoresis. Paresthesia, fasciculations, and muscle spasms may occur. Severe myocardial injury also has been reported.

Spiders belonging to the genus *Phoneutria* are found in South America, Costa Rica, and, most notably and clinically important, Brazil. Bites cause localized pain of varying severity that radiates proximally from the bite. Ninety percent of cases show at least mild systemic envenomation. Patients are symptomatic with nausea, vomiting, dizziness, tachycardia, hypertension, diaphoresis, visual changes, and priapism. Severe envenomation results in pulmonary edema and shock. Antivenin therapy is available.

Tegenaria agrestis is found in basements in the Pacific Northwest. In Europe, it exists as a rural spider, because *Tegenaria gigantea* and *Tegenaria domestica* compete for home habitats. Most reactions are mild, although some dermonecrotic reactions have been attributed to these spiders. Tarantulas can cause contact urticaria and ophthalmia nodosa related to hairs that become embedded in the cornea.

SCORPIONS

Local and systemic symptoms of scorpion stings are typically out of proportion to cutaneous signs. *Centruroides sculpturatus* produces somewhat more severe envenomation in the American Southwest, but the most dangerous Buthid scorpions are not found in the United States.[6] Most fatalities are caused by cardiorespiratory manifestations such as cardiogenic shock and pulmonary edema after envenomation and involve children younger than 10 years of age. Pancreatitis is an important cause of morbidity after scorpion envenomation. Toxic Buthid scorpions occur in Asia, Africa, and Latin America. Prazosin reverses the autonomic storm characteristic of the Indian red scorpion (*Mesobuthus tamulus*), and accelerated recovery with preserved myocardial function has been demonstrated when it is used in combination with antivenin.

Infection via Pentastomida, Chilopoda, Diplopoda, and Crustacea
TONGUE WORM (PENTASTOMIASIS)

Pentastomiasis is a zoonotic infestation that sometimes affects humans. The pentastomids *Armillifer* and *Linguatula* are wormlike arthropods endemic to Asia and Africa. They commonly infest the respiratory tracts of birds, reptiles, and small mammals. In humans, severe inflammation associated with the infestation can result in coughing, hemoptysis, lacrimation, coryza, and facial edema. Rarely, asphyxiation has been reported. This syndrome is known as *halzoun* or *marrara,* meaning suffocation.

CENTIPEDES AND MILLIPEDES

Centipedes have powerful jaws that inject a neurotoxic venom. Centipede bites may produce pain, paresthesia, erythema, edema, and profuse bleeding. Rarely, bites have been associated with coronary ischemia, rhabdomyolysis, proteinuria, and renal failure. Millipedes do not bite, but cause arcuate chemical burns via a caustic substance that they secrete when threatened. They may be found in line-dried clothing and the resulting burns may mimic signs of child abuse.

CRUSTACEANS AS A SOURCE OF INFECTION

Copepods are tiny aquatic crustaceans that serve as the intermediate hosts for nematodes including the guinea worm *Dracunculus medinensis* and the sushi worm *Gnathostoma spinigerum.* They may also transmit the cestodes *Spirometra mansonoides* and *Diphyllobothrium latum.*

Pediculosis

Pediculosis is the result of infestation by sucking lice of the phylum Arthropoda, class Insecta, order Phthiraptera, suborder Anoplura, family Pediculidae, or family Pthiridae. Lice are obligate ectoparasites, and three types infest humans: *Pediculus humanus capitis* (the head louse), *Pediculus humanus* (the body louse), and *Pthirus pubis* (the crab louse).

HEAD LICE

EPIDEMIOLOGY

Head lice affect 6 to 12 million people per year in the United States alone. Worldwide, much of the human population is affected, with highest prevalence among children between the ages of 3 and 12. Transmission occurs by means of direct contact or close contact of hats and scarves.

DIAGNOSIS

Head louse infestation should be suspected in any child with scalp pruritus and cervical adenopathy. Visual inspection can demonstrate nits, especially in the retroauricular area. Small bites and crusts of blood are common on the scalp. Definitive diagnosis involves finding at least one live louse on visual inspection of the scalp.

TREATMENT Rx

Current recommendations favor agents that kill lice by occlusion of the respiratory spiracles. One such agent (Ulesfia lotion) uses benzyl alcohol to stun the spiracle open and allow occlusion. For routine infection, a single, 10-minute, at-home application of ivermectin 0.5% lotion is 95% effective at 1 day, 85% effective at 7 days, and 74% effective at 14 days after treatment for eliminating head-louse infestations.[A1] For difficult-to-treat head lice infestation in children, oral ivermectin (400 μg/kg), given twice at a 7-day interval, had superior efficacy compared with topical 0.5% malathion lotion, suggesting that it could be an alternative treatment.[A2]

Malathion is a prescription organophosphate that acts by interfering with acetylcholinesterase. In the United States, it is marketed in a flammable vehicle that contributes substantially to its efficacy. There is relatively little resistance to this agent, but the trend is away from the use of neurotoxins in children.

Lindane is an organochloride compound that is still available by prescription. Central nervous system toxicity appears rare but together with environmental concerns resulted in banning of the product in California.

BODY LICE

EPIDEMIOLOGY

Body louse infestation is common in refugee situations, during war, and among the homeless in urban areas. This is a major public health concern because the louse can serve as a vector for at least three intracellular disease-causing bacteria: *Bartonella quintana* (causing trench fever and endocarditis), *Rickettsia prowazekii* (causing epidemic typhus), *and Borrelia recurrentis* (causing louse-borne relapsing fever).

CLINICAL MANIFESTATIONS

Early infestation produces a widespread dermatitis that may mimic atopic dermatitis, allergic contact dermatitis, or a viral exanthem. In patients with widespread excoriations, the most likely differential diagnosis is scabies. The diagnosis is made by finding bluish hued maculae cerulea (Fig. 359-6), prompting a search for body lice or nits in the seams of clothing.

TREATMENT Rx

Washing and hot drying or ironing of clothing will kill lice. Permethrin has also been used on clothing; however, a pediculocide is not always necessary.

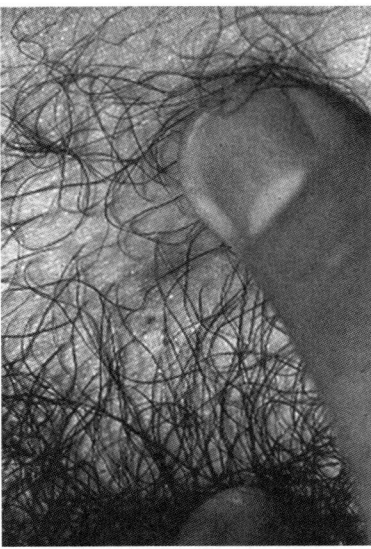

FIGURE 359-6. Maculae cerulae are bluish red spots that represent sites where body lice have fed.

CRAB LICE

PATHOBIOLOGY

Crab louse infestation is spread as a sexually transmitted disease. Roughly 30% of patients will have another concurrent sexually transmitted disease and adolescents with pubic lice are twice as likely as uninfested adolescents to have chlamydial or gonorrheal infection.

CLINICAL MANIFESTATIONS

Patients present with intense itching, and both lice and nits may be found on pubic hairs as well as hair on the chest, abdomen, and legs. Pubic lice occasionally may cause scalp infestation in patients with thick curly hair. They also may infest the eyelashes, causing phthiriasis palpebrarum infection. When observed in children, sexual exposure should be considered.

TREATMENT Rx

Treatment is by means of shaving or with topical agents used to treat head lice. Oral ivermectin has also been used at a dose of 200 to 400 µg/kg, repeated in 10 days.

Beetle-Related Dermatitis

Blister beetles (order Coleoptera) are widespread throughout the world and include members of the families Meloidae and Staphylinidae. Members of the family Oedemeridae are classified as "false" blister beetles, but can produce similar skin manifestations. Cantharidin accumulates during the larval stages of the beetle and gives it protection from predatory birds. When threatened, the beetles protect themselves by exuding a cantharidin-containing liquid. Contact with blister beetles results in vesicles and bullae. "Nairobi eye," or rove beetle dermatitis, in Northern Kenya is caused by *Paederus eximius*. Rove beetles were implicated in a recent epidemic of pustular eruption among U.S. forces in Pakistan. Treatment for all manifestations of blister beetles is largely symptomatic.

FLEAS

Fleas (order Siphonaptera) are ubiquitous among pets and wild animals. They serve as vectors for endemic typhus, bubonic plague, brucellosis, melioidosis and erysipeloid. The most common flea on dogs is the cat flea, *Ctenocephalides felis. Pulex irritans,* the human flea, can be found on dogs and became a major plague vector during the great epidemics. Flea bites cluster on the lower legs and present as intensely pruritic papulovesicles. Tungiasis is caused by the jigger or sand flea, *Tunga penetrans*. It typically presents with a necrotic pustule adjacent to the great toenail.

A veterinarian should be consulted about agents for flea control, including lufenuron and fipronil. Beach areas should restrict pets to prevent infestation.

FLIES

Mosquitoes and other flies belong to the order Diptera and represent major disease vectors. *Anopheles* mosquitoes bite mostly at night and are the major vectors of malaria. They also transmit filariasis. *Aedes* mosquitoes bite during the day and transmit dengue, viral encephalitis, yellow fever, and filariasis. *Culex* mosquitoes bite at night and transmit West Nile encephalitis, filariasis, and viral encephalitis. Culex mosquitoes also bite at dusk or early evening. Many arthropod diseases have a principal vector but also can be spread by other vectors. For example, although *Culex* mosquitoes are the major vector for West Nile virus in the United States, *Aedes* and *Anopheles* spp also can spread the disease. *Simulium* flies (black flies, humpback flies, buffalo gnats, turkey gnats) transmit onchocerciasis. *Lutzomyia* and *Phlebotomus* sandflies transmit leishmaniasis, *Bartonella bacilliformis,* and sandfly fever. Biting midges (punkies, gnats, no-see-ums) are small enough to pass through screens and cause papulovesicular and nodular reactions in sensitive individuals. Tabanid flies include the horse flies, deer flies, and greenheads. As a group, they are large and colorful and deliver painful bites. *Chrysops* deer flies transmit loiasis in Africa and tularemia in the United States. *Glossina* tsetse flies transmit trypanosomiasis.

Furuncular myiasis caused by the botfly is common in Latin America. *Dermatobia hominis,* glues its eggs to a mosquito, which serves as an intermediate vector. *Cordylobia anthropophaga,* the mango fly, tumbu fly, putzi fly, or skin maggot fly, is native to Africa and lays its eggs on drying clothing. It produces plaque-type myiasis with many maggots. *Cochliomyia hominivorax,* the screwworm, lays its eggs on wounds or mucous membranes. Screwworms are feared because they leave necrotic flesh and continue to travel through viable tissue. Sarcophagid flies deposit their living larvae on the hosts, where they produce a type of larva migrans. Myiasis is treated by means of mechanical removal with tweezers or by incision of the wound. Covering the embedded larvae with an occlusive substance such as surgical lubricant, petrolatum, or bacon encourages them to move upward facilitating removal.

Prevention of vector-borne disease requires control of standing water, use of screening and mosquito netting, and personal protection with repellents. Screening impregnated with pyrethroids is more effective than untreated screening. Secondary prevention includes malaria chemoprophylaxis and early treatment of illness. Other interventions include insecticidal sprays, and gas-powered mosquito traps. Most types of mosquito traps generate carbon dioxide and use chemical attractants such as octenol and butanone. Some *Culex* mosquitoes are repelled by octenol.

N,N-diethyl-3-methylbenzamide (DEET) remains the most widely used insect repellent, although picaridin is widely used in Europe and is gaining market share in the United States. IR3535, KBR 3023, and *para*-menthane diol are also used as repellents for application to skin. Permethrin is largely used for fabric impregnation. DEET has a long safety record, but occasionally can cause bullous dermatitis, anaphylaxis, or toxic encephalopathy. The American Academy of Pediatrics recommends slow-release products below 30% concentration. Neem oil products perform reasonably well against various mosquitoes, but citronella has limited efficacy.

HEMIPTERA: TRUE BUGS

Bedbugs have become pandemic and are increasingly recognized in suburban homes, hotels, and, especially, on college campuses.[7] They are red-brown and about the size of small ticks (Fig. 359-7). The wings are vestigial. *Cimex lectularius* and *C. hemipterus* (the tropical bedbug) parasitize birds and bats, who introduce them into buildings. They also spread readily via luggage. These organisms hide in cracks and crevices of beds, particularly along the seams of mattresses. Hepatitis B has been found in bedbugs, but they have not shown vector competence to transmit human disease. Bites are characteristically found on the face, neck, and arms. In covered areas, a string of bites termed "breakfast, lunch, and dinner" is typical (Fig. 359-8). Treatment of bites is with topical corticosteroids. Disinfestation involves extermination, washing and drying of all bedding on a hot setting, and placing the mattress and box spring in a zippered plastic case. Room hyperthermia has proved to be a viable alternative.

Triatome reduviids are important vectors for American trypanosomiasis (Chagas disease). Their wings overlap and are sclerotic proximally. The striped abdomen is visible lateral to the wings. Unilateral eyelid swelling (Romana sign) is caused by a conjunctival reaction to the bite and to triatome feces infected with trypanosomes.

HYMENOPTERA STINGS

Hymenoptera include membranous winged insects such as wasps, bees, and fire ants. They all result in painful stings and present a potential for anaphylactic reactions.[8] Unexpected stings occur frequently; therefore, allergic individuals must always carry a source of epinephrine such as an EpiPen auto-injector. Bees are eviscerated during the sting and the venom gland

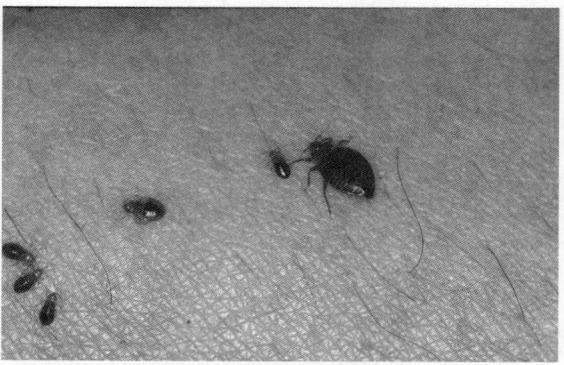

FIGURE 359-7. Bedbugs are red-brown and about the size of small ticks.

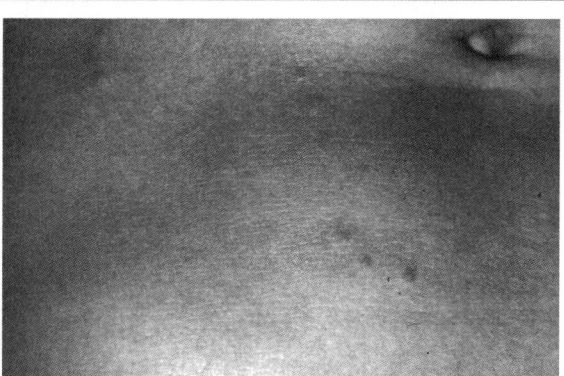

FIGURE 359-8. Bedbug bites are often arranged in a characteristic "breakfast, lunch, and dinner" pattern.

continues to inject additional venom. Therefore, bee stingers should be removed as rapidly as possible, with little concern for the exact method of removal. Venom immunotherapy can improve quality of life. Rush immunotherapy (a method for rapidly desensitizing patients to allergens) can be performed in those with severe reactions. Omalizumab has been used in conjunction with immunotherapy and has shown clinical effectiveness but further investigation is warranted to determine its exact role.

LEPIDOPTERIDS

Moths and caterpillars may have toxic hairs that may contain histamine, kinins, plasminogen activators, and other proteinaceous toxins. The reactions are usually toxic rather than allergic in effects. Clinical manifestations include pain, erythema, swelling, and hemorrhage. Systemic reactions may include renal failure. *Lonomia* caterpillars may cause a fatal bleeding diathesis with intracranial hemorrhage. Ocular reactions to hairs include ophthalmia nodosa, keratoconjunctivitis, subconjunctival nodules, iritis, and vitreoretinal involvement. Children who ingest caterpillars may develop edema of the lips, tongue, and buccal mucosa. Esophageal and tracheobronchial involvement occurs less commonly.

● DELUSIONS OF PARASITOSIS

Patients with delusions of parasitosis present with an unshakable belief that they are infested with pathogens such as insects, worms, bacteria, parasites, or fungi.[9] Some believe they are infested with inanimate materials such as hairs, filaments, fibers, and particles. It is difficult to help them. A careful evaluation should exclude formications secondary to cocaine addiction and pruritus related to systemic diseases such as renal failure or hyperthyroidism. Although delusions of parasitosis have traditionally been treated with pimozide, newer atypical antipsychotic agents such as risperidone, olanzapine, quetiapine, ziprasidone, and aripiprazole reduce the need for electrocardiographic monitoring.

● LEECHES AND OTHER ANNELIDS

Leeches occur in fresh water and may be associated with *Pseudomonas* or *Aeromonas* wound infections. Leeches contain anticoagulants, and the attachment sites may bleed freely when the leech is removed. More serious coagulation disorders with massive bleeding have been reported. Saturated salt solutions have been used to facilitate leech removal, but do not reduce the risk for infection.

 Grade A References

A1. Pariser DM, Meinking TL, Bell M, et al. Topical 0.5% ivermectin lotion for treatment of head lice. *N Engl J Med.* 2012;367:1687-1693.
A2. Chosidow O, Giraudeau B, Cottrell J, et al. Oral ivermectin versus malathion lotion for difficult-to-treat head lice. *N Engl J Med.* 2010;362:896-905.

GENERAL REFERENCES

For the General References and other additional features, please visit Expert Consult at https://expertconsult.inkling.com.

360

ANTIVIRAL THERAPY (NON-HIV)

JOHN H. BEIGEL

Although some viral infections are self-limited, others can cause significant morbidity and mortality. Effective therapy is available for many of these infections. This chapter reviews currently available antiviral agents for the treatment of infections caused by viruses other than human immunodeficiency virus (HIV). Not all agents discussed are licensed in all countries.

Currently available agents can be classified into those that directly inhibit viral replication at the cellular level (antivirals), those that modify the host response to infection (immunomodulators), and those that directly inactivate viral particles (microbicides/virucides). Antiviral agents can be classified based on their mechanism of action. For example, nucleic acid analogues inhibit viral DNA or RNA synthesis by competing with endogenous nucleic acids and block the viral DNA polymerase or RNA transcriptases. By comparison, protease inhibitors prevent viral replication by binding to the enzymes that cleave viral protein precursors into active proteins.

Antiviral strategies that are not covered in this chapter include local destructive measures that destroy both host tissues and virus simultaneously, such as cryotherapy, laser, and podophyllin treatment of warts. Although effective, such measures are useful only for discrete or localized mucocutaneous infections.

● ANTIVIRALS FOR HEPATITIS B VIRUS INFECTIONS

Acute hepatitis B infection (Chapter 148) generally does not require antiviral treatment. Currently approved antivirals for chronic hepatitis B (Chapter 149) include five nucleic acid analogues (adefovir, entecavir, lamivudine, telbivudine, and tenofovir) and two immune modulators (interferon alfa-2b and pegylated [PEG]-interferon alfa-2a) (Tables 360-1 to 360-3). Treatment may be initiated with any approved antiviral medications, but tenofovir, entecavir, and PEG-interferon alfa-2a are generally the preferred agents.[1] Tenofovir or entecavir is preferred for patients with compensated cirrhosis (Chapter 153).

TABLE 360-1	**ANTIVIRALS FOR HEPATITIS VIRUS INFECTIONS**		
VIRAL INFECTION	**DRUG**	**ROUTE**	**USUAL ADULT DOSAGE**
Chronic hepatitis B	Tenofovir	PO	300 mg/day
	Entecavir		
	Naïve virus	PO	0.5 mg daily; optimal duration of therapy unknown
	Lamivudine-resistant virus	PO	1 mg daily; optimal duration of therapy unknown
	Interferon alfa-2b	SC	6 MU/m² (up to 10 MU) 3 times weekly for 16-24 wk
	PEG-interferon alfa-2a	SC	180 μg weekly for 48 weeks
	Adefovir	PO	10 mg/day
	Lamivudine	PO	100 mg/day
	Telbivudine	PO	600 mg/day
Chronic hepatitis C	Ledipasvir/Sofosbuvir	PO	90 mg/400 mg once daily for 12-24 weeks
	Ombitasvir/ Paritaprevir/ Ritonavir plus Dasabuvir	PO	12.5 mg/75 mg/50 mg once daily plus dasabuvir 250 mg twice daily
	Sofosbuvir	PO	400 mg once daily for 12-24 weeks
	Simeprevir	PO	150 mg once daily for 12 weeks
	Boceprevir	PO	800 mg every 8 hours for 24-44 weeks
	PEG-interferon alfa-2a	SC	180 μg weekly for 48 weeks
	or PEG-interferon alfa-2b	SC	1.5 μg/kg weekly for 48 weeks
	plus Ribavirin	PO	800-1200 mg/day, depending on weight

TABLE 360-2 MECHANISMS OF EXCRETION AND THRESHOLDS FOR DOSE ADJUSTMENT

	MAJOR ROUTE OF ELIMINATION	THRESHOLD FOR ADJUSTMENT IN RENAL INSUFFICIENCY OR FAILURE	ADJUSTMENT FOR HEPATIC FAILURE	SPECIAL ADJUSTMENT FOR ELDERLY
Adefovir	Renal	CrCl < 50 mL/min	No adjustment	
Entecavir	Renal	CrCl < 50 mL/min	No adjustment	
Lamivudine	Renal	CrCl < 50 mL/min	No adjustment	
Ledipasvir/Sofosbuvir	Renal	CrCl < 20 mL/min	No adjustment	
Ombitasvir/Paritaprevir/ Ritonavir plus Dasabuvir	Renal	No adjustment	No adjustment	
Ribavirin	Renal	CrCl < 50 mL/min	No adjustment	
PEG-interferon alfa-2a	Renal	CrCl < 50 mL/min	Progressive rise in alanine transaminase	>60 years, consider reduction
Telbivudine	Renal	CrCl < 50 mL/min	No adjustment	
Sofosbuvir	Renal	CrCl < 50 mL/min	No adjustment	
Simeprevir	Hepatic	No adjustment	No adjustment	
Boceprevir	Hepatic	No adjustment	No adjustment	

TABLE 360-3 SIGNIFICANT ADVERSE EFFECTS (U.S. FDA BLACK BOX WARNING)

DRUG	BLACK BOX SYNOPSIS
Adefovir	Severe acute exacerbations of hepatitis B may occur with cessation of therapy. Nephrotoxicity may occur in patients at risk for or undergoing renal dysfunction. Lactic acidosis and severe hepatomegaly with steatosis
Entecavir	Lactic acidosis and severe hepatomegaly with steatosis; severe acute exacerbations of hepatitis B may occur with cessation of therapy.
Lamivudine	Severe acute exacerbations of hepatitis B may occur with cessation of therapy. Lactic acidosis and severe hepatomegaly with steatosis
Ribavirin	Monotherapy for hepatitis C is not effective. Hemolytic anemia Teratogenic and embryocidal
Interferon alfa	May cause or aggravate neuropsychiatric, autoimmune, ischemic, and infectious disorders
Telbivudine	Severe acute exacerbation of hepatitis B may occur with cessation of therapy; lactic acidosis and severe hepatomegaly with steatosis.

Patients with chronic hepatitis B (hepatitis B surface antigen [HBsAg] positive for > 6 months, detectable serum hepatitis B virus (HBV) DNA > 20,000 IU/mL, and an alanine aminotransferase [ALT] level > twice the normal level) should be evaluated for treatment. Patients with clinically decompensated hepatitis B (e.g., icterus or other signs) generally require antiviral treatment. Therapy in hepatitis B e antigen (HBeAg)-positive chronic hepatitis B should be continued until the patient has achieved HBeAg seroconversion and serum HBV DNA is undetectable, followed by at least 6 months of additional treatment after the appearance of anti-HBe. Therapy in HBeAg-negative chronic hepatitis B should continue for at least a year. Patients with decompensated cirrhosis or recurrent hepatitis B after liver transplantation should receive lifelong treatment.

Tenofovir

Tenofovir, which is a nucleotide analogue of adenosine monophosphate, was first approved for the treatment of HIV infection. The commercially available agent, tenofovir disoproxil fumarate, is an ester prodrug of tenofovir, with an effective tenofovir bioavailability of 25%. Administration following a high-fat meal increases the oral bioavailability.

Clinical Uses

Tenofovir is approved for the treatment of chronic hepatitis B in adults with evidence of active viral replication and either persistent elevations in serum aminotransferase levels or histologically active disease. Treatment with tenofovir is more effective than adefovir in producing histologic improvement and viral suppression in patients with HBeAg-negative or HBeAg-positive chronic hepatitis B.[A1] Tenofovir also has demonstrated efficacy in patients with lamivudine-resistant HBV.[A2][A3]

Toxicity

Tenofovir is generally safe and well tolerated for up to 5 years.[2] The most common side effects are nausea, diarrhea, vomiting, and anorexia. Lactic acidosis with hepatic steatosis has been reported, primarily when it is used in combination with other nucleoside analogues. Acute exacerbations of hepatitis B have been reported after discontinuation of tenofovir in patients who are coinfected with HIV and HBV.

Antiviral Resistance

Mutations in HBV polymerase that confer reduced susceptibility to tenofovir occur during prolonged use (>12 months). In vitro studies showed that adefovir-resistant HBV mutations are associated with three- to five-fold decrease in response to tenofovir, though clinical implications are not known.

Entecavir

Entecavir, which is a deoxyguanosine nucleoside analogue with specific antiviral activity for hepadnaviruses, is more potent than lamivudine and retains some activity against lamivudine-resistant HBV variants. It is well absorbed after oral administration, and its prolonged half-life (128 to 149 hours) allows once-daily dosing.

Clinical Uses

Entecavir is approved for the treatment of chronic hepatitis B in adults with evidence of active viral replication and either persistent elevations in serum aminotransferases or histologically active disease. Compared with lamivudine or telbivudine, entecavir is more efficacious in reducing HBV DNA levels and normalizing serum aminotransferases, as well as in improving histologic abnormalities.[A4][A5] Like tenofovir, entecavir can be used for lamivudine-resistant HBV infections, but higher doses and longer durations of therapy are needed.

Toxicity

Adverse effects reported during entecavir therapy include headache, fatigue, dizziness, nausea, abdominal pain, rhinitis, fever, diarrhea, cough, and myalgia. Lactic acidosis and severe hepatomegaly with steatosis have been reported. Severe exacerbations of hepatitis B have been observed after cessation of therapy.

Antiviral Resistance

Virologic breakthrough can occur in up to 4% of patients but is usually not indicative of resistant virus. True entecavir resistance, which is caused by specific mutations in HBV polymerase, is uncommon (1.2% after 5 years of treatment). In vitro studies show that entecavir-resistant mutations are susceptible to adefovir and tenofovir, but there is very little supportive clinical data.

Interferons

Interferons are glycoprotein cytokines with a complex array of antiviral, immunomodulating, and antineoplastic properties. Interferons are currently classified as alfa, beta, or gamma. The natural sources of these classes in general are leukocytes, fibroblasts, and lymphocytes, but they now can be produced by recombinant DNA technology. Although the full mechanism of

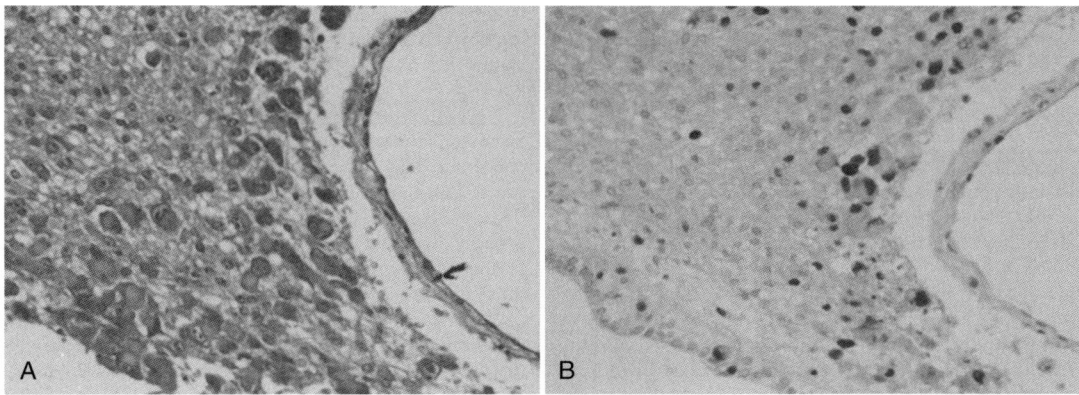

FIGURE 370-1. Pathology of CMV encephalitis. A, Large cells are seen in the perivascular region, some are multinucleated. B, The cytomegalic inclusions are present in the nucleus and stain with an antibody to CMV *(brown)*. Magnification is 40×. (Courtesy Martha Quezado, National Institutes of Health, Bethesda, MD.)

sphincter incontinence is common. Variable sensory findings are typically overshadowed by weakness. Babinski signs and diminished sensation below a discrete level across the trunk are evidence of an associated myelitis. With time, symptoms progress by ascending to involve the upper limbs and sometimes the cranial nerves. CSF examination generally shows polymorphonuclear pleocytosis, prominent elevation of protein levels, and a low glucose level. Spinal magnetic resonance imaging (MRI) may be normal or show enhancement of the conus medullaris, cauda equina, meninges, and nerve roots. Electrophysiologic studies reveal axonal neuropathy with evidence of acute denervation. Variable slowing of nerve conduction may occur.

The appearance of acute cauda equina syndrome in a patient with AIDS or in a solid organ or bone marrow transplant recipient is suggestive of CMV infection when a polymorphonuclear pleocytosis is present in CSF; however, the syndrome is not pathognomonic. Other conditions that may produce a cauda equina syndrome in AIDS patients include lymphomatous meningitis, syphilis, toxoplasmosis, other herpesvirus infections, and cryptococcal or bacterial meningitis. Progressive multifocal motor and sensory neuropathy that evolves during a period of weeks to months has also been seen in patients with CMV infection. Paresthesia and dysesthesia are quickly followed by prominent motor weakness involving both the upper and lower limbs asymmetrically. Neurogenic atrophy may be prominent. Nerve biopsy reveals necrotizing neuritis with mononuclear and polymorphonuclear infiltrates and cytomegalocytes localized around endoneurial capillaries in the nerve trunks and roots. Some patients may have necrotizing arteritis. PCR for CMV in CSF and comparison of levels of antibody to CMV in the serum and CSF may be useful in establishing the diagnosis.

TREATMENT   Rx

CMV neurologic complications should be treated with ganciclovir (5 mg/kg intravenously every 12 hours) plus foscarnet (60 mg/kg intravenously every 8 hours or 90 mg/kg intravenously every 12 hours until symptomatic improvement), followed by maintenance therapy with oral valganciclovir (900 mg daily) and intravenous foscarnet (90 to 120 mg/kg intravenously during 2 hours, every 24 hours); however, evidence of efficacy in these conditions is limited chiefly to case reports and small series. Cidofovir is a second-line agent (5 mg/kg by intravenous infusion during 1 hour once a week for 2 consecutive weeks, with saline hydration and probenecid, 2 g orally 3 hours before the dose and 1 g orally at 2 hours and 8 hours after the dose). CMV strains resistant to these agents have emerged, and CMV encephalitis has developed in the presence of maintenance ganciclovir therapy for CMV retinitis. Combination therapy (foscarnet and ganciclovir) or different drugs should be considered in patients already undergoing suppressive monotherapy or in those with persistent CSF pleocytosis. Maintenance therapy, which is the same regimen given every other week, is required unless the patient experiences immune reconstitution, such as after highly active antiretroviral therapy (HAART) in an AIDS patient or discontinuation of immunosuppressive regimens in a transplant or cancer patient. CMV retinitis can be treated with intravitreal ganciclovir or fomivirsen.

PROGNOSIS

The prognosis for long-term survival, especially with AIDS, is very poor, and most patients have only limited neurologic recovery.

● EPSTEIN-BARR VIRUS INFECTION

Epstein-Barr virus (EBV), the major cause of infectious mononucleosis (Chapter 377), is distributed worldwide. Individuals in areas of high population density and lower social strata acquire the virus in early childhood. However, seroepidemiologic studies indicate that virtually all persons are infected by EBV by 30 years of age.

Neurologic manifestations occur in 1 to 5% of patients with primary EBV infection and may be the predominant clinical finding. The most common neurologic disorder associated with infectious mononucleosis is meningoencephalitis, which is rare in early childhood and is most often observed in persons between the ages of 15 and 25 years. Its onset may be gradual during a span of several days or be explosive. Fever, headache, mild stiff neck, confusion, lethargy, seizures, and hyperreflexia are the most typical features. Some patients may present predominantly with ataxia, cerebellitis, or other focal neurologic features, including hemiparesis, focal seizures, and brain stem findings. Hyperintense signal abnormalities on T2-weighted and fluid attenuated inversion recovery (FLAIR) cranial MRI are frequently observed but are nondiagnostic. PCR for EBV in CSF and comparison of levels of antibody to EBV in the serum and CSF may be diagnostically useful.

Ganciclovir treatment (10 mg/kg/day intravenously for 3 weeks followed by 1000 mg/day orally for another 3 weeks or until the virus is cleared) has been used in some cases but is of unproven value. The prognosis for patients with EBV meningoencephalitis is excellent, with complete resolution anticipated in 1 to 2 weeks.

● SLOW VIRUS INFECTIONS OF THE CENTRAL NERVOUS SYSTEM

Human T-Lymphotropic Virus Type 1 and Human Immunodeficiency Virus

These viruses and their neurologic sequelae are considered in Chapters 378 and 394, respectively.

Subacute Sclerosing Panencephalitis

EPIDEMIOLOGY AND PATHOBIOLOGY

Subacute sclerosing panencephalitis (SSPE), which is caused by the measles virus (Chapter 367), usually affects children but can present in young adulthood. Patients generally have a history of measles within the first 2 years of life, and it is speculated that such early host exposure allows the emergence of persistent but defective virus replication because the SSPE virus genome, particularly the matrix gene, differs from wild-type measles. SSPE occurs after a latency period of months to years following acute measles infection. As a result of effective vaccination strategies against measles virus, the incidence of SSPE has decreased markedly to about 4 to 5 cases per year in the United States, but it remains 21 cases per million population in India.[2]

Gray matter is most prominently involved. The pathologic features of SSPE include gliosis, loss of myelin, and perivascular infiltrates of lymphocytes and plasma cells in white and gray matter. Neuronal cell loss is seen in later stages of the illness. Intranuclear Cowdry type A inclusions containing viral nucleocapsids are identified in neurons and glia.

CLINICAL MANIFESTATIONS AND DIAGNOSIS

SSPE usually begins with cognitive and behavioral changes, and cortical blindness is often an early feature. Progression is associated with motor dysfunction, including prominent myoclonus, cognitive decline, choreoathetosis, dystonia, and rigidity. Its course progresses during a period of 1 to 3 years to rigid quadriparesis and a vegetative state, frequently accompanied by autonomic features, such as hyperthermia, excessive sweating, and altered pulse and blood pressure. The condition is more common in rural settings and affects boys more often than girls. Retinal changes such as macular retinitis and pigmentary changes can precede the neurologic manifestations by several months.

The electroencephalogram typically reveals unilateral or bilateral periodic complexes with synchronous bursts of two or three high-amplitude slow waves per second, with recurrence at regular intervals of 5 to 8 seconds and a 1 : 1 relationship with myoclonic jerks.[3] MRI of the brain shows high signal intensity lesions that are diffuse in the subcortical and periventricular white matter with cortical atrophy, but also rarely may involve the basal ganglia and brain stem. In early stages of the illness, the MRI may be normal. Computed tomography (CT) of the brain shows generalized atrophy. CSF protein, glucose, and cell levels are usually normal; CSF is characterized by a high immunoglobulin concentration, oligoclonal bands, and intrathecal synthesis of antibody to measles virus antigens. Serum measles antibody titers are also high. These findings are usually sufficiently characteristic for diagnosis, but measles RNA can be detected in the brain by PCR. Rarely, brain biopsy is needed for definitive diagnosis in atypical cases. Measles virus may also cause subacute encephalitis in an immunocompromised host. The prominence of cognitive and motor dysfunction in these patients resembles that of SSPE, but in the clinical setting, its subacute onset and more rapid evolution and the presence of generalized seizures rather than myoclonus are distinctive. Brain abnormalities include abundant intranuclear inclusions, but inflammation is minimal, and neither serum nor CSF antibody titers against measles virus are high. For this reason, brain biopsy is generally needed for diagnosis.

TREATMENT AND PROGNOSIS   Rx

There is no established, unequivocally effective treatment of SSPE, but arrest of the disease has been reported in some patients with SSPE after long-term treatment with intrathecal interferon-α with intravenous ribavirin or oral inosine pranobex. About 5% of patients remit spontaneously, but SSPE progresses inexorably to coma, brain stem involvement, and death in 2 to 5 years in the remainder of patients. In immunosuppressed children, such as those with HIV infection, SSPE may be fulminant and may result in death over weeks to 3 to 4 months.

Progressive Rubella Panencephalitis

Progressive rubella panencephalitis is a rare disorder resembling SSPE but caused by rubella virus (Chapter 368). It occurs as a complication of congenital rubella syndrome or, more typically, after childhood rubella. With the advent of widespread rubella immunization, this disorder has been nearly eliminated in the United States.

A hiatus of years separates early infection from the onset of neurologic deterioration, which is characterized by behavioral changes, cognitive impairment, cerebellar ataxia, spasticity, and sometimes seizures. Myoclonus is a less prominent feature than it is in SSPE. Serology or isolation of the virus from brain or peripheral blood lymphocytes confirms the cause. There is no effective treatment, and the prognosis is similar to that for SSPE.

Progressive Multifocal Leukoencephalopathy
DEFINITION

This demyelinating disease is associated with infection of oligodendrocytes by JC virus, a papovavirus that is widely distributed in humans and must undergo genetic rearrangements in its noncoding control region to enable it to replicate efficiently in glial tissue.[4] Progressive multifocal leukoencephalopathy (PML) was the first demyelinating disease to be unequivocally associated with a viral infection.

EPIDEMIOLOGY

Serologic studies indicate that the infection predominantly occurs during childhood, and more than half of the population has been infected by age 20 years. Lesser increments of JC virus seropositivity are observed in each decade thereafter. Despite the wide dissemination of JC virus infection, PML is rarely observed in the absence of underlying cellular immunosuppression. It is also rarely observed in childhood. Until the AIDS epidemic, PML was most commonly observed in patients with lymphoproliferative disorders (62% of cases) and less commonly with myeloproliferative diseases (7%), carcinomatous diseases (2%), other immunodeficiency states, and granulomatous disorders such as tuberculosis and sarcoidosis. The prevalence of PML has increased dramatically during the AIDS pandemic: as many as 5% of AIDS patients develop PML, and AIDS is now the most common underlying disorder associated with it. PML also occurs in association with the administration of monoclonal antibodies for diseases that had not previously been associated with it, including natalizumab, an α4β1 and α4β7 integrin inhibitor used in the treatment of multiple sclerosis (Chapter 411) and Crohn's disease (Chapter 141), and efalizumab, an anti-CD11a antibody that is effective in the treatment of psoriasis (Chapter 438). Other therapeutic agents (e.g., rituximab, an anti-CD20 antibody; brentuximab vedotin, a monoclonal antibody used in treatment of lymphoproliferative disorders; and mycophenolate mofetil) have also been associated with PML, but usually when used to treat disorders that already carry a risk for PML and with incidence rates that are orders of magnitude lower than are seen with natalizumab.[5]

PATHOBIOLOGY

The cardinal feature of PML is demyelination, which is typically multifocal but occasionally unifocal (Fig. 370-2). These lesions may occur in any location in the white matter but have a predilection for the parieto-occipital regions. The lesions range in size from 1 mm to several centimeters; larger lesions may reflect the coalescence of multiple smaller lesions. The other histopathologic hallmark of PML is the presence of hyperchromatic, enlarged oligodendroglial nuclei and enlarged bizarre astrocytes with lobulated hyperchromatic nuclei. Electron microscopic examination reveals the JC virions, which are 28 to 45 nm in diameter and appear singly or in dense crystalline arrays in oligodendroglial cells and, less frequently, in reactive astrocytes. Inflammatory infiltrates are typically absent, except in patients who have reconstitution of their immune system, such as HIV-infected patients being treated with HAART, in whom macrophages and lymphocytes may be found.

CLINICAL MANIFESTATIONS

The clinical hallmark of PML is the presence of focal neurologic symptoms and signs associated with radiographic evidence of white matter disease in the absence of a mass effect.[6] The most common initial symptoms include weakness, speech and language abnormalities, and behavioral and cognitive disturbances. Gait disturbances, sensory loss, and visual impairment all occur in approximately 20 to 30%. Seizures and brain stem symptoms are less common. Signs noted on physical examination parallel the reported symptoms, with weakness, typically a hemiparesis, detected in more than half of patients at initial evaluation. Gait abnormalities, cognitive problems, and speech and language disorders (i.e., dysarthria and dysphasia) are observed in about 25% of patients at initial contact. Limb and trunk ataxia, which reflects cerebellar involvement, is detected in as many as 10% of patients but may occasionally result from severe impairment in position sense (i.e., sensory ataxia). Neuro-ophthalmic symptoms occur in 50% of patients with PML and are often the initial manifestation of the disorder. The most common visual deficit is homonymous hemianopia or quadrantanopia secondary to lesions of the optic radiations. Cortical blindness may develop. Other neuro-ophthalmic manifestations include optic agnosia, alexia without agraphia, and oculomotor abnormalities. Sensory disturbances occur with PML but are distinctly less common than impairment of strength or visual function.

DIAGNOSIS

The diagnosis of PML may be strongly suggested by the clinical manifestations and the radiographic imaging. When the clinical manifestations are coupled with a positive JC virus PCR finding in CSF, the diagnosis of PML is virtually certain. Brain biopsy with demonstration of the characteristic

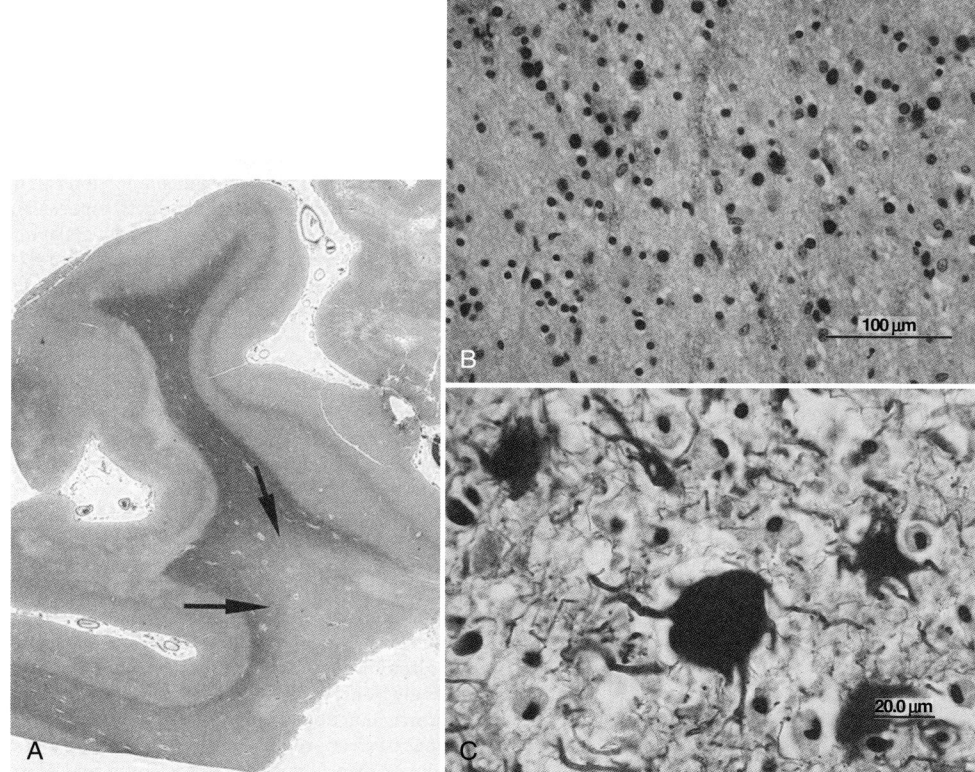

FIGURE 370-2. Pathology of progressive multifocal leukoencephalopathy. **A,** An area of demyelination is seen in the white matter that fails to stain with Luxol fast blue dye. **B,** Immunohistochemical staining with antibody to papovavirus shows brown-staining nuclei in oligodendrocytes, indicative of JC virus infection. **C,** Immunohistochemical staining for glial fibrillary acidic protein shows large bizarre astrocytes. (Courtesy Dr. Carlos Pardo, Johns Hopkins University, Baltimore, MD.)

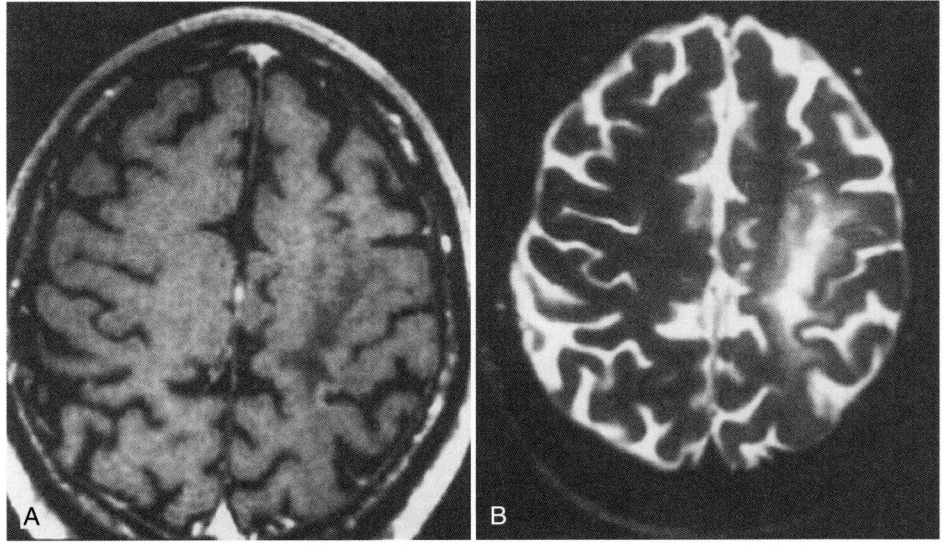

FIGURE 370-3. Cranial magnetic resonance images of progressive multifocal leukoencephalopathy. **A,** A T1-weighted image shows a hypointense signal abnormality of the left frontal lobe white matter. **B,** On T2-weighted imaging, the lesion is hyperintense.

histopathologic triad of PML coupled with immunohistochemical or electron microscopic evidence of JC virus remains the "gold standard" for diagnosis.

CT of the brain reveals hypodense lesions of the affected white matter that generally have a "scalloped" appearance because of involvement of the subcortical arcuate fibers lying directly beneath the cortex. Cranial MRI shows a hyperintense lesion on T2-weighted or FLAIR images in the affected regions (Fig. 370-3) and usually shows a hypointense lesion on T1-weighted images. Faint contrast enhancement, typically at the periphery of lesions, is seen in approximately 5 to 10% of pathologically confirmed cases of AIDS-associated PML and in 40 to 50% of natalizumab-associated PML on MRI. Intense intralesional nodular enhancement may be seen in patients with immune reconstitution. Frontal and parieto-occipital lobe lesions predominate, but the lesions may be observed in other sites, including the basal ganglia, the internal and external capsules, and the posterior fossa structures (i.e., cerebellum and brain stem).

The results of routine analysis of CSF are not diagnostic, but CSF protein may be elevated. CSF PCR for JC virus is of great value in diagnosis. Currently employed ultrasensitive quantitative PCR for JC virus in the CSF is not only highly sensitive but also specific.[7]

PROGNOSIS

Previously, PML was regarded as a fatal illness, with survival averaging 3 to 4 months in the typical patient. After the introduction of HAART, approximately 50% of patients with AIDS-associated PML survive for more than 12 months, often with partial or nearly complete clinical and radiographic recovery.[10] Factors associated with a more benign course include the presence of PML as the heralding manifestation of AIDS, high or climbing CD4+ T-lymphocyte counts, contrast enhancement of the lesions on radiographic studies, and any clinical or radiographic evidence of recovery. JC virus–specific T lymphocytes appear to be critical for control of the infection.

GENERAL REFERENCES

For the General References and other additional features, please visit Expert Consult at https://expertconsult.inkling.com.

371

PARVOVIRUS

NEAL S. YOUNG

DEFINITION

B19 parvovirus, which was discovered in the mid-1970s by electron microscopic observation of an anomalous precipitin reaction of a normal blood donor's serum (occupying position 19 in plate B), was first linked to human disease by the observation of virus-specific immunoglobulin M (IgM) antibody or the virus itself in the sera of sickle cell disease patients suffering transient aplastic crisis (Chapter 163). The common illness caused by the virus was identified later during outbreaks of fifth disease, a highly contagious rash illness of childhood long suspected of having a viral etiology. The ability of parvovirus to persist and to be manifested as an isolated hematologic syndrome was demonstrated by the presence of the virus in fetal liver at autopsy of hydropic newborns and in immunosuppressed patients with chronic pure red cell aplasia (Chapter 165).

The Pathogen

The parvoviruses form small icosahedral capsids of about 25 nm. They have a limited genome of single-stranded DNA. The approximately 5600 nucleotides of B19 parvovirus show remarkably little sequence variation among isolates; two variants, V9 and A6, are of uncertain clinical significance.

The Parvoviridae family contains many pathogenic animal viruses: feline panleukopenia virus, the cause of a fatal agranulocytosis in cats; canine parvovirus, which probably arose from the cat virus as a host range variant in the 1970s to produce a global pandemic and can cause fatal myocarditis in puppies; Aleutian mink virus infection, a model of immune complex disease; and porcine parvovirus, responsible for fetal wastage in pig litters. Antibodies to human adeno-associated viruses, which are dependoparvoviruses that are used as gene therapy vectors, occur naturally in humans, but B19 is the only parvovirus known to be pathogenic in humans.

EPIDEMIOLOGY

B19 infection is global; infectivity rates, inferred from the presence of anti-parvovirus IgG antibody in sera, are similar worldwide. Only isolated populations, Amazonian tribesman, and residents of remote islands off the coast of Africa have escaped exposure. B19 parvovirus infection is common in childhood, and half of 15-year-old adolescents have specific antiparvovirus B19 antibodies. Infection continues throughout adult life, and most elderly people are seropositive. In temperate climates, most infections occur in the spring, with small epidemics every few years being typical. Transmission is respiratory by droplet spread, and secondary infection rates among household contacts are high. Nosocomial infection can occur, and B19 parvovirus has been transmitted in blood products, especially pooled components such as factor VIII and IX concentrates. Producers of plasma derivatives now voluntarily screen by quantitative measurement of B19 DNA to reduce the risk for iatrogenic transmission.[1] The lack of a lipid envelope and the stable DNA genome make parvoviruses notoriously resistant to heat inactivation and solvent detergents.

PATHOBIOLOGY

The biology of the Parvoviridae makes them especially dependent on helper function from host cells or other viruses.[2] The autonomous parvoviruses propagate in actively dividing cells; the family Parvoviridae includes disease-causing animal parvoviruses. Adeno-associated viruses grow in tissue cultures infected with adenoviruses and herpesviruses and are popular vectors for gene transduction and therapy. B19 is the type member of the *Erythrovirus* genus, which includes very similar simian viruses, all of which are best propagated in the erythroid progenitor cells that are responsible for red blood cell production in the bone marrow. Active replication of virus can be detected by the presence of double-stranded intermediate forms by simple DNA hybridization methods. The transcription map of the erythroviruses differs markedly from that of other Parvoviridae. Only three genes produce proteins of known function. Many antigenic determinants recognized by the host immune system are located in helical loops that form the surface of each capsomere. Most of the capsid is composed of a major structural protein, called VP2, but about 5% of the capsid is the minor structural protein, VP1, which differs from VP2 only by an additional 226 amino acids at the amino terminus; this VP1 unique region is located external to the capsid surface and contains linear epitopes recognized by neutralizing antibodies.

The only known natural host cell of B19 parvovirus is the human erythroid progenitor. The tropism of the virus for an erythroid cell host results from its cellular receptor, globoside, a neutral glycolipid also known as erythrocyte P antigen. Rare individuals with the p phenotype, who congenitally lack globoside on their erythrocytes, are genetically insusceptible to B19 parvovirus infection; they show no serologic evidence of previous infection, and their marrow erythroid progenitors proliferate normally in the presence of high concentrations of virus. Parvovirus kills erythroid progenitors by expression of its nonstructural protein, and it is possible that some cells, such as megakaryocytes, may be lysed by restricted expression of viral proteins in the absence of viral propagation. B19 can be efficiently propagated in tissue culture of primary human hematopoietic cells in which erythropoietic differentiation is stimulated by erythropoietin.

The humoral immune response is dominant in B19 parvovirus infection. Natural antibody production correlates with disappearance of the virus from blood, and the presence of IgG appears to confer lasting protection against a second infection. Parvovirus infection can persist if immunoglobulin production is defective such that antibody fails to neutralize the virus; reactivity of antibodies to the unique amino-terminal region of VP1 is especially important.

CLINICAL MANIFESTATIONS

Fifth Disease

Most B19 parvovirus infections are asymptomatic. The most common clinical manifestation of infection is erythema infectiosum, or fifth disease, a rash illness of childhood characterized by a "slapped cheek" appearance (Fig. 371-1). In adult volunteers inoculated intranasally with B19, nonspecific influenza-like complaints occurred early along with viremia; the cutaneous eruption a week later corresponded to the appearance of antiviral antibodies. These more specific symptoms of B19 parvovirus infection are secondary to immune complex formation and deposition. Serologic testing generally shows seroconversion, IgM antibody or the appearance of IgG antibody to parvovirus. The rash of fifth disease may be evanescent, and recurrences can be provoked by sunlight, heat, emotion, or exercise. Fifth disease can be confused with rubella. In adults, the rash is less characteristic, can present as palpable purpura, may be associated with pruritus in up to 50% of patients,[3] and can be difficult to visualize in dark-skinned individuals.

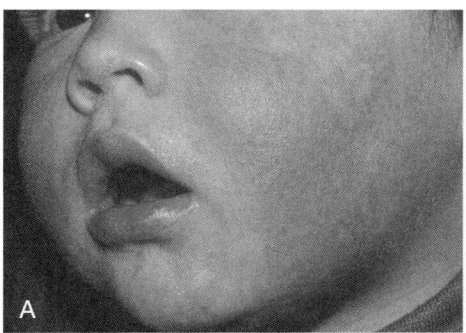

FIGURE 371-1. Erythema infectiosum. In this infection by parvovirus B19, a child will develop prominent erythema of the cheeks, "slapped cheeks" (A), followed by a lacelike erythema on the extremities (B) and buttocks. It is also known as fifth disease.

B19 Arthropathy

In contrast to the mild course in children with fifth disease, acute parvovirus infection in adults, particularly middle-aged women, may cause significant arthropathy.[4] Not only arthralgia but also a true inflammatory arthritis occurs in about 50% of older patients. Symmetrical joint involvement of the hands, ankles, knees, and wrists can resemble rheumatoid arthritis (Chapter 264), and the test result for rheumatoid factor may be positive. B19 arthropathy usually resolves within a few weeks; joint destruction does not occur. Parvovirus is not the cause of rheumatoid arthritis, but case reports suggest that B19 infection may mimic, precipitate, or worsen a variety of rheumatologic diseases, including juvenile rheumatoid arthritis, systemic lupus erythematosus, and fibromyalgia.

Transient Aplastic Crisis

In persons with underlying hemolysis or a high demand for production of circulating erythrocytes, acute B19 parvovirus infection causes transient aplastic crisis, an abrupt cessation of red blood cell production that exacerbates or, in previously compensated states, provokes severe anemia. Erythropoiesis is temporarily suppressed in all B19 parvovirus infections, but hemoglobin levels remain stable because of the long lifespan of erythrocytes. The anemic crises associated with low or absent reticulocytes in hereditary spherocytosis and sickle cell disease are virtually always secondary to B19 parvovirus infection. Parvoviremia is present in patients with transient aplastic crisis, and red cell production resumes once antibodies to the virus are produced and the infection is cleared. Transient aplastic crisis is generally a unique event in the patient's life, thus suggesting induction of long-lasting protective immunity. Although it is self-limited, aplastic crisis often requires transfusion and can lead to severe, occasionally fatal anemia that precipitates congestive heart failure and cerebrovascular accidents. Transient aplastic crisis is associated with a stereotypical bone marrow morphology, absence of maturing erythroid precursors, and the presence of "giant pronormoblasts" (Fig. 371-2) that are the cytopathic effect of parvovirus infection.

White blood cell and platelet counts may fall modestly during transient aplastic crisis, especially in patients with functioning spleens. Occasional cases of agranulocytosis may be due to B19; thrombocytopenia and pancytopenia have been reported, and B19 can precipitate a benign virus-associated hemophagocytic syndrome.

Persistent Infection

In patients who cannot mount an appropriate host antibody response, B19 parvovirus persists in the circulation, often at extremely high levels ($>10^{12}$ genome copies per milliliter). Patients do not develop the clinical features of fifth disease but instead have an entirely hematologic syndrome of pure red cell aplasia. The anemia is severe and requires transfusion; reticulocytes are absent from blood, as are erythroid precursors from marrow. Observation of giant pronormoblasts in the marrow may lead to the diagnosis. The failure to produce neutralizing antibodies to B19 parvovirus occurs in patients with congenital immunodeficiency (Nezelof's syndrome), with iatrogenic immunodeficiency (chemotherapy or immunosuppressive drugs), and with acquired immunodeficiency. Pure red cell aplasia secondary to parvovirus may be the first manifestation of the acquired immunodeficiency syndrome (AIDS), but this presentation is less common in the era of highly active antiretroviral therapy. Epidemiologic studies have suggested that parvovirus

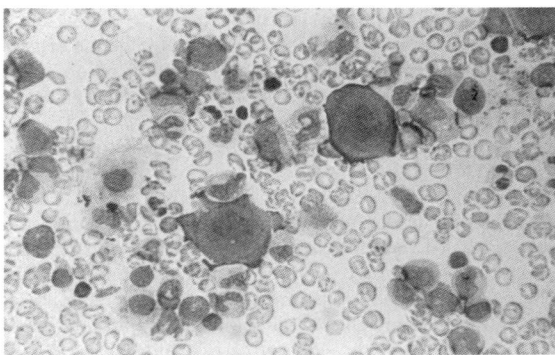

FIGURE 371-2. Bone marrow aspirate of a patient with chronic pure red cell aplasia secondary to persistent B19 parvovirus infection. Mature erythroid precursors are absent, and the prominent giant pronormoblasts are typical of B19 infection.

infection may worsen the manifestations of malaria (Chapter 345), especially the severity of anemia.[5]

Hydrops Fetalis

B19 parvovirus infection of the pregnant mother followed by transplacental transmission to the fetus can lead to an adverse outcome, either miscarriage or hydrops fetalis.[6] Parvovirus infects the fetal liver, the site of erythrocyte production during early development. Hydrops is the result of severe anemia as well as perhaps myocarditis, contributing to congestive heart failure. Prospective studies have led to an estimated 30% risk for transplacental infection and 9% risk for fetal loss in women who are exposed to B19 during pregnancy. Infection during the second trimester poses the greatest risk for birth of a hydropic infant; B19 parvovirus accounts for 10 to 20% of all cases of nonimmune hydrops fetalis. The risk for spontaneous abortion resulting from first-trimester infections has been more difficult to quantitate. The likelihood of an infection increases in epidemic years and correlates with the level of contact of the pregnant woman with children. Although most B19 infections during pregnancy probably do not lead to either loss of the fetus or congenital anomalies, B19 infection is a cause of fetal death. Congenital malformations have not been consistently associated with intrauterine parvovirus infection. However, severe anemia at birth with bone marrow histology consistent with either constitutional pure red cell aplasia (Diamond-Blackfan anemia) or congenital dyserythropoietic anemia has occurred in infants salvaged by in utero blood transfusions or exchange transfusion at birth.

Other Syndromes

Elevated hepatic aminotransferase levels can accompany fifth disease, and parvovirus infection has been associated with severe but usually self-limited hepatitis in some children.[7] The presence of B19 genetic sequences in cardiac tissue has led to a diagnosis of parvovirus myocarditis.[8] Serologic and DNA evidence of B19 infection implicated parvovirus in some patients with necrotizing vasculitis, Kawasaki disease, Henoch-Schönlein purpura, and giant cell arteritis. Glove-and-sock syndrome, an exanthem localized to the hands and feet and consisting of edema, erythema, paresthesia, and pruritus has

TABLE 371-1   DIAGNOSIS OF PARVOVIRUS B19

DISEASE	IgM	IgG	B19 DOT BLOT*	B19 PCR
Fifth disease	+++	++	−	+
Polyarthropathy syndrome	++	+	−	+
Transient aplastic crisis	+/−	+/−	++	++
Persistent anemia	+/−	+/−	++	++
Hydrops/congenital infection	+/−	+	+/−	++
Previous infection	−	++	−	+/−

*Sensitivity about 10^6 genome copies per milliliter.
Ig = immunoglobulin; PCR = polymerase chain reaction.

been linked to B19. Chronic fatigue syndrome may follow parvovirus infection. Meningitis, encephalitis, and a variety of neurologic complications may occur with fifth disease and parvovirus infection.[9]

False-positive results arise when the diagnosis of infection rests on detection of amplified B19 genome by polymerase chain reaction, and, furthermore, B19 parvovirus can persist at low levels in normal individuals for many months after infection.

DIAGNOSIS

Laboratory diagnosis relies on serologic and DNA tests[10] (Table 371-1). Virus-specific antibodies are measured in standardized commercial solid-phase enzyme-labeled immunoassays, generally using recombinant capsid proteins. "Capture" formats are preferred to detect serum IgM, which is first bound to a solid phase coated with anti-μ-chain antibodies, followed by the addition of viral antigen and an antiviral monoclonal antibody. IgM antibodies are diagnostically positive in almost all cases of fifth disease at initial evaluation and appear within a few days of the onset of transient aplastic crisis; IgM may persist for months after acute infection. IgG is usually assayed in conventional indirect assays. IgG circulates later than IgM, generally at the end of the first week of illness. Although titers of IgG are generally highest in the year after an acute infection, substantial interindividual variation and the presence of IgG in a large proportion of the population make measurement of IgG less helpful than other tests for diagnosis of parvovirus. DNA assays are required for persistent B19 infection, in which antibody production is absent or minimal. Parvovirus can also be found in the sera of patients with early transient aplastic crisis. Direct hybridization methods are reliable, and they detect clinically relevant viral titers of greater than 10^6 international units (orders of magnitude below levels present in both acute and persistent infection). Gene amplification methods are more sensitive but less reliable because of false-positive results. Virus can be detected in amniotic fluid, and both virus and IgM antibody to B19 are found in umbilical cord blood; the mother's serum will show seroconversion during pregnancy, but maternal IgM may be absent at the onset of hydrops fetalis.

PREVENTION

Effective vaccines exist for animal parvoviruses, and human B19 infection can also probably be prevented. A recombinant immunogen in development for the human virus lacks DNA and is therefore noninfectious; the empty capsids have been engineered to overexpress the highly immunogenic minor structural protein VP1, and a single 2.5-μg dose of empty capsids elicited excellent neutralizing antibody responses in normal volunteers. Vaccination could prevent transient aplastic crisis in patients with sickle cell disease and other hemolytic anemias, pure red cell aplasia in some immunodeficient individuals, and hydrops if seronegative mothers were inoculated early in pregnancy.

TREATMENT   Rx

Most parvovirus infections in normal children and adults do not require specific therapy. Isolation of infected individuals is impractical, with the exception of hospitalized cases. Pure red cell aplasia and the underlying persistent B19 parvovirus infection can be dramatically terminated by discontinuation of immunosuppressive therapy or institution of effective antiretroviral drugs in patients with AIDS. Commercial immunoglobulins are a good source of antibodies to parvovirus, and persistent B19 infection responds to a 5- or 10-day

course of IgG at 0.4 g/kg with a prompt decline in serum viral DNA, as measured by hybridization methods, accompanied by reticulocytosis and increased hemoglobin levels. This regimen has been curative in congenital immunodeficiency, but parvovirus in AIDS patients can persist at lower levels, and relapses of anemia may require repeated IgG administration. Immunoglobulin therapy can precipitate fifth disease rash and arthralgia.[11] Hydrops fetalis may resolve spontaneously, but intrauterine blood transfusions have been used with apparent success. Chronic arthropathy has been treated symptomatically with anti-inflammatory drugs, and there is not a role for the administration of immunoglobulin. As important as recognizing parvovirus infection is avoiding misinterpretation of laboratory studies, such as positive IgG serology or borderline IgM and DNA test results, and misguided maneuvers that delay appropriate alternative treatments.

GENERAL REFERENCES

For the General References and other additional features, please visit Expert Consult at https://expertconsult.inkling.com.

372

SMALLPOX, MONKEYPOX, AND OTHER POXVIRUS INFECTIONS

INGER K. DAMON

DEFINITION

Human illness caused by a poxvirus is characterized by a cutaneous manifestation; illness may be localized or systemic, depending on the particular poxvirus and the route of introduction. DNA-based assays, including DNA sequencing, are the most precise methods for identification and differentiation of poxvirus genera, species, strains, and variants. The guanosine plus cytosine content of orthopoxviruses, yatapoxviruses, molluscum contagiosum virus, and parapoxviruses is approximately 33%, 32%, 60%, and 63%, respectively.

The Pathogens

All poxviruses described in this chapter (Table 372-1) belong to the family Poxviridae, subfamily Chordopoxvirinae.

EPIDEMIOLOGY

Recognition of the epidemiologic characteristics of poxvirus diseases is valuable in assessing the potential etiologic agent of a particular suspected poxvirus lesion. Knowledge of zoonotic reservoirs, geographic localizations, and capacity for epidemic transmission is critical for clinical assessment and control measures. All human poxvirus infections are zoonotic in nature, with the exception of molluscum contagiosum and variola, which are solely human pathogens. Transmission of virus to humans and to animals is through direct contact with lesions or by fomites.

Parapoxvirus and molluscipoxvirus infections are endemic worldwide; orthopoxvirus and yatapoxvirus infections are geographically restricted, probably by the distribution of competent reservoir hosts. With the exception of variola virus (the causative agent of smallpox, a disease declared eradicated in 1980), none of these diseases is required to be reported to public health systems; furthermore, diagnostics are not widely available, so it is difficult to estimate disease incidence and prevalence with any certainty. In addition to variola virus, Congo Basin clade monkeypox viruses are considered to be select agents by the U.S. government; they must be reported and appropriately handled if discovered and if samples are maintained in the United States.

Orthopoxvirus

The epidemiology of smallpox, caused by the orthopoxvirus variola, is understood through detailed studies conducted during the end of the eradication campaign. Interhuman transmission of variola virus generally occurred through the inhalation of large airborne respiratory droplets of infectious

TABLE 372-1	TAXONOMY OF POXVIRUSES KNOWN TO INFECT HUMANS
GENUS	**SPECIES**
Orthopoxvirus	Variola virus, vaccinia virus, cowpox virus, monkeypox virus
Parapoxvirus	Orf virus, milker's node virus, bovine papular stomatitis virus, sealpox virus
Yatapoxvirus	Tanapox virus (Yaba-like disease virus), Yaba monkey tumor virus
Molluscipoxvirus	Molluscum contagiosum virus

variola virus. Transmission usually required prolonged face-to-face or other close contact, although airborne transmission over longer distances had been reported. Transmission by fomites or contact with infectious material from the rash also occurred. Aggregate data, collected during the smallpox eradication campaign, suggest a secondary attack rate of 58.4% in unvaccinated close or household contacts and a secondary attack rate of 3.8% in previously vaccinated close or household contacts. Case-fatality rates for variola major varied with the type of disease manifested, but aggregate rates of 10 to 30% in various outbreaks have been recorded. Severity of disease correlated with rash burden and was also more severe in children and pregnant women. Variola alastrim minor, a variant of variola with a case-fatality rate of less than 1%, has similar human-to-human disease transmission characteristics.

Monkeypox has a more complex epidemiology. The virus is zoonotic, and two genetically discrete virus clades have been described, each with apparent distinct clinical and epidemiologic parameters. Human infections in western and central Africa were first identified in 1970. Investigations in the Congo basin country Zaire, now the Democratic Republic of Congo, demonstrated that human-to-human transmission of monkeypox was less prevalent than that of smallpox. The secondary attack rate in unvaccinated contacts of monkeypox cases was calculated to be 9.3% versus 37 to 88% for smallpox. Previous smallpox vaccination (3 to 19 years previously) appeared to be 85% protective in preventing disease acquisition in contacts and also ameliorated the severity of disease. Overall, most identified cases acquired disease from presumed animal exposure; only 28% of cases were ascribed to person-to-person transmission. A case-fatality rate of approximately 10% was observed in unvaccinated persons, and the majority of fatalities and the most severe disease manifestations were observed in children younger than 5 years. Serosurveys suggested that subclinical infection may have occurred in up to 28% of close contacts of monkeypox patients in some communities; this relatively low rate may contribute to the rarity of sustained generations of human-to-human transmission in household and other close contact situations.

Among primary cases, recent close contact—through hunting, skinning, killing, cooking, or playing with carcasses—was identified with *Cercopithicus*, *Colobus*, and *Cercocebus* (primate); *Cricetomys* (terrestrial rodent); and *Funisciurus* and *Heliosciurus* (squirrel species). Samples of animals collected in areas of western and central Africa surrounding human cases demonstrated orthopoxvirus and sometimes monkeypox-specific seroprevalence in various members of these species, except in *Cricetomys* species. The prevailing hypothesis was that squirrel species were the probable reservoir of disease.

The disease reemerged in 1996 in the Democratic Republic of Congo, this time with 88% of cases derived from secondary human-to-human contact presumed to be because of the cessation of routine smallpox vaccination in 1980 after the eradication of smallpox. Mortality was only 1%. Ecologic serosurveys showed orthopoxvirus seroprevalence in terrestrial rodents (*Cricetomys emini*) and in one domestic pig (*Sus scrofa*).

Monkeypox virus was introduced to the United States in 2003 through a consignment of animals from the West African country of Ghana. The virus was identified as belonging to a distinct clade of monkeypox that included previous West African monkeypox isolates as well as isolates derived from earlier outbreaks in primate colonies. The U.S. cases had a less pronounced rash and a less severe illness, with no mortality or human-to-human transmission. When cases in the United States (2003) were compared with cases in Congo Basin (1980 to 1986), disease in the United States was less severe based on clinical criteria, the extent of the rash, and the case-fatality rate after controlling for age and vaccination status.[1] These data, along with comparison of the genomes of West African and Congo Basin monkeypox viruses, suggest at least two populations or clades of monkeypox virus. The apparent decreased pathogenicity and transmissibility of West African clade

monkeypox virus infection led, in part, to its declassification as a U.S. select agent in 2013.

Cowpox virus is found in Europe and Asia and is maintained in rodents; in Britain, the reservoirs are bank voles and wood mice. Human infection is a zoonosis. The domestic cat has been a common source of human infection, which probably explains the occurrence of cases in children; 26% of 54 cases occurred in children younger than 12 years. Most feline and human cases occur between July and October, with only occasional cases between January and June. Recent outbreaks in Europe have documented pet rats, or feeder rats, to be a source of transmission to humans. No case of bovine cowpox has been detected since 1976. Cowpox virus also is prevalent in European zoos, where cheetahs, lions, anteaters, rhinoceros, elephants, and okapi have occasionally transmitted infection to animal handlers.

Vaccinia is the live virus contained in preparations of the smallpox vaccines used to eradicate smallpox. In the United States, the vaccine is recommended for laboratory workers who use replicative orthopoxviruses and for selected military personnel. Contacts of vaccinees occasionally develop vaccinia infections. The origin of vaccinia is unknown, and no natural host for the virus is known. Recent studies have further distinguished cowpox and vaccinia viruses, both of which have been used as smallpox vaccines, and have identified at least three groups of cowpox and most vaccinia viruses group with one of these cowpox clades.[2] Vaccinia "variants" have been described, including buffalopox from contact with infected animals in India and vaccinia viruses in cattle handlers in Brazil.

Parapoxvirus

Human infection is an occupational hazard of farm workers, abattoir workers, veterinary surgeons, and students. It is most common in the lambing and calving seasons and among sheep workers.

Factors responsible for ongoing transmission have been attributed both to the environmental stability of orf virus in scab material and to the manifestation of chronic infections in some animals. A new parapoxvirus has been identified in deer hunters found to have cutaneous lesions after hunting and field dressing deer.[3]

Molluscipoxvirus

Molluscum contagiosum virus occurs worldwide, and increasing reports of the disease have paralleled the number of reported cases of acquired immunodeficiency syndrome (AIDS).[4] Traditional modes of transmission are associated with mild skin trauma such as abrasions, direct contact with a lesion, and fomites (e.g., shared towels) in some cases. However, the disease appears to be sexually transmitted, and genital lesions are more common than lesions elsewhere on the body. Children in daycare or school situations may transmit the disease to other children. Secondary spread of lesions may occur by autoinoculation (excoriation of primary lesions and spread to areas of normal skin) as well as by shaving. No known animal reservoir exists.

Yatapoxvirus

Tanapox virus is restricted to Africa, principally to Kenya and the Democratic Republic of Congo, and probably has a simian reservoir. Direct primate-to-human transmission through a break in skin has rarely been described in animal handlers, but an insect or arthropod intermediary may be involved in the transmission of tanapox virus to humans. No human-to-human transmission has been reported. Yaba monkey tumor virus causes localized infections after contact with infected primate lesions. Little is known about the epidemiology of this virus.

PATHOBIOLOGY

The majority of smallpox infections were initiated by inhalation of respiratory droplets and implantation of virus on the oropharyngeal and respiratory mucosa. No primary localized site of infection was evident if the route of exposure was by inhalation. Disease could also be introduced through suspensions of virus obtained from scabs of patients that were introduced percutaneously and constituted the practice of variolation. In these cases (when skillfully administered), illness was usually less virulent, a localized primary infectious lesion was present, and the asymptomatic incubation period was truncated.

After entry, virus moves to local lymph nodes and then disseminates to the reticuloendothelial system to replicate further. At this time, the individual is asymptomatic. In 10 to 14 days, secondary viremia occurs and heralds the prodrome of symptomatic illness. During this time, virus seeds the oropharynx and epidermis. The absence of a keratinized structure in the mucosa of the oropharynx leads to ulceration and release of virus in saliva; virus replicates in the epidermis to cause the characteristic macular, papular, and vesicular eruptions of smallpox.

In experiments in monkeys, high levels of type I interferons, interleukin-6, and interferon-γ are seen; D-dimers and thrombocytopenia suggest disseminated intravascular coagulation. Apoptosis with loss of T cells in lymphoid organs was also observed. Of note, tumor necrosis factor-α (TNF-α) levels were minimal in the infected animals, with a notable decrease in the expression of genes regulated by nuclear factor κB and TNF-α.

In humans, the viral lesions characteristic of illness primarily develop in the epidermis, where the cells of the malpighian layer swell and vacuolate to undergo ballooning degeneration. The cytoplasm continues to enlarge, loss of nuclear material is noted, and coalescence of vacuoles through cell rupture creates reticulating degeneration of the middle and upper layers of the stratum spinosum. In the next stages, the vesicle is formed. High titers of virus are found within the lesions. In mucosal surfaces, the absence of a horny layer allows the necrosis caused by proliferation of virus within the epithelium to create ulcers and leads to liberation of large quantities of virus into the oropharynx. Evaluation of other organs in human smallpox has been done only in select autopsy cases. Mild pathologic changes are seen in the lungs.

CLINICAL MANIFESTATIONS
Orthopoxvirus
Smallpox
Naturally acquired variola virus infection is characterized by fever and a distinctive rash, with several different clinical presentations (Table 372-2).[5] When the disease still existed, an asymptomatic incubation period of 10 to 14 days (range, 7 to 17) was followed by a fever that quickly rose to about 103° F (38° to 40° C), sometimes with dermal petechiae. Associated constitutional symptoms included backache, headache, vomiting, and prostration. Within a day or two after incubation, a systemic rash with a characteristic centrifugal distribution (i.e., lesions present in greater numbers on the oral mucosa, face, and extremities than on the trunk) appeared. The fever typically abated as the rash developed. Lesions commonly appeared on the palms and soles. The rash lesions were initially macular and then advanced to the papular stage, at which point they enlarged and progressed to a vesicle by day 4 to 5 and a pustule by day 7. When lesions became pustular, the fever typically returned. Lesions became encrusted and scabbed by day 14 and then sloughed off. Skin lesions in the vesicular and pustular stages were deep seated and in the same stage of development in any one area of the body (Fig. 372-1). The ordinary disease type was subgrouped into three categories based on the extent of rash on the face and the body: confluent, semiconfluent, and discrete. In ordinary confluent disease, no area of skin was visible between vesiculopustular rash lesions on the trunk or the face. In ordinary semiconfluent and discrete disease, patches of normal skin were visible between rash lesions on the trunk and face, respectively. Less severe manifestations (modified smallpox or variola sine eruptione) occurred in both unvaccinated and, more commonly, vaccinated individuals. The mortality rate correlated with the rash burden.

Four main clinical types of variola can be subgrouped according to the World Health Organization (WHO) classification schema: ordinary smallpox

(≈90% of cases) produced viremia, fever, prostration, and rash, and mortality rates were generally proportional to the extent of rash and ranged as described earlier; (vaccine) modified smallpox (5% of cases) produced a mild prodrome with few skin lesions in previously vaccinated people and had a mortality rate well below 10%; flat smallpox (≈5% of hospitalized cases) produced slowly developing lesions that were difficult to ascertain because they appeared flush with the (edematous) skin at the vesicular stage, and it was almost always fatal; and hemorrhagic smallpox (<1% of cases) induced bleeding into the skin and the mucous membranes and was invariably fatal. A discrete type of the ordinary form, with a typical febrile prodrome and rash, resulted from alastrim variola minor infection. Individuals with this form of disease were not nearly as moribund or "toxemic" as individuals with variola major infection. Previous vaccination was not necessarily protective against the hemorrhagic forms of disease but seemed to be protective against flat forms of disease.

In flat smallpox, illness was heralded by the abrupt onset of fever with temperatures of 38.3° to 38.9° C and the appearance of the rash after 3 to 4 days. The oral enanthem was often confluent, and sloughing of rectal mucosal membranes was also reported. At the papulovesicular stage of disease, lesions appeared as small indentations (day 6) with hemorrhages in the bases and were surrounded by an erythematous ring. By day 7 or 8, the lesions appeared flat. Bullous lesions that would slough were reported. Fever persisted throughout the disease course, and respiratory complications were often observed by day 7 or 8 of illness. Thrombocytopenia, neutropenia, and lymphocytosis were reported.

In hemorrhagic forms of smallpox, illness began with fever and typical prodromal symptoms; the fever never abated. Early after the onset of fever, petechiae and purpuric rashes became apparent; subconjunctival hemorrhages, hematuria, and vaginal bleeding were also seen. Patients usually died by day 6 of illness, well before any classic vesiculopustular rash was evident. In late hemorrhagic disease, after the onset of fever, typical maculopapular lesions developed, but the fever did not abate. The lesion evolved slowly, and areas of hemorrhage were evident at the base of the lesions. Bleeding occurred in the mucous membranes, thrombocytopenia was profound, and death occurred between days 8 and 10 of illness.

Monkeypox
After an incubation period of 7 to 17 days (mean, 12 days), a prodrome of fever, headache, backache, and fatigue begins.[6] The cutaneous eruption evolves similar to that of smallpox. Lesions evolve in the same stage in any one part of the body from macules, papules, and vesicles to pustules, and then they crust and scar (Fig. 372-2). After resolution of the rash, hypopigmentation is followed by hyperpigmentation of the scarred lesions. Pronounced

TABLE 372-2	WORLD HEALTH ORGANIZATION SMALLPOX TYPES
WHO SMALLPOX TYPE	**CLINICAL DEFINITION**
Variola sine eruptione	Fever, no rash
Modified	Like ordinary, with an accelerated course
Ordinary discrete	Fever, rash; areas of normal skin between pustules, even on the face
Ordinary semiconfluent	Fever, rash; pustules confluent on the face, discrete elsewhere
Ordinary confluent	Fever, rash; pustules confluent on the face and forearms
Flat	Fever, erythema, and edema of the skin; vesicles soft, flat, and bullous
Hemorrhagic, early	Fever (persistent), hemorrhages and petechiae, purpuric rash at illness onset
Hemorrhagic, late	Fever (persistent), rash, hemorrhage into the base of vesicles late in illness

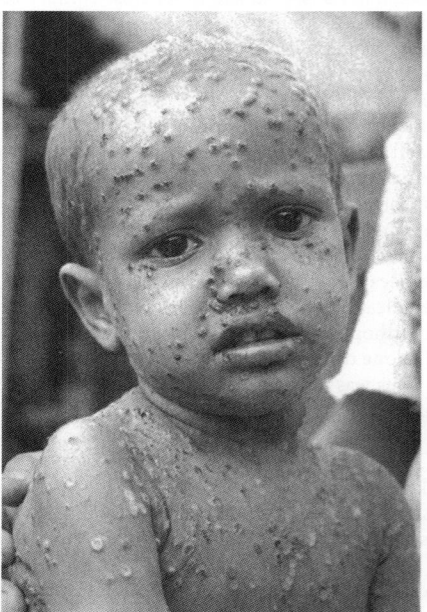

FIGURE 372-1. Pustular lesions of smallpox and beginning of scarring on the face and upper part of the torso. (From the Centers for Disease Control and Prevention Public Health Image Library, ID #: 7055. Photograph by Stan Foster.)

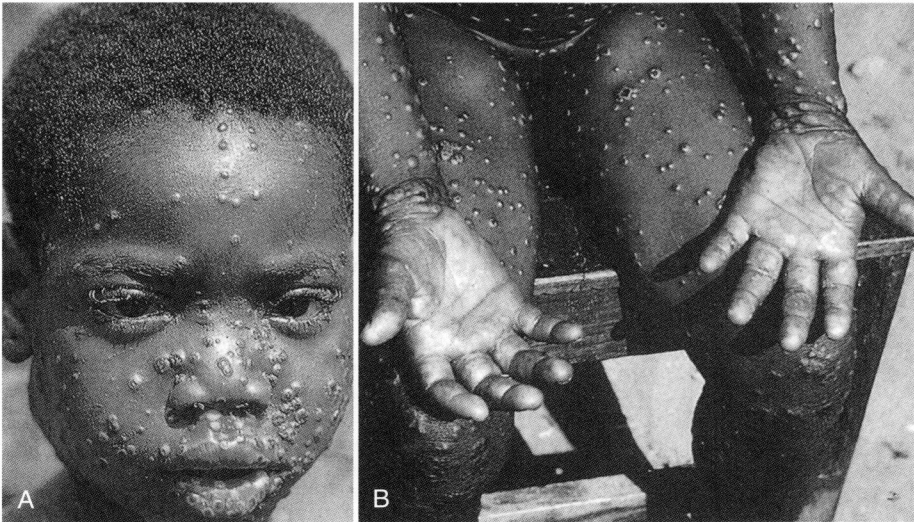

FIGURE 372-2. Rash of monkeypox of the head (A) and extremities (B) in a 7-year-old girl in central Zaire. (From Peters W, Pasvol G. *Tropical Medicine and Parasitology.* 5th ed. New York: Mosby; 2002:238.)

cervical, postauricular, submandibular, and inguinal lymphadenopathy clinically distinguishes monkeypox from smallpox.

Vaccinia

Multiple-puncture vaccinia virus infection by a bifurcated needle is the current smallpox vaccination regimen used for laboratory personnel working with orthopoxviruses, public health care personnel, and military in the United States. Most commonly, the infection progresses through a standard course of events from vesicle to pustule. However, of all vaccines used today, the smallpox vaccine, which is composed of live, replicative vaccinia virus, has one of the highest rates of adverse events. Major complications include progressive vaccinia, eczema vaccinatum, generalized vaccinia, postvaccinial encephalitis, accidental infection, and carditis.[7]

Progressive vaccinia, which is a rare and often fatal vaccine complication in persons with severe deficiencies in cellular immunity, occurs in about 1 per million vaccines, with a case-fatality rate of about 35%. Progressive vaccinia is characterized by frequently painless growth and spread of the vaccine virus beyond the inoculation site, often leading to necrosis and sometimes metastases to other body sites. The possibility of progressive vaccinia should be considered if the vaccination site lesion continues to progress and expand without apparent healing more than 15 days after vaccination.

Eczema vaccinatum[8] can occur in people with a history of atopic dermatitis (eczema), irrespective of its severity or activity, owing to local spread or dissemination from the primary vaccination site or contact with the unscabbed vaccination site of another person. A localized or generalized papular, vesicular, or pustular rash can develop anywhere on the body or be localized to previous eczematous lesions. Systemic illness with fever, malaise, and lymphadenopathy may occur. In the 1968 national U.S. surveillance of smallpox vaccination, there were 66 cases (no deaths) of eczema vaccinatum among 14.5 million vaccinees (4.6 cases/million) and 60 cases (1 death) among their several million contacts.

Generalized vaccinia describes the vesicular rash that develops after vaccination. Excluding dissemination associated with eczema vaccinatum and progressive vaccinia, it has been extremely rare to document virus in these lesions. True generalized vaccinia is believed to represent the end product of viremic spread of virus, and no predisposing factors have been identified. Generalized vaccinia was estimated to occur in about 242 of every million primary vaccinations. Studies done during the vaccination program in 2002 in the United States indicate that the majority of cases previously reported to be generalized vaccinia likely were generalized rashes caused by inflammatory or allergic responses to the vaccine, and not true generalized vaccinia. *Postvaccination encephalomyelitis* is a rare but serious complication that usually occurs only in primary vaccinees. Patients have variably displayed clinical and diagnostic features suggestive of a postimmunization demyelinating encephalomyelitis or direct viral invasion of the nervous system. This postvaccination reaction typically occurs 11 to 15 days after vaccination. Symptoms include

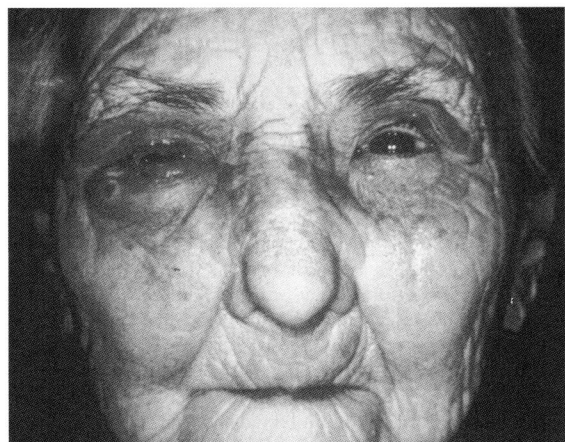

FIGURE 372-3. Vaccinia autoinoculation of an eye. (From the Centers for Disease Control and Prevention Public Health Image Library, ID #: 3322.)

fever, headache, vomiting, confusion, delirium, disorientation, restlessness, drowsiness or lethargy, seizures, and coma. Cerebrospinal fluid can demonstrate elevated pressure but generally has a normal cell count and chemistry profile. The diagnosis is one of exclusion, and no specific tests are available to confirm it. However, a few cases have been demonstrated to have anti-orthopoxvirus immunoglobulin M (IgM) or IgG responses in their cerebrospinal fluid.

Accidental infection occurs when virus from the vaccination site is transferred to another site or to another person through intimate skin contact. This complication generally occurs with primary vaccinees rather than revaccinees. Accidental self-inoculation, which most commonly occurs on the face, mouth, lips, or genitalia, is not usually serious and requires no specific treatment. Inoculation of the eye or eyelid is more serious and can be sight threatening if it is not evaluated and treated appropriately (Fig. 372-3). Between 1963 and 1968, ocular vaccinia was observed in 348 persons, including 22 who had evidence of corneal involvement and 11 who experienced permanent defects.

With buffalopox viruses in India and the Cantagalo virus in Brazil, up to 10 lesions have been described on the hands or arms of human handlers; fever, lymphadenopathy, backache, and fatigue are also associated symptoms. Transmission is believed to occur by unprotected contact with active lesions present on animal teats and udders. Interhuman transmission of buffalopox to family members has been reported to occur through contact.

Cowpox

Cowpox lesions are generally restricted to the hands and face; most patients (72%) have only one lesion. Multiple lesions may be caused by multiple primary inoculations, by autoinoculation, and very infrequently by lymphatic or viremic spread. The cowpox lesion passes through macular, papular, vesicular, and pustular stages before forming a hard black crust. The lesion is generally very painful, and erythema and edema are common at the late vesicular and pustular stages. Patients usually have lymphadenitis, fever, and general malaise. These features are generally severe in children, and absence from school or work is common. About 30% may be hospitalized. Most patients take 6 to 8 weeks to recover, but up to 12 weeks may be required. On occasion, a very severe infection and death may occur, typically in immunosuppressed individuals. Scarring is usually permanent.

Parapoxvirus

Lesions, such as from the orf virus, start as erythematous papules and progress in 1 to 2 weeks to target lesions with a red center surrounded by a white halo and an outer inflamed halo. Lesions then progress to a nodular and then a papillomatous stage, which often has a "weeping" surface. In some patients, lesions may enlarge and persist for weeks before resolving by a crusting stage, which also may persist for weeks. Very large granulomatous lesions may occasionally require surgical removal.

Most patients have only one lesion, but multiple primary lesions may develop. Systemic reaction is relatively uncommon, and the lesion is often not particularly painful. Lymphadenopathy is present in some patients, and lymphangitis is relatively uncommon. Erythema multiforme (Chapter 439) can develop in up to one third of patients.

Molluscum Contagiosum Virus

Molluscum infection occurs when molluscum contagiosum virus comes into contact with nonintact skin. The characteristic lesion begins as a small papule and, when mature, is a discrete, 2- to 5-mm-diameter, smooth, dome-shaped, pearly or flesh-colored nodule that is often umbilicated (see Fig. 440-9 in Chapter 440). A cheesy, off-white or yellowish material is easily expressed from lesions. Most patients have 1 to 20 lesions, but hundreds of lesions may occasionally be present. Because of multiple simultaneous infections or mechanical spread, the lesions may become confluent along the line of a scratch, and satellite lesions are sometimes seen.

In children, molluscum lesions occur mainly on the trunk and proximal ends of the extremities; in adults, lesions tend to occur on the trunk, pubic area, and thighs. In all cases, however, infection can be transmitted to other areas by autoinoculation. In men infected with human immunodeficiency virus (HIV), molluscum lesions can occur along the beard line and result in ocular involvement.

Individual lesions persist for about 2 months, but the disease usually persists for 6 to 9 months. Individuals with impaired cell-mediated immunity, including persons with HIV infection, tend to have more severe and prolonged infection.

Yatapoxvirus

Tanapox infection begins with a short febrile (38° to 39° C) illness that persists for 2 to 4 days and is sometimes accompanied by headache, backache, or prostration. The eruption of a lesion is frequently heralded by pruritus at the site of the outbreak. The lesion appears as a hyperpigmented macule, which often has central elevation and evolves to a papule with palpable induration. About 80% have a solitary nodule, but as many as 10 lesions can occur. Most lesions (72%) occur on the lower extremities, and the fewest occur on the face and areas normally covered by clothing.

Fever and systemic symptoms wane as the lesion erupts. The papule then becomes more "pocklike" but contains no fluid; umbilication or a pseudocrust may develop. Typically, the papule evolves into a firm, deep-seated, elevated nodule. At the end of the first week, the lesion is surrounded by erythema and indurated skin, and regional lymphangitis is common. Lesions then either ulcerate or become larger nodules (up to 2 cm in diameter) within about 2 weeks, after which the local inflammatory response wanes and the lesions began to granulate. Resolution of lesions occurs within 6 weeks. Infection appears to confer lifelong immunity.

DIAGNOSIS

Before its eradication, smallpox was relatively easy to recognize. Chickenpox (Chapter 375) produces a centripetally distributed rash and rarely appears

on the palms and soles; in chickenpox, prodromal fever and systemic manifestations are mild, the lesions are superficial in nature, and lesions in different developmental stages may be present in the same area of the body. Other diseases and conditions that could be confused with vesicular-stage smallpox include monkeypox, generalized vaccinia, disseminated herpes zoster or herpes simplex virus infection (Chapters 374 and 375), drug reactions (eruptions), erythema multiforme (Chapter 439), enteroviral infections (Chapter 379), scabies (Chapter 359), insect bites, impetigo (Chapter 439), and molluscum contagiosum. Diseases confused with hemorrhagic smallpox included acute leukemia (Chapter 183), meningococcemia (Chapter 298), and idiopathic thrombocytopenic purpura (Chapter 172). The Centers for Disease Control and Prevention have developed a protocol for evaluation of patients for potential smallpox (available at http://emergency.cdc.gov/agent/smallpox/diagnosis/evalposter.asp) and an algorithm for laboratory assessment of the vesiculopustular stage of rash (available at http://emergency.cdc.gov/agent/smallpox/diagnosis/pdf/poxalgorithm1-5-12.pdf).

Orthopoxvirus

Viral culture or electron microscopic evaluation of virion particles from clinical rash specimens has been the approach to diagnosis of orthopoxvirus infections. Serologic tests are largely genus specific, detect IgG, and usually cannot differentiate among species, although IgM levels can help differentiate recent orthopoxvirus infection from remote vaccination. Nucleic acid–based tests and polymerase chain reaction (PCR) assays are other options. If the diagnosis of smallpox is being considered, viral culture requires a biosafety level 4 (BSL-4) containment facility that is sanctioned by the World Health Organization to use variola virus.

Parapoxvirus

The differential diagnosis of parapoxvirus lesions can include ecthyma gangrenosum as a result of a *Pseudomonas aeruginosa* infection (Chapter 306), vaccinia or cowpox infection, cutaneous anthrax (Chapter 294), erysipeloid (Chapter 295), tularemia (Chapter 311), and tumor. Farm workers recognize the infection and tend not to seek medical attention for routine cases, so about 45% of reported cases may have no known contact with infected animals, and the clinical diagnosis of such cases may be difficult. With negative-stain electron microscopy, virions with the characteristic morphology of parapoxviruses are usually seen easily in lesion extracts, thereby providing a rapid, certain diagnosis of the genus. The virus can be grown in cell culture, and PCR detection can be performed. Species-specific and species-generic protein-based diagnostics have also been developed for parapoxviruses.

Molluscum Contagiosum Virus

The clinical appearance of molluscum lesions usually is sufficiently characteristic to permit a clinical diagnosis. Brick-shaped virions typically can be seen in large numbers if the cheesy material expressed from the lesion is examined by electron microscopy. The virus has not been cultured in standard tissue culture systems. The characteristic histopathology of these lesions is diagnostic, but PCR methods can also identify molluscum contagiosum.

Yatapoxvirus

The limited geographic distribution of tanapox virus and the patient's travel history help with the diagnosis of tanapox infection. Unique clinical features that differentiate tanapox from other orthopoxvirus infections are the nodular nature of the rash lesion, the paucity of lesions, the benign disease course, and the protracted resolution of the rash. The solid nodular and ulcerated lesions are larger and develop more slowly than those of monkeypox, but they are smaller and develop more rapidly than those of tropical ulcers.

Tanapox virus can be detected by electron microscopy, but the appearance of the virions cannot exclude infection with other morphologically similar brick-shaped poxviruses. Nucleic acid testing or cell line culture can make the definitive diagnosis.

TREATMENT AND PREVENTION ℞

Orthopoxvirus

Vaccination with smallpox vaccine is the mainstay for prevention of orthopoxvirus infection and was the primary method used to eradicate smallpox. Stockpiles of vaccine are available should smallpox recur. In the United States, however, smallpox vaccine is currently recommended only for laboratory personnel who work with infectious orthopoxvirus, certain public health personnel, and certain members of the military. In part because of stringent prescreening procedures, recent adverse events are rare with vaccination, but myocarditis or pericarditis was documented in 18 of 230,734 (8 per million) U.S. military primary vaccinees immunized in 2002 and 2003. In recent trials, both an attenuated tissue-cultured smallpox vaccine (LC16m8) and a replication-deficient smallpox vaccine (MVA) were about 95% effective both in newly vaccinated adults and as a booster.[A1][A2] Animal studies have demonstrated protective efficacy against a lethal monkeypox challenge.[9]

Currently, no antiviral drugs are licensed to treat orthopoxvirus or other poxvirus illnesses. Early administration of vaccinia immune globulin (VIG) may reduce the mortality of eczema vaccinatum from 30 to 40% to 7%, and VIG may also be useful for other complications (e.g., progressive vaccinia, severe generalized vaccinia, or contact infection) of vaccinia (smallpox) vaccine administration and for other orthopoxvirus infections. However, VIG alone has no clear benefit for treatment of smallpox infection itself.

Antiviral compounds (Chapter 360) with in vitro and in vivo activity against poxviruses include specifically 5-iodo-2′-deoxyuridine, adenine arabinoside, and trifluorothymidine. Because of their systemic toxicity, these compounds have been used topically for the treatment of orthopoxvirus ocular infections. In vitro, cidofovir is active against cowpox, vaccinia, monkeypox, and variola; in vivo, it protects challenged animals when it is given prophylactically or early in the evolution of disease. Cidofovir has known renal toxicity and is administered with hydration and probenecid. CMX-001/brincidofovir has been effective in treatment of systemic rabbitpox infection in rabbits and was used as part of a multidrug regimen to treat a case of progressive vaccinia.

Tecovirimat is an effective small-molecule antiviral in animal models of systemic orthopoxvirus infection[10] and has been used successfully as part of a multidrug regimen to treat a human case of eczema vaccinatum and a case of progressive vaccinia. Although not currently licensed, it is part of the U.S. Strategic National Stockpile and available for compassionate use to treat orthopoxvirus infections, including smallpox, as an investigational new drug sponsored by the Centers for Disease Control and Prevention.

Parapoxvirus

Most workers at risk for parapoxvirus become infected, and reinfection also occurs. The vaccine used to control orf in sheep is fully virulent and has caused human infection. Treatment options are limited; anecdotal reports have described the use of topical cidofovir, and other options may be topical formulations of interferon-modulating compounds such as imiquimod.

Molluscum Contagiosum Virus

Molluscum contagiosum infection is benign, and recovery is usually spontaneous, but treatment may be sought for cosmetic reasons, particularly for facial or multiple lesions. Options include cryotherapy, mechanical curettage, and chemical treatments such as podophyllin or podofilox, cantharidin, iodine, and tretinoin. Irritation has been a side effect of many of the chemical treatments. Topical application of a 3% cidofovir antiviral cream or suspension has been reported to be beneficial, as has the use of potentially immune-modulating cimetidine or topical imiquimod therapy. However, no therapy is documented to be beneficial by well-controlled randomized trials,[A3] although topical 10% potassium hydroxide solution, applied twice daily, is sometimes recommended. Covering of lesions and the use of proper hand hygiene after contact with lesions should prevent transmission in most situations. For individuals with AIDS and molluscum, highly active antiretroviral therapy with a resulting improvement in the CD4$^+$ cell count appears to be efficacious.[11]

PROGNOSIS

Monkeypox and smallpox both cause human illness, with mortality rates ranging from 10 to 40%; variola minor variants, however, have mortality rates of less than 1%. Yatapoxvirus infections are self-limited, and the illness resolves in the course of a few weeks. Parapoxvirus infections are manifested chiefly by localized symptoms, and the lesions resolve within a month or so in nonimmunocompetent hosts. Molluscum contagiosum infection is benign, usually with a spontaneous recovery, but the infection can persist for months. Variola minor has a mortality rate of less than 1%.

Grade A References

A1. Saito T, Fujii T, Kanatani Y, et al. Clinical and immunological response to attenuated tissue-cultured smallpox vaccine LC16m8. *JAMA.* 2009;301:1025-1033.

A2. von Krempelhuber A, Vollmar J, Pokorny R, et al. A randomized, double-blind, dose-finding Phase II study to evaluate immunogenicity and safety of the third generation smallpox vaccine candidate IMVAMUNE. *Vaccine.* 2010;28:1209-1216.

A3. van der Wouden JC, van der Sande R, van Suijlekom-Smit LW, et al. Interventions for cutaneous molluscum contagiosum. *Cochrane Database Syst Rev.* 2009;4:CD004767.

GENERAL REFERENCES

For the General References and other additional features, please visit Expert Consult at https://expertconsult.inkling.com.

373

PAPILLOMAVIRUS

JOHN M. DOUGLAS, Jr.

DEFINITION

Human papillomaviruses (HPVs) are a group of small DNA viruses that cause a variety of benign and malignant lesions of the skin and mucous membranes. The most commonly recognized HPV-associated diseases include warts (Chapter 440) at anogenital sites (condyloma acuminatum), other skin surfaces (common warts or verruca vulgaris), and the plantar surface of the foot (verruca plantaris). In addition, HPV infection causes squamous intraepithelial lesions of the cervix, also known as cervical intraepithelial neoplasia (CIN), and of other anogenital sites. It is considered the etiologic agent of a variety of cancers, especially cervical cancer.

The Pathogen

HPV is a member of the family Papillomaviridae. Like all papillomaviruses, HPV is nonenveloped, measures 55 nm in diameter, and has a double-stranded circular DNA genome of approximately 7900 base pairs enclosed by an icosahedral capsid. The HPV genome contains three functional regions: early genes (six total—E1, E2, E4, E5, E6, E7), which are expressed soon after infection and control replication, transcription, and cellular proliferation; late genes (two total—L1, L2), which are expressed in later stages of infection and encode the structural capsid proteins; and the long control region, which contains regulatory sequences that control the replication and transcription of early and late genes. Papillomaviruses complete their life cycle only in terminally differentiated epithelial cells and thus are difficult to grow in cell culture. Papillomavirus taxonomy is based on a genotyping system involving the use of DNA sequence relatedness of the gene encoding L1, the major capsid protein, with different types defined as having less than 90% homology.[1]

Papillomaviruses are classified taxonomically by genus (Greek letters) and species (numbered), each containing one or more types. Most HPV types are included in three large genera: alpha (primarily mucosal or genital types), beta, and gamma (both of which cause cutaneous lesions). Currently, more than 150 types of HPV have been identified, over 40 of which infect genital skin and mucosa. Of the genital types, approximately 15 are considered high risk because they are associated with high-grade squamous intraepithelial lesions and cancers of the cervix, anus, penis, vulva, vagina, and oropharynx, whereas others are considered low risk because they are largely associated with genital warts and low-grade squamous intraepithelial lesions.

EPIDEMIOLOGY

HPV infections are primarily transmitted by direct contact of skin or mucous membranes with an infected lesion. Genital HPV infection is typically contracted through sexual intercourse, although nonpenetrative genital contact, oral-genital contact, and manual-genital contact are also possible routes of transmission. In addition, genital HPV infection can be transmitted to the mouth and upper respiratory tract perinatally from infected mothers to newborns. For nongenital HPV infection, personal skin-to-skin contact also plays a primary role, although for plantar warts, fomite transmission from moist surfaces is likely to be an important source of infection. Both genital and nongenital infection can be transmitted to new sites by autoinoculation.

Regarding genital HPV, in the United States, an estimated 80 million or so persons are infected and about 14 million new infections occur annually, thereby making genital HPV the most common sexually transmitted infection.[2] The prevalence of anogenital warts is estimated to be approximately 1% in the sexually active adult population. Acquisition of infection begins shortly after sexual debut, with an estimated 40 to 60% incidence of at least one type within 2 years of initiation of sex. Risk factors for infection include variables related to probable exposure (e.g., younger age at onset of sexual activity, increased number of recent and lifetime partners, and number of partners of the sex partners), susceptibility (e.g., lack of circumcision for men), and absence of prevention factors (e.g., lack of consistent condom use or immunization). Most infections are asymptomatic and clear without treatment; only 10% are estimated to persist longer than 2 years.[3] The incidence of genital HPV infection and genital warts appears to be declining in some countries that have initiated immunization programs.[4]

Oral HPV infection is usually asymptomatic. Its prevalence in U.S. adults is approximately 5 to 7%, almost half of which are high-risk types.[5] Newly acquired oral oncogenic HPV infections are rare in healthy men, and most are cleared within 1 year.[6] Cutaneous HPV infection is most typically recognized as common and plantar warts, especially in children, in whom annual incidence rates of up to 30% have been reported.

All types and manifestations of HPV infection are more common in persons with impaired cell-mediated immunity, such as those infected with human immunodeficiency virus (HIV) or receiving immunosuppressive therapy. Among HIV-infected men who have sex with men, the prevalence of anal high-grade squamous intraepithelial lesions is almost 30%, and the anal cancer incidence is 46 per 100,000.[7] Of note, genital HPV infection may increase susceptibility to HIV infection, analogous to other sexually transmitted infections, raising the possibility that HPV vaccines could help prevent HIV infection.

Cervical cancer has declined in developed countries since the initiation of cytologic screening programs, although an estimated 12,000 cases and 4000 deaths still occur in the United States annually.[8] However, the disease is a major problem in the developing world, where screening is limited, and it is the third most common cancer in women worldwide, with an estimated 500,000 cases annually. Considering all anatomic sites, it is estimated that more than 600,000 HPV-associated cancers (5% of all cancers) occur globally each year.[9] In the United States, HPV causes about 18,000 cancers annually among females and about 8000 annually among males. HPV-associated oral cancers have been rising in the United States and are projected to become the most common HPV-associated cancer by 2020.[10]

PATHOBIOLOGY

HPV infections cause disease by producing aberrant cell growth. In the case of cutaneous and low-risk types, lesions such as warts result from HPV-induced benign proliferation of epidermal layers. For high-risk genital types, precancerous and cancerous lesions result from replacement of the epithelium by undifferentiated cells as a result of HPV-induced interference with normal cellular growth.

Infection begins in the lowest and least well-differentiated layer of the epithelium, the basal cells, where exposure is facilitated by microtrauma. Transcription and protein expression are highly coordinated with the level of cellular differentiation. In the basal layer, the viral genome becomes established in the nucleus as an episome that replicates in tandem with cellular replication, thus maintaining a stable copy number of viral genomes. As basal cells migrate up and differentiate in the superficial layers of the epithelium, full vegetative viral DNA replication and expression of structural proteins occur, with assembly of infectious virions in the most superficial layer of the epithelium, where they are released with the sloughing of dead cells during normal cellular turnover.

Persistent infection with various high-risk types of genital HPV is firmly established as the cause of squamous cell carcinoma and adenocarcinoma of the cervix, and HPV 16 in particular plays a causal role in other anogenital and oropharyngeal squamous cell cancers. There are also associations of beta-HPV types with squamous cell cancer of the skin. HPV DNA can be detected in more than 99% of cervical cancer cases, with 70% of cancers caused by the two most common high-risk types, HPV 16 and 18. The pathogenesis of HPV-induced cancer involves viral integration into the host genome with resulting disruption of the E2 transcription regulatory gene and increased expression of E6 and E7 proteins. These proteins have oncogenic activity and affect cell growth by binding with tumor suppressor proteins, E6 with p53 and E7 with the retinoblastoma tumor suppressor protein, thereby disrupting apoptosis and cell cycle regulation.

Although persistent infection with high-risk types is "necessary" for the development of cervical cancer, it is not considered "sufficient" because cancer does not develop in most infected women. Possible cofactors include cigarette smoking, prolonged hormonal contraceptive use, multiparity, micronutrient deficiency, immunodeficiency (e.g., HIV infection), and other infections, (i.e., *Chlamydia trachomatis* and herpes simplex virus type 2). In addition, data supporting a familial risk for cervical cancer point to possible genetic factors, including genes controlling the immune response (e.g., *HLA*, *TNF*) and cell cycle (e.g., *p53*).

Cervical cancers (Chapter 199) most commonly arise in the cervical transformation zone, the border between the squamous epithelium of the ectocervix and columnar epithelium of the endocervix. Analogously, anal cancer (Chapter 145) occurs primarily at the anatomically similar anocolumnar transition zone.

The immune response to HPV infection is less robust than for most viral infections. Viral proteins and infectious virions develop in superficial cells with limited contact with the immune system, and there is no cell lysis or viremia to trigger an inflammatory response. In addition, HPV suppresses several components of the immune response, including the interferon pathway and the expression of inflammatory cytokines and major histocompatibility complex class I. Antibody to HPV develops in only an estimated 60% of infected individuals, often as long as 6 to 12 months after infection. In contrast, the dynamics of the immune response are quite different after immunization, with almost 100% seroconversion within several months and antibody levels many-fold higher than those after natural infection. The high efficacy of HPV vaccines, which are believed to produce primarily humoral immunity, supports the importance of the antibody response in protection from infection. In contrast, once infection occurs, cellular immunity appears to be critical for clearance of infection.

The histopathologic changes of warts include epithelial papillomatosis and acanthosis, with hyperkeratosis, parakeratosis, and hyperplasia of the parabasal cells. A characteristic feature is the presence of koilocytes, which are large atypical keratinocytes with irregular, hyperchromatic nuclei surrounded by a perinuclear halo, in the upper epidermis. Squamous intraepithelial lesions are characterized by hyperkeratosis, parakeratosis, koilocytosis, and epidermal hyperplasia, with increased mitotic figures in the upper half of the epidermis. Several classification systems have been used to classify these lesions and their risk for progression based on the proportion of the epithelium replaced by undifferentiated cells. The CIN system grades lesions as CIN 1 (with undifferentiated cells occupying the lower third), CIN 2 (with undifferentiated cells in the lower third to two thirds), and CIN 3/carcinoma in situ (CIS, with undifferentiated cells across the full thickness of the epithelium). Alternatively, the Bethesda system, originally developed for use with cytology but increasingly used for histologic classification, includes only two categories: low-grade squamous intraepithelial lesions (equivalent to CIN 1) and high-grade squamous intraepithelial lesions (equivalent to CIN 2 and CIN 3/CIS).

CLINICAL MANIFESTATIONS

The clinical manifestations of HPV infection vary by anatomic site and viral type. Common warts are exophytic, hyperkeratotic papules that typically occur on the hands but can appear on any skin surface, including the genital skin; they are most commonly caused by HPV types 1, 2, 4, 27, and 57. Plantar warts, which are caused by similar types of HPV, are hyperkeratotic, endophytic, and often very painful. In contrast, flat warts (verruca plana), which are small flat-topped papules that occur more commonly on the face, hands, and legs, are caused by a different group of nongenital HPV types (e.g., types 3, 10, 28, 38, 42, 49, 75, and 76).

Epidermodysplasia verruciformis is an uncommon autosomal recessive disease that is usually manifested in childhood as diffuse warts that respond poorly to treatment and typically are caused by beta-HPV types, most commonly type 5, that are uniquely associated with it. This disease, which is thought to be due to a selective defect in cell-mediated immunity because other opportunistic infections do not occur, is associated with two types of lesions: flat warts caused by the same HPV types as in normal hosts, and scaly tinea versicolor–type lesions caused by epidermodysplasia verruciformis–associated types. The latter are associated with the development of squamous cell cancer in sun-exposed areas in 30 to 70% of persons. Similar skin lesions and, rarely, associated skin cancers can develop in other patients with acquired defects in cell-mediated immunity.

The most common clinical manifestations of oral HPV infection include oral squamous cell papillomas and condyloma acuminatum, which are caused by HPV types 6 and 11. Less frequent are common skin warts and focal epithelial hyperplasia, which are round, flat papules caused by HPV types 13 and 32. Warts caused by genital HPV types can also rarely occur in the upper respiratory tract, where they can cause a serious condition known as recurrent respiratory papillomatosis, which can result in hoarseness and even airway compromise. Oral leukoplakia (Chapters 190 and 425), which presents as a white patch or plaque and is considered to have premalignant potential, has been associated with HPV 16 and 18 infection.

Anogenital warts are papillomatous growths that occur throughout the anogenital skin and mucosa, typically at sites of genital friction. Most such warts are caused by HPV types 6 and 11, with approximately half of infected persons developing warts. Perianal warts are most common in persons with a history of anal intercourse and are often associated with intra-anal warts, but they also can occur without such contact, presumably through autoinoculation. Anogenital warts can range from flat or papular lesions to the classic pedunculated, cauliflower-shaped condyloma acuminatum. Warts are typically asymptomatic, noticed either by the patient as a "bump" or inadvertently during a genital examination, although they can cause itching, burning, pain, or, rarely, bleeding or mechanical obstruction of the birth canal in pregnant women.

Squamous intraepithelial lesions are most commonly found on the cervix as a result of screening for cervical cancer precursors by cytology (Papanicolaou [Pap] test) or HPV molecular testing, with confirmation by colposcopy and biopsy. Like warts, they also occur at other anogenital sites; and like cervical lesions, they are categorized either as low-grade or high-grade squamous intraepithelial lesions or as various stages of intraepithelial neoplasia (e.g., vulva—VIN; vagina—VaIN; anus—AIN; penis—PIN). Low-grade squamous intraepithelial lesions can be caused by either low- or high-risk types, whereas high-grade squamous intraepithelial lesions are primarily due to high-risk types. Most squamous intraepithelial lesions are not visible on mucosal surfaces without the application of 3 to 5% acetic acid and magnification, although they can appear as flat hyperpigmented papules known as bowenoid papulosis on the external genitalia.

DIAGNOSIS

Both cutaneous (Fig. 373-1) and genital (Fig. 373-2) warts generally present an easily recognized clinical picture and can be diagnosed by history and physical examination without laboratory testing. The application of 3 to 5% acetic acid causes whitening of HPV lesions on genital mucosa ("acetowhitening") and may be useful with magnification in women; however, because sensitivity and specificity of this application have not been defined, it is not recommended for routine use. Oral lesions are also generally recognized by physical examination.

The differential diagnosis of cutaneous warts includes seborrheic and solar keratoses, nevi, irritated acrochordons, clavi, and squamous cell carcinoma (Chapters 203 and 440); lichen planus (Chapter 438) can mimic flat warts and calluses of the foot or plantar warts. Genital warts must also be distinguished from the condyloma latum lesions of secondary syphilis (Chapter 319) and molluscum contagiosum (Chapters 372 and 440). Biopsy for histopathologic examination may be helpful for lesions at all anatomic sites that are atypical or not responsive to therapy, those suggestive of high-grade

squamous intraepithelial lesions or cancer (e.g., pigmented, indurated, fixed, bleeding, or ulcerated), or lesions in immunocompromised patients.

Cervical squamous intraepithelial lesions have traditionally been detected by cervical cytology through Pap tests, with assessment of abnormal results by colposcopy and biopsy for histopathologic examination. However, molecular testing for high-risk HPV is beginning to be used both for screening and for management of low-grade cytologic abnormalities.[11,12] Several large comparative trials have shown HPV testing to be more sensitive than Pap tests for detection of CIN 2/3 and more effective in prevention of cervical cancer.[A1][A2] HPV testing in combination with cytology (co-testing) has been approved to enhance the sensitivity of screening in women older than 30 years. HPV tests are also recommended for triage of women whose Pap test results show atypical squamous cells of undetermined significance, which is an equivocal test result. Although HPV testing has been recently approved by the U.S. Food and Drug Administration as a single test for primary cervical cancer screening, at present, its use as a single test in the absence of cytology is not recommended. Furthermore, HPV screening is not recommended for detecting possible infection at other sites (e.g., anus, oropharynx).

TREATMENT Rx

Management of HPV infection is directed toward diagnosis and treatment of the lesions themselves because there are no virus-specific therapies. Many lesions resolve spontaneously, so the goal of treatment is amelioration or

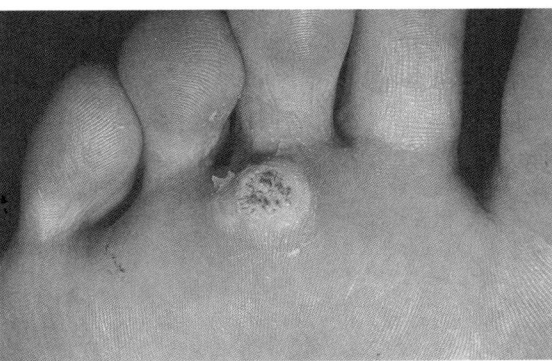

FIGURE 373-1. **Plantar wart.** A hyperkeratotic, verrucous papule or plaque beneath a pressure point on the sole of the foot is characteristic. Human papillomavirus types 1 (myrmecia), 2 (mosaic), and 4 are most common. Because plantar warts are driven into the skin by the pressure of walking or standing, they are usually the most treatment resistant.

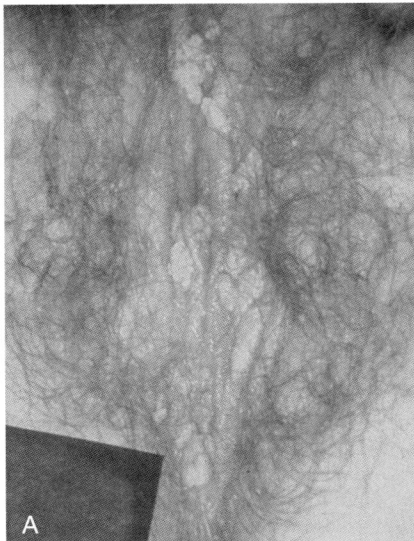

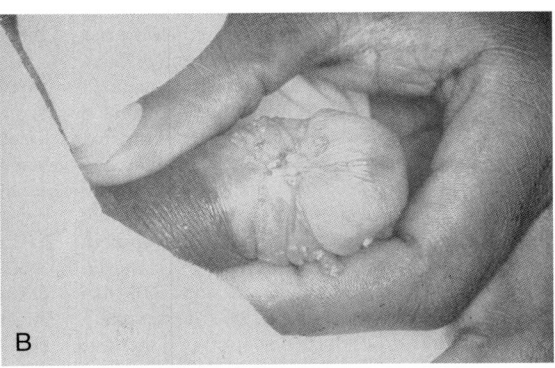

FIGURE 373-2. Genital human papillomavirus (HPV) infection. A, Vulvovaginal HPV infection. B, Penile HPV infection. (From Vermund SH, Bhatta MP. Papillomavirus infections. In: Cohen J, Powderly WG, eds. *Infectious Diseases,* 2nd ed. St Louis: Mosby; 2004.)

TABLE 373-1 RECOMMENDED TREATMENT OF GENITAL WARTS

PATIENT APPLIED

Podophyllotoxin (podofilox) 0.5% solution or gel; to be applied in up to 4 weekly cycles (twice daily for 3 days, followed by 4 days without treatment)

Imiquimod 3.75% cream (to be applied once daily at bedtime) or 5% cream (to be applied once daily at bedtime 3 times per week) for 6 to 10 hours for up to 16 weeks

Sinecatechins 15% ointment; to be applied 3 times daily for up to 16 weeks

PROVIDER ADMINISTERED

Cryotherapy with liquid nitrogen or cryoprobe; to be applied once every 1 to 2 weeks*

Trichloroacetic or bichloroacetic acid 80 to 90% solution; to be applied once weekly*

Office surgery* (excision, electrocautery, curettage)

*Safe for use in pregnancy.
Modified from Workowski KA; Centers for Disease Control and Prevention. Sexually transmitted disease treatment guidelines, 2014. *MMWR Morb Mortal Wkly Rep.* 2014 (in press).

TABLE 373-2 U.S. ADVISORY COMMITTEE ON IMMUNIZATION PRACTICES RECOMMENDATIONS FOR QUADRIVALENT (HPV 6, 11, 16, 18) AND BIVALENT (HPV 16, 18) HPV VACCINES

FEMALES

- Routine vaccination with three-dose series of quadrivalent or bivalent vaccine recommended in females aged 11 to 12 years, starting as young as 9 years
- Catch-up vaccination recommended in females aged 13 to 26 years who have not previously received full vaccine series

MALES

- Routine vaccination with three-dose series of quadrivalent vaccine recommended in males aged 11 to 12 years, starting as young as 9 years
- Catch-up vaccination recommended in immunocompromised persons and in males aged 13 to 21 years who have not previously received full vaccine series
- Catch-up vaccination recommended in men who have sex with men through age 26 years who have not previously received full vaccine series

Recommended dosage and schedule: 0.5 mL intramuscularly at 0, 2, and 6 months

Schedule modifications: if doses are missed, series does not need to be restarted, but second and third doses should be given as soon as possible.

Cervical cancer screening: no change in recommended interval

Special situations: females with genital warts, abnormal Papanicolaou test results, or positive human papillomavirus test results are unlikely to be infected with all four vaccine types and should be immunized per other recommendations; males with genital warts should also be immunized per other recommendations.

Pregnant and lactating women: not recommended for use in pregnancy based on lack of data; may be used in lactating women

Immunocompromised persons: no safety concerns because vaccine is noninfectious, but immune response and effectiveness might be reduced

Not recommended for females or males <9 and >26 years of age

Modified from Markowitz LE, Dunne EF, Saraiya M, et al; Centers for Disease Control and Prevention. Human papillomavirus vaccination. Recommendations of the Advisory Committee on Immunization Practices. *MMWR.* 2014;63:1-30.

---

prevention of symptoms or, in the case of high-grade squamous intraepithelial lesions, prevention of progression to cancer. Treatment involves destruction of lesions by physical techniques or topically applied or injected cytotoxic agents. Because treatment does not eradicate infection in surrounding tissues, recurrent lesions are common.

Treatment of warts depends on their location and size, the patient's preferences, and the provider's experience. Recommended first-line treatment of common, flat, and plantar warts includes the application of topical salicylic acid and cryotherapy; second-line treatment of recalcitrant lesions includes topical imiquimod (5% cream applied once daily at bedtime three times a week for up to 16 weeks), intralesional bleomycin, pulsed dye laser therapy, and surgical excision.[A3] Recommended treatment of genital warts (Table 373-1) includes patient-applied podophyllotoxin (0.5 or 0.15% solution or gel applied twice a day for 3 days, repeated weekly for four cycles), imiquimod, or sinecatechins, as well as provider-administered cryotherapy, trichloroacetic acid, or surgical excision; alternative treatments include intralesional interferon and laser surgery.[13] Oral lesions can be treated by locally destructive physical techniques.

For cervical lesions, treatment depends on histologic staging after colposcopy and biopsy and clinical context. Because CIN 1 usually regresses spontaneously, follow-up (by cytology, HPV test, and/or colposcopy) without treatment is recommended.[14] Treatment is generally recommended for all CIN 2/3 lesions, except in pregnant women, who have higher rates of spontaneous regression and a greater risk for reproductive tract complications after treatment, and in young woman with CIN 2. Treatment options include a variety of ablative and excisional techniques, such as cryosurgery, loop electrosurgical excision procedure, and laser surgery. Treatment is 90 to 95% effective in preventing the recurrence of lesions, and comparative clinical trials have shown similar efficacy for different treatment modalities.[A4]

PREVENTION

Primary Prevention

Primary prevention of HPV infection depends on avoidance of contact with infectious lesions and reduction of susceptibility through immunization. For example, the use of footwear in locker rooms may prevent plantar warts. For genital HPV infection, correct and consistent condom use can reduce the risk for both HPV infection and the HPV-associated diseases of genital warts, cervical squamous intraepithelial lesions, and cervical cancer. Male circumcision reduces the prevalence of both high-risk and low-risk types of genital HPV infection in men and transmission of HPV to their sex partners.[A5][A6]

Of greatest importance for prevention are HPV vaccines (Chapter 18), which are composed of virus-like particles assembled from the major capsid protein, L1. Recommendations have been made for two currently licensed vaccines, a quadrivalent vaccine (types 6, 11, 16, and 18) and a bivalent vaccine (types 16 and 18). Recommendations are pending for a newly-licensed 9-valent vaccine (types 6, 11, 16, 18, 31, 33, 45, 52, and 58) which could prevent a higher proportion of HPV-associated disease outcomes.[15,16] The quadrivalent vaccine, given in three doses during a period of 6 months, is highly effective. In women, it prevent CIN 1 and CIN 2/3 as well as genital warts, VaIN, and VIN caused by any of the four types.[A7] In men, it prevent genital warts and AIN.[A8][A9] The bivalent vaccine provides a high

level of protection against CIN but not genital wart.[A10] Both vaccines are recommended for routine immunization of 11- to 12-year-old girls as well as females 13 t 26 years of age (Table 373-2). However, these vaccines provide protection against only two of the types of HPV that are associated with cancer, so immunized women continue to need cervical cancer screening.

The quadrivalent vaccine is also recommended for routine immunization of 11- to 12-year-old boys as well as males aged 13 to 21 years of age for prevention of genital warts (Chapter 18). Among men who have sex with men, immunization is recommended up to 26 years of age because of the additional benefit of preventing AIN (see Table 373-2). Both girls and boys 9 to 10 years of age may also be vaccinated at the discretion of the provider.

These vaccines have no therapeutic benefit against existing infection or lesions, and they are most effective if given before initiation of sexual activity. Because the HPV vaccines contain no live virus, they can be safely given to persons with impaired immunity (e.g., HIV infection). Research priorities include determining the duration of immunity after immunization, the efficacy of a two-dose regimen,[17] the extent of cross-protection against nonvaccine types, and benefit in prevention of nongenital HPV–associated cancers.

Secondary Prevention

Screening plus treatment of high-grade cervical squamous intraepithelial lesions is one of the most successful of all cancer prevention strategies. Screening has been conventionally conducted using Pap tests, but HPV tests are increasingly used as well for both primary screening and management of low-grade cytologic abnormalities. Current guidelines in the United States have evolved and now recommend screening at 3-year intervals beginning at age 21 years.[18] HPV testing is not recommended in younger women because of the high prevalence of often recently acquired and likely transient HPV infection. In contrast, among women older than 30 years, co-testing with HPV plus cytology is a recommended alternative to cytology alone because its enhanced sensitivity allows extension of screening to 5-year intervals (Chapter 199). Women with negative cytology who test HPV positive can be followed with repeat co-testing in 1 year or triaged by use of an HPV

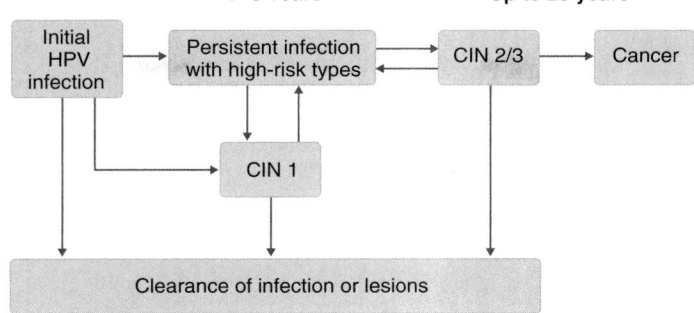

1–5 Years **Up to 20 years**

Risk factors for infection
- Younger age
- Increasing number of lifetime sex partners
- Lack of circumcision
- Lack of consistent condom use
- Not immunized

Initial HPV infection → Persistent infection with high-risk types → CIN 2/3 → Cancer

CIN 1

Clearance of infection or lesions

Cofactors for disease progression
- Hormonal exposure (long-term oral contraceptive use)
- Multiparity
- Other STIs (e.g., *Chlamydia trachomatis*, HSV-2)
- Smoking
- Nutritional deficiency
- Host genetics (e.g., polymorphisms in HLA and other genes)
- Deficiency of cell-mediated immunity
- Lack of Pap test screening

FIGURE 373-3. Natural history of genital human papillomavirus (HPV) infection and cervical cancer. CIN = cervical intraepithelial neoplasia; HSV = herpes simplex virus; STIs = sexually transmitted infections.

16/18 test. Management of other abnormalities is based on the degree of cytologic finding and age, with a higher threshold for treating younger women in whom abnormalities are more likely to resolve. With improvement in screening tests, a major prevention challenge remains increasing access to and use of screening services because approximately half of cervical cancers in the United States occur in women who were infrequently or never screened.

The value of cytologic screening for anal intraepithelial lesions in HIV-positive men who have sex with men is controversial but not currently recommended because of limited data on the natural history of these precursor lesions, the reliability of screening methods, and the safety and effectiveness of treatment.[13]

PROGNOSIS

Although the natural history of HPV infection is not fully characterized, the large majority of infections and premalignant lesions are self-limited in most immunocompetent patients. Whether infections no longer detectable have been cleared by the immune system or remain latent in the basal layer of the epithelium with the potential for reactivation is not clear, but the higher prevalence of detectable infection in advanced than in early HIV infection supports the possibility of long-term infection. Many if not most clinical lesions resolve spontaneously after the patient develops cell-mediated immunity. Spontaneous regression is estimated to occur in 25% of genital warts and more than 50% of common warts in children.

The natural history of CIN has been most intensively studied because of its relationship to cervical cancer, although many questions remain unanswered. Estimates of the likelihood of regression versus the risk for progression to invasive cancer are 90% and 1% for CIN 1, 40% and 5% for CIN 2, and 32% and 30% for CIN 3. The various stages of precursor lesions were traditionally viewed as a biologic continuum, with CIN 1 progressing through higher grades to cancer. However, newer data indicate that low-grade and high-grade squamous intraepithelial lesions may be distinct processes, in which low-grade lesions (CIN 1) represent a usually transient infection characterized by production of capsid protein (and probably infectious virions) and only minor cellular abnormalities, whereas high-grade lesions (CIN 2/3) represent proliferation of immature cells as a result of the activity of oncogenic proteins of high-risk types (Fig. 373-3). Initial infection frequently leads to a transient low-grade squamous intraepithelial lesion, with persistent infection in less than 10% of cases. Persistent infection can, in turn, lead directly to high-grade squamous intraepithelial lesions within several years of initial infection and can progress to invasive cancer after several decades. The natural history of squamous intraepithelial lesions at other anogenital sites is less well defined, but they may be associated with higher rates of spontaneous regression.

The majority of patients with HPV infection have an excellent prognosis, with the most serious outcomes of cancer occurring infrequently among the large number of persons infected. Treatment can hasten the resolution of cutaneous and genital warts and is highly effective for cervical lesions. Among women with CIN 3, long-term studies indicate that a 30% risk for cancer in untreated women can be reduced to less than 1% with treatment.

Grade A References

A1. Ronco G, Dillner J, Elfstrom KM, et al. Efficacy of HPV-based screening for prevention of invasive cervical cancer: follow-up of four European randomised controlled trials. *Lancet.* 2014;383:524-532.
A2. Bouchard-Fortier G, Hajifathalian K, McKnight MD, et al. Co-testing for detection of high-grade cervical intraepithelial neoplasia and cancer compared with cytology alone: a meta-analysis of randomized controlled trials. *J Public Health (Oxf).* 2014;36:46-55.
A3. Kwok CS, Gibbs S, Bennett C, et al. Topical treatments for cutaneous warts. *Cochrane Database Syst Rev.* 2012;9:CD001781.
A4. Martin-Hirsch PP, Paraskevaidis E, Bryant A, et al. Surgery for cervical intraepithelial neoplasia. *Cochrane Database Syst Rev.* 2013;12:CD001318.
A5. Tobian AAR, Serwadda D, Quinn TC, et al. Male circumcision for the prevention of HSV-2 and HPV infections and syphilis. *N Engl J Med.* 2009;360:1298-1309.
A6. Wawer MJ, Tobian AA, Kigozi G, et al. Effect of circumcision of HIV-negative men on transmission of human papillomavirus to HIV-negative women: a randomised trial in Rakai, Uganda. *Lancet.* 2011;377:209-218.
A7. Munoz N, Kjaer SK, Sigurdsson K, et al. Impact of human papillomavirus (HPV)-6/11/16/18 vaccine on all HPV-associated genital diseases in young women. *J Nat Cancer Inst.* 2010;102:325-339.
A8. Giuliano AR, Palefsky JM, Goldstone S, et al. Efficacy of quadrivalent HPV vaccine against HPV infection and disease in males. *N Engl J Med.* 2011;364:401-411.
A9. Palefsky JM, Giuliano AR, Goldstone S, et al. HPV vaccine against anal HPV infection and anal intraepithelial neoplasia. *N Engl J Med.* 2011;365:1576-1585.
A10. Lehtinen M, Paavonen J, Wheeler CM, et al. Overall efficacy of HPV-16/18 AS04-adjuvanted vaccine against grade 3 or greater cervical intraepithelial neoplasia: 4-year end-of-study analysis of the randomised, double-blind PATRICIA trial. *Lancet Oncol.* 2012;13:89-99.

GENERAL REFERENCES

For the General References and other additional features, please visit Expert Consult at https://expertconsult.inkling.com.

374

HERPES SIMPLEX VIRUS INFECTIONS

RICHARD J. WHITLEY

DEFINITION
The Pathogen

Herpes simplex virus (HSV), a member of the family Herpesviridae, has been implicated in human infections since descriptions of cutaneous spreading lesions in ancient Greek times. In 1968, well-defined antigenic and biologic differences were demonstrated between HSV type 1 (HSV-1) and HSV type 2 (HSV-2). Of all the herpesviruses, HSV-1 and HSV-2 are most closely related, with approximately 60% genomic homology. Historically, HSV-1 was more frequently associated with nongenital infection and HSV-2 with genital

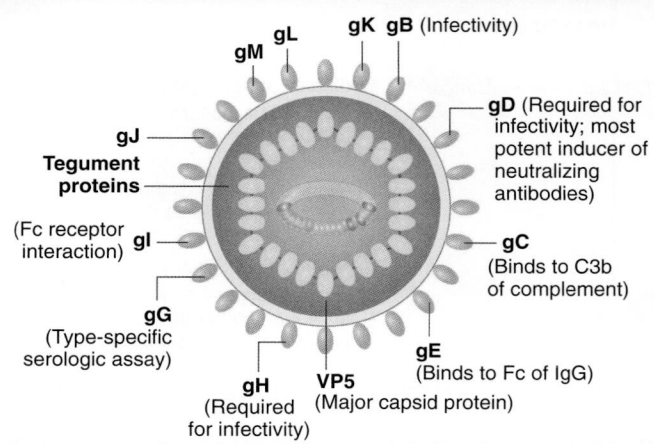

FIGURE 374-1. Schematic diagram of the herpes simplex virion. IgG = immunoglobulin G.

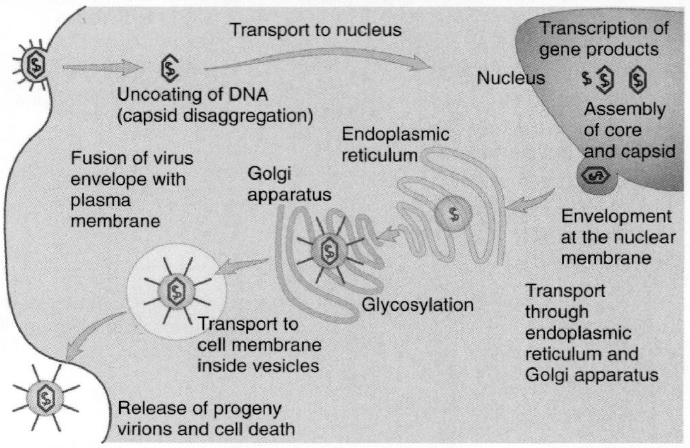

FIGURE 374-2. Schematic diagram of replication of herpes simplex virus.

disease, but these distinctions are much less relevant now that HSV-1 causes more than 50% of genital infection in some populations. These two viruses can be distinguished most reliably by DNA restriction enzyme analysis, but differences in antigen expression and biologic properties also serve as methods for differentiation.

Inclusion in the family Herpesviridae is based on the structure of the virion (Fig. 374-1). HSV contains double-stranded DNA at its central core, has a molecular weight of approximately 100 million, and encodes at least 80 polypeptides. The DNA core is surrounded by a capsid that consists of 162 capsomers arranged in icosapentahedral symmetry. The capsid is 100 to 110 nm in diameter. Tightly adherent to the capsid is the tegument, which consists of amorphous material. Loosely surrounding the capsid and tegument is a lipid bilayer envelope derived from host cell membranes. The envelope consists of polyamines, lipids, and glycoproteins. These glycoproteins confer distinctive properties to the virus and provide unique antigens to which the host is capable of responding. Notably, glycoprotein G (gG) provides antigenic specificity to HSV and therefore results in an antibody response that allows distinction between HSV-1 (gG-1) and HSV-2 (gG-2).

EPIDEMIOLOGY

HSV infections occur worldwide and have been reported in both developed and developing countries. Animal vectors for human HSV infections have not been described, and there is no seasonal variation in the incidence of HSV infections. HSV is transmitted from infected to susceptible individuals during close personal contact, and the virus must come in contact with mucosal surfaces or abraded skin for infection to be initiated. Because approximately a third of the world's population has recurrent HSV infections and because infection is rarely fatal, a large reservoir of HSV exists in the community.

Seroprevalence studies have demonstrated that acquisition of HSV-1 infection is related to socioeconomic factors. Antibodies, which indicate past infection, are found early in life among individuals of lower socioeconomic groups, presumably a consequence of crowded living conditions that provide a greater opportunity for direct contact with infected individuals. Antibodies develop in as many as 75 to 90% of individuals from lower socioeconomic populations by the end of the first decade of life. In contrast, only 30 to 40% of persons in the middle and upper socioeconomic groups are seropositive by the middle of the second decade of life.

Because infections with HSV-2 are usually acquired through sexual contact, antibodies to this virus are rarely found until the onset of sexual activity. There is a progressive increase in infection rates with HSV-2 in all populations beginning in adolescence. Overall, about one in five Americans has genital HSV-2 infection. As with HSV-1 infections, the rate of acquisition of HSV-2 infection appears to be related to socioeconomic factors. The number of sexual partners is also an important risk factor for the acquisition of HSV-2. Genital herpes infection has been found to be a risk factor for another sexually transmitted virus, human immunodeficiency virus (HIV; Chapter 386).

Localized, recurrent HSV-2 infection is the most common form of HSV infection during gestation. Transmission of infection to the fetus is most frequently related to shedding of the virus at the time of delivery. The incidence of cervical shedding in pregnant women with asymptomatic HSV infection is approximately 1%. Most infants in whom neonatal disease develops are born to women who are completely asymptomatic for genital HSV infection at the time of delivery and who have neither a past history of genital herpes nor a sexual partner reporting a genital vesicular rash. These women account for 60 to 80% of all women whose children acquire neonatal HSV infection. Women who experience a symptomatic or asymptomatic primary infection in the third trimester of gestation have a 30 to 50% risk for transmitting infection to the child.

PATHOBIOLOGY

Replication of HSV is a multistep process (Fig. 374-2). After the onset of infection, DNA is uncoated and transported to the nucleus of the host cell. This step is followed by transcription of immediate-early genes, which encode the regulatory proteins, and is followed by the expression of proteins encoded by early and then late genes.[1] These proteins include enzymes necessary for viral replication and structural proteins.

Assembly of the viral core and capsid takes place within the nucleus. Envelopment at the nuclear membrane and transport out of the nucleus occur through the endoplasmic reticulum and the Golgi apparatus. Glycosylation of the viral membrane occurs in the Golgi apparatus. Mature virions are transported to the outer membrane of the host cell inside vesicles. Release of progeny virus is accompanied by cell death. Replication for all herpesviruses is considered inefficient, with a high ratio of noninfectious to infectious viral particles.

A critical factor for transmission of HSV, regardless of virus type, is intimate contact between a person who is shedding virus and a susceptible host. With inoculation onto skin or mucous membranes, HSV replicates in epithelial cells; the incubation period is 4 to 6 days (Fig. 374-3). As replication continues, cell lysis and local inflammation ensue and result in the characteristic vesicles on an erythematous base. Regional lymphatics and lymph nodes become involved as a result of draining of infected secretions from the area of viral replication. Viremia and visceral dissemination may develop, depending on the immunologic competence of the host. In all hosts, the virus generally ascends peripheral sensory nerves to reach the dorsal root ganglia. Replication of HSV within neural tissue is followed by spread of the virus to other mucosal and skin surfaces by means of peripheral sensory nerves. HSV replicates further in epithelial cells and reproduces the lesions of the initial infection until infection is contained through host immune responses.

The histopathologic changes induced by HSV replication are similar in both primary and recurrent infection. Changes induced by viral infection include ballooning of infected cells and the appearance of condensed chromatin within the nuclei of cells, followed by subsequent degeneration of cellular nuclei. Cells lose intact plasma membranes and form multinucleated giant cells. They may also demonstrate intranuclear inclusions known as Cowdry type A bodies, which are suggestive but not diagnostic of HSV infection. With cell lysis, clear vesicular fluid containing large quantities of virus accumulates between the epidermis and dermal layer. The dermis reveals an intense inflammatory response, more so with primary infection than with recurrent disease. As healing progresses, the clear vesicular fluid becomes

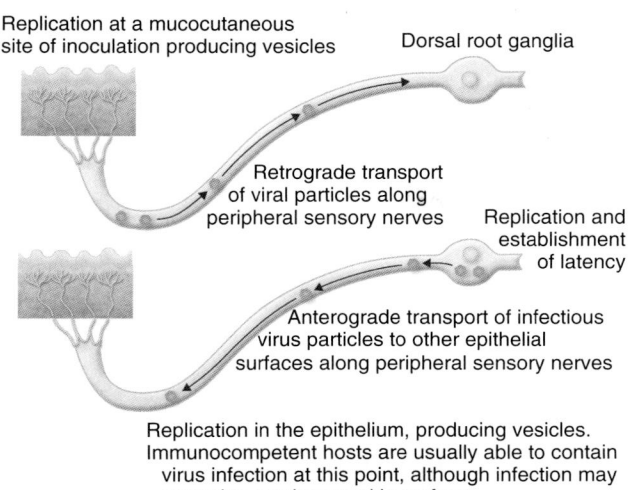

FIGURE 374-3. Schematic diagram of primary herpes simplex virus infection.

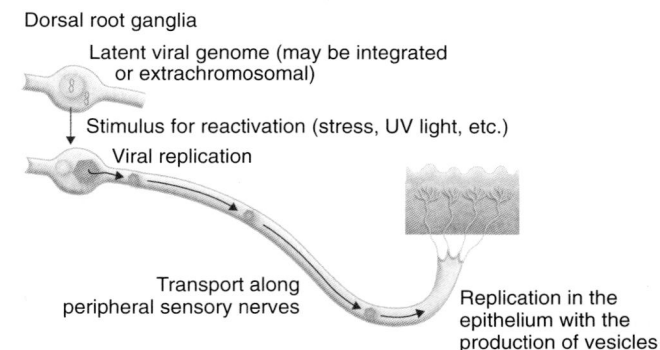

FIGURE 374-4. Schematic diagram of herpes simplex virus latency and reactivation. UV = ultraviolet.

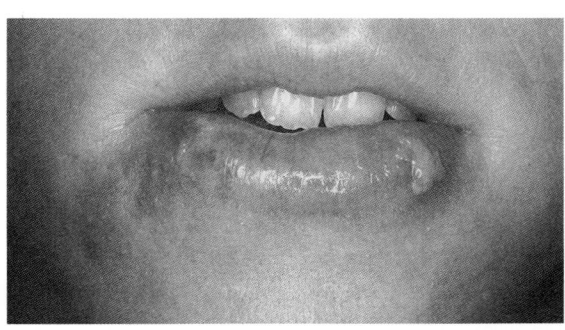

FIGURE 374-5. Herpes labialis, classic grouped blisters.

pustular with the recruitment of inflammatory cells. The pustule then forms a scab; scarring is uncommon.

Vascular changes in the area of infection include perivascular cuffing and hemorrhagic necrosis. These changes are particularly prominent when organs other than skin are involved, as is the case with herpes simplex encephalitis or disseminated neonatal HSV infection. Local lymphatics can show evidence of infection with intrusion of inflammatory cells because of draining of infected secretions from the area of viral replication. As host defenses are mounted, an influx of mononuclear cells can be detected in infected tissue.

A unique characteristic of all herpesviruses is their ability to establish latent infection, to persist in an apparently inactive state for varying lengths of time, and then to be reactivated (Fig. 374-4).[2] The latent viral genome may be either extrachromosomal or integrated into host cell DNA, depending on the virus.

Latency is established when HSV reaches the dorsal root ganglia after retrograde transmission through sensory nerve pathways. Latent virus may be reactivated and enter a replicative cycle at any point in time. Reactivation of latent virus is a well-recognized biologic phenomenon but not one that is understood from a molecular standpoint. Stimuli associated with the reactivation of latent HSV have included stress, fever, menstruation, and exposure to ultraviolet light. Precisely how these factors interact at the level of the ganglia remains to be defined. Reactivation may be clinically asymptomatic, or it may produce life-threatening disease.

CLINICAL MANIFESTATIONS
Gingivostomatitis
Gingivostomatitis (usually caused by HSV-1) occurs most frequently in children younger than 5 years. Illness is characterized by fever, sore throat, pharyngeal edema, and erythema, followed by the development of vesicular or ulcerative lesions on the oral and pharyngeal mucosa. Recurrent HSV-1 infections of the oropharynx are most frequently manifested as herpes simplex labialis (cold sores) and usually appear on the vermilion border of the lip (Fig. 374-5). Recurrences are triggered by fever, stress, and exposure to ultraviolet light as well as by other factors. Intraoral lesions as a manifestation of recurrent disease are uncommon.

Genital Herpes
Genital herpes is often caused by HSV-2, but approximately 50% of all new primary cases in young adults are caused by HSV-1. Primary infection in women usually involves the vulva, vagina, and cervix. In men, initial infection is most often associated with lesions on the glans penis, prepuce, or penile shaft. In individuals of either gender, primary disease is associated with fever, malaise, anorexia, and bilateral inguinal adenopathy. Women frequently have dysuria and urinary retention as a result of urethral involvement. Aseptic meningitis develops in as many as 10% of individuals with primary infection. Sacral radiculomyelitis may occur in both men and women and results in neuralgias, urinary retention, or obstipation. Complete healing of primary infection may take several weeks. The first episode of genital infection is less

severe in individuals who have previously had HSV-1 infections at other sites. Antibodies to HSV-1 appear to ameliorate the expression of HSV-2 clinical disease, although this effect is controversial.

Recurrent genital infections in either men or women can be particularly distressing. The frequency of recurrence varies significantly from one individual to another. Of note, viral DNA can be detected by polymerase chain reaction (PCR) in genital secretions three- to four-fold more frequently than symptomatic recurrences. Furthermore, recurrences detected by PCR can occur frequently during 24 hours and persist for brief periods. A third of infected individuals have virtually no or few clinical recurrences, a third have approximately three recurrences per year, and another third have more than three per year. Several seroepidemiologic studies have found that between 25 and 65% of individuals in the United States have antibodies to HSV-2 and that seroprevalence is correlated with the number of sexual partners.

Shedding of HSV from the genital tract can be either symptomatic or, more frequently, asymptomatic. Transmission can occur in the absence of symptoms. Genital ulcerative disease attributed to HSV is a risk factor for the acquisition of HIV infection.

Herpetic Keratitis
Herpes simplex keratitis (Chapter 423) is usually caused by HSV-1 and is accompanied by conjunctivitis in many cases. It is considered the most common infectious cause of blindness in the United States. The characteristic lesions of HSV keratoconjunctivitis are dendritic ulcers best detected by fluorescein staining of the cornea. Deep stromal involvement has also been reported and may result in visual impairment.

Other Cutaneous Manifestations
HSV infections can occur at any skin site. Common among health care workers are lesions on abraded skin or the fingers, known as herpetic whitlow. Similarly, in wrestlers, disseminated cutaneous lesions known as herpes gladiatorum may develop as a result of physical contact.

HERPES SIMPLEX VIRUS INFECTIONS IN IMMUNOCOMPROMISED HOSTS
HSV infections in immunocompromised hosts, including patients with acquired immunodeficiency syndrome, are usually due to reactivation of

latent infection and are clinically more severe, may be progressive, and require a longer time to heal. Manifestations of HSV infections in this population of patients include pneumonitis, esophagitis, hepatitis, colitis, and disseminated cutaneous disease. Individuals suffering from HIV infection may have extensive perineal or orofacial ulcerations. HSV infections are also noted to be of increased severity in individuals with extensive burns.

DIAGNOSIS

Definitive diagnosis of HSV infection requires detection of viral DNA by PCR testing or isolation of the virus. DNA amplification has become the diagnostic method of choice in assessing cerebrospinal fluid (CSF) specimens for evidence of HSV infection of the central nervous system and has significantly improved sensitivity for confirmation of HSV as the cause of lip and genital herpes infection. The main role for viral cultures is to assess possible resistance to antiviral therapy.

In the absence of PCR or diagnostic virologic facilities, cytologic examination of cells scraped from a clinical lesion may be useful in making a presumptive diagnosis of HSV infection. Material obtained from scraping the base of a lesion should be smeared on a glass slide and promptly fixed in cold ethanol. The slide can be stained according to the methods of Papanicolaou, Giemsa, or Wright. The presence of intranuclear inclusions and multinucleated giant cells is indicative but not diagnostic of HSV infection. This method has a sensitivity of only 60 to 70% and should not be the sole diagnostic method used.

In addition to new tests for viral DNA, type-specific serologic assays are commercially available. These tests are based on differences between HSV-1 and HSV-2.

TREATMENT   Rx

For *immunocompromised* patients, such as patients who have cancer or are receiving immunosuppressive drugs, patients with disseminated mucocutaneous infections, or patients with herpes encephalitis, the treatment of choice is intravenous acyclovir (5 to 10 mg/kg every 8 hours for 5 to 7 days).[A1] Caution must be exercised when acyclovir is used intravenously because it may crystallize in the renal tubules when it is given too rapidly or to dehydrated patients. Valacyclovir (500 to 1000 mg two or three times daily) and famciclovir (250 to 500 mg three times daily), depending on severity, are equally efficacious[A2] and have improved pharmacokinetics, as demonstrated by improved biodistribution and less frequent dosing intervals compared with oral acyclovir. Thus, they should preferentially be used for the treatment of non-life-threatening HSV infection.[3] For life-threatening disease, only intravenous medications should be given. Immunocompromised individuals with non-life-threatening mucocutaneous HSV infections can be given oral valacyclovir (500 to 1000 mg once or twice daily for 5 to 7 days), famciclovir (250 to 500 mg three times daily for 7 days), or acyclovir (400 mg two or three times daily for 7 to 10 days).

High-risk immunocompromised hosts are at risk for developing an acyclovir-resistant infection, usually as a consequence of either an altered or deficient thymidine kinase enzyme that activates acyclovir in infected cells. Such patients can be managed with foscarnet or cidofovir, continued until there is evidence of healing, with the doses based on renal function (see Tables 360-4 and 360-5 in Chapter 360).

In *immunocompetent* hosts with mucocutaneous infections, oral acyclovir (200 mg five times daily for 5 days) reduces lesions and speeds recovery. Oral valacyclovir (1 g/day for 5 days or 500 mg twice daily for 3 days) and oral famciclovir (1 g twice daily for 1 day) are equally effective.[A3][A4] Pritelivir (an inhibitor of the viral helicase-primase complex at 25 to 75 mg daily or 400 mg weekly) has recently been shown to reduce viral shedding and the duration of genital lesions in men and women, but is on clinical hold on the part of the FDA because of potential toxicity issues.[A5] Topical acyclovir is not as reliable as oral acyclovir and is not recommended.[4]

HSV has been used for experimental gene therapy. By removal of the $\gamma_1 34.5$ gene, both neurovirulence and the propensity to establish latency are ablated. These engineered viruses are being experimentally tested in patients with glioblastoma multiforme and colorectal metastases to liver.

PREVENTION

Some patients with particularly disabling oral recurrences or genital recurrences are candidates for chronic suppressive therapy. Potential regimens include oral acyclovir 400 mg twice daily, oral valacyclovir 500 mg or 1 g/day, and oral famciclovir 250 mg twice daily. Such regimens are approved by the U.S. Food and Drug Administration for genital herpes but not for herpes labialis. However, such therapy does not prevent recurrent HSV-2 meningitis.[A6]

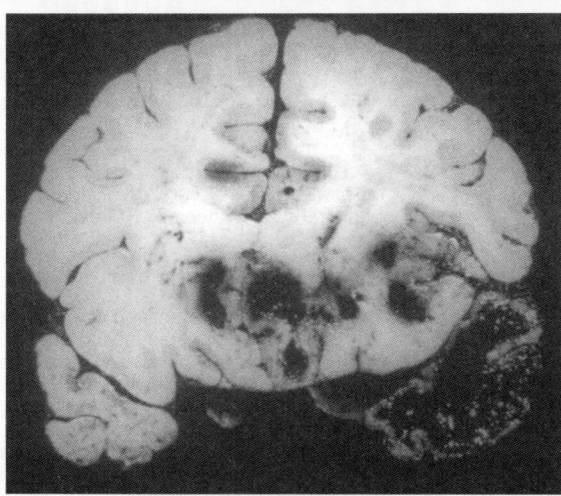

FIGURE 374-6. Hemorrhagic necrosis in herpes simplex encephalitis.

At present, experimental vaccines for HSV-1 and HSV-2 remain under investigation.[5] Acyclovir, valacyclovir, and famciclovir are given to recipients of solid organ and bone marrow transplants in the immediate post-transplantation period in an effort to prevent reactivation of latent disease at the doses noted previously. Valacyclovir (500 mg daily) decreases person-to-person transmission of HSV-2. Suppressive therapy of an HSV-2-infected but HIV-seronegative patient does not prevent HIV acquisition from HIV-seropositive partners.[6]

HERPES SIMPLEX ENCEPHALITIS

Herpes simplex encephalitis[7] is characterized by hemorrhagic necrosis of the temporal lobe (Chapter 414). Disease begins unilaterally and spreads to the contralateral temporal lobe (Fig. 374-6). It is the most common cause of focal, sporadic encephalitis in the United States today and occurs in approximately 1 in 150,000 individuals. Most cases are caused by HSV-1. The actual pathogenesis of herpes simplex encephalitis requires further clarification, although it has been speculated that primary or recurrent virus can reach the temporal lobe by ascending neural pathways, such as the trigeminal tracts or the olfactory nerves.

CLINICAL MANIFESTATIONS AND DIAGNOSIS

Clinical manifestations of herpes simplex encephalitis are characteristic of temporal lobe involvement and include headache, fever, altered consciousness, aphasia, and behavioral abnormalities. Focal seizures also may occur. CSF findings in these patients are variable but usually consist of a pleocytosis with both polymorphonuclear leukocytes and monocytes present. The protein concentration is characteristically elevated, and the glucose level is usually normal. Magnetic resonance imaging can suggest the diagnosis by demonstrating edema of either temporal lobe. Diagnosis can be confirmed by PCR detection of HSV DNA in the CSF by experienced laboratories.

TREATMENT AND PROGNOSIS   Rx

Mortality and morbidity are high, even with appropriate acyclovir antiviral therapy. At present, the mortality rate is approximately 30% 1 year after treatment. In addition, approximately 60% of survivors have moderate or severe neurologic impairment.

NEONATAL HERPES SIMPLEX VIRUS INFECTION

Neonatal HSV infection is estimated to occur in approximately 1 in 3500 deliveries in the United States each year.[8] Approximately 70% of cases are caused by HSV-2 and usually result from contact of the fetus with infected maternal genital secretions at the time of delivery. Manifestations of neonatal HSV infection can be divided into three categories: skin, eye, and mouth disease; encephalitis; and disseminated infection. As the name implies, skin, eye, and mouth disease consists of cutaneous lesions and does not involve other organ systems. Involvement of the central nervous system may occur with encephalitis or disseminated infection and generally results in diffuse encephalitis. CSF assay characteristically reveals elevated protein levels and mononuclear pleocytosis. Disseminated infection involves multiple organ systems and can cause disseminated intravascular coagulation, hemorrhagic pneumonitis, encephalitis, and cutaneous lesions. Diagnosis is difficult in the absence of skin lesions, which occurs in as many as 36% of cases. The mortality rate for each disease classification varies from zero for skin, eye, and mouth disease to 5% for encephalitis and 25% for neonates with disseminated infection, even with appropriate antiviral treatment. In addition to the high mortality associated with these infections, morbidity is significant in that children with encephalitis or disseminated disease develop normally in only 40% of cases, even with appropriate antiviral therapy (acyclovir, 20 mg/kg every 8 hours for 14 days for skin, eye, and mouth infections and 21 days for central nervous system or disseminated disease).

Grade A References

A1. Glenny AM, Fernandez Mauleffinch LM, Pavitt S, et al. Interventions for the prevention and treatment of herpes simplex virus in patients being treated for cancer. *Cochrane Database Syst Rev.* 2009;1:CD006706.
A2. Cernik C, Gallina K, Brodell RT. The treatment of herpes simplex infections: an evidence-based review. *Arch Intern Med.* 2008;168:1137-1144.
A3. Abudalu M, Tyring S, Koltun W, et al. Single-day, patient-initiated famciclovir therapy versus 3-day valacyclovir regimen for recurrent genital herpes: a randomized, double-blind, comparative trial. *Clin Infect Dis.* 2008;47:651-658.
A4. Corey L, Wald A, Patel R, et al. Once-daily valacyclovir to reduce the risk of transmission of genital herpes. *N Engl J Med.* 2004;350:11-20.
A5. Wald A, Corey L, Timmler B, et al. Helicase-primase inhibitor pritelivir for HSV-2 infection. *N Engl J Med.* 2014;370:201-210.
A6. Aurelius E, Franzen-Rohl E, Glimaker M, et al. Long-term valacyclovir suppressive treatment after herpes simplex virus type 2 meningitis: a double-blind, randomized controlled trial. *Clin Infect Dis.* 2012;54:1304-1313.

GENERAL REFERENCES

For the General References and other additional features, please visit Expert Consult at https://expertconsult.inkling.com.

375

VARICELLA-ZOSTER VIRUS (CHICKENPOX, SHINGLES)

JEFFREY COHEN

DEFINITION

Primary infection with varicella-zoster virus (VZV) results in the rash of varicella (chickenpox). The virus establishes a latent infection in the nervous system and can reactivate later in life to cause zoster (shingles).[1]

The Pathogen

VZV is a member of the alpha herpesvirus family and has a DNA core surrounded by a nucleocapsid, which is in turn surrounded by a viral envelope that is studded with glycoproteins. Antibody to viral glycoproteins is important for neutralizing the virus's infectivity and for protecting against primary infection. The virus encodes a thymidine kinase, which phosphorylates acyclovir, which in turn inhibits viral DNA replication by inhibiting the VZV DNA polymerase.

EPIDEMIOLOGY

Before the advent of an effective vaccine, more than 95% of children in temperate climates were infected with VZV. By comparison, infection is usually delayed until adulthood in tropical climates. Varicella usually occurs in children younger than 5 years. Zoster is less common in tropical areas, probably because of a delay in acquisition of varicella. Varicella is more common in the winter and spring, whereas zoster has no seasonal predilection.

Primary varicella infection can occur after exposure to either chickenpox or zoster. The virus is spread by droplets and aerosols from patients or by contact with vesicular lesions. Persons are infectious beginning about 2 days before the rash appears and continuing until all lesions have crusted. Although 60 to 90% of susceptible household contacts develop varicella, only 20 to 30% of susceptible persons exposed to zoster become infected. More than 95% of primary infections result in the symptoms of varicella, and second episodes of varicella are rare. Varicella is more severe in persons with impaired cellular immunity, including patients with acquired immunodeficiency syndrome (AIDS) and infants whose mothers present with varicella 5 days before to 2 days after delivery.

About 50% of persons who have had varicella and live to age 85 years will develop zoster. The risk for zoster rises with increasing age (especially 50 years and older) and with increasing impairment of cellular immunity. For example, men with AIDS have a 20-fold higher risk for development of zoster than age-matched controls. Less than 5% of persons have a second episode of zoster, but recurrent zoster is more common in persons with impaired cellular immunity.

PATHOBIOLOGY

Varicella is transmitted by the respiratory route. The virus is thought to infect epithelial cells and lymphocytes in the oropharynx and upper respiratory tract or in the conjunctiva, and then infected lymphocytes subsequently spread the virus throughout the body. The virus then enters the skin through endothelial cells in blood vessels and spreads to epithelial cells, where it causes the vesicular rash of varicella. Lesions initially are vesicular but become pustular after the infiltration of inflammatory cells. Later the lesions break open and dry to form crusts that usually heal without scarring. During primary infection, neurons in cranial nerve ganglia and dorsal root ganglia become latently infected with the virus.

If VZV-specific cellular immunity declines, the virus can reactivate from a ganglion, travel down the axon, and replicate in epithelial cells to cause dermatomal zoster. In highly immunocompromised persons, high-grade viremia during reactivation causes disseminated zoster.

Antibodies, which usually are present at the time varicella presents clinically, persist for life. Antibody is important for protection against varicella, as evidenced by the ability of varicella immune globulin to attenuate the disease. Cytotoxic T cells are present within 2 to 3 days after the onset of varicella and limit its severity. Varicella is more severe in persons with impaired cellular immunity but not in patients with hypogammaglobulinemia. Cellular immunity, not antibody, is required to prevent reactivation of virus and zoster.

CLINICAL MANIFESTATIONS

Varicella

Varicella begins with fever and malaise followed 1 to 2 days later by a disseminated, pruritic, vesicular rash (Fig. 375-1).[2] The usual incubation period for varicella is 2 weeks (range, 10 to 21 days) after exposure to an infected person. The lesions begin as papules that become vesicles, followed by pustules and then crusts. Lesions appear on the head and then spread to the trunk and then to the extremities; the mucosa can also be involved. There are typically 200 to 500 lesions in different stages on the skin. New lesions occur for up to 5 days in normal hosts, and crusting is complete within 2 weeks.

The most common complication of varicella is bacterial superinfection of skin lesions. Group A streptococcus (Chapter 290) or *Staphylococcus aureus* (Chapter 288) infections can cause cellulitis, bacteremia, and necrotizing fasciitis. Other complications include cerebellar ataxia, viral pneumonitis, hepatitis, and thrombocytopenia. Less frequent complications include viral meningitis, encephalitis, vasculopathy (which presents as a stroke), disseminated intravascular coagulopathy (Chapter 175), and Reye syndrome (more common in children receiving aspirin). Complications involving the lungs and liver are more common in children with impaired cellular immunity including those receiving systemic steroids, children with chronic pulmonary or skin disease, adults, and pregnant women during the third trimester. The fetal varicella syndrome, which occurs in fetuses infected during the first trimester, is characterized by atrophy of limbs with scarring of skin, chorioretinitis or cataracts, and central nervous system abnormalities. Patients with AIDS and moderately reduced CD4 cell counts may develop recurrent varicella lesions in the absence of new exposures, and patients with CD4 cell counts below 200/μL may develop progressive varicella with new lesions occurring for at least 1 month or chronic verrucous lesions.

Zoster

In healthy persons, zoster presents with localized pain and increased sensation for 1 to 3 days before the development of a dermatomal vesicular rash

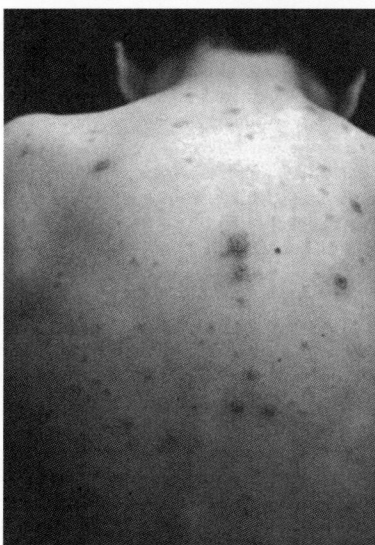

FIGURE 375-1. Child with varicella. (Courtesy of Centers for Disease Control and Prevention.)

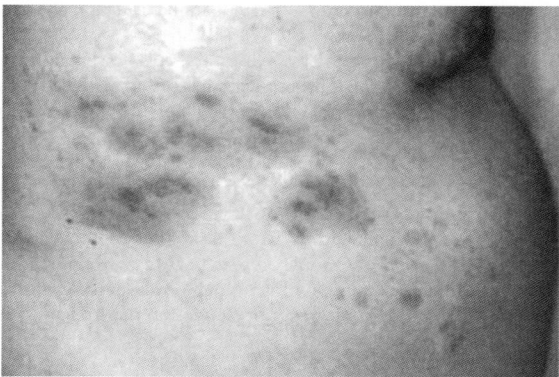

FIGURE 375-2. Dermatomal zoster. (Courtesy of Centers for Disease Control and Prevention.)

that does not cross the midline (Fig. 375-2). Zoster most frequently presents in the dermatomes innervated by trigeminal or thoracic ganglia. The rash is usually accompanied by itching, tingling, or pain. The lesions evolve from vesicles to pustules, and crusting is usually complete by 10 days. In normal hosts, a few lesions may develop outside of the dermatome owing to low-grade viremia. Some patients with zoster sine herpete never develop a rash. In persons with very impaired cellular immunity, reactivation is often associated with high-grade viremia with dissemination to large areas of the skin and involvement of multiple organs. As a result, patients with underlying malignancies are more likely to develop more serious complications from their zoster infections.[3]

A dreaded complication of zoster is post-herpetic neuralgia (Chapter 30) with pain persisting for at least 1 month after the rash has resolved. Patients may have allodynia (sensation of pain after nonpainful stimuli), paresthesias, dysesthesias, or severe neuropathic pain. Post-herpetic neuralgia is more common in persons older than 50 years. Other complications of zoster include bacterial superinfection; ocular disease, involving any of the structures of the eye, due to reactivation in the ophthalmic branch of the trigeminal ganglia; facial palsy caused by reactivation in the VII cranial nerve; Ramsay Hunt syndrome, with pain and vesicles in the ear, numbness of the anterior tongue, and ipsilateral facial palsy due to reactivation in the geniculate ganglion of the VII cranial nerve; motor neuropathy; and meningitis. Zoster vasculopathy, occurring at the time of zoster or a few months later, can present with stroke due to inflammation of the cerebral arteries.

Progressive outer retinal necrosis, with few inflammatory ocular cells, occurs when VZV reactivates in the eye of severely immunocompromised persons, including patients with AIDS and low CD4 cell counts. In contrast, acute retinal necrosis with a marked inflammatory response occurs when the virus reactivates in otherwise healthy persons. Patients with AIDS or recipients of hematopoietic stem cell transplants can have pancreatitis, hepatitis, and pneumonitis in the absence of or preceding a rash.

DIAGNOSIS

Most cases of varicella and zoster are diagnosed on the basis of their clinical presentation. A disseminated vesicular rash with lesions in various stages of evolution is usually sufficient for a diagnosis of varicella. The differential diagnosis includes impetigo (Chapter 441), enterovirus infections (Chapter 379), herpes simplex (Chapter 374), Stevens-Johnson syndrome (Chapter 440), and guttate psoriasis (Chapter 438). A dermatomal vesicular rash that does not cross the midline in a patient with a prior history of pain in the area is usually diagnostic of zoster. Herpes simplex is the most common disease that resembles zoster.

When the diagnosis of varicella or zoster must be confirmed definitively, polymerase chain reaction (PCR) for VZV from vesicular fluid is the most sensitive and specific test. PCR for VZV in the blood can be useful for diagnosis of visceral zoster in highly immunocompromised persons before the onset of rash. PCR for VZV in the cerebrospinal fluid and intrathecal synthesis of VZV-specific antibody is useful for diagnosis of VZV neurologic diseases. Culture is less sensitive than PCR because the virus is very labile. Direct fluorescent antibody testing of vesicle fluid is rapid but less sensitive than PCR. Detection of multinucleated giant cells (Tzanck smear) is less specific because lesions of herpes simplex virus have a similar appearance. Biopsy specimens show eosinophilic intranuclear inclusion bodies and multinucleate giant cells.

Serology for VZV is useful to determine the need for postexposure prophylaxis in persons who are at high risk for disease after exposure to varicella or zoster. Enzyme-linked immunosorbent assay tests are less sensitive than latex agglutination assays and may not detect antibodies in vaccinees.

TREATMENT   Rx

Varicella

Symptomatic treatment includes acetaminophen for fever and lotion or baths for pruritus. Although acyclovir is licensed for the treatment of varicella, the drug is not recommended for otherwise healthy children because it only modestly decreases symptoms by about 1 day.[A1] Acyclovir reduces visceral dissemination in immunocompromised persons, in whom intravenous acyclovir (500 mg/m² every 8 hours for children, 10 mg/kg every 8 hours for adults) is recommended for 7 to 10 days or until all lesions have crusted. Oral acyclovir (20 mg/kg four times daily for children or 800 mg five times daily for adults) given within 24 hours after the onset of rash reduces the duration of symptoms and is recommended for treatment of adolescents, adults, newborns whose mothers developed varicella near the time of delivery, immunocompromised persons, children with chronic pulmonary or skin disease, and persons with complications of varicella. Acyclovir also should be considered for household contacts of persons with varicella or for pregnant women in the third trimester; these patients often have more severe disease. Oral valacyclovir is also approved for treatment of children ages 2 years to <18 years with varicella (20 mg/kg three times daily with a maximum dose of 1 g). Oral valacyclovir, 1 g three times daily, or famciclovir, 500 mg three times daily result in higher antiviral drug levels than does oral acyclovir and can be used in nonpregnant adults.

Zoster

Acyclovir, valacyclovir, and famciclovir (for 7 days at the same doses as for varicella) are licensed for the treatment of zoster. Oral valacyclovir and famciclovir result in higher levels of antiviral activity than oral acyclovir does. Although therapy should be started within 3 days of the rash, therapy may still be of benefit if new lesions continue to occur after this time. Because patients younger than 50 years usually have little pain associated with zoster, antiviral therapy is often not used in these patients unless they have moderate to severe pain, have disease involving the eye, have other complications, or are immunocompromised. Antiviral drugs (see earlier) reduce the duration of lesions and zoster-associated pain but not the incidence of post-herpetic neuralgia.[A2] In severely immunocompromised persons, intravenous acyclovir (7 to 10 days or until all lesions have crusted) reduces the risk for visceral dissemination. Oral valacyclovir or famciclovir may be used in persons who are less severely immunocompromised.

Corticosteroids (e.g., prednisone, 60 mg/day and tapered over 21 days), in combination with acyclovir, reduce acute pain and improve the quality of life in persons older than 50 years but do not reduce the risk for post-herpetic neuralgia. Patients with moderate to severe pain often require narcotics.

Treatment of post-herpetic neuralgia is challenging.[4] Gabapentin (initiated at a dose of 300 mg at bedtime and titrated to a maximum dose of 1200 mg three times daily) or pregabalin (initiated at a dose of 75 mg at bedtime and titrated to a maximum dose of 300 mg twice daily) may reduce pain. Additional agents include nortriptyline (initiated at a dose of 25 mg at bedtime and titrated to a maximum dose of 150 mg daily), lidocaine patches, and topical capsaicin (which itself causes pain that is not tolerated in up to one third of patients). Opioid analgesics (see Table 30-5) may be needed, but there are concerns about long-term efficacy and safety.

Treatment of VZV Complications and Acyclovir-Resistant VZV

Intravenous acyclovir is recommended for persons with acute retinal necrosis. Corticosteroids (e.g., prednisone, 1 mg/kg per day for 3 to 5 days) and intravenous acyclovir (10 to 15 mg/kg every 8 hours for 14 days) are recommended for nonimmunocompromised persons with VZV vasculopathy. Zoster involving the eye should be evaluated by an ophthalmologist to assess the potential value of topical or intraocular therapy, such as the need to reduce intraocular pressure to treat glaucoma or to use mydriatics to prevent synechiae.

Acyclovir-resistant VZV infections are rare and are limited almost exclusively to patients with AIDS or recipients of transplants. Foscarnet (40 mg/kg every 8 hours) for 2 weeks or until all lesions have crusted is the treatment of choice for acyclovir-resistant VZV.

PREVENTION

Varicella

Patients with varicella or zoster are considered infectious until all lesions have completely crusted. Airborne and contact precautions are recommended for varicella, whereas only contact precautions are necessary for immunocompetent persons with localized zoster.

The live attenuated varicella vaccine is recommended for children aged 1 to 12 years and for persons 13 years and older without immunity to the virus. The vaccine is 75 to 90% effective in protection against symptomatic varicella and more than 95% effective in protecting against severe disease.[A3] Two doses of vaccine are given subcutaneously. The varicella vaccine is also given as part of a combined measles, mumps, rubella vaccine (MMRV) for children 1 to 12 years of age in the United States. The rate of disease due to varicella declined by 90% in the United States during the first 13 years after the vaccine was licensed.[5]

The most common complications of varicella vaccination are pain at the injection site, fever, and a mild rash within 2 weeks after vaccination. The rash is usually localized to the area of vaccination and is often papular; in some healthy persons, the rash can be disseminated, although there are fewer lesions and symptoms are much less severe than with wild-type virus. In persons with severely impaired cellular immunity, rash is more common, can be extensive, and may be accompanied by organ dysfunction. The varicella vaccine establishes latency and can cause shingles, although this complication occurs less commonly with vaccine virus than with wild-type virus. The vaccine strain of varicella has been transmitted to third parties only by vaccinees who developed a rash. Varicella vaccine is contraindicated in pregnant women and persons receiving high-dose immunosuppressive therapy (e.g., ≥2 mg/kg of prednisone daily) or with hematologic malignant neoplasms. Vaccination should be considered for human immunodeficiency virus (HIV)–infected children with age-specific CD4+ T cells of 15% or more and adolescents and adults with CD4+ T-cell counts of 200 cells/μL or higher. Serologic testing to verify immunity is not recommended for health care workers who have received two doses of vaccine because the currently available commercial antibody assays are not sensitive enough to detect protective levels of antibody.

Zoster

Zoster vaccine is approved by the U.S. Food and Drug Administration (FDA) for persons 50 years of age or older[A4] and recommended by the Advisory Committee on Immunization Practices for persons 60 years of age or older (Chapter 18). This vaccine is similar to the varicella vaccine, except that the titer of virus is about 14-fold higher. The vaccine is about 50% protective in preventing zoster and 66% effective in preventing post-herpetic neuralgia.[6] Although the vaccine's efficacy to prevent zoster declines in persons older than 70 years, efficacy to prevent post-herpetic neuralgia does not decline.[A5] Transient pain and erythema at the injection site are not uncommon, but serious complications attributable to the vaccine have not been reported. The

vaccine also can be given safely to adults with a prior history of zoster.[7] The vaccine is contraindicated in persons with hematologic malignant neoplasms, AIDS, or HIV infection with CD4 count of 200/μL or lower and in persons receiving high-dose immunosuppressive therapy (e.g., ≥20 mg of prednisone daily) or anti–tumor necrosis factor-α therapy.

Postexposure Prophylaxis

In persons exposed to varicella, three options are available. Varicella vaccine is preferred if exposure occurred within the prior 3 days and the patient is not immunocompromised.[A6] Vaccine is estimated to be 70 to 90% effective in healthy persons. VariZIG (formerly available as varicella immune globulin) prevents or attenuates varicella in 90% of susceptible persons if it is given within 4 days of exposure. The FDA recently approved VariZIG for use within 10 days of exposure, but it should be given as soon as possible after exposure.[8] VariZIG (given intramuscularly at 125 units/10 kg body weight, up to a maximum of 625 units) is indicated for susceptible persons at risk for severe varicella (e.g., pregnant women, preterm infants, neonates whose mothers have varicella between 5 days before and 2 days after delivery, immunocompromised persons) who are in close contact with patients with varicella or zoster. VariZIG has no effect in the treatment of zoster.

Oral acyclovir (40 to 80 mg/kg for 1 week beginning 7 to 9 days after exposure) is estimated to be 80 to 85% effective as postexposure prophylaxis. It is often used when the exposure occurred too long ago for vaccination or VariZIG.

PROGNOSIS

Before vaccination, about 100 children died of varicella each year in the United States. Now varicella is the underlying cause of death in an average of less than 3 Americans younger than 20 years annually.

Grade A References

A1. Klassen TP, Hartling L, Wiebe N, et al. Acyclovir for treating varicella in otherwise healthy children and adolescents. *Cochrane Database Syst Rev.* 2005;4:CD002980.

A2. Chen N, Li Q, Yang J, et al. Antiviral treatment for preventing postherpetic neuralgia. *Cochrane Database Syst Rev.* 2014;2:CD006866.

A3. Committee on Infectious Diseases. Policy statement. Prevention of varicella: update of recommendations for use of quadrivalent and monovalent varicella vaccines in children. *Pediatrics.* 2011;128:630-632.

A4. Schmader KE, Levin MJ, Gnann JW Jr, et al. Efficacy, safety, and tolerability of herpes zoster vaccine in persons aged 50-59 years. *Clin Infect Dis.* 2012;54:922-928.

A5. Gagliardi AM, Gomes Silva BN, Torloni MR, et al. Vaccines for preventing herpes zoster in older adults. *Cochrane Database Syst Rev.* 2012;10:CD008858.

A6. Macartney K, McIntyre P. Vaccines for post-exposure prophylaxis against varicella (chickenpox) in children and adults. *Cochrane Database Syst Rev.* 2014;6:CD001833.

GENERAL REFERENCES

For the General References and other additional features, please visit Expert Consult at https://expertconsult.inkling.com.

376

CYTOMEGALOVIRUS

W. LAWRENCE DREW

DEFINITION

Cytomegalovirus (CMV) is a member of the herpesvirus family and shares, with the other members, the ability to establish a long-lived latent infection. Most of the clinical disease caused by this virus results from reactivation of latent virus in immune-impaired patients, although primary infection in such patients can also be devastating.

The Pathogen

CMV has a linear, double-stranded DNA genome with about 250,000 base pairs that encode about 160 proteins. On microscopic examination, the hallmark of CMV infection is a large (cytomegalic), 25- to 35-μm cell containing

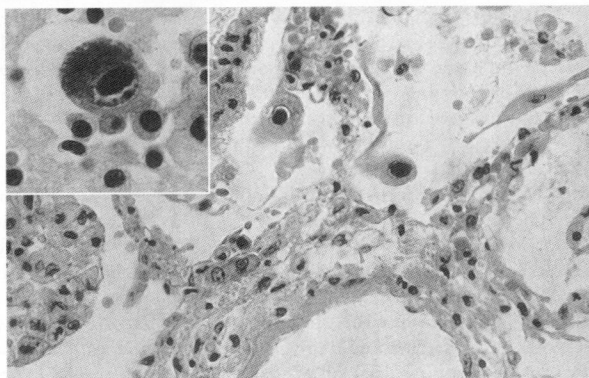

FIGURE 376-1. Cytomegalovirus (CMV) pneumonia. A lung biopsy specimen was stained with hematoxylin and eosin and magnified 250-fold. The *inset* shows a CMV "owl's eye" inclusion.

a large central, basophilic intranuclear inclusion (Fig. 376-1), referred to as an owl's eye.

EPIDEMIOLOGY

Multiple mechanisms account for the spread of this virus, including vertical (in utero, during vaginal delivery, and by breast milk) and horizontal (saliva, genital, urine) contact. These routes of transmission lead, collectively, to a 15 to 20% seroprevalence by 15 years of age in developed countries, with a higher seroprevalence in lower socioeconomic settings.[1] From that age on, there is a steady upward trend of 1 to 2% per year that is due in part to sexual transmission. As a result, approximately 50% of the general population of the United States is antibody positive by 35 years of age, and a 1% per year rate of increase occurs thereafter. In underdeveloped countries, up to 90% of persons may be seropositive by 2 years of age. Presumably, crowded living conditions permit spread of the virus through close contact with body fluids. A recent study showed that CMV was viable on metal and wood for up to 1 hour, glass and plastic to 3 hours, and rubber, cloth, and crackers to 6 hours.[2] CMV was more likely to be isolated from wet, highly absorbent surfaces. These considerations were felt to be particularly important because children may actively shed CMV in saliva and urine for months to years, and exposure to bodily fluids from young children poses substantial risk for CMV exposure among women of reproductive age. Two additional mechanisms of transmission are blood transfusion and organ transplantation. A final important epidemiologic fact is that reinfection with a different strain of CMV may occur in CMV-seropositive persons, especially those who are immunocompromised, pregnant, or sexually promiscuous.

PATHOBIOLOGY

In fully immunocompetent individuals, CMV rarely causes clinically evident end-organ disease. When immune mechanisms are deficient, especially those mediated by CD4+ and CD8+ lymphocytes, latent virus replicates and causes both direct and indirect effects.[3] Examples of direct virally mediated diseases are necrotizing CMV retinitis and esophagitis. In contrast, CMV pneumonitis is frequently manifested as subtle histologic alterations accompanied by limited viral replication, thus suggesting that immune-mediated injury may be the primary pathologic mechanism. Such injury may result from the upregulation and release of cytokines, including tumor necrosis factor-α, interferon-γ, and interleukin-2. Immune-mediated tissue injury may also be effected by CD8+ cytotoxic T lymphocytes directed against CMV-infected target cells. The clinical manifestations of CMV infection, including meningoencephalitis, retinitis, enteritis, vasculitis, pneumonitis, myocarditis, lymphadenitis, hepatitis, adrenalitis, and pancreatitis, reflect the range of cell types that CMV is capable of infecting.

The immune response to CMV infection involves both the humoral and cell-mediated arms, but the CD8+ cytotoxic T-cell response appears to be the most important. The CMV envelope glycoproteins that participate in viral entry are gB, gH/gL, and gCII. Humoral immunity directed at gB has been detected in convalescent phase sera and has been shown to block viral entry, cell-to-cell transmission, and syncytium formation in CMV-infected cells.

Fundamental to the pathogenesis of CMV is latency, or persistence of the viral genome in host cells without evidence of productive viral replication. It is thought that monocytes and bone marrow progenitor cells are sites of human CMV latency. Reactivation from the latent state has classically been associated with immunosuppression. Exposure to a rich milieu of cytokines and growth factors results in the activation of signal transduction pathways, generation of increased levels of intracellular transcription factors, and production of viable virus.

CLINICAL MANIFESTATIONS
Congenital and Neonatal Infection

In the developed world, congenital infection occurs in approximately 0.2 to 0.7% of newborns.[4] Thus in the United States each year, approximately 40,000 infants are born excreting CMV, and about 4000 (or ~10%) of these newborns show clinical evidence of congenital disease, such as microcephaly, intracerebral calcification, hepatosplenomegaly, and rash. About 90% of these clinically infected newborns will survive, but half of the survivors will have unilateral or bilateral hearing loss, mental retardation, or both. Mothers of most infants with these stigmata had a primary infection during pregnancy, although it is now well known that clinically evident congenital infection also occurs in infants born to mothers with past as well as with primary CMV infection.

Infection in Immunocompetent Persons

Virtually all CMV infections occurring in immunocompetent persons are asymptomatic. In some patients, a clinical illness resembling infectious mononucleosis may develop (Chapter 377), but with minimal pharyngitis and lymphadenopathy. Atypical lymphocytosis develops in these patients, similar to Epstein-Barr virus infection, but they have a negative heterophil antibody test result. CMV reactivation is common (33%) in critically ill immunocompetent patients, in whom it is associated with prolonged hospitalization and mortality, but whether it causes these effects is unclear.

Infection in Transplant Recipients

When a CMV-seronegative recipient receives a solid organ from a CMV-seropositive donor, the resulting illnesses include the "CMV syndrome," characterized by fever, neutropenia, atypical lymphocytes, and often hepatosplenomegaly. CMV disease may also develop in the transplanted organ. For example, CMV hepatitis in liver transplant recipients is associated with fever, hyperbilirubinemia, and elevated liver enzymes; liver failure may ensue and necessitate retransplantation. CMV-seropositive recipients of a solid organ transplant may develop CMV disease by either reactivation of latent infection or by transmission of CMV from a seropositive donor. Disease in CMV-seropositive recipients is, fortunately, less severe than that resulting from primary infection. CMV infection occurs more commonly in recipients of lung or liver transplants than in recipients of kidney transplants.

CMV pneumonia may occur after solid organ transplantation but is most common after stem cell transplantation. Fever, nonproductive cough, and dyspnea can progress rapidly. The diagnosis is suggested by interstitial to nodular infiltrates rather than by alveolar densities on chest radiographs. In contrast to solid organ transplantation, CMV disease after stem cell transplantation usually results from reactivation of latent CMV in a seropositive recipient rather than from a new, primary infection.

CMV may cause disease throughout the gastrointestinal tract. Colitis, which is a common syndrome in transplant recipients, is manifested as diarrhea, weight loss, and fever. It is characterized by diffuse submucosal hemorrhages and ulcerations.

Infection in Patients with Acquired Immunodeficiency Syndrome

In the era before highly active antiretroviral therapy, CMV retinitis occurred in approximately one third of patients with acquired immunodeficiency syndrome (AIDS), most often in those with CD4 counts below 50/mm³. It usually begins unilaterally with visual blurring, floaters, decreased acuity, and loss of visual fields and progresses to blindness if it is untreated. The retinal examination is abnormal, and the finding of apparent hemorrhages and exudates is the best diagnostic test (Fig. 376-2). CMV colitis is similar to that seen in transplant recipients, but esophagitis is also common and characterized by distal ulceration, which may be single but extensive. CMV neurologic disease occurs in multiple forms, including encephalitis and a polyradiculopathy/myelitis syndrome. With the efficacy of combination antiretroviral therapy, the incidence of all of these CMV syndromes has decreased dramatically, but they are still seen before HIV treatment or when such treatment is interrupted or ineffective.

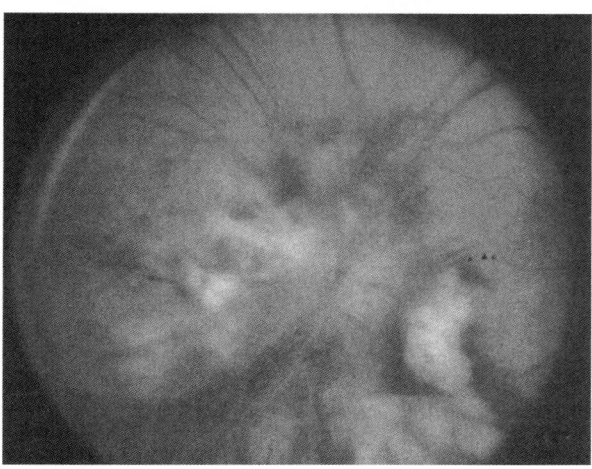

FIGURE 376-2. Cytomegalovirus retinitis as seen by direct ophthalmoscopic examination.

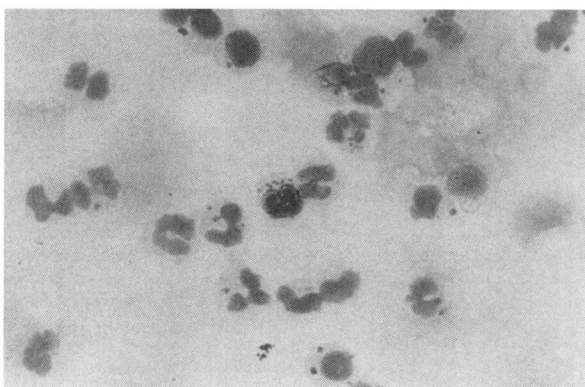

FIGURE 376-3. Peripheral blood leukocytes stained with monoclonal antibody to cytomegalovirus pp65 antigen by the immunoperoxidase technique (magnification ×500).

DIAGNOSIS

Assay of viral DNA by the polymerase chain reaction (PCR) is more sensitive than viral culture and is the best assay for the early detection of CMV disease. The assay can quantify the CMV viremia and thereby help to determine its clinical significance and to monitor therapy. Monoclonal antibodies can also be used to quantify viremia by counting CMV antigen–positive cells directly in peripheral blood leukocytes (antigenemia) (Fig. 376-3).

Seroconversion is an excellent marker for primary CMV infection, but increases in immunoglobulin G (IgG) titers, even four-fold or greater, are not diagnostic of newly acquired infection. CMV-specific IgM antibody develops during primary infection but may reappear during reactivation of latent CMV. The presence of IgG antibody is a sensitive marker of past infection and is used to screen transplant recipients and donors as well as certain blood product recipients and donors. An avidity assay can help in determining whether an infection is recent.

Viral culture, which was the prior "gold standard" for diagnosing CMV, has been supplanted by the assays described previously. Routine culture may require at least 4 to 6 weeks, whereas newer methods incorporating immunofluorescence can yield results in several days. The clinical significance of positive CMV cultures may be difficult to ascertain, particularly in immunosuppressed patients. For example, CMV may be present in the saliva or urine of up to 60 to 90% of transplant recipients and patients with AIDS, and virus in these sites does not prove that CMV is the cause of a patient's illness. Cytologic and histologic abnormalities are not sensitive measures of CMV infection, but they are specific and indicative of CMV disease.

PREVENTION

A nonviable CMV vaccine, containing the gB antigen, decreases primary infection in young women by 50% but is not commercially available. Other vaccine candidates are being developed but remain experimental.

Because CMV is transmitted by exchange of secretions or excretions, infection can be diminished by reducing exposure to body fluids. For example, transmission by both vaginal and anal intercourse, which are bidirectional risks, can be diminished by "safe sex." Similarly, limiting the contact of seronegative pregnant women with the secretions and excretions of children, especially preschoolers in daycare, can decrease primary infection and, in turn, congenital disease.

The risk for acquiring CMV disease can be reduced in seronegative, immunosuppressed patients through the use of blood products or organ grafts from CMV-seronegative donors. Valganciclovir and ganciclovir provide effective prophylaxis in solid organ transplantation.[A1][A2],5 Prophylaxis has been uncommon for stem cell transplant recipients, and these patients typically have been monitored weekly (from day 10 to day 100 after transplantation) for CMV DNA or antigenemia, with antiviral therapy introduced preemptively if seroconversion occurs or PCR testing is positive.[A3] With this strategy, infection is not prevented, but end-organ disease is avoided. However, late-onset CMV end-organ disease may occur when the antiviral is eventually discontinued.[6] More recently, letermovir, a CMV terminase substitute, at a dose of 120 mg or 240 mg daily has been shown to reduce the incidence of CMV infection in such patients.[A4] CMV-specific hyperimmune globulin (CMVIG) may be effective in treating pregnant women with primary CMV infection and preventing congenital infection, but controlled trials are needed. CMVIG has also been used prophylactically in high-risk seronegative organ transplant recipients, in whom it reduced CMV disease and CMV mortality. It is very expensive, however, and antivirals are more commonly used alternatives.

TREATMENT ℞

Oral valganciclovir, intravenous ganciclovir, intravenous ganciclovir followed by oral valganciclovir, intravenous foscarnet, intravenous cidofovir, and ganciclovir intraocular injection coupled with valganciclovir are all effective treatments of CMV syndromes (Table 376-1).

Ganciclovir (dihydroxypropoxymethylguanosine [DHPG], Cytovene) is given intravenously, 5 mg/kg two times daily during initial induction (2 to 3 weeks); maintenance therapy consists of 5 mg/kg once daily (Chapter 360). Valganciclovir achieves levels comparable to intravenous ganciclovir at 5 mg/kg when it is given orally in a 900-mg dose. Initial response in retinitis (improvement or stabilization of vision or ophthalmoscopic appearance) occurs in approximately 75% of patients treated with ganciclovir or valganciclovir.[A5] CMV retinitis can also be treated locally by intraocular ganciclovir injection, but this approach should be accompanied by valganciclovir to treat and/or prevent extraocular end-organ disease. Ganciclovir together with CMV hyperimmune globulin may reduce the mortality of CMV pneumonia after stem cell transplantation from approximately 85 to 40%, although the benefit of the antibody is unproved. Ganciclovir resistance may occur as a result of mutations in the phosphorylating gene (*UL97*) and/or in the DNA polymerase gene (*UL54*).[7] Granulocyte colony-stimulating factor may be needed to offset neutropenia.

Foscarnet, or phosphonoformic acid, blocks the pyrophosphate-binding site of viral DNA polymerase, thereby preventing cleavage of pyrophosphate from deoxyadenosine triphosphate. The recommended initial therapy with foscarnet is 60 mg/kg intravenously every 8 hours or 90 mg/kg every 12 hours. The maintenance dose ranges from 90 to 120 mg/kg daily. Adverse effects include renal impairment, anemia, hypocalcemia (especially ionized calcium), hypomagnesemia, and hypophosphatemia. Resistance to foscarnet can develop because of mutations in DNA polymerase. Although it is effective for treating CMV retinitis, its toxicity and the absence of an oral formulation make foscarnet a second choice for treatment of CMV disease. It is sometimes used in combination with ganciclovir for infections such as central nervous system disease or for treatment of ganciclovir-resistant virus.[8]

Cidofovir, or 3-hydroxy-2-phosphonomethoxypropyl cytosine (HPMPC), appears to the cell as a nucleotide and does not require phosphorylation by virus-encoded enzyme. It is therefore active against ganciclovir-resistant CMV strains that have resistance mutations only in *UL97*, the phosphorylating gene. When DNA polymerase (*UL54*) mutations occur in ganciclovir-treated patients, cross-resistance to cidofovir is frequent. These resistance mutations also occur in patients treated with cidofovir alone. The drug has an extremely long half-life that permits intravenous administration as infrequently as every 2 weeks during maintenance treatment.

Cidofovir is nephrotoxic, especially to the proximal renal tubule, but this side effect appears to be diminished by prehydration and concomitant probenecid therapy. Cidofovir toxicities make it a second- or third-line agent for CMV. Other drugs under investigation include brincidofovir, maribavir, and letermovir.[9]

TABLE 376-1	TREATMENT OF CYTOMEGALOVIRUS INFECTION	
	PREFERRED THERAPY	**ALTERNATIVE THERAPY**
Cytomegalovirus (CMV) retinitis* Sight-threatening lesions	Valganciclovir 900 mg bid PO plus ganciclovir intraocular injection	Ganciclovir IV; foscarnet IV; plus ganciclovir intraocular injection
Peripheral lesions	Valganciclovir 900 mg bid PO	Ganciclovir IV or foscarnet IV
Maintenance therapy	Valganciclovir 900 mg od PO	Ganciclovir IV or foscarnet IV
Relapsing	Reinduction with ganciclovir IV or valganciclovir 900 mg bid PO ± ganciclovir intraocular injection	
Ganciclovir resistant	Foscarnet IV ± ganciclovir intraocular injection	Cidofovir (if only UL97 mutation)
CMV gastrointestinal disease	Ganciclovir IV for 3-6 wk or valganciclovir 900 mg bid PO for 3-6 wk	Foscarnet IV for 3-6 wk
CMV neurologic disease	Ganciclovir IV + foscarnet IV	
CMV viremia syndrome	Valganciclovir 900 mg bid PO or ganciclovir IV until viremia clears	Foscarnet IV
Ganciclovir resistant	Foscarnet IV	

*If not already begun, antiretroviral therapy should be initiated concurrently with anti-CMV therapy, except possibly when treating central nervous system disease. For retinitis, anti-CMV therapy should be continued until the CD4 count has exceeded 100-150 cells/mm^3 for ≥6 months and the retinitis is inactive. If anti-CMV therapy is discontinued, regular monthly eye examinations should be continued. Early relapses of CMV retinitis in patients treated systemically are usually due to inadequate drug penetration, and reinduction with the same drug is often effective. Drug resistance may occur in patients treated for ≥3 months. Therapy of these patients may be guided by antiviral susceptibility testing.
Adapted from Drew WL, Erlich KS. Management of herpesvirus infections (cytomegalovirus, herpes simplex virus, and varicella-zoster virus). In: Volberding PA, Greene WC , Lange J, et al, eds. *HIV/AIDS Medicine Medical Management of AIDS 2012*. Philadelphia: Saunders Elsevier; 2012:433.

PROGNOSIS

In immunocompetent patients, the mononucleosis-like CMV syndrome resolves spontaneously. Infections in immunocompromised patients are much more serious and may result in failure of a transplanted solid organ and/or systemic CMV disease. For CMV pneumonia, death often occurs even with antiviral therapy, especially after stem cell transplantation. In AIDS patients, CMV infection generally resolves when CD4 counts exceed 100/mm^3, but it is a grave prognostic sign if counts do not recover to those levels.

Grade A References

A1. Hodson EM, Ladhani M, Webster AC, et al. Antiviral medications for preventing cytomegalovirus disease in solid organ transplant recipients. *Cochrane Database Syst Rev*. 2013;2:CD003774.
A2. Owers DS, Webster AC, Strippoli GF, et al. Pre-emptive treatment for cytomegalovirus viraemia to prevent cytomegalovirus disease in solid organ transplant recipients. *Cochrane Database Syst Rev*. 2013;2:CD005133.
A3. Boeckh M, Nichols WG, Chemaly RF, et al. Valganciclovir for the prevention of complications of late cytomegalovirus infection after allogeneic hematopoietic cell transplantation: a randomized trial. *Ann Intern Med*. 2015;162:1-10.
A4. Chemaly RF, Ullmann AJ, Stoelben S, et al. Letermovir for cytomegalovirus prophylaxis in hematopoietic-cell transplantation. *N Engl J Med*. 2014;370:1781-1789.
A5. Martin DF, Sierra-Madero J, Walmsley S, et al. A controlled trial of valganciclovir as induction therapy for cytomegalovirus retinitis. *N Engl J Med*. 2002;346:1119-1126.

GENERAL REFERENCES

For the General References and other additional features, please visit Expert Consult at https://expertconsult.inkling.com.

377

EPSTEIN-BARR VIRUS INFECTION

ROBERT T. SCHOOLEY

DEFINITION

Epstein-Barr virus (EBV), a member of the gamma human herpesvirus family, is the etiologic agent of infectious mononucleosis and of a diverse assortment of neoplastic syndromes.

EPIDEMIOLOGY

Ubiquitous in the human population, EBV is found in 90 to 95% of adults throughout the world. As in the case of other herpesviruses, infection with EBV is lifelong. The virus resides in B lymphocytes and is intermittently shed asymptomatically in oropharyngeal secretions, which accounts for the bulk of its transmission in the human population. The virus is not highly contagious; it is usually acquired during early childhood through sharing of saliva-bearing fomites or during adolescence through kissing, although it can be acquired at any decade of life. Thus, for example, EBV-seronegative platonic roommates of patients with acute infectious mononucleosis in college dormitory settings are not at higher risk for acquiring the virus than others in the college population. In addition to oropharyngeal spread, the virus can be transmitted by blood transfusion or through organ donation.

Most childhood EBV infections are clinically silent, but infection of adolescents and adults results in the clinical syndrome of infectious mononucleosis between 25 and 50% of the time, depending on the setting. The incidence of infectious mononucleosis is highest in the 15- to 24-year-old age group. Incidence rates in men and women are equal, but the peak incidence is 2 years earlier in women than in men. Incidence rates are lower in lower socioeconomic populations, in whom the likelihood of acquisition is greater in childhood than in adolescence.

PATHOBIOLOGY

EBV enters B lymphocytes through the CD21 molecule (also known as the C3d receptor) on the surface of B cells or nasopharyngeal epithelial cells. Major histocompatibility complex class II molecules serve as secondary receptors on B cells. Once inside the cell, the virus expresses several nuclear proteins (termed Epstein-Barr nuclear antigens [EBNAs]) that activate EBV-encoded latent membrane proteins and other gene products responsible for regulation of B-cell growth. These events are associated with the transformation or immortalization of the B cell that is the phenotypic hallmark of B-cell infection. EBV-transformed B cells proliferate vigorously and maintain EBV DNA within progeny cell nuclei in an episomal state. During acute EBV infection, up to 20% of peripheral blood B cells express EBNA.

The host response to acute EBV infection consists of a vigorous and coordinated cellular and humoral immune response. The humoral immune response includes IgM and IgG antibodies directed at the viral capsid (VCA) and to EBNA, as well as *heterophile* antibodies to surface antigens of sheep red blood cells. Heterophile antibodies are useful diagnostically and are present at some point in up to 90% of cases. These antibodies are an epiphenomenon in host defense and are not cross-reactive with any known viral antigens.

The cellular immune response includes both natural killer (NK) and EBV-specific CD4$^+$ and CD8$^+$ T lymphocytes. The expansion of the CD8$^+$ subset of T lymphocytes during acute EBV infection includes a subset of large, activated cells demonstrable on standard peripheral blood smears as "atypical" lymphocytes. This vigorous cellular immune response is associated with an outpouring of cytokines, including tumor necrosis factor, interleukin-1, and interleukin-6, that are responsible for many of the symptoms and signs of infectious mononucleosis. Over a period of 4 to 6 weeks after initial evaluation in most patients, immune response mechanisms gain control of the EBV-driven B-cell proliferation, and the virus enters into a lifelong period of symbiosis with the host. The virus is asymptomatically shed approximately 15% of the time in the oropharyngeal fluids of healthy human immunodeficiency virus type 1 (HIV-1)-seronegative adolescents and adults. The shedding rate increases significantly in patients with defects in cellular immunity, such as those that occur with HIV-1 infection or immunosuppression associated with organ allografts.

CLINICAL MANIFESTATIONS

Most cases of acute EBV infection are clinically silent. The syndrome of infectious mononucleosis consists of the clinical triad of fever, sore throat (Chapter 429), and lymphadenopathy, in association with an atypical lymphocytosis and the transient appearance of heterophile antibodies. The incubation period between exposure and the onset of symptoms is generally 30 to 50 days. The onset of symptoms may be abrupt, or it may be heralded by a several-day nonspecific prodrome of malaise and low-grade fever. Although the classic syndrome includes fever, sore throat, and adenopathy, the findings may be dominated by only one or any combination of these symptoms. Other common clinical manifestations include headache, malaise, and anorexia. On physical examination, patients are usually febrile. Pharyngeal erythema, tonsillar enlargement (see Fig. 429-5 in Chapter 429), and cervical adenopathy are generally present. Mild periorbital edema may also be observed. Abdominal findings may include splenomegaly or hepatomegaly, or both. Splenomegaly can be demonstrated by ultrasonographic examination in virtually all patients with infectious mononucleosis, although palpable splenomegaly is only present in about 20% of patients. Splenic enlargement is usually maximal in the second or third week of illness and might not be detectable at the initial presentation. Adenopathy may be observed in noncervical regions, but it is usually much less prominent than in cervical regions. Approximately 5% of patients will exhibit a rash that may be macular, scarlatiniform, or urticarial in nature. If patients with acute EBV infection are given ampicillin or its derivatives, a pruritic maculopapular eruption will develop in 90 to 100% of them. Patients with an ampicillin-induced rash during acute EBV infection generally tolerate the drug and other penicillin products when administered later in life.

DIAGNOSIS

Because clinical manifestations of acute EBV infection are variable and other organisms may cause similar clinical syndromes, laboratory tools are required to confirm an etiologic diagnosis. Heterophile antibodies to sheep red blood cells are classically used to diagnosis EBV-induced infectious mononucleosis. Although ultimately demonstrable in approximately 90% of symptomatic acute EBV infections, these antibodies are present in only about two thirds of patients at initial encounter. If antibodies are negative at the outset and clinical suspicion is high, repeat testing in the second or third week of the illness is warranted. Although EBV-specific antibodies remain the "gold standard" for the diagnosis of acute EBV infection, if heterophile antibodies are demonstrated in a straightforward case of infectious mononucleosis, it is not generally necessary to order EBV-specific serologic studies. IgM antibodies to the EBV capsid antigen (VCA) are the most useful serologic study in the diagnosis of acute EBV infection. Relatively high titers of IgG antibodies to VCA persist for life after initial infection and are not useful in making the diagnosis of acute EBV infection. Antibodies to EBNA are slower to arise than those to capsid antigens, and acute infection may be diagnosed by demonstration of seroconversion to this antigen. If the diagnosis is based on the emergence of antibodies to EBNA, both tests should be performed in the same laboratory.

Among pathogens causing clinical syndromes that can be mistaken for acute EBV infection, cytomegalovirus (Chapter 376) is the most frequent. Patients with cytomegalovirus infection are less likely to have an acute onset of illness, and pharyngitis is less frequently a prominent manifestation of the illness. *Toxoplasma gondii* (Chapter 349) infection can also present as a nonspecific febrile illness that can be confused with infectious mononucleosis. Streptococcal pharyngitis (Chapter 290) and primary herpes stomatitis (Chapter 374) may occasionally cause symptoms that are mistaken for acute EBV infection. None of these syndromes is associated with heterophile antibodies or with other serologic evidence of acute EBV infection. The differential diagnosis is generally made by serologic studies directed at these organisms or by culture. Nonetheless, physicians should be cognizant that organisms such as group A β-hemolytic streptococci (Chapter 290) and herpes simplex virus are also common in the human population and may be demonstrated in people whose symptoms are nonetheless due to acute EBV infection.

PREVENTION AND TREATMENT

Because the virus is usually transmitted by asymptomatic oral shedders and is so common in the human population, epidemiologic interventions to prevent spread are not practical. No vaccine yet has been developed. The clinical course is generally self-limited and does not usually require specific therapeutic intervention beyond the use of aspirin or acetaminophen for antipyresis and mild pain relief, except in the presence of specific complications such as when lymphadenopathy threatens the airway or in certain cases of autoimmune hemolytic anemia (Chapter 160) or thrombocytopenia (Chapter 172). Short courses of corticosteroids have been used to hasten symptomatic recovery in cases in which the symptoms are severe or refractory.[A1] Corticosteroids should not, however, be used routinely and should be given for no longer than a 10- to 14-day tapering course that begins at a dose equivalent of 0.5mg/kg of prednisone. Although EBV replication can be inhibited in vitro or in vivo by acyclovir and related antiviral agents, the symptoms of infectious mononucleosis are primarily driven by the immune response to the virus and come later than the time of maximal viral replication. Antiviral agents have not been demonstrated to significantly accelerate resolution of symptoms or prevent complications of the disease. One small randomized trial has reported 1-day reduction in length of hospital stay when patients with severe infectious mononucleosis are given metronidazole, but confirmatory data are required before this therapy becomes routine.[1]

PROGNOSIS

Most patients recover uneventfully from the acute symptoms and signs of infectious mononucleosis over a 2- to 3-week period, although many patients may have a variable period of malaise and fatigue that can last for another 3 to 4 weeks. Some patients may take longer to make a full recovery and experience fatigue and difficulty concentrating for up to 6 months after diagnosis. Symptoms often wax and wane and can be extremely troublesome. Reassurance is usually the best approach to these patients. Corticosteroids are not of benefit in this setting. Recovery may be less straightforward in patients with certain specific complications of acute EBV infection (outlined in the next section). Death from infectious mononucleosis is rare. When it does occur, it is most frequently associated with neurologic complications of the illness, splenic rupture, or the X-linked lymphoproliferative syndrome (discussed later).

Complications

Although most patients recover spontaneously from acute EBV infection, a number of complications may arise. In some patients, these complications dominate the clinical findings, and seroconversion to EBV may be the only evidence of acute EBV infection. The most serious complication of acute EBV infection arises in individuals with the X-linked lymphoproliferative syndrome. This syndrome occurs in males with mutations in the signaling lymphocyte activation molecule (SLAM)-associated protein (SAP) that regulates T and natural killer cells. These otherwise healthy individuals have severe clinical symptoms, a large lymphocytosis consisting of T and B cells, and severe hepatitis. If patients survive the acute infection, the syndrome may evolve into progressive agammaglobulinemia or lymphoma in the following months. The genetic defect associated with this syndrome can be diagnosed in utero, and early bone marrow transplantation has been recommended for the prevention of the devastating clinical syndrome associated with acquired EBV infection.

A number of less severe, organ system–specific complications are seen substantially more frequently than the X-linked lymphoproliferative syndrome. Patients should specifically be warned about splenic rupture, a complication attributable to splenomegaly (Chapter 168) and associated stretching of the splenic capsule that occurs most frequently in the second or third week of the illness, when other symptoms of the disease are abating. It may be accompanied by major or minor trauma but may also occur without an obvious antecedent event. Patients should be counseled against activities that might result in abdominal trauma for 6 to 8 weeks after the onset of symptoms. Left upper quadrant pain, especially pain radiating to the subscapular region, should raise this diagnostic consideration. As with other complications of acute EBV infection, splenic rupture may occur occasionally in patients without other prominent clinical manifestations of acute EBV infection. Other hematologic complications include autoimmune hemolytic anemia (Chapter 160), thrombocytopenia (Chapter 172), and neutropenia (Chapter 167). These complications usually arise from a combination of self-reactive antibodies and hypersplenism and are generally self-limited and resolve with resolution of the illness. Corticosteroids may be of benefit in more severe cases of autoimmune hemolytic anemia or thrombocytopenia.

A variety of neurologic syndromes are unusual complications of acute EBV infection. EBV DNA has been detected in brain tissue from rare patients with clinical manifestations compatible with herpes simplex encephalitis (Chapter 414). Although these patients have a much better prognosis than patients with herpes simplex encephalitis, they should receive parenteral acyclovir or ganciclovir as for herpes simplex (Chapters 360 and 414). Other neurologic complications include aseptic meningitis (Chapter 412), cerebellitis, mononeuritis multiplex (Chapter 420), Bell's palsy (Chapter 420), Guillain-Barré syndrome (Chapter 420), and transverse myelitis (Chapters 400 and 411). These complications may be clinically dramatic but are usually self-limited and associated with full recovery in 85% of patients without specific antiviral therapy.

Mild hepatomegaly can occur in acute infectious mononucleosis, and biochemical evidence of hepatitis (Chapter 148) should be expected in virtually every case of acute infection. More severe hepatic complications are uncommon, and renal, cardiac, pulmonary, and skeletal muscle complications are rare.

OTHER CLINICAL MANIFESTATIONS

In addition to infectious mononucleosis, EBV is also associated with neoplasia and lymphoproliferative disorders, which are seen most frequently in patients with defects in cellular immunity but are not restricted to such patients.

Post-transplantation Lymphoproliferative Disease

EBV-driven B-cell proliferation that is insufficiently regulated in the presence of prolonged periods of severe T-cell immunodeficiency may result in a polyclonal proliferation of B cells that is initially similar to that seen in acute infectious mononucleosis. Although most frequently occurring in the setting of organ transplantation, especially when patients are immunosuppressed with agents directed specifically at T lymphocytes, such as anti-CD3 antibodies or cyclosporine, this syndrome can be seen in other conditions with similar levels and durations of immunodeficiency such as HIV-1 infection. Post-transplantation lymphoproliferative disease (PTLD)[2] is seen more often when the donor is EBV seropositive and the recipient is seronegative, with the more intense immunosuppression of hematopoietic stem cell transplantation[3] (Chapter 178) in association with graft-versus-host disease, in patients who undergo splenectomy before transplantation, and in patient-donor pairs with higher degrees of HLA mismatch. These tumors are less frequently seen in the current era, in which allograft-associated immunosuppression is better targeted and less intense.

Patients with PTLD often present with fever, adenopathy, and splenomegaly. If the immunodeficiency persists, these disorders often proceed from a polyclonal stage, which can be reversed with restoration of immunity, to a monoclonal or oligoclonal stage that is progressive despite restoration of cellular immunodeficiency.

The diagnosis is not generally difficult to make in the appropriate clinical setting and can be made histopathologically. Elevated plasma levels of EBV DNA are associated with increased risk for PTLD after hematopoietic stem cell transplantation,[4] but their predictive value is less well established after solid organ transplantation.

There is some evidence that PTLD may be less frequent in patients who have received acyclovir or ganciclovir after transplantation, but these agents are less useful after the syndrome develops. Successful management depends on the extent to which the immunosuppressive condition can be reversed before the evolution of restricted clonality. Therapy with anti-CD20[5] antibodies with or without chemotherapy[6] is the treatment of choice for PTLD (Chapter 185). Radiation therapy is also used in some patients.

Burkitt's Lymphoma

EBV was initially described in patients with African Burkitt's lymphoma (Chapter 185). The tumor is composed of small, noncleaved B cells and, unless aggressively treated, is rapidly fatal. This aggressive B-cell lymphoma with a predilection for the head and neck is endemic in equatorial Africa and is geographically linked to *Plasmodium falciparum* malaria. EBV DNA is readily demonstrable in tumor biopsy specimens, and high titers of antibodies to EBV structural antigens are found in plasma. Sporadic cases of abdominal B-cell lymphomas with a histologic appearance compatible with Burkitt's lymphoma are also observed but are associated with EBV only about 25% of the time. The tumor is likewise seen in patients with HIV-1 infection. Although an etiologic role for EBV in Burkitt's lymphoma is widely accepted, the molecular basis by which EBV causes the neoplasm has not yet been fully delineated.

The risk for HIV-associated Burkitt's lymphoma increases with advancing immunodeficiency, but it may also be seen in patients with relatively preserved CD4 cell counts. Antiretroviral therapy reduces but does not eliminate the risk for Burkitt's lymphoma in HIV-1-infected persons. Despite the high-grade clinical behavior of the tumor, it should be vigorously treated because it is usually quite responsive to combination chemotherapy with or without radiation therapy (Chapter 185).

Hodgkin's Lymphoma

EBV is also associated with a subset of Hodgkin's lymphomas (Chapter 186), especially those of the lymphocyte-depleted or mixed-cellularity histologic subtypes. EBV DNA and proteins are detected in the Reed-Sternberg cells that are characteristic of Hodgkin's lymphoma. Therapy for EBV-associated Hodgkin's lymphoma is directed at the tumor's histology and stage (Chapter 186) and is not determined by whether it is related to EBV.

Central Nervous System Lymphoma

EBV is also associated with central nervous system (CNS) lymphoma (Chapter 185).[7] This tumor was most frequently observed in the post-transplantation setting before the HIV epidemic but is now the most frequent CNS neoplasm in HIV-1-infected individuals. The major differential diagnostic challenge is with *T. gondii* infection (Chapter 349). Although a tissue-based diagnosis is definitive, noninvasive neurodiagnostic approaches, coupled with the demonstration of EBV DNA in cerebrospinal fluid by polymerase chain reaction, can strongly support the diagnosis of lymphoma over that of *T. gondii* infection. Radiation therapy may be used, but its effects are generally palliative.

Nasopharyngeal Carcinoma

EBV has also been associated with certain cases of nasopharyngeal carcinoma (Chapter 190). This tumor is rare in Western countries, but it is much more frequent in southern China and in the Inuit population of Alaska. EBV-associated cases are generally less histologically differentiated than sporadic forms of nasopharyngeal carcinoma. EBV DNA is demonstrable in tumor tissue, and high titers of immunoglobulin A (IgA) and IgG antibodies to the EBV capsid antigens are found in plasma. The prognosis for this tumor is poor, although it is often treated with radiation therapy (Chapter 190).

Other EBV-Associated Neoplasms

EBV collaborates with another human gamma-herpesvirus, human herpesvirus type 8, to cause lymphoma in the HIV-1-infected population. These aggressive tumors present in body cavities such as the pleural, peritoneal, and pericardial spaces.

EBV DNA may also be found in moderate to slowly progressive destructive midline facial angiocentric tumors of T- and NK-cell phenotypes. This neoplasm presents clinically as a syndrome that was previously known as lethal midline granuloma (Chapter 185). EBV also plays a key role in the pathogenesis of an angiocentric EBV-associated B-cell tumor that presents clinically as lymphomatoid granulomatosis (Chapter 270).

Oral Hairy Leukoplakia

This clinical manifestation of EBV infection is characterized by a corrugated or "hairy" plaquelike lesion that extends around the lateral aspects of the tongue (Chapter 425). Oral hairy leukoplakia is most often observed in individuals with chronic forms of cellular immunodeficiency, especially those with HIV-1 infection and CD4 cell counts less than 200/μL. It is most often clinically confused with mucocutaneous candidiasis (Chapter 338) but can be differentiated because its distribution is restricted to the lateral surface of the tongue. Unlike thrush, it does not involve the buccal mucosa, palate, or pharynx and is not readily removed by superficial scraping. Biopsies demonstrate a characteristic histopathologic pattern, as well as the presence of EBV antigens and DNA within squamous epithelial cells. Although the lesions may be cosmetically troublesome, they are not generally painful. In the case of HIV-1-associated oral hairy leukoplakia, the lesions resolve with successful antiretroviral chemotherapy. If the immunosuppression cannot be reversed, oral hairy leukoplakia usually responds to valacyclovir, valganciclovir, or foscarnet (Chapter 425).

Chronic Active EBV Infection

Infrequent patients with no apparent defect in cellular immunity have been described in which chronic EBV infection has been associated with persistent or intermittent hepatitis or interstitial pulmonary disease (or both). These rare patients with bona fide organ system disease should not be confused with patients who have chronic fatigue syndrome or fibromyalgia rheumatica (Chapter 274), which have no relationship with EBV.

A1. Candy B, Hotopf M. Steroids for symptom control in infectious mononucleosis. *Cochrane Database Syst Rev.* 2006;3:CD004402.

GENERAL REFERENCES

For the General References and other additional features, please visit Expert Consult at https://expertconsult.inkling.com.

378

RETROVIRUSES OTHER THAN HUMAN IMMUNODEFICIENCY VIRUS

WILLIAM A. BLATTNER

TABLE 378-1 TRANSMISSION OF HTLV-1 AND HTLV-2

MODE OF TRANSMISSION	HTLV-1	HTLV-2
MOTHER TO INFANT		
Transplacental	Yes	Not known
Breast milk	Yes	Probable
SEXUAL		
Male to female	Yes	Yes
Female to male	Yes	Yes
Male to male	Yes	Not known
PARENTERAL		
Blood transfusion	Yes	Yes
Intravenous drug use	Yes	Yes
COFACTORS		
Ulcerative genital lesions	Yes	Not known
Cellular transfusion products	Yes	Yes
Sharing of "works"*	Yes	Yes
ELEVATED VIRUS LOAD		
Mother to infant	Yes	Not known
Heterosexual	Yes	Not known

*Intravenous paraphernalia, such as needles.

DEFINITION

There are now four members of the human T-lymphotropic virus (HTLV) family: HTLV-1, discovered in 1979; HTLV-2, discovered in 1982; and HTLV-3 and HTLV-4, discovered in 2005. HTLV-1 has been causally linked to adult T-cell leukemia/lymphoma (ATL) and to several chronic degenerative conditions, most notably HTLV-1–associated myelopathy/tropical spastic paraparesis (HAM/TSP), whereas disease associated with HTLV-2 is rare, and no disease associations have been established with HTLV-3 or HTLV-4.

The Pathogens

Within the taxa of RNA reverse transcribing viruses, the HTLV viruses, along with bovine leukemia virus, are classified in the subfamily Retroviridae within the genus Deltaretrovirus (formerly termed *oncovirus*). The oncogenic properties of these viruses and their molecular structure distinguish them from the human immunodeficiency retroviruses HIV-1 and HIV-2 (Chapter 386), which are members of the genus Lentivirus. Both deltaretroviruses and lentiviruses are capable of prolonged asymptomatic infection. In vitro, however, HIV-1 and HIV-2 have cytopathic effects on human T cells, whereas HTLV-1 and HTLV-2 are capable of transforming T cells into immortalized cell lines. The HTLVs are diploid single-stranded RNA viruses that replicate through cDNA, a proviral intermediate, by reverse transcriptase, a viral polymerase.

EPIDEMIOLOGY

HTLV-1 is widely disseminated worldwide and is estimated to infect 10 to 25 million persons, with the aggressive T-cell malignant neoplasm ATL developing in 2 to 6% and chronic inflammatory diseases, mainly HAM/TSP, developing in another 1 to 5% in their lifetime.[1] Similar to HIV, molecular epidemiology suggests that the four major subtypes of HTLV identified in humans arose from separate interspecies transmission from simians to humans. The discovery of HTLV-3 and HTLV-4 was made in Cameroon, where closely related viruses in nonhuman primates led to discovery in humans with exposure as bush meat hunters. Related to such interspecies transmission, there are four major geographic subtypes of HTLV-1: Cosmopolitan subtype A, Central African subtype B, Australo-Melanesian (Papua New Guinea, Melanesia, and Australian aborigines) subtype C, and Central African/Pygmies subtype D. Central Africa also carries a few rare subtypes (E, F, G). Within the cosmopolitan group are four subgroups: transcontinental, Japanese, West African, and North African. The virus from Australio-Melanesia differs molecularly from the Japanese and African strains by 5 to 10%, the result of independent evolution of the virus in these populations separated for tens of thousands of years. The stability of HTLV-1 in comparison to HIV-1 reflects the observation that HTLV favors viral expansion through proliferation of proviral DNA-harboring cells rather than infection of new cells by cell-free virions. The HTLV subtypes differ phylogenetically by approximately 30 to 40% among each other.

HTLV-1 is not universally present in all human populations but rather clusters geographically: southern Japan; Melanesia; Australia, in aboriginal peoples; West Africa and, by the slave trade from Africa, the Caribbean and the United States in African Americans; Central and South America; and the Mashhad region of Iran. In the United States, HTLV-1 infection is often found in persons who migrate from these regions. HTLV-2 is found in Native American people throughout North, Central, and South America and in West Africa. Most HTLV-2 infections in the United States and Europe occur in injection drug users, in whom the virus is spread by needle sharing and other injection practices. HTLV-3 and HTLV-4 were originally detected in Cameroon, but their extent in West Africa is not yet known.

Routes of Transmission

HTLV, like HIV-1, is transmitted sexually, perinatally, and by transfusion or injection drug use (Table 378-1).

Sexual Transmission

Sexual transmission of HTLV-1 from male to female and from female to male as well as from male to male has been documented. HTLV-1 transmission is cell associated and appears to be at least an order of magnitude less infectious than HIV-1. Coincidental infection with other sexually transmitted diseases, particularly those associated with ulcerative and inflammatory genital lesions, amplifies the risk of transmission. For HTLV-1, elevated viral load is linked to heightened transmission. In regions endemic for the virus, there is a characteristic age-dependent rise in HTLV-1 seroprevalence. This increase first becomes evident in the adolescent years; it is steeper in women than in men and continues in women after 40 years of age, whereas rates in men plateau around the age of 40 years. This pattern reflects more efficient male-to-female transmission. For HTLV-2, the rates for both genders are equal, thus suggesting that there may be differences in the kinetics of transmission between the two viruses.

Perinatal Transmission

For HTLV-1, transmission through breast-feeding is more efficient than in utero or perinatal transmission. Major risk factors that increase the efficiency of transmission include high proviral loads and increased duration of breast-feeding (>6 months). On average, 20% of infants breast-fed by HTLV-1–positive mothers seroconvert to HTLV-1, whereas only 1 to 2% of bottle-fed infants of HTLV-1–positive mothers become infected. In contrast, in utero and perinatal transmission accounts for virtually all HIV-1 transmission in the West, and breast-feeding accounts for an additional 15 to 20% of infant HIV infection in Africa. This difference may reflect the fact that maternal antibody to HTLV-1 transmitted across the placenta appears to neutralize perinatal HTLV-1 but not the highly mutable HIV-1. HTLV-2 is detectable in breast milk and, similar to HTLV-1, accounts for many childhood infections.

Transfusion and Injection Drug Use

Parenteral transmission, through either transfusion or injection drug use, is a major source of HTLV infection. Among blood donors in the United States, more than half of HTLV infections are due to HTLV-2. Among injection drug users, most infections are due to HTLV-2, and HTLV-2 is more efficiently transmitted by this route than HTLV-1 is.

Both HTLV-1 and HTLV-2 are transmitted in association with cellular components through a "virologic synapse,"[2] unlike HIV-1, which is transmitted by cells, plasma, or plasma products. Approximately 50% of the recipients of HTLV-1/HTLV-2–positive blood seroconvert, compared with more than 95% for HIV-1.

The only documented illness linked to HTLV-1 or HTLV-2 transfusion-associated transmission is the HTLV-associated demyelinating neurologic syndrome HAM/TSP. Leukemia has not been associated with transfusion of HTLV-positive blood. Among U.S. blood donors who are confirmed to be HTLV positive (slightly less than half are HTLV-1 positive and the others are HTLV-2 positive), the major risk factors are intravenous drug use, birthplace in an area in the Caribbean or Japan endemic for the virus, and sexual contact with a person with this profile.

Coinfection with HTLV-1 and HIV-1 appears to increase the progression to acquired immunodeficiency syndrome (AIDS) through unexplained mechanisms, possibly related to the cell-proliferative effects of HTLV-1 on HIV-1–infected T cells. Such a relationship has not been shown for HTLV-2. Other modes of transmission involving "casual contact" are not a source of infection. Health care and laboratory workers who experience a needlestick or skin or mucous membrane exposure in the absence of protective barriers have little or no risk for infection but should be monitored.

PATHOBIOLOGY

Virology

The HTLV viruses, which are single-stranded RNA viruses that contain a diploid genome, replicate through a DNA intermediary that integrates into the genome of the target T cell as a provirus, thereby resulting in lifelong infection. HTLV-1 is approximately 100 nm in diameter and has a thin, electron-dense outer envelope and an electron-dense, roughly spherical core. The total provirus genome contains 9032 nucleotides with two identical sequences termed *long terminal repeats* (LTRs) at the 5′ and 3′ ends of the genome, which contain regulatory elements that control virus expression and virion production. The retroviral structural genes (*gag* and *pol*) code for large overlapping polyproteins that are later processed into functional peptide products by virally encoded protease and cellular proteases. The encoding genes of the virus are *gag* (group-specific antigen), *pol* (polymerase/integrase/protease), and *env* (envelope), and it has a series of regulatory genes, *tax* and *rex*, and several smaller gene products that regulate infection and virus expression. A newly discovered viral gene is the basic leucine zipper factor (*HBZ*) gene, encoded by the minus strand of the HTLV-1 provirus and transcribed from the 3′ LTR. Tax protein plays a central role in enhancing the transcription of viral and cellular gene products that promote viral replication and transformation of human T lymphocytes. Through binding to the LTR, Tax promotes transcriptional activation of the viral genome, and by binding to key regulatory proteins of the NF-κB signaling pathway, it promotes cell activation and disease pathogenesis. Through binding to regulatory enhancers of the cell and through abrogation of key suppressor genes, Tax initiates the immortalization of the infected T cells. However, the Tax gene is susceptible to genetic mutations and is expressed in only about 60% of ATL cases. Rex stabilizes viral mRNA, essential for export of full-length Gag/Pol and single-spliced Env mRNA from the nucleus to the cytoplasm. *HBZ*, which is the only viral gene consistently expressed in all ATL patients, appears to be essential for persistent HTLV-1 infection.[3] HBZ inhibits the Tax-mediated activation of viral gene transcription through the 5′ LTR, which ultimately represses expression of viral proteins while simultaneously promoting the proliferation and survival of infected cells, regardless of Tax expression. An estimated 500 to 5000 HTLV clones exist in persons with asymptomatic infection, with a large proportion of clones detectable during years of follow-up.[4]

Viral Life Cycle

The initial stage of HTLV infection engages several mechanisms: *viral synapse*, cell-to-cell contact; *cellular conduits*, transient membrane extensions; *extracellular viral assembly*, membrane-bound virus; and *transinfection through dendritic cells*, virus captured on the cell surface of dendritic cells. After infection, the viral life cycle involves membrane fusion, followed by reverse transcription from an RNA template to a circular DNA provirus that is transported to the cell nucleus and integrated into the host genome. After the cell is infected, viral expansion is primarily achieved through proliferation of proviral DNA-harboring cells rather than through repeated cycles of cell-to-cell infection. For viral entry, HTLV-1 uses three distinct molecules for infection of activated CD4+ cells: heparin sulfate proteoglycans, neuropilin 1, and glucose transporter 1. HTLV-2 uses neuropilin 1 and glucose transporter 1 for entry into activated CD8+ T cells. After uptake and uncoating, viral RNA is transcribed by reverse transcriptase, an RNA-dependent DNA polymerase complexed to the RNA in the core of the virus particle, into double-stranded DNA. This double-stranded viral DNA is integrated into the host cell nucleus by the virally encoded integrase, which results in lifelong cell infection. The viral LTR elements are essential for integration and regulation of viral genome expression, which is controlled mainly by Tax and HBZ.

Pathogenesis of Adult T-Cell Leukemia

HTLV-1 is integrally involved in the pathogenesis of ATL through a multistage process that includes clonal integration of virus (sometimes including partial viral sequences that always include *HBZ*) into active cellular gene sequences. Interestingly, the *HBZ* gene is always present in ATL, and its quantification may be a useful marker for monitoring of the response to treatment. The clonal pattern of integration indicates that ATL is derived from a single transformed tumor cell that evolved from a virus infection *before* transformation rather than afterward as a passenger virus. Tax is an oncoprotein that interacts with numerous cellular proteins to reprogram cellular processes to alter transcription, cell cycle regulation, DNA repair, and apoptosis, thereby allowing cells with potential carcinogenic mutations to survive and to escape cell death. HBZ is also emerging as a key oncogenic protein involved in modulating cellular pathways related to cell growth, immune response, and T-cell differentiation.

In some healthy carriers, T-cell polyclonal and oligoclonal proliferations develop that can later progress to malignant transformation or may disappear spontaneously. Morphologically distinct "flower cells" (Fig. 378-1), which represent T cells with deeply lobulated nuclei resembling ATL leukemic cells, are seen on peripheral blood smears of healthy carriers, and increased numbers are detected in persons with higher HTLV viral loads.

Pathogenesis of Myelopathy/Spastic Paraparesis

Viral overproduction, as measured by high viral loads, appears to result from defective host immune responses characterized by very high levels of cytotoxic T cells. Local pathologic changes in neuronal tissue may result from immune-mediated damage caused by misdirected responses to molecular mimics of viral proteins or by local damage due to cytokine-induced damage of neuronal tissue as HTLV-1 cells infiltrate the perivascular space and the neurons of the central nervous system (CNS), particularly the spinal cord.

ADULT T-CELL LEUKEMIA/LYMPHOMA

EPIDEMIOLOGY AND PATHOBIOLOGY

The cumulative lifetime incidence of adult T-cell leukemia/lymphoma (ATL) in persons infected with HTLV-1 is between 2 and 6%, so about 2500 to 5000 cases per year occur in the approximately 10 to 25 million infected persons worldwide. The latency period is approximately 20 to 30 years after infection, with a slightly higher risk among HTLV-infected males. The age-adjusted incidence rate of ATL in the United States is 0.05 case for men and 0.03 for women per 100,000 people.[5] In areas endemic for HTLV-1, such as southern Japan and the Caribbean Islands, ATL accounts for half or more of adult lymphoid malignant neoplasms. ATL is rarely seen in children, but in one series of pediatric cases of ATL, four of the eight patients shared a homozygous deletion in the p16 gene locus, and deletion of exons 7 and 8 of p53 was detected in another child, thereby suggesting that a genetic predisposition interacts with viral infection to accelerate the progression of the disease.

CLINICAL MANIFESTATIONS

The most common disease caused by HTLV-1 is ATL, a type of T/natural killer–cell lymphoma in the new World Health Organization classification (Table 378-2). ATL is a high-grade lymphoma (Chapter 185), usually of large, medium, or pleiotropic morphology (or combined morphology) and advanced clinical stage.

The acute form of ATL, which accounts for about 55% of cases, is characterized by an aggressive, mature T-cell lymphoma that presents with a high

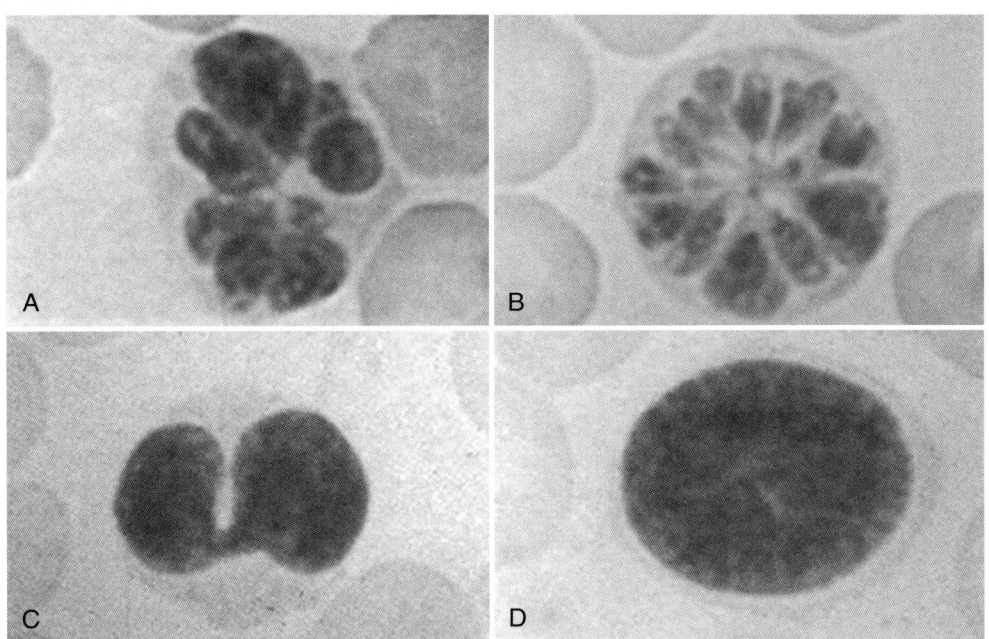

FIGURE 378-1. Photomicrographs demonstrating the morphologic features of leukemic cells observed in different subtypes of adult T-cell leukemia/lymphoma (ATL). A and B, Polylobulated morphology of the acute type, with the highly characteristic "flower cell" shown in B. C, Typical cleaved cell seen in chronic-type ATL. D, Typical morphology of smoldering ATL. (Courtesy K. Yamaguchi and K. Takatsuki.)

TABLE 378-2   HTLV-ASSOCIATED DISEASES

DIAGNOSIS	NATURE OF SYNDROME	STRENGTH OF ASSOCIATION
HTLV-1–ASSOCIATED DISEASES		
Adult T-cell leukemia/lymphoma	Aggressive lymphoproliferative malignant disease of mature T lymphocytes	Strong
HTLV-associated myelopathy/tropical spastic paraparesis (HAM/TSP)	Chronic progressive demyelinating syndrome of long motor tracts of spinal cord	Strong
Polymyositis	Degenerative inflammatory syndrome of skeletal muscles	Probable
Sporadic inclusion body myositis	Recently described HTLV-associated inflammatory muscle disease	Possible
Infective dermatitis	Chronic generalized eczema in adults and children; potential for pre-leukemia and immunodeficiency	Strong
Uveitis	Inflammatory infiltration of the uvea of the eye	Strong
Sjögren syndrome/keratoconjunctivitis sicca	Loss of tear production and dry eyes and dry mouth	Probable
Pulmonary lymphocyte alveolitis/ cryptogenic fibrosing alveolitis	Pulmonary infiltrate involving T lymphocytosis in lungs of patients with HAM/TSP and HTLV uveitis	Possible
HTLV-associated arthritis	Large-joint polyarthropathy; rheumatoid factor positive, with HTLV-1–positive cells infiltrating the synovia	Probable
Immunodeficiency	Subclinical (e.g., decreased PPD response) or clinical (e.g., association with clinical tuberculosis and poor response to therapy for symptomatic strongyloidiasis)	Probable
Miscellaneous clinical conditions	Case reports of small cell lung cancer with monoclonal HTLV-1 integration and invasive cervical cancer	Uncertain
HTLV-2–ASSOCIATED DISEASES		
HTLV-associated myelopathy	Increased numbers of cases among blood donors	Definite but rare

PPD = purified protein derivative.

white blood cell count, hypercalcemia, and cutaneous involvement. Lymphoma type (about 20% of cases) shares all features of acute ATL except for peripheral blood involvement. Other cases resemble T-prolymphocytic leukemia and are termed *chronic ATL* (about 20% of cases). A subset of patients with chronic ATL and with high serum levels of lactate dehydrogenase (LDH) and blood urea nitrogen (BUN) and low levels of albumin have a poor response to treatment, and their survival rates are similar to those of patients with the more aggressive acute and lymphoma types of ATL. Smoldering ATL (about 5%) may clinically resemble mycosis fungoides/Sézary syndrome (Chapter 185), with cutaneous involvement manifested as erythema or as infiltrative plaques or tumors (Fig. 378-2). A long prodrome of

signs (e.g., cutaneous rashes) and symptoms (e.g., fevers) is sometimes noted in chronic and smoldering ATL before transformation to an acute or lymphoma-type ATL that is rapidly fatal.

DIAGNOSIS

The diagnosis should be considered in an adult with mature T-cell lymphoma and hypercalcemia or cutaneous involvement (or both) with characteristic flower cells (see Fig. 378-1), particularly if the individual is from a known risk group or endemic region. The diagnosis is established by testing of serum for HTLV-1 antibodies. Polymerase chain reaction (PCR) can detect infection and distinguish the type of virus. The cytologically distinct flower cell,

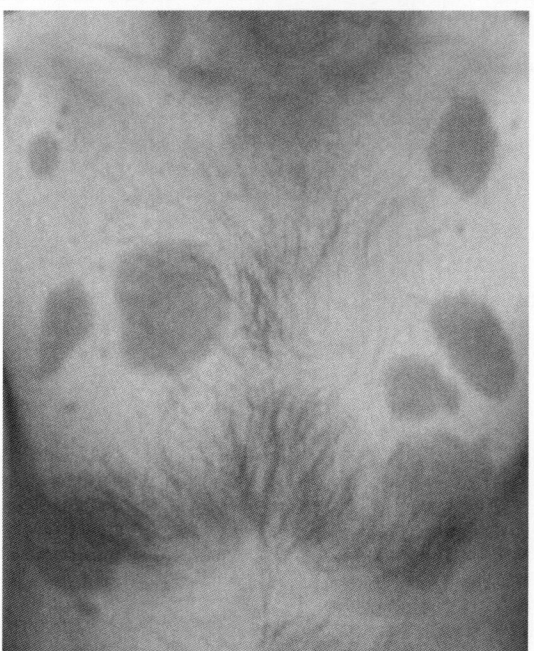

FIGURE 378-2. Cutaneous involvement in adult T-cell leukemia/lymphoma. (From Tomita H, Fumihide O, Kuwatsuka S, et al. Attenuation of an adult T-cell leukemia lesion after treatment of a concomitant simplex infection: a case study. *Virol J.* 2012;9:224. *http://www.virologyj.com/content/9/1/224.* Creative Commons Attribution License).

a sine qua non of HTLV-1–associated leukemia, is also seen in apparently healthy carriers. Occasional cases with characteristic clinical features are antibody negative but provirus positive as detected by PCR in blood cells or in biopsy specimens.

TREATMENT Rx

Treatment is based on the type of ATL and its natural history, but it is also influenced by the patient's age and the presence of selected biomarkers.

Smoldering and Chronic ATL

Watchful waiting traditionally has been recommended for patients with smoldering ATL and some patients with chronic ATL with a favorable biomarker profile (normal LDH, BUN, and albumin levels) because cytoablative therapy increases the risk of lethal opportunistic infections. Some observational data suggest, however, that 5-year survival could be improved by treating smoldering and selected chronic ATL with high doses of the antiviral agent zidovudine (800 to 1000 mg/day in divided dosage) in combination with interferon alfa (6 to 9 million units)[6] on a daily basis for 30 to 60 days, but controlled trials are needed to define the optimal dose and regimen.[7]

Acute, Lymphoma-type, and Aggressive Chronic ATL

In a randomized trial, a nine-drug regimen (vincristine, cyclophosphamide, doxorubicin, and prednisone [VCAP]; doxorubicin, ranimustine, and prednisone [AMP]; and vindesine, etoposide, carboplatin, and prednisone [VECP] [Chapter 185]) was significantly better than biweekly cyclophosphamide, doxorubicin, vincristine, and prednisone (CHOP) for inducing a complete remission.[A1] The nine-drug regimen provided nonsignificant improvements in progression-free survival at 1 year (28% vs. 16%), in median survival time (13 months vs. 11 months), and in 3-year overall survival (24% vs. 13%), but it was associated with more hematologic and infectious complications. Retrospective case series report a long-term survival of 20 to 40% after allogeneic hematopoietic stem cell transplantation (Chapter 178) but with significant treatment-related mortality.[8] Small case series have reported some benefit with zidovudine and interferon alfa, with potentially incremental benefit from the addition of arsenic triphosphate. Newer therapies, such as defucosylated humanized anti-CCR4 antibody (mogamulizumab) and denileukin diftitox (interleukin-2–diphtheria toxin conjugate), that target the high-affinity interleukin-2 receptor on ATL cells have shown some promise but need further study. In the absence of definitive data from randomized trials, a reasonable approach for patients with aggressive forms of ATL and favorable prognostic factors is VCAP-AMP-VECP alone. For patients with an unfavorable prognostic profile (thrombocytopenia, eosinophilia, bone marrow involvement, elevated LDH levels, high interleukin-5 serum level, C-C chemokine receptor 4 expression, lung resistance–related protein, p53 mutation, or p16 deletion), however, VCAP-AMP-VECP chemotherapy followed by allogeneic stem cell transplantation is recommended.

PROGNOSIS

Smoldering ATL has a relatively good prognosis, with a 5-year survival rate of 70%. For the chronic subtype, the 5-year survival is only 20%, even including the more favorable subset of patients with normal LDH, BUN, and albumin levels. For the aggressive forms of acute and lymphoma-type ATL, median disease-free survival is 0.6 year, with an overall survival of 0.8 year with high mortality linked to rapid tumor growth, infectious complications, and metabolic complications, especially hypercalcemia. Significant negative prognostic factors also include poor performance status at diagnosis, older age, advanced stage, and elevated serum LDH levels. Death usually results from rapid growth of tumor cells, hypercalcemia, bacterial sepsis, and opportunistic and other infectious complications.

HTLV-ASSOCIATED MYELOPATHY/TROPICAL SPASTIC PARAPARESIS

EPIDEMIOLOGY AND PATHOBIOLOGY

HTLV-1 causes an inflammatory neurologic syndrome known as HAM/TSP.[9] The lifetime incidence is approximately half the rate for ATL, with approximately 1 to 2% of carriers affected. HAM/TSP is approximately two times more likely to develop in females. The majority of adult cases occur in the 30- to 50-year age group, but cases have occurred in children as young as 3 years. These patterns suggest that the latency period for HAM/TSP is shorter than that for ATL and that both early-life and adult exposure causes disease. More than a dozen HAM/TSP cases associated with HTLV-2 have been reported, but the occurrence is infrequent compared with HTLV-1 carriers.

The pathogenesis results from trafficking of infected T cells in the perivascular areas and parenchyma of the spinal cord, where they cause astrocytosis. Ongoing inflammation of spinal gray and white matter results in a progressive and preferential demyelination and degeneration of the lateral and posterior columns, followed over time by loss of myelin and axons in the anterior columns.

CLINICAL MANIFESTATIONS

Symptoms include stiff gait, spasticity, lower extremity weakness, back pain, urinary incontinence and impotence, and (rarely) ataxia. The presenting symptom is stiff gait that progresses (usually slowly) to increasing spasticity and weakness, with incontinence and impotence developing later. In contrast to classic multiple sclerosis (Chapter 411), HAM/TSP is characterized by a generally slow and progressive course, absence of waxing and waning symptoms, and demyelination of long motor neurons rather than the CNS. However, some cases are acutely progressive, especially those associated with transfusion of HTLV-1–positive blood. It is not uncommon for other manifestations of HTLV-1–associated "autoimmune" disease to present coincident with the neurologic syndrome.

DIAGNOSIS

The diagnosis is suspected in patients with unexplained CNS disease and loss of pyramidal tract functions and is confirmed by testing of sera for HTLV-1 antibodies. Oligoclonal immunoglobulin bands in the cerebrospinal fluid (CSF) of patients with HAM/TSP react to HTLV-1 antigens, and the CSF to serum ratio of HTLV-1 antibodies is greater than 1. PCR quantification of the HTLV-1 cell-associated provirus in the CSF is also diagnostic. Spinal cord lesions often appear hyperintense on T2-weighted magnetic resonance imaging.

TREATMENT Rx

Corticosteroids (e.g., intravenous methylprednisolone 1.5 g for 3 consecutive days in the first week, 2 consecutive days in the second week, 1 day in the third week, and then monthly for 6 months; an alternative is oral prednisone, 1 mg/kg/day in tapering doses for 2 to 4 months) reduce symptoms in approximately 40% of cases, especially in early disease or in patients who are progressing rapidly. Studies evaluating antiviral drugs, such as lamivudine and zidovudine, have been inconclusive. Interferon alfa (3 MU three times per week) can improve neurologic symptoms. Pentoxifylline (400 to 1200 mg daily) decreases tumor necrosis factor-α and interferon-γ levels and has improved motor disability, especially spasticity, in uncontrolled trials. Cyclophosphamide also benefits some patients. Spasticity can be treated with tizanidine (2 to 12 mg daily) and botulinum toxin injection (100 to 400 IU every 4 to 6 months). Urinary incontinence is treated with oxybutynin (5 to 30 mg daily), imipramine (10 to 75 mg daily), or doxazosin mesylate (1 to 6 mg daily), and urinary retention is treated with bethanechol (10 to 50 mg daily). Treatment with danazol (100 to 400 mg daily in two divided doses) has resulted in improvement in urinary and fecal incontinence but not in the underlying neurologic deficit. Clinical trials are under way with Hu-Mik-(Beta)1, a genetically engineered antibody that blocks the action of interleukin-15 with the goal of blunting the autoimmune response that results in HAM/TSP.

PROGNOSIS

The prognosis of HAM/TSP is poor, with inexorable progression of neurologic deterioration.

OTHER HTLV-ASSOCIATED CONDITIONS

HAM/TSP is the prototype for a series of immune-mediated syndromes characterized by a high viral load, immune activation, and an indirect pathogenic mechanism produced by virally induced perturbations in immune function. Examples include skeletal muscle polymyositis, sporadic inclusion body myositis, uveitis (30 to 40% of cases in areas endemic for HTLV), large-joint arthropathy, pulmonary lymphocyte alveolitis/cryptogenic fibrosing alveolitis, Sjögren syndrome/keratoconjunctivitis sicca, and infective dermatitis, which is a pediatric syndrome characterized by inability to clear saprophytic skin infections (see Table 378-2). Carriers of HTLV-1 also have elevated rates of invasive cervical cancer, tuberculosis, parasitic infestations (e.g., strongyloidiasis), scabies, and refractory generalized eczema associated with infective dermatitis. One prospective study of HTLV-2–positive drug users showed an excess of asthma-related deaths and an increased frequency of skin and soft tissue infections.

PREVENTION

Patients often seek medical attention when confronted with a positive HTLV test result based on blood bank screening.[10] Confirmation with Western blot or PCR is needed. Confirmed positive patients must be told that complications related to HTLV-1 infection are rare and that HTLV-2 is hardly ever responsible for clinical disease. Second, it should be emphasized that these viruses are not easily transmitted. Third, the patient should be clearly counseled concerning the distinction between HTLV and HIV because the greatest fear that patients may experience is that they have the "AIDS virus." Other guidelines for prevention include the following:

- Blood for donation should be screened before transfusion, and positive donors should be deferred from donating.
- HTLV-1/HTLV-2–positive mothers should be discouraged from breast-feeding to prevent mother-to-infant transmission (except in particular settings, such as in the tropics, where diarrheal disease in non–breast-fed infants presents a high risk for morbidity and mortality).
- Condoms should be used by discordant couples, but given the relatively low frequency of sexual transmission per sexual encounter, couples who desire a pregnancy could time unprotected sexual intercourse to coincide with periods of maximal fertility. Such decisions, however, require careful discussion between the physician and the patient.

Postexposure prophylaxis with zidovudine is not recommended because the efficacy of such prophylaxis for HTLV infection has not been established. Vaccines containing whole virus and recombinant HTLV-1 envelope antigens have successfully prevented HTLV-1 infection in monkeys and in a rabbit model. However, a vaccine for humans is unlikely to be a high priority because of the relatively low incidence of clinical disease.

 Grade A Reference

A1. Tsukasaki K, Utsunomiya A, Fukuda H, et al. VCAP-AMP-VECP compared with biweekly CHOP for adult T-cell leukemia-lymphoma: Japan Clinical Oncology Group Study JCOG9801. *J Clin Oncol.* 2007;25:5458-5464.

GENERAL REFERENCES

For the General References and other additional features, please visit Expert Consult at https://expertconsult.inkling.com.

379

ENTEROVIRUSES

JOSÉ R. ROMERO

DEFINITION

The enteroviruses belong to the genus Enterovirus in the family Picornaviridae. With the advent of molecular virology, the more than 100 recognized strains are classified on the basis of phylogenetic analysis of the nucleic acid sequence of VP1, the major enteroviral capsid protein (Table 379-1).

The Pathogens

Enteroviruses are small (30 nm in diameter), nonenveloped, icosahedral-shaped viruses. The viral capsid is composed of four viral proteins (VP1 to VP4). The enteroviruses possess an approximately 7.4-kilobase positive-sense single-stranded RNA genome. The 5′ end of the genome is covalently linked to a small protein, VPg. The genome is organized into a long (about 740 nucleotides) 5′ nontranslated region that precedes a single continuous open reading frame measuring about 6.63 kilobases. The open reading frame, which is followed by a short 3′ nontranslated region and a terminal polyadenylate tail, yields a single large polyprotein that is post-translationally modified to produce four capsid proteins, seven nonstructural proteins, and several functional protein intermediates. The 5′ and 3′ nontranslated regions of VPg participate in replication of the viral genome. The 5′ nontranslated region of the enterovirus is essential for translation and contains determinants of neurovirulence in the polioviruses.

EPIDEMIOLOGY

Worldwide, an estimated 1 billion or more enteroviral infections occur annually. In the United States, about 30 to 50 million annual infections result in approximately 10 to 15 million symptomatic cases, with coxsackievirus B1, echovirus 6, echovirus 9, echovirus 18, and coxsackievirus A9 accounting for more than 50% of these enteroviral infections.[1]

Humans are the only known reservoir for enteroviruses. Enteroviral infections are seasonal, and the majority of infections occur during the summer and early autumn in temperate regions. For example, more than 80% of infections occur in the United States from June through October. However, winter outbreaks highlight their panseasonal occurrence. In tropical and subtropical regions, infections continue year-round, with an increased incidence during the rainy season.

Globally, the dominant circulating enterovirus serotypes may vary annually by geographic region. In the United States, 15 serotypes accounted for about 90% of all isolates reported (Table 379-2).

SPECIES	SEROTYPES
TABLE 379-1	**CLASSIFICATION OF ENTEROVIRUSES**
Enterovirus A	CV- A2-A8, A10, A12, A14, A16 EV- A71, A76, A90, A91, A92, A114, A119, A120
Enterovirus B	CV- A9 CV- B1-B6 E- 1-7, 9, 11-21, 24-27, 29-33 EV- B69, B73-B75, B77, B78, B79-B88, B93, B97, B98, B100, B101, B106, B107, B110, B111
Enterovirus C	PV- 1-3 CV- A1, A11, A13, A17, A19-A22, A24 EV- C95, C96, C99, C102, C104, C105, C109, C113, C116-C118
Enterovirus D	EV- D68, D70, D94, D111

TABLE 379-2 THE 14 MOST COMMON ENTEROVIRUS SEROTYPES REPORTED BY NATIONAL ENTEROVIRAL SURVEILLANCE SYSTEM LABORATORIES TO THE CDC, 2006-2008

ENTEROVIRUS SEROTYPE	PERCENTAGE
Coxsackievirus B1	16.5
Echovirus 6	10.7
Echovirus 9	10.7
Echovirus 18	8.8
Coxsackievirus A9	7.5
Coxsackievirus B4	6.7
Echovirus 11	5.8
Coxsackievirus B3	5.4
Echovirus 30	4.5
Coxsackievirus B5	4.4
Coxsackievirus B2	3.4
Echovirus 25	1.8
Echovirus 7	1.7
Coxsackievirus A16	1.7
Total	89.6

From Centers for Disease Control and Prevention (CDC). Nonpolio enterovirus and human parechovirus surveillance—United States, 2006-2008. *MMWR Morb Mortal Wkly Rep.* 2010;59:1577-1580.

viral replication, which is thought to occur in the mucosal tissues of the nasopharynx and intestinal tract (i.e., tonsils and Peyer patches), leads to seeding of the deep cervical and mesenteric lymph nodes. Further replication at these sites results in a minor viremia with seeding of multiple organs, including the liver, lungs, heart, and central nervous system (CNS). Viral replication at these sites causes many of the clinical manifestations of infection and is followed by a major viremia that may infect the CNS if it was spared during the initial viremia. The virus is cleared by type-specific neutralizing antibodies directed at the capsid proteins by day 7 to 10 after infection. IgA antibodies appear in the respiratory and gastrointestinal tracts 2 to 4 weeks after infection.

The host humoral immune response is pivotal in the prevention and eradication of enteroviral infections. Congenital or acquired B-cell immunodeficiencies may result in chronic or prolonged infection. Experimental evidence suggests that the interferons are important in limiting the spread of poliovirus once infection has occurred. Natural killer cells and gamma or delta T cells may play roles in regulating the host T-cell response.

Histopathologic findings in patients who died of poliomyelitis reveal neuronal necrosis in association with mononuclear and polymorphonuclear infiltrates that are initially perivascular in distribution but are later found diffusely within the gray matter of the anterior horns of the spinal cord, the reticular formation of the hindbrain, the vestibular nuclei, and the roof nuclei of the cerebellum. In nonpolio enterovirus CNS infections in immunocompetent hosts, findings include edema of the meninges and cerebral parenchyma, with microscopic perivascular lymphocytic infiltration, increased numbers of oligodendrocytes, and focal areas of necrosis and hemorrhage. In cases of enteroviral myocarditis (Chapter 60), a mononuclear cell inflammation is associated with widespread myocardial necrosis followed by fibrosis, which may be focal but results in myocardial damage.

CLINICAL MANIFESTATIONS

The incubation period for enterovirus infections is generally 3 to 6 days, with a range of 2 days to 2 weeks. Depending on serotype and the age of the patient, as many as 90% of infected individuals may have subclinical infections. The enteroviruses are responsible for a wide array of clinical syndromes affecting nearly every organ system, and no enterovirus serotype is uniquely associated with a single disease or clinical syndrome (Table 379-3).

The most frequent enteroviral syndrome, seen in about 50 to 80% of cases, is nonspecific febrile illness, which occurs most commonly in infants, toddlers, and young children. The onset of illness is abrupt, with fever, poor appetite, lethargy, irritability, emesis, diarrhea, and upper respiratory tract symptoms. Physical findings are minimal and consist of mild pharyngeal and conjunctival injection and lymphadenopathy. Exanthems may be present in about 25% of cases.

DIAGNOSIS

Nucleic acid amplification techniques (e.g., reverse transcription–polymerase chain reaction [RT-PCR] and nucleic acid–based sequence amplification) are the preferred methods for detection and identification of all enteroviruses. Multiple studies have documented that nucleic acid amplification techniques are more sensitive and rapid than cell culture for the detection of enteroviruses in cerebrospinal fluid (CSF). RT-PCR can detect enteroviruses in CSF, blood, tissue, stool, and other body fluids within hours, and the results can shorten hospitalizations, decrease the use of antibiotics, and reduce health care costs.

Serologic testing is of limited use, although a four-fold change in antibody titer to a specific serotype of enterovirus in paired acute and convalescent sera can establish the diagnosis. Cell culture is not recommended because of limited sensitivity, prolonged positivity even after the related clinical syndrome may have resolved, and the several days required for viral detection.

More than 80% of infections occur in individuals younger than 20 years, with the highest incidence in infants and children 4 years and younger. Nearly 45% of all infections occur in infants younger than 1 year. Among household members of infected children, clinical or serologic evidence of secondary infection can be seen in more than 50% of susceptible individuals. A male preponderance is noted in persons younger than 20 years (male-to-female ratio of 1.4 : 1), but not in older individuals.

Localized enteroviral outbreaks have been reported in neonatal units, nurseries, daycare centers, schools, camps, and sports teams. Community-wide outbreaks are common. Extensive regional outbreaks of EV-A71 have occurred in the Asia-Pacific region. Occasional pandemics, such as acute hemorrhagic conjunctivitis caused by EV-D70 and CV-A24, also have occurred.

Effective antipolio immunization programs have eradicated wild-type poliovirus serotype 2 worldwide and have also eradicated serotypes 1 and 3 from almost all countries except Afghanistan, Pakistan, and Nigeria, where they unfortunately remain endemic.[2] As a result, sporadic poliovirus outbreaks continue to occur in Africa, west Asia, China,[3] and war-torn Syria[4] from local reservoirs or imported infections. The use of live attenuated poliovirus vaccines has led to the problem of vaccine-derived polioviruses (VDPVs) as a result of the excretion of neurorevertant vaccine (Sabin) strains from individuals who have primary humoral immunodeficiencies, but not secondary humoral or other immunodeficiencies, or as a result of natural recombination between Sabin strains and members of the Enterovirus C species.[5] VDPVs that can circulate in the environment with evidence of person-to-person transmission have been termed circulating vaccine-derived polioviruses (cVDPVs). A third group of VDPVs, designated ambiguous VDPVs, are clinical isolates from individuals without known immunodeficiency or sewage isolates whose ultimate source is unknown. Similar to wild-type poliovirus, cVDPVs can cause acute flaccid paralysis in unimmunized or incompletely immunized individuals and have caused multiple outbreaks worldwide.

PATHOBIOLOGY

The polioviruses and the majority of the nonpolio enteroviruses are transmitted through a fecal-oral route. Notable exceptions include CV-A21 and EV-D68, which are spread by the respiratory route, and EV-D70, which may spread by contaminated fomites or ocular and respiratory secretions. Evidence also supports transplacental transmission of the enteroviruses.

Ingestion of the enteroviruses results in infection of cells of the pharynx and, because the virus is acid resistant, the lower gastrointestinal tract. Initial

TREATMENT AND PROGNOSIS   Rx

Nonspecific febrile enteroviral infections generally resolve in less than 5 days without sequelae. Because of concern for possible occult bacterial infection, however, significant numbers of young infants and children are hospitalized for evaluation and empirical therapy. After infection, virus may be shed into the nasopharynx for 2 to 6 weeks and in feces for several months.

TABLE 379-3 CLINICAL MANIFESTATIONS OF NONPOLIO ENTEROVIRUS INFECTIONS*

CLINICAL SYNDROME	GROUP A COXSACKIEVIRUSES†	GROUP B COXSACKIEVIRUSES	ECHOVIRUSES	ENTEROVIRUSES
Asymptomatic infection	All serotypes	All serotypes	All serotypes	All serotypes
Undifferentiated febrile illness ("summer grippe") with or without respiratory symptoms	All serotypes	All serotypes	All serotypes	68, 70, 71
Aseptic meningitis (often associated with an exanthem)	1, 2, 3, 4, 5, 6, 7, 8, 9, 10, 11, 14, 16, 17, 18, 22, 24	1, 2, 3, 4, 5, 6	1, 2, 3, 4, 5, 6, 7, 8, 9, 10, 11, 12, 14, 16, 17, 18, 19, 20, 21, 25, 30, 31, 33	70, 71
Encephalitis	2, 4, 5, 6, 7, 9, 10, 16	1, 2, 3, 4, 5	2, 3, 4, 6, 7, 9, 11, 14, 17, 18, 19, 25, 30, 33	70, 71
Acute flaccid paralysis (poliomyelitis-like)	4, 5, 6, 7, 9, 10, 11, 14, 16, 21, 24	1, 2, 3, 4, 5, 6	1, 2, 4, 6, 7, 9, 11, 14, 16, 17, 18, 19, 30	68, 70, 71
Myopericarditis	1, 2, 4, 5, 7, 8, 9, 14, 16	1, 2, 3, 4, 5, 6	1, 2, 3, 4, 6, 7, 8, 9, 11, 14, 16, 17, 19, 25, 30	
Pleurodynia	1, 2, 4, 6, 9, 10, 16	1, 2, 3, 4, 5, 6	1, 2, 3, 6, 7, 8, 9, 11, 12, 14, 16, 19, 25, 30	
Herpangina	1, 2, 3, 4, 5, 6, 7, 8, 9, 10, 16, 22	1, 2, 3, 4, 5	6, 9, 11, 16, 17, [22], 25	71
Hand-foot-and-mouth disease	4, 5, 6, 7, 9, 10, 16	2, 5	7	71
Exanthems	2, 4, 5, 6, 7, 9, 10, 16	1, 2, 3, 4, 5	2, 4, 5, 6, 9, 11, 16, 18, 25	71
Common cold	2, 10, 21, 24	1, 2, 3, 4, 5	2, 4, 8, 9, 11, 20, 25	
Lower respiratory tract infections (bronchiolitis, pneumonia)	7, 9, 16	1, 2, 3, 4, 5	4, 8, 9, 11, 12, 14, 19, 20, 21, 25, 30	68, 71, 104
Acute hemorrhagic conjunctivitis§	24			70
Generalized disease of the newborn	3, 9, 16	1, 2, 3, 4, 5	3, 4, 6, 7, 9, 11, 12, 14, 17, 18, 19, 20, 21, 30	

*A great many enterovirus serotypes have been implicated in most of these syndromes, at least in sporadic cases. The serotypes listed are those that have been clearly or frequently implicated. Serotypes with a strong association are underlined.
†Because detection of many of the group A coxsackieviruses originally required suckling mouse inoculation, they are likely to be underreported as causes of illness.
§Conjunctivitis without hemorrhage is frequently seen in association with other manifestations in patients infected with many group A and group B coxsackieviruses and echoviruses, especially coxsackieviruses A9, A16, and B1 to B5 and echoviruses 2, 7, 9, 11, 16, and 30. From Modlin JR. Enterovirus. *Cecil Textbook of Medicine*. 23rd ed. Philadelphia: WB Saunders; 2008, with minor changes.

SPECIFIC CLINICAL SYNDROMES
Central Nervous System Infections
ACUTE FLACCID PARALYSIS

CLINICAL MANIFESTATIONS AND DIAGNOSIS

During poliovirus epidemics, 90 to 95% of infections are subclinical. In another 4 to 8% of patients, infection results in fever, fatigue, headache, anorexia, myalgia, and sore throat, which resolve in 2 to 3 days. Paralytic polio develops in less than 1 to 2% of infected individuals.

Sporadic cases of acute flaccid paralysis can also be seen with other enteroviruses, especially coxsackievirus CV-A7 and enterovirus EV-A71 and occasionally EV-D68. With the exception of EV-A71, the paralysis associated with nonpolio enteroviruses tends to be milder, and fever is absent at the time of onset of the paralysis.[6] The upper extremities and face are more commonly involved. Sensory pathways remain intact.

CSF may reveal a mild lymphocytic pleocytosis (<100 cells/µL) in association with mildly increased protein and normal glucose concentrations. Neuroimaging is not generally useful, but increased signal may be seen on T2-weighted magnetic resonance imaging in the anterior horn regions of the spinal cord in patients whose acute flaccid paralysis is caused by poliovirus and nonpolio enteroviruses.

TREATMENT AND PROGNOSIS Rx

No specific therapy exists. Efforts should focus on monitoring for the development of respiratory failure or airway compromise as well as control of pain associated with muscle spasms.

The mortality associated with spinal poliomyelitis is about 5%. The mortality rates for enteroviruses associated with nonpolio enteroviral acute flaccid paralysis are not known. Before modern methods of respiratory and cardiovascular support, mortality rates higher than 50% were common in patients with bulbar or medullary poliomyelitis. The ultimate outcome of the paralysis is highly variable and can range from complete resolution to lifelong persistence. The greatest gains in recovery of strength occur during the first 6 months of convalescence. Paralytic limbs become atrophic, thereby leading to skeletal deformities. Patients with nonpolio enteroviruses usually have a more rapid recovery and less atrophy than do those with classic polio.

A syndrome of postpoliomyelitis muscle atrophy, which may be seen in 25 to 85% of individuals 2 to 3 decades after recovery from paralytic disease, is characterized by the gradual development of weakness, pain, and atrophy. Possible mechanisms include aging and neuronal dropout in compromised neuromuscular connections[7] or, less likely, reactivation/ongoing poliovirus infection.

MENINGITIS
The enteroviruses, especially echoviruses and group B coxsackieviruses, are the dominant cause of viral meningitis (Chapter 412) in all ages.[8]

CLINICAL MANIFESTATIONS AND DIAGNOSIS

The clinical picture varies with age. The predominant symptoms of meningitis in neonates are nonspecific fever, irritability, lethargy, and poor feeding, often with a full fontanelle and a generalized rash. In neonates with meningoencephalitis, clinical findings may consist of fever, lethargy, seizures, full fontanelle, and focal neurologic abnormalities. Hepatitis, myocarditis, or pneumonitis, singly or in combination, may be present in severe cases.

In older infants and children, an abrupt onset of fever is the most frequent initial symptom. The fever may persist for 1 to 5 days and may exhibit a biphasic pattern. Irritability or lethargy is common. Other nonspecific symptoms include poor feeding, vomiting, diarrhea, and rash. Headache is present in nearly all children old enough to report it. Rash, malaise, sore throat, abdominal pain, and myalgia are common, and photophobia may be reported. Seizures occur in less than 5% of cases. Examination may reveal a full fontanelle. Signs of meningeal irritation (i.e., nuchal rigidity, Brudzinski and Kernig signs) occur in less than 10% of infants younger than 3 months and increase with age.

In adolescents and adults, headache is nearly always present and severe enough to require narcotic analgesics for control. Some patients report temporary relief of headache after lumbar puncture. Fever is not universal, but photophobia, signs of meningeal irritation, nausea, emesis, and neck stiffness occur in more than two thirds of patients. Myalgia is reported in 20 to 90% of patients. Less frequent findings include rash and abdominal pain.

CSF analysis generally reveals a mild to moderate lymphocytic pleocytosis (<500 cells/µL). Some patients, however, may have lymphocyte counts higher than 1000 or have neutrophilic pleocytosis early in the course of illness and then progress to a predominance of lymphocytes hours to days later. In a small percentage of patients, particularly infants, no pleocytosis is present even though enterovirus can be detected. The protein concentration may be increased. Although the glucose concentration is generally normal, hypoglycorrhachia may occur, particularly in association with group B coxsackievirus meningitis. Neuroimaging in cases of meningitis is generally unrevealing. Nucleic acid amplification testing can detect enteroviruses in CSF. The serotypes most frequently identified from CSF specimens are, in descending order, E-9, E-11, E-30, CV-B5, E-6, CV-B2, CV-A9, E-4, CV-B4, E-7, E-18, E-5, and E-13.

TREATMENT AND PROGNOSIS   Rx

Treatment is supportive, with control of fever and pain. Currently available antiviral agents are not helpful. Hospitalization may not be necessary in adolescents and adults who appear well if a bacterial cause can be confidently excluded. In children and infants or when bacterial infection cannot be confidently excluded in adults, hospitalization and initial empirical antimicrobial therapy are advisable (Chapter 412) while awaiting the results of bacterial cultures of blood and CSF. Intravenous fluids may be required to prevent dehydration. Control of headache pain may require narcotic analgesics. Uncommon complications in all ages include coma, increased intracranial pressure, and inappropriate secretion of antidiuretic hormone.

The overwhelming majority of patients recover fully. The duration of illness in infants and children is generally less than 1 week. In adults, full recovery may take up to 3 weeks.

ENCEPHALITIS

The enteroviruses are responsible for up to 22% of identifiable causes of viral encephalitis (Chapter 414). In the single largest report of enterovirus-related encephalitis, 73% of confirmed cases occurred in individuals younger than 20 years, including about 40% of cases in patients younger than 10 years.

CLINICAL MANIFESTATIONS AND DIAGNOSIS

The onset of neurologic findings may be abrupt or be preceded by fever, headache, malaise, myalgia, upper respiratory symptoms, rash, nausea, emesis, or diarrhea. Somnolence, lethargy, and altered consciousness are common. Patients may exhibit irritability, changes in personality, or hallucinations. Generalized or focal seizures occur in up to 30% of patients, and a minority of patients may progress to coma. Neck stiffness and ataxia are frequent physical findings. Focal neurologic findings such as hemiplegia, hemichorea, and paresthesias are reported in nearly 30% of patients. The focal nature of the seizures and abnormal neurologic findings may be reminiscent of herpes simplex virus encephalitis (Chapter 374).

Among enteroviral encephalitides, EV-A71 is uniquely associated with severe brain stem encephalitis (rhombencephalitis), primarily in children. The initial manifestation may be a prodrome of either hand-foot-and-mouth disease or herpangina, which is followed by myoclonus that may be associated with ataxia, tremors, or cranial nerve abnormalities and a rapid onset of neurogenic pulmonary edema, shock, coma, and apnea.

Evaluation of CSF may reveal mild to moderate lymphocytic pleocytosis (<500 cells/μL), but the CSF white cell count may be normal. The protein concentration may be increased and may be the sole abnormality. The glucose concentration is generally normal. Enteroviruses may frequently be detectable by nucleic acid amplification testing of CSF.

TREATMENT AND PROGNOSIS   Rx

Management is supportive, with monitoring for the development of respiratory failure or airway compromise. Nearly 50% of patients require intensive care. In patients with focal neurologic findings, empirical acyclovir (10 to 15 mg/kg every 8 hours) is warranted until herpes simplex virus is excluded.

The median duration of hospitalization is less than 1 week, and mortality is below 10%. For severe EV-A71 rhombencephalitis, however, mortality may approach 70%. Long-term sequelae after rhombencephalitis include myoclonus, abducens nerve palsy, facial diplegia, ataxia, dysarthria, internuclear ophthalmoplegia, and central apnea.

Myopericarditis

Members of the Enterovirus B species and especially the group B coxsackieviruses are responsible for approximately a third of cases of acute myocarditis (Chapter 60). The majority of cases occur in young adults.

CLINICAL MANIFESTATIONS AND DIAGNOSIS

An upper respiratory tract infection may precede the onset of cardiac symptoms by 1 to 2 weeks. Fever may be present, and common initial symptoms include dyspnea, chest pain, and fatigue. Physical examination may reveal a gallop rhythm or a pericardial friction rub.

Cardiomegaly may be seen on the chest radiograph. Electrocardiographic findings vary and include low-voltage QRS complexes, ST segment depression, T wave inversion, pathologic Q waves, ventricular arrhythmias, and heart block. Echocardiographic findings include a decreased ejection fraction, ventricular dilation, and pericardial effusion. Blood troponin levels are frequently elevated. Cardiac magnetic resonance imaging may help localize areas of myocarditis. Myocardial biopsy is recommended in selected patients who have refractory heart failure or suspected giant cell myocarditis (Chapter 60); enterovirus can be detected by nucleic acid amplification tests.

TREATMENT AND PROGNOSIS   Rx

Supportive treatment includes bedrest and management of heart failure (Chapter 59), arrhythmias (Chapters 64 and 65), and pericarditis with or without pericardial effusion (Chapter 77). Immunosuppressive therapy is not generally recommended (Chapter 60). In approximately a third of patients with acute myocarditis, chronic dilated cardiomyopathy develops. In patients with pericarditis, recurrent pericardial effusions or chronic constrictive pericarditis may develop in the future.

Exanthems and Enanthems

Enterovirus infections may result in a wide spectrum of febrile exanthems and enanthems, including macular, papular, maculopapular, morbilliform, rubelliform, vesicular, urticarial, papulopustular, and scarlatiniform types. Exanthems are more commonly observed in children 15 years or younger. Any serotype is capable of causing several different rashes. With the exception of CV-A16, no serotype is associated with a unique rash. Echovirus 9 and CV-A9 can cause petechial or purpuric rashes reminiscent of meningococcemia (Chapter 298).

Hand-Foot-and-Mouth Disease and Herpangina

Hand-foot-and-mouth disease is typically associated with Enterovirus A species, particularly CV-A16, CV-A6, and EV-A71.[9] Herpangina is also most commonly caused by the group A coxsackieviruses in the Enterovirus A species, but it has also been associated with group B coxsackieviruses, echoviruses, and enteroviruses from the Enterovirus B species.

CLINICAL MANIFESTATIONS AND DIAGNOSIS

Hand-foot-and-mouth disease begins with low-grade fever, malaise, anorexia, and oral soreness. In 1 to 2 days, oral macules appear and then rapidly vesiculate and ulcerate. Oral lesions are typically distributed on the buccal mucosa and tongue, but they may also occur on the palate, uvula, anterior pillars, and gums. In approximately two thirds of patients, the enanthem is accompanied by an exanthem, with tender 3- to 7-mm vesicles on the dorsum of the hands and feet, frequently involving the palms and soles. Lesions may appear on the buttocks but tend not to be vesicular. Hand-foot-and-mouth disease associated with CV-A6 has a wider distribution of skin lesions that enlarge and vesiculate. Onychomadesis (loss of fingernails) can occur 1 to 2 months after the infection.

Herpangina begins with high fever, particularly in young patients. Additional findings include sore throat, mild cervical lymphadenopathy, sialorrhea, anorexia, dysphagia, abdominal pain, and emesis. Examination of the mouth and throat reveals 1- to 2-mm papulovesicular, grayish white lesions with an areola of erythema, primarily located on the anterior pillars of the tonsillar fauces. The soft palate, uvula, and tonsils may also be involved. Rarely, the posterior buccal surfaces and dorsal tip of the tongue may be involved. During a period of 2 to 3 days, the lesions increase to 3 to 4 mm in size. On average, five lesions are present.

TREATMENT AND PROGNOSIS   Rx

Hand-foot-and-mouth disease usually resolves in less than 1 week and herpangina generally resolves in 10 days, both typically uneventfully, without the need for hospitalization and without sequelae. Infants and young children may require hospitalization for administration of parenteral fluids. Disease associated with CV-A6 has a higher rate of hospitalization. Hand-foot-and-mouth disease due to EV-A71 may precede the development of life-threatening rhombencephalitis (see Encephalitis).

Acute Hemorrhagic Conjunctivitis

Acute hemorrhagic conjunctivitis (Chapter 423) is associated with EV-D70 and CV-A24. The illnesses caused by the two serotypes are indistinguishable from each other. However, acute hemorrhagic conjunctivitis caused by CV-A24 may be more commonly accompanied by upper respiratory and systemic symptoms and may be associated with less severe conjunctival hemorrhage. High secondary attack rates within households are common. Other enteroviruses can cause acute conjunctivitis or keratoconjunctivitis but generally without hemorrhagic manifestations.

CLINICAL MANIFESTATIONS

An incubation period of about 1 to 2 days precedes the rapid onset of palpebral swelling associated with lacrimation, photophobia, blurring of vision, and severe ocular pain. The hallmark subconjunctival hemorrhages vary in size from petechiae to large blotches. Although transient keratitis occurs frequently, it seldom results in subepithelial opacities. Preauricular adenopathy is common, but fever is not. An ocular mucopurulent discharge may occasionally be present.

TREATMENT AND PROGNOSIS ℞

Management is supportive. The illness usually persists for 1 to 2 weeks, but complete recovery is generally the rule. A transient lumbar radiculomyelopathy and acute flaccid paralysis–like illness may develop in some patients.

Respiratory Tract Syndromes

The enteroviruses may cause upper and lower respiratory tract syndromes, alone or accompanying other syndromes. As determined by nucleic acid amplification testing, enteroviruses are responsible for up to 15% of upper respiratory tract syndromes. They also cause 18% of lower respiratory tract syndromes in hospitalized children and 25% of hospitalizations in patients with acute wheezing. Recently, EV-D68 and EV-C104 are increasingly recognized as causes of respiratory tract disease.

CLINICAL MANIFESTATIONS AND DIAGNOSIS

The enterovirus "summer cold" (Chapter 361) consists of nasal congestion, rhinorrhea, and sneezing. Malaise and cough may be present. Fever and sore throat are typically absent or minimal.

Pharyngitis, tonsillitis, or pharyngotonsillitis begins abruptly with fever and sore throat. The nasopharynx, tonsils, uvula, and soft palate demonstrate erythema and inflammation. Petechiae may be present, and cervical lymphadenitis is common. Other syndromes associated with the enteroviruses include bronchitis (Chapter 96) and bronchiolitis.

Enteroviral pneumonias begin gradually with coryza, anorexia, and low-grade fever. A nonproductive cough, tachypnea, retractions, nasal flaring, and wheezing may be present. In severe cases, cyanosis may develop. The chest radiograph may demonstrate perihilar infiltrates, patchy consolidation, air trapping, and atelectasis. Recently, EV-D68 has become a cause of significant respiratory disease, primarily in young children and infants but also in adolescents and adults. An underlying pulmonary condition such as asthma or wheezing has been reported in 70% to 80% of cases. EV-D68-associated respiratory syndromes include pneumonia, bronchiolitis, asthmatic bronchitis, asthma exacerbation, and wheezing. Signs and symptoms include cough, wheezing, dyspnea, tachycardia, and inter- and subcostal retractions. Acute flaccid paralysis is a rare complication. Interestingly, fever may be absent, but hypoxia is common. The chest radiograph may show infiltrates and atelectasis.[10]

TREATMENT AND PROGNOSIS ℞

Treatment is supportive and consists of control of fever and pain. In older children and adults, hospitalization is not usually required. Resolution occurs in 7 days or less. Hospitalization and admission to an intensive care unit may be required for respiratory support of EV-D68 infection. Death is uncommon but does occur.

Myositis
PLEURODYNIA

The group B coxsackieviruses are the major cause of sporadic and epidemic pleurodynia, but the syndrome may also be caused by a limited number of echoviruses and group A coxsackieviruses within the Enterovirus A and B species.

CLINICAL MANIFESTATIONS AND DIAGNOSIS

The onset of illness is abrupt in approximately 75% of patients. In the remainder, the onset of pleuritic chest pain is preceded by a prodrome of headache, malaise, anorexia, and vague myalgia lasting up to 10 days. Pain may be referred to the lower ribs or the sternum, and it can radiate to the shoulders, neck, or scapula. Pain is exacerbated by deep breathing, coughing, sneezing, or movement. During paroxysms, patients tend to be tachypneic and to have shallow breathing. Additional findings can include abdominal pain, headache, cough, anorexia, nausea, vomiting, and diarrhea. Fever may be biphasic.

Physical examination does not generally reveal muscle tenderness, obvious myositis, or muscle swelling. A pleural friction rub may be present in 25% of patients. The chest radiograph is typically normal.

TREATMENT AND PROGNOSIS ℞

Treatment is supportive, with an emphasis on nonsteroidal analgesics (e.g., ibuprofen, 200 to 400 mg per dose every 4 to 6 hours) or hydrocodone (5 to 10 mg four times per day) alone or in combination with acetaminophen to control pain. The symptoms may persist for 1 to 14 days (mean of 3.5 days) and resolve without sequelae, although recurrent symptoms may occur in 25% of patients.

INFLAMMATORY MYOSITIS

Multiple enteroviral serotypes are associated with focal or generalized myositis. In patients with B-cell immunodeficiencies, a dermatomyositis-like syndrome may develop.

CLINICAL MANIFESTATIONS AND DIAGNOSIS

Nonspecific findings include fever and chills. Involved muscles may be weak, tender, and edematous. Chemical evidence of myositis may be evidenced by elevated serum levels of creatine kinase, myoglobinemia, and myoglobinuria.

TREATMENT AND PROGNOSIS ℞

Treatment is supportive. With the exception of patients with B-cell immunodeficiencies, recovery is complete and rapid.

Enterovirus Infections in Special Populations
PATIENTS WITH B-CELL IMMUNODEFICIENCIES

Nonpolio enteroviruses and polioviruses may result in chronic or prolonged infections in patients with congenital or acquired B-cell immunodeficiencies (Chapter 250), such as those with X-linked agammaglobulinemia, hyper-IgM syndrome, severe combined immunodeficiency syndrome, or common variable immunodeficiency, or in patients receiving chemotherapy or immunomodulatory therapies, especially rituximab, who are undergoing bone marrow or solid organ transplantation.

CLINICAL MANIFESTATIONS AND DIAGNOSIS

Meningoencephalitis, pulmonary infections, and severe gastroenteritis can occur. The initial symptoms may consist of only persistent headaches and lethargy. As the disease progresses, additional neurologic findings develop and may include ataxia, loss of cognitive skills and memory, dementia, emotional lability, paresthesias, weakness, dysarthria, and seizures. Non-CNS manifestations include a dermatomyositis-like syndrome, edema, exanthems, and hepatitis. CSF demonstrates a persistently elevated protein concentration and pleocytosis. Enterovirus is detectable in CSF by RT-PCR.

TREATMENT AND PROGNOSIS

Children with humoral immunodeficiency (Chapter 250) should receive life-long immunoglobulin replacement therapy in an attempt to prevent chronic infection. However, chronic meningoencephalitis develops in some patients and is usually ultimately fatal. Severe or fatal enteroviral infections have been reported in individuals receiving rituximab.

PREVENTION

Handwashing is the primary method for the prevention of enteroviral infections. Only poliovirus infections are currently preventable through vaccination. However, successful trials of inactivated EV-A71 vaccines have been completed in China.[A1][A2] These vaccines could significantly reduce the incidence of severe EV-A71 CNS disease in China. Whether the vaccine will be effective in other regions of the world will depend on its ability to protect from disease caused by the different genotypes found worldwide.

Grade A References

A1. Zhu FC, Meng FY, Li JX, et al. Efficacy, safety, and immunology of an inactivated alum-adjuvant enterovirus 71 vaccine in children in China: a multicentre, randomised, double-blind, placebo-controlled, phase 3 trial. *Lancet.* 2013;381:2024-2032.
A2. Zhu F, Xu W, Xia J, et al. Efficacy, safety, and immunogenicity of an enterovirus 71 vaccine in China. *N Engl J Med.* 2014;370:818-828.

GENERAL REFERENCES

For the General References and other additional features, please visit Expert Consult at https://expertconsult.inkling.com.

380

ROTAVIRUSES, NOROVIRUSES, AND OTHER GASTROINTESTINAL VIRUSES

MANUEL A. FRANCO AND HARRY B. GREENBERG

DEFINITION

Viruses are a principal cause of acute infectious gastroenteritis, a syndrome of vomiting, watery diarrhea, or both that begins abruptly in otherwise healthy persons. Two distinct viruses account for the majority of cases. Rotaviruses are the most frequent cause of sporadic, severe gastroenteritis in young children and are responsible for the death of approximately 1200 children daily worldwide,[1] mainly in developing countries. Noroviruses are the primary cause of epidemic infectious gastroenteritis in both infants and adults in developed countries. For example, outbreaks of gastroenteritis in closed settings, such as cruise ships and nursing homes, are a typical manifestation of norovirus infections. However, noroviruses are also a common cause of sporadic, severe gastroenteritis in young children.[2]

The Pathogens
Noroviruses

Noroviruses, which are one of the five genera of the Caliciviridae family, are nonenveloped, icosahedral viruses with a relatively small, positive-sense, single-stranded RNA genome. The norovirus genus is further classified into five genogroups (GI to GV), only three of which (GI, GII, and GIV) are known to infect humans. GIII and GV viruses infect bovines and mice, respectively, and to date these animal viruses have not been shown to infect humans. Viruses in each genogroup are further divided into genotypes (more than 25 have been described) and subgroups. Norwalk virus is a prototype genogroup I genotype 1 (GI.1) virus. The norovirus genome is approximately 7.7 kilobases in size and consists of three open reading frames, the first of which encodes the nonstructural proteins that are essential for virus

replication. The second open reading frame encodes the major capsid protein, viral protein 1 (VP1). When it is expressed as a recombinant protein, 180 molecules of VP1 autoassemble into virus-like particles (VLPs) that are critical to the study of noroviral epidemiology and immunity. Human noroviruses have not yet been adapted to cell culture, so diagnosis generally depends on amplification of virus genes by the polymerase chain reaction (PCR; see later) or use of VLPs as recombinant antigens for serologic analysis.

Rotavirus

Rotaviruses, which belong to the family Reoviridae, are large, icosahedral, nonenveloped viruses with a segmented, double-stranded RNA genome and a triple-layered protein coat. Rotaviruses are classified into groups A through G on the basis of the presence of cross-reactive antigenic epitopes and their overall genetic relatedness. Group A rotaviruses are the most commonly encountered viral enteric pathogens of young humans and many other species. Group B viruses have been identified sporadically in outbreaks of adult diarrheal illness in China and more recently in studies of children with sporadic gastroenteritis, principally in India. Group C rotaviruses are primarily veterinary pathogens and are infrequently associated with diarrheal disease in humans and animals around the world compared with group A rotaviruses. Groups D through G rotaviruses have been isolated only from animals, primarily avian species. Rotaviruses are 100-nm particles that have three concentric layers of proteins: the core is composed of VP1, VP2, and VP3 and the segmented, double-stranded RNA genome; the intermediate layer is formed by VP6, the most abundant and antigenic structural viral protein; and the external layer is composed of VP7 and VP4. The genome, which is composed of 11 segments of double-stranded RNA that together are approximately 18 kilobases in length, encodes six structural and six nonstructural proteins. As is the case among virtually all other RNA viruses, the rotavirus RNA polymerase is error prone and, along with selective pressure such as the evolution of immunity, drives viral diversity. For rotaviruses, gene reassortment, which is the mixing of gene segments from different parental viruses in cells coinfected by two or more strains, and rearrangement of the viral genome also contribute to genetic diversity. Reassortment of gene segments between animal and human rotavirus strains also occurs in natural settings, especially in less developed countries.

Other Agents

Other viral agents that cause human acute infectious gastroenteritis that is difficult to distinguish from disease caused by rotaviruses and noroviruses include the sapovirus (like norovirus, a member of the Caliciviridae family), enteric adenoviruses (Chapter 365) belonging to types 40 and 41, and astroviruses (Table 380-1). The frequency of detection (by PCR assays) of these viruses in individuals with acute gastroenteritis depends on the setting, but they are almost always detected much less frequently than are rotaviruses and noroviruses.[3] Coronaviruses (Chapter 366), toroviruses, picobirnaviruses, picornavirus (Chapter 379), bocavirus, parechoviruses, and pestiviruses have also been isolated occasionally from persons with acute gastroenteritis, but their roles as causative agents of enteric disease remain uncertain. Among patients with acute gastroenteritis, no etiologic agent is found in approximately 25 to 50% of cases.

EPIDEMIOLOGY
Norovirus

Over time, noroviruses appear to undergo antigenic drift in response to the acquisition of immunity in the general population, much like influenza viruses.[4] At present, gastroenteritis cases around the world are most frequently caused by the GII.4 norovirus strain, but new strains generally evolve every 2 to 4 years owing to antigenic drift. Outbreaks frequently take place in settings of close human contact, such as military establishments, cruise ships, nursing homes, and schools, especially in cold and dry weather (see Table 380-1). Viral spread is enhanced by the very high level of infectivity of noroviruses, as data suggest that 1 to 10 particles constitute an infectious dose.

Noroviruses of genotypes GII.4 and GII.3 also are responsible for about 12% of sporadic gastroenteritis in children younger than 5 years in both developed and developing countries. In the United States, noroviruses have recently surpassed rotavirus as the principal cause of medically attended visits for gastroenteritis in children younger than 5 years.[5] In the United States, noroviruses cause an estimated average of 570 to 800 deaths, 56,000 to 71,000 hospitalizations, 400,000 emergency department visits, 1.7 to 1.9 million outpatient visits, and 19 to 21 million total illnesses per year. The

TABLE 380-1 EPIDEMIOLOGIC AND CLINICAL FEATURES OF NOROVIRUS AND ROTAVIRUS

	NOROVIRUS	ROTAVIRUS	ASTROVIRUS
Epidemics	Occurs year-round; outbreaks tend to peak in cold weather	Year-round in equatorial countries; winter peak in others	Winter epidemics in children and endemic year-round
Key driver of epidemics	Antigenic drift strains promoted by population-based immunologic pressure	Size of the susceptible birth cohort	Unknown
Transmission	Fecal-oral, water, and food-borne outbreaks	Fecal-oral	Fecal-oral
Severity of diarrhea in children	Generally mild but can be severe	Most severe	Milder than rotavirus or noroviruses
Reservoir	Humans are the only known reservoir of noroviruses that infect humans	Mostly humans, but rotaviruses from farm animals and pets (especially in developing countries) infect humans	Humans are the only known reservoir of astroviruses that infect humans
Prevention	Viral protein 1–based vaccine in development	Several vaccines available	No vaccine in development
Age predisposition	All ages	Children <5 years; disease transmission in older family contacts is low (<25%)	Generally children, but adults may also get disease

death toll principally occurs in the elderly, and the health care costs principally occur in children younger than 5 years.[6]

Rotavirus

The incidence of rotaviral disease is similar in children in both developed and developing countries, suggesting that measures such as access to clean water will not replace the need for an effective vaccine. Before the introduction of an effective vaccine, rotavirus was estimated to be responsible for about 600,000 annual deaths worldwide. In developed countries, rotavirus rarely is fatal; but before the introduction of vaccines in the United States, it resulted in hospitalization for rotavirus-mediated gastroenteritis in about 1 in 75 children by 5 years of age.

In the temperate zones of the world, rotaviral infection occurs primarily during epidemic peaks in the cooler months of the year (see Table 380-1). This pattern is not seen, however, in countries within 10 degrees of the equator, where infection occurs in an endemic fashion year-round. Before the introduction of rotavirus vaccination, a yearly wave of rotaviral illness spread across the United States and Europe following peculiar spatiotemporal patterns. In the United States, this pattern of spread has been correlated with variation in birth rates, thereby suggesting that the number of babies experiencing their first infection is one of the primary drivers of rotavirus epidemics. The high birth rates in developing countries may also influence the differential epidemiologic distribution of rotaviruses. The widespread use of rotavirus vaccine has greatly reduced or eliminated this spatiotemporal spread of rotavirus in the United States.

Antibodies against the outer capsid proteins are the basis of serotypic classification of rotaviruses into G (glycoprotein, VP7) and P (protease-sensitive, VP4) serotypes. For technical reasons, P serotyping reagents are infrequently available, and classification is based on the P genotype (provided in brackets). Worldwide, most human infections are caused by five types of group A rotavirus; P[8]G1 is by far the most common (approximately 53% of strains), followed by P[8]G3, P[4]G2, P[8]G9, and P[8]G4. In some developing areas like India, Brazil, and Africa, P[6]G9, G5, and G8 rotaviruses, respectively, are frequently encountered. Some human rotavirus strains may have arisen after reassortment with bovine or porcine rotaviruses. A high prevalence of G12 viruses has recently been observed in several countries, thereby suggesting that this serotype may be an emerging rotavirus strain. Results from a large multicenter study in sub-Saharan Africa and south Asia, where most of the gastroenteritis deaths in children younger than 5 years of age occur, confirmed that rotavirus is the most common etiologic agent of this syndrome and causes an important nutritional burden in children.[7]

PATHOBIOLOGY

Norovirus

Histo-blood group antigens (HBGAs) are the receptors for noroviruses and determine susceptibility to disease in a strain-specific manner. The HBGAs are complex carbohydrate oligosaccharides linked to proteins or lipids that are expressed on the mucosal epithelia of the digestive tract. All three major families of HBGA, the ABO, Lewis, and secretor families, are involved in binding noroviruses. The secretor status of a person is controlled by the fucosyltransferase 2 (*FUT2*) gene. Secretor-negative individuals are specifically resistant to infection with the Norwalk virus (GI.1) and some GII viruses.

Although norovirus RNA has been detected in the blood stream of up to 15% of patients with norovirus gastroenteritis, the site of primary viral replication is most probably in the gastrointestinal tract. Consistent with the strong association of vomiting with norovirus disease, gastric emptying is delayed. Proximal jejunal biopsy specimens show blunting of the villi with crypt cell hyperplasia and cytoplasmic vacuolation, sometimes with an increase in epithelial cell apoptosis. A functional alteration of the epithelial barrier is likely to occur. Unknown at present is the effectiveness and persistence of long-term immunity in the context of natural infection, in which the infectious dose is generally quite low.

Rotavirus

For rotaviruses, HBGAs have also been recently proposed as receptors that determine susceptibility to disease in a strain-specific manner. Rotaviruses replicate in the villus tip cells of the small bowel, where the pathologic process includes shortening and atrophy of the villi, vacuolization of enterocytes, mononuclear infiltration in the lamina propria, and distention of the cisternae of the endoplasmic reticulum. However, the severity of clinical disease has not been directly related to the extent of intestinal disease; rather, it is related to levels of viral RNA in stool.

During the initial phases of the disease, altered intestinal secretion, motility, and permeability contribute to the pathophysiologic mechanism of diarrhea. Later in the course of disease, malabsorption can occur. Rotaviral NSP4, encoded by rotavirus gene 10, is a viral enterotoxin that mediates, at least in part, the early secretory components of the diarrhea. It has also been postulated that viral infection increases intestinal motility by stimulating the enteric nervous system, possibly through NSP4. Whether and to what degree the enterotoxic effect of NSP4 is clinically relevant in children or other animal species remains to be determined. Infected individuals have a short period of viremia, but its clinical consequences are unclear other than correlating with the level of fever. However, most rotavirus-infected children have mild elevations in hepatic enzymes, thereby suggesting that low-level hepatitis is a common occurrence.[8]

Rotavirus serum IgA levels measured shortly after natural infection in children generally correlate with intestinal IgA levels and appear to correlate with protection.[9] One explanation for recurrent rotavirus (and norovirus) infections is that protection from reinfection is mediated by intestinal IgA, which is not long-lasting in humans. Another explanation is that protection is dependent on neutralizing antibodies to one or both of the highly variable outer rotaviral proteins. However, a monovalent P[8]G1 vaccine induces significant protection against strains with different serotypes, thereby supporting the conclusion that protective immunity to rotavirus infection is, in large part, heterotypic.

CLINICAL MANIFESTATIONS

Norovirus

The clinical manifestations of norovirus infection are variable and depend in part on the age of the individual infected. About one third of infections are asymptomatic, but symptoms include diarrhea, nausea, vomiting, abdominal cramps, fever, and malaise that generally persist for 1 to 3 days. In children younger than 11 years, disease typically begins with the sudden onset of vomiting and can last 4 to 6 days. Virus can be shed in low titers for up to 8 weeks from otherwise healthy individuals and for more than a year in patients with severe immunodeficiency syndromes. In neonates and premature infants, vomiting often is not a symptom, and infection has been associated with necrotizing enterocolitis. To support the diagnosis of norovirus outbreaks, the following four criteria have been proposed: (1) vomiting in more than half of affected persons; (2) mean (or median) incubation period of 24 to 48 hours; (3) mean (or median) duration of illness of 12 to 60 hours; and (4) absence of bacterial pathogens in stool culture.

Rotavirus

Rotavirus diarrhea and dehydration tend to be more severe than illness caused by the other childhood enteric pathogens. Rotavirus diarrhea is watery, persists for approximately 5 days, is often preceded by the sudden onset of vomiting, and is frequently accompanied by fever and dehydration. The incubation period of rotavirus is estimated to be less than 48 hours. Viral excretion in feces persists for 10 days in the majority of children and can persist for up to 57 days. Excretion times are longer on examination by sensitive PCR-based assays rather than solid-phase immunoassay. By the age of 5 years, virtually all children have acquired immunity to rotavirus, and severe disease after this age is uncommon.

DIAGNOSIS

Norovirus

Reverse transcription–PCR (RT-PCR) is currently the procedure of choice to detect norovirus in clinical specimens, in food, and in water. Although enzyme-linked immunosorbent assays (ELISAs) to detect noroviruses are available in Europe, their sensitivity is genotype dependent, and diagnostic specificity and sensitivity vary on the basis of the diversity of the circulating strains in the population. Moreover, these immunoassays are not easily adaptable for detection of new strains. Norovirus RNA is detected by RT-PCR in stool samples of up to 16% of healthy individuals, a finding that complicates the diagnosis of norovirus gastroenteritis. Although the relationship between disease symptoms and viral load has not been fully established, a quantitative real-time RT-PCR has been proposed to establish a relative threshold of positivity for attributing disease to norovirus.

Rotavirus

Before the introduction of the rotavirus vaccine in developed countries, well above 50% of the moderate to severe diarrheal episodes in young children during the rotavirus "season" were due to rotavirus. In tropical countries, the presence of other enteric pathogens and the absence of seasonal occurrence of rotaviral disease make it more difficult to determine which diarrheal episodes are caused by rotavirus without a diagnostic assay. Numerous ELISAs for rotavirus are commercially available, and these are generally sensitive, specific, and easy to use under most conditions. PCR has increased sensitivity for detection of rotavirus and has permitted easy typing of viruses. With PCR-based methods, however, up to 29% of healthy children younger than 1 year may be rotavirus positive, so it is difficult to associate the detection of the virus with gastroenteritis. Thus, ELISA or quantitative RT-PCR (using a threshold level as for norovirus) is preferable for diagnosis of rotavirus gastroenteritis.

PREVENTION

Norovirus

The development of a norovirus vaccine for humans is likely to be a challenge owing to the antigenic heterogeneity among circulating strains, the propensity of noroviruses to undergo antigenic drift, waning immunity, and the lack of well-established correlates of protection. Nevertheless, a new VLP-based vaccine candidate has recently shown promising efficacy in the experimental viral challenge setting.[A1]

High percentage alcohol-based sanitizers (99.5% ethanol) and 10% povidone-iodine antiseptics are superior to other alcohol-based sanitizers at reducing norovirus contamination. Simple household antimicrobial hand soap and handwashing with tap water also decrease viral contamination.

Rotavirus

The first vaccine (Rotashield [Wyeth-Lederle]), which was a quadrivalent mixture of rhesus-human rotavirus reassortants, each containing a G protein from a common human rotavirus serotype, was licensed for use in the United States but subsequently withdrawn from the market because of its association with intussusception. Subsequently, two second-generation vaccines were shown in large studies to be safe, effective, and cost-effective in developed and developing countries. The two current rotavirus vaccines have been

based on two different approaches. One type of vaccine (RV5, RotaTeq [Merck]) uses a modified pentavalent vaccine made of a mixture of bovine and human reassortant rotaviruses.[A2] Another approach (RV1, Rotarix [GlaxoSmithKline]) is a monovalent attenuated human virus vaccine.[A3-A5] Neither type of vaccine prevents subsequent rotavirus infection or mild illness, but both types effectively prevent severe illness, especially in developed countries.

Protection rates in developed and middle-income countries for each rotavirus vaccine are similar, varying from 70 to 80% against any rotavirus disease and 90 to 100% against severe gastroenteritis. Recent evidence suggests that both licensed vaccines slightly increase the risk of intussusception,[10,11] but their benefits far outweigh this low-level risk. Even in the United States, where the burden of severe disease from rotavirus is lowest, the rotavirus vaccine has significantly reduced health care utilization and expenses for diarrhea in children.

In the United States, vaccination also has had an unexpected effect on rotavirus-induced diarrhea among unvaccinated persons, thereby suggesting the induction of herd immunity. The U.S. Advisory Committee on Immunization Practices (Chapter 18) and the World Health Organization[12] now recommend the routine use of these vaccines.

Currently available vaccines are only about 50% efficacious against severe diseases in the poorest developing countries.[A6-A9] Even with this reduced effectiveness, however, the two licensed vaccines are still cost-effective in the less developed world.

TREATMENT   Rx

Because both norovirus and rotavirus disease resolves within days without treatment, the basic therapeutic goal is to prevent acute dehydration. The recommended oral rehydration salts solution, which now has an osmolarity of 331 mmol/L, is as effective as higher osmolarity solutions.[A10] After rehydration, rapid age-appropriate refeeding is recommended. Rotavirus disease induces self-limited intestinal lactase deficiency, but lactose-containing products, particularly maternal milk, should not be withheld.

Passive oral immunotherapy with diverse preparations of immunoglobulins can shorten the duration of rotavirus infection but probably is economically feasible only for immunodeficient patients or low-birthweight infants in the developed world. Recently in Bangladesh, llama-derived, heavy-chain antibody fragment specific for rotavirus was able to reduce stool output in male infants with severe rotavirus-associated diarrhea.[A11] *Lactobacillus*, a bacterium present in yogurt, is safe and, in limited studies, appears moderately effective for treatment of acute rotavirus gastroenteritis. Nonetheless, different preparations of lactobacilli vary greatly in dose of bacteria, and a general recommendation on their use has not been issued. Several studies in developing countries have shown that zinc supplementation (10 mg/day for infants younger than 6 months and 20 mg/day for older children) is useful for the treatment and prevention of diarrhea, but further studies are needed to determine whether treatment will be useful in all developing and developed countries.

At present, no pharmacologic treatment of rotavirus or norovirus diarrhea is recommended.[13] Racecadotril (4.5 mg/kg per day), an enkephalinase inhibitor that acts on the enteric nervous system, has been shown to be useful as an adjunct to treat rotaviral diarrhea in several small studies. Ondansetron (0.15 mg/kg per day), a serotonin antagonist, is effective in reducing the emesis from gastroenteritis during the phase of oral rehydration. In several small studies, nitazoxanide (15 mg/kg per day) was helpful in the treatment of rotavirus gastroenteritis. More studies are needed before any of these various preparations can be generally recommended for treatment of rotavirus diarrhea.

Grade A References

A1. Atmar RL, Bernstein DI, Harro CD, et al. Norovirus vaccine against experimental human Norwalk virus illness. *N Engl J Med.* 2011;365:2178-2187.
A2. Vesikari T, Matson DO, Dennehy P, et al. Safety and efficacy of a pentavalent human-bovine (WC3) reassortant rotavirus vaccine. *N Engl J Med.* 2006;354:23-33.
A3. Vesikari T, Karvonen A, Prymula R, et al. Efficacy of human rotavirus vaccine against rotavirus gastroenteritis during the first 2 years of life in European infants: randomised, double-blind controlled study. *Lancet.* 2007;370:1757-1763.
A4. Ruiz-Palacios GM, Pérez-Schael I, Velázquez FR, et al. Safety and efficacy of an attenuated vaccine against severe rotavirus gastroenteritis. *N Engl J Med.* 2006;354:11-22.
A5. Linhares AC, Velázquez FR, Pérez-Schael I, et al. Efficacy and safety of an oral live attenuated human rotavirus vaccine against rotavirus gastroenteritis during the first 2 years of life in Latin American infants: a randomised, double-blind, placebo-controlled phase III study. *Lancet.* 2008;371:1181-1189.
A6. Madhi SA, Cunliffe NA, Steele D, et al. Effect of human rotavirus vaccine on severe diarrhea in African infants. *N Engl J Med.* 2010;362:289-298.

A7. Zaman K, Dang DA, Victor JC, et al. Efficacy of pentavalent rotavirus vaccine against severe rotavirus gastroenteritis in infants in developing countries in Asia: a randomised, double-blind, placebo-controlled trial. *Lancet.* 2010;376:615-623.

A8. Armah GE, Sow SO, Breiman RF, et al. Efficacy of pentavalent rotavirus vaccine against severe rotavirus gastroenteritis in infants in developing countries in sub-Saharan Africa: a randomised, double-blind, placebo-controlled trial. *Lancet.* 2010;376:606-614.

A9. Bhandari N, Rongsen-Chandola T, Bavdekar A, et al. Efficacy of a monovalent human-bovine (116E) rotavirus vaccine in Indian infants: a randomised, double-blind, placebo-controlled trial. *Lancet.* 2014;383:2136-2143.

A10. CHOICE Study Group. Multicenter, randomized, double-blind clinical trial to evaluate the efficacy and safety of a reduced osmolarity oral rehydration salts solution in children with acute watery diarrhea. *Pediatrics.* 2001;107:613-618.

A11. Sarker SA, Jäkel M, Sultana S, et al. Anti-rotavirus protein reduces stool output in infants with diarrhea: a randomized placebo-controlled trial. *Gastroenterology.* 2013;145:740-748.

GENERAL REFERENCES

For the General References and other additional features, please visit Expert Consult at https://expertconsult.inkling.com.

381

VIRAL HEMORRHAGIC FEVERS

DANIEL G. BAUSCH

DEFINITION

Viral hemorrhagic fever is an acute systemic illness classically involving fever, a constellation of initially nonspecific signs and symptoms, and a propensity for bleeding and shock. It may be caused by more than 30 different viruses from four taxonomic families, Filoviridae, Arenaviridae, Bunyaviridae, and Flaviviridae (Table 381-1), although not every virus in these families causes the syndrome. Hemorrhagic fever viruses are often named after the site of the first recognized case. All are single-stranded lipid-enveloped RNA viruses with small genomes (10 to 19 kilobases) that can be relatively easily inactivated in the environment. Pathogenicity varies widely by the specific virus and sometimes among strains of the same virus. Many of the hemorrhagic fever viruses have been placed on the Centers for Disease Control and Prevention select agents list of pathogens that pose a potential bioterrorism threat (Chapter 21).

EPIDEMIOLOGY

Maintenance in Nature and Transmission to Humans

With the exception of dengue virus, for which humans can now be considered the reservoir, hemorrhagic fever viruses are zoonotic, maintained in nature in mammalian reservoirs (see Table 381-1). Although viral hemorrhagic fevers collectively can be found worldwide, the endemic area of any given hemorrhagic fever virus is usually smaller than the extent of its natural reservoir or arthropod vector. With the exception of dengue and some hantaviruses, human infection is generally infrequent. Humans are dead-end hosts.

Hemorrhagic fever viruses may be transmitted to humans by usually inadvertent, direct exposure of mucous membranes or broken skin to the infected blood or excreta of its animal reservoir or, in the case of the flaviviruses and most of the bunyaviruses, by the bite of an arthropod vector. The infectious dose for most hemorrhagic fever viruses appears to be low, sometimes on the order of just a few virions. Aerosol transmission is not a predominant mode of spread, if it occurs at all, but studies in nonhuman primates show that transmission of many hemorrhagic fever viruses is possible through artificial aerosols, thereby raising the possibility of their potential use as bioweapons (Chapter 21).

Bat-Borne Viruses

The filoviruses (from the Latin *filo,* "thread," referring to their filamentous shape), Marburg and Ebola, are perhaps the most feared of all hemorrhagic fever viruses.[1] Fruit bats appear to be the filovirus reservoir, with transmission to humans likely from exposure to infected bat excreta or saliva. Nonhuman primates, especially gorillas and chimpanzees, and other wild animals may become infected, presumably from similar bat exposure, and transmit filoviruses to humans through contact with blood and body fluids of these animals, usually in association with hunting. Nonhuman primates, which are also dead-end hosts who develop severe and usually fatal disease similar to that seen in humans, may be easier prey for hunters when sick. Because hemorrhagic fever viruses are rapidly inactivated by heating, infection probably occurs by exposure during butchering and preparation. In the Philippines, Ebola Reston virus has been isolated from pigs that were presumably infected from exposure to bats.

In the recent outbreak in West Africa, which began in March, 2014, more than 20,000 cases and 8,000 deaths were confirmed by the end of the calendar year—numbers that dwarf all prior Ebola outbreaks combined.[2] The response has been hampered by limited facilities and trained medical personnel, some of whom have themselves become infected and died.

Rodent-Borne Viruses

Arenaviruses (from the Latin *arena,* "sand," referring to their sandy appearance on electron microscopy) are divided into two groups: the Old World (or lymphocytic choriomeningitis/Lassa) complex and the New World (or Tacaribe) complex.[3] Lassa virus and Lujo virus are found in Africa, whereas Junín, Machupo, Guanarito, Sabiá, and Chapare viruses are found in South America. Although there may be subtle differences among the syndromes produced by the New World arenaviruses, they are usually grouped together simply as the South American hemorrhagic fevers.

The genus Hantavirus of the Bunyaviridae family is similarly divided into Old and New World groups. The Old World hantaviruses, such as Hantaan, Seoul, and Puumala, among many others, cause hemorrhagic fevers with prominent renal involvement across Europe and Asia. New World hantaviruses, such as Sin Nombre and Andes, among many others, cause a viral hemorrhagic fever named hantavirus pulmonary syndrome, sometimes also called hantavirus cardiopulmonary syndrome to emphasize the significant cardiogenic component of this disease.

Pathogenic arenaviruses and hantaviruses are maintained in nature through chronic asymptomatic infection in rodents of the *Muridae* family, with a strict pairing between the specific virus and rodent species. Transmission between rodents may be by vertical or horizontal transmission or both, depending on the specific virus. Transmission to humans occurs through exposure to rodent excreta, either from aerosols produced when rodents urinate or by direct inoculation to the mucous membranes. Secondary aerosol generation is notoriously inefficient, so disturbing shed urine is a less likely mechanism of infection. In West Africa, Lassa virus is sometimes contracted when rodents are trapped and prepared for consumption or, more rarely, through a rodent bite. Experimental data suggest that humans may be infected with arenaviruses by the oral route.

The rodents that transmit Lassa, Machupo, and many of the Old World hantaviruses commonly invade the peridomestic environment, thereby putting housewives, children, and others who spend time at home at risk. In contrast, the reservoirs for Junín, Guanarito, and most of the New World hantaviruses typically inhabit agricultural fields, wood lots, or other rural habitats, thereby putting outdoor workers, campers, and hikers at risk.

Mosquito-Borne Viruses

Rift Valley fever virus is maintained in domestic livestock, such as cattle, buffalo, sheep, goats, and camels, in which it often provokes spontaneous abortion. The virus may be transmitted to humans by direct exposure to these animals, especially during parturition, or by mosquitoes. Farmers, abattoir workers, and veterinarians are at particular risk.[4]

Yellow fever virus is maintained in a cycle between monkeys and forest canopy mosquitoes. Sporadic cases occur when humans are bitten by these mosquitoes. Larger outbreaks occur when humans bring the virus back to more settled environments, where the urban mosquito *Aedes aegypti* can spread the virus directly between humans. *Ae. aegypti,* which typically lay eggs in artificial containers around the home and bite during the day, become infective a few weeks after feeding on a viremic monkey or human. Sanitation and mosquito control measures have virtually eliminated urban yellow fever in the Americas, but urban outbreaks continue to occur in Africa. For example, 849 cases and 171 deaths were reported in a recent outbreak in Sudan.[5]

Although nonhuman primates are also a reservoir for sylvatic strains of dengue, the virus is now largely maintained in humans, with a regular transmission cycle akin to that of urban yellow fever. Despite the presence of dengue virus in the tropics worldwide, less than 10% of infected persons develop hemorrhagic fever, primarily children between the ages of 4 and 12 years.

TABLE 381-1   PRINCIPAL VIRUSES CAUSING HEMORRHAGIC FEVER

VIRUS	DISEASE	GEOGRAPHIC DISTRIBUTION OF DISEASE	PRINCIPAL RESERVOIR/VECTOR	ANNUAL CASES	CASE TO INFECTION RATIO	HUMAN-TO-HUMAN TRANSMISSIBILITY
FILOVIRIDAE						
Ebolavirus[a]	Ebola HF	Sub-Saharan Africa	Fruit bat?	—[b]	1:1	High
Marburgvirus	Marburg HF	Sub-Saharan Africa	Fruit bat: Egyptian fruit bat (*Rousettus aegyptiacus*), perhaps others	—[b]	1:1	High
ARENAVIRIDAE[c,d]						
Old World Group						
Lassa	Lassa fever	West Africa	Rodent: natal mastomys or multimammate rat (*Mastomys natalensis*)	50,000-100,000	1:5-10	Moderate
Lujo[e]	Lujo HF	Zambia	Unknown, presumed rodent	Unknown	Unknown	Moderate to high
New World Group						
Junin	Argentine HF	Argentine pampas	Rodent: corn mouse (*Calomys musculinus*)	≈100	1:1.5	Low
Machupo	Bolivian HF	Beni department, Bolivia	Rodent: large vesper mouse (*Calomys callosus*)	≤50	1:1.5	Low
Guanarito	Venezuelan HF	Portuguesa state, Venezuela	Rodent: cane mouse (*Zygodontomys brevicauda*)	≤50	1:1.5	Low
Sabiá[f]	Proposed name: Brazilian HF	Rural area near São Paulo, Brazil?	Unknown, presumed rodent	Unknown	1:1.5	Low?
Chapare[g]	Chapare HF	Cochabamba, Bolivia	Unknown, presumed rodent	Unknown	Unknown	Unknown
BUNYAVIRIDAE[c]						
Old World Group						
Hantaan, Seoul, Puumala, Dobrava-Belgrade, others	HF with renal syndrome	Hantaan: northeast Asia Seoul: urban areas worldwide Puumala and Dobrava-Belgrade: Europe	Rodent Hantaan: striped field mouse (*Apodemus agrarius*) Seoul: brown or Norway rat (*Rattus norvegicus*) Puumala: bank vole (*Clethrionomys glareolus*) Dobrava-Belgrade: yellow-necked field mouse (*Apodemus flavicollis*)	50,000-150,000	Hantaan: 1:1.5 Others: 1:20	None

	Disease	Geographic Distribution	Natural Host/Vector	Estimated Cases/Year	Case-Fatality Ratio	Person-to-Person Transmission
New World Group						
Sin Nombre, Andes, Laguna Negra, others	Hantavirus cardiopulmonary syndrome	Americas	Rodent Sin Nombre: deer mouse (*Peromyscus maniculatus*) Andes: long-tailed colilargo (*Oligoryzomys longicaudatus*) Laguna Negra: little laucha or small vesper mouse (*Calomys laucha*)	50,000-150,000	Sin Nombre: 1:1 Others: up to 1:20	None, except for Andes virus
Rift Valley fever	Rift Valley fever	Sub-Saharan Africa, Madagascar, Saudi Arabia, Yemen	Domestic livestock/mosquitoes (sylvatic *Aedes* and others)	100-100,000[b,h]	1:100	None
Crimean-Congo HF	Crimean-Congo HF	Africa, Balkans, southern Russia, Middle East, India, Pakistan, Afghanistan, western China	Wild and domestic vertebrates/tick (primarily *Hyalomma* species)	≈500	1:1-2	High
FLAVIVIRIDAE						
Yellow fever	Yellow fever	Sub-Saharan Africa, South America up to Panama	Monkey/mosquito (*Aedes aegypti*, other *Aedes* and *Haemagogus* species)	5000-200,000[i]	1:2-20	None
Dengue	Dengue HF	Tropics and subtropics worldwide	Human/mosquito (*Ae. aegypti* and *albopictus*)	100,000-200,000[i]	1:10-100, depending on age, previous infection, genetic background, and infecting serotype	None
Omsk HF	Omsk HF	Western Siberia	Rodent/tick (primarily *Dermacentor* and *Ixodes* species)	100-200	Unknown	Not reported
Kyasanur Forest disease	Kyasanur Forest disease	Karnataka state, India; Yunnan Province, China; Saudi Arabia	Vertebrate (rodents, bats, birds, monkeys, others)/tick (*Haemaphysalis* species and others)	≈500	Unknown	Not reported, but laboratory infections have occurred
Alkhumra HF[j]	Proposed name: Alkhumra HF	Saudi Arabia, Egypt	Ticks?	≤50	Unknown	Not reported

[a] Six species or subtypes of Ebolavirus are recognized with varying associated case-fatality ratios (see Table 381-2). All are endemic to sub-Saharan Africa, with the exceptions of Reston ebolavirus, which is found in the Philippines, and Lloviu ebolavirus, which was detected in bats in Spain.

[b] Although some endemic transmission of the filoviruses (Ebolavirus > Marburgvirus) and Rift Valley fever virus occurs, these viruses have most often been associated with outbreaks.

[c] The virus families Arenaviridae and Bunyaviridae are serologically, phylogenetically, and geographically divided into Old World (i.e., Africa) and New World (i.e., the Americas) complexes.

[d] In addition to the arenaviruses listed in the table, Flexal and Tacaribe viruses have caused human disease as a result of laboratory accidents. Another arenavirus, Whitewater Arroyo, has been noted in sick persons in California, but its role as a pathogen has not been clearly established.

[e] Discovered in 2008. Only five cases (four of them fatal) from one outbreak have been noted. The index case came to South Africa from Zambia.

[f] Discovered in 1990. Only three cases (one fatal) have been noted, two of them from laboratory accidents.

[g] Discovered in 2003 from a small outbreak from which blood was obtained from one fatal case and Chapare virus isolated. Few other details have been reported.

[h] Although Rift Valley fever virus can be found throughout sub-Saharan Africa, large outbreaks usually occur in East Africa's Rift Valley region.

[i] Based on estimates from the World Health Organization. Incidence may fluctuate widely in place and time. Significant underreporting occurs.

[j] Alkhumra is considered by some to be a variant of Kyasanur Forest disease virus. Disagreement exists over the proper spelling of the virus, written as Alkhurma in some publications.

HF = hemorrhagic fever.

Tick-Borne Viruses

The viruses that cause Crimean-Congo hemorrhagic fever, Omsk hemorrhagic fever,[6] Kyasanur Forest disease, and Alkhumra hemorrhagic fever are maintained in small mammals, such as rodents, hares, and hedgehogs, among which the viruses are spread by ticks. Humans are infected either by tick bites or by exposure to contaminated blood or excreta of the reservoir animals. Ticks also spread Crimean-Congo hemorrhagic fever virus to large mammals, including cattle and other domestic livestock, whose transient and asymptomatic viremia puts farmers, abattoir workers, and veterinarians at risk.

Human-to-Human Transmission

Secondary human-to-human transmission occurs with many of the hemorrhagic fever viruses, but tertiary transmission is unusual and often associated with milder disease (see Table 381-1). Secondary attack rates for hemorrhagic fever viruses are generally low (15 to 20% for Ebola Zaire virus), probably because transmission between humans requires direct contact with contaminated blood or body fluids. Human-to-human infection probably usually occurs through oral or mucous membrane exposure, most often in the context of providing care to a sick family member (community) or patient (nosocomial transmission), and occasionally during funeral rituals that entail the touching of the corpse, especially for the filoviruses. Infection through fomites cannot be excluded. Aerosol infection is thought to be rare or non-existent. Large outbreaks almost always involve amplification in health care settings in which basic infection control measures have broken down, usually owing to extreme poverty or civil strife.

With the exception of hantaviruses and some of the flaviviruses, infectivity generally parallels the clinical state. Persons are generally most infectious late in the course of severe disease, especially when bleeding. The risk of transmission during the incubation period or from asymptomatic persons is negligible, although a case of Argentine hemorrhagic fever occurred from blood transfusion from an asymptomatic donor. Rarely, Ebola, Marburg, Lassa, and Junín viruses have been sexually transmitted during the first 3 months of convalescence owing to delayed viral clearance from the gonads, which is an immunologically protected site. Despite modern-day travel, imported cases of viral hemorrhagic fever remain extremely rare.

PATHOBIOLOGY

Although the precise mechanism varies with the specific virus, microvascular instability and impaired hemostasis are the pathobiologic hallmarks of viral hemorrhagic fever. Data from animal models suggest that cardiac inotropy may also be directly or indirectly inhibited in some viral hemorrhagic fevers, especially Lassa fever.

After inoculation, virus first replicates in dendritic cells and other local tissues, with subsequent migration to regional lymph nodes and then dissemination through the lymph and blood monocytes to a broad range of tissues and organs, including the liver, spleen, lymph nodes, adrenal glands, lungs, and endothelium. Migration of tissue macrophages results in secondary infection of permissive parenchymal cells. During the acute illness, virus can be found in a wide variety of body fluids, including blood, saliva, stool, and breast milk.

The interaction of virus with immune cells, especially macrophages and endothelial cells, results directly or indirectly (through soluble mediators) in cell activation and the unleashing of an inflammatory and vasoactive process consistent with the systemic inflammatory response syndrome. The synthesis of cell surface tissue factor triggers the extrinsic coagulation pathway. Impaired hemostasis may entail endothelial cell, platelet, or coagulation factor dysfunction. Disseminated intravascular coagulopathy (DIC) is frequently noted, especially with Ebola, Marburg, and Crimean-Congo hemorrhagic fever virus infections.

Tissue damage may be mediated through direct necrosis of infected cells or indirectly through apoptosis of immune cells, as seen in other forms of septic shock. The most affected organs vary with the virus (Table 381-2). For example, renal tubular necrosis and retroperitoneal edema are seen in hemorrhagic fevers with renal syndrome, whereas interstitial pneumonitis and myocardial depression are the hallmarks of hantavirus pulmonary syndrome. The liver is particularly affected in yellow fever, with fatty degeneration, coagulative midzonal necrosis of hepatocytes, and the presence of Councilman bodies. The brain and meninges are particularly affected in Kyasanur Forest disease and Omsk hemorrhagic fever and often in the South American hemorrhagic fevers as well. Reticuloendothelial proliferation is seen in Kyasanur Forest disease, with marked erythrophagocytosis in the spleen.

With the exception of disease caused by the hantaviruses and some of the flaviviruses, the pathogenesis of viral hemorrhagic fever appears to be related to unchecked viremia, with most fatal cases failing to mount a significant antibody response. By comparison, virus is cleared rapidly from the blood in survivors. Inflammatory cell infiltrates, which are usually mild, consist of a mix of mononuclear cells and neutrophils. In some viral hemorrhagic fevers, such as Ebola, virus replication and dissemination are facilitated by virus-induced suppression of the host adaptive immune response. For example, failure of the immune response to adequately respond appears to be a major determinant of severity in Lassa fever.[7]

In dengue, yellow fever, and hantavirus infections, in which viremia is usually cleared before the most severe phase of the disease, the host immune response may play a detrimental role. The unique process of antibody-mediated immune enhancement, in which secondary infection with a different dengue virus serotype is more severe than the primary one, may play a role in the pathogenesis of dengue hemorrhagic fever.

CLINICAL MANIFESTATIONS

Viral hemorrhagic fever is seen in both genders and all age groups, with a spectrum from relatively mild or even asymptomatic infection to severe vascular permeability resulting in shock, multiorgan system failure, and death. Although the clinical presentation may differ for each viral hemorrhagic fever as disease progresses, the limited data do not permit clear distinctions in most cases, especially in the early phases of disease. Dengue and Rift Valley fever viruses cause a range of syndromes, including rash and central nervous system involvement (Chapters 382 and 383). Hemorrhagic fever occurs in a minority of infections with these viruses.

After an incubation period ranging from days to weeks, most patients present with nonspecific signs and symptoms difficult to distinguish from a host of other febrile illnesses (see Table 381-2)[8], including fever, general malaise, anorexia, headache, chest or retrosternal pain, sore throat, myalgia, arthralgia, and lumbosacral pain. Conjunctival injection or hemorrhage is frequent but is not accompanied by itching, discharge, or rhinitis (Fig. 381-1). Relative bradycardia (Faget sign) and orthostatic hypotension may be noted, especially in yellow fever and dengue virus infections. The pharynx may be erythemic or, less frequently, exudative, especially in Lassa fever, and incorrectly lead to a diagnosis of streptococcal pharyngitis or mononucleosis. Gastrointestinal signs and symptoms readily ensue, including nausea, vomiting, epigastric and abdominal pain, abdominal tenderness (especially over the liver in filovirus infection), and nonbloody diarrhea or constipation. A misdiagnosis of appendicitis or other acute abdominal emergency (Chapter 142) sometimes prompts potentially hazardous surgical interventions.

In the recent Ebola outbreak in West Africa, the incubation period averaged 6 to 8 days. Most patients presented with some combination of fever (90%), headache (80%), diarrhea (50%), or vomiting (35%), often associated with myalgias, weakness, or abdominal pain. Hiccups also may be seen early in Ebola hemorrhagic fever.[9]

Neck pain and stiffness, retro-orbital pain, photophobia, and other meningeal signs are common in Rift Valley fever, Kyasanur Forest disease, and Omsk hemorrhagic fever. A dry cough, sometimes accompanied by a few scattered rales on auscultation, is common, but prominent pulmonary symptoms are uncommon early in the course of the disease, except with hantavirus pulmonary syndrome. Pregnant women often present with spontaneous abortion and vaginal bleeding. With the exception of yellow fever, jaundice is not typical except in patients with underlying Gilbert syndrome, drug reactions, or coinfection. Hepatosplenomegaly is frequent, but whether it is specific to the viral hemorrhagic fever or simply represents the high underlying prevalence of hepatosplenomegaly in populations in sub-Saharan Africa is unknown.

Various forms of rash, including morbilliform, maculopapular, petechial, and ecchymotic, may be seen (see Table 381-2). A maculopapular rash on the torso or face may be one early and relatively specific although insensitive indicator of Ebola or Marburg hemorrhagic fever. Rash almost always occurs in fair-skinned persons with Lassa fever but, for unclear reasons, rarely in blacks.

In severe cases, patients progress after 7 to 10 days of illness to vascular instability, which may be manifested by conjunctival injection and hemorrhage, facial flushing, edema, bleeding, hypotension, shock, and proteinuria. Facial and neck swelling are classic and relatively specific signs of Lassa fever and Lujo hemorrhagic fever.[10] The likelihood of clinically discernible hemorrhage varies with the infecting virus (see Table 381-2) and may be manifested as hematemesis, melena, hematochezia, metrorrhagia, petechiae, purpura,

TABLE 381-2 PATHOBIOLOGIC AND CLINICAL ASPECTS OF VIRAL HEMORRHAGIC FEVERS

DISEASE	INCUBATION PERIOD (DAYS)	ONSET	BLEEDING	RASH	JAUNDICE	HEART	LUNG	KIDNEY	CENTRAL NERVOUS SYSTEM	EYE	CASE-FATALITY RATIO	CLINICAL MANAGEMENT
FILOVIRIDAE												
Ebola HF	3-21	Variable	++	+++	+	++?	+	+	+	+	40-85%[a]	Supportive
Marburg HF	3-21	Abrupt	++	+++	+	++?	+	+	+	+	22-85%[b]	Supportive
ARENAVIRIDAE												
Lassa fever	5-16	Gradual	+	+[c]	0	++	+	0	+	0	20%	Ribavirin
Lujo HF	9-13	Abrupt	++	+	0	?	+	+	+	0	80%	Ribavirin
South American HFs[d]	4-14	Gradual	+++	+	0	++	+	0	+++	0	15-40%	Ribavirin, convalescent plasma
BUNYAVIRIDAE												
Hemorrhagic fever with renal syndrome	9-35	Abrupt	+++	0	0	++	+	+++	+	0	<1-50%. depending on specific virus	Ribavirin
Hantavirus pulmonary syndrome	7-35	Gradual	0 (except for Andes virus infection)	0	0	+++	+++	+	+	0	<1-50%. depending on specific virus	Supportive, ECMO?
Rift Valley fever[e]	2-5	Abrupt	++	+	++	+?	0	+	++	++	Up to 50% in severe forms	Ribavirin?
Crimean-Congo HF	1-12[f]	Abrupt	+++	0	++	+?	+	0	+	0	15-30%	Ribavirin
FLAVIVIRIDAE												
Yellow fever	3-6	Abrupt	+++	0	+++	++	+	++	++	0	20-50%	Supportive
Dengue HF	3-15	Abrupt	++	+++	+	++	+	0	+	0	Untreated: 10-15% Treated: ≤1%	Supportive
Omsk HF	3-8	Abrupt	++	0	0	+	++	0	+++	+	1-3%	Supportive
Kyasanur forest disease	3-8	Abrupt	++	0	0	+	++	0	+++	+	3-5%	Supportive
Alkhumra HF[g]	3-8	Abrupt	++	+	+	+	+	0	++	+	20-25%	Supportive

[a]Six species or subtypes of Ebolavirus are recognized with varying associated case-fatality ratios: Zaire, 85%; Sudan, 55%; Bundibugyo, 40%; Tai Forest (also called Côte d'Ivoire), 0% (only one recognized case, who survived); Reston, 0% (not pathogenic to humans); Lloviu, no human infections recognized.
[b]The case-fatality ratio was 22% in the first recognized outbreak of Marburg HF in Germany and Yugoslavia in 1967 but has been consistently above 80% in outbreaks in central Africa, where the virus is endemic. Possible reasons for this discrepancy include differences in quality of care, strain pathogenicity, route and dose of infection, underlying prevalence of immunodeficiency and comorbid illnesses, and genetic susceptibility.
[c]A morbilliform or maculopapular rash almost always occurs in persons with lighter skin, who are usually expatriates, but for unclear reasons is rarely present in darker-skinned Africans from the endemic area.
[d]Data are insufficient to distinguish between the syndromes produced by the various arenaviruses found in the Americas. They are thus frequently grouped as the South American hemorrhagic fevers.
[e]Hemorrhagic fever, encephalitis, and retinitis may be seen in Rift Valley fever independently of each other.
[f]The incubation period of Crimean-Congo HF varies with the mode of transmission: typically 1 to 3 days after tick bite and 5 to 6 days after contact with infected animal blood or tissues.
[g]Based on preliminary observations. Fewer than 100 cases have been reported.
ECMO = extracorporeal membrane oxygenation; HF = hemorrhagic fever; 0 = sign not typically noted/organ not typically affected; + = sign occasionally noted/organ occasionally affected; ++ = sign commonly noted/organ commonly affected; +++ = sign characteristic/organ involvement severe.

epistaxis, and bleeding from the gums and venipuncture sites (Fig. 381-2). Hemoptysis and hematuria are infrequent. Hemorrhage is almost never present in the first few days of illness. Large ecchymoses are characteristic of Crimean-Congo hemorrhagic fever. Central nervous system manifestations, including delirium, tremor, gait anomalies, convulsions, and hiccups, may be noted in end-stage disease, especially in Kyasanur Forest disease, Omsk hemorrhagic fever, and the South American hemorrhagic fevers, particularly Argentine hemorrhagic fever. Nevertheless, the cerebrospinal fluid findings are usually normal, with the exception of patients who have meningoencephalitis due to Kyasanur Forest disease and Omsk hemorrhagic fever, in which an elevated protein level is common. Renal insufficiency or failure is common, especially in hemorrhagic fever with renal syndrome.

Biphasic illnesses are classically noted for the flavivirus hemorrhagic fevers, in which a quiescent period of days (yellow fever, dengue hemorrhagic fever, and Rift Valley fever) to weeks (Kyasanur Forest disease and Omsk hemorrhagic fever) precedes the most severe manifestations, including hemorrhage, shock, renal failure, and meningoencephalitis. Distinct progressive phases of disease and recovery are classically described for hemorrhagic fever with renal syndrome (prodrome, hypotension, oliguria/renal failure, diuresis, and convalescence) and yellow fever (infection, intoxication, recovery) but are not seen in all cases. The initial manifestations for hantavirus pulmonary syndrome may be mild and nonspecific, but the disease may progress to require mechanical ventilation and pressor support within 24 hours; sinus bradycardia and ventricular tachycardia or fibrillation may occur. Encephali-

tis and retinitis may develop in Rift Valley fever independently of the presence or absence of viral hemorrhagic fever.

Bilateral noncardiogenic interstitial pulmonary edema consistent with the adult respiratory distress syndrome (ARDS) is the hallmark of hantavirus pulmonary syndrome, although chest radiographs may be normal early in the disease even when the patients complain of shortness of breath. Only about 30% of patients with hantavirus pulmonary syndrome have radiographic evidence of pulmonary edema on initial evaluation, although it develops in virtually all persons within 48 hours.

DIAGNOSIS

Because of their associated severity, risk of secondary spread, high degree of public scrutiny, and unfamiliarity to most physicians, consultation with a specialist who has experience with viral hemorrhagic fevers should be sought as soon as the diagnosis is considered. When to "sound the alarm" of viral hemorrhagic fever is a case-by-case decision left to the treating physician in consultation with experts in the field. Most viral hemorrhagic fevers are rare, and routinely practiced universal precautions are protective in most cases.

The early nonspecific presentation of viral hemorrhagic fevers makes them extremely difficult to diagnose clinically, especially outside of the setting of a recognized outbreak, which is usually detected when clusters of cases occur, especially when they involve health care workers. The differential diagnosis includes a broad array of febrile illnesses that varies by geographic region (Table 381-3). A complete epidemiologic history (including details of travel,

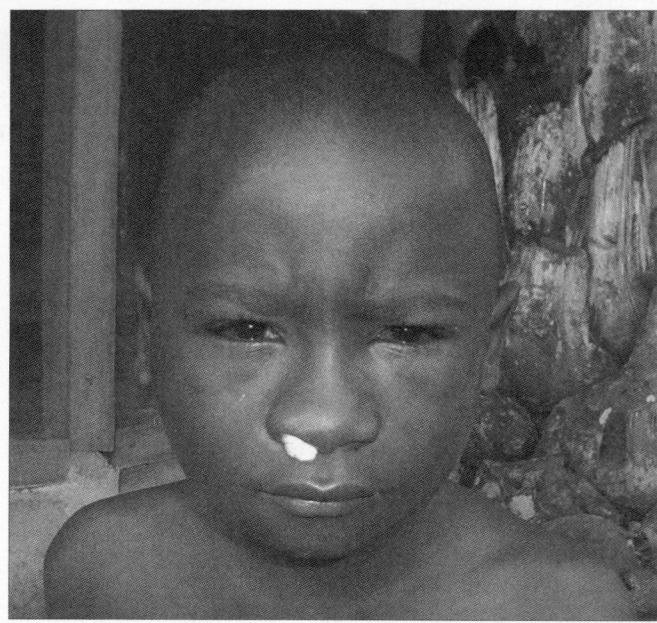

FIGURE 381-1. Subconjunctival hemorrhage and facial swelling in a boy with Lassa fever in Sierra Leone.

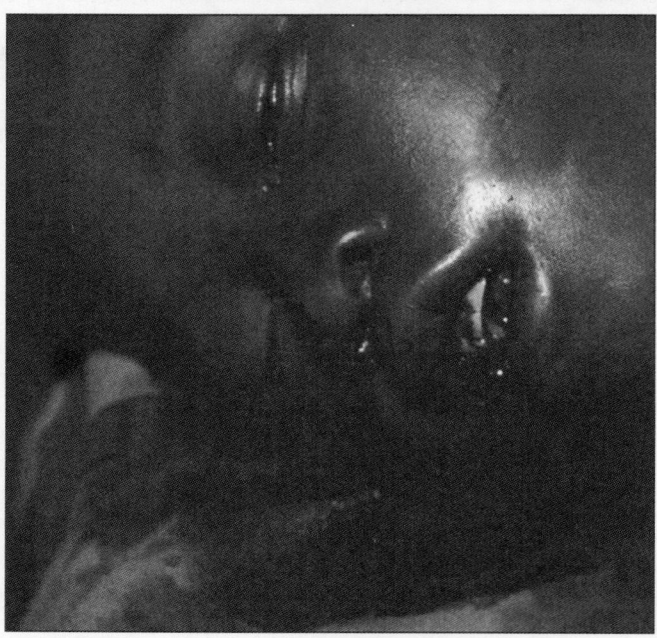

FIGURE 381-2. Bleeding in a patient with Ebola hemorrhagic fever. (From Bausch DG. Viral hemorrhagic fevers. In: Schlossberg D, ed. *Clinical Infectious Disease*. New York: Cambridge University Press; 2008.)

TABLE 381-3   DIFFERENTIAL DIAGNOSIS OF THE VIRAL HEMORRHAGIC FEVERS

DISEASE	DISTINGUISHING CHARACTERISTICS AND COMMENTS
PARASITES	
Malaria	Classically shows paroxysms of fever and chills; hemorrhagic manifestations less common; malaria smears or rapid test result usually positive; coinfection (or baseline asymptomatic parasitemia) common; responds to antimalarials
Amebiasis	Hemorrhagic manifestations other than bloody diarrhea generally not seen; amebic trophozoites identified in the stool by microscopy or antigen assays; responds to antiparasitics
Giardiasis	Positive stool antigen test result or identification of trophozoites or cysts in stool; responds to antiparasitics
African trypanosomiasis (acute stages)	Especially the East African form; examination of peripheral blood smear/buffy coat may show trypanosomes
BACTERIA (INCLUDING SPIROCHETES, RICKETTSIA, EHRLICHIA, AND COXIELLA)	
Typhoid fever	Hemorrhagic manifestations other than bloody diarrhea generally not seen; responds to antibiotics
Bacillary dysentery (including shigellosis, campylobacteriosis, salmonellosis, and enterohemorrhagic *Escherichia coli* and others)	Hemorrhagic manifestations other than bloody diarrhea generally not seen; responds to antibiotics
Capnocytophaga canimorsus	Associated with dog and cat bites, typically in persons with underlying immunodeficiency, notably asplenic patients; responds to antibiotics
Meningococcemia	Bacterial-induced DIC may mimic the bleeding diathesis of VHF; bleeding within the first 24-48 hours after onset of illness and rapidly progressive illness typical; large ecchymoses typical of meningococcemia are unusual in the VHFs except for Crimean-Congo HF; rapid serum latex agglutination tests can be used to detect bacterial antigen in meningococcal septicemia; may respond to antibiotics (critical to administer early)
Staphylococcemia	Bacterial-induced DIC may mimic the bleeding diathesis of VHF; may respond to antibiotics
Septic abortion	History of pregnancy and positive pregnancy test
Septicemic or pneumonic plague	Bacterial-induced DIC may mimic the bleeding diathesis of VHF; large ecchymoses typical of plague are unusual in the VHFs except for Crimean-Congo HF; pneumonic plague may mimic hantavirus pulmonary syndrome; may respond to antibiotics
Streptococcal or Epstein-Barr virus pharyngitis	May mimic the exudative pharyngitis sometimes seen in Lassa fever
Tuberculosis	Hemoptysis of advanced pulmonary tuberculosis may suggest VHF, but tuberculosis generally has a much slower disease evolution
Tularemia	Ulceroglandular and pneumonic forms more common; responds to antibiotics
Acute abdominal emergencies	Appendicitis, peritonitis, and bleeding upper gastrointestinal ulcer
Pyelonephritis and post-streptococcal glomerulonephritis	May mimic HF with renal syndrome
Anthrax (inhalation or gastrointestinal)	Prominent pulmonary manifestations and widened mediastinum on chest radiograph in inhalation form; responds to antibiotics
Atypical bacterial pneumonia (*Legionella, Mycoplasma, Chlamydophila pneumoniae* and *C. psittaci*, others)	May mimic hantavirus pulmonary syndrome; exposure to birds; symptoms often not present until late in the illness in psittacosis; responds to antibiotics

TABLE 381-3 DIFFERENTIAL DIAGNOSIS OF THE VIRAL HEMORRHAGIC FEVERS—cont'd

DISEASE	DISTINGUISHING CHARACTERISTICS AND COMMENTS
Relapsing fever	Recurrent fevers and influenza-like symptoms, with direct neurologic involvement and splenomegaly; spirochetes visible in blood while febrile; responds to antibiotics
Leptospirosis	Jaundice, renal failure, and myocarditis in severe cases; responds to antibiotics
Spotted fever group rickettsiae (including African tick bite fever, boutonneuse fever, Rocky Mountain spotted fever)	Incubation period of 7-10 days after tick bite, compared with 1-3 days in Crimean-Congo HF; necrotic lesions (eschar) typically seen at site of tick bite in some rickettsial diseases, whereas there may be only slight bruising at the bite site in Crimean-Congo HF; rash (if present) of rickettsial infection classically involves palms and soles
Q fever (*Coxiella burnetii*)	Broad spectrum of illness, including hepatitis, pneumonitis, encephalitis, and multisystem disease with bleeding; responds to antibiotics
Ehrlichiosis	Diagnosis by serology and PCR; blood film may be useful; responds to antibiotics
VIRUSES	
Influenza	Prominent respiratory component to clinical presentation; no hemorrhagic manifestations; influenza rapid test result may be positive; may respond to anti-influenza drugs
Arbovirus infection (including dengue and West Nile fever)	Encephalitis unusual but when present may mimic the VHFs with significant neurologic involvement (Kyasanur Forest disease, Omsk HF); usually less severe than VHF; hemorrhage not reported
Viral hepatitis (including hepatitis A, B, and E; Epstein-Barr; and cytomegalovirus)	Jaundice atypical in HF except yellow fever; test results for hepatitis antigens positive; fulminant infection resembling VHF may be seen in persons with underlying immune deficiencies
Herpes simplex or varicella-zoster	Fulminant infection with hepatitis (with or without vesicular rash); elevated transaminases and leukopenia typical; disseminated disease may be noted in otherwise healthy persons; poor response to acyclovir drugs unless recognized early
HIV/AIDS	Seroconversion syndrome or HIV/AIDS with secondary infections, especially septicemia
Measles	Rash may mimic that seen in early stages of some VHFs and may sometimes be hemorrhagic; prominence of coryza and upper respiratory symptoms in measles should help differentiate; vaccine preventable
Rubella	Rash may mimic that seen in early stages of some VHFs; usually a mild disease; vaccine preventable
Hemorrhagic or flat smallpox	Diffuse hemorrhagic or macular lesions; in contrast to the VHFs, the rash may involve the oral mucosa, palms, and soles; smallpox in the wild has been eradicated
Alphavirus infection (including chikungunya and o'nyong-nyong)	Joint pain typically a predominant feature
FUNGI	
Histoplasmosis	Pulmonary disease may mimic hantavirus pulmonary syndrome; recent entry into mines or caves
NONINFECTIOUS ETIOLOGIES	
Heat stroke	History for extreme heat exposure; absence of sweating; bleeding not typical, but DIC may occur
Idiopathic and thrombotic thrombocytopenic purpura (ITP/TTP)	Presentation usually less acute than in VHF; may have prominent neurologic symptoms in TTP; coagulation factors normal and DIC absent; often respond to corticosteroids (ITP) or plasma exchange (TTP)
Acute glaucoma	May mimic the acute ocular manifestations of Rift Valley fever
Hematologic malignant neoplasms (leukemia, lymphoma)	May resemble leukemoid reaction occasionally seen in HF with renal syndrome
Drug sensitivity or overdose	Stevens-Johnson syndrome and anticoagulant (warfarin) overdose
Industrial and agricultural chemical poisoning	Especially anticoagulants, although other symptoms of VHF absent
Hematoxic snake bite envenomation	History of snake bite

DIC = disseminated intravascular coagulopathy; HF = hemorrhagic fever; PCR, polymerase chain reaction; VHF, viral hemorrhagic fever.

possible exposures, occupational risks, and the progression of illness), physical examination, and preliminary basic laboratory results (Table 381-4) are critical. A diagnosis of viral hemorrhagic fever should be considered in patients with a clinically compatible syndrome who, within the incubation period for the particular viral hemorrhagic fever in question, (1) reside in or traveled to an endemic area (see Table 381-1); (2) had potential direct contact with blood or body fluids of someone who was ill with an acute viral hemorrhagic fever, such as health care workers, persons caring for family members at home or preparing bodies for burial, and laboratory personnel; (3) had contact with live or recently killed wild animals (especially nonhuman primates) in or recently arriving from an area where a viral hemorrhagic fever is endemic (although direct contact with the animal reservoir is not usually reported even in confirmed cases); (4) worked in a laboratory or animal facility where hemorrhagic fever viruses are handled; or (5) had sexual relations with someone recovering from a viral hemorrhagic fever in the last 3 months.

The index of suspicion should be especially high for persons in specific high-risk occupations, including health care workers, abattoir workers, veterinarians, farm workers, hunters, taxidermists, and travelers who have recently returned from endemic areas.[11] ARDS (Chapter 104) or other respiratory compromise in a person living in an endemic area for New World hantaviruses should prompt consideration of hantavirus pulmonary syndrome. Risk of tick infection, including physical examination for an eschar, should be

assessed if a tick-borne viral hemorrhagic fever is suspected. However, most viral hemorrhagic fevers are rare even in persons possessing one of the risk factors, so alternative diagnoses should always be aggressively sought, especially malaria and typhoid fever in areas where they are endemic. Acts of bioterrorism (Chapter 21) must be considered if viral hemorrhagic fever is strongly suspected in a patient without any of the aforementioned risk factors, especially if clusters of cases occur. All cases should be immediately reported to local, state, and federal health authorities.

Laboratory Testing

Prompt laboratory confirmation is imperative, but testing is unfortunately only available in a few specialized laboratories except for kits with varying sensitivity and specificity for the serologic diagnosis of dengue fever and hantavirus pulmonary syndrome. Assays commonly used in the diagnosis of viral hemorrhagic fever include polymerase chain reaction,[12] enzyme-linked immunosorbent assays for viral antigen and immunoglobulin M antibody, virus culture, and immunohistochemistry on postmortem tissues. These assays generally appear to have sensitivities and specificities above 90%, although serologic diagnosis of flavivirus infection is often complicated by cross-reactions. In the United States, testing can be arranged through the Centers for Disease Control and Prevention (phone: 404-639-1115, after hours: 770-488-7100; e-mail: dvd-1spath@cdc.gov).

TABLE 381-4 INDICATED CLINICAL LABORATORY TESTS AND CHARACTERISTIC FINDINGS IN PATIENTS WITH VIRAL HEMORRHAGIC FEVER

TEST	CHARACTERISTIC FINDINGS AND COMMENTS
Leukocyte count	Early: moderate leukopenia (except for hantavirus infection, in which early leukocytosis with immunoblasts is classically noted) Later: leukocytosis with left shift; granulocytosis more suggestive of bacterial infection
Hemoglobin and hematocrit	Hemoconcentration (especially noted in hemorrhagic fever with renal syndrome and hantavirus pulmonary syndrome)
Platelet count	Mild to moderate thrombocytopenia
Electrolytes	Sodium, potassium, and acid-base perturbations, depending on fluid balance and stage of disease
BUN/creatinine	Renal failure may occur late in disease.
Serum chemistries (AST, ALT, amylase, γ-glutamyltransferase, alkaline phosphatase, creatinine kinase, lactate dehydrogenase, lactate)	Usually increased, especially in severe disease; AST > ALT A lactate level >4 mmol/L (36 mg/dL) may indicate persistent hypoperfusion and sepsis. Lactate dehydrogenase is typically markedly increased in hantavirus pulmonary syndrome.
Sedimentation rate	Normal or increased
Blood gas	Metabolic acidosis may be indicative of shock and hypoperfusion
Coagulation studies (PT, PTT, fibrinogen, fibrin split products, platelets, D-dimer)	DIC common in Ebola, Marburg, Lujo virus, Crimean-Congo HF, and New World arenavirus infections
Urinalysis	Proteinuria common; hematuria may be occasionally noted Sediment may show hyaline-granular casts and round cells with cytoplasmic inclusions.
Blood culture	Useful early to exclude VHF and later to evaluate for secondary bacterial infection Blood should be drawn before antibiotic therapy is instituted.
Stool culture	Useful to exclude VHF (in favor of hemorrhagic bacillary dysentery)
Thick and thin blood smears	May aid in the diagnosis of blood parasites (malaria and trypanosomes), bacterial sepsis (meningococcus, capnocytophaga, and anthrax), and ehrlichiosis All negative in VHF unless coinfection
Rapid test, PCR, or other assay for malaria	Negative in VHF unless coinfection with malaria

ALT = alanine aminotransferase; AST = aspartate aminotransferase; BUN = blood urea nitrogen; DIC = disseminated intravascular coagulation; PCR, polymerase chain reaction; PT = prothrombin time; PTT = partial thromboplastin time; VHF = viral hemorrhagic fever.

TREATMENT   Rx

The rarity of most viral hemorrhagic fevers and their typical occurrence in remote and resource-poor settings make controlled studies on treatment difficult. Treatment guidelines generally follow those recommended for septic shock (Chapter 108). Patients should be placed in isolation in an intensive care unit. Intramuscular and subcutaneous injections should be minimized because of the risk of hematoma.

Clinical Management Guidelines
Fluid and Electrolyte Management
Severe microvascular instability, often complicated by vomiting, severe and sometimes voluminous diarrhea, and decreased fluid intake, typically requires aggressive fluid replacement to prevent shock. In the recent Ebola outbreak, patients often required up to 5 liters of intravenous fluids daily and potassium supplementation in addition to oral rehydration.[13,14] However, overaggressive and unmonitored rehydration may lead to significant third-spacing and pulmonary edema, especially in hantavirus pulmonary syndrome.

Early goal-directed therapies with crystalloids, blood products, and vasopressors can mitigate organ dysfunction and probably reduce mortality (Chapter 108). Peritoneal dialysis and hemodialysis (Chapter 131) have been extensively used in patients with hemorrhagic fever with renal syndrome

without frequent complications, but there is little published experience with the other viral hemorrhagic fevers. Specific World Health Organization guidelines for the fluid management of dengue shock syndrome in resource-limited environments specify a more conservative fluid repletion strategy because of the inability to monitor hydration status carefully and the resulting risk of fluid overload or pulmonary edema in this syndrome. Significant electrolyte imbalance may be noted, and hypokalemia often requires potassium supplementation.

Blood Products and Management of Disseminated Intravascular Coagulation
Although bleeding may be profuse in some viral hemorrhagic fevers, especially Crimean-Congo hemorrhagic fever and Ebola and Marburg hemorrhagic fevers, blood products should not be given empirically but only to meet defined clinical and laboratory parameters in the face of clinically significant hemorrhage. Transfusions, preferably with packed red blood cells, should be used to maintain a hemoglobin concentration above 7.0 g/dL while avoiding volume overload, taking into account that chronic anemia due to malaria and malnutrition may be frequent in patients in certain geographic areas. Whole blood is a reasonable alternative if packed cells are not available.

The possibility of DIC (Chapter 175) should be assessed by the relevant laboratory parameters (see Table 381-4), such as D-dimer levels. Transfusion of platelet concentrate (1 to 2 U/10 kg) should be considered when the platelet count is less than 50,000/μL in a bleeding patient or less than 20,000/μL without bleeding. The platelet count should generally rise by at least 2000/μL per unit of platelets transfused, although the response may be less if there is ongoing DIC and platelet consumption. Impaired platelet aggregation may promote hemorrhage in some viral hemorrhagic fevers, especially Lassa fever, even when platelet counts are not drastically low. Transfusion of fresh-frozen plasma (FFP) (15 to 20 mL/kg) should be considered when bleeding is present and fibrinogen levels are less than 100 mg/dL. Fibrinogen concentrate (total dose of 2 to 3 g) or cryoprecipitate (1 U/10 kg) may be administered instead of FFP, although FFP has the theoretical advantage of containing all coagulation factors and inhibitors deficient in DIC but no activated coagulation factors. Vitamin K (10 mg intravenously or orally on 3 consecutive days) may be given, especially if underlying malnutrition or liver disease is suspected. Folic acid has also sometimes been added to prevent the detrimental effect of acute folate deficiency on platelet production, especially in malnourished patients, although the efficacy of this treatment is unknown.

Oxygenation and Ventilation
In the early phases of disease and in the absence of iatrogenic pulmonary edema, most patients can be supported with oxygen administered by nasal cannula or face mask. The exception is hantavirus pulmonary syndrome, for which early endotracheal intubation and mechanical ventilation (Chapter 105) are often life-saving. Patients with viral hemorrhagic fever have an elevated risk of ventilator-induced lung injury (i.e., barotrauma) and pulmonary hemorrhage. In neurologically intact patients with hypoxemia, noninvasive positive-pressure ventilation may be a useful adjunct to forestall intubation. When mechanical ventilation is required, lung-protective tidal volumes of 6 to 8 mL/kg of ideal body weight should be employed. Extracorporeal membrane oxygenation has been used with apparent benefit in hantavirus pulmonary syndrome. Because of the risk of bleeding, arterial puncture for blood gas determination should be kept to a minimum.

Antibiotics and Secondary Infection
Patients should be immediately covered with appropriate antibacterial or antiparasitic therapy, with specific consideration of malaria (Chapter 345) and tick-borne rickettsial diseases (Chapter 327), until a diagnosis of viral hemorrhagic fever can be confirmed. These drugs should then be stopped unless there is evidence of coinfection. Secondary bacterial infection should be suspected when patients have persistent or new fever after about 2 weeks of illness, a time when most viral hemorrhagic fevers either have resulted in death or are resolving.

Antiviral Therapy
The only currently available specific antiviral therapy for any viral hemorrhagic fever is the guanosine analogue ribavirin, although it is not approved by the Food and Drug Administration for this indication (Table 381-5). The best data are for Lassa fever and hemorrhagic fever with renal syndrome,[A1] for which early treatment is imperative for maximum benefit. Anecdotal data suggest efficacy in other arenavirus hemorrhagic fevers, but controversial controlled trials of ribavirin in Crimean-Congo hemorrhagic fever and Rift Valley fever[A2] did not show efficacy. In vitro data generally show activity of ribavirin against dengue, yellow fever, and Omsk hemorrhagic fever viruses, but clinical studies have not been performed. The drug is not efficacious and should not be used for Ebola or Marburg hemorrhagic fevers. The main side effects of intravenous ribavirin are a mild to moderate hemolytic anemia, which infrequently necessitates transfusion and disappears with cessation of treatment, and rigors when the drug is infused too rapidly. ZMapp, which is a combination of three monoclonal antibodies, is effective for treating Ebola virus in non-human primates.[15] It has also been used in humans on a compassionate

TABLE 381-5 RIBAVIRIN THERAPY FOR VIRAL HEMORRHAGIC FEVER

INDICATION	ROUTE	DOSE[a]	INTERVAL
Treatment	IV[b]	30 mg/kg (maximum 2 g)[c]	Loading dose, followed by:
	IV[b]	15 mg/kg (maximum 1 g)[c]	every 6 hours for 4 days, followed by:
	IV[b]	7.5 mg/kg (maximum 500 mg)[c]	every 8 hours for 6 days
Prophylaxis	PO	35 mg/kg (maximum 2.5 g)[c]	Loading dose, followed by:
	PO	15 mg/kg (maximum 1 g)[c]	every 8 hours for 10 days:

[a]Pharmacokinetic and sensitivity testing for ribavirin has not been extensively performed for each viral hemorrhagic fever. The intravenous dose used is derived from that found efficacious in Lassa fever. Oral ribavirin has also been reported to be efficacious in many viral hemorrhagic fevers, especially for Crimean-Congo hemorrhagic fever, but few controlled data are available. Intravenous administration is strongly suggested whenever possible.
[b]The drug should be diluted in 150 mL of 0.9% saline and infused slowly.
[c]Reduce the dose in persons known to have significant renal insufficiency (creatinine clearance of less than 50 mL/minute).

use basis, but controlled trials to demonstrate efficacy definitively have not yet been performed. Other experimental therapies include TKM-Ebola (an RNA inhibitor), brincidofovir, and favipiravir.

A number of experimental antiviral drugs have shown in vitro activity and, in some cases, therapeutic benefit in animal studies, including various nucleoside analogues, inhibitors of S-adenosyl-L-homocysteine hydrolase, small interfering RNAs, phosphorodiamidate morpholino oligomers, antisense compounds, tyrosine kinase inhibitors, and other small molecules.[16] The Chinese drug chongcao shenkang has been reported to be efficacious in hemorrhagic fever with renal syndrome. None of these drugs are yet widely approved or available for treatment of viral hemorrhagic fever in humans.

Convalescent Plasma and Antibody Therapy

Although cellular immunity is thought to be the primary protection in most viral hemorrhagic fevers, transfusion of appropriately titered convalescent plasma within the first 8 days of illness has been reported to reduce the case-fatality of Argentine hemorrhagic fever from 15 to 30% to less than 1%. However, this therapy has been associated with a convalescent phase neurologic syndrome characterized by fever, cerebellar signs, and cranial nerve palsies in 10% of treated patients. Animal studies show convalescent plasma to be efficacious in Lassa fever as well, but only if it contains a high titer of neutralizing antibody and if there is a close antigenic match between the infecting viruses of the donor and recipient. Convalescent plasma also appears to be efficacious for Crimean-Congo hemorrhagic fever and Rift Valley fever, but there are no controlled data. Convalescent plasma or blood has been given to numerous patients with Ebola hemorrhagic fever, but its efficacy is still unknown. Because of the significant medical and logistical challenges to the use of convalescent immune plasma, including risk of concomitant transmission of other blood-borne pathogens, this therapy should be reserved for Argentine hemorrhagic fever and for severe and refractory cases when ribavirin is not an option. Numerous monoclonal and polyclonal antibody preparations have shown promise in animal models and may soon be ready for safety trials in humans.

Coagulation and Immune Modulators

A growing body of literature suggests that disturbances in the procoagulant-anticoagulant balance play an important role in the mediation of septic shock. A modest survival benefit (33%) was seen in monkeys treated with rNAPc2, a potent experimental recombinant inhibitor of the tissue factor/factor VIIa coagulation pathway.

Various immune modulators, including ibuprofen, corticosteroids, anti–tumor necrosis factor-α, nitric oxide inhibitors, statins, and interleukins, have not shown conclusive benefit in the treatment of sepsis. In a small study, recombinant interleukin-2 reduced the degree of acute renal insufficiency in hemorrhagic fever with renal syndrome, but further studies are needed before it can be considered the standard of care. Clinical trials of corticosteroids in hemorrhagic fever with renal syndrome have shown mixed results. Corticosteroids (e.g., 200 mg intravenous hydrocortisone per day, divided into two to four daily doses or administered by continuous infusion) are not recommended unless adrenal insufficiency is strongly suspected, the target blood pressure is not maintained despite adequate fluid repletion and vasopressors, or cerebral edema is suspected.

Management of Pregnancy

Uterine evacuation in pregnant patients appears to lower maternal mortality and should be considered, given the extremely high maternal and fetal mortality associated with viral hemorrhagic fever. However, this procedure must be performed with extreme caution because it can be considered high risk with regard to potential nosocomial transmission. Although it is technically contraindicated in pregnancy (Food and Drug Administration Category

X), ribavirin should nevertheless be considered, in consultation with the patient, as a life-saving measure for the mother who has a viral hemorrhagic fever for which the drug is efficacious (see Tables 381-2 and 381-5).

Other Considerations

Oral or parenteral acetaminophen, tramadol, opiates, or other analgesics should be used as needed for pain control (see Tables 30-4 and 30-5), adjusting as necessary for hepatic insufficiency. Use of salicylates and nonsteroidal anti-inflammatory drugs should be avoided because of the risk of bleeding. Prophylactic therapy for gastrointestinal stress ulcers with proton pump inhibitors or histamine H_2-receptor antagonists is recommended (see Table 138-1). Antiemetics, such as the phenothiazines, are frequently warranted. Seizures can usually be managed with standard medications (Chapter 403).

PREVENTION

Patient Isolation, Personal Protective Equipment, and Nursing Precautions

Normal barrier nursing precautions to prevent parenteral and droplet exposure to blood and body fluids suffice in most instances. Once the diagnosis is suspected, however, precautions should be upgraded to "viral hemorrhagic fever precautions," which include patient isolation and the use of surgical masks, face shields, double gloves, gowns, head and shoe covers, and protective aprons.[17] It is prudent to place the patient in a negative airflow room if it is available, but hermetically sealed isolation chambers are not required. Insecticide-treated bed nets and room screens should be used in open-air settings to prevent transmission of arthropod-borne hemorrhagic fever viruses. Access to the patient should be limited to a small number of designated staff and family members with specific instructions and training on infection control guidelines and the use of personal protective equipment. Small-particle aerosol precautions should be used when procedures are performed that may generate aerosols, such as endotracheal intubation. Disinfection with bleach or a number of other commercially available disinfectants is advised, including chemical or heat inactivation of human waste.

Contact Tracing

The early nonspecific presentation of the viral hemorrhagic fevers poses a serious challenge to effective epidemiologic surveillance. Fortunately, the low secondary attack rates afford a measure of reassurance even when cases go unrecognized as long as proper barrier nursing is maintained. Furthermore, because mild cases, which may be still more difficult to recognize, are usually not very infectious, missed or delayed diagnosis of these patients is unlikely to pose a problem from an infection control standpoint.

Persons with unprotected direct contact with a patient during the symptomatic phase of a human-to-human communicable viral hemorrhagic fever should be monitored daily for evidence of disease for the duration of the longest possible incubation period, starting after their last contact (see Table 381-2). Given the generally low secondary attack rates, especially outside of caretakers, widespread contact tracing, laboratory testing, and postexposure prophylaxis are not indicated for casual contacts. Contacts should check their temperature daily and record the results in a log. Despite lack of evidence for transmission during the incubation period, it is usually recommended that exposed persons avoid close contact with household members that might result in exposure to body fluids, such as sex, kissing, and sharing of utensils for the duration of the incubation period. Confinement of asymptomatic persons is not warranted, but persons who develop fever or other signs and symptoms suggestive of viral hemorrhagic fever should be immediately isolated until the diagnosis can be ruled out.

Vaccines

Vaccines for viral hemorrhagic fevers are at various stages of development. The 17D live attenuated yellow fever vaccine has a generally excellent protection and safety profile, despite recent recognition of rare serious adverse events in elderly persons.[A3] Confirmed previous vaccination with 17D should essentially exclude the diagnosis of yellow fever unless the patient was immunocompromised at the time of vaccination. A highly efficacious live attenuated vaccine, Candid 1, also exists for Argentine hemorrhagic fever,[A4] although it is licensed only in Argentina. Candid 1 may also be effective in Bolivian hemorrhagic fever but does not protect against other arenavirus infections. Experimental vaccines for hemorrhagic fever with renal syndrome, Rift Valley fever, Omsk hemorrhagic fever, and Kyasanur Forest disease may be efficacious, although most have not been widely tested and are not widely approved or available. A number of vaccine candidates have recently been shown to be efficacious in animal models of Ebola, Marburg, and Lassa virus infection.[18] Clinical trials of various Ebola vaccines are underway, with early results suggesting that they can safely elicit immunogenicity.[19]

Postexposure Prophylaxis

Postexposure prophylaxis should be considered only in persons with distinct high-risk exposure, defined as follows: (1) penetration of skin by a contaminated sharp instrument (e.g., needlestick injury); (2) exposure of mucous membranes or broken skin to blood or body secretions (e.g., blood splashing in the eyes or mouth); (3) participation in emergency procedures without appropriate personal protective equipment (e.g., resuscitation after cardiac arrest, intubation, or suctioning); and (4) prolonged (i.e., hours) and continuous contact in an enclosed space without appropriate personal protective equipment. The most infectious patients are those with severe clinical conditions, usually late in the course of illness. Prophylaxis should not be used when the only exposure was during the incubation period or after fever has subsided.

Postexposure prophylaxis with oral ribavirin has been recommended for Lassa fever, other arenavirus infections, and Crimean-Congo hemorrhagic fever, although no systematic data are available on its efficacy, and the frequent minor adverse events sometimes can be mistaken for the early signs of disease.[20] Oral ribavirin should be started immediately after the exposure, but not before counseling between the patient and the physician. The drug should be taken with food. Baseline hemoglobin, hematocrit, bilirubin, and creatinine levels should be determined, and therapy should be adjusted or reconsidered if significant anemia or renal insufficiency develops.

Convalescent plasma is given as postexposure prophylaxis for Argentine hemorrhagic fever. Numerous experimental vaccines, monoclonal antibodies, and other compounds have shown efficacy as postexposure prophylaxis in animal models, especially for filovirus infections, but are not yet approved for use in humans.

Reservoir and Vector Control

Avoiding contact with bats, primarily by avoiding entry into caves and mines in endemic areas, is a key prevention measure for Ebola and Marburg viruses. Personal protective equipment may be indicated for miners and other persons who work in these environments. Humans should also avoid exposure to fresh blood, body fluids, or meat of wild animals, especially nonhuman primates.

For rodent-borne viruses whose reservoirs often colonize human dwellings, improved "village hygiene" is recommended, such as eliminating unprotected storage of garbage and foodstuffs and plugging holes that allow rodents to enter homes. Prevention of the mosquito-borne hemorrhagic fever viruses hinges on controlling *Aedes* mosquitoes in and around the home, primarily by elimination of clean standing water containers that serve as larval habitats and by use of screened windows and doors, insecticide-treated bed nets, protective clothing, mosquito repellent, and aerosol bomb insecticides in enclosed spaces. Analogous measures can help protect against tick bites.

▏PROGNOSIS

The clinical course of viral hemorrhagic fever unfolds quite rapidly. In fatal cases, death usually occurs within 7 to 10 days after the onset of hemorrhagic fever symptoms in filovirus infection and in about 2 weeks with the arenaviruses and some of the other viruses. Mortality usually does not result directly from exsanguination, and external bleeding is seen in a minority of cases of viral hemorrhagic fever. Most deaths result from an intense inflammatory process akin to septic shock (Chapter 108) when insufficient effective circulating intravascular volume leads to hypotension, cellular dysfunction, and multiorgan system failure.

Common indicators of a poor prognosis include shock, bleeding, neurologic manifestations, high levels of viremia (or surrogate measurements of antigen or genome copies), elevated levels of aspartate aminotransferase (>150 IU/L), and pregnancy, especially during the third trimester, in which maternal and fetal mortality may be above 90%.

However, mild and even asymptomatic cases have been reported for what are considered the most virulent viral hemorrhagic fevers. Reasons for this heterogeneity are largely unknown, although differences in route and dose of infection, underlying comorbid illness, and host genetic predisposition have been postulated.

Survivors usually suffer no obvious long-term sequelae. Notable exceptions include deafness in up to 30% of patients after Lassa fever and sometimes after Venezuelan hemorrhagic fever and optic retinopathy with vision loss in Rift Valley fever. Nevertheless, convalescence may be prolonged, especially for Ebola and Marburg hemorrhagic fevers, with persistent myalgia,

arthralgia, anorexia, weight loss, alopecia, pancreatitis, uveitis, and orchitis up to a year after infection. The psychological effects of viral hemorrhagic fever may include significant irritability, depression, post-traumatic stress disorder, and social stigmatization. For Ebola virus, mortality rates have been about 70% in West Africa.[21] In contrast, a very high proportion of patients who have been treated in the U.S. and Europe have survived with modern supportive care and experimental therapies.[22] Because these patients received multiple therapies in combination and in an uncontrolled fashion, the efficacy of any one therapy cannot be assessed.

Clinical management during convalescence includes the use of warm packs, acetaminophen, nonsteroidal anti-inflammatory drugs, cosmetics, hair growth stimulants, anxiolytics, antidepressants, nutritional supplements, and nutritional and psychological counseling as indicated. Uveitis in patients recovering from Ebola hemorrhagic fever, recently renamed Ebola virus disease, responds to topical steroids and atropine.

Because the patient's clinical status and infectivity generally correlate with the level of viremia, patients who have recovered from their acute illness can safely be assumed to have cleared their viremia and discharged from the hospital without concern of subsequent transmission at home. RT-PCR testing of blood and other body fluids has sometimes revealed residual nucleic acids, but their significance is unclear without cell culture confirmation of the presence of infectious virus. Clearance of virus may be delayed for weeks to months from a few immunologically protected sites, such as the central nervous system, chambers of the eye, and gonads, with the last resulting in rare sexual transmission months after recovery from acute disease. Consequently, abstinence or condom use is recommended for 3 months after acute illness. Although transmission through toilet facilities or ocular secretions has not been noted, simple precautions to avoid contact with these potentially infected body fluids are prudent, including separate toilet facilities and regular handwashing. Breast-feeding should be avoided during convalescence unless there is no other way to support the baby.

Grade A References

A1. Huggins JW, Hsiang CM, Cosgriff TM, et al. Prospective, double-blind, concurrent, placebo-controlled clinical trial of intravenous ribavirin therapy of hemorrhagic fever with renal syndrome. *J Infect Dis.* 1991;164:1119-1127.

A2. Koksal I, Yilmaz G, Aksoy F, et al. The efficacy of ribavirin in the treatment of Crimean-Congo hemorrhagic fever in Eastern Black Sea region in Turkey. *J Clin Virol.* 2010;47:65-68.

A3. Gotuzzo E, Yactayo S, Cordova E. Efficacy and duration of immunity after yellow fever vaccination: systematic review on the need for a booster every 10 years. *Am J Trop Med Hyg.* 2013;89: 434-444.

A4. Enria DA, Ambrosio AM, Briggiler AM, et al. Candid#1 vaccine against Argentine hemorrhagic fever produced in Argentina. Immunogenicity and safety. *Medicina (B Aires).* 2010;70: 215-222.

▏GENERAL REFERENCES

For the General References and other additional features, please visit Expert Consult at https://expertconsult.inkling.com.

ARBOVIRUSES CAUSING FEVER AND RASH SYNDROMES

STANLEY J. NAIDES

● COLORADO TICK FEVER

▏DEFINITION

Colorado tick fever (mountain fever, American mountain fever) is an acute, often self-limited, typically biphasic febrile illness that is common in the Rocky Mountain areas, the Sierra Nevada and Wasatch ranges, and the Black Hills mountain areas.[1] The virus is transmitted through the bite of the hard-shelled tick *Dermacentor andersoni* (Rocky Mountain wood tick), and the disease's range corresponds to the vector's range. Other coltiviruses, such as the Salmon River, Eyach, Banna, Beijing, and Gansu viruses, have also been implicated in human disease.

The Pathogen

The causative agent, Colorado tick fever virus, is a member of the genus Coltivirus, family Reoviridae. Coltiviruses have a genome consisting of 12 double-stranded RNA segments. Colorado tick fever virus is the prototype member.

EPIDEMIOLOGY

D. andersoni is found at elevations of 4000 to 10,000 ft. Seasonal temperatures tend to influence the range, with the vector being found at higher elevations in warmer seasons and at lower elevations in colder seasons. Human exposure usually occurs during outdoor recreational activities in these areas. Occasional exposure occurs in nonendemic areas from ticks exported out of the endemic region in clothes, hiking equipment, or baggage. Infections generally take place between March and September, when the adult tick is most plentiful. Ticks are most abundant in south-facing dry and rocky slope habitats that favor small rodents (e.g., chipmunks, ground squirrels, marmosets), with underbrush cover, burrows, and humidity for the ticks. Colorado tick fever virus is found in nymphal and adult ticks that overwinter on the rodent host, in which viremia persists for weeks to months. In the endemic area, as many as 14% of *D. andersoni* ticks carry Colorado tick fever virus. Humans are an incidental host. Fewer than 50 cases have been reported annually in Colorado beginning in 1992. The actual number of cases is probably significantly larger and includes subclinical, mild, and unreported cases.

The geographic range of Colorado tick fever may be larger than the well-recognized endemic mountain areas. Serologically confirmed cases in California have been attributed to the Colorado tick fever–related virus S1-14-03, which is transmitted by *Dermacentor variabilis* (American dog tick). Salmon River virus causes a Colorado tick fever–like illness in rafters on the Salmon River in Idaho. Another similar virus, Eyach virus, has been implicated in neurologic illness in France and Germany and has been isolated from the deer ticks *Ixodes ricinus* and *Ixodes ventalloi*. Colorado tick fever has been reported rarely in mainland China.

PATHOBIOLOGY

Colorado tick fever virus replicates in CD34$^+$ stem cells in bone marrow and leads to mild to moderate leukopenia and thrombocytopenia. The virus also replicates in committed erythrocyte precursors and may be detected in circulating erythrocytes up to 4 weeks after infection.

CLINICAL MANIFESTATIONS

Patients report a tick bite or exposure in 90% of cases, but there is no notable local reaction to the tick bite. After a mean incubation of 3 to 4 days (range, 0 to 14 days), sudden-onset fever develops in association with malaise, chills, myalgia, weakness, headache, photophobia, retro-orbital pain, and cutaneous hyperesthesia. Conjunctival and oropharyngeal injection, palatal enanthem, lymphadenopathy, and splenomegaly may be present. The absence of prominent respiratory and gastrointestinal symptoms helps exclude other febrile illnesses. A petechial or maculopapular exanthem, found in 15% of patients, may be confused with the rash of Rocky Mountain spotted fever (Chapter 327). The illness has a "saddleback" fever pattern consisting of resolution of the initial fever within 1 week and recrudescence after a 2- to 3-day hiatus. A third fever episode may occur.

Leukopenia develops 5 to 6 days after onset of the illness. Mild thrombocytopenia and anemia may occur.

Myocarditis, pneumonitis, hepatitis, orchitis, and epididymitis may complicate adult infection, and aseptic meningitis or encephalitis may occur in up to 10% of childhood infections.

DIAGNOSIS

Clinical diagnosis is confirmed by demonstration of the Colorado tick fever viral genome or specific acute phase IgM antibody. The viral genome may be detected up to 6 weeks after infection by nucleic acid–based methods such as reverse transcription–polymerase chain reaction (RT-PCR) on blood or stored blood clots. Virions in circulating erythrocytes may be detected by immunofluorescent antibody labeling. Anti–Colorado tick fever virus IgM antibody is detected by antibody capture enzyme-linked immunosorbent assay (ELISA) or complement fixation. Neutralization assays using Vero or BHK-21 cells have been helpful.

Differentiating Colorado tick fever from Rocky Mountain spotted fever (Chapter 327) may be difficult before the appearance of the typical rash of the latter. However, Rocky Mountain spotted fever does not have a

saddleback fever pattern and is 20 times less common than Colorado tick fever in the western endemic area.

PROGNOSIS

Extreme weakness and malaise may persist for weeks to months after final resolution of the fever. Older patients have a prolonged recovery. Seventy percent of patients older than 30 years may still have fatigue 3 weeks after the fever, whereas children and adolescents may recover completely within a week. Rare instances of maternal-fetal transmission have been reported. Full recovery eventually occurs, except when the disease course is complicated by neurologic insult. Patients should refrain from donating blood for 6 months.

DENGUE

DEFINITION

Dengue is an acute febrile illness characterized by severe muscle and joint pain, rash, malaise, and lymphadenopathy. The severity of the musculoskeletal complaints gave rise to the sobriquet *breakbone fever*. Dengue occurs in the tropical and subtropical climes of the Caribbean, Central and South America, Asia, and Africa. The mosquito range extends into the southeastern part of the United States, where dengue reemerged in the 1980s. After World War II, a spreading global pandemic has been associated with erosion of mosquito control programs, human population spread into rural settings, increased air travel, deterioration in public health infrastructure, and global warming. Each year, more than 200 million people worldwide are infected with dengue.[2]

The Pathogen

Dengue virus is a member of the Flaviviridae family, which consists of single-stranded RNA viruses with a lipid envelope approximately 50 nm in diameter. There are four serotypes of dengue: DEN-1, DEN-2, DEN-3, and DEN-4. No cross-protection is seen among the serotypes, so dengue can develop after infection with another serotype. Infection with a second serotype places the individual at risk for the development of hemorrhagic fever (Chapter 381).

EPIDEMIOLOGY

Dengue is transmitted to humans by the bite of female *Aedes aegypti* and *Aedes albopictus* mosquitoes. *A. albopictus* has become the dominant pest mosquito in many urban centers. Members of the two mosquito species acquire dengue virus by biting humans, typically during the day. The mosquitoes nest in stagnant water around human dwellings; they are not typically encountered in the forest. In the human host, dengue virus may reach a titer of greater than 10^8 median infectious doses per milliliter. The mosquito becomes infected when taking its meal from a viremic host. The virus continues replication in the midgut epithelium and salivary glands of female mosquitoes, which remain infectious for life. Within 8 to 12 days of the initial infection, the mosquito's salivary glands become infected, and virus is shed with saliva during the next blood meal. A given mosquito may infect multiple individuals, especially in view of its skittishness during feeding—slight movement of the host interrupts its meal, after which it returns to the original or another host. Zoonotic life cycles involving nonhuman primates (i.e., chimpanzees, gibbons, and macaques) and canopy-dwelling forest *Aedes* species have been demonstrated in western Africa and Malaysia.

The incubation period is typically 4 to 7 days but may range from 3 to 14 days. During outbreaks in the southeastern United States and Puerto Rico, the risk for infection may be as high as 79% in naïve hosts, and clinical disease may develop in up to 20%. Immunity against the infecting serotype is probably lifelong, but individuals remain susceptible to the remaining serotypes. Peak transmission occurs after increased rainfall, when rainwater collected in household containers allows expansion of mosquito populations. Epidemics tend to occur in 3- to 5-year cycles, but interepidemic cases occur regularly.

Dengue is a particular risk to visitors to the tropics and is a leading cause of pediatric morbidity and mortality in endemic areas.[3] Globalization and climate change have contributed to expansion of the geographic range. In one study of people who now live in the United States but who were born, lived in, or traveled to dengue-endemic countries, 19% had IgG antibodies to dengue but 85% of them had no clinical history of dengue. Dengue accounts for approximately 2% of the febrile illnesses in travelers returning to the United States.

PATHOBIOLOGY

Dengue hemorrhagic fever (Chapter 381) and dengue shock syndrome are forms of dengue reinfection characterized by capillary leakage and hemorrhage. Previous infection with an alternative serotype allows antibody to the previously encountered serotype to combine with the newly infecting serotype. Although the first exposed serotype antibody is not neutralizing, it does allow enhanced antibody-mediated macrophage uptake, thereby leading to macrophage activation and increasing viral replication and viral load. Excretion of vasoactive inflammatory mediators by macrophages results in vascular leakage; severe vascular leak causes shock. Endothelial cell swelling and perivascular edema may occur. Rarely, dengue shock syndrome may occur with primary infection. Variation in a strain's ability to generate enhancing antibody, as well as differences in virulence, may account for differences in clinical behavior.

CLINICAL MANIFESTATIONS

Dengue infection is often subclinical. When it is symptomatic, dengue may be manifested as classic dengue, dengue hemorrhagic fever, or dengue shock syndrome. Patients may also have mild illness characterized by nonspecific fever, anorexia, and headache.

Classic dengue, which typically occurs in nonindigenous older children and adults, is characterized by sudden-onset fever, severe frontal headache, retro-orbital pain, myalgia, and, in many cases, nausea, vomiting, rash, lymphadenopathy, and arthralgia.[4] Patients may experience generalized weakness, altered taste, rigors, and cutaneous hyperesthesia. Classic dengue is self-limited, but some patients progress to dengue hemorrhagic fever or dengue shock syndrome, which is characterized by capillary leakage, hypotension, narrowed pulse pressure, and shock. Dengue in pregnancy may be severe.[5]

Physical examination demonstrates fever, relative bradycardia, scleral injection, ocular pressure tenderness, and pharyngeal injection. A transient macular rash appears on days 1 or 2 of illness. On days 2 and 3 of illness, fever and other symptoms may improve. The fever is typically but not consistently biphasic. After a hiatus of typically 2 days, fever and other symptoms recrudesce, although less severely. Generalized, nontender lymphadenopathy of the posterior cervical, epitrochlear, and inguinal regions may develop. Rash also recurs and appears as 2- to 5-mm speckles of pallor surrounded by erythema and occasionally accompanied by burning dysesthesia of the palms and soles. The rash may desquamate.

DIAGNOSIS

An adequate travel history and knowledge of occurrence of disease in the community can lead to consideration of dengue in the differential diagnosis. Viremia is of adequate intensity in infections with DEN-1, DEN-2, and DEN-3 to allow viral isolation. Viremia in DEN-4 infections is often less intense and more difficult to detect through inoculation of mosquito cells in vitro. Specific IgM antibody appears 3 to 5 days after infection. IgG antibody appears 9 to 10 days after infection. Cross-reactivity with other flaviviruses prevents serotype-specific diagnosis. Neutralization testing with hemagglutination inhibition is more specific, and complement fixation testing for IgG in paired sera is helpful. PCR-based assays are available.

Leukopenia develops by the second day of fever, falling to a low of 1000 to 2000 cells/mL by day 5 or 6, and is associated with granulocytopenia. In dengue hemorrhagic fever, thrombocytopenia of less than 100,000 cells/mL and a prolonged prothrombin time are characteristic.[6] Mild to moderate proteinuria and a few casts may be detected. Aspartate transaminase levels may be increased.

TREATMENT, PREVENTION, AND PROGNOSIS   Rx

Classic dengue resolves abruptly in 5 to 7 days, but fatigue and depression may linger for weeks; survival is uniform. The prognosis of patients with dengue hemorrhagic fever (Chapter 381) and dengue shock syndrome depends on early diagnosis and the introduction of supportive measures. Treatment is supportive and consists of antipyretics and analgesics. Initial resuscitation of patients with shock syndrome (Chapter 106) with crystalloid and colloidal solutions is indicated in those with moderately severe dengue shock syndrome. Fresh-frozen plasma and blood products are used as necessary.

A new tetravalent dengue vaccine can prevent about two-thirds of cases of dengue and about 95% of severe cases.[A1] Most infected patients recover fully, but the overall mortality rate is about 1% because of the poorer outcome of dengue shock and hemorrhagic fever (Chapter 381).

WEST NILE FEVER VIRUS

DEFINITION

West Nile fever is an acute febrile illness associated with malaise, rash, headache, myalgia, and lymphadenopathy. Infection involves a bird-mosquito-human cycle.[7] Viremia develops in all varieties of birds. Bats, cats, chipmunks, domestic rabbits, horses, skunks, squirrels, dogs, sheep, llamas, and alpacas may be infected.

The Pathogen

West Nile fever virus, which is the most widely distributed flavivirus, is transmitted by a variety of mosquito species. The mosquito vector varies: *Culex univittatus*, *Culex pipiens*, and *Culex molestus* in the Middle East and Africa; *Mansonia metallicus* in Uganda; and *Culex tritaeniorhynchus* in Asia. After introduction into the New York City area in 1999, *C. pipiens* became the most important vector in the United States. Other mosquito species may carry the virus.

EPIDEMIOLOGY

Viral transmission involves mosquitoes and wild birds, with mammals, including humans, being incidental end-stage hosts. In endemic areas, more than 60% of young adults have antibodies, thus suggesting a high prevalence of inapparent or undifferentiated febrile illness in children. There is no gender predominance. Between 0.5 and 1% of infected individuals experience a more severe illness. Incubation is typically 3 to 15 days but may be as short as 1 day. West Nile virus emerged in the United States in New York and has spread throughout the continental United States, Canada, Mexico, the Caribbean, and Central and South America. In America, birds of the Corvidae family (e.g., crows, jackdaws, ravens) are often infected, and recognition of increased death in crow populations continues to serve as a sentinel for the presence of West Nile virus. In addition to mosquito transmission, the virus has been transmitted by a transplanted organ, through blood transfusion, transplacentally, and in the laboratory. From 1999 to 2004, almost 17,000 neuroinvasive cases were reported to the Centers for Disease Control and Prevention.

Zika virus, a flavivirus related to dengue and West Nile virus, has emerged in Africa, Asia, and the Yap Islands of the southwestern Pacific. It causes outbreaks of fever, rash, arthralgia, and conjunctivitis.

PATHOBIOLOGY

West Nile virus grows in a variety of cells in vitro and produces cytopathic effects in *A. albopictus* cells. Individuals in whom encephalitis develops show evidence of diffuse brain inflammation and neuronal degeneration, with virus detected early in multiple sites. The virus initially replicates in keratinocytes and skin-resident dendritic cells, which then migrate to local lymph nodes, where replication generates viremia and organ dissemination. Either immune cell trafficking or disruption of the blood-brain barrier allows neuroinvasion.

CLINICAL MANIFESTATIONS

Approximately 80% of infections are asymptomatic, and most of the remaining infections are mild and manifested by fever, malaise, headache, nausea, anorexia, generalized lymphadenopathy, and myalgia.[8] Aseptic meningitis or encephalitis (Chapter 383) may occur in the elderly and, less commonly, in the very young. Severe neurologic disease, including meningitis, myelitis, encephalitis, and flaccid paralysis of the limbs and respiratory muscles, can develop. Like Colorado tick fever and dengue, West Nile fever may be biphasic. Nonpruritic, maculopapular, or roseolar rash occurs on the chest, back, and arms in half the patients, beginning during or with resolution of the fever. The rash persists for up to 1 week and then resolves with desquamation. Patients may experience vomiting, diarrhea, abdominal pain, and pharyngitis. Anterior myelitis or hepatitis may also occur. Disease is usually milder in children than in adults.

DIAGNOSIS

West Nile virus may be isolated from up to 77% of patients with West Nile fever on the first day of illness, but viral isolation is less common in patients with encephalitis (Chapter 383). Low-titer viremia may persist for the first 5 days of illness. Tests in acute and convalescent phase serum for virus-specific antibody using ELISA or immunofluorescence are diagnostic. However, virus-specific IgM may persist in the serum at 1 year after infection in a minority of patients. Detection of West Nile virus–specific IgM in cerebrospinal fluid is diagnostic of neuroinvasion because IgM normally does not cross the blood-brain barrier. Neutralization assays help distinguish cross-reactive antibodies to other flaviviruses. RT-PCR may detect viral RNA in human samples and in avian and insect specimens.

TREATMENT Rx

Treatment is supportive. The clinical value of antiviral agents is unknown. Infection is controlled by the endogenous development of neutralizing antibodies to protein E, the viral envelope protein.

PROGNOSIS

Illness generally persists 3 to 6 days before rapid recovery. The prognosis is excellent, but mortality rates of 10% or higher occur in patients with encephalitis (Chapter 383).

PHLEBOTOMUS FEVER

DEFINITION

Phlebotomus fever (i.e., sandfly fever, pappataci, and 3-day fever) is an acute, mild, self-limited febrile illness transmitted through the bite of *Phlebotomus* flies.

The Pathogen

Phlebotomus fever viruses are members of the genus Phlebovirus, family Bunyaviridae. The latter consists of a group of single-stranded RNA viruses that are 80 to 120 nm in diameter, possess a lipid envelope, and have three segments in the genome. A related virus, the Toscana virus hosted by *Phlebotomus perniciosus* and *Phlebotomus perfiliewi*, causes a similar illness in countries surrounding the northern Mediterranean basin and is emerging in western Europe. The related Punique, Granada, and sandfly fever Turkey viruses may cause similar febrile illnesses, acute meningitis, or meningoencephalitis.

EPIDEMIOLOGY

The virus's distribution parallels the distribution of *Phlebotomus* flies found throughout the Mediterranean basin, Middle East, and western India and Pakistan. In Central America, *Lutzomyia* fly species may transmit the virus. These tiny sandflies pass through mosquito netting to feed in the early evenings. Virus is maintained by transovarial and transstadial transmission. During outbreaks, humans may serve as a reservoir. Human infection is more common in rural areas during the summer months.[9] The incubation period is 2 to 6 days. Sandflies spread by hopping, thus limiting their travel range. Use of insect sprays locally is effective in decreasing risk.

CLINICAL MANIFESTATIONS

Sandfly fever virus causes an acute febrile illness associated with malaise, headache, photophobia, ocular pain, altered taste, myalgia, and arthralgia. The myalgias may be localized to specific regions (e.g., the chest) and simulate regional syndromes such as pleurodynia. A macular or urticarial rash may appear. Examination may show relative bradycardia after the first day, conjunctival injection, mild papilledema, or small palatal vesicles. Fever lasts 2 to 4 days and then subsides. Weakness and malaise may persist during convalescence. About 15% of patients experience recrudescence in 2 to 12 weeks. Aseptic meningitis may occur with mild cerebrospinal fluid pleocytosis. Peripheral leukopenia and lymphopenia may be present early in the illness. However, leukopenia may be delayed in some patients until the third day of illness, and a rebound relative lymphocytosis may be encountered.[10]

DIAGNOSIS

The diagnosis of phlebotomus fever is confirmed by isolation of virus after intracerebral inoculation of suckling mice, detection of the viral genome by RT-PCR, or detection of specific IgM antibody by ELISA.

TREATMENT AND PROGNOSIS Rx

Treatment is supportive, and recovery is complete. Ribavirin (Chapter 360) has been proposed as a therapeutic option.

RIFT VALLEY FEVER

Rift Valley fever, which is an acute-onset, febrile illness, is often associated with epizootic waves of spontaneous abortion in livestock.[11]

DEFINITION

The Rift Valley fever virus is a member of the family Bunyaviridae, genus Phlebovirus, but unlike other members of the genus, it is transmitted by *Aedes* mosquitoes.

EPIDEMIOLOGY

Rift Valley fever occurs throughout most of Africa, with the majority of epizootic outbreaks occurring in eastern and southern Africa, although outbreaks occurred in Saudi Arabia and Yemen in 2000 and Mauritania in 1998, 2003, 2010, and 2012. The principal initial vectors are probably the *Aedes* species associated with flooding, although *Stomoxys* flies have been shown to transmit virus as well. Shallow pools along rivers and streams play an important role as mosquito breeding sites. Feeding on nearby livestock allows a local epizootic outbreak and amplification of the virus in local mosquito populations, including *C. pipiens* in Egypt and *Culex theileri* in eastern Africa. Exposure to aborted livestock increases human risk of infection.

Hemorrhagic fever in humans is typically seen 1 to 2 weeks after a wave of abortion in livestock. Initial human cases usually occur in those who have close contact with livestock. The virus is highly transmissible through aerosolization. Although the risk for severe human infection is less than 1%, the extensive exposure associated with outbreaks can lead to significant morbidity and mortality. For example, in the 1977-1978 Egyptian outbreak associated with movement of camels from Sudan, an estimated 200,000 people were infected, with 600 deaths. Zinga virus, isolated in central Africa and Madagascar and shown to be responsible for mild human illness, is a strain of Rift Valley fever virus.

PATHOBIOLOGY

Rift Valley fever virus grows well in a variety of cell cultures and has cytopathic effects. After infection by a mosquito bite, virus is transported through the lymphatics to regional lymph nodes, where replication allows amplification of the input inoculum and development of viremia with systemic spread. Viral replication in liver, spleen, lymph node, adrenal, lung, and kidney tissues is highly cytopathic. In severe cases, hepatic necrosis and, rarely, focal brain necrosis may occur. Encephalitis is not associated with viremia, thus suggesting that this sequela is immune mediated rather than a direct viral effect. Inflammatory cell infiltration is associated with focal necrosis in the brain. Spontaneous abortion is common in livestock, but fetal loss in humans is not clearly correlated with viral infection.

CLINICAL MANIFESTATIONS

Most human infections are mild, with an abrupt onset of fever, chills, malaise, and arthralgia following a 2- to 6-day incubation. Despite the development of neutralizing antibodies, however, about 1 to 2% of infections progress to more severe disease, including a severe hemorrhagic fever associated with hepatic necrosis and disseminated intravascular coagulopathy. Recovery is complicated by retinal vasculitis or encephalitis, which occurs in less than 0.5% of patients 1 to 4 weeks after recovery and is associated with recurrent fever. In severe cases, focal brain necrosis and encephalitis may lead to hallucinations, stupor, coma, and death.

DIAGNOSIS

Intense viremia allows detection of virus by quantitative real-time RT-PCR. Specific IgM and IgG are detectable by ELISA applied to acute and convalescent (after 1 to 2 weeks) paired sera.

TREATMENT, PREVENTION, AND PROGNOSIS   Rx

Treatment is supportive. Ribavirin (see Table 381-5 and Chapter 360) has been proposed as a therapeutic option but exhibits limited penetration of the blood-brain barrier. Favipiravir, a selective inhibitor of RNA-dependent RNA polymerase, is also a candidate therapeutic under study. In endemic areas, vaccination of livestock is the most effective preventive measure.

The prognosis is good in the absence of retinitis or encephalitis. A high viral load at initial evaluation is a prognostic indicator for a poor outcome.

CHIKUNGUNYA FEVER

DEFINITION

Chikungunya fever is a febrile arthritis that occurs in sporadic cases and in epidemics.[12]

The Pathogen

Chikungunya, an enveloped, single-stranded RNA virus 60 to 70 nm in diameter, is a member of the family Togaviridae, genus Alphavirus. Chikungunya virus is transmitted by mosquitoes, principally *Aedes* species, but also by *Mansonia africana* and other genera. Known animal reservoirs are monkeys, baboons, and, in Senegal, *Scotophilus* bat species. During outbreaks, humans are the major reservoir.

EPIDEMIOLOGY

Chikungunya, which is endemic in sub-Sahara Africa, India, the Philippines, and Southeast Asia, spread in 2004-2005 to the Seychelles, Mauritius, and Mayotte islands with a genotype better adapted to *A. albopictus*. This genotype then spread to India, where the outbreak continues with millions being affected. The global emergence of this disease is exemplified by outbreaks in Réunion Island, Bhutan, Papua New Guinea, and Italy as well as by recently reported cases in several Caribbean islands.[13] Non-travel related cases have been reported in Florida, United States.[14] Outbreaks typically develop after heavy rains. In urban settings, outbreaks are explosive. In endemic areas, seroprevalence rates may be as high as 90%, thus suggesting that time required for loss of herd immunity is the reason for the prolonged absence of cases in a region after an outbreak. Globalization may contribute to increasing propensity for spread. After inoculation, the incubation period is typically 2 to 3 days but ranges from 1 to 12 days.

PATHOBIOLOGY

Intense viremia develops within 48 hours of the mosquito bite and wanes 2 to 3 days later. Onset of hemagglutination inhibition and neutralizing antibodies clears the viremia. Superficial capillaries in rash-involved skin demonstrate erythrocyte extravasation and perivascular cuffing. The virus adsorbs to human platelets and causes them to aggregate. Synovitis probably results from direct chikungunya viral infection of synovium.[15]

CLINICAL MANIFESTATIONS

Chikungunya fever is characterized by an explosive onset of fever and severe arthralgia. Constitutional symptoms, fever (temperature to 40° C), rigors, headache, photophobia, retro-orbital pain, conjunctival injection, pharyngitis, anorexia, nausea, vomiting, abdominal pain, tense lymphadenopathy, and myalgia are common. A maculopapular rash located on the torso, extremities, and occasionally the face, palms, and soles occurs in most patients 1 to 10 days after onset of the illness. Appearance of the rash is often associated temporally with initial defervescence; the rash may recur with fever and may be pruritic. Isolated petechiae and mucosal bleeding may occur, but significant hemorrhage is rare. Desquamation may take place when the rash resolves. The initial acute illness may last 2 to 3 days (range, 1 to 7 days). Fever may recrudesce after a 1- to 2-day hiatus. The polyarthralgia is migratory and predominantly affects the small joints of the hands, wrists, feet, and ankles, with less prominent involvement of the large joints.[16] Previously injured joints may be more severely affected. Stiffness and swelling may occur, but large effusions are uncommon. Synovial fluid shows decreased viscosity with poor mucin clot and 2000 to 5000 white blood cells per milliliter. Symptoms, including arthralgia, arthritis, and tenosynovitis, may persist for months to years. Maternal-fetal transmission may result in severe neonatal infection.

DIAGNOSIS

Chikungunya fever must be differentiated from dengue and o'nyong-nyong fever. Chikungunya virus may be isolated from blood during the initial 2 to 4 days of illness. In some patients, viral antigen may be detected in acute sera by hemagglutination assay as a result of the intensity of the viremia. Commercially available real-time RT-PCR assays on acute phase serum may be used to confirm the diagnosis. Specific IgM antibody may be detected for 6 months or longer. Hemagglutination inhibition and neutralization antibodies develop as the viremia is cleared. Complement fixation antibodies are positive by the third week and slowly decrease during the subsequent year.

TREATMENT AND PROGNOSIS   Rx

Treatment is supportive. Nonsteroidal anti-inflammatory agents are useful. During the acute arthritis, range of motion exercises lessen the stiffness. In most cases, mild joint symptoms may persist for months. Destructive arthropathy is rare and may be associated with low-titer rheumatoid factor, thus suggesting an unrelated, underlying inflammatory arthritis. Following the outbreak on Réunion Island in 2006, 70% of affected patients had episodic arthralgia, typically symmetric and incapacitating, with joint swelling in 63% at 3 years after infection.[17] In children, arthralgia and arthritis are milder and briefer in duration. A safe, immunogenic vaccine is currently under investigation.[18]

O'NYONG-NYONG FEVER

DEFINITION

O'nyong-nyong means "joint breaker" in the Acholi dialect of northwestern Uganda, where o'nyong-nyong fever first appeared in February 1959.

The Pathogen

O'nyong-nyong fever is clinically similar to chikungunya fever, and the viruses share antigenic similarity. O'nyong-nyong virus is also a member of the family Togaviridae, genus Alphavirus.

EPIDEMIOLOGY

Within 2 years of its appearance in 1959, the o'nyong-nyong fever virus spread through Uganda and eastern Africa and affected 2 million people. Serologically determined attack rates ranged from 50 to 60%, with case rates of 9 to 78%. Disease spread at a rate of 2 to 3 km daily. After the epidemic, the virus was not detected again until it was isolated from *Anopheles funestus* mosquitoes in Kenya in 1978. *Anopheles gambiae* also serves as a vector. Serologic surveys suggested that o'nyong-nyong virus is endogenous, but cases were not detected again until 1996-1997, during an outbreak in south central Uganda. An outbreak in western Côte d'Ivoire occurred in 2003. The nonhuman vertebrate reservoir for o'nyong-nyong virus is not known. The incubation period lasts at least 8 days. O'nyong-nyong fever virus vectors include *A. funestus*, *A. gambiae*, and other species.

Igbo-ora (meaning "the disease that breaks your wings") virus is a variant of o'nyong-nyong, with 98.5% homology between the two at the genomic level. Igbo-ora is serologically similar to the chikungunya and o'nyong-nyong viruses. In 1984, an epidemic of fever, rash, arthralgia, and myalgia occurred in four villages on the Ivory Coast. The virus was isolated from *A. funestus* and *A. gambiae* mosquitoes and from affected individuals.

PATHOBIOLOGY

Little is known about the pathobiology of o'nyong-nyong fever.

CLINICAL MANIFESTATIONS

Illness begins with a sudden onset of polyarthralgia and polyarthritis. Between 4 and 7 days later, rash begins with improvement in joint symptoms. The rash is uniform in nature, begins on the face, and then spreads to the torso and extremities and occasionally to the palms. The rash lasts 4 to 7 days before fading. Fever is not prominent, but postcervical lymphadenopathy may be marked. Arthralgia is incapacitating in most patients for up to a week, but residual joint pain may persist for months.

DIAGNOSIS

O'nyong-nyong fever is difficult to differentiate from chikungunya fever and may also be mistaken for measles. Specific hemagglutination inhibition and complement fixation tests are available. Mouse antisera raised against chikungunya virus react equally well with o'nyong-nyong virus, but o'nyong-nyong antisera do not react well with chikungunya virus. O'nyong-nyong–specific RT-PCR is available in reference laboratories.

TREATMENT AND PROGNOSIS   Rx

Treatment is symptomatic. Although residual joint pain often persists, there do not appear to be any long-term sequelae.

MAYARO FEVER

DEFINITION

Mayaro fever is an acute febrile illness characterized by fever, rash, arthralgia, and arthritis. Mayaro virus was first recognized in Trinidad in 1954. It has caused recorded outbreaks in Bolivia and Brazil and is endemic in the rain forest region where Bolivia, Brazil, and Peru share borders. Mayaro virus has a monkey reservoir and is transmitted to humans by *Haemagogus* mosquitoes dwelling in the tropical rain forest canopy.

The Pathogen

Mayaro virus is a member of the family Togaviridae, genus Alphavirus.

EPIDEMIOLOGY

Mayaro virus was responsible for an outbreak in Belterra, Brazil, in 1988. Eight hundred of 4000 exposed latex gatherers became infected, with a clinical attack rate of 80%. Forest workers and hunters continue to be at greatest risk. Cases of imported Mayaro virus infection have been documented in the United States and in Europe after travel to the endemic Brazil-Bolivia-Peru interborder region.[19] The virus has been isolated from a bird in Louisiana, thus raising the specter of emergence in North America.

PATHOBIOLOGY

Viremia occurs during the first 1 to 2 days of illness.

CLINICAL MANIFESTATIONS

Illness is characterized by a sudden onset of fever, headache, dizziness, chills, and arthralgia in the small joints of the hands and feet. About 20% of patients have joint swelling. Unilateral inguinal lymphadenopathy is seen occasionally. Leukopenia is common. Fever resolves after 3 to 7 days, but a maculopapular rash then develops on the trunk and extremities of about two thirds of patients and lasts about 3 days.

DIAGNOSIS

Mayaro virus may be isolated from blood by growth in Vero or C6/36 cells. RT-PCR with ELISA is available. A specific IgM is also available as an antibody capture ELISA.

TREATMENT AND PROGNOSIS   Rx

Treatment is supportive. Recovery is complete, although some patients have persistent arthralgia 6 months later.

ROSS RIVER FEVER VIRUS (EPIDEMIC FEBRILE POLYARTHRITIS)

Ross River fever virus causes an acute-onset, febrile illness characterized by rash and arthralgia. Ross River virus is a member of the family Togaviridae, genus Alphavirus.

EPIDEMIOLOGY

Epidemics of fever and rash have been observed in Australia since 1928. Isolation of Ross River virus from mosquitoes, its serologic association with epidemic polyarthritis, and isolation of the virus from epidemic polyarthritis patients in Australia confirmed Ross River virus as the etiologic agent of epidemic polyarthritis. Seroprevalence has been observed in endogenous populations in Papua New Guinea, western New Guinea, the Bismarck Archipelago, Rossel Island, and the Solomon Islands. An outbreak in the Fiji Islands affected more than 40,000 individuals in 1979 to 1980. A similar epidemic occurred in the Cook Islands early in 1980. Antibodies to Ross River virus are not found in individuals west of Weber's line, a hypothetical line separating the Australian geographic zone from the Asiatic zone. Endemic cases and epidemics occur in tropical and temperate regions in Australia. Queensland and New South Wales have a particularly high annual incidence associated with higher rainfall. High rainfall usually precedes epidemic periods, with cases subsequently occurring from spring through fall. Seroprevalence may reach just 6 to 15% in temperate coastal zones but is 27 to 39% in the plains of the Murray Valley river system. In Queensland, annual rates of disease range from 31.5 to 288.3 per 100,000 person-years. From 1992 to 2006, 55,000 cases of Ross River virus infection were reported in Australia.

Aedes vigilax is the major vector on the eastern coast of Australia and *Aedes camptorhynchus* in the salt marshes of southern Australia. *Culex annulirostris* is a freshwater breeding vector. Other Australian *Aedes* species and *Mansonia uniformis* may also serve as vectors. In outbreaks on the Pacific islands, *Aedes polynesiensis*, *A. aegypti*, *A. vigilax*, and *C. annulirostris* may have contributed to transmission. Domestic animals, rodents, and marsupials may serve as intermediate hosts. Virus may persist in *Aedes* mosquitoes.

There is a predominance of women among infected individuals. Children have a case attack rate ratio lower than that of adults. The incubation period is 7 to 11 days.

Barmah Forest virus, another alphavirus found in Australia in 1986, may be manifested in a fashion similar to epidemic febrile polyarthritis. The number of cases reported annually has been increasing since its initial discovery.

PATHOBIOLOGY

Ross River viral antigen may be detected in monocytes and macrophages early in infection, but intact virus is not identifiable by electron microscopy or cell culture. Dermal vessels show mild perivascular mononuclear cell infiltrates, mostly T lymphocytic, in erythematous and purpuric areas. Vessels in purpuric areas also show erythrocyte extravasation. Antigen can be demonstrated in epithelial cells in erythematous or purpuric skin and in the perivascular zone in erythematous skin. However, viral antigens have not been found in normal skin. Synovium undergoes lining cell hypertrophy and sublining vascular proliferation and mononuclear cell infiltration. Viral RNA can be identified by RT-PCR. Synovial fluid cell counts range from 1500 to 13,800 cells/mL and consist of monocytes, vacuolated macrophages, and a few neutrophils. Animal models of infection indicate that Ross River virus targets bone, joint, and skeletal muscle and elicits an inflammatory response mediated by the innate immune system.

CLINICAL MANIFESTATIONS

Arthralgia typically occurs abruptly, followed in 1 to 2 days by a macular, papular, or maculopapular rash that may be pruritic.[20] Three fourths of patients have severe, incapacitating arthralgia in an asymmetrical and migratory distribution. Commonly affected joints are the metacarpophalangeal joints, finger interphalangeal joints, wrists, knees, and ankles. The shoulder, elbow, toe, spine, hip, and temporomandibular joints may also be affected. Arthralgias are worse in the morning and after periods of inactivity. A third of patients have synovitis. Polyarticular swelling and tenosynovitis are common. Up to a third of patients have paresthesias or palm or sole pain. Classic carpal tunnel syndrome may occur.

In some individuals, rash may precede or follow the joint symptoms by 11 or 15 days, respectively. On occasion, vesicles, papules, or petechiae are seen. The trunk and extremities are typically involved, but the palms, soles, and face may also be affected. The rash resolves by fading to a brownish discoloration or by desquamation. Fever tends to be mild to moderate and lasts 1 to 3 days. Headache, nausea, and myalgia are common. Mild photophobia, respiratory symptoms, and lymphadenopathy may occur.

DIAGNOSIS

In the Australian epidemics before 1979, patients were antibody positive at the time of initial evaluation. However, in the Pacific island epidemics of 1979 to 1980, patients remained viremic and serologically negative for up to a week after the onset of symptoms. Virus in serum is stable for up to a month at 0° to −10° C. Current testing in Australia is performed with an indirect ELISA. The presence of specific IgM or evidence of seroconversion to IgG positivity supports a recent infection.

383

TREATMENT AND PROGNOSIS Rx

Treatment is supportive. Nonsteroidal anti-inflammatory drugs provide relief of joint pain. Half of all patients return to activities of daily living within 4 weeks despite residual polyarthralgia. Joint symptoms may recur, but episodes gradually resolve. In some patients, joint symptoms may persist for up to 3 years. Mild exercise tends to improve the joint symptoms.

SINDBIS

Sindbis virus causes a sudden-onset, febrile illness associated with arthralgia and rash. It is known as Ockelbo disease in Sweden, Pogosta disease in Finland, and Karelian fever in the Karelian Isthmus of Russia. *Aedes, Culex,* and *Culiseta* mosquitoes transmit the virus to humans, with birds serving as intermediate hosts.

EPIDEMIOLOGY

The virus was first isolated from *Culex* mosquitoes in the Egyptian village of Sindbis in 1952. Outbreaks frequently occur in the forested areas of Sweden, Finland, and the Karelian Isthmus, but sporadic cases and small outbreaks have occurred in Uganda, South Africa, Zimbabwe, central Africa, and Australia. Individuals involved in outdoor activities or occupations are at greatest risk. In northern Sweden, 2.9% of the population has Sindbis virus–specific serum IgG positivity indicative of prior infection.[21]

PATHOBIOLOGY

Skin lesions show perivascular hemorrhage, lymphocytic infiltrates, edema, and areas of necrosis. Virus has been isolated from skin lesions. Antiviral IgM may persist for years, thus raising the possibility that Sindbis virus arthritis is associated with viral persistence and a direct viral effect on the synovium. Autophagy, an evolutionarily conserved intracellular mechanism for recycling cytoplasmic material to lysosomes for degradation during times of stress, may be disrupted in neurons by Sindbis virus infection, thereby leading to programmed cell death or apoptosis.

CLINICAL MANIFESTATIONS

Arthralgia and rash are the initial symptoms, although one may precede the other by a few days. Arthralgia and arthritis involve the small joints of the hands and feet, wrists, elbows, ankles, and knees. On occasion, arthralgia affects the spine. Tendinitis is common and often involves the Achilles and hand extensor tendons. Fever, if present, tends to be mild to moderate. Constitutional symptoms, headache, fatigue, malaise, nausea, vomiting, pharyngitis, and paresthesias may be present but are not usually severe. Macular rash typically begins on the torso and then involves the arms, legs, palms, soles, and occasionally the head. Macules evolve to papules that have a tendency to vesiculate. Vesiculation is prominent on pressure points, including the palms and soles. As the eruption fades, a brownish discoloration is left. Vesicles on the palms and soles may become hemorrhagic. Rash may recur during convalescence.

DIAGNOSIS

Specific IgM detected by enzyme immunoassay supports a diagnosis of Sindbis virus infection. IgM titers may wane during a period of 3 to 4 years.

TREATMENT AND PROGNOSIS Rx

Treatment is supportive. Nonerosive chronic arthropathy is common in Sweden and Finland, with up to half of all patients having joint symptoms 2.5 years after infection. In a few cases, symptoms may persist for up to 6 years.

 Grade A Reference

A1. Villar L, Dayan GH, Arredondo-Garcia JL, et al, Efficacy of a tetravalent dengue vaccine in children in Latin America. *N Engl J Med.* 2015;372:113-123.

GENERAL REFERENCES

For the General References and other additional features, please visit Expert Consult at https://expertconsult.inkling.com.

ARBOVIRUSES AFFECTING THE CENTRAL NERVOUS SYSTEM

THOMAS P. BLECK

Arboviruses, which are also termed *arthropod-borne viruses,* can affect the central nervous system (CNS). These viruses share a number of clinical and epidemiologic similarities and have an RNA genome, but they do not form a formal virologic taxonomic group. Arboviruses generally have avian or small mammalian reservoirs and are transmitted to humans and other large mammals incidentally when an infected mosquito or other arthropod obtains a blood meal.

EPIDEMIOLOGY

Most human disease is subclinical; a few patients have a brief febrile illness resembling influenza, and a small percentage, usually at the extremes of age, suffer meningitis or encephalitis. The diseases (Table 383-1) reflect the quotidian and seasonal characteristics of their insect vectors. Other viruses of the same genera cause hemorrhagic fever (Chapter 381), and other less frequently encountered arboviruses are also capable of producing encephalitis.

Many of these agents cause notifiable disease in the United States: St. Louis, West Nile, Powassan, eastern equine, western equine, and the California serogroup encephalitis viruses. Case definitions and additional information are available at http://www.cdc.gov/ncidod/dvbid/arbor/index.htm.

The diseases described here are zoonoses (Chapter 328), that is, illnesses caused by viruses transmitted from animals to humans. They are more prevalent in the tropics and subtropics and are usually localized because of ecologic restrictions on their transmission.

PATHOBIOLOGY

Two pathologic processes are common to the arboviral encephalitides: neuronal and glial damage mediated by intracellular viral infection; and migration of immunologically active cells into the perivascular space and brain parenchyma. Endothelial cell swelling and proliferation, destruction of myelin sheaths in deep white matter areas, and vasculitis are present in some arboviral encephalitides.

After a bite by an infected arthropod, viral replication occurs in local tissues and regional lymph nodes. Viremia, which seeds extraneural tissues, occurs and persists, depending on the extent of replication in extraneural sites, the rate of viral clearance by the reticuloendothelial system, and the appearance of humoral antibodies. The sites of extraneural infection vary among the viruses. Many alphaviruses and flaviviruses involve striated muscle and endothelium, whereas Venezuelan encephalitis virus is associated with myeloid and lymphoid tissue invasion. During viremia, the neural parenchyma may be invaded, but the mode of penetration of virus across the blood-brain barrier is not completely understood. Possible mechanisms include passive movement of virus across vascular membranes and viral replication in the cerebral capillary endothelium. Factors that increase vascular permeability or disrupt the blood-brain barrier promote invasion of the nervous system. Infected monocytes may also bring the virus into the CNS. In experimental animal infection, flaviviruses enter the CNS through the olfactory epithelium.

The immune response to flaviviruses starts with an innate interferon response to viral replication. Neurons then produce chemokines that recruit various components of the cellular immune response. The induced T-cell and monocyte trafficking is needed to clear the virus from the CNS, but it can also damage neurons.

The immature brain is more susceptible to damage by western equine, Venezuelan equine, and California serogroup encephalitis viruses (Table 383-2). St. Louis encephalitis and West Nile encephalitis principally affect the elderly, whereas Japanese encephalitis and eastern equine encephalitis have a bimodal incidence and strike both children and elderly persons. In endemic areas, immunity accumulated with increasing age may reduce the incidence of disease in older persons for some viruses; however, the reasons for the increased severity of illness with other viruses remain unknown.

TABLE 383-1 ARTHROPOD-BORNE VIRUSES ASSOCIATED WITH HUMAN ENCEPHALITIS

VIRUS	INSECT VECTOR	COMMON VERTEBRATE HOSTS	GEOGRAPHIC DISTRIBUTION
TOGAVIRIDAE			
Alphaviruses	Mosquitoes		
Eastern equine encephalitis	*Culiseta* spp, *Aedes* spp, *Coquillettidia* spp		Eastern United States and Gulf Coast, Caribbean region, South America
Western equine encephalitis	*Culiseta* spp, *Culex* spp		Western United States, Canada
Venezuelan equine encephalitis	*Aedes* spp, *Culex* spp, *Psorophora* spp, and *Mansonia* spp		South America, Central America, Florida and southwestern United States
FLAVIVIRIDAE			
Japanese serocluster	Mosquitoes		
Japanese encephalitis	*Culex* and *Aedes* spp		East and Southeast Asia, India, Australia
West Nile encephalitis	*Aedes* spp, *Culex* spp, and others		Africa, Middle East, North America
St. Louis encephalitis	*Culex* spp		Western Hemisphere
Murray Valley encephalitis	*Culex* spp		Australia
Tick-borne encephalitis complex			
Central European encephalitis	*Ixodes* spp	Goats, sheep	Europe, Russia
Russian spring-summer encephalitis	*Ixodes* spp		Europe, northern and central Asia
Kyasanur Forest disease	*Haemaphysalis spinigera*	Rodents, insectivores	India
Omsk hemorrhagic fever	*Dermacentor reticulatus*	Rodents	Central Asia
Powassan	*Ixodes* spp	Squirrels, groundhogs	North America, Russia
Louping ill	*Ixodes ricinus*	Small mammals, sheep, birds	British Isles
Langat	*Ixodes* spp	Rodents	Malaysia, Thailand, parts of former Soviet Union
BUNYAVIRIDAE			
California encephalitis	*Aedes melanimon*, *Aedes dorsalis*	Rodents, rabbits	California
La Crosse encephalitis	*Aedes triseriatus*	Chipmunks, squirrels	Eastern and Midwestern United States

TABLE 383-2 FEATURES OF ARBOVIRAL ENCEPHALITIDES IMPORTANT IN THE UNITED STATES

	EASTERN EQUINE ENCEPHALITIS	WESTERN EQUINE ENCEPHALITIS	VENEZUELAN EQUINE ENCEPHALITIS	WEST NILE ENCEPHALITIS	ST. LOUIS ENCEPHALITIS	CALIFORNIA SEROGROUP ENCEPHALITIS
Annual U.S. cases of symptomatic disease	10	0-2 cases, mostly infants and children	Rare, mostly children	Up to 3000, mostly >40 years	0-2000, mostly >50 years	10-50, mostly children
Time of year	Late summer, early fall	Early and mid summer	Summer	Summer, fall	Mid to late summer	July-September
Case-fatality rate	50-70%, highest in children <15 years and adults >55 years	3-5% in children	35% in children, <10% in older persons	14-19%, 30% in adults >70 years	9% overall; 0% <20 years, 30% >65 years	<1%
Residual damage	30-50%, especially in children	33% in infants	Frequent in children	50%, more frequent in elderly	Frequent in elderly	Probably rare
Cerebrospinal fluid findings (cells/μL)	500-2000 cells, predominantly neutrophils	<500 cells, predominantly lymphocytes	<500 cells, predominantly lymphocytes	<500 cells, predominantly lymphocytes	<500 cells, predominantly lymphocytes	<500 cells, predominantly lymphocytes

CLINICAL MANIFESTATIONS

Clinical symptoms and signs vary among the viral causes (see later), although all share common signs and symptoms of encephalitis (Chapter 414).

DIAGNOSIS

Diagnosis depends on a careful history that includes exposure to vertebrate animals and arthropod vectors, age, season, and travel, including the geographic site of exposure. Laboratory confirmation of infection is essential. The virus may be isolated from acute phase serum or whole blood in laboratory animals or in tissue culture. Neutralization, complement fixation (CF), hemagglutination inhibition (HI), fluorescent antibody, and enzyme-linked immunosorbent assay (ELISA) of acute and 3-week convalescent sera can also produce the correct diagnosis. Antigen detection and IgM capture ELISA often permit diagnosis on initial evaluation and within a week of the onset of illness in most cases. Sensitive nucleic amplification assays using reverse transcription–polymerase chain reaction (RT-PCR) are under development for a number of the arboviruses and may lead to earlier diagnosis.

Differential Diagnosis

The most important initial consideration is to differentiate arboviral encephalitides from other acute CNS infections, including infections other than encephalitis (Chapters 412 and 413), treatable causes of encephalitis (Chapter 414), and paraneoplastic and autoimmune encephalitis (Chapters 412 and 414). Anti–N-methyl-D-aspartate (NMDA) receptor encephalitis, which is as common as most viral causes of encephalitis in parts of the United States,[1] is an important part of the differential diagnosis, particularly in young women and especially because—unlike arboviral infections—it often responds to immunosuppressive treatment.

The early prodrome resembles influenza (Chapter 364). Bacterial meningitis (Chapter 412; especially early or partially treated), infective bacterial endocarditis (Chapter 76), brain abscess (Chapter 413), subdural empyema (Chapter 413), and cerebral thrombophlebitis may mimic viral encephalitis, and the cerebrospinal fluid (CSF) profile is sometimes similar. Other infections that occasionally cause meningoencephalitis that may resemble arthropod-borne viral encephalitis include tuberculosis (Chapter 324), cryptococcosis (Chapter 336), histoplasmosis (Chapter 332), coccidioidomycosis (Chapter 333), Rocky Mountain spotted fever (Chapter 327), leptospirosis (Chapter 323), falciparum malaria (Chapter 345), trichinosis (Chapter 357), *Naegleria* meningitis (Chapter 412), typhoid fever (Chapter 308), Lyme disease (Chapter 321), and *Mycoplasma* pneumonia (Chapter 317).

Acute meningoencephalitis may result from infections with other viruses, including herpesviruses (Chapter 374), human immunodeficiency virus (Chapter 386), mumps virus (Chapter 369), enteroviruses (Chapter 379), lymphocytic choriomeningitis virus (Chapter 412), rabies (Chapter 414), influenza (Chapter 364), and the exanthematous viral infections of childhood (Chapters 367 and 368). The exposure history, the presence of similar disease in the community, and the summer-fall occurrence are principal clues to an arboviral etiology. Enteroviruses (Chapter 379) also cause summer-fall outbreaks, but the predominant syndrome is aseptic meningitis, and the concomitant occurrence of rash or pleurodynia is a helpful clue. Herpes simplex encephalitis (Chapter 414) presents an important diagnostic challenge because effective therapy is available and should be started quickly. The presence of localizing neurologic signs, localizing findings on computed tomography (CT) or magnetic resonance imaging (MRI), and detection of herpes simplex DNA in CSF by PCR help distinguish herpes simplex encephalitis from the arboviral encephalitides.

Noninfectious diseases of the CNS, such as stroke (Chapter 407), may rarely be confused with viral encephalitis. Subarachnoid hemorrhage (Chapter 408) produces meningismus, fever, headache, and neurologic signs that mimic an infectious etiology. Metabolic encephalopathies occasionally have features suggesting infectious encephalitis. Neoplastic or granulomatous diseases involving the CNS and a variety of diseases of uncertain etiology (Behçet disease [Chapter 270], Reye syndrome, acute multiple sclerosis [Chapter 411], and systemic lupus erythematosus [Chapter 266]) must be considered in the differential diagnosis as well.

PREVENTION

Control can be achieved by interruption of the cycle, including vaccination of reservoir animals, vector control, and education on vector avoidance. Practical measures include wearing long-sleeved clothing, using insect repellents, limiting outdoor activities during peak mosquito season, and eliminating standing pools of water. Vaccines are currently available for Japanese encephalitis.

TREATMENT   Rx

Treatment is symptomatic and may include bedrest, antipyretics, and analgesics. Early empirical treatment of herpes simplex encephalitis (Chapter 374) may be appropriate while the diagnostic evaluation to document arboviral encephalitis proceeds. To date, no immunologic therapy has demonstrated a useful effect in humans.

● EASTERN EQUINE ENCEPHALITIS

EPIDEMIOLOGY

Human disease is relatively rare, with fewer than 10 cases occurring each year in the Gulf Coast and Atlantic states, usually in association with an equine epizootic involving 100 to 300 animals. Outbreaks generally occur during the late summer and early fall. The occurrence of equine cases or outbreaks of fatal encephalitis in penned exotic birds precedes the appearance of human cases by several weeks or more. Epizootics of eastern equine encephalitis have been reported in the Caribbean (Hispaniola) and South America.[2]

In temperate areas, eastern equine encephalitis virus circulates between wild birds and *Culiseta melanura* mosquitoes in a freshwater swamp habitat. Equine epizootics and associated human cases result from extension of the transmission cycle to involve *Aedes* and *Coquillettidia* mosquitoes, which feed on horses and humans.[3]

PATHOBIOLOGY

The brain is grossly edematous and congested, and the inflammatory response is predominantly polymorphonuclear. The areas most affected are the basal ganglia, thalamus, hippocampus, and frontal and occipital cortices. Focal vasculitis, endothelial cell swelling, intravenous and arteriolar thrombus formation, demyelination, necrosis, neuronolysis, and neuronophagia are prominent. Eastern equine encephalitis virus appears to make use of host micro-RNAs to limit replication in myeloid cells, thereby restricting the host immune response and causing more severe neurologic damage.[4]

CLINICAL MANIFESTATIONS

Onset is abrupt, with high fever, vomiting, and somnolence. Stupor, coma, myoclonus, and generalized convulsions appear within 24 hours to as long as 10 days later. Autonomic disturbances (sialorrhea) may be prominent, and respiratory difficulty and cyanosis are frequent. In children, facial, periorbital, or generalized edema may be present.

A striking peripheral leukocytosis with immature neutrophils occurs frequently in patients with eastern equine encephalitis. CSF examination reveals 500 to 2000 white blood cells/μL (predominantly neutrophils). As the total cell count falls, neutrophils may persist as a significant fraction. Red blood cells may be present, protein concentration is elevated, and the glucose level is normal.

DIAGNOSIS

Brain CT and MRI are frequently abnormal and reveal lesions in the basal ganglia, thalami, and brain stem. The virus can rarely be isolated from blood or CSF. Serologic diagnosis by demonstration of a rise in antibody titer in appropriately timed paired sera is the most practical and available test. Because of the rapid course of the clinical disease, sera should be obtained at 2- to 3-day intervals during the acute phase of illness.

PREVENTION

An experimental formalin-inactivated chick embryo cell culture vaccine is used to protect laboratory and field workers. Reduction of mosquito populations by appropriate use of insecticides may be effective in threatened or established outbreaks.

TREATMENT   Rx

Treatment is supportive. Control of fever, intracranial pressure, seizures, fluid and electrolyte disturbances, and the airway is critical. Although attempts at immunologic therapy have been reported, no controlled data are available.

PROGNOSIS

The case-fatality rate is 50 to 70%. Mortality, like incidence, is highest in children younger than 15 years and in persons older than 55 years, with no gender predilection. Death usually occurs during the first week; in surviving patients, recovery begins during the second week and may progress rapidly. Good functional recovery is associated with a long prodromal course and absence of coma. Residual damage, found in 30 to 50% of patients, is often severe, especially in children, and is characterized by mental retardation, spastic paralysis, and radiographic evidence of brain atrophy.

● WESTERN EQUINE ENCEPHALITIS

EPIDEMIOLOGY

Few cases of western equine encephalitis have been reported in recent decades; the most recent epidemic occurred in Colorado in 1987. Epidemics occur in early or mid summer and may follow heavy snow melt or flooding, conditions favorable for breeding of mosquitoes. Cases of encephalitis in equines often precede the appearance of human disease. The illness principally affects residents of rural communities, and the incidence is higher in males than in females.

The ratio of inapparent to apparent infection is also age dependent and ranges from about 1 : 1 in infants younger than 1 year, to 58 : 1 in children 1 to 4 years old, to more than 1000 : 1 in persons older than 14 years. Western equine encephalitis virus also occurs in South America. Equine epizootics in Argentina have been associated with human cases.

Western equine encephalitis virus circulates between wild birds and *Culex tarsalis* mosquitoes. *Cx. tarsalis* is responsible for infection of humans and equines, which have low or undetectable viremia and do not perpetuate the chain of transmission. In temperate areas, transmission ceases during the winter months.

PATHOBIOLOGY

Pathologic examination of the brains of infants reveals massive parenchymal destruction; children dying months or years after the acute insult often have large cystic lesions in many areas of the brain. In older children and adults, acute western equine encephalitis is characterized by focal necrosis and perivascular cuffing, predominantly in the basal ganglia and thalami but also in deep cerebral white matter.

CLINICAL MANIFESTATIONS

The disease usually begins with an influenza-like illness consisting of fever, headache, malaise, and myalgia lasting 1 to 4 days. Somnolence, lethargy, photophobia, vomiting, and neck stiffness may follow; neurologic involvement may rapidly progress to stupor, coma, and seizures. Pareses, cranial nerve deficits, tremors, and abnormal reflexes may be present. In fatal cases, patients die 1 to 2 days after coma develops. Congenital infections have been documented and result in severe and progressive neurologic deterioration.

Leukocytosis and a shift to the left are common. The CSF contains fewer than 500 white blood cells/µL (at first polymorphonuclear, then mononuclear) and an elevated protein concentration (usually 90 to 110 mg/dL).

DIAGNOSIS

Viral isolation from blood or CSF is almost never successful. Diagnosis is achieved by demonstration of a rise in HI, fluorescent antibody, CF, ELISA, or neutralizing antibody titers in appropriately timed (10 to 14 days apart) paired sera. Demonstration of IgM antibodies in serum or CSF by ELISA provides a presumptive diagnosis.

PREVENTION

An experimental formalin-inactivated vaccine grown in chick embryo cell culture has been used to protect laboratory workers but is not indicated for others. In threatened or ongoing epidemics, residents should be advised to use protective clothing, insect repellents, and window screens and to restrict outdoor activity in the early morning, late afternoon, and evening (times of greatest mosquito activity). Public health measures include spraying insecticides aimed at the adult *Cx. tarsalis* vector.

TREATMENT Rx

There is no specific therapy for western equine encephalitis. Supportive therapy is similar to that discussed earlier for eastern equine encephalitis.

PROGNOSIS

Western equine encephalitis is most severe in infants and young children. The case-fatality rate is between 3 and 5%. Survivors generally experience sudden and rapid recovery. However, about a third of surviving infants suffer mental retardation, cerebellar damage, choreoathetosis, and spastic paralysis. Children with protracted illnesses in whom convulsions develop during the acute stage are more likely to suffer long-term neurologic sequelae. Adults may have a prolonged convalescent syndrome, but objective residua are rare.

VENEZUELAN EQUINE ENCEPHALITIS

Six antigenic subtypes of Venezuelan equine encephalitis virus (I to VI) with several antigenic variants of subtypes I and III are recognized serologically. Subtypes IAB and IC are responsible for epidemics involving humans and equines. In Florida, subtype II is enzootic and produces sporadic human disease. Methods of transmitting Venezuelan equine encephalitis virus as a biologic warfare agent were developed in the 1960s; an epidemic of Venezuelan equine encephalitis, especially if humans and horses become ill simultaneously, could represent an attack rather than naturally occurring illness.

EPIDEMIOLOGY

Before 1973, large equine epizootics occurred at 5- to 10-year intervals in Venezuela, Colombia, Ecuador, and Peru and involved many thousands of animals with mortality rates as high as 40%. Associated human morbidity was also great (up to 32,000 clinical cases). The disease was quiescent for several years but has reemerged in the Gulf Coast region of Mexico in the past decade. The last major outbreak occurred in Venezuela and Colombia in 1995, with more than 85,000 human cases. Laboratory infections are common in unvaccinated persons who work with the virus or infected animals.

A large variety of mosquito vectors, including species of the genera *Aedes*, *Psorophora*, and *Mansonia*, transmit subtypes IAB and IC during epizootic epidemics. Equines are the principal viremic hosts. Virus may be present in the pharyngeal excretions of human patients; contact or aerosol person-to-person spread, although possible, is not epidemiologically important.

The other members of the Venezuelan equine encephalitis viral complex, including subtype II in Florida, have enzootic transmission cycles involving *Culex* mosquitoes and small forest rodents and marsupials. Human disease is sporadic and relatively uncommon.

PATHOBIOLOGY

Pathologic changes in the CNS include edema, congestion, meningeal and perivascular inflammation, intracerebral hemorrhage, neuronal degeneration,

and vasculitis. In addition, hepatocellular degeneration and necrosis, widespread lymphoid depletion and follicular necrosis, and interstitial pneumonitis are frequent. Congenitally infected fetuses demonstrate massive and widespread necrosis of brain tissue, hemorrhage, and resorption of brain material resulting in hydranencephaly.

CLINICAL MANIFESTATIONS

The predominant syndrome is a self-limited influenza-like illness; encephalitis develops in only about 4% of infected persons, principally children younger than 15 years. Subclinical infections are rare.

After an incubation period of 2 to 5 days, there is a sudden onset of fever, chills, malaise, and headache, followed by myalgias, nausea, vomiting, and occasionally diarrhea. Physical examination reveals fever, tachycardia, conjunctival injection, and, in some cases, nonexudative pharyngitis. The acute illness generally subsides in 4 to 6 days, and convalescent symptoms may last up to 3 weeks. A biphasic course has sometimes been noted; acute symptoms can reappear after a brief remission, within a week after initial onset.

When it occurs, severe encephalitis is characterized by meningeal signs, seizures, tremor, stupor, coma, spastic paralysis, abnormal reflexes, cranial nerve palsies, and central respiratory failure. Residual neurologic damage occurs in severe cases. Infections of pregnant women acquired during the first and second trimester may result in fetal encephalitis and death.

The peripheral leukocyte count is often low, with a decrease in both lymphocytes and neutrophils, or normal with relative lymphopenia. In patients with CNS signs, the CSF contains up to 500 cells/µL, predominantly lymphocytes. Serum lactate dehydrogenase and aspartate aminotransferase concentrations may be elevated.

DIAGNOSIS

In contrast to the other arboviral encephalitides, Venezuelan equine encephalitis virus can be isolated from blood or from throat swabs or washings during the first 3 or 4 days of illness. Serodiagnosis is usually more practical and is achieved by testing appropriately timed paired sera by HI, CF, ELISA, neutralization, or IgM immunoassay.

PREVENTION

An experimental live attenuated vaccine made from subtype IAB is used for adult laboratory personnel. It provides solid immunity to subtypes IAB and IC but incomplete protection against heterologous Venezuelan equine encephalitis viruses. Epidemics and epizootics can be prevented by effective vaccination of equines. Spraying insecticides to reduce adult (infective) mosquito populations is the only means of immediate control in the face of an ongoing epidemic. Individual protection against mosquitoes is advised.

TREATMENT Rx

No specific therapy is available, and treatment of encephalitis cases is supportive.

PROGNOSIS

The case-fatality rate in children 5 years or younger with encephalitis is approximately 35%, but it is less than 10% in older persons.

JAPANESE ENCEPHALITIS

EPIDEMIOLOGY

Japanese encephalitis virus is a flavivirus that causes epizootics of clinical encephalitis in equines. The disease occurs throughout Asia, including Japan, China, the Korean peninsula, Taiwan, Okinawa, Vietnam, the Philippines, Burma, Malaysia, Bangladesh, east and south India, Sri Lanka, Thailand, and Indonesia. More than 30,000 clinical cases occur annually, about one third of which are fatal. Japanese encephalitis is a summertime disease in temperate areas but occurs sporadically year-round in the tropics. Several species of *Culex* mosquitos can transmit the virus, most notably *Cx. tritaeniorhynchus*.

Epidemics are most frequent at the northern fringe of the tropical zone, with a high incidence noted in southern China.[5] It is a predominantly rural disease, and the incidence in males is often higher than in females. In hyperendemic areas, more than 70% of adult populations surveyed have antibodies, and children younger than 15 years are principally affected by the disease.

In areas without a high prevalence of background immunity (e.g., northern India), however, all age groups are affected. In Japan, where schoolchildren have been protected by vaccination campaigns targeted at this age group, encephalitis has become prominent in the elderly. The ratio of clinically inapparent to apparent infection is higher than 500 : 1 in children and decreases with age; in Korea, the ratio in American servicemen was estimated at 25 : 1.

PATHOBIOLOGY

Neuropathologic changes and the distribution of lesions are similar to those described for St. Louis encephalitis (see later).

CLINICAL MANIFESTATIONS

Manifestations of Japanese encephalitis include abrupt fever, headache, and gastrointestinal symptoms. Meningeal irritation develops within 24 hours and is followed on the second or third day by the appearance of irritability, impaired consciousness, seizures (especially in children), muscle rigidity, parkinsonian findings, ataxia, coarse tremor, involuntary movements, cranial nerve deficits, paresis, hyperactive deep tendon reflexes, and pathologic reflexes. Weight loss and dehydration are often striking findings. In mild cases, fever subsides after the first week, and neurologic signs resolve by the end of the second week after onset. In severe cases, hyperpyrexia, progressive neurologic dysfunction, and coma result in death, usually between the seventh and tenth days. About 25% of patients undergo a prolonged recovery, with permanent sequelae often remaining. The occurrence of such sequelae correlates with severity of the acute stage of illness, and young children are most susceptible. Cardiorespiratory complications are frequent during the acute stage in these patients. A poor prognosis is associated with protracted high fever, frequent or prolonged seizures, high protein content in CSF, Babinski signs, and early respiratory depression. Fetal death from transplacental Japanese encephalitis infection has been reported.

DIAGNOSIS

Moderate peripheral leukocytosis and neutrophilia occur early in the disease. Pleocytosis (predominantly lymphocytic), protein elevation, and normal glucose concentration in CSF are usual findings.

MRI in Japanese encephalitis reveals edema in the basal ganglia, thalami, and focal areas of the cerebral cortex; evidence of hemorrhage in these areas may likewise be present. Enhancement may also be noted in the meninges, brain stem, and spinal cord.

Virus is rarely isolated from blood. Virus is also rarely recovered from the CSF of patients who live but may be recovered from the CSF of a third of patients who die. HI and neutralizing antibodies appear during the first week, and CF antibodies appear during the second week. Cross-reactions with other flaviviruses make serodiagnosis difficult. Specific IgM antibodies in serum or CSF are detectable by immunoassays in more than three fourths of patients at the time of hospital admission.

PREVENTION

Newer inactivated Vero cell culture–derived vaccines, including IC51 (marketed as Ixiaro and Jespect), CC-JEV (marketed as Encevac), and Jenvac, are available for use in persons older than 17 years[A1] and have recently been shown to be safe in children.[A2] They are more immunogenic than the older inactivated mouse brain–derived vaccine. A combined yellow fever–Japanese encephalitis vaccine (ChimeriVax-JE) is available in Australia and Thailand. A new chimeric vaccine, which is effective when it is administered concomitantly with measles-mumps-rubella vaccine, holds promise for children in endemic areas.[A3] In China, a live attenuated vaccine (SA14-14-2) is commonly used.

Ixiaro is licensed in the United States for individuals aged 2 months and older traveling to high-risk areas.[6] Generalized urticaria and angioedema may occur in 0.3%. Because two doses of the inactivated vaccine are used and approximately 1 month is required to confer protection, vaccination is not a practical measure in the event of an ongoing epidemic.[7]

Reduction of vector mosquito populations by the application of insecticides may help abort outbreaks. Immunization of swine is an ancillary control strategy.

TREATMENT   Rx

Treatment is supportive (see Eastern Equine Encephalitis). A randomized trial of interferon alfa showed no benefit.

PROGNOSIS

The case-fatality rate is probably about 25%. Sequelae such as mental impairment, emotional lability, choreoathetosis, tremor, parkinsonism, autonomic disturbances, paralysis, and psychiatric disturbances have been reported in up to 75% of patients.

● WEST NILE FEVER AND ENCEPHALITIS

Before 1996, the predominant clinical manifestation of West Nile virus was a brief influenza-like illness, sometimes with a rash (Chapter 382) but infrequently with neurologic manifestations. Epidemics since then in Romania, Israel, and North America have added meningitis, meningoencephalitis, and myelitis to the list of disorders attributable to the virus.[8] Sequence analyses of various isolates of the virus indicate two lineages. The first includes viruses from North America, Europe, Israel, western Africa, India, Russia, and Australia; the second includes viruses from sub-Saharan Africa and Madagascar.

EPIDEMIOLOGY

See Chapter 382. The incidence of neuroinvasive West Nile disease varies in different parts of the United States but can be seen nearly everywhere.[9] In a recent outbreak in Dallas, Texas, the incidence rate for West Nile encephalitis was 7.3 per 100,000 residents, with cases clustered in neighborhoods with high housing density.[10]

CLINICAL MANIFESTATIONS

The majority of infected people are asymptomatic. Fever develops in about 20%, and CNS manifestations are seen in less than 1%, although this percentage is higher in the elderly (Chapter 382). In those in whom clinical manifestations develop, an incubation period of 1 to 6 days is followed by the abrupt onset of symptoms, usually without a prodrome. The temperature rises quickly to 38.3° to 40.0° C, with rigors in a third of patients. Symptoms include drowsiness, severe frontal headache, ocular pain, myalgia, and pain in the abdomen and back. A small number of patients have dryness of the throat, anorexia, and nausea. Cough is common. Examination shows facial flushing, conjunctival injection, and coating of the tongue. Generalized lymphadenopathy had been a prominent feature in past epidemics but is no longer commonly reported. The spleen and liver are occasionally slightly enlarged. The temperature curve may be biphasic. A pale roseolar maculopapular rash, predominantly on the trunk and upper part of the arms, may appear from the second to fifth day but is now less common as well; it may be evanescent (several hours) or persist until defervescence, and it does not desquamate. Vesicular lesions occur rarely. The illness lasts 3 to 5 days in 80% of patients. Clinical manifestations appear to be more frequent in organ transplant recipients.

In the past decade, the incidence of CNS disease has increased in several epidemics, apparently because of a true increase in the invasiveness and neurovirulence of the virus. The virus causes a syndrome resembling poliomyelitis (Chapter 379), with prominent lower motor neuron dysfunction (acute flaccid paralysis with asymmetrical weakness and decreased deep tendon reflexes but preserved sensory function), which may be seen independently or with signs of meningoencephalitis. In some patients, prolonged, possibly permanent ventilatory failure requiring mechanical ventilation develops. About 95% of patients present with neuroinvasive disease and a significant neurologic defect; about 50% have weakness, 35% have tremor, and 15% have cranial neuropathies.[11] Some patients may have seizures, cranial nerve involvement, ataxia, tremors, or myoclonus. Acute inflammatory polyneuropathy (e.g., Guillain-Barré syndrome; Chapter 420) has also been reported. Other rare complications include myocarditis, pancreatitis, and hepatitis. Convalescence is often prolonged, lasting several weeks with prominent symptoms of fatigue. Lymph node enlargement requires several months to regress. Laboratory findings often include leukocytosis, whereas 10 to 15% of patients have leukopenia.

DIAGNOSIS

CSF examination may reveal a lymphocytic pleocytosis (<1800 cells/μL) with some increase in protein but a normal glucose concentration. Although West Nile virus may be isolated from the blood of three fourths of patients with West Nile fever on the first day of illness (Chapter 382), patients with West Nile encephalitis appear less likely to be viremic, and isolation of virus from CSF is infrequent. Viral RNA is detected in CSF by RT-PCR in about 50% of cases (Fig. 383-1). IgM antibody capture immunoassay, which is the test of choice, is more sensitive than RT-PCR. IgM antibodies may remain

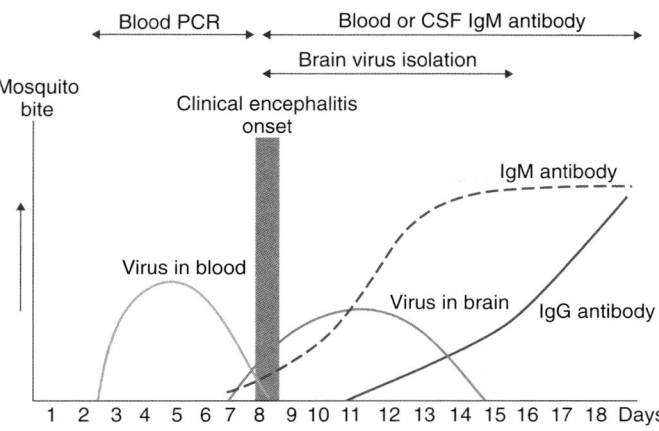

FIGURE 383-1. Typical time course for development of West Nile virus in blood and brain and occurrence of IgG and IgM antibodies in humans after West Nile virus infection. CSF = cerebrospinal fluid; PCR = polymerase chain reaction. (Reproduced from Davis LE, Beckham JD, Tyler KL. North American encephalitic arboviruses. *Neurol Clin.* 2008;26:727-757.)

detectable for up to 500 days after infection, so their presence should suggest acute infection only with compatible clinical manifestations. In some situations, cross-reactions with other flaviviruses, particularly St. Louis encephalitis virus, may complicate the interpretation of IgM immunoassays.

PREVENTION

Two phase II clinical trials of a live attenuated human chimeric vaccine (ChimeriVax-WN02) have demonstrated safety and both durable neutralizing antibody and cytotoxic T-cell responses.[12] A phase I trial of another chimeric vaccine (rWN/DEN4Δ30) also suggests promise. Because West Nile virus may be transmitted by organ transplantation, it is important to consider the possibility of this infection in organ donors.[13]

TREATMENT Rx

Treatment is symptomatic and similar to that suggested for eastern equine encephalitis. Patients may require prolonged mechanical ventilation for either the polio-like syndrome or Guillain-Barré syndrome. The Guillain-Barré syndrome seen in West Nile patients does not appear to respond to plasma exchange. A trial of intravenous human immunoglobulin with high-titer anti–West Nile virus activity could not be completed because of the unpredictable annual geographic shifts in the activity of the disease. A recombinant humanized monoclonal antibody appeared safe in a phase I trial but has not been tested further. Ribavirin has activity against West Nile virus, but its clinical utility remains unknown.

PROGNOSIS

The overall case-fatality rate is 4 to 14%, but it is higher in the elderly. Risk factors for death include more severe weakness or coma, immunocompromise, and failure to produce virus-specific IgM. The prognosis for neurologic recovery is generally good; most U.S. patients regain physical and mental function by 1 year, but about half the patients in some series still report difficulties 1 year after the illness.

● ST. LOUIS ENCEPHALITIS

ETIOLOGY

St. Louis encephalitis virus, a member of the family Flaviviridae,[14] shares close antigenic relationships with Japanese encephalitis, Murray Valley encephalitis, and West Nile viruses and is related to yellow fever (Chapter 381) and dengue (Chapter 382) viruses. Strains associated with *Culex pipiens*–borne epidemics in the northern United States are distinct from endemic strains transmitted by *Cx. tarsalis* in the western states.

EPIDEMIOLOGY

The virus is present in all parts of the Western Hemisphere, but epidemics occur only in North America and some Caribbean islands. During epidemic years, the virus has been responsible for up to 80% of all reported cases of

encephalitis of known etiology in the United States. Epidemics of up to 2000 cases have taken place, mainly in urban-suburban localities of the Ohio-Mississippi River basin and in eastern and central Texas and Florida. Small outbreaks have also occurred in the western United States. Epidemics generally take place between July and September but may arise later in the year in warm areas such as Florida. Previous exposure and immunity to dengue may provide a degree of cross-protection against clinical St. Louis encephalitis. The ratio of inapparent to apparent infection is 800 : 1 in children up to 9 years of age, 400 : 1 in persons aged 10 to 49 years, and 85 : 1 in persons older than 60 years.

In most of the eastern United States, St. Louis encephalitis virus circulates between wild birds and *Cx. pipiens* mosquitoes, which breed in polluted water. In Florida and in parts of the Caribbean, *Cx. nigripalpus* is the principal vector. The cycle in the western United States also involves wild birds, but the vector is *Cx. tarsalis*, also that of western equine encephalitis. Because of the similar ecology of St. Louis encephalitis and western equine encephalitis viruses in the West, mixed outbreaks occur, mostly in rural, agricultural areas.

Above-average summer temperatures and conditions such as deficient rainfall, which create stagnant pools suitable for *Cx. pipiens* breeding, are associated with epidemics in the eastern United States. St. Louis encephalitis in the western states is favored by warm spring temperatures, heavy snow melt, and flooding.

PATHOBIOLOGY

Pathologic changes in fatal cases are limited to microscopic findings. Leptomeningitis is characterized by lymphocytic inflammation. Parenchymal changes consist of lymphocytic perivascular cuffing, cellular nodule formation, and neuronal degeneration.

CLINICAL MANIFESTATIONS

Three clinical syndromes are recognized: febrile headache, aseptic meningitis, and encephalitis. After an incubation period of 4 to 21 days, a variable period of nonspecific symptoms, including fever (temperature of 38° to 41° C), headache, malaise, drowsiness, myalgia, and sore throat, may be followed by an acute or subacute onset of meningeal or encephalitic signs, or both. Nausea, vomiting, and photophobia are common.

Neurologic abnormalities occur in up to 25% of patients. Extrapyramidal abnormalities and altered consciousness are the most significant findings. Other findings include meningismus, cranial nerve deficits (particularly the facial nerve), abnormal reflexes, tremors, myoclonic twitching, nystagmus, and ataxia. Motor abnormalities are infrequent, and sensory changes are extremely uncommon. Seizures occur in 10% of patients and are a poor prognostic sign, as is a persistent high temperature of 40° to 41° C. Signs of markedly increased intracranial pressure are unusual. A Guillain-Barré–like syndrome (Chapter 420) has occasionally been associated with St. Louis encephalitis, both as an acute manifestation and during the convalescent period.

In uncomplicated cases of St. Louis encephalitis, a moderate peripheral neutrophilic leukocytosis and shift to the left are noted. CSF pressure is elevated, protein level is mildly elevated, and glucose concentration is normal; a pleocytosis of up to 500 cells/μL is present, with an early neutrophilia predominance changing to lymphocytes within days. Serum creatine kinase, aspartate aminotransferase, and aldolase levels are frequently elevated. The electroencephalogram typically shows polymorphic delta activity, most prominently in the frontal and temporal regions; electrographic seizures are common. CT scans are normal, but MRI may show edema involving deep structures such as the substantia nigra. Hypo-osmolality, presumably as a result of the syndrome of inappropriate antidiuretic hormone secretion (Chapter 225), is noted in a third of patients.

Genitourinary tract symptoms (urgency, frequency, incontinence, and retention), microscopic hematuria, pyuria, proteinuria, and elevated blood urea nitrogen are frequent. St. Louis encephalitis viral antigen in cells of the urinary sediment has been detected by fluorescent techniques, and virus-like particles have been detected in urine by immunoelectron microscopy.

DIAGNOSIS

St. Louis encephalitis virus is rarely isolated from blood or CSF obtained during the acute phase of illness. Serologic diagnosis is achieved by demonstration of changing antibody titers; the HI, fluorescent, ELISA, and neutralizing tests demonstrate antibody within the first week after onset, and titers rise during the ensuing 2 weeks. CF antibodies appear 10 to 20 days after onset. Rapid, early diagnosis is possible by detection of IgM antibodies by ELISA in serum and CSF. Serologic cross-reactions may occur in persons with previous exposure to dengue, West Nile, and other related flaviviruses. RT-PCR provides a more specific diagnosis, but its sensitivity is uncertain.

No vaccine is available for St. Louis encephalitis. Surveillance of viral activity in vectors and avian hosts is used to define the risk for human infection and to initiate vector control efforts. In an established outbreak, avoidance of mosquito bites and spraying to reduce infected adult mosquitoes are the only effective means of control.

TREATMENT Rx

Treatment is supportive.

PROGNOSIS

A convalescent syndrome characterized by weakness, fatigue, nervousness, tremulousness, sleeplessness, irritability, depression, difficulty concentrating, and headaches occurs in 30 to 50% of older persons and clears in 80% of them within 3 years. The overall case-fatality rate is approximately 9%. Mortality is negligible in persons younger than 20 years but rises steeply after 55 years to approximately 30% in patients older than 65 years. Approximately 50% of the deaths occur during the first week, and 80% occur within 2 weeks after onset.

MURRAY VALLEY ENCEPHALITIS AND ROCIO ENCEPHALITIS

Murray Valley encephalitis and Rocio encephalitis, which are similar to Japanese encephalitis in their pathogenesis and clinical features, are caused by closely related flaviviruses. Murray Valley encephalitis has occurred in small epidemics in the Murray and Darling River valleys of Victoria and New South Wales, Australia. The virus is endemic in northern Australia and New Guinea, where it is maintained in a bird-mosquito cycle. Rocio encephalitis has caused epidemics of 1000 or more cases in São Paulo State, Brazil.

TICK-BORNE ENCEPHALITIS

PATHOGENS

A complex of six antigenically related tick-borne flaviviruses cause encephalitis: Powassan, tick-borne encephalitis, louping ill, Kyasanur Forest disease, Omsk hemorrhagic fever, and Langat viruses. The predominant syndrome is hemorrhagic fever (Chapter 381), but meningoencephalitis may be a component of the disease spectrum. Two subtypes of tick-borne encephalitis virus (central European encephalitis and Russian spring-summer encephalitis) are distinguished by serologic tests, are ecologically distinct, and differ in virulence for humans. Powassan and louping ill viruses are rare causes of encephalitis in North America and the British Isles, respectively. These viruses are easily distinguished serologically from mosquito-borne flaviviruses but induce cross-reactions within the complex.

EPIDEMIOLOGY

Tick-borne encephalitis occurs in Europe (including eastern Europe and Ukraine), southern Scandinavia, and far eastern Russia during the summer months, which corresponds to peak tick vector populations.[15] Several hundred to more than 2000 cases are reported annually, with morbidity rates of up to 20 per 100,000 inhabitants. Adults older than 20 years are mainly affected, and persons frequenting wooded areas that are heavily tick infested are at highest risk. In Europe, the disease is relatively mild (case-fatality rate of 1 to 2%), but in the Far East, it is severe (20 to 25%).

The vector of tick-borne encephalitis is *Ixodes ricinus* in Europe and *Ixodes persulcatus* in the Far East. The tick vector also serves as a reservoir for the virus. Larval ticks parasitize small rodents, which serve as amplifying viremic hosts during the spring and summer. Large vertebrates (goats, sheep, cattle) are hosts for nymphal and adult ticks. Outbreaks have occurred in families or groups of individuals ingesting unpasteurized milk or cheese from goats or sheep.

CLINICAL MANIFESTATIONS

Inapparent infections are common. Symptomatic tick-borne encephalitis in Europe typically (but not invariably) has a biphasic course beginning 7 to 14 days after exposure with an influenza-like illness that lasts 1 week, followed by a period of clinical remission for several days and then an abrupt onset of aseptic meningitis or meningoencephalitis. The meningoencephalitis is usually benign, although severe paralytic illness, myelitis, myeloradiculitis, and bulbar forms may occur.

In the Far East, tick-borne encephalitis begins suddenly with fever, headache, and gastrointestinal symptoms, followed rapidly by the appearance of depressed sensorium, coma, convulsions, and paralysis. Bulbar paralysis and cervical myelitis are frequent findings. In fatal cases, death occurs in the first week after onset. Aseptic meningitis and milder forms of encephalitis also occur. Chronic forms of tick-borne encephalitis have been described, with active clinical and pathologic abnormalities present a year or more after onset.

DIAGNOSIS

Brain MRI in patients with tick-borne encephalitis shows evidence of edema in the basal ganglia, thalami, and brain stem in about 20% of cases. MRI of the spinal cord may show anterior horn cell lesions corresponding to lower motor neuron weakness on examination.

Isolation of virus from blood is also possible during the early phase of illness. Serologic diagnosis is achieved by the HI, CF, neutralization, or ELISA techniques.

PREVENTION

In eastern Europe and the former Soviet Union, vaccines are used in high-risk groups (forestry and agricultural workers, military personnel). In Austria, immunization of the general population has resulted in a marked decline in incidence. Avoidance of tick exposure by wearing of protective clothing and use of repellents may be recommended in areas of high tick-borne encephalitis activity.

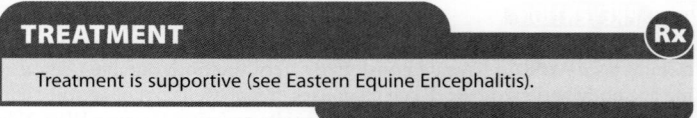

TREATMENT Rx

Treatment is supportive (see Eastern Equine Encephalitis).

PROGNOSIS

In European tick-borne encephalitis, convalescence is often prolonged, and residual paralysis may follow in severe cases. In the Far East, survivors frequently have residual paralysis, especially lower motor neuron paralysis of the upper extremities or shoulder girdle as a result of spinal cord involvement.

Louping Ill Encephalitis

Louping ill causes encephalitis in sheep (rarely in cattle, horses, and swine) in Scotland, northern England, and Ireland. Sporadic human cases have been recognized. Louping ill virus is maintained in nature by *I. ricinus* ticks and a variety of hosts, including small mammals, ground-dwelling birds (grouse), and probably sheep. The clinical features of louping ill resemble the European form of tick-borne encephalitis.

Powassan Virus Encephalitis

Powassan virus encephalitis has been documented in a small number of cases in the northeastern United States and eastern Canada. The virus is not associated with animal disease. The transmission cycle of Powassan virus involves *Ixodes cookei*, *Ixodes marxi*, and possibly other tick species along with mammals, particularly rodents and carnivores. Powassan encephalitis is characterized by fever and nonspecific symptoms, followed by encephalitic signs, which are frequently severe. Peripheral blood and CSF changes are similar to those described for other forms of flaviviral encephalitis. The case-fatality rate is about 50%, and residual paralysis may persist in survivors.

CALIFORNIA SEROGROUP ENCEPHALITIS

At least four members of the California serogroup of the Bunyaviridae family (Bunyavirus genus)—La Crosse, California encephalitis, Jamestown Canyon, and snowshoe hare viruses—cause encephalitis. California encephalitis virus occurs in the western United States (California, New Mexico, Utah, Texas) and has been implicated only rarely in human infections. In contrast, La Crosse virus, distributed more widely in the eastern half of the United States and southern Canada, is a major human pathogen. Jamestown Canyon and snowshoe hare viruses have also been implicated in sporadic cases of human encephalitis in the north central United States and Canada. California serogroup viruses have been implicated in human disease in China and the former Soviet Union.

EPIDEMIOLOGY

California serogroup encephalitis occurs as an endemic rather than an epidemic disease, with individual or small clusters of cases scattered across affected areas. Seventy to 120 cases are reported each year, generally between July and September, with a peak incidence in August. The virus primarily affects persons younger than 15 years living in rural and suburban areas characterized by deciduous hardwood forests. It is most prevalent in the north central states, where it is responsible for as many as 20% of cases of acute CNS infection in children. Focal "hot spots" (communities, even backyards) of recurrent summertime viral activity are recognized. The ratio of inapparent to apparent infection has been estimated variably at between 26 : 1 and 157 : 1.

The vector of La Crosse virus is *Aedes triseriatus*, which breeds both in forest tree holes and in artificial containers, notably discarded tires. This vector also serves as a reservoir for La Crosse virus. Wild rodents (squirrels, chipmunks) contribute to the cycle of transmission as viremic hosts. Humans acquire the disease by being bitten by an infected mosquito. *Aedes communis, Aedes stimulans, A. triseriatus,* and possibly anopheline mosquitoes are involved in transmitting Jamestown Canyon virus, and deer are the principal vertebrate hosts.

PATHOBIOLOGY

Histopathologic features in the CNS are qualitatively similar to those of other viral encephalitides. However, absence of inflammatory lesions in the cerebellum, medulla, and spinal cord may be a distinguishing feature of La Crosse infection.

CLINICAL MANIFESTATIONS

The clinical spectrum of California serogroup virus infection includes non-specific febrile illness, aseptic meningitis, and meningoencephalitis. The disease begins with fever, headache, sore throat, and gastrointestinal symptoms. In mild cases, CNS signs appear on the third day after onset and subside within 7 to 8 days. In the more severe form, neurologic signs appear within 24 to 48 hours of onset, usually in the form of generalized seizures, elevated intracranial pressure, and altered consciousness, and persist longer. Encephalitis may be severe in the acute stage, but the disease is almost always self-limited; death is extremely rare.

The peripheral white blood cell count is elevated, with a predominance of polymorphonuclear cells and a shift to the left. CSF contains up to 500 lymphocytes/μL; the protein level is normal or mildly elevated, and the glucose concentration is normal. The electroencephalogram reveals generalized slowing in the delta and theta range; focal delta wave activity related to cortical destruction and focal seizures are also common findings.

DIAGNOSIS

In contrast to the other arboviral encephalitides, brain MRI in patients with California serogroup encephalitides may show lesions involving the temporal lobe in a pattern similar to that of herpes simplex encephalitis. The virus cannot be recovered from blood or CSF obtained during the acute phase. Diagnosis is best achieved by counterimmunoelectrophoresis, HI, CF, fluorescent, ELISA, and neutralization tests for antibody in paired acute and convalescent sera. The most practical, sensitive, and reliable methods are the HI test with La Crosse viral antigen and IgM antibody capture ELISA. Viral RNA can be detected in CSF or brain tissue by RT-PCR, although the sensitivity of the test remains to be determined.

PREVENTION

There is no vaccine for California encephalitis, although research involving DNA-based vaccines appears promising. Vector control methods are of uncertain usefulness in this disease. In defined hot spots of recurrent viral activity, breeding sites for *A. triseriatus* should be eliminated, particularly by draining or eliminating standing water (e.g., discarded tires or birdbaths) and filling holes in trees. Parents should protect children by limiting exposure and using mosquito repellents.

TREATMENT Rx

Treatment is supportive.

PROGNOSIS

The case-fatality rate is less than 1%. The risk for permanent neuropsychiatric sequelae is unclear, but hemiparesis and persistent seizure disorders have been reported.

Grade A References

A1. Feroldi E, Pancharoen C, Kosalaraksa P, et al. Single-dose, live-attenuated Japanese encephalitis vaccine in children aged 12-18 months: randomized, controlled phase 3 immunogenicity and safety trial. *Hum Vaccin Immunother.* 2012;8:929-937.

A2. Miyazaki C, Okada K, Ozaki T, et al. Phase III clinical trials comparing the immunogenicity and safety of the Vero cell–derived Japanese encephalitis vaccine Encevac with those of mouse brain–derived vaccine by using the Beijing-1 strain. *Clin Vaccine Immunol.* 2014;21:188-195.

A3. Huang LM, Lin TY, Chiu CH, et al. Concomitant administration of live attenuated Japanese encephalitis chimeric virus vaccine (JE-CV) and measles, mumps, rubella (MMR) vaccine: randomized study in toddlers in Taiwan. *Vaccine.* 2014;32:5363-5369.

GENERAL REFERENCES

For the General References and other additional features, please visit Expert Consult at https://expertconsult.inkling.com.

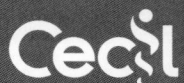

XXIV

HUMAN IMMUNODEFICIENCY VIRUS AND THE ACQUIRED IMMUNODEFICIENCY SYNDROME

384

EPIDEMIOLOGY AND DIAGNOSIS OF HUMAN IMMUNODEFICIENCY VIRUS INFECTION AND ACQUIRED IMMUNODEFICIENCY SYNDROME

THOMAS C. QUINN

GLOBAL STATISTICS

By 2014, approximately 80 million people had become infected with HIV since the beginning of the epidemic in 1981. Of these individuals, more than 45 million people had already died of AIDS, and it became ranked as one of the leading causes of death throughout the world.[1,2] According to estimates by the Joint United Nations Program on HIV/AIDS, 35 million people were living with HIV by 2013 (Fig. 384-1 and Table 384-1). In 2013 alone, 2.1 million people became newly infected, half of whom were young individuals between the ages of 15 and 24 years. The continuing rise in the population of people living with HIV infection reflects the combined effects of continued high rates of HIV infection and the beneficial impact of antiretroviral therapy (ART) resulting in fewer deaths[3] (Fig. 384-2).

The latest epidemiologic data indicate that globally, the spread of HIV appears to have peaked in 1996, when 3.5 million new HIV infections occurred.[4] In 2013, the estimated number of new HIV infections was approximately 35% lower than at the epidemic's peak about 15 years earlier. The epidemic appears to have stabilized in most regions, with new infections decreasing by 50% or more in 25 countries. Half of these reductions in the past 2 years have been among children. Despite these gains in some countries, prevalence continues to increase in Eastern Europe, Central Asia, and other parts of Asia because of the high rates of HIV infection. Sub-Saharan Africa remains the most heavily affected region and accounted for 72% of all new HIV infections in 2013.

Nearly 90% of all new infections occurred in developing countries; 50% occurred in women; and the major mode of transmission was heterosexual transmission, although infections continue to spread at high rates among men who have sex with men (MSM). Resurgence of the epidemic among MSM in high-income countries is increasingly well documented.[2] Differences are apparent in all regions, with some national epidemics continuing to expand even as the overall regional incidence of HIV infection stabilizes. Epidemic patterns have been changing over time. Perinatal transmission continues to occur in developing countries, where access to antiretroviral drugs to prevent mother-to-infant transmission is limited. In 2013, 240,000 children became newly infected, and 25 million children have been orphaned by the premature deaths of their parents from AIDS. In 2013, 1.5 million people died of AIDS, including 230,000 children.

DEMOGRAPHIC, SOCIAL, AND ECONOMIC IMPACT

For the first two decades of the epidemic, fatality rates from AIDS steadily increased and the average life expectancy in some countries in sub-Saharan Africa declined from 62 to 47 years of age. In Haiti, life expectancy was nearly 6 years less than it would have been in the absence of AIDS. Cambodia experienced a reduction in life expectancy of more than 4 years. However, the scaling up of antiretroviral therapy in low- and middle-income countries, as described later, has transformed national AIDS responses and generated broad-based health gains (Fig. 384-3). Since 1995, antiretroviral therapy has saved 14 million life-years in low- and middle-income countries, including 9 million in sub-Saharan Africa. As programmatic scale-up has continued, health gains have accelerated, with the number of life-years saved by antiretroviral therapy in Sub-Saharan Africa quadrupling in the last 4 years. Experience in the hyperendemic KwaZulu-Natal Province in South Africa illustrates the macroeconomic and household livelihood benefits of expanded treatment access, with employment prospects sharply increasing among individuals receiving antiretroviral therapy.[5,6]

THE GLOBAL RESPONSE

At a 2001 special session of the United Nations General Assembly on AIDS, 189 nations agreed that AIDS was a national and international security issue of the highest priority. The Global Fund for AIDS, Tuberculosis, and Malaria raised funds from private donations and industrialized countries to help support access to care and treatment in developing countries. This initiative was complemented by the U.S. government's Emergency Plan for AIDS Relief, now committed over a 10-year period through the Bush and Obama administrations to provide treatment and care for HIV-infected individuals, as well as additional resources for enhancing prevention efforts to prevent further transmission. As of 2014, approximately 13.6 million people in low- and middle-income countries were receiving antiretroviral therapy (ART)—a more than 25-fold increase since 2003 (see Fig. 384-3). The rapid expansion of antiretroviral therapy is one of the most remarkable achievements in recent public health history. ART coverage rose from 7% in 2003 to 54% in 2012 for individuals with CD4 counts less than 350 cells/mm³, with especially high coverage achieved in Latin America (68%), the Caribbean (67%), Oceania (69%), and Eastern and Southern Africa (56%). Sixty-three percent of all people now receiving treatment in low- and middle-income countries are living in Sub-Saharan Africa, compared with 25% in late 2003. Coverage remains low in Eastern Europe and Central Asia (25%) and in the Middle East and North Africa (15%).

Unfortunately, not all have equal access to therapy, even within countries with middle to high prevalence. For example, an estimated 800,000 children younger than 15 years now require ART, but only 200,000 are receiving treatment. Children account for approximately 14% of AIDS deaths. Nearly 90% of children infected with HIV are African. The median proportion of HIV-infected children receiving treatment is just 28% in Sub-Saharan Africa. Similarly, less than 40% of HIV-infected pregnant women in low- and middle-income countries are benefiting from antiretroviral prophylaxis despite success in certain countries, such as Botswana, Brazil, and Thailand, and the virtual elimination of pediatric HIV disease in the industrialized world. Likewise, in Eastern Europe and Central Asia, injection drug use accounts for more than 70% of HIV-positive persons. However, only 25% of treatment recipients in this region are injection drug users. In years to come, additional resources will be required to reach the additional millions of HIV-infected people who require treatment with antiretroviral drugs, especially in light of recent recommendations to expand access to all HIV-infected adults who have a CD4+ count of less than 500/mm³ based on the finding that early initiation of ART reduces mortality and incident tuberculosis.

REGIONAL EPIDEMICS

Sub-Saharan Africa

Sub-Saharan Africa represents the epicenter of the global HIV/AIDS pandemic (see Table 384-1). Studies in the late 1990s and early 2000s support the theory that HIV originated in Africa and that humans probably became infected sometime in the mid-20th century from a similar, related retrovirus in chimpanzees and sooty mangabey monkeys. For years, the infection remained limited to remote rural regions of Africa, but with urbanization, infected individuals migrated to major urban centers, where transmission was amplified and HIV spread to thousands of individuals within a relatively short period.

Seventy-five percent of all women infected with HIV live in Sub-Saharan Africa. In Côte d'Ivoire, home to the most serious epidemic in West Africa, HIV prevalence in females (6.4%) was more than twice as high than in males (2.9%). In Sub-Saharan Africa as a whole, women account for 60% of the estimated HIV infections. The risk for becoming infected is disproportionate for girls and young women. In Kenya, young women between 15 and 19 are three times more likely to be infected than their male counterparts, whereas 20- to 24-year-old women are 5.5 times more likely than men in their age cohort to be living with HIV infection. Among people aged 15 to 24 in Tanzania, females are four times more likely than males to be living with HIV. In the nine countries of Southern Africa most affected by HIV, the prevalence in young women 15 to 24 was on average three times higher than that in men of the same age.

Women's vulnerability to HIV in Sub-Saharan Africa stems not only from their greater physiologic susceptibility to heterosexual transmission but also from the severe social, legal, and economic disadvantages they often confront. HIV prevalence generally tends to peak at a younger age for women than for men. The very young are often at extremely high risk for infection through mother-to-child transmission.

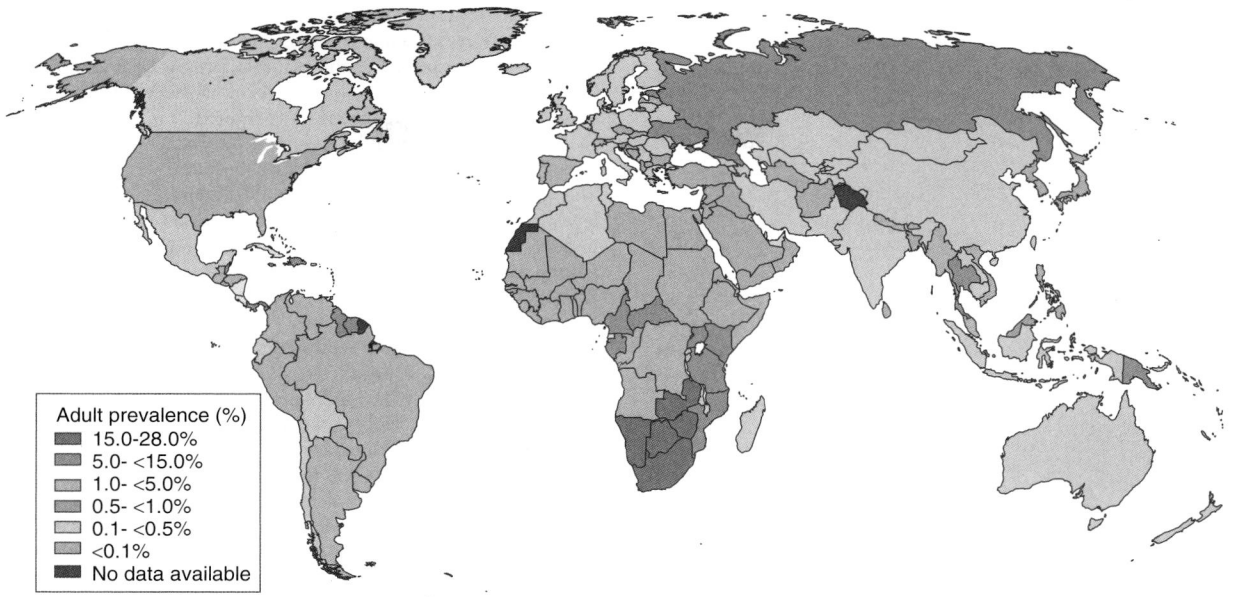

FIGURE 384-1. A total of 35.0 million people (33.2 to 37.2 million) were living with HIV infection in 2013. The adult prevalence of HIV infection is shown by country. (Data from UNAIDS GAP Report. UNAIDS; 2014.)

TABLE 384-1 REGIONAL HUMAN IMMUNODEFICIENCY VIRUS AND ACQUIRED IMMUNODEFICIENCY SYNDROME STATISTICS AND FEATURES AT THE END OF 2013

REGION	ADULTS AND CHILDREN LIVING WITH HIV/AIDS	ADULTS AND CHILDREN NEWLY INFECTED WITH HIV	ADULT PREVALENCE RATE* (%)	MAIN MODES OF TRANSMISSION FOR ADULTS LIVING WITH HIV/AIDS
Sub-Saharan Africa	24,700,000	1,500,000	4.9	Hetero
North Africa and Middle East	230,000	25,000	0.2	Hetero, IDU
Asia and the Pacific	4,800,000	350,000	0.3	Hetero, IDU
Latin America	1,600,000	94,000	0.4	MSM, IDU, Hetero
Caribbean	250,000	12,000	1.0	Hetero, MSM
Eastern Europe and Central Asia	1,100,000	110,000	1.0	IDU, Hetero, MSM
Western Europe	1,100,000	30,000	0.2	MSM, IDU, Hetero
North America	1,300,000	55,000	0.6	MSM, IDU, Hetero
Total	35,000,000	2,100,000	0.8	

*The proportion of adults (15 to 49 years of age) living with HIV infection or AIDS in 2013 using 2013 population numbers.
AIDS = acquired immunodeficiency syndrome; Hetero = heterosexual transmission; HIV = human immunodeficiency virus; IDU = transmission through injection drug use; MSM = sexual transmission among men who have sex with men.

Unfortunately, progress has been strikingly uneven in gaining access to ART in Sub-Saharan Africa, with coverage reaching or exceeding 50% in some countries (Botswana, Namibia, and Uganda) but remaining below 20% in most others.

Although some countries in Sub-Saharan Africa such as Kenya, Uganda, and Zimbabwe have shown recent declines in HIV prevalence, there is no evidence of any decline in Southern Africa, including the Republic of South Africa, Botswana, Namibia, and Swaziland, where exceptionally high infection levels continue. Southern Africa remains the area most heavily affected by the epidemic. The nine countries with the highest HIV prevalence worldwide are all located in this subregion, with each of these countries experiencing adult HIV prevalence greater than 10%; prevalence was as high as 26% in Swaziland, 24% in Botswana, and 23% in Lesotho. The Republic of South Africa is home to the world's largest population of people living with HIV (6.3 million), with a prevalence of 17.3%. Almost one in three pregnant women attending public antenatal clinics were infected with HIV. South Africa accounts for a large percentage of the treatment scale-up in sub-Saharan Africa, but as of 2013, antiretroviral therapy was only reaching 55% of South Africans eligible for treatment.

In Botswana, more than a third of pregnant women attending antenatal clinics and close to 50% of women 30 to 34 years of age were infected with HIV in 2013. Similarly, Lesotho has a national adult HIV prevalence of 23%, with 27% documented in women attending antenatal clinics. A third of pregnant women 25 to 34 years of age were infected. In Namibia, the prevalence of HIV infection is 13.4% in all adults, with an HIV prevalence of 42% in antenatal clinics in selected areas. In neighboring Mozambique, Malawi, and Zambia, HIV prevalence has been documented to be between 10% and 14%. There is wide geographic variation, however, with HIV infection rates in pregnant women ranging from less than 10% in some places to as high as 30% in others.

In the countries of Eastern Africa, HIV prevalence has either decreased or remained stable in the past several years. In Uganda, which saw a steep decline in HIV prevalence during the mid and late 1990s, adult HIV prevalence was estimated to be 6.7% in 2005. However, recent trends suggest that HIV prevalence may be increasing in selected areas (nationally at 7.2%), in part because of a decrease in mortality with access to ART but potentially also because of increasing incident rates as a result of decreasing condom use and an increased percentage of multiple partners. In neighboring Kenya, Eritrea, Tanzania,

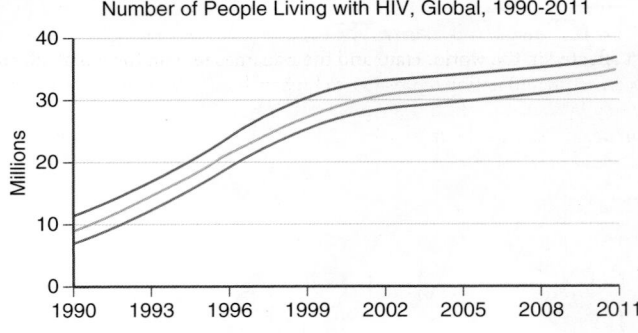

Number of People Living with HIV, Global, 1990-2011

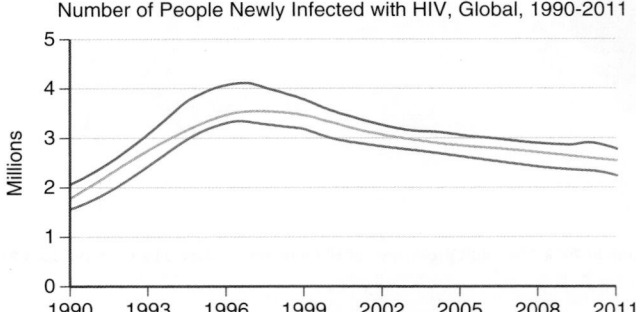

Number of People Newly Infected with HIV, Global, 1990-2011

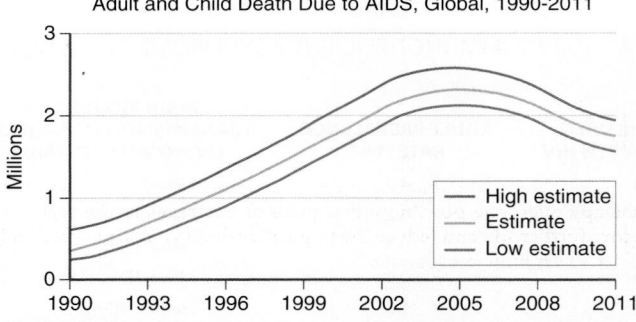

Adult and Child Death Due to AIDS, Global, 1990-2011

FIGURE 384-2. Global HIV trends in number of people living with HIV, new infections and fatalities, from 1990 to 2011. (Data from UNAIDS Global Report. *UNAIDS Report on the Global AIDS Epidemic 2012.* Geneva: UNAIDS; 2013.)

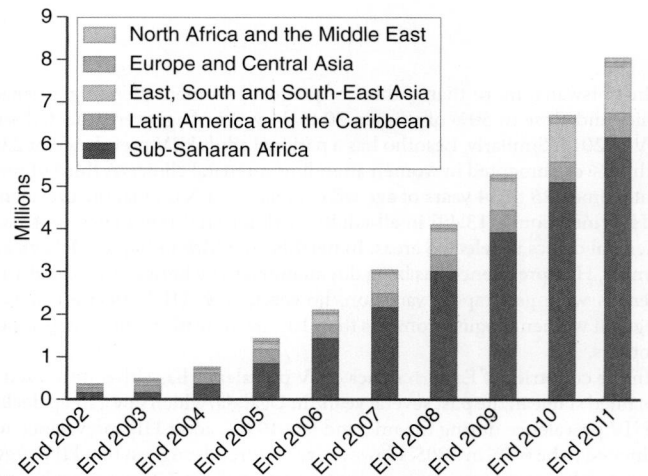

FIGURE 384-3. Estimated number of people receiving antiretroviral therapy in low- and middle-income countries from 2002 through 2011. (Data from UNAIDS Global Report. *UNAIDS Report on the Global AIDS Epidemic 2012.* Geneva: UNAIDS; 2013.)

Burundi, and Rwanda, the HIV epidemic has been stable in recent years, with prevalence rates ranging from 1% in Eritrea to 6% in Kenya, Tanzania, Burundi, and Rwanda. In Ethiopia, HIV prevalence (1.4%) has stabilized in urban areas but appears to be increasing in more distant rural areas, where access to treatment and care is more limited.

Western Africa is less severely affected than other parts of Sub-Saharan Africa, with national adult HIV prevalence rates of 2% in several countries. The highest rate in the region is in Côte d'Ivoire, at 3.0%. In Nigeria, infection levels vary radically across the country from 2.6% in the southwest to 6.1% in the north central zones (nationally 3.7%). HIV continues to spread rapidly among female sex workers and their clients, as well as in the general population. In some urban populations, more than 10% of adults are infected and the annual incidence is as high as 3%.

Despite the scale-up of treatment, AIDS is still one of the leading causes of death and years of productive life lost throughout the continent. Excess deaths attributable to HIV are highest in the 25- to 34-year-old group, usually a group with low mortality. Nearly 90% of deaths in this age group are in excess of background rates and were attributable to HIV. Because AIDS deaths are concentrated in childhood and young adult age groups, their effects are substantial, with life expectancy reduced markedly in several countries. HIV or AIDS cases will put an increasing strain on health care systems, which are already overburdened, and on individual households that are trying to manage with limited economic resources. Care and support for children orphaned by AIDS will become a growing concern throughout the region.

Asia and the Pacific

After Sub-Saharan Africa, Asia and the Pacific, home to 60% of the world's population, have the second largest number of HIV-infected individuals in the world, estimated at 4.8 million. In 2013, 350,000 adults and children became newly infected, in part because of growth of the HIV epidemic in China, India, and several other countries in Southeast Asia. With the exception of Thailand, national HIV prevalence levels remain comparatively low in most countries of Asia and the Pacific, with HIV prevalence being less than 1%, to some extent due to their large population base. Thus, because of the region's large population, Asia's comparatively low HIV prevalence translates into a substantial portion of the global HIV burden. India's national adult HIV prevalence rate of 0.3% offers little indication of the serious situation facing the country. An estimated 4.8 million people were living with HIV at the end of 2013—one of the highest figures in the world after South Africa.

Throughout the region, injection drug use remains one of the most prominent modes of transmission of HIV. More than 50% of injection drug users have already acquired HIV in Malaysia, Myanmar, Nepal, Thailand, Indonesia, Manipur, and Southern China. Very high rates of needle sharing have been documented among users in Bangladesh and Vietnam, along with evidence that a considerable proportion of sex workers in Vietnam also inject drugs. More recently, the epidemic in many parts of Asia is steadily expanding into lower risk populations through transmission to the sexual partners of those most at risk. In China, where the epidemic was previously driven by transmission through injection drug use, heterosexual transmission has become the predominant mode of HIV transmission.

China, with a fifth of the world's population, has also witnessed a dramatic escalation of the HIV epidemic in the past decade. A total of 780,000 Chinese individuals are estimated to be living with HIV. The HIV epidemic is particularly severe among injection drug users, who account for a quarter of all HIV infections. To compound the tragedy of the epidemic in China, reports from Henan province in Central China demonstrate that tens of thousands and possibly more rural villagers became infected by selling their blood to collecting centers that did not follow basic blood donation safety procedures. It has been estimated that 150,000 people have been infected through these practices. There are new signs of heterosexually transmitted HIV epidemics in at least three provinces—Guangdong, Guangxi, and Yunnan. Several other factors highlight the swift escalation of HIV infection in China. STDs quadrupled between 1997 and 2002, thus suggesting that unprotected sex with non-monogamous partners is increasing in China. There is massive population mobility. Approximately 100 million Chinese are temporarily or permanently away from their registered addresses, and increasing socioeconomic disparities add to the likelihood of the spread of HIV.

Indonesia, the world's fourth most populous country, is another example of how quickly the AIDS epidemic can emerge. After more than 10 years of negligible HIV prevalence, the infection rate in injection drug users, sex workers, and blood donors in some regions is rapidly increasing, with a 25% increase between 2001 and 2013. Papua New Guinea also has reported the highest HIV infection rates among the Pacific Island countries and territories. Even though the Philippines has maintained a low HIV prevalence, higher rates of STDs among Filipino sex workers, their clients, and MSM indicate low levels of condom use and the potential for rapid spread of HIV.

In some countries of Southeast Asia where HIV prevalence rose rapidly in the 1990s, strong prevention programs have limited the spread, most notably in Thailand, Cambodia, and Myanmar. Furthermore, the increased access to ART has coincided with a drastic drop in AIDS-related deaths. Despite these advances, AIDS is still a leading cause of death in Thailand and 1.2% of the country's population is infected with HIV. Although STDs and heterosexual transmission have declined as a result of the government's prevention programs, HIV continues to spread rapidly among injection drug users and MSM.

Treatment scale-up in Asia has been mixed. As of December 2013, 47% of those in South and Southeast Asia needing ART were receiving it, but only 18% were receiving it in East Asia, much lower than the global average (54%) for all low- and middle-income countries. In 2013, only one country in the Asia Pacific region (Cambodia) reached more than 80% coverage of antiretroviral therapy, whereas in Pakistan less than 20% of eligible infected persons received therapy. In Oceania, an estimated 69% received therapy.

Eastern Europe and Central Asia

The HIV epidemic has increased faster in Eastern Europe and Central Asia between 2000 and 2013 than in any other area of the world. In 2013 there were an estimated 1.1 million people living with HIV, a 20-fold increase in less than a decade. In recent years, the Russian Federation has experienced an exceptionally steep rise in reported HIV infections, 90% of which have been attributed to injection drug use. It is estimated that nearly 1% of the young people in Eastern Europe and Central Asia are injecting drugs, which places these individuals and their sex partners at high risk for becoming infected with HIV. In countries such as Azerbaijan, Georgia, Tajikistan, and Uzbekistan, HIV has experienced explosive growth. Similar explosive high rates of HIV are being documented in injection drug users and heterosexuals at risk for STDs in other countries of the Commonwealth of Independent States, in the Baltic States, and in Romania.

In Estonia, Latvia, and Lithuania, major HIV outbreaks are also occurring in selected populations, such as prison inmates. In one prison in Lithuania, 15% of the inmates were HIV positive, thus confirming the role of prisons in the spread of HIV in many countries of the region. The concentration of large numbers of young people in overcrowded prisons or juvenile justice facilities, often marked by an abundance of drugs but a scarcity of HIV information, clean needles, or condoms, provides fertile ground for the rapid spread of HIV among inmates and, on their eventual release, into the wider population.

Initially driven by injection drug use in young people, heterosexual transmission of HIV has become a prominent mode of spread in Belarus and Ukraine. With an estimated adult HIV prevalence rate of 0.8%, Ukraine is one of the most severely affected countries in the region. Three fourths of HIV infections in Ukraine are related to injection drug use, with a prevalence of 21.5% in injection drug users, and the proportion of sexually transmitted infection (STIs) is increasing, suggesting potential spread heterosexually and among MSM. Although many of these infections may occur in sex partners of injection drug users, the trend also may indicate spread into the wider population of these countries. In the Russian Federation and the Ukraine, up to 30% of female injection drug users are also involved in commercial sex work. In Odessa, 67% of sex workers who inject drugs were HIV positive. The public health efforts to stem the tide of the epidemic in these countries are limited and, in some cases, nonexistent. In contrast, HIV prevalence remains low in Poland, the Czech Republic, Hungary, and Slovenia, where well-designed national HIV/AIDS programs are in operation.

A number of countries in the region have expanded access to ART, although treatment coverage remains relatively low. By December 2013, only 25% of adults in need of therapy were receiving it—a level much less than the global average. Injection drug users, the population most at risk for HIV in Eastern Europe and Central Asia, are often least likely to receive ART when they are medically eligible. If effective interventions are not implemented in the more severely affected countries, it is likely that the situation will become dramatically worse over the next 5 years.

Latin America and the Caribbean

An estimated 1.6 million adults and children are living with HIV in Latin America and the Caribbean. Twelve countries in this region have an estimated HIV prevalence of 1% or greater in pregnant women. In several Caribbean countries, adult HIV prevalence rates are surpassed only by the rates experienced in sub-Saharan Africa, which makes this region the second most affected in the world. Haiti and the Bahamas remain the worst affected, with an estimated national prevalence higher than 1.8% in Haiti and a prevalence of 2.8% in the Bahamas. AIDS is the leading cause of death in some countries of the Caribbean basin. In Haiti, the Bahamas, and Guyana, the number of deaths in 15- to 34-year-olds is 2.5 times higher than it would have been in the absence of AIDS.

Homosexual and heterosexual transmission continues to be the major mode of transmission throughout the region, although there is evidence that spread of HIV is increasing through sharing of infected drug equipment. Population mobility, spurred by high rates of unemployment and poverty, is emerging as a significant factor in the epidemic's growth in this region. Central America's geographic position also makes it an important transit zone for people moving between the rest of the region and North American countries. Appropriately, protecting vulnerable populations on the move, including adolescent girls and young women, is now the focus of a regional prevention program in Central America. In Mexico, adult HIV prevalence in the wider population is still well under 1%, but prevalence rates are higher in specific population groups—6% in injection drug users and 15% in MSM. There is significant overlap between injection drug users and MSM, especially in Brazil and the southern Latin American countries, where injection drug use is a growing social phenomenon. Injection drug use is also a major route of HIV transmission in Argentina, Chile, and Uruguay.

Despite many constraints, the region has made progress in the provision of treatment and care. By reducing HIV-related morbidity through treatment, Brazil's treatment and care program is estimated to have avoided 234,000 hospitalizations in a 4-year period, thereby demonstrating a cost-effective approach to care. Argentina, Costa Rica, Uruguay, and Cuba now guarantee free and universal access to drugs through the public sector, and sharp reductions have recently been secured in Honduras and Panama. Treatment coverage has risen from 10% of those in need in 2004 to 68% in 2012. Similarly, pediatric antiretroviral coverage in the Caribbean was high (>60%) in comparison to the global average for children of 28%. Consistent with the evolving guidelines of HIV treatment, a growing number of people living with HIV in Latin America are starting treatment earlier at CD4+ cell counts of 350 or lower rather than waiting until the count drops below 200. Earlier initiation of therapy offers the possibility that medical outcomes in the region may improve further still and reduce the population-level viral load, which might result in lower transmission rates.

Western Europe

More than 1.1 million HIV-infected individuals reside in Western Europe, with trends similar to those witnessed in the United States, Australia, and New Zealand. Longer survival of people infected with HIV has led to a steady increase in the number of people living with the virus in high-income countries. In a multicountry study in Europe, Australia, and Canada, mortality rates in people living with HIV now approach those in the non–HIV-infected population, although excess mortality in HIV-infected people increases with the duration of infection. In the United Kingdom, half of all people living with HIV are receiving ART, with no appreciable increase in the number of patients with virologic failure or resistance to the drugs.

The HIV epidemic in Western Europe is a result of a multitude of epidemics that differ in their timing, scale, and effects on populations. A larger proportion of new HIV diagnoses in Western European countries occur through heterosexual intercourse. More than half of the new HIV infections in the United Kingdom in 2013 resulted from heterosexual sex, compared with 33% in 1998. In Ireland, a similar trend is visible, with numbers of heterosexually transmitted HIV infection increasing four-fold between 1998 and 2001. Unsafe sex between men remains an important factor for spread in most European countries, particularly in the United Kingdom, Germany, the Netherlands, and Spain. Injection drug use remains a major mode of transmission in Spain, France, and Portugal, but like in other countries in Europe, approximately a fourth of all HIV infections are now heterosexually transmitted. Most data from high-income countries demonstrate that the epidemic has shifted to the poor and marginalized sections of society. Underscoring the need for renewed prevention efforts, especially in young people, are findings of increases in high-risk behavior, less frequent condom use, and higher rates of STDs in several countries. In the United Kingdom, for example, rates of gonorrhea, syphilis, and chlamydial infections have more than doubled since 1995, and increases have been found in other Western European countries as well.

The United States

By 2013, more than 1.2 million people were living in the United States with HIV (see Table 384-1). Nationally, the adult HIV prevalence was estimated to be 0.6%. This increase reflects mixed results in the United States' effort to combat its epidemic. More people infected with HIV are living longer because of antiretroviral therapy, but unfortunately, the early gains made in prevention have not been sustained (Fig. 384-4). The number of newly recorded HIV cases in 46 states with confidential name–based reporting has varied only slightly since the late 1990s. In 2006, the annual incidence of HIV infection was estimated at 56,300, which was approximately 40% higher than previously estimated. The CDC estimates that approximately 50,000 people in the United States are newly infected with HIV each year. In 2011, there were an estimated 50,007 new HIV infections. Nearly two thirds of these new infections occurred in MSM; 18% were women who acquired HIV via heterosexual contact, 10% were men who also acquired HIV by heterosexual contact (Figs. 384-5 and 384-6), and 11% acquired HIV via injection drug use. The estimated rate of diagnosis of HIV infection for the United States was 16.1 in 100,000, with 31.4 in 100,000 in men and 8.0 in 100,000 in women.[7] In the United States, more than 620,000 people with AIDS have died since the epidemic began.

More women are being infected with HIV through unprotected heterosexual exposure (86%) and injection drug use (14%).[8] The main risk factor for women who acquire HIV during sex is the risk behavior of their male partners, such as injection drug use, commercial sex, or sex with other men. As in Latin America, women living in impoverished and marginal circumstances appear to be at disproportionate risk for HIV infection. In North Carolina, HIV-positive women were considerably more likely to be unemployed, requiring public assistance, and exchanging sex for money and gifts.

As the U.S. epidemic evolves, it is becoming more an epidemic of African Americans and other minorities (see Fig. 384-5). African Americans make up 12% of the U.S. population but account for 47% of new HIV diagnoses. Hispanics represent 17% of the population but account for 21% of new HIV diagnoses. Among African Americans and Hispanics, most men infected with HIV were exposed during sex with other men (72% and 79%, respectively), whereas most women with HIV become infected heterosexually (89% and 86%, respectively). African American women are more than 10 times more likely to be infected with HIV than are white women. AIDS continues to be one of the leading causes of death in African American women aged 25 to 34 years and ranks in the top three causes of death in African American men aged 25 to 54 years. In the United States, the challenge of slowing the rate of new HIV infections overlaps with the need to provide diagnosis, treatment, and care services more equitably. The number of AIDS-related deaths was 69% lower than in 1994. However, further declines in mortality will require greater success in encouraging timely diagnosis of HIV infection. An estimated 21% of people living with HIV are unaware of their HIV status[9] (Fig. 384-7). Moreover, in 36% of people in whom HIV was diagnosed, AIDS was diagnosed within 12 months. With the aim of increasing the percentage of people who receive a timely diagnosis of HIV, the Centers for Disease Control and Prevention recommends routine voluntary HIV testing in all health care settings unless the patient "opts out," to not be tested.

With an epidemic that is nearly into its third decade, complacency has increased and prevention efforts have dwindled as a result of declining mortality. Multiple studies illustrate that prevention efforts are not reaching the large number of at-risk individuals who engage in unsafe sex. Increased rates of STIs among MSM have been documented in the United States, Australia, Great Britain, Canada, and other developed countries. Rates of gonorrhea, syphilis, and chlamydia have more than doubled in the past 5 years among MSM in selected U.S. and European cities. Renewed efforts to enhance prevention efforts, particularly in HIV care clinics, are being echoed throughout all these countries.

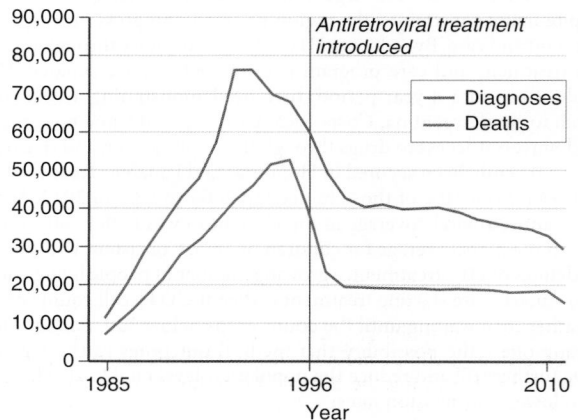

FIGURE 384-4. AIDS diagnosis and deaths in the United States from 1985 to 2010. (Data from Centers for Disease Control and Prevention. HIV Surveillance—United States, 1981-2008. *MMWR*. 2011;60:689-693.)

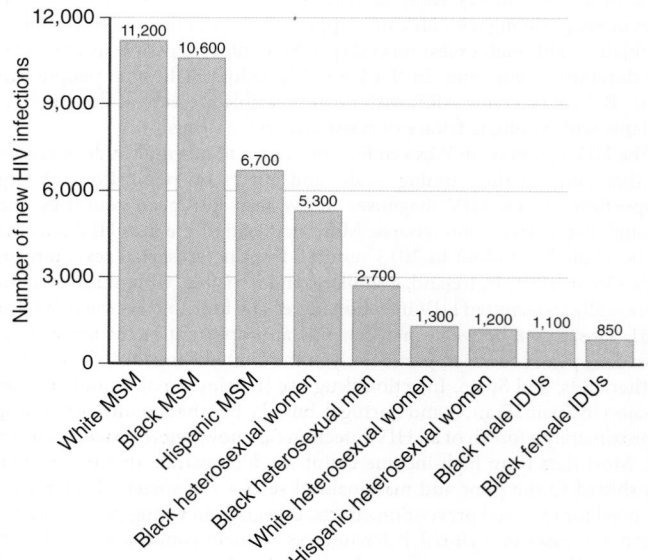

FIGURE 384-5. Estimated new HIV infections in the United States, 2010, for the most-affected subpopulations. IDUs = injection drug users; MSM = men who have sex with men. (Data from Centers for Disease Control and Prevention. Estimated HIV incidence in the United States, 2007-2010. *HIV Surveillance Suppl Rep.* 2012;17:4.)

DIAGNOSIS

Screening for HIV Infection

The history and physical examination are of limited value in making the diagnosis of early HIV infection,[10] so laboratory testing is key to making the diagnosis. The U.S. Preventive Services Task Force on HIV screening recommends that clinicians screen for HIV infection in all adolescents and adults aged 15 to 65 years.[11] Younger adults and older adults who are at increased risk also should be screened.[12] In addition, they recommended that clinicians screen all pregnant women for HIV, including those who present in labor who are untested and whose HIV status is unknown. These updated recommendations were based on increasing evidence of the benefits of early antiretroviral therapy for HIV-infected persons[A1] and its effectiveness in preventing HIV transmission.[A2] This recommendation for increased screening was based on

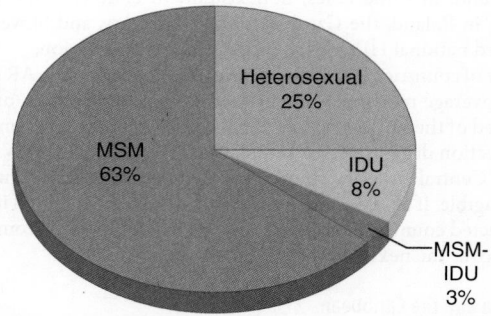

FIGURE 384-6. Estimated new HIV infections in 2010 in the United States by transmission category. IDUs = injection drug users; MSM = men who have sex with men. (Data from Centers for Disease Control and Prevention. Estimated HIV incidence in the United States, 2007-2010. *HIV Surveillance Suppl Rep.* 2012;17:4.)

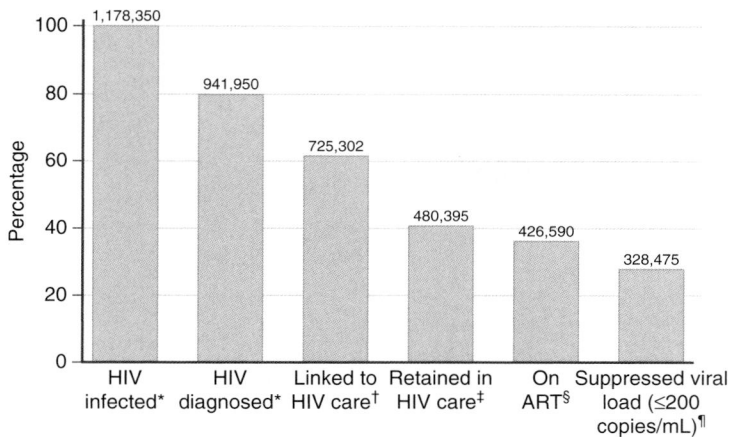

FIGURE 384-7. Number and percentage of HIV-infected persons engaged in selected stages of the continuum of HIV care in the United States. HIV = human immunodeficiency virus; ART = antiretroviral therapy. (Data from Centers for Disease Control and Prevention. Vital signs: HIV prevention through care and treatment—United States. *MMWR.* 2011;60:1618-1623.)
*HIV-infected, n = 1,178,350; HIV-diagnosed, n = 941,950.
†Calculated as estimated number diagnosed (941,950) × estimated percentage linked to care (77%); n = 725,302
‡Calculated as estimated number diagnosed (941,950) × estimated percentage retained in care (51%); n = 480,395.
§Calculated as estimated number retained in care (480,395) × percentage prescribed ART in the Medical Monitoring Project (MMP) (88.8%); n = 426,590.
¶Calculated as estimated number on ART (426,590) × percentage with suppressed viral load in MMP (77.0%); n = 328,475 (28% of the estimated 1,178,350 persons in the United States who are infected with HIV).

the fact that over 20% of HIV-infected individuals have never been tested and are unaware of their infection, and based on evidence that identification and treatment of HIV infection are associated with a markedly reduced risk for progression to AIDS, AIDS-related events, and deaths in individuals with immunologically advanced disease. One randomized trial (HPTN 052) clearly demonstrated that the use of antiretroviral therapy is associated with substantially decreased risk for transmission from HIV-positive persons to uninfected sexual partners. Furthermore, evidence also demonstrates that the identification and treatment of pregnant women dramatically reduces rates of mother-to-child transmission.[A3] The overall benefits of screening for HIV infection in adolescents, adults, and pregnant women are substantial.

On the basis of HIV prevalence data, MSM and active injection drug users are at very high risk for new HIV infection and would qualify for increased HIV screening. Behavioral risk factors for HIV infection include having unprotected vaginal or anal intercourse; having sexual partners who are HIV infected, bisexual, or injection drug users; or exchanging sex for drugs or money. Other persons considered at high risk include those who have acquired or request testing for other STIs. Patients may request HIV testing in the absence of reported risk factors. Individuals not at increased risk for HIV infection include persons who are not sexually active, those who are sexually active in exclusive monogamous relationships with uninfected partners, and those who do not fall into any of the previously mentioned categories. It is recognized that these risk categories are not mutually exclusive, the degree of sexual risk is a continuum, and individuals may not be aware of their sexual partner's risk factors for HIV infection. For patients younger than 15 years and older than 65 years, it would be reasonable for clinicians to consider HIV risk factors on an individual basis, especially those with new sex partners. However, clinicians should bear in mind that adolescent and adult patients may also be reluctant to disclose having HIV risk factors even when asked.

The evidence is insufficient to determine optimum time intervals for HIV screening. One reasonable approach would be a one-time screening of adolescents and adult patients to identify persons who are already HIV positive with repeated screening of those who are known to be at risk for HIV infection, those who are actively engaged in risky behaviors, and those who live or receive medical care in a high-prevalence setting (HIV seroprevalence > 1%). High-prevalence settings include STD clinics, correction facilities, homeless shelters, tuberculosis clinics, clinics serving MSM, and adolescent health clinics with high prevalence of STDs. Currently, a reasonable approach may be to re-screen groups at *very high* risk for new HIV infection at least annually and individuals at *increased risk* at slightly longer intervals (3 to 5

years). Women screened for HIV during previous pregnancies should be re-screened for HIV at all subsequent pregnancies. The CDC also recommends that all persons aged 13 to 65 years be screened for HIV in health care settings located in areas where the prevalence of undiagnosed HIV infection is greater than 0.1% and that persons with increased risk for HIV be re-tested at least annually.

Laboratory Assays

Diagnosis of HIV infection is usually based on serologic detection of immunoglobulin G (IgG) antibodies to HIV-specific proteins. A conventional serum test for diagnosing HIV infection is the repeatedly reactive immunoassay followed by a confirmatory Western blot or immunofluorescence assay. The combined tests are highly accurate with sensitivity and specificity greater than 99.5%. Results are available within 1 to 2 days for most commercial laboratories. New and improved assays are now available for early detection and confirmation of acute HIV infection, including combination tests (p24 antigen and HIV antibodies) and qualitative and quantitative HIV-1 RNA assays.

The diagnostic accuracy of HIV infection has improved with each generation of serologic assays. Whereas the first-generation tests were based on whole viral lysate and an indirect enzyme immunoassay, second-generation tests use synthetic and recombinant peptide antigens that have improved sensitivity and specificity. Third-generation assays have used "sandwich" assay formats that allow simultaneous detection of IgM and IgG antibodies. Now, fourth-generation assays combine antibody and antigen testing within the same diagnostic test format. With increasing sensitivity of these diagnostic assays, the "window period" wherein HIV antibodies may not be detected because of acute or very recent infection has gradually shortened from 6 weeks to less than 3 weeks.[11] This shortening of the window is particularly important when acute infection may not be suspected. In patients with symptoms and signs of acute HIV infection, direct testing with sensitive assays such as nucleic acid testing for HIV RNA may be used.

Rapid tests represent a major advance in HIV serologic testing. Rapid HIV testing may use either blood or oral fluid specimens and can provide results in 5 to 40 minutes. The sensitivity and specificity of the rapid tests are also greater than 99.5%; however, initially positive results require confirmation with conventional methods. Rapid testing can be offered on site in a variety of settings, including clinics, mobile vans, health fairs, and places of worship. Rapid testing is becoming the test of choice for all patients who request screening for immediate feedback and opportunities for quick intervention and counseling. Rapid tests are particularly important in management decisions of occupational or nonoccupational exposures, when patients are unlikely to return for results and seroprevalence rates are high, such as STD clinics or emergency departments, and when patients with an acute illness in which HIV-related complication is being considered and serostatus is not known.

In 2012, the U.S. Food and Drug Administration (FDA) approved the OraQuick in-home HIV test, the first self-administered HIV test kit to detect antibodies to both HIV-1 and HIV-2. The test is available for consumers in drugstores, and individuals may obtain test results within 20 to 40 minutes after collecting an oral fluid sample by swabbing the upper and lower gums inside the mouth and placing the sample into a developer vial provided as part of the kit. As with all rapid HIV assays, positive test results are preliminary and need to be confirmed with a standard HIV antibody test. In clinical trials, self-testing with this rapid HIV assay had a sensitivity of 92% and a specificity of 99.98% compared with the standard enzyme immunoassay (EIA) screening assay. An alternative to home testing is the home access HIV test system, which allows blood samples to be taken at home using a fingerstick test strip that is mailed to a laboratory for screening and confirmation. Results are obtained by phone using an individual identifier code supplied with the product.

Other methods to establish HIV infection include viral isolation or qualitative or quantitative detection of HIV nucleic acid through polymerase chain reaction techniques, branch-chain DNA testing, or nucleic acid sequence–based amplification. Limitations of these assays include cost, the requirement for venipuncture and more laboratory technology, and the time interval between sample collection and test results. None of these tests is considered superior to routine serologic testing. However, viral detection is useful in specific situations such as diagnosis of neonatal HIV infection when maternal antibody is passively transferred to the fetus, potentially providing a false-positive serologic result in uninfected infants and in patients with indeterminate serologic results or in those who may be in the window period before HIV seroconversion.[14]

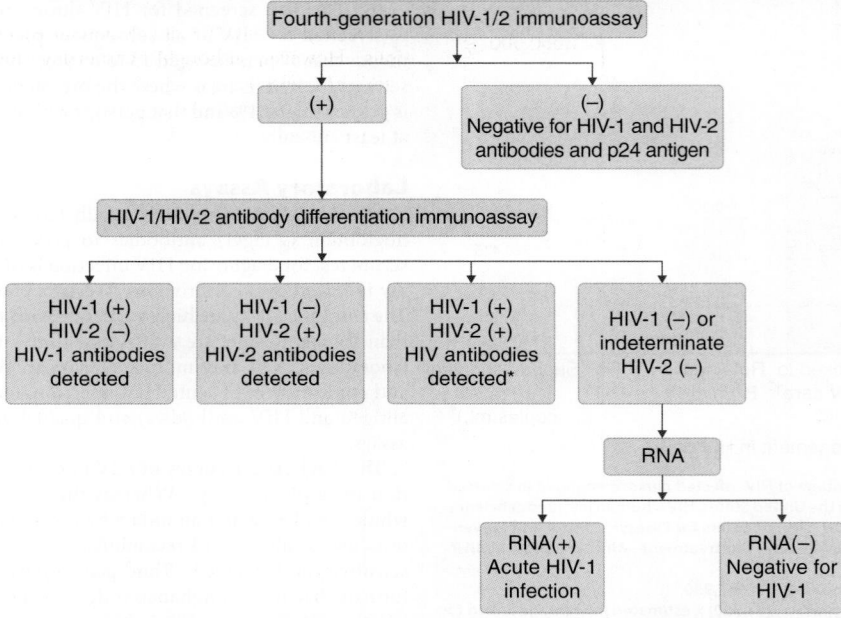

FIGURE 384-8. New HIV diagnostic testing algorithm evaluated in the United States, 2011-2013 HIV = human immunodeficiency virus. (From Centers for Disease Control and Prevention. Detection of acute HIV infection in two evaluations of a new HIV diagnostic testing algorithm—United States, 2011-2013. *MMWR.* 2013;62:489-494. *Additional testing required to rule out dual infection with HIV-1 and HIV-2.

In 2013, the CDC evaluated and later offered an alternative-testing algorithm for the diagnosis of HIV infection[15] (Fig. 384-8). In this algorithm, all initial testing of serum is performed by an FDA-approved fourth-generation HIV-1/2 immunoassay. Specimens that are reactive on the fourth-generation assay should be re-tested/confirmed with an FDA-approved second-generation antibody assay that differentiates HIV-1 antibodies from other HIV antibodies, providing a definitive diagnosis of either HIV-1 or HIV-2. Seropositive individuals should initiate medical care that includes additional laboratory tests such as viral load, CD4 determination, and antiretroviral resistance assays to stage HIV disease and for the selection of initial antiretroviral drug regimens. Specimens that are reactive on the fourth-generation assay but negative on the HIV-1/HIV-2 antibody differentiation assay should be re-tested with an FDA-approved nucleic acid test for HIV-1 RNA. Under these circumstances a reactive nucleic acid test indicates the presence of acute HIV infection. A negative result would indicate the absence of HIV-1, and either a false-positive result on the initial fourth-generation assay or rarely recent HIV-2 infection. If HIV-2 infection is a possibility, a nucleic acid amplification test (NAAT) for HIV-2 DNA can be considered. However, HIV-2 infection is rare in the United States and there is no FDA NAAT for HIV-2. If a fourth-generation screening assay is not available, a third-generation HIV-1/2 immunoassay can be used as the initial test, followed by subsequent testing as specified in the algorithm. This alternative will miss some acute HIV infections in antibody-negative persons.

The previously described algorithm emphasizes high sensitivity during initial testing with the fourth-generation immunoassay, in which false-positive antibody-negative test results might occur, but these can be resolved during subsequent laboratory testing as recommended as part of initial clinical evaluation. The new diagnostic algorithm replaces the Western blot with an HIV-1/HIV-2 antibody differentiation assay as the supplemental test and includes an RNA test to resolve reactive immunoassays with negative supplemental test results. In retrospective studies, this algorithm performed better than Western blot at identifying HIV antibody-positive persons, detecting acute HIV infections, and diagnosing unsuspected HIV-2 infections.

Grade A References

A1. Severe P, Juste MA, Ambroise A, et al. Early versus standard antiretroviral therapy for HIV-infected adults in Haiti. *N Engl J Med.* 2010;363:257-265.
A2. Cohen MS, Chen YQ, McCauley M, et al. HPTN 052 Study Team. Prevention of HIV-1 infection with early antiretroviral therapy. *N Engl J Med.* 2011;365:493-505.

A3. De Vicenzi I. Kesho Bora Study Group. Triple antiretroviral compared with zidovudine and single-dose nevirapine prophylaxis during pregnant and breast-feeding for prevention of mother-to-child transmission of HIV-1 (Kesho Bora study): a randomized controlled trial. *Lancet Infect Dis.* 2011;11:171-180.

GENERAL REFERENCES

For the General References and other additional features, please visit Expert Consult at https://expertconsult.inkling.com.

385

IMMUNOPATHOGENESIS OF HUMAN IMMUNODEFICIENCY VIRUS INFECTION

JOEL N. BLANKSON AND ROBERT F. SILICIANO

Human immunodeficiency virus type 1 (HIV-1) infection results in a progressive state of immune system dysregulation that ultimately leads to the acquired immunodeficiency syndrome (AIDS), which is characterized by profound depletion of CD4+ T lymphocytes and the inability to control infections by opportunistic pathogens that do not cause disease in individuals with a normal immune system. Despite decades of research on this condition, the basic pathogenic mechanisms are still incompletely understood. This chapter reviews current understanding of the mechanisms involved in HIV-1 immunopathogenesis.

PRIMARY INFECTION

The natural history of HIV-1 infection is illustrated in Figure 385-1. During acute HIV-1 infection, massive viral replication occurs in CD4+ T lymphocytes in the absence of an adaptive immune response. CD4+ T cells in the gut-associated lymphoid tissue and other mucosal sites express high levels of the HIV coreceptor CCR5 and are thus particularly prone to infection and depletion by the commonly transmitted R5 variants of HIV-1. In animal models, it has been shown that approximately 30% of memory CD4+ T cells are infected and depleted by 4 days after infection. This is in contrast to chronic infection, in which less than 1% of all CD4+ T cells are productively

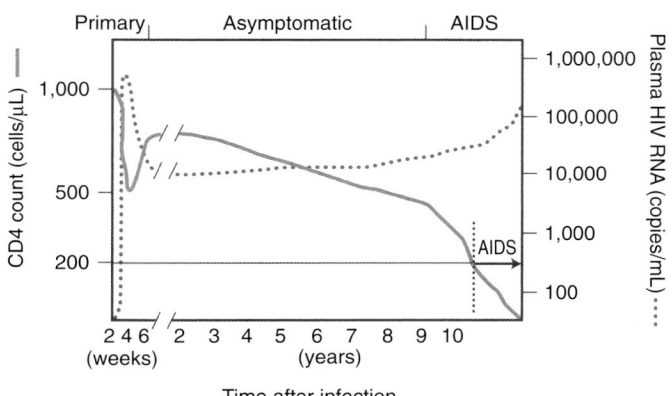

FIGURE 385-1. Natural history of HIV-1 infection. CD4 counts and viral load are shown in the three phases of infection. AIDS = acquired immunodeficiency syndrome.

infected at any given time. As a result of this massive early infection, plasma levels of virion-associated HIV-1 RNA of more than 1 million copies per milliliter are typically seen in plasma within 2 weeks of infection and patients tend to experience a constellation of signs and symptoms known as the *acute retroviral syndrome*. There can be significant declines in peripheral CD4+ T-cell counts in primary infection resulting in opportunistic infections. Within several weeks, the development of an effective HIV-1–specific cytolytic T-lymphocyte response results in the partial control of viral replication, and the plasma HIV-1 RNA level (commonly known as the viral load) falls and reaches a steady-state level known as the *set point*. The magnitude of the set point viral load during the second asymptomatic phase of the infection reflects a dynamic equilibrium between viral replication and the HIV-1–specific immune response. This set point determines the rate of progression to the final phase, clinical AIDS. The median set point is approximately 30,000 HIV-1 RNA copies per milliliter, and most patients who have this level of viremia will develop AIDS in a 5- to 10-year period if they are left untreated. Patients with much higher set point viral loads will tend to be rapid progressors who develop AIDS much more quickly; patients with much lower viral loads tend to be long-term nonprogressors.

SPECIFIC IMMUNITY FOR HUMAN IMMUNODEFICIENCY VIRUS

The host mounts a vigorous immune response to HIV-1 infection. The virus is thought to activate plasmacytoid dendritic cells through toll-like receptors, resulting in the secretion of type I interferons and other inflammatory cytokines. Whereas type I interferons have direct antiviral properties and enhance the HIV-1–specific immune response, excessive secretion may play a key role in pathogenic immune activation of CD4+ and CD8+ T cells (Fig. 385-2). Natural killer (NK) cells are important effector cells in the innate immune response that become activated when infection of target cells by HIV-1 or other viruses results in the downregulation of HLA molecules. Patients expressing certain NK receptor alleles are more likely to become long-term nonprogressors, suggesting that these cells may play a protective role possibly by controlling early HIV-1 replication, leading to the development of an effective adaptive immune response. Myeloid dendritic cells play a key role in the presentation of HIV-1 antigens to HIV-1–specific CD4+ and CD8+ T cells, which results in initiation of the adaptive immune response. They express CD4 molecules and have been shown to bind HIV-1. It is thought that in the process of presenting antigen, these cells may inadvertently transmit HIV-1 to clusters of activated CD4+ T cells.

The role of the humoral response in HIV-1 infection is not clear. HIV-1–specific antibodies, which are used to diagnose HIV-1 infection, do not develop until after peak viremia occurs. There is thus a window period in primary HIV-1 infection during which viremia is present in the absence of detectable antibodies. A subset of the antibodies that eventually appear are capable of preventing infection by blocking the interaction of the HIV-1 envelope protein gp120 with CD4 and coreceptor proteins on the surface of target cells. These so-called neutralizing antibodies are present at relatively low titers and have limited access to the critical regions of gp120. Recent studies suggest that the most effective neutralizing antibodies do not

develop until 2 to 3 years after infection.[1] These broadly neutralizing antibodies may eventually form the basis of a vaccine by preventing new infections. However, although neutralizing antibodies in general can exert significant selective pressure on the virus, immunologic escape through rapid viral evolution is common, and the bulk of evidence suggests that these antibodies do not play a major role in the control of viral replication in most long-term nonprogressors.

The selective depletion of CD4+ T cells is the main reason that HIV-1 infection results in such profound immunosuppression; these so-called helper T cells play a major role in every facet of the adaptive immune response. The ability of HIV-1–specific CD4+ T cells to proliferate and to secrete key cytokines such as interleukin-2 (IL-2) is lost shortly after primary infection, setting up the entire HIV-1–specific response for failure.

CD8+ T cells contribute to the control of HIV-1 infection by the direct lysis of infected cells and by the secretion of soluble factors such as macrophage inflammatory protein 1β that bind to chemokine receptors, thereby preventing HIV-1 entry into target cells.[2] However, the HIV-1–specific CD8+ T-cell response that partially controls HIV-1 replication after peak viremia in primary infection does not achieve sterilizing immunity, partly because of a reservoir of latent virus in resting memory CD4+ T cells that develops shortly after infection. These quiescent cells probably do not make HIV-1 proteins and thus are not recognized by cytolytic T lymphocytes. Furthermore, the cytolytic T-lymphocyte response in patients with progressive disease is of poor quality with limited proliferative capacity. Most importantly, the low fidelity of HIV-1 reverse transcriptase results in the development of mutations with each round of replication. Mutations that lead to escape from cytolytic T-lymphocyte responses have a selective advantage and are thus selected for rapidly.

THE EFFECT OF HUMAN IMMUNODEFICIENCY VIRUS-1 REPLICATION ON THE IMMUNE SYSTEM

Whereas the HIV-1–specific immune response helps limit the rate of viral replication, sterilizing immunity is never achieved and ongoing viral replication has a negative impact on the immune system. Continuous viral replication results in chronic immune activation (see Fig. 385-2).[3] The mechanism is not understood. The chronic immune response to the virus may lead to nonspecific inflammation, and microbial translocation resulting from the depletion of CD4+ T cells in the gut-associated lymphoid tissue also may be important. Whatever the mechanism, immune activation appears to drive the depletion of CD4+ T cells. The level of immune activation markers on CD8+ T cells correlates better with the rate of CD4 decline than does the magnitude of the viral load in untreated patients.

Increased levels of activation markers are seen on NK cells, B cells, CD4+ T cells, and CD8+ T cells. Activation is accompanied by an increase in the turnover rate of these cells. The function of NK cells is compromised, which may predispose to the poor control of other viruses. B-cell defects result in hypergammaglobulinemia and the production of autoantibodies. Poor antibody responses to vaccines are also seen as CD4+ T cells decline.

Studies of viral dynamics make it clear that most productively infected cells live only a short time (~1 day) before succumbing to viral cytopathic effects or host cytolytic T lymphocytes or NK cells. Although the loss of infected CD4+ T cells contributes to CD4 depletion, there is marked depletion of CD4+ T cells even though at any given time during chronic infection only 1% or less of these cells is productively infected. However, recent studies have suggested that non-productively infected CD4+ T cells are also susceptible to cell death by a pro-apoptotic and proinflammatory host response. Thus, it is currently thought that death of non-productively infected CD4+ T cells and chronic immune activation leading to the death of noninfected CD4+ T cells are the principle mechanisms for CD4 depletion.[4,5] Support for this idea comes from studies of the closely related simian immunodeficiency virus that replicates in natural simian hosts without causing immune activation or CD4 depletion. In addition to the quantitative loss of CD4+ T cells in HIV-1 infection, marked skewing of the CD4 T-cell repertoire is seen, and there is a diminished qualitative memory response to recall antigens long before the CD4+ T-cell count drops to 200 cells/μL. The chronic activation and high turnover rate of these cells eventually result in the progressive CD4 decline that is characteristic of HIV-1 infection.

There is evidence of immune exhaustion for both CD4+ and CD8+ T cells, and there is decline in the qualitative features of the CD8+ T-cell response to other chronic viruses such as cytomegalovirus and Epstein-Barr virus. This may be the result of anergy or depletion of the CD4+ T cells that are needed to sustain functional CD8+ T-cell responses.

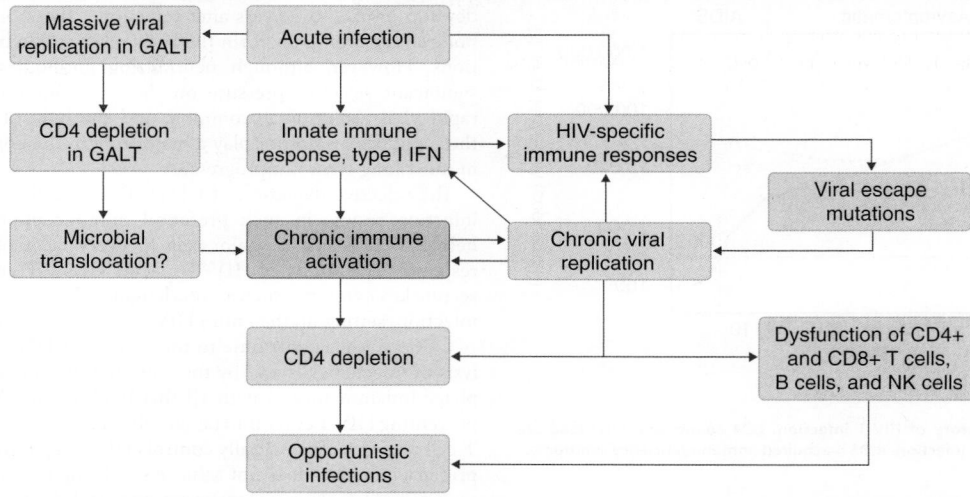

FIGURE 385-2. Parameters involved in chronic immune activation and CD4+ T-cell depletion. GALT = gut-associated lymphoid tissue; IFN = interferon; NK = natural killer.

CLINICAL CONSEQUENCES OF HUMAN IMMUNODEFICIENCY VIRUS INFECTION

Clinical immunodeficiency is associated with the late stages of HIV-1 infection, when profound CD4+ T-cell depletion has occurred. However, some level of immunodeficiency may be present shortly after infection because of qualitative changes in the immune response related to ongoing viral replication. As a result, patients are more susceptible to infections such as *Mycobacterium tuberculosis* infection before the CD4 count reaches the 200 cells/μL threshold that defines AIDS. Patients are also much more susceptible to malignant neoplasms such as non-Hodgkin's lymphoma at any CD4+ T-cell count. Other opportunistic infections arise at fairly predictable CD4+ T-cell counts. *Pneumocystis jiroveci* infections occur at CD4 counts of lower than 200 cells/μL, *Cryptococcus neoformans* and *Toxoplasma gondii* infections occur at CD4 counts of lower than 100 cells/μL, and *Mycobacterium avium* complex and cytomegalovirus infections occur at CD4 counts below 50 cells/μL. Whereas these infections are a consequence of diminished cellular immunity, there is also a marked increase in invasive pneumococcal infections in HIV-1–infected patients, possibly because of defects in humoral immunity.

The Response to Antiretroviral Therapy

Treatment with selected combinations of antiretroviral drugs, which is known as highly active antiretroviral therapy (HAART), suppresses viral replication to below the limits of detection of current commercial assays (50 copies of HIV-1 RNA per milliliter of plasma). Current evidence suggests that HAART produces a complete or nearly complete arrest in viral replication in adherent patients, but trace amounts of viremia persist because of stable viral reservoirs, including the latent reservoir in resting CD4+ T cells. This suppression of viral replication is usually accompanied by a substantial increase in CD4+ T-cell counts. The initial rise in CD4+ T-cell counts occurs mostly as a consequence of migration of cells from lymph nodes (where 98% of all CD4 T cells reside) to the peripheral blood as inflammation diminishes in lymphoid tissue. Subsequently, there is an increase in the production of memory CD4+ T cells in most individuals. Naïve T-cell production is also sometimes seen at lower levels. Clinical studies have shown that patients who experience significant immune reconstitution[6] can safely discontinue prophylactic therapy for opportunistic infections. However, it is not clear whether patients who maintain undetectable viral loads while receiving HAART yet do not achieve significant CD4 T-cell immune reconstitution are still at risk for opportunistic infections. Two large studies have shown that although the use of IL-2 treatment in conjunction with HAART will cause a significant increase in CD4+ T-cell counts in these patients, the enhanced immune reconstitution is not associated with any clinical benefit.

Just as a decline is seen in the functional CD4+ T-cell response shortly after primary infection, there is a qualitative improvement in CD4+ T-cell function shortly after HAART is initiated. In some cases, there are exaggerated immune responses to opportunistic infections leading to the immune reconstitution inflammatory syndrome (IRIS; Chapter 395), particularly when there is rapid control of viral replication after the initiation of HAART. IRIS usually presents as a paradoxical worsening of a disease process a few weeks after HAART is started and can occur even before there are significant changes in the absolute CD4+ T-cell counts. IRIS has been reported for virtually all known opportunistic infections, and in some cases it can occur in response to previously unrecognized infections. There have not been clinical trials looking at treatment of this condition, but nonsteroidal anti-inflammatory drugs and corticosteroids have been routinely used with varying degrees of success (Chapter 395).

GENERAL REFERENCES

For the General References and other additional features, please visit Expert Consult at https://expertconsult.inkling.com.

386

BIOLOGY OF HUMAN IMMUNODEFICIENCY VIRUSES

FRANK MALDARELLI

Human immunodeficiency virus (HIV) causes progressive immune deficiency and death from opportunistic infections or neoplastic diseases. Over 34 million individuals worldwide are currently infected with HIV, and over 30 million have died since the disease was first recognized in 1981. Developments in diagnosis, prevention, and treatment have reduced morbidity and mortality from HIV, but the epidemic remains substantial; in 2012, 2.3 million new HIV infections occurred and 1.6 million people died from HIV and acquired immunodeficiency syndrome (AIDS).[1] Improvements in HIV care grew from an understanding of the discovery, characterization, and elucidation of replication of HIV. Continued research led to discoveries of cellular processes, mechanisms of pathogenesis, and new concepts of host antiviral immunity. Here we summarize basic concepts of HIV biology. Our understanding of HIV remains incomplete, and efforts are ongoing to improve testing, characterize viral replication and pathogenesis, identify novel antiviral targets, and develop innovative strategies to eradicate HIV infection.

CLASSIFICATION AND ORIGIN

HIV belongs to the lentivirus genus of the Orthoretrovirinae subfamily of Retroviridae; all retroviruses are defined by the presence of a specific enzyme, reverse transcriptase, that catalyzes the synthesis of DNA from an RNA template, the central and unique event in retrovirus replication permitting integration of the viral DNA into the host genome. Retroviridae is a large family of viruses infecting diverse vertebrate hosts, mostly mammals and birds, and to a lesser degree, reptiles and fish. Retroviruses are responsible for a spectrum of diseases, including immunodeficiencies and neoplastic, neurologic, hematologic, encephalitic, and inflammatory disorders. Members of the lentivirus genus cause chronic, recurrent, or progressive diseases, including immunodeficiencies in various mammal species.

The origin of HIV variants currently circulating in humans has been traced by analyzing nucleic acid sequences of HIV and closely related viruses in primates; these analyses strongly indicate HIV emerged from zoonotic transmissions from primates to humans during the period 1890 to 1930 in Central and West Africa.[2] Zoonotic transmission requires close contact of blood and body fluid; scratches, bites, and butchery of captured infected animals provide ready mechanisms for transmission. Such opportunities for zoonotic transmission have likely taken place for thousands of years, and the reasons why an epidemic spread did not occur until recently are unclear. A number of factors may have contributed to epidemic spread during the late 19th and 20th centuries, including profound increases in human population density, habitat destruction forcing more contact between humans and other primates, malnutrition contributing to underlying immunodeficiency, population shifts due to political upheaval, and the development of infrastructure, such as roads, facilitating human travel over long distances.

The viral etiology of AIDS was first identified after intensive investigation of patients identified with AIDS. Cell cultures inoculated with plasma or co-cultured with lymphocytes from individuals with AIDS resulted in marked cytopathic effect; cell-free material transmitted the infection to fresh uninfected cultures and reproduced cytopathology; cultures contained both reverse transcriptase enzymatic activity and virions with morphology characteristic of lentiviruses. The virus was initially named HTLV-III because of its apparent relationship to the other human retroviruses HTLV-I and II; subsequent study demonstrated the virus responsible for AIDS was only distantly related to HTLV, and the new virus was renamed HIV. Molecular clones were constructed that reproduced cellular cytopathology. Plasma from infected individuals contained substantial antibodies to the virus, permitting development of robust new enzyme-linked immunosorbent assay (ELISA) and Western blot detection assays useful for patient diagnosis, epidemiologic surveillance, and blood product protection.

Following the development of the first tools for laboratory diagnosis of HIV infection, additional analysis identified individuals with symptomatic AIDS but who did not have serologic responses characteristic of HIV, leading to the identification of a second distinct immunodeficiency virus, denoted HIV-2. HIV-2 had a distribution restricted largely to West Africa and to countries having close economic, political, or cultural ties to West Africa.

Further genetic analysis and sampling of nonhuman primate species shed new light on sources of the HIV epidemic. HIV-1 can be classified using nucleic acid sequence analysis into four distinct groups: a large group of viruses found throughout the world (M, for "main"), a relatively small group of viruses in central Africa (O, for "other"), and two small groups in individuals with West African origin, comprising only fewer than 20 total infections, denoted N (not M, not O) and P. Phylogenetic reconstructions demonstrate distinct lineages for HIV-1 groups, indicating each is the result of a distinct zoonotic event (Fig. 386-1), which in the case of HIV-1 M, has spread worldwide. M viruses are closely related to a similar virus, simian immunodeficiency virus, present in chimpanzee species (denoted SIV$_{cpz}$ simian immunodeficiency virus, cpz to indicate the specific animal reservoir). Group O is most closely related to the SIV present in gorillas and in chimpanzees. In contrast, HIV-2 is highly related to SIV$_{smm}$, a lentivirus commonly present in the sooty mangabey, which has a geographic range including West and Central Africa, where HIV-2 was identified.

Group M viruses represent the great majority of infections in humans and are quite diverse, with at least nine subtypes, denoted A to D, F to H, J, and K. Analysis of the relationships of the nucleic acid sequences reveals an overall "starlike" phylogeny (see Fig. 386-1), indicating that, in general, all the current variants emerged from a common ancestor. Studies of the earliest viral sequences identified revealed it is likely that HIV underwent diversification early after transmission from animal reservoirs. Recombination among these subtypes may occur (see Fig. 386-1, *A/D*; and see later), yielding new recombinant viruses that are classified as circulating recombinant forms. Dual HIV-1/HIV-2 infections are also possible in geographic regions where viruses co-circulate, typically from West Africa.

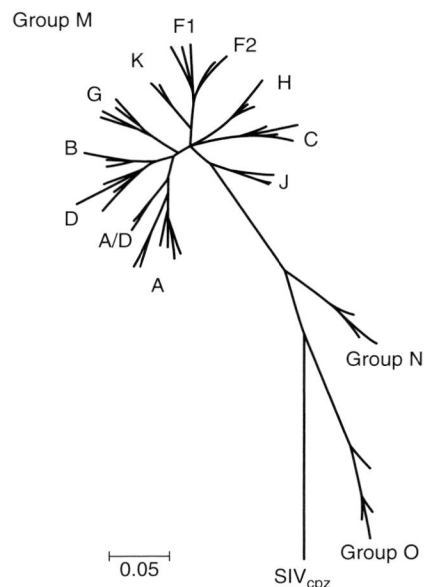

FIGURE 386-1. Phylogenetic relationships of HIV-1 groups and subtypes. Reference sequences of HIV RT were aligned in maximum likelihood phylogenetic trees constructed and rooted on the distant ancestor, SIV chimpanzee sequence (SIV$_{cpz}$). Group M viruses radiate in a starlike fashion, consistent with a common ancestor. An example of recombinant sequences (A/D) containing portions of parental subtypes A and D are identified as intermediate between the parental subtypes. Group O and N are distantly related to group M and likely represent independent zoonotic events. Marker = genetic distance depicting percent difference. HIV Sequence Database, http://www.hiv.lanl.gov/.

Once AIDS emerged, HIV spread rapidly throughout the world; while Africa maintained a highly diverse group of viruses, founder effects resulted in spread of one or a limited number of subtype viruses in countries outside Africa. The epidemic in the United States began with subtype B virus; although initially attributed to single case reports of individuals, careful and exhaustive analyses traced the HIV epidemic from Africa to the United States through Haiti. Importantly, current laboratory methods to detect HIV identify *all* HIV-1 and HIV-2 variants. In individuals from relevant geographic origin, especially West Africa, it is of paramount importance to characterize the infection precisely to target therapy appropriately; HIV-2 and group O HIV-1 are naturally resistant to non-nucleoside reverse transcriptase inhibitors and to fusion inhibitors.[3] As dual HIV-1/HIV-2 infections are possible, it is imperative that all individuals from endemic areas for these two viruses (especially West Africa) be tested for *both* HIV-1 and HIV-2.

STRUCTURE AND MOLECULAR BIOLOGY

Genome Structure and Organization

Like all retroviruses, HIV replicates via a DNA intermediate. The virion contains two copies of single-stranded (+) sense RNA (denoted viral RNA), and the stably infected cell contains double-stranded viral DNA integrated into the host genome (denoted the provirus). Viral RNA and the provirus have distinct genomic organization in untranslated 3′ and 5′ regions. Untranslated regions at each end of the genome contain a short terminal repeat, as well as unique sequences at the 5′ (U5) and 3′ (U3) regions that are duplicated during replication, generating a longer duplicated sequence termed the *long terminal repeat* at each end of the provirus.

HIV encodes nine genes whose products are required for structural, enzymatic, regulatory, and innate immune neutralization functions. By convention, HIV genes are denoted in lower italics (*gag, pol,* etc.) with names that broadly reflect their function, location in the virion, or a historical vestige of prior viral classification (e.g., *gag,* "group antigen"). Additional genes were characterized that function in regulation or replication (*tat, rev, vpr*) or in blocking immune responses to HIV (*vif, vpu, nef*); all are critical for HIV infection in vivo.

Virion Structure

The HIV virion contains viral gene products and cellular components essential to transmit infection and establish the proviral state. HIV virions are roughly spherical particles with a diameter of 80 to 120 nm and are composed of a viral core enveloped by a lipid membrane (Fig. 386-2).

The core of the mature virion is a conelike structure,[4] composed of the HIV p24 capsid (CA), which encapsidates components necessary for replication: two copies of HIV genomic RNA template complexed with HIV p6 nucleocapsid (NC); tRNA^{lys} primer; HIV enzymes reverse transcriptase, protease, and integrase; and HIV Vif. The viral envelope, which is derived from the plasma membrane of the host cell as HIV undergoes budding, contains viral proteins Gp120 (SU) and Gp41 (TM), as well as a structural matrix protein, MA.

HIV Virion

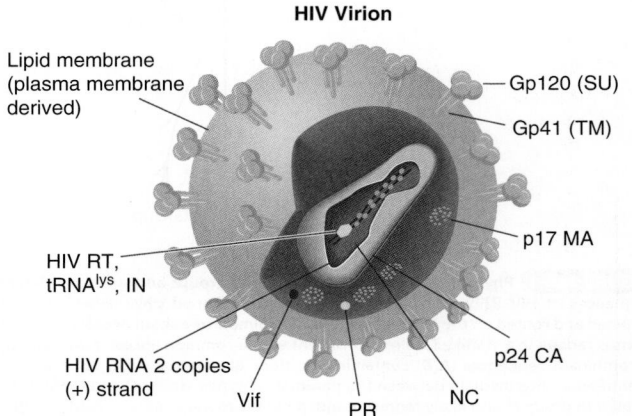

Lipid membrane (plasma membrane derived)
Gp120 (SU)
Gp41 (TM)
p17 MA
HIV RT, tRNA^{lys}, IN
HIV RNA 2 copies (+) strand
p24 CA
Vif
PR
NC

FIGURE 386-2. The HIV virion. HIV is an enveloped virus consisting of two (+) sense copies of viral RNA, enzymes required for replication contained in a viral core enveloped in a membrane derived by budding from the infected cell.

Replication Cycle
Early Events in Replication
Attachment and Fusion

Virus replication is initiated by direct contact of virions or infected cells with susceptible host cells (Fig. 386-3). Productive infection requires specific and essential interactions mediated by surface Env glycoprotein trimeric complexes consisting of HIV sp120 SU noncovalently bound to HIV gp41 TM.[5] The attachment phase is mediated exclusively by SU, which engages two distinct cell surface proteins for attachment, a receptor and a coreceptor (see Fig. 386-3). HIV initially binds CD4, resulting in conformational change in Env, which facilitates coreceptor binding. Typically, SU proteins use either the human chemokine receptor 5 (CCR5) or the human chemokine receptor 4 (CXCR4), to infect CD4+ T cells, but CCR5/CXCR4 dual tropic viruses circulate as well. Although virus infection can be propagated with either CCR5 or CXXCR4 as coreceptor, initial infection likely requires CCR5 tropic virus. Human populations have a significant population of individuals encoding a mutant CCR5 gene, who do not synthesize functional CCR5. HIV infection of individuals homozygous for CCR5 mutation is exceedingly rare, suggesting that initiation of infection virtually always requires interactions with CCR5. Inhibition of SU-coreceptor interactions has been achieved pharmacologically, and the U.S. Food and Drug Administration–approved coreceptor inhibitor maraviroc has potent anti-HIV activity.[6]

Engaging both receptor and coreceptor results in conformational change in Gp41, which reorganizes its structure and provides sufficient energy to drive membrane fusion. TM-mediated membrane fusion can be inhibited using specific peptide inhibitors that bind to Gp41; one such peptide fusion inhibitor, enfuvirtide, is in clinical practice.

Uncoating

Following entry into CD4 cells, HIV cores undergo uncoating (see Fig. 386-3) to release virion nucleic acid into the cytoplasm. Uncoating represents a critical checkpoint for innate antiviral activity that can strongly

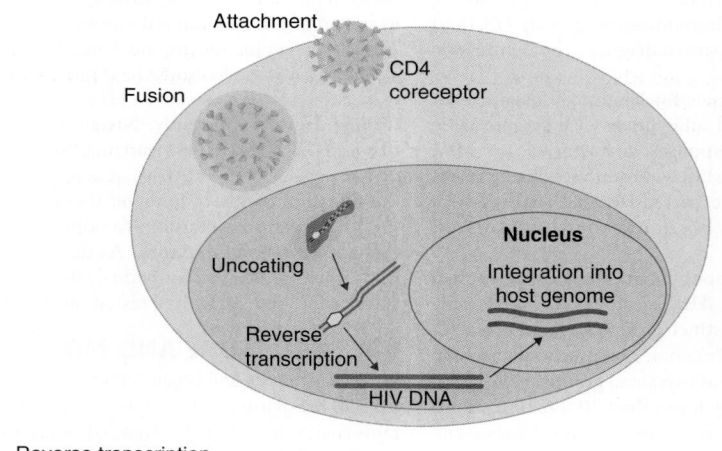

Attachment
Fusion
CD4
coreceptor
Uncoating
Nucleus
Integration into host genome
Reverse transcription
HIV DNA

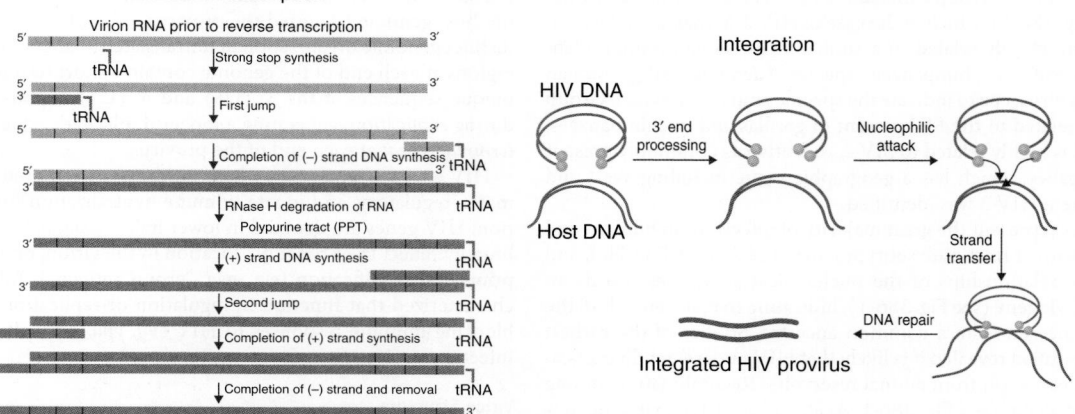

Reverse transcription
Virion RNA prior to reverse transcription
5′ 3′
tRNA
Strong stop synthesis
5′ 3′
3′
tRNA
First jump
5′ 3′
Completion of (−) strand DNA synthesis tRNA
5′ 3′ tRNA
3′
RNase H degradation of RNA tRNA
Polypurine tract (PPT)
3′ tRNA
(+) strand DNA synthesis tRNA
3′ tRNA
Second jump tRNA
Completion of (+) strand synthesis tRNA
Completion of (−) strand and removal tRNA
5′ 3′

Integration
HIV DNA
3′ end processing
Nucleophilic attack
Host DNA
Strand transfer
DNA repair
Integrated HIV provirus

FIGURE 386-3. Early events in HIV replication include attachment, fusion, uncoating, reverse transcription, and integration into the host genome. Details of HIV reverse transcription and integration are depicted.

restrict infectivity.[7,8] An interferon-inducible host protein, TRIM5-alpha, can block uncoating of a number of viruses through interactions with the viral core; unfortunately, TRIM5-alpha cannot restrict either HIV-1 or HIV-2. TRIM5-alpha is under substantial genetic selection, with one of the fastest rates of positive selection of any human gene. Studies suggest that the current version of TRIM5-alpha present in human populations may have been selected during a previous epidemic to protect against an ancient retroviral infection. In this model, simply summarized as "generals are always fighting the last war, especially if they have won it," the current TRIM5-alpha was selected in the past to prevent a retroviral infection. Unfortunately, the current TRIM5-alpha is unable to restrict HIV and uncoating takes place unabated in human cells.

Reverse Transcription: Viral Genome Replication
Following uncoating, HIV has fresh access to nucleoside triphosphates, permitting reverse transcription to take place in the cytoplasm (see Fig. 386-3).[9] The (+)-strand template strands of HIV RNA are complexed with reverse transcriptase and a specific tRNA[lys] that functions as a primer located at a specific primer binding site near the 5′ end of the template RNA and HIV RNA. Reverse transcription is a multistep process (see Fig. 386-3) that first synthesizes a DNA copy of the RNA genome and then excises the RNA from the RNA-DNA hybrid using an RNase H function of reverse transcriptase; RNA removal is incomplete, and residual RNA in a region denoted the polypurine tract (see Fig. 386-3) then serves to prime the next round of DNA synthesis. During reverse transcription a number of strand transfer events occur, permitting opportunities for frequent recombination. Reverse transcriptase is highly error prone, with only a rudimentary editing function. As a result, complete reverse transcription yields at least one mutation per virion synthesized per replication cycle. The replication cycle for HIV, estimated as 1 to 2 days, is relatively short, and the replicating population size is substantial. The combination of rapid and error-prone synthesis in a large replicating population results in a genetically diverse population that can respond rapidly to immune- or drug-selective pressure. Thus, rapid error-prone replication, combined with recombination, represents an important pathogenic determinant for HIV.

Reverse transcription was the first target for antiretroviral therapy, and a number of direct and allosteric inhibitors of reverse transcription have been developed. All reverse transcription inhibitors inhibit RNA-dependent DNA synthesis or DNA-dependent DNA synthesis. Nucleoside and nucleotide reverse transcriptase inhibitors are dideoxy analogues of deoxynucleotides that are incorporated as the template is copied and act as chain terminators, blocking additional nucleic acid synthesis. Non-nucleoside inhibitors of reverse transcription bind to reverse transcriptase in a hydrophobic domain proximal to the active site, deforming the enzyme structure and disrupting nucleic acid synthesis.

Nuclear Transport and Integration
Newly synthesized HIV DNA transports to the nucleus for integration into the host genome. A complex of the HIV protein integrase, newly synthesized HIV DNA, and associated proteins has been labeled an *intasome*. Structural studies have revealed a tetramer of integrase molecules bound to the ends of the retroviral DNA, bringing the DNA ends in close proximity, poised for integration into the genome in a multistep process (see Fig. 386-3). Integration is a highly successful target for antiretroviral therapy and inhibitors that block the transfer of HIV DNA strand into the host genome are now in clinical practice.

Early Evasion of Intracellular Immunity: Vif and Vpu
HIV infection triggers a complex set of immune responses, and several viral factors function to counteract innate and adaptive immunity. As described earlier, HIV is able to infect human cells because an otherwise effective restriction mechanism blocking uncoating by TRIM5-alpha is unable to detect the incoming virus. Infection results in activation of two additional interferon-induced genes, the ABOBEC family of nucleic acid editing enzymes and BST-2 (tetherin). HIV in turn encodes specific functions to counteract such antiviral mechanisms.

The interferon-induced APOBEC family (apolipoprotein B mRNA editing enzyme, catalytic polypeptide-like) of proteins are nucleic acid editing enzymes capable of catalyzing the removal of amino groups from the cytosine portion of cytidine; on copying, these deaminated cytidines base pair with adenosine, not guanine, and the net result is the introduction of multiple G-to-A mutations, resulting in hypermutation and complete viral inactiva-

tion. APOBEC can, in the absence of viral factors, be incorporated into new virions. As a result, during the next round of infection, after HIV enters a new host cell, APOBEC proceeds to hypermutate the newly reverse transcribed HIV genome. To block APOBEC-mediated inactivation of HIV, a viral gene product, Vif, directly binds to APOBEC proteins, redirecting it to degradation by ubiquitination pathways. Redirecting APOBEC for elimination rather than virion incorporation effectively neutralizes a potent innate immune response.

A second product of interferon induction is the bone marrow stromal antigen 2 (BST-2), CD317, or tetherin. BST-2 is tethered to the plasma membrane at both its amino and carboxy terminus and is enriched at virion budding. Tetherin can block the budding process directly; newly budding virions may contain one end of the tetherin molecule in the virion membrane, while the other end of tetherin remains on the cellular membrane, thereby effectively blocking virion release. To counter this host mechanism, the HIV-encoded protein Vpu effectively blocks tetherin by a number of mechanisms, including direct binding and redirecting the protein to intracellular degradation.

Late Steps in Replication
Transcription and Translation: Exploiting Cellular Processes to Balance Production of Viral Gene Products
Once the proviral state is established, HIV produces viral RNA and proteins using viral factors in concert with cellular mechanisms of transcription and translation. Thus, HIV replicates not by dismantling cell functions but rather by employing specific interactions between host factors, which ensures a balanced abundance of viral gene products.

Transcription
The integrated provirus is expressed in the context of host chromatin. The U3 portion of the HIV long terminal repeat contains binding sites for transcription factors common in lymphocytes and macrophage-monocyte lineages, including activator protein 1 (AP-1), specificity protein 1 (SP-1), nuclear factor kappa B (NF-κB), and nuclear factor of activated T cells (NFAT) binding sites. The presence of the viral transcription factor transactivator of transcription (Tat)[10,11] markedly stimulates transcription through binding to a specific RNA enhancer, denoted the transactivating region (TAR), and recruiting additional transcription factors (Fig. 386-4).

Post-transcriptional Processing
Retroviruses transcribe all of their genes from a single promoter. Full-length HIV RNA is processed for expression of all nine gene products and encapsidated as the viral genome into virions. To provide sufficient mRNA species to express all HIV proteins, RNA processing is highly regulated by alternative splicing and differential RNA transport (see Fig. 386-4).

Full-length RNA consists of a primary capped mRNA of approximately 9.2 kb that undergoes alternative splicing to produce three broad classes of RNA species: 9.2-kb unspliced RNA, responsible for translation of *gag/pol*; a number of distinct 4.5-kb singly spliced RNA species, responsible for translation of *vif, vpr*, and *vpu/env*; and 1.8-kb multiply spliced species, responsible for *tat, rev*, and *nef*. Multiply spliced 1.8-kb RNAs are constitutively expressed, but unspliced and singly spliced HIV mRNAs require specific transport out of the nucleus. The mechanism of retention in the nucleus is unclear, but the presence of cis regulatory sequences present in *gag/pol* and *env* result in nuclear retention. To export unspliced and singly spliced HIV RNAs, the viral protein Rev binds to a specific region in the *env* portion of the unspliced and singly spliced RNA, denoted as the Rev responsive element (RRE); the RRE is a sequence of c.240 nt that folds into a specific structure to which Rev binds. The Rev-RNA complex then engages the nuclear host CRM-1 transport apparatus, which transports RNA out of the nucleus. Engaging appropriate host elements therefore results in a balance of 9.2-, 4.5-, and 1.8-kb mRNA species.[12]

Translation of mRNA
All HIV RNAs are translated by cellular ribosomes on either smooth or rough endoplasmic reticulae. Abundance of several HIV proteins is regulated by translational mechanisms and post-translational modifications mediated by host mechanisms that are critical for viral protein function.

Full-length HIV RNA serves as RNA for encapsidation into the virion, and for Gag/Pol synthesis. Gag is synthesized as a 55-kd polyprotein precursor in relatively abundant amounts; Gag protein is N-myristoylated, permitting the protein to bind cellular membranes. The *pol* gene products are translated

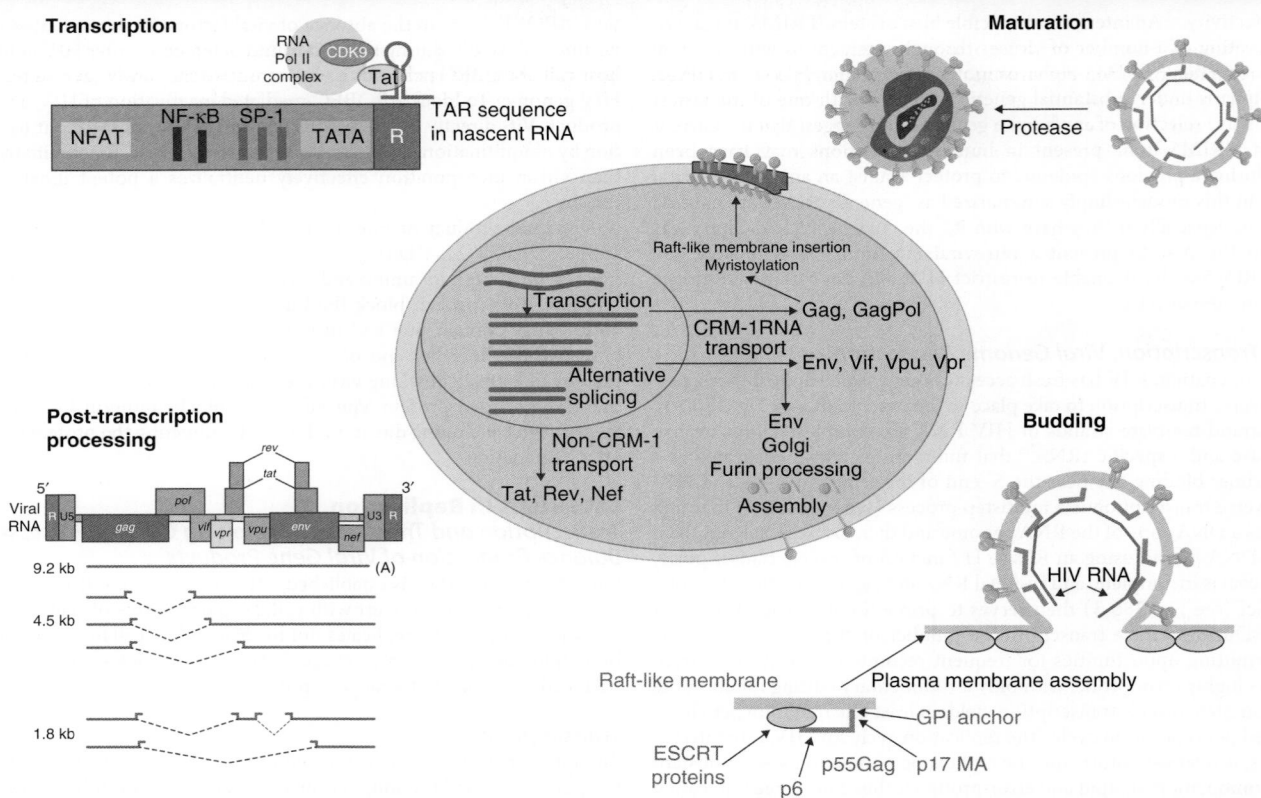

FIGURE 386-4. Late events in HIV replication. Following establishment of the provirus, transcription, post-transcriptional processing translation, virion assembly, budding, and virion maturation take place by co-opting cellular processes.

though frameshifting mechanisms.[13] Frameshifting is relatively inefficient, and the relative abundance of *pol* enzyme gene products is substantially lower than Gag proteins, effectively controlling the levels of enzymes in favor of an abundance of structural proteins.

HIV Vpu and Env proteins are translated from a 4.5-kb bicistronic mRNA, permitting effective production of both Vpu and Env proteins. As Vpu sequesters CD4 by direct protein-protein interactions on intracellular membranes (see later), it prevents CD4-Env interactions that would arrest Env within the cell. Thus, the coordinated expression of Vpu with Env ensures efficient expression of Env. Env is synthesized as a gp160 precursor of Env SU and TM, cotranslationally inserted into the lumen of rough endoplasmic reticulum membranes and glycoslylated predominantly at a number of canonical N glycosylation sites.

Multiply spliced mRNA species encoding *tat, rev,* and *nef* are translated earliest after infection; Tat and Rev are transported to the nucleus, where they activate transcription, and transport (see earlier). Nef serves a number of cytoplasmic functions in evasion of host immunity by binding MHC-1 and CD4, redirecting them away from plasma membranes. Thus, at an early time in the infectious cycle, immune molecules that help identify and target virus-infected cells are downregulated from the cell surface of infected cells, facilitating virus replication.

Transport and Assembly of Virion Components: An Elegant Dance

The late steps in virus replication are complex, but dissecting the individual steps has identified a number of critical interactions between host and virion components that represent active areas for development of useful therapeutics.

HIV virion proteins and virion RNA species traffic to the plasma membrane, where virion assembly takes place. Nascent Gag and GagPol polyprotein precursors undergo cotranslational modifications that target Gag to membranes.[14] Gag has self-assembly properties, but correct initial assembly of the virion core into a hexagonal lattice includes incorporation of virion RNA and additional factors. Virion RNA undergoes dimerization largely through direct RNA-RNA interactions that require specialized RNA sequences, denoted psi sequences, at the 5′ region of the genome favoring incorporation of only unspliced HIV RNA species. Gag polyprotein

precursor can bind HIV RNA directly, providing a potential mechanism for transport to the cell membrane. Gag also accumulates in specialized membrane microdomains enriched with sphingomyelin-saturated phospholipids and cholesterol typical of lipid rafts and binds components of the endosomal sorting complexes required for transport (ESCRT) pathway (see Fig. 386-4). The ESCRT pathway is normally involved in intracellular membrane remodeling and scission events necessary for events such as organelle biogenesis, lysosome formation, and cytokinesis; by recruiting ESCRT to sites of HIV assembly on the plasma membrane, HIV engages a highly specialized pathway to execute budding. Elegant studies of HIV transmission have suggested these events may also participate in cell-cell transmission of HIV at "virologic synapses," specialized areas of cell-cell contact.

During the budding process, HIV undergoes several maturation events, including proteolytic processing of the Gag and GagPol precursor proteins by HIV protease (see Fig. 386-4). Protease is embedded as part of the GagPol precursor, cleaves itself from the precursor and then proceeds to process Gag and GagPol into component proteins. Processing is essential for virion infectivity, and protease inhibitors are highly effective agents in HIV therapy. During processing, the core lattice begins to bend by introducing pentamers of CA at critical points of the hexagonal lattice, effectively folding the structure into a fullerene-like cone that encapsidates dimeric HIV RNA-tRNA[lys] and HIV enzymes. Proteolytic cleavage at the CA-SP1 site is critical; the development of maturation inhibitors that block cleavage by binding Gag instead of inhibiting protease represent a new antiviral target.

HIV Env precursor glycoprotein is processed by a cellular furin-like protease into mature products, gp120 (SU) and gp41, which traffic to plasma membranes through Golgi and post-Golgi membranes. Because the cellular receptor CD4 is also processed through similar mechanisms, intracellular Env-CD4 binding can effectively block Env from reaching the cell surface. The HIV Vpu protein, which directly binds and redirects CD4 to proteolytic degradation, thereby increases the proportion of Env reaching the cell surface and sites of HIV budding.

⬤ SUMMARY

By the completion of the infectious cycle, HIV has produced progeny for the next round of infection, obstructed adaptive and innate immune responses, and established a proviral state in the infected cell. Despite multiple mechanisms of immune evasion, the majority of infected cells (>99.9%) die within 1 to 2 days of infection. Thus, the virus has a strikingly short period to engage critical cell pathways to complete replication, while the cells are undergoing destruction. A minority of cells survive infection and persist for prolonged periods. As a consequence, current antiretroviral therapy that targets active steps in HIV replication does not eradicate HIV infection. Mechanisms of persistence remain poorly understood, but likely include transcriptional and immunologic mechanisms.[15] Additional research will be essential to determine mechanisms of persistence and to identify new strategies to cure HIV infection.

GENERAL REFERENCES

For the General References and other additional features, please visit Expert Consult at https://expertconsult.inkling.com.

387

PREVENTION OF HUMAN IMMUNODEFICIENCY VIRUS INFECTION

CARLOS DEL RIO AND MYRON S. COHEN

More than 30 years have passed since the first report of a case of human immunodeficiency virus (HIV) infection, and the pandemic has spread worldwide and infected more than 70,000,000 people, of whom approximately 35,000,000 have died as a consequence of acquired immunodeficiency virus (AIDS). HIV prevention efforts have been "front and center" since the virus was discovered as the cause of AIDS, as summarized in Figure 387-1. Behavioral interventions focused on HIV-negative persons have likely played a role in the falling population level incidence in some countries reported by the United Nations Program in HIV/AIDS (UNAIDS) in their 2012 report; however, approximately 2.7 million new infections still occur each year, and we have made little progress in reducing HIV incidence in the groups at highest risk. In the past few years, several promising new prevention strategies have demonstrated efficacy in clinical trials and are now being implemented,[1] leading President Obama to look toward an "AIDS-free generation." This chapter will provide a detailed view of HIV prevention approaches that are useful to the practicing clinician.

MODES OF TRANSMISSION AND PREVENTION

Sexual Transmission

The primary mode of HIV transmission throughout the world is sexual contact. However, the geographic distribution of cases attributable to homosexual or heterosexual transmission varies markedly. In the United States, most sexually transmitted cases of HIV are observed in men who have sex with men (MSM), and heterosexual transmission accounts for a smaller number of new infections except among women. However, heterosexual transmission is the leading mode of transmission worldwide and remains the primary mode of disease acquisition in Africa. Sexual transmission of HIV is relatively inefficient, but behavioral and biologic factors influence the likelihood of HIV transmission in a given sexual encounter. In particular, coinfection with classical sexually transmitted infections (STIs) (especially genital ulcerative diseases such as herpes simplex) greatly increases the infectiousness and the susceptibility of an individual. STIs increase the concentration of HIV in genital secretions, which increases the likelihood for transmission.

The risk for acquisition of HIV per coital act has been estimated to be 5 per 10,000 for insertive unprotected penile-vaginal intercourse to 50 per 10,000 for receptive unprotected anal intercourse. However, the risk is not stable and varies depending on the stage of infection and other amplifying cofactors. HIV transmission risk is highest in early HIV infection and in advanced infection (Fig. 387-2), demonstrating that the viral concentration in the genital secretions is the strongest predictor of the risk for transmission.

Prevention Strategies

Traditional strategies for the prevention of sexual transmission of HIV have focused on encouraging abstinence, reducing unsafe sexual behaviors (especially unprotected anal intercourse and concurrent relationships), encouraging proper condom use, and treating STIs. These interventions primarily focus on HIV-negative persons.

In situations in which a decision to engage in sexual activity has been made and the HIV status of the partner is positive, unknown, or in doubt, safe sexual practices ("safe sex") should be implemented. Consistent use of latex condoms has been shown to be effective in preventing HIV transmission at both individual and population levels. The condom should be made of latex and must be used properly. Natural skin condoms should not be used because they do not prevent transmission of HIV. Petroleum-based lubricants enhance the likelihood of rupture of latex condoms and should be avoided. If needed, water-based lubricants such as K-Y jelly should be used.

The effectiveness of condoms in preventing heterosexual transmission of HIV has been estimated to be 87%, but it may be as low as 60% or as high as 96%. The effectiveness of condoms during anal intercourse is probably lower because the frequency of condom breakage and slippage may be considerably higher than during vaginal intercourse. Circumcision represents an alternative strategy to protect men from HIV. Three randomized clinical trials have demonstrated a protective benefit of male circumcision, with the risk for acquisition of HIV infection through heterosexual intercourse decreasing by approximately 60%, with increasing reduction in HIV acquisition over time. However, this benefit has not been confirmed for MSM.

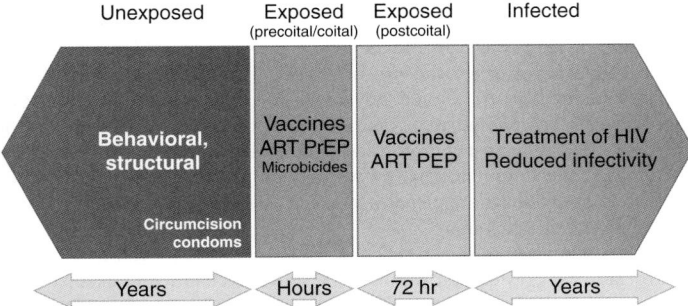

FIGURE 387-1. Opportunities for HIV prevention. ART = antiretroviral therapy; PEP = postexposure prophylaxis; PrEP = pre-exposure prophylaxis. (Modified from Cohen MS. Recent developments in HIV prevention. *AIDS* 2008, Abstract TUPL0102.)

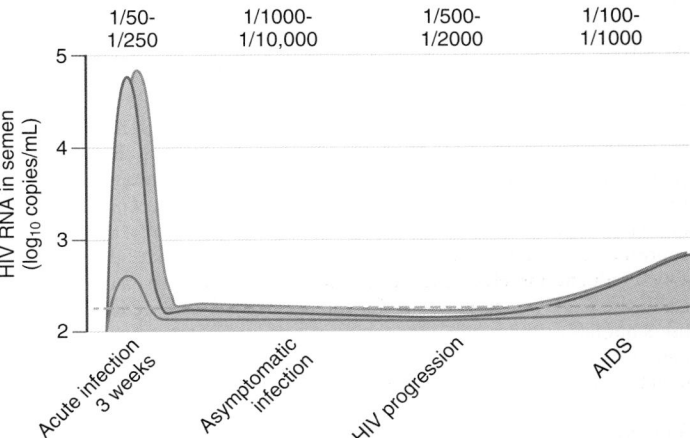

FIGURE 387-2. Prediction of the efficiency of HIV transmission according to HIV burden in the genital tract. Probability of male-to-female HIV transmission per coital act, as a function of HIV disease stage in the index case. Dashed line = a potential threshold for HIV transmission; orange = theoretical effect of a biologic intervention designed to reduce viral excretion; blue = expected distribution of viral burden in semen among men over time. (Modified from Cohen MS, Pilcher CD. Amplified HIV transmission and new approaches to HIV prevention. *J Infect Dis.* 2005;191:1391-1393.)

Antiretroviral therapy may influence infectivity and the subsequent risk for transmission through sexual contact. In the HPTN 052 study, early antiretroviral therapy of HIV-infected patients beginning at a CD4 count of 350 to 550 cells/mm^3 reduced sexual transmission of HIV-1 by 96%.[A1] Observational studies suggest that broader antiretroviral use at a population level can reduce HIV incidence. Antiretrovirals also are effective for the prevention of HIV when administered prophylactically to HIV-uninfected at-risk individuals as pre-exposure prophylaxis (PrEP). In a randomized trial, daily administration of co-formulated tenofovir plus emtricitabine as pre-exposure prophylaxis of MSM decreased the risk for HIV infection by 44%.[A2] Other studies using tenofovir with emtricitabine show a decrease of as much as two thirds in infections,[2] although findings have varied across studies dependings on adherence.[A3-A5] Based on these studies, in 2013 the U.S. Food and Drug Administration approved the use of co-formulated tenofovir plus emtricitabine for pre-exposure prophylaxis to prevent sexual transmission of HIV. The Centers for Disease Control and Prevention (CDC) has issued guidelines for clinicians for pre-exposure prophylaxis with antiretroviral drugs for the prevention of HIV-infection in the United States.[3] Similarly, a tenofovir-containing vaginal gel led to a 39% reduction in the risk for HIV infection among women, but a tenofovir vaginal gel is not currently available commercially.[A6] In addition, antiretrovirals can be given after exposure to prevent HIV acquisition (postexposure prophylaxis [PEP]). The CDC and professional organizations have published guidelines for antiretroviral postexposure prophylaxis after sexual, injection drug use, and other nonoccupational exposures to HIV.[4] In these guidelines it is recommended that persons seek care 72 hours or sooner after nonoccupational exposure to the blood, genital secretions, or other potentially infected body fluids of a person known to have HIV infection be offered a 28-day course of antiretroviral therapy.

Transmission in Injection Drug Users

The primary mode of HIV transmission in injection drug users is sharing of contaminated needles and syringes. Sharing of injection paraphernalia ("works") is commonplace among injection drug users and is reinforced by the cultural, economic, and legal environment in that community. The risk for transmission of HIV is highest in injection drug users who share needles and use drugs that are injected more frequently, such as cocaine or methamphetamines.

Prevention Strategies

The primary mode of preventing HIV transmission in PWID is to stop the use of intravenous drugs. Education programs that are culturally sensitive and geared to young audiences have the best chance of preventing drug use. Access to treatment centers for injection drug users is the best approach. However, approximately 80% of active drug users in the United States are not in substance abuse treatment because of either choice or the unavailability of treatment centers. For injection drug users who do not wish to seek treatment or who are unable to gain access to treatment, the most effective way to prevent HIV infection is to avoid sharing needles and paraphernalia. Some communities have adopted programs that provide free needles and syringes for injection drug users, and there is strong evidence that these programs, when implemented properly, are effective in reducing HIV transmission and do not result in increased drug use among participants. Where supplies cannot be obtained, needles and syringes should be cleaned after each use, preferably with readily accessible virucidal cleansers such as chlorine bleach (diluted 1 : 10). As with sexual transmission, preliminary data from Vancouver, Canada, suggest that antiretroviral treatment of injection drug users decreases incidence of HIV among drug users. Most recently, a randomized controlled trial conducted in injection drug users in Thailand demonstrated a 49% reduction in HIV acquisition when tenofovir was given as PrEP. As a result the CDC issued guidance for the use of PrEP among injection drug users but has recommended the use of co-formulated tenofovir plus emtricitabine rather than tenofovir alone as the preferred PrEP regimen among injection drug users.[5] However, this is an off-label indication.

Transmission through Blood Products and Other Tissues

HIV has been transmitted through the transfusion of single-donor blood and blood products, including whole blood, fresh-frozen plasma, packed red blood cells, cryoprecipitate, clotting factors, and platelets. Confidential donor exclusion, as well as the institution of HIV antibody screening in 1985, followed by additional testing for antibodies to HIV-2 and p24 antigen in 1996 and nucleic acid testing in 2002, has reduced the risk for HIV infection through the transfusion of blood or blood products to approximately 1 in 2,135,000. Transmission of HIV by liver, heart, kidney, pancreas, bone, and possibly skin transplantation has been reported. In contrast, relatively avascular tissues such as corneas and processed tissues have not been associated with transmission.

Prevention Strategies

The institution of HIV antibody testing of donated blood and blood products in 1985 has had the most dramatic effect on lowering the incidence of transfusion-related transmission. When combined with voluntary self-deferral and nucleic acid testing, the blood supply in most countries has become virtually free of HIV. Heat inactivation processes for cryoprecipitate and clotting factor concentrates has eliminated transmission of HIV through use of these products. Other products, such as immunoglobulin preparations and hepatitis B vaccines, are produced by fractionation methods that remove HIV and have never been associated with transmission of HIV. Organ and tissue donors should be evaluated and serologically screened in a manner similar to blood donors. In addition, donations of semen and bone from a living donor may be quarantined until subsequent testing has definitively ruled out the possibility of delayed seroconversion in the donor.

Transmission to Health Care Workers

Detailed studies examining the risk associated with specific exposures to health care workers, such as needlestick injuries and mucous membrane exposure, have demonstrated low risk for acquisition of disease in the workplace. More than 3628 health care workers have been prospectively examined in carefully designed surveillance studies at 10 high-incidence medical centers. The overall risk for seroconversion after a percutaneous needlestick from a known HIV-infected source is 0.3% per exposure. A retrospective study conducted by the CDC found that the risk for transmission of HIV to health care workers is increased when the device causing the injury is visibly contaminated with blood, when the device has been used for insertion into a vein or artery, when the device causes a deep injury, or when the source patient dies within 2 months after the exposure. Exposure of mucous membranes to HIV-infected blood has resulted in seroconversion only rarely, and the risk for transmission is estimated to be 0.09% per exposure.

Prevention Strategies

In August 1987, the CDC published guidelines recommending that the principles of "universal precautions" be incorporated into health care settings to minimize exposure of health care workers to blood and body fluids that may be infected with blood-borne pathogens such as HIV. Universal precautions are based on the premise that any patient may be infected with blood-borne infectious agents and it may be difficult, if not impossible, to differentiate those with infection from their uninfected counterparts. All specimens containing blood or blood-tinged fluids obtained from *any* patient should be considered hazardous and handled as such. The use of universal precautions helps minimize the transmission of many transmissible diseases in addition to HIV.

Gowns, protective eyewear, and masks are not usually needed except in circumstances in which splattering or splashing of blood-containing fluids is likely to occur. Health care workers with denuded skin, open lesions, or active dermatitis should avoid direct patient contact and should not process contaminated equipment or materials. Handling of sharp instruments ("sharps") represents the greatest risk for transmission of HIV to health care workers. Although injuries from sharps cannot be eliminated entirely, the number of exposures can be reduced substantially by adhering to guidelines put forth in universal precautions. Before a sharp instrument is used, thought should be given to where the instrument will be disposed after use. Impervious containers should be readily available in all patient care areas and identified by the health care worker *before* the use of sharps. These containers should be checked frequently and should not be allowed to overfill. Used needles should never be manipulated, bent, broken, or recapped. Recapping of needles is the single most common activity that results in needlestick injuries. Technologic developments that do not rely on health care worker compliance, such as self-sheathing needles, also have been important in decreasing the risk for needlestick injury.

Antiretroviral agents are also used for PEP in health care workers. A case-control study suggested that risk for HIV seroconversion after occupational exposure was decreased by approximately 81% with the use of zidovudine alone. Subsequent recommendations have incorporated the newer antiretroviral drugs, as well as risk stratification for the type of exposure, in the management of occupational exposure to HIV. In 2013, the CDC issued revised recommendations for the use of PEP after exposure to HIV among health care workers.[6] The essential elements of management of a health care worker after a needlestick or mucous membrane exposure include appropriately evaluating the donor (patient) and recipient (health care worker) at the time of exposure, counseling of the health care worker, and providing follow-up HIV testing. There is no longer the need to determine the severity of exposure to direct the number of antiretroviral drugs to be used; a regimen containing three or more drugs is now recommended with co-formulated tenofovir/emtricitabine plus raltegravir as the preferred regimen. Antiretroviral drugs for PEP should be initiated within 72 hours of exposure and continued for 4 weeks. The U.S. Public Health Service has established a National Clinicians' Post-Exposure Prophylaxis Hotline (PEPline) to provide expert consultation about the management of health care workers with potential HIV exposure. The PEPline can be accessed at 1-888-448-4911 or through the Internet at http://www.ucsf.edu/hivcntr/Hotlines/PEPline.

PREVENTION INTERVENTIONS FOR INFECTED INDIVIDUALS

Antiretroviral therapy administered to HIV-infected individuals decreases the risk for HIV transmission by over 96%, and thus suppression of HIV replication to undetectable levels is the most effective intervention to decrease HIV transmission from an HIV-infected person. As a result, the U.S. Department of Health and Human Services Antiretroviral treatment guidelines now recommend initiation of antiretroviral treatment regardless of the CD4 cell count and monitoring for viral suppression.

In addition, the CDC, Health Resources and Services Administration, National Institutes of Health, and Infectious Diseases Society of America have published joint recommendations for incorporating HIV prevention into the HIV medical care setting. These guidelines reflect four basic priorities: (1) screening for risky behavior and STIs; (2) providing general and tailored risk reduction messages to patients; (3) when indicated, referring patients for additional risk reduction services and other services that may affect risk reduction (e.g., substance abuse treatment); and (4) ensuring that patients are provided with partner counseling and referral services. HIV-infected persons should be screened and treated for STIs. The CDC's 2010 sexually transmitted disease treatment guidelines recommend that all patients with newly diagnosed HIV infection undergo screening for gonorrhea, chlamydial infection, hepatitis B and C virus infection, and syphilis. Screening for curable STIs (gonorrhea, chlamydial infection, and syphilis) should be performed at least annually in sexually active patients. More frequent screening for STI's might be appropriate depending on individual risk behaviors, the local epidemiology of STIs and whether incident STIs are detected by screening or by presence of symptoms.

PREVENTION IN DEVELOPMENT

As shown in Figure 387-1, many prevention strategies are available, and some are in development. Vaccine strategies are increasingly focused on the generation of different types of antibodies. Broad neutralizing antibodies offer almost compete protection in macaques from infection for several months, suggesting the feasibility of a protective vaccine.[7] Injectable antiretroviral agents in different classes may serve as an advance for PEP and PrEP, and such agents are in phase 2 testing. Delivering of slow-release topical tenofovir from a cervical ring is being examined in two clinical trials.

Grade A References

A1. Cohen MS, Chen YQ, McCauley M, et al. Prevention of HIV-1 infection with early antiretroviral therapy. N Engl J Med. 2011;365:493-505.
A2. Grant RM, Lama JR, Anderson PL, et al. Preexposure chemoprophylaxis for HIV prevention in men who have sex with men. N Engl J Med. 2010;363:2587-2599.
A3. Baeten JM, Donnell D, Ndase P, et al. Antiretroviral prophylaxis for HIV prevention in heterosexual men and women. N Engl J Med. 2012;367:399-410.
A4. Thigpen MC, Kebaabetswe PM, Paxton LA, et al. Antiretroviral preexposure prophylaxis for heterosexual HIV transmission in Botswana. N Engl J Med. 2012;367:423-434.
A5. Choopanya K, Martin M, Sutharasami P, et al. Antiretroviral prophylaxis for HIV infection among people who inject drugs in Bangkok, Thailand: a randomized, double-blind, placebo-controlled trial. Lancet. 2013;381:2083-2090.
A6. Abdool Karim Q, Abdoool Karim SS, Frohlich JA, et al. Effectiveness and safety of tenofovir gel, an antiretroviral microbicide, for the prevention of HIV infection in women. Science. 2010;329:1168-1174.

GENERAL REFERENCES

For the General References and other additional features, please visit Expert Consult at https://expertconsult.inkling.com.

388

ANTIRETROVIRAL THERAPY OF HUMAN IMMUNODEFICIENCY VIRUS AND ACQUIRED IMMUNODEFICIENCY SYNDROME

ROY M. GULICK

The development of effective antiretroviral therapy (ART) for human immunodeficiency virus (HIV) infection is one of the most notable achievements in modern medicine. The first cases of acquired immunodeficiency syndrome (AIDS) were reported from Los Angeles in 1981. In the early to mid-1980s, without any available antiretroviral treatments, the life expectancy of an individual diagnosed with AIDS was only approximately 6 to 12 months. The first antiretroviral drug, zidovudine (azidothymidine, AZT) was approved by the U.S. Food and Drug Administration (FDA) in 1987 on the basis of a short-term survival benefit. Triple-drug therapy was first introduced in the mid-1990s and resulted in a two-thirds decrease in HIV-related deaths within 2 years in developed countries. Today, there are a total of 28 antiretroviral drugs that are approved by the FDA and three-drug combination regimens are the standard of care. The benefits of ART were extended to developing countries, and an estimated over 14 million people currently are taking ART worldwide. The life expectancy of an HIV-infected individual appropriately treated with ART is now estimated to be nearly that of the general population, both in developed[1] and developing countries.[2]

WHEN TO START ART?

The rationale for starting ART early in someone with HIV infection is based on several principles: (1) untreated infection causes progressive immunodeficiency resulting in opportunistic diseases and death; (2) current ART regimens decrease plasma HIV RNA (viral load) levels and the risk for the emergence of drug resistance, as well as increase CD4+ T-lymphocyte counts and general immune function; and (3) current treatment results in years of virologic suppression. In addition, it is now appreciated that ART reduces inflammation and immune activation that leads to end-organ diseases (cardiac, hepatic, neurologic, oncologic, and renal) and that ART reduces HIV transmission.[A1] The rationale for delaying ART traditionally centered on practical factors: medication adherence can be challenging; drug toxicities occur, and the long-term side effects of antiretroviral drugs are not known; and the risk for clinical progression is low in early disease. Additionally, although ART can prevent HIV transmission, drug-resistant virus can be transmitted in the community. In fact, the U.S. Centers for Disease Control and Prevention estimates at least 15% of Americans newly diagnosed with HIV are infected with drug-resistant virus.[3]

Whereas before 2008, U.S. treatment guidelines recommended waiting to start antiretroviral treatment, current guidelines from both the U.S. Department of Health and Human Services and the International Antiviral Society–USA recommend starting ART in *all* HIV-infected patients, regardless of CD4 cell count number, because of both clinical benefits to the patient and reduction in HIV transmission to others.[4,5] This recommendation is supported by the fact that current ART regimens are potent, convenient, and generally well-tolerated, as well as by supportive clinical cohort data[6] and randomized controlled clinical trials.[A2] There are no randomized clinical trial data to support starting ART in patients with CD4 counts greater than 550 cells/μL, and thus some controversy in the field remains, as evidenced by British, European, and World Health Organization treatment guidelines that do not routinely recommend ART in patients with CD4 cell counts greater than 500/μL (Table 388-1).

WHAT TO START?

Since 1987, the FDA has approved 28 antiretroviral drugs from six mechanistic classes (Table 388-2). The goal of ART is to suppress viral replication, prevent the emergence of drug-resistant viral strains, enhance immunologic responses, decrease clinical events, and prolong healthy life. Antiretroviral drugs interfere with individual steps in the HIV replication cycle (Fig. 388-1). The first step of the life cycle is HIV entry, a three-step process

TABLE 388-1 WHEN TO START ANTIRETROVIRAL THERAPY

ANTIRETROVIRAL TREATMENT GUIDELINE AND YEAR (REFERENCE)	AIDS/ SYMPTOMS	ASYMPTOMATIC			
		CD4 <200	CD4 200-349	CD4 350-499	CD4 ≥500
U.S. Department of Health and Human Services (DHHS) 2014 http://www.aidsinfo.nih.gov	Yes	Yes	Yes	Yes	Yes
International Antiviral Society–USA 2014 *JAMA.* 2014;312:390	Yes	Yes	Yes	Yes	Yes
British HIV Association (BHIVA) 2013 *HIV Med.* 2014;15(suppl 1):1-85 http://www.bhiva.org	Yes	Yes	Yes	Certain patients	Certain patients
European AIDS Clinical Society (EACS) 2014 http://www.europeanaidsclinicalsociety.org/	Yes	Yes	Yes	Certain patients	Certain patients
World Health Organization (WHO) 2013 http://www.who.int/hiv/pub/guidelines/arv2013/en/index.html	Yes	Yes	Yes	Yes	No

TABLE 388-2 ANTIRETROVIRAL DRUGS

MECHANISTIC DRUG CLASS	GENERIC NAME	ABBREVIATION(S)	TRADE NAME	YEAR OF U.S. FDA APPROVAL
HIV NUCLEOSIDE ANALOGUE REVERSE TRANSCRIPTASE INHIBITORS (NRTIs)				
	zidovudine	ZDV, AZT	Retrovir	1987
	didanosine	ddI	Videx	1991
	zalcitabine	ddC	Hivid	1992*
	stavudine	d4T	Zerit	1994
	lamivudine	3TC	Epivir	1995
	abacavir	ABC	Ziagen	1998
	tenofovir	TDF	Viread	2001
	emtricitabine	FTC	Emtriva	2003
HIV NON-NUCLEOSIDE ANALOGUE REVERSE TRANSCRIPTASE INHIBITORS (NNRTIs)				
	nevirapine	NVP	Viramune	1996
	delavirdine	DLV	Rescriptor	1997
	efavirenz	EFV	Sustiva	1998
	etravirine	ETR	Intelence	2008
	rilpivirine	RPV	Edurant	2010
HIV PROTEASE INHIBITORS (PIs)				
	saquinavir	SQV	Invirase	1995
	ritonavir	RTV	Norvir	1996
	indinavir	IDV	Crixivan	1996
	nelfinavir	NFV	Viracept	1997
	amprenavir	APV	Agenerase	1999*
	lopinavir/ritonavir	LPV/r	Kaletra	2000
	atazanavir	ATV	Reyataz	2003
	fosamprenavir	FPV	Lexiva	2003
	tipranavir	TPV	Aptivus	2005
	darunavir	DRV	Prezista	2006
HIV ENTRY INHIBITORS (EIs)				
Fusion inhibitor	enfuvirtide	ENF, T-20	Fuzeon	2003
CCR5 antagonist	maraviroc	MVC	Selzentry	2007
HIV INTEGRASE INHIBITORS (INSTIs)				
	raltegravir	RAL	Isentress	2007
	elvitegravir	EVG	Viteka	2011
	dolutegravir	DTG	Tivicay	2013

*Withdrawn.
U.S. FDA = U.S. Food and Drug Administration; HIV = human immunodeficiency virus.

starting with binding of the HIV external membrane glycoprotein (gp120) to the CD4 receptor on the surface of the T lymphocyte. This binding induces a conformational change in gp120 permitting the second step of HIV entry, binding to a second cellular receptor, the chemokine receptor, either CCR5 (bound by R5 viruses) or CXCR4 (bound by X4 viruses). Some HIV strains are dual-tropic and can bind to either the CCR5 or CXCR4 receptor, and some individuals are infected with a mixed population of R5 and X4 viral strains. Binding to the chemokine receptor induces an additional conformational change allowing the viral protein gp41 to pierce the target cell membrane and then fold in on itself in a coil-on-coil interaction, leading to fusion of the viral and cellular membranes and extrusion of the viral particle contents (viral RNA, viral proteins) into the cytoplasm of the cell.

Inside the cell, viral RNA is transcribed to viral DNA by a viral-specific enzyme called *HIV reverse transcriptase.* Following transcription, two strands of viral DNA form a double-stranded complex catalyzed by a second viral-specific enzyme called *HIV integrase,* which also promotes transport of the viral DNA complex into the nucleus of the cell and strand transfer—the random integration of the viral DNA into the cellular genome. At the point of viral DNA integration, the cell is infected for life. It may enter a latent period, with a cellular lifespan as long as 60 years, or may be activated to transcribe both cellular and viral DNA into RNA and then translate RNA into proteins, including viral proteins, which assemble at the surface of the cell and then bud off into new viral particles. After budding, a third viral-specific enzyme, *HIV protease,* cleaves viral precursor proteins, a step that is necessary

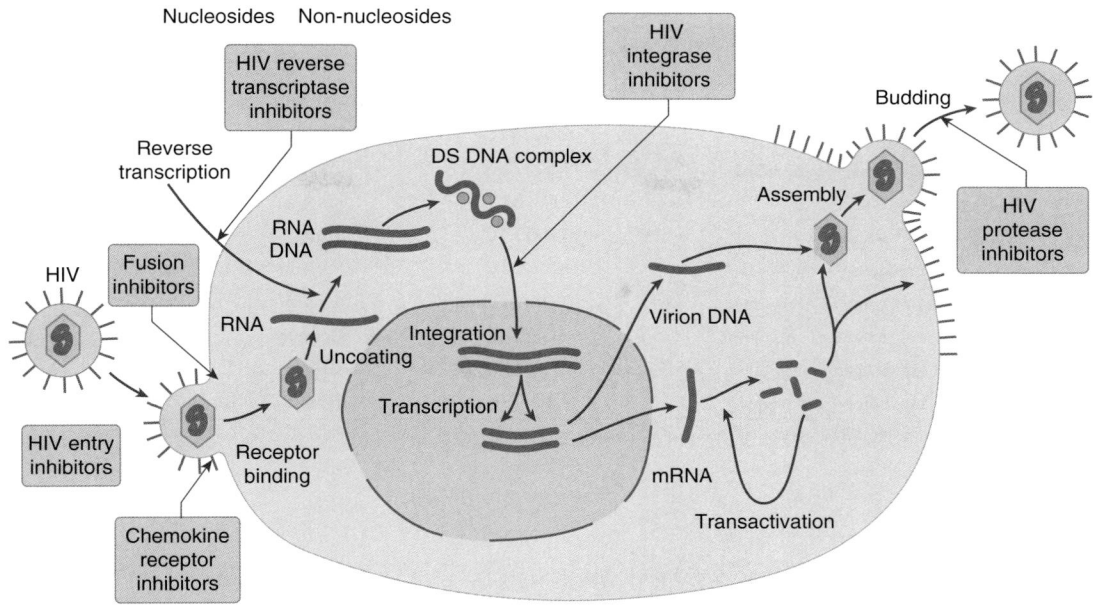

FIGURE 388-1. Life cycle of human immunodeficiency virus (*HIV*) and mechanisms of action of the six antiretroviral drug classes. See text (What to Start? section) for details.

for viral maturation and infectivity. One infected cell can produce hundreds to thousands of viral particles, and many will be capable of starting the process again on encountering another CD4+ T lymphocyte.

Antiretroviral drugs inhibit different steps of the HIV replication cycle (see Fig. 388-1). Two kinds of HIV entry inhibitors target the first step in the HIV life cycle, viral entry, by inhibiting either CCR5 chemokine receptor binding (CCR5 antagonists) or membrane fusion (fusion inhibitors). The nucleoside analogue reverse transcriptase inhibitors (NRTIs) target the viral-specific enzyme *HIV reverse transcriptase.* A second class of HIV reverse transcriptase inhibitors are the non-nucleoside analogue reverse transcriptase inhibitors (NNRTIs), which bind to a different part of the same enzyme. The integrase strand transfer inhibitors (INSTIs) inhibit the viral-specific enzyme *HIV integrase* by specifically targeting the transfer of viral DNA to the host cell genome. The HIV protease inhibitors (PIs) bind to the active site of the *HIV protease* enzyme and prevent precursor protein cleavage, viral maturation, and infectivity.

Initially, single nucleoside analogue therapy was studied for the treatment of HIV infection. However, virologic suppression, immune enhancement, and clinical benefits were only transient and drug-resistant virus emerged (Fig. 388-2). When more than one drug was available, dual nucleoside analogue therapy was studied and found to be better than single-drug therapy, but virologic, immunologic, and clinical benefits again were only temporary. A three-drug regimen was superior to two-drug therapy and led to essentially complete virologic suppression, preventing the emergence of drug-resistant viral strains and increasing CD4 cell counts, and resulted in durable effects. With potent virologic suppression and immunologic recovery came dramatic decreases in HIV-related illnesses and prolonged survival.

Despite their life-saving potential, early antiretroviral drug regimens had significant associated side effects and toxicities and were complicated to take. Some early drugs were associated with anemia and leukopenia (zidovudine), peripheral neuropathy (didanosine, zalcitabine, stavudine), pancreatitis (didanosine, stavudine), kidney stones (indinavir), nausea and vomiting (ritonavir), diarrhea (nelfinavir), and Stevens-Johnson syndrome (nevirapine). A common three-drug regimen in 1996 consisted of 20 pills, divided for dosing every 8 hours. Whereas the first decade of ART developed effective regimens that controlled viral replication, the second decade was about developing potent, well-tolerated, and convenient regimens to enable long-term use. Use of low-dose ritonavir or the newer drug cobicistat inhibits the cytochrome P450 3A4 isoenzyme, decreasing the metabolism of most protease inhibitors and the integrase inhibitor elvitegravir, allowing once- or twice-daily dosing; this strategy is known as pharmacokinetic boosting. Additional antiretroviral drugs were approved, and co-formulations (more than one

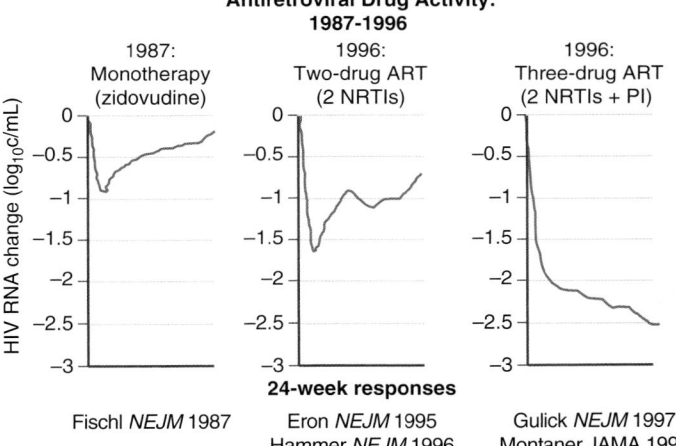

FIGURE 388-2. Antiretroviral drug (*ART*) activity: 1987 to 1996. Major clinical trials leading to finding of sustained efficacy of three-drug antiretroviral therapy. NRTI = nucleoside analogue reverse transcriptase inhibitors; PI = protease inhibitor. (1987: Fischl MA, et al. *N Engl J Med.* 1987;317:185-191; 1994: Eron JJ, et al. *N Engl J Med.* 1995;333:1662-1669 and Hammer SM, et al. *N Engl J Med.* 1996;335:1081-1090; 1996: Gulick RM, et al. *N Engl J Med.* 1997; 337:734-739 and Montaner JS, et al. 1998;279: 930-937.)

medicine in a single pill) were developed such that one-pill, once-daily HIV treatment was possible (Table 388-3).[A3-A6]

Currently, there are four FDA-approved, one-pill, once-daily regimens; these are popular with providers and patients and lead to excellent adherence, with virologic suppression rates over 85% in some groups. Potency, convenience, and tolerability are essential qualities of current antiretroviral drug regimens and account for the durable clinical benefits. Current recommended initial regimens in the U.S. ART guidelines (Table 388-4) are combinations of two nucleoside analogues together with a third drug (non-nucleoside reverse transcriptase inhibitor, protease inhibitor, or integrase inhibitor). Globally, the most widely used antiretroviral regimen is two nucleoside analogues combined with a non-nucleoside analogue (NNRTI). A study from Denmark estimated that the life expectancy of someone with HIV infection who is appropriately treated and is free from comorbidities (hepatitis C infection, injection drug use) is now that of the age-matched general population.

TABLE 388-3 ANTIRETROVIRAL FIXED-DOSE COMBINATIONS

DRUG CLASS(ES)	GENERIC NAMES	ABBREVIATION(S)	TRADE NAMES	DOSING	YEAR OF U.S. FDA APPROVAL
2 NRTI	zidovudine + lamivudine	ZDV/3TC	Combivir	Twice daily	1997
3 NRTI	abacavir + zidovudine + lamivudine	ABC/ZDV/3TC	Trizivir	Twice daily	2000
Boosted PI	lopinavir + ritonavir	LPV/RTV	Kaletra	Once or twice daily	2000
2 NRTI	tenofovir + emtricitabine	TDF/FTC	Truvada	Once daily	2004
2 NRTI	abacavir + lamivudine	ABC/3TC	Epzicom	Once daily	2004
2 NRTI + NNRTI	tenofovir + emtricitabine + efavirenz	TDF/FTC/EFV	Atripla	Once daily	2006
2 NRTI + NNRTI	tenofovir + emtricitabine + rilpivirine	TDF/FTC/RPV	Complera	Once daily	2011
2 NRTI + boosted INSTI	tenofovir + emtricitabine + elvitegravir + cobicistat	TDF/FTC/EVG/c	Stribild	Once daily	2012
2 NRTI + INSTI	abacavir + lamivudine + dolutegravir	ABC/3TC/DTG	Triumeq	Once daily	2014

NNRTI = non-nucleoside reverse transcriptase inhibitor; NRTI = nucleoside analogue reverse transcriptase inhibitor; PI = protease inhibitor.

TABLE 388-4 RECOMMENDED INITIAL ANTIRETROVIRAL DRUG REGIMENS

REGIMEN*	DRUGS
Non-nucleoside (NNRTI)-based	tenofovir/emtricitabine/efavirenz (co-formulated)
	tenofovir/emtricitabine (co-formulated) + atazanavir/ritonavir[†]
	abacavir/emtricitabine + efavirenz[‡]
	tenofovir/emtricitabine/rilpivirine (co-formulated)[§]
Protease inhibitor (PI)-based	tenofovir/emtricitabine (co-formulated) + darunavir/ritonavir[†]
	abacavir/lamivudine + atazanavir/ritonavir[†]
Integrase strand transfer inhibitor (INSTI)-based	tenofovir/emtricitabine (co-formulated) + raltegravir
	tenofovir/emtricitabine/elvitegravir/cobicistat (co-formulated)
	tenofovir/emtricitabine + dolutegravir
	abacavir/lamivudine + dolutegravir

*From Panel on Antiretroviral Guidelines for Adults and Adolescents. Guidelines for the use of antiretroviral agents in HIV-1-infected adults and adolescents. Department of Health and Human Services. http://aidsinfo.nih.gov/contentfiles/lvguidelines/AdultandAdolescentGL.pdf. November 13, 2014.
[†]Ritonavir and cobicistat are each used as pharmacokinetic boosters.
[‡]Only for baseline HIV RNA <100,000 copies/ml.
[§]Only for baseline HIV RNA <100,000 copies/ml and CD4 >200 cells/uL.

⬤ WHEN TO CHANGE ANTIRETROVIRAL THERAPY?

In a stable patient on ART, HIV RNA should be monitored every 3 to 6 months. Even with virologic suppression rates of over 85%, some patients will experience antiretroviral treatment failure, most commonly presenting as virologic failure, with a once-suppressed viral load level now being detectable above the limit of the HIV RNA assay (20, 40, or 50 copies/mL). The reasons for regimen failure can include suboptimal adherence, baseline drug resistance or cross-resistance, prior use of ART, use of less potent antiretroviral drug regimens, drug levels and drug-drug interactions, penetration into tissue reservoirs (e.g., genital tract, central nervous system [CNS]), suboptimal provider experience, and other, unknown reasons. Also, more than one factor may play a role in an individual patient. One of the challenges with treatment failure is to try to determine the cause of failure and then select the next regimen that can address and overcome the reason for failure.

U.S. ART guidelines suggest focusing on virologic failure and changing antiretroviral regimens promptly when failure is confirmed. Virologic failure can be defined as repeated detection of HIV RNA levels in a drug-adherent patient. HIV RNA levels suppressed below the level of detection of the assay are unlikely to result in the emergence of drug-resistant viral strains. Levels greater than 200 copies/mL (and certainly 500 copies/mL) will lead to the selection of drug-resistant viral strains and result in treatment failure. More controversial are HIV RNA levels between the level of detection and 200 copies/mL that may represent a higher virologic set point rather than ongoing viral replication and may not necessitate treatment change.

HIV is prone to errors in gene replication, and thus an individual is infected not with just one virus but a "swarm" of related viral strains with distinct genetic mutational patterns. Drug resistance is conferred by viral strains with specific amino acid substitutions in viral proteins (HIV reverse transcriptase, HIV protease, HIV integrase) that are selected for in the presence of an antiretroviral drug. For example, with ongoing replication in the presence of the

nucleoside analogue emtricitabine or lamivudine, a viral strain with the substitution of valine for methionine at amino acid position 184 (M184V) of HIV reverse transcriptase will be selected and confer complete resistance to these drugs. Drugs with which single substitutions confer resistance are considered to have a low barrier to resistance and include the nucleoside analogues emtricitabine and lamivudine, the NNRTIs efavirenz and nevirapine, and the integrase inhibitors elvitegravir and raltegravir. Drugs that require multiple substitutions are considered to have a high barrier to resistance, including the nucleoside analogue zidovudine and most of the HIV protease inhibitors. Drugs with overlapping resistance patterns lead to cross resistance. For example, a patient who develops resistance to emtricitabine with the M184V substitution will have complete cross resistance to lamivudine, even though the patient never took lamivudine. Drug resistance can be assessed by an HIV genotype (that identifies amino acid substitutions that must be correlated with drug resistance) or an HIV phenotype (that assesses viral growth in the presence of each of the drugs).[7]

Another common clinical conundrum is immunologic failure—a patient taking ART who achieves virologic suppression but fails to increase the CD4 cell count. The causes of immunologic failure are not clear, but associations with various factors, including CD4 count less than 200 cells/μL at the time of ART initiation, older age, coinfections, medications (e.g., zidovudine; the combination of didanosine and tenofovir), persistent immune activation, and loss of regenerative potential have been reported. There is no accepted treatment for immunologic failure. Neither changing nor adding antiretroviral drugs results in an improved CD4 cell response. Immune-based therapies have been studied but are not effective. In two large randomized clinical trials, interleukin-2 was associated with increased CD4 cell counts, but failed to demonstrate associated clinical benefits. Current management is to continue antiretroviral therapy, optimize opportunistic infection prophylaxes, and follow the patient closely.

WHAT ANTIRETROVIRAL THERAPPY TO CHANGE TO?

The current goal for all HIV-infected patients taking ART, regardless of treatment experience, is to maximally suppress the viral load level below the level of assay detection.[4] In a treatment-experienced patient, this is done by reviewing the ART history with a focus on adherence, tolerability, and possible drug-drug interactions; conduct drug-resistance testing (HIV genotype for first or second failure; HIV genotype and phenotype for more advanced failure); identify susceptible drugs and drug classes and, ultimately, design a subsequent regimen with at least two (and preferably three) fully active antiretroviral agents.[4]

In the last 10 years, a number of newer antiretroviral drugs have made this goal possible, including drugs in existing mechanistic classes with activity against class-resistant virus (the HIV protease inhibitors darunavir and tipranavir and the HIV NNRTI etravirine) and drugs with new mechanisms of action (the fusion inhibitor enfuvirtide; the CCR5 antagonist maraviroc; and the HIV integrase inhibitors raltegravir, elvitegravir, and dolutegravir). Several recent studies in treatment-experienced patients show that new active antiretroviral regimens result in virologic suppression rates that are nearly the same as those for treatment-naïve patients.[8] A recent study found that including nucleoside analogues in subsequent regimens is not necessary if the regimen contains more than two active antiretroviral drugs.

SIDE EFFECTS AND TOXICITY

Antiretroviral drugs (like all drugs) are associated with side effects and toxicity.[4] Probably the most common side effect of ART as a group is gastrointestinal (nausea, vomiting, diarrhea), although some drugs are more associated than others (e.g., zidovudine, ritonavir). Toxicities may be divided according to seriousness and drug classes. Life-threatening toxicities occur and include drug-related hepatitis associated with NNRTIs and protease inhibitors. Of these, the NNRTI nevirapine is unique in causing drug-related hepatitis more frequently in patients with higher CD4 counts (>250 cells/µL in women and > 400 cells/µL in men), likely due to an immunologic mechanism. A hypersensitivity reaction characterized by rash and constitutional symptoms is associated with the nucleoside analogue abacavir and the NNRTIs etravirine and nevirapine. An elegant study linked the abacavir-associated hypersensitivity reaction to a genetic locus that can be screened for in patients (HLA-B*5701, at a cost of approximately $50); if the drug is avoided in patients with the genetic marker, the risk for HSR is minimized.[A7] Lactic acidosis has been associated with the nucleoside analogue class (particularly stavudine and zalcitabine). The NNRTIs, although structurally unrelated, all are associated with rash; Stevens-Johnson syndrome is rarely described with etravirine or nevirapine. Teratogenicity is described with efavirenz (FDA pregnancy category D); however, newer U.S. recommendations allow continuing the drug in a pregnant woman with maximal virologic suppression, although the drug should not be started in a pregnant woman.[9]

Acute side effects can be troubling to the patient and can lead to suboptimal adherence. Providers should be in close contact with a patient starting a new antiretroviral regimen and have a low threshold to substitute offending drugs for side effects or toxicities. As noted, probably the most common side effect of antiretroviral drugs is gastrointestinal toxicity, though this often can be managed by taking ART with food. Zidovudine causes anemia, neutropenia, and fatigue. Efavirenz causes CNS side effects (e.g., vivid dreams, somnolence) in up to 50% of people and should be dosed at bedtime. Atazanavir causes increased indirect bilirubin by inhibiting uridine 5'-diphosphoglucuronosyltransferase, which can be associated with frank jaundice but is not associated with other liver test abnormalities.

With the current expectation that ART is life-long, chronic and cumulative toxicities also are important. Increased cardiovascular events are associated with some protease inhibitors[10] and controversially with abacavir. Indinavir and atazanavir cause renal stones. Metabolic changes, including hyperglycemia and frank diabetes, hyperlactatemia, and/or hyperlipidemia, are associated with stavudine and some protease inhibitors. Morphologic changes occur and can be very distressing for patients, including lipoatrophy (loss of fat in the face and extremities) associated with stavudine and zidovudine, and lipoaccumulation (gain of fat in the breasts, abdomen, and dorsocervical fat bad [buffalo hump]) associated with some protease inhibitors. Some NRTIs, including didanosine and stavudine, cause a progressive toxic peripheral neuropathy. Tenofovir is associated with proximal renal tubular dysfunction characterized by hypophosphatemia, proteinuria, glycosuria, and eventually, elevated creatinine. Tenofovir also has been associated with loss of bone mineral density over the first year of treatment that appears to stabilize thereafter. Newer antiretroviral drugs and investigational antiretroviral agents often are developed and selected for less toxicity.

SPECIAL POPULATIONS

Acute Infection

Previously debated, it is now recommended that an individual identified with acute HIV infection start three-drug ART. ART reduces signs and symptoms of acute HIV and also prevents ongoing HIV transmission. Because of the risk for acquiring drug-resistant HIV, ART should be started while awaiting the results of the HIV genotype. Many experts would start a protease inhibitor–containing regimen and then adjust when the genotypic results are available.

Acute Opportunistic Infection

A patient presenting with an acute opportunistic infection who was not previously known to have HIV infection prompts the question of the optimal time to start ART. Despite prior concerns of drug-drug interactions and precipitating the immune reconstitution inflammatory syndrome (IRIS) (Chapter 395), ART demonstrates benefits in patients with acute opportunistic infections. One study of patients with a treatable opportunistic infection diagnosed in the prior 2 weeks (the majority with *Pneumocystis* pneumonia) randomized them to start ART within 48 hours or to wait at least 4 weeks.[A8] There were significantly fewer clinical events (disease progression and death) in the group that started ART earlier. Additional studies of patients with tuberculosis also demonstrated clinical benefits to starting ART earlier, particularly in patients with CD4 counts less than 50 cells/µL.[A9-A11] Starting ART within 2 weeks of an opportunistic infection is now considered the standard of care. An exception is CNS opportunistic infections (e.g., cryptococcal or tuberculous meningitis) in which studies demonstrated increased mortality in patients who started ART earlier.[11,12]

Coinfection with Hepatitis B

If treatment is started for either infection, both need to be treated optimally: two active drugs for hepatitis B and three active drugs for HIV. The antiretroviral drugs emtricitabine, lamivudine, and tenofovir have activity against both viruses; thus, a suitable regimen to treat both infections would be tenofovir, emtricitabine (or lamivudine), and a third antiretroviral drug. Stopping drugs with activity against hepatitis B may result in a serious hepatitis flare.

Coinfection with Hepatitis C

The optimal time to treat hepatitis C infection in a patient with HIV infection is not known. The hepatitis C drug ribavirin has significant interactions with the antiretroviral drugs didanosine, stavudine, and zidovudine, and these combinations should be avoided. The newer hepatitis C protease inhibitors are unrelated to the HIV protease inhibitors and have no activity against HIV but may have significant drug interactions with HIV NNRTIs and protease inhibitors, and this is an active area of research.

Pregnancy

The recently updated U.S. Perinatal Treatment Guidelines recommend ART for prevention of mother-to-child transmission of HIV for all pregnant women, regardless of CD4 cell count or HIV RNA level. Based on their safety records, recommended drugs in pregnancy include the NRTIs lamivudine and zidovudine; the NNRTI nevirapine; and the PIs atazanavir, lopinavir, and ritonavir. Other drugs are considered alternatives (e.g., the NRTIs abacavir and tenofovir and the PI darunavir), although insufficient data are available on newer drugs (the NNRTIs etravirine and rilpivirine, and the CCR5 antagonist maraviroc). Efavirenz is teratogenic and should not be started in pregnant women; however, updated guidelines recommend continuing efavirenz in a women found to be pregnant if she is maximally virologically suppressed.

ANTIRETROVIRAL THERAPY FOR PREVENTION

One of the most successful HIV prevention strategies is the use of ART, both in HIV-infected and HIV-uninfected people. The first example of this was the prevention of HIV-infected mother-to-child transmission by giving the mother ART. In a classic study, the use of a single drug, zidovudine, in an HIV-infected mother reduced the risk for transmission to her infant from 25 to 8%. Current standard of care is to treat the mother with three-drug ART, with a resultant reduction in the risk for transmission to less than 1%.

A recent study randomized HIV-infected individuals with CD4 counts of 350 to 550/μL who were members of a committed couple with an HIV-uninfected individual to start ART immediately or to wait until the CD4 count decreased to less than 250 cells/μL and followed the seronegative partners for HIV seroconversion. Of 28 linked cases, 27 occurred in the group not on ART versus only 1 in an individual on ART (who had only recently started); thus, treating the infected individual with ART was associated with a 96% reduction in transmission to the HIV-uninfected partner.

Giving ART to at-risk HIV-uninfected individuals to avoid infection also is a strategy that has been explored. Postexposure prophylaxis is recommended on the basis of an older case-control study of health care workers exposed to HIV in which taking zidovudine was associated with an 81% decrease in the risk for seroconversion compared to no prophylaxis. The U.S. Centers for Disease Control and Prevention (CDC) recommends administering three-drug ART for 4 weeks following significant exposure (occupational or nonoccupational) to HIV.[13,14]

Pre-exposure prophylaxis (PrEP)[15] is a newer strategy in which one- or two-drug ART is given to HIV-uninfected individuals who are at risk for acquiring HIV infection on the basis of published studies in men who have sex with men,[A12] serodiscordant heterosexual couples,[A13] sexually active heterosexuals,[A14] and, most recently, injection drug users.[A15] Notably, two other PrEP studies in African women failed to show a benefit, although this may have been due to suboptimal adherence.[A16] Current U.S. CDC guidance recommends PrEP for high-risk individuals with two-drug ART with tenofovir-emtricitabine (coformulated) following exclusion of acute or chronic HIV infection, ongoing monitoring of HIV status and renal function, screening for sexually transmitted diseases, and risk reduction counseling and condom distribution.

CURE

Although current ART is highly effective, it is not curative. Soon after infection, HIV establishes a latent-CD4+ T-lymphocyte cell reservoir that can persist for an estimated 60 years. Even with years of ART-induced prolonged virologic suppression, the latent-cell reservoir does not decrease significantly. Strategies of intensification of ART by changing or adding additional antiretroviral drugs have not been successful in decreasing the reservoir. In 2009, the first known cure of HIV infection was reported: a 40 year-old man with HIV infection well controlled on ART developed acute myelogenous leukemia and underwent radiation, cytotoxic chemotherapy, and ultimately a bone marrow transplant from a donor with a deletion in the gene that codes for the CCR5 receptor that is required for HIV entry.[16] The patient's course was complicated by transplant rejection, administration of antirejection medications, cessation of ART, and a second bone marrow transplant. Ultimately, his HIV RNA remained suppressed below detection in the plasma in the absence of ART, his CD4 cell count returned to normal levels, and additional intensive investigations failed to identify replication-competent virus. After more than 5 years off of ART, he is considered to be cured. This case report is intriguing in that the cause of the cure is not clear (radiotherapy, chemotherapy, the CCR5-negative transplants, graft rejection, antirejection medications, or a combination of these), but the fact that it occurred is stimulating an intense research agenda for HIV cure.

Grade A References

A1. Cohen MS, Chen YQ, McCauley M, et al. Prevention of HIV-1 infection with early antiretroviral therapy. N Engl J Med. 2011;365:493-505.

A2. Severe P, Juste MA, Ambroise A, et al. Early versus standard antiretroviral therapy for HIV-infected adults in Haiti. N Engl J Med. 2010;363:257-265.

A3. Cohen CJ, Andrade-Villanueva J, Clotet B, et al. Rilpivirine versus efavirenz with two background nucleoside or nucleotide reverse transcriptase inhibitors in treatment-naïve adults infected with HIV-1 (THRIVE): a phase 3, randomised, non-inferiority trial. Lancet. 2011;378:229-237.

A4. Molina JM, Cahn P, Grinsztejn B, et al. Rilpivirine versus efavirenz with tenofovir and emtricitabine in treatment-naïve adults infected with HIV-1 (ECHO): a phase 3 randomised double-blind active-controlled trial. Lancet. 2011;378:238-246.

A5. DeJesus E, Rockstroh JK, Henry K, et al. Co-formulated elvitegravir, cobicistat, emtricitabine, and tenofovir disoproxil fumarate versus ritonavir-boosted atazanavir plus co-formulated emtricitabine and tenofovir disoproxil fumarate for initial treatment of HIV-1 infection: a randomised, double-blind, phase 3, non-inferiority trial. Lancet. 2012;379:2429-2438.

A6. Sax PE, DeJesus E, Mills A, et al. Co-formulated elvitegravir, cobicistat, emtricitabine, and tenofovir versus co-formulated efavirenz, emtricitabine, and tenofovir for initial treatment of HIV-1 infection: a randomised, double-blind, phase 3 trial, analysis of results after 48 weeks. Lancet. 2012;379:2439-2448.

A7. Mallal S, Phillips E, Carosi G, et al. HLA-B*5701 screening for hypersensitivity to abacavir. N Engl J Med. 2008;358:568-579.

A8. Zolopa A, Andersen J, Powderly W, et al. Early antiretroviral therapy reduces AIDS progression/death in individuals with acute opportunistic infections: a multicenter randomized strategy trial. PLoS ONE. 2009;4:e5575.

A9. Abdool Karim SS, Naidoo K, Grobler A, et al. Integration of antiretroviral therapy with tuberculosis treatment. N Engl J Med. 2011;365:1492-1501.

A10. Blanc FX, Sok T, Laureillard D, et al. Earlier versus later start of antiretroviral therapy in HIV-infected adults with tuberculosis. N Engl J Med. 2011;365:1471-1481.

A11. Havlir DV, Kendall MA, Ive P, et al. Timing of antiretroviral therapy for HIV-1 infection and tuberculosis. N Engl J Med. 2011;365:1482-1491.

A12. Grant RM, Lama JR, Anderson PL, et al. Preexposure chemoprophylaxis for HIV prevention in men who have sex with men. N Engl J Med. 2010;363:2587-2599.

A13. Baeten JM, Donnell D, Ndase P, et al. Antiretroviral prophylaxis for HIV prevention in heterosexual men and women. N Engl J Med. 2012;367:399-410.

A14. Thigpen MC, Kebaabetswe PM, Paxton LA, et al. Antiretroviral preexposure prophylaxis for heterosexual HIV transmission in Botswana. N Engl J Med. 2012;367:423-434.

A15. Choopanya K, Martin M, Suntharasamai P, et al. Antiretroviral prophylaxis for HIV infection in injecting drug users in Bangkok, Thailand (the Bangkok Tenofovir Study): a randomised, double-blind, placebo-controlled phase 3 trial. Lancet. 2013;381:2083-2090.

A16. Van Damme L, Corneli A, Ahmed K, et al. Preexposure prophylaxis for HIV infection among African women. N Engl J Med. 2012;367:411-422.

GENERAL REFERENCES

For the General References and other additional features, please visit Expert Consult at https://expertconsult.inkling.com.

389

INFECTIOUS AND METABOLIC COMPLICATIONS OF HUMAN IMMUNODEFICIENCY VIRUS AND ACQUIRED IMMUNODEFICIENCY SYNDROME

HENRY MASUR, LETHA M. HEALEY, AND COLLEEN HADIGAN

INFECTIOUS COMPLICATIONS

The initial cases of the acquired immunodeficiency syndrome (AIDS) were identified when unusual infectious diseases occurred in patients who had no prior diagnosis of an immunodeficiency. *Pneumocystis* pneumonia (PCP), toxoplasma encephalitis, cytomegalovirus (CMV) retinitis, and *Mycobacterium avium* bacteremia, as well as Kaposi sarcoma and central nervous system (CNS) lymphoma were so unusual in previously healthy patients that suspicion was quickly raised that the patients must have had some new form of immune deficit, especially when individual patients manifested several such infections either serially or concurrently, and when the number of such patients rapidly increased. The specific infectious syndromes were so characteristic of this new syndrome that their occurrence in previously healthy patients was soon considered as "AIDS defining" until the retroviral etiology of the syndrome was discovered and diagnostic tests for human immunodeficiency virus (HIV) became available for widespread clinical testing.

Despite the widespread availability of effective antiretroviral regimens in the United States since the late 1990s, AIDS-related opportunistic infections are still seen frequently at many health care facilities, especially those serving populations with poor access to health care. In the United States, opportunistic infections occur in two distinct populations: those who are not under effective care and those in whom effective antiretroviral therapy (ART) has recently been started.[1]

At least 25% of HIV-infected patients in the United States are unaware of their retroviral infection. This group often presents to health care facilities with opportunistic infections as their initial clue that they have HIV infection. A substantial number of patients, additionally, are aware of their HIV infection but are not in care as a result of economic, behavioral, or social factors. These patients also present with initial or serial opportunistic infections because they are not benefitting from stable and effective ART.

A second population who develop opportunistic infections includes patients who have access to care and are durably suppressed virologically. In this group, opportunistic infections develop when the initiation of ART unmasks the presence of opportunistic pathogens, creating symptomatic clinical syndromes. In addition, immune reconstitution inflammatory syndromes occur in the first few weeks or months after initiation of ART, representing exaggerated immune responses to viable organisms or to antigen (Chapter 395).

In addition to the relatively acute opportunistic infections that have been traditionally associated with AIDS, as patients live longer they are developing increasing morbidity and mortality due to certain viruses such as hepatitis C virus (HCV), and hepatitis B virus (HBV) (Chapter 149), as well as human papillomavirus (HPV) (Chapter 373).[2] HCV and HBV progression is accelerated in HIV-infected patients compared to HIV-uninfected patients, leading to earlier development of cirrhosis, liver failure, and hepatoma.[3,4] HPV is associated with cervical carcinoma and anal carcinoma, as well as oral cancers.

In addition to opportunistic infections and malignant neoplasms, an unexpected complication of chronic HIV disease in patients who have suppressed HIV viral loads has been a persistent inflammatory state that appears to be related to low-level HIV viremia. This viremia is usually below the level of detection of standard clinical assays for blood and may be related to viral replication in poorly understood reservoirs. The persistent inflammatory state appears to accelerate atherosclerotic cardiovascular and cerebrovascular disease, renal disease, and hepatic disease. This persistent inflammatory state interacts with the AIDS-related metabolic dysfunctions, including dysglycemias and dyslipidemias, which exacerbate and complicate the inflammation-induced accelerated atherosclerosis.[5,6]

PATHOBIOLOGY

HIV infection causes cellular immune dysfunction by multifaceted mechanisms that include reducing the number and function of CD4 lymphocytes. The immune defect in patients with HIV infection is unique: in no other population do PCP, toxoplasma encephalitis, CMV retinitis, cryptococcal meningitis, cryptosporidiosis, microsporidiosis, and Kaposi sarcoma occur so frequently and with such characteristic presentations. The opportunistic infections that occur in patients with HIV infection differ substantially in their prevalence and natural history compared with patients with other immunodeficiencies. They differ in subtle ways in terms of response to therapy and prevention from the syndromes and causative organisms that occur in patients with other immunologic disorders due to corticosteroids or calcineurin inhibitors, for instance, or from immunologic and inflammatory defects associated with neutropenia or antibody deficiency or complement disorders.

The number of circulating CD4 cells is an excellent indicator of patient prognosis and of susceptibility to opportunistic infection for patients with HIV/AIDS (Fig. 389-1). Monitoring CD4 counts prospectively has thus become a cornerstone of patient management. The blood HIV viral load is also an independent predictor of host susceptibility to opportunistic infection, but is not nearly as sensitive and specific for estimating survival or for

assessing susceptibility to opportunistic infection as are CD4 counts.[7] Although CD4 cells are enormously important to host defenses in all persons, the circulating CD4 count is not nearly as specific and sensitive a predictor of opportunistic infection susceptibility in any other patient population as they are in patients with HIV infection.

The specific opportunistic infections that an HIV-infected patient develops are influenced not only by the patient's specific immunologic defects but also by environmental and behavioral factors. For instance, in areas of the world where exposure to *M. tuberculosis* is common, tuberculosis is a major cause of morbidity and mortality in patients with AIDS regardless of CD4 count, although the incidence of disease increases as the CD4 count declines. In contrast, however, in areas of the world such as the United States where tuberculosis exposure is relatively uncommon, tuberculosis is rarely seen except in immigrants and persons exposed to special populations, such as those in prisons or homeless shelters. Other mycobacteria, such as the environmental pathogen *Mycobacterium avium,* have become much more common than tuberculosis. Similarly, in many areas of the developing world, salmonellosis is a common complication of HIV infection and often causes diarrhea and life-threatening bacteremic disease. In the developed world, however, salmonella exposure is much less frequent and thus enteric disease is more likely to be caused by microsporidia, cryptosporidia, or nonopportunistic pathogens such as *Clostridium difficile* than by *Salmonella.*

Behavioral factors are also important determinants of which opportunistic infections occur. Patients with a history of intravenous drug abuse are more likely to be infected with HCV and HBV than matched patients without substance abuse histories. They are also more likely to develop nonopportunistic processes such as *Staphylococcal* sepsis because of their parenteral exposures. Men who have sex with men who develop proctitis or colitis are more likely to have lymphogranuloma venereum proctitis or gonococcal proctitis than patients with different risk factors.

The pathogens that cause active disease in patients with HIV infection may be organisms that were acquired recently or may represent reactivation of latent organisms acquired months or years previously. *Mycobacterium tuberculosis, Pneumocystis jiroveci, Trypanosoma cruzi, Leishmania donovani, Histoplasma capsulatum,* and *Coccidioides immitis* are examples of pathogens that can cause acute disease either soon after exposure or after many months or years of latency as assessed by molecular typing or clinical epidemiology. Thus, many pathogens need to be considered as possible etiologic agents despite exposure that may have occurred in the distant past.

CLINICAL MANIFESTATIONS

One of the early observations about clinical disease in patients with AIDS was that the clinical manifestations of opportunistic infections were not identical to the presentations in other immunosuppressed patients. In patients with AIDS, for instance, PCP is much more likely to manifest with subacute symptoms over weeks or months than in HIV-uninfected patients with cancer or transplant recipients who most often present acutely over a few days. When patients are diagnosed with PCP, those with AIDS are usually less hypoxemic and have less impressive radiographic infiltrates despite the longer duration of symptoms before diagnosis. The number of organisms found in sputum or bronchoalveolar lavage specimens is also greater in patients with AIDS than in other immunosuppressed individuals, such as patients with cancer or transplant recipients, despite the less severe symptoms. Patients with AIDS also are more likely to develop treatment-limiting toxicity associated with trimethoprim-sulfamethoxazole than patients with cancer or transplant recipients. Patients with AIDS are also more likely to have multiple recurrences if they are not treated with chemoprophylaxis than other immunosuppressed populations.

For infections due to *Toxoplasma gondii,* patients with HIV/AIDS characteristically develop toxoplasma encephalitis. Other immunosuppressed populations more often develop disseminated visceral disease involving the liver, spleen, or kidneys. Similarly, CMV in patients with HIV/AIDS causes retinitis and colitis. In patients with stem cell transplants, however, retinitis is relatively uncommon and pneumonia is frequent.

Some pathogens that have been recognized to cause frequent disease among patients with HIV/AIDS, such as *M. avium, Cryptosporidium, Microsporidium,* and *Bartonella,* were rarely recognized as causes of life-threatening human disease before the HIV/AIDS epidemic. Even as diagnostic studies have improved for these pathogens, they are far more often recognized among patients with HIV/AIDS than among other highly immunosuppressed patient populations. Conversely, some pathogens that were deemed likely to be AIDS associated based on the mechanisms for host

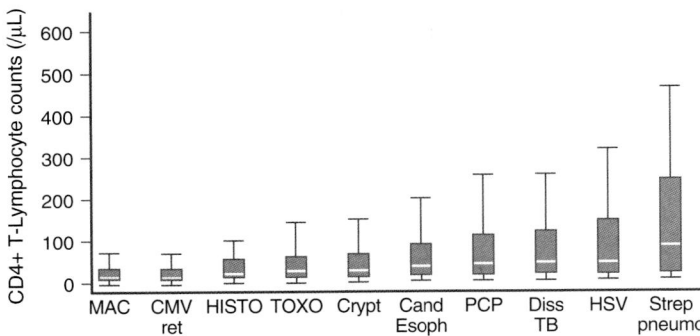

FIGURE 389-1. Distribution of CD4+ lymphocyte counts at diagnosis of opportunistic infection

immune response, such as *Listeria monocytogenes* and disseminated *Strongyloides stercoralis*, are rarely seen in patients with HIV/AIDS. The reasons why some pathogens are unexpectedly frequent, or unexpectedly unusual despite similar environmental exposures, have not been fully elucidated.

DIAGNOSIS

For any infection in any patient population, management is likely to be more effective and to be associated with fewer complications if the specific cause is conclusively identified, the appropriate therapy is started quickly, and unnecessary drugs are avoided. For patients with HIV infection, such an approach is especially appropriate given the broad range of opportunistic and nonopportunistic infections that could cause a particular syndrome, as well as the noninfectious causes, including drug toxicities, that can masquerade as infections.

Although the diagnostic approach always should be individualized to the specific patient considering the current CD4 count, past and current exposures, prior infections, the history, physical findings, and routine laboratory tests of the current illness, certain tests are consistently useful. Blood cultures for routine bacteria and fungi, a serum cryptococcal antigen test, or a syphilis serologic test often provide useful information. If the patient has pulmonary dysfunction, Gram stain and routine culture of expectorated or induced sputum is usually useful. If a history of appropriate geographic exposure is present, serum and urine histoplasma antigen and Coccidioides antibodies also can be useful, as can a *Toxoplasma* IgG test.

The utility of specific tests needs to be validated in each patient population to determine their positive and negative predictive value. Certain tests that are useful in other patient populations or for research purposes are not necessarily useful to clinically diagnose opportunistic infections. For instance, serum polymerase chain reaction (PCR) for CMV is very useful for managing patients who have received stem cell transplants, because their positive and negative predictive values are high. However, serum CMV PCR in patients with HIV infections correlates mainly with the degree of immunosuppression and does not have sufficient positive and negative predictive value to be useful for assessing the cause of end organ disease. Serum PCR for Epstein-Barr virus (EBV), varicella zoster virus (VZV), or herpes simplex virus (HSV) also would not be useful in most circumstances for similar reasons. An increasing number of laboratories are offering other molecular tests for opportunistic pathogens, but care must be taken to be certain that the predictive value of these tests is proved. For instance, PCR for *Pneumocystis* in bronchoalveolar lavage may have excellent negative predictive value, but its positive predictive value is very low because many immunosuppressed patients appear to be colonized with *Pneumocystis* and thus a positive result does not prove with any confidence that *Pneumocystis* is the cause of the pulmonary dysfunction.

Imaging is an important aspect of patient evaluation. Patients with HIV infection may have pathologic processes despite a paucity of symptoms or normal readings on routine chest radiographs, for example. Thus, computerized tomography (CT) of the lungs may reveal unexpected pathologic findings such as diffuse interstitial infiltrates suggestive of PCP despite the absence of cough, shortness of breath, or oxygen desaturation. Such a finding could lead to an induced sputum or bronchoalveolar lavage diagnosis of the process at a time when disease is mild and the likelihood of successful treatment is high. CT of the abdomen also should be considered in patients with low CD4 counts even in the absence of abdominal symptoms, because such a study may reveal unexpected adenopathy or organ infiltration that could be readily biopsied more feasibly than other more obvious clinical manifestations. Positron emission tomography and nuclear scans have roles for identifying the etiology of infectious syndromes.

TREATMENT   Rx

Empirical Management

For the initial management of a presumed infectious syndrome in a patient with HIV infection or AIDS, clinicians need to determine the urgency of starting therapy before the specific causative process is definitively identified. Given the range of processes that can cause disease in patients with HIV infection or AIDS, the optimal approach is to establish the specific cause before starting therapy. However, some patients will be too sick or deteriorating too quickly to permit withholding therapy until a diagnosis can be established. Thus, for some patients, empirical therapy may be the best management strategy, with careful monitoring of the patient to determine if the therapy is effective.

When assessing an HIV-infected patient with any clinical syndrome, especially a syndrome associated with fever, opportunistic infections are immediate considerations. However, the likelihood of an opportunistic infection depends on the current CD4 count: if the patient's current CD4 count is greater than 200 to 300 cells/µL, the likelihood of most opportunistic infections (other than tuberculosis) is low (but not zero). For any patient, regardless of CD4 count, common community-acquired, nonopportunistic infections also must be considered because HIV-infected patients are equally susceptible to these as their HIV-uninfected counterparts. In addition, noninfectious syndromes must be considered, especially as the patient population ages and congestive heart failure, cerebrovascular disease, or chronic renal disease occur, potentially accelerated by the HIV-related inflammatory state. Patients also may have more than one process occurring concurrently. A familiar scenario, for instance, for a patient with documented PCP, would be the failure to recognize that the reason for pulmonary deterioration is not progressive PCP, but superimposed congestive heart failure, pulmonary hypertension, pulmonary emboli, or secondary lung infection due to methicillin-resistant *Staphylococcus aureus* (MRSA), *Streptococcus pneumoniae*, or *Cryptococcus neoformans*.

For some syndromes, empirical therapy is appropriate in most patients, with response to therapy providing a presumptive diagnosis. For instance, an empiric 2-week course of pyrimethamine plus sulfadiazine would be appropriate for a patient with AIDS with a CNS mass lesion, CD4 count less than 100 cells/µL, and positive antitoxoplasma serum immunoglobulin G (IgG), before a brain biopsy would be performed. Given the potential morbidity of a brain biopsy, and the high probability that a patient with AIDS with cerebral toxoplasmosis would demonstrate clinical and radiologic improvement within 14 days, such an approach has been considered preferred compared to immediate brain biopsy or even, in some circumstances, lumbar puncture. Similarly, for a patient with a CD4 count less than 200 cells/µL who presents with fever, cough, shortness of breath, severe hypoxemia, and diffuse bilateral interstitial pulmonary infiltrates, empirical therapy with ceftriaxone or vancomycin, plus azithromycin, plus trimethoprim-sulfamethoxazole to adequately provide coverage against common causes of community-acquired pneumonia as well as PCP would often be appropriate if the patient were too unstable to tolerate bronchoscopy without a high risk for intubation.

Definitive Therapy

The NIH-CDC-HIVMA Guidelines for the Prevention and Treatment of Opportunistic Infections in HIV-Infected Adults and Adolescents and other chapters in this text provide details on the diagnostic, therapeutic, and preventive approaches to specific syndromes. The drugs of choice are also listed in Table 389-1, adapted from the CDC-NIH-IDSA Guideline on Management of Opportunistic Infections in Adults and Adolescents, which is updated regularly online throughout the year (http://www.aidsinfo.nih.gov).

The treatments for opportunistic infections change as new drugs and new data become available.[8] Thus major AIDS guidelines are now updated promptly on-line (www.aidsinfo.nih.gov). For hepatitis-C, recommendations are changing so rapidly that the on-line site should be consulted before therapy is initiated unless the provider is very familiar with current data (www.hcvguidelines.org).

The institution of therapeutic or preventive drugs requires careful considerations of pharmacokinetics and drug-drug interactions. Patients with HIV infection often have organ dysfunction that may alter absorption or excretion of drugs. These patients are also often on multiple drugs (both AIDS related and AIDS unrelated) that can interact with clinically important consequences for drug effectiveness or toxicity. Such therapy thus requires considerable experience and consultation with up-to-date references for guidance.

When a patient with HIV/AIDS who has not been receiving ART develops an opportunistic infection, prospective studies demonstrate that the patient will have longer survival and fewer AIDS-defining complications if the patient is put promptly on ART. The definition of "prompt," that is, the decision as to how soon to start ART, is a complex analysis that must factor in the patient's willingness and ability to take ART, the evolution of the opportunistic infection if ART is not initiated, access to medical care and drugs after hospitalization, ability to absorb the drugs, potential interactions of ART with other drugs, including those used to treat the opportunistic infection, the patient's ability to tolerate potential drug toxicities, and the possible consequences if immune reconstitution inflammatory syndrome occurs.[9] The general principle is to start ART as soon as possible, but each patient will require individual assessment to determine the optimal interval between recognition of an opportunistic infection and initiation of ART.

When patients who are already receiving ART develop an opportunistic infection or any other complication not directly related to the drug itself, ART should be continued. The regimen should be reassessed to ensure that it is optimal in terms of antiviral activity, tolerability, potential toxicity and drug interactions, and the patient's ability to attain adequate serum levels given their ability to absorb oral drugs.

TABLE 389-1 PROPHYLAXIS TO PREVENT FIRST EPISODE OF OPPORTUNISTIC DISEASE

OPPORTUNISTIC INFECTIONS	INDICATION	PREFERRED	ALTERNATIVE
Streptococcus pneumoniae	For individuals who have not received any pneumococcal vaccine, regardless of CD4 count, followed by: • If CD4 count ≥ 200 cells/μL • If CD4 count < 200 cells/μL For individuals who have previously received PPV23 *Revaccination* • If age 19-64 yr and ≥ 5 yr since the first PPV23 dose • If age ≥ 65 yr and if ≥ 5 yr since the previous PPV23 dose	PCV13 0.5 mL IM × 1 PPV23 0.5 mL IM at least 8 wk after the PCV13 vaccine PPV23 can be offered at least 8 wk after receiving PCV13 or can wait until CD4 count increased to > 200 cells/μL One dose of PCV13 should be given at least 1 yr after the last receipt of PPV23 PPV23 0.5 mL IM × 1 PPV23 0.5 mL IM × 1	PPV23 0.5 mL IM × 1
Influenza A and B virus	All HIV-infected patients	Inactivated influenza vaccine annually (per recommendation for the season) Live-attenuated influenza vaccine is contraindicated in HIV-infected patients	
Syphilis	For individuals exposed to a sex partner with a diagnosis of primary, secondary, or early latent syphilis within past 90 days Or For individuals exposed to a sex partner > 90 days before syphilis diagnosis in the partner, if serologic test results are not available immediately and the opportunity for follow-up is uncertain	Benzathine penicillin G 2.4 million U IM for 1 dose	*For penicillin-allergic patients:* • Doxycycline 100 mg PO q12h for 14 days Or • Ceftriaxone 1 g/day IM or IV for 8-10 days Or • Azithromycin 2 g PO for 1 dose; not recommended for MSM or pregnant women
Histoplasma capsulatum	CD4 count ≤ 150 cells/μL and at high risk because of occupational exposure or lives in a community with a hyperendemic rate of histoplasmosis (>10 cases/100 patient-years)	Itraconazole 200 mg/day PO	

(Guidelines for the Prevention and Treatment of Opportunistic Infections in HIV-Infected Adults and Adolescents. *http://aidsinfo.nih.gov/guidelines.*)
HIV = human immunodeficiency virus; IM = intramuscularly; IV = intravenously; MSM = men who have sex with men; PO = orally.

PREVENTION

Soon after the initial recognition of AIDS, before the era of ART or pathogen specific chemoprophylaxis, clinicians recognized that PCP ultimately occurred in 60 to 80% of patients in North America. Moreover, many of the patients who survived their first episode of PCP had one or more subsequent episodes. One of the first interventions demonstrated to prolong life was the institution of anti-*Pneumocystis* prophylaxis for patients who had oral thrush, oral hairy leukoplakia, a prior episode of PCP, or a CD4 count less than 200 cells/mm³. Subsequently, the concept of primary and secondary chemoprophylaxis was extended to other pathogens such as *M. avium* complex (MAC) and toxoplasma.

These observations about *Pneumocystis*, MAC, and toxoplasma led to the development of a comprehensive preventive strategy to minimize the impact of opportunistic infections on those HIV-infected individuals who are immunologically vulnerable as measured by their CD4 count and viral load or by prior experience with an opportunistic infection (CDC-NIH-IDSA Guideline on Management of Opportunistic Infections in Adults and Adolescents, http://www.aidsinfo.nih.gov). Specific chemotherapy for primary prevention is indicated for the duration of immunosuppression, with the CD4 count thresholds depending on the pathogen. Chronic suppressive therapy should be continued for durations that depend on the pathogen and the patient's CD4 count. Recommendations for primary prophylaxis are summarized in Table 389-2; more complete information on primary and secondary prophylaxis is available in the CDC-NIH-IDSA Guideline on Management of Opportunistic Infections in Adults and Adolescents (http://www.aidsinfo.nih.gov).

Although immune reconstitution with ART is the most effective method to prevent opportunistic infections, many patients with low CD4 counts and uncontrolled viremia will continue to benefit from chemoprophylaxis. These efforts should be modified when patients have had a durable suppression of their viremia and increase in their circulating CD4 counts.

Preventive strategies focus not only on chemoprophylaxis but also on immunization and reducing exposure to opportunistic pathogens. Examples of exposure reduction interventions likely to be effective would be reducing exposure of patients to puppies and kittens from commercial breeders and reducing consumption of untreated surface water to prevent cryptosporidiosis. Other useful interventions would include precautions in travel to the Southwest United States to avoid coccidioidomycosis and avoiding exposure to outdoor cats and rare meat to reduce the likelihood of toxoplasmosis.

Immunizations such as pneumococcal vaccine, HPV vaccine, and hepatitis B vaccine also can be important, although host response to vaccines is reduced when patients are immunosuppressed. Live virus vaccines must be avoided in patients with low CD4 counts.

METABOLIC DISORDERS

With effective and well-tolerated ART, HIV-infected patients have a survival that is almost as long as HIV-uninfected persons.[10] It has become clear that patients with HIV infection experience increased incidence of cardiovascular and cerebrovascular disease; metabolic diseases, including diabetes mellitus; chronic kidney and liver disease; and perhaps accelerated neurocognitive decline, compared to HIV-uninfected patients. The proposed etiology for these disorders appears to be multifactorial and includes various ART-associated toxicities, immune dysregulation, and chronic inflammation related to chronic retroviral disease, even in the context of durable viral suppression.

Text continued on p. 2302

TABLE 389-2   TREATMENT OF ACQUIRED IMMUNODEFICIENCY VIRUS–ASSOCIATED OPPORTUNISTIC INFECTIONS (INCLUDES RECOMMENDATIONS FOR ACUTE TREATMENT AND SECONDARY PROPHYLAXIS/CHRONIC SUPPRESSIVE/MAINTENANCE THERAPY)

OPPORTUNISTIC INFECTION	PREFERRED THERAPY	ALTERNATIVE THERAPY	OTHER COMMENTS
Pneumocystis pneumonia (PCP) infection	Patients who develop PCP despite TMP-SMX prophylaxis usually can be treated with standard doses of TMP-SMX. Duration of PCP treatment: 21 days *For moderate-to-severe PCP:* • TMP-SMX: (TMP 15-20 mg and SMX 75-100 mg)/kg/day q6h or q8h IV; can switch to PO after clinical improvement *For mild-to-moderate PCP:* • TMP-SMX: (TMP 15-20 mg and SMX 75-100 mg)/kg/day, given PO in three divided doses *Or* • TMP-SMX: (160 mg/800 mg or DS) 2 tablets q8h PO *Secondary prophylaxis, after completion of PCP treatment:* • TMP-SMX DS: 1 tablet/day PO *Or* • TMP-SMX (80 mg/400 mg or SS): 1 tablet/day PO	*For moderate-to-severe PCP:* • Pentamidine 4 mg/kg/day IV infused over ≥ 60 min; can reduce dose to 3 mg/kg/day IV because of toxicities *Or* • Primaquine 30 mg (base)/day PO + (clindamycin 600 mg q6h IV or 900 mg q8h IV) or (clindamycin 300 mg q6h PO or 450 mg q8h PO) *For mild-to-moderate PCP:* • Dapsone 100 mg/day PO + TMP 5 mg/kg q8h PO *Or* • Primaquine 30 mg (base)/day PO + (clindamycin 300 mg q6h or 450 mg q8h PO) *Or* • Atovaquone 750 mg q12h PO with food *Secondary prophylaxis, after completion of PCP treatment:* • TMP-SMX DS: 1 tablet PO three times weekly *Or* • Dapsone 100 mg/day PO *Or* • Dapsone 50 mg/day PO + (pyrimethamine 50 mg + leucovorin 25 mg)/wk PO *Or* • (Dapsone 200 mg + pyrimethamine 75 mg + leucovorin 25 mg)/week PO *Or* • Aerosolized pentamidine 300 mg/mo via Respirgard II nebulizer *Or* • Atovaquone 1500 mg/day PO *Or* • (Atovaquone 1500 mg + pyrimethamine 25 mg + leucovorin 10 mg)/day PO	*Indications for adjunctive corticosteroids:* • Pao₂ < 70 mm Hg at room air Or • Alveolar-arterial O₂ gradient > 35 mm Hg *Prednisone doses (beginning as early as possible and within 72 hours of PCP therapy):* • Days 1-5: 40 mg q12h PO • Days 6-10: 40 mg/day PO • Days 11-21: 20 mg/day PO IV methylprednisolone can be administered as 75% of prednisone dose. Benefit of corticosteroid if started after 72 hr of treatment is unknown, but some clinicians will use it for moderate-to-severe PCP. Whenever possible, patients should be tested for G6PD before use of dapsone or primaquine. Alternative therapy should be used in patients found to have G6PD deficiency. Patients who are receiving pyrimethamine/sulfadiazine for treatment or suppression of toxoplasmosis do not require additional PCP prophylaxis. If TMP-SMX is discontinued because of a mild adverse reaction, reinstitution should be considered after the reaction resolves. The dose can be increased gradually (desensitization) or reduced or the frequency modified. TMP-SMX should be permanently discontinued in patients with possible or definite Stevens-Johnson syndrome or toxic epidermal necrosis.

Toxoplasma gondii encephalitis

Treatment of acute infection:

- Pyrimethamine 200 mg PO 1 time, followed by weight-based therapy as follows:
  - If < 60 kg, pyrimethamine 50 mg/day PO + sulfadiazine 1000 mg q6h PO + leucovorin 10-25 mg/day PO
  - If > 60 kg, pyrimethamine 75 mg/day PO + sulfadiazine 1500 mg q6h PO + leucovorin 10-25 mg/day PO
  - Leucovorin dose can be increased to 50 mg q12h or q24h

Duration for acute therapy:

- At least 6 wk; longer duration if clinical or radiologic disease is extensive or response is incomplete at 6 wk

Chronic maintenance therapy:

- Pyrimethamine 25-50 mg/day PO + sulfadiazine 2000-4000 mg/day PO (in two to four divided doses) + leucovorin 10-25 mg/day PO

Treatment of acute infection:

- Pyrimethamine (leucovorin)* + clindamycin 600 mg q6h IV or PO

  Or
- TMP-SMX (TMP 5 mg/kg and SMX 25 mg/kg) q12h IV or PO

  Or
- Atovaquone 1500 mg q12h PO with food + pyrimethamine (leucovorin)*

  Or
- Atovaquone 1500 mg q12h PO with food + sulfadiazine 1000-1500 mg q6h PO (weight-based dosing, as in preferred therapy)

  Or
- Atovaquone 1500 mg q12h PO with food

  Or
- Pyrimethamine (leucovorin)* + azithromycin 900-1200 mg/day PO

Chronic maintenance therapy:

- Clindamycin 600 mg q8h PO + (pyrimethamine 25-50 mg + leucovorin)

  Or
- TMP-SMX DS 1 tablet q12h

  Or
- Atovaquone 750-1500 mg q12h PO + (pyrimethamine 25 mg + leucovorin 10 mg)/day PO

  Or
- Atovaquone 750-1500 mg q12h PO + sulfadiazine 2000-4000 mg/day PO (in two to four divided doses)

  Or
- Atovaquone 750-1500 mg q12h PO with food
- Pyrimethamine and leucovorin doses are the same as for preferred therapy.

Adjunctive corticosteroids (e.g., dexamethasone) should be administered only when clinically indicated to treat mass effect associated with focal lesions or associated edema; discontinue as soon as clinically feasible.

Anticonvulsants should be administered to patients with a history of seizures and continued through acute treatment, but should not be used as seizure prophylaxis.

If clindamycin is used in place of sulfadiazine, additional therapy must be added to prevent PCP.

Mycobacterium tuberculosis (TB) disease

After collecting specimen for culture and molecular diagnostic tests, empirical TB treatment should be started in individuals with clinical and radiographic presentation suggestive of TB.

Initial phase (2 mo, given daily, 5-7 times/wk by DOT):

- INH + [RIF or RFB] + PZA + EMB,

Continuation phase:

- INH + (RIF or RFB) daily (5-7 times/wk) or three times weekly

Total duration of therapy (for drug-susceptible TB):

- Pulmonary TB: 6 mo
- Pulmonary TB and culture-positive after 2 mo of TB treatment: 9 mo
- Extrapulmonary TB with a CNS infection: 9-12 mo
- Extrapulmonary TB with bone or joint involvement: 6-9 mo
- Extrapulmonary TB in other sites: 6 mo

Total duration of therapy should be based on number of doses received, not on calendar time.

Treatment for Drug-Resistant TB

Resistant to INH:

- (RIF or RFB) + EMB + PZA + (moxifloxacin or levofloxacin) for 2 mo; followed by (RIF or RFB) + EMB + (moxifloxacin or levofloxacin) for 7 mo

Resistant to rifamycin + 1 other drug:

- Regimen and duration of treatment should be individualized based on resistance pattern, clinical and microbiologic responses, and in close consultation with experienced specialists.

Adjunctive corticosteroid improves survival for TB meningitis and pericarditis.

RIF is *not recommended* for patients receiving HIV PI because of its induction of PI metabolism.

RFB is a less potent CYP3A4 inducer than RIF and is preferred in patients receiving PIs.

Once weekly rifapentine can result in development of rifamycin resistance in HIV-infected patients and is *not recommended.*

Therapeutic drug monitoring should be considered in patients receiving rifamycin and interacting ART.

Paradoxical IRIS that is not severe can be treated with NSAIDs without a change in TB or HIV therapy.

For severe IRIS reaction, consider prednisone and taper over 4 wk based on clinical symptoms.

For example:

- If receiving RIF: prednisone 1.5 mg/kg/day for 2 wk, then 0.75 mg/kg/day for 2 wk
- If receiving RFB: prednisone 1 mg/kg/day for 2 wk, then 0.5 mg/kg/day for 2 wk

A more gradual tapering schedule over a few months may be necessary for some patients.

TABLE 389-2 TREATMENT OF ACQUIRED IMMUNODEFICIENCY VIRUS–ASSOCIATED OPPORTUNISTIC INFECTIONS (INCLUDES RECOMMENDATIONS FOR ACUTE TREATMENT AND SECONDARY PROPHYLAXIS/CHRONIC SUPPRESSIVE/MAINTENANCE THERAPY)—cont'd

OPPORTUNISTIC INFECTION	PREFERRED THERAPY	ALTERNATIVE THERAPY	OTHER COMMENTS
Disseminated *Mycobacterium avium* complex (MAC) disease	*At least two drugs as initial therapy with:* • Clarithromycin 500 mg q12h PO + ethambutol 15 mg/kg/day PO Or • Azithromycin 500-600 mg + ethambutol 15 mg/kg/day PO if drug interaction or intolerance precludes the use of clarithromycin Duration: • At least 12 mo of therapy, can discontinue if no signs and symptoms of MAC disease and sustained (>6 mo) CD4 count>100 cells/μL in response to ART	Addition of a third or fourth drug should be considered for patients with advanced immunosuppression (CD4 counts < 50 cells/μL), with high mycobacterial loads (>2 log CFU/mL of blood), or in the absence of effective ART. *Third or fourth drug options may include:* • RFB 300 mg/day PO (dosage adjustment may be necessary based on drug interactions) Or • Amikacin 10-15 mg/kg/day IV Or • Streptomycin 1 g/day IV or IM Or • Moxifloxacin 400 mg/day PO or levofloxacin 500 mg/day PO	Testing of susceptibility to clarithromycin and azithromycin is recommended. NSAIDs can be used for patients who experience moderate-to-severe symptoms attributed to IRIS. If IRIS symptoms persist, short-term (4-8 wk) systemic corticosteroids (equivalent to 20-40 mg prednisone) can be used.
Salmonellosis	All HIV-infected patients with salmonellosis should be treated because of high risk for bacteremia. • Ciprofloxacin 500-750 mg q12h PO (or 400 mg q12h IV) if susceptible *Duration of therapy:* For gastroenteritis without bacteremia: • If CD4 count ≥ 200 cells/μL: 7-14 days • If CD4 count < 200 cells/μL: 2-6 wk For gastroenteritis with bacteremia: • If CD4 count ≥ 200/μL: 14 days; longer duration if bacteremia persists or if the infection is complicated (eg, if metastatic foci of infection are present) • If CD4 count < 200 cells/μL: 2-6 wk *Secondary prophylaxis should be considered for:* • Patients with recurrent Salmonella gastroenteritis ± bacteremia Or • Patients with CD4 < 200 cells/μL with severe diarrhea	• Levofloxacin 750 mg q24h PO or IV Or • Moxifloxacin 400 mg q24h PO or IV Or • TMP, 160 mg, SMX 800 mg q12h (PO or IV) Or • Ceftriaxone 1 g q24h IV Or • Cefotaxime 1 g q8h IV	Oral or intravenous rehydration if indicated. Antimotility agents should be avoided. The role of long-term secondary prophylaxis in patients with recurrent *Salmonella* bacteremia is not well established. Must weigh benefit against risks for long-term antibiotic exposure. Effective ART may reduce the frequency, severity, and recurrence of *Salmonella* infections.
Mucocutaneous candidiasis	*For oropharyngeal candidiasis; initial episodes (for 7-14 days):* Oral therapy: • Fluconazole 100 mg/day PO Or Topical therapy: • Clotrimazole troches, 10 mg PO five times daily Or • Miconazole mucoadhesive buccal 50-mg tablet—apply to mucosal surface over the canine fossa once daily (do not swallow, chew, or crush) *For esophageal candidiasis (for 14-21 days):* • Fluconazole 100 mg (up to 400 mg)/day PO or IV Or • Itraconazole oral solution 200 mg/day PO *For uncomplicated vulvovaginal candidiasis:* • Oral fluconazole 150 mg for 1 dose Or • Topical azoles (clotrimazole, butoconazole, miconazole, tioconazole, or terconazole) for 3-7 days *For severe or recurrent vulvovaginal candidiasis:* • Fluconazole 100-200 mg/day PO for ≥ 7 days Or • Topical antifungal ≥ 7 days	*For oropharyngeal candidiasis; initial episodes (for 7-14 days):* Oral therapy: • Itraconazole oral solution 200 mg/day PO Or • Posaconazole oral solution 400 mg q12h PO for 1 day, then 400 mg/day Topical therapy: • Nystatin suspension 4-6 mL q6h 1-2 flavored pastilles four or five times daily *For esophageal candidiasis (for 14-21 days):* • Voriconazole 200 mg q12h PO or IV Or • Posaconazole 400 mg q12h PO Or • Anidulafungin 100 mg IV 1 time, then 50 mg/day IV Or • Caspofungin 50 mg/day IV Or • Micafungin 150 mg/day IV Or • Amphotericin B deoxycholate 0.6 mg/kg/day IV Or • Lipid formulation of amphotericin B 3-4 mg/kg/day IV *For uncomplicated vulvovaginal candidiasis:* • Itraconazole oral solution 200 mg/day PO for 3-7 days	Chronic or prolonged use of azoles may promote development of resistance. Higher relapse rate for esophageal candidiasis seen with echinocandins than with fluconazole use. Suppressive therapy usually not recommended unless patients have frequent or severe recurrences. *If decision is to use suppressive therapy:* Oropharyngeal candidiasis: • Fluconazole 100 mg/day PO or three times weekly • Itraconazole oral solution 200 mg/day PO weekly Esophageal candidiasis: • Fluconazole 100-200 mg/day PO • Posaconazole 400 mg q12h PO Vulvovaginal candidiasis: • Fluconazole 150 mg PO once weekly

Cryptococcosis	*Cryptococcal meningitis:* Induction therapy (for at least 2 wk, followed by consolidation therapy): • Liposomal amphotericin B 3-4 mg/kg/day IV + flucytosine 25 mg/kg PO QID (NOTE: Flucytosine dose should be adjusted in patients with renal dysfunction.) Consolidation therapy (for at least 8 wk, followed by maintenance therapy): • Fluconazole 400 mg/day PO (or IV) Maintenance therapy Liposomal: • Fluconazole 200 mg/day PO for at least 12 mo *For non-CNS, extrapulmonary cryptococcosis and diffuse pulmonary disease:* • Treatment same as for cryptococcal meningitis *Non-CNS cryptococcosis with mild-to-moderate symptoms and focal pulmonary infiltrates:* • Fluconazole, 400 mg/day PO for 12 mo	*Cryptococcal meningitis:* Induction therapy (for at least 2 wk, followed by consolidation therapy): • Amphotericin B deoxycholate 0.7 mg/kg/day IV + flucytosine 25 mg/kg q6h PO Or • Amphotericin B lipid complex 5 mg/kg/day IV + flucytosine 25 mg/kg q6h PO Or • Liposomal amphotericin B 3-4 mg/kg/day IV + fluconazole 800 mg/day PO or IV Or • Amphotericin B deoxycholate 0.7 mg/kg/day IV + fluconazole 800 mg/day PO or IV Or • Fluconazole 400-800 mg/day PO or IV + flucytosine 25 mg/kg q6h PO Or • Fluconazole 1200 mg/day PO or IV Consolidation therapy (for at least 8 wk, followed by maintenance therapy): • Itraconazole 200 mg q12h PO for 8 wk—less effective than fluconazole Maintenance therapy: • No alternative therapy recommendation	Addition of flucytosine to amphotericin B has been associated with more rapid sterilization of CSF and decreased risk for subsequent relapse. Patients receiving flucytosine should have either blood levels monitored (peak level 2 hr after dose should be 30-80 μg/mL) or close monitoring of blood counts for development of cytopenia. Dosage should be adjusted in patients with renal insufficiency. Opening pressure should always be measured when an LP is performed. Repeated LPs or CSF shunting are essential to effectively manage increased ICP. Corticosteroids and mannitol are ineffective in reducing ICP and are **not recommended**. Some specialists recommend a brief course of corticosteroid for management of severe IRIS symptoms.
Histoplasmosis	*Moderately severe to severe disseminated disease:* Induction therapy (for at least 2 wk or until clinically improved): • Liposomal amphotericin B 3 mg/kg/day IV Maintenance therapy: • Itraconazole 200 mg q8h PO for 3 days, then 200 mg q12h PO *Less severe disseminated disease:* Induction and maintenance therapy: • Itraconazole 200 mg q8h PO for 3 days, then 200 mg q12h PO Duration of therapy: • At least 12 mo *Meningitis:* Induction therapy (4-6 wk): • Liposomal amphotericin B 5 mg/kg/day Maintenance therapy: • Itraconazole 200 mg q8h to q12h PO to for ≥ 1 yr and until resolution of abnormal CSF findings Long-term suppression therapy: For patients with severe disseminated or CNS infection after completion of at least 12 mo of therapy and those who relapse despite appropriate therapy: • Itraconazole 200 mg/day PO	*Moderately severe to severe disseminated disease:* Induction therapy (for at least 2 wk or until clinically improved): • Amphotericin B lipid complex 3 mg/kg/day IV Or • Amphotericin B cholesteryl sulfate complete 3 mg/kg/day IV Alternatives to itraconazole for maintenance therapy or treatment of less severe disease: • Voriconazole 400 mg q12h PO for 1 day, then 200 mg q12h Or • Posaconazole 400 mg q12h PO • Fluconazole 800 mg/day PO *Meningitis:* • No alternative therapy recommendation Long-term suppression therapy: • Fluconazole 400 mg/day PO	Itraconazole, posaconazole, and voriconazole may have significant interactions with certain ARV agents. These interactions are complex and can be bi-directional. Therapeutic drug monitoring and dosage adjustment may be necessary to ensure triazole antifungal and ARV efficacy and reduce concentration-related toxicities. Random serum concentration of itraconazole + hydroxy itraconazole should be > 1 μg/mL. Clinical experience with voriconazole or posaconazole in the treatment of histoplasmosis is limited. Acute pulmonary histoplasmosis in HIV-infected patients with CD4 counts > 300 cells/μL should be managed as in nonimmunocompromised host.

TABLE 389-2 TREATMENT OF ACQUIRED IMMUNODEFICIENCY VIRUS–ASSOCIATED OPPORTUNISTIC INFECTIONS (INCLUDES RECOMMENDATIONS FOR ACUTE TREATMENT AND SECONDARY PROPHYLAXIS/CHRONIC SUPPRESSIVE/MAINTENANCE THERAPY)—cont'd

OPPORTUNISTIC INFECTION	PREFERRED THERAPY	ALTERNATIVE THERAPY	OTHER COMMENTS
Cytomegalovirus (CMV) disease	*CMV retinitis:* Induction therapy: For immediate sight-threatening lesions (adjacent to the optic nerve or fovea): • Intravitreal injections of ganciclovir (2 mg) or foscarnet (2.4 mg) for one to four doses over a period of 7-10 days to achieve high intraocular concentration faster • Plus one of the listed preferred or alternative systemic therapy: Preferred systemic induction therapy: Valganciclovir 900 mg q12h PO for 14-21 days For peripheral lesions: Administer one of the preferred or alternative systemic therapy Chronic maintenance (secondary prophylaxis): Valganciclovir 900 mg/day PO *CMV esophagitis or colitis:* • Ganciclovir 5 mg/kg q12h IV; may switch to valganciclovir 900 mg q12h PO once the patient can tolerate oral therapy • Duration: 21-42 days or until symptoms have resolved • Maintenance therapy is usually not necessary, but should be considered after relapses *Well-documented, histologically confirmed CMV pneumonia:* • Experience for treating CMV pneumonitis in patients with HIV is limited. Use of IV ganciclovir or IV foscarnet is reasonable (doses same as for CMV retinitis) • The optimal duration of therapy and the role of oral valganciclovir have not been established *CMV neurologic disease:* (NOTE: **Treatment should be initiated promptly.**) • Ganciclovir 5 mg/kg q12h IV + (foscarnet 90 mg/kg q12h IV or 60 mg/kg q8h IV) to stabilize disease and maximize response, continue until symptomatic improvement and resolution of neurologic symptoms • The optimal duration of therapy and the role of oral valganciclovir have not been established	*CMV retinitis:* Alternative systemic induction therapy: • Ganciclovir 5 mg/kg q12h IV for 14-21 days Or • Foscarnet 90 mg/kg q12h IV or 60 mg/kg q8h for 14-21 days Or • Cidofovir 5 mg/kg/wk IV for 2 wk; saline hydration before and after therapy and probenecid, 2 g PO 3 hr before dose, followed by 1 g PO 2 hr and 8 hours after the dose (total of 4 g). (NOTE: This regimen should be avoided in patients with sulfa allergy because of cross sensitivity with probenecid.) Chronic maintenance (secondary prophylaxis): • Ganciclovir 5 mg/kg IV 5-7 times weekly Or • Foscarnet 90-120 mg/kg IV once daily Or • Cidofovir 5 mg/kg IV every other week with saline hydration and probenecid as above *CMV esophagitis or colitis:* • Foscarnet 90 mg/ kg q12h IV or 60 mg/kg q8h for patients with treatment-limiting toxicities to ganciclovir or with ganciclovir resistance Or • Valganciclovir 900 mg q12h PO in milder disease and if able to tolerate PO therapy Or • For mild cases, if ART can be initiated without delay, consider withholding CMV therapy. • Duration: 21-42 days or until symptoms have resolved	The choice of therapy for CMV retinitis should be individualized, based on location and severity of the lesions, level of immunosuppression, and other factors (e.g., concomitant medications and ability to adhere to treatment). The ganciclovir ocular implant, which is effective for treatment of CMV retinitis is no longer available. For sight-threatening retinitis, intravitreal injections of ganciclovir or foscarnet can be given to achieve higher ocular concentration faster. The choice of chronic maintenance therapy (route of administration and drug choices) should be made in consultation with an ophthalmologist. Considerations should include the anatomic location of the retinal lesion, vision in the contralateral eye, the patients' immunologic and virologic status and response to ART. Patients with CMV retinitis who discontinue maintenance therapy should undergo regular eye examinations—normally every 3 mo—for early detection of relapse IRU, and then annually after immune reconstitution. IRU may develop in the setting of immune reconstitution. *Treatment of IRU:* • Periocular corticosteroid or short courses of systemic steroid Initial therapy in patients with CMV retinitis, esophagitis, colitis, and pneumonitis should include initiation or optimization of ART.

Herpes simplex virus (HSV) disease	**Orolabial lesions (for 5-10 days):** • Valacyclovir 1 g q12h PO Or • Famciclovir 500 mg q12h PO Or • Acyclovir 400 mg q8h PO **Initial or recurrent genital HSV (For 5-14 days):** • Valacyclovir 1 g q12h PO Or • Famciclovir 500 mg q12h PO Or • Acyclovir 400 mg q8h PO **Severe mucocutaneous HSV:** • Initial therapy acyclovir 5 mg/kg q8h IV • After lesions begin to regress, change to PO therapy, as above. Continue until lesions are completely healed. **Chronic suppressive therapy:** For patients with severe recurrences of genital herpes or patients who want to minimize frequency of recurrences: • Valacyclovir 500 mg q12h PO • Famciclovir 500 mg q12h PO • Acyclovir 400 mg q12h PO • Continue indefinitely regardless of CD4 cell count.	*For acyclovir-resistant HSV:* Preferred therapy: • Foscarnet 80-120 mg/kg/day IV in two or three divided doses until clinical response Alternative therapy: • IV cidofovir (dosage as in CMV retinitis) Or • Topical trifluridine Or • Topical cidofovir Or • Topical imiquimod • Duration of therapy: 21-28 days or longer Patients with HSV infections can be treated with episodic therapy when symptomatic lesions occur or with daily suppressive therapy to prevent recurrences. Topical formulations of trifluridine and cidofovir are not commercially available. Extemporaneous compounding of topical products can be prepared using trifluridine ophthalmic solution and the IV formulation of cidofovir.
Varicella zoster virus (VZV) disease	*Primary varicella infection (chickenpox):* Uncomplicated cases (for 5-7 days): • Valacyclovir 1 g q8h PO Or • Famciclovir 500 mg q8h PO Severe or complicated cases: • Acyclovir 10-15 mg/kg q8h IV for 7-10 days • Can switch to oral valacyclovir, famciclovir, or acyclovir after defervescence if no evidence of visceral involvement. *Herpes zoster (shingles):* Acute localized dermatomal: • For 7-10 days; consider longer duration if lesions are slow to resolve • Valacyclovir 1 g q8h PO Or • Famciclovir 500 mg q8h Extensive cutaneous lesions or visceral involvement: • Acyclovir 10-15 q8h mg/kg IV until clinical improvement is evident • Can switch to PO therapy (valacyclovir, famciclovir, or acyclovir) after clinical improvement (i.e., when no new vesicle formation or improvement of signs and symptoms of visceral VZV), to complete a 10-14 day course. Progressive outer retinal necrosis (PORN): • (Ganciclovir 5 mg/kg ± foscarnet 90 mg/kg) q12h IV + (ganciclovir 2 mg/0.05 mL ± foscarnet 1.2 mg/0.05 mL) intravitreal injection twice weekly • Initiate or optimize ART Acute retinal necrosis (ARN): • (Acyclovir 10-15 mg/kg q8h IV) + (ganciclovir 2 mg/0.05 mL intravitreal injection twice weekly × 1-2 doses) for 10-14 days, followed by valacyclovir 1 g q8h PO for 6 wk	*Primary varicella infection (chickenpox):* Uncomplicated cases (for 5-7 days): • Acyclovir 800 mg PO 5 times per day *Herpes zoster (shingles)* Acute localized dermatomal: • For 7-10 days; consider longer duration if lesions are slow to resolve • Acyclovir 800 mg PO 5 times per day In managing VZV retinitis, consultation with an ophthalmologist experienced in management of VZV retinitis is strongly recommended. Duration of therapy for VZV retinitis is not well defined, and should be determined based on clinical, virologic, and immunologic responses and ophthalmologic responses. Optimization of ART is recommended for serious and difficult-to-treat VZV infections (e.g., retinitis, encephalitis).

ART = antiretroviral therapy; ARV = antiretroviral; CNS = central nervous system; DOT = directly observed therapy; EMB = ethambutol; ICP = intracranial pressure; IRIS = immune reconstitution inflammatory syndrome; IRU = immune recovery uveitis; NSAIDs = nonsteroidal antiinflammatory drugs; PI = protease inhibitor; PZA = pyrazinamide; RFB = rifabutin; RIF = rifampicin; TMP-SMX = trimethoprim/sulfamethoxazole.

Numerous studies have now demonstrated an increased risk for coronary heart disease (CHD) among HIV-infected populations compared to uninfected contemporaries.[11] Although much of this increased risk is attributable to traditional CHD risk factors, such as diabetes, hypertension, dyslipidemia, and smoking, HIV-specific factors such as ART exposure, chronic inflammation, and immune dysfunction are also likely to be contributory. ART-associated increases in lipids as well as nonspecific ART toxicities account for a portion of the observed increased CHD in HIV. Some of the more compelling data on this topic were obtained from the Strategies for Management of Antiretroviral Therapy (SMART) study, which was designed to test whether CD4 T-cell guided reductions in exposure to ART would result in decreased cardiovascular events. Unexpectedly, there was an apparent increase in cardiovascular events observed with drug conservation. A subsequent nested case-control analysis of these data showed strong associations between elevated markers of inflammation at baseline, such as interleukin 6 and D-dimer and all-cause mortality,[12] highlighting the contribution of inflammation and immune activation in the context of chronic viral infection.

Careful identification and management of CHD risk factors is warranted in HIV care. Smoking, which is often enriched in populations with HIV infection, is an important modifiable risk factor that may be addressed to provide CHD risk reduction. As in the general population, smoking cessation in HIV-infected patients is accompanied by a reduction in incident CHD.[13] Dyslipidemia, a commonly identified condition among HIV-infected patients, caused in part by certain protease inhibitors and non-nucleoside reverse transcriptase inhibitors, is another target for CHD reduction. Selection of ART agents with limited effects on dyslipidemia is one potential approach to optimize lipid levels, but use of direct lipid-lowering therapy is often indicated. However, observational data suggests that standard therapy with 3-hydroxy-3-methylglutaryl-coenzyme A (HMG-CoA) reductase inhibitors (statins) may be less effective for preventing cardiovascular disease[14] in the context of HIV despite their demonstrated ability to reduce markers of inflammation.[15] In addition, careful attention to potential drug-drug for preventing cardiovascular disease interactions is required when coadministering various protease inhibitors and statins due to effects on CYP3A4 activity that can lead to increased levels of statins.

Diabetes, insulin resistance, kidney injury, and neurocognitive dysfunction are also increased in HIV-infected populations. Similar to in the general population, the presence of chronic HCV infection is associated with an increased risk for diabetes and the development of chronic kidney disease[16] among individuals with HIV. However, immune dysfunction and toxicities associated with certain ART medications also increase the risk for diabetes and kidney injury in HIV.[17] Finally, the risk for developing HIV-associated neurocognitive dysfunction (HAND) has declined in the era of widespread ART use; however, longer survival and the increasing age of the HIV-infected population has led to a rise in the overall prevalence of HAND.[18] Indeed, with increased life expectancy, attentive care directed toward the recognition and management of metabolic, cardiovascular, and neurodegenerative conditions will become increasingly important in the health care approach to individuals living with HIV infection.

GENERAL REFERENCES

For the General References and other additional features, please visit Expert Consult at https://expertconsult.inkling.com.

390

GASTROINTESTINAL MANIFESTATIONS OF HIV AND AIDS

TAMSIN A. KNOX AND CHRISTINE WANKE

INTRODUCTION

Gastrointestinal (GI) diseases were among the leading causes of morbidity and mortality in persons infected with human immunodeficiency virus (HIV) before the advent of highly active antiretroviral therapy (HAART) in 1996. Profound wasting and chronic diarrhea are still manifestations of end-stage acquired immunodeficiency syndrome (AIDS) in persons who are not receiving or are resistant to antiretroviral therapy (ART). However, the common GI problems found today in persons receiving effective ART have shifted away from the enteric and hepatobiliary infections associated with low CD4+ counts. Current GI issues are mainly due to side effects of antiretroviral medications, to nutritional and metabolic disorders associated with chronic HIV disease and therapy, and to liver disease from coinfection with hepatitis B virus (HBV) and hepatitis C virus (HCV).

The degree of immunosuppression, measured by the CD4+ count, is the most important determinant of the likelihood of a GI illness, the type of disease, and its severity. The more profound the CD4+ count suppression, the more likely a GI disease will be present.

The route of transmission of HIV may affect GI function; men who have sex with men (MSM) have higher rates of diarrhea and Kaposi sarcoma than do those who acquired HIV from intravenous drug use (IVDU). Alcohol abuse or IVDU predisposes to liver disease. Regional exposures may increase the risk for disease. In resource-limited settings, lack of ART, increased exposure to pathogens, lack of clean water, poverty, and hunger are associated with increased prevalence and severity of GI disease. In contrast, nutritional and metabolic diseases such as obesity, metabolic syndrome, and fatty liver are seen in HIV populations with high caloric and fat intake and lack of exercise. GI complications of HIV infection and recommendations for their treatment are summarized in Table 390-1.

GASTROINTESTINAL DISEASES FOUND WITH CD4+ COUNTS GREATER THAN 200 TO 500 CELLS/μL

The GI diseases discussed in this section may also be seen with more advanced HIV infection.

Side Effects of Medications

Adverse effects of medications are frequently seen in the course of HIV treatment and may be due to ART[A1] or to the medications required for treatment or prevention of opportunistic infections. Gastric effects, including nausea, vomiting, loss of appetite, and dyspepsia, may occur as a symptom of the HIV infection itself or in response to ART regimens, particularly those with zidovudine, didanosine, ritonavir, amprenavir, or indinavir. Hypersensitivity reactions to ART, such as occurs in persons with the HLA-B5701 haplotype who take abacavir, may also be manifested as fever, abdominal pain, and rash. Didanosine, stavudine, and pentamidine may cause acute pancreatitis.

Lactic acidosis is a life-threatening condition caused by mitochondrial toxicity from nucleoside reverse transcriptase inhibitors (NRTIs), particularly stavudine, didanosine, and zidovudine. Early discontinuation of NRTIs and supportive care are key to recovery, but the syndrome may be difficult to diagnose because of nonspecific findings such as fatigue, nausea, muscle aches, weight loss, or abdominal pain. Blood lactate levels are usually greater than 5 mmol/mL. Nevirapine has been associated with liver toxicity when used in men and women with CD4+ counts higher than 250 and 400 cells/μL, respectively. One of the most common adverse effects of atazanavir has been asymptomatic elevation in indirect bilirubin. Some ART agents have also been associated with the development of significant elevations in triglycerides (to levels > 1000 mg/dL) and the associated development of pancreatitis.

Although all antiretrovirals have been associated with diarrhea, nelfinavir is particularly known to cause a secretory form of diarrhea. Although antiretroviral therapy is now likely the most common cause of diarrhea in treated HIV-infected patients, intestinal pathogens should still be sought in stool examinations, despite a normal CD4+ count or low HIV load.

Nutritional and Metabolic Disorders

With the advent of effective ART and the conversion of HIV to a chronic manageable disease, overnutrition and obesity have become frequent complications of HIV infection. Lifestyle factors and poor dietary choices may help promote the development of overweight/obesity, but some weight gain and increases in visceral fat may be related to the use of specific ART agents. HIV-associated lipodystrophy syndrome,[1] which was recognized after the introduction of effective triple ART regimens, is a complex of four distinct components: visceral fat accumulation, subcutaneous fat atrophy, atherogenic lipid profiles, and glucose intolerance. The pathogenesis remains unclear, but nutritional intake probably contributes to all components except fat atrophy. Chronic inflammation caused by long-term HIV infection and selected antiretrovirals has been implicated as well, particularly the protease

TABLE 390-1 RELATIONSHIP OF GASTROINTESTINAL DISEASES TO CD4+ COUNTS IN HIV-INFECTED PATIENTS

CD4+ COUNT	SYSTEM	SYMPTOMS AND DISEASES	TREATMENT
>200-500 cells/μL	GI and pancreas	**Nausea, vomiting, abdominal pain**	Changes in antiretroviral regimen
		Side effects of medications	Lipid-lowering agents, low-fat diet, no alcohol
		Pancreatitis	Treat specific pathogens, if present
		Diarrhea	Antimotility agents and fiber
	Nutritional and metabolic	**Lactic acidosis**	Stop nucleoside reverse transcriptase inhibitors
		Stavudine, didanosine, zidovudine	
		Changes in body shape	
		Obesity	Diet, exercise
		Metabolic syndrome	Diet, exercise, lipid-lowering agents, insulin-sensitizing agents
		Visceral obesity	hGH/GHRH in clinical trials
	Liver	**Liver function abnormalities, cirrhosis**	
		Chronic hepatitis with HCV	Combination of direct-acting agents against HCV
		Chronic HBV infection	Nucleosides/-tides for HBV infection
		Hepatotoxicity	Stop implicated antiretrovirals
	Oral lesions (≈400-500 cells/μL)	**Plaques, pain**	
		Oral thrush	Clotrimazole troche, nystatin, oral azoles
		Hairy leukoplakia	Acyclovir
		Herpes simplex-1	Acyclovir, famciclovir, valacyclovir
		Idiopathic ulcers	Corticosteroids, thalidomide (men)
		Gingivitis	Topical chlorhexidine, oral metronidazole
		Kaposi sarcoma	Radiation, intralesional injection, systemic chemotherapy
	Anorectal lesions	**Anorectal pain, mass, discharge, tenesmus**	
		Anal fissure, fistula, or perirectal abscess	Local care, surgery
		Foreign body in rectum	Endoscopic or surgical removal
		Sexually transmitted disease:	
		Gonorrhea, *Chlamydia trachomatis*, syphilis	Specific antibiotic therapy
		Herpes simplex infection	Acyclovir, famciclovir, valacyclovir
		Condyloma	Podophyllin, surgical excision, or ablation
		Anal cancer	Surgery, chemoradiation therapy
<200 cells/μL	Esophagus	**Dysphagia, odynophagia**	
	<200 cells/μL	*Candida*	Fluconazole, itraconazole, (voriconazole)
	<50 cells/μL	CMV	Ganciclovir
		Idiopathic ulcers	Oral corticosteroids, thalidomide (men)
		HSV	Acyclovir, famciclovir, valacyclovir
<100 cells/μL	Intestine	**Diarrhea**	
		Bacterial, viral, or protozoal infection	Treat specific pathogens
		AIDS enteropathy	Antimotility agents, nutritional support, ART
		Abdominal pain, fever	
		CMV	Treat specific pathogens
		Mycobacterium tuberculosis, MAC, *Histoplasma Cryptosporidium*	Surgery if perforation or dead bowel
	Malignancy	**GI bleeding, weight loss, or abdominal pain**	
		Kaposi sarcoma	As above
		Lymphoma	Systemic chemotherapy
<50 cells/μL	Wasting	**Weight loss**	
		Increased metabolic demands (infection, HIV)	Treat HIV and underlying infections
		Decreased oral intake	Appetite stimulants
		Malabsorption	Anabolic steroids, hGH
	Hepatobiliary	**Hepatomegaly, elevated liver function test results**	
		Opportunistic infections—MAC, fungal	Consider liver biopsy
		Lymphoma	
		Jaundice, RUQ pain, elevated liver function test results	
		AIDS cholangiopathy	ERCP and sphincterotomy
		Acalculous cholecystitis	Laparoscopic cholecystectomy

AIDS = acquired immunodeficiency syndrome; ART = antiretroviral therapy; CMV = cytomegalovirus; ERCP = endoscopic retrograde cholangiopancreatography; GHRH = growth hormone–releasing hormone; GI = gastrointestinal; HBV = hepatitis B virus; HCV = hepatitis C virus; hGH = human growth hormone; HIV = human immunodeficiency syndrome; HSV = herpes simplex virus; MAC = *Mycobacterium avium* complex; RUQ = right upper quadrant.

inhibitors. Host factors (e.g., genetics) also probably play a role in producing these syndromes. The co-occurrence of visceral fat accumulation, atherogenic lipid profiles, and glucose intolerance defines metabolic syndrome, the diagnosis of which requires three of the following factors: high triglyceride levels, low high-density lipoprotein levels, hypertension, elevated waist circumference, and glucose intolerance. The prevalence of metabolic syndrome has increased dramatically in HIV-infected individuals, and there is concern that it may contribute to the increased risk for cardiovascular disease in persons infected with HIV.[1,2]

Liver Disease
Liver disease is now the second leading cause of death in those with HIV infection, owing to the prevalence of coinfection with chronic viral hepatitis

(Chapter 149). Coinfection with HCV is present in approximately 25%, depending on the HIV transmission category: 50 to 90% of IVDUs and hemophiliacs, 10 to 20% of heterosexuals, and 5 to 10% of MSM.[3] Chronic HBV infection, defined by the presence of hepatitis B surface antigen (HBsAg), is found in approximately 10% of persons with HIV, and some have more than one viral coinfection. Hepatic fibrosis progresses more rapidly in HIV-infected individuals and leads to cirrhosis, decompensated liver disease, or hepatic failure (Chapter 154). This may be further accelerated by alcohol use, steatosis, or fatty liver disease and by hepatotoxicity from ART. Coinfection with HCV or HBV increases the risk for death by four- to six-fold over HIV infection alone and increases the risk of hepatic decompensation.[4] Mortality from liver disease increases as CD4+ cells decline, more markedly with CD4+ counts lower than 100 cells/μL. Early diagnosis and treatment of HCV and HBV may arrest or slow the progression of hepatic fibrosis and reduce the hepatotoxicity associated with antiretroviral treatment.

All persons with HIV infection should be screened for coinfection with HBV and HCV.[5] A positive serologic test for HBsAg indicates chronic HBV infection and should be followed by tests for HBV DNA and hepatitis B e antigen. Those without chronic HBV infection and with no protective antibody to HBV surface antigen (negative anti-HBs) should be vaccinated against HBV. If treatment of hepatitis B is to be initiated in the absence of ART, a dual regimen of telbivudine and adefovir is appropriate because these agents will not select for HIV resistance. A positive test for HCV antibody should prompt testing for HCV RNA, which determines whether chronic HCV infection is present. Noninvasive markers of hepatic fibrosis, serum biomarkers, and hepatic elastography (to measure hepatic stiffness) are being developed to replace liver biopsy. The prevalence of hepatocellular carcinoma (HCC) (Chapter 196) is increased in those with HIV coinfection; it is found at a younger age and is more aggressive in HIV-infected patients. Regular 6-month screening for HCC by serum α-fetoprotein levels and ultrasound imaging of the liver in persons with cirrhosis may help identify lesions earlier.

Randomized clinical trials have shown that anti-HCV therapy can induce a sustained virologic response (SVR)—that is, undetectable levels of HCV RNA measured 6 months after the end of treatment. However, SVR rates are approximately 60 to 80% of those achieved in persons with HCV monoinfection. Newer drug regimens in development with direct-acting antivirals hold promise for improved SVR rates without the side-effects of pegylated interferon.[6] To avoid drug interactions, neither didanosine (lactic acidosis) nor zidovudine (anemia) should be given with ribavirin.

Hepatotoxicity from ART occurs in up to 12% of patients started on a new ART regimen. Risk factors for hepatotoxicity include chronic HCV or HBV infection, female sex, and the use of ritonavir or nevirapine in the regimen. Effective ART has been associated with reduced hepatic inflammation, less progression of hepatic fibrosis, and decreased mortality from liver disease.

Oral Lesions

New oral lesions should raise suspicion for HIV disease. The lesions may be unsightly but asymptomatic or cause discomfort and difficulty eating. Thrush appears as white plaques, usually on the buccal mucosa. Oral hairy leukoplakia (Figure 425-5 in Chapter 425), which is associated with Epstein-Barr virus, consists of raised shaggy, dirty white patches on the sides of the tongue but is not premalignant.

Oral ulcers (Chapter 425) are caused by infection with herpes simplex virus type 1 (HSV-1) and tend to be more severe and persistent than ulcers in immunocompetent hosts. Idiopathic ulcers similar to those found in the esophagus are found in patients with advanced HIV disease. These deep necrotic ulcers are most commonly found on the buccal and pharyngeal mucosa. They respond to systemic corticosteroids or thalidomide. Gingivitis and periodontal disease appear as linear or diffuse erythema of the gums. With declining CD4+ counts, they may progress to necrotizing gingivitis with pain and hemorrhage. There is increasing concern that these bacterial diseases may contribute to systemic inflammation and more rapid progression of HIV disease.

Kaposi sarcoma (Chapter 393), a multicentric malignancy of endothelial cells caused by human herpesvirus 8 infection, is more common in MSM with HIV infection in the United States but is also prevalent in Africa. Oral lesions are found in half of persons with other sites of Kaposi sarcoma and appear on the palate or gums as raised reddish or bluish nodules.

Anorectal Diseases

Anorectal disorders in HIV-infected individuals are more prevalent in MSM. Anal fissures, fistulas, abscesses, and foreign objects may be found on anal examination as a consequence of receptive anal intercourse or manipulation. Proctitis caused by gonorrhea (Neisseria gonorrhoeae) (Chapter 299) is characterized by mucopurulent discharge from the anus, tenesmus, and bleeding. Chlamydia trachomatis infection (Chapter 318) also causes proctitis and inguinal lymphadenopathy. Cultures and swabs of the discharge are diagnostic.

Primary syphilis (Chapter 319) is manifested as an anal chancre or ulcer that may be tender because of its location. Secondary syphilis appears 2 to 6 months later as condylomata lata, or warty masses around the anus. Perianal shallow, painful ulcers caused by HSV (Chapter 374) evolve as the initial vesicles rupture. These ulcerations may be cultured for HSV, or scrapings will show viral inclusions. Patients may have concurrent herpes proctitis.

Anal condylomata or warts are caused by infection with human papillomavirus (HPV) (Chapter 373) and appear as white, pink, or gray painless lesions around the anus and in the anal canal. HPV types 16 and 18 are associated with the development of dysplasia and squamous cell cancer of the anus, which is manifested as bleeding or a mass. The prevalence of anal dysplasia may be as high as 50% in HIV-positive MSM, and the incidence of anal cancer has increased more than six-fold in the past two decades. Screening via anal cytology is being pioneered for high-risk individuals.

⬤ GASTROINTESTINAL DISEASES MORE COMMONLY SEEN WITH CD4+ COUNTS LESS THAN 200 CELLS/μL

GI illness increases in prevalence and severity as the CD4+ count declines. With marked immunosuppression, there may be multiple concurrent infections. Although specific antimicrobial therapy may control the infection, HAART is the most effective therapy.

Esophageal Diseases

Candidal esophagitis (Chapter 338) is the most common esophageal infection in HIV-infected individuals. The combination of oral thrush and dysphagia has a positive predictive value of 90% for esophageal candidiasis. If the symptoms do not resolve with treatment in 7 days, endoscopy is indicated.[7] Cytomegalovirus (CMV) (Chapter 376) and idiopathic esophageal ulcerations may appear when the CD4+ count falls below 50 cells/μL. Odynophagia, or severe pain on swallowing, is the initial symptom. Endoscopy shows large ulcerations with elevated margins, and CMV inclusions are seen in biopsy samples. HSV infections are much less common and appear as confluent shallow ulcerations in the esophagus. Idiopathic ulceration is diagnosed by the absence of viral inclusions on biopsy specimens.

Diarrhea

Diarrhea remains a common illness in HIV-infected individuals, even in the era of effective ART. Infections of the small intestine are accompanied by large-volume watery diarrhea. Colonic disease may be manifested as bloody, inflammatory, or small-volume diarrhea and tenesmus. Routine bacterial pathogens, including Salmonella, Campylobacter, and Shigella, have all been documented to cause diarrhea in HIV-infected patients. Enteroaggregative Escherichia coli has been identified as a cause of persistent diarrhea in HIV-infected individuals. The use of multiple antibiotics in HIV-infected patients has led to the frequent occurrence of Clostridium difficile colitis (Chapter 296). Mycobacterial infections with either Mycobacterium tuberculosis or atypical mycobacteria, most commonly Mycobacterium avium complex (MAC), may infiltrate the small bowel in HIV-infected patients. Although M. tuberculosis infection occurs with exposure in individuals with moderate CD4+ cell depletion, disseminated MAC disease occurs only in individuals with CD4+ counts lower than 50 cells/μL.

Most often, viral diarrheas are similar in manifestation to those in the general population, pathogens are not routinely identified in the clinical setting, and disease is self-limited. However, CMV may cause disease throughout the length of the GI tract in HIV-infected patients with CD4+ counts lower than 50 cells/μL. In the small bowel, CMV may cause a watery diarrhea, and in the colon, a colitis with blood and signs of inflammation on endoscopy. Biopsy with identification of virus in tissue is required to make the diagnosis of CMV enteric disease.

Parasitic causes of diarrhea are common in HIV-infected individuals.[8] Opportunistic parasitic pathogens include Cryptosporidium parvum, the microsporidial organisms Enterocytozoon bieneusi and Encephalitozoon intestinalis, and Cyclospora cayetanensis. Persistent diarrhea caused by cryptosporidiosis (Chapter 350) occurs when the CD4+ count is less than 200 cells/μL, and the most effective control of this pathogen is treatment of HIV.

Pathogens are not found in up to half of cases of diarrhea in HIV-infected patients, even after a full diagnostic evaluation. This condition has been called AIDS enteropathy and is associated with chronic diarrhea, malnutrition, and wasting.[9] It is possible that some of the chronic diarrhea is caused by pathogens that are not yet recognized or by noninfectious causes such as lymphoma. It is also likely that some of these pathogen-negative diarrheas are caused by HIV itself, which may infect the enterocyte as well as lymphoid tissue within the gut.

Malignancy

Kaposi sarcoma (Chapter 393) may develop at any location in the GI tract. Kaposi lesions appear endoscopically as raised reddish nodules that may bleed spontaneously. Non-Hodgkin lymphomas may involve any portion of the GI tract, as well as the liver, and are manifested as bleeding, obstruction, weight loss, or abdominal pain.

Wasting

Wasting in HIV-infected individuals is defined by the World Health Organization as a body mass index of less than 18.5 kg/m^2. Weight loss and wasting are still seen in patients with treated HIV infection, and even modest weight loss of 3% or greater increases mortality.

In uncontrolled HIV infection, multiple factors contribute to wasting. Caloric requirements are increased by the metabolic demands of HIV replication, concurrent opportunistic infections, and fever. Oral intake may be poor because of nausea, anorexia, dysphagia, odynophagia, or chronic diarrhea or as a result of food insecurity, depression, or dementia.[10] Weight loss is exacerbated by malabsorption of nutrients from small intestinal or pancreatic disease. HIV-infected persons may not be able to increase caloric intake to overcome the loss of nutrients in stool and meet the metabolic demands of their illness. Targeted approaches to wasting and weight loss include treatment of HIV or opportunistic infections, frequent small meals, and use of appetite stimulants (megestrol acetate, dronabinol), anabolic steroids (testosterone, oxandrolone, nandrolone[A2]), or recombinant human growth hormone, as indicated. With control of HIV replication, nutritional status and weight generally improve, although they may not return to premorbid levels if the wasting was severe.

Hepatobiliary Disease

Hepatobiliary disease is associated with very low CD4$^+$ counts, often less than 20 cells/μL. Evaluation of abnormalities in liver function should initially exclude HBV and HCV infection and drug-induced hepatotoxicity, particularly that involving antiretroviral or sulfa-containing medications. The presence of hepatomegaly suggests an infiltrative process such as MAC or fungal infection or lymphoma. Alkaline phosphatase is disproportionately elevated. Liver imaging often does not show a localized lesion but determines whether biliary dilation is present, a finding suggestive of extrahepatic disease. Liver biopsy with special stains and cultures may be definitive.

In contrast, the presence of right upper quadrant pain with or without jaundice indicates biliary tract disease (Chapter 155). AIDS cholangiopathy[11] includes a sclerosing cholangitis–like process with diffuse biliary strictures and dilations and papillary stenosis with narrowing of the distal common bile duct at the entrance to the duodenum. In papillary stenosis, the common bile duct is dilated proximal to the stenosis. Acalculous cholecystitis may also be seen. These changes are caused by infection of the biliary tree with *Cryptosporidium*, microsporidia, *Isospora belli*, or CMV in the setting of profound immunosuppression. Endoscopic retrograde cholangiopancreatography can be performed to establish the diagnosis, obtain brushings for examination, and treat papillary stenosis by sphincterotomy. Treatment of the specific organism seldom eradicates infection because of the degree of immunosuppression. However, treatment with ART can result in marked improvements in biliary findings.

APPROACH TO GASTROINTESTINAL DISEASES

The GI tract is host to a myriad of infectious and infiltrative diseases in HIV-infected persons. Even so, routine GI diseases such as diverticulitis, choledocholithiasis, or peptic ulcer disease must be considered, particularly in those treated with ART. The clinician is guided by the symptom complex, as laid out in Table 390-1, to identify the probable organisms or tumors by clinical findings. The CD4$^+$ count influences the likelihood of the type of GI infection. It is important to remember that multiple illnesses may occur simultaneously with HIV infection and that finding one cause of a symptom or complaint may not be sufficient.

With diarrhea, careful stool evaluations should include cultures for *Salmonella*, *Shigella*, and *Campylobacter*; assay for *Clostridium difficile* toxin; and at least three examinations for parasites, including acid-fast stains for MAC and *Cryptosporidium*. If these measures are unrevealing, upper GI endoscopy with biopsy of the small intestine is indicated to diagnose protozoal infections with *Cryptosporidium*, *Isospora belli*, or microsporidia. Signs of colitis are best evaluated by flexible sigmoidoscopy or colonoscopy with biopsy and cultures. Examination and biopsy of the terminal ileum with acid-fast stain is necessary to confirm the diagnosis of pathogens such as *M. tuberculosis* or MAC.

All persons with HIV should be screened for coinfection with HBV and HCV and vaccinated against hepatitis A and B if not immune. Finally, close attention to serial measurement of weight and calculation of the body mass index is crucial to identify those who may have poor outcomes as a result of weight loss or excessive weight gain.

Grade A References

A1. Malan N, Su J, Mancini M, et al. Gastrointestinal tolerability and quality of life in antiretroviral-naive HIV-1-infected patients: data from the CASTLE study. *AIDS Care*. 2010;22:677-686.
A2. Sardar P, Jha A, Roy D, et al. Therapeutic effects of nandrolone and testosterone in adult male HIV patients with AIDS wasting syndrome (AWS): a randomized, double-blind, placebo-controlled trial. *HIV Clin Trials*. 2010;11:220-229.

GENERAL REFERENCES

For the General References and other additional features, please visit Expert Consult at https://expertconsult.inkling.com.

391

PULMONARY MANIFESTATIONS OF HUMAN IMMUNODEFICIENCY VIRUS AND THE ACQUIRED IMMUNODEFICIENCY SYNDROME

KRISTINA CROTHERS AND ALISON MORRIS

INTRODUCTION

Pulmonary disease has historically been a leading cause of morbidity and mortality in patients with human immunodeficiency virus (HIV) and the acquired immunodeficiency syndrome (AIDS). Case reports of the previously rare *Pneumocystis* pneumonia (PCP) were the first harbingers of the AIDS epidemic in the 1980s, and in the early era of HIV, pulmonary infections such as bacterial pneumonia, PCP, and tuberculosis (TB) were frequently encountered. Pulmonary malignancies such as Kaposi sarcoma and lymphoma were also common. Prognosis for persons with HIV has changed dramatically with introduction of chemoprophylaxis for common infections such as PCP and with combination antiretroviral therapy (ART). The range of pulmonary diseases encountered in the HIV-infected patient has also changed over the course of the HIV epidemic and now includes fewer opportunistic infections with potential increases in diseases such as chronic obstructive pulmonary disease (COPD).

Pathobiology of HIV and Effects on Pulmonary Immunity

HIV infection in the absence of ART is characterized by immune dysfunction, dysregulation, and progressive immunodeficiency that results in a substantially increased risk for infections and other complications (Fig. 391-1). Early after initial infection, CD4 lymphocytes are depleted from mucosal-associated lymphoid tissue. During the chronic phase of untreated HIV, generalized immune activation and systemic CD4 lymphocyte depletion occurs, and remaining T cells may mount abnormal responses to antigens. Accompanying B-cell dysfunction results in abnormal polyclonal activation, hypergammaglobulinemia, and lack of specific antibody responses. Although ART decreases opportunistic infections and mortality in HIV-infected patients, persistent immune activation, dysfunction, and chronic low-level inflammation can persist and may contribute to the increased risk of several chronic comorbid diseases among HIV-infected individuals. The contribution of this chronic immune activation to pulmonary diseases such as COPD is currently unknown.

Within the lung parenchyma, HIV infection results in impaired innate and adaptive immune responses to pathogens.[1] Alveolar macrophages and lung CD4 T cells from HIV-infected individuals have deficiencies and impaired responses in pathogen recognition (e.g., influenza, *Mycobacterium tuberculosis*).[2] HIV can also lead to other abnormalities in host defense of the lung, including mucociliary function and soluble defense molecules within respiratory secretions. Among individuals who initiate ART, lung HIV viral levels and inflammation generally decrease, mirroring responses in the systemic

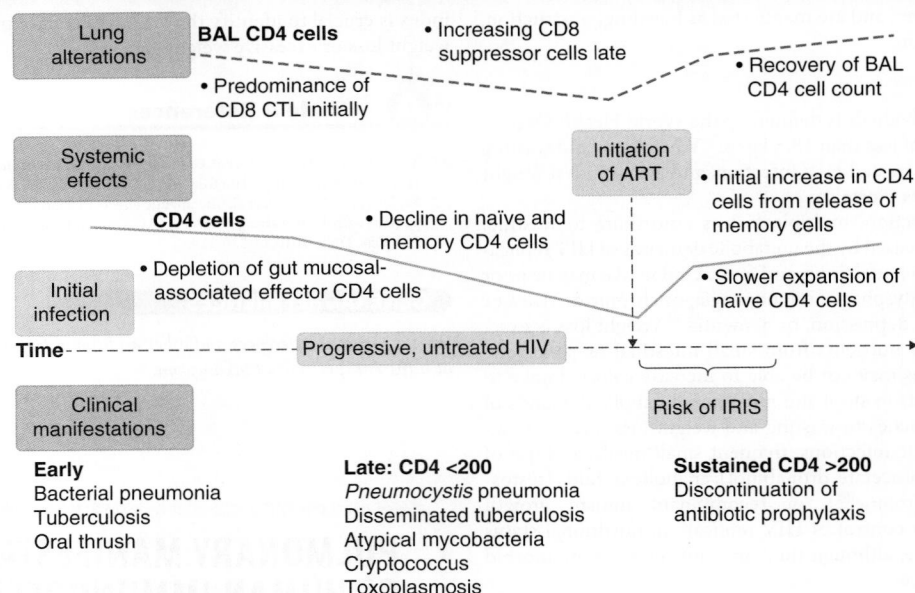

FIGURE 391-1. Systemic and lung alterations in T lymphocytes with HIV infection and initiation of antiretroviral therapy (ART). After initial HIV infection, CD4 lymphocytes of the effector memory type are depleted from mucosal-associated lymphoid tissue; the CD4 cells within the alveolar space appear to be spared but gradually decrease over time with progressive untreated HIV. During the chronic phase of HIV infection, there is progressive decline in the systemic CD4 cell count owing to decreased naïve and memory T cells. Within the alveolar space, HIV-specific cytotoxic CD8 T lymphocytes (CTL) predominate, although in late-stage disease these are replaced with CD8 suppressor lymphocytes. As discussed in the text, HIV infection is also associated with abnormal function of T cells, B-cell dysfunction, and within the lung, abnormalities in several other lines of host defense. With initiation of ART, CD4 cell counts increase systemically and in the lung. ART, antiretroviral therapy; BAL = bronchoalveolar lavage; IRIS, immune reconstitution inflammatory syndrome.

circulation. Nonetheless, HIV-infected individuals appear to have an increased risk of chronic lung diseases, although the mechanisms by which this increased risk occurs are not yet well understood.

EVALUATION OF THE HIV-INFECTED PATIENT WITH LUNG DISEASE

Respiratory disease is a common cause of both outpatient and inpatient visits in HIV-infected individuals. Pulmonary disease in this population can result from both infectious and noninfectious causes that are related to HIV infection or HIV medications, or that are unrelated to HIV. These pulmonary diseases often have characteristic clinical and radiographic manifestations, but there is also variability and overlap among them. In addition, HIV-infected patients often have more than one condition. For these reasons, definitive diagnosis of HIV-associated pulmonary diseases is encouraged when possible. The diagnostic evaluation should be guided by the constellation of the clinical signs and symptoms, laboratory testing, and radiographic appearance, as well as the severity of disease (Fig. 391-2A and 2B).

Clinical Findings

Often, the clinical history, physical examination, and laboratory testing can provide clues for a specific diagnosis (Table 391-1). For example, injection drug users have a greater risk of bacterial pneumonia and TB, whereas men who have sex with men have an increased risk of Kaposi sarcoma. As in the HIV-uninfected population, cigarette smoking is associated with bacterial pneumonia as well as COPD. In general, patients with a history of a previous opportunistic infection such as PCP are at increased risk of recurrence, although use of prophylaxis decreases disease incidence. Travel or place of residence also influences the risk of endemic fungal infections and TB. Certain extrapulmonary symptoms can also implicate specific diseases. For example, complaints of headache or altered mental status in a person with respiratory symptoms should prompt a search for *Cryptococcus* pneumonia and meningitis. Many diseases such as TB, malignancies, and fungal infections can cause extrapulmonary signs and symptoms such as lymphadenopathy, hepatic dysfunction, and bone marrow infiltration.

The CD4 cell count is one of the most critical pieces of information in determining the differential diagnosis of HIV-associated pulmonary disease (Table 391-2). Some diseases such as TB and bacterial pneumonia can occur at any CD4 cell count but are more common at lower counts, with a more atypical presentation of disease that is more likely to be disseminated. In contrast, disease such as pulmonary Kaposi sarcoma, *Toxoplasma gondii* pneumonia, and *Mycobacterium avium* complex are usually only seen if the

CD4 cell count is below 100 cells/μL, and more often below 50 cells/μL. PCP is uncommon above a count greater than 200 cells/μL and less common if the CD4 cell count is between 100 and 200 cells/μL in a person receiving ART. If available, the most recent CD4 cell count *prior to* hospitalization is often more useful in HIV-infected inpatients to guide decision making, because the CD4 count can fall in the setting of acute illness.

Radiographic Studies

The radiographic picture also provides important clues to the diagnosis of HIV-associated pulmonary disease (Table 391-3). Certain radiographic findings are "classic" for certain diseases such as bilateral perihilar diffuse infiltrates in PCP (Fig. 391-3), but atypical presentations of pulmonary disease are not uncommon. The radiographic presentation also varies with the CD4 cell count. For example, TB presents with upper lung zone infiltrates that are often cavitary in patients with CD4 cell counts above 200 cells/μL (Fig. 391-4), but cavitation is uncommon with TB in patients with low CD4 cell counts, and lower lobe consolidation mimicking bacterial pneumonia can be seen (Fig. 391-5).

PULMONARY INFECTIONS

Pulmonary infections remain a major cause of morbidity and mortality in HIV-infected populations. Although pulmonary infections are more common in individuals without access to ART, a study of over 9000 HIV-infected and HIV-uninfected individuals found incident pulmonary infections remained more common in the era of combination ART.[3] The CD4 cell count has significant impact on the epidemiology of pneumonia, and HIV-infected individuals with advanced immunosuppression are at risk of a large spectrum of infectious causes of pneumonia (Fig. 391-6). Individuals with higher CD4 cell counts also remain at increased risk of bacterial pneumonia and TB when compared to HIV-uninfected populations. The general approach to the HIV-infected patient with pneumonia is described above, and we discuss the three most common HIV-associated pulmonary infections in further detail below.

Bacterial Pneumonia

EPIDEMIOLOGY

Recurrent bacterial pneumonia, defined as two or more episodes within 12 months, is an AIDS-defining illness. The risk for bacterial pneumonia is substantially increased among HIV-infected individuals, and in contrast to other opportunistic infections, this elevated risk persists in the combination ART era. For example, in a study of HIV-infected veterans in the ART era, the incidence rate of bacterial pneumonia in HIV-infected individuals was 28.0

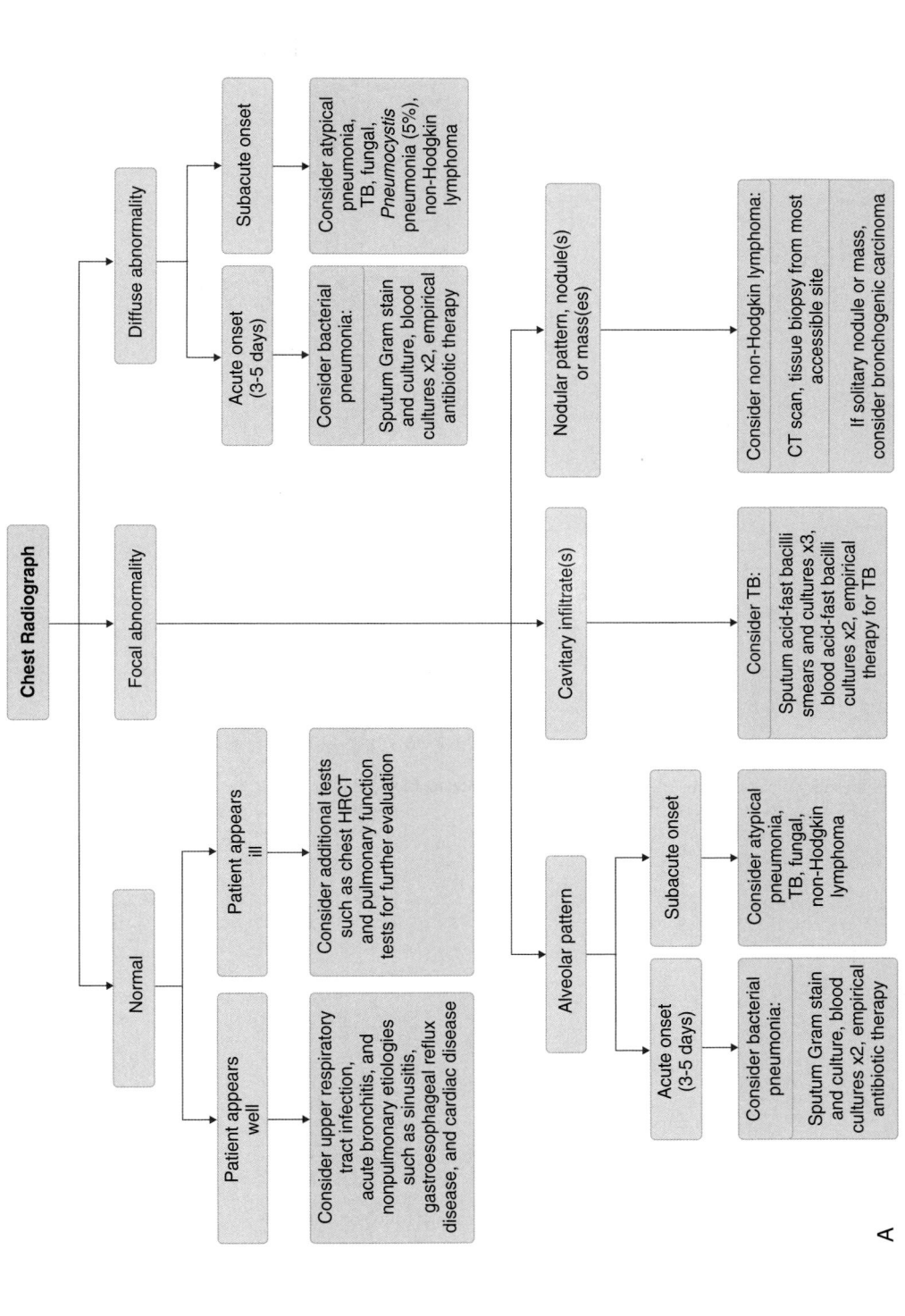

FIGURE 391-2. Diagnostic approach to the HIV-infected patient with clinical manifestations of possible pulmonary disease and a CD4 cell count greater than 200 cells/μL (A) and a CD4 cell count below 200 cells/μL (B). HRCT = high-resolution computed tomography; TB = tuberculosis.

Continued

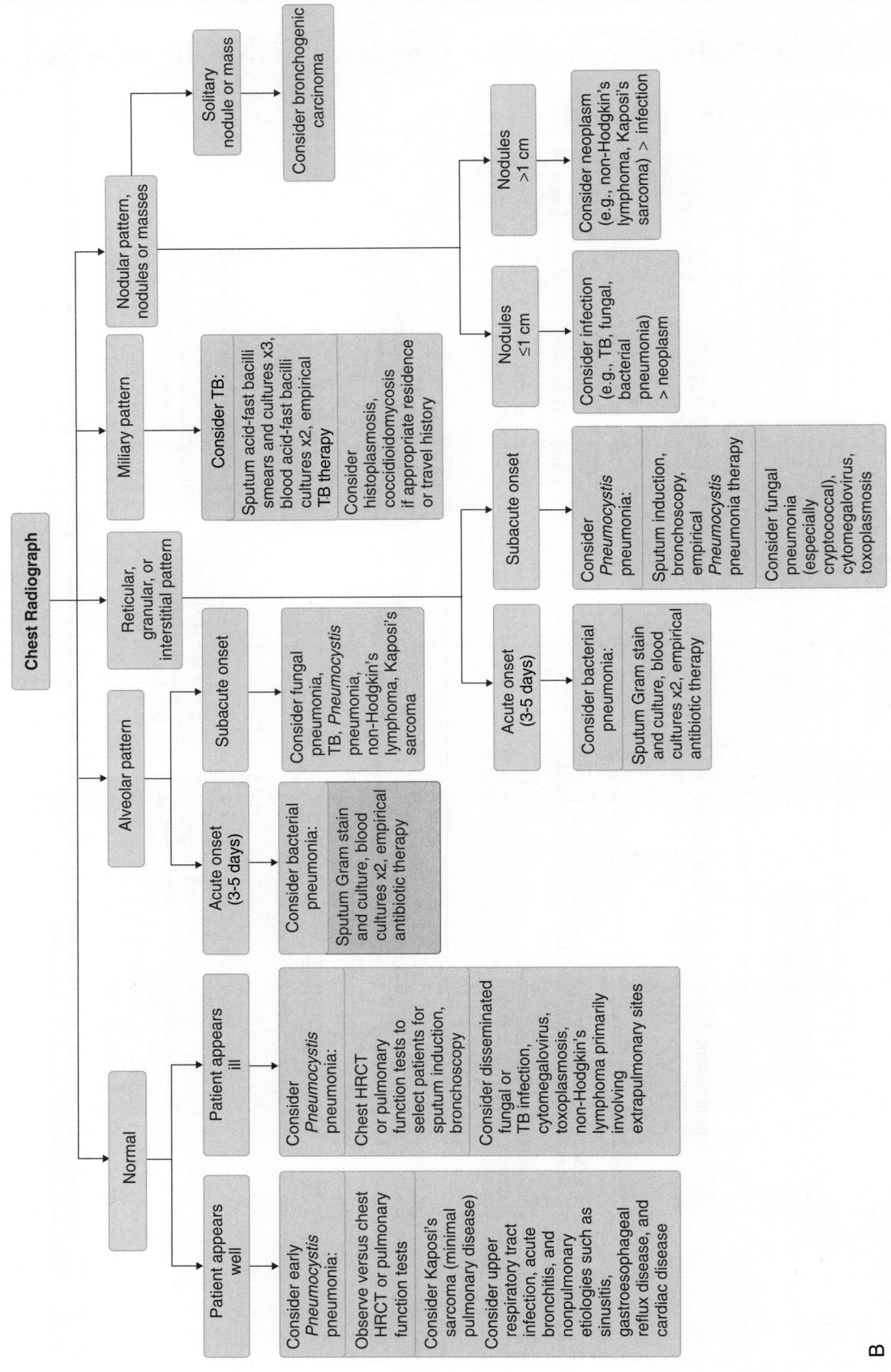

FIGURE 391-2, cont'd.

B

TABLE 391-1 DIAGNOSTIC CLUES TO ETIOLOGY OF HIV-ASSOCIATED PULMONARY DISEASES

CLINICAL SETTING

Ambulatory: URI > acute bronchitis > bacterial pneumonia > *Pneumocystis* pneumonia

Hospital: bacterial pneumonia > *Pneumocystis* pneumonia > TB > pulmonary KS

Intensive care unit: *Pneumocystis* pneumonia > bacterial pneumonia; non–AIDS associated conditions > AIDS-associated conditions

CD4 CELL COUNT (see Table 391-2)
PATIENT BACKGROUND

HIV transmission category: MSM—increased incidence of KS; IDU—increased incidence of bacterial pneumonia, TB

Habits: cigarettes—increased incidence of bacterial bronchitis, bacterial pneumonia, COPD, bronchogenic carcinoma

Travel and residence: assess risk for endemic fungal diseases, TB, NTM

MEDICAL BACKGROUND AND USE OF PROPHYLAXIS

Previous disease: increased incidence of recurrence of bacterial pneumonia, *Pneumocystis* pneumonia, fungal pneumonias

Prophylaxis/maintenance: decreased incidence of disease—*Pneumocystis* pneumonia, fungal pneumonias, TB (if PPD positive or positive interferon-γ release assay)

SYMPTOMS AND SIGNS

Respiratory symptoms: especially cough (productive or nonproductive) and symptom duration

Symptoms suggesting extrapulmonary or disseminated disease

Physical examination of the chest: focal or nonfocal findings

Signs suggesting extrapulmonary or disseminated disease

LABORATORY TESTS

WBC count: elevated or, if normal, elevated relative to baseline—bacterial pneumonia

Serum LDH: elevated—nonspecific but classically seen in *Pneumocystis* pneumonia

Arterial blood gas: nonspecific but useful for prognosis, management decisions (e.g., admission and whether corticosteroids are indicated for *Pneumocystis* pneumonia)

CHEST RADIOGRAPHY (see Table 391-3)

AIDS = acquired immunodeficiency syndrome; COPD = chronic obstructive pulmonary disease; HIV, human immunodeficiency virus; IDU = injection drug user; KS = Kaposi sarcoma; LDH = lactate dehydrogenase; MSM = men who have sex with men; NTM, nontuberculous mycobacteria; PPD = purified protein derivative (in an HIV-infected person, PPD is considered positive if ≥ 5-mm induration); TB = tuberculosis; URI = upper respiratory tract infection; WBC = white blood cell.

TABLE 391-2 CD4 CELL COUNT RANGES FOR HIV-ASSOCIATED PULMONARY DISEASES

ANY CD4 CELL COUNT

Bacterial pneumonia (most often *Streptococcus pneumoniae*, *Haemophilus* species)
Mycobacterium tuberculosis pneumonia
Influenza
Non-Hodgkin lymphoma
Lung cancer
Nonspecific interstitial pneumonitis
Lymphocytic interstitial pneumonitis
Pulmonary arterial hypertension
Chronic obstructive lung disease

CD4 CELL COUNT < 200 CELLS/μL

Pneumocystis pneumonia
Cryptococcus neoformans pneumonia

CD4 CELL COUNT < 100 CELLS/μL

Bacterial pneumonia caused by *Pseudomonas aeruginosa*
Toxoplasma gondii pneumonia
Pulmonary Kaposi sarcoma

CD4 CELL COUNT < 50 CELLS/μL

Mycobacterium avium complex—usually associated with disseminated disease
Histoplasma capsulatum—usually associated with disseminated disease
Coccidioides immitis—usually associated with disseminated disease
Aspergillus species (most often *Aspergillus fumigatus*) pneumonia
Cytomegalovirus pneumonia—usually associated with disseminated disease

TABLE 391-3 COMMON RADIOGRAPHIC FEATURES OF HIV-ASSOCIATED PULMONARY DISEASES

CONDITION	COMMON RADIOGRAPHIC FINDINGS
Pneumocystis pneumonia	Bilateral perihilar infiltrates Pneumatoceles, pneumothorax Ground-glass opacities Normal (chest radiograph) Upper lobe or asymmetrical infiltrates (less common)
Bacterial pneumonia	Focal infiltrates Pleural effusions Cavitary lesions
Mycobacterium tuberculosis	Focal infiltrates Normal (in extrapulmonary disease) Diffuse infiltrates/miliary pattern Nodules Cavitary lesions Intrathoracic adenopathy Pleural effusions Upper lobe involvement if high CD4 cell count
Mycobacterium kansasii	Consolidation Nodules Diffuse infiltrates Intrathoracic adenopathy Cavitary lesions Pleural effusions
Mycobacterium avium complex	Normal Intrathoracic adenopathy Focal pneumonia (rare)
Fungal pneumonia	Multifocal or diffuse infiltrates Focal infiltrate Normal Cystic lesions Nodules Intrathoracic adenopathy Pleural effusions (especially *Cryptococcus neoformans*)
Cytomegalovirus	Multifocal or diffuse infiltrates Reticular pattern Ground-glass opacities
Toxoplasma gondii	Bilateral infiltrates Pleural effusions
Non-Hodgkin lymphoma	Single or multiple nodules Focal infiltrates Diffuse interstitial infiltrates Pleural effusions Intrathoracic adenopathy
Kaposi sarcoma	Multifocal or diffuse infiltrates Bilateral central opacities Nodules Peribronchial cuffing, tram-track Kerley B lines Pleural effusions Intrathoracic adenopathy
Lung cancer	Masses Nodules Intrathoracic adenopathy Pleural effusions
COPD	Large lung volumes Flattened diaphragms Bullae Emphysema (chest CT)
Interstitial lung diseases	Normal (chest radiograph) Increased interstitial markings Small lung volumes Fibrosis Traction bronchiectasis Peribronchovascular nodules (sarcoidosis, LIP) Intrathoracic lymphadenopathy (sarcoidosis, rarely LIP)
Pulmonary hypertension	Normal Enlarged pulmonary arteries Vascular pruning Right heart enlargement

COPD = chronic obstructive pulmonary disease; CT = computed tomography; LIP = lymphocytic interstitial pneumonia

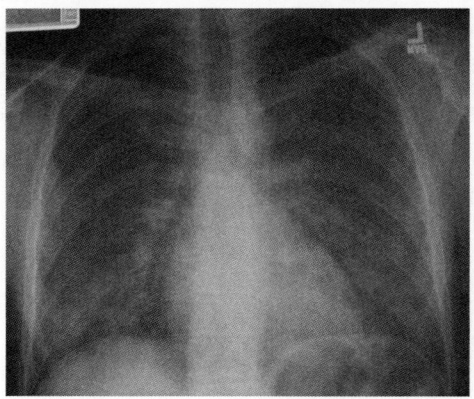

FIGURE 391-3. Chest radiograph of an HIV-infected person, CD4 cell count less than 200 cells/μL, demonstrating characteristic bilateral reticular-granular opacities of *Pneumocystis* pneumonia. Bronchoscopic alveolar lavage demonstrated *Pneumocystis* on Giemsa stain. Courtesy Laurence Huang, MD. Used with permission.

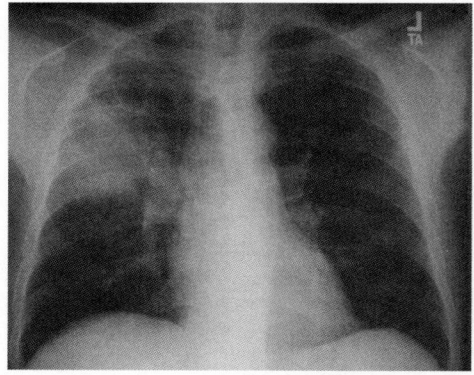

FIGURE 391-4. Chest radiograph of an HIV-infected person, CD4 cell count greater than 200 cells/μL, demonstrating a right upper lobe infiltrate with areas of cavitation. Sputum acid-fast bacillus stain was positive, and multiple sputum cultures grew *Mycobacterium tuberculosis*. Courtesy Laurence Huang, MD. Used with permission.

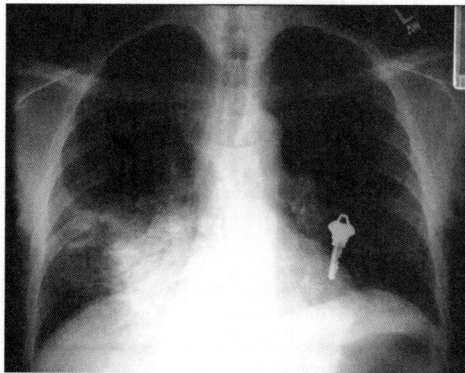

FIGURE 391-5. Chest radiograph of an HIV-infected person, CD4 cell count less than 200 cells/μL, revealing right lower lung zone consolidation with air bronchograms. Sputum culture grew *Mycobacterium tuberculosis* that was resistant to rifampin. Courtesy Laurence Huang, MD. Used with permission.

			CMV
			NTM
		Kaposi sarcoma	
		Other fungal infection	
		Cryptococcus	
		Pneumocystis pneumonia	
	Non-Hodgkin lymphoma ⟶		
Bacterial pneumonia ⟶ Bacteremia			
Reactivation TB	Primary TB	Atypical TB	
CD4 cells 500	200	100	50

Noninfectious complications (COPD, ARDS, lung cancer, etc.)

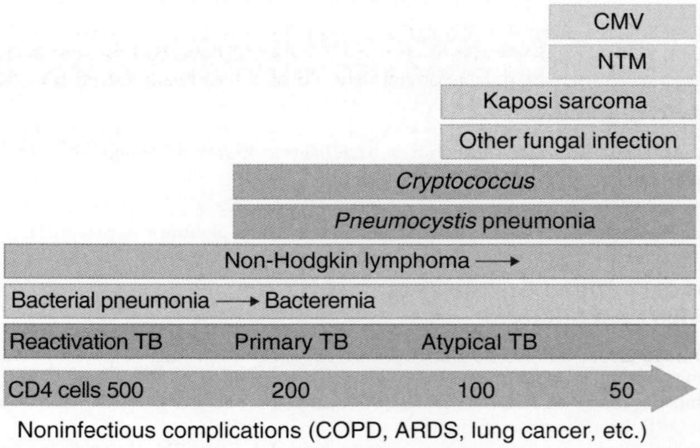

FIGURE 391-6. Risk of pulmonary complications by CD4 cell count. ARDS = acute respiratory distress syndrome; CMV = cytomegalovirus; COPD = chronic obstructive pulmonary disease; NTM = nontuberculous mycobacteria; TB = tuberculosis.

for bacterial pneumonia. Numerous bacteria may cause pneumonia in HIV. *Streptococcus pneumoniae* is the most commonly isolated cause of community-acquired bacterial pneumonia in HIV-infected populations and is often complicated by bacteremia and invasive disease. Other frequent causes of pneumonia in HIV-infected persons include *Haemophilus* species and *Staphylococcus aureus*, the latter of which can cause community-acquired pneumonia in patients both with and without a history of injection drug use. More unusual bacterial organisms that can cause pneumonia in HIV-infected persons include *Rhodococcus equi* and *Nocardia* species. Atypical causes of community-acquired bacterial pneumonia such as *Mycoplasma* or *Legionella* species do not seem to occur with increased frequency in HIV-infected compared to uninfected patients.

CLINICAL MANIFESTATIONS

Patients typically present with acute onset of symptoms over a few days, often with cough productive of purulent sputum, fever, systemic malaise, and leukocytosis with a neutrophilic predominance. Typical radiographic findings consist of segmental, lobar, or multilobar consolidation on chest radiograph, although more diffuse reticular or interstitial patterns can occur as well. Cavitary infiltrates may result from a number of different causes, including bacteria such as *S. aureus*, *Pseudomonas*, and *Nocardia* species. Numerous cavitary infiltrates, particularly from staphylococcal species, should prompt consideration of septic pulmonary emboli. The risk of invasive disease secondary to *S. pneumoniae* is increased in those who are not on ART and who have not received pneumococcal vaccine. Other risk factors for bacteremia secondary to *S. pneumoniae* include low CD4 cell count, alcohol abuse, current smoking, recent hospitalization, and other comorbid illnesses.

DIAGNOSIS

Blood cultures should be obtained, particularly in individuals with low CD4 cell counts, and sputum cultures considered. Thoracentesis should be considered for patients with pleural effusion, particularly if they are not responding appropriately to antimicrobial therapy.

per 1000 person-years compared with 5.8 per 1000 person-years in the HIV-uninfected group.[4] Bacterial pneumonia can occur throughout the course of HIV infection and at any CD4 lymphocyte count, although the incidence increases as the CD4 lymphocyte count declines. Additional risk factors for bacterial pneumonia include injection drug use and cigarette smoking.

PATHOBIOLOGY AND PATHOGENS

Immunodeficiency as reflected by circulating CD4 T-cell counts, as well as local abnormalities within the host defenses of the lung, confer increased risk

TREATMENT   Rx

The treatment of HIV-infected patients with community-acquired bacterial pneumonia should follow published guidelines.[5] Initial empirical therapy should include coverage against frequently identified organisms (e.g., *S. pneumoniae* and *Haemophilus* species) and should target both typical and atypical causes of bacterial pneumonia. Local drug resistance patterns should be taken into account, and monotherapy with a macrolide should be avoided if patients are already on macrolide prophylaxis. Macrolides should also be avoided if TB is in the differential, because resistance can develop. For patients with CD4 lymphocyte counts below 100 cells/μL or with recent hospitalization, neutropenia, broad-spectrum antimicrobial use, or underlying structural lung disease, consideration should be given to including coverage against *Pseudomonas aeruginosa*. For patients with recent health care contact, consideration should be given to antimicrobial therapy directed against microorganisms associated with health care–associated pneumonia (e.g., more resistant gram-positive and gram-negative organisms). Empirical coverage for methicillin-resistant *S. aureus* with vancomycin should also be considered in injection drug users and other high-risk populations.

PREVENTION

Pneumococcal vaccine should be given to HIV-infected patients. Current recommendations are for the 13-valent pneumococcal conjugate vaccine (PCV13) to be given first, followed by 23-valent pneumococcal polysaccharide vaccine (PPV23) at least 8 weeks or more later (Chapter 18). For those who have already received the PPV23, the PCV13 should be given at least 1 year later. Prevention of bacterial pneumonia also includes yearly administration of inactivated influenza vaccine to all HIV-infected individuals.

PROGNOSIS

Time to clinical stability and length of stay for HIV-infected patients with community-acquired bacterial pneumonia are generally similar to HIV-uninfected patients. Although 90-day mortality has overall improved among HIV-infected patients after an episode of pneumonia when comparing the early ART era to the current era, mortality rates remain substantially higher in patients during the 1 year following pneumonia. Risk factors for increased mortality following pneumonia include a CD4 cell count below 200 cells/µL, no ART use, older age, and greater burden of comorbid illness.

Mycobacterium Tuberculosis

EPIDEMIOLOGY

TB is the most common opportunistic infection seen in HIV infection worldwide (Chapter 324). A global explosion in TB cases has resulted from the AIDS epidemic, especially in low-income countries. In contrast to many other HIV-associated infections, TB can be transmitted from person to person via an airborne route, leading to disease in HIV-uninfected individuals as well. TB is often the first manifestation of HIV and is the leading cause of death. In the United States, although TB cases have declined, TB remains an important infectious complication in HIV-infected patients, particularly in high-risk groups such as those living in communal settings or who are incarcerated, foreign-born individuals, or those with a history of TB exposure. Multidrug-resistant (defined as resistance to at least isoniazid and rifampin) and extensively drug-resistant TB (defined as multidrug-resistant TB plus resistance to any fluoroquinolone and at least one second-line injectable drug) are increasing in the HIV population, and some studies find that HIV is an independent risk factor for drug resistance. Drug resistance is associated with decreased survival, especially in HIV-infected individuals with low CD4 cell counts or those not receiving ART. ART use significantly decreases the risk of TB.

CLINICAL MANIFESTATIONS

Although HIV-infected patients may present with characteristic symptoms of TB including fever, sweats, weight loss, and cough, individuals with more advanced immunosuppression (CD4 cell counts < 350 cells/µL) often have an atypical presentation with minimal symptoms. Patients with more advanced HIV are more likely to present with disseminated disease with risk increasing the lower the CD4 cell count. Other clinical history that is suggestive of TB is a history of recent or remote TB exposure or of latent TB without adequate treatment. On physical examination, patients may have signs of lung consolidation, lymphadenopathy, or hepatosplenomegaly. Laboratory testing is often nonspecific, but may reflect underlying organ involvement. The radiographic presentation depends on the degree of immunosuppression. Patients on ART with preserved CD4 cell counts usually have a chest radiographic pattern similar to that in the HIV-uninfected population with reactivation of TB, with upper lung zone infiltrates, often with cavitation (see Fig. 391-4). In patients with more advanced immunosuppression, the chest radiograph pattern is more consistent with primary TB (see Fig. 391-5). There are diffuse infiltrates, often in the middle and lower lung zones. Cavitation is uncommon in patients with a low CD4 cell count. A normal radiograph, miliary disease, or lymphadenopathy are also seen in HIV-infected patients with low CD4 cell counts. Pleural effusions may also be seen.

DIAGNOSIS

Definitive diagnosis by either culture of *M. tuberculosis* from an affected body site or identification by nucleic-acid amplification testing (NAA) is considered the gold standard. Visualization of acid-fast bacilli (AFB) on sputum smear may be the only feasible test in some resource-poor settings; however, HIV-infected individuals are more likely to have negative smears despite active disease. Current recommendations support obtaining three sputum specimens for AFB smear and culture with NAA testing of at least one sputum specimen. Use of NAA allows for rapid identification of the mycobacterial species in smear-positive specimens, allowing determination of TB versus nontuberculous mycobacteria. It is also able to identify *M. tuberculosis* in smear-negative patients more rapidly than culture. Because NAA testing does not provide information on drug sensitivity, it should always be paired with culture. Genotype testing can also be used and rapidly identifies drug resistance mutations, but it is not available in many settings. If three spontaneous sputum samples cannot be obtained, induced sputum or bronchoscopy should be performed. Specimens from other body sites such as cerebrospinal fluid, pleural fluid, and bone marrow aspirates can be evaluated. In patients with isolated pleural effusion where TB is suspected, pleural biopsy should be considered to obtain samples for culture and sensitivity. Mycobacterial blood cultures should be obtained, particularly in individuals with CD4 cell counts below 200 cells/µL.

TREATMENT   Rx

To prevent transmission of TB, empirical treatment should be started in any HIV-infected person suspected of having TB, even if smears are negative (Chapter 324). Patients with AFB detected on smears or culture should also be started on therapy directed against TB while waiting for identification of the mycobacterial species. The recommended regimen for HIV-infected individuals with suspected TB is isoniazid, rifampin, pyrazinamide, and ethambutol with pyridoxine (Table 391-4). Consultation with an expert in TB treatment is recommended in cases of drug resistance. Directly observed therapy is recommended for HIV-infected individuals with TB.

ART is an important adjunctive therapy in HIV-infected individuals with TB. Concurrent ART treatment is shown to decrease mortality, prolong AIDS-free survival, and decrease time to sputum conversion.[A1,A3] Patients receiving ART should be continued on it during TB treatment. In patients with a CD4 cell count below 50 cells/µL, randomized trials have shown that starting ART within 2 weeks of TB therapy is of benefit.[A4] In individuals with higher CD4 cell counts and severe clinical disease, ART should be initiated within 2 to 4 weeks. In all other individuals (except those with TB meningitis [who should have delayed ART]), ART should be started within 8 to 12 weeks. Initiation of ART can be difficult during TB treatment because there are a myriad of drug interactions. Immune reconstitution inflammatory syndrome (IRIS) can also be seen in about one third of individuals (Chapter 395). IRIS is a paradoxical reaction that presents with a temporary worsening of clinical symptoms or radiographic findings, resulting from increased immunity against TB (see later).

PREVENTION

Prevention of primary infection with TB consists of avoiding exposure. Prevention of transmission of drug-resistant TB is of particular importance. To decrease transmission to other patients or health care workers, HIV-infected patients with any suspicion of TB should be placed in isolation until three sputum smears are negative for AFB. Improved ventilation, rapid initiation of therapy and sensitivity testing, mask use, and shifts to outpatient therapy can help decrease nosocomial transmission.

HIV-infected individuals exposed to TB who develop latent infection are at high risk of reactivation, but this risk can be significantly decreased with appropriate prophylaxis. Prevention of reactivation disease involves testing for latent TB infection (LTBI) with either a tuberculin skin test or an interferon-γ release assay (IGRA). HIV-infected persons should be tested when first diagnosed and depending on the clinical situation (Table 391-5). Individuals testing positive (≥5 mm of induration on skin test or a positive IGRA) should receive a course of prophylaxis once active infection has been ruled out. Isoniazid (300 mg daily or 900 mg twice weekly) combined with pyridoxine should be given for 9 to 12 months.[A5] A recent randomized study demonstrated similar efficacy of a 3-month regimen of directly observed rifapentine and INH, with better completion rates.[A6] Other regimens can also be used (see Table 391-4).

Secondary prevention of TB after treatment of active infection is not generally recommended in the United States. Some studies have found that continuation of isoniazid after completion of 6 months of TB therapy decreases risk of recurrence in high-burden countries.

TABLE 391-4 TREATMENT AND PREVENTION REGIMENS FOR TUBERCULOSIS IN THE HIV-INFECTED PATIENT

	DRUGS	TOTAL DURATION	COMMENTS
Drug-susceptible pulmonary tuberculosis (TB)	*Initial phase (2 months):* Isoniazid + Rifampin or rifabutin + Pyrazinamide + Ethambutol *Continuation phase (4-7 months):* Isoniazid Rifampin or rifabutin	• 6 months • 9 months if culture positive after 2 months of TB therapy	• Give isoniazid with supplemental pyridoxine • Rifabutin preferred if patient is receiving protease inhibitor • Directly observed therapy 5-7 days/week recommended
Isoniazid-resistant pulmonary TB	*Initial phase (2 months):* Rifampin or rifabutin + Pyrazinamide + Ethambutol + Moxifloxacin or levofloxacin *Continuation phase (7 months):* Rifampin or rifabutin + Ethambutol + Moxifloxacin or levofloxacin	• 9 months	• Rifabutin preferred if patient is receiving protease inhibitor • Directly observed therapy recommended
Rifamycin-resistant or other drug-resistant pulmonary TB	Regimen per resistance pattern, clinical and microbiological responses		Consultation with experts recommended
Latent TB: preferred regimens	Isoniazid 300 mg PO daily *Or* Isoniazid 900 mg PO twice weekly	• 9 months	Latent TB defined as: 1. Screening test positive with no active disease and no previous history of treatment for active or latent TB *Or* 2. Close contact of person with infectious TB and no evidence of active disease • Give isoniazid with supplemental pyridoxine • Twice-weekly isoniazid regimen should be given by directly observed therapy
Latent TB: alternative regimens	Rifampin 600 mg PO daily or rifabutin (dose adjusted based on ART agents)	• 4 months	• Rifabutin preferred if patient receiving protease inhibitor

For detailed dosing and additional information, please see Reference 5.
ART = antiretroviral therapy.

TABLE 391-5 INDICATIONS FOR TESTING FOR LATENT TUBERCULOSIS IN HIV INFECTION

INDICATION	COMMENTS
When HIV first identified	Can use either tuberculin skin test or interferon-γ release assay to diagnose latent tuberculosis
Annually if patient at continuing risk of exposure to tuberculosis	
When individuals with a negative test have an increase in CD4 cell count to > 200 cells/μL with antiretroviral therapy	Active disease should be ruled out before starting therapy

PROGNOSIS

Response to therapy and time to negative cultures depends on the setting and the immunologic state of the patient. In the United States, response to therapy and time to convert sputum cultures in HIV-infected and HIV-uninfected individuals are similar. In contrast, the risk of death and relapse in sub-Saharan Africa is higher in HIV-infected individuals than in HIV-uninfected persons. HIV-infected patients with drug-resistant TB have decreased survival, particularly those with extensively drug-resistant TB, whose mortality may be as high as 90%.

Pneumocystis Pneumonia

EPIDEMIOLOGY

PCP was the first opportunistic infection described in the AIDS epidemic and was responsible for almost two thirds of AIDS-defining diagnoses (Chapter 341). With the widespread use of PCP prophylaxis followed by the introduction of ART, PCP incidence has decreased dramatically, although it remains the most common serious opportunistic infection in the United States. Some areas of the developing world such as Asia and South America have a high incidence of PCP, but the frequency of PCP in Africa may be lower, potentially because of geographic variations in *Pneumocystis* distribu-

tion, decreased susceptibility to PCP, lack of resources to detect *Pneumocystis*, or from competing risk of death from other infections (e.g., TB, bacterial pneumonia) that occur before HIV-infected individuals reach a CD4 cell count where they are susceptible to PCP.

Most cases of PCP occur in HIV-infected individuals who are not on ART, do not adhere to PCP prophylaxis, or are unaware of their HIV status. The primary risk factor is a CD4 cell count below 200 cells/μL, with the risk increasing as the CD4 cell count falls to lower levels. Risk of PCP is also higher in individuals with oropharyngeal candidiasis or a previous history of PCP. This risk can be reversed with successful ART. Individuals on ART also have a decreased risk of primary PCP if they have a suppressed HIV viral level with a CD4 cell count between 101 and 200 cells/μL.[6]

CLINICAL MANIFESTATIONS

The classic presentation of PCP in an HIV-infected patient is fever, a nonproductive cough, and dyspnea on exertion. The course of PCP in HIV infection may be subacute with duration of symptoms of 2 weeks or more, in contrast to the often fulminant disease in patients immunocompromised for reasons other than HIV, or in contrast to the acute course of bacterial pneumonia. Pleuritic chest pain and purulent sputum are much less common in PCP than in bacterial pneumonia. Complaints of hemoptysis should prompt investigation of other diagnoses. Physical examination in PCP is usually nonspecific, and the lungs are often normal on auscultation. Crackles are the most common abnormality, and signs of focal consolidation are less often seen. Patients are often hypoxic or desaturate with exertion, but this finding is nonspecific. A CD4 cell count below 200 cells/μL is usually seen. Serum lactate dehydrogenase (LDH) is often increased in patients with PCP, but an elevated serum LDH is not sufficiently specific to establish the diagnosis of PCP, nor is a normal LDH sufficiently sensitive to rule it out. A room air arterial blood gas should be measured if feasible to determine severity of disease, and an increase in the alveolar-arterial (A-a) oxygen gradient is common. The classic radiographic presentation is bilateral reticular or granular infiltrates (see Fig. 391-3). The infiltrates start in the perihilar region and extend toward the periphery with progressive disease. The opacities are

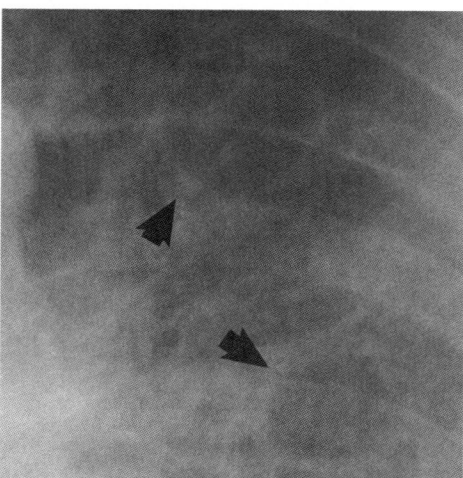

FIGURE 391-7. Close-up of the left lung from a chest radiograph of an HIV-infected person, CD4 cell count less than 200 cells/μL with *Pneumocystis* pneumonia. Two thin-walled cysts (*arrows*) are present. Courtesy Laurence Huang, MD. Used with permission.

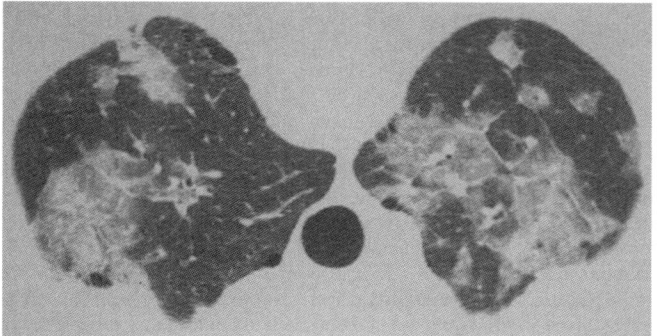

FIGURE 391-8. Chest high-resolution computed tomography (HRCT) in an HIV-infected person, CD4 cell count less than 200 cells/μL, whose chest radiograph showed normal findings. Because of clinical suspicion of *Pneumocystis* pneumonia (PCP), the patient underwent HRCT demonstrating characteristic patchy ground-glass opacities consistent with PCP. Courtesy Laurence Huang, MD. Used with permission.

TABLE 391-6	TREATMENT REGIMENS FOR *PNEUMOCYSTIS* PNEUMONIA IN HIV INFECTION*	
TREATMENT REGIMEN	**DOSE(S), FREQUENCY**	**TOXICITIES**
MILD PCP† (ARTERIAL Po₂ > 70 mm Hg *AND* ALVEOLAR-ARTERIAL O₂ DIFFERENCE < 35 mm Hg)		
Trimethoprim-sulfamethoxazole (TMP-SMX)	15-20 mg/kg (TMP component) daily (q6-8h or TMP-SMX 2 double strength tablets q8h)	Fever, dermatologic, gastrointestinal (GI), hematologic
TMP *plus*	15 mg/kg daily (q8h)	Dermatologic, GI, hematologic
Dapsone	100 mg once daily	
Clindamycin *plus*	1800 mg daily (q6-8h)	Dermatologic, GI, hematologic
Primaquine	30 mg (base) once daily	
Atovaquone	750 mg bid (with food)	Dermatologic, GI
MODERATE-SEVERE PCP‡ (ARTERIAL Po₂ < 70 mm Hg *OR* ALVEOLAR-ARTERIAL O₂ DIFFERENCE > 35 mm Hg)		
TMP-SMX	15-20 mg/kg (TMP component) daily (q6-8h)	Fever, dermatologic, GI, hematologic
Pentamidine	3-4 mg/kg once daily	Renal, pancreatic
Clindamycin *plus*	1800-2400 mg (q6-8h)	Dermatologic, GI, hematologic
Primaquine	30 mg (base) once daily	

*Recommended duration of therapy = 21 days.
†Oral route is preferred for patients with mild PCP who are treated as outpatients.
‡IV route is preferred (at least until clinical improvement) for patients with moderate-severe PCP. Adjunctive corticosteroids (prednisone 40 mg PO twice daily for 5 days, then 40 mg PO once daily for 5 days, then 20 mg PO once daily for 11 days or potency-equivalent methylprednisolone IV) should also be administered.
For detailed dosing and additional information, please see Reference 5.

typically symmetrical, but unilateral or asymmetrical disease can occur. Chest radiographs may also be normal, and atypical radiographic manifestations can occasionally be seen, including focal lobar consolidation, nodules, cavitary lesions, or miliary disease. In patients receiving aerosolized pentamidine for prophylaxis, upper lung infiltrates are more common owing to enhanced drug deposition in the lower lobes, and this presentation can be confused with TB. Pneumatoceles (thin-walled cysts) and pneumothoraces are common (Fig. 391-7). Pleural effusions and intrathoracic adenopathy are rare. Chest computed tomography (CT) can be a useful diagnostic study in patients who are suspected of having PCP, but present with a normal chest radiograph. In these patients, ground-glass opacities (Fig. 391-8) can suggest—but do not confirm—the diagnosis, because this finding is nonspecific; however, a normal high-resolution chest CT essentially rules out the diagnosis of PCP.

DIAGNOSIS

Empirical diagnosis is sometimes necessary in resource-limited settings, but definitive diagnosis with microscopic visualization of *Pneumocystis* in respiratory specimens is preferable. Because *Pneumocystis* culture cannot be performed, staining of respiratory samples is used to visualize organisms. Methenamine silver or toluidine blue O will stain the cyst wall. Giemsa and Diff-Quik staining will demonstrate both cystic and trophic forms. Immunofluorescence stains are also used and are more sensitive.

Spontaneously expectorated sputum cannot generally be used for PCP diagnosis, but induced sputum is often the first sample obtained in patients. Sensitivity of induced sputum varies by the clinical setting and experience of the institution. Repeated sputum samples are generally not obtained as they

are in TB. Because a negative induced sputum cannot rule out PCP, bronchoscopy with bronchoalveolar lavage (BAL) should be performed if the initial induced sputum is negative (Chapter 341). BAL has excellent sensitivity (>90%) in the HIV-infected population, and transbronchial biopsy is rarely needed to diagnose PCP.

Newer diagnostic techniques are being investigated and may become more widespread. Polymerase chain reaction (PCR) of respiratory specimens can be used to detect *Pneumocystis* DNA in various respiratory samples, including oral washes. It is very sensitive and specific for *Pneumocystis*, but it may be difficult to distinguish between colonization and disease and is not widely available. Tests to detect elevated levels of serum 1→3, β-D-glucan (a component of fungal cell walls) can be used to support a diagnosis of PCP, but levels can also be elevated in other fungal infections.[7]

TREATMENT   Rx

Anti-*Pneumocystis* Therapies

The first-line agent for treating PCP, regardless of severity, is trimethoprim-sulfamethoxazole (TMP-SMX) (Table 391-6). It is as effective as intravenous (IV) pentamidine but less toxic. Clinical resistance testing is not possible in PCP, but TMP-SMX can be used even if patients have been taking this agent for prophylaxis. Patients with mild PCP (PaO₂ > 70 mm Hg and A-a oxygen gradient < 35 mm Hg) who are able to tolerate oral medications can receive TMP-SMX by mouth. Patients who have moderate or severe PCP or who are unable to tolerate oral therapy should be given IV TMP-SMX. Therapy should be continued for a total duration of 21 days and may be switched to an oral regimen when the patient has clinically improved. Side effects of TMP-SMX are common in HIV-infected individuals. Frequent adverse effects include rash, nausea and vomiting, abnormal liver function tests, hyperkalemia, fever, and myelosuppression. Some toxicities of TMP-SMX can be life threatening, including Stevens-Johnson syndrome, toxic epidermal necrolysis, and a distributive shock syndrome that presents similarly to anaphylaxis, but these toxicities are rare. If side effects are mild, continuing treatment is recommended along with symptomatic treatment for adverse effects.

If patients cannot take TMP-SMX or if they develop a treatment-limiting side effect, several alternative regimens are available (see Table 391-6). IV pentamidine, clindamycin with primaquine, trimethoprim with dapsone, or atovaquone may be used. IV pentamidine is associated with a host of toxicities, including renal dysfunction, dysglycemias, pancreatitis, and torsades de pointes. Renal function and glucose levels need to be monitored during therapy; renal dysfunction and hypo- and hyperglycemia commonly occur. Clindamycin with primaquine has comparable efficacy to TMP-SMX or TMP-dapsone in mild to moderate disease. It may also be more effective than IV pentamidine in patients with severe disease. Because primaquine is administered orally, this regimen is less desirable if there is concern about effective gastrointestinal absorption. Dapsone with trimethoprim is recommended only in mild or moderate PCP. Oral atovaquone should not be given in moderate or severe PCP and is less effective than other regimens for mild disease.

Adjunctive Corticosteroids

Randomized studies have demonstrated an increase in survival when corticosteroids are used as adjunctive therapy in PCP. Patients with an initial room air PO_2 below 70 mm Hg or an A-a gradient above 35 mm Hg should receive corticosteroids (see Table 391-6). Corticosteroids should be started at the time of PCP treatment, or at least within 72 hours of starting treatment, because they work to decrease the inflammation produced by killing of Pneumocystis, thus preventing deterioration in oxygenation. Corticosteroids should not be held during treatment while awaiting confirmation of the diagnosis of PCP.

Antiretroviral Therapy

Many patients with PCP are not receiving ART at the time of diagnosis. Early initiation of ART during treatment for acute PCP is supported by a randomized trial demonstrating a decrease in the end-point of progression to AIDS or mortality when ART was started within 2 weeks of diagnosis of an opportunistic infection.[A7] This study did not include PCP patients with respiratory failure who required mechanical ventilation. Given the risk of IRIS in these patients, optimal timing of ART is not well-defined (see "Intensive Care of the HIV-Infected Patient").

Treatment Failure

Patients with PCP often show an initial clinical worsening during treatment, with worsening oxygenation, increased radiographic infiltrates, and fever as the host reacts to dying organisms. If the patient fails to demonstrate improvement after 4 to 8 days of therapy, treatment failure should be considered. Other causes of clinical worsening, such as fluid overload, development of a pneumothorax, or presence of another infection, should be sought before deciding to change treatment.

PREVENTION

Evidence of airborne transmission and clusters of PCP outbreaks suggest that isolation of patients with PCP might prevent transmission of infection, but current guidelines do not find sufficient evidence to support recommending respiratory isolation for HIV-infected individuals with PCP. Primary prophylaxis is instituted in HIV-infected individuals with a CD4 cell count below 200 cells/μL or in those with oral candidiasis. TMP-SMX is the preferred agent for prophylaxis (Table 391-7). Dapsone, atovaquone suspension, or aerosolized pentamidine can also be used. Secondary prophylaxis should be instituted in individuals after they complete PCP treatment. In general, secondary prophylaxis of PCP is similar to primary prophylaxis, except that aerosolized pentamidine has been associated with more breakthrough PCP

TABLE 391-7	PREVENTION REGIMENS FOR *PNEUMOCYSTIS* IN HIV INFECTION	
PREVENTION REGIMEN	ALTERNATIVE DOSING	COMMENTS
Trimethoprim-sulfamethoxazole 1 double-strength (DS) tablet daily	1 single-strength tablet daily 1 DS tablet thrice weekly	Also effective prophylaxis against *Toxoplasma gondii* and many bacterial pathogens
Dapsone 100 mg daily		Combine with pyrimethamine and leucovorin in persons who are *T. gondii* immunoglobulin G antibody positive. Consider combining with pyrimethamine and leucovorin when used for secondary prophylaxis.
Atovaquone suspension 1500 mg daily		Improved bioavailability compared to tablets
Aerosolized pentamidine 300 mg monthly via RespirGard II nebulizer		May be associated with increased risk of extrapulmonary disease

when used as secondary prophylaxis in individuals with a CD4 cell count below 100 cells/μL. Prophylaxis should be continued for life unless individuals experience immune reconstitution with ART. If the CD4 cell count is sustained above 200 cells/μL for at least 3 months, primary and secondary prophylaxis can be discontinued.

PROGNOSIS

Prognosis for persons with PCP has improved dramatically from the beginning of the AIDS epidemic. Improvements resulted first from use of corticosteroids in more severe disease. Whether use of ART has improved short-term prognosis from PCP is debated. Changes in intensive care unit (ICU) care (e.g., use of low-tidal-volume ventilation) have also improved outcomes of severe PCP. Overall mortality from PCP is around 10%, with mortality in patients requiring mechanical ventilation approximately 30%.[8] Studies have found that survival correlates with degree of hypoxemia, underlying comorbidities, younger patient age, higher albumin, and first episode of PCP.

Other Infections

FUNGAL INFECTIONS

Although *Pneumocystis* is the most common fungal cause of pneumonia in HIV-infected patients, other endemic and nonendemic fungi may cause disease, particularly in those who are more severely immunosuppressed (e.g., CD4 cell counts < 200 cells/μL, and more often when < 100 cells/μL). Histoplasmosis can be encountered in patients who have been to the U.S. Midwest, and coccidioidomycosis in patients from the Southwest. *Cryptococcus neoformans* is found throughout the world. Of note, although invasive aspergillosis is a well-documented complication of various immunosuppressive disorders, it is uncommon in patients with HIV disease. Risk factors for the development of aspergillosis in HIV-infected individuals include use of corticosteroids, neutropenia, marijuana, and broad-spectrum antimicrobial drugs.

In more severely immunodeficient HIV-infected patients, fungal infection is often disseminated. For example, the most commonly encountered manifestation of cryptococcal disease is meningitis. Coccidioidomycosis in HIV-infected persons can present with focal or diffuse pneumonia, as well as cutaneous disease, meningitis, liver or lymph node involvement, or disseminated disease. Disseminated histoplasmosis most often presents as a febrile wasting illness in HIV-infected persons. Isolated pulmonary disease secondary to fungal infection tends to be more rare but can occur, particularly with histoplasmosis and coccidioidomycosis; isolated or focal pulmonary disease is more likely in those with CD4 cell counts above 250 to 300 cells/μL. The most commonly encountered chest radiographic findings of cryptococcal, coccidioidal, and histoplasmosis infection consist of diffuse bilateral interstitial infiltrates that are often reticular or reticulonodular. Focal consolidation, nodular opacities, cavitation, pleural effusion, and hilar adenopathy are less frequent, but may also be seen (Fig. 391-9). Radiographic findings can mimic other diseases, particularly PCP and atypical bacterial infections.

Diagnosis of pulmonary fungal infection is usually established by culture of sputum or BAL fluid and occasionally of pleural fluid; however, serologic and antigen testing can aid in the diagnosis of a variety of fungal infections. Cryptococcal antigen is a sensitive and specific test performed on serum, cerebrospinal fluid, urine, BAL fluid, or pleural fluid. The *Histoplasma* antigen test is also a sensitive method for rapid diagnosis of disease and can be obtained on urine, serum, cerebrospinal fluid, or BAL fluid. Serologic tests are useful in evaluation of suspected coccidioidomycosis, with an estimated 80 to 90% sensitivity of complement fixation and tube precipitin test for diagnosis.

VIRAL INFECTIONS

Viral pneumonias are not frequently encountered in HIV-infected patients. Although often isolated in the BAL, cytomegalovirus (CMV) is a less common cause of pneumonia (Chapter 376). Most cases of CMV disease occur in patients with a CD4 lymphocyte count less than 50 cells/μL. Symptoms of CMV pneumonia are nonspecific; chest radiograph findings include reticular or ground-glass opacities, alveolar infiltrates, and nodules or nodular opacities. The diagnosis of CMV pulmonary disease can be challenging because BAL fluid culture is not specific. Definitive diagnosis requires biopsy and demonstration of widespread specific cytopathic changes in the lungs, but biopsies may not be feasible. Patients suspected of having CMV pneumonitis should undergo a careful evaluation for evidence of disseminated disease, particularly ocular involvement. Treatment of CMV pneumonia is the same as currently recommended for disseminated disease.

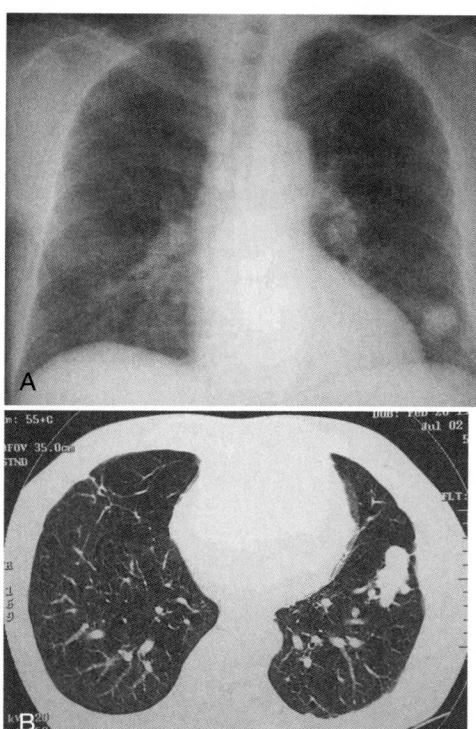

FIGURE 391-9. Chest radiograph (A) and chest computed tomography (CT) scan (B) of an HIV-infected individual, CD4 cell count less than 200 cells/μL. A multilobulated noncalcified mass measuring 4.6 × 2.4 cm is present in the left lower lobe, with multiple adjacent satellite nodules. Culture from CT-guided transthoracic needle aspiration revealed *Cryptococcus neoformans*. Courtesy Laurence Huang, MD. Used with permission.

Influenza generally presents similarly and has a comparable clinical course in HIV-infected as in HIV-uninfected adults (Chapter 364). HIV infection does not appear to increase the risk for influenza, although influenza-related mortality may be greater in those with AIDS compared to the general U.S. population. Prompt initiation of antiviral therapy directed against influenza is recommended. All HIV-infected persons should receive the inactivated influenza vaccine annually.

NONTUBERCULOUS MYCOBACTERIA

TB is the most common mycobacterial lung disease seen in HIV, but other nontuberculous mycobacterial pulmonary infections may occur. The two most common causes in HIV are *Mycobacterium avium* complex (MAC) and *Mycobacterium kansasii* (Chapter 325). Although the lungs may be a portal of entry for MAC, patients usually present with disseminated disease, and isolated pulmonary MAC in HIV is rare. When isolated pulmonary MAC is seen, it has been reported in patients receiving ART and thus may be a manifestation of immune reconstitution inflammatory syndrome. The chest radiograph is most often normal in MAC infection, even when cultures of respiratory specimens grow MAC. Focal infiltrates are rare. Endobronchial lesions containing MAC can sometimes be seen. MAC treatment consists of at least ethambutol and a macrolide. Additional agents can be considered in advanced immunosuppression, high mycobacterial burden, or inability to use ART. Primary MAC prophylaxis with azithromycin or clarithromycin is recommended in HIV-infected individuals with a CD4 cell count below 50 cells/μL. Secondary prophylaxis is recommended after a minimum of 12 months of treatment and can be discontinued when the CD4 cell count is above 100 cells/μL for at least 6 months.

M. kansasii is most common in the southern and central United States, with clusters of disease also reported in Europe, Asia, and Africa. It can occur at any CD4 cell count, but is most common in individuals with CD4 cell counts below 100 cells/μL. The clinical presentation and radiographic appearance of *M. kansasii* is similar to TB. Diagnostic work-up is also similar to that of TB, with the exception that identification of *M. kansasii* does not always indicate disease, because colonization can occur. Treatment consists of isoniazid, rifampin, and ethambutol with pyridoxine for a minimum of 12

months after cultures become negative. Rifabutin or a macrolide can be substituted for rifampin in patients taking a protease inhibitor or non-nucleoside reverse transcriptase inhibitor.

NONINFECTIOUS PULMONARY DISEASES
Chronic Obstructive Lung Disease

EPIDEMIOLOGY

HIV infection has been associated with several different manifestations of obstructive lung disease, including features of emphysema and chronic bronchitis, which together comprise COPD, as well as bronchial hyperresponsiveness, which characterizes asthma. Bronchiectasis causes an obstructive ventilatory defect and has been described in patients with HIV. COPD and bronchiectasis are known sequelae of severe or repeated opportunistic infection; however, evidence suggests that HIV infection is associated with an increase in COPD apart from the effects of opportunistic infections and after controlling for other traditional risk factors for COPD such as smoking and illicit drug use (Chapter 88).[9]

PATHOBIOLOGY

The pathogenesis of COPD in HIV infection is incompletely understood and likely involves multiple pathways. Respiratory tract infections, prior bacterial pneumonia or PCP, and colonization with microorganisms likely play an important role. The association of lung function with HIV specific markers suggests a potential pathogenic role for the virus itself. In comparison to HIV-uninfected persons, HIV-infected persons with poor viral control or greater degree of immunodeficiency have more severe diffusing capacity impairment.[10] Furthermore, a high viral load or low CD4 T-cell count (<100 cells/μL) have been associated with accelerated decline in airflow over time in a longitudinal cohort study of injection drug users.

CLINICAL MANIFESTATIONS

In general, the clinical presentation of chronic obstructive lung diseases is similar in HIV-infected as in uninfected persons. The majority of patients with COPD are cigarette smokers. HIV-infected individuals may be more likely to experience respiratory symptoms such as chronic cough, phlegm production, and dyspnea on exertion, for a given degree of impairment in pulmonary function, compared to HIV-uninfected individuals.

> **TREATMENT** Rx
>
> In general, treatment of asthma and COPD in patients with HIV infection is similar to that for the HIV-uninfected population, although no studies have specifically examined these treatments in persons with HIV. Smoking cessation should be prioritized. Protease inhibitors, particularly ritonavir, have been reported to increase systemic levels of inhaled or intranasal fluticasone. The use of high-dose inhaled corticosteroids for COPD in patients with HIV also requires careful monitoring for oral candidiasis and pneumonia.

PROGNOSIS

No studies have specifically addressed whether the prognosis for COPD in HIV-infected patients is similar to that in HIV-uninfected patients. COPD is likely to be a major cause of morbidity and mortality as HIV-infected patients are aging.

Lung Cancer

EPIDEMIOLOGY

Whereas AIDS-defining cancers such as Kaposi sarcoma and non-Hodgkin lymphoma have decreased, non-AIDS-defining cancers in HIV-infected patients have increased, primarily among those aged 50 years and older. Lung cancer is now the most common infection-unrelated non-AIDS-defining cancer and is a leading cause of mortality in HIV-infected persons. The incidence of lung cancer is greater among HIV-infected persons than among HIV-uninfected persons.[11]

PATHOBIOLOGY

Although lung cancer can develop at any CD4 lymphocyte count, immunodeficiency is postulated as a mechanism for the enhanced risk of lung cancer associated with HIV. Prior lung disease and infections, particularly bacterial pneumonia and TB, are also risk factors in epidemiologic studies. HIV viral load, CD4 cell count, and use of ART do not appear associated with lung cancer risk.

CLINICAL MANIFESTATIONS

Most HIV-infected patients who develop lung cancer are cigarette smokers. Although all pathologic types are seen, adenocarcinoma is the most frequent pathologic type reported; squamous cell carcinoma is the second most frequently observed pathologic type. The distribution of tumor stage at diagnosis and histologic type appear similar in HIV-infected as in uninfected patients. Radiographic appearance is also similar to that in the HIV-uninfected population.

TREATMENT Rx

Surgical resection should be considered for any patient who meets criteria based on stage of cancer and underlying medical condition. Chemotherapy and radiation may also be indicated. Significant decreases in CD4 cell counts and hematologic toxicity can occur with chemotherapy.

PROGNOSIS

Studies have been conflicting on the impact of HIV infection on survival for patients with lung cancer. Some studies suggest that survival is overall no different when stratified by stage of disease and propensity score adjustment, with an overall median survival for all stages of 7 months for HIV-uninfected controls versus 8 months for HIV-infected patients. Other studies have shown that when controlling for confounders and competing risks, HIV infection was associated with a greater risk of lung cancer–specific death, with an overall median survival of 6 months among non–small cell lung cancer patients with HIV compared to 20 months in patients without evidence of HIV. HIV-infected patients may less frequently receive lung cancer treatments, potentially accounting for survival differences. Whether lung cancer screening with an annual low-dose CT scan will have a beneficial effect on mortality in HIV-infected smokers, as it has in older HIV-uninfected heavy smokers, is not yet known.[12,13]

Other Thoracic Malignancies

The most common HIV-associated malignancy is Kaposi sarcoma (KS), although its incidence has decreased dramatically with combination ART. KS is an angioproliferative tumor and most commonly presents with mucocutaneous involvement. The lymph nodes, gastrointestinal tract, and lungs can also be involved. HIV-associated KS is substantially more likely in men who have sex with men than in other HIV risk groups. Human herpesvirus 8 (HHV-8) has been found in all forms of KS and appears to play a central role in pathogenesis.

Pulmonary KS presents in most patients when their CD4 T-cell counts are below 200 cells/μL. Respiratory symptoms typically are nonspecific and include nonproductive cough, dyspnea, and fever. Most but not all patients with pulmonary KS have concomitant mucocutaneous disease. Typical chest radiograph findings of pulmonary KS consist of bilateral perihilar or central opacities, as well as linear densities, nodular opacities, pleural effusions, and intrathoracic lymphadenopathy (Fig. 391-10A). The diagnosis of pulmonary KS can often be established by visualization of characteristic lesions on bronchoscopy. Endobronchial lesions from KS are flat or slightly raised, red or violaceous lesions (see Fig. 391-10B), and their presence is often sufficient to establish a presumptive diagnosis without requiring biopsy. HHV-8 may be detected in BAL. Tumors can regress in size and number in response to ART, and therefore all patients with KS should receive combination ART if no other contraindications exist. Treatment of more advanced systemic disease also includes chemotherapy. Of malignancies, KS is the most likely to be associated with IRIS in patients who initiate ART.

Almost all HIV-associated non-Hodgkin lymphomas (NHL) are of B-cell origin (Chapter 185). The majority are associated with Epstein-Barr virus (EBV) infection. As with KS, the incidence of NHL has declined dramatically in the era of combination ART. Most HIV-infected patients with NHL present with disseminated disease and extranodal involvement at diagnosis. Clinically apparent pulmonary involvement occurs in up to 30% of patients with AIDS-related NHL. Occasionally, the lung is the only site involved. Although NHL can present at a wide range of CD4 lymphocyte counts, most patients have advanced HIV infection, with median CD4 T-cell counts around 100 cells/μL.

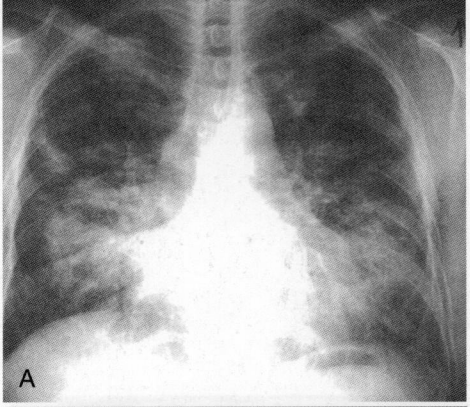

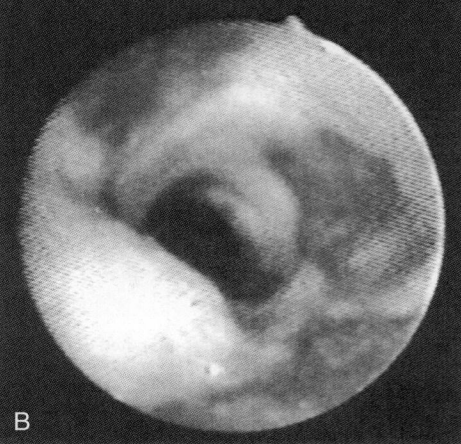

FIGURE 391-10. Chest radiograph (A) of an HIV-infected patient, CD4 cell count less than 100 cells/μL, with characteristic bilateral middle and lower lung zone, predominantly central, distribution of abnormalities of Kaposi sarcoma. The patient had no evidence of mucocutaneous disease, and the diagnosis was made by visualization of characteristic erythematous violaceous Kaposi sarcoma throughout the airways on bronchoscopy (B). B, courtesy Laurence Huang, MD. Used with permission.

Common presenting features of thoracic involvement with NHL are nonspecific and include cough and dyspnea. Systemic symptoms such as fever, sweats, and weight loss are common. Chest radiograph findings typically include single or multiple nodules, nodular opacities or masses, lobar infiltrates, and diffuse interstitial infiltrates; pleural effusions and intrathoracic lymphadenopathy are common accompanying findings. The diagnosis of NHL requires demonstration of malignant lymphocytes on cytology or biopsy specimens. Most often, the diagnosis is made by biopsy of an extrathoracic site. The yield of pleural cytology is significantly higher in HIV-associated pulmonary lymphoma as opposed to HIV-uninfected cases. Pulmonary involvement in NHL is treated as part of the systemic disease (Chapter 185).

Interstitial Lung Disease
EPIDEMIOLOGY

Interstitial lung disease is a less common cause of pulmonary disease than infections, malignancies, or obstructive lung diseases. HIV-infected individuals may develop a number of diagnoses seen in the general population such as nonspecific interstitial pneumonitis (NSIP), sarcoidosis, and hypersensitivity pneumonitis. Sarcoidosis is sometimes associated with initiation of ART, and it is debated whether it is a manifestation of IRIS. Lymphocytic interstitial pneumonia (LIP) is a disease entity that is more common in HIV-infected children than adults, and its incidence has decreased significantly since introduction of ART.

PATHOBIOLOGY

Causes of interstitial lung diseases are poorly understood. Pathology is similar to that seen in the HIV-uninfected population (Chapter 92). It is unclear whether LIP represents a unique pathologic disorder or results from multiple causes that lead to similar lung pathology. Lung biopsy in LIP demonstrates interstitial lymphocytes with spreading into the alveolar septae.

CLINICAL MANIFESTATIONS

Manifestations vary depending on the specific diagnosis, but symptoms often include progressive shortness of breath and nonproductive cough. Patients may be febrile. Physical examination may reveal crackles on lung examination. Systemic findings such as lymphadenopathy in sarcoidosis can provide clues to specific etiologies. Radiographic manifestations vary with the disease. Pulmonary function testing generally shows a pattern consistent with restrictive lung disease, and diffusing capacity for carbon monoxide is often impaired.

DIAGNOSIS

BAL is a useful initial procedure for ruling out infectious causes of lung disease, but definitive diagnosis of interstitial lung disease generally requires a lung biopsy. In most cases, a video-assisted thoracoscopic lung biopsy is preferred to transbronchial biopsy, although in the case of sarcoidosis, transbronchial biopsies are useful in establishing a diagnosis.

TREATMENT Rx

There have been no treatment trials of interstitial lung diseases in HIV-infected patients, and treatment should generally follow guidelines for the HIV-uninfected population (Chapter 92). In LIP, initiation of ART is recommended, with consideration of corticosteroids depending on the clinical severity.

PROGNOSIS

Prognosis is generally the same as that in the HIV-uninfected population. In a small number of cases, LIP may be a precursor to lymphoma, which carries a worse outcome, however LIP usually has a better prognosis in HIV infection because it may respond to initiation of ART.

Pulmonary Hypertension

EPIDEMIOLOGY

HIV is recognized as a cause of World Health Organization (WHO) Group 1 pulmonary arterial hypertension (PAH). PAH has been reported to occur with a prevalence of 0.5% in the HIV-infected population, compared to 1 to 2 cases per million in HIV-uninfected individuals.[14] HIV-infected individuals also may have additional risk factors for PAH, including IV drug use or liver disease.

PATHOBIOLOGY

The hallmark pathologic manifestation of HIV-PAH is the plexiform lesion. More subtle changes such as medial hypertrophy and intimal hyperplasia of pulmonary arterioles can also be seen. The exact causes of PAH in HIV are not well understood, but may involve genetic or environmental insults in addition to HIV.

CLINICAL MANIFESTATIONS

PAH in the HIV-infected patient presents similarly to PAH in the HIV-uninfected individual, although patients are often younger and have a better New York Heart Association functional class at presentation. Initial symptoms are often nonspecific, but patients eventually may report symptoms of dyspnea with exertion, syncope, or exertional chest pain. Physical examination can be normal or suggestive of right-sided heart failure.

DIAGNOSIS

The gold standard for diagnosis of PAH is right heart catheterization. Echocardiography is often performed as a screening test, but pulmonary arterial pressures on echocardiography may not correlate with pressures on catheterization. Other causes of pulmonary hypertension such as underlying lung disease, left-sided heart failure, or cirrhosis should be evaluated as well.

TREATMENT Rx

There have been few trials of standard PAH agents in HIV-infected populations, but in general, guidelines for PAH treatment in the HIV-uninfected population should be followed (Chapter 68). Epoprostenol may be associated

with a higher risk of intravascular infections in HIV-infected individuals, especially those who are active IV drug users. Sildenafil levels can increase when used in combination with antiretrovirals, particularly with regimens that include ritonavir. Tadalafil appears to have less interaction with ritonavir. Treatment with warfarin can also be used in addition to PAH-specific therapies. Although results of studies are conflicting, there may be some benefit to ART in this disease, and patients should be started on ART if they are not already receiving it.

PROGNOSIS

One-year survival for HIV-infected individuals with PAH is 58 to 88% and varies with the cohort studied. Lower CD4 cell count and higher HIV viral levels are associated with worse survival.

Intensive Care of the HIV-Infected Patient

The epidemiology of ICU care for HIV-infected ICU patients has shifted multiple times over the course of the AIDS epidemic. A recent study of HIV-infected veterans with a first ICU admission between 2002 and 2010 found that 15% of HIV-infected individuals had a medical or cardiac ICU admission, compared to 10% of HIV-uninfected individuals.[15] HIV-infected patients were also younger, had a longer length of stay, and were more likely to require mechanical ventilation. Another study of over 2500 HIV-infected individuals found that 4.2% required ICU admission over a median of 2.2 years of follow-up from an AIDS diagnosis; a diagnosis of HIV after the CD4 cell count had fallen below 350 cells/μL and low CD4 cell count were associated with increased incidence of ICU admission.[16] ART use was protective for ICU admission.

HIV-infected patients may be admitted to the ICU with conditions related to their HIV, with side effects of ART, or for reasons unrelated to HIV. Currently, about half of ICU admission diagnoses in this population are directly related to HIV (e.g., opportunistic infections, malignancies). HIV-infected individuals may also be admitted with common conditions such as myocardial infarction, the risk for which may be increased in HIV-infected individuals on ART. Life-threatening complications of ART such as lactic acidosis or severe IRIS can also precipitate ICU admission. In recent series, respiratory failure is still the most common cause of ICU admission, with PCP, TB, and bacterial pneumonia causing varying degrees of disease depending on the population. The outcome of HIV-infected ICU patients with acute respiratory distress syndrome (Chapter 104) now is similar to HIV-negative patients.[17] In about 20 to 40% of cases, HIV infection is not known at the time of ICU admission, and providers need to consider HIV infection in their differential even if HIV infection has not been confirmed.

Antiretroviral Therapy Use

Among HIV-infected patients admitted to the ICU, clinicians need to be aware of numerous antiretroviral drug toxicities, drug-drug interactions, and concerns regarding absorption and metabolism of specific medications. Side effects of ART are numerous. Several toxicities secondary to ART that may require ICU admission include acute liver failure, lactic acidosis, pancreatitis, and hypersensitivity reactions.

In HIV-infected ICU patients, clinicians need to decide whether to continue or initiate ART. In general, expert opinion is that ART should be continued in the ICU for critically ill HIV-infected patients already on ART, if ART can be safely administered with minimal drug-drug interactions or risk of toxicities while receiving ICU medications. For patients admitted to the ICU for AIDS-related diseases, initiation of ART should be strongly considered in consultation with an infectious disease specialist. Survival is improved when ART is started concurrently with or in close proximity to treatment of opportunistic infection, but existing data do not include critically ill patients with respiratory failure that is severe enough to require mechanical ventilation. Nevertheless, HIV-infected patients admitted for non-AIDS-related conditions but with prolonged ICU hospitalizations or severely decreased CD4 T-cell count should also be considered for ART initiation.

HIV-infected patients who initiate ART, particularly in close proximity to treatment for an opportunistic infection, are at risk for development of IRIS. IRIS is a paradoxical worsening of clinical status typically related to recovery of the immune system after immunosuppression (Chapter 395). IRIS occurs as a result of host inflammatory responses to previously recognized or subclinical infections, or to cancer or self-antigens. Manifestations of IRIS that can result in critical illness include pneumonitis, meningitis, hepatitis, and pericarditis. Respiratory failure secondary to IRIS is most often associated with TB and PCP. Other causes of clinical worsening such as a new infection, treatment failure, or drug reaction should be ruled out. IRIS is usually self-limited, and ART should be continued. Nonsteroidal anti-inflammatories can provide symptomatic relief.[A8]

Grade A References

A1. Abdool Karim SS, Naidoo K, Grobler A, et al. Integration of antiretroviral therapy with tuberculosis treatment. *N Engl J Med.* 2011;365:1492-1501.

A2. Abdool Karim SS, Naidoo K, Grobler A, et al. Timing of initiation of antiretroviral drugs during tuberculosis therapy. *N Engl J Med.* 2010;362:697-706.

A3. Blanc FX, Sok T, Laureillard D, et al. Earlier versus later start of antiretroviral therapy in HIV-infected adults with tuberculosis. *N Engl J Med.* 2011;365:1471-1481.

A4. Havlir DV, Kendall MA, Ive P, et al. Timing of antiretroviral therapy for HIV-1 infection and tuberculosis. *N Engl J Med.* 2011;365:1482-1491.

A5. Rangaka MX, Wilkinson RJ, Boulle A, et al. Isoniazid plus antiretroviral therapy to prevent tuberculosis: a randomised double-blind, placebo-controlled trial. *Lancet.* 2014;384:682-690.

A6. Sterling TR, Villarino ME, Borisov AS, et al. Three months of rifapentine and isoniazid for latent tuberculosis infection. *N Engl J Med.* 2011;365:2155-2166.

A7. Zolopa A, Andersen J, Powderly W, et al. Early antiretroviral therapy reduces AIDS progression/death in individuals with acute opportunistic infections: a multicenter randomized strategy trial. *PLoS ONE.* 2009;4:e5575.

A8. Meintjes G, Wilkinson RJ, Morroni C, et al. Randomized placebo-controlled trial of prednisone for paradoxical tuberculosis-associated immune reconstitution inflammatory syndrome. *AIDS.* 2010; 24:2381-2390.

GENERAL REFERENCES

For the General References and other additional features, please visit Expert Consult at https://expertconsult.inkling.com.

392

SKIN MANIFESTATIONS IN PATIENTS WITH HUMAN IMMUNODEFICIENCY VIRUS INFECTION

TOBY MAURER

From the beginning of the epidemic, skin disease has often been the initial feature of infection with human immunodeficiency virus (HIV). Cutaneous manifestations are often predictive of the stage of immunosuppression and long-term prognosis.[1] Morbidity from skin diseases, particularly from opportunistic infections, has decreased with the advent of antiretroviral therapy (ART), although there are still significant dermatologic problems for patients in the post-ART era (Table 392-1). Cutaneous manifestations seen in patients with HIV may be categorized as infectious, neoplastic, inflammatory, or related to ART.

● INFECTIOUS MANIFESTATIONS
HIV Seroconversion Exanthem

Acute retroviral syndrome (ARS) is an infectious mononucleosis–like illness consisting of fever, lymphadenopathy, pharyngitis, and neurologic symptoms.[2] It can be the presenting sign of primary HIV infection in 40 to 90% of patients. The rash typically presents as a nonspecific morbilliform eruption

affecting the upper part of the trunk and face, with relative sparing of the peripheries. It is often accompanied by aphthous and penile ulcerations. There is evidence that very early after infection, HIV goes to dendritic cells in skin and causes an inflammatory response, which may explain the rash. Patients with primary HIV infection may be highly infectious because of the presence of a high viral burden in blood and genital secretions. The HIV antibody test, however, is likely to be negative because ARS precedes sero-conversion by 2 to 6 weeks. Confirmation of ARS can be made by finding positive plasma HIV RNA in the setting of a negative HIV antibody. The potential benefits to public and individual health may now justify treatment of patients with acute HIV infection, particularly those who are symptomatic.[3] Initiation of ART in this phase may decrease disease severity, alter the initial viral set point, and decrease viral replication so as to reduce the risk HIV transmission.

Viruses
HERPES ZOSTER

Herpes zoster is 10 times more common in HIV patients than in the general population.[4] Because varicella virus (VZV) reactivation can be observed even at relatively normal CD4+ counts, herpes zoster may be the first feature of HIV infection. Herpes zoster in the setting of HIV may affect more than one dermatome, involve unusual locations, or become disseminated. Cutaneous dissemination often presents with multiple and monomorphic vesicular skin lesions in a generalized distribution. These can affect a number of distinct dermatomes and often cross the midline. Complications such as blindness (when the cranial nerve V1 distribution is affected), post-herpetic neuralgia, myelitis, encephalitis, and visceral involvement can cause significant morbidity. HIV patients with limited disease usually respond well to oral antiviral therapy, and antiviral treatment should be started at any time during the disease course (not only within the first 48 hours, as with herpes zoster not associated with HIV). Intravenous acyclovir should be considered for disseminated disease or for lesions involving the eye. There have been a few reports of a verrucous chronic form of zoster occurring in severely immunosuppressed patients; this form of zoster is usually associated with acyclovir resistance. Zoster has been one of the more commonly reported diseases in the immune reconstitution inflammatory syndrome (IRIS) (Chapter 395) and typically appears during the second stage (≈3 months after initiation of ART). The zoster vaccine is not recommended in patients with CD4 counts below 200 cells/µL. Use of the vaccine in patients with CD4 counts above 200 cells/µL is controversial because the safety and efficacy of zoster vaccination in this population has not been demonstrated.[5]

HERPES SIMPLEX VIRUS

Infection with herpes simplex virus (HSV) should always be considered in HIV patients with mucocutaneous ulcerations (Fig. 392-1), particularly when localized to the anogenital area. The presentation is generally typical and characterized by multiple tiny vesicles, punched-out erosions, or crusts. Atypical or extensive ulcerative, vegetative, or tumor-like lesions may also occur. Patients with CD4+ counts below 200 cells/µL may require higher doses of acyclovir to treat the infection. Patients who fail to respond may have HSV with acyclovir resistance, and alternative agents such as foscarnet or cidofovir may be required. In those unable to tolerate the toxicity profile of

TABLE 392-1	SKIN CONDITIONS COMMON IN PATIENTS WITH CD4+ COUNTS LESS THAN 200 CELLS/µL AND NOT RECEIVING ANTIRETROVIRAL THERAPY

Photodermatitis
Psoriasis, difficult to control or involving more than 50% of the body
Pruritic papular eruption associated with HIV infection
Prurigo nodularis
Oral hairy leukoplakia
Molluscum contagiosum
Eosinophilic folliculitis

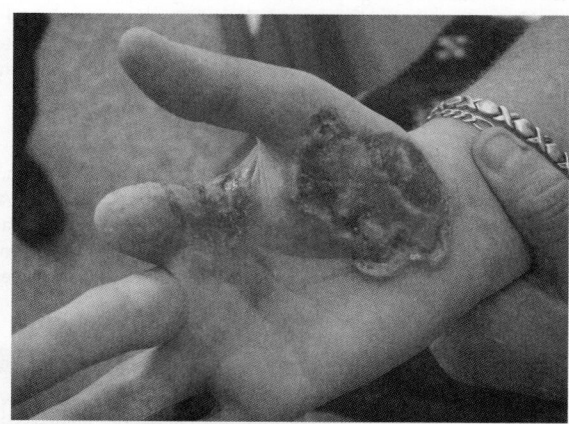

FIGURE 392-1. Chronic herpes simplex infection.

HUMAN PAPILLOMAVIRUS

Human papillomavirus (HPV) infection (Chapter 373) is very common in all stages of HIV infection. Common, flat, genital, and plantar warts are all seen with increased frequency. Lesions are often more extensive and more difficult to treat than in immunocompetent patients. The warts themselves are rarely symptomatic unless they are on the soles of the feet or around the fingernails, where they may cause excruciating pain. Severely immunosuppressed patients may have extensive warts that are recalcitrant to standard treatment. Although the advent of ART has not reduced the number or severity of warts, most patients commencing on ART often notice considerable improvement or resolution of existing lesions. Some patients receiving ART will not clear their warts despite improvement in the CD4+ count, suppression of viral load, and resolution of all other opportunistic infections. The reasons for this observation remain obscure. Treatment modalities include cryotherapy, surgery, laser, topical salicylic acid preparations, podophyllin, intralesional bleomycin, and contact sensitization immunotherapy; immunomodulatory therapy in the form of imiquimod has had less promising results in HIV patients. Topical cidofovir has been used, but the high cost of formulation limits its use. Owing to the frequent presence of high-risk HPV types, there is a risk of malignant transformation in HIV-infected patients. Anal carcinoma and anal intraepithelial neoplasia (AIN) are frequent (men and women) and may develop more rapidly in this population. Regular screening for cervical neoplasia should be performed in HIV-infected women, and screening anal and pap smears may be helpful in identifying anal dysplasia in men. HPV vaccination appears to be safe and immunogenic in the presence of HIV and is reasonable to consider in persons aged 9 to 26 years (as is suggested in the HIV-uninfected population). Investigations are ongoing as to whether HPV vaccination will demonstrate benefit in the broad group of HIV-infected patients older than 26.

MOLLUSCUM CONTAGIOSUM

Molluscum contagiosum is a poxvirus that causes a self-limited papular umbilicated eruption commonly seen in children. It is rarer to see in adults, and when on the face, persistent, or severe, it raises the possibility of HIV coinfection. It tends to occur when the CD4+ count falls below 200. First-line treatment is ART because molluscum contagiosum is invariably cleared with rising CD4+ counts. Ablative treatments such as cryotherapy or curettage will treat individual lesions more expeditiously; however, without ART, the lesions are likely to recur.

EPSTEIN-BARR VIRUS (ORAL HAIRY LEUKOPLAKIA)

Oral hairy leukoplakia (OHL) is characterized by nonpainful white plaques with a feathered edge, particularly on the lateral border of the tongue. It is associated with Epstein-Barr virus and is very rare in immunocompetent hosts. OHL can occur at any CD4+ count and may therefore be the initial feature of HIV infection. Table 392-2 lists diseases not affected by the CD4+ count. The appearance of OHL was a poor prognostic indicator before ART. There is no specific treatment of OHL, although it tends to resolve when patients are taking ART. Superinfection with Candida species should be considered if the lesions are painful.

Bacteria

STAPHYLOCOCCUS AUREUS

Infections with Staphylococcus aureus are commonly seen in HIV disease. Staphylococcal folliculitis (Fig. 392-2) tends to be more severe or refractory to treatment than in patients who are HIV negative. Other cutaneous manifestations of staphylococcal infection include cellulitis, bullous impetigo, abscesses, ecthyma (necrotic plaques), or rarely, botryomycosis. HIV-infected persons are at a heightened risk of infection with methicillin-resistant S. aureus (MRSA) and appear to have increased susceptibility for recurrence. Choice of treatment is dictated by location and severity of infection. The use of antiseptic washes such as benzoyl peroxide or chlorhexidine solution may have a role in the treatment of S. aureus folliculitis, but these agents can dry out the skin and lead to eczematous eruptions prone to secondary bacterial infections. Systemic antibiotics can be used, and susceptibility testing (or knowledge of local resistance patterns) should guide antibiotic selection. The use of topical mupirocin to reduce MRSA carriage is controversial because it does not appear to reduce infection rates. Abscesses should be incised and drained. Rifampin can be used in combination with other antibiotics to reduce carriage rates of S. aureus, but caution should be used in patients receiving ART, because rifampin is a potent inducer of cytochrome P-450 and will therefore interfere with protease inhibitors. More severe infections may require intravenous antibiotics.

BARTONELLA

Bacillary angiomatosis (BA) is caused by Bartonella species (most commonly Bartonella henselae and Bartonella quintana). The cutaneous lesions appear as angiomatous lesions that can present in papular, nodular, or verrucous forms. Clinically, they may resemble lesions of Kaposi sarcoma (KS) and may also be confused with pyogenic granuloma or cutaneous lymphoma. Systemic involvement is common; visceral disease may present as osseous lesions, hepatic and splenic tumors, lymph node disease, pulmonary lesions, brain lesions, bone marrow infiltration, and widespread fatal systemic involvement. BA can present with unexplained fever, bacteremia, or endocarditis and should be considered in any HIV-infected patient with fever of unknown origin. Suspicious cutaneous lesions should always be biopsied and examined with hematoxylin, eosin, and Warthin-Starry silver staining. Blood and tissue cultures should be obtained, and indirect fluorescent antibody testing is useful when available. Polymerase chain reaction (PCR)-based tests play an important role and can be performed on biopsy and serum samples. Immunohistochemical staining for anti-HHV8 can be used to differentiate KS from BA. Bacillary angiomatosis responds to antibiotics such as erythromycin or doxycycline. Although cutaneous lesions resolve in 3 to 4 weeks, the treatment should be continued for at least 3 months. Severely ill patients should be treated with intravenous doxycycline combined with either gentamicin or rifampin for at least 3 months.

SYPHILIS

Syphilis (Chapter 319) is frequently seen in patients with HIV infection. Given the increasing number of reported syphilis cases, regular screening for syphilis, even in asymptomatic HIV-infected patients, is recommended. Its cutaneous manifestations are protean, and therefore syphilis should be

these agents, topical or intralesional cidofovir has been reported to be beneficial.[6]

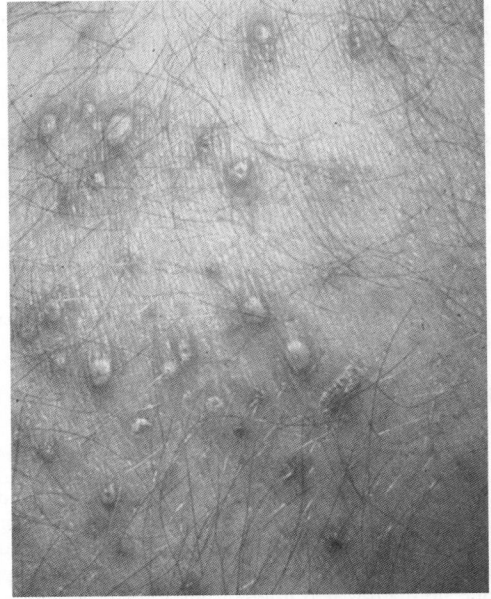

FIGURE 392-2. Staphylococcal folliculitis.

TABLE 392-2 SKIN CONDITIONS THAT CAN OCCUR AT ANY CD4+ COUNT
Eczema
Xerosis
Tinea/onychomycosis
Kaposi sarcoma
Warts
Syphilis

considered in any patient infected with HIV who has a new cutaneous eruption. An example of a secondary syphilis exanthem is shown in Figure 392-3. Primary, secondary, and tertiary forms of syphilis may be manifested clinically as they are in HIV-negative individuals, although atypical findings are not uncommon. Central nervous system (CNS) involvement may occur early in HIV patients, and relapse in the CNS may be more common after standard treatment. In most HIV patients, serologic tests are accurate and reliable for the diagnosis of syphilis and to monitor response to treatment. Atypical results can occur, and the use of other tests (biopsy and darkfield microscopy) should be considered when clinical findings do not match clinical findings.[8] First-line treatment is with benzathine penicillin G, 2.4 million units in a single dose. Azithromycin resistance is becoming more common. Close follow-up is essential, and titers of syphilis serology should be documented to ensure adequate treatment and CNS clearance. HIV-infected patients who meet criteria for treatment failure should be managed in the same manner as HIV-uninfected patients, because serologic clearance of syphilis appears largely unaffected by the use of ART. CSF examination and retreatment should be strongly considered for patients whose non-treponemal test titers do not decrease appropriately within 6 to 12 months of treatment.

Fungi

CANDIDA

Oral candidiasis is a common and localized infection caused by the yeast *Candida albicans*. It is commonly seen in patients with immunodeficiency, including HIV infection. It is characterized by white cheesy plaques and papules, loosely adherent to the tongue and oropharynx. Topical therapies include clotrimazole troches and nystatin oral suspension. Fluconazole is recommended for moderate to severe disease, but resistance has been noted in the setting of advanced HIV with extensive prior triazole use. Second-line treatment is with oral itraconazole, although it is unclear whether pulsed therapy is preferable.

DERMATOPHYTES

Cutaneous dermatophyte infections are common in HIV-infected patients, but it is not clear if these are any more frequent than in the non–HIV-infected population. Tinea infections follow a normal pattern and can involve the hands, feet, lower trunk, groin, and buttocks. The dermatophyte can spread to hair-bearing areas and present with plaques of folliculitis known as Majocchi granuloma. In those with advanced HIV, tinea infections can be atypical, diffuse, and severe. Tinea of the palms, soles, and other areas can be treated with topical imidazoles or terbinafine. If extensive areas are involved, oral antifungals are usually a more effective alternative and should be continued for approximately 1 month in cases of Majocchi granuloma. Treatment of onychomycosis with oral antifungals is standard but should be used selectively after risks and benefits of treatment are considered.

OTHER FUNGI

Cryptococcus neoformans is an encapsulated yeast that is a well-recognized opportunistic infection in advanced HIV (CD4+ count < 200 cells/μL). Clinical manifestations most commonly involve the lungs and CNS, but cutaneous dissemination can be seen in approximately 10% of patients.[9] Skin lesions can occur anywhere on the body and present as pearly 2- to 5-mm

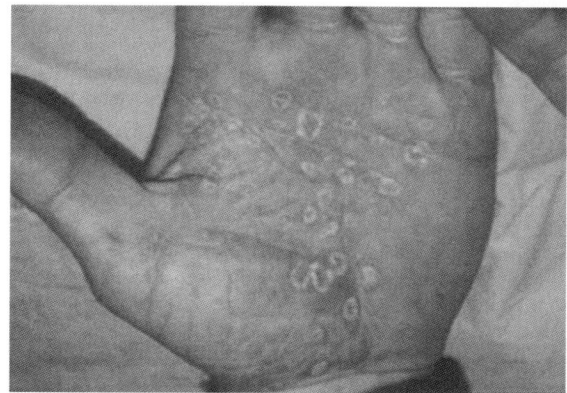

FIGURE 392-3. Secondary syphilis.

molluscum-appearing papules. Unlike molluscum, however, they develop over a short period of time. Large gelatinous plaques with umbilicated areas may also occur. Diagnosis is established by skin biopsy and culture. *Cryptococcus* on the skin in HIV is always associated with systemic cryptococcal infection and a serum cryptococcal antigen will be positive. *Histoplasma capsulatum* and *Penicillium marneffei* may morphologically resemble molluscum. Patients who have had these diseases should be evaluated for long-term suppressive doses of antifungal medications.

Infestations

SCABIES

Scabies is caused by infestation with the mite *Sarcoptes scabiei* and is commonly seen in HIV infection. It can be manifested as the classic rash of scabies, with burrows affecting the finger and toe webs and widespread excoriated papules with a predilection for the axillae, nipples, and genitalia. With advancing immunosuppression, the infestation can become more widespread and refractory to treatment. Crusted scabies can develop with advanced HIV and presents with thick crusts that are teeming with mites. Combination treatment with a topical agent such as permethrin or benzoyl benzoate and systemic treatment with ivermectin tablets is recommended for crusted scabies. Topical agents may be sufficient for classic scabies. Lindane lotion is often used to treat scabies, but there have been reports of lindane-resistant scabies and neurologic side effects attributed to this treatment.

TUMORS

Kaposi Sarcoma

KS is the most common HIV-associated malignancy, but since the introduction of ART, there has been a significant decrease in its incidence. It is characterized by dusky purple nodules and plaques with a predilection for the extremities and oral mucosa (Fig. 392-4). Poor prognostic factors include lymphedema and internal organ involvement. It is caused by HHV8, also known as Kaposi sarcoma–associated virus. The virus may be transmitted vertically, sexually, or casually, and its presence is necessary for the development of KS. Immune reconstitution with ART is the first-line treatment for early disease. Chemotherapy can be added for aggressive or unresponsive KS.

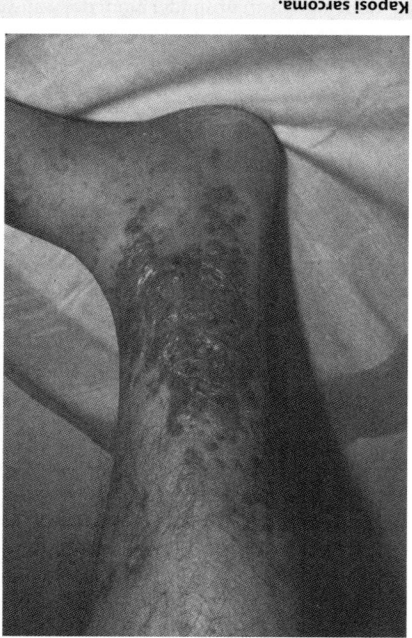

FIGURE 392-4. Kaposi sarcoma.

Malignant Melanoma

Malignant melanoma occurs with increased incidence in HIV-positive patients. Melanoma behavior can be more aggressive because HIV patients are more likely to present with metastases and have worse outcomes. High-risk patients should be screened annually, and those with a history of malignant melanoma should be followed closely for recurrence or early evidence of metastasis.[10]

Nonmelanoma Skin Cancer

Persons with AIDS have a three- to five-fold increased risk of developing a nonmelanoma skin cancer. The clinical manifestations of squamous cell carcinoma (SCC) and basal cell carcinoma (BCC) are identical to those seen in the uninfected population. Cutaneous SCC may be dangerous in the context of HIV infection, because lesions can present at a younger age and are associated with a high risk for local recurrence, metastasis, and increased mortality. Management of SCC is surgical excision, whereas curettage and electrodessication may be appropriate for BCC lesions on the extremities or trunk. Surgical excision should be the treatment of choice for BCC on the face.

INFLAMMATORY MANIFESTATIONS

Immune Reconstitution Inflammatory Syndrome

Most patients benefit substantially after the commencement of ART with a large reduction in morbidity and mortality. However, a subset of patients experience unmasking of new skin disease or paradoxical worsening of existing dermatologic conditions, attributable to IRIS (Chapter 395). Risk factors for developing IRIS include starting ART with a low CD4 nadir (<200 cells/μL) and the presence of subclinical opportunistic or other infections at the time of ART initiation. The most common skin manifestations of early IRIS include varicella-zoster reactivation and eosinophilic folliculitis. KS can present with organ involvement during IRIS. Other cutaneous manifestations include HPV (presenting as genital, flat, or common warts), reactivation of HSV or cytomegalovirus, cutaneous mycobacterial infection, or molluscum contagiosum. Leprosy, fungal infections, and parasitic infections such as leishmaniasis have also been reported. IRIS is most effectively treated by identifying and treating any underlying infection.

Seborrheic Dermatitis

Seborrheic dermatitis is a common dermatosis in the general population, but it has a strikingly increased prevalence in HIV-infected patients. Although more common in those with advanced HIV, the condition can be seen in all stages of immunosuppression. It appears as orange-red scaly patches affecting the scalp, eyebrows, nose, and cheeks. Seborrheic dermatitis can also affect the central portion of the chest and genitalia. ART appears to make seborrheic dermatitis more responsive to the standard therapy consisting of combinations of topical antifungals (econazole or ketoconazole) and low-potency corticosteroids.

Atopic Dermatitis

Atopic dermatitis (AD) is common in HIV-infected patients. The condition is characterized by pruritic scaly plaques that are classically localized to flexural areas. The distribution, however, can vary with ethnicity; AD in black Africans often involves the extensor surfaces. Treatment for AD is the same in the non–HIV-infected population. Frequent application with emollients should be emphasized. Topical steroids and sedating antihistamines are useful for flares. Topical pimecrolimus and tacrolimus are licensed for the treatment of atopic dermatitis, but their safety has not been demonstrated in HIV infection. As with other dermatoses, AD improves with ART, but in patients who had a CD4+ nadir less than 200 cells/μL it tends to be more persistent even with ART.

Psoriasis

Psoriasis may appear early in HIV infection. The severity ranges from mild to severe, with more severe disease correlating with worsening immunosuppression. This observation is paradoxical because psoriasis is thought to be a T-cell–mediated disease but may be explained by immune dysregulation. All psoriasis subtypes occur in the setting of HIV, but inverse (flexural), guttate, and erythrodermic forms are seen most often. Psoriatic arthritis is more common and severe than in the non-HIV population. Treatment should be tailored to disease severity. First-line therapy for mild to moderate psoriasis includes topical steroids, calcipotriol, and retinoids (tazarotene). In those with moderate to severe disease, ultraviolet therapy (UVB, PUVA) and ART are the first-line treatments. Oral retinoids are an appropriate second-line agent. Immunosuppressive agents such as methotrexate and cyclosporine can be used for severe or refractory disease. Patients on these agents should be followed closely, and concomitant prophylaxis for opportunistic infections should be considered. Given the limited evidence and risks associated with their use (particularly in the HIV-infected population), tumor necrosis factor (TNF)-α inhibitors should be reserved for patients with very refractory psoriasis and those with debilitating arthritis. ART invariably reduces the severity of psoriasis and is considered a first-line treatment in those with moderate to severe disease.

Papular Pruritic Eruption of HIV

Papular pruritic eruption (PPE) is commonly seen in Africa and Asia in association with HIV. The condition presents with excoriated papules that initially appear on the extensor extremities but subsequently extend to involve the trunk and face. Pruritus can be severe. Because its presentation is nondescript, other itchy skin diseases such as eczema or eosinophilic folliculitis should be considered in the differential diagnosis. Skin biopsies have been considered to be important to distinguish between PPE and other itchy papular eruptions.[11] When present, PPE is highly predictive of HIV infection and is often the presenting sign. It has been hypothesized that this condition represents a hyperactive immune response to arthropod bites. Treatment is difficult, but potent topical corticosteroids and UVB may be of some benefit. Because PPE presents at CD4 counts of 350 cells/μL or less, it may be an indication for ART initiation. The condition has been reported to improve dramatically with effective ART.

Eosinophilic Folliculitis

Eosinophilic folliculitis is characterized by urticarial follicular-based papules and pustules located primarily on the scalp, face, neck, and upper chest (Fig. 392-5). These lesions are intensely itchy, and skin biopsy is helpful in ruling out other causes of folliculitis. Eosinophilic folliculitis tends to be seen when CD4+ counts are less than 200 cells/μL. It can also be seen as part of the immune reconstitution syndrome within the first 16 weeks of starting ART. Treatments include topical corticosteroids, antihistamines, itraconazole, metronidazole, oral retinoids, and UV light therapy. If immune reconstitution is implicated, these agents can be given for an 8- to 12-week period while immune restoration stabilizes.

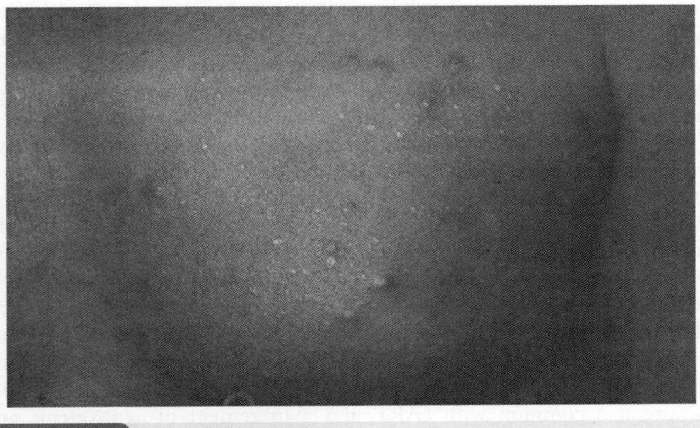

FIGURE 392-5 Eosinophilic folliculitis.

Prurigo Nodularis

Prurigo nodularis is characterized by pruritic dome-shaped nodules that initially develop on photoexposed areas of the extremities but eventually extend to involve the trunk. Development of prurigo nodularis is associated with background skin pigment and CD4 counts below 100 cells/mm². Standard treatment options include emollients, potent topical steroids, and sedating antihistamines such as chlorpheniramine or hydroxyzine. Thalidomide is often effective in recalcitrant cases but requires careful monitoring for peripheral neuropathy, and women of childbearing potential require effective contraception. Immune reconstitution and reduction of viremia with ART are helpful. Regimens that include raltegravir may be useful in refractory cases.[12]

Photodermatitis

HIV-infected patients have a tendency toward photosensitivity, a phenomenon that is poorly understood. Patients are commonly on photosensitizing medications like trimethoprim-sulfa and dapsone for prophylaxis and treatment of concurrent infections. But even in the absence of classic photosensitizing drugs, HIV itself and pigmented skin are risk factors for photodermatitis. Photodermatitis presents with pruritic plaques or indurated plaques in photoexposed areas of the skin like the cheeks, ears, lower lip, tip of the nose, and dorsal hands. Sunscreen and sun avoidance are the treatments.

METABOLIC MANIFESTATIONS

HIV Lipodystrophy Syndrome

Lipodystrophy syndrome was first described in 1998 and consists of peripheral lipoatrophy, central lipohypertrophy, lipid abnormalities, and insulin resistance. It is likely that it is caused by a number of factors, including ART, although it is unlikely that a single agent is responsible. Cutaneous facial lipoatrophy tends to be the most problematic dermatologic aspect, with significant associated psychological morbidity (Fig. 392-6). Currently, no treatments are effective for lipodystrophy syndrome, although surgical correction with dermal fillers may improve the cosmetic appearance.

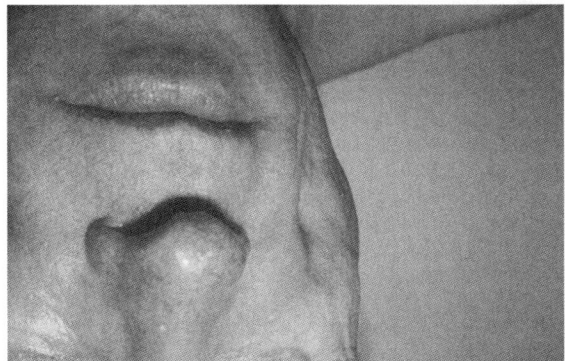

FIGURE 392-6. HIV-associated facial lipoatrophy.

GENERAL REFERENCES

For the General References and other additional features, please visit Expert Consult at https://expertconsult.inkling.com.

393
HEMATOLOGY AND ONCOLOGY IN PATIENTS WITH HUMAN IMMUNODEFICIENCY VIRUS INFECTION

THOMAS S. ULDRICK AND ROBERT YARCHOAN

Patients with human immunodeficiency virus (HIV) infection or acquired immunodeficiency syndrome (AIDS) have a substantially increased risk of developing a number of cancers. Three of these cancers, Kaposi sarcoma (KS), certain non-Hodgkin lymphomas (NHLs), and cervical cancer, confer a diagnosis of AIDS when they arise in an HIV-infected patient and are referred to as AIDS-defining malignancies (ADMs). HIV increases the risk for a number of other tumors, including classic Hodgkin lymphoma (cHL), and nonmelanoma skin cancer. These other HIV-associated tumors are referred to as non–AIDS-defining malignancies (NADMs) (Table 393-1).[1] Cytopenias and coagulation abnormalities are also common in patients with AIDS.

Effective combination antiretroviral therapy (cART) for HIV became broadly available in 1996. Its widespread use dramatically reduced opportunistic infections (OIs) and increased the longevity of patients with HIV infection. In part for these reasons, the number of persons living with HIV in the United States has approximately doubled since 1996. The use of cART also decreased the incidence of KS and NHL in the HIV-infected population. Nonetheless, these tumors remain important causes of morbidity and mortality. However, as the HIV-infected population ages, NADM, as well as other cancers not associated with HIV, are becoming increasingly common, and cancer is now a leading cause of death of HIV-infected persons. Cytopenias are also less common with cART, and management of neutropenia and anemia has shifted from growth factor support to effective treatment of HIV.

Still, HIV increases the risk of hematologic abnormalities, which continue to cause diagnostic and therapeutic challenges. With more than 1 million people in the United States and 30 million people globally infected with HIV, management of HIV-infected patients with cancers and blood disorders is increasingly important.

CANCERS IN HIV-INFECTED PATIENTS

Care of the HIV-infected patient with cancer requires integration of oncologic and infectious disease expertise, including evaluation of comorbidities, planning of timing and selection of cART, and OI prophylaxis. Although patients with advanced AIDS may tolerate chemotherapeutic regimens poorly, patients whose HIV is controlled with cART can often receive full-dose regimens and do as well as their HIV-negative counterparts. There are 30-plus approved antiretroviral agents. Consideration of potential pharmacokinetic interactions between antiviral drugs and cancer therapy is required.

EPIDEMIOLOGY

The standardized incidence ratios of KS and certain aggressive B-cell NHLs are markedly increased in patients with HIV, especially those with low CD4 counts. KS, certain NHLs, cervical cancer, and a number of other NADMs are directly or indirectly caused by oncogenic viruses, especially Kaposi sarcoma herpesvirus (KSHV, also called human herpesvirus 8 [HHV-8]), Epstein-Barr virus (EBV), human papillomavirus (HPV), hepatitis C virus (HCV), and hepatitis B virus (HBV) (see Table 393-1). Many of these viruses are prevalent in various HIV-infected populations and are poorly controlled in the setting of immunosuppression. HIV-infected individuals also often have increased exposure to other cancer risk factors, such as cigarette smoke.

Substantial changes in the patterns of cancer in the U.S. AIDS epidemic have been noted since the introduction of cART. The incidence of KS and NHL have decreased relative to their peak, while the burden of NADMs, most of which develop over a longer period of time, is rising. Whereas most cancers developing in HIV patients were ADMs early in the epidemic, these cancers are now divided approximately evenly between ADM and other cancers (Fig. 393-1).[2] Overall, cancer is one of the leading causes of death in HIV-infected patients in countries where cART is widely available, in part because fewer patients are dying from other causes, such as OIs associated with low CD4 counts or AIDS itself. Also, HIV-associated cancers, especially ADMs, are a major public health concern in many resource-limited regions, such as sub-Saharan Africa.

PREVENTION AND SCREENING

Several chemopreventive strategies and behavioral interventions should be used to prevent HIV-associated malignancies. The risk of KS and NHL in patients with HIV is decreased with cART.[3] Some studies show that improved immunity with cART also can reduce the prevalence of premalignant HPV-associated cervical[3] and anal squamous intraepithelial neoplasia and lesions. Vaccination against HBV and antiviral therapy against HBV and HCV decrease the risk of hepatocellular carcinoma in many HIV-uninfected populations and are warranted. Smoking is prevalent in many HIV-infected populations, and smoking cessation interventions are advised. Nonmelanoma skin cancer is increased with HIV, and reduction of exposure to ultraviolet radiation is prudent.

HPV vaccines can reduce the risk of HPV-associated cancers and premalignant conditions. They should optimally be administered in early adolescence before the onset of sexual activity and exposure to HPV infection. A concern in this area is that the rate of uptake of the HPV vaccine is now low in the United States, especially in boys. Recent studies suggest that there may also be value in vaccination after the onset of sexual activity, in part to prevent reinfection after clearance of high-risk strains. The HPV vaccine has been shown to be safe in HIV-infected children and adults, and those with relatively preserved immune function can develop antibodies to the vaccine; however, it has not been shown whether the vaccine is protective in this population. Women with HIV infection, squamous intraepithelial lesions (SIL), and/or poor control of oncogenic HPV subtypes need more frequent gynecologic evaluation than low-risk women (see section on cervical cancer). Given the markedly increased risk of anal cancer in women and men with HIV (see Table 393-1), programs have been developed employing cytologic examination of anal mucosa to screen for and treat high-grade squamous intraepithelial lesions (HSIL).[4] A National Cancer Institute (NCI)-funded prospective study is planned to evaluate whether this approach is effective in preventing anal cancer.

TABLE 393-1 AIDS-DEFINING MALIGNANCIES AND COMMON NON–AIDS-DEFINING MALIGNANCIES IN PERSONS WITH HIV IN THE COMBINED ANTIRETROVIRAL THERAPY ERA

MALIGNANCIES	STANDARD INCIDENCE RATIO (HIV ONLY / AIDS)	ESTIMATED % OF ALL CANCERS 2004-2007 IN HIV/AIDS IN UNITED STATES	VIRAL ASSOCIATIONS	OTHER IMPORTANT RISK FACTORS
AIDS-DEFINING MALIGNANCIES				
Non-Hodgkin lymphoma				
Systemic	10-15 / 30-60	25.9%	EBV, KSHV*	
Primary CNS lymphoma	250 / 1020	3%	EBV	
Kaposi sarcoma	1300 / 3640	18.5%	KSHV	
Cervical cancer	2.9 / 5.3	2.4%	HPV	Smoking
NON–AIDS-DEFINING MALIGNANCIES				
Lung cancer	2.6 / 2.6	10%	—	Smoking
Anal cancer	9.2 / 20	5.7%	HPV	Smoking
Classic Hodgkin lymphoma	5.6 / 14	4.4%	EBV	
Oropharyngeal carcinoma	1.7 / 2.1	2.5%	HPV	Smoking, alcohol
Hepatocellular carcinoma	2.7 / 3.3	2.3%	HBV, HCV	Alcohol, aflatoxins, tobacco

*EBV associations vary with different AIDS-related lymphomas; approximately 30% Burkitt lymphomas, approximately 30-60% diffuse large B-cell lymphomas, and 100% of plasmablastic lymphomas. KSHV is associated with primary effusion lymphoma (≈80% coinfected with EBV) and large cell lymphoma arising in the setting of KSHV-associated multicentric Castleman disease (EBV negative).
CNS = central nervous system; EBV = Epstein-Barr virus; HBV = hepatitis B virus; HCV = hepatitis C virus; HPV = human papillomavirus; KSHV = Kaposi sarcoma herpesvirus.
From HIV/AIDS Cancer Match Study: standardized incidence rates in people with HIV but not AIDS at baseline versus AIDS at baseline, each compared to the general U.S. population. HIV estimates from Engels EA, et al. *Int J Cancer.* 2008;123:187-194. AIDS estimates from Engels EA, et al. *AIDS.* 2006;20:1645-1654. Percentage of total cancers of based on 34 states included in HACM, from Shiels MS, Pfeiffer RM, Gail MH, et al. Cancer burden in the HIV-infected population in the United States. *J Natl Cancer Inst.* 2011;103:753-762.

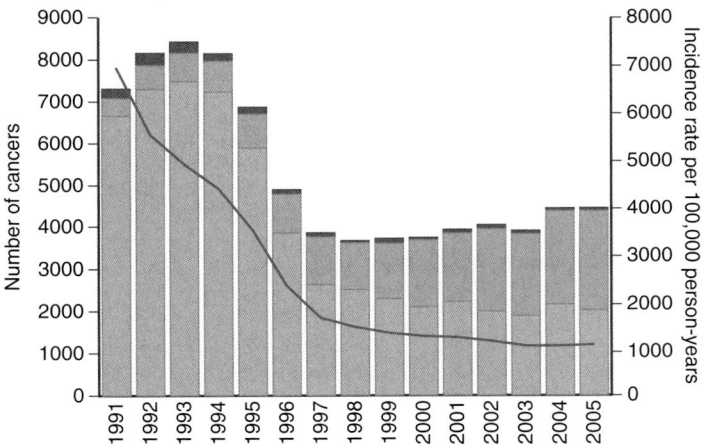

FIGURE 393-1. Trends in AIDS-defining malignancies (*orange bars*) and other malignancies (*green bars*) in persons with HIV/AIDS in the United States in the years 1991-2005. Blue = poorly classified cancers; line represents incidence rate. From Shiels MS, Pfeiffer RM, Gail MH, et al. Cancer burden in the HIV-infected population in the United States. *J Natl Cancer Inst.* 2011;103:753-762.

Although they have not been specifically evaluated in patients with HIV, routine recommended cancer screening, such as stool guaiac examinations or colonoscopy, mammography, and perhaps low-dose chest computed tomography (CT)[5] should be offered based on indications for the general population. In addition to these preventive measures, physicians caring for HIV-infected patients should be aware of cancers associated with HIV infection (see Table 393-1) and be alert for their development.

Non-Hodgkin Lymphoma and Classic Hodgkin Lymphoma in HIV

The Centers for Disease Control and Prevention (CDC) 1993 definition of AIDS considers Burkitt (or equivalent), immunoblastic (or equivalent), or primary brain lymphoma as AIDS defining. This classification is outdated, however. Using the current World Health Organization classification, patients with HIV are at substantially increased risk for eight distinct lymphomas or lymphoproliferative disorders. In this chapter, we use the term AIDS-related lymphoma (ARL) to collectively describe the NHLs with substantially increased standardized incidence ratios in patients with HIV/AIDS.[6]

EPIDEMIOLOGY

ARLs are aggressive mature B-cell lymphomas, including diffuse large B-cell lymphoma (DLBCL) with centroblastic (germinal center) or immunoblastic (activated B-cell) phenotypes, Burkitt lymphoma (BL), plasmablastic lymphoma (PBL), primary diffuse large B-cell lymphoma of the central nervous system (PCNSL), primary effusion lymphoma, and large cell lymphoma arising in the setting of KSHV-associated multicentric Castleman disease (KSHV-MCD). Classic Hodgkin lympoma (cHL) and KSHV-MCD also occur with markedly increased frequency in HIV-infected patients, although these are not NHLs and thus are not usually categorized as ARL. HIV testing should be considered in a patient with any of these tumors. ARL risk increases with immunosuppression and HIV viremia. With cART, ARL incidence decreased in the United States by 50%, mainly because of decreases in subtypes occurring at low CD4+ counts. Still, ARL risk is greatly elevated. The estimated U.S. incidence is 97 per 100,000 person-years. ARL is a major public health problem in sub-Saharan Africa.

PATHOBIOLOGY

Many aggressive mature B-cell lymphomas (ARLs) are caused by the gamma-herpesviruses EBV or KSHV, and for these, poor viral immune control related to global and in some cases virus-specific immune defects contributes to lymphomagenesis (see Table 393-1). EBV and KSHV encode for a number of genes, including mimics of human immune genes that are important for viral survival and transmission but are also implicated in lymphomagenesis. Examples include EBV-encoded CD40-like latent membrane protein (LMP-1) and KSHV-encoded viral FLICE-like inhibitory protein (vFLIP). Furthermore, chronic B-cell immune activation, especially in the setting of uncontrolled HIV, appears important, especially for NHL subtypes that occur at relatively preserved CD4+ counts. Activation-induced cytidine deaminase (AICDA), an enzyme required for germinal center class switch recombination and somatic hypermutation, also induces mutations and pathogenic translocations. Importantly, *c-myc/Ig* translocations are seen in Burkitt lymphoma (BL), a majority of EBV-positive plasmablastic lymphoma (PBLs), and 24% of DLBCLs, likely accounting for the high proliferative rate and aggressive nature of these tumors.

CLINICAL MANIFESTATIONS

ARL and classic Hodgkin lympoma (cHL) often present with adenopathy or "B" symptoms (fever, night sweats, or weight loss in excess of 10% body weight). Involvement of bone marrow, liver, gastrointestinal (GI) tract, and CNS are common. HIV patients with cHL often have EBV-associated disease with either mixed cellularity or lymphocyte-depleted subtypes, present with high-risk disease, and also may present with extranodal involvement. PBL classically presents as an oral-cavity mass; however, other nodal or extranodal presentations are common. Primary effusion lymphoma often presents with pleural, peritoneal, or pericardial effusions but may have extracavitary presentations. Patients with primary effusion lymphoma commonly have concurrent KS or KSHV-MCD. Edema, hypoalbuminemia, and cytopenias are also common in primary effusion lymphoma and largely related to the underlying KSHV-associated malignancy rather than HIV.

DIAGNOSIS

Staging Evaluation of Systemic Lymphoma and Classic Hodgkin Lymphoma

Diagnosis of aggressive mature B-cell lymphoma (ARL) or cHL requires biopsy of a lymph node or involved extranodal lesion. Immunohistochemical markers are required for classification and include a combination of B-cell lineage markers and KSHV-encoded latency-associated nuclear antigen (LANA) and *in situ* hybridization for EBV-encoded small RNAs (EBER). Evaluation for *c-myc/Ig* translocations is warranted. Viral markers are particularly important for the CD20-negative large cell lymphomas plasmablastic lymphoma (PBL), and primary effusion lymphoma.

Staging includes CT of the neck, chest, abdomen, and pelvis; (^{18}F)-fluorodeoxyglucose positron emission tomography (^{18}FDG-PET) when available; and bone marrow biopsy. For ARL, CNS imaging by magnetic resonance imaging (MRI) with gadolinium (preferred) or CT with contrast and lumbar puncture with cerebrospinal fluid (CSF) cytology and flow cytometry are required. CNS imaging and CSF evaluation are not standard for cHL, although in HIV-associated cases, the CNS can be involved.

Baseline laboratory tests include HIV viral load, CD4 count, lactate dehydrogenase (LDH), complete blood cell count with differential, evaluation of renal and liver function, HBV surface and core antibody and surface antigen, and HCV serology or HCV RNA viral load. Patients with detectable HBV core antibody or surface antigen require a quantitative HBV viral load. Evaluation of cardiac function is recommended.

TREATMENT   Rx

General Approach to Supportive Care

Supportive care and combination antiretroviral therapy (cART) deserve special consideration. The survival of patients with ARL and cHL has improved in the cART era, and use of cART during ARL therapy may improve long-term outcomes. However, cART is not always essential during chemotherapy; 85 to 90% long-term survival rates have been obtained for the germinal center phenotype of DLBCL and BL with regimens that involved withholding cART.[7,8] Pharmacokinetic and toxicity interactions between cART and chemotherapeutic agents must be considered. Protease inhibitors (especially ritonavir) and cobicistat, a pharmacologic booster used in some cART formulations, inhibit CYP3A4, decrease metabolism of many chemotherapeutic agents, potentially increase toxicity, and should be avoided if possible. Zidovudine has overlapping hematotoxicity, and tenofovir requires renal monitoring. Often, cART is continued in patients on effective regimens when feasible, preferably with a protease inhibitor–sparing regimen; a new cART regimen need not necessarily be introduced before initiating lymphoma therapy. In patients with toxicities due to drug-drug interactions during curative-intent therapy, temporary suspension of nonessential drugs, including cART, is important.

OI prophylaxis is important, especially in patients with CD4 counts of less than 100 cells/mm^3. Regardless of baseline CD4 count, patients should receive *Pneumocystis jiroveci* pneumonia (PCP) prophylaxis, preferably trimethoprim-sulfamethoxazole (TMP-SMX). Patients with less than 100 CD4 cells/mm^3 also require prophylaxis against atypical mycobacterial infections with azithromycin 1200 mg weekly. Prophylaxis against herpes simplex virus and varicella zoster reactivation using valacyclovir should be strongly considered. Patients with active HBV require anti-HBV therapy. Prophylactic antifungals should be considered to prevent oral candidiasis, but azoles should be avoided during chemotherapy administration. Monitoring for OIs in patients with AIDS is important. Patients with HIV undergoing lymphoma therapy remain immunosuppressed beyond the end of therapy. Extension of these OI prophylaxis recommendations for at least 6 months beyond the end of therapy, and until CD4 cells adequately recover, is reasonable.

PERIPHERAL LYMPHOMA IN HIV

TREATMENT AND PROGNOSIS   Rx

Diffuse Large B-cell Lymphoma

In the cART era, lymphoma-specific characteristics and treatment-related factors are important in determining disease-free survival. The age-adjusted International Prognostic Index (based on stage, performance status, and LDH), CD4 cut-off of 100 cells/mm^3, and HCV status provide additional prognostic information for overall survival. Most patients, even with low CD4 counts and poor performance status, should be approached with curative intent. For CD20-positive tumors, the anti-CD20 monoclonal antibody rituximab substantially improves long-term cancer outcomes, but patients with CD4$^+$ counts less

than 50 cells/mm^3 remain at high risk of infectious complications[9] and do no better overall.[A2] The best-studied regimens for DLBCL are DA-EPOCH-R (rituximab; continuous-infusion etoposide, doxorubicin, and vincristine; oral prednisone; bolus cyclophosphamide; and filgrastim), short-course DA-EPOCH with dose-dense rituximab (SC-EPOCH-RR), and R-CHOP (rituximab, cyclophosphamide, doxorubicin, vincristine, and prednisone).[10] Pooled data suggest that EPOCH provides a better backbone regimen than CHOP for HIV-associated DLBCL as long as the CD4$^+$ count is above 50 cells/mm^3.[A3]

Burkitt Lymphoma

For BL, CHOP is inadequate. Preliminary results from a study of modified CODOX-M/IVAC combined with rituximab in HIV-associated BL demonstrated 1-year overall survival of 83% but 9% treatment-related mortality. A recent study reported 90% long-term overall survival for BL in a small number of HIV-infected patients treated with SC-EPOCH-RR with intrathecal methotrexate and deferred cART. EPOCH has a better toxicity profile than CODOX-M/IVAC. During the first cycle, BL patients require allopurinol and adequate hydration to avoid tumor lysis syndrome.

Plasmablastic Lymphoma

PBL is a recently recognized CD20-negative aggressive large B-cell lymphoma. Retrospective data suggest that outcomes are poor with CHOP or localized disease treated with radiation, with median survival less than 2 years. Recently, *c-myc/Ig* translocations have been noted in a majority of cases. Regimens effective in NHL with high proliferative rates, such as DA-EPOCH, are recommended.

KSHV-Associated Lymphomas, Including Primary Effusion Lymphoma

There is no established therapy for KSHV-associated NHL. Anthracycline-based regimens may be curative in some cases. Concurrent KSHV-MCD requires specific treatment.

CNS Prophylaxis and Treatment

CNS involvement in ARL is common and confers a poor prognosis. Routine CNS prophylaxis is required for BL and is commonly included for other ARLs. Treatment includes intrathecal methotrexate and/or cytosine arabinoside. Intensive intraventricular or intrathecal therapy is required for patients with leptomeningeal disease at the time of diagnosis.

Resource-Limited Settings

Physicians treating ARL in resource-limited settings face many challenges, often including a shortage of pathologists and laboratory support required to make an accurate diagnosis. Lower-cost regimens that are easy to administer and do not require extensive supportive care are often used. CHOP is a commonly used regimen for DLBCL and other ARLs in resource-limited settings but may be challenging to administer. HIV-associated BL in Africa is often treated with a cyclophosphamide-based combination regimen.

Classic Hodgkin Lymphoma

Despite some biological differences in cHL between HIV-infected and uninfected patients, outcomes appear comparable in the cART-era. ABVD (doxorubicin, bleomycin, vinblastine, and dacarbazine) or risk-adapted therapy are often used. In a retrospective study of ABVD, 5-year progression-free survival and overall survival were 59 and 81%, respectively. In a prospective study of risk-adapted therapy, 2-year progression-free survival and overall survival were 91 and 92%, respectively. However, treatment-related mortality was 6% with the more intensive regimen BEACOPP (bleomycin, etoposide, cyclophosphamide, vincristine, procarbazine, and prednisone).

PRIMARY CENTRAL NERVOUS SYSTEM LYMPHOMA (PCNSL)

DIAGNOSIS

AIDS-related PCNSL almost always arises in patients with CD4 counts of less than 50 cells/mm^3, many of whom are not aware they have AIDS or for other reasons have not been controlled with cART. Patients with AIDS-related PCNSL usually present with focal neurologic symptoms, seizures, or headaches related to the CNS mass. Outcomes remain poor in the cART era, with a 2-year overall survival of less than 25%. This is in part due to difficulty in diagnosis, neurologic comorbidities, and delayed or inadequate lymphoma treatment.[11] Patients with AIDS and CNS masses require urgent evaluation to minimize lag time to definitive therapy. Brain MRI with gadolinium demonstrates single or multiple contrast-enhancing masses in PCNSL that are not reliably distinguishable from toxoplasmosis. Prior to effective treatment for HIV, a course of empirical antibiotics for toxoplasmosis was sometimes an initial step in managing patients with AIDS with ring-enhancing CNS masses; however, empirical therapy for toxoplasmosis without concomitant CNS evaluation should not be considered an initial diagnostic maneuver for patients in the cART era. Nuclear imaging with ^{201}Tl-SPECT or ^{18}FDG-PET generally differentiates infections from malignancies. Imaging of the neck, chest, abdomen, and pelvis is required to exclude systemic malignancy. Lumbar puncture should be undertaken when safe to evaluate CSF cell count, glucose, protein, cytopathology, flow cytometry, EBV, JC virus, toxoplasmosis, and cryptococcal antigen. Definitive diagnosis requires biopsy. However, in patients with less than 50 CD4 cells/mm^3, a combination of a ring-enhancing brain mass on MRI, positive ^{201}Tl-SPECT or ^{18}FDG-PET, and a high CSF EBV viral load is adequate to institute therapy for presumptive AIDS-related PCNSL if a biopsy is not feasible. Staging requires ophthalmologic evaluation.

TREATMENT [Rx]

Whole-brain radiation has often been used but can have severe neurologic toxicities. With cART availability, radiation-sparing therapy may be preferable, with promising preliminary results demonstrated in one clinical trial to date.

Kaposi Sarcoma
EPIDEMIOLOGY

There are four epidemiologic categories of KS: (1) classic, commonly seen in elderly Mediterranean men (2) endemic, seen in African men, women, and children (3) iatrogenic, seen in transplant or other patients on chronic immunosuppressive medications, and (4) epidemic AIDS related. KSHV is the causative agent for all epidemiologic forms, but in the absence of immunosuppression, relatively few KSHV-infected patients develop KS. HIV coinfection or other immunosuppression dramatically enhances the risk of KS in KSHV-infected persons. Transmission of KSHV appears to be largely due to saliva exchange, and transmission may be increased in the setting of uncontrolled HIV or other infections such as malaria. KSHV seroprevalence is high in gay men in the United States but lower in injection drug users and less than 10% in the general population. In sub-Saharan Africa, seroprevalence ranges from 40 to 80%.

In the United States, KS incidence initially decreased by 84% with introduction of cART. Further declines have been more modest, and estimated incidence has recently stabilized at about 62 cases per 100,000 person-years. KS is now the second most common tumor in persons with HIV in the United States. In parts of sub-Saharan Africa, KS is the most common tumor in men overall, and second most common in women.

PATHOBIOLOGY

KS is an angioproliferative tumor with abnormal vascularity and infiltrating inflammatory cells. The pathognomonic KS spindle cells are generally poly- or oligoclonal and KSHV infected. KSHV encodes several micro-RNA and viral homologues of human genes that effect immune signaling and angiogenesis. Most KSHV-infected spindle cells express a limited set of latent viral proteins, such as LANA, which provide a proliferative advantage and suppress apoptosis. A minority (2 to 3%) of cells also express lytic KSHV-proteins, such as KSHV-encoded viral interleukin-6 (vIL-6) and viral G-protein–coupled receptor (vGPCR), which amplify production of angiogenic and immune modulatory factors that affect the tumor microenvironment and appear important in KS pathogenesis. Defective immune surveillance of KSHV-infected cells in HIV-infected patients is permissive for the development of KS. HIV may promote KS by other mechanisms as well. For example, the Tat protein of HIV can enhance infection of target cells by KSHV.

CLINICAL MANIFESTATIONS

KS generally presents as multiple painless, cutaneous, purplish or brown lesions that are initially flat and can become nodular and congruent (Fig. 440-19). KS often presents in the feet (Fig. 393-2) but can involve other areas of the skin as well. Advanced KS can have associated edema, ulceration, pain, and superinfection. KS frequently involves the oral palate. It can involve lymph nodes, the GI system, lungs, and may have associated pleural effusions. Pulmonary KS can be life threatening. GI disease is often asymptomatic, but occult blood loss is common. Involvement of the liver, bones, or soft tissues has been described. Visceral-only disease may be seen. KS may wax and wane with immune status. Progressive disease has been described after starting cART, and an immune reconstitution inflammatory syndrome (IRIS) (Chapter 395) has been proposed. KS may also progress

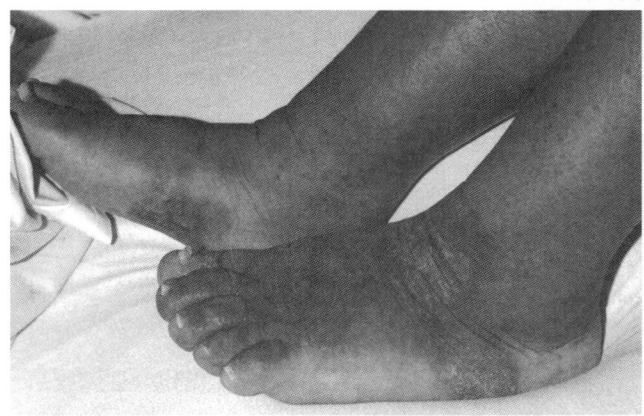

FIGURE 393-2. Kaposi sarcoma involving the feet.

in the setting of uncontrolled KSHV-associated multicentric Castleman disease (KSHV-MCD) or primary effusion lymphoma.

DIAGNOSIS AND STAGING

KS is diagnosed by biopsy. An estimate of the extent of cutaneous disease and evaluation for complications of advanced cutaneous disease is required. Evaluation for visceral disease includes fecal occult blood testing and chest imaging. Abnormalities require endoscopic evaluation. Pulmonary KS is diagnosed based on visualization of typical endobronchial lesions, with endobronchial biopsy generally deferred because of bleeding risk. KS in a lymph node biopsy often requires evaluation for concurrent lymphoma or KSHV-MCD.

KS is staged by the AIDS Clinical Trials Group (ACTG) TIS system, which is based on tumor burden ($T_{0\ or\ 1}$), immune status ($I_{0\ or\ 1}$), and presence of any systemic illness ($S_{0\ or\ 1}$). Poor risk (subscript 1) is defined by extensive oral disease, tumor-associated edema or ulceration, or non-nodal visceral disease (T_1); CD4 below 150 cells/mm^3 (I_1); and the presence of OIs, constitutional symptoms, or poor performance status (S_1).

TREATMENT [Rx]

cART is fundamental in treating HIV-associated KS. Immunosuppressive medications such as steroids, cyclosporine, and rituximab should be avoided when possible, and surgery has little role except for purpose of biopsy. Limited (T_0) HIV-associated KS is often managed with cART alone, which can induce KS regression over several months. KS-specific therapy is generally reserved for cases causing morbidity or other patient distress. Local therapies, such as topical alitretinoin gel, intralesional injection of vinblastine, laser therapy, or cryotherapy can be effective but are associated with local toxicities. They are occasionally used for very localized disease. Most patients who require KS-specific therapy are now given systemic therapy. Chemotherapy may be required urgently for symptomatic pulmonary KS. Progressive KS in patients who have recently initiated cART is often an indication for specific KS therapy, and chemotherapy plus cART is better than cART alone. Generally, KS is treated until remission or response plateau is attained. The number of cycles required is variable. The main objective of therapy is long-term remission or durable control. Because KSHV cannot be eradicated, KS is not considered curable, and relapses can occur.

Liposomal anthracyclines (doxorubicin and daunorubicin) and paclitaxel are approved by the U.S. Food and Drug Administration (FDA) for use in KS. Liposomal doxorubicin 20 mg/m^2 every 3 weeks is the most commonly used therapy. In the cART era, response rates of 45 to 80% may be anticipated. The FDA warns against cumulative lifetime doses exceeding 550 mg/m^2, although risk of cardiotoxicity is believed to be lower with liposomal formulations than with bolus non-liposomal anthracyclines. Paclitaxel should be considered in patients who have inadequate KS regression, cannot tolerate liposomal anthracyclines, or have reached their cumulative lifetime dose. A randomized trial comparing liposomal doxorubicin 20 mg/m^2 every 3 weeks with paclitaxel 100 mg/m^2 every 2 weeks in persons with advanced KS showed comparable efficacy, but increased toxicity in the paclitaxel arm.

Interferon-α can be effective in patients with preserved CD4$^+$ counts but is generally not used owing to poor tolerability of side effects. Several available targeted therapies have recently been evaluated in KS. In renal transplant–associated KS, modification of immunosuppression from cyclosporine to the mTOR inhibitor sirolimus leads to tumor regression. However, in a study of sirolimus in AIDS-related KS, responses were limited, and drug interactions with ritonavir complicated dosing. Bevacizumab and imatinib have shown activity but alone appear inferior to cytotoxic agents. Thalidomide is active at high doses that are associated with toxicities. Studies of the thalidomide analogs (IMiDs) lenalidomide and pomalidomide are underway.

Low-cost agents that are easy to administer are required for KS treatment in sub-Saharan Africa. Vincristine, doxorubicin, bleomycin, and etoposide all are used in this setting. Oral etoposide was associated with an overall response rate of 36% in previously treated patients, the majority of whom were not on cART. In a randomized study of ABV (doxorubicin, bleomycin, vincristine) combined with cART versus cART alone in treatment-naïve patients, most with advanced KS, early addition of chemotherapy was feasible and effective in this setting, with an increase of 1-year overall response rate from 39 to 66%.[A6] To reduce risk of cardiac toxicity, some practitioners exclude doxorubicin and use BV in combination with cART.

PROGNOSIS

The prognosis for patients with AIDS-related KS has improved dramatically with cART. There are two main risk groups: good risk (T_0S_0, T_1S_0, or T_0S_1) versus poor risk (T_1S_1). Pulmonary involvement increases risk of death, and women with have a worse prognosis independent of other TIS risk factors. Poor CD4 immune reconstitution is often associated with need for recurrent therapy.

Multicentric Castleman Disease

MCD describes a group of lymphoproliferative disorders associated with dysregulated IL-6. The plasmablastic variant is often caused by KSHV, and nearly all MCD in patients with HIV is KSHV-MCD.

PATHOBIOLOGY

KSHV-MCD is a polyclonal lymphoproliferative disorder of KSHV-infected B cells with plasmablastic morphology. Symptoms are associated with KSHV-lytic activation and vIL-6 upregulation. Marked elevations in human IL-6 and IL-10 are noted, and along with KSHV are strongly implicated in disease pathogenesis.

CLINICAL MANIFESTATIONS AND DIAGNOSIS

KSHV-MCD is characterized by intermittent severe inflammatory symptoms, including fevers, night sweats, fatigue and cachexia, and edema, as well as lymphadenopathy and splenomegaly. GI and respiratory symptoms are common; rheumatologic, neurologic, and dermatologic manifestations may also be present. Laboratory abnormalities include anemia, thrombocytopenia, hyponatremia, hypoalbuminemia, and elevated KSHV viral load. Most patients requiring therapy have an elevated C-reactive protein, and this can be a useful test to include in the initial evaluation of patients with suspected KSHV-MCD. Diagnosis requires pathologic confirmation, usually from a lymph node. Patients should be evaluated for concurrent KS and lymphoma. Although KSHV-MCD has been considered rare, its diagnosis is often missed and may thus be underreported. Indeed, there is evidence that the incidence of KSHV-MCD is increasing in the cART era. KSHV-MCD should be considered in HIV patients with unexplained fever, anemia, or other manifestations, especially if they have KS or are at risk for KSHV infection. Severe inflammatory symptoms similar to KSHV-MCD that are also related to excess cytokines, especially IL-6, have been described in KSHV-infected patients without KSHV-MCD.[12] Many of these patients also have KS or primary effusion lymphoma. The term KSHV inflammatory cytokine syndrome (KICS) has been proposed for such patients.

TREATMENT   Rx

The best-studied treatment for KSHV-MCD is rituximab 375 mg/m^2 weekly for 4 weeks, which leads to resolution of symptoms in most patients. However, it may be insufficient in advanced disease and is associated with worsening KS. Approximately 30% of patients will relapse within 1 year. Rituximab combined with liposomal doxorubicin appears promising for patients with concurrent KS or severe symptoms.[13] Corticosteroids are sometimes administered transiently to help control acute life-threatening symptoms, but they do not appear to treat the underlying disease and can be associated with worsening KS and increased risk of infections, so should be avoided when possible. High-dose zidovudine with valganciclovir is active, although not as effective as rituximab for severe inflammatory symptoms and cytopenias. Chemotherapy regimens used in NHL and/or splenectomy have been used but are largely replaced by targeted approaches. HIV-infected patients require cART. Length of KSHV-MCD treatment, role of maintenance therapy, and evaluation and

management of concurrent malignancies remain an active area of investigation. Patients are treated to resolution of symptoms and improvement in laboratory abnormalities.

PROGNOSIS

Without treatment, the prognosis of KSHV-MCD prognosis is poor, with patients succumbing to inflammatory manifestations, infections, or lymphoma. With effective therapy, 1-year survival is greater than 85%, and long-term remissions are possible.

Cervical Cancer

HIV-infected patients are at increased risk of chronic infection with high-risk genotypes of HPV, cervical HSIL, and development of cervical cancer compared to HIV-negative women. In the United States, cervical cancer screening guidelines for HIV-negative women are currently based on periodic cervical cytology, or Papanicolaou (Pap) testing, with the option of co-testing for high risk-HPV in women aged 30 and older. Because of the increased risk and persistence of HPV in HIV-infected women, the current U.S. Department of Health and Human Services (DHHS) guidelines for cervical cancer screening include only cytology and not high-risk HPV testing.[14] These guidelines recommend that HIV-infected women should be screened for cervical cancer with Pap testing at the time of HIV diagnosis, and Pap testing should be repeated in 6 months. Provided both Pap tests are normal, cervical cancer screening should be continued with annual Pap tests. In general, a Pap test with cytologic abnormalities should prompt referral for a colposcopic evaluation of the cervix as well as the vagina and vulva with directed biopsies. However, for a Pap test showing atypical squamous cells of uncertain significance (ASC-US), options include either immediate referral to colposcopy or repeat cytology in 6 to 12 months. If a cervical biopsy shows HSIL, then the patient should undergo treatment to prevent malignant transformation. Treatment options are similar to those for HIV-negative women, involving either ablative (with cryotherapy or laser) or excisional therapies (with conization by loop electrosurgical excisional procedure (LEEP) or cold-knife). Because HIV-infected women, especially those with low CD4 counts and those not on cART, have high rates of persistent and recurrent SIL post treatment, these women must be followed closely with cytology and colposcopy, as indicated, and treated for recurrences. Cervical cancer screening guidelines in the general population have been updated frequently in the past two decades, and physicians should be alert for changes in screening recommendations for HIV-infected women.

In resource-limited settings, cervical cancer is a leading cause of cancer-related mortality in women. "Screen-and-treat" approaches based on cervical visual inspection with acetic acid (VIA) or rapid HPV testing with immediate treatment are being evaluated.[A7] Treatment of cervical cancer in HIV-infected patients is similar to its treatment in the general population. Patients whose HIV is well controlled on cART generally tolerate therapy and have similar outcomes to HIV-uninfected patients.

Non–AIDS-Defining Malignancies

The term non–AIDS-defining malignancy (NADM) is used to categorize cancers with increased standardized incidence ratios in HIV-infected populations that are not considered AIDS-defining by the CDC. Like AIDS-defining malignancies, many are caused by oncogenic viruses. The commonest NADMs are lung cancer, anal cancer (Fig. 393-3A) (caused by HPV), classic Hodgkin lymphoma (Fig. 393-3B) (caused by EBV), oropharyngeal cancers (caused by HPV), and liver cancer (often caused by HBV or HCV). Less common NADMs include vulvar and penile cancer (caused by HPV), Merkel cell carcinoma (caused by Merkel cell polyomavirus), and conjunctival carcinoma, which is seen especially in sub-Saharan Africa. Increased prevalence of smoking contributes to lung cancer risk, as well as risk for some other NADMs. However, HIV remains a risk factor for lung cancer independent of smoking, perhaps as a result of chronic inflammation or recurrent lung infections. HIV viremia is an independent risk factor for at least some virus-associated NADMs, including anal cancer and cHL.[15] Increased longevity in HIV patients with chronic liver disease from HBV, HCV, or other causes appears to account for an increasing number of hepatocellular carcinomas in HIV patients. In addition to NADM, incidental cancers whose risk is not increased by HIV, such as breast or colon cancer, are also increasing in number as the number of HIV-infected persons increases and this population ages.

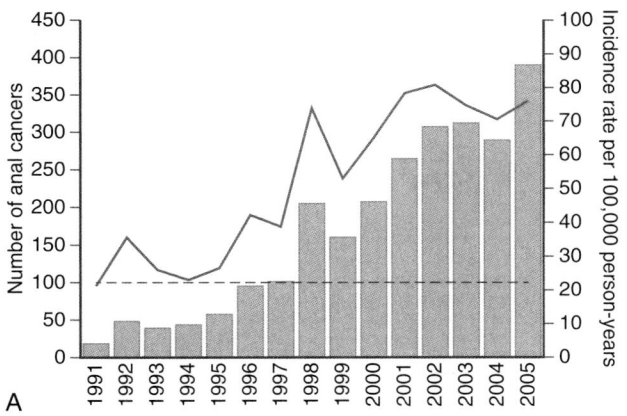

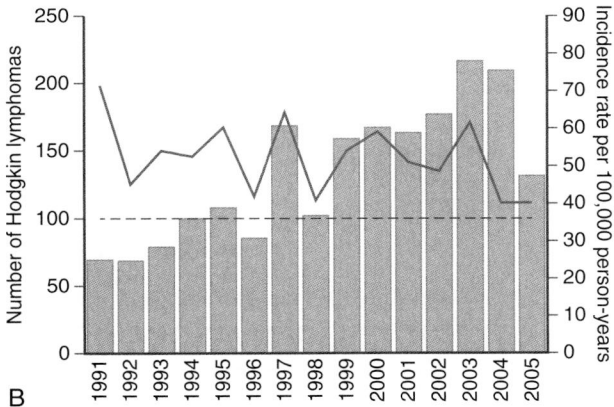

FIGURE 393-3. Trends in (A) anal cancer and (B) classic Hodgkin lymphoma in persons with HIV/AIDS in the United States in the years 1991-2005. Bars represent number of cases, line represents incidence rate. From Shiels MS, Pfeiffer RM, Gail MH, et al. Cancer burden in the HIV-infected population in the United States. *J Natl Cancer Inst.* 2011;103:753-762.

TABLE 393-2	DIFFERENTIAL DIAGNOSIS OF ANEMIA IN HIV-INFECTED PATIENTS

CAUSED BY PREDOMINANTLY DECREASED RED BLOOD CELL PRODUCTION

Anemia of chronic inflammation
Malignancies
    Non-Hodgkin lymphoma
    Classic Hodgkin lymphoma
    Kaposi sarcoma herpesvirus-associated multicentric Castleman disease
Infections
    Parvovirus B-19
    Mycobacterial infections
    Fungal infections (*Cryptococcus neoformans*, histoplasmosis)
    Bartonella infections
Nutritional deficiencies
    B_{12} deficiency
    Folate deficiency
    Iron deficiency
Drug effects
    Zidovudine
    Trimethoprim-sulfamethoxazole
    Cytotoxic chemotherapy
    Hepatitis C therapy (interferon-α/ribavirin)

CAUSED BY PREDOMINANTLY INCREASED RED BLOOD CELL DESTRUCTION OR BLOOD LOSS

Hemophagocytic syndrome, generally associated with infectious agents
    Epstein-Barr–virus associated diseases (e.g., classic Hodgkin lymphoma)
    Kaposi sarcoma herpesvirus-associated diseases
    Cytomegalovirus
    Mycobacterium tuberculosis
    Histoplasmosis
Autoimmune anemia
    Kaposi sarcoma herpesvirus-associated multicentric Castleman disease
    Lymphomas
    Idiopathic
Hemolysis
    Inherited hemoglobinopathy
    Glucose-6-phosphate dehydrogenase deficiency and exposure to offending drugs
    Malaria
Microangiopathic hemolytic anemia
    Thrombotic thrombocytopenia purpura with low ADAMTS13 activity
    Idiopathic
Gastrointestinal blood loss

The approach to management of NADM in patients with HIV is generally comparable to HIV-negative patients and should be based on performance status and stage in patients without serious HIV-associated comorbidities. With cART, many HIV-infected patients tolerate standard cancer therapy, including chemoradiation with intensity-modulated radiation therapy for localized cervical cancer or anal cancer, liver transplant for hepatocellular carcinoma, and allogeneic stem cell transplantation for hematologic malignancies. Attention to potential pharmacokinetic interactions between cART and chemotherapy is required. $CD4^+$ counts and HIV viral load should be monitored and appropriate OI prophylaxis administered.

HEMATOLOGIC ABNORMALITIES IN HIV-INFECTED PATIENTS

Red Blood Cell Disorders and Anemia

Anemia is common in patients with HIV and has a broad differential diagnosis (Table 393-2). Many patients have anemia of chronic inflammation.

EPIDEMIOLOGY

HIV-associated anemia is associated with decreased $CD4^+$ count, complications of AIDS, and HIV itself. Although less common in patients treated with cART, mild anemia is still seen in over 25% of persons with HIV and over 70% with advanced AIDS. More severe anemia (hemoglobin < 10 mg/dL) is seen in 5 to 10% of patients on cART and is also related to low CD4 count. Anemia may be a sign of comorbidities such as poor nutrition or undiagnosed cancer, as well as a marker of poor HIV control. Anemia is an important independent predictor of mortality.[16]

PATHOBIOLOGY

Anemia may be related to multiple factors in patients with HIV (see Table 393-2). Anemia of chronic inflammation is common (Chapter 158). Hepcidin, a mediator of the anemia of inflammation, is inversely correlated with $CD4^+$ count. HIV may also decrease the number of erythroid progenitor cells and affect erythropoietin signaling through a direct effect of inflammatory cytokines such as IL-1 and IL-6.

DIAGNOSIS

Patients with anemia despite effective cART should be evaluated for underlying causes; the etiology may be multifactorial. Medications should be reviewed for bone marrow suppressive agents, such as chemotherapy or TMP-SMX. Zidovudine causes macrocytic anemia, but newer cART regimens rarely cause anemia. Complete blood cell counts, reticulocyte count, and mean corpuscular volume (MCV) will direct additional evaluation. Iron studies including serum ferritin help differentiate anemia of inflammation from iron deficiency. Deficiencies of vitamin B_{12} or folic acid should be considered. Patients with HIV often have a positive direct Coombs test, but this is not generally associated with hemolysis. KSHV-MCD should be considered, especially in patients with KS or at risk for KSHV infection. Patients with hemolysis require evaluation for an etiology such as medications (e.g., dapsone in glucose-6-phosphate dehydrogenase deficiency) or lymphoproliferative disorders. Occult GI bleeding (e.g., caused by KS or lymphoma of the GI tract) should be ruled out by testing for stool blood and GI endoscopy as indicated. Severe anemia of unclear etiology requires bone marrow biopsy with evaluation for malignancy, hemophagocytic syndrome, or infection.

TREATMENT

Treatment of anemic HIV patients requires cART, which alone can be corrective. Additional therapy is based on the management of other underlying causes. Recombinant erythropoietin is rarely indicated.

White Blood Cell Disorders

A hallmark of HIV infection is a decrease in the CD4$^+$ T-lymphocyte count, which occurs largely in the setting of uncontrolled HIV. CD8$^+$ cells are often relatively preserved. Neutropenia is common in AIDS. Especially in patients with CD4 counts less than 200 cells/mm^3 not on cART, absolute neutrophil counts less than 1000×10^6/L increases risk for bacterial infections. However, patients of African descent may have benign ethnic neutropenia associated with a polymorphism in Duffy antigen/receptor chemokine gene (*DARC*), which does not appear to increase infection risk. Neutropenic patients should be evaluated for HIV viremia, nutritional deficiencies, and hematotoxic medications. Neutropenia often improves with cART and immune reconstitution. HIV-associated and ethnic neutropenia responds to filgrastim if needed to support delivery of chemotherapy.

Thrombocytopenia

Thrombocytopenia is common with uncontrolled HIV and often related to platelet destruction due to platelet activation, immune thrombocytopenia, or (rarely) thrombotic thrombocytopenia purpura (TTP). Patients with immune thrombocytopenia should be evaluated for underlying causes. TTP with decreased ADAMTS13 activity and anti-ADAMTS13 antibodies, as well as idiopathic HIV-associated thrombotic microangiopathies have been described. The differential diagnosis of thrombocytopenia in HIV also includes medications, OIs, malignancy, KSHV-MCD, HCV infection, liver disease, disseminated intravascular coagulation, and heparin-induced thrombocytopenia.

HIV-associated thrombocytopenia usually improves with cART, whereas that from other causes may require specific therapies. Severe immune thrombocytopenia responds to steroids, rituximab, intravenous immunoglobulin, or anti-D globulin. Splenectomy should generally be avoided because of risk of infections in splenectomized HIV-infected patients. TTP with low ADAMTS13 activity usually responds to cART and plasma exchange.

Thrombosis

Estimated venous thromboembolism incidence in HIV is 2.6 to 5.7 per 1000 person-years. The incidence is increased in hospitalized patients. It is associated with lower CD4$^+$ counts and is commonly related to surgery, catheters, OIs, underlying malignancy (including KS or PCNSL), or medications. However, correcting for known venous thromboembolism risk factors, HIV itself further increases risk by about 25%. Management of thrombosis in patients with HIV should generally follow standard guidelines (Chapter 38). However, interactions between specific antiretroviral agents and warfarin have been reported with cART and may be related to CYP2C9 inhibition. Also, HIV may specifically increase the risk of heparin-induced thrombocytopenia.

FUTURE DIRECTIONS

With increased use of cART worldwide, continued aging of the HIV-infected population, and changes in the prevalence of other cancer risk factors, the epidemiology of cancer and hematologic disorders in the setting of HIV will continue to evolve. In addition to treating HIV, there may be opportunities to reduce the risk of some HIV-associated cancers by preventing or treating specific associated oncogenic viruses. HBV and HPV vaccines hold the potential to dramatically reduce the incidence of hepatocellular, anogenital, and oropharyngeal cancers. An ongoing trial should clarify the role of screening for and treatment of anal high-grade squamous intraepithelial lesions in preventing anal cancer. Prevention strategies are particularly important for sub-Saharan Africa.

In the last decade, AIDS-defining malignancies have continued to be an important cause of morbidity and mortality, while non-AIDS defining malignancies and incidental tumors are increasingly common. Although outcomes for patients with HIV and cancer can be similar to the general population, they are generally more complex to treat. Looking forward, improved understanding of the safety and tolerability of specific cancer drugs and immunotherapies in patients with HIV is required. Targeted therapies for less common subtypes of lymphoma as well as KS may improve outcomes and decrease toxicity. There is an NCI initiative to encourage enrollment of HIV-infected patients in NCI-funded trials whenever possible. Advances in treatment of AIDS-defining malignancies in resource-limited settings will require improved diagnostics, training capacity, and infrastructure. Low-cost regimens and preferably oral agents for common cancers are urgently needed. Evaluation of the effect of HIV on hematopoietic progenitor cells is an area

of active research, especially in relation to allogeneic stem cell transplant and other cell therapies[17] that are being evaluated for a potential HIV cure.[18]

Grade A References

A1. Silverberg MJ, Neuhaus J, Bower M, et al. Risk of cancers during interrupted antiretroviral therapy in the SMART study. *AIDS.* 2007;21:1957-1963.
A2. Kaplan LD, Lee JY, Ambinder RF, et al. Rituximab does not improve clinical outcome in a randomized phase III trial of CHOP with or without rituximab in patients with HIV-associated non-Hodgkin's lymphoma: AIDS-malignancies consortium trial 010. *Blood.* 2005;106:1538-1543.
A3. Sparano JA, Lee JY, Kaplan LD, et al. Rituximab plus concurrent infusional EPOCH chemotherapy is highly effective in HIV-associated B-cell non-Hodgkin lymphoma. *Blood.* 2010;115:3008-3016.
A4. Gbabe OF, Okwundu CI, Dedicoat M, et al. Treatment of severe or progressive Kaposi's sarcoma in HIV-infected adults. *Cochrane Database Syst Rev.* 2014;8:CD003256.
A5. Cianfrocca M, Lee S, Von Roenn J, et al. Randomized trial of paclitaxel versus pegylated liposomal doxorubicin for advanced human immunodeficiency virus–associated Kaposi sarcoma: evidence of symptom palliation from chemotherapy. *Cancer.* 2010;116:3969-3977.
A6. Mosam A, Shaik F, Uldrick TS, et al. A randomized controlled trial of highly active antiretroviral therapy versus highly active antiretroviral therapy and chemotherapy in therapy-naive patients with HIV-associated Kaposi sarcoma in South Africa. *J Acquir Immune Defic Syndr.* 2012;60:150-157.
A7. Kuhn L, Wang C, Tsai WY, et al. Efficacy of human papillomavirus–based screen-and-treat for cervical cancer prevention among HIV-infected women. *AIDS.* 2010;24:2553-2561.

GENERAL REFERENCES

For the General References and other additional features, please visit Expert Consult at https://expertconsult.inkling.com.

394

NEUROLOGIC COMPLICATIONS OF HUMAN IMMUNODEFICIENCY VIRUS INFECTION

JOSEPH R. BERGER AND AVINDRA NATH

The neurologic complications of human immunodeficiency virus (HIV) infection can affect any portion of the neuraxis. They can be broadly divided into two large groups: those that are the consequence of HIV infection and those that are secondary in nature and occur chiefly as a result of the associated immunosuppression (Table 394-1). With respect to the former group, some of these disorders, such as acute HIV meningitis, are relatively rare, whereas others, such as HIV-associated neurocognitive disorders (HAND) and HIV-associated peripheral neuropathy, are common. HIV meningitis generally occurs at the time of seroconversion, but other disorders, such as HAND, HIV myelopathy, and HIV peripheral neuropathy, are typically not observed until advanced stages of immunosuppression.

The most common neurologic complications occurring as a secondary consequence of the virus are opportunistic infections. The most frequent of such infections are central nervous system (CNS) toxoplasmosis (Chapter 349), cryptococcosis (Chapter 336), tuberculosis (Chapter 324), cytomegalovirus encephalitis (Chapter 376), JC virus infection that results in progressive multifocal leukoencephalopathy (Chapter 370), and varicella-zoster virus encephalitis or myelitis (Chapter 375). However, many noninfectious

TABLE 394-1 CLASSIFICATION OF THE NEUROLOGIC COMPLICATIONS OF HIV INFECTION

DIRECT (HIV ASSOCIATED)	INDIRECT
Acute meningitis	Opportunistic infections
Chronic meningitis	Neoplasms
Encephalopathy	Toxic/metabolic
Myelopathy	Drug effects
Peripheral neuropathy	Cerebrovascular disease
Myositis/myopathy	
Neurocognitive disorders	

complications occur as well. The incidence of primary CNS lymphoma is remarkably high. Unlike non–AIDS-associated primary CNS lymphoma, in which Epstein-Barr virus can be recovered from only 50% of tumors (Chapter 185), all AIDS-related primary CNS lymphomas have been associated with Epstein-Barr virus infection (Chapter 393). A wide variety of toxic and metabolic complications have been observed in HIV-infected patients, including Wernicke encephalopathy and vitamin B$_{12}$ deficiency. Drugs, particularly antiretroviral agents, have also been associated with neurologic complications. Certain nucleoside analogues (e.g., the "d" drugs didanosine [ddI], dideoxycytidine [ddC], and stavudine [d4T]; see Table 394-5) are frequently associated with peripheral neuropathy. Finally, a wide variety of cerebrovascular disorders have been associated with HIV infection. Thrombotic ischemic stroke in this population has been attributed to an as yet undefined procoagulant tendency. Certain infections seen with increased frequency in patients infected with HIV, such as syphilis, tuberculosis, and cryptococcosis, may be associated with stroke. In addition, CNS vasculitis has occasionally been observed with HIV infection, either from HIV or from an associated varicella-zoster infection.

In recent years, it is being increasingly recognized that in a few weeks or months after initiation of combination antiretroviral therapy (ART), some patients will clinically deteriorate even when there is a robust drop in plasma viral load and recovery of CD4 cell counts. In these patients, the recovery of immune function may result in an inflammatory syndrome termed *immune reconstitution inflammatory syndrome* (IRIS; Chapter 395). This most often occurs when a patient has an underlying opportunistic infection, in which case the inflammation is targeted to the site of the infection. On occasion, IRIS may occur in the brain without any identifiable opportunistic infection and is attributable to a restoration of a robust immune response to HIV itself.

Few HIV-infected individuals will escape experiencing one or more of these complications during their lifetime.[1] They are responsible for a significant amount of morbidity and mortality. Not infrequently, more than one neurologic condition coexists in the same patient, which is often a source of confusion because one of the illnesses may be appropriately diagnosed and treated, yet the patient continues to deteriorate. Furthermore, one must also consider that any neurologic abnormalities observed are the consequence of more pedestrian disorders, such as radiculopathy secondary to disc herniation, and are unrelated to the HIV infection. In patients not responding to appropriate therapy for a proven disorder, careful clinical reevaluation is essential.

● HIV-ASSOCIATED NEUROCOGNITIVE DISORDERS

DEFINITION

HIV dementia has been referred to by a number of names, including subacute encephalitis, multinucleated giant cell encephalitis, AIDS dementia complex, and HIV-associated neurocognitive disorders (HAND).

A spectrum of increasing cognitive impairment has been described in association with HIV infection. An acquired impairment in cognitive function involving two ability domains, with a performance at least 1.0 standard deviations (SD) below the mean for norms on standardized neuropsychological tests but no cognitive impairment in everyday function, has been referred to as asymptomatic neurocognitive impairment. Patients with mild neurocognitive disorder have a similar disorder on neuropsychological testing but exhibit problems with daily functions. Those with HIV dementia have marked impairment (≥2 SD) on at least two domains in neuropsychological testing and marked interference in day-to-day activities because of cognitive impairment. By definition, the diagnosis of HAND requires that there be no delirium and no other etiology to explain the deficit.

EPIDEMIOLOGY

In the pre-ART era, HIV dementia was observed more commonly. Early studies suggested that it was evident in more than 50% of preterminal patients. The Multicenter AIDS Cohort Study found an incidence of 4% coincident with the diagnosis of AIDS, and dementia developed in 7% within 1 year of the development of AIDS and in 14% within 2 years. Other studies have found slightly higher rates. After the introduction of combination ART in 1996, the incidence rate of HIV dementia declined substantially, but the prevalence of the disorder increased; this finding may be the result of prolonged survival of affected patients.[2] Studies suggest that the cumulative incidence of HAND may be climbing to involve as many as 50% of patients with HIV infection, but most patients have milder forms of cognitive impairment.[3]

Risk factors for HAND include low CD4 cell counts, concurrent anemia, extremes of age, and history of substance abuse or addiction. Depression is also a common comorbidity. Congenitally or perinatally infected children may exhibit delayed development. Genetic factors such as *APOE4* and polymorphisms in chemokine monocyte chemotactic protein-1 (CCL-2) and tumor necrosis factor receptor have been identified as risk factors for the development of HAND.

PATHOBIOLOGY

HIV enters the brain early after the initial infection. In all likelihood, the virus enters the brain in infected mononuclear cells, although it is possible that it also enters as cell-free virus. HIV can be demonstrated in the brain as early as 2 weeks after infection. The viral infection predominates in invading macrophages in the brain, microglial cells, and multinucleated giant cells, usually in perivascular areas. HIV can also infect astrocytes, and studies suggest that in patients with cognitive impairment, 16 to 19% of astrocytes may be infected. HIV may remain latent for extended periods. Infection of other cell types is a rare event. The brain may thus be an important reservoir for HIV and a potential source for the emergence of drug-resistant viruses. Certain proteins of the virus, Tat and gp120, have been demonstrated to have a significant pernicious effect on neuronal function and viability either through direct toxic effects on neurons or by stimulation of glial cells, which in turn produce neurotoxic metabolites—cytokines and chemokines—or induce oxidative stress. Similarly, the perivascular HIV-infected inflammatory cells produce a wide variety of chemokines and cytokines that also have similar deleterious effects. Therefore, there appear to be parallel paths, direct viral neurotoxicity and toxicity from inflammatory byproducts, that lead to the development of HAND.[4] Drugs of abuse, such as opiates, cocaine, and methamphetamine, can stimulate HIV replication in glial cells and synergize with the HIV proteins to cause neurotoxicity and glial cell activation.

On gross examination, the brain typically exhibits cortical atrophy, sulcal widening, and ventricular dilation. Histopathologic examination shows multinucleated giant cells, microglial nodules, white matter pallor, astrogliosis, and perivascular inflammation (Fig. 394-1). The multinucleated giant cell, which is a syncytium of macrophages, has been regarded as the hallmark of infection, but it is not uniformly present in patients with HAND. The pathologic changes are most prominent in the basal ganglia, prefrontal cortex, and hippocampus. Concomitant vacuolar myelopathy is seen in as many as 40% of patients, although it has become less common since the introduction of ART.

CLINICAL MANIFESTATIONS

Most commonly, patients describe impaired memory, poor concentration, impairment of executive function, and difficulty reading. They often find it difficult to recall a passage recently read. Other frequent symptoms include gait problems, depression, and tremors, and patients may appear apathetic and slow or become socially withdrawn. Headaches, fatigue, and sexual dysfunction are frequent. The most commonly observed physical findings are psychomotor slowing with bradyphrenia and impaired rapid repetitive and alternating movements, hyperreflexia, increased tone, facial masking, frontal release signs (snout, glabellar, involuntary grasp), and abnormal ocular motility with breakdown of smooth pursuit. The dementia has the features of a subcortical dementia not inconsistent with the relatively marked disease burden observed in dopaminergic basal ganglia. Screening tools for HAND have been proposed (Table 394-2) and a battery of specific neuropsychological tests used (Table 394-3). Staging of the disease along a continuum has been widely adopted (Table 394-4).

DIAGNOSIS

Computed tomography of the head typically shows brain atrophy, but findings may be normal. Central atrophy is generally more pronounced than cortical atrophy. In children, calcification of the basal ganglia is often observed. Similar findings are seen on magnetic resonance imaging (MRI). Basal ganglia hyperintensity is seen rarely on T2-weighted images and may resolve during the course of ART. White matter hyperintensities are also commonly detected on T2-weighted images and fluid-attenuated inversion recovery (FLAIR) sequences (Fig. 394-2). These lesions may be discrete and focal or large and confluent. They are generally symmetrically distributed and may be confused with lesions of progressive multifocal leukoencephalopathy. Unlike progressive multifocal leukoencephalopathy lesions, they are typically not hypointense on T1-weighted sequences.

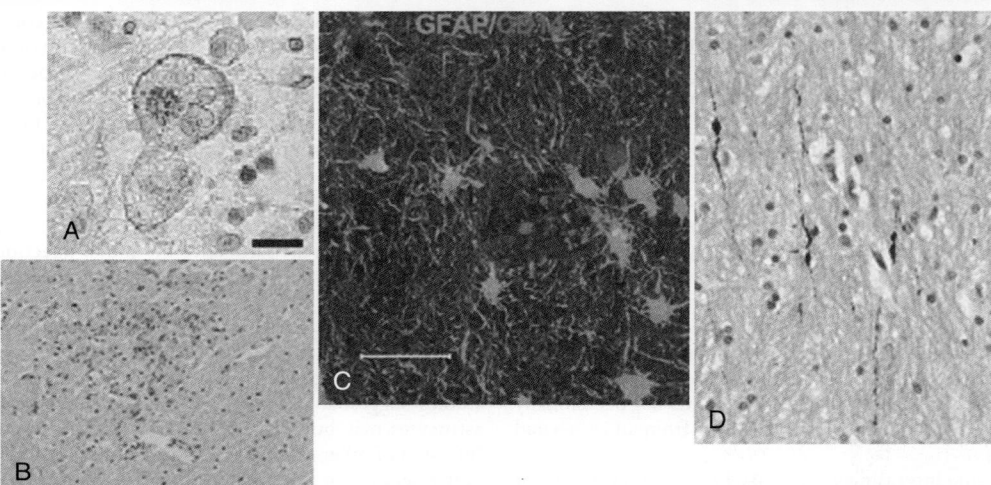

FIGURE 394-1. Histopathology of HIV dementia. **A,** Multinucleated giant cell immunostaining for HIV antigen. **B,** A microglia nodule shows a collection of inflammatory cells. The HIV-infected cells are immunostained for HIV antigen and are brown. **C,** A confocal photomicrograph shows astrocytosis. The astrocytes are stained blue with antibody to glial acidic fibrillary protein (GAFP). The macrophages are immunostained with antibody to CD14 (*red*). **D,** In neurons immunostained with antibody to amyloid precursor protein, beading of the neuritis suggests interruption of axonal flow. (**C,** Courtesy Carlos Pardo, Johns Hopkins University, Baltimore, MD; **D,** Courtesy Chris Zink, Johns Hopkins University, Baltimore, MD.)

TABLE 394-2 SCREENING TEST FOR HIV-ASSOCIATED NEUROCOGNITIVE DISORDERS

MAXIMUM SCORE	SCORE	
		MEMORY REGISTRATION
		Give 4 words to recall (dog, hat, green, peach), 1 second to say each. Then ask the patient all 4 after you have said them.
4	( )	**ATTENTION**
		Antisaccadic eye movements: 20 commands _____ errors of 20 trials
		≤3 errors = 4; 4 errors = 3; 5 errors = 2; 6 errors = 1; >6 errors = 0
6	( )	**PSYCHOMOTOR SPEED**
		Ask patient to write the alphabet in uppercase letters horizontally across the page (use the back of this form) and record the time: _____ sec
		≤21 sec = 6; 21.1-24 sec = 5; 24.1-27 sec = 4; 27.1-30 sec = 3; 30.1-33 sec = 2; 33.1-36 sec = 1; >36 sec = 0
4	( )	**MEMORY RECALL**
		Ask for 4 words from Registration above. Give 1 point for each correct.
		For words not recalled, prompt with a "semantic" clue, as follows: animal (dog); piece of clothing (hat), color (green), fruit (peach). Give ½ point for each correct after prompting.
2	( )	**CONSTRUCTION**
		Copy a cube; record the time: _____ sec
		<25 sec = 2; 25-35 sec = 1; 35 sec = 0
TOTAL SCORE: _____ /16		

From Power C, Selnes OA, Grim JA, McArthur JC. HIV dementia scale: a rapid screening test. *J Acquir Immune Defic Syndr Hum Retrovirol.* 1995;8:273-278.

TABLE 394-3 NEUROPSYCHOLOGICAL BATTERY PROPOSED FOR EVALUATION OF HIV-ASSOCIATED NEUROCOGNITIVE DISORDERS

Fine motor control
  Grooved pegboard
  Finger tapping

Rapid sequential problem solving
  Trail making A and B
  Digit symbol

Visuospatial problem solving
  Block design

Spontaneity
  Verbal fluency

Visual memory
  Visual reproduction

TABLE 394-4 MEMORIAL SLOAN-KETTERING SCALE FOR HIV-ASSOCIATED NEUROCOGNITIVE DISORDERS

Stage 0 (normal)	Normal mental and motor function
Stage 0.5 (equivocal or subclinical)	Absent, minimal, or equivocal symptoms without impairment of work or capacity to perform activities of daily living
Stage 1 (mild)	Able to perform all but the more demanding aspects of work or activities of daily living
Stage 2 (moderate)	Able to perform all the basic activities of daily self-care but cannot work or maintain the more demanding aspects of daily life
Stage 3 (severe)	Major intellectual incapacity or motor disability with slowing
Stage 4 (end stage)	Nearly vegetative

From Price RW, Brew BJ. The AIDS dementia complex. *J Infect Dis.* 1988;158:1079-1083.

TREATMENT   Rx

Whether ART needs to cross the blood-brain barrier for a better neurocognitive outcome remains uncertain. Higher cerebrospinal fluid (CSF) penetrant ability is associated with lower levels of HIV RNA in the CSF.[5] Prudence dictates that highly CNS-penetrant ARTs would best be used, although other factors should be considered (e.g., the drug's pharmacokinetics, protein binding, and IC$_{95}$). Brain HIV RNA levels have been demonstrated to be significantly higher in patients with HIV encephalopathy.[6] Newer CCR5 antagonists, maraviroc and vicriviroc, demonstrate good CSF penetration and may be uniquely suited for the treatment of HAND. Table 394-5 provides a list of ARTs with their respective CSF-to-plasma ratios, which may provide a proxy for CNS penetration. A variety of other therapies have been proposed for the treatment of HAND that chiefly addresses the proposed inflammatory pathway of the pathogenesis of the disorder. To date, none has been established to be effective. The flow chart in Figure 394-3 provides an algorithm for the management of HAND. Careful attention to treatment of comorbidities is also essential. Special consideration needs to be given to the choice of anticonvulsants, since drug-drug interactions are common owing to induction of hepatic enzymes or serum albumin binding properties that may alter drug levels of ARTs.

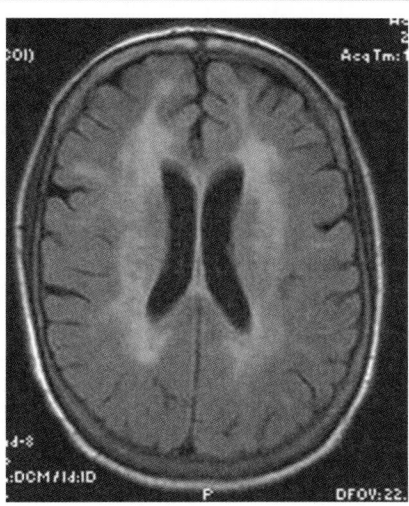

FIGURE 394-2. Magnetic resonance image of the brain in HIV dementia. The FLAIR image shows confluent areas of signal hyperintensity adjacent to ventricles.

TABLE 394-5	CEREBROSPINAL FLUID–TO-PLASMA RATIOS FOR ANTIRETROVIRAL THERAPIES
	CEREBROSPINAL FLUID–TO-PLASMA RATIO
NUCLEOSIDE REVERSE TRANSCRIPTASE INHIBITORS	
Zidovudine (AZT)	0.3-1.35
Stavudine (d4T)	0.16-0.97
Abacavir (ABC)	0.3-0.42
Didanosine (ddI)	0.16-0.19
Lamivudine (3TC)	0.11
Zalcitabine (ddC)	0.09-0.37
Emtricitabine	0.04
NUCLEOTIDE REVERSE TRANSCRIPTASE INHIBITORS	
Tenofovir	<0.05
FUSION INHIBITORS	
Enfuvirtide	NA
NON-NUCLEOSIDE REVERSE TRANSCRIPTASE INHIBITORS	
Nevirapine (NVP)	0.28-0.45
Delavirdine	0.02
Efavirenz	0.01
PROTEASE INHIBITORS	
Indinavir	0.02-0.76
Saquinavir	<0.05
Nelfinavir	<0.05
Ritonavir	<0.05
Amprenavir	<0.05
Lopinavir	<0.05
Atazanavir	0.0021-0.0226
Fosamprenavir	<0.05

Adapted from McArthur JC, Haughey N, Gartner S, et al. Human immunodeficiency virus–associated dementia: an evolving disease. *J Neurovirol.* 2003;9:205-221.

PROGNOSIS

In the pre-ART era, the life expectancy of patients with HIV dementia was less than 6 months. The institution of effective ART has considerably increased the life expectancy of affected patients, and partial recovery of neurocognitive deficits may be seen.

HIV MYELOPATHY

A broad spectrum of myelopathies occurs with HIV infection (Table 394-6). HIV causes a distinct myelopathy referred to as HIV vacuolar myelopathy. Evident in 20 to 55% of autopsies, this myelopathy is under-recognized clinically. It is characterized by an insidious onset of leg weakness and gait abnormality that usually occurs during the course of advanced HIV infection. Sensory complaints include vague leg discomfort and distal paresthesias. Bowel and bladder dysfunction is frequent. Physical examination reveals spastic paraparesis with lower extremity hyperreflexia, a spastic-ataxic gait,

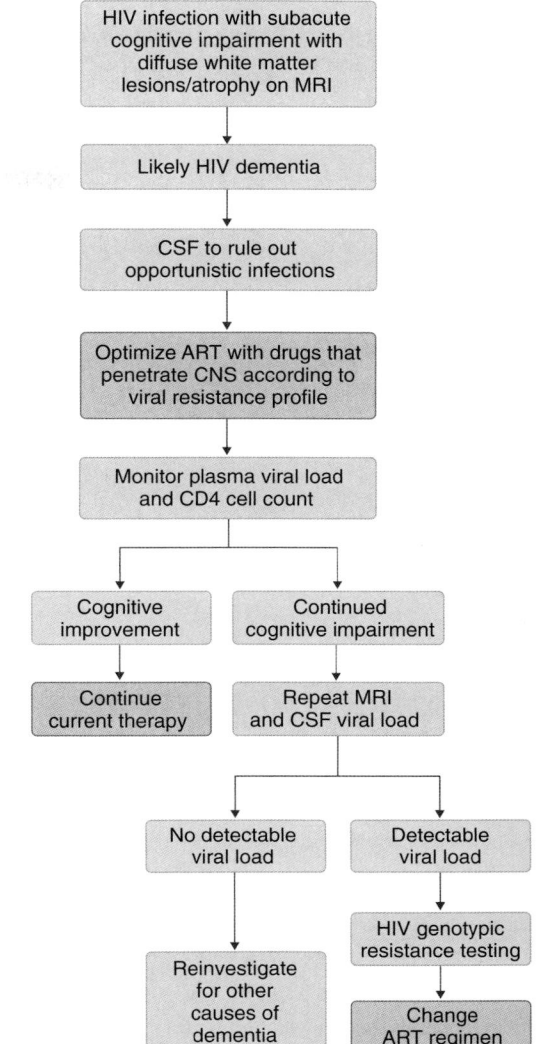

FIGURE 394-3. Flow chart for the treatment of HIV dementia. ART = antiretroviral therapy; CNS = central nervous system; CSF = cerebrospinal fluid; HIV = human immunodeficiency virus; MRI = magnetic resonance imaging.

and impaired sensation with vibratory and position perception disproportionately affected. The sensory loss may be asymmetrical, but the presence of a discrete sensory level should suggest an alternative cause of the myelopathy. MRI of the spinal cord is usually normal but may show cord atrophy or hyperintense signal abnormalities within the cord on T2-weighted images. The value of spinal MRI lies in exclusion of other diagnostic possibilities, particularly structural abnormalities of the cord. Somatosensory evoked potentials generally demonstrate delayed conduction. Although findings on gross examination of the cord and dura are usually normal, histopathologic examination typically reveals loss of myelin with spongy degeneration, axonal preservation, microglial nodules, and multinucleated giant cells involving the lateral and posterior columns of the spinal cord. The pathogenesis of this disorder remains obscure. The clinical and pathologic features are suggestive of vitamin B_{12} deficiency (Chapter 164), but no consistent abnormalities are found in serum levels of vitamin B_{12} or its metabolites, and replacement therapy with cyanocobalamin or S-methyl-L-methionine has not proved to be beneficial. The most effective management appears to be ART coupled with physical therapy.

HIV PERIPHERAL NEUROPATHY

Although a large number of peripheral neuropathies have been described in association with HIV infection, the one most commonly observed is a distal symmetrical sensorimotor peripheral neuropathy that ultimately affects at least a third of all HIV-infected persons. This neuropathy is seen more often in advanced disease. The patient typically complains of "burning feet." Distal paresthesias and numbness are reported, and the pain may be debilitating.

TABLE 394-6   SPECTRUM OF MYELOPATHIES IN HIV INFECTION

HIV ASSOCIATED

Vacuolar myelopathy
Acute myelitis
Relapsing remitting encephalomyelitis
Spinal myoclonus

VIRAL

Cytomegalovirus
HTLV-1 and HTLV-2
Varicella-zoster virus
Measles virus
Progressive multifocal leukoencephalopathy

BACTERIAL

Mycobacterium tuberculosis
Treponema pallidum
Pseudomonas cepacia

FUNGAL

Cryptococcus immitis
Aspergillus spp.
Nocardia

PARASITIC

Toxoplasma gondii
Schistosoma

MALIGNANCY

Primary CNS lymphoma
Metastatic CNS lymphoma
Other tumors (e.g., glioma)

VASCULAR

Necrotizing vasculitis
Disseminated intravascular coagulation

TOXIC/METABOLIC

Vitamin B_{12} deficiency
Protease inhibitor epidural lipomatosis

CNS = central nervous system; HTLV = human T-lymphotropic virus.

Distal vibratory, pinprick, and temperature sensory perceptions are diminished, and the Romberg sign is often abnormal. Ankle jerks are depressed or absent, and mild weakness of the toes with associated atrophy of the intrinsic muscles of the foot is frequently noted. Nerve conduction studies show reduced sensory nerve action potentials and conduction velocities. Nerve conduction amplitudes are reduced disproportionately to the reduction in conduction velocity. Electromyography may demonstrate features consistent with either acute or chronic denervation. Skin biopsy shows a reduction in cutaneous nerve fibers.

A clinically indistinguishable neuropathy may be seen with some of the antiretroviral agents, particularly with ddI, ddC, and d4T. The neuropathy associated with these agents appears to be dose dependent. Other drugs used in treatment of AIDS or its complications, such as hydroxyurea, isoniazid, vincristine, and thalidomide, may result in a similar peripheral neuropathy. Discontinuation of the use of these drugs should result in improvement in the neuropathic features; however, a phenomenon referred to as coasting, in which continued worsening of the neuropathy occurs after discontinuation of the offending agent, may be observed for a period of several months.

Shortly after seroconversion, a demyelinating peripheral neuropathy may be observed that is identical to Guillain-Barré syndrome or chronic inflammatory polyradiculoneuropathy (Chapter 420) if it progresses for a duration of 3 weeks or more. An autoimmune process is the probable pathogenesis, and these neuropathies respond to therapy routinely used in the treatment of these conditions. In rare instances, mononeuritis multiplex (Chapter 420) may be seen with HIV infection.

HIV MYOPATHY

Several forms of muscle disease occur with HIV infection and, like other neurologic disorders, may be due to HIV or be secondary to other processes. Among the latter are myopathies associated with drugs such as zidovudine and cholesterol-lowering agents, opportunistic infections, neoplastic infiltrates, and vasculopathies. HIV myopathy mirrors the clinical and laboratory findings of classic polymyositis (Chapter 269). It is characterized by a progressive symmetrical weakness of the limb girdle and neck flexor muscles. Fatigue, myalgias, and wasting are observed in up to 50% of affected persons. Muscle enzymes, including creatine kinase and aldolase, are elevated, and the electromyogram shows short, brief, polyphasic unit action potentials. Muscle biopsy reveals myofibrillar necrosis, phagocytosis, variation in fiber size, and regeneration and degeneration, typically with endomysial inflammatory infiltrates. This myopathy is rare, with an incidence of less than 1%, and has been observed in any stage of HIV infection. All patients with weakness who are taking a nucleoside reverse transcriptase inhibitor (NRTI) should have blood lactate levels measured because of an association between a recently described neuromuscular weakness syndrome and lactic acidosis in patients taking NRTIs. The contribution of zidovudine to the genesis of HIV-associated myopathy remains controversial. As in non-HIV polymyositis, corticosteroid therapy is beneficial and can be administered with tolerable side effects.

HIV-ASSOCIATED CENTRAL NERVOUS SYSTEM IRIS

Some individuals may develop a subacute encephalopathy following the introduction of ARTs. Symptoms include impairment in neurocognitive function, seizures, and ultimately impairment of consciousness and coma; if untreated, the syndrome may result in death.[7] Risk factors include a low CD4 lymphocyte nadir (usually < 50 cells/mm^3) or a rapid decline in viral load following initiation of ART. Although the exact mechanism is unclear, the syndrome is associated with immune restoration (Chapter 395) and infiltration of CD8 cytotoxic T cells into the brain. MRI may show diffuse multifocal white matter hyperintensities on FLAIR and T2-weighted images suggestive of edema. CSF shows a mild lymphocytosis. In some of these patients, the CSF HIV viral load is greater than that in the plasma. It thus appears that the target of the immune restoration may be the viral reservoir in the brain. A second type of CNS IRIS, with HIV infection manifesting as a fulminant focal encephalitis associated with demyelination, has also been described. This resembles the Marburg variant of multiple sclerosis. Successful treatment with corticosteroids has been described for both forms of IRIS (Chapter 395), although no clinical trials have been performed.

GENERAL REFERENCES

For the General References and other additional features, please visit Expert Consult at https://expertconsult.inkling.com.

395

IMMUNE RECONSTITUTION INFLAMMATORY SYNDROME IN HIV/AIDS

ROBERT COLEBUNDERS AND MARTYN A. FRENCH

DEFINITION

Treatment of human immunodeficiency virus (HIV) infection with combination antiretroviral therapy (ART) results in the restoration of protective pathogen-specific immune responses and the regression or prevention of opportunistic infections (OIs) and cancers in most individuals (Chapter 389). However, restoration of an immune response against a pathogen may also result in immunopathology at body sites infected by the pathogen. This has been referred to as immune restoration disease (IRD) to differentiate it from immunodeficiency disease, but it is now commonly known as immune reconstitution inflammatory syndrome (IRIS), because an inflammatory illness is the most common clinical feature.[1]

Essentially any pathogen that causes an infection as a result of HIV-induced cellular immunodeficiency may be associated with IRIS after ART is commenced. However, the clinical characteristics and severity of IRIS associated with each type of pathogen vary greatly (Table 395-1). For example, IRIS associated with *Mycobacterium tuberculosis*, cryptococcal, or JC polyomavirus (JCV) infection is manifested differently from an OI caused by these

TABLE 395-1   EXAMPLES OF IMMUNE RECONSTITUTION INFLAMMATORY SYNDROME

PATHOGEN	NOMENCLATURE	TYPICAL CHARACTERISTICS OF THE DISEASE
Mycobacterium tuberculosis	TB-IRIS	Paradoxical exacerbation of TB
Nontuberculous mycobacteria (NTM)	NTM immune reconstitution syndrome	Mainly lymphadenitis, also pulmonary disease and hepatitis
Bacille Calmette-Guérin (BCG)	BCG-IRIS	Necrotizing regional lymphadenitis
Mycobacterium leprae	Leprosy-related IRIS	Borderline and type 1 reactional state
Cryptococcus neoformans	Cryptococcal-IRIS	Mainly meningitis, also lymphadenitis
Pneumocystis jiroveci	*Pneumocystis*-IRIS	Paradoxical exacerbation of pneumonitis
Cytomegalovirus (CMV)	CMV retinitis after ART or immune recovery uveitis	Acute retinitis after commencing ART or uveitis
JC polyomavirus	Inflammatory PML	Multifocal leukoencephalopathy with inflammatory features
Human herpesvirus 8	KS-IRIS	Rapid progression of existing and/or new KS lesions
Hepatitis B or C virus	Some cases of ART-associated hepatotoxicity	Hepatitis flare and/or liver enzyme elevation
Herpes zoster virus		Mainly dermatomal or multidermatomal zoster, occasionally myelitis
Molluscum contagiosum virus	Inflammatory molluscum contagiosum	Inflamed molluscum lesions
Malassezia spp.	Inflammatory seborrheic dermatitis	Abnormally inflamed seborrheic dermatitis

ART = antiretroviral therapy; IRIS = immune reconstitution inflammatory syndrome; KS = Kaposi's sarcoma; PML = progressive multifocal leukoencephalopathy; TB = tuberculosis.

gens, which has been demonstrated by measuring delayed-type hypersensitivity skin test responses or the frequency of circulating antigen-specific T cells that produce interferon (IFN)-γ. However, there is increasing evidence that innate immune responses by myeloid cells (monocytes, macrophages, and neutrophils) and their mediators also contribute to the immunopathology, particularly in paradoxical tuberculosis (TB)-IRIS. The immunopathogenesis of IRIS associated with other pathogens is less well understood and appears to vary depending on the provoking pathogen. For example, IRIS associated with JCV infection (inflammatory progressive multifocal leukoencephalopathy [PML]) is characterized by an inflammatory cell infiltrate dominated by CD8+ T cells in affected areas of the brain.

CLINICAL MANIFESTATIONS

The clinical manifestations of IRIS are different for each associated pathogen and will therefore be described for each pathogen. Only disease that presents a significant patient management problem will be discussed.

Mycobacterium tuberculosis

M. tuberculosis is the most common pathogen involved in IRIS, with estimates of incidence ranging from 7 to 43% of patients with HIV infection and treated TB. Most TB-IRIS develops within the first 3 months after the initiation of ART. Patients in whom paradoxical TB-IRIS develops typically give a history of having improved with treatment of TB before initiation of ART. After starting ART, recurrent, worsening, or new clinical or radiologic manifestations of TB develop. Common manifestations include fever, enlargement of lymph nodes, and worsening radiographic pulmonary infiltrates. Tracheal compression by intrathoracic lymph nodes or massive pleural effusions can cause life-threatening dyspnea. Respiratory failure as a result of worsening pulmonary infiltrates and acute respiratory distress syndrome have occasionally been reported. In a large prospective cohort of HIV-TB coinfected patients in Mozambique, TB-IRIS occurrence within 12 weeks of starting ART was independently associated with the mortality of HIV-TB coinfected patients at 48 weeks post ART initiation.[3] In a prospective case series from South Africa, neurologic TB-IRIS accounted for 12% of cases of paradoxical TB-IRIS. Meningitis, tuberculoma, or both were the most common manifestations. TB-IRIS should be considered as a potential cause of hepatitis, especially in patients with disseminated TB who are being treated with a combination of anti-TB therapy and ART. Peritonitis secondary to bowel perforation and splenic rupture are other unusual findings. Though usually negative, mycobacterial cultures may be positive, particularly if IRIS occurs early during anti-TB therapy and in patients with multidrug-resistant TB. Histologic examination often reveals necrotizing granulomas.

High rates of TB have been reported during ART, especially in the initial months of treatment in ART programs in resource-limited settings. This type of TB has been referred to as ART-associated TB because the mechanisms underlying the manifestations of TB after initiating ART are likely to be heterogeneous. Diagnoses of active TB before initiation of ART may be missed because of the inherent insensitivity of TB diagnostics in this patient group and only later be diagnosed during ART. Because ART-induced immune recovery is a time-dependent process and some patients fail to respond immunologically, a proportion of cases may develop as a result of persisting immunodeficiency. Other patients may have active subclinical disease at the time of ART initiation, and progression to symptomatic disease may be accelerated by ART-induced restoration of a cellular immune response against *M. tuberculosis* antigens. Of patients in this latter group, some have exuberant inflammatory clinical features that are consistent with a diagnosis of TB-IRIS.

Nontuberculous Mycobacteria

Atypical manifestations of *Mycobacterium avium* complex (MAC) disease in patients who had commenced zidovudine monotherapy were the first indication that IRIS may be a complication of ART. MAC and other nontuberculous mycobacteria have been associated with IRIS in 3 to 4% of patients who commence combination ART with a CD4+ T-cell count lower than 100/μL. Disease is usually localized, as opposed to the disseminated nontuberculous mycobacterial disease of patients with acquired immunodeficiency syndrome (AIDS), and is most commonly manifested as fever, night sweats, and lymphadenitis. Unmasking disease is most common. Peripheral lymphadenitis may suppurate and sometimes cause chronically discharging fistulas to the skin. Abdominal disease frequently causes pain, which is usually associated with lymphadenitis and occasionally with omental masses, hepatitis, and inflammation of the spleen (Fig. 395-1). Pulmonary and thoracic disease usually

pathogens, and the resulting illness is often severe and may result in death. In contrast, herpes zoster after ART is usually indistinguishable from that occurring before ART, and it is only the timing of onset that suggests that it results from IRIS.

IRIS develops mainly during the first 3 months of ART but occasionally later. Two patterns are recognized. Paradoxical IRIS refers to the worsening or atypical manifestation (or both) of an established OI after ART is commenced. In most cases the infection had been treated before ART was initiated, and the immune response appears to be against residual antigens of the pathogen. Unmasking IRIS refers to disease that occurs for the first time after ART is commenced and appears to result from an immune response against a subclinical infection by an opportunistic pathogen.[2]

EPIDEMIOLOGY

The reported incidence of IRIS has varied from 8% to over 40% in different studies. To some extent, the large variation reflects the lack of universally accepted diagnostic criteria. It also probably reflects differences in risk factors in the populations of patients studied. The most important risk factors for IRIS are a low CD4+ T-cell count when ART is initiated and, in patients in whom paradoxical IRIS develops, disseminated infection and a short time between treatment of the infection and commencement of ART.

PATHOBIOLOGY

Information about the pathogenesis of IRIS has been obtained mostly by studying patients who experience disease associated with a mycobacterial infection.[3] Both clinicopathologic and immunologic studies have shown an association with a T$_H$1 cellular immune response against mycobacterial anti-

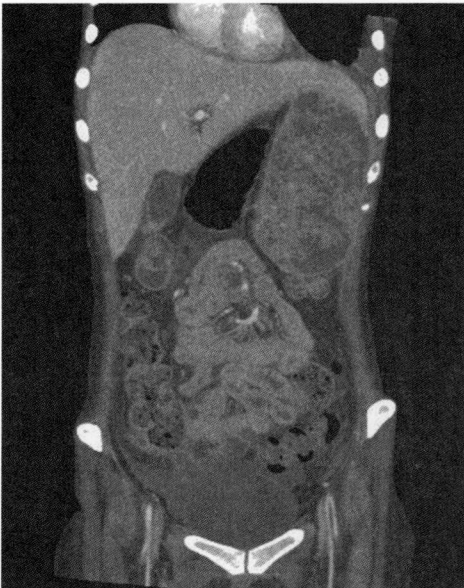

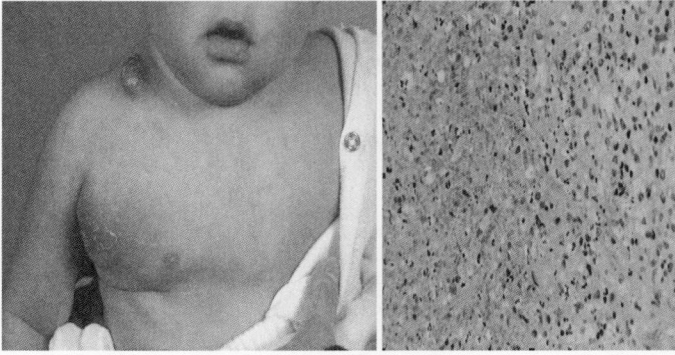

FIGURE 395-2. Bacille Calmette-Guérin (BCG)-associated immune reconstitution inflammatory syndrome after antiretroviral therapy for HIV infection in a child who received BCG vaccination shortly after birth. A biopsy specimen from the larger lesion demonstrated necrotizing granulomatous inflammation.

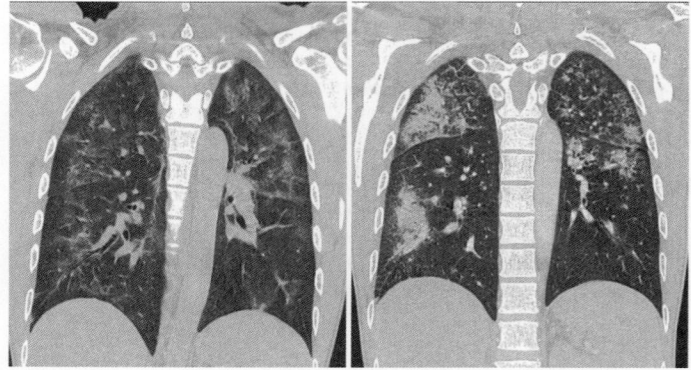

FIGURE 395-1. *Mycobacterium avium* complex–associated immune reconstitution inflammatory syndrome manifested as necrotizing inflammation in the spleen and abdominal lymph nodes.

FIGURE 395-3. *Pneumocystis jiroveci*–associated immune reconstitution inflammatory syndrome. *Left,* Before treatment of the *P. jiroveci* infection. *Right,* After treatment of the *P. jiroveci* infection and commencing antiretroviral therapy.

causes cough that is sometimes associated with chest pain. Bronchoscopy may reveal endobronchial lesions. Microscopic examination of biopsy material or aspirates from affected tissues often reveals mycobacteria, but these may not be cultured.

In HIV-seropositive children vaccinated with bacille Calmette-Guérin (BCG), a BCG-associated lymphadenitis and abscesses may develop after starting highly active antiretroviral therapy (HAART) (Fig. 395-2).

Leprosy-related IRIS is usually manifested as unmasking of previous subclinical *Mycobacterium leprae* infection, with a borderline and a type I reactional state.

Cryptococci

The proportion of patients with HIV infection and treated cryptococcosis in whom cryptococcosis-IRIS develops ranges from 8 to 42%. The majority represent a recurrence of previously treated cryptococcal meningitis. Inflammatory reactions to quiescent meningeal infection during the first few weeks of ART have also been reported. The time at onset of cryptococcosis-IRIS varies from 4 days after initiation of ART to around 3 years. Central nervous system (CNS) features of cryptococcosis-IRIS include intracranial cryptococcoma or abscesses, spinal cord abscesses, recalcitrant raised intracranial pressure, optic disc swelling, cranial nerve lesions, dysarthria, hemiparesis, and paraparesis. Extracranial manifestations of cryptococcosis-IRIS include lymphadenitis, eye disease, suppurating soft tissue lesions, and pulmonary disease that may include cavitating or nodular lesions.

At the diagnosis of cryptococcal meningitis, cerebrospinal fluid (CSF) white blood cell counts of 25 cells/μL or less and protein levels of 50 mg/dL or less are associated with the development of IRIS. On the other hand, CSF profiles at the moment of paradoxical cryptococcosis-IRIS may show an increased white blood cell count and an increased opening pressure of greater than 25 cm H_2O, but these features overlap significantly with those observed in patients with non–IRIS-related relapses of cryptococcal meningitis. The value of determining serum and CSF cryptococcal antigen titers in predicting or diagnosing cryptococcosis-IRIS is unclear, but a positive CSF cryptococcal culture prior to commencing ART is a predictor. Cultures of CSF or tissue samples obtained at the time of paradoxical cryptococcosis-IRIS may be negative even when cryptococci can be seen on microscopy.

Pneumocystis jiroveci

Patients who have been treated for *P. jiroveci* pneumonitis (PJP) may experience pulmonary inflammation after ART is commenced. It is usually characterized by fever, cough, dyspnea, chest discomfort, and patchy alveolar infiltrates on the chest radiograph (Fig. 395-3). In some patients, organizing pneumonia develops.

JC Polyomavirus

Progressive PML of the brain occurs when cellular immune responses fail to control JCV infection of oligodendrocytes and astrocytes. It is characterized by a paucity of inflammatory cells in brain lesions. ART is the only effective therapy, presumably because it enhances cellular immune responses against JCV antigens. However, ART may also result in a paradoxical worsening of established PML or in unmasking of subclinical JCV infection and appearance of PML for the first time. These manifestations of PML are often atypical in that imaging studies of the brain demonstrate changes associated with inflammation, and brain biopsy specimens demonstrate inflammatory cell infiltrates with a prominence of CD8$^+$ T cells. Between 19 and 23% of cases of PML in HIV-infected patients are due to paradoxical or unmasking IRIS. The median time at onset is 7 weeks, and most cases occur within the first 3 months of ART but very occasionally as late as 26 months after commencing ART. Predictors of PML-IRIS have not been identified.

Human Herpesvirus 8

A prospective study of Kaposi's sarcoma (KS) in patients from Mozambique commencing ART found that paradoxical KS-IRIS developed in 31% of patients with pre-ART KS, and that unmasking KS-IRIS developed in 7% of patients without pre-ART KS. Clinical manifestations included an increased number of preexisting skin lesions that sometimes exhibited increased nodularity and ulceration, new skin or mucosal lesions, and lymphedema. Independent risk factors for the development of KS-IRIS were KS before ART, human herpesvirus 8 DNA detectable in plasma, a hematocrit of less than 30%, and a plasma HIV RNA level greater than 5 log$_{10}$ copies/mL.

Some cases of KS-IRIS will resolve without treatment, but chemotherapy is usually necessary. Doxorubicin has been used most often.

Cytomegalovirus

Eye disease is the most common manifestation of IRIS associated with cytomegalovirus (CMV) infection. Retinitis usually develops during the first few weeks of ART as a "paradoxical" worsening of treated retinitis or as a new manifestation of CMV retinitis. Previously treated CMV infection is the most common cause of immune recovery uveitis (IRU), which presumably results from the restoration of an immune response against residual CMV antigens in the eye. The risk for development of CMV-associated IRU is greatest in patients who had a large proportion of the retina affected by CMV infection. It may develop up to 21 months after ART is commenced, and the clinical manifestations vary in severity from a transient vitreitis to persistent uveitis, papillitis, cystoid macular edema, and epiretinal membranes.

Hepatitis B and C Viruses

Hepatotoxicity manifested as elevated serum liver enzyme levels occurs in up to 18% of patients after ART is initiated. Several causes have been defined, but the most important risk factor is concomitant infection with hepatitis B virus (HBV) or hepatitis C virus (HCV). Prospective studies of patients with HIV infection who are coinfected with HBV, HCV, or both, who commenced ART demonstrated that 22 to 24% of patients with HBV coinfection, 13.5% of patients with HCV coinfection, and 50% of patients with both HBV and HCV coinfection experienced a "flare" of hepatitis. Flares of HBV hepatitis were associated with increased plasma levels of several immune mediators, thus suggesting that it was a manifestation of IRIS in the liver. Patients who experienced flares of HBV hepatitis had higher plasma HBV DNA levels and serum alanine transaminase levels before ART was commenced. Severe hepatitis after ART in patients with HIV infection and coinfection with HBV or HCV is uncommon but can occasionally result in liver decompensation and death.

Herpes Simplex Virus

Exacerbation of mucocutaneous herpes simplex virus (HSV) disease may occur after ART is initiated. Sometimes, lesions become hemorrhagic and exhibit tissue necrosis. Rarely, HSV infection of the brain may be unmasked by commencing ART and be manifested as encephalitis.

DIAGNOSIS

Immunologic tests for diagnosing IRIS are currently not available for routine use. In the absence of diagnostic tests, IRIS may be established with diagnostic criteria that take into consideration the timing, clinical characteristics, and pathology of the disease, as well as the virologic response to the ART.

TREATMENT Rx

The general approach to the treatment of IRIS is to continue ART and provide antimicrobial therapy for the provoking infection when it is active (usually in unmasking IRIS).[4] Cessation of ART should be considered only in patients with life-threatening disease when all other measures have failed. Anti-inflammatory therapy should not be given routinely but be reserved for patients with severe inflammation, particularly when it is life-threatening. Corticosteroid therapy is used most often, but its effectiveness may vary from one type of IRIS to another. Thus, a randomized controlled trial in South Africa demonstrated that corticosteroids (prednisone 1.5 mg/kg/day for 2 weeks, then 0.75 mg/kg/day for 2 weeks) are a safe and effective treatment option for paradoxical TB-IRIS.[A1] In contrast, in an analysis of data from previously reported cases of PML-IRIS, it was suggested that corticosteroid therapy is not effective, although it was indicated that only early use of corticosteroid therapy is likely to be effective. There is anecdotal evidence suggesting that corticosteroid therapy can be effective in other types of IRIS, but there are potential risks to using corticosteroid therapy in HIV patients who are very immunodeficient, and it should only be used after weighing all considerations and should be based on evidence from clinical trials if available. Corticosteroid therapy for IRIS affecting the eye should be supervised by an ophthalmologist.

PREVENTION

Given that a low CD4$^+$ T-cell count is a major risk factor for the development of IRIS, commencing ART at a CD4$^+$ T-cell count higher than 350/µL, as recommended by many treatment guidelines, will prevent most cases. However, this is not possible in patients who are seen for the first time with an OI or in many patients from countries with limited resources. Other strategies to prevent paradoxical IRIS are therefore under investigation.

Several observations indicate that a high pathogen load is an important risk factor for IRIS, including the association with disseminated and drug-resistant TB, a shorter duration of treatment of TB or cryptococcal meningitis, and positive CSF cultures for cryptococcal infection prior to commencing ART. Therefore, delaying the introduction of ART so that the OI can be fully treated might be beneficial.[5,6] However, doing so may increase the risk for development of other OIs or cancers. The results of the AIDS Clinical Trial Group study A5164 provided evidence supporting the introduction of ART at the same time as antimicrobial therapy, particularly in patients with PJP.[A2] In addition, the results of three randomized controlled trials (SAPiT,[A3] CAMELIA,[A4] and STRIDE[A5]) demonstrated that for HIV/TB-coinfected patients with advanced immunosuppression, the survival benefit of starting ART within the first 2 weeks of TB therapy might outweigh the risk for IRIS and other adverse events. Nevertheless, a more recent clinical trial of the effect of timing of ART initiation on TB treatment outcomes for HIV-positive patients with CD4 counts of 220 cells/µL or more showed that ART can be delayed until after completion of 6 months of TB treatment in this population.[A6] In contrast, commencing ART at the same time as treatment of cryptococcal meningitis has been shown to reduce long-term survival when compared with delaying ART until the meningitis has been treated.[A7] It seems probable that IRIS affecting the CNS is more likely than other types of IRIS to result in morbidity and mortality. Therefore, a single approach to this issue may not be possible, and a strategy for commencing antimicrobial therapy and ART may have to be determined for each pathogen or for infections of the CNS.

PROGNOSIS

The prognosis for patients in whom IRIS develops is highly variable because of differences in the extent of the infection by the provoking pathogen, the characteristics of the immunopathology caused by the restored immune response, and the body site affected. Most cases of IRIS are self-limited, and outcomes are usually good. However, mortality rates of up to 66% have been reported for cryptococcosis-IRIS. The mortality rate for TB-IRIS is much lower, but hospital admissions are common. Mortality and hospitalization rates are particularly high when TB- or cryptococcosis-IRIS affects the CNS. Indeed, involvement of the CNS by any type of IRIS may result in death or permanent neurologic disability.[7-9] For example, mortality rates of 53% have been reported for paradoxical PML-IRIS and 31% for unmasking PML-IRIS. Furthermore, patients who survive PML-IRIS may have neurologic sequelae such as hemiparesis or seizures. Patients with lymphadenitis resulting from TB-IRIS and those with meningitis resulting from cryptococcosis-IRIS occasionally undergo recurrent relapses and can become steroid dependent.

Autoimmune Disease and Sarcoidosis

Patients with HIV infection who are receiving ART have an increased susceptibility to some autoimmune diseases, mainly Graves disease, and sarcoidosis. Although sometimes referred to as types of IRIS, they appear to have a different immunopathogenesis.

Grade A References

A1. Meintjes G, Wilkinson RJ, Morroni C, et al. Randomized placebo-controlled trial of prednisone for paradoxical tuberculosis-associated immune reconstitution inflammatory syndrome. AIDS. 2010; 24:2381-2390.
A2. Zolopa A, Andersen J, Powderly W, et al. Early antiretroviral therapy reduces AIDS progression/death in individuals with acute opportunistic infections: a multicenter randomized strategy trial. PLoS ONE. 2009;4:e5575.
A3. Abdool Karim SS, Naidoo K, Grobler A, et al. Timing of initiation of antiretroviral drugs during tuberculosis therapy. N Engl J Med. 2010;362:697-706.
A4. Blanc FX, Sok T, Laureillard D, et al; CAMELIA (ANRS 1295–CIPRA KH001) Study Team. Earlier versus later start of antiretroviral therapy in HIV-infected adults with tuberculosis. N Engl J Med. 2011;365:1471-1481.
A5. Havlir DV, Kendall MA, Ive P, et al; AIDS Clinical Trials Group Study A5221. Timing of antiretroviral therapy for HIV-1 infection and tuberculosis. N Engl J Med. 2011;365:1482-1491.
A6. Mfinanga SG, Kirenga BJ, Chanda DM, et al. Early versus delayed initiation of highly active antiretroviral therapy for HIV-positive adults with newly diagnosed pulmonary tuberculosis (TB-HAART): a prospective, international, randomized, placebo-controlled trial. Lancet Infect Dis. 2014;14: 563-571.
A7. Boulware DR, Meya DB, Muzoora C, et al. Timing of antiretroviral therapy after diagnosis of cryptococcal meningitis. N Engl J Med. 2014;370:2487-2498.

GENERAL REFERENCES

For the General References and other additional features, please visit Expert Consult at https://expertconsult.inkling.com.

XXV

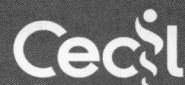

NEUROLOGY

396

APPROACH TO THE PATIENT WITH NEUROLOGIC DISEASE

ROBERT C. GRIGGS, RALPH F. JÓZEFOWICZ, AND
MICHAEL J. AMINOFF

CLINICAL MANIFESTATIONS

Many symptoms of nervous system diseases are a part of everyday experience for most normal people. Slips of the tongue, headaches, backache and other pains, dizziness, lightheadedness, numbness, muscle twitches, jerks, cramps, and tremors all occur in totally healthy persons. Mood swings with feelings of elation and depression, paranoia, and displays of temper are equally a part of the behavior of completely normal people. The rapid increase in information about neurologic diseases, coupled with the intense interest of people in all walks of life in medical matters, has focused public attention on both common and rare neurologic conditions.

Most older people are concerned that they or their spouse have or are developing Alzheimer disease or stroke. The almost ubiquitous tremor of the elderly prompts concern about Parkinson disease. Many younger patients are concerned about multiple sclerosis or brain tumor, and few normal people lack one or more symptoms suggesting the diagnosis of a serious neurologic disease. For most of these and other common diagnoses, the results of imaging and other tests are typically normal when symptoms first appear, and such tests should not be performed to reassure the patient or physician. Moreover, the widespread availability of neurodiagnostic imaging and electrophysiologic, biochemical, and genetic testing has led to the detection of "abnormalities" in many young and most elderly persons. In evaluating a patient's symptoms, it is imperative that a clinical diagnosis be reached without reference to a neurodiagnostic laboratory finding. Patients with disorders such as headache, anxiety, and depression do not usually have abnormal laboratory results. Abnormalities noted on various neurodiagnostic studies are often incidental findings whose treatment may be justified and necessary, but such treatment will not improve the patient's symptoms. Abnormalities detected incidentally that are not accompanied by signs or symptoms may, as for disorders such as hypertension, require aggressive evaluation and treatment, but in general, the adage that it is difficult to improve an asymptomatic patient should be kept in mind. Thus, in elderly patients, few imaging or electrophysiologic studies are interpreted as "normal," but in the absence of specific complaints consistent with the findings, treatment and even further evaluation should reflect an estimate of the specificity and sensitivity of the test as well as the likelihood that the patient will require and benefit from treatment. It is a good rule of thumb that one should never perform (or refer to the result of) a neurodiagnostic procedure without a specific diagnosis or at least a differential diagnosis in mind.

It is important to allow patients to describe any symptoms in their own words. Direct questions are often necessary to fully characterize the problem, but suggested terms or descriptors for symptoms are frequently grasped by a patient unfamiliar with medical terminology and then parroted to subsequent interviewers. The patient's terms should always be used in recording symptoms. Terms such as *lameness, weakness, numbness, heaviness, cramps,* and *tiredness* may each mean pain, weakness, or alteration of sensation to some patients.

DIAGNOSIS

History

In neurologic diagnosis, the history usually indicates the nature of the disease or the diagnosis, whereas the neurologic examination localizes it and quantitates its severity. For many diseases, the history is almost the only avenue to explore. Examples of such disorders include headaches, seizures, developmental disorders, memory disorders, and behavioral diseases. In arriving at a diagnosis, the following points are useful. Consider the entire medical history of the patient. Early life events or long-standing processes such as head or spine trauma, unilateral hearing or visual loss, poor prowess in sports, poor performance in school, spinal curvature, and bone anomalies are easily overlooked but may point to the underlying disease process.

Consider the tempo and duration of the symptoms. Have the symptoms been progressive without remission, or have there been plateaus or periods of return to normal? Cerebral mass lesions (tumor, subdural) tend to have a progressive but fluctuating course; seizures and migraine, an episodic course; and strokes, an abrupt ictal onset with worsening for 3 to 5 days, followed by partial or complete recovery.

Can one disease account for all of the symptoms and signs? The clinician should formulate a diagnostic opinion in anatomic terms. Is the history suggestive of a single (e.g., stroke or tumor) focus or multiple sites of nervous system involvement (e.g., multiple sclerosis), or is the process a disease of a system (vitamin B_{12} deficiency, myopathy, or polyneuropathy)?

The neurologic history is the most important component of neurologic diagnosis. A careful history frequently determines the cause and allows one to begin localizing the lesions, which aids in establishing whether the disease is diffuse or focal. Symptoms of acute onset suggest a vascular cause or seizure; symptoms that are subacute in onset suggest a mass lesion such as a tumor or abscess; symptoms that have a waxing and waning course with exacerbations and remissions suggest a demyelinating cause; and symptoms that are chronic and progressive suggest a degenerative disorder.

The history is often the only way of diagnosing neurologic illnesses that typically have normal or nonfocal findings on neurologic examination. These illnesses include many seizure disorders, narcolepsy, migraine and most other headache syndromes, the various causes of dizziness, and most types of dementia. The neurologic history may often provide the first clues that a symptom is psychological in origin. The following are points to consider in obtaining a neurologic history.

- *Carefully identify the chief complaint or problem.* Not only is the chief complaint important in providing the first clue to the physician about the differential diagnosis, but it is also the reason the patient is seeking medical advice and treatment. If the chief complaint is not properly identified and addressed, the proper diagnosis may be missed and an inappropriate diagnostic work-up may be undertaken. Establishing a diagnosis that does not incorporate the chief complaint frequently focuses attention on a coincidental process irrelevant to the patient's concerns.

- *Listen carefully to the patient for as long as necessary.* A good rule of thumb is to listen initially for at least 5 minutes without interrupting the patient. The patient often volunteers the most important information at the start of the history. During this time, the examiner can also assess mental status, including speech, language, fund of knowledge, and affect, and observe the patient for facial asymmetry, abnormalities in ocular movements, and an increase or a paucity of spontaneous movements as seen with movement disorders.

- *Steer the patient away from discussions of previous diagnostic test results and the opinions of previous caregivers.* Abnormal results of laboratory studies may be incidental to the patient's primary problem or may simply represent a normal variant.

- *Take a careful medical history, medication history, psychiatric history, family history, and social and occupational history.* Many neurologic illnesses are complications of underlying medical disorders or are due to adverse effects of drugs. For example, parkinsonism is a frequent complication of the use of metoclopramide and most neuroleptic agents. A large number of neurologic disorders are hereditary, and a positive family history may establish the diagnosis in many instances. Occupation plays a major role in various neurologic disorders such as carpal tunnel syndrome (in machine operators and people who use computer keyboards) and peripheral neuropathy (caused by exposure to lead or other toxins).

- *Interview surrogate historians.* Because patients with dementia or altered mental status are generally unable to provide exact details of the history, a family member may need to provide the key details required to make an accurate diagnosis. This situation is especially common with patients who have dementia and certain right hemispheric lesions with various agnosias (lack of awareness of disease) that may interfere with their ability to provide a cogent history. Surrogate historians also provide missing historical details for patients with episodic loss of consciousness, such as syncope and epilepsy.

- *Summarize the history for the patient.* Summarizing the history is an effective way to ensure that all details were covered sufficiently for a tentative diagnosis to be made. Summarizing also allows the physician to fill in historical gaps that may not have been apparent when the history was initially taken. In addition, the patient or surrogate may correct any historical misinformation at this time.

- *End by asking what the patient thinks is wrong.* This question allows the physician to evaluate the patient's concerns about and insight into the condition. Some patients have a specific diagnosis in mind that spurs them to seek medical attention. Multiple sclerosis, amyotrophic lateral sclerosis, Alzheimer disease, and brain tumors are diseases that patients often suspect may be the cause of their neurologic symptoms. This discussion will also help guide how to discuss prognosis, especially in patients with advanced neurologic disease.[1]

Diagnostic Challenges

Two common situations provide special challenges to the diagnostic skills of the physician.

Physical Abuse as a Cause of Neurologic Symptoms

Traumatic injury inflicted by family members or others is usually difficult to detect by the medical history and examination. Physically battered babies, abused children, battered women, and traumatized seniors are often unable or unwilling to complain of this cause or contribution to symptoms. The only method to prevent overlooking this frequent cause of common problems is systematic consideration of the possibility in every patient and awareness of the often subtle signs that suggest physical trauma: ecchymoses or fractures (often attributed to a logical cause), denial of expected symptoms, failure to keep appointments, and unexplained intensification of neurologic symptoms (headache, dizziness, ringing in the ears, blackouts).

Alcoholism and Drug Abuse

See Chapters 33 and 34. A host of neurologic disorders can be the result of intentional ingestion of toxins (Chapter 110). Patients do not give an accurate account of their use of these agents. Consequently, physical signs and laboratory screening test results that give evidence of drug-related hepatic and other metabolic abnormalities may point to a major underlying problem.

⬤ ACUTE NEUROLOGIC DISORDERS REQUIRING IMMEDIATE DIAGNOSIS AND TREATMENT

Most neurologic diagnoses are arrived at by a careful, thorough history and an appropriately complete examination. However, the tempo of illness and the availability of life-saving treatment that is effective only if it is administered within minutes of first evaluating a patient dictate rapid action in several specific circumstances.[2] Coma (Chapter 404), repetitive seizures (Chapter 403), acute stroke (Chapters 407 and 408), suspected meningitis and encephalitis (Chapters 412 and 414), head and spine trauma (Chapter 399), and acute spinal cord compression are diagnosed by clinical and laboratory assessment, and urgent treatment must be instituted as soon as ventilation and cardiac status are stabilized.

⬤ NEUROLOGIC EXAMINATION

The neurologic examination is always tailored to the clinical setting of the patient. The approach to an ambulatory office patient is very different than the approach to a critically ill patient.[3] A complete neurologic examination of a child is much different from that of an elderly adult, and the examination of a patient with specific complaints focuses on findings pertinent to that patient. Thus, more detailed testing of cognition is indicated in patients with behavioral or memory disturbance, and more detailed testing of sensation should be performed in patients with complaints of pain, numbness, or weakness.

However, many tests of neurologic function are routinely indicated in all patients because they provide a baseline for future examination and are frequently helpful in detecting unsuspected neurologic disease in apparently normal persons or in patients whose symptoms initially suggest disease outside the nervous system. It is particularly important to perform all routine tests in patients with abnormalities in one sphere of neurologic dysfunction; otherwise, erroneous localization of a lesion or disease process is likely. For deviations from normal to be recognized and quantitated, it is essential for a physician to have extensive experience in the routine assessment of normal persons.

The General Examination

Specific neurologic symptoms or signs should prompt attention to the assessment of general findings. Head circumference should be measured in patients with central nervous system (CNS) or spinal cord disease (normally 55 ± 5 cm in adults). Head enlargement is occasionally a normal, often hereditary variant but should suggest a long-standing anomaly of the brain or spinal

cord. The skin should be inspected for café au lait maculae, adenoma sebaceum, vascular malformations, lipomas, neurofibromas, and other lesions (Chapter 417). Neck range of motion, straight leg raising, and spinal curvature (scoliosis) should be assessed. Carotid auscultation for bruits is indicated in all older adults; carotid palpation is seldom informative. In patients with bladder, bowel, or leg symptoms, a rectal sphincter examination for tone and ability to contract voluntarily is usually indicated. Limitation of joint range of motion or painless swelling of joints is often a sign of an unsuspected neurologic lesion.

Neurologic Examination

The various aspects of the detailed neurologic examination are considered in specific symptom and disease sections noted later. The five major divisions of the examination should be assessed in all patients. During a careful medical history, mental status is often adequately assessed: level of consciousness, orientation, memory, language function, affect, and judgment. If any of these functions are abnormal, more detailed testing is needed. Cranial nerve function that should be tested in all patients includes visual acuity (with and without correction); optic fundi; visual fields; pupils (size and reactivity to direct and consensual light); ocular motility; jaw, facial, palatal, neck, and tongue movement; and hearing.

Examination of the motor system (Chapter 421) is essential in all patients because incipient weakness is generally overlooked by the patient. Muscle tone (flaccid, spastic, or rigid), muscle size (atrophy or hypertrophy), and muscle strength can be assessed rapidly. Muscle strength testing should always assess specific functional activities, including the ability to walk on heel and toe, to sit up from a supine position, to rise from a deep knee bend or deep chair, to lift the arms over the head, and to make a tight fist. Gait, stance, and coordination are assessed. The patient should be observed for tremor and other abnormal movements and the muscles inspected for fasciculations.

Sensory testing (Chapter 420) need not be detailed unless there are sensory symptoms. However, vibration perception in the toes and the normality of perception of pain, temperature, and light touch in the hands and feet should be assessed.

Muscle stretch reflexes and plantar responses should always be assessed by evaluating right-left symmetry and disparity between proximal and distal reflexes or arm and leg reflexes. Biceps, triceps, brachioradialis, quadriceps, and ankle reflexes should be quantitated from 1 to 4 (4 = clonus; 3 = spread; 2 = brisk; 1 = hypoactive).

The Comatose Patient

The rapid examination required for a patient with an altered state of consciousness is much different from that of an alert, aware individual (Chapter 404). Many aspects of the neurologic examination cannot be tested: cognitive function, subtleties of sensory perception, specific motor functions, coordination, gait, and stance. Moreover, the muscle stretch reflexes are likely to fluctuate from one moment to the next, and minor asymmetries are much less important than in an awake patient. Instead, attention should focus on examination of the level of consciousness, respiratory pattern, eyelid position and eye movements, pupils, corneal reflexes, optic fundi, and motor responses. Particular elements of the general examination must also be assessed quickly: evidence of cranial and spinal trauma, tenderness of the skull to percussion, nuchal rigidity (but not in patients with head or neck trauma), and evidence of physical abuse.

⬤ COMMON COMPLAINTS OF POSSIBLE NEUROLOGIC ORIGIN

Weakness

It is axiomatic that patients typically have motor signs before motor symptoms and, conversely, sensory symptoms before sensory signs. Thus, patients with even severe weakness may not report symptoms of weakness. Somewhat paradoxically, patients who complain of "weakness" often do not have confirmatory findings on examination that document the presence of weakness.

Weakness, when it is actually a symptom of neurologic disease, is frequently caused by diseases of the motor unit (Chapters 419, 421, and 422) and is usually reported by a patient in terms of loss of specific functions—for example, difficulty with tasks such as climbing stairs, rising from a chair, sitting up, lifting objects onto a high shelf, or opening jars. Symptoms may also reflect the consequences of weakness, such as frequent falls or tripping. Such symptoms can be remarkably quantitative. A patient with leg muscle

TABLE 396-1	DISORDERS COMMONLY ACCOMPANIED BY WEAKNESS

Disorders of the motor unit
Upper motor neuron lesions—spasticity
Basal ganglia disorders—rigidity
General medical conditions
    Heart failure
    Respiratory insufficiency
    Renal, hepatic, and other metabolic disease
    Alcoholism and other toxin-related disease
Psychiatric and behavioral disorders
    Depression
    Malingering

weakness who is falling even as infrequently as once a month almost invariably has severe weakness of the knee extensor muscles and can be shown on examination to have a knee extension lag, an inability to lift the leg fully against gravity and lock the knee.

The symptom of weakness without findings of weakness on examination is not generally the result of neuromuscular disease but can be a sign of neurologic disease outside the motor unit or, more commonly, a symptom of disease outside the nervous system altogether (Table 396-1).

Episodic and Intermittent Weakness
The complaint of attacks of severe weakness or paralysis occurring in a patient with baseline normal strength is an uncommon symptom. It is typical of the periodic paralyses and may also be seen with episodic ataxias and myotonic disorders (Chapter 421). All these disorders are ion channelopathies. These channelopathies (e.g., the calcium channelopathy hypokalemic periodic paralysis) are rare but treatable disorders (Chapter 421). Episodic weakness is also seen in patients with neuromuscular junction disorders such as myasthenia gravis and the myasthenic syndrome (Chapter 422). On occasion, patients with narcolepsy complain of intermittent paralysis as a reflection of sleep paralysis (Chapter 405).

Fatigue
Complaints of fatigue, tiredness, and lack of energy are even less likely than the symptom of weakness to reflect definable neurologic disease. With the exception of neuromuscular junction disorders such as myasthenia gravis, fatigue is rarely a complaint of diseases of the motor unit. Fatigue can be a sign of upper motor neuron disease (corticospinal pathways) and is a common complaint of established multiple sclerosis and other multifocal CNS disease. Similarly, any process that produces bilateral corticospinal tract or extrapyramidal disease can cause fatigue. Examples include motor neuron disease (Chapter 419), spinal cord disease in the cervical cord region (Chapter 400), and Parkinson disease (Chapter 409). In addition, disorders that impair sleep (Chapter 405) may include fatigue as a complaint.

Fatigue, like weakness, is much more often than not a sign of disease outside the central and peripheral nervous system. Depression and other psychiatric and behavioral disorders (Chapter 397) as well as the medical illnesses associated with a complaint of weakness are all frequent causes of fatigue.

Chronic fatigue syndrome and many cases of fibromyalgia (Chapter 274) have fatigue as a dominant disabling symptom. These disorders are defined in part by the absence of consistent neurologic findings and lack of demonstrable disease in the nervous system.

Spontaneous Movements
Muscle tremors, jerks, twitches, cramps, and spasms (Chapter 410) are frequent symptoms. The cause of spontaneous movements can reside at any level of the nervous system. In general, movements that occur in an entire limb or in more than one muscle group concurrently are caused by CNS disease. Movements confined to a single muscle are likely to be a reflection of disease of the motor unit (including the motor neurons of the brain stem and spinal cord). When spontaneous movements of a muscle are associated with severe pain, patients often use the term *cramp*. Cramp is a medically defined disorder that reflects the intense contraction of a large group of motor units. Leg cramps are occasionally a sign of an underlying disease of the

anterior horn cell, nerve roots, or peripheral nerve; however, cramps are frequent in normal persons and particularly common in older patients, and they are usually benign. When they are severe, cramps can produce such intense muscle contraction that muscle injury is caused and muscle enzyme (e.g., creatine kinase) levels are elevated in blood.

The rare muscle diseases in which an enzyme deficiency interferes with substrate use as fuel for exercise (e.g., McArdle disease) are often associated with severe exercise-provoked muscle contractures. These contractures are electrically silent on electromyography, in contrast to the intense motor unit activity seen with cramps. Such contractures should not be confused with the limitation of joint range of motion resulting from long-standing joint disease or long-standing weakness, also termed contractures.

The intense muscle contractions of tetany are frequently painful. Although tetany is usually a reflection of hypocalcemia (Chapter 245), it can occasionally be seen without demonstrable electrolyte disturbance. Tetany results from hyperexcitability of peripheral nerves. Similarly, in the syndrome of tetanus produced by a clostridial toxin (Chapter 296), intensely painful life-threatening muscle contractions arise from hyperexcitable peripheral nerves. A number of toxic disorders, such as strychnine poisoning and black widow spider envenomation, produce similar neurogenic spasms.

Muscle Pain
Acute muscle pain in the absence of abnormal muscle contractions is an extremely common symptom. When such pain occurs after strenuous exercise or in the context of an acute viral illness (e.g., influenza), it probably reflects muscle injury. In such patients, the serum creatine kinase level is often raised. It is uncommon for this frequent and essentially normal sign of muscle injury to be associated with weakness or demonstrable ongoing muscle disease. Chronic muscle pain is a common symptom but is seldom related to a definable disease of muscle.

Loss of Balance
Unsteadiness of gait is a common symptom. When it is associated with complaints of dizziness or vertigo (Chapter 428), disease of the labyrinth, vestibular nerve, brain stem, or cerebellum is a probable cause. When unsteadiness and loss of balance are unassociated with dizziness, particularly if the unsteadiness appears to be out of proportion to other symptoms of the patient, a widespread disorder of sensation or motor function is likely.

Abnormal Gait and Posture
The ability to stand and walk in a well-coordinated, effortless fashion requires integrity of the entire nervous system.[4] Relatively subtle deficits localized to one part of the central or peripheral nervous system produce characteristic abnormalities (Table 396-2).

Sensory Symptoms
Sensory symptoms can be negative or positive. Negative symptoms represent a loss of sensation, such as a feeling of numbness. Positive symptoms, by contrast, consist of sensory phenomena that occur without normal stimulation of receptors and include paresthesias and dysesthesias. Paresthesias may include a feeling of tingling, crawling, itching, compression, tightness, cold, or heat and are sometimes associated with a feeling of heaviness. The term *dysesthesias* is used correctly to refer to abnormal sensations—often tingling, painful, or uncomfortable—that occur after innocuous stimuli, whereas *allodynia* refers to painful perception from a stimulus that is not normally painful. For some patients, it may be difficult to distinguish paresthesias and dysesthesias from pain. *Hypesthesia* denotes a loss or impairment of touch, whereas *hypalgesia* denotes a loss of pain sensibility. By comparison, *hyperesthesia* and *hyperalgesia* indicate a lowered threshold to tactile or painful stimuli such that there is increased sensitivity to such stimuli.[5]

With the use of a wisp of cotton, a single-use pin, and a tuning fork, the trunk and extremities are examined for regions of abnormal or absent sensation. Special instruments are available for quantifying sensory function, such as the computer-assisted sensory examination, which is based on the detection of touch, pressure, vibratory, and thermal sensation thresholds.

Alterations in pain and tactile sensibility can generally be detected by clinical examination. It is important to localize the distribution of any such sensory loss to distinguish between nerve, root, and central dysfunction. Similarly, abnormalities in proprioception can be detected by clinical examination when patients are unable to detect the direction in which a joint is

TABLE 396-2 CHARACTERISTIC GAIT DISORDERS

SPECIFIC DISORDER	LOCATION OF LESION	CHARACTERISTICS
Spastic gait	Bilateral corticospinal pathways within the thoracic or cervical cord or in the brain	Legs stiff, feet turning inward, "scissoring"
Hemiparetic gait	Unilateral central nervous system, cervical cord, or brain	Affected leg circumducted, foot extended, arm flexed
Sensory ataxia	Posterior columns of the spinal cord or peripheral nerve	Wide-based, high steps; Romberg sign present
Cerebellar ataxia	Brain stem or cerebellum	Wide-based steps; Romberg sign absent
Parkinsonian gait	Basal ganglia	Shuffling, small steps
Dystonic gait	Basal ganglia; also corticospinal pathways	Abnormal posture of the arms, head, neck
Gait disorder of the elderly	Multifactorial: bihemispheric disease, spinal cord disease, impaired proprioception, muscle weakness	Stooped posture, wide-based steps; often retropulsion
Steppage gait	Distal muscle weakness	High steps ("steppage")
Waddling gait	Proximal muscle weakness	Both legs circumducted to allow locking of the knees
Antalgic gait	Non-neurologic; reflects disease of joints, bones, or soft tissue	Minimizes pain in the hip, spine, leg
Hysterical gait	Psychiatric or behavioral disorder	Reeling side to side, associated astasia-abasia, bizarre arm and trunk movements

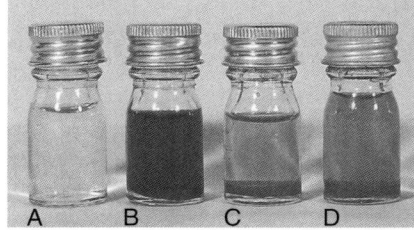

FIGURE 396-1. **Cerebrospinal fluid (CSF) examination. A,** Normal crystal-clear CSF. **B,** Blood in the CSF, which could result from a traumatic (bloody) tap or from subarachnoid hemorrhage. In a traumatic tap, subsequent tubes of CSF are usually less bloody. **C,** Centrifuged CSF in a traumatic tap. The supernatant is nearly clear. **D,** CSF from a patient with subarachnoid hemorrhage. There is blood at the bottom of the tube and the supernatant is yellow (xanthochromic) as a result of breakdown of blood cells in the CSF before the lumbar puncture. (From Forbes CD, Jackson WD. *Color Atlas and Text of Clinical Medicine.* 3rd ed. London: Mosby; 2003, with permission.)

moved. With severe loss of proprioception, patients may develop pseudoathetoid movements of the outstretched hands, sensory ataxia, or postural and action tremors.

Disorders of peripheral nerves commonly lead to sensory disturbances that depend on the population of affected nerve fibers (Chapter 420). Some neuropathies are predominantly large-fiber neuropathies. Appreciation of movement and position is impaired, and paresthesias are common. Examination reveals that vibration and position sensations are impaired, and movement becomes clumsy and ataxic. Pain and temperature appreciation is relatively preserved. The tendon reflexes are lost early. In other neuropathies, small fibers are selectively affected: spontaneous pain is common and may be burning, lancinating, or aching in quality. Pain and temperature appreciation is disproportionately affected in these neuropathies, and autonomic dysfunction may be present. Examples of small-fiber neuropathies include diabetes (Chapter 229) and alcoholism (Chapter 33). Most sensory neuropathies are characterized by a distal distribution of sensory loss, whereas sensory neuronopathies are characterized by sensory loss that may also involve the trunk and face and tends to be particularly severe. Sensory changes in a radiculopathy conform to a root territory; in cauda equina syndromes, sensory deficits involve multiple roots and may lead to saddle anesthesia and loss of the normal sensation associated with the passage of urine or feces.

Lesions of the posterolateral columns of the cord, such as occur in multiple sclerosis (Chapter 411), vitamin B_{12} deficiency (Chapter 416), and cervical spondylosis (Chapter 400), often lead to a feeling of compression in the affected region and to a Lhermitte sign (paresthesias radiating down the back and legs on neck flexion). Examination reveals ipsilateral impairment of vibration and joint position senses, with preservation of pain and temperature appreciation. Conversely, lesions of the anterolateral region of the cord (as by cordotomy) or central lesions interrupting fibers crossing to join the spinothalamic pathways (as in syringomyelia; Chapter 417) lead to impairment in pain and temperature appreciation with relative preservation of vibration, joint position sense, and light touch. Motor deficits may also be present and help localize the lesion. Upper motor neuron dysfunction

(Chapter 400) from cervical lesions leads to quadriplegia, whereas more caudal lesions lead to paraplegia; lesions below the level of the first lumbar vertebra may simply compress the cauda equina and result in lower motor neuron deficits from a polyradiculopathy as well as impairment of sphincter and sexual function.

NEUROLOGIC DIAGNOSTIC PROCEDURES

Lumbar Puncture

Sampling of cerebrospinal fluid (CSF) by lumbar puncture is crucial for accurate diagnosis of meningeal infections and carcinomatosis (Fig. 396-1). Ultrasound imaging can reduce the risk of an unsuccessful or traumatic lumbar puncture. CSF analysis is also helpful in evaluating patients with central or peripheral nervous system demyelinating disorders and with intracranial hemorrhage, particularly when imaging studies are inconclusive.

The CSF formula often provides an important clue to the pathologic process involved (Table 396-3). An elevated white blood cell count is seen with infections and other inflammatory diseases as well as with carcinomatosis. The differential white blood cell count may point to a specific class of pathogen; polymorphonuclear leukocytes suggest a bacterial process, whereas mononuclear cells suggest a viral, fungal, or immunologic cause. The CSF glucose concentration is typically reduced in bacterial and fungal infections as well as with certain viral infections (e.g., mumps virus) and sarcoidosis. The CSF protein concentration is elevated in a variety of disorders, including most infections and demyelinating neuropathies.

Specialized tests that can be performed on CSF include oligoclonal bands, a pathologic pattern of bands on CSF electrophoresis that is seen in up to 90% of patients with multiple sclerosis. The bands, which represent monoclonal immunoglobulins that are locally synthesized in the CNS, are not specific for multiple sclerosis and may be seen with other inflammatory and noninflammatory conditions, including systemic lupus erythematosus, human immunodeficiency virus infection, and stroke.

CSF polymerase chain reaction is a rapid, sensitive, and specific test for the diagnosis of herpes simplex encephalitis (Chapter 414), for which it has replaced brain biopsy as the diagnostic procedure of choice. The CSF VDRL (Venereal Disease Research Laboratory) assay is a specific although insensitive test for neurosyphilis (Chapter 319).

A lumbar puncture should not be performed in patients who have an obstructive noncommunicating hydrocephalus or a focal CNS mass lesion causing raised intracranial pressure, because reducing CSF pressure acutely in these settings by lumbar puncture may result in cerebral or cerebellar herniation. Lumbar puncture may be safely performed in patients with a communicating hydrocephalus, such as with idiopathic intracranial hypertension (pseudotumor cerebri), and it may even be an effective treatment in selected patients with this condition.

Electroencephalography

Electroencephalography is the recording and measurement of scalp electrical potentials to evaluate baseline brain functioning and paroxysmal brain electrical activity suggestive of a seizure disorder.

Electroencephalography is performed by securing 20 electrodes to the scalp at predetermined locations based on an international system that uses

TABLE 396-3 CHARACTERISTIC CEREBROSPINAL FLUID FORMULAS

	TURBIDITY AND COLOR	OPENING PRESSURE	WBC COUNT	DIFFERENTIAL CELLS	RBC COUNT	PROTEIN	GLUCOSE
Normal	Clear, colorless	70-180 mm H₂O	0-5 cells/µL	Mononuclear	0	<60 mg/dL	>⅔ serum
Bacterial meningitis	Cloudy, straw colored	↑	↑↑	PMNs	0	↑↑	↓
Viral meningitis	Clear or cloudy, colorless	↑	↑	Lymphocytes	0	↑	Normal
Fungal and tuberculous meningitis	Cloudy, straw colored	↑	↑	Lymphocytes	0	↑↑	↓↓
Viral encephalitis	Clear or cloudy, straw colored	Normal to ↑	↑	Lymphocytes	0 (herpes ↑)	Normal to ↑	Normal
Subarachnoid hemorrhage	Cloudy, pink	↑	↑	PMNs and lymphocytes	↑↑	↑	Normal (early); ↓ (late)
Guillain-Barré syndrome	Clear, yellow	Normal to ↑	0-5 cells/µL	Mononuclear	0	↑	Normal

PMN = polymorphonuclear leukocyte; RBC = red blood cell; WBC = white blood cell.

standardized percentages of the head circumference, the "10-20 system." Each electrode is labeled with a letter and a number, the letter identifying the skull region (Fp = frontopolar; F = frontal; P = parietal; C = central; T = temporal; O = occipital) and the number identifying the specific location, with odd numbers representing left-sided electrodes, even numbers representing right-sided electrodes, and zero representing midline placements. These electrodes are then connected in various combinations of pairs to generate voltage potential differences, and the potentials are displayed on a computer screen.

To delineate the spatial distribution of the changing electrical field for an electroencephalogram (EEG), an orderly arrangement of electrode pairs is used, and each specific arrangement is known as a montage. Montages are generally of two types: referential, in which each electrode is connected to a single reference electrode such as the ear; and bipolar, in which electrodes are connected sequentially to one another to form a chain. A standard EEG generally records about 30 minutes of brain activity, both in the awake state and in the first two stages of sleep. Various activating procedures are used during the recording of an EEG, including hyperventilation and photic stimulation. These activating procedures may precipitate seizure discharges in some patients with seizure disorders, thereby increasing the sensitivity of the test.

The amplitudes of scalp electrical potentials are low, averaging 30 to 100 µV. They represent a summation of excitatory postsynaptic potentials and inhibitory postsynaptic potentials that are largely generated by the pyramidal cells in layer 4 of the cerebral cortex. Action potentials are of too brief a duration to have an effect on the EEG.

The EEG is analyzed with respect to symmetry between each hemisphere, wave frequency and amplitude, and the presence of spikes (20 to 70 milliseconds) and sharp waves (70 to 200 milliseconds), which may indicate a seizure focus. Electroencephalographic frequencies are divided into four categories as follows: delta (<4 Hz), theta (4-7 Hz), alpha (8-13 Hz), and beta (>13 Hz).

The normal waking EEG (Fig. 396-2A) in a patient with eyes closed contains rhythms of alpha frequency in the occipital leads and beta frequency in the frontal leads. Normal sleep causes a generalized slowing of EEG frequencies and an increase in amplitude in each stage of sleep, such that stage N3 sleep consists of more than 50% large-amplitude delta rhythms. EEG abnormalities are of two types: abnormalities in background rhythm and abnormalities of a paroxysmal nature (Table 396-4).[6]

The major usefulness of the EEG is for diagnosis and categorization of a seizure disorder (see Fig. 396-2B).[7] EEGs are neither highly sensitive nor completely specific for a diagnosis of seizures. Because seizures are paroxysmal events, it is not unusual for an EEG to be normal—or only minimally abnormal—in a patient with epilepsy if it is recorded during an interictal phase (the period between seizures). Only about 50% of patients with seizures show epileptiform activity on the first EEG. Repeating the EEG with provocative maneuvers such as sleep deprivation, hyperventilation, and photic stimulation may increase this percentage to 90%. Conversely, about 1% of adults and 3.5% of children who are neurologically normal and who never had a seizure have epileptiform activity on an EEG.

The EEG may provide clues to the diagnosis of certain neurologic conditions, including viral encephalitis, prion disorders, and some forms of coma. In each of these situations, the EEG can have specific patterns that suggest a specific neurologic diagnosis. In herpes simplex encephalitis, periodic lateralizing epileptiform discharges emanating from the temporal lobes are frequently present. Triphasic slow waves are common in hepatic encephalopathy (see Fig. 396-2C) but are a nonspecific finding. Creutzfeldt-Jakob disease is characterized by the presence of bilateral synchronous repetitive sharp waves. The EEG is also helpful in evaluating comatose patients, in confirming brain death when an apnea test cannot be performed because of cardiac instability, and for staging sleep in polysomnography.

In the past, the EEG was often used to localize neurologic lesions such as stroke, brain tumor, and abscess. With the advent of neuroimaging, EEG is almost never used for these purposes in developed countries.

Nerve Conduction Study

A nerve conduction study (NCS) is the recording and measurement of the compound nerve and muscle action potentials elicited in response to an electrical stimulus. To perform a motor NCS, a surface (active) recording electrode is placed over the belly of a distal muscle that is innervated by the nerve in question. A reference electrode is placed distally over the tendon. The nerve is then supramaximally stimulated at a predetermined distance proximal to the active electrode, and the resultant compound motor action potential (CMAP) is recorded. The terminal latency, amplitude, and duration of the evoked potential are measured directly, and the conduction velocity is calculated from the latencies of the evoked potentials with stimulation at two different points; the distance between the two points (conduction distance) is divided by the difference between the corresponding latencies (conduction time) to derive a calculated velocity (conduction velocity = distance ÷ time).

To perform a sensory NCS, the active recording electrode is placed over the portion of the skin innervated by the nerve in question, and a sensory nerve action potential is recorded after electrical stimulation of the nerve, similar to that noted for a motor NCS. NCS abnormalities include reduced amplitudes, prolonged terminal latencies, conduction block, and slowed conduction velocities (Table 396-5).

The NCS is helpful in documenting the existence of a neuropathy, quantifying its severity, and noting its distribution (i.e., whether it is distal, proximal, or diffuse). In addition, the NCS can provide information on the modality involved (i.e., motor versus sensory) and can suggest whether the lesion is axonal or demyelinating. The NCS is also helpful in diagnosis of compressive mononeuropathies, such as carpal tunnel syndrome, ulnar palsy, peroneal nerve palsy, and tarsal tunnel syndrome.

F Wave and H Reflex

The F wave and H reflex are ways of looking at the conduction characteristics for proximal portions of nerves, including the nerve roots. The F wave is a late CMAP evoked intermittently from a muscle by a supramaximal electrical stimulus to the nerve, and it is due to antidromic activation (backfiring) of alpha motor neurons. F waves can be elicited from practically all distal motor nerves. The H reflex is a late CMAP that is evoked regularly from a muscle by a submaximal stimulus to a nerve, and it is due to stimulation of Ia afferent fibers (a spinal reflex). The H reflex can be routinely obtained from calf muscles only with stimulation of the tibial nerve in the popliteal fossa.

F waves are helpful in diagnosis of Guillain-Barré syndrome, in which demyelination is often confined to the proximal portions of nerves early in the course of the disease. The H reflex is often absent in patients with acute S1 radiculopathy.

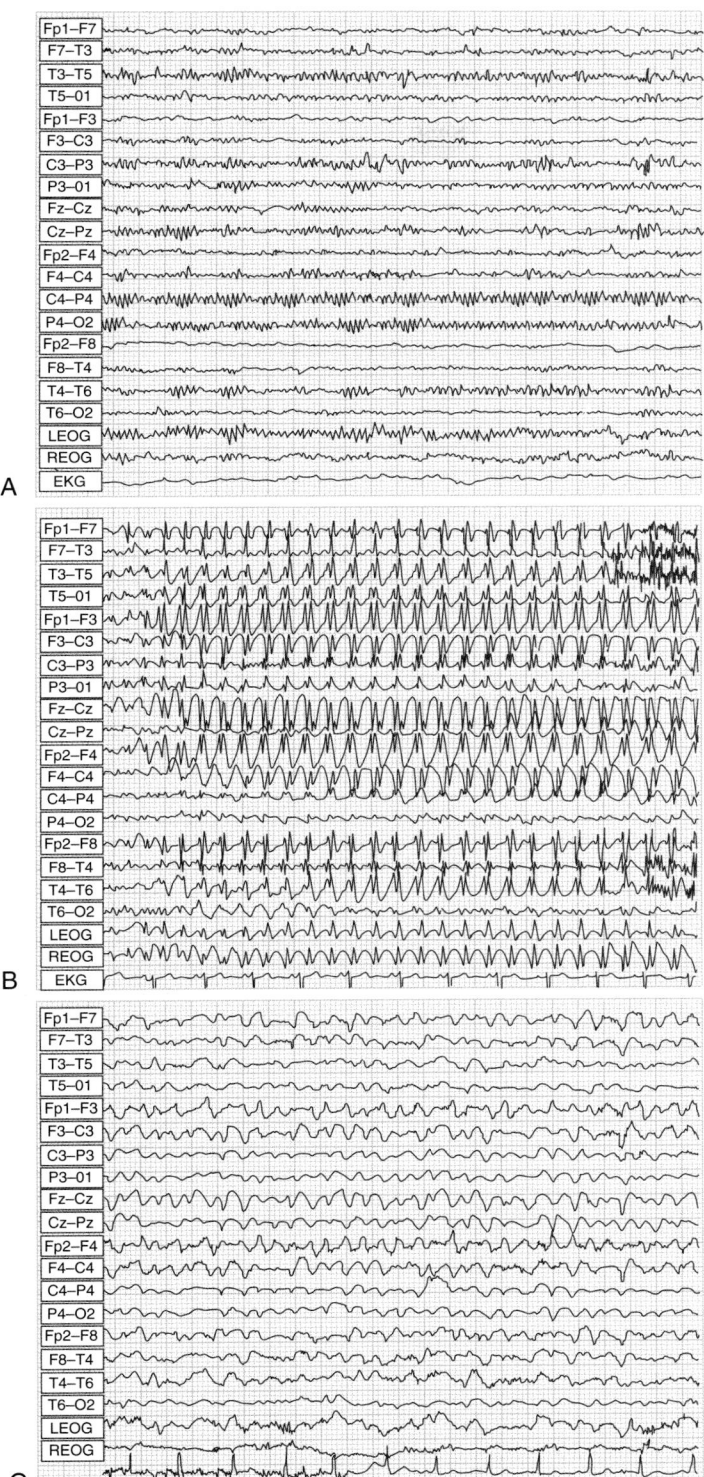

FIGURE 396-2. Normal and abnormal electroencephalograms. **A,** The EEG of a normal awake adult. **B,** A 3-Hz spike and wave activity, a pattern seen in absence epilepsy. In each record, channels 1 through 8 and 11 through 18 represent left- and right-sided bipolar electrode placements, respectively. Channels 9 and 10 represent midline bipolar electrode placements, and channels 19 and 20 represent the left and right electro-oculograms (eye movements). Each major horizontal division represents 1 second. **C,** Triphasic slow waves, a pattern seen in hepatic or other metabolic encephalopathies.

TABLE 396-4 ELECTROENCEPHALOGRAPHIC ABNORMALITIES

ELECTROENCEPHALOGRAPHIC ABNORMALITY	CLINICAL CORRELATE
BACKGROUND RHYTHM ABNORMALITIES	
Generalized slowing	Most metabolic encephalopathies
Triphasic waves	Hepatic, renal, and other metabolic encephalopathies
Focal slowing	Large mass lesions (tumor, large stroke)
Electrocerebral inactivity with lack of response to all stimuli	Neocortical death, hypothermia, drug overdose
PAROXYSMAL ABNORMALITIES	
3-Hz spike and wave, augmented by hyperventilation	Absence epilepsy
3- to 4-Hz spike and wave in light sleep or with photic stimulation	Primary generalized epilepsy
Central to midtemporal spikes	Benign rolandic epilepsy, other partial epilepsies
Anterior temporal spikes or sharp waves	Simple or complex focal (partial) seizures of mesial temporal origin
Hypsarrhythmia (high-voltage chaotic slowing with multifocal spikes)	Infantile spasms (West syndrome)
Burst suppression	Severe anoxic brain injury, barbiturate coma

TABLE 396-5 NERVE CONDUCTION STUDY ABNORMALITIES

ABNORMALITY	CLINICAL CORRELATE
Reduced CMAP amplitude	Axonal neuropathy
Prolonged terminal latency	Demyelinating neuropathy Distal compressive neuropathy
Conduction block	Severe focal compressive neuropathy Severe demyelinating neuropathy
Slowed conduction velocity	Demyelinating neuropathy

CMAP = compound muscle action potential.

Repetitive Stimulation Study

A repetitive stimulation study is a method of measuring electrical conduction properties at the neuromuscular junction. To perform a repetitive stimulation study, a surface recording electrode is placed over a muscle belly, and the nerve innervating that muscle is electrically stimulated with a supramaximal stimulus at a certain frequency. A series of electrical potentials are then recorded whose amplitude is roughly proportional to the number of muscle fibers being activated.

A repetitive stimulation study is helpful in diagnosis of neuromuscular junction disorders such as myasthenia gravis and myasthenic syndrome (Lambert-Eaton syndrome). In myasthenia gravis, the amplitudes of evoked potentials become progressively smaller with repetitive stimulation in clinically involved muscles. Clinically uninvolved muscles often do not demonstrate this decrement. In myasthenic syndrome, an increment is seen in the amplitudes of evoked potentials with rapid repetitive electrical stimulation.

Electromyography

Electromyography (EMG) is the recording and study of insertional, spontaneous, and voluntary electrical activity of muscle.[8] It allows physiologic evaluation of the motor unit, including the anterior horn cell, peripheral nerve, and muscle.

EMG is performed by insertion of a needle electrode into the muscle in question and evaluation of the motor unit action potentials both visually (on a computer screen) and aurally (over a loudspeaker). Muscles are typically studied at rest and during voluntary contraction. During EMG, the electrical activity of muscle is studied in four settings (Table 396-6): insertional activity (occurring within the first second of needle insertion), spontaneous activity (electrical activity at rest), voluntary activity (electrical activity with muscle contraction), and recruitment pattern (change in electrical activity with maximal contraction).

EMG is helpful in evaluation of patients with weakness in that it can help determine whether the weakness is due to anterior horn cell disease, nerve root disease, peripheral neuropathy, or an intrinsic disease of muscle itself (myopathy). EMG can differentiate acute denervation from chronic denervation and may thus give an indication about the time course of the lesion causing the neuropathy. In addition, on the basis of which muscles have an abnormal EMG pattern, it is possible to determine whether the neuropathy is due to a lesion of a nerve root (radiculopathy), the brachial or lumbosacral plexus (plexopathy), an individual peripheral nerve (mononeuropathy), or multiple peripheral nerves (polyneuropathy).

EMG is also helpful in differentiating active (inflammatory) myopathies from chronic myopathies. Active myopathies include dermatomyositis, polymyositis, inclusion body myositis, and some forms of muscular dystrophy (e.g., Duchenne dystrophy). Chronic myopathies include the other muscular dystrophies, the congenital myopathies, and some metabolic myopathies.

TABLE 396-6   ELECTROMYOGRAPHIC ABNORMALITIES

ABNORMALITY	CLINICAL CORRELATE
INSERTIONAL ACTIVITY	
Prolonged	Acute denervation Active (usually inflammatory) myopathy
SPONTANEOUS ACTIVITY	
Fibrillations and positive waves	Acute denervation Active (usually inflammatory) myopathy
Fasciculations	Chronic neuropathies Motor neuron disease (rare fasciculations may be normal)
Myotonic discharges	Myotonic disorders Acid maltase deficiency
VOLUNTARY ACTIVITY	
Neuropathic potentials: large-amplitude, long-duration, polyphasic potentials	Chronic neuropathies and anterior horn cell diseases
Myopathic potentials: small-amplitude, short-duration, polyphasic potentials	Chronic myopathies Neuromuscular junction disorders
RECRUITMENT	
Reduced	Chronic neuropathic disorders
Rapid	Chronic myopathies

Myotonic dystrophy and myotonia congenita produce characteristic myotonic discharges.

It may take several weeks for a muscle to develop EMG signs of acute denervation after nerve transection. For this reason, EMG performed in the acute setting after nerve injury should be interpreted with caution, and it may need to be repeated at a later date.

Evoked Potentials

Evoked potentials are ways of measuring conduction velocities for sensory pathways in the CNS by means of computerized averaging techniques. Three types of evoked potentials are routinely performed: visual, brain stem auditory, and somatosensory.

Pattern Reversal Visual Evoked Potentials

The pattern reversal visual evoked potential (PVEP) assesses the function of central visual pathways, in particular the optic nerves. To perform this test, EEG electrodes are placed over the occipital regions of the scalp, and the patient is asked to look at the center of a black-and-white checkerboard screen with one eye patched. The color of the checks alternates about twice per second, a process known as pattern reversal. The scalp potentials elicited by approximately 100 such pattern reversals are then recorded and signal averaged by a computer. This signal averaging cancels the random EEG activity and differentially amplifies the evoked potential, which consists of a major positivity with a latency of about 100 milliseconds (the so-called P100 response). This response is recorded for each eye, and its latency is measured. A prolonged P100 latency in one eye, in the absence of ocular disease, implies slowed conduction velocity in the optic nerve and suggests demyelination of that nerve. PVEP testing is helpful when multiple sclerosis is suspected clinically and it is necessary to document the presence of a second demyelinating lesion in the CNS that may not be clinically evident (Fig. 396-3).

Brain Stem Auditory Evoked Potentials

The brain stem auditory evoked potentials (BAEP) assess function in the central auditory pathways in the brain stem. EEG electrodes are placed over the vertex and mastoid process, and a series of clicks at a frequency of 5 Hz are delivered to each ear separately for 3 minutes. The scalp potentials elicited by the clicks are then recorded and signal averaged by a computer. This signal averaging cancels the random EEG activity and differentially amplifies the evoked potential. A series of five waves are recorded for each ear, and each wave corresponds to a different point in the central auditory pathway (Table 396-7). The wave latencies for the right and left ears are compared, and a delay in any of the latencies suggests a lesion at that point in the central brain stem auditory pathway. BAEP testing is helpful in diagnosis of acoustic schwannoma and other tumors in the cerebellopontine angle.

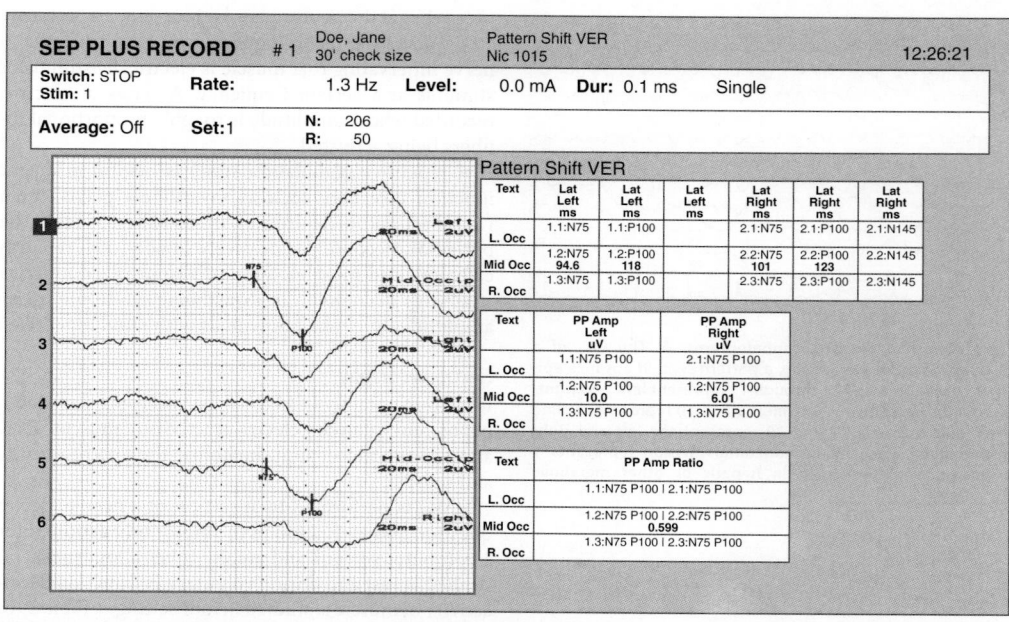

FIGURE 396-3. Abnormal pattern reversal visual evoked potential in a patient with multiple sclerosis. The prolonged P100 wave latency with left eye stimulation suggests a conduction defect in the left optic nerve. The top three channels represent right eye stimulation, and the bottom three channels represent left eye stimulation. Each horizontal division represents 20 milliseconds.

Somatosensory Evoked Potentials

The somatosensory evoked potential (SEP) assesses conduction in the central somatosensory pathways in the posterior columns of the spinal cord, brain stem, thalamus, and primary sensory cortex in the parietal lobes. To perform SEP testing, recording electrodes are placed over Erb point and the cervical spine (for medial or ulnar nerve stimulation), over the popliteal fossa and lumbar spine (for peroneal or tibial nerve stimulation), and over the scalp. A series of 1000 to 2000 electric shocks at a frequency of 5 Hz are delivered to the median or ulnar nerve (for an upper extremity SEP) or to the fibular (peroneal) or tibial nerve (for a lower extremity SEP). The scalp potentials elicited by the electric shocks are then recorded and signal averaged by a computer. This signal averaging cancels the random EEG activity and differentially amplifies the evoked potential. A series of waves are recorded for each nerve stimulated, with each wave corresponding to a different point in the somatosensory pathways in the spinal cord, brain stem, and cerebral cortex. The wave latencies for the right and left limbs are compared, and a delay in any of the latencies suggests a lesion at that point in the somatosensory pathways.

SEP testing, like PVEP, is helpful when multiple sclerosis is suspected clinically and it is necessary to document the presence of a second demyelinating lesion in the CNS that may not be clinically evident. SEP testing is also useful for prognostication in comatose patients and for monitoring of spinal cord function intraoperatively in patients undergoing spinal surgery.

Electronystagmography

Electronystagmography accurately records eye movements and nystagmus after certain provocative maneuvers. To perform this test, disc electrodes are placed over the bridge of the nose and lateral to each outer canthus, and the electrical leads from these discs are connected to an oscilloscope. Because the cornea is electropositive and the retina is electronegative, these electrodes accurately record lateral eye movements. The patient is first observed for spontaneous nystagmus with the eyes open and closed and then for nystagmus evoked by lateral gaze, for nystagmus induced by hot and cold air instilled in the outer ears (caloric induced), and for positional nystagmus. The last is performed by rotating the patient in a specialized chair. Spontaneous nystagmus suggests a vestibular pathologic lesion, as does an imbalance in the nystagmus evoked by these maneuvers in the right and left ears.

Imaging

On the basis of the relative advantages and disadvantages of computed tomography (CT), magnetic resonance imaging (MRI), and other neuroimaging modalities, different clinical entities can and should be assessed differently (Table 396-8). In acute ischemic stroke (Chapter 407) without bleeding, CT abnormalities typically appear within 4 to 12 hours and are seen even earlier with larger infarctions and embolic infarctions. CT detects hemorrhagic stroke (Chapter 408) acutely and can estimate its age. CT is also the preferred initial imaging modality for detection of intraparenchymal hemorrhage and subarachnoid hemorrhage, and it often suggests whether an aneurysm is the likely cause. Either CT angiography or magnetic resonance angiography can display the three-dimensional anatomy of aneurysms with sufficient detail for therapy to be planned, but surgical treatment generally

TABLE 396-7 BRAIN STEM AUDITORY EVOKED POTENTIAL WAVE GENERATORS

WAVE	LOCATION
I	Auditory nerve
II	Cochlear nucleus
III	Superior olivary nucleus
IV	Lateral lemniscus
V	Inferior colliculus

TABLE 396-8 STRENGTHS AND WEAKNESSES OF SELECTED IMAGING MODALITIES

MODALITY	STRENGTHS	WEAKNESSES
Computed tomography (CT)	Fast; best test for acute intraparenchymal or subarachnoid hemorrhage and calcification; easy to monitor patients; excellent for bones	Less sensitive to parenchymal lesions than MRI; potential for significant reaction to contrast material; radiation exposure
Conventional angiography	Best imaging modality for aneurysms, vascular malformations, and vasculitis	Invasive and often lengthy; risk of stroke and other complications
Conventional myelography	Good images of nerve roots and small osteophytic lesions; accurate for bony stenosis; useful in patients with contraindications to MRI	Invasive, with risk of complications from lumbar puncture and instillation of contrast material; does not image intramedullary lesions well
CT myelography	Excellent for imaging nerve roots and detecting root compression from degenerative processes	Invasive, with risk of complications from lumbar puncture and instillation of contrast material
Magnetic resonance imaging (MRI)	Noninvasive; no radiation; multiplanar; extremely sensitive, safe contrast agent	Less sensitive than CT for detection of subarachnoid hemorrhage and calcification; less sensitive for bony skull fractures; contraindicated in patients with implanted metallic devices or foreign bodies; the patient must be able to cooperate and tolerate confined space; time-consuming relative to CT
Magnetic resonance angiography (MRA)	Noninvasive; good for screening for extracranial and intracranial vascular disease; may be performed with or without contrast agent	Need cooperative patient; technically demanding; may overestimate the degree of vascular stenosis (noncontrast MRA); cannot image distal vessels optimally without contrast agent; may miss small lesions (e.g., aneurysms)
Positron emission tomography (PET)	Limited role in helping to distinguish radiation necrosis from tumor; sometimes helpful in the diagnosis of Alzheimer disease and epilepsy	Requires a cyclotron to generate radioisotopes with a short half-life; lower resolution and less available than MRI or CT
Single-photon emission computed tomography (SPECT)	Occasionally useful in epilepsy; sensitive for diffuse pathologic processes; easier to use than PET	Lower resolution than PET, MRI, or CT
Proton magnetic resonance spectroscopy	Localization of seizure focus; may help diagnose and classify dementias such as Alzheimer disease; may distinguish brain tumors from other mass lesions; may distinguish radiation necrosis from recurrent tumor	Specificity not yet determined; not routinely available; lower resolution; time-consuming
Ultrasonography	Fast; easy to use; can be performed at the bedside to assess vessel patency	Does not assess the vertebral arteries; less sensitive and specific than MRA; cannot visualize vessels in the upper neck and cranial base
Transcranial Doppler (TCD)	Fast; easy to use; assesses vascular velocities quantitatively; can assess cerebral vasospasm and occluded vessels	Does not provide images of vessels

Reproduced and modified from Hackney D. Radiologic imaging procedures. In: Goldman L, Ausiello D, eds. *Cecil Medicine*, 23rd ed. Philadelphia: Saunders Elsevier; 2008:2623-2627.

requires preprocedure catheter arteriography. CT is the first-line method for evaluation of brain trauma and diagnosis of a subdural or epidural hematoma (Chapter 399), usually without requiring intravenous contrast material. However, MRI is better than CT to delineate the anatomy of a subdural hematoma and to estimate the age of the lesion. Many brain tumors are initially recognized on CT scans, but MRI is the preferred modality for detection and characterization of all brain tumors (Chapter 189), including those that might be the cause of new-onset seizures in adults.[9]

Grade A Reference

○───○

A1. Shaikh F, Brzezinski J, Alexander S, et al. Ultrasound imaging for lumbar punctures and epidural catheterisations: systematic review and meta-analysis. *BMJ.* 2013;346:f1720.

GENERAL REFERENCES

For the General References and other additional features, please visit Expert Consult at https://expertconsult.inkling.com.

397

PSYCHIATRIC DISORDERS IN MEDICAL PRACTICE

JEFFREY M. LYNESS

OVERVIEW

Disorders in Psychiatry

Psychiatric disorders, also known as mental illnesses, are extraordinarily common and have a profound impact on well-being and functional status. Collectively, psychiatric disorders account for more aggregate disability than do those involving any other organ system, with depression alone being second only to cardiovascular disorders.

Psychiatric disorders are defined as disorders of the psyche—that is, conditions that affect thoughts, feelings, or behaviors. By definition, such mental disturbances must be sufficient to produce significant distress in the patient or impairment in role or other functioning. Because the pathogeneses of most psychiatric disorders are incompletely understood, classification is based on clinical syndromes that are defined by diagnostic criteria with high inter-rater reliability because they emphasize discrete reportable or observable symptoms and signs. Interestingly, however, underlying genetic variations and pathophysiologic mechanisms seem to cut across these descriptive diagnostic categories,[1] although such underlying findings do not yet aid in predicting the clinical course of disease or therapeutic decision making.

Specific Syndromes

Because many psychiatric disorders result from the direct influence of neurologic conditions, systemic diseases, or drugs on brain functioning, assessment of any new or worsened psychiatric condition must include evaluation for their potential contributions (Table 397-1). Delirium (Chapter 28) and dementia (Chapter 402), which are neurocognitive disorders defined by impairment in intellectual functions such as attention, memory, or language, are always the result of neurologic abnormalities, systemic illnesses, or drugs. Although intellectual impairment is the hallmark of neurocognitive disorders, these conditions also may manifest as alterations in other aspects of mental status, including mood, thought content, thought process, and behavior. If a noncognitive psychiatric syndrome is caused by an identifiable underlying condition, it is known as a secondary psychiatric disorder (e.g., depression secondary to hypothyroidism).

The major nonsecondary, noncognitive psychiatric syndromes (Table 397-2)[2] can coexist with multiple syndromes; for example, a patient suffering major depression with psychotic features may have depressive, anxiety, and psychotic syndromes simultaneously. Addictive disorders are considered in Chapters 33 and 34.

TABLE 397-1	IMPORTANT CAUSES OF PSYCHIATRIC SYNDROMES
CENTRAL NERVOUS SYSTEM DISEASES	

Trauma
Tumor
Toxins
Seizures
Vascular
Infections
Genetic/congenital malformations
Demyelinating diseases
Neurodegenerative diseases
Hydrocephalus

SYSTEMIC DISEASES

Cardiovascular
Pulmonary
Endocrine
Metabolic
Nutritional
Infections
Cancer

DRUGS (e.g., recreational, prescription, or over-the-counter drugs)

Drug intoxication
Drug withdrawal

Comorbid Conditions in Psychiatry

It is common for persons who suffer from mental disorders to meet the diagnostic criteria for more than one condition. Although such comorbidity may reflect the limitations of current approaches to diagnosis, psychiatric comorbidity influences the choices or sequence of indicated treatments and may worsen the overall prognosis. Comorbidity with other medical conditions also is common, probably reflecting complex bidirectional causal relationships between physical and mental illnesses, and such comorbidity also often worsens the prognosis for both conditions.

Treatments in Psychiatry

Treatments in psychiatry are intended to reduce or eliminate symptoms, thereby improving the patient's distress and dysfunction and averting suicidal behavior. Pharmacotherapy remains an evidence-based mainstay of the treatment of many psychiatric conditions. The evidence for a number of forms of psychotherapy administered in individual, group, or family modalities supports its use as primary treatment or co-treatment of many conditions. Other psychosocial interventions, ranging from self-help groups to the use of structured treatment or residential programs, are often important adjuncts to treatment. Nonpharmacologic evidence-based somatic therapies include electroconvulsive therapy, light therapy, and vagal nerve stimulation for particular forms of major depression. Encouraging data are emerging to support deep brain stimulation for selected cases of severe depressive or obsessive-compulsive disorders.

Mood Disorders

Mood disorders are categorized as either depressive (also termed *unipolar*), characterized by depressive episodes only, or bipolar, characterized by manic or hypomanic episodes, typically with depressive episodes as well.

MAJOR DEPRESSIVE DISORDER

DEFINITION

Major depressive disorder is characterized by one or more episodes of idiopathic major depressive syndrome (Table 397-3).

EPIDEMIOLOGY

In the United States, major depression has a 12-month prevalence of approximately 7%, and it is at least 1.5 times more common in females than males. Lifetime prevalence is up to 10% in males and 20 to 25% in females. New depressive episodes have an annual incidence of approximately 3%. Depression accounts for more than twice as much disability in midlife as any other medical condition, and its overall cumulative burden is greater than that from all but cardiovascular disorders. The economic impact is also enormous, with U.S. estimates of annual costs for depression exceeding $12 billion for

TABLE 397-2 IMPORTANT PSYCHIATRIC SYNDROMES AND DISORDERS

SYNDROME	MAIN SYMPTOMS AND SIGNS	MAY OCCUR AS PART OF THESE DISORDERS
Neurocognitive	Deficits in intellectual functions (e.g., level of consciousness, orientation, attention, memory, language, praxis, visuospatial, executive functions)	Neurocognitive disorders Intellectual disability (if onset in childhood)
Mood: depressive	Lowered mood, anhedonia, negativistic thoughts, neurovegetative symptoms	Neurocognitive disorders Mood disorders (bipolar or depressive) (primary or secondary) Psychotic disorders (schizoaffective disorder)
Mood: manic	Elevated or irritable mood, grandiosity, goal-directed hyperactivity with increased energy, pressured speech, decreased sleep need	Neurocognitive disorders Bipolar disorder (primary or secondary) Psychotic disorders (schizoaffective disorder)
Anxiety	All include anxious mood and associated physiologic symptoms (e.g., palpitations, tremors, diaphoresis). May include various types of dysfunctional thoughts (e.g., catastrophic fears, obsessions, flashbacks) and behavior (e.g., compulsions, avoidance behavior).	Neurocognitive disorders Mood disorders (bipolar or depressive) (primary or secondary) Psychotic disorders (primary or secondary) Anxiety disorders (primary or secondary) Obsessive-compulsive and related disorders
Psychotic	Impairments in reality testing: delusions, hallucinations, thought process derailments	Neurocognitive disorders Mood disorders (bipolar or depressive) (primary or secondary) Psychotic disorders
Somatic symptom syndromes	Somatic symptoms with associated distressing thoughts, feelings, or behaviors	Mood disorders (bipolar or depressive) (primary or secondary) Anxiety disorders (primary or secondary) Obsessive-compulsive and related disorders Trauma-related disorders Somatic symptom disorders
Personality pathology	Enduring patterns of dysfunctional emotional regulation, thought patterns, interpersonal behavior, impulse regulation	Neurocognitive disorders (dementia) Personality change due to another medical condition Personality disorders

Author summary based on categories and criteria from American Psychiatric Association. *Diagnostic and Statistical Manual of Mental Disorders.* 5th ed. (DSM-5) Washington, DC: American Psychiatric Association; 2013.

treatment, $8 billion for associated morbidity, and $33 billion for lost earnings and work productivity.

PATHOBIOLOGY

Major depression is probably not a single disease entity but rather a heterogeneous group of conditions with multiple pathogenic mechanisms. It is both multifactorial and polygenic: genetic factors account for approximately 40% of the risk for depression, but multiple gene loci, most of which are currently unknown, are probably involved in a complex interplay with developmental and environmental influences. Alterations in the brain's noradrenergic and serotonergic systems are likely related to the efficacy of current antidepressant medications. The hypothalamic-pituitary-adrenal axis is hyperactive in depression, as evidenced by a nonsuppressed response to the dexamethasone suppression test, although this test is too insensitive and nonspecific for clinical use as a diagnostic tool. Neuroimaging studies in subjects with depression show an array of findings, including smaller hippocampal volumes that may be the result of exposure to chronically elevated cortisol levels, and altered cerebral metabolic activity in regions including frontal-striatal circuitry and the anterior cingulate cortex. Cognitive psychology studies have demonstrated dysfunctional patterns of negative thinking, with distorted thoughts about self, the future, and the environment. Poor quality or absence of social relationships, and stressful life events, particularly events such as deaths, separations, or functional impairment, are powerfully associated with depression as well.

CLINICAL MANIFESTATIONS

The symptoms of depression (see Table 397-3) may be conceptually grouped as alterations in mood, ideation (i.e., thought content), and somatic/neurovegetative functioning. Importantly, patients with depressive illness may be seen without a depressed mood, albeit by definition they then must have loss of interest or pleasure in their usually desired activities. They may also exhibit prominent anxiety, irritability, or somatization. Although mild forms of major depression in the community often remit spontaneously within a few months without medical care, patients may have persistent symptoms for months or years before seeking treatment.

DIAGNOSIS

The diagnosis is made clinically by elicitation of findings from the history and mental status examination to determine the presence of major depressive syndrome. The differential diagnosis includes other idiopathic disorders with episodes of major depression, such as bipolar disorder (distinguished by a

history of manic episodes) and schizoaffective disorder (distinguished by a history of psychotic episodes in the absence of depression). Major depression may accompany delirium or dementia, and secondary depression also commonly accompanies serious medical illnesses in the elderly;[3] these comorbid conditions require careful, well-coordinated care. Screening instruments (see Table 27-3 in Chapter 27) can help identify cases of depression. For example, using the two-item version of the Patient Health Questionnaire, the screener asks the patient: Over the past 2 weeks, how often have you (1) Had little interest or pleasure in doing things, or (2) Been feeling down, depressed, or hopeless. Responses for each question are scored as: 0 = not at all, 1 = several days, 2 = more than half the days, 3 = nearly every day. A score of 3 points or higher on the two-item screen is associated with 75% probability of having a depressive disorder.

TREATMENT Rx

The three phases of treatment include (1) acute, in which treatment is provided to resolve the major depressive episode; (2) continuation, in which the acute treatment is continued for at least 4 to 8 months to prevent relapse; and (3) maintenance, for those with two to three or more episodes of recurrent depression, for whom treatment is maintained indefinitely to reduce the frequency and severity of future recurrences.[4] Combinations of psychotherapy and medication are used for more complex or severe clinical conditions.

Acute treatment of depression includes focused psychotherapies (Table 397-4), which are more efficacious than usual care and equivalent to medications when used for patients in primary care settings.[A1] Based on the patient's preference, psychotherapy rather than medication may be the initial treatment of mild to moderate major depression with prominent psychosocial stressors. Involvement of family members for education, support, and sometimes formal family therapy may be an important adjunctive or primary therapeutic approach. These therapies may be administered with decreased frequency during the continuation or maintenance phases of treatment. However, psychotherapies alone are insufficient for more severe forms of depression, including major depression with psychotic features. Meta-analyses suggest that the combination of medication with psychotherapy is more effective than medication alone in the initial treatment of mild to moderate major depression.[A2]

Medications should be used as initial treatment for most patients with more severe forms of major depression. Antidepressant medications (Table 397-5) are also effective for acute, continuation, and maintenance therapy. A meta-analysis found that sertraline and escitalopram have the best profiles of efficacy and tolerability, whereas mirtazapine and venlafaxine also have strong efficacy in head-to-head comparisons with other antidepressants.[A3] Overall,

TABLE 397-3 SYMPTOMS/SIGNS OF AN EPISODE OF MAJOR DEPRESSIVE SYNDROME

DIAGNOSTIC CRITERIA (*must be present for a minimum of 2 consecutive weeks*)

Depressed mood (may be irritable mood in children and adolescents) most of the day, nearly every day, *OR*

Markedly diminished interest or pleasure most of the day, nearly every day *AND*

Weight loss or gain, or change in appetite (decrease or increase) nearly every day

Change in sleep (insomnia or hypersomnia) nearly every day

Psychomotor agitation or retardation nearly every day

Fatigue or loss of energy nearly every day

Feeling of worthlessness or guilt nearly every day

Diminished concentration or indecisiveness nearly every day

Recurrent thoughts of death or suicidal ideation, or a suicide attempt, or a specific suicide plan

MNEMONIC TO AID RECALL OF DIAGNOSTIC CRITERIA: *"SIG: E CAPS"* (*i.e., prescribe energy capsules*) for depressed mood

Sleep change
Interests decreased
Guilt
Energy decreased
Concentration decreased
Appetite/weight disturbance
Psychomotor changes
Suicide thoughts

DEPRESSIVE SYMPTOMS/SIGNS GROUPED CONCEPTUALLY, WITH ADDITIONAL COMMON PHENOMENA

Emotional

Depressed mood, sadness, tearfulness
Irritability (seen in all ages, perhaps most commonly in children/adolescents and the elderly)
Anxiety
Loss of interests or pleasure (anhedonia)

Ideational

Worthlessness/lowered self-esteem
Guilt
Hopelessness/nihilism
Helplessness
Thoughts of death, dying, suicide

Somatic/Neurovegetative

Change in appetite/weight
Change in sleep
Anergia
Decreased libido
Trouble concentrating
Diurnal variation in symptoms (*mornings—worst pattern is most characteristic*)

Other

Ruminative thinking (*tendency to dwell on one [negativistic] theme*)
Somatoform symptoms or somatic worry
Psychotic symptoms (*negativistic delusions most characteristic*)—defines the subtype "Major Depression with Psychotic Features"

Based on criteria from American Psychiatric Association. *Diagnostic and Statistical Manual of Mental Disorders.* 5th ed. (DSM-5) Washington, DC: American Psychiatric Association; 2013.

TABLE 397-4 TREATMENTS FOR DEPRESSION

NAME OF PSYCHOTHERAPY	APPROACH
Cognitive psychotherapy	Identify and correct negativistic patterns of thinking
Interpersonal psychotherapy	Identify and work through role transitions or interpersonal losses, conflicts, or deficits
Problem-solving therapy	Identify and prioritize situational problems; plan and implement strategies to deal with top-priority problems
Psychodynamic psychotherapy	Use therapeutic relationship to maximize use of the healthiest defense mechanisms and coping strategies

however, data suggest that no second-generation agent is predictably better than others,[A4] although agents targeting noradrenergic as well as serotonergic systems may be more efficacious in more severe depression. Because antidepressant medications typically do not begin to improve symptoms for at least 1 to 2 weeks, with maximal benefit accruing up to at least 6 to 8 weeks, it is crucial to see patients regularly (every 1 to 2 weeks initially) to monitor their clinical status, provide support and education, and foster adherence. Antidepressant medications appear to increase the relative risk for suicidal behavior in adolescents and young adults, so such patients require careful benefit/risk assessments and close monitoring. By comparison, the relative risk for suicidal behavior is not increased by drug treatment in individuals older than age 25 and is substantially lowered in older adults. For patients with a psychotic depression, the addition of an antipsychotic medication (see later) to an antidepressant may be more efficacious than either alone.[A5] A single intravenous dose of ketamine may rapidly reduce severe depressive symptoms within 24 hours, although its use must be considered investigational at the present time.[A6] Electroconvulsive therapy is preferred for the most severe forms of major depression, including major depression with psychotic features, and is also used for depression refractory to other forms of treatment. Deep brain stimulation is an investigational therapy for otherwise refractory depression.

Optimal care for depression in primary care and other treatment settings may be enhanced by the use of collaborative chronic care models. However, despite considerable evidence supporting such models,[A7] lack of reimbursement mechanisms has limited their implementation in most communities and clinical settings.

PROGNOSIS

Optimal guideline-based treatment of major depression results in full remission in up to 80% of patients, and the expectation is that patients with major depression will return to baseline functioning after resolution of the depressive episodes. However, at least 50 to 70% of patients will suffer recurrent episodes, up to 20% may experience chronic major depression, and many more will achieve only partial remission with persistent lower-level symptoms because of a variety of factors, including limited access to care, nonadherence, or insufficiently assertive treatments.

BIPOLAR DISORDER

DEFINITION AND EPIDEMIOLOGY

Bipolar disorder is characterized by recurrent episodes of idiopathic mania. Most persons with bipolar disorder also have recurrent episodes of major depression.[5]

The 12-month prevalence of bipolar disorder is approximately 0.6%. Males are affected slightly more often than females. The average age at first onset is late adolescence or early adulthood. Childhood onset is possible, but diagnosis may be difficult because of symptomatic overlap with other conditions of childhood, including attention-deficit/hyperactivity disorder. Onset in midlife to late life is also possible, although most late-onset mania is secondary to other medical conditions or drugs rather than idiopathic bipolar disorder.

PATHOBIOLOGY

Even though the pathogenesis of bipolar disorder remains unclear, genetic factors play a greater role than in unipolar depressive conditions. Heritability has been traced to several specific loci in rare families, but genetic screening is not yet clinically useful, and the gene associations have to date revealed no unifying pathophysiologic themes. Most cases of bipolar disorder are polygenic and multifactorial, with genetic factors accounting for approximately 50% of the risk for the disorder. Dysregulation of the frontostriatal systems is probably involved in the manifestations of the illness. Though not specific enough to be diagnostic, structural neuroimaging studies show increased ventricular-brain ratios suggestive of parenchymal atrophy. Phase advance of central circadian rhythms can precipitate episodes of mania, so the decreased sleep need of persons with incipient mania may produce a vicious cycle in which phase-advanced circadian cycles lead to a further decreased need for sleep, thereby resulting in further phase advancement. Psychosocial stressors also often play a role in precipitating episodes of both mania and depression.

CLINICAL MANIFESTATIONS AND DIAGNOSIS

The symptoms of mania include a distinct period of abnormally and persistently elevated (euphoric) or irritable mood; goal-directed hyperactivity, often for pleasurable activities, with poor judgment that leads to long-lasting adverse financial, psychosocial, or medical consequences (e.g., sprees of

TABLE 397-5 COMMONLY USED ANTIDEPRESSANT MEDICATIONS*

NAME OF CLASS/ SPECIFIC MEDICATION	IMMEDIATE MECHANISM OF ACTION	INITIAL ADULT DOSE	TARGET ADULT DOSE RANGE[†]	SIDE EFFECTS	COMMENTS
SSRIs (selective serotonin reuptake inhibitors)	Inhibit presynaptic reuptake of serotonin			Nausea, diarrhea, sexual dysfunction, serotonin syndrome	
Citalopram		20 mg daily	20-40 mg daily (maximum 20 mg daily in patients age > 60 yr)	Risk of QTc prolongation/ torsade de pointes in at-risk patients	Few drug-drug interactions
Escitalopram		10 mg daily	10-20 mg daily		Enantiomer of citalopram
Fluoxetine		20 mg daily	20-40 mg daily (depression), up to 80 mg daily (OCD)		Long half-life; tends to be activating
Paroxetine		20 mg daily	20-50 mg daily	Anticholinergic effects	Tends to be sedating
Sertraline		25-50 mg daily	50-200 mg daily		Few drug-drug interactions
SNRIs (serotonin and norepinephrine reuptake inhibitors)	Inhibit presynaptic reuptake of serotonin and norepinephrine			Nausea, diarrhea, serotonin syndrome, sinus tachycardia, mild elevation in blood pressure, tremor	
Duloxetine		30-60 mg daily	30-60 mg daily on a twice-daily schedule, maximum of 120 mg/day		
Venlafaxine		37.5 mg bid	150-375 mg/day on bid schedule		XR form allows once-daily dosing
Desvenlafaxine		50 mg daily	50 mg daily, maximum of 100 mg ER daily		Metabolite of venlafaxine
TCAs (tricyclic antidepressants)	Inhibit presynaptic reuptake of serotonin and norepinephrine (in varying proportions depending on the specific TCA)			Anticholinergic effects, sedation, orthostatic hypotension, tremor, cardiac conduction delays, ventricular arrhythmias	
Amitriptyline		25-75 mg qhs	150-300 mg qhs		Strongly anticholinergic and sedating; aim for combined amitriptyline/nortriptyline blood level of 120-250 ng/mL
Desipramine		25-75 mg daily	150-300 mg daily		Aim for blood level of 115-250 ng/mL
Doxepin		25-75 mg qhs	150-300 mg qhs		Strongly sedating
Imipramine		25-75 mg daily	150-300 mg daily		Strongly anticholinergic; aim for combined imipramine/ desipramine blood level of 180-350 ng/mL
Nortriptyline		25-50 mg qhs	50-150 mg qhs		Aim for blood level of 50-150 ng/mL; least anticholinergic of the TCAs
MAOIs (monoamine oxidase inhibitors)	Inhibit monoamine oxidase, the enzyme that catalyzes oxidative metabolism of monoamine neurotransmitters			Need for tyramine-free diet to avoid sympathomimetic (hypertensive) crisis; sedation, anticholinergic effects, tremor, orthostatic hypotension	
Isocarboxazid		10 mg bid	20-60 mg/day in bid-qid dosing		
Phenelzine		15 mg tid	45-90 mg/day in tid or qid dosing		
Selegiline	(selective MAO-B inhibitor)	5 mg bid	5 mg bid	Tyramine-free diet not required	Take with meals
Tranylcypromine		10 mg tid	30-60 mg/day in tid dosing		
Other					
Bupropion	Unknown, although it is a weak inhibitor of presynaptic reuptake of norepinephrine and dopamine	75-150 mg/ day	300-450 mg/day	Activating; risk for seizures reduced by divided dosing and careful dosage titration	Divided dosing required unless using SR or XL forms
Mirtazapine	Antagonist at α_2 and 5-HT$_2$ receptors	15 mg qhs	30-45 mg qhs; maximum of 45 mg qhs	Sedation, hyperphagia	Becomes more stimulating at higher doses
Trazodone	Inhibits presynaptic reuptake of serotonin; antagonist at 5-HT$_2$ and 5-HT$_3$ receptors	25-50 mg qhs	300-600 mg qhs for depression, 25-100 mg qhs for insomnia	Sedation, priapism	Few sexual side effects
Vilazodone	Inhibits presynaptic reuptake of serotonin; agonist at 5-HT$_{1A}$ receptors	10 mg daily	40 mg daily	Nausea, diarrhea, sexual side effects	Dosage must be increased slowly

*Patients on any of these medications must be monitored for suicidal thoughts.
[†]Target doses in the elderly may be lower.
ER = extended release; 5-HT$_2$ = 5-hydroxytryptamine; OCD = obsessive-compulsive disorder; qhs = at bedtime; SR = sustained release; XR = extended release.

TABLE 397-6 SYMPTOMS/SIGNS OF AN EPISODE OF MANIA

DIAGNOSTIC CRITERIA

A distinct period of abnormally; persistently elevated, expansive, or irritable mood; and abnormally and persistently increased goal-directed activity or energy lasting ≥ 1 week and present most of the day, nearly every day, _AND_

3 or more of the following symptoms/signs (4 or more if the mood abnormality is only irritability):

Inflated self-esteem/grandiosity
Decreased need for sleep
More talkative or pressure to keep talking
Subjective experience of racing thoughts or flight of ideas observed on examination
Distractibility
Increase in goal-directed activity or psychomotor agitation
Excessive involvement in activities with a high potential for painful consequences

MANIC SYMPTOMS/SIGNS GROUPED CONCEPTUALLY, WITH ADDITIONAL COMMON PHENOMENA

Emotional

Euphoria
Irritability
Labile affect

Ideational

Grandiosity

Somatic/Neurovegetative

Increased energy
Psychomotor agitation
Decreased need for sleep
Distractibility

Other

Goal-directed hyperactivity
Pressured speech
Impaired judgment
Flight of ideas
Psychotic symptoms (may include delusions, hallucinations, or derailment of thought processes such as loose associations)—defines the subtype "mania with psychotic features"

From _Diagnostic and Statistical Manual of Mental Disorders._ 5th ed. (DSM-5) Washington, DC: American Psychiatric Association, 2013, with permission.

spending, sexual activity, or gambling); increased energy; decreased need for sleep; pressured speech; and distractibility.[6]

As with major depression, the diagnosis is based on findings from the history and examination revealing a pattern of recurrent manic episodes (Table 397-6) that are usually interspersed with major depressive episodes and cannot be explained by other medical conditions, medications, or other substances. Although persons with bipolar disorder may become psychotic while in manic or depressed states, a history of psychotic symptoms in the absence of mania or depression indicates a diagnosis other than bipolar disorder. Manic and depressive episodes may also be seen in the course of delirium (Chapter 28) and dementia (Chapter 402), in which case the psychiatric symptoms are accompanied by the neurocognitive impairment that is the hallmark of the latter conditions.

TREATMENT   Rx

The mainstay of treatment for bipolar disorder is mood stabilizer medications to reduce the frequency and severity of recurrent manic and depressive episodes.[7] Traditional mood stabilizers with substantial evidence base to support their use include lithium (typical dose of 600 to 1500 mg/day or higher given in two or three divided doses as needed to achieve plasma levels of 0.6 to 1.2 mEq/L [up to 1.4 mEq/L in acute mania]), valproic acid (typical dose of 500 to 1500 mg/day or higher as tolerated to achieve plasma levels of 50 to 100 µg/mL), and carbamazepine (typical dose of 400 to 1200 mg/day as tolerated to achieve plasma levels of 4 to 12 µg/mL). The combination of lithium plus valproate is superior to valproate alone for prevention of relapses.[A3] A number of other anticonvulsants have been tried but generally with less empirical support for their use, although lamotrigine (starting at 25 mg/day, maximum dose of 200 mg/day, titrated slowly to minimize the risk for Stevens-Johnson syndrome) can be used for prophylaxis against depressive

episodes. Even though several second-generation antipsychotic medications have received approval by the U.S. Food and Drug Administration (FDA) for their mood-stabilizing properties, their potential to precipitate metabolic syndrome (and to a lesser extent, tardive dyskinesia) should limit their use as maintenance medications to patients for whom other mood stabilizers are inefficacious or poorly tolerated. For acute episodes of mania, second- or first-generation antipsychotics are more rapidly efficacious than mood stabilizers, with doses similar to their use for acute psychosis (see Table 397-12). For acute treatment of depressive episodes, antidepressants may be required, but they may precipitate mania. Therefore, patients should receive therapeutic doses of a mood stabilizer first, and exposure to antidepressant medication should be for the minimum dose and duration required. Electroconvulsive therapy is useful for refractory mania or depression and for patients with relative contraindications to medications, such as pregnant women. Standard psychotherapies for unipolar depression also may be used for bipolar depression. Ongoing psychotherapy may be important to encourage compliance with maintenance treatments and help patients manage psychosocial stressors, thereby minimizing their impact on precipitating mania or depression.

PROGNOSIS

Although the classically described course of bipolar disorder includes return to baseline functioning between episodes, some patients may experience frequent debilitating episodes (known as "rapid cycling," defined as four or more episodes per year), and others may experience deterioration in overall functioning over time.

OTHER MOOD DISORDERS

Although the diagnosis of chronic major depression should be made in patients with long-lasting major depressive episodes, others may have chronic (≥2 years) lower-level depressive symptoms known as persistent depressive disorder (dysthymia), a significant minority of whom will improve with a combination of antidepressant medication and psychotherapy. Other patients may have "less than major depression" of shorter duration, often referred to as "subsyndromal" or "subthreshold" depression. Growing evidence suggests that broad psychosocial interventions (e.g., bibliotherapy, social activation) may prevent progression to full-fledged major depression in such patients. Premenstrual dysphoric disorder manifests as cyclical depressive and anxiety symptoms that resolve in the week post menses and recur in the week before the onset of menses; this is the only mood disorder that may respond to brief cyclical administration of antidepressant medication.

Less severe bipolar-related disorders include bipolar II disorder, which is characterized by episodes of hypomania (i.e., low-level manic symptoms without substantial functional impairment and without psychosis) and episodes of major depression. Such patients typically seek care during depressive episodes rather than during hypomania, but antidepressant medication may worsen the manic symptoms. It is therefore imperative to ask about a history of manic or hypomanic symptoms in the evaluation of all patients with depression. Cyclothymic disorder, which includes episodes of hypomania and low-level depressive episodes, may be difficult to distinguish from the mood instability seen in "cluster B" personality disorders (see later).

ANXIETY DISORDERS

DEFINITION

The anxiety disorders (Table 397-7) are a group of conditions whose hallmark is idiopathic anxiety, typically accompanied by psychological (i.e., thought content) and somatic symptoms. Anxiety is a common accompanying symptom in many other psychiatric disorders, but the primary anxiety disorders lack the neurocognitive deficits, depressive or manic symptoms, or psychosis seen in the other disorders. Trauma-related and obsessive-compulsive disorders are now classified separately from the anxiety disorders.

EPIDEMIOLOGY

Anxiety disorders are a worldwide problem.[8] Panic disorder has a 12-month prevalence of 2 to 3%. Generalized anxiety disorder has a 12-month prevalence of approximately 3%, and the phobias collectively have a prevalence of 10 to 15% in the adult population. Clear data on incidence rates are not available. Most primary anxiety disorders have an age at first onset in adolescence through the mid-30s, with generalized anxiety disorder toward the older end of that range. Most anxiety symptoms with new onset in later life are due to mood or neurocognitive disorders or are secondary to medical illnesses or

TABLE 397-7 TYPES OF ANXIETY DISORDERS

ANXIETY DISORDER	MAJOR CLINICAL CHARACTERISTICS
Panic disorder	Recurrent unexpected panic attacks, typically with anticipatory anxiety and avoidance behavior
Generalized anxiety disorder	Excessive anxiety and worry, not meeting the criteria for other anxiety disorders, lasting ≥ 6 months
Phobias:	
Agoraphobia	Anxiety about or avoidance of places or situations from which escape might be difficult or embarrassing or in which help might not be available in the event of panic symptoms
Social phobia (social anxiety disorder)	Anxiety provoked by exposure to social situations, typically with ensuing avoidance behavior; may be generalized (i.e., in response to many interpersonal situations) or specific in response to a particular social situation (e.g., using a public restroom, public speaking)
Specific phobia	Anxiety provoked by exposure to a specific feared object or (nonsocial) situation, typically with ensuing avoidance behavior

Author summary based on categories and criteria from American Psychiatric Association. *Diagnostic and Statistical Manual of Mental Disorders.* 5th ed. (DSM-5) Washington, DC: American Psychiatric Association; 2013.

TABLE 397-8 COMMON SOMATIC MANIFESTATIONS OF ANXIETY

CARDIORESPIRATORY

Palpitations
Chest pain
Dyspnea or sensation of being smothered

GASTROINTESTINAL

Sensation of choking
Dyspepsia
Nausea
Diarrhea
Abdominal bloating or pain

GENITOURINARY

Urinary frequency or urgency

NEUROLOGIC/AUTONOMIC

Diaphoresis
Warm flushes or chills
Dizziness or presyncope
Paresthesias
Tremor
Headache

---

drugs; true late-onset primary anxiety disorders are often triggered by traumatic or other stressful life events.

PATHOBIOLOGY

Anxiety may be understood in part as inappropriate triggering of the stress response system, commonly referred to as the "fight-or-flight" response. However, it is important to recognize that the responses involve a wide range of cognitive, motor, neuroendocrine, and autonomic systems and thus are not limited to manifestations of sympathetic nervous system activity. The central nucleus of the amygdala is believed to play a crucial role in coordinating the anxiety response. The amygdala receives excitatory glutamatergic input from several cortical areas and from the thalamus, thereby allowing it to respond to a wide variety of stimuli, including sensory input from the external world, as well as stressors that are processed and recognized by cortical association areas. The amygdala in turn projects to the many brain regions that subserve the clinical manifestations of the anxiety response, in part through its direct projections to the important centers of monoaminergic systems: dopaminergic neurons of the ventral tegmental area in the midbrain, noradrenergic neurons in the locus caeruleus, and serotonergic neurons in the raphe nuclei.

From a cognitive psychology perspective, the pathogenesis of many anxiety disorders, particularly panic, may be understood as catastrophic misinterpretations of normal somatic sensations. A vulnerable individual may become aware of a normal or minimally abnormal body sensation, which is interpreted as something concerning, thereby leading to sympathetic and other autonomic arousal, which in turn leads to further somatic sensations (e.g., tachycardia, sweating) in what becomes a vicious cycle of thoughts and somatic symptoms.

CLINICAL MANIFESTATIONS

Most individuals experience one or more somatic symptoms (Table 397-8) that accompany psychic anxiety, regardless of whether the anxiety is normal or part of a pathologic condition. Such somatic symptoms may be referable to virtually every body organ system.

Many anxiety disorders include acute, discrete periods of symptoms known as panic attacks. In a panic attack, the patient experiences an abrupt surge in anxiety, fear-related thoughts, and somatic symptoms in the space of a few minutes ("crescendo onset"). The acute symptoms resolve quickly, typically within an hour or less.

Panic Disorder

Panic disorder consists of recurrent panic attacks. Although some panic attacks may be precipitated by situations known to be stressful, at least some attacks must be unexpected ("out of the blue"). Patients also exhibit anticipatory anxiety in which they experience ongoing psychic distress by worrying about their next panic attack or the attack's effects (e.g., humiliation if the attack were to happen in public view). In addition, patients manifest

avoidance behavior by staying away from known triggers or from situations in which having a panic attack might be dangerous (e.g., driving) or particularly distressing (e.g., in public spaces). For many patients, the anticipatory anxiety and avoidance behavior may be more disabling than the panic attacks themselves. Avoidance behavior may overlap with agoraphobia, which is defined as a distressing and disabling fear of places or situations from which escape might be difficult or embarrassing or from which help might not be available in the event of panic-like symptoms. Common agoraphobic foci include being outside one's home alone, being on bridges or in tunnels, traveling by vehicle, or being in crowds or lines. A third or more of patients with panic disorder have comorbid agoraphobia, whereas others have agoraphobia alone or comorbid with other conditions.

Generalized Anxiety Disorder

This more heterogeneous condition is defined by the presence of clinically significant anxiety and associated somatic symptoms for 6 or more months. Generalized anxiety disorder is often "trumped" in the diagnostic hierarchy by other conditions that produce anxiety.

Phobias

The phobias are a group of conditions defined by the consistent ability of a specific environmental stimulus to elicit a pathologic anxiety response. Exposure to such a stimulus nearly always produces this response, so the patient avoids the stimulus whenever possible or endures the stimulus with considerable distress. In addition to agoraphobia, the other main types of phobias are social phobia (social anxiety disorder) and specific phobias (see Table 397-7).

DIAGNOSIS

Diagnosis of anxiety disorders must rest on consideration of both syndromic and etiologic perspectives.[9] From a syndromic perspective, a careful history and mental status examination are required to determine the pattern of anxiety and associated symptoms and to determine whether the phenomenology fits the pattern for any of the anxiety disorders as described earlier. The history and mental status examination must also assess for the presence of any other psychiatric disorder that might truly be comorbid with the anxiety disorder but might also supersede the anxiety disorder in the diagnostic hierarchy. For example, generalized anxiety may be seen as part of neurocognitive disorders (delirium or dementia), depressive or bipolar disorders, and psychotic disorders.

From an etiologic perspective, it is important to determine whether the anxiety disorder is primary (idiopathic) or secondary to a systemic or neurologic condition (see Table 397-1), drug intoxication, or withdrawal state. The evaluation should include laboratory tests (e.g., toxic drug screen) as guided by the differential diagnosis generated from the clinical evaluation.

TABLE 397-9 SELECTED ANTIANXIETY AND HYPNOTIC DRUGS*

DRUG	TRADE NAME	INITIAL DOSE	TARGET DOSE RANGE†	SIDE EFFECTS	COMMENTS
Benzodiazepines				Sedation, ataxia, risk for falls	Potential for abuse/dependence
Lorazepam	Ativan	0.5 mg bid-qid	2-6 mg/day, tid-qid dosing		Reliable IM absorption
Diazepam	Valium	2-5 mg bid-tid	10-40 mg/day, bid-tid dosing		Long half-life of drug and active metabolites
Triazolam	Halcion	0.125 mg qhs	0.125-0.25 mg qhs	Rebound insomnia	Used as hypnotic
Chlordiazepoxide	Librium	5 mg bid-tid	10-40 mg/day, bid-tid dosing		Long half-life of drug and active metabolites
Temazepam	Restoril	7.5 mg qhs	7.5-30 mg qhs		Used as hypnotic
Alprazolam	Xanax	0.25 mg tid-qid	2-8 mg/day, tid-qid dosing	Possibly greater addictive potential	
Clorazepate	Tranxene	7.5-15 mg bid-tid	15-60 mg/day, bid-tid dosing		
Flurazepam	Dalmane	15-30 mg qhs	15-30 mg qhs	Daytime somnolence	Used as hypnotic
Oxazepam	Serax	10-15 mg tid-qid	10-30 mg tid-qid		
Clonazepam	Klonopin	0.5 mg bid-tid	0.5-5 mg bid-tid		Long duration of action
Zaleplon	Sonata	5-10 mg qhs	5-20 mg qhs		"Nonbenzodiazepine" hypnotic
Zolpidem	Ambien	5-10 mg qhs	5-10 mg qhs		"Nonbenzodiazepine" hypnotic
Eszopiclone	Lunesta	1-2 mg qhs	1-3 mg qhs		"Nonbenzodiazepine" hypnotic
β-Blockers					
Propranolol	Inderal	20 mg bid	Individualize, 40-120 mg/day	Bradycardia, hypotension, potential for mental slowing	Only helps with sympathetically mediated somatic symptoms of anxiety

*Antidepressants (see Table 397-5) are often first-line agents of choice for primary anxiety disorders.
†Target doses in the elderly may be lower.
qhs = at bedtime.

TREATMENT Rx

Empirical evidence from controlled trials demonstrates the efficacy of cognitive-behavioral psychotherapies for most of the anxiety disorders.[A9] Such therapies, which use the principles of learning theory to extinguish unhelpful behavior and positively reinforce more functional behavior, help the patient learn to identify and correct the dysfunctional patterns of thinking ("automatic thoughts") that underlie or trigger the cognitive-physiologic cascade of pathologic anxiety responses. Cognitive behavioral therapy may be used as sole therapy, particularly for specific phobias, or in combination with pharmacotherapy. Frequently, cognitive behavioral therapy may be administered as part of family therapy (e.g., to help family members avoid behavior that inadvertently reinforces the patient's symptoms) or in group therapy settings.

Although anxiolytic drugs such as the benzodiazepines (Table 397-9) will usually relieve acute anxiety symptoms, concerns about their long-term efficacy and side effects (e.g., risk for abuse, risk for neurocognitive impairment or falls) make antidepressant medications the more attractive pharmacologic agents for most anxiety disorders (see Table 397-5). Most antidepressants, with the probable exception of bupropion, are helpful for panic disorder, generalized anxiety disorder, and social phobia.

PROGNOSIS

In general, most persons with ongoing anxiety disorders tend to have a chronic course of waxing and waning symptoms. Maintenance therapies should often be used for patients with more chronic anxiety disorders, although evidence to support long-term therapies is not as robust as for mood and psychotic disorders.

Obsessive-Compulsive Disorder

The fifth edition of the *Diagnostic and Statistical Manual of Mental Disorders* (DSM-5) has created a new category of "Obsessive-Compulsive and Related Disorders" in recognition that obsessive-compulsive disorder (OCD) has a distinct pathogenesis from other anxiety disorders. OCD is likely related to other conditions such as body dysmorphic disorder, hoarding disorder, trichotillomania (hair-pulling), and excoriation (skin-picking) disorder.

Patients with OCD have recurrent obsessions or compulsions (Table 397-10), and most patients have both.[10] OCD should not be confused with obsessive-compulsive personality traits or disorder, described later under "Personality Disorders." Obsessions, not to be confused with obsessing (ruminating) on a topic, are recurrent, persistent, and typically distressing thoughts that at some point during the course of the disorder are experienced as intrusive and unwanted. The latter quality may be described in language such as "I don't know where this thought comes from" or "I don't know why I have this thought, I would never actually do such a thing!" Compulsions are repetitive behaviors or mental acts the individual feels

TABLE 397-10 COMMON TYPES OF OBSESSIONS AND COMPULSIONS IN OBSESSIVE-COMPULSIVE DISORDER

OBSESSIONS

Aggressive (fears of harming self or others, of blurting out obscenities, or of other unwanted aggressive acts; unwanted violent or horrific images)
Contamination (concerns about dirt, germs, body waste or secretions, environmental contaminants, or animals/insects)
Sexual (concerns about unwanted sexual images or impulses)
Hoarding/saving
Religious (scrupulosity) (excessive concerns about sacrilege, blasphemy, right/wrong, morality)
Need for symmetry/exactness
Somatic (excessive concern about illness, body part, or appearance)

COMPULSIONS

Cleaning/washing (excessive or ritualized handwashing, showering, or other grooming)
Checking (checking locks, stove, appliances; checking body in relation to somatic obsessions; checking that did not or will not harm self or others)
Repeating rituals (rereading or rewriting; routine activities such as going through a door or arising from a chair)
Counting
Ordering/arranging
Hoarding/saving

Adapted from Goodman WK, Price LH, Rasmussen SA, et al. The Yale-Brown Obsessive Compulsive Scale. I. Development, use, and reliability. *Arch Gen Psychiatry.* 1989;46:1006-1011.

driven to perform in response to an obsession or according to rigid rules. For example, compulsive handwashing may relate to obsessional thoughts about germs or contamination. Patients with OCD typically attempt to ignore, suppress, or neutralize their obsessions, but doing so causes great psychic distress. OCD patients may spend many hours per day related to their obsessions and compulsions.

The 12-month prevalence of OCD is approximately 1%, with onset typically in childhood, adolescence, or young adulthood. Remission rates are low in adults, with most persons experiencing a chronic waxing and waning course. Pathogenesis probably involves altered functioning of the striatofrontal systems, as well as a prominent role for central serotonergic systems. Obsessions and compulsions may represent inappropriate triggering of neural "scripts" involving thoughts and behaviors that have been analogized to the scripts involved in animal grooming and other complex but stereotypical behaviors.

The only efficacious antidepressants in OCD are those with strong activity on serotonergic systems, such as the selective serotonin reuptake inhibitors and the tricyclic compound clomipramine. Cognitive-behavioral therapies also have well-demonstrated efficacy. Deep brain stimulation (DBS)[11] targeting the ventral capsule/ventral striatum is FDA approved (as a humanitarian device exemption) for severe treatment-refractory OCD. Although early studies are relatively encouraging, the role of DBS in clinical practice remains to be defined.

Acute Stress Disorder and Post-traumatic Stress Disorder

Acute stress disorder and post-traumatic stress disorder (PTSD) are specific manifestations of symptoms referable to an extremely traumatic event. The event by definition must involve exposure to actual or threatened death, serious injury, or sexual violence, as reported directly by the patient or by family members or friends. Patients suffer from repeated or extreme exposure to aversive details of the event. It is important to recognize that acute stress disorder or PTSD does not develop in all individuals exposed to a common traumatic event (e.g., a natural or man-made disaster). Some individuals may instead develop other anxiety disorders, major depression, mania, or psychosis, and diagnosable psychopathology may never develop at all in some or many others.

PTSD symptoms by definition persist for more than 1 month after the traumatic event and include the following types of clinical phenomena: (1) intrusion, such as intrusive memories, dreams, flashbacks, or intensely distressing psychological or physiologic responses to reminders of the trauma; (2) avoidance of distressing memories or external reminders of the trauma; (3) negative cognitions and mood, such as amnesia for aspects of the event, negativistic thoughts about oneself in general or blame related to the event, persistent negative emotions, diminished interests or activities, or feelings of detachment; and (4) alterations in arousal and reactivity. Acute stress disorder by definition resolves in less than 1 month, with symptoms of intrusion, avoidance, or arousal as well as negative mood or dissociative symptoms (e.g., "in a daze").

The 12-month prevalence of PTSD in the United States is about 3%, with projected lifetime risk approaching 9%. About half of adults with PTSD have complete recovery within 3 months, but PTSD may persist for many months or years. Both cognitive-behavioral and psychodynamic psychology perspectives are useful in informing psychotherapeutic treatments.[12] Antidepressants also have demonstrated efficacy in PTSD.

⬤ PSYCHOTIC DISORDERS

Psychotic symptoms, defined as a loss of reality testing, include delusions (fixed false beliefs), hallucinations (false sensory perceptions), and major derailments in thought processes (e.g., loose associations). Psychotic symptoms may be seen in the course of neurocognitive, secondary, and mood disorders. The psychotic disorders are defined by the presence of psychotic symptoms in the absence of prominent mood disturbance, or of neurocognitive deficits at the level seen in delirium or dementia. In general, the diagnosis and treatment of patients with psychotic disorders should be conducted in mental health specialty settings, but primary care settings are common points of entry to care.

Schizophrenia

DEFINITION AND EPIDEMIOLOGY

Schizophrenia, the prototypical psychotic disorder, necessarily includes symptoms of psychosis ("positive" symptoms) and also often includes "negative symptoms" such as affective flattening, abulia, apathy, and social withdrawal. The level of functioning is impaired in one or more realms (e.g., occupational, interpersonal, or self-care). The lifetime prevalence of schizophrenia is slightly less than 1%, and its chronic debilitating course takes a considerable toll on patients, families, and society. Peak onset is in late adolescence to young adulthood, slightly younger for males than females. The annual incidence is approximately 15 per 100,000, but with marked variability across study samples and populations. When narrowly defined as above, the condition is slightly more common in males than in females.

PATHOBIOLOGY

The pathogenesis of schizophrenia remains unknown. Twin studies show that the disease is multifactorial. Genetic factors account for up to 50% of the risk, and multiple gene loci appear to be involved. Studies of postmortem brains indicate a nongliotic neuropathologic process with subtle disruptions of cortical cytoarchitecture. It is likely that psychosocial factors and neurodevelopment interact with a nonlocalizable brain "lesion" that is either present at birth or acquired early in life. The dopaminergic mesocortical and mesolimbic pathways are important in the production of psychotic symptoms.

TABLE 397-11	SYMPTOMS AND SIGNS OF MAJOR PSYCHOTIC DISORDERS

SCHIZOPHRENIA

Delusions
Hallucinations
Disorganized speech (i.e., thought process derailments)
Grossly disorganized or catatonic behavior
Negative symptoms: affective flattening, alogia, avolition
Major impairment in social or occupational functioning
Duration of at least 6 months

SCHIZOAFFECTIVE DISORDER

During the course of illness, at least one episode of schizophrenia-like psychotic symptoms *PLUS* a mood syndrome (either major depression or mania) *AND*
During the course of illness, at least 2 weeks of schizophrenia-like psychotic symptoms *in the absence of* a mood syndrome

DELUSIONAL DISORDER

One or more delusions for at least 1 month, most often nonbizarre (i.e., potentially plausible, such as delusions of being followed, poisoned, infected, loved at a distance, deceived by a spouse or lover, or having a disease)
Not meeting full criteria for an acute episode of schizophrenia
Functioning *not* markedly impaired other than as related to the impact of the delusion(s) and its ramifications

Based on criteria from American Psychiatric Association. *Diagnostic and Statistical Manual of Mental Disorders.* 5th ed. (DSM-5) Washington, DC: American Psychiatric Association; 2013.

DIAGNOSIS

The diagnosis of schizophrenia is based on the presence of delusions, hallucinations, and disorganized speech and behavior, often accompanied by apathy and social withdrawal and resulting in major impairment in functioning for at least 6 months (Table 397-11). In patients with single schizophrenia-like psychotic episodes of briefer duration, with subsequent return to asymptomatic baseline functioning, brief psychotic disorder (<1 month) or schizophreniform disorder (1 to 6 months) may be diagnosed.

TREATMENT   Rx

Antipsychotic medications (Table 397-12), often with adjunctive benzodiazepines, are used to treat acute psychotic episodes, commonly in acute inpatient settings so that the patient can be managed safely until the acute symptoms improve.[13] Although maintenance antipsychotic medications help reduce the severity and frequency of acute psychotic episodes,[A10] comprehensive psychosocial rehabilitation programs are required to help patients manage interpersonal and other stressors and to improve overall clinical outcomes. Second-generation ("atypical") antipsychotic medications have replaced first-generation antipsychotics in common U.S. practice because of their lower rates of extrapyramidal side effects, including tardive dyskinesia, although their efficacy is better than that of first-generation drugs. However, second-generation drugs contribute to the increase in obesity and metabolic syndrome in patients with chronic schizophrenia (Chapter 434). One trial found that oral long-chain ω-3 polyunsaturated fatty acids reduced the rate of onset of psychosis by more than four fifths during a 1-year follow-up of adolescents and young adults with especially high-risk profiles for incipient psychosis. Unfortunately, programs that include compulsory supervision to ensure adherence to outpatient medication regimens have not reduced subsequent readmission rates for psychotic patients.[A11]

PROGNOSIS

The prognosis of individuals with schizophrenia is often poor, with recurrent episodes of psychotic exacerbations superimposed on progressively deteriorating baseline functioning. However, antipsychotic drugs significantly reduce relapse rates at 1 year from 64 to 27%.[A12] Some patients have a more favorable course, and a small number of individuals may recover completely. Male sex, prominent negative symptoms, younger age at first onset, and enduring psychosocial stressors and family discord all predict poorer outcomes. Although many patients with schizophrenia survive into later life, overall life expectancy is shortened by at least 10 to 15 years because of poor health behaviors, higher rates of other medical disorders including metabolic syndrome, and a lifetime suicide risk of approximately 5 to 6%.

TABLE 397-12   COMMONLY USED ANTIPSYCHOTIC MEDICATIONS

DRUG NAME	INITIAL DOSE FOR PSYCHOSIS IN SCHIZOPHRENIA*	TARGET DOSE FOR PSYCHOSIS IN SCHIZOPHRENIA†	SIDE EFFECTS	CHLORPROMAZINE DOSAGE EQUIVALENCE (FIRST-GENERATION DRUGS ONLY)/ OTHER COMMENTS
First-generation drugs			Low-potency drugs: anticholinergic effects, orthostatic hypotension, prolongation of QT interval, cholestatic jaundice High-potency drugs: extrapyramidal side effects (dystonias, akathisia, parkinsonism, neuroleptic malignant syndrome), hyperprolactinemia with galactorrhea	
Chlorpromazine	100 mg daily	300-1000 mg/day, daily-bid dosing		100 mg
Thioridazine	50-100 mg daily	300-800 mg/day, daily-bid dosing	Pigmentary retinopathy at higher doses	100 mg
Thiothixene	2-5 mg daily	5-60 mg/day, daily-bid dosing		5 mg
Trifluoperazine	2-5 mg daily	5-40 mg/day, daily-bid dosing		5 mg
Perphenazine	4-8 mg daily	8-64 mg/day, daily-tid dosing		8 mg
Haloperidol	0.5-2 mg daily	2-10 mg/day (up to 40 mg/day or higher in refractory cases), daily-bid dosing		2 mg; available in depot IM form
Fluphenazine	1-2.5 mg daily	2.5-10 mg/day (up to 40 mg/day in refractory cases), daily-bid dosing		2 mg; available in depot IM form
Second-generation drugs			Metabolic syndrome, risk for stroke and mortality in older patients with dementia, QT prolongation	
Risperidone	0.5-1 mg daily-bid	2-4 mg/day, daily-bid dosing	Extrapyramidal side effects at higher doses	Available in depot IM form
Olanzapine	5 mg daily	5-10 mg daily (up to 20 mg/day in refractory cases)		
Ziprasidone	20 mg bid	20-80 mg bid		
Quetiapine	25-50 mg bid-tid	300-800 mg/day, bid-tid dosing		Extended-release form for daily dosing
Asenapine	5 mg bid	5-10 mg bid		Sublingual form only
Paliperidone	3-6 mg daily	6-12 mg daily		
Iloperidone	1 mg bid	2-12 mg daily		
Lurasidone	40 mg daily	40-160 mg daily		
Aripiprazole	10-15 mg daily	10-30 mg daily		Partial agonist/antagonist at D_2 receptors
Clozapine	12.5 mg daily-bid	300-900 mg/day, daily-bid (titrate dose slowly by 25-50 mg/day every 3-7 days)	Risk for agranulocytosis, requires ongoing monitoring of complete blood count	Efficacy superior to that of other antipsychotics, but hematologic risks and need for monitoring limit its use

*Doses for other indications, such as agitation in delirium or dementia, may be much lower.
†Target doses in the elderly may be lower.

Schizoaffective Disorder

Schizoaffective disorder is a chronic recurrent disorder with a lifetime prevalence of approximately 0.3%. It is characterized by episodes of psychosis in the absence of mania or depression, and also by mood episodes (manic or depressed) with psychotic features. As a result, the diagnosis of schizoaffective disorder requires knowledge of the patient's course over time and cannot be based on the patient's clinical findings at any one point in time. Treatment is symptomatic and involves the use of antipsychotic medications (see Table 397-12), mood stabilizers (see the Treatment box for bipolar disorders), and antidepressant medications (see Table 397-5) to target specific psychotic and mood symptoms. The outcomes of schizoaffective disorder are heterogeneous but on average intermediate between those of schizophrenia and mood disorders.

Delusional Disorder

Delusional disorders are characterized by one or more delusions in the absence of a thought process disorder, prominent hallucinations, or the negative symptoms seen in schizophrenia. The most characteristic types of delusions are potentially plausible ("nonbizarre"), such as unfounded beliefs of a partner's infidelity. Delusional disorder has a lifetime prevalence of approximately 0.2%. The pathogenesis of delusional disorder remains largely unknown. It is often only partially responsive to antipsychotic medications (see Table 397-12), but patients' functioning may be largely unimpaired if they are able, with the aid of antipsychotics and psychotherapy, to avoid acting on their delusions.

SOMATIC SYMPTOM AND RELATED DISORDERS

Formerly termed *somatoform disorders*, the somatic symptom disorders include both somatic symptoms and associated thoughts, feelings, or behaviors that are distressing and disabling (Table 397-13). Although identifiable physical disease is insufficient to explain the patient's presentation fully, in all these conditions (other than factitious disorder) the patient's distress and dysfunction are *not* consciously produced and thus are just as distressing and baffling to patients as would be similar symptoms produced by physical disease. Malingering is the conscious feigning of illness for conscious gain and is therefore not in this category; indeed, malingering is not considered to be a mental disorder at all.

TREATMENT

Management of patients with somatic symptom disorders is often difficult because physicians must simultaneously maintain an appropriate level of vigilance for undiagnosed physical illness while avoiding unnecessary tools and therapies. Keys to ongoing care include maintaining an ongoing therapeutic alliance, setting regular office visits, conveying empathy for the patient's very real distress without colluding with the patient's belief in an identifiable physical disorder, and assertively treating depression, anxiety, or other comorbid psychopathology. Antidepressant medications may benefit selected patients (e.g., some chronic pain syndromes), even in the absence of comorbid psychiatric disorders.

TABLE 397-13 SOMATIC SYMPTOM & RELATED DISORDERS

TYPE	MAIN CLINICAL MANIFESTATIONS
Somatic symptom disorder	One or more distressing somatic symptoms, together with excessive thoughts, feelings, or behaviors related to these symptoms; subsumes most of the former terms somatization disorder, pain disorder, undifferentiated somatoform disorder, and many with the former diagnosis of hypochondriasis.
Illness anxiety disorder	Illness preoccupation and excessive health-related behaviors, in the absence of or disproportionate to somatic symptoms; subsumes some patients with the former diagnosis of hypochondriasis.
Conversion disorder (functional neurologic symptom disorder)	Neurologic somatoform symptoms (other than pain) with clinical evidence incompatible with recognized neurologic or general medical conditions (e.g., paralysis, blindness, dyscoordination, convulsion-like phenomena, memory or other neurocognitive complaints)
Psychological factors affecting other medical conditions	Psychological factors adversely affecting a (non-mental disorder) medical symptom or condition by worsening the course, interfering with treatment, adding to known health risks, or influencing underlying pathophysiology
Factitious disorder (commonly called Munchausen)	Falsification of physical or psychological signs or symptoms, with health- or help-seeking behaviors, in the absence of clear external rewards

Author summary based on criteria from American Psychiatric Association. *Diagnostic and Statistical Manual of Mental Disorders*. 5th ed. (DSM-5) Washington, DC: American Psychiatric Association; 2013.

TABLE 397-14 PERSONALITY DISORDERS

TYPE OF PERSONALITY DISORDER	MAIN IDENTIFYING CHARACTERISTICS
CLUSTER A: ODD/ECCENTRIC	
Schizoid personality disorder	Detachment from social relationships, restricted emotional expression
Schizotypal personality disorder	Discomfort with close relationships, cognitive or perceptual distortions, eccentric behavior
Paranoid personality disorder	Pervasive distrust and suspiciousness of others' motives as malevolent
CLUSTER B: DRAMATIC/EMOTIONAL/ERRATIC	
Borderline personality disorder	Instability of interpersonal relationships, self-image, and affects, and marked impulsivity
Narcissistic personality disorder	Grandiosity, need for admiration, and lack of empathy
Antisocial personality disorder	Pervasive disregard for and violation of the rights of others, lack of true remorse ("conscience")
Histrionic personality disorder	Pervasive excessive emotionality (theatricality) and attention seeking
CLUSTER C: ANXIOUS/FEARFUL	
Avoidant personality disorder	Social inhibition, feelings of inadequacy, and sensitivity to negative views from others
Dependent personality disorder	Pervasive and excessive need to be taken care of, resulting in submissive and clinging behavior and fears of separation
Obsessive-compulsive personality disorder	Pervasive preoccupation with orderliness, perfectionism, and mental and interpersonal control

Author summary based on criteria from American Psychiatric Association. *Diagnostic and Statistical Manual of Mental Disorders*. 5th ed. (DSM-5) Washington, DC: American Psychiatric Association; 2013.

PERSONALITY DISORDERS

Personality is defined as the repertoire of enduring patterns of inner mental experience and behavior, including affect and impulse regulation, defense and coping mechanisms, and interpersonal relatedness.[14] Dimensional models of personality (i.e., using multiple continuous measures of constructs such as neuroticism, extraversion, and openness to experience) likely are a more accurate representation of the spectrum of human personality, but categorical diagnostic categories (i.e., personality disorders) are more useful for clinicians to determine prognosis and treatments. Personality and personality disorders are the result of complex interactions among genetic, environmental, and developmental factors. The cumulative point prevalence of all personality disorders in the general adult population is approximately 10 to 15%, with rates as high as 50% in patients receiving care in psychiatric treatment settings.

CLINICAL MANIFESTATIONS AND DIAGNOSIS

A personality disorder is diagnosed when enduring personality traits lead to pervasive (if variable) distress or dysfunction in a broad range of personal and social situations (Table 397-14). In diagnosing personality disorders, care must be taken to distinguish personality *traits*, which by definition are enduring, from time-limited *states*. Most persons can regress to more primitive personality styles not characteristic of their baseline personality traits under the influence of substantial psychosocial stressors.

TREATMENT Rx

In most circumstances, the goal is not to alter fundamental personality structure but rather to help the patient maximize use of their personality strengths (e.g., optimal defense and coping mechanisms) while minimizing the harmful effects of emotional dysregulation, dysfunctional defenses, and destructive behavior. Dialectic behavior therapy is an evidence-based, focused psychotherapy that is based on specific cognitive-behavioral techniques and has been demonstrated to reduce self-injurious behavior and suicidality in patients with borderline personality disorder.

Although pharmacotherapy is not the mainstay of treatment of most personality disorders, drugs can be useful in selected patients. Antipsychotic drugs may be used to target escalating paranoia in paranoid personality disorder or for short-term reduction in emotional and impulse regulation with a

wide range of (often cluster B, see Table 397-14) personality disorders in times of crisis. For longer-term treatment of emotional dysregulation in borderline and other cluster B personality disorders, mood stabilizers or antidepressants may be used.

SUICIDE AND EVALUATION OF SUICIDALITY

Suicide is a leading cause of death worldwide. Suicide rates in the United States average approximately 11 per 100,000 per year, with considerable variability geographically and demographically. Of all age-, gender-, and race-based demographic groups, the highest U.S. suicide rates occur in older white men, while suicide is the third leading cause of death in adolescents and young adults and the tenth leading cause of death in the population overall. Suicide attempts, which outnumber completed suicides by a factor of up to 11 : 1, lead to considerable morbidity and utilization of health care resources. Persons who attempt suicide represent an overlapping but distinct population from those who die by suicide. Nonetheless, a previous history of a suicide attempt is a powerful risk for subsequent death by suicide. Suicide attempts and verbal threats should always be evaluated carefully and never dismissed as "gestures" or "attention-seeking" behavior.

Suicide is a potentially preventable cause of death, but despite considerable research on risks for suicidal behavior, specific predictions about an individual's behavior cannot be made with certainty. Nonetheless, the linchpin of clinical evaluation is a methodical assessment of risks for suicide (Table 397-15), together with direct questioning of the patient regarding thoughts of death, dying, and suicide; specific plans (in ideation or action) for suicide; and the details of any attempts. Patients at significantly increased risk for suicide should immediately be referred for psychiatric evaluation, with emergency referral if the risk is deemed to be imminent or increasing.

WHEN TO REFER A PATIENT FOR PSYCHIATRIC EVALUATION

Clinical decisions to refer a patient for specialty psychiatric evaluation must be made on an individual basis by taking into account the patient's clinical findings, including any previous history and immediate needs, and the

TABLE 397-15   SOME IMPORTANT RISKS FOR SUICIDE AND SUICIDE ATTEMPTS

Mental disorder, particularly depression, bipolar, substance use, psychotic, and personality disorders

Other symptoms of acute psychic distress, particularly hopelessness and panic attacks

Previous history of suicide attempt

Family history of suicide or suicide attempt (and, to a lesser degree, of any mental disorder)

Family violence, including physical or sexual abuse

Access to firearms or other lethal methods

Incarceration

Exposure to suicidal behavior of others (family, peers, public figures)

Social isolation

Interpersonal discord or other psychosocial stressors

Demographic factors, including male, non-Hispanic white or American Indian/ Alaska Native race, older age

TABLE 397-16   GENERAL CONSIDERATIONS IN DECIDING TO REFER A PATIENT FOR PSYCHIATRIC SPECIALTY CARE

Diagnosis or ongoing care of severe/chronic mental disorders, including bipolar disorder, psychotic disorders such as schizophrenia, and psychotic symptoms in other disorders

Management of more severe forms of other mental disorders and those refractory to treatment, including depression, anxiety disorders, and substance use disorders

Need for safety evaluation or management, including suicidality, homicidality or other aggressivity, or inability to care for self

Diagnostic uncertainty

Psychiatric comorbid conditions complicating diagnosis or treatment, including personality and substance use disorders coexisting with other psychiatric disorders

Psychiatric-medical comorbid conditions complicating diagnosis or treatment, including management of psychiatric disorders during pregnancy

Need for expertise in psychopharmacologic treatment

Need for expertise in other somatic therapies (e.g., electroconvulsive therapy, light therapy)

Need for expertise in psychotherapy or other psychosocial interventions

clinician's own experience and expertise in assessing and managing the disorder (Table 397-16).

Grade A References

A1. Bortolotti B, Menchetti M, Bellini F, et al. Psychological interventions for major depression in primary care: a meta-analytic review of randomized controlled trials. Gen Hosp Psychiatry. 2008;30:293-302.

A2. Cuijpers P, Sijbrandij M, Koole SL, et al. Adding psychotherapy to antidepressant medication in depression and anxiety disorders: a meta-analysis. World Psychiatry. 2014;13:56-67.

A3. Cipriani A, Furukawa TA, Salanti G, et al. Comparative efficacy and acceptability of 12 new-generation antidepressants: a multiple-treatments meta-analysis. Lancet. 2009;373:746-758.

A4. Gartlehner G, Hansen RA, Morgan LC, et al. Comparative benefits and harms of second-generation antidepressants for treating major depressive disorder: an updated meta-analysis. Ann Intern Med. 2011;155:772-785.

A5. Wijkstra J, Lijmer J, Burger H, et al. Pharmacological treatment for psychotic depression. Cochrane Database Syst Rev. 2013;11:CD004044.

A6. Murrough JW, Iosifescu DV, Chang LC, et al. Antidepressant efficacy of ketamine in treatment-resistant major depression: a two-site randomized controlled trial. Am J Psychiatry. 2013;170:1134-1142.

A7. Woltmann E, Grogan-Kaylor A, Perron B, et al. Comparative effectiveness of collaborative chronic care models for mental health conditions across primary, specialty, and behavioral health care settings: systematic review and meta-analysis. Am J Psychiatry. 2012;169:790-804.

A8. BALANCE investigators and collaborators. Lithium plus valproate combination therapy versus monotherapy for relapse in bipolar I disorder (BALANCE): a randomized open-label trial. Lancet. 2010;375:385-395.

A9. Cuijpers P, Sijbrandij M, Koole S, et al. Psychological treatment of generalized anxiety disorder: a meta-analysis. Clin Psychol Rev. 2014;34:130-140.

A10. Leucht S, Cipriani A, Spineli L, et al. Comparative efficacy and tolerability of 15 antipsychotic drugs in schizophrenia: a multiple-treatments meta-analysis. Lancet. 2013;382:951-962.

A11. Burns T, Rugkasa J, Molodynski A, et al. Community treatment orders for patients with psychosis (OCTET): a randomised controlled trial. Lancet. 2013;381:1627-1633.

A12. Leucht S, Tardy M, Komossa K, et al. Antipsychotic drugs versus placebo for relapse prevention in schizophrenia: a systematic review and meta-analysis. Lancet. 2012;379:2063-2071.

GENERAL REFERENCES

For the General References and other additional features, please visit Expert Consult at https://expertconsult.inkling.com.

398

HEADACHES AND OTHER HEAD PAIN

KATHLEEN B. DIGRE

DEFINITION

Headache, which is a very common symptom, can be secondary to a serious underlying abnormality but is usually a primary headache disorder such as migraine headache, tension-type headache, cluster headache, and paroxysmal hemicrania.[1]

EPIDEMIOLOGY

About 90% of all adults experience headache at some time in their lives, and over 75% of children have complained of headaches by the age of 15 years. In the United States, the direct and indirect costs associated with migraine are over $20 billion annually. Patients at most risk for lost days of employment are those with transformed migraine and daily headache.

In large population-based studies, the relative risk of having migraine, tension-type headaches, or cluster headaches increases up to four times if a first-degree relative has the same kind of headaches. Studies of twins, especially identical twins, also show a similar susceptibility.

PATHOBIOLOGY

Headache pain is initiated by primary trigeminal afferents that innervate the blood vessels, mucosa, muscles, and tissues. Fibers from these sources coalesce in the trigeminal ganglion, especially the first division. The trigeminal afferents terminate in the primary sensory nucleus of cranial nerve V and its spinal nucleus, which has several small subnuclei, the most important of which is the subnucleus caudalis. This subnucleus receives afferents from meningeal vessels, dura-sensitive neurons, and even the upper cervical cord and then projects them to the lateral and medial thalamus by way of the spinothalamic tract and to diencephalic and brain stem regions that are involved in the regulation of autonomic functions. Thalamic nociceptive information ascends to the sensory cortex, as well as to other areas of the brain.

Although secondary headaches may stimulate the pathway by way of processes such as inflammation and compression, primary headache disorders occur spontaneously by means of chemical mediators. The sequence of events commences with peripheral activation caused by neurogenic plasma extravasation activated spontaneously or by cortical spreading depression. The trigeminocervical complex, especially the nucleus caudalis, is then activated, and patients can experience allodynia, a condition in which a nonnoxious stimulus is sensed as painful.

Aura is defined as a focal visual, sensory, or motor neurologic disturbance that may occur with or without headache. Aura is thought to occur when cortical spreading depression causes depolarization of membranes. Both neurons and glia can cause both constriction and dilation of blood vessels. Migraine headache clearly has a genetic component. Familial hemiplegic migraine can be caused by mutations in the *CACNA1A* gene, which is located on chromosome 19p13.2-p13.1 and encodes for voltage-gated neuronal calcium channels. Mutations in the *CACNA1A* gene also cause episodic ataxia and epilepsy. Another mutation is in *ATP1A2*, also called the familial hemiplegia migraine 2 (*FHM2*) gene, which is located on chromosome 1q21-q23 and encodes for the sodium-potassium adenosine triphosphatase (Na^+,K^+-ATPase) transport protein. A third genetic locus is the *SCN1A* gene on chromosome 2q24.3, which is a voltage-gated sodium channel. In addition, many single nucleotide polymorphisms have been associated with migraine. Although there are linkages to many genetic loci for more common forms of migraine, migraine and other headaches probably have multiple gene interactions with environmental factors, and it is clear that the genetic contributions are complex.

CLINICAL MANIFESTATIONS

Patients with headache may describe the pain as throbbing, bandlike, or aching. The pain is frequently unilateral but can be bilateral. Migraine headache is often associated with nausea, vomiting, photophobia, and phonophobia. It is invariably moderate to severe and interferes with activities. Other autonomic manifestations that can accompany migraine, cluster, and other headache variants include ptosis, conjunctival injection, tearing, rhinorrhea, Horner syndrome, and facial edema. Secondary headaches sometimes may appear to be similar to tension-type or migraine headaches, but "red flags" may suggest a secondary rather than a primary headache disorder (Table 398-1). Particular attention should be paid to the sudden onset of severe headaches, which frequently have an underlying secondary cause.[2]

DIAGNOSIS

Evaluation of an individual's headache is five elements of the history. The family history helps determine whether a person has a genetic predisposition to headache. The life history of headache determines whether the headache is new or has evolved over the course of a lifetime. The attack history provides the clinical features of the headache or headaches. The medical and psychiatric history determines whether there are comorbid conditions that can cause or worsen the headache. The medication and drug history determines whether the headache could be caused by or worsened by medications or drugs the person has ingested.

Diagnosis of the type of headache is based on the type of pain, the duration of headache, and accompanying features (Table 398-2). Secondary headaches are usually due to an underlying condition such as a brain tumor (Chapter 189), increased or low intracranial pressure, sinus disease (Chapter 426), or a vascular malformation (Chapter 408); on removing the cause, the headache generally improves. Headaches that occur at a frequency of less than 15 days a month are called episodic, whereas headaches that occur more than 15 days a month are considered chronic.

The diagnostic evaluation for headache depends on the clinical findings. If there is a typical history without any reason for further diagnostic evaluation and if the findings on neurologic examination are completely normal, no further evaluation is needed. The features of the history that are most likely to predict migraine headache without a secondary disorder include a pulsating quality, duration of 4 to 72 hours, unilateral location, nausea, and disabling nature. However, if there are atypical features of the history or any abnormality on neurologic examination, further evaluation is indicated. Patients with cluster headache types and headaches of undetermined cause need imaging to exclude secondary causes.[3]

In patients with acute headache, computed tomography (CT) is best for assessing acute hemorrhage as the cause of the headache, whereas magnetic resonance imaging (MRI) is best for assessing most persistent headaches to look for mass lesions, evidence of intracranial hypertension or hypotension, hemosiderin (old hemorrhage), and congenital abnormalities (e.g., Chiari malformation). In individuals older than 60 years with an unexplained new or unusual headache, the erythrocyte sedimentation rate (ESR) and/or C-reactive protein (CRP) level should be measured to evaluate for giant cell arteritis (Chapter 78). Cerebrospinal fluid (CSF) analysis, including opening pressure, protein, glucose, cells, culture, and cytology, is indicated in patients with suspected intracranial hypertension or meningitis.

TREATMENT   Rx

Treatment of acute headache depends on the type and severity of the headache. For mild headaches, simple analgesics such as acetaminophen[A1] (500 to 1000 mg), acetaminophen with caffeine,[A2] aspirin (250 to 1000 mg),[A3] and nonsteroidal anti-inflammatory drugs[A4] (NSAIDs, e.g., ibuprofen, 400 to 800 mg; naproxen sodium, 220 to 500 mg) will suffice.

PREVENTION

Preventive medications are recommended when headaches are frequent or severe enough to interfere with quality of life. The choice of medications should be based on the type of headache (migraine, tension type), their side-effect profiles, and the patient's comorbid conditions (Table 398-3).

PROGNOSIS

The natural history of headache depends on many factors, including the type of headache, comorbid conditions that accompany the headache, and success of treatment. Risk factors for chronic headache include female sex, migraine-type headaches, frequent headaches, obesity, low education and socioeconomic level, overuse of medication, depression, anxiety, stressful life events, and sleep apnea.

TABLE 398-1	REASONS FOR FURTHER EVALUATION TO LOOK FOR SECONDARY HEADACHES

Beginning of headaches at an older age, without a previous history or a positive family history

Unexplainable and abnormal worsening of previously existing migraines

Dramatic or unusual change in character of the prodrome or the headache previously present

Headaches awakening the patient in the middle of the night (except for a cluster headache)

Headaches much worse when recumbent or with coughing, sneezing, or the Valsalva maneuver

Unusually severe headache of sudden onset ("worst headache of my life")

Focal deficits that do not disappear after the headache is over

Any abnormal neurologic or new psychiatric finding on examination

A new headache in a patient with human immunodeficiency virus infection, malignancy, or pregnancy

---

TABLE 398-2	DIFFERENTIAL DIAGNOSIS OF HEADACHE

HEADACHE TYPE	GENETICS	EPIDEMIOLOGY	CHARACTERISTIC FEATURES	LENGTH	ACCOMPANYING SYMPTOMS
Migraine headache	Complex genetics but usually a family history	More frequent in women	Unilateral, bilateral; throbbing; moderate to severe; worsens with activity	Hours to days	Photophobia, phonophobia, nausea and/or vomiting
Tension-type headache	Usually a family history	Equal frequency in men and women	Tight band–like pain; bilateral; pain may be mild to moderate; improves with activity	Hours to days	No nausea or vomiting; small amount of light or sound sensitivity, but not both
Cluster headache	May have a family history	More frequent in men	Unilateral severe pain in the face	Minutes to hours	Ipsilateral ptosis, miosis, rhinorrhea, eyelid edema, tearing
Paroxysmal hemicrania	Usually no family history	More frequent in women	Unilateral pain in the face	Minutes	Ipsilateral ptosis, miosis, rhinorrhea, eyelid edema, tearing; responds to indomethacin
Short unilateral headache with conjunctival injection, tearing	No family history	More frequent in men	Unilateral eye pain; orbit pain	Seconds to 240 seconds	Conjunctival injection, tearing
Hemicrania continua	No family history	More frequent in women	Unilateral continuous headache with episodic stabbing pains	Continuous	Ipsilateral autonomic features: ptosis, miosis, rhinorrhea, eyelid edema, tearing

TABLE 398-3 PREVENTIVE MEDICATIONS FOR HEADACHE

DRUG	RATIONAL USE	DOSAGE	SIDE EFFECTS	CONTRAINDICATIONS/CAUTION
β-Blockers (e.g., propranolol, nadolol, timolol)	Migraine, anyone with elevated blood pressure	20-80 mg; may increase	Lethargy, depression	Asthma, low blood pressure
Calcium-channel antagonists: verapamil, amlodipine	Cluster headache, elevated blood pressure	Verapamil, 120 to 480 mg/day	Low blood pressure	
Nonsteroidal anti-inflammatory drugs:				
naproxen, ibuprofen	Migraine, tension-type, and menstrual migraine	Naproxen, 200-600 mg/day; ibuprofen, 600-800 mg bid-tid	Gastrointestinal	Ulcers, sensitivity, allergy
Indomethacin	Paroxysmal hemicrania, hemicrania continua	25 mg tid	Gastrointestinal	Ulcers
Tricyclic antidepressants: amitriptyline, nortriptyline, imipramine	Migraine, tension-type headache, anyone with poor sleep	10-25 mg qhs; may increase	Dry mouth, orthostatic hypotension, weight gain	Sensitivity
Anticonvulsants: topiramate valproate	Migraine, cluster headache	Topiramate, 25-50 mg bid; valproate, 250-500 mg bid	Topiramate: weight loss, kidney stones, intra-ocular hypertension Valproate: weight gain	Pregnancy—both U.S. FDA classification D

MIGRAINE HEADACHE

DEFINITION

Migraine is an inherited headache disorder that is typically unilateral but sometimes bilateral, moderate to severe, worsens by routine physical activity, associated with nausea and/or vomiting, and accompanied by photophobia and phonophobia. The headache occurs anytime and persists from 4 to 72 hours. It may occur with or without an aura (a focal neurologic symptom that may be visual, sensory, or motor). Visual auras may have positive (photopsias) and negative (scotomas) features.

EPIDEMIOLOGY

The prevalence of migraine is 15 to 20% in women and 4 to 7% in men. In children the prevalence may be as high as 17% and is equal in boys and girls. At puberty, the prevalence rises in girls and remains higher throughout their lifespan. The highest prevalence occurs between the ages of 25 and 55. Migraine with aura affects 5% of the adult population, and 90% of auras are visual. Migraine is more prevalent in white persons and in those with a lower socioeconomic status or income.

Comorbid conditions that may be associated with migraine headache include epilepsy, stroke, depression, anxiety, myocardial infarction, patent foramen ovale, Raynaud phenomenon, irritable bowel syndrome, and pain disorders such as fibromyalgia. Menstruation and ovulation may increase the frequency of headache.

PATHOBIOLOGY

The aura of a migraine headache is thought to be due in part to cortical spreading depression, which is associated with a brief reduction in blood flow followed by hyperemia. These changes do not seem to correlate with the phase of the headache. Pain occurs when trigeminal afferents of the dura are stimulated.

CLINICAL MANIFESTATIONS

Migraine headache often begins with a prodrome that may persist for hours to days, when patients note difficulty concentrating or fatigue without headache. An aura may or may not occur but is generally present before the headache begins. The headache may be unilateral or bilateral, throbbing, moderate to severe, and worsened with activity. Accompanying clinical features include nausea, vomiting, and sensitivity to light and sound. Other clinical features include neck pain, occasionally dizziness, osmophobia (sensitivity to odors), and difficulty thinking clearly.

The migraine aura is generally visual but can be sensory or include aphasia or vertigo. Migraine aura without headache begins with a neurologic disturbance (e.g., a visual phenomenon), but without a subsequent headache. Although an aura is traditionally thought to precede the headache, it can be present during the headache phase.

DIAGNOSIS

The diagnosis of migraine is based on the history. The differential diagnosis includes tension-type headache, but most moderate to severe headaches are migraine. In patients with a history suggestive of a secondary headache, further evaluation with MRI should be considered (see Table 398-2). However, if the headache is typical of migraine and the findings on neurologic examination are normal, no further studies are needed.

TREATMENT   Rx

Treatment of migraine is divided into treatment of the acute headache and prevention of subsequent migraine attacks. Acute treatment is most effectively accomplished with migraine-specific care: a nonspecific analgesic agent or combination analgesic therapy for milder migraine, and most frequently aggressive migraine-specific therapy for migraine (Table 398-4). For example, mild attacks can generally be treated successfully with over-the-counter analgesics such as acetaminophen (suggested dose, 650 to 1000 mg) or NSAIDs (aspirin, 900 to 1000 mg; ibuprofen, 1000 to 1200 mg; naproxen, 500 to 825 mg; or ketoprofen, 75 mg). If the migraine headaches are moderate to severe, patients benefit from migraine-specific therapies (see Table 398-4) such as triptans (sumatriptan, zolmitriptan, rizatriptan, almotriptan, naratriptan, frovatriptan, and eletriptan), ergotamine (dihydroergotamine, ergotamine tartrate), or isometheptene,[A4] and the combination of naproxen plus sumatriptan may be better than either alone[A5] (see Table 398-4).

During pregnancy, mild to moderate attacks can be treated with acetaminophen. Moderate headaches may respond to the combination of acetaminophen, isometheptene mucate (a mild vasoconstrictor, 65 mg), and dichloralphenazone (a mild sedative, 100 mg). Antinausea agents include prochlorperazine (10 to 25 mg) and metoclopramide (2.5 to 10 mg).

Stratification of care, including tailoring the treatment according to the type of headache, results in fewer days of disability and use of medications.[A6] Which migraine-specific drug will work for any individual patient depends on the patient. It is important to avoid overuse of analgesic and other medications (especially opiates) because overuse can cause chronic daily headache in susceptible individuals. Prompt treatment improves the outcome of headache when compared with late treatment. Contraindications to use of triptans (see Table 398-4) include uncontrolled hypertension, clinical evidence of ischemic heart disease, and Prinzmetal angina.

Opioids such as N-acetyl-p-aminophenol (APAP) with codeine, or butorphanol, benefit some patients, but meperidine is not effective. Oral opiates should not be used for chronic recurrent, primary headaches, although sometimes opiates (e.g., acetaminophen, 325 mg, with codeine, 30 mg) are often the only option during pregnancy or in patients with severe vascular disease. When opiates are used, caution is required, and the associated risks of rebound headache and dependency must be recognized by both the patient and physician. Barbiturates (with caffeine and aspirin) have not been efficacious in controlled trials but may be helpful in individual patients in whom other migraine-specific drugs cannot be used.

For moderate to severe attacks, options include dihydroergotamine (1 to 2 mg intranasally)[A7]; oral, intranasal, or subcutaneous administration of

TABLE 398-4 SPECIFIC TRIPTAN MEDICATIONS FOR THE TREATMENT OF ACUTE MIGRAINE

	SUMATRIPTAN	ZOLMITRIPTAN	NARATRIPTAN	RIZATRIPTAN	ALMOTRIPTAN	FROVATRIPTAN	ELETRIPTAN
Trade name	Imitrex	Zomig	Amerge	Maxalt	Axert	Frova	Relpax
Forms	SC, nasal (NS), oral	Oral: tablet/ZMT, NS	Oral	Oral: tablet/MLT	Oral	Oral	Oral
Dose	Oral: 50-100 mg (200 mg/24 hr max.) SC: 4-6 mg (12 mg/ 24 hr max.) NS: 5-20 mg (40 mg/ 24 hr max.)	2.5-5 mg (10 mg/ 24 hr max.) 5 mg (10 mg/ 24 hr max.)	1-2.5 mg (5 mg/ 24 hr max.)	5-10 mg (30 mg/ 24 hr max.)	6.25-12.5 mg (25 mg/24 hr max.)	2.5 mg (7.5 mg/24 hr max.)	20-40 mg (80 mg/ 24 hr max.)
Half-life	2-3 hr	3-4 hr	6-8 hr	2-3 hr	3-4 hr	26 hr	4-6 hr
Crosses blood-brain barrier	–	+	+	+	+	+	+
Use with monoamine oxidase inhibitor (MAOI)	–	–	+	–	+	+	–
Good for recurrences	–	–	+	–	–	+	–
Rapid response	SC, 10-15 min NS, 15-20 min Oral, 30 min	30 min	1-4 hr	30 min	60 min	1-4 hr	20-30 min
Menstrual migraine	+	+	+	+	+	+	+
Other	Now in combination with naproxen (Treximet)			Decrease dose by half with propranolol			Do not use with CYP3A4 drugs (ketoconazole and some macrolide antibiotics)

NS = nasal spray; SC = subcutaneous.

sumatriptan (25 to 100 mg orally, 20 mg intranasally, or 4 to 6 mg subcutaneously); or other triptans (e.g., naratriptan, 2.5 mg; zolmitriptan, 5 mg; rizatriptan, 10 mg; eletriptan, 40 mg; frovatriptan, 2.5 mg; or almotriptan, 12.5 mg).[A8] Ergotamine (2 mg sublingually or 1 to 2 mg orally), when given early in the migraine attack, can be effective if the associated nausea and peripheral vasoconstriction are tolerable.

For very severe attacks, dihydroergotamine (1 mg subcutaneously or 0.5 to 1 mg intravenously) is usually effective but generally requires an antiemetic (e.g., promethazine, 25 mg) before IV use.[4,5] Ketorolac (60 mg IM or 30 mg IV), prochlorperazine (10 to 25 mg IM or 10 mg IV[A9] delivered over a 5-minute period), or metoclopramide (10 mg IV)[A10] are useful for patients who are nonresponsive or have contraindications to vasoactive abortive agents.

PREVENTION

Preventive treatment (see Table 398-3) is often recommended when the headaches interfere with activities on 3 or more days per month, the headaches are severe or prolonged, or migraine is complicated by events such as cerebral infarction.[A11] Prophylactic options include β-adrenergic blockers, calcium-channel antagonists, NSAIDs, tricyclic antidepressants, valproate,[A12] and topiramate.[A13] Topiramate, divalproex, timolol, propranolol, metoprolol, atenolol, nadolol, acebutolol, captopril, lisinopril, and candesartan reduce migraine frequency by 50% or more compared with placebo, with no statistically significant differences among them.[A14] Other alternatives include the serotonergic drug cyproheptadine (4 to 20 mg) or the monoamine oxidase inhibitor phenelzine (30 to 60 mg). Acupuncture and biofeedback have been used successfully. OnabotulinumtoxinA injection is also effective for prophylaxis of chronic migraine.[A15]

PROGNOSIS

The prognosis for patients with migraine is variable. In many patients, headaches decrease in severity with age, but migraine aura without headache becomes more frequent with older age. Modification of inciting factors such as avoiding dietary triggers (tyramine, phenylethylamine, ethanol), amelio-rating or preventing insomnia, and averting environmental triggers (light, sound, odor) may improve outcome. Migraines may become chronic, defined as more than 15 days per month, especially when associated with obesity, snoring, depression, and low socioeconomic status.[6]

TENSION-TYPE HEADACHE

DEFINITION

Tension-type headache is defined as a mild or moderate holocranial headache without nausea or vomiting. Patients may have either photophobia or phonophobia but not both, and the headache does not worsen with activity.

EPIDEMIOLOGY

The 1-year prevalence is 14 to 93 per 100,000 individuals for episodic tension-type headache and 8.1 per 100,000 for chronic tension-type headache. Tension-type headaches are more common in women than in men, regardless of age, race, and educational level. Tension-type headaches are more common in Western countries and less frequent in Asian countries, and they are more common in white persons than in African Americans.

PATHOBIOLOGY

The pathophysiology of tension-type headache is less well understood than that of the other types of headache. Myofascial tenderness is increased, especially in chronic tension-type headache. Genetic factors are uncertain. Migraine and tension-type headache often coexist. Although tension-type headaches are not due to emotion or muscle contraction, triggers of a tension-type headache are similar to those associated with migraine: stress, fatigue, and lack of sleep. Comorbid conditions in patients with tension-type headache include depression and anxiety in more than 50% of individuals.

CLINICAL MANIFESTATIONS

Tension-type headaches are usually mild to moderate in severity, and most individuals do not seek care. Tension-type headache can be episodic (occurring < 15 days per month) or chronic (occurring > 15 days per month). In many patients headaches remain episodic, but about 25% progress to chronic headache. Of the patients with chronic tension-type headache, about a quarter to a third continue as chronic, half can improve to episodic, and in about a quarter medication overuse headache can develop. Episodic tension-type headaches can last minutes, hours, or days.

DIAGNOSIS

Headaches that can be misdiagnosed as tension-type headache include migraine, hemicrania continua, new daily persistent headache, and headaches caused by brain tumors, elevated or low intracranial pressure, or giant cell arteritis. A careful history is the best way to distinguish other types of headaches.

TREATMENT   Rx

Episodic tension-type headaches are generally treated successfully[7] with acetaminophen (650 to 1000 mg) or NSAIDs (aspirin, 900 to 1000 mg; naproxen, 250 to 500 mg; ibuprofen, 200 to 800 mg; or ketoprofen, 12.5 to 75 mg). However, analgesic use for more than 3 days per week can worsen headaches and lead to medication-induced headache.

PREVENTION

Chronic tension-type headaches may benefit from prophylactic treatment with amitriptyline (starting with 10 mg at bedtime and increased slowly up to 100 mg until the patient improves or intolerable side effects develop), nortriptyline (25 to 100 mg each evening), doxepin (25 to 75 mg/day), maprotiline (10 to 25/mg/day), or fluoxetine (10 to 20 mg/day). Tricyclics are generally more efficacious than serotonin reuptake inhibitors.[A16] Muscle relaxants, physical therapy, localized botulinum toxin injection, and acupuncture can be useful.[A17]

PROGNOSIS

Tension-type headache has a variable prognosis. Adolescents with tension-type headache and two or more psychiatric factors (e.g., depression and anxiety) have a worse prognosis.

CLUSTER HEADACHE AND OTHER TRIGEMINAL AUTONOMIC CEPHALALGIAS

DEFINITION

Trigeminal autonomic cephalalgias, including cluster headaches, are unilateral headaches associated with ipsilateral autonomic features. Other trigeminal autonomic cephalalgias include paroxysmal hemicrania, which is characterized by bouts of headache that persist for 5 to 30 minutes, is generally unilateral, and usually occurs in women; they typically respond to indomethacin. Hemicrania continua, another indomethacin-responsive headache seen in both men and women, is characterized by continuous unilateral pain

and mild associated autonomic features; it frequently coexists with a form of chronic daily headache. Short unilateral neuralgiform headache with conjunctival injection and tearing is a rare trigeminal autonomic cephalalgia that occurs in men; individual headaches persist for only a short time (seconds to 2 minutes).

EPIDEMIOLOGY

Cluster headache occurs in 56 to 401 per 100,000 persons and is more frequent in men (3 : 1 to 7 : 1). Attacks usually begin between 20 and 30 years of age. Paroxysmal hemicrania occurs in 56 to 381 per 100,000 persons; it affects women more often (2 : 1) and can begin at any age but usually commences at 34 to 41 years. Short unilateral neuralgiform headache with conjunctival injection and tearing is rare, with a slight male preponderance (2 : 1).

PATHOBIOLOGY

Cluster headache may have a genetic predisposition. Imaging studies such as positron emission tomography and functional MRI show inferior posterior hypothalamic activation at the onset of cluster headache and other trigeminal autonomic cephalalgias. In addition, the trigeminovascular complex and the cranial autonomic system are activated. The pathophysiology of hemicrania continua is unknown, and there is debate whether it is associated with hypothalamic involvement or whether it resembles migraine.

CLINICAL MANIFESTATIONS

Cluster headache is almost always unilateral, rarely bilateral, and has characteristic ipsilateral autonomic features, commonly including lacrimation and conjunctival injection and occasionally nasal congestion, rhinorrhea, ptosis, miosis, flushing, and eyelid edema (Table 398-5). The location of the pain is usually behind or above the eye or in the temple but can include the forehead, cheek, teeth, or jaw. The pain reaches its maximum intensity in about 9 minutes and tends to end abruptly. Attacks occur one to eight times a day and are usually described as "boring" or "stabbing" excruciating pain that persists for 15 minutes to 2 hours. Migraine symptoms may coexist, including unilateral photophobia, phonophobia, and rarely, an aura. Unlike migraine patients, who usually try to rest, patients with cluster headaches pace and are unable to sit or lie down. Cluster headaches, often precipitated by alcohol, histamine, or nitroglycerin, have a daily periodicity and may also have a seasonal periodicity. For example, episodic cluster headache may occur annually or every 2 years, often in the same season each time. Chronic cluster headache occurs without a remission.

Paroxysmal hemicrania is pain of short duration, usually 2 to 30 minutes, and occurs unilaterally around the eye, temple, or maxillary region, sometimes precipitated by head movements. Autonomic features similar to cluster headache can occur. The usual attack rate is up to 40 episodes each day. Bouts of pain may be episodic, separated by a remission, but most patients have daily chronic paroxysmal hemicrania without a remission.

Short unilateral neuralgiform headache with conjunctival injection and tearing attacks are unilateral and consistently on the same side. Although the

TABLE 398-5 DISTINGUISHING CHARACTERISTICS OF THE TRIGEMINAL AUTONOMIC CEPHALALGIAS

CHARACTERISTIC	CLUSTER	PAROXYSMAL HEMICRANIA	HEMICRANIA CONTINUA	SHORT UNILATERAL NEURALGIFORM HEADACHE WITH CONJUNCTIVAL INJECTION AND TEARING
Sex—F:M	1:3-7	2:1	2:1	1:2
Unilateral	+	+	+	+
Attack frequency	1-8/day	1-40/day		3-200/day
Attack duration	15-80 min	2-30 min	Continuous with episodic exacerbations	5-240 sec
Autonomic features	+	+	+ with exacerbations	+
Indomethacin effect	−	+++	+++	−
Acute treatment at onset	Oxygen, sumatriptan SC, DHE nasal spray; sumatriptan or zolmitriptan nasal spray (A-level evidence)	None	None	None
Preventive medications	Verapamil, lithium, corticosteroids, anticonvulsants (A level)	Indomethacin (A level)	Indomethacin (A level)	Lamotrigine, topiramate, gabapentin (B level)

DHE = dihydroergotamine; SC = subcutaneous.

pain is excruciating, the attack is brief, usually seconds; most patients are free of pain between attacks, although a dull ache can be present. Associated autonomic features include ipsilateral conjunctival injection and tearing.

DIAGNOSIS

The diagnostic criteria for cluster headache include severe unilateral orbital, supraorbital, or temporal pain persisting for 15 to 180 minutes with at least one of the following: ipsilateral conjunctival injection or lacrimation, nasal congestion or rhinorrhea, eyelid edema, forehead and facial sweating, miosis with or without ptosis, and restlessness or agitation. Attacks occur between once and as often as eight times each day. There is no other cause of the disorder.

Paroxysmal hemicrania is defined by unilateral pain persisting for 2 to 30 minutes, about 5 times each day, with one or more autonomic features such as conjunctival injection, nasal congestion, eyelid edema, forehead and facial sweating, and miosis or ptosis (or both). Complete prevention may be achieved with indomethacin.

Hemicrania continua is a unilateral headache that occurs daily and continuously without pain-free periods; its intensity is moderate, with exacerbations of severe pain. During the exacerbations, at least one ipsilateral autonomic feature is present: conjunctival redness, lacrimation, nasal congestion, ptosis, or miosis. It responds to indomethacin.

Short unilateral neuralgiform headache with conjunctival injection and tearing is diagnosed by unilateral orbital, supraorbital, temporal stabbing pain persisting for 5 to 240 seconds at a frequency of 3 to 200 per day. It is associated with conjunctival injection and tearing.

An imaging procedure such as MRI is indicated for all patients at the onset of cluster headaches or other trigeminal autonomic cephalalgias, because they can be the result of infection (Chapters 412 to 414), vascular malformation (Chapter 408), or neoplasm, especially a pituitary tumor (Chapter 189). Other possibilities in the differential diagnosis include migraine, hypnic headache (rare short-lasting headaches exclusively during sleep in the elderly), and trigeminal neuralgia.

TREATMENT   Rx

Because the course of the headache is brief, oral medications take too long to work to be effective.[8] The use of 100% oxygen at 7 to 10 L/min for 15 to 30 minutes benefits some patients.[A18] Sumatriptan or zolmitriptan nasal spray or sumatriptan subcutaneously (4 to 6 mg) can be helpful.[A19] Dihydroergotamine can be helpful when given nasally, intramuscularly, or even intravenously. Refractory cases may respond to occipital nerve stimulation. Chronic paroxysmal hemicranias and hemicrania continua are characterized by a response to indomethacin, 25 to 50 mg three times daily. Short unilateral neuralgiform headache with conjunctival injection and tearing attacks is so brief that there are no medications to treat it acutely.

PREVENTION

Preventive medications should be started at the beginning of a cluster bout. Verapamil, 240 to 480 mg, is the drug of choice. Lithium (300 mg twice daily) is an alternative. Corticosteroids (e.g., prednisone, 40 mg/day, or dexamethasone, 4 mg twice daily for 2 weeks) act rapidly as a bridge to prevent cluster headache while other preventive medications are started. Valproic acid (500 to 1500 mg/day in divided doses), topiramate (50 to 100 mg/day), melatonin (4 mg at bedtime), and gabapentin (300 mg three times daily) are sometimes beneficial. Surgical approaches, including suboccipital steroid injections,[A20] occipital nerve stimulators, sphenopalatine ganglion stimulation, hypothalamic stimulation, and destructive procedures, are sometimes necessary for this disabling headache.

Paroxysmal hemicrania and hemicrania continua respond to daily indomethacin (25 to 50 mg three times daily). If the patient cannot tolerate indomethacin, calcium-channel blockers (e.g., verapamil, 240 to 480 mg/day) or melatonin may be helpful. Preventive treatment of short unilateral neuralgiform headache with conjunctival injection and tearing includes lamotrigine (100 to 400 mg/day), topiramate (50 to 100 mg), gabapentin (300 to 900 mg), or IV lidocaine (starting at 2 mg/minute with cardiac monitoring).[9]

Short unilateral neuralgiform headache with conjunctival injection and tearing is regarded as a more difficult headache to prevent. Lamotrigine and topiramate may be helpful.

PROGNOSIS

Cluster headache is often a lifelong problem, but remissions may persist for longer periods as the patient ages. The other trigeminal autonomic cephalalgias are probably lifelong; nevertheless, symptomatic treatment combined with preventive medications is helpful.

CHRONIC DAILY HEADACHE

DEFINITION

Though not a specific disorder, chronic daily headache, defined as a headache that is present on more than 15 days per month, is challenging for both patients and physicians. These headaches may be chronic migraine, chronic tension-type headache, new daily persistent headache, or chronic cluster headache, with or without overuse of medications.

EPIDEMIOLOGY

Up to 5% of the population suffers from chronic daily headache, most commonly chronic tension type or chronic migraine. Trigger factors such as a previous infection, mild head injury, or stressful life event are present in 40 to 60% of patients with new daily persistent headache. Risk factors for chronic daily headache include medication overuse, history of migraine headache, frequent headache, depression, female sex, obesity, snoring, stressful life events, and low educational level.

PATHOBIOLOGY

Chronic daily headache is probably related to migraine, with both central and peripheral abnormalities. Once migraine has been prolonged and headache occurs on a daily basis, allodynia, a sense that a usually nonpainful stimulus is becoming painful, often develops. Use of an opiate for more than 8 days per month, especially in men, use of barbiturates for more than 5 days per month, especially in women, or use of triptans for more than 10 to 14 days per month can often lead to chronic migraine headache or at least worsening of headaches.

CLINICAL MANIFESTATIONS

New daily persistent headache is characterized by daily occurrence, onset at specific time, and an unrelenting course. It is generally bilateral, nonpulsating, mild to moderate, and associated with features of migraine, photophobia, phonophobia, or nausea. Severe nausea or vomiting is rare. New daily persistent headache can be disabling and is difficult to treat. Chronic daily headache is often associated with profound psychiatric comorbidity, especially depression and anxiety; such psychiatric comorbidity predicts intractability.

DIAGNOSIS

Diagnosis of chronic daily headache is based on the history. It is important to identify the underlying type of primary chronic daily headache: chronic migraine, chronic tension-type headache, new daily persistent headache, or hemicrania continua. Headaches of less than 4 hours' duration can also be chronic and daily: cluster headache, paroxysmal hemicrania, hypnic headaches occurring every night (usually in the elderly), and episodic stabbing headache. It is most important to exclude secondary headaches (including post-traumatic headache), headaches associated with vascular disorders (e.g., giant cell arteritis, arteriovenous malformations, carotid and vertebral artery dissections), and headaches associated with nonvascular disorders (e.g., intracranial hypertension, intracranial hypotension, infections). MRI and laboratory studies (e.g., ESR in an elderly individual) are commonly recommended. Lumbar puncture (LP) to assess intracranial pressure may also be indicated in selected patients.

TREATMENT   Rx

The most common cause of chronic daily headache is overuse of medications, so patients must be weaned off the overused symptomatic medication. Treatment of underlying depression, anxiety, and pain may also be helpful. Occasionally, hospital admission is necessary to break the headache cycle. Acute migraine-specific treatments (see earlier), especially IV dihydroergotamine (0.5 to 2 mg), are helpful in terminating migrainous attacks.

PREVENTION

Medications that are helpful in preventing chronic daily headache include tricyclic antidepressants, selective serotonin reuptake inhibitors if patients are depressed, anticonvulsants, β-blockers, and calcium-channel blockers (see Tables 398-3 and 398-4). For hemicrania continua, indomethacin (25 to 50 mg three times daily) is the preferred treatment.

PROGNOSIS

The prognosis depends on the underlying headache diagnosis. If medication overuse is the cause and the patient is successfully detoxified, about 75% of patients improve when treated with preventive medications. Treatment may fail if the diagnosis is incorrect or because of continued overuse of medications, overuse of caffeine, lack of sleep, dietary or other life triggers, hormonal factors, or psychiatric factors. Explaining medication overuse headache to the patient, in-patient and out-patient detoxification, and multidisciplinary care treatments have been found helpful.

● SECONDARY CAUSES OF HEADACHES
Sinus Headache

Rhinosinusitis (Chapter 426) is characterized by inflammation or infection of the nasal mucosa and sinuses. The sinuses themselves are relatively insensate, but ducts, turbinates, blood vessels, and ostia are the painful structures.[10]

Headaches attributed to rhinosinusitis are frontal headaches with pain in the face, ears, or teeth. The onset of pain is simultaneous with the rhinosinusitis, and the headache and face pain resolve within 7 days after successful treatment. The diagnosis requires imaging and clinical evidence that support the diagnosis of acute rhinosinusitis. Many acute and most chronic headaches that are initially thought to result from sinus disease are found to be migraine or tension-type headache.

The headache should resolve with treatment of acute sinusitis (Chapter 426). If it does not, an underlying primary headache disorder is likely.

Temporal (Giant Cell) Arteritis

Temporal arteritis (Chapter 271) is an inflammatory process seen almost exclusively in elderly individuals. Headache, especially pain in the jaw when chewing, is one of the most common features. Its incidence is approximately 12 per 100,000 and increases with age to 51 per 100,000 in individuals older than 80. It affects women more often than men (3:1) and is more common in white individuals, especially those of Scandinavian and British descent. It is associated with polymyalgia rheumatica.

The headache has no specific feature, but the pain is usually continuous, generalized, and occasionally throbbing. The temples are generally painful, and patients complain of pain when performing certain activities of daily living, such as chewing food or combing their hair. Transient monocular blindness, permanent blindness, and diplopia can occur.

Elevation of the ESR and C-reactive protein occurs almost invariably. The diagnosis is made by finding giant cells in a temporal artery biopsy specimen. Immediate treatment with corticosteroids, sometimes before the biopsy result is available, is necessary in doses between 40 and 80 mg daily, with the dose then titrated downward while monitoring the ESR or CRP. Used early enough, corticosteroids (Chapter 271) generally prevent the complications of temporal arteritis, including blindness. The disorder can be long lasting.

Intracranial Hypertension and Pseudotumor Cerebri

Intracranial hypertension can be primary and idiopathic or secondary to cerebral venous thrombosis (Chapter 407), a mass in the brain (Chapter 189), hydrocephalus, or other intracranial processes. *Pseudotumor cerebri* is an all-encompassing term referring to increased intracranial pressure without obvious mass lesions.[11] Primary idiopathic intracranial hypertension occurs in obese women of childbearing age. Secondary pseudotumor cerebri causes a similar syndrome but is due to an offending agent such as medications (e.g., tetracycline, minocycline, lithium, vitamin A–related medications, growth hormone), endocrine disorders (e.g., parathyroid dysfunction), and sleep apnea.

Idiopathic increased intracranial pressure occurs in 1 to 2 per 100,000 individuals but in 19 to 20 per 100,000 individuals (15 to 55 years of age) who are obese. Women are affected more frequently than men (6-8:1). Onset is usually in young adulthood.

The cause of the increased pressure is either poor CSF absorption, as is thought to be the problem in idiopathic intracranial hypertension; venous hypertension, as is seen in venous thrombosis; or a mass that causes an increase in pressure. A genetic component is also likely because there are reports of the condition occurring in families.

CLINICAL MANIFESTATIONS

Idiopathic intracranial hypertension is characterized by headache in more than 90% of individuals, about 90% of whom are obese. The headache may be pulsatile and is frequently felt behind the eyes. Patients often report neck pain, upper back pain, or even radicular pain. The intensity of headache does not correlate with the height of the intracranial pressure. Pulse-synchronous tinnitus is a frequent accompaniment, as are transient visual obscurations and diplopia.

On examination, papilledema (Chapter 423, Fig. 423-27) may be found. The remainder of the general and neurologic examination is usually normal in patients with idiopathic intracranial hypertension, but abnormalities on examination may point to a secondary cause, such as underlying venous sinus thrombosis (Chapter 407), ischemic stroke, central nervous system infection (Chapters 412 and 413), or brain tumor (Chapter 189). Although idiopathic intracranial hypertension often persists for years, the condition can be self-limited. In about a third of patients, there are permanent visual sequelae related to the effect of papilledema.

DIAGNOSIS

The diagnosis of intracranial pressure is made by the symptoms and signs such as papilledema (Chapter 423, Fig. 423-27). MRI is necessary to exclude secondary causes of increased intracranial pressure. MR or CT venography is often needed to exclude venous sinus thrombosis (Chapter 407). LP must be performed unless patients have a contraindication such as an intracranial mass lesion, and CSF pressure should be measured. The diagnosis can be made if the pressure is elevated (CSF > 250 mm H_2O) and the fluid itself is normal in terms of its protein level, glucose level, and cell count. Visual fields must be examined formally because visual acuity is not affected until late in the course of the disorder.

TREATMENT   Rx

Acetazolamide (doses ranging from 500 to 4000 mg daily) combined with a weight loss program is more efficacious for individuals with idiopathic intracranial hypertension and mild to moderate visual loss than is placebo.[A21] Any underlying secondary cause should also be treated (e.g., stopping an offending medication, treatment of sleep apnea [Chapter 100]). Weight loss is beneficial in obese subjects. If visual loss progresses, surgical procedures should be considered. Optic nerve sheath fenestration allows CSF to escape through slits or windows in the orbit; sometimes the treatment of one side decreases the optic disc swelling on the other side as well. Complications include visual loss or diplopia, so visual fields must be followed carefully to anticipate and prevent visual loss. Lumbar or ventricular peritoneal diversion procedures also reduce intracranial pressure, but their complications include infection and shunt obstruction.

PROGNOSIS

The prognosis of patients with idiopathic intracranial hypertension is good with treatment, but up to a third of inadequately treated patients can experience permanent defects of visual fields or loss of visual acuity. Individuals are susceptible to recurrence if they suddenly gain weight.

Intracranial Hypotension

Intracranial hypotension (or CSF hypovolemia) causes a headache that is characteristically better when the patient is supine and worse when the patient is upright. It can be primary (spontaneous) or secondary to another underlying cause, most commonly a previous LP.[12]

Intracranial hypotension was once considered rare, but modern imaging techniques suggest an incidence of about 5 per 100,000 per year; it is slightly more common in women than men. The onset is usually at about 40 years of age, but it can occur in children and the elderly. Post-LP headaches occur more commonly but only infrequently persist.

PATHOBIOLOGY

The cause of primary intracranial hypotension is thought to be a small leak or tear in the dura, usually in the lumbar region around cystic structures called Tarlov cysts. The cause of intracranial hypotension may not be the tear itself but rather the low CSF volume and low epidural venous pressure that assists in development of the lower pressure and hence the leak. The leaks frequently occur in the thoracic and cervicothoracic junction spine. Previous trauma history is reported in only one third of cases. Genetic and connective tissue disorders (e.g., Ehlers-Danlos syndrome, Marfan syndrome [Chapter 260]) may predispose individuals to have these leaks.

CLINICAL MANIFESTATIONS

Intracranial hypotension is characterized clinically by a positional headache. The location of the pain is variable, and the most constant characteristic is the orthostatic change in the pain. If the leak is untreated for a long time, the headache may lose the orthostatic characteristic. Posterior neck pain can also occur. Changes in hearing, taste, and balance, as well as blurred vision and diplopia, can develop if hindbrain herniation occurs. If very severe hindbrain herniation occurs, changes in consciousness, subdural hygromas, ataxia, a pseudo-frontotemporal dementia can occur.

DIAGNOSIS

The diagnosis of intracranial hypotension is made by MRI showing pachymeningeal enhancement, venous engorgement, dural thickening, pituitary fossa enlargement, and herniation of the hindbrain (Fig. 398-1). Hindbrain herniation appears as a downward descent of the posterior fossa along with loss of the prechiasmatic cistern, flattening of the pons against the clivus, and descent of the cerebellar tonsils, which is often misconstrued as a Chiari I malformation. LP may also show low (<50 mm H_2O) CSF pressure, but it also may be normal. The diagnosis is most commonly made by clinical characteristics and imaging, so the decision as to whether or not to do an LP should be made on a case-by-case basis because there is at least a theoretical risk of more hindbrain herniation. The differential diagnosis includes new daily persistent headache, chronic migraine, or another secondary headache. The diagnosis is confirmed if a CSF leak is demonstrated by isotope studies, CT myelography, or MR myelography.[13]

TREATMENT AND PROGNOSIS [Rx]

For spontaneous intracranial hypotension, the recommended treatment is bed rest and an epidural blood patch (blind or directed). Treatment of CSF leaks includes bed rest, caffeine (200 to 300 mg two to three times daily), an abdominal binder wrapped around the abdomen to increase central pressure, and generous intake of oral fluids.[14] For post–dural puncture headache and most spontaneous episodes, an epidural blood patch usually improves the symptoms within days.[A22] Surgical repair is rarely required. With treatment, the symptoms and MRI findings should resolve completely. Recurrence is infrequent.

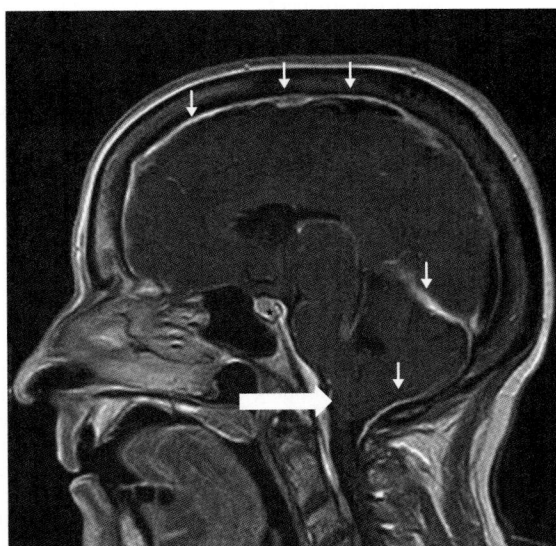

FIGURE 398-1. Intracranial hypotension. This 56-year-old woman had headaches that initially were positional. Gadolinium-enhanced magnetic resonance imaging shows characteristic findings of engorgement of the pituitary (*), slumping of the posterior fossa with tonsillar herniation (*large arrow*), and meningeal enhancement (*smaller arrows*).

Trigeminal Neuralgia

Trigeminal neuralgia is a distinct, excruciatingly painful condition provoked by sensory stimuli in the distribution of the trigeminal nerve.[15] Trigeminal neuralgia occurs in 4 per 100,000 individuals, most commonly in persons between 50 and 70 years of age and in women slightly more than in men (1.5 : 1).

In younger individuals, multiple sclerosis (Chapter 411) can be associated with the condition. In older individuals, an ectatic artery in the vertebrobasilar system often causes the syndrome. The trigeminal nerve root entry zone is thought to be the site of pathology. Either demyelination or compression of this region increases the firing of trigeminal afferents. When a specific cause can be defined, the term *symptomatic trigeminal neuralgia* is often used.

CLINICAL MANIFESTATIONS

Trigeminal neuralgia pain is characteristically sharp, lancinating (shooting), and electric shock–like in the distribution of the trigeminal nerve: cheek (V2), chin or lower teeth (V3), and around the eyes (V1). A combination of V2 and V3 is the most common. The paroxysms are brief—usually seconds but up to 2 minutes. Some patients have a dull and continuous interictal pain, whereas most have only staccato-like volleys of pain. Pain is usually triggered by stimuli such as touching the face, brushing the teeth, air moving across the face, or masticating food. Once a volley of pain is triggered, there is usually a refractory period in which pain will not occur.

DIAGNOSIS

Diagnostic criteria include paroxysmal attacks of pain persisting for a second to 2 minutes and affecting one or more divisions of the trigeminal nerve. To make the diagnosis, the pain must be intensely sharp, stabbing, or precipitated by a trigger. Each attack is stereotypical, and there are usually no other neurologic defects. Idiopathic trigeminal neuralgia by definition has no causative lesion, whereas symptomatic trigeminal neuralgia has a cause such as vascular compression of the trigeminal nerve root exit zone. The differential diagnosis includes trigeminal autonomic cephalgia, which has autonomic accompaniments that are not associated with trigeminal neuralgia. Atypical facial pain, idiopathic stabbing headache, and Tolosa-Hunt syndrome, an inflammatory syndrome of the anterior cavernous sinus, are also included in the differential. MRI is recommended to evaluate possible secondary causes of trigeminal neuralgia, such as demyelination, tumors, and vascular loops on the trigeminal nerve exit zone.

TREATMENT [Rx]

Trigeminal neuralgia is treated with medications or surgery. Carbamazepine (400 to 1200 mg) is considered the first-line agent for the neuralgia.[A23] Phenytoin (200 to 300 mg), baclofen (40 to 80 mg), clonazepam (2 to 6 mg), valproic acid (500 to 1500 mg), lamotrigine (100 to 400 mg), gabapentin (900 to 1800 mg), oxcarbazepine (300 to 1800 mg), levetiracetam 2 to 4 g), and topiramate (50 to 200 mg) are also used. Botulinum toxin may be a novel treatment for this disorder. Surgical treatments include microvascular decompression, which may alleviate the symptoms and preserve sensory function. Other treatments include partial destruction of the trigeminal nerve with heat (radio frequency lesions) or with glycerol (chemical destruction).[16]

PROGNOSIS

Patients with trigeminal neuralgia can have spontaneous or medication-induced remissions. Microvascular decompression is often curative. In patients whose pain is triggered by mastication, weight loss and inanition may develop; prompt treatment is essential.

Glossopharyngeal Neuralgia

Less common than trigeminal neuralgia, glossopharyngeal neuralgia is unilateral pain in the distribution of the glossopharyngeal and vagal nerves in the ear, jaw, throat, and base of the tongue.[17] This neuralgia is rare, with a prevalence of less than 1/100,000. The cause is thought to be compression of the glossopharyngeal nerve by blood vessels, tumor, or aneurysm and demyelination or infection.

The pains are paroxysmal and persist for less than seconds to 2 minutes, but patients can experience 30 to 40 attacks in a day. Like trigeminal neuralgia, the pain is triggered by chewing, swallowing, or talking.

The diagnosis is made clinically. MRI should be done to evaluate the glossopharyngeal nerve to exclude a tumor or vascular abnormality. The differential diagnosis includes trigeminal neuralgia, geniculate neuralgia, and atypical pain syndrome.

Pharmacologic therapy is similar to that for trigeminal neuralgia, and carbamazepine 200 to 800 mg) is usually the drug of choice. Surgical therapy and microvascular decompression or radio frequency ablation should be considered in patients whose weight loss does not respond promptly to medication.[18]

Grade A References

A1. Prior MJ, Codispoti JR, Fu M. A randomized, placebo-controlled trial of acetaminophen for treatment of migraine headache. *Headache.* 2010;50:819-833.

A2. Pini LA, Guerzoni S, Cainazzo M, et al. Comparison of tolerability and efficacy of a combination of paracetamol + caffeine and sumatriptan in the treatment of migraine attack: a randomized, double-blind, double-dummy, cross-over study. *J Headache Pain.* 2012;13:669-675.

A3. Kirthi V, Derry S, Moore RA. Aspirin with or without an antiemetic for acute migraine headaches in adults. *Cochrane Database Syst Rev.* 2013;4:CD008041.

A4. Evers S, Afra J, Frese A, et al. EFNS guideline on the drug treatment of migraine—revised report of an EFNS task force. *Eur J Neurol.* 2009;16:968-981.

A5. Law S, Derry S, Moore RA. Sumatriptan plus naproxen for acute migraine attacks in adults. *Cochrane Database Syst Rev.* 2013;10:CD008541.

A6. Lipton RB, Stewart WF, Stone AM, et al. Disability in Strategies of Care Study Group. Stratified care vs step care strategies for migraine: the Disability in Strategies of Care (DISC) Study: a randomized trial. *JAMA.* 2000;284:2599-2605.

A7. Aurora SK, Silberstein SD, Kori SH, et al. MAP0004, orally inhaled DHE: a randomized, controlled study in the acute treatment of migraine. *Headache.* 2011;51:507-517.

A8. Thorlund K, Mills EJ, Wu P, et al. Comparative efficacy of triptans for the abortive treatment of migraine: a multiple treatment comparison meta-analysis. *Cephalalgia.* 2014;34:258-267.

A9. Kostic MA, Gutierrez FJ, Rieg TS, et al. A prospective, randomized trial of intravenous prochlorperazine versus subcutaneous sumatriptan in acute migraine therapy in the emergency department. *Ann Emerg Med.* 2010;56:1-6.

A10. Friedman BW, Garber L, Yoon A, et al. Randomized trial of IV valproate vs metoclopramide vs ketorolac for acute migraine. *Neurology.* 2014;82:976-983.

A11. Silberstein SD, Holland S, Freitag F, et al. Evidence-based guideline update: pharmacologic treatment for episodic migraine prevention in adults: report of the Quality Standards Subcommittee of the American Academy of Neurology and the American Headache Society. *Neurology.* 2012;78:1337-1345.

A12. Linde M, Mulleners WM, Chronicle EP, et al. Valproate (valproic acid or sodium valproate or a combination of the two) for the prophylaxis of episodic migraine in adults. *Cochrane Database Syst Rev.* 2013;6:CD010611.

A13. Linde M, Mulleners WM, Chronicle EP, et al. Topiramate for the prophylaxis of episodic migraine in adults. *Cochrane Database Syst Rev.* 2013;6:CD010610.

A14. Shamliyan TA, Choi JY, Ramakrishnan R, et al. Preventive pharmacologic treatments for episodic migraine in adults. *J Gen Intern Med.* 2013;28:1225-1237.

A15. Aurora SK, Dodick DW, Diener HC, et al. OnabotulinumtoxinA for chronic migraine: efficacy, safety, and tolerability in patients who received all five treatment cycles in the PREEMPT clinical program. *Acta Neurol Scand.* 2014;129:61-70.

A16. Jackson JL, Shimeall W, Sessums L, et al. Tricyclic antidepressants and headaches: systematic review and meta-analysis. *BMJ.* 2010;341:c5222.

A17. Schiapparelli P, Allais G, Rolando S, et al. Acupuncture in primary headache treatment. *Neurol Sci.* 2011;32(suppl 1):S15-S18.

A18. Cohen AS, Burns B, Goadsby PJ. High-flow oxygen for treatment of cluster headache: a randomized trial. *JAMA.* 2009;302:2451-2457.

A19. Law S, Derry S, Moore RA. Triptans for acute cluster headache. *Cochrane Database Syst Rev.* 2013;7:CD008042.

A20. Leroux E, Valade D, Taifas I, et al. Suboccipital steroid injections for transitional treatment of patients with more than two cluster headache attacks per day: a randomised, double-blind, placebo-controlled trial. *Lancet Neurol.* 2011;10:891-897.

A21. Wall M, McDermott MP, Kieburtz KD, et al. Effect of acetazolamide on visual function in patients with idiopathic intracranial hypertension and mild visual loss: the idiopathic intracranial hypertension treatment trial. *JAMA.* 2014;311:1641-1651.

A22. Bradbury CL, Singh SI, Badder SR, et al. Prevention of post-dural puncture headache in parturients: a systematic review and meta-analysis. *Acta Anaesthesiol Scand.* 2013;57:417-430.

A23. Gronseth G, Cruccu G, Alksne J, et al. Practice parameter: the diagnostic evaluation and treatment of trigeminal neuralgia (an evidence-based review): report of the Quality Standards Subcommittee of the American Academy of Neurology and the European Federation of Neurological Societies. *Neurology.* 2008;71:1183-1190.

GENERAL REFERENCES

For the General References and other additional features, please visit Expert Consult at https://expertconsult.inkling.com.

399

TRAUMATIC BRAIN INJURY AND SPINAL CORD INJURY

GEOFFREY S.F. LING

EPIDEMIOLOGY

Traumatic brain injury and traumatic spinal cord injury are common preventable diseases. Approximately 1.4 million cases of traumatic brain injury are reported annually in the United States, but this number is widely recognized as a gross underestimation. Concussions and milder brain injuries occur in many millions of individuals each year. In the U.S. military alone, over 25,000 service members suffered traumatic brain injuries in 2013, of which about 85% were mild concussions. Moderate to severe traumatic brain injury results directly in about 52,000 deaths in the United States annually—almost a third of all injury-related deaths—and is the single leading cause of traumatic death and disability (Chapter 111). The majority of traumatic brain injuries are due to falls (Chapter 25), motor vehicle accidents, and assaults. An additional approximately 11,000 cases of severe spinal cord injury occur each year in the United States, resulting from of motor vehicle accidents, falls, sports-related injuries, and work-related accidents (Chapter 111). The majority of patients with traumatic brain and spinal cord injuries are young adult males.

Over the past 20 years, overall mortality associated with traumatic brain and spinal cord injuries has decreased because of prompt neurosurgical intervention, improved care in intensive care units (ICUs), and prevention of complications such as deep vein thrombosis and decubitus ulcers. The almost 5.5 million survivors of traumatic brain and spinal cord injuries in the United States often require extended rehabilitation.[1] Because the majority of these patients are young and otherwise in good physical health at the time of injury, many need chronic care for decades. Even relatively minor injury can lead to major disability. If untreated, many patients with mild to moderate traumatic brain injury continue to have residual symptoms months later, and many are unable to return to gainful employment.[2]

PATHOBIOLOGY

Traumatic injury to the central nervous system has two phases. The first is neuronal injury and occurs as a direct result of the initiating traumatic event. The second or late phase, caused by multiple neuropathologic processes, can continue for days to weeks after the initial injury.

Primary Injury Phase

The primary injury phase is immediate, and its damage, which can cause death almost instantaneously, is often complete by the time medical care can be instituted. In closed compartment injury to the head or spine, the direct impact of neuronal tissue against the bony vault and shearing of neurovascular structures result in brain damage. Because brain neuronal structures reside in a fluid-filled compartment, these structures can lag behind the bony structure as it moves during sudden stopping of the body in motion. Thus, the structures will strike both anteriorly and posteriorly against the inner bony table, and a coup-contrecoup lesion will result. If a rotational component is present, the structures will torque, twist, and shear, thereby causing diffuse axonal injury. Motor vehicle accidents are particularly injurious because of the sudden deceleration. In penetrating lesions, the moving projectile tears neural, vascular, and support structures as it traverses through the brain or spinal cord. A projectile moving at high velocity (e.g., bullet) creates a vacuum that can cause tissue cavitation in its wake. The temporary cavity, which will ultimately collapse, may be many-fold larger than that of the projectile itself. The transient expansion of surrounding tissue can cause substantial irreversible damage.

Secondary Injury Phase

The delayed secondary phase of injury, which begins immediately after the primary phase and can continue for a prolonged period, involves both neurons and glia. Most neurologic injury may be related to this secondary injury, when "neuron suicide" is caused by processes such as hypoxia, ischemia, inflammation, and the effects of free radicals, excitatory amino acids, and certain ions (e.g., calcium). The injured brain is more susceptible to hypoxic-ischemic states. The most commonly affected areas are the hippocampus and "watershed" areas. It has been hypothesized that much of the delayed neurologic compromise can be attributed to delayed ischemia.

Diffuse microvascular damage is due to early loss of cerebral vascular autoregulation and loss of integrity of the blood-brain barrier, with resulting endothelial changes such as the formation of intraluminal microvilli. Although the clinical significance of this injury is uncertain, it may play a role in the development of cerebral edema.

Diffuse axonal injury, which consists of shearing of axons in cerebral white matter, causes neurologic deficits such as nonfocal encephalopathy. The consequences of this type of injury can be delayed for up to 12 hours after the initial trauma.

Following a single concussion, these same processes probably occur but not to the degree that they cause detectable permanent damage. If multiple concussions are sustained during a patient's lifetime, however, chronic traumatic encephalopathy may develop and result in dementia and other neurodegenerative disorders. One potential mechanism is an accumulation of tau proteins.

CLINICAL MANIFESTATIONS

Traumatic Brain Injury

The signs and symptoms of traumatic brain injury vary with its severity. Patients suffering from mild traumatic brain injury, oftentimes called a *mild concussion*, often experience transient loss of consciousness, headache, difficulty concentrating, anxiety, and disrupted sleep. Chronic traumatic encephalopathy can present with alterations in mood and behavior or with cognitive impairment.[3]

The clinical examination is typically normal, but detailed neuropsychological testing may reveal mild cognitive abnormalities. With moderate traumatic brain injury, patients may have an abnormal sensorium, motor and sensory involvement, and impaired language; the results of neurologic examination will be abnormal. In severe traumatic brain injury, patients are comatose; at best, they may exhibit some eye opening and decorticate or decerebrate posturing to stimulation. Traumatic brain injury may be accompanied by a transient increase in systemic arterial pressure, and some patients may become apneic.

Focal injuries cause neurologic deficits related to the site of impact. The orbitofrontal and anterior temporal lobes are most commonly affected. Extreme vigilance is needed to recognize the development of delayed hematomas and edema, which can be manifested days later.

Traumatic Spinal Cord Injury

Spinal Cord Syndromes

There are three main spinal cord syndromes: Brown-Séquard, central cord, and anterior cord syndromes. In Brown-Séquard syndrome, the deficits are referable to a lesion of a lateral half of the cord; findings consist of loss of ipsilateral motor, touch, proprioception, and vibration sensation, as well as contralateral loss of pain and temperature sensation. Central cord syndrome is manifested as bilateral loss of motor function involving the upper extremities but sparing the lower extremities and is sometimes referred to as "man in a barrel syndrome." Proximal weakness is greater than distal weakness. Pain and temperature sensation is reduced, whereas proprioception and vibration are usually spared. Anterior cord syndrome is manifested by deficits referable to bilateral anterior and lateral spinal cord columns or funiculi. There is loss of touch, pain, and temperature sensation and motor function below the level of the lesion, but the posterior column functions of proprioception and vibratory sensation remain intact.

Spinal Shock

After acute traumatic spinal cord injury, patients may suffer from spinal shock or temporary loss of spinal reflexes below the level of injury, including loss of muscle stretch reflexes, the bulbocavernosus reflex, and the anal wink. In high cervical injuries, the lower reflexes (bulbocavernosus and anal wink) may be preserved. Some patients demonstrate the Schiff-Sherrington phenomenon, in which reflexes are affected above the level of injury. Patients with spinal shock also may lose autonomic reflexes, thereby leading to neurogenic hypotension, ileus, and urinary retention.

DIAGNOSIS

Traumatic Brain Injury

Point-of-injury standardized clinical tools, such as the Standardized Assessment of Concussion (Table 399-1), can help first responders identify patients at risk of having suffered a mild traumatic brain injury or concussion. The diagnosis of traumatic brain injury is still made clinically by a physician.

For more severe injury, the Glasgow Coma Scale score (Table 399-2) should be calculated promptly, and a detailed neurologic examination should be performed to determine the extent of injury and the severity of impairment. Important clinical signs of occult injury may be revealed on a general physical examination. For example, a scalp laceration should be palpated for evidence of an underlying skull fracture. Periorbital ecchymosis ("raccoon

---

TABLE 399-1 ASSESSING BRAIN INJURY

Neurologic screening: loss of consciousness, incoordination, memory loss, blank look, facial injury

Neck examination: describe range of motion, tenderness, upper and lower limb sensation and strength

Balance examination: double leg stance, single leg stance, tandem stance

Coordination examination: finger to nose

Orientation:

What month is it?

What is the date today?

What is the day of the week?

What year is it?

What time is it right now? (within 1 hour)

Immediate memory

Word list:	Alternate lists:		
elbow	candle	baby	finger
apple	paper	monkey	penny
carpet	sugar	perfume	blanket
saddle	sandwich	sunset	lemon
bubble	wagon	iron	insect

Concentration: digits backward

4-9-3	6-2-9	5-2-6	4-1-5
3-8-1-4	3-2-7-9	1-7-9-5	4-9-6-8
6-2-9-7-1	1-5-2-8-6	3-8-5-2-7	6-1-8-4-3
7-1-8-4-6-2	5-3-9-1-4-8	8-3-1-9-6-4	7-2-4-8-5-6

Concentration: months of the year in reverse order

Delayed recall: memory (administered after physical examinations, same word list as before)

Table modified from McCrea M. Standardized mental status assessment of sports concussion. *Clin J Sport Med.* 2001;11:176-181; and SCAT3. *Br J Sports Med.* 2013;47:259.

TABLE 399-2 GLASGOW COMA SCALE SCORE

BEST EYE RESPONSE	BEST VERBAL RESPONSE	BEST MOTOR RESPONSE
1 = No eye opening	1 = No verbal response	1 = No motor response
2 = Eye opening to pain	2 = Incomprehensible sounds	2 = Extension to pain
3 = Eye opening to verbal command	3 = Inappropriate words	3 = Flexion to pain
4 = Eyes open spontaneously	4 = Confused	4 = Withdrawal from pain
	5 = Oriented	5 = Localizing pain
		6 = Obeys commands

To calculate the score, sum the numbers from each of the three columns.

TABLE 399-3 DECISION RULES FOR DETERMINING INDICATIONS FOR CT SCAN IN PATIENTS WITH MINOR HEAD INJURY

STUDY	POPULATION OF PATIENTS	INDICATIONS FOR CT SCAN	REPORTED ACCURACY (%)* SENSITIVITY	SPECIFICITY
Canadian CT Head Rule[†]	GCS score of 13-15, loss of consciousness, no neurologic deficit, age ≥ 16 yr	High-risk patients: GCS score <15 at 2 hr after injury, suspected skull fracture, any sign of basal skull fracture, vomiting (≥2 times), age ≥ 65 yr[‡]	100	69
		Medium-risk patients: retrograde amnesia > 30 min, dangerous mechanism (pedestrian vs. motor vehicle, ejection from motor vehicle, fall from height > 1 m or 5 stairs)[§]	98	50
New Orleans Criteria[§]	GCS score of 15, loss of consciousness, no neurologic deficit, no seizure, no anticoagulation, age ≥ 3 yr	Headache, vomiting, seizure, intoxication, short-term memory deficit, age > 60 yr, or injury above the clavicles	100	25

*Validity for identifying patients with traumatic CT findings.
[†]Stiell IG, Wells GA, Vandemheen K, et al. The Canadian CT Head Rule for patients with minor head injury. *Lancet.* 2001;357:1391-1396.
[‡]High-risk patients in whom a CT scan is mandatory.
[§]Medium-risk patients in whom a CT scan is recommended but close clinical observation is an alternative.
[§]Haydel MJ, Preston CA, Mills TJ, et al. Indications for computed tomography in patients with minor head injury. *N Engl J Med.* 2000;343:100-105.
CT = computed tomography; GCS = Glasgow Coma Scale.

TABLE 399-4 AMERICAN ACADEMY OF NEUROLOGY: DIAGNOSIS AND MANAGEMENT OF CONCUSSION

CRITICAL STEPS	SUPPORTING INFORMATION
Immediately remove from play or work	Adherence to state concussion laws
First responders should use a validated clinical tool to determine risk of concussion	(See Table 399-1)
Diagnosis and clinical care is made by LHCP	Clinical practice guidelines for treatment of symptoms
Return to play or work only after detailed evaluation and written authorization by LHCP	Graded physical activity that does not exacerbate symptoms
Cognitive restructuring through education, reassurance, reattribution of symptoms
Retirement from activity counseling by LHCP	Retirement counseling for patients with history of multiple concussions with subjective neurobehavioral symptoms should begin a discussion with the patient about retirement

LHCP = Licensed health care provider, an individual who has acquired knowledge and skills relevant to evaluation and management of sports concussions and is practicing within the scope of his or her training and experience.
Adapted from Giza CC, Kutcher JS, Ashwal S, et al. Summary of evidence-based guideline update: evaluation and management of concussion in sports: report of the Guideline Development Subcommittee of the American Academy of Neurology. *Neurology.* 2013;80:2250-2257.

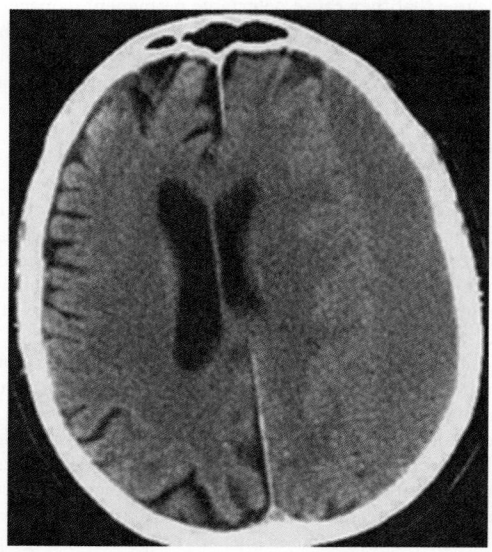

FIGURE 399-1. Subdural hematoma.

eyes") and postauricular ecchymosis ("Battle sign") suggest a basal skull fracture. A clear or blood-tinged watery discharge from the nose or ear may be a cerebrospinal fluid leak.

Intracranial bleeding caused by traumatic brain injury includes subdural hematoma, epidural hematoma, intraparenchymal hemorrhage, contusion, and traumatic subarachnoid hemorrhage (Chapter 408). The most common is subdural hematoma, which is the basis of approximately 50% of admissions for head injury. Epidural hematoma accounts for about 3%. An associated skull fracture, especially at the temporoparietal junction, increases the incidence of epidural hematoma, usually by disruption of the middle meningeal artery.

Imaging
A computed tomography (CT) scan without contrast should be obtained as soon as possible after the initial clinical assessment. The need for neuroimaging is best determined by using the Glasgow Coma Scale score and a validated clinical prediction instrument such as the Canadian CT Head Rule (Table 399-3). In any patient suspected of having suffered a head injury, the severity of the concussion should be assessed (Table 399-4). A subdural hematoma (Fig. 399-1) is blood that accumulates above the brain but below the dura; on CT imaging it appears as a crescentic or concave opacity overlying the

brain. An epidural hematoma (Fig. 399-2) is blood that accumulates below the skull but above the dura; it appears as a convex or lenticular opacity on CT imaging. Skull fractures are best diagnosed with the use of CT bone windows.

Traumatic Spinal Cord Injury
A detailed neurologic examination is needed to identify the level of the injury and the severity of any deficits, as well as to document the degree of neurologic dysfunction at the earliest time possible. The level of the injury is the lowest spinal cord segment with intact motor and sensory function. Normal neurologic findings in patients with a clear sensorium obviate the need for imaging studies. However, any complaints of pain over the spine, numbness, tingling, or weakness should raise suspicion of spinal cord injury. In particular, a complaint of "burning hands" suggests traumatic spinal cord injury.

The time of injury should be recorded as accurately as possible. The prognosis for neurologic improvement is better if the lesion is incomplete as opposed to complete. During the acute period, serial examinations must be performed frequently.

If spinal cord injury is suspected, the patient should be appropriately immobilized, such as with a rigid collar and back board. In patients who are able to cooperate with a neurologic examination, are not intoxicated, and do not have painful distracting injuries (e.g., femoral fracture, which would interfere with the leg motor and sensory examination), normal neurologic findings effectively rule out cervical spine disease.

Imaging

In patients who are alert and stable, the Canadian C-Spine Rule (Fig. 399-3) can be used to reduce unnecessary spinal imaging without any adverse effect on patients' outcomes.[A1] In other patients, the radiologic evaluation should begin with plain radiographs of the bony spine, with further neuroimaging of any abnormalities that are found. Bony vertebrae should be examined with CT, whereas the spinal cord and intervertebral and paravertebral soft tissue are best studied with MRI. A chest radiograph is usually indicated to provide images of the lower cervical and thoracic vertebrae; the presence of a pleural effusion in the setting of a possible thoracic spine injury suggests a hemothorax.

Ligamentous Injury versus Spinal Cord Injury

If plain radiographs of the cervical spine are normal but the patient still complains of neck pain, a ligamentous injury should be considered. Ligamentous injury can be evaluated by flexion-extension radiographs of the cervical spine. If pain prevents an adequate study, patients should be kept in a rigid cervical collar for 3 to 5 days until the pain and muscle spasm resolve. If studies at that time are normal, the patient will no longer require the collar. Conversely, abnormal results warrant surgical evaluation to determine whether further immobilization or surgical correction is necessary.

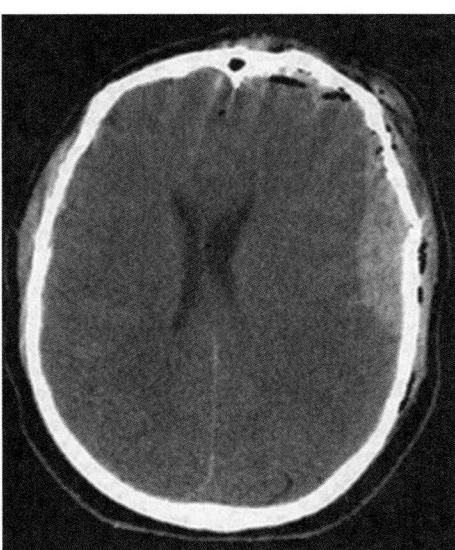

FIGURE 399-2. Epidural hematoma.

TREATMENT   Rx

The immediate goals of therapy are to arrest ongoing injury, preserve and if possible restore neurologic function, and avoid secondary medical complications. To achieve this goal, an organized team approach is essential. Despite major research efforts, current clinical treatment is largely confined to supportive measures: maintaining perfusion pressure, minimizing intracompartment hypertension (e.g., increased intracranial pressure [ICP]), and indirectly treating edema.

Traumatic Brain Injury
Initial Management

It is crucial that prehospital providers optimize perfusion and oxygenation; the duration and severity of hypoxia and hypotension in this critical early period have dramatic consequences on clinical outcome. Treatment begins with immediate attention to airway and cardiopulmonary function, early

---

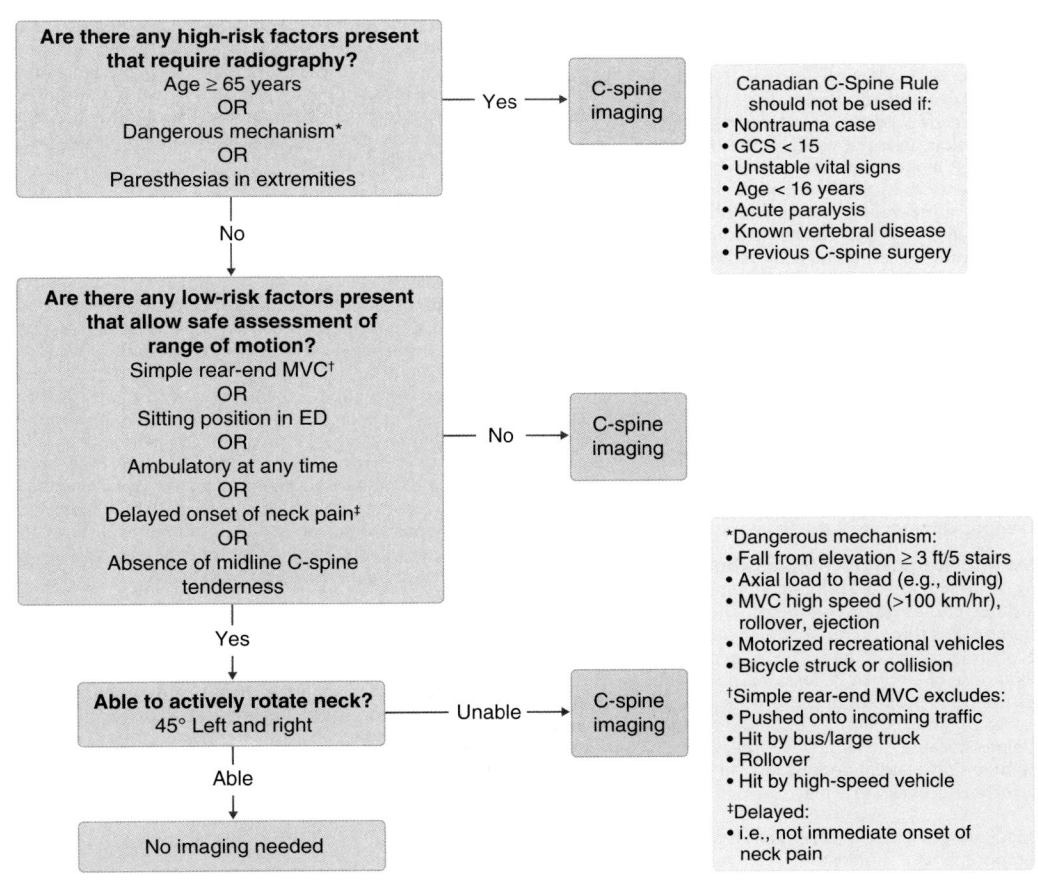

FIGURE 399-3. Canadian C-Spine Rule. For alert (Glasgow Coma Scale ≥ 15) and stable trauma patients in whom cervical spine injury is a concern. ED = emergency department; GCS = Glasgow Coma Scale (see Table 399-2); MVC = motor vehicle collision. (Modified from Stiell IG, Clement CM, McKnight RD, et al. Comparative validation of the Canadian C-Spine Rule and the NEXUS low-risk criteria in alert and stable patients. *N Engl J Med.* 2003;349:2510-2518; and Stiell IG, Wells GA, Vandemheen KL, et al. The Canadian C-Spine Rule for radiography in alert and stable trauma patients. *JAMA.* 2001;286:1841-1848).

identification of the potential for traumatic brain injury, and minimization of secondary insults such as hypoxia and ischemia.[4]

Individuals with a suspected concussion immediately should be removed from play or work[5] and by law should not return until a detailed evaluation with written authorization can be made by an appropriate and experienced physician expert.[6] Patients with mild or moderate traumatic brain injury often have returned to normal or are rapidly recovering by the time they reach advanced medical care. The critical element is the duration of altered mental status, amnesia, or loss of consciousness (see Table 399-4). Longer periods of abnormal sensorium are associated with higher grades of concussion, and higher grades of concussion necessitate longer periods of convalescence.

Severe Traumatic Brain Injury

Patients with Glasgow Coma Scale scores of 8 or less are considered to have severe traumatic brain injury. With this level of impaired consciousness, even with an intact gag reflex, patients are unable to protect their airway adequately. Intubation should be performed with either an endotracheal or a nasotracheal tube, depending on clinical circumstances. The patient should be in a rigid neck collar with the head elevated 30 degrees. The neck collar is used not only to protect the cervical spine until appropriate imaging can be performed but also to keep the head midline to avoid compromising venous drainage.

Certain lesions require prompt surgical intervention, whereas others do not. Penetrating wounds, intracerebral hemorrhage with a mass effect (including subdural and epidural blood), and bone injury (e.g., displaced fracture and vertebral subluxation) require emergency surgical evaluation for intervention. However, focal hypoxic-anoxic, diffuse axonal, and diffuse microvascular injuries do not warrant surgical intervention; treatment remains primarily with the critical care clinician. Skull fractures and intracranial hemorrhages require neurosurgical evaluation. In general, if a fracture is displaced more than the thickness of the skull, it needs to be elevated.

If a surgical lesion is not identified, the patient should be admitted to an ICU. When intracranial hypertension is suspected, a 30-mL intravenous (IV) dose of 23% hypertonic saline through a central venous catheter[A2] may be better than mannitol (at a dose of 0.5 to 1 g/kg IV) to reduce it. IV steroids are of no benefit acutely and increase mortality at 2 weeks after the injury.[A3] Continuous infusion of 3% hypertonic saline through a central venous catheter may be started at a rate of 75 to 100 mL/hour, with the goal of a serum sodium level of 150 to 155 mM/L to maintain ICP below 20 mm Hg. Hyperventilation also may be tried but has a potential to exacerbate ischemia; if used, the goal should be hyperventilation to a PCO_2 of 34 to 36 mm Hg. Induced hypothermia for traumatic brain injury remains controversial, but high-quality randomized trials show no benefit and perhaps even deleterious effects.[A4] For closed head injury, a transfusion threshold of 7 g/dL is preferable to a threshold of 10 g/dL.[A5]

In addition to ICP control, cerebral perfusion must be maintained. The goal is to maintain cerebral perfusion pressure, which is the difference between mean arterial pressure and ICP, higher than 60 mm Hg. Volume resuscitation is the first therapeutic intervention, with the aim of achieving euvolemia or only slight hypervolemia to a central venous pressure (CVP) goal of 4 to 6 mm Hg. For fluid resuscitation, saline is preferred over albumin.[A6] If a cerebral perfusion pressure above 60 mm Hg cannot be achieved with IV fluids alone, vasoactive pharmacologic agents such as norepinephrine (beginning at 2 µg/minute by continuous IV infusion) and phenylephrine (100 µg/minute) may be required. Invasive hemodynamic monitoring with an arterial pressure line and CVP catheter may be needed.

Regular neurologic examinations and appropriate brain imaging are useful to guide ongoing therapy. In one randomized trial, ICP monitoring to maintain a pressure of 20 mm Hg or less was no better than care based on imaging and clinical examination.[A7] If the patient is still at a Glasgow Coma Scale score of 8 or less, however, U.S. guidelines recommend that an ICP-monitoring device be used. An intraventricular catheter provides the most reliable data. It is also a treatment option because it allows drainage of cerebrospinal fluid. However, a subdural bolt and fiberoptic catheter are less invasive alternatives.

Pharmacologic Coma and Surgical Decompression

If ICP remains poorly controlled after the aforementioned efforts, pharmacologic coma or surgical decompression is considered. The postulated effect of pharmacologic coma on ICP is through reduction of cerebral metabolism. If the decision to use pharmacologic coma is made, pentobarbital can be administered at a loading dose of 5 mg/kg IV, followed by an infusion of 1 to 3 mg/kg/hour. Another option is propofol (loading dose of 2 mg/kg IV, followed by an infusion of up to 5 mg/kg/hour). Continuous electroencephalographic monitoring is helpful because the target response is burst suppression. Barbiturates and propofol are myocardial depressants, so aggressive cardiovascular management is often necessary to achieve the desired cerebral perfusion pressure.

Recalcitrant elevated ICP despite these interventions is an ominous sign. In such cases, bifrontotemporoparietal craniectomy can reduce ICP and the length of ICU stay but has not been shown to improve outcomes.[A8][A9]

Complications

If the patient is agitated, an evaluation should be made to determine whether the patient is in pain or poorly tolerating mechanical ventilation. If

pain is a concern, a narcotic analgesic such as fentanyl (50 to 100 µg IV) or morphine (1 to 2 mg IV) should be administered. Because these agents are easily reversed by naloxone, periodic reassessment of neurologic status can be performed. If agitation alone is the issue, haloperidol (0.5 to 2 mg IV), a nonsedating agent that still maintains the ability to perform a neurologic examination, should be considered.

The PO_2 level should be maintained at approximately 100 mm Hg. Phenytoin (loading dose of 1000 mg IV, followed by a maintenance dose of 300 mg/day IV) reduces seizures during the first week after traumatic brain injury, but its later usefulness is less clear. Fever greatly increases cerebral metabolism; antipyretic interventions such as acetaminophen and cooling blankets should be used as needed. Gastric stress ulcers may be prevented with H_2 antagonists such as ranitidine (50 mg IV three times daily) or proton pump inhibitors such as omeprazole (20 mg/day orally [PO]). Low-dose heparin (5000 units subcutaneously [SC] twice daily) or a low-molecular-weight heparin such as enoxaparin (40 mg/day SC) and pneumatic stockings should be instituted to avoid deep vein thrombosis. A nasogastric or orogastric tube should be placed for nutrition. Feeding should be initiated as soon as practical, usually on the second day after injury. Because cerebral edema is a concern, hyperosmotic feeding should be instituted. If ileus is present, total parenteral nutrition (TPN; Chapter 217) should be given.

After the first 6 to 12 hours, effort should be made to reduce hyperventilation. Otherwise, the metabolic compensation to chronic hyperventilation negates the ameliorative effects of the respiratory alkalosis.

Regular neurologic examinations and monitoring of ICP and cerebral perfusion pressure are useful to guide ongoing therapy. Generally, the peak period of cerebral edema is from 48 to 96 hours after traumatic brain injury. Thereafter, cerebral edema spontaneously resolves, often associated with clinical improvement.

Recovery

Recovering patients may experience "postconcussive syndrome," which is primarily manifested as headache. Other symptoms may include difficulty concentrating, changes in appetite, sleep abnormalities, and irritability. In general, postconcussive syndrome lasts a few weeks after injury, but it can persist beyond a year or more. Amantadine (100 mg twice daily and increasing up to 200 mg twice daily) can accelerate early recovery after severe traumatic brain injury but may not improve the ultimate outcome.[A10]

Therapies are based on the patient's symptoms.[7] For headache, nonsteroidal anti-inflammatory agents (e.g., ibuprofen, 400 to 600 mg PO), migraine drugs (e.g., sumatriptan, 25 to 50 mg PO), and biofeedback may be considered. For cognitive dysfunction, neuropsychological testing may be helpful in determining appropriate intervention. Amantadine (100 mg twice daily) is effective for reducing irritability and aggression in post-head trauma patients with normal renal function.[A11]

Traumatic Spinal Cord Injury
Initial Management

Emergency management of traumatic injury to the spinal cord begins with the basics of airway, breathing, and circulation.[8] A secure airway is essential. For patients suffering from high cervical lesions, spontaneous ventilation will be lost. Cervical lesions below C5 may also be associated with impaired ventilatory capability. If there is any concern that the airway or ventilatory effort is compromised, emergency intubation is required. In a patient in whom the cervical spine has not been imaged, the preferred method is nasotracheal intubation under fiberoptic guidance. Other approaches are nasotracheal (blind) or orotracheal intubation, provided in-line traction is applied.

Other immediate concerns are bleeding and circulation. Hypotension may be due to either neurogenic shock or hypovolemia. For neurogenic shock, vasopressive pharmacologic agents such as phenylephrine (beginning as a continuous IV infusion at 100 µg/minute with titration to clinical effect) may be needed. If tachycardia is present, hypovolemia is more likely, so fluid resuscitation would be more appropriate.

Targeted Therapy

Methylprednisolone is no longer advocated for the treatment of acute spinal cord injury. The decision for surgical intervention should be based on the stability of the anterior, middle, and posterior vertebral columns. The anterior column consists of the anterior half of the vertebral body and the vertebral disc. The middle column is the posterior half of the body and the disc. The posterior column is composed of the arch, facets, and ligaments. In general, if two of the three columns are damaged, surgical stabilization is needed. If immediate surgery is not indicated, the patient should be admitted to the ICU for further management.

Acute and Subacute Management

Patients with severe spinal cord injuries require close cardiovascular and ventilatory care, supportive care for bladder and bowel function, approaches to avoid pressure ulcers (Chapter 25), and general measures similar to those used for patients with traumatic brain injury.

Neurogenic Shock and Dysautonomia

After traumatic spinal cord injury, patients are at risk for neurogenic shock and dysautonomia. Lesions of the cervical and thoracic spine disrupt the descending sympathetic pathways to the intermediolateral cell column of the thoracolumbar spinal cord, thereby leading to peripheral vasodilation and hypotension. If the lesion is at T3 or above, sympathetic tone to the heart is compromised. In this setting, hypotension is accompanied by bradycardia, thus producing the neurogenic shock triad of bradycardia, hypotension, and peripheral vasodilation.

Initial therapy for dysautonomia should be fluid administration to restore an adequate circulating volume with a target CVP of 4 to 6 mm Hg. A hematocrit of 30 is optimal for perfusion of the central nervous system, so blood can be used if the patient is anemic. If blood is not required, either colloid (e.g., albumin solutions) or crystalloid (e.g., normal saline) may be used. If there is a suspicion of cardiac or pulmonary disease, a pulmonary artery catheter may be needed briefly to assess fluid status and the relationship between pulmonary pressure and CVP.

Once adequate circulating volume has been achieved, hypotension should be managed with vasopressive agents such as phenylephrine (see earlier), norepinephrine (see earlier), or dopamine (beginning at 1 μg/kg/minute by continuous IV infusion) (Chapter 106), with the goal of a mean arterial pressure of 85 mm Hg or greater. Symptomatic bradycardia can be treated with atropine (1 mg IV).

Ventilatory Compromise

An injury at C5 or higher results in diaphragmatic denervation and requires complete ventilatory assistance.[9] Proper management requires endotracheal or nasotracheal intubation and mechanical ventilation, with an appropriate tidal volume (6 to 10 mL/kg), an FIO_2 to achieve a PO_2 between 80 and 100 mm Hg, and a rate to give a PCO_2 of 40 mm Hg. Positive end-expiratory pressure should also be given to minimize atelectasis (Chapter 90). If the patient does not show signs of ventilatory recovery within 2 weeks of intubation, a tracheostomy should be considered.

Lesions below C5 may also be associated with inadequate spontaneous ventilation. Midcervical lesions may be associated with intact but compromised diaphragm function. If suspected, a "sniff" test under fluoroscopy can be performed to determine whether both hemidiaphragms are functioning properly. If not, intubation/tracheostomy with volume-controlled ventilation may be needed. If intact, pressure support ventilation may be sufficient (Chapter 105) to achieve an appropriate tidal volume.

Cervical lesions at C6 and below spare the phrenic nerves but may disrupt innervation of the intercostal muscles. The primary finding is decreased cough and an inability to increase ventilation when needed, thereby leading to atelectasis and pneumonia; assisted elimination of tracheal secretions is essential.

Thromboembolic Disease

Thromboembolic disease (Chapters 81 and 98) is a leading cause of morbidity and mortality after traumatic spinal cord injury. Prolonged immobility of the lower extremities leads to deep venous thrombosis in up to 70% of spinal cord–injured patients. Patients should receive prophylaxis with low-molecular-weight heparin (e.g., enoxaparin 30 mg twice daily SC) within 72 hours of injury. Anticoagulation can be held on the day of surgery but should be resumed 24 hours after surgery. A less effective alternative is intermittent compression devices (e.g., pneumatic stockings) with low-dose unfractionated heparin. An inferior vena cava filter may be placed if anticoagulation therapy is contraindicated.

Visceral Function

The abdominal wall musculature is innervated by T7 to T12. The stomach, small bowel, liver, pancreas, and proximal two thirds of the colon receive innervation from T5 to L2. Spinal cord injury at these levels or above may impair visceral function. For ileus, a nasogastric tube should be placed to decompress the stomach. Parental nutrition should be started as soon as possible. Enteral feeding should be delayed until gastrointestinal motility returns, usually within 2 to 3 weeks. In comparison with conservative bowel management, transanal irrigation improves constipation, fecal incontinence, and symptom-related quality of life in patients with spinal cord-injuries.[A12]

Stress-induced peptic ulcer disease occurs in nearly a third of patients without prophylaxis. H_2-receptor antagonists such as ranitidine (50 mg IV three times daily) or a proton pump inhibitor such as omeprazole (20 mg/day PO) reduce the incidence of ulcers.

Bladder tone may be lost because of spinal shock. A Foley catheter should be placed for a minimum of 5 to 7 days to drain the bladder and evaluate volume and renal status. After spinal shock has resolved, autonomic dysreflexia may occur as a result of bladder distention. Clinical signs such as sweating, skin flushing, and hypertension may be present. Clinical examination with palpation and percussion will reveal a distended bladder, which can be treated by bladder training or intermittent catheterization.

Nutrition

Until enteral feeding can begin, parenteral nutrition should be used. Ideally, TPN should be started. However, if TPN is not possible, peripheral parenteral nutrition should be used until TPN (Chapter 217) can begin. Energy expenditures of 19 kcal/kg/day for high cervical injuries to 35.8 kcal/kg/day for injuries at T10 and below have been reported. A caloric level of 80% of the Harris-Benedict prediction should be used for quadriplegic patients. The full Harris-Benedict predicted amount should be used in patients with thoracic spine injuries and below. Indirect calorimetry should be used to determine the caloric needs of each patient so as to optimize nutritional support.

Other Therapy

In a randomized trial, pregabalin, 150 to 600 mg/day, was effective in reducing central neuropathic pain after spinal cord injury.[A13] Patients with traumatic spinal cord injury have a propensity for the development of decubitus ulcers and pressure sores (Chapter 25). Mechanical kinetic beds, regular log rolling (every 2 hours), and padded orthotics are all useful in minimizing this complication. Orthotics, physical therapy, and occupational therapy (for cervical cord injury) are also important to minimize contractures and begin the rehabilitation process.

PROGNOSIS

Traumatic Brain Injury

The most useful prognostic indicator after traumatic brain injury is the neurologic examination at initial evaluation. For patients with severe traumatic brain injury, the initial Glasgow Coma Scale score is the most reliable prognostic indicator. The lower the initial Glasgow Coma Scale score, the less likely a patient will have meaningful neurologic or functional recovery. After traumatic brain injury, 40% of patients with a score of 8 have a good recovery versus only 7% when the score is 3. Furthermore, only 27% of patients with a score of 3 survive versus 88% of patients with a score of 8. Patients in whom the Glasgow Coma Scale score remains the same or worsens over a period of 6 hours do worse clinically than those whose score improves. Further prognostic stratification at 24 hours can be based on pupillary responses, motor responses, and age (Chapter 404). Substantial increases of CSF α-synuclein may indicate widespread neurodegeneration and reflect secondary neuropathologic events after severe traumatic brain injury.[10]

A subsequent head injury before full recovery from even a mild traumatic brain injury may occasionally result in "second impact syndrome," which can worsen the clinical outcome. When seen (mostly in children and adolescents), coma develops rapidly after the second injury, often within minutes. There is decreased autoregulation, diffuse cerebral edema, and intracranial hypertension. Second impact syndrome is associated with high mortality.

Traumatic Spinal Cord Injury

For traumatic spinal cord injury, the completeness of the injury is the most useful predictor (Table 399-5). A grade "A" or complete motor and sensory deficit below the lesion has a poor prognosis. If such a lesion persists for 24 hours, there is little likelihood of meaningful recovery. On the other hand, even severe partial injuries have a higher probability of recovery.

TABLE 399-5 AMERICAN SPINAL INJURY ASSOCIATION IMPAIRMENT SCALE

GRADE	INJURY TYPE	DEFINITION	LIKELIHOOD OF RECOVERY*
A	Complete	No motor or sensory function below the lesion	15.5% (cervical) and 7% (thoracic)
B	Incomplete	Sensory but no motor function	47%
C	Incomplete	Some motor strength (<3)	84%
D	Incomplete	Motor strength > 3	84%
E	None	Sensory and motor function normal	100%

*Data from Coleman WP, Geisler FH. Injury severity as primary predictor of outcome in acute spinal cord injury: retrospective results from a large multicenter clinical trial. *Spine J.* 2004;4:373-378.

Grade A References

A1. Stiell IG, Clement CM, Grimshaw J, et al. Implementation of the Canadian C-Spine Rule: prospective 12 centre cluster randomised trial. *BMJ.* 2009;339:b4146.
A2. Wakai A, McCabe A, Roberts I, et al. Mannitol for acute traumatic brain injury. *Cochrane Database Syst Rev.* 2013;8:CD001049.
A3. Edwards P, Arango M, Balica L, et al. Final results of MRC CRASH, a randomised placebo-controlled trial of intravenous corticosteroid in adults with head injury–outcomes at 6 months. *Lancet.* 2005;365:1957-1959.
A4. Georgiou AP, Manara AR. Role of therapeutic hypothermia in improving outcome after traumatic brain injury: a systematic review. *Br J Anaesth.* 2013;110:357-367.
A5. Robertson CS, Hannay HJ, Yamal JM, et al. Effect of erythropoietin and transfusion threshold on neurological recovery after traumatic brain injury: a randomized clinical trial. *JAMA.* 2014;312:36-47.
A6. Myburgh J, Cooper DJ, Finfer S, et al. Saline or albumin for fluid resuscitation in patients with traumatic brain injury. *N Engl J Med.* 2007;357:874-884.
A7. Chesnut RM, Temkin N, Carney N, et al. A trial of intracranial-pressure monitoring in traumatic brain injury. *N Engl J Med.* 2012;367:2471-2481.
A8. Timmons SD, Ullman JS, Eisenberg HM. Craniectomy in diffuse traumatic brain injury. *N Engl J Med.* 2011;365:373.
A9. Cooper DJ, Rosenfeld JV, Murray L, et al. Decompressive craniectomy in diffuse traumatic brain injury. *N Engl J Med.* 2011;364:1493-1502.
A10. Giacino JT, Whyte J, Bagiella E, et al. Placebo-controlled trial of amantadine for severe traumatic brain injury. *N Engl J Med.* 2012;366:819-826.
A11. Hammond FM, Bickett AK, Norton JH, et al. Effectiveness of amantadine hydrochloride in the reduction of chronic traumatic brain injury irritability and aggression. *J Head Trauma Rehabil.* 2014;29:391-399.
A12. Christensen P, Bazzocchi G, Coggrave M, et al. A randomized, controlled trial of transanal irrigation versus conservative bowel management in spinal cord-injured patients. *Gastroenterology.* 2006;131:738-747.
A13. Cardenas DD, Nieshoff EC, Suda K, et al. A randomized trial of pregabalin in patients with neuropathic pain due to spinal cord injury. *Neurology.* 2013;80:533-539.

GENERAL REFERENCES

For the General References and other additional features, please visit Expert Consult at https://expertconsult.inkling.com.

400

MECHANICAL AND OTHER LESIONS OF THE SPINE, NERVE ROOTS, AND SPINAL CORD

RICHARD L. BARBANO

DEFINITION

Disorders of the spine, nerve roots, and spinal cord are frequent reasons for a patient to visit a physician. Many of these disorders either initially or eventually involve more than one element of the vertebra–spinal cord–nerve root unit, so there is much overlap in the pathobiology and clinical manifestations of these diseases.

The spine consists of 30 vertebrae: 7 cervical (C), 12 thoracic (T), 5 lumbar (L), 5 sacral (S), and the coccyx (Fig. 400-1). The ring shape of the bony vertebrae forms a protective circle around the spinal cord while leaving ample room to allow the cord to move within this canal during flexion and extension of the spine. The vertebral bodies help bear the compressive weight of the body and provide the surface area to support the intervertebral discs, which act to cushion the axial force along the spine. The overlapping facet joints and multiple sets of longitudinal ligaments give the spine stability during its many ranges of motion. The posteriorly placed foramina allow the exit of spinal nerves.

The spinal cord consists of 31 spinal segments, with one more cervical cord segment (8) than vertebrae; each gives rise to a bilateral pair of spinal nerves. Spinal nerves C1 to C7 exit the canal above their corresponding vertebral body, the C8 nerve exits below the C7 vertebra, and subsequent inferior nerves also exit below the numbered vertebrae. The spinal segments of the cord itself, however, lie progressively superior to the vertebrae, so that the end of the spinal cord, the conus medullaris, in adults is approximately adjacent to the L1 vertebra. The more caudal spinal nerves travel as the cauda equina in the subarachnoid space within the spinal canal before exiting their

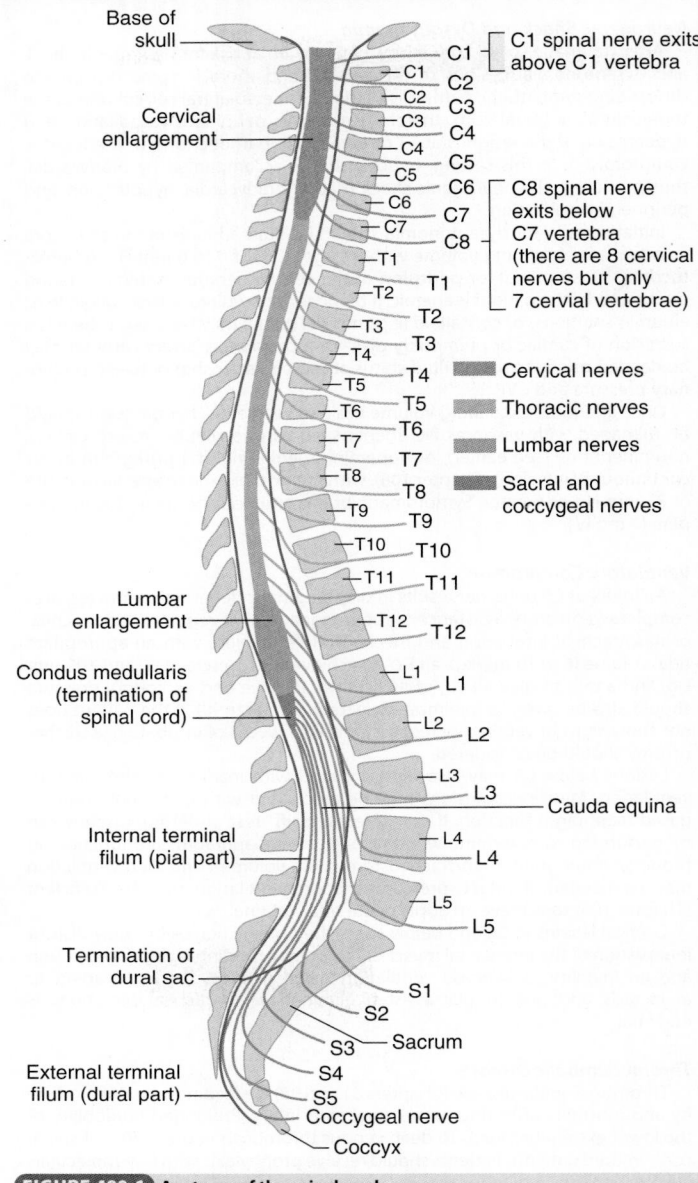

FIGURE 400-1. Anatomy of the spinal cord.

respective foramina. The spinal cord does not have a uniform diameter; the cervical and lumbar segments are wider compared with the thoracic and lower sacral areas because the increased motor and sensory neurons supplying the arms and legs enlarge the cord.

Spinal nerves are formed by the joining of the anterior and posterior spinal roots, which directly exit and enter the spinal cord. The anterior root derives from axons of the anterior horn cells and lateral columns, and it serves motor and autonomic efferent pathways; the posterior root mostly derives from the axons from the dorsal root ganglion and carries afferent sensory signals (Fig. 400-2). The sensory root is twice the thickness of the motor root and lies in a more anterior and inferior location as it crosses the foramen.

CLINICAL MANIFESTATIONS

Disorders of the spinal nerve root produce signs and symptoms referable to the corresponding dermatome or myotome. By far the most frequent complaint is localized neck or back pain, but compromise of the nerve roots or spinal cord will cause symptoms such as abnormal or painful sensations (paresthesias or dysesthesias), loss of sensation, weakness, and autonomic dysfunction (most commonly bladder or bowel incontinence).

When it affects a myotome (the group of muscles served by motor neurons of a spinal cord segment; Fig. 400-3), the motor deficit associated with a spinal root disorder is of the lower motor neuron type. Typical findings are weakness, hypotonia, depressed or absent reflexes, and, if the syndrome has

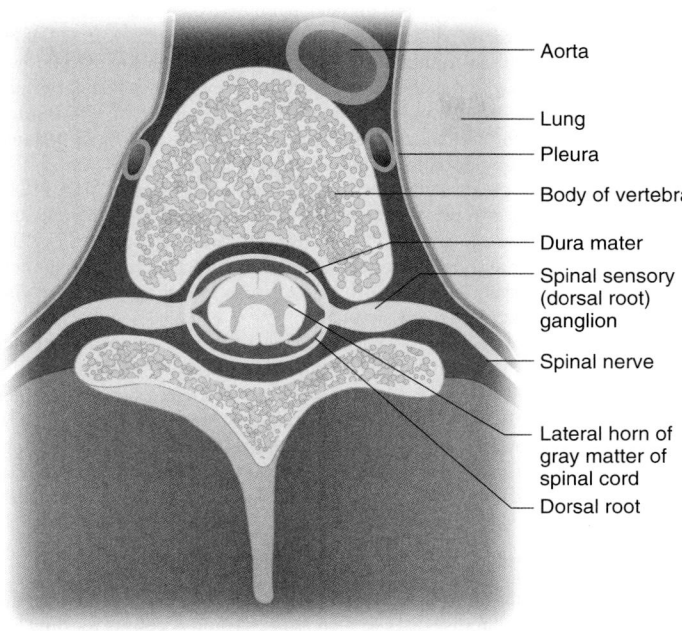

FIGURE 400-2. Anatomy of the spinal cord: section through a thoracic vertebra.

persisted for at least several weeks, atrophy with or without fasciculations. Sensation at the root level is diminished or absent for all modalities, but sensation below the affected root level is intact.

Conversely, disorders of the spinal cord produce a "level" below which sensation is abnormal and motor deficits are of the upper motor neuron type, with weakness without atrophy (unless complicated by disuse), hypertonia, and increased reflexes. At the level of a spinal cord lesion, the motor deficits can be of the lower motor neuron type as the anterior horn cell bodies or exiting fibers are affected; below this level, an upper motor neuron syndrome will predominate. With strokes (Chapter 406) and other central nervous system (CNS) disorders, the full upper motor neuron syndrome may not be present in the acute phase of cord injury and can take time to appear.

DIAGNOSIS

The clinical history can help localize the patient's symptoms, especially complaints of pain and sensory alterations that may exist in the absence of objective sensory loss on probing with light touch, pinprick, and vibration stimuli. The neurologic examination should include evaluation of the sensory, motor (Table 400-1), and reflex (Table 400-2) functions. Careful side-to-side comparisons can help assess subtle deficits. For example, elderly patients often have decreased or absent ankle jerks, so contralateral comparison is necessary. However, all muscles receive innervation from more than one root/spinal cord level, and all roots send fibers to multiple muscles. The clinical implication of this anatomic pattern is that individual muscles are rarely profoundly weak, and patients rarely report isolated muscle weakness in single root involvement syndromes. Likewise, overlap of the sensory dermatomes (see Fig. 400-3) explains why sharp demarcations in the sensory examination rarely occur.

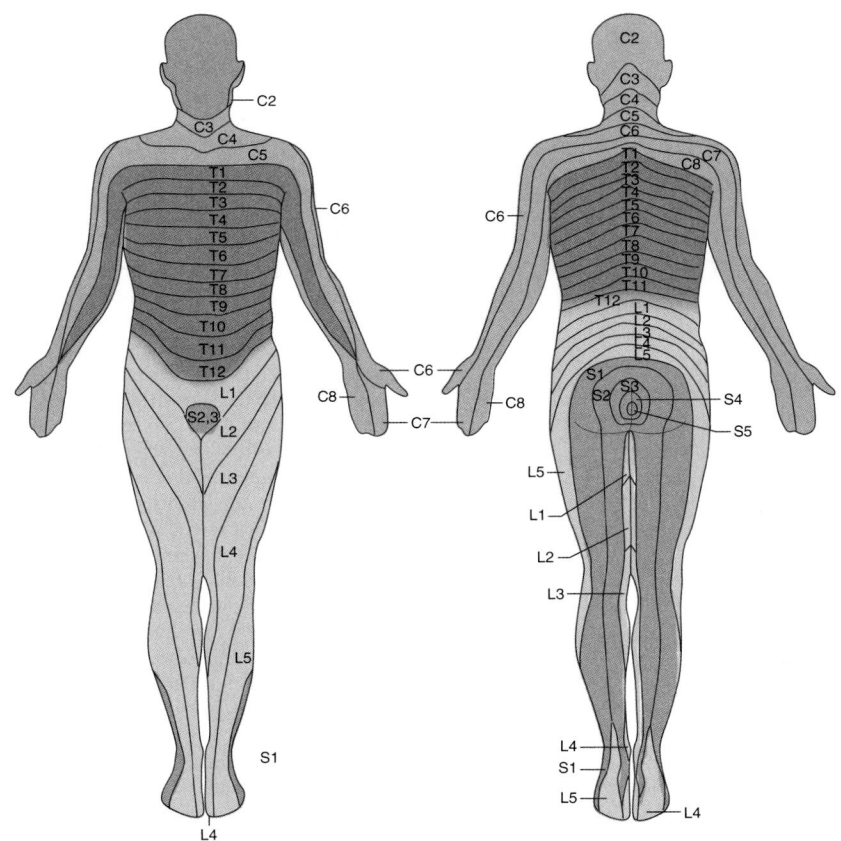

Levels of principal dermatomes

C5	Clavicles	T10	Level of umbilicus
C5,6,7	Lateral parts of upper limbs	T12	Inguinal or groin regions
C8, T1	Medial sides of upper limbs	L1,2,3,4	Anterior and inner surfaces of lower limbs
C6	Thumb	L4,5 S1	Foot
C6,7,8	Hand	L4	Medial side of great toe
C8	Ring and little fingers	S1,2, L5	Posterior and outer surfaces of lower limbs
T4	Level of nipples	S1	Lateral margin of foot and little toe
		S2,3,4	Perineum

FIGURE 400-3. Schematic demarcation of levels of principal dermatomes shown as distinct segments. There is actually considerable overlap between any two adjacent dermatomes.

TABLE 400-1   ESSENTIAL MUSCLE TESTING

ROOT	MUSCLES	ACTION/TESTING
ARM		
C5	Deltoid	Abducts arm
	Infraspinatus	Externally rotates arm with elbow flexed
C6	Brachioradialis	Flexes elbow (along with biceps [C5-6])
C7	Triceps	Extends elbow
	Extensor digitorum	Extends fingers
C8	Flexor digitorum	Flexes fingers (both superficialis and profundus)
	Flexor pollicis longus	Flexes distal phalanx of thumb
T1	Interossei	Spread fingers
LEG		
L1-2	Iliacus	Flexes hip
L2-3	Adductor magnus	Adducts thigh (as part of adductor group)
L3-4	Quadriceps	Extends knee
L4	Tibialis anterior	Dorsiflexes foot
L5	Extensor hallucis longus	Great toe extension
	Extensor digitorum longus	Toe extension
S1	Hamstrings	Flex knee
	Flexor hallucis longus	Flexes great toe (along with S2)

TABLE 400-2   ESSENTIAL REFLEX EXAMINATION

REFLEX	EFFECT	ROOT/IMPLICATION
Jaw jerk	Jaw closes with tap on slightly opened jaw	Cranial nerve V; implies lesion above cervical cord
Biceps	Tap tendon: elbow flexion	C5-6; musculocutaneous nerve
Brachioradialis	Tap tendon over distal radius with elbow flexed and mid pronation: elbow flexion	C5-6; radial nerve
Triceps	Tap tendon: elbow extension	C6 < C7
Finger flexion	Tap partially flexed fingertips: finger flexion	C6-T1; when hyperactive, may imply lesion above midcervical spinal cord
Patella	Tap patella: quadriceps contraction (knee extension)	L2-4
Achilles	Tap Achilles tendon: foot plantar flexion	S1-2
Babinski	Scratch sole: great toe flexion	Great toe extension implies lesion of cord (or brain) above L4
Anal wink	Scratch perineum: external anal sphincter contraction	Absence of contraction implies S2-4 lesion

DISORDERS OF THE SPINE
Neck and Back Pain

DEFINITION

Most neck and back pain is mechanical, that is, theoretically emanating from the spine's structural elements, which are the vertebrae, discs, ligaments, tendons, and muscles. The location of pain is either axial, which means it is located along the spine itself, or referred. The term *perceived pain* is sometimes used when the pain from a spinal lesion is felt elsewhere by the patient, whereas *referred pain* is often used to describe pain that is experienced by the patient in the spinal area but caused by nonspinal structures. If the pain follows a dermatomal (nerve root) distribution, it is referred to as *radicular pain*, which is likely to involve the nerve root.

EPIDEMIOLOGY

Neck and back pain is a frequent reason for visits to a primary care physician. Low back pain is more common than neck pain, but both are common. The thoracic spine, possibly because of rib attachments and limited range of

motion, is an uncommon location for back pain. An exception to this general rule is the condition of diffuse idiopathic skeletal hyperostosis (DISH; Chapter 273), which is a noninflammatory age-related condition of unknown etiology, characterized by ossification of paravertebral ligaments and peripheral entheses. It is more common in men, with a prevalence of 30% in men by age 65. Pain in the thoracic spine region occurs in up to 80% of patients and is accompanied by notable decreased range of motion.

In the general population, the incidence of self-reported neck pain is 213 per 1000; the 12-month prevalence of any pain is typically between 30 and 50%, and pain severe enough to limit activity is between 1.7 and 11.5%. The prevalence is higher among women. Risk factors for neck pain include inherited factors, poor psychological health, and tobacco use; the presence of disc degeneration is not a significant factor.

More than 70% of people will experience low back pain significant enough to inhibit their participation in daily activities at some time in their life. The highest prevalence is in the 45- to 64-year age group. There is less of a gender difference than with neck pain, although tobacco use is an associated risk factor. Physical work–related factors (e.g., heavy lifting, prolonged sitting, repetitive twisting) increase risk; prospective studies show that psychosocial issues such as work monotony and job dissatisfaction also are major predisposing factors.

PATHOBIOLOGY

Although the popular impression is that the disc is the source of most spine pain, it is estimated that disc disease such as protrusion accounts for only 5% of all low back problems. Degenerative changes are a much more common cause of both acute and chronic spine pain. There is a genetic predisposition to intervertebral disc degeneration, with heritability estimates in the range of 34 to 61%.

Degenerative changes can result in spondylosis, a condition that includes degenerative disc disease with bulging and occasionally herniation. The condition is often accompanied by the formation of osteophytes, ligamentous hypertrophy, and sometimes facet fracture and vertebral subluxation. Spondylosis, which is a consequence of age-related disc disease, is exemplified by the fact that almost everybody has at least anterior osteophytes by the age of 40 years, and it is not necessarily painful. Spondylosis probably starts with age-related disc desiccation and loss of elasticity of the annulus fibrosus. Tension of the longitudinal ligaments results in the formation of hypertrophic osteophytes. Compromise of microvascular supply may also contribute. Eventually, the facet joints can ride over one another, thereby leading to instability, formation of more osteophytes, and inflammation of the synovial joints. If there is fracture of the pars interarticularis, the term *spondylolysis* is used. Further instability between the intervertebral segments leads to spondylolisthesis, in which one vertebral body shifts sagittally in relation to its adjacent vertebra. Spondylolisthesis is graded by the amount of shift as measured with flexion and extension lateral spine films.

DISH is characterized by calcification and ossification of the anterior longitudinal spinal ligament and less frequently the posterior longitudinal ligament. The latter can compromise spinal cord roots as well as the spinal cord itself, especially in the cervical region.[1]

Whiplash, an acute flexion-extension injury of the cervical spine, is common after motor vehicle accidents and other situations of rapid deceleration. Although specific acute and chronic manifestations are controversial, the acute syndrome is generally accepted to be a result of mechanical irritation of pain-sensitive structures in the cervical spine, with or without nerve root injury. More severe trauma can cause fracture and vertebral instability, both of which require rapid surgical evaluation.

CLINICAL MANIFESTATIONS

Acute neck pain and low back pain are commonly limited to the axial region, although radicular signs and symptoms can occur in the presence of nerve root irritation. The most common radicular pain occurs in the distribution of a dermatome. Other radicular signs and symptoms can include dysesthesias or sensory loss in the affected dermatome, decreased strength in muscles of the affected myotome, and decreased reflex. Cranial nerve findings, diffuse weakness throughout a limb or in more than one limb, hemisensory symptoms, autonomic symptoms, and increased reflexes are not manifestations of spine disease and should prompt more extensive evaluation for other conditions that affect the brain or brain stem. Bowel and bladder symptoms should prompt urgent evaluation of a cauda equina or myelopathy syndrome (see later).

Acute spine problems can also cause referred or perceived pain at sites other than their anatomic source. For example, mechanical low back pain may include aching in the buttocks or thigh, most often posteriorly and occasionally the hip region but rarely below the knee. More commonly, however, the term *referred pain* denotes the situation in which other structures, usually internal organs, refer pain to the spine or back. Areas of referred pain usually share the same embryologic origin and, during development, the same sensory pathways. Differentiation of referred pain from localized back pain depends on the history and examination. Mechanical pain is often exacerbated by movement such as twisting, bending, extension, or flexion, whereas referred pain tends to be independent of such activities.

Chronic spine disorders lead to chronic back pain directly and as a secondary complication. For example, chronic degenerative arthropathy can lead to degenerative lumbar scoliosis with secondary involvement of neural structures. Back pain and radiculopathy are the most prominent symptoms, present in upward of 80% of patients, but symptoms of neurogenic claudication also develop in about 50% of patients.

DIAGNOSIS

History and Clinical Examination

The history and examination are essential for the initial evaluation and triage of patients with neck and back pain. Patients with so-called red flags (Table 400-3) merit special attention, as does any patient who awakens from sleep because of pain or has pain that is constant and unchanged by position, is unremitting and progressive, or is accompanied by any systemic signs or symptoms.

As part of the history in the setting of acute neck trauma, well-established screening protocols such as the Canadian C-Spine Rule and the NEXUS Low-Risk Criteria (Fig. 400-4) are validated ways to detect cervical spine fracture and direct appropriate radiographic evaluation. In such a setting, a computed tomographic (CT) scan of the cervical spine would be the imaging test of choice.

On clinical examination, inspection should assess evidence of trauma, muscle wasting, fasciculations, erythema, rashes, and scars. Palpation is directed to areas of point tenderness during evaluation for more diffusely tender regions, muscle spasm, and masses. If light percussion of the spinous process evokes significant pain, a focal process, such as fracture, malignant neoplasm (Chapter 189), or infection (Chapter 413), should be considered because such a finding is unusual in typical mechanical spine pain. Finally, the active and passive range of motion for flexion, extension, rotation, and tilt should be noted. Many provocative tests have been described for the evaluation of neck and back pain, but few have undergone formal evaluation of their diagnostic accuracy. For neck pain, contralateral rotation of the neck with extension of the arm and fingers suggests cervical root involvement, particularly in combination with other provocative tests, such as the Spurling maneuver, in which the patient's head is rotated 45 degrees to the contralateral side, with the neck in slight extension to minimize the foraminal opening. Downward pressure on the top of the head by the examiner will reproduce arm dysesthesias. Provocative tests also can diminish symptoms. For example, in the cervical distraction test, the examiner's hands are placed under the jaw and occiput; gentle upward pulling of the head will temporarily reduce or alleviate the symptoms.

For low back pain, the straight leg raise has sensitivity of 0.85 to 0.91 but a specificity of only 0.26 to 0.52 for the diagnosis of sciatica due to a herniated disc. The crossed straight leg raise test has a lower sensitivity of 0.23 to 0.34 but a much higher specificity of 0.86 to 0.90. The seated straight leg raise can

be used for confirmation of root irritation as the spine-leg angle is increased to 90 degrees. A negative result of the seated straight leg raise in the setting of a positive result of the straight leg raise suggests the possibility of a nonorganic component, although a mechanical alteration of the root exit zone in this position should also be considered.

Ancillary Testing

For neck pain (Fig. 400-5), plain radiography and CT scanning, which are the mainstays of cervical spine imaging, allow adequate view of the bony structures. Magnetic resonance imaging (MRI) has largely replaced myelography, which is still used occasionally to provide information about the spinal cord and nerve roots. However, MR abnormalities are common and can have a high false-positive rate; for example, 12 to 17% of patients younger than 30 years and 86 to 89% of patients aged 60 have disc degeneration as evidenced by loss of signal intensity, disc protrusion, narrowing of the disc space, or foraminal stenosis. Cervical discography also has a high false-positive rate and cannot be recommended as a diagnostic test in the assessment of neck pain.

Uncomplicated acute low back pain, with or without radiculopathy, is generally self-limited, and imaging studies are unnecessary unless any of the red flags (see Table 400-3) are present.[A1] The American College of Physicians recommends MRI only in patients who have major or progressive neurologic deficits, in whom a serious underlying condition is expected, or in whom surgery or epidural steroids are being considered.[2] For trauma, osteoporosis, or patients older than 70 years, plain radiography may suffice if the results are normal and no other abnormalities are present. Otherwise, with few exceptions, MRI is the test of choice given its superiority in evaluating soft tissue structures and its lack of radiation exposure. Care must be taken, however, to ensure correlation with the clinical syndrome, because 28% of asymptomatic volunteers with a mean age of 42 have herniated discs, 52% have bulging discs, and 14% have annular tears. The percentage of imaging abnormalities increases even more in asymptomatic volunteers older than 60 years; 57% have significantly abnormal scans, with 36% showing herniated discs and close to 98% showing disc degeneration. Abnormalities of the Modic end plate, anterolisthesis, and disc extrusion are more strongly associated with

---

TABLE 400-3 "RED FLAGS" IN THE EVALUATION OF SPINE PAIN

Recent significant trauma or minor trauma at age > 50 years
Unexplained weight loss
Unexplained fever
Immunosuppression
History of cancer
History of prior local surgery
Systemic disorder, bone or arthritic disorder
Intravenous drug use
Prolonged use of corticosteroids or osteoporosis
Age > 70 years
Focal neurologic deficit with progressive symptoms
Duration > 6 weeks
Thoracic spine pain

Modified from Davis PC, Wippold FJ, Brunberg JA, et al. ACR Appropriateness Criteria on low back pain. *J Am Coll Radiol.* 2009;6:401-407.

The NEXUS Low Risk Criteria (NLC) Algorithm for screening of neck injuries

- No posterior midline cervical spine tenderness—Midline posterior bony cervical-spine tenderness is present if the patient reports pain on palpation of the posterior midline neck from the nuchal ridge to the prominence of the first thoracic vertebrae, or if the patient evinces pain with direct palpation of any cervical spinous process.
- No evidence of intoxication—Patients should be considered intoxicated if they have either of the following: a recent history provided by the patient, or an observer of intoxication or intoxicating ingestion, or evidence of intoxication on physical examination such as an odor of alcohol, slurred speech, ataxia, dysmetria, or other cerebellar findings, or any behavior consistent with intoxication. Patients may also be considered to be intoxicated if tests of bodily secretions are positive for alcohol or drugs that affect level of alertness.
- A normal level of alertness—An altered level of alertness can include the following: a Glasgow Coma Scale score of 14 or less; disorientation to person, place, time, or events; an inability to remember three objects at five minutes; a delayed or inappropriate response to external stimuli; or other findings.
- No focal neurological deficit—A focal neurological deficit is any focal neurological finding on motor or sensory examination.
- No painful distracting injuries—No precise definition of painful distracting injury is possible. This category includes any condition thought by the clinician to be producing pain sufficient to distract the patient from a second (neck) injury. Such injuries may include, but are not limited to, any long-bone fracture; a visceral injury requiring surgical consultation; a large laceration, degloving injury, or crush injury; large burns; or any other injury causing acute functional impairment. Physicians may also classify any injury as distracting if it is thought to have the potential to impair the patient's ability to appreciate other injuries.

FIGURE 400-4. The NEXUS Low-Risk Criteria (NLC) algorithm for screening of neck injuries. (Reproduced from Hoffman JR, Mower WR, Wolfson AB, et al. Validity of a set of clinical criteria to rule out injury to the cervical spine in patients with blunt trauma. National Emergency X-Radiography Utilization Study Group. *N Engl J Med.* 2000;343: 94-99.)

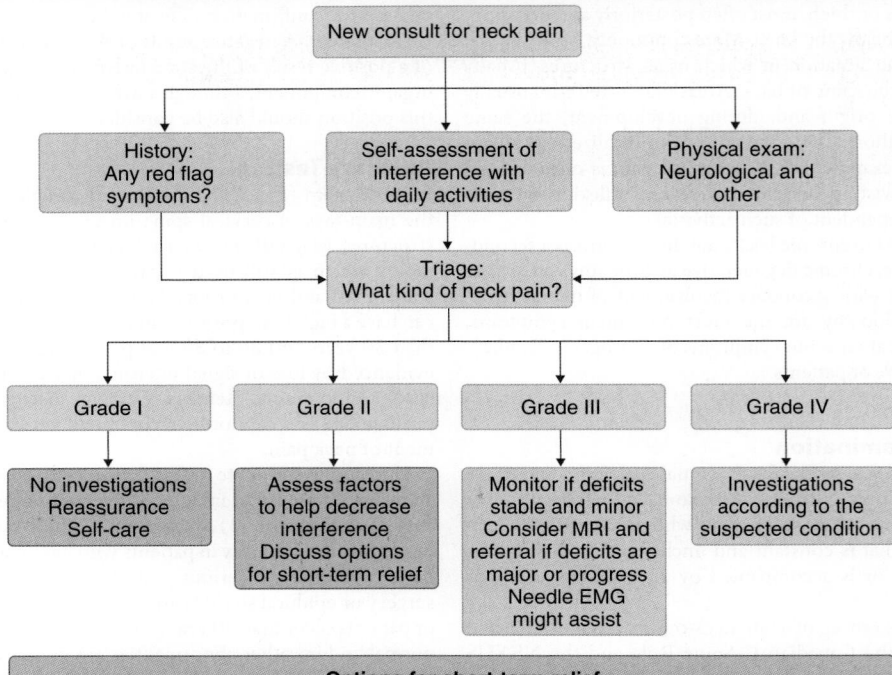

FIGURE 400-5. Approach to new-onset neck pain. EMG = electromyography; MRI = magnetic resonance imaging. (Modified from Guzman J, Haldeman S, Carroll LJ, et al. Clinical practice implications of the Bone and Joint Decade 2000-2010 Task Force on Neck Pain and Its Associated Disorders. From concepts and findings to recommendations. *Spine.* 2008;33:S199-S213.)

TABLE 400-4	MECHANICAL NECK PAIN				
	NECK STRAIN	**HERNIATED NUCLEUS PULPOSUS**	**OSTEOARTHRITIS**	**MYELOPATHY**	**WHIPLASH**
Age (yr)	20-40	30-50	>50	>60	30-40
Pain location	Neck	Arm	Neck	Arm/leg	Neck
Onset	Acute	Acute	Insidious	Insidious	Acute
Flexion	+	+	−	−	+
Extension	−	+/−	+	+	+
Plain radiography	−	−	+	+	−

+ = present; − = absent.
From Borenstein DG, Wiesel SW, Boden SD. *Neck Pain: Medical Diagnosis and Comprehensive Management.* Philadelphia: WB Saunders; 1996.

low back pain than is disc degeneration without end plate changes. Situations in which alternative imaging should be considered include spondylosis and stress fracture, for which bone scintigraphy with single-photon emission CT (SPECT) is more sensitive than MRI. CT can also be useful when MRI is contraindicated or to evaluate scoliosis, bone graft integrity, surgical fusion, and instrumentation. For back and neck pain that persists for 6 weeks, electrodiagnostic testing can demonstrate compromise of spinal root function but is not usually helpful in axial spine pain without neurologic symptoms.

Differential Diagnosis
Mechanical or idiopathic pain explains up to 97% of cases of neck pain (Table 400-4) and low back pain (Table 400-5); the remaining 3% is nonmechanical in origin and includes referred pain and other conditions. Acute mechanical neck pain is most often caused by a neck strain, a herniated nucleus pulposus, or whiplash; for pain of insidious onset, osteoarthritis and myelopathy are the leading causes. For back pain, muscle strain and a herniated nucleus pulposus are acute causes; insidious causes include osteoarthritis, spinal stenosis, spondylolisthesis, and scoliosis. Queries regarding the red flags will identify serious and nonmechanical causes of neck and back pain (Fig. 400-6).

Abdominal and pelvic structures can refer pain to the low back (referred pain). Abdominal aortic aneurysms (Chapter 78) can present with a mid- to low back ache that may radiate to the hips or anterior thighs. Cholecystitis (Chapter 155) can cause pain in the midthoracic area; pancreatic disease (Chapter 144) can cause pain in the L1 region; and diverticulitis (Chapter 142) in the left lower quadrant can cause diffuse low back pain. Genitourinary disorders (Chapter 123) can cause colicky referred pain to the flanks and costovertebral angle. Bladder disorders (Chapter 123) may occasionally refer pain to the sacral area, as can prostate problems (Chapter 129). Pelvic disorders in women that can cause referred low back pain include endometriosis (Chapter 236), ectopic pregnancy, and pelvic inflammatory disease (Chapters 299 and 318). Most of these disorders have additional signs and symptoms to aid in the diagnosis.

Myocardial ischemia (Chapters 71 to 73) can be associated with anterior neck pain, although less commonly than with left arm or jaw pain. Arterial dissections (Chapter 78) are more commonly associated with neck pain; for example, up to 20% of patients with carotid dissections complain of anterolateral pain, and about 80% of patients with vertebral dissections have posterior or occipital pain. Patients with arterial dissections frequently but not necessarily have signs and symptoms of stroke (Chapter 407). Disorders of the esophagus (Chapter 138) and mass lesions of the throat (Chapters 190 and 429) can also present as neck pain.

Acute spine pain can precede the rash in herpes zoster (Chapter 375) or can be seen in the vaso-occlusive crisis of sickle cell anemia (Chapter 163). Infections of the disc (Chapter 413) cause sharp back pain worsened by

TABLE 400-5 MECHANICAL LOW BACK PAIN

	MUSCLE STRAIN	HERNIATED NUCLEUS PULPOSUS	OSTEOARTHRITIS	SPINAL STENOSIS	SPONDYLOLISTHESIS	SCOLIOSIS
Age (yr)	20-40	30-50	>50	>60	20	30
Pain pattern location	Back (unilateral)	Back (unilateral)	Back (unilateral)	Leg (bilateral)	Back	Back
Onset	Acute	Acute (prior episodes)	Insidious	Insidious	Insidious	Insidious
Standing	↑	↓	↑	↑	↑	↑
Sitting	↓	↑	↓	↓	↓	↓
Bending	↑	↑	↓	↓	↑	↑
Straight leg	−	+	−	+ (stress)	−	−
Plain radiography	−	−	+	+	+	+

From Borenstein DG, Wiesel SW, Boden SD. *Low Back Pain: Medical Diagnosis and Comprehensive Management.* 2nd ed. Philadelphia: WB Saunders; 1995.

movement. Arachnoiditis (Chapter 412), an inflammatory process of the arachnoid space, can cause diffuse chronic back pain, often after the introduction of foreign substances or manipulation of the intrathecal space. Finally, 20 to 50% of patients with depression (Chapter 397) will complain of back pain that often is diffuse and described in emotionally laden terms. Complaints of low back pain are also common in malingering patients.

TREATMENT Rx

Treatment options vary according to the severity of pain, presence of radicular signs or symptoms, and any underlying disease. Acute nontraumatic neck pain is common and usually benign. Beneficial treatments include nonsteroidal anti-inflammatory drugs (NSAIDs, e.g., ibuprofen 600-800 mg three times daily for 2 weeks), exercise, and physical therapy.[A2] The low risk of myocardial infarction or upper gastrointestinal bleed from NSAIDs must be weighed against pain relief and the relative benignity of the condition. Chiropractic manipulation is of benefit but has the rare complication of posterior circulation stroke from arterial dissection, especially in patients younger than 45 years. Low-level laser therapy[A3] and acupuncture[A4] are also of short-term benefit. Cervical collars and traction are not of established benefit. Even in the absence of radicular pain, surgical intervention for neck pain is indicated in cases of vertebral instability, such as caused by fracture or dislocation. Surgery, including fusion, may be needed for stabilization after surgery for lesions such as tumors, infections, or hemorrhages. For neck pain that is accompanied by signs or symptoms of radiculopathy, surgery should be considered but is not usually the initial therapy (see later). If a cervical spine lesion is causing spinal cord compression, emergent evaluation for possible surgery is indicated (see later). For chronic neck pain, yoga therapy yields significant pain relief with the possible added benefits of improving quality of life and psychological well-being.[A5]

Because acute low back pain is generally benign, invasive therapy should be avoided in the first 3 months. Conservative treatment includes NSAIDs (e.g., ibuprofen 600-800 mg three times daily as needed) and controlled physical activity; strict bed rest for longer than 2 days is no better than restricted physical activity.[A6] Acetaminophen is no better than placebo.[A7] Other options include local heat and massage. Spinal manipulation, exercise therapy, massage, and cognitive-behavioral therapy are moderately effective.[A8-A10] True acupuncture appears no better than sham acupuncture.[A11]

For chronic nonradicular low back pain, exercise and cognitive-behavioral therapy are recommended; yoga should also be considered.[A12] Prolotherapy, in which a mild irritant is injected into a tendon or ligament to increase blood flow and promote healing, and facet joint injections can be helpful, but intradiscal steroid injections and percutaneous intradiscal radiofrequency thermocoagulation are not effective.[A13] Transcutaneous electrical neurostimulation (TENS) does not appear to provide any functional improvement in patients with chronic lumbar pain.[A14] Oral analgesic medications are frequently offered and include NSAIDs; duloxetine (30 to 60 mg daily) may be a reasonable alternative. In one randomized trial, tanezumab (10 to 20 mg intravenously, repeated 8 weeks later), a humanized monoclonal antibody that specifically inhibits nerve growth factor, reduced pain better than naproxen or placebo.[A15]

When persistent nonradicular low back pain is accompanied by associated degenerative spine changes, surgical fusion is of benefit but not superior to interdisciplinary rehabilitation.[A16] If degenerative changes lead to lumbar scoliosis with or without neurologic signs, however, decompressive surgery with or without fusion appears effective for at least 5 years for the majority of patients. Outcomes after instrumented lumbar spinal fusion are improved if rehabilitation is delayed for 12 weeks after the operation. In more focal disor-

ders, surgery to remove disc material pressure from pain-sensitive structures can be considered; techniques include open, laser, and microdiskectomy approaches, with little evidence to favor one option over the other.

PROGNOSIS

Between 50 and 85% of patients who have neck pain that persists for more than 1 day report recurrence of symptoms in 1- and 5-year follow-up. Slightly more than 50% of patients recover within 3 months, and those who remain symptomatic generally have relatively little pain and disability.[3] Patients younger than 45 years have less recurrence, and patients aged 45 to 59 have the highest risk. Prior neck injury or pain, coexistent low back pain, and self-perceived poor general health are risk factors for symptoms persisting past 3 months or recurrence.

Mechanical spine pain, even with radicular symptoms, resolves without specific intervention within 30 days in many patients and within 3 months in 90% of patients. Recurrence is frequent, however, especially in patients with spondylosis, because the underlying process persists and further degeneration of the spinal elements can be expected.

Long-term disability is more common with obesity, low education level, tobacco use, high levels of pain at the onset, tendency to somatization, job dissatisfaction, lack of availability of light-duty employment, and need to perform significant lifting at work. The strongest factors affecting outcome are psychological, especially worrying, fear avoidance, anger, and frustration.[4] Genetic variability, such as in polymorphisms of catechol O-methyltransferase, also may play a role in the development of chronic pain.

Spinal Stenosis

DEFINITION

Spinal stenosis, which is a narrowing of the spinal canal, results in compression of neural structures in the cervical and lumbar regions, where the diameter of the spinal cord is largest. Signs and symptoms of spinal stenosis are referable to these levels. In the lumbar region, L4-5 is the most common level of stenosis, followed by L3-4 and L5-S1.

EPIDEMIOLOGY

The annual incidence of spinal stenosis in the United States is about 1 to 2 per 100,000 for the cervical region and 5 per 100,000 for the lumbar region.[5] Spinal stenosis often coexists in the cervical and lumbar regions, and the incidence is higher in patients with more complex degenerative anatomy.

PATHOBIOLOGY

Primary spinal stenosis is due to a congenital narrowing of the spinal canal. Causes of secondary stenosis include chronic degenerative conditions such as spondylosis and thickening of the ligamenta flava and longitudinale posterius neoplasia, osteomyelitis, and rheumatoid arthritis. In patients receiving corticosteroids long term, epidural lipomatosis is a cause predominantly at the thoracic level. The underlying cause of symptoms may be multifactorial, with direct nerve pressure, duration of the pressure, capillary restriction, venous congestion, and reliance on the anastomosis of cerebrospinal fluid for metabolic homeostasis all potentially playing a role.

In spinal stenosis, myelopathy results from compression of the veins that drain the canal, thereby leading to capillary stasis and edema, which result in

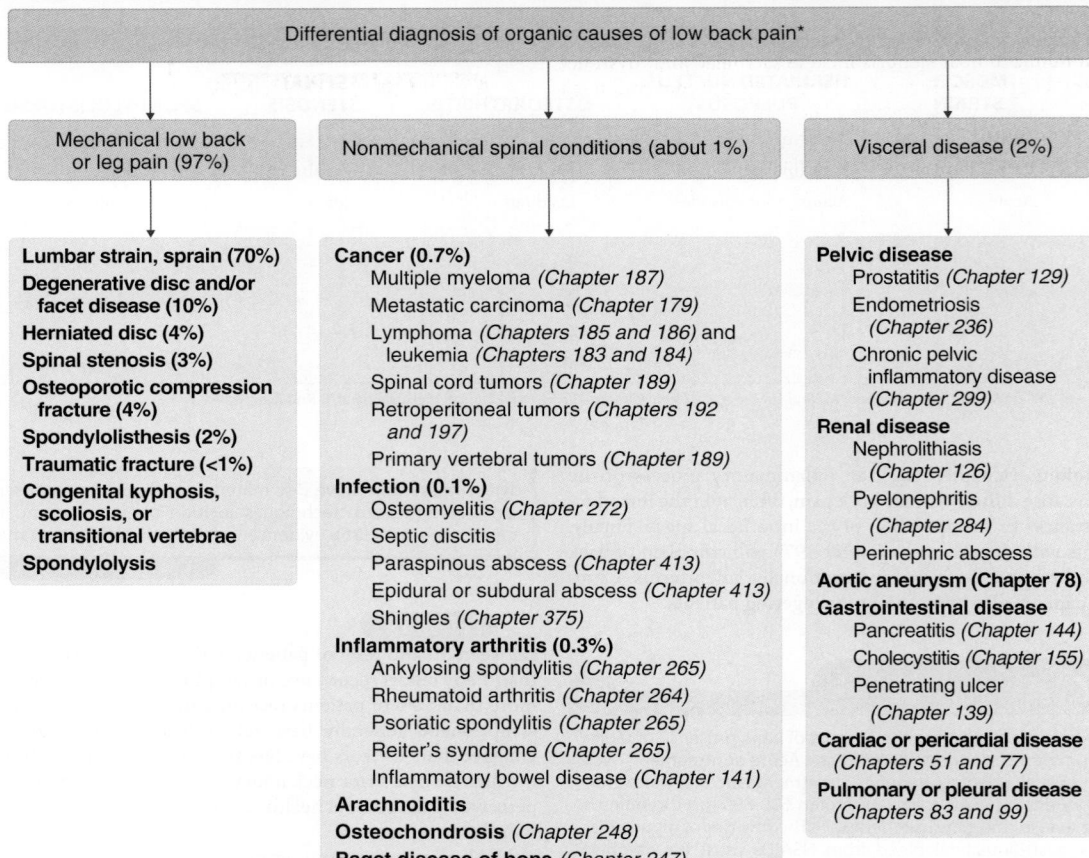

FIGURE 400-6. Differential diagnosis of organic causes of low back pain. * Percentages are approximations and may vary substantially in different practices. (Data from Deyo RA, Weinstein JN. Low back pain. *N Engl J Med.* 2001;344:363-370.)

further compromise of the spinal cord. If the anterior spinal artery is also occluded intermittently or chronically, ischemic gliosis develops. The cord itself can be compressing, and dynamic injury can occur during flexion and extension, especially in chronic degenerative conditions associated with thickening and buckling of the ligamentum flavum. Superimposed trauma, such as severe flexion-extension from whiplash injury or falls, can cause the central cord syndrome (see later, Disorders of the Spinal Cord).

CLINICAL MANIFESTATIONS

Cervical stenosis, which usually results from spondylosis (cervical spondylotic myelopathy) and degenerative spine changes superimposed on congenital stenosis, can be manifested in a number of ways. At the C5-8 level, both the cord and roots are involved, and patients develop lower motor neuron findings in the arms and upper motor neuron signs in the legs; the result is the slow onset of painless atrophy of the weakened hand muscles, accompanied by gait abnormalities. Above the C5 level, the arms may become numb and clumsy, but there is little atrophy. Gait problems are frequently described as leg stiffness, heaviness, or incoordination, and patients may complain of falls or fear of falling, difficulty walking on uneven surfaces, and needing to watch where they are walking. In general, neck pain is not as prominent a complaint as is low back pain in lumbar spinal stenosis, but radicular pain occurs in about one third of patients. On examination, a Lhermitte's sign, which is a shock-like tingling traveling down the spine with neck flexion or less commonly with extension, may be elicited. Sensation to pinprick examination will often be decreased in the hands, but this finding may be patchy and not well demarcated. Increased muscle tone will predominate in the legs, and reflexes will likely be increased; the Babinski sign is often present. The stance and gait may be wide based, with slow, short steps. Romberg's sign may be present.

Lumbar spinal stenosis can present with intermittent or persistent signs and symptoms referable to both cord and roots; axial neck or back pain is almost always present. However, the correlation between symptoms and the diameter of the canal is poor. The pain can also radiate in a pseudoradicular pattern from the lumbar region into the gluteal region, groin, and one or both upper legs, but pain rarely radiates distal to the knee unless spinal root involvement occurs. Lumbar neurogenic claudication is perhaps the most specific; symptoms are precipitated by compressive effects on the spinal cord and exiting roots and are characterized by increasing leg paresthesias and weakness as the patient remains standing and gravity pulls the lumbar cord enlargement into the narrowed spinal segment. As opposed to vascular claudication (Chapter 79), symptoms occur even at rest and can be relieved only by bending at the waist or sitting; the patient will characteristically report improved ability to walk if bent at the waist. Other features that suggest neurogenic claudication rather than vascular claudication include back pain, paresthesias, numbness, weakness, and prolonged presence of symptoms after changing position (seconds to 1 to 2 minutes in vascular claudication but 2 to 20 minutes in neurogenic claudication).

DIAGNOSIS

Although MRI can localize and quantify the severity of the stenosis, the degree of stenosis does not correlate well with the degree of symptoms. The normal diameter of the lumbar canal is approximately 22 to 25 mm, relative lumbar stenosis is 10 to 12 mm diameter, and a diameter of less than 10 mm is considered absolute stenosis. MRI also can identify any comorbid spinal disease, such as degenerative changes and spondylolisthesis. However, CT myelography, which provides the details needed for surgical treatment, is another alternative. Electromyography (EMG) is not generally useful in the diagnosis of spinal stenosis except in assessment of comorbid conditions (e.g., localized radiculopathy) that might be important for surgical planning, as well as for detection of other potentially significant disorders, such as polyneuropathy.

The differential diagnosis of lumbar spinal stenosis includes vascular claudication from peripheral vascular disease (Chapter 79) and abdominal aortic aneurysm (Chapter 78).[6] The symptoms of vascular claudication are activity dependent, unlike the positional dependency of the spinal stenosis. Other conditions that can mimic lumbar stenosis include sacroiliac joint dysfunction, radiculopathy or disc prolapse, polyneuropathy, tethered cord, and spina bifida. Hip pathology, including avascular necrosis, should also be considered. Because cervical stenosis can cause both arm and leg symptoms, the differential diagnosis also includes multiple sclerosis (Chapter 411), syringomyelia (Chapter 417), Arnold-Chiari malformation (Chapter 417), cerebrovascular disease (Chapters 407 and 408), normal-pressure hydrocephalus (Chapter 189), and motor neuron disorders (Chapter 419).

TREATMENT   Rx

Spinal stenosis is not necessarily an indication for surgery. Conservative therapy with NSAIDs (e.g., ibuprofen 400-800 mg four times daily (max 3.2 gm/d) or acetaminophen 650 mg every 4 to 6 hrs (max 3.25 gm/d), muscle relaxants, physical therapy, and a hard cervical collar can help many patients. Epidural injection of lidocaine is as effective as injection of lidocaine plus steroids in patients whose pain is disabling.[A17] For spinal stenosis, epidural injection with etanercept, a tumor necrosis factor (TNF)-α inhibitor, has an analgesic effect that may be superior to steroids.[A18] However, surgery should be considered in patients with severe symptoms and signs of progressive myelopathy. Decompressive laminectomy, with or without fusion, is superior to nonsurgical therapy for improvement of pain and function for at least a year in patients with lumbar spinal stenosis.[A19]

PROGNOSIS

Because spinal stenosis is usually degenerative, it is often a slowly progressive condition without rapid deterioration. Nevertheless, up to 50% of patients are stable in the long term. After symptoms develop and the condition is affecting quality of life, decompressive surgery should be considered. Because the underlying condition itself is progressive, however, surgery is not a permanent cure, and symptoms often recur.

DISORDERS OF THE NERVE ROOTS

DEFINITION

Disorders of the nerve root, termed *radiculopathy*, lead to symptoms referable to a dermatome or myotome. Either the ventral (anterior, motor) or posterior (dorsal, sensory) root can be involved independently or after they join to form the spinal nerve. Symptoms will follow the anatomic location. Because the root must traverse the vertebral foramen, it is prone to disorders of the spine at these locations. *Sciatica*, which is a commonly used but poorly defined term, often connotes low back pain with radiation into the ipsilateral leg, thereby implying pain radiating along the sciatic nerve, which anatomically contains fibers originating in the L4-S2 roots. The cauda equina syndrome results from disease involving the roots of the lower lumbar and sacral spinal cord levels as they traverse inside the spinal canal on their way to exit below their respective vertebral bodies.

PATHOBIOLOGY

Irritation of the spinal sensory nerve root or dorsal root ganglion causes symptoms referable to that dermatome. Spontaneous dysesthesias are hypothesized to result from ectopic discharges from the injured nerve; sensitization of the injured nerve leads to tactile evoked dysesthesias in the same distribution. Mechanical compression of the nerve contributes to the syndrome. In addition, inflammatory cytokines leak from the nucleus pulposus into the epidural space, where they result in endoneurial edema and pain. The pro-inflammatory cytokine TNF-α is a likely main contributor. Rupture of the nucleus pulposus releases phospholipase A_2, which also plays an important role in the inflammatory process. The inflammatory process itself can cause pain even in the absence of frank root compression.

The nerve root exits through the intervertebral foramen, where it is subject to compression and injury. The proximal portion of the nerve root has a small region of decreased vascular supply, where it is especially prone to edema, which can exacerbate the effect of the original injury. Treatment of this edema is one of the potential therapeutic effects of corticosteroid injections. The S1 root is the most susceptible to injury at the foramen because it is the largest-diameter spinal nerve and exits through the narrowest lumbar foramen. In addition, because it is traveling inferiorly from the S1 spinal cord level to pass out of the foramen under the S1 vertebral body, it passes through the superior, most narrow part of the foramen. The superior location of the sensory

root on these nerves may account for the early predominance of sensory symptoms versus motor symptoms.

CLINICAL MANIFESTATIONS

The symptoms of radiculopathy depend on the affected root. Root involvement is likely if pain radiates beyond the shoulder or the knee. In the thoracic region, root involvement often produces symptoms that "wrap around" the trunk. Radicular pain is often worsened by activities that increase intraspinal pressure, such as coughing, sneezing, straining, and other Valsalva maneuvers. The characteristics of the pain vary, but when they are exacerbated by such provocation, they are often described as sharp, shooting, electrical, and tingling. When reporting the symptoms, patients may point to or rub the distal dermatome where they are experiencing the discomfort (perceived pain). Patients also may report specific positions that increase or decrease pain; for example, sitting will often worsen the pain of acute lumbar disc herniation, and neck extension can produce radiating pain in cervical disc herniation or other processes that narrow the foramen.

It is uncommon for patients to spontaneously note anesthesia, but they often note dysesthesias in radiculopathy, even in the absence of spine pain. The localization of these dysesthesias often follows the dermatome but also may be described diffusely by the patient. Likewise, complaints of weakness may be difficult to isolate to a particular muscle; however, exceptions exist, such as when the patient complains of a weak grip or a foot drop.

On examination, side-by-side strength testing of specific muscles (Chapter 421, Table 421-3) can help identify slight weakness. Slight weakness may also be identified by evaluating for pronator drift in the arms or asking patients to walk on their toes, walk on their heels, and do shallow knee bends on each leg independently. Sensory examination should test all potential root distributions; pinprick is often sufficient, and it is helpful to ask the patient to report any abnormalities, not just frank hypesthesia. Hyperreflexia in the arms is not expected in a spinal nerve disorder and, if unexplained, should be further investigated for an injury to the spinal cord or brain (Chapter 399). Patients who are older than 65 years or who have a peripheral neuropathy (Chapter 420) might have reduced or even absent ankle jerks.

The cauda equina syndrome is manifested as unilateral or bilateral leg weakness, saddle anesthesia, urinary dysfunction with hesitancy or retention, and, less commonly, bowel dysfunction. Depending on the cause, it is frequently accompanied by low back pain. The syndrome can be accompanied by severe sciatica, which can be unilateral or bilateral but also involve perineal pain. The weakness of the legs, which may be asymmetrical, is of the lower motor neuron type. The major causes of the cauda equina syndrome include lumbar disc herniation, neoplasm, and lumbar spinal stenosis.

DIAGNOSIS

The history and physical examination are similar to the evaluation of neck and back pain (see earlier), with special emphasis on finding evidence of nerve root involvement.

The patient should be queried about bowel and bladder dysfunction. Frank incontinence needs to be investigated for either the cauda equina syndrome or a myelopathy. If the patient has any loss of perineal sensation, such as might be noted during or after voiding or bowel movement, the examination should test perianal sensation, anal sphincter tone, and anal wink reflex. Because the cauda equina syndrome involves nerve roots, reflexes should be normal or decreased; hyperactive reflexes or a Babinski sign would indicate a myelopathy (see later).

Ancillary Testing

Imaging to evaluate a potential radiculopathy is similar to the evaluation for neck and back pain (see above), but MRIs must be interpreted judiciously. For example, MRI performed 1 year after disc herniation with sciatica cannot determine which patients continue to be symptomatic and which are symptom free.[7] Alternatively, EMG can localize radicular abnormalities and their severity as well as assess possible comorbid neurologic diseases, such as diffuse peripheral or entrapment neuropathies. EMG electrodiagnostic localization can be extremely helpful in determining whether a finding on MRI is truly associated with neurologic impairment, and it has a high sensitivity and specificity for identification of acute and chronic denervation when the motor (anterior) aspect of the root is involved. However, EMG is less sensitive (about 30 to 70%) if only the sensory (posterior) limb of the root is involved by the lesion. MRI with its high sensitivity and EMG with its high specificity should be considered complementary tests.

Differential Diagnosis

Many mechanical processes can injure the spinal nerve root (see earlier, Neck and Back Pain), and most of the causes of spine pain can cause root disorders. Spinal cord compression may accompany radiculopathy.

In addition to conditions that can affect the nerve root as it leaves the spinal column, intracolumn abnormalities below the level of the conus medullaris can affect the lumbar and sacral roots before they exit, thereby resulting in the cauda equina syndrome. Most commonly, the cauda equina syndrome is caused by extrinsic compression of the caudal sac by a mass, such as a large and centrally herniated lumbar disc, metastatic tumor, abscess, or epidural hematoma, but arachnoiditis or chronic meningitis must be considered.

Disorders of the brachial or lumbosacral plexus can cause pain radiating down a limb in a radicular or polyradicular pattern. Painful peripheral neuropathies (Chapter 420) can also resemble a radiculopathy. Non-neurologic disorders, such as fibromyalgia (Chapter 274) and polymyalgia rheumatica (Chapter 271), can cause axial pain that mimics a radiculopathy. Cervical radiculopathy also can be mimicked by acromioclavicular joint arthropathy, shoulder bursitis, and the shoulder impingement syndrome; lumbar radiculopathy can be mimicked by hip arthritis, trochanteric bursitis, iliotibial band syndrome, and hamstring tendinitis (Chapter 263).

TREATMENT Rx

Acute neck and back pain, even with radicular symptoms, is usually self-limited and resolves.[8] If radiculopathy is associated with an underlying non-structural lesion, such as infection or tumor, treatment should be directed toward that underlying lesion (see also later, Metastatic Spinal Cord Compression). If symptoms or neurologic dysfunction progress or persist for more than 6 weeks, interventional options should be considered. Surgery is indicated for spinal instability, progressive neurologic deficits, or severe radicular pain that persists for more than 3 months despite conservative therapy, especially in patients with spinal stenosis and herniated discs.

In cervical radiculopathy, either foraminal or epidural corticosteroid injection may be of benefit. A series of injections, usually between one and three, provides short-term relief of radicular symptoms, with an acceptable adverse event profile. Although minor events, such as increased neck pain, headache, and vasovagal reactions, are relatively frequent (5 to 20%), serious events, such as epidural hematoma or abscess, are uncommon (<1%). In cervical spondylopathy with radiculopathy, surgery provides more rapid pain relief than does physiotherapy but little additional benefit in the long term.[A20] Anterior cervical discectomy, with or without fusion, is beneficial. Cervical anterior discectomy and arthroplasty result in a lower risk of postoperative dysphagia compared with discectomy and fusion, but more complicated surgeries are not of established benefit.

In lumbar radiculopathic pain, epidural steroid injections may provide relatively minor short-term symptom relief for 2 to 6 weeks, but they do not improve function or relieve pain beyond 3 months. They usually will not delay or avoid surgery and therefore are not routinely recommended.[A21] Chemonucleolysis of a lumbar disc is moderately superior to placebo but inferior to surgery.

For symptomatic radiculopathy associated with a herniated disc, either open surgical discectomy or microdiskectomy is superior to nonsurgical therapy for at least 3 months.[9] If the condition is isolated to a single disc and no significant degenerative changes are present, longer periods of benefit are more likely. Patients who derive a greater benefit from surgery include those with radiculopathy in which the MRI shows a herniated disc with a resultant compression of the thecal sac of one third or more, or those with nerve root compression.[10] Systematic reviews suggest that conservative discectomy allows a quicker return to work and has less long-term back pain than does more aggressive surgery,[11,12] but with the downside of an increased risk of recurrent disc herniation.

DISH can cause symptomatic radiculopathy.[13] When progressive or associated with myelopathy, surgical decompression of the ossified posterior longitudinal ligament should be considered. No particular surgical approach has been shown to be superior, and each case must be approached based on individual factors.[14]

DISORDERS OF THE SPINAL CORD

DEFINITION AND GENERAL OVERVIEW

A disorder of the spinal cord itself is termed a *myelopathy*. A myelopathy can be intramedullary, as the result of a disorder intrinsic to the cord, or extramedullary, as the result of an abnormality that is extrinsic to the cord but compressing it.

EPIDEMIOLOGY AND PATHOBIOLOGY

Spinal cord disorders can be caused by a wide range of conditions (Table 400-6).

The functional elements of the spinal cord (Fig. 400-7) include descending tracts largely to motor and autonomic neurons, motor neurons, autonomic neurons, and sensory ascending tracts. The anterior horn cell motor neuron is the cell body for the axon that will become the anterior nerve root and continue directly to innervate the muscle. The cell bodies for the primary sensory neurons reside in the dorsal root ganglion outside the spinal cord itself.

CLINICAL MANIFESTATIONS

The clinical manifestations of myelopathy result from the spinal level of the lesion. The majority of signs will be bilateral, but asymmetry, or even unilaterality, does not exclude a spinal cord lesion.

In general, the three major functions affected are motor, sensory, and autonomic, especially bowel, bladder, and erectile function. If anterior horn cells are involved at the lesion level, the corresponding myotome will exhibit lower motor neuron function (hypotonic weakness), and reflexes may be decreased at that level. Below the lesion, however, patients will have hypertonic weakness that can progress to spastic paralysis, hyperreflexion, and Babinski sign. Sensation will be decreased from the level of the lesion and distally. Because increased tone and spasticity often develop over time, they may not be dramatic at the initial clinical presentation. If the posterior columns are compromised, patients may lose joint position sense and develop ataxia, especially of gait. If the posterior columns of the cervical cord are impaired, patients may have pseudoathetosis of the fingers, manifested as unconscious athetotic movements of the fingers of the outstretched arm when the eyes are closed.

The anterior cord syndrome is manifested as lower motor neuron weakness at the level of the lesion (anterior horn); upper motor neuron weakness and spasticity below the lesion (corticospinal tracts); autonomic dysfunction below the level of the lesion (lateral horn), most often bowel and bladder dysfunction; and loss of pain and temperature sensation below the level of the lesion (spinothalamic tract). Vibration and joint position sense remain intact (posterior columns). The major causes of this syndrome are vascular, such as an anterior spinal artery, or an anteriorly impinging mass lesion, such as disc or vertebral body mass.

The central cord syndrome is manifested as lower motor neuron signs and symptoms at the level of the lesion (anterior horn cells) and upper motor neuron signs and symptoms below the lesion (corticospinal tracts), urinary retention, and a band of loss of temperature and pain sensation at the level of the lesion (anterior white commissure decussation of these fibers). In the midcervical level, this syndrome is typical of syringomyelia (Chapter 417). Other major causes include intramedullary tumors (Chapter 189) and post-traumatic cervical injury (Chapter 399) in patients with disc herniation or preexisting cervical spondylosis.

TABLE 400-6	CAUSES OF MYELOPATHY
Trauma/compression	**Neoplastic**
Direct ± vertebral spine disease	Metastatic cord compression
Spondylotic myelopathy/stenosis	Spinal tumors
Post-traumatic syrinx	Paraneoplastic
Arachnoid cyst	**Infectious**
Vascular	Epidural abscess
Cord infarction	Syphilis
Dural arteriovenous malformation	Lyme disease
Inflammatory/autoimmune	Tuberculosis
Multiple sclerosis	HIV infection
Devic disease	Tropical spastic paraparesis
Acute disseminating encephalomyelitis	Herpes zoster
Adrenomyeloneuropathy	**Toxic/metabolic**
Systemic lupus erythematosus	Post-radiation myelopathy
Sjögren syndrome	Vitamin B$_{12}$ deficiency
Mixed connective tissue disease	Vitamin E deficiency
Postinfectious/postvaccination	Heroin
Arachnoiditis	Epidural lipomatosis
	Congenital/hereditary
	Chiari malformation
	Syringomyelia

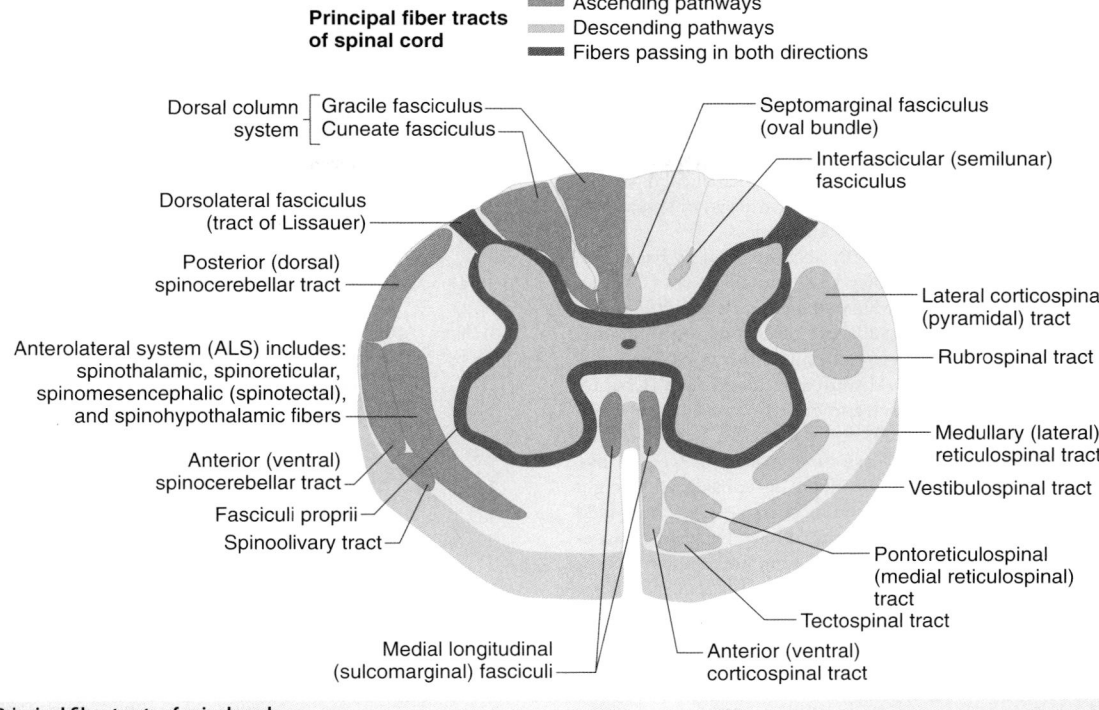

FIGURE 400-7. Principal fiber tracts of spinal cord.

The posterior cord syndrome is manifested as complaints of imbalance, especially in the dark or with eyes closed, and an examination notable for ataxia, presence of Romberg's sign, and loss of vibration sense and proprioception below the level of the lesion (posterior columns), with preservation of pain and temperature sensation. Patients are seldom weak. Posterior compression may be caused by spondylotic disease, but other major causes include deficiencies of vitamin B$_{12}$ or vitamin E (Chapters 218 and 416), syphilis (Chapter 319), AIDS-associated vacuolar myelopathy (Chapter 394), and nitrous oxide inhalation (Chapter 432).

The Brown-Séquard (cord hemisection) syndrome combines features of these syndromes. At the level of the lesion, patients exhibit ipsilateral lower motor weakness (anterior horn) and loss of all sensation (posterior root entry zone). Below the level of the lesion, patients have ipsilateral upper motor weakness and spasticity (corticospinal tract) and ipsilateral loss of vibration sense and proprioception (posterior columns), with contralateral loss of pain and temperature (spinothalamic tract, the fibers of which have crossed from the opposite side through the anterior white commissure). The Brown-Séquard syndrome is often caused by trauma (Chapter 399) or eccentric compression.

The conus medullaris syndrome refers to dysfunction of the distal-most tapered portion of the spinal cord, which anatomically lies at approximately the T12-L1 vertebral spine level. The arms are normal; weakness in the legs is variable but often symmetrical when it is present. The main signs and symptoms are sexual dysfunction, loss of bowel and bladder control, and perianal anesthesia with loss of the anal wink reflex. The major causes are disc herniation, lumbar stenosis, and neoplasm.

DIAGNOSIS

Symptoms of bilateral involvement of the arms or legs suggest a myelopathy, although bilateral leg involvement can be seen in lumbar spinal stenosis and the cauda equina syndrome. Complaints of leg stiffness or incoordination suggest spasticity from myelopathy. Other symptoms include a recent change in bowel or bladder function, erectile dysfunction, imbalance (especially in the dark or with eyes closed), and catching of feet when walking. These central symptoms can also reflect lesions of the brain stem and higher, so the patient should be queried about cortical and brain stem symptoms (e.g., cognitive function, vision, facial strength, sensation, and swallowing). Focal back pain supports a myelopathy.

Examination for a potential myelopathy must include an evaluation of anal tone and perineal sensation. The patient should be examined in a gown to allow inspection of the spine as well as the overlying skin. A sensory level, which represents a point where distal (inferior) sensation is altered, should also be sought, but a spinal cord lesion rarely causes a sharp line of sensory demarcation. Joint position sense can be diminished if the posterior columns are involved. A tandem gait will assess possible gait ataxia. Finally, the patient should be examined for distal hypertonicity, if not frank spasticity, by assessment for hyperreflexia and Babinski signs. In acute spinal cord lesions, however, a state of "spinal shock" can cause hyporeflexia or even a flaccid paralysis.

Ancillary Testing

MRI is the test of choice because it provides anatomic detail of the spine and subarachnoid space as well as the spinal cord. MRI may also show evidence of demyelinating or metastatic disease. Plain films are not adequate to evaluate the spinal cord. If the MRI is normal, lumbar puncture is sometimes useful for evaluation of conditions that resemble myelopathy: Guillain-Barré syndrome (Chapter 420), infectious or carcinomatous meningitis (Chapter 412), arachnoiditis, and transverse myelitis.

Differential Diagnosis

The many causes of myelopathy (see Table 400-6) can typically occur at any spinal level, but certain conditions predominate at specific spinal levels.

Any lesion that has an upper cervical location must be evaluated for disorders of the craniocervical junction, especially disorders that can produce atlantoaxial instability, such as rheumatoid arthritis (Chapter 264); after trauma, cervical or odontoid fracture must be excluded. Disorders at the base of the skull, such as Chiari I and other congenital malformations (Chapter 417), can sometimes affect the upper cervical cord. Syringomyelia (Chapter 417), which may or may not be associated with Chiari malformation, also has a predilection for the cervical cord.

The thoracic cord is relatively protected from all but direct trauma, but it is the most common site for metastatic cord compression. Transverse myelitis is most commonly thoracic, and the thoracic cord also is particularly vulnerable to a watershed ischemic myelopathy due to severe hypotension. Epidural lipomatosis often is most symptomatic at the thoracic level. DISH also has a predilection for the thoracic cord and can produce spinal cord compression by ossification of the posterior longitudinal ligament.

The lumbar-conus region is the most common site for disc herniations. In addition, ependymomas are relatively more common in this region, as are metastases from more caudal locations and compression from arachnoiditis.

The rapidity of onset helps in diagnosis. Acute or relatively acute myelopathy suggests vascular causes, trauma, demyelinating lesions, or sudden decompensation of a preexisting lesion, such as a pathologic fracture. In a young person with no other comorbid illnesses, a demyelinating illness, such as multiple sclerosis (Chapter 411) or acute disseminated encephalomyelitis (Chapter 414), is suggested; other CNS lesions separated in space with white matter signal abnormalities on MRI would increase the likelihood of this diagnosis. In older persons or patients with known vascular risk factors, hypotension, or an onset in the immediate postoperative period, a spinal cord infarction is possible. Sudden sharp back pain suggests mechanical disorders (e.g., pathologic fracture, sudden worsening spondylolisthesis) or spinal cord infarction, whereas demyelinating lesions are often painless.

Myelopathy developing subacutely, especially accompanied by back pain, can be caused by metastatic disease (Chapter 189) and abscesses (Chapter 413). Both of these conditions must be evaluated and treated as true emergencies to prevent permanent paralysis. Subacute or chronic myelopathies include vitamin B$_{12}$ deficiency (Chapter 416), although nitrous oxide inhalation may cause an acute expression of the disorder; syringomyelia (Chapter 417); and more slowly growing tumors, such as meningiomas (Chapter 189), lipomas, and neurofibromas (Chapter 417).

In the setting of known malignant disease or unexplained weight loss, metastatic cord compression (Chapter 189) must be considered. Weight loss, back pain, and fever can be seen in infection (Chapters 412 and 413) and occasionally spondyloarthropathies (Chapter 265). Infectious causes also include tropical spastic paraparesis (human T-lymphotropic virus type 1 [HTLV-1; Chapter 378]). Syphilis (Chapter 319) is the cause of tabes dorsalis; patients may have other signs and symptoms, such as lancinating pains, ataxia, depressed leg reflexes, and Argyll Robertson pupils. Myelopathies that follow an infectious illness include acute disseminated encephalomyelitis and progressive necrotizing myelopathy. Transverse myelitis can follow viral infections, such as herpes zoster (Chapter 375). Myelopathy accompanied by evidence of multifocal cortical dysfunction would likely be multiple sclerosis or acute disseminated encephalomyelitis (Chapter 414). An accompanied peripheral neuropathy is seen in vitamin B$_{12}$ deficiency myelopathy (Chapter 416), which tends to cause gait ataxia. Rheumatoid arthritis (Chapter 264) causes progressive loss of cartilage and bone destruction, potentially leading to atlantoaxial instability and cervical subluxation. Other systemic illnesses, such as systemic lupus erythematosus (Chapter 266), Behçet syndrome (Chapter 270), and sarcoidosis (Chapter 95), can also cause myelopathies. In patients with exogenous or endogenous hypercortisolemia (Chapter 227), epidural deposition of unencapsulated fat can cause epidural lipomatosis that compresses the spinal column. Patients with a distant history of trauma might be evaluated for post-traumatic syringomyelia. Patients with a history of lumbar puncture, surgery, or intrathecal injections can develop arachnoiditis.

Younger patients are more likely to be symptomatic from congenital disorders, ankylosing spondylitis, or multiple sclerosis. In patients older than 55 years, cervical spondylotic myelopathy is the most common cause of myelopathic symptoms.

TREATMENT AND PROGNOSIS Rx

High-dose steroids should be used in cord compression from metastatic tumors (Chapter 189). Steroids are also frequently used in transverse myelitis, although no controlled trials have been performed. Steroids are no longer recommended for acute spinal cord trauma (Chapter 399).

Patients with spinal cord lesions must be assessed emergently for any potential complications. With high cervical spine lesions, paresis or paralysis of the diaphragm and respiratory depression can occur. Although not emergent, higher cervical or medulla extension of inflammatory myelopathies can cause distressing hiccups and nausea. In lesions at the thoracic level or above, interruption of the lateral column autonomic pathways can lead to autonomic instability, including altered blood pressure responses. At almost any level, but especially at the conus and cauda equina, acute urinary retention may require catheterization. Long-term complications of spinal cord injury include osteoporosis (Chapter 243), orthostatic hypotension (Chapters 51 and 62), and chronic neuropathic pain (Chapter 420), all of which may require specific therapy. Other aspects of treatment and prognosis depend on the specific cause.

Specific Causes of Myelopathy
VASCULAR MYELOPATHIES

The CNS tissue of the spinal cord is as intolerant of ischemia as the brain is. Vascular myelopathy occurs when there is loss of blood flow to the spinal

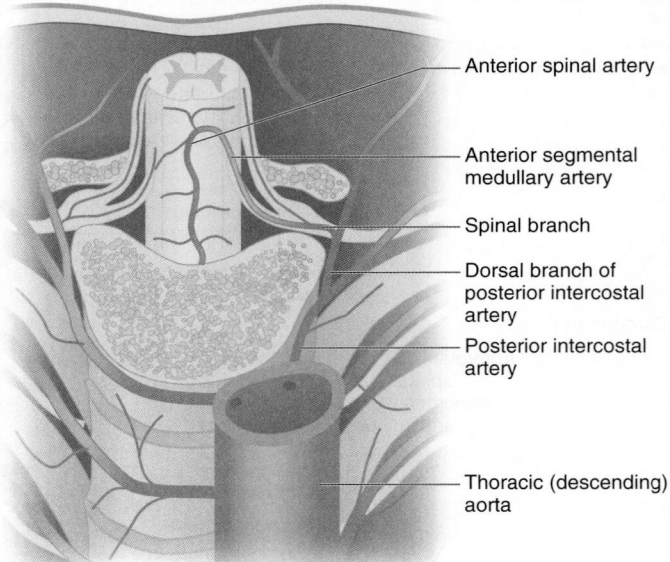

- Anterior spinal artery
- Anterior segmental medullary artery
- Spinal branch
- Dorsal branch of posterior intercostal artery
- Posterior intercostal artery
- Thoracic (descending) aorta

FIGURE 400-8. Blood supply of the spinal cord: section through thoracic level, anterosuperior view.

cord, whether it is acute or chronic and whether the cause is ischemic or hemorrhagic.

The blood supply to the spinal cord comes from the anterior and posterior spinal arteries that run longitudinally along the length of the spinal cord (Fig. 400-8). The paired posterior spinal arteries are derived in their most rostral origin as branches of the vertebral arteries at the level of the medulla and then run inferiorly along the posterolateral surface of the spinal cord. Along their course, they are fed by a series of small arteries that enter the spinal canal through the intervertebral foramina. Inside the canal, they anastomose extensively to provide redundancy. The anterior spinal artery is formed superiorly when branches of the vertebral artery join to form a single anterior spinal artery, which then runs down the midline of the anterior surface of the spinal cord. It also receives feeders along its length, but not to the same extent as the posterior segmental branches do. A large anterior radicular artery at C5-6 supplies the cervical enlargement. The main caudal anterior blood supply, however, is from the large artery of Adamkiewicz that enters the spinal canal between the cord levels of T9 and L2 and serves as the main blood supply to the anterior spinal artery, which supplies the lumbar enlargement, the lower thoracic cord, and the conus medullaris.

Compromise of the microvascular supply to the cord underlies the gliotic changes in many slowly progressive myelopathies such as spondylotic myelopathy. Ischemic causes include general hypotension, atherosclerotic disease, embolic events, vasculitis, and vascular steal; hemorrhagic events usually result from rupture of abnormal vascular malformations.

Severe global hypotension or aortic dissection or surgery can cause ischemic myelopathy, especially in watershed areas of the spinal cord, notably the thoracic region. Atherosclerosis, especially of the artery of Adamkiewicz, can lead to ischemic infarction of the cord by either decreased perfusion or thromboembolic events. Ischemia has also been reported to be a result of compression of the anterior spinal artery by a centrally herniated T12-L1 disc.

Embolic events and local thrombosis can occur in pregnancy and sickle cell disease (Chapter 163). During decompression sickness (Chapter 94), nitrogen bubbles cause microvascular emboli and ischemia. Vasculitis affecting the spinal cord is rare, but granulomatous angiitis of the CNS and polyarteritis nodosa (Chapter 270) can lead to infarction.

Spinal dural arteriovenous fistulas are the most common type of vascular malformation of the spinal cord. Arteriovenous malformations are most common in the thoracic cord, especially in patients older than 30 years. Vascular malformations can cause myelopathy by being mass lesions that compress local structures, by interfering with normal venous drainage, by diverting blood as part of a vascular steal with exercise of muscles that compete for blood flow, or by hemorrhage.

Spinal cord hemorrhage, which is rare, can occur intramedullary in the cord itself or in subarachnoid, subdural, or epidural locations. Intramedullary hemorrhage is most often caused by trauma, although bleeding can also occur into a tumor or from an intramedullary vascular malformation. Bleeding from a malformation that enters the subarachnoid space can cause back pain and headache. Epidural hematomas, which cause extramedullary cord compression, can occur as a complication of surgery, myelography, or lumbar puncture, particularly in patients with bleeding diatheses.

CLINICAL MANIFESTATIONS

Occlusion of the artery of Adamkiewicz usually presents with signs of thoracic watershed ischemia—paraplegia with relative sparing of the sacral roots. Infarction in the anterior spinal artery distribution results in dysfunction of the anterior two thirds of the cord, including the anterior horns, spinothalamic tracts, and corticospinal tracts; patients usually present with acute paraparesis and impaired bowel and bladder function. Sharp and sometimes circumferential pain at the level of the infarct is often described. Below the level of the lesion, temperature and pain sensation are lost, but vibration and position sense (posterior columns) are preserved.

Infarction of the posterior arteries is less common because of their better collateral circulation. Clinical manifestations, which are less dramatic, include loss of vibratory and position sense, ataxia, gait coordination problems, and Romberg sign; reflexes may be depressed at the level of the infarction.

The central cord vasculature syndrome is similar clinically to a traumatic central cord syndrome (Chapter 399). It may occur as a watershed lesion between the territories of the anterior and posterior spinal circulation and is most common in the cervical cord in older patients with preexisting cervical spondylotic disease.

Vascular malformations most often have a chronic progressive clinical course. Pain is common. Arteriovenous fistulas, commonly in the thoracic cord, present as progressive paraplegia. Patients may have exacerbations of symptoms with exercise and certain postures, and sudden worsening usually indicates hemorrhage.

DIAGNOSIS

Vascular malformations are initially evaluated by MRI, which also can assess the health of the surrounding tissue. When the vascular malformation is connected to the dura (arteriovenous fistula), myelography can occasionally detect lesions that are not seen or are poorly defined by MRI. If embolization or surgery is being considered, spinal angiography is needed to identify feeding and draining vessels, although the test carries a small risk of infarction. Intramedullary arteriovenous malformations are more commonly found in the cervical and thoracic levels and may require angiography to be visualized. When imaging is equivocal, lumbar puncture can be considered; an elevated leukocyte count (>10 cells/μL) suggests an inflammatory myelopathy rather than a vascular lesion.

TREATMENT AND PROGNOSIS [Rx]

Treatment options are limited and include reversal of the cause of ischemia, such as by correcting hypotension (Chapter 106) or treating for emergent sickle crisis (Chapter 163). Prognosis for most cases of spinal cord infarct is poor unless blood flow is restored rapidly. In one study, for example, 3-year mortality was 23%, 42% of survivors needed wheelchairs, but 40% of those in wheelchairs at hospital discharge were able to walk at a 3-year follow-up.[15]

Arteriovenous fistulas are treated by occluding the shunt with embolization or surgery. Successful treatment may arrest and occasionally improve symptoms. Patients with suspected epidural hematomas (Chapter 399) require emergency treatment and surgery if there is progressive neurologic dysfunction.

INFLAMMATORY AND METABOLIC MYELOPATHIES

Transverse myelitis, multiple sclerosis, and other demyelinating diseases are considered in Chapter 411. Metabolic myelopathies can be caused by vitamin B$_{12}$, vitamin E, and copper deficiencies (Chapter 218).

Acute disseminated encephalomyelitis is mostly a monophasic disorder of demyelination of the spinal cord and brain. If it is isolated to the spinal cord, it might best be termed *transverse myelitis*. Parainfectious or postvaccination causes account for at least 75% of cases. Postvaccination acute disseminated encephalomyelitis is associated with measles-mumps-rubella vaccinations

and diphtheria-tetanus-polio vaccinations, as well as with vaccinations for influenza, hepatitis B, pertussis, and Japanese B encephalitis.

Connective tissue diseases can infrequently be a cause of myelopathy. Systemic lupus erythematosus (Chapter 266), with or without antiphospholipid antibody, can include myelitis in 1 to 3% of patients. Sjögren syndrome (Chapter 268), Behçet syndrome (Chapter 270), sarcoidosis (Chapter 95), ankylosing spondylitis (Chapter 265), mixed connective tissue disease (Chapter 270), and systemic sclerosis (Chapter 267) can be associated with inflammatory myelitis.

Human T-lymphotropic virus type 1 (HTLV-1)–associated myelopathy/tropical spastic paraparesis (Chapter 378) is a chronic progressive myelopathy that causes leg weakness, spasticity, loss of vibratory sense, and bladder dysfunction. More than 90% of infected persons remain asymptomatic, with transformation to a symptomatic condition thought to be largely related to the host's inflammatory response. Other neurologic dysfunctions associated with HTLV-1 infection include mild cognitive impairment, sensory neuropathy, and erectile dysfunction. There is no effective therapy.

DIAGNOSIS

In general, diagnosis of the inflammatory myelopathies is based on the clinical examination. MRI often shows a high T2 signal focal enlargement of the cord.

TREATMENT AND SECONDARY PREVENTION [Rx]

Intravenous corticosteroid infusions (e.g., methylprednisolone, 1 g intravenously daily for 5 days) are usually the mainstay for treatment of acute attacks of inflammatory myelopathies.

In patients who do not respond to corticosteroids, plasma exchange is effective in the acute treatment of CNS demyelinating disorders; about 60% of patients show improvement at 6 months. Factors predicting improvement are initiation of treatment within 15 days of the onset of symptoms and evidence of early improvement.

METASTATIC SPINAL CORD COMPRESSION

When metastatic cancer invades the spine or epidural space, the resultant destruction and growth compress the spinal cord and lead to a myelopathy. The prevalence of metastatic spinal cord compression may be as high as 5% in patients with cancer, depending on the type of malignant neoplasm and its tendency to metastasize to bone. Prostate (Chapter 201), breast (Chapter 198), and lung (Chapter 191) cancers each account for approximately 15 to 20% of cases, and non-Hodgkin lymphoma (Chapter 185), renal cell cancer (Chapter 197), and multiple myeloma (Chapter 187) account for about 5 to 10% each.

Most metastatic disease causes compression as a result of an extradural lesion, although a smaller number of metastatic lesions can be intradural-extramedullary disease. Intramedullary metastases are rare. Symptoms can be caused by direct compression of the cord and roots in the epidural space as the result of direct extension from hematogenous metastasis to the vertebral body. However, some tumors (e.g., lymphomas) may grow through the intervertebral foramen without causing significant bone destruction; the accompanying edema can compromise the local vasculature and cause ischemic damage in addition to direct compression. Vertebral destruction can make the spine unstable and cause pathologic fractures that can lead to cord and root damage.

CLINICAL MANIFESTATIONS

About 90% of patients present with pain that is classically worse on lying down and increases with the Valsalva maneuver. If the nerve root is involved, the pain will have a radicular component; if there is bone collapse, pain can be made worse by movement. Muscle weakness is present in 35 to 75% of patients at the time of diagnosis, sensory deficits in 50 to 70% of patients, and autonomic dysfunction in 50 to 60% of patients. The range of signs will depend on the level of compression.

DIAGNOSIS

Spinal cord compression, which must be suspected when any patient with cancer complains of spine pain even in the absence of neurologic signs or symptoms, is a neurologic emergency. MRI is the test of choice because plain films, which might recognize bone metastases and vertebral collapse, will miss soft tissue tumors that are in the epidural space and yield no information about the spinal cord itself. Conventional myelography should be used if MRI cannot be performed because of availability or the presence of metallic implants in the patient. Because up to 35% of patients have more than one site of metastasis, care should be taken to image the entire spine by MRI, myelography, or isotope bone scanning.

Differential Diagnosis

For extradural lesions, the differential diagnosis includes lipomas, fibromas, meningiomas, and chordomas as well as vascular malformations and abscesses. Intradural-extramedullary lesions include neurofibromas (Chapter 417), neurinomas, meningiomas, vascular malformations, and (less often) metastases. Arachnoid cysts, although benign, can cause compression through pressure effect. Finally, intramedullary lesions that can present as myelopathy and must be considered in the differential of metastatic cord compression include intramedullary vascular malformations, ependymomas, astrocytomas, and syringomyelia.

TREATMENT   Rx

Prompt initiation of corticosteroids (e.g., dexamethasone, loading dose of 10 to 16 mg followed by tapering over 10 to 14 days) and radiation therapy are the mainstays of initial therapy. Surgical decompressive surgery plus radiation therapy is better than radiation therapy alone for maintaining ambulation[A22] in patients who have a radioinsensitive tumor, have displacement of the spinal cord on MRI, have a single site of cord compression, and have not been totally paraplegic for more than 48 hours.

PROGNOSIS

Metastatic spinal cord compression usually occurs in the setting of metastases to multiple locations, and the expected survival prognosis is generally less than 6 months. Prognosis is improved in patients with malignant neoplasms that are sensitive to steroid therapy (especially lymphoma and leukemia) or are radiosensitive (e.g., multiple myeloma, small cell lung cancer). Patients who are ambulatory at the time of diagnosis, have a single site of compression, and had a less rapid onset of symptoms also generally have a better prognosis.

Grade A References

A1. Chou R, Fu R, Carrino JA, et al. Imaging strategies for low-back pain: systemic review and meta-analysis. *Lancet.* 2009;373:463-472.
A2. Gross A, Miller J, D'Sylva J, et al. Manipulation or mobilization for neck pain. *Cochrane Database Syst Rev.* 2010;5:CD004249.
A3. Chow RT, Johnson MI, Lopes-Martins RA, et al. Efficacy of low-level laser therapy in the management of neck pain: a systematic review and meta-analysis of randomised placebo or active-treatment controlled trials. *Lancet.* 2009;374:1897-1908.
A4. Fu LM, Li JT, Wu WS. Randomized controlled trials of acupuncture for neck pain: systematic review and meta-analysis. *J Altern Complement Med.* 2009;15:133-145.
A5. Michalsen A, Traitteur H, Ludtke R, et al. Yoga for chronic neck pain: a pilot randomized controlled clinical trial. *J Pain.* 2012;13:1122-1130.
A6. Dahm KT, Brurberg KG, Jamtvedt G, et al. Advice to rest in bed versus advice to stay active for acute low-back pain and sciatica. *Cochrane Database Syst Rev.* 2010;6:CD007612.
A7. Williams CM, Maher CG, Latimer J, et al. Efficacy of paracetamol for acute low-back pain: a double-blind, randomised controlled trial. *Lancet.* 2014;384:1586-1596.
A8. Chou R, Huffman LH, American Pain Society, American College of Physicians. Nonpharmacologic therapies for acute and chronic low back pain: a review of the evidence for an American Pain Society/American College of Physicians clinical practice guideline. *Ann Intern Med.* 2007;147:492-504.
A9. Cherkin DC, Sherman KJ, Kahn J, et al. A comparison of the effects of 2 types of massage and usual care on chronic low back pain: a randomized, controlled trial. *Ann Intern Med.* 2011;155:1-9.
A10. Bronfort G, Evans R, Anderson AV, et al. Spinal manipulation, medication, or home exercise with advice for acute and subacute neck pain: a randomized trial. *Ann Intern Med.* 2012;156:1-10.
A11. Vas J, Aranda JM, Modesto M, et al. Acupuncture in patients with acute low back pain: a multicentre randomised controlled clinical trial. *Pain.* 2012;153:1883-1889.
A12. Tilbrook HE, Cox H, Hewitt CE, et al. Yoga for chronic low back pain: a randomized trial. *Ann Intern Med.* 2011;155:569-578.
A13. Chou R, Atlas SJ, Stanos SP, et al. Nonsurgical interventional therapies for low back pain. A review of the evidence for an American Pain Society Clinical Practice Guideline. *Spine.* 2009;34:1078-1093.
A14. Buchmuller A, Navez M, Milletre-Bernardin M, et al. Value of TENS for relief of chronic low back pain with or without radicular pain. *Eur J Pain.* 2012;16:656-665.
A15. Kivitz AJ, Gimbel JS, Bramson C, et al. Efficacy and safety of tanezumab versus naproxen in the treatment of chronic low back pain. *Pain.* 2013;154:1009-1021.
A16. Wang X, Wanyan P, Tian JH, et al. Meta-analysis of randomized trials comparing fusion surgery to non-surgical treatment for discogenic chronic low back pain. *J Back Musculoskelet Rehabil.* 2014; [Epub ahead of print].
A17. Friedly JL, Comstock BA, Turner JA, et al. A randomized trial of epidural glucocorticoid injections for spinal stenosis. *N Engl J Med.* 2014;371:11-21.
A18. Ohtori S, Miyagi M, Eguchi Y, et al. Epidural administration of spinal nerves with the tumor necrosis factor-alpha inhibitor, etanercept, compared with dexamethasone for treatment of sciatica in patients with lumbar spinal stenosis: a prospective randomized study. *Spine (Phila Pa 1976).* 2012;37:439-444.
A19. Weinstein JN, Tosteson TD, Lurie JD, et al. Surgical versus nonsurgical therapy for lumbar spinal stenosis. *N Engl J Med.* 2008;358:794-810.
A20. Nikolaidis I, Fouyas IP, Sandercock PA, et al. Surgery for cervical radiculopathy or myelopathy. *Cochrane Database Syst Rev.* 2010;1:CD001466.
A21. Bicket MC, Horowitz JM, Benzon HT, et al. Epidural injections in prevention of surgery for spinal pain: systematic review and meta-analysis of randomized controlled trials. *Spine J.* 2015;15:348-362.
A22. Patchell RA, Tibbs PA, Regine WF, et al. Direct decompressive surgical resection in the treatment of spinal cord compression caused by metastatic cancer: a randomized trial. *Lancet.* 2005;366:643-648.

GENERAL REFERENCES

For the General References and other additional features, please visit Expert Consult at https://expertconsult.inkling.com.

401

REGIONAL CEREBRAL DYSFUNCTION: HIGHER MENTAL FUNCTIONS

DAVID S. KNOPMAN

DEFINITION

Higher mental function is at the core of what defines competent, independent individuals. Impairment of higher mental function can be broadly classified into four categories. Intellectual developmental disorder is a form of cognitive impairment that is present from infancy. Acquired forms of cognitive impairment are delirium, dementia, and focal cognitive disorders. Delirium (Chapter 28) is defined by its acute or subacute onset and coexistent alterations in alertness. Dementia (Chapter 402) represents an acquired cognitive impairment that is usually gradual in onset and not associated with alterations in alertness. Focal cognitive disorders involve only one aspect of cognition: memory, language, visuospatial cognition, or executive cognitive functioning, each of which is supported by a different cerebral region.

For the majority of patients in a non-neurology practice, a global description such as "normal mental function" or "cognitively impaired" will suffice. Cognitive impairment then becomes a diagnosis that subsumes all forms of altered higher mental function regardless of which domains are affected or how severely they are affected.

CLINICAL MANIFESTATIONS AND DIAGNOSIS

An informal conversation with a patient lacks sensitivity for detecting cognitive impairment. If cognitive impairment is suspected from the patient's history, formal assessments should be performed. Bedside evaluations of orientation, memory, language, reasoning, and visuospatial function can be used to derive an overall view of cognitive function but do not automatically translate into diagnoses, because alertness, cooperation, education, native language, sensorimotor function, and mood must be taken into account. Although scores on bedside mental status examinations correlate strongly with severity and prognosis, they provide only rough guides to cognitive ability and cannot localize a cognitive deficit anatomically in the brain. The Mini-Cog Test (Chapter 27, Table 27-5) is among the most brief of available bedside examinations. If cognitive dysfunction is discovered in the course of the bedside examination, further exploration of individual cognitive domains must be undertaken.

MEMORY FUNCTION AND AMNESIC DISORDERS

DEFINITION

Human memory operates over a wide time range, from seconds to decades, and with quantities of information ranging from a single word to a lifetime's experience. Each neural system that achieves this monumental dynamic range has its own brain localization[1,2] (Table 401-1).

TABLE 401-1 DESCRIPTION OF MEMORY SYSTEMS

TYPE OF MEMORY FUNCTION	REGIONAL LOCALIZATION	LEARNING EFFICIENCY	TIME SPAN UNTIL EFFECTIVE RETRIEVAL	CAPACITY	CLINICAL TESTING TECHNIQUES	EXAMPLES IN DAILY LIFE
Declarative episodic memory	Hippocampus, medial thalamus	Single exposure	Decades	Very large, with rehearsal and elaboration	Recall of 3-4 words after 5 minutes	Recall of recent events and conversations
Declarative semantic memory	Temporal-parietal association cortices	Capable of single exposure; enhanced with repetition	Decades	Very large, perhaps limitless	Confrontation naming, general knowledge	Vocabulary, knowledge of life events from remote past
Attention span, "immediate memory"	Primary auditory or visual cortex	Single exposure only	Seconds	Very small: 7 ± 2 digits (auditory)	Digit span	Dialing a telephone number after hearing it or reading it
Working memory	Lateral frontal cortex	Single exposure only	Seconds	Small	Digits backward	Supporting many mental activities, such as mental arithmetic, abstract reasoning
Procedural memory	Basal ganglia, probably association neocortices	Requires extensive training	Decades	Moderate	Experimental laboratory methods only	Retention of motor skills (e.g., riding a bicycle, typing)

Declarative memory describes the type of learning and retrieval of facts and information that occur with conscious attention and intent; examples include remembering conversations, events, and intentions. Declarative memory has semantic and episodic components. Semantic memory refers to the brain's storehouse of knowledge, words, and facts. Episodic memory refers to learning and recall of specific events. Retention of information for more than a few seconds in the face of exposure to additional facts, details, or events requires declarative episodic memory to store and organize the information suitable for later recall. It is this declarative episodic memory system that is assessed as "memory" in the clinical setting. Anterograde amnesia is the clinical manifestation of disturbances in declarative episodic memory. Anterograde refers to failure to learn, and hence recall, new information on an ongoing basis. Most disorders of memory also exhibit retrograde amnesia, a disturbance of the ability to retrieve information from the past.

Immediate recall of information with zero delay and zero intervening information is a very short-term declarative memory function. Immediate memory is capable of storing an image of an auditory message in exact form, but only a small amount and for a short period. The fidelity of immediate memory recall accuracy drops off dramatically over seconds, particularly if intervening sensory stimuli attract attention. A comparable system exists in the visual modality in that the memory acts like a photograph that fades rapidly. From a clinical perspective, immediate memory is separate from declarative episodic memory. Immediate recall is generally used as a marker of attention and alertness and not memory per se.

PATHOBIOLOGY

The hippocampal formations are the anatomic structures of importance for the declarative episodic memory system. The hippocampal formations are imaged well with magnetic resonance imaging (MRI) (Fig. 401-1). The principal input to the hippocampus comes through the entorhinal cortex from multimodal association areas in the frontal, parietal, and temporal neocortices. A second important input is a cholinergic pathway that originates in the septum of the medial-orbital frontal lobe. There are two principal output circuits of the hippocampal formations. One is via the subiculum back to multimodal association areas. The other hippocampal efferent pathway projects via the fornix to the mammillary bodies. The projection from the mammillary bodies passes through the medial thalamus to the ventral anterior nucleus of the thalamus, then to the posterior cingulate, and then back to the entorhinal cortex. The hippocampal circuit is believed to facilitate the formation of memory in association neocortices. The hippocampus does not store a particular learned fact, but rather it enables the appropriate region in a multimodal association cortical region to do so.

Lesions in one hippocampal formation will not generally have as devastating an impact on episodic memory as bilateral lesions will. However, in older persons who may have subclinical bilateral hippocampal pathology, a unilateral lesion, particularly in the dominant hemisphere, may produce a dense

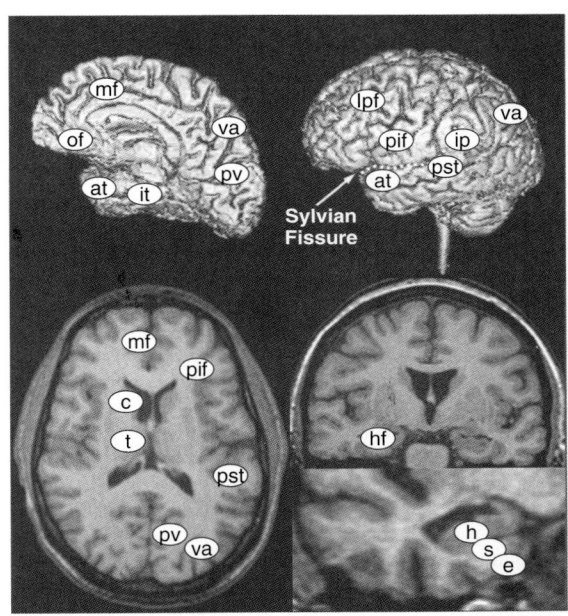

FIGURE 401-1. **Magnetic resonance images of a normal brain.** *Upper left,* Midsagittal view; *upper right,* left lateral view; *lower left,* axial view through the head of the caudate and body of the thalamus; *lower right,* coronal view through the mammillary bodies, with a magnified view of the medial temporal lobe. at = anterior temporal; c = caudate nucleus; e = entorhinal cortex; h = hippocampus; hf = hippocampal formation; ip = inferior parietal cortex; it = inferior temporal; lpf = lateral prefrontal cortex; mf = medial frontal cortex; of = orbital frontal cortex; pif = posterior inferior frontal cortex (Broca's area); pst = posterior superior temporal; pv = primary visual cortex (area 17); s = subiculum; t = temporal; va = visual association cortex (areas 18 and 19). (Courtesy Maria Shiung and Clifford Jack, MD.)

anterograde amnesia. Lesions in the columns of the fornix, mammillary bodies, and medial thalamus have also been linked to anterograde amnesia.

CLINICAL MANIFESTATIONS

Patients with anterograde amnesia have poor or no recollection of events, conversations, or observations. Family members report that patients repeat themselves in conversation or re-ask the same questions over the course of a few minutes to hours. Patients will generally forget important events and conversations, even when they were fully engaged in them. They will lose track of the date and time of day. They will forget appointments, even with reminders. Generally, patients with anterograde amnesia will fail to encode most events and happenings around them. The consequences of such memory failure are usually more evident to the family and acquaintances of patients with the disorder than they are to the patients themselves. Anosognosia (lack of awareness) for the deficit of anterograde amnesia is very common, though not universal. Patients who most vehemently complain of memory loss are often suffering from depression rather than focal cognitive dysfunction.

Because some degree of forgetting is ubiquitous in human experience, it is challenging to distinguish between "everyday" forgetting and forgetting that is pathologic. All adults occasionally misplace important items, overlook an appointment, or forget some part of a conversation. In cognitively normal individuals, distraction, preoccupation, inattention, exhaustion, sleep deprivation, or other major life stressors inevitably produce some instances of excess forgetting. Pathologic forgetting as a result of a brain disorder produces a much greater degree of forgetting than occurs in the course of normal daily life, but there is no formulaic description of the boundary at which normal forgetting ends and pathologic forgetting begins.

DIAGNOSIS

The diagnosis of anterograde amnesia begins with a complaint of memory impairment from the patient or someone close to the patient. Testing of memory can be performed at the bedside in alert patients. The patient is asked to learn three or four words and recall them after 1 or 2 minutes. A patient with severe anterograde amnesia will recall none or at most one of the words, whereas individuals with normal memory can recall all of the words or all but one.

In patients with questionable memory difficulties, assessment by an experienced neuropsychologist is often a necessary part of the evaluation. Standardized tests of memory have greater precision and reliability and involve the use of lengthier material to be remembered and a longer delay between learning and recall.

Determining the Cause

Alzheimer's disease is the most common disorder in which anterograde amnesia occurs (Chapter 402). In Alzheimer's disease, anterograde amnesia is usually the dominant cognitive symptom, particularly early in the illness. Hippocampal atrophy is common (Chapter 402, Fig. 402-3). Anterograde amnesia also occurs in other dementing illnesses, such as vascular dementia and dementia with Lewy bodies.

Strokes can damage regions involved in episodic memory. Occlusion of the medial temporal branch of the posterior cerebral artery causes infarction of the hippocampus. Infarction in the territory of penetrating branches of the tip of the basilar artery causes bilateral medial thalamic infarcts.

Anterograde amnesia may be a major residual deficit after herpes simplex encephalitis (Chapter 374). Herpes simplex encephalitis has a predilection for damaging structures at the base of the cerebral hemispheres; frequently, the temporal lobes are severely damaged. Korsakoff's syndrome, the residual of the encephalopathy of thiamine deficiency (Chapter 416), is characterized by profound anterograde amnesia. Hemorrhagic necrosis of the mammillary bodies occurs in Korsakoff's syndrome. Survivors of closed head injuries (Chapter 399) may have anterograde amnesia because the medial temporal lobes are vulnerable to trauma as a result of their close proximity to the temporal bone. Survivors of an episode of anoxic-ischemic encephalopathy may also have dense anterograde amnesia. The pyramidal neurons of the CA1 region of the hippocampus are particularly vulnerable to hypoxic injury.

The syndrome of transient global amnesia involves anterograde amnesia, but the duration of the amnesia is a matter of 6 to 12 hours rather than the weeks or months seen in post-traumatic amnesia or the permanent deficits in patients with Alzheimer's disease or Korsakoff's syndrome. Patients with transient global amnesia remain alert though inattentive; the key element of the syndrome is that they lay down no new memories during the event. As a consequence, they are amnestic for the several hours of the episode. Transient global amnesia generally affects middle-aged or elderly individuals. Its cause is not known, although it is not usually due to typical cerebrovascular disease or epilepsy. Electroencephalography is typically not specifically abnormal, but diffusion-weighed MRI often shows distinctive abnormalities of the hippocampus a day or more after the onset of transient global amnesia.

THE APHASIAS

DEFINITION

Aphasia is a disorder of language at the conceptual level. Aphasics may have difficulty producing language, comprehending language, or both.

PATHOBIOLOGY

In more than 99% of right-handed individuals, language is localized to the left hemisphere. In left-handed individuals, language is also predominantly localized to the left hemisphere, although varying degrees of bilateral or rarely right hemispheric dominance may be seen. The hemisphere involved in language is referred to as the dominant hemisphere. Anatomic differences in the temporal and parietal lobes of the dominant hemisphere versus the other hemisphere also reflect its specialization for language.

Different aspects of language processing can be localized to specific regions within the dominant hemisphere. Experimental studies with positron emission tomography and functional magnetic resonance imaging can provide a rather detailed perspective on localization of various language subfunctions,[3] but the clinical neuroanatomy of language is less precise. Conceptualizing language functions as receptive or expressive, there are a few major clinical-anatomic relationships. Lesions in the dominant hemisphere's auditory association areas cause receptive language dysfunction. The critical regions are located in the superior temporal lobes adjacent to the primary auditory cortex and in the adjacent supramarginal and angular gyri of the inferior parietal lobule, an area known as Wernicke's area. Lesions in the dominant hemisphere's lateral inferior posterior frontal lobes, often referred to as Broca's area, result in expressive language deficits. Loss of access to one's vocabulary for either understanding spoken language or expressing oneself results from lesions in any portion of the region of the dominant hemisphere around the sylvian fissure, including the lateral posterior inferior frontal lobe, the inferior parietal lobule, and the superior and middle temporal gyri. Coronal and axial MRI scans give a detailed view of the critical language regions (see Fig. 401-1).

In clinical practice, aphasia may be caused by cerebrovascular or neurodegenerative diseases, especially frontotemporal lobar degenerations and Alzheimer's disease[4,5] (Chapter 402). Less commonly, space-occupying lesions such as brain tumors (Chapter 189) or brain abscesses (Chapter 413) can cause aphasic syndromes.

CLINICAL MANIFESTATIONS

The language comprehension difficulties in persons with aphasia must be distinguished from hearing disorders (Chapter 428), and the motor speech dysfunction in aphasia must be distinguished from dysarthria. Errors of articulation in persons with aphasia reflect altered conceptual selection of what is to be said. In aphasia, mispronunciation of a sound within one word may be followed by perfect pronunciation of the same sound in a different word. In dysarthria, by comparison, the errors in articulation or phonation are consistent.

Aphasia has three principal components: impaired verbal comprehension, disordered verbal expression, and impaired naming. Disorders of reading, writing, and sentence repetition are additional elements of the aphasia syndrome. The disordered verbal comprehension may range from profound to mild. When profound, patients are unable to grasp the meaning of single words. In milder forms of disordered comprehension, patients may be able to follow one-step but not two- or three-step commands. Usually, the comprehension difficulty involves both spoken and written language, but each can be affected separately. Anomia, which is an inability to produce names of people or objects, is common in almost all aphasic syndromes.

In expressive aphasic syndromes, written material and spoken speech are most often affected in parallel. Speech is labored in the expressive aphasias, and it lacks the normal melody and variation in intonation that characterize normal speaking. Melody and intonation are referred to as the prosody of speech. Speech is often grammatically impoverished. The number of words per utterance is greatly reduced, thus giving the speech a choppy, staccato character. These features are referred to as speech apraxia. *Nonfluency* is a related term that describes the reduced number of words and the terseness of verbal output. In some aphasic syndromes, speech is often degraded by anomia and paraphasic errors (word or syllable substitutions), even when fluency, melody, and intonation are preserved.

Specific Aphasic Syndromes

Specific common aphasic syndromes exhibit various combinations of receptive and expressive difficulty (Table 401-2).

WERNICKE'S APHASIA

In Wernicke's aphasia, verbal comprehension of both written and verbal language is severely impaired. Patients with Wernicke's aphasia have difficulty

TABLE 401-2 MAJOR APHASIC SYNDROMES

APHASIA SYNDROME	REGIONAL LOCALIZATION	SPONTANEOUS SPEECH ABNORMALITIES	AUDITORY COMPREHENSION	CONFRONTATION NAMING	SENTENCE REPETITION
Broca's aphasia	Lateral inferior frontal lobe	Nonfluent, labored, agrammatic	Preserved	Poor	Poor
Wernicke's aphasia	Posterior superior temporal-parietal supramarginal gyrus	Fluent, many paraphasic errors, very little information content	Very impaired	Poor	Poor
Global aphasia	Major portions of the frontoparietal operculum and superior temporal lobe	Nonfluent or virtually absent	Very impaired	Poor	Poor
Anomic aphasia	Small lesion somewhere in the perisylvian region	Fluent, may contain some paraphasias	Normal or mildly impaired	Poor to moderately impaired	Preserved or impaired

understanding the meaning of individual words and may not be able to follow any command consisting of greater than one step. Their speech is fluent but marred by paraphasia and anomia. Wernicke's aphasics tend to lack awareness of the extent of their communicative difficulties and are often unaware that the words they are uttering are fundamentally incorrect. Embolic strokes are the most common cause of Wernicke's aphasia. The location that typically causes Wernicke's aphasia is the dominant posterior superior temporal lobe or inferior supramarginal gyrus (see Fig. 401-1).

SEMANTIC VARIANT OF PRIMARY PROGRESSIVE APHASIA
The aphasic disturbance of semantic variant of primary progressive aphasia is characterized by a loss of access to the meaning of words. Spontaneous speech melody, intonation, and grammatical integrity are preserved, but patients have marked difficulties with production of nouns and verbs. This condition is usually caused by left anterior temporal lobe degeneration owing to one of the frontotemporal lobar degenerations (Chapter 402).

BROCA'S APHASIA
Broca's aphasia is a syndrome in which expressive language is prominently affected. Patients with Broca's aphasia have nonfluent labored speech. The location of the lesion that typically causes Broca's aphasia is the dominant posterior inferior frontal lobe (see Fig. 401-1). The typical syndrome is usually due to embolic strokes. Patients with Broca's aphasia have largely preserved comprehension and as a result are acutely aware of their difficulties and become frustrated with them. Depression is common in Broca's aphasics.

NONFLUENT/AGRAMMATIC VARIANT OF PRIMARY PROGRESSIVE APHASIA
The nonfluent/agrammatic variant of primary progressive aphasia is characterized by the gradual onset of labored, hesitant, sparse speech that is often grammatically impoverished. Comprehension of spoken speech is typically preserved. This syndrome is usually caused by one of the frontotemporal lobar degenerations (Chapter 402).

GLOBAL APHASIA
Global aphasia occurs when both expressive and receptive problems are present. Global aphasia often appears acutely after a major infarction, hemorrhage, or traumatic brain injury involving the dominant hemisphere. Global aphasia may also be present in the context of severe dementia.

ANOMIA
Anomia is at the milder end of the spectrum of language disorders. Some anomic aphasics also have difficulty with sentence repetition, even in the presence of relatively preserved comprehension and verbal expressive abilities. There is some controversy whether this latter syndrome, called conduction aphasia, represents a disconnection between the perisylvian centers for comprehension and expression or whether it represents a lesion in the cortical auditory areas involved in immediate auditory memory.

IDEOMOTOR APRAXIA
Ideomotor apraxia is a disorder at the interface between comprehension and execution of facial or limb motor actions. Patients with ideomotor apraxia have no paresis of the face or limb musculature and are able to carry out simple tasks, but they are unable to execute more complex tasks or commands. For example, in a woman who is able to name a comb and use her right hand to point to parts of her body, ideomotor apraxia can be demonstrated if she is unable to indicate through her actions how she would use the comb.

STUTTERING
The left pars opercularis is a locus where the intrinsic functional architecture of speech-language processes is altered in patients with persistent developmental stuttering.[6]

DIAGNOSIS
The diagnosis of aphasia is made by listening to the patient speak and by examining comprehension, naming ability, reading, and writing in a standardized fashion. Frequently the diagnosis of aphasia is made during attempts to obtain a history from the patient. It is helpful to prompt patients to speak about a neutral topic such as what they had for their last meal or what they did the previous day. Listening to their spontaneous speech allows the examiner to characterize its fluency, grammatical form, articulation, melody, and intonation, as well as difficulty finding words, the presence of paraphasias, and the overall information content.

Comprehension should be examined formally by asking the patient to perform tasks that range from one to at least three steps. Naming can be tested by asking the patient to name a series of common objects, such as the parts of the hand and arm (e.g., thumb, palm, knuckles, wrist, elbow). In general, the more commonly a word is used in the language, the easier it will be to name, whereas infrequent words are harder for aphasics. Reading and writing should also be tested.

Portions of the dominant perisylvian cerebral cortex may be damaged by infarction (Chapters 407 and 408), hemorrhage, and other space-occupying brain lesions such as neoplasms (Chapter 189) and abscesses (Chapter 413). Aphasia secondary to stroke has an abrupt onset, usually with some subsequent improvement. Recovery from aphasia after a stroke may occur as ischemic zones around an infarction eventually regain function. Regions remote from the infarction may also be synaptically depressed acutely after a stroke (diaschisis) but eventually regain function. Finally, regions in the nondominant hemisphere may become more active over the course of recovery. Aphasia that has a gradual and slowly progressive onset occurs in the degenerative dementia syndromes of progressive aphasia and semantic dementia (Chapter 402).

TREATMENT Rx
Speech therapy may be helpful for patients in the first few months after a brain injury that causes aphasia.

CORTICAL DISORDERS OF VISUAL FUNCTION AND HEMISPATIAL NEGLECT

DEFINITIONS
Cortical disorders of vision and spatial cognition are caused by lesions in the occipitoinferotemporal or occipitoposteroparietal lobes. The principal disorders of cortical visual functioning are alexia (impaired reading), object agnosia (impaired recognition of visual forms), and prosopagnosia (impaired face recognition). The principal disorders of spatial cognition are simultanagnosia (impaired integration of complex visual scenes), dressing apraxia, and visual hemispatial neglect (lack of awareness of the personal or extrapersonal hemispace). Diagnosis of a cortical visual disorder requires integrity of primary visual function from the cornea to the lateral geniculate nuclei.

PATHOBIOLOGY

Higher visual function is localized to a network centered in the occipital lobe and includes the inferior temporal and posterior parietal lobes[7] (see Fig. 401-1). From area 17, processing of visual information passes to visual association areas 18 and 19. From there it proceeds in several directions. Disorders of higher visual function can be related to a ventral or dorsal pathway. The ventral pathway from the visual centers to the medial temporal lobe links visual information to meaning ("What is the object?"). The dorsal visual processing pathway has several target regions. One links the visual centers to the parietal lobes and is concerned with locating objects in space and determining spatial relationships among objects in order to grasp a complete visual scene ("Where is the object?"). Another integral part of the dorsal visual processing stream is the cortical control of the extraocular muscles in the parietal and prefrontal regions, whereby the eyes are directed to various elements of a visual scene so that the individual elements are synthesized into a coherent ensemble. Yet a third part of the dorsal visual pathway leads to premotor areas that, in conjunction with eye movement control, facilitate visually guided limb motor actions.

Alexia occurs as a result of lesions in the ventral pathway of the dominant hemisphere. Object agnosia may also occur with lesions, usually bilateral, in the ventral pathway. Alexia and object agnosia occur with neurodegenerative diseases that affect the parieto-occipital cortex (Fig. 401-2). Simultanagnosia, dressing apraxia, and hemispatial neglect are syndromes caused by lesions in the dorsal pathway. Limb apraxia and impaired visuomotor activities may result from disruption of the premotor pathways that interact with the dorsal visual system. Simultanagnosia usually requires bilateral posterior parietal lesions. Dressing apraxia and hemispatial neglect arise from unilateral lesions, most often in the nondominant hemisphere. Cortical blindness is a consequence of bilateral occipitoparietal pathology.

CLINICAL MANIFESTATIONS

Alexia may occur as an isolated deficit, or it may occur in the context of other evidence of aphasia. Patients may be able to recognize individual letters but are unable to recognize a string of letters as a word. In pure alexia, auditory comprehension of words and sentences is preserved. Patients with object agnosia may be unable to identify objects visually, but they will be able to recognize the object based on its characteristic sound or how it feels to touch. In simultanagnosia, patients may be able to identify small objects easily if they happen to appear within the narrow viewing area at the center of their visual field. At the same time, such patients will fail to grasp the bigger visual picture. They may appear to be functionally blind. This clinical picture is referred to as Balint's syndrome.

Patients with cortical disorders usually have difficulty with visuoconstructional tasks such as copying figures or drawing simple objects such as a flower, house, or clock. Dressing apraxia represents a deficit of practical significance in which patients are unable to comprehend the orientation of articles such as a shirt or a blouse and to manipulate them.

The most severe form of a cortical disorder of visuospatial processing is cortical blindness. In this condition, in which the anterior visual pathways can be reasonably believed to be intact, patients appear functionally blind.

On occasion, they also exhibit anosognosia for the blindness and claim they can see. This latter condition is referred to as Anton's syndrome.

Hemispatial neglect occurs in the setting of acute strokes involving the nondominant perisylvian region. Even when there is no hemianopia as measured by single visual stimuli, presentation of double simultaneous stimuli to the patient reveals unawareness in the nondominant field. Hemispatial neglect can be demonstrated at the bedside with a task such as drawing a clock. A patient with hemispatial neglect will fail to place the numbers on the nondominant side (i.e., the left side in a right-handed person). Patients with hemispatial neglect may sometimes deny that their paretic limb belongs to them.

DIAGNOSIS

Information about visual functioning can be obtained from the history. The patient or the patient's informant may report that the patient cannot read, cannot read a clock, or cannot find objects when asked to get something off a table or out of a cupboard. There is often a history of motor vehicle accidents in which the patient failed to see another vehicle, the curb, or the side of a garage. Patients may report difficulty recognizing people's faces even though they are able to recognize them by their voices or by other cues.

Bedside tests that screen for visuospatial deficits include either copying a simple geometric design or drawing an object. Intersecting pentagons and a cube are objects used clinically. Clock drawing is a brief but informative exercise. Reading of words or commands and naming of objects can be done at the bedside as well. Face recognition is more difficult to assess at the bedside. Formal testing of visuospatial function in the neuropsychology laboratory involves the use of specially designed instruments to characterize visual processing.

The etiology of lesions that cause deficits in cortical vision and spatial cognition ranges from focal cerebrovascular disease, neoplasms, infectious processes, and brain trauma to neurodegenerative disorders. When a stroke causes a disorder of cortical visuospatial processing or hemispatial neglect, it is usually abrupt in onset. Space-occupying brain lesions such as neoplasms or brain abscesses that cause cortical visual disorders do so on a subacute basis. Disordered visuospatial function may also appear insidiously when caused by the degenerative disorder posterior cortical atrophy. Patients with posterior cortical atrophy, which is usually due to Alzheimer's disease, show marked atrophy of the occipital lobe (see Fig. 401-2).

● EXECUTIVE COGNITIVE DYSFUNCTION AND CONTROL OF PERSONAL BEHAVIOR

DEFINITIONS

Integrative abilities that are broadly referred to as executive cognitive function include mental agility, abstract reasoning, and problem solving. Executive cognitive function represents processes that support mental flexibility, adaptability, focus, and tenacity. Control of personal actions and regulation of interpersonal relationships are also closely related to executive cognitive dysfunction. The term *comportment* denotes how a person behaves, particularly toward other people.

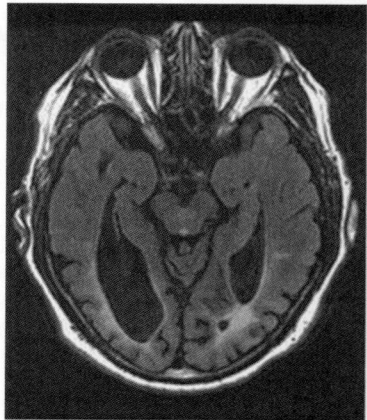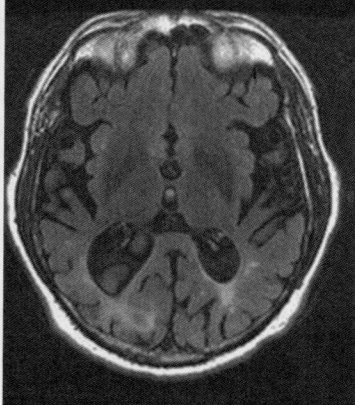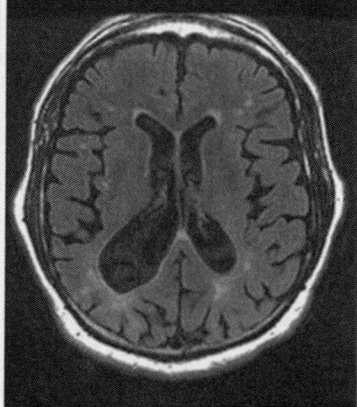

FIGURE 401-2. Magnetic resonance (MR) scans of a patient with the syndrome of posterior cortical atrophy caused by Alzheimer's disease. The MR scan shows marked atrophy of the primary visual areas and parieto-occipital association areas. The right hemisphere is more affected than the left.

PATHOBIOLOGY

The anatomic basis of executive cognitive function and comportment is a network of brain regions anchored by the prefrontal and anterior temporal lobe neocortex[8,9] (see Fig. 401-1). These regions receive input from multiple cortical and subcortical regions. The caudate nucleus is the site of a major frontal lobe efferent pathway. The medial thalamus is a major afferent source to the frontal lobes. The anterior temporal lobes are also part of the same integrative circuitry as the prefrontal regions. Lesions in the lateral prefrontal regions are associated with slowing of cognitive processing, difficulty with set shifting (switching from one idea or task to another), difficulty initiating tasks, and loss of mental flexibility. The frontal and anterior temporal lobes are involved in the modulation of personal behavior and interpersonal relationships. Patients with lesions in the medial prefrontal lobes are often apathetic and lack initiative. Patients with lesions in the orbital frontal or right anterior temporal lobe may exhibit disinhibition, impulsivity, and a striking loss of ability to interpret or predict the feelings of others.

Traumatic brain injury (Chapter 399) is a common cause of frontal lobe and anterior temporal damage. The orbital frontal, frontal polar, and anterior temporal regions are particularly vulnerable to contusions because of their proximity to the skull (Fig. 401-3). Patients with traumatic brain injuries may also suffer diffuse white matter damage as a result of shear injuries. Disconnection of the frontal and anterior temporal lobes from other parts of the brain can produce executive cognitive dysfunction and altered control of personal behavior.

CLINICAL MANIFESTATIONS

Executive cognitive functioning and control and regulation of behavior are usually affected concurrently. Patients with executive dysfunction are deficient in goal-oriented behavior; they lose the ability to predict the consequences of their actions or words. Patients with executive dysfunction also exhibit poor mental agility and inflexibility in their thinking and control of their actions. They are easily distracted and exhibit a tendency to perseverate, in which the answer to a prior question is repeated in response to subsequent questions. They are disinhibited; as a consequence, when asked to recall a specific event, they may glibly answer with a fabrication, a phenomenon referred to as confabulation.

Patients with lateral prefrontal pathology exhibit poor performance on tests of abstract reasoning and mental agility. In a test such as verbal similarities, they tend to be very concrete and narrowly focused. They become easily distracted and are slow in performing tasks that require sustained attention. Because of their mental rigidity and difficulty in set shifting, they do poorly on tests that require the ability to vary their response strategies, such as verbal fluency tests.

Patients with medial frontal lesions are often profoundly apathetic and lack initiative and motivation. They may be laconic and completely unable to express emotion, whether it be anger, sadness, or elation. They tend to be indifferent to their surroundings, a state referred to as abulia. The majority of patients with substantial prefrontal or anterior temporal lobe pathology lack insight into the extent of their inappropriate behavior.

In contrast, other patients with altered comportment exhibit different manifestations of dysregulation of personal actions and interpersonal behavior. These alterations may include difficulty controlling impulsivity, poor social graces (manifested as rude behavior or caustic comments), a disregard for the feelings of others (loss of empathy), and a general failure to understand what constitutes acceptable behavior in a particular social context. If the underlying disease is progressive, gross alterations in table manners and loss of interest in maintaining personal hygiene may appear. Inappropriate sexual behavior may occur. Patients with prominent disease of the frontal lobes may also exhibit hyperorality, which is a compulsion to put nonfood objects into their mouths. Hyperorality can be life-threatening, depending on the substance ingested.

DIAGNOSIS

The clinical history is essential for documenting the characteristic changes in personality, behavior, and interpersonal relationships. The history must almost always be obtained from an informant who knows the patient well, because the patient may assert that there are no problems.

Mental status examination is an integral part of the diagnosis of an executive cognitive disorder. Simply interacting with the patient may be quite revealing. The patient may exhibit abulia, disinhibition, socially inappropriate behavior, or easy distractibility. Tests of executive cognitive function that are suitable for bedside use include verbal similarities and differences, the digits backward test, reciting the months of the year backward, or spelling a word backward. Verbal fluency, which is a very useful test of mental flexibility and set shifting, is tested by asking patients to produce as many words as they can that begin with a particular letter of the alphabet in 60 seconds. Frequently, a patient with a frontal lesion will quickly produce two or three words and then stop.

Bedside testing of executive cognitive dysfunction provides only a superficial view of the cognitive domain. Assessment in the neuropsychology laboratory gives a more refined estimate of the degree of executive dysfunction.

Space-occupying lesions of the frontal lobes (e.g., neoplasms, brain abscesses) can lead to the cognitive and behavioral syndromes of frontal lobe dysfunction. With these diseases, executive cognitive dysfunction and alteration of control of personal behavior develop over a period of weeks.

In patients with acute brain trauma (Chapter 399), brain imaging at the time of initial medical and surgical evaluation will reveal whether the brain suffered acute traumatic lesions. Chronically, traumatic brain injury may later lead to encephalomalacia of the frontal lobes (see Fig. 401-3).

Neurodegenerative diseases such as frontotemporal lobar degeneration (Chapter 402) are associated with dysfunction and brain loss in the prefrontal (Chapter 402, Fig. 402-7) and anterior temporal lobes (Chapter 402, Fig. 402-8). These disorders may produce the entire spectrum of executive cognitive dysfunction and altered control of personal behavior over a period of a year or longer.

Some diseases that do not directly damage the frontal or anterior temporal neocortex may cause executive cognitive dysfunction and alteration of control of personal behavior because of the interconnectedness of the frontal and anterior temporal lobes with other cortical and subcortical regions. Multiple sclerosis (Chapter 411), a disorder of white matter pathways, may cause abnormalities in cognition and behavior of the frontal type. Similarly, Huntington's disease (Chapter 410) and progressive supranuclear palsy, which affect the caudate nuclei, may also resemble a frontal cognitive and behavioral

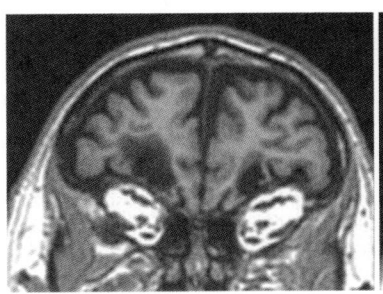
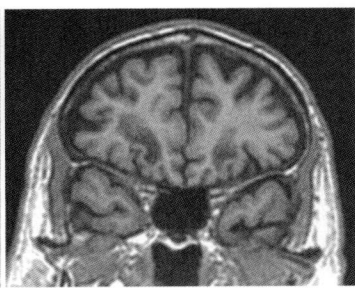
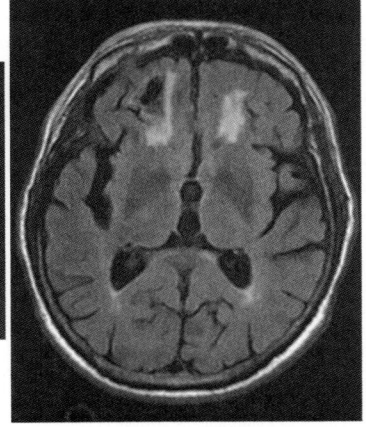

FIGURE 401-3. Coronal (*left and middle*) and axial magnetic resonance images of frontal brain trauma. This patient who suffered a closed head injury several years ago now has encephalomalacia in the orbital frontal cortices bilaterally.

syndrome and result in executive cognitive dysfunction and alterations in comportment.

TREATMENT   Rx

Cognitive-behavioral therapies offer modest but definite benefit for patients with aphasia and for those with mild attention deficits and mild memory deficits caused by brain injury.

FUTURE DIRECTIONS

The assessment of cognition is being supplemented by new imaging techniques. Functional magnetic resonance imaging can provide an unprecedented view into cortical connectivity patterns, which are influenced by aging and disease.[10]

GENERAL REFERENCES

For the General References and other additional features, please visit Expert Consult at https://expertconsult.inkling.com.

402

ALZHEIMER DISEASE AND OTHER DEMENTIAS

DAVID S. KNOPMAN

DEMENTIA

DEFINITION

Dementia, which is a disorder of cognition, interferes with daily functioning and results in loss of independence (Table 402-1). The majority of dementias are of gradual onset, are progressive in course, and occur in persons with previously normal cognition. However, none of these features are necessary aspects of the definition of dementia. Some dementias, such as those caused by an acute neurologic illness secondary to stroke, encephalitis, or head trauma, may begin abruptly and then remain static for long periods. Conversely, a small subset of dementias, such as Creutzfeldt-Jakob disease (Chapter 415), have a rapid onset and a course that can run for less than a year. Dementia may also occur in persons with developmental disabilities and long-standing cognitive deficits.

TABLE 402-1   DEFINITION OF DEMENTIA

Dementia is cognitive impairment that interferes with the ability to function at work or at usual activities; *and*

It represents a decline from prior levels of functioning and performing; *and*
The cognitive impairment and impaired functioning are not explained by delirium or major psychiatric disorder.

The cognitive impairment of dementia is detected and diagnosed through a combination of:
(a) History-taking from the patient and a knowledgeable informant; *and*
(b) Objective cognitive assessment, either a "bedside" mental status examination or neuropsychological testing.

The cognitive or behavioral impairment of dementia involves **at least two** of the following domains:
   Impaired ability to acquire and remember new information
   Impaired reasoning and handling of complex tasks; poor judgment
   Impaired visuospatial abilities
   Impaired language functions (speaking, reading, writing)
   Changes in personality, behavior, or comportment

Adapted from McKhann GM, Knopman DS, Chertkow H, et al. The diagnosis of dementia due to Alzheimer's disease: recommendations from the National Institute on Aging-Alzheimer's Association workgroups on diagnostic guidelines for Alzheimer's disease. *Alzheimers Dement.* 2011;7:263-269.

EPIDEMIOLOGY

The prevalence and incidence of dementia increase with advancing age. Dementia is uncommon before 50 years of age.[1] In individuals older than 65 years, the prevalence of dementia of all types is about 7%. In the age range of 65 to 69, the prevalence of dementia is only 1 to 2%, but it increases to 20 to 25% in the 85- to 89-year age range and continues to rise steadily thereafter. The incidence of new cases of dementia is about 1 per 100 per year at the age of 70 and rises to about 2 to 3 new cases per 100 per year by about the age of 80. Incidence rates continue to rise into the ninth and tenth decades of life. With the dramatic increase in longevity in North America, the societal burden of dementia has risen substantially.

In absolute numbers, far more women than men have dementia, because women live longer. However, men and women have an equal age-adjusted risk for the development of dementia. There are no racial or ethnic differences in the risk for dementia.

PATHOBIOLOGY

Dementia is the culmination of dysfunction in the cerebral hemispheres, especially the association cortices, hippocampal formations, their supporting subcortical nuclear structures (e.g., caudate nuclei, thalamus), and their white matter interconnections (see Fig. 401-1). Specific diseases that cause dementia do so by affecting particular parts of the cerebral cortex, subcortical nuclei, or the underlying white matter pathways linking different cortical regions.

CLINICAL MANIFESTATIONS

Any of the major domains of cognition—declarative episodic memory, executive cognitive functioning, visuospatial function, or language—may be affected in dementia (Chapter 401). Because Alzheimer disease is the most common dementia, anterograde amnesia is typically present first and most intensely in the majority of dementia patients. In other dementing illnesses, deficits in the other cognitive domains may be dominant. A pervasive and nearly invariant aspect of dementia is a loss of insight (anosognosia) into the extent of one's cognitive and functional losses.

Neuropsychiatric symptoms are also common in dementia. Apathy and loss of initiative are almost always present. Depression and anxiety are frequent, as are irritability, paranoia, delusional thinking, and hallucinations. Daily functioning of patients with dementia is compromised. In early dementia, difficulty is likely to be present in management of finances and medications, independent travel, preparation of meals, and keeping of appointments. In more advanced disease, difficulty becomes evident in basic activities of daily living such as bathing, dressing, toileting, and feeding oneself. Dementias secondary to cerebrovascular or Lewy body disease are often associated with specific abnormalities in strength, coordination, gait, or balance. Alzheimer disease, the most common dementia, typically has no associated motor abnormalities.

DIAGNOSIS

Clinical Examination

Dementia is strictly a clinical diagnosis based on evidence of cognitive dysfunction in both the history and the mental status examination.[2] The key elements of the history flow from the definition of dementia: What is the evidence for impairment in one or more domains of cognition? What is the evidence that daily functioning is affected? The mental status examination is necessary to establish that alertness is preserved (i.e., the patient does not have delirium [Chapter 28]) and to determine what specific areas of cognition exhibit directly observable impairment. For diagnosis of the syndrome of dementia, no laboratory test supersedes the clinical history and mental status examination. Laboratory testing is critical, however, to determine the cause of the dementia.

Bedside testing of mental status is based on the principles of cognitive neurology (Chapter 401). For moderate or severe dementia to be distinguished from normal cognitive states, a bedside mental status examination such as the Mini-Cog test (Chapter 27, Table 27-5) is accurate. However, for mild dementia, bedside mental status examinations lack sensitivity (i.e., they fail to diagnose some cases of mild dementia). For patients with suspected mild dementia,[3] neuropsychometric testing is a useful adjunct to the bedside examination. The neurologic examination is also important for evaluation of signs of specific causes of dementia, including signs of cerebrovascular disease (e.g., hemiparesis [Chapter 406]) and signs of extrapyramidal disease (e.g., rigidity, bradykinesia, resting tremor [Chapter 409]).

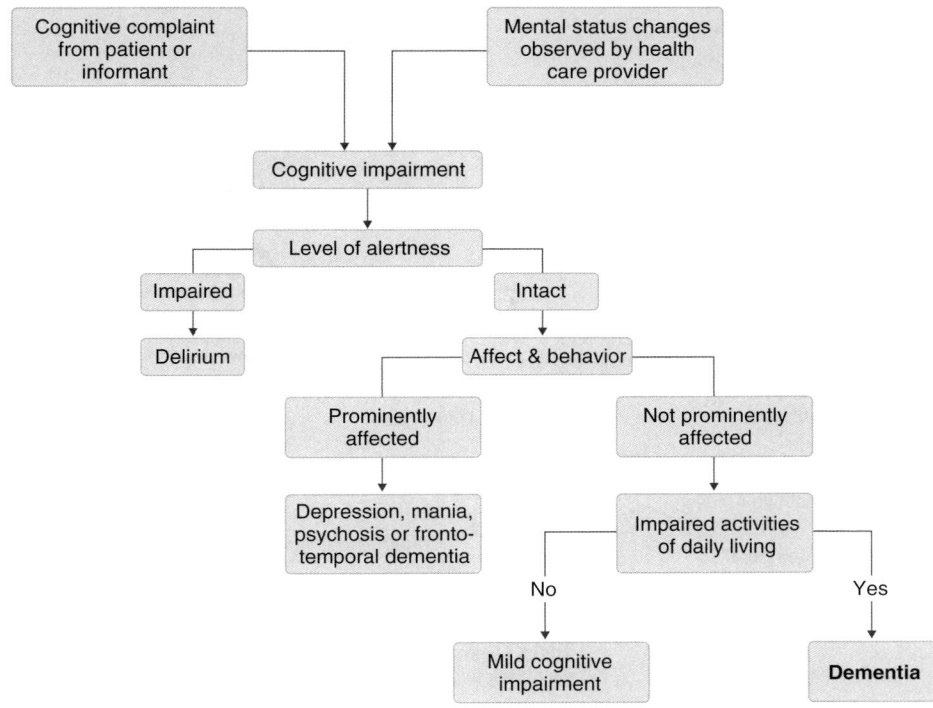

FIGURE 402-1. Flow diagram to establish the diagnosis of dementia.

Differential Diagnosis

Dementia must be distinguished from other disorders of cognition (Fig. 402-1). Delirium (Chapter 28) also affects cognition directly; key features distinguishing it from dementia include impaired arousal and attention. Delirium is almost always of sudden onset, whereas the majority of cases of dementia are of gradual onset.

Primary psychiatric diseases (Chapter 397) such as major depression, bipolar disorder, and schizophrenia may also impair cognition. In dementia, however, the impairment in cognition is typically equivalent to or more pervasive than the changes in mood and behavior.

The principal diseases that cause dementia are three neurodegenerative diseases—Alzheimer disease, Lewy body disease, and frontotemporal lobar degeneration—and cerebrovascular disease (Fig. 402-2). The neurodegenerative diseases that cause dementia are typically slow and insidious in onset and inexorably progressive. Dementia secondary to cerebrovascular disease may be of either sudden or gradual onset.

Many much less common secondary causes account for less than 2% of all dementias. Drug intoxication (Chapters 34 and 416), metabolic disorders (Chapter 205), central nervous system infections (Chapters 412 to 414), and brain structural lesions (Chapter 401) are typically subacute in onset; if they are diagnosed and treated early, the cognitive deficits improve or resolve completely. A number of medications such as sedatives, pain medications, corticosteroids, digoxin, and others cause mental confusion, particularly but not always at toxic levels (Chapter 110). Metabolic disorders that may also cause subacute confusion and produce a cognitive disorder include hypothyroidism or hyperthyroidism (Chapter 226), vitamin B_{12} deficiency (Chapter 416), chronic liver disease (Chapter 153), chronic renal failure (Chapter 130), and hypocalcemia or hypercalcemia (Chapter 245). Chronic viral infections of the brain, especially human immunodeficiency virus infection, frequently cause dementia (Chapter 394). Chronic meningitides in the differential diagnosis of dementia include cryptococcal meningitis (Chapter 336), tuberculous meningitis (Chapter 324), and tertiary syphilis (Chapter 319). Finally, structural lesions of the brain, including primary and metastatic tumors (Chapter 189), chronic subdural hematomas (Chapter 399), and normal-pressure hydrocephalus (Chapter 189), can cause a syndrome resembling dementia that consists of a subacute or slowly progressive decline in cognition with few or no other neurologic symptoms or signs.

PROGNOSIS
Except for the secondary causes of dementia and the rare dementing illnesses caused by single episodes of brain injury (e.g., severe head trauma, anoxic

encephalopathy), dementia is a condition that invariably leads to worsening of cognition and function. Almost all dementia patients progress from mild stages to severe dementia during the course of several years if they do not die prematurely. The rate of cognitive decline is variable among individuals and, of course, also varies with the specific disease. In general, dementia can be said to decrease life expectancy by half compared with the life expectancy of nondemented individuals.

End-of-Life Care
The terminal stage and end-of-life care issues (Chapter 3) associated with the common dementias are usually similar. Dementia itself does not directly cause death, but it is strongly linked to reduced survival. Patients with dementia typically die of the same illnesses that affect debilitated individuals, such as sepsis, pneumonia, pulmonary embolism, or heart disease.

Most patients with dementia experience their terminal illnesses in hospitals or extended care facilities. Given the inexorably progressive nature of most dementing illnesses and their likelihood of producing severe and completely disabling cognitive and functional impairment, it is widely accepted that patients with end-stage dementia should receive conservative care. Feeding tubes and ventilatory support should not generally be considered.

MILD COGNITIVE IMPAIRMENT

DEFINITION
Mild cognitive impairment represents the transition between the state of normal cognition and dementia.[4] Patients with mild cognitive impairment have abnormalities in a specific aspect of cognition to such an extent that it is clearly different from normal performance but does not interfere with daily functioning to any appreciable degree. More than one domain of cognition may be affected. The amnesic form of mild cognitive impairment, in which declarative episodic memory is impaired, is the most common. Alterations in attention, concentration, and mental agility may also be seen (Table 402-2). The term *cognitively impaired, not demented* includes patients whose mild cognitive impairment may progress to dementia but also encompasses anyone who is neither cognitively normal nor demented, such as individuals with stable lifelong cognitive impairment.

EPIDEMIOLOGY
The prevalence and incidence of mild cognitive impairment are about the same as those of dementia. Both increase with advancing age.

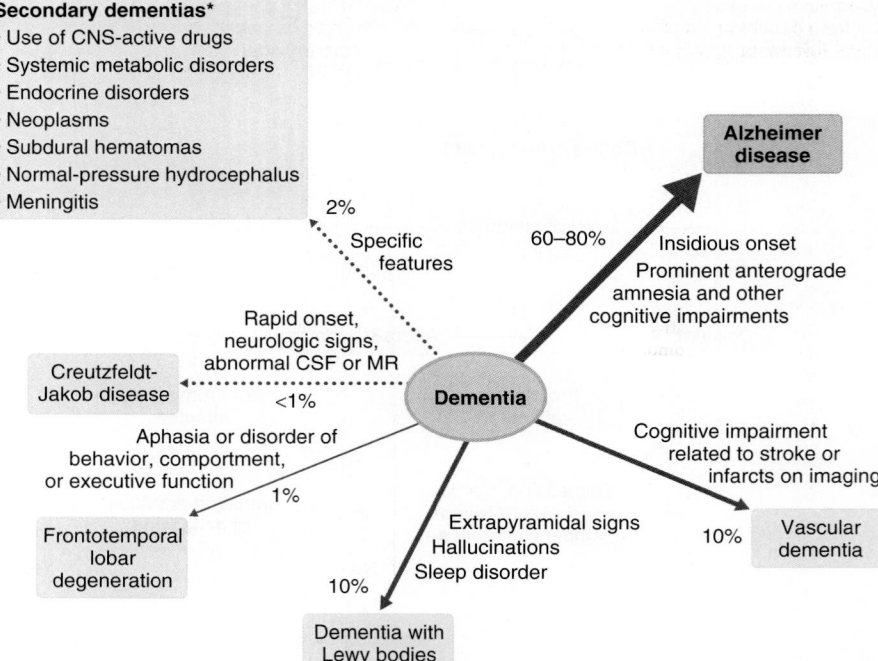

Secondary dementias*
- Use of CNS-active drugs
- Systemic metabolic disorders
- Endocrine disorders
- Neoplasms
- Subdural hematomas
- Normal-pressure hydrocephalus
- Meningitis

FIGURE 402-2. Flow diagram for the differential diagnosis of dementia. The percentage contributions of various diagnoses are approximate. *The list of secondary causes of dementia is not exhaustive. CNS = central nervous system; CSF = cerebrospinal fluid; MR = magnetic resonance imaging.

TABLE 402-2	DIAGNOSTIC CRITERIA FOR AMNESIC MILD COGNITIVE IMPAIRMENT

The presence of a new memory complaint, preferably corroborated by an informant

Objective evidence of an impairment in episodic declarative memory (for age)

Normal general cognitive functions

No substantial interference with work, usual social activities, or other activities of daily living

No dementia

Adapted from Albert MS, DeKosky ST, Dickson D, et al. The diagnosis of mild cognitive impairment due to Alzheimer's disease: recommendations from the National Institute on Aging-Alzheimer's Association workgroups on diagnostic guidelines for Alzheimer's disease. *Alzheimers Dement.* 2011;7:270-279.

PATHOBIOLOGY

Mild cognitive impairment is a risk state for the subsequent development of dementia. Alzheimer disease, followed by cerebrovascular disease and Lewy body disease, is the most common underlying cause.

CLINICAL MANIFESTATIONS

Patients with mild cognitive impairment may have more insight into their emerging cognitive difficulties than do patients with dementia. Hence, some patients with mild cognitive impairment may themselves seek medical consultation because of concern about their memory or their thinking. They or their family members may report a milder extent of many of the symptoms of dementia. Patients with mild cognitive impairment forget recent events and conversations or have trouble with mental flexibility, multitasking, problem solving, or completing mentally challenging activities at the speed they once did. Mental status testing will sometimes corroborate the complaints, but neuropsychometric testing may be needed to document impairment. Other patients with mild cognitive impairment may have virtually no insight into their memory loss, but the impairment is diagnosed after family members force the patient to undergo an evaluation.

DIAGNOSIS

When mild cognitive impairment is suspected, the principal alternative diagnosis is that the person is cognitively intact or that the person has dementia. The diagnosis of normal function should be straightforward when the patient and family have no complaints of cognitive impairment and the patient scores normally on bedside cognitive testing. However, a number of circumstances may cloud the issue, including very low or very high levels of prior educational and occupational achievement, instances in which English (or whatever the dominant language is) was a second language, severe hearing loss or blindness, and major alterations in mood or major motor disabilities that interfere with daily functioning. In such circumstances, the history of cognitive difficulty and the examination of cognitive status may be so confounded by these other phenomena that distinguishing between normal cognitive function and mild cognitive impairment is challenging. Conversely, distinguishing between mild cognitive impairment and dementia may be straightforward when daily functioning is obviously impaired. In other circumstances, it may be difficult to ascertain whether a person is functioning fully independently or not. For example, many older adults reside in assisted living facilities that provide services such as cooking and housekeeping. In such individuals with few daily responsibilities, it is difficult to determine whether they are functionally impaired.

TREATMENT   Rx

As of 2014, no treatments have been approved for mild cognitive impairment, although a randomized trial demonstrated that donepezil therapy, 10 mg/day, significantly reduced the rate of development of dementia secondary to Alzheimer disease at 1 year but not at 3 years.[A1] Physical activity appears to provide a modest slowing of cognitive decline.[A2]

PROGNOSIS

Mild cognitive impairment should be viewed as a risk state for the subsequent development of dementia. With use of the definition of amnesic mild cognitive impairment in Table 402-2, the rate of evolution from mild cognitive impairment to dementia is 15% per year. Mild (relative risk, 1.2) and moderate (relative risk, 1.4) cognitive impairment are also associated with increased all-cause mortality.

ALZHEIMER DISEASE

DEFINITION

Alzheimer disease, which is a pathophysiologic process involving β-amyloidosis and limbic and isocortical neurodegeneration, produces a

DIAGNOSTIC CRITERIA FOR PROBABLE ALZHEIMER DISEASE DEMENTIA

The clinical diagnosis of probable Alzheimer disease dementia is made when:

Criteria for dementia met (see Table 402-1), and the illness has the following characteristics:

Insidious onset: symptoms have a gradual onset over months to years; *and*
Clear-cut history of worsening of cognition by report or observation; *and*
The initial and most prominent cognitive deficits are evident on history and examination consistent with an amnestic disorder (most common) or a nonamnestic cognitive disorder (less common) (aphasia, visuospatial disorder, or behavioral/dysexecutive disorder).

The diagnosis of probable Alzheimer disease dementia **should not** be applied when there is substantial evidence for another neurodegenerative disease, extensive cerebrovascular disease, or a non-neurologic medical comorbidity or medication use that could have a substantial impact on cognition.

Research criteria for probable Alzheimer disease dementia with higher certainty when imaging or cerebrospinal fluid biomarkers are available:

Probable Alzheimer disease dementia is present based on above clinical criteria, and the following neuroimaging and cerebrospinal fluid (CSF) biomarker profiles are present:

Highest-probability biomarker profile: β-amyloid marker (CSF or imaging) "positive" *and* neuronal injury marker (CSF tau, FDG-PET or structural MR) "positive"
Intermediate probability biomarker profile: β-amyloid marker "positive" *and* neuronal injury marker "negative" or indeterminate
Highest probability: probable Alzheimer disease dementia is present based on above clinical criteria, and a known pathogenic mutation is present in *APP*, *PSEN1*, or *PSEN2*

FDG-PET = ^{18}fluoro-deoxyglucose positron emission tomography; MR = magnetic resonance.
Adapted from McKhann GM, Knopman DS, Chertkow H, et al. The diagnosis of dementia due to Alzheimer's disease: recommendations from the National Institute on Aging-Alzheimer's Association workgroups on diagnostic guidelines for Alzheimer's disease. *Alzheimers Dement.* 2011;7:263-269.

dementing illness in which anterograde amnesia is a dominant symptom (Table 402-3). The clinical diagnosis implies that the causative pathologic process is of the Alzheimer type, whereas the pathologic diagnosis rests on the findings of characteristic histopathologic features.

EPIDEMIOLOGY

Between 60 and 80% of all dementing illness is due to Alzheimer disease. Among all individuals older than 65 years, the prevalence of Alzheimer disease is estimated to be about 5%. As with dementia in general, the prevalence doubles in every 5-year interval after age 65, and the incidence continues to rise into the 10th and 11th decades of life. Men and women may be equally affected, although on an absolute basis, far more women have prevalent Alzheimer disease because women live longer than men. There are no ethnic or racial differences in the predilection for Alzheimer disease.

Risk Factors

Established risk factors for Alzheimer disease include advancing age and a family history. Putative risk factors include diabetes mellitus, hypertension, cardiovascular disease, and head trauma. Evidence for and against each of these four conditions is inconclusive, but the consensus is that at least diabetes and hypertension may play a role in the pathogenesis of Alzheimer disease. Low educational achievement is also a consistent risk factor, but most experts believe educational level is a proxy for some other factor, such as socioeconomic status or the early childhood medical and psychosocial environment. Protective factors have also been proposed, but their status is much debated.

PATHOBIOLOGY

The histopathologic diagnosis of Alzheimer disease is based on the joint presence of a substantial cerebral burden of neuritic plaques and neurofibrillary tangles.[5] Neuritic plaques consist of a core of aggregated β-amyloid peptide surrounded by degenerating neurites, which are fragments of axons and dendrites. β-Amyloid contains 39 to 42 amino acids and is proteolytically derived from a larger protein, the amyloid precursor protein. Neurofibrillary tangles are intracellular aggregations of an excessively phosphorylated form of the microtubule-associated protein tau. The altered tau protein self-aggregates and forms neurofibrillary tangles. In a low-powered microscopic section of frontal, temporal, or parietal cortex, at least six neuritic plaques and

neurofibrillary tangles should be visible for the diagnosis of Alzheimer disease to be made.

Pathophysiology

The progression of changes of β-amyloidosis follows a roughly predictable pattern in Alzheimer disease. Positron emission tomographic (PET) imaging with ligands that bind to β-amyloid shows that β-amyloid begins to accumulate in the neocortex as long as 20 years before dementia occurs. Soluble aggregates of β-amyloid in oligomeric (consisting of a small number of monomers) forms may be the key pathogenic molecules that eventually induce or accelerate neuronal injury. By the time clinical dementia due to Alzheimer disease is present, large numbers of β-amyloid peptide–containing deposits invariably are found in neuritic plaques in the neocortex. Neuritic plaques represent the end stage of the Alzheimer process. Because β-amyloidosis begins well before clinical symptoms appear and probably reaches a plateau in terms of abundance, the amount of β-amyloidosis does not closely mirror the severity of dementia in Alzheimer disease.

The regional extent of neurofibrillary tangles in Alzheimer disease grows as the disease progresses. Neurofibrillary tangles appear in the medial temporal lobe and brain stem in cognitively normal persons by the fourth decade of life. In persons destined to develop Alzheimer disease, a critical part of the pathophysiology involves transsynaptic spread of neurofibrillary tangle pathology to cortical association areas. At the time clinical symptoms develop, neurofibrillary tangles are found in association neocortices of the frontal, parietal, and temporal lobes. It is only in the most severe and final stages that neurofibrillary tangles are found in the occipital lobes and primary motor and sensory cortices. The location of neurofibrillary tangles corresponds faithfully to the clinical evolution of specific symptoms and severity of Alzheimer disease. In mild cognitive impairment, the earliest clinical manifestation of Alzheimer disease, the most intense burden of neurofibrillary tangles is in the entorhinal cortex and hippocampi, precisely the regions involved in declarative episodic memory. Hippocampal atrophy is characteristic, and reductions in hippocampal volumes may be observed on magnetic resonance imaging (MRI; Fig. 402-3). Involvement of the association neocortices with neurofibrillary tangles represents the histopathologic correlate of the progression to dementia. Quantitative MRI in patients with mild cognitive impairment who later progress to dementia shows increasing atrophy of key cortical association areas, such as the lateral temporal lobes, inferior parietal lobes, posterior cingulate cortex, and lateral frontal lobes. Reflecting the spread to association neocortex, language functions, visuospatial functions, and executive cognitive functions typically become impaired some time after declarative episodic memory dysfunction occurs.

The most consistent neurotransmitter deficit in Alzheimer disease is in cholinergic neurotransmission. The cells of origin of hippocampal and neocortical cholinergic projections are located in the septum, diagonal band, and nucleus basalis. Neurofibrillary tangles accumulate in the neurons in these regions as Alzheimer disease develops, but there is also neurochemical evidence that these neurons are stressed much earlier in the disease.

Genetics

The overwhelming majority of Alzheimer disease is due to sporadic (not genetic) disease. However, in a very small number of instances, Alzheimer disease occurs as an autosomal dominant disease. The three known genes involved in autosomal dominant Alzheimer disease all are directly involved in the production of β-amyloid peptide. The first is the amyloid precursor protein (*APP*) gene, located on chromosome 21q21.3. Eighteen known mutations in this gene lead to excess production of β-amyloid and are reliably associated with a very early onset (20 to 50 years of age) of Alzheimer disease. Another line of evidence implicating the *APP* gene in Alzheimer disease is the invariable appearance of the pathologic process of Alzheimer disease in individuals with Down syndrome (trisomy 21 [Chapter 41]), who have an extra copy of the *APP* gene as a result of the trisomy.

The other two genes associated with autosomal dominant Alzheimer disease are the presenilin 1 and 2 genes, located on chromosomes 14q24.3 and 1q31.42. A large number of presenilin 1 mutations account for the majority of autosomal dominant Alzheimer disease. Both genes code for a similar protein known as presenilin. Presenilin is involved in degradation of the APP molecule at the gamma cleavage site. It is believed that the Alzheimer disease–causing mutations in presenilin 1 and 2 lead to a "toxic gain of function" that produces excess β-amyloid peptide. The presenilin mutations are also associated with early-onset (age 40 to 60) Alzheimer disease.

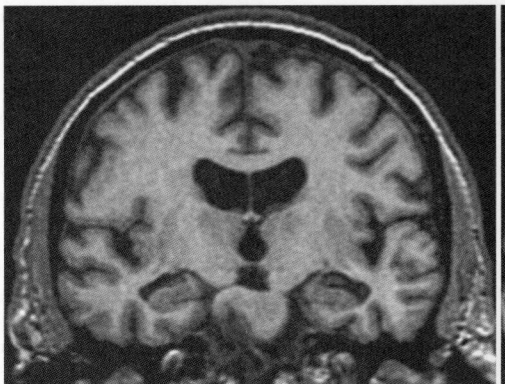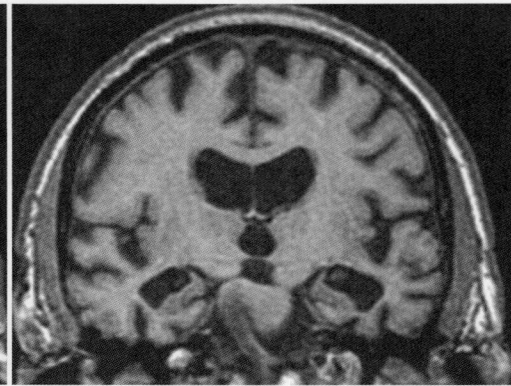

FIGURE 402-3. Serial coronal images from magnetic resonance imaging of a patient with Alzheimer disease. The scan on the left was performed when the patient was clinically normal. The scan on the right was performed 11 years later when the patient was demented. Hippocampal atrophy has increased dramatically from the first to the subsequent scan. (Courtesy Maria Shiung and Clifford Jack.)

Studies of the familial aggregation of Alzheimer disease have shown that later-onset disease also displays genetic risks, but only a few genes have been definitively linked to later-onset Alzheimer disease. The most prominent gene related to later-onset Alzheimer disease, located on chromosome 19q13.2, encodes apolipoprotein E (apo E), a protein involved in lipid transport. In humans, three allelic variants of apolipoprotein gene (*APOE*) are determined by differences in the amino acids cysteine and arginine at positions 112 and 158 of the 299–amino acid protein. One of the allelic variants, with arginine at both positions, designated the ε4 variant, is strongly associated with a 14-fold increased risk for Alzheimer disease in homozygotes and a three-fold increase in heterozygotes. In many series, almost 50% of Alzheimer disease patients but only about 25% of nondemented controls have at least one copy of the *APOE* ε4 allele. The presence of an *APOE* ε4 allele does not always cause Alzheimer disease in that the disease never develops in some carriers of the genotype. The mechanism by which the *APOE* ε4 allele predisposes to Alzheimer disease is not established, but the tertiary structure of the APOE protein with arginine at positions 112 and 158 may lead to impaired binding to β-amyloid, which in turn reduces the clearance of β-amyloid from cells.

A rare missense mutation in the *TREM2* gene also increases the risk of Alzheimer disease.[6] The pathophysiology appears to be impaired containment of inflammatory processes rather than a direct effect on neurologic function.

CLINICAL MANIFESTATIONS

The early course of Alzheimer disease is dominated by difficulties with anterograde amnesia. Some of the usual complaints include forgetting recent events and conversations, misplacing items, problems with keeping track of the date, getting lost in familiar surroundings, and problems with remembering to complete tasks. The frequency and severity of the memory lapses progress from occasional difficulty to more pervasive and consistent failure.

In mild Alzheimer disease, declarative episodic memory function may be lost. Familiarity and access to previous knowledge may allow patients to function in their usual daily routines as long as nothing out of the ordinary is required of them. They may still retain the ability to prepare simple meals and take walks in their neighborhood without getting lost. However, even in mild Alzheimer disease, medication-taking errors and difficulty managing money or balancing a checkbook are likely to occur. Traveling to unfamiliar places often accentuates confusion. Changes in personality commonly accompany the cognitive losses. Apathy, loss of initiative, and loss of interest in previous hobbies and pastimes are ubiquitous in early Alzheimer disease.

As the disease progresses, the ability to perform necessary daily tasks becomes more and more difficult to the point that the patient will need assistance preparing meals, paying bills, taking transportation, and keeping house. As the disease moves into the severe stages, assistance and supervision in basic activities such as bathing, dressing, toileting, and eating become necessary.

In the terminal stages of the disease, all communicative abilities may be lost. Mobility may still be preserved until late in the disease. Alzheimer disease patients commonly die of illnesses that strike other debilitated elderly individuals, such as sepsis, pneumonia, and congestive heart failure.

The duration of the course of clinical Alzheimer disease is long but variable. The time from mild dementia to death may be as short as 2 to 3 years or may be well over a decade. For patients in whom mild dementia is diagnosed, about 10% per year reach the stage of severe dementia.

Rarely, Alzheimer disease is associated with prominent symptoms in cognitive domains other than memory. The most common of the atypical syndromes is one in which profound visuospatial deficits occur without the typical severe anterograde amnesia. This syndrome is referred to as posterior cortical atrophy.

DIAGNOSIS

The diagnosis of Alzheimer disease, like that of dementia itself, is largely a clinical one based on the history and examination. The key elements in the history are a gradual onset and insidious progression of cognitive impairment, especially anterograde amnesia. The mental status examination should demonstrate impairment in short-term memory and other cognitive deficits. Alzheimer disease should be thought of as a diagnosis of inclusion: if the history and examination are compatible with Alzheimer disease and if certain exclusions can be verified, the diagnosis can be made with confidence.

The pathophysiology of Alzheimer disease in patients with mild cognitive impairment or dementia can be assessed with cerebrospinal fluid (CSF) protein markers (β-amyloid and tau) (see Table 402-3)[7] and with brain imaging (structural MRI, [18]fluoro-deoxyglucose PET,[8] and amyloid positron emission tomography[9]) (Figs. 402-4 and 402-5). PET imaging of abnormal deposition of tau protein, now available for research purposes, may enhance the accurate diagnosis of Alzheimer disease.[10] Efforts are now underway to diagnose Alzheimer disease while individuals are still asymptomatic.

Differential Diagnosis

A number of other conditions that bear similarity to Alzheimer disease must be excluded on clinical or laboratory grounds (see Fig. 402-2). One is dementia with Lewy bodies, which is suggested by the presence of parkinsonism, prominent visual hallucinations, and a specific sleep disorder. At autopsy, the pathologic processes of Lewy body disease and Alzheimer disease often coexist, thus suggesting that the diagnoses overlap. Frontotemporal lobar degeneration is suggested by prominent behavioral and personality changes or by prominent language difficulties early in the course. Hippocampal sclerosis has unique neuropathologic findings but is virtually impossible to distinguish from Alzheimer disease by clinical features. Other neurodegenerative conditions in the differential diagnosis of Alzheimer disease include Huntington disease (Chapter 410), progressive supranuclear palsy (Chapter 410), corticobasal degeneration (Chapter 410), amyotrophic lateral sclerosis (Chapter 419), and Wilson disease (Chapter 211); however, these diseases invariably have prominent motor manifestations early in their course. Normal-pressure hydrocephalus (Chapter 189; see later) is a rare cause of dementia associated with a gait disorder.

It is particularly challenging to distinguish dementia caused by cerebrovascular disease from Alzheimer disease (see later). The fact that Alzheimer disease and cerebrovascular disease often coexist requires clinicians to consider both simultaneously.

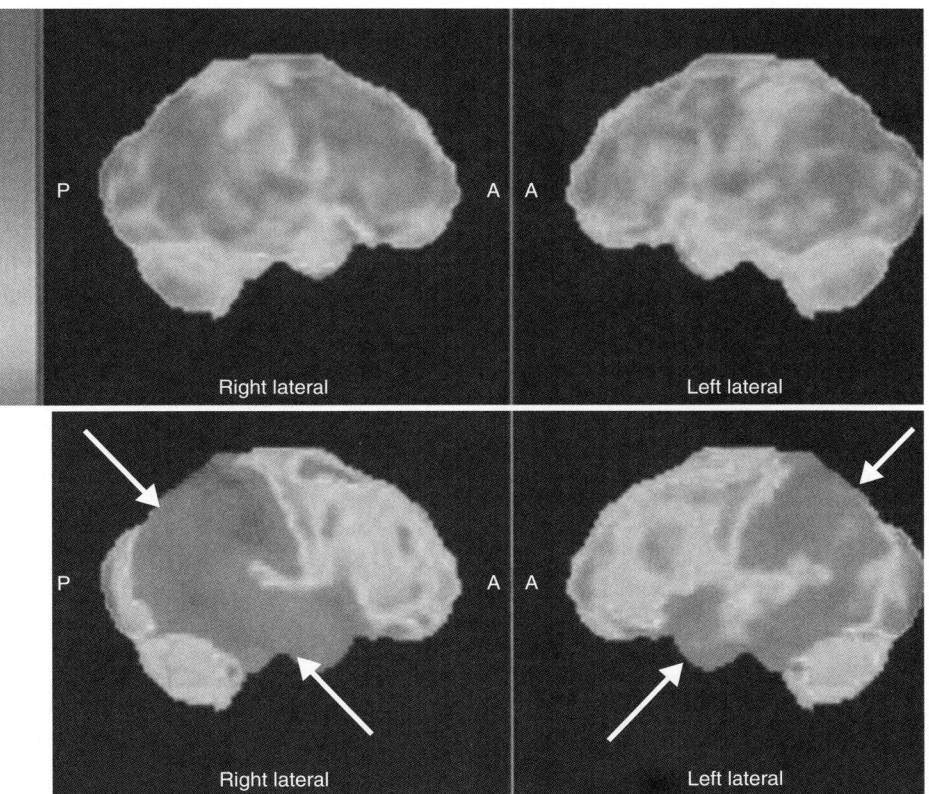

FIGURE 402-4. ¹⁸Fluoro-deoxyglucose positron emission tomographic scan of a patient with Alzheimer disease dementia. Computerized reconstructions of the regional glucose uptake ratio (using pons as reference) of the cortical surface show hotter colors (*yellow and orange*) in areas of normal glucose uptake, whereas cooler colors (*green and blue*) indicate hypometabolism. The scan on the top is from a normal individual of the same age. The scan on the bottom is from a patient with typical Alzheimer disease dementia, and it shows hypometabolism in the temporal and parietal cortical regions (*arrows*).

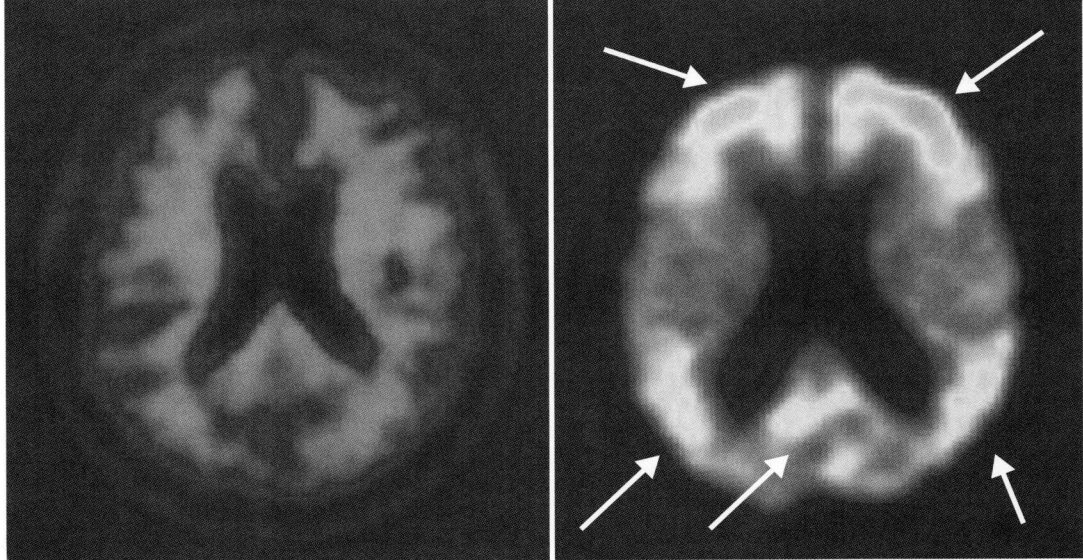

FIGURE 402-5. Amyloid positron emission tomographic (PET) scan of a patient with Alzheimer disease dementia. On this axial image of a ¹¹C Pittsburgh compound B PET scan, the left scan is from an individual with no cortical amyloid retention. The green signal represents low levels of nonspecific white matter binding. On the right, a scan of a patient with Alzheimer disease dementia shows the prominent retention of the amyloid imaging agent in the frontal, parietal, and posterior cingulate cortices (*arrows*).

PREVENTION AND TREATMENT   Rx

There are no established preventive therapies. Although a healthy diet, physical exercise, and stimulating cognitive leisure activities are sensible, they have not been shown to protect against Alzheimer disease. Except in patients who have folate or vitamin B₁₂ deficiency, vitamin B supplementation is not effective in slowing cognitive decline.[A3] Treatment of diabetes (Chapter 229) and hypertension (Chapter 67) is beneficial for other reasons, but it is not clear that such treatment alters the course of Alzheimer disease. Antidepressants generally are ineffective and increase adverse events when used to treat patients with Alzheimer disease.[A4]

Once Alzheimer disease becomes symptomatic, support for family caregivers is a critical intervention that cannot be overemphasized. Support groups through the Alzheimer Association (available at *www.alz.org*) can benefit families coping with the disease.

Important safety issues include supervision of medications, supervision of finances, and close scrutiny of motor vehicle operation. Operation of other potentially dangerous tools, firearms, appliances, and equipment should also be carefully monitored or avoided. Patients with Alzheimer disease often wander and can become lost long distances from home. Identification of patients can prevent tragic occurrences.

Evidence-Based Treatments

Two classes of drugs are approved for the treatment of Alzheimer disease: cholinesterase inhibitors and memantine, a glutamate receptor antagonist.[11] The rationale for use of cholinomimetic drugs (donepezil, 5 or 10 mg/day; galantamine, 16 or 24 mg/day; or rivastigmine, (6-12 mg/day orally or 4.5-9 mg/day by skin patch) is the reduced levels of cholinergic markers in the neocortex of patients dying of Alzheimer disease. All three agents delay the progression of symptoms to a statistically significant but clinically marginal extent at 6 to 12 months in patients with mild to moderate Alzheimer disease.[A5-A8] In community-dwelling patients who had been treated with donepezil for at least 3 months and who had moderate or severe Alzheimer disease, those who continued donepezil at 10 mg daily had clinically important functional benefits over the next 12 months compared with those who discontinued it. There is no compelling evidence that these agents alter its biological progression. Individual patients often do not show any clear benefits of treatment. Memantine, which is a low- to moderate-affinity uncompetitive *N*-methyl-D-aspartate receptor antagonist that acts on glutamate neurotransmission, appears to delay the progression of functional decline in patients with moderate to severe Alzheimer disease at a dose of 10 mg twice daily.[A9]

One study of patients with moderately severe Alzheimer disease showed that vitamin E was effective in delaying progression, and recent studies in patients with mild to moderate Alzheimer disease also suggest a benefit.[A10] Multivitamins are not efficacious,[A11] nor are humanized monoclonal antibodies that bind soluble forms of amyloid[A12][A13] or inhibit the formation of amyloid plaques.[A14]

PROGNOSIS

Alzheimer disease is inevitably progressive, and severe cognitive impairment and complete dependence on others develop in virtually all patients unless they die prematurely. Alzheimer disease also contributes to premature death; the mortality rate in patients with Alzheimer disease is about 10% per year. In patients with advanced dementia, the 6-month mortality is about 55%; pneumonia, fever, and eating problems are associated with poor prognosis.

● VASCULAR DEMENTIA

DEFINITION

Vascular dementia is a dementing illness in which the underlying cause is cerebral infarction. For a cognitive disorder to be attributed to cerebrovascular disease from a neuropathologic perspective, there must be sufficient cerebral infarction in locations known to be responsible for the cognitive deficits in the absence of other neurodegenerative neuropathologic changes (Table 402-4). When cerebrovascular disease produces cognitive impairment that is not severe enough to meet the criteria for dementia, it is referred to as vascular cognitive impairment.

TABLE 402-4	DIAGNOSTIC CRITERIA FOR THE SYNDROME OF DEMENTIA CAUSED BY CEREBROVASCULAR DISEASE (VASCULAR DEMENTIA)

Dementia as defined in Table 402-1

Clinically important cerebrovascular disease is demonstrable by *either* of the following:

    Onset of the cognitive disturbance or dramatic worsening of an existing disturbance that occurred within 3 months of a stroke, where stroke is defined as a focal neurologic deficit of acute onset in which the symptoms and signs persist for more than 24 hours

    Neuroimaging evidence of bilateral brain infarctions rostral to but including the thalamus

EPIDEMIOLOGY

In clinical studies, as many as 20% of dementia patients have cerebrovascular disease. Like Alzheimer disease, it is less common in patients younger than 65 years and increases steadily thereafter. In neuropathologic studies, about 25% of all cases of dementia have some vascular component. Roughly half that number are relatively pure vascular dementia; the remainder consists of vascular disease mixed with Alzheimer disease. Men and women are equally affected.

Risk Factors

Risk factors for vascular dementia include cardiovascular disease, atrial fibrillation,[12] higher glucose levels,[13] diabetes, and hypertension. There are no known protective factors other than treatment of these risk factors. Populations with high rates of generalized vascular disease should have higher rates of vascular dementia, but competing mortality from cardiovascular disease may obscure part of the relationship. Microinfarcts contribute to brain atrophy and cognitive impairment, particularly before dementia is clinically evident. In the first year after a stroke, the risk for development of dementia is about nine-fold higher than the rate in persons without a stroke; the risk remains about two-fold higher in subsequent years.

PATHOBIOLOGY

The majority of vascular disease causing cognitive impairment is due to atherosclerosis. One mechanism is through large infarctions, such as those secondary to occlusive disease in major cerebral vessels, including the carotid arteries and the anterior, middle, and posterior cerebral arteries (Chapter 407). A second mechanism of infarction is at the arteriolar level, with lacunar infarctions in the thalamus, basal ganglia, and subcortical white matter. Both these processes can be detected by brain MRI. Infarcts in the hippocampal formations, medial thalamus, caudate nuclei, and parietal association areas are highly likely to produce cognitive impairment but not necessarily dementia. Microinfarcts, which are small zones of infarction that are not visible to the naked eye but can be observed with light microscopy, may also contribute to the dementia. The simultaneous presence of Alzheimer disease is common in vascular dementia.

There are other uncommon causes of vascular dementia. Cerebral autosomal dominant arteriopathy with subcortical infarcts and leukoencephalopathy (CADASIL) is a very rare inherited disease that usually becomes clinically evident between the ages of 30 and 50 years and causes severe white matter disease, headaches, and dementia. The cause of CADASIL is mutations in the *notch3* gene on chromosome 19q12. Cerebral amyloid angiopathy, a β-amyloidosis in which the β-amyloid peptide accumulates in the media of small to medium-sized arteries in the leptomeninges and superficial cortex, causes cerebral hemorrhages that may lead to dementia if it occurs in sufficient number and in critical locations. Cerebral amyloid angiopathy is also seen in Alzheimer disease, but its hemorrhagic manifestations may occur in individuals with little evidence of Alzheimer disease clinically and modest evidence pathologically. Cerebral vasculitis (Chapter 270) is a very rare cause of dementia.

CLINICAL MANIFESTATIONS

The spectrum of cognitive changes in patients with cerebrovascular disease is broad. The more common cognitive syndromes in cerebrovascular disease include mild cognitive impairment, a dementia with prominent anterograde amnesia, and a dementia with prominent changes in personality and executive function. Some patients with vascular cognitive impairment without dementia may have deficits in only one domain (Chapter 401). A number of aphasia syndromes are a result of cerebral infarction or hemorrhage in the perisylvian regions of the dominant hemisphere. Infarction or hemorrhage in the occipitotemporal or occipitoparietal regions may produce one of the disorders of visual cognition, such as alexia or visual agnosia. Infarcts in the caudate nuclei, particularly if they are bilateral, may produce a cognitive syndrome that includes both amnesia and disordered executive function, thus mimicking dementia. Large infarcts in the right parietal lobe can also produce dementia. Infarcts in the medial thalami or in the hippocampal formations can produce isolated amnesia.

The evolution of symptoms in vascular dementia does not follow a stereotypical pattern. In some, the dementia syndrome may remain static. In others, new strokes may lead to substantial declines in cognition and function. Some patients with vascular dementia may experience a gradually declining illness. Patients with vascular cognitive impairment without dementia or vascular

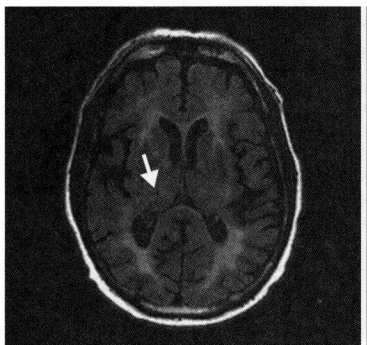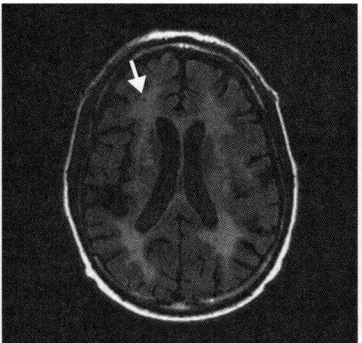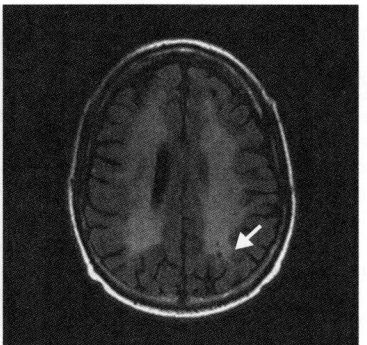

FIGURE 402-6. Axial magnetic resonance images of a patient with extensive cerebrovascular disease. The images show extensive white matter hyperintensities bilaterally. There are also lacunar infarcts (*arrows*).

dementia may also have other neurologic signs typical of patients with cerebrovascular disease, such as hemiparesis, hemianopia, hemisensory changes, or cranial nerve abnormalities.

DIAGNOSIS

The diagnosis of vascular dementia is based on the neurologic history and examination. Brain imaging, preferably with MRI, is essential to establish the presence of infarcts. The cardinal diagnostic features of vascular dementia are that (1) the cognitive disorder should have begun within 3 months of a clinical stroke event and (2) there should be multiple bilateral infarcts in the cerebral hemispheres visible on brain imaging studies (Fig. 402-6). A temporal link between the onset or worsening of cognitive impairment and a stroke is important in demonstrating that cerebrovascular disease is etiologically relevant to the cognitive impairment. Brain imaging of infarcts in the cerebral cortex, basal ganglia, thalamus, and cerebral white matter has obvious value for establishment of cerebrovascular disease. In contrast to actual infarcts on imaging, the presence of white matter hyperintensities without infarcts on brain MRI is much less specific.

The accuracy of the clinical diagnosis of vascular dementia is generally lower than that of Alzheimer disease. The combination of (1) a temporal relationship between dementia and a stroke and (2) imaging evidence of bilateral infarcts is diagnostically specific for vascular dementia but is insensitive. Broader diagnostic criteria (see Table 402-4) are more sensitive but less specific. The usual alternative diagnosis is Alzheimer disease, and there is typically no way to be certain whether and how much Alzheimer disease is simultaneously present.

PREVENTION AND TREATMENT   Rx

Some cases of vascular dementia should be preventable. With early lifelong aggressive treatment of diabetes (Chapter 229), hypertension (Chapter 67), and hyperlipidemia (Chapter 206), the number of cerebral infarcts should be reduced, with a corresponding reduction in the number of cases of vascular dementia. Evidence for this link comes from large-scale studies in which the treatment of hypertension reduced the frequency of strokes and incident dementia. Once vascular dementia develops, cholinesterase inhibitors have shown some benefit,[A15] but the major goal is to prevent future strokes.

PROGNOSIS

Patients with vascular dementia can often be expected to have severe cardiovascular disease and a greater likelihood of future strokes and cardiac ischemic events. Survival of patients with vascular dementia is poorer than that of patients with Alzheimer disease.

DEMENTIA WITH LEWY BODIES

DEFINITION

Dementia with Lewy bodies is a multifaceted dementing disorder in which the underlying pathologic process includes Lewy bodies in limbic and cortical structures (Table 402-5). Some clinicians make a distinction between patients in whom parkinsonism preceded the cognitive disorder and those in whom the cognitive disorder occurred either simultaneously with or before

TABLE 402-5	DIAGNOSTIC CRITERIA FOR THE DEMENTIA SYNDROME ASSOCIATED WITH LEWY BODY PATHOLOGY

Dementia as defined in Table 402-1

The cognitive disturbance is of insidious onset and is progressive, based on evidence from the history or serial cognitive examination.

The presence of **at least two** of the following:
Parkinsonism (rigidity, resting tremor, bradykinesia, postural instability, parkinsonian gait disorder)
Prominent, fully formed visual hallucinations
Substantial fluctuations in alertness or cognition
Rapid eye movement sleep behavior disorder (Chapter 405)
Severe worsening of parkinsonism by antipsychotic drugs

The disturbance is not better accounted for by a systemic disease or another brain disease.

Adapted from McKeith IG, Dickson DW, Lowe J, et al. Diagnosis and management of dementia with Lewy bodies: third report of the DLB Consortium. *Neurology.* 2005;65:1863-1872.

the movement disorder. This distinction may be somewhat useful in clinical practice, but there are few clinical or neuropathologic differences based on different sequences of signs and symptoms. The diagnosis of dementia with Lewy bodies is similar in principle to diagnosis of both dementia and Parkinson disease (Chapter 409) in the same individual, but *dementia with Lewy bodies* is a term with broader connotations because of other features (hallucinations, fluctuations, and sleep disorder) that may be more apparent than the movement disorder.

EPIDEMIOLOGY

Dementia with Lewy bodies is about a quarter as common as Alzheimer disease.[14] Lewy body disease becomes more common with advancing age, and the prevalence of dementia with Lewy bodies increases with advancing age as well. As with the other dementias, there are no known ethnic or racial differences, but dementia with Lewy bodies may be more common in men. There are no known risk factors for dementia with Lewy bodies. Dementia develops in up to 30% of patients with Parkinson disease, and advancing age is the major risk factor.

PATHOBIOLOGY

The pathology of dementia with Lewy bodies is a mixture of Lewy body disease and Alzheimer disease. In general, the more intense the Lewy body disease, the less abundant the Alzheimer disease. Lewy bodies, which are intraneuronal inclusions that contain α-synuclein, are found in the nucleus basalis, pars compacta of the substantia nigra, locus caeruleus, other brain stem structures, amygdala, cingulate gyrus, and neocortex. The earliest locations of Lewy bodies are the brain stem, where they affect nuclei involved in sleep and arousal, and the substantia nigra, the locus caeruleus, and cranial nerve nuclei IX and X. Typically, the nucleus basalis, transentorhinal cortex, cingulate gyrus, and neocortex become involved later.

In Lewy body disease, the α-synuclein protein becomes misfolded and aggregates intraneuronally. Mutations in the α-synuclein gene have been seen in a few families with autosomal dominant Parkinson disease, but most cases of dementia with Lewy bodies are sporadic.

CLINICAL MANIFESTATIONS

The clinical manifestations of dementia with Lewy bodies include four major abnormalities: the cognitive disorder, the neuropsychiatric disorder, the motor disorder, and the disorder of sleep and wakefulness. The cognitive disorder may differ from Alzheimer disease, although there is considerable overlap.[15] In a typical patient with dementia with Lewy bodies, visuospatial deficits, impaired concentration, and impaired attention dominate the picture. In some patients, the deficits in executive functions may be similar to what is seen in frontotemporal lobar degeneration. Anterograde amnesia is usually present but milder than in Alzheimer disease. Language deficits are not prominent. The neuropsychiatric manifestations of dementia with Lewy bodies, including prominent apathy, loss of initiative, and depression, may be more disabling than the cognitive symptoms. The motor manifestations include bradykinesia, gait disturbances, postural disturbances, and rigidity. Rest tremor is less common in dementia with Lewy bodies in patients in whom the cognitive disorder appears before the parkinsonism. Visual hallucinations, fluctuations in alertness, and rapid eye movement (REM) sleep disorders are part of a broader disorder of the regulation of sleep and wakefulness. Visual hallucinations are often graphic, detailed, and bizarre, perhaps because the sleep phenomenon of dreaming intrudes into wakefulness. Patients with dementia with Lewy bodies have large fluctuations in their alertness and arousal from day to day.

REM sleep behavior disorder (Chapter 405) is a parasomnia in which patients exhibit dream enactment behavior, often with violent, threatening overtones. Patients typically relate that they feel as though they are being chased by something or someone. Their behavior while they are asleep consists of excessive talking, calling out or shouting, and thrashing about, often to the point of striking a bed partner or falling out of bed. The REM sleep behavior disorder may precede the development of Parkinson disease and dementia with Lewy bodies by years.

DIAGNOSIS

The diagnosis of dementia with Lewy bodies is based on clinical information that corroborates the presence of abnormalities in cognition, motor function, neuropsychiatric behavior, and regulation of sleep and wakefulness. Formal neuropsychological testing is often helpful in evaluating memory, executive function, and visuospatial function in a detailed manner. Neuroimaging has only a limited role in the diagnosis of dementia with Lewy bodies.

Differential Diagnosis

Other disorders that must be considered in patients with dementia and a movement disorder include progressive supranuclear palsy (Chapter 410), which can resemble dementia with Lewy bodies in terms of both the dementia and the motor disorder. In progressive supranuclear palsy, patients are much less likely to have disorders of arousal and typically have other distinctive signs and symptoms, including the characteristic supranuclear gaze palsy and other brain stem findings. The corticobasal degenerations, which are members of the family of frontotemporal lobar dementias (see later), may also produce a movement disorder and dementia. Huntington disease (Chapter 410) is associated with dementia and a movement disorder, but the movement disorder of Huntington disease includes prominent chorea and athetosis, neither of which is present in dementia with Lewy bodies.

Normal-pressure hydrocephalus (Chapter 189) is a rare disorder typically characterized by the triad of a gait disorder, dementia, and urinary incontinence. Altered dynamics of CSF flow in the ventricular system appear to reduce periventricular metabolism and also induce damage in periventricular axons.[16] Normal-pressure hydrocephalus can be suspected when computed tomography or MRI shows ventricular enlargement that is out of proportion to the amount of sulcal widening. Predicting a favorable response to ventriculoperitoneal shunting in suspected normal-pressure hydrocephalus has proved to be difficult. Imaging studies that measure CSF flow through the aqueduct of Sylvius or that measure flow of radiolabeled CSF with radionuclide cisternography have not been useful. Clinical response to the removal of a high volume (e.g., 30 mL) of CSF through lumbar puncture is sometimes used to select patients for surgery, although its positive and negative predictive value is unclear. Normal-pressure hydrocephalus is very rare relative to dementia with Lewy bodies and Alzheimer disease.

TREATMENT   Rx

Management of patients with dementia with Lewy bodies is challenging because of the simultaneous appearance of a cognitive disorder, a neuropsychiatric disorder, a motor disorder, and a sleep and wakefulness disorder. Treatment of the motor disorder is accomplished with antiparkinsonian drugs such as levodopa and dopaminergic agonists (Chapter 409). Treatment with these agents should be instituted for dementia with Lewy bodies if there are prominent gait or balance problems that threaten safety and interfere with independence. These medications may worsen hallucinations and exacerbate confusional states, but this concern should not preclude a treatment trial if the motor symptoms pose safety risks or interfere with independence.

Cholinesterase inhibitors, which do not exacerbate parkinsonian symptoms, have a beneficial effect on neuropsychiatric symptoms and perhaps on the cognitive disorder.[A16] Autonomic disturbances such as urinary incontinence can be challenging to treat in persons with dementia with Lewy bodies, because the usually prescribed medications have anticholinergic pharmacologic profiles. Anticholinergic drugs have a definite risk of increasing confusion.

Hallucinations and agitation impair quality of life for the patient and family and often require treatment. Some antipsychotic agents that might otherwise control these symptoms dramatically exacerbate the parkinsonism in dementia with Lewy bodies. Atypical antipsychotics are usually recommended, but there is insufficient experience from controlled clinical trials. Many movement disorder specialists prefer to use quetiapine in doses of 25 to 200 mg/day or clozapine at 6.25 to 50 mg/day because these agents appear to have the lowest rate of extrapyramidal side effects. However, it is not possible to make any strong statements about the relative efficacy of atypical antipsychotics in treating the hallucinations in dementia with Lewy bodies, especially in view of the possibility that atypical antipsychotic agents may be associated with higher-than-expected mortality.

REM sleep behavior disorder (Chapter 405) can be disabling, but there are no controlled clinical trials to inform treatment. Some sleep disorder specialists typically use either melatonin, 3 to 12 mg, or clonazepam, 0.5 to 2 mg, at bedtime.

Treatment of depressive symptoms may substantially improve a patient's functioning. Use of one of the newer-generation antidepressants, such as sertraline (25 to 100 mg/day) or citalopram (10 to 20 mg/day), may be beneficial and does not necessarily interfere with management of the other symptoms (Chapter 397).

PROGNOSIS

As opposed to patients with Alzheimer disease, some studies show that patients with dementia with Lewy bodies have a more rapidly progressive course and poorer survival. As a result of the combination of manifestations, patients with dementia with Lewy bodies may become disabled sooner in their course.

● FRONTOTEMPORAL LOBAR DEGENERATION

DEFINITION

The frontotemporal lobar degenerations are a group of neurodegenerative disorders with distinctive clinical manifestations and a predilection for the prefrontal and anterior temporal neocortices. The most common clinical syndrome is a disorder of behavior and personal relationships (comportment) with a loss of executive functions (Table 402-6). This syndrome is referred to as behavior-variant frontotemporal dementia. Other syndromes in the clinical spectrum of frontotemporal lobar degeneration involve different aspects of language or motor dysfunction of the limbs.

EPIDEMIOLOGY

Unlike Alzheimer disease, the frontotemporal lobar degenerations have a peak age at onset in the 50- to 70-year range, and the incidence declines after the age of 70. In patients with dementia who are younger than 70 years, frontotemporal lobar degeneration makes up 10 to 20% of cases.[17] However, across the entire age spectrum, the frontotemporal lobar degenerations are much less common than Alzheimer disease, dementia with Lewy bodies, or vascular dementia. Both men and women are affected equally. There are no known risk factors for the frontotemporal lobar degenerations except a family history.

PATHOBIOLOGY

The clinical syndrome in frontotemporal lobar degeneration is determined by the lobar location of the pathologic process. Right prefrontal or anterior

TABLE 402-6   DIAGNOSTIC CRITERIA FOR BEHAVIOR-VARIANT FRONTOTEMPORAL DEMENTIA

The following symptom must be present to meet criteria for behavior-variant frontotemporal dementia:

Shows progressive deterioration of behavior and/or cognition by observation or history (as provided by a knowledgeable informant)

Three of the following behavioral/cognitive symptoms that are persistent or recurrent must be present **within 3 years of onset** to meet criteria for **possible** behavior-variant frontotemporal dementia:

Early behavioral disinhibition such as socially inappropriate behavior, loss of manners or decorum, or impulsive, rash, or careless actions

Early apathy or inertia

Early loss of sympathy or empathy

Early perseverative, stereotyped, or compulsive/ritualistic behavior

Hyperorality and dietary changes such as altered food preferences, binge eating, increased consumption of alcohol or cigarettes, or oral exploration or consumption of inedible objects

Neuropsychological profile exhibits executive/generation deficits with relative sparing of memory and visuospatial functions

Probable behavior-variant frontotemporal dementia is diagnosed when **all of the following** are present:

Criteria met for possible behavior-variant frontotemporal dementia

Significant functional decline present by caregiver report

Imaging results that demonstrate frontal and/or anterior temporal atrophy on MRI or CT, or frontal hypoperfusion or hypometabolism on PET or SPECT

The diagnosis of behavior-variant frontotemporal dementia **should not** be applied when the pattern of deficits is better explained by a psychiatric diagnosis, other non-degenerative nervous system disorders, or medical disorders.

CT = computed tomography; MRI = magnetic resonance imaging; PET = positron emission tomography; SPECT = single-photon emission computed tomography.
Adapted from Rascovsky K, Hodges JR, Knopman D, et al. Sensitivity of revised diagnostic criteria for the behavioural variant of frontotemporal dementia. *Brain*. 2011;134:2456-2477.

temporal disease and brain atrophy produce behavioral syndromes like frontotemporal dementia. Left frontal involvement tends to produce progressive nonfluent aphasia. Predominant left anterior temporal lobe involvement may produce semantic dementia.

On histopathologic grounds, patients with frontotemporal lobar degeneration can be divided into three groups: those whose inclusions contain the microtubule-associated protein tau, those whose inclusions contain the TAR DNA-binding protein 43 (TDP-43), and those whose inclusions contain the fused in sarcoma (FUS) protein, another ribonucleic acid–binding protein. The latter is much less common than the first two. Each type includes both genetically determined and sporadic forms.

Among the tau-positive varieties are Pick disease, in which intracellular tau-positive inclusions known as Pick bodies are seen. Several other pathologic tau-positive subtypes occur, including progressive supranuclear palsy, corticobasal degeneration, and the disorder associated with mutations in the tau gene. Nearly 50 mutations in the *MAPT* gene on chromosome 17q21 are associated with autosomal dominant frontotemporal lobar degeneration syndromes, each with a slightly different clinical and neuropathologic phenotype.[18] The most common is a proline-to-leucine mutation at codon 301, located in exon 10. The tau gene undergoes alternative splicing, resulting in six isoforms of the tau protein. Pathologic mutations appear to disrupt splicing of alternative isoforms of tau protein, which in turn adversely affects the binding of tau to microtubules in neurons. Reduced binding of tau to microtubules is deleterious to microtubule function and neuronal integrity.

The TDP-43–positive frontotemporal lobar degenerations are almost equally common. Immunostaining shows that there are distinctive TDP-43–containing inclusions. Mutations in the granulin (*GRN*) gene, also located on chromosome 17q21, cause familial autosomal dominant forms of frontotemporal lobar degeneration with TDP-43–positive inclusions. Nearly 70 different mutations in the granulin gene are linked to frontotemporal lobar degenerations. All of the mutations lead to premature degradation of the messenger RNA, a process termed *haploinsufficiency*. Granulin mutation carriers have an abnormally low amount of the protein progranulin. The normal function of granulin in the brain is unclear, and the pathophysiologic basis for dementia in persons with granulin gene mutations is unknown. The link between alterations in TDP-43 and *GRN* mutations is also unknown at this time.

A third important gene mutation involved in frontotemporal lobar degenerations associated with TDP-43 inclusions is the hexanucleotide repeat expansion in *C9ORF7* gene located on chromosome 9p21. This latter mutation is the most common of the mutations causing frontotemporal lobar degeneration.[19]

Frontotemporal lobar degenerations that are FUS positive are much less common. At this time, all FUS-positive cases have had the behavioral variant of frontotemporal dementia.

CLINICAL MANIFESTATIONS

The clinical manifestations of the syndrome of frontotemporal dementia begin insidiously. Apathy, loss of initiative, and flattening of affect are common early symptoms. As the disease progresses, the entire spectrum of behavioral changes associated with dysfunction of the frontal and anterior temporal lobes appears.[20] On cognitive assessments, patients may have preserved memory functions, but they typically have difficulty with tests of executive cognitive function. When frontotemporal dementia progresses to moderate or severe stages, the behavioral changes remain prominent, but the disease becomes more difficult to distinguish from other dementias such as Alzheimer disease. The neuropathology of behavior-variant frontotemporal dementia may be either tau positive or TDP-43 positive.

In some patients with frontotemporal lobar degeneration, signs and symptoms of motor neuron disease (Chapter 419) develop, such as weakness, atrophy, and fasciculation in the limbs or the bulbar musculature. In other patients with frontotemporal lobar degeneration, asymmetrical limb apraxia develops that is part of the corticobasal syndrome. Features of progressive supranuclear palsy may also appear in patients with behavior-variant frontotemporal dementia.

Aphasic disturbances are often the presenting manifestation of patients with frontotemporal lobar degeneration. The two most characteristic syndromes are a nonfluent/agrammatic variant of primary progressive aphasia or the semantic variant of primary progressive aphasia. The nonfluent/agrammatic primary progressive aphasia variant is seen in patients who exhibit hesitancy in selecting words in their speech, a problem that may be difficult for others to appreciate at first. Anomia is an early sign. Gradually, the patient's speech becomes laconic and labored. Eventually, a nonfluent, apractic, agrammatic speech develops. In other cognitive domains, patients often have no deficits. Other nonfluent/agrammatic primary progressive aphasic patients may eventually become virtually mute even though they may appear to have preserved memory and visuospatial functions. Patients with nonfluent/agrammatic primary progressive aphasia often have tau-positive neuropathologic findings.

The semantic variant of primary progressive aphasia, previously known as semantic dementia, is a disorder that involves dissolution of the meaning of words or objects. A patient with semantic variant primary progressive aphasia may also become unable to access knowledge about objects (object agnosia) and people's faces (prosopagnosia). The most striking demonstration of the deficit in semantic variant primary progressive aphasia is when a patient can produce the name of an object—a watch, for example—but then cannot say what a watch is for when asked. Often, patients with semantic variant primary progressive aphasia have preservation of the ability to learn a list of words, even if their knowledge of the meaning of the words is diminished. Patients with semantic variant primary progressive aphasia usually have TDP-43–positive neuropathologic findings.

Not all patients with primary progressive aphasia fit neatly into a well-delineated syndrome. Although the semantic and nonfluent/agrammatic variants of primary progressive aphasia are almost always due to frontotemporal lobar degenerations, other variants, especially one in which word-finding problems predominate (the logopenic variant of primary progressive aphasia), may be due to Alzheimer disease.

DIAGNOSIS

Frontotemporal lobar degeneration must first be suspected on clinical grounds, based on the appearance of one of the distinctive clinical syndromes such as frontotemporal dementia (see Table 402-6) or one of the aphasic subtypes.[21,22] Neuropsychological testing can also aid in the diagnosis by detecting abnormalities in executive function and verifying that memory function is preserved, as it often is. For all frontotemporal lobar degeneration syndromes, MRI showing focal atrophy of the frontal (Fig. 402-7) or temporal lobes (Fig. 402-8) is highly likely to be diagnostic. Imaging with fluorodeoxyglucose-enhanced PET can also be useful when the clinical diagnosis is uncertain and MRI is nondiagnostic.

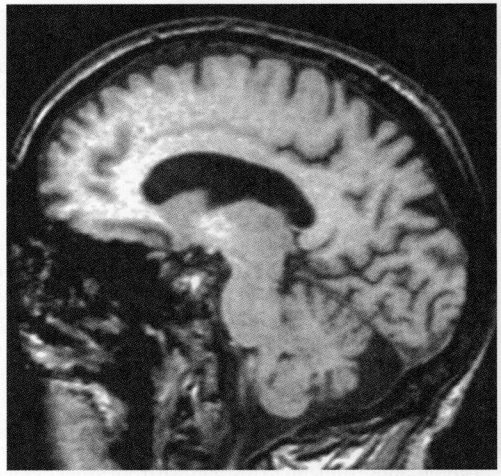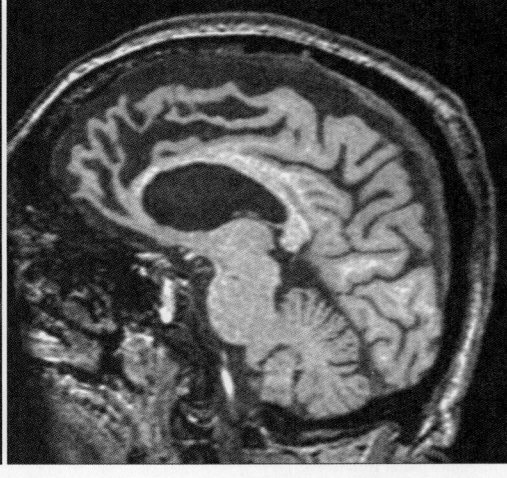

FIGURE 402-7. Parasagittal image from magnetic resonance imaging of a patient with frontotemporal dementia (*left*). Atrophy of the frontal lobes is dramatic compared with the brain of a normal individual (*right*). (Courtesy Maria Shiung and Clifford Jack.)

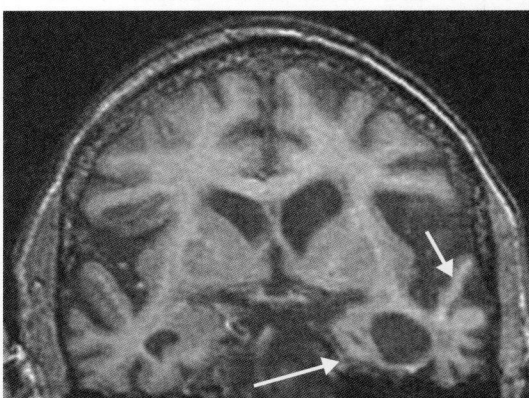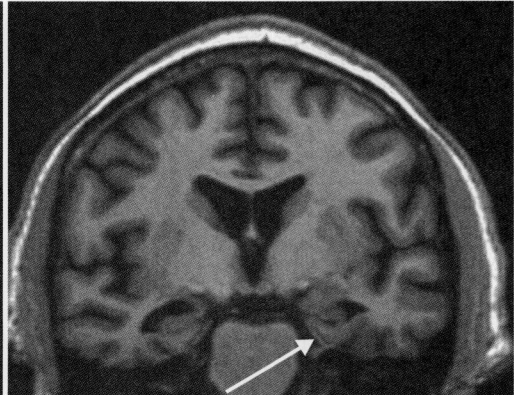

FIGURE 402-8. Coronal images from magnetic resonance imaging of a patient with semantic variant of primary progressive aphasia (*left*). There is prominent asymmetrical atrophy of the left anterior temporal lobe involving the amygdala, head of the hippocampus, and the lateral temporal lobe neocortex. By comparison, on the scan of a patient with Alzheimer disease dementia (*right*), the neocortex is preserved even though there is atrophy involving the amygdala and head of the hippocampus (*arrows*).

TREATMENT   Rx

There is no symptomatic therapy specifically for frontotemporal lobar degeneration. In patients with agitation, paranoia, delusions, or obsessive behavior, atypical antipsychotics (e.g., quetiapine, 25 to 200 mg/day) are used, but no controlled clinical trials are available. There are no preventive or disease-modifying treatments of frontotemporal lobar degeneration.

PROGNOSIS

Specific frontotemporal lobar degeneration syndromes have dramatic differences in their clinical course and outcome. In patients with motor neuron signs and symptoms, the prognosis is usually poor, with survival of only about 2 years from the time of diagnosis. Patients with semantic variant and nonfluent variant primary progressive aphasia have much more protracted and gradual trajectories; survival for more than 10 years is not uncommon. Behavior variant frontotemporal dementia itself can also exhibit a more protracted course.

 Grade A References

A1. Petersen RC, Thomas RG, Grundman M, et al. Vitamin E and donepezil for the treatment of mild cognitive impairment. *N Engl J Med.* 2005;352:2379-2388.
A2. Lautenschlager NT, Cox KL, Flicker L, et al. Effect of physical activity on cognitive function in older adults at risk for Alzheimer disease: a randomized trial. *JAMA.* 2008;300:1027-1037.
A3. Aisen PS, Schneider LS, Sano M, et al. High-dose B vitamin supplementation and cognitive decline in Alzheimer disease: a randomized controlled trial. *JAMA.* 2008;300:1774-1783.
A4. Banerjee S, Hellier J, Dewey M, et al. Sertraline or mirtazapine for depression in dementia (HTA-SADD): a randomised, multicentre, double-blind, placebo-controlled trial. *Lancet.* 2011;378:408-411.
A5. Courtney C, Farrell D, Gray R, et al. AD2000 Collaborative Group. Long-term donepezil treatment in 565 patients with Alzheimer's disease (AD2000): randomised double-blind trial. *Lancet.* 2004;363:2105-2115.
A6. Raina P, Santaguida P, Ismaila A, et al. Effectiveness of cholinesterase inhibitors and memantine for treating dementia: evidence review for a clinical practice guideline. *Ann Intern Med.* 2008;148:379-397.
A7. Howard R, McShane R, Lindesay J, et al. Donepezil and memantine for moderate-to-severe Alzheimer's disease. *N Engl J Med.* 2012;366:893-903.
A8. Winblad B, Kilander L, Eriksson S, et al. Donepezil in patients with severe Alzheimer's disease: double-blind, parallel-group, placebo-controlled study. *Lancet.* 2006;367:1057-1065.
A9. Reisberg B, Doody R, Stoffler A, et al. Memantine in moderate-to-severe Alzheimer's disease. *N Engl J Med.* 2003;348:1333-1341.
A10. Dysken MW, Sano M, Asthana S, et al. Effect of vitamin E and memantine on functional decline in Alzheimer disease: the TEAM-AD VA cooperative randomized trial. *JAMA.* 2014;311:33-44.
A11. Grodstein F, O'Brien J, Kang JH, et al. Long-term multivitamin supplementation and cognitive function in men: a randomized trial. *Ann Intern Med.* 2013;159:806-814.
A12. Doody RS, Thomas RG, Farlow M, et al. Phase 3 trials of solanezumab for mild-to-moderate Alzheimer's disease. *N Engl J Med.* 2014;370:311-321.
A13. Salloway S, Sperling R, Fox NC, et al. Two phase 3 trials of bapineuzumab in mild-to-moderate Alzheimer's disease. *N Engl J Med.* 2014;370:322-333.
A14. Doody RS, Raman R, Farlow M, et al. A phase 3 trial of semagacestat for treatment of Alzheimer's disease. *N Engl J Med.* 2013;369:341-350.
A15. Erkinjuntti T, Kurz A, Gauthier S, et al. Efficacy of galantamine in probable vascular dementia and Alzheimer's disease combined with cerebrovascular disease: a randomised trial. *Lancet.* 2002;359:1283-1290.
A16. Rolinski M, Fox C, Maidment I, et al. Cholinesterase inhibitors for dementia with Lewy bodies, Parkinson's disease dementia and cognitive impairment in Parkinson's disease. *Cochrane Database Syst Rev.* 2012;3:CD006504.

GENERAL REFERENCES

For the General References and other additional features, please visit Expert Consult at https://expertconsult.inkling.com.

403

THE EPILEPSIES

SAMUEL WIEBE

DEFINITION

A seizure is defined by transient focal or generalized signs or symptoms due to abnormal excessive or synchronous neuronal activity in the brain. Focal seizures, which originate within neuronal networks limited to one cerebral hemisphere, produce signs and symptoms corresponding to the specific region of the brain affected by the seizure. Generalized seizures rapidly affect extensive neuronal networks on both cerebral hemispheres, and their signs and symptoms are consistent with substantial involvement of both sides of the brain.

Seizures are not synonymous with epilepsy. The epilepsies should be distinguished from situations in which acute brain insults (e.g., infections, trauma, intoxication, metabolic disturbances) cause one or more seizures without a resulting chronic seizure tendency. Acute symptomatic seizures, or provoked seizures, constitute about 40% of all incident cases of nonfebrile seizures, typically respond to treatment of the provoking factor, and do not require long-term treatment with antiepileptic drugs.

The epilepsies are a group of conditions in which an underlying neurologic disorder results in a chronic tendency to have recurrent unprovoked seizures. Under these circumstances, the diagnosis of epilepsy is established if (1) two or more unprovoked seizures occur, or (2) one seizure occurs in a person whose risk of recurrence is at least 60%, or (3) one or more seizures occur in the context of a known epilepsy syndrome.[1] The causes, types, and clinical expression of the epilepsies are numerous and varied. However, some of the epilepsies conform into identifiable epileptic syndromes, which consist of clusters of clinical and electroencephalographic (EEG) features that have specific causes, respond to particular treatments, and may have specific prognostic implications.

EPIDEMIOLOGY

Incidence and Prevalence

Seizures are common in the general population, and about 1 in 10 people will experience a seizure in their lifetime. Most of these seizures are provoked by acute events and are not related to epilepsy. The overall annual incidence of acute symptomatic seizures, excluding febrile seizures, in developed countries is about 39 per 100,000 people. The incidence is higher in men and follows a bimodal age distribution. Incidence is at its highest peak in the first year of life (up to 300 per 100,000), reaches a nadir of 15 per 100,000 in the third and fourth decades of life, and rises again to 123 per 100,000 after 75 years of age. These differences are attributable to the high incidence of acute symptomatic seizures associated with metabolic, infectious, and encephalopathic causes during the neonatal period, and of cerebrovascular and degenerative diseases in elderly persons.

The epilepsies are common and affect humans of any age. After headache, the epilepsies are the most frequent chronic neurologic condition seen in general practice worldwide. In developed countries, the prevalence of active epilepsy ranges from 5 to 7 per 1000 persons, and the median annual incidence is 45 per 100,000 (range, 30 to 67), varying by age and socioeconomic status.[2] One in 26 people will develop epilepsy during their lifetime (1 in 21 males and 1 in 28 females).[3] The incidence of epilepsy peaks in children younger than 5 years at 60 to 70 per 100,000, decreases throughout adolescence to 30 per 100,000 in early adulthood, and rises again after the sixth decade, reaching a peak of 150 to 200 per 100,000 persons older than 75 years. Overall, the incidence and prevalence of the epilepsies are higher in developing countries, largely owing to a higher frequency of perinatal insults, trauma, and infectious disorders of the brain and to suboptimal treatment. In these countries, the median prevalence of active epilepsy is 12.5 per 1000 (range, 5 to 57 per 1000), and the annual incidence ranges from 78 to 190 per 100,000. Furthermore, the patterns of age-specific incidence are quite different in developing countries, where incidence peaks in young adults, not in elderly persons.

Risk Factors

Among all age groups, the top five risk factors for developing acute symptomatic seizures are head trauma (16%), stroke (16%), infectious disorders

TABLE 403-1	COMMON CAUSES OF ACUTE SYMPTOMATIC (PROVOKED) SEIZURES

METABOLIC

Hypernatremia, hyponatremia, hypocalcemia, hypoxia, hypoglycemia, nonketotic hyperosmolar hyperglycemia, renal failure

DRUG INDUCED

Theophylline, meperidine, tricyclic antidepressants, ephedra, gingko, phenothiazines, quinolones, β-lactams, isoniazid, antihistamines, cyclosporine, interferons, tacrolimus, cocaine, lithium, amphetamines

DRUG WITHDRAWAL

Alcohol, benzodiazepines, barbiturates

ENDOCRINE

Hyperthyroidism, hypothyroidism, peripartum

OTHER SYSTEMIC CONDITIONS

Sickle cell crisis, hypertensive encephalopathy, systemic lupus erythematosus, polyarteritis, eclampsia, high fever

CENTRAL NERVOUS SYSTEM DISORDERS

Trauma, stroke, intracerebral hemorrhage, encephalitis, abscess, bacterial meningitis

(15%), toxic-metabolic disorders (15%), and drug and alcohol withdrawal (14%) (Table 403-1).

The risk factors for developing epilepsy differ in adults and children. In childhood, excluding inherited epilepsies, the risk is increased by febrile seizures, head trauma, infections of the brain, mental retardation, cerebral palsy, and attention-deficit/hyperactivity disorder. Perinatal insults do not carry an increased risk for epilepsy unless they are accompanied by mental retardation or cerebral palsy.

In adults, risk factors for developing epilepsy can be identified in only one third of patients, in whom head trauma, brain infections, stroke, and Alzheimer disease are the most common. The risk of developing epilepsy is increased more than 500-fold by a history of a military head injury, 30-fold by a severe civilian head injury (Chapter 399), 20-fold each by stroke (Chapter 407) and brain infections (Chapters 412 to 414),[4] and 10-fold each for Alzheimer disease (Chapter 402), migraine headache (Chapter 398), and hypertension. In Latin America, the most frequently identified risk factor is brain infection. In endemic areas, neurocysticercosis (Chapter 354) accounts for about 10% of all newly diagnosed cases of epilepsy.

Pathobiology

Pathogenesis

The pathologic substrates and mechanisms underpinning initiation and propagation differ for focal and generalized seizures. In focal seizures, an aggregate of cortical or subcortical neurons develop high-frequency bursts of sodium-dependent action potentials caused by a shift in calcium conductance, thereby resulting in the typical EEG spike discharge (Fig. 403-1). Spread of bursting activity to other neurons is normally prevented by surrounding inhibitory mechanisms, such as hyperpolarization and inhibitory interneurons. When a sufficient number of neurons are engaged in sustained bursting, further excitatory phenomena ensue, including the increased release of excitatory neurotransmitters owing to presynaptic accumulation of Ca^{2+}, depolarization of surrounding neurons owing to increased extracellular K^+, and further neuronal activation caused by depolarization-induced activation of N-methyl-D-aspartate (NMDA) receptors. As excitation increases and inhibition decreases, additional neurons are recruited regionally and distantly, thereby resulting in seizure propagation. The mechanisms by which neurons develop a tendency toward anomalous bursting activity include alterations in neurotransmitters, membrane receptors, ion channels, second-messenger systems, and gene expression of various proteins.

Considerably less is known about the basic mechanisms underlying generalized seizures, which depend prominently on thalamocortical circuits. In absence seizures, the classic generalized spike-and-wave discharges seen on EEG are related to alterations in oscillatory rhythms generated by circuits that connect the thalamus and cortex and that involve T-type Ca^{2+} channels, which are located in the reticular nucleus of the thalamus. In generalized convulsive seizures, cortical neurons exhibit prolonged depolarization during the tonic phase, followed by rhythmic depolarization and

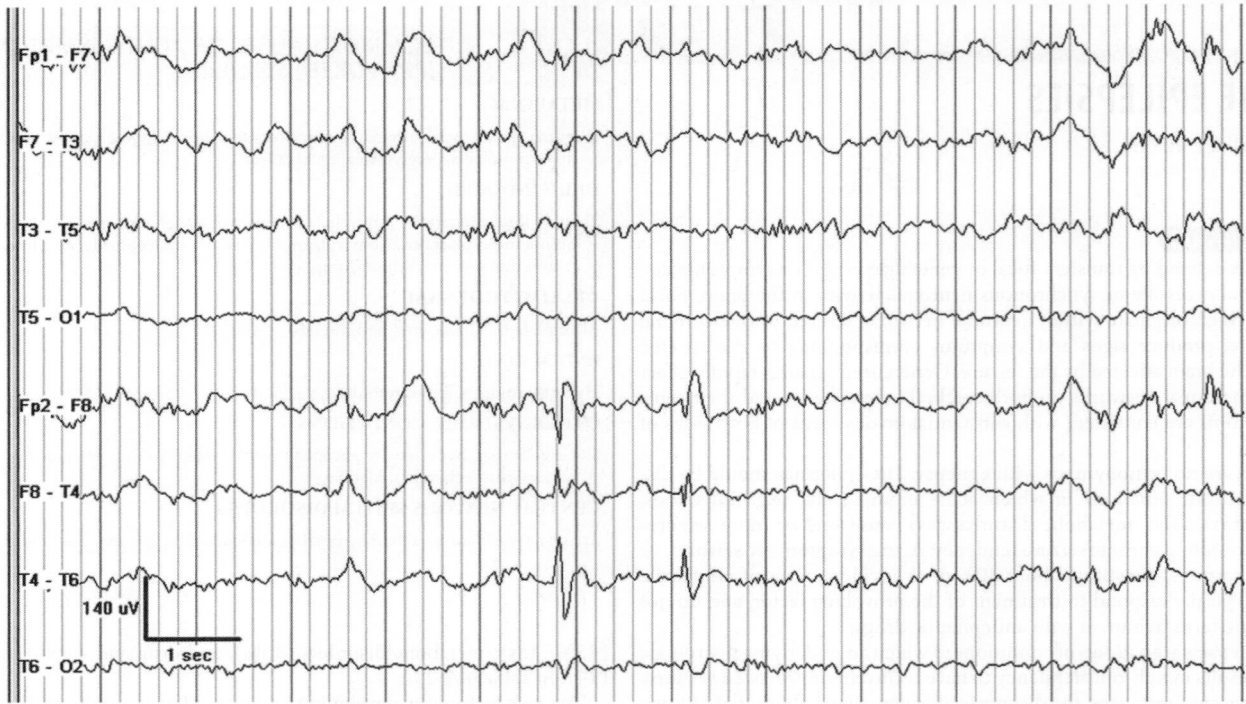

FIGURE 403-1. Selected electroencephalogram channels showing a typical right anterior temporal spike, the archetypal interictal footprint of temporal lobe epilepsy. The patient had right hippocampal sclerosis.

repolarization during the clonic phase. Activation of NMDA receptors increases calcium Ca^{2+} influx, thereby leading to further neuronal excitation. The initiation and modulation of generalized convulsive seizures involve cholinergic, noradrenergic, serotonergic, and histaminergic afferents from the brain stem and basal forebrain structures, which modulate excitability of hemispheric motor mechanisms.

Genetics

Only 15% of patients have one or more first-degree relatives who also suffer from epilepsy, and of those, about 75% have just one affected relative. However, the risk is still higher in first-degree relatives of patients with epilepsy than in the general population. In a large population-based study, the cumulative incidence of epilepsy to age 20 years was 2.5-fold higher in siblings and 3.4-fold higher in offspring of patients with epilepsy.

The genetics of epilepsy is evolving rapidly and can be categorized into three large groups[5]:

1. Conditions in which epilepsy forms part of a mendelian disorder include over 200 rare conditions that encompass neurocutaneous disorders (Chapter 417), neurodegenerative disorders, inherited malformations of cortical development (Chapter 417), and inherited metabolic disorders. For example, genes have been identified in progressive myoclonic epilepsies (e.g., Unverricht-Lundborg disease, Lafora disease, and the neuronal ceroid lipofuscinosis), X-linked myoclonic epilepsy with mental retardation, and cortical malformation syndromes (e.g., polymicrogyria, pachygyria, periventricular nodular heterotopia).

2. Epilepsies that can be directly explained by single gene mutations are rare and account for only about 1% of all epilepsy cases. Over 30 genes have been identified involving the following 15 epilepsy syndromes: genetic epilepsy with febrile seizures plus, severe myoclonic epilepsy of infancy and related syndromes, benign familial neonatal convulsions, benign familial neonatal-infantile seizures, benign familial infantile seizures, juvenile myoclonic epilepsy, childhood absence epilepsy, West syndrome, early infantile epileptic encephalopathy with suppression burst, malignant migrating partial seizures of infancy, autosomal dominant nocturnal frontal lobe epilepsy, familial infantile myoclonic epilepsy, epilepsy + paroxysmal exercise-induced dyskinesia, familial lateral temporal lobe epilepsy, and familial focal epilepsy with variable foci. Genetic mutations may affect neuronal excitability, neuronal metabolism, synaptic function, or network development. Although most of these gene mutations affect ion channels (SCN1A, SCN1B, SCN2A, KCNQ2, KCNQ 3, KCNT1, KCTD7), other cellular functions affected include neurotransmitter release (STXBP1), neurotransmitter receptors (CHRNA, CHRNB, GABRD, GABRG2, GRIN2A, GRIN2B), synaptic function (SYN1), glucose transport (SLC2A1), glutamate transport (SLC25A22), gene regulation and transcription (ARX), cell adhesion (PCDH19), cell membrane function (PRRT2, TBC1D24, DEPDC5), protein kinase and cell energy function (CDKL5, BCKDK, ATP1A2), and neuronal signaling (EFHC1, LGI1, PLCB1). An increased genetic predisposition for epilepsy is associated with specific genotypes (MTHFR C677T) in patients who develop post-traumatic epilepsy. Transcranial magnetic stimulation shows increased cortical excitability in siblings of patients with epilepsy, even when these epilepsies are acquired.

3. In some patients, the epilepsy is associated with "complex" disease genes. In this large group, which constitutes about 50% of all patients with epilepsy, multiple genes with individually small but additive effects act in combination with environmental factors to produce an increased risk for epilepsy.

CLINICAL MANIFESTATIONS

The clinical expression of seizures varies widely depending on the type of seizure and the areas of the brain involved by the epileptic activity. Accurate identification of the specific types of seizures determines the syndrome and dictates the type of drug the patient should receive.

Focal Seizures

Focal seizures originate within neuronal networks limited to one area of one cerebral hemisphere and produce signs and symptoms corresponding to the function subserved by the area of cerebral cortex engaged by the seizure (Table 403-2). Focal seizures are now subclassified according to their clinical expression; if consciousness or awareness is predominantly impaired, they are referred to as dyscognitive seizures. For example, patients who formerly were classified as having simple partial seizures now are classified as having focal seizures with preserved consciousness.

An aura consists of sensory, autonomic, or psychic symptoms that are experienced at the start of an observable seizure. The aura is a focal seizure itself, and it is often missed because patients and clinicians focus on the more dramatic dyscognitive or convulsive seizure that follows. Careful inquiry about the occurrence of an aura is of crucial importance for three reasons. First, it points to a focal as opposed to a generalized onset, thereby implying an underlying focal structural or functional brain abnormality (e.g., a tumor) that requires further investigation. Second, focal seizures have important implications for therapy and for prognosis (see later). Third, the nature of the

TABLE 403-2 CLINICAL MANIFESTATIONS OF DIFFERENT TYPES OF FOCAL SEIZURES AND AREAS OF THE BRAIN INVOLVED

SEIZURE TYPE	AREAS OF BRAIN INVOLVED	CLINICAL EXPRESSION
Somatosensory	Postcentral rolandic; parietal	Contralateral intermittent or prolonged tingling, numbness, sense of movement, desire to move, heat, cold, electric shock. Sensation may spread to other body segments.
	Parietal	Contralateral agnosia of a limb, phantom limb, distortion of size or position of body part
	Second sensory; supplementary sensory-motor	Ipsilateral or bilateral facial, truncal or limb tingling, numbness, or pain. Often involve lips, tongue, fingertips, feet
Motor	Precentral rolandic	Contralateral regional clonic jerking, usually rhythmic, may spread to other body segments in jacksonian motor march. Often accompanied by sensory symptoms in same area
	Supplementary sensory-motor	Bilateral tonic contraction of limbs causing postural changes, may exhibit classic fencing posture, may have speech arrest or vocalization
	Frontal	Contralateral head and eye version, salivation, speech arrest or vocalization; may be combined with other motor signs (as above) depending on seizure spread
Auditory	Heschl gyrus—auditory cortex in superior temporal lobe	Bilateral or contralateral buzzing, drumming, single tones, muffled sounds
Olfactory	Orbitofrontal; mesial temporal cortex	Often described as unpleasant odor
Gustatory	Parietal; rolandic operculum; insula; temporal lobe	Often unpleasant taste, acidic, metallic, salty, sweet, smoky
Vertiginous	Occipitotemporal-parietal junction; frontal lobe	Sensation of body displacement in various directions
Visual	Occipital	Contralateral static, moving, or flashing colored or uncolored lights, shapes, or spots. Contralateral or bilateral, partial or complete loss of vision.
	Temporal; occipitotemporal-parietal junction	Formed visual scenes, faces, people, objects, animals
Limbic	Limbic structures: amygdala, hippocampus, cingulum, olfactory cortex, hypothalamus	Autonomic: abdominal rising sensation, nausea, borborygmi, flushing, pallor, piloerection, perspiration, heart rate changes, chest pain, shortness of breath, cephalic sensation, lightheadedness, genital sensation, orgasm Psychic: déjà vu, jamais vu, depersonalization, derealization, dreamlike state, forced memory or forced thinking, fear, elation, sadness, sexual pleasure, hallucinations or illusions of visual, auditory, or olfactory nature
Dyscognitive	Usually bilateral involvement of limbic structures (see above)	Previously known as "complex partial seizures", characterized by a predominant alteration of consciousness or awareness. The current definition requires involvement of at least two of five components of cognition: perception, attention, emotion, memory, and executive function.

NOTE: Focal seizures may evolve into bilateral convulsive seizures.

TABLE 403-3 GENERALIZED SEIZURES: CLASSIFICATION AND CLINICAL EXPRESSION

SEIZURE TYPE	SUBTYPE	CLINICAL EXPRESSION
Absence	Typical	Abrupt cessation of activities, motionless, blank stare and loss of awareness lasting about 10 seconds. Attack ends suddenly, and patient resumes normal activities immediately.
	Atypical	Longer duration than typical absence, often accompanied by myoclonic, tonic, atonic, and autonomic features as well as automatisms
	With myoclonus	Absence with myoclonic components of variable intensity
Myoclonic	Myoclonic	Sudden, brief (<100 msec), shock-like, involuntary, single or multiple contractions of muscle groups of various locations
	Myoclonic atonic	A sequence consisting of a myoclonic followed by an atonic phase
	Myoclonic tonic	A sequence consisting of a myoclonic followed by a tonic phase
Tonic		Sustained increase in muscle contraction lasting a few seconds to minutes
Clonic		Prolonged regularly repetitive contractions involving the same muscle groups at a rate of 2-3 cycles per second
Atonic		Sudden loss or diminution of muscle tone lasting 1-2 seconds, involving head, trunk, jaw or limb musculature
Tonic-clonic		A sequence consisting of a tonic followed by a clonic phase

symptoms points to the area of the brain that gives rise to the seizure and that could be a target for surgical treatment.

The neuronal discharge causing the focal seizure may remain confined to the region where it began (as an aura or more objective focal event), or it may spread to involve additional brain areas. Thus, a focal seizure originating in the cortical area that represents sensation of the hand (rolandic area) may begin with contralateral hand tingling and then progress to involve additional cortical regions ipsilaterally, producing more extensive sensory symptoms as well as clonic motor signs. Seizures of rolandic origin in particular exhibit a peculiar type of propagation, in which the seizure activity "marches" from hand to arm to leg area ipsilaterally, a process referred to as a jacksonian march. After the clonic motor activity ends, patients are often weak; a post-ictal or Todd paralysis may last hours or even a day or 2, with gradual resolution. The seizure may also propagate to distant ipsilateral or contralateral regions along known anatomic pathways.

In dyscognitive seizures, seizure propagation sufficiently involves limbic and bilateral structures to cause alteration of consciousness. Focal seizures originating from any region can become dyscognitive seizures, and unilateral focal seizures can progress to involve bilateral brain areas and cause a convulsive seizure. Such convulsive seizures usually take the form of generalized

tonic-clonic events rather than another type of generalized seizure (Table 403-3).

The evolution of the focal clinical seizure reflects the evolution of the EEG changes, which in turn reflects the pathophysiology of the process. A simultaneous rhythmic, localized discharge (often in the 4- to 7-Hz range) becomes higher in amplitude and lower in frequency as the seizure continues. Some seizures that begin in the association cortex (e.g., frontal or parietal lobes) have bizarre or extremely brief clinical manifestations without postictal deficits and create diagnostic challenges. The stereotyped nature of the clinical events, with identification of EEG changes if present, may be the only way to make an appropriate diagnosis. The diagnosis can be even more challenging if the seizure spreads to different cortical regions during different seizure episodes, thereby producing variable constellations of clinical findings at different times.

Focal seizures with or without dyscognitive features can also occur as a series of single events without intervening normal behavior, thereby resulting in focal status epilepticus. Focal status epilepticus with dyscognitive seizures is characterized by prolonged confused behavior. EEG findings may be normal in a focal seizure without altered awareness, even in patients with status epilepticus, but the diagnosis is usually evident from the clinical

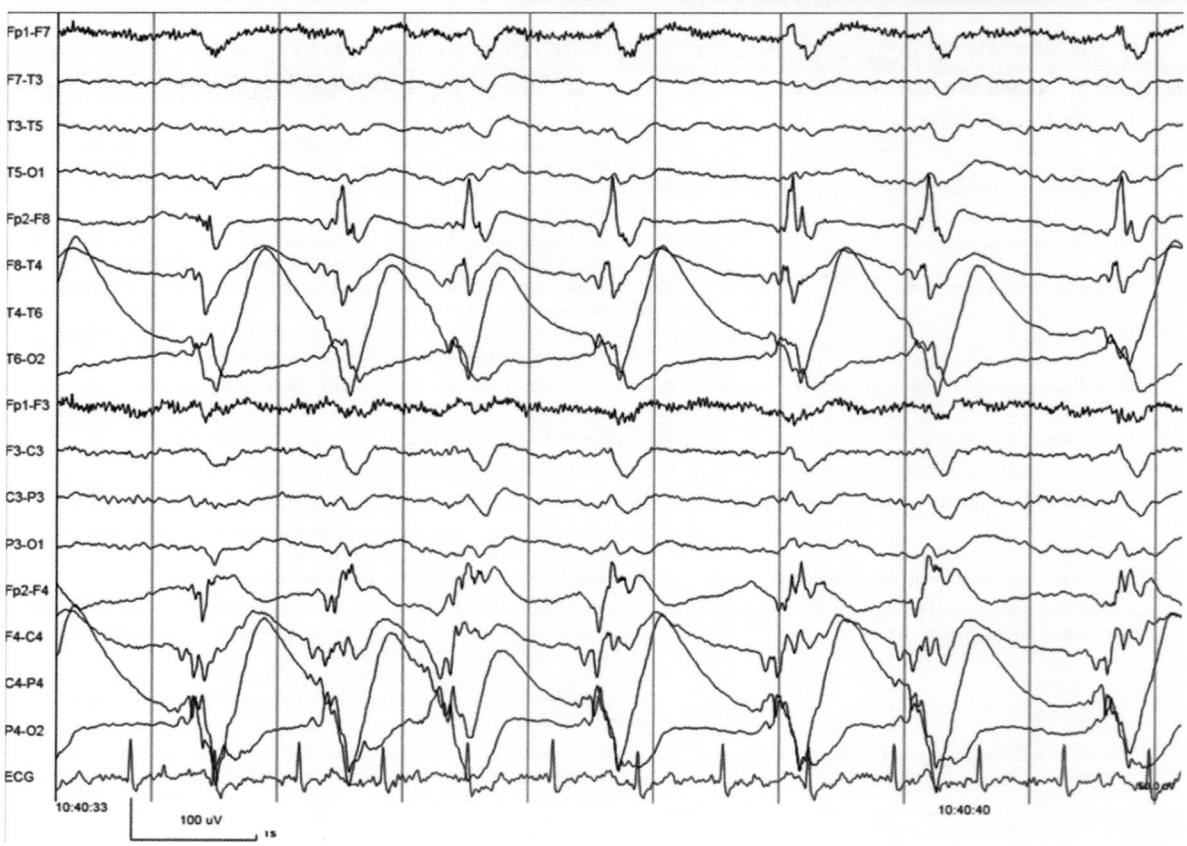

FIGURE 403-2. Focal right hemisphere nonconvulsive status epilepticus in a comatose patient with a large right hemisphere infarct.

features. In status epilepticus of focal dyscognitive seizures, EEG recordings show continuous abnormalities that are not of the same nature as seen in single seizures in that individual. The most common are a slow background with superimposed rhythmic high-amplitude sharp waves or repetitive rhythmic seizure discharges (Fig. 403-2). This type of status epilepticus is most frequent with frontal lobe seizures but can occur in temporal lobe seizures as well. The factors that precipitate status epilepticus are not well defined, nor are the implications for treatment or prognosis.

Nonconvulsive status epilepticus consists of a state of confusion or impaired mental status in patients with various neurologic diagnoses (i.e., trauma, stroke) in the acute intensive care unit setting. It also denotes a condition that can occur de novo in older adults without a precipitating cause and that is characterized by prolonged confusional episodes, which are caused by generalized slow spike-and-wave status epilepticus. Clinical suspicion should prompt an EEG study, which is essential for diagnosis.

Generalized Seizures

Generalized seizures rapidly affect both cerebral hemispheres, and their clinical expression is consistent with substantial involvement of both sides of the brain (see Table 403-3). Convulsive seizures, which are also referred to as grand mal seizures, consist of excessive abnormal muscle contractions that may be sustained or interrupted and usually are a combination of tonic and clonic phases (generalized tonic-clonic seizures). This type of seizure may involve both hemispheres at the onset or may result from propagation of a focal seizure. These dramatic seizures often frighten witnesses and cause severe disruption of social interaction and development. They may begin with a "cry" as a result of abrupt air movement across the glottis from sudden tonic muscle contraction. The patient becomes diffusely stiff, usually with limb and body extension. Breathing is suspended, cyanosis occurs, and urinary incontinence is common. After 15 to 45 seconds, the tonic activity gives way to clonic, rhythmic, sometimes asymmetrical jerking of all four extremities. The rhythmic contractions gradually become slower in frequency until the event stops; the patient is apneic, comatose, and diaphoretic, but breathing with stridor and gasping begins within 60 seconds. Patients who have generalized tonic-clonic seizures in public often prompt bystanders to initiate resuscitation efforts, although such patients begin spontaneous

respiration within 1 minute or so. Postictal stupor persists for a variable length of time. The patient generally sleeps for 2 to 8 hours and then complains of severe headache, sore muscles, a bitten tongue, and the inability to concentrate for a day or more. After generalized tonic-clonic seizures, some individuals have severe memory loss that gradually improves, sometimes over a period of weeks. Generalized tonic-clonic seizures also are a common expression of many metabolic, toxic, traumatic, or ischemic insults (see Table 403-1), but these provoked seizures do not qualify for the diagnosis of epilepsy.

Absence seizures, or petit mal seizures, are the second most common type of generalized seizure. Patients experience an abrupt onset and termination of a momentary lapse of awareness. Patients have no perception of any aspect of the event and may or may not realize that some time was lost, although individuals often lose their train of thought. Because consciousness is abruptly lost and immediately regained, there is neither an aura nor residual postictal symptoms. These seizures begin in childhood, and school teachers are often the first to notice them. In absence seizures, patients stop abruptly, stare vacantly, may have brief eye blinking or myoclonic movements (see Table 403-3), particularly if the event extends beyond 10 seconds (as judged by EEG), and regain function instantly. These seizures can occur many times a day but are not associated with progressive neurologic disease. They can also occur in a more continuous form as nonconvulsive status epilepticus with resultant confusion.

Some patients with extensive bilateral brain disease have a variation of absence seizures known as atypical absence. The event is similar in terms of loss of contact, but there is more motor, autonomic, or automatic activity, and the EEG demonstrates discharges that are slower than the 3-Hz spike and wave of typical absence seizures.

Myoclonic seizures consist of brief episodes of sudden motor contraction (see Table 403-3) that can be focal, with one arm involved, or bilateral and massive, with involvement of the face, both upper extremities, and the trunk. Consciousness is preserved but can be difficult to evaluate because of the brevity of these seizures. Myoclonic seizures form part of three main clinical constellations: juvenile myoclonic epilepsy, which starts in childhood or adolescence and often persists into adulthood; epilepsy with various combinations of absence and myoclonic seizures; and epilepsy in

TABLE 403-4 DISORDERS RESEMBLING SEIZURES

VASCULAR AND PERFUSION DISORDERS

Migraine, syncope, transient ischemic attack, transient global amnesia, arrhythmia/hypoperfusion

PSYCHIATRIC DISORDERS

Psychogenic nonepileptic seizures, panic disorder, dissociative disorder

MOVEMENT DISORDERS

Tics, paroxysmal dystonia, paroxysmal choreoathetosis, paroxysmal ataxia

SLEEP DISORDERS

Night terrors, sleep walking, sleep myoclonus, narcolepsy/cataplexy, rapid eye movement sleep intrusions

METABOLIC DISTURBANCES

Alcoholic blackouts, delirium tremens, hypoglycemia, hallucinogenic drugs

OTHER

Breath-holding spells, paroxysmal vertigo, migraine with recurrent abdominal pain and cyclic vomiting

TABLE 403-5 CLINICAL FEATURES THAT HELP DISTINGUISH A GENERALIZED TONIC CLONIC SEIZURE FROM SYNCOPE

	SEIZURE	SYNCOPE
Clinical context and circumstances	Neurologic or systemic conditions that predispose to seizures, family history of seizures. Mental fatigue, sleep deprivation, alcohol use or withdrawal, systemic illness	Cardiovascular disorders, dehydration, anemia. Family history of syncope
Triggers	Usually none (unless reflex epilepsy)	Orthostatic hypotension, venipuncture, painful and noxious stimuli, emotional stress, micturition, Valsalva maneuver
Clinical features		
Onset	No warning unless there is an aura. Abrupt loss of consciousness, generalized stiffening, and fall. Occurs in any position.	Tiredness, nausea, diaphoresis, tunneling of vision. Loss of consciousness over few seconds and fall. Occurs usually standing.
Course	Prominent tonic phase then clonic movements lasting about 1 minute, cyanosis, labored breathing, may bite tongue or cheeks, sometimes urinary incontinence	Usually loss of tone, pallor, multifocal myoclonic jerks lasting < 15 seconds, sometimes urinary incontinence, usually no tongue or cheek biting
Offset	Postictal sleepiness and confusion lasting up to hours, headache, myalgia	Rapid recovery over seconds to less than few minutes, no confusion, headache or myalgia. May have fatigue.

the setting of degenerative or inherited syndromes with bilateral cerebral involvement and abnormal cerebral function. Myoclonic seizures most commonly occur in the morning after awakening and often increase in frequency to culminate in a generalized tonic-clonic seizure.

Atonic and tonic seizures are brief but extremely disabling motor events that are characterized by a sudden increase or decrease in muscle tone. The result is falls and injuries with variable impairment of awareness. Such seizures frequently begin in children with diffuse central nervous system (CNS) disease and multiple types of seizures, but they persist during adulthood.

DIAGNOSIS

The basic diagnosis of seizures is established by the clinical history. Although EEG, imaging, and laboratory studies are commonly required to determine the type of epilepsy, epilepsy syndrome, site of origin of focal seizures, and occurrence of nonepileptic seizures, the answer to the basic question of whether the patient's episodes are seizures or not rests almost entirely on a careful clinical history. The diagnosis of epilepsy can also be established by history, because epilepsy is defined as the occurrence of two unprovoked seizures or one unprovoked seizure in the context of a high underlying risk of recurrence or an epileptic syndrome.

Differential Diagnosis

The first question facing clinicians is whether the episodes under consideration are indeed seizures. The diverse clinical expression of seizures entails a large differential diagnosis among conditions that produce episodic neurologic dysfunction (Table 403-4). Common conditions resembling seizures include syncope (Chapters 51 and 62), transient ischemic attacks (Chapter 407), migraine (Chapter 398), movement disorders (Chapter 410), and psychogenic nonepileptic seizures (see Table 403-4).

A number of historical elements dramatically change the likelihood of this diagnosis. Three essential elements help determine whether an episode is a seizure (Table 403-5) and distinguish seizures from other causes of temporary loss of consciousness, especially syncope (Chapters 51 and 62):

1. The clinical context, including medical and family history and circumstances under which the episode occurred
2. Specific triggers or provoking factors
3. A detailed clinical description of the event, including four key components:
   - What is the first symptom or sign (presence and type of aura, evidence of focal seizure at onset)?
   - How does it evolve after onset (what happens during the seizure proper, what are the signs or symptoms, how long does it last)?
   - How does it end (gradually or abruptly)?
   - Are there any neurologic deficits after the seizure ends?

Because patients have limited or no recall, the history from others is crucial. Observers can contribute important information about the patient's activity, responses, and appearance, including changes in color, diaphoresis, respirations, vocalization, and muscle tone. This information is often essential to characterize the type of seizure and to distinguish seizures from conditions that resemble seizures.

Migraine (Chapter 398) and focal seizures not only resemble each other but also coexist as comorbid conditions and share genetic susceptibility loci. Features that favor a diagnosis of seizures over classic migraine include an inconsistent occurrence of headache during the event, a brief duration, and the occurrence of more severe seizures. Myoclonus (Chapter 410) occurs in a variety of settings (e.g., metabolic encephalopathies) without any association with epilepsy or the EEG changes seen in myoclonic epilepsy.

Frontal lobe seizures arise predominantly during sleep and can have dramatic motor expression. They can be confused with nonepileptic psychogenic seizures, sleep disorders (Chapter 405), or movement disorders (Chapters 409 and 410). Video EEG monitoring may be necessary for diagnosis.

Patients with panic attacks (Chapter 397) can experience events that mimic focal seizures with autonomic and psychic features. However, panic attacks usually have a longer duration, do not progress to more severe seizures, and can be linked to specific circumstances. Nevertheless, focal seizures with limbic symptoms are often misdiagnosed as panic attacks.

Psychogenic nonepileptic seizures are behaviors that resemble seizures and are often part of a conversion reaction (Chapter 397) precipitated by underlying psychological distress. Psychogenic seizures can be difficult to diagnose because they can mimic almost any type of seizure, and they often coexist with epilepsy in the same patient. An erroneous diagnosis of nonepileptic seizures poses a risk for inappropriate discontinuation of medication, with resulting status epilepticus. Conversely, an erroneous diagnosis of seizures can result in iatrogenic illness owing to unnecessary therapy, excessive sedation, and cardiorespiratory depression. Features suggesting nonepileptic seizures include variable clinical manifestations across episodes, frequent and prolonged episodes, lack of response to antiseizure medication, out-of-phase upper and lower body movements, prominent pelvic thrusting, and lack of rigidity. Secondary gain is usually evident, and there is often a history of sexual abuse. Nevertheless, the peculiarities of these attacks may require continuous video EEG monitoring for diagnosis.

Diagnostic Investigations

A detailed history, EEG recordings, and magnetic resonance imaging (MRI) can lead to a definitive diagnosis of epilepsy and its cause in up to 50% of patients. In other patients, the information is insufficient or inconsistent, but the physiologic and CNS abnormalities surrounding the actual event allow it to be placed provisionally into a specific diagnostic category in about another 30% of patients. Continuous video EEG monitoring in an inpatient epilepsy unit can increase diagnostic sensitivity and specificity.

Single Seizures

Acute symptomatic seizures (see Table 403-1) are the known consequence of an acute condition, and investigations should be directed at the possible cause of these seizures. When no known cause is readily apparent, the seizures are considered to be unprovoked. Evaluation of patients who present with a first unprovoked seizure includes either brain computed tomography (CT) or MRI, which reveals a possible cause in about 10% of patients. An EEG obtained after the seizure will demonstrate abnormalities with prognostic significance in 20 to 25% of these patients. Blood tests (including levels of serum electrolytes, glucose, calcium, and magnesium; tests of liver and kidney function; a complete blood cell count; and screening for suspected toxins) will reveal abnormalities in up to 15% of these patients but are often nonspecific. Lumbar puncture is indicated if CNS infections are suspected and in all patients infected with human immunodeficiency virus (HIV), even in the absence of clinical findings suggestive of infection.

Epilepsy
Electroencephalogram

The EEG is the keystone investigation in all patients with seizures and epilepsy. Between seizures, the EEG can assess overall brain function and the type, location, and amount of epileptiform (spike) discharges. The EEG is crucial in determining the epilepsy syndrome and choosing appropriate antiepileptic drugs. In focal epilepsies, the EEG often demonstrates focal slowing and spike discharges in the area of abnormality.

The EEG can establish the definitive diagnosis of epilepsy if electrical changes consistent with a seizure are recorded during a clinical seizure. However, the EEG may fail to demonstrate electrical changes during a typical clinical seizure if the seizure focus is too small (at least 6 cm^2 of cortical involvement is needed to create an EEG epileptiform change), if the seizure focus is deep or in the mesial or inferior surfaces of the brain, or if the event in question is not an epileptic seizure. The EEG is always abnormal during generalized convulsive and absence seizures.

The initial EEG is normal in up to 60% of people with known epilepsy. However, epileptiform abnormalities occur in more than 80% of individuals with focal epilepsy if three or more interictal EEG studies are performed. In generalized epilepsies, interictal epileptiform discharges are more common and are easier to capture in the EEG.

The type of abnormality points to the epileptic syndrome. For example, the EEG can show hypsarrhythmia in West syndrome (see later) or the classic 3-Hz generalized spike wave in generalized epilepsies with absence seizures (see Table 403-3).

In some circumstances, it is imperative to record seizures, such as in the evaluation of patients for epilepsy surgery and when the diagnosis of seizures is in question. Continuous video EEG monitoring for prolonged periods has made it possible to capture these events. Continuous EEG is also used in comatose patients in the intensive care unit setting when nonconvulsive seizure or status epilepticus is suspected.

Magnetoencephalography

Magnetoencephalography measures the small magnetic fields that are generated by electrical activity in the brain and approximates their location using mathematical models. Its use is largely restricted to the evaluation of patients for epilepsy surgery, in whom it is used for mapping interictal discharges and the localization of brain function when superimposed on brain MRI.

Imaging Studies

Brain MRI, which can demonstrate lesions in most patients whose epilepsy is associated with a structural cause, should be performed in essentially all patients with new-onset seizures. The most common lesions in adults with new-onset focal seizures are post-stroke or post-traumatic gliosis or encephalomalacia (50%), tumors (15%), vascular abnormalities (15%), developmental abnormalities (15%), and mesial temporal sclerosis (9%).[6] The use of fluid-attenuated inversion recovery (FLAIR) (Fig. 403-3A) sequences increases the sensitivity to detect abnormalities of cortical development as well as hippocampal sclerosis, which point to the need for chronic anticonvulsant therapy or possible surgical treatment. Functional imaging

procedures such as positron emission tomography (PET) for analysis of metabolism and single-photon emission computed tomography (SPECT) (see Fig. 403-3B) for determination of blood flow are also used to help localize areas of the brain to be targeted with epilepsy surgery.

Genetic Testing

Based on genetic test accuracy, implications for diagnosis and management, and ability to offer genetic counseling, an international consensus panel has identified eight epilepsy syndromes of genetic origin for which genetic testing of patients is most useful: Ohtahara syndrome, early-onset infantile spasms, X-linked infantile spasms, Dravet syndrome, epilepsy and mental retardation limited to females, early-onset absence epilepsy, autosomal dominant nocturnal frontal lobe epilepsy, and epilepsy with paroxysmal exercised-induced dyskinesia. As with other conditions, the ethical aspects and potential harms and benefits of genetic testing must be carefully considered.

Epileptic Syndromes and Constellations

Epileptic syndromes include 27 age-related syndromes, of which all but 6 begin or occur in infancy and childhood (Table 403-6). In addition, specific clinical constellations represent diagnostically meaningful forms of epilepsy, with specific implications for treatment, especially surgery, and also categorize for structural-metabolic causes, epilepsies of unknown cause, and conditions characterized by seizures that are not a form of epilepsy (e.g., febrile seizures). The diagnosis of epileptic syndromes and constellations is based on the types of seizures, the setting in which seizures occur, the patient's neurologic and cognitive status, age at onset, family history, and results of diagnostic studies, including EEG and MRI. The selection of specific drug and surgical treatment depends on the types of seizures present (Table 403-7). The need for lifelong treatment, the risk for genetic transmission, the likelihood of concurrent neurologic diseases, the risk for comorbid conditions, and the long-term prognosis are critical factors that can be addressed only with knowledge of the specific epileptic syndrome or constellation.

Some Specific Seizure Syndromes and Constellations
Neonatal and Infantile Epilepsy Syndromes

Benign neonatal convulsions occur in previously healthy newborns on about day 5 as focal or generalized tonic seizures. Mutations in two potassium channel genes (KCNQ2, KCNQ3) have been associated with this syndrome. Potassium channel regulation may be age dependent and therefore account for the age-related appearance of the seizures. The EEG shows rhythmic slow-wave activity or spiking with seizures. The seizures are refractory to treatment, are recurrent over a brief interval, and disappear within a month. About 90% of such infants subsequently have normal development, whereas 10 to 20% have subsequent seizures.[7]

Genetic epilepsy with febrile seizures plus (GEFS+) is a syndrome that consists of febrile seizures in combination with other nonfebrile types of seizures, including myoclonic, absence, atonic, tonic-clonic, and focal seizures. Mutations in at least three genes for voltage-gated ion sodium channels (SCN1A, SCN1B, SCN2A), two for GABA receptors (GABRD, GABRG2), and one for cell adhesion function (PCDH19) have been identified.

Dravet syndrome (severe myoclonic epilepsy of infancy) starts in the first year of life with myoclonic seizures plus other seizure types, including absence, atonic, and focal. In this devastating syndrome, the seizures are resistant to treatment and are accompanied by developmental and cognitive decline. Mutations in the SCN1A sodium channel have been identified.

West syndrome comprises a triad of epileptic spasms, developmental arrest, and an EEG pattern called hypsarrhythmia (a markedly abnormal EEG pattern with high-amplitude slowing and superimposed multifocal spikes, polyspikes, and spike and slow-wave complexes). It appears before the age of 12 months and ceases by 5 years of age, often to be replaced by other epilepsy syndromes such as Lennox-Gastaut syndrome. Tuberous sclerosis (Chapter 417) and hypoxia are among the common causes, but a cause may not be found. Associated abnormalities often include developmental delay, porencephaly, atrophic lesions, calcifications, and agenesis of the corpus callosum. West syndrome and early infantile epileptic encephalopathy have been associated with mutations in genes involved in a number of neurotransmitter and cellular functions (ARX, CDKL5, STXBP1).

Childhood Epilepsy Syndromes

Childhood absence epilepsy begins before age 12 years, and its onset peaks at age 5 to 7 years, with a strong genetic tendency. It is more common in girls

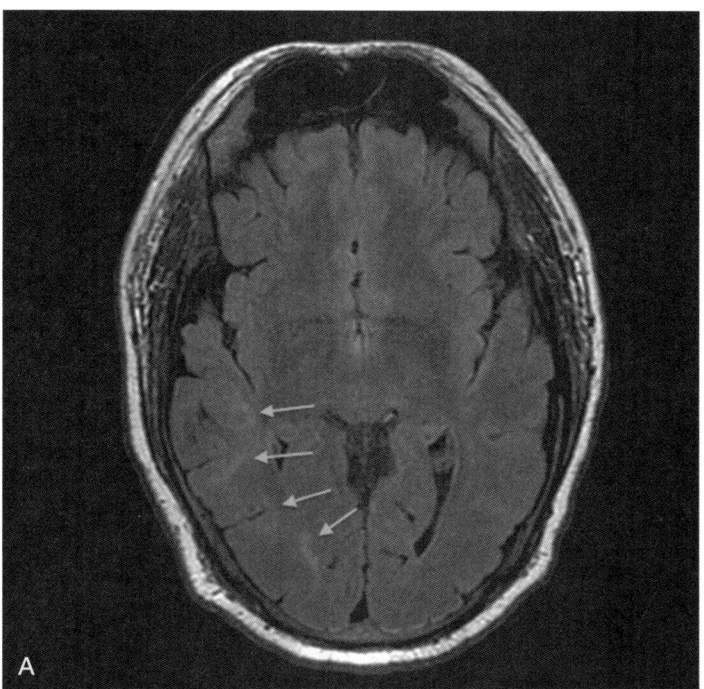

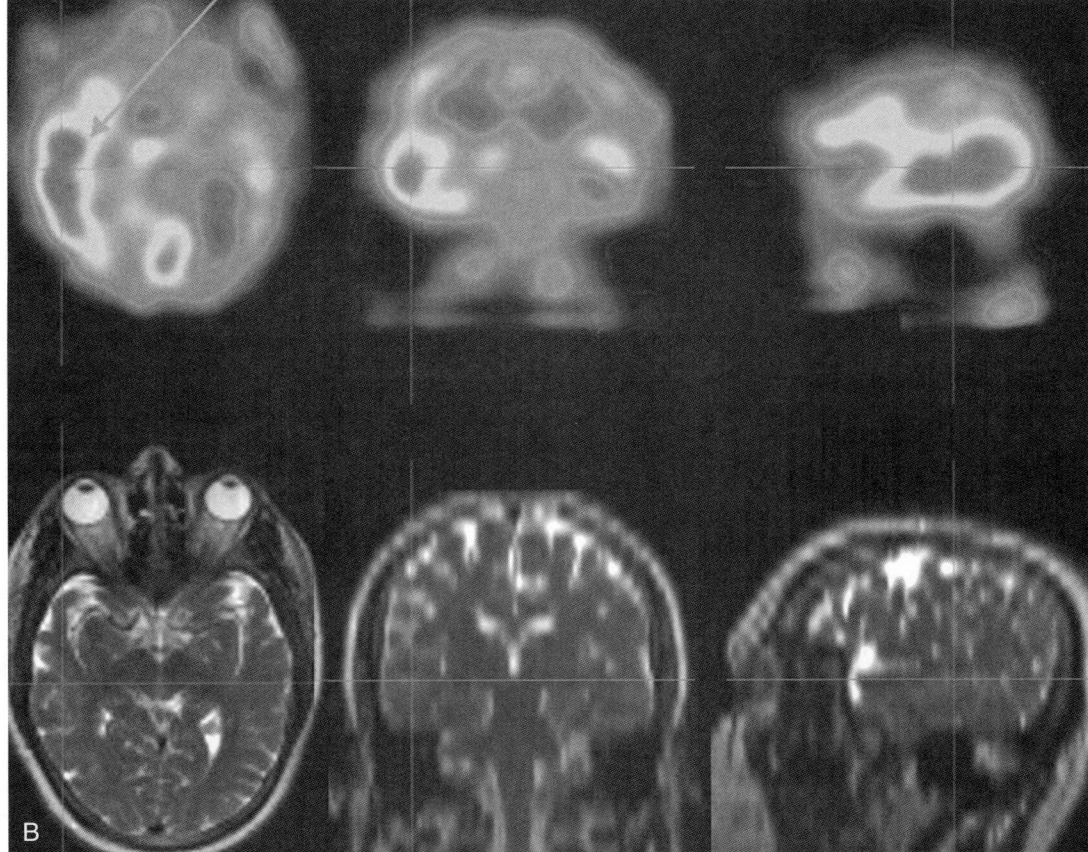

FIGURE 403-3. Imaging studies from a patient with dramatic motor seizures that were initially attributed incorrectly to psychogenic nonepileptic events. **A,** Fluid-attenuated inversion recovery (FLAIR) axial magnetic resonance image (MRI) demonstrating a large developmental cortical abnormality involving the mid-posterior right temporal lobe. **B,** Ictal SPECT demonstrating an area of hyperperfusion during a seizure that corresponds to the abnormality seen on the MRI and confirms the area of seizure origin.

than boys and is characterized by very frequent daily absence seizures (up to hundreds per day), rarely with other types of generalized seizures. It occurs in the setting of otherwise normal brain structure and function, and it is self-limited in about 40% of cases. The seizures are accompanied by a characteristic 3-Hz spike-and-wave EEG discharge, which appears in short bursts between seizures and in continuous runs during seizures. Remission usually occurs before the age of 12 years, but generalized tonic-clonic seizures occasionally may develop in adolescence. In early-onset absence epilepsy, mutations have been found in genes related to GABA receptors (*GABRA1, GABRG2*) and glucose transport (*SLC2A1*).

TABLE 403-6 EPILEPTIC SYNDROMES AND CONSTELLATIONS ACCORDING TO THE NEW INTERNATIONAL CLASSIFICATION

BY AGE AT ONSET

Neonatal Period
Benign familial neonatal epilepsy
Early myoclonic encephalopathy
Ohtahara syndrome

Infancy
Epilepsy of infancy with migrating partial seizures
West syndrome
Myoclonic epilepsy in infancy
Benign infantile epilepsy
Benign familial infantile epilepsy
Dravet syndrome
Myoclonic encephalopathy in nonprogressive disorders

Childhood
Febrile seizures plus (can start in infancy)
Panayiotopoulos syndrome
Epilepsy with myoclonic atonic (previously astatic) seizures
Benign epilepsy with centrotemporal spikes
Autosomal dominant nocturnal frontal lobe epilepsy
Late-onset childhood occipital epilepsy
Epilepsy with myoclonic absences
Lennox-Gastaut syndrome
Epileptic encephalopathy with continuous spike and wave during sleep
Landau-Kleffner syndrome
Childhood absence epilepsy

Adolescence-Adult
Juvenile absence epilepsy
Juvenile myoclonic epilepsy
Epilepsy with generalized tonic-clonic seizures alone
Progressive myoclonus epilepsies
Autosomal dominant partial epilepsy with auditory features
Other familial temporal lobe epilepsies

LESS SPECIFIC AGE RELATIONSHIP

Familial focal epilepsy with variable foci (childhood to adult)
Reflex epilepsies

DISTINCTIVE CONSTELLATIONS

Mesial temporal lobe epilepsy with hippocampal sclerosis
Rasmussen syndrome
Gelastic seizures with hypothalamic hamartoma
Hemiconvulsion-hemiplegia-epilepsy

Lennox-Gastaut syndrome is one of the most severe childhood epilepsies. It starts before age 8 years (peak from 3 to 5 years) and is characterized by a triad of mental retardation, multiple types of generalized seizures (atypical absence, generalized tonic-clonic, tonic, atonic), focal seizures that are highly resistant to treatment, and a typical EEG pattern of slow spike and wave (slower than the typical 3 Hz associated with absence seizures) and bursts of fast rhythms at 10 to 12 Hz during sleep. It often follows the resolution of West syndrome.

Benign epilepsy with centrotemporal spikes (benign rolandic epilepsy) starts between 3 and 13 years of age and is characterized by almost exclusively nocturnal focal motor or sensory seizures that have a facial or oral onset and often evolve to convulsive seizures. Nearly 50% of cases have a family history of epilepsy, but most patients have no known brain abnormality. The EEG shows spiking in the centrotemporal region. In some cases, the disorder may not require treatment because it usually remits spontaneously.

Adolescence and Adult Epilepsy Syndromes and Constellations

Juvenile myoclonic epilepsy usually starts in the second decade with generalized tonic-clonic and myoclonic seizures. Mutations in γ-aminobutyric acid (GABA) receptors (*GABRG1*) and in genes related to neuronal signaling (*EFHC1*) can be found. Seizures typically occur in the morning immediately after awakening. The seizures are especially linked to sleep deprivation and tend to appear in college students. A proportion of these patients have had absence seizures as well. The EEG typically shows fast (4 to 6 Hz) generalized spike and wave. Lifetime treatment is generally needed.

Mesial temporal lobe epilepsy with hippocampal sclerosis is the most common epilepsy to produce focal dyscognitive seizures in adults. It is characterized by recurrent focal limbic seizures (see Table 403-2), with and without impaired awareness, that originate in mesial temporal and limbic structures. Up to 70% of patients have a risk factor such as lengthy and complicated seizures before the age of 4 years, frequently associated with fever or encephalitis, meningitis, or trauma. However, the characteristic seizures generally begin some years later. Although most cases are sporadic, familial forms of mesial temporal lobe epilepsy have been associated with a novel susceptibility locus on chromosome 18(P11.31).

Various components of the mesial temporal limbic network (including the hippocampus, entorhinal cortex, amygdala, neocortical areas of the frontal and temporal lobes, and dorsal medial thalamus) are probably involved in the pathogenesis of these seizures. Mesial temporal sclerosis, also called hippocampal sclerosis, is characterized by neuronal loss and gliosis, mostly in the CA1 and CA3 regions of the hippocampus, with mossy fiber reorganization that is seen as sprouting of neuropeptide Y and dynorphin interneurons into the inner third of the dentate molecular layer. Whether hippocampal sclerosis is the cause or the result of seizures (or both) is not known. However, up to 12% of children with febrile status epilepticus have MR evidence of hippocampal injury, thereby suggesting a causal association.[8] The seizures of mesial temporal lobe epilepsy often begin at 5 to 15 years of age. Seizures are typically dyscognitive with limbic symptoms; they begin with an aura of a rising epigastric sensation or a feeling of déjà vu, followed by oral and alimentary automatisms and later by contralateral arm dystonia and ipsilateral arm automatisms. The seizures are lengthy (lasting several minutes), rarely generalize, and typically occur three to five times a month. Auras without subsequent seizures are common. Hippocampal atrophy and increased hippocampal signal are best seen on T2-weighted and FLAIR coronal MRI sequences, and widespread interictal hypometabolism is seen in the temporal lobe on PET. Material-specific (verbal or visual) memory impairment corresponds to primary involvement of the dominant or nondominant hippocampus. EEG recordings show temporal lobe spikes interictally as well as rhythmic 4- to 7-Hz discharges over the appropriate temporal lobe during seizures.

Seizures with Less Specific Age Relationship

Reflex seizures are triggered reliably by specific simple (e.g., flashing lights, sound) or elaborate (e.g., reading) stimuli. The mechanisms are diverse and may involve cortical and brain stem pathways, cortical dysregulation of extracellular calcium concentrations, and an imbalance between excitatory and inhibitory neurotransmitters. Visual-sensitive seizures (triggered by light or visual patterns) are the most common type of reflex seizures. They occur most commonly in females, and their incidence peaks around puberty, when they represent up to 10% of all new cases of epilepsy. Other triggers of reflex seizures include specific thoughts, actions, reading, tactile stimuli, adopting certain positions, eating, listening to music, startle, and contact with hot water. The triggered seizures can be myoclonic, convulsive, atonic, or focal, depending on the triggering stimulus. Avoiding the offending stimulus is crucial to avoid seizures, emphasizing the importance of careful questioning about seizure triggers in patients with epilepsy.

TREATMENT   Rx

The treatment of seizures and epilepsy is guided by accurate knowledge of the type of seizure and epileptic syndrome, the probability of recurrent seizures, the likelihood and severity of psychosocial or physical consequences with further seizures, and whether the benefit from treatment substantially outweighs the risks for side effects. It is important to identify and correct any environmental, physiologic, or lifestyle factors, such as sleep deprivation and irregular sleep habits, and alcohol abuse, which can lower the seizure threshold and trigger seizures in patients with epilepsy.

Single Unprovoked Seizures

The decision to treat single unprovoked seizures depends on the likelihood of recurrence according to prognostic variables (see Prognosis) and on the individual patient's profile and preference. A meta-analysis demonstrated that antiepileptic drug treatment after a first seizure reduces the absolute risk of having a second seizure in the short term by 33%, corresponding to a number needed to treat (NNT) of 3. However, at least two randomized trials have shown that treatment of the first seizure with antiepileptic drugs does not prevent the development of epilepsy in the long term.[A1] Therefore, the decision to treat the first seizure should be individualized based on the patient's

TABLE 403-7 ANTIEPILEPTIC DRUG SELECTION BY SEIZURE TYPE

SEIZURE TYPE	COMMONLY USED (ALPHABETICAL ORDER)	LESS COMMONLY USED (ALPHABETICAL ORDER)	EFFECTIVENESS (GRADE A RECOMMENDATION)	
			NEW-ONSET SEIZURES	REFRACTORY SEIZURES
Focal seizures with or without dyscognitive features or evolution to convulsions	Carbamazepine (CBZ) Gabapentin (GBP) Lamotrigine (LTG) Levetiracetam (LEV) Oxcarbazepine (OXC) Phenytoin (PHT) Tiagabine (TIAG) Topiramate (TPM) Valproate (VPA) Zonisamide (ZNS) Lacosamide (LAC)	Acetazolamide (ACZ) Clonazepam (CLN) Clorazepate (CLZ) Phenobarbital (PB) Primidone (PRM) Felbamate (FBM)	CBZ*§ GBP*§ LEV§ LTG*§ OXC*§ PB* PHT*§ TPM* VPA* ZNS§	CBZ† GBP* LAM* LEV* OXC* PB† PHT† TIAG* TPM* VPA† ZNS*
Generalized convulsive seizures (clonic, tonic or tonic-clonic seizures)	Carbamazepine Lamotrigine Levetiracetam Oxcarbazepine Phenytoin Topiramate Valproate Zonisamide	Acetazolamide Clonazepam Clorazepate Felbamate Phenobarbital Primidone	CBZ† LEV* LTG* PHT† VPA*	CBZ† LAM* LEV* PHT† TPM* VPA*
Absence seizures	Ethosuximide (ESM) Lamotrigine Valproate Topiramate	Acetazolamide Clonazepam Phenobarbital Primidone	ESM*§ LTG* VPA*§	
Myoclonic seizures	Clonazepam Levetiracetam Valproate Zonisamide	Phenobarbital	VPA†	

*Supported by class I evidence, American Academy of Neurology.
§Supported by class I evidence for initial monotherapy, International League Against Epilepsy.
†Often the "standard" of comparison, without evidence of effectiveness by randomized controlled trials.

preference, the risk for and impact of recurrent seizures (e.g., driving and employment), and the risk for medication side effects.

Acute Symptomatic (Provoked) Seizures

Seizures that are provoked by specific exposures are usually self-limited and not associated with an enduring seizure tendency, so the primary therapeutic consideration should be identification and treatment of the underlying disorder (see Table 403-1). However, the risk of developing epilepsy after febrile seizures is about 10 times that of the general population. If antiepileptic drugs are needed to treat seizures acutely, they usually can be discontinued after the patient has recovered from the primary illness. Some acute conditions like stroke (Chapter 407), brain infections (Chapters 412 to 414), and trauma (Chapter 399) can produce both acute symptomatic seizures and an enduring seizure tendency, so it would seem logical to use long-term antiepileptic drug treatment. To date, however, randomized controlled trials have not been able to demonstrate that antiepileptic drugs prevent the development of epilepsy in these conditions, so long-term therapy is not recommended unless epilepsy develops.

Epilepsy Syndromes with a Favorable Course

In syndromes such as benign epilepsy of childhood with centrotemporal spikes and some types of childhood occipital epilepsy, seizures are mild, infrequent, or exclusively nocturnal, and they remit spontaneously, thereby making treatment generally unnecessary. In selected cases, treatment may be desirable to prevent recurrences and to help alleviate parental concerns. In such cases, drug treatment is usually limited to 1 to 2 years regardless of interictal EEG abnormalities, which can persist long after seizures have remitted. The recommended antiepileptic drugs are those used in focal epilepsy in children, including oxcarbazepine, carbamazepine, valproate, gabapentin, lamotrigine, and topiramate (Table 403-8). Some patients with reflex seizures may require antiseizure medication, which should be chosen according to seizure type (see Table 403-7).

Choice of Antiepileptic Drugs

The ultimate goal of treatment is to obtain complete freedom from seizures without side effects. Some of the newer antiepileptic drugs (see Table 403-8) are better tolerated and have better pharmacokinetics than older drugs, but there is no robust evidence to support superior efficacy of one drug over another. The choice of medication depends on the type of seizure and epilepsy syndrome (thereby making a correct diagnosis crucial) and the medication's side effects, cost, and ease of use. Specific drugs are effective for specific types of seizures, and some drugs can worsen other types of seizures. Knowledge of individual drugs as they relate to age, sex, comorbid conditions, drug interactions, sedation, tolerance, mood, and withdrawal is critical in the drug selection process (see Table 403-7). For example, ethosuximide and valproic acid are more effective than lamotrigine for the treatment of childhood absence epilepsy.

Drugs that cause enzyme induction (e.g., carbamazepine, phenytoin, phenobarbital, oxcarbazepine, topiramate) or inhibition (e.g., valproic acid) can be difficult to manage when additional medications, such as oral contraceptives, are used for independent conditions. For these clinical settings and in elderly patients, gabapentin and levetiracetam are particularly useful because they have no appreciable drug interactions.

In patients with newly diagnosed focal epilepsy, the underlying cause influences the response to antiepileptic drugs. The likelihood of achieving seizure freedom is higher for patients with vascular malformations, stroke, and tumors (63 to 78%), and lower for patients with hippocampal sclerosis and malformations of cortical development (40 to 50%). Among patients presenting with a new diagnosis of epilepsy, about 65% achieve seizure remission on antiepileptic drug treatment. Of these patients, about 45 to 50% achieve seizure remission with the first antiepileptic drug, 10 to 15% with the second, 1% with the third, and 3% with a combination of two or more antiepileptic drugs. Because the likelihood of achieving subsequent seizure remission is small if two drug trials fail, the 35% or so of patients who fail adequate trials of two antiepileptic drugs are considered to be drug resistant. In these patients, other forms of treatment, including surgery, should be considered. The first consideration in managing apparently drug-resistant patients is to ensure that the diagnosis is correct and the antiepileptic drug is appropriate. Other common causes of a poor response to drugs include poor adherence to antiepileptic drugs, sleep deprivation, alcohol use, fatigue, emotional stress, systemic illnesses, use of concurrent medications, and nonepileptic seizures. After addressing these factors, patients who remain drug resistant should be considered potential candidates for surgical therapy.[9]

Surgical Treatment

Surgical treatment entails resection or disconnection of the cerebral region that contains the seizure focus. Removal of an epileptogenic region requires accurate identification of the region as well as documentation of a lack of functional consequences after its removal. Video EEG monitoring with seizure recording from scalp electrodes, MRI protocols with special attention to areas

TABLE 403-8 CHARACTERISTICS OF MAJOR ANTIEPILEPTIC DRUGS

NAME	TOTAL MILLIGRAMS PER DAY (USUAL SCHEDULE)	THERAPEUTIC RANGE (µg/mL)	PROMINENT SIDE EFFECTS	OTHER EFFECTS	OTHER ISSUES
Carbamazepine	400-1600 (bid)	4-12	Diplopia, fatigue, hyponatremia	Mood stabilizer	Enzyme inducer
Ethosuximide	750-1250 (daily, bid)	40-100	Ataxia, lethargy	Rash, bone marrow suppression	
Gabapentin	600-6000 (tid, qid)	2-12	Fatigue	Treatment of pain	No drug interactions
Lamotrigine	100-600 (bid)	4-18	Insomnia, headache, tremor, anxiety	Mood stabilizer	Risk for Stevens-Johnson syndrome; slow start-up
Lacosamide	200-400 (bid)	Not well established	Dizziness, diplopia, tremor,	Minor prolongation of PR interval	Low risk of drug interaction
Levetiracetam	500-3000 (bid)	3-63	Mood change, irritability, lethargy		No drug interactions
Oxcarbazepine	300-2400 (tid)	6-40	Diplopia, hyponatremia, sedation	Mood stabilizer	
Phenobarbital	60-240 (at bedtime)	15-40	Fatigue, depression, sedation	Joint pain	Enzyme inducer
Phenytoin	200-600 (bid)	10-20	Fatigue, hirsutism, gingival hypertrophy	Treatment of some pain	Enzyme inducer
Topiramate	50-600 (bid)	2-12	Anorexia, weight loss, kidney stones, speech disturbance, distal paresthesias	Headache prophylaxis, mood stabilizer	Enzyme inducer
Valproate	4000 (bid or tid)	50-100	Weight gain, hair loss, tremor	Headache prophylaxis, mood stabilizer	Enzyme inhibitor, parkinsonian effects in elderly patients
Zonisamide	100-600 (at bedtime)	10-40	Anorexia, kidney stones, dizziness, distal paresthesias	Mood stabilizer	

commonly associated with refractory seizures (e.g., the medial temporal and frontal lobes), and functional neuroimaging, including PET and SPECT, are used to make the assessment. In temporal lobe epilepsy, neuropsychological evaluation is essential to localize dysfunction and establish the level of function in the region considered for resection. EEG localization of the region of seizure onset and mapping of brain function may require the surgical implantation of intracranial electrodes for recording and for stimulating cortical tissue. These procedures are performed by multidisciplinary teams in specialized epilepsy centers.

Epilepsy surgery interventions that have been subjected to rigorous randomized trials include temporal lobe resection compared with medical therapy for mesial temporal lobe epilepsy, comparison of different amounts of temporal lobe resection, different intensities of vagus nerve stimulation, and thalamic stimulation compared with medical therapy. The most dramatic surgical effect is seen for temporal lobe resection compared with medical therapy. In one randomized trial, 58% of surgical patients and only 8% of medical patients became seizure free at 1 year. Among these patients, clinically meaningful improvement in quality of life was achieved in 56% of patients treated surgically compared with only 11% of patients treated medically.[A2] In another small randomized trial of patients with drug-resistant temporal lobe epilepsy, surgery plus continued antiepileptic medications was successful in eliminating seizures in 11 of 15 patients at 2 years, whereas all medically treated patients continued to have seizures at 2 years.[A3] As a result, patients with drug-resistant temporal lobe epilepsy should be evaluated for epilepsy surgery. Nonrandomized studies demonstrate enduring freedom from seizures at 10 years or more after hemispheric disconnection (61%), temporal lobe resection (64%), parieto-occipital resection (46%), and frontal lobe resection (27%). Palliative surgical procedures such as callosotomy and multiple subpial transections have lower success rates and are used when surgical resection of the seizure focus is not possible. In the long term, about 65% of patients undergoing surgery achieve sustained seizure freedom (40 to 50% immediately after surgery, and 15% after a period of initial seizures), 16% have a fluctuating course of relapsing-remitting seizures, and 18% never become seizure free.[10,11] Promising surgical therapies for epilepsy include radiosurgery and various types of electrical stimulation of the brain.[12]

Status Epilepticus

Status epilepticus is a medical emergency in which seizures occur continuously or repeatedly without intervening resumption of consciousness for 30 minutes. However, even 5 minutes of generalized tonic-clonic seizures cause hypoxia, lactic acidosis, muscle breakdown, and neuronal damage. Most episodes of status epilepticus are caused by an acute brain insult in persons without underlying epilepsy, so a cause should be sought promptly. After securing the airway and stabilizing cardiovascular function, immediate intervention with parenteral agents is needed to stop the seizures. In a randomized trial of adults in status epilepticus treated before arriving at the hospital, 10 mg of intramuscular midazolam was more effective and at least as safe as 4 mg of intravenous (IV) lorazepam for stopping seizures.[A4] In the emergency department, options include IV lorazepam (0.1 mg/kg given at 2 mg/minute),[A5] a continuous IV midazolam (0.1 to 2 mg/kg/hour) followed by IV phenytoin (15 mg/kg at a rate of 50 mg/minute) or fosphenytoin (15-20 mg/kg at a rate of 150 mg/minute) to provide a more long-lasting effect. If seizures continue for 10 to 15 minutes, options include phenobarbital (20 mg/kg IV) or continuous IV midazolam (0.1 to 2 mg/kg/hour), pentobarbital (0.5 to 3 mg/kg/hour), or propofol (2 to 4 mg/kg/hour), most appropriately in an intensive care setting. In refractory cases, general anesthesia for 24 hours is used. In children, convulsive status epilepticus can be controlled within 10 minutes in 70 to 75% of patients treated with either IV diazepam (0.2 mg/kg) or IV lorazepam (0.1 mg/kg).[A6]

Considerations in Women

Changes in hormone levels during the menstrual cycle may aggravate seizures perimenstrually in some women (i.e., catamenial epilepsy). The administration of oral contraceptives (Chapter 238), Depo-Provera, acetazolamide (250 to 500 mg/day), or clobazam (10 to 20 mg/day) may reduce perimenstrual seizures. Enzyme-inducing antiepileptic drugs (see Table 403-8) that reduce estrogen levels by enhancing its metabolism require patients to be treated with higher doses of estrogen or alternative methods of contraception.

Pregnancy poses challenges with regard to seizure control, teratogenesis, and outcomes of pregnancy. Nevertheless, pregnancy itself has no consistent effect on the frequency of seizures, and more than 90% of pregnancies in women with epilepsy are safe and successful. Freedom from seizures for at least 9 months preceding pregnancy is associated with a high probability of freedom from seizures during the pregnancy. Serum levels of lamotrigine, phenytoin, carbamazepine, levetiracetam, and oxcarbazepine may change during pregnancy and should be monitored. Valproate carries a higher risk for major congenital malformations and an enduring reduction in cognitive abilities in children exposed to this medication in utero; therefore its use should be avoided during pregnancy if seizure control permits it. Similarly, polytherapy and high doses of antiepileptic drugs should be avoided if possible, but antiepileptic drugs should not be discontinued. There is no increased risk for cesarean section or premature contractions, and epilepsy itself does not increase the risk for cognitive impairment in the child. Supplementation with at least 0.4 mg of folic acid daily should be given before conception and during pregnancy to reduce the risk for neural tube defects.[13]

Discontinuing Antiepileptic Drugs

About 60% of patients have seizures that are easy to control with antiepileptic drugs. Medications may be slowly tapered over 4 to 6 months in patients who have remained free of seizures for 2 years or longer, have had few seizures before treatment started, and who have a normal neurologic examination and EEG. However, the increased absolute risk for recurrent seizures after withdrawal of medication is about 20% (number needed to harm of 5). The consequences of a recurrent seizure, the costs and side effects of drugs, and aspects such as personal preferences influence the decision to withdraw antiepileptic drugs in patients who have been free of seizures.

PROGNOSIS

The prognosis is favorable in the majority of patients who experience either unprovoked seizures or one of the epilepsies.

Prognosis after Febrile Seizures

Febrile seizures are common and usually consist of generalized tonic-clonic seizures. They are provoked by fever and therefore are not considered epilepsy. The seizures begin after 6 months of age and stop before 6 years of age. Usually, febrile seizures are left untreated because the prognosis is benign.[14] When febrile seizures occur in the setting of a neurologic abnormality or are prolonged or complicated, the risk for later epilepsy is increased.

Prognosis after a Single Unprovoked Seizure

The risk of experiencing recurrent seizures after a first unprovoked seizure ranges from 21 to 69% at 2 years and from 34 to 70% at 5 years. The risk is lower in the general population than in hospital-based studies (36% at 1 year and 45% at 2 years). The probability of a relapse decreases with time; about 50% of recurrences occur within 6 months of the initial seizure, and 76 to 96% occur within 2 years. The two most consistent predictors of recurrence are the presence of a neurologic cause for the seizure, which is often uncovered on brain MRI or by the neurologic examination and history, and an epileptiform or slow EEG. The 2-year risk for recurrence is lowest for patients without an identified neurologic cause and with a normal EEG (about 25%), intermediate for patients with an identified neurologic cause or without a cause but with an abnormal EEG (48%), and highest for those with a neurologic cause and an abnormal EEG (about 65%). The risk rises dramatically if more than one seizure has occurred; after a second unprovoked seizure, the risk for a third seizure is 73%, and after a third seizure, the risk for a fourth seizure is 76%.

Prognosis of Epilepsy

The natural history of untreated epilepsy, mostly in developing countries, shows that 30 to 40% of patients obtain 5- to 10-year remissions without treatment. In developed countries, where treatment is generally started after two unprovoked seizures have occurred, the likelihood of 5-year remission is about 60% when patients are followed for 10 years, and about 70% when patients are followed for 20 years. The rate of 5-year remission in children is about 75%. In the long term, sustained freedom from seizures is achieved in about 60% of patients (early remission in about 35 to 40% of patients, and late remission in about 20 to 25%), about 16% of patients fluctuate between relapses and remissions, and about 25% never achieve seizure remission.[15] Epilepsy is considered to be resolved in patients who had an age-dependent epilepsy syndrome and are now past the applicable age, or in patients who have been seizure free for at least 10 years, with no seizure medications for the last 5 years.

Conversely, the duration of active epilepsy before achieving control is one of the most powerful predictors of remission. If seizures remain uncontrolled during the first year after diagnosis, the chance of ever achieving control is only 60%. If the period of uncontrolled seizures extends to 4 years, the chance of ever achieving control is only 10%. The presence of multiple seizure types and frequent generalized tonic-clonic seizures is associated with a lower likelihood of remission. Less than 40% of patients with newly diagnosed mesial temporal lobe epilepsy will be controlled with medications, although familial cases are more easily managed medically.

Children whose seizures remain uncontrolled are at risk of developing cognitive impairment, especially at a younger age, thereby emphasizing the importance of prompt seizure control. In children with absence epilepsy, the 12-month probability of seizure control and remaining on medication is about 35 to 40% overall, but it is higher for ethosuximide (45%) and valproic acid (44%) than for lamotrigine (21%).[AG] In longitudinal population studies of children with newly diagnosed epilepsy, quality of life improves over time in about 50%, remains stable in 30%, and deteriorates in 20%.

Patients with epilepsy are at risk for poor psychosocial outcomes, depression, and increased mortality.[16] The risk for death is two to three times higher in epilepsy than in the general population, and it can be up to five times higher in patients with frequent generalized convulsions and drug-resistant epilepsy.[17] The major causes of death are underlying conditions such as stroke and pneumonia. Sudden unexpected death in epilepsy occurs in 1 per 1000 patient-years and is particularly devastating because it affects young individuals with frequent uncontrolled seizures.

Grade A References

A1. Glauser T, Ben-Menachem E, Bourgeois B, et al. Updated ILAE evidence review of antiepileptic drug efficacy and effectiveness as initial monotherapy for epileptic seizures and syndromes. *Epilepsia.* 2013;54:551-563.
A2. Fiest KM, Sajobi TT, Wiebe S. Epilepsy surgery and meaningful improvements in quality of life: Results from a randomized controlled trial. *Epilepsia.* 2014;55:886-892.
A3. Engel J Jr, McDermott MP, Wiebe S, et al. Early surgical therapy for drug-resistant temporal lobe epilepsy: a randomized trial. *JAMA.* 2012;307:922-930.
A4. Silbergleit R, Durkalski V, Lowenstein D, et al. Intramuscular versus intravenous therapy for prehospital status epilepticus. *N Engl J Med.* 2012;366:591-600.
A5. Prasad M, Krishnan PR, Sequeira R, et al. Anticonvulsant therapy for status epilepticus. *Cochrane Database Syst Rev.* 2014;9:CD003723.
A6. Chamberlain JM, Okada P, Holsti M, et al. Lorazepam vs diazepam for pediatric status epilepticus: a randomized clinical trial. *JAMA.* 2014;311:1652-1660.
A7. Glauser TA, Cnaan A, Shinnar S, et al. Ethosuximide, valproic acid, and lamotrigine in childhood absence epilepsy: initial monotherapy outcomes at 12 months. *Epilepsia.* 2013;54:141-155.

GENERAL REFERENCES

For the General References and other additional features, please visit Expert Consult at https://expertconsult.inkling.com.

404

COMA, VEGETATIVE STATE, AND BRAIN DEATH

JAMES L. BERNAT AND EELCO F.M. WIJDICKS

The assessment and treatment of a comatose patient are among the most challenging activities in clinical medicine. Physicians must systematically and rapidly identify the cause of coma while simultaneously supporting vital systems and taking action to reverse the pathologic process. If coma is caused by a major medical illness, the damage to the brain may be irreversible. For example, resuscitation from cardiac arrest (Chapter 63) is successful only if the brain has not been irreversibly damaged by the hypoxic-ischemic injury. Many patients in acute coma have a hemispheric lesion that causes a mass effect. In such situations the mass effect may need to be reduced medically, or the mass may need to be removed to avoid permanent secondary brain stem injury.

Consciousness is usually considered a global brain function. Focal cerebral hemispheric lesions (Chapters 396 and 406) that alter fragments of consciousness may produce cognitive disturbances such as aphasia, apraxia, or agnosia (Chapter 401). Although language, praxis, and gnosis are elements of normal consciousness, their selective loss does not usually result in a diminution of the quantity of consciousness, so these focal syndromes are not classified as disorders of consciousness.

Disorders of consciousness (Table 404-1) must be distinguished from brain death and locked-in syndrome or other causes of unresponsiveness such as catatonia or psychogenic stupor (Chapter 397). Human consciousness has two measurable clinical dimensions that correspond to two distinct brain neuronal systems: (1) wakefulness, which is the organism's arousal and readiness to respond to internal or external stimuli and which is provided by the reticular system of the rostral brain stem and its thalamic and forebrain ascending projections; and (2) awareness of self and environment, which is provided by a diffuse parallel network of thalamocortical and corticocortical circuits. Wakefulness is a prerequisite for awareness, but as exemplified by patients in a vegetative state, awareness may be lost despite maintained wakefulness.

COMA

Coma is a pathologic state of eyes-closed unresponsiveness in which the patient has neither awareness nor wakefulness and from which the patient cannot be aroused to awareness or wakefulness by vigorous stimuli. Stupor is a similar disorder in which stimuli can temporarily arouse the patient to limited responsiveness, but in the absence of stimuli the patient returns to an unresponsive state. Sleep, by contrast, is a normal state of active cyclic unconsciousness from which subjects can be fully and persistently aroused to full normal consciousness.

TABLE 404-1 COMPARISON OF DISORDERS OF CONSCIOUSNESS*

	AWARENESS	WAKEFULNESS	BRAIN STEM/RESPIRATORY	MOTOR	EEG	EVOKED POTENTIALS	PET/fMRI	PROGNOSIS
Brain death	Absent	Absent	Absent	Absent	ECS	Absent	Absent cortical metabolism	The person has died
Coma	Absent	Absent	Depressed, variable	Reflex or posturing	Polymorphic delta, burst suppression	BAER variable; cortical ERPs often absent	Resting < 50%	Variable
Vegetative state	Absent	Present, intact sleep-wake cycles	Intact	Reflex, nonpurposeful	Delta, theta, or ECS	BAER preserved; cortical ERPs variable	Resting < 50%; primary areas stimulatable	Poor, when chronic
Minimally conscious state	Intact but poorly responsive	Intact	Intact	Variable with purposeful movements	Nonspecific slowing	BAER preserved; cortical ERPs often preserved	Reduced; secondary areas also stimulatable	Variable
Locked-in syndrome	Intact but communication difficult	Intact	Intact breathing; often brain stem signs	Quadriplegia, pseudobulbar palsy	Usually normal	BAER variable; cortical ERPs normal	Normal or nearly normal	Poor

*The table lists typical findings, which are not necessarily present in all patients. Locked-in syndrome may be mistaken for a disorder of consciousness.
BAER = brain stem auditory evoked response; ECS = electrocerebral silence; EEG = encephalography; ERP = event-related potential; fMRI = functional magnetic resonance imaging; PET = positron emission tomography.
From Bernat JL. *Ethical Issues in Neurology.* 3rd ed. Philadelphia: Lippincott Williams & Wilkins; 2008:292.

Coma is not a univocal state; it has levels of depth depending on the degree of reflex response to stimulation. Disorders of consciousness comprise a continuum from the mildest state of lethargy to the deepest stage of coma.

EPIDEMIOLOGY

The frequencies of the various causes of coma vary widely depending on the setting. In most settings, however, post-traumatic, metabolic, anoxic, and toxic causes are the most common (Table 404-2).

PATHOBIOLOGY

Wakefulness is provided by a network of neurons and their connections in the central tegmentum of the pons and midbrain (reticular system) that receives input at each level as it ascends into the central basal forebrain, thalamus, and cerebral cortex. Damage to this neuronal network by trauma, ischemia, hypoxia, edema, or metabolic or toxic insults leads to coma because the ascending arousal mechanism is disturbed.

Awareness of self and environment requires not only wakefulness but also normal functioning of massive parallel reverberating neuronal circuits between the thalamus and multiple cortical regions to provide an integrated and unified experience. These structures and their connections can be damaged by the same pathologic conditions that affect the arousal system, but thalamic and cortical neurons are more susceptible to damage because of their higher metabolic demands. A given global brain insult, such as systemic hypoxia and ischemia suffered during cardiac arrest, can selectively damage the cortical and thalamic neurons necessary for awareness while largely sparing the phylogenetically older and less metabolically demanding neurons of the arousal network of the reticular system. This selective damage can result in the vegetative state, which is characterized by wakefulness without awareness.

Coma can be caused by (1) structural damage as a result of brain trauma, edema, inflammation, ischemia, or mass lesions or (2) diffuse metabolic and toxic effects on brain neurons. Structural lesions can affect the arousal neuronal network of the brain stem and basal forebrain directly through local neuronal damage or indirectly by downward or lateral pressure or displacement that causes local ischemia. Metabolic and toxic encephalopathies diffusely affect all brain neurons, particularly the metabolically sensitive cortical and thalamic neurons. However, acute metabolic derangements or toxicities also can cause structural brain injury by altering blood pressure or oxygenation (e.g., opioid toxicity [Chapter 34]), brain edema (e.g., acute liver failure [Chapter 154]), or acute demyelination (e.g., from too rapid correction of chronic hyponatremia [Chapter 116]).

Structural lesions that cause coma typically produce clinically recognizable syndromes of cerebral "herniation" in which intracranial pressure shifts produce caudal displacement and ischemia of the midbrain and medial temporal lobe through the tentorial incisura that induces dysfunction of cranial nerves, breathing, and motor systems. Central transtentorial herniation from slowly expanding axial lesions is uncommon; more common is uncal herniation from rapidly expanding and laterally placed lesions that trap the

TABLE 404-2 CAUSES OF STUPOR AND COMA

Traumatic brain injury*
  Contusion
  Intracerebral, epidural, subdural, or subarachnoid hemorrhage
  Raised intracranial pressure
Neoplasms and other mass lesions
Infections
  Meningitis
  Encephalitis
  Brain abscess or empyema
  Sepsis or other infection, especially in the elderly or a demented patient*
Cerebrovascular disease
  Subarachnoid hemorrhage
  Infarction in the brain stem or cerebellum or large hemispheric infarction
  Hemorrhage in the brain stem or cerebellum or large hemispheric hemorrhage
  Vasculitis, disseminated intravascular coagulation, thrombotic thrombocytopenic purpura
Seizures
  Status epilepticus
  Spike-wave stupor
  Postictal state
Metabolic encephalopathies*
  Hypoglycemia, hyperglycemia
  Hypercalcemia
  Hyponatremia, hypernatremia
  Hypoxemia, including anoxia after cardiac arrest
  Acidosis
  Organ system failure: hepatic, renal, pulmonary, cardiac
  Endocrinopathy (e.g., myxedema coma)
Toxic encephalopathies
  Drug intoxications*: alcohol, barbiturates, benzodiazepines, opioids, stimulants, salicylates, anticonvulsants, anticholinergics, psychotropic drugs, or others
  Poisoning: carbon monoxide, industrial toxins
Other encephalopathies
  Hypertensive encephalopathy
  Acute hydrocephalus
  Pituitary apoplexy
Other
  Conversion, malingering, catatonia

*Most common causes.

ipsilateral oculomotor nerve against the uncus of the temporal lobe. Lateral displacement of brain structures can supplement or exceed downward displacement. The ascending arousal system also can be damaged directly by primary brain stem catastrophes such as pontomesencephalic hemorrhage and infarction, or indirectly by downward-directed pressure waves produced by hemispheric mass lesions such as from brain trauma (Chapter 399) or supratentorial neoplasms (Chapter 189), abscesses (Chapter 413), hemorrhages (Chapter 408), or large infarctions (Chapter 407).

Metabolic encephalopathies disturb the neuronal microenvironment by altering the precise metabolic conditions necessary for normal neuronal excitability. Disturbances in the neuronal milieu can be caused by alterations in blood flow, oxygen delivery, glucose concentration, temperature, electrolyte concentrations, and intracranial pressure, as well as by meningitis, seizures, and organ failure. The depth of the resulting alteration of consciousness depends on the severity of the metabolic disturbance: mild metabolic encephalopathies can cause slowness or lethargy, whereas severe metabolic encephalopathies can produce deep coma. The rapidity of onset is of particular importance. A sudden drop in the serum sodium concentration (Chapter 116) may result in coma and seizures, whereas a slow decline to an equivalent level may not. Toxic encephalopathies can be caused by poisoning with exogenous agents such as depressant drugs or by endogenous toxins resulting, for example, from renal or hepatic failure and produce the same continuum of severity. Acute meningeal inflammation, caused most commonly by bacterial meningitis, induces coma by a combination of inflammatory and vascular changes.

CLINICAL MANIFESTATIONS

A comatose patient is unresponsive and cannot be aroused to awareness or wakefulness. The level of consciousness can be assessed by loudly speaking the patient's name directly in the ear. Patients should be asked to look up and down to test for locked-in syndrome, in which vertical eye movements may be the only remaining voluntary movement. Noxious stimuli can be used to elicit motor responses. Stimulation of nasal hair and the nasal septum with a cotton-tipped swab may elicit airway protective reflexes. Acceptable examples of nontraumatic noxious stimuli that can elicit a rapid response if present include compression of the supraorbital nerve, temporomandibular joints, or nail beds, or a sternal rub with fingers or knuckles. Motor responses to these stimuli usually can be graded as localization, withdrawal, reflex extensor posturing, and none.

DIAGNOSIS

The diagnosis of coma requires a detailed history, physical, and neurologic examination (Table 404-3), laboratory tests, and neuroimaging studies.[1] Immediate attention should be paid to whether the patient has signs of meningitis (e.g., fever, nuchal rigidity) or head trauma (Chapter 399) or has focal findings suggestive of a mass, lesion, bleeding, or ischemic injury.

Coma assessment scales are useful to describe the depth of coma, serially assess changes, and estimate prognosis. The widely used Glasgow Coma Scale (Chapter 399, Table 399-1) was devised to assess patients with traumatic brain injury and is a combination of three responses. The FOUR Score (Table 404-4) is more useful for all causes of coma, because it more accurately assesses brain stem function and quantifies awareness.

The relevant history includes eyewitness accounts of any preceding headache, vomiting, confusional state, prescription and street drug use, alcohol consumption, diabetes, fever, head trauma, seizure activity, and medical illnesses, especially atrial fibrillation. The rate at which neurologic function declined can be especially helpful.

After determining the level of consciousness, the neurologic examination focuses on four systems whose careful assessment can distinguish structural from metabolic causes of coma and delineate the functional brain level caused by the pathologic process: (1) the respiratory rate and pattern; (2) the pupils' size, shape, and reactivity; (3) spontaneous eye movements and elicited vestibuloocular reflexes; and (4) motor responses to stimuli (Table 404-5).

The respiratory rate and pattern should be observed. Cheyne-Stokes respiration is a periodic form of breathing whose amplitude forms a sine wave, with 5- to 45-second periods of apnea punctuating periods of hyperpnea; it is seen in metabolic encephalopathies, especially those caused by heart failure, and during sleep. Central neurogenic hyperventilation, which is continuous hyperpnea and tachypnea that produces a pure respiratory alkalosis, occurs with lesions of the rostral brain stem tegmentum at the midbrain level; rapid deep breathing (Kussmaul) that is compensating for a severe metabolic acidosis (Chapter 118) looks similar. Irregular breathing patterns with apneic periods may indicate severe brain stem involvement and can be agonal.

Pupillary size and reactivity to a bright light stimulus can be assessed to evaluate the integrity of the optic and oculomotor nerves, midbrain, and sympathetic nerves. The reactivity of the pupils to light is an important sign that discriminates structural coma from metabolic-toxic coma. The pupils usually remain reactive through varying depths of metabolic-toxic coma, often until apnea ensues, whereas pupillary reflexes are lost earlier in structural coma caused by transtentorial herniation. The pupils are small, equal, and reactive in patients with metabolic encephalopathies. When the oculomotor nerve or the midbrain is involved, the ipsilateral pupil becomes unreactive to light because of damage to the parasympathetic pupilloconstrictors and dilates because of the unopposed sympathetic pupillodilators. When herniation proceeds further, the brain stem sympathetic tracts are also damaged so the affected pupil(s) returns to midposition and becomes unreactive to light or dark. Lesions that affect only the pons and not the midbrain (e.g., pontine hemorrhage, infarction) can cause pinpoint pupils whose intact

TABLE 404-3	SOME INITIAL CLINICAL CLUES TO THE DIAGNOSIS OF STUPOR AND COMA

STRUCTURAL CAUSES

History
  Abrupt onset of unconsciousness
  Sudden headache
  Vomiting
Examination
  Focal neurologic signs (hemiparesis, posturing, asymmetrical reflexes)
  Abnormal pupillary light reflexes

METABOLIC OR TOXIC CAUSES

History
  Gradual onset of unconsciousness
  Preceding confusional state
  Seizures
  Known cognitive impairment
  Taking insulin or street drugs
Examination
  Absence of focal neurologic signs
  Presence of frontal release signs
  Intact pupillary light reflexes
  Tremor, asterixis, or multifocal myoclonus
  Evidence of systemic infection
  Needle tracks

MENINGITIS

History
  Worsening headache
  Neck stiffness and pain
  Fever, chills
  Progressive stupor and coma
Examination
  Fever, rigors
  Nuchal rigidity and signs of meningeal inflammation

TABLE 404-4	FOUR SCORE COMA ASSESSMENT SCALE*

EYE RESPONSE

E4 = Eyelids open or unopened, tracking or blinking to command
E3 = Eyelids open but not tracking
E2 = Eyelids closed but open to pain
E1 = Eyelids remain closed with pain stimuli

MOTOR RESPONSE

M4 = Thumbs up, fist, or peace sign
M3 = Localizing to pain
M2 = Flexion response to pain
M1 = Extension response to pain
M0 = No response to pain or generalized myoclonic status epilepticus

BRAIN STEM REFLEXES

B4 = Pupillary and corneal reflexes present
B3 = One pupil dilated and unreactive to light
B2 = Pupillary or corneal reflexes absent
B1 = Pupillary and corneal reflexes absent
B0 = Absent pupillary, corneal, or cough reflexes

RESPIRATION

R4 = Regular breathing pattern
R3 = Cheyne-Stokes breathing pattern
R2 = Irregular breathing pattern
R1 = Triggers or breathes above the ventilator rate
R0 = Apnea or breathes at the ventilator rate

*For nontraumatic coma and other disorders of consciousness.
From Wijdicks EFM. *The Comatose Patient*. 2ed. New York: Oxford University Press; 2014.

TABLE 404-5   BRAIN FUNCTIONAL LEVELS DETERMINED BY FINDINGS IN CLINICAL SYSTEMS

FUNCTIONAL LEVEL	CONSCIOUSNESS	RESPIRATION	PUPILS	VESTIBULO-OCULAR REFLEXES	MOTOR RESPONSES
CENTRAL TRANSTENTORIAL HERNIATION					
High diencephalic	Light stupor	Eupnea, yawning, post-hyperventilation apnea	Small, reactive	Loss of checking component	Paratonia, grasp
Low diencephalic	Deep stupor	Cheyne-Stokes	Small, reactive	Loss of checking component	Decorticate posturing
Midbrain	Coma	Central neurogenic hyperventilation	Midposition, fixed	Loss of medial rectus function	Decerebrate posturing
Upper pons	Coma	Central neurogenic hyperventilation	Midposition, fixed	Loss of medial rectus function	Decerebrate posturing
Lower pons	Coma	Ataxic	Midposition, fixed	Absent	Flaccid
Medulla	Coma	Apnea	Midposition, fixed	Absent	Flaccid
UNCAL TRANSTENTORIAL HERNIATION					
Early third nerve	Unreliable	Normal	Ipsilateral dilated, fixed	Normal	Contralateral hemiparesis
Late third nerve	Coma	Cheyne-Stokes or central neurogenic hyperventilation	Ipsilateral dilated, fixed; contralateral dilated, fixed	Medial rectus dysfunction	Ipsilateral hemiparesis and contralateral decerebrate posturing
Midbrain-pons	Coma	Central neurogenic hyperventilation or ataxic	Midposition, fixed	Absent	Bilateral decerebrate posturing

reaction to light can be seen with a magnifying glass. Preexisting disease (e.g., diabetes) or locally applied eye medications can also impair pupillary reflexes.

Spontaneous eye movements may have localizing value. Conjugate horizontal eye deviation points to the side of brain lesions rostral to the brain stem (usually in the cerebral hemispheres) but to the side opposite brain stem lesions. Tonic downward eye deviation suggests acute lesions of the thalamus or dorsal midbrain. Tonic upward eye deviation is unusual but is seen in patients with hypoxic-ischemic lesions. Ocular bobbing with a rapid downward movement followed by a slow return upward suggests a pontine lesion. Reverse ocular bobbing with a slow downward and rapid upward movement ("ocular dipping") has poor localizing value but may be seen after hypoxic-ischemic insults and metabolic disorders. "Ping-pong" gaze with alternating conjugate horizontal eye movements is nonspecific, but a slower and otherwise similar disorder called periodic alternating gaze is seen in patients with portosystemic encephalopathy (Chapter 153). Ocular skew deviation, in which one eye is higher than the other on primary gaze, suggests a brain stem lesion.

The vestibuloocular reflex assesses brain stem and cerebral hemispheric function by reflexively inducing eye movements. First, the external auditory canal should be inspected to exclude perforation of the tympanic membrane and obstruction by cerumen. Ice water is then injected into the canal (10 mL for usual assessment but 50 mL for assessment of brain death), and the induced reflex eye movements are observed (see Table 404-5). In patients with normal consciousness, such as in psychogenic coma, marked horizontal nystagmus is produced. In patients with stupor at a diencephalic level, such as from metabolic encephalopathy, the fast component of nystagmus is suppressed, so the patient responds with full tonic conjugate eye movements toward the injected ear. With lesions of the oculomotor or abducens nerves or lesions of the midbrain or pons, ophthalmoplegia of localizing value is observed. In brain death or total brain stem failure, no response is observed. The vestibuloocular reflexes may be ablated after treatment with ototoxic antibiotics.

Motor responses are observed after noxious stimulation. At lower functional levels of structural coma, limb posturing is often observed. Limb posturing is a unilateral or bilateral, stereotyped, tonic brain stem reflex movement induced by stimulation, especially noxious stimuli. Decorticate posturing, in which the arm is flexed and the ipsilateral leg is extended, suggests a midbrain functional level. Decerebrate posturing, in which both the arm and the ipsilateral leg are extended, suggests a pontine functional level. When the entire brain stem is destroyed, as in brain death, all limbs remain flaccid during stimulation. Metabolic-toxic encephalopathies usually produce symmetrical motor signs, whereas structural causes of coma frequently produce asymmetrical motor signs. Hypoglycemia and acute hyponatremia are exceptions in which aphasia, gaze paresis, and hemiparesis may be seen. Myoclonic seizures with continuous or intermittent rhythmic clonic movements frequently develop in patients who have suffered hypoxic-ischemic neuronal damage during cardiopulmonary arrest. Myoclonic status epilepticus is a poor prognostic sign.

On the general physical examination, assessment of vital signs, otoscopy, optic funduscopy, and inspection for head trauma, nuchal rigidity, and needle tracks can provide key findings. Emergency laboratory testing should generally include a complete blood cell count, serum electrolytes, a blood glucose level, tests of renal and liver function, coagulation tests, thyroid function tests, arterial blood gas analysis, a blood alcohol concentration, a urine drug screen, and an electrocardiogram. If intoxication is likely, particularly in the absence of ketones, uremia, or an abnormal lactate level, the anion gap (Chapter 118) and osmolar gap should be measured. Routine toxicologic testing rarely changes acute management and usually adds little to the diagnostic evaluation, except in patients with a normal CT scan and no lateralizing signs or physical examination.

If signs of meningitis are present, blood cultures and a lumbar puncture should be performed without the delay of obtaining brain imaging if no marked focal signs (e.g., hemiparesis) are present. Brain computed tomography (CT) should be performed urgently in nearly every patient in coma. When a CT scan is normal in a comatose patient with no clear lateralizing neurologic signs, the coma is usually the result of intoxication. Pesticides (Chapter 110), ethanol, atypical alcohols, opioids (including heroin [Chapter 34]), and benzodiazepine intoxication (Chapter 397) should be considered.

After the neurologic examination, screening laboratory tests, brain CT, and lumbar puncture have been accomplished, a tentative diagnosis can be made in most patients. If focal signs are present despite normal findings on CT, consideration should be given to an acute stroke involving the posterior circulation (Chapters 407 and 408). Brain CT angiography or magnetic resonance imaging (MRI) can clarify the diagnosis. If lateralizing signs are absent, metabolic and toxic causes are most likely. An electroencephalogram (EEG) is useful in patients in whom nonconvulsive seizure activity may be causing stupor or coma.

TREATMENT

Management of coma requires simultaneous diagnostic, supportive, and treatment measures (Table 404-6). Specific treatments, which depend on the causative diagnosis, include urgent attention to any head trauma (Chapter 399). Emergency stabilization of respiration and circulation and control of seizures are critical for all patients. In patients without focal findings or obvious meningitis, 50% dextrose (25 g intravenously [IV]), thiamine (50 mg IV), naloxone (0.4 to 2 mg IV), and flumazenil (0.2 mg IV) can be administered during the diagnostic assessment. If fever, nuchal rigidity, or leukocytosis is present, the patient should be treated presumptively for bacterial meningitis (Chapter 412) with IV antibiotics before neuroimaging and lumbar puncture.

Elevated intracranial pressure must be lowered urgently. Treatments include hyperventilation by bag or ventilator, IV hyperosmolar agents such as mannitol, and IV glucocorticoid drugs for patients with vasogenic edema from brain tumors (Chapter 189), abscesses (Chapter 413), or bacterial meningitis (Chapter 412). Therapeutically induced mild hypothermia for several days improves outcomes in patients who are in coma after diffuse hypoxic-ischemic neuronal

TABLE 404-6	EMERGENCY MANAGEMENT OF COMATOSE PATIENTS

1. Ensure oxygenation
2. Maintain the circulation
3. Administer 50% dextrose, 25 g IV, and control glucose
4. Lower raised intracranial pressure
5. Stop seizures with lorazepam, 1-2 mg IV
6. Search for and treat infections
7. Restore acid-base and electrolyte balance
8. Normalize body temperature
9. Administer thiamine, 50 mg IV, and multivitamins
10. Consider administration of opioid antagonists (naloxone, 0.4-2 mg IV)
11. Consider administration of benzodiazepine antagonists (flumazenil, 0.2 mg IV)
12. Control agitation
13. Protect the eyes
14. Consider inducing therapeutic hypothermia for diffuse hypoxic-ischemic causes

Modified from Posner JB, Saper CB, Schiff ND, et al. *Plum and Posner's Diagnosis of Stupor and Coma.* 4th ed. New York: Oxford University Press; 2007:311.

TABLE 404-7	DIAGNOSIS OF THE VEGETATIVE STATE

I. Absence of:
  Awareness of self or environment
  Purposeful or voluntary behavioral response to all stimuli
  Language comprehension or expression

II. Presence of:
  Intermittent wakefulness manifested by the presence of sleep-wake cycles
  Autonomic functions
  Cranial nerve and spinal reflexes

III. Potential behavioral repertoire:
  Breathe spontaneously
  Spontaneous roving eye movements
  Utter sounds but no words
  Grimace to pain, make facial expressions
  Yawn, make chewing jaw movements, swallow saliva
  Move limbs nonpurposefully, arch back, decorticate limb posturing
  Flexion withdrawal from noxious stimuli
  Move head or eyes briefly toward sound or movement
  Auditory startle

damage caused by cardiac arrest,[A1] and a temperature target of 36° C is as good as 33° C.[A2] Neurosurgical removal of expanding mass lesions and unroofing the skull (hemicraniectomy) can be life-saving in selected patients.[A3]

PROGNOSIS

The prognosis of coma is highly variable[2] and depends on the cause, stage, degree of structural brain damage, and potential reversibility. The majority of surviving patients who undergo therapeutic hypothermia after cardiac arrest have preserved cognitive function and are able to return to work.[3] Prediction rules for recovery apply only to a specific cause. The prognosis after traumatic brain injury can be predicted by the Glasgow Coma Score (Chapter 399, Table 399-1). In patients who have survived cardiopulmonary arrest and resuscitation and in whom toxic and metabolic factors (e.g., sedation, neuromuscular blockade, hypothermia, organ failure, and shock) are not present, the likelihood for recovery of awareness is less than 1% if the following signs are present:

  Day 1: presence of myoclonic status epilepticus
  Days 1 to 3: bilateral absence of the N20 response of the somatosensory evoked potential
  Days 1 to 3: serum neuron-specific enolase concentration higher than 33 µg/L
  Day 3: absent pupillary or corneal reflexes; extensor or absent motor responses

If the patient remains comatose on day 3 without these findings and without a contribution from a potentially reversible metabolic or toxic encephalopathy, the probability of recovery of awareness is below 10% if there is no withdrawal response to painful stimuli and below 40% if the patient withdraws to painful stimuli but lacks spontaneous eye opening.

Some patients may appear to recover completely within days after an episode of impaired cerebral oxygenation but then regress days to weeks later with the syndrome of delayed posthypoxic leukoencephalopathy, which is caused by demyelination. Neuroimaging typically shows diffuse hemispheric demyelination that spares the cerebellum and brain stem. The cerebrospinal fluid may show an elevated myelin basic protein level, and biopsy can confirm leukoencephalopathy. Some patients slowly recover over 3 to 12 months, but usually with substantial neurologic sequelae.[4] Others may linger in a vegetative or minimally conscious state (see below).

THE VEGETATIVE STATE

The vegetative state is a disorder of consciousness in which wakefulness is retained but awareness of self and environment is entirely absent to the extent that it can be tested clinically.[5] The vegetative state may be a transient stage during spontaneous recovery from coma to awareness, or it may be a chronic unchanging state. Adjectives such as "persistent" or "permanent" should be avoided because they generate confusion by confounding the diagnosis and prognosis.

EPIDEMIOLOGY AND PATHOBIOLOGY

The vegetative state is caused by diffuse or multifocal brain lesions that disconnect the polymodal cerebral cortices from the thalami but spare the brain stem and hypothalamus. The prevalence of a transient vegetative state after brain injury is unknown. The prevalence of a chronic stable vegetative state is 19 per million.

Causative lesions can be located bilaterally in the thalami, diffusely in the cerebral cortex, or diffusely in the white matter that connects the thalami to the cortex. Two clinical disorders are most commonly responsible: diffuse hypoxic-ischemic neuronal damage to the thalami and cortex suffered during cardiopulmonary arrest and diffuse axonal injury from a traumatic injury caused by a torque force. These two disorders have different pathologies: hypoxic-ischemic injury affects cortical, thalamic, and cerebellar neurons, whereas diffuse axonal injury shears and disconnects the axons at the gray matter–white matter junction diffusely or multifocally in the cortex.

CLINICAL MANIFESTATIONS AND DIAGNOSIS

The clinical features of the vegetative state (Table 404-7) are dominated by what patients do. A careful neurologic examination must be performed to search for any evidence of awareness, because up to 40% of patients in whom a vegetative state is initially diagnosed are actually in a minimally conscious state (see later).

The vegetative state is a clinical syndrome with a spectrum of severity. The typical patient has diffuse slow-wave activity on the EEG, but the most severely affected patients have isoelectric EEGs. However, some patients who are entirely unresponsive generate appropriate EEG responses to distinct commands, thereby suggesting they have residual cognitive function and conscious awareness. As determined by functional neuroimaging studies, a subset of patients with a clinically diagnosed vegetative state possess awareness as evidenced by their ability to perform ideational tasks on command.[6] Such functional neuroimaging tests are not yet part of routine clinical practice but may become standard clinical assessment tools for patients who are suspected to be in a vegetative state.

TREATMENT AND PROGNOSIS Rx

No treatments reverse or improve a long-standing stable vegetative state. The aggressiveness of medical treatment of patients in the vegetative state should ideally be guided by their previously stated wishes. Patients require the same medical and nursing care, physical therapy, and nutritional needs as patients in coma. Patients should be referred to specialized neurorehabilitation units when possible.

People who recover after a prolonged anoxic vegetative state usually have an initially preserved pupillary light reflex and nociceptive response, paroxysmal sympathetic hyperactivity, and median nerve somatosensory evoked potentials.[7] Patients who are in a vegetative state from nontraumatic causes and who do not regain awareness within 3 months of the insult have less than a 1% chance of experiencing significant neurologic recovery and often raise serious ethical and moral dilemmas for their families and caregivers.[8] After traumatic brain injury, the prognosis cannot be estimated with a similar degree of certainty until after 1 year, although functional neuroimaging is a promising approach to identify patients who are destined to recover awareness.

TABLE 404-8 DIAGNOSIS OF THE MINIMALLY CONSCIOUS STATE

Globally impaired responsiveness

Limited but discernable evidence of awareness of self and environment as demonstrated by the presence of one or more of the following behaviors that occur in a contingent relationship to relevant environmental stimuli and are not simply reflexive movements:

    Follow simple commands

    Gesture yes/no answers

    Make intelligible vocalizations or gestures in direct response to a question's linguistic content

    Reach for objects that demonstrates a clear relationship between object location and direction of reach

    Touch and hold objects in a manner that accommodates the size and shape of the object

    Sustain visual pursuit to moving stimuli

    Smile or cry appropriately to linguistic or visual content of emotional but not to affectively neutral topics or stimuli

THE MINIMALLY CONSCIOUS STATE

The minimally conscious state (Table 404-8) is a disorder of altered consciousness characterized by a profound lack of responsiveness but with partial or intermittent evidence of awareness of self and environment. Patients typically may have suffered less severe injuries than patients in the vegetative state. The minimally conscious state is much more common than the vegetative state, from which it must be distinguished. When compared with patients in the vegetative state, patients in the minimally conscious state are more likely to respond to environmental and sensory stimuli and to stimulant medications such as levodopa or dopamine agonists (which stimulate thalamic dopaminergic neurons and are prescribed in the same dose ranges as for the treatment of Parkinson disease [Chapter 409]). In patients who are minimally conscious or in a vegetative state at 4 to 16 weeks after traumatic brain injury, amantadine (starting at 100 mg twice daily and increasing up to 200 mg twice daily) can accelerate the early pace of rehabilitative recovery but may not improve ultimate recovery.[A4] Patients in the minimally conscious state require the same specialized neurorehabilitation services as those in the vegetative state. There are no good prognostic data for the minimally conscious state other than for recovery of the subset of patients after traumatic brain injury (Chapter 399).

THE LOCKED-IN SYNDROME

The locked-in syndrome, a state of profound paralysis, is not a disorder of consciousness but may be mistaken for one. In its classic form, it is produced when a large infarction or hemorrhage in the pontine tegmentum and base produces quadriplegia, pseudobulbar palsy, and paralysis of horizontal eye movements. Once the acute encephalopathy resolves, locked-in patients usually remain awake and alert, breathe spontaneously, and have normal consciousness and cognition, to the extent that they can be tested accurately. Inexperienced examiners may incorrectly diagnose locked-in patients as being comatose because of their profound paralysis, pinpoint pupils, and seeming unresponsiveness. A similar state of profound global paralysis with intact cognition can be produced by advanced amyotrophic lateral sclerosis (Chapter 419), Guillain-Barré syndrome (Chapter 420), or critical illness polyneuropathy (Chapter 420).

Patients can be taught to communicate with voluntary vertical eye movements and eyelid movements, which are typically their only retained volitional movements, because they are controlled rostral to the pons. Most affected patients, particularly older patients with comorbid illnesses, die within a few months, but some otherwise healthy young patients who have become locked in as a result of basilar artery occlusion have survived for many years. Occasional patients may recover function to become independent. Computerized systems targeting remaining voluntary eye movements can help patients communicate.

BRAIN DEATH

Brain death is the term popularly applied to the determination of human death based on tests that show irreversible cessation of all clinical brain functions. Once illness or injury has destroyed the brain or rendered its clinical functions irreversibly lost, a human being is dead.[9] Brain death is a medically and legally accepted determination of human death throughout North America, Europe, Australia, most of the developed world, and much of the developing world.[10] Brain-dead patients serve as ideal multiorgan donors.

TABLE 404-9 TESTS FOR BRAIN DEATH IN ADULTS

I. Preconditions showing irreversibility: all necessary
- Presence of a structural brain lesion sufficient to produce all the clinical signs
- Absence of reversible significant toxic or metabolic encephalopathy:
  - No depressant drug intoxication
  - No neuromuscular blockade (use electroneurography if uncertain)
  - No severe hypothermia
  - No severe hypotension
- Sequential repeated testing or one test followed by a confirmatory blood flow test

II. Signs showing complete cessation of all clinical brain functions: all necessary
- Coma: no spontaneous movements, no response to any stimuli, and no reflex movements integrated by the brain
- Apnea: no breathing or respiratory effort when the $P_{ACO_2} \geq 60$ mm Hg while protecting the P_{AO_2}
- Brain stem areflexia: all necessary
  - Absent pupillary light and dark reflexes
  - Absent corneal touch reflexes
  - Absent facial movement to noxious stimuli
  - Absent vestibulo-ocular reflexes tested by caloric irrigation of the external auditory canal with 50 mL of ice water
  - Absent pharyngeal and tracheal reflexes to endotracheal tube suctioning

III. Confirmatory tests: optional but desirable; neuroimaging preferred
- Neuroimaging that shows complete absence of intracranial blood flow; one test
  - Intravenous radionuclide angiography
  - Transcranial Doppler ultrasound
  - Computed tomographic angiography
  - Magnetic resonance angiography or diffusion
  - Single-photon emission computed tomography
- Electrophysiologic testing (use only if intracranial pressure is not elevated)
  - Electroencephalography + brain stem auditory evoked responses + somatosensory evoked responses: all isoelectric

EPIDEMIOLOGY AND PATHOBIOLOGY

Most cases of brain death result from massive traumatic brain injury (Chapter 399), intracranial hemorrhage (Chapter 408), meningitis (Chapter 412), or diffuse hypoxic-ischemic neuronal damage as a result of cardiac arrest (Chapter 63) or asphyxia. Marked cerebral edema from the primary injury or illness produces severe intracranial hypertension. When intracranial pressure exceeds mean arterial blood pressure (or systolic blood pressure in some cases), intracranial blood flow ceases and widespread ischemic death of brain neurons ensues.

CLINICAL MANIFESTATIONS AND DIAGNOSIS

Brain-dead patients have no brain functions measurable at the bedside. The diagnosis should be suspected in any patient who is deeply comatose, is unresponsive to stimuli, has absent pupillary light reflexes, and is apneic and completely ventilator dependent. The diagnosis requires a comprehensive evaluation (Table 404-9). In the United States, one examination typically suffices, but diagnostic criteria in several states and many countries require two examinations, and some require two physicians to certify the findings.

TREATMENT

Once the diagnosis has been made, the patient is declared dead. If the family has agreed to allow the deceased patient to serve as an organ donor, the ventilator is reattached following the apnea test, and the patient is moved to the surgical suite. If the patient is not an organ donor, the ventilator is not reattached, and all lines and monitors are discontinued. Physicians should be knowledgeable about local laws that may restrict making the diagnosis in patients belonging to certain religious groups that do not accept brain death as human death.

Grade A References

A1. Arrich J, Holzer M, Havel C, et al. Hypothermia for neuroprotection in adults after cardiopulmonary resuscitation. *Cochrane Database Syst Rev.* 2012;9:CD004128.

A2. Nielsen N, Wetterslev J, Cronberg T, et al. Targeted temperature management at 33 degrees C versus 36 degrees C after cardiac arrest. *N Engl J Med.* 2013;369:2197-2206.

A3. Jüttler E, Unterberg A, Woitzik J, et al. Hemicraniectomy in older patients with extensive middle-cerebral-artery stroke. *N Engl J Med.* 2014;370:1091-1100.

A4. Giacino JT, Whyte J, Bagiella E, et al. Placebo-controlled trial of amantadine for severe traumatic brain injury. *N Engl J Med.* 2012;366:819-826.

GENERAL REFERENCES

For the General References and other additional features, please visit Expert Consult at https://expertconsult.inkling.com.

405

DISORDERS OF SLEEP

BRADLEY V. VAUGHN

DEFINITION

Sleep is essential to good health and a sense of well-being. This normal state of decreased responsiveness promotes good function of bodily processes, restores the properties of alertness, and promotes memory storage and learning.[1] Conversely, the disruption of sleep is associated with a variety of complaints and physiologic consequences. Second in frequency only to pain, sleep-wake complaints lead over one in three individuals to seek medical attention. Sleep disruption frequently manifests as intrusion of components of the sleep state into periods of wakefulness. Untreated sleep disorders cause various health issues, impair job performance, and affect psychosocial interactions. Sleep disruption may also exacerbate symptoms of other diseases by worsening a preexisting disorder or impairing the ability to cope with the symptoms of the original disease. It is often difficult to recognize that such signs are related to dysfunctional sleep.

PATHOBIOLOGY

Complex humoral, neurochemical, and neuronal networks affect the sleep-wake state. Dynamic in organization, sleep is composed of non–rapid eye movement (NREM) sleep and rapid eye movement (REM) sleep. NREM is divided into three stages (N1, N2, and N3) and REM is denoted as stage R. Each stage has a distinct physiologic regulation. Each of these sleep stages may have specific contributions to health, and the stages also interact.

Wakefulness involves activation of the monoaminergic neuronal groups, basal forebrain cholinergic neurons, and the brain stem reticular activating system. These areas work in concert to promote the brain's ability to respond to stimuli. The reticular activating system promotes the relay of sensory information to the cerebral hemispheres, while the forebrain cholinergic and monoaminergic neurons promote attention of the hemispheric networks to sensory information.

With the onset of sleep, information from two major drives (homeostatic and circadian) influences the ventral lateral preoptic area to suppress the networks of wakefulness and allow the initiation of NREM sleep. NREM sleep typically starts as stage N1, with mild slowing of the electroencephalogram (EEG) and slow eye movements (Table 405-1). Stage N1 is associated with the feeling of drowsiness. Although minimal sensory processing can occur, memory is not stored. Blood pressure may decrease slightly, and breathing becomes more periodic. Stage N1 represents about 5% of the night.

The hallmark of stage N2 sleep is the presence of characteristic sleep spindles and K complexes on the EEG. Although stage N2 is considered light sleep, this stage is associated with less responsiveness to stimuli than stage N1 and less responsiveness to elevated CO_2 and low oxygen. Stage N2 typically represents about 50% of a night's sleep.

Stage N3 is characterized by slow waves (0.5 to 2.0 Hz, >75uV) on the EEG. These slow waves are more prominent in brain areas that are more heavily used during the preceding waking period and may be related to reorganization of neuronal synapses. In stage N3, which constitutes 20% of the night, the individual is difficult to arouse and has rhythmic breathing that is slightly less responsive to elevated CO_2 and low oxygen than during stage N2.

REM sleep (stage R) is primarily generated by cholinergic neurons in the subcaeruleus nucleus in the brain stem, which then activate other neuronal groups to produce the rapid eye movements, active theta and alpha frequency EEG waveforms, loss of muscle tone, sensory processing, and reduced temperature regulation associated with stage R. Most vivid dreaming occurs in stage R, but dreams can occur in other stages. Despite the vivid dreams during stage R, most muscles are paralyzed. Ventilation is solely dependent upon the diaphragm, yet this stage is associated with the least amount of responsiveness to low oxygen and elevated CO_2. Stage R typically encompasses about 20% of the night and is ended by activation of norepinephrine and serotonergic neurons. Age influences sleep. REM sleep occupies 50% of sleep at birth and then gradually declines to 20 to 25% by age 3 years. Slow wave sleep is prominent in children and declines in men in their late 20s and in women by age 40 to 50 years.

Sleep stages graphed through the night demonstrate the dynamic interplay of the various stages. As seen in a hypnogram, sleep has repeating cycles of approximately 90 minutes. These cycles show a predominance of stage N3 in the first two cycles, and a gradual lengthening of the periods of stage R sleep in the latter half of the sleep period. The reason for this progression is unknown, but these features suggest other complex drivers are at work.

Many models that consider the array of neurochemical pathways that influence sleep can theoretically explain its physiologic regulation. The most accepted two-driver model uses the homeostatic and circadian drivers to

TABLE 405-1 SLEEP STAGE PARAMETERS*

STAGE	EEG FINDINGS	EYE MOVEMENTS (EOG)	SUBMENTAL EMG	ASSOCIATED PHYSIOLOGY
Wakefulness (W)	**More than 50% of an epoch has alpha rhythm over occipital region (posterior dominant rhythm).**	**Rapid eye movements** to slow movements. **Blinking** may be present.	**Normal to high muscle tone**	Memory registration, voluntary control over breathing
Stage N1	**Attenuation of the posterior dominant rhythm for > 50% of the epoch, replaced with mixed theta frequency low-amplitude activity.** *Vertex sharp waves.* N1 continues until beginning of N2 or arousal.	*Slow rolling eye movements*	*Variable but less than wake*	Automatic behavior can occur, mild cognitive processing, periodic breathing
Stage N2	**K-complexes and/or sleep spindles.** *Low-amplitude mixed-frequency EEG.* N2 persists until transition to N3, R, or an arousal.	*No eye movements, but slow eye movements may persist.*	*Variable amplitude, typically lower than W and higher than R*	No memory, decreased arousal to stimuli, less response to elevated CO_2 and low oxygen
Stage N3	**Slow wave activity (0.5-2 Hz, >75 µV) for > 20% of an epoch.** Sleep spindles may persist. N3 persists until transition to N2, R, or an arousal.	*No eye movements seen*	*Variable amplitude, typically lower than N2 and can be as low as R*	No memory, least responsive to arousing stimuli, less response to elevated CO_2 and low oxygen, but monotonous breathing pattern
Stage R (REM sleep)	**Low-amplitude mixed-frequency EEG.** *Sawtooth waves.* R persists until transition to N1, transition to N2, between K complexes without eye movements, or an arousal.	**Rapid eye movements**	**Low muscle tone**	Similar response to stimuli as light sleep, irregular breathing pattern, least response to elevated CO_2 and low oxygen

*Sleep staging requirements. **Boldfaced** items are requirements for staging. *Italicized* items are non-required associated findings that may be present in that stage.
EEG = electroencephalogram; EMG = electromyogram; EOG = electro-oculogram.
Adapted from the American Academy of Sleep Medicine. *The AASM Manual for the Scoring of Sleep and Associated Events.* 2nd ed. version 2.1. Westchester, IL: American Academy of Sleep Medicine; 2014.

explain sleep-wake state.[2] Other issues such as psychological status also play a role. In the two-driver model, the homeostatic drive is the accumulation of substances that promote sleepiness while the person is awake. These substances are metabolized during sleep. Mental and physical activities increase this drive by producing neuronal byproducts (e.g., adenosine), whereas caffeine blunts this drive by blocking adenosine. In contrast, the circadian rhythm drive promotes wakefulness and, through its predictable cycle, prepares the body for anticipated activities. The circadian rhythm is a naturally occurring rhythm that is slightly longer than 24 hours but is readjusted each day to maintain alignment with the natural day-night cycle. The circadian rhythm is primarily adjusted by bright light and to a lesser extent by other factors such as exercise, food, and social interactions. The hormone melatonin, which is released in response to darkness, can also influence the phase of the circadian rhythm. Throughout the 24-hour period, the homeostatic and circadian drives maintain balance between the sleep and wake states. When the circadian rhythm is stronger than the homeostatic drive, the person is awake, and when the homeostatic drive is stronger than the circadian rhythm, the person is sleepy (Fig. 405-1). This theoretical model helps explain aspects of sleep-wake regulation, such as the periods of post-lunch sleepiness or evening wakefulness.

CLINICAL MANIFESTATIONS

Most patients who seek medical help for sleep issues present with one of three complaints: (1) excessive sleepiness, (2) difficulty attaining or sustaining sleep, (3) or unusual events associated with sleep. Excessive sleepiness may be confused with fatigue or lack of energy. Common symptoms include morning headaches, lapses of attention, or diffuse muscle aches. Difficulty with sleep at night may be a clue to daytime issues, and nocturnal events may be a clue to brain issues.

DIAGNOSIS

Both subjective information and objective tests are used to investigate sleep complaints. Questionnaires such as the Pittsburgh Sleep Quality Index

(Fig. 405-2) can provide a broad overview of sleep symptoms, including bedtime, wake time, activities, medications, and other substances that could influence sleep.

Objective testing of sleep includes actigraphy, polysomnography, multiple sleep latency testing, and maintenance of wakefulness testing. Actigraphy monitors movement, typically of a nondominant extremity, over 7 to 28 days. When combined with a sleep diary, actigraphy estimates total sleep time and assesses the sleep-wake schedule. Polysomnography (Chapter 100, Fig. 100-1) assesses both sleep stage and associated physiology. Sleep stage is determined by EEG, electro-oculogram, and submental electromyogram activity. Measures assessing physiology include respiratory function (flow, effort, and gas exchange), limb muscle activity, electrocardiogram, and sometimes esophageal pH or core body temperature. Polysomnography is most useful for sleep disruption such as sleep apnea (Chapter 100), excessive movements, parasomnias, or for unexplained excessive sleepiness[3] (Table 405-2). More limited overnight recordings may focus on strictly respiratory

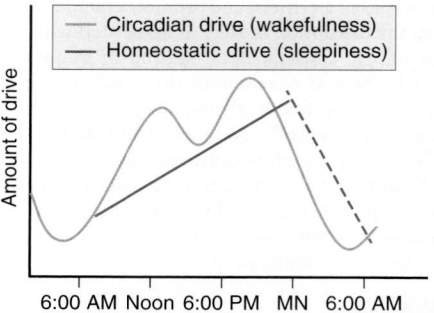

FIGURE 405-1. Idealized graph depicting the two-process model. The circadian driver promotes wakefulness (*orange*), and the homeostatic drive promotes sleep (*blue*). The dynamic interaction of the two drives is shown.

TWO WEEK SLEEP DIARY

INSTRUCTIONS:
1. Write the date, day of the week, and type of day: Work, School, Day Off, or Vacation.
2. Put the letter "C" in the box when you have coffee, cola or tea. Put "M" when you take any medicine. Put "A" when you drink alcohol. Put "E" when you exercise.
3. Put a line (l) to show when you go to bed. Shade in the box that shows when you think you fell asleep.
4. Shade in all the boxes that show when you are asleep at night or when you take a nap during the day.
5. Leave boxes unshaded to show when you wake up at night and when you are awake during the day.

SAMPLE ENTRY BELOW: On a Monday when I worked, I jogged on my lunch break at 1 PM, had a glass of wine with dinner at 6 PM, fell asleep watching TV from 7 to 8 PM, went to bed at 10:30 PM, fell asleep around Midnight, woke up and couldn't got back to sleep at about 4 AM, went back to sleep from 5 to 7 AM, and had coffee and medicine at 7:00 in the morning.

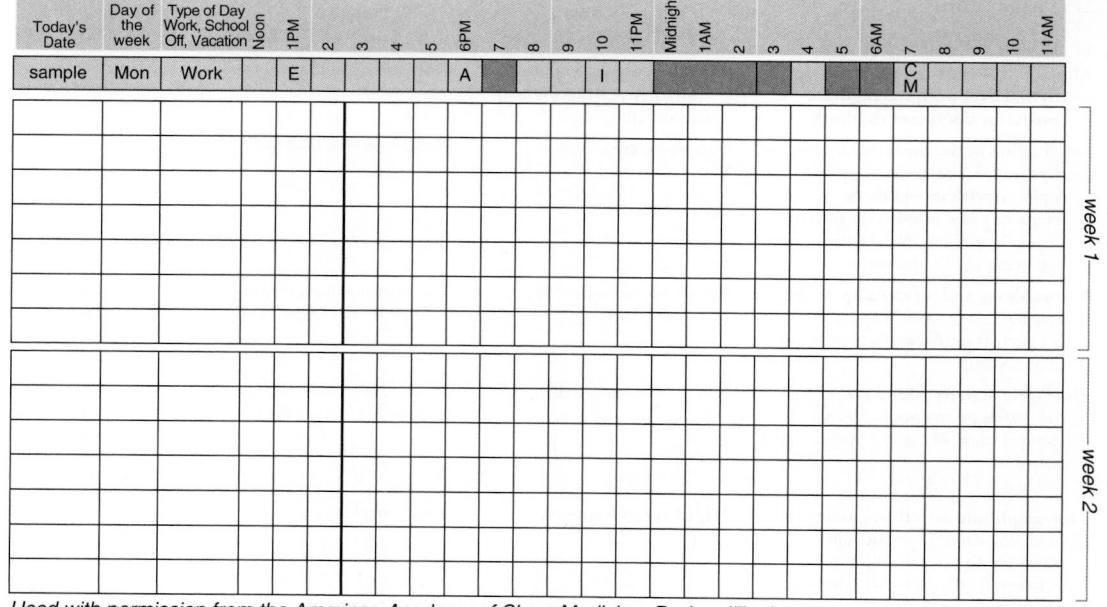

Used with permission from the American Academy of Sleep Medicine, Darien, Illinois.

FIGURE 405-2. Example of a sleep diary. Patients record their daily schedule, work, and medications.

TABLE 405-2 INDICATIONS FOR POLYSOMNOGRAPHY

POLYSOMNOGRAPHY IS ROUTINELY INDICATED FOR:

Diagnosis of sleep-related breathing disorders (SRBD), including suspected obstructive sleep apnea (OSA) in patients with coronary heart disease, history of stroke or transient ischemic attacks, or significant tachyarrhythmias or bradyarrhythmias

Positive airway pressure (PAP) titration in patients with sleep-related breathing disorders

A preoperative clinical evaluation to evaluate for the presence of OSA before upper airway surgery for snoring or OSA

Patients with heart failure if they have nocturnal symptoms suggestive of sleep-related breathing disorders (disturbed sleep, nocturnal dyspnea, snoring) or if they remain symptomatic despite optimal medical management

Patients with neuromuscular disorders and sleep-related symptoms

Patients suspected of periodic limb movement disorder

Polysomnography and multiple sleep latency test on the ensuing day for patients suspected of having narcolepsy

Follow-up polysomnography:

  After titration of oral appliance treatment in patients with moderate to severe OSA

  Following surgical treatment of patients with moderate to severe OSA

  After surgical or dental treatment of patients with SRBDs whose symptoms return

  Substantial weight gain or loss in patients on PAP for SRBD

  Insufficient clinical response to PAP therapy

  Assessment of oral appliance after final fitting (guideline)

Evaluation of patients with sleep behaviors suggestive of unusual or atypical parasomnias or in which specific motor patterns are in question

POLYSOMNOGRAPHY IS OPTIONAL FOR:

Evaluation of sleep behaviors suggestive of potentially injurious parasomnias

POLYSOMNOGRAPHY IS *NOT* ROUTINELY INDICATED FOR:

Patients whose symptoms resolve with continuous positive airway pressure (CPAP) treatment

Diagnosis of chronic lung disease

Diagnosis of typical, uncomplicated, and noninjurious parasomnias when the diagnosis is clearly delineated

Patients with a seizure disorder who have no specific complaints consistent with a sleep disorder

Diagnosis or treatment of restless legs syndrome, except where diagnostic uncertainty exists

Establishing the diagnosis of depression

Diagnosis of circadian rhythm sleep disorders

measurements. Two tests quantify the ability to fall asleep and stay awake: the multiple sleep latency test and maintenance of wakefulness test. The multiple sleep latency test quantifies objective sleepiness based upon the time to onset of sleep across five daytime naps. The multiple sleep latency test is useful for narcolepsy, but there is overlap between normal individuals and patients with sleep disruption. The maintenance of wakefulness test quantifies the propensity to stay awake across four 40-minute epochs, and it can provide objective evidence of the daytime efficacy of stimulant therapy.

HYPERSOMNIA

Sleepiness is normal just prior to a typical sleep period or after prolonged wakefulness. In 5 to 20% of adults, sleep is excessive because it occurs in inappropriate settings. When mild, sleepiness may have a minor effect on quality of life. When severe, however, sleepiness intrudes on activities such as driving, conversation, or eating, and it may cause lapses of attention or diminished cognitive abilities, such as missing an exit on the highway. The perception of sleepiness is reduced with prolonged sleep deprivation, so that chronically sleep-deprived individuals become accustomed to their impairment and fail to recognize their degree of sleepiness.

DIAGNOSIS

Clinicians should question hypersomnic patients for clues about sleep debt, dyssomnia, brain issues, or medical or psychiatric causes (Fig. 405-3). Patients should be queried regarding their schedule during the week and weekends. Information regarding sleep habits and environment may disclose important factors contributing to the sleepiness. Patients with sleep apnea (Chapter 100), narcolepsy, excessive periodic limb movements, circadian rhythm disorders, and parasomnias may have excessive daytime sleepiness as their main complaint. A history of snoring, observed apnea, morning headaches, cataplexy, sleep paralysis, hypnogogic hallucinations, or altered sleep schedule suggests contributions of a specific sleep disorder. Excessive sleepiness can also result from many medical disorders and medications. Patients with heart (Chapter 58), kidney (Chapter 131), or liver failure (Chapter 153), rheumatologic disease, or endocrinologic disorders such as hypothyroidism (Chapter 226) and diabetes (Chapter 229) may note sleepiness and fatigue. Neurologic disorders such as stroke (Chapters 407 and 408), tumor (Chapter 189), demyelinating disease (Chapter 411), and head trauma (Chapter 399) can cause excessive sleepiness.

Sleepiness can be quantified subjectively by questionnaires or by physiologic measures such as a multiple sleep latency test. The Epworth Sleepiness

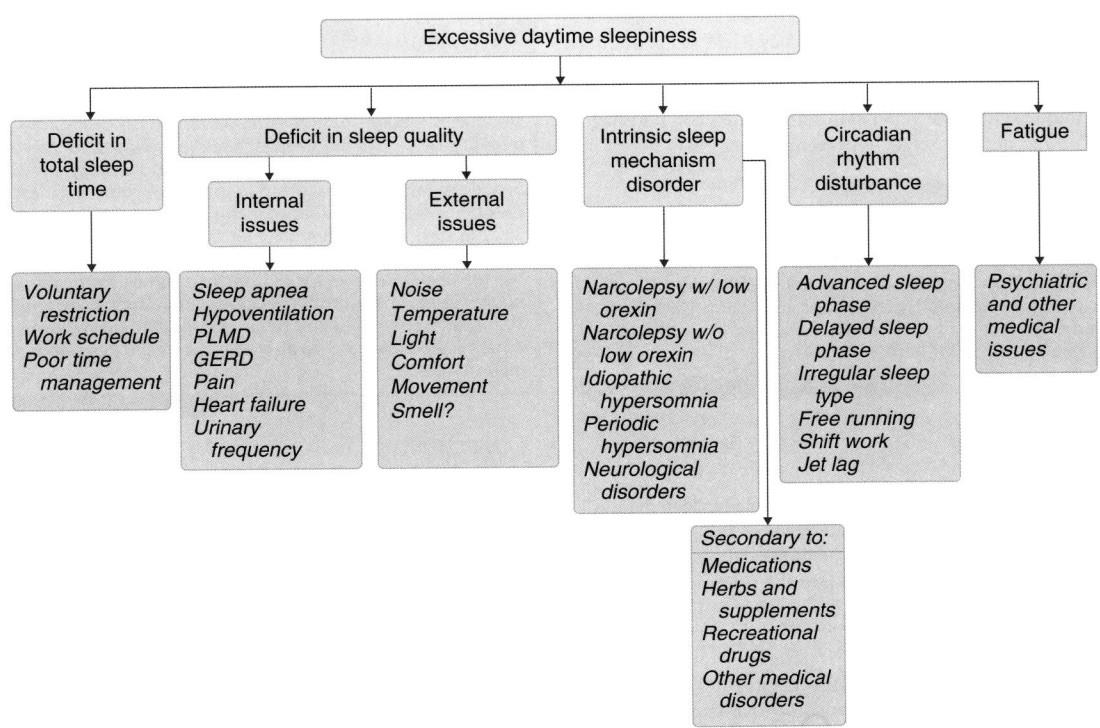

FIGURE 405-3. Differential diagnosis of excessive daytime sleepiness. GERD = gastroesophageal reflux disease; PLMD = periodic limb movement disorder.

TABLE 405-3 EPWORTH SLEEPINESS SCALE

How likely are you to doze off or fall asleep in the following situations, in contrast to just feeling tired? This refers to your usual way of life in recent time. Even if you have not done some of these things recently, try to work out how they would have affected you. Use the following scale to choose the most appropriate number for each situation.

0 = would never doze
1 = slight chance of dozing
2 = moderate chance of dozing
3 = high chance of dozing

SITUATION	CHANCE OF DOZING
Sitting and reading	_____
Watching TV	_____
Sitting and inactive in a public place (theater or meeting)	_____
As a passenger in a car for an hour without a break	_____
Lying down to rest in the afternoon when circumstances permit	_____
Sitting and talking to someone	_____
Sitting quietly after lunch (without alcohol)	_____
In a car, while stopped for a few minutes in traffic	_____
Total	_____

Adapted from Johns MW. A new method for measuring daytime sleepiness: the Epworth Sleepiness Scale. *Sleep.* 1991;14:540-545.

Scale quantifies sleepiness by asking the subject to rate on a scale of 0 to 3 (0, no chance; 3, high likelihood) the chance of dozing in eight situations (Table 405-3). A score of 7 is considered average, whereas a score of 10 or more is consistent with subjective sleepiness. This score has a modest correlation with physiologic measures of sleepiness but a better correlation with the respiratory disturbance index in patients with obstructive sleep apnea (Chapter 100). Daytime studies, the multiple sleep latency test, and the maintenance of wakefulness test, may be used to assess sleepiness or wakefulness across a series of trial "naps." The multiple sleep latency test is validated as a test for narcolepsy, whereas the maintenance of wakefulness test gives a snapshot of the patient's ability to stay awake.

Other Hypersomnias

Idiopathic hypersomnia is a disorder in which hypersomnia cannot be explained by another disorder, is characterized by unrelenting hypersomnia, and is only minimally improved with therapy. Patients find that their symptoms persist despite long sleeping periods. These patients have average sleep latencies of less than 8 minutes, typically do not display REM sleep, but may have stage N3 on their multiple sleep latency test studies. Fluctuating symptoms of hypersomnia can also occur in other disorders such as in Kleine-Levin syndrome (a unique syndrome of periodic hypersomnia, hyperphagia, and hypersexuality) and in perimenstrual hypersomnia.

TREATMENT Rx

Treatment of sleepiness should focus on correcting the underlying cause of sleepiness.[4] Stimulants such as modafinil (200 to 400 mg)[A1] should be used only in individuals who are impaired by the symptoms and in whom other therapies have failed to correct the hypersomnia. Some patients with Kleine-Levin syndrome respond to lithium (Chapter 397).

Narcolepsy
DEFINITION

Narcolepsy includes a tetrad of excessive sleepiness, cataplexy, sleep paralysis, and hypnogogic hallucinations. In the past, narcolepsy was divided into patients with cataplexy (type 1) and patients without it (type 2), but the subtypes of narcolepsy are also defined based upon the presence or absence of the neurotransmitter hypocretin-1.

EPIDEMIOLOGY

Narcolepsy with cataplexy (narcolepsy type 1) affects1 in 2000 to 6000 individuals; 40 to 80% have the complete tetrad, and approximately 50% complain of sleep disruption. Over 90% of individuals in the United States with cataplexy have the HLA-DQB1*0602 gene,[5] and a similar percentage have

low CSF hypocretin-1 levels. Narcolepsy without cataplexy (narcolepsy type 2) occurs in about 2 per 1000 individuals; approximately 40% have the HLA-DQB1*0602 gene, and fewer exhibit low CSF hypocretin-1 levels. Despite the connection to a gene, the risk to first-degree relatives is only 1 to 2%, or about a 10- to 50-fold increased risk compared with the general population.

PATHOBIOLOGY

Narcolepsy with cataplexy (narcolepsy type 1) reflects the loss of hypocretin-producing neurons in the lateral hypothalamus. This neurotransmitter is important for stabilizing the sleep-wake state and for motor control. Thus the manifestations of the disease are related to frequent stage shifts and intrusion of REM sleep atonia into wakefulness. Why these neurons are lost is not known, but immune mechanisms are postulated.[6]

CLINICAL MANIFESTATIONS

The tetrad of excessive sleepiness, cataplexy, hypnogogic hallucinations, and sleep paralysis are the major clinical manifestations. Cataplexy is abrupt loss of muscle tone triggered by strong emotional stimuli such as laughter, surprise, or anger. Patients are aware of their surroundings but lose muscle control, first in the face and neck, followed by the arms and then the trunk and legs. Hypnogogic (sleep-onset) and hypnopompic (sleep-offset) hallucinations are vivid and often frightening visual or auditory events. Sleep paralysis is an inability to move or speak, typically during the transition out of sleep when individuals have complete or partial awareness of their surroundings. Patients may describe a strong feeling of impending doom, being chased, or having to escape imminent danger. Patients with narcolepsy are often considered perpetually sleepy, but most have normal sleep duration over a 24-hour period. However, their sleep is fragmented, with sleep intruding into daily activities and interrupted at night with wakefulness. Sleep paralysis and hypnogogic hallucinations can occur in normal individuals, especially after sleep deprivation, but cataplexy is virtually pathognomonic for narcolepsy.

DIAGNOSIS

The diagnosis of narcolepsy type 1 and type 2 is based upon a mean sleep latency of less than 8 minutes and the presence of REM sleep on at least two of the five naps of a multiple sleep latency test. The multiple sleep latency test is predicated on the documentation of at least 6 hours of sleep prior to the study. The previous night's polysomnography must also not show other sleep pathologies. A low cerebrospinal fluid hypocretin level in the setting of excessive sleepiness can also confirm of the diagnosis of narcolepsy type 1, but this finding is not seen in type 2.

TREATMENT Rx

Treatment of narcolepsy focuses on improving symptoms of excessive sleepiness, cataplexy, and REM sleep intrusion into wakefulness (Table 405-4). Sleepiness requires a three-pronged approach of improving the quality and quantity of nighttime sleep, scheduling naps, and prescribing stimulants. Nighttime sleep may be improved with sodium oxybate (20 to 40 mg/kg in divided nighttime doses), which improves daytime alertness and reduces cataplexy.[A2] Stimulants such as modafinil (100 to 600 mg/day), armodafinil (50 to 250 mg/day), methylphenidate (5 to 60 mg/day), and dextroamphetamine (5 to 60 mg/day) improve daytime function but do not return the patient to a normal level.[7] Patients should not use stimulants in the evening and night hours. Selective serotonin reuptake inhibitors (SSRIs) (Chapter 397, Table 397-5) and combined serotonin-norepinephrine reuptake inhibitors (SNRIs) (Chapter 397, Table 397-5) also reduce cataplexy as well as sleep paralysis and hallucinations.

PROGNOSIS

Narcolepsy is lifelong disorder. Patients who present in adolescence or young adulthood may progress to more severe symptoms, but the disorder does not affect longevity.

SLEEP-RELATED BREATHING DISORDERS
Sleep Apnea

Sleep apnea (Chapter 100) is defined by repetitive breathing pauses that may interrupt sleep hundreds of times per night. The patient's bed partner may note that the patient's breathing has stopped or that the individual "holds their breath," but most patients are unaware of the events. In the sleep laboratory, apneas are defined by cessation of breathing for more than 10

TABLE 405-4 THERAPIES FOR NARCOLEPSY

MODALITY	STARTING DOSE	HIGHEST DOSE	DOSE AT
Scheduled naps	10-15 minutes	15 minutes	Just prior to time needing to be awake
OVER-THE-COUNTER STIMULANT			
Caffeine	25 mg	300 mg	AM
STIMULANTS			
Modafinil	100-200 mg	600 mg	AM and noon
Armodafinil	50-150 mg	250 mg	AM
Methylphenidate	5-10 mg	120 mg	AM and noon
Methylphenidate ER	10-20 mg	120 mg	AM
Dextroamphetamine	5-10 mg	60 mg	AM and noon
Combination dextroamphetamine/amphetamine	5-10 mg	60 mg	AM and noon
IMPROVE NIGHTTIME SLEEP, DAYTIME ALERTNESS, AND CATAPLEXY			
Sodium oxybate	225 mg	900 mg	Bedtime and 4 hr into sleep
THERAPIES FOR CATAPLEXY (NOT FDA APPROVED)			
Fluoxetine	10-20 mg	40 mg	AM
Venlafaxine	75 mg	225 mg	AM at lower dose or divided
Protriptyline	5 mg	40 mg	AM at lower dose or divided

seconds and are usually associated with oxygen desaturation and arousal occurring more frequently than five events per hour of sleep. Sleep apnea is classified as two major forms: obstructive and central. Obstructive apnea is defined as the loss of flow due to obstruction, typically in the upper airway, whereas central apnea is the absence of airflow due to the absence of effort.

Obstructive apnea is the most common form of sleep apnea. Approximately 50% of patients with sleep apnea have daytime sleepiness, but other symptoms such as insomnia and parasomnia events may be clues to underlying obstructive sleep apnea. Standardized questionnaires (Table 405-5) can help select patients for definitive polysomnography (Chapter 100, Fig. 100-1). Treatment typically involves the use of continuous positive airway pressure (CPAP), an oral appliance, or surgery. Neither supplemental oxygen[A3] nor medication[A4] provide substantial benefit.

Central apnea is the absence of ventilation without an effort to breath (Chapter 86). These patients have respiratory pauses that are associated with oxygen desaturation and arousals. Central apneas can be caused by cardiac disease, narcotics, or neurologic abnormalities that result in dysregulation of respiration. Cheyne-Stokes breathing, which may have features of both central and obstructive apnea, often occurs only during sleep. The classical Cheyne-Stokes pattern of crescendo-decrescendo breathing with central apnea can be seen in individuals with heart failure, neurologic lesions, and metabolic or toxic encephalopathies. Central apneas can be diagnosed by overnight polysomnography. The addition of a CO_2 monitor can distinguish between apnea related to normal or low CO_2 versus high CO_2 and help direct treatment. Low CO_2 levels in the presence of apnea may suggest a high CO_2 apnea threshold that may respond to increasing CO_2 levels, whereas apnea in the setting of an elevated CO_2 level would suggest failure of the respiratory control mechanism, as seen in patients who are taking narcotics. Therapy depends upon the etiology but can include reduction or elimination of respiratory suppressants (narcotics), CPAP, bilevel PAP, nocturnal ventilation, and respiratory stimulants.

HYPOVENTILATION

Hypoventilation, as defined by elevated CO_2 levels (Chapter 86), may occur solely during sleep. Patients may note daytime sleepiness, fatigue, morning headache, or unrefreshing sleep. Although the prevalence is unknown, hypoventilation is common in individuals with central obesity, neuromuscular disease, pulmonary disease, and narcotic use. Although typically worse in REM sleep, the elevation of CO_2 and commonly coexisting drop in oxygen saturation is more prolonged than the pattern seen with sleep apnea. Hypoventilation syndrome is treated with positive airway pressure or noninvasive ventilation.

Insomnia
DEFINITION

Insomnia is the complaint of difficulty initiating or maintaining sleep, or of unrefreshing sleep that results in daytime symptoms of excessive fatigue or

TABLE 405-5 STOP-BANG QUESTIONNAIRE FOR OBSTRUCTIVE SLEEP APNEA

Snoring		
Do you snore loudly? (louder than talking or loud enough to be heard through closed doors)	Yes	No
Tired		
Do you often feel tired, fatigued, or sleepy during the daytime?	Yes	No
Observed		
Has anyone observed you stop breathing during your sleep?	Yes	No
Blood pressure		
Do you have or are you being treated for high blood pressure?	Yes	No
Body Mass Index (BMI)		
BMI more than 35 kg/m²?	Yes	No
Age		
Age older than 50 yr?	Yes	No
Neck circumference		
Neck circumference greater than 40 cm?	Yes	No
Gender		
Gender male?	Yes	No
Elevated risk of OSA: answering yes to three or more items		
Low risk of OSA: answering yes to less than three items		

Adapted from Chung F, Yegneswaran B, Liao P, et al. STOP questionnaire: a tool to screen patients for obstructive sleep apnea. *Anesthesiology.* 2008;108:812-821.

impairment of performance.[8] Daytime sequelae differentiate individuals with a limited need for sleep from individuals with insomnia. Chronic insomnia is defined by symptoms that persist more than 1 month.

EPIDEMIOLOGY

Most individuals have occasional nights with difficulty falling asleep or maintaining sleep, often provoked by psychological challenges or sudden changes in their environment. Approximately 35% of individuals complain of intermittent difficulty with sleep, and approximately 10% have chronic insomnia. Women, older individuals, and patients with psychiatric or chronic medical illness are predisposed to develop insomnia. Insomnia is also more common in individuals with lower socioeconomic status and poor education. Patients with behavioral traits such as obsessive-compulsive tendency, frequent rumination, or poor coping strategies are also at greater risk for insomnia. Lack of "good-quality" sleep disrupts life and may lead to other symptoms.

PATHOBIOLOGY

Patients with insomnia frequently give historical clues directed toward the mechanisms behind their insomnia. Studies on patients with insomnia show these individuals are in a state of hyperarousal. Increased brain metabolic rates during NREM sleep may provide a neurophysiologic basis for chronic insomnia. Most patients have multiple factors that contribute to the insomnia, including features that predispose them to insomnia, events that precipitated the insomnia, and behaviors that perpetuate the insomnia. Effective treatment requires identifying these contributing factors. Many patients have a coincident psychiatric disorder (Chapter 397) or psychological or medical issues. Patients with depression or anxiety may have insomnia for years prior to the presentation of the affective disorder. Patients with heart (Chapter 58), liver (Chapter 153), or renal (Chapter 131) failure or disturbances of the gastrointestinal or respiratory systems commonly complain of insomnia. Patients with heart failure may note difficulty remaining in bed owing to breathing issues. Restless legs syndrome frequently presents as insomnia. Pain of any origin can interrupt sleep, and patients with limited mobility, such as muscular dystrophy (Chapter 421) or Parkinson disease (Chapter 409), may have pressure points that awaken them. Sleep schedules may be influenced by disease (e.g., patients with dementia [Chapter 402] in whom circadian rhythm abnormalities promote nighttime awakenings).

CLINICAL MANIFESTATIONS

The patient's symptom complex may give clues to a poor sleep environment, maladaptive behaviors, psychological stress, psychiatric or neurologic disease, primary sleep disorder, or other medical issues. Insomnia may be initiated by events that shift schedules or by a change in medications. Initiating events may play little role in long-term insomnia but give important clues to preventing further recurrence of the insomnia. If insomnia persists, many patients adopt behaviors that perpetuate the insomnia. Maladaptive habits that may occur during the day or night include heavy daytime caffeine or alcohol use, watching television or playing video games while in bed, or eating or exercising during the usual sleep period. A subgroup of patients may develop sleep phobias or have anxiety about the oncoming sleep period. This expectation of poor sleep promotes apprehension about sleep and may perpetuate counterproductive sleep rituals. These maladaptive behaviors become the predominant feature of the subtype of psychophysiologic insomnia (Table 405-6). Some patients exaggerate their symptoms, whereas other patients may not perceive that they are asleep. Individuals with paradoxical insomnia have normal physiologic sleep but do not recognize that they have been asleep. Other patients may have the unrealistic expectation that sleep should not be interrupted by any arousals or that they must sleep a set number of hours. Rarely, idiopathic insomnia starts in childhood and continues as a lifelong difficulty of sleep. These patients may have defective sleep mechanisms. Noting the timing of the insomnia during the sleep period may also be helpful. Difficulty with the onset of sleep suggests an underlying delayed sleep phase, and insomnia with early morning arousal suggests underlying depression or advanced sleep phase. Documentation of schedule changes (e.g., from jet lag or shift work) can be useful in determining links to circadian rhythm issues.

DIAGNOSIS

The diagnosis of insomnia is based upon the patient's history that difficulty with sleep results in daytime sequelae (Fig. 405-4). Frequently, more than one subtype occurs in the same patient, and there is little evidence that subtypes direct therapy.

TABLE 405-6 CLASSIFICATION OF ADULT INSOMNIA
INSOMNIA
Subtypes:
Psychophysiologic insomnia—maladaptive behaviors conditioned in response to associating the bed environment or thoughts of bedtime with heightened arousal; patients typically sleep better in a different environment, such as away on vacation.
Idiopathic insomnia—insomnia beginning in infancy or childhood, with a persistent unremitting course and no improvement with change in environment
Paradoxical insomnia (sleep state misperception)—insomnia characterized by a marked mismatch between the patient's description of sleep duration and objective polysomnographic findings
INSOMNIA ASSOCIATED WITH
Adjustment insomnia—associated with an acute or active psychosocial stressor
Inadequate sleep hygiene—associated with lifestyle habits that impair the ability to sleep
Insomnia comorbid with a psychiatric disorder—associated with an active psychiatric disorder such as anxiety or depression
Insomnia comorbid with a medical condition—associated with a condition such as renal failure, hepatic failure, chronic pain, nocturnal cough or dyspnea, or hot flashes
Insomnia caused by a drug or substance—secondary to consumption or discontinuation of medications, drugs of abuse, alcohol, or caffeine

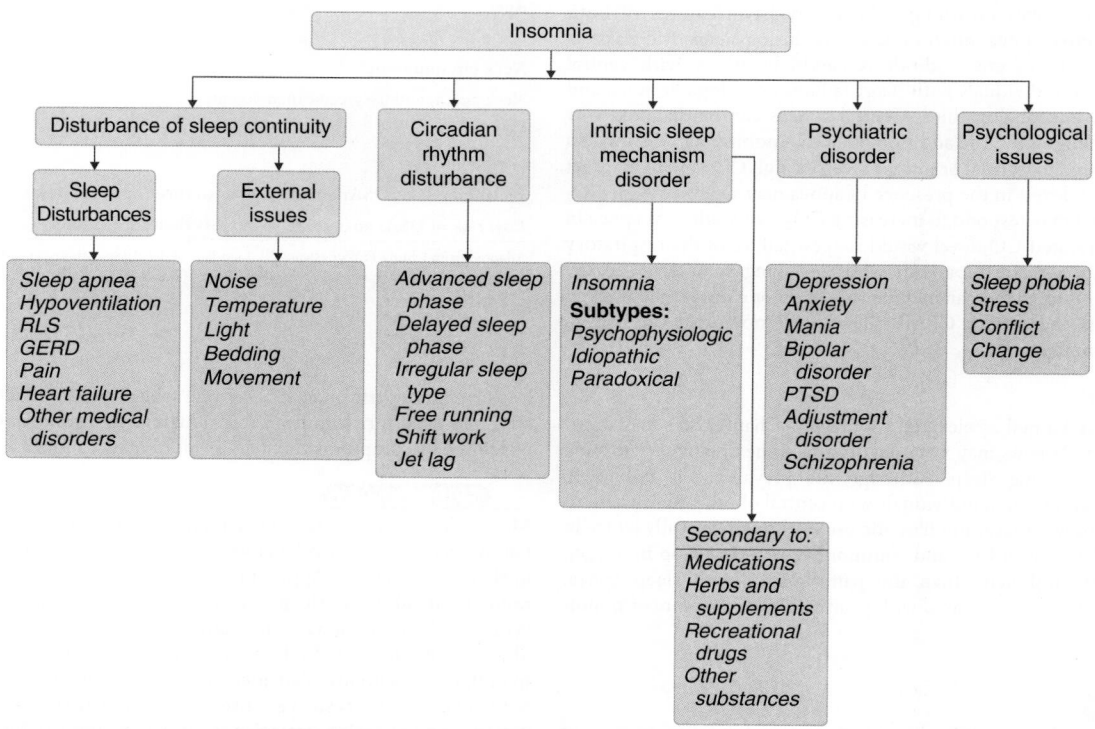

FIGURE 405-4. Differential diagnosis of insomnia. GERD = gastroesophageal reflux disease; PTSD = post-traumatic stress disorder; RLS = restless leg syndrome.

The history should include a review of the patient's 24-hour schedule, meals, caffeine, tobacco and medicine intake, sleep environment, attitudes about sleep, and the sleep experience. In addition, a thorough history from the bed partner may disclose features the patient is unaware of, such as snoring, limb movements, and sleep habits. Patients should be asked to keep a diary of their daily events for at least 3 weeks. This diary will often show specific patterns or clues the patient is unaware of. Actigraphy can also help determine the patient's sleep-wake schedule. Polysomnography should be considered only if the patient has symptoms of sleep apnea or has failed multiple therapeutic trials.

TREATMENT Rx

Insomnia is generally treated as a single disorder even though it has been divided into subtypes (see Table 405-6), but effective treatment requires identifying factors that contribute to insomnia. Treatment is multipronged and includes improving behaviors that promote sleep, addressing the perpetuating factors, and deciding if hypnotic medication is appropriate. Every patient with insomnia needs to develop good sleep hygiene habits that should be reviewed with the patient and bed partner. Cognitive behavioral therapy provides long-term success for insomnia (Table 405-7), but a combination of cognitive behavioral therapy with hypnotics outperforms either alone. The cognitive portion focuses on restructuring beliefs about sleep, whereas behavioral therapies focus on actions that may mitigate maladaptive behaviors and promote better sleep behaviors: progressive relaxation techniques, stimulus control, sleep or time-in-bed restriction, and factors that accentuate homeostatic and circadian drives.

Hypnotics are best used for short-term treatment while starting cognitive behavioral therapy (Table 405-8). The benzodiazepine receptor agonists zolpidem (5 to 10 mg [CR form, 6.25 to 12.5 mg]), zaleplon (5 to 10 mg), and longer-acting eszopiclone (1 to 3 mg) are the usual initial therapies. Agents with rapid onset and a short half-life are used for difficulties initiating sleep. Agents with a longer half-life or continuous-release agents are used for sleep maintenance. Melatonin[AS] or a melatonin receptor agonist (ramelteon 8 mg) improves the initiation and maintenance of sleep. Antidepressant medications (Chapter 397, Table 397-5) are also used for insomnia. Low-dose doxepin (3 and 6 mg) promotes sleep by blocking the effects of central nervous system histamine. In patients with insomnia and an underlying affective disorder, the combination of the short-term use of a hypnotic, such as a benzodiazepine receptor agonist, and long-term antidepressant or anxiolytic is better for both the insomnia and affective disorder than either therapy alone.

PROGNOSIS

Most patients will improve, although some will relapse. Intractable insomnia often heralds an affective disorder (Chapter 397). Except for very rare patients with the prion-induced fatal familial insomnia (Chapter 415), patients with insomnia have only a slightly lower life expectancy, primarily from cardiovascular disease.[9]

Circadian Rhythm Disorders

DEFINITION

Circadian rhythm disorders cause misalignment of the person's sleep-wake cycle and the naturally occurring day-night cycle. Pathologic symptoms must be persistent or recurrent, and the patient must incur some social, occupational, or additional impairment. Individuals may note insomnia, excessive daytime sleepiness, or both. Circadian rhythm sleep-wake disorder is typically classified by comparing the patient's rhythm to the naturally occurring day. Circadian rhythm sleep-wake disorders are subtyped into advanced phase type (early to bed and rise), delayed phase type (late to bed and rise), irregular type (no clear pattern), and free-running type (no entrainment to the environment). Additionally, the inciting situation is included (e.g., jet lag type or shift work type). Another disorder related to circadian rhythm involves the gastrointestinal cycle: night eating syndrome, in which individuals consume over half of their caloric intake after 9 PM.

TABLE 405-7 NONPHARMACOLOGIC THERAPIES FOR INSOMNIA

COGNITIVE BEHAVIORAL THERAPY with or without relaxation therapy (Standard)
The combination of multiple modalities noted below
STIMULUS-CONTROL THERAPY (Standard)
Go to bed only when sleepy.
Use the bedroom only for sleeping and sex.
Go to another room when unable to sleep in 15 to 20 minutes, read or engage in other quiet activities, and return to bed only when sleepy; repeat if necessary.
Have a regular wake time regardless of the duration of sleep.
Avoid daytime napping.
SLEEP-RESTRICTION THERAPY (Guideline)
Reduce time in bed to the estimated total sleep time (minimum, 5 hr).
Increase time in bed by 15 minutes every week when the patient estimates the sleep efficiency is at least 85% (ratio of time asleep to time in bed).
RELAXATION THERAPY (Standard)
Physical component: progressive muscle relaxation, autogenic training
Mental component: reducing intrusive thoughts through imagery training, meditation, or hypnosis
PARADOXICAL INTENTION (Guideline for sleep-onset difficulties)
Instruct the patient to remain passively awake in bed and avoid any effort to fall asleep.
COGNITIVE THERAPY (Insufficient evidence as a single therapy)
Education to alter maladaptive or unrealistic beliefs and attitudes about sleep, such as that a minimum of 8 hours of sleep per night is required for health.
SLEEP HYGIENE EDUCATION (Insufficient evidence as a single therapy)
Correction of extrinsic factors and behaviors that affect sleep, such as environmental disruption (pets, music, or television); bedroom temperature; fixation on the bedside clock; use of alcohol, nicotine, or caffeine; lack of exercise or exercise too close to bedtime.

TABLE 405-8 MEDICATIONS FOR INSOMNIA

NAME	DOSE	TIME OF DOSE	FDA INDICATION	COMMON SIDE EFFECTS	HALF-LIFE	MECHANISM
Melatonin	0.25-6 mg	Evening 1-3 hr before bed	No	Grogginess, headache	30-50 min	Melatonin receptor agonist (dark)
Tryptophan	1-15 g	Evening	No	Drowsiness, headaches, dizziness	1-3 hr	Modulates serotonin
Zolpidem SL	1.75-10 mg	Bedtime	Yes	Sleepiness, amnesia, falls parasomnias	1-2 hr	Benzodiazepine receptor agonist (BZRA)
Zolpidem reg	5-10 mg	Bedtime	Yes	Sleepiness amnesia, falls, parasomnias	1-2 hr	BZRA
Zolpidem CR	6.25-12.5 mg	Bedtime	Yes	Sleepiness, amnesia, falls	1-2 hr but continued release	BZRA
Zaleplon	5-20 mg	Bedtime	Yes	Sleepiness, dizziness, parasomnias	1 hr	BZRA
Eszopiclone	1-3 mg	Bedtime	Yes	Sleepiness, dizziness	4-8 hr	BZRA
Doxepin	3-6 mg	Bedtime	Yes	Drowsiness, dizziness, nausea	17 hr	Histamine receptor antagonist
Mirtazapine	7.5-15 mg	Bedtime	No	Drowsiness, dizziness, weight gain	20 hr	Histamine receptor antagonist
Ramelteon	4-8 mg	Bedtime	Yes	Sleepiness, headache	1-2 hr	Melatonin receptor agonist

FDA = U.S. Food and Drug Administration.

The prevalence of circadian rhythm disorders is not known. Some patterns of sleep are inherent in specific age groups. Advanced sleep phase issues are more common in the elderly, and delayed sleep phase issues are more common in adolescents, but these stereotypes may not indicate the true prevalence of the disorder. Purposeful shifting of the circadian rhythm, such as with shift work or jet lag, is common, but although 28% of the U.S. work-force works nights or rotating shifts, only one third of these individuals have this disorder. A free-running circadian rhythm is more common among blind persons, of whom about 25% have the disorder.

PATHOBIOLOGY

Circadian rhythm sleep-wake disorders may be more prevalent in today's "24-hour society," which offers constant stimuli to remain awake. Teens are more vulnerable to the phase delaying effects of light in the evening. The human "master clock" resides in the suprachiasmatic nucleus of the hypothalamus, but peripheral tissues also generate a self-sustained circadian rhythm based upon clock gene expression. About 2 to 10% of genes are expressed with circadian rhythmicity. Abnormalities in genetic clock genes may contribute to circadian rhythm disorders.[10] Variations in the *Clock*, *Per2*, and *Per3* genes appear to influence the morning/evening preference. Advance sleep phase type has been associated with the *Per2* S662G mutation and the *Ck1d* T44A mutation, whereas delayed sleep phase type is associated with the *Per3* V647G and *Ck1e* S408N mutations. The latter mutation is also associated with free-running type. Free-running type in individuals who are blind appears to be related to the loss of the photoreceptive ganglion cell input to the hypothalamus and not into the retina itself.

CLINICAL MANIFESTATIONS

Circadian rhythm disorders cause insomnia and/or excessive sleepiness. Patients may incur sleep deprivation by trying to maintain schedules that are not consistent with their inherent clocks. Some individuals "catch up" on the weekends by sleeping during their preferred times. Once asleep, the patient has sound sleep. Circadian rhythm sleep-wake disorders are associated with an increased risk of accidents and impair quality of life.

Delayed phase–type patients typically have trouble falling asleep and may not fall sleep for over 2 hours later than the conventional bedtime. They then have trouble arousing in the morning, preferring late wake times. Advanced phase–type patients fall asleep early in the evening and awaken several hours earlier than the conventional morning awakening. Patients complain of early morning awakening and the inability to maintain wakefulness during evening activities. Free-running type individuals have a circadian rhythm that continues to run on the 24.3- to 25-hour cycle. In this disorder, also known as non-24-hour sleep-wake rhythm disorder, patients have alternating episodes of insomnia and excessive sleepiness, depending upon the phase of the endogenous sleep-wake cycle. This disorder can be easily confused with a periodic hypersomnia. Irregular-type patients have both excessive sleepiness and insomnia, with deceased functioning during the waking period.

Jet lag–type patients are affected by temporary changes in the environment owing to travel across time zones. Most find travel west easier than travel east because of the inherent nature of the clock being longer than 24 hours.

Shift work–type patients suffer from circadian misalignment because most shift workers try to resume a typical diurnal pattern on their days off despite nocturnal waking on their work days. This schedule predisposes the worker to poor adaptation.

DIAGNOSIS

The diagnosis of a circadian rhythm disorder is made by history and a 14-day sleep diary or actigraphy recording.[11] Normal individuals have a tendency toward "morningness" or "eveningness," so the diagnosis requires documentation of a negative impact of circadian rhythm on quality of life.

TREATMENT   Rx

Most therapy is directed toward aligning the circadian rhythm with the desired sleep-wake schedule, commonly by gradually shifting the sleep-wake schedule and then maintaining the schedule in the correct phase. Shifting the schedule, known as chronotherapy, can be accomplished by allowing a gradual delay or free running of the inherent schedule (promoted with the use of time clues) to move the phase of the circadian rhythm to the desired time.

Time clues may also be used to fix a circadian rhythm into a specific phase, but the circadian rhythm is susceptible to such clues only if they are given at an appropriate time of the endogenous circadian rhythm. For example, bright light given to a normal individual in the evening delays the cycle, whereas bright light in the morning may advance the cycle. A reliable point of reference is the nadir of the temperature cycle, which typically occurs approximately 2 hours prior to the natural wake up time. Typically, bright light, exercise, food, and social interactions delivered prior to the temperature nadir will delay the cycle, whereas these stimuli delivered after the temperature nadir will advance the cycle. Melatonin has an opposite effect and typically advances the cycle if given 2 to 4 hours prior to the onset of sleep and may delay the cycle if used after the temperature nadir.

After chronotherapy realigns the circadian rhythm, patients with delayed phase type may benefit from morning bright light or from melatonin in the evening. These individuals are subject to relapses, and the schedule should be strictly maintained. Patients with advanced phase type may be misdiagnosed with depression,[12] but they may benefit from evening bright light to delay the onset of sleep. Jet lag can be improved by appropriate use of time clues in reference to the endogenous cycle. Although short-term hypnotics and stimulants are commonly used to help adjustment, these do not realign the circadian rhythm any faster than the usual one time zone per day.

For shift-work disordered sleep, modafinil 100 to 200 mg at the start of the shift may help maintain alertness.[A6] Patients can wear sunglasses to minimize the phase shifting effects of the morning light. Melatonin once they return home and short-term use of a hypnotic may increase sleep duration. Alternatively, some shift workers may find a modified shift in their sleep schedule more appealing—sleeping 8 AM to 4 PM on their work days and 4 AM to noon on their days off. With this schedule, the circadian rhythm shifts by only 4 hours, so patients experience fewer total of hours shifting in any period.

Parasomnia

DEFINITION

Parasomnias are undesirable behavioral events or experiential phenomena occurring during entry into, within, or as part of arousal from sleep. These events include abnormal movements, behaviors, emotions, perceptions, dreaming, and activities of the autonomic nervous system. Parasomnias are typically subdivided into disorders of arousal from NREM sleep, REM sleep-related parasomnias, and other parasomnias. The disorders of arousal include disorders of sleepwalking, sleep terrors, and confusional arousal. REM-related parasomnias include nightmare disorder, REM sleep behavior disorder, and recurrent sleep paralysis. Other parasomnias include sleep-related eating, catathrenia (repetitive nocturnal groaning), or exploding head syndrome.

EPIDEMIOLOGY

Approximately 3% of adults and 15% of children have a sleep-related behavior. Although some parasomnias, such as disorders of arousal from NREM sleep (sleepwalking, sleep terrors, and confusional arousals) are more common in children, others have no age predilection or are more common in older individuals. REM-related parasomnias, such as nightmare disorder, are common among all ages and especially individuals with post-traumatic stress disorder (Chapter 397). REM sleep behavior disorder, which is another REM sleep–related parasomnia, is more common in the elderly, but the exact prevalence is unknown.

CLINICAL MANIFESTATIONS

Individuals and bed partners may complain of frequent movement during sleep. This complaint may be more concerning to the bed partner than the patient. Some individuals will complain of being active sleepers.

DIAGNOSIS

The history is the mainstay of the diagnosis of most parasomnias. Key features include age of onset, time of night of the events, memory for the events, and family history (Table 405-9). Stereotypical behavior, the same behavior with each event, can also help in categorizing the events. Events such as periodic limb movements, rhythmical movement disorder, or epileptic seizures are stereotypical, whereas sleepwalking, sleep or night terrors, and dream enactment have different behavior with each event. Although historical features can help distinguish among these disorders, many patients may require polysomnography to delineate the cause (see Table 405-9).

DISORDERS OF AROUSAL FROM NREM SLEEP

These disorders include a spectrum of behaviors that occur as a partial arousal from deep NREM sleep: sleep walking, sleep terrors, and confusional arousals. Although probably a continuum, the individual symptoms distinguish the

TABLE 405-9 KEY FEATURES OF NOCTURNAL EVENTS

DISORDER	SYMPTOMS	TIME OF NIGHT	DURATION	FREQUENCY	STEREOTYPICAL	MEMORY	POLYSOMNOGRAPHIC FINDINGS
Sleepwalking	Slow, deliberate, complex behaviors	First half of sleep period	Seconds to minutes	Less than one per night to fewer	No	No or partial vague memory	Arousal from slow wave sleep
Sleep terrors	Piercing scream, followed by fight or flight response	First half	Seconds to minutes	Less than one per night or fewer	No	No or partial vague memory	Arousal from slow wave sleep
Confusional arousals	Variety of unusual behaviors upon sudden awakening	Anytime	Seconds to minutes	Less than one per night or fewer	No	No or partial vague memory	Arousal from slow wave sleep
Sleep-related eating	Eating of high-calorie or strange foods in a messy manner	First half	Minutes	May occur nightly	No	No or partial vague memory	Arousal typically from NREM sleep
Nightmares	Frightening dreams associated with anxiety	Latter half	Seconds to minutes	Variable	No, but may have a common theme	Yes	Events occur in REM sleep
REM sleep behavior disorder	Dream enactment, may be violent	Latter half	Seconds	Multiple times per night	No	Yes	Excessive EMG activity in REM sleep
Rhythmic movement disorder	Rocking, head banging	Near sleep onset but may be throughout the night	Minutes to hours	Multiple times per night	Yes	Yes	Rhythmic movement in transition from waking to sleeping
Catathrenia	Nocturnal prolonged moaning	Intermittent throughout the night	Minutes to hours	Multiple	Yes	No	Prolonged expiratory moans and groans, with slowed respiratory rate
Exploding head syndrome	Loud painless sound of explosion inside the head	Near the onset of sleep	Seconds	Rare, typically infrequent	Yes	Yes	Typically events are close to sleep onset

EMG = electromyogram; NREM = non–rapid eye movement; REM = rapid eye movement.

disorders. Individuals with sleepwalking have ambulation as part of their episodes, whereas sleep terrors are accompanied by a piercing scream or cry and expression of intense fear. Confusional arousals are characterized by disorientation, slow speech, and mentation or inappropriate behavior such as eating, fighting, or sexual intimacy. Pathobiologically, these individuals have NREM sleep simultaneously with the awake state. These events are more common in the first third of the night, are associated with no or little memory for the event, and are not stereotypical. Events are more likely to occur after sleep deprivation, alcohol ingestion, sleeping in strange environments, or coincidental conditions such as sleep apnea that evoke arousals. Patients are neurologically and psychiatrically normal during wakefulness. Polysomnography shows the episodes occur during slow wave sleep, with some features of wakefulness. Therapy includes ensuring safety for those who may injure themselves or others (e.g., placing the bed on the floor, blocking windows, or moving the patient's bedroom to the ground floor), decreasing factors that may cause arousals, and avoiding inciting factors such as sleep deprivation or alcohol. There are no established medications, but treatment of sleep apnea (Chapter 100) appears to reduce events. Other treatments, such as clonazepam 0.5 to 2 mg and tricyclic antidepressants (Chapter 397, Table 397-5), have been tried with varying success.

REM SLEEP BEHAVIOR DISORDER
In REM sleep behavior disorder, patients lose the characteristic sleep and muscle atonia of REM sleep and act out during their dreams.[13] REM sleep behavior disorder can be violent, with patients injuring themselves or bed partners. This elaborate motor activity is often associated with vivid recall of a dream that correlates with the witnessed behavior. Patients can have single or multiple events, commonly in the latter half of the night. REM sleep behavior disorder usually begins in late adulthood, but it can occur in children. This behavior disorder can be induced by medications such as tricyclic antidepressants, monoamine oxidase inhibitors, and serotonin reuptake inhibitors. Chronic REM sleep behavior disorder has been linked to alpha-synucleinopathies and the subsequent development of disorders such as Parkinson disease (Chapter 409), multiple system atrophy (Chapter 409), and Lewy body dementia (Chapter 402); over two thirds of adult patients with REM sleep behavior disorder eventually develop a neurodegenerative disease. The diagnosis is based upon the presence of excessive electromyographic

activity during REM sleep and the history of dream enactment. Patients should be evaluated for signs of degenerative disorders (Chapters 402 and 409), strokes (Chapters 407 and 408), posterior fossa tumors (Chapter 189), or demyelinating disease (Chapter 411). Most patients respond well to clonazepam (0.25 to 3 mg) or melatonin (1 to 9 mg).

NIGHTMARES
Nightmares or recurrent disturbing dreams can be a presenting symptom of a sleep disturbance. Nightmares are emotionally intense dreaming associated with fear, anxiety, anger, sadness, or other negative emotions. Individuals awaken from stage R or light NREM sleep to full alertness and usually recall the event immediately. Nightmares are most commonly associated with a psychologically disturbing event, but they also may occur as a result of anti-hypertensive medications, antidepressants, or dopamine agonists. If related to medication, treatment starts with removal of the provocative substance. Prazosin (5 to 20 mg) and imagery rehearsal may be effective.

OTHER PARASOMNIAS
Individuals with sleep-related eating disorder consume high-calorie, sometimes bizarre, foods during sleep and have no or little memory for the consumption. They have morning anorexia and unexplained weight gain. Catathrenia is a rare disorder characterized by repetitive nocturnal groaning. Bed partners usually express concern because the patient has long expiratory groans that sound mournful. These patients respond to CPAP. Rhythmic movement disorder includes a variety of stereotyped movements, usually involving large muscles, that are sustained into light sleep. Movements may include head banging, body rocking, leg rolling, humming, and chanting. Patients are unaware of the movement or describe the movement as a compulsion prior to sleep. This behavior is difficult to treat but diminishes with age. Exploding head syndrome is an abrupt sensation or perceived loud sound of an explosion near the onset of sleep. It is painless, and the events are not a harbinger of other underlying pathology.

RESTLESS LEGS SYNDROME
Restless legs syndrome (Chapter 420) is characterized by four essential features: discomfort or urge to move, worse with rest, better with movement, and worse in the evening.[14] Patients may complain of an unpleasant crawling

or deep unusual sensation in the legs or arms, with improvement after moving the extremities. Patients with restless legs syndrome may relay that the discomfort can be debilitating and cause them to walk or continuously move their legs until the early morning hours. Some patients note that their legs will move or dance on their own, thereby indicating periodic limb movements in wakefulness. About 85 to 90% of restless legs syndrome patients will have periodic limb movements in sleep, but only a minority of patients with periodic limb movements in sleep will meet the clinical criteria of restless legs syndrome.

FDA-approved therapies for restless legs syndrome are dopamine agonists (pramipexole 0.125 to 1.5 mg or ropinirole 0.25 to 3 mg), transdermal rotigotine (1 to 3 patch/24 hours), and gabapentinoid medications (e.g., gabapentin-encarbil 600 to 1800 mg).[15] Augmentation, in which a dopamine agonist increases the severity of symptoms, is treated by carefully substituting another agent, such as pregabalin (300 mg daily),[A7] for the dopamine agonist. In some patients, restless legs syndrome has linked to low iron in the central nervous system. Some patients improve with oral iron therapy (e.g., 325 mg ferrous sulfate two to three times per day for 3 to 4 months until ferritin levels exceed 50 mg/L and iron saturations exceed 20%), and some require more aggressive intravenous iron therapy. More intractable patients may require chronic narcotics (Chapter 30, Table 30-4).[A8]

Grade A References

A1. Philip P, Chaufton C, Taillard J, et al. Modafinil improves real driving performance in patients with hypersomnia: a randomized double-blind placebo-controlled crossover clinical trial. *Sleep.* 2014;37:483-487.

A2. Alshaikh MK, Tricco AC, Tashkandi M, et al. Sodium oxybate for narcolepsy with cataplexy: systematic review and meta-analysis. *J Clin Sleep Med.* 2012;8:451-458.

A3. Gottlieb DJ, Punjabi NM, Mehra R, et al. CPAP versus oxygen in obstructive sleep apnea. *N Engl J Med.* 2014;370:2276-2285.

A4. Mason M, Welsh EJ, Smith I. Drug therapy for obstructive sleep apnoea in adults. *Cochrane Database Syst Rev.* 2013;5:CD003002.

A5. Ferracioli-Oda E, Qawasmi A, Bloch MH. Meta-analysis: melatonin for the treatment of primary sleep disorders. *PLoS ONE.* 2013;8:e63773.

A6. Liira J, Verbeek JH, Costa G, et al. Pharmacological interventions for sleepiness and sleep disturbances caused by shift work. *Cochrane Database Syst Rev.* 2014;8:CD009776.

A7. Allen RP, Chen C, Garcia-Borreguero D, et al. Comparison of pregabalin with pramipexole for restless legs syndrome. *N Engl J Med.* 2014;370:621-631.

A8. Trenkwalder C, Benes H, Grote L, et al. Prolonged release oxycodone-naloxone for treatment of severe restless legs syndrome after failure of previous treatment: a double-blind, randomised, placebo-controlled trial with an open-label extension. *Lancet Neurol.* 2013;12:1141-1150.

GENERAL REFERENCES

For the General References and other additional features, please visit Expert Consult at https://expertconsult.inkling.com.

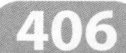

406

APPROACH TO CEREBROVASCULAR DISEASES

LARRY B. GOLDSTEIN

DEFINITION

The term *cerebrovascular disease* refers to a group of conditions in which injury to the brain or spinal cord occurs from a vascular cause. The onset is generally abrupt, but it also can be insidious. Clinical manifestations depend on the location and extent of damage to neural structures. Although risk factors and treatments may overlap, cerebrovascular diseases are pathophysiologically divided into those in which an insufficiency in the blood supply causes ischemic injury and those in which bleeding, either into the parenchyma (intracerebral or much more rarely intraspinal hemorrhage) or into the space between the pial and arachnoid coverings over the brain or spinal cord (subarachnoid hemorrhage), causes direct neural injury, leads to secondary ischemic injury, or acts as a space-occupying lesion. Cerebrovascular disease is often both preventable and treatable.

EPIDEMIOLOGY

Nearly 800,000 Americans have a stroke each year, and about 75% are first strokes. Measured in terms of disease-attributed healthy years of life lost, cerebrovascular disease ranks second in the United States and third worldwide.[1] Stroke, which is a generic term for cerebrovascular disease, has fallen from the third to the fourth leading cause of death in the United States (behind heart disease, cancer, and lung and respiratory diseases), primarily because of a dramatic reduction in stroke-related mortality. From 2000 to 2010, the annual stroke death rate in the United States fell by about 36%, with the actual number of stroke-related deaths falling by about 23%.[2] Stroke is the underlying cause of death of about 130,000 Americans each year, corresponding to approximately 1 in 19 deaths in the country. About 60% of stroke deaths occur in women, but the rates are actually highest in African American men. It is estimated that someone in the United States has a stroke about once every 40 seconds.

The overall prevalence of stroke is estimated at 2.8%, with 6.8 million American adults having had a stroke.[2] Even though the incidence of stroke has been declining substantially, largely because of better prevention, the declining case-fatality rate has kept the population prevalence reasonably stable.

The risk of stroke generally increases with age, and it doubles for every decade after the age of 55 years. In addition, blacks, people with lower levels of education, individuals who reside in the southeastern portion of the country (the "Stroke Belt"), and individuals with a first-degree relative who had a stroke before the age of 65 years have a higher risk of stroke and of stroke-related mortality. Poor diet, lack of exercise (Chapter 16), cigarette smoking (Chapter 32), exposure to environmental tobacco smoke, obesity (Chapter 220), and excess alcohol consumption (Chapter 33) are lifestyle factors that greatly increase the risk of stroke. Of the medical conditions that increase the risk of stroke, hypertension (Chapter 67) has the highest population-attributable risk. Other stroke risk factors include atrial fibrillation (Chapter 64), diabetes (Chapter 229), dyslipidemia (Chapter 206), inflammatory states, elevated homocysteine levels, high lipoprotein (a), carotid artery stenosis, patent foramen ovale (Chapter 69), other congenital heart defects, and sleep apnea (Chapter 100).[3] Coagulation disorders (Chapter 176), oral contraceptive agents (Chapter 238), and migraine headache with aura (Chapter 398) also may contribute to the risk. Mendelian diseases associated with stroke include sickle cell disease (Chapter 163); mitochondrial encephalopathy, lactic acidosis, and stroke (MELAS); cerebral autosomal dominant arteriopathy with subcortical infarcts and leukoencephalopathy (CADASIL; Chapter 402); Fabry disease (Chapters 208 and 275); and Marfan syndrome (Chapter 260). In addition, autosomal dominant polycystic kidney disease (Chapter 127) is associated with intracranial aneurysms and fibromuscular dysplasia. Ehlers-Danlos type IV (Chapter 260) is also associated with intracranial aneurysms as well as cervical arterial dissection. Several genetic polymorphisms also have been associated with stroke (e.g., variants on chromosome 9p21 and 4q25), although these genetic markers are not yet clinically relevant.

PATHOBIOLOGY

Anatomy

An understanding of vascular anatomy and its normal variants as well as their relationships to functional neuroanatomy can provide important clues for identifying the cause of cerebrovascular symptoms and signs in individual patients and can also help guide treatment.

Aortic Arch

Paired carotid and vertebral arteries normally supply the brain (Fig. 406-1). The right common carotid artery arises from the brachiocephalic trunk (innominate artery), which then gives rise to the right subclavian artery. The right vertebral artery generally arises from the proximal portion of the right subclavian artery. The left common carotid artery usually arises directly from the aortic arch; but in some individuals, it may arise from the proximal portion of the brachiocephalic trunk ("bovine" anatomy). The left subclavian artery originates from the aortic arch distal to the left common carotid artery and also supplies the left vertebral artery.

Internal Carotid Arteries

The common carotid arteries bifurcate into the internal carotid artery and external carotid artery in the neck, generally at the level of the thyroid cartilage. The bifurcation may less commonly occur above the lower level of the

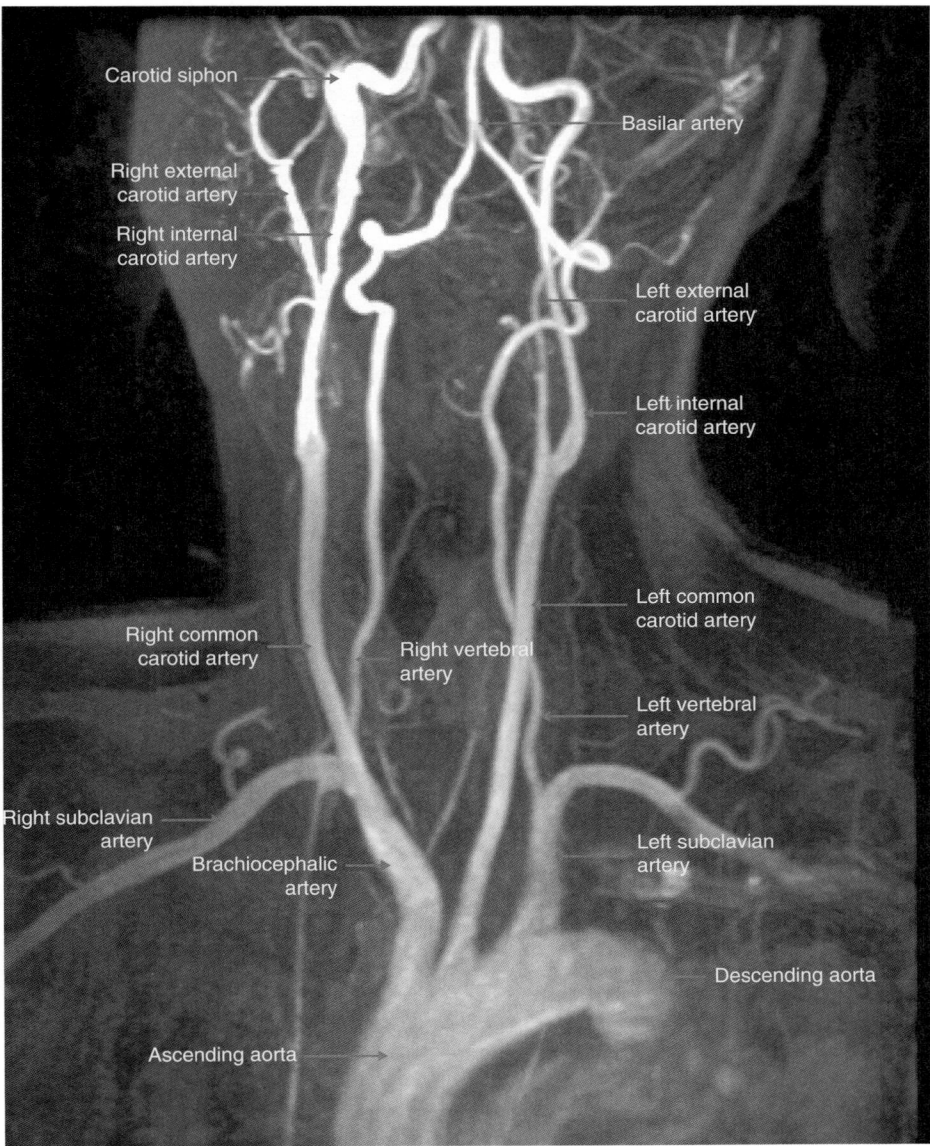

FIGURE 406-1. Magnetic resonance angiogram of normally configured aortic arch.

mandible or lower in the neck. The internal carotid artery enters the skull through the foramen lacerum and travels through the petrous bone adjacent to the inner ear. It then enters the cavernous sinus, ascends in an S shape (carotid siphon), penetrates the dura, and finally divides into the anterior cerebral artery and middle cerebral artery (Fig. 406-2). The ophthalmic artery can originate from the internal carotid artery in the carotid siphon, but it more commonly arises from the supraclinoid internal carotid artery, followed by the posterior communicating and anterior choroidal arteries.

External Carotid Arteries

In contrast to the internal carotid arteries, the external carotid arteries have extracranial branches. The superficial temporal arteries (palpable anterior to the ears) and facial arteries can anastomose with the intracranial circulation through branches of the ophthalmic artery and can be clinically important in the setting of a proximal internal carotid artery occlusion.

Vertebral Arteries

Although the vertebral arteries generally arise from the subclavian arteries, they can also originate from the aortic arch or thyrocervical trunk. They most commonly enter the C6 transverse process but may also enter at the C4, C5, or C7 levels. They exit the transverse processes at C1, turn posteriorly behind the atlantoaxial joint, and then pass through the dura at the foramen magnum.

Intracranially, they typically join at the pontomedullary junction to form the single basilar artery, although the vertebral artery can end in the posterior inferior cerebellar artery in some individuals (Fig. 406-3). The portion of the vertebral artery between its origin and its entry into the transverse process is referred to as the V1 segment. The V2 segment refers to the portion of the artery traveling through the transverse foramina; the V3 segment, the portion between where the artery exits the transverse foramina and penetrates the dura; and the V4 segment, the intracranial portion of the artery. One vertebral artery may be hypoplastic. Clues are that the ipsilateral transverse foramina are generally smaller on the side of the hypoplastic artery and that the proximal portion of the basilar artery can be displaced ipsilateral to the hypoplastic artery. The V3 segment is particularly vulnerable to mechanical injury that can lead to dissection. The vertebral arteries have medial branches that unite to form the anterior spinal artery and lateral branches that supply the dorsolateral medulla and inferior portion of the cerebellum, which also supplies the vestibular nuclei (Fig. 406-4). Other medial branches of the vertebral artery supply the medullary pyramid, inferior olivary nucleus, medial lemniscus, and hypoglossal nerve fibers. Longer circumferential branches from the vertebral arteries and posterior cerebral arteries supply the spinothalamic tracts and sympathetic fibers as they traverse the medulla, the sensory nuclei, and the descending tracts from cranial nerve V as well as emerging fibers from the vagus and glossopharyngeal nerves.

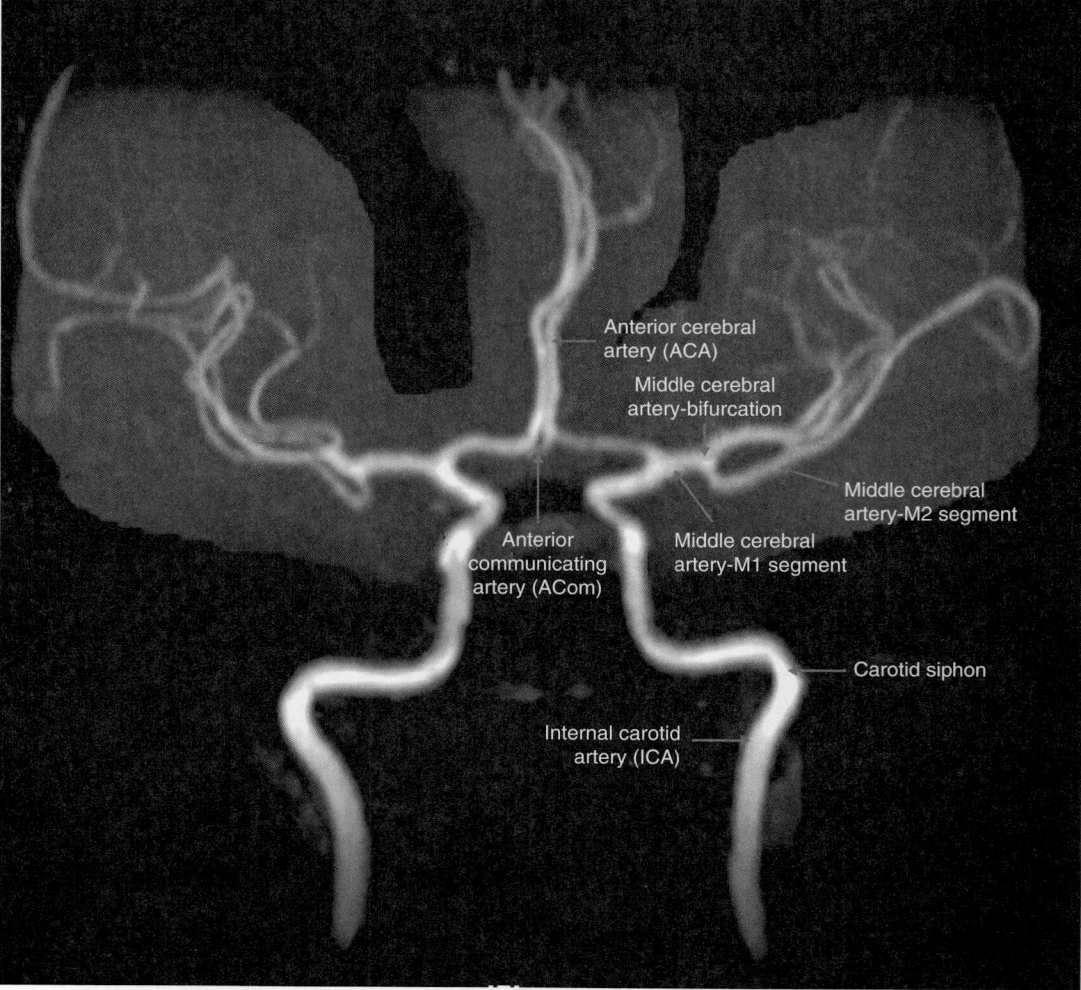

FIGURE 406-2. Magnetic resonance angiogram of the intracranial portion of the internal carotid artery and its main branches.

Basilar Artery

The basilar artery has small penetrating branches supplying the dorsal portions of the pons and midbrain (see Figs. 406-3 and 406-4). The anterior inferior cerebellar arteries originate from the mid–basilar artery. They supply portions of the cerebellar hemispheres in addition to the lateral pons; cranial nerves V, VII, and VIII; and pontine portions of the spinothalamic tracts and sympathetic fibers. The two superior cerebellar arteries arise from the distal basilar artery at the level of the midbrain proximal to the common origin of the two posterior cerebral arteries. The oculomotor nerve exits the midbrain between the superior cerebellar artery and posterior cerebral artery. The superior cerebellar arteries give branches supplying the dorsal midbrain, including the colliculi and the superior portions of the cerebellar hemispheres and vermis. The long circumferential vessels also supply the dorsolateral brain stem.

In addition to the anterior inferior cerebellar artery and superior cerebellar artery, the basilar artery has paramedian vessels supplying the middle portion of the basis pontis and midline pontine structures, including the corticospinal tracts, medial longitudinal fasciculus, and pontine reticular nuclei. At the midbrain level, paramedian branches of the basilar artery supply the cerebral peduncles, cranial nerve III nuclei and fibers, and medial portions of the red nucleus and medial lemniscus. Short circumferential branches supply the ventrolateral pons and midbrain.

Circle of Willis

The anastomosis at the base of the brain is termed the circle of Willis. The two anterior cerebral arteries are connected by the anterior communicating artery. The posterior communicating arteries connect the supraclinoid internal carotid arteries with the proximal posterior cerebral arteries. In persons with an intact circle of Willis, the entire intracranial circulation can be sup-

plied by a single patent internal carotid artery or vertebral artery. The majority of individuals, however, have an incomplete circle of Willis (see Fig. 406-2). One common variant is for the portion of the anterior cerebral artery between the internal carotid artery and the anterior communicating artery (A1 segment) to be hypoplastic or absent. In this case, both anterior cerebral arteries can be supplied from a single internal carotid artery. Another common variant is for the portion of the posterior cerebral artery between its normal origin from the basilar artery and the posterior communicating artery (P1 segment) to be absent or hypoplastic (termed a "fetal" posterior cerebral artery). In these individuals, the distal posterior cerebral artery territory is supplied by the carotid rather than by the vertebrobasilar arteries.

Anterior Cerebral Arteries

The anterior cerebral arteries travel anteriorly and then turn posteriorly with leptomeningeal branches supplying the medial portions of the frontal and parietal lobes (Figs. 406-5 to 406-7; see also Fig. 406-2). In about half of people, the anterior cerebral artery divides into pericallosal and callosal marginal branches. Terminal portions of the latter artery supply the medial cortex between the parietal and occipital lobes. Damage to this area can be confused with "watershed" hypoperfusion injury. A series of small lenticulostriate arteries originate from the A1 and A2 (between the anterior communicating artery and corpus callosum) segments of the anterior cerebral artery. The recurrent artery of Heubner is a large, important medial striate artery that provides blood supply to the anterior and inferior portions of the anterior limb of the internal capsule, anterior and inferior portions of the caudate nucleus, anterior globus pallidus, putamen, hypothalamus, olfactory bulbs and tracts, and uncinate fasciculus. It can be inadvertently damaged during surgical clipping of an anterior communicating artery aneurysm.

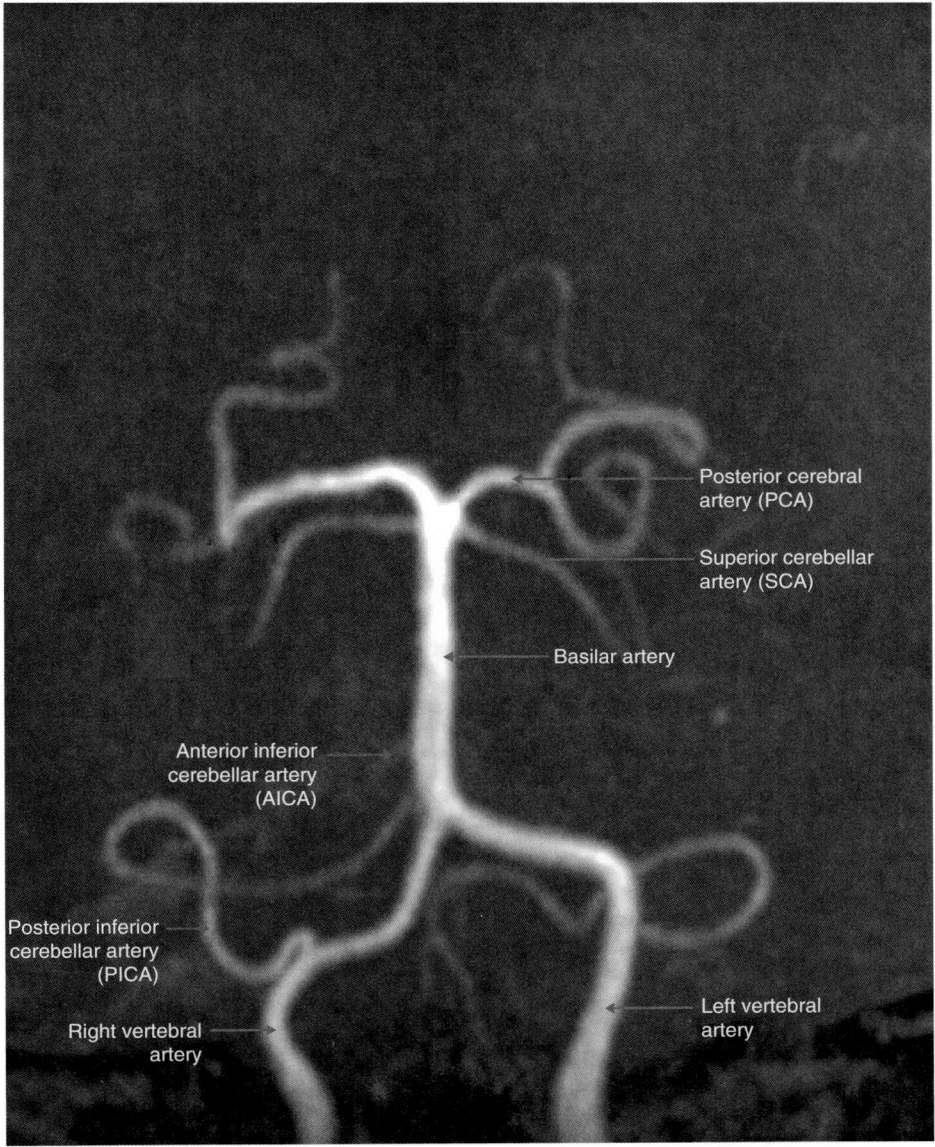

FIGURE 406-3. Magnetic resonance angiogram of the intracranial portion of the vertebrobasilar system.

Anterior Choroidal Artery

The anterior choroidal artery (medial striate artery) commonly arises from the supraclinoid internal carotid artery distal to the posterior communicating artery. It travels posteriorly over the medial optic tract and enters the brain at the choroidal fissure. It gives branches to the optic tract, anterior hippocampus, amygdala, tail of the caudate nucleus, geniculate body, and inferior portion of the posterior limb of the internal capsule (see Fig. 406-7). Ischemic lesions in this area can be confused with lesions arising from the middle cerebral artery.

Middle Cerebral Artery

The middle cerebral artery supplies the bulk of the frontal, parietal, and lateral portions of the temporal lobes (Figs. 406-8 and 406-9; see also Figs. 406-6 and 406-7). The M1 segment refers to the portion of the middle cerebral artery between its origin from the supraclinoid internal carotid artery and its distal branches (see Fig. 406-2). The middle cerebral artery bifurcates in the sylvian fissure in 20 to 30% of individuals and trifurcates in about 70% of individuals. The superior division supplies the frontal and parietal lobes, and the inferior division supplies the lateral portion of the temporal lobe. The M1 segment gives rise to some medial and all of the lateral lenticulostriate arteries. These arteries supply the head and body of the caudate nucleus, the putamen, and the globus pallidus as well as the anterior limb,

genu, and superior portions of the posterior limb of the internal capsule (see Fig. 406-7).

Posterior Cerebral Artery

The distal portion of the posterior cerebral artery divides into an anterior and a posterior division (see Fig. 406-3). The anterior division supplies the inferior and medial portions of the temporal lobe into the middle cranial fossa with distal branches anastomosing with those of the middle cerebral artery. The posterior division supplies the occipital lobe, including the calcarine cortex, with terminal branches anastomosing with those of the middle cerebral artery and anterior cerebral artery. The proximal portions of both the posterior cerebral artery and the posterior communicating artery give off small penetrating arteries to the thalamus (thalamoperforators). In some individuals, a single common artery arising from the P1 segment (artery of Percheron) can supply both thalami. Unless the posterior cerebral artery has a fetal-type origin from the internal carotid artery, thalamic strokes are generally related to the vertebrobasilar circulation. Two posterior choroidal arteries arise separately from the posterior cerebral artery and supply the choroid plexus, posterior thalamus, fornix, and midbrain tectum. Posterior cerebral artery perforators also supply the medial portions of the cerebral peduncles, substantia nigra, red nuclei, hippocampus, and posterior hypothalamus.

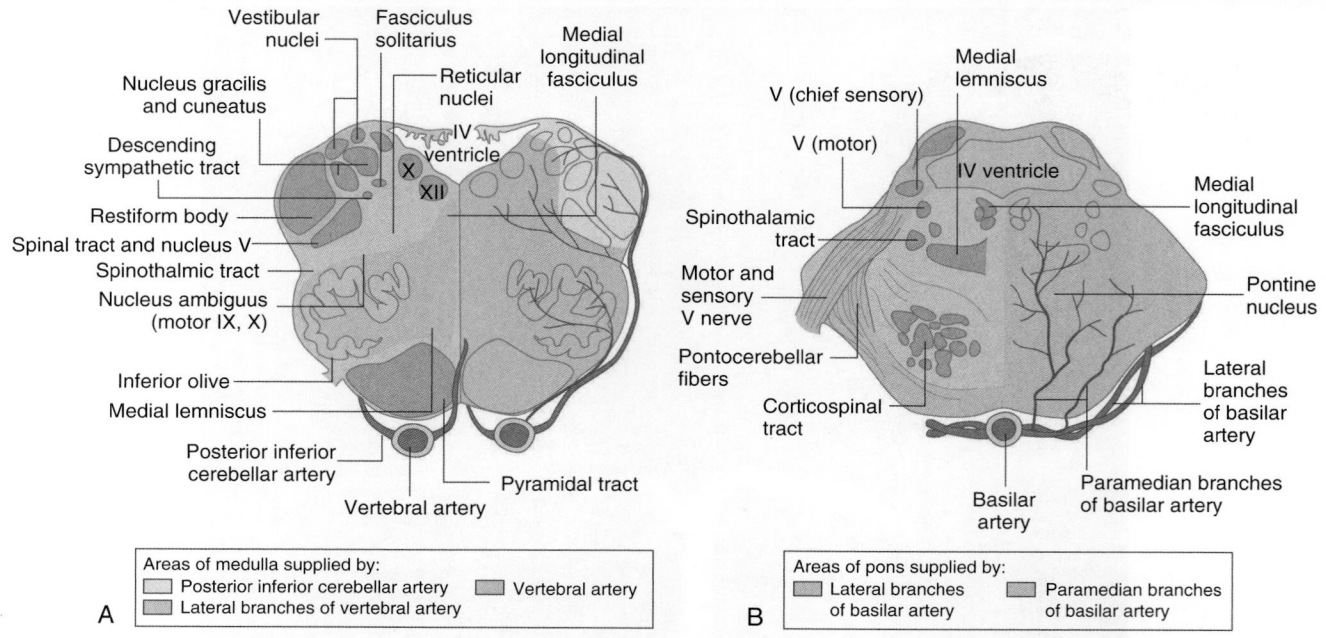

FIGURE 406-4. Brain stem blood supply. **A,** Cross section of the medulla oblongata at the level of the hypoglossal nuclei (cranial nerve XII). Short branches of the vertebral and anterior spinal arteries supply the medulla. Longer circumferential branches, including the posterior inferior cerebellar artery, supply the lateral portions of the medulla. **B,** Cross section of the midpons region. The medial portion receives blood supply from short, perforating basilar artery branches. More laterally, the blood supply comes from lateral basilar artery branches. (From Zivin JA. Approach to cerebrovascular diseases. In: Goldman L, Schafer AI. *Goldman's Cecil Medicine.* 24th ed. Philadelphia: Elsevier Saunders; 2012.)

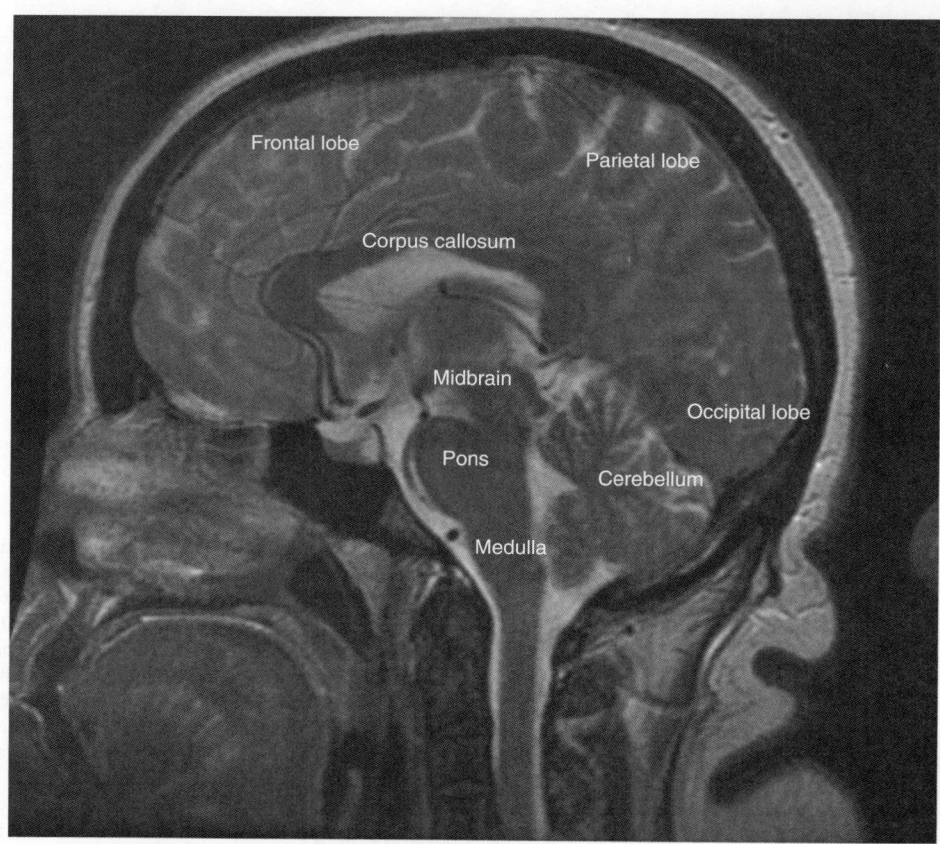

FIGURE 406-5. Parasagittal T2-weighted magnetic resonance image showing midline structures.

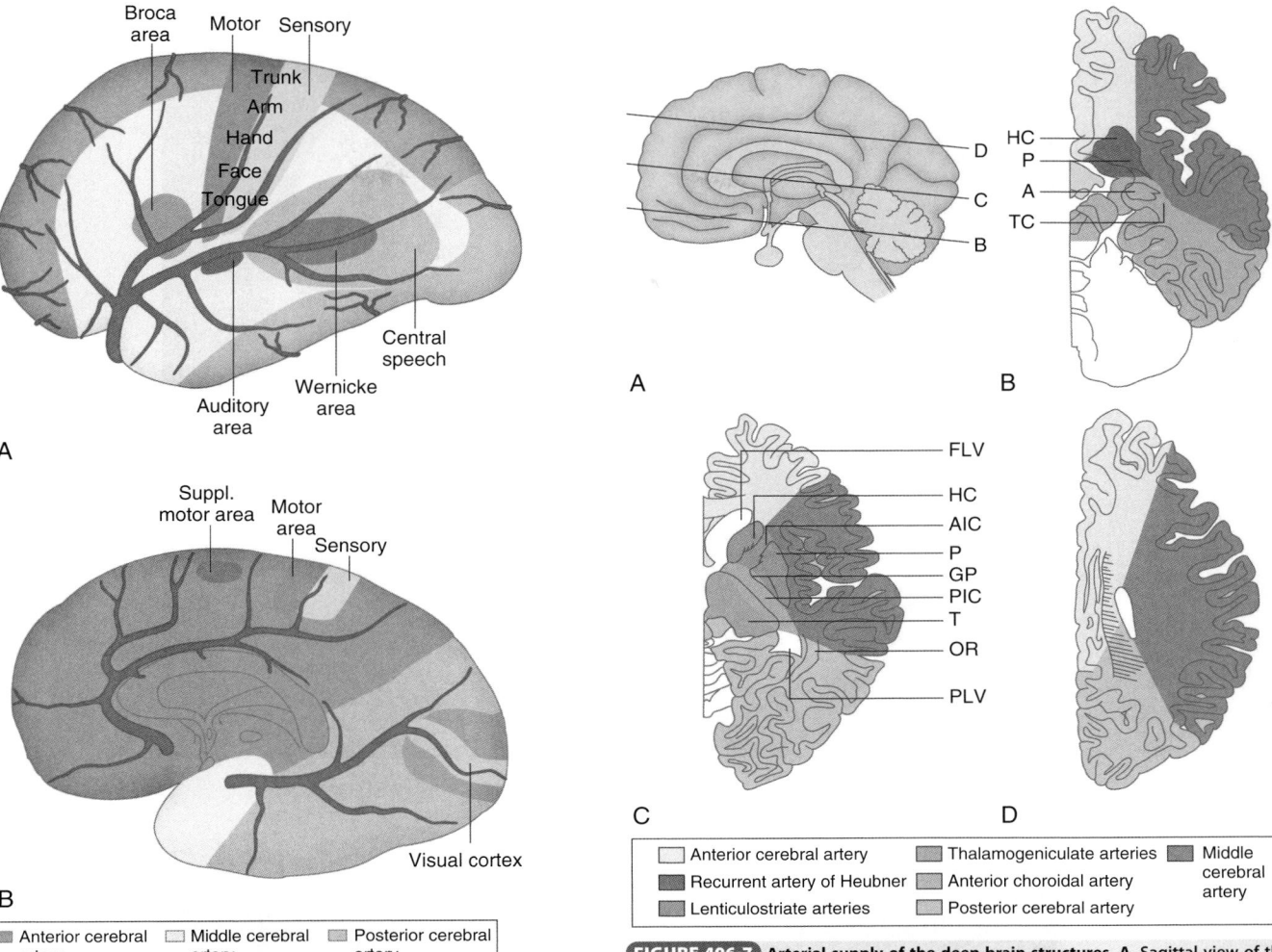

FIGURE 406-6. Surface cerebral arterial anatomy. Lateral (A) and medial (B) views of the cerebral hemisphere show the surface distributions of the anterior, middle, and posterior cerebral arteries. (From Zivin JA. Approach to cerebrovascular diseases. In: Goldman L, Schafer AI. *Goldman's Cecil Medicine.* 24th ed. Philadelphia: Elsevier Saunders; 2012.)

FIGURE 406-7. Arterial supply of the deep brain structures. A, Sagittal view of the brain showing the computed tomographic (CT) planes through which views B, C, and D were taken. B, CT plane through the head of the caudate nucleus (HC), putamen (P), amygdala (A), tail of the caudate nucleus (TC), hypothalamus, temporal lobe, midbrain, and cerebellum. C, CT plane through the frontal horn of the lateral ventricle (FLV), head of the caudate nucleus (HC), anterior and posterior limbs of the internal capsule (AIC, PIC), putamen (P), globus pallidus (GP), thalamus (T), optic radiations (OR), and posterior horn of the lateral ventricle (PLV). D, CT plane through the centrum semiovale. (Modified from De Armond S, Fusco MM, Dewey MM. *Structure of the Human Brain, a Photographic Atlas.* 3rd ed. New York: Oxford University Press; 1989, with permission.)

Venous System

The venous drainage of the brain is divided into superficial and deep systems (Figs. 406-10 and 406-11). Deep structures drain into the inferior sagittal sinus and vein of Galen that join to form the straight sinus, which runs along the tentorium to join the superior sagittal sinus at the torculum. The cerebral veins drain into the sagittal sinus. The two transverse sinuses extend laterally from the torculum into the sigmoid sinus, which then forms the jugular vein. Oftentimes, one hypoplastic transverse sinus can cause confusion if a sinus thrombosis is suspected. In these cases, the jugular notch in the occipital bone and jugular foramen may be smaller on the side of the hypoplastic transverse sinus. Each cavernous sinus surrounds the ipsilateral internal carotid artery. Fibers from cranial nerve VI run within the cavernous sinus inferior to the carotid artery, with fibers from cranial nerves III, IV, V1, and V2 running in its lateral wall. The two cavernous sinuses connect to each other and drain into the petrosal sinus and then the sagittal sinus.

Physiology
Cerebral Blood Flow

The brain, which is among the body's most metabolically active tissues, receives about 14% of resting cardiac output. Normal resting metabolism of brain tissue requires 140 µmol of oxygen and 24 µmol of glucose per 100 g of tissue per minute. Although total blood flow to the brain remains constant in normal conditions, regional flow changes with mental activity, often manifested by changes in synaptic activity, and provides the basis for functional

magnetic resonance imaging or positron emission tomography imaging studies. Approximately 80% of glucose is used to generate energy, with the remainder metabolized to lactate or used for synthetic activities. Little glucose is stored in the brain, and the brain's high metabolic demand makes it particularly vulnerable to reductions in oxygen and blood supply. Cerebral blood flow at rest averages 50 to 100 mL per 100 g of brain tissue per minute. If blood flow falls below this level, normal neuronal function is suppressed (i.e., neurons become electrically quiescent). If the deficit persists, irrevocable neural injury can result.

Cerebral blood flow is regulated though a variety of mechanisms in addition to mental activity. Constant, overall cerebral blood flow is maintained through autoregulation. This autoregulatory relationship is reflected in the equation cerebral blood flow = cerebrovascular resistance/mean arterial pressure. If the mean arterial pressure is decreased, there is a compensatory decrease in cerebrovascular resistance (through dilation of cerebral arterioles) to maintain cerebral blood flow constant. If the mean arterial pressure is increased, there is a compensatory increase in cerebrovascular resistance (through constriction of cerebral arterioles). There are, however, limits to cerebral autoregulation. At mean arterial pressures greater than about 150 mm Hg, cerebral arterioles are maximally constricted, and cerebral blood flow rises. At mean arterial pressures below about 50 mm Hg, cerebral arterioles are maximally dilated, and cerebral blood flow falls. In the setting of

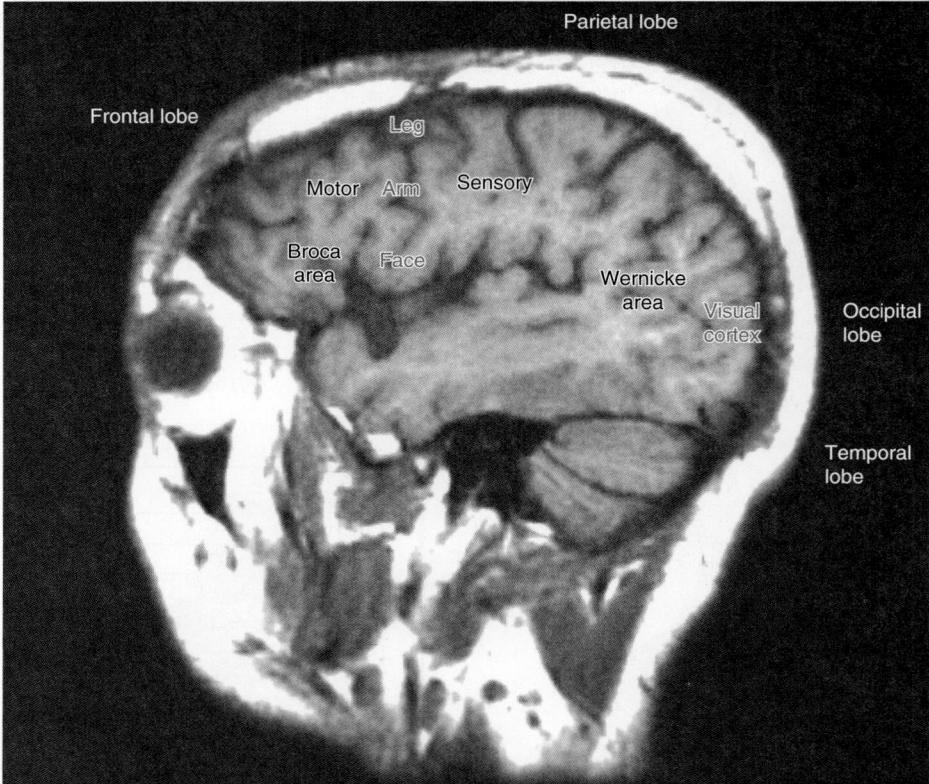

FIGURE 406-8. Sagittal, lateral T1-weighted magnetic resonance image showing cortical motor, sensory, visual, and language areas.

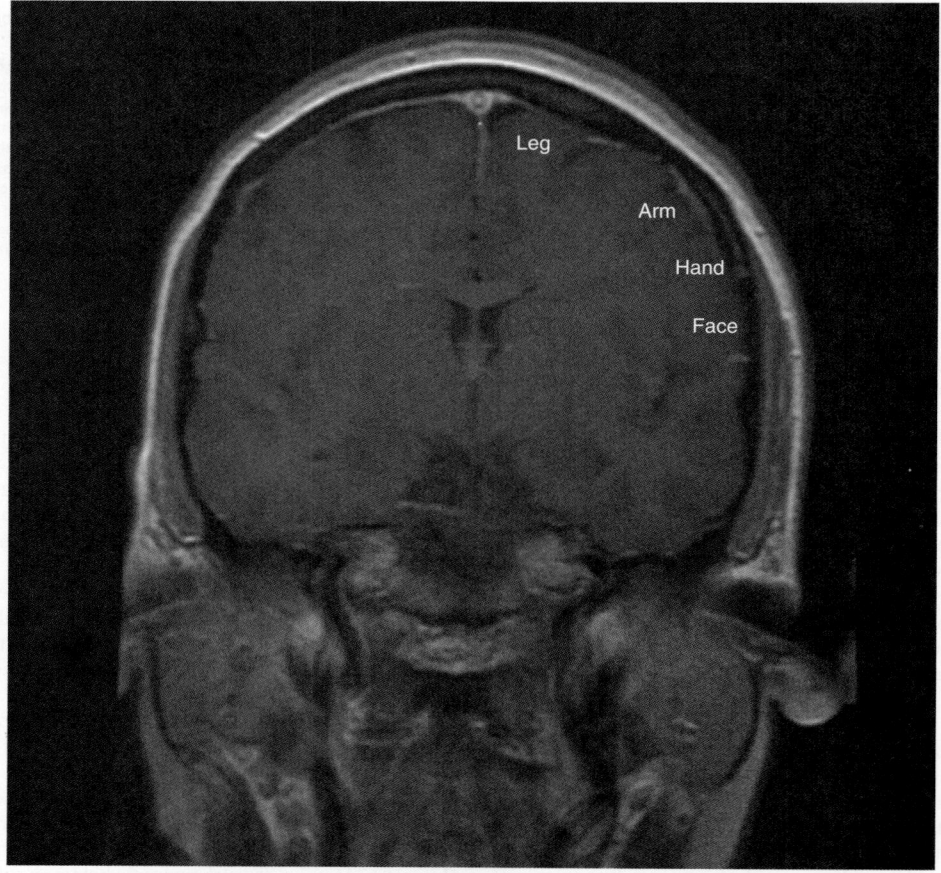

FIGURE 406-9. Coronal T1-weighted magnetic resonance image showing cortical areas for the leg, arm, hand, and face.

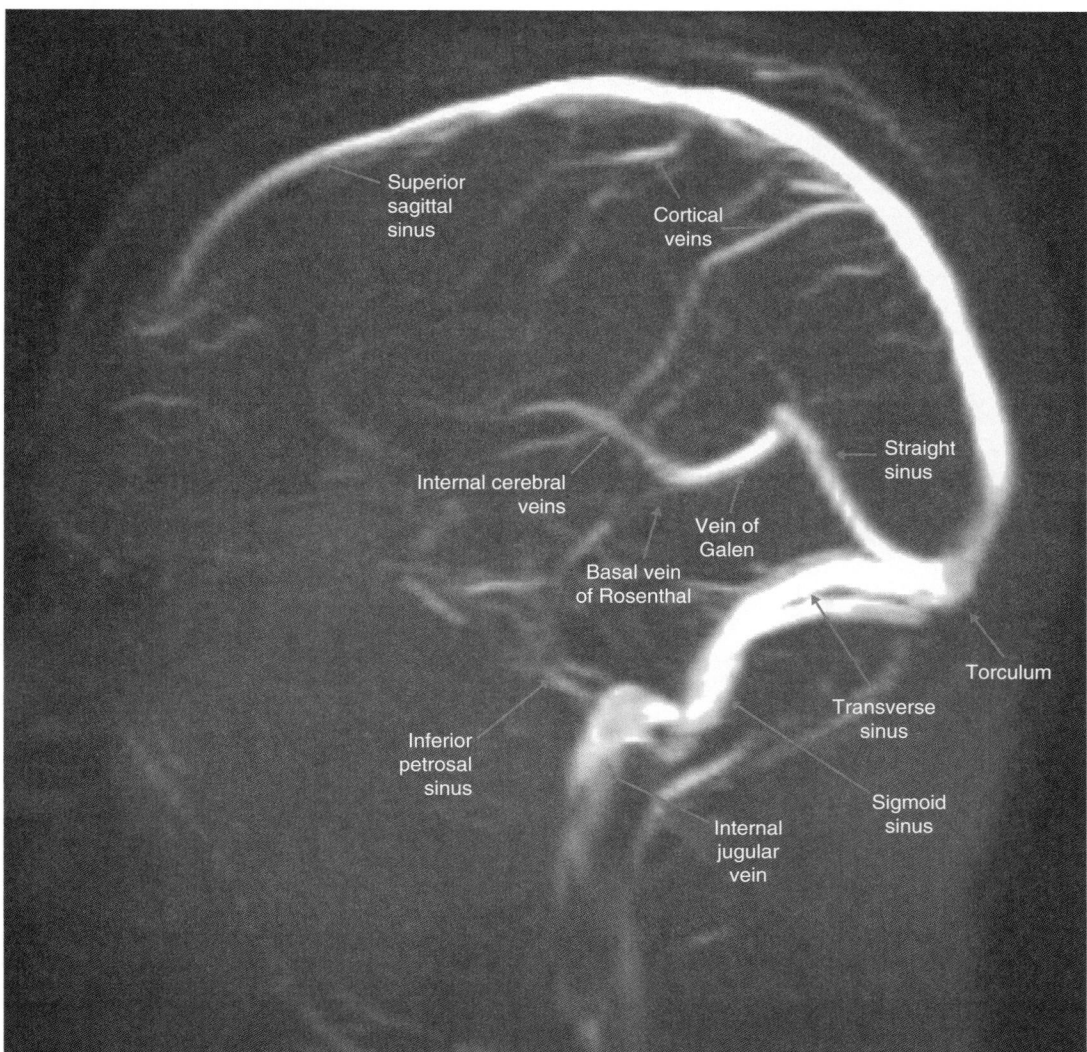

FIGURE 406-10. Parasagittal magnetic resonance venogram showing venous structures.

chronic hypertension, the autoregulatory relationship between cerebrovascular resistance and mean arterial pressure is shifted to higher critical mean arterial pressures (i.e., cerebral blood flow falls at a higher mean arterial pressure).

Metabolic factors can also affect cerebral blood flow. Hypercapnia causes cerebral vasodilation, and hypocapnia causes cerebral vasoconstriction that is mediated by changes in the pH of the brain's extracellular fluid. Cerebral blood flow declines by approximately 2% for every 1 mm Hg decline in P_{CO_2}. In patients who have increased intracranial pressure and threatened herniation, a short period of hyperventilation (target arterial P_{CO_2} of 30 to 35 mm Hg) can be used as a temporary measure until more definitive treatment can be instituted. The response is only transient because of compensation by the choroid plexus, and a rebound increase in Pa_{CO_2} can lead to a rise in intracranial pressure when hyperventilation is discontinued.

Blood-Brain Barrier
The triggering of a neuronal action potential depends on the relative concentrations of Na^+, K^+, and Ca^{2+}, and it is also modulated by Mg^{2+} and a variety of neurotransmitters. The blood-brain barrier is critical for maintaining the environment necessary for normal neuronal function.[4] The blood-brain barrier consists anatomically of the capillary endothelial cells, a basement membrane with pericytes, and astrocytic perivascular footplates. The brain's vascular endothelial cells, which are the principal component of the blood-brain barrier, are joined by tight junctions and generally lack the transport channels found elsewhere in the body. As a result, the blood-brain barrier prevents hydrophilic polar and large molecules in the blood from entering the brain. By comparison, oxygen and carbon dioxide rapidly cross the blood-brain barrier. Nutrients, toxins, and drugs can cross the blood-brain barrier by simple diffusion, by transport through carrier molecules based on concentration gradients (facilitated transport), or by energy-dependent mechanisms (active transport). Glucose is the brain's sole source of energy. Glucose transport into the brain is through non–energy-dependent facilitated transport (glucose transporter isotype 1, Glut1). In the setting of ischemia, endothelial cell function can be compromised, and the blood-brain barrier can fail.

The Neurovascular Unit
The concept of the neurovascular unit has become important for understanding the complex relationships between anatomic structures and the integrity of brain function. The term reflects the physiologic interrelatedness of the brain's various components, including endothelial cells, vascular smooth muscle, adventitial cells, glia, and neurons. The concept reflects the observation that local pH as well as neural activity can affect local cerebral blood flow. In addition to linking neural activity with blood flow and maintaining the blood-brain barrier, the neurovascular unit can secrete a variety of immunologic and neurotrophic factors that further affect both normal function and the brain's response to injury.

● CEREBRAL ISCHEMIA
Because of its high metabolic demands, brain function is completely dependent on its supply of blood and oxygen. Clinical symptoms ensue when global or regional blood supply falls below the critical 50 mL per 100 g per minute. Permanent neural injury does not occur if the supply of blood and oxygen is

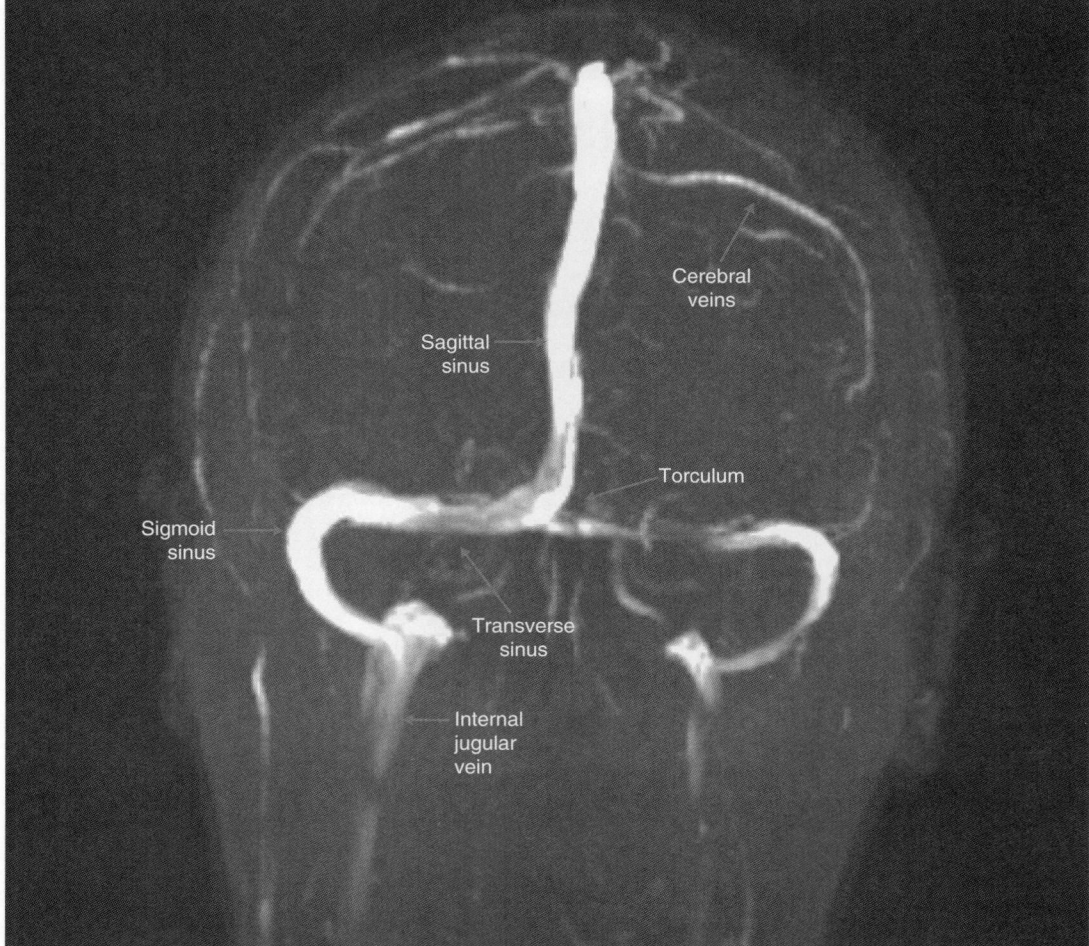

FIGURE 406-11. Anteroposterior magnetic resonance venogram showing venous structures.

quickly restored, such as with a faint (Chapter 62) in the setting of a global reduction in the supply of blood or oxygen or a transient ischemic attack (Chapter 407) with brief, local reductions in cerebral blood flow. Certain groups of neurons may be particularly vulnerable to hypoxic-ischemic injury (i.e., regions of the hippocampus, cerebellar Purkinje cells, and neocortical layers III, V, and possibly VI). Hypoxic-ischemic injury can be global, diffuse, or focal.

Global Ischemic Injury

Global ischemic injury occurs in the setting of complete cardiovascular collapse, such as with ventricular fibrillation, electromechanical dissociation, and asystole (Chapter 63). Some neurons are particularly vulnerable to ischemic injury and will be selectively damaged, whereas neurons only millimeters away may be spared.[5] In the setting of hypotension, areas of brain between the territories of major arteries (i.e., between the anterior cerebral artery and middle cerebral artery in the frontal cortex and adjacent subcortical white matter), between the middle cerebral artery and posterior cerebral artery (in the parieto-occipital cortex and adjacent subcortical white matter), and between penetrating arteries from distal branches of the middle cerebral artery and lenticulostriate arteries (deep hemispheric white matter, centrum semiovale) are especially vulnerable and are termed watershed areas.

The duration of anoxia, the duration of cardiopulmonary resuscitation (CPR), and the cause of cardiac arrest are related to poor outcome after CPR (Chapters 63 and 404), but none of these factors accurately discriminate between poor and favorable outcomes. Prognosis also cannot be based on the circumstances of CPR or on elevated body temperature alone. Myoclonus or status epilepticus within the first day after cardiac arrest implies a poor prognosis, as does the absence of pupillary or corneal reflexes or extensor motor responses 3 days after cardiac arrest in patients who remain comatose. Bilateral absence of cortical somatosensory evoked responses within 1 to 3 days also portends a poor prognosis.

Out-of-hospital cardiac arrest carries a poor prognosis if effective CPR is not rapidly instituted. A period of therapeutic hypothermia may improve neurologic outcome after resuscitated cardiac arrest if it can be instituted rapidly (Chapter 63).[A1] If the cerebral cortex is irreversibly damaged but the relatively resistant brain stem control of respiration and cardiovascular regulation is preserved, the patient can enter a persistent vegetative state (Chapter 404).

Diffuse Hypoxic Injury

Diffuse hypoxia can alter cognition, cause confusion, impair consciousness, and lead to coma, which can be irreversible. Causes include travel to high altitudes, severe anemia, and pulmonary disease. Symptoms are generally present when the PaO_2 abruptly falls to less than 40 mm Hg. Increases in cerebral blood flow can partially compensate for slow declines in PaO_2, which may still cause symptoms with further or rapid reductions.

Focal Ischemic Injury

Focal ischemic injury is caused by occlusion of a cervical or intracranial artery that supplies the brain. Although this injury can occur from many causes (including infection, inflammation, metabolic disorders, trauma, and hematologic disorders), the majority of strokes are related to thrombotic or embolic occlusion (Fig. 406-12). If flow is not restored within minutes, a core area of irreversible brain injury is commonly produced. A surrounding area of variable size, depending on the artery involved and the integrity of collaterals in which blood flow is reduced, will suffer injury that is not irreversible. The brain in this area, termed the penumbra, is electrically quiescent and contributes to the resulting neurologic deficit. Because the pH of the extracellular fluid in the penumbral zone is low, vessels are maximally dilated and the cerebral autoregulatory response is inoperative. Because cerebrovascular resistance in the penumbral zone is fixed, any decline in mean arterial pressure can further reduce its cerebral blood flow, thereby extending the volume

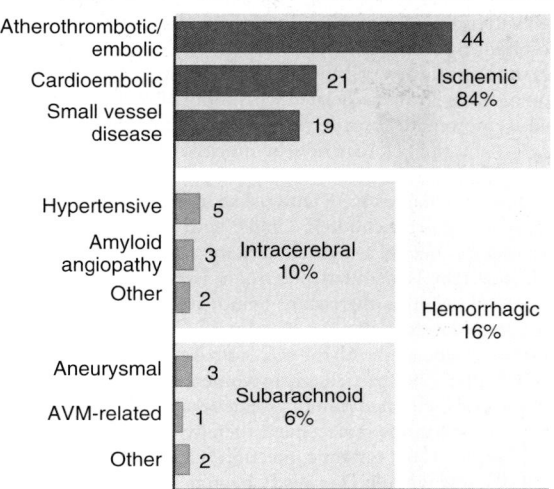

FIGURE 406-12. Classification of cerebrovascular disease by cause. AVM = arteriovenous malformation. (From Zivin JA. Approach to cerebrovascular diseases. In: Goldman L, Schafer AI. *Goldman's Cecil Medicine.* 24th ed. Philadelphia: Elsevier Saunders; 2012.)

of infarcted brain tissue. A variety of neuroimaging techniques can help distinguish penumbral from infarcted brain tissue (i.e., magnetic resonance diffusion-perfusion mismatch, computed tomographic perfusion imaging) but have not been standardized and have not yet proved useful for clinical decisions regarding the use of reperfusion therapy. Many putative neuroprotective strategies aimed at preserving ischemic brain tissue until it can be reperfused through collateral flow have failed in clinical trials.

PATHOLOGY

Permanent occlusion of a cerebral artery results in necrosis of its supplied neurons, glia, and endothelial cells (pan-necrosis). In gross appearance, the area of infarcted brain may be pale or hemorrhagic if secondary bleeding occurred. Over time, the lesion becomes cavitary (encephalomalacia). On microscopic examination, ischemic neurons initially appear small and angular. The cytoplasm becomes homogeneously eosinophilic, and the nucleus becomes dark and pyknotic. As endothelial cells die, associated areas of petechial hemorrhage may appear. An initial inflammatory reaction may lead to microvascular occlusions, such that flow to ischemic tissue may not be restored even if a proximal thrombus is removed (no-reflow phenomenon). Leukocytes that infiltrate ischemic tissue can also release interleukins and cytokines, which can contribute to cytotoxic injury. Blood macrophages begin to reach the infarcted tissue, and neovascularization peaks after about 2 weeks. Macrophage-mediated removal of cellular debris peaks at about 3 to 4 weeks after the infarct. Astrocytes then form a glial scar around the area of infarction.

PATHOPHYSIOLOGY

Because the brain has no reserve energy supply, energy-dependent neuronal and glial processes stop soon after acute deprivation of blood and oxygen. Calcium ions enter depolarized neurons and glia, where they activate second messengers, including lipases and proteases, thereby releasing free fatty acids and generating free radicals that degrade cellular organelles and membranes. Depolarized neurons also release high levels of excitatory neurotransmitters, such as glutamate into synapses, which leads to further neuronal depolarization and calcium entry. Once this cascade has been initiated, neurons may still degenerate over time by apoptosis (programmed cell death) even if blood flow is restored. Although promising in the laboratory, all attempts to block the ischemic cascade pharmacologically have failed in clinical trials to date.

● CEREBRAL HEMORRHAGE

Subarachnoid hemorrhage, which is bleeding between the pial and arachnoid coverings over the brain, is most commonly related to a ruptured aneurysm

(Chapter 408).[6] Cerebral aneurysms may occur spontaneously or be acquired as a result of infection or trauma. They are more common in first-degree relatives of patients who have a cerebral aneurysm and with certain conditions, such as autosomal dominant polycystic kidney disease (Chapter 127) and type IV Ehlers-Danlos syndrome (Chapter 260). Noninfectious aneurysms are typically situated at branch points of major cerebral arteries: anterior cerebral artery–anterior communicating artery, internal carotid artery–posterior communicating artery, middle cerebral artery bifurcation, basilar artery tip. Initial brain injury can be caused by an acute increase in intracranial pressure, with delayed ischemic injury related to the development of vasospasm after 7 to 10 days. Interference with the absorption of cerebrospinal fluid though the arachnoid granulations can lead to communicating hydrocephalus. Clot within the third or fourth ventricle or cerebral aqueducts can cause obstructive hydrocephalus.

The most common causes of intracerebral parenchymal brain hemorrhages are hypertension (Chapter 67) and cerebral amyloid angiopathy. Myriad other potential vascular and nonvascular causes, including vascular malformations, vasculitis (Chapter 270), venous sinus thrombosis, and coagulopathies (Chapters 172, 173, and 174), are less common. Some tumors (e.g., melanoma [Chapter 203] and renal cell carcinoma [Chapter 197]) can be manifested as an intracerebral hemorrhage. Hypertension-related intracerebral hemorrhage occurs in typical areas of the brain (i.e., basal ganglia, thalamus, basis pontis, and cerebellum). In contrast, intracerebral hemorrhage related to cerebral amyloid angiopathy is typically lobar and located closer to the cortical surface. Without sequential neuroimaging studies showing an initial area of ischemic injury, lobar hemorrhages may be difficult to distinguish from a hemorrhagic infarction. Susceptibility-weighted brain magnetic resonance imaging sequences may reveal prior microhemorrhages at the gray-white junction in patients with cerebral amyloid angiopathy.

● CEREBRAL EDEMA

When neurons and glia are injured by ischemia, energy metabolism fails and the cells can no longer maintain normal ion gradients between the intracellular and extracellular compartments. The result is cytotoxic edema, in which cells swell soon after the injury. Neurons, glia, and endothelial cells can be affected. Vasogenic edema, which may occur as a result of disruption of the blood-brain barrier due to injury to the endothelium, allows large molecules to pass through the blood-brain barrier and to gain access to the brain. Edema generally peaks between 48 and 72 hours after the onset of ischemic injury. In patients with ischemic stroke, the development of cytotoxic edema can lead to an increase in intracranial pressure and, when severe, herniation. In selected patients, craniotomy can be considered to relieve the pressure until the edema subsides.

Neurons, glia, and endothelial cells are also damaged in the setting of intracerebral hemorrhage. The hemorrhage itself is a space-occupying lesion that can also be associated with both cytotoxic and vasogenic edema. Mass effect from cerebellar hemorrhages can compress the fourth ventricle (thereby leading to obstructive hydrocephalus), compress the brain stem (thereby compromising the reticular activating system and impairing consciousness), or cause herniation. Surgical evacuation of intracerebral hemorrhage is not of proven value (Chapter 408), but emergent evacuation of cerebellar hemorrhages can be life-saving and leave surviving patients with little or no long-term functional impairment.

  Grade A Reference

A1. Arrich J, Holzer M, Havel C, et al. Hypothermia for neuroprotection in adults after cardiopulmonary resuscitation. *Cochrane Database Syst Rev.* 2012;9:CD004128.

GENERAL REFERENCES

For the General References and other additional features, please visit Expert Consult at https://expertconsult.inkling.com.

407

ISCHEMIC CEREBROVASCULAR DISEASE

LARRY B. GOLDSTEIN

DEFINITION

Ischemic cerebrovascular disease is caused by an impairment of blood supply to the brain. The injury may be focal (related to occlusion of a single artery), multifocal (related to occlusion of several arteries), or diffuse. Although certain clinical features (e.g., severe hypertension, headache, impaired consciousness) may suggest brain hemorrhage (Chapter 408) rather than ischemia, it is not possible to differentiate the two sets of conditions without a brain imaging study. In the absence of an inflammatory disease such as vasculitis or other rare conditions, simultaneous involvement of more than one vascular distribution suggests a proximal source of embolism (i.e., a cardiogenic or a proximal arterial source). Involvement of a single vascular territory may be due to either local steno-occlusive disease (e.g., atherosclerosis) or a proximal source of embolism. Involvement in the distribution of a single penetrating artery suggests small-vessel type intracranial disease, but ischemic strokes in this distribution may also be caused by proximal arterial steno-occlusive disease or embolism.

The definition of ischemic stroke is brain, spinal cord, or retinal cell death attributable to ischemia with neuropathologic, neuroimaging, or clinical evidence of permanent injury.[1] Overall, approximately 85% of strokes are related to ischemic disease, with 44% attributable to atherosclerosis (Chapter 70), 21% to cardiogenic embolism, and 20% to small-vessel disease.

Transient ischemic attack (TIA) is defined as a brief episode of neurologic dysfunction resulting from focal cerebral ischemia with no evidence of corresponding tissue injury. Symptoms are similar to those of ischemic stroke. Previously characterized as a transient deficit with symptoms persisting for less than 24 hours, evidence of corresponding tissue injury can be seen on brain magnetic resonance imaging (MRI) in 30 to 40% of patients who otherwise fulfill the clinical definition of TIA.

EPIDEMIOLOGY

Stroke (ischemic and hemorrhagic) is the second leading cause of death worldwide and the fourth leading cause of death in the United States.[2] It is also one of the leading causes of adult disability. In addition to age, race or ethnicity, and family history, a variety of lifestyle factors and medical conditions increase the risk of stroke (Chapter 406; Table 407-1). Of these, hypertension is the single most important (Chapter 67; Table 407-1), and the risk of stroke increases with increasing blood pressure with no threshold effect. Diabetes (Chapter 229) is associated with an approximate doubling of the risk of stroke (Table 407-1). Atrial fibrillation (Chapter 64; Table 407-1) is

TABLE 407-1 COMMON STROKE RISK FACTORS

FACTOR	POPULATION-ATTRIBUTABLE RISK	RISK REDUCTION WITH TREATMENT
LIFESTYLE		
Cigarette smoking	12-14%	50% within 1 year of quitting
Physical inactivity	30%	?
Excess alcohol consumption	7%	?
MEDICAL		
Hypertension	>90%	32%
Diabetes	5-27%	—
Atrial fibrillation	2-24%	64%
Carotid stenosis	2-7%	50%
Sickle cell disease	—	91% with transfusion therapy in children

Data from Goldstein LB, Bushnell CD, Adams RJ, et al. Guidelines for the primary prevention of stroke: a guideline for healthcare professionals from the American Heart Association/American Stroke Association. *Stroke.* 2011;42:517-584.

associated with up to 25% of ischemic strokes, with the absolute risk varying by concomitant risk factors.

Extracranial carotid artery stenosis is found in up to 5 to 10% of individuals older than 65 years and is associated with about 10% of all ischemic strokes. Untreated asymptomatic carotid stenosis carries only about a 1 to 2% annual risk of stroke, and the risk may now be much lower, perhaps as low as 0.5% annually, with standard medical therapy. Stroke is also a complication of sickle cell disease (Chapter 163), with risk dramatically reduced with transfusion therapy in high-risk children. Unlike with coronary heart disease, the overall association between high cholesterol concentration and the risk of stroke is less certain. Ischemic stroke risk is associated with higher levels of total cholesterol, whereas the risk of hemorrhagic stroke is increased with lower cholesterol levels.

Other factors associated with the risk of stroke include migraine headaches with aura (Chapter 398), particularly in women who smoke and are receiving oral contraceptives; elevated homocysteine level; high lipoprotein (a) level; postmenopausal hormone replacement therapy (Chapter 240); coagulation disorders (Chapter 176); systemic infection (Chapter 76); renal impairment (Chapter 130); low vitamin D levels (Chapters 218 and 244); and a variety of environmental factors, including high levels of air pollution.

PATHOBIOLOGY

For patients who have a TIA and who are by definition at increased risk of having an ischemic stroke during the next few days or weeks or who have an ischemic stroke, distinguishing among the major pathophysiologic causes (i.e., atherothrombotic, cardioembolic, small vessel) is critical to guide secondary prevention. Atherothrombosis due to atherosclerosis (Chapter 70) is the most common cause of a TIA or stroke that is related to steno-occlusive disease in a single artery.[3] The ischemia may be caused when progressive stenosis at the site of an atherosclerotic plaque leads to hemodynamic compromise affecting distal brain tissue. Sometimes bleeding into the plaque can lead to abrupt arterial occlusion, and sometimes a thrombus that has formed on an ulcerated plaque may embolize and occlude a distal artery. Occlusion of a cerebral artery, however, does not necessarily lead to ischemic brain injury. Blood may still reach the supplied territory through collaterals, either through the circle of Willis or from extracranial-intracranial anastomoses.

Arterial dissection, previously thought to occur only rarely and usually to result in major stroke, is now recognized more frequently on the basis of noninvasive vascular imaging such as MR angiography or computed tomography (CT) angiography. Other arteriopathies, such as fibromuscular dysplasia (Chapters 67, 80, and 125), may also lead to single, large-vessel distribution, ischemic stroke. Atherosclerosis of the ascending aorta or aortic arch can lead to the formation of thrombus, which can then embolize to a cerebral artery.

Atrial fibrillation is the single most common cause of cardioembolic stroke, with annual risks of 3 to 5% if it is not treated with anticoagulation but declining to about one fourth of that risk with anticoagulation (Chapter 64). The use of extended cardiac rhythm monitoring (i.e., 30-day event-triggered loop monitoring; Chapter 62) reveals occult atrial fibrillation in up to 25% of patients with an otherwise cryptogenic stroke. Other cardiac causes of cerebral embolism include clots or vegetations in patients with valvular heart disease (Chapter 75), such as mechanical prosthetic heart valves (Chapter 75), infectious endocarditis (Chapter 76), and nonbacterial endocarditis (Chapter 76); and mural thrombi in patients with a cardiomyopathy (Chapter 60) or myocardial infarction (MI), particularly anteroseptal MI (Chapter 73). Paradoxical embolism of a venous clot across a congenital heart defect, such as a patent foramen ovale or an atrial septal defect (Chapter 69), is another potential cause of embolic stroke.[4]

Small-vessel intracranial disease may result in ischemic stroke in the distribution of a single penetrating vessel. These strokes commonly affect deep structures (e.g., centrum semiovale, basal ganglia, thalamus, internal capsule, pons) and occur more frequently in patients with hypertension and diabetes. Classically, small-vessel strokes are caused by lipohyalinosis, which is a thickening of the vessel wall resulting in a diminished luminal area, but they also can be caused by atherothrombotic embolism.

Symptoms of ischemic stroke may worsen during the first hours or days through various mechanisms. For example, decreases in systemic blood pressure may decrease cerebral blood flow to marginally perfused, ischemic brain. In the setting of atherothrombotic disease, a partially occluded artery may progress to complete occlusion. Recurrent embolism may occur from a proximal arterial or cardiac source. Cerebral edema may develop during the first few days after an ischemic stroke, and the resulting mass effect can lead to

TABLE 407-2 CLINICAL MANIFESTATIONS OF ISCHEMIC CEREBROVASCULAR DISEASE

OCCLUDED ARTERY	TYPICAL MAJOR CLINICAL MANIFESTATIONS*
Internal carotid artery	Ipsilateral visual loss Ipsilateral middle cerebral artery syndrome
Anterior choroidal artery	Contralateral hemiparesis Contralateral sensory impairment Contralateral visual field defect
Anterior cerebral artery	Contralateral leg > arm paresis Contralateral leg > arm sensory deficit
Middle cerebral artery	Contralateral hemiparesis affecting face and arm > leg Contralateral sensory deficit affecting face and arm > leg Contralateral visual field defect Aphasia (dominant hemisphere) Contralateral hemispatial neglect (nondominant or dominant hemisphere)
Posterior cerebral artery	Contralateral homonymous hemianopia (or homonymous superior or inferior quadrantanopia) Contralateral sensory deficits (thalamic involvement)
Basilar artery tip	Bilateral central visual loss Confusion
Basilar artery	Ipsilateral cranial nerve deficit Contralateral hemiparesis Contralateral sensory impairment affecting arm and/or leg Coordination deficit
Vertebral artery, posterior inferior cerebellar artery	Ipsilateral sensory impairment over the face Dysphagia Ipsilateral Horner syndrome Ataxia
Superior cerebellar artery	Gait ataxia Ipsilateral limb ataxia Variable contralateral limb weakness

*Note: not all may be present.

clinical deterioration (Chapter 406). Secondary bleeding can occur in an area that was primarily the site of an ischemic injury when reperfusion, either through collateral vessels or as the result of a therapeutic intervention, restores blood flow into vessels in which the endothelium was damaged by the original ischemic insult.

CLINICAL MANIFESTATIONS

Neurologic deficits that occur in the setting of ischemic stroke depend on the involved vascular territory (Table 407-2) and underlying cause. Embolic stroke is generally characterized by the presence of a maximal deficit at onset, whereas the onset may be more gradual or stuttering in the setting of an atherothrombotic stroke. The distinction, however, is not of great use for diagnosis in individual patients. Transient symptoms in the same distribution can be caused by TIA if there is no permanent tissue injury.

Internal Carotid Artery

The bifurcation of the common carotid artery into the internal and external carotid arteries in the neck is a common site of atherosclerotic disease (see Fig. 406-1). With occlusion of the internal carotid artery, patients who have an incomplete circle of Willis can suffer profound contralateral loss of motor and sensory function affecting the face, arm, and leg. In patients with an intact anterior communicating artery that can supply the ipsilateral anterior cerebral artery, the leg may be relatively spared, and an internal carotid artery occlusion may be clinically indistinguishable from a middle cerebral artery occlusion. If the anterior communicating artery is absent on the side opposite an internal carotid artery occlusion, the ipsilateral leg may also be affected, and the presentation may be confused with a cardioembolic cause because both hemispheres are involved. Occlusion of the ipsilateral ophthalmic artery can lead to blindness in that eye. Transient symptoms of retinal ischemia, classically described by patients as a "shade coming down over my vision," indicate amaurosis fugax. Other common symptoms include a darkening or blurring of vision in the affected eye. Transient hypoperfusion ipsilateral to a high-grade internal carotid artery stenosis can cause limb-shaking TIAs that can be confused with seizures. Systemic hypotension in the setting of a high-grade carotid stenosis can lead to ischemic injury in watershed zones between

the major intracranial arteries and in the border zone between the distal territories of cortical and lenticulostriate penetrating vessels.

Anterior Choroidal Artery

The anterior choroidal artery generally arises from the supraclinoid portion of the internal carotid artery (see Fig. 406-7). Causes of occlusion of the anterior choroidal artery are similar to those of occlusion of the small intracranial arteries. Symptoms can include contralateral motor and sensory deficits and contralateral visual field deficits, the latter of which can occur in isolation.

Cerebral Arteries

About 2% of strokes are related to isolated occlusion of the anterior cerebral artery (see Figs. 406-6 and 406-7). Occlusion of the A1 segment in patients in whom the contralateral A1 segment is hypoplastic or absent can lead to bilateral leg involvement, abulia, and urinary incontinence because of infarction of both frontal lobes.

The middle cerebral artery is the most common artery involved in occlusions related to cardiogenic embolism. It supplies the lateral portions of the frontal, parietal, and temporal lobes as well as the basal ganglia and the anterior limb and genu of the internal capsule. Middle cerebral artery occlusions are characterized by involvement of the contralateral face and arm to a greater extent than of the leg (see Figs. 406-6, 406-8, and 406-9), often accompanied by a contralateral hemispatial neglect. When the dominant hemisphere is involved, the patient may have an aphasia. With frontal lobe involvement, patients often have an ipsilateral, conjugate deviation of the eyes, which can be forced past the midline with vigorous encouragement, oculocephalic maneuvers, or caloric stimulation.

Branch middle cerebral artery occlusions can result in partial syndromes. For example, a branch middle cerebral artery occlusion with intact collaterals can cause a global aphasia without an accompanying motor deficit. Anterior branch, dominant hemisphere middle cerebral artery occlusions can cause an expressive, cortical-type motor (Broca) aphasia with sparing of comprehension. Occlusion of the angular branch of the middle cerebral artery can cause receptive, cortical-type (Wernicke) aphasia. Borderzone infarcts can result in transcortical aphasias, characterized by relatively preserved repetitions.

Both posterior cerebral arteries arise from the basilar artery in about 75% of people. In the other 25%, one or both P1 segments are hypoplastic or absent, with the posterior cerebral arteries arising from the ipsilateral internal carotid artery (so-called fetal circulation). Without vascular imaging, it is not possible to determine if a posterior cerebral artery distribution infarct (see Figs. 406-6 to 406-8) is related to carotid or vertebrobasilar circulation disease. The posterior cerebral artery and posterior communicating arteries supply the thalamus. Thalamic infarctions can result in contralateral hemianesthesia and ataxia. Contralateral hemiballismus can result if the subthalamic nucleus is damaged. Infarction of the ipsilateral occipital lobe causes a contralateral homonymous hemianopia that can be partial, depending on the extent of injury. The visual field deficit tends to become more congruous in the two eyes as the area of injury becomes more posterior (i.e., the closer to the occipital pole).

Vertebral and Basilar Arteries

Occlusion of the basilar artery (see Figs. 406-3 and 406-4B) can lead to "locked-in syndrome" (Chapter 404) in which the patient is awake and alert, because the periaqueductal gray can receive a separate blood supply, but unable to move or to communicate except for vertical eye movements, because of sparing of the collicular nuclei in the midbrain. The tip of the basilar artery is a common location for embolic occlusion. Symptoms can include visual field defects due to unilateral or bilateral occipital injury and confusional states due to thalamic involvement.

Occlusions of penetrating and circumferential branches of the basilar artery and vertebral artery can produce a variety of symptoms (see Table 407-2), depending on the portion of the artery involved, several of which constitute eponymous midbrain, pontine, or medullary syndromes. Occlusion of the superior cerebellar artery can cause truncal ataxia because of infarction of the cerebellar vermis, with or without ataxia of the ipsilateral limbs, which can be caused by infarction of the ipsilateral cerebellar hemisphere.

Small Vessels

Occlusion of a small penetrating intracranial vessel can result in one of the classic lacunar syndromes (Table 407-3). These syndromes are not otherwise localizing and can occur with occlusions of small penetrating vessels in either the anterior or vertebrobasilar circulations. Lacunar syndromes are not pathognomonic of small-vessel intracranial disease and can be caused by a variety of other conditions, including emboli from a more proximal arterial or cardioembolic source or brain hemorrhage (Chapter 408).

DIAGNOSIS

The diagnosis of ischemic stroke depends on acquiring an accurate history, eliciting key findings on general and neurologic examinations, and obtaining supporting data from selected laboratory studies (Fig. 407-1). An initial anatomic and pathophysiologic differential diagnosis is usually established on the basis of the patient's history. Findings on physical and neurologic examinations can support or refute initial conclusions based on the history and can further refine the differential diagnosis.

History

The abrupt onset of a focal neurologic deficit in the distribution of a specific vascular territory is the hallmark of acute ischemic stroke. The differential and most likely diagnosis can often be determined on the basis of history alone. For example, a patient with a history of atrial fibrillation who abruptly develops word-finding difficulties associated with a right hemiparesis and sensory impairment most likely had a cardiogenic embolus to the left middle cerebral artery. A patient with the acute onset of diplopia, vertigo, and a hemiparesis most likely has a lesion in the brain stem.

Goals of the immediate history include determining the exact time when symptoms began or the last time the patient was known to be well, concomitant medical illnesses, risk factors, medications, allergies, and other potential causes for symptoms that might mimic acute ischemic stroke. Because a stroke may affect a patient's ability to communicate, the history may require input from a witness. Additional details of the patient's past medical, family, and social history may need to be deferred in the emergent setting, but these issues can be explored if the information is important for acute treatment decisions.

Physical Examination

Severely elevated blood pressures in the setting of neurologic deficits referable to the basal ganglia, thalamus, pons, or cerebellum increase the

TABLE 407-3	LACUNAR SYNDROMES
Pure motor stroke	
Pure sensory stroke	
Ataxic hemiparesis	
Clumsy hand–dysarthria	

likelihood of a brain hemorrhage (Chapter 408). In a patient with transient vertigo associated with left arm movement, a reduced blood pressure in that arm suggests subclavian steal syndrome. Detection of an anterior cervical bruit contralateral to symptoms and signs indicative of a middle cerebral artery distribution infarct increase the likelihood of symptomatic carotid stenosis. An irregularly irregular heart rhythm with or without a cardiac murmur may indicate atrial fibrillation and a cardioembolic etiology. Finding a cholesterol embolus on funduscopic examination can be consistent with a proximal source of atheroembolism. Funduscopy can also show evidence of a small-vessel disease related to diabetes or hypertension (see Figs. 423-24 and 423-26).

A general neurologic examination (Chapter 396) including evaluations of cognition, language, spatial neglect, cranial nerves, motor function, sensation, coordination, gait, and reflexes is important both for documenting stroke-related deficits and for providing information critical for determining the area of the brain affected by the stroke and the severity of the injury. The use of a standardized graded neurologic impairment assessment provides a tool for measuring the severity of the stroke, determining the risks and benefits of treatment interventions, assessing prognosis, and observing patients objectively over time. The National Institutes of Health Stroke Scale (Table 407-4), which is the most commonly used approach, is both reliable and well validated. The individual items are summed to provide a total score.

Initial Laboratory Tests

Laboratory testing can help exclude conditions that may mimic, complicate, or lead to an acute ischemic stroke (Table 407-5).[5] Tests that should be obtained in all patients with suspected ischemic stroke include a complete blood count and platelet count, prothrombin time/international normalized ratio (INR), activated partial thromboplastin time, blood glucose level, serum electrolytes, tests of renal function, troponin level, and oxygen saturation. An electrocardiogram should be obtained urgently, and the patient should be sent for a CT brain scan or MRI as soon as he or she is stable enough. Additional tests are indicated in selected patients. For example, women of childbearing age should have a pregnancy test. A toxicology screen and blood alcohol levels should be obtained if drug or alcohol abuse is suspected. In patients who may be receiving a direct thrombin inhibitor or a factor Xa inhibitor, a thrombin time or ecarin clot time may be helpful in determining whether the patient is anticoagulated. An elevated erythrocyte sedimentation rate may point to an inflammatory cause or systemic infection.

The complete blood count can provide information about both the potential cause of the stroke and possible therapeutic interventions. An elevated white blood cell count may indicate an infectious cause of stroke, such as infective endocarditis (Chapter 76). Systemic infection may also cause a recrudescence of prior stroke symptoms in a patient who had previously

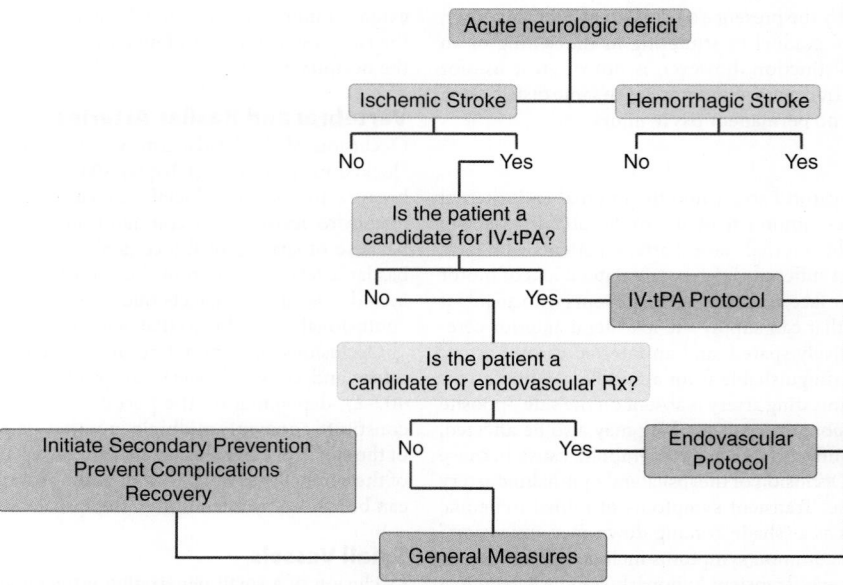

FIGURE 407-1. Approach to ischemic stroke. IV-tPA = intravenous tissue plasminogen activator; Rx = therapy. (From Goldstein LB. Modern medical management of acute ischemic stroke. *Methodist DeBakey Cardiovasc J.* 2014;10:99-104.)

TABLE 407-4 NATIONAL INSTITUTES OF HEALTH STROKE SCALE

Administer stroke scale items in the order listed. Record performance in each category after each subscale exam. Do not go back and change scores. Follow directions provided for each exam technique. Scores should reflect what the patient does, not what the clinician thinks the patient can do. The clinician should record answers while administering the exam and work quickly. Except where indicated, the patient should not be coached (i.e., repeated requests to patient to make a special effort).

INSTRUCTIONS	SCALE DEFINITION	SCORE
1a. **Level of Consciousness:** The investigator must choose a response if a full evaluation is prevented by such obstacles as an endotracheal tube, language barrier, orotracheal trauma/bandages. A 3 is scored only if the patient makes no movement (other than reflexive posturing) in response to noxious stimulation.	0 = **Alert**; keenly responsive. 1 = **Not alert**; but arousable by minor stimulation to obey, answer, or respond. 2 = **Not alert**; requires repeated stimulation to attend, or is obtunded and requires strong or painful stimulation to make movements (not stereotyped). 3 = Responds only with reflex motor or autonomic effects or totally unresponsive, flaccid, and areflexic.	_____
1b. **LOC Questions:** The patient is asked the month and his/her age. The answer must be correct—there is no partial credit for being close. Aphasic and stuporous patients who do not comprehend the questions will score 2. Patients unable to speak because of endotracheal intubation, orotracheal trauma, severe dysarthria from any cause, language barrier, or any other problem not secondary to aphasia are given a 1. It is important that only the initial answer be graded and that the examiner not "help" the patient with verbal or nonverbal cues.	0 = **Answers** both questions correctly. 1 = **Answers** one question correctly. 2 = **Answers** neither question correctly.	_____
1c. **LOC Commands:** The patient is asked to open and close the eyes and then to grip and release the nonparetic hand. Substitute another one-step command if the hands cannot be used. Credit is given if an unequivocal attempt is made but not completed due to weakness. If the patient does not respond to command, the task should be demonstrated to him or her (pantomime), and the result scored (i.e., follows none, one, or two commands). Patients with trauma, amputation, or other physical impediments should be given suitable one-step commands. Only the first attempt is scored.	0 = **Performs** both tasks correctly. 1 = **Performs** one task correctly. 2 = **Performs** neither task correctly.	_____
2. **Best Gaze:** Only horizontal eye movements will be tested. Voluntary or reflexive (oculocephalic) eye movements will be scored, but caloric testing is not done. If the patient has a conjugate deviation of the eyes that can be overcome by voluntary or reflexive activity, the score will be 1. If a patient has an isolated peripheral nerve paresis (CN III, IV, or VI), score a 1. Gaze is testable in all aphasic patients. Patients with ocular trauma, bandages, preexisting blindness, or other disorder of visual acuity or fields should be tested with reflexive movements, and a choice made by the investigator. Establishing eye contact and then moving about the patient from side to side will occasionally clarify the presence of a partial gaze palsy.	0 = **Normal**. 1 = **Partial gaze palsy**; gaze is abnormal in one or both eyes, but forced deviation or total gaze paresis is not present. 2 = **Forced deviation**, or total gaze paresis not overcome by the oculocephalic maneuver.	_____
3. **Visual:** Visual fields (upper and lower quadrants) are tested by confrontation, using finger counting or visual threat, as appropriate. Patients may be encouraged, but if they look at the side of the moving fingers appropriately, this can be scored as normal. If there is unilateral blindness or enucleation, visual fields in the remaining eye are scored. Score 1 only if a clear-cut asymmetry, including quadrantanopia, is found. If patient is blind from any cause, score 3. Double simultaneous stimulation is performed at this point. If there is extinction, patient receives a 1, and the results are used to respond to item 11.	0 = **No visual loss**. 1 = **Partial hemianopia**. 2 = **Complete hemianopia**. 3 = **Bilateral hemianopia** (blind including cortical blindness).	_____
4. **Facial Palsy:** Ask—or use pantomime to encourage—the patient to show teeth or raise eyebrows and close eyes. Score symmetry of grimace in response to noxious stimuli in the poorly responsive or noncomprehending patient. If facial trauma/bandages, orotracheal tube, tape, or other physical barriers obscure the face, these should be removed to the extent possible.	0 = **Normal** symmetrical movements. 1 = **Minor paralysis** (flattened nasolabial fold, asymmetry on smiling). 2 = **Partial paralysis** (total or near-total paralysis of lower face). 3 = **Complete paralysis** of one or both sides (absence of facial movement in the upper and lower face).	_____
5. **Motor Arm:** The limb is placed in the appropriate position: extend the arms (palms down) 90 degrees (if sitting) or 45 degrees (if supine). Drift is scored if the arm falls before 10 seconds. The aphasic patient is encouraged using urgency in the voice and pantomime, but not noxious stimulation. Each limb is tested in turn, beginning with the nonparetic arm. Only in the case of amputation or joint fusion at the shoulder, the examiner should record the score as untestable (UN) and clearly write the explanation for this choice.	0 = **No drift**; limb holds 90 (or 45) degrees for full 10 seconds. 1 = **Drift**; limb holds 90 (or 45) degrees, but drifts down before full 10 seconds; does not hit bed or other support. 2 = **Some effort against gravity**; limb cannot get to or maintain (if cued) 90 (or 45) degrees, drifts down to bed, but has some effort against gravity. 3 = **No effort against gravity**; limb falls. 4 = **No movement**. UN = **Amputation** or joint fusion, explain: _____ 5a. **Left Arm** 5b. **Right Arm**	_____
6. **Motor Leg:** The limb is placed in the appropriate position: hold the leg at 30 degrees (always tested supine). Drift is scored if the leg falls before 5 seconds. The aphasic patient is encouraged using urgency in the voice and pantomime, but not noxious stimulation. Each limb is tested in turn, beginning with the nonparetic leg. Only in the case of amputation or joint fusion at the hip, the examiner should record the score as untestable (UN) and clearly write the explanation for this choice.	0 = **No drift**; leg holds 30-degree position for full 5 seconds. 1 = **Drift**; leg falls by the end of the 5-second period but does not hit bed. 2 = **Some effort against gravity**; leg falls to bed by 5 seconds, but has some effort against gravity. 3 = **No effort against gravity**; leg falls to bed immediately. 4 = **No movement**. UN = **Amputation** or joint fusion, explain: _____ 6a. **Left Leg** 6b. **Right Leg**	_____

TABLE 407-4 NATIONAL INSTITUTES OF HEALTH STROKE SCALE—cont'd

INSTRUCTIONS	SCALE DEFINITION	SCORE
7. **Limb Ataxia:** This item is aimed at finding evidence of a unilateral cerebellar lesion. Test with eyes open. In case of visual defect, ensure testing is done in intact visual field. The finger-nose-finger and heel-shin tests are performed on both sides, and ataxia is scored only if present out of proportion to weakness. Ataxia is absent in the patient who cannot understand or is paralyzed. Only in the case of amputation or joint fusion, the examiner should record the score as untestable (UN) and clearly write the explanation for this choice. In case of blindness, test by having the patient touch nose from extended arm position.	0 = **Absent**. 1 = **Present in one limb**. 2 = **Present in two limbs**. UN = **Amputation** or joint fusion, explain: _____	_____
8. **Sensory:** Sensation or grimace to pinprick when tested, or withdrawal from noxious stimulus in the obtunded or aphasic patient. Only sensory loss attributed to stroke is scored as abnormal, and the examiner should test as many body areas (arms [not hands], legs, trunk, face) as needed to accurately check for hemisensory loss. A score of 2, "severe or total sensory loss," should only be given when a severe or total loss of sensation can be clearly demonstrated. Stuporous and aphasic patients will, therefore, probably score 1 or 0. The patient with brain stem stroke who has bilateral loss of sensation is scored 2. If the patient does not respond and is quadriplegic, score 2. Patients in a coma (item 1a = 3) are automatically given a 2 on this item.	0 = **Normal**; no sensory loss. 1 = **Mild-to-moderate sensory loss**; patient feels pinprick is less sharp or is dull on the affected side; or there is a loss of superficial pain with pinprick, but patient is aware of being touched. 2 = **Severe to total sensory loss**; patient is not aware of being touched in the face, arm, and leg.	_____
9. **Best Language:** A great deal of information about comprehension will be obtained during the preceding sections of the examination. For this scale item, the patient is asked to describe what is happening in the attached picture, to name the items on the attached naming sheet, and to read from the attached list of sentences. Comprehension is judged from responses here, as well as to all of the commands in the preceding general neurological exam. If visual loss interferes with the tests, ask the patient to identify objects placed in the hand, repeat, and produce speech. The intubated patient should be asked to write. The patient in a coma (item 1a = 3) will automatically score 3 on this item. The examiner must choose a score for the patient with stupor or limited cooperation, but a score of 3 should be used only if the patient is mute and follows no one-step commands.	0 = **No aphasia**; normal. 1 = **Mild-to-moderate aphasia**; some obvious loss of fluency or facility of comprehension, without significant limitation on ideas expressed or form of expression. Reduction of speech and/or comprehension, however, makes conversation about provided materials difficult or impossible. For example, in conversation about provided materials, examiner can identify picture or naming card content from patient's response. 2 = **Severe aphasia**; all communication is through fragmentary expression; great need for inference, questioning, and guessing by the listener. Range of information that can be exchanged is limited; listener carries burden of communication. Examiner cannot identify materials provided from patient response. 3 = **Mute, global aphasia**; no usable speech or auditory comprehension.	_____
10. **Dysarthria:** If patient is thought to be normal, an adequate sample of speech must be obtained by asking patient to read or repeat words from the attached list. If the patient has severe aphasia, the clarity of articulation of spontaneous speech can be rated. Only if the patient is intubated or has other physical barriers to producing speech, the examiner should record the score as untestable (UN) and clearly write an explanation for this choice. Do not tell the patient why he or she is being tested.	0 = **Normal**. 1 = **Mild-to-moderate dysarthria**; patient slurs at least some words and, at worst, can be understood with some difficulty. 2 = **Severe dysarthria**; patient's speech is so slurred as to be unintelligible in the absence of or out of proportion to any dysphasia, or is mute/anarthric. UN = **Intubated** or other physical barrier, explain:_____	_____
11. **Extinction and Inattention (formerly Neglect):** Sufficient information to identify neglect may be obtained during the prior testing. If the patient has a severe visual loss preventing visual double simultaneous stimulation, and the cutaneous stimuli are normal, the score is normal. If the patient has aphasia but does appear to attend to both sides, the score is normal. The presence of visual spatial neglect or anosognosia may also be taken as evidence of abnormality. Since the abnormality is scored only if present, the item is never untestable.	0 = **No abnormality**. 1 = **Visual, tactile, auditory, spatial, or personal inattention** or extinction to bilateral simultaneous stimulation in one of the sensory modalities. 2 = **Profound hemi-inattention or extinction to more than one modality**; does not recognize own hand or orients to only one side of space.	_____

From http://www.ninds.nih.gov/doctors/nih_stroke_scale.pdf. Accessed February 26, 2015.

recovered or in whom a stroke had not been previously recognized. Polycythemia (Chapter 166) can cause hyperviscosity that leads to occlusion of small intracranial vessels. Thrombocytopenia, either primary or secondary, can lead to platelet thrombi. The prothrombin time/INR and activated thromboplastin time provide indices that may reveal an underlying coagulation disorder, and thrombocytopenia and coagulation disorders may preclude treatment with intravenous recombinant tissue plasminogen activator (rtPA).

Both hypoglycemia (Chapter 230) and hyperglycemia (Chapter 229) may cause strokelike symptoms. Impaired renal function (Chapter 130) is a risk factor for ischemic stroke and may increase the risks of using thrombolytic and anticoagulant medications. Abnormalities of other serum electrolytes (e.g., hyponatremia; Chapter 116) can also cause neurologic symptoms.

The electrocardiogram may reveal changes suggestive of acute myocardial ischemia as well as atrial fibrillation, the most common cause of embolic stroke. Stroke may also cause a variety of cardiac arrhythmias. Acute MI, especially anteroseptal MI, is associated with a higher risk of cardiogenic embolism, and an acute stroke may also precipitate an MI. A troponin level is usually adequate for this purpose, especially because it remains elevated for several days after the MI when embolism from a mural thrombus is most likely to occur. Patients with acute stroke should be placed on telemetry monitoring. Urgent echocardiography is used selectively.

Brain Imaging

CT or MRI brain imaging is an essential part of the evaluation of all patients with suspected ischemic stroke. Imaging can locate the area of damage, distinguish a brain hemorrhage from an ischemic stroke, and identify mass lesions such as tumor (Chapter 189), abscess (Chapter 413), or subdural hematoma that can present acutely and mimic a stroke. Brain CT is widely and rapidly available and provides the information necessary for the treatment of most patients with acute stroke. Brain MRI can detect areas of acute ischemic injury not apparent on CT brain imaging (Fig. 407-2), but it cannot be performed in patients with metal implants and devices such as cardiac pacemakers and is a challenge to perform in unstable patients.

The changes on brain CT, such as loss of gray-white distinction, loss of the insular ribbon, and blurring of the borders of the basal ganglia, can be subtle. The area of ischemic injury on brain CT scan appears as a relative hypodensity (Fig. 407-3), in contrast to brain hemorrhage, which appears hyperdense compared with the surrounding brain parenchyma (see Fig. 408-2). CT can also show acute hemorrhage in the subarachnoid space, which can be indicative of aneurysmal rupture (see Fig. 408-1). The dense middle cerebral artery sign or the dot sign, in which an artery in the sylvian fissure may appear dense, can indicate thrombus in these vessels.

The findings on CT are often normal in the acute phase of ischemic stroke, and MRI is more sensitive for detecting acute ischemic injury (Fig. 407-4). Because brain CT imaging of posterior fossa structures is often obscured by beam hardening artifact from the petrous bones, MRI is also more sensitive for visualizing the brain stem and cerebellum. MRI signal patterns also can

distinguish acute from subacute and remote ischemic injury, distinguish acute and remote brain hemorrhage, and identify other nonvascular conditions. However, MRI is not required before treatment with intravenous rtPA because CT can reliably exclude parenchymal brain hemorrhage and can detect other common conditions that may mimic a stroke, such as a mass lesion.

Lumbar Puncture

Lumbar puncture is rarely necessary in the evaluation of patients with acute stroke. In occasional patients, meningitis, especially septic meningitis from

TABLE 407-5	IMMEDIATE DIAGNOSTIC STUDIES: EVALUATION OF A PATIENT WITH SUSPECTED ACUTE ISCHEMIC STROKE

ALL PATIENTS

Noncontrast brain CT or brain MRI
Blood glucose
Oxygen saturation
Serum electrolytes/renal function tests*
Complete blood count, including platelet count*
Markers of cardiac ischemia*
Prothrombin time/INR*
Partial thromboplastin time*
ECG*

SELECTED PATIENTS

Thrombin time and/or ecarin clotting time if it is suspected the patient is taking direct thrombin inhibitors or direct factor Xa inhibitors
Hepatic function tests
Toxicology screen
Blood alcohol level
Pregnancy test
Arterial blood gas tests (if hypoxia is suspected)
Chest radiography (if lung disease is suspected)
Lumbar puncture (if meningitis is suspected or subarachnoid hemorrhage is suspected but the CT scan is negative for blood)
Electroencephalogram (if seizures are suspected)

*Although it is desirable to know the results of these tests before giving intravenous recombinant tissue-type plasminogen activator, fibrinolytic therapy should not be delayed while awaiting the results unless (1) there is clinical suspicion of a bleeding abnormality or thrombocytopenia, (2) the patient has received heparin or warfarin, or (3) the patient has received other anticoagulants (direct thrombin inhibitors or direct factor Xa inhibitors).
CT = computed tomography; ECG = electrocardiogram; INR = international normalized ratio; MRI = magnetic resonance imaging.
From Jauch EC, Saver JL, Adams HP Jr, et al. Guidelines for the early management of patients with acute ischemic stroke: a guideline for healthcare professionals from the American Heart Association/American Stroke Association. *Stroke.* 2013;44:870-947.

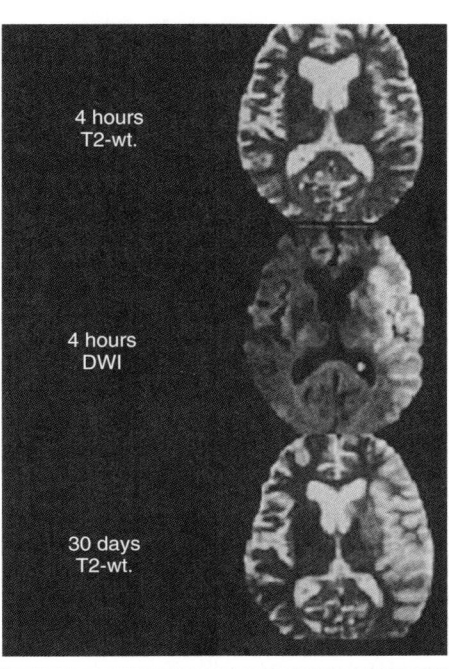

FIGURE 407-2. Magnetic resonance imaging (MRI) showing possible advantages of diffusion-weighted imaging (DWI) relative to conventional MRI at early times after vascular occlusion. *Top,* Conventional T2-weighted MRI 4 hours after symptom onset that appears normal. *Middle,* At the same time, a DWI scan shows abnormalities in the left hemisphere. *Bottom,* Repeated T2-weighted MRI 1 month later showed an infarction in the same location as the initial DWI scan. (Courtesy Gregory W. Albers, Stanford University, Stanford, Calif.)

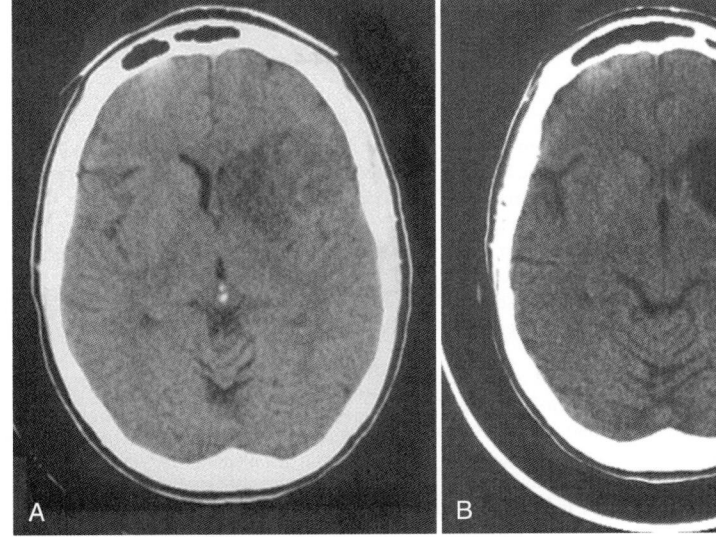

FIGURE 407-3. Computed tomographic imaging. **A,** A computed tomography (CT) scan of a patient with a left hemisphere infarction 6 to 24 hours after the onset of symptoms shows a hypodense area in the basal ganglia region and compression of the frontal horn of the lateral ventricle. **B,** A CT scan shows the chronic infarction 1 year later; atrophy and loss of tissue volume are visible. (Courtesy Gregory W. Albers, Stanford University, Stanford, Calif.)

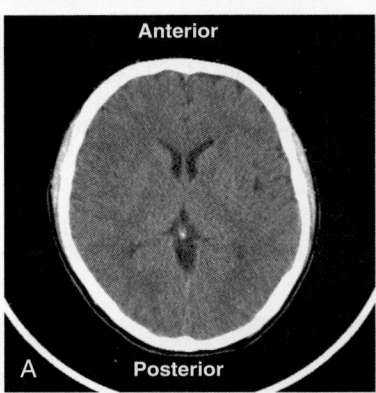
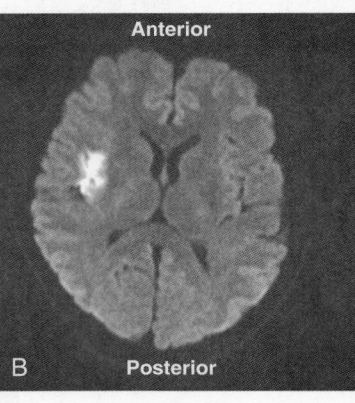
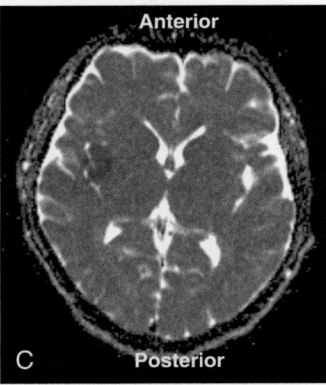

FIGURE 407-4. A, Computed tomographic imaging. B, Magnetic resonance imaging, diffusion sequence. C, Magnetic resonance imaging, apparent diffusion coefficient (ADC) map. Computed tomography shows no evidence of ischemic injury. There is an obvious area of restricted diffusion in the right frontotemporal cortex that is dark on the ADC map, consistent with an area of acute ischemic injury.

cardiogenic embolism in a patient with infective endocarditis, may cause stroke or strokelike symptoms and be an indicator for an urgent lumbar puncture. Brain CT usually demonstrates blood in the subarachnoid space in patients presenting with symptoms and signs of subarachnoid hemorrhage (Chapter 408), such as headache and meningismus. If, however, brain CT fails to visualize a subarachnoid hemorrhage in a patient in whom the clinical suspicion of subarachnoid hemorrhage is high, lumbar puncture should still be obtained.

Other Imaging

Carotid duplex ultrasonography, which combines B-mode vascular imaging with measures of blood flow velocity, is commonly used to screen for extracranial carotid artery stenosis but is rarely indicated in the acute setting. Both CT and MR angiography provide noninvasive vascular imaging of the extracranial and intracranial cerebral circulation, and either study can be obtained in conjunction with parenchymal imaging in the acute setting. CT or MR angiography may be helpful in identifying cervical artery dissections in a patient with headache, neck pain, and symptoms and signs consistent with ipsilateral ischemic injury. Venous sinuses should be imaged if a sinus thrombosis is being considered. In patients who are not candidates for intravenous rtPA but who may be considered for acute endovascular therapy, these studies can be used to identify a proximal arterial occlusion. Transcranial Doppler ultrasonography is an alternative for evaluating the proximal cerebral vessels, but it cannot be obtained in some patients because of inadequate sonographic windows.

Diagnostic catheter angiography carries about a 0.5 to 1.5% risk of causing a stroke and has largely been supplanted in the acute setting by noninvasive vascular imaging. Catheter angiography is, however, superior to CT or MR angiography for visualizing smaller intracranial vessels and for detecting intracranial vasculopathies such as vasculitis (Chapter 270).

Differential Diagnosis

The hallmark of acute ischemic stroke is the abrupt onset of a focal neurologic deficit, frequently attributable to an area of brain supplied by a specific artery or arteries. In some patients, however, the onset of ischemic stroke may be stuttering, and the stroke symptoms may have been heralded by a prior TIA. The detection of an ipsilateral cervical artery bruit may also support the diagnosis. Embolic stroke typically has its maximal severity at onset, but it can involve multiple vascular territories. The diagnosis of an embolic stroke may be further suggested by finding a cardiac murmur, an irregularly irregular heart rhythm, or signs of emboli in other vascular territories.

A variety of other neurologic conditions may also be manifested acutely. Migraine with aura (Chapter 398) can be associated with focal neurologic deficits, including speech impairment, visual changes, vertigo, weakness, numbness, and imbalance. Partial seizures (Chapter 403) may have negative symptoms, including aphasia and paresis, and a patient with a postictal Todd paralysis may appear to have had a stroke. As a further challenge in diagnosis, seizures may occur in patients who are having an acute stroke. In a patient without a previous diagnosis, the first episode of multiple sclerosis (Chapter 411) can mimic a stroke. Mass lesions such as neoplasms (Chapter 189) and abscesses (Chapter 413) are generally associated with a slowly progressive

TABLE 407-6	TIME GOALS FOR EVALUATION AND TREATMENT OF PATIENTS WITH ACUTE ISCHEMIC STROKE
TIME AFTER EMERGENCY DEPARTMENT ARRIVAL	**GOALS**
10 minutes	Assess ABCs, vital signs
	Provide oxygen if hypoxemic
	Obtain intravenous access
	Obtain laboratory studies
	CBC, coagulation, electrolytes
	Check glucose level, treat if indicated
	Perform screening neurologic assessment
	Activate stroke team
	Order "stroke code" brain CT or MRI
	Obtain 12-lead ECG
25 minutes	Review history
	Establish time at onset or last known normal
	Perform neurologic examination
	NIH Stroke Scale
45 minutes	Review laboratory studies
	Review brain CT or MRI results
	Evaluate inclusion and exclusion criteria (see Tables 407-8 and 407-9)
60 minutes	Review risks and benefits
	Obtain consent
	Begin infusion

ABCs = airway, breathing, circulation; CBC = complete blood count; CT = computed tomography; ECG = electrocardiogram; MRI = magnetic resonance imaging; NIH = National Institutes of Health.

worsening of neurologic symptoms but may occasionally be manifested acutely. Metabolic disorders such as hypoglycemia (Chapter 230) or hyperglycemia (Chapter 229), toxin exposures (Chapters 22 and 110), and drug intoxications (Chapter 34) can cause focal symptoms similar to stroke. Strokelike symptoms may also be a manifestation of malingering, a conversion disorder, or other psychiatric illness.

TREATMENT

Intravenous rtPA

After initial respiratory and hemodynamic stabilization, the management of patients with acute ischemic stroke is directed at determining expeditiously (Table 407-7; see also Fig. 407-1) whether treatment with intravenous rtPA is appropriate (Table 407-7; see also Fig. 407-1). Intravenous rtPA, administered within 4.5 hours of the onset of symptoms,[A1] does not reduce mortality but results in a higher odds of a better neurologic outcome at 3 months compared with placebo. The benefit of rtPA declines over time within this 4.5-hour treatment window, with the odds ratio for a favorable 3-month outcome declining from 2.55 for treatment within 0 to 90 minutes, to 1.64 for 91 to 180 minutes, to 1.26 for 181 to 270 minutes, and to no statistical benefit for treatment

TABLE 407-7   ADMINISTRATION OF rtPA FOR ACUTE ISCHEMIC STROKE

Infuse 0.9 mg/kg (maximum dose 90 mg) over 60 minutes, with 10% of the dose given as a bolus over 1 minute.

Admit the patient to an intensive care or stroke unit for monitoring.

If the patient develops severe headache, acute hypertension, nausea, or vomiting or has a worsening neurological examination, discontinue the infusion (if IV rtPA is being administered) and obtain emergent CT scan.

Measure blood pressure and perform neurological assessments every 15 minutes during and after IV rtPA infusion for 2 hours, then every 30 minutes for 6 hours, then hourly until 24 hours after IV rtPA treatment.

Increase the frequency of blood pressure measurements if systolic blood pressure is >180 mm Hg or if diastolic blood pressure is >105 mm Hg; administer antihypertensive medications to maintain blood pressure at or below these levels (Table 407-10).

Delay placement of nasogastric tubes, indwelling bladder catheters, or intra-arterial pressure catheters if the patient can be safely managed without them.

Obtain a follow-up CT or MRI scan at 24 hours after IV rtPA before starting anticoagulants or antiplatelet agents.

CT = computed tomography; IV = intravenous; MRI = magnetic resonance imaging; rtPA = recombinant tissue plasminogen activator.
From Jauch EC, Saver JL, Adams HP Jr, et al. Guidelines for the early management of patients with acute ischemic stroke: a guideline for healthcare professionals from the American Heart Association/American Stroke Association. *Stroke.* 2013;44:870-947.

---

beyond 4.5 hours. Registry studies support a benefit in routine clinical practice similar to that in randomized trials.[6] As a result, current guidelines recommend that treatment with intravenous rtPA (Food and Drug Administration approved up to 3 hours after symptom onset) not be given if more than 4.5 hours have elapsed since the onset of symptoms. Treatment with rtPA is efficacious and safe among patients who are chronically treated with warfarin, provided their INR is 1.7 or lower, and is contraindicated with an INR higher than 1.7.[A2] Treatment increases the risk of intracranial hemorrhage, but the overall benefit includes these adverse events, which do not significantly increase in frequency during the 4.5-hour treatment window. Some patients have absolute exclusion criteria against treatment with intravenous rtPA (Table 407-8), with additional relative contraindications for treatment between 3 and 4.5 hours (Table 407-9). In patients without contraindications, treatment should begin as soon as possible in either treatment window.

Endovascular Therapy

Although strokes caused by large proximal occlusions tend to benefit less from treatment with intravenous rtPA compared with more distal or small-vessel obstructions, no randomized trials show additional benefit of infusing rtPA directly into the thrombus or of other endovascular treatments compared with intravenous rtPA alone, even though several devices are Food and Drug Administration approved to remove clots from brain blood vessels. As a result, current guidelines recommend treatment with intravenous rtPA even if intra-arterial treatments are available. Endovascular therapy can be considered in selected patients who cannot be treated with intravenous rtPA, such as patients who had a recent surgical procedure and who present up to 6 hours after a middle cerebral artery occlusion and perhaps longer after basilar artery occlusion.

Other Treatments

Regardless of whether the patient received intravenous rtPA or endovascular therapy, care in a comprehensive specialized stroke unit that incorporates rehabilitation is associated with better patient outcomes. Urgent anticoagulation to prevent recurrent stroke, to prevent worsening, or to improve functional outcome of patients with acute ischemic stroke is not recommended. Aspirin should not be started within 24 hours of treatment with intravenous rtPA, but aspirin should be started at 325 mg daily within 24 to 48 hours after the onset of stroke.[A3] Hemicraniectomy can increase survival in patients with extensive middle cerebral artery strokes, but most survivors will require assistance with their body needs.[A4]

Antihypertensive medications to reduce blood pressure acutely by 10 to 25% in the first 24 hours with a goal of blood pressure to below 140/90 mm Hg by 1 week does not improve outcomes compared with discontinuation of all antihypertensive medications.[A5] Current guidelines recommend that antihypertensive medications not be given unless the blood pressure rises to more than 220/120 mm Hg or higher in the absence of other indications. An exception is that blood pressure can be lowered in patients who are otherwise candidates for intravenous rtPA with a goal of maintaining blood pressures below 180/105 mm Hg after treatment (Fig. 407-5).

Several potential complications of acute stroke can often be avoided. Patients with stroke in any vascular distribution are at risk of aspiration

TABLE 407-8   INCLUSION AND EXCLUSION CHARACTERISTICS OF PATIENTS WITH ISCHEMIC STROKE WHO COULD BE TREATED WITH IV rtPA WITHIN 3 HOURS FROM SYMPTOM ONSET

INCLUSION CRITERIA

Diagnosis of ischemic stroke causing measurable neurological deficit
Onset of symptoms <3 hours before beginning treatment
Aged ≥18 years

EXCLUSION CRITERIA

Significant head trauma or prior stroke in previous 3 months
Symptoms suggest subarachnoid hemorrhage
Arterial puncture at noncompressible site in previous 7 days
History of previous intracranial hemorrhage
Intracranial neoplasm, arteriovenous malformation, or aneurysm
Recent intracranial or intraspinal surgery
Elevated blood pressure (systolic >185 mm Hg or diastolic >110 mm Hg)
Active internal bleeding
Acute bleeding diathesis, including but not limited to
   Platelet count <100,000/mm^3
   Heparin received within 48 hours, resulting in aPTT greater than the upper limit of normal
   Current use of anticoagulant with INR >1.7 or PT >15 seconds
   Current use of direct thrombin inhibitors or direct factor Xa inhibitors with elevated sensitive laboratory tests (such as aPTT, INR, platelet count, and ECT; TT; or appropriate factor Xa activity assays)
Blood glucose concentration <50 mg/dL (2.7 mmol/L)
CT demonstrates multilobar infarction (hypodensity >⅓ cerebral hemisphere)

RELATIVE EXCLUSION CRITERIA

Recent experience suggests that under some circumstances—with careful consideration and weighting of risk to benefit—patients may receive fibrinolytic therapy despite 1 or more relative contraindications. Consider risk to benefit of IV rtPA administration carefully if any of these relative contraindications are present:
   Only minor or rapidly improving stroke symptoms (clearing spontaneously)
   Pregnancy
   Seizure at onset with postictal residual neurological impairments
   Major surgery or serious trauma within previous 14 days
   Recent gastrointestinal or urinary tract hemorrhage (within previous 21 days)
   Recent acute myocardial infarction (within previous 3 months)

NOTES:

- The checklist includes some FDA-approved indications and contraindications for administration of IV rtPA for acute ischemic stroke. Recent guideline revisions have modified the original FDA-approved indications. A physician with expertise in acute stroke care may modify this list.
- Onset time is defined as either the witnessed onset of symptoms or the time last known normal if symptom onset was not witnessed.
- In patients without recent use of oral anticoagulants or heparin, treatment with IV rtPA can be initiated before availability of coagulation test results but should be discontinued if INR is >1.7 or PT is abnormally elevated by local laboratory standards.
- In patients without history of thrombocytopenia, treatment with IV rtPA can be initiated before availability of platelet count but should be discontinued if platelet count is <100,000/mm^3.

aPTT = activated partial thromboplastin time; CT = computed tomography; ECT = ecarin clotting time; FDA = Food and Drug Administration; INR = international normalized ratio; IV = intravenous; PT = partial thromboplastin time; rtPA = recombinant tissue plasminogen activator; TT = thrombin time.
From Jauch EC, Saver JL, Adams HP Jr, et al. Guidelines for the early management of patients with acute ischemic stroke: a guideline for healthcare professionals from the American Heart Association/American Stroke Association. *Stroke.* 2013;44:870-947.

---

pneumonia (Chapter 97). Stroke patients should not receive oral medications or nutrition until their ability to swallow safely has been assessed. Urinary tract infections (Chapter 284) are a potential complication; the routine placement of indwelling bladder catheters should be avoided, and patients who require an indwelling bladder catheter should have it removed as soon as feasible. Any infectious complications should be treated aggressively, and antipyretics should be used to maintain euthermia because fever is associated with more ischemic injury and poorer outcomes. Immobilized patients should receive deep venous thrombosis prophylaxis with subcutaneous unfractionated heparin or low-molecular-weight heparin (see Table 38-2) if it is not contraindicated, with mechanical intermittent pneumatic compression if anticoagulation is contraindicated,[A6] or with both.

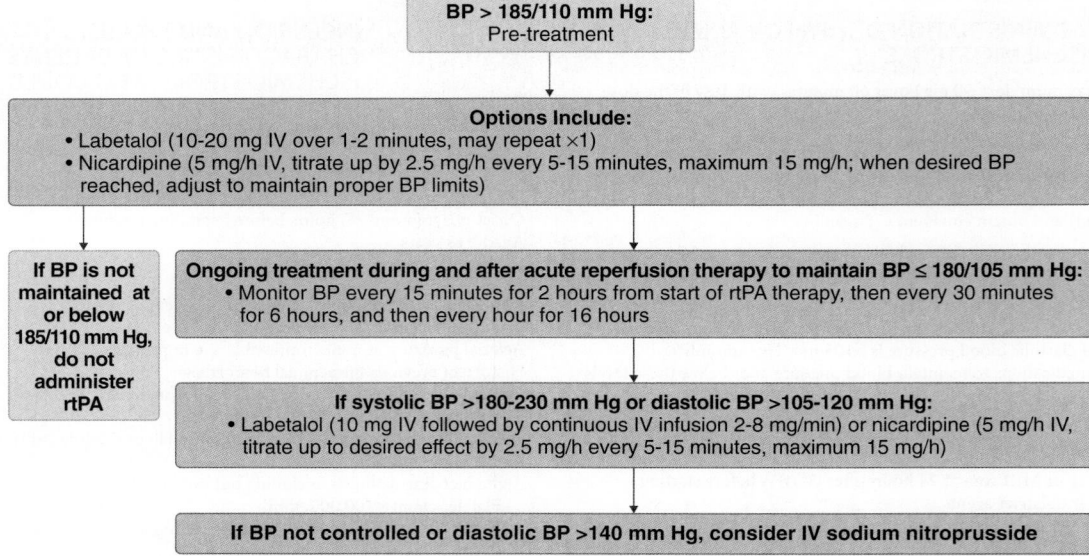

Abbreviations: BP, blood pressure; IV, intravenously; and rtPA, recombinant tissue plasminogen activator.

Adapted from Jauch EC, Saver JL, Adams HP, Jr., et al. Guidelines for the early management of patients with acute ischemic stroke: a guideline for healthcare professionals from the American Heart Association/ American Stroke Association. *Stroke.* 2013;44:870–947.

FIGURE 407-5. Potential Approaches to Arterial Hypertension in Acute Ischemic Stroke Patients Who are Candidates for Acute Reperfusion Therapy.

TABLE 407-9 RELATIVE CONTRAINDICATIONS TO IV rtPA IN PATIENTS WITHIN 3 TO 4.5 HOURS AFTER ONSET OF SYMPTOMS OF ACUTE ISCHEMIC STROKE

National Institutes of Health Stroke Scale >25 (see Table 407-4)
Age > 80 years old
Taking an oral anticoagulant regardless of INR
History of diabetes *and* a prior ischemic stroke

INR, international normalized ratio; IV, intravenous; and rtPA, recombinant tissue plasminogen activator.
Adapted from Jauch EC, Saver JL, Adams HP, Jr., et al. Guidelines for the early management of patients with acute ischemic stroke: a guideline for healthcare professionals from the American Heart Association/American Stroke Association. *Stroke.* 2013;44:870-947.

UNUSUAL CAUSES OF STROKE

Ischemic strokes may be caused by a variety of rarer conditions. Specific treatments, many of which are not supported by extensive clinical trial data, vary accordingly (Table 407-10).

Cerebral Venous Thrombosis

Thrombosis of a cerebral venous sinus can cause headache, focal strokelike manifestations, seizures, altered mental status, and papilledema.[7] With superior sagittal sinus obstruction (see Fig. 406-10), patients can develop bilateral leg weakness and sensory changes. Obstruction of a transverse sinus or one of the major veins over the cerebral convexity (see Fig. 406-11) can also produce symptoms, depending on the area of the brain that is injured. Cerebral venous sinus thrombosis is an uncommon condition that is usually seen in patients with coagulopathies, disseminated cancer, or a prior inner ear infection. It can also occur in the peripartum period. Venous obstruction can mimic an ischemic arterial stroke, but symptoms and signs are often more diffuse and resemble encephalitis (Chapter 414) or meningitis (Chapter 412). The diagnosis can be suspected on routine CT or MRI and confirmed by CT or MR venography (Fig. 407-6). Initial acute treatment options include either body weight–adjusted subcutaneous low-molecular-weight heparin (see Table 38-2) or dose-adjusted intravenous heparin (see Table 81-4), even if patients have some degree of hemorrhage,[8] and one small randomized trial found that treatment with low-molecular-weight heparin was associated with lower mortality.[A7] Oral warfarin anticoagulation should be started and continued for at least 3 months, with an INR target of 2.0 to 3.0. Longer periods of anticoagulation may be considered, depending on the cause of the sinus thrombosis.

Cervical Artery Dissection

A cervical artery dissection or cerebral artery dissection, each of which is caused by the formation and subsequent longitudinal extension of an intramural hematoma, can narrow or obstruct the arterial lumen. These dissections can be spontaneous, or they can be associated with major neck injury, relatively minor trauma (such as a chiropractic neck manipulation or neck hyperextension), or otherwise innocuous activities, such as coughing, sneezing, or lifting. Patients may have underlying fibromuscular dysplasia (Chapters 67 and 80); inherited conditions, such as Marfan syndrome (Chapter 260), Ehlers-Danlos syndrome, or tuberous sclerosis (Chapter 417); an elevated blood homocysteine level; or no identified underlying cause. The diagnosis can be challenging but should be considered especially in an otherwise healthy young patient who has neck or facial pain in conjunction with a stroke. MR angiography may show a hyperintense mass adjacent to a flow void, and MR angiography or catheter angiography can show a tapered lumen leading to an obstruction or even a double lumen. Treatment may include thrombolysis, anticoagulation, or endovascular or surgical repair, depending on individual circumstances, but no randomized trials are available to guide such decisions.

Vasculitis (Chapters 266, 270, and 271) can cause focal or multifocal cerebral ischemia due to local inflammation, stenosis, and even necrosis of extracranial or intracranial blood vessels.[9] Patients can have preexisting or concurrent headaches, cognitive changes, and seizures. Because vasculitis often involves multiple arteries, multiple foci of ischemic injury on neuroimaging studies may mimic multiple emboli. Cerebral angiography classically shows multiple areas of beadlike segmental narrowing, but findings may be normal. Similar findings may occur with other causes of intracranial vasculopathy, and the angiographic appearance is not specific. The diagnosis may require leptomeningeal/cortical biopsy, which may be negative because the inflammatory process can be multifocal rather than diffuse. Examples of vasculitides that can cause strokelike symptoms include primary central nervous system vasculitis, systemic lupus erythematosus (Chapter 266), rheumatoid vasculitis (Chapter 264), Behçet disease (Chapter 270), Takayasu arteritis (Chapters 78 and 270), temporal arteritis (Chapter 271), fibromuscular dysplasia (Chapters 67 and 80), granulomatosis with angiitis (Chapter 270), sarcoidosis (Chapter 95), meningovascular syphilis (Chapter 319), and lymphomatoid angioendotheliomatosis.

TABLE 407-10 USUAL CAUSES OF ISCHEMIC STROKE

CAUSE	SETTING	NOTES	POSSIBLE TREATMENT
Vasculitis (Chapter 270)	Patients commonly but not always have a prior known vasculitic condition	Vasculitis can be manifested with headache, cognitive impairment, multiple areas of infarction, or hemorrhage. Vasculitis affecting the cerebral vasculature can occur in the setting of systemic vasculitis or be confined to the central nervous system (primary vasculitis of the central nervous system). Diagnosis is supported by evidence of an inflammatory response in the spinal fluid, meningeal enhancement on MRI, and a typical pattern of focal stenoses on cerebral angiography. Brain/meningeal biopsy is often necessary to exclude other causes.	Steroids, immunosuppression
Sickle cell disease (Chapter 163)	Patients with known sickle cell disease; persons of African, Indian, and Mediterranean descent	Sickle cell disease can cause stroke by occlusion of small brain vessels or by intimal fibrosis leading to large-vessel occlusion. Patients with sickle cell disease can be monitored with transcranial Doppler ultrasound.	Transfusions to reduce hemoglobin S to <30% to 50% of total hemoglobin, hydroxyurea
Atrial myxoma (Chapter 60)	Usually not previously diagnosed; may be suspected on physical examination but usually otherwise asymptomatic and discovered on echocardiography	Atrial myxoma is the most common primary cardiac tumor and can lead to emboli.	Surgical removal of the tumor
Coagulation disorders (Chapter 176)	Young people with stroke of unknown cause or history suggesting coagulopathy, such as prior venous thrombosis, pulmonary embolism, multiple (particularly late) miscarriages	Prothrombotic coagulopathies can be inherited or acquired. These are more commonly associated with venous thrombosis and can lead to stroke in patients with a right to left shunt as paradoxical emboli. Late miscarriages in women or unprovoked deep venous thrombosis may be clues to an underlying coagulopathy. In addition to abnormalities of fibrinogen occurring in patients with cancer, anticardiolipin/antiphospholipid antibodies, and lupus anticoagulants are most commonly associated with ischemic stroke. Coagulopathies need to be considered in all patients with a cerebral venous sinus thrombosis.	Platelet antiaggregants or anticoagulation
Hyperviscosity	Usually caused by polycythemia vera, macroglobulinemia, or multiple myeloma	Hyperviscosity can cause ischemic stroke through occlusion of small intracranial vessels.	Treatment of underlying hematologic disorder
Cervical artery dissection	Often in otherwise healthy younger individuals	Dissections can be caused by trauma or occur spontaneously. Underlying causes include fibromuscular dysplasia (which can also affect renal arteries), Marfan syndrome, Ehlers-Danlos type IV, and tuberous sclerosis.	Dissections often heal spontaneously with no evidence of residual vascular injury. A period of anticoagulation is commonly used in patients with stroke related to dissection; however, data showing the benefit of the approach are lacking.
Aortic dissection (Chapter 78)	Marfan syndrome, Ehlers-Danlos syndrome	Aortic dissection can be manifested with chest pain radiating to the back.	Emergency surgical repair
Moyamoya	Usually discovered with intracranial vascular imaging, such as CT angiography, MR angiography, or catheter angiography	Moyamoya refers to neovascularization in patients with occlusion of the distal intracranial internal carotid arteries or proximal middle cerebral arteries. Moyamoya can be the result of other conditions (moyamoya syndrome) or occur without identifiable cause (moyamoya disease). Moyamoya can be associated with both ischemic stroke and brain hemorrhage.	Extracranial-intracranial bypass
Fabry disease (Chapter 208)	Stroke in the setting of typical historic features and physical examination findings; may be considered in young persons with stroke of unknown cause	Fabry disease is an X-linked disorder causing reduction in α-galactosidase. In addition to stroke, Fabry disease can cause angiokeratomas, acroparesthesias, hypohidrosis, corneal opacities, and renal and cardiac disease.	Enzyme replacement therapy is available but has not been shown to reduce stroke risk.

CT = computed tomography; MR = magnetic resonance.

Strokes occur in about 8 to 17% of patients with sickle cell disease and in about 2% of individuals with sickle cell trait (Chapter 163). Ischemic strokes are more common in children, whereas hemorrhagic strokes are more common in adults. Transfusion therapy can markedly reduce the risk of a first or recurrent stroke.[A8]

Drug-Related Causes of Stroke

A variety of legal and illicit drugs (Chapter 34) can precipitate an ischemic stroke. Intravenous drug users are more likely to develop bacterial endocarditis (Chapter 76), which can cause embolic stroke. Solid adulterants in injected material can reach the brain through an existing shunt, such as a patent foramen ovale, or they can cause local pulmonary arteriolitis that damages the endothelium and results in arteriovenous shunts through which microemboli can reach the brain. Potent vasoconstricting drugs (e.g., cocaine, ephedrine, phenylpropanolamine, and fenoxazoline) and dietary supplements (e.g., ephedra) may precipitate cerebral vasospasm and ischemic stroke, although hemorrhagic strokes are more common (Chapter 408). These drugs

have been used in high doses as appetite suppressants, and case reports suggest that stroke may occur even after the first use of these products.

Rare Genetic Causes

A number of relatively rare genetic diseases can cause ischemic stroke. *Cerebral autosomal dominant arteriopathy with small subcortical infarcts and leukoencephalopathy* (CADASIL) can cause multiple deep infarcts and dementia in patients without other risk factors for stroke. A mutation in the Notch3 receptor gene on the short arm of chromosome 19 leads to an accumulation of Notch3 protein in vascular smooth muscle cells. The mean age at onset is about 40 years, although migraine with aura often antedates strokes by several years. Dementia usually develops within 10 to 15 years. Antenatal diagnosis is recommended in affected families. Treatment is symptomatic, with CADASIL-associated headaches potentially responding to acetazolamide (125 to 500 mg daily).

X-linked *Fabry disease* (angiokeratoma corporis diffusum) (Chapter 208) frequently includes cerebrovascular occlusion due to the accumulation of

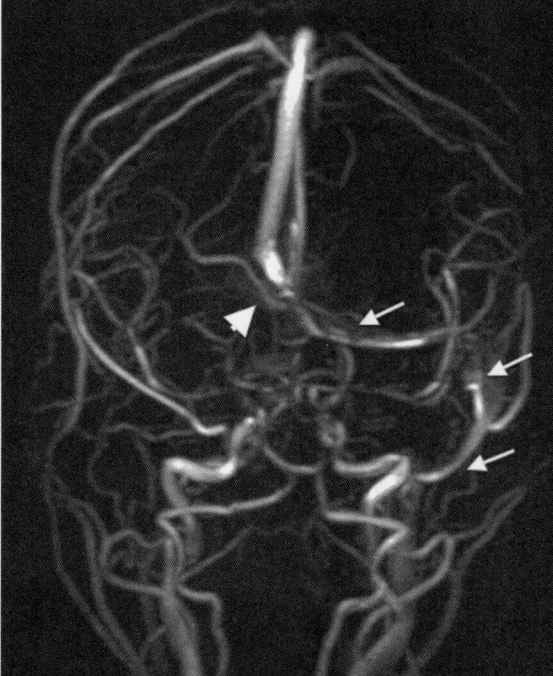

FIGURE 407-6. Magnetic resonance venogram showing absent flow in the right transverse sinus (*arrowhead*) and sigmoid sinus and intact flow in the left transverse sinus and sigmoid sinus (*arrows*).

glycolipids in small and medium-sized arteries. Enzyme replacement therapy is recommended, although it is not proven to reduce the risk of stroke. *Neurofibromatosis* (Chapter 417) can occlude the internal carotid arteries or the proximal part of the anterior cerebral circulation. Marfan syndrome (Chapter 260) can cause ischemic stroke due to dissection of the carotid arteries or related valvular heart disease.

Fat Embolism

Fat embolism (Chapter 98) after trauma to the long bones (Chapter 111), orthopedic procedures, and even severe trauma to large fat deposits can cause a stroke, usually several days later. Diffuse embolization can produce encephalopathy or seizures, but more focal emboli can be manifested as an ischemic stroke.

Cryptogenic Stroke

An echocardiogram may reveal an undiagnosed patent foramen ovale (Chapter 68) as a potential cause of a cryptogenic stroke. Despite a comprehensive evaluation, however, no definitive cause of stroke is found in 15 to 40% of patients with strokes. Randomized trials confirm that prolonged ECG monitoring with an event-triggered recorder or an insertable monitor increases the detection of atrial fibrillation to 9 to 16% compared with 1 to 3% with just 24-hour monitoring.[A9][A10] Other initially cryptogenic strokes may be due to embolism from either a cardiac or other proximal arterial source.[10] Clinical trials are needed to determine the most appropriate antithrombotic management of these patients.

RECOVERY/REHABILITATION

The process of recovery begins even before the sequelae of acute brain injury have resolved. Multidisciplinary physiotherapy should include assessments by speech pathologists, physical therapists, and occupational therapists. Organized inpatient multidisciplinary rehabilitation is associated with a 34% lower odds of death, a 30% lower odds of death or institutionalization, and a 35% lower odds of death or dependency for patients with deficits warranting these services. All patients with stroke-related deficits should be assessed for rehabilitative interventions. Because depression can complicate stroke and affect recovery, all patients should be screened for depression.

PREVENTION   Rx

Primary Prevention

Because more than 75% of strokes are first events, primary prevention of stroke is of paramount importance.[11,12] Following a healthy lifestyle (not smoking, following a diet low in sodium and rich in fruits and vegetables, getting at least 30 minutes of moderate or vigorous physical activity daily, having a body mass index below 25 kg/m², and consumption of no more than one alcoholic drink per day for women and one or two for men) is associated with an 80% lower risk of a first stroke compared with people who do not follow these lifestyles. The effect is graded, with increasing benefit depending on the number of healthy lifestyles an individual follows. There is no evidence that prophylactic treatment with aspirin or other antiplatelet drugs reduces the risk of stroke in low-risk individuals.

Risk factors that are amenable to treatment (see Table 407-1) include hypertension, diabetes, atrial fibrillation, and carotid stenosis. Treatment of hypertension dramatically reduces the risk of stroke.[13] Regular blood pressure screening and treatment of hypertension (see Tables 67-7 and 67-9) with a goal below 140/90 mm Hg are recommended. Blood pressure treatment and the use of a statin in patients with diabetes (Chapter 229) are recommended to lower the risk of a first stroke. Statins (Chapter 206) are also recommended to prevent a first ischemic stroke in patients with coronary heart disease. Although microvascular complications of diabetes are reduced with adequate glycemic control (target glycated hemoglobin level <7%), there is no evidence that tight control reduces the risk of stroke or coronary heart events. Patients who have atrial fibrillation are at increased risk of embolism and benefit from treatment with warfarin or a novel oral anticoagulant (Chapter 64).[14] Anticoagulation with warfarin is indicated for stroke prevention in patients with a mechanical prosthetic heart valve (Chapter 75). The U.S. Preventive Services Task Force recommends against screening for asymptomatic carotid artery stenosis.[15]

Prevention of Stroke in the Patient with Asymptomatic Carotid Stenosis

The benefit of carotid endarterectomy for patients with asymptomatic carotid stenosis is currently uncertain because of advances in medical therapy.[16] The risk of ipsilateral stroke associated with an asymptomatic carotid stenosis may be considerably less than 1% per year on the basis of older observational studies and clinical trials,[17] and the reported benefit of carotid endarterectomy depends on surgical success and complication rates that may not be widely achievable outside of randomized trials. Clinical trials are in progress comparing carotid revascularization in asymptomatic patients with current best medical therapy. Population screening for asymptomatic carotid stenosis is not recommended.

Secondary Prevention after a Transient Ischemic Attack or Stroke

Although clinical trials demonstrating the efficacy of lifestyle interventions for secondary stroke prevention are generally lacking, the same lifestyle behaviors associated with a reduced risk of a first stroke are an essential part of secondary stroke prevention.[18] Patients should routinely be prescribed an antiplatelet agent unless there are contraindications. Short-term dual antiplatelet therapy with aspirin and clopidogrel is more efficacious than single-agent therapy,[A12] but long-term therapy is not and may cause more serious bleeding.[A11] The choice of agent needs to be individualized, but aspirin (50 to 325 mg daily), clopidogrel (75 mg daily), or aspirin plus sustained-release dipyridamole (25/200 mg twice daily) are proven options.[19] The exception is the patient who has a specific indication for treatment with an anticoagulant, such as atrial fibrillation or a prosthetic heart valve, or in whom antithrombotic therapy is contraindicated.

Blood pressure reduction is recommended to lower the risk of recurrent stroke and other vascular events.[20] The precise timing of initiation of antihypertensive therapy after ischemic stroke is not established, but it can begin once the patient is stabilized after the acute period, generally after at least 24 hours. An average reduction of 10/5 mm Hg is associated with about a 25% reduction in the risk of recurrent stroke. In a randomized trial of patients with MRI-defined symptomatic lacunar infarctions, reducing systolic blood pressure to a target of less than 130 mm Hg starting 2 weeks later significantly reduced the rate of intracerebral hemorrhage and insignificantly reduced all subsequent stroke compared with a target of 130 to 149 mm Hg.[A13] The choice of a specific antihypertensive regimen for secondary prevention should be individualized (see Tables 67-7 and 67-8); some data suggest that increased blood pressure variability, which is more common with β-blockers, blunts the benefit of blood pressure reduction for preventing recurrent stroke.

Patients with a prior stroke or TIA and known atherosclerotic disease, diabetes, or hyperlipidemia meeting criteria for statin therapy should be treated with a high-potency statin (e.g., 40 to 80 mg of atorvastatin or 20 to 40 mg of rosuvastatin daily; see also Table 206-5), unless contraindicated, to reduce the risk of recurrent stroke and of other cardiovascular events.[21] Stopping a statin in the setting of an acute ischemic stroke is associated with increased morbidity and mortality.

In addition to these general measures, additional specific treatment for secondary stroke prevention depends on the cause of the stroke. Atrial fibrillation–related stroke is associated with a high risk of recurrence (i.e., 6 to 10% annually). Patients with atrial fibrillation–related stroke should be treated with warfarin or a novel oral anticoagulant (e.g., direct thrombin inhibitor, factor Xa inhibitor). Anticoagulation with warfarin is indicated in patients with stroke related to acute MI.

Procedures and Devices

The rate of recurrent stroke after stroke or TIA related to a high-grade (70 to 99%) extracranial carotid artery stenosis may be as high as 25% during the next 2 years, with the highest risk in the first weeks after the index event. Because this risk of recurrence is decreased by 50% with successful carotid revascularization, selected patients with stroke associated with 70 to 99% extracranial carotid artery stenosis within the prior 6 months benefit from carotid revascularization, provided the procedure can be performed with less than 6% morbidity. Depending on characteristics such as age, gender, comorbid conditions, and increasing time since the index event, patients with a 50 to 69% extracranial carotid stenosis may also benefit from revascularization. Patients with less than 50% carotid stenosis do not benefit from carotid revascularization. Extracranial-intracranial bypass does not reduce the risk of recurrent strokes in patients with complete occlusion of an extracranial carotid artery.[A14]

Stroke related to a high-grade (i.e., 50 to 99%) intracranial stenosis is associated with a high risk of recurrence. Aspirin is preferred to warfarin in these patients because it is as efficacious and is associated with fewer complications. Intracranial angioplasty/stenting is no better than medical treatment (e.g., aggressive lifestyle modification, platelet antiaggregant therapy, and a high-potency statin) for the prevention of a recurrent stroke in this setting.[A15]

Stenting is generally not as efficacious as endarterectomy for secondary stroke prevention in patients with carotid stenosis,[A16] although younger patients may have a lower combined risk of stroke, MI, and death with stenting and older patients may do better with endarterectomy.[22]

Intention-to-treat analysis of data from three prospective randomized trials of transcatheter closure of a patent foramen ovale in patients with cryptogenic stroke found a nonsignificant reduction in the combined risk of stroke and TIA and in the risk of stroke with closure compared with medical therapy alone.[A17] There remains no Food and Drug Administration–approved device for this purpose, and additional clinical trials are in progress.

PROGNOSIS

TIA is a major risk factor for stroke and requires urgent evaluation to detect specific causes that may require immediate treatment. Overall, approximately 10% of patients who have a TIA will have a stroke within 90 days, with almost half occurring within 2 days. The strokes that occur are frequently disabling or fatal. Factors associated with higher risk include age older than 60 years, diabetes, impaired speech or weakness, symptoms lasting more than 10 minutes, and evidence of ischemic injury on brain MRI. After the acute period, about 20% of patients who had a TIA will have a stroke during the next 10 years.

Stroke-related mortality varies by age. The 30-day stroke mortality rate is estimated to be 9% for patients aged 65 to 74 years, 13% for patients aged 74 to 84 years, and 23% for patients older than 85 years. About 30% of patients who have had a stroke will have a recurrent stroke within 5 years. Stroke is also a leading cause of disability. Among stroke survivors, approximately 45% have cognitive deficits, 30% are unable to walk without assistance, 25% are institutionalized, and 25% are dependent in activities of daily living after 6 months.

Grade A References

A1. Emberson J, Lees KR, Lyden P, et al. Effect of treatment delay, age, and stroke severity on the effects of intravenous thrombolysis with alteplase for acute ischaemic stroke: a meta-analysis of individual patient data from randomised trials. *Lancet.* 2014;384:1929-1935.

A2. Xian Y, Liang L, Smith EE, et al. Risks of intracranial hemorrhage among patients with acute ischemic stroke receiving warfarin and treated with intravenous tissue plasminogen activator. *JAMA.* 2012;307:2600-2608.

A3. Sandercock PA, Counsell C, Tseng MC, et al. Oral antiplatelet therapy for acute ischaemic stroke. *Cochrane Database Syst Rev.* 2014;3:CD000029.

A4. Jüttler E, Unterberg A, Woitzik J, et al. Hemicraniectomy in older patients with extensive middle-cerebral-artery stroke. *N Engl J Med.* 2014;370:1091-1100.

A5. He J, Zhang Y, Xu T, et al. Effects of immediate blood pressure reduction on death and major disability in patients with acute ischemic stroke: the CATIS randomized clinical trial. *JAMA.* 2014;311:479-489.

A6. Dennis M, Sandercock P, Reid J, et al. Effectiveness of intermittent pneumatic compression in reduction of risk of deep vein thrombosis in patients who have had a stroke (CLOTS 3): a multi-centre randomised controlled trial. *Lancet.* 2013;382:516-524.

A7. Misra UK, Kalita J, Chandra S, et al. Low molecular weight heparin versus unfractionated heparin in cerebral venous sinus thrombosis: a randomized controlled trial. *Eur J Neurol.* 2012;19:1030-1036.

A8. Wang WC, Dwan K. Blood transfusion for preventing primary and secondary stroke in people with sickle cell disease. *Cochrane Database Syst Rev.* 2013;11:CD003146.

A9. Gladstone DJ, Spring M, Dorian P, et al. Atrial fibrillation in patients with cryptogenic stroke. *N Engl J Med.* 2014;370:2467-2477.

A10. Sanna T, Diener HC, Passman RS, et al. Cryptogenic stroke and underlying atrial fibrillation. *N Engl J Med.* 2014;370:2478-2486.

A11. Lee M, Saver JL, Hong KS, et al. Risk-benefit profile of long-term dual- versus single-antiplatelet therapy among patients with ischemic stroke: a systematic review and meta-analysis. *Ann Intern Med.* 2013;159:463-470.

A12. Wang Y, Wang Y, Zhao X, et al. Clopidogrel with aspirin in acute minor stroke or transient ischemic attack. *N Engl J Med.* 2013;369:11-19.

A13. Benavente OR, Coffey CS, Conwit R, et al. Blood-pressure targets in patients with recent lacunar stroke: the SPS3 randomised trial. *Lancet.* 2013;382:507-515.

A14. Powers WJ, Clarke WR, Grubb RL Jr, et al. Extracranial-intracranial bypass surgery for stroke prevention in hemodynamic cerebral ischemia: the Carotid Occlusion Surgery Study randomized trial. *JAMA.* 2011;306:1983-1992.

A15. Derdeyn CP, Chimowitz MI, Lynn MJ, et al. Aggressive medical treatment with or without stenting in high-risk patients with intracranial artery stenosis (SAMMPRIS): the final results of a randomised trial. *Lancet.* 2014;383:333-341.

A16. Liu ZJ, Fu WG, Guo ZY, et al. Updated systematic review and meta-analysis of randomized clinical trials comparing carotid artery stenting and carotid endarterectomy in the treatment of carotid stenosis. *Ann Vasc Surg.* 2012;26:576-590.

A17. Pineda AM, Nascimento FO, Yang SC, et al. A meta-analysis of transcatheter closure of patent foramen ovale versus medical therapy for prevention of recurrent thromboembolic events in patients with cryptogenic cerebrovascular events. *Catheter Cardiovasc Interv.* 2013;82:968-975.

GENERAL REFERENCES

For the General References and other additional features, please visit Expert Consult at https://expertconsult.inkling.com.

408

HEMORRHAGIC CEREBROVASCULAR DISEASE

STEPHAN A. MAYER

Approximately 20% of all strokes are due to spontaneous intracranial hemorrhage, of which about three quarters are caused by intracerebral hemorrhage and one quarter by subarachnoid hemorrhage. Intracerebral hemorrhage, which is most frequently caused by the rupture of small penetrating arteries, results in a focal collection of clot within the brain parenchyma. By comparison, subarachnoid hemorrhage is caused by rupture of vessels on the brain's surface, most often due to a congenital aneurysm, and results in diffusion of blood throughout the cerebrospinal fluid (CSF) spaces. In about 40% of either form of hemorrhagic stroke, blood extends into the brain's ventricles, a devastating complication known as intraventricular hemorrhage. Both types of hemorrhagic stroke have high mortality rates, but recovery and survival have improved in recent decades owing to advances in neurocritical care.

SUBARACHNOID HEMORRHAGE

EPIDEMIOLOGY AND PATHOBIOLOGY

About 30,000 new cases of spontaneous subarachnoid hemorrhage occur each year in the United States, predominantly involving young adults. Subarachnoid hemorrhage accounts for 5% of all strokes, with an incidence of approximately 1 in 10,000 individuals annually. Women are affected more than men are, and the rate is twice as high in African Americans as in whites. About 10% of patients with subarachnoid hemorrhage have a first-degree relative who has also had a subarachnoid hemorrhage, even in the absence of an identifiable genetic predisposition such as polycystic kidney disease (Chapter 127), Marfan syndrome (Chapter 260), or Ehlers-Danlos syndrome (Chapter 260). Modifiable risk factors for subarachnoid hemorrhage include cigarette smoking, heavy alcohol use, chronic and poorly controlled hypertension, and use of sympathomimetic agents such as cocaine and phenylpropanolamine. The use of warfarin, especially if the international

TABLE 408-1	NONANEURYSMAL CAUSES OF SUBARACHNOID HEMORRHAGE (IN APPROXIMATE ORDER OF FREQUENCY)

Trauma
Idiopathic perimesencephalic subarachnoid hemorrhage
Arteriovenous malformation
Intracranial arterial dissection (Chapter 407)
Cocaine and amphetamine use (Chapter 34)
Mycotic aneurysm (Chapter 76)
Pituitary apoplexy (Chapter 224)
Moyamoya disease (Chapter 407)
Central nervous system vasculitis (Chapter 270)
Sickle cell disease (Chapter 163)
Coagulation disorders (Chapters 172, 174, and 175)
Primary or metastatic neoplasm (Chapter 189)

normalized ratio (INR) is higher than 3, but not of aspirin is associated with an increased risk of intracerebral hemorrhage compared with no therapy.[1]

In 80% of cases, subarachnoid hemorrhage is caused by a rupture of an intracranial saccular or berry aneurysm. In about half of subarachnoid hemorrhages in which an aneurysm is not identified, the blood has a focal perimesencephalic distribution around the midbrain or anterior to the pons. In these cases, the source of bleeding is probably venous. In the remainder of cases of nonaneurysmal subarachnoid hemorrhage, the bleeding source is usually a thin-walled arterial "blister." Other causes include arteriovenous malformations; mycotic aneurysms (Chapter 76); vasculitis (Chapter 270); tumors (Chapter 189); and severe coagulation disorders, such as hemophilia (Chapter 174), marked thrombocytopenia (Chapter 172), and disseminated intravascular coagulation (Chapter 175) (Table 408-1).

CLINICAL MANIFESTATIONS

The classic symptom of subarachnoid hemorrhage is a rapidly developing, severe "thunderclap" headache, which the patient typically refers to as the "worst headache of my life." The headache is usually generalized, but focal pain may refer to the site of aneurysmal rupture (e.g., periorbital pain related to an ophthalmic artery aneurysm). Commonly associated symptoms include stiff neck, loss of consciousness, nausea, vomiting, back or leg pain, and photophobia. In patients who lose consciousness, tonic posturing may occur and may be difficult to differentiate from a seizure. Although aneurysmal rupture often occurs during periods of exercise or physical stress, subarachnoid hemorrhage can occur at any time, including sleep. More than one third of patients give a history of a premonitory, "sentinel headache" in the days to weeks before presenting with subarachnoid hemorrhage. These prodromal symptoms are usually caused by minor leaks of blood from the aneurysm, but they also may be caused by acute thrombosis or expansion of an aneurysm.

About 5% of patients with subarachnoid hemorrhage present with signs related to local compression of the cranial nerves or brain stem from a large aneurysm and have focal neurologic signs that may point to the site of bleeding and clot formation. The most common syndrome is a third cranial nerve palsy, which is manifested as ptosis, exodeviation of the eye, and anisocoria due to compression from a large posterior communicating artery aneurysm. Large fusiform dolichoectatic aneurysms most frequently occur in the basilar artery and can be manifested with signs and symptoms related to brain stem or cranial nerve compression. Hemiparesis or aphasia suggests a middle cerebral artery aneurysm, and paraparesis or abulia suggests an aneurysm of the proximal anterior cerebral artery.

DIAGNOSIS

In about 15% of patients, subarachnoid hemorrhage is initially misdiagnosed as a migraine headache or viral syndrome, especially in patients with milder symptoms. Neck stiffness, seizures, diastolic blood pressure above 110 mm Hg, vomiting, and headache increase the likelihood of a hemorrhagic stroke rather than an ischemic stroke, but neuroimaging is required for reliable diagnosis.[2] Approximately 40% of misdiagnosed patients experience subsequent neurologic deterioration due to rebleeding, hydrocephalus, or vasospasm before returning to medical attention. A high degree of vigilance is required to establish the diagnosis of subarachnoid hemorrhage, by either computed tomography (CT) or lumbar puncture if the initial CT scan is normal.

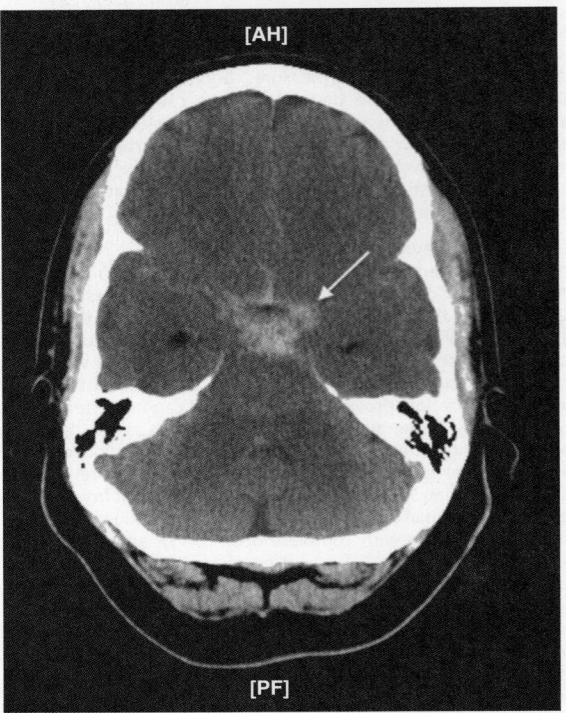

FIGURE 408-1. Computed tomographic imaging. Subarachnoid hemorrhage (note hyperintensity in the suprasellar cistern, *arrow*). (Courtesy Dr. Larry B. Goldstein.)

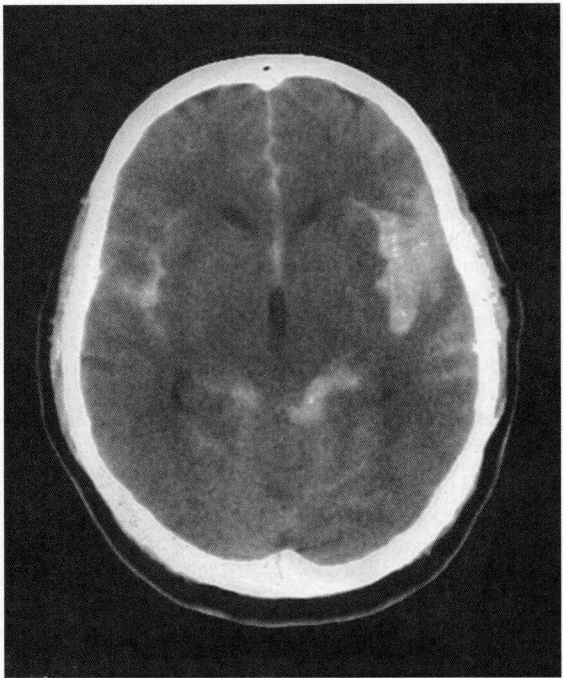

FIGURE 408-2. Computed tomographic scan showing a diffuse, thick subarachnoid hemorrhage.

Computed Tomography

Any patient with suspected subarachnoid hemorrhage should then be sent immediately for an emergency CT scan, which will almost always reveal blood within the basal cisterns if it is performed within 24 hours of the onset of symptoms (Fig. 408-1). More severe hemorrhage can extend into the interhemispheric and bilateral sylvian fissures (Fig. 408-2). The sensitivity of CT declines, however, as time passes from the clinical onset of bleeding, and

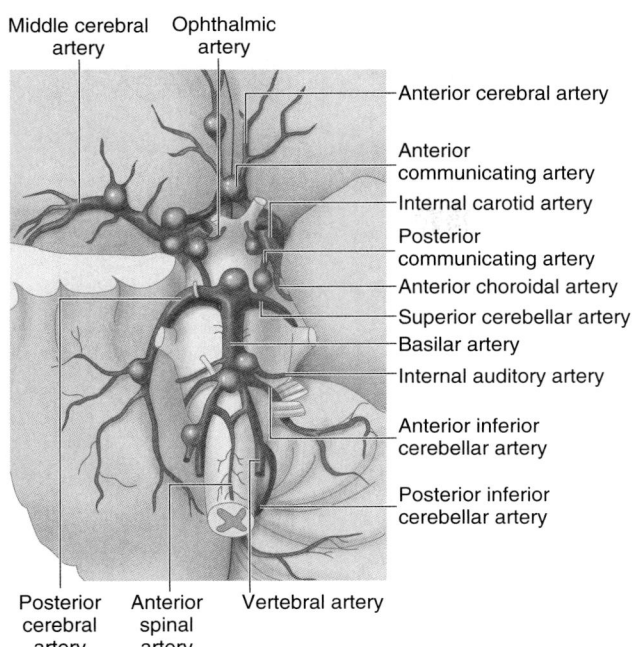

FIGURE 408-3. Saccular aneurysms. Saccular or berry aneurysms typically develop at the bifurcations of arteries on the undersurface of the brain. (Courtesy Dr. Justin Zivin.)

TABLE 408-2	MORTALITY ACCORDING TO THE HUNT-HESS GRADING SCALE FOR ANEURYSMAL SUBARACHNOID HEMORRHAGE	
GRADE	**CLINICAL FINDINGS**	**HOSPITAL MORTALITY (%)**
I	Asymptomatic or mild headache	5
II	Moderate to severe headache, or oculomotor palsy	5
III	Confused, drowsy, or mild focal signs	10
IV	Stupor (localizes to pain)	34
V	Coma (posturing or no motor response to pain)	52
Total		20

Data are from patients treated at Columbia University Medical Center.

the sensitivity of CT is only about 75% by 48 hours after the onset of symptoms. As a result, lumbar puncture is mandatory if the CT scan is normal but the index of clinical suspicion remains high.

Lumbar Puncture

The CSF is usually grossly bloody. Subarachnoid hemorrhage can be differentiated from a traumatic tap by the xanthochromic (yellow-tinged) appearance of the supernatant fluid after centrifugation. However, xanthochromia may not be present until up to 12 hours after the subarachnoid hemorrhage. The CSF pressure is nearly always high, and the protein level is elevated. Initially, the proportion of CSF leukocytes to erythrocytes is that of peripheral blood, with a usual ratio of 1 : 700; after several days, however, a sterile chemical meningitis caused by blood in the CSF may induce a reactive leukocytosis with a low CSF glucose level. Red blood cells and xanthochromia disappear in about 2 weeks unless hemorrhage recurs.

Angiography

Cerebral angiography is the definitive diagnostic procedure to detect intracranial aneurysms and to define their anatomy (Fig. 408-3). Although the increasing availability and image quality of CT and magnetic resonance angiography have allowed some centers to use these tests to make the initial diagnosis, four-vessel (bilateral internal carotid and vertebral artery injections) angiography is mandatory when results of those tests are negative. In approximately 20% of cases of subarachnoid hemorrhage, the initial angiogram is normal. Vasospasm, local thrombosis, or poor technique can lead to a false-negative angiogram. For this reason, patients with an initially normal angiogram should have a follow-up study 1 to 2 weeks later; an aneurysm will be demonstrated in about 5% of these cases. The exception to this rule is found in patients with perimesencephalic subarachnoid hemorrhage, who do not require follow-up angiography.

Magnetic Resonance Imaging

Conventional magnetic resonance imaging (MRI) sequences (T1- or T2-weighted scans) are generally less sensitive than CT scans for detecting blood. Susceptibility-weighted imaging may be useful for documenting a completely thrombosed aneurysm in selected patients who have subarachnoid hemorrhage but a normal angiogram.

Laboratory Testing

In addition to routine admission laboratory tests, care should be taken to check an INR, partial thromboplastin time, and platelet count to diagnose a coagulopathy; an electrocardiogram and serum troponin level to diagnose

sympathetically mediated cardiac injury; and a chest radiograph to look for neurogenic pulmonary edema or aspiration pneumonitis.

TREATMENT ℞

The initial goals of treatment are to minimize acute primary brain injury in poor-grade patients with a depressed level of consciousness (Hunt-Hess grades III to V; Table 408-2), to manage secondary complications, and to prevent rebleeding.[3] Mortality after subarachnoid hemorrhage is substantially lower when patients are treated at high-volume regional centers with access to skilled interventionalists and specialized neurocritical care.

Severe primary brain injury related to the acute effects of hemorrhage is the leading cause of death and disability after subarachnoid hemorrhage, and comprehensive management can reduce both morbidity and mortality (Table 408-3). In poor-grade patients, the immediate concern in the emergency department is reducing intracranial pressure (ICP) and preventing secondary cerebral hypoxic-ischemic injury. Patients with an impaired ability to protect the airway should be intubated with supplemental oxygen given as needed. Hypotension should be treated aggressively with fluids and vasopressors to maintain a mean arterial pressure of 90 mm Hg (Chapter 106). Stuporous or comatose patients with extensive subarachnoid blood, intraventricular hemorrhage, acute obstructive hydrocephalus, or global cerebral edema should be empirically treated for intracranial hypertension with 1.0 g/kg of 20% mannitol before emergent placement of an external ventricular drain. Repeated doses of mannitol or 0.5 to 2.0 mL of 23.4% hypertonic saline can be repeated hourly as needed to reduce ICP to less than 20 mm Hg or to reverse signs of transtentorial herniation, with careful monitoring of serum sodium, osmolality, and volume status.

Cerebral Aneurysms

Recurrent bleeding is a devastating complication of subarachnoid hemorrhage. Preventive strategies depend on the cause, which is usually a cerebral aneurysm, and the site of the initial bleed.

Saccular or berry aneurysms most often occur at the circle of Willis or its major branches, especially at bifurcations. They arise where the arterial elastic lamina and tunica media are defective, tend to enlarge with age, and can become paper-thin. Because saccular aneurysms are rarely detected in children and the incidence of subarachnoid hemorrhage increases with age, it seems clear that congenital wall defects develop into aneurysms only over time. The site of rupture is usually through the dome of the aneurysm. Approximately 15% of patients who present with subarachnoid hemorrhage from an identifiable aneurysm also harbor another unruptured intracranial aneurysm.

Intracranial aneurysms are seen in about 2% of adults, thereby suggesting that approximately 2 to 3 million Americans have an aneurysm. However, more than 90% of these aneurysms are small (<10 mm) and remain asymptomatic throughout life. The annual risk of rupture of an asymptomatic intracranial aneurysm is approximately 0.7%. Important risk factors for the initial rupture of an intracranial aneurysm include increasing size, prior subarachnoid hemorrhage from another aneurysm, active cigarette smoking, and location in the basilar apex and posterior communicating artery. CT angiography is a sensitive (97%) and specific (98%) test for the diagnosis of cerebral aneurysms.[4]

If an aneurysm rebleeds, approximately 50% of patients die immediately, and another 30% suffer incremental brain injury. The risk of rebleeding is highest within the first 24 hours after the initial aneurysmal rupture (4%) and remains elevated (approximately 1% to 2% per day) for the next 4 weeks (Fig. 408-4). The cumulative risk of rebleeding in untreated patients is 20% at 2

TABLE 408-3 MANAGEMENT PROTOCOL FOR ACUTE SUBARACHNOID HEMORRHAGE

Blood pressure	• Control elevated blood pressure during the preoperative phase (systolic blood pressure <160 mm Hg) with IV labetalol or nicardipine (see Table 67-14) to prevent rebleeding.
Rebleeding prophylaxis	• ε-Aminocaproic acid 4 g IV on diagnosis followed by 1 g/hr until aneurysm repair, for a maximum of up to 72 hours after ictus
Intravenous hydration	• Normal (0.9%) saline at 1.0-1.5 mL/kg/hr
Laboratory testing	• Periodically check complete blood count and electrolytes. • Obtain serial ECGs and check admission cardiac troponin level to evaluate for cardiac injury; perform echocardiography in patients with abnormal ECG findings or elevated troponin levels.
Seizure prophylaxis	• Fosphenytoin or phenytoin IV load (15-20 mg/kg); discontinue on postoperative day 1 unless patient has seized, is poor grade, or has focal cortical disease or is otherwise unstable. Starting dose is 300 mg daily IV adjusted to maintain therapeutic levels of 10-20 mg/dL.
Vasospasm prophylaxis	• Nimodipine 60 mg orally every 4 hours until day SAH 21 or discharge
Physiologic homeostasis	• Cooling blankets to maintain temperature ≤37.5°C • Insulin drip to maintain glucose 100-120 mg/dL • Transfuse to maintain hemoglobin >7.0 g/dL (in the absence or active cerebral or cardiac ischemia)
Cerebral edema	• Mannitol 1.0 g/kg IV or 30 mL of 23.4% hypertonic saline solution as needed to maintain ICP <20 mm Hg
Hydrocephalus	• Emergent external ventricular drain placement in all stuporous/comatose patients (Hunt-Hess IV/V) as well as lethargic patients with hydrocephalus
Vasospasm diagnosis	• Transcranial Doppler sonography every 1 or 2 days until the tenth day after SAH • Computed tomography angiography and perfusion on day 4-8 after SAH or for neuroworsening
Therapy for symptomatic vasospasm	• Place patient in Trendelenburg (head down) position. • Infuse 1 liter normal saline during 30 minutes. • If the deficit persists, raise the systolic blood pressure with phenylephrine or norepinephrine until the deficit resolves (target 180-220 mm Hg). • If refractory, monitor cardiac output and add dobutamine or milrinone to maintain cardiac index ≥4.0 L/min/m². • Transfuse to maintain hemoglobin >10.0 g/dL. • Emergency angiography for intra-arterial verapamil or cerebral angioplasty unless the patient responds well to the above measures.

ECG = electrocardiogram; ICP = intracranial pressure; SAH = subarachnoid hemorrhage.

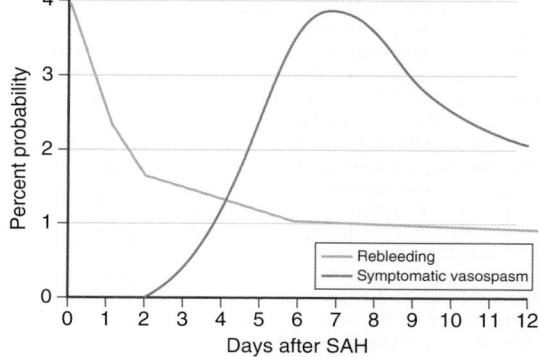

FIGURE 408-4. The daily percentage probability for the development of symptomatic vasospasm or rebleeding after subarachnoid hemorrhage (SAH). Day 0 denotes day of onset of subarachnoid hemorrhage.

weeks and 30% at 1 month. Poor clinical grade and larger aneurysms are the strongest risk factors for in-hospital rebleeding.

Prolonged infusion (i.e., 2 weeks) of antifibrinolytic agents such as ε-aminocaproic acid or tranexamic acid reduces the risk of rebleeding but does not improve outcomes because of an increased risk of cerebral ischemia.[A1] However, very short-term therapy (e.g., ε-aminocaproic acid 4 g followed by 1 g/hour until 4 hours before angiography for a maximum of 72 hours after the onset of hemorrhage) appears to be beneficial.[A2] Control of arterial hypertension (maintain systolic blood pressure <160 mm Hg) and administration of an anticonvulsant to minimize the risk of acute seizure activity (phenytoin 20 mg/kg intravenously is most commonly used) may also reduce acute rebleeding, although trials to support this practice are lacking.

Complete obliteration of a ruptured saccular aneurysm by either endovascular coiling or surgical clipping is the definitive treatment for the prevention of rebleeding and should be performed as an emergency procedure. For small to medium-sized anterior circulation aneurysms in good-grade patients, endovascular coil embolization results in better 6-month outcomes than does surgical clipping,[A3] with a 23% lower likelihood of death or disability at 1 year. The only exception to this rule is Hunt-Hess grade V patients, who have an extremely poor neurologic prognosis. In addition to preventing rebleeding, early aneurysm repair permits treatment of symptomatic vasospasm with hypertensive hypervolemic therapy, which is not feasible with an unprotected aneurysm.

Endovascular coil embolization involves packing of the ruptured aneurysm with soft, thrombogenic detachable platinum coils. This procedure leads to complete obliteration of small to medium-sized aneurysms (<10 mm in diameter) in 80 to 90% of cases, with an acceptable complication rate of approximately 10%. About 5% of coiled patients develop recurrent dilation at the neck of the original aneurysm and require repeated coil embolization or delayed surgical clipping.

Surgical clipping requires a craniotomy to expose the aneurysm, after which the neck of the aneurysm is clipped under an operating microscope to exclude it entirely from the parent artery. Surgical repair carries a 5 to 15% risk of major morbidity or mortality, especially a stroke due to inadvertent occlusion of an adjacent vessel or intraoperative rebleeding. The risk of surgery increases with larger aneurysms and is lower in the hands of more experienced operators. Clipping is preferred and sometimes the only option for treatment of widenecked aneurysms that are unable to safely contain a coil mass without migration onto the parent artery.

Fusiform Aneurysms

Fusiform aneurysms are elongated, atherosclerotic ectasias of large arteries. They are usually in the basilar artery but can be seen in the internal, middle, and anterior cerebral arteries. As fusiform aneurysms progressively dilate, they compress surrounding structures and cause focal neurologic dysfunction, such as facial pain (cranial nerve V), hemifacial spasm (cranial nerve VII), and hearing loss with vertigo (cranial nerve VIII). Fusiform aneurysms even can mimic pituitary (Chapter 224) and suprasellar mass lesions or cerebellopontine angle tumors (Chapter 189). Fortunately, fusiform aneurysms rarely rupture; but if they do, total occlusion is usually required because their stiff walls and shape make surgical clipping difficult.

Mycotic Aneurysms

An infected embolism, usually from infectious endocarditis (Chapter 76), may lodge in a distal branch of a cerebral artery, where it causes microinfarction or microabscesses. The artery may rupture acutely, or focal arteritis and mycotic aneurysms may develop. Up to 10% of these aneurysms, which are often multiple and in distal cerebral arteries, may eventually rupture, but treatment other than as for the endocarditis itself is uncertain. As a result, diagnostic imaging usually is undertaken only after symptoms appear, and the potential value of serial imaging is controversial. Anticoagulation is contraindicated in the setting of acute septic emboli to the brain because of the high risk of hemorrhagic complications.

Other Causes of Subarachnoid Hemorrhage

In patients who suffer subarachnoid hemorrhage from other causes, treatment is aimed at the underlying condition. In patients with an idiopathic perimesencephalic venous subarachnoid hemorrhage, rebleeding is rare, symptomatic vasospasm does not occur, and no specific treatment is

TABLE 408-4 MODIFIED FISHER COMPUTED TOMOGRAPHY RATING SCALE FOR THE PREDICTION OF SYMPTOMATIC VASOSPASM

GRADE	CRITERIA	PERCENTAGE OF AFFECTED PATIENTS	Delayed Cerebral Ischemia*	Infarction
			FREQUENCY OF	
0	No SAH or IVH	5%	0%	0%
1	Minimal/thin SAH, no biventricular IVH	30%	12%	6%
2	Minimal/thin SAH, *with* biventricular IVH	5%	21%	14%
3	Thick SAH,† no biventricular IVH	43%	19%	12%
4	Thick SAH, *with* biventricular IVH	17%	40%	28%
	All patients	100%	20%	12%

IVH = intraventricular hemorrhage; SAH = subarachnoid hemorrhage.
*Delayed cerebral ischemia is defined as symptomatic deterioration, cerebral infarction, or both resulting from vasospasm.
†Thick SAH is defined as completely filling at least one cistern or fissure.
From Claassen J, Bernardini GL, Kreiter K, et al. Effect of cisternal and ventricular blood on risk of delayed cerebral ischemia after subarachnoid hemorrhage: the Fisher scale revisited. *Stroke.* 2001;32:2012-2020, with permission.

indicated. Coagulation and platelet disorders require prompt treatment (Chapters 173 and 174) to prevent further bleeding. Arteriovenous malformations, which more commonly cause intracerebral rather than subarachnoid hemorrhage, are discussed later.

Prevention, Diagnosis, and Treatment of Vasospasm

Delayed cerebral ischemia from vasospasm accounts for a large proportion of morbidity and mortality after subarachnoid hemorrhage.[5] Progressive arterial narrowing develops in approximately 70% of patients, but delayed ischemic deficits develop in only 20 to 30%. The process begins 3 to 5 days after the hemorrhage, becomes maximal at 5 to 14 days, and gradually resolves during 2 to 4 weeks (see Fig. 408-4). The most important risk factor for symptomatic vasospasm is thick cisternal or intraventricular clot, which can be graded by the modified Fisher scale (Table 408-4).

Blood pressure control can be liberalized once the aneurysm has been repaired and brain perfusion becomes the dominant consideration. The calcium-channel blocker nimodipine (60 mg orally every 4 hours) reduces the frequency of delayed ischemic deterioration and infarction by about 30%.[A4] Patients should receive isotonic fluid resuscitation (i.e., 1 mL/kg/hour of 0.9% saline) to maintain a euvolemic state guided by total fluid balance, a central venous pressure above 5 mm Hg, and other measures of volume status, such as inferior vena cava ultrasound and cardiac output monitoring.

Symptomatic vasospasm usually involves a decrease in the level of consciousness, hemiparesis, or both. Transcranial Doppler ultrasonography is widely used to diagnose vasospasm of the larger cerebral arteries after subarachnoid hemorrhage but has important limitations. CT angiography and perfusion are rapidly gaining acceptance as more useful tests to diagnose large-vessel spasm and reductions in tissue blood flow.

Treatment of acute symptomatic vasospasm relies on antispasmodic medication and on increasing blood volume, blood pressure, and cardiac output in an attempt to improve cerebral blood flow through arteries that have lost the capacity to autoregulate. Pressors such as norepinephrine (starting at 2.5 µg/kg/minute) and phenylephrine (starting at 10 µg/minute) should be titrated as needed to elevate systolic blood pressure to levels as high as 180 to 220 mm Hg. Short-term clinical improvement occurs in about 70% of patients. Cerebral angioplasty can lead to dramatic improvement in patients who have severe deficits that are refractory to hemodynamic augmentation.

Cerebral Edema

Brain edema after subarachnoid hemorrhage may be focal and related to a space-occupying hematoma, or it can be global, which is an ominous pattern that implies severe primary brain injury and a poor prognosis. Treatment, which should be guided by continuous ICP monitoring targeted at a goal of less than 20 mm Hg, incorporates CSF drainage, sedation, cerebral perfusion pressure optimization (target of 60 to 90 mm Hg), bolus osmotherapy with mannitol or hypertonic saline, hyperventilation, and, in the most severe cases, induced hypothermia (see Table 408-3). There is no evidence supporting the use of dexamethasone or other corticosteroids for the treatment of brain swelling after subarachnoid hemorrhage.

Hydrocephalus

Patients with subarachnoid hemorrhage may present acutely with obstructive hydrocephalus, which can lead to dangerous elevations in ICP and precipitate transtentorial herniation. Later in the disease course, the majority of patients with acute hydrocephalus transition to a treatable form of normal-pressure hydrocephalus. These patients have persistent psychomotor slowing, confusion, and gait instability that respond to permanent ventriculoperitoneal shunting.

Seizures

Generalized tonic-clonic seizures occur in about 10% of patients after subarachnoid hemorrhage: about 5% at onset and about 5% during the hospitalization. Prehospital seizures and focal pathologic changes on CT (i.e., subdural hematoma or cerebral infarction) are risk factors for in-hospital seizures. Antiepileptic therapy (see Table 408-3) is typically started at the time of diagnosis to minimize the risk of rebleeding caused by surges in arterial blood pressure and cerebral blood flow but can be safely discontinued in good-grade patients on postoperative day 1. Prophylactic antiepileptic therapy until discharge from the intensive care unit is a treatment option for comatose patients who remain at risk for nonconvulsive seizures, which occur in 15% of comatose patients monitored with continuous electroencephalography.

Medical Complications

Subarachnoid hemorrhage places patients at risk for a variety of common medical complications that occur as a consequence of homeostatic derangements. The most common are fever, anemia, hyperglycemia, and hyponatremia. The extent and severity of these derangements are independently correlated with poor outcome and should be actively managed according to an established protocol (see Table 408-3). Many poor-grade patients develop acute cardiopulmonary dysfunction due to massive sympathetic outflow at the time of bleeding. Electrocardiographic QT segment prolongation with T-wave inversion and minor elevations in troponin levels signal the possibility of cardiac injury. The most common important clinical manifestations are pulmonary edema (Chapter 59) and left ventricular neurogenic stunning (Chapters 59 and 107) that resolve during the first week. Treatment is supportive.

PREVENTION

Approximately 15% of patients who suffer a subarachnoid hemorrhage have two or more aneurysms. Secondary prevention of subarachnoid hemorrhage requires surgical or endovascular repair of any unruptured aneurysms because they are at high risk to bleed in the future. Other important measures to reduce the risk of aneurysm formation or bleeding from an unruptured aneurysm include blood pressure control (Chapter 67), cessation of cigarette smoking, and abstaining from alcohol.

Patients will sometimes present with an incidental and asymptomatic unruptured intracranial aneurysm discovered by neuroimaging. The risk-benefit tradeoff of treatment versus observation in these cases is complex and warrants referral to an experienced neurologist or neurosurgeon. Large size is the most important risk factor for subsequent aneurysm rupture, followed by symptoms related to expansion or compression, cigarette smoking, midline location, family history of subarachnoid hemorrhage, and postmenopausal status.[6] Small unruptured aneurysms of the internal carotid artery, by contrast, are at extremely low risk of bleeding and should be managed conservatively.

PROGNOSIS

Approximately 20% of patients with subarachnoid hemorrhage treated at high-volume centers do not survive to discharge. The most important determinant of outcome after subarachnoid hemorrhage is the patient's neurologic condition on arrival to the hospital. On the modified Hunt-Hess grading scale (see Table 408-2), patients who are classified as grade I or grade II have a relatively good prognosis; grade III carries an intermediate prognosis, and grade IV and grade V have a poor prognosis. The severity of the clinical grade on admission generally correlates with the overall extent of bleeding and obstructive hydrocephalus. Other risk factors for mortality include advanced age, large aneurysm size, aneurysm rebleeding, cerebral infarction from vasospasm, and global cerebral edema.[7]

About 50% of survivors remain disabled by a neurocognitive syndrome that includes prominent memory loss, fatigue, inability to concentrate, depression, and anxiety. Cognitive and physical rehabilitation are essential for maximizing recovery in severely affected patients.

The rate of rupture among previously unruptured cerebral aneurysms is about 1% per year overall but ranges from 0.34% per year for aneurysms smaller than 5 mm to about 3% per year for aneurysms 10 to 24 mm and about 20% per year for aneurysms 25 mm or larger.[8] By comparison, patients who have an idiopathic perimesencephalic subarachnoid hemorrhage usually recover fully. For other less common causes, prognosis depends on the underlying condition. One-year survivors of subarachnoid hemorrhage have a two-fold higher rate of death as they age compared with the matched general population.[9]

⬤ INTRACEREBRAL HEMORRHAGE

Intracerebral hemorrhage is defined as acute spontaneous bleeding into the brain parenchyma. Primary intracerebral hemorrhage results from microscopic small-artery degeneration in the brain, caused by either chronic, poorly controlled hypertension (80% of cases) or amyloid angiopathy (20% of cases). Secondary intracerebral hemorrhage refers to intraparenchymal bleeding from a diagnosable anatomic vascular lesion or coagulopathy (Table 408-5).

EPIDEMIOLOGY

Intracerebral hemorrhage is responsible for 10 to 15% of all strokes in Western countries but up to 20 to 30% of strokes among Asian populations. The incidence of intracerebral hemorrhage in the United States is approximately 60,000 per year. By far the most important risk factor for intracerebral hemorrhage is hypertension, particularly when it is poorly controlled. The risk of intracerebral hemorrhage is about 40% higher in blacks than in whites. Worldwide, the incidence of intracerebral hemorrhage ranges from 10 to 40 per 1 million people, with the rate in Japan being at the top end of this range. Age-adjusted rates for men are about 50% higher than those for women. Other risk factors for intracerebral hemorrhage include heavy alcohol use, coagulopathy, and low serum cholesterol levels.

PATHOBIOLOGY

Primary intracerebral hemorrhage typically consists of a large, space-occupying confluent area of blood that has clotted within the brain parenchyma (Fig. 408-5). Abrupt arterial rupture leads to rapid accumulation of blood within the brain parenchyma, thereby causing increased local tissue pressure, physical distortion, and displacement of the brain. After the bleeding has stopped, the blood clots. Plasma that is rich in thrombin and other clotting factors then seeps into the surrounding brain tissue, where it triggers a cascade of secondary brain injury that evolves during days to weeks. This unique form of *neurohemoinflammation* causes local brain edema, programmed neuronal and glial apoptotic cell death, and breakdown of the brain-blood barrier.

The arterial disease that results in primary intracerebral hemorrhage is microscopic. Poorly controlled chronic hypertension (Chapter 67) causes a

small-vessel vasculopathy characterized by fragmentation, degeneration, and the eventual rupture of penetrating arteries within the brain. The most commonly affected structures are the basal ganglia and thalamus (50%), followed by the lobar regions (33%) and the brain stem and cerebellum (17%) (Fig. 408-6). In 40% of cases, blood also ruptures into the ventricular system, thereby causing intraventricular hemorrhage.

Cerebral *amyloid angiopathy*, which is a distinctive cause of nonhypertensive lobar intracerebral hemorrhage in the elderly, is characterized by the deposition of β-amyloid protein in small to medium-sized blood vessels of the brain and leptomeninges. Amyloid can be demonstrated when microscopic examination of brain tissue demonstrates birefringence after application of Congo red stain. Amyloid angiopathy usually occurs as a sporadic disorder, and it is unrelated to systemic amyloidosis (Chapter 188). In addition to lobar intracerebral hemorrhage, patients may present with dementia, gait disturbance, complex partial seizures due to multiple microbleeds, or small multifocal white matter demyelinating lesions that are thought to

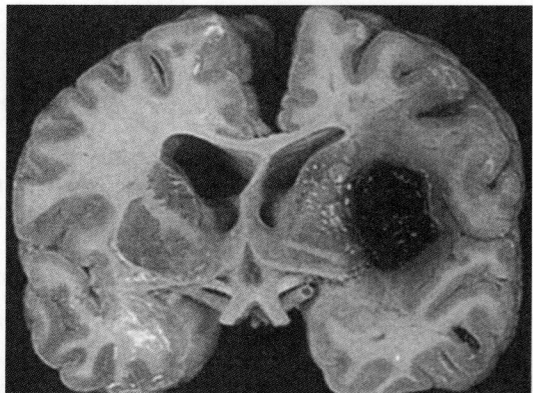

FIGURE 408-5. Pathology specimen showing a large basal ganglia parenchymal hemorrhage in the left hemisphere. (Courtesy Gregory W. Albers, Stanford University, Stanford, Calif.)

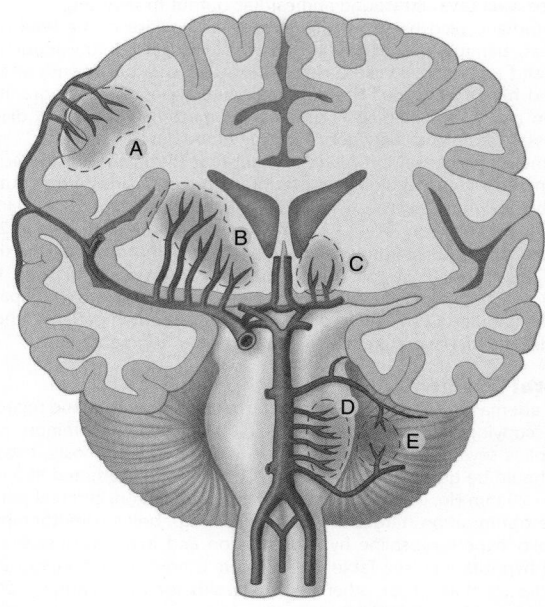

FIGURE 408-6. Typical sites and sources of intracerebral hemorrhage. Intracerebral hemorrhages most commonly involve the cerebral lobes and originate from penetrating cortical branches of the anterior, middle, or posterior cerebral arteries (*A*); the basal ganglia and originate from ascending lenticulostriate branches of the middle cerebral artery (*B*); the thalamus and originate from ascending thalamogeniculate branches of the posterior cerebral artery (*C*); the pons and originate from paramedian branches of the basilar artery (*D*); and the cerebellum and originate from penetrating branches of the posterior inferior, anterior inferior, and superior cerebellar arteries (*E*). (From Qureshi AI, Tuhrim S, Broderick JP, et al. Spontaneous intracerebral hemorrhage. *N Engl J Med.* 2001;344:1450-1460.)

TABLE 408-5	CAUSES OF SECONDARY INTRACEREBRAL HEMORRHAGE

Trauma
Arteriovenous malformation
Intracranial aneurysm
Coagulopathy
Hemorrhagic conversion of cerebral infarct
Dural sinus thrombosis
Intracranial neoplasm
Cavernous angioma
Dural arteriovenous fistula
Venous angioma
Cocaine or sympathomimetic drug exposure
Central nervous system vasculitis

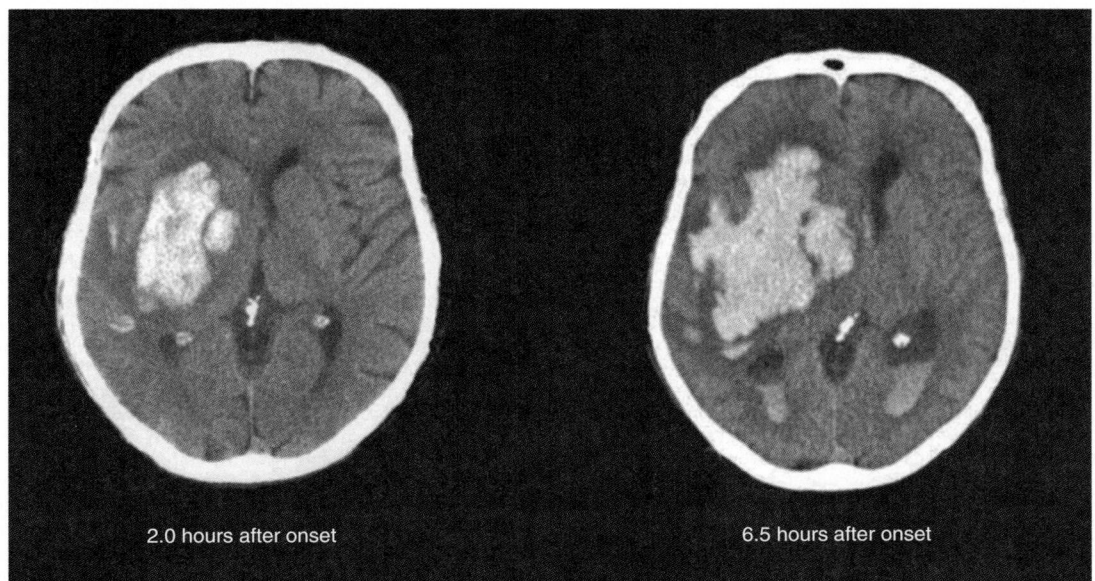

2.0 hours after onset

6.5 hours after onset

FIGURE 408-7. Early hematoma growth in a 48-year-old chronically hypertensive woman. *Left,* The baseline computed tomography scan shows a moderate-sized intracerebral hemorrhage in the right putamen. At this point, she is stuporous with a left hemiparesis. *Right,* A follow-up computed tomography scan performed after she deteriorated to coma with bilateral decerebrate posturing shows massive expansion of the hematoma as well as new intraventricular hemorrhage and obstructive hydrocephalus. Within 24 hours, she was declared brain dead. (From Mayer SA, Rincon F. Treatment of intracerebral haemorrhage. *Lancet Neurol.* 2005;4:662-672.)

represent an autoimmune response to β-amyloid and that may engender an inflammatory response.

CLINICAL MANIFESTATIONS

Primary intracerebral hemorrhage usually is manifested as an acute focal neurologic deficit. It is clinically indistinguishable from ischemic stroke (Chapter 407), except that the onset and evolution of the deficit tend to be more violent. Unlike an aneurysmal subarachnoid hemorrhage, which often causes a dramatic surge in ICP with sudden loss of consciousness at its onset, intracerebral hemorrhage tends to produce progressive headache, vomiting, and a depressed level of consciousness during several hours. In fulminant cases, however, catastrophic bleeding can lead to a massive hematoma and brain death within 6 hours of onset.

The *putamen* is the site most frequently affected. When the expanding hematoma involves the adjacent internal capsule, patients develop dense contralateral hemiparesis, usually with hemianesthesia and hemianopia. Larger hemorrhages progressively affect the overlying cortex, thereby resulting in aphasia, hemispatial neglect, and contralateral gaze paresis. When the hemorrhage arises in the *thalamus,* hemianesthesia can initially precede the hemiparesis. The completed syndrome is usually characterized by a dense contralateral sensorimotor deficit that may be accompanied by a contralateral visual field deficit, impaired upward gaze, or both.

Lobar hemorrhages, which usually originate at the junctions between gray and white matter in the cerebral hemispheres, may result from either hypertension or amyloid angiopathy. The clinical manifestation depends on the location of the hemorrhage.

In 40% of cases, deep parenchymal cerebral bleeding ruptures into the ventricular system, thereby causing intraventricular hemorrhage. Blood in the third or fourth ventricle blocks the normal anterograde flow of CSF through the ventricular system, thereby resulting in acute hydrocephalus and intracranial hypertension. Left untreated, massive intraventricular hemorrhage results in rapid descent into coma with motor posturing and rostrocaudal loss of brain stem reflexes.

Pontine hemorrhage typically causes coma with quadriparesis, grossly disconjugate ocular motility disorders, and miotic pupils, although small hemorrhages may mimic syndromes of infarction. *Cerebellar hemorrhage* usually begins abruptly with vomiting and ataxia that usually is severe enough to prevent standing and walking. It is occasionally accompanied by dysarthria, adjacent cranial nerve (mostly sixth and seventh) dysfunction, and paralysis of conjugate ipsilateral gaze.

Seizures complicate the course of intracerebral hemorrhage in about 12% of patients. Although the risk is higher when the cortex is the primary site of bleeding, seizures can complicate deep intracerebral hemorrhage as well.

Expansion of the hematoma due to active, ongoing bleeding is an important cause of early neurologic deterioration after an intracerebral hemorrhage (Fig. 408-7). When the initial CT scan is obtained within 3 hours of the onset of symptoms, follow-up imaging reveals obvious enlargement of the hematoma in nearly 40% of patients, even in the absence of a coagulopathy. The likelihood of progression is even higher if the first CT scan is obtained earlier but minimal when the initial CT scan is obtained more than 6 hours after the onset of the bleed. Enlargement of the mass usually does not change the clinical picture until there is enough brain stem compression to precipitate coma, which can happen abruptly.

DIAGNOSIS

Intracerebral hemorrhage cannot be distinguished from ischemic stroke (Chapter 407) on the basis of clinical findings alone. Nonenhanced CT imaging of the brain is the method of choice for making the emergency diagnosis of intracerebral hemorrhage (see Fig. 408-7). CT readily demonstrates the size and location of the hematoma, any extension into the ventricular system, the degree of surrounding edema, and tissue displacement, such as a midline shift, due to mass effect. CT angiography may reveal secondary intracerebral hemorrhage due to an aneurysm or arteriovenous malformation or active extravasation of contrast material into the clot ("spot sign"), which implies an increased risk of early growth of the hematoma when it is identified soon after the onset of symptoms.

MRI techniques such as gradient-echo are highly sensitive for the diagnosis of intracerebral hemorrhage as well. The diagnosis of probable amyloid angiopathy is made clinically in patients with the appropriate clinical picture of lobar hemorrhages when gradient MRI reveals multiple cortical microbleeds. Conventional diagnostic cerebral angiography should be reserved for patients in whom secondary causes of intracerebral hemorrhage, such as aneurysms, arteriovenous malformations, cortical vein or dural sinus thrombosis, or vasculitis, are suspected.

TREATMENT   Rx

Treatment in an intensive care unit or stroke unit is strongly recommended for at least the first 24 hours after the onset of an intracerebral hemorrhage because the risk of neurologic deterioration is highest during this time. The most urgent treatment consideration is whether to proceed emergently with surgical evacuation or the placement of a ventricular drain.

Surgical Management

Although intracerebral hemorrhage has traditionally been considered a neurosurgical problem, randomized controlled trials have shown that craniotomy and surgical evacuation of the hematoma within 24 hours do not improve outcome compared with initial medical management,[A5] even with larger bleeds within 1 cm of the cortical surface.[A6] However, these trials did not enroll patients if their physician thought that emergency surgery was a life-saving intervention, and many experts still believe that urgent craniotomy can improve the outcome of younger patients with large lobar hemorrhages and a deteriorating course due to mass effect.

In contrast to supratentorial intracerebral hemorrhage, it is widely accepted that patients with cerebellar hemorrhages exceeding 3 cm in diameter benefit from emergent surgical evacuation. Because abrupt and dramatic deterioration to coma can occur within the first 24 hours of the onset of symptoms in these patients, surgery should be performed promptly before further clinical deterioration occurs.

Ventricular Drainage

External ventricular drainage is indicated in all stuporous or comatose patients with intraventricular hemorrhage and ventricular enlargement in whom aggressive support is indicated. This life-saving procedure, which can be performed at the bedside, decompresses the intracranial vault and arrests the process of downward brain stem herniation by allowing drainage of bloody CSF into a drainage receptacle. Connecting the drainage system to a pressure transducer also allows measurement of ICP.

Reverse of Anticoagulation

Fifteen percent of intracerebral hemorrhages are associated with the use of oral anticoagulants, and these patients face a high risk of progressive bleeding during a prolonged time window of many hours. For warfarin-associated intracerebral hemorrhage, failure to correct the INR promptly to below 1.4 further increases the risk of progressive bleeding and is associated with increased mortality. Patients who are taking warfarin and who present with an intracerebral hemorrhage should be treated immediately with a four-factor prothrombin complex concentrate and intravenous vitamin K (Table 408-6), a regimen that results in a substantially faster correction of the INR in a greater proportion of patients.[A7] A single dose of recombinant activated factor VIIa (3 to 6 mg by intravenous push) normalizes the INR within minutes, promotes hemostasis, and is an attractive option for expediting life-saving neurosurgical intervention when minutes count, but at the cost of a 5% risk of a thromboembolic complication such as myocardial infarction or stroke. Patients with intracerebral hemorrhage anticoagulated with unfractionated or low-molecular weight heparin should be reversed with protamine sulfate

(Chapters 38 and 174). Patients with thrombocytopenia or platelet dysfunction can be treated with a single dose of desmopressin, platelet transfusions, or both, but evidence for efficacy is lacking. Treatment options for intracerebral hemorrhage associated with novel oral anticoagulants (e.g., rivaroxaban, dabigatran, apixaban, and edoxaban) are extremely limited (Chapter 38). If anticoagulation must be restarted after recovery, the risk of recurrent intracranial hemorrhage is about 2.5 per 100 patient-years.[10]

Blood Pressure Control

Acute intracerebral hemorrhage often leads to extreme arterial hypertension. Aggressive blood pressure reductions in the setting of impaired autoregulation can result in exacerbation of ischemic injury, whereas lack of blood pressure control can theoretically exacerbate the early growth of the hematoma and the risk of vasogenic edema. Although current guidelines[11] recommend a systolic blood pressure target of less than 180 mm Hg and a mean blood pressure target of 160 mm Hg,[A8] lowering of systolic blood pressure to less than 140 mm Hg within 6 hours of onset of symptoms does not reduce mortality and provides only borderline improvement in the extent of disability among survivors compared with a goal of less than 180 mm Hg.[A9] Given the need to precisely control blood pressure levels in the setting of impaired autoregulation, use of fast-acting continuous infusion agents with intra-arterial monitoring is recommended. Agents of choice are labetalol, a combined α- and β-blocker, and nicardipine, which is a calcium-channel blocker (see Table 67-14). Sodium nitroprusside should be avoided because of its lack of a reliable dose-response effect and its capacity to directly increase ICP.

Cerebral Edema

Brain swelling can progress for many days after the onset of intracerebral hemorrhage, but it most often causes neurologic deterioration within the first 72 hours in patients with hemorrhages exceeding 30 mL in volume. Management of cerebral edema should be guided by measurement of the ICP with an external ventricular drain or parenchymal monitor, with efforts directed at maintaining ICP below 20 mm Hg and cerebral perfusion pressure above 70 mm Hg. As is the case with subarachnoid hemorrhage, therapy should be directed by an approach that includes sedation, blood pressure optimization, bolus osmotherapy, controlled hyperventilation, mild hypothermia, and, as a last resort, salvage hemicraniectomy in selected younger patients (Chapter 399). Dexamethasone and other corticosteroids do not effectively treat intracerebral hemorrhage–related brain edema and are contraindicated. Hypotonic intravenous fluids (i.e., 0.45% saline or 5% dextrose in water) should be strictly avoided because the free water in these solutions can aggravate brain edema.

Medical and Neurologic Complications

To combat malnutrition and muscle wasting, early enteral feeding (Chapter 216) should be initiated through a nasoduodenal feeding tube in patients who lack the capacity to swallow. Body temperature and the blood glucose level should be maintained in the normal to slightly elevated range with surface cooling and continuous insulin infusion. About 12% of patients with intracerebral hemorrhage experience convulsive seizures during their hospitalization, and risk is increased with lobar location. Prophylactic anticonvulsant therapy with phenytoin (20 mg/kg intravenously) or a similar agent is reasonable for high-risk stuporous or comatose patients. If seizures have not occurred, anticonvulsants should be discontinued at discharge because they can hamper neurologic recovery during rehabilitation. Even with anticonvulsant therapy, continuous electroencephalographic monitoring reveals electrographic seizure activity in 20% of comatose patients. It is unclear whether midazolam infusion or other aggressive measures to eliminate these seizures (Chapter 403) can improve outcome.

TABLE 408-6	MEDICAL MANAGEMENT PROTOCOL FOR ACUTE INTRACEREBRAL HEMORRHAGE
Blood pressure	• Maintain mean arterial pressure <140 mm Hg with continuous infusion of labetalol (2-10 mg/min) or nicardipine (5-15 mg/hr). • If stuporous or comatose, measure ICP and maintain CPP >70 mm Hg.

Reversal of anticoagulation	• For elevated INR: vitamin K 10 mg IVP *and* 4F-PCC
	    INR 2 to <4: 25 units/kg; not to exceed 2500 units
	    INR 4-6: 35 units/kg; not to exceed 3500 units
	    INR >6: 50 units/kg; not to exceed 5000 units
	• For heparin: protamine sulfate 10 to 50 mg slow IV push (1 mg reverses approximately 100 units of heparin)
	• For thrombocytopenia or platelet dysfunction: desmopressin 0.3 µg/kg IVP and/or transfuse 6 units of platelets
	• Expedited INR reversal for life-saving neurosurgical intervention: recombinant activated factor VIIa 40-80 µg/kg (approximately 3.0-6.0 mg) IVP

Intracranial hypertension	• Elevate head of bed to 30 degrees • Mannitol 1.0-1.5 g IV • Hyperventilate to P_{CO_2} of 30 mm Hg
Fluids and nutrition	• Normal (0.9%) saline at 1.0 mL/kg/hr • Begin enteral feeding through nasoduodenal tube within 24 hours
Seizure prophylaxis	• For coma with intracranial hypertension or acute seizures: fosphenytoin or phenytoin IV load (15-20 mg/kg); 300 mg IV daily for 7 days
Physiologic homeostasis	• Cooling blankets to maintain temperature ≤37.5° C • Insulin drip to maintain glucose 120-180 mg/dL

4F-PCC = four-factor prothrombin complex concentrate containing factors II, VII, IX, and X; CPP = cerebral perfusion pressure; ICP = intracranial pressure; INR = international normalized ratio; IVP = intravenous push.

PREVENTION

Blood pressure reduction (Chapter 67), which significantly decreases the risk of intracerebral hemorrhage and other forms of stroke, is by far the most effective method for preventing recurrent intracerebral hemorrhage. Angiotensin-converting enzyme inhibitors are particularly effective (see Table 67-7). Antiplatelet agents and anticoagulants of all types should be meticulously avoided in patients with multiple lobar microbleeds caused by amyloid angiopathy.

PROGNOSIS

Factors that consistently predict death or functional disability at 30 days include a large volume of intracerebral hemorrhage, depressed level of consciousness, intraventricular hemorrhage, infratentorial location, and older age. The volume of the hematoma can be easily calculated from CT scan images by use of the "ABC ÷ 2 method," which involves multiplying the diameter of the hematoma in three dimensions and dividing by two. A simple clinical grading scale incorporates these variables and can give a reliable prediction of mortality risk at 30 days.

Except in the most severe cases, however, caution is warranted in communicating a hopeless prognosis before aggressive efforts have been made to resuscitate victims of intracerebral hemorrhage. Physicians tend to underestimate the chances of a good outcome, and many poor outcomes result from self-fulfilling prophesies of doom. Mortality after intracerebral hemorrhage is lower among patients in specialty neurologic intensive care units, presumably because of adherence to best medical practices, early transition to rehabilitation, and cautious optimism when setbacks occur.

● BRAIN VASCULAR MALFORMATIONS

Brain vascular malformations are space-occupying congenital anomalies that can often exist for a lifetime without symptoms. The most feared and dangerous complication is rupture, which can be manifested as intracerebral hemorrhage, as intraventricular hemorrhage, or less often as subarachnoid hemorrhage.

EPIDEMIOLOGY

About 10% of intracerebral hemorrhages but only about 1% of strokes are caused by vascular malformations. The prevalence of an arteriovenous malformation is about 0.5%, and the annual incidence of hemorrhage is between 1 and 3 cases per 100,000 people. Hemorrhage from an arteriovenous malformation is most common during the second through fourth decades. The risk of rebleeding is about 7% acutely. For the next 5 years, the risk of bleeding is about 2% per year, and it then falls to about 1 to 2% annually thereafter. Over a lifetime, a young person therefore has a 50 to 60% probability of another hemorrhage, each of which carries a 10 to 15% risk of acute death. Unlike with some causes of cerebral hemorrhage, preexisting hypertension does not seem to be a risk factor.

PATHOBIOLOGY

Cerebrovascular malformations are characterized on the basis of their histologic appearance and the intervening neural parenchyma. The most frequent type of vascular malformation is an arteriovenous malformation, in which a core or nidus of dysplastic vessels is fed by arteries and drained by veins without intervening capillaries. The result is a low-resistance, high-flow shunt that leads to progressive arterial dilation and venous wall thickening. The nidus usually does not contain any intervening neural tissue. Bleeding from a feeding artery aneurysm usually results in subarachnoid hemorrhage, bleeding from the nidus itself usually results in intracerebral hemorrhage, and bleeding from a draining vein usually is manifested as intraventricular hemorrhage.

The next most common vascular malformations are cavernous angiomas or hemangiomas. These malformations, which also do not contain neural tissue, are composed of small-caliber sinusoidal vascular channels that are commonly thrombosed.

Dural arteriovenous fistulas are typically acquired lesions that result from the formation of small arteriovenous shunts in the wall of a cavernous sinus as a consequence of dural sinus thrombosis. Over time, flow through the fistula increases, leading to pulsatile expansion of regional veins and subsequent rupture. Rare familial cases have been described.

CLINICAL MANIFESTATIONS

About 50% of arteriovenous malformations are manifested with intracranial hemorrhage, about 30% initially are manifested as seizures, and about 20% may be manifested with progressive neurologic disability. An increasing proportion, however, are now detected by brain imaging as part of the evaluation of headaches (Chapter 398), to which arteriovenous malformations may or may not be causally related.

Because an arteriovenous malformation can bleed into the subarachnoid space, the brain parenchyma, or the ventricular system, symptoms and signs depend on the location and severity of bleed. Post-bleeding cerebral vasospasm, which is less common than aneurysmal bleeding, occurs in less than 5% of cases and is typically linked to thick cisternal clot or extensive intraventricular hemorrhage.

Patients who develop seizures as a result of these arteriovenous malformations often have focal seizures (Chapter 403). Even without seizures, patients can develop focal neurologic deficits due to vascular thrombosis or the shunting of blood through the malformation rather than allowing it to perfuse normal brain tissue.

DIAGNOSIS

A noncontrast CT scan may show bleeding, sometimes in a location that is unusual for a primary intracerebral hemorrhage or a ruptured aneurysm. Contrast-enhanced CT may show marked enhancement of the feeding arteries and draining veins. Another option is MRI with signal void on T1- or T2-weighted images.[12] However, angiography is the definitive test to identify an arteriovenous malformation and to delineate its size, gross morphology, feeding arteries, and draining veins. Even if an arteriovenous malformation is found by unilateral carotid injection, four-vessel angiography is indicated because malformations can be multiple and can be associated with saccular aneurysms.

When cavernous angiomas or hemangiomas hemorrhage, they tend to produce minor focal syndromes that appear on MRI as a classic target lesion that results from multiple previous minor bleeding events. The low flow rate through these lesions makes them difficult to detect by angiography.

TREATMENT Rx

In a patient who survives the initial hemorrhage, the two therapeutic goals are to avoid neurologic deterioration and to remove the arteriovenous malformation completely. General medical treatment measures for intracranial hemorrhage related to arteriovenous malformation are the same as for intracerebral hemorrhage (see Table 408-6). Removal of the arteriovenous malformation can be curative, but surgery is challenging for malformations in critical neurologic areas. Options include selective embolization of the feeding arteries, surgical resection, and radiation-induced thrombosis, alone or sometimes in combination. Selective embolization can reduce the size of the malformation and blood flow through it but rarely can obliterate it completely. Stereotactic radiosurgery is used only for small lesions, and its therapeutic effect depends on the gradual shrinkage of abnormal vessels after the procedure.

Microsurgical removal of an arteriovenous malformation is often performed in stages until a postoperative angiogram shows no residual malformation. However, recanalization and recurrent hemorrhage can occur, and long-term success rates are unknown.

PREVENTION AND PROGNOSIS

The prognosis of an unruptured arteriovenous malformation varies according to its location, size, and morphology. In a randomized trial, medical management emphasizing control of hypertension, avoidance of anticoagulants, and use of anticonvulsants to control seizures was superior to multimodality intervention with surgery, embolization, or radiotherapy, with a 10% rate of death or stroke at 33 months compared with a 30% risk in the intervention group.[A10] Until further data are available, routine interventional treatment of unruptured arteriovenous malformations is not justified.[13]

Grade A References

A1. Baharoglu MI, Germans MR, Rinkel GJ, et al. Antifibrinolytic therapy for aneurysmal subarachnoid haemorrhage. *Cochrane Database Syst Rev*. 2013;8:CD001245.

A2. Gaberel T, Magheru C, Emery E, et al. Antifibrinolytic therapy in the management of aneurismal subarachnoid hemorrhage revisited. A meta-analysis. *Acta Neurochir (Wien)*. 2012;154:1-9.

A3. Molyneux AJ, Kerr RS, Yu LM, et al. International subarachnoid aneurysm trial (ISAT) of neurosurgical clipping versus endovascular coiling in 2143 patients with ruptured intracranial aneurysms: a randomised comparison of effects on survival, dependency, seizures, rebleeding, subgroups, and aneurysm occlusion. *Lancet*. 2005;366:809-817.

A4. Feigin VL, Rinkel GJ, Algra A, et al. Calcium antagonists in patients with aneurysmal subarachnoid hemorrhage: a systematic review. *Neurology*. 1998;50:876-883.

A5. Mendelow AD, Gregson BA, Fernandes HM, et al. Early surgery versus initial conservative treatment in patients with spontaneous supratentorial intracerebral haematomas in the International Surgical Trial in Intracerebral Haemorrhage (STICH): a randomised trial. *Lancet*. 2005;365: 387-397.

A6. Mendelow AD, Gregson BA, Rowan EN, et al. Early surgery versus initial conservative treatment in patients with spontaneous supratentorial lobar intracerebral haematomas (STICH II): a randomised trial. *Lancet*. 2013;382:397-408.

A7. Sarode R, Milling TJ Jr, Refaai MA, et al. Efficacy and safety of a 4-factor prothrombin complex concentrate in patients on vitamin K antagonists presenting with major bleeding: a randomized, plasma-controlled, phase IIIb study. *Circulation*. 2013;128:1234-1243.

A8. Tsivgoulis G, Katsanos AH, Butcher KS, et al. Intensive blood pressure reduction in acute intracerebral hemorrhage: a meta-analysis. *Neurology*. 2014;83:1523-1529.

A9. Anderson CS, Heeley E, Huang Y, et al. Rapid blood-pressure lowering in patients with acute intracerebral hemorrhage. *N Engl J Med*. 2013;368:2355-2365.

A10. Mohr JP, Parides MK, Stapf C, et al. Medical management with or without interventional therapy for unruptured brain arteriovenous malformations (ARUBA): a multicentre, non-blinded, randomised trial. *Lancet*. 2014;383:614-621.

GENERAL REFERENCES

For the General References and other additional features, please visit Expert Consult at https://expertconsult.inkling.com.

409

PARKINSONISM

ANTHONY E. LANG

Parkinsonism is a clinical syndrome that consists of four cardinal signs: tremor, rigidity, akinesia, and postural disturbances (TRAP). Parkinson disease is a common cause of the TRAP syndrome, but there are numerous other causes (Table 409-1).

TABLE 409-1　DIFFERENTIAL DIAGNOSIS OF PARKINSONISM

PARKINSON DISEASE

Sporadic
Genetic
　Autosomal dominant (e.g., α-synuclein gene mutations, duplications, triplications; *LRRK2* mutations)
　Autosomal recessive (e.g., *parkin, DJ1, PINK1*)

SECONDARY PARKINSONISM

Neurodegenerative diseases (sporadic or genetic)
　Progressive supranuclear palsy*
　Multiple system atrophy*
　Corticobasal degeneration*
　Dementia with Lewy bodies*
　Alzheimer disease*
　ALS-parkinsonism-dementia complex of Guam
　Huntington disease
　Rapid-onset dystonia-parkinsonism
　Pallidopyramidal degeneration (including PARK9 and PARK15)
　Neuroacanthocytosis
　Spinocerebellar ataxias (e.g., SCA-3, SCA-2)
　Wilson disease
　Pantothenate kinase–associated neurodegeneration (Hallervorden-Spatz syndrome)
　Neuroferritinopathy
　Calcification of the basal ganglia (Fahr disease)
　Dopa-responsive dystonia (not a degenerative disorder)
Drugs*
　Neuroleptics, metoclopramide, prochlorperazine, tetrabenazine, reserpine, cinnarizine, flunarizine, α-methyldopa, lithium
Toxic
　MPTP, manganese (including illicit use of ephedrone), carbon monoxide, mercury
Infectious
　Encephalitis lethargica
　Other encephalitis, including HIV associated
　Subacute sclerosing panencephalitis
　Creutzfeldt-Jakob disease
Vascular*
　Atherosclerosis
　Amyloid angiopathy
Neoplastic
　Brain tumor
　Other mass lesions
Normal-pressure hydrocephalus*
Head trauma
Multiple sclerosis

*See Table 409-4 for additional details.
ALS = amyotrophic lateral sclerosis; HIV = human immunodeficiency virus; MPTP = 1-methyl-4-phenyl-1,2,3,6-tetrahydropyridine.
Modified from Cloutier M, Lang AE. Movement disorders: an overview. In: Factor SA, Lang AE, Weiner WJ, eds. *Drug Induced Movement Disorders*. Malden, Mass: Blackwell; 2005:3-19.

PARKINSON DISEASE

EPIDEMIOLOGY

Parkinson disease, which is the second most common neurodegenerative disorder after Alzheimer disease, occurs in approximately 1 in 1000 in the general population and in 1% of persons older than 65 years. Men are affected slightly more often than women (3 : 2).

PATHOBIOLOGY

The cause of Parkinson disease is believed to be a variable combination of poorly understood genetic[1] and environmental factors.[2] Both autosomal dominant and recessive genes can cause classic Parkinson disease. The protein α-synuclein, which is the chief constituent of the hallmark cytoplasmic inclusion, the Lewy body (Chapter 402), is critical in the pathogenesis of Parkinson disease. Abnormal aggregation of the protein, either from mutations in the α-synuclein gene or as a result of excessive production of the normal protein because of gene duplications or triplications, is associated with varying disease phenotypes. Other defined genetic abnormalities may be associated with classic later-onset Parkinson disease, including *LRRK2*, which is currently the most common cause of autosomal dominantly inherited Parkinson disease, or with early-onset parkinsonism, typically found in the autosomal recessive forms associated with *parkin, DJ1*, and *PINK1*. Other genes in which mutations may increase the risk for development of Parkinson disease include the glucocerebrosidase gene (*GBA*).

Strong support for the "environmental hypothesis" of sporadic Parkinson disease relates to the observation that the selective neurotoxin 1-methyl-4-phenyl-1,2,3,6-tetrahydropyridine (MPTP) causes acute parkinsonism due to loss of dopamine neurons in the substantia nigra pars compacta (SNc). MPTP is oxidized to the active toxin MPP^+, which is a selective inhibitor of complex I of the mitochondrial electron transport chain. This knowledge, combined with recognition of the importance of dopamine (see later), has implicated oxidative stress in the pathogenesis of Parkinson disease. Other proposed pathogenetic factors include mitochondrial dysfunction, protein misfolding or aggregation, excitotoxicity, inflammation, apoptotic cell death, and loss of trophic support.

Pathology

Many of the features of Parkinson disease are due to loss of dopamine in the neostriatum (especially the putamen) secondary to loss of pigmented dopaminergic neurons in the SNc of the midbrain. Approximately 60% of these dopaminergic neurons will have degenerated before clinical features of the disease develop.[3]

In addition to the prominent degenerative changes in the SNc (cell loss, gliosis, abnormal deposition of aggregated α-synuclein as Lewy bodies and Lewy neurites), pathologic changes are also evident in other brain stem nuclei, in cortical regions, and in peripheral autonomic neurons. Indeed, it has been suggested that Parkinson disease may begin in the lower brain stem and the olfactory system, where it causes early loss of the sense of smell and only later involves the substantia nigra. Independent of the order of involvement, it is likely that the widespread extranigral neurodegenerative changes account for the many symptoms that do not respond to dopamine replacement and that become increasingly problematic as the disease progresses. How the disease progresses and spreads in the nervous system is unknown. Studies suggest the possibility of cell-to-cell transmission of a form of α-synuclein that may then induce abnormal folding and aggregation of the normal protein in a "permissive templating" fashion similar to prion diseases (Chapter 415).[4]

CLINICAL MANIFESTATIONS

Typically, the symptoms begin in one limb. This asymmetry often persists into later stages of the disease.

Motor Symptoms
Tremor
The classic "resting tremor" of Parkinson disease has characteristic clinical features.[5] The tremor has a frequency of 4 to 6 cycles per second, typically with a "pill-rolling" character when it involves the hand. It is generally present with the limb in complete repose and typically subsides when the limb moves and takes up a new position, although the tremor may reemerge ("reemergent tremor") within a short time after maintaining the new position. Because resting tremor diminishes or subsides with action, it may not be disabling but can be embarrassing and may be associated with aching or

fatigue of the affected limb. Resting tremor is usually accentuated by stress (e.g., by asking the patient to perform mental calculations). It is also characteristically present in the upper limbs while walking. A higher-frequency (e.g., 7 to 10 Hz) postural and kinetic tremor is also common in patients with various causes of parkinsonism.

Rigidity

Rigidity is a form of increased muscle tone appreciated best on slow passive movements. It may be characterized as "cogwheel" when a tremor is superimposed or as "lead pipe" when it is not. Rigidity is "activated" or accentuated on examination by asking the patient to move the limb opposite the one being tested. Patients may complain of stiffness, but the rigidity is not usually disabling.

Akinesia

Akinesia or bradykinesia comprises a variety of disturbances in movement, including slowness, reduced amplitude, fatiguing, and interruptions in ongoing movement. This disabling aspect of parkinsonism interferes with all voluntary activities and accounts for many of the well-known features of parkinsonism: lack of facial expression with reduced blinking (hypomimia or masked facies—the "reptilian stare"), soft monotonous speech (hypophonia), impaired swallowing resulting in drooling (sialorrhea), small handwriting (micrographia), reduced arm swing while walking, shortened stride and shuffling gait, difficulty arising from a low chair, and problems turning over in bed. Arrest in ongoing movement ("motor block") can interfere with a variety of activities, but it is best appreciated as freezing of gait. Bradykinesia is evident on inspection and elicited by testing rapid repetitive and alternating movements: finger tapping, opening and closing the fist, pronating and supinating the wrist, and toe and heel tapping.

Postural Disturbances

Postural disturbances include a flexed posture in the limbs and trunk (stooped, simian posture) as well as postural instability resulting in imbalance and falls. Patients may complain of being unable to stop themselves from going forward (propulsion) or backward (retropulsion). Clinical assessment of postural instability includes the "pull test," in which the examiner abruptly pulls the patient off balance while being ready to catch the patient in the event of a fall.

Other Symptoms

In addition to the motor features of parkinsonism, a variety of non–motor-related features are extremely common. These include pain and other sensory disturbances; dysautonomic complaints, such as urinary urgency and frequency; orthostatic faintness; constipation; male erectile dysfunction; sleep abnormalities, including rapid eye movement behavioral disorder (Chapter 405); anxiety; fatigue; depression; and cognitive disturbances, including dementia.[6] As the disease progresses, more resistant features develop, including "axial" motor disturbances (speech and swallowing abnormalities, freezing, and postural instability) as well as neurobehavioral and cognitive dysfunction.

Complications

In addition to the manifestations of the disease itself, complications of drug therapy include motor- and non–motor-related fluctuations and psychiatric or behavioral disturbances.[7] Thus, in the later stages of the disease, the clinical picture often fluctuates from hour to hour and even from minute to minute. Accordingly, patients exhibit a mixture of the classic features of parkinsonism, which may improve considerably in response to medication; symptoms that persist despite the peak benefit of medication; and symptoms that occur as a complication of dopaminergic medication (Table 409-2).

DIAGNOSIS

Testing for monogenetic forms of Parkinson disease (e.g., *parkin*) is becoming available, but guidelines for its use have not yet been developed. Given the classic clinical manifestations, the diagnostic evaluation focuses largely on ways to exclude other causes of parkinsonism (Table 409-3).[8] Young-onset patients should have Wilson disease excluded by determination of 24-hour urine copper and serum ceruloplasmin and by slit lamp examination (Chapter 211). Findings on magnetic resonance imaging are generally normal in Parkinson disease, but it is indicated to exclude other diagnoses (Table 409-4).[9] Positron emission tomography, which can assess the presynaptic and postsynaptic sides of the nigrostriatal dopamine system, is useful

TABLE 409-2	PROBLEMS IN LATE-STAGE PARKINSON DISEASE	
PROBLEM	**SYMPTOMS**	
LATER TREATMENT-RESISTANT SYMPTOMS		
Motor	Dysarthria Dysphagia Freezing of gait (on-period freezing) Postural instability with falls	
Non–motor	Dysautonomia, weight loss Sensory symptoms, including pain (some may be responsive to levodopa) Changes in mood or behavior (depression, anxiety), sleep disturbances (excessive daytime sleepiness often caused by or aggravated by dopaminergic medication) Rapid eye movement sleep behavior disorder (may develop before parkinsonism) Fatigue Cognitive dysfunction and dementia	
RELATED TO TREATMENT AND DISEASE		
Motor fluctuations	Wearing off of drug effect (predictable end-of-dose deterioration, morning akinesia), increased latency to benefit ("delayed-on"), dose failures ("no-on") On-off phenomenon, more rapid and unpredictable fluctuations Concomitant fluctuations of non–motor-related symptoms ("non-motor fluctuations") that may be as disabling as motor symptoms (or more so)	
Dyskinesias (abnormal involuntary movements)	Peak-dose dyskinesias: chorea, athetosis, and, less often, more prolonged dystonia, typically worse on the initially affected side Diphasic dyskinesia ("beginning-of-dose" and "end-of-dose" dyskinesias): mixtures of choreoathetosis, ballism, dystonia, alternating movements (especially in the legs) Off-period dystonia: most often involving the legs and feet (including morning foot dystonia)	
Psychiatric disturbances	Vivid dreams and nightmares Visual hallucinations with a clear sensorium Hallucinations with confusion Mania, impulse control disorders (e.g., hypersexuality, problem gambling), dopaminergic drug addiction Paranoid psychosis	

Modified from Lang AE, Lozano AM. Parkinson's disease—second of two parts. *N Engl J Med.* 1998;339:1130-1143.

TABLE 409-3	CLINICAL CLUES TO AN ALTERNATIVE (NON–PARKINSON DISEASE) CAUSE OF PARKINSONIAN SIGNS AND SYMPTOMS

Extraocular movements—e.g., nystagmus, limitation of vertical gaze, especially with slowing of downward saccadic eye movements

Early and prominent dysarthria or dysphagia

Prominent or early abnormal neck postures: flexion or extension

Ataxia—limb, gait (impaired tandem gait)

Lower body distribution with relative sparing of upper limb function

Early postural instability, falls, or freezing

Dysautonomia (early and prominent), prominent hypotensive response to dopaminergic medication

Pyramidal tract signs—very brisk reflexes, clonus, extensor plantar responses

Peripheral nerve dysfunction—loss of reflexes, distal sensory loss, weakness

Apraxia and cortical sensory changes

Early severe dementia

Poor response to levodopa

for research, but the most common ligand, [18F]fluorodopa, does not reliably distinguish Parkinson disease from many other neurodegenerative diseases that mimic it. The same limitations apply to evaluation of the dopamine transporter by single-photon emission computed tomography, which is available for clinical use. The finding of increased echogenicity in the SNc of the midbrain on transcranial ultrasound may be more specific in diagnosing Parkinson disease, but the data are not conclusive.

TABLE 409-4 DISEASES THAT MUST BE DISTINGUISHED FROM PARKINSON DISEASE

DIAGNOSIS	IMPORTANT DISTINGUISHING CLINICAL FEATURES	RESPONSE TO LEVODOPA/COMMENTS (INCLUDING IMAGING)
Multiple system atrophy (MSA) (includes older terms: striatonigral degeneration, sporadic olivopontocerebellar atrophy, and Shy-Drager syndrome) (a "synucleinopathy")	Early dysautonomia (including orthostatic hypotension and sexual impotence) and bladder dysfunction (with autonomic and nonautonomic components) Cerebellar dysfunction	Good response initially evident in 20% and sustained partial response in ≈15% Dyskinesias or motor fluctuations possible; cranial dystonia may be prominent Patient is wheelchair bound despite response to levodopa (early loss of postural reflexes, with or without ataxia)
MSA-P, a predominant parkinsonian manifestation	Pyramidal tract signs Stimulus-sensitive myoclonus of the hands and face	MRI (including diffusion-weighted imaging and gradient-echo sequences) often shows diagnostic changes in the striatum in MSA-P and "hot cross bun sign" in the pons and hyperintensity in middle cerebellar peduncles in MSA-C
MSA-C, a predominant cerebellar manifestation (mixed features are common)	Extreme forward neck flexion (anterocollis) Mottled, cold hands Inspiratory stridor Prominent dysarthria	
Progressive supranuclear palsy (a "tauopathy")	Supranuclear vertical ophthalmoplegia Other oculomotor and eyelid disturbances Axial rigidity greater than limb rigidity Early falls, speech and swallowing disturbances Nuchal extension Cognitive or behavioral changes Progressive nonfluent aphasia Possibly a higher incidence of hypertension than in Parkinson disease and other neurodegenerative causes of parkinsonism	Good response rarely evident; benefit only for classic parkinsonian features, such as limb rigidity, classic bradykinesia with fatiguing of amplitude of repetitive movements, and rare examples of tremor at rest MRI often demonstrates profound midbrain atrophy ("hummingbird sign" on a midline sagittal view, "morning glory sign" on axial view)
Corticobasal (cortical-basal ganglionic) degeneration (a "tauopathy")	Apraxia, cortical sensory loss, alien limb phenomenon Pronounced asymmetrical rigidity Limb dystonia Stimulus-sensitive myoclonus Aphasia (progressive nonfluent aphasia) Cognitive dysfunction (frontotemporal dementia)	Usually negligible MRI may show pronounced asymmetrical cortical atrophy
Vascular parkinsonism	"Lower-half" parkinsonism with gait disturbances predominating, often with minimal or much milder upper body involvement Additional neurologic deficits (e.g., pyramidal tract signs, pseudobulbar palsy)	Usually poor, but some respond well Imaging demonstrates multiple infarcts involving the basal ganglia and subcortical white matter
Dementia with Lewy bodies (a "synucleinopathy")	Early dementia (cognitive profile somewhat different from that of Alzheimer disease) Spontaneous hallucinations, fluctuating cognitive status, falls, orthostatic hypotension, RBD Pronounced sensitivity to the extrapyramidal side effects of neuroleptic drugs Parkinsonism may be similar to typical Parkinson disease, although rigidity may be more prominent than bradykinesia or tremor	Motor features may respond well; psychiatric side effects of dopaminergic drugs are typically dose limiting
Alzheimer disease	Early dementia (memory loss, apraxia, aphasia) Tremor uncommon Spontaneous hallucinations less common than in dementia with Lewy bodies	Poor
Normal-pressure hydrocephalus	"Lower-half" parkinsonism ("gait apraxia") Urinary complaints (frequency, urgency, incontinence) Cognitive disturbances	Generally poor Imaging demonstrates ventriculomegaly out of proportion to cortical atrophy
Drug-induced parkinsonism	All the classic features of parkinsonism (tremor may be less common than in Parkinson disease) Usually symmetrical signs and symptoms Other drug-induced movement disorders (e.g., tardive dyskinesia with neuroleptics)	Usually poor because of ongoing dopamine receptor blockade; may aggravate movements of tardive dyskinesia

MRI = magnetic resonance imaging; RBD = rapid eye movement sleep behavior disorder.

TREATMENT   Rx

Treatment of Parkinson disease is directed at slowing its progression ("neuroprotective" or "disease-modifying" treatments); improving symptoms, typically by restoring dopaminergic tone medically or by correcting basal ganglia neurophysiology surgically ("symptomatic"); or attempting to restore or to regenerate the damaged neurons ("neurorestorative" or "neuroregenerative" therapy).

Exercises may provide benefit. In one randomized trial, for example, tai chi training reduced balance impairments and lowered the incidence of falls in patients with mild to moderate Parkinson disease better than did stretching training.[A1] Another trial of three different forms of exercise showed variable benefit in all groups, possibly more with treadmill and resistance exercises.[A2]

Medical Treatment

To date, no medical treatment (Table 409-5) has been proved to modify the progressive course of Parkinson disease. The selective monoamine oxidase B inhibitors selegiline and rasagiline[A3] may exert disease-modifying effects, and

the potential effects of agents such as the calcium-channel blocker isradipine, the pro-urate agent inosine, the peroxisome proliferator-activated receptor γ agonist pioglitazone, and the nicotine patch (encouraged by the lower incidence of Parkinson disease in smokers) are currently under study.

Early treatment in a patient with little or no disability may entail only education, psychological support, encouragement to remain active and to become involved in an exercise program, and ongoing follow-up. There is some evidence that early treatment, even when patients are only mildly symptomatic, may preserve quality of life. A treatment philosophy that still requires evidence-based support involves the early initiation of symptomatic therapy to bolster the brain's compensatory mechanisms that have begun to fail as the physical symptoms of parkinsonism become manifested.

When symptoms begin to interfere with function, mildly effective drugs such as a monoamine oxidase B inhibitor, amantadine, and anticholinergics (the last predominantly for tremor in younger patients) may provide adequate benefit (see Table 409-5).[10] When symptoms are more pronounced or inadequately controlled with these approaches, dopaminergic therapy should be introduced. In patients younger than 65 years who are cognitively intact and

TABLE 409-5 DRUGS FOR PARKINSON DISEASE

CLASS	DRUG	USUAL STARTING DOSE	USUAL FINAL DOSAGE	IMPORTANT ADVERSE EFFECTS	COMMENTS	INDICATIONS
Anticholinergic	Many (e.g., benztropine, trihexyphenidyl)	Benztropine or trihexyphenidyl, 1-2 mg 2-3 times per day	Varied	Peripheral effects, e.g., dry mouth, blurred vision, constipation, difficulty with urination Central effects, e.g., confusion, memory problems, hallucinations	Relatively contraindicated in the elderly and contraindicated in patients with cognitive disturbances	Early treatment of tremor
Miscellaneous	Amantadine	100 mg once per day	100 mg 2 or 3 times per day	Confusion, visual hallucinations; livedo reticularis, swelling of the ankles; dose reduction or drug withdrawal necessary in patients with renal failure	Previously considered a dopaminergic drug, now thought to act primarily through NMDA antagonist effects	Early treatment; later for dyskinesias
	Memantine	5 mg once daily	10 mg twice daily	Confusion, fatigue, dizziness, headache	NMDA antagonist	Possibly effective for cognitive dysfunction in PDD
Dopamine precursor	Levodopa given with peripheral dopa decarboxylase inhibitor (DDCI) (carbidopa [in 4:1 and 10:1 ratios] or benserazide [4:1]*)	50 (levodopa)/12.5 (DDCI) mg (4:1 preparation) 3 times per day (with meals to reduce nausea and vomiting)	Varied; begin with 3-times-daily schedule (controlled-release levodopa-carbidopa may be given twice daily at first); late in the disease, patients may require multiple doses per day (sometimes >2 g/day) Initially give with meals to reduce GI upset; later avoid meals to improve absorption and reliability of response	Peripheral and central dopaminergic side effects Peripheral: nausea, vomiting, and orthostatic hypotension Central: motor fluctuations, dyskinesias, psychiatric disturbances	Peripheral side effects often controlled by additional carbidopa or the peripheral dopamine receptor blocker domperidone* Controlled-release formulations often less bioavailable with less reliable absorption (more "dose failures" later on)	Formulations: immediate-release—for early and later treatment Controlled-release (with carbidopa [4:1] or benserazide [4:1]*)—for predictable motor fluctuations (wearing off) and nighttime akinesia Stalevo (with carbidopa and entacapone)—for wearing off Parcopa (orally disintegrating tablets for faster absorption)—for patients with problematic long latency to benefit with individual doses Melevodopa* (methyl ester of levodopa; effervescent prodrug with much higher water solubility than tablets of levodopa; available in Italy) Duodopa* (used with a pump for duodenal infusions)—for problematic motor fluctuations

TABLE 409-5 DRUGS FOR PARKINSON DISEASE—cont'd

CLASS	DRUG	USUAL STARTING DOSE	USUAL FINAL DOSAGE	IMPORTANT ADVERSE EFFECTS	COMMENTS	INDICATIONS
Dopamine agonists Ergot derived	Bromocriptine	1.25 mg 3 times per day with meals	30-40 mg/day	Peripheral and central dopaminergic side effects; pedal edema, excessive daytime sleepiness Pleuropulmonary reaction, retroperitoneal fibrosis, erythromelalgia Impulse control disorders probably equally common with all dopamine agonists	Peripheral side effects often well controlled with domperidone* Rare pulmonary, retroperitoneal, and skin effects possibly caused by ergot derivation (drug withdrawal usually required)	Early and adjunctive therapy
	Pergolide	0.05 mg once per day × 2 days, increasing slowly thereafter	3-5 mg/day	As for bromocriptine; cardiac valvulopathy	As for bromocriptine	Not the first agonist because it causes restrictive cardiac valve disease
	Cabergoline*	0.5-1 mg once per day	2-6 mg/day	As for pergolide	As for pergolide Long half-life allows once-daily dosage	As for pergolide, although advantage of a long half-life may outweigh this concern
	Lisuride*	0.1-0.2 mg 1-3 times per day	2-5 mg/day	As for bromocriptine	As for bromocriptine	Uncertain whether cardiac valve abnormalities occur Parenteral formulations allow chronic infusion (pump) therapy
Non-ergot derived	Ropinirole	0.25 mg 3 times per day	Up to 24 mg/day in 3 divided doses Once-daily extended/ prolonged-release formulation available	Peripheral and central dopaminergic side effects similar to those of ergot-derived dopamine agonists, with the probable exceptions of pleuropulmonary reaction, retroperitoneal fibrosis, erythromelalgia, and cardiac valvulopathy	Effective as first-line and adjunctive therapy; dopamine D_3 agonist effects may contribute to efficacy Some patients withdrawing from the drug (especially those with impulse control disorders) experience symptoms similar to an addictive drug withdrawal ("dopamine agonist withdrawal syndrome")	De novo therapy shown to be associated with fewer motor complications than with levodopa Implications of less progressive loss of dopamine terminal function on imaging uncertain
	Pramipexole	0.125 mg 3 times per day	Up to 4.5 mg/day in 3 divided doses Once-daily extended/ prolonged-release formulation available	As for ropinirole	As for ropinirole, possibly greater "D_3-preferring" effects—may account for antidepressant effect	As for ropinirole
	Rotigotine	Nominal dose: 2.0 mg/day (10 cm² containing 4.5 mg)	Transdermal patch nominal dose 4.0-16 mg/day (patch content 9-36 mg; 20-80 cm²)	As for ropinirole Additional adverse effects related to skin patch application (dermatitis)	May be effective for both first-line and adjunctive therapy	
	Piribedil*	50 mg once/day	150-250 mg/day (in 3-5 doses per day)	As for ropinirole	As for ropinirole	
	Apomorphine	3-5 mg SC injection	Parenteral agent given as needed or as continuous infusion	Peripheral and central dopaminergic side effects Local skin reactions, including nodule formation	Concomitant antiemetic (eg, domperidone,* trimethobenzamide) needed	Late-stage problematic motor fluctuations Long-term use of infusions may reduce dyskinesias as well as motor fluctuations

Class	Agent	Starting Dose	Usual Dose	Side Effects	Comments	Indications
Monoamine oxidase B inhibitors	Selegiline	5 mg once per day	5 mg 2 times per day	Dopaminergic effects of other drugs possibly accentuated, insomnia, confusion	Last dose given at midday to avoid insomnia	Early mild disease; Some controversial evidence suggesting disease-modifying effects; Predictable motor fluctuations (wearing off)
	Zydis selegiline	1.25 mg once per day	1.25 or 2.5 mg/day (wafer formulation)	As for selegiline	As for selegiline; Absorbed from the buccal mucosa, thereby avoiding first-pass hepatic metabolism and methamphetamine metabolite of selegiline	As for selegiline
	Rasagiline	1 mg once per day	1-2 mg once per day	As for selegiline	As for selegiline	Possible disease-modifying effects; As for selegiline
Catechol O-methyltransferase (COMT) inhibitors	Tolcapone	100 mg 3 times per day	100 or 200 mg 3 times per day (at 6-hour intervals)	Effects of levodopa accentuated; Diarrhea in approximately 5% of patients; Hepatotoxicity; Urine discoloration	Dose of levodopa may have to be reduced by as much as 25%; diarrhea (sometimes explosive) typically forces discontinuation; Ongoing monitoring of liver function tests required (second-line COMT inhibitor)	Motor fluctuations, especially wearing off (probably more effective than entacapone)
	Entacapone	200 mg with each dose of levodopa	200 mg 4-10 times per day (given with doses of levodopa)	Effects of levodopa accentuated; 10% note brown/orange urine discoloration	As for tolcapone; diarrhea possibly less frequent; Liver function monitoring unnecessary	As for tolcapone; Available in a combination tablet with levodopa/carbidopa (Stalevo)
A$_{2A}$ antagonist	Istradefylline* (Japan only)	20 mg once per day	20 mg once per day	Increased dyskinesias		
Atypical neuroleptics	Clozapine	12.5 mg hs	Wide range (6.25-150 mg/day), usually <75 mg/day	Agranulocytosis, sedation, hypotension, sialorrhea	Very low risk of worsening parkinsonism; agranulocytosis rare (<1%) and reversible if discovered early (requires regular monitoring of complete blood count)	Drug-induced psychosis; Other "off-label" indications include drug-resistant tremor and possibly levodopa-induced dyskinesias
	Quetiapine	12.5-25 mg hs	25-150 mg/day	Sedation; May worsen parkinsonism	Probably less effective than clozapine	Drug-induced psychosis
Acetylcholinesterase inhibitors	Donepezil	5 mg once per day	5-10 mg/day	Peripheral cholinergic side effects: nausea, vomiting, diarrhea, syncope, bradycardia; Increased tremor, worsening of other Parkinson features		Dementia; Possibly effective for psychotic symptoms, especially hallucinations
	Rivastigmine	1.5 mg twice per day	3-12 mg/day	As for donepezil	Patch formulation available for transdermal administration—tolerability may be improved over oral formulation	As for donepezil

*Unavailable in the United States.

GI = gastrointestinal; NMDA = N-methyl-D-aspartate; PDD = Parkinson disease dementia.

For evidence-based treatment recommendations, see Suchowersky O, Gronseth G, Perlmutter J, et al. Practice parameter: neuroprotective strategies and alternative therapies for Parkinson disease (an evidence-based review): report of the Quality Standards Subcommittee of the American Academy of Neurology. Neurology. 2006;66:976-982; Pahwa R, Factor SA, Lyons KE, et al. Practice parameter: treatment of Parkinson disease with motor fluctuations and dyskinesia (an evidence-based review): report of the Quality Standards Subcommittee of the American Academy of Neurology. Neurology. 2006;66:983-995; and Miyasaki JM, Shannon K, Voon V, et al. Practice parameter: evaluation and treatment of depression, psychosis, and dementia in Parkinson disease (an evidence-based review): report of the Quality Standards Subcommittee of the American Academy of Neurology. Neurology. 2006;66:996-1002.

lack other major medical problems, initial therapy with a dopamine agonist may delay the development of motor complications. However, these drugs result in more excessive sleepiness, leg edema, "impulse control disorders" (such as pathologic gambling, hypersexuality, binge eating, and shopping), and hallucinations than levodopa does. If a full dose of a dopamine agonist does not provide adequate clinical benefit or has intolerable side effects, levodopa should be initiated. In older patients, in those with cognitive dysfunction (more prone to hallucinations with dopamine agonists), and in circumstances that require more rapid improvement of pronounced disability, levodopa should be the initial drug used.

Alleviating Symptoms

Levodopa is the most effective treatment of Parkinson disease, but it is associated with a variety of side effects (see Table 409-2). For the first year or more, the benefit of levodopa lasts throughout the day with little symptomatic variability. However, in time, the duration of benefit declines, with worsening of symptoms the first thing in the morning (morning akinesia) and for a variable time before scheduled daytime doses (wearing-off/end-of-dose akinesia). Within 2 to 5 years of initiation of treatment, up to 50% of patients may also experience involuntary movements (chorea, athetosis, dystonia), most often at the peak action of the medication. These complications, which are generally more prominent and occur earlier in patients with an onset of disease at a younger age, reflect the short half-life of levodopa combined with the underlying progressive loss of presynaptic dopamine neurons and result in nonphysiologic "pulsatile" stimulation of striatal dopamine receptors, which then induces "neuroplastic" changes in postsynaptic striatal neurons. Initially, these complications rarely cause major disability.

Although initiation of therapy with a dopamine agonist rather than with levodopa may be associated with a delay in the onset of these motor problems, the clinical benefit is generally less than with levodopa,[A4] and all patients eventually require the addition of levodopa to control symptoms. No data support delaying treatment with levodopa, and some data suggest that levodopa could have a neuroprotective effect. Even as Parkinson disease progresses, most of the classic features continue to respond after 20 years or more of treatment. It is not clear that delaying motor complications in the first 5 years of treatment by the initial use of a dopamine agonist improves long-term outcome or quality of life; indeed, clinical status, including the incidence of motor complications, may be no different after 10 years of treatment in those initiating therapy with a dopamine agonist and those starting with levodopa.

There is no clear advantage to starting initial treatment with a controlled-release rather than with an immediate-release preparation of levodopa or combining levodopa with a catechol O-methyltransferase inhibitor. When motor fluctuations develop during levodopa therapy, however, they can be managed by a number of approaches (see Table 409-5), including increasing the frequency of the dose, using a controlled-release preparation, prolonging the action by blocking metabolism (monoamine oxidase B or catechol O-methyltransferase inhibition), or adding a dopamine agonist. For example, adding rasagiline or entacapone to levodopa provides significant incremental benefits.

Newer levodopa formulations that provide more reliable, sustained plasma levels are in active development.[A5] A formulation that provides continuous infusion into the duodenum (Duodopa) can significantly improve symptoms during "off" time without increasing dyskinesias compared with immediate-release levodopa[A6]; this formulation is available in most European countries and was recently approved in Canada and the United States for patients with problematic motor fluctuations. Dyskinesias improve when doses of dopaminergic medications are reduced, but the parkinsonism often increases to an intolerable level. Amantadine may improve the dyskinesias without worsening the parkinsonism. Newer agents under study include the α_2-adrenergic receptor antagonist fipamezole[A7] and antagonists of the metabotropic glutamate receptor mGluR5, such as AFQ056,[A8] but these medications are not yet approved for use. Antagonists of the adenosine A_{2A} receptor are being actively studied but with variable results. One of these, istradefylline, is marked in Japan for the treatment of wearing-off phenomenon.

Medical management of Parkinson disease often includes a variety of other agents, including medications directed at the treatment of orthostatic hypotension (Chapter 62), depression (Chapter 397), anxiety (Chapter 397), urinary frequency and urgency (Chapters 26 and 129), and male erectile dysfunction (Chapter 234).[11] Management of late-stage Parkinson disease requires skill in polypharmacy and an understanding of the complicated benefit-risk ratios of the many drugs needed.

Surgical Treatment

Bilateral deep brain stimulation of the subthalamic nucleus or globus pallidus improves the symptoms of Parkinson disease, often permits lower doses of antiparkinson medications to be used, improves self-reported quality of life, and is about twice as effective as medical therapy despite the adverse effects associated with the procedure.[A9-A11] Early use of subthalamic nucleus deep brain stimulation, at a time when patients are just beginning to develop motor complications (mean duration of disease, 7.5 years), provides significantly greater benefit than best medical therapy. Thalamic deep brain stimulation is of limited utility because it is effective only for tremor. The best predictor of a good response to deep brain stimulation of the subthalamic nucleus is the patient's ongoing clinical response to levodopa.[12] Apart from tremor, which may be resistant to the highest tolerable dose of levodopa but generally responds well to surgery, symptoms that are resistant to the peak effect of levodopa (e.g., dysarthria, postural instability with falls) also fail to respond to deep brain stimulation. The typical good candidate for deep brain stimulation of the subthalamic nucleus is an otherwise healthy, relatively young, cognitively intact, and psychiatrically stable patient who still responds well to levodopa (apart from tremor) but is suffering from disabling motor fluctuations and dyskinesias.

Double-blind randomized trials of transplantation of fetal substantia nigra into the striatum have failed to show significant efficacy and also have been associated with the side effect of transplant-induced off-medication dyskinesias. Postmortem assessments in a small number of patients surviving for more than 10 years after fetal transplants have shown Lewy bodies in the transplanted dopamine neurons, thus suggesting that the pathologic process can be "transmitted" to neurons placed in the diseased host.[13] Nevertheless, some patients treated with fetal transplants have responded well for many years, and research in this field is ongoing.

A sham-controlled study demonstrated significant benefit with gene transfer of glutamic acid decarboxylase (AAV-GAD) into the subthalamic nucleus in patients with advanced Parkinson disease.[A12] By comparison, double-blind randomized trials of bilateral intraputamenal infusion of glial-derived neurotrophic factor and gene therapy with AAV-neurturin (administered into the putamen and the substantia nigra) failed to confirm the benefits that were suggested by unblinded studies.[14]

PROGNOSIS

Parkinson disease progresses inexorably during a period of many years; the speed and course of progression vary considerably from patient to patient. So far, genotypic information has not helped predict outcomes.[15] Some patients maintain an excellent response to treatment and seem to change very little during prolonged follow-up, but most note increasing disability, with the development of many symptoms that are poorly responsive to medications. Factors such as poor postural stability, falls, dysarthria, dysphagia, dysautonomia, excessive daytime sleepiness, and dementia contribute to the disability and increased mortality.

FUTURE DIRECTIONS

Gene therapies directed at either modifying neurotransmitter function or inducing neuroregeneration and other cell-based therapies are under development. Future treatments must also address the widespread, multisystemic nature of the disease, especially symptoms that are unrelated to nigrostriatal dopamine deficiency and that fail to respond to current therapies.

OTHER CAUSES OF PARKINSONISM

The numerous causes of parkinsonism (see Table 409-1) are sometimes termed akinetic-rigid syndrome, Parkinson syndrome, atypical parkinsonism, or even Parkinson-plus syndrome to emphasize that these patients commonly demonstrate additional clinical features indicative of the more widespread and particularly more severe pathologic involvement of areas beyond the dopaminergic SNc. These other parkinsonism conditions are generally associated with "postsynaptic" changes that result in a poor or unsustained response to levodopa, and this unresponsiveness serves as one of the most important of several clues that the parkinsonism features are caused by conditions other than Parkinson disease (see Table 409-4) (i.e., "parkinsonism minus" a levodopa response; see Table 409-3).

 Grade A References

A1. Li F, Harmer P, Fitzgerald K, et al. Tai chi and postural stability in patients with Parkinson's disease. *N Engl J Med.* 2012;366:511-519.

A2. Shulman LM, Katzel LI, Ivey FM, et al. Randomized clinical trial of 3 types of physical exercise for patients with Parkinson disease. *JAMA Neurol.* 2013;7:183-190.

A3. Olanow CW, Rascol O, Hauser R, et al. A double-blind, delayed start trial of rasagiline in Parkinson's disease. *N Engl J Med.* 2009;361:1268-1278.

A4. Gray R, Ives N, Rick C, et al. Long-term effectiveness of dopamine agonists and monoamine oxidase B inhibitors compared with levodopa as initial treatment for Parkinson's disease (PD MED): a large, open-label, pragmatic randomised trial. *Lancet.* 2014;384:1196-1205.

A5. Hauser RA, Hsu A, Kell S, et al. Extended-release carbidopa-levodopa (IPX066) compared with immediate-release carbidopa-levodopa in patients with Parkinson's disease and motor fluctuations: a phase 3 randomised, double-blind trial. *Lancet Neurol.* 2013;12:346-356.

A6. Olanow CW, Kieburtz K, Odin P, et al. Continuous intrajejunal infusion of levodopa-carbidopa intestinal gel for patients with advanced Parkinson's disease: a randomised, controlled, double-blind, double-dummy study. *Lancet Neurol.* 2014;13:141-149.

A7. Lewitt PA, Hauser RA, Lu M, et al. Randomized clinical trial of fipamezole for dyskinesia in Parkinson disease (FJORD study). *Neurology.* 2012;79:163-169.

A8. Stocchi F, Rascol O, Destee A, et al. AFQ056 in Parkinson patients with levodopa-induced dyskinesia: 13-week, randomized, dose-finding study. *Mov Disord.* 2013;28:1838-1846.
A9. Deuschl G, Schade-Brittinger C, Krack P, et al. A randomized trial of deep-brain stimulation for Parkinson's disease. *N Engl J Med.* 2006;355:896-908.
A10. Schuepbach WM, Rau J, Knudsen K, et al. Neurostimulation for Parkinson's disease with early motor complications. *N Engl J Med.* 2013;368:610-622.
A11. Weaver FM, Follett KA, Stern M, et al. Randomized trial of deep brain stimulation for Parkinson disease: thirty-six-month outcomes. *Neurology.* 2012;79:55-65.
A12. LeWitt PA, Rezai AR, Leehey MA, et al. AAV2-GAD gene therapy for advanced Parkinson's disease: a double-blind, sham-surgery controlled, randomised trial. *Lancet Neurol.* 2011;10:309-319.

GENERAL REFERENCES

For the General References and other additional features, please visit Expert Consult at https://expertconsult.inkling.com.

410

OTHER MOVEMENT DISORDERS

ANTHONY E. LANG

DEFINITION

Movement disorders are first divided into hypokinetic and hyperkinetic categories. *Hypokinetic disorders,* which are characterized by akinesia, bradykinesia, and rigidity, are parkinsonian syndromes and are discussed elsewhere (Chapter 409). The common *hyperkinetic movement* disorders (Table 410-1) are defined by their specific clinical phenomena.

CLINICAL MANIFESTATIONS AND DIAGNOSTIC APPROACH

The traditional approach to a neurologic symptom is first to address localization within the nervous system (i.e., "Where is the lesion?"), followed by an evaluation of the origin ("What is the lesion?").[1] The neurologic examination is critical in determining the localization of the lesion, and generally the history, including the nature of onset and the progression of the symptoms, determines the most likely diagnosis. However, when a movement disorder is the predominant problem, the approach is somewhat different. The pathophysiology of most movement disorders is complex and often poorly understood. Many of these disorders are the result of dysfunction of different circuits in the brain, and it is often impossible to ascertain a specific anatomic localization. Instead, an accurate appreciation of the clinical phenomena is the first important step in evaluating these patients. The clinician must observe and examine the patient to define the type of movement disorder that best describes the clinical picture. This accurate characterization then allows the generation of a differential diagnosis for the specific movement disorder. The age and nature of onset, the distribution, the progression of symptoms, a family history of similar or related symptoms, and the presence of other neurologic and systemic signs then help to determine the most likely explanation for that movement disorder.

TREMOR

Tremor, which is a rhythmic, sinusoidal movement of a body part, is caused by regular, either synchronous or alternating, contractions of reciprocally innervated muscles.[2] Tremors are classified based on whether they occur at rest (weight fully supported against gravity) or in action. Resting tremors are typically seen in Parkinson disease and other parkinsonism syndromes (see Table 409-1). Action tremors are further divided into postural, kinetic, or intention tremors. A postural tremor is seen with the maintenance of a posture against gravity (e.g., when the arms are outstretched in front of the body). A *kinetic tremor* is seen with a voluntary movement of the limb (e.g., a tremor in an upper limb when performing the finger-to-nose test). An intention tremor increases in amplitude on approaching a target.

CLINICAL MANIFESTATIONS

Most action tremors (Table 410-2) combine postural and kinetic components. All tremors worsen with stress, including performing an affected activity in public. Initially, a tremor may be evident only when one attempts fine, dexterous tasks such as threading a needle, soldering, or using a screwdriver. More severe tremors interfere with activities such as handwriting, fastening buttons, shaving, eating soup with a spoon, or drinking from a cup. Patients

TABLE 410-1 HYPERKINETIC MOVEMENT DISORDERS

| Tremor |
| Chorea |
| Ballism |
| Dystonia |
| Athetosis |
| Tics |
| Myoclonus |
| Startle |
| Stereotypies |
| Miscellaneous |

TABLE 410-2 DIFFERENTIAL DIAGNOSIS OF TREMOR AND RHYTHMIC MOVEMENT DISORDERS

ENHANCED PHYSIOLOGIC TREMOR

Metabolic disorders
  Hyperthyroidism
  Hyperparathyroidism
  Hypoglycemia
  Pheochromocytoma
Drugs
  Caffeine
  Theophylline
  Amphetamines
  Lithium
  Valproic acid
  Antidepressants
  Amiodarone
  β-Agonists
  Others
Withdrawal of drugs
  Benzodiazepines
  Alcohol
  Others
Fever, sepsis
Anxiety, stress, fatigue

PRIMARY OR IDIOPATHIC TREMOR

Essential tremor
Task-specific tremor
Orthostatic tremor
Idiopathic palatal tremor

TREMOR ASSOCIATED WITH CENTRAL NERVOUS SYSTEM DISEASES

Tremor with parkinsonian syndromes
  Idiopathic Parkinson disease
  Multiple system atrophy
  Progressive supranuclear palsy
  Corticobasal degeneration
  Neuroleptic-induced parkinsonism
Wilson disease
Multiple sclerosis
Fragile X premutation-tremor/ataxia syndrome
Stroke
Arteriovenous malformation
Tumor
Head trauma
Midbrain tremor (Holmes tremor)

TREMOR ASSOCIATED WITH PERIPHERAL NEUROPATHIES

PSYCHOGENIC TREMOR

OTHER RHYTHMIC MOVEMENT DISORDERS

Rhythmic movements in dystonia (dystonic tremor)
Rhythmic myoclonus (including myoclonic tremor)
Asterixis
Clonus
Epilepsia partialis continua
Hereditary chin quivering
Spasmus nutans
Head bobbing with hydrocephalus
Nystagmus

Modified from Cloutier M, Lang AE. Movement disorders: an overview. In: Factor SA, Lang AE, Weiner WJ, eds. *Drug Induced Movement Disorders.* Malden, Mass: Blackwell; 2005:3-19.

often adapt or use compensatory measures, such as switching an activity to a less affected hand (e.g., shaving with the nondominant hand), using two hands to drink, drinking only from an incompletely filled glass or cup, or completely avoiding more challenging feeding activities in public. Severe action and intention tremors can cause handwriting to become completely illegible and can result in dependence on others for care.

Head tremors, which may be side to side, up and down, or mixed, are rarely disabling but are often a source of embarrassment. Tremor of the larynx, which causes the voice to quaver, is best appreciated by asking the patient to sustain a note. Action tremor of the lower limbs is assessed by having the patient hold the foot up to a target (e.g., the examiner's hand) and then perform a heel-knee-shin test.

Most upper limb action tremors affect many activities to a similar extent. Less commonly, tremors can affect a single task in isolation (task-specific tremors), the most common being a primary writing tremor. Orthostatic tremor is apparent in the legs and in antigravity muscles only when the patient is standing in one spot and subsides during walking or leaning against a wall; these patients commonly complain of a tremendous sense of insecurity while standing and a fear of falling. Electrophysiologic assessment demonstrates a very characteristic high-frequency tremor (14 to 16 Hz).

Enhanced Physiologic Tremor

A 7- to 12-Hz tremor is detectable in everyone with electrophysiologic recording. This physiologic tremor is enhanced and may become symptomatic in a variety of circumstances, including fatigue, anxiety, and excitement. This same tremor may be accentuated by drugs and systemic processes.

Essential Tremor

Essential tremor affects up to 5% of the general population after the age of 60 years. Essential tremor is often inherited in an autosomal dominant fashion, with the phenotype showing genetic heterogeneity from at least three different genes, most recently *LINGO1*,[3] as well as environmental influences. Recent pathology studies have variably demonstrated microscopic abnormalities of cerebellar Purkinje cells. The age of onset may be as early as the first or second decade of life, but senile tremor may be delayed until the mid-60s. Patients first become aware of a mild postural and action tremor in the hands, which is indistinguishable from an enhanced physiologic tremor and may result in little functional impairment for many years until it gradually interferes with activities. Older patients with large-amplitude, lower frequency tremors can have a resting component that is often misdiagnosed as Parkinson disease (see Table 409-1).

TREATMENT ℞

Treatment of essential tremor does not influence the course of the illness and therefore is justified only when the tremor interferes with function. At least 50% of patients note improvement or complete amelioration of tremor following the ingestion of a small amount of ethanol.

First-line drug treatment includes trials of a noncardioselective β-adrenergic blocker (e.g., propranolol, ≤ 320 mg/day), primidone (starting in a low dose of 25 to 62.5 mg at night and increasing to 500 to 750 mg/day), or topiramate (≤400 mg/day).[A1] Other drugs that have been shown probably to be effective in double-blind crossover trials include gabapentin (1200 to 1800 mg/day), atenolol (50 to 150 mg/day), alprazolam (0.125 to 3 mg/day), and sotalol (75 to 200 mg/day). However, sotalol is associated with ventricular arrhythmias and dose-related QT interval prolongation, so it is not routinely considered as treatment of essential tremor. The medications that have been shown to be of possible benefit include nadolol (120 to 240 mg/day), nimodipine (120 mg/day), and clonazepam (0.5 to 6 mg/day), but many patients remain resistant to all drugs. Botulinum toxin may be effective, but it also may result in dose-dependent weakness and pain at the injection site. If disability is substantial, thalamic deep brain stimulation or thalamotomy can be of major benefit, with 60 to 90% reductions following bilateral treatment.[4] However, a few patients suffer permanent neurologic sequelae, such as speech problems, owing to intracranial hemorrhage or other postoperative complications, even with unilateral procedures, and even more suffer such problems after bilateral procedures. Newer approaches to thalamotomy include gamma knife and focused ultrasound.[5]

CHOREA

Chorea (Table 410-3) consists of irregular, random, brief, flowing movements that often flit from one body part to another in an unpredictable and purposeless sequence. Patients may incorporate choreiform movements into a voluntary movement to mask them. The severity varies from the appearance

TABLE 410-3   DIFFERENTIAL DIAGNOSIS OF CHOREA

GENETIC DISORDERS

Benign hereditary chorea
Huntington disease
Huntington-like conditions
Neuroferritinopathy
Neuroacanthocytosis, including McLeod syndrome
Dentatorubropallidoluysian atrophy
Wilson disease
Neurodegeneration with brain iron accumulation 1 (NBIA 1) (previously Hallervorden Spatz disease)
Spinocerebellar ataxias
Ataxia-telangiectasia
Ataxia-oculomotor apraxia type 1
Tuberous sclerosis

INFECTIONS/PARAINFECTIOUS CAUSES

Sydenham chorea
Acquired immunodeficiency syndrome (including complications)
Encephalitis and postencephalitic disorders
Creutzfeldt-Jakob disease

DRUGS

Levodopa
Dopaminergic agonists used for Parkinson disease
Amphetamines
Anticholinergics
Anticonvulsants (especially phenytoin)
Neuroleptics
Tricyclic antidepressants
Selective serotonin reuptake inhibitors (occasionally)
Oral contraceptives (typically in patients with a prior history of Sydenham chorea)
Antihistaminics

ENDOCRINOLOGIC/METABOLIC CONDITIONS

Hyperthyroidism
Hypoparathyroidism
Chorea gravidarum
Acquired hepatolenticular degeneration

IMMUNOLOGIC DISORDERS

Systemic lupus erythematosus
Antiphospholipid syndrome
Henoch-Schönlein purpura

VASCULAR DISORDERS

Stroke
Hemorrhage
Arteriovenous malformation
Polycythemia rubra vera

OTHER CONDITIONS

Cerebral palsy
Kernicterus
Head trauma
Cardiopulmonary bypass with hypothermia
Neoplastic and paraneoplastic syndromes
Paroxysmal dyskinesias

Modified from Cloutier M, Lang AE. Movement disorders: an overview. In: Factor SA, Lang AE, Weiner WJ, eds. *Drug Induced Movement Disorders*. Malden, Mass: Blackwell; 2005:3-19.

of being slightly fidgety or restless, to striking, continuous movements involving the whole body. Many patients with chorea seem unaware of their movements, whereas others can be very troubled and disabled.

Huntington Disease

DEFINITION AND EPIDEMIOLOGY

Huntington disease is a fully penetrant autosomal dominant neurodegenerative disorder caused by an expanded trinucleotide (CAG) repeat in the gene for the protein huntingtin. The worldwide 2.71 per 100,000 prevalence ranges from 5.7 per 100,000 for individuals of European descent to 0.4 per 100,000 for Asians.[6] The age at diagnosis is driven by the longest expanded allele and as yet unidentified genetic or environmental factors.

PATHOBIOLOGY

Huntington disease is characterized neuropathologically by neuronal loss accompanied by intraneuronal inclusions and gliosis, especially in the caudate nucleus and putamen (the striatum) and the cerebral cortex. Understanding how these changes result from the expanded polyglutamine tract in the mutated huntingtin protein is the goal of current research.

CLINICAL MANIFESTATIONS

Symptoms typically begin between the ages of 30 and 55 years, but 5 to 10% of patients have an onset before the age of 20 years (juvenile Huntington disease) and a few patients begin to have symptoms quite late in life. Symptoms include a combination of a movement disorder, psychiatric disturbances, and cognitive dysfunction. Early on, the movement disorder is predominantly chorea, but parkinsonism and dystonia develop later. Some patients, especially those with juvenile onset, have a more rapidly progressive akinetic-rigid and dystonic form (the Westphal variant). Psychiatric manifestations, which are universal but widely variable, include personality changes, impulsiveness, aggressive behavior, depression, and paranoid psychosis. These psychiatric symptoms may precede the motor manifestations, and psychotropic drug therapy may be incorrectly blamed for the subsequent development of the movement disorder. Cognitive changes result in progressive subcortical dementia with disturbed attention, concentration, judgment, and problem-solving that differs from the typical cortical dementia of Alzheimer disease. Oculomotor dysfunction, most often manifested by difficulties with refixating the gaze and a resulting tendency to use blinks and head thrusts, is another common feature.

DIAGNOSIS

The diagnosis is confirmed by genetic testing. Normal alleles of the *IT15* gene have fewer than 30 CAG repeats, whereas 40 or more repeats invariably result in clinical illness. An earlier age of onset correlates with larger numbers of CAG repeats. Patients with intermediate alleles (27 to 35) have more behavioral abnormalities, such as apathy and suicidal ideation, than unaffected individuals.

TREATMENT AND PROGNOSIS ℞

Current care for patients with Huntington disease involves a multidisciplinary team of clinical geneticists, neurologists, psychiatrists, psychologists, social workers, occupational and physical therapists, speech therapists, nutritionists, and nurses. Genetic counseling for patients and family members is critical. Chorea may be extremely responsive to drugs that reduce central dopamine activity, especially tetrabenazine, starting at 12.5 mg two or three times daily and gradually increasing to up to 100 to 200 mg/day. Amantadine (300 to 400 mg/day) and possibly riluzole (200 mg/day) may reduce chorea. Other potential agents that work by blocking dopamine receptors include haloperidol (3 to 30 mg/day), pimozide (0.5 to 10 mg/day), fluphenazine (0.5 to 20 mg/day), and reserpine (0.75 to 5 mg/day). These agents should be reserved for patients with disabling chorea because they may be associated with increased parkinsonism, postural instability, depression, sedation, and other adverse effects. Unfortunately, physical function may not improve significantly even when the chorea is controlled. Psychiatric symptoms (e.g., anxiety, psychosis, depression) can be managed effectively with the same strategies as in other psychiatric diseases (Chapter 397). Disease-modifying strategies are under active development.[7]

Progression can be monitored by following changes in gray matter volumes in both premanifest and early-stage patients.[8] Patients inexorably decline at a relatively constant rate,[9] and the disease progresses to institutionalization and death over the course of approximately 15 years.

Other Choreas

Most of the non-neurodegenerative causes of chorea (see Table 410-3) can be excluded by a careful history (including a detailed drug history) and a focused set of investigations, including, in appropriate circumstances, wet preparation of peripheral blood for acanthocytes (which are associated with neurodegeneration), immunologic studies (including anticardiolipin antibodies), endocrine assessment (hyperthyroidism, pregnancy), and neuroimaging. Among 36 adult cases of autoimmune chorea seen at one institution in 5 years, 50% had a coexisting autoimmune disorder, especially systemic lupus erythematosus (Chapter 266), and most of the remainder had a paraneoplastic cause, especially small cell carcinoma of the lung and adenocarcinoma.[10]

Sydenham chorea, which is a late component of rheumatic fever (Chapter 290), is presumably the result of immunologic cross-reactivity between the causative group A β-hemolytic streptococcus and the basal ganglia. This disorder is infrequently seen in North America but is more common in developing countries. Sydenham chorea usually affects children and young adults,

TABLE 410-4 DIFFERENTIAL DIAGNOSIS OF BALLISM

Focal lesions in basal ganglia
    Vascular: Stroke (including infarction and hemorrhage), cavernous angioma, postsurgical complications
    Neoplastic: Metastases, primary central nervous system tumors
    Infections: Cryptococcosis, toxoplasmosis, tuberculoma
    Inflammatory: Multiple sclerosis
    Iatrogenic: Subthalamotomy, thalamotomy

Immunologic: Systemic lupus erythematosus, scleroderma; Behçet's disease
Nonketotic hyperglycemia (high-intensity lesions in striatum on T1 MRI)
Hypoglycemia
Sydenham's chorea
Head injury

Drugs
    Anticonvulsants
    Oral contraceptives
    Levodopa

Modified from Cloutier M, Lang AE. Movement disorders: an overview. In: Factor SA, Lang AE, Weiner WJ, eds. *Drug Induced Movement Disorders.* Malden, Mass: Blackwell; 2005:3-19.
MRI = magnetic resonance imaging.

and it is more common in girls before puberty. Adults with a history of Sydenham chorea in childhood may develop chorea during pregnancy or in response to taking oral contraceptive agents or estrogen preparations. They also may have a higher rate of subsequent psychiatric disturbances and impaired executive neurologic function even when in remission.[11] Drugs that can cause chorea should be withdrawn if possible.

Ballism

Ballism, which is considered an extreme form of chorea, involves large-amplitude, random, often violent flinging movements of the proximal limbs (Table 410-4). It is most often a consequence of an acute cerebral insult, such as a stroke, and it usually involves one side of the body, particularly the arm, hence the term *hemiballism*. When a causative lesion can be demonstrated, it typically involves the region of the subthalamic nucleus or the striatum. When the condition is caused by a stroke, movements usually subside spontaneously over days to weeks, although they may persist indefinitely in some patients. Treatment often requires the use of medication that antagonizes the effects of dopamine in the brain, including dopamine receptor blockers (neuroleptics such as haloperidol, 3 to 30 mg/day) or dopamine depleters (e.g., tetrabenazine, 50 to 200 mg/day). Functional neurosurgery (e.g., pallidotomy, deep brain stimulation) can be considered in patients with refractory, persistent symptoms.

● DYSTONIA

DEFINITION AND PATHOBIOLOGY

In dystonia, sustained muscle contractions, often initiated or worsened by voluntary action, result in repetitive twisting and sometimes tremulous movements and abnormal postures. Dystonia can be classified as primary dystonia, dystonia-plus, secondary dystonia, and heredogenerative dystonias (Table 410-5). Recently, a new classification uses five descriptors to specify the clinical characteristics: age at onset, body distribution, temporal pattern, whether dystonia occurs in isolation (or only accompanied by tremor; "pure dystonia") or coexists with other movement disorders (typically parkinsonism and myoclonus).[12] *Etiology* is defined as the presence or absence of degenerative or structural nervous system pathologic process and by whether the mode of inheritance is autosomal dominant, autosomal recessive, X-linked recessive, mitochondrial, or acquired. A commonly used classification scheme for the genetic dystonias involves applying the "DYT" prefix followed by a number (e.g., 1 to 25); however, several shortcomings have encouraged an active reevaluation of this approach. Acquired causes include drugs, toxins, infections, vascular disease, neoplasia, trauma, and psychogenic.

CLINICAL MANIFESTATIONS

Common forms of dystonia include eyelid closure (blepharospasm), jaw opening or closing (oromandibular dystonia), pulling or turning of the neck in any one or combination of directions (cervical dystonia: rotatory torticollis, laterocollis, retrocollis, anterocollis), hyperadduction and less often excessive abduction of the vocal cords (laryngeal dystonia or spasmodic

TABLE 410-5 CLASSIFICATION AND CAUSES OF DYSTONIA

PRIMARY DYSTONIAS (PRIMARY TORSION DYSTONIA)	HEREDODEGENERATIVE DYSTONIAS

Familial (several genetic causes and types)
Sporadic, usually adult onset, focal, or segmental
	X-linked
	  Lubag disease
	  Deafness-dystonia-optic atrophy (Mohr-Tranebjaerg) syndrome
	  Pelizaeus-Merzbacher disease
	  Lesch-Nyhan syndrome
	Autosomal dominant
	  Rapid-onset dystonia-parkinsonism
	  Juvenile parkinsonism (e.g., from mutations in the *parkin* gene)
	  Huntington disease
	  Machado-Joseph disease (SCA3) and other SCAs
	  Dentatorubropallidoluysian atrophy

DYSTONIA-PLUS	

Dystonia with parkinsonism
  Dopa-responsive dystonia
  Dopamine agonist–responsive dystonia (e.g., aromatic acid decarboxylase deficiency)
Myoclonus dystonia	

PRIMARY DYSTONIAS (PRIMARY TORSION DYSTONIA) / DYSTONIA-PLUS / SECONDARY DYSTONIAS	HEREDODEGENERATIVE DYSTONIAS

SECONDARY DYSTONIAS
Perinatal cerebral injury
  Athetoid cerebral palsy
  Delayed-onset dystonia
  Pachygyria
  Kernicterus
Encephalitis
  Reye syndrome
  Subacute sclerosing leukoencephalopathy
  Wasp sting
  Creutzfeldt-Jakob disease
  Human immunodeficiency virus infection
Head trauma
Thalamotomy
Brain stem lesion
Primary antiphospholipid syndrome
Stroke
Arteriovenous malformation
Hypoxia
Brain tumor
Multiple sclerosis
Central pontine myelinolysis
Cervical cord injury
Peripheral injury
Drugs
Toxins
Hypoparathyroidism
Psychogenic conditions
	Autosomal recessive
	  Wilson disease
	  Niemann-Pick disease type C
	  GM$_1$ gangliosidosis
	  GM$_2$ gangliosidosis
	  Metachromatic leukodystrophy
	  Homocystinuria
	  Glutaric acidemia
	  Triose-phosphate isomerase deficiency
	  Hartnup disease
	  Ataxia-telangiectasia
	  Neurodegeneration with brain iron accumulation (NBIA 1) (previously Hallervorden Spatz disease)
	  Juvenile neuronal ceroid lipofuscinosis
	  Neuroacanthocytosis
	  Intranuclear hyaline inclusion disease
	  Hereditary spastic paraplegia with dystonia
	Probably autosomal recessive
	  Familial basal ganglia calcifications (also dominantly inherited)
	  Progressive pallidal degeneration
	  Rett syndrome
	Mitochondrial
	  Leigh disease
	  Leber disease
	  Other mitochondrial cytopathies
	Sporadic, with parkinsonism
	  Parkinson disease
	  Progressive supranuclear palsy
	  Multiple system atrophy
	  Corticobasal degeneration

Modified from Cloutier M, Lang AE. Movement disorders: an overview. In: Factor SA, Lang AE, Weiner WJ, eds. *Drug Induced Movement Disorders.* Malden, Mass: Blackwell; 2005:3-19.

dysphonia), abnormal posturing and tightness of the hand while writing or using the hand for other tasks (writer's cramp, manual dystonia), abnormal posturing of the trunk or pelvis (axial dystonia), or abnormal posturing of the lower limb, including plantar flexion and inversion of the foot. The movements are often slow and sustained, although they also may be rapid (dystonic spasms). Slower, sinuous writhing dystonic movements, particularly present in the distal limbs, are referred to as *athetosis*. Dystonia is often made worse by activity (action dystonia), and a unique aspect of dystonia is that only selected acts may be affected, with complete sparing of all other activities in the same limb (task-specific dystonia, including writer's cramp and musician's cramp). In some patients, dystonia remains isolated and action specific over many years; in others, it progresses to involve adjacent muscles (overflow dystonia) and may eventually be present at rest, in which case joint contractures may result. Another common feature of dystonia is its transient improvement with the use of a sensory trick (geste antagoniste), such as lightly touching the chin to relieve severe cervical dystonia or the lid to relieve disabling blepharospasm. Patients with dystonia, independent of cause, often have additional postural and action tremors, phenotypically similar to those in essential tremor. Some patients also demonstrate more irregular, coarse, lower frequency rhythmic movements called *dystonic tremor*.

Dystonia is often classified according to the site of involvement: focal, only one body part (e.g., blepharospasm, cervical dystonia, writer's cramp); segmental, two or more contiguous body parts; multifocal, two or more noncontiguous body parts; generalized, trunk and at least two other sites (with or without leg involvement); and hemidystonia, unilateral (generally a causative focal brain lesion is found most often involving the putamen).

DIAGNOSIS AND PROGNOSIS

For diagnostic and prognostic purposes, dystonia also may be distinguished by age of onset as childhood-onset, adolescent-onset, or adult-onset dystonia. The younger the age of onset, the more likely a cause can be defined. Conversely, isolated dystonia beginning in adult life is most often an idiopathic disorder; further investigations are typically unrewarding and are usually not indicated. Likewise, independent of the cause, dystonia beginning in childhood commonly progresses to segmental or generalized involvement whereas adult-onset dystonia usually remains focal or segmental.

Specific Dystonias
PRIMARY (IDIOPATHIC) OR ISOLATED DYSTONIAS

Primary dystonia accounts for up to 90% of patients with a pure dystonic syndrome, in which dystonia either is the only motor feature or is accompanied only by tremor. To date, no consistent neuropathologic changes have been found in the small numbers of brains affected by primary dystonia that have been studied.

When symptoms begin in childhood, a definable genetic cause is often identified, the most common being DYT1, usually resulting from the autosomal dominant inheritance of a GAG deletion in the *torsin A* gene (Oppenheim dystonia). This disorder is more common in persons of Ashkenazi Jewish descent. The dystonia often begins in the first decade of life and can progress to severe disability, although the spectrum of disease, even within the same family, can be quite varied and penetrance is relatively low (~40%). Other genetic forms of dystonia include *THAP1* mutations for DYT6 and *TUBB4A* mutations for DYT4 or "whispering dystonia." Genetic testing is available but in the case of DYT1 is recommended only when the age of onset in the patient or another affected family member is less than 26 years.

ADULT-ONSET IDIOPATHIC DYSTONIA

Adult-onset idiopathic dystonia is the most common type of dystonia seen in general neurologic practice. The dystonia typically begins in the face, neck, or arm and may remain focal and nonprogressive or spread only to contiguous muscles after many years.[13] The cause of this disorder is not known, although a positive family history may be noted if multiple family members can be examined. Genetic forms of adult-onset focal or segmental dystonia include *ANO3* and *GNAL* mutations for craniocervical dystonia and possibly *CIZ1* mutations for cervical dystonia.

DYSTONIA-PLUS

The term *dystonia-plus* refers to a small number of disorders characterized by dystonia with other neurologic signs that result from a known or presumed genetic defect without an underlying progressive neurodegenerative process. In the newer classification, these conditions are included in the group of disorders with dystonia combined with other neurologic features.

Dopa-responsive dystonia, which usually results in dystonia beginning in the first decade of life, most often in the lower limbs, sometimes can be mistaken for hereditary spastic paraplegia or cerebral palsy. Most patients with dopa-responsive dystonia have a mutation in the *GCH1* gene, which results in reduced production of dopamine. Approximately 75% of patients have notable worsening of dystonia as the day progresses (diurnal variation). Exercise often aggravates the dystonia. Patients commonly demonstrate some degree of bradykinesia (especially in the legs) and postural instability. Rare adult-onset disease may result in a pure parkinsonian phenotype. Dopa-responsive dystonia should be considered in all children with dystonia. Symptoms are exquisitely sensitive to low doses of levodopa (typically as little as 50 mg/day of levodopa), and this treatment allows patients to live a normal life without the usual complications seen in Parkinson disease (Chapter 409).

Myoclonus dystonia, which usually begins within the first decade of life, combines dystonia with separate multifocal myoclonic jerks. Myoclonus dystonia is genetically heterogeneous; the most common definable cause is a mutation in the *e-sarcoglycan* gene. The dystonia in these patients most often involves the neck or upper limbs, is mild, and is often overlooked. The disorder also can include psychopathology, such as obsessive-compulsive behavior. A characteristic feature of this disorder is the marked ameliorative effect of ethanol on both the myoclonus and the dystonia, a feature that sometimes results in alcohol abuse.

OTHER DYSTONIAS

Dystonia may be a symptom of many diseases. The nature and extent of the investigations undertaken depend on such factors as age at onset, clues provided on the history, and additional neurologic or systemic features on examination. Wilson disease (Chapter 211) is an important consideration in the diagnosis of dystonia beginning in children and young adults. Another potentially treatable form of dystonia caused by a mutation in the *SLC30A10* gene, which codes for a manganese transporter.[14] The phenotype is similar to that of Wilson disease, with generalized dystonia, cirrhosis, and hyperintensities in the basal ganglia on T1 MRI scans.

Some patients with dystonia, chorea, or a mixture of the two (choreoathetosis) have intermittent symptoms (paroxysmal dyskinesias) and may be normal between episodes. The duration of symptoms can be as brief as a few seconds to a few minutes or persist for several hours. Symptoms triggered by sudden movement, which are termed *kinesigenic,* are typically brief; prolonged episodes are commonly triggered by exercise, stress, fatigue, caffeine, or alcohol. Paroxysmal dyskinesias may be genetically determined, idiopathic, the manifestation of another disorder (e.g., head injury, brain tumor, or stroke), or even psychologically based. A mutation of the *PRRT2* gene has been described in a large proportion of genetically determined paroxysmal kinesigenic dystonia.

TREATMENT ℞

Ideally, treatment is directed at the underlying cause, such as dopa-responsive dystonia, which is treated with levodopa (usually up to 300 mg/day) or Wilson disease (Chapter 211). Patients with mutations in the manganese transporter gene may benefit from chelation with ethylenediaminetetraacetic acid (EDTA) (see Table 22-1). Unfortunately, cause-specific treatment usually is not possible, so a variety of symptomatic treatments may be tried, often unsuccessfully, in an attempt to reduce disability.

Focal injections of botulinum toxin are now usually the first choice for treatment of focal and segmental dystonias.[A3] This approach can improve symptoms of patients with cranial (blepharospasm, oromandibular dystonia) and cervical dystonia. Patients with task-specific limb dystonias (e.g., writer's cramp) often benefit less because weakness of the treated muscles, which is the most common side effect of this therapy, can impair other important upper limb functions.

Young patients in particular can tolerate and benefit from high doses of anticholinergic drugs such as trihexyphenidyl (6 to 40 mg/day, but sometimes as much as 100 mg/day). Muscle relaxants, including benzodiazepines (diazepam, 5 to as much as 100 mg/day) and baclofen (40 to 120 mg/day), may provide some benefit. Dopamine-depleting (e.g., tetrabenazine, 50 to 200 mg/day) and dopamine-blocking (e.g., haloperidol, 3 to 30 mg/day) agents are occasionally helpful (more often effective in tardive dystonia than in other types). Paroxysmal kinesigenic dyskinesia usually responds well to anticonvulsant drugs. Paroxysmal exercise-induced dyskinesias are associated with mutations in the *SLC2A1* gene, which encodes the glucose transporter GLUT1, and may respond to a ketogenic diet. Neurosurgical treatments, particularly deep brain stimulation of the internal segment of the globus pallidus,[A4] can be considered in medically refractory, disabling dystonia, especially in patients with idiopathic dystonia (e.g., DYT1, adult-onset cervical dystonia).[15]

TICS

EPIDEMIOLOGY AND PATHOBIOLOGY

Tics are repetitive, stereotyped movements (motor tics) or vocalizations (vocal tics). Transient tics are extremely common in childhood, and simple tics may begin in childhood and persist throughout adult life.[16] Most tics (Table 410-6) are primary or idiopathic and have no identifiable cause. Secondary tics are caused by a defined underlying brain disease or environmental factor.

CLINICAL MANIFESTATIONS

Tics vary in terms of complexity, from abrupt, brief, meaningless movements or sounds (simple motor tics such as eye blinking, nose wrinkling, or head jerking; simple vocal-phonic tics such as sniffing, throat clearing, or grunting) to more sustained, more deliberate, almost meaningful gestures or utterances (complex motor tics such as touching, hand shaking, and jumping; complex vocal tics such as echolalia [repeating others], palilalia [repeating oneself], and coprolalia [uttering profanities]). The frequency of the tics in an individual patient varies markedly over minutes, hours, days, weeks, and years.

DIAGNOSIS

Various characteristics help to differentiate tics from other abnormal movements. Tics are often described by patients as being "semivoluntary" in response to an inner, irresistible urge. Premonitory sensory symptoms occasionally precede the tic, usually in the same general anatomic area as the tic itself. Relief is often associated with the production of the tic. Tics can be partially or completely voluntarily suppressed for variable periods, but often at the expense of mounting inner tension and psychological discomfort. Performing the tic or sometimes even substituting another more acceptable behavior for the socially inappropriate tic alleviates the tension. Many patients report that some tics occur in response to a typical urge, whereas the same or different tics may be unexpected and totally involuntary.

Tourette Syndrome
EPIDEMIOLOGY AND PATHOBIOLOGY

The exact relationship between childhood tics and Gilles de la Tourette syndrome remains uncertain. Tourette's syndrome is a common disorder, with an overall prevalence of 7.7 per 1000 children. There is a male preponderance of 3:1 for the classic syndrome, but female patients manifest obsessive-compulsive features more often than tics. A functional mutation in the *HDC* gene encoding L-histidine decarboxylase can be a rare cause of Tourette syndrome, thereby suggesting a role for histaminic neurotransmission in its pathogenesis.

CLINICAL MANIFESTATIONS AND DIAGNOSIS

The criteria for this disorder include the presence of multiple motor and at least one vocal tic beginning before the age of 21 years (typically between ages 2 and 10 years) and lasting for more than 1 year, waxing and waning symptoms over time (new tics replacing old ones; previous tics sometimes recurring years after they had originally resolved), and the absence of other

TABLE 410-6 ETIOLOGIC CLASSIFICATION OF TICS

PRIMARY OR IDIOPATHIC TICS

Transient motor or phonic tics
Chronic motor or phonic tics
Adult-onset tics
Tourette syndrome

SECONDARY TICS

Genetic disorders
  Neuroacanthocytosis
  Huntington disease
  Neurodegeneration with brain iron accumulation 1 (NBIA 1) (previously
    Hallervorden-Spatz disease)
  Idiopathic dystonia*
  Tuberous sclerosis*
Chromosomal disorders
Infections
  Sydenham chorea
  PANDAS†
  Encephalitis and postencephalitic disorders
  Creutzfeldt-Jakob disease
  Neurosyphilis
Drugs
  Methylphenidate
  Amphetamines
  Cocaine
  Levodopa
  Carbamazepine
  Phenytoin
  Phenobarbital
  Lamotrigine
  Neuroleptics
Developmental disorders
  Mental retardation
  Pervasive developmental disorders/autism
Other causes
  Head trauma
  Stroke
  Carbon monoxide poisoning
  Cardiopulmonary bypass with hypothermia

RELATED DISORDERS

Mannerisms, stereotypies
Compulsions
Self-injurious behavior

Modified from Cloutier M, Lang AE. Movement disorders: an overview. In: Factor SA, Lang AE, Weiner WJ, eds. *Drug Induced Movement Disorders*. Malden, Mass: Blackwell; 2005:3-19.
*Tics have been described with these conditions but may simply be coincidental.
†Pediatric autoimmune neuropsychiatric disorders associated with streptococcal infections. The existence of this disorder remains somewhat controversial.

explanatory medical conditions. Involuntary swearing (coprolalia), a highly publicized feature of the syndrome, is present in fewer than 10% of patients and is usually manifested by aborted forms such as "fu" and "shi." Patients commonly exhibit a variety of comorbid disorders including obsessive-compulsive disorder, attention-deficit disorder (with or without hyperactivity), impulse control problems, and other behavioral disturbances.

TREATMENT   Rx

Most patients who fulfill diagnostic criteria for Tourette syndrome have mild symptoms that do not require drug treatment; education, reassurance, behavioral therapy,[15] and follow-up are often sufficient.[17] When tics (isolated or as part of Tourette syndrome) interfere with social and physical function, low-dose clonazepam (0.5 to 4 mg/day) may be effective. Clonidine (0.05 to 0.5 mg/day) is variably effective in controlling tics and may be useful for impulse control and symptoms of attention-deficit/hyperactivity disorder (ADHD); alternatively, guanfacine (0.5 to 4 mg/day) can be used. The most effective treatments for disabling tics are the dopamine receptor blockers such as risperidone (0.5 to 16 mg/day), haloperidol (0.5 to 20 mg/day), pimozide (0.5 to 10 mg/day), fluphenazine (0.5 to 20 mg/day), and aripiprazole (5 to 15 mg/day), but caution is required in view of the potential for important side effects, including tardive dyskinesia, with long-term use. An alternative without this complication is the dopamine depleter tetrabenazine (50 to 200 mg/day). Injected botulinum toxin may be effective for simple motor tics of the face and neck and may also reduce the urge to perform the tic. More aggressive use of botulinum toxin in neck muscles should be considered in

patients with very forceful neck tics, which have rarely been associated with complications such as noncompressive myelopathy and vertebral artery dissection. Comorbid ADHD can be treated safely with stimulant therapy (e.g., methylphenidate, 2.5 to 60 mg/day) without increasing the severity of tics. Obsessive-compulsive symptoms may respond well to selective serotonin reuptake inhibitors (e.g., clomipramine, 25 to 250 mg/day; paroxetine, 10 to 60 mg/day; or citalopram, 10 to 40 mg/day). Behavioral disorders, which remain a major therapeutic challenge, may require a variety of psychotherapeutic or behavioral modification approaches. Even in the absence of behavioral disturbances, comprehensive behavioral intervention, which incorporates habit reversal training, can be very effective as first-line therapy for tic disorders. For this approach to be generalized, however, more trained providers will be needed. Promising preliminary reports of deep brain stimulation require confirmation in controlled clinical trials.

PROGNOSIS

The natural history of Tourette syndrome is to stabilize and often improve in adolescence. Approximately 50% of patients have a complete or partial remission at this time.

MYOCLONUS

DEFINITION

Myoclonus (or myoclonic jerks) consists of sudden, brief, shocklike, involuntary movements that result from both active muscle contraction (positive myoclonic jerks) and brief inhibition of ongoing muscle activity (negative myoclonic jerks). The most common form of negative myoclonic jerk is asterixis.

PATHOBIOLOGY

Myoclonus generally arises in the central nervous system, although rare peripheral causes are described, and it is distinct from abnormal muscle activity associated with peripheral nervous system diseases, such as fasciculations or myokymia. Myoclonus can be classified according to origin (Table 410-7), including physiologic, essential, epileptic, and symptomatic forms. Physiologic myoclonus, such as hypnic (sleep) jerks and hiccups, occurs in normal healthy subjects. Patients with essential myoclonus, which may be sporadic or inherited, often have additional postural tremor or dystonia, and this disorder is probably the same as what is now referred to as myoclonus dystonia (see Dystonias, earlier). Epileptic myoclonus arises in the context of seizures (Chapter 403), including many inherited generalized epileptic syndromes and the progressive myoclonic epilepsies. Symptomatic myoclonus occurs in association with a large number of encephalopathic states.

CLINICAL MANIFESTATIONS AND DIAGNOSIS

Myoclonic jerks are very short, typically lasting less than 150 msec. Myoclonus can be spontaneous, action induced, reflex (induced by various sensory stimuli), or a combination. Spontaneous myoclonus occurs at rest, without any provocation. Action myoclonus occurs during purposeful movement and is often very disabling owing to its interference with volitional activity. Reflex myoclonus can be triggered by visual, auditory, or somesthetic stimuli. The distribution of myoclonus may be focal, segmental, multifocal, or generalized. When myoclonus involves more than one body area, the movements may be synchronous or asynchronous. Myoclonus can be intermittent or repetitive, and it sometimes is rhythmic (e.g., usually originating in the brain stem or spinal cord). Palatal myoclonus, now referred to as palatal tremor, is a rhythmic movement disorder originating in the brain stem and involving the soft palate as well as the eyes, facial muscles, neck, and limbs; it is commonly the result of a focal lesion (e.g., stroke, demyelination) in the connections between the dentate nucleus of the cerebellum and the inferior olives of the medulla (symptomatic palatal tremor).

DIAGNOSIS

Myoclonus can be classified according to the anatomic site of origin, usually with the assistance of detailed electrophysiologic assessments.[18] These sites may be cortical, subcortical (e.g., thalamus; lower brain stem [reticular myoclonus]), or spinal (two types: spinal segmental and propriospinal).

TREATMENT   Rx

Management of myoclonus, when possible, should be directed specifically at the underlying cause. Drug treatment includes a variety of anticonvulsant

TABLE 410-7 CLASSIFICATION AND CAUSES OF MYOCLONUS

PHYSIOLOGIC MYOCLONUS

Sleep myoclonus
Anxiety-induced myoclonus
Exercise-induced myoclonus
Hiccups
Benign infantile myoclonus during feeding

ESSENTIAL MYOCLONUS

Essential myoclonus*
  Hereditary
  Sporadic
Myoclonus dystonia*

EPILEPTIC MYOCLONUS

Fragments of epilepsy
  Isolated epileptic myoclonic jerks
  Photosensitive myoclonus
  Myoclonic absences
  Epilepsia partialis continua
  Idiopathic stimulus-sensitive myoclonus
Childhood myoclonic epilepsies
  Infantile spasms
  Lennox-Gastaut syndrome
  Cryptogenic myoclonus epilepsy
  Juvenile myoclonic epilepsy of Janz
Benign familial myoclonic epilepsy
Baltic myoclonus (Unverricht-Lundborg)

SYMPTOMATIC MYOCLONUS

Storage disease
  Lafora body disease
  Lipidoses
  Neuronal ceroid lipofuscinosis
  Sialidosis
Spinocerebellar degeneration
  Friedreich ataxia
  Ataxia-telangiectasia
  Other spinocerebellar degenerations
Basal ganglia degenerations
  Wilson disease
  Idiopathic torsion dystonia
  Neurodegeneration with brain iron accumulation 1 (NBIA 1) (Hallervorden-Spatz disease)
  Progressive supranuclear palsy
  Corticobasal degeneration
  Parkinson disease
  Multiple system atrophy
  Huntington disease
  Dentatorubropallidoluysian atrophy

Mitochondrial cytopathies
Dementias
  Alzheimer disease
  Creutzfeldt-Jakob disease
  Dementia with Lewy bodies
  Frontotemporal lobar degeneration with TDP-43 positive inclusions
Viral encephalopathies
  Subacute sclerosing panencephalitis
  Encephalitis lethargica
  Herpes simplex encephalitis
  Arbovirus encephalitis
  Human immunodeficiency virus infection
  Postinfectious encephalitis
Metabolic disorders
  Hepatic failure
  Renal failure
  Dialysis dysequilibrium syndrome
  Hyponatremia
  Hypoglycemia
  Nonketotic hyperglycemia
  Infantile myoclonic encephalopathy
  Multiple carboxylase deficiency
  Biotin deficiency
Toxins
  Bismuth
  Heavy-metal poisoning
  Methylbromide, dichlorodiphenyltrichloroethane (DDT)
  Drugs (multiple)
Physical encephalopathies
  Posthypoxic myoclonus (Lance-Adams)
  Post-traumatic status
  Heat stroke
  Electric shock
  Decompression injury
Focal central nervous system damage
  Stroke
  Post-thalamotomy status
  Tumor
  Trauma
  Spinal cord lesions
Peripheral myoclonus (lesions of peripheral nerve, plexus, or nerve root)
Whipple disease
Paraneoplastic syndromes
Psychogenic myoclonus

Modified from Cloutier M, Lang AE. Movement disorders: an overview. In: Factor SA, Lang AE, Weiner WJ, eds. *Drug Induced Movement Disorders*. Malden, Mass: Blackwell; 2005:3-19.
*Probably represents the same entity.

medications, most notably clonazepam (1.5 to 15 mg/day), valproic acid (10 to 15 mg/kg/day), carbamazepine (600 to 1200 mg/day), and levetiracetam (1000 to 4000 mg/day). Lacosamide (200 to 400 mg/day) is also effective in select patients. Postanoxic action myoclonus (the Lance-Adams syndrome) in some patients who survive severe cerebral anoxia also may respond to 5-hydroxytryptophan (400 to 2800 mg/day) given with carbidopa (75 to 300 mg/day). Acetazolamide (250 to 1000 mg/day) may be useful for patients with action myoclonus.

HYPEREXPLEXIA

Hyperexplexia, which is a disorder related to myoclonus, manifests as an excessive startle response to tactile, visual, and/or auditory stimulations. Genetic causes are mainly abnormalities in synaptic transmission of the inhibitory neurotransmitter glycine, including glycine receptor α_1 gene (*GLRA1*), glycine receptor subunit gene (*GLRB*), and the presynaptic glycine transporter 2 gene *SLC6A5*. Some patients demonstrate only generalized body jerking or an exaggerated startle response that habituates poorly after repeated stimuli. By comparison, other patients experience disabling stiffness in response to sudden unexpected stimuli, such as loud sound. The disorder typically responds well to clonazepam (1.5 to 15 mg/day) therapy.

Additional medications that have been tried with mixed results include clobazam, levetiracetam, valproic acid, and phenobarbital.

OTHER MOVEMENT DISORDERS
Drug-Induced Movement Disorders

All the movements listed in Table 410-1 can be induced by medications. Neuroleptic drugs, which block postsynaptic dopamine receptors, particularly the D2 subtype, can result in a variety of movement disorder syndromes, including acute dystonic reactions, akathisia, drug-induced parkinsonism (including "the rabbit syndrome" with perinasal and perioral rest tremor), the neuroleptic malignant syndrome, and a variety of later-onset, often persistent, movements referred to as tardive dyskinesia.

ACUTE DYSTONIC REACTIONS

Acute dystonic reactions (Chapter 434) are most often seen in young patients who are receiving potent antipsychotic agents (e.g., young male patients receiving high doses of haloperidol for acute psychosis), but they also occur in patients receiving dopamine receptor blockers, including metoclopramide as antiemetic therapy. Symptoms range from overt dystonic postures of the face and neck, to involuntary prolonged deviation of the eyes (oculogyric crises), to simple slurring of speech and difficulty coordinating the tongue.

Symptoms often vary from moment to moment and can increase with anxiety and improve with relaxation or reassurance. Acute dystonic reactions are self-limited and respond rapidly to a parenteral injection of an anticholinergic drug such as benztropine (2 mg intravenously [IV] followed by 2 mg three orally [PO] times daily for a variable duration depending on neuroleptic use) or an antihistaminic such as diphenhydramine (50 mg IV followed by oral benztropine).

AKATHISIA

Akathisia refers to a sense of restlessness and a need to move. Typically, the patient performs a variety of purposeful or semipurposeful, often complex, movements in response to an uncomfortable subjective restlessness, including pacing when standing, marching in place, rocking, shifting weight, moving legs when sitting, picking at clothing or hair, rubbing body parts with hands, and other similar movements. Akathisia is most often a side effect of medications, especially neuroleptic drugs and selective serotonin reuptake inhibitors (Chapter 397). Symptoms occur in a dose-related fashion and usually resolve on drug withdrawal. Akathisia is a common reason for psychiatric patients to comply poorly with their medications; management includes adjustment of the dose or type of antipsychotic agent and trials of β-blockers (e.g., propranolol, 80 mg/day) or antiparkinson agents, such as anticholinergics (e.g., benztropine (6 mg/day) or amantadine (200 to 300 mg/day). Rare patients experience a very disabling and persistent form referred to as tardive akathisia. Akathisia is also sometimes seen in patients with Parkinson disease.

NEUROLEPTIC MALIGNANT SYNDROME

The neuroleptic malignant syndrome (Chapters 432 and 434) is an uncommon but severe, sometimes fatal, complication of neuroleptic therapy. Patients usually manifest a combination of features including fever, marked rigidity, changes in level of arousal, and autonomic instability. Laboratory abnormalities include a marked increase in the serum creatine kinase level and the blood leukocyte count. Management involves early recognition, withdrawal of the causative agent, systemic supportive therapy, a dopamine agonist (most experience has been with the older agent bromocriptine, ≤ 60 mg/day), and, when necessary, dantrolene sodium (50 to 600 mg/day PO or ≤ 10 mg/kg/day IV) to reduce muscle contraction.

TARDIVE DYSKINESIA
Epidemiology and Pathobiology

The term *tardive dyskinesia* encompasses a wide variety of abnormal movements caused by chronic neuroleptic therapy (Chapter 434). The cumulative 5-year incidence rate in patients taking classic neuroleptics is approximately 25%, and the incidence may continue to increase almost linearly beyond that point. The annualized risk is estimated to be 5% in haloperidol-treated patients compared with 2% in patients treated with atypical neuroleptics. The pathophysiology commonly has been attributed to hypersensitivity or upregulation of dopamine D2 receptors induced by chronic blockade. However, this explanation is generally felt to be inadequate, especially for more persistent symptoms, and other proposed mechanisms include oxidative stress from increased dopamine turnover and a maladaptive synaptic plasticity.

CLINICAL MANIFESTATIONS

Tardive dyskinesia generally begins after a minimum of 6 weeks of treatment. One of the most common forms involves the lower facial muscles and has been given a variety of names, including orobuccolinguomasticatory dyskinesia. The movements generally include repetitive chewing and smacking movements with the tongue either protruding between the lips (fly-catching movements) or pushing into the cheek (bonbon sign). Although the movements are somewhat choreic, they are not as random as true chorea. The more stereotypical, repetitive nature of the movements, involving not only face but also the limbs (e.g., piano playing movements of the fingers, rocking or thrusting of the pelvis), has encouraged the more recent term tardive stereotypies. This term, however, fails to fulfill the definition of stereotypy owing to the lack of distractibility and the unpredictability of the sequence of movements. Many patients with classic orofacial tardive dyskinesia seem unaware of the presence of the movements and are not disabled by them, but others are embarrassed or otherwise impaired.

Tardive akathisia and tardive dystonia are less common but particularly disabling subtypes of tardive dyskinesia. Rarer forms include tardive tics (tourettism), tardive tremor, tardive myoclonus, and even tardive oral or genital pain.

TREATMENT AND PROGNOSIS   Rx

Treatment is often unsatisfactory, but the dopamine depleter tetrabenazine (50 to 200 mg/day) can be very effective. Other drugs that possibly provide benefit include amantadine, propranolol, zolpidem, ginkgo biloba, and clonazepam.[19] Consideration should be given to discontinuing concurrent anticholinergic medications. Prevention is the most important consideration. The physician must regularly reassess the need for ongoing neuroleptic therapy, consider switching to an atypical agent when possible (particularly quetiapine and clozapine; Chapter 397), and routinely evaluate the patient for the presence of early subtle clinical features, such as mild pursing of the lips or rolling movements of the tongue in the mouth. Unfortunately, tardive dyskinesia may persist for many years despite withdrawal of neuroleptic treatment in up to 50% of patients. Several atypical neuroleptics, such as risperidone and olanzapine, nevertheless block dopamine D2 receptors sufficiently to cause drug-induced parkinsonism and tardive dyskinesias.

Restless Legs Syndrome
EPIDEMIOLOGY

Restless legs syndrome (Chapter 405) is now recognized as an extremely common disorder affecting between 3 and 29% of the general population. Women are affected more frequently than men. Although the incidence increases with age, it also can affect children, in whom it may be confused with "growing pains" or ADHD.

PATHOBIOLOGY

Restless legs syndrome is most often primary or idiopathic, in which case it is frequently inherited in an autosomal dominant fashion. Eight genetic loci associated with restless legs syndrome include variants in *MEIS1, BTBD9, MAP2K5/LBXCOR1, PTPRD,* and *PCDHA3,* as well as loci on 2p14 and 16q12.1. Restless legs syndrome also may be secondary to other causes, including peripheral neuropathy, uremia, pregnancy, and iron deficiency, and it may occur more commonly than by chance in some neurodegenerative disorders such as Parkinson disease. The pathophysiology of restless legs syndrome is uncertain, but central iron dysregulation may somehow alter central dopamine. Serum ferritin levels are often low, even in the presence of normal values of hemoglobin, hematocrit, iron, and iron-binding capacity.

CLINICAL MANIFESTATIONS AND DIAGNOSIS

In restless legs syndrome, as in akathisia, movements occur because of the subjective need to move. However, unlike in akathisia, the patient typically complains of a variety of sensory disturbances in the legs, including pins and needles, creeping or crawling sensations, aching, itching, stabbing, heaviness, tension, burning, or coldness. Occasionally, similar symptoms are appreciated in the upper limbs or other areas of the body. These symptoms are usually experienced during periods of prolonged inactivity, especially with recumbency in the evening, and are often associated with insomnia (Chapter 405). The discomfort appears particularly during the transition from wake to sleep in the evening and often follows a circadian pattern, peaking between midnight and 4 AM. Symptoms are typically relieved only by movement or stimulation of the legs; although these maneuvers are effective while they are being performed, the discomfort usually returns as soon as the individual becomes inactive or returns to bed to try to sleep. Patients often have significant problems with immobility during long automobile drives or plane flights.

In approximately 80% of patients, this condition is associated with another movement disorder, periodic leg movements in sleep, sometimes inappropriately called nocturnal myoclonus. These periodic, slow, sustained (1 to 2 seconds) movements range from synchronous or asynchronous dorsiflexion of the toes and feet to triple flexion of one or both legs. In 15% of patients, more rapid myoclonic movements or slower, prolonged dystonic-like movements of the feet and legs are present while patients are awake. In the absence of evidence of a secondary cause of restless legs syndrome, the only useful routine test is a serum ferritin level.

TREATMENT   Rx

Dopamine agonists (e.g., pramipexole, 0.125 to 1.5 mg at bedtime), ropinirole (0.25 to 3 mg at bedtime), and transdermal rotigotine (1 to 3 mg/24 hours) are the treatments of choice in moderate-to-severe restless legs syndrome and can be very effective. Levodopa preparations (100 to 300 mg of levodopa at bedtime; consider controlled-release preparation) are also effective but are more often associated with disabling rebound symptoms early in the morning or during the day (augmentation). Gabapentin enacarbil (a gabapentin prodrug at 600 mg to 1200 mg/day) is also effective and approved in the United States at the 600-mg dose.[A7] Patients with milder symptoms may respond to gabapentin (300 to 2400 mg/day). Opiate agonists (e.g., oxycodone, 5 mg at bedtime; codeine, 30 mg at bedtime; propoxyphene, 65 mg or N-100 mg at bedtime) and less often benzodiazepines (e.g., clonazepam, 0.5 to 2 mg at bedtime) also may be effective. Tolerance or loss of original benefit may occur with all these treatments. Iron replacement is indicated in patients with reduced serum ferritin levels (325 mg ferrous sulfate two or three times per day for 3 to 4 months until ferritin levels exceed 50 mg/L and iron saturations exceed 20%).

Painful Legs and Moving Toes

Another uncommon but well-defined movement disorder of the lower limbs has been termed *painful legs and moving toes*. Patients typically complain of a deep pulling or searing pain in the lower limbs, associated with continuous involuntary wriggling or writhing of the toes. Occasionally, the ankle and less commonly more proximal muscles of the legs are involved. Rarely, a similar problem is seen in the upper limbs as well. Although a peripheral nerve trigger, such as a radiculopathy, may be evident, the pain and movements probably are generated centrally in the spinal cord or brain stem. Various treatments have been tried without much benefit to the pain, which is typically the major concern of the patient.

Other Abnormal Movements

Numerous abnormal movements are caused by dysfunction of the peripheral nerves (e.g., fasciculations, myokymia); these movements are usually easily separated from the movement disorders described earlier. *Hemifacial spasm* is a common disorder in which irregular clonic and tonic movements involve the muscles innervated by the facial nerve, usually owing to compression of the seventh nerve as it exits the brain stem, most often by a normal small artery or vein and less often by a mass lesion or inflammatory process. Eyelid twitching is usually the first symptom, followed at variable intervals by lower facial muscle involvement. Magnetic resonance imaging (MRI) with careful assessment of the posterior fossa is necessary to exclude secondary causes. Treatment usually involves injections of botulinum toxin into selected facial muscles, although surgical decompression can be curative.

Cerebellar Ataxias and Spastic Paraplegias

There are an extremely large number of causes of cerebellar ataxia (Table 410-8). Many are hereditary, with the full spectrum of possible inheritance patterns. Sporadic or noninherited ataxias are common; in many cases, a cause can be defined and treatment may be effective in halting or even reversing the process. However, a large proportion of ataxias in adults are progressive, presumably owing to a degenerative cause, many of which remain to be determined.

TABLE 410-8	DIFFERENTIAL DIAGNOSIS OF ADULT-ONSET ATAXIA

Inherited
  Autosomal dominant, including the spinocerebellar ataxias (SCAs)
  Autosomal recessive, including Friedreich ataxia
  X-linked, including fragile X tremor ataxia syndrome (FXTAS)
  Mitochondrial
  Episodic ataxias
Autoimmune (e.g., paraneoplastic, anti-GAD antibodies, postinfectious)
Degenerative (e.g., multiple system atrophy [MSA-C])
Demyelinating (e.g., multiple sclerosis)
Infectious
Metabolic (e.g., hypothyroidism, vitamin E deficiency)
Stroke
Trauma (e.g., closed head injury)
Toxic (e.g., alcoholic cerebellar degeneration, lithium)
Tumor: Primary and secondary brain tumors

GAD = glutamate decarboxylase.

HEREDITARY CEREBELLAR ATAXIAS

The hereditary cerebellar ataxias, which may begin in childhood or adulthood, can progress at widely varying rates. These ataxias are divided into early-onset ataxias, which are usually inherited as autosomal recessive disorders,[20] and adult-onset ataxias, which are usually autosomal dominant. A small number are X-linked. Because most of these ataxias are untreatable, it is important to recognize the rare causes of treatable or preventable progressive ataxias.

Friedreich Ataxia

EPIDEMIOLOGY AND PATHOBIOLOGY

The most common progressive inherited ataxia in children is Friedreich ataxia. Friedreich ataxia is a trinucleotide-repeat disorder that affects the central and peripheral nervous systems, the heart, and many other organs. Friedreich ataxia is an autosomal recessive disorder with no anticipation. It has an estimated carrier frequency in the population of approximately 1 in 100 and a resulting disease prevalence of approximately 1 per 50,000.

The normal length of the GAA repeat on the long arm of chromosome 9 (9q13-q21) is 10 to 21 copies, but expansion in individuals with Friedreich ataxia results in 200 to 900 copies and disrupts the expression of the protein frataxin. GAA unstable expansion, which occurs on an intron, leads to gene silencing rather than to the production of an abnormal protein. Higher numbers of copies correlate with more severe neurologic deficits. Frataxin appears to be critical for iron export and mitochondrial function. Because accumulation of mitochondrial iron affects the production of oxygen radicals, loss of frataxin may lead to oxidative mitochondrial damage. The pathology of Friedreich ataxia includes spinal cord atrophy, which often is evident on MRI, with loss of neurons in Clarke columns and the dorsal root ganglia. Degeneration occurs in spinocerebellar tracts, pyramidal tracts, dorsal column tracts, and peripheral nerves, with minor cell loss in the brain stem and cerebellum. Cardiomyopathy is associated with ventricular hypertrophy and chronic interstitial myocardial fibrosis.

CLINICAL MANIFESTATIONS AND DIAGNOSIS

Typical Friedreich ataxia first manifests clinically during puberty with progressive ataxia, loss of lower extremity deep tendon reflexes, and extensor plantar responses (i.e., Babinski signs). Other common clinical features include nystagmus, dysarthria, stocking-glove sensory loss, and weakness in the lower extremities. Patients frequently have kyphosis, scoliosis, and pes cavus. Interstitial myocardial disease may cause a typical hypertrophic cardiomyopathy (Chapter 60). A small number of patients have a later onset and less severely progressive course, sometimes with retained or even brisk reflexes.

The diagnosis is made by genetic testing for the trinucleotide repeat expansion, which usually is present on at least one allele. Point mutations are sometimes present in the other allele and are more difficult to detect. Potentially treatable conditions with similar clinical manifestations include vitamin B$_{12}$ deficiency (Chapter 218), abetalipoproteinemia (Chapter 140), and a selective defect in vitamin E absorption (Chapter 218).

TREATMENT AND PROGNOSIS ℞

No effective disease-modifying treatments are available, so treatment consists of supportive measures. Intensive inpatient rehabilitation can improve overall function. Nicotinamide can increase frataxin concentrations,[21] but whether it alters the clinical course of the disease is unproven. Future treatments may include histone deacetylase inhibitors that may increase frataxin gene expression. The disorder is progressive, and patients usually are wheelchair bound by their mid-20s. The average age at death is 37 years, and the major cause of death is hypertrophic cardiomyopathy (Chapter 60).

Other Spinocerebellar Ataxias

The hereditary spinocerebellar ataxias are routinely classified by their specific molecular diagnosis. At least 20 autosomal recessive and more than 35 autosomal dominant cerebellar ataxias have been identified. Clinical features, ethnic origin, and family history may suggest an autosomal recessive, autosomal dominant, or X-linked inheritance and often narrow the search for the genetic mutation. As the molecular pathogenesis of many of the hereditary ataxias is unraveled, the current numerical classification, which largely reflects the chronology of the identification of causative mutations, is likely to be replaced by a gene-specific or pathophysiologic approach. Spinocerebellar ataxias 1, 2, 3, 6, 7, and 17 are caused by trinucleotide expansions in or adjacent to a protein-coding region of a gene. These expansions result in polyglutamine expansions in the protein product, which likely results in a toxic gain of function in a manner analogous to the pathogenesis of Huntington disease.

CLINICAL MANIFESTATIONS AND DIAGNOSIS

The predominant clinical features of the spinocerebellar ataxias are ataxia and dysarthria. Other cerebellar signs include titubation, dysdiadochokinesia, and dysmetria. With increasing ataxia, patients can become wheelchair bound. Additional clinical signs include ophthalmoplegia, dementia, optic atrophy, retinal pigmentary degeneration, deafness, dysphagia, and peripheral neuropathy. Extrapyramidal features include masked facies, cogwheel rigidity, dystonia, athetosis, and chorea. Levodopa-responsive parkinsonism (Chapter 409) may be seen in some patients, particularly in spinocerebellar ataxias 2 and 3. Pyramidal dysfunction includes spastic limbs, especially legs; hyperreflexia; and Babinski response. Diagnosis is based on genetic testing.

TREATMENT AND PROGNOSIS Rx

In a small randomized trial, varenicline (a partial agonist of 24β2 neuronal nicotinic acetylcholine receptors, at 1 mg/day for 2 weeks then 2 mg/day) improved gait, stance, and timed 25-foot walk but did not improve appendicular function, except for rapid alternating movements, in adults with genetically confirmed SCA3.[A8] However, these results have not been reproduced, and the drug is often poorly tolerated. No treatment is currently available for the other spinocerebellar ataxias, although preliminary data indicate that physiotherapy may improve gait and balance. The spinocerebellar ataxias are progressive, with worsening gait, hand coordination, speech, and eye movements, but with preserved mental function in most forms. Pneumonia is a common cause of death.

HEREDITARY SPASTIC PARAPLEGIAS

Hereditary spastic paraplegias, also known as Strümpell disease, are a group of clinically and genetically heterogeneous monogenic neurodegenerative disorders.[22] The prevalence is approximately 1 per 10,000 in the population. Over 70 different genetic loci have been identified; approximately 20 autosomal dominant, over 45 autosomal recessive, 5 X-linked, and one a maternal trait of inheritance. The most common forms of hereditary spastic paraplegia are autosomal dominant mutations in one of four proteins: spastin (SPG4), atlastin-1 (SPG3A), *REEP1* (SPG31), and reticulon-2 (SPG12). These proteins are involved in the endoplasmic reticulum network, whose morphology and distribution in neurons has a special importance for their normal function. Defects of ganglioside biosyntheses and defects in glucocerebrosidase functions are present in some forms. At autopsy, patients with hereditary spastic paraplegia have axonal degeneration of the pyramidal tracts and dorsal column tracts with lesser involvement of the spinocerebellar tracts. The neurons of origin are intact. The peripheral nervous system is unaffected.

CLINICAL MANIFESTATIONS

Patients with hereditary spastic paraplegia have a progressive gait disturbance with spasticity of lower extremities, hyperreflexia, clonus, and extensor plantar responses. Cranial nerves, speech, swallowing, and upper extremities remain normal. Although patients can experience weakness of their lower extremities, spasticity is usually the disabling component. The progressively increased leg spasticity results in tripping and an inability to run. Pain is infrequent, and sensation is normal. Other clinical features include pes cavus (30 to 50%), decreased vibratory sensation, and urinary frequency, urgency, and hesitancy. Pure hereditary spastic paraplegia is limited to symptoms and signs of spasticity, whereas complex or complicated hereditary spastic paraplegia can include cognitive impairment, dementia, epilepsy, extrapyramidal disturbances, cerebellar involvement, retinopathy, optic atrophy, deafness, polyneuropathy, or skin lesions.

DIAGNOSIS

Hereditary spastic paraplegia is diagnosed when patients meet clinical criteria and when other causes of spasticity are excluded. MRI may show spinal cord

TABLE 410-9	DIFFERENTIAL DIAGNOSIS OF SPASTIC PARAPLEGIAS

Hereditary
    Dopa-responsive dystonia
    Spinocerebellar ataxias
    Adult-onset adrenoleukodystrophy (Chapters 227 and 411)
Structural lesions of the spinal cord (Chapter 400)
Cervical spondylosis (Chapter 400)
Tumor (Chapter 179)
Arteriovenous malformation (Chapter 408)
Syringomyelia (Chapter 417)
Multiple sclerosis (Chapter 411)
Primary lateral sclerosis (Chapter 419)
Vitamin B_{12} deficiency (Chapter 416)
Copper deficiency (Chapter 416)
Infections
    Human immunodeficiency virus (Chapter 394)
    Human T-lymphotropic virus type 1 (Chapter 378)
    Tertiary syphilis (Chapter 319)

atrophy, but cerebrospinal fluid analysis and nerve conduction studies are normal. The differential diagnosis of spastic paraplegia includes other genetic conditions, spinal cord disease from structural lesions, multiple sclerosis, and vitamin deficiencies or retroviral infections (Table 410-9). Even a positive family history does not obviate the need to exclude potentially treatable alternative diagnoses.

TREATMENT AND PROGNOSIS Rx

No specific treatment is available. Symptomatic therapy is aimed at decreasing disability and preventing complications, such as contractures. Antispastic agents, such as oral baclofen (usually 10 to 20 mg three times daily), improve spasticity but should be used with caution because they may worsen weakness. Some reports suggested an improved therapeutic response to intrathecal baclofen, but no controlled trials have addressed this issue. Preliminary data also raise the possible utility of injected botulinum neurotoxin type A injections for improving spasticity. Most patients become non-ambulatory between 60 and 70 years of age. Patients with complicated hereditary spastic paraplegia often have other disabling features. Some patients with parkinsonism may benefit from dopaminergic therapies such as levodopa.

Grade A References

A1. Zappia M, Albanese A, Bruno E, et al. Treatment of essential tremor: a systematic review of evidence and recommendations from the Italian Movement Disorders Association. *J Neurol.* 2013;260: 714-740.

A2. Armstrong MJ, Miyasaki JM. Evidence-based guideline: pharmacologic treatment of chorea in Huntington disease: report of the Guideline Development Subcommittee of the American Academy of Neurology. *Neurology.* 2012;79:597-603.

A3. Hallett M, Albanese A, Dressler D, et al. Evidence-based review and assessment of botulinum neurotoxin for the treatment of movement disorders. *Toxicon.* 2013;67:94-114.

A4. Volkmann J, Wolters A, Kupsch A, et al. Pallidal deep brain stimulation in patients with primary generalised or segmental dystonia: 5-year follow-up of a randomised trial. *Lancet Neurol.* 2012; 11:1029-1038.

A5. Piacentini J, Woods DW, Scahill L, et al. Behavior therapy for children with Tourette disorder: a randomized controlled trial. *JAMA.* 2010;303:1929-1937.

A6. Wilt TJ, MacDonald R, Ouellette J, et al. Pharmacologic therapy for primary restless legs syndrome: a systematic review and meta-analysis. *JAMA Intern Med.* 2013;173:496-505.

A7. Kume A. Gabapentin enacarbil for the treatment of moderate to severe primary restless legs syndrome (Willis-Ekbom disease): 600 or 1,200 mg dose? *Neuropsychiatr Dis Treat.* 2014;10:249-262.

A8. Zesiewicz TA, Greenstein PE, Sullivan KL, et al. A randomized trial of varenicline (Chantix) for the treatment of spinocerebellar ataxia type 3. *Neurology.* 2012;78:545-550.

GENERAL REFERENCES

For the General References and other additional features, please visit Expert Consult at https://expertconsult.inkling.com.

411

MULTIPLE SCLEROSIS AND DEMYELINATING CONDITIONS OF THE CENTRAL NERVOUS SYSTEM

PETER A. CALABRESI

The disorders of myelin encompass a wide range of diseases in which either myelin is not formed in a normal fashion (dysmyelinating disease) or normally formed myelin is destroyed or not maintained appropriately (demyelinating disease) (Table 411-1). *Dysmyelinating* diseases are uncommon and include an array of leukodystrophies that have a genetic basis. *Demyelinating* diseases are much more common and include multiple sclerosis (MS), which represents more than 95% of all types of disorders of central nervous system (CNS) myelin.

Some disorders of myelin have a distinct pathogenesis in which the disruption of myelin is secondary. Further, in many of the diseases of myelin, the axon degenerates as a result of decreased trophic support from loss of myelin, impaired health of the oligodendrocyte, or increased susceptibility to injury in the absence of myelin. This observation led to the recent hypothesis that axonal loss is the underlying substrate for permanent disability in MS, adrenoleukodystrophy, and perhaps other diseases of myelin.[1]

 MULTIPLE SCLEROSIS

DEFINITION

MS is a disease characterized by multifocal areas of demyelination in the brain and spinal cord, with associated inflammatory cell infiltrates, reactive gliosis, and axonal degeneration. It typically manifests in young adults with episodic neurologic dysfunction. Although the exact origin of MS remains enigmatic, evidence suggests that it is an immune-mediated attack on myelin, with secondary disruption of axons leading to progressive disability over time in most afflicted patients.

TABLE 411-1 DISEASES OF MYELIN

IDIOPATHIC

Recurrent or chronic progressive demyelination (multiple sclerosis and its variants)
Monophasic demyelination (may be the first clinical episode of multiple sclerosis)
Optic neuritis
Acute transverse myelitis
Acute disseminated encephalomyelitis; acute hemorrhagic leukoencephalopathy

VIRAL INFECTIONS

Progressive multifocal leukoencephalopathy
Subacute sclerosing panencephalitis (Chapter 370)

NUTRITIONAL AND METABOLIC DISORDERS (Chapter 416)

Combined systems disease (vitamin B_{12} deficiency)
Copper deficiency (dorsal columns and subacute optic neuropathy)
Demyelination of the corpus callosum (Marchiafava-Bignami disease)
Central pontine myelinolysis

ANOXIC-ISCHEMIC SEQUELAE (Chapter 404)

Delayed postanoxic cerebral demyelination
Progressive subcortical ischemic encephalopathy

LEUKODYSTROPHIES PRIMARILY AFFECTING CENTRAL NERVOUS SYSTEM MYELIN

Adrenoleukodystrophy (Schilder disease)
Pelizaeus-Merzbacher disease (sudanophilic leukodystrophies)
Spongy degeneration
Vanishing white matter disease
Others (Alexander disease, Canavan disease)
Leukodystrophies of the central and peripheral nervous system
Metachromatic leukodystrophy
Globoid cell leukodystrophy (Krabbe disease)

EPIDEMIOLOGY

The annual incidence of MS varies by location and ranges between 1.5 and 11 per 100,000 people. MS is second only to trauma as the most common cause of neurologic disability in young adults. Recent studies suggest that the incidence rate has increased, in part because of recognition of more cases at an earlier stage, but probably also because of a truly rising incidence, especially in women. The prevalence is estimated at 350,000 to 400,000 in the United States and more than 1,000,000 worldwide, but these numbers may be underestimates owing to incomplete recognition of the disease, even in developed countries, and the increased incidence since these estimates were made.

MS occurs 2- to 2.5-fold more frequently in women than in men, a sex predilection that is common in autoimmune diseases. The disease most often manifests in the third to fourth decades of life, but with an incidence age range from postpubertal teenagers to persons in their 50s. Rare cases occur in infants or in patients in their 60s, but extreme caution is warranted in these situations to exclude alternative processes. In many of the late-onset MS cases, symptoms were present in younger years and were attributed to other causes.

MS is most common in people of Northern European descent. In many areas of the world, MS is more prevalent in temperate latitudes (approaching 1 in 500 in some locations) and becomes less common toward the equator (1 in 20,000 or rare case reports only in some locations), perhaps explained in part by migration patterns of people with the same gene pools. However, the absence of complete genetic penetrance in monozygotic twin studies and recent increases in incidence in genetically stable populations strongly suggest an environmental component to the disease. Indeed, an outbreak of MS was documented on the Faroe Islands following World War II, and numerous other clusters have been reported, although a single environmental trigger has not been identified.[2]

Several studies have linked cigarette smoking with risk for MS. High levels of vitamin D and early exposure to excessive sunlight (sunburns) have been linked with lower risk for MS, possibly related to the beneficial effects of cholecalciferol on regulating immune cell responses.

PATHOBIOLOGY AND GENETICS

Monozygotic twins with MS show a concordance rate of between 15 and 50%, compared with only 3 to 5% concordance in dizygotic twins, consistent with a strong but incomplete role for genes in causing MS. The lifetime risk for MS is increased to 2 to 4% in individuals with a first-degree relative with MS, compared with the general population risk of 0.1%. In addition, between 10 and 20% of patients with MS have a first-degree relative with another autoimmune disease, commonly rheumatoid arthritis, systemic lupus erythematosus, or autoimmune thyroid disease. Psoriasis (Chapter 438) and inflammatory bowel disease (Chapter 141) also may be more common in patients with MS. Genetic modeling of the disease strongly argues against a single MS gene and suggests that many different genes predispose to MS and account for its many phenotypes and its overlap with other autoimmune diseases.[3] Linkage and association studies have identified the human leukocyte antigen (HLA) or major histocompatibility complex (MHC) region on chromosome 6p21 as one genetic determinant for MS. The MHC class II region, involved in presentation of antigen to CD4+ T cells, is the most strongly associated locus. The HLA-DR2 allele and, more specifically, the molecular haplotype HLA-DRB*1501 allele have repeatedly been implicated. Multiple single-nucleotide polymorphisms (SNPs) in the interleukin-2 (IL-2) receptor-α gene and the IL-7 receptor-α gene also appear to be associated with a higher risk for MS. Over 100 other gene SNPs have been identified, most of which are related to immune function. Although patterns are emerging to suggest dysregulation of differing immune cell subsets, the associations to date are not strong enough to have clinical predictive value.

PATHOLOGY

Most cases are characterized by multifocal areas of demyelination and gross gliotic scar in the brain and spinal cord. Classic locations of these lesions, called *plaques*, are the optic nerves, periventricular white matter, deep white matter, juxtacortical white matter, corpus callosum, cerebellar peduncles, and dorsolateral spinal cord. However, there is a bias toward recognition of lesions in white matter because of the relative ease of detecting demyelination and inflammation in white compared with gray matter. Indeed, more recent pathologic studies have confirmed demyelination, neuritic damage, and atrophy in the cerebral cortex (pial surface and intracortical) and deep gray matter structures. At the microscopic level, one usually sees multiple areas of perivenular inflammatory cell infiltrates with extravasation into the surrounding tissue parenchyma. In the acute active plaque, CD4 helper T (T_H) cells are prominent in the perivenular areas. Proinflammatory cytokines released from T_H1 (interferon-γ [IFN-γ]) and T_H17 (IL-17, TNF, and granulocyte-macrophage colony-stimulating factor [GM-CSF]) cells are thought to mediate damage. Increasingly, large numbers of CD8 cytotoxic T cells have been documented in brain tissue, especially in the parenchyma, and these cells may mediate direct damage to axons and oligodendrocytes through release of proteases such as granzyme B. Most parenchymal inflammatory cells, especially in chronic plaques, are CD68+ macrophages and microglia. In addition to the influx of circulating immune cells, prominent astroglial activation and in some cases oligodendrocyte precursor cell differentiation occurs in response to injury. Over time, the inflammation becomes less prominent in the center of the plaque, but a chronic active rim of inflammation with microglial activation exists at a well-demarcated border between abnormal and normal unharmed myelin. This characteristic of MS is seldom seen in other disorders of myelin. Although oligodendrocytes may survive, proliferate, and result in partial remyelination (shadow plaques) in some early cases, this process is hardly ever complete in MS. Over time, remyelination is less successful, and oligodendrocyte precursor cells appear unable to differentiate into mature myelinating oligodendrocytes.[4]

The number of damaged axons correlates with the extent of inflammation. Further, axonal damage and even neuronal apoptosis and loss are seen in the cortex and retina. Atrophy of both the brain and spinal cord, which occurs more rapidly in MS than in normal aging, reflects loss of both myelin and axons.

No consistent microbial cause has been discerned from careful examination of MS tissues for known infectious pathogens. Differential expression of human herpesvirus type 6, which is acquired by most people in childhood, has been noted in oligodendrocytes of patients with MS, but whether this virus is a cofactor in demyelination or just a bystander remains unclear. Evidence suggests the possibility that the earliest event in MS may be an insult to the oligodendrocytes, with subsequent activation of resident immune cells and secondary recruitment of other immune cells only at later stages.

Some pathologists believe that four distinct subtypes of MS can be discerned, in which the pathologic characteristics are consistent in every lesion, thereby allowing classification of patients with differing pathologic categories rather than just describing evolution of lesions over time. Type I lesions are characterized by typical perivenular inflammatory infiltrates consisting mainly of T cells, with early preservation of oligodendrocytes. Type II lesions are similar to type I but have an additional humoral component with immunoglobulin G (IgG) deposition and complement activation. Type III lesions are distinguished by not being based around venules and by prominent loss of myelin-associated glycoprotein, with evidence for oligodendrocyte apoptosis. Type IV lesions have inflammatory infiltrates more similar to those in types I and II but also have oligodendrocyte loss as in type III. These varying pathologic features may begin to explain clinical subtypes of the disease.

PATHOGENESIS

It remains possible that the autoimmune hypothesis is wrong and that the inflammation observed in MS is secondary to an as yet uncharacterized primary degenerative process. Proponents of this theory cite evidence from pathologic features of hyperacute cases, in which the oligodendrocytes appear to die before any systemic immune response occurs, as well as recent data revealing neuronal and axonal death or demyelination in the absence of inflammation.

Macrophages and microglia, which make up the majority of cells within the parenchymal infiltrate in chronic MS plaques, are potent antigen-presenting cells and express HLA and costimulatory molecules. Activated macrophages and microglia also have effector functions, including release of cytokines that are partly (IL-6, tumor necrosis factor-α) or completely distinct from the T cells (IL-1β, IL-12, and IL-23). In high concentrations, these cytokines may damage oligodendrocytes and neurons and activate T cells.

CLINICAL MANIFESTATIONS
Presenting Symptoms

MS, which can manifest in many ways across a broad age range, may initially masquerade as a variety of different illnesses (Table 411-2; see Table 411-1). In a classic presentation, a young white person, more often a woman, will have the acute to subacute onset of impaired vision or sensation. Fatigue, depression, bladder urgency, weakness, impaired balance, and impaired

TABLE 411-2	CONDITIONS THAT CAN BE MISTAKEN FOR MULTIPLE SCLEROSIS AND OTHER DISEASES OF MYELIN

VASCULAR DISEASE

Small-vessel cerebrovascular disease
Vasculitides
Arteriovenous malformation
CADASIL
Antiphospholipid antibody syndrome

STRUCTURAL LESIONS

Craniocervical junction, posterior fossa, or spinal tumors
Cervical spondylosis or disc herniation
Chiari malformation or syrinx

DEGENERATIVE DISEASES

Hereditary myelopathy
Spinocerebellar degeneration

INFECTIONS

HTLV-1 infection
HIV myelopathy or HIV-related cerebritis
Neuroborreliosis (e.g., Lyme disease)
JC virus/progressive multifocal leukoencephalopathy
Neurosyphilis

OTHER INFLAMMATORY CONDITIONS

Systemic lupus erythematosus
Sjögren syndrome
Sarcoidosis

MONOFOCAL OR MONOPHASIC DEMYELINATING SYNDROMES

Transverse myelitis
Optic neuritis
Neuromyelitis optica/Devic disease
Acute disseminated encephalomyelitis

OTHER CONDITIONS

Hashimoto thyroiditis with or without encephalopathy
Nonspecific MRI abnormalities related to migraine, aging, or trauma

CADASIL = cerebral autosomal dominant arteriopathy with subcortical infarcts and leukoencephalopathy; HIV = human immunodeficiency virus; HTLV = human T-cell lymphotropic virus; MRI = magnetic resonance imaging.

coordination also are common symptoms. The often remarkably mild nature of the first symptoms often dissuades the patient from seeking medical attention or is insufficiently impressive to stimulate the physician to order diagnostic tests. Furthermore, patients may initially have few objective neurologic findings, especially between attacks.

Paresthesias of a limb that are circumferential and do not follow a dermatome suggest a spinal cord lesion; these symptoms often manifest distally and then ascend to involve more proximal parts of the limb, spread to the contralateral limb, or progress from a leg to an arm. Similarly, bandlike sensations around a limb or the torso also suggest a myelopathic process.

Incomplete transverse myelitis is a focal (partial) spinal cord syndrome that is usually inflammatory and does not follow vascular territories. It is a common presentation of MS.

Lhermitte sign, an electrical sensation moving down the spine into the limbs on flexion of the neck, is characteristic of cervical myelitis from any cause, including MS. Frank loss of sensation is less common as an early symptom or sign but is seen in more advanced cases. Burning, electrical, or deep aching sensations are also common in MS.

Sensory Abnormalities

On examination, the most common sensory findings are loss of vibration perception, most prominent in the feet, and incomplete spinal cord levels to pinprick or vibration, which are often more notable in a graded fashion rather than at a distinct level. Such sensory levels may be asymmetrical and differ by sensory modality because of isolated demyelination in the dorsal columns compared with the spinothalamic tracts. Patchy or seemingly nonanatomic focal areas of impaired sensation can occur, and some patients describe bizarre sensations such as water dripping or bugs crawling on an area of the body.

Visual Effects

Optic neuritis (Chapter 424) is a classic manifesting syndrome, typically with visual symptoms in one eye. In optic neuritis, patients often complain of pain over the temporal eyebrow and worsening on lateral eye movement. The visual impairment may be described as looking through frosted glass or a veil. The scotoma or area of greatest loss often can be mapped in a centrocecal distribution (central focal point to the blind spot laterally), which in mild cases may be evident only as desaturation to red color using the head of a pin. More severe cases may result in total loss of light perception. In most acute cases of optic neuritis, the inflammation is retrobulbar (behind the disc), so no immediate changes are visible on the optic disc, thereby leading to the aphorism "the patient sees nothing, and the doctor sees nothing." However, there should be a relative afferent papillary defect (Marcus-Gunn pupil; Chapter 424) with paradoxical dilation of the affected eye to direct light on swinging a flashlight from the unaffected eye in which consensual constriction was induced. In cases of bilateral optic neuritis (new or old), this abnormality may not be seen. Patients usually spontaneously recover substantial vision after weeks to months. Later, the optic disc may become pale, especially in the temporal region, a finding reflecting damage to the axons following inflammation and demyelination, even with recovery of normal visual acuity. Patients often have more subtle chronic visual impairment for colors, low contrast visual acuity, and contrast sensitivity. Visual testing using low contrast letter acuity charts commonly reveals substantial visual loss after clinical optic neuritis.

Visual impairment from impaired tracking of eye movements owing to brain stem or cerebellar disease most commonly occurs in the setting of an acute lesion affecting the medial longitudinal fasciculus, which is the neurologic pathway that yokes the eyes together on lateral saccades. Patients may experience frank diplopia or just blurred vision, especially when they look off to one side rapidly, such as when looking over one's shoulder while driving. The neurologic sign of this problem is called *internuclear ophthalmoplegia* (Chapter 424) and manifests as slowed or absent adduction of one eye with abducting nystagmus of the other eye. It may occur bilaterally or may exist in milder forms, such that the adduction lag is imperceptible to the human observer. Blurred vision from cerebellar damage with nystagmus is very common in MS and is often worse on extreme lateral or vertical gaze. *Oscillopsia*, the sensation that the environment is moving when it actually is not, is another symptom of impaired cerebellar coordination of the eyes. Saccadic eye movement or loss of smooth pursuit is common in MS and also can be seen in numerous neurologic conditions or with aging.

Motor Symptoms

The most common motor symptoms of MS are weakness and impaired coordination in a leg, with ascending involvement from distal to proximal and commonly spreading to the contralateral leg or ipsilateral arm. The lesion causing these symptoms is more commonly in the cervical spinal cord rather than the thoracic spinal cord, even when the first sign is partial footdrop. It is likely that axons that must conduct impulses over the longest distance (entire length of the spinal cord) from a site of inflammatory demyelination will become symptomatic before axons delivering signals to closer synapses (adjacent anterior horn cells in the cervical cord). Clinically, the weakness may be severe and may result in an obvious paralysis or be so subtle as to be undetectable. Heat-induced fatigue and weakness, as manifested by focal symptoms (slapping of a foot or dragging a leg) occurring after 15 to 20 minutes of exercise and resolving with rest, are characteristic of early demyelinating disease. The early absence of associated hyperreflexia and plantar extensor responses (Babinski sign) may make it difficult to document corticospinal tract involvement. Later, in more established MS, classic corticospinal tract signs are often evident and manifest clinically as spastic gait (either hemiparetic or paraparetic), muscle cramps, and clonus (sustained reflex loop), sometimes occurring with positional changes and mistaken for signs of a cerebellar tremor.

Ataxia may occur as a result of impaired delivery of sensory information up the spinal cord or from demyelination of cerebellar pathways in the brain stem or cerebellum. Often, the two are mixed and may be confounded further by visual loss and impaired ability to compensate by fixing on the environment; this combination commonly causes dizziness in crowds, in which fixation may be further obscured. Appendicular dysmetria resulting in tremor on reaching for an object is a common cause of impaired coordination and dexterity. Lower extremity and truncal ataxia may result in a wide-based (drunk) gait. Other movement disorders, such as postural tremor and titubation

(head tremor), are much less common in MS. *Myokymia* (wormlike muscle movements) under the skin, especially around the face, however, is fairly common. Pseudoathetosis and parkinsonism can be seen in severe cases.

Cognitive and Behavioral Symptoms

Over 50% of patients with MS experience bouts of moderate-to-severe depression (Chapter 397). There is also increased incidence of bipolar disease, which may manifest after treatment of depression or treatment with corticosteroids. Pseudobulbar affect, either pathologic laughing or crying, is seen in patients with more advanced disease. Numerous cognitive symptoms, including short-term memory loss, word-finding difficulty, trouble with multitasking, and cognitive fatigue, may be mistaken for depression but are well-recognized primary symptoms of MS pathology. Most patients do not progress to dementia (Chapter 402), but cognitive and behavioral impairments are major causes of losing employment and marital discord.

Organ Dysfunction

Bladder symptoms are extremely common, but often are not volunteered, so specific questions must be asked concerning urinary frequency, urgency, incontinence, or retention. Careful discrimination of a spastic bladder (detrusor muscle spasm) causing incontinence from an atonic bladder or spasm of the external sphincter (the latter two causing retention) leading to overflow incontinence is critical to designing treatment (Chapter 26). Urinary tract infections (Chapter 284) owing to bladder dysfunction may aggravate symptoms of MS.

Bowel dysfunction commonly manifests as constipation (Chapter 136), which may be primary (related to spinal cord involvement) or secondary (related to self-induced dehydration to manage urinary frequency or to side effects of anticholinergic drugs). Bowel incontinence secondary to an incompetent anal sphincter is less common and most often occurs as an isolated episode of fecal urgency, sometimes related to dietary change or diarrheal illness.

Sexual dysfunction is common and underdiscussed in MS. In men, erectile dysfunction is frequent. In women and men, loss of libido and inability to achieve orgasm can occur as a result of medication, loss of sensation, heat-induced worsening of symptoms, physical barriers to intercourse (impaired mucosal moisture, spasticity, and pain), depression, or disorders of body image.

Systemic Symptoms

Fatigue is common in MS. It may be linked to depression but often occurs independently and can be the most disabling symptom of the disease. A sleep history is important to exclude daytime fatigue resulting from disrupted sleep secondary to pain, cramps, bladder frequency, sleep apnea, periodic limb movements, depression, or disrupted sleep-wake cycles. Daytime fatigue even after a good night of sleep may occur in mid-afternoon and may be described as being "unplugged" or completely drained. Many patients obtain benefit from a short daytime nap.

Sensitivity to heat, which is a classic symptom of MS, occurs only in some patients. Even minor elevations of the body temperature can dramatically worsen symptoms (Uhthoff phenomenon). Some patients complain of worsened symptoms in cold weather, likely related to increased dysfunction of already stiff muscles or signal blockade consistent with the known physiology of nerve conduction, which has an inverted U-shaped temperature versus conduction curve.

Pregnancy

Women with MS may have children, and the activity of MS lessens during the course of pregnancy, especially by the third trimester, when the frequency of exacerbations is reduced by approximately two thirds.[5] Relapses are more frequent in the first 6 postpartum months, but no evidence indicates that pregnancy changes the natural history of the disease. Whether breast-feeding alters the course of MS is unclear, but it is contraindicated for patients who resume disease-modifying drugs following delivery.

Types of Multiple Sclerosis

The three major clinical types of MS are relapsing remitting, secondary progressive, and primary progressive. Approximately 85 to 90% of patients present with relapsing-remitting MS, characterized by acute or subacute episodes of new or worsening old neurologic symptoms that increase in severity, plateau, and then partly or completely remit. Patients may have no detectable residual deficit, or they may accumulate significant permanent disability from an attack. Most patients with relapsing-remitting MS convert to secondary progressive MS after 20 to 40 years. This stage of the disease, which is characterized by at least 6 months of progressive worsening without evidence of a relapse, can be diagnosed with confidence only retrospectively. Some patients with secondary progressive MS also have interposed relapses distinct from their periods of progressive worsening, although these episodes become less frequent with time. Primary progressive MS, which is characterized by progressive deterioration from the onset for at least 1 year without a history of distinct relapses, occurs in approximately 10 to 15% of patients. It is more common in middle-aged men and typically has more involvement of the spinal cord and fewer inflammatory brain lesions. Other uncommon types of MS also are described. Progressive relapsing MS refers to a fairly uncommon variant of MS (6%), in which a relapse ensues after an initially primary progressive course. Acute progressive MS (Marburg disease) causes acute or subacute progressive neurologic deterioration leading to severe disability within days to a month in a patient with no prior history of MS. This rare form of the disease may progress to a quadriplegic, obtunded state with death as a result of intercurrent infection, aspiration, or respiratory failure from brain stem involvement.

DIAGNOSIS

The diagnosis of MS rests on demonstrating evidence of at least two inflammatory demyelinating lesions referable to different locations within the CNS, occurring at different times (usually ≥ 1 month apart), and for which no better explanation exists.[6] Diagnostic criteria allow for the diagnosis to be made on clinical grounds alone as long as appropriate exclusionary testing is performed (Table 411-3). Clinical evidence of a lesion requires objective findings on examination, not just a symptom. Further, repeated episodes of neurologic dysfunction that could be explained based on one lesion (e.g., a cervicomedullary junction lesion causing brain stem, cerebellar, and corticospinal tract dysfunction) is not enough evidence to diagnose MS.

Magnetic Resonance Imaging

No definitive diagnostic laboratory test exists for MS, but magnetic resonance imaging (MRI) of the brain is extremely useful and should be performed in all patients in whom MS is a diagnostic consideration.[7] More than 95% of patients with clinically definite MS have an abnormal brain MRI, and the presence of high-signal, bright lesions is so characteristic of MS that a

normal brain MRI should suggest an alternative diagnosis. Brain MRI is also useful in predicting future MS at the time of a clinically isolated demyelinating syndrome. Specific MRI findings allow for confirmation of disease disseminated in time and space (different parts of the brain or spinal cord) and fulfilling evidence for dissemination in time (Table 411-4). MS plaques typically appear as high-signal (white) areas on fluid attenuation inversion recovery (FLAIR) T2-weighted images, which allow for the best discrimination of the supratentorial lesions by suppressing high signal from cerebrospinal fluid (CSF) in the ventricles (Fig. 411-1). Lesions generally range in size from 2 mm to 2 cm; larger plaques occasionally resemble a tumor. Features of an MRI lesion suggesting MS include an elliptical shape, discrete borders, lack of mass effect, and gadolinium enhancement. Typical locations include the periventricular area (perpendicular to or abutting the walls of the ventricles) (Fig. 411-2), the corpus callosum, the cerebellar peduncles, the brain stem, the juxtacortical area, and the dorsolateral spinal cord (Fig. 411-3). Cortical

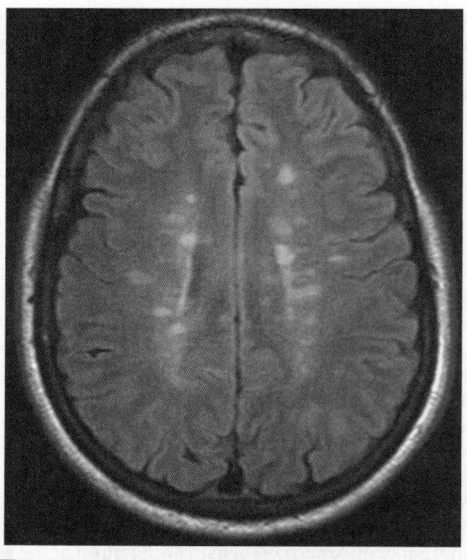

FIGURE 411-1. Axial fluid attenuation inversion recovery image of the brain from a patient with multiple sclerosis revealing classic multiple periventricular and deep white matter high signal lesions.

TABLE 411-3	2010 REVISIONS TO THE MCDONALD DIAGNOSTIC CRITERIA FOR MULTIPLE SCLEROSIS
CLINICAL PRESENTATION	**ADDITIONAL DATA NEEDED FOR DIAGNOSIS OF MULTIPLE SCLEROSIS**
Two or more attacks; objective clinical evidence of two or more lesions; or one lesion with a prior attack	None*
Two or more attacks; objective clinical evidence of one lesion	Dissemination in space, demonstrated by: 1. MRI (see Table 411-4), or 2. Two or more MRI-detected lesions consistent with MS plus positive CSF, or 3. Await further clinical attack implicating a different site
One attack; objective clinical evidence of two or more lesions	Dissemination in time, demonstrated by: 1. MRI (see Table 411-4), or 2. Second clinical attack
One attack; objective clinical evidence of one lesion (monosymptomatic presentation; clinically isolated syndrome)	1. Dissemination in space, demonstrated by: a. MRI (see Table 411-4), or b. Two or more MRI-detected lesions consistent with MS plus positive CSF, and 2. Dissemination in time, demonstrated by: a. MRI (see Table 411-4), or b. Second clinical attack

Modified from Polman CH, Reingold SC, Banwell B, et al. Diagnostic criteria for multiple sclerosis: 2010 revisions to the McDonald criteria. *Ann Neurol.* 2011;69:292-302.
*Must rule out other causes (e.g., see Table 411-2).
CSF = cerebrospinal fluid; MRI = magnetic resonance imaging; MS = multiple sclerosis.

TABLE 411-4	MAGNETIC RESONANCE IMAGING CRITERIA IN MULTIPLE SCLEROSIS (INTERNATIONAL PANEL RECOMMENDATIONS: 2010)

DISSEMINATION IN TIME

Detection of a new T2 or gadolinium-enhancing lesion if it appears at any time compared with a reference scan*
Simultaneous presence of asymptomatic gadolinium-enhancing and nonenhancing lesions at any time

DISSEMINATION IN SPACE

At least one gadolinium-enhancing lesion in at least two of four areas:
  Periventricular
  Juxtacortical
  Infratentorial
  Spinal cord

DIAGNOSIS OF PRIMARY PROGRESSIVE MULTIPLE SCLEROSIS

One year of disease progression (retrospectively or prospectively determined) plus two of the following:
  a. Positive brain magnetic resonance imaging (≥1 T2 lesion in at least one characteristic area: periventricular, juxtacortical, or infratentorial)
  b. Positive spinal cord magnetic resonance imaging (two focal T2 lesions)
  c. Positive cerebrospinal fluid (isoelectric focusing evidence of oligoclonal immunoglobulin G bands or increased immunoglobulin G index, or both)

From Polman Ch, Reingold SC, Banwell G, et al. Diagnostic criteria for multiple sclerosis: 2010 revisions to the McDonald criteria. *Ann Neurol.* 2011;49:292-302.
*CAUTION: Determination that a T2 lesion is indeed new can be challenging. A new T2 lesion must be of sufficient size and location to reflect one that could not have been missed previously for technical reasons of slice orientation, thickness or spacing, tissue contract, patient motion, or other artifacts. This judgment requires standardized scanning procedures, with emphasis on careful repositioning, as well as input from qualified evaluators experienced in multiple sclerosis imaging.

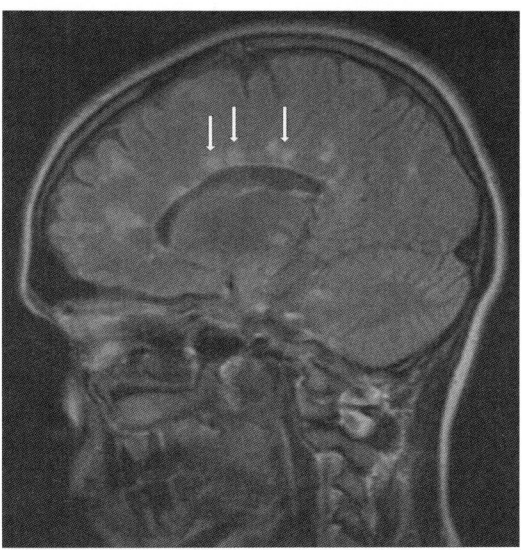

FIGURE 411-2. Sagittal fluid attenuation inversion recovery image of the brain from a patient with multiple sclerosis revealing classic periventricular lesions radiating outward from the ventricles (*arrows*).

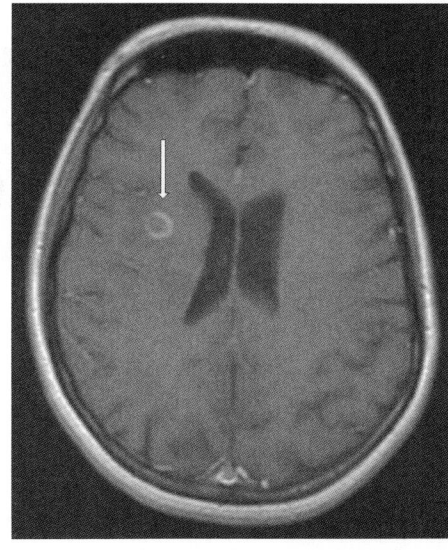

FIGURE 411-4. Axial T1-weighted image after gadolinium contrast showing an actively inflamed ring-enhancing lesion (*arrow*) in a patient with multiple sclerosis.

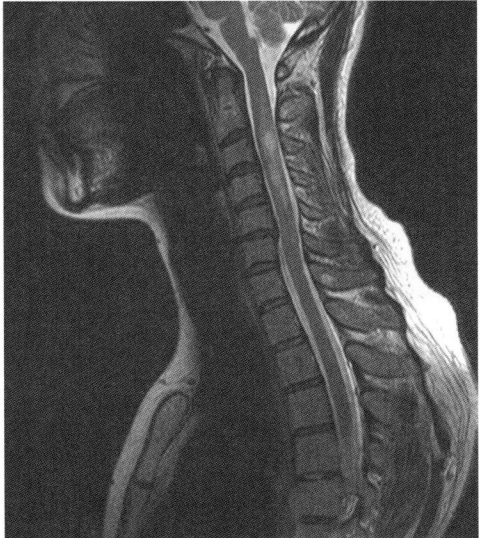

FIGURE 411-3. Sagittal T2-weighted image of the brain and cervical spine from a patient with multiple sclerosis. The image shows a high-signal plaque from C3-C5 in the spinal cord.

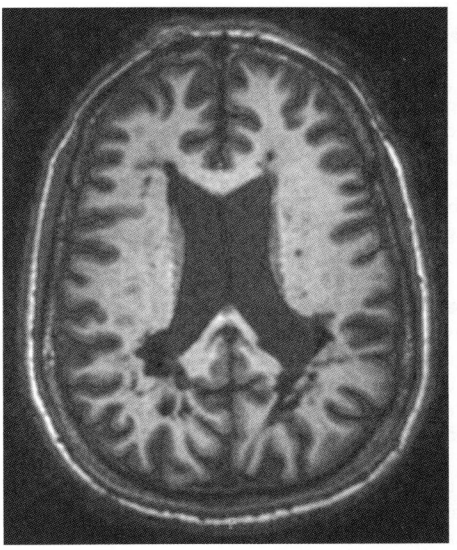

FIGURE 411-5. Axial T1-weighted image showing numerous areas of T1 low signal ("black holes"), ventricular enlargement, and diffuse atrophy.

and deep gray matter lesions also occur but are less clearly seen on conventional MRI. Gadolinium enhancement, which suggests permeability of the blood-brain barrier, is correlated with new or active inflammation in lesions (Fig. 411-4). Lesions that enhance on a T1-weighted sequence usually have a concomitant lesion in the same location on a T2-weighted image. However, T2-weighted lesions may form without evident enhancement. Gadolinium enhancement typically persists for 2 to 8 weeks and thus may be missed on intermittent scans. Persistent areas of low signal on T1-weighted images before contrast ("black holes") correlate with pathologic evidence of axonal loss and atrophy (Fig. 411-5).

Cerebrospinal Fluid
Examination of the CSF is useful in many cases but is not mandatory in patients with a typical clinical presentation and MRI evidence of disseminated disease. CSF evaluation includes cell counts, total protein, glucose, oligoclonal bands with a paired serum sample, and an IgG index. The presence of myelin basic protein is not specific for MS because it can be elevated secondary to any disruption of CNS tissue. Oligoclonal IgG bands in the CSF or an elevated IgG index provides evidence for intrathecal production of immunoglobulins. However, although oligoclonal bands are common in MS, they also can occur with infection or other immune-mediated processes. As

a result, the test lacks specificity for MS and has a sensitivity of only approximately 85 to 90% of patients with clinically definite MS. In clinically isolated demyelinating syndromes (see later), the sensitivity is even lower (~50%). Further, the sensitivity depends on local laboratory techniques.

CSF evaluation is generally recommended if an alternative diagnosis is considered, especially if one suspects an infectious or neoplastic process (e.g., fever, sweats, unusual travel history, tick bite, or rash). CSF analysis also may be useful if clinical or MRI criteria are incomplete to provide confirmation of the diagnosis.

Evoked Potential Tests
Evoked potentials (Chapter 396) may be useful in some situations to document objective evidence of slowed conduction owing to demyelination in locations different from those recognized clinically. However, visual evoked potentials (VEPs), brain stem auditory evoked potentials, and somatosensory evoked potentials are less sensitive and less specific for MS than is high-resolution MRI. Multifocal VEPs may be more sensitive than global VEPs in revealing focal areas of abnormal conduction along the optic nerve.

Optical Coherence Tomography
Optical coherence tomography is performed with an office-based device that uses the reflection of infrared light (from an exogenous source directed

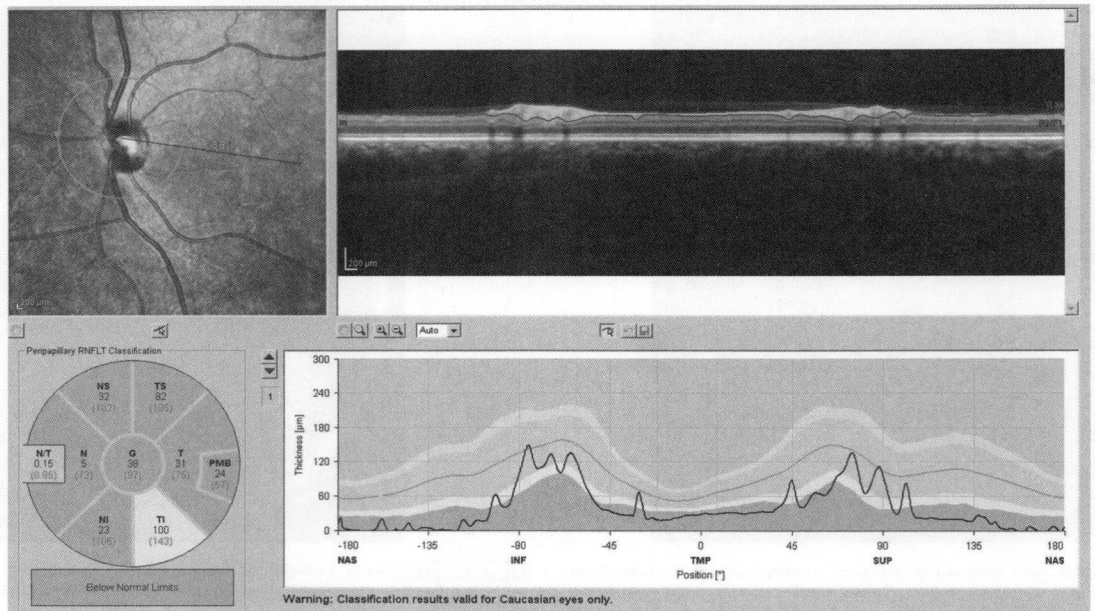

FIGURE 411-6. High-resolution spectral domain optical coherence tomography scan. The scan is from the retina of a patient with multiple sclerosis and history of optic neuritis in the scanned eye. The *upper left* is a fundus photo; the *upper right* is the tomogram map of the peripapillary retinal nerve fiber layer. *Lower panels* show regional quantitative data and color maps based on percentile compared to age- and sex-matched healthy controls (*green* is 5th to 95th percentile, *yellow* is 5th percentile, and *red* is first percentile).

through the pupil) off the back of the eye to quantify the thickness of retinal tissues, including the peripapillary retinal nerve fiber layer and macular layers. This test, which has been widely used in glaucoma, can monitor axonal and retinal ganglion cell damage, both in the setting of acute optic neuritis and in detecting subclinical neuroaxonal damage (Fig. 411-6). Retinal nerve fiber layer thinning correlates with brain atrophy and may be useful as a surrogate marker of more global neurodegeneration in MS.

Differential Diagnosis

The diagnosis of MS may be so clear that it is recognized by the patient and is readily confirmed by the primary physician or so obscure that even experienced specialists disagree.[8] Many processes (see Table 411-2) can mimic the clinical, radiologic, and CSF findings associated with MS, and there is no "gold standard" diagnostic test that is 100% sensitive and specific for the disease.

Processes that mimic MS include structural lesions, especially of the base of the brain and of the spinal cord, in which one lesion can cause symptoms referable to many different tracts and at different perceived locations in the body. Chiari malformations with or without syrinx (Chapter 417), disc herniation (Chapter 400), cervical spondylosis, and low-grade tumors (Chapter 189) can produce symptoms of MS both in newly presenting patients and in patients who truly have MS but who also have a second process.

Various infectious diseases can mimic MS. Examples include human T-cell lymphotropic virus types I and II (virally associated myelopathy or tropical spastic paraparesis; Chapter 378), human immunodeficiency virus (neuropathy, myelopathy, cognitive impairment, CNS white matter changes; Chapter 394), neuroborreliosis (Lyme disease; Chapter 321), neurosyphilis (Chapter 319), Epstein-Barr virus (Chapter 377), cytomegalovirus (Chapter 376), herpes simplex virus (Chapter 374), varicella-zoster virus myelitis (Chapter 375), and JC virus (progressive multifocal leukoencephalopathy; Chapter 370).

Inflammatory diseases that usually involve other parts of the body can concomitantly affect or, rarely, manifest in the CNS. Examples include sarcoidosis (Chapter 95), systemic lupus erythematosus (Chapter 266), Sjögren syndrome (Chapter 268), and vasculitides (Chapter 270). Ischemic vascular disease secondary to any cause also can resemble MS. Metabolic and nutritional disorders that can mimic MS include vitamin B_{12} deficiency and methylmalonic acidemia (in some cases distinct from cyanocobalamin deficiency). Rarely, central pontine myelinolysis (Chapters 116 and 416) is mistaken for MS. Thyroid disease (Chapter 226) may mimic the fatigue of MS and may cause dysesthesias and disorders of the optic nerve and muscles. Nutritional deficiency (Chapter 215) and malabsorption have been associated with demyelination and may mimic MS. Copper deficiency can cause dorsal column pathology, neuropathy, anemia, and optic neuropathy. Vitamin D

deficiency (Chapter 244), which is becoming increasingly common, can cause proximal weakness, fatigue, asthenia, bone loss, and impaired immune function. Vitamin A deficiency, although not common in industrialized countries, can cause night blindness and immune dysfunction.

Monophasic demyelinating syndromes with or without multiple other lesions often, but not always, progress to become MS (see later). Spinocerebellar atrophy and hereditary myelopathy cause slowly progressive disease but do not cause sensory and visual abnormalities.

Hereditary diseases are increasingly recognized as mimicking MS. Spinocerebellar atrophy may manifest as progressive myelopathy and ataxia. A variety of genetic neuropathies (type 2 CMT mitofusinopathies, adult-onset polyglucosan body disorder; Chapter 420), ataxias (Friedreich, ataxia telangiectasia; Chapter 410), mitochondrial diseases (progressive optic atrophy, Leber, MELAS, MERRF; Chapter 421), and metabolic diseases (urea cycle disorders; Chapter 205) can have CNS manifestations that could lead to misdiagnosis.

TREATMENT ⟨Rx⟩

The treatment of MS can be divided into drugs designed to relieve symptoms, drugs designed to modify the course of the disease, and nondrug measures.[9] Numerous drugs target specific aspects of MS: depression, fatigue, muscle spasticity, pain, insomnia, and bladder, bowel, and sexual dysfunction. Before considering a symptomatic therapy, the patient should be educated about the purpose of the drug and its side-effect profile. On learning that these drugs have no long-term impact on disease activity, patients may elect not to use them for relief of symptoms alone. Symptomatic therapies are best started at low doses and frequently require titration to obtain the optimal balance between efficacy and side effects.

Treatment of Specific Symptoms

Depression and emotional lability are common symptoms of MS. In addition to appropriate supportive care and counseling, antidepressant therapy with one of the "activating" serotonergic or noradrenergic drugs (fluoxetine, sertraline, citalopram, escitalopram, venlafaxine, or bupropion) can be of benefit (see Table 397-5). If anxiety and panic symptoms predominate, a less activating drug such as paroxetine may be preferable. Patients with pain or insomnia may benefit more from a sedating antidepressant (amitriptyline, nortriptyline, or trazodone) given at bedtime, which may have the added anticholinergic benefits on urinary bladder urgency.

Spasticity can be managed by physical therapy, stretching, and institution of either baclofen (5 to 160 mg in divided doses) or tizanidine (2 to 32 mg in divided doses). Either drug should be started as a single agent at a low dose at bedtime, gradually increasing to three to four times daily, with a larger dose at bedtime to target nocturnal symptoms. Decreasing muscle tone can result in weakness. Baclofen should never be discontinued abruptly because of the potential for a severe withdrawal reaction.

Bladder urgency resulting from detrusor muscle spasm can be managed effectively with anticholinergics such as oxybutynin (5 to 20 mg in divided doses) or tolterodine (1 to 4 mg) or focal injections of botulinum toxin, but these agents can cause temporary urinary hesitancy or retention. Bladder ultrasonography permits accurate bedside assessment of postvoid residual volume to determine whether a patient is retaining excessive amounts of urine. Urinary retention may be improved by removing drugs known to induce it (e.g., anticholinergics and opioids). Primary urinary retention is difficult to treat with drugs, but external sphincter spasm can be treated with α_{1a}-adrenergic receptor blockers such as tamsulosin (0.4 to 0.8 mg) and doxazosin (1 to 8 mg). Bethanechol (10 to 150 mg in divided doses) may be tried for an atonic bladder, but intermittent catheterization is often required. Alternative causes of bladder symptoms such as urinary tract infections, prostatic enlargement, or anatomic changes following pregnancy should be considered and managed separately. Prolonged urinary retention predisposes to infections, structural damage to the bladder and kidneys, and malignancy. Persistent postvoiding residual volumes greater than 300 cc should be treated medically, with intermittent straight catheterization recommended for patients with large volume retention refractory to medical therapy.

Painful dysesthesias and paroxysmal dystonic spasms may be managed effectively with antiepileptic drugs (gabapentin, 300 to 5400 mg/day in divided doses; pregabalin, 75 to 600 mg/day in divided doses; or carbamazepine, 100 to 2400 mg/day in divided doses) or tricyclic antidepressants (amitriptyline, 10 to 150 mg; or nortriptyline, 10 to 50 mg). Patients with trigeminal neuralgia (Chapter 398) may respond to these drugs or to baclofen, misoprostol, botulinum toxin, or decompression surgery.

Sexual dysfunction in MS is often multifactorial. Patients with erectile dysfunction usually respond well to the phosphodiesterase inhibitors, which enhance penile vasodilation (Chapter 234). Education regarding the use of lubrication, alternative sensory stimulation, and the adverse effect of heat, can improve sexual function.

Symptoms related to heat sensitivity may improve on cooling. Cooling devices can prevent this phenomenon, but there is no persistent benefit of inducing hypothermia.

Systemic Treatments

Corticosteroids (e.g., methylprednisolone, 1 g/day IV for 3 to 5 days) shorten the duration and severity of symptoms from an acute exacerbation but have no proved effect on long-term disability. Oral corticosteroids used in equivalent dosage are probably equally efficacious and safe. Intravenous immunoglobulin and plasma exchange may occasionally to benefit steroid-refractory patients, but large randomized placebo-controlled trials in relapsing MS have failed to show consistent benefits, perhaps because only patients with type II disease (humoral component) are likely to respond.

Approved Disease-Modifying Treatments

Twelve disease-modifying agents have been approved by the U.S. Food and Drug Administration (FDA): IFN-β1b (Betaseron and Extavia), IFN-β1a (Avonex), IFN-β1a (Rebif), pegylated interferon (Plegridy), glatiramer acetate (Copaxone), natalizumab (Tysabri), alemtuzumab (Lemtrada), mitoxantrone (Novantrone), fingolimod (Gilenya), teriflunomide (Aubagio), and dimethyl fumarate (Tecfidera). All of these agents are approved for relapsing-remitting MS, and mitoxantrone is indicated for worsening forms of MS and for secondary progressive MS.

The four IFN-β drugs reduce the relapse rate by approximately one third.[A1] IFN-β1b (8 million international units [IU], subcutaneously [SC] every other day [Betaseron and Extavia]) and IFN-β1a (30 μg intramuscularly [IM] weekly [Avonex] or 22 to 44 μg SC three times weekly [Rebif]) appear to have a more rapid onset of action, perhaps based on their dosing regimen, compared with weekly IFN-β1a (30 μg IM weekly). However, weekly IFN-β1a Avonex is less immunogenic and results in only a 3% incidence of neutralizing antibodies, which reduce efficacy, compared with 20 to 30% for the other IFN-β preparations. The major side effects of IFN-β are a flulike reaction (low-grade fever, chills, and myalgias 6 to 24 hours after the injection), local reactions at the injection site (pain, erythema, and rarely necrosis), and elevated aminotransferase levels (rarely severe hepatitis). These side effects can be managed by initiating the drug slowly and by prophylaxis with acetaminophen and nonsteroidal anti-inflammatory agents, and they improve in most patients after 3 to 6 months. A long-acting pegylated version of IFN-β1a dosed at 125 μg SC every 2 weeks reduced the annualized relapse rate by 38% and gadolinium-enhancing MRI lesions by 82% versus placebo in a phase 3 trial.[A2] Side effects remained typical of the interferon-β drugs and were not prolonged.

Glatiramer acetate is a copolymer of four amino acids designed to mimic myelin basic protein; given as 20 mg/day SC or as 40 mg SC three times a week, it also reduces relapses by about one third and is well tolerated by most patients.[A3] Major side effects are local reactions at the injection site, (swelling, hives, and delayed lipoatrophy), and a rare, self-limited (15 to 20 minutes) systemic reaction consisting of chest pain, palpitations, and anxiety. No

monitoring of blood tests is required for this medication. The effect of glatiramer acetate on MRI T2-weighted and gadolinium-enhancing lesions is less dramatic than for the interferons (30% reduction), perhaps because its primary effect is not at the blood-brain barrier.

Natalizumab is a monoclonal antibody directed against the α_4-integrin chain of the leukocyte adhesion molecule VLA-4. In a large phase 3 trial, this drug, at a dose of 300 mg intravenously (IV) every 4 weeks, reduced relapses by 68% compared with placebo and reduced gadolinium-enhancing lesions by 92%.[A4] However, approximately 1 in 500 patients develop JC virus brain infection (Chapter 370) after 24 months of exposure, which causes progressive multifocal leukoencephalopathy (PML). The risk for PML appears to be in higher in patients with JC virus serum antibody titers greater than 0.9 compared with low-titer or seronegative patients, although the results may change over time so patients require repeated testing.

Alemtuzumab, a monoclonal antibody that targets CD52 on lymphocytes and monocytes, reduces annualized relapse rates by approximately 50% and also can reduce the progression of disability compared with IFN-β1a.[A5][A6] The drug is given as yearly courses at 12 or 24 mg daily for 5 consecutive days in year 1 and for 3 days in years 2 and 3. Serious side effects associated with alemtuzumab include a 20 to 25% risk for developing autoimmune thyroid disease and rare cases of immune thrombocytopenic purpura (Chapter 172), autoimmune hemolytic anemia (Chapter 160), autoimmune neutropenia (Chapter 167), and Goodpasture syndrome (Chapter 121).

Mitoxantrone, which is an anthracenedione antineoplastic agent with potent immunosuppressive activity, is approved to slow the progression of neurologic disability and reduce the relapse rate in patients with relapsing-remitting MS and secondary progressive MS.[A7] The recommended dose is 5 to 10 mg/m² intravenous infusion every 3 months, and the lifetime use of this drug is limited to 2 to 3 years (or a cumulative dose of 120 to 140 mg/m²) because of its cardiotoxicity.

Fingolimod is a sphingosine-1 phosphate receptor modulator that is given orally once daily at 0.5 mg. Fingolimod reduces relapse rates and the progression of disease compared with placebo[A8] and compared with interferon therapy.[A9] However, it generally is not considered first-line therapy because its risks, including type 2 heart block and herpes encephalitis, are concerning, especially in young, otherwise healthy people with MS. Fingolimod side effects include first-dose bradycardia, macular edema, and respiratory infections.

Teriflunomide is approved as an oral agent for MS based on two phase 3 trials in which the annualized relapse rate was reduced by 31% compared with placebo, and disability also was reduced.[A10] It is dosed at 7 or 14 mg/day PO and requires monitoring of blood tests for rare liver and kidney toxicities.

Oral dimethyl fumarate (240 mg twice daily) reduces the annualized relapse rate (49 to 55%) and disease progression in addition to suppressing active MRI lesions.[A11][A12] A differently formulated drug that is a combination of monomethyl fumarate and dimethyl fumarate has been marketed in Germany for psoriasis since 1994. Four cases of PML have been reported in patients who had received the German formulation and were either exposed to other drugs associated with PML or had alternative risk factors such as preexisting or drug-induced leukopenia. Dimethyl fumarate results in severe leukopenia in 3% of patients.

No specific treatment algorithm can be recommended because the disease is heterogeneous, there are few head-to-head studies between medications, and reported effect sizes of the approved drugs versus placebo depend on the varying characteristics of patients in different trials. As a result, the treatment decision is best made in conjunction with the patient based on the patient's disease, the side-effect and safety profiles of the various drugs, and the physician's assessment of severity and prognosis.[10] Older drugs such as IFN-β or glatiramer acetate have provided variable responses, with some patients doing well for many years. For the typical newly diagnosed patient with relapsing MS but no early signs of poor prognosis (e.g., high relapse rate with early accrual of disability, African American ancestry, high lesion load, T1 black holes on MRI, multiple spinal cord lesions), one reasonable strategy is to start with one of the older, relatively safe drugs such as IFN-β1b or glatiramer acetate and then switch to the other if the patient experiences a severe relapse, multiple small relapses, or new MRI lesions, before escalating to one of the newer, more potent drugs associated with more potential risk.

Other Therapies

Rituximab (1000 mg IV 2 weeks apart repeated every 6 months) is a monoclonal antibody that depletes B-cell lymphocytes and can significantly reduce inflammatory brain lesions and relapse by approximately 50% for up to 48 weeks in patients with relapsing-remitting MS.[A13] However, it has not been effective in primary progressive MS. Newer, fully humanized anti-CD20 monoclonal antibodies (ocrelizumab and ofatumumab) have shown equal or better efficacy in phase 2 trials of relapsing MS.

Daclizumab (an anti-CD52 [IL-2 receptor-α] monclonal antibody dosed at 150 to 300 mg SC every 4 weeks) reduced annualized relapse rate by 50 to 60% and MRI activity in two phase 2 trials A.[A14] Cladribine (2-chlorodeoxyadenosine, 3.5 or 5.25 mg/kg/day) given as a short course once per year reduced the annualized relapse rate by 55% and disease progression by one third compared with placebo in a phase 3 trial.[A15] Both these drugs may have a role in treating MS, but they also have global immunosuppressive effects that increase the risk for serious infections and possibly other systemic complications.

In a phase 2 trial, treatment with 0.6 mg/day of laquinimod, a novel oral immunomodulatory agent, resulted in a 40% decrease in MRI lesions in relapsing-remitting multiple sclerosis at 36 weeks.[A16] In a subsequent large randomized trial of patients with relapsing-remitting multiple sclerosis, laquinimod (0.6 mg/day PO) reduced the relapse rate, the progression of disability, and the MRI lesions.[A17] However, this drug has not been approved in the United States because of concerns about its long-term side effects.

In a randomized trial, sustained-release dalfampridine, a potassium-channel blocker at 10 mg twice daily, improved walking in 35% of patients compared with only 8% of patients receiving placebo, leading to its approval by the FDA as a symptomatic therapy for MS.[A18] Although only a subset of patients appear to benefit, the effect is fairly rapid and likely extends beyond just ambulation in those who are responders. Dalfampridine is contraindicated in patients with a history of seizures and may cause dizziness, insomnia, and an increase in paresthesias.

Other forms of immunosuppression, including methotrexate, azathioprine, mycophenolate mofetil, and cyclophosphamide, may have some efficacy in MS, although either no definitive clinical trials have been done with these agents or safety profiles have outweighed risks, and none is as yet approved for MS by the FDA.

Other Approaches to Well-Being

Patients with MS are at high risk for developing osteopenia or osteoporosis (Chapter 243), so prophylaxis with vitamin D and calcium and treatment with bisphosphonates or other proved approaches should be considered. Patients with suboptimal 25-OH vitamin D levels (<30 ng/mL) on standard 1000-IU cholecalciferol replacement therapy should consider increasing to 4000 to 5000 IU/day or 50,000 IU every other week or, in some cases, weekly, with appropriate monitoring of vitamin D and serum plus urine calcium levels. If osteoporosis has already been diagnosed, bisphosphonate therapy, such as alendronate (10 mg/day or 70 mg/week) or a similar drug, is generally indicated.

Nonmedical treatment of MS is a critical part of managing the disease. Patients derive benefit from a health care team approach consisting of an experienced MS physician, nurse, social worker, therapist, and counselor, with appropriate referral to other subspecialties as needed. Alternative and complementary therapies (Chapter 39) are commonly used by patients with MS, and the risks and benefits of these approaches must be discussed with the patient.

PROGNOSIS

The average lifespan of patients with MS is approximately 8 years less than normal, a finding reflecting a bimodal distribution in which many patients live a normal lifespan and a few die earlier owing to aggressive disease, severe disability, infection, or suicide.[11] Most patients presenting with relapsing-remitting MS convert to secondary progressive MS after 20 to 40 years. Only one third of patients will require use of a wheelchair, but 50% may need assistive devices and nearly two thirds will have disability that prevents them from working. African Americans and men of all races tend to have a more aggressive course and are more likely to become disabled. Immunomodulating therapy early in the course of the disease appears to slow progression of disability, but long-term follow-up data are open-label and uncontrolled, so it is difficult to quantify the extent of this benefit.

OTHER DISEASES OF MYELIN
Monofocal and Monophasic Demyelinating Processes

OPTIC NEURITIS AND TRANSVERSE MYELITIS

Optic neuritis (Chapter 424) and transverse myelitis are inflammatory processes that can occur as entities distinct from MS or as part of MS (see earlier).[12] In addition, optic neuritis and transverse myelitis can occur together in the syndrome called *neuromyelitis optica* (Devic disease).

Optic Neuritis

Optic neuritis (Chapter 424) is an inflammatory disease that usually involves the retrobulbar portion of the optic nerve and sometimes parts of the optic chiasm. Although optic neuritis is most often associated with MS (50 to 75%), it also can be seen as an isolated idiopathic disorder (25 to 50%), as part of neuromyelitis optica, or associated with other inflammatory and infectious diseases such as chronic relapsing inflammatory optic neuropathy, systemic lupus erythematosus, Sjögren syndrome, sarcoidosis, Lyme disease, syphilis, and human immunodeficiency virus infection. The pathobiologic features are thought to be similar to those of MS and are characterized by

idiopathic inflammatory demyelination followed by secondary axonal injury. Hereditary optic neuropathies may be unmasked during periods of stress and manifest as an acute monocular visual loss.

CLINICAL MANIFESTATIONS AND DIAGNOSIS

The clinical presentation, which typically is monocular visual loss with pain over the brow that worsens with lateral eye movement, is similar regardless of whether it manifests as part of MS (see the earlier discussion of the visual effects of MS) or not. When it involves the optic nerve head, it is called *papillitis* and, in bilateral cases, can be impossible to differentiate from papilledema. Optic neuritis also can be mimicked by anterior segment, choroidal, or retinal diseases. Optic neuritis is distinguished from optic neuropathy, which is a chronic, generally noninflammatory condition of the optic nerve caused by tobacco or nutritional amblyopia, ischemia, Leber disease, Charcot Marie Tooth type 2a (mitofusinopathy; Chapter 420), or a number of other rare hereditary diseases (Chapter 424). Subclinical optic neuropathy in the absence of painful monocular visual loss may result in retinal nerve fiber layer thinning over time.

TREATMENT   Rx

Among patients with optic neuritis, the 15-year risk for developing MS is 25% in patients without lesions on their baseline brain MRI but 72% in patients with one or more baseline MRI lesions. Treatment with intravenous methylprednisolone as in MS may shorten the duration and severity of the attack, but no definitive evidence indicates that it changes the long-term outcome. Oral prednisone alone, without prior treatment with intravenous methylprednisolone, may increase the risk for recurrent optic neuritis and should be avoided. Data support the use of IFN-β drugs and glatiramer acetate in patients whose optic neuritis is at high risk for conversion to MS (one or more typical brain MRI lesions).

Transverse Myelitis

Transverse myelitis is a rare (~1 in 100,000 people) monophasic inflammatory process of the spinal cord that is usually distinct from MS in that it either involves the entire cross section or is longitudinally extensive along three vertebral body segments rostrocaudally.[13] Transverse myelitis or myelopathy may be idiopathic or associated with inflammatory diseases (systemic lupus erythematosus, Sjögren syndrome, vasculitis, or MS), infectious diseases, or vascular diseases (antiphospholipid antibody syndrome or dural venous fistula).

CLINICAL MANIFESTATIONS AND DIAGNOSIS

In its fulminant form, transverse myelitis causes complete loss of motor and sensory function below the affected level of the spinal cord and causes concomitant bowel, bladder, and sexual dysfunction. Autonomic involvement can be seen in cervical and high thoracic spine cases. Transverse myelitis also may manifest in an incomplete or partial form, which is more commonly associated with MS. In older patients, patients with vascular risk factors, or patients with central cord edema pattern on MRI, spinal angiography should be considered to exclude spinal cord ischemia or infarction (Chapter 400).

TREATMENT AND PROGNOSIS   Rx

Treatment of the inflammatory process is usually with methylprednisolone (1000 mg IV for 3 to 5 days), followed by specific treatment of any identifiable underlying disease process. The prognosis is worse than in MS in that significant recovery is seen in fewer than 50% of patients and many patients remain completely paralyzed after the initial attack. Plasma exchange or cyclophosphamide may be considered in steroid-refractory cases.

NEUROMYELITIS OPTICA

Neuromyelitis optica (NMO) is now recognized as an entity distinct from MS and is characterized by an optic neuritis, often bilateral and temporally associated with a fulminant multilevel transverse myelitis. A specific serum IgG (NMO-IgG) directed against aquaporin 4 strongly predicts this process. Brain lesions may be seen on MRI and have a predilection for the brain stem. Neuromyelitis optica may be similar to what is called *opticospinal MS* in Japan, although the latter overlaps with MS. There is no proved effective treatment, but patients are usually given anti-inflammatory and immunosuppressive medications (e.g., azathioprine 2 to 3 mg/kg or prednisone 1 mg/

kg). Therapies directed against B cells (anti–CD-20 or anti-CD19 monoclonal antibodies), humoral factors (complement), or nonpathogenic antibody blockers of aquaporin 4–IgG binding also have shown efficacy, but no placebo-controlled trials have been completed as yet. The prognosis is generally poor; if not treated, most patients develop sustained disabling visual loss and weakness.

ACUTE DISSEMINATED ENCEPHALOMYELITIS

Acute disseminated encephalomyelitis and its hyperacute form, acute necrotizing hemorrhagic encephalopathy, are thought to be forms of monophasic immune-mediated inflammatory demyelination. They differ from MS in that they are typically monophasic, whereas MS is by definition multiphasic or chronically progressive. However, no reliable clinical or pathologic criteria are available to differentiate the two processes, which may represent a continuum. Patients may present with fever, headache, meningeal signs, and altered consciousness, which are exceedingly rare in MS. There is no known effective treatment. Large numbers of patients, especially children, make remarkable recoveries, but the necrotizing form can be severely disabling or fatal. Relapsing forms of the disease in children are more likely to become MS.

Leukodystrophies

The leukodystrophies represent a variety of diseases formerly characterized by their common clinical and pathologic characteristics of white matter and, presumably, myelin. Many of these diseases now have a defined biochemical and genetic basis, and some (e.g., Alexander disease) are no longer considered dysmyelinating diseases.[14]

ADRENOLEUKODYSTROPHY AND ADRENOMYELONEUROPATHY

Adrenoleukodystrophy and adrenomyeloneuropathy, which are caused by impaired ability of the peroxisomes to metabolize very-long-chain fatty acids, represent different phenotypes resulting from the same X-linked, incompletely recessive genetic defect. Impaired oxidation of very-long-chain fatty acids results from deficient function of the enzyme lignoceroyl–coenzyme A ligase. The defective gene maps to Xq28 and codes for a peroxisomal membrane protein (ALDP), which is a member of a large family of proteins referred to as the adenosine triphosphate–binding cassette (ABC) transporters, specifically *ABCD1*.

Childhood cerebral adrenoleukodystrophy, which is the most common form of the disorder, represents 45% of all cases; it is seen only in male patients, with an onset at ages 4 to 11 years. Adolescent (5%) and adult (3%) cerebral forms progress at a similar or slower rate than the childhood form.

CLINICAL MANIFESTATIONS

Adrenomyeloneuropathy begins in young men as slowly progressive paraparesis with hypogonadism, impotence, sphincter disturbances, variable adrenal insufficiency, and axonal neuropathy affecting mainly the lower extremities. A rare acute inflammatory form with rapid progression and dementia may occur. A similar, but usually milder, disorder can be seen in up to 20% of women who are hemizygous for the disease.

DIAGNOSIS

Diagnosis is established in male patients by finding elevated very-long-chain fatty acids in the plasma. DNA-based diagnosis in carriers is reliable and is recommended in women because of false-negative results using the plasma assay.

TREATMENT   Rx

Treatment is unsatisfactory. A 4 : 1 mixture of glyceryl trioleate and glyceryl trierucate (i.e., "Lorenzo oil") normalizes plasma very-long-chain fatty acids within 4 weeks and has few side effects. Although clinical trials suggested that treatment in presymptomatic patients delayed or prevented the onset of disease, this treatment is ineffective after symptoms have begun and the disease progresses relentlessly.

Pelizaeus-Merzbacher Disease

Pelizaeus-Merzbacher disease is a rare, chronic, familial leukodystrophy usually caused by a genetic defect in the X-linked myelin proteolipid protein (PLP) gene. In classic Pelizaeus-Merzbacher disease, age at onset varies between 3 months and 9 years, and the age at death varies between 6 years and 25 years. However, milder forms of spastic paraplegia 2 are now well recognized in adults. The disease manifests as a slowly progressive myelopathy, often with cerebellar and cognitive involvement, and the diagnosis is established by genetic testing for mutations in the *PLP* gene. A variety of different types of PLP mutations account for the variability in clinical phenotypes. An autosomal recessive disease called Pelizaeus-Merzbacher–like disease 1 and the less-severe spastic paraplegia 44, caused by mutations of the gap junction protein gamma-2 gene (*GJC2*), are recognized variants. No specific treatment exists beyond supportive therapy.

Metachromatic Leukodystrophy

Metachromatic leukodystrophy usually results from a recessively inherited defect in the lysosomal enzyme arylsulfatase A. Absence of arylsulfatase A results in the accumulation of sulfatide in both central and peripheral myelin and myelin-forming cells; instability of the myelin membranes results in the breakdown of myelin. Metachromatic leukodystrophy is generally divided into four subtypes: congenital, late infantile (most common), juvenile, and adult. It appears in all ethnic groups and has an overall frequency of 1 in 40,000.

The clinical manifestations are variable and may include progressive spastic paraparesis, extrapyramidal signs, seizures, and peripheral neuropathy. Brain MRI usually shows large confluent symmetrical high-signal areas in the cerebral white matter, brain stem, and cerebellum, but a more patchy appearance resembling MS is occasionally seen in adult cases. At present, no satisfactory treatment exists. Some evidence suggests that bone marrow transplantation delays the onset in presymptomatic patients and may slow progression of the disease.

Globoid Cell Leukodystrophy

Globoid cell leukodystrophy (Krabbe disease; Chapter 208) is characterized biochemically by accumulation of galactocerebroside in cerebral white matter as a result of deficient galactocerebroside β-galactosidase activity. The disease is transmitted as an autosomal recessive trait and affects infants in the first 2 to 3 months of life, initially manifesting with behavioral changes and failure to achieve developmental milestones. Rare late-onset cases manifest with progressive motor impairment and, less frequently, visual failure. Neuropathologic examination reveals marked loss of myelin throughout the brain, with the presence of round or oval macrophages and large, irregular, multinucleated cells, termed *globoid cells*, that are filled with galactocerebroside. Accumulation of galactosylsphingosine (psychosine) is thought to cause destruction of oligodendrocytes and marked reduction of myelin formation.

Canavan Disease

Canavan disease is a fatal, progressive leukodystrophy with an autosomal recessive inheritance, caused by mutations in the gene for aspartoacylase, an enzyme that hydrolyzes *N*-acetylaspartate into L-aspartate and acetate. Aspartoacylase deficiency results in elevated levels of its substrate molecule, *N*-acetylaspartate, brain edema, and dysmyelination. Clinically, the disease manifests with retardation, seizures, and diffuse, symmetrical white matter degeneration in the subcortical areas, with involvement of the globus pallidum on MRI. No treatment is available.

Vanishing White Matter Disease

Vanishing white matter disease is an increasingly recognized autosomal recessive disorder with a broad range of clinical manifestations from rapidly progressive presentations in infants to slowly progressive disease in adults. The disease is caused by mutations in the eukaryotic translation initiation factor 2B (*eIF2B*) genes 1 to 5, which code for proteins involved in the integrated stress response of cells. Pathologic characteristics include vacuolated myelin with cystic appearance on MRI. No specific therapy, other than avoidance of stress, is known.

Grade A References

A1. Filippini G, Del Giovane C, Vacchi L, et al. Immunomodulators and immunosuppressants for multiple sclerosis: a network meta-analysis. *Cochrane Database Syst Rev.* 2013;6:CD008933.

A2. Calabresi PA, Kieseier BC, Arnold DL, et al. Pegylated interferon beta-1a for relapsing-remitting multiple sclerosis (ADVANCE): a randomised, phase 3, double-blind study. *Lancet Neurol.* 2014;13:657-665.

A3. Johnson KP, Brooks BR, Cohen JA, et al. Copolymer 1 reduces relapse rate and improves disability in relapsing-remitting multiple sclerosis: results of a phase III multicenter, double-blind placebo-controlled trial. *Neurology.* 1995;45:1268-1276.

A4. Polman C, O'Connor PW, Havrdovra E, et al. A randomized, placebo-controlled trial of natalizumab for relapsing multiple sclerosis. *N Engl J Med.* 2006;354:899-910.

A5. Cohen JA, Coles AJ, Arnold DL, et al. Alemtuzumab versus interferon beta 1a as first-line treatment for patients with relapsing-remitting multiple sclerosis: a randomised controlled phase 3 trial. *Lancet.* 2012;380:1819-1828.

A6. Coles AJ, Twyman CL, Arnold DL, et al. Alemtuzumab for patients with relapsing multiple sclerosis after disease-modifying therapy: a randomised controlled phase 3 trial. *Lancet.* 2012; 380:1829-1839.

A7. Hartung H-P, Gonsette R, Konig N, et al. Mitoxantrone in progressive multiple sclerosis: a placebo-controlled, double-blind, randomized, multicentre trial. *Lancet.* 2002;360:2018-2025.

A8. Kappos L, Radue EW, O'Connor P, et al. A placebo-controlled trial of oral fingolimod in relapsing multiple sclerosis. *N Engl J Med.* 2010;362:387-401.

A9. Calabresi PA, Radue EW, Goodin D, et al. Safety and efficacy of fingolimod in patients with relapsing-remitting multiple sclerosis (FREEDOMS II): a double-blind, randomised, placebo-controlled, phase 3 trial. *Lancet Neurol.* 2014;13:545-556.

A10. O'Connor P, Wolinsky JS, Confavreux C, et al. Randomized trial of oral teriflunomide for relapsing multiple sclerosis. *N Engl J Med.* 2011;365:1293-1303.

A11. Fox RJ, Miller DH, Phillips JT, et al. Placebo-controlled phase 3 study of oral BG-12 or glatiramer in multiple sclerosis. *N Engl J Med.* 2012;367:1087-1097.

A12. Gold R, Kappos L, Arnold DL, et al. Placebo-controlled phase 3 study of oral BG-12 for relapsing multiple sclerosis. *N Engl J Med.* 2012;367:1098-1107.

A13. Castillo-Trivino T, Braithwaite D, Bacchetti P, et al. Rituximab in relapsing and progressive forms of multiple sclerosis: a systematic review. *PLoS ONE.* 2013;8:e66308.

A14. Gold R, Giovannoni G, Selmaj K, et al. Daclizumab high-yield process in relapsing-remitting multiple sclerosis (SELECT): a randomised, double-blind, placebo-controlled trial. *Lancet.* 2013;381: 2167-2175.

A15. Giovannoni G, Comi G, Cook S, et al. A placebo-controlled trial of oral cladribine for relapsing multiple sclerosis. *N Engl J Med.* 2010;362:416-426.

A16. Comi G, Jeffery D, Kappos L, et al. Placebo-controlled trial of oral laquinimod for multiple sclerosis. *N Engl J Med.* 2012;366:1000-1009.

A17. Vollmer TL, Sorensen PS, Selmaj K, et al. A randomized placebo-controlled phase III trial of oral laquinimod for multiple sclerosis. *J Neurol.* 2014;261:773-783.

A18. Goodman AD, Brown TR, Krupp LG, et al. Sustained-release oral fampridine in multiple sclerosis: a randomised, double-blind, controlled trial. *Lancet.* 2009;373:732-738.

GENERAL REFERENCES

For the General References and other additional features, please visit Expert Consult at https://expertconsult.inkling.com.

412

MENINGITIS: BACTERIAL, VIRAL, AND OTHER

AVINDRA NATH

BACTERIAL MENINGITIS

DEFINITION

Meningitis is an inflammation of the arachnoid membrane, the pia mater, and the intervening cerebrospinal fluid (CSF). The inflammatory process extends throughout the subarachnoid space around the brain and spinal cord and involves the ventricles. Pyogenic meningitis is usually an acute bacterial infection that evokes a polymorphonuclear response in CSF. By comparison, tuberculous meningitis (Chapter 324) is often subacute and characterized initially by a modest polymorphonuclear pleocytosis that rapidly evolves to lymphocytic predominance.

EPIDEMIOLOGY

The incidence of bacterial meningitis has dropped dramatically in developed countries since the introduction of vaccines against bacterial pathogens such as *Haemophilus influenzae* type b (Chapter 300), *Streptococcus pneumoniae* (Chapter 289), and *Neisseria meningitidis* (Chapter 298).[1] Since the advent of the *Haemophilus* vaccine, the incidence of bacterial meningitis in the United States has decreased by approximately 30%, *S. pneumoniae* has become the most common pathogen, and the disease is now more common in older adults than children; mortality rates (~15%) have not changed.[2] Worldwide, however, bacterial meningitis remains a major cause of mortality and morbidity. Although all human microbes have the potential to cause meningitis, only a few organisms account for most cases of bacterial meningitis.

The clinical setting in which meningitis develops may provide a clue to the specific bacterial cause. *H. influenzae* (Chapter 300) affects primarily children, whereas *S. pneumoniae* (Chapter 289) causes meningitis in adults, especially those older than 50 years with comorbid conditions. Meningococcal

meningitis (Chapter 298) most often occurs in outbreaks. In developed countries, *Listeria monocytogenes* (Chapter 293) is emerging as the most common cause of bacterial meningitis, with peak frequencies in the neonatal period and in persons 60 years of age and older. Simultaneous mixed bacterial meningitis is rare but occurs in the setting of neurosurgical procedures, penetrating head injury, head trauma with fracture of the cribriform plate, erosion of the skull or vertebrae by adjacent neoplasm, extension of osteomyelitis, or intraventricular rupture of a cerebral abscess; isolation of anaerobes should strongly suggest the latter two of these situations. Meningitis involving anaerobes also may occur very rarely as a result of an intestinal-meningeal fistula following surgery and radiation therapy for colorectal cancer. In approximately 10% of patients with pyogenic meningitis, the bacterial cause cannot be defined.

Over the past several decades, gram-negative bacillary meningitis has doubled in frequency in adults, a change reflecting more frequent and extensive neurosurgical procedures, as well as other nosocomial factors. *L. monocytogenes* has increased 8- to 10-fold as a cause of bacterial meningitis in large urban general hospitals. *Listeria* infections are most often food-borne via dairy products, processed meats, uncooked vegetables, and precut salads. Although *Listeria* meningitis may occur in immunocompetent individuals, it occurs mostly in organ transplant recipients, patients undergoing hemodialysis, patients receiving corticosteroids or cytotoxic drugs for treatment of cancer or autoimmune diseases, patients with liver disease, alcoholic patients, pregnant women, and neonates. Meningitis caused by coagulase-negative staphylococci, which represents approximately 3% of cases in large urban hospitals, occurs as a complication of neurosurgical procedures and is often caused by methicillin-resistant strains. Viridans streptococci, *Pseudomonas*, and other gram-negative bacteria are the agents most often associated with meningitis that complicates diagnostic myelography and percutaneous trigeminal rhizotomy.

In large tertiary care hospitals, approximately 40% of cases of bacterial meningitis in adults are of nosocomial origin.[3] The leading causes are gram-negative bacilli (primarily *Escherichia coli* and *Klebsiella*), which account for approximately 40% of nosocomial episodes, as well as various streptococci, *Staphylococcus aureus*, and coagulase-negative staphylococci, each responsible for approximately 10% of nosocomial cases.[4]

Meningococcal disease, including meningitis, may occur sporadically and in cyclic outbreaks. High-risk groups include individuals who live in close quarters such as crowded classrooms, college dormitories, military barracks, or jails. In children the greatest risk is in the first year of life. In industrialized countries, serogroups B and C account for the majority of infections. In developing countries, serogroups A and, to a lesser extent, C are dominant. In sub-Saharan Africa, the so-called meningitis belt, recurrent yearly waves of serogroup A meningococcal infections can occur. The incidence of meningococcal meningitis was probably underestimated historically when the diagnosis was based on isolation of the organism. Polymerase chain reaction (PCR) testing suggests twice the number of cases.

Predisposing factors for the development of pneumococcal meningitis include acute otitis media (Chapters 289 and 426), with or without mastoiditis, which is seen in approximately 20% of adult patients. Pneumonia is present in approximately 15% of patients with pneumococcal meningitis, a much higher frequency than in meningitis caused by *H. influenzae* or *N. meningitidis*. Acute pneumococcal sinusitis (Chapter 426) is occasionally the initial focus from which infection spreads to the meninges. A recent or remote major head injury (Chapter 399) precedes approximately 10% of episodes of pneumococcal meningitis, and CSF rhinorrhea (usually caused by a defect or fracture in the cribriform plate) is present in approximately 5% of patients. Cochlear implants, particularly those that include a positioner, have been implicated in cases of childhood bacterial meningitis, especially episodes resulting from *S. pneumoniae*. Occasionally, meningitis caused by *S. pneumoniae* develops in patients with central nervous system (CNS) shunts. Splenectomy or splenic dysfunction, as in sickle cell anemia (Chapter 163) cirrhosis (Chapter 153) with portal hypertension, or defects in humoral immunity also predispose patients to pneumococcal meningitis. Alcoholism (Chapter 33) is an underlying risk factor in 10 to 25% of adults with pneumococcal meningitis in urban hospitals. The estimated annual incidence of bacterial meningitis (primarily pneumococcal) in patients infected with human immunodeficiency virus (HIV) is 150-fold higher than in the general population.

S. aureus meningitis is seen most commonly as a complication of a neurosurgical procedure, after penetrating skull trauma, or occasionally secondary to staphylococcal bacteremia and endocarditis. Meningitis attributable to gram-negative bacilli takes one of three forms: neonatal meningitis, meningitis after trauma or neurosurgery, or spontaneous meningitis in adults (e.g., bacteremic *Klebsiella* meningitis in a patient with diabetes mellitus). The most common causes of gram-negative bacillary meningitis in adults are *E. coli* (≈30%) and *Klebsiella-Enterobacter* (≈40%). Meningitis caused by group A streptococci is uncommon but occasionally occurs after acute otitis media, more often in children than in adults. *H. influenzae* type b meningitis in an adult suggests an underlying anatomic or immunologic defect.

Patients with defects in cell-mediated immunity are susceptible to the development of CNS infections with intracellular organisms such as *L. monocytogenes*. Patients with defective humoral immunity and an inadequate antibody response are particularly vulnerable to meningitis with *S. pneumoniae* and *H. influenzae*. Patients with neutropenia are at higher risk for meningitis with *Pseudomonas aeruginosa* and members of the Enterobacteriaceae family.

PATHOBIOLOGY

Pathology
On gross examination, purulent exudate in the subarachnoid space is most abundant in the cisterns at the base of the brain and over the convexities of the rolandic and sylvian sulci, which are expansions of the subarachnoid space. Although neither the infecting organism nor the inflammatory exudate directly invades cerebral tissue, the subjacent brain becomes congested and edematous. The effectiveness of the pial barrier generally prevents bacterial meningitis from causing a cerebral abscess; when these two processes coexist, the sequence is usually that an initial abscess leaks its contents into the ventricular system and produces secondary ventriculitis and meningitis.

The inflammatory exudate can extend around the perivascular spaces to adjacent structures, especially the arteries and veins that carry a layer of pia mater and arachnoid membrane as they enter the brain from the cortical surface. *Cortical thrombophlebitis* results from venous stasis and adjacent meningeal inflammation. Infarction of cerebral tissue may follow. *Involvement of cortical and pial arteries* by peripheral aneurysm formation and vascular occlusion or narrowing (related to spasm, arteritis, or both) of the supraclinoid portion of the internal carotid artery at the base of the brain occurs in approximately 15% of patients with meningitis. The anterior and middle cerebral arteries may have markedly increased intracerebral blood flow velocity (an index of stenosis or arterial spasm) on transcranial Doppler ultrasonography, a finding corresponding to focal cerebral signs. In fulminating cases, particularly meningococcal meningitis, *cerebral edema* may be marked even though the pleocytosis is only moderate. Rarely, temporal lobe herniation through the tentorium develops in such patients and compresses the midbrain, thereby leading to ipsilateral third nerve palsy and contralateral hemiparesis or cerebellar herniation through the foramen magnum with compression of the medulla, which results in apnea, hemodynamic instability, and coma. *Damage to cranial nerves* occurs in areas where dense exudate accumulates around the nerves; the third and sixth cranial nerves are also vulnerable to damage by increased intracranial pressure. *Ventriculitis* accompanies most cases of bacterial meningitis and may rarely progress to *ventricular empyema*. As the exudates continue to accumulate, obstruction of the flow of CSF may result in *hydrocephalus*. Obstruction of the foramina of Magendie and Luschka at the base of the fourth ventricle results in noncommunicating or obstructive hydrocephalus, whereas obstruction at the level of the arachnoid granulations in the venous sinuses results in communicating hydrocephalus. *Subdural effusions* are sterile transudates that develop over the cerebral cortex and can be demonstrated readily by computed tomography (CT) as low-density areas about the cerebrum; rarely, such effusions become infected and produce subdural empyema.

Pathogenesis
Bacteria may gain access to the meninges by several routes: (1) hematogenous spread from a distant site, (2) direct ingress from the upper respiratory tract or skin through an anatomic defect (e.g., skull fracture, meningocele, sequela of surgery), (3) passage intracranially through venules in the nasopharynx, or (4) spread from a contiguous focus of infection (infection of the paranasal sinuses, leakage of a brain abscess). Bacteremic spread of *H. influenzae*, *N. meningitidis*, and *S. pneumoniae* is probably the most frequent path of infection. Bacteremia is usually initiated by pharyngeal adhesion and colonization by an infecting strain. Adhesion of such strains, as well as of *S. pneumoniae*, to mucosal surfaces is abetted by their capacity to produce proteases that cleave immunoglobulin A, thus inactivating this local antibody defense. Adhesion of *N. meningitidis* to nasopharyngeal cells is affected by

fimbriae or pili and promoted by previous damage to ciliated cells such as from smoking or viral infections. Meningococci invade the nasopharyngeal mucosal cells by means of endocytosis and are transported to the abluminal side in membrane-bound vacuoles. *H. influenzae*, in contrast, invades intercellularly by causing separation of the apical tight junctions between columnar epithelial cells. When these meningeal pathogens gain access to the blood stream, their intravascular survival is aided by the presence of polysaccharide capsules that inhibit phagocytosis and confer resistance to complement-mediated bactericidal activity.

Bacteria also may travel along nerve tracts to invade the brain. For example, *L. monocytogenes* invades the intestine, and animal models suggest that these bacteria can travel along the vagus nerve to the brain stem, from where they also may invade the meninges in the posterior fossa.

The mechanism by which bacteria gain access to the subarachnoid spaces from blood appears to be related to specific adhesion molecules on brain endothelial cells. Once established in any part of the meninges, infection quickly extends throughout the subarachnoid space. Bacterial replication proceeds relatively unhindered because the low CSF levels of immunoglobulin and complement early in meningeal inflammation result in minimal or no opsonic or bactericidal activity and because surface phagocytosis of unopsonized organisms is meager in such a fluid environment. During meningitis, the concentrations of immunoglobulins in CSF increase but still remain relatively low. Secondary bacteremia may follow meningeal infection and may itself contribute to continuing further inoculation of CSF.

Bacterial meningitis following head trauma occurs because of a dural fistula from the nasal cavity, paranasal sinuses, or middle ear to the subarachnoid space. The most frequent site is at the cribriform plate, where the bone is thin and the dura is tightly adherent to the bone. Leakage of CSF results in CSF rhinorrhea and loss of smell.

Bacterial components (e.g., pneumococcal cell walls or lipoteichoic acid, *H. influenzae* lipo-oligosaccharide) are major elicitors of meningeal inflammation by causing release into the subarachnoid space of various pro-inflammatory cytokines such as interleukin-1 and tumor necrosis factor (TNF) from endothelial and meningeal cells, macrophages, and microglia. Cytokines appear to enhance the passage of leukocytes by inducing several families of adhesion molecules that interact with the corresponding receptors on leukocytes. Cytokines also can increase the binding affinity of a leukocyte selectin, leukocyte adhesion molecule, for its endothelial cell receptor and may thereby further contribute to trafficking of neutrophils into the subarachnoid space.

In bacterial meningitis, neutrophils move into the subarachnoid space but are not able to control the bacterial infection because their phagocytic properties are inefficient as a result of a lack of opsonic and bactericidal activity. Within the subarachnoid space, neutrophils release prostaglandins, matrix metalloproteinases, and free radicals that disrupt the endothelial intercellular tight junctions and the subendothelial basal lamina. The increased local vascular permeability of the blood-brain barrier may cause cerebral edema, which also can be caused by increased CSF pressure as a result of obstruction of CSF outflow because of interstitial inflammation at the level of the arachnoidal villi.

Cerebral blood flow, which depends on mean arterial pressure, appears to be increased in the early stages of meningitis, but it subsequently decreases, substantially in some patients, and this decreased blood flow itself may cause ischemic neurologic injury. Localized regions of marked hypoperfusion, attributable to focal vascular inflammation or thrombosis, can occur in patients with normal blood flow. Impairment of cerebral blood flow autoregulation, as measured by transcranial Doppler ultrasonography of the middle cerebral artery, occurs early in acute bacterial meningitis and causes cerebral blood flow to correspond directly to mean arterial blood pressure, with attendant hyperperfusion or hypoperfusion of the brain. On recovery, the ability of the cerebral vasculature to maintain a constant level of perfusion despite variations in mean arterial pressure is restored.

CLINICAL MANIFESTATIONS

History
Acute-onset fever, generalized headache, vomiting, and stiff neck are common to many types of meningitis (Table 412-1). Most patients with community-acquired pyogenic meningitis have had an antecedent or accompanying upper respiratory tract infection or nonspecific febrile illness, acute otitis (or mastoiditis), or pneumonia. Myalgia, particularly in patients with meningococcal disease, backache, and generalized weakness are common symptoms. The illness usually progresses rapidly, with the development of confusion,

TABLE 412-1   SYMPTOMS AND SIGNS OF BACTERIAL MENINGITIS*

CHARACTERISTIC	EPISODES OF MENINGITIS
Duration of symptoms < 24 hr	48%
Predisposing conditions	
Otitis or sinusitis	25%
Pneumonia	12%
Immunocompromise†	16%
Symptoms at initial evaluation	
Headache	87%
Nausea	74%
Neck stiffness	83%
Triad of fever, neck stiffness, and change in mental status	44%
Focal neurologic deficits	33%
Aphasia	23%
Hemiparesis	7%
Indices of CSF inflammation	
Opening pressure (mm H_2O)‡	370 ± 130
White cell count§	
Mean (cells/µL)	$7753 \pm 14,736$
<100/µL	7%
100-999/µL	14%
>999/µL	78%
Protein (g/L)	4.9 ± 4.5
CSF/blood glucose ratio	0.2 ± 0.2
Positive blood culture‖	66%
Blood tests	
ESR (mm/hr)¶	46 ± 37
C-reactive protein (g/L)**	225 ± 132
Platelet count (platelets/µL)††	$198,000 \pm 100,000$

*Data from 696 cases reported in van de Beek D, de Gans J, Spanjaard L, et al. Clinical features and prognostic factors in adults with bacterial meningitis. *N Engl J Med.* 2004;351:1849-1859. The study included 671 patients who had a total of 696 episodes of community-acquired meningitis. Plus-minus values are means ± standard deviation.
†Immunocompromise was defined by the use of immunosuppressive drugs, a history of splenectomy, or the presence of diabetes mellitus or alcoholism, as well as patients infected with human immunodeficiency virus.
‡CSF pressure was measured in 216 patients.
§The CSF leukocyte count was determined in 659 patients; CSF specimens from 14 patients had too many leukocytes for an exact count to be performed.
‖Blood culture was performed in 611 patients.
¶The ESR was determined in 549 patients.
**C-reactive protein levels were determined in 394 patients.
††The thrombocyte count was determined in 653 patients.
CSF = cerebrospinal fluid; ESR = erythrocyte sedimentation rate.

obtundation, and loss of consciousness. Occasionally, the onset may be less acute, with meningeal signs being present for several days to a week.

General Physical Findings

Evidence of meningeal irritation is usually present, as evidenced by a stiff neck, Kernig sign (inability to straighten the leg when the hip is flexed to 90 degrees), and Brudzinski sign (involuntary flexion of the hip and knee when the neck is passively flexed). Neck stiffness, Kernig sign, and Brudzinski sign each have sensitivities of approximately 30% or lower for diagnosing acute bacterial meningitis in adults.[5] Although the classic triad of fever, stiff neck, and change in mental status is initially present in only 44% of episodes, a combination of two of four symptoms (headache, fever, stiff neck, and altered mental status) is found in 95% of patients. The findings of meningitis may be easily overlooked in infants, obtunded patients, elderly patients with heart failure or pneumonia, or immunosuppressed individuals, who may have meningitis without prominent meningeal signs; in such patients, lethargy should be investigated carefully, meningeal signs should be sought, and examination of CSF is indicated if any doubt exists. In elderly patients, neck stiffness may be difficult to evaluate because of osteoarthritis in the neck or stiffness of neck muscles secondary to basal ganglia disorders. When neck stiffness is caused by meningitis, the neck resists flexion but can be rotated passively from side to side; with cervical spine disease, however, resistance is present in all directions of neck movement. Neck stiffness disappears during coma.

The presence of a petechial or ecchymotic rash (see Fig. 298-3) in a patient with meningeal findings almost always indicates meningococcal infection and requires prompt treatment because of the rapidity with which this infection can progress (Chapter 298). Rarely, extensive petechial and ecchymotic lesions occur in meningitis caused by *S. pneumoniae, H. influenzae,* or echovirus type 9. Very rarely, skin lesions almost indistinguishable from those of meningococcal bacteremia occur in patients who have acute *S. aureus* endocarditis (see Fig. 76-1) and who also have meningeal signs and pleocytosis (secondary to either staphylococcal meningitis or embolic cerebral infarction). Usually, one or two of the lesions in such a patient represent purulent purpura; aspiration of material reveals staphylococci on Gram staining. In the summer, viral aseptic meningitis may produce meningeal signs, macular and petechial skin lesions, and a pleocytosis of several hundred cells, sometimes with neutrophils predominating initially.

Fulminant meningococcal septicemia may cause hemorrhages within the adrenal glands and result in Waterhouse-Friderichsen syndrome (Chapter 227), a condition characterized by the sudden onset of a febrile illness, large petechial hemorrhages in the mucous membranes and skin, cardiovascular collapse, and disseminated intravascular coagulation. In contrast, hyponatremia and the syndrome of inappropriate secretion of antidiuretic hormone may develop in patients with meningitis attributable to *H. influenzae.* A concurrent respiratory tract infection or acute otitis media may be present with either *H. influenzae* or *S. pneumoniae.*

In patients with a basilar skull fracture, the potential for development of a dural fistula and bacterial meningitis is indicated by the presence of CSF rhinorrhea, periorbital ecchymoses, bruising behind the ear (Battle sign), hemotympanum, or blood in the external auditory canal. Meningitis complicating neurosurgical procedures may be insidious in onset and difficult to distinguish from the altered consciousness and signs of meningeal irritation that are expected in the postoperative period. However, fever or prolonged obtundation is an indication for evaluation of CSF.

Neurologic Findings and Complications

Neurologic complications in patients with inadequately treated bacterial meningitis can be severe and disabling. Cranial nerve abnormalities, involving principally the third, fourth, sixth, or seventh nerve, occur in 5 to 10% of adults with community-acquired meningitis and usually disappear shortly after recovery. Persistent sensorineural hearing loss occurs in 10% of children with bacterial meningitis, and another 16% have transient conductive hearing loss. The most likely sites of involvement in patients with persistent sensorineural deafness appear to be the inner ear (infection or toxic products possibly spreading from the subarachnoid space along the cochlear aqueduct) and the acoustic nerve. In children, permanent hearing impairment is more common after meningitis caused by *S. pneumoniae* than by *H. influenzae* or *N. meningitidis.*

Seizures (focal or generalized; Chapter 403) occur in 20 to 30% of patients and may result from reversible causes (high fever or hypoglycemia in infants, penicillin neurotoxicity when large doses are administered intravenously (IV) to patients with renal failure) or, more commonly, from focal cerebral injury related to arterial hypoperfusion and infarction, cortical venous thrombosis, or focal edema and cerebritis. Seizures can occur during the first few days or can appear with associated focal neurologic deficits caused by vascular inflammation some days after onset of the meningitis. In adults with seizures accompanying meningitis, *S. pneumoniae* is more commonly the cause, but alcohol withdrawal is a confounding factor.

Increased CSF pressure, which can be caused by brain swelling or hydrocephalus, is associated with seizures, vomiting, sixth and third nerve dysfunction, abnormal reflexes, reduced consciousness or coma, dilated and poorly reactive pupils, and the Cushing response of decerebrate posturing, hypertension, bradycardia, and irregular respirations. In approximately a fourth of fatal cases of community-acquired meningitis in adults, cerebral edema accompanied by temporal lobe herniation is observed at autopsy.

Papilledema (see Fig. 423-27) occurs in less than 1% of patients with bacterial meningitis, even with high CSF pressure, probably because the patient is seen early in the process before changes in the nerve head have occurred. The presence of this sign should indicate the possibility of another associated or independent suppurative intracranial process, such as subdural empyema or brain abscess. Marked central hyperpnea sometimes occurs in patients with severe bacterial meningitis; CSF acidosis, which is principally due to increased lactic acid levels, provides much of the respiratory stimulus.

Focal cerebral signs (principally hemiparesis, dysphasia, visual field defects, and gaze preference) occur in approximately a third of adults with community-acquired bacterial meningitis. These signs may develop because of arterial or venous occlusion. In addition, cerebral blood flow velocity may be decreased in patients with increased intracranial pressure and may lead to temporary or lasting neurologic dysfunction. It is important to distinguish these vascular effects from postictal changes (Todd paralysis), which usually persist for less than a day. Meningitis may cause the syndrome of inappropriate secretion of antidiuretic hormone.

DIAGNOSIS

Bacterial meningitis is a medical emergency that requires immediate diagnosis and rapid institution of antimicrobial therapy. Delay in treatment is the most critical factor in determining the morbidity and mortality of patients with bacterial meningitis. The diagnosis of bacterial meningitis is not difficult in a febrile patient with meningeal symptoms and signs developing in the setting of a predisposing illness. The diagnosis may be less obvious in an elderly, obtunded patient with pneumonia or a confused alcoholic patient in impending delirium tremens.

When the diagnosis of bacterial meningitis is entertained, blood cultures should be performed, CSF examined and cultured, and antimicrobial therapy instituted promptly. If a mass lesion (cerebral abscess, subdural empyema) is suspected from the history, clinical setting, or physical findings (papilledema, focal cerebral signs), CT with or without contrast enhancement or magnetic resonance imaging (MRI) should be performed because of the danger of brain herniation with lumbar puncture. Antibiotics can and commonly should be started immediately, even before performing lumbar puncture, because it takes approximately 2 hours for antibiotics to affect CSF cultures. Diagnostic lumbar puncture should not be delayed to perform CT or MRI except in patients who have focal neurologic findings suggestive of a parameningeal collection or other intracranial mass lesions; in such patients, it is critical to initiate antimicrobial therapy for meningitis of unknown origin or brain abscess before CT or MRI is performed. Patients with community-acquired meningitis rarely have important abnormalities detected on CT in the absence of focal neurologic findings.

Laboratory Findings
Cerebrospinal Fluid Examination

Initial CSF pressure is usually moderately elevated (200 to 300 mm H_2O in adults). Striking elevations ($\geq$450 mm H_2O) occur in occasional patients with acute brain swelling complicating meningitis in the absence of an associated mass lesion. Findings on CSF analysis are strikingly abnormal in patients with meningitis, and such findings help suggest the cause even before the results of culture are available (Table 412-2). In patients with skull fractures, CSF rhinorrhea can be distinguished from nasal secretions by the presence of glucose.

Gram-Stained Smear

By the time of hospitalization, most patients with pyogenic meningitis have large numbers ($\geq10^5$/mL) of bacteria in their CSF. Careful examination of the Gram-stained smear of the spun sediment of CSF reveals the etiologic agent in 60 to 80% of cases. In most instances in which gram-positive diplococci (or short-chain cocci) are observed on a stained CSF smear, they are pneumococci. *Enterococcus*, an occasional cause of nosocomial meningitis, is detected by latex particle agglutination. Rarely, three species may morphologically mimic *Neisseria* in CSF or may suggest a mixed infection with short gram-negative rods and meningococci: *Acinetobacter baumannii*, *Moraxella* sp, and *Pasteurella multocida*. Culture of CSF reveals the etiologic agent in 80 to 90% of patients with bacterial meningitis if CSF is obtained before or within 1 to 2 hours of the initiation of antibiotics.

Special Testing Procedures

Broad-range PCR, which can be performed on CSF within 1.5 hours, can diagnose bacterial meningitis in patients in whom antimicrobial therapy was begun before lumbar puncture or when cultures are negative and a bacterial origin is still suspected. However, the sensitivity of PCR for bacterial infections ranges from approximately 80 to 95%, so a negative result does not exclude the diagnosis. In resource-poor countries, a reagent strip that detects cells, proteins, and glucose has a sensitivity and specificity above 96% for diagnosing bacterial meningitis.[6] In many parts of the world, it may be especially useful for distinguishing bacterial meningitis from CNS malaria (Chapter 345).

Cell Count

Cells counts should be determined promptly because the cells will begin to lyse after 90 minutes. The normal CSF white blood cell count is less than 5/μL (all mononuclear). The cell count in untreated meningitis usually ranges between 100 and 10,000/μL, with polymorphonuclear leukocytes predominating initially (>80%) and lymphocytes appearing subsequently.

The cell count in *L. monocytogenes* meningitis tends to be lower (median, 585/μL) than in other types of community-acquired pyogenic meningitis. Extremely high cell counts (>50,000/μL) should raise the possibility of intraventricular rupture of a cerebral abscess. Cell counts as low as 10 to 20/μL may be observed early in bacterial meningitis, particularly that caused by *N. meningitidis* and *H. influenzae*. Occasionally, in granulocytopenic patients or in elderly persons with overwhelming pneumococcal meningitis, CSF may contain very few leukocytes and yet may appear grossly turbid because of the presence of a myriad of organisms and an elevated protein level. Meningitis caused by several bacterial species (*Mycobacterium tuberculosis*, *Borrelia burgdorferi*, *Treponema pallidum*, *Leptospira* sp, *Francisella tularensis*, *Brucella* sp) is characteristically associated with a lymphocytic pleocytosis. With *L. monocytogenes* meningitis in an adult, there is usually a polymorphonuclear response but lymphocytes may predominate in rare instances.

Glucose

CSF glucose is reduced to values of 40 mg/dL or less (or < 50% of the simultaneous blood level) in 50% of patients with bacterial meningitis; this finding helps distinguish bacterial meningitis from most viral meningitides or parameningeal infections. However, a normal CSF glucose value does not exclude the diagnosis of bacterial meningitis. The blood glucose level should be determined simultaneously because patients with diabetes mellitus (or those who are receiving intravenous glucose infusions) have an elevated CSF glucose level that can be appreciated only by comparison with the simultaneous blood level; however, it may take 90 to 120 minutes for equilibration to occur after major shifts in the level of glucose in the circulation. The hypoglycorrhachia characteristic of pyogenic meningitis appears to result from interference with normal carrier-facilitated diffusion of glucose and increased utilization of glucose by host cells.

Protein

The level of protein in lumbar CSF is usually elevated to greater than 100 mg/dL, and higher values are more commonly observed in pneumococcal meningitis. Extreme elevations, 1000 mg/dL or greater, may indicate subarachnoid block with obstruction of CSF flow. Values higher than 15 mg/dL in ventricular CSF are considered abnormal. If the lumbar puncture is traumatic, the CSF protein level is corrected by subtracting 1 mg/dL for every 1000 red blood cells.

TABLE 412-2	COMMON CEREBROSPINAL FLUID FINDINGS IN PATIENTS WITH MENINGITIS			
MICROORGANISM	**CSF OPENING PRESSURE (cm H_2O)**	**CELL COUNT (CELLS/μL)**	**PROTEIN (mg/dL)**	**GLUCOSE (mg/dL)**
Bacteria*	>20	>1000	>100	<10
Mycobacterium tuberculosis	>20	100-500	>100	10-45
Borrelia burgdorferi	<20	100-500	50-150	10-45
Treponema pallidum	<20	5-500	50-150	10-45
Fungi	<20	5-500	>100	10-45
Viruses	<20	5-500	50-150	Normal

Modified from Kim KS. Acute bacterial meningitis in infants and children. *Lancet Infect Dis.* 2010;10:32-42.
*Group B streptococci, *Escherichia coli*, *Listeria monocytogenes*, *Streptococcus pneumoniae*, *Neisseria meningitidis*, and *Haemophilus influenzae* type b.
CSF = cerebrospinal fluid.

Other Abnormalities

Elevated levels of lactic acid occur in pyogenic meningitis. The diagnostic accuracy of a CSF lactate level is at least as good as a cell count for differentiating bacterial from aseptic meningitis,[7] and a value above 3.0 mmol/L has a sensitivity and specificity of 94 to 95% for bacterial meningitis.[8] However, the CSF lactate level is less useful in patients who have received antibiotics and it also may be increased in other conditions such as cerebral ischemia, stroke, and head trauma. Although lactate dehydrogenase levels are higher in patients with bacterial meningitis than in patients with viral infections of the CNS, these alterations are not helpful in determining the specific etiologic agent.

Blood and Respiratory Tract Cultures

Bacteremia is demonstrable in approximately 80% of patients with *H. influenzae* meningitis, 50% of patients with pneumococcal meningitis, and 30 to 40% of patients with meningococcal meningitis. Hence, blood cultures should be performed routinely in patients suspected of having bacterial meningitis. Cultures of the upper respiratory tract are not helpful in establishing an etiologic diagnosis.

Determination of serum creatinine and electrolyte levels is important in view of the gravity of the illness, the occurrence of specific abnormalities secondary to the meningitis (syndrome of inappropriate secretion of antidiuretic hormone), and problems with therapy in patients with renal dysfunction (seizures and hyperkalemia with high-dose penicillin therapy). In patients with extensive petechial and purpuric skin lesions, evaluation for coagulopathy is indicated. Elevated serum procalcitonin levels have been used to distinguish bacterial meningitis from that of viral origin, but CSF examination (Gram stain, white blood cell count, glucose, culture) usually provides more direct and specific information.

Radiologic Studies

Because of the frequency with which pyogenic meningitis is associated with primary foci of infection in the chest, nasal sinuses, or mastoid, radiographs of these areas should be taken when clinically indicated at the appropriate time after antimicrobial therapy is begun. Initial head CT or MRI is not indicated in most patients with bacterial meningitis. For example, in patients who undergo head CT or MRI before lumbar puncture for suspected meningitis, only approximately 5% have a mass effect identified on CT. Baseline clinical features associated with abnormal findings on CT include age older than 60 years, history of CNS disease, seizure within the previous week, abnormal level of consciousness, abnormal visual fields, limb drift, and aphasia. In patients without any of these clinical findings, only approximately 1% have a mass effect identified on CT or MRI that would raise concern regarding lumbar puncture.

Specific changes that may be observed on CT or MRI during meningitis include cerebral edema and enlargement of the subarachnoid spaces, contrast enhancement of the leptomeninges and the ependyma, or patchy areas of diminished density as a result of associated cerebritis and necrosis. In patients with meningitis whose clinical status deteriorates or fails to improve, CT or MRI may help demonstrate suspected complications—that is, sterile subdural collections or empyema; ventricular enlargement secondary to communicating or obstructive hydrocephalus; prominent persisting basilar meningitis; extensive areas of cerebral infarction resulting from occlusion of major cerebral arteries, veins, or venous sinuses; or marked ventricular wall enhancement suggesting ventriculitis or ventricular empyema. MRI is superior to CT for visualizing these abnormalities. Rarely, cerebral hemorrhage identifiable on CT may complicate acute bacterial meningitis in adults. In approximately 10% of adults with bacterial meningitis, findings on cranial CT (mastoid or sinus wall defect, eroding retrobulbar mass, pneumocephalus) are indicative of disruption of the dural barrier.

Rarely, paraparesis or tetraparesis resulting from myelitis may complicate bacterial meningitis. In this situation, T2-weighted or short tau inversion recovery (STIR) sequences on MRI can be helpful to exclude spinal cord compression by an extramedullary mass.

Differential Diagnosis

Headache, fever, stiff neck, confusion, vomiting, and pleocytosis are features of meningeal inflammation and are common to many types of meningitis (e.g., bacterial, fungal, viral, chemical) and also some parameningeal processes. The CSF findings are most helpful in distinguishing among these processes (Chapters 413 and 414).[9] Although a lymphocyte-predominant pleocytosis without hypoglycorrhachia is characteristic of viral (usually enteroviral or herpes simplex virus type 2 [HSV-2]) meningitis or meningoencephalitis (HSV-1), the initial CSF finding may be a polymorphonuclear response (of ≤ 60%) that quickly becomes mononuclear. HSV-1 encephalitis is suggested by neurologic findings (dysphasia, hemiparesis, olfactory hallucinations, other temporal lobe signs, seizures), abnormalities in the orbitofrontal and medial temporal lobes on MRI, and distinctive electroencephalographic changes in the temporal lobe or lobes. The rash, fever, and headache of Rocky Mountain spotted fever (Chapter 327) may suggest meningococcal infection, but the geographic and seasonal predilections of the former can provide clues. Approximately 10% of patients hospitalized with Rocky Mountain spotted fever have CSF cell counts higher than 100/μL (>70% polymorphonuclear), and thus the condition initially may be confused with bacterial meningitis. The rash associated with enteroviral infections typically consists of erythematous macules and papules on the face, neck, and trunk. Acute subarachnoid hemorrhage (Chapter 408) may be confused with bacterial meningitis because of headache, stiff neck, and vomiting. However, subarachnoid hemorrhage usually has a more abrupt onset without a prodromal fever but with evidence of subarachnoid blood on CT or CSF examination. In patients with neuroleptic malignant syndrome (Chapters 410 and 418), fever, generalized rigidity, and a fluctuating level of consciousness with autonomic instability and leukocytosis may develop. The most specific laboratory abnormality in these patients is a markedly elevated creatine kinase level.

In a patient with meningitis but whose CSF does not reveal the etiologic agent on a Gram-stained smear, particularly when the CSF glucose level is normal and the polymorphonuclear pleocytosis is atypical, certain treatable processes that can mimic bacterial meningitis should be considered in the differential diagnosis:

1. *Parameningeal infections.* The presence of infections (chronic ear or nasal accessory sinus infections, lung abscess) predisposing to brain abscess, epidural (cerebral or spinal) abscess, subdural empyema, or pyogenic venous sinus phlebitis should be sought (Chapter 413). Neurologic symptoms may appear in the course of primary bacterial meningitis, but their presence should alert the physician to the need for close scrutiny for the presence of a space-occupying infectious process in the CNS. Neurologic symptoms or findings antedating the onset of meningeal symptoms should suggest the possibility of a parameningeal infection. Isolation of an anaerobic organism should suggest the possibility of intraventricular leakage of a cerebral abscess.

2. *Bacterial endocarditis.* Bacterial meningitis may occur during bacterial endocarditis (Chapter 76) caused by pyogenic organisms such as *S. aureus* and enterococci. In subacute bacterial endocarditis, sterile embolic infarctions of the brain may produce meningeal signs and a pleocytosis consisting of several hundred cells, including polymorphonuclear leukocytes. A history of dental manipulation, fever, and anorexia antedating the meningitis should be sought; careful examination for heart murmurs and peripheral stigmata of endocarditis is indicated.

3. *"Chemical" meningitis.* The clinical and CSF findings (polymorphonuclear pleocytosis and even reduced glucose level) of bacterial meningitis may be produced by chemically induced inflammation. Acute meningitis after diagnostic lumbar puncture or spinal anesthesia may result from bacterial or chemical contamination of equipment or anesthetic agent. Chemical meningitis, characterized by polymorphonuclear pleocytosis, hypoglycorrhachia, and a latent period of 3 to 24 hours, occurs after 1% of metrizamide myelograms. Endogenous chemical meningitis resulting from material from an epidermoid tumor or a craniopharyngioma leaking into the subarachnoid space, a glioblastoma invading the ventricles (Chapter 189), or carcinomatous meningitis (see later) can produce polymorphonuclear pleocytosis and hypoglycorrhachia.

Complications
Non-neurologic Complications
Shock

When shock occurs in patients with pyogenic meningitis, it is usually a manifestation of the accompanying intense bacteremia, as in fulminant meningococcemia, rather than a manifestation of the meningitis itself. Management is guided by the principles of septic shock therapy (Chapter 108), with appropriate modifications in patients with heart failure (Chapter 59).

Coagulation Disorders

Coagulopathies (Chapter 174) are frequently associated with the intense bacteremia (usually meningococcal, occasionally pneumococcal) and hypotension that can accompany meningitis. The changes may be mild, such as thrombocytopenia (with or without prolongation of the prothrombin and partial thromboplastin times), or more marked, with clinical evidence of disseminated intravascular coagulation (Chapter 175).

Septic Complications
Endocarditis
In patients with pneumococcal meningitis, particularly those with concomitant bacteremia and pneumonia, acute endocarditis (Chapter 76) can develop, most commonly on the aortic valve. In such patients, febrile relapse and a new cardiac murmur may appear shortly after the completion of antimicrobial therapy for meningitis.

Pyogenic Arthritis
Septic arthritis may result from the bacteremia associated with meningitis caused by *S. pneumoniae*, *N. meningitidis*, or *H. influenzae*.

Prolonged Fever
With appropriate antimicrobial treatment of community-acquired bacterial meningitis, patients become afebrile within 2 to 5 days. Sometimes, however, the fever persists or recurs after an afebrile period. In a patient with persisting headache, obtundation, and cerebral findings, inadequate drug therapy or neurologic sequelae (cortical venous thrombophlebitis, ventriculitis, subdural collections) are important considerations. Re-evaluation of CSF, particularly Gram-stained smear and culture, is essential in these circumstances. Drug-induced fever (Chapters 254 and 280) should be suspected in patients who continue to show clinical improvement in all other respects. Metastatic infection (septic arthritis, purulent pericarditis, thoracic empyema, endocarditis) may be the cause of continuing or recurrent fever. A syndrome, probably immunologic, consisting of fever, arthritis, and pericarditis 3 to 6 days after the initiation of effective antimicrobial therapy for meningococcal meningitis occurs in approximately 10% of patients (Chapter 298).

Recurrent Meningitis
Repeated episodes of bacterial meningitis generally indicate a host defect, either in local anatomy or in antibacterial and immunologic defenses (e.g., recurrent *N. meningitidis* infections in patients with congenital or acquired deficiencies of complement, particularly the late-acting components). Approximately 10% of episodes of pneumococcal meningitis in adults are recurrent meningitis, but only 0.5% of patients with community-acquired meningitis caused by other microorganisms have recurrent attacks. *S. pneumoniae* is the cause of a third of episodes of community-acquired recurrent meningitis; various streptococci, *H. influenzae*, and *N. meningitidis* are the cause of another third of episodes. In contrast, in nosocomial recurrent meningitis, gram-negative bacilli and *S. aureus* are the cause of approximately 60% of episodes. A history of head trauma is frequent in patients with recurrent meningitis. Organisms may enter the subarachnoid space directly, through a defect in the cribriform plate (the most common site), in association with the empty sella syndrome, by means of a basilar skull fracture, through an erosive sequestrum of the mastoid, through congenital dermal defects along the craniospinal axis (usually evident before adult life), or as a consequence of penetrating cranial trauma or neurosurgical procedures. The anatomic defect may produce a frank CSF leak (rhinorrhea or, less commonly, otorrhea) or may entrap a vascular cuff of meninges that may subsequently serve as a direct route for organisms to reach the meninges. CSF rhinorrhea may be intermittent, and meningitis may occur months or years after head injury.

Any patient with bacterial meningitis, particularly if the meningitis is recurrent, should be evaluated carefully for congenital or post-traumatic defects. The presence of CSF rhinorrhea should be sought at admission and subsequently (rhinorrhea may clear during active meningitis only to recur when the inflammation has resolved). Clinical clues suggesting the presence of a CSF fistula through the cribriform plate, pericranial air sinuses, or temporal bone include (1) a salty taste in the throat, (2) positionally dependent rhinorrhea (rhinorrhea only in the lateral recumbent or prone position suggests an otic or sphenoid origin), (3) anosmia (cribriform plate leak), and (4) hearing loss or full feeling in the ear, often with a finding of fluid or bubbles behind the tympanic membrane (leakage into the middle ear). Quantitative determination of the glucose and chloride content of nasal secretions and detection of a transferrin band unique to CSF by protein electrophoresis can definitively establish the presence of CSF rhinorrhea.

Recurrent pneumococcal meningitis may develop without apparent predisposing circumstances, and cryptic CSF leaks should be sought actively in such patients by CT of the frontal and mastoid regions and by radioisotope techniques. Radioiodine-labeled albumin is introduced intrathecally, and pledgets of cotton placed in the nares are subsequently examined for the radionuclide. Intrathecal introduction of fluorescein as a visual tracer (under ultraviolet light) can similarly be used to detect active leaks. Surgical closure of CSF fistulas should be performed to prevent further episodes of meningitis. Extracranial approaches through the ethmoidal sinuses can be used to repair cribriform plate or sphenoidal sinus dural defects and avoid the higher morbidity associated with craniotomy.

In most patients with CSF otorrhea and rhinorrhea after an acute head injury, the leak ceases in 1 or 2 weeks. *Persistent rhinorrhea for more than 4 to 6 weeks is an indication for surgical repair.* Prolonged administration of penicillin does not prevent pneumococcal meningitis and may encourage infection with more drug-resistant species.

TREATMENT   Rx

Antimicrobial Agents
Antimicrobial therapy should be initiated promptly in this life-threatening emergency. Subsequent management should be undertaken with close monitoring, often in an intensive care unit. Treatment should be aimed at the most likely causes based on clinical clues, such as the age of the patient, the presence of a petechial or purpuric rash, a recent neurosurgical procedure, and CSF rhinorrhea. However, it is difficult to distinguish among the various causes of bacterial meningitis on clinical grounds alone, although patients with pneumococcal meningitis frequently have altered mental status and progress rapidly to coma, often with recurrent seizures and the rapid development of focal neurologic deficits. If the infecting organism is observed on examination of a Gram-stained smear of the CSF sediment, specific therapy is initiated. If the etiologic agent is not seen on a smear from a patient with suspected bacterial meningitis or if lumbar puncture is delayed because head CT is needed, empirical antimicrobial therapy should be initiated (Table 412-3).

Adequate CSF bactericidal activity, which is critical to cure the meningitis, depends on the ability of the antibiotic to penetrate CSF and maintain its activity in the purulent exudate, as well as on its metabolism and rate of clearance from CSF. The ability of the antibiotic to penetrate CSF depends on its lipid solubility, protein binding in serum, molecular size, and the status of the blood-CSF barrier. For example, chloramphenicol has very high lipid solubility, whereas β-lactam antibiotics have poor solubility. With the exception of rifampin and chloramphenicol, the commonly used antimicrobial agents do not readily penetrate the normal blood-brain barrier, but the passage of penicillin and other antimicrobial agents is enhanced in the presence of meningeal inflammation (Table 412-4). Antimicrobial drugs should be administered IV throughout the treatment period; the dose should not be reduced as the patient improves because normalization of the blood-brain barrier during recovery reduces the achievable CSF drug levels. Bactericidal drugs (penicillin, ampicillin, third-generation cephalosporins) are preferred whenever possible, and CSF levels of antibiotics at least 10 to 20 times the minimal bactericidal concentration are needed for optimal therapy. Some antibiotics are removed from CSF by active transport into blood via the epithelium of the choroid plexus; by comparison, third-generation cephalosporin antibiotics persist in CSF for longer periods. First- or second-generation cephalosporins and clindamycin do not provide effective levels in CSF and should not be used.

Empirical Treatment
Initial treatment of presumed bacterial meningitis when the etiologic agent cannot be identified on a Gram-stained smear of CSF is based on the available clinical clues.[10] In older children and adults, therapy with vancomycin and a third-generation cephalosporin (cefotaxime or ceftriaxone) is recommended (see Table 412-3). In adults older than 50 years and in high-risk groups, ampicillin is also added because of the possibility of the presence of *L. monocytogenes*, which is susceptible to ampicillin or amoxicillin but not to third-generation cephalosporins. In a penicillin-allergic individual, trimethoprim-sulfamethoxazole is a suitable alternative for *Listeria* meningitis. In special settings, such as nosocomial meningitis associated with neurosurgical procedures or penetrating head trauma, more resistant species such as methicillin-resistant *S. aureus* (MRSA), coagulase-negative staphylococci, and *P. aeruginosa* may be responsible; in these situations, vancomycin in addition to cefepime is indicated as initial therapy.

Meningitis of Specific Bacterial Cause
Pneumococcal Meningitis
The treatment of choice for pneumococcal meningitis in adults has historically been penicillin, with vancomycin (or chloramphenicol) being a reasonable alternative in patients allergic to penicillin (see later). However, penicillin-resistant pneumococcal strains are found worldwide, including 25% of clinical isolates in the United States. Thus, antimicrobial susceptibilities should be determined for all pneumococcal isolates from CSF, blood, or sterile body fluids (see Table 412-4). Approximately 9% of pneumococcal isolates

TABLE 412-3 INITIAL EMPIRICAL THERAPY FOR COMMUNITY-ACQUIRED AND NOSOCOMIAL PURULENT MENINGITIS BASED ON AGE AND CLINICAL SETTING (see Table 412-7 for dosing schedules)

PREDISPOSITIONS	LIKELY PATHOGENS	PREFERRED ANTIMICROBIALS	ALTERNATIVE ANTIMICROBIALS
Age			
<1 mo	Group B streptococcus, *Escherichia coli*, *Listeria monocytogenes*	Amoxicillin/ampicillin plus cefotaxime	Amoxicillin/ampicillin plus aminoglycoside
1-23 mo	*Streptococcus pneumoniae*, *Neisseria meningitidis*, group B streptococci, *Haemophilus influenzae*, *E. coli*	Vancomycin* plus ceftriaxone or cefotaxime	Meropenem (? plus vancomycin*)
2-50 yr	*N. meningitidis*, *S. pneumoniae*	Vancomycin* plus ceftriaxone or cefotaxime	Meropenem (? plus vancomycin*)
>50 yr	*S. pneumoniae*, *N. meningitidis*, *L. monocytogenes*	Vancomycin* plus ceftriaxone or cefotaxime plus ampicillin	Vancomycin* plus ceftriaxone or cefotaxime plus trimethoprim-sulfamethoxazole
Impaired immunity	*L. monocytogenes*, gram-negative bacilli, *S. pneumoniae*	Ampicillin plus ceftazidime or meropenem plus vancomycin*	Trimethoprim-sulfamethoxazole plus meropenem
Cerebrospinal fluid leak or basilar skull fracture	*S. pneumoniae*, various streptococci, *H. influenzae*	Vancomycin* plus cefotaxime or ceftriaxone	Vancomycin* plus meropenem
After neurosurgery or penetrating trauma	*S. aureus*, coagulase-negative staphylococci, aerobic gram-negative bacilli (including *P. aeruginosa*)	Vancomycin* plus cefepime	Vancomycin* plus ceftazidime or vancomycin* plus meropenem
Cerebrospinal fluid shunts (external or internal)	Coagulase-negative staphylococci, *S. aureus*, aerobic gram-negative bacilli (including *P. aeruginosa*), *Propionibacterium acnes*	Vancomycin* plus cefepime	Vancomycin* plus ceftazidime or vancomycin* plus meropenem

Modified from Tunkel AR, Hartman BJ, Kaplan SL, et al. Practice guidelines for the management of bacterial meningitis. *Clin Infect Dis.* 2004;39:1267-1284.
*If dexamethasone is also administered, consideration should be given to the addition of rifampin.

TABLE 412-4 PERMEABILITY OF ANTIBIOTICS INTO CEREBROSPINAL FLUID

GOOD CONCENTRATIONS IN CSF WITH AND WITHOUT MENINGITIS	ADEQUATE CONCENTRATIONS IN CSF IN MENINGITIS	FAIR TO POOR CONCENTRATIONS IN CSF IN MENINGITIS
Chloramphenicol	Penicillin	Early cephalosporins
Sulfonamides	Ampicillin	Cephalothin
Cephalosporins	Methicillin	Cefoxitin
Cefotaxime	Oxacillin	Aminoglycosides
Ceftriaxone	Nafcillin	Gentamicin
Ceftazidime	Carbenicillin	Tobramycin
Moxalactam	Ticarcillin	Amikacin
Cefepime	Tetracycline	Clindamycin
Metronidazole	Erythromycin	Benzathine penicillin
Trimethoprim-sulfamethoxazole	Ethambutol	
Isoniazid	Rifampin	
	Vancomycin	
	Meropenem	

Courtesy Allen Aksamit, Mayo Clinic, Rochester, Minn.
CSF = cerebrospinal fluid.

from patients with meningitis in the United States are resistant to third-generation cephalosporins, with a minimal inhibitory concentration of 2 μg/mL or greater. If the minimal inhibitory concentration for cefotaxime or ceftriaxone (≤1.0 μg/mL) indicates a susceptible isolate, cefotaxime or ceftriaxone would be the drug of choice. If the isolate is highly penicillin resistant or is resistant to 1 μg/mL ceftriaxone or cefotaxime, alternative therapy (vancomycin with or without rifampin IV) is indicated. Because of the increasingly wide distribution of highly resistant strains, initial therapy (pending susceptibility testing) with cefotaxime (or ceftriaxone) in addition to vancomycin IV is recommended. When initial adjunctive therapy with dexamethasone is used (see later) along with vancomycin, it should be borne in mind that vancomycin levels in CSF may be reduced by concomitant corticosteroid use.

Although resistance to chloramphenicol is unusual in pneumococcal isolates from the United States, chloramphenicol has poor bactericidal activity against penicillin-resistant isolates from children with meningitis in South Africa. The relative chloramphenicol resistance of such strains may not be discerned on usual laboratory testing, but it is revealed when the minimum bactericidal concentration is determined. For this reason, vancomycin is preferred over chloramphenicol for the initial treatment of pneumococcal meningitis in a highly penicillin-allergic patient.

The β-lactam antibiotic meropenem is as effective as cefotaxime for meningitis caused by *S. pneumoniae*, *N. meningitidis*, and *H. influenzae* in adults and in children. Cefepime is also similar to ceftriaxone and cefotaxime for infection with *S. pneumoniae*, *N. meningitidis*, and *H. influenzae*, and it has greater activity than these antibiotics against *Enterobacter* sp and *P. aeruginosa* (Table 412-5).

Meningococcal Meningitis

Intravenous administration of penicillin G and ampicillin, in doses used to treat meningitis caused by penicillin-susceptible pneumococci, successfully treats *N. meningitidis* meningitis resulting from susceptible strains. Meningococci resistant to penicillin have occasionally been isolated in Spain (≤50% of strains), South Africa, and Canada but rarely in the United States. Most of these isolates have been only intermediately resistant to penicillin (minimal inhibitory concentration of 0.1 to 1.0 μg/mL), although rare strains have had high-level resistance related to β-lactamase production and require third-generation cephalosporins such as ceftriaxone, which is as effective as the potentially more toxic chloramphenicol. Nevertheless, "meningitis doses" of penicillin or ampicillin may provide CSF levels that are sufficient for infections with some strains of intermediately penicillin-resistant *N. meningitidis*. Usually, a 7-day course of antibiotics is sufficient.

Haemophilus influenzae Meningitis

At present, 25 to 35% of isolates of *H. influenzae* type b in the United States are β-lactamase producers and are ampicillin resistant; cefotaxime or ceftriaxone is the initial therapy of choice (see Table 412-5). Alternatives include cefepime or the combination of chloramphenicol and ampicillin; if the isolate proves susceptible to ampicillin, chloramphenicol may be discontinued. Although more than 50% of isolates are chloramphenicol resistant in some areas of Spain, less than 1% of isolates have been found to be resistant in the United States. A 10-day course of antibiotics is usually sufficient.

Staphylococcal Meningitis

For the treatment of adult meningitis caused by MRSA or in a penicillin-allergic patient, vancomycin is the alternative of choice (Tables 412-6 and 412-7). Because penetration of vancomycin into CSF is limited, adjunctive intrathecal (or intraventricular) therapy with vancomycin (without preservative) is occasionally used when CSF cultures have remained positive after 48 hours of intravenous therapy alone and CSF levels can be monitored. For adult meningitis caused by MRSA, intravenous vancomycin (with adjunctive intra-

TABLE 412-5 ANTIMICROBIAL THERAPY FOR COMMUNITY-ACQUIRED BACTERIAL MENINGITIS OF KNOWN CAUSE IN ADULTS OR CHILDREN (See Table 412-7 for Dosing Schedules)

ORGANISM	PREFERRED ANTIMICROBIAL THERAPY	ALTERNATIVE ANTIMICROBIAL THERAPY
Streptococcus pneumoniae		
Penicillin MIC < 0.1 µg/mL	Penicillin G or ampicillin	Cefotaxime, or ceftriaxone, or vancomycin, or chloramphenicol
Penicillin MIC 0.1-1 µg/mL	Ceftriaxone or cefotaxime	Vancomycin,* or meropenem, or cefepime
Penicillin MIC ≥ 2.0 µg/mL	Vancomycin* (plus cefotaxime or ceftriaxone)	Moxifloxacin or gatifloxacin
Cefotaxime or ceftriaxone MIC ≥ 1.0 µg/mL	Vancomycin* (plus cefotaxime or ceftriaxone)	Moxifloxacin or gatifloxacin
Neisseria meningitidis		
Penicillin MIC < 0.1 µg/mL	Penicillin G or ampicillin	Ceftriaxone, or cefotaxime, or chloramphenicol
Penicillin MIC 0.1-1.0 µg/mL	Ceftriaxone or cefotaxime	Chloramphenicol, or meropenem, or gatifloxacin, or moxifloxacin
Haemophilus influenzae		
β-Lactamase negative	Ampicillin	Ceftriaxone, or cefotaxime, or cefepime, or chloramphenicol
β-Lactamase positive	Ceftriaxone or cefotaxime	Cefepime, or chloramphenicol, or gatifloxacin, or moxifloxacin
Listeria monocytogenes	Ampicillin† or penicillin G†	Trimethoprim-sulfamethoxazole or meropenem
Streptococcus agalactiae (group B streptococci)	Ampicillin† or penicillin G†	Cefotaxime or ceftriaxone

*Addition of rifampin should be considered. Consider intrathecal (or intraventricular vancomycin, 5 to 20 mg/day) if not responding to intravenous therapy.
†Addition of intravenous gentamicin should be considered.
MIC = minimal inhibitory concentration.

TABLE 412-6 THERAPY FOR NOSOCOMIAL MENINGITIS OF KNOWN BACTERIAL CAUSE IN ADULTS

ORGANISM	THERAPY OF CHOICE	ALTERNATIVE THERAPY
Staphylococcus aureus		
Methicillin susceptible	Nafcillin or oxacillin; in difficult cases may add rifampin	Vancomycin or meropenem
Methicillin resistant	Vancomycin; in difficult cases may add rifampin	Daptomycin, ceftaroline, or trimethoprim-sulfamethoxazole
Coagulase negative	Vancomycin; may consider addition of rifampin	Daptomycin
Enterococcus sp		
Ampicillin susceptible	Ampicillin plus gentamicin	Vancomycin plus gentamicin
Ampicillin resistant	Vancomycin plus gentamicin	Daptomycin
Ampicillin and vancomycin resistant	Daptomycin	
Escherichia coli and other	Cefotaxime, ceftriaxone, or cefepime	Meropenem or aztreonam or ampicillin or trimethoprim-sulfamethoxazole
Enterobacteriaceae*		
*Pseudomonas aeruginosa**	Cefepime or ceftazidime	Meropenem or aztreonam or ciprofloxacin

Modified from van de Beek D, Drake JM, Tunkel AR. Nosocomial bacterial meningitis. *N Engl J Med.* 2010;362:146-154.
*Selection of specific antimicrobial drug should be based on in vitro susceptibility results, with consideration given to the addition of an aminoglycoside (e.g., tobramycin, gentamicin, or amikacin).

thecal vancomycin as needed) is the treatment of choice. In severe or refractory cases, the addition of rifampin is warranted.

Listeria Meningitis
Ampicillin is the drug of choice for *Listeria* meningitis. When combined with gentamicin, it can have a synergistic bactericidal effect. Third-generation cephalosporins and vancomycin are not effective. In patients allergic to ampicillin, intravenous trimethoprim-sulfamethoxazole may be used, followed by oral trimethoprim alone.

Gram-Negative Bacillary Meningitis
Cefotaxime or ceftriaxone (see Tables 412-6 and 412-7) is used to treat meningitis known to be caused by susceptible gram-negative bacilli (e.g., *E. coli, Klebsiella, Proteus*), but they should not be used to treat meningitis caused by less susceptible species such as *P. aeruginosa* and *Acinetobacter*. After identifying the specific pathogen and determining its drug susceptibilities, alterations in antimicrobial therapy may be indicated. Although experience is limited, fluoroquinolones can also be used. If the organism is *P. aeruginosa*, ceftazidime or cefepime is recommended and may be combined with vancomycin (see Tables 412-6 and 412-7).

Zoonotic Meningitis
Brucella meningitis (Chapter 310) is a subacute or chronic process that is often accompanied by other manifestations of neurobrucellosis (encephalitis, polyradiculitis, myelitis). Infection is transmitted to humans in endemic areas (Central and South America, Mediterranean littoral, Arabian peninsula) from the ingestion of unpasteurized milk or cheese or direct contact with domestic animals. Neurobrucellosis occurs in 2 to 5% of patients with brucellosis. CSF findings consist of a lymphocytic pleocytosis (<500 cells/µL), hypoglycorrhachia, and an elevated protein level, findings that could mistakenly suggest tuberculous meningitis. The diagnosis is based on demonstration of antibody in serum and CSF or by isolation of *Brucella* from blood; the microorganism is isolated from CSF in only a minority of cases. Treatment of adults involves the three-drug combination of doxycycline (200 mg/day), rifampin (600 mg/day), and trimethoprim-sulfamethoxazole (20 mg/kg/day IV, based on trimethoprim

component, in 6-hour aliquots) for several months, depending on the clinical and CSF responses.

Streptococcus suis is an uncommon cause of meningitis seen in pig breeders, butchers, and abattoir workers in Europe, Canada, and China. *S. suis* meningitis, which is an acute illness with a brisk neutrophilic pleocytosis, is often initially mistaken for pneumococcal meningitis on the basis of Gram stain of CSF. Treatment of adults consists of penicillin (12 to 24 million units [U]/day in 4-hour aliquots) or ampicillin (12 g/day in 4-hour aliquots) IV for 10 to 14 days.

Bacillus anthracis (Chapter 294) is a rare cause of meningitis that most often develops as a complication of inhalation anthrax following exposure to aerosols of anthrax spores in the setting of large-scale processing of wool and hides or a bioterrorism attack (Chapter 21). Anthrax meningitis is an acute process characterized by hemorrhagic or serohemorrhagic CSF with a neutrophilic predominance (several thousand cells per cubic millimeter), hypoglycorrhachia, an elevated protein level, and prominent large gram-positive bacilli on stained smear. Treatment of adults initially includes ciprofloxacin (400 mg at 12-hour intervals) in addition to penicillin (24 million U/day in 4-hour aliquots) and chloramphenicol (4 g/day in 6-hour aliquots) IV. Alternatively, treatment could substitute levo- or moxifloxacin for ciprofloxacin, meropenem for penicillin, and linezolid or chloramphenicol (Chapter 278). Whether all drugs are continued (or treatment is narrowed to one or two antimicrobials) and the duration of treatment depend on whether the meningitis is of suspected bioterrorist origin (Chapter 21) or caused by cutaneous anthrax resulting from animal (or animal product) exposure (Chapter 294). Consultation with infectious disease and public health authorities should be sought.

Duration of Therapy
The frequency of CSF examination depends on the clinical course, but examination should be repeated in 24 to 48 hours if there has not been satisfactory improvement or if the causative microorganism is a more resistant gram-negative bacillus or a highly penicillin-resistant (or cephalosporin-resistant) *S. pneumoniae* strain, especially in patients who are receiving adjunctive dexamethasone therapy. Routine "end-of-treatment" CSF examination is unnecessary in most patients with the common types of community-acquired bacterial meningitis. Although 5 days of ceftriaxone treatment is as good as

TABLE 412-7 DOSES OF ANTIMICROBIAL DRUGS FOR TREATMENT OF BACTERIAL MENINGITIS*

ANTIMICROBIAL DRUG	ADULTS (24-HR DOSE)	INFANTS AND CHILDREN (24-HR DOSE)
β-LACTAMS		
Penicillin G	24 million U, q4h aliquots	300,000 U/kg, q4h aliquots
Ampicillin	12 g, q4h aliquots	300 mg/kg, q4h aliquots
Nafcillin	10-12 g, q4h aliquots	200 mg/kg, q4h aliquots
Oxacillin	10-12 g, q4h aliquots	200 mg/kg, q4h aliquots
Aztreonam (a monobactam)	6-8 g, q6-8h aliquots	
Meropenem (a carbapenem[†])	6 g, q8h aliquots	120 mg/kg, q8h aliquots
CEPHALOSPORINS		
Cefotaxime	12 g, q4h aliquots	200-300 mg/kg, q6h aliquots
Ceftriaxone[‡]	4 g, q12h aliquots	80-100 mg/kg, q12h aliquots
Ceftazidime	6 g, q8h aliquots	150 mg/kg, q8h aliquots
Cefepime	6 g, q6-8h aliquots	150 mg/kg, q8h aliquots
Ceftaroline	600 mg, q12h aliquots	Safety not established in children
AMINOGLYCOSIDES		
Gentamicin[§]	5 mg/kg, q8h aliquots	7.5 mg/kg, q8h aliquots
Tobramycin[§]	5 mg/kg, q8h aliquots	7.5 mg/kg, q8h aliquots
Amikacin[§]	15 mg/kg, q8h aliquots	20-25 mg/kg, q8h aliquots
FLUOROQUINOLONES		
Ciprofloxacin	800-1200 mg, q8-12h aliquots	—
Gatifloxacin[‖]	400 mg, q24h dosing	—
Moxifloxacin[‖]	400 mg, q24h dosing	—
OTHERS		
Chloramphenicol	4-6 g, q6h aliquots	75-100 mg/kg, q6h aliquots
Vancomycin[¶]	2-3 g, q6-8h aliquots	50-60 mg/kg, q6h aliquots
Rifampin	600 mg, q24h dosing	10-20 mg/kg, q12-24h aliquots
Trimethoprim-sulfamethoxazole**	20 mg/kg, q6h aliquots	20 mg/kg, q6h aliquots
Daptomycin	6 mg/kg, q24h dosing	6 mg/kg, q24h dosing

*Dosages are intravenous and for patients with normal renal and hepatic function.
[†]Use may be associated with seizures, but much less so than with imipenem.
[‡]Four-gram maximum daily dose.
[§]Peak and trough serum levels should be monitored.
[‖]No data are available on the optimal dosage required for bacterial meningitis.
[¶]Monitoring of trough serum levels is advisable; they should be maintained at concentrations of 15 to 20 µg/mL. If the patient is not responding well, one may need to monitor cerebrospinal fluid levels and, if low, temporarily increase the daily dose accordingly or add adjuvant intrathecal vancomycin (5 to 20 mg), as for the treatment of methicillin-resistant *Staphylococcus aureus* meningitis.
**Dosage based on the trimethoprim component of the combination.

10 days in children who are stable at 5 days,[A1] longer courses are still recommended in adults. Meningococci are rapidly eliminated from the circulation and CSF with appropriate antimicrobial therapy, which should be continued for 4 to 7 days after the patient becomes afebrile. If the patient has responded well, a follow-up lumbar puncture is not necessary. *H. influenzae* meningitis should be treated for 7 to 10 days. Follow-up CSF examination may be omitted in patients who have responded with rapid clinical resolution of the meningitis. In pneumococcal meningitis, antimicrobial treatment should be continued for 10 to 14 days and follow-up examination of CSF should be performed, particularly when the patient has coexistent mastoiditis. More prolonged therapy is indicated with concomitant parameningeal infection. Meningitis caused by *L. monocytogenes* should be treated for 21 days. Treatment of gram-negative bacillary meningitis with parenteral antimicrobials is prolonged, usually for a minimum of 3 weeks (particularly in patients after a recent neurosurgical procedure) to prevent relapse. Repeated examinations of CSF are necessary both during and at the conclusion of treatment to determine whether bacteriologic cure has been achieved.

Other Aspects of Treatment
Adjunctive Corticosteroids
In children, the routine use of dexamethasone administered IV (either 0.15 mg/kg every 6 hours for 4 days or 0.4 mg/kg every 12 hours for 2 days), either at the time of or 10 to 20 minutes before initiating antimicrobial therapy (third-generation cephalosporin), has no effect on mortality but reduces the incidence of neurologic sequelae (primarily bilateral sensorineural hearing loss). In adults with community-acquired bacterial meningitis, adjunctive dexamethasone therapy (10 mg every 6 hours IV or 4 days) significantly reduced the proportion of patients with an unfavorable neurologic outcome from 25 to 15% or a fatal outcome from 15 to 7%.[A2] Adverse events were not increased in those receiving dexamethasone. Notably, the risk for gastrointestinal bleeding was not increased in the dexamethasone-treated group. The beneficial effect of dexamethasone was most evident in the subgroup of patients with pneumococcal meningitis, in whom the rate of unfavorable outcomes was reduced from 52 to 26% and deaths from 34 to 14%. In a study of adolescents and adults with bacterial meningitis in Vietnam, dexamethasone significantly reduced death and disability by approximately 54% at 6 months in patients with confirmed disease but not in those with suspected disease.[A3] By comparison, adjunctive corticosteroids were not effective in treating bacterial meningitis in a large trial of predominantly HIV-positive patients in sub-Saharan Africa.[A4] Based on these data, adjunctive dexamethasone (0.15 mg/kg every 6 hours for 2 to 4 days, with the initial dose given 10 to 20 minutes before or simultaneously with the initial dose of antimicrobial therapy) is recommended in adults with suspected or demonstrated pneumococcal meningitis and perhaps routinely in all cases of bacterial meningitis, at least in non–HIV-infected patients in high-income countries,[A5] and its benefits extend for at least 13 years after the event.[A6] When vancomycin is used for treatment of meningitis resulting from highly cephalosporin-resistant *S. pneumoniae*, as is recommended in the United States, the addition of rifampin should be considered because dexamethasone may reduce the CSF concentration of vancomycin (see Table 412-4).

Elevated Cerebrospinal Fluid Pressure (Brain Swelling)
Occasional patients with acute bacterial meningitis experience marked brain swelling (CSF pressure > 450 mm H_2O), which may lead to temporal lobe or cerebellar herniation after lumbar puncture. To decrease the possibility of this complication when the pressure is found to be this high, only a small amount of CSF should be removed for analysis (the amount present in the manometer), and a 20% solution of mannitol (0.25 to 0.5 g/kg IV) should be infused over a period of 20 to 30 minutes while monitoring (if possible) for a decline in CSF pressure to a lower level before the spinal needle is removed. Continued control of increased intracranial pressure, if needed thereafter, may be effected with additional mannitol; dexamethasone (10 mg IV, followed by 0.15 mg/kg every 6 hours) should be used in patients with brain swelling regardless of the suspected bacteriologic cause of meningitis.

In a stuporous patient or one with respiratory insufficiency and markedly increased intracranial pressure, use of a ventilator to reduce the arterial carbon dioxide pressure to between 25 and 32 mm Hg is reasonable, and the patient's head should be elevated 30 to 45 degrees. Intubation should be performed with minimal stimulation to avoid an appreciable further rise in pressure; pharmacologic aids to intubation are recommended, such as succinylcholine and opioids, with the possible use of adjunctive intravenous lidocaine. Subsequently, transient increases in intracranial pressure associated with hyperactive airway reflexes can be mitigated by intratracheal instillation of lidocaine before vigorous suctioning. With continued marked and fluctuating elevations in intracranial pressure, use of a continuous intracranial monitoring device may be warranted. Induced hypothermia is not beneficial and may be harmful.[A7]

Hypotension

Initial hypovolemia or hypotension, if present, should be treated with fluid to prevent significantly decreased cerebral blood flow. Over the next 24 to 48 hours, inappropriate secretion of antidiuretic hormone may contribute to further brain swelling; in such cases, fluid should be restricted to 1200 to 1500 mL daily in adults if possible, although a study in children suggests that routine fluid restriction does not improve outcome and that the resulting decrease in extracellular water may increase the likelihood of hypovolemia and an adverse outcome.

Supportive Care

Patients with acute bacterial meningitis should receive constant nursing attention in an intensive care unit to ensure prompt recognition of seizures and to prevent aspiration. If seizures occur, they should be treated acutely in adults with diazepam (administered slowly IV at a dose of 5 to 10 mg) or lorazepam (4 to 8 mg). Maintenance anticonvulsant therapy can be continued thereafter with intravenous phenytoin (Chapter 403) until the medication can be administered orally (PO). Sedation should be avoided because of the danger of respiratory depression and aspiration.

Surgery

Surgical treatment of an accompanying pyogenic focus such as mastoiditis should be undertaken when recovery from the meningitis is as complete as possible but under continuing antibiotic administration. Rarely, the mastoid infection (e.g., Bezold abscess) is so hyperacute that early drainage may be required after 48 hours or so of antibiotic therapy when the acute meningeal process has subsided somewhat.

PROGNOSIS

Prompt treatment of bacterial meningitis usually results in rapid recovery of neurologic function. Persistent or late-onset obtundation and coma without focal findings suggest brain swelling, subdural effusion, hydrocephalus, loculated ventriculitis, cortical thrombophlebitis, or sagittal sinus thrombosis. The last three conditions are commonly associated with fever and continuing pleocytosis.

The mortality rate for community-acquired bacterial meningitis in adults varies with the etiologic agent and clinical circumstances. With current antimicrobial therapy, the mortality rate for *H. influenzae* meningitis is less than 5% and that for meningococcal meningitis is approximately 10%. The highest mortality is seen with pneumococcal (20%) and *L. monocytogenes* (20 to 30%) meningitis.

The mortality rate for gram-negative bacillary meningitis, commonly nosocomial in origin, has been 20 to 30% in adults, but may be decreasing. The mortality rate for recurrent community-acquired meningitis in adults (≈5%) is lower than the 20% rate for nonrecurrent episodes. Poor prognostic factors include advanced age, the presence of other foci of infection, underlying diseases (leukemia, alcoholism), obtundation, seizures within the first 24 hours, and delay in instituting appropriate therapy.

Residual neurologic damage is seen in 10 to 20% of patients who recover from bacterial meningitis. Approximately 25% of adults considered clinically well recovered (expected to function independently and resume activities of daily life, including work) from pneumococcal meningitis show neuropsychological abnormalities, mainly loss of cognitive speed, when they are examined 6 to 24 months after hospital discharge. Developmental delay and speech defects are each observed in approximately 5% of children, and bacterial meningitis is associated with lower subsequent educational achievement and economic self-sufficiency in adulthood.[11]

PREVENTION

Vaccination

The meningococcal vaccine is approximately 85% protective against only four of the strains that cause illness: A, C, Y, and W-135 (Chapters 18 and 298). Making a universal vaccine against the B strains has been challenging because there are many types that cause illness in different parts of the world. All 11- to 12-year-olds should be vaccinated with meningococcal conjugate vaccine, and a booster dose should be given at age 16 years (Chapter 18). For adolescents who receive the first dose at age 13 through 15 years, a one-time booster dose should be administered, preferably at age 16 through 18 years, before the peak in increased risk. Adolescents who receive their first dose of quadrivalent meningococcal conjugate vaccine at or after age 16 years do not need a booster dose. Effective vaccines are now available for many subtypes of *H. influenzae* type b (Chapter 300). Adher-

ence to recommended vaccination (Chapter 18) substantially reduces meningitis from each of these organisms.

Chemoprophylaxis

Prompt prophylaxis of close contacts (individuals who frequently slept and ate in the same household with the patient, girlfriend, or boyfriend) is warranted because up to a third of secondary cases of meningococcal disease develop within 2 to 5 days of illness in the initial case. Only hospital personnel who were in close contact with a patient (mouth-to-mouth resuscitation, initial examination before institution of respiratory precautions) are at special risk. Commonly, oral rifampin is used for prophylaxis: for adults (other than pregnant women), 600 mg twice daily for 2 days; for children, 10 mg/kg twice daily for 2 days. Alternatively, for adults, ciprofloxacin (500 mg), ofloxacin (400 mg), or azithromycin (500 mg), each given PO as a single dose, may be used. Another choice is ceftriaxone intramuscularly as a single dose in adults (250 mg) or children (125 mg).

Widespread use of *H. influenzae* type b polysaccharide protein-conjugate vaccine in developed countries has largely eliminated the need for chemoprophylaxis of close childhood contacts of patients with *H. influenzae* meningitis or invasive infection. However, prophylaxis would be indicated for unimmunized close household contacts of an index patient (e.g., recent immigrant) younger than 6 years. If two or more cases of invasive *H. influenzae* type b disease occur in children at a daycare center, prophylaxis of other unimmunized attendees is warranted with rifampin (20 mg/kg/day PO) for 4 days.

VIRAL MENINGITIS

DEFINITION

The nonspecific term *aseptic meningitis* describes an inflammatory process involving the meninges, usually accompanied by a mononuclear pleocytosis, without evidence of pyogenic bacterial infection on Gram stain or culture. The definition encompasses various processes that produce similar clinical pictures and inflammatory responses: viral meningitis, atypical and nonpyogenic bacterial and fungal meningitis, chemically induced meningitis, drug-induced meningitis, neoplastic meningitis, meningeal inflammation caused by adjacent pyogenic infections, and meningitis associated with autoimmune hypersensitivity diseases. Aseptic meningitis, which is usually an acute or subacute process, can be further divided into types by the duration of illness (chronic versus chronic-intermittent) and distinctive cellular responses in CSF (e.g., eosinophilic meningitis).

Many of the viruses causing meningitis also may cause infection of the brain parenchyma (encephalitis; Chapter 414) or spinal cord. Sometimes, parenchymatous involvement and meningeal involvement occur simultaneously in the same patient and are referred to as meningoencephalitis and meningomyelitis.

EPIDEMIOLOGY

Most cases of community-acquired aseptic meningitis are the result of viruses, principally enteroviruses, which account for more than 60% of viral meningitides and for 90% of those for which an etiologic agent is identified (Table 412-8). Enteroviruses are members of the Picornaviridae (small RNA) family, which consists of more than 60 serotypes: 28 echoviruses, 23 group A and 6 group B coxsackieviruses, 4 numbered enteroviruses (68 to 71), and 3 polioviruses. The most common serotypes implicated in viral meningitis from year to year have been echoviruses 4, 6, 9, 11, 16, and 30 (most recently 13 and 33) and coxsackie B serotypes 2 to 5. Currently, poliovirus infections (Chapter 379) are limited to parts of Asia and Africa, although rare cases occur secondary to attenuated vaccine strains.

Many viruses that produce the clinical picture of aseptic meningitis, such as arthropod-borne viruses, HSV-1, enterovirus 71, lymphocytic choriomeningitis virus, mumps virus, HIV-1, cytomegalovirus, and Epstein-Barr virus, also can produce the clinical picture of meningoencephalitis and encephalitis (Chapter 414). In addition, some viruses involve the spinal cord, including the anterior horn cells (poliovirus, West Nile virus) or the dorsal root ganglia (HSV-2).

Enterovirus

An estimated 10 to 15 million clinical enteroviral infections (Chapter 379) occur annually in the United States, and these include an estimated 50,000 to 75,000 cases of enteroviral meningitis. In temperate climates, enteroviral meningitis peaks during the summer and fall, especially in children. Serotypes tend to cycle with varying periodicity, and outbreaks are related to lack

TABLE 412-8 AGENTS OF VIRAL MENINGITIS

COMMON

Nonarthropod Viruses

Picornavirus (RNA)
  Enterovirus
    Echovirus
    Coxsackie A
    Coxsackie B
    Enterovirus 70, 71
    Poliovirus
Herpes simplex virus type 2 (HSV-2) (DNA)

Arthropod-Borne Viruses (Arboviruses)

Togavirus (alphavirus, RNA)
  Eastern equine encephalitis (EEE)
  Western equine encephalitis (WEE)
  Venezuelan equine encephalitis (VEE)
Flavivirus (RNA)
  St. Louis encephalitis (SLE)
  West Nile virus (WNV)
Bunyavirus (RNA)
  California encephalitis

UNCOMMON

Arenavirus (RNA)
  Lymphocytic choriomeningitis (LCM)
Paramyxovirus (RNA)
  Mumps
Retrovirus (RNA)
  Human immunodeficiency virus (HIV-1)

RARE

Herpesvirus (DNA)
  Herpes simplex virus type 1 (HSV-1)
  Epstein-Barr virus (EBV)
  Cytomegalovirus (CMV)
  Varicella-zoster virus (VZV)
  Human herpesvirus type 6 (HHV-6)
Adenovirus (DNA)
Coltivirus (RNA)
  Colorado tick fever
Bunyavirus (RNA)
  Toscana virus (a Phlebovirus)

of previous exposure to a particular serotype. Serotype-specific protective antibodies develop following infection, so subsequent episodes of enteroviral meningitis are uncommon and are caused by a different serotype.

Humans are the only known reservoir of enteroviruses. Enteroviral infection is spread predominantly by the fecal-oral route and occasionally by the respiratory route.

Herpes Simplex Virus

HSV (Chapter 374) accounts for 1 to 3% of all episodes of aseptic meningitis and occurs most commonly in sexually active adults or adolescents. In individuals with primary genital herpes (HSV-2) infection, up to 36% of women and 13% of men have symptoms of aseptic meningitis. Recurrences of genital herpes are common and are sometimes accompanied by aseptic meningitis. More than 80% of cases of benign recurrent aseptic meningitis are caused by HSV-2. In contrast, HSV-1 CNS infection almost always manifests as encephalitis rather than aseptic meningitis. Herpesviruses also may be reactivated in patients taking immunomodulatory drugs, which are often used to treat autoimmune diseases.

Arboviruses

Although the most common form of CNS infection caused by arboviruses (Chapters 383 and 414) is encephalitis, aseptic meningitis also may occur. These vector-borne viruses are introduced subcutaneously by a mosquito (e.g., West Nile virus, Japanese B encephalitis), tick (e.g., Colorado tick fever), or sandfly (e.g., Toscana virus). Birds, which are vectors of mosquito-borne arboviruses, may not be obviously sick, although West Nile virus may cause prominent die-offs of corvine species, especially crows and blue jays, which can provide clues to an outbreak affecting humans.

The geographic spread of alphavirus infections (Eastern equine encephalitis, Western equine encephalitis, Venezuela equine encephalitis) in the

United States is determined by the range of their individual mosquito vectors. Eastern equine encephalitis occurs sporadically or as focal outbreaks in the summer in the eastern and Gulf coasts, most frequently in children and elderly persons. Western equine encephalitis occurs predominantly in the western states, and Venezuela equine encephalitis is found in Florida. St. Louis encephalitis infections were originally recognized in the Midwest, but sporadic cases and outbreaks have occurred more recently in most parts of the United States; it is the most common arbovirus causing aseptic meningitis in the United States. West Nile virus infections first appeared in the United States in 1999 and now account for approximately 3000 cases of meningitis and another 3000 cases of encephalitis annually.

Mumps

Mumps virus (Chapter 369) was the leading identifiable cause of viral meningitis before widespread immunization in the 1960s. Episodes occurred most frequently in the winter and spring. It is now an uncommon cause of viral meningitis in the United States.

Lymphocytic Choriomeningitis

Lymphocytic choriomeningitis virus is transmitted to humans by rodents through direct contact, through ingestion of animal-contaminated food, or via aerosol or an animal bite. Cases tend to occur in early winter when mice seek shelter in homes. Outbreaks have occurred following exposure to pet or laboratory hamsters. Currently, lymphocytic choriomeningitis virus is infrequently a cause of aseptic meningitis.

PATHOBIOLOGY

The two basic routes for virus to gain access to the CNS are hematogenous (enteroviral infection) or neuronal (HSV infection). Enteroviruses pass through the stomach, where they resist the acid pH, and proceed to the lower gastrointestinal tract. Some virus also undergoes replication in the nasopharynx and spreads to regional lymphatics. After presumably binding to specific enterocyte receptors, the virus breaches the epithelial lining and undergoes primary replication in a permissive cell. From there, the virus progresses to Peyer patches, where further replication occurs. A minor enterovirus viremia then seeds the CNS, heart, liver, and reticuloendothelial system. Following extensive replication at the latter sites, a major viremia ensues, often accompanying the onset of clinical illness. The mechanism by which enterovirus enters the CNS is presumed to involve crossing the blood-CSF barrier's tight endothelial junctions and then entering CSF, probably at the choroid plexus.

In contrast, HSV infections may reach the CNS via the neuronal route: in HSV-1 encephalitis, from oral sites via the trigeminal and olfactory nerve; in HSV-2 (and the rare HSV-1) aseptic meningitis, by spread from a primary genital lesion and ascent along the sacral nerve roots to the meninges. After subsidence of the primary infection, HSV-1 may remain dormant in the trigeminal or olfactory root ganglia only to reactivate at a later date, enter the temporal lobe, and produce encephalitis. Similarly, HSV-2 may remain latent in the sacral root ganglia until subsequent reactivation causes later episodes of aseptic meningitis.

CLINICAL MANIFESTATIONS

Enteroviral Meningitis

The clinical features of enteroviral meningitis (Chapter 379) in older children and adults often begin abruptly with headache (85 to 100%), fever (80 to 100%), and stiff neck (50 to 80%). In some patients the course is biphasic, with the initial prodromal phase being characterized by low-grade fever and nonspecific symptoms (malaise, sore throat, diarrhea), followed by a second phase at which time the meninges are seeded, with the development of higher fever, nausea, vomiting, myalgia, photophobia, and stiff neck. Other enteroviral syndromes may coexist, particularly pleurodynia or pericarditis resulting from coxsackieviruses. Rash may be a manifestation of infections caused by echoviruses, particularly echovirus type 9, coxsackieviruses A9 and A16, and enterovirus 71; the latter three cause hand-foot-and-mouth disease, which may occur alone or accompany aseptic meningitis. Echovirus 9 epidemics often produce syndromes of exanthem, enanthem (small, grayish white lesions resembling Koplik spots on the buccal mucosa), and aseptic meningitis, either alone or in combination; a macular and petechial rash in the presence of a meningitic syndrome must be differentiated from meningococcal meningitis.

Neurologic abnormalities affecting the cerebrum are rarely observed because such cases would be defined as encephalitis or meningoencephalitis rather than enteroviral meningitis. In agammaglobulinemic individuals in whom enteroviral CNS infection develops, meningitis may progress to a chronic meningoencephalitis with multiple neurologic features, including headache, seizures, ataxia, weakness, hearing loss, obtundation, and coma.

The clinical course of enteroviral meningitis is benign, even in the minority of patients in whom the onset is acute and even fulminant. Symptoms subside within a week in children but may continue for several weeks in adults.

Herpes Simplex Virus Type 2 Meningitis

Aseptic meningitis is a common complication of primary genital HSV-2 infection (Chapter 374); up to 36% of women and 13% of men have headache (developing over 2 to 3 days), stiff neck, and photophobia. Clinical features of meningitis occur 3 to 12 days after the appearance of genital lesions and usually last for 4 to 7 days. Neurologic complications occur in up to 37% of patients and include dysesthesia or paresthesia in the perineum or sacral area, urinary retention, and constipation; evidence of transverse myelitis with motor weakness in the lower extremities, hyporeflexia, and paraparesis occasionally ensues. Recurrent episodes of HSV-2 meningitis may occur at intervals of months or years in 20% of patients. In recurrent HSV-2 meningitis, fever may develop but is not as prominent as in bacterial or acute enteroviral meningitis. Recurrent vesicular lesions, paresthesia, or dysesthesia in areas of previous genital herpes may or may not precede individual recurrences of meningitis. Between recurrences, CSF findings and clinical manifestations return to normal. In patients who have had neurologic complications with a first episode of HSV-2 meningitis, the findings subside within 6 months.

Mumps Meningitis

Symptomatic CNS disease, principally meningitis or meningoencephalitis, occurs in 1 to 10% of patients with mumps parotitis (Chapter 369), but pleocytosis occurs in more than 50% of patients with mumps, most of whom lack CNS symptoms. When meningitis occurs in patients with mumps, it usually follows parotitis by 4 to 10 days, but it may precede parotitis by up to 1 week. The typical features of viral meningitis (headache, fever, vomiting) are each present in 50 to 100% of patients. Stiff neck (40 to 90%) is common, and abdominal pain (perhaps complicating pancreatitis or oophoritis) or orchitis (in ≤ 20% of men with mumps) may be present. Other complications of mumps may involve the nervous system (eighth nerve damage, transient facial nerve paralysis, and rarely, fifth nerve palsy) but are usually independent of mumps meningitis or meningoencephalitis. The incubation period for mumps is 18 to 21 days. When mumps meningitis occurs in the absence of clinical parotitis, it is difficult to distinguish it from other forms of viral meningitis.

When meningitis complicates mumps, fever, which had been low grade, rises to 103° F or higher and persists at this level for 3 or 4 days. Most cases are uncomplicated, with approximately a 10-day duration of illness and then complete recovery. However, symptomatic mumps meningitis may persist for more than 14 days in some patients.

Meningitis Caused by Lymphocytic Choriomeningitis Virus

Lymphocytic choriomeningitis virus infections are uncommon, and clinical illness occurs after an incubation period of 1 to 3 weeks. Illness begins with a grippe-like syndrome of fever, rigors, malaise, myalgia, anorexia, and photophobia. Sore throat and arthralgia or arthritis of the digits are noted by some patients. Orchitis or parotitis occurs rarely. This grippe-like illness lasts 1 to 3 weeks in humans, but 15% of patients have a biphasic illness consisting of transient improvement and then recrudescence, 1 to 2 days later, of fever, photophobia, and more prominent headache. Meningeal signs are observed during the second phase. The duration of meningitis caused by lymphocytic choriomeningitis virus, like that of mumps meningitis, tends to be longer than the 7 to 10 days for enteroviral meningitis.

Meningitis Caused by Human Immunodeficiency Virus

Initial infection with HIV-1 (Chapter 384) is symptomatic in 40 to 90% of patients but is frequently overlooked. The interval between exposure and onset of symptoms is 2 to 4 weeks. This acute illness resembles mononucleosis, with fever, malaise, lymphadenopathy, arthralgia, myalgia, anorexia, nausea, headache, and morbilliform rash. A few patients with this initial syndrome have manifestations of aseptic meningitis (headache, photophobia, nausea, vomiting, and stiff neck). Occasionally, encephalopathy or cranial nerve palsies (seventh, eighth, and fifth) develop. Symptoms of the initial HIV-1 aseptic meningitis syndrome last several weeks and then subside. Occasionally, manifestations similar to those of the initial infection may appear later in the course of untreated infection.

DIAGNOSIS

Cerebrospinal Fluid Examination

CSF findings in all types of viral meningitis are similar and consist of a predominantly lymphocytic pleocytosis, usually 50 to 1000/μL but occasionally up to several thousand per cubic millimeter, a normal glucose concentration, and a mildly elevated protein level, usually less than 150 mg/dL. During the first 24 to 48 hours of enteroviral meningitis, a predominance of neutrophils (55 to ≤ 90%) is observed in approximately 50% of patients; subsequently, the principal cells in CSF change to lymphocytes. Occasionally, no pleocytosis is noted in patients proved by culture or PCR to have early enteroviral meningitis. Rarely, hypoglycorrhachia occurs in meningitis resulting from mumps or lymphocytic choriomeningitis virus or in infants with enterovirus.

Polymerase Chain Reaction versus Culture or Antibody Detection

The recent development of reverse-transcription PCR for enteroviruses can reduce detection time to as little as 5 hours, thereby shortening hospital stay and minimizing the unnecessary use of antimicrobial agents. Its sensitivity in CSF is 85 to 100%, with a specificity of 90 to 100%, depending on the laboratory.[12] By comparison, viral culture of enterovirus from CSF has a sensitivity of only 65 to 75% and takes 4 to 8 days.

HSV-2 can be cultured from CSF in approximately 75% of patients with aseptic meningitis during an initial episode of genital HSV-2 infection, but it is rarely isolated from CSF during meningitis associated with recurrent genital herpes. PCR for HSV-2 DNA is usually positive in the CSF of patients with initial episodes of meningitis and is positive in approximately 80% of patients with benign recurrent meningitis caused by lymphocytic choriomeningitis virus.

The diagnosis can be made retrospectively by demonstrating seroconversion in antibody to gG-2 antigen in HSV-2 meningitis. A four-fold rise in titer to mumps or lymphocytic choriomeningitis virus between acute and convalescent sera is also diagnostic. Serodiagnosis is not practical for sporadic enteroviral meningitis because of the lack of specificity of antibodies to individual serotypes.

Differential Diagnosis

The most important process to distinguish from viral meningitis is bacterial meningitis. A predominance of CSF neutrophils, hypoglycorrhachia, and bacteria on Gram-stained smear or culture indicate bacterial meningitis. An early neutrophilic predominance in CSF combined with a macular and petechial rash in enteroviral meningitis may mimic meningococcemia with meningitis. Occasional bacteria and fungi cause meningitis with a predominantly lymphocytic pleocytosis similar to that of most viral meningitides (Table 412-9). Epidemiologic considerations and clinical findings aid in distinguish-

TABLE 412-9	NONVIRAL INFECTIOUS CAUSES OF ASEPTIC MENINGITIS	
UNCOMMON	**RARE**
BACTERIAL	
Leptospira interrogans serovars	*Mycoplasma pneumoniae*
Borrelia burgdorferi	*Ehrlichia chaffeensis*
Treponema pallidum	*Listeria monocytogenes*
Mycobacterium tuberculosis	*Borrelia recurrentis* and *Borrelia hermsii*
Brucella sp	*Chlamydia psittaci*
Parameningeal infections	Staphylococcal enterotoxin or TSST-1
Subacute bacterial endocarditis	*Rickettsia rickettsii* and *Rickettsia prowazekii*
Partially treated bacterial (pyogenic) meningitis	
FUNGAL	
Cryptococcus neoformans	*Blastomyces dermatitidis*
Coccidioides immitis	*Sporothrix schenckii*
Histoplasma capsulatum	*Candida* sp
PROTOZOAN	
	Trypanosoma brucei sp
	Toxoplasma gondii
	Acanthamoeba sp

TSST-1 = toxic shock syndrome toxin 1.

ing leptospiral, Lyme *Borrelia,* and syphilitic meningitis, whereas hypoglycorrhachia suggests tuberculous and cryptococcal meningitis.

PREVENTION AND TREATMENT

The introduction of live attenuated mumps vaccine in the United States reduced mumps from the leading cause of aseptic meningitis and meningoencephalitis to the point at which it occurs only rarely. Chronic enteroviral meningitis and meningoencephalitis in agammaglobulinemic patients have been controlled by parenteral (even intrathecal) administration of immune globulin.

No approved antiviral chemotherapy is available for enteroviral meningitis. Pleconaril, a drug that prevents attachment of virus to host cells, can produce clinical improvement in agammaglobulinemic patients with chronic enteroviral meningoencephalitis.

Intravenous acyclovir (5 to 10 mg/kg three times daily) is used to treat hospitalized, symptomatic patients with HSV-2 meningitis, particularly when the disease is associated with primary genital herpes, although it has not been shown in clinical trials to alter the course of illness. In patients with frequent recurrences of HSV meningitis, it is reasonable to attempt prophylaxis with oral antivirals: valacyclovir (500 mg/day),[A8] famciclovir (250 mg twice daily), or acyclovir (400 mg twice daily).

PROGNOSIS

The course and outcome in patients with enteroviral meningitis are almost always benign, although approximately 1% of patients have subsequent abnormalities, probably reflecting a meningoencephalitic process. Most viral meningitides are self-limited, but some cause chronic or recurrent illness. Persistent meningitis or meningoencephalitis, sometimes fatal, can occur in individuals with hereditary (usually X-linked agammaglobulinemia or common variable immunodeficiency) deficiencies in B-lymphocyte function. HIV-1 may produce a prolonged meningeal inflammation. HSV-2 infection is the most common viral cause of recurrent episodes of aseptic meningitis.

OTHER MENINGITIDES
Nonviral Infectious Causes of Aseptic Meningitis

Categories of aseptic meningitis other than the viral meningitides include nonviral infectious processes (see Table 412-9), noninfectious processes (Table 412-10), chronic meningitides (Table 412-11), recurrent meningitis (Table 412-12), and eosinophilic meningitis (Table 412-13). Nonviral infectious causes are uncommon or rare in comparison to viral or acute suppurative meningitis. Some of the bacterial causes (e.g., *Leptospira* serovars, *B. burgdorferi, Brucella* sp, *T. pallidum*) produce a lymphocytic pleocytosis; others (partially treated bacterial meningitis, subacute bacterial endocarditis

TABLE 412-10 NONINFECTIOUS CAUSES OF ASEPTIC MENINGITIS

Drug hypersensitivity

Systemic disease
  Systemic lupus erythematosus
  Familial Mediterranean fever
  Behçet syndrome
  Granulomatosis with polyangiitis (formerly Wegener)
  Cogan syndrome
  Sarcoidosis
  Still disease
  Kawasaki disease
  Lead poisoning

Neoplastic disease
  Metastatic carcinomatous meningitis
  Central nervous system tumors (meningeal gliomatosis, dysgerminomas, ependymomas)
  Tumors that leak inflammatory material into cerebrospinal fluid (squamous cells in epidermoid tumors of the posterior fossa, cholesteatomas)

Inflammatory processes involving central nervous system structures primarily
  Chemical meningitis following myelography (water-soluble nonionic contrast material)
  Continuous spinal and epidural anesthesia, inflammation after neurosurgery
  Granulomatous cerebral vasculitis
  Vogt-Koyanagi-Harada syndrome

with embolic cerebral infarcts) produce a mixed neutrophilic-mononuclear pleocytosis; and *M. tuberculosis,* though producing a lymphocytic response with developing hypoglycorrhachia, may show a predominantly neutrophilic response in a minority of patients early in the disease. Although patients with *L. monocytogenes* infection usually have neutrophilic pleocytosis, this

TABLE 412-11 INFECTIOUS CAUSES OF CHRONIC (PERSISTENT) LYMPHOCYTIC MENINGITIS

CAUSATIVE CONDITIONS	OTHER CSF FINDINGS
BACTERIAL	
Mycobacterium tuberculosis	Usually < 500 white blood cells/μL, low glucose, high protein
Borrelia burgdorferi (Lyme disease)	Normal glucose, elevated protein
Treponema pallidum (secondary syphilitic meningitis, tertiary meningovascular syphilis)	Elevated protein; Venereal Disease Research Laboratory positive in CSF and serum
Brucella sp (uncommon)	Often low glucose; elevated protein
Tropheryma whippelii (rare)	Cells positive for periodic acid–Schiff on meningeal biopsy
Partially treated bacterial meningitis	Mixture of PMNs and lymphocytes, bacteria on Gram stain and culture
Parameningeal infections	Lymphocytes or mixed lymphocytic-PMN response, normal glucose
FUNGAL	
Cryptococcus neoformans	Low glucose, elevated protein, budding yeast on fungal wet mount, antigen detectable
Coccidioides immitis	Often low glucose, may have 10-20% eosinophils, elevated protein, presence of complement-fixing antibody
Histoplasma capsulatum	Low glucose; complement-fixing antibodies in CSF; antigen detectable in urine, CSF, serum
Blastomyces dermatitidis	Low glucose
Candida sp	Low glucose, may have PMN or lymphocyte predominance, fungal stain may be positive
Aspergillus sp	Lymphocytes or PMNs predominate
Sporothrix schenckii (sporotrichosis)	Low glucose; protein, 200-800 mg/dL
PROTOZOAL	
Toxoplasma gondii	Usually, picture is that of an encephalitis; often in patients with AIDS; pleocytosis is mild (<60 cells/μL) and protein is mildly elevated
Trypanosoma gambiense or *Trypanosoma rhodesiense*	Meningoencephalitis is stage II of disease, elevated protein and immunoglobulin M, trypanosomes on Giemsa-stained smear
VIRAL	
Mumps	Rarely, low glucose
Lymphocytic choriomeningitis	Rarely, low glucose
Echovirus (in patients with congenital agammaglobulinemia)	Occasionally, low glucose
HIV-1	Cell counts lower (10-20/μL) than in acute self-limited meningitis at clinical onset of HIV infection or may develop during course of AIDS

AIDS = acquired immunodeficiency syndrome; CSF = cerebrospinal fluid; HIV = human immunodeficiency virus; PMN = polymorphonuclear leukocyte.

TABLE 412-12 CAUSES OF CHRONIC (RECURRENT) MENINGITIS

Infections
  Herpes simplex virus type 2

Leakage of contents from central nervous system tumors (chemical meningitis)
  Epidermoid tumors
  Craniopharyngiomas
  Cholesteatomas

Drug hypersensitivity with repeated use of agent

Inflammatory processes
  Behçet syndrome
  Systemic lupus erythematosus
  Mollaret meningitis
  Vogt-Koyanagi-Harada syndrome

TABLE 412-13	CAUSES OF EOSINOPHILIC MENINGITIS*
CAUSATIVE CONDITIONS	**SOURCE**
PARASITIC DISEASE	
Angiostrongylus cantonensis	Ingestion of raw shellfish; Pacific
Taenia solium (cysticercosis)	Fecal-oral transmission of *T. solium* eggs
Gnathostoma spinigerum	Ingestion of raw fish; Japan, Southeast Asia
Baylisascaris procyonis	Accidental ingestion of *B. procyonis* eggs from raccoon feces
Trichinella spiralis (trichinosis)	Ingestion of poorly cooked pork
Schistosoma sp	Exposure of skin to fresh water; Africa, Middle East
Echinococcus granulosus	Contact with infected dogs passing eggs in feces
Toxoplasma gondii	Ingestion of meat containing cysts or food contaminated with oocysts from cat feces
Toxocara canis (visceral larva migrans)	Ingestion of infective eggs from dog feces
FUNGAL INFECTIONS	
Coccidioides immitis	Southwestern United States
NEOPLASTIC DISEASE	
Lymphoma, leukemia, metastatic carcinoma	
Hypereosinophilic syndrome (myeloproliferative disorder)	
INFLAMMATORY PROCESSES	
Sarcoidosis	
Drug hypersensitivity	
Presence of foreign body in the central nervous system	

*The percentage of eosinophils varies from as little as 6% to the majority of cells.

infection may suggest aseptic meningitis because of its sometimes indolent onset and, occasionally, an early predominantly lymphocytic response in young children. Fungal (e.g., *Cryptococcus neoformans, Coccidioides immitis, Histoplasma capsulatum*) meningitides are associated with a predominantly mononuclear response, sometimes with a small percentage of eosinophils, particularly in coccidioidal meningitis (Chapter 333). Patients with Rocky Mountain spotted fever (Chapter 327), an acute disease with a macular and petechial rash, may exhibit confusion. When examined, the CSF in approximately 20% of such patients shows a pleocytosis of 10 to 100 or more cells/μL, with either a neutrophilic or lymphocytic predominance. The clinical picture may suggest either enteroviral or meningococcal disease.

Epidemiologic factors are important in raising suspicion for nonviral aseptic meningitis. Leptospirosis (Chapter 323) may be suggested by a history of recent direct or indirect exposure to animals (e.g., dogs, rodents, dairy cattle) and their urine. Neurobrucellosis (Chapter 310) is suggested by the recent ingestion of unpasteurized cheese from the Mediterranean littoral, Middle East, or Mexico or by work as a veterinarian or in an abattoir. Specific endemic mycoses may be a consideration with residence in the southwestern United States (coccidioidomycosis; Chapter 333) and the Mississippi River valley (histoplasmosis; Chapter 332). The setting of immunosuppression by drugs or illness such as acquired immunodeficiency syndrome would raise the possibility of *C. neoformans* (Chapter 336) or *L. monocytogenes* (Chapter 293). Sexual promiscuity and the macular rash of secondary syphilis could suggest *T. pallidum* (Chapter 319) as the cause in a patient with lymphocytic meningitis.

Noninfectious Causes of Aseptic Meningitis

Noninfectious causes fall into four principal categories (see Table 412-10): drug hypersensitivity; systemic processes such as systemic lupus erythematosus and other collagen-vascular diseases; neoplastic disease, primary or metastatic, infiltrating the leptomeninges; and inflammatory processes primarily involving the CNS. Although a mononuclear cell predominance is found in the CSF in most noninfectious aseptic meningitides, there are several important exceptions. Drug hypersensitivity meningitis usually causes a neutrophilic response, although occasionally mononuclear cells or eosinophils predominate. In systemic lupus erythematosus (Chapter 266), the pleocytosis may be predominantly lymphocytic or neutrophilic (sometimes several thousand per cubic millimeter) with a normal CSF glucose level. Hypoglycorrhachia is a feature of few noninfectious aseptic meningitides and suggests malignant disease or sarcoidosis. Various drugs, most

commonly the nonsteroidal anti-inflammatory drugs, have also been implicated in aseptic meningitis.

Chronic (Persistent) Meningitis

Chronic meningitis is defined by the clinical syndrome of headache, stiff neck, altered mental status, nausea and vomiting, evidence of myelopathy or radiculopathy with or without cranial nerve palsies (e.g., III, IV, VI, VII, VIII), and an inflammatory response in the CSF for 4 weeks or longer. Obstruction of CSF flow may produce hydrocephalus and papilledema.

Infectious Causes

Among the more common bacterial causes of chronic meningitis, *M. tuberculosis* (Chapter 324) is the most important to identify because if untreated, it is almost always fatal within 4 to 8 weeks (see Table 412-11).[13] Similarly, parameningeal infections (Chapter 413) must be recognized and treated promptly because surgery often is necessary to provide a specific bacteriologic diagnosis and prevent neurologic residua. Tuberculosis should be suspected in patients with a previous history of a tuberculous illness, a history of recent exposure, HIV infection or another immunosuppressed state, particularly the use of drugs and biologics that block TNF-α and that are often used to treat autoimmune diseases. Clinical manifestations include fever and night sweats, sixth cranial nerve palsies, stroke related to arteritis, or lesions on the chest radiograph. The purified protein derivative skin test may be negative in patients who are severely immunosuppressed or who have recently acquired or overwhelming disease. Acid-fast smear and culture of concentrated CSF can provide the diagnosis, and PCR can be very helpful despite its low sensitivity of only about 70%.[14] As a result, it may be difficult to establish an early diagnosis. When clinical and CSF findings suggest the diagnosis, treatment (Chapter 324) should be initiated while awaiting the culture results. Drug resistance and coinfection with HIV infection can be major impediments to adequate treatment. Rifampicin resistance can be easily detected by PCR, because almost all the mutations that confer rifampicin resistance are contained within a well-defined segment of the *rpoB* gene. Resistance to other drugs is less easily detected by these methods.

Parameningeal infections (Chapter 413) should be suspected when chronic meningitis with focal neurologic signs develops in the setting of chronic otitis media or sinusitis, pleuropulmonary infection, or right-to-left cardiopulmonary shunting. Contrast-enhanced CT or MRI of the head is important to delineate brain abscess, sinus infection, and epidural or subdural infections.

Meningitis may accompany the skin, mucous membrane, and lymph node features of secondary syphilis (Chapter 319), or it may occur alone. Individual cranial nerves (II to VII) may be involved; visual abnormalities, hearing loss, and facial palsy are most frequent. The fluorescent treponema antibody absorption test or microhemagglutination *T. pallidum* serologic studies are helpful in distinguishing the process from biologic false-positive Venereal Disease Research Laboratory (or rapid plasma reagent) results in serum.

Lyme disease meningitis (Chapter 321) should be suspected on the basis of epidemiologic grounds (geographic location, season, tick exposure) and associated clinical features (erythema migrans rash, Bell palsy, radiculopathy). The diagnosis is made by enzyme-linked immunosorbent assay with Western blot confirmation.

A variety of fungal infections can cause a chronic meningitis. Cryptococcal meningitis (Chapter 336) is common in immunosuppressed individuals and can be diagnosed by detection of cryptococcal antigen in the CSF. Histoplasmosis (Chapter 332) should be suspected in endemic regions. Aspergillosis (Chapter 339) is angiocentric and can cause associated cerebral infarcts. Mucormycocis (Chaper 340) is common in patients with poorly controlled diabetes mellitus. Flucytosine is superior to fluconazole when used with amphotericin B for treatment of cryptococcal meningitis (Chapter 336).

Noninfectious Causes

Noninfectious causes of meningitis include malignant disease, chemical meningitis, and primary inflammatory conditions (Table 412-14). Malignant disease may be diagnosed by cytologic examination of large volumes of CSF. Contrast-enhanced MRI may disclose thickening of the meninges and nerve roots, but meningeal biopsy may be required for diagnosis. Chemical meningitis from previous subarachnoid injection may persist, with xanthochromia noted in CSF; meningeal inflammation may be identified on contrast-enhanced CT or MRI.

Meningeal or CNS sarcoid (Chapter 95) may be isolated or occur with other organ involvement, such as pulmonary granulomas, lymphadenopathy, or myopathy. Neurologic findings can include diabetes insipidus and cranial

TABLE 412-14　NONINFECTIOUS CAUSES OF CHRONIC (PERSISTENT) LYMPHOCYTIC MENINGITIS

CAUSATIVE CONDITIONS	OTHER CSF FINDINGS
NEOPLASMS	
Metastatic: Lung, breast, stomach, pancreas, lymphoma, melanoma, leukemia	Low glucose; elevated protein, cytologic examination; polarizing microscopy; clonal lymphocyte markers
Central nervous system: Meningeal gliomatosis, meningeal sarcoma, cerebral dysgerminoma; epidermoid tumors/cysts	
CHEMICAL INFLAMMATION	
Endogenous: Epidermoid tumor, craniopharyngioma	Low glucose, elevated protein
Exogenous: Recent injection into the subarachnoid space	Low glucose, elevated protein
PRIMARY INFLAMMATORY PROCESSES	
Central nervous system sarcoid	Often low glucose, elevated protein, elevated angiotensin-converting enzyme levels in CSF (and serum)
Granulomatosis with polyangiitis (formerly Wegener)	Elevated protein
Behçet syndrome	Elevated protein
Isolated granulomatous angiitis of the central nervous system	Elevated protein
Systemic lupus erythematosus	Elevated protein
?Chronic idiopathic benign meningitis	Elevated protein

CSF = cerebrospinal fluid.

TABLE 412-15　CAUSES OF CHRONIC (PERSISTENT) MENINGITIS WITH NEUTROPHIL PREDOMINANCE

UNCOMMON	OTHER CSF FINDINGS
BACTERIAL	
Nocardia asteroides	Low glucose, markedly elevated protein, culture positive
Actinomyces israelii	Low glucose, elevated protein, anaerobic culture positive
Arachnia propionica	Low glucose, elevated protein, anaerobic culture positive
FUNGAL	
Candida sp	Low glucose, elevated protein, culture positive
Aspergillus sp	Low glucose, elevated protein, enzyme immunoassay or enzyme-linked immunosorbent assay for Aspergillus galactomannan
Zygomycetes	Low glucose, elevated protein
Dematiaceous fungi	Low glucose, protein may be markedly elevated
NONINFECTIOUS	
Systemic lupus erythematosus	Low glucose, elevated protein
Chemical meningitis	Low glucose, protein may be markedly elevated
VERY RARE	
Bacterial	
Brucella sp	Low glucose, elevated protein
Mycobacterium tuberculosis	Low glucose, elevated protein, polymerase chain reaction positive for M. tuberculosis DNA
Fungal	
Pseudoallescheria boydii	Low glucose, protein may be markedly elevated
Coccidioides immitis	Low glucose, elevated protein, presence of complement-fixing antibody
Blastomyces dermatitidis	Low glucose, protein elevated, antigen detection possible in CSF and urine
Histoplasma capsulatum	Low glucose; protein mildly elevated; complement-fixing antibodies in CSF; antigen detectable in CSF, urine, serum

CSF = cerebrospinal fluid.

nerve palsies. Granulomatosis with polyangiitis (Chapter 270) may produce meningeal inflammation and cranial nerve palsies, often in association with air sinus disease. The diagnosis is suggested by lesions on the chest radiograph, microscopic hematuria, skin lesions, peripheral neuropathy, and serum antineutrophil cytoplasmic antibodies. Aseptic meningitis associated with systemic lupus erythematosus (Chapter 266) may be accompanied by other neurologic manifestations (seizures, encephalopathy, stroke, transverse myelopathy), systemic manifestations (rash, arthritis), and antinuclear and anti-DNA antibodies.

Chronic (Intermittent) Meningitis

In chronic intermittent meningitis, all clinical and CSF abnormalities resolve completely between episodes without antimicrobial therapy (see Table 412-11). Uncommonly, a patient may have several episodes resulting from different viral agents. The major causes of recurrent aseptic meningitis are infections (almost always viral and resulting from HSV-2), endogenous chemical meningitis, drug hypersensitivity (including the use of intravenous immunoglobulins) with meningitis following each use, and inflammatory and autoimmune diseases.

In HSV-2 recurrent meningitis, lymphocytes predominate, with the cell numbers being approximately 40% higher in the initial episode than in recurrences. Leakage of material from intracranial epidermoid cysts produces 1000 to 5000 cells/μL (≈80% polymorphonuclear leukocytes) initially, with a subsequent mononuclear cell predominance. Occasionally, polarizing microscopy may demonstrate keratin and cholesterol crystals in the CSF of patients with endogenous chemical meningitis. In Behçet syndrome (Chapter 270), the CSF may have predominantly mononuclear cells or polymorphonuclear leukocytes. Mollaret meningitis, a syndrome of benign recurrent meningitis usually caused by HSV-2, is initially associated with neutrophils and monocytes in the CSF without hypoglycorrhachia but subsequently transitions to a predominantly lymphocytic pleocytosis. However, prolonged treatment with valcyclovir 1 g/day does not prevent recurrences of HSV-2–associated meningitis. Vogt-Koyanagi-Harada syndrome, a rare uveomeningoencephalitis, consists of recurrent meningitis/meningoencephalitis and anterior or posterior uveitis, followed by vitiligo, poliosis, alopecia, and dysacousia; the CSF cellular response is mononuclear, and an autoimmune origin, directed against a melanocyte antigen, has been suggested.

Chronic Meningitis with Predominantly Neutrophilic Pleocytosis

Chronic persistent neutrophilic meningitis (Table 412-15) is defined by the following combination: (1) clinical features consistent with meningitis; (2) initial CSF examination showing greater than 50% neutrophils, hypoglycorrhachia, and elevated protein concentration; (3) antimicrobial therapy that would be appropriate for the usual causes of bacterial meningitis; (4) negative smears and cultures for bacteria on the initial CSF specimen; and (5) repeated CSF examination 7 days or more after initial analysis showing 50% or greater neutrophils, hypoglycorrhachia, and elevated protein concentration.

Among the bacterial causes (see Table 412-15) are organisms (Actinomyces israelii and Arachnia propionica [Chapter 329]) that can be isolated by culture only under anaerobic conditions. Coexisting pulmonary lesions may suggest Nocardia (Chapter 330) or M. tuberculosis (Chapter 324) as the cause, although the initial polymorphonuclear pleocytosis present in some cases uncommonly persists much beyond a week before changing to a lymphocytic predominance. Brucella (Chapter 310) and endemic invasive mycotic infections would be suggested by epidemiologic considerations. Other fungal causes may be diagnosed, particularly in immunocompromised patients, by antigen testing with enzyme-linked immunosorbent assay (Aspergillus sp galactomannan; Chapter 339), or meningeal biopsy may be required.

Occasionally, exogenous chemical meningitis secondary to intrathecal injection of antimicrobials, chemotherapeutic agents, or contrast media may produce persisting pleocytosis and hypoglycorrhachia resulting from sclerosing arachnoiditis well after the inciting medication has been withdrawn. Systemic lupus erythematosus (Chapter 266) can produce a variety of meningitides, including acute lymphocytic or neutrophilic aseptic meningitis, as well as chronic persistent lymphocytic or neutrophilic CSF responses.

Eosinophilic Meningitis

The presence of 5% or greater eosinophils in CSF is uncommon and suggests parasitic disease, certain fungal infections such as coccidioidal or candidal meningitis, neoplastic diseases, or a few inflammatory processes (see Table 412-13).[15] In most cases, eosinophils are mixed with lymphocytes, which predominate; the highest percentage of eosinophils is seen with meningitis caused by migrating larvae of the raccoon ascarid *Baylisascaris procyonis* (Chapter 357) and the rat lung worm *Angiostrongylus cantonensis* (Chapter 357). In fungal meningitides, particularly those resulting from *C. immitis* (Chapter 333), the CSF response is primarily mononuclear with 6 to 20% eosinophils; hypoglycorrhachia may be a feature of *C. immitis* and *Candida* meningitis (Chapter 338) and of neoplastic processes and sarcoid.

Most patients with eosinophilic meningitis, except those with cases resulting from trichinosis (Chapter 357) or drug hypersensitivity, have prolonged symptoms suggesting chronic meningitis. Most patients with meningitis of parasitic or neoplastic origin have evidence of cerebral involvement as well.

Grade A References

A1. Molyneux E, Nizami SQ, Saha S, et al. 5 versus 10 days of treatment with ceftriaxone for bacterial meningitis in children: a double-blind randomised equivalence study. *Lancet*. 2011;377: 1837-1845.

A2. van de Beek D, Farrar JJ, de Gans J, et al. Adjunctive dexamethasone in bacterial meningitis: a meta-analysis of individual patient data. *Lancet Neurol*. 2010;9:254-263.

A3. Nguyen TH, Tran TH, Thwaites G, et al. Dexamethasone in Vietnamese adolescents and adults with bacterial meningitis. *N Engl J Med*. 2007;357:2431-2440.

A4. Scarborough M, Gordon SB, Whitty CJ, et al. Corticosteroids for bacterial meningitis in adults in sub-Saharan Africa. *N Engl J Med*. 2007;357:2441-2450.

A5. Brouwer MC, McIntyre P, Prasad K, et al. Corticosteroids for acute bacterial meningitis. *Cochrane Database Syst Rev*. 2013;6:CD004405.

A6. Fritz D, Brouwer MC, van de Beek D. Dexamethasone and long-term survival in bacterial meningitis. *Neurology*. 2012;79:2177-2179.

A7. Mourvillier B, Tubach F, van de Beek D, et al. Induced hypothermia in severe bacterial meningitis: a randomized clinical trial. *JAMA*. 2013;310:2174-2183.

A8. Aurelius E, Franzen-Rohl E, Glimaker M, et al. Long-term valacyclovir suppressive treatment after herpes simplex virus type 2 meningitis: a double-blind, randomized controlled trial. *Clin Infect Dis*. 2012;54:1304-1313.

A9. Day JN, Chau TT, Wolbers M, et al. Combination antifungal therapy for cryptococcal meningitis. *N Engl J Med*. 2013;368:1291-1302.

GENERAL REFERENCES

For the General References and other additional features, please visit Expert Consult at https://expertconsult.inkling.com.

413

BRAIN ABSCESS AND PARAMENINGEAL INFECTIONS

AVINDRA NATH AND JOSEPH BERGER

Brain abscess affects the brain's parenchyma directly, whereas parameningeal infections produce suppuration in potential spaces covering the brain and spinal cord (epidural abscess and subdural empyema) or produce occlusion of the contiguous venous sinuses and cerebral veins (cerebral venous sinus thrombosis).

BRAIN ABSCESS

EPIDEMIOLOGY

The frequency of various causes of brain abscess (Table 413-1) in the population has been difficult to ascertain because of wide variations among case series, in part as a result of referral patterns. In addition, children with brain abscesses often have cyanotic congenital heart disease or otogenic infection. Cryptogenic abscesses account for a greater percentage of cases in more recent series, perhaps related to the presence of a patent foramen ovale. On average, 90% of brain abscesses occur as a consequence of a focus of suppuration elsewhere in the body, with the remainder due to introduction of the infection from head wounds or neurosurgical procedures. Males predominate in virtually all series of brain abscess. Terminally ill patients in whom medical care is withdrawn may be found to have abscesses at autopsy, but these abscesses are of little clinical importance.

PATHOBIOLOGY

Brain abscesses are collections of purulent material (neutrophils and necrotic tissue) caused by infection with a variety of bacterial, fungal, and parasitic

organisms. Infection arising from other sites typically seeds the brain hematogenously. When contiguous to the brain, infection enters the brain by direct extension or by traveling along veins with associated thrombophlebitis of pial veins and sinuses. Within the brain, the infection begins as a cerebritis with perivascular infiltrates and infiltration of neutrophils into the brain parenchyma. With time, the developing abscess is characterized by a purulent exudate that includes necrotic brain tissue as well as viable and necrotic neutrophils. Granulation tissue develops at the interface between necrotic and viable tissue, and eventually, the abscess is walled off by a fibrous capsule. Formation of the capsule depends on the virulence of the organism and the immune status of the individual. More virulent organisms are associated with larger lesions, more necrosis, earlier ependymitis, and a greater degree of inflammation outside the collagen capsule.

CLINICAL MANIFESTATIONS

The clinical picture reflects a triad of the infectious nature of the lesion, focal brain involvement, and an increasing intracranial mass effect (Table 413-2).[1] One or two elements may be absent in a given case, particularly early in the course. Among infectious symptoms, fever is present at onset or early in the course in only about 60% of cases. Neck stiffness is an infrequent complaint, and meningeal signs are elicited in about 30% of cases. The absence of classical signs may delay diagnosis.[2]

Focal neurologic deficits depend on the site and size of the lesion, which in turn will be determined by the causal or predisposing condition. In some patients, seizures precede the diagnosis. The early deficits in patients with temporal lobe lesions, which are typically caused by spread of an otogenic

TABLE 413-1	CONDITIONS THAT PREDISPOSE TO THE DEVELOPMENT OF BRAIN ABSCESS
Otogenic	
Otitis media	
Mastoiditis	
Dental	
Cardiac	
Cyanotic heart disease	
Tetralogy of Fallot	
Patent foramen ovale	
Infective endocarditis	
Pulmonary	
Pulmonary arteriovenous fistula	
Lung infection	
Lung abscess	
Bronchiectasis	
Esophageal strictures	
Cerebral infarcts and tumors	
Penetrating and nonpenetrating head injury	
Postoperative neurosurgical procedure (trauma and nontrauma related)	
Dermal sinus tracts	
Sepsis	
Immunosuppression	
Unknown mechanism	

TABLE 413-2	BRAIN ABSCESS: INITIAL FEATURES IN 123 CASES
Headache	55%
Disturbed consciousness	48%
Fever	58%
Nuchal rigidity	29%
Nausea, vomiting	32%
Seizures	19%
Visual disturbance	15%
Dysarthria	20%
Hemiparesis	48%
Sepsis	17%

abscess, are contralateral homonymous superior quadrantic visual field defects and, if in the dominant hemisphere, aphasia. Motor deficits eventually occur in 40 to 50% of supratentorial abscesses. Cerebellar abscesses, which are often caused by aural-mastoid infections, are characterized by ipsilateral limb ataxia; there may also be abnormal head positioning (forward and away from the side of the lesion) and nystagmus that is slow and coarse on gaze to the side of the abscess and rapid in the opposite direction. Patients with multiple brain abscesses may have multifocal signs or encephalopathy. Patients with *Toxoplasma* species (Chapter 349) brain abscesses often have movement disorders because these abscesses frequently localize to the basal ganglia. In fact, nearly all patients with human immunodeficiency virus (HIV) infection in whom hemiballism or hemichorea is present have *Toxoplasma* species brain abscesses.

Headache is an important initial symptom in 80 to 90% of patients with bacterial abscess but is less frequent (≈20%) in patients with fungal abscesses. Symptoms of increased intracranial pressure, such as nausea, depressed level of consciousness, and papilledema, occur less often. The development of headache in a patient with a known chronic anaerobic infection, such as aural-mastoid, paranasal sinus, or pulmonary suppuration, suggests the possibility of brain abscess. Similarly, the development of headache in a child with cyanotic congenital heart disease is often related to a brain abscess. Tetralogy of Fallot (Chapter 69) is the most common congenital heart anomaly associated with brain abscess.

DIAGNOSIS

Examination of the cranium, ears, paranasal sinuses, oral cavity, heart, and lungs may provide important clues to the etiology, as may overt signs of infection at other sites. Cultures of blood and sputum may identify the organism and its antimicrobial sensitivity. In patients with signs of raised intracranial pressure, lumbar puncture may be contraindicated because of the risk of herniation.

Magnetic resonance imaging (MRI) can detect early changes such as brain edema and is preferable to computed tomography (CT).[3] In the early cerebritis stage, T2-weighted MRI shows abnormally high signal intensity corresponding to low signal intensity on the T1-weighted images. The fluid-attenuated inversion recovery (FLAIR) sequence provides superior visualization of brain edema. On T1-weighted images, the area of cerebritis that is seen initially as a low-signal-intensity, ill-defined area later progresses to a central cavity with slightly higher signal intensity than cerebrospinal fluid (CSF), surrounded by edema that is slightly hypointense in comparison to brain parenchyma. Later stages of infection show central necrosis and formation of a rim of slightly high signal intensity on T1-weighted images (Fig. 413-1). With gadolinium administration, there is a ring-enhancing lesion. Diffusion-weighted imaging helps differentiate abscesses from brain tumors; an abscess cavity demonstrates high signal with decreased apparent diffusion coefficient values, whereas necrotic tumor cavities demonstrate the opposite.

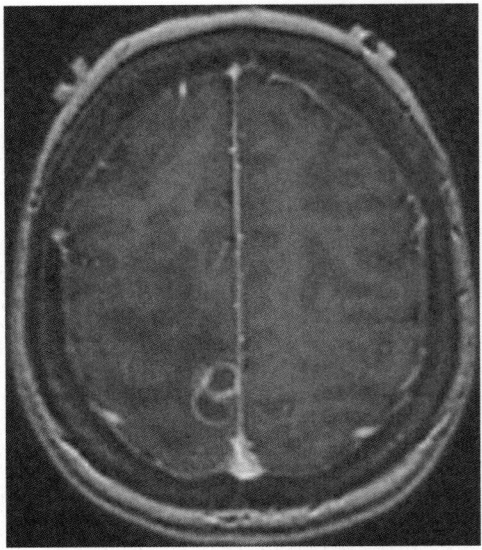

FIGURE 413-1. Brain abscess. Magnetic resonance imaging with gadolinium shows a multiloculated ring-enhancing lesion caused by *Nocardia* species infection.

Surgical aspiration or excision of the lesion may be necessary to establish a microbial diagnosis. Gram stain and culture from abscess fluid, with proper handling, have high yield, with or without previous antibiotic therapy. If immediate surgery is planned, antibiotics can be deferred until culture material has been acquired. Multiplex polymerase chain reaction testing is being developed for rapid identification of bacterial organisms and detection of antibiotic resistance genes.

TREATMENT   Rx

Brain abscess requires urgent intervention.[4] Because of the risk for cerebral herniation with large lesions, treatment of cerebral edema (intravenous (IV) dexamethasone, 16 to 24 mg/day in four divided doses) may be needed even while initiating surgical intervention. Corticosteroids often decrease edema within 8 hours but may retard the formation of a capsule around the brain abscess, suppress the immune response to the infection, and decrease penetration of antibiotics. Hence, they should be used for short periods, usually only until surgical decompression by needle drainage or surgical removal is possible. Empirical antibiotic therapy (Table 413-3) is recommended prior to surgery, based on the likely source of infection.

Successful antibiotic management of brain abscess is based on knowledge of proved or suspected pathogens as well as familiarity with a drug's spectrum of activity and penetration into the central nervous system. When surgery cannot be performed, empirical antibiotic therapy must be initiated. A trial of nonsurgical treatment may be considered in patients with (1) small lesion size, (2) an already identified pathogen, (3) no symptoms or signs of increased intracranial pressure requiring neurosurgical intervention, (4) a deep or inaccessible lesion, (5) multiple abscesses, (6) a contraindication to surgery (e.g., a bleeding diathesis), (7) a short duration of symptoms, which suggests that the lesion is in the cerebritis stage, and (8) availability of monitoring with MRI.[5]

In patients who are suspected of having a brain stem abscess, the possibility of listerial infection (Chapter 293) should be considered (Fig. 413-2), even in the absence of a clear immunodeficiency. Empirical parenteral antibiotics to cover *Listeria* species should be started (Chapter 293).

Brain abscesses caused by *Toxoplasma* species (Chapter 349) usually occur in immunocompromised patients (e.g., patients with HIV infection), are not accompanied by capsule formation, and hence respond well to antibiotic therapy alone. As a result, patients with acquired immunodeficiency syndrome and suspected cerebral toxoplasmosis (Chapter 349) should receive antimicrobial therapy initially.

TABLE 413-3	COMMON PATHOGENS AND EMPIRICAL THERAPY FOR BRAIN ABSCESS	
PREDISPOSING CONDITION	**COMMON PATHOGENS**	**ANTIMICROBIAL AGENTS***
Dental abscess	Streptococci, *Bacteroides fragilis*	Penicillin + metronidazole
Chronic otitis	*Bacteroides fragilis*; *Pseudomonas, Proteus, Klebsiella* species	Cefotaxime or ceftriaxone + metronidazole; ceftazidime or cefepime for *Pseudomonas* species
Sinusitis	Streptococci; *Haemophilus, Staphylococcus* species	Cefotaxime, ceftriaxone, or nafcillin + metronidazole
Penetrating trauma or postsurgical	*Staphylococcus, Pseudomonas, Enterobacter* species; streptococci	Nafcillin or vancomycin + ceftriaxone or cefotaxime + metronidazole
Bacterial endocarditis or drug use	Mixed flora, streptococci, *Staphylococcus* species	Nafcillin or vancomycin + ceftriaxone or cefotaxime + metronidazole
Congenital heart disease	Streptococci	Cefotaxime or ceftriaxone
Pulmonary infection	*Nocardia* species, *Bacteroides fragilis*, streptococci, mixed flora	Penicillin + metronidazole + trimethoprim-sulfamethoxazole
HIV infection	*Toxoplasma gondii*	Pyrimethamine + sulfadiazine + folinic acid

*See Table 287-4 in Chapter 287 for dosing schedules.

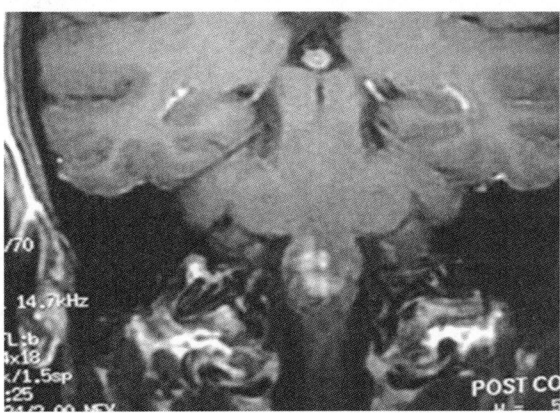

FIGURE 413-2. Brain stem abscess. Magnetic resonance imaging with gadolinium shows an enhancing lesion in the brain stem caused by *Listeria* species infection.

TABLE 413-4 INITIAL CHARACTERISTICS OF 915 PATIENTS WITH SPINAL EPIDURAL ABSCESS

STAGE 1	
Back pain	71%
Fever	66%
STAGE 2	
Radicular pain	20%
STAGE 3	
Muscle weakness	26%
Sphincter incontinence	24%
Sensory deficits	13%
STAGE 4	
Paralysis	31%
Quadriplegia	3%

From Reihsaus E, Waldbaur H, Seeling W. Spinal epidural abscess: a meta-analysis of 915 patients. *Neurosurg Rev.* 2000;23:175-204.

PROGNOSIS

Before the CT scan era, the mortality of brain abscesses ranged from 40 to 60%, and even with the drastic reduction in mortality in the era of modern neuroimaging, the mortality rate remains about 10%.[6] About 70% of patients recover fully. In post-transplantation patients and those with deep hemispheric or brain stem abscesses, mortality rates may exceed 80%. Other factors associated with a poor prognosis include extremes of age, multiple abscesses, and diagnostic delay in the absence of systemic signs of infection. Impaired level of consciousness is a poor prognostic sign even with early hospitalization and rapid diagnosis. Anaerobic and gram-negative organisms and culture-negative cases also have a poor prognosis. Seizures (Chapter 403) develop in up to 50% of patients, sometimes after latencies as long as 5 years.

SPINAL EPIDURAL ABSCESS

DEFINITION

Infection within the epidural space around the spinal cord is an uncommon but often readily treatable potential cause of paralysis and death. The epidural space surrounds the dural sac and is limited by the posterior longitudinal ligament anteriorly, the ligamenta flava and the periosteum of the laminae posteriorly, and the pedicles of the spinal column and the intervertebral foramina containing their neural elements laterally. The space communicates with the paravertebral space through the intervertebral foramina. Superiorly, the space is closed at the foramen magnum. Caudally, the space is closed by the sacrococcygeal ligament. The epidural space contains loose areolar connective tissue, semiliquid fat, lymphatics, arteries, an extensive plexus of veins, and the spinal nerve roots.

EPIDEMIOLOGY

Spinal epidural abscesses can result from hematogenous spread of infection; risk factors include IV drug use, organ transplantation, chronic steroid use, malignancy, and diabetes. Local infection after acupuncture for back pain or epidural analgesia can also cause epidural abscesses. Cutaneous sites of infection are the most common remote sources, especially in IV drug users. Abdominal, respiratory tract, and urinary sources are also common. Osteomyelitis may be a cause of either direct extension or hematogenous spread, particularly when associated with sepsis. Contiguous spread may occur from epidurally placed catheters, psoas abscesses, decubitus ulceration, perinephric and retropharyngeal abscesses, or surgical sites. Minor back trauma has been implicated in causing a paraspinal hematoma, which may subsequently be seeded hematogenously. *Staphylococcus aureus* is the most common organism isolated from spinal epidural abscesses. In 2012, an outbreak of fungal paraspinal infections was attributed to epidural injections of contaminated methylprednisolone.[7]

PATHOBIOLOGY

Because the dura mater around the cord is adherent to the vertebral column anteriorly, more epidural abscesses lie posteriorly, and because no anatomic barriers separate the spinal segments in the posterior epidural space, such abscesses usually extend over several vertebral segments. Spinal cord dysfunction probably reflects toxic processes secondary to inflammation, as well as venous thrombosis, thrombophlebitis, ischemia secondary to compression of the spinal arteries, and edema.

CLINICAL MANIFESTATIONS

The presence of a risk factor (>80% of patients) in the setting of neurologic deficits or back or radicular pain should suggest a spinal epidural abscess. The clinical manifestations can be divided into four stages (Table 413-4). Back pain (71%), fever (66%), tenderness of the spine with focal percussion (17%), spinal irritation (20%), and headache (3%) are common.[8] Radicular pain can be mistaken for sciatica, a visceral abdominal process, chest wall pain, or cervical disc disease. Clinical signs are often substantially greater than would be predicted from the anatomic extent of pus or granulation tissue.

Unfortunately, the diagnosis often is missed initially. If the condition goes unrecognized at an early stage, the symptoms can evolve over a period of hours to days to paralysis below the spinal level of infection.

DIAGNOSIS

The differential diagnosis includes compressive and inflammatory processes involving the spinal cord: transverse myelitis (Chapter 411), herniation of an intervertebral disc (Chapter 400), epidural hemorrhage (Chapter 400), or metastatic tumor (Chapter 189), none of which are associated with evidence of systemic infection. Blood leukocytosis may not be present, but the sedimentation rate is often elevated. Other infectious processes that may produce back or neck pain or tenderness must be excluded: bacterial meningitis (Chapter 412), perinephric abscess, disc space infection, and bacterial endocarditis (Chapter 76).

Lumbar puncture should be avoided in patients suspected of having a spinal epidural abscess, for fear of spreading the infection to the subarachnoid space and causing meningitis. Gadolinium-enhanced MRI (Fig. 413-3) is the method of choice for diagnosis,[9] but MRI findings in patients undergoing epidural analgesia can resemble those of epidural spinal abscess even when no infection is present.

TREATMENT   Rx

Patients with a progressing neurologic deficit should undergo urgent surgical drainage; CT-guided aspiration may be useful, and antibiotics plus percutaneously guided needle aspiration may be as therapeutically effective as antibiotics plus surgery. Unless culture results and sensitivities dictate otherwise, empirical therapy should cover *S. aureus* (nafcillin, 2 g every 6 hours; vancomycin, 1 g every 12 hours for methicillin-resistant strains). Additional gram-negative coverage with a third-generation cephalosporin (e.g., cefotaxime, 2 g every 6 hours, or ceftriaxone, 2 g every 12 hours) or a quinolone (e.g., ciprofloxacin, 400 mg every 12 hours) should be considered for severe disease. Rifampin (300 mg every 12 hours) may be added because of its ability to penetrate the abscess cavity. IV therapy should be continued for 3 to 4 weeks except in the presence of osteomyelitis (6 to 8 weeks).

PROGNOSIS

The mortality rate associated with spinal epidural abscess is about 15%. Approximately 50% of survivors have residual neurologic deficits. More severe preoperative neurologic deficits and deficits of longer duration are associated with a worse prognosis. In general, patients who develop paralysis that persists for longer than 36 hours do not recover function.

SUBDURAL EMPYEMA

Subdural empyema is an infection in the space between the dura and the arachnoid. It usually results from infected paranasal sinuses and rarely from infected mastoid sinuses by extension of thrombophlebitis from the sinuses into the subdural space. The infection is most commonly unilateral because bilateral spread is prevented by the falx. The empyema may evolve to cause cortical vein thrombosis, cerebral abscesses, or purulent meningitis.

CLINICAL FEATURES AND DIAGNOSIS

The most common symptoms are headache, fever, a neurologic deficit, and a stiff neck. However, subdural empyema may progress and cause signs of raised intracranial pressure, such as vomiting, altered level of consciousness, seizures, and papilledema. A high degree of suspicion is needed to establish the diagnosis early in the course of the illness. In patients with sinusitis (Chapter 426), the symptoms of subdural empyema may be incorrectly attributed to the sinusitis.

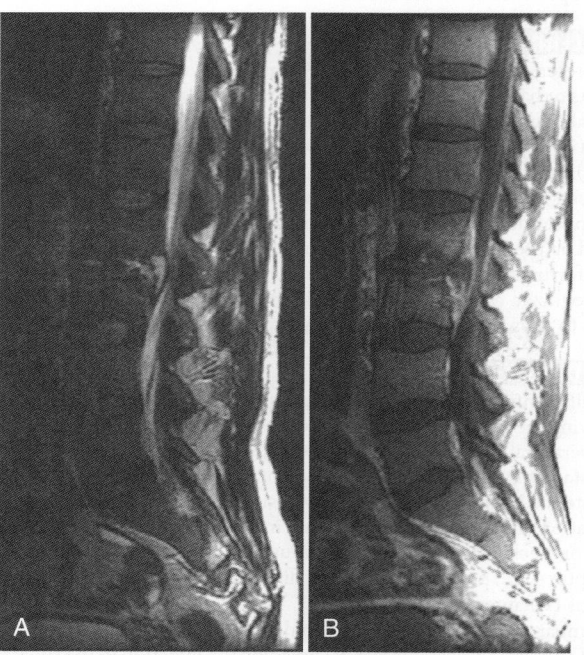

FIGURE 413-3. Spinal epidural abscess. A and B, Magnetic resonance images of the lumbosacral spine show a lesion in the epidural space compressing the thecal sac.

MRI with gadolinium enhancement and diffusion-weighted images is particularly useful in visualizing the subdural infection as a crescent-shaped mass with an enhancing rim over the cerebral convexities and below the inner table of the skull (Fig. 413-4). CSF evaluation is useful only if there is accompanying meningitis. In a patient with signs of raised intracranial pressure, lumbar puncture should be avoided because of the risk for herniation.

TREATMENT ▸ Rx

Surgical drainage of the empyema is mandatory. IV antibiotic therapy is also necessary and is based on the organisms isolated at the time of craniotomy.

PROGNOSIS

Mortality rates in most series are about 25%, with severe neurologic sequelae remaining in 20% of survivors. Accompanying venous sinus thrombosis or brain abscess carries a poor prognosis.

VENOUS SINUS THROMBOSIS SECONDARY TO INFECTION

The venous sinus system (Fig. 413-5) lacks valves, thereby permitting retrograde propagation of clots or infections that emanate from structures located in the central portion of the face or the middle ear.[10]

Septic Cavernous Sinus Thrombosis
DEFINITION

The cavernous sinuses are the most caudal dural venous chambers at the base of the skull. The paired structures lie on either side of the pituitary fossa immediately above the midline sphenoid sinus. The cavernous sinus encloses the "cavernous portion" of the internal carotid artery as well as the third, fourth, and sixth cranial nerves en route to the apex of the orbit.

EPIDEMIOLOGY AND PATHOBIOLOGY

The infection usually spreads from the paranasal sinuses, dental abscesses, or other infections affecting the orbit or middle third of the face. *S. aureus* is the most common organism. Streptococci, pneumococci, and gram-negative bacilli are less common; anaerobic infection has also been reported. Many cases of idiopathic intracranial hypertension (Chapters 189 and 398) are due to thrombosis in the lateral sinuses.

CLINICAL MANIFESTATIONS

Cavernous sinus thrombosis may be manifested as an acute fulminant disease or have an indolent subacute manifestation. Fever and other systemic symptoms from sepsis may be present. Clinical symptoms and signs are related to anatomic structures within the cavernous sinuses or drained by them: unilateral periorbital edema, headache, photophobia, proptosis, ophthalmoplegia, pupillary dilation, decreased corneal reflex, and periorbital sensory loss. Obstruction of venous drainage from the retina can result in papilledema, retinal hemorrhages, and visual loss. The infection can spread rapidly (24 to 48 hours) through the intercavernous sinuses to the contralateral cavernous sinus. Thrombus can extend to other dural venous sinuses, adjacent vascular structures, or the brain parenchyma.

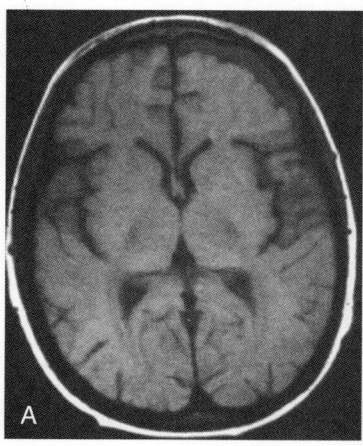
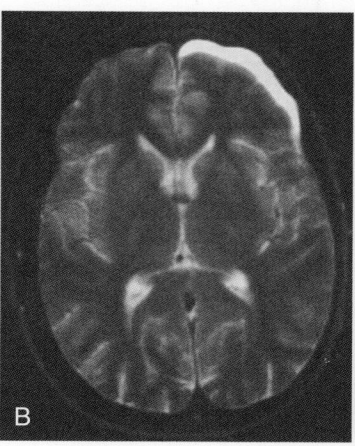
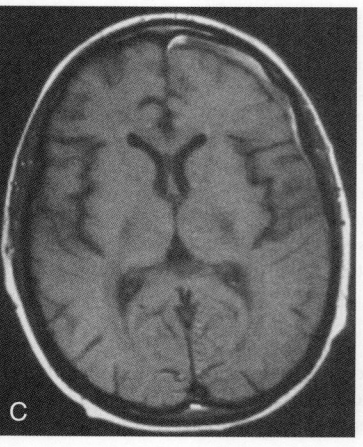

FIGURE 413-4. Subdural abscess. A, T1-weighted MRI shows a hypodense area in the left frontal region. B, T2-weighted image shows increased signal intensity in the same region. C, A contrast scan shows enhancement in the same region.

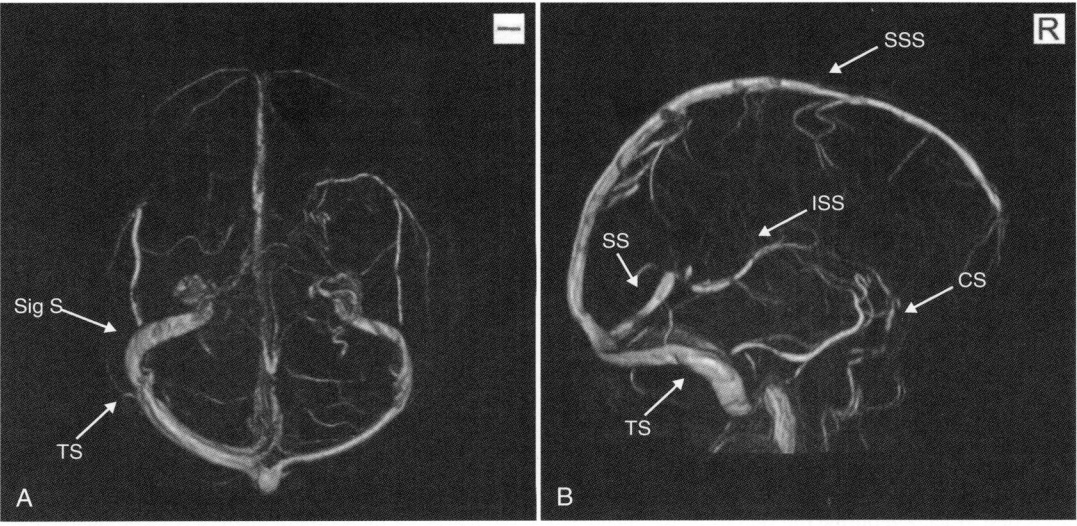

FIGURE 413-5. Anatomy of major venous sinuses. Magnetic resonance venography of the brain shows the normal venous sinuses. A shows sigmoid sinus (Sig S) and transverse sinus (TS). B shows superior sagittal sinus (SSS), inferior sagittal sinus (ISS), straight sinus (SS), transverse sinus (TS), and cavernous sinus (CS).

DIAGNOSIS

The diagnosis is made on clinical findings and confirmed by radiographic studies. Radiologic evaluation includes sinus imaging, particularly the sphenoid and ethmoid sinuses. MRI using flow parameters and MR venogram is sensitive and may reveal deformity of the cavernous portion of the internal carotid artery, a heterogeneous signal from the abnormal cavernous sinus, and an obvious hyperintense signal of thrombosed vascular sinuses. MRI with IV gadolinium can demonstrate venous thrombosis by illustrating a lack of the normal "flow void" within vascular structures. Cranial CT scans are less helpful but may show a subtle increase in the size and enhancement of the thrombosed sinus. MR angiography may demonstrate extrinsic narrowing of the intracavernous portion of the internal carotid artery.

TREATMENT AND PROGNOSIS   Rx

Blood cultures are often negative, so delays in diagnosis are common. Even when the diagnosis is established, empirical antimicrobial treatment may not provide full coverage.

Treatment consists of prompt drainage of infected paranasal sinuses or other identifiable source of infection, as well as specific antistaphylococcal agents (Chapter 288). Heparin anticoagulation without a loading dose is sometimes initiated to reduce morbidity from associated brain ischemia, but experience in septic venous thrombosis is limited compared with the more frequent use of anticoagulation in nonseptic venous thromboses. Hemorrhage caused by anticoagulation is rare in this setting. Despite modern therapy, mortality rates remain as high as 44%.

Lateral Sinus Thrombosis

Septic thrombosis of the lateral sinus results from acute or chronic infections of the middle ear.

CLINICAL MANIFESTATIONS AND DIAGNOSIS

Symptoms consist of ear pain and fever followed by headache, nausea, vomiting, loss of hearing, and vertigo, usually evolving over a period of several weeks. Symptoms or signs suggestive of otitis media (Chapter 426), including mastoid swelling, may be seen. Sixth cranial nerve palsies can occur, but other focal neurologic signs are rare. In some patients with nonseptic lateral sinus thrombosis, headache may be the only symptom. Papilledema occurs in 50% of cases, and elevated CSF pressure is present in most, especially with occlusion of the right lateral sinus, which is the major venous conduit from the superior sagittal sinus (Fig. 413-6).

CSF is usually normal, although a parameningeal inflammatory profile (mild pleocytosis, slight elevation in protein level, and a normal glucose level) may be seen. The diagnosis is confirmed by MR venography.

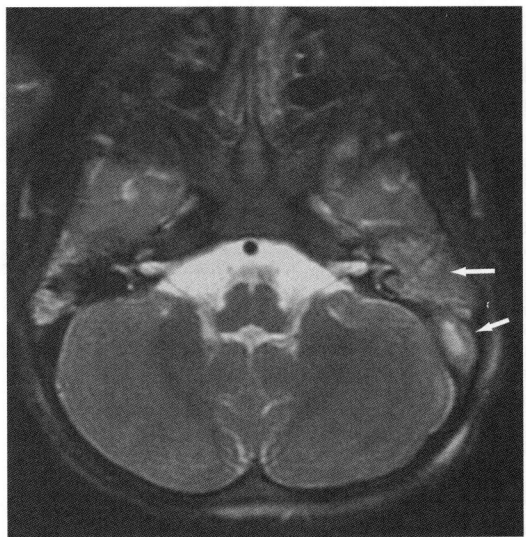

FIGURE 413-6. Lateral sinus thrombosis. Magnetic resonance imaging shows a thrombus in the lateral sinus (*short arrow*) with accompanying mastoiditis (*long arrow*).

TREATMENT   Rx

Treatment includes IV antibiotics to cover staphylococci, anaerobes, and gram-negative bacilli such as *Proteus* species and *Escherichia coli* (nafcillin, 2 g every 6 hours, or vancomycin, 1 g every 12 hours; plus cefotaxime, 2 g every 6 hours, or ceftriaxone, 2 g every 12 hours; plus metronidazole, 7.5 mg/kg every 6 hours, or clindamycin, 300 mg every 6 hours; plus ciprofloxacin, 400 mg every 12 hours). Surgical drainage (mastoidectomy or tympanoplasty) may be required to eradicate the nidus of infection and determine the antibiotic susceptibility of the organism. If the sinus contains pus, it must be opened so the septic thrombus can be removed. Unless vision is compromised, increased intracranial pressure seldom requires specific treatment such as drainage or placement of a shunt.

PROGNOSIS

Broad IV antibiotic coverage and eradication of the perisinus infection, which may require surgical drainage, early in the course of the illness lead to a good prognosis. Neurologic sequelae may include a sixth nerve palsy, ataxia, and hearing loss.

Septic Sagittal Sinus Thrombosis

Although superior sagittal sinus thrombosis is the most common form of venous sinus thrombosis and is frequently associated with the use of oral contraceptives, septic sagittal sinus thrombosis is an uncommon condition that occurs as a consequence of purulent meningitis, infections of the ethmoid or maxillary sinuses spreading through venous channels, compound infected skull fractures, or (rarely) neurosurgical wound infections.

CLINICAL MANIFESTATIONS AND DIAGNOSIS

Symptoms are primarily related to the elevated intracranial pressure and can evolve rapidly to stupor and coma. Seizures and hemiparesis may result from cortical infarction. Early recognition and treatment are necessary because septic sagittal sinus thrombosis carries a high mortality rate. The rate of progression, severity of symptoms, and prognosis are all related to the location of thrombosis. Obstruction of the anterior third of the sinus produces less intense symptoms and evolves more slowly.

CSF abnormalities are frequent, including enough red blood cells that the CSF can sometimes be mistaken for a subarachnoid hemorrhage; the opening pressure is increased in proportion to the extent of sagittal sinus involvement. A septic sagittal sinus is best visualized during the venous phase of cerebral angiography or MR venography. The diagnosis can also be made by MRI, which demonstrates an abnormal increase in signal intensity (absent flow void) within the affected venous sinus. Contrast-enhanced CT scanning may reveal a contrast void lying at the junction of the transverse and sagittal sinuses (the region of the torcular); this so-called delta sign is an intraluminal clot surrounded by contrast material.

TREATMENT   Rx

IV antibiotics should be directed at organisms recovered from the meningeal process or the meningeal site. *S. aureus* (Chapter 288), β-hemolytic streptococci (Chapter 290), pneumococci (Chapter 289), and gram-negative aerobes such as *Klebsiella* species (Chapter 306) are the most common organisms. Associated paranasal sinusitis should be drained surgically.

PROGNOSIS

If the thrombosis progresses to involve the middle and posterior thirds of the sinus, deterioration progresses rapidly. The prognosis is poor, with a mortality rate of nearly 30%.

NEUROLOGIC COMPLICATIONS OF INFECTIOUS ENDOCARDITIS

Neurologic complications develop in nearly one third of patients with infective endocarditis (Chapter 76), and neurologic manifestations are the initial symptom in 20% of patients with infective endocarditis. In nearly 30% of patients, the neurologic complications occur within 2 weeks after the initiation of treatment. Stroke is the most common manifestation; most strokes are due to cerebral emboli, and others are due to intracerebral hemorrhage. Infective endocarditis should always be considered in a patient with a fever and stroke.

PATHOBIOLOGY

Cerebral embolization occurs as a result of dislodgement or disruption of the cardiac vegetations and frequently causes occlusion of cerebral blood vessels. Emboli occurring before the initiation or completion of treatment with antibiotics may contain microorganisms capable of causing metastatic infections such as abscesses, arteritis, meningitis, or mycotic aneurysms. Most cerebral emboli involve small or moderate-sized blood vessels, and multiple cerebral emboli are common. Intracranial hemorrhage is usually due to rupture of a mycotic aneurysm (Chapter 408), septic erosion of the arterial wall without the formation of an aneurysm, or hemorrhagic transformation of a large cerebral infarct. Mycotic aneurysms are observed in approximately 2 to 3% of patients with infective endocarditis. About 20% of patients with mycotic aneurysms have multiple aneurysms; involvement of the middle cerebral artery and its branches occurs in more than 75% of patients, unlike congenital aneurysms, which occur predominantly in the circle of Willis. Mycotic aneurysms develop as a result of either septic embolization into the vasa vasorum or direct penetration of the microorganism into the wall of the artery. Streptococci and staphylococci account for nearly 90% of all mycotic aneurysms.

CLINICAL MANIFESTATIONS

The nature of the clinical manifestations depends on the underlying pathophysiology.[11] Embolic stroke typically causes the acute onset of a focal neurologic deficit. Seizures may also occur. Multiple microemboli result in an altered or fluctuating level of consciousness not adequately explained by other abnormalities.

Most patients with mycotic aneurysms have a sudden, often fatal, subarachnoid or intracerebral hemorrhage without warning signs. Warning signs, if present, include severe localized headache, ischemic events, seizures, and cranial nerve abnormalities. In some patients, mycotic aneurysms may be asymptomatic and resolve with antibiotic therapy. Some patients develop micro- or macroabscesses, septic or aseptic meningitis (Chapter 412), or a generalized toxic metabolic encephalopathy.

DIAGNOSIS

MRI is the modality of choice for the diagnosis of cerebral infarcts and brain abscesses related to endocarditis. Gradient echo sequences on the MRI may be more sensitive than a CT scan for detecting intracranial hemorrhage and also can detect microbleeds. MRI should also include diffusion-weighted sequences for detection of infarcts. An MR angiogram is preferred for diagnosing an aneurysm. CSF evaluation is useful if accompanying meningitis or a slow leak from an aneurysm is suspected but not visualized with these imaging tests.

TREATMENT   Rx

Treatment of patients with infective endocarditis and cerebral emboli requires prevention of embolization with appropriate antibiotic therapy and sometimes cardiac surgery (Chapter 76). Anticoagulation is contraindicated in patients with cerebral infarcts and septic emboli because of the high risk for complications from intracerebral bleeding.

Patients with unruptured aneurysms smaller than 7 mm in diameter, proximal aneurysms, multiple aneurysms, ruptured aneurysms without an intracerebral hematoma, and aneurysms for which excision is likely to cause a neurologic deficit can be monitored conservatively with serial MRI and MR angiography. All other aneurysms require surgical excision of the aneurysm and the adjacent septic vessel wall. Patients who cannot undergo surgery may be candidates for endovascular embolization of the aneurysmal vessel.

PROGNOSIS

Mortality rates in patients with infective endocarditis and cerebral emboli range from 30 to 80%.[12] Mortality is high if there is hemorrhagic transformation of the infarct. Mortality in patients with ruptured mycotic aneurysms is 80%, and even patients with unruptured aneurysms have a mortality rate of 30%.

GENERAL REFERENCES

For the General References and other additional features, please visit Expert Consult at https://expertconsult.inkling.com.

414

ACUTE VIRAL ENCEPHALITIS

ALLEN J. AKSAMIT JR.

DEFINITION

Encephalitis is a diffuse or focal inflammation of the parenchyma of the brain. The term *encephalitis* indicates that the predominant clinical syndrome arises from infection and inflammation in the parenchyma of the brain rather than in the leptomeninges. When both the leptomeninges and brain parenchyma are involved, the term *meningoencephalitis* is used.

EPIDEMIOLOGY

Viral encephalitis has an estimated incidence of 7 per 100,000 per year. In general, a specific cause is identified in less than 50% of patients in the United

TABLE 414-1 COMMON CAUSES OF ENCEPHALITIS IN THE UNITED STATES

I. Causes of viral encephalitis
 A. Nonseasonal
  Herpes simplex virus type 1 (herpes simplex encephalitis)
  Herpes simplex virus type 2 (neonatal encephalitis or adult meningoencephalitis)
 B. Seasonal—summer and fall—arboviruses (arthropod borne)
  West Nile virus
  St. Louis encephalitis virus
  Eastern equine encephalitis virus
  Western equine encephalitis virus
  La Crosse/California encephalitis virus
 C. Seasonal—non–arthropod borne
  Summer and fall: enteroviruses (including coxsackieviruses, echoviruses, polioviruses, and enterovirus 71)
  Winter: influenza virus
 D. Immunosuppressed patients
  Human immunodeficiency virus (chronic HIV encephalitis)
  Varicella-zoster virus (subacute encephalitis)
  JC virus (progressive multifocal leukoencephalopathy)
  Cytomegalovirus (ventriculitis or encephalitis)
  Human herpesvirus 6 (subacute encephalitis)
  Epstein-Barr virus (subacute encephalitis)

II. Uncommon causes in the United States
  Powassan fever encephalitis virus
  Lymphotropic choriomeningitis virus
  Rabies
  Measles (subacute sclerosing panencephalitis)
  Mumps
  Adenovirus
  Herpes B virus (of monkeys)
  Rubella (progressive rubella panencephalitis)

III. Causes outside the United States
  Tick-borne encephalitis virus (Russia, Asia)
  Japanese encephalitis virus (Japan, Southeast Asia, Malaysia)
  Venezuelan equine encephalitis virus (Central and South America)
  Dengue virus (Southern Asia, Africa, South America)
  Rift Valley fever virus (east central Africa)
  Murray Valley encephalitis virus (Australia)
  Powassan fever encephalitis virus (Canada)
  Nipah virus (Malaysia and Bangladesh)

States. Many viruses (Table 414-1) are implicated, and testing by serologic or nucleic acid identification (by polymerase chain reaction [PCR]) is required to identify the specific virus.[1] The epidemiology of each virus responsible for central nervous system infection (see Table 414-1) is distinct in terms of the patients who are at highest risk, geographic distribution, and seasonal occurrence, especially the arboviruses (Chapter 383) and enteroviruses (Chapter 379), which are covered in separate chapters.

In the United States, the most common cause of nonepidemic encephalitis is herpes simplex encephalitis, which is caused by herpes simplex virus type 1 (Chapter 374). The most common epidemic virus in the United States is now West Nile virus (Chapter 383), which is a mosquito-transmitted Flavivirus related to St. Louis encephalitis virus and its Asian counterpart Japanese encephalitis virus. There is serologic cross-reactivity between St. Louis encephalitis, Japanese encephalitis, and West Nile viruses.

PATHOBIOLOGY

In general, gross pathologic inspection of an encephalitic brain does not reveal purulence visible to the naked eye. If focal purulence is present, *cerebritis* is the more correct term. If frank necrosis and purulence are present, the correct pathologic term is *brain abscess* (Chapter 413). Encephalitis, however, can be associated with substantial necrosis, and patients with severe acute viral encephalitides frequently have microscopic evidence of necrosis. Certain viral encephalitides, such as herpes simplex encephalitis, can be both focal and hemorrhagic. Viruses that cause acute encephalitis may often also cause meningitis (Chapter 412). Indeed, patients with encephalitis virtually always have some microscopic inflammatory changes in the leptomeninges. Conversely, patients with viral meningitis will inevitably have some component of microscopic encephalitis. The degree of inflammatory change present in the brain is determined by the individual viral pathogen and by host immune factors, which are responsible for the reaction to the invading virus.[2]

CLINICAL MANIFESTATIONS

The clinical findings in patients with acute viral encephalitis start with a prodrome of fever, headache, malaise, myalgia, and nonspecific symptoms.[3] Nausea, vomiting, diarrhea, cough, sore throat, and rash can precede the neurologic symptoms as part of the systemic initial manifestations of the infection. Invasion of the nervous system is typically accompanied by headache, photophobia, and altered consciousness, with symptoms progressing over a period of several days. Seizures are also a common heralding symptom. Signs of meningeal irritation may be present and are an unreliable finding in encephalitis.

Focal brain dysfunction is seen with some viruses. For example, West Nile virus (Chapter 383) can cause a brain stem encephalitis with an early onset of coma. Herpes simplex virus (Chapter 374) tends to cause focal cortical neurologic deficits, including hemiparesis, aphasia, and seizures. Limbic parts of the brain commonly involved by herpes simplex encephalitis or rabies can lead to prominent behavioral changes at the beginning of the illness before the patient's level of consciousness is depressed. Focal or generalized seizures are particularly common when encephalitis affects the hippocampus and limbic system. Rabies is typically associated with brain stem–mediated laryngospasm, hydrophobia, and depressed consciousness. Because of spinal cord anterior horn cell involvement, West Nile virus, St. Louis encephalitis virus, poliovirus, and rabies virus infections can cause focal or asymmetrical weakness with areflexia.

DIAGNOSIS

In patients with coma or focal deficits, computed tomography (CT) of the head should usually be performed before spinal fluid analysis to exclude a substantial mass effect and to avoid the risk of herniation during lumbar puncture.[4] In patients without focal findings, however, lumbar puncture should be performed immediately to establish the diagnosis and allow early empirical treatment. Opening pressures should be measured because increased intracranial pressure can occur with all forms of viral encephalitis and may need additional treatment.[5]

Spinal fluid analysis typically reveals an elevated protein level, which usually is less than 120 mg/dL. The cerebrospinal fluid (CSF) glucose level is typically normal and greater than 40% of the coincident serum value, but rare patients may have a low CSF glucose level suggestive of a bacterial infection (Chapter 412). The CSF white blood cell count is typically elevated, usually in the range of 10 to 500 cells/μL. The cell type is usually a lymphocytic predominance. However, a polymorphonuclear predominance is seen in some cases of West Nile encephalitis and cytomegalovirus ventriculitis.

Serologic or PCR testing on spinal fluid is helpful (Table 414-2). PCR testing has the added advantage of proving direct viral infection within the central nervous system, but serologic testing is more appropriate for some infections like West Nile virus encephalitis, which is best confirmed by an IgM antibody response in spinal fluid.

Magnetic resonance imaging (MRI) of the brain is the most sensitive technique for defining abnormalities in patients with viral encephalitis.[6] However, frank viral encephalitis can occur with normal findings on MRI. MRI findings also can suggest the responsible virus. For example, herpes simplex encephalitis has a characteristic pattern involving the mesiotemporal, inferofrontal, and insular cortices, usually unilateral or asymmetrically bilateral.

Differential Diagnosis

A number of nonviral pathogens can cause encephalitis that is clinically and pathologically indistinguishable from viral encephalitis.[7] Examples include *Rickettsia* (Chapter 327), *Borrelia* (Chapter 322), Whipple disease (Chapters 140 and 275), *Toxoplasma* (Chapter 349), *Mycoplasma* (Chapter 317) and *Acanthamoeba* (Chapter 352). Other forms of infectious non-viral causes mimicking viral encephalitis include bacterial cerebritis, meningovascular syphilis, and cerebral cysticercosis.

Additionally, autoimmune encephalitides can mimic viral encephalitis, including limbic paraneoplastic encephalitis, especially associated with antibodies against the voltage-gated potassium channel complex, Hashimoto encephalopathy associated with autoimmune thyroiditis (Chapter 226), and encephalitis associated with anti–N-methyl-D-aspartate (NMDA) receptor antibodies.[8] In parainfectious encephalitis, a systemic viral infection is associated with a febrile encephalopathy, sometimes with inflammatory spinal fluid but without direct evidence of brain invasion by the organism. Examples of parainfectious encephalitis include infection and encephalopathy associated with influenza virus (Chapter 364), varicella virus (Chapter 375), and

TABLE 414-2   SELECTED TESTS FOR VIRAL ENCEPHALITIS

ORGANISM/ SYNDROME	TEST	COMMENT
WEST NILE VIRUS		
West Nile encephalitis	IgM in CSF	Diagnostic of CNS invasive disease including encephalitis or acute flaccid paralysis
HERPES SIMPLEX VIRUS TYPE 1		
Herpes simplex encephalitis	PCR in CSF	Sensitive and specific in the acute phase
HERPES SIMPLEX VIRUS TYPE 2		
Neonatal encephalitis	PCR in CSF	Confirmatory, high sensitivity
Relapsing meningitis	PCR in CSF	Sensitive and specific in first 3 days of illness
HUMAN HERPESVIRUS 6		
Limbic encephalitis	PCR in CSF	Confirmatory, sensitivity unknown
VARICELLA-ZOSTER VIRUS		
Meningoencephalitis	PCR in CSF	Confirmatory when used with clinical and spinal fluid findings; sensitivity unclear
EPSTEIN-BARR VIRUS		
EBV encephalitis	PCR in CSF	Suggests CNS invasion by virus
JC VIRUS		
Progressive multifocal leukoencephalopathy	PCR in CSF	Diagnostic but incompletely (70%) sensitive
CYTOMEGALOVIRUS		
CMV ventriculitis	PCR in CSF	Sensitive and specific

CNS = central nervous system; CSF = cerebrospinal fluid; IgM = immunoglobulin M; PCR = polymerase chain reaction.

Epstein-Barr virus (Chapter 377). Furthermore, primary demyelinating disease (Chapter 411), particularly in the form of acute disseminated encephalomyelitis, overlaps clinically with viral encephalitis.

SELECTED SPECIFIC VIRUSES
Herpes Simplex Encephalitis
EPIDEMIOLOGY

Herpes simplex (Chapter 374) encephalitis, which is second only to West Nile encephalitis (Chapter 383) as the most common form of encephalitis in the United States, has an annual incidence of two to four cases per million people per year. There is no seasonal or gender predisposition. The encephalitis can strike older children but is most commonly a disease of adults.

PATHOBIOLOGY

Herpes simplex encephalitis usually occurs in immunocompetent patients, but immunosuppressed patients may also be affected. Patients who are deficient in toll-like receptor 3 in the immune system may be selectively vulnerable to herpes simplex encephalitis.

Herpes simplex virus type 1 infects and establishes latency in the majority of the population. Whether herpes simplex encephalitis arises from reactivation of a latent viral infection in the trigeminal ganglion or is a primary nasopharyngeal infection that ascends into the olfactory nervous system is uncertain.

The pathology of herpes simplex encephalitis is a necrotizing hemorrhagic inflammatory encephalitis in a characteristic pattern affecting the mesiotemporal, inferofrontal, and insular cortices, with gray matter predominance. Even if the brain is affected bilaterally, the pathologic features are usually asymmetrical, a pattern that helps distinguish herpes simplex from other forms of limbic encephalitis.

CLINICAL MANIFESTATIONS

The clinical manifestations of herpes simplex encephalitis usually begin with a nonspecific febrile prodrome that is followed within hours to days by the symptoms of headache, malaise, nausea, and vomiting. A reduced level of consciousness may occur early. Seizures may be the first manifestation of this encephalitis. Focal neurologic deficits, such as hemiparesis or aphasia, appear early and can be mistaken for stroke. More specific manifestations of herpes simplex encephalitis are symptoms of limbic system–associated behavioral changes, such as behavioral or emotional lability and inappropriateness. Memory is affected early if consciousness is preserved. As the encephalitis progresses, symptoms of increased intracranial pressure, lethargy, and coma are usual. Focal findings alone in the context of clinical encephalitis are not sufficient to confirm a diagnosis of herpes simplex encephalitis.

DIAGNOSIS

Spinal fluid analysis is necessary in the diagnosis of herpes simplex encephalitis. In a patient with focal encephalitis or coma, however, CT of the brain should be performed before spinal fluid analysis to avoid the risk of herniation. Elevation of the CSF protein level and the white blood cell count, with a predominance of lymphocytes, is the most frequent pattern; red blood cells are also commonly seen. The CSF glucose level is usually normal but is less than 50% of the blood glucose level in about 5% of patients.

The best and most accurate test for proof of herpes simplex encephalitis is the presence of herpes simplex virus type 1 DNA amplified by PCR in the spinal fluid. Herpes simplex virus type 1 can be distinguished from herpes simplex virus type 2 by specific primer amplification, applied as part of the PCR analysis. Because herpes simplex type 2 can cause encephalitis in neonates and meningoencephalitis in adults, this distinction may guide therapy.

MRI typically shows characteristic focal involvement with increased T2 and fluid-attenuated inversion recovery (FLAIR) signal in the mesiotemporal lobes (including the amygdala, hippocampus, and uncus), the inferofrontal lobes (cingulate gyrus and orbital frontal cortex), and the insular cortex (Fig. 414-1). MRI abnormalities are often unilateral but can be bilateral and asymmetrical. Focal MRI abnormalities must be distinguished from brain abscess (Chapter 413), cerebral infarction (Chapter 407), cerebral hemorrhage (Chapter 408), brain tumors (Chapter 189), and paraneoplastic limbic encephalitis. Radiographically detected involvement of the mesiotemporal rather than the lateral temporal areas and involvement of the gray matter rather than the white matter suggest herpes simplex encephalitis as the diagnosis. Early gadolinium contrast enhancement may occur but is not universal.

CT of the head is less sensitive than MRI for detecting mild cases of herpes encephalitis. However, because herpes simplex encephalitis can be hemorrhagic, CT may sometimes identify the hemorrhage more accurately than MRI can.

Electroencephalography is an adjunctive test that can show periodic lateralized epileptiform discharges ipsilateral to the involved temporal lobe. However, the findings are not specific for herpes simplex encephalitis and commonly occur in patients with cerebral infarction (Chapter 407) and occasionally other forms of viral encephalitis.

> **TREATMENT**   **Rx**
>
> Multicenter prospective trials emphasize that early treatment affects outcome. When suspicion for herpes simplex encephalitis is raised in the acute setting by the presence of focal signs or symptoms, early empirical treatment is recommended even while the diagnostic evaluation is proceeding.
> Intravenous acyclovir (10 mg/kg every 8 hours for 14 to 21 days) is the therapy of choice. No prospective data support a longer duration of therapy or higher doses of acyclovir to improve neurologic outcomes.

Rabies

Human rabies is an encephalitic illness caused by the rabies virus, usually transmitted by an animal bite. It produces a fatal encephalitis, although the latency between animal bite exposure and occurrence of neurologic symptoms may sometimes obscure the diagnosis.

EPIDEMIOLOGY AND PATHOBIOLOGY

Rabies is a rare illness in the United States and developed world.[9] However, initially unsuspected cases have been transmitted via trivial bites by infected bats, which are widely distributed in every state in the United States except Hawaii. Rabies virus variants in bats are now responsible for the majority of recent human cases in the United States and Canada. Raccoon rabies has extended from Florida into Georgia, Alabama, and South Carolina.

Canine rabies is still endemic in much of the developing world, including Africa, Latin America, Eastern Europe, and Asia, and the vast majority of

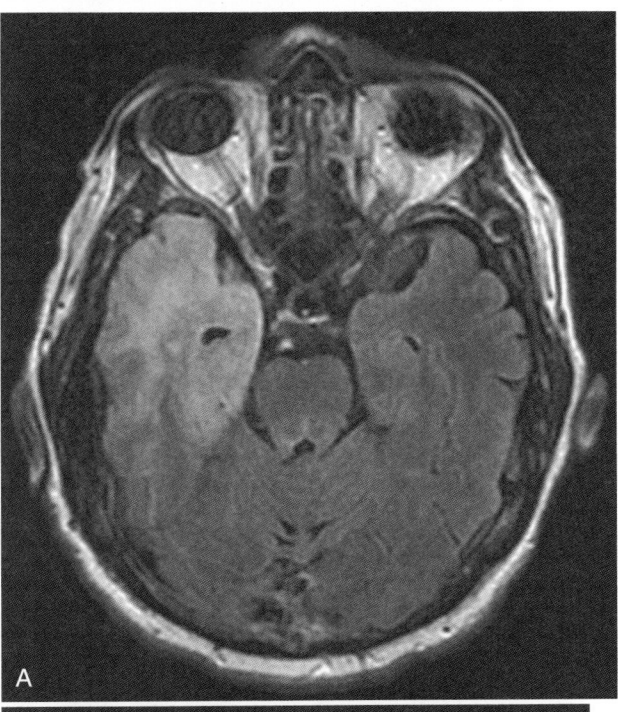

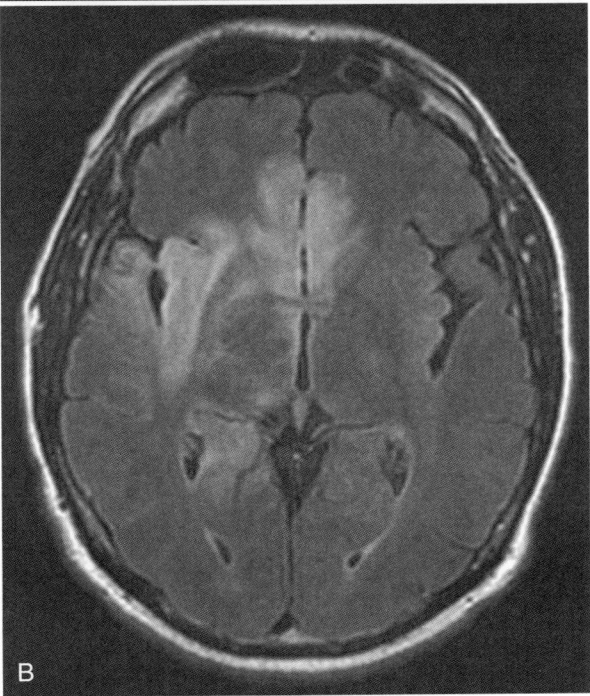

FIGURE 414-1. Magnetic resonance imaging (MRI) in herpes simplex encephalitis. Fluid-attenuated inversion recovery (FLAIR) MRI scan of the brain, showing increased signal (A) in the right mesiotemporal lobe (including the amygdala, hippocampus, and uncus), and (B) in the bilateral inferofrontal lobes (cingulate gyrus and orbital frontal cortex) and the right insular cortex.

the pathologic diagnosis. Because the disorder tends to be a brain stem encephalitis, the bulbar cardiovascular and respiratory centers are affected.

CLINICAL MANIFESTATIONS

Human rabies usually develops 20 to 90 days after a bite, although rarely disease develops after only a few days or after a year or more following bite exposure. Multiple bites and facial bites are associated with shorter incubation times.

Nonspecific prodromal symptoms include fever, chills, malaise, fatigue, insomnia, anorexia, headache, and irritability. In the majority of patients, pain or paresthesias will develop in the limb that was affected by the bite. Following the prodromal illness, an encephalitic form develops in about 80% of patients and causes behaviors ranging from episodes of agitated arousal to quiet lethargy. Fever is a common accompaniment but not universal at this phase. Disinhibition of brain stem reflexes leads to hydrophobia with laryngospasm and an inability to deal with salivation, swallowing of water, or other oral intake. When the brain stem encephalitis affects the bulbar, cardiovascular, and respiratory centers, autonomic dysfunction, cardiopulmonary complications, and respiratory failure may occur.

Another form of rabies that affects up to a third of patients is known as paralytic rabies. This form of rabies is manifested as acute flaccid paralysis, which may be multifocal and affect both the limbs and the bulbar musculature, thereby resembling poliomyelitis (Chapter 379) because of its multifocality. It also can be confused with Guillain-Barré syndrome (Chapter 420). Paralytic rabies typically occurs in conjunction with febrile encephalitis.

DIAGNOSIS

Findings on spinal fluid analysis may be abnormal in human rabies. A lymphocytic pleocytosis, usually less than 100 white cells/μL, is found in more than 50% of patients in the first week of illness. The CSF protein concentration usually is mildly elevated, and the glucose level is usually normal.

Imaging of patients with rabies is sometimes useful. MRI may show gray matter involvement, particularly involvement of the brain stem, with increased T2 signal, commonly without enhancement. Spinal cord MRI in patients with paralytic rabies may show multifocal increased T2 signal mimicking acute disseminated encephalomyelitis. Involvement of brain gray matter, including the hippocampus and basal ganglia structures, indicates the gray matter predilection and often bilateral involvement of supratentorial structures. However, MRI cannot be relied on to exclude rabies.

Serum antibodies against rabies virus are not usually present in unimmunized patients until the second week of illness, and patients can die before having a detectable serum antibody level. Serum antibodies may also be present in spinal fluid, but their absence is unreliable in excluding the diagnosis. Classically, staining a skin biopsy sample taken from an area near the nape of the neck for rabies antigen in the sensory nerves can confirm the diagnosis of rabies. Alternatively, small amounts of rabies RNA can be detected by PCR testing. Typical specimens to detect virus include saliva, brain tissue, or spinal fluid. A positive result confirms the diagnosis, but the exclusionary value of negative results is unknown.

TREATMENT   Rx

After an animal bite, local treatment with antirabies immunoglobulin and systemic treatment with vaccination are typically offered. Rabies postexposure prophylaxis includes local wound cleansing, passive immunization with immunoglobulin, and active immunization with rabies vaccine.[10] Inactivated cell culture rabies vaccines are used for active immunization, and the risk for vaccination-induced acute disseminated encephalomyelitis has been markedly reduced by the use of these vaccines. However, once rabies encephalitis is manifested, it is unclear whether vaccination, though regularly used, has any role in improving outcome. Antiviral therapy and a variety of immunotherapies, including ribavirin and interferon alfa, have been tried in the treatment of rabies, usually without success. Although one patient has survived with the use of therapeutic coma without vaccination, subsequent reports of patients treated in similar fashion have been associated with a fatal outcome. Treatment is otherwise supportive, and outcome is essentially always fatal.[11]

Rare Causes of Encephalitis

Lymphocytic choriomeningitis (Chapter 412) virus is a human infection acquired from mice. Typically, humans acquire the infection by contact with food or dust that is contaminated by excreta of the common house mouse. Most commonly, human disease occurs in winter, when the natural host

human rabies cases occur as a result of untreated dog bites from endemic areas. Dog rabies came under control in the United States during the 1950s and was associated with a marked reduction in the number of human cases transmitted by dogs. Much of the dog-related clinical rabies seen in the United States is the result of dog bites that occurred in developing countries, before the patient migrated to the United States. Rare cases of transmission of rabies to transplant organ recipients have occurred in the United States.

The presence of Negri bodies (intracytoplasmic viral inclusions) in neurons of the brain stem, cerebellum (especially the Purkinje cells), or hippocampus defines rabies pathologically. These inclusions are often not present, but detection of antigen by immunohistochemical means can aid in tends to move indoors. It can also be acquired as a consequence of laboratory exposure by human caretakers.

Mumps virus (Chapter 369) is typically acquired by the respiratory route. Infection can occur throughout the year, but the incidence is higher during the spring. Although mumps virus infects both sexes equally, meningoencephalitis develops in males three times more frequently than in females. Vaccination programs in the United States have made mumps encephalitis rare.

TREATMENT   Rx

Effective antiviral therapy does not exist for most forms of viral encephalitis, except for herpes simplex encephalitis.[12] However, because of the usual delay in establishing or excluding the diagnosis of herpes simplex encephalitis, patients suspected of having encephalitis should start acyclovir therapy (10 mg/kg intravenously every 8 hours for 2 weeks) even while specific serologic and spinal fluid analyses are being performed to make a specific diagnosis.

Supportive measures for patients with encephalitis typically include intensive care unit monitoring and treatment in the initial phases of the illness. Seizures are common and frequently refractory to antiepileptic drugs; however, the seizures themselves can increase morbidity and mortality, so vigorous treatment attempts are required (Chapter 403).

In patients who are immunosuppressed (see Table 414-1), the spectrum of possible infections is broader and potentially more treatable. Examples include varicella-zoster virus (Chapter 375), with acyclovir administered at doses similar to those used for herpes simplex virus, and cytomegalovirus (Chapters 370 and 376), with ganciclovir administered at 5 mg/kg intravenously every 12 hours for 2 weeks or cidofovir administered at 5 mg/kg intravenously weekly for 2 weeks, although some patients require long-term oral valganciclovir (900 mg every 24 hours) or intravenous cidofovir (5 mg/kg every 2 weeks). HIV encephalitis (Chapter 394) responds in variable degree to triple antiretroviral therapy. By comparison, no specific treatments are currently effective for Epstein-Barr virus (Chapters 370 and 377) and JC virus (progressive multifocal leukoencephalopathy [Chapter 370]). Variable success has been reported for treatment of HHV-6 encephalitis in hematopoietic stem cell transplant recipients using ganciclovir, foscarnet, or valganciclovir alone or in combination (Chapter 360, Table 360-4).[13]

PROGNOSIS

The prognosis of encephalitis is dependent on the cause, with an overall mortality rate of about 6% in the U.S.[14] Herpes simplex encephalitis, even with adequate treatment, has a 20% mortality, and the likelihood of major persistent morbidity with seizures or defects in memory and behavior is 35 to 40%. Each of the arboviruses has a different mortality rate, with eastern equine encephalitis virus associated with the highest mortality. La Crosse encephalitis virus has the lowest mortality and is the most benign. Some forms of encephalitis have specific sequelae, such as sensorineural deafness or hydrocephalus associated with mumps encephalitis.

GENERAL REFERENCES

For the General References and other additional features, please visit Expert Consult at https://expertconsult.inkling.com.

415

PRION DISEASES

PATRICK J. BOSQUE

DEFINITION

Prion diseases are a group of closely related neurodegenerative conditions of humans and other mammals. They are caused by an accumulation of abnormally aggregated forms of the prion protein (PrP), a protein that is normally produced in the central nervous system (CNS). This abnormal form of the protein can act as an infectious agent called a prion and transmit disease to another host. The prion is thus an infectious protein conformation that contains no specific nucleic acid. The name *Creutzfeldt-Jakob disease* (CJD) is

applied to most human forms of prion disease, although other names are used for some forms.

EPIDEMIOLOGY

Prion diseases occur worldwide, with an incidence of about one case per million annually. These conditions can be acquired sporadically, genetically, or infectiously, but sporadic disease accounts for about 90% of cases, and genetic forms account for almost all the remainder. Both dietary and iatrogenic exposure have transmitted prion disease to humans, but these infectiously acquired forms represent less than 1% of cases in most human populations.

Two human outbreaks of prion disease, kuru and variant CJD, were caused by dietary exposure.[1] Kuru was epidemic in tribes of the Fore language group in the highlands of New Guinea. It probably arose as a case of sporadic prion disease, and then was spread by the practice of ritual cannibalism. The last exposures are thought to have occurred in the late 1950s, but new clinical cases have occurred as recently as 2009, thereby indicating an incubation period of more than 50 years.

Variant CJD is caused by eating meat from cattle infected with the prion disease known as bovine spongiform encephalopathy (BSE). Variant CJD first arose in Great Britain in 1994, about 10 years after an outbreak of a massive BSE epidemic there. Despite the exposure of millions of people to meat contaminated with BSE prions, fewer than 200 people worldwide have contracted variant CJD. The incidence of variant CJD has decreased in recent years as the BSE outbreak in cattle has been contained and the entry of contaminated meat into the food supply restricted.[2]

Contaminated cadaveric dura mater allografts and pituitary-derived growth hormone injections have each caused more than 200 iatrogenic cases of CJD.[3] Most dura mater–associated cases have been from a single product, Lyodura, manufactured before May 1987. All growth hormone cases involve product derived from cadaveric pituitaries before recombinant growth hormone became available in the 1980s. Blood and blood products derived from donors with variant CJD have transmitted the illness, but perhaps surprisingly, sporadic CJD seems not to have been transmitted through blood products. Other modes of iatrogenic spread of CJD are quite rare. Contaminated surgical instruments are persuasively documented to have transmitted CJD on six occasions, and corneal transplants have been documented to transmit CJD only twice.

PATHOBIOLOGY

PrP is a cell surface glycoprotein normally produced in the brain and several other tissues. Its function is unknown, but it may play a role in copper metabolism. An abnormally aggregated form of PrP termed *PrP^{Sc}* accumulates in the brain in prion disease. Remarkably, PrP^{Sc} is able to recruit the normal form of PrP into the pathologic aggregate. The precise structure of PrP^{Sc} aggregates and the mechanism of prion propagation are incompletely understood, but a basic conceptual model proposes that the normally α-helical regions of PrP directly interact with the β sheets of PrP^{Sc}, lose their normal α-helical structure, and then join the aggregate. At some point, the growing aggregate fractures, thereby creating additional aggregate particles. In this way, an aggregate of PrP^{Sc} can propagate as an infectious agent. A curious feature of prion diseases is that more than one aggregated structure of PrP^{Sc} can be stably propagated, and these various "strains" of prions can give rise to distinct clinical manifestations.

Predominantly β-sheet aggregates of other proteins are implicated as the causes of more common neurodegenerative diseases (e.g., the β-amyloid protein in Alzheimer disease [Chapter 402] and synuclein in Parkinson disease [Chapter 409]).[4] Although these other diseases are not infectiously transmitted, recent studies suggest that a mechanism of self-propagation like that described above for prion diseases may play a role in their pathogenesis.

What precisely initiates sporadic or genetic prion diseases is not known. In infectious forms of prion disease that are transmitted by the alimentary route, prions first replicate in the enteric lymphatic system, including Peyer patches. From the lymphatic system, prions spread to the CNS via sympathetic nerves in lymphatic tissue. Once in the CNS, prions appear to spread trans-synaptically. As with other neurodegenerative diseases associated with accumulations of aggregated proteins, the mechanism by which the PrP aggregates cause neuronal dysfunction and death is unknown.

Pathology

Traditionally, prion diseases are recognized by a combination of vacuolization (status spongiosus) of the gray matter, astrocytic gliosis, and loss of neurons. In modern practice, they are diagnosed by demonstrating the presence of PrP^{Sc}, using techniques that exploit the enhanced resistance to degradation displayed by these PrP aggregates. In the biochemical method, homogenized brain tissue is treated with a protease that dissolves the normal form of PrP but leaves a resistant core of PrP^{Sc} intact. This protease-resistant core can then be identified by Western blotting. The histologic technique involves hydrolyzing proteins on tissue sections. Normal PrP is dissolved, but PrP^{Sc} can still be identified immunohistochemically. Certain forms of prion disease have a distinct and characteristic histochemical appearance. For example, variant CJD produces a peculiar type of amyloid plaque surrounded by vacuoles, the so-called florid plaque.

Genetics

All inherited forms of prion disease are caused by mutations in the PrP coding sequence of the gene *PRNP*.[5] Mutations associated with familial forms of prion disease include more than 20 missense mutations, two premature stop mutations, and a series of insertions in a region of a repeated eight–amino acid sequence. Genetic forms of prion disease are transmitted in an autosomal dominant pattern, usually with high but incomplete penetrance. Three distinctive forms of prion disease are associated with certain *PRNP* mutations. First, the Gerstmann-Sträussler-Scheinker syndrome is caused by any of several mutations in *PRNP*, the most common of which codes for a substitution of leucine for proline at codon 102 (P102L). Pathologically, there are accumulations of plaques of PrP amyloid in the brain, especially in the cerebellum. Second, fatal familial insomnia is caused by a D178N mutation on the same allele as a methionine at the polymorphic codon 129 of *PRNP*. Pathologically, there is neuronal loss and accumulation of PrP^{Sc} in the thalamus. In contrast, the D178N mutation on an allele with valine at codon 129 causes a disease that is indistinguishable from sporadic CJD. Third, some *PRNP* mutations cause slowly progressive dementia. The most common of these mutations are large expansions of the octapeptide repeat region.

Certain common genotypes affect susceptibility to prion disease. Codon 129 of *PRNP* is polymorphic, with alleles coding for either valine or methionine. Persons who are homozygous (129VV or 129MM) at this allele are overrepresented among victims of sporadic CJD, and all victims of variant CJD carry 129M on both *PRNP* alleles.

CLINICAL MANIFESTATIONS

Sporadic CJD is the most common form of human prion disease. It typically begins in later midlife at an average of about 60 years of age, although onset as young as 17 years and as old as 80 years has been reported. In about 25% of cases, patients or their families report a prodrome of a psychiatric disturbance such as anxiety, depression, or altered sleep.[6] Cognitive dysfunction is usually the most prominent neurologic sign. Unlike Alzheimer disease, however, prion disease typically causes motor signs (e.g., ataxia, bradykinesia, spasticity), vague somatic sensory disturbances, or alterations in visual perception. Myoclonus is a characteristic but not pathognomonic sign. Perhaps the most distinctive feature of prion disease is the pace of its progression. Typically, clear decrements in neurologic function can be observed over a period of weeks.

Variations on this typical presentation can occur in sporadic cases and are more common in genetic and infectiously transmitted disease. At least some of these variations are probably caused by the propagation of prion strains that are different from the strain usually associated with sporadic CJD. Recently, a sporadic form of prion disease termed *variable protease encephalopathy* has been characterized; behavioral disorders related to frontal lobe dysfunction are common, and the PrP^{Sc} found in the brain of victims is generally more sensitive to protease digestion than is typical of PrP^{Sc}.[6,7] Slowly progressive CJD may have clinical manifestations similar to those of familial Alzheimer disease (Chapter 402) or resemble Huntington disease (Chapter 410).

In Gerstmann-Sträussler-Scheinker syndrome, the clinical signs are prominent ataxia, a slower rate of progression than occurs with sporadic CJD (typically 5 to 6 years from onset to death), and late dementia. Fatal familial insomnia begins with anxiety, depression, and sleep disturbance. Ataxia or other motor signs may also develop early in the disease course. Dementia occurs relatively late in the condition. Very rarely, a sporadic form of CJD will be manifested as a clinical syndrome of fatal insomnia. A family with a *PRNP* Y163X truncation has been reported to have prion protein amyloid throughout their peripheral organs, including bowel and peripheral nerves. Patients developed diarrhea, a severe autoimmune neuropathy, cortical amyloid plaques, and cerebral amyloid angiopathy.[8]

Variant CJD acquired by exposure to BSE prions is distinguished clinically from sporadic CJD by a much younger mean age at onset (mean, 26 years; range, 12 to 74 years), the prominence of psychiatric and sensory signs early in the disease, and the later emergence of dementia and motor signs, typically more than 6 months after the first symptoms. Iatrogenic CJD usually resembles sporadic CJD, but a subset of patients may have an ataxic form that clinically and pathologically shares some features with Gerstmann-Sträussler-Scheinker syndrome. Kuru begins with limb pain followed by cerebellar ataxia and tremor ("kuru" means "shiver" in the Fore language). Overt dementia occurs late in the disease course.

DIAGNOSIS

The diagnosis of prion disease should be considered in patients with relatively rapidly progressive dementia, but certain treatable structural, inflammatory, metabolic, endocrine, and nutritional causes of rapidly progressive dementia entities can mimic prion disease (Table 415-1).[9] In particular, any signs of inflammation in the cerebrospinal fluid (CSF) should prompt consideration of a diagnosis other than prion disease. The clinician may also need to consider special tests to search for some rare but treatable conditions (Table 415-2).

If the initial evaluation fails to yield an alternative diagnosis, a number of available tests further support the diagnosis of prion disease. However, prion diseases are rare, and ancillary tests have less-than-perfect specificity and sensitivity; if they are applied indiscriminately, these tests will frequently yield false-positive results. The presence of either elevated CSF levels of the proteins 14-3-3[10] or CSF[11] or blood levels of tau[12] is relatively specific for CJD if inflammatory and ischemic causes of dementia are excluded. An unusual hyperintensity of the deep gray matter (basal ganglia and thalamus)

TABLE 415-1	DIFFERENTIAL DIAGNOSIS OF RAPIDLY PROGRESSIVE DEMENTIA
Neurodegenerative diseases that may mimic CJD	Alzheimer disease (Chapter 402), diffuse Lewy body disease (Chapter 402), frontotemporal dementia (Chapter 402), corticobasal ganglion degeneration (Chapter 402), progressive supranuclear palsy (Chapter 409)
Some less common treatable diseases that mimic CJD	**Autoimmune:** CNS vasculitis (Chapter 270), limbic encephalitis (Chapter 414), Hashimoto encephalopathy (Chapter 414), anti–voltage-gated potassium channel encephalopathy, sarcoidosis (Chapter 95), steroid-responsive autoimmune encephalopathy (Chapter 414) **Infections:** viral encephalitis (Chapter 414), chronic meningitis (Chapter 412), Whipple disease (Chapter 275) **Neoplasms:** primary CNS lymphoma (Chapter 185), intravascular lymphoma (Chapter 185) **Nutritional:** Wernicke encephalopathy (Chapter 416) **Toxicities:** lithium, bismuth, methotrexate **Structural:** Normal-pressure hydrocephalus (Chapter 189)

CJD = Creutzfeldt-Jakob disease; CNS = central nervous system.

TABLE 415-2	EVALUATION OF RAPIDLY PROGRESSIVE DEMENTIA
Initial screening	**Serum tests:** glucose, sodium, calcium, blood urea nitrogen, creatinine, hepatic aminotransferases, albumin, prothrombin time, TSH, antinuclear antigen, vitamin B_{12}, HIV and syphilis serology **Imaging:** brain MRI **CSF:** glucose, protein, cell counts, VDRL
Further tests to consider	**Serum:** antibodies against thyroglobulin, thyroid peroxidase, voltage-gated potassium channel, Hu (ANNA-1) **CSF:** cytology, flow cytometry **Brain biopsy**
Test findings supporting a diagnosis of prion disease	**MRI:** T2 hyperintensity in the basal ganglia, sometimes in the cortex **CSF 14-3-3 protein:** elevated levels fairly specific for CJD **EEG:** Periodic sharp wave complexes

CJD = Creutzfeldt-Jakob disease; CSF = cerebrospinal fluid; EEG = electroencephalography; HIV = human immunodeficiency virus; MRI = magnetic resonance imaging; TSH = thyroid-stimulating hormone; VDRL = Venereal Disease Research Laboratory test.

and sometimes the cortical gray matter on certain magnetic resonance imaging sequences (T2-weighted, fluid-attenuated inversion recovery, and diffusion-weighted weighting) occurs in about two thirds of CJD cases. The electroencephalogram in patients with CJD may show a pattern of periodic large-amplitude triphasic complexes. New methods for amplifying prions *in vitro* may enable clinicians to diagnose prion disease from urine,[13] nasal brushings,[14] and other tissues.

The definite diagnosis of prion disease can be made by brain biopsy. National or regional specialized prion disease centers, such as the National Prion Disorders Pathology Service Center (available at http://www.cjdsurveillance.com) in the United States, can assist pathologists in tissue analysis. In patients with a family history of neurodegenerative disease consistent with prion disease, determining the sequence of the protein-coding region of the prion protein gene can be diagnostic if a mutation is found.

TREATMENT AND PROGNOSIS   Rx

Prion diseases are incurable, and no treatment significantly improves the course of disease. Most patients with sporadic CJD die within a year of the onset of symptoms. Patients with Gerstmann-Sträussler-Scheinker syndrome and certain other genetic or variant forms of prion disease may live longer. Excellent animal models of prion disease exist, and a number of novel therapeutic approaches are under active investigation. It is worthwhile to consider enrollment in experimental clinical trials if they are available (http://clinicaltrials.gov).

PREVENTION

Most cases of prion disease occur sporadically and cannot be prevented. Genetic cases can potentially be prevented through genetic counseling and prenatal testing, although whether such measures are warranted to prevent a disease that may not manifest until midlife or later is an ethically complex question. Infectiously transmitted cases are currently amenable to preventive measures, including avoidance of surgical transmission as a result of contaminated instruments or tissue grafts and protection of the human food supply from meat products contaminated with BSE or other ruminant prions. Chronic wasting disease is epidemic among deer and elk in certain regions of the United States, and scrapie, which affects sheep and goats, is endemic at low levels in the United States and many other countries. Neither of these prion diseases has been convincingly linked to human illness, but prudence dictates that humans should avoid eating any prion-infected animal.

GENERAL REFERENCES

For the General References and other additional features, please visit Expert Consult at https://expertconsult.inkling.com.

416

NUTRITIONAL AND ALCOHOL-RELATED NEUROLOGIC DISORDERS

BARBARA S. KOPPEL

An adequate supply of vitamins and minerals is necessary for embryonic and early development as well as subsequent maintenance of metabolic function of both the central and peripheral nervous systems. Deficiencies of vitamins and minerals can cause a variety of neurologic syndromes (Table 416-1), each with well-described constellations of symptoms that are dependent on the location of the resulting pathologic changes within the nervous system.[1]

Vitamin deficiency (Chapter 218) can be caused by either malnutrition (Chapter 215) or malabsorption (Chapter 140). In addition to the insufficient intake of needed elements, functional deficiency can also result from increased demand owing to sepsis, chronic inflammatory conditions, dialysis, and problems incorporating the element or delivering it to its site of action. Exposure to alcohol or other neurotoxins in the setting of certain vitamin deficiencies (usually B_1) synergistically contributes to neuropathology. In malnourished patients, multiple simultaneous vitamin deficiencies can result in complex symptoms owing to overlapping areas of nervous

system involvement. Malnutrition is the most common cause of vitamin deficiency in economically disadvantaged countries. Overdependence on single food sources that may be neurotoxic (e.g., cassava, grass peas, spoiled grains) may complicate the presentation. Another example of this phenomenon is the alcoholic (Chapter 33) who obtains calories from alcohol, which is neurotoxic, and fails to take in micronutrients and vitamins. Even when adequate food supplies are readily available, malnutrition may be caused by inadequate consumption due to mechanical obstruction from cancer of the mouth or gastrointestinal tract, unbalanced ("fad") diets, fasting, anorexia, chronic nausea, or recurrent or persistent vomiting. Rarely, deficiencies arise in patients with genetic diseases that block intestinal absorption, transport across the blood-brain barrier, or uptake into mitochondria, neurons, and glia.

Iatrogenic causes include failure to feed patients who are comatose, not self-sufficient (from dementia, brain injury, psychiatric illness), or dysphagic, as can occur following a stroke or spinal cord injury. Vitamin deficiency can also result from failure to include adequate amounts of vitamin and mineral supplements in parenteral or liquid enteral diets.

As bariatric surgery becomes more common in the treatment of morbid obesity (Chapter 220), it has become a common cause of neurologic disorders associated with many vitamin deficiencies. Patients who have undergone restrictive ("lap band," gastric stapling) or especially bypass procedures require lifelong, not just perioperative, supplementation and monitoring of vitamin levels.

DEFICIENCY OF WATER-SOLUBLE VITAMINS
Thiamine (Vitamin B₁) Deficiency

Thiamine is converted to thiamine pyrophosphate, which serves as a coenzyme in glucose and lipid metabolism and in the synthesis of neurotransmitters from branched-chain amino acids (Chapter 218). To avoid deficiency, thiamine must be consumed regularly in adequate amounts, at least 0.33 mg per 1000 calories, or about 1 mg/day (more during pregnancy or lactation). Food sources include whole grains, legumes, meat, and fortified bread or cereals.

BERI-BERI

In developing countries, the most common manifestation of thiamine deficiency is beri-beri, which is characterized by a peripheral sensorimotor axonal neuropathy with numbness, paresthesias, or burning pain, occasionally accompanied by heart failure ("wet beri-beri"). Other causes of thiamine deficiency include reliance on foods in which the vitamin has been inactivated by processing (e.g., polished rice), overcooking, or eating foods that contain thiaminase-producing bacteria (e.g., raw fish).

WERNICKE ENCEPHALOPATHY

Even short-term (<3 weeks) thiamine deficiency can result in Wernicke encephalopathy, a syndrome characterized by insidious development and progression (over days to weeks) of confusion or delirium, abnormal eye movements, and ataxia.[2] Fewer than one third of patients develop all three elements of this triad. Wernicke encephalopathy occurs most often in the setting of poor nutrition and prolonged vomiting in patients with chronic alcohol abuse. Based on pathologic changes discovered at autopsy, about 12% of heavy alcohol users and 60% of patients dying of alcohol-related causes have Wernicke encephalopathy. The symptoms and signs of Wernicke encephalopathy reflect the preferential dysfunction of brain regions that have a high demand for thiamine, a cofactor in energy-producing cycles. These areas include the blood-brain barrier, anterior and centromedian thalamus, mammillary bodies, periaqueductal gray matter, superior and inferior colliculi, and floor of the fourth ventricle. The most common pathologic changes in these regions include neuronal swelling and microscopic hemorrhages, followed by gliosis. Rarely, the cerebral cortex and hypothalamus may be involved as well. Deficiency of α-ketoglutamate dehydrogenase activity in astrocytes leads to microglial activation and glutamatergic toxicity.

CLINICAL MANIFESTATIONS AND DIAGNOSIS

The full triad of mental status change, abnormal eye movements, and ataxia occurs in only about one third of cases. Acute symptoms may be provoked if intravenous (IV) glucose or food is given before thiamine has been replaced. Because a medical history may be unobtainable until the patient's confusion clears, physical signs of chronic alcoholism (e.g., gynecomastia, skin angiomata, pulmonary erythema, ascites, jaundice) (Chapters 146 and 152) must be sought.

TABLE 416-1 SUMMARY OF VITAMIN AND MINERAL DEFICIENCIES

VITAMIN AND MINERAL DEFICIENCIES	NEUROLOGIC SYNDROME(S)	SUPPORTING TESTS	TREATMENT	CAUSES (OTHER THAN MALNUTRITION)
A (Retinol)	Blindness from retinal or corneal damage	Visual fields, visual acuity; Serum level < 30-65 µg/dL	30,000 IU vitamin A daily × 1 wk	Hypothyroidism, diabetes, renal or liver failure
B_1 (thiamine)	Wernicke encephalopathy: ataxia, nystagmus, ophthalmoparesis, confusion, delirium; Korsakoff syndrome: amnesia, confabulation; Beri-beri: axonal neuropathy	MRI: symmetrical lesions of midbrain (periaqueductal area), pons, hypothalamus, thalamus, cerebellum; MRI: necrosis of mamillary bodies, dorsomedial and anterior thalamus; Nerve conduction tests: decreased amplitude; Serum thiamine level < 20 ng/dL; Decreased erythrocyte transketolase	Prevent by 100 mg PO daily before and 1 year after bariatric surgery, 100 mg IV before glucose administration or refeeding after starvation; Treat Wernicke encephalopathy with 5 days of thiamine, 100-500 mg IV or IM daily, until improvement stabilizes, then PO 100 mg daily; Antioxidants (N-acetylcysteine)	Alcoholism, bariatric or other major GI surgery, prolonged vomiting, hemodialysis, diuretic treatment of heart failure, cachexia, 5-fluorouracil, other blockers of thiamine phosphate production
B_3 (niacin)	Pellagra: confusion, dementia, weakness, ataxia, spasticity, myoclonus, glossitis, dermatitis, photosensitivity	Erythrocyte NAD, plasma niacin, urinary N1-methylnicotinamide	Nicotinic acid, 50 mg PO tid or 25 mg IV tid; nicotinamide, 50-100 mg IM or PO tid	Alcoholism, corn- or cereal-based diet, Hartnup syndrome, carcinoid syndrome
B_5 (pantothenic acid)	Dysesthesias, foot paresthesias	Deficient coenzyme A	5 mg PO daily	Severe malnutrition
B_6 (pyridoxine)	Neuropathy, sensory ataxia, depression; Infantile pyridoxine-deficient epilepsy	Plasma PLP < 27 nmol/L; urinary 4-pyridoxic acid, < 3 nmol; ↑ Homocysteine after methionine loading challenge; ↑ α-AASA in urine, plasma, CSF	50-100 mg PO daily for neuropathy (preventive use if taking B_6 antagonist); 100-200 mg daily for adult epilepsy	Diverticulosis, isoniazid, cycloserine, other antagonists; Genetic defects in antiquitin (aldehyde dehydrogenase), pyridoxal synthesis
B_{12} (cobalamin)	Myelopathy with spastic paraparesis and sensory ataxia, peripheral neuropathy, optic neuropathy, memory loss, dementia; indirect contributor to stroke	Blood level < 200 pg/mL; ↑ Methylmalonic acid > 145 nmol/L; Intrinsic factor antibodies; Schilling test, megaloblastic anemia; Delayed somatosensory evoked potentials; ↑ Homocysteine, total > 12.5 µmol/L	IM B_{12}, 1000 µg daily for 1 week, then weekly for 1 month, then monthly; or oral B_{12}, 1000 µg daily; or nasal B_{12}, 500 µg weekly for lifetime if abnormal absorption, 50-100 µg daily if normal absorption	Achlorhydria, gastric or ileal resection, blind loop syndrome, sprue, HIV infection, nitrous oxide anesthesia (especially abuse), fish tapeworm, vegan diet
D (calciferol)	Proximal myopathy, often painful; cognitive impairment; Secondary compression of spinal cord, plexus, or peripheral nerves from rickets or osteomalacia	25-(OH) vitamin D_3 level < 10 ng/mL in urine; Serum calcium; ↑ PTH > 54 pg/mL; Osteopenia/porosis on bone densitometry	Daily supplementation with 400 IU, >50,000 IU 3 times per wk if malabsorption; use blood level or urine calcium excretion to guide (should be > 100 mg/day)	Lack of exposure to sunlight, including sunblock protection; chronic antiepileptic drug use
E (tocopherol)	Spinal and cerebellar ataxia, Babinski sign, ophthalmoplegia, peripheral neuropathy, retinitis pigmentosa	Vitamin E level < 2.5 mg/L (normal, 6-15 with normal lipid level); ↑ A-β-lipoprotein levels, antigliadin antibodies; Genetic analysis to rule out other spinocerebellar ataxias such as Friedreich ataxia	Supplement with 6-800 IU, 5-10 mg/kg twice daily, for ataxia of genetic causes, water-soluble 200 mg/kg/day or IM α-tocopherol for malabsorption	Biliary atresia, celiac sprue, Genetic: ↓ α-tocopherol transport protein (8q13), microsomal triglyceride transfer protein
Folate	Dementia, B_{12} deficiency, stroke	↑ Homocysteine, plasma level < 2.5 µg/L	1 mg 3 times daily until normal level, then maintenance of 1 mg/day; Pregnancy: additional 0.4 mg/day if taking a folate antagonist	Malabsorption or use of antagonist (methotrexate) or antiepileptic medication
K (phytonadione)	Intracranial hemorrhage	INR or PT elevation	IM phytonadione at birth, maternal vitamin K for last month of pregnancy	Medication use that increases metabolism (e.g., phenytoin)
Copper	Myelopathy, neuropathy	Serum Cu < 75 µg/dL, ↓ urinary Cu, ceruloplasmin < 23 mg/dL; MRI: ↑ T2 signal in cervical cord, dorsal column; Mutation in ATP7A gene (Menkes disease)	Elemental Cu, 8 mg/day PO week 1, 6 mg/day week 2, 4 mg/day week 3, 2 mg/day ongoing malabsorption; Menkes disease: 250 mg SC bid	Wilson disease, Menkes disease, alcoholism, malabsorption, gastric bypass, zinc toxicity
Magnesium	Seizures, encephalopathy	Serum magnesium < 1.5 mg/dL, correct for low albumin	Magnesium sulfate IV or PO; Avoid magnesium-wasting drugs	Alcoholism, especially beer
Potassium	Muscle weakness, chronic, acute	Serum potassium < 3.5 mEq/L, ECG	IV or PO KCl until normalized	Diuretic use, bulimia

AASA = aminoadipic semialdehyde; CSF = cerebrospinal fluid; ECG, electrocardiography; GI = gastrointestinal; INR = international normalized ratio; MRI = magnetic resonance imaging; NAD = nicotinamide adenine dinucleotide; PLP = pyridoxal-5-phosphate (active coenzyme of pyridoxine); PT = prothrombin time; PTH = parathyroid hormone.

Mental status changes range from mild memory impairment or inattention to delirium, often with apathy or abulia. Eye movement abnormalities include nystagmus, dysconjugate gaze, and gaze palsies[3]. Ataxia can affect the limbs (legs more than arms), trunk, and gait. Patients with Wernicke encephalopathy can also have autonomic and hypothalamic dysfunction, with bradycardia and hypothermia as well as papilledema, optic neuropathy, seizures, and myoclonus.

In symptomatic patients, T2-weighted magnetic resonance imaging (MRI) can be normal but often demonstrates symmetrical increased signal due to edema or hemorrhage in affected areas, most often periventricular thalamus, periaqueductal regions in the floor of the fourth ventricle or cerebellum, and in the mamillary bodies. Low thiamine levels (<50 mg/mL) are common, although levels may be normal in about 10% of cases. Because thiamine deficiency disrupts carbohydrate metabolism, serum levels of lactate and pyruvate can be elevated.

KORSAKOFF SYNDROME

Korsakoff syndrome becomes apparent in up to 80% of patients who survive Wernicke encephalopathy. It is more likely to follow Wernicke encephalopathy in the setting of alcoholism than in nutritional deficiency alone, thereby implying a synergistic mechanism that may be due to repeated episodes of alcohol withdrawal with associated glutamate neurotoxicity, compounded by lack of thiamine. The primary pathologic findings occur in the limbic system, especially the mamillary bodies, amygdala, and dorsomedial and anterior thalamus. Cortical involvement may be related to alcohol neurotoxicity rather than thiamine deficiency.

As confusion and delirium of Wernicke syndrome improve, an amnestic state in which patients are often unaware of their memory impairment becomes apparent. Korsakoff syndrome can be reliably identified only following resolution of acute delirium and global confusional states. It is characterized by disproportionate retrograde and anterograde episodic amnesia, transient confabulation, and hallucinations. Occasionally, Korsakoff psychosis is present clinically or pathologically without documented episodes of Wernicke encephalopathy, perhaps because Wernicke encephalopathy was subclinical or was not recognized acutely.

The memory deficit, which precludes learning new information or acquisition of new memories, is disproportionately severe in relation to other aspects of cognitive function. For example, alertness, attention, social interactions, and motor learning (procedural memory) are generally well preserved. There may be mild disorientation with respect to time and place, and sometimes apathy and other emotional changes are present. Confabulation, in which the intrusion of errors in response to questions leads to fabrication of answers without the intention to deceive, is sometimes present spontaneously in the first weeks after Wernicke encephalopathy. Confabulation may be a compensatory mechanism, and it usually lessens over time. Neuropsychological testing frequently demonstrates emotional changes and mild problems in executive function, which are indicative of frontal lobe involvement.

TREATMENT AND PROGNOSIS   Rx

Untreated, Wernicke encephalopathy is fatal in 90% of cases. However, timely thiamine replacement (see Table 416-1) can prevent or treat Wernicke encephalopathy as well as beri-beri. In the acute setting, high-dose IV or IM thiamine, which is recommended to circumvent any problems with swallowing or absorption, will lead rapidly—often within hours—to complete resolution of nystagmus and oculomotor paresis, followed by resolution of the ataxia and eventually of the mental status changes attributable to thiamine deficiency. However, many alcoholic patients may have residual ataxia and cognitive impairment, including memory dysfunction, owing to the toxic effects of alcohol itself (see later).[4] Because Korsakoff syndrome does not respond to thiamine replacement, prevention by timely recognition and treatment of Wernicke encephalopathy is essential. Magnesium (Chapter 119) must also be replaced if deficient.

Cobalamin (Vitamin B$_{12}$) Deficiency

Cobalamin is involved in methionine pathways that regulate myelination during development and maintain myelin throughout life (Chapter 218). Deficiency results in combined system disease (peripheral neuropathy and spinal cord degeneration) or subacute combined degeneration of the dorsal (sensory) and lateral (motor) tracts (i.e., myelopathy).[5] The spinal cord tracts that are dysfunctional result in impaired position and vibratory sensation and spastic paraparesis.

Cobalamin deficiency (Chapters 164 and 218) is most common in individuals older than 60, because the incidence of atrophic gastritis (Chapter 139) and achlorhydria rises in older individuals, and acid is required for B$_{12}$ processing. Long-term use of proton pump inhibitors may play a role in development of B$_{12}$ deficiency, as does a lack of gastric intrinsic factor needed for absorption of vitamin B$_{12}$. Cobalamin deficiency is rarely due to inadequate dietary intake (e.g., a vegan diet for several years), because it is stored in fat. A more common cause in recent years is bypass surgery for weight loss. Nitrous oxide ("laughing gas") toxicity, usually from illicit use rather than

administration as an anesthetic, can cause cobalamin deficiency by inactivating the cobalamin-dependent enzyme methionine synthase. Long-term treatment of diabetes with metformin also can lower B$_{12}$ levels. Low vitamin B$_{12}$ levels have been associated with increased homocysteine levels, but a relationship to vascular disease or vascular dementia has not been established.

CLINICAL MANIFESTATIONS

Demyelination of the dorsal columns causes proprioceptive loss that can result in sensory ataxia owing to loss of position sense in the feet.[6] Romberg sign (failure to maintain balance with the eyes closed) distinguishes sensory from cerebellar ataxia. An axonal peripheral neuropathy with numbness and tingling in the hands and feet is almost always present. Motor function eventually becomes impaired as well. The optic nerve can be involved, and vagal neuropathy has been reported. Signs of cerebral involvement include memory loss, personality changes, and occasionally hallucinations and psychosis. Encephalopathy and dementia may be present, but B$_{12}$ deficiency may be a secondary phenomenon in a patient with another cause of memory impairment, or both conditions may coexist without a causative relationship. Neurologic abnormalities may be present without anemia, especially because the anemia can be corrected by high-dose folate replacement. Symptoms generally progress slowly, but they can appear rapidly after exposure to nitrous oxide anesthesia in individuals with preexisting subclinical cobalamin deficiency.

DIAGNOSIS

Serum vitamin B$_{12}$ levels are usually low (<300 pg/mL) but can rarely be normal in symptomatic patients. In such cases, serum levels of methylmalonic acid and homocysteine are useful ancillary tests because these levels are increased as a result of impaired cobalamin-dependent reactions. Pernicious anemia (Chapter 164) is severe in about 20% of patients. However, both the hematocrit and mean corpuscular volume are sometimes normal because the hematologic effects of cobalamin deficiency can be partially masked by folate supplementation.

Low levels of cobalamin are sometimes present in normal people, especially the elderly, in which dementia, peripheral polyneuropathy, and myelopathy may be due to a myriad of causes. Therefore, a low cobalamin level may reflect poor nutrition or absorption rather than being the cause of these conditions. Causality is definitively confirmed by clinical improvement after cobalamin replacement, which usually begins after several weeks and may continue for up to a year.

TREATMENT   Rx

Treatment usually begins with a subcutaneous or intramuscular (IM) injection of 500 to 1000 μg of cobalamin daily for 1 week and then weekly for 1 month. After that time, oral supplementation with 50 to 100 μg daily of cyanocobalamin usually suffices in patients with achlorhydria or other causes of malabsorption; 1000 μg daily should be used in patients with intrinsic factor antibodies.[A1] Sublingual, transdermal patch, and nasal gel forms (500 μg weekly) can also be effective.

PROGNOSIS

Neurologic symptoms, especially paresthesias, typically improve to some extent within 3 months of achieving adequate B$_{12}$ serum levels. Numbness and areflexia often persist, especially if treatment is delayed. If there is no improvement whatsoever, vitamin B$_{12}$ deficiency is unlikely to be the cause of the condition. For example, human immunodeficiency virus–associated myelopathy, which can have a similar clinical manifestation, does not reverse with supplemental vitamin B$_{12}$ because it is caused by disruption of transmethylation pathways, not low cobalamin levels (see Table 416-1).

Folate Deficiency

Folate is an important coenzyme in the metabolism of nucleic and amino acids (Chapter 218). Folate deficiency is an important risk factor for neural tube defects in utero. In Cuban adults, especially alcoholic men, a crop failure led to semistarvation and an epidemic of blindness that resolved with folate and B vitamin supplementation. Folate deficiency also results in elevated levels of homocysteine, which is associated with an increased risk for ischemic heart disease and stroke. Folate and B vitamin supplementation in patients with elevated homocysteine levels but without classic homocysteinemia did not reduce adverse vascular events in clinical trials. Patients with genetic folate deficiency due to lack of methylenetetrahydrofolate reductase, which converts ingested folate to the active metabolic cofactor, have an increased risk of intracerebral hemorrhage.

The supplementation of flour with folate has greatly reduced the risk of folate deficiency, and all pregnant women are now prescribed supplemental folate. Women of child-bearing age should be treated even before pregnancy if they have any conditions that predispose to folate deficiency.

Folate deficiency also leads to megaloblastic anemia (Chapter 164). Before correction of megaloblastic anemia with folate alone, vitamin B_{12} levels should be checked to avoid ongoing neurologic injury resulting from unrecognized cobalamin deficiency. Folate deficiency is treated with 1 mg three times daily for 1 month, followed by 1 mg daily.

Pyridoxine (Vitamin B_6) Deficiency

Pyridoxine is a coenzyme in multiple reactions that involve gluconeogenesis, biosynthesis of neurotransmitters, and the metabolism of amino acids, nucleic acids, and lipids. Pyridoxine deficiency can be caused by genetic defects, such as defective antiquitin, that lead to increased utilization of pyridoxine. In adults, low serum levels of pyridoxine are well tolerated, so symptomatic deficiency is rare. However, symptomatic deficiency can occur in the setting of renal failure (Chapter 130), dialysis (Chapter 131), or cirrhosis (Chapter 153), or with medications such as isoniazid for antitubercular therapy (Chapter 324) or hydralazine for heart failure (Chapter 59) if patients do not receive concurrent supplementation. Deficiency is also seen with extreme malnutrition, especially diets consisting predominantly of white rice.

CLINICAL MANIFESTATIONS AND DIAGNOSIS

Prolonged pyridoxine deficiency causes a painful peripheral axonal neuropathy that leads to weakness and sensory ataxia. Some patients have skin thickening, seborrheic dermatitis, or glossitis, which can suggest pellagra. Serum levels of the active form of pyridoxine, pyridoxal 5′-phosphate, and urine levels of the metabolite 4-pyridoxic acid are low. Ancillary tests include nerve conduction studies, which show significantly reduced amplitudes in sensory and motor action potentials with normal conduction velocity times, typical of an axonal neuropathy.

In epilepsy caused by pyridoxine deficiency, seizures begin in the neonatal period and may persist, along with intellectual disability. Electroencephalography shows a highly disorganized pattern with excessive slow frequency activity and abundant multifocal and generalized spikes resembling hypsarrhythmia. Pyridoxine deficiency in pregnancy can be caused by hyperemesis gravidarum and may rarely produce neurologic disease in offspring, but routine supplementation is not recommended for all pregnancies.

Toxicity due to excess pyridoxine intake (>100 mg daily) leads to a ganglioneuropathy manifested by pure sensory symptoms, including sensory loss, ataxia, areflexia, and the presence of Romberg sign. However, this syndrome, which can result from an overdosing of vitamin supplements, is less common than deficiency-related neurologic disease.

TREATMENT   Rx

Patients in whom symptoms of pyridoxine deficiency develop or who take pyridoxine antagonists should receive supplemental pyridoxine (50 to 100 mg daily). Children with pyridoxine-dependent epilepsy require immediate and lifelong supplementation with 100 mg of pyridoxine daily.

For pyridoxine toxicity, simply stopping excess oral vitamin intake will eventually completely reverse the damage. The only exception is if a very large IV dose was administered, in which case neuropathy is not reversible.

DEFICIENCY OF FAT-SOLUBLE VITAMINS
Vitamin E (Tocopherol) Deficiency

Although vitamin E is composed of several tocopherols, it is the α form that is biologically active in humans and contained in most foods. Because it is so widely available, deficiency is almost never due to inadequate dietary consumption. Rather, vitamin E deficiency is almost always the result of malabsorption because of such conditions as biliary and pancreatic disease (Chapters 155 and 144), cystic fibrosis (Chapter 89), celiac disease (Chapter 140), Crohn disease (Chapter 141), extensive small bowel resection, and blind loop syndrome (Chapter 140). In addition, vitamin E deficiency is associated with genetic defects in the α-tocopherol transfer protein,

hypolipoproteinemia and abetalipoproteinemia, chylomicron retention disease, and ataxia with vitamin E deficiency.

CLINICAL MANIFESTATIONS AND DIAGNOSIS

Neurologic manifestations of vitamin E deficiency include a spinocerebellar syndrome with ataxia, loss of vibration and position senses, hyporeflexia, extensor plantar responses, and rarely myopathy. Other findings can include ptosis, abducens paresis, nystagmus, and retinopathy.

Serum levels of vitamin E can vary with the serum lipid levels. In extreme hyperlipidemia, such as cholestasis, the ratio of vitamin E to cholesterol will be more reliable than the absolute vitamin E level, which can be normal despite a low ratio of vitamin E to cholesterol.

Although generally not toxic, excessive intake of vitamin E causes bleeding, including hemorrhagic infarcts, in adults, probably owing to its effects on platelet function. During pregnancy, high doses of vitamin E can interfere with oxidation in the fetus and cause growth retardation.

TREATMENT

The amount of vitamin E replacement required depends on the cause of the deficiency. Malabsorption syndromes require 1000 to 2000 mg daily for infants and 10 to 20 g daily for adults. Genetic causes can be treated with 5 to 10 g/day. After bariatric surgery, supplementation with 300 mg daily is recommended. For vitamin E, 1 mg is equivalent to 1.49 IU. Although the mechanism is unknown, 2000 IU/day of α-tocopherol may slow functional decline in patients with moderate to severe Alzheimer disease.

Vitamin D (Calciferol) Deficiency

Vitamin D deficiency (Chapter 218) results from inadequate exposure to sunlight, dietary insufficiency, or malabsorption caused by celiac disease, inflammatory bowel disease, or extensive small bowel resection. The average multivitamin contains 400 IU of combined D_2 (ergocalciferol) and D_3 (cholecalciferol), whereas 20 minutes of full-body summer sun exposure provides 10,000 IU of D_3, the form used in the body. Vitamin D deficiency causes rickets in children and osteomalacia (Chapter 244) in adults. Bone remodeling may lead to compression of the spinal cord or roots (Chapter 400) owing to changes in vertebral bodies and foramina. Abrupt lack of vitamin D causes hypocalcemia with secondary hyperparathyroidism (Chapter 245). Hypocalcemia, in turn, can cause tetany, encephalopathy and generalized seizures.[7] Deficiency also causes proximal myopathy, worse in the legs than the arms, which can lead to peculiar patterns of gait as a result of weakness and fear of falling. It is associated with sleep disorders and fibromyalgia. Vitamin D plays a role in immune modulation of regulatory T cells, which may explain the relationship of vitamin D deficiency to a later risk of developing multiple sclerosis[8] (Chapter 411) and narcolepsy. Vitamin D deficiency is also associated with an increased incidence of Alzheimer and all-cause dementia.[9]

Individuals whose dietary absorption is normal require 400 to 600 IU (10 to 15 μg) of vitamin D_3 daily, but persons with malabsorption may need more than twice that amount. Reliance on sunlight is not recommended owing to risks of skin cancer (Chapter 203) as well as variability in personal environmental exposure. The eventual dose of supplementation, either weekly with 50,000 units (1.25 mg) of ergocalciferol (D_2) or daily with 400 to 800 IU of cholecalciferol (D_3), should be titrated to produce a serum 25-hydroxyvitamin D level of at least 20 ng/mL.

Toxicity from excess absorption of vitamin D, as is seen in sarcoidosis (Chapter 95) or granulomatous conditions or from excessive intake, is rare. Like deficiency states, vitamin D toxicity causes muscle and bone pain (Chapter 245).

Vitamin A Deficiency

Vitamin A deficiency, which is most often associated with retinal dysfunction ("night blindness" [Chapter 423]), can also impair the ability to taste and has rarely been associated with raised intracranial pressure in children. Malabsorption seldom leads to vitamin A deficiency, because it is stored in the body for long periods. Vitamin A toxicity, which is occasionally a complication of using isotretinoin for acne or excessive dietary consumption of liver (especially from fish-eating mammals such as polar bear, seal, and walrus), can cause idiopathic intracranial hypertension (Chapters 189 and 398) with headache and papilledema that leads to diminished vision or even blindness in severe cases.

Vitamin K Deficiency

Vitamin K deficiency, a rare consequence of malabsorption, is most often seen in patients who have compromised liver synthesis or who are taking the antagonist warfarin (Chapter 218). Vitamin K deficiency causes excessive bleeding and increases the risk of intracerebral hemorrhage (Chapter 408), especially in newborns whose mothers are taking antagonists such as phenytoin. Now that newborns are routinely given injections of vitamin K, maternal supplementation using 5 mg daily for the last month of pregnancy is reserved for women on vitamin K antagonists.

● DEFICIENCY OF MISCELLANEOUS ELEMENTS AND NUTRIENTS

Copper Deficiency

Acquired copper deficiency (Chapter 218) is rare and can be difficult to recognize. It occurs most often in premature or malnourished infants and in patients with malabsorption due to celiac disease, cystic fibrosis (Chapter 89), Crohn disease (Chapter 141), or intestinal blind loops after surgery (e.g., a Whipple procedure for pancreatic cancer or other malignancy, or bypass surgery for weight loss). It can also occur in patients with nephrotic syndrome (Chapter 121) and intestinal bacterial overgrowth (Chapter 140). Copper deficiency is also a well-recognized consequence of excessive intake of zinc, which upregulates copper chelation. Excessive zinc exposure usually results from overuse of zinc-containing products, such as denture cream or herbal preparations to treat rhinitis and sinusitis, or as a consequence of parenteral overload during hemodialysis (Chapter 131).

The most common neurologic complication of copper deficiency is a myelopathy that is clinically very similar to that seen with cobalamin deficiency.[10] The most prominent features are spastic paraparesis and sensory ataxia. A peripheral polyneuropathy of the axonal type is usually present as well. Optic neuropathy, wrist drop, and foot drop have also been reported. Copper levels, including excreted urinary copper, should be measured in patients who are suspected of having vitamin B_{12} deficiency but fail to respond to cyanocobalamin replacement. Treatment consists of oral copper supplementation, 8 mg/day tapering weekly over 3 weeks, followed by maintenance of 2 mg/day for life.

Wilson disease (Chapter 211) is an autosomal recessive disorder caused by mutation in the *ATP7B* gene that encodes ceruloplasmin, a copper-transporting protein. Symptoms result from excessive copper accumulation, primarily in the liver and brain, as a result of failed transport and impaired copper excretion. Psychiatric features such as personality change, disinhibition, depression, and psychosis sometimes overshadow neurologic manifestations such as dementia, dysarthria, chorea, tremor, and dystonia. Deposition of copper in Descemet membrane causes the characteristic Kayser-Fleischer ring, which is seen in the iris in over 95% of patients (Chapter 211, Fig. 211-2). Serum ceruloplasmin levels are low. Accumulation of copper in the liver leads to chronic liver failure. Wilson disease is treated by copper chelation (Chapter 211) and by minimizing dietary intake.

Menkes disease, an X-linked recessive copper deficiency caused by mutations in the *ATP7A* gene needed for absorption, is characterized by severe intellectual disability and kinky hair. The diagnosis is made by finding low serum copper levels or changes in the ratio of dopamine to norepinephrine. Large doses of copper histidine (250 mg twice daily until age 1, then daily until age 3) must be delivered subcutaneously, but improvement is variable. Patients survive to adulthood only if copper injections are begun in the neonatal period.

Other Nutritional Disorders

Biotin deficiency is caused by lack of protein in the diet, unsupplemented total parenteral nutrition, and an autosomal recessive disorder affecting biotinidase, which prevents biotin from being accessible for use. Genetic causes result in developmental delay, seizures, ataxia, and deafness if supplementation is not begun in the newborn period. Dietary deficiencies lead to lethargy, myalgias, and paresthesias, along with rash.

Some epidemics of peripheral neuropathy or optic neuropathy, such as Strachan Jamaican neuropathy and Cuban tobacco-alcohol amblyopia, which have occurred in the setting of malnutrition or overdependence on one source of food, have responded to replacement of B vitamins or folate and are therefore presumed to be due to deficiencies of these nutrients. Cyanide poisoning (Chapter 110) from smoking or consumption of sugarcane may contribute to toxicity. Iodine deficiency leads to hypothyroidism (Chapter 226), which causes varying degrees of cretinism.

Overreliance on one hardy food source (grass peas, chick peas) may lead to spastic paraparesis from lathyrism owing to oxalyldiaminoproprionic acid, which is a neurotoxic glutamate agonist. In older Nigerian men, cassava tuberis (konzo), which can potentiate neurotoxicity from cyanate and glucoside (Chapter 110), causes sensory neuropathy, ataxia, optic atrophy, and sensorineural deafness. In contrast, women and children develop spasticity, presumably from the same toxin. Amyotrophic lateral sclerosis and Parkinson-dementia complex in Guam are probably caused by cycad toxins in flour.

● ALCOHOL-RELATED DISORDERS

Alcohol (Chapter 33) is responsible for a wide spectrum of neurologic disorders. At one extreme, it can cause irreversible dementia, cerebellar degeneration, optic neuropathy, and peripheral polyneuropathy. After chronic overuse, withdrawal from alcohol causes transient neurologic overexcitation syndromes such as seizures, tremors, hallucinosis, and delirium tremens. Acute intoxication can range from mild euphoria to vestibular and cerebellar dysfunction to coma and death. It can also contribute to falls, accidents, behavioral dyscontrol with violence, and subsequent trauma. When alcohol is the main source of calories, it contributes to nutritional deficiency syndromes such as Wernicke-Korsakoff syndrome, beri-beri, and pellagra. Alcohol-induced liver toxicity results in hepatic encephalopathy and non-Wilsonian hepatolenticular degeneration. Coagulopathy caused by liver disease or suppressed platelet production raises the risk for subdural or intracranial hematoma (Fig. 416-1). Fetal alcohol syndrome reflects the vulnerability of the developing nervous system to the toxic effects of alcohol.

Signs of intoxication correlate with blood alcohol levels: 50 mg/dL for personality changes; 150 mg/dL for ataxia, vestibular dysfunction, and nystagmus; 300 mg/dL for stupor; 400 mg/dL for coma; and up to 500 mg/dL for respiratory depression or apnea. However, the effects vary greatly depending on the chronicity of intake and the rate at which high levels develop. Intoxication alone should never be assumed to be the sole cause of a depressed mental state, because alcoholics are at increased risk for other causes of coma (Chapter 404).

Specific Clinical Syndromes

Seizures and status epilepticus (Chapter 403) can be a direct consequence of intoxication, withdrawal, hyponatremia (Chapter 116), and hypomagnesemia (Chapter 119), or they can result from epileptogenic foci owing to previous head trauma or stroke. Even in patients with delirium tremens, other causes of seizures should be investigated and treated appropriately.

Hepatic encephalopathy is most often seen in patients with alcoholic cirrhosis (Chapter 153), especially patients who have bleeding esophageal varices. It is characterized by irritability alternating with depressed mental status, seizures, tremor, and asterixis. Although temporary reversal of encephalopathy with flumazenil (2 mg IV) can confirm the diagnosis, treatment focuses on trying to reduce the serum ammonia level, usually with lactulose (15 to 30 mL orally twice daily) and nonabsorbable antibiotics such as rifaximin (550 mg twice daily), neomycin (500 mg to 1 g three times daily), or metronidazole (250 mg two to four times daily).[11] Closure of spontaneous portosystemic shunts by embolization may be effective for reducing intractable encephalopathy in some patients.[12]

Dementia develops even when nutrition is well maintained because of alcohol's direct neurotoxic effects, although the absolute amounts of alcohol necessary to produce dementia are unclear.[13] In younger patients with dementia, 10 to 25% of cases are attributed to alcohol. In the elderly, excessive alcohol consumption is associated with faster cognitive decline compared with light to moderate alcohol consumption.[14] Frontal lobe dysfunction results in executive dysfunction (planning, abstract reasoning) rather than the amnesia that is prominent in Wernicke-Korsakoff syndrome. Contributing factors include head injury, status epilepticus, and cerebrovascular disease. The appearance of cerebral atrophy is further evidence of alcohol's deleterious effect involving both gray and white matter. The dementia is probably not reversible, although case reports credit the NMDA receptor antagonist memantine (28 mg XR daily) with improving scores on the mini–mental status examination, and small studies have reported improved cognition in patients taking rivastigmine (306 mg twice daily), an acetylcholinesterase inhibitor.

Wernicke encephalopathy and Korsakoff syndrome are described in the section on thiamine.

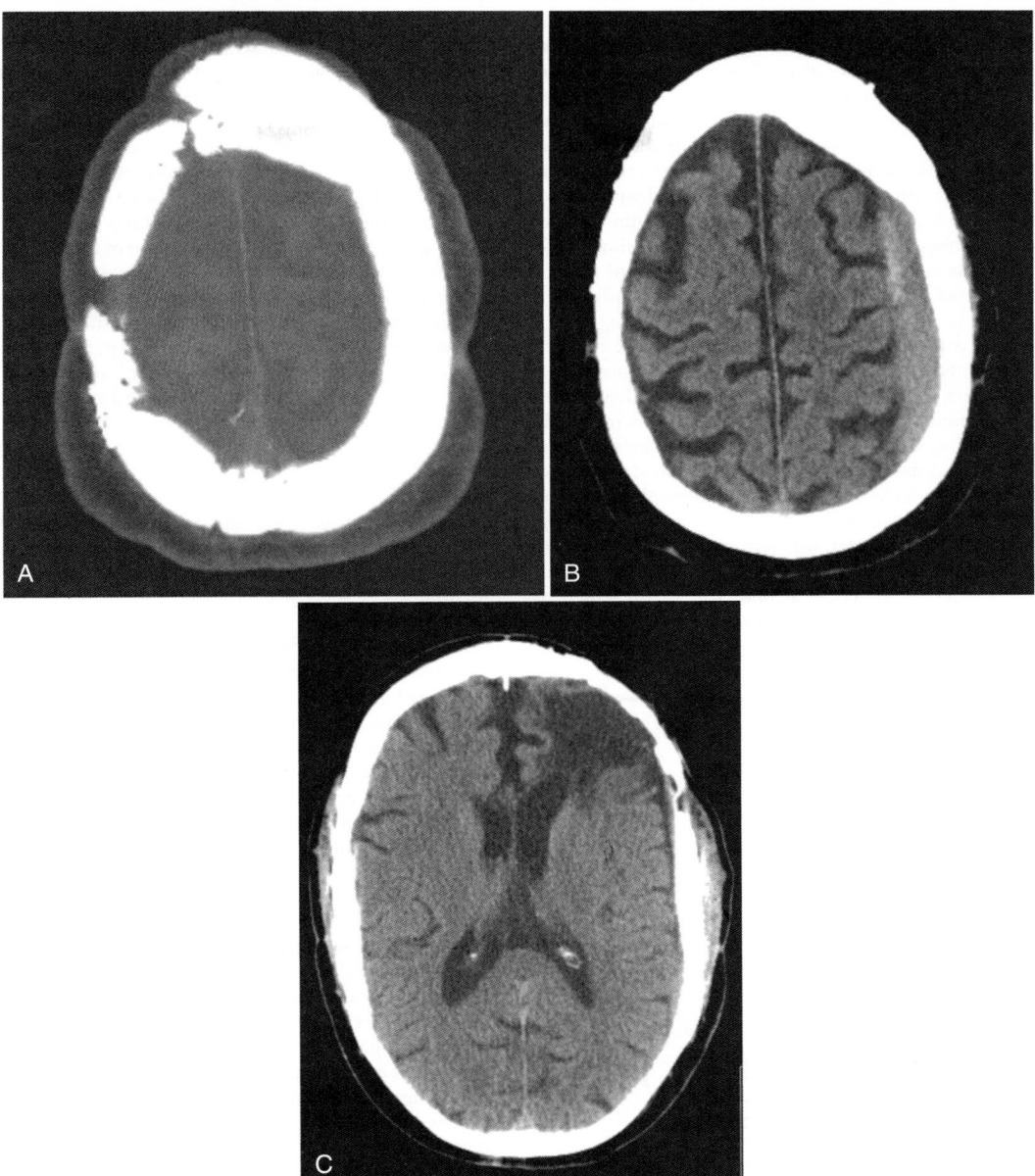

FIGURE 416-1. Alcoholic man admitted after a seizure, with no clinical signs of head trauma, lateralized weakness, or aphasia, but drowsy several hours after receiving lorazepam 2 mg intravenously. Computerized tomography axial brain scan shows (**A**) craniotomy defect on right, (**B**) mixed chronic and acute subdural hematoma on left, and (**C**) left frontal encephalomalacia from prior trauma.

Marchiafava-Bignami syndrome was first described in postmortem studies of Italian chianti drinkers but can occur in persons who consume any type of alcohol. Acute signs include coma, seizures, hemiparesis, rigidity, and sometimes death. The most severe pathology involves demyelination and necrosis of the corpus callosum. Findings on MRI include increased T2- and diffusion-weighted signals in the corpus callosum, especially the splenium.

Cerebellar degeneration and ataxia result from alcohol-induced loss of Purkinje cells, mainly in the anterior superior part of the cerebellar vermis; the cerebellar hemispheres are less affected. As a result, the clinical picture is one of mainly truncal and gait ataxia, with a wide-based unsteady gait and inability to walk tandem. The arms are much less involved if affected at all. Intention tremor, nystagmus, and dysarthria are rare. Findings are exacerbated by concurrent thiamine deficiency, leading to Wernicke encephalopathy. Alcohol may activate antibodies against Purkinje cells in individuals with gluten intolerance.

Optic neuropathy, which occurs with severe chronic alcohol abuse, is manifested as progressive painless visual loss as a result of damage to the optic nerve fibers. The macular region is most affected. Similar findings, first described in Cuban men who were heavy cigar smokers, have also been attributed to tobacco. However, neither alcohol nor tobacco is apparently directly responsible for the optic nerve damage, so it is more likely the syndrome results from malnutrition and deficiencies of multiple vitamins, including vitamins A and B.

Peripheral neuropathy (Chapter 420) ("alcoholic neuropathy") is the most common neurologic complication of chronic alcoholism. It is an axonal sensorimotor neuropathy that causes dysfunction of small nerve fibers, thereby leading to distal painful sensory symptoms such as burning dysesthesias and paresthesias of the soles of the feet. The typical numbness develops in a stocking-glove distribution, with loss of ankle reflexes. Mild distal weakness eventually occurs in some patients. Involvement of the autonomic nervous system frequently causes impotence as well as urinary or bowel complaints. Although vitamin supplements, especially thiamine and pyridoxine, may lead to some improvement, especially in the painful paresthesias, complete resolution is rare. If abstinence from alcohol is not also achieved, the symptoms persist, thereby implying that a direct toxic effect of alcohol is likely.

Compressive neuropathies, especially of the radial nerve ("Saturday night palsy") and peroneal nerve, can result after prolonged pressure on a nerve while the patient is obtunded from heavy alcohol consumption. Recovery takes many weeks but is generally complete.

Myopathy occurs in binge drinkers, in whom severe muscle injury with rhabdomyolysis (Chapter 113) can develop, especially in the setting of fasting and prolonged absence of movement. Myoglobinuria can result in kidney damage. Heavy alcohol consumption is also associated with cardiomyopathy (Chapter 60), which can lead to arrhythmias even in the absence of hypokalemia. Chronic alcohol abuse causes a symmetrical proximal weakness (Chapter 421), which is not usually severe enough to prevent walking or standing. It can be detected in up to 50% of heavy users, but only with a careful examination.

Fetal alcohol syndrome is recognized at birth in infants whose mothers consumed significant amounts of alcohol in the early stages of pregnancy, but the quantity required to place a fetus at risk has not been definitively determined. The characteristic findings are growth retardation, microcephaly, hypotonia, skeletal and cardiac anomalies, and characteristic facial features (micrognathia, small palpebral fissures). Recently, migration defects have been demonstrated by diffusion-weighted MRI and tractography. Exposure of the developing brain to alcohol can also lead to subtle or severe neurocognitive defects and attention deficit disorder, which may not be detected until later in childhood. Although malnutrition and excess alcohol have synergistic deleterious effects, the teratogenic effects of alcohol are not prevented by adequate amounts of thiamine, folate, and other vitamins.

 Grade A Reference

A1. Andres E, Fothergill H, Mecili M. Efficacy of oral cobalamin (vitamin B$_{12}$) therapy. *Expert Opin Pharmacother.* 2010;11:249-256.

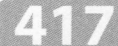
GENERAL REFERENCES

For the General References and other additional features, please visit Expert Consult at https://expertconsult.inkling.com.

417

CONGENITAL, DEVELOPMENTAL, AND NEUROCUTANEOUS DISORDERS

JONATHAN W. MINK

CONGENITAL DISORDERS
Malformations of Cerebral Cortex

Developmental malformations of the cerebral cortex arise from a wide variety of etiologies, including genetic mutations, intrauterine infections, intrauterine ischemia, and toxic exposures.[1] These malformations are heterogeneous and can result from disrupted neuronal proliferation, migration, or cortical organization. In general, disorders that arise early in development are more severe than those that arise after the basic architecture of the brain has developed. When small areas of the brain are involved, the patient may have minor impairment of neurologic function. When larger areas of the brain are involved, patients often have cognitive deficits and more severe neurologic dysfunction. Epilepsy (Chapter 403), which is the most common manifestation of abnormal cortical development, may occur with or without other neurologic signs or symptoms.

Disorders of Neuronal Proliferation

Neuronal proliferation can be abnormally increased or decreased owing to a variety of mechanisms. These disorders can manifest with megalencephaly or microcephaly, or head size can be normal. Abnormal proliferation can involve specific cell types, thereby resulting in focal or multifocal areas of dysplasia or in the formation of hamartomas (see Tuberous Sclerosis, later).

FOCAL CORTICAL DYSPLASIA WITH BALLOON CELLS

Focal cortical dysplasia is caused by abnormal proliferation of both neurons and glia. Its neuropathology is characterized by the presence of giant dysmorphic neurons and "balloon cells" associated with altered cortical lamination, but some lesions have abnormal cortical layering with ectopic neurons in white matter. Affected patients typically present with partial seizures that are often intractable to medical therapy. These seizures can begin at any age but most commonly present during childhood or adolescence. The type of seizure depends on the anatomic location of the dysplasia. Other neurologic manifestations such as sensory, motor, or cognitive impairments depend on the extent of the dysplasia and whether multiple brain regions are affected. The diagnosis of focal cortical dysplasia is usually made with brain magnetic resonance imaging (MRI), which demonstrates focal thickening of a gyrus or alteration of the gray–white matter junction. Management includes medical treatment of seizures, but surgical resection of the epileptic focus may be required for complete remission (Chapter 403).

Disorders of Neuronal Migration

Disorders of neuronal migration typically result in disruption of the normal laminar organization of the cerebral cortex. Defects include impaired initiation of neuronal migration, impaired orderly migration, and impaired termination of migration. All result in abnormal cortical organization and function.

LISSENCEPHALY AND BAND HETEROTOPIA

The lissencephalies (smooth brain) are a group of disorders that are caused by arrested migration of neurons to the cerebral cortex. Lissencephaly, which is typically diagnosed in infancy or early childhood, is usually accompanied by microcephaly, severe global developmental delay, cerebral palsy,[2] and intractable epilepsy. Lissencephaly genes include *PAFAH1B1* (also known as *LIS1* on chromosome 17p13.3), *DCX* (on chromosome Xq22), and *TUBA1A* (on chromosome 12), all of which are involved in the regulation of microtubule organization and function. Individuals with mutations of *LIS1* typically have severe malformations that are most prominent in the posterior cerebrum. More extensive mutations in the region of *LIS1* result in Miller-Dieker syndrome, a condition characterized by lissencephaly and distinctive facial features that include a prominent forehead, midface hypoplasia, low-set and abnormally shaped ears, and a small jaw. Males with *DCX* mutations typically have a severe lissencephaly that is most prominent in the anterior cerebrum. Individuals with *TUBA1A* mutations may have isolated lissencephaly or may have lissencephaly with cerebellar hypoplasia. Diagnosis of lissencephaly is made by brain MRI that shows a smooth cortex with minimal sulcation. Genetic testing for *LIS1*, *DCX*, and *TUBA1A* is available. Management consists of seizure control, genetic counseling, and supportive care.

Band heterotopia (double cortex) is a less severe form of lissencephaly that is usually seen in women with *DCX* mutation. Clinical manifestations of band heterotopia range from mild to severe and include seizures, intellectual disability, and developmental delay. Women with a *DCX* mutation are at risk of having male children with severe lissencephaly. Brain MRI demonstrates a band of gray matter underlying a nearly normal-appearing cerebral cortex. Management consists of seizure control and genetic counseling.

NODULAR HETEROTOPIA

Nodular heterotopias are characterized by nodular ectopic collections of neurons and glia in the subependyma or in the subcortical white matter. The most important form is subependymal nodular heterotopia, a condition characterized by multiple gray matter nodules in the walls of the lateral ventricles bilaterally. This X-linked condition is due to a mutation in *FLNA* (chromosome Xq28), which codes for filamin A, an actin-cross-linking phosphoprotein that is critical for the initiation of migration. As a result of this mutation, many neurons do not migrate out of the subventricular zone. Most affected individuals are heterozygous females. Males are severely affected and often die in infancy. Most affected females present with seizures during childhood or adolescence. Females may be intellectually normal or have mild disability. Individuals with subependymal nodular heterotopia appear to be at increased risk for aortic or carotid dissection and for cardiac valvular abnormalities.

The diagnosis is based on brain MRI, which shows gray matter nodules along the walls of the lateral ventricles. Genetic testing for *FLNA* is available. Management consists of seizure control and genetic counseling.

Disorders of Cortical Organization

Disorders of cortical organization include conditions such as polymicrogyria and schizencephaly. These disorders are not due to abnormal numbers of neurons or impaired migration but instead include abnormalities of gyration, sulcation, connectivity, or synaptogenesis. The best-understood of these disorders are polymicrogyria and schizencephaly.

POLYMICROGYRIA

Polymicrogyria is characterized by regions of complex cortical convolutions with miniature gyri that are fused and superimposed together. Polymicrogyria is caused by failure of cortical organization as a result of in utero injury or genetic mutation; it has been associated with prenatal infections (e.g., cytomegalovirus) and possible vascular abnormalities, but often it is idiopathic. A single gene, *GPR56* (chromosome 16q13), has been associated with bilateral frontoparietal polymicrogyria. *GPR56* codes for a G protein–coupled receptor that appears to be important for human cerebral cortical development. Clinical manifestations include epilepsy, developmental delay, cerebral palsy, and intellectual disability, depending on the location and extent of the abnormality. The diagnosis of polymicrogyria is made by brain MRI. Clinical management consists of seizure management and supportive therapies.

SCHIZENCEPHALY

Schizencephaly is characterized by infolding of cortical gray matter along a hemispheric cleft near the primary cerebral fissures. It is thought to represent a more extensive injury than what leads to polymicrogyria. In most cases, the cause cannot be determined, but it has been associated with in utero insult. A rare familial form has been described, but no gene has been identified. Clinical features include developmental delay, cerebral palsy, dysarthria, and epilepsy. The clinical abnormalities are more severe with large open-lip schizencephaly and with bilateral lesions than with small unilateral closed-lip schizencephaly. Diagnosis is made by brain MRI. Management consists of seizure control and supportive therapies when indicated.

Malformations of Cerebellum and Brain Stem

Developmental abnormalities of the hindbrain are less well understood than are abnormalities of cerebral cortical development.[3] Two of the better known and important syndromes are Joubert syndrome and Dandy-Walker malformation.

JOUBERT SYNDROME

Joubert syndrome is characterized by a distinctive pattern of cerebellar and brain stem developmental malformation. Four causative genes (*NPHP1*, *CEP290*, *AHI1*, and *TMEM67* [*MKS3*]) together account for approximately 30% of cases. Clinical features include hypotonia, truncal ataxia, developmental delay, abnormal eye movements, and disordered breathing. The combination of signs and severity can be variable. Some individuals with Joubert syndrome also have retinal dystrophy, renal disease, ocular colobomas, occipital encephalocele, or hepatic fibrosis. No formal diagnostic criteria exist. The diagnosis is usually based on the combination of hypotonia in infancy with later development of ataxia, intellectual impairment, and abnormal breathing pattern, or abnormal eye movements in combination with a characteristic MRI finding known as the molar tooth sign. The molar tooth sign results from hypoplasia of the cerebellar vermis and accompanying brain stem abnormalities on axial imaging through the junction of the midbrain and pons. Genetic testing is available for the four identified genes. Management is supportive. Caffeine can be helpful for periodic hypoventilation, but some patients require tracheostomy.

DANDY-WALKER MALFORMATION

Dandy-Walker malformation is characterized by cerebellar vermis hypoplasia and cystic dilation of the fourth ventricle. Rare familial cases have been reported, but a genetic basis has not been identified. This heterogeneous disorder is usually accompanied by hypotonia, delayed motor development, and ataxia. Intellectual disability is present in about 50% of affected individuals. In some cases, hydrocephalus requires shunting. Diagnosis is based on characteristic findings on brain MRI. Treatment is supportive, with cerebrospinal fluid (CSF) shunting when indicated.

CHIARI MALFORMATIONS

Four types of Chiari malformation have been described. The most common of these are Chiari types I and II. Chiari I malformations are most often

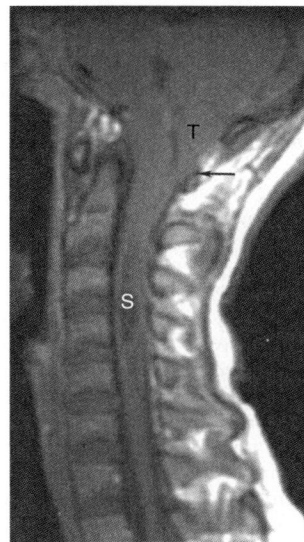

FIGURE 417-1. Chiari I malformation. A sagittal magnetic resonance image shows low, pointed cerebellar tonsils (i.e., Chiari I malformation, T) that extend to the level of C1 (*arrow*) and a dilated central canal of the spinal cord (i.e., syringohydromyelia [S]). (From Barkovich AJ, Kuzniecky RI. Congenital, developmental, and neurocutaneous disorders. In Goldman L, Ausiello D, eds. *Cecil Textbook of Medicine.* 23rd ed. Philadelphia: Saunders Elsevier; 2008:2790.)

diagnosed in adulthood, whereas Chiari II malformations are associated with spina bifida and are usually diagnosed in childhood.

Chiari I malformations are characterized by downward displacement of the cerebellar tonsils through the foramen magnum, often first accompanied by compression of the tonsils. Chiari I is a developmental abnormality that is thought to be congenital in most cases, even though symptoms may not present until adulthood, typically in the third or fourth decade of life. The abnormality is often asymptomatic and discovered only as an incidental finding. However, clinical manifestations can result from compression of neural structures at the cranial-cervical junction or obstruction of CSF flow. Signs and symptoms include headaches that worsen with straining or coughing, lower cranial nerve findings, downbeat nystagmus, ataxia, or long-tract signs. Chiari I malformations are accompanied by syringomyelia (see later) in up to 80% of cases. Diagnosis is made with brain MRI, which shows the cerebellar tonsils extending through the foramen magnum 5 mm or more (Fig. 417-1). Surgical treatment with craniocervical decompression is recommended for symptomatic patients but usually not for asymptomatic individuals or patients whose only symptom is headache.[4]

Chiari II malformations, commonly called Arnold-Chiari malformations, are characterized by descent of the cerebellar tonsils, the inferior vermis, and portions of the cerebellar hemispheres into the spinal canal, along with elongation and displacement of the brain stem and fourth ventricle. Chiari II malformations are almost always associated with meningomyelocele and spina bifida. Hydrocephalus requiring shunting occurs in most cases. Brain stem dysfunction may result from intrinsic malformation or from compression of neural structures at the craniocervical junction. Treatment is surgical repair of the myelomeningocele, relief of hydrocephalus, and occasionally cervical bone decompression. The prognosis depends on the level and extent of the myelomeningocele and on the severity of brain anomalies.

Malformations of Spinal Cord

TETHERED SPINAL CORD

Tethered spinal cord syndrome is a disorder caused by an anomalous filum terminale that restricts the normal ascent of the conus medullaris and limits the movement of the spinal cord within the spinal column. The result is an abnormal stretching of the spinal cord, with neurologic symptoms referable to the lower spinal cord. Tethering may also develop after spinal cord injury. Associated spinal anomalies are common and may include diastematomyelia, spinal lipomas, dermal sinuses, and fibrolipomas of the filum terminale. Symptoms can occur at any age but usually develop during periods of rapid growth in childhood or adolescence. However, tethered spinal cord syndrome may go undiagnosed until adulthood, when sensory and motor problems and loss of bowel and bladder control emerge. Erectile dysfunction may occur in males. Symptoms are typically progressive. Diagnosis is made with MRI, which shows a low conus medullaris (i.e., below the bottom of the L2 vertebral body) or a thickened or fat-containing filum terminale. Diminished pulsations of the spinal cord may also be seen. Treatment consists of surgical release of the tethered cord. With successful surgery, symptoms typically do not progress and may improve.

SYRINGOHYDROMYELIA

Syringohydromyelia is a condition in which the central canal of the spinal cord (hydromyelia) or the substance of the spinal cord (syringomyelia) is expanded by the accumulation of CSF. In many cases, both hydromyelia and syringomyelia are present (syringohydromyelia). The proximate cause of syringes probably is altered flow of CSF, with variations in pressure in different parts of the subarachnoid space. The pressure variations create forces that drive CSF into the spinal cord. Possible causes include narrowing of the foramen magnum, Chiari I and II malformations, intramedullary and extramedullary spinal cord tumors, and subarachnoid scarring. Subsequent extension of the cyst may result from rapid changes in intraspinal pressure owing to such events as coughing or sneezing. Symptoms of syringohydromyelia most commonly begin in late adolescence or early adulthood and progress irregularly, with long periods of stability. The classic presentation is asymmetrical weakness and atrophy in the upper extremities, loss of upper limb deep tendon reflexes, and loss of pain and temperature sensation (with preservation of vibration and proprioception) in the neck, arms, and upper part of the trunk. With progression, spasticity and hyperreflexia develop in the lower extremities. Progressive ascending and descending levels of weakness and sensory impairment typically occur over time. The diagnosis is made by spinal MRI (see Fig. 417-1). If syringohydromyelia is identified, it is important to perform a brain MRI to look for associated abnormalities of the craniocervical junction. Occasionally, mild central canal dilation is discovered incidentally in patients without spinal cord symptoms or signs. If no associated cause is found, the prognosis of such incidentally discovered anomalies is generally good. Treatment is directed at the cause if one can be identified. Syringopleural or syringoperitoneal shunting is sometimes performed, with variable benefit.

DEVELOPMENTAL DISORDERS

Disorders that result from impaired postnatal neurodevelopmental function range from specific disorders such as fragile X syndrome and Rett syndrome, to complex syndromes such as autism, to nonspecific developmental delay and learning disabilities.

Fragile X Syndrome

Fragile X syndrome is an X-linked trinucleotide repeat disorder that is characterized by nonsyndromic intellectual disability in most affected males. It is the most common genetic cause of intellectual disability, affecting 1/4000 males and 1/8000 females. The pathogenesis of fragile X syndrome is not well understood. The classic disorder is seen in males with full mutations (>200 repeats) in the *FMR1* gene.[5] Fragile X syndrome may present as only moderate to severe intellectual disability, but it is often associated with a prominent forehead, large ears, prominent jaw, and macro-orchidism. Postpubertal males often have poor impulse control, perseveration, and poor eye contact. Up to 25% of affected males have autism. Heterozygous females may be asymptomatic or may have a syndrome similar to what is seen in males, depending on repeat size and random X-inactivation.

Other disorders associated with *FMR1* include the fragile X ataxia syndrome, which is characterized by the late onset, usually after age 50 years, of progressive cerebellar ataxia and intention tremor in individuals who have an *FMR1* premutation (60 to 200 repeats). It occurs equally in males and females. Diagnosis of *FMR1* disorders is by molecular genetic testing. Cytogenetic testing for fragile sites is no longer recommended because it is less sensitive and more expensive than molecular testing. Treatment is symptomatic and supportive. Genetic counseling is recommended for affected individuals and their families.

Rett Syndrome

Rett syndrome is a neurodevelopmental disorder that occurs classically in females with mutations in the *MECP2* gene. *MECP2* mutations are generally lethal in male embryos, but Rett syndrome has been reported in males with XXY karyotype or with somatic mosaicism. *MECP2* is thought to mediate transcriptional silencing of methylated DNA. Most mutations are probably de novo or may reflect germline mosaicism; 99% of cases represent a single

occurrence within a family. Affected girls are usually normal at birth and have apparently normal development for the first 6 to 18 months of life. Brain growth decelerates, and development stagnates, followed by rapid regression of language and motor skills. A classic feature of Rett syndrome is the loss of purposeful hand use and the development of repetitive stereotyped hand movements that usually have the appearance of wringing or clapping. Other features present to variable degree are bruxism, episodic apnea and hyperpnea, seizures, gait disorders, and tremor.[6] Non-neurologic features include growth failure and wasting, bowel dysmotility, scoliosis, osteopenia, and vasomotor changes in the limbs. Diagnosis is by clinical criteria followed by molecular genetic testing. Treatment is symptomatic.

Autism

Autism or autism spectrum disorder is characterized by impaired social communication and interactions as well as restricted and repetitive behaviors. Autism is associated with many different causes and is often idiopathic.[7] Fragile X syndrome and tuberous sclerosis are two important entities in which an autistic phenotype can occur and in which autism may be the most prominent feature.

Symptoms typically present before 3 years of age and persist into adulthood. Autism is a spectrum ranging from severe, with impairment in all domains, to mild with normal intellect and language but with impaired social interactions and repetitive behaviors or restricted interests. Autism has many causes but in most cases is idiopathic. Epilepsy is common in autism. Diagnosis is based on careful diagnostic interview and examination (Table 417-1). When epilepsy is present, treatment with antiepileptic medications is indicated. Behavioral therapy can help individuals learn rules for social interaction and can improve communication. It can also help with problematic behavior. Educational support is important. Medications such as atypical antipsychotics, selective serotonin reuptake inhibitors, and anxiolytics (Chapter 397) can help with aggressive behavior, repetitive behaviors, and anxiety.

NEUROCUTANEOUS DISORDERS

Neurocutaneous disorders are congenital syndromes characterized by dysplastic and neoplastic lesions primarily involving the nervous system and skin. The more than 40 described syndromes include neurofibromatosis, tuberous sclerosis, Sturge-Weber syndrome, and von Hippel-Lindau disease.

Neurofibromatosis

Neurofibromatosis encompasses a spectrum of syndromes with distinctive neural and cutaneous lesions. The two major forms of neurofibromatosis are genetically and clinically distinct.

NEUROFIBROMATOSIS TYPE 1

Neurofibromatosis type 1, which is the classic disorder described by von Recklinghausen, is an autosomal dominant condition with an incidence of

TABLE 417-1	DIAGNOSTIC CRITERIA FOR AUTISM SPECTRUM DISORDER

1. Deficits in Social Communication/Interaction (must have all three criteria):
   a. Problems reciprocating social or emotional interaction, including difficulty establishing or maintaining back-and-forth conversations and interactions, inability to initiate an interaction, and problems with shared attention or sharing of emotions and interests with others
   b. Severe problems maintaining relationships—ranges from lack of interest in other people to difficulties in pretend play and engaging in age-appropriate social activities, and problems adjusting to different social expectations
   c. Nonverbal communication problems such as abnormal eye contact, posture, facial expressions, tone of voice and gestures, as well as an inability to understand these

2. Restricted and Repetitive Behavior (at least 2 criteria must be met):
   a. Stereotyped or repetitive speech, motor movements or use of objects
   b. Excessive adherence to routines, ritualized patterns of verbal or nonverbal behavior, or excessive resistance to change
   c. Highly restricted interests that are abnormal in intensity or focus
   d. Hyper- or hyporeactivity to sensory input or unusual interest in sensory aspects of the environment

Symptoms must be present in early childhood but may not become fully manifest until social demands exceed capacities. Symptoms need to be *functionally impairing* and not better described by another DSM-5 diagnosis.

From American Psychiatric Association. *Diagnostic and Statistical Manual of Mental Disorders.* 5th ed. Arlington, VA: American Psychiatric Publishing, 2013.

1 per 2500 to 3000 births.[8] Although it is an autosomal dominant disease, approximately 50% of cases are due to new mutations. Most mutations in *NF1* occur in the parental germline. The *NF1* gene, which is located on chromosome 17q11.2, codes a protein called neurofibromin, which is thought to function as a tumor suppressor by acting as a negative regulator of the Ras signaling pathway. Neurofibromatosis type 1 is characterized by multiple café au lait spots, axillary and inguinal freckling, multiple discrete cutaneous neurofibromas (Fig. 417-2), and Lisch nodules (Table 417-2). Subcutaneous neurofibromas may be painful or disfiguring. Learning disabilities are present in at least 50% of individuals. Other manifestations include plexiform neurofibromas, optic nerve and other central nervous system (CNS) gliomas, malignant peripheral nerve sheath tumors, tibial dysplasia, and vasculopathy.

Management of patients depends on the specific manifestations and often requires multidisciplinary collaboration. Most patients with neurofibromatosis type 1 do not require treatment, but all require surveillance (Table 417-3). Subcutaneous, intraspinal, and intracranial tumors can be treated surgically. Optic nerve gliomas may be treated with chemotherapy; both cisplatin and temozolomide have shown some benefit. Radiation is not recommended. Genetic counseling should be provided to all patients and their families.

NEUROFIBROMATOSIS TYPE 2

Neurofibromatosis type 2, which is often referred to as central neurofibromatosis, is an autosomal dominant condition with an incidence of approximately

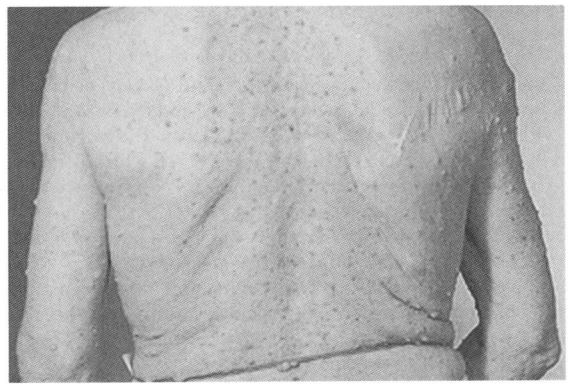

FIGURE 417-2. Multiple neurofibromas covering the back of a patient with neurofibromatosis type 1.

TABLE 417-2	DIAGNOSTIC CRITERIA FOR NEUROFIBROMATOSIS TYPE 1

Two or more of the following clinical features signify the presence of neurofibromatosis type 1:
  Six or more café au lait macules (>0.5 cm at largest diameter in prepubertal individuals or >1.5 cm in individuals past puberty)
  Axillary freckling or freckling in inguinal regions
  Two or more neurofibromas of any type or ≥ 1 plexiform neurofibroma
  Two or more Lisch nodules (iris hamartomas)
  A distinctive osseous lesion
  A first-degree relative with neurofibromatosis type 1 diagnosed by using the above-listed criteria

TABLE 417-3	RECOMMENDED SURVEILLANCE IN PATIENTS WITH NEUROFIBROMATOSIS TYPE 1

Annual physical examination by a physician who is familiar with the individual and with the disease

Annual ophthalmologic examination in early childhood, less frequent examination in older children and adults

Regular developmental assessment by screening questionnaire (in childhood)

Regular blood pressure monitoring

Other studies only as indicated on the basis of clinically apparent signs or symptoms

Monitoring of those who have abnormalities of the central nervous system, skeletal system, or cardiovascular system by an appropriate specialist

1 in 25,000 individuals.[9] The *NF2* gene is located on chromosome 22q12.2. Its gene product merlin is a cytoskeletal protein thought to act as a membrane-stabilizing protein. The specific function of merlin is unknown. Neurofibromatosis type 2 is characterized by bilateral vestibular schwannomas, which usually present with symptoms of tinnitus, hearing loss, and imbalance. The age at onset is usually in young adulthood, but some individuals may develop posterior subcapsular lens opacities or mononeuropathy in childhood. Almost all affected individuals develop bilateral vestibular schwannomas by age 30 (Table 417-4). Affected individuals may also develop schwannomas of other cranial and peripheral nerves, meningiomas, and (rarely) ependymomas or astrocytomas. Posterior subcapsular lens opacities are the most common ocular abnormality.

Management is dependent on the specific manifestations and complications. In individuals who either have tested positive for known *NF2* mutations or have a family history of neurofibromatosis type 2 and whose genetic status cannot be determined with genetic testing, annual brain MRI is recommended starting between ages 10 and 12 years and continuing until at least age 40 years. Hearing evaluations may be useful in detecting changes in auditory nerve function before changes can be visualized by MRI. Routine complete eye examinations should be part of the care of all individuals.

Bevacizumab, a vascular endothelial growth factor inhibitor (5 mg/kg intravenously every 2 weeks), can improve hearing in some patients with neurofibromatosis type 2 and vestibular schwannomas. Surgical treatment of schwannomas and meningiomas may be indicated to preserve function or to relieve compression of adjacent structures, especially in patients with intramedullary spinal tumors. Genetic counseling should be provided to affected individuals and their families.

Tuberous Sclerosis

Tuberous sclerosis complex is characterized by abnormalities of the brain, kidney, and heart.[10] Tuberous sclerosis may occur as an autosomal dominant syndrome or result from spontaneous mutation. Two tuberous sclerosis genes have been identified. *TSC1* (chromosome 9q34) codes for a protein called hamartin, a protein that interacts with the product of the *TSC2* gene to inhibit the mammalian target of rapamycin (mTOR). *TSC2* (chromosome 16p13) codes for tuberin, which interacts with hamartin. *TSC2* mutations account for about 60% of individuals with clinical tuberous sclerosis.[11]

Specific findings vary across individuals, and severity ranges from minimal to severe. Skin lesions are seen in almost 100% of affected individuals, but CNS lesions are the leading cause of morbidity and mortality. Epilepsy is seen in as many as 80% of patients with CNS lesions. Intellectual impairment and developmental delay are common, and up to 40% of patients have an autism spectrum disorder. Giant cell astrocytoma is the leading cause of death. Up to 80% of children with tuberous sclerosis have an identifiable renal lesion (Chapter 197) by 10.5 years of age, and renal disease is the second leading cause of early death in individuals with tuberous sclerosis. Cardiac rhabdomyomas, which can occur in up to 50% of patients, are usually present at birth and typically regress over time. Diagnosis of tuberous sclerosis (Table 417-5) is usually clinical and confirmed by identification of calcified or uncalcified hamartomas on imaging studies (Fig. 417-3).

Treatment is directed at complications of the disease, particularly epilepsy (Chapter 403). Neurosurgical intervention may sometimes be indicated for epilepsy and for symptomatic treatment of complications such as hydrocephalus, which results from midline giant cell tumors. In a randomized

TABLE 417-4	DIAGNOSTIC CRITERIA FOR NEUROFIBROMATOSIS TYPE 2

Presence of one or more of the following makes the diagnosis of neurofibromatosis type 2:
  • Bilateral vestibular schwannomas
  • A first-degree relative with neurofibromatosis type 2, *and*
      Unilateral vestibular schwannoma, *or*
      Any two of: meningioma, schwannoma, glioma, neurofibroma, posterior subcapsular lenticular opacities*
  • Unilateral vestibular schwannoma, *and*
      Any two of: meningioma, schwannoma, glioma, neurofibroma, posterior subcapsular lenticular opacities*
  • Multiple meningiomas, *and*
      Unilateral vestibular schwannoma, *or*
      Any two of: schwannoma, glioma, neurofibroma, cataract*

*"Any two of" refers to two individual tumors or cataracts.

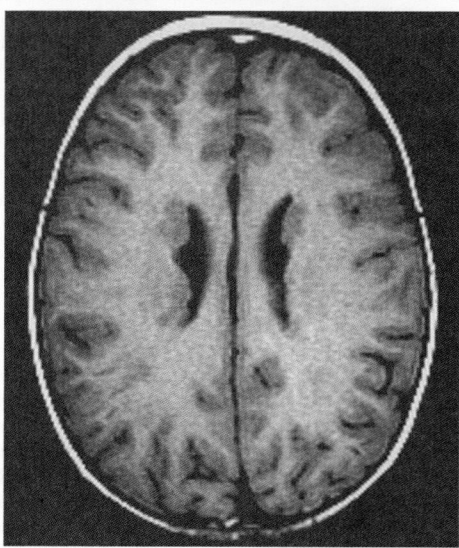

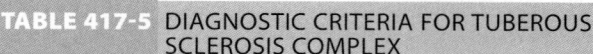

FIGURE 417-3. Subependymal nodules and multiple cortical tubers in a patient with tuberous sclerosis.

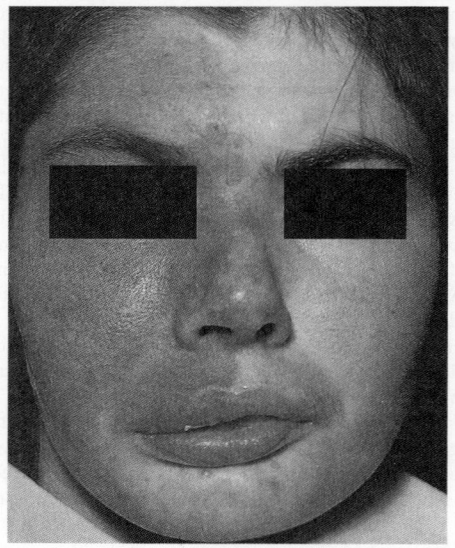

FIGURE 417-4. Sturge-Weber syndrome. This patient has a classic diffuse capillary hemangioma in the distribution of the ophthalmic, nasociliary, and maxillary branches of the trigeminal nerve. The lesion extends backward over the anterior two thirds of the crown of the head. (From Forbes CD, Jackson WD. *Color Atlas and Text of Clinical Medicine.* 2nd ed. London: Mosby; 1996.)

TABLE 417-5	DIAGNOSTIC CRITERIA FOR TUBEROUS SCLEROSIS COMPLEX

Definite—Two major features or one major feature plus two minor features
Probable—One major feature plus one minor feature
Possible—One major feature or two or more minor features

MAJOR FEATURES

Facial angiofibromas or forehead plaque
Nontraumatic ungual or periungual fibromas
More than three hypomelanotic macules (ash leaf spots)
Shagreen patch (connective tissue nevus)
Multiple retinal nodular hamartomas
Cortical tuber
Subependymal nodule
Subependymal giant cell astrocytoma
Cardiac rhabdomyoma, single or multiple
Lymphangiomyomatosis
Renal angiomyolipoma

MINOR FEATURES

Multiple dental enamel pits
Hamartomatous rectal polyps
Bone cysts
Cerebral white matter radial migration lines
Gingival fibromas
Nonrenal hamartoma
Retinal achromic patch
"Confetti" skin lesions
Multiple renal cysts

controlled trial, treatment with everolimus (10 mg/day) reduced the size of the angiomyolipomas in 42% percent of participants receiving active drug as compared with 0% of participants receiving placebo.[A2] In another double-blind placebo controlled trial, everolimus titrated to a concentration of 5 to 15 ng/mL was effective in reducing the size subependymal giant cell astrocytomas by at least 50% in 35% of participants receiving active drug as compared with 0% of participants receiving placebo.[A3] At similar doses, everolimus also can change fractional anisotropy and radial diffusivity, suggesting that the genetic defect of tuberous sclerosis complex in the brain may be modified pharmacologically. Serial brain MRI and renal ultrasound screening may be indicated in some patients because benign tumors of these organs may enlarge rapidly. Genetic counseling is an important part of management.

Sturge-Weber Syndrome

Sturge-Weber syndrome is a sporadic disorder characterized by facial vascular nevi, epilepsy, cognitive impairment, and sometimes hemiparesis, hemianopsia, or glaucoma. It is most commonly due to somatic mutation in *GNAQ* (chromosome 9q21).[12] The characteristic CNS feature of this disorder is capillary angiomatosis of the pia mater. Cerebral cortical calcifications are generally seen in a pericapillary distribution and are progressive. Most patients with Sturge-Weber syndrome have epilepsy. The diagnosis is usually based on the presence of a facial nevus (Fig. 417-4), which is manifested as a typical port-wine stain, and confirmatory imaging on a contrast brain MRI showing leptomeningeal enhancement.

Regular ophthalmologic examination is warranted because of the risk for glaucoma. Treatment is usually aimed at the epilepsy, which can be medically intractable. In patients with intractable epilepsy and infantile-onset hemiplegia, hemispherectomy can improve the seizures and the neurodevelopmental outcome.

Von Hippel-Lindau Disease

Von Hippel-Lindau disease (i.e., CNS angiomatosis) is an autosomal dominant disorder caused by a defective tumor suppressor gene (*VHL*) at chromosome 3p25-p26.[13] It is characterized by retinal angiomas, brain (usually cerebellar) and spinal cord hemangioblastomas, renal cell carcinomas, endolymphatic sac tumors, pheochromocytomas, papillary cystadenomas of the epididymis, angiomas of the liver and kidney, and cysts of the pancreas, kidney, liver, and epididymis. Both sexes are affected equally.

Symptoms typically begin during the third or fourth decade. Retinal inflammation with exudate, hemorrhage, and retinal detachment from the retinal angiomas typically precedes the cerebellar complaints, but the order is not constant. The ocular findings are nonspecific, and the retinal detachment may mask the underlying lesion. Headache, vertigo, and vomiting result from cerebellar tumors. Cerebellar signs such as ataxia, dysdiadochokinesis, and dysmetria are common. Rare patients present with symptoms of spinal cord or visceral lesions, or may have hearing loss from tumors of the endolymphatic sac.

Clinical diagnosis is established if the patient has more than one CNS hemangioblastoma, one hemangioblastoma with a visceral manifestation of the disease, or one manifestation of the disease and a known family history. Molecular genetic testing detects mutations in the *VHL* gene in nearly 100% of affected individuals.

For patients with von Hippel-Lindau disease and for those with a disease-causing VHL mutation, surveillance is recommended with annual ophthalmologic examination, annual blood pressure monitoring, measurement of urinary catecholamine metabolites beginning at age 5 years in families with pheochromocytoma, and annual abdominal ultrasound examination beginning at age 16 years, with evaluation of suspicious lesions by computed tomography or MRI. Treatment is symptomatic. Retinal detachments and tumors are treated by laser therapy. Large brain tumors (Chapter 189), renal cell carcinomas (Chapter 197), pheochromocytomas (Chapter 228), epididymal tumors (Chapter 200), and endolymphatic sac tumors are treated surgically; smaller CNS tumors may be treated by gamma knife.

Grade A References

A1. Plotkin SR, Stemmer-Rachamimov AO, Barker FG 2nd, et al. Hearing improvement after bevacizumab in patients with neurofibromatosis type 2. *N Engl J Med.* 2009;361:358-367.
A2. Bissler JJ, Kingswood JC, Radzikowska E, et al. Everolimus for angiomyolipoma associated with tuberous sclerosis complex or sporadic lymphangioleiomyomatosis (EXIST-2): a multicentre, randomised, double-blind, placebo-controlled trial. *Lancet.* 2013;381:817-824.
A3. Franz DN, Belousova E, Sparagana S, et al. Efficacy and safety of everolimus for subependymal giant cell astrocytomas associated with tuberous sclerosis complex (EXIST-1): a multicentre, randomised, placebo-controlled phase 3 trial. *Lancet.* 2013;381:125-132.

GENERAL REFERENCES

For the General References and other additional features, please visit Expert Consult at https://expertconsult.inkling.com.

418

AUTONOMIC DISORDERS AND THEIR MANAGEMENT

WILLIAM P. CHESHIRE, JR.

The peripheral autonomic nervous system and the central integration of autonomic reflexes maintain homeostasis and modulate the complex physiologic responses at the interface between the internal milieu and the external world. Autonomic activity, which generally occurs below the level of conscious control, regulates cardiovascular, thermal, metabolic, gastrointestinal (GI), urinary, and reproductive functions and coordinates the adaptive response to stress.

Many diseases can involve the autonomic nervous system, which in turn can involve all organ systems. Examples include brain lesions that affect any part of the central autonomic network, disorders that damage peripheral nerve function, and systemic illnesses that impair autonomic responses.

EPIDEMIOLOGY

The most frequently disabling manifestation of autonomic failure is orthostatic hypotension, which increases in prevalence with aging and is associated with a two-fold increased risk for falls, fractures, syncope, transient ischemic attacks, and decreased functional capacity in elderly individuals. The prevalence of orthostatic hypotension is 5 to 20% among all elderly persons, but it rises to 30% in persons older than 75 years and to greater than 50% in frail individuals who live in nursing homes. Neurally mediated syncope (vasodepressor, vasovagal), as well as various situational syncopes that occur in response to emotional distress, micturition, defecation, coughing, carotid sinus stimulation, and other factors, accounts for 1 to 3% of all emergency room visits. The lifetime prevalence of syncope is about 20%. Another common autonomic syndrome is postprandial hypotension, which occurs in 20 to 60% of elderly individuals and is associated with an increased risk for mortality.

Diabetes mellitus (Chapter 229) is the most common cause of autonomic neuropathy in the developed world. Within 10 to 15 years of the onset of diabetes, laboratory evidence of autonomic neuropathy can be detected in about 30% of patients, and symptomatic autonomic failure with orthostatic hypotension can be detected in about 5% of patients.[1] Other autonomic symptoms in diabetics include constipation in 40 to 60% of patients, gastroparesis in 20 to 40%, bladder dysfunction in 30 to 80%, erectile impotence in more than 30% of males, and occasionally intermittent diarrhea.

Hyperhidrosis involving the palms and soles represents the most common form of essential hyperhidrosis and affects about 1% of the population. Although excessive sweating is usually symptomatic, anhidrosis may go unnoticed unless it interferes with the thermoregulatory response to heat stress. Impaired thermoregulation can increase mortality during heat waves or in times of heat stress (Chapter 109).

PATHOBIOLOGY

The peripheral autonomic nervous system comprises three main divisions: (1) the sympathetic outflow from the thoracolumbar segments of the spinal cord, (2) the parasympathetic outflow from cranial nerves III, VII, IX, and X and the sacral spinal segments, and (3) the enteric ganglionated plexuses intrinsic to the wall of the gut. Disorders of the autonomic nervous system may occur suddenly or evolve gradually. They may affect specific or multiple autonomic pathways, depending on their pathogenesis and localization. Orthostatic hypotension, a hallmark of autonomic disorders, results from sympathetic vasomotor denervation, which renders a standing patient unable to constrict the splanchnic and other peripheral vascular beds in response to the pooling of blood volume (300 to 800 mL) owing to gravity.

Physiologic effects of sympathetic activation include pupillary dilation, increased heart rate and contractility, increased peripheral vascular resistance, bronchodilation, increased glandular secretions, decreased GI motility, increased sweating, decreased function of reproductive organs, and mobilization of energy substrates. The effects of parasympathetic activation include pupillary constriction, lacrimal and salivary secretion, decreased heart rate and contractility, bronchoconstriction, increased GI motility, and contraction of the detrusor muscle of the bladder. Sympathetic and parasympathetic responses, though generally antagonistic, are not always equally counterbalanced among organ systems.

Sympathetic preganglionic neurons, which use acetylcholine as their primary neurotransmitter, originate in the segmentally organized intermediolateral column of the spinal cord and exit via the ventral roots to pass through the white rami communicans and reach the paravertebral sympathetic chain ganglia, which innervate all organs and tissues except those of the abdomen and pelvis. The superior cervical ganglion, for example, innervates cranial structures, and the stellate ganglion innervates the upper limb. Sympathetic preganglionic axons also form the splanchnic nerves, which innervate the celiac, superior mesenteric, and hypogastric ganglia, as well as the adrenal medulla. With the exception of neurons that innervate the sweat glands, which are cholinergic, all other sympathetic postganglionic neurons are adrenergic neurons with norepinephrine as their primary transmitter.

Preganglionic innervation of parasympathetic neurons is also cholinergic; however, in contrast to their sympathetic counterparts, the major postganglionic parasympathetic neurotransmitter is acetylcholine. Parasympathetic preganglionic fibers originate in the Edinger-Westphal, salivatory, and vagal dorsal motor nuclei in the brain stem. The ciliary, sphenopalatine, otic, submandibular, sublingual, and pelvic ganglia send postganglionic parasympathetic fibers to their target organs. Cranial nerves IX and X, which constitute the afferent limbs of the baroreceptor reflex, relay beat-to-beat information about systemic arterial pressure to the nucleus of the solitary tract.

The GI tract contains neural plexuses, the most prominent of which are the myenteric (Auerbach) plexus found between the two layers of the muscularis externa and the submucosal (Meissner) plexus. Disorders of the enteric nervous system mainly affect GI motility or sphincter control rather than absorptive or secretory functions.

BRAIN DISORDERS

Important disease targets involved in central autonomic regulation include the interrelated neuronal cell groups of the hypothalamus, as well as the ventrolateral medulla, nucleus of the solitary tract, parabrachial nucleus, periaqueductal gray matter, amygdala, and insular and prefrontal cortices. Together, these relay systems and integrative centers compose the central autonomic network, which when impaired, fails to activate or modulate sympathetic and parasympathetic tone and neurohumoral responses.

A number of neurodegenerative disorders disrupt the central pathways of autonomic regulation. The most severe form is multiple system atrophy, a sporadic adult-onset disease in which severe autonomic failure accompanies and may precede parkinsonism (Shy-Drager syndrome; Chapter 409) or cerebellar ataxia (Chapter 410). In multiple system atrophy, degeneration of the striatum, pigmented nuclei, pontine nuclei, inferior olives, cerebellar Purkinje cells, and dorsal vagal and vestibular nuclei is associated with oligodendroglial cytoplasmic inclusions composed of α-synuclein filamentous aggregates. Autonomic dysfunction also occurs in dementia with Lewy bodies (Chapter 402) and to a lesser degree in Parkinson disease,[2] both of which also involve abnormal neuronal accumulation of α-synuclein.

Essential to the integration of behavioral, autonomic, and neuroendocrine responses is the tightly packed interwoven group of cells that constitute the hypothalamus. Lesions of the anterior hypothalamus may alter thirst perception and sodium regulation. Dysfunction of the magnocellular arginine vasopressin neurons of the supraoptic and supraventricular nuclei can be manifested as decreased secretion of antidiuretic hormone, thereby resulting in diabetes insipidus (Chapter 225) with hypovolemia, or as inappropriately increased secretion of antidiuretic hormone, thereby resulting in hyponatremia. Medial preoptic–anterior hypothalamic dysfunction associated with dysgenesis of the corpus callosum (Shapiro syndrome) is characterized by episodic hyperhidrosis and hypothermia. Lesions of the posterior hypothalamus can result from hypothermia, Wernicke-Korsakoff syndrome (Chapter 416), acute traumatic brain injury (Chapter 399), multiple sclerosis (Chapter 411), mesodiencephalic hematoma, and toluene toxicity.

Catastrophic neurologic conditions such as subarachnoid hemorrhage (Chapter 408), head trauma (Chapter 399), status epilepticus (Chapter 403), and acute hydrocephalus with increased intracranial pressure can profoundly stimulate sympathetic responses with cardiovascular consequence. Release of the hypothalamus as a result of cortical inhibition is the presumed mechanism. These paroxysmal sympathetic storms (diencephalic syndrome) are characterized by episodic sympathetic hyperactivity with hypertension, tachycardia, hyperventilation, pupillary dilation, flushing, and diaphoresis. Communicating hydrocephalus, structural lesions affecting the medial frontal cortex, and degenerative conditions affecting the frontobasal ganglia can cause urinary incontinence with uninhibited bladder contractions.

Autonomic responses are closely linked to emotional states. Portions of the insular and anterior cingulate cortices mediate the autonomic responses to emotional stress. Because cardioregulatory function is represented within the insular cortex, insular strokes have been associated with destabilization of sympathoregulatory balance and occasional adverse cardiac events. Correlations of electroencephalography and electrocardiography have shown that seizures arising from the mesial temporal lobe may induce ictal tachycardia or, more rarely, bradycardia or asystole.

Lesions of the brain stem may also be manifested as autonomic dysfunction. Damage to the medulla oblongata may give rise to hypertension, orthostatic hypotension, or syncope. Medullary ischemia or compression can cause acute neurogenic hypertension (Cushing response). Lateral medullary infarction (Wallenberg syndrome) typically produces ipsilateral Horner syndrome and occasionally more extensive dysautonomia, including bradycardia, acute hypertension, supine hypotension, or central hypoventilation.

● SPINAL CORD DISORDERS

Lesions of the spinal cord (Chapter 400), whether compressive, demyelinating, vascular, or neoplastic, commonly result in an overactive bladder (Chapter 26) with symptoms of frequency, urgency, and sometimes incontinence. Lesions that involve the sacral cord segments or cauda equina result in an underactive bladder with incomplete emptying, overflow incontinence, sphincter atonia, and sexual dysfunction.

After spinal cord injuries above the level of splanchnic sympathetic outflow at T5, sprouting of afferent fibers in the thoracolumbar dorsal horns and necrosis of the descending white matter connections to sympathetic preganglionic neurons result in autonomic dysreflexia. In these patients, strong peripheral sensory stimuli such as bladder or bowel distention can induce a reversible state of sympathetic hyperresponsiveness that may present with hypertension, diaphoresis, flushing, or headache.

● PERIPHERAL GANGLIONOPATHIES AND NEUROPATHIES

Autonomic dysfunction can arise at the level of the autonomic ganglia or peripheral nerves (Table 418-1). Peripheral autonomic nerves are generally small in caliber and unmyelinated or thinly myelinated. Peripheral neuropathies that selectively involve small nerve fibers can cause various combinations of sensory, sympathetic, or parasympathetic signs and symptoms.

Among the peripheral dysautonomias is the syndrome of pure autonomic failure, which is defined as the insidious onset of severe generalized autonomic failure as the sole clinical feature in the absence of any signs of extrapyramidal, cerebellar, or sensory or motor peripheral nerve dysfunction. Pathologic studies have found Lewy body accumulation in autonomic ganglia, peripheral autonomic nerves, the substantia nigra, and the locus ceruleus.

Diabetic neuropathy involves autonomic nerves early in its course, and about 20% of patients advance to a clinically consequential cardiovascular autonomic neuropathy, which is a marker for and increased risk of cardiovascular mortality and morbidity.[3] The incidence increases with the duration of diabetes and advancing age. In diabetic patients, microvascular ischemia causes progressive peripheral nerve damage, although an autoimmune mechanism may also play a role in a subset of patients. Glycemic burden appears to represent a continuum of risk for autonomic neuropathy, because some patients with impaired glucose regulation or newly diagnosed diabetes already have evidence of small fiber neuropathy.

Other syndromes of neurologic autoimmunity (Table 418-2) include Guillain-Barré syndrome, in which antiganglioside antibodies mediate an

TABLE 418-1	SOME CAUSES OF PERIPHERAL AUTONOMIC NEUROPATHY
Metabolic	Diabetes mellitus
	Alcohol
	Acute intermittent porphyria
	Uremia
Autoimmune	Autoimmune autonomic ganglionopathy
	Guillain-Barré syndrome
	Morvan syndrome
	Lambert-Eaton myasthenic syndrome
	Chronic inflammatory demyelinating polyradiculoneuropathy
	Sjögren syndrome
	Systemic lupus erythematosus
	Mixed connective tissue diseases
Paraproteinemic	Amyloidosis
Nutritional	Cyanocobalamin deficiency
	Thiamine deficiency
	Gluten-sensitive neuropathy
Toxic	Heavy metals
	Organic solvents
	Organophosphates
	Vacor
	Acrylamide
Drug induced	Cisplatin
	Vincristine
	Amiodarone
	Metronidazole
	Perhexiline
	Paclitaxel
Infectious	Human immunodeficiency virus
	Leprosy
	Chagas disease
	Botulism
	Diphtheria
	Lyme disease
Genetic	Hereditary sensory and autonomic neuropathies
	Types I and II
	Type III (familial dysautonomia)
	Type IV (congenital insensitivity to pain)
	Type V
	Fabry disease
Idiopathic	Adie syndrome
	Ross syndrome
	Acute cholinergic neuropathy
	Chronic idiopathic anhidrosis
	Amyotrophic lateral sclerosis

TABLE 418-2 AUTOIMMUNE AUTONOMIC NEUROPATHIES	
CLINICAL SYNDROME	ASSOCIATED AUTOANTIBODY
Autoimmune autonomic ganglionopathy	Anti-GAChR
Guillain-Barré syndrome	Anti-GM1, anti-GM3
Paraneoplastic autonomic neuropathy	ANNA-1 (anti-Hu), PCA-2, CRMP-5
Lambert-Eaton myasthenic syndrome	Anti-VGCC
Morvan syndrome	Anti-VGKC
Sjögren syndrome	SSA (anti-Ro), SSB (anti-La)
Intestinal dysmotility syndromes	Anti-GnRH

ANNA-1 = antineuronal nuclear antibody; anti-GAChR = nicotinic ganglionic acetylcholine receptor antibody; anti-GM1, anti-GM3 = antiganglioside antibody; anti-GnRH = gonadotropin-releasing hormone antibody; anti-VGCC = P/Q-type voltage-gated calcium-channel antibody; anti-VGKC = voltage-gated potassium-channel antibody; CRMP-5 = collapsin response mediator protein 5; PCA-2 = Purkinje cell cytoplasmic antibody type 2.

acute inflammatory demyelinating polyradiculoneuropathy that may be associated with tachycardia, blood pressure lability, and pupillomotor, sudomotor, and vasomotor disturbances (Chapter 420). The syndrome of acute pandysautonomia typically develops dramatically over a period of days to weeks as combined sympathetic and parasympathetic failure with GI dysmotility and, in contrast to Guillain-Barré syndrome, sparing of the somatic nerves. An antecedent (presumably viral) infection is reported in about 50%

of cases. The finding of antibodies against the nicotinic acetylcholine receptor in the autonomic ganglia in many of these patients has established autoimmune autonomic ganglionopathy as a definable disease entity.[4] Ganglionic acetylcholine receptor antibodies occur in some patients with lung cancer or thymoma. Low levels of these antibodies have also been found in a subset of patients with isolated GI dysmotility.

Autoimmune neuromyotonia is characterized by peripheral nerve hyperexcitability, insomnia, fluctuating delirium, and prominent dysautonomia with hyperhidrosis and orthostatic intolerance. Most patients have antibodies to voltage-gated potassium channels (Chapter 422).

Paraneoplastic autonomic neuropathies, which can predate the diagnosis of malignancy, are a rare epiphenomenon of malignancy, most frequently small cell lung carcinoma (Chapter 191), and can also occur in association with ovarian carcinoma (Chapter 199), breast carcinoma (Chapter 198), thymoma, lymphoma (Chapter 185), and other cancers. The most commonly encountered paraneoplastic antibody is antineuronal nuclear antibody type 1 (ANNA-1 or anti-Hu), which binds to a 35- to 40-kD family of neuronal nuclear RNA-binding proteins, including those in autonomic and enteric ganglia. Antibodies against collapsing response mediator proteins (CRMP-5 or anti-CV2) have also been associated with paraneoplastic autonomic neuropathy. Dysautonomia occurs in approximately 10 to 30% of patients with ANNA-1 and in 30% of patients with CRMP-5 seropositivity. Small cell lung cancer (Chapter 191) has been found in more than 80% of patients seropositive for ANNA-1 or CRMP-5.

Hereditary sensory and autonomic neuropathy (HSAN) type I, which is due to mutations of the gene for serine palmitoyltransferase, is inherited in an autosomal dominant pattern and is characterized by distal anhidrosis with loss of nociception and thermal perception. Mutations in *HSN2* have been linked to HSAN type II, an autosomal recessive neuropathy that causes distal anhidrosis and sensory loss. Sural nerve biopsy specimens disclose virtual absence of myelinated fibers and decreased numbers of unmyelinated fibers. Autonomic involvement is most prominent in HSAN type III, commonly known as familial dysautonomia or Riley-Day syndrome. This autosomal recessive disorder, which affects 1 in 3600 live births in parents of Ashkenazi Jewish descent, has been linked to mutations in the I-κB kinase–associated protein gene (*IKBKAP*). Pathologic studies disclose severely depleted sympathetic preganglionic and postganglionic neuronal populations with preservation of parasympathetic neurons. Affected children cry without tears, feed poorly, lack lingual fungiform papillae, have depressed patellar reflexes, and are subject to orthostatic hypotension and autonomic storms owing to impaired baroreflex afferent neurons.

HSAN type IV, or congenital insensitivity to pain with anhidrosis, is an autosomal recessive disorder that is associated with mental retardation and repeated episodes of fever. HSAN type IV results from mutations in the gene for neurotrophic tyrosine kinase receptor type 1 (*NTRK1*), which is important for inducing neurite outgrowth in embryonic sensory and sympathetic neurons. Peripheral nerve biopsy discloses virtual absence of unmyelinated fibers.

HSAN type V is an autosomal recessive disorder characterized by loss of pain and thermal sensation. It is caused by mutations in the nerve growth factor beta subunit (*NGFB*) gene.

The age-related decline in baroreflex sensitivity, adrenergic responses to sympathetic activation, parasympathetic control of heart rate, esophageal and GI motility, and efficient thermoregulation predisposes the elderly to orthostatic, postprandial, and drug-induced hypotension. Pheochromocytomas (Chapter 228) cause paroxysmal autonomic symptoms, including blood pressure lability, and carcinoid syndrome (Chapter 232) causes flushing.

CLINICAL MANIFESTATIONS

Several distinct patterns of autonomic dysfunction help in identifying underlying causes.

Generalized Autonomic Failure

Early symptoms of adrenergic failure typically include lightheadedness on arising in the morning or following a warm shower, physical exercise, or a large meal. Other common symptoms include male erectile dysfunction, decreased sweating, dry mouth, constipation, and bladder dysfunction. Severe orthostatic hypotension without pulse acceleration (Chapter 62), which is the hallmark of severe generalized autonomic failure, occurs in at least 50% of patients and may be accompanied by supine and nocturnal hypertension, in which the normal diurnal decrease in blood pressure during sleep is reversed.

Acute Autonomic Syndromes

Acute or subacute manifestations of autonomic dysfunction may result from rapidly developing disease or from decompensation of chronic autonomic disease. An abrupt onset of new focal autonomic signs, particularly when accompanied by headache or motor or sensory deficits, should prompt a detailed neurologic assessment for an acute cerebral or spinal syndrome, which may be caused by vascular, traumatic, inflammatory, neoplastic, or infectious diseases.

Chronic Autonomic Syndromes

The clinical spectrum of chronic autonomic neuropathies includes distal small fiber neuropathies with a stocking-and-glove distribution of anhidrosis, often combined with loss of pain and temperature sensibility. Other symptoms include orthostatic hypotension and impaired exercise tolerance, with either an increased resting heart rate due to a parasympathetic cardiovagal neuropathy or a fixed heart rate that does not increase adequately in response to physiologic demands as a result of the involvement of sympathetic fibers. Some patients with distal sudomotor neuropathy will complain of spontaneous or gustatory proximal hyperhidrosis with episodic sweating involving the face, head, and upper part of the trunk.

Gastroparesis, which is a common feature of autonomic neuropathies, is characterized by delayed gastric emptying, which may be manifested as early satiety, nausea, anorexia, bloating, and sometimes pain and weight loss. Intestinal dysmotility may cause severe constipation (Chapter 136). In advanced peripheral neuropathies (Chapter 420), in ganglionopathies in which involvement is not length dependent, and in central degenerative disorders, the loss of sweating may extend to proximal body regions or globally. Widespread anhidrosis may result in impaired thermoregulatory sweating and the potential for hyperthermia in conditions of heat stress (Chapter 109).

Paroxysmal Dysautonomias

Paroxysmal and episodic autonomic symptoms include postprandial hypotension, which is a reduction in systolic blood pressure of at least 20 mm Hg within 2 hours of the start of a meal, typically one high in carbohydrate content. Postprandial hypotension may occur in elderly individuals with or without orthostatic hypotension.

Dysfunction of the afferent limb of the baroreflex system leads to volatile blood pressure in patients with acute inflammatory demyelinating polyneuropathy and syndromes of arterial baroreflex failure. Additional causes of aberrant activation of autonomic reflexes include epilepsy, diencephalic syndrome, subarachnoid hemorrhage, acute head trauma, pheochromocytoma, intoxication, drug withdrawal, neurally mediated syncope, and panic disorder.

Selective Autonomic Syndromes

Regional autonomic disorders are characterized by focal or system-selective autonomic dysfunction. An example is harlequin syndrome, in which heat stress, exercise, or sudden emotion in a patient with hemifacial cutaneous sympathetic denervation evokes a dramatic facial division in which the denervated half remains pale and dry and the intact half flushes red. Oculosympathetic paresis (Horner syndrome) may also be present. Harlequin syndrome may occur in patients with Holmes-Adie syndrome, which consists of tonic pupils with asymmetrical or absent tendon reflexes, and has been described in patients with Ross syndrome, a partial dysautonomia consisting of the clinical triad of unilateral or bilateral tonic pupils, tendon hyporeflexia, and segmental body anhidrosis.

Other Specific Syndromes

Baroreflex failure is commonly the result of damage to the carotid sinus baroreceptors or the glossopharyngeal nerves. Similarly, interruption of vagal input from the aortic arch baroreceptors to the nucleus of the solitary tract can impair baroreflex responses. Baroreflex failure also occurs in patients who have undergone surgery or irradiation of the neck. These patients will exhibit severe and labile hypertension with concomitant tachycardia, palpitations, headache, diaphoresis, and emotional lability.[5] Takotsubo cardiomyopathy (Chapter 60) is a stress-induced syndrome of typically reversible left ventricular myocardial dysfunction brought on by a catecholamine surge.

Serotonin syndrome develops within hours or days of the addition of a new serotonergic agent to a drug regimen that already enhances serotonergic neurotransmission, on overdose with a selective serotonin reuptake inhibitor, or from abuse of psychostimulants such as amphetamine, methamphetamine, and 3,4-methylenedioxymetamphetamine (MDMA or "ecstasy"). Manifestations include agitation, hypervigilance, confusion, hyperthermia, increased sweating, fluctuating blood pressure, hyperreflexia, and myoclonus.

Neuroleptic malignant syndrome (Chapter 432) is a potentially life-threatening hypermetabolic condition that develops within days to weeks in 0.2% of patients who receive drugs that block dopamine 2 receptors. The clinical findings consist of hyperthermia, profuse sweating, muscle rigidity, bradykinesia, and delirium. If the offending medication is not withheld, the syndrome may progress to tachycardia, tachypnea, labile blood pressure, myoclonus, obtundation, and catatonia.

Among the infectious neuropathies, tetanus infection (Chapter 296) causes sympathetic overactivity in a third of patients because of the exotoxin tetanospasmin, which is taken up by peripheral nerve terminals and transported across synaptic junctions to reach the central nervous system. There it binds to gangliosides at presynaptic junctions to disinhibit preganglionic neurons and damages autonomic brain stem nuclei. Sympathetic hyperactivity results in labile or persistent hypertension or hypotension, tachyarrhythmias, peripheral vasoconstriction, fever, and profuse sweating. Diphtheritic neuropathy (Chapter 292) causes bulbar weakness and may be associated with cardiovagal impairment but not usually with orthostatic hypotension.

The acute cholinergic neuropathy of botulism (Chapter 296) occurs along with bulbar and generalized neuromuscular paralysis 12 to 36 hours after the ingestion of food contaminated with the gram-positive anaerobic bacterium *Clostridium botulinum*. Botulinum toxin binds with high affinity to presynaptic receptors of cholinergic nerve terminals and inhibits the release of acetylcholine, thereby blocking neuromuscular and cholinergic autonomic transmission. Autonomic manifestations include anhidrosis, dry eyes, dry mouth, paralytic ileus, gastric dilation, urinary retention, and sometimes orthostatic hypotension with fluctuating blood pressure and vasomotor tone.

Human immunodeficiency virus infection commonly causes autonomic disturbances, particularly in its advanced stages. Manifestations can include orthostatic hypotension, tachycardia, urinary dysfunction, impotency, diarrhea, and cardiac conduction defects. Perivascular mononuclear inflammatory infiltrates and neuronal degeneration in biopsy specimens of sympathetic ganglia suggest an autoimmune pathogenesis.

Chagas disease (Chapter 347) causes a predominantly parasympathetic neuropathy characterized by megaesophagus, megaduodenum, and megacolon, as well as sympathetic cardiovascular failure with cardiomegaly and conduction defects. The autonomic neuropathy has an autoimmune basis and develops years to decades following primary infection with *Trypanosoma cruzi*.

Leprosy (Chapter 326), one of the most common causes of neuropathy worldwide, frequently causes peripheral autonomic neuropathy as a result of an immune reaction against *Mycobacterium leprae*. Focal anhidrosis occurs in areas of hypopigmented and hypoesthetic skin. Cardiac denervation and orthostatic hypotension have been described.

Toxins known to cause autonomic neuropathy include the rodenticide Vacor, as well as thallium, arsenic, mercury, acrylamide, and organic solvents such as carbon disulfide and hexacarbon. Organophosphate poisoning (Chapter 110) induces miosis and copious secretions. Ergot poisoning from rye contaminated with the fungus *Claviceps purpurea* results in intense vasoconstriction, paresthesia, seizures, and diarrhea. Poisoning with muscarine, which is present in certain poisonous mushrooms (Chapter 110), results in increased salivation, sweating, and lacrimation followed by nausea, abdominal pain, and diarrhea.

Medicinal drugs that may induce an autonomic peripheral neuropathy include cisplatin, vincristine, amiodarone, metronidazole, perhexiline maleate, and paclitaxel. Many drugs are capable of increasing or decreasing sweating (Table 418-3).

Nutritional deficiencies that lead to autonomic dysfunction include alcoholic neuropathy, which is a dying-back neuropathy identical to that of beriberi that is caused by thiamine deficiency (Chapter 416). Distal parts of the vagus nerve are affected early, and orthostatic hypotension may occur in more advanced stages. Subacute combined degeneration from vitamin B_{12} deficiency (Chapter 218) results in axonal degeneration and is occasionally manifested as orthostatic hypotension. Autonomic neuropathy has been described in some cases of celiac disease (Chapter 140).

Amyloidosis (Chapter 188) results from the focal deposition of insoluble fibrillary proteins arranged in β-pleated sheet configurations within the extracellular space of various tissues, which may include the vasculature of peripheral autonomic nerves and sympathetic ganglia. Amyloid neuropathy is typically manifested as a painful distal small fiber sensory and severe autonomic neuropathy. autonomic dysfunction frequently occurs in primary AL

TABLE 418-3 SOME COMMONLY PRESCRIBED DRUGS THAT AFFECT SWEATING

Drugs that increase sweating
Opioids
Serotonin reuptake inhibitors
Anticholinesterases
Cholinergic agonists

Drugs that decrease sweating
M_3 anticholinergics
Carbonic anhydrase inhibitors
Tricyclic antidepressants
Neuroleptics
Antihistamines
Central α-adrenergic agonists
Botulinum toxin

(amyloid light-chain), immunoglobulin light chain–associated disease, and hereditary amyloidosis, but only rarely in reactive or AA (amyloid A) amyloidosis.

Functional Dysautonomias

A functional autonomic disorder is a medical condition that impairs normal autonomic function in some way but in the absence of a known structural neurologic deficit. Examples include neurally mediated syncope (Chapter 62), irritable bowel syndrome (Chapter 137), and some forms of orthostatic intolerance and pain, the molecular basis of which await discovery. Syndromic features can help to disambiguate functional dysautonomias from psychosomatic disorders (Chapter 397), which also may manifest autonomic symptoms just as they may manifest sensory or motor symptoms.

DIAGNOSIS

Clinical evaluation of autonomic dysfunction begins with a careful history. It is important to distinguish chronic and stable conditions from progressive and episodic phenomena and to recognize the circumstances that provoke or modify symptoms. Orthostatic hypotension, for example, is typically worse in the morning and may be aggravated by dehydration, deconditioning, prolonged standing, physical exertion, heat, carbohydrate ingestion, or menstruation (Table 418-4).[6]

Bedside Evaluation

The skin examination should assess turgor, pallor, flushing, and acral cyanosis, as well as any asymmetry of sweating, which may be more palpable than visible. Signs of pupillary asymmetry, ptosis, mucosal dryness, distal sensory or reflex changes, bradykinesia, or rigidity should be noted.

Blood pressure and heart rate should be measured with the patient supine and again after standing for 1 to 3 minutes and correlated with symptoms. Orthostatic hypotension is defined as a reduction in systolic blood pressure of at least 20 mm Hg or a reduction in diastolic blood pressure of at least 10 mm Hg, with or without symptoms, within 1 to 3 minutes of assuming an erect posture.[7] Neurogenic orthostatic hypotension is typically sustained with continued standing. Measurements taken immediately on standing can be misleading because some healthy young persons without orthostatic hypotension will exhibit transient hypotension within 30 seconds of standing but then recover. Except in patients treated with β-blockers, orthostatic hypotension without reflex tachycardia is evidence of generalized adrenergic failure. If reflex tachycardia occurs, dehydration or excessive venous pooling should be considered.

Some patients with orthostatic intolerance experience an abnormal increase in heart rate rather than a drop in blood pressure on standing. Postural tachycardia syndrome[8] is defined as an increase in heart rate by more than 30 beats per minute in adults (40 beats per minute in adolescents) and to consistently greater than 120 beats per minute when standing.

Laboratory Evaluation

Appropriate laboratory testing depends on the type and distribution of autonomic dysfunction. Investigations may include a complete blood cell count, fasting glucose, electrolytes, morning cortisol, thyroid function testing, vitamin B_{12} level, and when indicated, autoimmune markers. Creatine kinase should be checked in patients with hyperthermia.

In a patient with an autonomic neuropathy, seropositivity for any of the characterized paraneoplastic autoantibodies should prompt a careful search for an underlying malignancy, even if the results of routine imaging studies

TABLE 418-4 GRADING OF ORTHOSTATIC INTOLERANCE

	SYMPTOM FREQUENCY	ACTIVITIES OF DAILY LIVING IN THE UPRIGHT POSTURE	STANDING TIME (ON MOST OCCASIONS)	ORTHOSTATIC BLOOD PRESSURE
Grade I	Infrequent orthostatic symptoms developing only under conditions of increased stress*	Unrestricted	>15 min	May or may not be abnormal
Grade II	Intermittent orthostatic symptoms occurring at least weekly	Some limitation	>5 min	Some changes in cardiovascular indices, e.g., oscillations, or decrease in pulse pressure by > 50%
Grade III	Frequent orthostatic symptoms occurring on most occasions	Marked limitation	>1 min	Orthostatic hypotension is present > 50% of the time, recorded on different days
Grade IV	Orthostatic symptoms are consistently present	Incapacitated and unable to stand without presyncope or syncope developing	<1 min	Orthostatic hypotension is severe and consistently present

*Conditions that increase orthostatic stress include dehydration, deconditioning from prolonged bedrest, physical exertion, heat stress, and medications that lower blood pressure or impair adrenergic function.
Adapted from Low PA, Singer W. Update on management of neurogenic orthostatic hypotension. *Lancet Neurol.* 2008;7:451-458.

are normal. Positron emission tomography is more sensitive than computed tomography in detecting small tumor foci. In patients with suspected pheochromocytoma, the most sensitive screening test is the free metanephrine level (Chapter 228).

Pupillary responses to the instillation of dilute pilocarpine, epinephrine, and cocaine can assist in the localization of oculosympathetic and oculoparasympathetic deficits. Lacrimal secretion may be quantified by the Schirmer and rose bengal tests (Chapter 268). Sialography may be useful to quantify salivary flow. Salivary gland biopsy may be necessary to diagnose Sjögren syndrome, particularly the seronegative form.

Manometry and scintigraphic studies are useful in the diagnosis of disorders of GI motility. Postvoiding residual volumes or urodynamic studies can elaborate patterns of urinary bladder dysfunction (Chapter 26). Suspected amyloid may require biopsy (Chapter 188).

Ambulatory blood pressure testing (Chapter 67), usually over a period of 24 hours, is useful to detect patterns of nocturnal hypertension, postprandial hypotension, and the labile hypertension of baroreflex failure. Adrenergic function can be assessed noninvasively by tilt table testing (Chapter 62). Adrenergic failure can also be defined by deficient recovery and overshoot of arterial pressure following 15 seconds of expiration at 40 mm Hg. The Valsalva ratio, defined as the maximum heart rate generated by the Valsalva maneuver divided by the lowest heart rate within 30 seconds of the peak, is a measure of parasympathetic cardiovagal function. A sensitive index of cardiovagal function is the heart rate response to sinusoidal deep breathing, which quantifies respiratory sinus arrhythmia.

Noninvasive tests of sudomotor function, such as the quantitative sudomotor axon reflex test, the Silastic sweat imprint, or the thermatoregulatory sweat test, can assess sweating function. These tests as well as skin biopsies to examine intraepidermal nerve fiber density can be useful in detecting autonomic involvement in small fiber neuropathies.[9,10]

TREATMENT Rx

Treatment begins with educating patients about the underlying physiology, helping them avoid exacerbations, and managing their symptoms. In cases of mild dysautonomia, medications may not be needed. Elderly patients may be able to compensate for some of the age-associated decline in autonomic function through regular exercise.

Efforts at treating the underlying cause of an autonomic neuropathy should be pursued. Good control of glucose in patients with diabetes mellitus (Chapter 229) reduces the rate of complications, including neuropathy. Meticulous foot care can prevent cutaneous and joint trauma, ulceration, and infection of desensitized skin.

Orthostatic Intolerance

The goals of treatment are to increase the time the patient is able to stand without orthostatic symptoms developing, while simultaneously avoiding excessive recumbent hypertension. Mild orthostatic hypotension and syncope may respond to conservative measures such as increasing oral hydration (2 to 2.5 L/day), drinking sports beverages, and adding dietary salt or sodium tablets to increase daily salt intake to 10 to 20 g. Prolonged bedrest and medications that could potentially exacerbate orthostatic hypotension should be avoided if possible. Elevating the head of the bed by inserting 4- to 6-inch blocks under the head posts can improve orthostatic tolerance

in some patients by reducing nocturnal natriuresis and stimulating release of renin.

Water bolus treatment (drinking 16 oz of water) can increase systolic blood pressure by 20 mm Hg for about 2 hours by a sympathetic reflex.[A1][A2] The addition of either glucose or salt is counterproductive in that both attenuate the systemic vasoconstriction produced by pure water. Lower extremity resistance strength training combined with education about physical countermaneuvers (leg crossing, squatting, bending forward, or placing one foot on a chair) can help patients increase venous return to the heart and improve orthostatic tolerance by activating leg muscles.[A3] Compressive stockings are effective if they are tightly fitting, especially if they provide abdominal compression in addition to leg compression.[A4] However, they may be poorly tolerated in warm climates and are cumbersome to apply.

Pharmacologic measures are of variable benefit, and patients commonly stop taking them soon after they are prescribed.[11] Examples include midodrine (5 to 10 mg three times daily) to constrict capacitance vessels,[A5] fludrocortisone (0.1 to 0.4 mg/day) to expand plasma volume and sensitize peripheral vascular α-adrenergic receptors,[A6] and pyridostigmine (30 to 60 mg two or three times daily) to enhance ganglionic transmission during orthostatic stress.[A7] Yohimbine (5.4 mg three times daily) improves orthostatic hypotension by engaging residual sympathetic tone.[A8] Pyridostigmine has a more modest pressor effect but has the advantage of inducing less supine hypertension. Droxidopa (100 to 600 mg three times daily), an orally active synthetic precursor of norepinephrine, has recently been approved in the U.S. for the treatment of symptoms of neurogenic orthostatic hypotension.[A9] Aldose reductase inhibitors (e.g., epalrestat [50 mg three times daily]) may provide some benefit for patients with diabetic cardiovascular autonomic neuropathy,[12] but no such drugs are currently approved by the U.S. Food and Drug Administration.

Postprandial hypotension may be managed by dividing meals to avoid large carbohydrate loads. Caffeine or midodrine with breakfast may be helpful.

Sweating Disorders

Initial therapy for palmar hyperhidrosis begins with tap water iontophoresis, in which a low-level electric current applied to the skin surface blocks sweat ducts at the level of the stratum corneum; for severe cases, endoscopic thoracic sympathotomy is effective. Focal hyperhidrosis, such as gustatory sweating caused by aberrant innervation of the facial sweat glands by regenerating parasympathetic fibers of the facial nerve, responds well to botulinum toxin injections. Generalized hyperhidrosis can be suppressed by oral anticholinergic drugs (e.g., glycopyrrolate, 1 to 2 mg one to three times daily), which tends to be better tolerated than other anticholinergic agents because very little crosses the blood-brain barrier; dry mouth is an invariable side effect. Aluminum chloride hexahydrate (20%) in anhydrous ethyl alcohol applied topically to dry skin at bedtime), oral belladonna (0.2 mg 1 to 2 times daily), propantheline (15 mg three times daily), topiramate (beginning at 25 mg twice daily), and clonidine (0.1 mg three times daily orally or by transdermal patch) may also be helpful for hyperhidrosis. Botulinum toxin types A and B, injected intradermally, are effective for axillary hyperhidrosis.

In a patient who is unable to sweat, hyperthermia cannot be prevented by drinking more water. Seeking shade, avoidance of exertion in hot weather, moistening the skin with a wet washcloth, and the use of portable fans can be effective. Carbonic anhydrase inhibitors, such as topiramate and zonisamide, and anticholinergic medications can inhibit thermoregulatory sweating and should be avoided if patients experience heat intolerance.

Hyperadrenergic Disorders

Nocturnal hypertension may be minimized by avoiding pressor agents within several hours of bedtime, elevating the head of the bed, or having a nighttime snack. In severe cases, bedtime hydralazine (25 mg), nifedipine (10 mg), amlodipine (2.5 to 5 mg), or a nitroglycerin patch (0.1 mg/hour) may be needed. Paroxysmal and labile hypertension in patients with arterial baroreflex denervation may respond to clonidine (0.1 mg three times daily orally or by transdermal patch).

PROGNOSIS

The prognosis depends on the nature of the autonomic disorder. In general, the development of orthostatic hypotension worsens the prognosis.

A diagnosis of multiple system atrophy carries an estimated life expectancy of 7 to 9 years.[13] A patient with pure autonomic failure may have a prolonged and stable clinical course, but this syndrome may progress years later to a phenotype of multiple system atrophy or dementia with Lewy bodies. Amyloid neuropathy portends a median survival of less than 1 year if orthostatic hypotension is present. Diabetic autonomic neuropathy is associated with an approximately two-fold increased risk for silent myocardial ischemia and overall mortality.

Regional Sympathetic Dysfunction

Regional sympathetic dysfunction may accompany the pain that sometimes follows peripheral nerve injuries. For example, sympathetic activation can occur as a normal physiologic response to any painful state.

Complex regional pain syndrome is characterized by severe ongoing neuropathic pain that is disproportionate in intensity, duration, and distribution to the expected sequela of limb trauma.[14] In this syndrome, allodynia (pain in response to normally nonpainful stimuli, such as light touch or cold) or hyperalgesia (increased sensitivity to painful stimuli) accompany cutaneous vasomotor or sudomotor abnormalities. The vasomotor changes are manifested as vasodilation with a warm, red, or swollen limb, or alternatively as vasoconstriction with a cold pale limb. The sudomotor findings range from regional hyperhidrosis to anhidrosis. Regional dystrophic changes, such as dry atrophic skin, sparse or coarse hair, brittle nails, and osteopenia, may also develop. Although sympathetic dysfunction may be pronounced, it does not appear to cause the pain. The mechanisms of pain and sympathetic dysfunction in this condition are incompletely understood and may result from crosstalk among aberrantly regenerated peripheral nerve fibers, expression of new α-adrenergic receptors on sensory nerve fibers and sweat glands, release of substance P and pro-inflammatory peptides at the site of injury, and sensitization of pain-mediating structures at multiple levels within the central nervous system.

Mobilization of the affected limb is of paramount importance in the early treatment of complex regional pain syndrome.[15] A primary goal of analgesic medication or regional anesthesia in early treatment is to facilitate participation in physical therapy. No therapy is supported by consistent data from properly sized and conducted randomized trails.[A10] Small trials report improvement with the use of bisphosphonates (e.g., alendronate, 40 mg orally or 7.5 mg intravenously daily), steroids (e.g., prednisone, 40 mg daily, or methylprednisolone, 8 mg four times daily initially and then tapered), dimethyl sulfoxide (50% cream one to four times daily), epidural clonidine (300 to 700 µg daily), intrathecal baclofen (25 to 75 µg daily), and epidural spinal cord stimulation. Intravenous immunoglobulin (0.5 g/kg) has also been used with variable results.

Grade A References

A1. Shannon JR, Diedrich A, Biaggioni I, et al. Water drinking as a treatment for orthostatic syndromes. *Am J Med.* 2002;112:355-360.
A2. Young TM, Mathias CJ. The effects of water ingestion on orthostatic hypotension in two groups of chronic autonomic failure: multiple system atrophy and pure autonomic failure. *J Neurol Neurosurg Psychiatry.* 2004;75:1737-1741.
A3. Winker R, Barth A, Bidmon D, et al. Endurance exercise training in orthostatic intolerance: a randomized, controlled trial. *Hypertension.* 2005;45:291-298.
A4. Podoleanu C, Maggi R, Brignole M, et al. Lower limb and abdominal compression bandages prevent progressive orthostatic hypotension in elderly persons: a randomized single-blind controlled study. *J Am Coll Cardiol.* 2006;58:1425-1432.
A5. Izcovich A, González Malla C, Manzotti M, et al. Midodrine for orthostatic hypotension and recurrent reflex syncope: a systematic review. *Neurology.* 2014;83:1170-1177.
A6. Ong AC, Myint PK, Shepstone L, et al. A systematic review of the pharmacological management of orthostatic hypotension. *Int J Clin Pract.* 2013;67:633-646.
A7. Logan IC, Witham MD. Efficacy of treatments for orthostatic hypotension: a systematic review. *Age Ageing.* 2012;41:587-594.
A8. Shibao C, Okamoto LE, Gamboa A, et al. Comparative efficacy of yohimbine against pyridostigmine for the treatment of orthostatic hypotension in autonomic failure. *Hypertension.* 2010;56:847-851.
A9. Kaufmann H, Freeman R, Biaggioni I, et al. Droxidopa for neurogenic orthostatic hypotension: a randomized, placebo-controlled, phase 3 trial. *Neurology.* 2014;83:328-335.
A10. O'Connell NE, Wand BM, McAuley J, et al. Interventions for treating pain and disability in adults with complex regional pain syndrome. *Cochrane Database Syst Rev.* 2013;4:CD009416.

GENERAL REFERENCES

For the General References and other additional features, please visit Expert Consult at https://expertconsult.inkling.com.

419

AMYOTROPHIC LATERAL SCLEROSIS AND OTHER MOTOR NEURON DISEASES

PAMELA J. SHAW

DEFINITION

The motor neuron diseases (Table 419-1) are a heterogeneous group of disorders in which selective loss of function of upper motor neurons, lower motor neurons, or both results in impairment of the nervous system's control of voluntary movement. The most common acquired motor neuron disease, amyotrophic lateral sclerosis (ALS), is a combined upper and lower motor neuron disorder. The features of lower motor neuron involvement are muscle wasting, fasciculations, and flaccid weakness, with normal or depressed tendon reflexes. Upper motor neuron dysfunction may cause increased muscle tone, clonus, weakness in a pyramidal distribution, and extensor plantar responses. Recent advances in the molecular genetics of hereditary motor neuron diseases have improved their classification and enhanced the careful diagnosis that is essential for genetic counseling, guidance, treatment, and advising patients about prognosis.

AMYOTROPHIC LATERAL SCLEROSIS

EPIDEMIOLOGY

ALS is a neurodegenerative disorder that causes progressive injury and cell death of lower motor neurons in the brain stem and spinal cord, as well as upper motor neurons in the motor cortex. ALS has an incidence of about 2 per 100,000 and a prevalence of 6 to 8 per 100,000. The global incidence is fairly uniform, with the exception of a few high-incidence foci such as the Western Pacific island of Guam. The disease affects predominantly middle-aged and elderly individuals, with a mean age at onset of 55 to 60 years, although younger individuals can also be affected. Increasing age, male sex (male/female ratio ≈ 1.6 : 1), and genetic susceptibility are the only proven risk factors, although ongoing research is assessing the effects of athleticism/physical exercise and other potential environmental risk factors. Approximately 90% of cases of ALS occur sporadically, but 5 to 10% are familial, usually with an autosomal dominant mode of inheritance.

PATHOBIOLOGY

The process of neuronal degeneration in ALS is complex. The subtype of disease caused by *SOD1* mutations accounts for 20% of familial ALS cases and 2% of ALS overall. Mutant *SOD1* appears to trigger a complex interplay of multiple pathogenic processes, including oxidative stress, protein aggregation, mitochondrial dysfunction, excitotoxicity, and impaired axonal transport.[1] Non-neuronal cells in the vicinity of motor neurons may contribute importantly to neuronal injury. Genetically engineered mouse models of *SOD1*-related ALS have shown that normal astrocytes can protect motor neurons expressing mutant *SOD1* and that removing the expression of mutant *SOD1* from microglia or astrocytes slows the progression of disease in these murine models. Astrocytes expressing mutant *SOD1* exert toxic effects on neighboring motor neurons through as yet undefined mechanisms.[2]

Familial motor neuron disease has been linked to mutations in multiple genes, including *SOD1*, alsin, senataxin, angiogenin, *VAPB*, dynactin, *TARDBP*, and *FUS/TLS*. Accumulating evidence suggests that defective RNA processing likely plays a key role in the pathogenesis of ALS. A very important recent discovery is the finding of GGGGCC hexanucleotide

TABLE 419-1 CLASSIFICATION OF MOTOR NEURON DISORDERS

COMBINED UPPER AND LOWER MOTOR NEURON DISORDERS

Amyotrophic lateral sclerosis
  Familial adult onset
  Familial juvenile onset
  Sporadic
  ALS-plus syndromes
    ALS with frontotemporal dementia
    Western Pacific ALS–parkinsonism-dementia complex

UPPER MOTOR NEURON DISORDERS

Primary lateral sclerosis
Hereditary spastic paraplegias
Neurolathyrism
Konzo

LOWER MOTOR NEURON DISORDERS

Hereditary
  Spinal muscular atrophies (SMAs)
    Proximal autosomal recessive SMA (associated with *SMN* mutations) types I to IV
    Other forms of SMA not associated with *SMN* mutations
    Distal spinal muscular atrophies/hereditary motor neuronopathies
      Kennedy disease (X-linked spinobulbar neuronopathy)
      Hexosaminidase deficiency (GM2 gangliosidosis)
Acquired
  Monomelic focal and segmental spinal muscular atrophies
  Multifocal motor neuropathies
  Acute motor axonal neuropathy (AMAN)
  Postpolio syndrome
  Postirradiation syndrome
Infective disorders
  Acute poliomyelitis
  West Nile fever
  Other viral infections (e.g., enterovirus 71 and rabies virus)
  Human immunodeficiency virus–associated motor neuron disorder
  Lyme disease
  Creutzfeldt-Jakob disease (amyotrophic forms)

DISORDERS OF THE BULBAR MOTOR SYSTEM

Kennedy disease (X-linked bulbospinal neuronopathy)
Brown-Vialetto-Van Laere syndrome
Fazio-Londe disease

TOXIC DISORDERS OF THE MOTOR NEURON

Neurolathyrism
Konzo
Heavy metal toxicity (lead, mercury)
Western Pacific ALS–parkinsonism-dementia complex
Postirradiation motor neuron injury

DISORDERS OF MOTOR NEURON OVERACTIVITY

Neuromyotonia
Stiff person syndrome

MISCELLANEOUS MOTOR NEURON DISORDERS

Endocrinopathies (e.g., hyperthyroidism, hyperparathyroidism, hypoglycemia)
Copper deficiency syndrome
Benign cramp-fasciculation syndrome

---

intronic expansions in the chromosome 9 *C9ORF72* gene. Such changes account for up to 40% of familial ALS cases, and up to 7% of sporadic ALS.[3] *SMN1* gene duplications are associated with a two-fold increased risk of sporadic ALS. In the sporadic disease, associations have been reported with alterations in at least eight other genes.

Pathology

At autopsy, the gross pathologic features of ALS consist of atrophy of the cerebral precentral gyrus, as well as sclerosis and pallor of the corticospinal tracts of the spinal cord. Thinning of the hypoglossal nerves and ventral spinal roots may be observed, and muscle atrophy is obvious. Microscopically, ALS patients will typically have lost at least 50% of their spinal motor neurons and have diffuse astrocytic gliosis in the spinal gray matter. By comparison, motor neurons in Onuf nucleus in the sacral spinal cord (which innervate the pelvic floor muscles) and the motor nuclei of cranial nerves III, IV, and VI (which

control eye movements) are relatively preserved. A cardinal feature in residual motor neurons is the presence of ubiquitinated proteinaceous inclusions, which may be compact or skein-like. TDP-43 has been recognized as a major protein constituent of these aggregates. In the motor cortex, there is variable loss of upper motor neurons and astrocytic gliosis. In the descending corticospinal tracts, axonal loss, myelin pallor, and gliosis are seen. The atrophied skeletal muscle shows clusters of angular atrophic fibers and fiber-type grouping that results from serial denervation and reinnervation. The selectivity of the disease process for the motor system is now recognized to be relative, and involvement of extramotor parts of the central nervous system can be found, especially in the sensory and spinocerebellar pathways, substantia nigra neurons, and dentate granule cells in the hippocampus. In the newly described ALS variant caused by C9ORF72 expansions, the characteristic extramotor system pathology demonstrates cerebellar and hippocampal inclusions that are P62+ and TDP-43-negative by immunostaining. Some of these inclusions comprise dipeptide proteins generated by aberrant translation of the G4C2 repeats.[4]

CLINICAL MANIFESTATIONS

ALS is characterized by a combination of upper and lower motor neuron degeneration. Lower motor neuron degeneration causes weakness, atrophy, and fasciculation of the limb and bulbar musculature. Features of upper motor neuron dysfunction include the incongruous presence of active or brisk tendon reflexes in a wasted limb, increased muscle tone, and sometimes the presence of Babinski sign. Upper motor neuron bulbar disease causes pseudobulbar palsy, with emotional lability, a brisk jaw jerk, slowing of repetitive tongue movements, and strained effortful speech. Fatigue and weight loss are also common symptoms. With end-stage disease, most patients will have features of upper and lower motor neuron dysfunction affecting all four limbs and the bulbar musculature.

In approximately 75% of patients, the disease starts distally, focally, and asymmetrically in an upper or lower limb, followed by progressive spread of injury in an anatomically logical progression to contiguous groups of motor neurons. Affected individuals may notice weakness, wasting or clumsiness of one hand, or unilateral footdrop. Muscle cramps may precede other clinical features, and fasciculations are most noticeable in the large proximal limb muscles. In the upper limbs, the thenar and intrinsic hand muscles tend to be severely affected, whereas the triceps and finger flexors are relatively spared until late in the disease. In the lower limbs, the pattern of weakness is often in a pyramidal distribution (flexors weaker than extensors), with early weakness of hip flexion and ankle dorsiflexion and severe involvement of the distal muscles.

Bulbar symptoms, which are the initial feature in approximately 25% of patients, are especially common in elderly women with ALS. The first problem is usually slurring of speech, initially apparent only when the individual is tired. Patients often have a mixed spastic/flaccid dysarthria in which speech develops a tight strangled quality because of the upper motor neuron component, with a superimposed nasal quality as a result of the flaccid lower motor neuron weakness of the palate and nasopharynx. In patients with bulbar disease, examination often reveals weakness of the facial muscles; a spastic, weak, wasted, and fasciculating tongue; and a brisk jaw jerk. Dysphagia, initially more pronounced for liquids than for solids, usually follows the dysarthria within a few weeks or months. Complications include weight loss and prolonged and arduous meal times with frequent episodes of coughing, drooling of saliva, and aspiration pneumonia.

Respiratory muscle weakness is rarely the initial feature of ALS. More commonly, respiratory muscle weakness develops insidiously and causes dyspnea and orthopnea. Diaphragmatic weakness may be apparent from the paradoxical movement of the abdominal wall during inspiration and a marked decline in forced vital capacity in the supine position. Symptoms of nocturnal carbon dioxide retention may develop, including interrupted sleep, morning headaches, anorexia, and daytime somnolence.

Neck muscle weakness, which is common later in the course of disease, causes difficulty holding the head upright (dropped head syndrome). Eye movements tend to be spared even in advanced disease, thereby permitting limited communication by movements of the eyes. Similarly, the strength of the pelvic floor muscles is relatively preserved, so patients with ALS usually remain continent throughout the course of the disease.

Overt features of frontotemporal dementia (Chapter 402), with progressive deterioration in personality and behavior, will develop in approximately 5% of patients with ALS. Cognitive dysfunction may precede, follow, or coincide with the features of motor dysfunction. Up to 50% of ALS patients without overt dementia may show more subtle features of frontal lobe dysfunction.[5] The C9ORF72-ALS variant causes both ALS and/or fronto-temporal dementia (Chapter 402), and patients with this subtype of ALS are more likely to have cognitive disturbances as well as a family history of dementia or psychosis.[6]

About 5 to 10% of ALS patients have the progressive muscular atrophy variant with clinical features reflecting only degeneration of lower motor neuron groups in the spinal cord. In primary lateral sclerosis, patients have pure upper motor neuron degeneration. Although severe spastic spinobulbar paresis ultimately develops in these patients, the duration of survival is commonly 10 to 15 years after the onset of symptoms. The progressive bulbar palsy variant usually progresses to involve the limbs, although limb signs may not be present initially.

Several ALS variants follow a more segmental pattern than is typical in ALS. Up to 10% of patients with ALS have flail arm syndrome, which is more common in men and is associated with a longer median survival than seen in those with typical ALS. A similar focal manifestation in the lower limbs, flail leg syndrome, is another recognized segmental variant.

DIAGNOSIS

The diagnosis of ALS is essentially clinical, and there is no specific diagnostic test. Diagnosis requires evidence of lower motor neuron degeneration by clinical, electrophysiologic (Chapter 396), or neuropathologic examination; upper motor neuron degeneration by clinical examination; and progressive spread of symptoms or signs within a region or to other regions, as determined by the history or examination. The diagnosis also requires the absence of other disease processes as determined by electrophysiologic testing, neuroimaging, and (if performed) biopsy. Generally accepted criteria (Table 419-2) classify patients as having definite, probable, or possible ALS. However, a number of other conditions may mimic ALS (Table 419-3), and

---

TABLE 419-2 AWAJI-SHIMA CONSENSUS CRITERIA FOR DIAGNOSING AMYOTROPHIC LATERAL SCLEROSIS

The diagnosis of ALS requires:
1. Evidence of LMN loss (reduced interferential pattern on full contraction and increased firing rate)
2. Evidence of reinnervation (motor units of large amplitude and longer duration)
3. Fibrillation and sharp waves or fasciculation potentials (fibrillation and sharp waves are required in weak limb muscles)

Number of muscles affected by region:
Cervical and lumbar-sacral region: a minimum of 2 muscles innervated by different roots and nerves
Bulbar and thoracic region: a minimum of 1 muscle

Diagnostic classification: Awaji-Shima Consensus Recommendations and the Revised El Escorial Criteria
Clinically definite ALS:
    clinical or electrophysiologic evidence of the presence of LMN as well as UMN signs in the bulbar region and at least 2 spinal regions or the presence of LMN and UMN signs in 3 spinal regions.
Clinically probable ALS:
    clinical or electrophysiologic evidence of LMN and UMN signs in at least 2 regions, with some UMN signs necessarily rostral to (above) the LMN signs.
Clinically possible ALS:
    clinical or electrophysiologic signs of UMN and LMN dysfunction are found in only 1 region, or UMN signs are found alone in ≥ 2 regions, or LMN signs are found rostral to UMN signs.

ALS = amyotrophic lateral sclerosis; LMN = lower motor neuron; UMN = upper motor neuron.

UMN signs: clonus, Babinski sign, absent abdominal reflexes, hypertonia, loss of dexterity.
LMN signs: atrophy, weakness. If only fasciculation, search with EMG for active denervation.
Regions reflect segmental motor neuron pools: bulbar, cervical, thoracic, and lumbosacral.

Adapted from Costa J, Swash M, de Carvalho M. Awaji criteria for the diagnosis of amyotrophic lateral sclerosis: a systematic review. *Arch Neurol.* 2012;69:1410-1416.

TABLE 419-3 DISORDERS THAT CAN MIMIC AMYOTROPHIC LATERAL SCLEROSIS/MOTOR NEURON DISEASE

FORM OF MOTOR NEURON DISEASE	MIMIC SYNDROMES	CLINICAL CLUES
Progressive muscular atrophy (PMA)/LMN-predominant phenotype	Multifocal motor neuropathy	Weakness out of proportion to wasting. Neurophysiology identifies conduction block. Anti-GM1 antibodies may be raised.
	Kennedy disease	Gynecomastia, distal sensory features, perioral fasciculation, indolent progression
	Spinal muscular atrophy	SMA can be adult onset. Pure LMN syndrome. Slower progression than PMA. Probably no family history.
	Chronic idiopathic demyelinating polyneuropathy	Electrophysiology identifies peripheral nerve demyelination.
	Benign cramp-fasciculation syndrome	Predominantly middle-aged men. Largely calf involvement. Failure to progress. No active denervation on EMG.
	Postpolio syndrome	Pure LMN syndrome. Past history of an illness compatible with poliomyelitis. Indolent progression.
	Lead poisoning	Extramotor clinical features, e.g., constipation, nail and buccal signs
	Acute motor axonal neuropathy (AMAN—a Guillain-Barré syndrome variant)	Acute onset, with progression ceasing after a few weeks. Nerve conduction studies show features of motor axonopathy.
	Hereditary motor neuropathies	Pure LMN syndrome. Family history, clinical signs indicating chronicity, slower rate of progression.
	Porphyria	Extramotor clinical features, family history, episodic exacerbations
	Compressive focal motor neuropathies	Pure motor disorders can result from compression of the deep palmar branch of the ulnar nerve and posterior interosseous branch of the radial nerve. Failure to extend beyond territory of one nerve. Electrophysiology with or without imaging helpful.
Amyotrophic lateral sclerosis	Multilevel spinal cord and root compression by discs, osteophytes, or tumor	Sensory symptoms and pain are common. UMN signs often caudal to LMN signs
	Thyrotoxicosis	Systemic symptoms and signs
	Combined peripheral neuropathy and cervical myelopathy	MRI of the spine and electrophysiology will differentiate
	Inclusion body myositis	Rarer than ALS. Characteristic pattern of weakness with early involvement of the long finger flexors and quadriceps.
	Paraneoplastic syndromes, especially lymphoma	History of malignancy or systemic features
	Sjögren syndrome	Non–motor-related symptoms
	Radiation myelopathy	History of radiotherapy
	Structural lesions of the bulbar region (e.g., tumor of the tongue base)	Pain, failure of features to extend outside the bulbar territory
Primary lateral sclerosis	Hereditary spastic paraplegia	Family history. Symptoms rarely extend beyond the lower limb territory. Prominent bladder dysfunction.
	Multiple sclerosis	Non–motor-related symptoms and signs (e.g., eye, bladder, cerebellar, and sensory involvement)
	Spinal cord compression by disc or tumor	Pain and sensory involvement usually present

ALS = amyotrophic lateral sclerosis; EMG = electromyography; LMN = lower motor neuron; MRI = magnetic resonance imaging; SMA = spinal muscular atrophy; UMN = upper motor neuron.

about 8% of patients in whom ALS is initially diagnosed have other lower motor neuron syndromes, such as multifocal motor neuropathy with conduction block, Kennedy disease, or mixed spinal cord and root compression (Chapter 400).[7] Conversely, 10 to 15% of patients in whom ALS is ultimately diagnosed may first undergo inappropriate surgery for presumed spinal cord or root compression abnormalities.

Blood tests that may be helpful in distinguishing ALS from mimic syndromes (see Table 419-3) include a complete blood count and serum calcium level, thyroid function tests, serum protein electrophoresis, Venereal Disease Research Laboratory test, creatine kinase level, inflammatory markers (erythrocyte sedimentation rate and C-reactive protein), and levels of anti-GM1 ganglioside and anti–myelin-associated glycoprotein (MAG) antibodies. Further testing, which is guided by the patient's clinical findings, might include acetylcholine receptor antibody; mutation screening in patients with familial disease, suspected Kennedy disease, or spinal muscular atrophy (SMA); heavy metal screening; urinary porphyrins; serum hexosaminidase A and B levels; *Borrelia* titers; and testing for human immunodeficiency virus.

Typical features of ALS on electromyography (EMG) include evidence of active denervation (i.e., positive sharp waves, fibrillation, and fasciculation potentials) and chronic denervation, as evidenced by large motor unit potentials that cannot be explained by a single nerve, root, or plexus lesion. Neuroimaging of the brain and spinal cord is usually needed to exclude structural pathology.

Baseline respiratory function tests should be performed on all patients. Muscle biopsy is indicated only in atypical cases when diagnostic uncertainty persists.

TREATMENT Rx

ALS is best managed in specialized centers that offer multidisciplinary care. Teams typically include a neurologist, nurse specialist, occupational therapist, physical therapist, speech and language therapist, and dietitian. During the course of the disease, patients frequently require referral for placement of a gastrostomy tube and to provide respiratory support.

No therapy currently has a dramatic effect in slowing the progression of ALS. Riluzole, a sodium channel blocker whose primary mechanism of action is to reduce excitotoxicity through inhibition of presynaptic glutamate release, prolongs survival by approximately 3 months when given at 50 mg twice daily.[A1] It may cause fatigue, nausea, and dizziness, but these effects are frequently transient. Liver function tests should be performed at baseline and monthly for the first 3 months of therapy. Other trials of potential neuroprotective therapies have so far proved negative. New experimental approaches include the use of gene therapy and antisense oligonucleotide technology to reduce the expression of disease-causing genes,[8] and cell-based therapy aimed primarily at providing a supportive environment to prolong the survival of endogenous motor neurons.[9]

Good clinical care must focus on symptoms and preservation of independence and quality of life. In patients with progressive bulbar problems, optimal positioning, attention to food and fluid consistency, and protective swallowing techniques are helpful. If weight loss continues, high-calorie nutritional supplements are added between meals. In ALS patients with dysphagia due to upper motor neuron impairment of the upper esophageal sphincter, local injection of botulinum toxin type A can significantly improve the dysphagia and may represent an alternative to percutaneous endoscopic gastrostomy.[A2] Placement of a gastrostomy tube via endoscopy or under radiologic guidance is recommended in patients in whom dehydration, weight loss of 10 to 15%, frequent distressing choking episodes, prolonged and tiring mealtimes, or aspiration pneumonia develop. Tube placement is higher risk in patients with respiratory insufficiency. Tubes should ideally be placed before the patient's forced vital capacity falls below 50% of expected. Some evidence suggests that radiologically guided gastrostomy insertion may be safer in frail patients in the late stages of ALS.[10]

Respiratory muscle weakness, which can develop insidiously during the course of ALS, causes breathlessness, orthopnea, daytime somnolence, morning headaches, and interrupted sleep. Management must emphasize detection and prevention of aspiration pneumonia, assistance in clearing of secretions by agents to reduce saliva production (e.g., anticholinergic drugs such as glycopyrrolate, 1 to 2 mg 3 to 4 times daily, or intrasalivary botulinum toxin injections), providing a suction machine, use of a mucolytic agent such as carbocisteine (in a dose of up to 750 mg three times daily), adoption of a semi-upright position for sleep, and aggressive antibiotic therapy for chest infection (Chapters 96 and 97). A small dose of sublingual lorazepam (0.5 to 1 mg) may be useful if the dyspnea is accompanied by extreme anxiety; opiate therapy (e.g., morphine, diamorphine, fentanyl [Chapter 30, Table 30-4]) may be given orally, transdermally, or by subcutaneous infusion to relieve respiratory distress during the later stages of the disease.

As respiratory function worsens, noninvasive ventilation can alleviate symptoms of chronic hypoventilation, significantly improve quality of life, and prolong survival,[A3] especially in patients with orthopnea, daytime hypercapnia, and nocturnal oxygen desaturation. Full 24-hour ventilation via a tracheostomy is an option that is chosen uncommonly by fully informed patients. Ongoing clinical research is evaluating the value of cough assist devices and diaphragm pacing, as well as the optimal way to manage respiratory symptoms at the end of life. Palliative care teams and hospices can contribute substantially to the care of ALS patients in the later stages of the disease. In the absence of ventilatory support, ALS patients will almost always die in their sleep from hypercapnic coma. In the terminal phases (Chapter 3), the aim of treatment is to ensure comfort by prescribing opiates and anxiolytic medications as required to alleviate discomfort or distress.

PROGNOSIS

Clinical features associated with a worse prognosis include older age at onset of symptoms, early compromise of respiratory function, bulbar symptoms, and more rapid presentation to medical attention. The mean duration from the onset of symptoms to death in patients with sporadic ALS ranges from 27 to 43 months. The average 5-year survival rate is 25%, and approximately 5% of patients will survive for more than 10 years. The usual cause of death is respiratory failure, which may be accompanied by bronchopneumonia.

SPINAL MUSCULAR ATROPHIES

DEFINITION

The term *spinal muscular atrophy* encompasses a group of pure lower motor neuron disorders that cause progressive symmetrical muscle weakness and wasting. Because the bulbar musculature may be affected, an alternative term, *hereditary motor neuronopathy*, has been proposed. The time of onset is variable and ranges from in utero to adult life.

EPIDEMIOLOGY AND PATHOBIOLOGY

The most common type of SMA is caused by mutations in the survival motor neuron (*SMN*) gene and is inherited as an autosomal recessive disorder. The estimated carrier frequency of an *SMN* mutation is 1 in 50. Type 1 SMA (Werdnig-Hoffmann disease) has an incidence of 1 in 8000 births. SMA is divided into subtypes I to IV according to age at onset and severity of the phenotype.

The human *SMN* gene on chromosome 5q13 exists in two forms, with 5–base pair differences between *SMN1* and its centromeric homologue *SMN2*. A change in exon 7 of *SMN2* leads to skipping of exon 7, and as a result, 80% of the protein encoded by *SMN2* is truncated and nonfunctional rather than full length. The majority of patients with SMA have homozygous absence of *SMN1* exon 7, but *SMN1* may be replaced by a copy of *SMN2* during DNA replication by a process known as gene conversion. An individual may have one to four copies of *SMN2*, with a proportional increase in the amount of full-length SMN protein. A molecular basis for the wide variation in the phenotypic severity of SMA, which can range from in utero onset (SMA type I) to adult onset (SMA type IV), is the number of copies of *SMN2* and the SMN protein levels, although other disease-modifying factors have also been implicated.

The SMN protein oligomerizes and associates with other proteins to form the SMN complex, which in turn has an important role in the assembly of spliceosomal small nuclear ribonucleoproteins that have a function in pre-mRNA splicing in the nucleus. These cellular processes are ubiquitous, so either the clinical features of SMA may be caused by a particular susceptibility of lower motor neurons to defects in RNA processing or SMN may have functions that are specific to the motor neuron, including axonal transport of mRNA molecules essential for the health of the distal axon. Recent work has highlighted the role of dysregulation of ubiquitin homeostasis and β-catenin signaling, as well as genes involved in motor neuron synaptogenesis in the pathophysiology of SMA.[11]

At autopsy, patients with SMA have atrophic spinal cords with loss of α-motor neurons and evidence of motor neuron degeneration and gliosis. The ventral roots are atrophic, and muscle atrophy is apparent with microscopic evidence of denervation and reinnervation.

CLINICAL MANIFESTATIONS

Type I SMA (Werdnig-Hoffman disease) is characterized by severe generalized muscle weakness and hypotonia at birth or by the age of 6 months;

affected children never sit or walk. Type II is an intermediate form with an onset of muscle weakness before the age of 18 months; patients can sit but are never able to walk unaided. Type III SMA (Wohlfart-Kugelberg-Welander disease) appears after 18 months of age; patients acquire the ability to stand and walk but often become wheelchair dependent in adolescence or adult life, although life expectancy is normal. Patients with type IV SMA have an onset of muscle weakness in adult life.

DIAGNOSIS

The diagnosis of SMA caused by changes in *SMN* can be made by genetic testing in a patient with appropriate clinical signs and symptoms; 95% of affected individuals have *SMN* deletions. Prenatal diagnosis is available. Electrophysiology and muscle biopsy reveal evidence of denervation.

Other disorders can present in infancy or childhood as hypotonia, and a pattern of weakness similar to *SMN*-related SMA can be distinguished by associated clinical features such as early respiratory distress or vocal cord paralysis, or an atypical distribution of motor features such as upper limb– or lower limb–predominant or scapuloperoneal involvement. The etiologic relationship of these disorders to classic SMA can be clarified by testing for *SMN* mutations.

It is important to distinguish SMA type I from infantile botulism, which can have a similar initial clinical picture. EMG with high-frequency repetitive nerve stimulation shows a decrement in botulism, and testing for the presence of botulinum toxin can confirm the diagnosis (Chapter 296). SMA II and SMA III can be distinguished from chronic inflammatory demyelinating polyneuropathy (Chapter 420) by the presence of normal cerebrospinal fluid protein and normal nerve conduction studies in SMA. Patients with SMA type III can have clinical features that are similar to those of the hereditary motor and sensory neuropathies, but it can be distinguished by neurophysiologic assessment and genetic testing.

TREATMENT AND PROGNOSIS Rx

No disease-modifying treatment of SMA is currently available,[A4][A5] although experimental approaches to upregulate expression of the SMN protein, enhance SMN2 exon 7 inclusion, or replace the deficient SMN protein using gene therapy are being actively explored.[12] In a randomized trial of children with SMA II and SMA III, initial results have indicated that oral olesoxime (10 mg/kg/day), which preserves mitochondrial function in stressed cells, slows the progressive loss of motor function. Another experimental approach is to alter splicing of the *SMN2* pre-mRNA to produce a functional SMN protein.[13] Such children may benefit from passive and active physical therapy, lightweight braces, surgical correction of scoliosis, and respiratory support measures.

Patients with type I SMA usually die by the age of 18 months, patients with type II typically survive into adolescence, and patients with type III and type IV have a normal life expectancy.

SPINOBULBAR MUSCULAR ATROPHY/KENNEDY DISEASE

EPIDEMIOLOGY

Kennedy disease, or spinobulbar muscular atrophy (SBMA), is an X-linked degenerative disorder of the lower motor neurons. Though rare, it is important not to miss the diagnosis because of the genetic implications for the family and a more benign course than occurs with ALS. The diagnosis should be considered in any male patient with a pure lower motor neuron disorder, particularly when the disease course is relatively indolent, gynecomastia is present, or there is evidence of a mild accompanying sensory neuropathy.

PATHOBIOLOGY

SBMA is a trinucleotide repeat disorder in which a CAG expansion encodes for a polyglutamine tract in the first exon of the androgen receptor gene on chromosome Xq11-12. The androgen receptor, which contains three functional domains, is transported to the nucleus, where it binds to DNA and acts as a transcription factor. Expansion of the polyglutamine tract results in reduced target gene transactivation, and neurodegeneration occurs when the

polyglutamine tract reaches a critical length of approximately 40 repeats. The neurodegeneration in patients with SBMA is considered to result from a ligand-dependent toxic gain of function of the mutant androgen receptor protein. Complete loss of its function, as seen in testicular feminization syndrome (Chapter 233), does not lead to motor neuron degeneration. The toxicity has not been fully characterized, but protein aggregation, impairment of protein degradation pathways, disruption of gene transcription, impairment of axonal transport, and neurotrophic factor signaling may all contribute.

Pathologic examination reveals mild spinal cord atrophy with ventral horn gliosis and loss of α-motor neurons. Misfolding of the polyglutamine (Q)-expanded protein leads to the formation of nuclear inclusions that contain the amino-terminal epitopes of the mutant androgen receptor within motor neurons and certain non-neuronal tissues.

CLINICAL MANIFESTATIONS AND DIAGNOSIS

The mean age at onset of SBMA is 30 years, with a range of 15 to 60 years, and the severity of the disease and its age at onset correlate with the size of the repeat expansion. Initial symptoms consist of hand tremors, fasciculations, and muscle cramps, followed by progressive weakness and atrophy of the limb and bulbar muscles. Limb muscle weakness tends to be proximal and predominantly involves the lower limbs. There are no clinical signs of upper motor neuron dysfunction. Weakness of the lower facial and tongue muscles causes dysarthria, and jaw weakness may cause the mouth to hang open. The presence of perioral fasciculations with quivering of the chin is a characteristic feature. Pharyngeal involvement can cause dysphagia, and respiratory muscle weakness causes breathlessness. Mild distal sensory loss is frequently present in the lower limbs. Features of mild androgen insensitivity are frequent: gynecomastia, testicular atrophy, and erectile dysfunction. Heterozygous female carriers of SBMA may show mild clinical manifestations of the disease.

EMG and muscle biopsy, which are often performed because the creatine kinase level tends to be elevated, reveal evidence of chronic denervation. Genetic screening for the CAG repeat expansion in exon 1 of the androgen receptor gene is diagnostic.

TREATMENT AND PROGNOSIS Rx

Because there are no established disease-modifying therapies for SBMA, current therapy consists of supportive care to prevent complications.[14] Recent human trials of the luteinizing hormone–releasing analogue leuprorelin and clenbuterol have not produced conclusive evidence of improvement. The course of the disease is slowly progressive in comparison to ALS and is compatible with normal life expectancy, although a proportion of patients may die of respiratory failure. Patients may become wheelchair dependent over a period of 2 to 3 decades, but some remain ambulatory until late in life.

Grade A References

A1. Miller RG, Mitchell JD, Moore DH. Riluzole for amyotrophic lateral sclerosis (ALS)/motor neuron disease (MND). *Cochrane Database Syst Rev*. 2012;3:CD001447.
A2. Restivo DA, Casabona A, Nicotra A, et al. ALS dysphagia pathophysiology: differential botulinum toxin response. *Neurology*. 2013;80:616-620.
A3. Bourke SC, Tomlinson M, Williams TL, et al. Effects of non-invasive ventilation on survival and quality of life in patients with amyotrophic lateral sclerosis: a randomized controlled trial. *Lancet Neurol*. 2006;5:140-147.
A4. Wadman RI, Bosboom WM, van der Pol WL, et al. Drug treatment for spinal muscular atrophy type I. *Cochrane Database Syst Rev*. 2012;4:CD006281.
A5. Wadman RI, Bosboom WM, van der Pol WL, et al. Drug treatment for spinal muscular atrophy types II and III. *Cochrane Database Syst Rev*. 2012;4:CD006282.

GENERAL REFERENCES

For the General References and other additional features, please visit Expert Consult at https://expertconsult.inkling.com.

420

PERIPHERAL NEUROPATHIES

MICHAEL E. SHY

APPROACH TO PERIPHERAL NEUROPATHIES

DEFINITION AND PATHOBIOLOGY

Peripheral neuropathy is a general term for disorders affecting peripheral nerves. The peripheral nervous system consists of motor, sensory, and autonomic neurons that extend outside the central nervous system (CNS) and are ensheathed by Schwann cells or ganglionic satellite cells. The peripheral nervous system includes the dorsal and ventral spinal roots, spinal and cranial nerves, sensory and motor terminals, and part of the autonomic nervous system. Motor neurons extend from their cell body in the ventral horn of the spinal cord to the neuromuscular junctions at the muscle that they innervate. The cell bodies of primary sensory neurons lie outside the spinal cord in the dorsal root ganglia, where they extend peripherally to specialized sensory end organs, including nociceptors, thermoreceptors, and mechanoreceptors. Central projections from dorsal root ganglia enter the spinal cord through the dorsal roots. At each spinal segment, the ventral roots, which carry motor axons, and the dorsal roots, which carry sensory axons, join to form mixed sensorimotor nerves. In the cervical, brachial, and lumbosacral areas, the mixed spinal nerves form plexuses from which arise the major anatomically defined limb nerves. Each mixed nerve is composed of large numbers of myelinated and nonmyelinated nerve fibers of varying diameter. The large myelinated axons include motor neurons and large fiber sensory nerves that mediate position and vibration sense. Small, thinly myelinated and nonmyelinated axons primarily provide nociception and autonomic functions. Preganglionic sympathetic autonomic fibers begin in the intermediolateral column of the spinal cord and synapse in ganglia of the sympathetic trunk. Preganglionic parasympathetic fibers travel long distances from their cell bodies in the brain stem or sacral spinal cord to reach terminal ganglia near the organs that the parasympathetic fibers innervate.

CLINICAL MANIFESTATIONS

Symptoms of peripheral neuropathy include weakness, sensory loss, abnormal balance, and autonomic dysfunction. Weakness is often distal and more severe in the legs than the arms. Deep and superficial muscles that are innervated by the peroneal nerve, such as the tibialis anterior and peroneus brevis and longus muscles, often cause more symptoms than do the plantar flexion muscles innervated by the tibial nerve, such as the gastrocnemius. As a result, tripping on a carpet or curb and ankle sprains are frequent symptoms. In the hands, symptoms typically involve fine movements, such as using buttons or zippers and inserting and turning keys in locks. Cramps, the painful knotting of a muscle, frequently occur with motor or sensorimotor neuropathies.

The sensory symptoms of neuropathy reflect disease of small, thinly myelinated or nonmyelinated fibers subserving pain and temperature, as well as large myelinated fibers subserving position sense. Common symptoms of small fiber sensory neuropathy include feeling as though the feet are "walking on pebbles" or "ice cold" and difficulty determining whether bath water is hot or cold with the foot. Painful dysesthesias, such as feeling as though the feet are "on fire," "on hot coals," or "stuck with pins," are also associated with small fiber abnormalities. Similar symptoms occur less frequently in the hands because most neuropathies are dependent on the length of the nerves; as a general rule, sensory symptoms appear in the hands after sensory symptoms in the legs have progressed up to the knee. An exception is when the patient also has carpal tunnel syndrome, which causes pain and tingling in the hands and can awaken patients from sleep. Large fiber sensory loss usually impairs balance, which may be worse at night when vision cannot overcome the loss of proprioception. Loss of proprioception is also frequently length dependent, so a patient may improve balance by lightly touching a wall with the hand to improve proprioceptive input to the brain.

Autonomic symptoms are frequent in neuropathies associated with diabetes or amyloidosis and include urinary retention or incontinence, abnormalities of sweating, constipation alternating with diarrhea, and lightheadedness when standing. Impotence is frequent.

DIAGNOSIS

Systematic Approach to Patients with Peripheral Neuropathy

Evaluation begins with the history and physical examination to demonstrate peripheral nerve disease and proceeds to neurophysiologic testing to characterize whether the process is demyelinating or axonal. Other specific tests are then ordered (Fig. 420-1). Peripheral neuropathies usually affect both motor and sensory nerves, causing both weakness and sensory loss. However, certain neuropathies are predominantly sensory, such as diabetes, or motor, such as multifocal motor neuropathy (Tables 420-1 and 420-2). Most neuropathies are symmetrical and length dependent. Pronounced asymmetries in symptoms suggest specific disorders, such as mononeuritis multiplex or hereditary neuropathy with liability to pressure palsies. It is also useful to know whether symptoms are acute (<1 month), subacute (<6 months), or

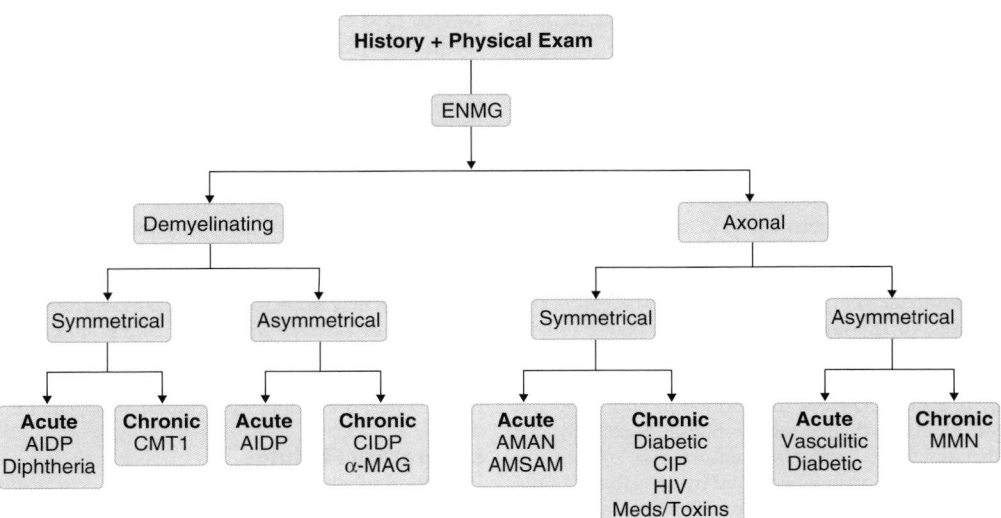

FIGURE 420-1. A systematic approach to evaluating neuropathy. The diseases listed are examples of neuropathies associated with specific neurophysiologic and clinical findings. Diabetic distal, predominantly sensory neuropathies are manifested as chronic axonal neuropathies; acute asymmetrical neuropathies can also occur with diabetes. Most neuropathies caused by toxins or by side effects of medication are chronic, symmetrical axonal neuropathies. AIDP, AMAN, and AMSAN are subtypes of Guillain-Barré syndrome. These and other examples are discussed in more detail in the text. AIDP = acute inflammatory demyelinating polyradiculoneuropathy; AMAN = acute motor axonal neuropathy; AMSAN = acute motor and sensory axonal neuropathy; CIDP = chronic inflammatory polyradiculoneuropathy; CIP = chronic illness polyneuropathy; CMT1 = Charcot-Marie-Tooth disease type 1, a genetic disorder; HIV = human immunodeficiency virus–related neuropathy; α-MAG = anti–myelin-associated glycoprotein; MMN = multifocal motor neuropathy.

TABLE 420-1   PREDOMINANTLY SENSORY NEUROPATHIES

CLASSIFICATION	SUBGROUP	TYPE	FIBERS
Genetic		HSAN	Large, small
Inflammatory/ immune	Monoclonal gammopathy	Anti-MAG (early on)	Mainly large
	Vasculitis	Sjögren syndrome	Large, small
	Paraneoplastic	Anti-Hu	Large
Metabolic	Diabetic	Distal symmetrical polyneuropathy	Large, small
Infectious	HIV	HIV neuropathy	Small
	Herpes zoster	Focal radiculoneuropathy	Small
	Leprosy	Tuberculoid	Small
Toxic/deficiency	Medications	Vincristine	Small
		Paclitaxel	Large
		Cisplatin	Large
		Thalidomide	Large
		NRTIs	Small
	Toxins	Thallium	Small
		Acrylamide	Large
		Pyridoxine (B_6)	Large, small
	Deficiency states	Vitamin B_1	Large, small
		Vitamin B_{12}	Large
		Vitamin E	Large
Idiopathic	Frequent		Large, small

HIV = human immunodeficiency virus; HSAN = hereditary sensory and autonomic neuropathy; MAG = myelin-associated glycoprotein; NRTIs = nucleoside reverse transcriptase inhibitors.

TABLE 420-2   PREDOMINANTLY MOTOR NEUROPATHIES

CLASSIFICATION	SUBGROUP	TYPE
Genetic		HMN
Inflammatory/immune	Guillain-Barré	AMAN
	Multifocal motor neuropathy	MMN
	Critical illness myopathy	CIM
Toxic/deficiency	Medications	Dapsone
	Toxins	Lead (adults)

AMAN = acute motor axonal neuropathy; HMN = hereditary motor neuropathy.

chronic (>6 months). For example, Guillain-Barré syndrome develops over a period of days to weeks, whereas chronic inflammatory demyelinating polyneuropathy (CIDP) evolves over months and inherited neuropathies may develop over years.

Neurologic Examination

Wasting of muscle is prominent in many sensorimotor or motor neuropathies, regardless of whether they are primary axonal or primary demyelinating disorders, because even demyelinating neuropathies are associated with secondary axonal degeneration. Atrophy frequently occurs in muscles of dorsiflexion, such as the tibialis anterior, and in intrinsic hand muscles, such as the first dorsal interosseus. Fasciculations, which appear as small twitches of the muscle, are sometimes present, particularly in axonal neuropathies.

Weakness is often most pronounced in foot dorsiflexion and eversion and in the intrinsic hand muscles. In the lower extremities, weakness usually progresses to the muscles of plantar flexion before more proximal muscles become involved.

Sensory loss is usually in a stocking-glove distribution in both large and small fiber neuropathies. Cold, erythematous, or bluish discolored feet suggest loss of small fiber function. Large fiber sensory loss, or "sensory ataxia," in the upper extremities can often be detected by an inability of the patient to locate the thumb accurately with the opposite index finger while the eyes are closed or by the presence of a characteristic irregular tremor (pseudoathetosis) of the outstretched fingers.

The sensory examination should include vibration, position, and light touch, as well as pain and temperature. It is important to determine the degree and extent of sensory loss, in addition to the pattern of deficits (symmetrical or asymmetrical; distal or generalized; focal, multifocal, or diffuse).

The complete absence of reflexes early in the course of a neuropathy suggests a demyelinating neuropathy (Chapter 411); for example, the absence of reflexes in early childhood is often the first detectable abnormality in children with inherited demyelinating neuropathies. Alternatively, the absence of ankle reflexes but the presence of normal patellar or upper extremity reflexes is common in "dying back" (length-dependent) axonal neuropathies, both acquired and inherited. Reflexes may be present in small fiber neuropathies.

On gait testing, subtle weakness in the feet can be detected by an inability of the patient to heel-walk. Sensory ataxia can be appreciated by a wide-based gait or inability to tandem-walk.

Neurologic Testing
Neurophysiology
Electromyography (EMG) and nerve conduction studies can determine whether a neuropathy is primarily demyelinating or axonal and can confirm whether the process is symmetrical or asymmetrical (Chapter 396).

Motor nerve conduction velocities measure conduction over the main body of nerves but not their proximal or distal portion. Distal motor latencies and F wave latencies measure velocities over the distal and proximal portions of the nerves. When slowing is roughly the same over the proximal, distal, and main portion of the nerve, the slowing is said to be uniform. When the slowing is multifocal or asymmetrical, either along the same nerve or between different nerves, the slowing is said to be nonuniform. Slowed conduction velocities (to less than 70% of normal) suggest that the neuropathy is primarily demyelinating.

The sensory nerve action potential is a summation of action potentials from individual large-diameter sensory axons. In axonal neuropathies, amplitudes of the compound muscle action potential or sensory nerve action potential are reduced. When there has been a loss of individual sensory axons, amplitudes of the sensory nerve action potential are reduced.

The presence of spontaneous activity on EMG, such as fibrillations or positive sharp waves, suggests that an acute or active process is damaging axons and denervating muscle. The presence of large, polyphasic motor units suggests partial reinnervation of muscle by regenerating axons (i.e., a more chronic process). Recruitment of motor units is also reduced in patients with demyelinating and axonal neuropathies.

Quantitative Sensory Testing
Quantitative sensory testing can assess and quantify vibratory, thermal, or painful sensory function in patients with peripheral neuropathies or other sensory disorders. Although the stimulus is an objective physical event, the response represents a subjective report and requires cooperation from the patient; as a result, this test by itself cannot diagnose sensory neuropathies or sensory loss.

Nerve and Skin Biopsy
Nerve biopsy is occasionally indicated to address specific questions, such as whether vasculitis, tumor, or another infiltrative or metabolic disorder is present. Biopsy of sural nerves is performed just above the ankle. After biopsy, patients lose sensation over the region on the lateral aspect of the foot that is innervated by the sural nerve, and transient painful dysesthesias may develop around the biopsy site. Teased sural nerve fiber analysis can demonstrate segmental demyelination or remyelination, and electron microscopy can demonstrate features of nerve regeneration and identify specific pathologic processes.

Epidermal skin biopsies with quantification of a loss of small epidermal nerve fibers may aid in the diagnosis of sensory neuropathies, particularly in neuropathies such as diabetes mellitus, human immunodeficiency virus (HIV) infection, or chemotherapeutic drugs. Skin biopsies can be used to evaluate myelinated sensory nerves, although these techniques are largely for research purposes rather than clinical management.

Laboratory Findings
Evaluation of all patients with suspected neuropathy should include blood glucose and creatinine levels, as well as a complete blood count (including red blood cell indices to detect possible macrocytosis). If the history and EMG are consistent with exposure to a toxin or a vitamin deficiency state, specific testing is indicated. Most patients should also have a vitamin B_{12} level measurement (Chapter 164), a test for syphilis (Chapter 319), and serum immunofixation electrophoresis for possible monoclonal gammopathy (Chapter 187). In unexplained sensory neuropathies, HIV testing should be considered

(Chapter 394). In selected patients, electrodiagnostic studies will suggest the need to test for specific antibodies, such as antibodies reacting to ganglioside GM_1 or myelin-associated glycoprotein (MAG). Genetic testing is most cost-effective when selection of candidate genes is based on the patient's nerve conduction studies, inheritance pattern, and clinical findings.

INHERITED NEUROPATHIES

DEFINITION

Inherited neuropathies are frequently called Charcot-Marie-Tooth (CMT) disease based on the three physicians who initially characterized the disorders in the late 19th century. They are also referred to as hereditary motor and sensory neuropathies, hereditary motor neuropathies, or hereditary sensory and autonomic neuropathies, depending on their clinical manifestation. Autosomal dominant forms are subdivided into demyelinating (CMT1) and axonal (CMT2) forms based on electrophysiologic and neuropathologic criteria. X-linked (CMTX) and autosomal recessive (CMT4) forms are also seen.[1] Each type of CMT is subdivided by the specific genetic cause of the neuropathy. For example, the most common form of CMT1, termed CMT1A, is caused by a duplication of a fragment of chromosome 17 containing the peripheral myelin protein 22-kD (PMP22) gene (see later). Mutations in more than 70 genes have been identified as causes of inherited neuropathies.

EPIDEMIOLOGY

The prevalence of CMT is about 1 in 2500, without ethnic predisposition. The 17p11.2 duplication causing CMT1A accounts for 60 to 70% of CMT1 patients, CMT1X for approximately 10 to 20% of CMT cases, CMT1B for less than 5% of patients, and CMT2 for about 20% of cases. The prevalence of hereditary neuropathy with liability to pressure palsies is not known, but about 85% of patients with clinical evidence of this syndrome have a chromosome 17p11.2 deletion.

PATHOBIOLOGY

Dysmyelination, demyelination, remyelination, and axonal loss are characteristic features of the demyelinating forms of CMT1. In Dejerine-Sottas neuropathy, myelin may never have formed normally. In CMT1, onion bulbs of concentric Schwann cell lamellae are usually present on nerve biopsies, with loss of both small- and large-diameter myelinated fibers and sometimes axons. Focal, sausage-like thickenings of the myelin sheath (tomacula) are characteristic of hereditary neuropathy with liability to pressure palsies (HNPP) but may also be found in other forms of CMT1, particularly CMT1B. In CMT1, disability typically correlates better with secondary axonal degeneration than with demyelination itself, thereby demonstrating the importance of Schwann cell–axonal interactions in demyelinating disease.

CLINICAL MANIFESTATIONS

Despite phenotypic variability, the typical clinical course of CMT1 and CMT2 patients includes normal development before weakness, and sensory loss appearing gradually within the first 2 decades of life. Affected children are often slow runners and have difficulty with activities that require balance (e.g., skating, walking across a log). Ankle-foot orthoses are frequently required by the third decade. Fine movements of the hands for activities such as turning a key or using buttons and zippers may be impaired, but the hands are rarely as affected as the feet. Most patients remain ambulatory throughout life and have a normal lifespan.

A minority of CMT patients have a more severe phenotype with delayed motor milestones and onset in infancy, termed *Dejerine-Sottas neuropathy*. Especially severe cases are classified as congenital hypomyelination if myelination appears to be disrupted during embryologic development. Many patients have de novo autosomal dominant disorders, and the term Dejerine-Sottas neuropathy is currently used primarily to denote severe early-onset clinical phenotypes regardless of the inheritance pattern. Patients with hereditary motor neuropathies sometimes have mild sensory abnormalities, and patients with hereditary sensory and autonomic neuropathies usually have some weakness. The same mutations in the same gene (GARS) cause both CMT2D and hereditary motor neuropathy type V.

DIAGNOSIS

Molecular testing, performed after the family history, neurologic examination, and neurophysiologic testing have suggested the probable candidate genes (GeneClinics—available at www.geneclinics.org), is the "gold standard" for the diagnosis of inherited neuropathies.[2] Nerve conduction velocity testing can distinguish between demyelinating and axonal neuropathies. Most CMT1 patients, particularly those with CMT1A, have a uniformly slow nerve conduction velocity of about 20 m/second. Asymmetrical slowing, which is characteristic of hereditary neuropathy with liability to pressure palsies, may be found in patients with missense mutations in PMP22, MPZ, EGR2, and GJB1. Although CMT2 is characterized by axonal loss and reduced compound muscle action potential or sensory nerve action potential amplitudes, virtually all forms of CMT1 have axonal loss as well as demyelination. Genetic testing should focus on specific possibilities.

Differential Diagnosis

Inherited neuropathies must be distinguished from acquired neuropathies (see later). Other genetic disorders of the CNS, such as hereditary spastic paraplegia (Chapter 410) or leukodystrophies (Chapter 411), may mimic inherited neuropathies by causing length-dependent weakness, sensory loss, and foot deformities such as pes cavus; these patients often have upper motor neuron signs, such as increased reflexes or Babinski signs, and do not have neurophysiologic evidence of neuropathy.

TREATMENT   Rx

There is no specific therapy for the inherited neuropathies, but clinical and genetic counseling and symptomatic and rehabilitative treatment are important. A detailed family history and often examination of family members are required for prognosis and genetic counseling.

Ankle-foot orthoses to correct footdrop may return gait and balance to normal for years. Foot surgery is sometimes offered to correct inverted feet, pes cavus, and hammertoes. Surgery may improve walking, alleviate pain over pressure points, and prevent plantar ulcers. Foot surgery, however, is generally unnecessary and does not improve weakness and sensory loss. Ascorbic acid, progesterone antagonists, and subcutaneous injections of neurotrophin 3 have improved animal models of CMT1A but have not improved patients with CMT1A or other forms of CMT.

INFLAMMATORY AND IMMUNOLOGIC NEUROPATHIES

Guillain-Barré Syndrome

DEFINITION

Guillain-Barré syndrome refers to acquired, inflammatory peripheral neuropathies that have (1) an acute onset, (2) elevated cerebrospinal fluid (CSF) protein levels with low CSF cell counts (cyto-albumologic dissociation), and (3) a monophasic illness with at least partial recovery.[3] Guillain-Barré syndrome is subdivided into acute inflammatory demyelinating polyneuropathy, acute motor and sensory axonal neuropathy, acute motor axonal neuropathy, and Miller-Fisher syndrome (Table 420-3).

EPIDEMIOLOGY

Acute inflammatory demyelinating polyneuropathy accounts for up to 97% of cases of Guillain-Barré syndrome in North America and Europe. It is a sporadic disorder with an incidence of 0.6 to 1.9 cases per 100,000 in North America and Europe. Men are more likely to be affected than women (1.4 : 1). In 60% of cases, acute inflammatory demyelinating polyneuropathy is preceded by a respiratory tract infection (e.g., cytomegalovirus [Chapter 376], Epstein-Barr virus [Chapter 377], or gastroenteritis [*Campylobacter jejuni*; Chapter 303]). In the Netherlands, 5% of cases have been attributed to a preceding hepatitis E infection.[4] Acute motor axonal neuropathy and acute motor and sensory axonal neuropathy are rare in North American and Europe but more frequent in China, Japan, Mexico, Korea, and India.[5]

PATHOBIOLOGY

All forms of Guillain-Barré syndrome probably result from postinfectious molecular mimicry in which nerve antigens are attacked by the immune system because they resemble antigens presented by microbes, in particular, *C. jejuni*. For example, the HS/0:19 serotype of *C. jejuni* is common in northern Chinese patients with Guillain-Barré syndrome and in other countries. Assays with antiganglioside antibodies, bacterial toxins, and lectins have characterized potential immunogenic regions of diarrhea-associated *C. jejuni* strains. However, it is not clear that molecular mimicry causes acute

TABLE 420-3 INFLAMMATORY AND IMMUNE-RELATED NEUROPATHIES

DISORDER	TYPE	CLINICAL TRAITS	PATHOBIOLOGY	TREATMENT*
Guillain-Barré syndrome	AIDP	Acute flaccid weakness, sensory loss	Demyelination, lymphocyte infiltration	Plasma exchange, IVIG
	AMAN/AMSAN	Acute flaccid weakness, no sensory loss in AMAN	Molecular mimicry, association with *Campylobacter jejuni*	? Plasma exchange or IVIG
	Fisher syndrome	Acute ataxia, ophthalmoparesis and areflexia	Anti-GQ1b antibodies	? Plasma exchange or IVIG
CIDP		Slower onset of weakness, sensory loss	Inflammatory/immune-mediated demyelination	Corticosteroids, plasma exchange, IVIG
Monoclonal gammopathy	IgM	Sensory > motor	Particularly anti-MAG	Immune suppression (Chapter 187)
	IgG	Sensorimotor	Many probably chance associations, osteosclerotic myeloma, solitary plasmacytoma; POEMS may be immune mediated	Treatment of myeloma
Multifocal motor neuropathy		Pure motor	Focal demyelination, antibodies to GM_1 frequent	IVIG

*Typical regimens: IVIG, 0.4 g/kg/day × 5 days for a total of 2 g/kg; may be repeated monthly as needed. Corticosteroids: prednisone, 60 to 80 mg/day for up to 3 months, followed by gradual tapering, depending on the clinical response, with a goal to about 20 mg on an alternate-day regimen.
AIDP = acute idiopathic demyelinating polyneuropathy; AMAN = acute motor axonal neuropathy; AMSAN = acute motor and sensory axonal neuropathy; CIDP = chronic inflammatory polyradiculoneuropathy; Ig = immunoglobulin; IVIG = intravenous immune globulin; MAG = myelin-associated glycoprotein; POEMS = polyneuropathy, organomegaly, M protein, skin changes.

inflammatory demyelinating polyneuropathy, which is the most common form in the United States and Europe.

CLINICAL MANIFESTATIONS

Weakness, the most common initial symptom in both acute inflammatory demyelinating polyneuropathy and acute motor and sensory axonal neuropathy, can be mild, such as difficulty walking, or severe, such as total quadriplegia and respiratory failure. Bilateral weakness of facial muscles (facial diplegia) occurs in about 50% of cases. The most common manifestation is leg weakness that progresses into the arms. Although Guillain-Barré syndrome has been described as an "ascending paralysis," proximal weakness is common, and 5% of cases have isolated cranial nerve involvement that subsequently descends into the limbs. Slight sensory loss occurs in most patients. The autonomic nervous system is involved in about 65% of patients.

Length-dependent weakness without sensory loss develops in patients with acute motor axonal neuropathy, including cranial nerve involvement in about 25%. Miller-Fisher syndrome consists of the triad of ophthalmoplegia, ataxia, and areflexia. Facial weakness, ptosis, and pupillary abnormalities may be present. Nerve conduction velocities in Miller-Fisher syndrome are generally normal, unlike the case with acute inflammatory demyelinating polyneuropathy.

DIAGNOSIS

The diagnosis of acute inflammatory demyelinating polyneuropathy and acute motor and sensory axonal neuropathy is based on the history, physical examination, and CSF evaluation. Deep tendon reflexes are decreased or absent, and the CSF is abnormal, with a high protein level but a paucity of white blood cells. The weakness is symmetrical. The presence of CNS abnormalities should cast doubt on the diagnosis. Acute inflammatory demyelinating polyneuropathy is distinguished from acute motor and sensory axonal neuropathy by nerve conduction studies. In both acute inflammatory demyelinating polyneuropathy and acute motor and sensory axonal neuropathy, the CSF should have fewer than five white blood cells (WBCs)/mL. If the CSF cell count is greater than 50 WBCs/mL, another diagnosis, such as HIV infection (Chapter 394) or Lyme disease (Chapter 321), should be considered. Elevated CSF protein may not be apparent in the first 7 to 10 days of the illness; in up to 10% of cases, CSF protein levels remain normal. Approximately 5% of patients with Guillain-Barré syndrome have Miller-Fisher syndrome, and more than 85% of these patients have polyclonal antibodies that react with the ganglioside GQ_{1b}.

Differential Diagnosis

The differential diagnosis varies in different parts of the world. Historically, poliomyelitis (Chapter 379) was the major cause of acute flaccid quadriparesis. In North America, polio has been eradicated, but other viral illnesses may induce polio-like syndromes: ECHO 70 (Chapter 379), coxsackievirus (Chapter 379), West Nile virus (Chapter 383), and rarely, rabies (Chapter 414). Because these diseases are not demyelinating disorders, they can be distinguished from acute inflammatory demyelinating polyneuropathy by their normal nerve conduction velocity. However, the results of electrodiagnostic studies are similar in both acute motor axonal neuropathy and the polio-like syndromes, thus making distinction between acute motor axonal neuropathy and these viral syndromes difficult.

Tick paralysis (Chapter 359), caused by a toxin within the tick, can mimic Guillain-Barré syndrome, particularly in children. Usually, removal of the tick is associated with improvement within hours, although progression can occur. Progression is particularly likely in Australia, where the toxin differs from that found in North America.

Botulism (Chapters 296 and 422) rapidly produces a flaccid paralysis. Patients have ophthalmoplegia, bulbar weakness, dry mouth, constipation, and orthostatic hypotension, but sensory symptoms do not develop. Other entities that can mimic Guillain-Barré syndrome are acute spinal cord compression (Chapter 400), acute transverse myelitis (Chapter 411), and vascular myelopathies, all of which are characterized by decreased reflexes before the development of upper motor neuron signs such as increased reflexes. Carcinomatous or lymphomatous meningitis can also cause a rapidly developing quadriparesis, but both are associated with elevated CSF WBC counts.

TREATMENT   Rx

Patients with Guillain-Barré syndrome require hospitalization because of the potential for respiratory compromise. Pulmonary function tests should be performed frequently; a vital capacity of less than 1 L or a negative inspiratory force of less than −70 suggests the need for ventilator support in an intensive care unit. Autonomic instability and difficulty swallowing should be monitored. Therapies directed at modulating the immune system are effective in Guillain-Barré syndrome. Although intravenous immunoglobulin (IVIG; 2 g/kg divided over 2 to 5 days in the first 2 weeks)[A1] and plasma exchange[A2] are equally effective,[A3] at least in the first 2 weeks, IVIG is preferred because of its convenience unless there are contraindications, such as low serum immunoglobulin A (IgA) levels, renal failure, or severe hypertension. Plasma exchange, usually four exchanges of 1.5 L of plasma spread over a 10-day period, is also effective. Two plasma exchanges may be sufficient in mild cases, and six exchanges are not superior to four in severely affected patients. This therapy should be administered within the first 2 weeks and not later than 4 weeks after the onset of clinical disease. Intravenous corticosteroids alone are not beneficial.[A4] Methylprednisolone (500 mg/day for 5 days) in association with IVIG has a slight initial advantage over IVIG alone but no benefit in terms of long-term disability.[A5]

Ten percent of patients with Guillain-Barré syndrome relapse after initially responding to plasma exchange or IVIG. These patients usually respond to a second cycle of the previously effective treatment. The combined use of plasma exchange followed by IVIG does not improve the prognosis.

PROGNOSIS

Fifty percent of patients progress to their nadir, or maximum disability, within 2 weeks, 75% within 3 weeks, and more than 90% within 4 weeks of the onset of symptoms. With supportive care, mortality in Guillain-Barré is 3% at 6 months, primarily in the elderly and severely affected patients, and especially during the recovery phase.[6] After a brief period of stabilization, slow spontaneous recovery occurs over a period of weeks or months. Most patients recover completely or are left with minor sequelae; about 20% have a persistent disability. The long-term prognosis depends at least in part on the extent of axonal loss.[7] Patients with low compound muscle action potential amplitudes in the upper extremities are more likely to have a poor prognosis.

Patients with acute motor axonal neuropathy will recover after approximately 2 months, but the extent of recovery may be less than in Guillain-Barré syndrome. In general, the prognosis in Miller-Fisher syndrome is excellent.

Chronic Inflammatory Demyelinating Polyradiculoneuropathy

DEFINITION

CIDP is a chronic acquired demyelinating sensorimotor neuropathy that may be monophasic, relapsing, or progressive. By definition, CIDP develops over at least a 2-month period, which is slower than for acute inflammatory demyelinating polyneuropathy, which it otherwise resembles.

EPIDEMIOLOGY

CIDP occurs in all age groups, with a mean age range of 30 to 50 years. Women are more likely to be affected than men. Antecedent events are less common than in Guillain-Barré syndrome; they occur in about 30% of patients and include upper respiratory infections, gastrointestinal infections, vaccinations, surgery, and trauma.

PATHOBIOLOGY

CIDP is considered an autoimmune disorder based on pathologic findings in nerve biopsy samples from patients and on animal models, such as experimental allergic neuritis, in which a similar disorder follows immunization with peripheral nervous system myelin components and Freund adjuvant. Nerve biopsy shows macrophage-mediated segmental demyelination, occasional endoneurial lymphocytic T-cell infiltrates, and endoneurial edema. The major histocompatibility complex class I and II antigens are upregulated, and there are often deposits of immunoglobulins and complement split products on the outer Schwann cell membranes or myelin sheaths. CIDP can be passively transferred to animals by patient sera, but no clear autoantigen has been identified.

CLINICAL MANIFESTATIONS

Weakness and sensory loss begin insidiously and progress over a period of months to years.[8] Weakness is commonly proximal as well as distal. Patients can become bedridden. Loss of proprioception from damage to large-diameter sensory nerves may affect balance and result in an action tremor. Deep tendon reflexes are usually absent or markedly decreased. Facial weakness (15%), ptosis or ophthalmoparesis (5%), and papilledema occur occasionally. Variant forms include pure motor, pure sensory, and multifocal disease.

DIAGNOSIS

Diagnosis is based on clinical symptoms and signs, electrodiagnostic studies, and CSF examination. Nonuniform, asymmetrical slowing on nerve conduction studies is characteristic. One portion of a nerve may have different conduction than another. For example, if damage is primarily in the spinal roots, proximal conduction velocities and F wave latencies may be most affected. Compound muscle action potentials are generally reduced because of the concomitant axonal degeneration that occurs with demyelinating neuropathies. However, temporal dispersion and conduction block may also reduce the amplitude of muscle action potential in any demyelinating neuropathy. Sensory nerve conduction is also slow in CIDP, but because sensory nerve action potentials are often not detectable, sensory conduction velocity may be unmeasurable.

CSF results resemble those of acute inflammatory demyelinating polyneuropathy: WBC counts are usually less than 10 cells/μL, and protein levels are higher than 60 mg/dL. CSF cell counts greater than 50/μL suggest another diagnosis, such as HIV infection or hematologic malignancy. CSF protein levels may be normal early in the course of CIDP.

Differential Diagnosis

CIDP is distinguished from acute inflammatory demyelinating polyneuropathy by its time course. CIDP can also occur in diabetes, lymphoma, monoclonal gammopathies (see later), and asymmetrical inherited neuropathies (see earlier).

TREATMENT   Rx

Corticosteroids, IVIG (as used for the Guillain-Barré syndrome except that it often needs to be repeated on an approximately monthly basis for up to and sometimes exceeding 6 months), and plasma exchange appear to be equally effective[A6] treatments for CIDP, with about two thirds of patients responding. For steroids, a standard approach is oral prednisone (1 mg/kg/day) for 6 to 8 weeks, followed by slow tapering over a 3- to 12-month period to a maintenance level of about 0.1 mg/kg/day. A response to prednisone may take months to occur, and occasional patients may worsen before they respond. Other alternatives are pulsed dexamethasone (6 cycles of 40 mg/day orally for 4 days) or short-term prednisolone (60 mg/day for 5 weeks, then tapering to zero), which is equally effective for CIDP.[A7] Plasma exchange is also effective. Because of the side effects or inadequate response to long-term corticosteroids, azathioprine, cyclosporine, cyclophosphamide, methotrexate, mycophenolate mofetil, rituximab, and interferon-α or -β have been used with variable success in uncontrolled reports.[9]

Neuropathy Associated with Monoclonal Gammopathy

DEFINITION

Monoclonal gammopathy refers to the presence in the β-γ region of serum protein electrophoresis of an abnormal spike (variably termed a paraprotein, monoclonal protein, or M protein) consisting of immunoglobulins of the same isotype, all produced by a single clone of abnormally proliferating lymphocyte/plasma cells. In some cases, the M protein is part of a malignant lymphoproliferative disease such as multiple myeloma, solitary plasmacytoma (IgG and IgA), Waldenström IgM macroglobulinemia (Chapter 187), lymphoma (Chapter 185), chronic lymphocytic leukemia (Chapter 184), primary amyloidosis (Chapter 188), or cryoglobulinemia (Chapter 187). In most instances, however, monoclonal gammopathy is not initially associated with any of these disorders and is classified as a monoclonal gammopathy of uncertain significance (MGUS), although in patients with MGUS, the gammopathy may evolve into a malignant form (Chapter 187).

EPIDEMIOLOGY

Monoclonal gammopathy occurs in up to 8% of patients with peripheral neuropathy of unknown etiology. However, MGUS is frequent, being found in 1% of the population older than 50 years and in 3% older than 70 years, and most subjects with MGUS do not have neuropathy. In some cases, the co-occurrence of neuropathy and M protein may be a coincidence, but in other cases, the M protein is clearly related to the neuropathy.

The prevalence of neuropathy is higher in patients with IgM versus IgG or IgA M proteins. The prevalence of symptomatic neuropathy associated with IgM monoclonal gammopathy in patients older than 50 years is approximately 20 per 100,000. In half of such patients, the M protein reacts with either the HNK1 carbohydrate moiety of MAG or with other glycoproteins (MPZ, PMP22) and glycolipids (sulfoglucuronylparagloboside [SGPG] and lactosaminylparagloboside [SGLPG]). IgM M proteins associated with neuropathy may also bind to other neural antigens.

In patients with IgG monoclonal gammopathy and neuropathy, the relationship is less clear than with IgM. Although about 10% of patients with multiple myeloma have neuropathy, in most cases, the M protein does not react with a neural antigen, and patients do not improve with immunotherapy (see later). Conversely, approximately 50% of patients with the osteosclerotic form of myeloma have neuropathy, often associated with the non-neurologic manifestations of organomegaly, endocrine abnormalities, and brown, tannish discoloration of the skin). Collectively, the M protein, polyneuropathy and other features are referred to by the acronym POEMS (Chapter 187).[10] Similarly, about 50% of patients with light chain amyloidosis have neuropathy.

PATHOBIOLOGY

In patients with IgM M proteins that immunoreact with MAG, nerve biopsies demonstrate segmental demyelination with deposits of M protein and complement. The myelin lamellae are often widened on sural nerve biopsies, but a biopsy is not necessary for diagnosis. High titers (>1 : 10,000) of anti-MAG IgM antibodies are associated with neuropathy, and intraneural or systemic injection of anti-MAG IgM M proteins causes complement-mediated demyelination of nerves in animals.

CLINICAL MANIFESTATIONS

Most patients with anti-MAG neuropathies are initially seen in their sixth to seventh decade of life with dysesthesias and paresthesias in their legs and unsteadiness while walking because of loss of proprioception. Physical examination shows a length-dependent large fiber sensory neuropathy. Weakness may develop later.

DIAGNOSIS

Nerve conduction velocities are slow (about 25 m/second) with pronounced delays in distal motor latencies, thus prompting the designation *distal acquired demyelinating symmetrical neuropathy* to distinguish the disorder from CIDP.

TREATMENT Rx

Treatment of neuropathies associated with monoclonal gammopathy is similar to that for CIDP (see earlier). However, patients with anti-MAG-related neuropathies do not respond as well to treatment as do patients with CIDP. Anecdotal data support the benefit of rituximab (375 mg/m^2 weekly for 4 weeks) in some patients.

PROGNOSIS

Progression of the neuropathy of monoclonal gammopathy disables about 25% of patients after 10 years and 50% after 15 years. The course of patients with osteosclerotic myeloma and neuropathy depends on the response to treatment of the myeloma. In patients whose myeloma responds to treatment, more than 50% have improvement in neuropathy. In other patients with sensorimotor neuropathies associated with plasma cell dyscrasias, the course is variable, and the M protein may not be related to their neuropathy.

Multifocal Motor Neuropathy and Lewis-Sumner Syndrome

DEFINITION

Multifocal motor neuropathy is characterized by progressive, distal more than proximal, asymmetrical limb weakness, mostly affecting the upper limbs with minimal or no sensory impairment.

EPIDEMIOLOGY

The prevalence of multifocal motor neuropathy is estimated at 2 per 100,000. Men are more frequently affected than women (2.6 : 1). Initial symptoms develop in 80% between the ages of 20 and 50 years, with a mean age at onset of 40 years. Lewis-Sumner syndrome occurs less frequently than multifocal motor neuropathy.

PATHOBIOLOGY

Multifocal motor neuropathy is considered to be an autoimmune neuropathy based on its clinical improvement with immunologically based therapies and because of a frequent association with antiglycolipid antibodies. Patients with MMN often have serum antibodies that react with ganglioside GM$_1$, and these titers decrease during effective treatment. GM$_1$ is highly represented in neural membranes at the nodes of Ranvier, compact myelin, and the motor end plate at the neuromuscular junction. A blocking effect on mouse distal motor nerve conduction has been induced in vitro by sera from multifocal motor neuropathy patients with and without high anti-GM$_1$ antibody titers. These data support the presence of serum factors responsible for conduction block in the sera of patients with multifocal motor neuropathy, although these factors are not invariably related to anti-GM$_1$ antibodies. Lewis-Sumner syndrome, however, is not associated with antiganglioside antibodies.

CLINICAL MANIFESTATIONS

The usual pattern is progressive, distal, asymmetrical arm weakness, often in the distribution of a single nerve. In a minority of patients, weakness may start proximally or in the legs. The disease will frequently affect other nerves, occasionally with a crossed distribution (i.e., one arm and the contralateral leg). Asymmetry and predominance of arm weakness may become less evident as the disease progresses. Localized muscle atrophy may be mild or

absent in the early stage of the disease but can become prominent later as a result of axonal degeneration.

Fasciculations, cramps, and myokymia occur in patients with multifocal motor neuropathy and those with amyotrophic lateral sclerosis (Chapter 419), thereby making distinction between the two disorders difficult. Marked asymmetry in the degree of clinical findings and electrophysiologic abnormalities between contiguous nerves is suggestive of multifocal motor neuropathy rather than amyotrophic lateral sclerosis. Cranial nerve involvement or respiratory failure as a result of unilateral or bilateral phrenic nerve palsy rarely occurs in multifocal motor neuropathy. The presence of sensory loss suggests Lewis-Sumner syndrome.

DIAGNOSIS

The diagnosis is established by the presence of multifocal, persistent partial conduction blocks on motor but not sensory nerve conduction studies. Lewis-Sumner syndrome has sensory loss as well as weakness, with conduction block in both sensory and motor nerves.

TREATMENT

IVIG (2 g/kg) is the initial treatment for multifocal motor neuropathy, and almost 80% of patients respond within a week. However, improvement is typically brief (3 to 6 weeks), so repeated treatments are required indefinitely.[11] Clinical improvement is often accompanied by a reduction or resolution of the motor conduction block in some nerves, but it does not consistently correlate with a reduction in antiganglioside antibody titers. Patients may eventually become refractory to IVIG, and another agent may be needed, such as rituximab (e.g., 375 mg/m^2 weekly for 4 weeks) or azathioprine (2 to 3 mg/kg/day). Plasma exchange and corticosteroids are generally ineffective and have been associated with worsening neuropathy in some patients. Lewis-Sumner syndrome, which is a multifocal variant of CIDP, responds to the same treatments as CIDP.

PARANEOPLASTIC NEUROPATHIES

DEFINITION

Paraneoplastic neuropathies (Chapter 179) are a "remote effect of cancer" not caused by metastatic invasion of neural tissue; radiation therapy or chemotherapy; metabolic, vascular, or hormonal disturbances; or opportunistic infections. It is hypothesized that they are the result of host immune responses to a tumor antigen or antigens that are also present in neural tissues.

EPIDEMIOLOGY

Paraneoplastic syndromes occur in less than 1% of patients with cancer; peripheral neuropathy is only one of the paraneoplastic syndromes. Although more than 25% of patients with cancer have evident neuropathy on neurologic examination, the relationship to malignancy is unclear in most. Paraneoplastic neuropathy may develop before, during, or after the tumor is diagnosed. In certain tumors, neuropathies are distinctive and should prompt a thorough investigation for cancer. Small cell carcinoma of the lung (Chapter 191) is by far the most common underlying neoplasm, followed by carcinoma of the stomach, breast, colon, rectum, ovary, and prostate.

PATHOBIOLOGY

Subacute sensory neuropathy, the most characteristic paraneoplastic neuropathy, results from an immune-mediated ganglionitis that destroys sensory neurons in the dorsal root ganglia. Mononuclear inflammatory infiltrates composed of CD4$^+$ and prominent CD8$^+$ T cells, along with plasma cells, are found in the stroma surrounding the dorsal root ganglion neurons. Other findings include atrophy of the dorsal roots; loss of sensory neurons, which appear to be replaced by a proliferation of satellite cells (Nageotte nodule); axonal degeneration; and secondary degeneration of the dorsal column of the spinal cord. Inflammatory infiltrates can also be found in peripheral nerves or muscle. Sural nerve biopsies typically reveal only loss of myelinated nerve fibers and are not useful for diagnosis.

CLINICAL MANIFESTATIONS

Subacute sensory neuropathy is characterized by subacute, progressive impairment of all sensory modalities and is associated with severe sensory ataxia and areflexia.[12] Subacute sensory neuropathy may precede the diagnosis of tumor by months or even years. At onset, patients may have shooting pain and burning sensations. Other symptoms include numbness, tingling, and a progressive sensory loss that may be asymmetrical. Symptoms usually progress rapidly to involve all four limbs, the trunk, and face. Findings may then stabilize, although by this time the patient is often totally disabled. Occasional patients have an indolent course.

Neurologic examination reveals loss of deep tendon reflexes and involvement of all modalities of sensation; large fiber modalities such as vibration and joint position sense are most severely affected. The loss of position sense may lead to severe sensory ataxia with pseudoathetoid movements of the hands and an inability to walk despite normal strength. Cranial nerve involvement includes sensorineural deafness, loss of taste, and facial numbness. The asymmetrical pattern of symptoms sometimes suggests a radiculopathy or plexopathy.

A paraneoplastic encephalomyelitis characterized by patchy, multifocal neuronal loss in regions of the cerebral hemispheres, the limbic system, the cerebellum, the brain stem, the spinal cord, and autonomic ganglia often develops in patients with subacute sensory neuropathy. Autonomic symptoms include impotence, dry mouth, and constipation.

DIAGNOSIS

The diagnosis is based on recognizing the typical neuropathy in the setting of malignancy.[13] The results of routine laboratory studies are generally normal. The diagnosis is supported by finding serum polyclonal IgG anti-Hu antibodies, also called antineuronal antibodies type 1, or by indirect immunofluorescence or immunohistochemistry and confirmed by Western blot analysis.

Subacute painful, asymmetrical neuropathy or neuronopathy in an elderly patient should prompt a search for carcinoma of the lung because small cell lung cancer (Chapter 191) accounts for more than 80% of the associated tumors. Subacute sensory neuropathy has also been reported in patients with adenocarcinoma of the lung, breast, ovary, stomach, colon, rectum, and prostate, as well as Hodgkin and non-Hodgkin lymphoma. In patients with no evidence of cancer, detection of anti-Hu antibodies should prompt a computed tomography study of the chest with special attention to the mediastinal lymph nodes. The use of whole body positron emission tomography with fluorodeoxyglucose has been advocated for early diagnosis in patients with anti-Hu antibodies or clinical suspicion of subacute sensory neuropathy because it may reveal neoplastic adenopathy months before computed tomography or magnetic resonance imaging.

TREATMENT Rx

Subacute sensory neuropathy responds poorly to plasma exchange, IVIG, or immunosuppressant medications, even when such treatment is started early in the course of the disease. Successful treatment of the tumor rarely induces remission of subacute sensory neuropathy but may stabilize symptoms.

Other Neuropathies Possibly Associated with Cancer
SENSORIMOTOR NEUROPATHY
Sensorimotor neuropathy occurs in approximately 25% of patients with all types of tumors. The neuropathy can have an acute or subacute onset, with a progressive or relapsing-remitting course. Because no antineuronal antibody has been specifically associated with these neuropathies, their paraneoplastic nature is not established. Severe or relapsing neuropathies often precede the diagnosis of cancer, but the search for malignancy is generally limited to a chest radiograph, stool samples for blood, and routine blood tests. There are no specific treatments for these neuropathies, and their progression does not necessarily correlate with that of the malignancy.

PARANEOPLASTIC VASCULITIS OF NERVES
A nonsystemic vasculitic neuropathy, which may also involve muscle, occurs with various types of tumor, including small cell lung cancer, lymphoma, and carcinoma of the kidney, stomach, and prostate. Neurologic symptoms may develop either before or after the tumor is diagnosed. The neuropathy is subacute and progressive and usually affects older men. Like many paraneoplastic disorders, these neuropathies often respond poorly to treatment.

VASCULITIC NEUROPATHIES

DEFINITION
Vasculitic neuropathies (Table 420-4) typically present as painful acute or semiacute axonal mononeuritis multiplex. There is acute motor and sensory loss in multiple nerve territories. The number of nerves involved may be extensive enough to make the distinction between a multifocal and diffuse neuropathy difficult. Occasionally, vasculitic neuropathy can present as sensory neuropathy, trigeminal neuropathy, compressive neuropathy, or autonomic neuropathy. Neuropathy can occur in systemic vasculitis associated with other organ systems, as well as in nonsystemic vasculitis affecting just nerve and muscle.

EPIDEMIOLOGY
Systemic vasculitic neuropathy is more common than nonsystemic vasculitic neuropathy. Peak ages at onset of both are the fifth to eighth decades, but vasculitis can occur at any age. Neuropathy, particularly mononeuritis multiplex, is common in several forms of systemic vasculitis. Rheumatoid arthritis (Chapter 264) evolves into systemic rheumatoid vasculitis in 5 to 15% of patients, and vasculitic neuropathy will develop in about 50% of these patients. More than 50% of patients with Churg-Strauss syndrome (Chapter 270), 40 to 50% with granulomatosis with polyangiitis (Chapter 270), 35 to 75% with polyarteritis nodosa (Chapter 270), and a majority of patients with mixed cryoglobulinemia (Chapter 187) have neuropathy. Patients with Sjögren syndrome (Chapter 268) are often initially found to have sensory neuropathies. Neuropathies are uncommon in systemic lupus erythematosus.

PATHOBIOLOGY
In patients with mononeuritis multiplex, axonal degeneration develops as a result of nerve ischemia caused by the vasculitic process. Immune-mediated inflammation and necrosis of blood vessel walls occlude the vessel's lumen, thereby resulting in ischemic damage. Small arteries or arterioles (50 to 300 μm) are most commonly affected, particularly those that occur in watershed areas between the distribution of the major nutrient arteries of proximal nerves. True nerve infarcts are rare.

TABLE 420-4	SYSTEMIC VASCULITIS AND NEUROPATHY			
TYPE	SEROLOGY FEATURES	ASSOCIATED FEATURES	USUAL NEUROPATHY TYPE	NEUROPATHY PREVALENCE
Rheumatoid arthritis	RF 80–90%	Arthralgias, arthritis frequent; multiple organs	Mononeuritis multiplex and sensorimotor neuropathy	50% of patients with vasculitis
Churg-Strauss	c-ANCA <30% p-ANCA <50%	Eosinophilia Asthma	Mononeuritis multiplex	20% of patients
Granulomatosis with polyangiitis	c-ANCA 75-90% p-ANCA <20%	Pulmonary and renal	Mononeuritis multiplex	15% of patients
Polyarteritis nodosa	c- and p-ANCA rare	Multiple organs, 30% hepatitis B	Mononeuritis multiplex	60% of patients
Mixed cryoglobulinemia	No	Hepatitis C, purpura frequent	Mononeuritis multiplex	20-90% of patients
Sjögren syndrome	α-Ro/SS-A 60%, α-La/SS-B 50%	Dry eyes, dry mouth; women 90%	Sensory	25% of patients
Systemic lupus erythematosus	ANA screen >90%	Multiorgan	Sensorimotor neuropathy	5-20% of patients

ANA = antinuclear antibodies; p- and c-ANCA = perinuclear and cytoplasmic antineutrophil cytoplasmic antibodies; RF = rheumatoid factor; α-Ro/SS-A and α-La/SS-B = antibodies to the Ro/SS-A and La/SS-B antigens.

The immune-mediated inflammation is associated with antibody-antigen complexes that are deposited in the wall of the blood vessel. Antibodies also bind directly to endothelial cell antigens. In both circumstances, complement is activated, as evidenced by deposition of membrane attack complex. Chemotactic factors then recruit neutrophils, which release proteolytic enzymes and generate toxic oxygen free radicals.

The sensory neuropathy of Sjögren syndrome probably results from the infiltration of dorsal root ganglia by cytotoxic T cells. Some patients with systemic vasculitis have symmetrical neuropathies rather than mononeuritis. The pathogenesis of such cases is not defined.

CLINICAL MANIFESTATIONS

Patients typically have a relatively sudden onset of painful, focal or multifocal weakness, or sensory loss. These symptoms reflect ischemia anywhere along the length of the nerve or nerves, generally in the lower extremities.

DIAGNOSIS

Nerve biopsy of clinically affected sensory nerves (sural, superficial peroneal, or superficial radial) is often necessary because therapy may be aggressive and long-term. Superficial peroneal nerve biopsy may be combined with muscle biopsy from the same incision. Pathologic features diagnostic of vasculitis occur in 60% of patients, and less specific features such as multifocal loss of fibers occur in others. Findings diagnostic of vasculitis include destruction of the vessel and inflammation within the vessel wall. Fibrinoid necrosis, vessel wall scarring, recanalization, neovascularization, and hemosiderin are common but not essential histopathologic features of vasculitis.

Although nerve biopsy is the gold standard for diagnosis, clinical, serologic, and electrophysiologic findings can suggest the diagnosis. For example, EMG and nerve conduction velocity studies can distinguish between mononeuritis multiplex and a symmetrical neuropathy. It is essential to confirm nerve conduction velocity abnormalities in a nerve before biopsy. An acute or subacute onset of asymmetrical weakness or sensory loss in the distribution of individual nerves suggests mononeuritis multiplex, particularly in the setting of a known connective tissue disorder. Systemic symptoms, such as unexplained weight loss and purpura, or constitutional symptoms, such as fever, myalgias, arthralgias, pulmonary disease, abdominal complaints, rashes, or night sweats, suggest systemic vasculitis in a patient with mononeuritis multiplex.

The erythrocyte sedimentation rate is usually elevated in the systemic vasculitides but is normal in nonsystemic cases. Perinuclear and cytoplasmic antineutrophil cytoplasmic antibody (p-ANCA and c-ANCA) suggests granulomatosis with polyangiitis (Chapter 270) or Churg-Strauss syndrome (Chapter 270). Hepatitis C (Chapter 149) is usually associated with the presence of cryoglobulins. Serum complement levels, extractable nuclear antigen, angiotensin-converting enzyme levels, serum protein electrophoresis, and HIV serology are generally indicated. CSF analysis is not usually helpful in cases of vasculitic neuropathy but may be needed to exclude infectious (e.g., Lyme disease [Chapter 321]) or other inflammatory causes.

Differential Diagnosis

Acute or subacute mononeuritis multiplex may also result from diabetes, sarcoidosis, Lyme disease, and malignant infiltration of nerves. Multifocal motor neuropathy with conduction block and Lewis-Sumner syndrome can resemble vasculitic mononeuritis multiplex. Sensory neuropathies similar to those in Sjögren syndrome may occur in patients with diabetes, paraneoplastic syndromes associated with anti-Hu antibodies, and pyridoxine deficiency.

TREATMENT   Rx

Systemic Vasculitis

For most vasculitic neuropathies (Chapter 270), oral prednisone (1 mg/kg) is appropriate in relatively mild cases, but intravenous methylprednisolone (1000 mg/day for 3 to 5 days) may be indicated as initial treatment in severe cases. Daily dosing is commonly used for the first 2 months or longer if the disease remains active. Subsequently, the dose is gradually tapered, with a transition to alternate-day dosing and discontinuation depending on the clinical picture and associated systemic features.

Corticosteroid treatment may be adequate for Churg-Strauss syndrome, but additional medication is generally needed in other forms of systemic vasculitic neuropathy. In most cases of granulomatosis with polyangiitis, combined therapy with glucocorticoids and oral cyclophosphamide (2 mg/kg/day) or weekly oral methotrexate (7.5 mg/week) is used. Azathioprine (2 to 3 mg/kg/day) is an alternative.

Because patients with nonsystemic vasculitic neuropathy may recover spontaneously or have a relatively benign course, low-dose or alternate-day oral prednisone (60 to 80 mg/day) is often adequate therapy. Azathioprine or weekly methotrexate can be used as a glucocorticoid-sparing agent. Doses such as 60 mg of prednisone on alternate days, 2 to 3 mg/kg/day of azathioprine, or 7.5 to 15 mg/week of methotrexate are reasonable starting doses that can ultimately be decreased if the treatments prove effective.

PROGNOSIS

Most systemic and nonsystemic vasculitis cases respond at least partially to treatment. The prognosis of patients with nonsystemic vasculitis is better than that of patients with systemic vasculitis, with fewer episodes of nerve damage; the disease may be monophasic or relapsing-remitting over a period of years. Most patients recover the ability to walk.

CRITICAL ILLNESS NEUROPATHY

DEFINITION

Critical illness polyneuropathy is an acute or subacute axonal length–dependent neuropathy that occurs in critically ill patients, not as a direct consequence of their underlying illness. The neuropathy is monophasic and recovers, at least in part, if the patient survives the underlying illness.[14]

EPIDEMIOLOGY

The incidence of critical illness polyneuropathy is uncertain because of variable diagnostic criteria. Moreover, it frequently accompanies critical illness myopathy (Chapter 421), which may be indistinguishable from it. Critical illness polyneuropathy frequently occurs in patients with systemic inflammatory response syndrome (Chapters 106 and 108), a generalized inflammatory host response to severe illness; up to 70% of patients with sepsis develop length-dependent axonal neuropathy.

PATHOBIOLOGY

Nerve biopsies have identified perivascular lymphocytic infiltration, macrophages, and cytokines such as interleukin-1β, interferon-γ, and interleukin-12. Ischemia caused by a sepsis-induced abnormal distribution of capillary blood flow, nutritional deprivation, and hypoglycemia has also been implicated in critical illness polyneuropathy.

CLINICAL MANIFESTATIONS

The typical finding is rapid development of profound limb weakness days to weeks after acquiring a severe illness that necessitated intensive care unit admission and ventilator support. Respiratory muscles are often involved, thereby resulting in inability to wean from the ventilator. Elicitable deep tendon reflexes distinguish critical illness polyneuropathy from acute inflammatory demyelinating polyneuropathy. Sensory testing is difficult to perform in severely ill patients but is usually normal.

DIAGNOSIS

Laboratory studies are rarely helpful. CSF protein is normal, unlike acute inflammatory demyelinating polyneuropathy. A lack of cells excludes infectious or inflammatory disorders. Creatine kinase levels are normal, unlike critical illness myopathy, in which they may be elevated.

Motor conduction velocities are normal with reduced or absent compound muscle action potential amplitudes. Critical illness polyneuropathy is predominantly a motor disorder, so sensory conduction velocities and sensory nerve action potential amplitudes are normal. Abnormal spontaneous activity reflecting axonal damage may occur within 1 to 3 weeks of onset. The presence of neuropathic and myopathic abnormalities suggests that critical illness polyneuropathy and critical illness myopathy coexist.

Differential Diagnosis

Distinguishing between critical illness myopathy and critical illness polyneuropathy can be difficult. Glucocorticoids and neuromuscular blocking agents predispose to critical illness myopathy (Chapter 421), which occurs in up to 5% of critically ill patients and is also manifested as rapidly progressive weakness of the limbs and diaphragm. Muscle biopsy and special electrical techniques aid in the diagnosis of critical illness myopathy. Acute inflammatory demyelinating polyneuropathy can mimic critical illness polyneuropathy but can be distinguished by slow nerve conduction velocity and abnormal CSF. Acute motor axonal neuropathy or acute motor and sensory axonal neuropathy may be more difficult to distinguish, particularly if sepsis or another underlying disorder induces an abnormal CSF; nevertheless, the presence of antiganglioside antibodies may help distinguish these disorders from critical illness polyneuropathy. Myasthenia gravis (Chapter 422), botulinum toxin (Chapter 296), and other toxins can cause a similar clinical picture.

TREATMENT

Treatment is directed at the underlying disease or diseases, such as sepsis (Chapter 108). Glucocorticoids and neuromuscular blocking agents should be avoided if possible because both have been associated with critical illness myopathy.

PROGNOSIS

In-hospital mortality has been reported to be as high as 84% in patients with critical illness polyneuropathy compared with 50% in similarly ill patients without it. Although most patients improve if they survive their underlying illness, up to 10% have persistent severe limb weakness and are dependent on a ventilator. Most patients have some weakness 2 years after discharge.

DIABETIC AND OTHER METABOLIC NEUROPATHIES

DEFINITION

Diabetic peripheral neuropathies can be separated into two large groups: (1) symmetrical, predominantly sensory or autonomic neuropathies (or both); and (2) asymmetrical mononeuropathies or plexopathies.

EPIDEMIOLOGY

Diabetes (Chapter 229) is the most common cause of neuropathy in the Western world. Diabetic neuropathy occurs in 8 to 70% of patients with diabetes, depending on the criteria used to diagnose neuropathy, and patients with retinopathy or overt albuminuria are more than twice as likely to have neuropathy. Distal symmetrical polyneuropathies are the most common diabetic neuropathy, but distal autonomic neuropathy is also common.[15] For example, impotence develops in 20 to 60% of diabetic men, but widespread autonomic dysfunction develops in less than 5% of diabetic patients.

PATHOBIOLOGY
Distal Symmetrical Polyneuropathy and Autonomic Neuropathy

The pathogenesis of distal symmetrical polyneuropathy and autonomic neuropathy involves both microvascular and metabolic abnormalities, with a causal link between increased blood glucose levels and the development and progression of diabetic neuropathy. The mechanisms by which hyperglycemia causes nerve dysfunction may include activation of the polyol pathway, extensive glycation, altered diacylglycerol/protein kinase activity, and oxidative stress. Evidence from animal models suggests a role for neurotrophic factors, in particular, nerve growth factor, which selectively supports small fiber sensory and sympathetic neurons.

Acute Asymmetrical Neuropathies

The focal nature of these diabetic neuropathies is presumed to result from occlusion of endoneurial arterioles with resultant ischemic damage to the nerve. Changes suggestive of vasculitis are observed in epineurial and perineurial blood vessels in about 50% of cases, and perivascular lymphocytic infiltrates are common.

CLINICAL MANIFESTATIONS
Distal Sensory Polyneuropathy and Autonomic Neuropathy

Distal symmetrical polyneuropathy is typically manifested as insidious symmetrical sensory loss of small (pain and temperature) and large (proprioception) fiber modalities. Paresthesias or painful dysesthesias (e.g., burning or tingling feet) are common although not invariable. An unsteady gait may

be the initial finding. Weakness is usually minimal, even in the distal foot muscles. Ankle reflexes are generally absent, although patellar reflexes may be present. Feet and distal calves are often cold and erythematous. Slow distal proximal progression of sensory symptoms and signs is the rule. By the time that symptoms reach the knees, abnormalities often begin in the hands.

When sensory changes reach the level of the knees, symptoms of autonomic neuropathy often begin: gastroparesis, constipation that may alternate with diarrhea, orthostatic hypotension, anhidrosis, cardiac arrhythmias, and impotence. Autonomic abnormalities can be the most disabling component of diabetic neuropathy.

Acute Asymmetrical Neuropathies

Asymmetrical, acute neuropathies cause focal or multifocal symptoms, depending on the peripheral nerve or nerves affected. They are usually accompanied by acute pain in the afflicted region. The pain may be deep and aching or throbbing and lancinating. Most cases of acute focal or multifocal diabetic neuropathy eventually resolve, at least partially. Pain may resolve within a few months, whereas weakness may take a year or more to recover and may persist. Characteristic manifestations include the following:

Diabetic lumbosacral radiculoplexus neuropathy. Patients are frequently elderly with type 2 diabetes (Chapter 229). Asymmetrical pain in the upper part of the thigh is followed by progressive weakness and atrophy of the proximal leg muscles. Progression to the other leg frequently occurs. In about 50% of affected patients, autonomic symptoms (Chapter 418), including orthostatic, hypotension, and gastrointestinal and sexual dysfunction, also develop. Weakness may progress, and about 50% of patients require a wheelchair for ambulation. Many patients require opiates for pain. After the nadir, the patient will usually stabilize for several months, followed by progressive improvement. As many as 50% of patients do not regain full ambulation.

Truncal radiculopathy. An acute, focal onset of pain and sensory loss develop over a region of the trunk. In extreme cases, the abdominal wall muscles may become weak, resembling a hernia. As with diabetic lumbosacral radiculoplexus neuropathy, at least partial improvement will occurs after a period of months, but the pain is difficult to control.

Cranial neuropathies. The classic manifestation is an acute oculomotor nerve palsy in which retro-orbital pain is followed by diplopia and ptosis. Pupillary fibers are often spared, thereby distinguishing the disorder from lesions that compress the oculomotor nerve and cause a dilated pupil. Similar findings may occur with the trochlear or abducens nerves. Bell palsy is more frequent in diabetic patients and is less likely to involve taste than in patients without diabetes.

Compressive mononeuropathies. Compressive neuropathies, such as carpal tunnel syndrome, occur more frequently in diabetic patients for unclear reasons. It is not known whether the response of carpal tunnel syndrome to treatment is as effective as when these mononeuropathies occur independently of diabetes.

DIAGNOSIS
Distal Sensory Polyneuropathy

The diagnosis of distal symmetrical polyneuropathy is based on identification of a predominantly sensory length–dependent neuropathy in the presence of either type 1 or type 2 diabetes. Neuropathy can develop independently of good control of blood sugar. Clinically similar neuropathies occur in patients with glucose abnormalities that are detectable only by oral glucose tolerance testing. Nerve conduction studies usually show low-amplitude or nondetectable sensory nerve action potential amplitudes; when detectable, sensory conduction may be slightly slow. Compound muscle action potential amplitudes are often reduced. Motor conduction studies are slightly slowed even if there is only minimal motor involvement clinically. Needle EMG in distal muscles typically demonstrates changes characteristic of chronic denervation. Occasional fibrillations and positive sharp waves may also be present.

Acute Asymmetrical Neuropathy

The focal neuropathies tend to occur in older patients with type 2 diabetes. The characteristic syndromes are diagnosed on the basis of their clinical manifestations and association with diabetes. EMG may demonstrate pronounced denervation in affected muscles. Concomitant evidence of distal symmetrical polyneuropathy is often present clinically and by electrophysiologic studies.

TREATMENT

Distal Symmetrical Polyneuropathy

An important treatment goal in distal symmetrical polyneuropathy is prevention of osteomyelitis (Chapter 272) and the resultant amputation of toes and feet. Because patients often do not sense injuries to their feet, diligence in foot care is important. Specific treatments to reverse or halt progression of the distal symmetrical polyneuropathy in diabetic patients are not yet available. Current therapy is based on control of hyperglycemia, management of symptoms, and foot care. Careful control of blood glucose (Chapter 229) remains the only treatment proved to delay the onset and slow progression of distal symmetrical polyneuropathy. [A8] There is, however, no HbA$_{1c}$ threshold below which patients avoid risk for neuropathy. For the treatment of pain (Chapter 30), combination therapy with gabapentin (beginning at 300 mg three times a day but increasing up to more than 600 mg three times a day) and low doses of sustained-release morphine (e.g., 15 mg twice daily) is effective when less aggressive treatments fail. [A9] Pregabalin is effective at doses of 300 mg to 600 mg daily. [A10] Duloxetine (60 to 120 mg daily) [A11] and tricyclic antidepressant medications (e.g., amitriptyline 10 to 100 mg or nortriptyline 10 to 100 mg) may also be useful. [A12] Because of potential sedative side effects, these medications are usually begun with a low dose given at bedtime and then gradually increased based on benefits and toxicity.

Acute Asymmetrical Neuropathy

Although acute asymmetrical neuropathy generally improves spontaneously, improvement may take months and remain incomplete. Intravenous corticosteroids, IVIG, or plasma exchange may improve the speed and extent of recovery, but these treatments are not of established benefit. Pain management is similar to that for distal symmetrical polyneuropathy. Because the pain in patients with diabetic lumbosacral radiculoplexus neuropathy and truncal radiculopathy is focal, topical therapy with capsaicin may be effective.

● INFECTIOUS NEUROPATHIES

Neuropathies Associated with HIV Infection

The peripheral nervous system may be involved in all phases of HIV infection (Chapter 394). The most common peripheral neuropathy is a distal, painful, sensory axonal polyneuropathy that is similar to the toxic neuropathy caused by nucleoside reverse transcriptase inhibitors (NRTIs), including zidovudine, zalcitabine, didanosine, stavudine, and lamivudine. When an iatrogenic neuropathy is suspected, discontinuation of NRTIs may improve symptoms. Conversely, a neuropathy caused by HIV is likely to stabilize or improve with antiretroviral treatment.

Inflammatory neuropathies such as chronic or acute inflammatory demyelinating polyneuropathy can also occur in the early stages of HIV infection; the CSF cyto-albumin dissociation usually seen with these conditions may not be evident in these patients because of a mild CSF mononuclear pleocytosis. The response of these neuropathies to plasma exchange or IVIG is generally good. In later stages of HIV infection, cytomegalovirus (Chapter 376) may cause either an acute lumbosacral polyradiculopathy as a result of direct invasion of nerve roots or a mononeuritis multiplex through a vasculitic mechanism.

Neuropathies Associated with Herpes Zoster

Varicella-zoster virus (Chapter 375) usually remains latent in cranial or spinal ganglia after resolution of a systemic infection. Reactivation, which is more frequent in elderly and immunocompromised patients, causes a vesicular skin eruption accompanied by pruritus and dysesthesias. Herpes zoster resolves spontaneously but is frequently followed by post-herpetic neuralgia, which is characterized by severe pain persisting for more than 6 weeks after the rash appears. Early treatment with oral acyclovir (800 mg, five times daily for 7 days) may reduce both the duration of the acute phase and the risk for post-herpetic neuralgia. The use of concomitant corticosteroids in addition to acyclovir improves acute pain without exacerbating viral spread but does not reduce the incidence or severity of post-herpetic neuralgia.

Neuropathy Associated with Lyme Disease

Borrelia burgdorferi causes a disease with three stages (Chapter 321). In the first stage, shortly after and in the same area of a tick bite, a nonpruritic rash (erythema migrans) appears and spontaneously disappears after a few weeks. The second stage is frequently associated with neurologic complications such as lymphocytic meningitis and focal and multifocal peripheral and cranial neuropathies; characteristic manifestations are unilateral or bilateral facial palsy and radiculitis. The third stage is associated with severe neurologic

complications, including encephalopathy, encephalomyelitis, and a predominantly sensory axonal polyneuropathy. A lymphocytic pleocytosis in CSF and demonstration of *B. burgdorferi* infection in serum or CSF are the main laboratory findings. Treatment is discussed in Chapter 321.

Neuropathy Associated with Leprosy

Leprosy (Chapter 326) is infrequent in the United States but is the most common cause of peripheral neuropathy in some developing countries. Leprosy presents in different forms, depending on the host's immune system. Patients with normal cell-mediated immunity are more likely to have a tuberculoid form characterized by hypopigmented skin lesions associated with decreased sensation. In patients with abnormal cell-mediated immunity, the more severe lepromatous form with large disfiguring lesions may develop. A mononeuritis multiplex pattern with prominent superficial sensory loss is the most typical clinical manifestation of leprosy. If treated early, neuropathies in leprosy improve. World Health Organization recommendations call for combination therapy that includes dapsone (50 to 100 mg/day or 200 to 250 mg/week), rifampicin (600 mg monthly), and clofazimine (100 mg/day) (Chapter 326).

Neuropathy Associated with Diphtheria

Vaccination has made diphtheria (Chapter 292) rare in developed countries, but it is an important cause of subacute neuropathy in developing countries. Some strains of *Corynebacterium diphtheriae* produce a potent neurotoxin that causes palatal weakness, lens accommodation deficits, and extraocular palsies. These acute manifestations are followed by limb paralysis that resembles acute inflammatory demyelinating polyneuropathy (see earlier). The neuropathy caused by the neurotoxin usually resolves with resolution of the infection. The diphtheria organism can be eradicated by therapy with antibiotics such as erythromycin (2 g/day intravenously divided twice daily for adults) or penicillin (procaine penicillin G, 1.2 million U/day intramuscularly divided twice daily for 14 days). However, the neuropathy, as with other manifestations of the disease, generally requires treatment with diphtheria antitoxin, a hyperimmune antiserum produced in horses. Depending on the severity of the disease, antitoxin is administered intramuscularly or intravenously (80,000 to 120,000 units for extensive disease for 3 or more days; Chapter 292).

● TOXIC AND DEFICIENCY SYNDROMES

In Western countries, toxic neuropathies are frequently the side effects of medications[16] rather than a result of environmental exposure. In most cases, iatrogenic neuropathy is manifested as a length-dependent or "dying-back" axonal neuropathy. Treatment requires a correct diagnosis (Table 420-5) and discontinuation of the drug. Improvement often takes many months. In a randomized trial of patients with painful chemotherapy-induced peripheral neuropathy, duloxetine (30 mg orally once daily for 1 week, then 60 mg daily for 4 weeks) resulted in a greater reduction in pain compared with placebo. [A13]

Compressive Neuropathies

Peripheral nerves are vulnerable to chronic compression in many sites: median nerve compression at the wrist within the carpal tunnel (*carpal tunnel syndrome*), median nerve compression in the upper part of the forearm, ulnar nerve compression in the hand (*cubital tunnel syndrome*), ulnar nerve compression at the elbow or wrist, tibial nerve compression behind the medial malleolus (*tarsal tunnel syndrome*), and peroneal nerve compression over the lateral fibular head.

TABLE 420-5   TOXIC AND DEFICIENCY NEUROPATHIES

Associated with antineoplastic agents: vincristine, paclitaxel (Taxol), cisplatin, suramin, thalidomide

Associated with antimicrobials: chloroquine, dapsone, isoniazid, metronidazole, nitrofurantoin

Associated with cardiac medications: amiodarone, perhexiline, hydralazine

Associated with other medications: colchicine, tacrolimus, gold salts, phenytoin, disulfiram (Antabuse), pyridoxine (vitamin B$_6$)

Associated with heavy metals: lead, arsenic, mercury, thallium

Associated with chemical compounds: acrylamide, carbon disulfide, ethylene glycol, hexacarbons, organophosphate esters, vacor

Deficiency neuropathies: vitamin B$_1$ deficiency, vitamin B$_{12}$ deficiency, vitamin E deficiency

CARPAL TUNNEL SYNDROME

Entrapment of the median nerve at the wrist reflects the limited space available for the median nerve because of the surrounding bone, joint, ligaments, tendons, and synovium. Repetitive motion of the fingers is an exacerbating element. Other precipitating factors include trauma, osteoarthritis, synovial cysts, myxedema, and amyloid deposition. Symptoms typically include paresthesias of the first three fingers, often at night, and are relieved by shaking or elevating the hand. In severe disease, objective sensory loss in the median nerve distribution, weakness of median-innervated muscles such as the abductor pollicis brevis, and prolongation of nerve conduction across the carpal tunnel (prolonged distal latency) are characteristic. The diagnosis is supported by identification of *Tinel sign*, in which tapping the carpal tunnel elicits paresthesias in the median nerve distribution, and by paresthesias produced by sustained flexion of the wrist *(Phalen sign)*. Treatment begins with splinting of the wrist in slight dorsiflexion during sleep. Injection of corticosteroids into the carpal tunnel provides temporary benefit. Severe carpal tunnel syndrome is treated surgically by release of the carpal ligament.[A14]

Bell Palsy

Unilateral facial paralysis of acute onset frequently occurs on an idiopathic basis (Bell palsy). The diagnosis is one of exclusion. Facial nerve palsies also occur in the setting of *herpes zoster oticus* and are associated with otalgia and varicelliform lesions affecting the external ear, ear canal, or tympanic membrane. Facial paralysis of a lower motor neuron type can be caused by carcinomatous meningitis (Chapters 195 and 412), sarcoidosis (Chapter 95), Lyme disease (Chapter 321), and HIV infection (Chapter 394).

Primary tumors of the facial nerve can cause rapidly developing facial paralysis. Facial paralysis can also occur in *CNS disease* affecting the pontomedullary junction, such as stroke or multiple sclerosis (Chapter 411).

CLINICAL MANIFESTATIONS AND DIAGNOSIS

Most cases of facial paralysis are idiopathic. Patients typically notice facial paralysis on inspection in the mirror in the morning. Facial paralysis may be heralded or accompanied by pain behind the ear. The severity of paralysis varies widely.

TREATMENT   Rx

In a randomized trial, 10 days of oral corticosteroids (prednisolone 25 mg twice daily for 10 days) administered early in the course increased the return of facial function from 63 to 83% at 3 months in patients with idiopathic Bell palsy, but acyclovir was of no benefit.[A15] In severe cases, protection of the cornea from drying and injury is essential.

PROGNOSIS

Most patients improve, but about 10% of patients have little recovery. Aberrant regeneration of the facial nerve can cause synkinesias, such as "jaw winking" (when the eye is closed) or tearing accompanying salivation ("syndrome of crocodile tears").

Trigeminal Neuralgia (Tic Douloureux)

Trigeminal neuralgia and other painful cranial neuralgias are discussed in Chapter 398.

Grade A References

A1. Hughes RA, Swan AV, van Doorn PA. Intravenous immunoglobulin for Guillain-Barré syndrome. *Cochrane Database Syst Rev.* 2014;9:CD002063.
A2. Raphael JC, Chevret S, Hughes RA, et al. Plasma exchange for Guillain-Barré syndrome. *Cochrane Database Syst Rev.* 2012;7:CD001798.
A3. El-Bayoumi MA, El-Refaey AM, Abdelkader AM, et al. Comparison of intravenous immunoglobulin and plasma exchange in treatment of mechanically ventilated children with Guillain Barré syndrome: a randomized study. *Crit Care.* 2011;15:R164.
A4. Hughes RA, van Doorn PA. Corticosteroids for Guillain-Barré syndrome. *Cochrane Database Syst Rev.* 2012;8:CD001446.
A5. van Koningsveld R, Schmitz PI, Meche FG, et al. Effect of methylprednisolone when added to standard treatment with intravenous immunoglobulin for Guillain-Barré syndrome: randomised trial. *Lancet.* 2004;363:192-196.
A6. Eftimov F, Winer JB, Vermeulen M, et al. Intravenous immunoglobulin for chronic inflammatory demyelinating polyradiculoneuropathy. *Cochrane Database Syst Rev.* 2013;12:CD001797.
A7. Eftimov F, Vermeulen M, van Doorn PA, et al. Long-term remission of CIDP after pulsed dexamethasone or short-term prednisolone treatment. *Neurology.* 2012;78:1079-1084.
A8. Callaghan BC, Little AA, Feldman EL, et al. Enhanced glucose control for preventing and treating diabetic neuropathy. *Cochrane Database Syst Rev.* 2012;6:CD007543.
A9. Gilron I, Bailey JM, Tu D, et al. Morphine, gabapentin, or their combination for neuropathic pain. *N Engl J Med.* 2005;352:1324-1334.
A10. Moore RA, Straube S, Wiffen PJ, et al. Pregabalin for acute and chronic pain in adults. *Cochrane Database Syst Rev.* 2009;3:CD007076.
A11. Lunn MP, Hughes RA, Wiffen PJ. Duloxetine for treating painful neuropathy, chronic pain or fibromyalgia. *Cochrane Database Syst Rev.* 2014;1:CD007115.
A12. Griebeler ML, Morey-Vargas OL, Brito JP, et al. Pharmacologic interventions for painful diabetic neuropathy: an umbrella systematic review and comparative effectiveness network meta-analysis. *Ann Intern Med.* 2014;161:639-649.
A13. Smith EM, Pang H, Cirrincione C, et al. Effect of duloxetine on pain, function, and quality of life among patients with chemotherapy-induced painful peripheral neuropathy: a randomized clinical trial. *JAMA.* 2013;309:1359-1367.
A14. Jarvik JG, Comstock BA, Kliot M, et al. Surgery versus non-surgical therapy for carpal tunnel syndrome: a randomised parallel-group trial. *Lancet.* 2009;374:1074-1081.
A15. Gronseth GS, Paduga R. Evidence-based guideline update: steroids and antivirals for Bell palsy: report of the Guideline Development Subcommittee of the American Academy of Neurology. *Neurology.* 2012;79:2209-2213.

GENERAL REFERENCES

For the General References and other additional features, please visit Expert Consult at https://expertconsult.inkling.com.

421

MUSCLE DISEASES

DUYGU SELCEN

DEFINITION

Muscle diseases, which are also called myopathies, are disorders of skeletal muscle structure or function. Myopathies can be primary and occur in isolation, or they can be part of a multisystem disorder.

EPIDEMIOLOGY

Many muscle diseases (Table 421-1) are inherited as autosomal dominant, autosomal recessive, X-linked, or maternal (mitochondrial) conditions. Environmental factors that may precipitate myopathies include recent infection, foreign travel, exposure to medications such as statins, and alcohol abuse (Chapter 33). Exercise commonly precipitates symptoms in patients with metabolic myopathies, whereas exposure to cold and high carbohydrate or potassium-rich food can precipitate weakness in muscle channelopathies.

The prevalence of muscle disease is estimated to be about 1 per 1000 people, including acute and transient disorders (e.g., myositis owing to infectious or toxic causes) and chronic inflammatory or genetic disorders that cause substantial morbidity over decades or a lifetime. Myopathies can cause premature death owing to neuromuscular weakness and secondary respiratory infections or to involvement of other organs in multisystem diseases. Myocardial involvement, which is particularly common in some muscle diseases, can cause heart failure or life-threatening arrhythmias.

TABLE 421-1 CLASSIFICATION OF MYOPATHIES

HEREDITARY

Muscular dystrophies
Congenital myopathies
Myotonia and channelopathies
Metabolic myopathies
Mitochondrial myopathies

ACQUIRED

Inflammatory myopathies
Endocrine myopathies
Myopathies associated with systemic illness
Drug-induced/toxic myopathies

Adapted from Goldman L, Schafer AI, eds. *Cecil Medicine.* 24th ed. Philadelphia: Elsevier; 2012.

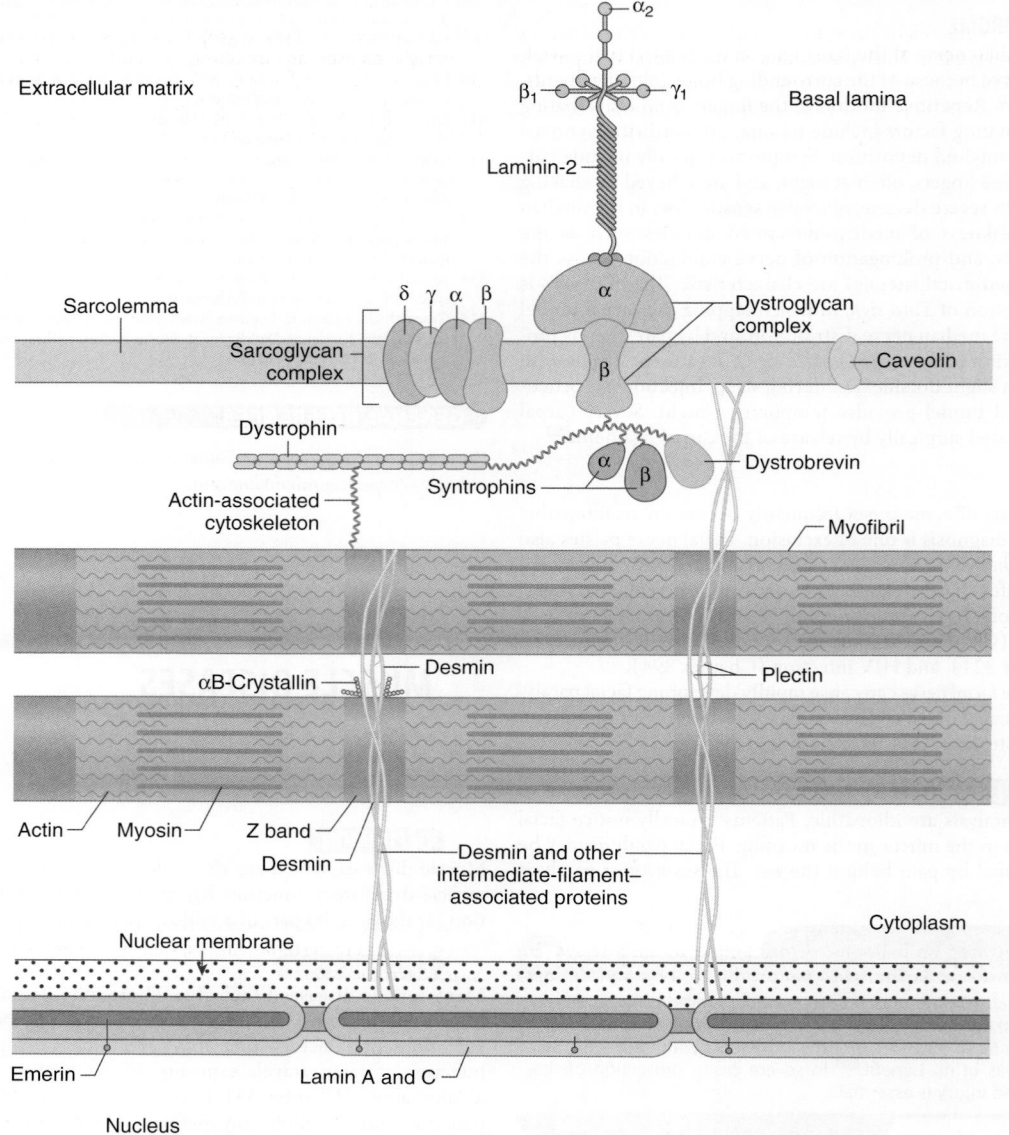

FIGURE 421-1. Muscle structure. (From Goldman L, Schafer AI, eds. *Cecil Medicine*. 24th ed. Philadelphia: Elsevier; 2012.)

PATHOBIOLOGY

Muscle disease can result from a perturbation in the anatomy or any of the physiologic processes required for muscle contraction or the genes that control them. Skeletal muscle is part of a motor unit, which is defined as the anterior horn cell body, its axon, the neuromuscular junction, and the skeletal muscle fibers innervated by the one axon. The motor unit is coordinated in a manner that allows efficient muscle contraction and function. The number of muscle fibers innervated by each motor unit varies from a few (e.g., in muscles controlling very precise movements, such as extraocular muscles) to more than 1000 (e.g., large and powerful but less precise muscles, such as quadriceps).

Skeletal muscle is composed of myriad muscle fibers. Muscle fibers, which are multinucleated cells formed by fusion of myoblasts during development, are surrounded by a plasma membrane, the sarcolemma, which is surrounded by a basal lamina and endomysial connective tissue. Groups of muscle fibers compose the fascicles, which are surrounded by perimysium, and the groups of fascicles in turn are surrounded by epimysium. Nerve branches, blood vessels, muscle spindles, and fat cells lie within the connective tissue of the muscle.

Each muscle fiber is composed of myofibrils, which themselves are composed of repeat units a few microns long called sarcomeres. The sarcomere consists of a highly organized protein network that gives the muscle fiber its characteristic striated appearance. Each sarcomere is flanked by two Z discs.

Z discs are composed of multiple proteins, including α-actinin. Emanating from the Z disc are thin filaments, composed of actin, troponin, and tropomyosin. Thick filaments consist of myosin. Other structures comprise subcellular organelles, including the mitochondria, which are the principal energy source, the endoplasmic reticulum, and the transverse tubules that communicate with the extracellular space.

Muscle function (Fig. 421-1) is dependent on chemical energy from adenosine triphosphate (ATP). In the first 30 minutes of sustained activity, ATP is produced by the breakdown of glycogen (glycolysis), and after 30 minutes ATP is produced by fatty acid β-oxidation and oxidative phosphorylation within the mitochondria. The process that leads to muscle contraction begins with the generation of the muscle fiber action potential (Chapter 53), which initiates muscle contraction after it is propagated into the interior of muscle fiber through the transverse tubular system. The release of calcium from the endoplasmic reticulum triggers a coordinated series of events that lead to the coupling of excitation to contraction. Calcium binds to troponin, which interacts with tropomyosin and results in actin-myosin binding. The repeated formation and cleavage of actin-tropomyosin cross-bridges, in an ATP-dependent process, results in sliding of thick and thin filaments and shortening of the sarcomere.

The structural integrity of the muscle fiber surface membrane is maintained by a network of proteins within the muscle. Dystrophin is a key component of the subsarcolemmal cytoskeleton. In combination with several glycoproteins called sarcoglycans (α, β, δ, γ), dystroglycans (α, β), and syntrophins (α, β1, β2), which form the dystrophin-sarcoglycan complex, it anchors the contractile elements of the muscle fiber to the sarcolemma and to the extracellular basal lamina. The basal lamina contains several important proteins, such as collagen, fibronectin, and laminin, which includes merosin and related proteins. The intermediate proteins, including desmin, connect the Z disc and other organelles to the subsarcolemmal cytoskeleton.

CLINICAL MANIFESTATIONS

Muscle diseases often present with localized or diffuse muscle weakness, reduced exercise tolerance, resting or exercise-induced muscle pain, muscle enlargement or atrophy, cramps, delayed relaxation, or rarely, myoglobinuria. These symptoms and signs can be masked by other neurologic or systemic features in patients with multisystem diseases.

History

The assessment of patients with neuromuscular diseases begins with a careful history, general physical examination, and detailed neurologic examination. The age of onset, the rate of progression, and whether the process is episodic, static, or progressive can provide important clues. Congenital and childhood onset myopathies can be associated with reduced fetal movements, breech delivery, weak cry or suck, and the delayed acquisition of motor milestones. Weakness is the most common presenting symptom, but other symptoms of muscle disease include muscle pain, reduced exercise intolerance, change in the muscle bulk (hypertrophy or atrophy), abnormal spontaneous muscle activity, delayed relaxation, fatigue, or myoglobinuria. Weakness may be relatively static as in some congenital myopathies, progressive as in muscular dystrophies, intermittent as in periodic paralysis, fluctuating as in neuromuscular junction disorders (Chapter 422), or exercise related as in metabolic myopathies. The most common distribution of weakness is proximal or limb-girdle weakness, which results in difficulties in getting out of low chairs, a bathtub, or a car seat; climbing up and down stairs; arising from squat; or getting off the floor. Proximal arm weakness manifests as difficulty reaching to shelves, washing or brushing hair, or raising arms to put on a shirt. Distal leg weakness can lead to difficulty walking on uneven surfaces, tripping over curbs, difficulty standing on the toes, or slapping feet owing to footdrop. Distal upper limb weakness results in difficulty opening jars, typing at a keyboard, writing, or buttoning clothes. Bilateral facial weakness can result in difficulty whistling, blowing up balloons, or drinking through a straw. Predominant involvement of ocular muscles can produce ptosis and diplopia. Weakness of the bulbar muscles manifests as difficulties with speech and swallowing, neck weakness that can lead to a dropped head, and respiratory muscle weakness that can lead to symptoms suggestive of nocturnal hypoventilation or respiratory failure. The early recognition of progressive respiratory failure is essential because it is treatable with noninvasive positive-pressure ventilation.

Fatigue and exercise intolerance can be presenting symptoms of muscle diseases, but they can also be multifactorial and nonspecific. In isolation, these symptoms usually do not indicate a primary muscle disease.

Muscle pain is another nonspecific symptom that can arise from many systemic and psychiatric conditions. Sometimes patients describe aching, stiffness, numbness, or burning as pain. Muscle diseases rarely cause diffuse, generalized, or persistent muscle pain. Muscle pain without muscle weakness is often a feature of fibromyalgia (Chapter 274) or chronic fatigue syndrome. Diffuse myalgia can occur in inflammatory muscle disease such as polymyo-

sitis or dermatomyositis, vasculitis, or viral or parasitic myositis. Muscle pain precipitated by exercise usually suggests a metabolic myopathy.

Muscle cramps are involuntary painful contractions that may occur in healthy individuals. Dehydration, renal failure (Chapter 130), and electrolyte imbalances (Chapters 116, 117, 119, and 245) can also produce muscle cramps. Muscle stiffness can occur in inflammatory, metabolic, and ion-channel diseases as well as in conditions such as multiple sclerosis (Chapter 411), polymyalgia rheumatica (Chapter 271), and connective tissue diseases (Chapter 256).

Fasciculations are caused by spontaneous firing of muscle fibers that are innervated by a single motor unit. Fasciculations may occur in normal persons, in whom they are usually exacerbated by stress and increased caffeine intake. Fasciculations in association with muscle weakness suggest anterior horn cell disease. Myotonia, often described as muscle stiffness, is characterized by prolonged contraction and delayed relaxation of muscle.

Myotonia can affect limb, facial, or bulbar muscles, and it can lead to persistent limb muscle contraction, eyelid closure, or dysphagia. Myotonic dystrophy is the most common muscle disease associated with myotonia, but patients usually complain more of weakness than the myotonia. Conversely, the myotonia associated with sodium and chloride channelopathies can be disabling. Patients who describe locking of their hands but do not have objective myotonia rarely have a physical explanation for their symptoms.

Tetany is the most severe form of sustained muscle contraction. Tetany occurs in patients with hypocalcemia and hypomagnesemia (Chapter 119), and it is aggravated by metabolic or respiratory alkalosis (Chapter 118).

Severe acute muscle damage, termed *rhabdomyolysis* (Chapters 113), results in myoglobinuria that presents as dark brown or red urine. Such discoloration must be distinguished from other causes of pigmenturia (Chapter 114) such as hemolysis or porphyria.

The detailed family history should include questions about muscle disease, including specific questions about the use of canes, braces, or wheelchairs. It also should assess whether family members have had a cardiomyopathy, unexpected sudden death, diabetes, or cataracts.

Physical Examination

A full physical examination must look for signs that may suggest any of the systemic diseases that are associated with myopathies. The skin examination can give clues to systemic illness, such as the heliotrope rash of dermatomyositis (Chapter 269).

A comprehensive neurologic examination should be performed in each patient to exclude possible central or peripheral nervous system disorders (Table 421-2). The examination begins as soon as the patient enters the examination room. Proximal leg muscle weakness may be evident if patients push themselves up on their thighs or have a waddling gait. Patients should be examined for possible facial muscle weakness or wasting, ptosis, or characteristic dysmorphic features, such as with myotonic dystrophy (Fig. 421-2), that can lead to an immediate clinical diagnosis.

Patients should be asked to rise from a squatting position and walk on their toes to assess possible calf weakness and on their heels to assess ankle dorsiflexion weakness. Patients should be asked to stand to assess posture and any evidence of rigidity or scoliosis. Joints should be moved passively to assess for contractures.

All muscle groups should be inspected for evidence of involuntary movements, atrophy, or hypertrophy. Muscles should be palpated for tenderness

TABLE 421-2	CLINICAL FINDINGS DIFFERENTIATING MUSCLE FROM NERVE DISEASE			
FINDING	**MYOPATHY**	**ANTERIOR HORN CELL DISEASE**	**PERIPHERAL NEUROPATHY**	**NEUROMUSCULAR JUNCTION DISEASE**
Distribution	Usually proximal and symmetrical but can be distal or asymmetrical at onset	Distal, asymmetrical, and bulbar	Distal, symmetrical	Extraocular, bulbar, proximal limb, but sometimes distal
Atrophy	Slight early, marked late	Marked early	Moderate	Absent
Fasciculations	Absent	Frequent	Sometimes present	Absent
Reflexes	Lost late	Variable, can be hyperreflexic	Lost early	Normal or hyporeflexic
Pain	Variable	Absent	Variable, distal when present	Absent
Cramps	Rare	Frequent	Occasional	Absent
Sensory loss	Absent	Absent	Usually present	Absent
Serum creatine kinase	Usually elevated	Occasionally mildly elevated	Normal	Normal

Adapted with revision from Goldman L, Schafer AI, eds. *Cecil Medicine*. 24th ed. Philadelphia: Elsevier; 2012.

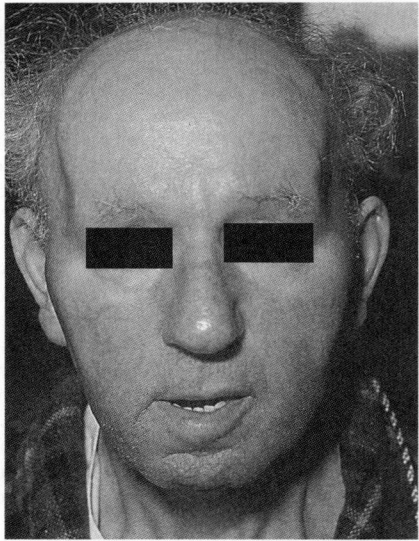

FIGURE 421-2. Myotonic dystrophy in a 50-year-old man. His appearance is typical with facial weakness, atrophy of the temporal muscles and sternocleidomastoids, and frontal baldness, which gives a monklike appearance. (From Goldman L, Schafer AI, eds. *Cecil Medicine.* 24th ed. Philadelphia: Elsevier; 2012.)

TABLE 421-3	MEDICAL RESEARCH COUNCIL SCALE OF MUSCLE STRENGTH

GRADE	DEGREE OF STRENGTH
5	Normal power
4	Active movement against gravity and resistance (often subdivided into 4−, 4, and 4+)
3	Active movement against gravity, but not against resistance
2	Active movement, with gravity eliminated
1	Observable muscle contraction, but not capable of initiating movement
0	No contraction

Adapted from Goldman L, Schafer AI, eds. *Cecil Medicine.* 24th ed. Philadelphia: Elsevier; 2012.

or unusual texture. Myotonia can be assessed by the inability to relax the muscle belly after percussion with a reflex hammer or the inability to relax the fingers from a firm grip.

Strength should be graded (Table 421-3) in each muscle group. Observing children and infants when they play with toys and how they stand up and walk usually reveals more than formal manual muscle strength testing. The pattern of muscle involvement can provide clues for the diagnosis of a specific myopathy.

DIAGNOSIS

Neurophysiologic testing, measurement of serum creatine kinase (CK), muscle biopsy, and genetic testing help guide the diagnosis of muscle diseases (Table 421-4).

A complete blood count and serum levels of alanine aminotransferase, aspartate aminotransferase, and creatinine can assess possible systemic involvement. An elevated erythrocyte sedimentation rate or C-reactive protein level is found in some inflammatory myopathies and is typical of connective tissue disorders (Chapters 256 and 257). Additional tests to evaluate patients suspected of having inflammatory myopathy or connective tissue disease can include antinuclear antibodies, extractable nuclear antigens, rheumatoid factor, antineutrophilic cytoplasmic antibodies, anti-Jo-1, anti-Mi2, anti-MDA5, anti-3-hydroxy-3-methylglutaryl-coenzyme A reductase, or anti–signal recognition particle antibodies (Chapter 257).

The muscle isoform (MM) of CK is frequently elevated in patients with muscle disease, although a normal level is seen in metabolic myopathies and in some chronic myopathies. A mild to moderate increase in the serum CK level can occur in patients with peripheral neuropathy, radiculopathy, and anterior horn cell diseases. The serum CK level is markedly increased in

TABLE 421-4	GUIDING PRINCIPLES FOR ASSESSING MUSCLE DISEASES

1. History
  Age of onset (most inherited and acquired disorders have a characteristic age of onset)
  Rate of progression (acute suggests an acquired, often inflammatory cause)
  Fluctuating weakness (may indicate a neuromuscular junction disorder, metabolic myopathy, or a channelopathy)
  Relationship to exercise (may indicate metabolic myopathy or channelopathy)
  Muscle pain (may indicate inflammatory or metabolic myopathy)
  Relevant multisystem involvement (may indicate a mitochondrial cytopathy or myotonic dystrophy)
  Family history (may indicate a genetically determined chronic muscle disease)

2. Pattern of weakness
  Limb-girdle weakness is relatively nonspecific.
  Inherited disorders often have specific patterns of muscle involvement.
  Fluctuating weakness may indicate a neuromuscular junction disorder, metabolic myopathy, or a channelopathy.

3. Testing
  The serum creatine kinase can be normal.
  Electromyography is often normal in metabolic myopathies.
  All patients with muscular dystrophy should have an electrocardiogram and echocardiogram to look for cardiomyopathy and/or conduction defect.
  Muscle magnetic resonance imaging is increasingly being used to guide muscle biopsy and may sometimes reveal diagnostic patterns of muscle involvement.
  Some inherited muscle diseases can be diagnosed clinically and confirmed by genetic testing without requiring other investigations (e.g., myotonic dystrophy; Duchenne, Becker, and facioscapulohumeral dystrophy).
  Muscle biopsy will reveal the cause in most cases; it identifies specific inflammatory myopathies and muscular dystrophies and often provides diagnostic clues for other muscle and neurogenetic disorders.

Adapted with revision from Goldman L, Schafer AI, eds. *Cecil Medicine.* 24th ed. Philadelphia: Elsevier; 2012.

dystrophinopathies, dysferlinopathy, some of the sarcoglycanopathies α-dystroglycanopathies, and during rhabdomyolysis (Chapter 113). However, it can decline later in muscular dystrophies as the disease progresses. When the serum CK level exceeds the upper limit of normal by about 10-fold, levels of alanine aminotransferase, aspartate aminotransferase, and lactate dehydrogenase also can be elevated, and some patients can be initially misdiagnosed as having hepatitis (Chapters 147 and 148) before the serum CK level is measured. The blood lactate level can be increased in patients with a mitochondrial myopathy, but a normal value does not exclude this diagnosis. In patients with acute muscle pain and/or weakness, electrolytes and thyroid function tests should be checked.

In patients who are diagnosed with dermatomyositis (Chapter 269), the evaluation should include a search for an underlying malignancy. In patients with suspected mitochondrial cytopathy, a serum and/or spinal fluid lactate level should be obtained. In patients with suspected fatty acid β-oxidation defects, blood acylcarnitine profile may be useful for the diagnosis.

Electromyography
Electromyography (EMG) consists of nerve conduction studies, repetitive nerve stimulation, and needle examination of muscles (Chapter 396). Nerve conduction studies (Chapter 420) are normal in patients with myopathies. In myopathies, the needle examination typically shows complex, polyphasic, low-amplitude motor unit potentials. Myotonia is caused by recurrent depolarization of the muscle fiber surface membrane and has characteristic waxing and waning rhythmical discharges or fibrillation potentials during the needle examination on an EMG. Contractures are electrically silent on EMGs, but muscle cramps are associated with high-amplitude, high-frequency bursts of motor unit activity. The EMG can be normal in some focal myopathies, such as inflammatory myositis, in metabolic myopathies, and in some congenital myopathies.

Genetic Testing
The widespread availability of molecular genetic testing has revolutionized the approach to patients who are suspected of having hereditary muscle disease. Dystrophin genetic testing can identify the defects in dystrophin in 90 to 95% of the patients with Duchene and Becker muscular dystrophy. Commercial test panels are available for muscle diseases such as limb-girdle

muscular dystrophies, congenital muscular dystrophies, myofibrillar myopathies, and congenital myopathies; however, the test panels have only about an 85% sensitivity because they do not cover the entire coding region (unlike whole exome sequencing) or genome (unlike whole genome sequencing). The sensitivity is higher if multiple affected and some unaffected family members and more than one family are analyzed at the same time. Novel genes causing muscular dystrophies are still being discovered using whole exome sequencing.

Muscle Biopsy

Despite advances in genetics and molecular biology, muscle biopsy remains a key component in the diagnosis of most muscle diseases. The biopsy site should be carefully chosen from a clinically affected but not too severely involved muscle. Fresh-frozen sections of the specimens should be used for histochemical studies because even marked morphologic alterations may be undetected in paraffin-embedded tissue. Immunocytochemical localization of specific proteins is useful and diagnostic in some forms of muscular dystrophies. Specific enzyme histochemistry and biochemistry can be used for metabolic myopathies. Genetic analysis of the muscle specimen can be more informative than blood specimens for mitochondrial myopathies.

Imaging

Muscle computed tomography (CT) and magnetic resonance imaging (MRI) are of limited utility for evaluating muscle diseases but can be very useful in excluding spinal cord abnormalities that may cause weakness. Some inherited myopathies are associated with patterns of atrophy and the replacement of muscle with fat. In patchy or focal inflammatory myopathy, MRI can guide muscle biopsy. Functional MRI is sometimes useful in patients with suspected mitochondrial disorders.

● SPECIFIC MUSCLE DISEASES
Inherited Muscle Diseases

The four main categories of inherited muscle diseases include muscular dystrophies (Table 421-5), congenital myopathies (Table 421-6), muscle ion-channel disorders (Table 421-7), and metabolic myopathies (Table 421-8). Some gene defects cause specific phenotypes that are instantly recognizable at the bedside by an experienced clinician, but less specific phenotypes can be caused by defects in more than one gene. A systematic approach is critical for an efficient and successful investigation of these disorders.

Muscular Dystrophies

The term *muscular dystrophy* refers to the primary degeneration of the muscle fiber, usually associated with an increase in fatty and fibrous connective tissue. The common clinical presentation is progressive muscle weakness.[1]

DYSTROPHINOPATHIES

Duchenne and Becker muscular dystrophies are caused by mutations in the dystrophin gene, which is located on the X chromosome. Female carriers can develop variable phenotypes, including a severe Duchenne-like presentation, mild adult-onset limb-girdle weakness, asymptomatic CK elevation, and cardiomyopathy.

Duchenne Muscular Dystrophy

Duchenne muscular dystrophy is the most common inherited muscle disease, with an incidence of about 1 in 5000 male births. About one third of patients carry a de novo mutation without a family history. In most patients, a frameshift mutation in the dystrophin gene results in a complete absence of the dystrophin protein. This absence of dystrophin disrupts the mechanical link between the sarcomere and the sarcolemma, thereby causing a calcium leak that leads to necrosis of muscle fibers.

CLINICAL MANIFESTATIONS

Duchenne dystrophy typically presents in young boys who are between 2 and 5 years of age with delayed motor milestones, difficulty running, increasing falls, and enlarged calves. The disorder is relentlessly progressive and can cause a cardiomyopathy (Chapter 60) that leads to heart failure and fatal arrhythmias. Intellectual disability, learning disorders, autism, and attention deficit hyperactivity disorder can be associated features. By 12 years of age, most affected individuals can no longer ambulate. By the age of 20 years, most patients develop joint contractures and kyphoscoliosis that lead to further respiratory compromise.

TABLE 421-5 MUSCULAR DYSTROPHIES

X-LINKED
Dystrophinopathies (Duchenne/Becker muscular dystrophy)
Emery-Dreifuss (Emerin)
FHL1-related (FHL1)

AUTOSOMAL DOMINANT
Facioscapulohumeral dystrophy (D4Z4 repeat deletions in 4q35 subtelomeric region in 95%; toxic gain of function in *DUX4* in 5%)
Myotonic dystrophy, type 1 (ctg repeats in *DMPK*)
Myotonic dystrophy, type 2 (cctg repeats in *ZNF9*)
Oculopharyngeal muscular dystrophy (*PABPN1*)
Myotilinopathy* (*MYOT*)
Laminopathy (*LMNA*)
Caveolinopathy (*CAV3*)
DNAJB6opathy* (*DNAJB6*)
Desminopathy* (*DES*)
Zaspopathy* (*ZASP*)
Bag3opathy* (*BAG3*)
Filaminopathy* (*FLNC*)
α-B-crystallinopathy* (*CRYAB*)
Titinopathy* (*TTN*)
VCPopathy† [valosin-containing protein] (*VCP*)
MYH7-myopathy†,‡ [Laing myopathy] (*MYH7*)
MYH2-myopathy† (*MYH2*)
Nesprinopathy (*SYNE1, SYNE2*)
TIA1opathy [Welander distal myopathy] (*TIA1*)
KLHL9opathy [kelch-like homologue-9] (*KLHL9*)

AUTOSOMAL RECESSIVE
Calpainopathy (*CAPN3*)
Dysferlinopathy (*DYSF*)
Anoctaminopathy (*ANO5*)
α-sarcoglycanopathy (*SGCA*)
β-sarcoglycanopathy (*SGCB*)
δ-sarcoglycanopathy (*SGCD*)
γ-sarcoglycanopathy (*SGCG*)
Telethoninopathy (*TCAP*)
TRIM32opathy (*TRIM32*)
α-Dystroglycanopathies§ (*FKRP, POMT1, POMT2, FKTN, POMGNT1, LARGE, DAG1, DPM2, DPM3*)
Titinopathy (*TTN*)
Laminopathy (*LMNA*)
Plectinopathy (*PLEC*)
Merosin deficiency§ (LAMA2)
Selenoproteinopathy‡,§ (*SEPN1*)
CollagenVIopathy§ (*COL6A1, COL6A2, COL6A3*)
With generalized lipodystrophy (*PTRF*)
Integrinα7opathy§ (*ITGA7*)
Integrinα9opathy§ (*ITGA9*)
With mitochondrial structural abnormalities§ (*CHKB*)
GNE-opathy† [glucosamine (UDP-N-acetyl)-2-epimerase/N-acetylmannosamine kinase] (*GNE*)
Matrin3opathy (*MATR3*)

*Associated with pathologic features of myofibrillar myopathy.
†Associated with pathologic features of inclusion body myopathy.
‡Can also cause congenital myopathy.
§Can also cause congenital muscular dystrophy.

TABLE 421-6 CONGENITAL MYOPATHIES

Central core, multi-minicore disease (*RYR1, SEPN1, MYH7, ACTA1, LMNA*)

Centronuclear myopathy (*MTM1, DNM2, RYR1, BIN1*)

Nemaline rod myopathy (*NEB, ACTA1, TPM3, TPM2, TNNT1, CFL2, KLHL40, KBTBD13*)

Congenital fiber-type disproportion (*ACTA1, SEPN1, RYR1, MYH7*)

Myosin storage myopathy (*MYH7*)

Other structural myopathies: Cap myopathy, zebra body myopathy, sarcotubular myopathy, spheroid body myopathy, fingerprint body myopathy, trilaminar myopathy, cylindrical spiral myopathy, myopathy with muscle spindle excess, myopathy with tubular aggregates.

DIAGNOSIS

Affected individuals have a 20- to 100-fold elevation of their serum CK level. Confirmation of diagnosis requires DNA analysis of the dystrophin gene. If genetic testing is negative, then a muscle biopsy is indicated. The pathologic features are typical of a chronic myopathy. Immunostaining shows an absence of dystrophin except in revertant fibers that express dystrophin (Fig. 421-3).

TREATMENT   Rx

Management requires a multidisciplinary team approach,[2] including physical therapy to prevent contractures and the timely provision of appropriate devices and wheelchairs. The cardiomyopathy is typically managed by using β-blockers and angiotensin-converting enzyme inhibitors (Chapter 59). An orthopedic surgeon should help with monitoring of scoliosis and spinal fusion if indicated. A pulmonologist should assess and follow respiratory function, including the initiation and monitoring of noninvasive ventilation. An endocrinologist can be helpful for managing osteoporosis and adrenal suppression during chronic steroid use. Ophthalmologic evaluation is needed to address cataract formation. Prednisone (0.75 mg/kg/day or weekend 10 mg/kg/day) prolongs the ability to ambulate[A1] despite its significant side effects (Chapter 35). Prednisone may also help respiratory function and slow the progression of scoliosis. Agents used for exon skipping and for read-through of premature stop codons are being tested clinical trials.[3]

TABLE 421-7　CHANNELOPATHIES AND RELATED DISORDERS

DISORDER	PATTERN OF CLINICAL FEATURES
Thomsen disease	Myotonia
Becker disease*	Myotonia and weakness
Paramyotonia congenita	Paramyotonia
Hyperkalemic periodic paralysis	Periodic paralysis, sometimes with myotonia and paramyotonia
Hypokalemic periodic paralysis	Periodic paralysis
Andersen-Tawil syndrome	Periodic paralysis, cardiac arrhythmias, skeletal abnormalities
Myotonia fluctuans	Myotonia
Myotonia permanens	Myotonia
Acetazolamide-responsive myotonia	Myotonia
Schwartz-Jampel syndrome* (Chondrodystrophic myotonia)	Pseudomyotonia, dysmorphism, blepharospasm
Rippling muscle disease	Muscle mounding/stiffness
Brody disease*	Delayed relaxation, no myotonia on electromyogram
Malignant hyperthermia	Anesthetic-induced excessive calcium release by sarcoplasmic reticulum

*Autosomal recessive; all other listed diseases are autosomal dominant.
Adapted with revision from Goldman L, Schafer AI, eds. *Cecil Medicine*. 24th ed. Philadelphia: Elsevier; 2012.

PROGNOSIS

With ventilatory support, patients often live well into the third or even fourth decades. Chronic respiratory failure is the primary cause of death in the late 20s or early 30s, with most patients succumbing to pneumonia, heart failure, or arrythmias.

Becker Muscular Dystrophy

Becker dystrophy is a milder form of Duchenne dystrophy caused by an in-frame mutation in the dystrophin gene.

CLINICAL MANIFESTATIONS AND DIAGNOSIS

Becker dystrophy can present in boys older than age 5 years, teenagers, or even in adults. Typical findings are symmetrical proximal weakness and prominent calf hypertrophy. Heart failure is common and may be the initial manifestation in some patients. The CK is elevated, although not to the same degree as seen in Duchenne dystrophy. Genetic testing for dystrophin gene is positive in about 90 to 95% of patients. If genetic testing is negative in a

TABLE 421-8　METABOLIC AND MITOCHONDRIAL MYOPATHIES

DISORDERS OF GLYCOGEN METABOLISM

Type II: α-1,4-Glucosidase (acid maltase) (*GAA*)
Type III: Debrancher (*AGL*)
Type IV: Branching (*GBE1*)
Type V: Myophosphorylase (*PYGM*)
Type VII: Phosphofructokinase (*PFKM*)
Type VIII: Phosphorylase b kinase (*PHBK*)
Type IX: Phosphoglycerate kinase (*PGK*)
Type X: Phosphoglycerate mutase (*PGAM-M*)
Type XI: Lactate dehydrogenase (*LDHA*)
Type XII: Aldolase A, (*ALDOA*)
Type XIII: β-Enolase (*ENO3*)
Type XIV: Phosphoglucomutase 1 (*PGM1*)

DISORDERS OF LIPID METABOLISM

Carnitine palmitoyltransferase II (*CPT2*)
Primary systemic carnitine deficiency (*SCL22A5*)
Secondary carnitine deficiency
Very long-chain acyl coenzyme A dehydrogenase deficiency (*ACADVL*)
Long-chain acyl coenzyme A dehydrogenase deficiency (*ACADL*)
Medium-chain acyl coenzyme A dehydrogenase deficiency (*ACADM*)
Short-chain acyl coenzyme A dehydrogenase deficiency (*ACADS*)
Long chain hydroxyl/acyl coenzyme A dehydrogenase deficiency (*LCHAD*)
Multiple acyl coenzyme A dehydrogenase deficiency (*ETFA*)
Medications (valproic acid)

MITOCHONDRIAL MYOPATHIES

Chronic progressive external ophthalmoplegia
Kearns-Sayre syndrome
Mitochondrial encephalopathy, lactic acidosis, and stroke-like episodes (MELAS)
Mitochondrial neurogastrointestinal encephalomyopathy (MNGIE)
Myoclonic epilepsy with ragged red fibers (MERRF)
Infantile myopathy and lactic acidosis
Cytochrome c oxidase deficiency

Adapted with revision from Goldman L, Schafer AI, eds. *Cecil Medicine*. 24th ed. Philadelphia: Elsevier; 2012.

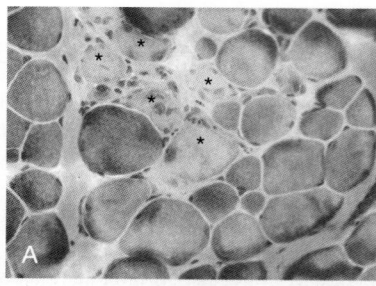 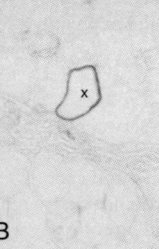 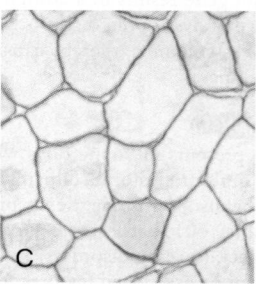

FIGURE 421-3. **Duchenne muscular dystrophy. A,** Trichromatically stained section of a specimen from a patient with Duchenne dystrophy displaying necrotic fibers (*) and increased endomysial and perimysial connective tissue. **B,** Dystrophin immunostain shows absent dystrophin reactivity in all fibers except for a revertant fiber (x). **C,** Normal sarcolemmal dystrophin reactivity in a control section.

patient suspected of having Becker dystrophy, a muscle biopsy is indicated. Muscle biopsy findings are similar to those of Duchenne dystrophy but less severe: immunohistochemistry shows decreased dystrophin expression, and immunoblotting reveals decreased expression and/or a lower molecular weight dystrophin protein.

TREATMENT AND PROGNOSIS   Rx

Management is largely supportive. Corticosteroids are rarely used. Similar to Duchenne dystrophy, screening for respiratory function and cardiac monitoring is indicated. Heart transplantation (Chapter 82) has been performed in patients with severe restrictive cardiomyopathy (Chapter 60).

Many patients have a normal lifespan, although some develop respiratory failure and have a shortened lifespan owing to respiratory complications. Heart failure and arrhythmias occur late in the course of disease.

Female Carriers of Duchenne or Becker Dystrophy

Female carriers of a dystrophin gene mutation are usually totally asymptomatic. However, about 2.5 to 10% of carriers can develop symptoms, including myalgias, proximal muscle weakness, and cardiomyopathy. Rarely, they present with a Duchenne phenotype owing to an XO karyotype (Turner syndrome) or skewed X-chromosome inactivation. If a specific mutation is identified in the family, targeted DNA analysis can confirm the diagnosis. Immunostaining of the muscle specimens shows a mosaic pattern, in which some fibers express dystrophin normally and others show decreased or even absent expression. Management of symptomatic carriers is similar to the management of Duchenne and Becker dystrophy patients with similar disease severities.

Facioscapulohumeral Muscular Dystrophy

Facioscapulohumeral muscular dystrophy is an autosomal dominant disorder with variable penetrance. It is the third most common dystrophy after the dystrophinopathies and myotonic muscular dystrophy, with a prevalence of about 1 in 15,000. About 95% of patients have a truncated D4Z4 tandem repeat region in chromosome 4q35.[4] The other 5% have hypomethylation of the D4Z4 region along with a mutation in the *SMCHD1* gene, which is critical for the structural maintenance of chromosome-flexible hinge-domain-containing protein 1.[5]

CLINICAL MANIFESTATIONS

Facioscapulohumeral muscular dystrophy has a highly variable penetrance within the same family. Severe proximal facial weakness can present in infancy, or mild and almost asymptomatic distal weakness can present in late adulthood. Some gene carriers never present with clinical symptoms or signs. The muscle weakness initially affects the face, where it causes difficulty smiling or whistling. Patients then develop scapular, humeral, truncal, and lower limb weakness leading to foot drop. Scapular winging is a typical feature. Muscle involvement is often asymmetrical.

Associated symptoms can include high-frequency hearing loss and retinal telangiectasia. Rare patients with retinal vascular abnormalities can develop retinal exudation leading to retinal detachment (Chapter 423). Infants with profound facial diplegia can also have intellectual disability and intractable epilepsy.

DIAGNOSIS

The CK level ranges from normal to mildly elevated. EMG shows typical myopathic features. Muscle biopsy shows chronic myopathic changes sometimes with an inflammatory exudate. Definite diagnosis is based on genetic testing.

TREATMENT AND PROGNOSIS   Rx

Management is supportive, and corticosteroids are of no benefit. Patients do benefit, however, from physical therapy for motion exercises for the shoulder girdle, molded ankle-foot orthoses for the footdrop, hearing aids for patients with hearing loss, and scapular fixation surgery to improve shoulder range of motion. Cardiac features are not prominent, and respiratory muscle weakness is a late feature. The prognosis is highly variable, depending on the severity and age of onset. Many patients have a normal lifespan.

Myotonic Dystrophies

Myotonic dystrophies, which are the second most common inherited muscle disease, affect about 1 in 8000 of the population. The two types, DM1 and DM2, are inherited in an autosomal dominant manner. Both cause multisystem disease and can be difficult to distinguish from each other. DM1 is caused by an abnormal expansion of CTG nucleotide repeats in an untranslated region of the dystrophia myotonica protein kinase (*DMPK*) gene on chromosome 19q. DM2 is caused by an abnormal expansion of CCTG nucleotide repeats in intron 1 of the zinc finger protein 9 (*ZNF9*) gene on chromosome 3q.

CLINICAL MANIFESTATIONS

Patients typically have frontal balding, ptosis, and temporal and masseter muscle wasting. Speech is nasal in quality, and patients display a high-steppage gait owing to their distal myopathy. On neurologic examination, myotonia is seen with percussion (inability to relax the muscle after percussion with a reflex hammer), after a grip (inability to relax the fingers after a firm grip), and in the eyelids (inability to open forcibly closed eyelids). Weakness in DM1 predominantly affects facial, oropharyngeal, forearm flexor, and foot dorsiflexor muscles. In DM2, weakness is predominantly proximal, although deep finger flexors are frequently affected. Muscle pain and stiffness are common in DM2 but can be seen in DM1 as well. Systemic features include premature subcapsular lens cataracts, testicular atrophy, intellectual disability, impotence, and hypersomnolence mediated by both central and neuromuscular mechanisms. Endocrine dysfunction is common, including diabetes mellitus and thyroid abnormalities. Dysphagia and constipation are common. Progressive cardiac conduction defects can lead to sudden death. Patients may require ventilation support after general anesthesia. Women who transmit DM1 are at high risk for having a child with a severe congenital form, including hypotonia at birth, respiratory failure, failure to thrive, and globally delayed developmental milestones with mild to severe intellectual disability.

DIAGNOSIS

Classical myotonic dystrophy usually can be diagnosed clinically by a patient's essentially pathognomonic facial features (see Fig. 421-2). The CK may be normal or mildly elevated. EMG, which is useful when the diagnosis is unsuspected or unclear, reveals myopathic features and myotonic discharges. Molecular genetic analysis of the nucleotide repeats confirms the diagnosis.[6]

TREATMENT   Rx

All patients should have an annual electrocardiogram and a Holter monitor to detect conduction system abnormalities (Chapter 62). An echocardiogram should be performed at diagnosis and repeated about every 2 to 4 years. Respiratory function testing also is usually recommended about every 2 to 4 years, and a sleep study is useful to detect nocturnal hypoventilation for symptomatic patients.

Mexilitene (150 to 200 mL three times daily) is well tolerated and can improve muscle relaxation.[A2] Hypersomnolence (Chapter 405) can be treated with overnight positive-pressure ventilation. Methylphenidate (200 mg daily)[A3] may be preferable to modafinil (300 mg daily) for excessive day-time sleepiness, but neither provides dramatic results.[7] Cardiac pacing, which is frequently required, can reduce the incidence of paroxysmal atrial fibrillation.[A4] Physical therapy can help to prevent contractures.

OTHER MUSCULAR DYSTROPHIES

Limb-girdle muscular dystrophies are a diverse group of myopathies caused by gene defects or deficiencies of muscle proteins that are critical for the normal function of the muscle cell membrane and especially the dystrophin-sarcoglycan complex.[8] Inheritance can be autosomal dominant or recessive. Although most patients have classical limb-girdle muscle weakness at the onset, some can present with distal leg muscle involvement that may initially be misdiagnosed as sensorimotor neuropathy. Some causes can be identified clinically by an experienced clinician. However, EMG can help to differentiate these conditions from neuropathies, and muscle biopsy, immunohistochemistry studies, and genetic analysis are often required to make a precise diagnosis.[9]

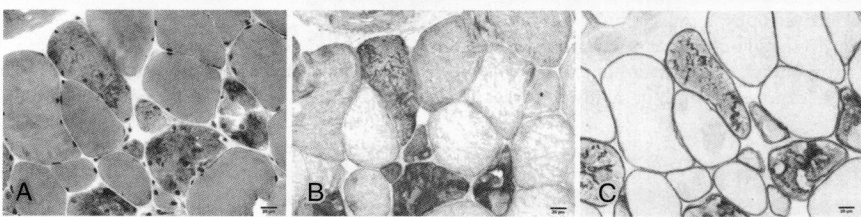

FIGURE 421-4. Myofibrillar myopathy. **A,** Trichromatically stained section of a specimen from a patient with myofibrillar myopathy displaying abnormal fibers with hyaline deposits or amorphous material and vacuoles. Abnormal fibers show abnormal and ectopic expression for desmin **(B)** and dystrophin **(C).**

Myofibrillar myopathies present with progressive distal or proximal muscle weakness and characteristic morphologic features on muscle biopsy (Fig. 421-4). Cardiomyopathy and neuropathy can be associated features.[10]

Emery-Dreifuss muscular dystrophy[11] was originally X-linked and was initially shown to be caused by mutations in the emerin gene, a nuclear membrane protein. However, mutations in five other genes can cause a similar phenotype. Patients have a distinctive phenotype, including progressive joint contractures, scapuloperoneal distribution weakness, and cardiomyopathy with a progressive cardiac conduction disorder. The CK is often elevated but can be normal. Cardiac function needs to be monitored periodically. As with the dystrophinopathies, female carriers of the X-linked forms may develop weakness and cardiac disease.

Oculopharyngeal muscular dystrophy is an autosomal dominant myopathy caused by a trinucleotide repeat expansion of the poly(A)-binding protein, nuclear 1 (*PABPN1*) gene. Onset typically occurs in the fifth or sixth decade of life with dysphagia and marked ptosis. Marked distal and proximal weakness occurs later in the disease course. Surgical correction of ptosis often yields excellent results, but the dysphagia can be more difficult to manage. Patients often have a normal lifespan.

CONGENITAL MUSCULAR DYSTROPHIES

Congenital muscular dystrophies (see Table 421-5) are a rare group of autosomal recessive muscle diseases that present in infancy or childhood with hypotonia and muscle weakness.[12,13] The main differential diagnosis is spinal muscular atrophy (Chapter 419) and congenital myasthenia (Chapter 422). Affected infants can have joint contractures, which can be severe at birth. Some have a pure muscle phenotype and survive into adulthood. Others have severe central nervous system and eye involvement, which are associated with hypoglycosylation of α-dystroglycan that may be fatal in early childhood.

Congenital Myopathies

Congenital myopathies are rare inherited muscle diseases that are generally less severe than congenital muscular dystrophies. Patients present at birth with hypotonia, myopathic facies, and delayed motor milestones. The weakness is usually slowly progressive.[14] Respiratory muscle weakness can occur, and patients can present with ventilator failure at birth or insidiously in adult life. The most severely affected patients present in utero with reduced fetal movements and polyhydramnios. Muscle biopsy is diagnostic.

Central core myopathy is usually due to mutations in the ryanodine receptor gene (*RYR1*) and is strongly associated with malignant hyperthermia (Chapter 432). *Nemaline myopathies* are caused by different gene defects, including nebulin (*NEB*), skeletal α-actin (*ACTA1*), -tropomyosin$_{slow}$ (*TPM3*), β-tropomyosin (*TPM2*), troponin T$_{slow}$ (*TNNT1*), cofilin (*CFL2*), kelch-like family member 40 (*KLHL40*), and kelch-repeat- and BTB-[POZ]-domain-containing 13 (*KBTBD13*). Characteristic nemaline rods are seen on muscle biopsy. *Centronuclear myopathy* can be X-linked owing to mutations in myotubularin (*MTM1*), dominant owing to mutations in dynamin 2 (*DNM2*), or recessive owing to mutations in *RYR1* or amphiphysin 2 (*BIN1*). Muscle biopsy is diagnostic.

No specific treatments are available. Management requires a multidisciplinary team approach similar to muscular dystrophies.[15]

Ion Channelopathies

Ion channelopathies (see Table 421-7) are genetically determined disorders in which the muscle membrane functions abnormally. The combined prevalence of the various skeletal muscle channelopathies is about 1.1 per 100,000.[16] Each has a specific molecular cause, but the phenotypes overlap.

CHLORIDE CHANNELOPATHIES

Mutations in the muscle chloride-channel gene *CLCN1* cause autosomal dominant (Thomson) and autosomal recessive (Becker) myotonia congenita. Patients present with painless myotonia, muscle stiffness that may be slightly worse in the cold and improves with exercise (the warm-up phenomenon), muscle hypertrophy, and grip and percussion myotonia. EMG shows myotonic discharges. The myotonia responds to mexiletine (150 to 200 mg up to three times a day).[A5] Patients have a normal lifespan.

SODIUM CHANNELOPATHIES

Mutations in *SCN4A*, which is the voltage-gated sodium-channel gene, cause a range of autosomal dominant phenotypes, including hyperkalemic periodic paralysis, paramyotonia congenita, and potassium aggravated myotonia. Periodic paralysis is typically precipitated by sustained exercise that leads to weakness during the rest period, by potassium-rich food, or sometimes by emotional stress or cold. The attacks can persist for hours, during which the patient can be quadriplegic with depressed tendon reflexes but normal sensation, eye movements, and respiration. The serum potassium level may be high or normal during the attack. The physical examination is usually normal between attacks, but some patients develop fixed proximal weakness later in the disease. In patients with paramyotonia, the muscle stiffness paradoxically increases with exercise and is often painful. Cold sensitivity is typically more extreme than that seen in myotonia congenita, and cold can precipitate the muscle weakness. The diagnosis is made clinically, although patients with fixed proximal muscle weakness, which can be confused with other myopathies, have vacuolar changes and sometimes tubular aggregates on muscle biopsy. For both phenotypes, management involves avoidance of precipitating factors such as cold or strenuous exercise. If the myotonia is disabling, medications that act on sodium channels such as dichlorphenamide (50 to 450 mg daily),[A6] acetazolamide (250 mg twice daily), mexiletine (150 mg three times a day), phenytoin (300 to 600 mg daily), and carbamazepine (400 to 800 mg daily) can be considered. Life expectancy is normal.

CALCIUM CHANNELOPATHIES

Hypokalemic periodic paralysis is usually caused by autosomal dominant mutations in the voltage-dependent calcium channel gene *CACNA1S* but in about 10% of cases is caused by dominant mutations in *SCN4A*. The attacks of weakness, which are usually more severe and prolonged than in hyperkalemic period paralysis, generally persist for hours to days before gradually resolving. Attacks occur spontaneously or during prolonged rest after vigorous exercise and also can be precipitated by a high carbohydrate meal. The serum potassium level is reduced or low-normal during the attack. Avoidance of high carbohydrate loads and treatment with acetazolamide (125 to 1000 mg/day)[A7] or dichlorphenamide (50 to 400 mg/day) is effective. Patients may develop permanent muscle weakness if they have frequent attacks.

OTHER FORMS OF PERIODIC PARALYSIS AND MUSCLE STIFFNESS

Periodic paralysis can occur in a wide range of metabolic and electrolyte disorders (Table 421-9). Mutations in the *KCNJ2* gene, which encodes the inward rectifier potassium channel Kir2.1, cause *Andersen-Tawil syndrome*, an autosomal dominant, usually hypokalemic, periodic paralysis that is associated with distinctive facial features, including hypertelorism and low-set ears, as well as a propensity for cardiac arrhythmias. Treatment includes acetazolamide (250 mg twice daily) and dichlorphenamide. For patients with sulfa allergy, potassium-sparing diuretics such as spironolactone (25 to 100 mg/day) or triamterene (25 to 100 mg/day) can be used. The patients should be

TABLE 421-9	SECONDARY CAUSES OF PERIODIC PARALYSIS

HYPOKALEMIC

Thyrotoxicosis
Primary hyperaldosteronism (Conn syndrome)
Renal tubular acidosis (e.g., Fanconi syndrome)
Juxtaglomerular apparatus hyperplasia (Bartter syndrome)
Gastrointestinal potassium wastage
Villous adenoma
Pancreatic non-insulin-secreting tumors with diarrhea
Nontropical sprue
Barium intoxication
Potassium-depleting diuretics
Amphotericin B
Licorice
Corticosteroids
Toluene toxicity
p-Aminosalicylic acid
Carbenoxolone

HYPERKALEMIC

Addison disease
Hypoaldosteronism
Excessive potassium supplementation
Potassium-sparing diuretics
Chronic renal failure

From Goldman L, Ausiello DA, eds. *Cecil Textbook of Medicine.* 23rd ed. Philadelphia: Elsevier; 2008.

treated as indicated for the cardiac arrhythmia and prolonged QT interval (Chapter 65). *Brody disease,* an autosomal recessive disorder caused by mutations in the SR calcium ATPase gene (*ATP2A1*), is characterized by exercise-induced muscle stiffness that is electrically silent on EMG. There are case reports of treatment with dantrolene, verapamil, or nifedipine with varying success.

Neuromyotonia (Isaac syndrome) is an autoimmune disorder associated with peripheral nerve hyperexcitability. It is caused by voltage-gated potassium-channel antibodies and is part of a spectrum of disorders, including limbic encephalitis. Oral immunomodulatory therapy, intravenous immunoglobulin, plasmapheresis, and symptomatic therapy with carbamazepine or phenytoin have been used with varying response. *Rippling muscle syndrome,* which can be caused by mutations in the *CAV3* gene, is characterized by rippling muscles triggered by exercise or percussion. Rippling muscle syndrome and neuromyotonia can be paraneoplastic phenomena, and a search for malignancy should be considered in these patients.

Metabolic Myopathies

Metabolic myopathies (see Table 421-8) are caused by enzyme defects that affect the three principal stages of muscle metabolism: (1) carbohydrate disorders due to a defect of glucose-glycogen metabolism; (2) disorders of fatty acid oxidation; and (3) disorders of mitochondrial oxidative phosphorylation. Muscle dysfunction can be acute, recurrent, and reversible, but the exercise intolerance can cause progressive weakness or even rhabdomyolysis (Chapter 113).

DISORDERS OF CARBOHYDRATE METABOLISM

Because glucose and glycogen are the primary energy sources for muscle contraction, any defects of glucose-glycogen metabolism cause muscle pain, cramps, contracture, and weakness within the first 30 minutes of exercise. The most common form is myophosphorylase deficiency (Chapter 207), and other forms are extremely rare. Most of these disorders are inherited autosomal recessively, although phosphoglycerate kinase deficiency is X-linked. Patients also note exercise intolerance and become deconditioned. Severe episodes are associated with very high CK levels, rhabdomyolysis, and myoglobinuria.

Phosphorylase Deficiency

Phosphorylase deficiency (McArdle disease, type IV glycogenosis) typically presents with muscle pain or cramps after short bursts of exercise. Some patients present with recurrent rhabdomyolysis. Persistent exercise beyond 30 minutes leads to the "second-wind" phenomenon, when fatty acids become the primary source of muscle energy. Clinical examination and the CK can be normal between the attacks, although some patients develop fixed proximal muscle weakness with myopathic features on EMG. Histochemical

and enzyme analysis of muscle confirms the diagnosis. High protein diet and 37 g oral sucrose shortly before exercise[A8] and graded exercise may improve symptoms, but patients are at risk for developing contractures. The life expectancy is normal.

Acid Maltase Deficiency

Acid maltase deficiency (type II glycogenosis, α-1,4-glucosidase), also called Pompe disease, may present in infancy as a very severe generalized muscle disease that is fatal before age 2 years, as a juvenile variant that causes muscle weakness and death by the second or third decade owing to respiratory failure, or as an adult-onset form that presents with limb-girdle muscle weakness or sometimes with respiratory failure (Chapter 208). In each type, EMG reveals myotonic discharges. Abnormal glycogen storage and acid phosphatase–positive vacuoles are seen on muscle biopsy. The disorder can be diagnosed by measuring the enzyme activity in leukocytes or in muscle, but the use of dried blood samples to measure enzyme activity is increasingly becoming the standard practice. Mutation analysis is also clinically available. Enzyme replacement therapy appears promising in children and in the late-onset form.[A9]

DISORDERS OF FATTY ACID METABOLISM

After about 30 minutes of exercise, when the muscle glycogen reserves become exhausted, fatty acids become the principal source of muscle energy. Fatty acid metabolism involves the transport of fatty acids from the serum into the muscle and mitochondria, where both carnitine and carnitine palmitoyltransferase are key components of the β-oxidation pathway.

Fatty acid oxidation disorders can present with a proximal myopathy, exercise intolerance, muscle pain, rhabdomyolysis, and cardiomyopathy. Other features can include neuropathy, pigmentary retinopathy, recurrent hypoketotic hypoglycemia, seizures, and intellectual disability. There may be a family history of sudden unexpected death syndrome. The most common fatty acid oxidation defect is *medium-chain acyl-CoA dehydrogenase (MCAD) deficiency. Carnitine palmitoyltransferase I deficiency* presents in childhood with an encephalopathy and liver failure associated with hypoglycemia and a high blood ammonia during metabolic crises. *Carnitine palmitoyltransferase II deficiency* can present as a fatal infantile onset form or more commonly between first to sixth decade of life with muscle pain, exercise intolerance, and myoglobinuria, typically after a long period of fasting or sustained exercise.

Carnitine deficiency can be primary or secondary. *Primary carnitine deficiency* causes myopathy, cardiomyopathy, and encephalopathy in association with hypoketotic hypoglycemia, although pure muscle presentations have been described. The diagnosis can be made by finding a low blood level, although prominent fat deposition in muscle is another clue. Other metabolic myopathies that can cause a secondary carnitine deficiency include disorders of β-oxidation and mitochondrial oxidative phosphorylation and may cause similar symptoms as the primary carnitine deficiency. Analysis of serum acylcarnitines, urine organic acids, and urine acylglycines and specific enzyme assays in fibroblasts can help to pinpoint the enzyme defect.

TREATMENT ℞

General treatment approach is avoidance of precipitating factors, such as prolonged fasting or prolonged exercise. Carbohydrate intake is advised before exercise, and patients should be prescribed a high carbohydrate, low fat diet with frequent feedings. Both primary and secondary carnitine deficiencies respond well to oral carnitine replacement (200 to 400 mg/kg/day in divided doses). Some patients have a multiple acyl-coenzyme A dehydrogenase deficiency (also called trifunctional enzyme deficiency, or glutaric aciduria type II), which responds well to riboflavin (100 mg daily).

DISORDERS OF MITOCHONDRIAL OXIDATIVE PHOSPHORYLATION

Disorders of mitochondrial oxidative phosphorylation (see Table 421-8), which are among the most common causes of inherited metabolic diseases, can present with isolated myopathy but often are multisystemic with cardiac involvement, diabetes mellitus, and both central and peripheral neurologic features.[17] Abnormal fatigability or exercise intolerance is a frequent complaint. Common CNS manifestations include epilepsy, migraine, strokelike episodes, myoclonus, ataxia, neuropathy, pigmentary retinopathy, dementia, and psychomotor regression.

Mitochondrial oxidative phosphorylation requires five respiratory chain complexes that are located on the inner mitochondrial membrane.[18]

Mitochondrial dysfunction results in energy deficits, which can lead to organ failure. Mitochondrial proteins can be coded by mitochondrial DNA (mtDNA), which is maternally inherited, and nuclear DNA, which can be inherited in an autosomal dominant, recessive, or X-linked manner. Phenotypic presentation of mtDNA defects depends on heteroplasmy, which is the amount and tissue distribution of the mutant mtDNA. If the amount of heteroplasmy exceeds a certain threshold, symptoms become apparent. Mitochondrial DNA disorders affect the structure or amount of the respiratory chain proteins, whereas nuclear DNA disorders can affect the proteins, the assembly of the respiratory chain, or the maintenance of mtDNA.

CLINICAL MANIFESTATIONS

Mitochondrial diseases should be considered in all patients who have a complex multisystemic myopathy, especially patients with neuromuscular, ocular, and endocrine involvement.

Mitochondrial encephalomyopathy with lactic acidosis and strokelike episodes (MELAS) is most frequently caused by a point mutation of mtDNA (m.3243A>G). Patients can have myopathy, cardiomyopathy, strokelike attacks, and encephalopathy. Some patients have one or only a few of these characteristics, some only have diabetes and deafness, and some only have cardiomyopathy.

Myoclonic epilepsy with ragged-red fibers (MERRF) is usually caused by a point mutation of mtDNA (m.8344A>G). It presents with a proximal myopathy associated with slowly progressive ataxia, epilepsy, peripheral neuropathy, and myoclonus.

Leber hereditary optic neuropathy (Chapter 424) predominantly affects young adult men, more than 95% of whom have mtDNA point mutations in m.3460G>A, m.11778G>A, or m.14484T>C. Patients develop subacute bilateral visual failure in both eyes within 2 to 3 months.

Chronic progressive external ophthalmoplegia with ptosis and gradual limitation of eye movements is seen in up to 20% of mitochondrial disorders. About 95% of patients have sporadic mtDNA point mutations or deletions, but the disease can be inherited as either an autosomal dominant or recessive trait. Mutations in *POLG* gene, which encodes the mitochondrial polymerase γ, are the most common causes of autosomal dominant or recessive progressive external ophthalmoplegia. *Kearns-Sayre syndrome* is characterized by the triad of external ophthalmoplegia, retinitis pigmentosa, and onset before the age of 20 years plus at least one of the following: heart block, cerebellar ataxia, or cerebrospinal fluid protein greater than 100 mg/dL. Kearns-Sayre syndrome is usually sporadic and caused by a single deletion of mtDNA.

Mitochondrial DNA depletion syndromes can present in neonatal period or infancy with subacute necrotizing encephalomyopathy (*Leigh syndrome*), hepatorenal failure, cardiomyopathy, and severe lactic acidosis. Children with *Pearson syndrome*, which is caused by accumulation of mtDNA deletions, typically present with pancytopenia, sideroblastic anemia, and exocrine pancreatic failure. *Primary coenzyme Q10 (ubiquinone) deficiency* is a rare autosomal recessive disorder that can present with encephalopathy, lipid storage myopathy, myoglobinuria, seizures, and cerebellar ataxia, or as an isolated nephrotic syndrome or an isolated myopathy.

DIAGNOSIS, TREATMENT, AND PROGNOSIS

The investigation of suspected mitochondrial disorders involves a systematic screen for multisystem complications, especially diabetes and cardiomyopathy; muscle biopsy to look for ragged red fibers, cytochrome c oxidase deficiency or biochemical evidence of respiratory chain dysfunction; search for mitochondrial deletion or depletion in muscle; and molecular genetic tests. Some primary mtDNA defects are not detectable in blood, so skeletal muscle is often required for the biochemical and genetic tests. For example, diagnosis of primary coenzyme Q10 (CoQ10) deficiency is made by measuring CoQ10 in muscle but not in blood.

Patients with primary CoQ10 deficiency can respond dramatically to CoQ10 supplementation (30 mg/kg/day in children and up to 2400 mg/day in adults in three divided doses). Vitamins and cofactors, including thiamine, riboflavin, and CoQ10, have shown varying degrees of benefit in different mitochondrial diseases. Management is largely supportive with monitoring and treatment of complications. Prognosis varies depending on the phenotype, ranging from the relatively normal life expectancy with chronic external ophthalmoplegia to a relatively rapid demise with Leigh syndrome.

OTHER METABOLIC AND TOXIC MYOPATHIES

Myopathy can complicate many metabolic disorders, including hypothyroidism (Chapter 226), Addison disease (Chapter 227), hyperaldosteronism

TABLE 421-10 TOXIC MYOPATHIES
INFLAMMATORY
Cimetidine
D-Penicillamine
Procainamide
L-Tryptophan
L-Dopa
NONINFLAMMATORY NECROTIZING OR VACUOLAR
Statins
Chloroquine
Colchicine
Emetine
ε-Aminocaproic acid
Labetalol
Cyclosporine
Tacrolimus
Isoretinoic acid (vitamin A analogue)
Vincristine
Alcohol
RHABDOMYOLYSIS AND MYOGLOBINURIA
Statins
Alcohol
Heroin
Amphetamine
Toluene
Cocaine
ε-Aminocaproic acid
Pentazocine
Phencyclidine
MALIGNANT HYPERTHERMIA
Halothane
Ethylene
Diethyl ether
Methoxyflurane
Ethyl chloride
Trichloroethylene
Gallamine
Succinylcholine
MITOCHONDRIAL
Zidovudine
MYOTONIA
2,4-D-Chlorophenoxylacetic acid
Anthracene-9-carboxylic acid
Cholesterol-lowering agents
Chloroquine
Cyclosporine
MYOSIN LOSS
Nondepolarizing neuromuscular blocking agents*
Intravenous glucocorticosteroids*

*In the setting of critical illness.
Adapted with revisions from Goldman L, Ausiello DA, eds. Cecil Textbook of Medicine, 23rd ed. Philadelphia: Elsevier; 2008.

(Chapter 227), hyperparathyroidism (Chapter 245), vitamin D deficiency (Chapter 244), and liver and renal failure (Chapters 130 and 153). The myopathy is often subtle, the CK level and EMG are often normal, and the muscle biopsy may be nonspecifically abnormal.

Many drugs cause myopathy (Table 421-10) with proximal muscle weakness, muscle pain, and exercise intolerance. The CK and EMG can be normal, and muscle biopsy findings may be nonspecific. The diagnosis may depend on the resolution of symptoms after the toxic agent is removed. Perhaps the most commonly incriminated medications are statins, which can cause muscle pain, an increased CK level, and rarely, myoglobinuria.

INFLAMMATORY MUSCLE DISEASES

Inflammatory myopathies are a heterogeneous group of acquired muscle diseases (Table 421-11) that usually present with muscle weakness and exercise intolerance, with or without pain. Most patients have an elevated CK level and an abnormal EMG. Muscle biopsy shows an inflammatory infiltrate. However, the inflammatory process can be patchy and missed on the EMG

TABLE 421-11 CLASSIFICATION OF INFLAMMATORY MYOPATHIES

IDIOPATHIC

Polymyositis
Dermatomyositis
Inclusion body myositis
Overlap syndromes with other connective tissue disease (scleroderma, systemic lupus erythematosus, mixed connective tissue disease, Sjögren syndrome, rheumatoid arthritis, polyarteritis nodosa)
Sarcoidosis and other granulomatous myositis
Behçet disease
Inflammatory myopathies and eosinophilia
  Eosinophilic polymyositis
  Diffuse fasciitis with eosinophilia
Focal myositis
Myositis ossificans

INFECTIOUS

Bacterial: *Staphylococcus aureus*, streptococci, *Escherichia coli*, *Yersinia* sp., *Legionella* sp., gas gangrene (*Clostridium welchii*), leprous myositis, Lyme disease (*Borrelia burgdorferi*)
Viral: acute myositis after influenza or other viral infections (adenovirus, coxsackievirus, echovirus, parainfluenza virus, Epstein-Barr virus, arbovirus, cytomegalovirus), retrovirus-related myopathies (HIV, HTLV-1), hepatitis B and C
Parasitic: trichinosis (*Trichinella spiralis*), toxoplasmosis (*Toxoplasma gondii*), cysticercosis, sarcosporidiosis, trypanosomiasis (*Taenia solium*)
Fungal: *Candida* sp., *Cryptococcus* sp., sporotrichosis, actinomycosis, histoplasmosis

HIV = human immunodeficiency virus; HTML-1 = human T-lymphotrophic virus 1.
From Goldman L, Ausiello DA, eds. *Cecil Textbook of Medicine*. 23rd ed. Philadelphia: Elsevier; 2008.

or muscle biopsy, especially if the specimen is small or if a clinically unaffected muscle is biopsied. Similarly, a short period of corticosteroid therapy can mask the findings. MRI guidance can help to identify high-yield locations for muscle biopsy.

Systemic diseases associated with an inflammatory myopathy include polymyositis, dermatomyositis, inclusion body myositis (Chapter 269), systemic lupus erythematosus (Chapter 266), mixed connective tissue disease (Chapter 266), Sjögren syndrome (Chapter 268), rheumatoid arthritis (Chapter 264), and sarcoidosis (Chapter 95). Systemic viral illnesses and other infectious microorganisms (see Table 421-11) frequently cause muscle pain and an elevated CK, which rarely are major clinical problems.

Sarcopenia and Muscle Wasting

Muscle wasting is a common problem in elderly people (Chapter 25), partly related to hormonal changes and largely related to underuse. Critically ill patients rapidly lose muscle owing to inactivity and reduced protein synthesis,[19,20] with some potential to slow this process with protein-calorie nutrition (Chapter 111). Sarcopenia is also a prominent feature of many cancers, end-stage heart failure (Chapter 58) and renal failure (Chapter 131), and eating disorders (Chapter 219).

Grade A References

A1. Manzur AY, Kuntzer T, Pike M, et al. Glucocorticoid corticosteroids for Duchenne muscular dystrophy. *Cochrane Database Syst Rev*. 2008;1:CD003725.
A2. Logigian EL, Martens WB, Moxley RT IV, et al. Mexiletine is an effective antimyotonia treatment in myotonic dystrophy type 1. *Neurology*. 2010;74:1441-1448.
A3. Puymirat J, Bouchard JP, Mathieu J. Efficacy and tolerability of a 20-mg dose of methylphenidate for the treatment of daytime sleepiness in adult patients with myotonic dystrophy type 1: a 2-center, randomized, double-blind, placebo-controlled, 3-week crossover trial. *Clin Ther*. 2012;34:1103-1111.
A4. Russo V, Rago A, Politano L, et al. The effect of atrial preference pacing on paroxysmal atrial fibrillation incidence in myotonic dystrophy type 1 patients: a prospective, randomized, single-bind cross-over study. *Europace*. 2012;14:486-489.
A5. Statland JM, Bundy BN, Wang Y, et al. Mexiletine for symptoms and signs of myotonia in nondystrophic myotonia: a randomized controlled trial. *JAMA*. 2012;308:1357-1365.
A6. Sansone V, Meola G, Links TP, et al. Treatment for periodic paralysis. *Cochrane Database Syst Rev*. 2008;1:CD005045.
A7. Matthews E, Portaro S, Ke Q, et al. Acetazolamide efficacy in hypokalemic periodic paralysis and the predictive role of genotype. *Neurology*. 2011;77:1960-1964.
A8. Andersen ST, Haller RG, Vissing J. Effect of oral sucrose shortly before exercise on work capacity in McArdle disease. *Arch Neurol*. 2008;65:786-789.
A9. van der Ploeg AT, Clemens PR, Corzo D, et al. A randomized study of alglucosidase alfa in late-onset Pompe's disease. *N Engl J Med*. 2010;362:1396-1406.

GENERAL REFERENCES

For the General References and other additional features, please visit Expert Consult at https://expertconsult.inkling.com.

422

DISORDERS OF NEUROMUSCULAR TRANSMISSION

AMELIA EVOLI AND ANGELA VINCENT

DEFINITION

Neuromuscular transmission depends on the release of acetylcholine from synaptic vesicles that are stored in the terminal boutons of the motor nerve axon (Fig. 422-1). Invasion of the motor nerve terminal by the action potential opens voltage-gated calcium channels, resulting in the Ca^{2+}-dependent release of the vesicular contents into the synaptic space. Acetylcholine binds to the acetylcholine-gated ion channels (acetylcholine receptors [AChRs]) on the postsynaptic membrane, thereby leading to the opening of these channels and a local depolarization, the end-plate potential. If the end-plate potential exceeds the critical firing threshold, voltage-gated sodium channels (sited at the bottom of the postsynaptic folds) open to generate the muscle action potential that propagates along the muscle fiber and activates muscle contraction. The action of acetylcholine is terminated by its dissociation from the AChRs, which close spontaneously after 1 to 4 milliseconds; hydrolysis of acetylcholine by acetylcholinesterase; and acetylcholine diffusion from the synaptic cleft. Meanwhile, in the motor nerve terminal, the voltage-gated calcium channels close spontaneously, and the resting membrane potential is restored through the transient opening of voltage-gated potassium channels.

The extent to which the amplitude of the end-plate potential exceeds the threshold for activation of the voltage-gated sodium channels is called the safety factor. In healthy individuals, the amplitude decreases during repeated activity but does not fall below this threshold; thus, neuromuscular transmission is not compromised. However, if there is an abnormally low end-plate potential amplitude, failure of neuromuscular transmission may occur. Causes include defects in the release of acetylcholine, the postsynaptic response to acetylcholine, or the number or sensitivity of the voltage-gated sodium channels. Morphologic changes to the presynaptic or postsynaptic components or to the basal lamina between them may also influence the efficacy of transmission. Although myasthenia gravis and some neurotoxic envenomations (Chapter 112) are the most common disorders of neuromuscular transmission, a number of conditions have been implicated (Table 422-1).

AUTOIMMUNE DISEASES

Myasthenia Gravis

EPIDEMIOLOGY

Myasthenia is the most common disorder of neuromuscular transmission, with a prevalence of about 15 per 100,000 in Western countries.[1] All races can be affected, and it can occur at any age from year 1 onward. There is a small peak in the incidence rate in women in the third decade and a larger peak, the majority males, at later ages. The annual incidence rises to about 5 per 100,000 after age 70 years. It is especially important to differentiate myasthenia gravis from other causes of limb or bulbar muscle weakness in elderly people.

Myasthenia gravis itself is heterogeneous and can be divided into different subtypes; the relative frequency of these different forms is not known, but relatively mild childhood forms are frequent in Asian countries. Neonatal myasthenia gravis, due to the placental transfer of maternal antibodies to the AChR or to muscle-specific kinase (MuSK), affects up to one in eight babies born to mothers with myasthenia gravis. Autoimmune myasthenia gravis must be distinguished from congenital myasthenic syndromes, which are caused by gene mutations.

PATHOBIOLOGY

Pathophysiology

Myasthenia gravis is the result of a defect in neuromuscular transmission. The postsynaptic response to acetylcholine, the end-plate potential, is reduced so

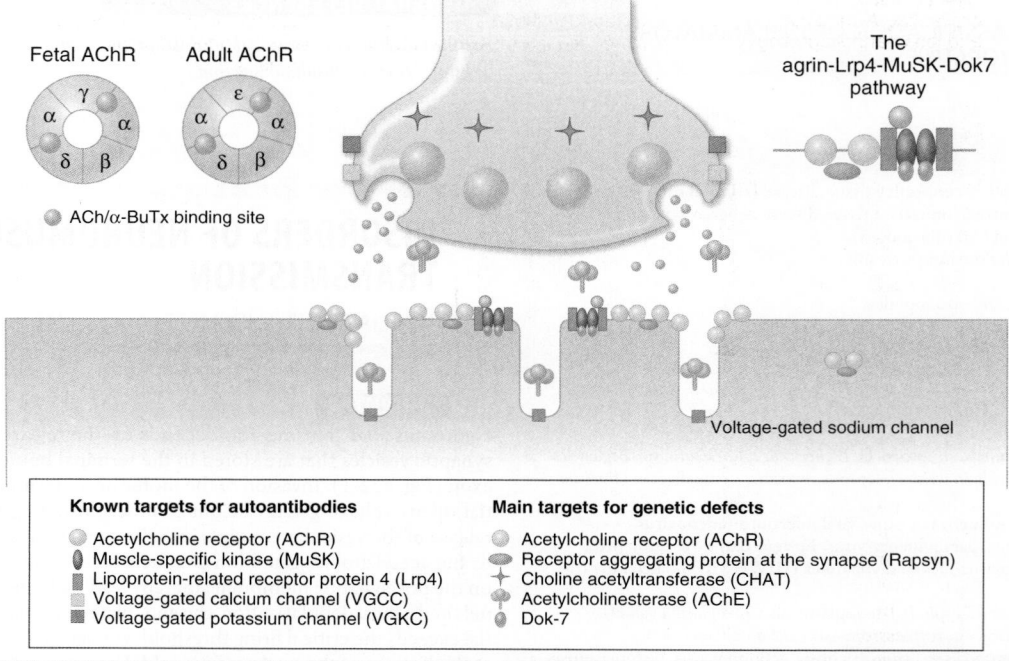

FIGURE 422-1. Diagrammatic representation of the neuromuscular junction, indicating the ion channels, receptors, enzymes, and associated proteins that are the most frequent targets for autoimmune diseases *(left)* or mutations in genetic diseases *(right)*. The acetylcholine receptor exists in fetal and adult isoforms as illustrated at *top left*. The replacement of the fetal form by the adult form takes place toward the end of gestation in humans. The agrin-Lrp4-MuSK-DOK7 pathway associated with AChRs on the postsynaptic membrane is illustrated at *top right*. α-BuTx, α-bungarotoxin, the snake toxin that binds with high specificity to the two Ach binding sites on the AChRs.

TABLE 422-1 DISORDERS OF NEUROMUSCULAR TRANSMISSION

DISEASE	TARGET	PATHOBIOLOGY
AUTOIMMUNE		
Myasthenia gravis	AChRs	Antibodies to AChR in 85% reduce AChR numbers and EPP amplitude
	MuSK	Antibodies to MuSK in 5-10%; mechanism not clear
	Lrp4	Antibodies to Lrp4 in a proportion of patients; mechanism not clear
Transient neonatal myasthenia	AChRs, MuSK	Maternal antibodies cause transient disease in neonate; not seen commonly if mother receiving treatment
Arthrogryposis	Fetal AChR	Maternal antibodies that inhibit fetal AChR function resulting in paralyses in the fetus in utero, leading to joint contractures and rarely arthrogryposis
Lambert-Eaton myasthenic syndrome	VGCCs	Antibodies to VGCC in 90% reduce VGCC numbers and ACh release and EPP amplitude
Acquired neuromyotonia	VGKCs	Antibodies to VGKC-complex in 40% lead to increased and spontaneous ACh release
GENETIC		
Acetylcholine receptor deficiency	AChR	Recessive mutations in AChR-subunit genes cause reduced AChR expression
Acetylcholine receptor deficiency		Recessive mutations in *RAPSYN* cause reduced anchoring of AChR on the postsynaptic membrane, or in *DOK-7* cause a synaptopathy
AChR kinetic abnormalities	AChR	Dominant or recessive mutations in AChR-subunit genes cause kinetic defects—"slow" and "fast" channel syndromes
Choline acetyltransferase deficiency	Choline acetyltransferase	Recessive mutations in the gene for choline acetyltransferase (*CHAT*) cause reduced ACh release
Acetylcholine esterase deficiency	AChE	Recessive mutations in the collagen tail (*COLQ*) that anchors AChE at the neuromuscular junction cause absence of AChE
Arthrogryposis, multiple pterygium, Escobar's syndrome	Can occur with rapsyn, δ- or γ-subunit AChR mutations	Fetal akinesia
NEUROTOXIC		
Botulism	Presynaptic ACh release	Botulinum toxin gains entry into the presynaptic motor nerve and cleaves proteins involved in ACh release mechanism
Envenomation following bites from snakes, spiders, scorpions, etc.	Varied sites of action	Neurotoxins specific for VGCCs, VGKCs, AChE, AChRs, voltage-gated sodium channels, and other targets are frequent in many animal venoms and generally inhibit function
Drugs and insecticides	Varied sites of action	Muscle relaxants and other drugs
		Many antibiotics and quinine-related drugs can alter neuromuscular transmission at high dose
		Organophosphates block AChE and have complicated acute and chronic actions

AChE = acetylcholinesterase; AChR = acetylcholine receptor; EPP = end-plate potential; MuSK = muscle-specific kinase; Lrp4 = low-density lipoprotein-related receptor protein 4; VGCC = voltage-gated calcium channel; VGKC-complex = voltage-gated potassium channel and associated proteins.

that the threshold for activation of the muscle action potential is not reached. At a severely affected end plate, this deficiency can occur at the initiation of contraction, but it is most common during repetitive activity when the end-plate potential naturally declines, despite a compensatory rise in the release of acetylcholine. This phenomenon, occurring across many end plates within a muscle, is responsible for the decrement in the amplitude of the compound

muscle action potential on repetitive nerve stimulation, a finding that is diagnostic of a disorder of neuromuscular transmission.

In myasthenia gravis, the reduced end-plate potentials result from loss of functional AChRs on the postsynaptic membrane and also from simplification of the postsynaptic folds, which contain the voltage-gated sodium channels. In most patients, these changes are caused by antibodies against the

Direct block of function
preventing ACh binding
and ion channel opening

Cross-linking of AChRs by
divalent antibodies leading to
increased internalization and
degradation

Complement-mediated lysis of
the postsynaptic membrane
leading to morphologic
damage and loss of AChRs

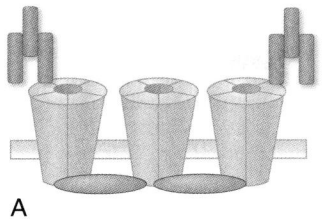
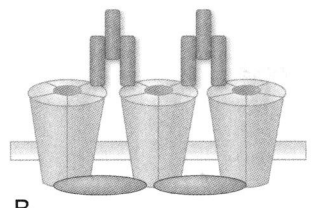
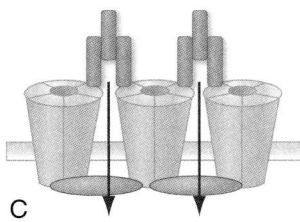

A   B   C

FIGURE 422-2. Mechanisms of loss of the acetylcholine receptor (AChR) at the neuromuscular junction. Antibodies can act (A) by directly blocking ACh binding or ion channel function; (B) by cross-linking the AChRs in the membrane, thereby leading to increased internalization and degradation; or (C) by complement-dependent lysis of the AChR-containing postsynaptic membrane. In myasthenia gravis, complement-dependent lysis is likely to be the most important mechanism overall. Interestingly, there is no evidence of complement-dependent mechanisms in either Lambert-Eaton myasthenic syndrome or acquired neuromyotonia, in which cross-linking of the respective ion channels with increased internalization seems to be the main mechanism.

AChRs. The pathophysiology in patients with antibodies to other postsynaptic proteins, such as MuSK and the low-density lipoprotein-related receptor protein 4 (Lrp4), involves different mechanisms that are not yet fully understood. Like most synapses, the neuromuscular junction is highly regulated. If the nerve is cut, leading to loss of neuromuscular transmission, the muscle responds by upregulating the expression of AChRs that revert to a fetal phenotype (see Fig. 422-1). Alternatively, if the activity of the postsynaptic muscle decreases, the motor nerve attempts to compensate. Consequently, the synthesis of AChRs in the muscle fiber and the release of acetylcholine from the motor nerve are increased in myasthenia gravis.

Pathogenesis
Myasthenia gravis is an antibody-mediated disease that is associated with other autoimmune disorders, especially thyroid disease (Chapter 226). Younger AChR antibody-positive patients have an increased prevalence of the human leukocyte antigen (HLA)-B8 and -DR3 haplotypes that are also frequently associated with autoimmunity. AChR antibodies are immunoglobulin G (IgG), have high affinity, are highly specific for the native human AChR, and act by three main mechanisms (Fig. 422-2). First, a few antibodies directly inhibit the binding of acetylcholine to the AChR, thereby causing a pharmacologic-like blockade of function.[2] Second, because of their divalence, antibodies can bind simultaneously to two adjacent AChRs, through the α-subunits that are present in duplicate in each receptor, to form AChR-antibody complexes that are internalized and degraded by the muscle fiber, thereby leading to loss of AChRs. Third, most of the antibodies are IgG1 subclass, which binds and activates complement. The result is activation of the membrane attack complex with destruction of the postsynaptic membrane and morphologic damage. All these effects are strictly limited to the neuromuscular junction; the remainder of the muscle fiber is essentially normal.

Specific antibody production requires helper T cells that can recognize AChR epitopes. The thymus gland, which is often abnormal in myasthenia, is thought to play a role in the immune response against AChR.[3] In patients with early-onset disease, the thymus is often the site of follicular hyperplasia, with T- and B-cell lymphocytic infiltrates in an expanded medulla. These infiltrates, which are very similar to the germinal centers found in lymph nodes, contain B cells that express surface immunoglobulin specific for AChRs and plasma cells that synthesize AChR antibodies. In the thymic medulla, muscle-like "myoid" cells have AChRs on their surface in both normal and myasthenic individuals; these cells may be an early target of complement and antibodies, thereby providing the antigenic stimulus responsible for chronic germinal center formation and AChR antibody production.

In late-onset myasthenia gravis and in patients with MuSK antibodies, the thymus is mostly normal for age. However, some patients without conventional AChR or MuSK antibodies have typical thymic hyperplasia and antibodies that bind to tightly clustered AChR on transfected cells.

Thymomas, which are epithelial cell tumors, occur in 10 to 15% of myasthenic patients and nearly always are associated with AChR antibodies. Thymomas associated with myasthenia gravis correspond mainly to the World Health Organization types B1 and B2 and are characterized by active thymopoiesis (i.e., the capacity to promote T-cell maturation and export). Thymoma epithelial cells express muscle antigens and AChR subunits, and they are

thought to be responsible for defective negative selection, with the export to the periphery of autoreactive T lymphocytes. Rarely, myasthenia gravis arises after removal of a thymoma.

About 40% of AChR antibody-negative patients have antibodies to MuSK, a muscle tyrosine kinase that is specifically expressed at the neuromuscular junction and plays a crucial role in the formation and maintenance of the postsynaptic membrane.[4] MuSK is activated by nerve-secreted agrin, through its coreceptor Lrp4; MuSK phosphorylation and dimerization induce an intracellular signaling cascade that leads to AChR clustering. In animal models, MuSK antibodies cause loss of AChR and reduced postsynaptic folds, as well as a lack of the normal compensatory presynaptic increase in the release of acetylcholine. However, MuSK antibodies are predominantly IgG4 and do not activate complement, so it is not yet clear how these antibodies cause the neuromuscular pathophysiology.

A small number of AChR and MuSK antibody-negative patients have serum antibodies to Lrp4.[5] Lrp4 antibodies interfere with Lrp4-agrin binding and reduce AChR expression in vitro, and their pathogenicity has been recently demonstrated in an animal model.

CLINICAL MANIFESTATIONS
Myasthenia gravis presents clinically with painless muscle weakness that increases with muscle use and improves after rest. In many patients, the weakness starts in the eye muscles, where it results in double vision and ptosis (drooping eyelids). In others, it may first affect bulbar muscles or limb muscles (Fig. 422-3). Virtually any skeletal muscle may be involved as the illness progresses. Typically, the weakness varies in distribution and severity from day to day or from week to week, and it is often worse in the evening. It may first appear following an infection. Established weakness can increase with anxiety, with infection, or with the menstrual period.

Ptosis, which is often asymmetrical, and diplopia initially can be transient and first noticed while driving, for example. Severity can range from mild unilateral ptosis or minimal diplopia to profound bilateral ptosis combined with almost complete ophthalmoplegia. Bulbar symptoms include weakness of facial muscles with difficulties in closing eyes and a "snarling" smile, difficulty in chewing, nasal or slurred speech that can noticeably deteriorate as speech continues, impaired swallowing sometimes associated with nasal regurgitation of fluids, reduced tongue movements, and head droop related to neck weakness.

Limb muscle involvement is common, and proximal muscles are usually more involved than distal. Weakness of the legs can lead to collapse when walking and can be misinterpreted as a functional (psychogenic) disorder. Weakness of elbow extension and of finger abduction may be prominent. By contrast, ankle dorsiflexion is rarely affected except in severe disease. Respiratory dysfunction is less common but can be life-threatening, especially if associated with dysphagia. Selective involvement of the diaphragm can cause severe breathlessness in the supine posture. Wasting is uncommon but can affect the facial muscles and tongue, for example, in long-standing disease. Tendon reflexes are typically brisk. Bladder disturbances are rare, and sensory symptoms do not occur.

Subtypes of Myasthenia Gravis
Several subgroups can be distinguished on the basis of clinical and pathologic criteria and can help to inform treatment.

Ocular Myasthenia Gravis

Ocular myasthenia gravis is confined to extraocular muscles; if it remains localized for at least 2 years, subsequent generalization is unlikely. AChR antibody levels are generally low and are undetectable in about 50% of patients. This subgroup rarely is associated with a thymoma. The neuromuscular junction of ocular muscles shows structural and physiologic differences from limb muscles. Ocular weakness is often the presenting symptom not only in myasthenia gravis but also in neurotoxin poisoning, for example, botulism (Chapter 296). Thus, physiologic factors or accessibility of the neuromuscular junctions of ocular muscles to circulating factors may make them particularly vulnerable to antibodies in myasthenia gravis.

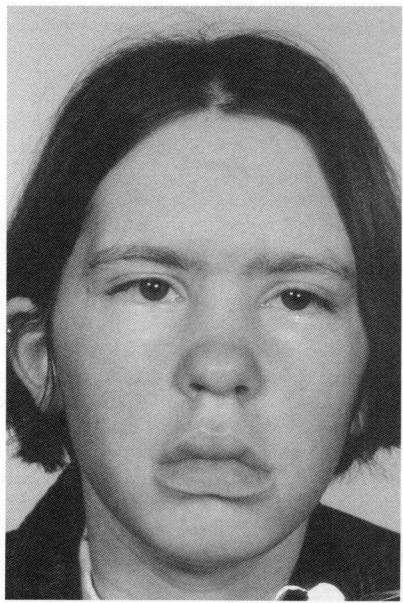

FIGURE 422-3. Marked ocular and facial muscle weakness in a young female with myasthenia gravis.

Generalized Myasthenia Gravis with Acetylcholine Receptor Antibodies

Among patients with generalized disease and AChR antibodies, there are three clinical subgroups. Early-onset myasthenia gravis is more frequent in females and associates strongly with HLA-A1, -B8, and -DR3. The thymus is generally hyperplastic. AChR antibody titers are usually high and decline to varying degrees after successful treatments, including thymectomy.

Late-onset myasthenia gravis is becoming increasingly common with the aging of the population and, when associated with bulbar weakness, may be mistaken for amyotrophic lateral sclerosis (Chapter 419) or brain stem cerebrovascular disease. Among older patients, males are more frequently affected.

Thymoma-associated myasthenia gravis is an important distinction because thymectomy or other specific tumor therapy is required. Most patients with thymomas and myasthenia gravis present between the ages of 30 and 60 years.

Myasthenia Gravis with Muscle-Specific Kinase Antibodies

About 15% of myasthenic patients with generalized symptoms do not have detectable AChR antibodies. Up to 40% of these patients have antibodies to MuSK.[6] MuSK antibodies are absent or very infrequent in patients with AChR antibodies, patients with persistent ocular symptoms, and patients with thymoma. Compared with typical myasthenia gravis, MuSK antibody-positive disease is characterized by high prevalence in younger females; predominant bulbar, neck, and respiratory muscle weakness; and an increased rate of facial and tongue muscle atrophy.

Myasthenia Gravis with Neither Acetylcholine Receptor nor Muscle-Specific Kinase Antibodies

Some patients with thymus hyperplasia and good response to treatment, including thymectomy, may have antibodies that bind only to clustered AChRs on AChR-expressing cells. A variable proportion of AChR and MuSK antibody-negative patients have Lrp4 antibodies. These antibodies have not been found associated with thymoma.

DIAGNOSIS

Diagnosis is based on the clinical features, serologic testing for specific antibodies, electromyography (EMG) and, if doubt still remains or specialized facilities are not available, the clinical response to anticholinesterase medication (Table 422-2).[7] Mediastinal imaging is needed to exclude a thymoma especially in patients with AChR antibodies.

TABLE 422-2 DIAGNOSTIC EVALUATION (EXCLUDES NEUROMYOTONIA)

	AChR MG	MuSK MG	Lrp4-MG SN-MG	NEONATAL MG	LEMS	CMS	BoTx	MM
Onset birth, recovery of muscle strength within 2 mo	–	–	–	+	–	AChR γ-subunit mutations, variable severity	–	–
Onset birth plus arthrogryposis	–	–	–	+	–	Rapsyn or AChR δ-subunit mutations	–	–
Onset at <1 yr and persistent	–	–	–	–	–	Any CMS Dok-7, rapsyn deficiency, and SCS may present later	+	+/–
Infantile apneas	–	–	–	+/–	–	Fast channel syndrome, rapsyn, or ChAT mutation		
AChR Ab positive	+	–	–	+/–	–	–	–	–
MuSK Ab positive	–	+	–	+/–	–	–	–	–
VGCC Ab positive	–	–	–	–	+	–	–	–
EMG decrement >10%	+	+/–	+/–	+	+	+	+/–	–
EMG jitter increased	+	+ Especially face muscles	+	+	+	+	+	+/–
Post-tetanic potentiation	–	–	–	–	+	–	+	–
AChE inhibitor response	+	Poor or deterioration	+	+	Often weak	Except SCS, COLQ, or DOK7 mutations	+/–	–
Thymoma	+/–	–	–	–	–	–	–	–

AChE = acetylcholinesterase; AChR = acetylcholine receptor; BoTx = botulism; ChAT = choline acetyltransferase; CMS = congenital myasthenic syndromes; Dok-7 = downstream of kinase 7; LEMS = Lambert-Eaton myasthenic syndrome; Lrp4 = low-density lipoprotein-related receptor protein 4; MG = myasthenia gravis; MM = mitochondrial myopathy; MuSK = muscle-specific kinase; SCS = slow-channel syndrome; SN = seronegative for AChR and MuSK antibodies.

If AChR antibodies are absent, especially in patients with generalized symptoms, testing for MuSK antibodies is recommended. Both AChR and MuSK antibodies are very specific, and their detection in symptomatic patients confirms the diagnosis. It is not yet clear whether testing for the rarer Lrp4 or clustered AChR antibodies, which is available in specialist centers, will prove helpful in patients with inconclusive clinical and EMG findings.

The electrophysiologic abnormality is an abnormally large decrement (>10%) in the amplitude of the compound muscle action potential on low-rate (3-Hz) repetitive nerve stimulation or increased jitter on single-fiber EMG. In patients with MuSK antibodies, EMG abnormalities may be detectable only in facial muscles. These EMG changes are not specific for myasthenia gravis but can occur in any disorder that interferes with neuromuscular transmission.

Intravenous administration of edrophonium (Tensilon), a short-acting cholinesterase inhibitor, transiently improves myasthenic weakness but requires an appropriate medical setting, including resuscitative facilities and the availability of atropine, because of the risk for adverse events and severe cholinergic reactions, including syncope. A test dose of 2 mg is given intravenously, followed 30 seconds later by 6 to 8 mg if no adverse event has occurred. The equivalent doses in children are a 20-μg/kg test dose followed by 60 to 80 μg/kg. Some patients improve sufficiently with the test dose, so it is not necessary to give the full dose. An alternative pharmacologic test in adults is a single dose of subcutaneous or intramuscular neostigmine (1 to 2.5 mg) or of oral pyridostigmine (60 mg).

Differential Diagnosis

Congenital myasthenic syndromes (see later) should be considered in patients who have clinical and EMG evidence of myasthenia but are seronegative on antibody assays. Lambert-Eaton myasthenic syndrome almost always begins with difficulty in walking; ocular symptoms are rare, and specific laboratory tests are available (see later). The ocular muscle involvement that characterizes Miller-Fisher syndrome is more rapid in onset than is usual in myasthenia gravis and is associated with GQ1b antibodies (Chapter 420). Mitochondrial myopathy may show signs that are similar to those of myasthenia gravis (e.g., asymmetrical ptosis and limitation of eye movements), and there may be increased jitter on single-fiber EMG, but this condition and oculopharyngeal dystrophy can be distinguished from myasthenia gravis by the nonfluctuating weakness and by muscle biopsy (Chapter 421). In neurasthenia and chronic fatigue syndrome (Chapter 274), the laboratory tests for myasthenia gravis are negative.

TREATMENT   Rx

Most patients with AChR antibodies respond to oral pyridostigmine, 30 to 60 mg four or five times daily; in patients with mild disease, this dose may adequately control symptoms.[8] Doses in excess of 90 mg are likely to cause gastrointestinal side effects, abdominal cramps and diarrhea, which can be controlled with oral propantheline bromide, 15 mg, or loperamide, 2 mg. Patients with MuSK antibodies generally have an unsatisfactory response.[9] In some of these patients, pyridostigmine, even at low doses, can increase weakness and cause nicotinic side effects (muscle cramps and diffuse fasciculations).

Neonatal Myasthenia Gravis
Pyridostigmine, 3 to 5 mg, can be given every 4 hours to about an hour before a feeding. Close monitoring and respiratory support in a special unit may be required.

Ocular Myasthenia
Diplopia can sometimes be helped by the use of prisms. Ocular symptoms that respond incompletely to pyridostigmine are generally improved by low-dose prednisone therapy (e.g., 5 mg every other day), increasing by 5 mg at weekly intervals either until symptoms are completely controlled or until a ceiling dose (e.g., 1 mg/kg) is reached.[10] When remission is established, the dose can be slowly reduced (e.g., by 5 mg at 2-weekly intervals) until symptoms recur and then adjusted upward to define the effective minimal dose. Full withdrawal of prednisone is usually followed by a symptomatic relapse. Thymectomy is not considered beneficial for nonthymomatous ocular myasthenia gravis. In patients who fail to respond adequately to prednisone or who are intolerant of the medication, the addition of azathioprine (2 to 2.5 mg/kg body weight) or ocular muscle surgery is an option. However, the diagnosis should be questioned in patients who show no improvement with high-dose prednisone treatment.

Thymoma
Thymoma is usually an indication for surgery, but removal of the tumor seldom improves muscle weakness. If the tumor is locally invasive, postoperative radiotherapy is indicated. If tumor spread is more extensive, chemotherapy with cisplatin-containing regimens can be considered. Thymoma-associated myasthenia gravis is generally severe, and most patients need long-term treatment with steroids and immunosuppressants (see below).[11]

Generalized Nonthymomatous Myasthenia Gravis
When generalized symptoms are inadequately controlled by pyridostigmine, thymectomy is often recommended even for patients without a thymoma, especially patients younger than age 50 years. On the basis of uncontrolled studies, thymectomy in early-onset patients with AChR antibodies appears to be associated with an increased rate of remission, and a randomized trial evaluating the efficacy of thymectomy for nonthymomatous myasthenia gravis is in progress. By comparison, thymectomy is not beneficial in patients who have MuSK antibodies and in whom the thymus is generally devoid of hyperplastic changes. As a general rule, thymectomy, even in the presence of a thymoma, should never be an emergency treatment but rather should be postponed until a stable control of myasthenic symptoms is achieved.

Immunosuppressive therapy with prednisone is usually administered in the initial phases of treatment owing to its short-latency effect.[A1] Most patients respond to alternate-day prednisone, started at a low dose (e.g., 10 mg every other day) and increasing by 5 to 10 mg per dose to 1.0 to 1.5 mg/kg. Because starting prednisone can temporarily exacerbate the disease, patients are usually best managed in the hospital, especially if they have bulbar or respiratory muscle involvement. When remission is established, the dose can be reduced by 5 to 10 mg every 2 weeks (or more slowly) to the effective minimal dose. Prophylactic treatment for osteoporosis (Chapter 243) and careful follow-up for other side effects is mandatory in all patients.

For long-term treatment, other immunosuppressive medication is required in patients who do not respond satisfactorily to prednisone or who need high maintenance doses. Because these agents have a long latency of effect, they are generally combined with prednisone (see earlier) during initial treatment and then used as monotherapy if steroids can be withdrawn or are contraindicated. Azathioprine (2.5 mg/kg/day) is the preferred treatment; compared with prednisone alone, combination treatment is better tolerated and associated with fewer relapses.[A2] Cyclosporine (3 to 5 mg/kg daily) is effective as monotherapy or combined with steroids[A3] and is frequently used as the second-choice immunosuppressant. Although the efficacy of mycophenolate mofetil in association with prednisone is questioned, this agent at the standard dose of 2000 mg/day is used in patients who are unresponsive to or intolerant of azathioprine. Tacrolimus is considered a third-line immunosuppressant.[A4] Methotrexate (5 to 15 mg weekly) has similar efficacy and safety as azathioprine as a steroid-sparing agent.[A5] When remission has been achieved, doses of these agents can be reduced slowly and cautiously; full withdrawal is likely to be followed by relapse.

Immunoglobulin infusion and plasmapheresis are equally efficacious[A6] for providing short-term improvement, typically persisting 4 to 6 weeks, and can be used in preparation for thymectomy, to cover the initiation of prednisone therapy, or to control disease exacerbations. An immunoglobulin infusion of 1 g/kg given on day 1 only is as effective as 1 g/kg given on day 1 and again on day 2. Because of the short-lived benefits of these therapies, they must be accompanied by additional immunosuppressive therapy (see earlier).

Inhibition of the production of acetylcholinesterase using a short antisense oligonucleotide was both effective and safe in a phase Ib study on AChR antibody-positive patients (a phase II study is underway). High-dose cyclophosphamide[A7] and two monoclonal antibodies, rituximab (which markedly reduces circulating B cells) and eculizumab (which binds C5 to preventing complement activation),[A8] have been used successfully in patients with refractory disease.

PROGNOSIS

The increasing use of immunosuppressive therapies, coupled with advances in critical care, has greatly improved the prognosis of myasthenia gravis. Patients with myasthenic crisis are at high risk for recurrences,[12] but many patients achieve optimal control of symptoms with a normal life expectancy. The prognosis is not as good, however, in patients with invasive thymoma, who have a 5-year survival rate of about 80%, or with invasive thymic carcinomas, who have a 5-year survival rate of only about 40%.

Lambert-Eaton Myasthenic Syndrome
DEFINITION AND EPIDEMIOLOGY

The Lambert-Eaton myasthenic syndrome, which is a rare disorder that affects all races, can occur in paraneoplastic and nonparaneoplastic forms. The incidence of the paraneoplastic form is higher, but its shorter survival results in a similar prevalence of the two types. The associated tumor is usually a small cell lung cancer (about 2% of patients with small cell lung cancer develop Lambert-Eaton myasthenic syndrome), and more rarely a lymphoma. The nonparaneoplastic form associates with HLA-A1, -B8, and -DR3, as in early-onset myasthenia gravis.

PATHOBIOLOGY

Lambert-Eaton myasthenic syndrome is an antibody-mediated presynaptic disorder characterized by a reduced number of acetylcholine quanta (vesicles) released by each nerve impulse. End-plate potentials recorded from intercostal muscle biopsies are consequently much reduced in amplitude. During high-frequency repetitive nerve stimulation, the end-plate potential amplitude increases, probably because build-up of calcium in the motor nerve terminal leads to increased release of acetylcholine. Freeze-fracture electron microscopic studies of motor nerve terminals show that the "active zone" particles, which correspond to voltage-gated calcium channels, are reduced in number and disorganized. The antibodies in Lambert-Eaton myasthenic syndrome bind to the presynaptic nerve terminal at the sites of acetylcholine release and appear to act principally by cross-linking the voltage-gated calcium channels, thereby leading to their clustering and internalization. The antibodies also interfere with transmitter release from postganglionic parasympathetic and sympathetic neurons in injected mice, providing an explanation for the autonomic dysfunction observed in many patients.

CLINICAL MANIFESTATIONS

Almost all patients present with difficulty in walking, which exhibits a rolling characteristic.[13] Weakness in ocular, bulbar, and respiratory muscles is less common than in myasthenia gravis. Weakness predominantly affects proximal muscles, which may show augmentation of strength during the first few seconds of a maximal contraction. Reflexes are absent or depressed but can increase after 10 seconds of maximal contraction of the muscle (post-tetanic potentiation). Autonomic symptoms such as dry mouth, constipation, and erectile dysfunction are present in most patients. Cerebellar ataxia may be present in association with small cell lung cancer. Patients with nonparaneoplastic Lambert-Eaton myasthenic syndrome may have other autoimmune diseases, notably vitiligo.

DIAGNOSIS

Diagnosis is based on the clinical features, on a positive serum voltage-gated calcium-channel antibody test, and on the characteristic EMG findings (see Table 422-2). Antibodies specific for the α1A (P/Q) subtype of voltage-gated calcium channels are found in 90% of patients, both with and without small cell lung cancer. Patients may not respond convincingly to intravenous edrophonium. On EMG, the amplitude of the resting compound muscle action potential is reduced. It decreases further during low-rate repetitive nerve stimulation but increases by more than 100% immediately after 10 seconds of voluntary contraction of the muscle or during high-frequency (40-Hz) nerve stimulation. Single-fiber EMG is less specific because an increased jitter does not distinguish between myasthenia gravis and Lambert-Eaton myasthenic syndrome.

On diagnosis, an extensive search for malignancy is necessary. All patients should undergo thoracic computed tomography scanning and fluorodeoxyglucose positron emission tomography (FDG-PET). If tumor screening is negative, it should be repeated periodically every 3 to 6 months for at least 2 years after the onset of neurologic symptoms.

Differential Diagnosis

Botulinum poisoning (Chapter 296) causes blockade of presynaptic transmitter release at the neuromuscular junction as well as EMG changes similar to those in the Lambert-Eaton myasthenic syndrome. Botulism is detected by finding the toxin in serum or the *Clostridium botulinum* bacteria in the wound or feces. Myopathies (Chapters 269 and 421) can mimic Lambert-Eaton myasthenic syndrome clinically, but autonomic changes do not occur, EMG findings are different, and muscle biopsy is abnormal.

TREATMENT   Rx

Plasmapheresis leads to clinical improvement within a few days in acutely ill patients, and most patients respond to immunosuppressive drugs or intravenous immunoglobulin therapy. Intravenous immunoglobulin therapy (1 g/kg for 2 days) improves strength, with an associated decline in specific

antibody.[14] Specific tumor treatment often leads to improvement of the neurologic disorder. Most patients respond to symptomatic treatment with 3,4-diaminopyridine (10 to 20 mg four times daily).[A3] However, 3,4-diaminopyridine has not yet been approved by the U.S. Food and Drug Administration, but a phosphate version of the drug has been licensed in Europe. Immunosuppressive treatment with prednisone, azathioprine, or cyclosporine may be required in patients with severe weakness, using doses similar to those prescribed for myasthenia gravis. Rituximab has been used in few patients with severe weakness.

PROGNOSIS

Prognosis mainly depends on that of the associated malignancy. Patients with paraneoplastic Lambert-Eaton myasthenic syndrome tend to have a progressive disease and a less satisfactory response to treatment.

ACQUIRED NEUROMYOTONIA

DEFINITION AND EPIDEMIOLOGY

Neuromyotonia, or Isaacs' syndrome, is a rare disorder primarily characterized by myokymia (spontaneous undulating muscle contractions) that can be intermittent or continuous and may be present during sleep or general anesthesia. It results from the hyperexcitability of motor nerves. A milder variant, the cramp-fasciculation syndrome, is more common.

PATHOBIOLOGY

Neuromyotonia may be associated with other autoimmune diseases or other autoantibodies, and cerebrospinal fluid analysis may show oligoclonal bands. In about 15% of patients, it is paraneoplastic, usually associated with thymoma and more rarely with lung cancer. Occasionally, neuromyotonia follows infection or allergic reactions, and it may improve spontaneously within weeks to months in these cases.

In neuromyotonia, peripheral nerve hyperexcitability is caused by dysfunction of voltage-gated potassium channel (Kv1), whose activation within milliseconds of nerve depolarization limits the depolarizing afterpotential and prevents the generation of repetitive discharges. In autoimmune neuromyotonia, pathogenic antibodies may induce loss of voltage-gated potassium channels and are often directed against contactin-associated protein-2, which is required for clustering Kv1 channels at the juxtaparanodal regions.

CLINICAL MANIFESTATIONS

The clinical presentation is variable but can include muscle stiffness, cramps, myokymia, fasciculations, pseudomyotonia (e.g., failure to relax after fist clenching), and weakness. Increased sweating is common. In the cramp-fasciculation syndrome, symptoms are milder and mostly induced by exertion. Some patients have sensory symptoms, including neuropathic-type pain, or less severe paresthesias, dysesthesia, and numbness, and a few have autonomic and central nervous system features of an encephalopathy, with insomnia, hallucinations, delusions, and mood change (Morvan's syndrome).

DIAGNOSIS

EMG shows spontaneous motor unit discharges: distinctive doublet, triplet, or multiplet bursts with high intraburst frequency (40 to 300 per second), longer continuous bursts, and postactivation contraction. The abnormal muscle activity may be generated at different sites throughout the length of the nerve but is usually distal. Many patients have serum antibodies to the voltage-gated potassium channel-complex (Kv1 channel and associated proteins), predominantly to contactin-associated protein-2.[15] The differential diagnosis includes neuromyotonia caused by acquired and inherited neuropathies and neuromyotonia—usually associated with episodic ataxia—caused by voltage-gated potassium-channel gene mutations (Kv1.1).

TREATMENT AND PROGNOSIS   Rx

Neuromyotonia can be improved by anticonvulsant drugs, such as carbamazepine (up to 800 to 1000 mg daily), phenytoin (up to 300 mg daily), or lamotrigine (up to 100 mg daily), that depress sodium channel function and reduce the hyperexcitability of nerves. Plasmapheresis and intravenous immunoglobulins, using the same regimen as for myasthenia gravis, may be followed by short-term improvement. Immunosuppressive medications (as for myasthenia gravis) are effective in some patients. Neuromyotonia is often a monophasic disease that can be successfully managed with symptomatic and immunodulating treatment. When it is associated with myasthenia gravis, the administration of pyridostigmine can increase symptoms of motor nerve hyperexcitability. Prognosis is less favorable in cases with central nervous system involvement, which may be associated with invasive thymomas.

GENETIC MYASTHENIC SYNDROMES

Congenital myasthenic syndromes (see Table 422-1) are inherited disorders that result from mutations in genes encoding key proteins at the neuromuscular junction. In the United Kingdom, their prevalence is at least 6 per 1 million population.

PATHOBIOLOGY

Congenital myasthenic syndromes are classified by the site of the mutated protein: presynaptic, synaptic, or postsynaptic. Postsynaptic disorders are more frequent and most commonly involve the AChR ε-subunit gene, in which single nucleotide missense substitutions or frameshift mutations result in complete loss of function of the AChR ε-subunit. Because this subunit replaces the AChR γ-subunit around the time of birth, infants are normal in development but show weakness during late pregnancy and in the neonatal period. Survival depends on the continued expression of the γ-subunit. By contrast, null mutations in non-epsilon subunits are probably lethal. AChR deficiency can also result from defects in the gene for rapsyn, a cytoplasmic protein required for the clustering of the AChRs at the neuromuscular junction. Single-nucleotide changes in genes for any of the AChR subunits can affect affinity for acetylcholine and gating efficiency, thereby leading to kinetic defects. In the fast-channel syndrome (recessive), AChR openings are abnormally brief, whereas the opposite occurs in the slow-channel syndrome (dominant), in which the channel opens for prolonged periods, thereby resulting in subsynaptic accumulation of cations and degenerative changes with loss of AChR.

Mutations in the *COLQ* gene, which gives rise to the collagen tail that anchors acetylcholinesterase in the synaptic cleft, are less common. The absence of acetylcholinesterase is responsible for reduced quantal release and for continuous exposure of the postsynaptic membrane to acetylcholine, thereby leading to cation overload and junctional fold degeneration. Mutations in choline acetyltransferase, the enzyme responsible for the synthesis of acetylcholine, do not always lead to dysfunction at rest; during repetitive activity, however, the amount of acetylcholine in each packet decreases, with consequent failure of neuromuscular transmission. Mutations in *DOK7* cause a "synaptopathy" with small, simplified neuromuscular junctions. Dok-7 binds MuSK, and the mutations are thought to impair the signaling that maintains the synaptic structure. Other gene mutations are less common (see Table 422-1).

CLINICAL MANIFESTATIONS

Clinical manifestations may vary from death in utero in severe cases to mild symptoms that present in adulthood.[16] Although most cases present in infancy with ptosis, hypotonia, and difficulties with feeding and breathing, the slightly different patterns of muscle weakness provide clues that point to which gene is involved. Arthrogryposis multiplex congenita, indicative of fetal akinesia, occurs with rapsyn mutations. Life-threatening episodic apnea can occur with mutations in choline acetyltransferase or rapsyn or in fast-channel syndromes. Severe ophthalmoplegia occurs in end-plate acetylcholinesterase deficiency, AChR deficiency due to AChR subunit mutations, and fast-channel syndromes, but is rarely seen in the other genetic syndromes. Motor symptoms with *DOK7* mutations usually appear at about 2 years of age after the child first learns to walk and are characterized by a limb-girdle weakness associated with ptosis and by facial and bulbar muscle involvement.

 DIAGNOSIS

A congenital myasthenic syndrome should be considered when symptoms are evident at birth or during early infancy and other relatives are affected. However, a negative family history does not exclude the diagnosis, and the onset can be later in the slow-channel syndrome, rapsyn, and *DOK7* mutations.

Impaired neuromuscular transmission can be detected by a decremental response on repetitive nerve stimulation and increased jitter on single-fiber EMG. In the slow-channel and acetylcholinesterase deficiency syndromes, the prolonged end-plate potential outlasts the refractory period of the muscle fiber, and a single nerve stimulus can be followed by a repetitive compound muscle action potential (double response) (see Table 422-2). Genetic analysis is essential to confirm the diagnosis and help in treatment, prognosis, and counseling, although the faulty gene has not been identified in many families.

The principal differential diagnoses are spinal muscular atrophy, infant botulism, hereditary neuropathies, and congenital myopathies or muscular dystrophies. Onset in early childhood, adolescence, or adulthood may lead to the incorrect diagnosis of seronegative myasthenia gravis.

 TREATMENT AND PROGNOSIS   Rx

Many of the congenital myasthenic syndromes respond to acetylcholinesterase inhibitors, as used for myasthenia gravis, and to 3,4-diaminopyridine (1 mg/kg/day in four divided doses). Patients with the slow-channel syndrome respond to quinidine (at doses corresponding to serum levels of 1 to 2.5 mg/L) or to fluoxetine (60 to 100 mg/day in adults though some patients may respond to doses as low as 20 mg), but the use of fluoxetine in children or adolescents requires psychiatric supervision. For syndromes in which the neuromuscular junction is destabilized or there are degenerative changes, such as for Dok-7 or end-plate acetylcholinesterase deficiency, treatment with ephedrine (45 to 100 mg/day in adults, 3 mg/kg/day in children) or salbutamol (0.5 to 4 mg, three times a day) can be remarkably effective. The beneficial effects of this treatment are not seen immediately but build up over a period of 6 months or more.

Although congenital disorders can be fatal during infancy, usually because of apneic episodes during infections, most tend to be nonprogressive or even may improve during adolescence or adult life. The exceptions are the slow-channel syndrome and acetylcholinesterase deficiency, which, owing to the excess AChR activations, can be associated with end-plate progressive degenerative changes, although this risk is largely mitigated with treatment.

 Grade A References

A1. Schneider-Gold C, Gajdos P, Toyka KV, et al. Corticosteroids for myasthenia gravis. *Cochrane Database Syst Rev.* 2005;2:CD002828.
A2. Palace J, Newsom-Davis J, Lecky B. A randomized double-blind trial of prednisolone alone or with azathioprine in myasthenia gravis. Myasthenia Gravis Study Group. *Neurology.* 1998;50: 1778-1783.
A3. Hart IK, Sathasivam S, Sharshar T. Immunosuppressive agents for myasthenia gravis. *Cochrane Database Syst Rev.* 2007;4:CD005224.
A4. Nagane Y, Utsugisawa K, Obara D, et al. Efficacy of low-dose FK506 in the treatment of myasthenia gravis: a randomized pilot study. *Eur Neurol.* 2005;53:146-150.
A5. Heckmann JM, Rawoot A, Bateman K, et al. A single-blinded trial of methotrexate versus azathioprine as steroid-sparing agents in generalized myasthenia gravis. *BMC Neurol.* 2011;11:97.
A6. Gajdos P, Chevret S, Toyka KV. Intravenous immunoglobulin for myasthenia gravis. *Cochrane Database Syst Rev.* 2012;12:CD002277.
A7. De Feo LG, Schottlender J, Martelli NA, et al. Use of intravenous pulsed cyclophosphamide in severe, generalized myasthenia gravis. *Muscle Nerve.* 2002;26:31-36.
A8. Howard JF Jr, Barohn RJ, Cutter GR, et al. A randomized, double-blind, placebo-controlled phase II study of eculizumab in patients with refractory generalized myasthenia gravis. *Muscle Nerve.* 2013;48:76-84.
A9. Keogh M, Sedehizadeh S, Maddison P. Treatment for Lambert-Eaton myasthenic syndrome. *Cochrane Database Syst Rev.* 2011;2:CD003279.

GENERAL REFERENCES

For the General References and other additional features, please visit Expert Consult at https://expertconsult.inkling.com.

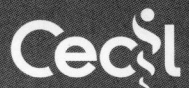

XXVI

EYE, EAR, NOSE, AND THROAT DISEASES

423

DISEASES OF THE VISUAL SYSTEM

MYRON YANOFF AND J. DOUGLAS CAMERON

The eye is a compact, complicated structure (Fig. 423-1) that is remarkably stable throughout life. Once the growth of the eye is complete, at approximately age 3 years, the structure of the eye changes very little for the next 60 to 80 years.

The eyelids physically protect the eye. The pathway of light through the eye, termed the *visual axis,* is transparent and contains no opaque structures such as blood vessels. Light passes through the tear film, cornea, intraocular aqueous, crystalline lens, vitreous, and retina, all of which, except for the crystalline lens, remain essentially transparent throughout life. Delicate intraocular structures are protected by a tough collagenous "eye wall" composed of the cornea and sclera. The optic nerve, which is composed of axons from the retinal ganglion cells, is supported by dura, arachnoid, and pia mater, which are contiguous with the brain. The optic nerve is long enough to allow free excursions of the eye through a 100-degree arc under the influence of six coordinated and critically placed rectus muscles. All these functional components are housed in a bony cavity, the orbit, which protects the eye from external injury.

The eyelid skin, only loosely connected to underlying structures, is among the thinnest of the body. The eyelid is unique because it contains the highest density of sebaceous glands in the body. These meibomian glands produce a sebaceous (lipid) material that is the principal evaporation retardant for the tear film. Malorientation of the eyelid margin or malorientation of the cilia (trichiasis) may cause extensive scarring of the anterior surface of the cornea, even to the point of blindness. The eyelid is opened by contraction of the levator muscle. The tendon of the levator tends to degenerate over time to produce mechanical ptosis. The soft tissue of the eyelid is separated from the soft tissue of the orbit by the orbital septum, a major collagenous barrier that protects intraorbital soft tissue from extension of preseptal eyelid inflammation. Extension of inflammation from preseptal cellulitis or ethmoiditis may cause septic optic neuropathy or cavernous sinus thrombosis. The elastic tissue supporting the skin of the anterior eyelid is reduced over time, thereby causing dermatochalasis ("baggy eyelids"). Redundant tissue may be sufficient in quantity to restrict the visual field, particularly superiorly.

The conjunctiva is a mucous membrane covered by stratified, nonkeratinizing squamous epithelium containing goblet cells. The epithelium is supported by delicate fibrovascular tissue that contains lymphatic channels. Squamous carcinoma or malignant melanoma originating in the conjunctiva may extend through these channels to regional lymph nodes or beyond. The conjunctival epithelium contains melanocytes. Immune processing cells are present in the epithelium (Langerhans cells) and in the stroma as collections of non-nodal B and T lymphocytes. Non-nodal primary lymphomas, which tend to have an indolent course in this location, may arise from this tissue. The aqueous portion of tears is formed constantly by accessory lacrimal glands in the conjunctiva and eyelid soft tissue as well as by reflex action from the lacrimal gland. Symptoms of itching and burning, as well as periodic disturbance of vision, may result from inadequacies of the tear film layer.

Tears drain through puncta at the nasal eyelid margin through the nasolacrimal duct to exits in the nasal cavity inferior to the inferior turbinate. The epithelium of the nasolacrimal duct also contains melanocytes and is supported by a resting lymphocyte population. Neoplasms including lymphoma, concretions (dacryoliths), and tissue injury from trauma may occlude the puncta in adults.

The cornea is avascular and lined both anteriorly and posteriorly by surface cells. Lack of an adequate tear film (dry eye syndrome) may seriously alter the ability of the cornea to transmit light, thereby affecting visual acuity. The posterior cellular lining of the cornea is a single layer of highly modified corneal endothelial cells that maintain tissue dehydration. Lack of effective pumping by the endothelial cells will allow excess hydration of the corneal stroma, that is, corneal edema. The corneal stroma is particularly sensitive to proteolysis from collagenases found with certain inflammatory conditions, such as herpes simplex keratitis. The cumulative effect of multiple episodes may be corneal thinning and possible perforation of the cornea.

Intraocular pressure is measured by applanation tomography. The amount of pressure necessary to flatten the central cornea is proportional to the intraocular pressure.

The anterior chamber is bounded by the posterior surface of the cornea, the anterior surface of the iris, and the anterior surface of the crystalline lens within the pupillary space. Aqueous material normally flows from the posterior chamber into the anterior chamber through the pupil and exits into the general circulation through the trabecular meshwork. Most causes of pathologically increased intraocular pressure and optic nerve damage (i.e. glaucoma) are due to abnormalities of filtration through the trabecular meshwork. The posterior chamber is bounded by the posterior surface of the iris, the ciliary body circumferentially, and the anterior surface of the vitreous. The crystalline lens is located entirely in the posterior chamber.

The anterior segment is composed of the cornea and the anterior and posterior chambers. Most of the anterior segment is derived from the skin and neural crest tissue. The posterior segment is the remainder of the eye. Most of the posterior segment structures are derived from the central nervous system and neural crest tissue.

When first formed, the crystalline lens is a totally cellular structure bounded by a true basement membrane. Throughout life, the new cells that are continuously added from the outer layer epithelial cells compress the central cells, thereby resulting in cell degeneration in the central core (nucleus). The lens doubles in volume from birth to age 70 years at the cost of both pliability (presbyopia) and clarity (cataract). The lens is suspended in the posterior chamber by fibers (zonules) attached to the ciliary body.

The ciliary body is the posterior extent of the iris. Its surface cells produce aqueous, and its muscles function in accommodation.

The vitreous is composed primarily of water and type II collagen. The vitreous makes up the majority of the volume and weight of the eye. It functions as a biochemical sink as well as to maintain neural retinal attachment. With time, the vitreous shrinks and separates from the retina (posterior vitreous detachment). Condensed and displaced vitreous casts a shadow on the retina, which is perceived by the patient as "floaters."

The retina is the site of photochemical conversion of light to electrical energy. Ganglion cells and their axons in the internal retina aggregate at the optic disc to form the optic nerve. Only the inner half of the retina is supplied by intraretinal vessels that are seen by ophthalmoscopy. The outer half of the retina is supplied by large-caliber capillary vessels in the choroid (the choriocapillaris). Only a 500-μm area of the posterior retina, the central macula (about 3 to 5% of the total retina), has the ability to resolve images to 20/20. The remainder of the retina has much less sensitive image resolution. Extensive biochemical support and control of stray light are performed by the retinal pigment epithelium located between the choriocapillaris and the photoreceptor outer segments. The blood-retinal barrier, which protects the biochemical integrity of the retina, is composed of anatomic attachments between neighboring retinal pigment epithelial cells, as well as attachments between vascular endothelial cells of the retinal circulation. The retina is held in place by physiologic forces that may be compromised by holes in the retina (rhegmatogenous retinal detachment) or by fluid accumulating in the subretinal space (serous retinal detachment).

The optic nerve is composed of approximately 1 million axons from retinal ganglion cells. Axons are separated into bundles by pial septa, which are in turn enclosed in an arachnoid layer. The dura is contiguous with the posterior sclera and the periosteum of the optic canal. Delicate vessels extending from the dura across the arachnoid to the pial septa supply the optic nerve. The central retinal artery is present in the axial layer of the optic nerve near the eye but does not supply blood to the optic nerve itself. The optic nerve axons travel through a collagenous sieve in the plane of the posterior sclera, the lamina cribrosa. The choroid is that portion of the uveal tract external to the retina. This layer is composed of various calibers of blood vessels that ultimately supply blood for the choriocapillaris. There are no lymphatic channels in the choroid.

The sclera is composed of dense, relatively disorganized collagen. It is opaque because of the nonhomogeneous structure of the collagen and the degree of hydration relative to the cornea. There are multiple scleral ostia for arteries, veins, and nerves, both posteriorly and anteriorly.

The orbit is composed of bones of the facial skeleton. Sutures between major bones exist in the superior nasal and superior temporal quadrants. Multiple vessels and nerves extend through the thin ethmoid bone from nasal sinus tissue medially. The orbital floor is poorly supported over the maxillary sinus and may rupture with increased intraorbital pressure. The nasolacrimal duct travels through a portion of the lacrimal bone. Portions of the sphenoid

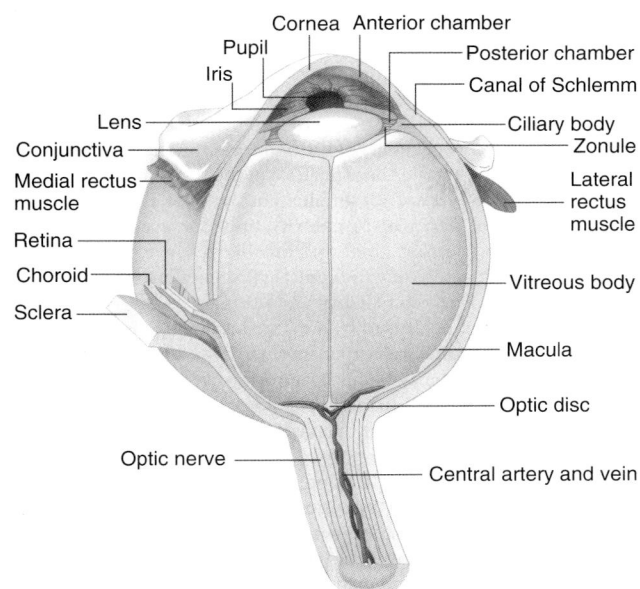

FIGURE 423-1. Anatomy of the eye.

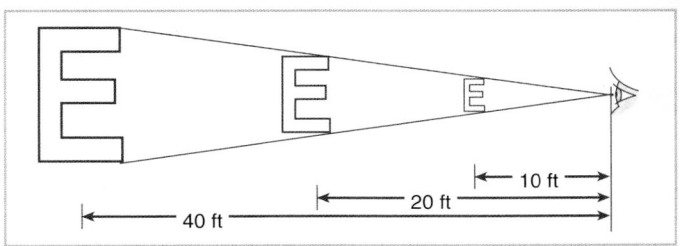

FIGURE 423-2. Snellen visual acuity. The most common test for visual acuity measures the eye's ability to resolve linear images at a test distance of 20 feet, approximating infinity (parallel rays of light). A 20/20 E subtends 5 minutes of arc at a distance of 20 feet, with each segment of the E subtending 1 minute of arc. The larger letters (e.g., 20/30, 20/40) are determined by the distance at which they subtend an angle of 5 minutes. Thus, an E that subtends 5 minutes at 40 feet, if viewed clearly at 20 feet, indicates 20/40 visual acuity.

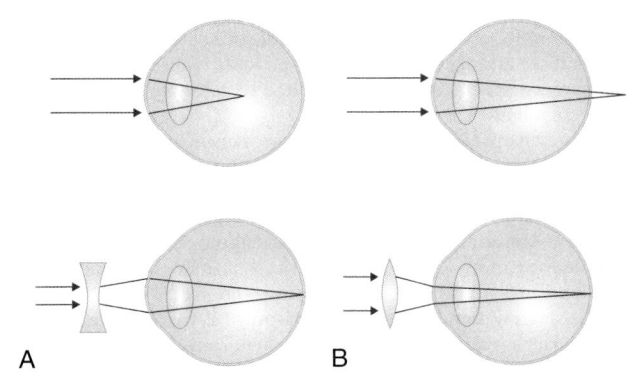

FIGURE 423-3. Myopia/hyperopia. A, In the myopic eye, parallel rays of light are focused anterior to the retina. A divergent lens can be used to compensate for the mismatch between refracting power and axial length. B, The hyperopic eye requires the additional power of a convergent lens to bring images into focus on the retina.

bone protect the optic nerve. Major cranial nerves travel through the adjacent superior orbital fissure, also a portion of the sphenoid bone. There is no normal lymphoid tissue in the orbit outside of the lacrimal gland. The rectus muscle may be enlarged by inflammation in thyroid eye disease, but the tendinous insertion into the sclera is not inflamed early in the course of the disease.

CLINICAL MANIFESTATIONS AND DIAGNOSIS

Patients may present with complaints of diminished vision, eye pain, red eyes, or pain around the eye. The causes may be primarily ophthalmic (e.g., cataract) or systemic (e.g., diabetic retinopathy). A comprehensive ophthalmologic examination also should evaluate for possible asymptomatic local (e.g., choroidal melanoma) or systemic (e.g., hypertensive retinopathy) abnormalities in patients with normal acuity and no subjective complaints.

Functional Evaluation

The most objective and common measure of ocular function is line letter acuity, with normal vision (Table 423-1) defined as the ability to see at 20 feet what a normal person sees at 20 feet (Fig. 423-2). Less than 20/20 vision can be caused by an abnormality anywhere from the tear film to the visual cortex of the occipital lobe (see Fig. 423-1). However, normal vision also includes other functions, such as the perception of color, motion, contrast, brightness, field, and depth, for which there is greater variation among individuals and no universally adopted, standardized scales. Normal visual acuity is potentially achievable in essentially all individuals, either naturally or with visual correction.

Correction of vision is based on the refraction of light (Fig. 423-3). The diopter (D) is the unit of measurement of the ability of an optical system to refract (bend) light. The normal human eye has the refractive capacity of approximately 60 D. If the eye is too short, light will be focused behind the eye (hyperopia). If the eye is too long, light will be focused in the vitreous in front the retina (myopia). Normally, a person can voluntarily control the crystalline lens, alternating between near and distant tasks. At approximately age 45 years, the lens becomes stiff, and the eye becomes set for distance (presbyopia). Refraction is the method of determining the amount of optical correction (strength of glasses) needed to establish 20/20 (6/6) vision.

Examination of pupillary response assesses whether neural function is intact (see Figs. 424-2 and 424-4). Confrontational visual field testing (see Fig. 424-1 in Chapter 424) should be performed in each eye to detect gross quadrantic defects. Extraocular motility should be assessed to exclude nerve or muscle abnormalities (see Table 424-4). Color vision testing plates are a sensitive indicator of optic nerve function.

Diagnostic testing during a routine eye examination also includes external examination of the lids and adnexa, applanation tonometry to determine intraocular pressure, biomicroscopy (slit lamp examination) of the anterior

TABLE 423-1	VISUAL ACUITIES REQUIRED FOR COMMON DAILY TASKS
20/20	Physiologic vision
20/30-20/100	Driver's license, varies by state
20/50	Newspaper print
20/70	Large-print *Reader's Digest*
20/100	Write a check
20/200	Legally blind
20/400	Paper currency

segment, and ophthalmoscopic examination of the ocular fundus. Other office tests when indicated include exophthalmometry (measurement of proptosis), visual field and electrophysiologic testing, and vascular imaging (fluorescein angiography, mainly in diabetic patients; ocular computed tomography [OCT] to investigate retinal macular disease); and corneal topography.

The conjunctiva, cornea, lens, and anterior chamber are evaluated using a slit lamp. The slit lamp is composed of a binocular microscope with variable magnification (40× and 80×) in conjunction with adjustable light sources. An increased concentration of protein can be detected in the anterior chamber because of the Tyndall (flare) effect, indicating vascular incompetence associated with either inflammation or ischemia. Even individual inflammatory cells can be resolved with the slit lamp. A cobalt blue filter can be used to detect fluorescein dye that accumulates in regions of abnormal epithelium (dendrite of herpes simplex keratitis or a corneal abrasion). The slit beam is used to examine the crystalline lens to determine the depth of the anterior chamber and the degree of opacification from a cataract. By using a green filter with the 90-D lens, the retinal vessels and retinal vascular abnormalities such as microaneurysm can be seen at relatively high magnification.

COMMON CLINICAL CONDITIONS
Chronic Abnormal Vision

MYOPIA

Nearsightedness (myopia; see Fig. 423-3) is usually discovered during childhood when children cannot perform distant tasks during school (reading the blackboard) or during school screening. Myopia usually progresses until the eye is fully developed, typically by age 20 to 25 years. Rapidly progressing myopia during childhood or at any time after age 25 years requires evaluation for juvenile glaucoma, diabetes mellitus (reversible metabolic changes in the crystalline lens), trauma (development of a cataract), or use of corticosteroids (development of a cataract). Myopia is usually fully correctable with glasses. Laser in situ keratomileusis (LASIK) is one of the refractive surgical procedures that may be used in adults to correct myopia and other refractive errors, with 95% of patients achieving visual acuity of 20/40 or better.[A1] Complications of LASIK include glare symptoms, dry eye, and undercorrection or overcorrection. Rare but serious complications include epithelial ingrowth, diffuse keratitis, and flap dislocation. In patients who undergo subsequent cataract surgery, special attention is needed to calculate the parameters for the intraocular lens.

Pathologic myopia is a heritable condition causing progressive weakening of the posterior sclera and resulting increases in the axial length of the eye. The posterior radius of curvature of the eye increases (posterior staphyloma). The refractive error is usually above −8 D and may be as high as −20 D in severe cases. Abnormal physical forces in pathologic myopia may lead to retinal hole formation, retinal detachment, or intraocular hemorrhage. The primary abnormality leading to loss of vision is choroidal neovascularization. Associated systemic conditions include trisomy 21, Cornelia de Lange's syndrome, Stickler's syndrome, and Marfan syndrome. Clinical surveillance must be maintained to watch for treatable complications such as retinal detachment. Pathologic myopia is usually treated with spectacles or contact lenses. Refractive procedures are less successful in pathologic myopia because of the severity of the refractive errors and the presence of posterior segment abnormalities. Surgical and laser procedures may be required to treat retinal and choroidal lesions (e.g., subretinal neovascularization).

HYPEROPIA

In hyperopia (farsightedness; see Fig. 423-3), in contrast to myopia, the eye tends to have a shorter than average axial length. Compensatory mechanisms of the crystalline lens may functionally correct small degrees of hyperopia until age 40 years, when the crystalline lens loses its pliability. The 40-year-old hyperopic changes from latent to manifest hyperopia simultaneously. The initial pair of glasses may have to correct for both distance and near tasks (bifocals). Refractive surgical procedures can correct up to 5 D of hyperopia.

ASTIGMATISM

Astigmatism usually is the result of irregularities in the radius of curvature of the cornea. Astigmatism is not a pathologic state, but rather a variation in anatomy; most people have some degree of astigmatism. Trauma to the cornea can cause alteration of structure, leading to irregular astigmatism. Symptoms are predominantly blurry vision and difficulty seeing fine detail. Regular astigmatism can be corrected with spectacle lenses or with rigid contact lenses, whereas irregular astigmatism requires rigid contact lenses. Some forms of astigmatism can also be corrected with laser ablation of the cornea.[1]

KERATOCONUS

Keratoconus is an acquired irregularity of corneal curvature; its cause is controversial but probably at least partly genetic. Onset generally is during adolescence, and the process often evolves over 5 years or so. The prevalence in the United States appears to be about 55 cases per 100,000 people but is probably greater when subclinical cases diagnosed by computerized videokeratography are considered.

Patients with keratoconus typically have astigmatism, which may be severe. The condition is usually bilateral but not symmetrical. Mild degrees of keratoconus can be corrected with glasses or contact lenses. Corneal collagen cross-linking can provide a sustained improvement in vision.[A2] For severe cases, corneal transplantation (graft) often is very successful.[2]

STRABISMUS

The control of simultaneous orientation of the two eyes to ensure that the visual axes of both eyes are aligned is not complete until several years following birth. Misalignments of the two eyes (strabismus) may be the result of abnormalities in the central nuclei of the brain, malfunction of one or several peripheral nerves, or intrinsic abnormalities of the rectus or oblique muscles (see Fig. 424-6). If the eyes are not simultaneously stimulated with the images of the same degree of clarity or complexity, only one eye will develop normally. The image processing ability of the blurred eye will not develop (amblyopia). In most cases, only the central vision is affected. The peripheral vision in both eyes is likely to be equal and normal.

Amblyopia also may be caused by a marked difference in refractive error between the two eyes (anisometropic amblyopia) or eyelid ptosis (deprivational amblyopia). Ptosis may be neurogenic or mechanical (e.g., congenital eyelid hemangioma). To avoid amblyopia, it is extremely important to refer a child with strabismus to an ophthalmologist as soon as the strabismus is noted.

Treatment options include patching or atropine eye drops, which are equally effective in providing good vision if patients are treated before age 7 years.[3] The outcome of treatment is more favorable if amblyopia is detected before age 2 to 3 years but may be successful into the teenage years.

Esotropia is deviation of one or both eyes inward. Esotropia may not be clinically evident until the child is 3 to 4 months of age. Delay in facial maturation (underdeveloped nasal bridge) may give the appearance of esotropia, even though the visual axes are correctly aligned. In true strabismus, the light reflex will be in the center of one cornea and decentered in the other.

Exotropia is deviation of one or both eyes outward. Exotropia tends to be intermittent and less likely to result in amblyopia.

Both esotropia and exotropia may be treated by using appropriate corrections of refractive error with glasses (occasionally bifocals). Occasionally extraocular muscle surgery is necessary to correct alignment. To allow the second eye to develop to its full potential, amblyopia is corrected by occluding the stronger eye with a patch or by pharmacologically occluding (blurring) the better eye with atropine. Success is directly related to compliance.

DIPLOPIA (DOUBLE VISION)

Acute onset of diplopia is an ominous sign suggestive of a third nerve palsy (Chapter 424). Diplopia of any kind is an intolerable symptom, but vertical diplopia is less tolerated than horizontal diplopia.

COLOR VISION CHANGE

Most cases of congenital color blindness go undetected for many years. Acquired color deficiency at any age may be caused by a cataract or optic nerve disease.

CHANGE IN VISION

If only one eye has a change in vision, the problem, such as a cataract or retinal detachment, is most likely in that eye. If both eyes have a change in vision, the problem generally is outside of the eye, such as homonymous hemianopia (Chapter 424). Improvement of near vision in middle age may be a sign of cataract ("second sight") or hyperglycemia. Transient complete unilateral or bilateral loss of vision may be caused by vascular abnormalities inside or outside of the eye (Table 423-2).

Acute Eye Abnormalities
PAIN

The most severe eye pain (Table 423-3), typically associated with a red eye, is caused by acute angle-closure glaucoma. Sharp, intermittent pain is usually caused by ocular surface abnormalities (e.g., corneal foreign body). Burning pain that clears with blinking generally relates to tear film abnormalities (dry eyes). Deep boring pain most often is associated with an ocular abnormality (e.g., uveitis).

RED EYE

A red or inflamed eye can be caused by conjunctivitis, iritis (anterior uveitis), acute glaucoma, corneal trauma, or infection (Table 423-4). Of these causes, all are typically painful, with the occasional exception of conjunctivitis.

DISTORTED VISION

Distorted vision (metamorphopsia), which is the perception that straight lines are distorted or bowed, results from macular dysfunction. Causes include fluid under the retina; exudative macular degeneration, which tends to elevate the retina; and an epiretinal membrane, which tends to contract the retina.

NIGHT BLINDNESS
Retinitis pigmentosa, vitamin A deficiency, and systemic medications such as phenothiazines can cause true night blindness, in which patients have difficulty seeing any stars in the sky on a clear night and may be unable to ambulate without assistance in a dark environment. Patients with cataracts may have difficulty driving at night because of excessive glare and visual distortion.

SENSATION OF FLASHING LIGHTS
The sudden onset of flashes in the peripheral visual field suggests a posterior vitreous detachment with resulting traction of the vitreous on the peripheral retina, sometimes with a resulting retinal tear. The flashes, which may be more pronounced in the dark and with rapid eye movement, may be associated with the sudden onset of floaters, which can indicate debris or blood in the vitreous cavity. Because a tear in the retina can lead to a retinal detachment, urgent consultation with an ophthalmologist is required.

Flashing light with a migraine (Chapter 398) is described as scintillations or zigzagging lights that march across the visual field for a few minutes or as long as 30 minutes, sometimes associated with transient visual field loss. Headache is not universal.

FLOATERS
Floaters, which are caused by small aggregates in the vitreous cavity, result from the normal aging of the vitreous. The acute onset of vitreous floaters may be associated with uveitis or with the sudden onset of bleeding in the vitreous cavity owing to diabetes or sickle cell anemia. Acute floaters, however, particularly if associated with flashing lights, may indicate a posterior vitreous detachment or a retinal tear with an impending retinal detachment. Urgent ophthalmic referral is essential.

PHOTOPHOBIA
Photophobia, particularly if associated with eye pain, redness, and decreased vision, is a symptom of uveitis or traumatic iritis. Photophobia is also typical of acute migraine and meningeal irritation. Prompt ophthalmologic referral is prudent.

HALOS AROUND LIGHTS
Patients with cataracts commonly see halos around lights, particularly when driving at night. Episodic decreased vision, redness, and halos around lights may be symptoms of impending angle-closure glaucoma. Halos also can occur as a complication of refractive eye surgery.

FOREIGN BODY SENSATION
A foreign body sensation is commonly caused by dry eyes. An entropion (Fig. 423-4) or misdirected lashes (trichiasis) also can cause a foreign body sensation. Most corneal abrasions cause severe pain, but minor corneal abrasions may be associated with a foreign body sensation rather than the severe pain that usually accompanies a more severe abrasion. An arc welder burn causes a punctate corneal keratopathy, and foreign body sensation may be a prominent symptom. A true conjunctival or corneal foreign body also may be present.

EXCESSIVE TEARING
Impairment of tear drainage can occur with an ectropion or any obstructions of the nasolacrimal drainage system. An entropion or abnormal lashes rubbing on the cornea (trichiasis) stimulate tear production.

EYELID TWITCHING
Any irritation of the conjunctiva or cornea can cause the eyelids to twitch. Occasional twitching of the lids usually is associated with stress or adrenergic stimulation. Benign essential blepharospasm is severe spasm of the lids leading to functional impairment. Multiple sclerosis (Chapter 411) also can cause lid spasm.

CONJUNCTIVITIS
Any ocular inflammation, including corneal ulcers, angle-closure glaucoma, endophthalmitis, and uveitis, can be associated with secondary

TABLE 423-2 DIFFERENTIAL DIAGNOSIS OF SUDDEN VISUAL LOSS

UNILATERAL	BILATERAL
Amaurosis fugax (carotid artery stenosis)	Eclampsia
Central retinal artery occlusion	Vertebrobasilar infarct
Occipital lobe infarct	Trauma
Temporal arteritis	
Nonarteritic anterior ischemic optic neuropathy	
Hemorrhage	
Preretinal (high altitude, Valsalva)	
Vitreous	
Aqueous (hyphema)	
Trauma	

TABLE 423-3 CAUSES OF EYE PAIN

Blepharitis	Glaucoma
Blocked tear duct	Hordeolum (stye)
Chalazion	Iritis
Conjunctivitis	Keratoconus
Corneal abrasion	Optic neuritis
Dry eyes	Scleritis
Ectropion	Trauma
Entropion	Uveitis
Foreign object	

TABLE 423-4 DIFFERENTIAL DIAGNOSIS OF COMMON CAUSES OF INFLAMED EYE*

FEATURE	ACUTE CONJUNCTIVITIS	ACUTE IRITIS[†]	ACUTE GLAUCOMA[‡]	CORNEAL TRAUMA OR INFECTION
Incidence	Extremely common	Common	Uncommon	Common
Discharge	Moderate to copious	None	None	Watery or purulent
Vision	No effect on vision	Slightly blurred	Markedly blurred	Usually blurred
Pain	None	Moderate	Severe	Moderate to severe
Conjunctival injection	Diffuse: more toward fornices	Mainly circumcorneal	Mainly circumcorneal	Mainly circumcorneal
Cornea	Clear	Usually clear	Steamy	Change in clarity related to cause
Pupil size	Normal	Small	Moderately dilated and fixed	Normal or small
Pupillary light response	Normal	Poor	None	Normal
Intraocular pressure	Normal	Normal	Elevated	Normal
Smear	Causative organisms	No organisms	No organisms	Organisms found only in corneal ulcers related to infection

*Other less common causes of red eyes include endophthalmitis, foreign body, episcleritis, and scleritis.
[†]Acute anterior uveitis.
[‡]Angle-closure glaucoma.

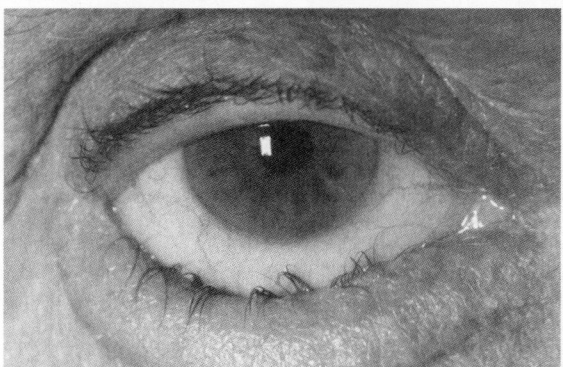

FIGURE 423-4. Involutional entropion. (From Palay DA, Krachmer JH. *Primary Care Ophthalmology,* 2nd ed. Philadelphia: Elsevier Mosby; 2005.)

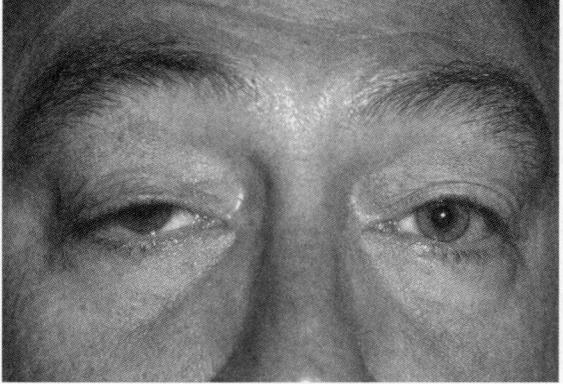

FIGURE 423-5. Ptosis of the right upper lid. (From Palay DA, Krachmer JH. *Primary Care Ophthalmology,* 2nd ed. Philadelphia: Elsevier Mosby; 2005.)

conjunctivitis. Conjunctivitis usually involves the entire conjunctiva, is associated with a discharge, and usually is not associated with pain (see Table 423-4).

PTOSIS (DROOPY EYELID)

Ptosis (Fig. 423-5) can be caused by a third nerve palsy, which usually is associated with diplopia and a reduction in elevation, depression, and medial movement of the pupil. Horner's syndrome (see Fig. 424-5) is associated with a small pupil. With myasthenia gravis (Chapter 422), other typical features of muscle weakness are usually present or can be elicited. Some patients have mild mechanical ptosis, especially after eye surgery.

PROPTOSIS (EXOPHTHALMOS)

Proptosis, or a prominent globe, can be a manifestation of thyroid abnormalities, especially Graves' disease (Chapter 226), in which proptosis is subacute and bilateral but sometimes asymmetrical (Fig. 423-6). An orbital pseudotumor can cause acute, usually unilateral proptosis, with severe pain, particularly with eye movement, and often with decreased vision. An optic nerve tumor causes chronic, unilateral proptosis associated with a slow onset of visual field loss. Acute cellulitis can be associated with unilateral proptosis, severe redness, and moderate to severe pain, commonly with sinusitis and an elevated white blood cell count.

SMALL PUPIL

A unilateral small pupil is best detected in dark conditions. Causes include Horner's syndrome, associated with ptosis on the same side; the bilaterally small, poorly reacting pupils of tertiary syphilis (Argyll Robertson pupils), which accommodate with normal constriction to a near object; miotic drops (e.g., pilocarpine); traumatic iritis; uveitis; and recent eye surgery.

LARGE PUPIL

Any α-adrenergic or anticholinergic agent placed into the eye can cause a large pupil. With eye trauma, the iris sphincter muscle can be damaged, and an abnormally large pupil can result. Tears in the iris sphincter can sometimes be appreciated on slit lamp examination. Third nerve palsy may cause a dilated pupil associated with ptosis and decreased elevation, depression, and medial eye movement. Adie's pupil (see Fig. 424-3) is an idiopathic, unilateral large pupil that is hypersensitive to weak cholinergic stimulation. Recent eye surgery, uveitis, closed-angle glaucoma, and traumatic iritis can cause a large pupil.

LEUKOKORIA

Leukokoria (white pupil) in a child is often a sign of retinoblastoma. However, any condition that changes transmission of ambient light to reflection of ambient light through the pupil may cause this sign. Some of the more common nonretinoblastoma conditions presenting with leukokoria (Table 423-5) include cataracts, retinal detachment, persistent hyperplastic primary vitreous (a developmental anomaly of the vitreous resulting in intraocular fibrosis and retinal detachment), Coats' disease (a developmental vascular malformation of the retina leading to retinal detachment), and ocular toxocariasis (a parasitic intraocular nematode infection, which leads to intraocular scarring and retinal detachment).

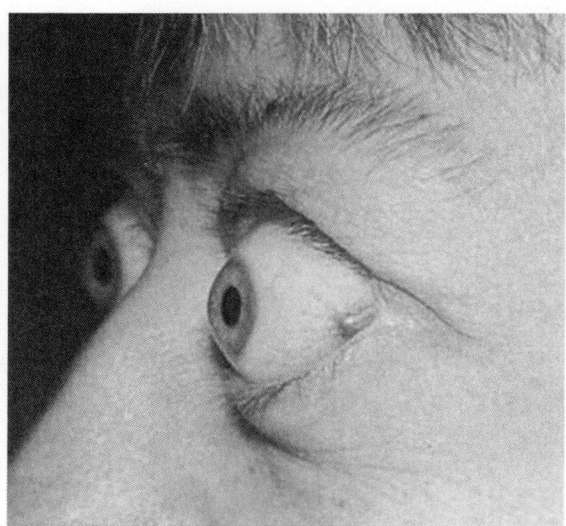

FIGURE 423-6. Graves' ophthalmopathy with characteristic exophthalmos and eyelid retraction.

TABLE 423-5 DIFFERENTIAL DIAGNOSIS OF LEUKOKORIA
Retinoblastoma
Cataract
Persistent hyperplastic primary vitreous
Retinopathy of prematurity (retrolental fibroplasia)
Coats' disease (retinal telangiectasia)
Retinal detachment
Toxocariasis
Familial exudative vitreoretinopathy (FEVR)

Eyelid Abnormalities
ECTROPION AND ENTROPION

An ectropion is an out-turning of the lower lid (Fig. 423-7), typically with the inner part of the lower end visible between the eye globe and the lid. Causes include aging, scarring, a mass on the lower lid, and seventh nerve palsy. Common symptoms include burning, itching, tearing, and the sense of a foreign body. Treatment is symptomatic, unless the underlying cause can be surgically corrected.

An entropion, which is an in-turning of the lower lid (see Fig. 423-4), is usually age-related and associated with irritation, burning, and a foreign body sensation. If it leads to trichiasis, in which the eyelashes rub or abrade the cornea, the lashes can be removed with forceps or surgery.

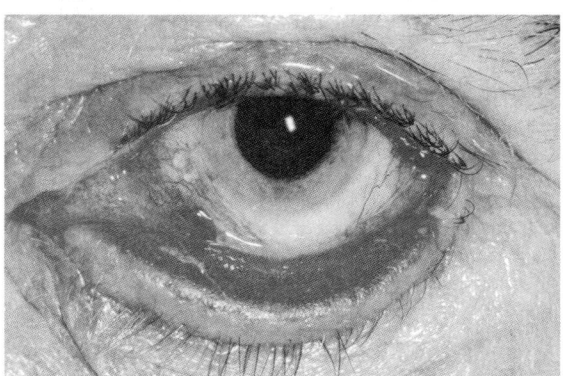

FIGURE 423-7. Involutional ectropion. (From Palay DA, Krachmer JH. *Primary Care Ophthalmology*, 2nd ed. Elsevier Mosby, Philadelphia, 2005.)

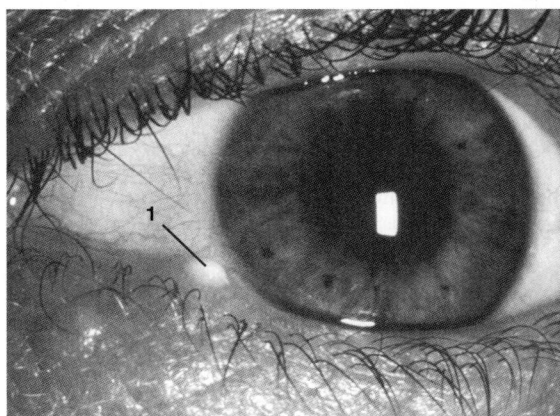

FIGURE 423-9. A lower lid stye *(1)*. (From Palay DA, Krachmer JH. *Primary Care Ophthalmology*, 2nd ed. Philadelphia: Elsevier Mosby; 2005.)

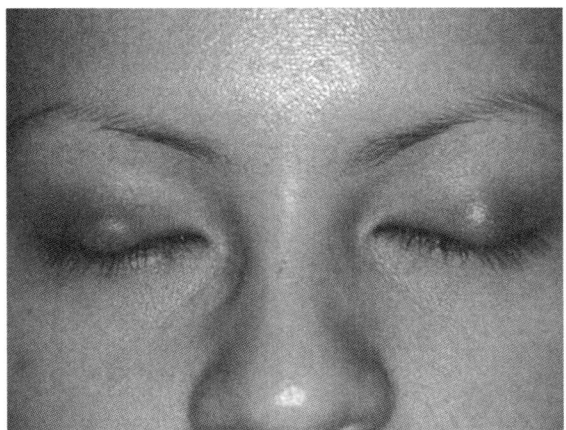

FIGURE 423-8. Bilateral chalazion in the upper eyelids.

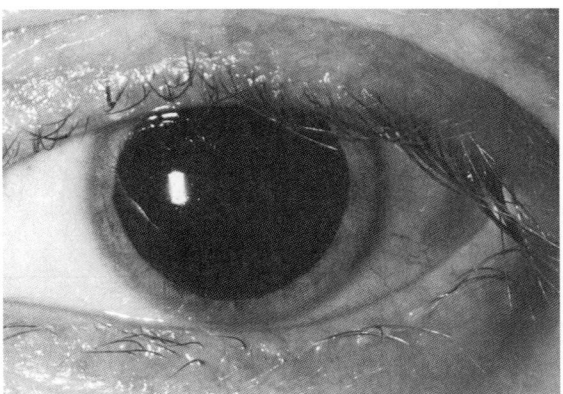

FIGURE 423-10. Staphylococcal blepharitis. The lid margins are very red and under high magnification demonstrate tiny ulcerations. (From Palay DA, Krachmer JH. *Primary Care Ophthalmology*, 2nd ed. Philadelphia: Elsevier Mosby; 2005.)

CHALAZION

A chalazion (Fig. 423-8) is a localized lipogranulomatous inflammation that results when the eyelid reacts to the contents of a ruptured sebaceous (meibomian) gland. The retained, lipid-rich sebaceous material acts as a foreign material that stimulates a lipogranulomatous foreign body inflammatory reaction. A painless or slightly tender, poorly demarcated, nonmobile nodule forms under the eyelid skin. Most lesions resolve over days to weeks with warm compresses or without specific treatment. Occasionally, an ophthalmologist may inject steroids to reduce inflammation or debulk the foreign material by incision and drainage through the tarsal conjunctiva. Some individuals may have recurrent chalazion.

HORDEOLUM (STYE)

A hordeolum (stye) (Fig. 423-9) is an extremely painful abscess in a hair or eyelash follicle or in a sebaceous gland. Styes are usually self-limited infections that respond to warm compresses and topical antibiotics (e.g., bacitracin or erythromycin ointment or moxifloxacin or gatifloxacin drops). An ophthalmologist may perform incision and drainage if symptoms do not improve within 48 hours.

BLEPHARITIS

Blepharitis (Fig. 423-10), which is a nonspecific inflammation of the eyelid skin, is common, particularly in men. The condition is usually bilateral and symmetrical. Rosacea (Chapter 439) is the most common associated cutaneous condition, and *Staphylococcus aureus* is the most common infectious agent. If untreated, blepharitis becomes chronic and may lead to corneal and conjunctival inflammation (blepharoconjunctivitis). Ophthalmic antibiotic ointment (e.g., bacitracin or erythromycin) is more efficacious than eye drops, but systemic antibiotics (e.g., minocycline, 50 to 100 mg, or doxycycline, 100 mg, once daily; tetracycline, 250 mg twice daily; or erythromycin, 250 mg three times daily) are recommended if there is any evidence of inflammation of the cornea or conjunctiva.

In seborrheic blepharitis, exfoliated keratinous debris accumulates along the eyelid margin, particularly at the follicles of the eyelashes, and irritates the conjunctiva. Treatment of this chronic condition is directed at mechanically removing the keratinous debris by scrubbing the eyelid and eyelashes daily with a mild detergent ("baby shampoo") in warm water applied with a soft cloth.

BENIGN EYELID NEOPLASMS

Skin tags, also known as squamous papillomas, are the most common benign skin lesions. Other skin lesions include seborrheic keratitis, actinic keratitis, inverted follicular keratitis, and benign lesions of the eccrine and apocrine systems. Most of these benign lesions are cured by simple excision.

SEBACEOUS CARCINOMA

Sebaceous carcinoma originates from sebaceous glands either in the tarsal plate (meibomian gland) or associated with eyelashes (glands of Zeis) and is capable of producing widespread metastasis resulting in death.[4] Muir-Torre syndrome is a syndrome of sebaceous tumors associated with visceral malignancy. Except for chronic, unilateral blepharitis, owing to the peculiar manner of spread of this tumor in the plane of the skin epithelium (pagetoid spread) without causing the formation of nodules, few symptoms occur early in the course of the disease. The tumor may progress to involve the tarsal conjunctiva, the bulbar conjunctiva, and even the corneal epithelium. A characteristic sign is regional loss of eyelashes. When the mass thickens, it may have the appearance of a chalazion, and a history of multiple chalazia in the same region of the eyelid is suggestive of sebaceous carcinoma.

Treatment is surgical removal. Surgical margins are difficult to estimate because of the intraepithelial extension of the tumor. Topical mitomycin C has been suggested as treatment for pagetoid invasion of the conjunctiva. In advanced cases, removal of the eyelids, eye, and orbital contents (exenteration) may be necessary.

BASAL CELL CARCINOMA

Basal cell carcinoma (Fig. 423-11), which originates from the basal cell layer of the epithelium, is a common cutaneous malignancy (Chapter 203). The lesion, which usually is asymptomatic, is often a well-demarcated, elevated nodule that may have a central region of ulceration and fine cutaneous vascular channels (telangiectasias). A common benign cutaneous lesion, sometimes confused clinically with basal cell carcinoma, is seborrheic keratosis (Chapter 440), which tends to be soft and appear hyperpigmented; the most common site is the lower eyelid, especially in the nasal quadrant. Basal cell carcinoma, particularly near the medial canthus, may extend posteriorly into the soft tissues of the orbit. Imaging before surgical excision for medial canthal lesions may be necessary to determine the true extent of the tumor. Basal cell carcinoma is treated by surgical excision, using Mohs' technique with intraoperative histologic evaluation to determine adequate margins of excision, if possible.[5]

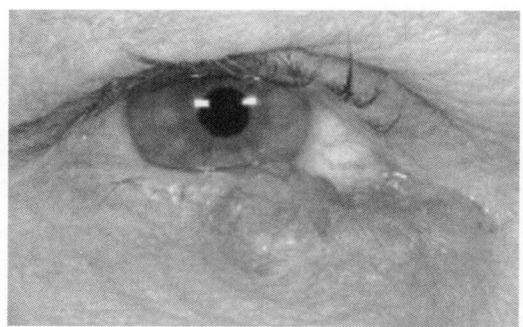

FIGURE 423-11. A typical nodular basal cell carcinoma. (From Palay DA, Krachmer JH. *Primary Care Ophthalmology*, 2nd ed. Philadelphia: Elsevier Mosby; 2005.)

Metastasis is extremely rare. With early detection and adequate excision of the local lesion, the prognosis is excellent.

EYELID SQUAMOUS CELL CARCINOMA

Eyelid squamous carcinoma, which is much less common than basal cell carcinoma, arises from the surface squamous epithelium. Ultraviolet light exposure is the major risk factor. In contrast to basal cell carcinoma, squamous cell carcinoma can metastasize, most often to regional lymph nodes. Treatment is surgical excision. Except in rare circumstances, such as in immunosuppressed patients or patients with xeroderma pigmentosa, the prognosis is excellent.

Ocular Surface Abnormalities
DRY EYES

Even minor disturbances in the tear film can cause itching, burning, pulling, and transient changes in vision. Dry eyes that cause conjunctival hyperemia without purulent discharge particularly disturb some patients. Paradoxically, decreased tearing can result in irritation and secondary increased (reflux) tearing.

Most daily tear production is not by the lacrimal gland but by small collections of lacrimal glands, mucus-producing glands, and sebaceous glands located throughout the conjunctiva, eyelid, and anterior orbital soft tissue. Over time, particularly in women, production of tear film diminishes. Because tear film production is lower during sleep, patients often note symptoms on awakening followed by slow resolution over minutes or hours. Wind and low humidity environments, such as in commercial airliners, can exacerbate symptoms. The reduction in aqueous components of tears is often associated with a compensatory increase in mucus production, which tends to blur vision until the patient blinks or uses supplemental tears. These symptoms are particularly prominent in persons who have rheumatoid arthritis (Chapter 264), Sjögren's syndrome (Chapter 268), Stevens-Johnson syndrome (Chapter 440), and ocular cicatricial pemphigoid (Fig. 423-12).

Treatment is not definitive and is rarely satisfactory. No medication increases the production of tears. Low-viscosity artificial tears (e.g., polyethylene glycol 400 0.4%), which do not tend to blur vision but have a short duration of action, are best used during visually important tasks.

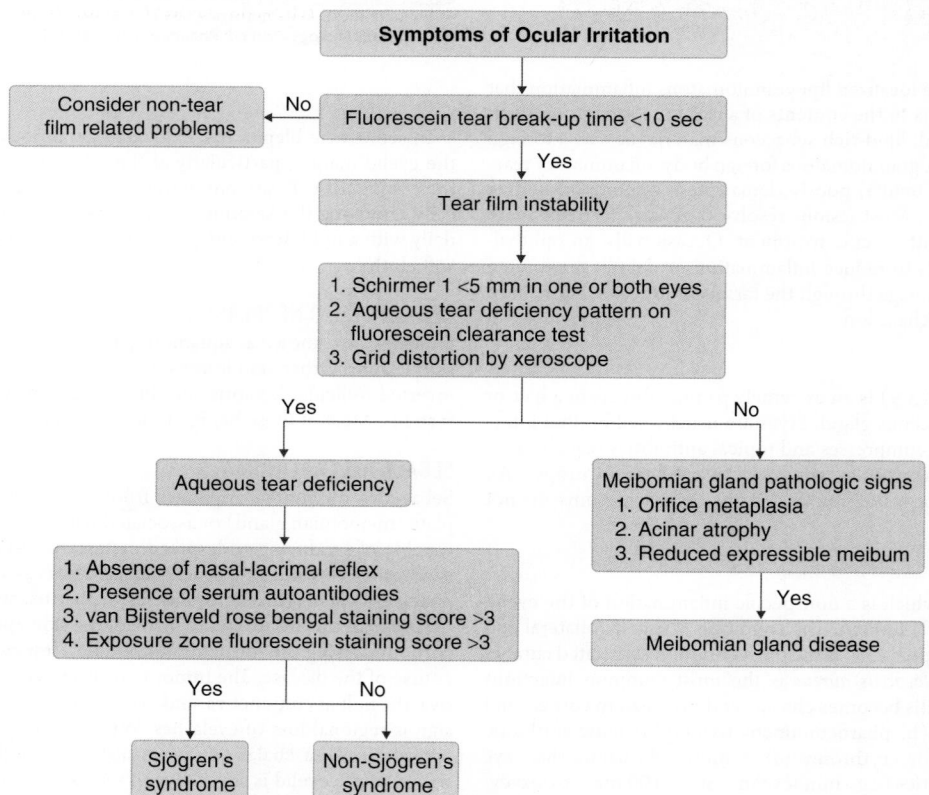

FIGURE 423-12. Diagnostic algorithm for ocular irritation. (Modified from Pflugfelder SC, Tseng SC, Sanabria O, et al. Evaluation of subjective assessments and objective diagnostic tests for diagnosing tear-film disorders known to cause ocular irritation. *Cornea.* 1998;17:38-56.)

High-viscosity tears (e.g., carboxymethylcellulose sodium) have a longer duration of action but tend to blur vision; they are best used at bedtime to maintain lubrication of the ocular surface during sleep. When artificial tears do not control symptoms, occlusion of the nasolacrimal duct with synthetic plugs or permanent surgical occlusion tends to retain the tears that are produced. Anti-inflammatory drugs (e.g., cyclosporine 0.05% drops, every 12 hours indefinitely) can preserve glandular tissue that may be affected by local inflammation. For patients with systemic disease associated with dry eyes, effective treatment of the systemic disease sometimes improves the eye abnormalities.

PINGUECULA AND PTERYGIUM

A pinguecula (Fig. 423-13) consists of a limbal (at junction of cornea and sclera) and bulbar conjunctival degenerative process caused by ultraviolet light damage to the subepithelial tissue. It is very common and rarely causes symptoms. If the supportive tissue degeneration extends into the cornea, it becomes a pterygium (Fig. 423-14), which may cause visual changes and require surgical excision. About 2 to 10% with a pterygium have a coexisting squamous carcinoma, which often is clinically unsuspected and diagnosed only by histopathologic examination.[6]

RECURRENT EROSION

Recurrent erosion of the cornea usually is a delayed reaction to minor traumatic corneal abrasion. The abrasion heals abnormally, resulting in a weakness of the epithelial attachment to underlying tissue. Weeks to months to years later, the patient is awakened in the middle of the night with extreme ocular pain on opening the eyelids. The epithelium has become "stuck" to the overlying upper lid and is mechanically abraded. The condition is treated with hyperosmotic drops and ointment. There is a tendency to recurrence.

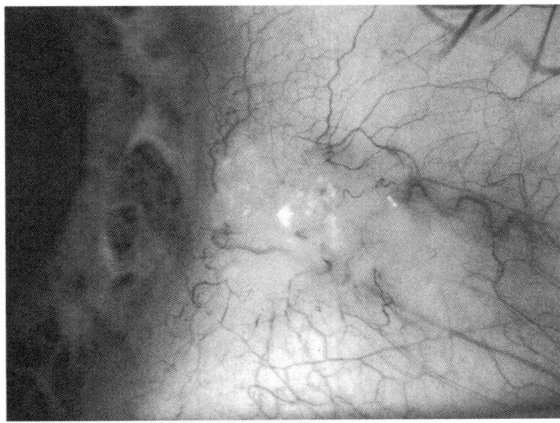

FIGURE 423-13. Pinguecula. These lesions are found at the 3-o'clock and 9-o'clock positions and are extremely common, especially in older patients. (From Palay DA, Krachmer JH. *Primary Care Ophthalmology,* 2nd ed. Philadelphia: Elsevier Mosby; 2005.)

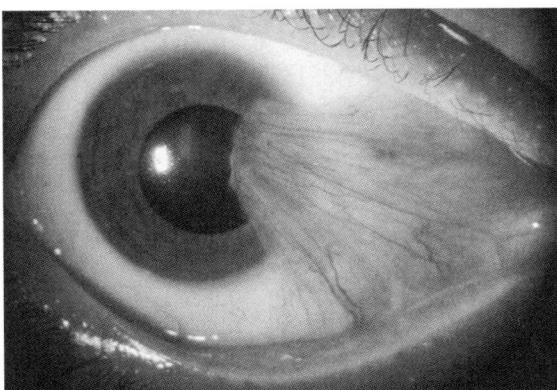

FIGURE 423-14. Pterygium. These lesions are found in the horizontal meridian, most common nasally. (From Palay DA, Krachmer JH. *Primary Care Ophthalmology,* 2nd ed. Philadelphia: Elsevier Mosby; 2005.)

ACCIDENTAL TRAUMA

With ocular trauma, many tissues of the eye can be easily disrupted, and the effects of trauma may not be manifest for months or even years after the episode of trauma. If the traumatic episode disrupts the eye wall (cornea and sclera), surgical repair is necessary, usually urgently. If the eye wall is intact, surgical treatment is often not necessary, at least initially.

CORNEAL ABRASION

Shearing trauma or hypoxia associated with overwearing of contact lenses may cause corneal abrasion, one of the most common forms of ocular injury. Symptoms are often intense and intolerable. Healing (i.e., re-epithelialization) of the cornea occurs within 24 to 48 hours. Rust from metallic fragments is toxic to the epithelium and should be removed. Fungal keratitis may complicate injuries from fingernails or vegetable matter, such as tree branches. Treatment usually consists of a topical antibiotic (e.g., erythromycin ointment, four times daily for 10 days) to prevent bacterial keratitis. Subsequent scarring usually does not occur unless deeper structures, such as Bowman's membrane, are affected. Topical anesthetics never should be prescribed to control pain because they increase the risk for microbial keratitis and scarring and may delay healing.

MAJOR OCULAR TRAUMA

Hyphema (Fig. 423-15) is hemorrhage into the anterior chamber caused by blunt trauma. If the patient is in an intensive care unit and supine, the blood will distribute uniformly over the iris to cause the appearance of increased pigmentation of the iris (heterochromia iridis). If the patient has been sitting, the blood may settle by gravity to form an aqueous-blood interface with the blood in the dependent portion of the anterior chamber. Hyphema, which is a sign of serious ocular damage, may lead to secondary glaucoma and blood staining of the cornea. It requires prompt evaluation by an ophthalmologist.

The most common site of rupture of a globe is at the limbus (junction of cornea and sclera), where a pigmented mass may be noted. The mass may be either a blood clot or an anteriorly displaced uveal tract (usually iris). Any manipulation of the globe may force the remaining intraocular tissue through the wound and may make the injury irreparable. Surgical repair is usually indicated.

Cataract and retinal detachment are not common except in severe accidental trauma. A unilateral cataract or unilateral glaucoma may occur decades after the injury, even when an injury is too minor to be recalled. Traumatic cataract and traumatic glaucoma are treated in the same manner as other forms of these conditions.

● INFLAMMATORY EYE DISORDERS
Uveitis

Inflammation of any part or parts of the uveal tract (iris, ciliary body, and choroid) may be called anterior or posterior uveitis, iritis, iridocyclitis, or choroiditis. Symptoms include a red eye (see Table 423-4), decreased vision, and photophobia. The inflammation is chronic, and a cause is rarely found. However, uveitis accompanies many autoimmune diseases, often without correlation with the activity of the systemic inflammation. Anterior

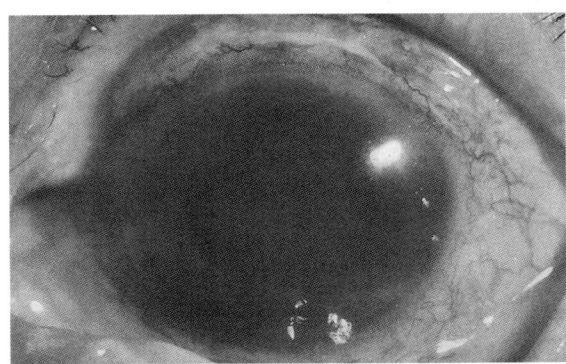

FIGURE 423-15. Hyphema following cataract surgery. (Courtesy of Dr. Myron Yanoff.)

uveitis or conjunctivitis is nearly universal in patients with reactive arthritis (Chapter 265). About 25% of patients with ankylosing spondylitis (Chapter 265) develop acute, recurrent anterior uveitis. Two to 12% of patients with inflammatory bowel disease (Chapter 141) develop anterior uveitis, which is also common with psoriatic arthritis but not with psoriasis alone (Chapters 265 and 438). Treatment with topical corticosteroids (e.g., prednisolone acetate 1%, one drop in the affected eye or eyes every 1 to 6 hours while awake) is usually sufficient to control the ocular disease.

Endophthalmitis

Endophthalmitis is extensive inflammation within the eye from any cause. Most cases of endophthalmitis involve a breach in the eye wall (cornea and sclera), associated with either accidental trauma (incidence of approximately 5%) or surgical procedures (incidence of approximately <0.03%).[7] The initial symptom is usually decreased vision followed by dull ocular pain. The initial sign is often evidence of inflammatory cells either within the aqueous (anterior uveitis) or within the vitreous (vitreitis). The cells can be seen only by slit lamp biomicroscopy. Common microbial organisms include toxin-producing gram-positive species and gram-negative species that are often associated with rapidly destructive course. Other organism of relatively low virulence, *Propionibacterium acnes* and *Staphylococcus epidermidis*, follow a more indolent course with less potential destruction. Metastatic endophthalmitis infection from a primary source outside of the eye is an unusual cause.

Diagnosis is established by sampling anterior chamber fluid or preferably vitreous fluid (vitreous tap) and evaluation of that fluid by Gram stain and culture. Prophylaxis against endophthalmitis includes preoperative topical instillation of povidone-iodine and intracameral antibiotic injection at the end of cataract surgery.

Systemic antibiotics are not effective, and patients benefit from vitrectomy only if the initial vision of the affected eye is light perception or worse. In severe cases, a vitrectomy through a pars plana incision reduces the microbial and inflammatory debris burden. Initial treatment is with topical antibiotics (e.g. commonly used but not limited to, vancomycin 1 mg/0.1 mL and ceftazidime 2.25 mg/0.1mL) and corticosteroids. Under certain circumstances, simultaneous intraocular antibiotics (vancomycin 1 mg and ceftazidime, 2.25 mg/0.1mL) minimize the destructive effects of retinal inflammation.

Allergic Conjunctivitis

Allergic conjunctivitis (Table 423-6) is commonly associated with atopy, hay fever, and allergic rhinitis (Chapter 251). Itching, a foreign body sensation, and a watery discharge are common. Treatment includes cool compresses and topical vasoconstrictors or antihistamines (e.g., naphazoline drops, four times daily during the allergic season, or levocabastine drops, four times daily). Long-term treatment with mast cell stabilizers (e.g., pemirolast drops, four times daily during the allergic season) or the combination of an antihistamine plus a mast cell stabilizer (e.g., olopatadine drops, two times daily during the allergic season) can be extremely effective in treating chronic symptoms.

INFECTIOUS EYE DISORDERS
Cellulitis

Preseptal cellulitis (Fig. 423-16) is soft tissue inflammation of the eyelid anterior to the orbital septum. The orbital septum divides the soft tissues of the eyelid from the soft tissues of the orbit. Orbital tissue is more susceptible to damage by the inflammation than is the preseptal tissue.

The clinical signs of preseptal cellulitis include soft tissue swelling, hyperemia, and conjunctival chemosis (edema). Movement of the eye is not restricted. Extension of inflammation posterior to the orbital septum is indicated by proptosis of the globe and ophthalmoplegia (restricted motion). Treatment of preseptal cellulitis includes oral antibiotics (e.g. commonly used but not limited to, amoxicillin-clavulanate, 500 mg orally every 8 hours for 10 days, or Bactrim 500 mg/PO, BID for cases of suspected Methicillin-resistant Staphylococcus aureus (MRSA)). Treatment of orbital cellulitis, which can lead to septic optic neuritis, intracranial spread, and cavernous sinus thrombosis, may require intravenous antibiotics and surgical drainage of a paraorbital abscess.

Adenoviral Conjunctivitis

Viral conjunctivitis (Fig. 423-17) is common (see Table 423-6), and adenoviral conjunctivitis (especially subtypes 7, 11, and 18) is the most common type.[8] The condition is highly contagious through direct contact or inhalation of respiratory particles. After an incubation period of 5 to 15 days, the patient presents with very red eyes (see Table 423-4), itching, burning, a foreign body sensation, and often a discharge and ocular discomfort (see Table 423-3), which persist for 5 to 15 days. Preauricular lymphadenopathy may be present,

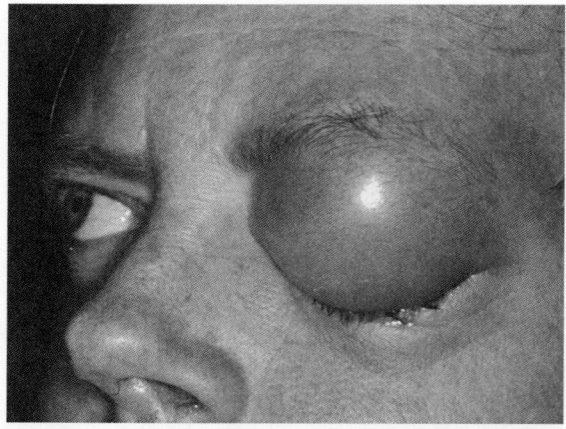

FIGURE 423-16. Eyelid abscess. Preseptal cellulitis, commonly resulting from minor penetrating trauma, may evolve into an abscess. Treatment requires incision and drainage followed by systemic antibiotics.

TABLE 423-6 OPHTHALMIC DISORDERS ASSOCIATED WITH CONJUNCTIVITIS

DISORDER	ACUTE OR CHRONIC	UNILATERAL OR BILATERAL	KEY SYMPTOMS	DEGREE OF INJECTION	DISCHARGE TYPE	OTHER FEATURES
Viral conjunctivitis	Acute	Bilateral, possibly asymmetrical	Itching, burning, soreness	4+	Watery	Preauricular lymphadenopathy
Bacterial conjunctivitis	Acute	Unilateral or bilateral	Burning	3+	Heavy, mucopurulent	Lids possibly adherent
Chlamydial conjunctivitis	Subacute, chronic	Usually unilateral	Burning, irritation	2+	Scant, mucopurulent	Usual occurrence in young, sexually active adults
Herpes simplex conjunctivitis	Acute	Unilateral	Photophobia, irritation	1-2+	None	Dendritic ulcer on the cornea or vesicles on the lid possible
Allergic conjunctivitis	Chronic	Bilateral	Itching	2+	Stringy, mucoid	Usual occurrence in atopic persons, possible seasonal symptoms
Blepharitis	Chronic	Bilateral	Itching, burning, foreign body sensation	1-2+	Usually none	Inflammation and crusting of lid margins
Dry eye	Chronic	Bilateral	Foreign body sensation	1+	Mucoid in severe cases	Punctate fluorescein staining of the cornea

Adapted from Palay DA, Krachmer JH. *Primary Care Ophthalmology*, 2nd ed. Philadelphia: Elsevier Mosby; 2005.

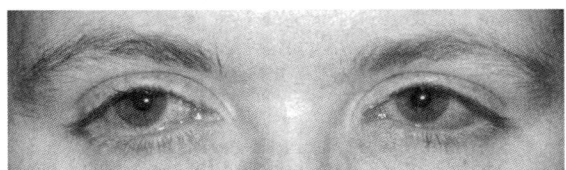

FIGURE 423-17. Diffuse injection of the conjunctiva with a watery discharge is evident in this case of viral conjunctivitis. (From Palay DA, Krachmer JH. *Primary Care Ophthalmology*, 2nd ed. Philadelphia: Elsevier Mosby; 2005.)

and a history of upper respiratory tract infection is common. The disease is self-limited, and treatment is aimed at patients' comfort. Cool compresses are often soothing. Patients are advised to wash their hands frequently. Topical antibiotics are not required, and topical corticosteroids are contraindicated.

Bacterial Conjunctivitis

Fewer than 5% of cases of conjunctivitis are caused by bacteria, mostly *Staphylococcus*, *Haemophilus*, or *Streptococcus* species. Patients have a mucoid or purulent discharge (Fig. 423-18), often with crusting and edema of the conjunctiva (chemosis) and lids. Bacterial conjunctivitis responds to broad-spectrum antibiotic solutions or ointments (e.g., topical erythromycin ointment three times daily for 2 weeks) (Table 423-7).

Chlamydial Conjunctivitis

Adult inclusion conjunctivitis is a chronic conjunctivitis caused by sexual transmission of *Chlamydia trachomatis* (Chapter 318). Patients often have preauricular lymphadenopathy. Oral erythromycin (500 mg orally, four times daily for 7 days) or azithromycin (1 g orally twice daily for 7 days) is required. Trachoma, which is a chronic cicatricial conjunctivitis after repeated chlamydial infection (Chapter 318), is the world's leading cause of corneal blindness. It causes an entropion, inversion of the eyelashes (trichiasis), corneal vascularization, and opacification. Topical erythromycin or tetracycline, twice daily for 3 to 4 weeks, can be effective, but surgical epilation or eyelid reconstruction may be required.

Herpes Simplex Keratitis

Herpes simplex keratitis is the most common cause of central corneal ulcer (Fig. 423-19).[9] Herpes simplex virus also can cause vesicular eyelid dermatitis. Initially, the main signs of primary herpes simplex keratitis are a red eye and a corneal epithelial dendritic ulcer. With appropriate antiviral therapy (e.g., ganciclovir 0.15% ophthalmic gel five times daily for at least 1 week or until healed),[A3] the keratitis usually heals without scarring. Recurrent herpes simplex keratitis may be precipitated by fever, menses, sunlight, irradiation, or stress. With recurrence, the disease may extend into the corneal stroma and cause a red eye, ocular discomfort, blurred vision, and corneal scarring. The treatment of stromal involvement is multifactorial and may not be successful. Corneal transplantation may be needed.

Herpes Zoster Ophthalmicus

Herpes zoster ophthalmicus (shingles, Chapter 375) has a propensity to involve one or more branches of the trigeminal nerve. The virus also can affect the uveal tract and, in immunosuppressed patients, the retina (i.e., acute retinal necrosis). When the trigeminal nerve is involved, spread to the inside of the eye (uveitis) is most likely if vesicles are present in the inner corner of the eyelids or on the nose, especially the tip of the nose. If the uvea is not involved, the skin lesions heal with some scarring but no long-term effects. In patients with moderate to severe skin involvement, treatment can be started with oral acyclovir (800 mg orally five times per day for 7 to 10 days). If uveitis develops, the treatment (e.g., prednisolone acetate drops 1% four times daily and atropine 1.0% once or twice daily) can be extended and difficult.

Pseudomonal and Gonococcal Keratitis

Keratitis, which is inflammation of the corneal stroma, can be caused by spread of pathogens internally from a corneal ulcer. *Pseudomonas aeruginosa* (Chapter 306), which causes a particularly virulent keratitis, is the most common gram-negative pathogen and is especially common in wearers of contact lenses. To avoid internal spread, urgent treatment is necessary (e.g., fortified tobramycin [9 mg/mL] or gentamicin [1.5 mg/mL], every hour, alternating with fortified cefazolin, 50 mg/mL every hour, so a treatment is

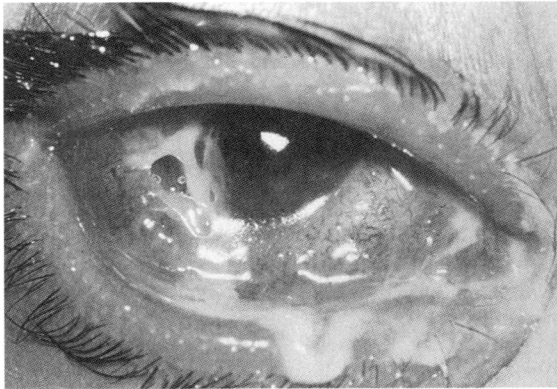

FIGURE 423-18. Bacterial conjunctivitis. Purulent discharge and conjunctival hyperemia suggest bacterial conjunctivitis. Viral conjunctivitis produces watery discharge, foreign body sensation, preauricular lymphadenopathy, and conjunctival follicles seen on slit lamp examination. (Reproduced with permission from the American Academy of Ophthalmology.)

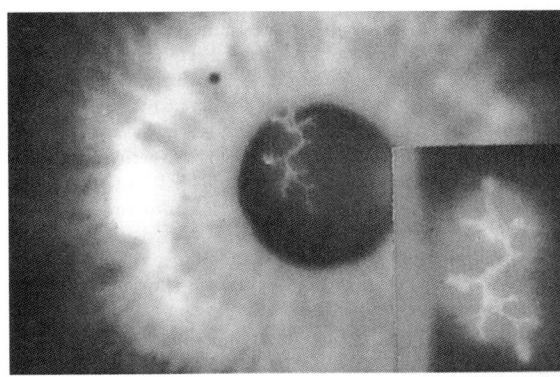

FIGURE 423-19. Herpes simplex corneal epithelial keratitis in diffuse light and in light passed through a cobalt blue filter after fluorescein staining *(inset)*. Note the dendritic staining pattern characteristic of herpes simplex.

TABLE 423-7		TOPICAL ANTIBIOTICS FOR EYE INFECTIONS	
DRUG	**TYPE**	**CONCENTRATION**	**DOSE**
Moxifloxacin	Drops	0.5%	1 drop BID × 7 days
Gatifloxacin	Drops	0.5%	1 drop q2H × 24 hours; then QID × 6 days
Ciprofloxacin	Drops	0.3%	1 drop q2H × 48 hours; then q4H × 5 days
Gentamicin	Drops	0.3%	1 drop 4 times daily
Ofloxacin	Drops	0.3%	1 drop 2H × 48H; then q2H × 5 days
Bacitracin	Ointment	500 U/g	Put in eye, for several days
Tobramycin	Ointment	0.3%	Put in eye, for several days
Erythromycin	Ointment	0.5%	Put in eye, for several days

given each one-half hour around the clock). The dosage and duration of the treatment depend on the response.

Another gram-negative cause of a virulent keratitis is *Neisseria gonorrhoeae* (Chapter 298). Corneal infection is accompanied by copious tearing and a characteristic hyperpurulent discharge. Prompt treatment is essential in preventing corneal perforation.

Cytomegalovirus Retinitis

Cytomegalovirus retinitis (Chapter 376) is unusual except in immunosuppressed patients, especially patients with human immunodeficiency virus infection. Clinically, a central retinochoroiditis is seen. The presumptive diagnosis is made on the characteristic intense, retinal, wedge-shaped reaction, with considerable exudates and hemorrhages, giving the terms "pizza pie retinitis" and "hemorrhagic cottage cheese retinitis" to the entity. Treatment is antiviral drugs: ganciclovir (5 mg/kg intravenously twice daily, two to three times per week), foscarnet (90 mg/kg intravenously twice daily, twice per week), or cidofovir (5 mg/kg intravenously, weekly for 3 weeks) with follow-up maintenance. Intravitreal injections using an appropriately reduced dose is also commonly used in selected cases.

Acanthamoeba Keratitis

Acanthamoeba species (Chapter 352) can cause a severe, blinding keratitis. Contact lens wearing is a major risk factor. A characteristic stromal ring infiltrate develops, and uveitis may occur. Using a confocal microscope, the acanthamebic parasite can be observed clinically as a pear-shaped cyst (11 to 15 μm). Numerous treatment protocols exist (e.g., polyhexamethyl biguanide 0.02% drops every hour).[10] The duration and dose depend on the response, but the ideal treatment is not yet in hand. Corneal transplantation may be necessary in cases of severe corneal scarring.

Toxoplasmic Retinitis

Toxoplasma gondii (Chapter 349) causes both a congenital and acquired retinochoroiditis, which is more common in immunosuppressed patients. The lesions begin as an acute retinitis that atrophies centrally and pigments peripherally as it heals. The protozoa are found both in free and encysted forms within the retina. The condition may be self-limited and diagnosed as a healed incidental finding that does not need treatment. Standard treatment of vision-threatening toxoplasmosis remains controversial.[11] When active lesions are in the macula or a severe vitreitis causes at least a two-line decrease in vision, 4 to 6 weeks of quadruple therapy (pyrimethamine, 200 mg oral loading dose then 25 mg orally daily; folinic acid, 10 mg orally every other day; sulfadiazine, 2 g oral loading dose then 1 g four times daily; and oral corticosteroids, e.g., prednisone, 20 to 60 mg orally daily beginning at least 24 hours after antibiotic therapy is started and tapered 10 days before stopping antibiotics) usually produces good results. Alternative regimens may include clindamycin (150 to 450 mg orally three to four times daily) or atovaquone (1 g oral loading dose then 500 mg daily).

Fungal Endophthalmitis

Fungal endophthalmitis is infrequent (7% of microbial endothalmitis)[12] but is a potentially disastrous infection of the inside of the eye, often leading to blindness. The primary organisms are *Candida, Coccidioides,* and *Aspergillus* species, which can gain access inside the eye either by traumatic introduction or through hematogenous spread. The patient presents with a red eye, ocular pain, and decreased vision. Multiple vitreous abscesses tend to be caused by fungi, whereas a solitary abscess is more likely caused by bacteria. Usually a vitreous "tap" (biopsy) is performed for culture and to guide therapy. Vitrectomy and intraocular fungal agents are indicated in advanced cases.

Tuberculosis

About 1% of patients with pulmonary tuberculosis (Chapter 324) have uveal involvement, usually as iridocyclitis or diffuse choroiditis. Painless progressive visual loss is the most common symptom. Small yellow choroidal lesions may be seen, and retinal periphlebitis may occur secondarily. Treatment is as for the primary disease.

Syphilis

About 5% of patients with secondary syphilis (Chapter 319) develop anterior uveitis or neuroretinitis. In tertiary syphilis, the miotic Argyll Robertson pupil reacts poorly to light but briskly to accommodation. Treatment is as for the systemic disease.

STRUCTURAL AND AGE-RELATED DISORDERS
Cataract

A cataract is an opacification of the crystalline lens. The lens doubles in volume between birth and age 70 years as new lens "fiber cells" are laid down on the external aspect of the lens cortex, beneath the lens capsule. The older fibers in the center of the lens cannot be desquamated into the surrounding aqueous and thus are compressed into the center of the lens. At birth, the lens is pliable and totally transparent. By age 45 years, the lens loses its pliability, which compromises near vision. As the process progresses, the lens loses its transparency, beginning at the center of the lens (nuclear sclerosis). The

concurrent change in density of the lens nucleus may alter the optical characteristics of the eye to cause acquired nearsightedness ("second sight"). Ultimately, the cataract may become so dense that cataract surgery is necessary to restore vision.

Symptoms are typically loss of vision, especially at night, and glare. Cataract surgery, performed as an outpatient, is elective and depends on how much the decreased vision interferes with the normal lifestyle of the patient. A synthetic intraocular lens implant is inserted into the eye during surgery. Prognosis for restoration of vision is excellent, depending on the function of the retina. In general, cataracts develop asymmetrically. The worst eye (vision-wise) should have surgery first. As the second eye's cataract worsens, decreasing vision and monocularity are indications for cataract surgery in the second eye.

Glaucoma

Glaucoma results from an imbalance between the production of aqueous fluid and the drainage of aqueous fluid. The aqueous is produced by the nonpigmented ciliary epithelium of the pars plicata of the ciliary body. Aqueous fluid leaves the eye through the trabecular meshwork into the venous circulation. If the drainage function does not match the production potential, the intraocular pressure increases. If the elevated intraocular pressure is high enough or is present long enough, ganglion cells in the retina are damaged, causing loss of their axons. Loss of axons can best be appreciated clinically at their normal exit from the eye, the optic disc. Bulk loss of axons will lead to enlargement of the optic cup, which is recorded as increase in the cup-to-disc ratio.

In open-angle glaucoma, there is apparent free anatomic access to the trabecular meshwork. In closed-angle glaucoma, there is a relative or absolute anatomic barrier to the flow of aqueous.

CHRONIC OPEN-ANGLE GLAUCOMA

The most common type of glaucoma in elderly people is chronic open-angle glaucoma. The first symptom is loss of peripheral visual field with retention of central visual function. The visual field may be reduced considerably before the patient notes loss of function. Most cases of chronic open-angle glaucoma are identified during routine eye examinations, either by discovery of abnormally high intraocular pressure[13] or by the presence of a high cup-to-disc ratio (Fig. 423-20). Average intraocular pressure is generally at or below 21 mm Hg, but exceptions exist depending on corneal thickness (causing artifacts of measurement in patients with excessively thin or thick corneas) and genetic disposition. The diagnosis of glaucoma is confirmed by characteristic visual field loss as determined by automated perimetry.

The treatment goal is to reduce intraocular pressure, initially with pharmacologic agents: β-blockers (e.g., betaxolol drops 0.5% twice daily), carbonic anhydrase inhibitors (e.g., dorzolamide drops twice daily), α-agonists (e.g., apraclonidine drops twice daily), and antiprostaglandins (e.g., latanoprost drops twice daily).[14] Generally, the drops are taken for a lifetime. Applying energy to the structures of the trabecular meshwork with a laser (laser trabeculoplasty) often results in years of control of intraocular pressure. In resistant cases, mechanical filtration is accomplished surgically by bypassing the trabecular meshwork either by creating a fistula (trabeculectomy) between the anterior chamber and the episcleral tissue or by implanting a synthetic filtration device (a tube-shunt) from the anterior chamber through the sclera into a collection reservoir located at the equator of the eye in the soft tissues of the orbit.

PSEUDOEXFOLIATIVE GLAUCOMA

Pseudoexfoliative glaucoma syndrome is a genetically determined biochemical abnormality of the basement membrane protein, fibrillin. The syndrome occurs among people throughout the world but is especially prominent in Scandinavians and Saudi Arabians. Affected individuals are identified by accumulation of abnormal fibrillin (exfoliative material) on the surface of the crystalline lens, most easily seen in the pupillary space. Pseudoexfoliative glaucoma increases the risk for developing open-angle glaucoma five-fold, to a lifetime risk of about 10%. Treatment is as for open-angle glaucoma.

ANGLE-CLOSURE GLAUCOMA

Angle-closure glaucoma (Fig. 423-21) may occur over a short period of time and cause extreme debilitating symptoms.[15] Alternatively, symptoms may develop over a long period of time with few specific symptoms.

The risk factors for angle-closure glaucoma are based on the anatomic configuration of the components of anterior chamber. Persons who are

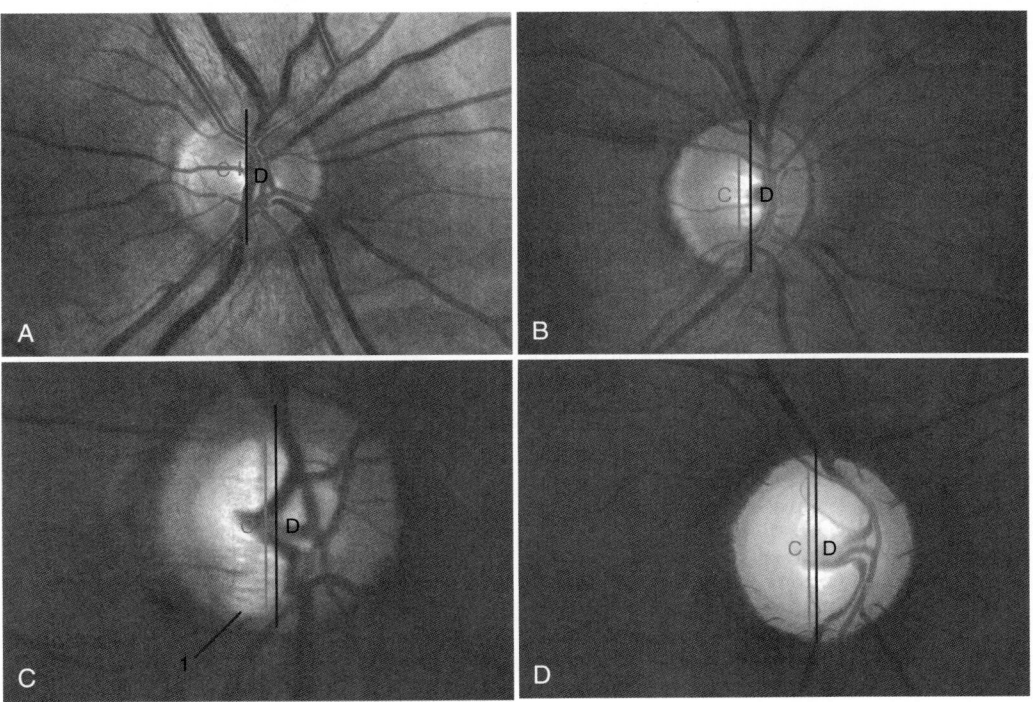

FIGURE 423-20. Cup-to-disc ratios. **A,** Normal cup-to-disc (C/D) ratio of 0.1. **B,** Likely normal C/D ratio of 0.5. **C,** C/D ratio of 0.8 vertically with inferior notching (1) of the nerve (glaucomatous change). **D,** C/D ratio of 0.90 vertically (glaucomatous change). C = cup; D = disc. (From Palay DA, Krachmer JH. *Primary Care Ophthalmology,* 2nd ed. Philadelphia: Elsevier Mosby; 2005.)

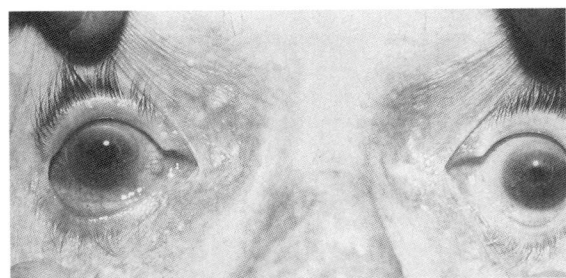

FIGURE 423-21. Acute angle-closure glaucoma. The left eye is normal. The red right eye has a nonreactive pupil. (Courtesy of Dr. Myron Yanoff.)

farsighted (hyperopia) have a shortened anterior-to-posterior axis of the eye, indicated clinically by a shallow anterior chamber. As the crystalline lens increases in volume with time, the iris is displaced anteriorly. At some point, the posterior surface of the iris may come in relatively tight contact with the anterior surface of the lens. Aqueous flow is restricted, and fluid accumulates in the posterior chamber, where it displaces the diaphanous peripheral iris anteriorly. When the peripheral iris comes in contact with the posterior cornea, the anterior chamber angle is suddenly occluded. Angle closure may be precipitated by pharmacologic dilation of the pupil. Patients who are far-sighted (hyperopia) or have cataracts should be dilated with caution. The intraocular pressure may increase from 21 mm Hg to 50 to 70 mm Hg (nearly equaling diastolic arterial pressure). The symptoms of acute angle closure may include extreme pain, which may be poorly localized to the eye, nausea, and vomiting. Persistent vomiting may cause abdominal pain, simulating an acute abdomen.

Initial treatment is with topical (e.g., timolol 0.5% in one dose) and systemic pressure-lowering agents (e.g., carbonic acetazolamide, 250 to 500 mg intravenously or two 250-mg tablets orally in one dose if intravenous access or drug is not available), followed by creation of a fistula in the peripheral iris with a laser (YAG laser iridectomy) between the posterior chamber and the anterior chamber to bypass the obstruction. Most patients require a laser iridectomy prophylactically in the second eye to prevent angle-closure glaucoma.

Secondary glaucoma may also occur after intraocular hemorrhage, intraocular trauma, and intraocular inflammation. Some developmentally related secondary glaucomas, such as the iridocorneal endothelial syndrome, may not become evident until adulthood.

Retinal Detachment

A retinal detachment is a separation of the neural (sensory) retina from the retinal pigment epithelium. The two main types are rhegmatogenous, caused by a retinal hole, as may occur with a posterior vitreous detachment, and nonrhegmatogenous, caused by traction, such as in proliferative diabetic retinopathy or by fluid accumulation under neural retina in conditions such as malignant hypertension or eclampsia of pregnancy.

The classic symptoms are a sensation of flashes of light, floaters in the field of the involved eye owing to the causative vitreous detachment, and a shadow. Urgent treatment usually is needed. Laser photocoagulation is used to treat small posterior detachments, whereas cryotherapy is used for more peripheral tears. Intravitreal injection of 125 μg ocriplasmin (a recombinant protease with activity against fibronectin and laminin, which are components of the vitreoretinal interface) can significantly improve outcomes in patients with vitreomacular traction and macular holes.[A1] More extensive detachments may be treated with the injection of air. The air bubble will locate in the superior portion of the globe and tamponade the hole while it heals; the patient's head must be in the correct position for the duration of treatment. Large rhegmatogenous and traction retinal detachments are treated by more involved surgical procedures (scleral buckle surgery or vitreous surgery), which in most cases require general anesthesia and are associated with a longer postoperative course. Serous retinal detachments generally resolve without direct intervention when the underlying cause is successfully treated.

Age-Related Macular Degeneration

Age-related macular degeneration is a neurodegenerative disease that affects the junction between the neural retina and the retinal pigment epithelium, mainly in the sixth to ninth decades of life. About 8.5% of the world's blindness is caused by age-related macular degeneration, mainly in industrialized countries. In the United States, age-related macular degeneration affects more than 1.75 million persons, and its prevalence increases with each decade after the age of 55 years. The genetic influence of age-related macular degeneration has not yet been determined, but abnormalities of complement factor H may play a role. Environmental factors such as smoking are known to accelerate this degenerative process.

Two types predominate: the "dry" or geographic type, and the "wet" or neovascular type. The wet type causes the most profound vision loss but is less common than the dry type.

The first sign of age-related macular degeneration is variation of the character and density of the retinal pigment epithelial pigment ("pigment dropout") in the posterior region of the retina, the macula. The pathologic process causes abnormal protein (lipofuscin) to accumulate between the retinal pigment epithelial cells and its basement membrane complex (Bruch's membrane), designated as *drusen*. The drusen of macular degeneration (soft drusen) are small (30 μm), hypopigmented, poorly defined areas in the deep retina. This stage, called dry age-related macular degeneration, may antedate subjective alteration in vision by several decades. The anticipated rate of progression is difficult to determine in individual cases.

The first symptom of age-related macular degeneration is loss of vision. Loss of vision corresponds with loss of photoreceptor outer segments. The effect is in the exact center of the most sensitive portion of the retina, the fovea. The peripheral retina is not involved. As the process progresses, individuals with advanced disease will be able to walk down a street without apparent difficulty (a peripheral retinal function) but will not be able to recognize facial features of people whom they meet (a macular retinal function). Visual aids and other devices, such as special glasses and television aids, may allow patients to continue with daily functions and to continue to live independently. This phase of the process, the "dry phase," advances at a slow rate (months to decades), during which patients develop retinal features of well-defined pigment loss (geographic retinal atrophy; Fig. 423-22). No current treatment exists for the dry phase of the disease, except for a possible positive influence of dietary supplements (antioxidants). Vitamin supplementation with vitamins C and E, β-carotene, zinc, and copper may retard the progression of moderate age-related macular degeneration to severe age-related macular degeneration.[AS] β-Carotene (a vitamin A precursor) of this quantity is not recommended for cigarette smokers because of an increased risk for lung cancer. Cessation of smoking, control of blood sugar, control of blood lipid levels, and control of systemic blood pressure are particularly important behavioral modifications.

In the "wet phase" of age-related macular degeneration (Fig. 423-23), frail, neovascular channels originating from the established vascular system of the choroid may extend through a breach in Bruch's membrane into the subretinal space (subretinal neovascularization). Spontaneous hemorrhage of the vessels adds to photoreceptor loss. Hemorrhage is accompanied by acute, and usually permanent, loss of central visual acuity (i.e., the wet phase of age-related macular degeneration). Both eyes are usually affected to a similar degree. Neovascularization can be identified by fluorescein angiography and OCT. Intraocular injections of antivascular endothelial growth factors (e.g., ranibizumab or bevacizumab) reduce the risk for visual loss in patients with neovascular age-related macular degeneration and can result in gains in vision.[16] Other treatments include argon laser photocoagulation or, in advanced cases, vitrectomy to remove subretinal neovascular membranes.

SYSTEMIC DISEASES WITH OCULAR SYMPTOMS DURING ADULTHOOD

Diabetes Mellitus

Diabetic retinopathy is one of the leading causes of blindness in the United States. More than 75% of the blind are women. Background diabetic retinopathy, with microaneurysms, hemorrhages, exudates (Fig. 423-24), and macular edema, accounts for most cases of decreased vision but rarely causes profound vision loss. Most diabetic patients never develop the more severe proliferative diabetic retinopathy (Fig. 423-25), which generally occurs only after 15 years or more of diabetes and causes a profound loss of vision.

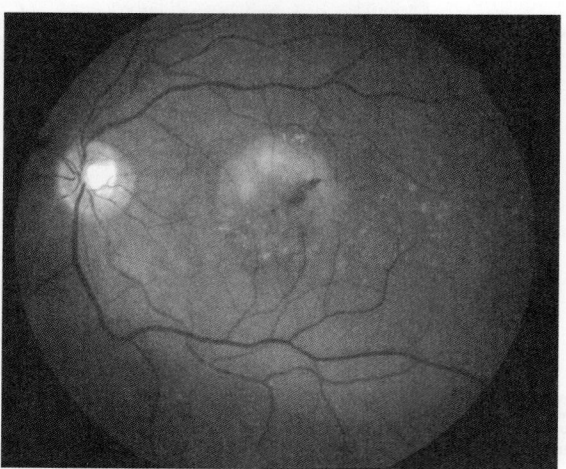

FIGURE 423-23. Wet age-related macular degeneration. A "dirty gray" neovascular membrane is present under the central macular area.

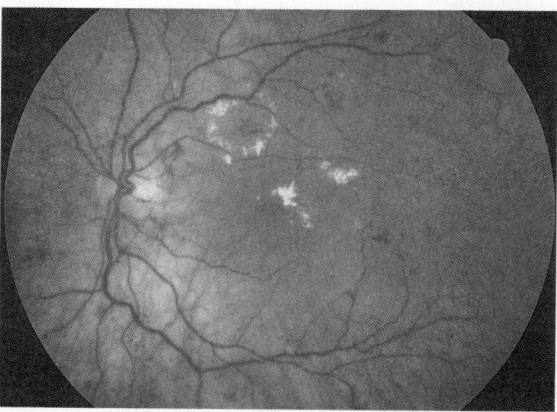

FIGURE 423-24. Background diabetic retinopathy. Exudates, microaneurysms, and small hemorrhages are seen in the posterior pole (right eye).

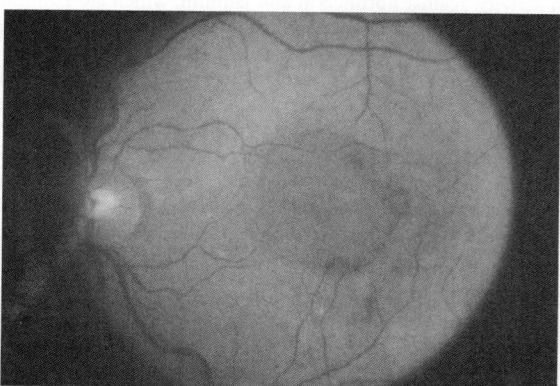

FIGURE 423-22. Dry age-related macular degeneration. Drusen are present in the posterior pole around a large area of geographic atrophy of the retinal pigment epithelium.

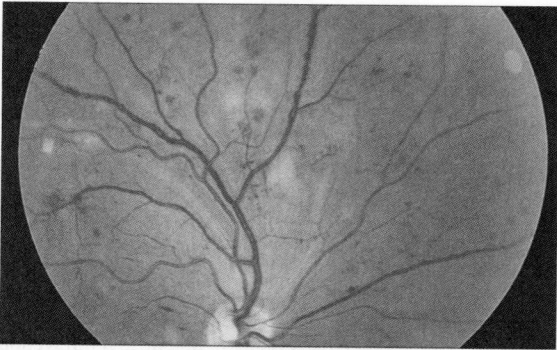

FIGURE 423-25. Severe proliferative diabetic retinopathy with cotton-wool spots, intraretinal microvascular abnormalities, and venous bleeding. (From Yanoff M, Duker JS, eds. *Ophthalmology*. Philadelphia: Mosby Elsevier; 2009.)

Diabetic retinopathy is closely correlated with the duration of diabetes mellitus (Chapter 229). The prevalence of diabetic retinopathy is about 27% among patients who have had type 1 diabetes for 5 to 10 years, 70 to 90% among patients who have had diabetes for more than 10 years, and 95% among patients who have had diabetes for 20 to 30 years. In patients with type 2 diabetes (Chapter 229), the prevalence of diabetic retinopathy is about 23% after 12 years and 60% after 16 years. Tight control of blood glucose greatly reduces the risk for the development of diabetic retinopathy.[17]

The treatment of diabetic retinopathy includes control of the diabetes and any hyperlipidemia,[A7] laser therapy for background diabetic retinopathy, and laser or surgical therapy to treat proliferative diabetic retinopathy.[A8] Antiangiogenic therapy (e.g., ranibizumab) may be superior to laser therapy for diabetic macular edema[A9]; intravitreal steroid injection is also beneficial.[A10] With acute hyperglycemia, accumulation of sorbitol may lead to lenticular swelling; secondary refractive errors may persist for 6 to 8 weeks.

Hypertension

In chronic hypertension (Chapter 67), the characteristic retinal vascular findings can assess the severity of hypertension. As the severity increases, patients develop arterial narrowing, arteriovenous nicking (Fig. 423-26), nerve fiber layer infarcts, and intraretinal hemorrhages. Moderately sclerosed arterioles have a "copper wiring" appearance, whereas severely sclerosed vessels demonstrate "silver wiring." Acute hypertension may cause optic nerve edema ("papilledema"; Fig. 423-27) and serous retinal detachments that usually resolve without significant sequelae if blood pressure is controlled.

Other Systemic Diseases

In bacterial endocarditis (Chapter 76), emboli may cause conjunctival hemorrhages or the characteristic Roth's spot (Fig. 423-28). Accumulation of copper in the posterior cornea may aid in the diagnosis of Wilson's disease (Chapter 211), although its clinical diagnosis usually precedes the characteristic Kayser-Fleischer ring (see Fig. 211-2), which fades after treatment. Tay-Sachs and Niemann-Pick diseases (Chapter 208) are associated with a foveal cherry-red spot owing to the accumulation of gangliosides within perifoveal ganglion cells. Pseudoxanthoma elasticum (Chapter 260) is often associated with characteristic angioid streaks of the retina.

VASCULAR ABNORMALITIES OF THE EYE

The major vessels of the retina enter the eye at a point of relative constriction in the tissues of the lamina cribrosa of the optic disc. In persons who have generalized vascular disease, particularly systemic hypertension, occlusion of either the artery or vein may lead to a sudden loss of vision. Partial occlusion of either the artery or vein is associated with less visual loss but still increases the risk for developing neovascular glaucoma.

Arterial occlusion of the central retinal artery (Fig. 423-29) presents as painless acute loss of vision. The ischemic posterior retina generally has a pale gray appearance except at the fovea, where the normal color is preserved (cherry-red spot). The clinical appearance of edema resolves over time, but vision generally does not recover.

Venous occlusion of the central retinal vein (Fig. 423-30) presents as painless loss of vision. The retina, however, is characterized by extreme, generalized hemorrhages, which resolve very slowly and are often associated with opaque areas of focal retinal ischemia (cotton-wool spots). This process destroys the full thickness of the retina. Usually, no vision returns without

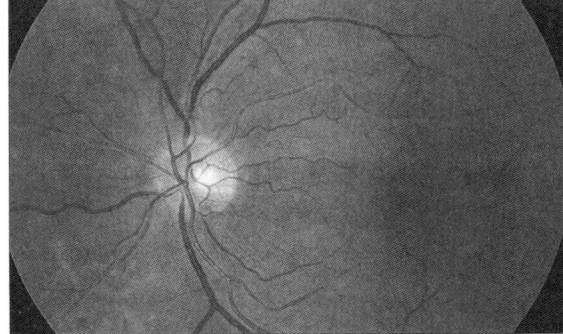

FIGURE 423-26. Hypertension retinopathy with narrowed arterioles whose sclerosed walls create the appearance of "nicking" when the arterioles cross venules. (From Yanoff M, Duker JS, eds. *Ophthalmology*. Philadelphia: Mosby Elsevier; 2009.)

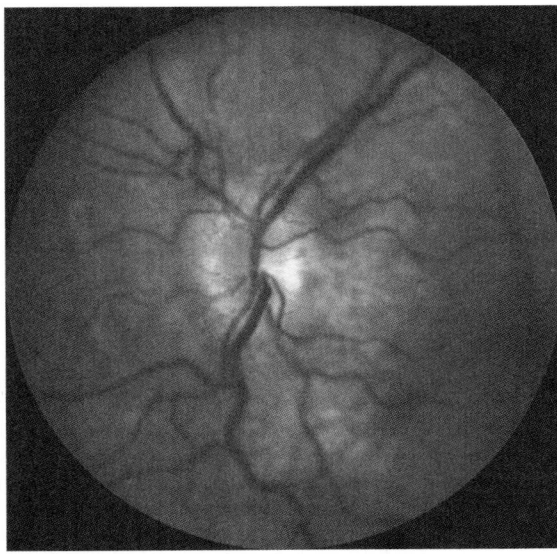

FIGURE 423-27. Papilledema. (Courtesy of Dr. Kathleen Digre.)

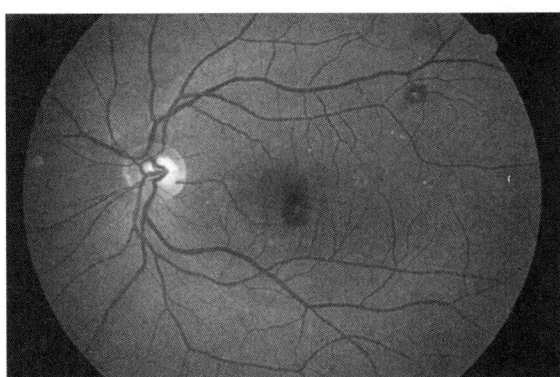

FIGURE 423-28. Roth's spots. Multiple white-centered hemorrhages in a man with recurrent subacute bacterial endocarditis. White-centered hemorrhages are also seen with leukemia and diabetes. The small white scars are probably the residua of previous episodes.

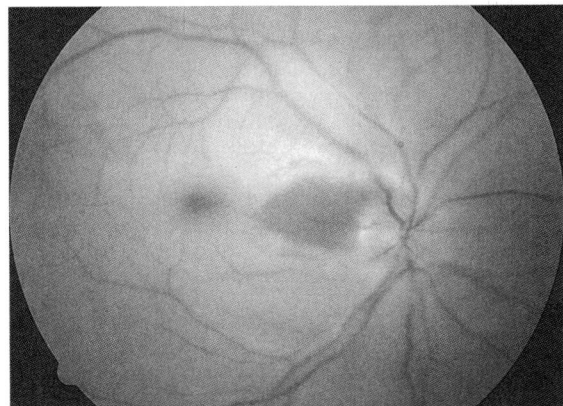

FIGURE 423-29. Central retinal artery occlusion. Fundus photograph shows diffuse retinal edema. The heavily pigmented fovea with its uniquely thin inner retina produces a cherry-red spot against the dusky macula. In this case, a small area of retina adjacent to the optic disc is spared, owing to the presence of a cilioretinal artery.

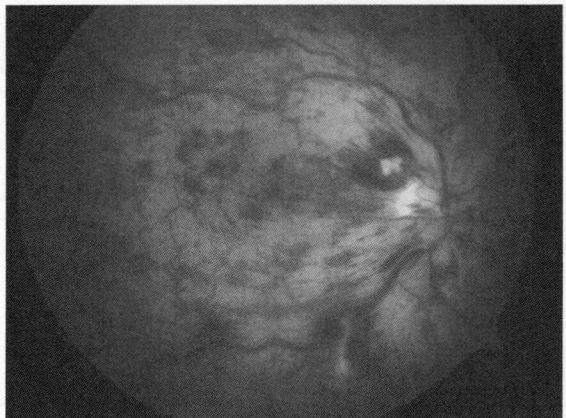

FIGURE 423-30. Central retinal vein occlusion with diffuse intraretinal hemorrhages in all four quadrants.

TABLE 423-8	PARTIAL LIST OF SYSTEMIC MEDICATIONS CAUSING DRY EYE	
MEDICATION	**CLASS**
Ibuprofen	Nonsteroidal anti-inflammatory
Diphenhydramine	Antihistamine
Triprolidine	Antihistamine
Chlorpheniramine	Antihistamine
Atenolol	β-Blocker
Metoprolol	β-Blocker
Propranolol	β-Blocker
Clonidine	α-Agonist
Scopolamine	Anticholinergic
Amiodarone	Antiarrhythmic
Thiabendazole	Antinematode
Isotretinoin*	Retinoid

*Severe, long-term dry eye with onset up to several years after treatment. All others tend to abate with cessation.
From Goldman L, Ausiello DA, eds. *Cecil Textbook of Medicine*, 23rd ed. Philadelphia: Saunders Elsevier; 2008:2852.

treatment, but intravitreal ranibizumab can provide significant and sustained visual improvement.▄▄ Central vein occlusion is associated with a major risk for developing secondary neovascular glaucoma.

Giant cell arteritis (temporal arteritis [Chapter 271]) is occlusion of the blood supply of the optic disc by inflammation of the short posterior ciliary arteries. Occlusion causes acute, painless loss of vision. Presenting symptoms before visual loss often include a vague sensation of fatigue, scalp tenderness, or jaw claudication. Diagnosis is suspected by classic characteristics and by an elevated erythrocyte sedimentation rate or elevated C-reactive protein level. Histologic confirmation is provided by a biopsy showing granulomatous inflammation in the region of the internal elastic lamina of the temporal artery. Emergent treatment, often protracted, with systemic steroids (Chapter 271) can prevent vascular occlusion and visual loss, but lost vision is not usually restored by treatment. There is a significant risk for the process developing in the second eye.

Nonarteritic optic neuropathy is caused by occlusion of the posterior ciliary arteries and infarction of the optic disc, resulting in acute, usually unilateral, painless loss of vision. There often are no antecedent symptoms except those systemic signs and symptoms associated with systemic nonarteritic vascular disease such as systemic hypertension. Occlusion is thought to be due to atherosclerosis or some other lumen-compromising mechanism. No treatment restores vision. There is a risk for the same process affecting the second eye.

● IDIOPATHIC INFLAMMATORY AND AUTOIMMUNE DISORDERS

Ocular or periocular tissues may be the primary focus of isolated idiopathic or autoimmune inflammation. Pain is common, and changes in vision may occur.

Keratoconjunctivitis Sicca

Keratoconjunctivitis sicca, or the dry eye syndrome, results from deficiency of any of the tear film layers. Symptoms include gritty, foreign body sensations, burning, photophobia, and decreased visual acuity. Idiopathic inflammation in keratoconjunctivitis sicca and xerostomia represents Sjögren's syndrome (Chapter 268). Recurrent corneal erosion, keratitis, and corneal opacification can occur. Many medications can also cause dry eyes (Table 423-8).

Artificial tears, up to four times daily, and lubricating ointments are helpful. Corticosteroids (e.g., loteprednol 0.5% eye-drops four times a day) are also effective as an initial treatment. Cyclosporine eye-drops (0.05%, one drop in each eye every 12 hours) are useful when other measures fail.

Scleritis

Episcleritis, which is an inflammation immediately underlying the conjunctiva, is distinguished from conjunctivitis because its radially oriented vessels do not move with the conjunctiva. Mild pain may be present. Episcleritis is self-limited. Instillation of 2.5% phenylephrine is helpful in making the diagnosis because it causes blanching in episcleritis but not in scleritis. Oral or topical nonsteroidal anti-inflammatory medications such as flurbiprofen or diclofenac may hasten resolution.

Scleritis, which presents as severe pain and redness, is associated with infectious or autoimmune connective tissue disease in about 50% of cases. Vision may be reduced if the posterior sclera is involved. Diffuse or sectoral hyperemia is nonmobile and does not blanch with instillation of phenylephrine. Secondary uveitis and keratitis may occur. Diagnostic evaluation includes ultrasonography or magnetic resonance imaging and laboratory tests to identify potential underlying conditions. Treatment may require topical or oral nonsteroidal anti-inflammatory medications or corticosteroids.

Mooren's Ulcer

Mooren's ulcer is idiopathic, progressive, peripheral corneal thinning, likely autoimmune. It can be unilateral or bilateral, and pain is common. Topical corticosteroids, mucolytics, and cytotoxic agents have been used. Bandage contact lenses and conjunctival recession or advancement have also been used with variable success.

Orbital Pseudotumor

Nonspecific, idiopathic orbital inflammation involving the lacrimal gland (dacryoadenitis), extraocular muscles (myositis), orbital fat, sclera, or optic nerve sheath (optic perineuritis) can be caused by orbital pseudotumor. Some of the cases of idiopathic orbital inflammation have been recently associated with immunoglobulin G4 autoimmune disease. Pain is frequent. Patients may present with proptosis, limited ocular movements, or decreased acuity. OCT or magnetic resonance imaging excludes a mass lesion. Patients respond dramatically to systemic corticosteroids within 24 hours, but the steroids must be tapered slowly over months to prevent recurrence.

Iritis

Iritis presents with pain, photophobia, and blurred vision, with about 50% of cases related to systemic disease. Slit lamp examination shows inflammatory cells and protein exudate in the anterior chamber. Symptomatic treatment is with prednisolone acetate 1% suspension four times a day and cycloplegic drugs (cyclopentolate 1 or 2% twice daily) is usually effective, but repeated episodes require evaluation for autoimmune and infectious causes.

Rheumatoid Arthritis

Juvenile rheumatoid arthritis (Chapter 264) is the most common specific childhood entity associated with uveitis. In adults, the ocular manifestations of rheumatoid arthritis mainly affect the anterior part of the eye, cornea, and sclera. Nearly 50% of patients who have peripheral ulcerative keratitis of the cornea have an associated systemic disease, mainly collagen vascular disease, and especially rheumatoid arthritis. Similarly, almost half of patients who have scleritis have an associated systemic disease, and about 15% of these are connective tissue diseases. Scleromalacia perforans, which is aseptic necrosis of the sclera, is associated with rheumatoid arthritis about 46% of the time.

Systemic Lupus Erythematosus

Systemic lupus erythematosus (Chapter 266) causes eye manifestations from both the primary disease and its treatment with derivatives of chloroquine. The retina may show a retinal vasculitis, and the optic nerve an optic neuritis, ischemic or nonischemic. Chloroquine therapy can cause a toxic retinal degeneration, but this complication is rare if the daily dose of chloroquine does not exceed 250 mg (and 6.5 mg/kg of body weight for hydroxychloroquine).

Sarcoidosis

About 25% of patients with sarcoidosis (Chapter 95) develop chronic uveitis. Sarcoid also can involve the lids, conjunctiva, optic nerve, cranial nerves, and lacrimal glands. Anterior uveitis is treated topically with prednisolone acetate in decreasing doses, depending on degree of inflammation, and with daily cycloplegics (cyclopentolate 2%, atropine 1%). Posterior uveitis, dacryoadenitis, and neurologic manifestations require systemic corticosteroids, but the doses have not been standardized.

Sympathetic Ophthalmia

Sympathetic ophthalmia is an autoimmune disease characterized by bilateral, granulomatous uveitis following trauma to one eye. The condition is very rare, occurring in less than 1 per 10,000 cases of ocular surgical procedures and 1 per 1000 cases of accidental trauma.[18]

The identified antigen within the eye is thought to be located in the outer retina. The disease is recognized clinically by signs of inflammation in the uninjured eye, generally 2 weeks or longer after the injury. Generally, removal of the injured eye within these 2 weeks will protect against the development of sympathetic ophthalmia in the uninjured eye, but once the uninjured eye is involved, removal of the originally injured eye is not likely to influence the process. Left untreated, inflammation may destroy the function of both eyes. When sympathetic ophthalmia is established, the patient will require anti-inflammation treatment (e.g., prednisolone, 1.0 to 1.5 mg/kg orally per day), most likely for an extended period. Most patients retain useful vision if treated at an early stage.

⬤ GENETICALLY DETERMINED DISEASES THAT MAY BECOME SYMPTOMATIC DURING ADULTHOOD
Corneal Stromal Dystrophy

Most corneal dystrophies are autosomal dominant and bilateral, progress slowly, and primarily affect one layer of an otherwise normal cornea. Common types of dystrophies are anterior basement membrane, macular, granular, lattice, and Fuchs' endothelial. Some result from mutations within the same gene. For example, the *BIGH3* on 5q31 is associated with granular and lattice dystrophy and corneal dystrophy of Bowman. The main symptom, caused by opaque corneal deposits, is blurred vision. If the decreased vision interferes with activities of normal living, a corneal transplantation can be performed.

Choroidal Dystrophy

Choroidal dystrophies are progressive, inherited disorders characterized by atrophy of the retinal pigment epithelium and choroid. The main entities are central areolar choroidal sclerosis (autosomal dominant or recessive), gyrate atrophy (deficiency of the mitochondrial matrix enzyme ornithine-δ-aminotransferase), and choroideremia (deficiency of component A of Rab geranylgeranyl transferase). No treatment exists for central areolar choroidal sclerosis or choroideremia. An arginine-restricted diet may be helpful in treating gyrate atrophy.

Retinitis Pigmentosa

Retinitis pigmentosa (Fig. 423-31) is bilateral and symmetrical, starts in early adult life, and is progressive. Retinitis pigmentosa can be an autosomal dominant or recessive disease, X-linked, digenic, mitochondrial, or sporadic. The primary defect, apoptotic in nature, appears to be in the neural retinal receptors. The main findings consist of the tetrad of bone-corpuscular retinal pigmentation; a pale, waxy optic nerve; attenuation of retinal arterioles; and a posterior subcapsular cataract. Night blindness is the primary symptom. The electroretinogram usually shows no electrical evidence of retinal function. Vitamin A palmitate supplementation (15,000 IU daily) may slow the rate of progression. Gene therapy is under investigation.

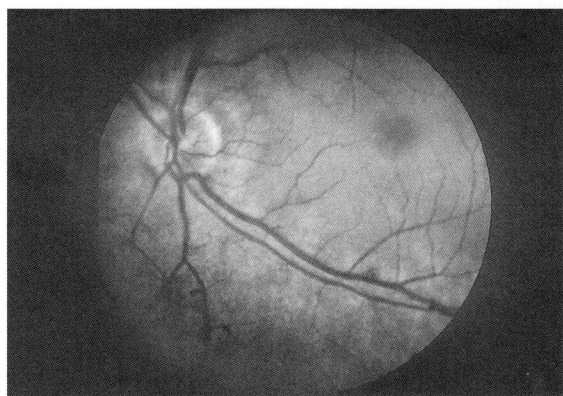

FIGURE 423-31. Retinitis pigmentosa. Fundus photograph shows "bone spicule" pigmentation of the midperipheral fundus, waxy pallor of the optic disc, and attenuated retinal vessels, the most consistent finding in retinitis pigmentosa. (Courtesy of Dr. John I. Loewenstein.)

⬤ COMMON PEDIATRIC OR ADOLESCENT DISEASES THAT MAY PERSIST INTO ADULTHOOD
Retinopathy of Prematurity

The peripheral retina, particularly the temporal retina, is not vascularized in premature infants (36 weeks or younger). In the premature infant, vessels of the immature retina may leave the plane of the retina and grow into the adjacent vitreous body, where tractional forces can cause total, irreversible retinal detachment. The detached retina forms a mass of fibrovascular tissue posterior to the crystalline lens, explaining the original name of this condition, *retrolental fibroplasia*. The primary risk factor for retinopathy of prematurity is the degree of prematurity of the infant and the use of supplemental oxygen. Early recognition and treatment of retinal neovascularization are essential for reestablishing normal retinal vascular development.

Hemangioma of the Eyelid

Hemangioma of the eyelid is a hamartomatous (tissue normally found in the area) malformation of vessels in the soft tissues of the eyelid. The abnormal vascular channel, which may not be clinically evident until several weeks after birth, can expand to enlarge the eyelid and cause mechanical ptosis. Eyelid hemangioma may involute over time, usually in 4 to 7 years, but in the interval there is risk for developing amblyopia. Traditional treatment includes intralesional steroid injection, laser photocoagulation, and, rarely, surgical debulking. Oral propanolol can result in complete regression of eyelid capillary hemangioma in 4 months[19] in patients who are younger than 1 year, which is when the risk for developing amblyopia is highest.

Congenital Cataract

Opacification of the crystalline lens occurs in many developmental and biochemical abnormalities. In congenital rubella (Chapter 368), the opacity is relatively limited to the fetal nucleus and has a pearl-like density. Cataract extraction is essential for dense cataracts of any type if amblyopia is to be prevented, but liberation of live rubella virus into the eye during cataract surgery may lead to necrotizing endophthalmitis and loss of the eye.

The cataract of galactosemia (Chapter 205) is potentially reversible with dietary restriction of galactose. Most other congenital cataracts do not progress. The degree of vision, which may be surprisingly adequate, cannot be accurately predicted by the clinical appearance of lens opacity.

⬤ TUMORS OF THE EYE
Retinoblastoma

Retinoblastoma, the most common intraocular malignant tumor of childhood, results from uncontrolled proliferation of retinoblasts, which are pluripotential neuroectodermal cells that will differentiate into the various components of mature retina. A genetic deletion of the *Rb* (retinoblastoma) gene occurs in the chromosomal region 13q14. The tumor initially proliferates in the plane of the retina but is capable of involving all structures within the eye. Retinoblastoma may spread to the central nervous system through the optic nerve and through blood vessels to tissues at distant sites.

Approximately 40% of cases of retinoblastoma are heritable and generally diagnosed before age 12 months, much earlier than the nonheritable form. In 80% of heritable retinoblastomas, retinal tumors are multiple in each eye and are bilateral. These patients have a significant risk for developing a secondary primary malignant tumor (e.g., osteogenic sarcoma).

The nonheritable, sporadic form arises spontaneously and represents about 60% of cases. The average age at presentation is 24 months. Generally only a single tumor occurs in one eye, unlike the heritable form, in which multiple tumors in one eye and bilateral tumors are common. No detectable chromosomal abnormality is present, thereby making the risk for retinoblastoma in succeeding generations low. These children have the same risk for second primary tumors as the general population.

Retinoblastoma is often discovered by parents or relatives who notice a light reflex in one eye relative to the other either (white or "cat's eye" reflex; leukokoria). Children with retinoblastoma also may present with strabismus, iris neovascularization, dilated fixed pupil, secondary glaucoma, or tumor accumulation in the anterior chamber (neoplastic hypopyon). More advanced cases may present with signs of intraocular inflammation or ruptured globe with orbital extension. In some of cases of regressed retinoblastoma, the sole clinical sign may be a small, calcified tumor in the plane of the retina with surrounding retinal pigment epithelial scarring. Magnetic resonance imaging is the diagnostic test of choice.[20]

Most children are treated with chemotherapy, sometimes also with intraocular laser therapy or radiation, or both. Enucleation is used for advanced cases with no visual potential.

Malignant Melanoma

Malignant melanoma (Chapter 203) of the conjunctiva is rare. The individuals at risk are middle aged and lightly pigmented. Melanoma of the conjunctiva may arise from a preexisting nevus or de novo, but most arise from unilateral, acquired, variably pigmented regional, flat, or slightly elevated lesions in which the degree and distribution of pigmentation tend to vary over time. The regions of greatest risk are in the conjunctiva at the limbus (junction of cornea and sclera), in the conjunctival fornix (deep peripheral recesses of the conjunctiva), and in the caruncle (elevated nodule between the nasal lid margins). Extensions onto the corneal surface or formation of a nodule or loss of pigmentation are indications for biopsy. Proliferation and hyperpigmentation of melanocytes without nuclear or cellular atypia is not associated with progression to melanoma, whereas associated nuclear or cellular atypia, particularly coupled with mitotic activity, is highly linked with progression to melanoma. Frank melanoma with a thickness of more than 0.8 mm is a risk factor for metastatic melanoma. Treatment is surgical excision, often supplemented with cryoablation. The long-term outcome is less favorable than for cutaneous melanoma because the tumor may metastasize early when the primary tumor is very small (e.g., 2 mm).

Malignant melanoma of the uveal tract is the most common primary intraocular malignancy of adults, but its incidence is only 2 to 6 per 1 million per year in high-risk populations (blue-eyed white people). The tumor, which arises from preexisting nevi or dendritic melanocytes anywhere in the uveal tract, is almost always unilateral, unicentric, and nodular and is usually diagnosed at an asymptomatic phase during routine screening examination of the dilated fundus. Symptomatic tumors arise near sensitive portions of the retina (e.g., the macula) or cause retinal detachment or cystoid macular edema. Iris tumors (Fig. 423-32) are generally pigmented and elevated above the surrounding contour, where they are recognized early in their course. Posterior tumors may be completely amelanotic and occasionally may have a bilobed appearance. Accuracy in diagnosing melanoma of the uveal tract by clinical means alone is greater than 98%. Treatment is controversial; options include enucleation of the eye, external beam and plaque (iodine-125) radiation, and en bloc resection. The overall survival rate is approximately 50% at 15 years. Risk factors for metastasis, most commonly to the liver, include tumor size, cell type, angiogenic mimicry, the presence of monosomy 3, and other genetic markers.

Orbital Tumors

Primary tumors in the orbit of adults include cavernous hemangioma, schwannomas, and various proliferations of fibrous tissue (solitary fibrous tumor). Rhabdomyosarcoma may arise from ectopic rests of mesenchyme rather than from mature rectus muscle. Orbital tumors usually are diagnosed

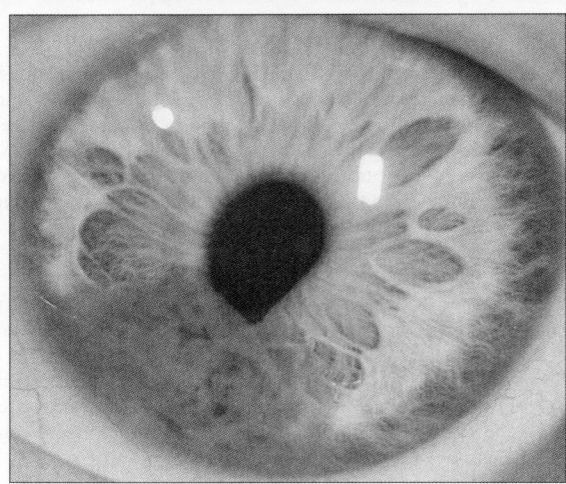

FIGURE 423-32. Iris melanoma that has prominent intrinsic blood vessels. Note peaking of the pupil toward the tumor. (From Yanoff M, Duker JS, eds. *Ophthalmology*. Philadelphia: Mosby Elsevier; 2009.)

by imaging techniques. The treatment is orbital exploration and surgical removal.

Lymphoma

Orbital and conjunctival lymphomas are usually small B-cell mucosa-associated lymphoid tissue tumors (Chapter 185). Approximately 50% of cases ultimately include systemic disease that may, however, be delayed by decades. External beam radiation is used to treat isolated periocular disease, whereas systemic chemotherapy is required for systemic involvement.

Large-cell B-cell lymphoma (Chapter 185) may present in the eye as a form of vitreitis (cells suspended in the vitreous) or a subretinal or intraretinal infiltrate before it is discovered in the central nervous system. The diagnosis may be verified by cytologic examination of vitrectomy specimens. Treatment is generally systemic, but the outcome is usually poor.

The eye may infrequently be involved in multiple myeloma (Chapter 187). Retinal hemorrhages and vitreous opacification may occur. Periorbital osteolytic lesions of bone may be present.

Lacrimal Gland Tumors

The lacrimal gland contains a resting population of non-nodal lymphocytes and is a second common site for lymphomas. Epithelial neoplasms may arise from components of the acini and ducts of the lacrimal gland. Malignant epithelial tumors (adenoid cystic carcinoma) may metastasize at an early stage through perineural spaces of large peripheral nerves to adjacent bone. Most epithelial tumors are treated with total surgical removal of the lacrimal gland because of the risk for recurrence and malignant transformation of residual tumor. The prognosis for malignant lacrimal gland tumors is generally poor.

Ocular Metastasis

Metastasis to the orbit in adults is very uncommon because of its relatively small vascular volume. Metastasis to the rectus muscles present with adult-onset strabismus. Metastasis to the orbit is more common in childhood leukemia than adult leukemia.

Metastasis to the uveal tract is common, especially from primary breast and lung tumors. Metastatic lesions often grow rapidly and disturb visual function; serous retinal detachment is common.

● OCULAR EFFECTS OF SYSTEMIC MEDICATIONS

Innumerable medications may cause ocular side effects (Table 423-9). Therefore, patients taking systemic medications often require periodic surveillance to identify ocular toxicity.

The most common cause of drug-induced glaucoma is topical corticosteroid therapy of more than 4 to 6 weeks' duration in the 5 to 6% of the population that is genetically predisposed. Nonsteroidal drugs usually cause narrow-angle glaucoma. Sulfa-containing drugs may induce glaucoma as an idiosyncratic reaction in persons with either narrow or open anterior chamber configuration. Treatment is the same as for non-drug-induced glaucoma.[21]

TABLE 423-9	SYSTEMIC MEDICATIONS WITH OCULAR EFFECTS
AGENT	**EFFECT**
Chloroquine	Dyschromatopsia, visual field defects
Hydroxychloroquine	Dyschromatopsia, visual field defects
Thioridazine	Blurred vision
Chlorpromazine	Blurred vision
Digoxin	Yellow vision
Ethambutol	Optic neuritis
Amiodarone	Corneal whorls, pigmentary retinopathy
Corticosteroids	Glaucoma, cataract
Plaquenil	Pigmentary maculopathy
Tamoxifen	Retinopathy
Neuroleptics	Nystagmus
Compazine	Oculogyric crisis
Vitamin A	Pseudotumor cerebri
5-Fluorouracil	Canalicular stenosis (tearing)
Isotretinoin	Severe dry eye (long-term effect)

From Goldman L, Ausiello DA, eds. *Cecil Textbook of Medicine*, 23rd ed. Philadelphia: Saunders Elsevier; 2008:2852.

Chloroquine and *hydroxychloroquine* may cause decreased color vision and visual field defects at high doses. Chloroquine toxicity is thought to occur after a cumulative dose of 300 g, whereas hydroxychloroquine may cause symptoms after long-term maintenance of 750 mg/day. The macular portion of the fundus develops a typical bull's-eye pattern of pigment disturbance. Corneal whorls composed of epithelial intracellular pigment may be seen. Vision loss from retinal toxicity is not reversible and tends to progress even after cessation of hydroxychloroquine treatment. Annual fundus examination with color testing, macular function tests, and automated visual field test may be indicated.

Ethambutol is often used for chronic pulmonary infection. The dose of drug is dependent on body weight. Ocular complications, toxic optic neuropathy, is rare but unpredictable in incidence and outcome. Careful follow up with close ophthalmic clinical surveillance is required.

Any of the commonly used antituberculous medications may cause optic neuropathy, although *ethambutol* carries the greatest risk. Pupillary response, color vision, acuity, and visual fields are the clinical parameters used to assess optic nerve function.

Cornea verticillata may be seen in patients taking *amiodarone* because of lysosomal accumulations within the epithelial basement membrane. *Fabry's disease* produces similar changes, as can other medications. Corneal whorls are usually reversible when caused by drug toxicity, and they rarely interfere with vision.

 Grade A References

A1. Shortt AJ, Allan BD, Evans JR. Laser-assisted in-situ keratomileusis (LASIK) versus photorefractive keratectomy (PRK) for myopia. *Cochrane Database Syst Rev.* 2013;1:CD005135.

A2. Wittig-Silva C, Chan E, Islam FM, et al. A randomized, controlled trial of corneal collagen cross-linking in progressive keratoconus: three-year results. *Ophthalmology.* 2014;121:812-821.

A3. Kaufman HE, Haw WH. Ganciclovir ophthalmic gel 0.15%: safety and efficacy of a new treatment for herpes simplex keratitis. *Curr Eye Res.* 2012;37:654-660.

A4. Stalmans P, Benz MS, Gandorfer A, et al. Enzymatic vitreolysis with ocriplasmin for vitreomacular traction and macular holes. *N Engl J Med.* 2012;367:606-615.

A5. Evans JR, Lawrenson JG. Antioxidant vitamin and mineral supplements for slowing the progression of age-related macular degeneration. *Cochrane Database Syst Rev.* 2012;11:CD000254.

A6. Chakravarthy U, Harding SP, Rogers CA, et al. Alternative treatments to inhibit VEGF in age-related choroidal neovascularisation: 2-year findings of the IVAN randomised controlled trial. *Lancet.* 2013;382:1258-1267.

A7. Chew EY, Ambrosius WT, Davis MD, et al., for the ACCORD Eye Study Group. Effects of medical therapies on retinopathy progression in type 2 diabetes. *N Engl J Med.* 2010;363:233-244.

A8. Hoerle S, Kroll P. Evidence-based therapy of diabetic retinopathy. *Ophthalmologica.* 2007;221:132-141.

A9. Régnier S, Malcolm W, Allen F, et al. Efficacy of anti-VEGF and laser photocoagulation in the treatment of visual impairment due to diabetic macular edema: a systematic review and network meta-analysis. *PLoS OnE.* 2014;9:e102309.

A10. Zhang Y, Ma J, Meng N, et al. Comparison of intravitreal triamcinolone acetonide with intravitreal bevacizumab for treatment of diabetic macular edema: a meta-analysis. *Curr Eye Res.* 2013;38:578-587.

A11. Tan MH, McAllister IL, Gillies ME, et al. Randomized controlled trial of intravitreal ranibizumab versus standard grid laser for macular edema following branch retinal vein occlusion. *Am J Ophthalmol.* 2014;157:237-247.

GENERAL REFERENCES

For the General References and other additional features, please visit Expert Consult at https://expertconsult.inkling.com.

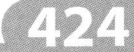

NEURO-OPHTHALMOLOGY

ROBERT W. BALOH AND JOANNA C. JEN

A mechanistic understanding of vision impairment along with disturbances in pupillary and oculomotor control lies close to the heart of diagnosing neurologic disorders.

● VISION

One of the most difficult diagnostic problems is vision loss that cannot be explained by obvious abnormalities of the eye. To evaluate such a patient properly, the examining physician must be familiar with the anatomy and physiology of the afferent visual system. The afferent visual pathways cross the major ascending sensory and descending motor systems of the cerebral hemispheres and in their anterior portion are intimately related to the vascular and bony structures at the base of the brain. Not surprisingly, localization of lesions within the afferent visual pathways has great value in neurologic diagnosis.

Anatomy of the Visual Pathways

Light entering the eye falls on the retinal rods and cones, which transduce the stimulus into neural impulses to be transmitted to the brain. The distribution of visual function across the retina takes a pattern of concentric zones increasing in sensitivity toward the center, the fovea. The fovea consists of a "rod-free" central grouping of approximately 100,000 slender cones. The ganglion cells subserving these cones send their axons directly to the temporal aspect of the optic disc, where they form the papillomacular bundle. Axons originating from ganglion cells in the temporal retina curve above and below the papillomacular bundle and form dense arcuate bands.

The arteries supplying the optic nerve and retina derive from branches of the ophthalmic artery. The central retinal artery approaches the eye along each optic nerve and pierces the inferior aspect of the dural sheath about 1 cm behind the globe to enter the center of the nerve. The artery emerges in the fundus at the center of the nerve head, from which it nourishes the inner two thirds of the retina by superior and inferior branches. Anastomotic branches derived from the choroidal and posterior ciliary arteries, the ciliary system, supply the choroid, optic nerve head, and outer retinal layers, including the photoreceptors. In about 10% of the population, the macula is supplied by a retinociliary artery, a branch of the ciliary system. Venous drainage from the retina and nerve head flows primarily through the central retinal vein, whose course of exit from the eye parallels that of entry of the artery.

What each eye "sees" is termed its *visual field* (Fig. 424-1). The nasal side of the left retina and the temporal side of the right see the left side of the world, and the upper half of each retina sees the lower half of the world. Behind the eyes, the optic nerves pass through the optic canal to form the optic chiasm. In the chiasm, nerves from the nasal half of each retina decussate and join the fibers from the temporal half of the contralateral retina. From the chiasm, the optic tracts pass around the cerebral peduncles to reach the lateral geniculate ganglia. The orientation of the visual field is rotated 90 degrees in the lateral geniculate such that images from the inferior visual field project to the medial half, whereas images from the superior visual field project to the lateral half. The geniculocalcarine radiation initially fans out into superolateral and inferolateral projections, the latter passing around the lateral ventricle and for a short distance into the temporal lobe (Meyer's loop) before turning posteriorly to reach the striate cortex of the occipital lobe. In the occipital lobe, the striate cortex (area 17) lies along the superior and inferior bands of the calcarine fissure, with macular fibers projecting most

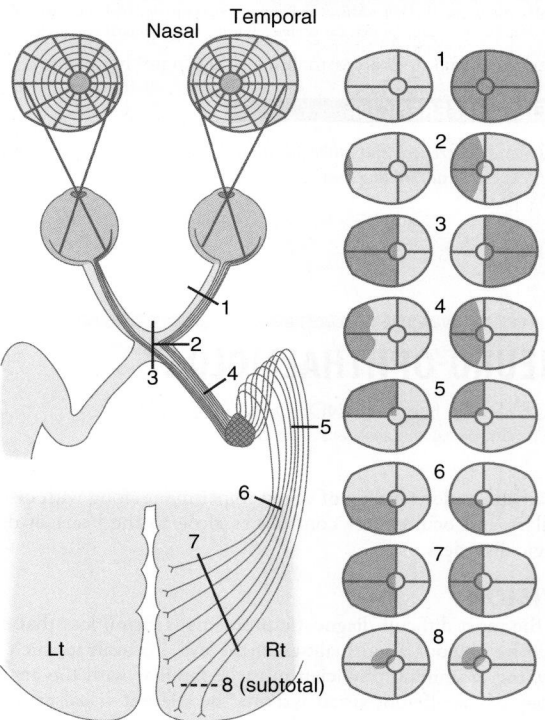

Nasal   Temporal

Lt   Rt

8 (subtotal)

FIGURE 424-1. Visual fields that accompany damage to the visual pathways. *1,* Optic nerve: unilateral amaurosis. *2,* Lateral optic chiasm: grossly incongruous, incomplete (contralateral) homonymous hemianopia. *3,* Central optic chiasm: bitemporal hemianopia. *4,* Optic tract: incongruous, incomplete homonymous hemianopia. *5,* Temporal (Meyer's) loop of the optic radiation: congruous partial or complete (contralateral) homonymous superior quadrantanopia. *6,* Parietal (superior) projection of the optic radiation: congruous partial or complete homonymous inferior quadrantanopia. *7,* Complete parieto-occipital interruption of the optic radiation: complete congruous homonymous hemianopia with psychophysical shift of the foveal point, often sparing central vision and resulting in "macular sparing." *8,* Incomplete damage to the visual cortex: congruous homonymous scotomas, usually encroaching at least acutely on central vision.

posteriorly to the occipital pole and more peripheral retinal projections lying more anteriorly.

Localization of Lesions within Visual Pathways

Monocular vision loss is due to a lesion in one eye or optic nerve. Binocular visual loss, on the other hand, can result from disease located anywhere in the visual pathways from the corneas to the occipital poles. Lesions involving the optic chiasm produce nonhomonymous visual abnormalities (e.g., the bitemporal hemianopia illustrated by lesion 3 in Fig. 424-1). Optic tract abnormalities are comparatively rare but produce characteristic visual changes. The fibers serving identical points in the homonymous half fields do not fully commingle in the optic tract, so lesions damaging this structure produce incongruous homonymous hemianopia. Lesions of the geniculate nuclei, optic radiations, or visual cortex produce congruent hemianopic field defects that may go unrecognized unless the hemianopia intrudes on macular vision. Postgeniculate visual loss can be differentiated from pregeniculate visual loss by (1) a normal funduscopic appearance, (2) intact pupillary light reactions, and (3) appropriate lesions on brain imaging.

Examination of the Afferent Visual System

Visual function is most commonly assessed by "best-corrected visual acuity" (Chapter 423). If visual acuity is not normal, it must be determined whether acuity can be improved with lenses or at least with the use of a pinhole. The normal reference is recognition of letters at an idealized 20 feet, and acuity charts are designed with even larger letters that are normally recognized at proportionally greater distances. Thus, if one reads letters at 20 feet no better than those normally perceived at 40 feet, vision is recorded as 20/40. Small visual charts that are easily carried in the physician's case permit quick and fairly accurate bedside appraisal of acuity.

Visual fields can be tested at the bedside by confrontation, and rough estimates of their integrity can be made even in patients with reduced

TABLE 424-1	COMMON CAUSES OF TRANSIENT MONOCULAR VISION LOSS	
CATEGORY (TYPICAL DURATION)	**CAUSES**	**DIFFERENTIAL FEATURES**
Thromboembolism (1-5 min)	Atherosclerosis	Other atherosclerotic vascular disease, associated crossed hemiparesis, angiography (carotid atheroma)
	Cardiac	Valvular disease, mural thrombi, atrial fibrillation, recent myocardial infarction
	Blood dyscrasia	Blood tests positive for sickle cell anemia, macroglobulinemia, multiple myeloma, polycythemia, other
Vasospasm (5-30 min)	Migraine	Ipsilateral headache, other classic aura, family history
Vascular compression (few seconds)	Increased intracranial pressure	Precipitated by position change, Valsalva maneuver, or pressure waves
	Tumor	Associated slowly progressive monocular visual loss
Vasculitis (1-5 min)	Temporal arteritis	Associated headache, polymyalgia rheumatica, palpable temporal artery, elevated sedimentation rate

alertness. The fields should be tested individually for each eye because the pattern of visual field defects can provide important localizing information. A quick screen of the visual fields can be made by having the patient fixate on the examiner's nose and identify the number of fingers flashed in each of the four visual field quadrants. With practice and a cooperative subject, accurate confrontation fields can be obtained that outline even scotomas. Ophthalmoscopic examination permits direct visualization of the retina and optic disc. Corneal, lenticular, or vitreous opacities severe enough to produce visual symptoms can almost always be detected with the ophthalmoscope.

Common Causes of Visual Loss
Eye

The cause of monocular vision loss secondary to ocular and retinal lesions can often be detected by ophthalmoscopic examination or by measurement of intraocular pressure (Chapter 423). *Glaucoma* caused by impaired absorption of aqueous humor results in a high intraocular pressure that usually produces gradual loss of peripheral vision, "halos" seen around lights, and occasionally, pain and redness in the affected eye. The diagnosis is made by tonometric measurement of high intraocular pressure and may be suspected by palpating an abnormally firm globe and observing a deep, pale optic cup and attenuated blood vessels. *Retinal tears* and *detachments* give rise to unilateral distortions of the visual image seen as sudden angulations or curves of objects containing straight lines (metamorphopsia). *Hemorrhages* into the vitreous humor or infections or inflammatory lesions of the retina can produce scotomas that resemble those resulting from primary disease of the central visual pathway.

Binocular vision loss secondary to retinal disease in younger subjects is often due to *heredodegenerative conditions.* Vascular diseases, diabetes (Chapter 229), and age-related macular degeneration are causes in older patients. In most cases of *pigmentary retinal degeneration,* visual loss begins peripherally and slowly proceeds centrally. By contrast, *macular degeneration* (see Figs. 423-22 and 423-23) impairs central vision early in its course. A common variant in the complement factor H (*CFH*) gene is associated with a markedly increased risk for the development of age-related macular degeneration. Ranibizumab and bevacizumab are about equally effective treatment for neovascular age-related macular degeneration. [A1]

Optic Nerve

Acute or subacute monocular vision loss (Table 424-1) as a result of optic nerve disease is most commonly produced by demyelinating disorders, vascular obstruction, neoplasm, or hereditary optic neuropathy. Demyelinating disease of the nerve head (*optic neuritis* or *papillitis*) produces disc edema along with loss of central vision in the affected eye only; subjectively unrecognized scotomas may sometimes be found in the other eye. Demyelination of the optic nerve behind the point where the retinal vein emerges (*retrobulbar neuritis*) initially leaves a normal-looking disc but a central or paracentral scotoma. With chronic demyelinating disorders, the optic disc becomes pale and atrophic. The clinical course and therapeutic response of optic neuritis depend on the underlying inflammatory mechanism. In more than 50% of patients initially seen with optic neuritis, typical symptoms and signs of multiple sclerosis eventually develop (Chapter 411). Optic neuritis caused by multiple sclerosis is not responsive to steroids, but optic neuritis related to systemic lupus erythematosus (Chapter 266), vasculitis (Chapter 270), or sarcoidosis (Chapter 95) may be steroid responsive.[1]

Optic neuritis with an associated transverse myelitis is the clinical hallmark of neuromyelitis optica, which is a severe demyelinating disease often mistaken for multiple sclerosis but now recognized to be caused by anti-aquaporin 4 autoantibodies. The recommended treatment options include rituximab (1 g infusions at an interval of 2 weeks) or azathioprine (3 mg/kg/day orally).[2] Doses should be adjusted based on response and immune suppression.

Intraocular arterial occlusion may produce either central visual loss or an altitudinal field defect (*ischemic optic neuropathy*). Tumors (Chapter 189) invading the optic nerve or space-occupying lesions compressing it anywhere between the orbit and chiasm cause gradually decreasing central vision or a sector defect of the peripheral visual field. With such chronic lesions, the affected optic nerve becomes visibly atrophic.

Acute binocular vision loss resulting from bilateral optic nerve disease is most often caused by demyelinating disease or by toxic (methanol, tobacco, isoniazid) or nutritional factors (B vitamin deficiency, particularly of thiamine) (Chapter 416). In younger persons and those lacking a clear history of toxic exposure, demyelinating lesions overwhelmingly predominate. Symptoms are of abrupt or subacute onset with visual blurring, which may progress rapidly to blindness within hours or days. There may be pain about the eyes, particularly with movement. *Leber's optic neuropathy*, caused by a mutation in mitochondrial DNA, typically begins painlessly and centrally in one eye, with the second eye affected weeks to months later.

Papilledema is disc edema secondary to increased intracranial pressure (Table 424-2).[3] Vision is normal except under one of two circumstances: (1) acute transient episodes of amaurosis lasting a few seconds and attributable to acute increases in intracranial pressure (plateau waves) and (2) progressive loss of peripheral vision with long-standing, severe papilledema caused by compression of the optic nerve head. Idiopathic intracranial hypertension (Chapter 189) is commonly seen in overweight women of childbearing age. Subacute or chronic binocular vision loss secondary to optic nerve disease can result from *toxic* and *nutritional* causes or from *inherited optic atrophy*. The latter sometimes accompanies spinocerebellar degeneration but may selectively affect the optic nerve. With either cause, visual loss is painless and primarily affects central vision; ophthalmoscopy shows optic atrophy.

Chiasm and Optic Tract

Patients with lesions of the optic chiasm or optic tract are often unaware of visual impairment until the deficit encroaches on central vision in one or both eyes. Intrinsic or extrinsic neoplasms and parachiasmal arterial aneurysms are the most common lesions in this location. Gliomas that arise within the chiasm or optic tract are rare in adulthood. Extrinsic lesions compressing the chiasm or tract include *pituitary adenomas* (Chapter 224), *dysgerminomas*, *craniopharyngiomas*, *meningiomas* (Chapter 189), and large *aneurysms* of the carotid or basilar artery (Chapter 408). The diagnosis rests on finding the characteristic visual field abnormalities (bitemporal hemianopia for chiasm and incongruous homonymous hemianopia for optic tract lesions) and identifying the lesion with computed tomography or magnetic resonance imaging. Pituitary apoplexy secondary to acute hemorrhage into the gland (Chapter 224) can result in sudden vision loss; prompt neurosurgical intervention under steroid coverage is required for most patients.

Visual Radiations and Occipital Cortex

Lesions involving the postgeniculate visual pathways most often result from *vascular damage, traumatic injuries, neoplasms,* or rarely, *inflammatory* or *degenerative disorders* involving the cerebral white matter. Their localization can be deduced by the resulting visual field defects. Vascular disease of the occipital lobes is the most common cause of homonymous visual field defects in middle-aged and elderly people. *Anton's syndrome* refers to cerebral visual loss with denial of a visual defect. Affected patients not only deny that they are blind but also confabulate details of their visual environment from memory. Anton's syndrome results from bilateral lesions involving the parieto-occipital lobes or in the setting of metabolic encephalopathy. The reversible *posterior leukoencephalopathy syndrome*, which is characterized by headache, seizures, confusion, and cortical visual loss, is associated with an abrupt increase in blood pressure, such as may be seen with eclampsia and with immunosuppressive therapy after transplantation.

⬤ PUPILLARY CONTROL

The neuromechanisms that control pupil size and reactivity are complex, yet they can be evaluated by simple clinical procedures. The diameter of the pupil is determined by the antagonistic actions of the iris sphincter and dilator muscles, with the latter playing a minor role. If the sphincter muscle is severed or ruptured, it does not retract toward one quadrant but rather continues to function, except in the altered segment. Therefore, pupillary response can be evaluated even in the presence of significant damage to the iris.

Anatomy and Localization of Lesions within Pupillary Pathways

The size of the pupil is governed by tonic balance between sympathetic and parasympathetic innervation of the muscles of the iris.[4] Sympathetic stimulation dilates the pupil, whereas parasympathetic stimulation constricts it. In the normal resting state, light entering the eye provides the major stimulus governing the size of the pupil (Fig. 424-2). Light activates the retinal rods and cones, with maximal sensitivity in the macular area. The optic nerve fibers follow the crossed and uncrossed visual pathways to the pregeniculate portion of the optic tracts, where the receptor fibers for light diverge to the pretectal nucleus located at the midbrain-diencephalic junction. Interneurons project from this nucleus to the Edinger-Westphal nuclei atop the midbrain third nerve nuclear complex of either side. From that point, paired parasympathetic efferents leave the midbrain in the third nerves, travel in the interpeduncular space across the petroclinoid ligament and edge of the tentorium, traverse the cavernous sinus, and then enter the orbit through the superior orbital fissure. In the orbit, the parasympathetic efferents synapse in the ciliary ganglion, from which ciliary nerves enter the eye to reach the pupillary muscles.

The principal sympathetic control of the pupil originates in the ventral lateral hypothalamus (first-order neuron), from which fibers descend ipsilaterally through the brain stem tegmentum and thence to the cervical cord, where they synapse with preganglionic neurons in the intermedial lateral column of the upper three thoracic segments. Preganglionic fibers (second-order neurons) emerge with the ventral roots of C8, T1, and T2 and ascend in the neck to synapse in the superior cervical ganglion adjacent to the base of the skull. Postganglionic (third-order neurons) pupillary fibers accompany the internal carotid artery through the skull and then leave it to follow the ophthalmic branch of the trigeminal nerve to reach the pupillodilator muscle of the eye.

Examination of the Pupil

The pupillary response to light should be examined in a dimly lighted room, where the pupils are naturally dilated. First, the size and symmetry of the pupils are assessed by shining a dim light onto the face from below so that both pupils are seen simultaneously in the indirect illumination. To test light reactivity, gaze is directed at a distant object (so that constriction secondary to convergence is minimal), and first one and then the other pupil is illuminated with a bright light source. If a pupil reacts poorly to direct light, it is

TABLE 424-2	DIFFERENTIATION OF OPTIC NEURITIS FROM PAPILLEDEMA	
	OPTIC NEURITIS	**PAPILLEDEMA**
Central-cecocentral vision loss	Present	Absent
Distribution	Usually unilateral	Usually bilateral
Ocular pain on movement	Present	Absent
Direct light reflex	±Reduced	Intact
CT and MRI of head	White matter plaques	Tumor, venous occlusion, etc.
Visual evoked responses	Abnormal	Normal
Lumbar puncture pressure	Normal	Elevated

CT = computed tomography; MRI = magnetic resonance imaging.

observed as the opposite eye is illuminated (consensual response). Pupils that react poorly to light should be tested for reactivity to the near reflex by first having the patient gaze at a distant object and then quickly fixate on an object just in front of his or her nose. *Light-near dissociation* refers to a pupil that does *not* react to light but does accommodate by constricting to a near target.

Common Causes of Pupillary Abnormalities

With so-called benign pupillary dilation or *physiologic anisocoria*, there is a long-standing difference in the size of the two pupils with normal reflex reactions; the disparity remains constant during constriction and dilation. Lesions compressing or damaging the pretectal region interrupt the afferent light reflex bilaterally to produce dilated and light-fixed pupils (e.g., lesion 2; see Fig. 424-2).[5] Pupillary constriction to the near response is preserved until late stages. Tumors of the pineal gland (e.g., dysgerminomas) and *localized infarctions* are the most common lesions in this location. *Adie's tonic pupil* (Fig. 424-3) is a medium to large (3 to 6 mm) pupil that constricts little or not at all to light and very slowly to accommodation but constricts with the instillation of dilute (0.125%) pilocarpine (Fig. 424-4). The condition usually affects one eye (occasionally both), is more common in women 25 to 45 years of age, and carries no serious implications. It most likely results from postviral denervation of the pupillary muscles. Unexplained unilateral or bilateral dilated pupils as an isolated finding can result from *accidental or intentional instillation of mydriatic drugs*. Transdermal scopolamine is a common cause. Failure of the pupil to constrict promptly with pilocarpine (1%) gives the diagnosis if the history is unclear. Interruption of the emerging third nerve in the ventral midbrain or along the proximal part of its course produces a dilated pupil 6 to 7 mm in diameter. Important causes of compression of the third nerve in this region are *aneurysms* (Chapter 408), *neoplasia* (Chapter 189), and *brain herniation* (Chapter 189) as a result of increased intracranial pressure. In nearly all cases, the pupillary involvement is associated with other signs of third nerve involvement (see later text).

Sympathetic paralysis of the eye with ptosis, anhidrosis, and miosis (Horner's syndrome; Fig. 424-5) can result from lesions anywhere along the pathway of the sympathetic innervation to the eye (Table 424-3). The diagnosis can sometimes be made by identifying associated signs in the

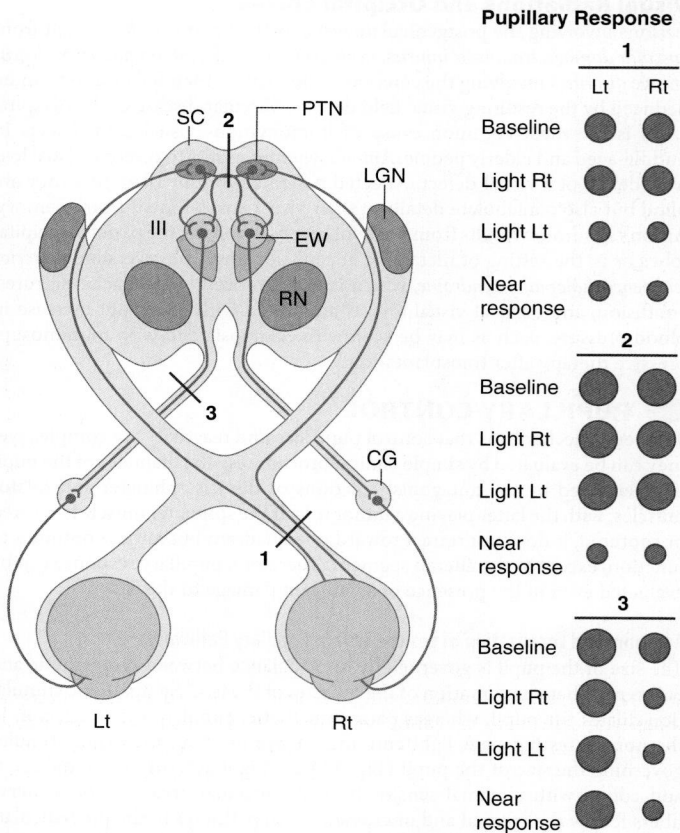

Pupillary Response

	Lt	Rt
1		
Baseline	●	●
Light Rt	●	●
Light Lt	●	●
Near response	●	●
2		
Baseline	●	●
Light Rt	●	●
Light Lt	●	●
Near response	●	●
3		
Baseline	●	●
Light Rt	●	●
Light Lt	●	●
Near response	●	●

FIGURE 424-2. Pupillary responses associated with lesions of the *(1)* optic nerve, *(2)* pretectum, and *(3)* oculomotor nerve. Baseline is obtained with fixation on a distant target and the near response with a target in front of the nose. CG = ciliary ganglion; EW = Edinger-Westphal nucleus; LGN = lateral geniculate nucleus; PTN = pretectal nucleus; RN = red nucleus; SC = superior colliculus.

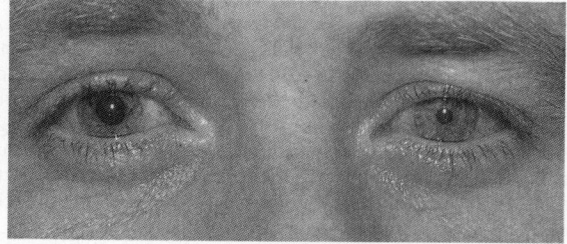

FIGURE 424-3. Adie's tonic pupil in the right eye of a young woman. The affected pupil is "tonic"; that is, it responds slowly to light and accommodation but on rapid testing appears unresponsive. The site of the lesion is usually obscure, but the condition is benign. There may be associated areflexia. (From Forbes CD, Jackson WF. *Color Atlas and Text of Clinical Medicine*, 3rd ed. London: Mosby; 2003.)

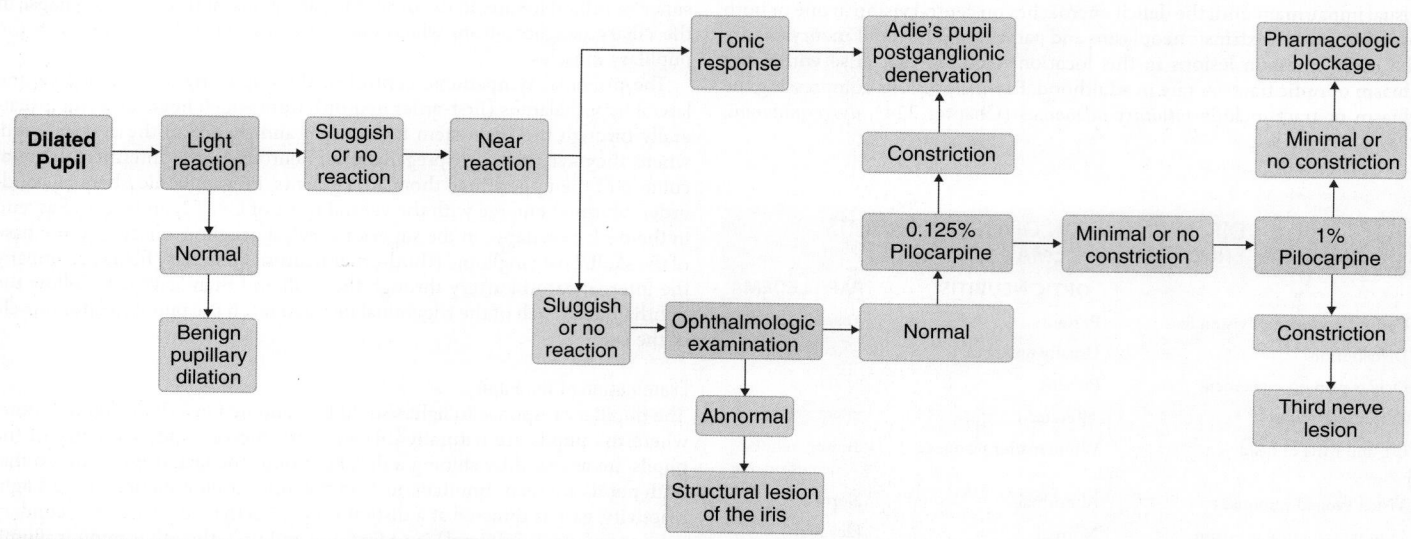

FIGURE 424-4. Use of pilocarpine to help differentiate between different causes of a dilated pupil.

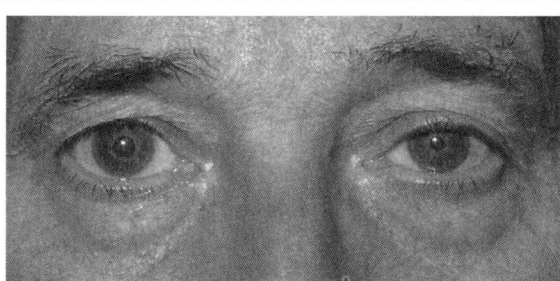

FIGURE 424-5. Horner's syndrome. Note the characteristic ptosis of the left eye associated with constriction of the pupil (miosis). This patient had syringomyelia, but Horner's syndrome has many possible causes. (From Forbes CD, Jackson WF. *Color Atlas and Text of Clinical Medicine,* 3rd ed. London: Mosby; 2003.)

TABLE 424-3 HORNER'S SYNDROME RESULTS FROM LESIONS IN MULTIPLE LOCATIONS

LOCATION OF LESION	NEURON INVOLVED	TYPE OF LESION	ASSOCIATED SYMPTOMS AND SIGNS
Lateral brain stem	1st order	Infarction, glioma	Vertigo, nystagmus, imbalance, numbness, weakness
Apex of lung	2nd order	Lung cancer, trauma	Often none
Neck	3rd order	Carotid dissection or inflammation	Pain, monocular visual loss, hemiparesis

TABLE 424-4 SUPRANUCLEAR OCULOMOTOR CONTROL SYSTEMS

SYSTEM	DESCRIPTION	FUNCTION	KEY ANATOMIC STRUCTURES
Saccade	Fast conjugate voluntary movements	Move the fovea to a new target of interest	Frontal eye field, superior colliculus, pretectum—vertical, pontine—horizontal cerebellar dentate nucleus
Smooth pursuit/ optokinetic	Slow conjugate tracking	Match eye velocity to target velocity	Occipital, parietal, pons, cerebellar flocculus
Vestibulo-ocular	Slow conjugate compensatory eye movements	Keep eyes stable when head moves	Pontomedullary region
Vergence	Slow disconjugate tracking	Focus on near and far targets	Pretectum, tectum

brain stem or neck or along the carotid artery. *Argyll Robertson pupils* are small (1 to 2 mm), unequal, irregular, and fixed to light; they constrict minimally to accommodation. Their principal cause is tertiary neurosyphilis (Chapter 319).

OCULOMOTOR CONTROL

Abnormal eye movements can result from disturbances at several levels. Disconjugate eye movements result from lesions in the individual ocular muscles, the myoneural junctions, the oculomotor nerves and their three paired nuclei in the brain stem, and the internuclear medial longitudinal fasciculus (MLF), which yokes the eyes in horizontal movements. Supranuclear lesions typically produce disorders of conjugate gaze (gaze palsies).

Anatomy and Localization of Lesions within the Oculomotor Pathways
Nuclear and Internuclear Pathways
The abducens (sixth) nerve supplies the lateral rectus muscle. Selective involvement of the abducens nerve anywhere along its pathway leads to isolated weakness of abduction of the affected eye. Destruction of the abducens nucleus in the brain stem results in a conjugate gaze paralysis (ipsilateral) because, in addition to oculomotor neurons, the nucleus contains interneurons destined for the contralateral medial rectus nucleus. The trochlear (fourth) nerve supplies the contralateral superior oblique muscle, which turns in and depresses the eye. Patients with superior oblique weakness note an increase in diplopia with head tilt toward the side of weakness and often tilt their head in the opposite direction. At rest, there is slight upward deviation of the involved eye, and downward movement is impaired when the affected eye is turned in. Patients typically complain of diplopia when reading or going down stairs. The third (oculomotor) cranial nerve supplies the remaining ocular muscles. Involvement of the third nerve nucleus in the midbrain always produces at least some bilateral oculomotor weakness; the superior rectus division of the nucleus supplies the contralateral superior rectus muscle (all other divisions supply ipsilateral muscles). Peripheral third nerve paralysis can result from lesions damaging the structure anywhere from its course within the ventral midbrain to where it enters the orbit through the superior orbital fissure. When complete, third nerve palsy produces a widely dilated pupil, severe ptosis, and an externally deviated eye held in position by unopposed contraction of the lateral rectus muscle. In such conditions, the continued trochlear action reveals itself by intorsion of the eye when the subject attempts to look down.

The MLF interconnects the abducens nucleus in the pons with the contralateral oculomotor nuclear complex in the midbrain. It terminates cephalad in the interstitial nucleus in the rostral midbrain and can be traced as far caudad as the thoracocervical region of the spinal cord (coordinating nuchal-ocular control). Lesions involving the MLF characteristically produce internuclear ophthalmoplegia, in which the eyes are conjugate in the primary position but disconjugate on lateral gaze. With fully developed internuclear ophthalmoplegia on lateral gaze away from the side of the lesion, the contralateral eye abducts and shows nystagmus, whereas the ipsilateral adducting eye does not move nasally because of failure of ascending impulses to reach the medial rectus division of the third nerve nucleus. Adduction for convergence is usually relatively maintained.

Supranuclear Pathways
Pathways descending from the frontal eye fields in the frontal lobe through the superior colliculi to the contralateral brain stem regulate rapid voluntary eye movements (*saccades*) (Table 424-4).[6] Pathways descending from the parieto-occipital and frontal regions to the ipsilateral brain stem subserve slow visual tracking (smooth pursuit—foveal target; optokinetic—full-field target). For the vestibulo-ocular reflex, primary afferent neurons in the inner ear synapse with neurons in the vestibular nuclei, which in turn synapse with appropriate oculomotor neurons to produce compensatory eye movements. The *convergence* center is located in the rostral-dorsal midbrain near the vertical gaze center.

Examination of Eye Movements
Fixation and gaze holding are tested by having the patient look center, right, left, up, and down. Each position should be held steady and unwavering with the observer carefully documenting abnormal movements or ocular disconjugacies. Each supranuclear oculomotor control system is examined separately. *Saccades* are tested by having the patient alternately fixate on two targets such as the examiner's finger and nose; the speed and accuracy are noted. *Smooth pursuit* is tested by slowly moving a target back and forth and up and down and observing the patient's ability to produce smooth tracking movements. If the target velocity is low, normal subjects should be able to pursue without requiring catch-up saccades. The *vestibulo-ocular reflex* is evaluated with the head-thrust test (Chapter 428). *Convergence* is tested by having the patient follow a target moving from far to near. The degree of convergence depends to some extent on the cooperation of the patient. A clear sign that the patient is attempting to converge is simultaneous pupillary constriction.

Common Causes of Abnormal Oculomotor Control
Strabismus (Ocular Misalignment)
A comitant (same in all directions of gaze) strabismus present since childhood is usually a benign *congenital disorder*. Latent congenital strabismus can become manifested in adulthood in association with a systemic illness. An acquired skew deviation (vertical displacement of the ocular axes) indicates a lesion within the otolith-ocular pathways (generally the brain stem). Incomitant strabismus can result from restrictive disease of the orbit or from

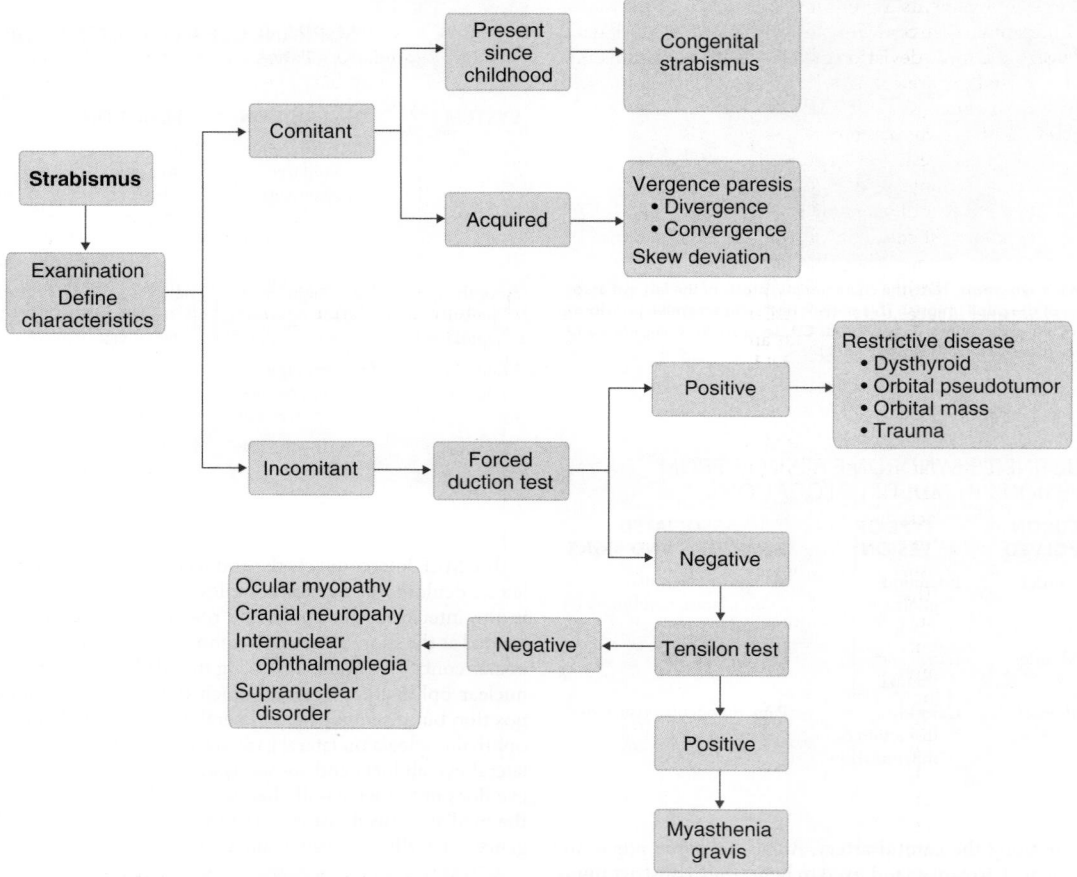

Diagnostic tests that help differentiate among common causes of strabismus.

abnormal muscle or oculomotor nerve function. The presence of mechanical restriction is confirmed by the use of forced duction testing (Fig. 424-6) (After a topical anesthetic is applied to the eye, the ophthalmologist grasps the muscle insertion with large blunt-toothed forceps. Failure of the eye to deviate fully in the pulled direction implies restriction.) Common causes of *orbital restrictive disease* include dysthyroid ophthalmopathy (Chapter 226), orbital pseudotumor, trauma, and orbital mass lesions (Chapter 423). Variable strabismus that increases with fatigue suggests *myasthenia gravis* (Chapter 422). A Tensilon test can usually confirm the diagnosis (see Fig. 424-6). If both restrictive disease and myasthenia gravis (Chapter 422) have been excluded, most patients with incomitant strabismus have processes affecting the oculomotor nuclei, their fascicles, or the cranial nerves themselves. Common causes of an *isolated third nerve palsy* in an adult include aneurysm (Chapter 408), small-vessel occlusive disease (including diabetes mellitus [Chapter 229], trauma [Chapter 399], and neoplasm. Typically, third nerve lesions secondary to vascular disease spare the pupil. Vascular disease and trauma are by far the most common causes of *isolated trochlear nerve palsy*. The abducens nerve is particularly vulnerable to isolated traumatic involvement because of its long pathway outside the brain stem. Lesions that produce increased intracranial pressure (Chapter 189) can lead to abducens nerve dysfunction regardless of the location and produce a "false localizing sign." Other common causes of *isolated sixth nerve palsy* are vascular disease (Chapter 407), trauma (Chapter 399), and neoplasm. About one fourth of cases of cranial nerve palsy (third, fourth, or sixth nerves) remain undiagnosed.

Internuclear Ophthalmoplegia

Internuclear ophthalmoplegia (Fig. 424-7) may be unilateral or bilateral, partial or complete, depending on the location of the lesion and the degree of damage to the MLF. *Demyelinating* and small *vascular lesions* are the most common causes of unilateral internuclear ophthalmoplegia unaccompanied by other ocular palsies or brain stem signs. Larger brain stem lesions that damage one or more oculomotor nuclei plus the MLF often produce

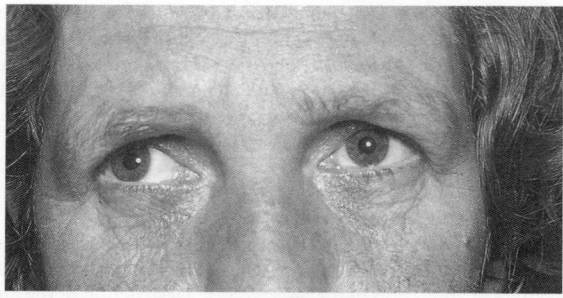

Internuclear ophthalmoplegia may be an initial feature of brain stem involvement in multiple sclerosis. On lateral gaze to the right, adduction of the left eye is incomplete. On convergence, eye movement was normal. The lesion is in the left medial longitudinal bundle, between the nucleus in the pons and the third nerve nucleus on the opposite side. (From Forbes CD, Jackson WF. *Color Atlas and Text of Clinical Medicine,* 3rd ed. London: Mosby; 2003.)

combinations of disconjugate eye movements coupled with nuclear oculomotor palsies. Myasthenia gravis (Chapter 422) can produce an ophthalmoparesis resembling internuclear ophthalmoplegia as a result of greater involvement of the medial rectus than the lateral rectus. Demyelinating diseases (Chapter 411) are the most common causes of bilateral internuclear ophthalmoplegia involvement.

Disorders of Conjugate Gaze

Acute lesions involving a frontal eye field (e.g., hemorrhage or infarction [Chapters 407 and 408]) result in a transient inability to direct the eyes contralaterally. Vertical eye movements are not affected by unilateral lesions. Bilateral damage to the frontal eye fields or their descending pathways may produce an inability to move the eyes voluntarily (horizontal or vertical) despite preserved reflex eye movements, a condition called *oculomotor apraxia*. Lesions involving the horizontal gaze center in the pons produce an ipsilateral paralysis of conjugate gaze and tonic deviation of the eyes to the contralateral side (Chapter 423). Lesions of the pretectum selectively impair vertical gaze, with the vertical upgaze center being slightly rostral and dorsal to the vertical downgaze center. Patients with the *dorsal midbrain syndrome* (Parinaud's syndrome) have a conjugate upgaze paresis. When they attempt to make upward saccades, convergence retraction nystagmus develops. As noted earlier, impaired convergence and light-near dissociation of the pupillary reflexes are also part of the syndrome. The most common causes of the dorsal midbrain syndrome include tumors of the pineal gland (Chapter 223) (dysgerminomas), hydrocephalus (Chapter 189), and localized infarction. With the so-called locked-in syndrome (secondary to basilar artery thrombosis [Chapter 404]), voluntary horizontal eye movements are absent; the patient's only remaining motor functions are vertical eye and lid movements.

Nystagmus

Spontaneous nystagmus can be congenital or acquired. *Congenital nystagmus* typically has a high frequency and variable waveform (usually pendular) and is highly fixation dependent. It generally remains horizontal in all positions of gaze. The lifelong history and lack of symptoms confirm the diagnosis. Spontaneous nystagmus resulting from a *peripheral vestibular* lesion (i.e., in the labyrinth or vestibular nerve) usually has combined horizontal and torsional components (Table 424-5). The nystagmus resolves within a few days of the acute lesion. Acquired persistent spontaneous nystagmus indicates a lesion in the brain stem or cerebellum, or both. The latter is often purely vertical, horizontal, or torsional. Spontaneous *downbeat nystagmus* is commonly seen with lesions of the cerebellum or cervicomedullary junction (e.g., Arnold-Chiari malformation [Chapter 417]).

Gaze-evoked nystagmus is always in the direction of gaze and is usually present with and without fixation. It is most commonly produced by the ingestion of *drugs* such as phenobarbital, phenytoin, alcohol, and diazepam (Chapter 110). It can also occur in patients with such varied conditions as myasthenia gravis (Chapter 422), multiple sclerosis (Chapter 411), and cerebellar atrophy. Asymmetrical horizontal gaze-evoked nystagmus is caused by a structural brain stem or cerebellar lesion (particularly at the cerebellopontine angle), with the lesion generally being on the side of the larger amplitude nystagmus (Bruns' nystagmus). *Rebound nystagmus* is a type of gaze-evoked nystagmus that either disappears or reverses direction as the eccentric gaze position is held. When the eyes are returned to the primary position, nystagmus occurs in the direction of the return saccade. Rebound nystagmus occurs in patients with cerebellar atrophy and focal structural lesions of the cerebellum; it is the only variety of nystagmus thought to be specific for cerebellar involvement. *Disconjugate gaze–evoked nystagmus* most commonly results from lesions of the MLF (see earlier discussion), but it can also occur with other lesions of the brain stem involving the oculomotor nuclei. Positional nystagmus is discussed in Chapter 428.

Other Ocular Oscillations

Ocular bobbing consists of a fast conjugate downward eye movement followed by a slow return to the primary position. The phenomenon accompanies

severe displacement or destruction of the pons or, less often, metabolic central nervous system depression. *Ocular myoclonus* consists of continuous rhythmic pendular oscillations, most often vertical, at a rate of 1 to 3 beats per second; it often accompanies palatal myoclonus and has a similar pathogenesis. *Square-wave jerks* and *ocular flutter* consist of brief, intermittent, horizontal oscillations (back-to-back saccades) arising from the primary gaze position. These types of ocular oscillation are most commonly seen with cerebellar disease but can also accompany more diffuse central nervous system disorders. *Opsoclonus* consists of rapid, chaotic, conjugate, repetitive saccadic eye movements (dancing eyes). Opsoclonus accompanies the cerebellar dysfunction, with the most chaotic varieties associated with brain stem encephalitis or the remote effects of systemic neoplasm, especially neuroblastoma in children. *Ocular dysmetria* refers to overshooting and undershooting of saccadic eye movements, often followed by multiple attempts at refixation. It reflects cerebellar dysfunction.

Grade A Reference

A1. Chakravarthy U, Harding SP, Rogers CA, et al. Ranibizumab versus bevacizumab to treat neovascular age-related macular degeneration: one-year findings from the IVAN randomized trial. *Ophthalmology*. 2012;119:1399-1411.

GENERAL REFERENCES

For the General References and other additional features, please visit Expert Consult at https://expertconsult.inkling.com.

425

DISEASES OF THE MOUTH AND SALIVARY GLANDS

TROY E. DANIELS AND RICHARD C. JORDAN

More than 200 primary lesions or diseases occur in the oral mucosa, gingiva, teeth, jaws, and minor or major salivary glands.[1] In addition, secondary abnormalities of the oral mucosa or salivary glands can be caused by systemic diseases or drugs. The most common or important of these diseases may be observed during physical examination and may be part of a systemic process.

ORAL MUCOSAL DISEASES
Acute Ulcerations

Painful short-term ulcerations can be caused by mechanical trauma, immunologic mechanisms, or bacterial or viral infections (Table 425-1). Soon after formation, oral mucosal ulcers become covered by a white to gray pseudomembrane, analogous to scabs on dry epidermis. Pseudomembrane-covered ulcers are distinguished from white hyperkeratotic lesions by their clinical features of pain, a flat surface, and an erythematous periphery. Traumatic ulcers are characteristically located on the tongue or inside the cheeks or lips, are close to the chewing surfaces of the teeth, and have irregular borders.

APHTHOUS STOMATITIS ("CANKER SORES")

These idiopathic recurrent ulcers, which afflict up to 20% of the population, are found on all nonkeratinized areas of the oral mucosa except the hard palate, gingiva, and vermilion, which are keratinized (Fig. 425-1).[2] They form well-defined circular lesions that may be single or multiple. There are three clinical forms: (1) minor, which are flat and less than 1 cm in diameter and last 5 to 10 days; (2) major, which have raised borders, are greater than 1 cm, and often last for weeks or months; and (3) herpetiform, which are usually clusters of very small ulcers that resemble recurrent herpetic lesions but are not preceded by vesicles and do not occur on keratinized mucosa. A viral or bacterial pathogenesis has not been established for any of these forms. Lesions clinically identical to minor aphthae occur in Behçet's syndrome (Chapter 270). Aphthae are occasionally associated with anemias or gluten-sensitive enteropathy and may become more frequent and severe in association with human immunodeficiency virus (HIV) infection (Table 425-2).

TABLE 424-5	KEY DISTINGUISHING FEATURES OF PERIPHERAL AND CENTRAL TYPES OF SPONTANEOUS AND POSITIONAL NYSTAGMUS	
TYPE OF NYSTAGMUS	**PERIPHERAL (END ORGAN AND NERVE)**	**CENTRAL (BRAIN STEM AND CEREBELLUM)**
Spontaneous	Unidirectional, fast phase away from the lesion, combined horizontal torsional, inhibited with fixation	Bidirectional or unidirectional; often pure horizontal, vertical, or torsional; *not* inhibited with fixation
Static positional	Fixed or changing direction, inhibited with fixation	Fixed or changing direction, *not* inhibited with fixation
Paroxysmal positional	Vertical-torsional, occasionally horizontal-torsional, vertigo prominent, fatigability, latency	Often pure vertical, vertigo less prominent, no latency, nonfatigable

TABLE 425-1   ORAL MUCOSAL ULCERS

TYPE/DISEASE	CLINICAL FEATURES
INSIDIOUS ONSET, CHRONIC	
Multiple or Bilateral	Shallow ulcers on mucosa, skin, or both
Pemphigus vulgaris	Begin as short-duration blisters
Mucous membrane pemphigoid	Begin as short-duration blisters
Lichen planus	Bilaterally symmetrical lesions (associated with hyperkeratosis and/or erythema)
Lupus erythematosus	Asymmetrical lesions, with or without systemic lupus (associated with hyperkeratoses and/or erythema)
Drug reaction	Variable lesions; appropriate history of drug use (e.g., penicillamine, gold)
Epidermolysis bullosa	Begin as blisters; lifelong history
Solitary	Indurated or cratered ulcers
Squamous cell carcinoma	Most common on tongue, oropharynx, lip, mouth floor
Adenocarcinomas, various	Most commonly on palate, cheeks, mouth floor
Tuberculosis	Usually painful
Actinomycosis	Often associated with draining sinus
Deep mycoses (particularly histoplasmosis, coccidioidomycosis)	Associated with systemic infection
Midline granuloma	Associated with necrosis, may perforate palate
Underlying osteonecrosis	Associated with prior cancer radiation therapy or bisphosphonate use
ACUTE ONSET, OFTEN SELF-LIMITING	
Clusters	Usually small and shallow ulcers; history of blisters
Primary herpes simplex	Any oral mucosal site, associated with fever, malaise
Recurrent herpes simplex	Only on gingiva, hard palate, or lip (keratinized mucosa)
Varicella-zoster	Unilateral lesions along neural distribution
Herpangina	Usually on oropharynx
Measles (rubeola)	Precede skin rash; associated with fever, malaise
Solitary or Multiple (without Clustering)	Variable, usually without history of blisters
Traumatic ulcers	Usually solitary; history of trauma
Aphthous stomatitis (canker sores)	Circular, often multiple, only on nonkeratinized mucosa
Behçet's syndrome	Oral lesions similar to recurrent aphthae
Erythema multiforme	Multiple lesions, often involve lower labial mucosa; can be recurrent or chronic
Drug reaction	Appropriate history of drug use
Necrotizing sialometaplasia	Deep ulcers, usually on palate
Primary syphilis	Solitary, indurated, painless, any site
Gonorrhea	Painful, surrounded by erythema, any site

TABLE 425-2   ORAL LESIONS ASSOCIATED WITH HUMAN IMMUNODEFICIENCY VIRUS INFECTION

Kaposi's sarcoma (human herpesvirus type 8)

Candidiasis (pseudomembranous, hyperplastic and/or erythematous lesions)

Other opportunistic fungal infections (e.g., histoplasmosis or coccidioidomycosis)

Aphthous ulcers (increased frequency, duration, or size)

Virus-associated epithelial hyperplasias
  Hairy leukoplakia (Epstein-Barr virus)
  Oral wart (human papillomavirus type 11 and other types)
  Focal epithelial hyperplasia (Heck's disease) (human papillomavirus types 13 and 32)
  Condyloma acuminatum (human papillomavirus types 6 and 11)

Herpes zoster (varicella-zoster virus)

Exaggerated forms of gingivitis and inflammatory periodontal disease

Decreased salivary gland function

Parotid gland enlargement (lymphoepithelial lesion)

Non-Hodgkin's lymphoma (e.g., plasmablastic lymphoma)

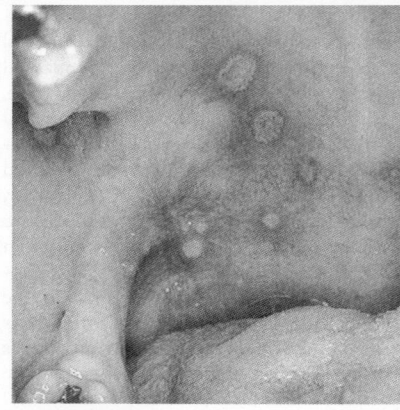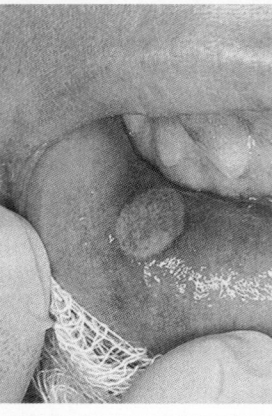

FIGURE 425-1. Aphthous ulcers. *Left,* A cluster of minor aphthae on the soft palate and buccal mucosa, present about 1 week. *Right,* A major aphthous ulcer on the labial mucosa, present about 3 weeks.

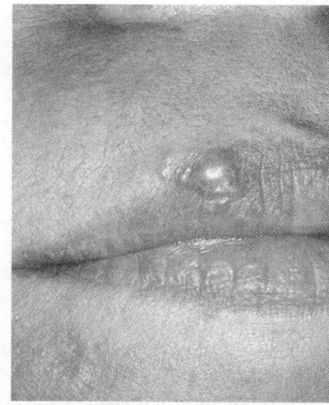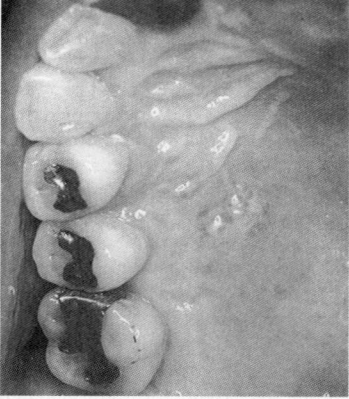

FIGURE 425-2. Clusters of recurrent herpes simplex vesicles. *Left,* on the lip; *right,* on the hard palate, both present 2 to 3 days, in different patients.

Minor or herpetiform aphthous ulcers may not require treatment unless they occur frequently.[A1] Topical steroids, such as fluocinonide gel or ointment, can reduce the severity and duration of the lesions only if applied with prodromal symptoms or earliest signs. A suspension of tetracycline or doxycycline in water used as a mouth rinse at the onset of symptoms also reduces the severity and duration of disease. None of these treatments prevent future lesions. Major aphthae usually require treatment with prednisone (e.g., 40 mg daily for 3 days); failure to respond significantly should prompt incisional biopsy to exclude neoplasia. Unfortunately, no treatment will cure a patient of recurrent aphthous stomatitis.[A2]

VIRAL ULCERS

Several types of virus (most commonly herpes simplex type 1; Chapter 374) cause multiple oral mucosal vesicles that last only a few hours or days and then become irregular shallow ulcers. In the initial infection by herpes simplex virus, usually in children, numerous vesicles may appear on any oral mucosal site (primary herpetic gingivostomatitis), accompanied by malaise, headache, fever, and cervical lymphadenopathy. Patients previously exposed to this virus may develop recurrent (secondary) lesions as clusters of small vesicles, most commonly on the lips (herpes labialis) and less commonly on the keratinized mucosa of the gingiva or hard palate (Fig. 425-2). Such lesions contain live virus and tend to recur at the same site but less frequently with increasing age.

Although widespread vaccination has reduced the incidence, similar mucosal vesicles may also accompany the initial infection by the varicella-zoster virus in children with chickenpox (Chapter 375), and unilateral lesions may occur if herpes zoster (Chapter 375) affects branches of the trigeminal nerve. Uncommonly, oral mucosal ulcers may be caused by different types of coxsackievirus (Chapter 379), appearing on any oral site in hand-foot-and-mouth disease or on the soft palate or pharynx in herpangina. After infection by the measles (rubeola) virus, small ulcers (Koplik's spots; see Fig. 367-1) may form on the inside of the cheeks 1 to 2 days before development of the skin rash (Chapter 367).

ERYTHEMA MULTIFORME

In this potentially recurrent disease, painful oral mucosal ulcerations develop rapidly, with or without target-like skin lesions. It may be associated with a previous viral infection or hypersensitivity to a food or drug. The affected patients, usually young adults with minimal or no systemic symptoms, have irregularly shaped ulcers that can be small and few or involve large areas of the mucosa; the most common sites are the lower labial mucosa and vermilion. On the vermillion, hemorrhagic crusting is a characteristic finding. These lesions can be distinguished from those of primary herpes by the absence of oral vesicles and systemic symptoms or by the presence of characteristic skin lesions (Chapter 439). A major variant of this disease is Stevens-Johnson syndrome, in which ocular, genital, and other lesions may accompany the oral lesions.

VENEREAL INFECTIONS

Primary syphilis may arise as a solitary, indurated, painless ulcer on the oral mucosa that resolves spontaneously in 4 to 6 weeks (Chapter 319). Uncommonly, *Neisseria gonorrhoeae* (Chapter 299) may cause oral ulcers, usually in the pharynx, which may be confused with oral ulcers of other causes.

Oral Squamous Cell Carcinoma

About 4% of all cancers occur in the mouth, commonly as squamous cell carcinomas of the mucosal epithelium (Chapter 190). Oral carcinoma occurs usually in the fifth decade or beyond, in men twice as frequently as in women, and is associated with long-term use of tobacco in more than 80% of cases.

Oral carcinoma usually arises as a chronic, indurated, cratered ulcer, but white (leukoplakia) and especially red (erythroplakia) macular lesions (Table 425-3; Fig. 425-3) frequently exhibit premalignant dysplasia or early carcinoma. Oral carcinomas spread to cervical lymph nodes. The overall 5-year survival rate is about 40%, but early treatment of small, localized lesions can lead to survival rates as high as 90%. Nevertheless, current guidelines find insufficient evidence to recommend for or against screening in asymptomatic adults.[3]

Over the past decade, there has been a rapid increase in a type of head and neck cancer associated with the human papillomavirus (HPV) type 16 (Chapter 373).[4] Occurring primarily at the base of tongue and tonsillar region of the oropharynx, this form of nonkeratinizing squamous cell carcinoma is seen in younger patients who typically lack the history of smoking and alcohol that is usually associated with more traditional forms of oral cancer. Other features of the disease include advanced stage at presentation and its good response to radiation and chemotherapy (Chapter 190). In the absence of concurrent tobacco use, the 5-year survival rate is 70 to 80%.

TABLE 425-3   WHITE AND RED/BLUE ORAL MUCOSAL LESIONS

WHITE LESIONS (PLAQUES)

Squamous cell carcinoma (early)
Frictional keratosis (buccal mucosa at dental occlusal line)
Leukoplakia (with or without dysplasia)
Smokeless tobacco–associated lesions
Nicotine stomatitis (palate)
Lichen planus (reticular and plaque types)
Pseudomembranous candidiasis (thrush)
Hyperplastic candidiasis (candidal leukoplakia)
Hairy leukoplakia (HIV associated; usually on lateral tongue)
Geographic tongue
Mucous patch or condyloma latum of secondary syphilis
Pseudomembrane-covered ulcers (see Table 425-1)

RED OR BLUE LESIONS (MACULAR, MACULOPAPULAR)

Squamous cell carcinoma (early)
Erythroplakia (epithelial dysplasia)
Erythematous (atrophic) candidiasis
Median rhomboid glossitis
Mucocutaneous diseases (see Table 425-1)
Angular cheilitis
Telangiectasias and purpuras (red to blue)
Kaposi's sarcoma (blue to purple)

HIV = human immunodeficiency virus.

Other Chronic Ulcerations

Prescription drugs that can be responsible for chronic oral mucosal ulcerations include barbiturates, β-blockers, nonsteroidal anti-inflammatory drugs, and many others.[5] Several mucocutaneous diseases can cause chronic multifocal oral mucosal lesions composed of ill-defined areas of erythema and ulceration. They are among the most difficult oral lesions to diagnose and are discussed later with the red lesions (see Table 425-3). Several microbial infections or underlying osteonecrosis (e.g., associated with bisphosphonate and other medication use) can lead to indurated, chronic oral mucosal ulcerations with moderate symptoms (see Table 425-1).

White Lesions

White plaques are commonly found in the mouth but, like ulcerations, have a wide variety of causes and outcomes (see Table 425-3). The clinical descriptor term *leukoplakia* applies to a white plaque that does not rub off and whose appearance does not indicate another disease. Leukoplakia can occur in any area of the mouth and usually exhibits benign hyperkeratosis on biopsy (see Fig. 190-1). On long-term follow-up, 2 to 6% of these lesions undergo malignant transformation into squamous cell carcinoma. Areas of leukoplakia with a corrugated surface or mixed with areas of erythema are often found in the lower labial or buccal vestibule of patients who use smokeless tobacco.

Frictional keratoses are often found posterior to the lower molar teeth as irregular white plaques and on the buccal mucosa as white lines adjacent to the dental occlusion. Unlike leukoplakia, these lesions rarely become malignant.

LICHEN PLANUS

Oral lesions of lichen planus (Chapter 438) occur in about 1% of the population, usually as multiple, bilaterally symmetrical reticular white plaques, with or without adjacent areas of erythema (atrophy or erosion) or irregular ulcers[6] (Fig. 425-4). The presence of mucosal atrophy, erosion, or ulceration usually causes pain and sensitivity to certain foods. Most lesions can be

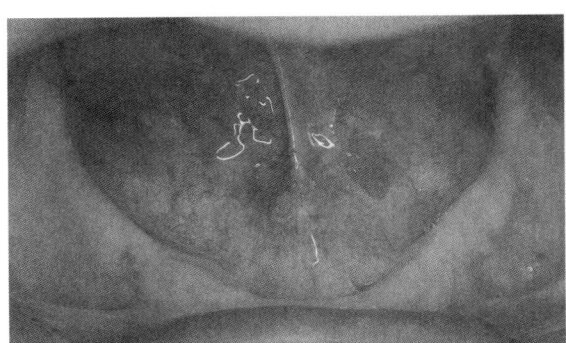

FIGURE 425-3. Squamous cell carcinoma. Biopsy of this area of erythroplakia with slight induration in the anterior mouth floor exhibited squamous cell carcinoma.

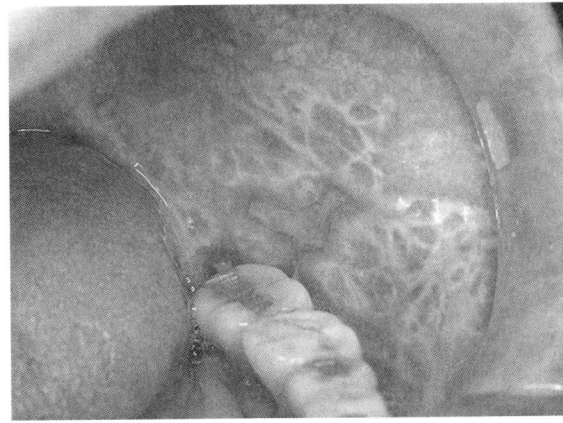

FIGURE 425-4. Lichen planus. A similar-appearing lesion is also present on the right buccal mucosa. Note central pseudomembrane-covered ulceration.

adequately controlled by topical application of fluocinonide or clobetasol gel or ointment (0.05%, three times a day) for periods of several weeks,[A3] although recurrence is common.

ORAL CANDIDIASIS

This common fungal disease (Chapter 338) has three clinical forms: pseudomembranous (thrush), erythematous (atrophic), and hyperplastic (candidal leukoplakia). Pseudomembranous candidiasis, usually of relatively short duration, occurs on any site and consists of white fungal plaques that can be rubbed off, leaving a red or bleeding base. Lesions of hyperplastic candidiasis are white, have fungal hyphae within the surface layers of hyperkeratotic epithelium, do not rub off, and are most often found on the anterior buccal mucosa or on the tongue. Erythematous candidiasis is discussed under Red Lesions. All forms of oral candidiasis represent overgrowth or superficial infection by *Candida* species from the oral flora, induced by a variety of causes, including suppression of bacterial flora by systemic antibiotics, chronic salivary dysfunction, uncontrolled diabetes mellitus or anemia, and immunosuppression (especially in HIV-infected patients). The condition can be managed with topical or systemic antifungal agents, although acquired resistance to fluconazole (200 mg on the first day, then 100 mg every day for 2 to 4 weeks) therapy can occur.

HAIRY LEUKOPLAKIA

The lesion of hairy leukoplakia, which is caused by Epstein-Barr virus, is a white plaque occurring most frequently on the lateral surfaces of the tongue bilaterally in immunosuppressed persons, usually HIV infected (Fig. 425-5). *Candida* may be present in the surface layers, but the lesion is not eliminated by effective antifungal therapy. The diagnosis of hairy leukoplakia by biopsy should raise suspicion of HIV infection or other forms of systemic or local immunosuppression.

GEOGRAPHIC TONGUE

Also called *benign migratory glossitis,* this benign idiopathic condition affects the dorsal tongue of about 2% of the population. It is characterized by well-defined areas of atrophied filiform papillae bordered by arcs of normal or hyperplastic filiform papillae and by gradual changes in the location of these lesions over time (Fig. 425-6). Treatment is usually not necessary.

SECONDARY SYPHILIS

Secondary syphilis may manifest as a well-defined white plaque on the labial or palatal mucosa, called *condyloma latum* (or "split papule," because of its lobulated periphery), or as a mucous patch.

Red Lesions

Solitary red macules or plaques (*erythroplakia*) are less common in the mouth than white lesions but should be viewed with concern because they may exhibit premalignant dysplasia, carcinoma in situ, or carcinoma (see Table 425-3 and Fig. 425-3). One exception is a red macule occurring in the midline of the posterior dorsal tongue, classified as *median rhomboid glossitis,* which is an idiopathic but uniformly benign condition that is often associated with localized overgrowth of *Candida* species.

ERYTHEMATOUS (ATROPHIC) ORAL CANDIDIASIS

Erythematous (atrophic) oral candidiasis is a chronic condition characterized by erythema and atrophy of the filiform papillae on the dorsal tongue or by patchy, ill-defined erythema on the palate, tongue, or buccal mucosa (Fig. 425-7). It is usually accompanied by symptoms of oral mucosal burning and sensitivity to spicy foods. It occurs most commonly in patients with chronic salivary hypofunction (e.g., Sjögren's syndrome or anticholinergic drug effects), but it also occurs in patients who wear removable dentures infected with *Candida,* in whom mucosal erythema is confined to the denture-bearing area.

For acute or chronic oral candidal infections, systemic or topical antifungal drugs are necessary to resolve the associated lesions. In patients who have clinically apparent salivary production, fluconazole (200 mg on the first day, then 100 mg every day for 2 to 4 weeks) is the drug of choice. However, systemic antifungal drugs may not be effective in patients who have severe salivary hypofunction and insufficient saliva to convey the drug from the bloodstream to oral mucosa. In such patients, with remaining natural teeth, *oral* antifungal preparations (troches or pastilles), all of which contain cariogenic amounts of sucrose or glucose, *must not be used* to avoid enhancing dental caries. Instead, slow oral dissolution (15 to 20 minutes for 2 weeks to 2 months) of vaginal nystatin tablets (twice daily) or miconazole tablets (50 mg daily), which contain little or no caries-supporting carbohydrates, is safe and effective; patients usually need frequent sips of water to aid in dissolving the tablets. Effective topical or systemic treatment significantly improves oral symptoms. Treatment of denture-associated candidiasis requires concurrent treatment of the denture.

The treatment end point is reached when mucosal burning symptoms cease, the patient can again tolerate acidic or spicy foods, and filiform papillae on the dorsal tongue have returned to normal; this recovery takes 2 to 12

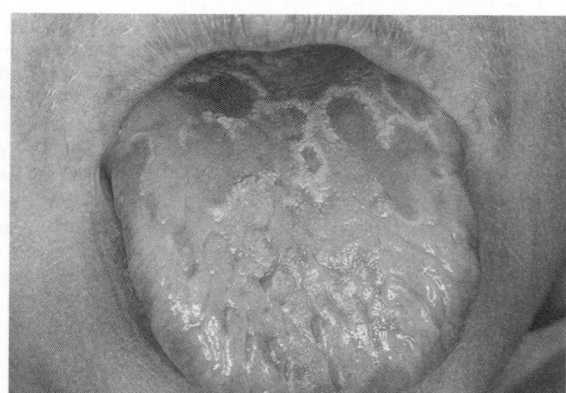

FIGURE 425-6. Geographic tongue. The distribution of these changes on the dorsal tongue may change over time, but they are asymptomatic and diagnosed by their characteristic appearance.

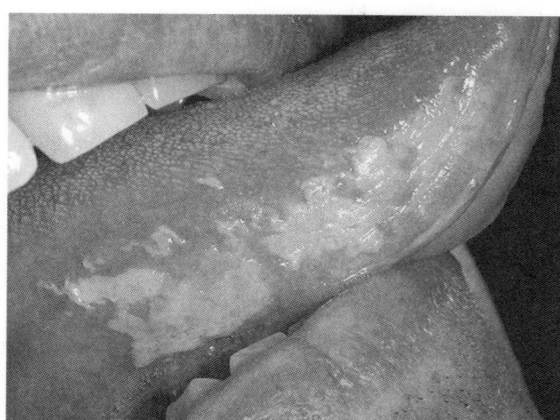

FIGURE 425-5. Hairy leukoplakia. These white plaques were the first visible sign of human immunodeficiency virus infection.

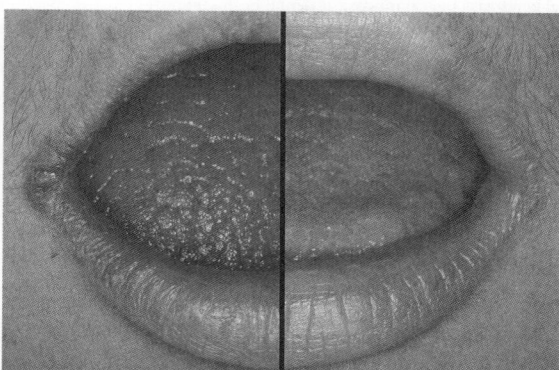

FIGURE 425-7. Erythematous oral candidiasis. *Left,* Erythematous candidiasis in a 26-year-old woman with primary Sjögren's syndrome, exhibiting symptomatic angular cheilitis, atrophic mucositis, and lingual papillary atrophy. *Right,* Asymptomatic and normal-appearing mucosa after treatment with appropriate topical antifungal drugs (see text).

weeks, depending on patients' salivary production and treatment compliance. Recurrence is common in patients with chronic salivary hypofunction or immunosuppression, which necessitates recurring or long-term treatment using a noncariogenic topical antifungal drug that provides a sufficient duration of oral mucosal contact (e.g., nystatin or miconazole tablets).

ANGULAR CHEILITIS

Erythema or crusting of the labial angles is usually caused by *Candida* species (see Fig. 425-7) and is usually associated with intraoral candidiasis. In such cases, topical treatment of the angular cheilitis with clotrimazole (1% cream) must be accompanied by intraoral or systemic antifungal treatment, as described previously.

MUCOCUTANEOUS DISEASES

The mucocutaneous diseases of pemphigus vulgaris, mucous membrane pemphigoid, atrophic or erosive lichen planus, and lupus erythematosus can cause similar-appearing oral lesions. Their diagnosis requires examination of a biopsy specimen by routine histopathology and direct immunofluorescence to identify characteristic deposits of various inflammatory proteins.

The first lesions of pemphigus vulgaris are usually oral mucosal vesicles that rapidly rupture, leaving painful erosions or ulcerations. These are followed by development of skin lesions. Rarely, the lesions remain confined to the mouth (Chapter 439).

Lesions of mucous membrane (cicatricial) pemphigoid are usually confined to the oral mucosa or conjunctivae and occur in patients older than 50 years. They begin as vesicles that quickly rupture, leaving ulcers that are chronic but only moderately symptomatic. Use of topical fluocinonide or clobetasol (0.05% gel or ointment, three times a day, 4 to 12 weeks) for several months, as described for lichen planus, is sometimes sufficient to treat the oral lesions, but some patients also need systemic treatment (Chapter 439).

Oral mucosal lesions of lupus may occur in patients who have systemic lupus erythematosus (SLE), in patients who do not have SLE but later develop that disease, or in patients who do not develop SLE (Chapter 266). In this latter group, the lesions of mucosal lupus may be analogous to the skin lesions of chronic discoid lupus. They take the form of reticular hyperkeratotic figures associated with erythema, often resembling lichen planus, but unlike lichen planus are usually solitary or bilaterally asymmetrical. They can be controlled by topical fluocinonide (0.05%, three times a day, 2 to 4 weeks) or intralesional triamcinolone suspension (5 mg/mL), or respond to systemic treatment of SLE.

Pigmentations

Brown or gray-black macules on the oral mucosa are relatively common and range from benign to highly malignant. They may be caused by localized increase in melanin production, proliferation of melanin-producing cells, or deposition of local or systemically distributed pigmented substances (Table 425-4). Mucosal pigmentation may occur after long-term administration of hydroxychloroquine, minocycline, ketoconazole, methyldopa, or cyclophosphamide. Malignant melanomas can occur at any oral mucosal site, but about 85% develop on the hard palatal mucosa or gingiva, or both. Diagnosis of any

of these conditions is usually established by biopsy and knowledge of relevant underlying conditions.

Lesions of Kaposi's sarcoma associated with HIV infection often appear first on the oral mucosa, especially the palate. They begin as macules with a blue or purple color, at which time they must be distinguished from purpura. Later, they spread radially and expand vertically (Chapter 393).

● ORAL SOFT TISSUE TUMORS

A range of oral benign soft tissue tumors should be treated by excisional biopsy.

Connective Tissue Hyperplasias

The most common oral soft tissue tumors are small, pedunculated masses of hyperplastic fibrous connective tissue covered by normal-appearing mucosa (Table 425-5). Solitary lesions are usually found on the inside of the cheeks or lips. Similar lesions may be present at the border of an ill-fitting denture or may occur in clusters on the hard palate under an ill-fitting denture (palatal papillomatosis).

Generalized or multifocal enlargement of the gingiva (gingival hyperplasia) may be caused by chronic administration of phenytoin, cyclosporine, and many of the calcium-channel blocking drugs (e.g., diltiazem, verapamil, or nifedipine; Fig. 425-8). It can also be associated with a hereditary defect or be caused by an infiltration of atypical white blood cells in some types of leukemia (particularly acute monocytic leukemia; Chapter 183) or by uncontrolled diabetes mellitus (Chapter 229).

Reactive Hyperplasias

Small masses with surfaces that are ulcerated or only partially covered by normal-appearing mucosa usually represent reactive lesions in the form of pyogenic granulomas (whose frequency increases during pregnancy), peripheral giant cell granulomas, or lymphoid hyperplasia of the lingual or other tonsillar tissue. The granulomas are most often located on the gingiva. Rarely, such lesions may represent a metastatic neoplasm.

Epithelial Proliferations

Small, white, wartlike epithelial masses are common and can occur in any area of the oral mucosa (Fig. 425-9). They are occasionally classified as epithelial neoplasms, but most do not continue to grow. Human papillomavirus types 2, 6, 11, 13, 32, and 57 have been identified in these wartlike

TABLE 425-4	PIGMENTATIONS OF THE ORAL MUCOSA (BROWN OR GRAY-BLACK IN COLOR)

INCREASED MELANIN PRODUCTION (FLAT LESIONS)

Oral melanotic macule
Ephelis (vermilion border)
Systemic diseases: Addison's disease, von Recklinghausen's disease of skin, Albright's syndrome, Peutz-Jeghers syndrome

PROLIFERATION OF MELANIN-PRODUCING CELLS (FLAT OR RAISED LESIONS)

Pigmented cellular nevi (benign and premalignant types)
Atypical melanocytic hyperplasia, melanoma in situ, radial growth phase of melanoma
Malignant melanoma

NONMELANIN PIGMENTATION

Amalgam tattoo
Focal deposition of systemically distributed metal (lead, bismuth, mercury, others) usually at sites of chronic inflammation
Systemically administered drugs (chloroquine, minocycline, ketoconazole, cyclophosphamide)

TABLE 425-5	ORAL SOFT TISSUE TUMORS

CONNECTIVE TISSUE HYPERPLASIA (NORMAL-APPEARING OVERLYING MUCOSA)

Irritation fibroma
Denture-associated hyperplasia
Palatal papillomatosis
Generalized gingival hyperplasia
Drug-induced (phenytoin, nifedipine, cyclosporine)
Hereditary

REACTIVE HYPERPLASIA (ERYTHEMATOUS OVERLYING MUCOSA)

Pyogenic granuloma/pregnancy tumor
Peripheral giant cell granuloma
Inflammatory gingival hyperplasia
Hyperplastic lingual tonsil

EPITHELIAL MASSES (USUALLY IRREGULAR WHITE SURFACE)

Papilloma/oral wart
Squamous cell carcinoma
Verrucous carcinoma
Focal epithelial hyperplasia (Heck's disease)
Condyloma acuminatum (venereal wart)
Keratoacanthoma (on lips)

SALIVARY DUCT OBSTRUCTION (MINOR SALIVARY GLANDS)

Mucocele/ranula (usually fluctuant)
Salivary stone (sialolith)

SUBEPITHELIAL NEOPLASMS

Primary connective tissue or salivary gland tumors
Metastatic lesions (especially in the mandible)
Lymphoma (especially in the palate or posterior mandible)
Focal or generalized leukemic infiltrates in the gingiva (especially with acute monocytic leukemia)

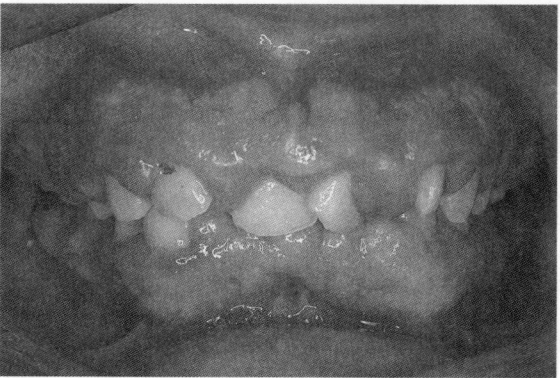

FIGURE 425-8. Drug-induced gingival hyperplasia. Similar clinical lesions may occur with prolonged use of various drugs or as a hereditary condition (see text).

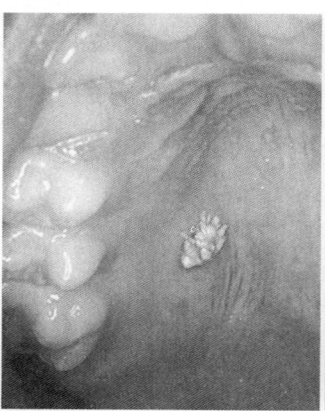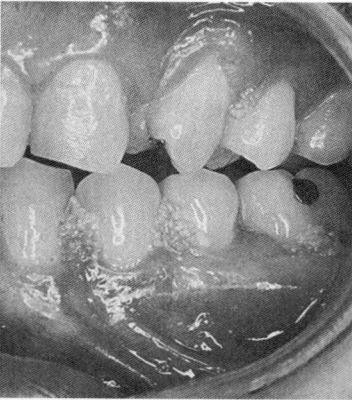

FIGURE 425-9. Papillary epithelial tumors. *Left,* A solitary squamous papilloma. *Right,* multiple gingival papillomas, occurring in all quadrants, from condyloma acuminatum, associated with papilloma virus subtype 6 or 11.

TABLE 425-6	CAUSES OF SALIVARY GLAND ENLARGEMENT

USUALLY UNILATERAL

Benign or malignant salivary gland neoplasms (more than 20 different histopathologic types)
Bacterial infection
Chronic sialadenitis (single gland)

USUALLY BILATERAL AND ASSOCIATED WITH SALIVARY HYPOFUNCTION

Viral infection (mumps, cytomegalovirus, influenza, Coxsackie A)
Sjögren's syndrome (benign lymphoepithelial lesion)
Chronic granulomatous diseases (sarcoidosis, tuberculosis, leprosy)
Recurrent parotitis of childhood
Human immunodeficiency virus infection/acquired immunodeficiency syndrome

BILATERALLY SYMMETRICAL, SOFT, NONTENDER, PAROTID ONLY

Sialadenosis (asymptomatic parotid enlargement), idiopathic or associated with:
  Diabetes mellitus
  Hyperlipoproteinemia
  Hepatic cirrhosis
  Anorexia/bulimia
  Chronic pancreatitis
  Acromegaly
  Gonadal hypofunction
  Phenylbutazone use

lesions, which are usually classified generically as squamous papillomas. A large wartlike lesion on the oral mucosa should raise suspicion of verrucous carcinoma.

Mucous Retention Lesions (Mucoceles)

Mucoceles are small, chronic, or recurring vesicles or bullae that occur commonly on the inside of the cheeks and lips, the posterior palate, and the mouth floor. They are caused by injury to one of the many submucosal minor salivary glands, resulting in extravasation of mucus, which causes granulomatous inflammation or blockage of the excretory duct, leading to cyst formation. Both types of lesions require conservative surgical excision because simple incision and drainage are usually followed by recurrence.

● SALIVARY GLAND DISEASES
Primary Diseases of Salivary Glands

Unilateral major salivary gland enlargement that is markedly painful or tender to palpation and has a purulent exudate or nothing expressible from the duct suggests bacterial sialadenitis. Any exudate should be cultured, and initial treatment should be with an oral penicillinase-resistant antibiotic, such as cloxacillin or dicloxacillin, 500 mg, every 6 hours.

More than 20 types of benign or malignant neoplasms appear as firm and nontender unilateral or bilateral enlargement of a major gland or as a firm submucosal nodule on the palate or the labial or buccal mucosa (Table 425-6). Their causes are unknown, except for Warthin's tumor (adenolymphoma), which has a strong association with cigarette smoking. Uncommonly, unilateral major gland enlargement may be reactive—for example, chronic sialadenitis from duct obstruction or inadequately treated bacterial sialadenitis.

Salivary gland tumors are relatively uncommon and usually present as a swelling in one of the major paired salivary glands or in one of the minor glands of the mouth. Most occur in the major glands, with approximately 90% developing in the parotid. The most common benign salivary gland

tumor is the pleomorphic adenoma. Most salivary gland tumors in the parotid gland are benign, in contrast to the sublingual gland, where more than 90% are malignant. Approximately half of tumors in the submandibular and minor glands are malignant. Benign tumors are generally slowly growing, not fixed to the skin, and do not show ulceration. Malignancies generally grow more quickly, are often fixed to the skin or adjacent normal structures, and tend to show ulceration. Adenoid cystic carcinoma has a characteristic local infiltration by perineural spread. Detection of any salivary gland mass lesions should be followed by appropriate imaging, cytology, and biopsy.[7] Both benign and malignant tumors are generally treated by surgery.[8]

Secondary Diseases of Salivary Glands
BILATERAL SALIVARY GLAND ENLARGEMENT AND DECREASED SALIVARY SECRETION ASSOCIATED WITH SYSTEMIC DISEASES

The best-known cause of bilateral salivary gland enlargement is infection by the mumps virus (Chapter 369) in children. However, the prevalence of mumps decreased in the United States by more than 98% after the introduction of an effective vaccine in 1967, and now there are only a few hundred to a few thousand cases per year. Uncommonly, a less acute, mumps-like illness may occur in adults in association with cytomegalovirus (Chapter 376), influenza (Chapter 364), or Coxsackie A (Chapter 379) virus infection.

About 15% of patients who meet the American College of Rheumatology classification criteria for Sjögren's syndrome[9] (Chapter 268) may gradually develop chronic bilateral enlargement of major salivary glands, which feel firm and nontender or only slightly tender to palpation. Histologically, the tumors begin as a benign lymphoepithelial lesion (myoepithelial sialadenitis), but after years of chronicity, some transform into an extranodal marginal zone lymphoma (Chapter 185).

In most patients with Sjögren's syndrome, gradually progressive salivary hypofunction can impair speech and swallowing and cause a characteristic pattern of progressive dental caries that leads to excessive tooth loss if not actively prevented. In severe cases, the oral mucosa becomes dry and sticky, saliva is not expressible from the major ducts, and about one third of patients have signs and symptoms of chronic erythematous candidiasis (see earlier discussion and Fig. 425-7).

The salivary component of Sjögren's syndrome is diagnosed from a labial salivary gland biopsy specimen that contains three to five minor glands and exhibits focal lymphocytic sialadenitis in the absence of nonspecific chronic sialadenitis or another disease, such as noncaseating granuloma.[10] A patient's symptoms of oral dryness (xerostomia) can be caused by a wide variety of conditions (Table 425-7).

Several chronic granulomatous diseases, such as sarcoidosis (Chapter 95), tuberculosis (Chapter 324), and leprosy (Chapter 326), can cause bilateral enlargement and decreased function of salivary glands. The clinical and serologic features of sarcoidosis may occasionally closely mimic those of Sjögren's syndrome, and the distinction is best made by minor salivary gland biopsy.

TABLE 425-7	CAUSES OF DECREASED SALIVARY SECRETION

TEMPORARY

Effects of short-term drug use (e.g., antihistamines)
Virus infections (e.g., mumps)
Dehydration
Psychogenic conditions (e.g., anxiety)

CHRONIC

Effects of chronically administered drugs (particularly antidepressants, monoamine
    oxidase inhibitors, neuroleptics, parasympatholytics, some combinations of drugs
    for treating hypertension)
Chronic diseases
    Sjögren's syndrome
    Sarcoidosis
    Human immunodeficiency virus or hepatitis C infection
    Depression
    Diabetes mellitus (uncontrolled)
    Amyloidosis (primary or secondary)
    Central nervous system diseases
Other effects of treatment
    Therapeutic radiation to the head and neck
    Graft-versus-host disease
Absent or malformed glands (rare)

A few adult patients with HIV infection and most children who are infected in utero develop major salivary gland enlargement and reduced salivary secretion that are caused by lymphocytic infiltration. Parotid gland enlargement usually represents a solid or cystic lymphoepithelial lesion (see Table 425-2).

Recurrent parotitis of childhood includes episodes of unilateral or bilateral parotid enlargement. During flares of this illness, salivary secretion may be reduced, but usually without prominent secondary symptoms or signs. This condition, of unknown cause, usually subsides after puberty.

ASYMPTOMATIC PAROTID ENLARGEMENT (SIALADENOSIS, SIALOSIS)

Parotid glands can develop bilateral, symmetrical enlargement that is soft and nontender to palpation and associated with normal salivary function (see Table 425-6). Diagnosis is established by this clinical presentation and the presence of one of the systemic diseases known to be associated with it: diabetes mellitus (Chapter 229), hyperlipoproteinemia (Chapter 206), hepatic cirrhosis (Chapter 153), anorexia or bulimia (Chapter 219), chronic pancreatitis (Chapter 144), acromegaly (Chapter 224), and gonadal hypofunction. It can also result from use of phenylbutazone or be a reaction to iodine-containing contrast media. Biopsy of the affected glands is not indicated for diagnosis.

Impaired Salivary Secretion without Gland Enlargement

The common symptom of dry mouth (xerostomia) is most often a side effect of chronically administered drugs. Many classes of drugs reduce unstimulated salivary secretion through anticholinergic or other mechanisms (see Table 425-7). Patients experience these symptoms soon after beginning to use the drug but produce enough saliva during a meal for normal chewing and swallowing. However, the symptoms and associated dental caries are dose dependent and gradually increase with prolonged use of the drug. The classes of drugs producing the most profound effects are most tricyclic antidepressants, most neuroleptics, monoamine oxidase inhibitors, and all anticholinergics. A combination of drugs for treatment of hypertension may also cause symptoms of dry mouth.

Several systemic diseases affect salivary secretion. As noted earlier, most patients with Sjögren's syndrome, some with sarcoidosis, and a few patients with HIV infection experience symptoms of dry mouth to various degrees, with or without salivary gland enlargement. In addition, patients who have primary or secondary *amyloidosis* with salivary gland amyloid deposits may develop impaired secretion. The symptom of xerostomia is more prevalent in individuals who exhibit symptoms of depression, even in those not taking drugs for its treatment. Studies done before the availability of antidepressant drugs showed that symptoms of depression were associated with decreased salivary secretion.

Irradiation of the head and neck region to treat a malignant tumor usually produces profound dry mouth during therapy. Secretory capacity recovers only slightly in the months after treatment for patients with solid tumors but

recovers significantly for those with multifocal tumors (e.g., Hodgkin's disease).

TREATMENT

Significant chronic salivary hypofunction from any cause produces a risk for dental caries (decay) in approximate proportion to the secretory impairment, but caries can largely be prevented if appropriate measures are taken as soon as the hypofunction begins. Remaining teeth should be protected by a comprehensive dental caries prevention program, monitored by a dentist and including frequent application of appropriate topical fluorides, removal of dental plaque, counseling on control of cariogenic dietary carbohydrates, and placement of appropriate dental restorations as necessary.

Symptomatic treatment of mild to moderately severe salivary hypofunction can include sialagogues such as sugar-free hard candies or chewing gum, regular sips of water, and use of saliva substitutes at night, but no topical therapy is reliably helpful.[A4] Symptoms of severe hypofunction can be improved by prescribing pilocarpine (5 mg four times a day), if not contraindicated, but such treatment alone will not prevent dental caries.

Chronic erythematous oral candidiasis is a frequent sequela of chronic salivary hypofunction, and its treatment and retreatment, as noted earlier, substantially improve the patient's oral symptoms.

PERIODONTAL DISEASE

Periodontal diseases are a group of oral infections that affect the periodontium, which are the tissues that support and maintain teeth in the jaws. A worldwide problem, it is the most common causes of tooth loss. Periodontal disease in its most prevalent form is associated with excessive build-up of plaque on teeth and roots. Most cases of periodontal disease begin with inflammation of the gingiva—termed *gingivitis*—that may progress to loss of the supporting bone around the roots of the teeth. Other subtypes of periodontal disease are recognized with differing risk factors and natural histories. The mainstay of treatment is the removal of subgingival calculus and biofilm deposits using mechanical methods (tooth brushing, flossing, scaling, and root planing). Referral for appropriate dental care is indicated. Despite ongoing concerns, there is no current evidence that periodontal disease is an independent risk factor for coronary artery disease.[11]

 Grade A References

A1. Femiano F, Buonaiuto C, Gombos F, et al. Pilot study on recurrent aphthous stomatitis (RAS): a randomized placebo-controlled trial for the comparative therapeutic effects of systemic prednisone and systemic montelukast in subjects unresponsive to topical therapy. *Oral Surg Oral Med Oral Pathol Oral Radiol Endod.* 2010;109:402-407.
A2. Brocklehurst P, Tickle M, Glenny AM, et al. Systemic interventions for recurrent aphthous stomatitis (mouth ulcers). *Cochrane Database Syst Rev.* 2012;9:CD005411.
A3. Davari P, Hsiao HH, Fazel N. Mucosal lichen planus: an evidence-based treatment update. *Am J Clin Dermatol.* 2014;15:181-195.
A4. Furness S, Worthington HV, Bryan G, et al. Interventions for the management of dry mouth: topical therapies. *Cochrane Database Syst Rev.* 2011;12:CD008934.

GENERAL REFERENCES

For the General References and other additional features, please visit Expert Consult at https://expertconsult.inkling.com.

426

APPROACH TO THE PATIENT WITH NOSE, SINUS, AND EAR DISORDERS

ANDREW H. MURR

Patients with nose, sinus, and ear disorders may have a variety of chief complaints. Nasal symptoms most commonly relate to rhinorrhea or congestion, both of which may be due to allergic, infectious, inflammatory, neoplastic, or structural causes. Sinus disorders, which commonly arise as a feeling of stuffiness or congestion but are sometimes also manifested as pain or even headache (Chapter 398), have a similar set of causes. Common ear complaints include pain, tinnitus, loss of hearing (Chapter 428), and vestibular symptoms (Chapter 428), commonly described by the patient as dizziness but recognized by the physician as vertigo that is different from the lightheadedness that characterizes presyncope and syncope (Chapters 51 and 62). Epistaxis, which is bleeding from the nose, is usually easy to distinguish from hemoptysis from the bronchial tree (Chapter 83) or hematemesis from the gastrointestinal tract (Chapter 135).

Loss of hearing (Chapter 428) and vestibular symptoms (Chapter 428) are discussed elsewhere, as are smell, the related sensation of taste (Chapter 427), and the details of head and neck tumors (Chapter 190). This chapter focuses on the approach to patients with other common nose, sinus, and ear complaints.

⬤ NASAL AND SINUS COMPLAINTS
Rhinitis and Sinusitis
▬ DEFINITION

Rhinitis is generally defined as any inflammatory process in the nose, with the common result being a sensation of excess mucous or nasal congestion. The patient may have a sensation of fluid dripping from the nose, either coming from the nose anteriorly or coming from the nose posteriorly. Anterior nasal drainage may be perceived by the patient as being accompanied by an activity such as eating (gustatory rhinitis) and may be visible to an observer. Posterior nasal drainage is more nebulous and subjective, but it is very common and is referred to as postnasal drip.

In general, acute rhinitis and sinusitis describe inflammatory conditions of the nose and sinuses that last less than 4 weeks. Chronic rhinitis and sinusitis persist for more than 3 months despite treatment. Recurrent acute rhinitis and sinusitis are defined by exacerbations that occur four or more times per year and last 7 to 10 days per episode. Subacute rhinitis and sinusitis define symptoms that persist between 4 and 12 weeks and resolve completely with treatment.

▬ EPIDEMIOLOGY

The most common reason for a patient to seek the advice of a physician in the United States concerns problems relating to rhinitis and sinusitis. More than 20 million visits by patients per year are devoted to this complaint, and billions of dollars are spent on medications that are expected to improve the condition.

▬ PATHOBIOLOGY

Humans normally produce about 2 L of mucus per day from their nasal lining. The nose functions primarily as a humidification and filtration system, with a clean and refreshed nasal mucous blanket serving to trap particulate matter and organisms. The nasal and sinus lining consists of ciliated respiratory epithelium; the cilia function in a highly organized and orderly fashion under normal circumstances to transport particulate matter trapped in the mucous blanket in a consistent fashion so that the mucus can be swallowed, thereby avoiding deposition in the bronchi. The nose also serves as the organ of olfaction (Chapter 427) to allow patients to discern tastes and avoid spoiled foods that could cause illness.

The parasympathetic nervous system controls both vascular tone and mucus production in the nose. Inflammatory conditions, such as the common cold, can cause the nasal and sinus lining to swell, thus highlighting the nasal cycle governed by parasympathetic neural control. In a normal state, one side of the nose is relatively decongested and one side is relatively congested because of vascular engorgement. This vascular dilation allows humidification and warming of inspired air and can also affect the ability to discern odors in the process of olfaction. During rhinitis, the inflammation exaggerates the normal relative comparison between the decongested and congested sides of the nose and can be perceived as an uncomfortable nasal stuffiness that shifts from side to side over a period of several hours.

Sinusitis differs from rhinitis in that the term implies an infectious cause rather than physiologic dysfunction. Nevertheless, many different mechanisms of inflammation besides infection may give rise to what is currently generally termed sinusitis.

▬ CLINICAL MANIFESTATIONS

When normal nasal mucosal function is lost, patients often complain of nasal crusting or obstruction, hypersecretion or postnasal drip, coughing, facial pressure, and fatigue. Nasal obstruction that shifts from side to side during

TABLE 426-1	MAJOR AND MINOR SINUSITIS FACTORS
MAJOR FACTORS	**MINOR FACTORS**
Facial pain or pressure (in conjunction with other nasal symptoms)	Headache
	Halitosis
Facial fullness	Fatigue
Nasal obstruction	Dental pain
Nasal discharge or purulence	Fever (in nonacute rhinosinusitis)
Fever (in acute rhinosinusitis)	Cough
	Ear pressure or fullness

the day is common in many types of rhinitis and may be considered an exaggeration of normal physiology.

Major symptoms of sinusitis (Table 426-1) include facial pressure, facial congestion or fullness, nasal obstruction, nasal discharge, and anosmia. Minor symptoms include headache, halitosis, fatigue, dental pain, cough, and ear pressure. Major signs include purulence in the nose noted on examination and, with acute sinusitis, fever. Pain is a frequent complaint with acute sinusitis but infrequent with chronic sinusitis. Patients with chronic sinusitis often note a dull facial pressure that seems to worsen with dependency. Patients with acute sinusitis may have discrete facial pain or dental pain but also have obvious purulent nasal discharge, often with a frank fever. It is important to note that facial pain is not a symptom of chronic sinusitis in the absence of other nasal signs and symptoms. Generally, sinusitis is thought to be present on the basis of at least two major factors, one major factor and two minor factors, or purulence on nasal examination.

▬ DIAGNOSIS
History

A thorough history should probe whether patients have tried over-the-counter or prescription medications, including antihistamines, decongestants, mucolytics, analgesics, mast cell stabilizers, and even steroids, and whether they have helped improve the condition. In addition, other prescription medications have side effects that affect nasal physiology, including birth control pills, antihypertensive medications that cause systemic vasodilation, aspirin, steroids, and antibiotics. Specific questions regarding allergies are important, including seasonality or environmental triggers, the presence or absence of pets, food sensitivities, recent changes in environment, and living conditions, with a focus on old or new carpets, mattresses, furnace filters, or freshly painted interior walls. A patient should be questioned about past allergy skin testing or other testing.

A recent history of other family members or coworkers being ill suggests an infectious process. An astute physician often suspects an infectious process by noting the similarity and time course of symptoms in other patients; this information can be related to patients so that they know what to expect in terms of time course and recovery. A careful past medical history should allow one to determine whether relevant conditions such as previous nasal surgery or trauma, granulomatous diseases, cystic fibrosis (Chapter 89), rheumatologic conditions, immune deficiencies (Chapter 250), or other problems may be contributing factors. Unilateral nasal congestion raises concern for either an anatomic abnormality, such as septal deviation, perhaps related to previous trauma, a polyp or other neoplastic mass, or perhaps even a foreign body.

Physical Examination

The nose should be inspected with a nasal speculum to assess nasal septal anatomy (Fig. 426-1), the most caudal aspect of the inferior turbinates (Fig. 426-2), and the possibility of large nasal polyps (Fig. 426-3) or other masses. In patients with allergic rhinitis, the physical examination may reveal pale and swollen inferior turbinates, whereas copious nasal secretions are more apparent with viral infections. By spraying the nose with a topical decongestant such as phenylephrine (Neo-Synephrine) or oxymetazoline, the middle meatus, which is the air space between the middle turbinate and lateral nasal wall, can often be visualized to assess for nasal polyps or purulent discharge. Examination of the mouth and oropharynx, including the posterior pharyngeal wall, with a tongue blade if necessary, can sometimes identify a stream of postnasal discharge or pus. Sinus palpation and transillumination, although part of the art of medicine, are not sufficiently reliable for diagnosis. The patient's ability to open the mouth without limitation helps exclude trismus, which can sometimes be caused by a deep neck infection.

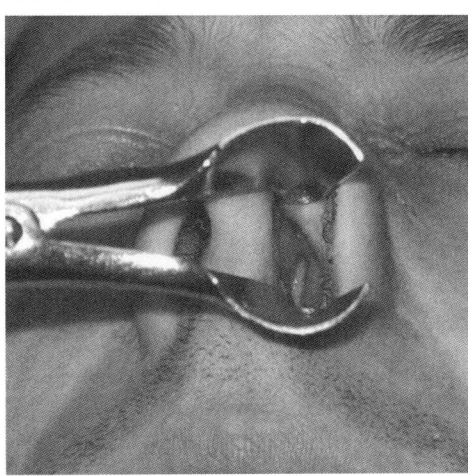

FIGURE 426-1. Purulent drainage from the middle meatus seen on anterior rhinoscopy.

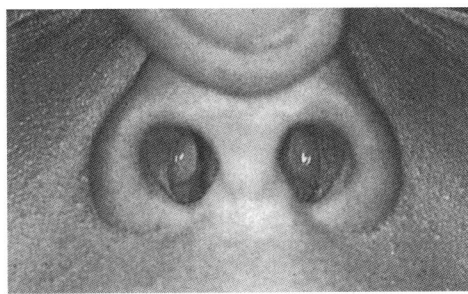

FIGURE 426-2. Edematous inferior turbinates narrowing the nasal airway in a patient with hay fever. Physical examination. (From Dhillon RS, East CA, eds. *Ear, Nose and Throat and Head and Neck Surgery*, 2nd ed. Edinburgh: Churchill Livingstone; 1994:34.)

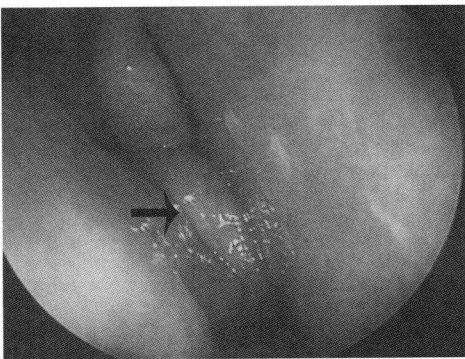

FIGURE 426-3. Nasal polyp in the right nasal cavity. A polyp is seen on the right side just inferior to the middle turbinate, next to the nasal septum. It is paler than the surrounding tissue.

A complete examination of the head and neck should be performed to look for signs of recent or old trauma such as ecchymosis under the eyelids, swelling of the soft tissue of the face, or deviation of the nasal dorsum. The neck should be palpated for adenopathy (Chapter 168) or other masses.

A basic eye examination should be performed to assess pupillary function, extraocular movements, and possible nystagmus (Chapter 424). An ear examination should be conducted to assess the tympanic membranes bilaterally. In patients with an abnormality of the tympanic membrane or concomitant complaints of hearing loss or disequilibrium (Chapter 428), pneumatoscopy using an air bulb attached to the otoscope can be used to

insufflate the ear canal and assess for mobility of the tympanic membrane; decreased mobility suggests a middle ear effusion. Weber and Rinne testing using a 512-Hz tuning fork screens for conductive hearing loss, especially unilateral loss.

Endoscopic examination of the nose, almost always performed by a specialist, is the "gold standard" for evaluating rhinitis and sinusitis. A flexible or rigid fiberoptic scope can allow fine inspection of the septum, turbinates, middle meatus, and sphenoethmoid recess, as well as direct inspection of the nasopharynx, orifice of the eustachian tube, and fossa of Rosenmüller, which is just rostral to the eustachian tube in the nasopharynx and is often the site of origin of nasopharyngeal carcinoma (Chapter 190). Flexible endoscopy can be used to further inspect the oropharynx, larynx, and most of the hypopharynx (Chapter 429).

Laboratory Findings
Cultures
Cultures of the nostril or lower nasal cavity are not typically useful and are not recommended. An endoscopically guided culture of the middle meatus by a specialist may help guide treatment for acutely ill immunocompromised patients, for patients suspected of having acute bacterial rhinosinusitis, for patients with refractory chronic rhinosinusitis, or for those whose sinusitis is suspected of causing secondary meningitis, epidural or subdural abscess, brain abscess, orbital involvement, or cavernous sinus thrombosis.

Other Tests
A nasal smear can reveal eosinophils, which is consistent with allergic rhinitis (Chapter 251). Likewise, skin testing or radioallergosorbent testing can help pinpoint allergic triggers (Chapter 249). In patients with acute sinusitis, a white blood cell count with differential may be useful. In patients with chronic sinusitis, serum immunoglobulin levels can be helpful: highly elevated immunoglobulin E (IgE) levels can raise suspicion for allergic fungal sinusitis, whereas low levels of IgG and other subclasses suggest immunodeficiency (Chapter 250). If the patient has chronic nasal crusting as a primary complaint, screening serologic tests for sarcoid (Chapter 95), granulomatosis with polyangiitis (formerly called Wegener's granulomatosis) (Chapter 270), T-cell lymphomas (Chapter 185), syphilis (Chapter 319), tuberculosis (Chapter 324), Sjögren's syndrome (Chapter 268), and other chronic inflammatory diseases can be considered. Relatively rare infections such as rhinoscleroma may also be present, so biopsy and cultures may be indicated to help reveal a diagnosis. Use of illicit substances should be considered because cocaine and other illicit drugs may cause chronic nasal crusting. In a patient with a lifelong history of sinusitis since childhood, cystic fibrosis should also be considered (Chapter 89).

Imaging
Non-contrast-enhanced computed tomography (CT) is indicated for patients with known or suspected rhinitis and sinusitis. CT is generally performed to document the presence of disease or the effects of treatment to improve the disease. A CT with contrast is used to evaluate complications of sinusitis. Finally, CT is critical before any surgical treatment of the sinuses because of the anatomic information that it provides the surgeon. Opacification or other findings on CT (Fig. 426-4) can sometimes differentiate among the various causes of sinusitis. Plain films have little utility and are not generally recommended. Magnetic resonance imaging (MRI) is occasionally helpful, especially when evaluating tumors or processes that erode bone and are proximate to the brain or eye.

Differential Diagnosis
A rapid onset of sinus-related symptoms suggests a viral upper respiratory infection, especially if the patient also has typical systemic symptoms, such as arthralgia, myalgia, fever, chills, gastrointestinal symptoms, and cough in addition to nasal congestion, postnasal drip, and headache. By comparison, acute bacterial rhinosinusitis causes facial pressure and purulent postnasal discharge. Viral disease can progress to a secondary bacterial infection, which can become chronic. An acute onset of inhalant allergy is often seasonal or can be traced to a particular precipitant (Chapter 251). Allergic rhinitis typically responds to an empirical trial of antihistamines, whereas viral or bacterial rhinitis does not.

Chronic sinusitis must be differentiated from rhinitis, which is not accompanied by the same degree of incessant inflammation. Types of rhinitis include gustatory rhinitis associated with eating, rhinitis of pregnancy, rhinitis related to abuse of topical vasoconstrictors (rhinitis medicamentosa),

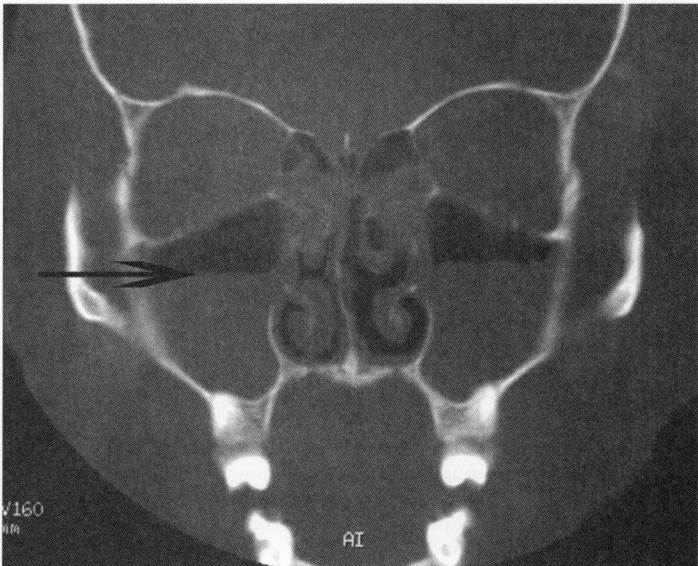

FIGURE 426-4. Coronal computed tomography showing bilateral acute pansinus-itis. There are bilateral fluid levels in the maxillary sinuses that, if aspirated, can be sent for microbiology.

rhinitis associated with illicit drug use (e.g., cocaine or methamphetamine), rhinitis of aging, vasomotor rhinitis presumably related to a hypersecretory state mediated by the parasympathetic nervous system, and perennial allergic rhinitis, whose hallmark is a lack of seasonality.

Chronic sinusitis may be caused by chronic viral infection, chronic bacterial infection, chronic fungal infection, and chronic allergy. It is often difficult to pinpoint a specific cause, but the common underlying factor is often inflammatory in nature. Although maxillary antral punctures were used for diagnosis and treatment in the pre-CT era, endoscopically guided culture techniques combined with CT are now the standard of care, except for acute bacterial maxillary sinusitis, for which surgical decompression is desirable, or for some cases of refractory sinusitis in immunocompromised patients or patients in the intensive care unit, where direct culture can guide antibiotic therapy.

CT can reveal mucoceles, which are blocked individual sinuses that continue to secrete mucus and can slowly erode bone, expand to involve the eye and brain, or become acutely infected. A mycetoma, which is an isolated "fungus ball" in a sinus, has a characteristic hyperdensity within a sinus opacification. Mycetomas (Chapter 342) are noninvasive but may erode bone through pressure necrosis over a long period.

Mucus retention cysts, often present in the maxillary sinus, are manifested as a spherical opacification; an estimated 10% of the population has a mucus retention cyst, which is usually asymptomatic.

TREATMENT   Rx

Medical Therapy
Infectious Rhinitis
Viral rhinitis is treated with supportive care, including fluid replacement and treatment of the febrile component of the syndrome with acetaminophen or nonsteroidal anti-inflammatory medications. Steam has a mild decongestant effect, and vitamin C and good nutrition may help hasten the resolution of symptoms. Oral decongestants (e.g., pseudoephedrine, 120 mg every 12 hours for several days), mucolytics (e.g., guaifenesin, 200 to 400 mg every 4 to 6 hours for several days), and ipratropium bromide (0.03 or 0.06%, two sprays on each side of the nose every 12 hours for several days) are of potential benefit.

For clinically diagnosed acute purulent rhinitis or acute rhinosinusitis of less than 10 days' duration, antibiotics are of little benefit because a diagnosis of bacterial rhinosinusitis based on the history and physical examination is quite inaccurate.[A1][A2] For example, a 10-day course of amoxicillin does not reduce symptoms at day 3 or 10 compared with placebo among patients with acute rhinosinusitis, and it only slightly improves symptoms at day 7.[A3]

Because the potential side effects of antibiotics are not trivial, they should be reserved for patients with a high probability of bacterial infection. The best clinical predictors of the presence of *acute* bacterial rhinosinusitis rather than

viral rhinosinusitis include persistent symptoms for 10 or more days without evidence of clinical improvement; high fever (>39° C or 102° F) with purulent nasal discharge or facial pain for at least 3 to 4 consecutive days; or the onset of worsening symptoms more than 5 days after the onset of an apparent viral upper respiratory tract infection. In patients who meet one or more of those three criteria, the Infectious Diseases Society of America[1] recommends empirical antibiotic therapy, preferably with amoxicillin-clavulanate (875 mg/125 mg orally twice daily, increasing to 2000 mg/125 mg orally twice daily in patients with fever greater than 39° C or 102° F, immunocompromise, or recent antibiotic use). In patients who are allergic to penicillin, the best alternatives are doxycycline (100 mg orally twice daily) or a fluoroquinolone (e.g., levofloxacin 500 mg orally daily or moxifloxacin 400 mg orally daily); by comparison, macrolides, trimethoprim-sulfamethoxazole, and second- and third-generation oral cephalosporins are not recommended because of high levels of resistance. The usual course of therapy is 5 to 7 days, regardless of the medication chosen. Intranasal saline irrigations, using either physiologic or hypertonic saline, may be a useful adjunct in patients with acute bacterial rhinosinusitis,[A4] but neither topical decongestants nor antihistamines are useful. If patients worsen despite 72 hours of treatment or do not improve after 5 to 7 days, further evaluation should include CT to localize the infection, and cultures—either by direct sinus aspiration or endoscopically guided cultures of the middle meatus; other cultures are unreliable.

Chronic sinusitis is a term that encompasses multiple pathophysiologic mechanisms and implies a prolonged course of sinus symptoms that have been refractory to symptomatic treatment over a period of at least 3 months. Chronic sinusitis presents with nasal congestion, nasal drainage, facial pressure, and sometimes anosmia. Unlike acute sinusitis, patients with chronic sinusitis do not typically have fever or severe headache. Corticosteroids, either in a topical spray (e.g., triamcinolone acetonide, two 55-µg sprays to each side of the nose every day; mometasone furoate, two 50-µg sprays to each naris every day; fluticasone propionate, two 50-µg sprays to each naris every day; or budesonide, two 32-µg sprays to each naris every day) for 6 weeks or delivered in an oral tapering dose (prednisone 40 mg per day for 5 days, followed by 30 mg per day for 5 days, followed by 20 mg per day for 5 days, followed by 10 mg per day for 5 days; or methylprednisolone 4 mg tablets beginning with 24 mg the first day and tapering by 4 mg each subsequent day for 6 days) are the mainstay of treating the symptoms of chronic rhinosinusitis. Endoscopically obtained cultures of the middle meatus can help define which patients may improve with culture-guided antibiotic treatment. Antifungal agents, including itraconazole in an oral or aerosolized form and amphotericin B in an aerosolized form, do not appear beneficial in the treatment of typical chronic sinusitis.[A5]

Allergic Rhinitis
Allergic rhinitis (Chapter 251) responds to various antihistamines, such as diphenhydramine hydrochloride (25 to 50 mg every 4 to 6 hours), loratadine (5 mg twice a day or 10 mg a day), cetirizine hydrochloride (10 mg a day), fexofenadine hydrochloride (60 mg twice a day or 120 mg/day), and topical nasal steroids, including triamcinolone acetonide (two sprays [55 µg] to each side of the nose every day), mometasone furoate (two sprays [50 µg] to each naris every day), fluticasone propionate (two sprays [50 µg] to each naris every day), and budesonide (two sprays [32 µg] to each naris every day). Oral steroids such as prednisone and methylprednisolone in various doses are sometimes useful as well. Allergic desensitization is sometimes recommended when a discrete allergen elicits a strong reaction in a patient. Allergic desensitization, through injections or the sublingual route, may specifically be beneficial for some inflammatory disorders, such as allergic rhinitis.

Topical nasal steroids may be of benefit when acute rhinosinusitis is confirmed by either radiography or nasal endoscopy.[A6] However, topical intranasal steroids are also not of proven benefit for treating sinusitis diagnosed by primary care physicians on purely clinical grounds[A7] or for treating the common cold.[A8] Topical nasal steroids are commonly used with good clinical effect in patients with chronic rhinosinusitis.

Surgical Therapy
Patients who have severe symptoms, who fail to respond to therapy, or who have unusual, or resistant, or recurrent infections should be sent to a specialist for further evaluation and treatment (Table 426-2). Surgery is recommended in patients with benign neoplasms, mucoceles, juvenile nasopharyngeal angiofibroma, and some types of malignancies. Surgery can correct septal deviations and anatomically related nasal obstruction. Surgery on the inferior turbinates may be beneficial for refractory rhinitis. Functional endoscopic surgery, which is designed to preserve mucociliary function and is performed with endoscopes through the nostril without skin incisions, can be useful for recurrent acute sinusitis and chronic rhinosinusitis.[A9]

Nasal Polyps

During the evaluation of symptoms of rhinitis or sinusitis, the physical examination may reveal nasal polyps. Nasal polyps often present with symptoms of

TABLE 426-2	WHEN TO REFER A PATIENT WITH PRESUMED BACTERIAL RHINOSINUSITIS TO AN ENT SPECIALIST

- Temperature >39°C (>102° F); orbital edema; severe headache, visual disturbance, altered mental status, meningeal signs
- Failure to respond to more than two courses of antimicrobial therapy
- Nosocomial infection, anatomic abnormalities
- Immunocompromise or multiple comorbidities
- Unusual or resistant pathogens
- Fungal sinusitis or granulomatous disease
- Recurrent episodes suggesting chronic sinusitis

Adapted from Chow AW, Benninger MS, Brook I, et al. IDSA clinical practice guideline for acute bacterial rhinosinusitis in children and adults. *Clin Infect Dis.* 2012;54:e72-e112.

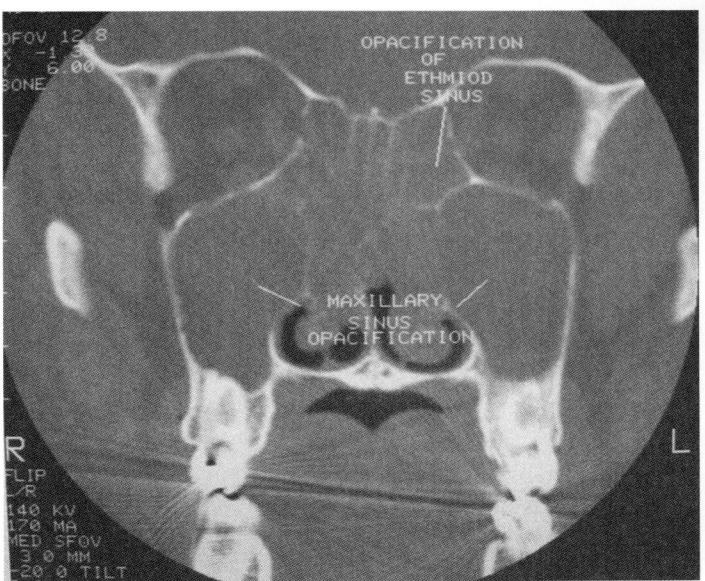

FIGURE 426-5. Computed tomography showing bilateral nasal polyposis of a chronic nature.

nasal blockage and anosmia along with typical symptoms of rhinitis. When polyps are present, the nasal congestion is often unrelenting. Sometimes, patients with prolonged symptoms will present with a visible mass in their nostril. Rarely, facial asymmetry or orbital involvement will be the presenting sign of long-ignored nasal polyps. Patient with nasal polyps may be more likely to complain of facial or ear pain than patients with rhinitis without polyps.[2]

Nasal polyps typically begin near the ethmoid sinuses in the middle meatus and extend into the nose, where they block the nasal airway and/or the sinuses. Nasal polyps may be caused by chronic inflammation and also often occur as part of a rare metabolic disorder of arachidonic acid metabolism triggered by exogenous aspirin intake—known as aspirin-exacerbated respiratory disease. Also known as Samter's triad, patients with this syndrome have asthma that is exacerbated by aspirin ingestion, a skin rash precipitated by aspirin, and often have difficult-to-control chronic nasal polyposis. This constellation of symptoms is thought to be caused by inflammation elicited by leukotrienes, which are upregulated by the prostaglandin blockade caused by aspirin and sometimes by other nonsteroidal anti-inflammatory drugs. Human papillomavirus (Chapter 373) may cause an inverted papilloma, which presents as a polyp causing unilateral nasal obstruction. This initially benign neoplasm responds to surgical excision but can transform to frank malignancy. Polyps are also seen in patients with cystic fibrosis, especially patients with the delta F508 mutation (Chapter 89). They are also seen in allergic fungal sinusitis, which is manifested by an elevated IgE level, positive fungal cultures (usually for aspergillosis), Charcot-Leyden crystals on histopathology, characteristic densities on CT, and nasal polyposis that is often, but not always, unilateral. Antral choanal polyps may extend into the nasal cavity or nasopharynx and cause obstruction.

Nasal polyps will be visible in a careful examination (see Fig. 426-3), and their extent can be shown on a CT scan (Fig. 426-5). Unilateral nasal polyposis is suggestive of antral choanal polyps, malignancy, inverted papilloma, or allergic fungal sinusitis; early biopsy is recommended.

Benign inflammatory nasal polyps frequently respond to oral steroids, either in a tapered burst dose or, in rare cases, in small amounts of titrated daily oral steroids such as prednisone (40 mg per day for 5 days, followed by 30 mg per day for 5 days, followed by 20 mg per day for 5 days, followed by 10 mg per day for 5 days) or methylprednisolone (beginning with 24 mg the first day and tapering by 4 mg each subsequent day for 6 days).[A10] Topical steroids are also efficacious for treating nasal polyps.[A11]

Surgery for benign nasal polyposis can improve symptomatic control and reduce the need for oral steroids. Surgery is always recommended for inverted papillomas, antral choanal polyps, and mucoceles, and surgery is likely to be helpful if acute sinusitis has caused central nervous system complications such as brain abscess (Chapter 413), meningitis (Chapter 412), epidural abscess, subdural abscess, or orbital abscess. Occasionally, surgery will be required when an untreated and aggressively growing polyp causes orbital or skull base erosion. Allergic fungal sinusitis is often treated with a combination of surgery, corticosteroids, and sometimes immunotherapy.

Epistaxis

For a patient with epistaxis, it is first critical to determine the severity of the blood loss. Persistent bleeding may result from warfarin, antiplatelet agents, or any underlying platelet (Chapters 172 and 173) or clotting deficiency (Chapter 174). Physical examination should focus on inspection of the anterior septum, which is the most frequent point of origin for epistaxis. Frequently, dilated blood vessels on the caudal septum can be seen with anterior

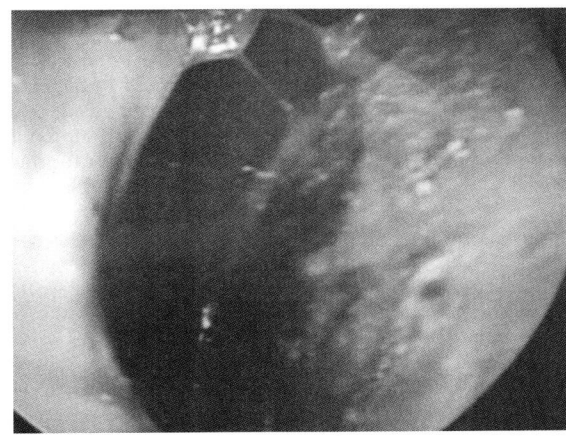

FIGURE 426-6. Dilated nasal vessels and crusting typical of a patient with epistaxis.

rhinoscopy (Fig. 426-6). The combination of unilateral otitis media, epistaxis, nasal congestion, and a neck mass would be concerning for nasopharyngeal carcinoma. Rare tumors that can arise with bleeding include juvenile nasopharyngeal angiofibromas in male patients.

Epistaxis can be treated by local pressure, packing (using nasal sponges, balloons, or by ½-inch by 72-inch gauze impregnated with petroleum jelly), humidification, and hydration. Hospitalization and transfusion are rarely required. Offending medications should be reduced in dose or discontinued temporarily if possible. Topical vasoconstrictive medication such as oxymetazoline spray, two sprays on each side of the nose every 12 hours for 3 days, can help prevent persistent epistaxis. Occasionally, lasers or other types of cautery are used to improve the problem. At times, surgical arterial clipping or interventional neuroradiologic arterial occlusion can address a specific bleeding area.

EAR PAIN

DEFINITION

Ear pain (Table 426-3) is discomfort perceived by a patient in the area of the temporal bone. Although the discomfort can often be localized by the patient, at times the cause of the discomfort may in fact be distant from the site where the pain is felt. This referred pain can be due to problems in the oral cavity, oropharynx, hypopharynx, or larynx.

TABLE 426-3	CAUSES OF OTALGIA		
CAUSES OF OTALGIA	EXTERNAL EAR	MIDDLE EAR	UPPER AERODIGESTIVE TRACT
Likely	Otitis externa Herpes zoster oticus Chondritis Foreign body	Acute otitis media Acute eardrum perforation Barotrauma Chronic otitis media with impending complication	Tonsillitis Tonsil abscess Deep neck abscess Tumor (especially base of the tongue, tonsil, hypopharynx, larynx, nasopharynx)
Unlikely	Malignant otitis externa Tumor	Tumor	

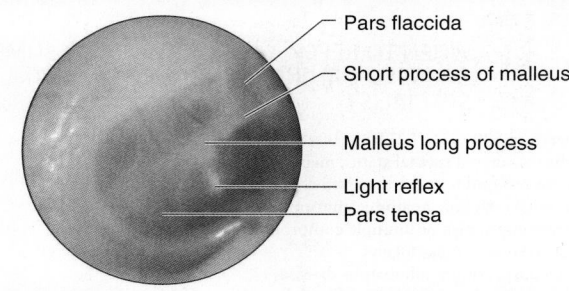

FIGURE 426-7. A normal tympanic membrane. (From Dhillon RS, East CA, eds. *Ear, Nose and Throat and Head and Neck Surgery*, 2nd ed. Edinburgh: Churchill Livingstone; 1994:2.)

Labels: Pars flaccida · Short process of malleus · Malleus long process · Light reflex · Pars tensa

PATHOBIOLOGY

The ear is well supplied with sensory nerves and is positioned on the side of the skull. The ear is divided into the outer ear, or pinna, and the ear canal; the middle ear, which encompasses the tympanic membrane and ossicles (Fig. 426-7); and the inner ear, which consists of the cochlea and the vestibular canals, including the utricle and saccule. In general, otalgia is due to problems in the outer or middle ear. The trigeminal nerve innervates the anterior-superior quadrant of the pinna, whereas the C2 and C3 cervical cutaneous nerves innervate the rest of the majority of the outer ear. However, there are contributions by the 9th and 10th nerves in the ear canal and even a small patch of sensory innervation by the 7th nerve in the posterior superior ear canal. It is the overlap in distribution of the 9th and 10th cranial nerves that establishes the anatomic basis for referred otalgia in diseases of the oral cavity, oropharynx, and larynx. Therefore, ear pain may be due to inflammatory conditions of the skin of the outer ear, the ear canal, or the middle ear, or it may be due to disease processes unrelated to the ear itself.

CLINICAL MANIFESTATIONS

Patients with ear pain often have complaints referable directly to the ear itself. In cases of otitis externa, frankly obvious erythema and swelling of the skin of the ear canal may be present. Even minute physical manipulation of the ear may be excruciating. In chondritis of the pinna, which may be related to rheumatologic disorders, infection, or trauma, the entire pinna may be swollen and painful. Hearing loss accompanying otalgia may indicate middle ear disease, especially otitis media. Patients sometimes complain of pain in the ear after air travel or driving from a mountainous region. Quick changes in pressure, such as encountered in scuba diving, may indicate barotrauma (Chapter 94), in which the eustachian tube is unable to compensate rapidly enough for the changes in pressure that are encountered. Pain may also be a post-traumatic symptom from relatively minor percussion injury, more severe head trauma, or percussion injury related to a blast. Pain related to noise exposure may also indicate damage to the middle ear or even the inner ear. Deep-seated boring pain over the temporal area accompanied by retro-orbital pain can be due to petrous apex disease, including petrous apicitis.

DIAGNOSIS

History

A patient with ear pain should be asked to reveal the location of the discomfort, the duration of the symptoms, and any activities related to onset of the condition. As an example, recent swimming would make otitis externa ("swimmer's ear") more likely, whereas a recent upper respiratory infection with hearing loss would suggest otitis media. Questions should address possible hearing loss, vertigo, otorrhea, hoarseness, voice change, dysphagia, odynophagia, dyspnea, hemoptysis, hematemesis, and weight loss. A social history with specific concentration on tobacco and alcohol use should be obtained. A possible family history of upper aerodigestive tract and nasopharyngeal carcinoma should be sought. A past surgical history can reveal distant ear or throat surgery.

Physical Examination

A complete head and neck examination, including general assessment for trauma and a basic eye examination, is required. The outer ear and pinna should be examined first. The ear canal should first be palpated and then

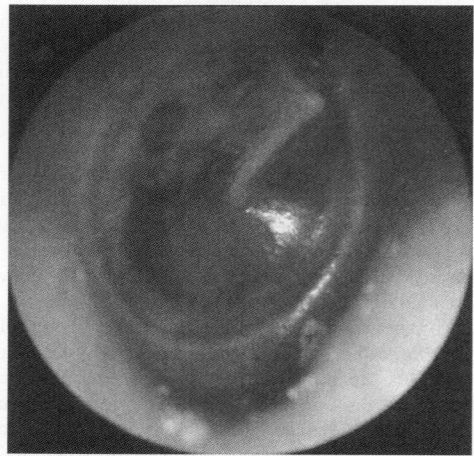

FIGURE 426-8. Otoscopic appearance in otitis media with effusion. The handle and short process of the malleus are brought into relief by retraction of the eardrum. There is a slightly yellow appearance of the eardrum related to the middle ear effusion. (From Dhillon RS, East CA, eds. *Ear, Nose and Throat and Head and Neck Surgery*, 2nd ed. Edinburgh: Churchill Livingstone; 1994:7.)

inspected. An otoscope with a pneumatic bulb attachment is critical to establish the presence or absence of a middle ear effusion. Inspection of the tympanic membrane should be accomplished with notations made about patency and perforation, translucency of the eardrum, position and definition of the malleus, and the eardrum's mobility with the ear canal sealed and a puff of air delivered by the pneumatic bulb. Abnormalities may be caused by infection (Fig. 426-8) or barotrauma (Fig. 426-9). Examination with a 512-Hz tuning fork should be performed to determine lateralization of the sound (Weber test) and whether air conduction is superior to bone conduction (Rinne test). Facial nerve function should be assessed (Chapter 396) by determining whether the patient can raise the eyebrows, close the eyes, wrinkle the nose, and purse the lips. The presence or absence of nystagmus should be recorded. Inspection of the nose, oral cavity, oropharynx, and neck should be accompanied by cranial nerve examination (Chapter 396). Palpation of the tongue and tonsils is especially important if the ear pain is intense and persistent. A careful neck examination should be performed to look for masses. Oral cavity infections (Chapter 425), such as a peritonsillar abscess or severe tonsillitis, may arise as ear pain, and the physical examination should reveal trismus, erythema, mass effect, and other common signs of pharyngitis.

Laboratory

An audiogram can assess hearing loss (Chapter 428). A tympanogram measures compliance of the middle ear system and is an accurate method for diagnosis of otitis media. Cultures are rarely performed because they require tympanocentesis, and cultures of the external ear can reveal a vast variety of organisms that are often treated empirically with antibiotics. If a fever and middle ear effusion are present and neck stiffness is found on physical examination, lumbar puncture may rarely be recommended.

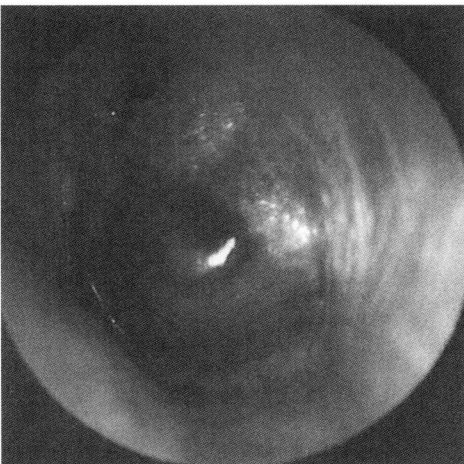

FIGURE 426-9. Blood in the middle ear (hemotympanum). Causes include otitic barotrauma, secretory otitis media, and a high jugular bulb. (From Dhillon RS, East CA, eds. *Ear, Nose and Throat and Head and Neck Surgery,* 2nd ed. Edinburgh: Churchill Livingstone; 1994:26.)

Imaging

In general, imaging is indicated if complications of acute or chronic otitis media are suspected or to look for occult causes of otalgia in the upper aerodigestive tract. If a patient is suspected of having meningitis, epidural or subdural abscess, brain abscess, or sagittal sinus thrombosis, imaging is mandatory. Imaging is also useful for operative planning in patients with chronic otitis media or (rarely) to evaluate for the presence of tumors in the middle or external ear.

Differential Diagnosis

Otitis externa, which is an infection of the skin of the ear canal, is often due to manipulating the ear after swimming or trying to scratch an ear canal that itches because of skin irritation. Patients exhibit erythema of the canal skin and extreme pain on manipulation of the ear canal. In the presence of concomitant cranial neuropathies, especially in diabetic or otherwise immunocompromised patients, malignant otitis externa with osteomyelitis should be suspected. Inspection of the tympanic membrane may reveal fluid consistent with otitis media; the tuning fork examination should support the presence of conductive hearing loss. Vesicles on the conchal portion of the pinna, especially when accompanied by facial nerve paralysis, strongly suggest herpes zoster oticus with Ramsay Hunt syndrome (Chapter 375). Perforation of the eardrum suggests either acute or chronic otitis media, traumatic perforation, or possibly cholesteatoma (Chapter 428) if the perforation is in the posterior-superior quadrant. Chronic draining otorrhea of long standing with a deep boring pain and perforation of the tympanic membrane suggests a complication of otitis media.

If findings on ear and cranial nerve examination are negative but the patient's complaints of otalgia are persistent, special effort needs to be made to visualize the upper aerodigestive tract, including the nasopharynx, oral cavity, oropharynx, larynx, and hypopharynx, to be sure that infection or tumor is not present in these hard-to-examine areas. MRI can be very useful in these cases.

TREATMENT Rx

Otitis externa is often treated with office suctioning of debris under a microscope and the application of antibiotic drops (ciprofloxacin, tobramycin, neomycin, polymyxin B), with or without hydrocortisone in various combinations.[3] Frequently, a small wick or sponge is placed in the ear canal to help maintain patency of the canal and allow facile application of the medications (Fig. 426-10). For otitis media, oral antibiotic treatment is directed at eradicating *Haemophilus influenzae, Moraxella catarrhalis, Streptococcus pneumoniae,* and *Staphylococcus aureus* with amoxicillin or erythromycin as for sinusitis. The benefit is notable for children 2 years or younger with bilateral otitis media and for older children with otitis plus otorrhea, whereas other patients can be observed without antibiotics. In general, antibiotics provide somewhat better short-term outcomes but at the expense of significantly more diarrhea and

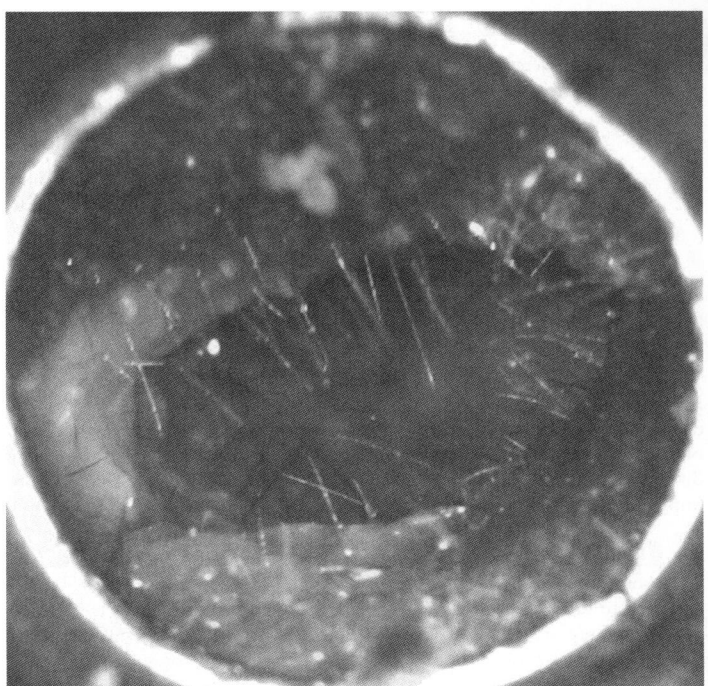

FIGURE 426-10. Otitis externa. Otitis externa in a patient's left ear with the tympanic membrane in the distance. Exudate and erythema are present. The ear canal is quite painful, and a wick may be necessary to maintain patency of the external auditory canal.

rashes.[A12][A13] Interestingly, the natural history of acute otitis media is acute perforation of the eardrum, which often results in otorrhea and relief of pain. Most middle ear effusions clear spontaneously within 3 months regardless of whether they are treated. Most perforations of an eardrum caused by trauma heal without surgical intervention, but if an eardrum perforation persists for more than about 3 months, surgical closure and the use of tympanoplasty with or without mastoidectomy can be contemplated. Chronic draining perforations, especially if located in the posterior-superior quadrant of the tympanic membrane, may portend the presence of cholesteatoma and may require tympanomastoid surgery.

In patients in whom herpes zoster is suspected, acyclovir can be started at 800 mg by mouth five times per day for 7 days, with or without prednisone (Chapter 375). Intracranial complications of otitis media often need to be addressed surgically.

  Grade A References

A1. Kenealy T, Arroll B. Antibiotics for the common cold and acute purulent rhinitis. *Cochrane Database Syst Rev.* 2013;6:CD000247.
A2. Lemiengre MB, van Driel ML, Merenstein D, et al. Antibiotics for clinically diagnosed acute rhinosinusitis in adults. *Cochrane Database Syst Rev.* 2012;10:CD006089.
A3. Garbutt JM, Banister C, Spitznagel E, et al. Amoxicillin for acute rhinosinusitis: a randomized controlled trial. *JAMA.* 2012;307:685-692.
A4. Wei CC, Adappa ND, Cohen NA. Use of topical nasal therapies in the management of chronic rhinosinusitis. *Laryngoscope.* 2013;123:2347-2359.
A5. Orlandi RR, Smith TL, Marple BF, et al. Update on evidence-based reviews with recommendations in adult chronic rhinosinusitis. *Int Forum Allergy Rhinol.* 2014;4(suppl 1):S1-S15.
A6. Zalmanovici TA, Yaphe J. Intranasal steroids for acute sinusitis. *Cochrane Database Syst Rev.* 2009;4:CD005149.
A7. Williamson IG, Rumsby K, Benge S, et al. Antibiotics and topical nasal steroid for treatment of acute maxillary sinusitis: a randomized controlled trial. *JAMA.* 2007;298:2487-2496.
A8. Hayward G, Thompson MJ, Perera R, et al. Corticosteroids for the common cold. *Cochrane Database Syst Rev.* 2012;8:CD008116.
A9. Smith TL, Kern R, Palmer JN, et al. Medical therapy vs surgery for chronic rhinosinusitis: a prospective, multi-institutional study with 1-year follow-up. *Int Forum Allergy Rhinol.* 2013;3:4-9.
A10. Poetker DM, Jakubowski LA, Lal D, et al. Oral corticosteroids in the management of adult chronic rhinosinusitis with and without nasal polyps: an evidence-based review with recommendations. *Int Forum Allergy Rhinol.* 2013;3:104-120.
A11. Rudmik L, Schlosser RJ, Smith TL, et al. Impact of topical nasal steroid therapy on symptoms of nasal polyposis: a meta-analysis. *Laryngoscope.* 2012;122:1431-1437.
A12. Tähtinen PA, Laine MK, Huovinen P, et al. A placebo-controlled trial of antimicrobial treatment for acute otitis media. *N Engl J Med.* 2011;364:116-126.
A13. Venekamp RP, Sanders S, Glasziou PP, et al. Antibiotics for acute otitis media in children. *Cochrane Database Syst Rev.* 2013;1:CD000219.

GENERAL REFERENCES

For the General References and other additional features, please visit Expert Consult at https://expertconsult.inkling.com.

427

SMELL AND TASTE

ROBERT W. BALOH AND JOANNA C. JEN

Millions of people suffer from disorders of taste and smell, but these disorders are often neglected because they are not fatal and, unlike abnormalities of vision and hearing, are not considered serious handicaps. Chemosensory disorders, however, often reduce the enjoyment and quality of life and are important to patients who suffer from them.

DEFINITION

The sensory receptor for taste, the taste bud, is made up of 50 to 150 cells arranged to form a pear-shaped organ. The lifespan of these cells is 10 to 14 days, and they are constantly being renewed from dividing epithelial cells surrounding the bud. Taste buds are located on the tongue, soft palate, pharynx, larynx, epiglottis, uvula, and upper third of the esophagus. The taste buds located on the anterior two thirds of the tongue and on the palate are innervated by the chorda tympani branch of the seventh cranial nerve. The ninth cranial nerve innervates the posterior third of the tongue. The ninth and tenth nerves innervate taste buds in the pharynx and larynx. Afferent signals from the taste buds project to the nucleus of the solitary tract in the medulla and then through a series of relays to the thalamus and postcentral somatosensory cerebral cortex (primary ipsilateral). Free nerve endings of the fifth cranial nerve are found on the tongue and in the oral cavity, and lesions involving these pathways can also alter taste perception.

Olfactory receptors lie in a roughly dime-sized area of specialized pigmented epithelium that arches along the superior aspect of each side of the nasal mucosa. Specialized bipolar sensory cells in this region thrust short receptor hairs into the overlying mucosa to detect aromatic molecules as they dissolve. Like taste buds, the specialized receptor portion of the bipolar neuron undergoes continuous renewal, with turnover occurring approximately every 30 days. Thin axons of the bipolar neurons course through small holes in the cribriform plate of the ethmoid bone to form connections in the overlying olfactory bulb on the ventral surface of the frontal lobe. From there, second- and third-order neurons project directly and indirectly to the prepiriform cortex and parts of the amygdaloid complex of both sides of the brain, which represents the primary olfactory cortex.

PATHOBIOLOGY
Pathology

Disorders of taste interfere with digestion because taste stimulants alter salivary and pancreatic flow, gastric contractions, and intestinal motility. Smell also contributes to the anticipation and ingestion of food because much of what is tasted is derived from olfactory stimulation during ingestion and chewing. An inability to detect noxious tastes and odors can result in food or gas poisoning, particularly in elderly subjects. In the extreme, chemosensory disorders can lead to overwhelming stress, anorexia, and depression. Genes that encode chemoreceptor proteins belong to the G protein–coupled receptor superfamily, which accounts for up to 1% of mammalian genomes.[1] Sequence diversity in these genes encodes unique structural motifs that bind to different ligands signaling different odors and tastes. Distinct and dedicated taste receptor cells express unique receptors to detect each of the five basic tastes: sweet (sensed by the heterodimers T1R1 and T1R3), umami (detected by the heterodimers T1R2 and T1R3), bitter (sensed by an estimated 30 T2Rs), sour (sensed by PKD2L1, with membrane-tethered carbonic anhydrase IV sensing carbonation), and salty (epithelial sodium channel). The taste receptor cells transform and transmit information to primary afferents through multiple cranial nerves (VII, IX, and X) that project to the solitary tract nucleus in the brain stem, with relay in the thalamus, and then onward to the primary cortex (Fig. 427-1).

Pathophysiology

Disorders of taste and smell can be divided into local, systemic, and neurologic categories (Table 427-1). The taste buds and the specialized receptor portion of the bipolar olfactory cells are constantly being renewed, and the

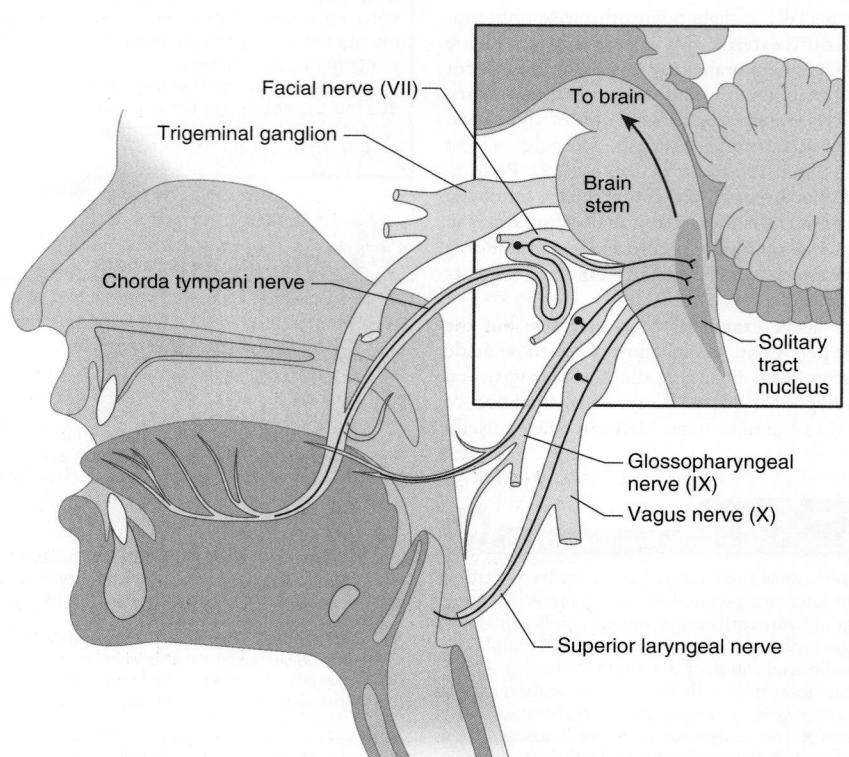

FIGURE 427-1. **Anatomy of peripheral taste pathways.** Taste information is transmitted from the mouth and the pharynx through multiple cranial nerves that project to the solitary tract nucleus in the brain stem, with relay in the thalamus before reaching the cortex. (Copyright 1999-2000 David Klemm. Reproduced from Bromley SM. Smell and taste disorders: a primary care approach. *Am Fam Physician.* 2000;61:427-436, 438.)

TABLE 427-1	COMMON CAUSES OF LOSS OF TASTE AND SMELL	
	TASTE	**SMELL**
Local	Radiation therapy, oral infections, dentures, dental procedures	Allergic rhinitis, sinusitis, nasal polyposis, upper respiratory infection
Systemic	Cancer, renal failure, hepatic failure, nutritional deficiency (vitamin B_3, zinc), Cushing's syndrome, hypothyroidism, diabetes mellitus, infection (viral), drugs (antirheumatic and antiproliferative, e.g., corticosteroids, cisplatin, carboplatin, cyclophosphamide, doxorubicin, and methotrexate)	Renal failure, hepatic failure, nutritional deficiency (vitamin B_{12}), Cushing's syndrome, hypothyroidism, diabetes mellitus, infection (viral hepatitis, influenza), drugs (nasal sprays, antihistamines, decongestants, antibiotics, and antirheumatic and antiproliferative drugs that affect taste)
Neurologic	Bell's palsy, familial dysautonomia, multiple sclerosis	Head trauma, multiple sclerosis, Parkinson's disease, Alzheimer's disease, frontal tumor

process of renewal can be affected by nutritional, metabolic, and hormonal states as well as by therapeutic radiation, drugs, and age. For example, with interruption of mitosis by antiproliferative agents, return of normal taste function takes a minimum of 10 days, whereas return to normal olfactory function takes more than 30 days. Diuretics can block apical ion channels on a taste bud, and antifungal drugs inhibit cytochrome P-450–dependent enzymes at the level of the receptors. Numerous local conditions, such as colds and allergies, chronic sinusitis, and nasal polyposis, can influence the sense of smell by restricting airway patency. Accidental blows to the head can shear the fine axons of the bipolar olfactory neurons and result in loss of smell. Lesions of the fifth, seventh (chorda tympani), and ninth nerves can lead to disordered taste sensation. Olfactory and gustatory disturbances can serve as important diagnostic signs for focal neurologic lesions (e.g., frontal lobe tumors). Hallucinations of smell and taste occur in persons with epileptogenic lesions affecting the mesial temporal lobe and insular region, respectively. Finally, olfactory disturbances and hallucinations occur with a number of psychiatric illnesses (particularly depressive illness and schizophrenia).

CLINICAL MANIFESTATIONS

The most frequently encountered causes of loss of smell are local obstructive disease, viral infections, head injuries (Chapter 399), and normal aging (Chapter 25).[2,3] Patients can lose their sense of smell not only from chronic allergies and sinusitis (Chapter 426) but also from the nasal sprays and drops that they use to treat these conditions. The most common causes of loss of the sense of taste are viral infections and drug ingestion, particularly antirheumatic and antiproliferative drugs (see Table 427-1). Many of the systemic disorders listed in Table 427-1 probably produce their effect by decreasing the rate of turnover of sensory receptors on the tongue and olfactory epithelia. Disturbances of smell and taste in malnourished patients may be due to specific deficiencies in vitamins and minerals, such as zinc. Viral illnesses, such as influenza (Chapter 364), viral hepatitis (Chapter 148), and allergic rhinitis (Chapter 251), are the most common causes of loss of both taste and smell.[4] Multifocal neurologic disorders such as multiple sclerosis (Chapter 411) and traumatic head injuries (Chapter 399) can affect the central olfactory and gustatory pathways at multiple levels; as a result, abnormalities in taste and smell are common in such patients. Loss of smell is increasingly being recognized in the early stages of many neurodegenerative disorders, including Parkinson's disease, Alzheimer's dementia, motor neuron disease, and Huntington's disease.[5] An irritative lesion from a neoplastic, inflammatory, or demyelinating process may lead to a persistent disturbance rather than to a loss of taste.

DIAGNOSIS

Olfaction can be tested grossly at the bedside with a few easily recognized odors, such as coffee, chocolate, and the roselike aroma of the compound phenylethyl alcohol. Nasal irritants should be avoided. Each nostril is tested separately to determine whether the problem is unilateral or bilateral. Gustatory sensation is typically tested with weak solutions of sugar, salt, and acetic

acid or vinegar. The patient must keep the tongue protruded and respond to questions by nodding the head or by pointing to names of the tastes written on cards. The anterior two thirds and posterior third of the tongue should be tested separately.

TREATMENT ℞

Treatment of olfactory dysfunction secondary to nasal disease is aimed at opening the air passageways while preserving the olfactory epithelium (Chapter 426). Intranasal steroids for rhinosinusitis (Chapter 426), antibiotics as needed for sinusitis, and therapies for seasonal allergies (Chapter 251) are useful in selected cases. Drugs known to affect taste or smell (see Table 427-1) should be discontinued for a trial. Vitamin and mineral therapies are of unproven benefit.

GENERAL REFERENCES

For the General References and other additional features, please visit Expert Consult at https://expertconsult.inkling.com.

428

HEARING AND EQUILIBRIUM

ROBERT W. BALOH AND JOANNA C. JEN

DEFINITION

The neural pathways subserving hearing and those most important for equilibrium and spatial orientation are anatomically proximate in much of their course from their end organs in the inner ear to their termination in the superior portion of the temporal lobe. Because of the close anatomic linkage, disorders that affect hearing often affect equilibrium, and vice versa. For this reason, they are considered together here.

PATHOBIOLOGY

Despite their anatomic propinquity, however, substantial pathophysiologic differences make clinical examination of the two systems different. The auditory system is physiologically relatively isolated, so that its function and dysfunction can be tested independently of other neural systems. The vestibular system, in contrast, has many close physiologic links with other neural systems (particularly the visual-oculomotor, somatosensory, and autonomic systems) and can be difficult to test in isolation of these other systems.

DIAGNOSIS

Abnormalities of the auditory system lead to only a few well-defined and unique symptoms (i.e., hearing loss or tinnitus). Abnormalities of the vestibular system can cause symptoms that mimic disorders of other neural structures. Such symptoms include dizziness, visual distortion (oscillopsia), imbalance, nausea, vomiting, and even syncope.

DISORDERS OF THE AUDITORY SYSTEM

DEFINITION
Anatomy and Physiology of Hearing

In normal hearing, sound waves are transmitted from the tympanic membrane through the three ossicles of the air-filled middle ear (air conduction) to the oval window and the basilar membrane of the fluid-sealed cochlea. The ossicles increase the gain from the tympanum to oval window about 18-fold, compensating for the loss that sound waves moving from air to fluid would otherwise suffer. In the absence of this system, sound may reach the cochlea by vibration of the temporal bone (bone conduction) but with much less efficiency (approximately 60-dB loss). Hair cells, tonotopically organized along the cochlear basilar membrane, detect the vibratory movement of that membrane and transduce vibration into nerve impulses. The nerve impulses are relayed by nerve cells that synapse at the base of hair cells and have their bodies in the spiral ganglion to the cochlear nucleus of the ipsilateral pontine tegmentum. The spiral cochlea mechanically analyzes the frequency content of sound. For high-frequency tones, only sensory cells in the basilar region are activated, whereas for low-frequency tones, all or nearly all sensory cells are activated. Therefore, with lesions of the cochlea and its afferent nerve, the hearing levels for different frequencies are usually unequal, typically resulting in better hearing sensitivity for low-frequency than for high-frequency tones. Within the brain stem, auditory signals ascend from the ventral and dorsal cochlear nuclei to reach the superior olivary nuclei of both sides. Thus, nervous system lesions central to the cochlear nucleus do not cause monaural hearing loss, and conversely, unilateral central lesions do not cause deafness. From these structures, the pathway projects by way of the lateral lemnisci to the inferior colliculi. Each inferior colliculus transmits to the other and to its ipsilateral medial geniculate body, which in turn sends the final projection to the transverse auditory gyrus lying in the superior portion of the ipsilateral temporal lobe.

The normal ear can detect sound frequencies ranging between 20 and 20,000 Hz; the upper range drops off fairly rapidly with advancing age. The ear is most sensitive between 500 and 4000 Hz, which roughly corresponds to the frequency range most important for understanding speech. The hearing level in this range has several practical implications in terms of the degree of handicap and the potential for useful correction with amplification. A 30- to 40-dB hearing level in the speech range would impair normal conversation, whereas an 80-dB hearing level would make everyday auditory communication almost impossible (the social definition of deafness).

EPIDEMIOLOGY

About 5% of the world population suffers from disabling hearing loss (defined by the World Health Organization as greater than 40 dB in the better hearing ear in adults and greater than 30 dB in the better hearing ear in children). The prevalence of disabling hearing loss is twice as high in poorer countries compared with richer countries. The prevalence increases with every age decade,[1] and it is higher in men than in women across all age decades. Hearing loss is independently associated with accelerated cognitive decline and incident cognitive impairment in community-dwelling older adults.

PATHOBIOLOGY

Localization of Lesions within the Auditory Pathways

Conductive hearing loss results from lesions involving the external or middle ear. It is typically characterized by an approximately equal loss of hearing at all frequencies and by well-preserved speech discrimination once the threshold for hearing is exceeded. Patients with conductive hearing loss can hear speech in a noisy background better than in a quiet background because they can understand loud speech as well as anyone.

Sensorineural hearing loss results from lesions of the cochlea or auditory division of the eighth cranial nerve, or both. With sensorineural hearing loss, the hearing levels for different frequencies are usually unequal, typically resulting in better hearing for low- than for high-frequency tones. Patients with sensorineural hearing loss often have difficulty in hearing speech that is mixed with background noise and may be annoyed by loud speech. Three important manifestations of sensorineural lesions are diplacusis, recruitment, and tone decay. Diplacusis and recruitment are common with cochlear lesions; tone decay usually accompanies eighth nerve involvement.

Central hearing disorders result from lesions of the central auditory pathways. As a rule, patients with central lesions do not have impaired hearing for pure tones, and they can understand speech as long as it is clearly spoken in a quiet environment. If the listener's task is made more difficult with the introduction of background noise or competing messages, performance deteriorates more markedly in patients with central lesions than in normal subjects.

DIAGNOSIS

Evaluation
Bedside Test

A quick test for hearing loss in the speech range is to observe the response to spoken commands at different intensities (whisper, conversation, shouting). Tuning fork tests permit a rough assessment of the hearing level for pure tones of known frequency. The clinician can use his or her own hearing level as a reference standard. In the Rinne test, nerve conduction is compared with bone conduction by holding a tuning fork (preferably 512 Hz) against the mastoid process until the sound can no longer be heard. It is then placed 1 inch from the ear and, in normal subjects, can be heard about twice as long

by air as by bone. If bone conduction is better than air conduction, the hearing loss is conductive, but care must be taken to ensure that the bone conduction is not heard in the normal ear. In the Weber test, the tuning fork is placed on the patient's forehead or upper teeth. Normally, this sound is referred to the center of the head. If it is referred to the side of unilateral hearing loss, the hearing loss is conductive; if it is referred away from the side of unilateral hearing loss, the loss is sensorineural.

Audiometry

Pure tone testing is the cornerstone of most auditory examinations. Pure tones at selected frequencies are presented through either earphones (air conduction) or a vibrator pressed against the mastoid portion of the temporal bone (bone conduction), and the minimal level that the subject can hear (threshold) is determined for each frequency. Two speech tests are routinely used. The *speech reception threshold* is the intensity at which the patient can correctly repeat 50% of the words presented. The speech reception threshold is a test of hearing sensitivity for speech and should reflect the hearing level for pure tones in the speech range. The *speech discrimination test* is a measure of the patient's ability to understand speech when it is presented at a level that is easily heard. In patients with eighth nerve lesions, speech discrimination scores can be severely reduced, even when pure tone thresholds are normal or nearly normal; by comparison, in patients with cochlear lesions, discrimination tends to be proportional to the magnitude of hearing loss.

Brain stem auditory evoked responses can be recorded from scalp electrodes at 0 to 10 msec (early), 10 to 50 msec (middle), and 50 to 500 msec (late) following a click (a high-frequency stimulus). The early potentials reflect electrical activity at the cochlea, eighth cranial nerve, and brain stem; the later potentials reflect cortical activity. Computer averaging of the responses to 1000 to 2000 clicks separates the evoked potential from background noise. Early evoked responses may be used to estimate the magnitude of hearing loss and to differentiate among cochlea, eighth nerve, and brain stem lesions.

Differential Diagnosis
Conductive Hearing Loss

The history, examination, and audiometry usually provide the key differential features for identifying common causes of hearing loss (Fig. 428-1). The most common cause of conductive hearing loss is *impacted cerumen* in the external canal. This benign condition is usually first noticed after bathing or swimming when a droplet of water closes the remaining tiny passageway. The most common serious cause of conductive hearing loss is inflammation of the middle ear, *otitis media*, either infective (suppurative; see Fig. 426-8) or noninfective (serous). Fluid accumulates in the middle ear, impairing the conduction of airborne sound to the cochlea. Because the air cavity of the middle ear is in direct connection with the mastoid air cells, infection can spread through the mastoid bone and, occasionally, into the intracranial cavity. Chronic otitis media with perforation of the tympanic membrane can result in an invasion of the middle ear and other pneumatized areas of the temporal bone by keratinizing squamous epithelium (*cholesteatoma*). Cholesteatomas can produce erosion of the ossicles and bony labyrinth, resulting in a mixed conductive and sensorineural hearing loss. Barotrauma to the middle ear arises with otalgia and hearing loss and can be associated with serous effusion or hematotympanum (see Fig. 426-9). *Otosclerosis* commonly produces progressive conductive hearing loss by immobilizing the stapes with new bone growth in front of and below the oval window. The hearing loss is typically conductive, although in some persons the cochlea may be invaded by foci of otosclerotic bone, producing an additional sensorineural hearing loss. Otosclerosis usually stabilizes when the hearing level reaches 50 to 60 dB and rarely progresses to deafness. Other common causes of conductive hearing loss include trauma, congenital malformations of the external and middle ear, and glomus body tumors.

Sensorineural Hearing Loss
Hereditary Deafness

Genetically determined deafness, usually from hair cell aplasia or deterioration, may be present at birth or may develop in adulthood. The diagnosis of *hereditary deafness* rests on the finding of a positive family history. Mutations in connexin 26, a key component of gap junctions in the inner ear, account for most cases of recessively inherited deafness. *Intrauterine factors* resulting in congenital hearing loss include infection (especially rubella); toxic, metabolic, and endocrine disorders; and anoxia associated with Rh incompatibility and difficult deliveries.

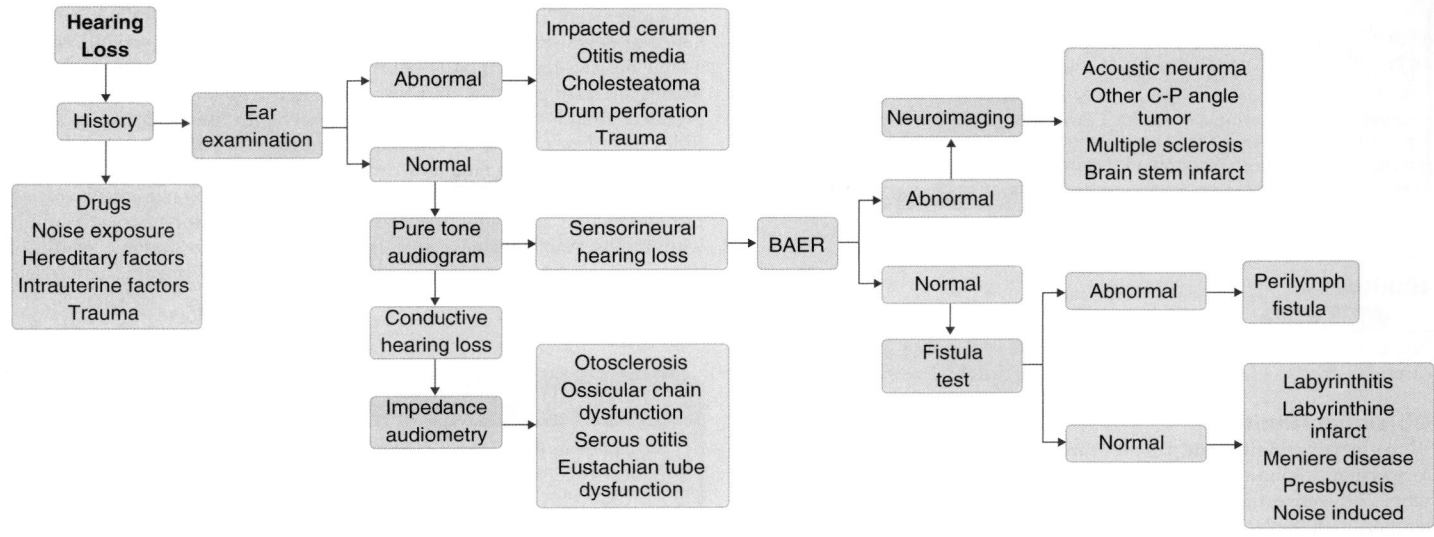

FIGURE 428-1. Evaluation of hearing loss. BAER = brain stem auditory evoked response; C-P = cerebellopontine.

Cochlear Damage

Acute unilateral deafness usually has a cochlear basis. *Bacterial or viral infections* of the labyrinth, *head trauma* with fracture or hemorrhage into the cochlea, or *vascular occlusion* of a terminal branch of the anterior inferior cerebellar artery can extensively damage the cochlea and the vestibular labyrinth. An isolated sudden unilateral sensorineural hearing loss is presumed to reflect a viral infection of the cochlea and auditory nerve terminals.[2] High-dose steroids followed by a rapid taper are recommended (see Treatment).

Sudden unilateral hearing loss often associated with vertigo and tinnitus can result from a *perilymphatic fistula*. Such fistulas may be congenital or may follow stapes surgery or head trauma.

Drugs

Drugs cause acute and subacute bilateral hearing impairment. Salicylates, furosemide, and ethacrynic acid have the potential to produce transient deafness when they are taken in high doses. More toxic to the cochlea are aminoglycoside antibiotics (gentamicin, tobramycin, amikacin, kanamycin, streptomycin, and neomycin). These agents can destroy cochlear hair cells in direct relation to their serum concentrations. Some antineoplastic chemotherapeutic agents, particularly cisplatin, cause severe ototoxicity.

Meniere Disease

Subacute relapsing cochlear deafness occurs with *Meniere disease,* a condition associated with fluctuating hearing loss and tinnitus, recurrent episodes of abrupt and often severe vertigo, and a sensation of fullness or pressure in the ear. Recurrent endolymphatic hypertension (hydrops) is believed to cause the episodes. On pathologic examination, the endolymphatic sac is dilated, and the hair cells become atrophic. The resulting deafness is subtle and reversible in the early stages but subsequently becomes permanent and is characterized by diplacusis and loudness recruitment. The disorder is usually unilateral, but in about 20 to 40% of patients, bilateral involvement occurs.

Presbycusis

The gradual, progressive, bilateral hearing loss commonly associated with advancing age is called presbycusis.[3] Presbycusis is not a distinct disease entity but rather represents multiple effects of aging on the auditory system. It may include conductive and central dysfunction, although the most consistent effect of aging is on the sensory cells and neurons of the cochlea. The typical audiogram of presbycusis is a symmetrical high-frequency hearing loss gradually sloping downward with increasing frequency. The most consistent pathologic finding associated with presbycusis is degeneration of sensory cells and nerve fibers at the base of the cochlea.

Noise

The recurrent trauma of *noise-induced hearing loss* affects approximately the same region at the base of the cochlea and is also common, particularly among those with exposure to loud explosive or industrial noises. Loud, blaring, modern music has become a recent offender. The loss almost always begins at 4000 Hz and does not affect speech discrimination until late in the disease process. With only brief exposure to loud noise (hours to days), there may be only a temporary threshold shift, but with continued exposure, permanent injury begins. The duration and intensity of exposure determine the degree of permanent injury.

Acoustic Neuroma

Progressive unilateral hearing loss, which arises insidiously, initially in the high frequencies, and worsens by almost imperceptible degrees, is characteristic of benign neoplasms of the cerebellopontine angle, most commonly *acoustic neuromas.* In about 10% of cases, the hearing loss can be acute, apparently due to either hemorrhage into the tumor or compression of the labyrinthine vasculature. Magnetic resonance imaging (MRI) with contrast enhancement reliably identifies small acoustic neuromas.

Central Hearing Loss

Central hearing loss is unilateral only if it results from damage to the pontine cochlear nuclei on one side of the brain stem from conditions such as *ischemic infarction* of the lateral brain stem (e.g., occlusion of the anterior inferior cerebellar artery [Chapter 407]), a plaque of *multiple sclerosis* (Chapter 411), or, rarely, invasion or compression of the lateral pons by a *neoplasm* or *hematoma* (Chapters 189 and 399). Bilateral *degeneration* of the cochlear nuclei accompanies some of the rare recessive inherited disorders of childhood. As noted, clinically important unilateral hearing loss never results from neurologic disease arising rostral to the cochlear nucleus. Although bilateral hearing loss could, in theory, result from bilateral destruction of central hearing pathways, in practice this is rare because involvement of neighboring structures in the brain stem or hemisphere would usually produce overwhelming neurologic disability.

TREATMENT Rx

If an underlying disorder has not yet destroyed the auditory system and can be ameliorated medically or surgically, hearing may be improved or preserved. Most patients with otosclerosis respond to stapedectomy. Closure of a perilymph fistula may improve hearing. Antibiotic and decongestive treatment of otitis media (Chapter 426) should prevent permanent hearing loss.

A brief course of high-dose steroids is commonly used for patients with idiopathic sudden unilateral sensorineural deafness, but the evidence to support this approach is limited.[A1] Intratympanic corticosteroid treatment (four doses of 40 mg/mL of methylprednisolone during 2 weeks) is not inferior to oral treatment (60 mg/day of oral prednisone followed by a 5-day taper) for idiopathic sudden sensorineural hearing loss,[A2] and combination oral and intratympanic therapy may be better than either alone.[A3] A low-salt diet and diuretics are effective in selected cases of Meniere disease. Folic acid supplementation appears to reduce the rate of hearing loss in the elderly.[A4] Hearing aids amplify sound, usually with the goal of making speech intelligible. Patients with conductive hearing loss require simple amplification, but those with sensorineural hearing loss often need frequency-selective amplification to make hearing aids useful. Cochlear implants can help patients with profound hearing loss if they have some intact auditory nerve fibers.[4] Intense postoperative speech recognition training is required.

Tinnitus

DIAGNOSIS

The evaluation of common causes of tinnitus (Fig. 428-2) begins with a careful history to identify common offending drugs.[5]

Objective Tinnitus

With objective tinnitus, the patient hears a sound arising external to the auditory system, a sound that can usually be heard by the examiner with a stethoscope. Objective tinnitus usually has benign causes, such as noise from temporomandibular joints, opening of eustachian tubes, or repetitive muscle contractions. Sometimes, in a quiet room, the patient can hear the pulsatile flow in the carotid artery or a continuous hum of normal venous outflow through the jugular vein. The latter can be obliterated by compression of the jugular vein or extreme lateral rotation of the neck. Pathologic objective tinnitus occurs when patients hear turbulent flow in vascular anomalies or tumors (e.g., glomus jugulare tumor). Objective tinnitus may also be an early sign of increased intracranial pressure. Such tinnitus, which probably arises from turbulent flow through compressed venous structures at the base of the brain, is usually overshadowed by other neurologic abnormalities.

Subjective Tinnitus

Subjective tinnitus can arise from sites anywhere in the auditory system. The sounds most frequently reported are metallic ringing, buzzing, blowing, roaring, or, less often, bizarre clanging, popping, or nonrhythmic beating. Tinnitus heard as a faint, moderately high pitched, metallic ring can be observed by almost anyone who concentrates attention on auditory events

in a quiet room. Sustained louder tinnitus accompanied by audiometric evidence of deafness occurs in association with both conductive and sensorineural hearing loss. Tinnitus observed with otosclerosis tends to have a roaring or hissing quality, and that associated with Meniere disease often produces sounds that vary widely in intensity with time and quality, sometimes including roaring or clanging. Tinnitus with auditory nerve lesions tends to be higher pitched and ringing in quality. Audiometric and brain stem evoked response testing can help distinguish between lesions involving the conducting apparatus, the cochlea, and the auditory nerve. Tinnitus without observable deafness appears sporadically and for variable lengths of time in many persons without other evidence of an ongoing pathologic process.

TREATMENT   Rx

Most patients with tinnitus can be helped by a careful evaluation to exclude serious underlying conditions and by subsequent reassurance when appropriate. Often, exacerbating factors such as chronic anxiety and depression can be treated. In patients with hearing loss and tinnitus, a hearing aid may improve tinnitus because the amplification of ambient sound may effectively mask the tinnitus. This mechanism probably explains the frequent observation that removal of cerumen from the external auditory canal to improve ambient hearing also improves tinnitus. Also, when cerumen is attached to the tympanic membrane, tinnitus may result from local mechanical effects on the conductive system. For patients who find their tinnitus most obtrusive when trying to sleep, recorded masking sounds (e.g., white noise, rainfall, mountain stream) can be helpful. A careful drug history should be taken (see Fig. 428-2), and a drug-free trial period should be considered when possible.

No medications are approved for the treatment of tinnitus in the United States or Europe. Benzodiazepines (e.g., diazepam, 2 to 5 mg every 8 hours) or tricyclic amines (e.g., amitriptyline, 25 to 75 mg at bedtime) may provide temporary symptomatic relief of tinnitus, but cognitive-behavioral therapy is a more effective long-term approach that can significantly decrease tinnitus and improve health-related quality of life.[A5] In patients with concomitant profound bilateral sensorineural hearing loss, cochlear implants can improve hearing and often decrease tinnitus.

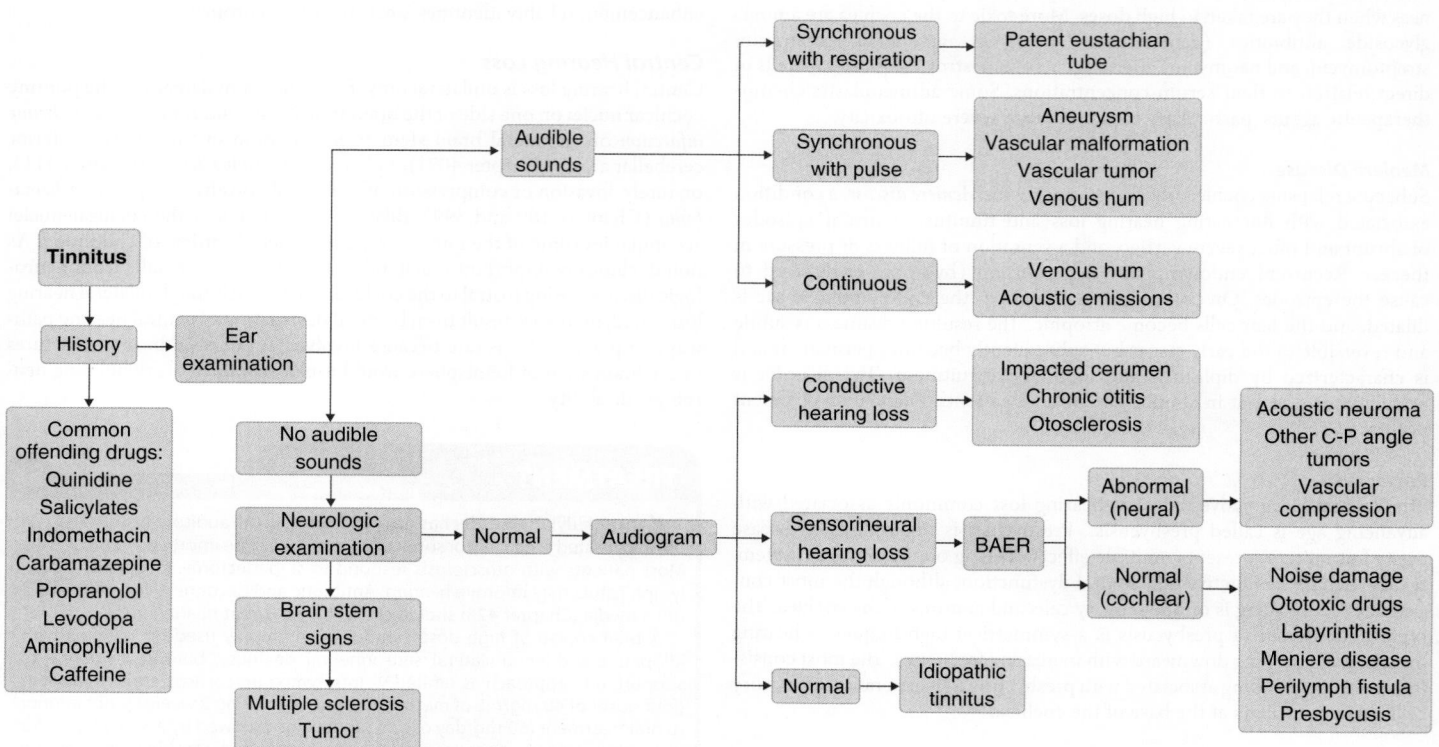

FIGURE 428-2. Evaluation of tinnitus. BAER = brain stem auditory evoked response; C-P = cerebellopontine.

EQUILIBRIUM–VESTIBULAR SYSTEM

PATHOBIOLOGY

Anatomy and Physiology of the Vestibular System

The paired vestibular end organs lie within the temporal bones next to the cochlea. Each organ consists of three semicircular canals that detect angular acceleration and two otolith structures, the utricle and saccule, that detect linear acceleration (including gravitational). Like the cochlea, these organs possess hair cells that act as force transducers, converting the forces associated with head acceleration into afferent nerve impulses. The hair cells of the three semicircular canals, each of which is oriented at right angles to the others, are located in the crista, where their cilia are embedded in a gelatinous mass called the *cupula*. Movement of the head causes the endolymph to flow either toward or away from the cupula, bending the cilia and, depending on the direction of endolymphatic movements, either exciting or inhibiting the afferent nerves at the base of the hair cells. Because the afferent nerves are tonically active, the baseline activity can be increased or decreased, depending on the direction of hair cell bending. Furthermore, the two sets of semicircular canals are approximately mirror images of each other, so that rotational movement of the head that excites one canal inhibits the analogous canal on the opposite side. The hair cells of the utricle and saccule are located in an area called the *macule*. The macule of the utricle lies approximately in the plane of the horizontal canal, and the macule of the saccule is approximately in the plane of the anterior canal. The hair cell cilia are embedded in a membrane that contains calcium carbonate crystals or otoliths; the density of otoliths is considerably greater than that of the endolymph. Linear accelerations of the head combine with the linear acceleration of gravity to distort the otolith membrane, thereby bending the cilia of the hair cells and modulating the activity of the afferent nerve terminals at the base of the hair cells.

The afferent vestibular nerves have their cell bodies in Scarpa's ganglion. The nerve fibers travel in the vestibular portion of the eighth cranial nerve contiguous to the acoustic portion. Fibers from different receptor organs terminate in different vestibular nuclei at the pontomedullary junction. There are also direct connections with many portions of the cerebellum, the greatest representation being in the flocculonodular lobe, the so-called vestibular cerebellum. Efferent fibers from the brain stem travel through the vestibular nerve to reach hair cells of the semicircular canals and macules, where they modulate afferent activities. From the vestibular nuclei, second-order neurons make important connections to the vestibular nuclei of the other side, to the cerebellum, to motor neurons of the spinal cord, to autonomic nuclei in the brain stem, and, most important for the examining clinician, to the nuclei of the oculomotor system. Fibers from the vestibular nuclei also ascend through the brain stem and thalamus to reach the cerebral cortex bilaterally.

DIAGNOSIS

Evaluation
History

Most vestibular problems presented to the physician are episodic, and often there are neither symptoms nor signs when the physician examines the patient. The history, therefore, can become paramount for identifying vestibular dysfunction. The history should attempt to distinguish vertigo (the illusion of movement in space) from lightheadedness (presyncope), ataxia (disequilibrium of the body without true movement in space), and psychogenic symptoms (the feeling of dissociation or, sometimes, disequilibrium).

About 12% of patients with vertigo have a central cause, and about 88% have a problem with the peripheral vestibular apparatus.[6] In general, peripheral vertigo is more severe, is more likely to be associated with hearing loss and tinnitus, and often leads to nausea and vomiting. Nystagmus associated with peripheral vertigo is usually inhibited by visual fixation. Central vertigo is generally less severe than peripheral vertigo and is often associated with other signs of central nervous system disease. The nystagmus of central vertigo is not inhibited by visual fixation and frequently is prominent when vertigo is mild or absent.

Common Causes of Vertigo
Physiologic Vertigo

Physiologic vertigo includes common disorders that occur in healthy people, such as *motion sickness, space sickness,* and *height vertigo* (Fig. 428-3). In these conditions, vertigo (defined as an illusion of movement) is minimal while autonomic symptoms predominate. With height vertigo, patients may experience acute anxiety and panic reaction. Individuals with motion sickness and space sickness typically develop perspiration, nausea, vomiting, increased salivation, yawning, and generalized malaise. Gastric motility is reduced and digestion impaired. Even the sight or smell of food is distressing. Hyperventilation is a common sign, and the resulting hypocapnia leads to changes in blood volume, with pooling in the lower parts of the body predisposing to postural hypotension and syncope. An unusual variant of motion-induced dizziness occurs when the subject returns to stationary conditions after prolonged exposure to motion (*mal de débarquement syndrome*). Typically, affected patients report that they feel the persistent rocking sensation of a boat long after returning to solid ground. Rarely, the syndrome can last for months to years after exposure to motion and can even be incapacitating. The cause is unknown.

Physiologic vertigo can often be suppressed by supplying sensory cues that help to match the signals originating from different sensory systems. Thus, motion sickness, which is caused by a mismatch of visual and vestibular signals, is exacerbated by sitting in a closed space or reading (giving the visual system the miscue that the environment is stationary). It may be improved by looking out at the horizon. Height vertigo, caused by a mismatch between

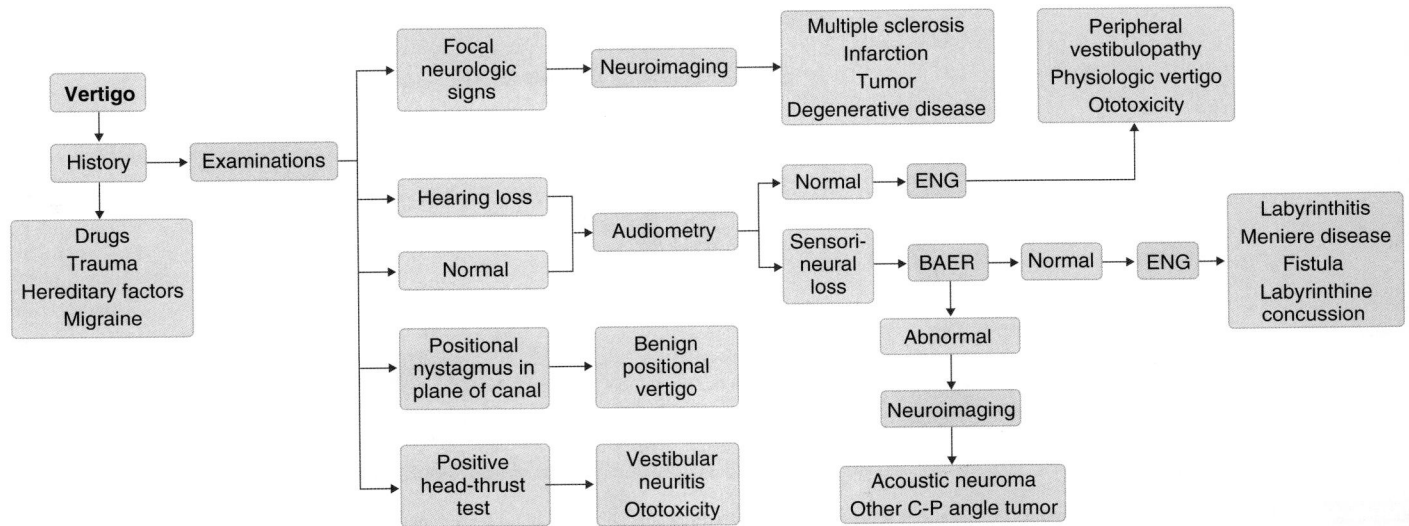

FIGURE 428-3. Evaluation of vertigo. BAER = brain stem auditory evoked response; C-P = cerebellopontine; ENG = electronystagmography.

sensation of normal body sway and lack of its visual detection, can often be relieved either by sitting or by visually fixating a nearby stationary object.

Benign Paroxysmal Positional Vertigo (Canalithiasis)

Benign paroxysmal positional vertigo is by far the most common cause of vertigo.[7] Patients with this condition develop brief episodes of vertigo (less than 1 minute) with position change, typically when turning over in bed, getting in and out of bed, bending over and straightening up, or extending the neck to look up (so-called top-shelf vertigo). Benign paroxysmal positional vertigo results when otolith debris inadvertently enters one of the semicircular canals. It can occur after head trauma or inner ear infection but most commonly occurs spontaneously in older people. The diagnosis rests on finding characteristic positional nystagmus in the plane of the affected canal (see later). It is important to recognize this syndrome because, in most patients, it can be cured by simple bedside maneuvers (Fig. 428-4). If the history or findings are atypical, the condition must be distinguished from other causes of positional vertigo that may occur with tumors or infarcts of the posterior fossa.

Acute Peripheral Vestibulopathy (Vestibular Neuritis)

One of the most common clinical neurologic syndromes at any age is the acute onset of vertigo, nausea, and vomiting lasting for several days and not associated with auditory or neurologic symptoms.[8] A viral origin is suspected, but attempts to isolate an agent have been unsuccessful, except for occasional findings of a herpes zoster infection. Pathologic studies showing atrophy of one or more vestibular nerve trunks, with or without atrophy of their associated sense organs, are evidence of a vestibular nerve site and, probably, viral cause for many patients with this syndrome. Many patients report an upper respiratory tract illness 1 to 2 weeks before the onset of vertigo. This syndrome occasionally occurs in epidemics (epidemic vertigo), may affect several members of the same family, and more often erupts in the spring and early summer. Most affected patients gradually improve during 1 to 2 weeks, but residual dizziness and imbalance can persist for months.

Meniere Disease

Meniere disease (see earlier) accounts for about 10% of all patients with vertigo.[9] The diagnosis is based on documenting episodic severe attacks accompanied by fluctuating hearing levels on audiometric testing beginning in the low frequencies.

Migraine

Vertigo is a common symptom with migraine (Chapter 398). It can occur with headaches or in separate isolated episodes, and it can predate the onset of headache. So-called benign paroxysmal vertigo of childhood is often the

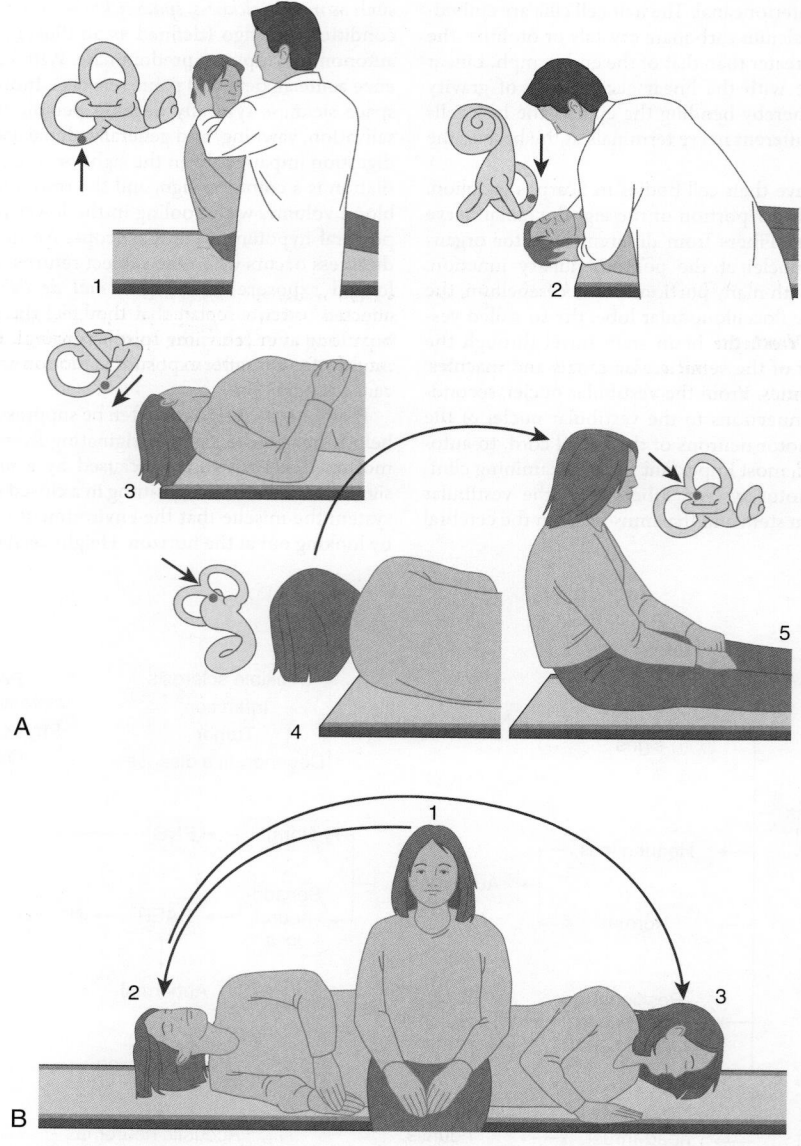

FIGURE 428-4. Modified Epley's (A) and Semont's (B) maneuvers for benign positional vertigo affecting the right posterior semicircular canal. The procedure is reversed to treat the left posterior semicircular canal. The entire sequence should be repeated until no nystagmus is elicited. (From Fife TD, Iverson DJ, Lempert T, et al. Practice parameter: therapies for benign paroxysmal positional vertigo [an evidence-based review]: report of the Quality Standards Subcommittee of the American Academy of Neurology. *Neurology.* 2008;70:2067-2074.)

first symptom of migraine. The mechanism of vertigo with migraine is not clear, but both peripheral and central types of nystagmus can occur with attacks. A few develop typical features of Meniere disease.

Post-traumatic Vertigo

Vertigo, hearing loss, and tinnitus often follow a blow to the head (Chapter 399) that does not result in temporal bone fracture, termed *labyrinthine concussion*. Although they are protected by a bone capsule, the delicate labyrinthine membranes are susceptible to blunt trauma. Blows to the occipital or mastoid region are particularly likely to produce labyrinthine damage. *Transverse fractures* of the temporal bone typically pass through the vestibule of the inner ear, tearing the membranous labyrinth and lacerating the vestibular and cochlear nerves. Complete loss of vestibular and cochlear function is the usual sequela, and the facial nerve is interrupted in approximately 50% of cases. Examination of the ear often reveals hemotympanum (see Fig. 426-9), but bleeding from the ear seldom occurs because the tympanic membrane usually remains intact. As noted earlier, *benign paroxysmal positional vertigo* is also a common sequela of head trauma. *Fistulas* of the oval and round windows can result from impact noise, deep-water diving, severe physical exertion, or blunt head injury without skull fracture. The mechanism of the rupture is a sudden negative or positive pressure change in the middle ear or a sudden increase in cerebrospinal fluid pressure transmitted to the inner ear through the cochlear aqueduct and internal auditory canal. Clinically, the rupture leads to the sudden onset of vertigo or hearing loss, or both. Surgical exploration of the middle ear is warranted when there is a clear relationship between the onset of vertigo or hearing loss, or both, and the onset of severe exertion, barometric change, head injury, or impact noise.

Postconcussion Syndrome

The so-called postconcussion syndrome refers to a vague dizziness (rarely vertigo) associated with anxiety, difficulty in concentrating, headache, and photophobia induced by a head injury resulting in concussion (Chapter 399). On occasion, similar but less pronounced symptoms are associated with mild head injury judged to be trivial at the time. The cause is unknown, but animal studies indicate that small multifocal brain lesions (petechiae) commonly occur after concussive brain injury.

Other Peripheral Causes of Vertigo

Vertigo can be associated with *chronic bacterial otomastoiditis*, either from direct invasion of the inner ear by the bacteria or by erosion of the labyrinth by a cholesteatoma. Radiographic studies of the temporal bone readily identify these disorders. *Autoimmune inner ear disease* typically arises with episodic vertigo and fluctuating hearing levels similar to Meniere disease, but it is more fulminant with early bilateral involvement. It can occur in isolation or with other systemic features of autoimmune disease. About two thirds of patients have antibodies directed against heat shock protein 70. The aminoglycosides streptomycin and gentamicin are remarkably selective for vestibular ototoxicity. The patient may suffer acute vertigo if the toxic effect is asymmetrical. More often, there is a progressive symmetrical loss of vestibular function leading to imbalance but not vertigo. Unfortunately, many patients being treated with ototoxic drugs are initially bedridden and unaware of the vestibular impairment until they recover from their acute illness and try to walk. They then discover that they are unsteady on their feet and that the environment tends to jiggle in front of their eyes (*oscillopsia*). The diagnosis can be made at the bedside with a head-thrust test (bilateral corrective saccades; see later). Caloric and rotational testing can document the degree of vestibular loss. The best treatment is prevention. If the drug is discontinued early during the course of symptoms, the disorder may stabilize or improve.

Vascular Insufficiency

Vertebrobasilar insufficiency is a common cause of vertigo in older people. Whether the vertigo originates from ischemia of the labyrinth, brain stem, or both structures is not always clear because the blood supplies to the labyrinth, eighth cranial nerve, and vestibular nuclei originate from the same source, the basilar vertebral circulation (Chapter 406). Vertigo with *vertebrobasilar insufficiency* is abrupt in onset, usually lasting several minutes, and is frequently associated with nausea and vomiting. Associated symptoms resulting from ischemia in the remaining territory supplied by the posterior circulation include visual illusions and hallucinations, drop attacks and weakness, visceral sensations, visual field defects, diplopia, and headache. These symptoms occur in episodes either in combination with the vertigo or alone. Vertigo may be an isolated initial symptom of vertebrobasilar ischemia, but repeated

episodes of vertigo without other symptoms should suggest another diagnosis. Vertebrobasilar insufficiency is usually caused by atherosclerosis of the subclavian, vertebral, and basilar arteries. On occasion, episodes of vertebrobasilar insufficiency are precipitated by postural hypotension, Stokes-Adams attacks, or mechanical compression from cervical spondylosis. MRI of the brain is usually normal because the vascular insufficiency is transient and function returns to normal between episodes. Magnetic resonance angiography can identify occlusive vascular disease most commonly involving the vertebral-basilar junction.

Vertigo is a common symptom with *infarction of the lateral brain stem or cerebellum* (Chapter 407), or both. The diagnosis is usually clear, based on the characteristic acute history and pattern of associated symptoms and neurologic findings. On occasion, cerebellar infarction or hemorrhage arises with severe vertigo, vomiting, and ataxia without associated brain stem symptoms and signs that might suggest the erroneous diagnosis of an acute peripheral vestibular disorder. The key differential is the finding of clear cerebellar signs (extremity and gait ataxia) and of direction-changing, gaze-evoked nystagmus. Such patients must be watched carefully for several days because they may develop progressive brain stem dysfunction due to compression by a swollen cerebellum.

Cerebellopontine Angle Tumors

Most tumors growing in the cerebellopontine angle (e.g., *acoustic neuroma, meningioma, epidermal cyst*) grow slowly, allowing the vestibular system to accommodate so that they produce only a vague sensation of disequilibrium rather than acute vertigo (Chapter 189). On occasion, however, episodic vertigo or positional vertigo heralds the presence of a cerebellopontine angle tumor. In virtually all patients, retrocochlear hearing loss is present, best identified by audiometric testing. MRI with contrast enhancement is the most sensitive diagnostic study for identifying a cerebellopontine angle tumor.

Other Central Causes of Vertigo

Acute vertigo may be the first symptom of *multiple sclerosis* (Chapter 411), although only a small percentage of young patients with acute vertigo eventually develop multiple sclerosis. Vertigo in multiple sclerosis is usually transient and often associated with other neurologic signs of brain stem disease, in particular, internuclear ophthalmoplegia or cerebellar dysfunction. Vertigo may also be a symptom of *parainfectious encephalomyelitis* or, rarely, *parainfectious cranial polyneuritis*. In this instance, the accompanying neurologic signs establish the diagnosis. The *Ramsay Hunt syndrome* (geniculate ganglion herpes) is characterized by vertigo and hearing loss associated with facial paralysis and, sometimes, pain in the ear. The typical lesions of herpes zoster (Chapter 375), which may follow the appearance of neurologic signs, are found in the external auditory canal and over the palate in some patients. Rarely is herpes zoster responsible for vertigo in the absence of the full-blown syndrome. *Granulomatous meningitis* (Chapter 412) or *leptomeningeal metastasis* and cerebral or systemic *vasculitis* (Chapter 270) may involve the eighth nerve, producing vertigo as an early symptom. In these disorders, cerebrospinal fluid analysis usually suggests the diagnosis (Chapter 396). Patients suffering from *temporal lobe epilepsy* (Chapter 403) occasionally experience vertigo as the aura. Vertigo in the absence of other neurologic signs or symptoms is never caused by epilepsy or other diseases of the cerebral hemispheres.

Bedside Tests
Hyperventilation

If the history is not clear, bedside provocative tests to mimic the symptom may assist in making a pathophysiologic diagnosis.[10] Hyperventilation, which lowers the arterial partial pressure of carbon dioxide ($Paco_2$) and decreases cerebral blood flow, causes a lightheaded sensation associated with syncope. Patients with compressive lesions of the vestibular nerve, such as with an acoustic neuroma or cholesteatoma, or with demyelination of the vestibular nerve root entry zone may develop vertigo and nystagmus after hyperventilation. Presumably, metabolic changes associated with hyperventilation trigger the partially damaged nerve to fire inappropriately.

Vestibulospinal Function

Bedside tests of vestibulospinal function are often insensitive because most patients can use vision and proprioceptive signals to compensate for any vestibular loss. Patients with acute unilateral peripheral vestibular lesions may past-point or fall toward the side of the lesion, but within a few days, balance returns to normal. Patients with bilateral peripheral vestibular loss have more

TABLE 428-1 DESCRIPTION, MECHANISM, AND FOCUS OF DIAGNOSTIC WORK-UP FOR COMMON TYPES OF DIZZINESS

TYPE OF DIZZINESS	DESCRIPTION	MECHANISM	FOCUS OF DIAGNOSTIC EVALUATION
Vertigo	Spinning (environment moves), tilt, drunkenness	Imbalance in tonic vestibular activity	Auditory and vestibular systems
Near-faint	Lightheaded, swimming	Decreased blood flow to entire brain	Cardiovascular system
Psychophysiologic	Dissociated from body, spinning inside (environment still)	Impaired central integration of sensory signals	Psychiatric assessment
Disequilibrium	Off balance, unsteady on feet	Loss of vestibulospinal, proprioceptive, cerebellar, or motor function	Neurologic assessment

difficulty compensating and usually show some imbalance on the Romberg and tandem walking tests (Chapter 396), particularly with eyes closed.

Doll's-Eye and Head-Thrust Tests

The vestibulo-ocular reflex can be tested at the bedside with the doll's-eye and head-thrust tests. In an alert human, rotating the head back and forth in the horizontal plane induces compensatory horizontal eye movements that are dependent on both the visual and vestibular systems. The doll's-eye test is a test of vestibular function in a comatose patient (Chapter 404) because such patients cannot generate pursuit or corrective fast components. In this setting, conjugate compensatory eye movements indicate normally functioning vestibulo-ocular pathways. Because the vestibulo-ocular reflex has a much higher frequency range than the smooth pursuit system, a qualitative bedside test of vestibular function can be made with the *head-thrust test*. It is performed by grasping the patient's head and applying brief, small-amplitude, high-acceleration head thrusts first to one side and then the other. The patient fixates on the examiner's nose and the examiner watches for corrective saccades, which are a sign of an inappropriate compensatory slow phase.

Caloric Test

The caloric test induces endolymphatic flow in the horizontal semicircular canal and horizontal nystagmus by creating a temperature gradient from one side of the canal to the other. With a cold caloric stimulus, the column of endolymph nearest the middle ear falls because of its increased density. This causes the cupula to deviate away from the utricle (ampullofugal flow) and produces horizontal nystagmus with the fast phase directed away from the stimulated ear. A warm stimulus produces the opposite effect, causing ampullopetal endolymph flow and nystagmus directed toward the stimulated ear (a mnemonic is COWS, meaning cold opposite, warm same). Because of its ready availability, ice water (approximately 0° C) can be used for bedside caloric testing. To bring the horizontal canal into the vertical plane, the patient lies in the supine position with head tilted 30 degrees forward. Infusion of 1 to 3 mL of ice water induces a burst of nystagmus usually lasting about a minute. Greater than a 20% asymmetry in nystagmus duration suggests a lesion on the side of the decreased response. The ice water caloric test is a useful way to test the integrity of the oculomotor pathways in a comatose patient. In this case, ice water induces only a slow tonic deviation toward the side of stimulation.

Positional Tests

Examination for pathologic vestibular nystagmus should include a search for spontaneous and positional nystagmus (see Table 424-5). Because vestibular nystagmus secondary to peripheral vestibular lesions is inhibited with fixation, the yield is increased by impairing fixation with +30 lenses (Frenzel glasses) or infrared video recordings. Two types of positional testing are typically performed: moving the patient from the sitting to head-hanging-right and head-hanging-left positions (Dix-Hallpike test) and turning the head to the right and left while the patient lies supine. Induced positional nystagmus may be paroxysmal or persistent, and it may be in the same direction in all positions or change directions in different positions. The most common cause of positional nystagmus is otolith debris in the semicircular canals, either free floating (paroxysmal) or attached to the cupula (persistent). This type of nystagmus always occurs in the plane of the affected canal—vertical torsional for the vertical canals and horizontal torsional for the horizontal canal. By contrast, central positional nystagmus is often pure vertical or horizontal and cannot be explained by stimulating a single semicircular canal.

Nystagmography

Nystagmography tests oculomotor control by inducing and recording eye movements. A standard test battery includes (1) tests of visual ocular control

(saccades, smooth pursuit, and optokinetic nystagmus), (2) a careful search for pathologic nystagmus with fixation and with eyes open in darkness, and (3) the measurement of induced vestibular nystagmus (caloric and rotational). Nystagmography can be helpful in identifying a vestibular lesion and localizing it within the peripheral and central pathways.

Evaluating the "Dizzy" Patient

The history is key because it determines the type of dizziness (vertigo, near-faint, psychophysiologic disequilibrium), associated symptoms (neurologic, audiologic, cardiac, psychiatric), precipitating factors (position change, trauma, stress, drug ingestion), and predisposing illness (systemic viral infection, cardiac disease, cerebrovascular disease). The history provides direction for both the examination and the diagnostic evaluation (Table 428-1). When focal neurologic signs are found, neuroimaging usually leads to a specific diagnosis. When vertigo is present without focal neurologic symptoms or signs, head-thrust and positional testing are key to localizing the lesion to the labyrinth or eighth nerve. Audiometry and nystagmography are useful if the cause of vertigo is not clear after the history and examination. Patients with psychophysiologic dizziness should be identified early so that needless tests are not obtained. A detailed cardiac evaluation (including loop monitoring) often identifies the cause of episodic near-fainting (Chapters 51 and 62).

TREATMENT

Treatment of vertigo can be divided into three general categories: specific, symptomatic, and rehabilitative. When possible, treatment should be directed at the underlying disorder (Table 428-2). Specific therapies include particle repositioning maneuvers (the Epley and Semont maneuvers; see Fig. 428-4) for benign paroxysmal positional vertigo.[A6-A8] For vestibular neuritis, steroids (e.g., methylprednisolone, 1 mg/kg/day for 5 days, then tapered during the next 15 days) are effective, at least for the short term,[A9] but antiviral agents are not. For Meniere disease, a low-salt diet and diuretics (e.g., 25 mg hydrochlorothiazide and 50 mg triamterene daily) are effective. Intratympanic gentamicin can significantly reduce vertigo in patients with unilateral Meniere disease who do not respond to medical treatment.[A10] Endolymphatic duct blockage is a potential option for medically refractory Meniere disease.[A11]

In many cases, however, symptomatic treatment either is combined with specific therapy or is the only treatment available. Many different classes of drugs have been found to have antivertiginous properties, and in most instances, the exact mechanism of action is uncertain. All these agents produce potentially unpleasant side effects, and the decision concerning which drug or combination to use is based on their known complications and on the severity and duration of the vertigo. An episode of prolonged, severe vertigo is one of the most distressing symptoms that a patient can experience. Affected patients prefer to lie still with eyes closed in a quiet, dark room. Antivertiginous drugs with sedation, such as promethazine HCl (25 mg) or diazepam (5 mg), may be helpful. Prochlorperazine suppositories (25 mg) may stop vomiting.

In more chronic vertiginous disorders, when the patient is trying to carry on normal activity, less sedating antivertiginous medications, such as meclizine (25 mg) or transdermal scopolamine (0.5 mg every 3 days), may provide relief. Chronic use of these drugs should be avoided.

Vestibular rehabilitation exercises are designed to help the patient compensate for permanent loss of vestibular function.[A12] As the acute stage of nausea and vomiting subsides, the patient should attempt to focus the eyes and to move and hold them in the direction that provokes the most dizziness. A useful exercise involves staring at a visual target while oscillating the head from side to side or up and down, slow at first and then fast. The patient should try to stand and walk, at first in contact with a wall or with an assistant, and make slow supported turns. As improvement occurs, head movements should be added while standing and walking.

TABLE 428-2	TREATMENT OF COMMON VERTIGO SYNDROMES
SYNDROME	**TREATMENT**
Benign positional vertigo	
Posterior canal variant	Epley's maneuver (see Fig. 428-4)
Horizontal canal variant	Barbecue roll toward normal side (side with less nystagmus), sleep with normal ear down
Vestibular neuritis	Methylprednisolone, 100 mg × 3 days, gradual taper during 22 days (must start within 3 days of onset)
Meniere disease	
Medical	Low salt (1-2 g salt/day) *and* either hydrochlorothiazide 25-50 mg/day *or* hydrochlorothiazide 25 mg/day plus triamterene 50 mg/day
Surgical	Intratympanic gentamicin, vestibular nerve section

Grade A References

A1. Wei BP, Stathopoulos D, O'Leary S. Steroids for idiopathic sudden sensorineural hearing loss. *Cochrane Database Syst Rev.* 2013;7:CD003998.
A2. Rauch SD, Halpin CF, Antonelli PJ, et al. Oral vs intratympanic corticosteroid therapy for idiopathic sudden sensorineural hearing loss: a randomized trial. *JAMA.* 2011;305:2071-2079.
A3. Gundogan O, Pinar E, Imre A, et al. Therapeutic efficacy of the combination of intratympanic methylprednisolone and oral steroid for idiopathic sudden deafness. *Otolaryngol Head Neck Surg.* 2013;149:753-758.
A4. Durga J, Verhoef P, Anteunis LJ, et al. Effects of folic acid supplementation on hearing in older adults: a randomized, controlled trial. *Lancet.* 2007;369:208-216.
A5. Cima RF, Maes IH, Joore MA, et al. Specialised treatment based on cognitive behaviour therapy versus usual care for tinnitus: a randomised controlled trial. *Lancet.* 2012;379:1951-1959.
A6. Hunt WT, Zimmermann EF, Hilton MP. Modifications of the Epley (canalith repositioning) manoeuvre for posterior canal benign paroxysmal positional vertigo (BPPV). *Cochrane Database Syst Rev.* 2012;4:CD008675.
A7. Kim JS, Oh SY, Lee SH, et al. Randomized clinical trial for apogeotropic horizontal canal benign paroxysmal positional vertigo. *Neurology.* 2012;78:159-166.
A8. Kim JS, Oh SY, Lee SH, et al. Randomized clinical trial for geotropic horizontal canal benign paroxysmal positional vertigo. *Neurology.* 2012;79:700-707.
A9. Fishman JM, Burgess C, Waddell A. Corticosteroids for the treatment of idiopathic acute vestibular dysfunction (vestibular neuritis). *Cochrane Database Syst Rev.* 2011;5:CD008607.
A10. Pullens B, van Benthem PP. Intratympanic gentamicin for Meniere's disease or syndrome. *Cochrane Database Syst Rev.* 2011;3:CD008234.
A11. Saliba I, Gabra N, Alzahrani M, et al. Endolymphatic Duct Blockage: A Randomized Controlled Trial of a Novel Surgical Technique for Ménière's Disease Treatment. *Otolaryngol Head Neck Surg.* 2015;152:122-129.
A12. Hillier SL, McDonnell M. Vestibular rehabilitation for unilateral peripheral vestibular dysfunction. *Cochrane Database Syst Rev.* 2011;2:CD005397.

GENERAL REFERENCES

For the General References and other additional features, please visit Expert Consult at https://expertconsult.inkling.com.

429
THROAT DISORDERS
PAUL W. FLINT

Nearly every systemic and infectious disease results in head and neck manifestations, with the majority affecting the upper aerodigestive tract. Diseases of the upper aerodigestive system include infection (acute and chronic; viral, bacterial, and fungal), systemic disease, and neoplasm (Chapter 190), some of which require urgent care or referral to an otolaryngologist.

Abnormalities of swallowing, respiratory function, voice, and speech are influenced by the anatomic site involved, the host's immune status and inflammatory response, the severity of the disease process, and the presence or absence of neurologic involvement.

In a patient with hoarseness, current clinical practice guidelines recommend visualization of the larynx for symptoms that persist for 3 months or longer; however, warning signs of a potentially serious or emergent throat condition warrant referral regardless of duration. These conditions include persistent throat pain with or without trismus, difficulty in swallowing, difficulty in breathing, hemoptysis, and ear pain with normal ear examination findings. Diagnostic testing options, which include fiberoptic examination, imaging, pulmonary function studies, and laboratory testing, are directed by history, symptoms, and physical findings.

ANATOMY OF THE UPPER AERODIGESTIVE TRACT

The pharynx is divided into three anatomic regions (Fig. 429-1). The *nasopharynx* is the region above the soft palate and uvula. Its anatomic components include the adenoids, the openings of the eustachian tubes, Rosenmüller's fossa at the junction of the posterior and lateral walls, and the posterior aspect of the inferior turbinates of the nasal cavity. Diseases of the nasopharynx typically produce few symptoms until the process is well advanced and causes nasal obstruction (Chapter 426), epistaxis (Chapter 426), ear pain (Chapter 426), headache (Chapter 398), or cranial nerve abnormalities due to extension to the skull base. The *oropharynx* begins at the level of the soft palate and extends inferiorly to the tip of the epiglottis. This region includes the faucial tonsils, the base of the tongue, the lingual tonsils, the soft palate, the uvula, and part of the posterior pharyngeal wall. The *hypopharynx*, which extends from the tip of the epiglottis to the upper esophagus (the cricopharyngeus muscle) below, includes the larynx (epiglottis, arytenoids, glottis or true vocal cords), the piriform sinuses (pharyngeal folds lateral to the larynx), and the posterior pharyngeal wall. The tip of the epiglottis can be visualized by an experienced examiner with use of a laryngeal mirror or sometimes even on a routine oral examination with just a flashlight and tongue blade. The nasopharynx and hypopharynx are best visualized with a flexible fiberoptic nasopharyngoscope.

INFECTIOUS DISEASES OF THE UPPER AERODIGESTIVE SYSTEM

Infectious disorders of the upper aerodigestive tract typically are manifested as sore throat (pharyngitis), changes in voice (laryngitis), or both. The clinical evaluation must differentiate among bacterial (usually streptococcus [Chapter 290]), viral, and other infections and systemic causes (Table 429-1). Clinical differentiation of sore throat is critical to primary care and emergency management of the airway.

Pharyngitis

Bacterial infection accounts for approximately 5 to 10% of pharyngitis in adults compared with 30 to 40% in children. Unfortunately, as many as two thirds of adults with a sore throat are prescribed antibiotics.

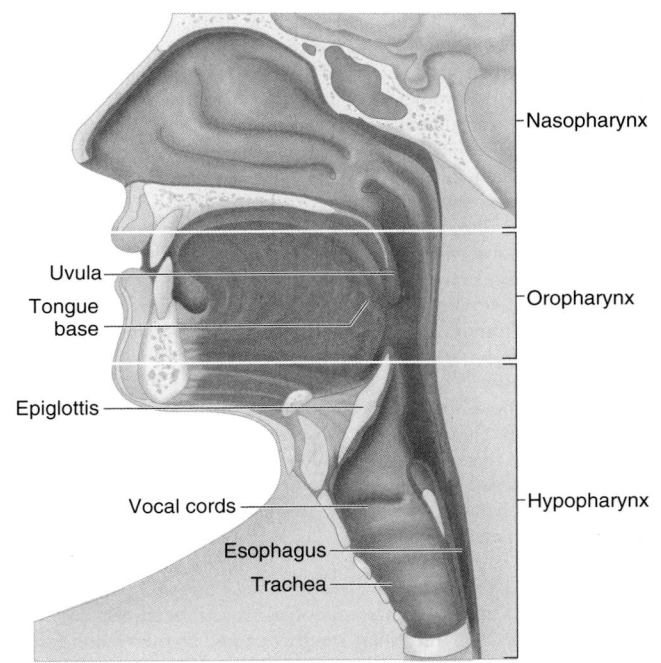
FIGURE 429-1. The pharynx (throat) is typically divided into three distinct anatomic regions (nasopharynx, oropharynx, and hypopharynx). (Courtesy Thomas A. Tami, MD.)

TABLE 429-1 CLINICAL DIFFERENTIATION OF COMMON CONDITIONS ARISING AS SORE THROAT

FEATURE	VIRAL PHARYNGITIS	BACTERIAL TONSILLITIS	PERITONSILLAR ABSCESS	EPIGLOTTITIS
Tonsillar enlargement	Usual	Rare	None	None
Tonsillar exudates	Occasional (infectious mononucleosis)	Usual	Often	None
Tonsillar asymmetry	None	None	Usual	None
Trismus (inability to open jaw)	None	None	Usual	None
Cervical adenopathy	Occasional	Usual (tender)	Usual (tender)	None
Tender larynx	Rare	None	None	Usual

From Tami TA. Throat disorders. In: Goldman L, Schafer AI, eds. *Goldman's Cecil Medicine.* 24th ed. Philadelphia: Elsevier Saunders; 2012.

STREPTOCOCCAL INFECTIONS

Group A beta-hemolytic *Streptococcus pyogenes* (Chapter 290) is the most common cause of bacterial pharyngitis in adults, although it accounts for only 10% of all pharyngitis in adults. Infection is manifested with the rapid onset of sore throat, often accompanied by pain with swallowing, fever, chills, malaise, headache, mild neck stiffness, and anorexia. Hypertrophic tonsils with exudates, foul breath, and tender cervical adenopathy are hallmark findings.[1] Some patients have palatal petechiae or a scarlatiniform rash. Rhinorrhea, hoarseness, cough, conjunctivitis, diarrhea, and ulcerative oral lesions are less common.

Untreated group A beta-hemolytic *S. pyogenes* pharyngitis usually resolves within 3 to 7 days. The administration of antibiotics within 24 to 48 hours reduces pain by approximately 1 day,[A1] whereas both immediate and delayed antibiotics reduce the risk of suppurative complications.[2] Antibiotics also reduce the contagious period from 2 weeks to 24 hours after administration. For prevention of rheumatic fever (Chapter 290), antibiotic therapy must be started within 10 days after the onset of symptoms. The risk of acute poststreptococcal glomerulonephritis (Chapter 121), however, is not affected by antibiotics.

To minimize the potential side effects and costs of unnecessary antibiotics, antibiotic therapy should be based on the presence of fever, tender anterior cervical adenopathy, tonsillar swelling or exudates, age, and the absence of cough (Table 429-2). If three or four of these criteria are present, the likelihood of group A beta-hemolytic streptococcal infection is 40 to 60%, whereas fewer criteria are associated with progressively lower probabilities. A rapid antigen test may be obtained because of the residual risk of false-positive or false-negative diagnoses, but its incremental diagnostic value is low, except in borderline cases.[3] If the rapid antigen test result is negative but the clinical suspicion remains high, a throat culture specimen should be obtained for confirmation.

Antibiotic options (Chapter 290) include penicillin (penicillin VK, 250 mg three times a day or 500 mg twice a day for 5 to 10 days), which is usually chosen to treat acute bacterial pharyngitis,[A2] although cefuroxime axetil (250 mg twice a day for 5 to 10 days) is even more effective for primary treatment and can be effective for persistent infection. In patients with proven recurrent infections, clindamycin (300 mg orally three times a day for 10 days) or amoxicillin–clavulanic acid (875 mg orally twice a day, or 500 mg three times a day for 10 days) is recommended. For patients who are allergic to penicillin, azithromycin (500 mg/day for 3 days or a single dose of 2 g)[A3] is another alternative. Evidence also suggests that a single dose of oral or intramuscular corticosteroids given at the start of treatment will reduce the pain of severe pharyngitis, especially in children.[A4] In patients with recurrent symptomatic episodes despite appropriate antimicrobial therapy, tonsillectomy can decrease future throat infections compared with continued observation.[A5]

Non–group A beta-hemolytic streptococcal infections (Chapter 290), including groups B, C, and G, can cause acute pharyngitis with a clinical picture that mirrors that of group A beta-hemolytic streptococcal pharyngitis. Glomerulonephritis is a known sequela, whereas rheumatic fever is not. Penicillin or clindamycin, as prescribed for group A beta-hemolytic streptococcus, provides adequate coverage.

NONSTREPTOCOCCAL BACTERIAL PHARYNGITIS

A variety of bacteria other than streptococci can infect the throat. *Staphylococcus aureus* (Chapter 288) infections, whether caused by methicillin-resistant (MRSA) or methicillin-sensitive (MSSA) strains, usually are manifested with chronic hoarseness. Laryngoscopy typically reveals thickened erythematous vocal folds with edema, whitish debris, and crusting, which may resemble

TABLE 429-2 GUIDELINES FOR THE MANAGEMENT OF PHARYNGITIS*

CENTOR SCORE[†]	PERCENTAGE POSITIVE FOR *STREPTOCOCCUS* INFECTION	ACP/CDC GUIDELINES
0	7%	Do not test, do not treat
1	12%	Do not test, do not treat
2	21%	Treat if rapid test result positive
3	38%	Option 1: treat if rapid test result positive Option 2: treat empirically
4	57%	Treat empirically

*As recommended by the American College of Physicians (ACP) and the Centers for Disease Control and Prevention (CDC). See *Arch Intern Med.* 2012;172:847-852.
[†]Calculated as follows: 1 point each for temperature >38°C, absence of cough, presence of swollen and tender anterior cervical nodes, tonsillar swelling or exudate, or age 3 to 14 years; and −1 point for age ≥45 years.

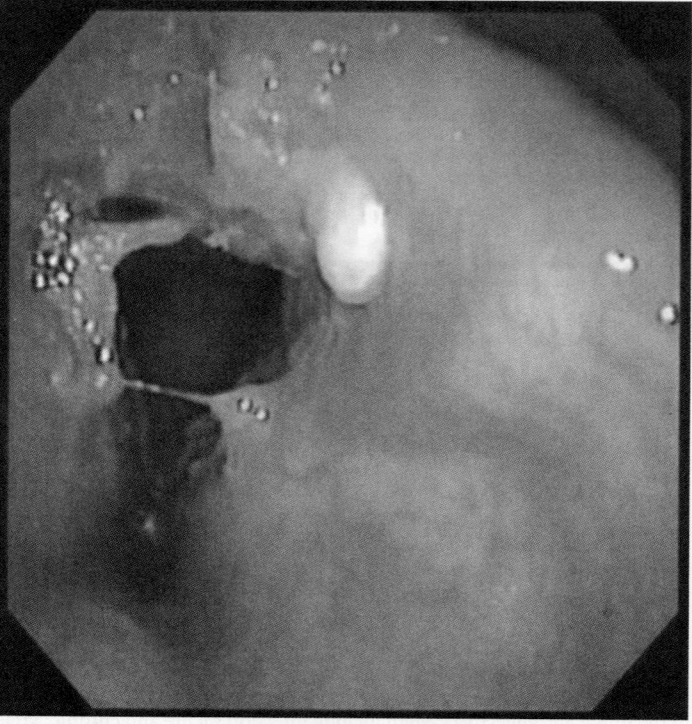

FIGURE 429-2. Fiberoptic laryngoscopy demonstrating chronic laryngitis secondary to methicillin-sensitive *S. aureus* infection. Diagnosis is based on culture and biopsy.

leukoplakia (Fig. 429-2). Trimethoprim-sulfamethoxazole (160 mg/800 mg twice daily for 2 to 4 weeks) has been shown to be effective,[4] although treatment should be guided by antibiotic sensitivities.

Bordetella pertussis (Chapter 313) infections have become more common in adults because of their gradual loss of immune protection after vaccination. Adults typically present with cough, often but not always accompanied by nonspecific upper respiratory symptoms, fever, and leukocytosis. A *B. pertussis* serum immunoglobulin G titer higher than 27 IU/mL is highly predictive of recent infection.[5] Erythromycin (500 mg four times a day for 14 days) or azithromycin (500 mg single dose orally on day 1, then 250 mg daily on days 2 through 5) is effective treatment.

Neisseria gonorrhoeae (Chapter 299) can cause sexually transmitted gingivitis, stomatitis, glossitis, and pharyngitis, especially in men who have sex with men. Treatment is the same as for urogenital disease and should include treatment for chlamydia. Options include ceftriaxone, 250 mg intramuscularly in a single dose; azithromycin, 1 g orally in a single dose; and doxycycline, 100 mg orally twice daily for 7 days. *Treponema pallidum* (Chapter 319) can cause oral and oropharyngeal ulcerations that involve the lips, tongue, and tonsil. Treatment is the same as that recommended for systemic disease. *Chlamydia* (Chapter 318), which is commonly associated with pneumonia and bronchitis, also can cause pharyngitis and hoarseness, sometimes as its presenting symptoms. *Mycoplasma pneumoniae* (Chapter 317), which frequently accounts for 15 to 20% of cases of community-acquired pneumonias, also can cause sore throat, nasal congestion, and coryza. Treatment of chlamydia and mycoplasma infections with tetracyclines, macrolides, and quinolones is the same as for the pneumonias they cause (Chapters 318 and 317).

Francisella tularensis (Chapter 311) is a gram-negative bacillus that causes tularemia. Oropharyngeal involvement is associated with fever, pharyngeal erythema, exudative tonsillitis, and tender lymphadenopathy. A false-positive monospot test result and atypical lymphocytosis can mimic infectious mononucleosis. The organism is sensitive to macrolides, fluoroquinolones, and tetracyclines.

Corynebacterium diphtheriae infection (Chapter 292) involves the mucosal surfaces of the upper respiratory tract, where it causes a patchy gray-black pseudomembrane in the nasopharynx, oropharynx, larynx, and trachea. About 75% of patients complain of throat pain. Airway obstruction and severe dysphagia are life-threatening sequelae. Antitoxin is given in combination with penicillin, erythromycin, tetracycline, clindamycin, or rifampin.

Arcanobacterium haemolyticum (Chapter 292) is a gram-positive bacillus that can cause pneumonia, meningitis, osteomyelitis, brain abscess, and peritonsillar abscess in both normal and immunocompromised patients. Uncomplicated pharyngitis may be treated with erythromycin (500 mg four times a day for 10 days). Complicated infections require intravenous dosing with vancomycin, clindamycin, or cephalexin, with or without gentamicin (see Table 287-4).

PERITONSILLAR ABSCESS AND DEEP SPACE INFECTIONS

Only about 1% of patients with acute bacterial pharyngitis develop serious suppurative complications.[6] The best predictors are severe tonsillar inflammation and severe earache, but most complications occur in patients with neither of these findings. Peritonsillar abscesses usually can be diagnosed on physical examination (Fig. 429-3) and managed by an otolaryngologist in an outpatient setting by surgical or needle drainage. Oral antibiotics, such as amoxicillin (500 mg orally twice a day for 10 days) plus metronidazole (500 mg orally three times a day for 10 days), clindamycin (300 to 600 mg three times a day for 14 days), or amoxicillin-clavulanate (875 mg orally twice a day for 10 days), are recommended.

By comparison, patients with deep neck abscesses often have swelling of the external neck, trismus, torticollis, and even a compromised airway due to infection that has spread to the fascial planes of the neck and chest. These infections require urgent evaluation, usually with a computed tomography scan with contrast enhancement. Aggressive management includes incision and drainage as well as broad-spectrum intravenous antibiotics that cover aerobic and anaerobic bacteria (e.g., clindamycin, 600 mg intravenously every 8 hours; ampicillin-sulbactam, 3 g every 6 hours; or penicillin G, 2 million units every 4 hours plus metronidazole 500 mg every 6 hours).[7]

Severe infections of the pharynx can cause septic thrombophlebitis of the internal jugular vein (Lemierre's syndrome), an uncommon but serious complication. Patients typically present with persistent fever, difficulty in swallowing, neck pain, and a neck mass due to an underlying peritonsillar, retropharyngeal, or parapharyngeal abscess.[8] Diagnosis is best established with a contrast-enhanced computed tomography scan of the neck. This potentially life-threatening condition is almost always associated with anaerobic infection, especially with *Fusobacterium necrophorum* or *A. haemolyticum* (Chapter 297). Infection can extend into the intrathoracic vasculature, and patients can develop bacteremia and septic pulmonary emboli. Treatment should be directed toward anaerobic coverage (e.g., clindamycin, 600 mg every 8 hours, or metronidazole, 500 mg every 6 hours). Anticoagulation with heparin is controversial and generally reserved for persistent septic emboli. Surgical intervention includes drainage of the abscess. Ligation or excision of the jugular vein may be indicated for persistent septic emboli unresponsive to medical management. Mortality rates can be as high as 5%.

VIRAL INFECTIONS

In adults, the common cold (Chapter 361) causes 30 to 60% of cases of pharyngitis, with rhinovirus (Chapter 361) accounting for the majority of cases, followed by coronavirus (Chapter 366) and parainfluenza (Chapter 363) (see Table 429-2). U.S. adults experience an average of 2.5 episodes per year of noninfluenza upper respiratory infections, each with a 7.4-day average duration of symptoms. For the entire U.S. population, these 500 million episodes cost an estimated $40 billion annually, in part because of associated systemic symptoms such as fever, cough, and sinusitis and in part because of associated exacerbations of allergies, asthma, and chronic obstructive pulmonary disease.

The viral infection that is most likely to be confused with a bacterial infection is mononucleosis. Mononucleosis is caused by Epstein-Barr virus (Chapter 377), which has a seroprevalence of 67% in U.S. children and adolescents aged 6 to 19 years.[9] After an incubation period of 3 to 7 weeks, patients present with initial malaise, fever, and chills followed by sore throat, fever, and anorexia. Some patients have associated abdominal discomfort due to splenomegaly or hepatomegaly, headache, stiff neck, and rash. On physical examination, patients have erythematous pharyngitis with exudative tonsillar hypertrophy (Fig. 429-4), prominent lingual tonsils, and adenoid hypertrophy (Waldeyer's ring). Aphthous-type ulcerations and petechiae may be seen, especially at the junction of the hard and soft palate. Impressive cervical adenopathy is typical, and 50% of patients have splenomegaly. Lymphoid hyperplasia can cause some degree of upper airway obstruction in about 5% of patients.

A blood count will show lymphocytosis, usually with more 10% atypical lymphocytes. The heterophil antibody test result is often positive, and Epstein-Barr virus–specific antibody tests are diagnostic. β-Lactam

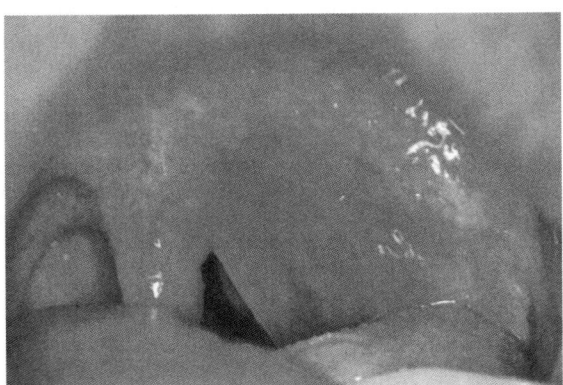

FIGURE 429-3. Left peritonsillar abscess identified by bulging anterior pillar and soft palate with midline shift. (Courtesy Thomas A. Tami, MD.)

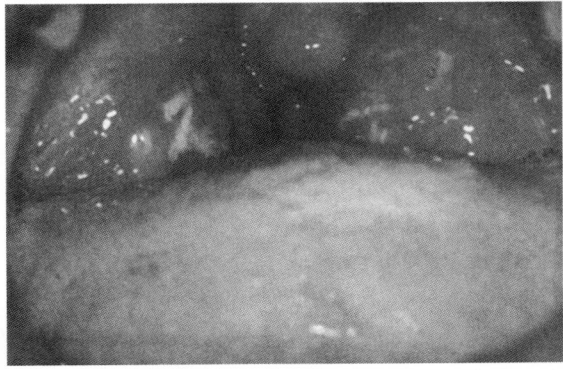

FIGURE 429-4. Mononucleosis with symmetrical exudative tonsillitis. (Courtesy Thomas A. Tami, MD.)

antibiotics, which may mistakenly be prescribed, will cause a maculopapular rash in 95% of patients. Laryngeal obstruction may require hospitalization and intravenous corticosteroids (e.g., dexamethasone, 8 to 10 mg intravenously three times a day).

Influenza virus infection can include nonexudative pharyngitis, but the predominant symptoms are tracheobronchial, usually accompanied by fever, headache, rhinorrhea, cough, and myalgia, without lymphadenopathy.[10] Adenovirus (Chapter 365) can cause pharyngitis associated with fever, nonproductive cough, nasal congestion, myalgia, headache, nausea, vomiting, and diarrhea, especially in outbreaks, such as among military recruits, or in immunocompromised patients.

Primary herpes simplex virus (Chapter 374) infection is characterized by pharyngitis with or without gingival stomatitis. Symptoms include sore throat, fever, and malaise; physical findings include erythema and hypertrophy of the tonsils with exudates, often with enlarged, tender cervical nodes. It may be difficult to distinguish clinically from group A beta-hemolytic streptococcal pharyngitis unless patients have herpes-like lesions of the oral cavity or oropharynx.

Human immunodeficiency virus infection (Chapter 384) can be manifested as an acute retroviral syndrome that mimics infectious mononucleosis and resolves in 1 to 2 weeks. The diagnosis must be considered in febrile patients with known risk factors. Once infection is established, oral and oropharyngeal infectious ulcerations may be due to herpes simplex virus, cytomegalovirus, syphilis, cryptococcus, histoplasmosis, or mycobacteria. Large, painful, noninfectious aphthous ulcers also can involve the tonsillar fossa, floor of mouth, hypopharynx, and epiglottis (Chapter 425).

FUNGAL INFECTIONS

By far, the most common fungal infection of the oropharynx and larynx is candidiasis. *Candida* (Chapter 338) is a normal commensal organism of the oral cavity and oropharynx, but it can be an opportunistic infectious agent in immunocompromised patients, patients who have received prior head and neck irradiation, patients with xerostomia or diabetes, and immunocompetent patients who have been treated with antibiotics or with systemic or inhaled steroids. *Candida* infection is manifested with sore throat, burning of the mouth and tongue, dysgeusia, dysphagia, and hoarseness. White pseudomembranes characteristic of thrush (Fig. 429-5) may involve the oral cavity, oropharynx, hypopharynx, larynx, and esophagus. Treatment includes oral hygiene, probiotics, and topical antifungals (Chapter 338). Fluconazole (200 mg orally once a day for 14 to 21 days) is indicated for laryngeal and esophageal involvement and for recurrent disease. Itraconazole (200 mg orally once a day for 14 to 21 days) should be considered for nonresponders.

Other fungal infections may affect the oropharynx and larynx in isolation or as part of a systemic infection. *Blastomycosis* (Chapter 334) involves the larynx in less than 5% of cases, in which it produces pseudoepitheliomatous hyperplasia and clinically resembles squamous cell carcinoma. *Histoplasmosis* (Chapter 332), which is endemic to the Ohio and Mississippi river valleys, can involve the oral cavity, oropharynx, and larynx in immunocompromised patients. *Cryptococcosis* (Chapter 336) can involve the larynx and occurs most often in an immunocompromised host, in whom pseudoepitheliomatous hyperplasia may occur.

Paracoccidioidomycosis (Chapter 335) is the leading cause of fungal laryngitis in South America, especially among farmers. It causes pseudoepitheliomatous hyperplasia that can be misdiagnosed initially as squamous cell carcinoma. *Coccidioidomycosis* (Chapter 333), which is endemic to southwestern United States, can involve the larynx, in which it results in hoarseness and throat pain and can progress to airway obstruction. For each of these fungal diseases, treatment is similar to what is recommended for the disseminated disease (Chapter 331) that usually accompanies pharyngeal and laryngeal disease.

MYCOBACTERIAL INFECTIONS

The risk that tuberculosis (Chapter 324) infection will involve the oropharynx and larynx is low, with only about 1 to 1.5% of infected tuberculosis patients having involvement of the tonsils or larynx. Tonsillar involvement, which most often occurs in the presence of systemic disease, is manifested as sore throat with exudative tonsillitis and cervical adenopathy. Other diseases that can have a similar clinical presentation include lymphoma (Chapter 185), squamous cell carcinoma (Chapter 190), and sarcoidosis (Chapter 95). Tuberculosis in the larynx is most likely to involve the vocal folds and supraglottis (false vocal folds). It is manifested with hoarseness and odynophagia, and its lesions mimic squamous cell carcinoma. Approximately 50% of cases occur in the presence of active disseminated disease, about one third occur with inactive disease, and the other 15% occur as primary laryngeal disease.[11]

In contrast, *Mycobacterium leprae* infection (Chapter 326) is manifested with laryngeal disease in one third of patients with systemic disease. The clinical picture is indistinguishable from that of laryngeal tuberculosis. Atypical mycobacteria rarely involve the larynx, and infection most often is manifested as cervical adenopathy.

CHRONIC TONSILLITIS

Patients may develop deep tonsillar crypts that accumulate debris, such as food or sloughed mucosa, thereby providing an ideal environment for the growth of bacteria, especially anaerobes. Such patients commonly complain of whitish or yellow pieces of semisolid debris on or emanating from their tonsils. These tonsilliths often have a foul taste and odor, and they can cause halitosis. Some patients have chronic sore throats because of the persistent infection. Treatment includes frequent gargling of a hydrogen peroxide mouthwash and occasionally expressing this debris from the tonsil manually. Long-term amoxicillin (500 mg three times a day for 21 days) or clindamycin (300 mg orally three times a day for 21 days) may be effective; however, the presence of *Actinomyces*, a commensal organism of the oral cavity and oropharynx, is indicative of chronic infection that requires tonsillectomy because even long-term antibiotics are unlikely to be effective.[12]

Epiglottitis

Epiglottitis (supraglottitis) is an uncommon problem in adults and has become even less common in children because of routine *Haemophilus influenzae* vaccination in children (Chapters 18 and 300). In adults, *Streptococcus pneumoniae* (Chapter 289) is now the most common organism,[13] and adults present with a severe sore throat, odynophagia, fever, and "hot potato" voice. Airway obstruction occurs less frequently than in children, although it should be considered a possibility. Palpation or movement of the larynx causes significant pain. On transnasal fiberoptic laryngoscopy, the larynx typically reveals swelling, erythema, and occasionally exudates of the epiglottis and other supraglottic structures. Patients with a confirmed diagnosis of epiglottitis require intravenous antibiotics (e.g., cefotaxime, 2 g every 6 hours, or ceftriaxone, 1 to 2 g/day, intravenously), and they should be observed in an intensive care unit setting until symptoms improve because of the risk of rapidly progressive airway obstruction.

⬤ NONINFECTIOUS PHARYNGITIS
Laryngopharyngeal Reflux

Patients with gastroesophageal reflux disease (Chapter 138) can develop laryngopharyngeal reflux with intermittent hoarseness, nighttime or chronic cough, postnasal drip, "globus" sensation, reactive airway disease, halitosis,

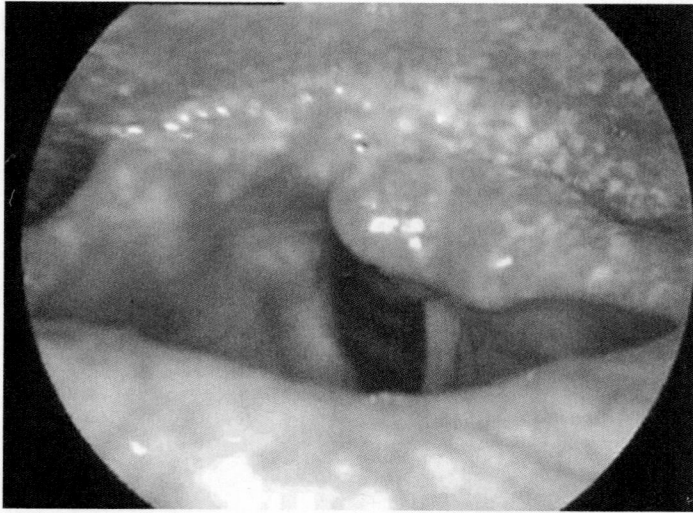

FIGURE 429-5. Fiberoptic laryngoscopy demonstrating characteristic erythema and white pseudomembrane secondary to *Candida* infection.

and brackish or acid taste in the back of the mouth and throat. Findings on laryngoscopy, although nonspecific, may include posterior laryngitis, with swollen and erythematous arytenoid cartilages, thickening of the vocal folds, interarytenoid edema, and thickening of the mucosa. In severe cases, spasm or thickening of the cricopharyngeus muscle, also known as the upper esophageal sphincter (Chapter 138), can cause dysphagia as a result of poor pharyngeal emptying or even spillage of secretions into the larynx with aspiration.[14]

Treatment should address dietary change, behavioral modification, elevation of the head of the bed at night, and a therapeutic trial of a proton pump inhibitor for up to 3 months (Chapter 138). Empirical treatment without laryngoscopy is reasonable in patients with classic symptoms, but patients who do not respond within 3 months or patients with warning signs (e.g., ear pain, trismus, or odynophagia) require laryngoscopy to exclude more serious causes of hoarseness. In patients with persistent symptoms and a positive pH probe or with evidence of Barrett's esophagitis, an antireflux procedure (Chapter 138) should be strongly considered.[15]

SYSTEMIC DISEASES OF THE THROAT AND LARYNGITIS

About 80% of patients with *pemphigus* (Chapter 439) will have symptoms affecting the nasal cavity, oral cavity, and oropharynx, and half of these patients will have laryngeal involvement.[16] Shallow ulcerations with fibrinous material and surrounding erythema are characteristic. Bullous lesions are less likely to be observed because the epithelial layer sloughs during swallowing. Laryngeal involvement may result in stenosis with airway obstruction due to scarring. Upper aerodigestive tract involvement occurs in 35% of patients with *pemphigoid* (Chapter 439), and 50% of these patients will have laryngeal involvement. Treatment in both disorders consists of high-dose steroids (prednisone, 75 to 100 mg orally per day until remission) during the attack phase and then tapered to a maintenance dose (25 to 50 mg orally every other day). Other immunosuppressive medications, such as azathioprine, cyclophosphamide, or cyclosporine (Chapter 35), may be required in the maintenance phase. Perilesional or intralesional triamcinolone acetonide injections are recommended during the maintenance phase for new lesions.[17]

Granulomatosis with polyangiitis (Chapter 270) includes laryngeal involvement in 20% of patients, with a predilection for the subglottis. Presenting symptoms may include hoarseness, cough, dyspnea, wheezing, and stridor. Flow-volume loops are useful and demonstrate flattening of both inspiratory and expiratory loops characteristic of a fixed extrathoracic obstruction. Patients presenting with airway obstruction require surgical intervention. Active disease with granulation tissue requiring airway management is treated with endoscopic dilation and steroid injection. Systemic immunosuppression is not effective for treatment of laryngeal involvement, so open resection may be required as the disease becomes chronic with the deposition of fibrous tissue.[18]

Relapsing polychondritis involves cartilage in the ear, nose, and upper and lower airway as well as in the articular joints and costal cartilage. About 50% of patients will develop dyspnea, cough, hoarseness, stridor, or wheezing due to the destruction of cartilage and the resulting loss of structural support of the airway.[19] Airway obstruction may necessitate stenting or tracheostomy.

About 25 to 30% of patients with rheumatoid arthritis (Chapter 264) develop hoarseness, globus symptoms, and difficulty in swallowing. Hoarseness may result from acute inflammation or chronic nodular formation. Bilateral arytenoid joint involvement may impair vocal fold motion and cause airway obstruction with stridor. Surgical intervention may be necessary to open the airway. The role of steroids (systemic or injectable) for airway stenosis in rheumatoid arthritis has not been established.

About 1 to 5% of all patients with *sarcoidosis* (Chapter 95) develop laryngeal involvement, usually manifested as hoarseness. As the disease progresses, however, it can cause a conical stenosis due to thickening of the soft tissue. Laryngeal paralysis can be caused by a mass effect or by adenopathy with peripheral nerve compression along the course of the vagus or recurrent laryngeal nerve. Vocal fold involvement responds to intralesional steroid injection, but endoscopic laser excision is recommended in patients with airway symptoms.

Amyloidosis (Chapter 188) may deposit anywhere in the upper aerodigestive tract. Hoarseness and cough are the most common symptoms in patients with laryngeal involvement, but pharyngeal involvement may be associated with pain. Airway obstruction is rare. Surgical debulking with or without external beam radiation can relieve symptoms and even resolve the lesions.

NEUROLOGIC DISORDERS AFFECTING THE THROAT

Neurologic disorders of the oropharynx, hypopharynx, and larynx may be due to focal diseases or be a local manifestation of generalized neurologic disease. Head and neck manifestations of neurologic and neuromuscular disorders are classified as hyperfunctional and hypofunctional disorders. Hyperfunctional disorders include muscle tension dysphonia, dystonia (Chapter 410), essential tremor (Chapter 410), myoclonus, and stuttering. Hypofunctional neurologic disorders include Parkinson's disease (Chapter 409), multiple sclerosis (Chapter 411), neuromuscular disorders (Chapters 419 and 422), postpolio syndrome (Chapter 379), myopathies (Chapter 421), medullary disorders, and laryngeal paralysis. Given the variety of disorders with head and neck manifestations, it is critical to identify and to classify the physical findings and associated symptoms. For example, a patient who complains about the sound of the voice may in fact have a normal voice but actually have severe dysarthria and hypernasality secondary to amyotrophic lateral sclerosis. The site of the lesion associated with the neurologic disorder will result in characteristic physical findings and facilitate establishment of a correct diagnosis (Table 429-3).

Hyperfunctional Neurologic Disorders

In *dystonia* (Chapter 410), spasmodic dysphonia fluctuates moment to moment and day to day. Adductor spasms of the vocal folds produce strained, strangled vocal quality with pitch breaks. Abductor spasms produce breathy hypophonic word breaks. Nonspeech sounds (laughter) and singing voice may be normal. This condition responds well to botulinum toxin injections.[20]

Muscle tension dysphonia, which may be difficult to distinguish from dystonia, can occur secondary to underlying weakness (paresis, aging) with compensatory hyperfunction. Speech has a rough strained quality, perhaps with pitch breaks, and does not fluctuate moment to moment. It generally responds to voice therapy.

Vocal tremor is seen in 30% of patients with *essential tremor* (Chapter 410) and may be associated with spastic dystonia. Patients have a tremulous, quavering vocal quality, with or without head or hand tremor. Because of involvement of pharyngeal and laryngeal muscles, botulinum toxin may not be effective.

Myoclonus (Chapter 410) causes rhythmic contraction of the palate, pharynx, or larynx at a rate of one or two per second. Patients may have audible clicking from the eustachian tube or larynx. Voice may or may not be affected. Palate and vocal folds may be treated with botulinum toxin.

Pseudobulbar palsy (Chapters 404 and 419) causes spasticity and hyperreflexia of the bulbar muscles (pharynx, palate, lips tongue, and larynx).

TABLE 429-3	CORRELATING SITE OF LESION WITH PHYSICAL FINDINGS IN NEUROLOGICAL DISORDERS AFFECTING THE THROAT
SITE OF LESION	**SIGNS**
Cortex	Aphasia Aphonia Dysarthria Dysphonia Stridor
Extrapyramidal system	Vocal strain and pitch breaks Tremor Hypophonia/tachyphemia Spasmodic movements Focal, regional, or generalized dystonia
Cerebellum	Ataxia Dysmetria Tremor Incoordination
Brain stem	Flaccid paralysis Associated dense sensory deficit
Peripheral	Focal paresis or paralysis Other cranial nerve ± Palate involvement defines location

Modified from Blitzer A, Alexander RE, Grant NN. Neurologic disorders of the larynx. In: Flint PW, Haughey BH, Lund VJ, et al, eds. *Cummings: Otolaryngology–Head and Neck Surgery.* 6th ed. Philadelphia: Mosby Elsevier; 2015.

Patients develop dysarthria, hypernasality, and a harsh strident strained vocal quality, which is more spastic than spasmodic.

Hypofunctional Neurologic Disorders

Parkinson's disease affects speech and swallowing in more than 80% of patients. Patients have dysarthria, prosody of speech, hypophonia, tachyphemia, monotonous pitch, and absence of vocal tremor.

Laryngeal examination shows bilateral vocal fold bowing with incomplete glottic closure. In advanced disease, vocal fold motion becomes hypokinetic. Pooling of secretions occurs as swallowing dysfunction progresses. Patients benefit from early intervention by speech-language therapists to address both voice and swallowing symptoms. In *progressive supranuclear palsy*, bulbar symptoms progress more rapidly, with pronounced speech and swallowing difficulty (Chapter 409). In *multiple system atrophy* (Chapter 409), progressive airway obstruction from bilateral vocal fold motion impairment may necessitate tracheostomy. In *myasthenia gravis* (Chapter 422), hypernasal speech, palatal weakness, and hypophonia may be accompanied by difficulties with swallowing and respiration. Some patients with *amyotrophic lateral sclerosis* (Chapter 419) present with bulbar symptoms that result from buccal-labial-lingual weakness, which produces speech and swallowing dysfunction, before the definitive diagnosis is made. In *multiple sclerosis* (Chapter 411), dysphonia and dysarthria are common.

LUMP IN THE THROAT

The sensation of a lump in the throat,[21] called *globus pharyngeus*, should prompt a careful history and physical examination by an otolaryngologist to exclude a serious diagnosis. When no underlying anatomic disease is found, possible causes include gastroesophageal reflux and spasm of the cricopharyngeus. Cognitive-behavioral therapy may be helpful.

HOARSENESS

Hoarseness, also called dysphonia, is characterized by altered voice quality, pitch, loudness, or vocal effort. Relevant history includes smoking status, occupation, and recent procedures involving the neck or affecting the recurrent laryngeal nerve. Symptomatic treatment should be considered in patients who have evidence suggesting a recent bacterial infectious process or gastroesophageal reflux without any historical features, such as ear pain, dysphagia, or odynophagia, or physical findings such as adenopathy or oral lesions suggestive of tumor. Additionally, there is no evidence to support the use of oral corticosteroids in patients with hoarseness. Hoarseness does not resolve within 3 months or the history or physical examination suggests a serious cause, prompt expert laryngoscopy is indicated.[22]

The symptom of hoarseness invariably points to the larynx as the site of disease. Benign lesions are most common, including vocal nodules (screamer's nodules), vocal cord cysts, vocal cord granulomas (usually resulting from intubation trauma or laryngeal hyperfunction), and vocal cord papillomas. Malignant neoplasms must be suspected (Chapter 190), especially in patients with a strong smoking history.

Of the malignant tumors that can occur in the hypopharynx and larynx, squamous cell carcinoma is the most common and is usually associated with tobacco and ethanol use. However, the incidence of human papillomavirus–related oropharyngeal squamous cell carcinoma is increasing and should be considered in the nonsmoking population. Squamous cell carcinoma (Chapter 190) can occur on essentially any mucosal surface in the head and neck. Symptoms can range from mild sore throat to hoarseness, severe dysphagia, and odynophagia. Pain is often referred to the jaw or ear. Associated cervical lymph node enlargement is also common in advanced disease. Successful management depends on early detection by a careful examination of the entire upper aerodigestive tract, biopsy with histopathologic examination, and aggressive treatment based on the clinical stage and site of the lesion.

LARYNGEAL PARALYSIS

Laryngeal paralysis most often is manifested as a unilateral paralysis as a result of a mediastinal tumor; surgical trauma during thyroid, carotid, or anterior cervical spine surgery; blunt or penetrating trauma; aortic aneurysm; progressive neurologic disease; or viral or idiopathic causes. The severity of impairment can be determined from subjective criteria based on the patient's symptoms, such as breathiness, aspiration, and exertional intolerance.

Unilateral vocal fold paralysis with a favorable prognosis occurs after blunt trauma, endotracheal intubation, idiopathic vocal fold paralysis, and paralysis associated with viral pathogens (Ramsay Hunt syndrome). In this setting, the severity of aspiration, dysphonia, and electromyographic findings can be used to determine the choice of procedure and timing of intervention. Temporary medialization with collagen injection is warranted in patients with unilateral paralysis and a good prognosis. Patients who have poor prognosis for recovery include those with injury after complete section of the nerve during a surgical resection of tumor, invasion of cranial nerves by a tumor, paralysis associated with thoracic aneurysm, or paralysis due to progressive neurologic disorders. In patients with a low likelihood of recovery, permanent medialization of the paralyzed vocal fold is warranted.

Bilateral vocal fold motion impairment, which is less common, has the same causes. Its management is most often directed toward improving the airway because the predominant symptom is airway obstruction.

Grade A References

A1. Spinks A, Glasziou PP, Del Mar CB. Antibiotics for sore throat. *Cochrane Database Syst Rev.* 2013;11:CD000023.

A2. van Driel ML, De Sutter AI, Keber N, et al. Different antibiotic treatments for group A streptococcal pharyngitis. *Cochrane Database Syst Rev.* 2013;4:CD004406.

A3. Jorgensen DM. Single-dose extended-release oral azithromycin vs. 3-day azithromycin for the treatment of group A beta-haemolytic streptococcal pharyngitis/tonsillitis in adults and adolescents: a double-blind, double-dummy study. *Clin Microbiol Infect.* 2009;15:1103-1110.

A4. Hayward G, Thompson MJ, Perera R, et al. Corticosteroids as stand alone or add-on treatment for sore throat. *Cochrane Database Syst Rev.* 2012;10:CD008268.

A5. Alho OP, Koivunen P, Penna T, et al. Tonsillectomy versus watchful waiting in recurrent streptococcal pharyngitis in adults: randomised controlled trial. *BMJ.* 2007;334:939.

GENERAL REFERENCES

For the General References and other additional features, please visit Expert Consult at https://expertconsult.inkling.com.

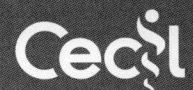

XXVII

MEDICAL CONSULTATION

430

PRINCIPLES OF MEDICAL CONSULTATION

GERALD W. SMETANA

APPROACH TO MEDICAL CONSULTATION

A general medical or subspecialty medical physician may receive a request to perform a consultation for a variety of purposes. In some settings, a single consultative encounter will be requested, or the consultant will determine that only one visit, either in the inpatient or in the outpatient setting, is necessary. More commonly, the approach will include one or more follow-up visits to meet the goals of the consultation from the perspectives of the requesting physician, patient, and consultant. The consultant generally assumes one of four roles: cognitive consultant, procedural consultant, comanager with shared care, or comanager with principal care. The consultant as a comanager continues to care for a component of the patient's needs in an ongoing fashion while being careful to coordinate this comanagement with the continuing role of the requesting physician. Finally, in some situations, it may be most appropriate for the physician who initially requested the consultation no longer to play an active role in the care of the patient but rather to transfer ongoing care exclusively to the consultant.

From a practical perspective, consulting medical physicians, whether they are generalists or subspecialists, enter into the consultative mode in a relatively limited number of ways. Surgeons may request a preoperative medical consultation to assess operative risk and obtain recommendations regarding perioperative care (Chapter 431) or, after surgery, to seek help in managing specific postoperative complications or assisting in the patient's long-term management. Both general medical physicians and medical subspecialists appropriately seek help from a subspecialist with particular knowledge in problems outside their own area of expertise to reduce uncertainty. Sometimes these requests are for specific medical procedures, but requests often seek cognitive guidance as well. Finally, noninternists may seek medical consultation for reasons other than perioperative care. For example, a psychiatrist may request a consultation to help determine whether the somatic symptoms of a particular patient represent important medical conditions (Chapter 434). In the peripartum setting, specific complications of pregnancy may require sophisticated medical consultation (Chapter 239).

Each of these settings raises different challenges for the medical consultant. In all settings, however, a number of general principles apply and can improve the effectiveness of consultations. Communication between physicians and other team members is critical to the process of consultation in all settings. The burgeoning patient safety movement has developed best practices for "hand-offs" that can be applied to consultations.

SETTING-SPECIFIC CONSULTATIVE ISSUES

An effective consultant must recognize the setting in which the consultation is requested and possess the required content knowledge. Distressingly, a number of studies have demonstrated that the requesting physician and the consultant often have different views on the reasons that a consultation was requested, and this initial disconnection, if present, will doom any medical consultation.

Preoperative Surgical Consultation

In the preoperative setting, the medical consultant should not "clear" a patient for surgery and must avoid the temptation to do so even if asked. Clearance may incorrectly imply that the procedure has no risk or that the medical consultant will take responsibility for having misled the patient and surgeon. Instead, the medical consultant should help determine the inherent risk associated with the proposed procedure for the particular patient, whether the patient is in the best possible condition for surgery, and whether any generic or patient-specific interventions would reduce the risk (Chapter 431). Effective consultation also requires a specialized knowledge base, whether the consultation is focusing on a particular organ system or on overall perioperative risk (Chapter 431). A poor consultant-patient interaction can have a substantial negative effect on a patient's confidence in the planned therapy.[1]

Postoperative Surgical Consultation

Surgeons typically request a postoperative medical consultation when a complication has developed that is beyond their area of expertise (Chapter 433). These problems are commonly urgent, so the goal is expeditious consultation and prompt intervention. Management of these problems does not usually differ from management in nonoperative settings. Another reason for a postoperative consultation is to obtain assistance in post-hospitalization care or to facilitate seamless discharge planning. Consultants should aid in the transition to the outpatient or long-term care setting by taking primary or consultative roles as appropriate.

Medical-Medical Consultations

Cross-consultations between medical subspecialists or between a subspecialist and a generalist, in either direction, are quintessential examples of collaboration. For subspecialty consultations, the key is to provide the requested expertise without overstepping into the domain of the expertise of the requesting physician. A growing example of medical-medical consultation is the situation in which a hospitalist assumes principal responsibility for an inpatient admission and then returns the patient to the primary care physician after discharge from the hospital. In this consultative interaction, close communication is critical because primary responsibility for the patient's care has shifted from the outpatient medical physician to the inpatient physician. This transfer of responsibility is not dissimilar to that occurring when a patient is submitted to the care of a subspecialist for a procedure such as cardiac catheterization or gastrointestinal endoscopy. Similar issues also arise when a critically ill patient with a condition such as a complicated myocardial infarction (Chapter 73) or shock (Chapters 106, 107, and 108) is managed principally by a critical care medical specialist and is then expected to return to the care of the primary physician after hospital discharge. However, a key difference is that the inpatient hospitalist physician, unlike the consulting subspecialist, will not typically have an ongoing comanagement role. Because of the higher risk for discontinuity, effective communication at the time of hospitalization, whenever key issues arise during hospitalization, and at the time of discharge, is even more important in the inpatient hospitalist model than in the other settings in which subspecialists may take on more of a comanagement role. Effective and comprehensive handoffs at the time of hospital discharge improve continuity and reduce the potential for errors and medicolegal liability.

Rapid Response Teams

A recent quality improvement initiative has been the development of rapid response teams. These teams aim to reduce the "failure to rescue," which often precedes an unplanned intensive care unit (ICU) transfer or non-ICU cardiac arrest. In this model, a prespecified consultative team urgently sees sick, hospitalized patients when a "trigger" abnormality indicates potential impending serious complications. The activation triggers for rapid response teams have varied somewhat among institutions, but there is substantial agreement on what constitutes an appropriate trigger (Table 430-1). Rapid response teams differ from traditional "code blue teams" in several important aspects, the most important of which is their goal to rescue patients before a crisis situation occurs (Table 430-2).

Although implementation of these teams has not consistently reduced hospital mortality, most trials have shown a reduction in unplanned ICU transfers and in hospital length of stay. For example, in a trial of 5391 patients at a single academic medical center, patients randomly assigned to a rapid response team had a shorter length of stay, fewer unplanned ICU transfers, and lower mortality in patients with unplanned ICU transfers.[A1] Other studies have shown a greater impact on unplanned ICU transfers and a reduction in hospital cardiac arrest rates.[2] In a systematic review, rapid response teams significantly reduced non-ICU cardiac arrests and total in-hospital adult mortality.[3]

This consultative strategy crosses specialties and may include general internal medicine, hospital medicine, and critical care physicians, as well as respiratory therapists and ICU nurses. When an emergency consultation is generated by a trigger event, the consultant's relationship is primarily with the patient rather than with the referring physician.

Consultations for Special Populations

When consulting for psychiatrists or in the peripartum period, the consultant requires special expertise to understand the different expressions of signs and symptoms in specific populations, as well as how and when to modify typical

TABLE 430-1 TRIGGERS: CRITERIA FOR MOBILIZING AN IN-HOSPITAL RAPID RESPONSE SERVICE

VITAL SIGNS

Heart rate
- Heart rate <40 beats/min, especially if symptoms
- Heart rate >140 beats/min

Blood pressure
- Systolic blood pressure <90 mm Hg or >30-40 mm Hg below patient's usual stable blood pressure
- Systolic blood pressure >200 mm Hg for >30 min
- Diastolic blood pressure >110 mm Hg with symptoms

Respiratory rate
- Respiratory rate <8 breaths/min or >35 breaths/min
- New onset of marked dyspnea, compromised airway, cyanosis

Oxygenation
- O_2 saturation <85% for >5 min (except patients with chronic severe hypoxemia)
- Need for 100% supplemental O_2 or a non-rebreathing O_2 mask

Temperature
- Body temperature >39° C or associated with acute decompensation

NEUROLOGIC STATUS

- Acute change in mental status
- New focal findings
- Prolonged or repeated seizures
- ≥2 Point decline in Glasgow coma scale score

GENERAL STATUS

- Uncontrollable bleeding
- Decreased urine output to <50 mL over 4 hr

Based on criteria of The Joint Commission and on other sources.

TABLE 430-2 FEATURES OF RAPID RESPONSE TEAMS AND TRADITIONAL CODE TEAMS

FEATURE	TRADITIONAL CODE TEAM	RAPID RESPONSE TEAM
Criteria for calling team	No pulse, blood pressure, or respiratory effort; unresponsive	Low blood pressure, rapid heart rate, respiratory distress, change in mental status
Typical conditions	Cardiac arrest, respiratory arrest, airway obstruction	Sepsis, pulmonary edema, arrhythmias, respiratory failure
Typical team composition	Anesthesia fellow, ICU fellow, internal medicine house staff, ICU nurse	ICU fellow, ICU nurse, respiratory therapist, internal medicine house staff
Typical call rate (number per 1000 admissions)	0.5-5	20-40
In-hospital mortality	70-90%	0-20%

ICU = intensive care unit.
Adapted from Jones DA, DeVita MA, Bellomo R. Rapid-response teams. *N Engl J Med.* 2011;365:139-146.

TABLE 430-3 REASONS TO CONSIDER A SUBSPECIALTY CONSULTATION

To provide ongoing comanagement: become a partner in inpatient care
- For an acute, unstable problem
- For a chronic condition

To perform a procedure (or advise on whether to perform it)
- Diagnostic
- Therapeutic

To provide one-time or periodic advice
- Diagnostic guidance
- Therapeutic guidance
- Reassurance
- Medicolegal issues

the same guidelines as those for general internists. However, because both the training and ongoing practices of such physicians may or may not include the same spectrum and complexity of disease encountered by typical general internists, the subspecialty consultant must use judgment regarding both the initial consultation and the advisability of ongoing comanagement.

STRATEGIES FOR EFFECTIVE CONSULTATION

It is critical that requesting and consulting physicians agree about the reason for the consultative request. For example, the nature of a preoperative medical consultant's evaluation would differ substantially if the request were (1) routine, (2) for advice on perioperative insulin management in a patient with type 1 diabetes, or (3) to assist in determining the risks and benefits of proceeding to vascular surgery in a high-risk patient with coronary artery disease and a previous stroke. Effective communication at the time of the request will improve the value of the consultation and clarify the question. When there is doubt regarding the reason for the consultation, the consultant should speak directly to the referring physician before completing the evaluation of the patient.

Common reasons for medical consultation include assessment of perioperative risk; interpretation of a laboratory abnormality; help in performing a procedure, in obtaining advice, or in selecting therapy; and aid in providing long-term care. Prophylactic strategies (venous thromboembolism, endocarditis, and surgical site infection) infrequently generate requests for medical consultation because they are commonly standardized to conform to practice guidelines at individual institutions.

Determining the question will also help narrow the scope of the consultant's advice and minimize the number of recommendations. Adherence by the requesting physician to any of the recommendations made by the consultant is higher for consultations with fewer recommendations. Another strategy to minimize the number of recommendations is to restrict advice to pertinent issues at the time, preferably in order of their importance. For example, a consultant who is asked to aid in the care of a critically ill pregnant patient with HELLP syndrome (hemolysis, elevated liver enzymes, and low platelet count) (Chapters 160 and 239) should not also make recommendations regarding the value of cigarette cessation (Chapter 32), even though this issue will be pertinent after the mother and child have survived the acute event.

Requesting physicians are also more likely to adhere to recommendations when the patient is sicker, when the consultation is performed promptly, when advice is given to institute specific therapy rather than perform more diagnostic testing, when the consultant writes frequent follow-up notes, and when computerized order entry support systems are used to convey recommendations. When giving advice about medications, consultants should indicate specific doses and duration of treatment. If a recommendation is likely to be controversial (e.g., postpone surgery), it is always preferable to speak directly to the requesting physician before writing a consultation note in the hope that direct conversation will provide an opportunity to develop a consensus that may then be reflected in the formal consultation note. In one study of 323 physicians, the three elements of greatest perceived importance for a high-quality consultation request were to frame the question, to indicate clearly whom to call with the response, and to establish urgency.[4]

Consultants should be careful to restrict their advice to their particular area of expertise. For example, unless a particular antipsychotic medication is contraindicated because of a medical issue (Chapter 434), it is wisest to defer decision making regarding psychiatric management to the psychiatrist. A

medical recommendations because of special circumstances (Chapters 239 and 434). Although these consultations occasionally result in long-term comanagement, more commonly they revolve around the resolution of an isolated problem. In addition, the medical consultant should not make assumptions about the requesting physician's knowledge base regarding the specific medical issues that generate the consultation. The written report and verbal communications should be comprehensive and commonly include more basic medical content and specific recommendations than may be typical of a consultation for a medical subspecialist.

Subspecialty consultations requested by primary care physicians may be for advice, a technical procedure, or ongoing comanagement (Table 430-3). Consultations for general practitioners or family physicians generally follow

TABLE 430-4	GUIDELINES TO HELP MAKE CONSULTATIONS EFFECTIVE

Determine whether the goal is to obtain advice (and, if so, specifically for what) or to aid in ongoing comanagement (see Table 430-2).

Understand the urgency of the consultation so that the consultation will be performed on a timely basis that meets the needs of the requesting physician and patient.

Perform a focused but careful history and physical examination—do not rely on information gathered by others.

Do not rehash information in an overly detailed note—emphasize the key issues your evaluation reinforced or discovered.

Be sure your recommendations are clearly listed and appropriately detailed—for example, indicate specific drugs, doses, and durations.

Limit the number of total number of recommendations to improve adherence.

Indicate how to monitor the effectiveness of your recommendations, as well as how to contact you urgently if problems arise.

Adjust your involvement (advice vs. comanagement) as appropriate, in concert with the requesting physician.

Serve as a peer—teach as appropriate but also seek to learn.

Remember that personal contact with the requesting physician, even if very brief, may be far more helpful than the best of written notes.

Do not disappear—follow the patient as frequently as appropriate, in coordination with the requesting physician.

For a more complete discussion of this topic, see Goldman L, Lee T, Rudd P. Ten commandments for effective consultations. *Arch Intern Med.* 1983;143:1753-1755 and Salerno SM, Hurst FP, Halvorson S, et al. Principles of effective consultation: an update for the 21st-century consultant. *Arch Intern Med.* 2007;167:271-275.

strongly worded consultation note that advises against a particular strategy will put another physician in a difficult medicolegal position if it differs from the physician's usual or recommended practice. The most important attributes of a consultative role are simple, concise recommendations and a clearly stated rationale for decision making. Detailed differential diagnosis is less important, and literature support is usually unnecessary.

Timely consultation reports improve physician satisfaction and patient care. For example, primary care physicians note that failure to receive timely reports from consultants limits their ability to provide high-quality care.[5]

Salerno and colleagues have proposed modifications of Goldman's original "Ten Commandments" for effective consultations (Table 430-4). These recommendations serve as a helpful guide for consultants to improve adherence to their advice and, as a result, improve patient outcomes. Specific interactive training on the principles of consultation can increase the effectiveness of consultative communication.[A2]

SPECIAL CONSULTATIVE SITUATIONS

Curbside Consultation

Informal consultations are commonly called "curbside" consultations. In the current era, ready access to online medical references may potentially reduce curbside requests. Consultants in "cognitive" specialties such as infectious diseases, rheumatology, and endocrinology provide a disproportionate amount of informal (compared with formal) consultations. Informal consultations may occur by telephone, by e-mail, or in person. Curbside consultation is ingrained into the fabric of medical care.

Both generalists and specialists participate in an average of three to four curbside consultations per week. These consultations commonly involve questions about diagnostic tests, treatment plans, and the potential value of a formal consultation (which follows about one third of curbside consultations) in the future. To be effective, curbside consultations should be brief, involve a single question, and require no direct examination of the patient or medical records.

An important limitation of curbside consultations is that the consultant must rely on limited, secondhand information from the requesting physician rather than primary data from direct evaluation of the patient. Consultants report that such indirect information is inaccurate in as many as half of curbside consultations.[6] This reality, along with lack of financial compensation, leads to a greater degree of dissatisfaction with the curbside process by consultants than by requesting physicians. Salaried consultants may view a request for a curbside consultation more favorably than might those whose livelihood depends on a fee-for-service model of care.

Although requesting physicians may perceive reduced medicolegal risk when they obtain and even document a curbside consultation, consultants may fear the risk for malpractice liability themselves when offering such advice. However, courts have consistently found that curbside consultants have no liability because no direct physician-patient relationship exists. Rather, the relationship is only between the requesting and consulting physicians.

Electronic Consultations

Increasingly, physicians are using electronic communication, either as part of a shared electronic medical record or by e-mail, to supplement formal consultation requests.[7] An obvious advantage of this approach is that the requesting and consulting physician can communicate on their own schedules. Potential benefits include saving time, reducing costs, and improving continuity and access to specialty care. However, the lack of reimbursement for such activities may be a barrier to e-consultations.

Mandatory Consultations

In some situations, mandatory consultations may help enforce a standard of care. For example, mandatory inpatient infectious disease consultations, as part of an antimicrobial stewardship program, can improve the rational use of antimicrobial agents in the hospital and after discharge. Similarly, instituting routine consultation for patients with certain sentinel conditions, such as diabetes, may improve outcomes.

Comanagement

A consultation that begins with an initial encounter or a limited number of follow-up visits may evolve into ongoing comanagement. In such an arrangement, the physician initially serving in a consultative role becomes at least coequal to the requesting physician in the provision of ongoing care. In some situations, the consultant may actually become the primary physician. This arrangement is obvious in situations in which the consultation was requested specifically for the provision of ongoing care. Other examples include situations in which an oncologist assumes principal care of a patient with a malignancy or a nephrologist assumes principal care of a patient with end-stage renal disease who is being maintained on dialysis. In some of these situations, a general internist who initially requested the consultation may now become the consultant and provide advice on preventive care and occasional help with intercurrent medical problems.

Comanagement is also increasingly common in the hospital setting. Medical consultants may become comanagers of postoperative surgical patients, with a potential for improving outcomes. In an early randomized trial of perioperative patients, formal comanagement, in which a medical physician took responsibility for managing medical problems rather than acting in a consultative role, reduced postoperative complications; in addition, both nurses and surgeons preferred this model. However, not all studies have shown that comanagement improves patient outcomes. In one study of comanagement on a neurosurgical service, for example, nursing staff perceived substantial improvement in the quality of patient care and costs were reduced, but there were no differences in mortality, readmission rates, or length of stay.[8] In some institutions, comanagement for orthopedic or other surgical patients has become routine and does not require a specific request for consultation. Internists currently comanage more than one third of surgical inpatients in some hospitals.

In some settings, the outpatient primary care physician may retain a comanagement role even as a cardiologist cares for a patient with acute myocardial infarction, a pulmonologist cares for a patient in the ICU, a hospitalist cares for a patient in the general medical setting, or a noninternist addresses a specific problem.

RESPONSIBILITIES OF THE CONSULTANT

The consultant is responsible to two parties: the patient and the referring physician. A paternalistic approach is not desirable. The consultant should not limit communication to the referring physician and must not withhold discussion and recommendations from the patient. However, the consultant should not usurp the role of the referring physician, who remains responsible for assembling information and advice from varied sources, as well as for developing an integrated plan with the patient. For example, in the preoperative setting, the consultant should not express a final opinion regarding the suitability of proceeding to surgery without first discussing all relevant considerations with the referring surgeon. In the trilateral deliberative model, the patient, referring physician, and consultant each have responsibilities and constraints inherent in their relationships (Fig. 430-1). Above all, the role of the consultant is to improve patient care and outcomes.

Relationships in Consultative Medicine

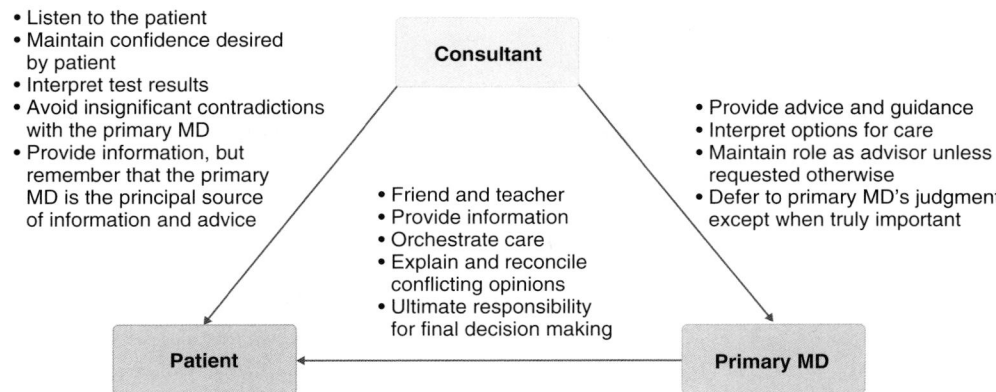

FIGURE 430-1. Consultative relationships. The consultant must execute his or her duty to the patient while acknowledging and hopefully conforming to the collegial professional model of advising the primary physician. If, however, the patient's safety or welfare is at stake, the consultant's duty is to be sure that the patient's needs always take precedence. (Based on Emanuel LL, Richter J. The consultant and the patient-physician relationship: a trilateral deliberative model. *Arch Intern Med.* 1994;154:1785-1790, and other sources.)

IMPACT OF CONSULTATIONS ON PATIENT OUTCOME

Few controlled trials have investigated the impact of medical consultations on outcomes. In one small study in the 1990s, an outpatient preoperative medical consultation reduced unnecessary admissions (those that did not result in surgery) compared with usual care (inpatient consultation at the discretion of the surgeon). Other reports indicate that anywhere from 5 to 50% of preoperative medical consultations result in changes in patient management. However, any potential benefit of preoperative medical consultation for improving important outcomes remains unproved.[9]

Grade A References

A1. Rothschild JM, Woolf W, Finn KM, et al. A controlled trial of a rapid response system in an academic medical center. *Jt Comm J Qual Patient Saf.* 2008;34:417-425.
A2. Kessler CS, Afshar Y, Sardar G, et al. A prospective, randomized, controlled study demonstrating a novel, effective model of transfer of care between physicians: the 5 Cs of consultation. *Acad Emerg Med.* 2012;19:968-974.

GENERAL REFERENCES

For the General References and other additional features, please visit Expert Consult at https://expertconsult.inkling.com.

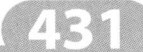

PREOPERATIVE EVALUATION

STEVEN L. COHN

Each year in the United States, more than 25 million inpatient surgical procedures and an additional 25 million outpatient procedures are performed. Although more than one third of these surgical patients are older than 65 years, overall morbidity and mortality are relatively low, in part because of modern anesthetic and surgical techniques. A crucial aspect of safety is careful preoperative evaluation of the patient not only by the surgeon and anesthesiologist but also, in many instances, by a general medical consultant or medical subspecialist.

OPERATIVE RISK ASSESSMENT

The components of perioperative risk include those related to the patient, procedure, provider, and anesthesia. Anesthetic risk is low, with mortality less than 0.03% in a normal healthy patient—American Society of Anesthesiology (ASA) class 1—but increasing to 0.2% in ASA class 2 (mild systemic

disease), 1.2% in class 3 (severe systemic disease), 8% in class 4 (severe systemic disease that is a constant threat to life), and 34% in class 5 (a moribund patient not expected to survive for 24 hours without surgery). Meta-analysis suggests that when feasible, neuraxial (spinal or epidural) anesthesia may reduce postoperative complications compared with general anesthesia (Chapter 432), but decisions regarding the anesthetic technique should be the responsibility of the anesthesiologist and not be part of the preoperative medical consultation. With respect to the provider, data support a "learning curve," with better outcomes when procedures are performed by more experienced, higher-volume surgeons.

GENERAL RISK ASSESSMENT

History and Physical Examination

The medical history and physical examination are the most important components in assessing a patient's risk for surgery. The consultation should focus on pertinent medical problems, particularly cardiopulmonary symptoms and diseases that are associated with risk and are likely to influence perioperative management (Chapter 430). The importance of the past surgical history is to determine whether the patient was able to undergo major surgery in the recent past or had any perioperative medical or anesthetic-related complications that could occur again. The social history should assess and quantify the amount, duration, and last use of tobacco, alcohol, or illicit substances. It is important to document allergies to medications, foods, and latex as well as to obtain an accurate list of the patient's current prescription and over-the-counter medications, including doses and adherence. The family history is relevant primarily for any genetically associated complications such as malignant hyperthermia or a bleeding disorder. The review of systems should include the presence or absence of chest pain and dyspnea and the patient's exercise capacity. The physical examination must include the vital signs, assessment of the airway and respiratory status, cardiovascular examination, and documentation of any neurologic deficit.

Preoperative Tests

Screening preoperative test results in otherwise healthy individuals are usually normal and, even when abnormal, rarely affect management (generally <1%) (Table 431-1).[1] Most significant abnormalities can be predicted from the clinical information obtained, which then guides selective testing based on the history, the physical findings, and the planned type of surgery and anesthesia. Most patients undergoing low-risk surgery with local anesthesia require no preoperative testing. Repeat testing should be avoided if recent (within 3 months) results were normal, unless the patient's condition or medications have changed.

Perioperative Medications

Decisions regarding whether to continue a medication perioperatively should consider the drug's pharmacokinetics (Chapter 29) as well as its effects on the primary disease and perioperative risk, including potential interactions with anesthetic agents. Some medications are essential to continue (e.g., cardiac medications and corticosteroids), whereas others must be

TABLE 431-1   RECOMMENDATIONS FOR PREOPERATIVE LABORATORY TESTING

TEST	% ABNORMAL	% INFLUENCING MANAGEMENT	INDICATIONS
Hemoglobin	1.8	0.1	Expected major blood loss, symptoms of anemia, chronic kidney disease
White blood count	0.7	0.0	Suspected infection, myeloproliferative disorder, myelotoxic medications
Platelet count	0.9	0.02	Bleeding diathesis, myeloproliferative disorder, myelotoxic medications
Prothrombin time/INR	0.3	0.0	Bleeding diathesis, liver disease, malnutrition, antibiotic use, anticoagulants
Partial thromboplastin time	6.5	0.1	Bleeding diathesis, anticoagulant use
Electrolytes	12.7	1.8	Renal disease, medications affecting electrolytes (e.g., diuretics, digoxin, ACE inhibitor, ARBs)
Glucose	9.3	0.5	Known DM, steroids, morbid obesity
Renal function	8.2	2.6	Renal disease, DM, HTN, major surgery, older age, medications affecting renal function
Liver function tests	0.4	0.1	Known liver disease, albumin level if at risk for needing postoperative parenteral nutrition
Urinalysis	19.1	1.4	No indication unless GU symptoms or instrumentation planned (although often requested before joint replacement or spine surgery)
Electrocardiogram (<50 years old)	29.6 (19.7)	2.6	Vascular surgery; intermediate risk surgery with at least 1 RCRI risk factor; not indicated in asymptomatic patients undergoing low-risk procedures or solely based on age
Chest radiograph (<50 years old)	21.2 (4.9)	3.0	Acute cardiopulmonary disease suspected based on history and physical examination; history of stable chronic cardiopulmonary disease in patient older than 70 years without a chest radiograph in the past 6 months.

ACE = angiotensin-converting enzyme; ARB = angiotensin receptor blocker; DM = diabetes mellitus; GU = genitourinary; HTN = hypertension; INR = international normalized ratio; RCRI = Revised Cardiac Risk Index (1 point each for coronary artery disease; heart failure; prior cerebrovascular accident or transient ischemic attack; diabetes mellitus on insulin; creatinine >2.0; and abdominal, thoracic, or suprainguinal vascular surgery) (see Table 431-3).
Modified from Smetana GW, Macpherson DS. The case against routine preoperative laboratory testing. *Med Clin North Am.* 2003;87:7-40.

discontinued (e.g., oral hypoglycemic agents) or have their dose altered (e.g., insulin and anticoagulants). Still other medications should be started prophylactically to minimize perioperative risk (e.g., anticoagulants for prophylaxis against venous thromboembolism [Chapter 81] and antibiotic prophylaxis for surgical site infection or endocarditis [Chapter 76]). Data are often lacking or conflicting. Table 431-2 briefly summarizes "consensus" perioperative recommendations for the major classes of drugs.

CARDIAC RISK ASSESSMENT

A significant proportion of patients who undergo surgery have either known coronary artery disease or risk factors for it, and postoperative cardiac complications are second only to direct surgical complications as a cause of perioperative mortality. The goal is to risk-stratify patients clinically and to determine whether additional testing, new medications, or cardiac interventions will be beneficial.

History and Physical Examination

Important information includes any history of previous cardiac disease (myocardial infarction [MI], angina, heart failure, arrhythmias, valvular disease), cardiac interventions (e.g., coronary artery bypass grafting; percutaneous coronary intervention, including date and type of stent placed), cardiac evaluation (noninvasive testing, angiography), risk factors (hypertension, diabetes mellitus, dyslipidemia, cigarette smoking), and associated diseases (peripheral arterial disease, stroke, chronic kidney disease, and chronic obstructive pulmonary disease [COPD]). Current status regarding chest pain or dyspnea, functional capacity, and medications should be assessed. The physical examination serves to confirm findings in the history as well as to assess severity and control of the disease (e.g., heart failure, hypertension, valvular disease). The preoperative electrocardiogram rarely changes management unless it demonstrates evidence of a recent or silent MI, but it can be useful as a baseline against which to compare postoperative tracings.

Cardiac Risk Indices

Over the years, a number of risk indices have been proposed to assist in preoperative cardiac evaluation. The most widely used, the revised cardiac risk index (RCRI; Table 431-3), was derived during the evaluation of several thousand patients, was validated in thousands more, and has been incorporated into the consensus guidelines developed by the American College of Cardiology and the American Heart Association. These guidelines, which are updated periodically, use a stepwise strategy based on clinical risk factors, surgery-specific risk, and exercise capacity, combined with a systematic approach to perioperative testing and treatment in patients with known or

suspected cardiac disease (Fig. 431-1). Because the RCRI may underestimate risk in major vascular surgery and did not include many types of lower-risk surgeries (Table 431-4), newer risk indices have been developed. Although these alternatives have not been widely validated, current American[2] and European[3] guidelines recommend either the RCRI or the National Surgical Quality Improvement (NSQIP) myocardial infarction/cardiac arrest risk calculator[4]. Preoperative levels of troponin[5] and of brain natriuretic peptide (BNP)[6] are independent predictors of postoperative cardiac complications, although it is unclear how to use these biomarkers and whether any intervention based on these numbers will improve outcome.

Noninvasive Tests

One emphasis of current guidelines is to minimize cardiac testing unless the results are likely to alter management. A resting echocardiogram (Chapter 55) is indicated to evaluate valvular heart disease in patients with clinically suspicious murmurs and to evaluate left ventricular function in patients with heart failure. Other than for the assessment of aortic stenosis (see later), resting echocardiography is not a reliable predictor of perioperative cardiac events.

Exercise testing (with or without imaging) is preferred to pharmacologic stress testing because it assesses functional capacity (see Table 51-3), but its use is often limited by a patient's inability to achieve the target heart rate. Furthermore, patients with adequate exercise capacity by history rarely require preoperative stress testing.

Pharmacologic Stress Testing

Pharmacologic stress testing (either dipyridamole or adenosine with nuclear imaging [Chapters 56 and 71] or dobutamine echocardiography [Chapters 55 and 71]) is indicated when a patient who needs a stress test cannot perform adequate exercise (see Table 71-6 and Fig. 71-3 in Chapter 71). Both tests have a similar sensitivity for predicting perioperative ischemic complications, whereas stress echocardiography has fewer false-positive results. Nevertheless, local expertise commonly influences which test is selected. Dipyridamole and adenosine can cause bronchospasm and are best avoided in patients with symptomatic or severe asthma or obstructive lung disease, but they are preferred in patients with left bundle branch block, in whom exercise or stress echocardiography is more likely to give false-positive results. Quantitatively, the number and extent of reperfusion defects or wall motion abnormalities correlate with the severity of disease, likelihood of complications, and need for further evaluation by angiography.

Patients whose clinical condition would warrant stress testing independent of planned surgery should have such testing before elective operations.

TABLE 431-2 PERIOPERATIVE MANAGEMENT OF MEDICATIONS

MEDICATION CLASS	RECOMMENDATION
Anticoagulants (heparins, warfarin NOACs [novel oral anticoagulants])*	Continue for minor surgery Discontinue at an appropriate interval before major surgery Consider bridging anticoagulation for patients at high risk for interim thrombosis (Chapter 38)
Antiplatelet drugs	Continue for minor surgery Discontinue clopidogrel and ticagrelor at least 5 days before surgery and prasugrel at least 7 days before surgery, except in patients with recent coronary stenting If discontinuing aspirin, do so 3-7 days before surgery
Cardiovascular medications	Continue most agents Consider starting β-blockers in patients at high risk for perioperative cardiac morbidity (vascular or high-risk surgery) Withhold diuretics on the morning of surgery, especially if signs of volume depletion are present Consider stopping ACE inhibitors or ARBs at least 12 hours before surgery unless patient has heart failure or uncontrolled hypertension Stop tamsulosin before cataract surgery (floppy iris syndrome)
Lipid-lowering agents	Continue "statins" Discontinue other agents
Pulmonary agents	Continue
Gastrointestinal agents	Continue
Diabetic agents (see text)	Withhold oral hypoglycemic agents on the morning of surgery; restart when the patient resumes eating For type 1 diabetes, continue some form of insulin (long acting or intravenous) at all times For type 2 diabetes, decrease the dose of morning intermediate insulin; continue basal insulin
Thyroid agents (hypothyroidism and hyperthyroidism) (see text)	Continue thyroid replacement Continue antithyroid medication and postpone surgery until the hyperthyroidism is controlled
Oral contraceptives, hormone replacement, and SERMs	May discontinue 3 weeks before surgery only in patients at high risk for perioperative venous thromboembolism; otherwise continue
Corticosteroids (see text)	Continue chronic corticosteroids; increase the dosage to account for surgical stress
Psychotropic agents	Continue SSRIs but consider withholding them several weeks before CNS surgery Continue tricyclic antidepressants, benzodiazepines, lithium, and antipsychotics Usually discontinue MAOIs 10-14 days before surgery
Chronic opioids	Continue; substitute equianalgesic or higher doses for surgical pain
Rheumatologic agents	Continue methotrexate Discontinue other DMARDs and anticytokines about 2 weeks before surgery Continue hypouricemic agents
Neurologic agents	Continue antiseizure medications Consider withholding antiparkinsonian agents briefly Continue agents for myasthenia gravis
Herbal agents	Discontinue all agents

*See also Tables 431-6 and 431-7 for more detail.
ARB = angiotensin receptor blocker; ACE = angiotensin-converting enzyme; CNS = central nervous system; DMARD = disease-modifying antirheumatic drug; MAOI = monoamine oxidase inhibitor; SERM = selective estrogen receptor modulator; SSRI = selective serotonin reuptake inhibitor.
Adapted from Cohn SL, Macpherson DS. Perioperative medication management. In: Cohn SL, Smetana GW, Weed HG, eds. *Perioperative Medicine: Just the Facts.* New York: McGraw-Hill; 2006.

TABLE 431-3 CLINICAL FACTORS IMPORTANT IN ASSESSING PERIOPERATIVE CARDIAC RISK

REVISED CARDIAC RISK INDEX CRITERIA*

Ischemic heart disease defined as history of myocardial infarction, positive exercise test, current complaint of chest pain considered secondary to myocardial ischemia, use of nitrate therapy, or pathological Q waves on the electrocardiogram
Or at least two of the following:
Heart failure defined as S₃ or bilateral rales on physical examination or pulmonary edema on chest radiograph
Cerebrovascular disease defined as history of transient ischemic attack or history of cerebrovascular accident
Insulin-dependent diabetes mellitus
Chronic renal insufficiency defined as baseline creatinine of 2.0 mg/dL or greater
High-risk surgery defined as intrathoracic, intra-abdominal, or suprainguinal vascular surgery

*Lee TH, Marcantonio ER, Mangione CM, et al. Derivation and prospective validation of a simple index for prediction of cardiac risk of major noncardiac surgery. *Circulation.* 1999;100:1043-1049.

TABLE 431-4 RISKS OF VARIOUS SURGICAL PROCEDURES

HIGH (VERY ELEVATED) RISK (CARDIAC RISK >5%)

Major vascular surgery
Emergent major operations
Prolonged procedures with large fluid shifts or significant blood loss

INTERMEDIATE (BUT ELEVATED) RISK (CARDIAC RISK 1-5%)

Intraperitoneal or intrathoracic procedures
Carotid endarterectomy
Endovascular aortic aneurysm repair
Head and neck surgery
Orthopedic procedures
Prostate surgery

LOW RISK (CARDIAC RISK <1%)

Superficial operations
Cataract surgery
Breast surgery
Ambulatory surgery

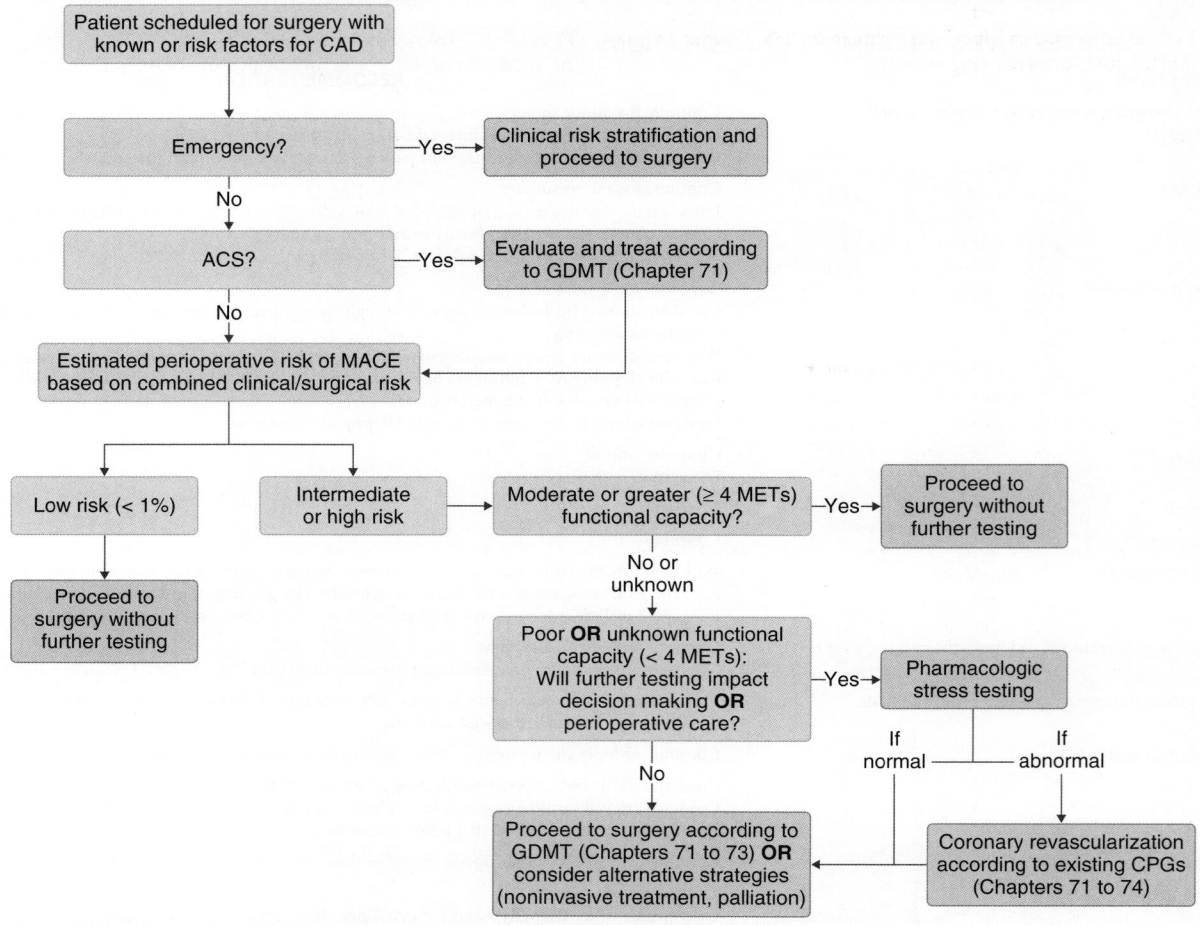

FIGURE 431-1. Stepwise approach to perioperative cardiac assessment for CAD. ACS = acute coronary syndrome (Chapter 72); CAD = coronary artery disease; CPGs = clinical practice guidelines; GDMT = guideline-directed medical therapy; MACE = major adverse cardiac event; METs = metabolic equivalents. Adapted from Fleisher LA, Fleischmann KE, Auerbach AD, et al. 2014 ACC/AHA Guideline on Perioperative Cardiovascular Evaluation and Management of Patients Undergoing Noncardiac Surgery: Executive Summary: A Report of the American College of Cardiology/American Heart Association Task Force on Practice Guidelines. *J Am Coll Cardiol.* 2014;64:2373-2405.

Otherwise, stress testing is recommended only in patients at elevated risk for noncardiac surgery and with poor functional capacity (defined as the inability to walk two to four blocks at 3-4 mph on level ground or to climb one flight of stairs; see Table 51-5) if the results will change management.

Risk Reduction Strategies for Ischemic Heart Disease
Medical Therapy
In by far the largest trial of prophylactic perioperative β-blockers, a high dose of extended-release metoprolol, started hours before surgery, reduced perioperative MI, but at the expense of increasing strokes and overall mortality, in part owing to more hypotension and bradycardia.[A1] Meta-analyses that exclude trials whose veracity has been called into question by ongoing institutional investigations of the primary author have reinforced that β-blockers can reduce perioperative MI but with the side effect of increasing stroke. The net result is no evidence for a reduction in overall mortality and probably increased risk in patients who do not have a very high risk for perioperative MI.[A2][A3] It may be reasonable to start β-blockers before surgery in patients with intermediate-high risk ischemia on stress testing or with 3 or more RCRI risk factors, but validated data to support this option are insufficient to make definitive recommendations.[7] Bisoprolol (5 mg daily) or atenolol (25 mg daily) may be preferable to metoprolol, and any benefits are more likely to be seen when β-blockers are started at least 1 week before surgery at a low dose and titrated to a heart rate of 55 to 70 beats per minute.[8] Until more evidence is available, it seems prudent to avoid starting β-blockers immediately before surgery and to avoid them in the settings of emergency surgery, prior cerebrovascular disease, or sepsis.

Neither clonidine[A4] nor aspirin[A5] is beneficial for reducing perioperative cardiac events. Limited data on prophylactic calcium antagonists or nitrates have not shown major benefits in preventing complications after noncardiac surgery. Statins (Chapter 206) reduce endovascular inflammation and stabilize endothelial plaque. Current data suggest that they should be continued perioperatively and also begun preoperatively in patients who meet criteria for their ongoing use (Chapter 206).[A6] Aggressive fluid management to optimize cardiac output is controversial, and recent studies show no clear advantage when added to standard medical therapy.[A7][A8]

Invasive Therapies
Prophylactic coronary revascularization in patients who have stable cardiac symptoms and no aortic stenosis and do not meet standard criteria for the procedure (Chapter 71) does not reduce perioperative myocardial infarction, death within 30 days, or long-term mortality at an average of 2.7 years in patients who receive appropriate medical therapy.[A9] Preoperative coronary revascularization is indicated only if the patient meets the criteria for coronary angiography or revascularization independent of the need for surgery.

For bare metal stents, data suggest that elective surgery should be delayed for 4 to 6 weeks after stenting because of the risk for in-stent thrombosis when dual antiplatelet therapy with aspirin and clopidogrel is discontinued early or because of the alternative risk for bleeding if surgery is performed in patients receiving such antiplatelet therapy (Chapter 74). For drug-eluting stents, elective surgery should be delayed for at least 6 months and preferably 12 months if possible[9] so that patients can complete an uninterrupted course of dual antiplatelet therapy. For balloon angioplasty without stenting, a delay of 2 weeks is generally recommended. If antiplatelet therapy has to be discontinued, clopidogrel is usually discontinued 5 to 7 days before the noncardiac procedure, prasugrel is stopped 7 days before, and ticagrelor is stopped

5 days before, whereas aspirin is continued, if possible.[10] If aspirin also must be discontinued, it is usually stopped approximately 5 to 7 days before surgery, but shorter durations are being evaluated.

Other Cardiovascular Diseases
Heart Failure
Heart failure, which is a major risk factor for surgery, requires treatment and optimization before surgery (Chapter 59). Routine use of *pulmonary artery catheters* does not reduce morbidity or mortality in patients undergoing elective noncardiac surgery.[A10] Although an elevated BNP level is a risk factor, there is no evidence that treatment to lower the BNP level or use of β-blockers will reduce postoperative complications in patients with heart failure.

Valvular Heart Disease
Patients with *symptomatic aortic stenosis* who meet the criteria for valve replacement (Chapter 75) independent of their need for surgery should undergo the valve replacement before the noncardiac surgery. However, patients usually survive noncardiac surgery with intensified care if they refuse valve replacement or time does not permit it. An asymptomatic aortic valve area of 1.0 to 1.5 cm^2 carries an increased risk for perioperative complications[11] but is an indication for more careful monitoring rather than valve surgery. Patients with severe mitral regurgitation also have higher risks for postoperative cardiovascular complications.[12] Endocarditis prophylaxis (Chapter 76) is appropriate for patients with mechanical heart valves, previous endocarditis, complex congenital heart disease, or valvular disease in a heart transplant recipient undergoing invasive dental or upper respiratory procedures (Chapter 76).

Hypertension
Hypertension with blood pressure lower than 110 mm Hg diastolic or 180 mm Hg systolic without significant target organ damage does not increase the risk for major perioperative cardiac complications. Even when the preoperative diastolic blood pressure is higher, limited data suggest that surgery is safe after additional antihypertensive therapy.

Arrhythmias
Although patients with arrhythmias have increased perioperative risk, the risk is increased because the arrhythmias are usually markers of more serious heart disease or cause hemodynamic problems. Patients with hemodynamically significant tachyarrhythmias and bradyarrhythmias should generally be treated as in the nonoperative setting (Chapters 64 and 65), except for the special circumstance of anticoagulation in the perioperative setting (Chapter 38).

● PULMONARY RISK ASSESSMENT
Postoperative pulmonary complications are as common as cardiac complications and are associated with significant morbidity and mortality. Major complications include respiratory failure (e.g., reintubation, prolonged mechanical ventilation), pneumonia, atelectasis requiring bronchoscopy, and to a lesser degree, bronchospasm or an exacerbation of COPD requiring treatment and prolonged length of stay. Many postoperative pulmonary complications are due to exaggerations of the usual postoperative changes in pulmonary function: decreased lung volumes, diaphragmatic dysfunction, ventilation-perfusion mismatches and shunting, hypoventilation, hypoxemia, and impaired defense mechanisms. Pulmonary risk factors can be divided into patient-related and procedure-related factors, the latter of which include the type of surgery, anesthesia, and related factors.[13]

Patient-Related Factors
COPD (Chapter 88) increases the risk for postoperative pulmonary complications approximately twofold, depending on its severity, whereas well-controlled *asthma* (Chapter 87) does not increase risk. Active cigarette smokers are at increased risk, mainly related to the number of pack years smoked; smoking cessation at least 4 to 8 weeks before surgery may reduce the risk. *Obstructive sleep apnea* (Chapter 100), typically associated with obesity, confers an increased risk for hypercapnia and hypoxemia, and obese patients are at increased risk for atelectasis.[14] Advanced age, poor functional status, pulmonary hypertension, an altered mental state, and suppressed immune status from chronic steroid use, alcohol use, or diabetes may also increase the risk for postoperative pulmonary complications. Pulmonary hypertension has also been associated with increased risk.

Procedure-Related Factors
The most important predictors of postoperative pulmonary complications are the type of surgery and proximity of the surgical incision to the diaphragm. Pulmonary function decreases by approximately 50% after intrathoracic surgery, upper abdominal procedures, and abdominal aortic aneurysm repair and does not fully return to normal for several weeks. Lower abdominal surgery is associated with a 25% decrease in pulmonary function. Laparoscopic procedures are usually associated with lower rates of postoperative pulmonary complications and shorter hospital stays than open procedures. Neuraxial anesthesia (epidural or spinal) may be associated with decreased risk when compared with general anesthesia, but the decision about which type of anesthesia to use is best left to the anesthesiologist. Emergency surgery, prolonged duration of anesthesia or surgery (>2 to 6 hours), and routine postoperative nasogastric tube use increase the risk for postoperative pulmonary complications.

Pulmonary Function Tests
In general, pulmonary function tests (Chapter 85) are no more predictive of pulmonary complications than is clinical risk assessment alone. Such testing may be more helpful in assessing risk for lung resection surgery when it can predict the function of the remaining lung mass. However, even a postoperative predicted forced expiratory volume in 1 second (FEV$_1$) of less than 800 mL for lung resection, which is thought to portend a very high risk for death or prolonged mechanical ventilation, is not an absolute contraindication to surgery. Preoperative arterial blood gas evaluation is also of little benefit in predicting postoperative pulmonary complications. Cardiopulmonary exercise testing for maximal oxygen consumption is useful for evaluating high-risk patients before lung resection surgery.

Risk Reduction Strategies
Unfortunately, many of the risk factors for postoperative pulmonary complications cannot be modified. Inhaled bronchodilators (β-agonists and anticholinergics) and steroids can optimize the respiratory status of patients with COPD and asthma. Broad-spectrum antibiotics should be used to treat exacerbations caused by bacterial infection. Chest physiotherapy may be helpful, particularly for thoracic surgery. Smoking should be stopped at least 8 weeks before surgery, if possible.

Lung expansion maneuvers (either incentive spirometry or deep-breathing exercises) can significantly improve pulmonary function, minimize atelectasis, and reduce risk, especially for thoracic and upper abdominal surgery. Pain control (Chapter 30) improves pulmonary function by allowing deeper breathing. Epidural analgesia and patient-controlled intravenous analgesia reduce postoperative pulmonary complications and, when possible, are preferable to parenteral narcotics. Long-acting neuromuscular blockers should be avoided, and the selective rather than the routine use of a nasogastric tube may also decrease risk.

● ENDOCRINE CONDITIONS
Diabetes Mellitus
The major risks associated with surgery in diabetic patients are cardiac complications and wound infections. Complications are probably related more to associated diseases and end-organ involvement (coronary artery disease, chronic kidney disease, and autonomic neuropathy) than to the glucose level itself. Significantly, elevated glucose levels may impair wound healing and interfere with leukocyte defense mechanisms. However, current recommendations suggest a glucose target level of 140 to 180 mg/dL rather than tight perioperative control.[15]

Patients whose diabetes is controlled by diet require only perioperative glucose monitoring (finger sticks) with short-acting insulin coverage on an as-needed basis. Patients taking oral hypoglycemic agents (Chapter 229) should not take them on the morning of surgery (chlorpropamide should be stopped 2 to 3 days before and metformin preferably 12 to 24 hours before major surgery) and should be monitored with sliding-scale insulin coverage as needed. Patients taking insulin are most often given one half to two thirds of their usual intermediate-acting insulin on the morning of surgery and are then given short-acting insulin on a sliding scale and correction dose based on finger stick monitoring (Chapter 229). Continuous intravenous insulin, which provides tighter glucose control but is associated with more episodes of hypoglycemia and requires a monitored setting, is typically used in patients undergoing cardiac surgery and in critically ill patients. There are no validated guidelines regarding the management of patients taking long-acting basal insulin (glargine). In general, it should be continued, but its dose may be reduced for ambulatory surgery or in patients with tight control or with chronic kidney disease. Regardless of the mode of treatment, frequent monitoring of the glucose level is critical.

Exogenous Corticosteroids and Adrenal Insufficiency

The stress of surgery activates the hypothalamic-pituitary-adrenal (HPA) axis, which in turn stimulates release of adrenocorticotropic hormone (ACTH) and subsequent secretion of cortisol (Chapter 227), but a patient who is taking exogenous corticosteroids may have suppression of the HPA axis and not be able to respond to this stress adequately. As a result, hypotension and shock may occur.

In general, a daily dose equivalent to 5 mg or less of prednisone (Chapter 227), alternate-day short-acting therapy, or corticosteroids given for less than 3 weeks do not cause clinically significant HPA suppression, so no supplemental therapy is indicated. Conversely, doses greater than 20 mg/day of prednisone for longer than 3 weeks usually suppress the HPA axis and warrant perioperative supplemental corticosteroids. In patients who are taking intermediate dosing regimens or who took large doses in the past year but are not taking corticosteroids or are taking lower doses now, the options are to perform an ACTH (cosyntropin) stimulation test, if time permits, and treat only patients with an inadequate response (Chapter 227) or to prescribe supplemental corticosteroids empirically.

Despite a lack of definitive evidence that supplemental steroids are required,[A11] when supplemental corticosteroids are felt to be appropriate, short-term therapy tailored to the level of expected stress can provide protection without adverse effects on wound healing and with only short-term problems with glucose intolerance and fluid retention. For minor procedures or local anesthesia, the recommended approach is to give the patient's usual dose before surgery without further supplementation. For moderate surgical stress (e.g., open cholecystectomy, lower extremity vascular surgery), a reasonable approach is 50 mg of hydrocortisone intravenously before surgery, followed by 25 mg every 8 hours for 1 to 2 days, and then the patient's usual dose. For major surgical stress, patients are typically given 75 to 100 mg of hydrocortisone intravenously before induction of anesthesia, followed by 50 mg every 8 hours for 1 to 3 days until the stressful period resolves, and then their usual dose.

Thyroid Disease

An inadequately treated or undiagnosed hyperthyroid patient is potentially at risk for thyroid storm postoperatively. Elective surgery should be postponed in patients who are symptomatic or have resting tachycardia until they are euthyroid. Treatment of a thyrotoxic patient undergoing urgent or emergency surgery includes a combination of β-blockers, antithyroid agents, and iodine to control the resting heart rate to less than 90 beats per minute, as well as prophylactic corticosteroid supplementation, as used for thyroid storm (Chapter 226).

Conversely, patients with mild to moderate hypothyroidism tolerate surgery reasonably well. Patients with markedly symptomatic hypothyroidism should be treated with oral levothyroxine (T_4) for several weeks before elective surgery. For emergency surgery, intravenous liothyronine (T_3) or T_4 (200 to 300 µg intravenously, then 50 to 100 µg/day) and supplemental corticosteroids (hydrocortisone, 100 mg intravenously, then 25 to 50 mg every 6 hours) should be given. Myxedema coma is a rare complication of surgery.

🔴 LIVER DISEASE

Routine preoperative testing of liver function is not recommended, but elective surgery should be avoided in patients with acute viral, alcoholic, or drug-induced hepatitis. Patients with stable mild chronic hepatitis tolerate surgery well.

Patients with alcoholic liver disease or cirrhosis are at risk for postoperative complications, including bleeding, infection, poor wound healing, and delirium.[16] The severity of disease as assessed by Child-Turcotte-Pugh criteria and the MELD (Model for End-Stage Liver Disease) score (Chapter 154) can be used to estimate risk; the MELD score is thought to be more predictive of outcome. Child's C class and MELD score greater than 15 portend very high risk, and elective surgery is usually contraindicated. Aggressive treatment of coagulopathy, ascites, and encephalopathy is indicated before surgery.

🔴 HEMATOLOGIC PROBLEMS

Preoperative anemia, even to a mild degree, is independently associated with an increased risk for 30-day morbidity and mortality in patients undergoing major noncardiac surgery,[17] but operative patients generally tolerate hemoglobin levels as low as 7 g/dL. Preoperative transfusion should not be triggered solely by the hemoglobin level but should also consider the expected blood loss from the surgical procedure and the patient's comorbid conditions. For patients with cardiopulmonary disease, however, a goal of 10 g/dL has typically been recommended for major surgery, although a trigger of 8 to 9 g/dL may be appropriate.[18]

Patients without a personal or family history of abnormal bleeding require no preoperative testing of coagulative function, but those with such a history should be evaluated. Ideally, the prothrombin time should be within 3 seconds of control (international normalized ratio <1.5), the partial thromboplastin time within 10 seconds of control, and the platelet count above a minimum of 50,000, depending on the type of surgery.

The approach to perioperative anticoagulation, both in terms of prevention of venous thromboembolism and for the management of a patient taking warfarin, aspirin, or other antithrombotic medications, is described elsewhere (Chapter 38). For patients already on anticoagulants, perioperative recommendations depend on the short-term risks for thromboembolism and bleeding (Table 431-5)[19] and provide additional guidelines regarding perioperative aspirin use in cardiac and noncardiac surgery. However, the need for bridging therapy has been questioned because the risk for bleeding with early postoperative anticoagulation may outweigh any potential benefit.[20] Use of the new oral anticoagulants (dabigatran, rivaroxaban, and apixaban) obviates the need for bridging therapy because of their shorter half-lives and more rapid onset of action compared with warfarin (Table 431-6). They can be stopped closer to the time of surgery but should be started postoperatively only after adequate hemostasis has been ensured, usually 48 to 72 hours after major surgery.

TABLE 431-5	SUGGESTED APPROACH TO ANTICOAGULATION IN THE PERIOPERATIVE PATIENT

Low thromboembolic risk/low bleeding risk
- Continue anticoagulant therapy with INR in therapeutic range.

Low thromboembolic risk/high bleeding risk
- Discontinue anticoagulant therapy 5 days before the procedure.
- Start LMWH prophylaxis once daily or UFH IV 1 day after acenocoumarol interruption and 2 days after warfarin interruption. Administer the last dose of LMWH at least 24 hr before the procedure or give UFH IV up to 4-6 hr before surgery.
- Resume LMWH or UFH at the preprocedural dose 1-2 days (at least 12 hr) after the procedure according to hemostatic status. Resume anticoagulant therapy 1 to 2 days after surgery at the preprocedural dose + 50% boost dose for 2 consecutive days according to the hemostatic status.
- LMWH or UFH is continued until the INR has returned to therapeutic levels.

High thromboembolic risk
- Discontinue anticoagulant therapy 5 days before the procedure.
- Start therapeutic LMWH twice daily or UFH IV 1 day after acenocoumarol interruption and 2 days after warfarin interruption. Administer the last dose of LMWH at least 24 hr before the procedure or give UFH IV up to 4-6 hr before surgery.
- Resume LMWH or UFH at the preprocedural dose 24-72 hr after the procedure depending on the risk of bleeding. Resume anticoagulant therapy 12-24 hr after surgery according to hemostatic status.
- LMWH or UFH is continued until the INR has returned to therapeutic levels.

LMWH = low-molecular-weight heparin; INR = international normalized ratio; IV = intravenous; UFH = unfractionated heparin.
Adapted from Poldermans D, Bax JJ, Boersma E, et al. Guidelines for pre-operative cardiac risk assessment and perioperative cardiac management in non-cardiac surgery. The Task Force for Preoperative Cardiac Risk Assessment and Perioperative Cardiac Management in Non-cardiac Surgery of the European Society of Cardiology (ESC) and endorsed by the European Society of Anaesthesiology (ESA). *Eur Heart J.* 2009;30:2769-2812 and Douketis JD, Spyropoulos AC, Spencer FA, et al. Perioperative management of antithrombotic therapy: Antithrombotic Therapy and Prevention of Thrombosis, 9th ed: American College of Chest Physicians Evidence-Based Clinical Practice Guidelines. *Chest.* 2012;141:e326S-350S.

TABLE 431-6 PREOPERATIVE MANAGEMENT OF THE NEW ORAL ANTICOAGULANTS

DRUG	CREATININE CLEARANCE (mL/min)	HALF-LIFE (hr)	TIMING OF LAST DOSE BEFORE SURGERY	
			Standard Bleeding Risk Surgery	High Bleeding Risk Surgery*
Dabigatran	>50	13-15	1 day	2 days
	31-50	18	2 days	3-4 days
	≤30	27	3-4 days	4-5 days
Rivaroxaban	>30	7-11	1 day	2 days
	≤30	?	2 days	3-4 days
Apixaban	>30	8-14	1 day	2 days
	≤30	?	2 days	3-4 days

*Examples include neurosurgery, spine surgery, cardiac, major abdominal, and vascular surgery.

RENAL DISORDERS

Chronic kidney disease is an independent risk factor for postoperative cardiovascular events and death.[21] Patients with chronic kidney disease typically have other comorbid diseases and may also have fluid and electrolyte abnormalities, anemia, and bleeding diatheses, which should be treated and optimized before surgery. Patients maintained on dialysis should ideally undergo dialysis the day before surgery to optimize their volume status, prevent hyperkalemia, and minimize acute shifts in acid-base balance.

NEUROLOGIC AND GERIATRIC PROBLEMS

The risk for a postoperative stroke in unselected patients after general surgery is less than 0.5%, but patients with a history of stroke, older patients, and those undergoing vascular surgery, especially carotid and cardiac surgery, have higher risk. Patients with symptomatic carotid bruits require further investigation and possible intervention before elective surgery (Chapter 407). Patients who newly receive perioperative β-blockers, particularly high doses of metoprolol, appear to be at increased risk for stroke, and the risk must be balanced against the protective effect of β-blockers for perioperative MI. However, there is no evidence that continuation of chronic β-blockade increases risk for postoperative stroke. There is no evidence to support preoperative intervention in patients with asymptomatic bruits before noncardiac surgery. The general recommendation is to delay elective surgery for at least 4 weeks after a stroke, although some data suggest waiting up to 9 months.[22]

The elderly are at higher risks for a variety of poor postoperative outcomes. Cognitive impairment (Chapters 27 and 28), frailty (Chapter 24), malnutrition, and prior institutionalization all are associated with a poorer prognosis.[23]

 Grade A References

A1. Devereaux PJ, Yang H, Yusuf S, et al. Effects of extended-release metoprolol succinate in patients undergoing non-cardiac surgery (POISE trial): a randomised controlled trial. *Lancet.* 2008;371:1839-1847.
A2. Bangalore S, Wetterslev J, Pranesh S, et al. Perioperative beta blockers in patients having non-cardiac surgery: a meta-analysis. *Lancet.* 2008;372:1962-1976.
A3. Nowbar AN, Cole GD, Shun-Shin MJ, et al. International RCT-based guidelines for use of preoperative stress testing and perioperative beta-blockers and statins in non-cardiac surgery. *Int J Cardiol.* 2014;172:138-143.
A4. Devereaux PJ, Sessler DI, Leslie K, et al. Clonidine in patients undergoing noncardiac surgery. *N Engl J Med.* 2014;370:1504-1513.
A5. Devereaux PJ, Mrkobrada M, Sessler DI, et al. Aspirin in patients undergoing noncardiac surgery. *N Engl J Med.* 2014;370:1494-1503.
A6. Sanders RD, Nicholson A, Lewis SR, et al. Perioperative statin therapy for improving outcomes during and after noncardiac vascular surgery. *Cochrane Database Syst Rev.* 2013;7:CD009971.
A7. Yealy DM, Kellum JA, Huang DT, et al. A randomized trial of protocol-based care for early septic shock. *N Engl J Med.* 2014;370:1683-1693.
A8. Pearse RM, Harrison DA, MacDonald N, et al. Effect of a perioperative, cardiac output-guided hemodynamic therapy algorithm on outcomes following major gastrointestinal surgery: a randomized clinical trial and systematic review. *JAMA.* 2014;311:2181-2190.
A9. McFalls EO, Ward HB, Moritz TE, et al. Coronary-artery revascularization before elective major vascular surgery. *N Engl J Med.* 2004;351:2795-2804.
A10. Sandham JD, Hull RD, Brant RF, et al. Canadian Critical Care Clinical Trials Group. A randomized, controlled trial of the use of pulmonary-artery catheters in high-risk surgical patients. *N Engl J Med.* 2003;348:5-14.
A11. Yong SL, Coulthard P, Wrzosek A. Supplemental perioperative steroids for surgical patients with adrenal insufficiency. *Cochrane Database Syst Rev.* 2012;12:CD005367.

GENERAL REFERENCES

For the General References and other additional features, please visit Expert Consult at https://expertconsult.inkling.com.

432

OVERVIEW OF ANESTHESIA

JEANINE P. WIENER-KRONISH AND LEE A. FLEISHER

In the United States, more than 40 million procedures, including outpatient procedures that require an anesthetic, are performed annually. Additionally, many invasive procedures outside of the operating room, such as in the gastrointestinal endoscopy and electrophysiology suites, are performed using deep sedation or general anesthesia. With modern techniques, anesthesia causes or contributes to mortality in about 1 per 20,000 healthy patients. Although the worldwide perioperative mortality attributable to anesthesia has declined by more than 90% in the past several decades,[1] the overall inpatient postoperative mortality rate remains about 4%, with large variations even among developed countries.[2]

PREOPERATIVE ASSESSMENT

Important aspects of preoperative risk assessment include the type of surgery to be performed, the patient's underlying medical condition, and the particular demands for anesthesia (Chapter 431). In addition, a number of other issues are relevant to management and anesthetic evaluation.

Airway Assessment

Assessment of the airway is always necessary, even if regional anesthesia or monitored anesthesia care (local anesthesia with sedation) is planned, because unexpected complications or compromise of airway reflexes may lead to an emergent need to support ventilation. The laryngeal mask airway device allows many patients to be ventilated easily, but it is important to assess the ability to intubate the patient as well as the ability to ventilate. The prevalence of difficult intubation is about 6% for nonobese patients, and reasons for difficulty include airway pathology (e.g., tumors, previous surgery), reduced mobility of the cervical spine, obstructive sleep apnea, or the anatomic relationship between the larynx and trachea.[3] In many such patients, endotracheal intubation can be accomplished by using a fiberoptic bronchoscope to place the endotracheal tube through either the nose or mouth. If this approach is not successful, a surgical airway must be created.

Criteria for extubation in postoperative patients are similar to those in other patients who receive mechanical ventilation (Chapter 105). Older patients with more severe, comorbid diseases, especially underlying cardiac or pulmonary disease, are more likely to require postoperative reintubation, which is associated with a nine-fold increase in mortality.[4]

MEDICATION REACTIONS

Malignant Hyperthermia

Malignant hyperthermia (Chapter 434) is characterized by acute hyperpyrexia developing during or immediately after general anesthesia.[5] The channels that regulate the duration and amplitude of calcium efflux from the sarcoplasmic reticulum are the ryanodine receptors, which exist as three isoforms. Gain-of-function mutations affecting RyR1, the receptor expressed primarily in skeletal muscle, are present in 1 per 15,000 to 50,000 people and are associated with enhanced sensitivity to halothane and caffeine and with malignant hyperthermia and central core disease. More than 80 distinct mutations have been detected, and mutation of the adult skeletal muscle sodium channel, SCN4A, may also cause the syndrome. Patients with mutations predisposing to malignant hyperthermia function normally at resting conditions, but exposure to volatile anesthetics, including halothane, isoflurane, enflurane, desflurane, and sevoflurane, or exposure to a depolarizing muscle relaxant, succinylcholine, can precipitate life-threatening muscle contractures, increases in heart rate and body temperature, rhabdomyolysis, myoglobinuria, and metabolic acidosis. The mortality rate is 80% in untreated patients but about 5% with current treatment. Note that succinylcholine causes a release of myoglobin from muscle in small amounts even in normal patients. Patients with malignant hyperthermia do not predictably respond to triggering agents, and some patients with malignant hyperthermia have had milder symptoms of malignant hyperthermia after the administration of nontriggering agents. Malignant hyperthermia now often occurs in muted forms, probably because of the decreased use of succinylcholine by anesthesiologists, the diagnostic awareness of malignant hyperthermia by anesthesiologists, the routine use of carbon dioxide monitors so that increases in end-expiratory carbon dioxide are detected quickly, and the availability of dantrolene. If malignant hyperthermia is suspected by obtaining a family history of adverse events with the administration of anesthesia or when a patient has a reaction suspicious for malignant hyperthermia, a muscle biopsy is usually obtained for in vitro contracture testing, which evaluates the muscle contracture responses to caffeine or halothane. Genetic investigations are also recommended, but malignant hyperthermia cannot be excluded on the basis of genetic testing alone because of the diversity of mutations and genes that can be involved in this syndrome. The Malignant Hyperthermia Association of the United States, www.mhaus.org, is available for information to the public, and all medical personnel can get information 24 hours every day on the malignant hyperthermia hotline, 1-800-MHHYPER or 1-800-644-9737.

Dantrolene is the drug of choice to prevent and to reverse the symptoms of malignant hyperthermia. Dantrolene decreases muscle sensitivity to caffeine, reduces the calcium release from the sarcoplasmic reticulum, and produces some muscle weakness. Dantrolene comes in 20-mg bottles and must be dissolved in sterile water; the recommended dose is 2.5 mg/kg given rapidly up to 10 mg/kg. Drug should be given every 5-10 minutes until symptoms subside. Other treatments for malignant hyperthermia include: discontinuing the use of any volatile anesthetics; hyperventilating the patient and administering 100% oxygen; administering bicarbonate for severe acidosis; controlling fevers; and maintaining a temperature below 39°C, without causing hypothermia by using iced fluids, surface cooling, and cooling of body cavities if necessary. Monitoring of temperature and vital signs, urinary output, muscle enzymes, glucose, coagulation studies, acid-base status, and gas exchange is recommended.

Two other rare congenital myopathies associated with mutations of the RyR1 include central core disease and multiminicore disease. Patients with central core disease present with infantile hypotonia; a muscle biopsy is needed for definitive diagnosis. Multiminicore disease is a nonprogressive congenital myopathy in which infants present with hypotonia, ophthalmoplegia, and arthrogryposis. These children develop scoliosis and eventually may require chronic ventilation. Avoidance of triggering agents is advised for these syndromes and for patients with other myopathies. Both malignant hyperthermia and central core disease are thought to be inherited as autosomal dominant diseases, but extensive genetic analysis has revealed overlapping phenotypes.

Monoamine Oxidase Inhibitors and Serotonin Toxicity
Anesthesiologists routinely ask if patients are taking a monoamine oxidase (MAO) inhibitor because of their many drug interactions with analgesics in perioperative patients. Also, serotonin toxicity has features similar to malignant hyperthermia and must be distinguished from it. Serotonin toxicity, characterized as a triad of neuromuscular hyperactivity (tremor, clonus, myoclonus, hyperreflexia, and pyramidal rigidity), autonomic hyperactivity (diaphoresis, fever, tachycardia, and tachypnea), and altered mental status (agitation, excitement, and confusion) can be precipitated by the coadministration of MAO inhibitors and selective serotonin reuptake inhibitors (SSRIs). Patients who are taking SSRIs have a higher overall perioperative mortality, a higher 30-day readmission rate, and a higher likelihood of bleeding.[6] Rigidity, increasing arterial carbon dioxide levels, and fever above 38.5°C are associated with life-threatening toxicity. Ecstasy, or 3,4-methylenedioxymethamphetamine (MDMA), combined with MAO inhibitors, including moclobemide, can lead to fatalities because it acts as a serotonin releaser. Tramadol, used for pain relief, and venlafaxine, an antidepressant, act as serotonin releasers and are associated with toxicity when used in patients who are taking MAO inhibitors.

Anaphylaxis in the Perioperative Period
The incidence of life-threatening hypersensitivity reactions during anesthesia is 1 : 4000 to 1 : 25,000. Anaphylaxis is caused by immunoglobulin E (IgE)-mediated reactions (Chapter 253), whereas anaphylactoid reactions produce the same clinical picture but are not mediated by IgE. Anaphylaxis during anesthesia can present as cardiovascular collapse, airway obstruction,

flushing, or edema of the skin, singly or in combination, so a careful history of any previous allergic reactions to medications and the nature of the reaction must be obtained by the anesthesiologist and other members of the perioperative team. Neuromuscular blocking agents, such as succinylcholine, and opioid analgesics can cause nonimmunologic release of histamine from mast cells and produce a similar clinical syndrome. Antibiotics, protamine, and blood transfusions (Chapter 177), all given routinely during operations, also can elicit a variety of systemic reactions. About 75% of perioperative hypersensitivity reactions appear to be due to muscle relaxants, especially rocuronium and vecuronium, with a mortality of 3 to 6%. In patients with apparent allergic reactions, skin testing is usually performed, and IgE levels are usually obtained to determine whether the patient had an allergic reaction to a perioperative medication.

Latex Allergies
For sensitized patients (Chapter 253), exposure to even low amounts of latex-containing particles is sufficient to induce a severe anaphylactic reaction. A latex-free operating environment, in which no latex gloves or latex accessories are used, is key in patients with known allergy. Skin prick tests with latex extracts should be considered in patients at high risk for latex allergy. Early aggressive treatment with epinephrine is critical if severe anaphylaxis occurs.

INTRAOPERATIVE MANAGEMENT
There are three general classes of anesthesia: general, regional, and monitored anesthesia care. The same drugs are often used for general anesthesia and monitored anesthesia care; achievement of the two different conditions requires knowledge of the pharmacokinetics of the drugs (Table 432-1).

General Anesthesia
General anesthesia can be achieved with a balanced drug regimen that induces a loss of consciousness, which can range from a deep sedation requiring only airway support to states requiring full ventilatory support because of weakness and loss of respiratory drive. Both intravenous and inhalational drugs can be used to induce and maintain general anesthesia. In contrast, monitored anesthesia care denotes a state in which patients can still control their airway, do not require ventilatory support, but are sleepy, have less pain, and may be amnestic.

Propofol
Propofol, an alkylphenol, is perhaps the most frequently used intravenous anesthetic for induction of anesthesia and is often used for maintenance of anesthesia during short procedures or to achieve deep sedation during monitored anesthesia care. It is lipid soluble and quickly cleared from the central

TABLE 432-1	COMMON ANESTHETIC APPROACHES FOR VARIOUS TYPES OF SURGERY

SURGERY ON INTRA-ABDOMINAL OR INTRATHORACIC ORGANS

Examples: cardiac surgery, lung resections, gastric bypass
  General anesthesia usually administered because mechanical ventilation is often required
  Drugs include premedication for anxiety with midazolam, general anesthesia with volatile anesthetics (desflurane, sevoflurane, nitrous oxide), neuromuscular blockade, and opioid analgesics*
  Epidural anesthesia and analgesia also used; examples include ropivacaine, lidocaine, with fentanyl

SURGERY ON LIMBS

Examples: hip replacement, knee replacement, foot or arm surgery
  Can perform with epidural or spinal anesthesia, depending on the limb. Examples of medications would include tetracaine, lidocaine, ropivacaine, and fentanyl or morphine.
  Can perform axillary or scalene block; examples include lidocaine and ropivacaine
  For postoperative pain control: can perform regional blocks that leave the catheter in place, including femoral nerve block, axillary nerve blocks

CATARACT SURGERY—LOCAL ANESTHESIA ON EYE WITH OR WITHOUT SEDATION

Examples of drugs used for sedation include midazolam and fentanyl

*Includes the use of opioids given intraoperatively with effects that extend into the postanesthesia care unit (PACU) or postoperative period, opioids given in the PACU, or opioids given or intended to be given after discharge from the PACU.

compartment, so it is rapidly eliminated even after long periods of continuous infusion. However, the clearance of propofol is changed by gender (men have lower clearance rates than women), size (children require higher doses), age (elderly patients have decreased clearance rates and experience increased effects with the drug), and narcotics, which decrease its clearance. Because of its predilection for causing apnea, propofol should be administered only by someone with expertise in airway management. Propofol also decreases arterial blood pressure, causes pain with injection, and can precipitate myoclonus. Large quantities of propofol can cause the propofol infusion syndrome, which is associated with cardiomyopathy, metabolic acidosis, skeletal myopathy, hyperkalemia, hepatomegaly, and lipemia. Despite these issues, propofol is frequently used because the recovery from propofol is within minutes, even after it is given as a prolonged continuous infusion, in contrast to the longer duration of drug effects seen after the administration of other intravenous sedatives.

Propofol is the preferred agent for healthy outpatients undergoing colonoscopy because it leads to earlier discharge and higher patient satisfaction compared with other agents.[A1] When combined with midazolam, sedation is deeper, patient satisfaction is higher, and time to discharge is no longer,[A2] even when administered by nonanesthesiologists.[A3]

Midazolam

Midazolam, a benzodiazepine that produces muscle relaxation through a central mechanism, is hypnotic, sedative, anxiolytic, amnesic, and anticonvulsant. Its amnesic and anticonvulsant effects are mediated through α_1-subunit-containing γ-aminobutyric acid A (GABA$_A$) receptors, and the anxiolytic and muscle relaxation are mediated through α_2-subunit-containing GABA$_A$ receptors. Only 20% receptor occupancy is needed to produce anxiolysis, whereas unconsciousness requires 60%. Long-term administration of benzodiazepines produces tolerance, which appears to decrease receptor binding and function. Benzodiazepines cause dose-related depression of the respiratory system, with a peak effect at 3 minutes and significant depression persisting for 60 to 120 minutes. The rate of administration of the drug affects the onset of depression: the faster the drug is given, the quicker the respiratory depression occurs. Benzodiazepines and opioids appear to produce additive respiratory depression, including apnea. Unlike propofol, benzodiazepines used alone decrease blood pressure only modestly. Other drugs, particularly drugs that affect the cytochrome P-450 3A4 enzyme (including azole antifungals, human immunodeficiency virus [HIV] protease inhibitors, and calcium-channel blockers), affect the clearance of midazolam and prolong its half-life significantly. There are several reports of prolonged amnesia in HIV patients who received midazolam for conscious sedation. Midazolam also has an active metabolite and is often associated with delirium in elderly patients (Chapter 28), perhaps because it impairs both implicit and relational memory.

Opioids

Opioids are classified as naturally occurring (morphine, codeine), semisynthetic (heroin), and synthetic (methadone, fentanyl, remfentanil). They can be administered both intravenously and in the neuraxial space (epidural or spinal). There are four opiate receptors (mu, kappa, delta, and nociceptin receptors), which are G protein–coupled receptors. Chronic exposure to agonists leads to cellular adaptation mechanisms that probably are involved in tolerance, dependence, and withdrawal. Clinically, mu agonists are used almost exclusively; mu agonists include morphine, fentanyl, and meperidine. Opioid analgesics are administered because they relieve pain, but they have other important effects, including respiratory depression, decreased gastric emptying, nausea and vomiting, sedation, constipation, pruritus, dependence, and tolerance, when given repeatedly. When opioids are given with propofol or benzodiazepines, there is a synergistic depressive effect on respiration, hence the rationale for monitoring patients who receive medications for conscious sedation.

Ketamine

Ketamine is unique among the intravenous agents because it has analgesic properties and decreases tolerance to opiates. Ketamine produces dose-related analgesia, which may be profound even when patients can keep their eyes open, breathe spontaneously, and protect their own airway with conserved swallowing and cough reflex. Side effects include increased lacrimation, salivation, and muscle tone. Ketamine increases cerebral blood flow, can increase seizure activity, and can produce undesirable psychological reactions; these side effects are dose related and may be minimized by the concomitant use of benzodiazepines. Ketamine is also a bronchial smooth muscle relaxant and can prevent experimentally induced bronchospasm. Ketamine is usually associated with an increase in blood pressure, heart rate, and cardiac output. These features make ketamine a useful drug for sedating patients with hemodynamic instability.

Dexmedetomidine

Dexmedetomidine is a highly selective α_2-agonist that is associated with less respiratory depression and more cooperative behavior than is propofol. Dexmedetomidine also causes hypnosis, analgesia, sympatholysis, and inhibition of insulin secretion. Dexmedetomidine induces sedation with a respiratory pattern and electroencephalographic changes similar to natural sleep. Even high concentrations of dexmedetomidine are associated with preservation of spontaneous respiration; however, when dexmedetomidine is administered in combination with sympatholytic or cholinergic agents, there is a high risk for extreme bradycardia and sinus arrest. Dexmedetomidine is associated with less amnesia than are benzodiazepines. Although propofol and benzodiazepines commonly have been used in critically ill patients to achieve sedation for procedures or for maintenance of mechanical ventilation, dexmedetomidine appears to have significant advantages over benzodiazepines because it causes less delirium and decreases the time that critical care patients spend on ventilators.[A4]

Volatile Anesthetics

Volatile (inhalational) anesthetics include desflurane, sevoflurane, isoflurane, and nitrous oxide, as well as halothane, which now is rarely used in the United States. Inhaled anesthetics are absorbed through the respiratory epithelium and mucous membranes of the respiratory tract, and they are excreted mainly by exhalation. Access to the circulation is almost instantaneous, owing to the large pulmonary surface area. The pharmacologic effects of inhaled anesthetics depend primarily on alveolar ventilation, the ventilation-perfusion ratio, coadministered gases, gas flow, and the physicochemical properties of the anesthetic gas rather than on the quantity of drug administered, the extent and rate of absorption, protein binding, excretion, secretion, or metabolism. Based on the available evidence, no inhalational agent appears to be superior to any other.

All inhalational agents, with the exception of nitrous oxide, cause dose-dependent cardiovascular depression. Severe hepatotoxicity, which led to the discontinuation of the use of chloroform, carbon tetrachloride, and trichloroethylene anesthetics, is seen as fatal hepatic necrosis with in 1 in 10,000 halothane anesthetics. This problem appears to occur much less frequently with isoflurane and desflurane. Mild halothane hepatoxicity is self-limited and can occur with a single exposure, whereas fulminant halothane hepatitis occurs only after multiple exposures to the drug, has a high mortality rate (50%), and is associated with antibodies to halothane-altered antigens.

Nitrous oxide, which is the only nonhalogenated agent still used, is not metabolized in human tissues. It irreversibly oxidizes the cobalt atom of vitamin B$_{12}$, thereby inhibiting the activity of the cobalamin-dependent enzyme methionine synthase. Individuals with vitamin B$_{12}$ deficiency or with mutations of methionine synthase may be at risk for neurologic injury from nitrous oxide, which should not be used in patients at risk. Exposure to high concentrations of more than 10^3 ppm may be associated with an increased incidence of abortions and decreased fertility, so exposure should be avoided in patients and personnel at risk. Nitrous oxide is safe in major non-cardiac surgery.[A5] General anesthesia can be achieved only by giving combinations of drugs along with nitrous oxide to achieve the desired effects. Based on the available evidence, no one general anesthetic appears to be superior to any other.

Neuromuscular Blockers

Neuromuscular blockers are used to paralyze muscles to facilitate endotracheal intubation and mechanical ventilation, to decrease shivering during induced hypothermia, or to improve conditions for optimal surgery. Succinylcholine causes prolonged depolarization of the neuromuscular junction, thereby resulting in failure to generate an action potential. Within 9 to 13 minutes after 1 mg/kg of succinylcholine, 90% of muscle strength is restored. The very rapid onset and rapid return of muscle function make succinylcholine a useful drug for difficult intubations. Side effects of succinylcholine include hyperkalemia, myalgia, masseter spasm, sinus bradycardia and nodal rhythms, and increased intraocular pressure.

Most of the other neuromuscular drugs used by anesthesiologists are nondepolarizing in that they compete with acetylcholine for the neuromuscular junction and can be reversed by increasing the quantity of acetylcholine.

These drugs are categorized by their chemical makeup: steroidal compounds, benzylisoquinolinium compounds, and other chemical compounds. Clinically, a drug is often chosen for its duration of action. Intermediate agents, which act for 20 to 50 minutes and are used most frequently, include vecuronium, rocuronium, atracurium, and cisatracurium. These drugs have different routes of metabolism, so the choice of agent depends in part on the presence of coexisting disease. Sugammadex, a recently developed direct antagonist to the neuromuscular blocking agents, is not approved for use in the United States at the time of this writing.

The chronic administration of neuromuscular blocking agents is associated with prolonged paralysis, particularly in patients given concomitant steroids. Other notable interactions with nondepolarizing agents include that antibiotics can increase neuromuscular blockade; magnesium sulfate potentiates neuromuscular blockade; lithium can potentiate neuromuscular blockade with succinylcholine and with pipecuronium; and antiepileptic drugs cause resistance to nondepolarizing muscle blockade so that larger doses must be administered to achieve paralysis; and patients receiving anticonvulsants have accelerated recovery from neuromuscular blockade.

Regional Anesthesia

Regional anesthesia involves the deposition of local anesthetics near nerves, including the deposition of local anesthetics in the epidural space and into the cerebral spinal fluid (CSF). Local anesthetics, which are aminoesters or aminoamides, affect cardiac function, as well as central nervous system function when administered systemically.

The binding of the local anesthetic to the sodium channels in the axoplasm prevents opening of the channels and conduction of nerve impulses. The rates of onset and recovery from nerve blockade are controlled by the diffusion of the local anesthetic into and out of the whole nerve.

Examples of regional anesthesia include neuraxial techniques, the deposition of local anesthetics near the brachial plexus to anesthetize the arms (axillary or intrascalene blocks), deposition near the femoral or sciatic nerves to anesthetize the legs, deposition near ulnar or radial nerves for lower arm blocks, deposition near the pudenal nerves for groin procedures, and deposition of local anesthesia in the caudal space for groin surgeries. Dentists employ this technique frequently when they inject local anesthesia near various nerves in the oral cavity. Many surgeries, including carotid surgery and the placement of fistulas for dialysis, can be performed with regional anesthesia. Regional anesthetics may also require supplementation with sedation or general anesthesia.

The dangers of regional anesthesia include the injection of local anesthesia into the systemic circulation. Systemic toxicity is manifested as convulsions and respiratory depression, which can require assisted ventilation. Tinnitus, visual and auditory disturbances, and dizziness are signs of milder central nervous toxicity. Cardiac toxicity can be manifested by decreases in heart rate, prolonged conduction times, and negative inotropic effects. Bupivacaine toxicity is associated with ventricular fibrillation. Intralipid 20% at various doses (1.5 ml/kg rapid bolus [~100mL in average adult] followed by infusion of 0.25 ml/kg/min for 10 minutes) has been reported in case reports and in animal studies to reverse these toxic effects, although the optimal dosing has yet to be determined. Furthermore, the prolonged duration of many of the local anesthetics may require the institution of cardiopulmonary bypass until the drugs are metabolized.

Neuraxial (Spinal and Epidural) Anesthesia and Analgesia

Spinal anesthesia is the instillation of local anesthetics into the CSF. Epidural anesthesia is the instillation of larger volumes of local anesthetics into the epidural space, which is the potential space that exists just before the CSF. Spinal anesthesia is associated with an increased incidence of headache in younger patients, so epidural anesthesia is often used in younger patients. Complications of epidural and spinal anesthesia and analgesia include failed blocks, postdural puncture headaches, and toxicity from the local anesthetics. Another major concern of neuraxial anesthesia is that patients on antiplatelet agents may develop epidural hematomas, although epidural hematoma remains a rare event, occurring in fewer than 1 in 150,000 operations even in the presence of potent antiplatelet agents. Other more rare complications of epidural and spinal anesthetics, in addition to the effects of local anesthesia outlined previously, include intracranial subdural hematoma, transverse myelitis, hypotension, and cardiac arrest.

Postoperative epidural analgesia, by which either local anesthesia or local anesthesia and narcotics are instilled into the epidural space for postoperative pain control, is associated with superior pain control, lower doses of opioids, improved bowel mobility, slightly decreased length of stay in the intensive care unit, and a slight decrease in the requirement for mechanical ventilation.[A6]

GENERAL VERSUS REGIONAL ANESTHESIA

The decision regarding what type of anesthesia should be administered often depends on the requirements of the surgery. For example, laparoscopic surgery requires general anesthesia because the insufflations of gases impair the ability to breathe adequately. General anesthesia is also required for surgeries on the airway or thorax because mechanical ventilation is usually needed to sustain adequate respiration. Low tidal volume and low positive end-expiratory pressure are preferred.[A7] Procedures that do not allow any movement (e.g., precise procedures in the brain) often require general anesthesia and paralysis. For patients in whom the intraoperative technique could include general anesthesia, regional anesthesia, or a combination of the two, regional anesthesia may minimize pulmonary complications, but the data are conflicting.

Side effects of general anesthesia depend on the drugs used to achieve anesthesia, whether neuromuscular blockade is administered, and whether mechanical ventilation is used. Complications of endotracheal intubation include local pain, trauma to the airway, swelling, vocal cord paralysis, increased bronchospasm, and death from improper placement. Volatile anesthetics are associated with postoperative atelectasis (Chapter 90), whereas regional anesthesia helps preserve respiratory dynamics. Postoperative cognitive dysfunction (Chapter 28) does not seem to depend on the type of anesthesia administered.

NAUSEA AND VOMITING

Postoperative nausea and vomiting are more likely with volatile anesthetics but also are common when perioperative opioids are administered. Prophylactic ondansetron, dexamethasone, and droperidol each reduce postoperative nausea and vomiting, independently, by about 26%, with the main predictor for efficacy being the patient's risk for nausea and vomiting.[A8] It should be noted that droperidol has received a "black box" warning from the U.S. Food and Drug Administration, so it is not used very often in the United States. Total intravenous anesthesia with propofol reduces postoperative nausea and vomiting by only about 20%, often because narcotics are still administered. The use of spinal or epidural anesthesia may decrease the incidence of nausea and vomiting. In addition to general anesthesia, risk factors for postoperative nausea and vomiting include female gender, a prior history of nausea and vomiting, a history of motion sickness, nonsmoking, and intended administration of opioids for postoperative analgesia. If three or more risk factors are present, patients generally are recommended to receive at least two prophylactic pharmacologic antiemetic agents of different classes (e.g., selected among ondansetron or another $5\text{-}HT_3$ antagonist, droperidol, dexamethasone, scopolamine, or phenothiazides) preoperatively for the prevention of nausea and vomiting.

Grade A References

A1. Wang D, Chen C, Chen J, et al. The use of propofol as a sedative agent in gastrointestinal endoscopy: a meta-analysis. PLoS ONE. 2013;8:e53311.

A2. Wang D, Wang S, Chen J, et al. Propofol combined with traditional sedative agents versus propofol-alone sedation for gastrointestinal endoscopy: a meta-analysis. Scand J Gastroenterol. 2013;48:101-110.

A3. Molina-Infante J, Dueñas-Sadornil C, Mateos-Rodríguez JM, et al. Nonanesthesiologist-administered propofol versus midazolam and propofol, titrated to moderate sedation, for colonoscopy: a randomized controlled trial. Dig Dis Sci. 2012;57:2385-2393.

A4. Riker RR, Shehabi Y, Bokesch PM, et al. Dexmedetomidine vs midazolam for sedation of critically ill patients. JAMA. 2009;301:489-499.

A5. Myles PS, Leslie K, Chan MT, et al. The safety of addition of nitrous oxide to general anaesthesia in at-risk patients having major non-cardiac surgery (ENIGMA-II): a randomised, single-blind trial. Lancet. 2014;384:1446-1454.

A6. Popping DM, Elia N, Van Aken HK, et al. Impact of epidural analgesia on mortality and morbidity after surgery: systematic review and meta-analysis of randomized controlled trials. Ann Surg. 2013;259:1056-1067.

A7. Hemmes SN, Gama de Abreu M, Pelosi P, et al. High versus low positive end-expiratory pressure during general anaesthesia for open abdominal surgery (PROVHILO trial): a multicentre randomised controlled trial. Lancet. 2014;384:495-503.

A8. Apfel CC, Korttila K, Abdalla M, et al. A factorial trial of six interventions for the prevention of postoperative nausea and vomiting. N Engl J Med. 2004;350:2441-2451.

GENERAL REFERENCES

For the General References and other additional features, please visit Expert Consult at https://expertconsult.inkling.com.

433

POSTOPERATIVE CARE AND COMPLICATIONS

DONALD A. REDELMEIER

POSTOPERATIVE CARE

Overview

Postoperative medical complications are common, potentially fatal, and variable across different settings. Large national studies show about a two-fold difference in risk for mortality between high- and low-ranked hospitals. However, analyses disagree about how much these differences reflect a greater incidence of each complication (failure of prevention around the time of surgery), a heightened lethality of each complication (failure to rescue in the aftermath of surgery), or the differences in the severity of disease or surgical skill. Regardless of the explanation, the purpose of medical consultation is to relieve human suffering by the prevention, detection, and correction of postoperative complications. The main constraint is that the consultant often has limited ongoing direct contact with the patient before or after the perioperative interval.

Effective Teamwork

The medical consultant (Chapter 430) in the postoperative setting must have both a knowledge of medicine and an appreciation of the team psychology that can improve the outcomes of patients.[1] In contrast to other settings, the internist is not the team leader, often does not maintain an ongoing relationship with the patient, and does not have the authority of the most responsible physician. Moreover, patients may be dispersed across diverse surgical services, each with its own orientation and culture. The challenges of coordination and communication are enormous, particularly given the multiple other health care professionals involved in complex surgical cases. Considerable tact is often needed to avoid antagonizing the surgeon, disrupting the team's dynamics, or inducing a cascade of cumbersome inopportune testing. The development and use of safety checklists can be an effective way for teamwork to improve outcomes.[2]

Focusing on Recovery

Facilitating the patient's recovery from surgery differs conceptually from managing patients with acute exacerbations of chronic disease. In the postoperative setting, many therapies need to be stopped at some point because the patient has recovered, such as discontinuing a urinary catheter because the patient can now void spontaneously or discontinuing a major tranquilizer because the patient is now oriented and coherent. Discontinuation of many other interventions requires substantial judgment, such as the decision when to discontinue intravenous access, supplemental oxygen, and intermittent laxatives. Much depends on experience and reconsideration of an individual patient's situation on a regular basis.

Reading Anesthesia Records

A focused review of the anesthesia record is essential because the consultant is rarely present during the operation. Perhaps the most basic information to identify is the date of surgery because the time elapsed helps in interpreting the patient's current state of recovery. Sometimes the date is not immediately evident if more than one surgery has been performed, a planned operation was canceled, or misquotations have arisen. Data about the duration of surgery, type of anesthesia (e.g., regional, spinal, or general [Chapter 432]), and major intraoperative events help establish reasonable expectations about the future course as well as the possibility of specific complications (e.g., epidural hematoma after spinal anesthesia). Sharing some of the basic data with the patient is often helpful because many individuals either benefit from repetition or are not otherwise informed.

Patterns of Mistakes

Medical errors (Chapter 12) that arise in postoperative care often seem mundane in retrospect yet can be lethal if undetected. Some patterns of mistakes have the feature of "double trouble," such as when a patient has both a potassium level of 2.0 mEq/L and an international normalized ratio of 2.0 but care focuses on only one of these abnormalities. Other mistakes occur because a single problem arises at an awkward moment, such as a patient in whom acute dyspnea develops when another patient is having a seizure. Still other mistakes relate to the fallibility of human memory and attention, such as when a normal blood glucose value in the morning leads clinicians to presume that the level is still normal at night. These errors can result in substantial harm, failures of clinicians to learn from past mistakes, and unprofessional reactions related to embarrassment. None of these patterns are unique to postoperative care, yet the fast and unfamiliar terrain of surgical settings can make even simple mistakes difficult to avoid.

Checking Orders

The first method for reducing errors after surgery is to check the postoperative orders already written for the patient. Such double-checking is a tedious task, and clinicians often direct insufficient attention to this review in the faulty belief that most of the work is already done. Ironically, checking orders written by another clinician requires more than customary attention because of the challenges of following someone else's legibility, sequencing, and preferences. The set of orders may need to be read twice: once for errors of commission (e.g., a calcium-channel blocker ordered at the wrong dose) and once for errors of omission (e.g., a β-blocker inadvertently not reordered after surgery). A classic mistake on postoperative orders is failure to follow through on interventions initiated immediately before surgery (e.g., delirium tremens prophylaxis). A particularly vexing issue is the need for repeated rechecking on subsequent days (e.g., new orders for sedative drugs).

Recommended Prophylaxis

Some complications are sufficiently frequent and serious that routine prophylaxis is merited in the postoperative setting. For example, systemic anticoagulation is indicated for most patients at risk for postoperative deep venous thrombosis (Chapters 38 and 81). The 2012 American College of Chest Physicians evidence-based clinical practice guidelines provide specific recommendations for both nonorthopedic[A1] and orthopedic[A2] surgery patients. Gastric acid suppression (Chapter 139) is justified for patients at high risk for postoperative gastric bleeding. Parenteral antibiotics are indicated for patients undergoing prosthetic joint replacement. In contrast, antibiotic prophylaxis is indicated only for selected patients who are at high risk for endocarditis (Chapter 76). The optimal method for gauging whether a patient is at high risk for each complication is contentious and thereby leads to variation in practice patterns across different settings.

Future Prevention

A postoperative consultant who maintains communication, facilitates the patient's recovery, and avoids postoperative mistakes also has the chance to initiate medical interventions for general medical care. Such opportunities for prevention might include influenza vaccination, colon cancer screening, and cholesterol reduction. The main advantage of such comprehensive care is that it conforms to the ideal of providing all services possible to the individual. The main disadvantage of such comprehensive care is the potential for creating unintended chaos, confusion, or misquotation (Chapter 430). Such unintended consequences distract the surgical team from the primary goal and also carry some risk for side effects at a time when the patient is trying to recover from surgery. Many effective postoperative consultants will defer such opportunities for prevention to the physicians who assume long-term responsibility for the patient's care.

COMPLICATIONS

Symptoms

Chest Pain

Chest pain is a common problem after surgery and has an extensive differential diagnosis (Chapter 51). In the postoperative setting, the immediate consideration is an acute ischemic myocardial event. The diagnosis of a perioperative myocardial infarction (MI) differs somewhat from community-acquired MI (Table 433-1). Interpretation of a patient's symptoms, examination findings, and electrocardiogram is often problematic because of changes related to surgery and anesthesia. Instead, diagnosis is heavily dependent on biomarkers, such as an elevated troponin level, especially because many postoperative MIs are painless. Among patients undergoing noncardiac surgery, the peak postoperative troponin level during the first 3 days after surgery is significantly associated with 30-day mortality, even if patients do not have any other evidence of an acute MI.[3] Management priorities include supplemental oxygen, heart rate control, and correction of severe anemia. Thrombolysis is often contraindicated, but percutaneous coronary intervention may be considered. In the absence of data from randomized trials, other therapies, such as aspirin, clopidogrel, nitrates, statins, and angiotensin-converting enzyme inhibitors, should be used on a case-by-case basis (Chapter 73).

Dyspnea

Shortness of breath (Chapter 83) after surgery has an extensive differential diagnosis (Table 433-2). The three key considerations are fluid overload/heart failure (Chapter 58), pulmonary embolism (Chapter 98), and air space disease (a continuum encompassing atelectasis [Chapter 90], bronchitis [Chapter 96], aspiration [Chapter 94], mucous plugging, and pneumonia).

TABLE 433-1 CRITERIA FOR DIAGNOSIS OF POSTOPERATIVE MYOCARDIAL INFARCTION

The diagnosis of perioperative MI requires any one of the following criteria.

Criterion 1: A typical rise in the troponin level or a typical fall in an elevated troponin level detected at its peak after surgery in a patient without a documented alternative explanation for an elevated troponin level (e.g., pulmonary embolism) or a rapid rise and fall in CK-MB only if troponin measurement is unavailable.*
This criterion requires that one of the following criteria be met:
   Ischemic signs or symptoms (e.g., chest, arm, or jaw discomfort; shortness of breath; pulmonary edema)
   Development of pathologic Q waves on an ECG
   Changes on an ECG indicative of ischemia
   Coronary artery intervention
   New or presumed new cardiac wall motion abnormality on echocardiography or new or presumed new fixed defect on radionuclide imaging

Criterion 2: Pathologic findings of acute or healing MI

Criterion 3: Development of new pathologic Q waves on an ECG if troponin levels were not obtained or were obtained at times that could have missed the clinical event

*Because CK-MB is both less sensitive and less specific than troponin levels in the perioperative setting than in other settings, it should be used for diagnostic purposes only when troponin levels are not obtainable.
CK-MB = creatine kinase MB isoenzyme; ECG = electrocardiogram; MI = myocardial infarction.
Reproduced with permission from Devereaux PJ, Goldman L, Yusuf S, et al. Surveillance and prevention of major perioperative ischemic cardiac events in patients undergoing noncardiac surgery: a review. CMAJ. 2005;173:779-788.

Distinguishing among these considerations requires focusing on the speed of onset, timing relative to surgery, vital signs, findings on oximetry, and physical examination findings (Chapter 83). Fluid overload is most commonly seen soon after the cessation of positive-pressure ventilation or vasodilating analgesia. It is also common 3 to 5 days postoperatively when fluid that had been "third spaced" is mobilized into the intravascular compartment. Interventions that are safe in most situations include administration of oxygen and withholding of sedation. The use of continuous positive airway pressure can reduce the rate of reintubation in hypoxemic postoperative patients.[A3] Other interventions that will be helpful or harmful, depending on the specific situation, include diuretics, opioids, elaborate medical imaging, and vigorous physiotherapy.

Anorexia

Loss of appetite (Chapter 132) after surgery has an extensive differential diagnosis that can be narrowed substantially if the patient was eating properly before surgery. The immediate priority is to search for and correct underlying contributors. Oral, enteral, or parenteral support is not the priority initially, although such support may become necessary. Drug toxicity is a particularly common, easily detected when considered, and a rapidly reversible contributor to postoperative anorexia. Anatomic abnormalities are usually evident by medical imaging studies. Other common metabolic contributors include abnormalities in electrolytes, calcium, phosphorus, and magnesium. Acalculous cholecystitis (Chapter 155) is an important postoperative complication that must be considered in a patient with right upper quadrant tenderness.

Vomiting

Vomiting is the extreme form of nausea in the postoperative setting, and the two symptoms share the same differential diagnosis. In most patients, vomiting is unexpected and merits immediate attention. Initial management is to ensure that the patient's airway is protected, to discontinue oral medications (and find parenteral substitutes if necessary), and to consider insertion of a nasogastric tube. In patients after gastrointestinal surgery, the priority considerations include the possibility of an anastomotic leak, peritoneal abscess, and other anatomic abnormality. In patients after operations on more remote parts of the body, the priorities are emetogenic medications (such

TABLE 433-2 DISTINGUISHING AMONG COMMON CAUSES OF ACUTE POSTOPERATIVE DYSPNEA

	PULMONARY AIR SPACE	FLUID OVERLOAD/HEART FAILURE	PULMONARY THROMBOEMBOLISM
CHARACTERISTICS OF TIMING			
Days since surgery	1-7 days	0-5 days	5-28 days
Speed of onset	1-3 days	1-24 hours	1-5 minutes
PREVIOUS HISTORY			
Previous lung disease	++		
Previous heart failure		++	
Previous venous thrombosis			++
ABNORMAL VITAL SIGNS			
Temperature			
Heart rate	+	+	+
Blood pressure	+	+	++
Respiratory rate	+	++	+
Oximetry	++		+
PHYSICAL EXAMINATION			
Jugular venous distention		+	+
Pulmonary rales	+	++	
S$_3$ gallop		++	
RESPONSE TO TREATMENT			
Oxygen	+	+	+
Anticholinergic bronchodilators	+	+	+
Withdrawal of sedatives	+	+	+
Aggressive physiotherapy	++		
Diuretics/afterload reduction		++	

as postoperative chemotherapy), gastroparesis associated with autonomic neuropathy, and fecal impaction. Multiple antinausea medications are available for symptomatic relief (e.g., prochlorperazine, ondansetron, dexamethasone, droperidol) and act in an additive manner when they are used in combination (e.g., prochlorperazine 5 mg intramuscularly plus ondansetron 4 mg intramuscularly). [A5] If no reversible contributor is identified, the default diagnosis is prolonged idiopathic ileus, and a therapeutic trial of intravenous neostigmine can be considered (e.g., neostigmine 2.5 mg intravenously during 5 minutes).

Diarrhea

Diarrhea (Chapter 140) is relatively rare after surgery and involves a limited number of possibilities if the patient's bowel movements were normal before surgery. In such cases, the situation represents an acute-onset diarrhea that is usually secretory in nature. The immediate priority is to exclude toxic megacolon, which is caused by overgrowth of toxigenic *Clostridium difficile* and is a potential emergency. Clinical evaluation for toxic megacolon requires assessment for tachycardia, hypotension, delirium, and other signs of sepsis rather than waiting on initial stool studies for confirmation of infection with *C. difficile*. Risk factors for antibiotic-associated diarrhea include advanced age, use of broad-spectrum antibiotics (e.g., third-generation cephalosporins), and unknown host susceptibility factors (e.g., past episodes of pseudomembranous colitis). A definitive diagnosis is frequently never established, and treatment focuses on feeding the patient a lactose-free diet while avoiding intestinal paralytics. Complete resolution is typical, provided adequate fluid and electrolyte levels are maintained.

Weakness

Generalized weakness after surgery is almost inevitable, but focal weakness may reflect nerve damage caused by intraoperative positioning (e.g., damage to the facial nerve after carotid endarterectomy) and rarely indicates a new intracranial event (e.g., intracerebral bleeding [Chapter 408] secondary to anticoagulation). Neurologic deficits are often overlooked during the initial postoperative interval and may become apparent only after the patient has regained strength elsewhere in the body. Conversely, new deficits that are evident early after surgery and resolve rapidly thereafter may reflect an old stroke that was fully compensated during less stressful circumstances. Medical imaging of the brain is worthwhile if no explanation is apparent on initial assessment. Nonfocal weakness commonly responds to physical therapy.

Delirium

Changes in mental status after surgery are common, especially in elderly patients (Chapter 28), and can be remarkably difficult to correct. The immediate priorities are to determine whether the impairment is acute or chronic and to detect easily reversible contributors (such as infection, hypoglycemia, and alkalosis). A complete assessment is often unnecessary if the patient had normal mental status before surgery because many dementia syndromes are thereby excluded (such as vitamin B_{12} deficiency, tertiary syphilis, and Alzheimer's disease). Immediate treatment usually focuses on discontinuation of medications such as anticholinergics, narcotics, and tranquilizers. The patient may also benefit from the continuous presence of friends and family members, who can provide frequent orientation and constant attention. A sense of patience is necessary because delirium rarely resolves instantly. The benefit of low-dose neuroleptics (e.g., risperidone, 0.5 mg by mouth twice daily) remains uncertain. Delirium after surgery is associated with a significant decline in cognitive ability during the next year, with a trajectory characterized by an initial decline and prolonged impairment.[4]

Seizures

The development of uncontrolled seizures (Chapter 403) after surgery is rare. The immediate priorities are to exclude status epilepticus, to uncover any past history of a seizure disorder, and to identify provocative factors. Neurosurgical patients typically undergo a standardized treatment protocol, including steroids and imaging. Other conditions that can cause abnormal movements must be excluded, such as septic rigors, delirium tremens, Parkinson's disease, major psychopathology, hypothermic shivering, and hypercapnic asterixis. Additional considerations include detection and correction of any underlying metabolic abnormalities, such as hypocalcemia, hypoxemia, hyponatremia, hypophosphatemia, and drug toxicity. Treatment focuses primarily on reversing the underlying precipitating cause and providing nonspecific care with benzodiazepines, phenytoin, and ongoing monitoring.

Signs

Hypertension

Hypertension may reflect a variety of disorders and must be treated in a manner that neither overreacts nor underreacts to the situation. Hypertension is particularly common after neurosurgical procedures or carotid endarterectomy. The initial assessment focuses on whether the patient has chronic hypertension based on the past history, current electrocardiogram, or findings on funduscopy. Other potential causes include undertreated pain, agitated delirium, fluid overload, alcohol withdrawal, and inadvertent discontinuation of chronic antihypertensive medications. In uncertain cases, systemic analgesia is often helpful, along with nitrates (e.g., nitroglycerin, 0.4 mg/hour transdermally) and β-blockers (e.g., metoprolol, 5 mg intravenously). The major complication of treatment is the potential for overcorrection and inadvertent hypotension; such errors are particularly common in patients with no evidence of past hypertension.

Hypotension

Hypotension (Chapter 8) after surgery is generally an emergency, and the immediate concern is internal bleeding, especially after intra-abdominal operations or when anticoagulation is used to prevent venous thrombosis. The initial stages of hypotension are frequently unrecognized because of biologic stress responses by patients, psychological denial by clinicians, and misattribution to the concurrent use of analgesia. Early hypotension is particularly easy to overlook if the patient has coexisting chronic hypertension and the apparently "normal" blood pressure is dismissed as unremarkable. Treatment usually entails volume supplementation,[5] vasopressors as needed (Chapters 107 and 108), serial assessments, and a search for underlying causes. An extensive differential diagnosis sometimes needs to be considered if no anatomic cause related to surgery is evident (Chapter 106). Routine use of pulmonary artery catheters to guide therapy is not helpful,[A5] whereas prompt echocardiography can almost always find the cause of severe hemodynamic instability.

Tachycardia

Tachycardia after surgery can be caused by myriad arrhythmias (Chapters 64 and 65) and may contribute to postoperative cardiac ischemia. Distinguishing between newly detected and newly incident tachycardia can sometimes be accomplished by determining whether the patient does or does not complain of palpitations. An initial assessment also requires review of the electrocardiogram to distinguish atrial fibrillation from other disorders. The goal of treatment is to identify and to correct precipitating factors, such as pain, blood loss, hypoxia, electrolyte abnormalities, fluid overload, volume depletion, pulmonary embolism, and drug withdrawal. Most arrhythmias respond to correction of the underlying abnormality. Specific antiarrhythmic treatment, when needed, is generally similar to that used in the nonoperative setting (Chapters 64 and 65). For atrial fibrillation, anticoagulation is sometimes contraindicated; in such situations, cardioversion within 48 hours merits consideration. Postoperative atrial fibrillation portends a 2-fold higher long-term risk of ischemic stroke.[6]

Fever

Fever (Chapter 280) after surgery is common, frequently perplexing, and often multifactorial. Worrisome possibilities include transfusion reactions (Chapter 177), hospital-acquired pneumonia (Chapter 97), urinary tract infection (Chapter 284), line sepsis (Chapter 282), and wound infection. In many cases, no definitive cause is found, the patient recovers spontaneously, and the default diagnosis is atelectasis. Detailed evaluation, when necessary, requires culture of blood, urine, and the surgical site to identify specific microbiologic organisms. Selection of empirical antibiotics is usually based on local practice patterns and hospital ecology, with the disadvantages of breeding resistant organisms. Hydration, nutrition, and general supportive care are important yet frequently neglected needs of patients with prolonged elevations in body temperature. Selective decontamination of the digestive tract and oropharynx appears to be beneficial but chlorhexidine is not.[A6]

Edema

Peripheral edema (Chapter 51), which is often first noticed by nursing staff after surgery, is rarely life-threatening unless it is treated with excessive diuretics. The cause is usually multifactorial and includes increased hydrostatic pressure (including heart failure and gravity from intraoperative positioning), decreased oncotic pressure (related to hypoalbuminemia from decreased liver production or increased losses), and capillary leak (potentially caused by medications or tissue reactions). Treatment focuses on correction of underlying abnormalities, maintenance of nutrition, judicious use of diuretics, monitoring of renal function, provision of systemic anticoagulation against deep venous thrombosis, and efforts toward mobilization of the patient. A low-salt diet, afterload reduction, and aldosterone antagonists (e.g., oral spironolactone, 25 mg once daily) may be helpful in patients in whom heart failure (Chapter 59) is the dominant mechanism.

Laboratory

Leukocytosis

An elevated white blood cell count (Chapter 167) can have many causes, but the immediate priority is to exclude a life-threatening septic process (Chapters 106 and 108). Direct microscopic examination of the peripheral blood smear (Chapter 157) can be helpful to check for toxic granulations (see Fig. 157-18), Döhle's bodies (see Fig. 157-19), and a shift toward primitive band cells. Many cases are due to noninfectious causes, including infarcted tissue (skin, heart, intestinal tract), inflammatory conditions (renal insufficiency, diabetic ketoacidosis, lupus erythematosus), and demargination stress reactions (dehydration, systemic corticosteroids, inotropic medications). In the absence of direct evidence, some clinicians may initiate antibiotics empirically, whereas others may elect waiting. Substantial controversy remains about the proper duration of an empirical trial of antibiotics when no cause is discovered and the patient is otherwise recovering.

Anemia

Anemia (Chapter 158) is common and sometimes underappreciated because coexisting volume depletion causes the blood hemoglobin concentration to underestimate the degree of blood loss. Major perioperative hemorrhage is associated with subsequent stroke and MI in patients undergoing noncardiac, non-neurologic surgery.[7] The initial priority is to differentiate bleeding at the surgical site from other causes. In many cases, the exact cause is unclear, and substantial uncertainty may arise over the need to initiate gastric acid suppression therapy or to interrupt systemic anticoagulation against venous thrombosis. In a large randomized trial, transfusion at a hemoglobin threshold of 10 g/dL was no better than transfusion for symptoms of anemia or at the physician's discretion for a hemoglobin level of below 8 g/dL.[A7] Guidelines for transfusion therapy depend on the patient's cardiac reserve as well as on the available blood bank supply at the particular medical center. A reasonable goal is to maintain a hemoglobin level of 7 mg/dL or higher, except in patients with cardiovascular disease, in whom a hemoglobin goal of 10 mg/dL is reasonable. The immediate postoperative interval is not usually the appropriate time to initiate erythropoietin, oral iron replacement, or detailed evaluations for other hematologic abnormalities.

Abnormalities in Platelet Count

Patients often have abnormal platelet counts after surgery yet rarely require further evaluation or treatment. In most cases, the thrombocytopenia is mild, does not require transfusion therapy, resolves in a few weeks, and is not a sign of an ominous disorder (e.g., sepsis or heparin-induced thrombocytopenia). Platelet transfusions are indicated if the decrease in platelet count is extreme, accompanied by evidence of major blood loss, or related to recent surgery on the central nervous system (including the eye). Thrombocytosis is also common about a month after surgery and is occasionally extreme. However, even postoperative thrombocytosis exceeding 1,000,000/mL rarely necessitates treatment, does not predispose patients to unwanted clotting disorders, and typically resolves spontaneously after a few weeks.

Abnormal Sodium Concentration

Both hyponatremia and hypernatremia (Chapter 116) are frequent complications in the postoperative setting. The immediate priorities are to assess the patient's intravascular volume status and to correct possible volume depletion. The causes of hyponatremia are multifactorial, including excessive use of diuretics, high levels of intrinsic antidiuretic hormone (as a result of factors such as drugs, pain, and mechanical ventilation), and unmeasured osmoles (e.g., intravenous contrast agents). This risk for postoperative hyponatremia may be reduced by the administration of isotonic saline rather than by water restriction.[A8] Once hyponatremia develops, vasopressin antagonists (Chapter 116) are effective for both hypervolemic and euvolemic hyponatremia.[A9] Hypernatremia is always due to free water deficiency, which may indicate severe cognitive impairment or other factors interfering with the ability to express thirst or to ingest water. Correction is similar to that in the nonoperative setting. Abnormalities in sodium concentration require careful follow-up, can recur at any point after an operation, yet are rarely the root cause of a patient's inability to recover from surgery.

Abnormal Serum Potassium Concentration

Hyperkalemia and hypokalemia (Chapter 117) are also frequent postoperative complications. The immediate priority is to assess and to stabilize the patient's electrocardiographic findings. Hyperkalemia is usually due to cellular shifts, renal failure, and tissue destruction (including hemolysis). Hyperkalemia will generally be corrected with treatments that shift potassium into cells (e.g., intravenous glucose with or without insulin) and enhance total excretion (e.g., gastrointestinal binding agents). Hypokalemia is usually due to inadequate intake, excessive loss, or cellular shifts. Hypokalemia will generally be corrected with replacement therapy and rarely requires aldosterone antagonism. Both abnormalities can usually be treated as in the nonoperative setting (Chapter 117). The prognosis is favorable if the patient's electrocardiogram shows no major dysrhythmias and if renal function is preserved.

Alkalosis

Systemic alkalosis (Chapter 118) typically requires volume supplementation because the cause is generally intravascular volume depletion. Blood gas determinations may be necessary in some cases to exclude the possibility of concurrent carbon dioxide retention with compensatory metabolic alkalosis. Untreated, alkalosis can result in altered mentation, cardiac arrhythmias, and delayed mobilization. Most patients with postoperative alkalosis do not require carbonic anhydrase inhibitors or intravenous acid. The prognosis is usually favorable, with gradual correction during a period of several days. Rapid correction of alkalosis, unlike rapid correction of hyponatremia, is not known to cause neurologic injury.

Azotemia

The initial assessment of an elevated serum creatinine concentration (Chapter 114) focuses on reviewing previous values (to distinguish acute from chronic renal insufficiency) and identifying contributing factors (such as prerenal volume depletion, intrarenal nephrotoxins, or postrenal urethral obstruction). A trial of intravenous fluids may be useful on both a diagnostic and therapeutic basis. Treatment is the same as in the nonoperative setting. Subsequent monitoring is always necessary, with serum creatinine measurements obtained on a daily basis. Serial measurements of urinary volume and body weight as well as a urine culture are occasionally helpful in selected cases. The prognosis is dependent on the underlying factors and is less favorable after cardiac surgery.

Hyperbilirubinemia

Elevations in serum bilirubin (Chapter 147) are rare after surgery, even though abnormalities in liver enzyme levels occur frequently with general anesthesia. The most benign explanation is Gilbert's syndrome, but the immediate priority is to assess for possible hepatic failure (especially in patients who have received halothane). As in the nonoperative setting, treatment involves withdrawing potential hepatotoxins, supporting the patient, and allowing time for liver function to recover (Chapter 153). Treatment of hepatic encephalopathy is particularly important because of the constipation and generalized catabolic state that also follow major surgery. Monitoring should include serial measurement of liver function on a daily basis because each component (e.g., bilirubin, albumen, prothrombin time) can be altered by factors unrelated to the liver. The prognosis is unfavorable if the patient's liver function fails to recover quickly.

Hypoalbuminemia

Reductions in serum albumin are common after surgery and are an ominous prognostic finding. The cause is rarely decreased production if the reduction in the albumin level occurs rapidly. Possible explanations include nephrotic syndrome, capillary leak into extravascular spaces, and occult catabolism in unrecognized sites. Treatment with albumin infusions does not usually normalize the biochemical abnormality and does not seem to improve patient mortality rates significantly. The main priorities are to continue nutritional support, to preserve skin integrity, to minimize the use of systemic diuretics, to correct any contributing factors, and to consider correlated serum protein deficiencies (such as reduced levels of immunoglobulins or antithrombin III). Hypoalbuminemia can also cause indirect harm by the loss of carrier proteins, which thereby predisposes patients to potential drug toxicity. The long-term prognosis is favorable for survivors because the serum albumin level will eventually fully return to normal.

Abnormalities in Blood Glucose Concentration

In patients with diabetes mellitus (Chapter 229), serum blood glucose concentrations often become unstable after surgery because of altered dietary intake, decreased physical activity, and the release of counter-regulatory hormones. The priority is to avoid hypoglycemia, severe hyperglycemia, diabetic ketoacidosis, cerebral damage, and repeated events. Intensive control of the blood glucose level increases the risk for severe hypoglycemia and death, so a target glucose level of about 140 to 200 mg/dL is recommended.[A10] Rapid reversal of sepsis or focal infection can lead to a precipitous decrease in insulin requirements; in such cases, vigilance is required because unsuspected hypoglycemia may cause permanent damage or be fatal in a patient who may otherwise seem to be sleeping. Patients need to be forewarned that temporary doses of subcutaneous insulin may be required but do not commit the patient to chronic insulin therapy. Monitoring involves serial measurement of blood glucose concentration until the patient is eating in a reliable manner.

Special Situations
Multiplicity

Some postoperative complications are difficult to classify because no single dominant problem is apparent by symptoms, signs, or laboratory test results. Instead, patients may have multiple problems that need to be addressed simultaneously. The immediate goal is to set priorities and to avoid the temptation to try to eliminate every possibility on the first day. The corollary is to continue to check progress during the subsequent days needed for a complete diagnosis and successful therapy. Because so many concerns require attention in the postoperative interval, the risk is that clinicians will lose track of a secondary issue and make an error that seems obvious in retrospect.

Redundancy

Postoperative complications sometimes generate multiple consultations with physicians who have overlapping abilities. An example might be a patient with a postoperative fever that prompts consultations from pulmonology, nephrology, dermatology, general medicine, and infectious disease specialists. In theory, gathering a critical mass of medical experts together should increase the likelihood of accurate diagnosis, timely treatment, and foolproof follow-up. In reality, however, coordination and communication are never perfect. Personal rivalries, diffusion of responsibility, and many other psychological factors may impede interactions among consultants. Opportunities for miscommunication may be further accentuated if the patient has an exotic diagnosis that is a special draw on the consultant's attention (e.g., pheochromocytoma). Arguing in front of the patient, in view of other professionals, or in the medical record can be demoralizing. The priority is to communicate effectively with the surgical team responsible for the patient and to encourage that team to make final decisions.

Ambiguity

Another vexation occurs when an urgent request is not connected to a clear rationale (Chapter 430). Diplomacy is needed to establish whether the motivation reflects medicolegal concerns rather than biologic changes in the patient. Sometimes the stimulus that drives the consultation can best be addressed by providing reassurance and confirmation. Sometimes the stimulus is an obscure preexisting disorder (e.g., moyamoya disease), and the surgical team has neither the experience nor the time to investigate how this unrelated medical condition can influence recovery from surgery. Sometimes the stimulus is an unspoken political wish to transfer the care of a burdensome patient from one physician to another. A consultant should develop an understanding of how to interact with other clinicians under such ambiguous circumstances.

Setting Priorities

Requests for consultation often arrive outside conventional working hours, are usually tinged with a sense of urgency, and sometimes cluster to encompass more than one patient. Developing an effective method for prioritizing patients is a crucial clinical skill. One communication strategy is to provide an objective estimated time of arrival for the initial request from the surgical team. An often helpful treatment strategy is to make some safe suggestions at the time of the initial request so that clear-cut recommendations can be instituted during the interval before the patient is seen and used later to help evaluate the patient's status and course.

Aftermath

In many postoperative cases, the original reason for consultation may resolve and no major issues remain. The situation now provides an opportunity to review the patient, particularly for the appropriate use of unrelated medications. The consultant may often detect excessive medications that were appropriate early in the hospital course but have ceased to be necessary, thereby justifying discontinuation (e.g., diuretics, antibiotics, bronchodilators). Discontinuing medications that have become superfluous requires initiative and wisdom, and the common mistake is to propagate unnecessary medications in stable patients under the rationale of "don't mess with success." The ability to watch the patient for several hours or for a day or two often presents an ideal opportunity for the safe withdrawal of medications. Ironically, discontinuing a treatment sometimes requires more skill, time, and initiative than starting it.

Grade A References

A1. Gould MK, Garcia DA, Wren SM, et al. Prevention of VTE in nonorthopedic surgical patients. Antithrombotic Therapy and Prevention of Thrombosis, 9th ed: American College of Chest Physicians Evidence-Based Clinical Practice Guidelines. *Chest.* 2012;141:e227S-e277S.
A2. Falck-Ytter Y, Francis CW, Johanson NA, et al. Prevention of VTE in orthopedic surgery patients. Antithrombotic Therapy and Prevention of Thrombosis, 9th ed: American College of Chest Physicians Evidence-Based Clinical Practice Guidelines. *Chest.* 2012;141:e278S-325S.
A3. Squadrone V, Coha M, Cerutti E, et al. Continuous positive airway pressure for treatment of postoperative hypoxemia: a randomized controlled trial. *JAMA.* 2005;293:589-595.
A4. Apfel CC, Korttila K, Abdalla M, et al. A factorial trial of six interventions for the prevention of postoperative nausea and vomiting. *N Engl J Med.* 2004;350:2441-2451.
A5. Sandham JD, Jull RD, Brant RF, et al. A randomized, controlled trial of the use of pulmonary-artery catheters in high-risk surgical patients. *N Engl J Med.* 2003;348:5-14.
A6. Price R, MacLennan G, Glen J. SuDDICU Collaboration. Selective digestive or oropharyngeal decontamination and topical oropharyngeal chlorhexidine for prevention of death in general intensive care: systematic review and network meta-analysis. *BMJ.* 2014;348:g2197.
A7. Carson JL, Terrin ML, Noveck H, et al. Liberal or restrictive transfusion in high-risk patients after hip surgery. *N Engl J Med.* 2011;365:2453-2462.
A8. Neville KA, Sandeman DJ, Rubinstein A, et al. Prevention of hyponatremia during maintenance intravenous fluid administration: a prospective randomized study of fluid type versus fluid rate. *J Pediatr.* 2010;156:313-319.
A9. Rozen-Svi B, Yahav D, Gheorghiade M, et al. Vasopressin receptor antagonists for the treatment of hyponatremia: systematic review and meta-analysis. *Am J Kidney Dis.* 2010;56:325-337.
A10. Kansagara D, Fu R, Freeman M, et al. Intensive insulin therapy in hospitalized patients: a systematic review. *Ann Intern Med.* 2011;154:268-282.

GENERAL REFERENCES

For the General References and other additional features, please visit Expert Consult at https://expertconsult.inkling.com.

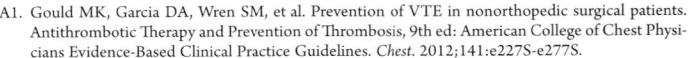

434

MEDICAL CONSULTATION IN PSYCHIATRY

PETER MANU

HEALTH STATUS IN PSYCHIATRIC PATIENTS

The physical health of psychiatric patients is poor, with a higher risk for death at an early age than in the mentally sane. Poverty, social neglect, substandard medical care, unhealthy life habits, and complications of psychiatric treatments are major contributors to the increased morbidity and mortality of patients with chronic psychiatric disorders, who have a 20-year average decline in life expectancy. Integrated care models that coordinate general medical care with psychiatric care can help meet the needs of patients with chronic psychiatric problems.[1]

MEDICAL EVALUATION IN PSYCHIATRIC SETTINGS

Inpatient psychiatric care is provided in the United States in 444 non-federal, self-standing psychiatric hospitals with a total of 101,500 beds and 1373 general hospitals with inpatient psychiatric units. Requirements for medical training in psychiatry vary. In the United States, psychiatric residents have up

TABLE 434-1 COMMON REASONS FOR TRANSFERRING PSYCHIATRIC INPATIENTS WITH ACUTE MEDICAL DETERIORATION TO A GENERAL HOSPITAL

Fever	17%
Neurologic deficits, seizures, alteration of consciousness	14%
Fall, head trauma	13%
Abdominal pain, gastrointestinal bleeding	10%
Dyspnea, hypoxia	10%
Chest pain	8%
Urinary retention, azotemia, electrolyte imbalance	7%
Arrhythmia, hypotension, syncope	6%
Edema, cellulitis	5%
All others	10%

From Manu P, Asif M, Khan S, et al. Risk factors for medical deterioration of psychiatric inpatients: opportunities for early recognition and prevention. *Compr Psychiatry.* 2012;53:968-974.

TABLE 434-2 MAJOR MEDICAL COMPLICATIONS OF PSYCHOTROPIC DRUGS

CARDIOVASCULAR	
Cardiomyopathy	Clozapine
Hypertension	MAO inhibitors, venlafaxine
Myocarditis	Clozapine
Orthostatic hypotension	Tricyclics, trazodone, antipsychotics
QTc prolongation	Antipsychotics, tricyclics
Venous thromboembolism	Clozapine, risperidone, phenothiazines
RESPIRATORY	
Choking	Antipsychotics, tricyclics
Laryngospasm	Antipsychotics
Respiratory depression	Benzodiazepines, barbiturates, methadone, antidepressants, atypical antipsychotics
GASTROINTESTINAL	
Bowel obstruction	Tricyclics, antipsychotics
Dysphagia	Tricyclics, antipsychotics
Hepatic impairment	Carbamazepine, valproic acid, phenothiazines, mirtazapine, nefazodone, quetiapine, olanzapine, clozapine, MAO inhibitors, naltrexone
Pancreatitis	Carbamazepine, valproic acid, clozapine, olanzapine
KIDNEY AND URINARY TRACT	
Renal insufficiency	Lithium, clozapine
Urinary retention	Antipsychotics, tricyclics
ENDOCRINE	
Hyperprolactinemia	First-generation antipsychotics, risperidone
Hypothyroidism	Lithium, quetiapine
Inappropriate ADH secretion	Serotonin reuptake inhibitors, methadone, tricyclics
Metabolic syndrome	Clozapine, olanzapine, risperidone, quetiapine
HEMATOLOGIC	
Leukocytosis	Lithium
Neutropenia	Clozapine, olanzapine, risperidone, carbamazepine, valproate, mirtazapine
Thrombocytopenia	Carbamazepine, valproate
MUSCULOSKELETAL	
Rhabdomyolysis*	Antipsychotics, serotonin reuptake inhibitors, MAO inhibitors
SKIN	
Stevens-Johnson syndrome	Lamotrigine, carbamazepine, barbiturates
OTHER	
Fever*	Antipsychotics, serotonin reuptake inhibitors, MAO inhibitors
Seizure	Bupropion, MAO inhibitors, tricyclics, phenothiazines

*Includes neuroleptic malignant syndrome and serotonin syndrome.
ADH = antidiuretic hormone; MAO = monoamine oxidase.

to 4 months of inpatient medical training. With such limited medical training, psychiatrists cannot be expected to be experts in assessing nonpsychiatric problems. Free-standing psychiatric facilities employ consultants to evaluate medical issues and to manage outpatient-level conditions, but they are not equipped to provide inpatient-level medical or surgical services. Patients who require a higher level of care are transferred to a medical, surgical, or medical/psychiatric unit of a general hospital.

As many as 15% of patients who are admitted for psychiatric care may be transferred to a general hospital for medical conditions that arise or deteriorate during inpatient psychiatric care.[2] Febrile illnesses, acute neurologic changes, and falls account for nearly half of the transfers (Table 434-1). Nearly half of the patients admitted for dementia with behavioral disturbance will develop a medical complication during an inpatient psychiatric stay, a rate that is two- to three-fold higher than for other psychiatric patients. Renal insufficiency, anemia, poor nutritional status, and older age are also independent predictors of medical deterioration.

Medical deterioration can have major adverse consequences for psychiatric inpatients. First, it may lead to life-threatening complications if the condition is not rapidly diagnosed and treated. Second, it interrupts behavioral interventions and may require the discontinuation of psychotropic drug treatment or electroconvulsive therapy (ECT). Third, it prolongs the length of stay and can add considerable expense to the episode of psychiatric illness, especially when patients are transferred from locked psychiatric units to a general hospital, where they require constant observation by qualified personnel.

EVALUATION OF CHIEF COMPLAINTS

Medical consultation for psychiatric patients creates unique challenges in evaluation of the chief complaint. Many patients with outpatient psychiatric disorders have somatic symptoms, such as fatigue, weakness, dizziness, headache, insomnia, widespread pain, and constipation. In most of these patients, the underlying mental illnesses are mood disorders (unipolar depression and dysthymia), anxiety disorders (panic disorder and generalized anxiety disorder), somatoform disorders, substance use disorders (most often alcohol, opiates, cocaine, and benzodiazepine), and borderline personality disorder. As a group, these patients have many physical complaints and resist a psychological explanation for their symptoms even when the medical evaluation fails to identify objective abnormalities. Standardized screening approaches can help clinicians and patients alike.[3]

In contrast, patients admitted for inpatient psychiatric treatment often have psychotic disorders, developmental abnormalities, or dementia with behavioral disturbance; they are frequently vague or silent about physical suffering and only rarely voice somatic delusions. Such patients may deny pain even after bowel perforation or myocardial infarction.

Medical consultation in psychiatry is not more difficult than in other clinical settings but must be informed by knowledge about the serious complications of psychiatric treatments (Table 434-2). A rigorous diagnostic evaluation is therefore required to avoid the errors of omission created by the weak correlation between complaints and disease. This evaluation should include consideration of physical disorders, drug effects (adverse reaction, toxicity, or withdrawal), cognitive impairment (delirium), sensory impairment (loss of vision, hearing, speech, or postural balance), and situational maladjustment (isolation, overload, or loss of privacy). Attribution of symptoms to the patient's psychiatric condition should remain a diagnosis of exclusion.

MEDICAL COMPLICATIONS OF PSYCHIATRIC TREATMENTS

Antipsychotic-Induced Metabolic Syndrome

Metabolic syndrome is more prevalent (range, 29 to 63%) in schizophrenic and other psychiatric patients treated with second-generation antipsychotics, especially clozapine but also olanzapine, risperidone, and quetiapine because they induce substantial weight gain. The mechanism of weight gain centers on the drug's affinity for the histamine$_1$ (H$_1$)–receptor and the neurobiologic mechanisms that regulate appetite and metabolism through the production and activity of serotonin, leptin, and tumor necrosis factor-α. As a result, up to 40% of patients receiving long-term treatment with antipsychotics have prediabetes, and about 10% have diabetes.[4]

Because the glucose intolerance often seen in patients treated with antipsychotic agents is due to insulin resistance (Chapter 229), it is best treated by aggressive weight reduction (Chapter 213), increasing physical activity (Chapter 16), and metformin (Chapter 229) or a combination of these. For example, in randomized trials, metformin, 850 mg twice daily, significantly reduced the weight gain and reversed the metabolic abnormalities associated with the initiation of second-generation antipsychotic drugs,[A1] and a single daily dose of 750 mg may prevent weight gain if it is initiated at the onset of olanzapine treatment.[A2] Another option is to switch from olanzapine, quetiapine, or risperidone to aripiprazole.[A3] In treating hypertension, β-adrenergic blockers should be used cautiously in patients receiving neuroleptics because they increase the potential for orthostatic hypotension, syncope, and falls. Smoking cessation programs combining transdermal or transmucosal nicotine replacement, bupropion, and cognitive-behavioral therapy should be strongly recommended despite the dismally high failure rates that have been reported in patients with chronic schizophrenia (Chapter 32).

Antipsychotic-Induced Myocarditis and Cardiomyopathy
Antipsychotic-induced myocarditis and cardiomyopathy (Chapter 60) are most common in patients treated with clozapine (0.9%) and fluphenazine (0.4%). In contrast, the risk for these complications is only 0.1% in patients receiving haloperidol, thioridazine, and risperidone.

The accepted pathophysiologic explanation for myocarditis is an immunoglobulin E–mediated acute hypersensitivity reaction, similar to the allergic myocarditis produced by penicillins, sulfonamides, and methyldopa. In a small number of patients, a competing hypothesis proposes that clozapine induces hypereosinophilic myocarditis, colitis, hepatitis, pancreatitis, alveolitis, and interstitial nephritis. A direct cardiotoxic effect of drug metabolites cannot be excluded.

In patients in whom myocarditis develops, the mortality rate is as high as 50%, with almost half the deaths occurring suddenly and unexpectedly. The average duration of exposure to clozapine before diagnosis or death is 21 days, and the dosage range is 50 to 725 mg/day. Common symptoms are fever (48%), dyspnea (35%), influenza-like illness (30%), chest pain (22%), and fatigue (17%). Laboratory features include left ventricular hypokinesia or reduced ejection fraction (48%) or pericardial effusion (17%) on echocardiography, nonspecific repolarization abnormalities on electrocardiography (35%), peripheral eosinophilia (35%), elevated creatine kinase and troponin levels (22%), and radiographic evidence of heart failure (13%). The diagnosis can be confirmed by endomyocardial biopsy showing fraying of myocytes and perivascular infiltrates with degranulated eosinophils. Among survivors, symptoms resolve or substantially improve after discontinuation of clozapine and treatment with high-dose corticosteroids (e.g., prednisone, 1 mg/kg/day for 4 days, tapered to 0.33 mg/kg/day for the following 4 days).

Clozapine-induced dilated cardiomyopathy may be caused by an evolving myocarditis or by chronic injury mediated by free radicals, similar to the myocarditis produced by doxorubicin (Chapter 60). The demographic features are similar to those of myocarditis, but the mean duration of treatment before diagnosis is much longer (9 months vs. 3 weeks), and the mortality rate is lower (22% vs. 51%). Patients have clinical or echocardiographic evidence of left ventricular dysfunction without eosinophilia or enzymatic evidence of myocardial necrosis.

Prolonged QTc Interval and Sudden Death
Significant prolongation of the QTc interval (Chapter 65) leading to ventricular tachyarrhythmias and sudden cardiac death (Chapter 63) can occur after antipsychotic treatment with the usual doses of thioridazine, haloperidol, and sertindole. Abnormal myocardial repolarization has been observed during treatment with most antipsychotic medications and after intentional or accidental overdoses of tricyclic antidepressants, lithium, and methadone (Chapter 110). All antipsychotics affect the cardiac potassium channel by blocking the rapidly activating component of the rectifier potassium current (Chapter 61). This effect translates into a dose-dependent increase in the duration of phase 3 of the action potential. The drug concentration that produces 50% inhibition of rapid potassium outflow varies for each drug (e.g., 1 nmol/L for haloperidol and 6 nmol/L for olanzapine). Compared with nonusers of antipsychotic drugs, the risk for sudden death is twice as high for current users of conventional (first-generation) antipsychotics and is 2.25 times higher for current users of atypical (second-generation) antipsychotics. All patients about to start antipsychotic drugs should be asked about a personal history of syncope and a family history of long QT syndrome or sudden death at a young age. A baseline electrocardiogram and serum electrolyte values should be obtained before starting of antipsychotic drug therapy, tricyclic antidepressants, and methadone. Interval electrocardiograms should be obtained after each increase in medication in older patients, patients with known heart disease, and those starting other drugs known to produce QTc prolongation or hypokalemia (Chapter 65). A QTc interval of 500 milliseconds or longer requires the discontinuation of all drugs that affect membrane repolarization. QTc intervals longer than 450 milliseconds in men and 470 milliseconds in women, QTc dispersion (difference between the longest and shortest QTc on a 12-lead electrocardiogram) longer than 100 milliseconds, and increase in QTc duration of more than 60 milliseconds in comparison to the baseline measurement should prompt re-evaluation of the risks and benefits associated with the drugs in question.

Choking and Laryngeal Dystonia
Asphyxia deaths from choking occur at a rate of 0.8% per 1000 psychiatric patients each year, a frequency that is more than 100 times greater than in the general population. In addition, videofluoroscopy demonstrates silent aspiration in 38% of psychiatric patients who survive a choking incident. Half the psychiatric patients with dysphagia have a fast-eating syndrome seen in association with restlessness, poor chewing skills, food pocketing in the cheeks, and attention deficits that characterize psychotic disorders and mental retardation. Bradykinetic dysphagia, which is seen in 25% of psychiatric patients with choking episodes, is due to the antidopaminergic and anticholinergic effects of psychotropic medications. This condition, which features reduced lingual range of motion, increased oral transit time, decreased pharyngeal peristalsis, and delayed initiation of the swallowing reflex, is seen in patients with neurologic features of drug-induced Parkinsonism (Chapter 409). Dyskinetic dysphagia (7% of choking cases), which generally occurs in patients maintained with long-term antipsychotic medication, is part of the clinical spectrum of tardive dyskinesia (Chapter 410). The examination reveals involuntary contractions of the tongue and perioral musculature, clumsiness of voluntary movements of the tongue, and discontinuous bolus propulsion in the oral stage. In the remaining patients, the dysphagia is due to cerebrovascular disease (11%) or to pharyngeal or esophageal disease (7%).

Laryngeal dystonia, which is a life-threatening complication of antipsychotic drug therapy, primarily with haloperidol and phenothiazines, is produced by acute spasmodic contraction of the adductor laryngeal muscles. Symptoms include respiratory distress, dysphonia, and stridor. Neuroleptic-induced bronchospasm may precede the onset of stridor. Patients typically indicate extreme subjective distress by clutching their anterior cervical area. Most patients also have other dystonias involving the head and neck, including torticollis, retrocollis, trismus, tongue protrusion, and deviation of the eyes (up, down, or sideward). In general, the symptoms and signs develop in the first week after starting or rapidly increasing the dose of neuroleptic medications. A reduction in the dose of anticholinergic or antiparkinsonian medication used to prevent or to treat extrapyramidal symptoms can also precipitate laryngeal dystonia. The condition is more common in young men and must be distinguished from epiglottitis, allergic or anaphylactic laryngeal edema or laryngospasm, mechanical obstruction, and psychogenic stridor. Intravenous administration of diphenhydramine (initial dose, 25 mg; may repeat after 5 minutes if symptoms persist) is the treatment of choice, and endotracheal intubation is seldom required.

Drug-Induced Neutropenia and Agranulocytosis
Drug-induced neutropenia with absolute neutrophil counts of less than 1500/μL has been observed during treatment with most second-generation antipsychotics (clozapine, olanzapine, risperidone, and quetiapine) and mood stabilizers (carbamazepine, valproic acid, and lamotrigine) as well as with some antidepressant drugs (tricyclic antidepressants and mirtazapine). Clozapine-induced neutropenia occurs in 4 to 5% of patients within 6 months after treatment is started and progresses to agranulocytosis in 10% or more of neutropenic patients if the drug is continued. In vitro, clozapine toxicity requires peroxide and peroxidase, and the defect in oxidation is related to abnormalities in the NQO2 (quinone oxidoreductase) gene involved in drug detoxification. Treatment with clozapine should be started only if the baseline absolute neutrophil count is higher than 1500/μL. The concomitant use of carbamazepine, angiotensin-converting enzyme inhibitors, sulfonamides, propylthiouracil, and mirtazapine should be avoided because they can produce neutropenia and increase the risk for agranulocytosis. Clozapine should be stopped and the patient evaluated immediately for fever, oral ulcerations, and symptoms or signs of infection. Complete blood counts should be obtained once a week for the first 26 weeks and every other week thereafter, and clozapine should be stopped and all medications reassessed if the absolute neutrophil count drops below 1500/μL. Clozapine-related agranulocytosis has been treated successfully with colony-stimulating factors (either granulocyte or granulocyte-macrophage colony-stimulating factor).

Neutropenia has also been associated with olanzapine, risperidone, and quetiapine in patients who have never received clozapine. Treatment with anticonvulsant mood stabilizers, particularly carbamazepine, is associated with a dose-dependent neutropenia and thrombocytopenia in approximately

TABLE 434-3	DIFFERENTIAL DIAGNOSIS OF NEUROLEPTIC MALIGNANT SYNDROME
Infection of the central nervous system	
Infection in patients with drug-induced Parkinsonism	
Drug overdose (psychostimulants, antidepressants, lithium, anticholinergics)	
Alcohol or drug withdrawal (benzodiazepines, barbiturates, antiparkinsonian drugs)	
Side effects of nonpsychotropic dopamine-depleting drugs (reserpine, metoclopramide, prochlorperazine, promethazine)	
Cholinergic rebound	
Serotonin syndrome	
Thyrotoxicosis	
Malignant hyperthermia	

TABLE 434-4	CLASSES OF MEDICATIONS THAT PRODUCE SEROTONIN SYNDROME IN PSYCHIATRIC PATIENTS
Selective serotonin reuptake inhibitors	
Monoamine oxidase inhibitors	
Atypical antipsychotics	
Heterocyclic antidepressants	
Trazodone	
Dual-uptake inhibitors	
Psychostimulants	
Buspirone	
Mood stabilizers	
Analgesics	
Antiemetics	
Cough suppressants	
Dietary supplements	

10% of patients in the first 6 months of treatment and should be monitored with complete blood counts twice each month during this period.

Neuroleptic Malignant Syndrome

Neuroleptic malignant syndrome, which occurs in approximately 0.2% of patients receiving neuroleptics, must be part of the differential diagnosis of fever and rhabdomyolysis (Chapter 113) in a psychiatric patient (Table 434-3). The frequency is greater in young men and patients who are malnourished or dehydrated, have Parkinson's disease, or are treated parenterally with large doses of neuroleptics during short periods. The main diagnostic criteria are elevated temperature (higher than 104°F [40°C] in 40% of patients) and diffuse muscle rigidity (ranging from mild hypertonicity to severe "lead pipe" stiffness). In addition, two or more of the following are required for a definitive diagnosis: (1) autonomic instability (tachycardia, elevated or labile blood pressure, postural hypotension, diaphoresis, sialorrhea, and urinary incontinence), (2) changes in mental status (ranging from confusion to mutism or coma), (3) leukocytosis (up to 20,000/mL), and (4) elevated creatine kinase (up to 100,000 IU/L). Other clinical manifestations include bradykinesia, chorea, dystonias, dysphagia, dysarthria or aphonia, seizures, and tremor. The severity of rhabdomyolysis correlates with the creatine kinase level and with the presence of myoglobinemia, myoglobinuria, metabolic acidosis, and azotemia. The electroencephalogram shows nonspecific slowing in slightly more than half of patients.

The time lag from starting of the drug to the onset of neuroleptic malignant syndrome is generally short, with 30% of cases developing within 48 hours and 96% within the first month of treatment. The exception appears to be clozapine-associated neuroleptic malignant syndrome, which has an average time lag of 50 days. Neuroleptic syndrome is sometimes confused with severe catatonia (Chapter 397), but the catatonic signs in neuroleptic malignant syndrome are usually restricted to mutism and akinesia. Furthermore, hyperthermia, rigidity, tremor, and rhabdomyolysis are not present in patients with catatonia. Nonetheless, close medical follow-up of severely catatonic patients is warranted because they are at very high risk (22%) for neuroleptic malignant syndrome.

Untreated, neuroleptic malignant syndrome has a mortality rate of 10% as a result of acute renal failure, aspiration pneumonia, adult respiratory distress syndrome, disseminated intravascular coagulation, and cerebellar neuronal degeneration. Most fatalities are avoidable if the diagnosis is made early, the neuroleptic agent is discontinued rapidly, and the patient is immediately transferred to an intensive care setting for supportive and specific therapy. Bromocriptine (2.5 mg three times daily orally or through a nasogastric tube; may increase by 2.5 mg three times daily to a maximal daily dose of 40 mg) or amantadine (100 mg orally or through a nasogastric tube twice daily; may increase to 300 mg/day in divided doses) should be used in moderately severe cases and continued until the muscle rigidity and metabolic abnormalities have significantly improved. The skeletal muscle relaxant dantrolene (starting with a dose of 1 mg/kg intravenously and titrated to a maximal dose of 10 mg/kg/day divided into three intravenous or oral doses) should be added to bromocriptine or amantadine in patients with fulminant hypermetabolic features and those with persistent muscle rigidity despite treatment with dopamine agonists. Refractory neuroleptic malignant syndrome improves after ECT.

Serotonin Syndrome

Serotonin syndrome (Chapter 432) is an adverse drug reaction primarily produced by excess serotonergic agonism of central nervous system and peripheral serotonin receptors by selected drugs (Table 434-4).[5] In postmarketing surveillance studies of the newer antidepressants, the syndrome has an incidence of 4 cases per 10,000 patient-months in patients who start taking nefazodone, a drug that inhibits neuronal uptake of serotonin and norepinephrine and also acts as a 5-hydroxytryptamine type 2 (5-HT$_2$) receptor antagonist. The syndrome also occurs in 15% of patients with intentional overdose of selective serotonin reuptake inhibitors (SSRIs). The serotonin syndrome is caused by overstimulation of 5-HT$_{1A}$ and possibly also 5-HT$_2$ receptors through excess of serotonin precursors or agonists, increased serotonin release, reduced serotonin uptake, and decreased serotonin metabolism. Severe cases of the syndrome have been more frequently reported in patients treated with monoamine oxidase inhibitors who took over-the-counter dextromethorphan or the illegal methylenedioxymethamphetamine (Ecstasy) or who started treatment with serotonin reuptake inhibitors, meperidine, or atypical antipsychotics such as aripiprazole.

Potentially life-threatening, the syndrome is characterized by changes in mental status (ranging from agitation to confusion and coma), autonomic instability (tachycardia, labile or high blood pressure, diaphoresis, and diarrhea), neuromuscular abnormalities (myoclonus, mydriasis, ocular clonus, rigidity, hyperreflexia, tremors, and shivering), and hyperthermia. The symptoms occur within the first 24 hours and sometimes within minutes after the initial use of medication, a change in dose, addition of a new drug, or overdose attempt. Death may occur as a consequence of rhabdomyolysis with renal failure, hyperkalemia, disseminated intravascular coagulation, and acute respiratory distress syndrome. The differential diagnosis includes neuroleptic malignant syndrome, viral or bacterial meningitis or encephalitis (Chapter 109), anticholinergic toxidrome (Chapter 110), and drug (Chapter 34) or alcohol (Chapter 33) withdrawal.

General management includes immediate discontinuation of serotonergic drugs, comprehensive supportive therapy, and benzodiazepines for control of agitation and myoclonus. Specific therapy relies on the use of cyproheptadine (an H$_1$-receptor antagonist with antiserotonergic and anticholinergic properties) and chlorpromazine (a 5-HT$_{1A}$ and 5-HT$_2$ receptor antagonist). Cyproheptadine should be started at a dose of 12 mg administered orally or through a nasogastric tube, with additional 2-mg doses given every 2 hours until symptoms improve or the maximal dose of 32 mg has been reached. The usual maintenance dose of cyproheptadine is 8 mg three times daily. Chlorpromazine (50 mg intramuscularly; may repeat three or four times daily and increase gradually to 400 mg/day in divided doses) is indicated in patients with severe symptoms who must be treated parenterally. Rapid improvement has also been observed after single doses of olanzapine (10 mg administered sublingually). Chlorpromazine and olanzapine should be used only after the possibility of neuroleptic malignant syndrome has been excluded.

Antipsychotic-Induced Hyperprolactinemia

Drug-induced hyperprolactinemia is produced by first-generation antipsychotic medications and by risperidone, but it is rare with other atypical antipsychotics such as aripiprazole, olanzapine, and ziprasidone. In patients treated with prolactin-raising antipsychotic medications, hormone levels are above the normal limit in 60% of women and 40% of men. Symptomatic hyperprolactinemia (Chapter 224) occurs in about one third of these patients and is generally associated with a 10-fold increase above baseline levels. Excess prolactin leads to dysfunction of target tissues (galactorrhea, oligomenorrhea and amenorrhea, infertility, sexual impairment, and gynecomastia) as well as an increased risk for breast cancer, osteoporosis, and cardiovascular disease. The mechanism of antipsychotic-related hyperprolactinemia is suppression of dopamine inhibition of lactotroph cells in the hypothalamus. Brain imaging is required in symptomatic patients and those with significant elevated prolactin levels to exclude tumors of the pituitary and hypothalamus.

Psychogenic Polydipsia and Drug-Induced Hyponatremia

Hyponatremia, which is present in approximately 6% of patients at the time of admission to inpatient psychiatric care and is more common in older patients and those with hypertension, approximately doubles the risk of medical deterioration.[6] The diagnosis is often delayed because traditional manifestations of hyponatremia, such as lethargy, restlessness, weakness, and disorientation, overlap with features of psychiatric disorders.

Patients with psychogenic polydipsia typically have serum hypo-osmolality and a maximally dilute urine (urine osmolality <100 mOsm/L).[7] The incidence of polydipsia is 20% and the incidence of water intoxication is 5% in inpatient psychiatric facilities. Urinary incontinence and nocturnal enuresis may be part of the clinical manifestation. The mechanism of increased thirst is poorly understood but may involve incomplete suppression of antidiuretic hormone (ADH) by the hypothalamus as well as response to the mouth dryness produced by the anticholinergic effect of many psychotropic drugs. The differential diagnosis includes diuretic effect, renal insufficiency, glucocorticoid deficiency, and hypothyroidism. Stringent measures to restrict fluid intake are generally effective in patients with moderate hyponatremia, and clozapine limits polydipsia and improves water intoxication in refractory cases.

Drug-induced syndrome of inappropriate antidiuretic hormone (SIADH) is predominantly related to SSRIs, and animal experiments have suggested that the excess serotonin stimulates release of ADH and will lead to hyponatremia, provided water intake is sufficient. Other drugs that are commonly used by psychiatric patients and that may produce SIADH include tricyclic antidepressants, monoamine oxidase inhibitors, carbamazepine, conventional and second-generation antipsychotics, benzodiazepines, methadone, and nicotine. Elderly patients, patients with a lower body mass index, and those with a baseline plasma sodium level of less than 138 mEq/L are at higher risk. The median time to diagnosis after SSRIs are started is 9 days. Urinary excretion of sodium usually is more than 20 mEq/L, and urine osmolality is higher than 300 mOsm/L. In patients with mild asymptomatic hyponatremia, SSRIs can be continued with careful monitoring while the patient is placed on supervised fluid restriction. For patients who cannot tolerate fluid restriction or have symptomatic hyponatremia with serum sodium levels of less than 125 mEq/L, the use of tolvaptan (initially 15 mg, titratable to 30 or 60 mg), a vasopressin V_2-receptor antagonist, is effective.[A4]

Risk Assessment before Electroconvulsive Therapy

ECT is highly effective for the treatment of drug-refractory major depression and other psychiatric disorders. The procedure requires a brief period of general anesthesia with sodium pentothal, etomidate, or propofol as well as muscle paralysis with succinylcholine, during which the patient receives bag-valve-mask ventilation with supplemental oxygen and is monitored with continuous electrocardiography and pulse oximetry. Bronchospasm may follow induction of anesthesia, particularly in patients already at risk for respiratory compromise. During electrical stimulation of the brain, parasympathetic activation can lead to bradycardia or several seconds of asystole, which can be avoided by premedicating the patient with intravenous glycopyrrolate. The parasympathetic effect lasts until onset of the akinetic seizure, when sympathetic tone increases and produces tachycardia, an elevation in blood pressure, and increased myocardial demand for oxygen. These changes can be corrected with intravenous esmolol. At the same time, because of the enhanced neuronal metabolic rate, augmented blood flow to the brain increases intracranial pressure. This elevated sympathetic tone causes ECT-related myocardial ischemia, tachyarrhythmias, and potential rupture of aortic or intracranial aneurysms. The elevated intracranial pressure may lead to brain herniation in patients with a space-occupying lesion. Older patients have a high rate of prolonged confusion, arrhythmias, and falls after ECT. A structured medical evaluation before ECT can address risks and the potential for complications (Fig. 434-1). Every effort must be made to optimize the patient's active medical conditions before ECT. For high-risk patients, one must require that ECT be performed in a

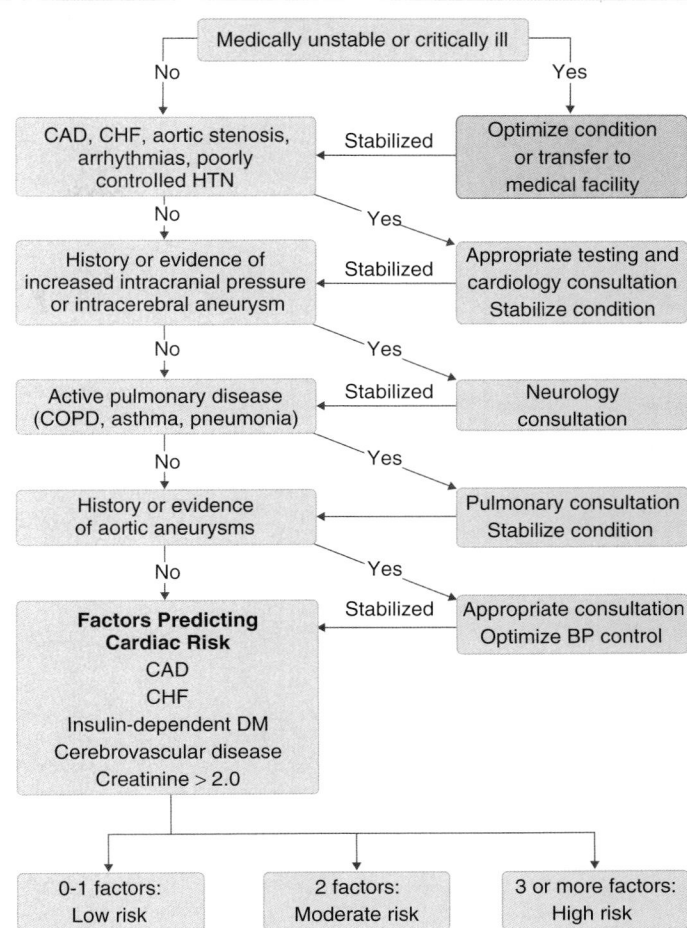

FIGURE 434-1. **Risk assessment before electroconvulsive therapy.** BP = blood pressure; CAD = coronary artery disease; CHF = congestive heart failure; COPD = chronic obstructive pulmonary disease; DM = diabetes mellitus; HTN = hypertension. (Modified from Frederickson A, Manu P. Risk assessment prior to electroconvulsive therapy. In Manu P, Suarez RE, Barnett BJ, eds. Handbook of Medicine in Psychiatry. Washington, DC: American Psychiatric Publishing; 2006:687-700.)

setting that allows immediate access to an intensive care unit rather than in the ECT suite of a self-standing psychiatric hospital. Essential medications should be administered with a small amount of fluid 6 hours before ECT. Drugs that can increase or decrease the seizure threshold, such as lidocaine, theophylline, phenothiazine, tricyclic antidepressants, and benzodiazepines, must be discontinued before ECT. Optimal pre-ECT risk assessment, careful anesthesia, and post-ECT monitoring result in a serious complication rate of only 0.9% and essentially no fatalities.

 Grade A References

A1. Chen CH, Huang MC, Kao CF, et al. Effects of adjunctive metformin on metabolic traits in nondiabetic clozapine-treated patients with schizophrenia and the effect of metformin discontinuation on body weight: a 24-week, randomized, double-blind, placebo-controlled study. *J Clin Psychiatry.* 2013;74:e424-e430.

A2. Wu RR, Zhao JP, Guo XF, et al. Metformin addition attenuates olanzapine-induced weight gain in drug-naïve first-episode schizophrenia patients: a double-blind, placebo-controlled study. *Am J Psychiatry.* 2008;165:352-358.

A3. Stroup TS, Byerly MJ, Nasrallah HA, et al. Effects of switching from olanzapine, quetiapine, and risperidone to aripiprazole on 10-year coronary heart disease risk and metabolic syndrome status: results from a randomized controlled trial. *Schizophr Res.* 2013;146:190-195.

A4. Josiassen RC, Goldman M, Jessani M, et al. Double-blind, placebo-controlled, multicenter trial of a vasopressin V_2-antagonist in patients with schizophrenia and hyponatremia. *Biol Psychiatry.* 2008;54:1097-1100.

GENERAL REFERENCES

For the General References and other additional features, please visit Expert Consult at https://expertconsult.inkling.com.

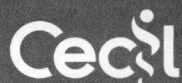

XXVIII

SKIN DISEASES

435

STRUCTURE AND FUNCTION OF THE SKIN

DAVID H. CHU

The skin, as the largest organ of the body, is a complex multifunctional entity with many regional specializations that provide its host both protection from, and interaction with, its environment. The skin is not just an impenetrable shield against external injury but rather a dynamic, intricate, integrated arrangement of cells, tissues, and matrix elements that together perform a variety of functions, as follows:

- *Physical/mechanical protection:* The epidermis, which is the selectively permeable layer outermost covering of the skin, helps regulate water loss and provides a physical barrier against external insults. The underlying dermis provides mechanical strength to the skin.
- *Thermoregulation:* Eccrine glands mediate the excretion of water, evaporation of which is critical for thermoregulation. The cutaneous vasculature also helps regulate heat exchange via vasoconstriction and vasodilatation.
- *Immunologic surveillance:* Resident and transient cells of the immune system provide some of the earliest defenses against infectious diseases, toxins, and malignantly transformed cells.
- *Sensation:* Nerve endings and specialized sensory apparatus embedded within the skin provide sensory inputs such as pain and itch.
- *External appearance:* The contours, texture, pigment, and regional variations of the skin are keys to an individual's external appearance and perception by others.

These various functions of the skin are mediated by one or more of its major regions—the epidermis, dermis, and subcutaneous fat (Fig. 435-1). These anatomic subdivisions are interdependent, functional units, each relying on and connected with its surrounding tissue for regulation and modulation of normal structure and function at molecular, cellular, and tissue levels of organization.

Whereas the epidermis and its outer stratum corneum constitute a large part of the physical barrier provided by the skin, the structural integrity of skin as a whole is primarily attributable to the dermis and subcutaneous fat. Antimicrobial activities are provided by the innate immune system and antigen-presenting Langerhans cells of the epidermis, by circulating immune cells that migrate from the blood vessels in the dermis, and by antigen-presenting dendritic cells of the dermis. The most superficial cells of the epidermis provide most of the protection from ultraviolet (UV) irradiation (Chapter 20). Sensation emanates from nerves that initially traverse the subcutaneous fat to the dermis and epidermis before ending in specialized receptive organs or free nerve endings. The largest blood vessels of the skin are found in the subcutaneous fat, where they transport nutrients and circulating immune cells. The cutaneous lymphatics, which also course through the dermis and subcutaneous fat, filter debris and regulate tissue hydration. The skin's pigmentation is regulated by melanocytes, whereas actinic damage and aging are influenced by the epidermis, the dermis, and the subcutaneous fat.

EPIDERMIS

Epidermal Differentiation

The epidermis, which is the outermost layer of the skin, is composed primarily of keratinocytes that differentiate to form a stratified squamous epithelium.[1] The epidermis is a continually renewing structure that gives rise to specialized derivatives called *appendages*—pilosebaceous units, sweat glands, and nails. The keratinocytes within the epidermis are organized into four layers, named for either their position or structural property (Fig. 435-2). Cells develop from the basal layer and then undergo programmed biochemical and morphologic changes that ultimately result in formation of the outermost stratum corneum, which serves as a hardened shield against the host environment. Melanocytes, Langerhans cells, and Merkel cells form the bulk of cells that reside within different layers of the epidermis. Some regional differences in the epidermis and its appendages are readily apparent (e.g., the thickness of palmoplantar and truncal skin compared with eyelid skin), whereas other differences are evident only at the microscopic or biochemical level (e.g., differential expression of keratins in dorsal compared with volar skin).

The Basal Layer

The basal layer, which is the germinative layer of the epidermis, contains proliferative cells that give rise to the more differentiated levels of the epidermis. Keratinocyte differentiation (keratinization) is a genetically programmed, regulated, complex series of morphologic and metabolic changes whose end point is a terminally differentiated, cornified envelope that consists of dead keratinocytes (corneocytes) and contains a protein-reinforced plasma membrane with surface-associated lipids.

All epithelial cells have intermediate filaments known as keratins. Keratins primarily serve a structural role, and they are expressed in region-specific and function-specific obligate heteropolymer pairs in a pattern that is determined by cell type, tissue type, developmental stage, differentiation stage, and disease condition. The critical role of these molecules is underscored by the numerous manifestations of disease that arise because of mutations in their genes.

Basal cells attach to their underlying basal lamina via keratin filaments at hemidesmosomes in the basement membrane zone. They also attach to each other and to other keratinocytes via desmosomes, which are specialized junctions required for epidermal integrity. Keratinocytes also contain melanosomes—vacuoles that contain pigment that is synthesized by melanocytes and transferred to keratinocytes via phagocytosis. This pigment helps protect against UV damage and contributes to macroscopic skin coloring.

In the epidermis, the greatest amount of mitotic activity occurs in the basal layer. Cell kinetic studies suggest that different basal keratinocytes have different proliferative potentials, and in vivo and in vitro studies suggest the existence of long-lived epidermal stem cells. Because basal cells can be expanded in tissue culture and used to reconstitute enough epidermis to cover the entire skin surface of burn patients, these long-lived stem cells appear to have extensive proliferative potential.

The Spinous Layer

The spinous layer is characterized by the presence of abundant desmosomes, which are critical for tight epidermal adhesion and resemble intercellular "spines" under light microscopy. The classic vesiculobullous disease pemphigus vulgaris (Chapter 439) results from desmosomal disruption.

The Granular Layer

The granular layer, so named because of the abundant keratohyalin granules contained in the cells that constitute it, represents an intermediate phase of keratinocyte differentiation. This layer is where a number of the structural components will form the cornified cell envelope of the epidermal barrier, as well as a number of proteins that process these components. Keratohyalin granules are composed primarily of profilaggrin, keratin filaments, and loricrin. Profilaggrin is cleaved into filaggrin monomers, which aggregate with keratin to form macrofilaments. Eventually, filaggrin is degraded into molecules that contribute to hydration of the stratum corneum and help filter UV radiation. Loricrin, which is a cysteine-rich protein, is released from keratohyalin granules and then binds to desmosomal structures. Loricrin is subsequently cross-linked to the plasma membrane by tissue transglutaminases to help form the cornified cell envelope.

The Stratum Corneum

The final stage of granular cell differentiation into a corneocyte involves the cell's own programmed destruction, a process during which almost all cellular contents are destroyed, with the exception of the keratin filaments and filaggrin matrix. The cells eventually extrude their nuclei and become a flattened stratum corneum that provides mechanical protection and a barrier to the loss of water or the entry of soluble substances from the environment.

The stratum corneum barrier is formed by a two-compartment system of lipid-depleted, protein-enriched corneocytes surrounded by a continuous extracellular lipid matrix. The extracellular lipid matrix is primarily responsible for the regulation of permeability, desquamation, antimicrobial peptide activity, toxin exclusion, and selective chemical absorption. By comparison, corneocytes provide mechanical reinforcement, hydration, cytokine-mediated initiation of inflammation, and protection from UV damage.

Mutations in the transglutaminase enzymes and in structural proteins such as filaggrin and loricrin cause the ichthyoses and keratodermas, which result when a poorly formed epidermal barrier, both functionally and structurally,

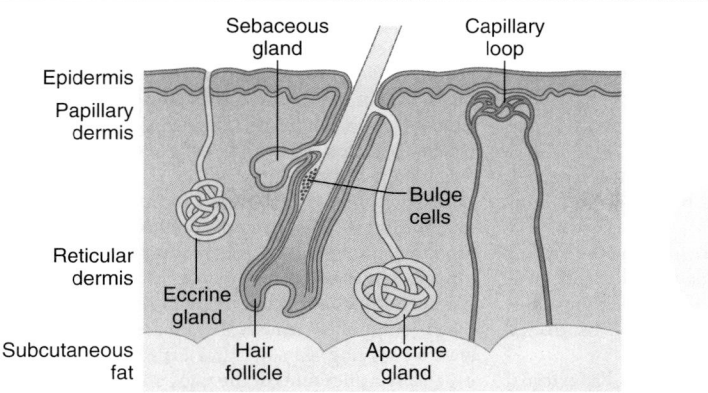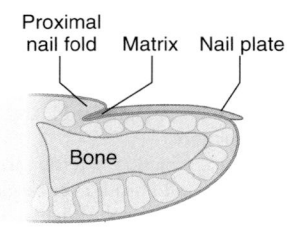

FIGURE 435-1. General structure of the skin and epidermal appendages. The epidermis is the outermost keratinized layer of skin, resting on top of the dermis via a basement membrane zone. The epidermal appendages are specialized structures and include the eccrine and apocrine sweat glands, sebaceous glands, hair, and nails. Capillary loops traverse the dermis to its most superficial aspect for diffusion and transport.

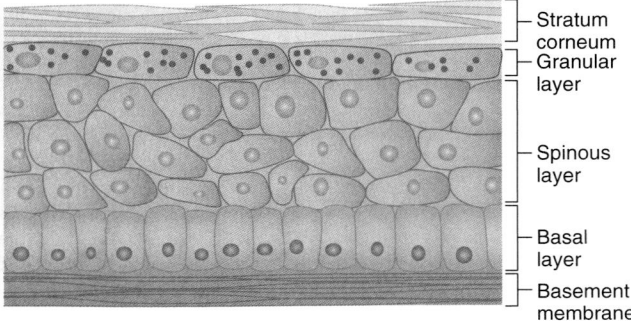

FIGURE 435-2. The epidermis and its layers of differentiation.

causes hyperkeratosis and scaling, derangements in water permeability and temperature regulation, and increased susceptibility to infections. Patients with filaggrin mutations are more susceptible to developing atopic dermatitis.[2] The sequelae of these mutations highlight the importance of the epidermis and stratum corneum for maintaining tissue and organism homeostasis.

Epidermal Adhesion
Keratinocytes are held together by a number of intercellular junctions, including tight junctions, gap junctions, adherens junctions, and desmosomes. Complex protein networks form each of these types of junctions, and genetic mutations can have significant effects on the function of the epidermis.

Tight junctions determine epidermal permeability by regulating the distribution of water-soluble molecules between adjacent cells. The primary structural proteins in these junctions are the claudins, and mutations in claudin 1 can cause a syndromic form of ichthyosis.

Gap junctions, formed primarily by connexins, allow small molecules and electric current to pass between adjacent cells. Connexin mutations can cause a number of phenotypes in genetic syndromes, such as the keratitis-ichthyosis deafness syndrome.

Adherens junctions are transmembrane structures that associate with the actin cytoskeleton. The extracellular interactions are calcium-dependent reactions between cadherins. These cadherin proteins associate with an intracellular complex including p120ctn, β-catenin, and plakoglobin. Plakoglobin and p-cadherin have been identified to be mutated in two genetic conditions, Naxos disease (plakoglobin) and hypotrichosis with juvenile macular dystrophy (p-cadherin).

Desmosomes are cell-cell junctions that provide strength and rigidity to cells. They also participate in skin and tissue differentiation and development. Three protein families make up desmosomes—the armadillo proteins (such as plakoglobin and plakophilins), cadherins (including desmocollins and desmogleins), and plakins (desmoplakin, envoplakin, periplakin, plectin, BPAG1, corneodesmosin, and microtubule actin cross-linking factor). A number of genetic conditions involve mutations within these protein-encoding genes,

such as ectodermal dysplasia–skin fragility syndrome (plakophilin 1). In addition, autoantibody diseases (e.g., bullous pemphigoid and pemphigus vulgaris) and bacterial infections (e.g., bullous impetigo and staphylococcal scalded skin syndrome) can inactivate these proteins, thereby resulting in numerous adhesion disorders that are manifested clinically as skin fragility and blistering conditions.

Calcium is an important mediator of cell adhesion, as evidenced by Hailey-Hailey and Darier's diseases, in which mutations in genes encoding calcium transporters disrupt calcium distribution, thereby resulting in characteristic epidermal dyscohesion and blistering. Many of the proteins involved in cell-cell adhesion also require calcium for their binding or adhesive properties.

Nonkeratinocytes of the Epidermis
Melanocytes synthesize the pigment molecule melanin, which performs a critical role in absorbing and mitigating UV damage to the skin and underlying tissues.[3] A number of enzymes convert the amino acid tyrosine into different forms of melanin, which then are sorted into membrane-bound organelles known as melanosomes. These melanosomes are then transported to the tips of melanocytic dendrites and subsequently transferred to adjacent keratinocytes. Melanocytes are neuroendocrine derived cells that are not intrinsic cells of the skin but migrate there early in development.

The function of melanocytes has been highlighted by disorders in melanocyte number or function. The classic dermatologic disease, vitiligo (Chapter 441), is caused by the autoimmune depletion of melanocytes, but disorders of pigmentation can be caused by dysfunction at any of the steps of melanogenesis. For example, various forms of oculocutaneous albinism result from defects in melanin synthesis, whereas the subtypes of Griscelli's syndrome (skin and hair hypopigmentation, ocular albinism, neurologic disorders) result from mutations involved in lysosomal and melanosomal transfer of pigment to keratinocytes. Keratinocyte-melanocyte interactions are critical for melanocyte homeostasis and differentiation, influencing proliferation, dendricity, and melanization.

Merkel cells, which are mechanoreceptors, are located in sites of high tactile sensitivity, including skin of the digits, lips, regions of the oral cavity, and the hair follicle. Ultrastructurally, Merkel cells are easily identified by the membrane-bounded, dense-core granules that contain neurotransmitter-like substances and markers of neuroendocrine cells. Merkel cell–derived neoplasms are particularly aggressive and difficult to treat.

Langerhans cells are dendritic antigen-processing and antigen-presenting cells in the epidermis, mostly in a suprabasal position. Although they are not unique to the epidermis, they form 2 to 8% of the total epidermal cell population. Langerhans cells, which present antigens to T cells of the epidermis, are implicated in allergic contact dermatitis, cutaneous leishmaniasis, and human immunodeficiency virus (HIV) infection. Langerhans cells are reduced in the epidermis of patients with conditions such as psoriasis, sarcoidosis, and contact dermatitis, and they are functionally impaired by UV radiation, especially UVB.

Nonresident Cells of the Epidermis
Circulating immune cells that pass through the skin play key roles in infection control and immune surveillance. The activation of γ-δ T cells in the

epidermis is an important step in wound healing. Recent advances in melanoma therapy (Chapter 203) target T-cell costimulatory molecules, thereby underscoring the importance of this subset of immune cells in host responses to malignancy.

Epidermal Appendages

The epidermal appendages, including the hair follicle, nails, sebaceous gland, eccrine gland, and apocrine gland (see Fig. 435-1), are specialized structures that have particular unique functions.

Eccrine glands occur throughout the skin, but they are found in the highest concentrations on the palms, soles, and head. Eccrine glands, which are critical for thermoregulation, secrete a watery solution that includes sodium chloride, urea, uric acid, potassium, and immunoglobulins. Secretion is controlled by cholinergic sympathetic nerves.

Apocrine glands, which are scent glands, are found in the axilla, external genitalia, areola, and perianal areas. Secretion by these glands is increased by fear, sexual excitement, and other situations that result in heightened tension.

The nail unit (Chapter 442) consists of a nail matrix, nail plate, and nail bed. The proximal nail matrix is an organized germinative epithelium that produces the keratinized nail plate. The nail bed, which is a specialized epithelium located under the nail plate, attaches the nail plate to the digit.

Sebaceous glands are found throughout the dermis except for the palms and soles. Many of these glands empty their contents through a duct into the lumen of hair follicles. In certain areas of the body, the glands occur in the absence of hairs (glans penis, lips, labia minora, and eyelids). Sebaceous secretions include triglycerides, waxy esters, squalene, cholesterol, and fatty acids.

Hair follicles undergo a carefully orchestrated program of cyclical differentiation and proliferation. The hair follicle bulge consists of pluripotent skin stem cells that can give rise to all the layers of the follicle and hair shaft, as well as the epidermis under certain conditions of wound repair. The hair cycle (Chapter 442) consists of the phases of growth (anagen), involution (catagen), resting (telogen), and eventual release (exogen) of the mature hair follicle.

THE DERMAL-EPIDERMAL JUNCTION

The dermal-epidermal junction is a basement membrane zone that forms the interface between the epidermis and dermis. The major functions of the dermal-epidermal junction are to attach the epidermis and dermis to each other and provide resistance against external shearing forces. This junction serves as a support for the epidermis, determines the polarity of growth, directs the organization of the cytoskeleton in basal cells, provides developmental signals, and serves as a semipermeable barrier.

The dermal-epidermal junction can be subdivided into three supramolecular networks: the hemidesmosome-anchoring filament complex, the basement membrane, and the anchoring fibrils. The critical role of this region in maintaining skin structural integrity is exemplified by the large number of mutations or functional inactivations that cause blistering diseases[4,5]. For example, basal keratinocyte cleavage within the superficial dermal-epidermal junction causes epidermolysis bullosa simplex. Abnormalities within the lamina lucida and lamina densa regions cause junctional epidermolysis bullosa, and abnormalities within the sublamina densa/anchoring filaments cause the deep blistering of dystrophic epidermolysis bullosa.

THE DERMIS

The dermis, which constitutes the bulk of the skin and provides its flexibility and mechanical strength, is an integrated system of connective tissue elements that accommodate networks of nerves and blood vessels. The dermis has two major regions: the upper papillary dermis and the deeper reticular dermis. The papillary dermis, which is usually no more than twice the thickness of the epidermis, runs just beneath it and undulates its contours. The reticular dermis, which forms the bulk of the dermal tissue, is composed primarily of collagen and elastin. The subpapillary plexus, a horizontal plane of vessels, marks the boundary between the papillary and reticular dermis. The lowest boundary of the reticular dermis is defined by the transition of its fibrous connective tissue to the adipose connective tissue of the subcutaneous fat.

Connective Tissue Matrix of the Dermis

Collagen, which forms the bulk of the acellular portion of the dermis, provides both tensile strength and elasticity. The periodically banded, interstitial collagens account for most of the collagen in the adult dermis (type I, 80 to 90%; III, 8 to 12%; and V, < 5%). Type IV collagen is confined to the basal

lamina of the dermal-epidermal junction, blood vessels, and epidermal appendages. Type VI collagen is associated with fibrils and interfibrillar spaces. Type VII collagen forms anchoring fibrils at the dermal-epidermal junction. The classic diseases of collagen function are the various subtypes of Ehlers-Danlos syndrome (Chapter 260),[6] a heterogeneous collection of disorders characterized by joint hypermobility, skin extensibility, abnormal scarring, and tissue friability.

Elastic connective tissue is a complex molecular mesh that includes elastin and fibrillin and that extends from the lamina densa of the dermal-epidermal junction throughout the dermis and into the connective tissue of the subcutaneous fat. Elastic fibers return the skin to its normal configuration after it has been stretched or deformed. Mutations in elastin, which is the elastic fiber matrix component, causes the disease cutis laxa, a condition that is characterized by sagging skin that has little extensibility and hangs in loose folds, especially noticeable on the neck and in the axillae and groin. Mutations in the gene encoding fibrillin, a microfibril component, are implicated in Marfan syndrome (Chapter 260). Elastic fibers are normally located between bundles of collagen fibers, although in certain pathologic conditions, such as Buschke-Ollendorff syndrome (dermatofibrosis lenticularis disseminata), both elastic and collagen fibers become assembled within the same bundle, thereby resulting in the formation of characteristic benign connective tissue nevi and osteopoikilosis.

Pseudoxanthoma elasticum (Chapter 260), which is characterized by loss of skin elasticity and calcified elastic fibers, results from mutations in ABCC6, a transmembrane transporter in the ATP-binding cassette transporter family, although the mechanisms responsible for the observed elastic fiber defects are not understood. In addition to genetic mutations, solar radiation and aging also damage elastic fibers.

The fibrous and cellular elements of the dermis are embedded within a more amorphous matrix that can bind water and regulate the compressibility of the dermis. Various glycoproteins interact with other matrix components via integrin receptors to facilitate cell migration, adhesion, morphogenesis, and differentiation. Fibronectin, which is synthesized by both epithelial and mesenchymal cells, covers collagen bundles and the elastic network. Vitronectin is present on all elastic fibers except for oxytalan. Tenascin is found around the smooth muscle of blood vessels, arrector pili muscles, and appendages such as sweat glands.

Cellular Components of the Dermis

Fibroblasts, macrophages, and mast cells are the regular residents of the dermis. Fibroblasts migrate through the tissue and are responsible for the synthesis and degradation of matrix proteins and a number of soluble factors in the fibrous and nonfibrous connective tissue. Fibroblasts provide a structural extracellular matrix framework and also promote interactions between the epidermis and the dermis. Fibroblasts are also instrumental in wound healing and scarring, increasing their proliferative and synthetic activity during these processes.

Monocytes, macrophages, and dermal dendrocytes constitute the mononuclear phagocytic system of cells in the skin. Macrophages are derived from precursors in the bone marrow, differentiate into circulating monocytes, and then migrate into the dermis to differentiate. These cells are phagocytic, antigen-processing and antigen-presenting, microbicidal, tumoricidal, secretory, and hematopoietic. They are also involved in coagulation, atherogenesis, wound healing, and tissue remodeling. The dermal dendrocyte is a phagocytic fixed connective tissue cell in the dermis of normal skin. These cells are particularly abundant in the papillary dermis and upper reticular dermis, where they function as antigen-presenting cells. They are also likely the cell of origin of a number of benign fibrotic proliferative conditions in the skin, such as dermatofibromas and fibroxanthomas.

Mast cells, which are the specialized secretory cells responsible for the immediate-type hypersensitivity reaction in skin, are also involved in subacute and chronic inflammatory processes. These processes are mediated by the histamine, heparin, tryptase, chymase, carboxypeptidase, neutrophil chemotactic factor, and eosinophilic chemotactic factor of anaphylaxis that are synthesized in their granules and released in response to various stimuli. Mast cells also can become hyperplastic and hyperproliferative in mastocytosis (Chapter 255).

SUBCUTANEOUS FAT

The subcutaneous fat insulates the body, serves as a reserve energy supply, cushions and protects the skin, and allows for its mobility over underlying structures. This fat is a key determinant of body contours and therefore plays an important cosmetic role as well. At the junction of the deep reticular dermis and the underlying fat layer is an abrupt transition from predominantly fibrous dermal connective tissue to primarily adipose tissue. Despite this anatomic contrast, the dermis and the subcutaneous fat are structurally and functionally integrated through networks of nerves and vessels, as well as in the continuity of epidermal appendages such as growing hair follicles and sweat glands.

Adipocytes, which form the bulk of the cells in the subcutaneous fat layer, are organized into lobules defined by septa of fibrous connective tissue. Within the septa run the nerves and vascular structures that supply the region. Fat synthesis and storage can occur by enhanced accumulation of lipid within, or proliferation of, existing adipocytes or by the creation of new adipocytes from undifferentiated mesenchyme. The hormone leptin (Chapter 223), secreted by adipocytes, regulates fat homeostasis. Leptin levels are higher in subcutaneous than omental adipose tissue, thereby suggesting a role for leptin in the distribution of adipose tissue.

The importance of the subcutaneous tissue is highlighted in conditions in which it is absent or abnormal. In Werner's syndrome (Chapter 205), the absence of subcutaneous fat over bone lesions results in ulcers and poor wound healing. In scleroderma (Chapter 267), the replacement of subcutaneous fat with dense fibrous connective tissue results in taut and painful skin. In both the hereditary and acquired lipodystrophies (Chapter 392), loss of subcutaneous fat disrupts glucose, triglyceride, and cholesterol regulation and can cause significant cosmetic alteration. Inflammation of the subcutaneous fat, termed panniculitis (Chapters 142 and 266), can be caused by many different tissue derangements and systemic conditions.

CUTANEOUS VASCULATURE

Blood Vessels

The rich vascular network of the skin is located at boundaries within the dermis and supplies the epidermal appendages. Dermal vessels branch from musculocutaneous arteries that penetrate the subcutaneous fat and enter the deep reticular dermis. At this point, they are organized into a horizontal arteriolar plexus. From this plexus, ascending arterioles extend toward the epidermis. At the junction between the papillary and reticular dermis, terminal arterioles form the subpapillary plexus. Capillary loops then extend from these terminal arterioles of the plexus into the more superficial papillary dermis. At the apex of each capillary loop, the thinnest portion of the vessel allows for diffusion and transport of material out of the capillary. The descending limbs of capillary loops drain into venous channels of the subpapillary plexus. The postcapillary venules of the subpapillary plexus are responsive to histamine and are therefore often the sites of inflammatory cells.

In the adult, the cutaneous vasculature normally remains quiescent, in part owing to inhibition of angiogenesis by factors such as thrombospondin. Pathogenic stimuli, such as from tumors or after a wound, sometimes result in secondary angiogenesis. One of the key mediators of such angiogenesis is vascular endothelial growth factor, which often is secreted by tumors or by keratinocytes.

Numerous disorders can manifest themselves within the cutaneous vasculature.[7] Leukocytoclastic vasculitis (Chapters 270 and 439), also called cutaneous necrotizing venulitis, occurs within the venules in response to a number of potential pathogenic mechanisms, including medication reactions, infections, neoplasms, and systemic inflammatory conditions. Stasis dermatitis (Chapter 436), urticaria (Chapters 252 and 440), polyarteritis nodosa (Chapter 270), thrombosis (Chapter 70), and thrombophlebitis (Chapter 81) all affect different-sized vessels in the skin, some by occlusion of vessels (vasculopathy) and others by inflammation of the vessels (vasculitis).

Lymphatics

The lymph channels of the skin are responsible for resorbing fluid released by vessels and clearing the tissues of cells, proteins, lipids, bacteria, and degraded substances.[8] These vessels begin in blind-ending loops in the papillary dermis and then continue to drain into successively larger plexuses deeper in the tissue. Lymphatic flow in the skin is propelled by arterial pulsations, muscle contractions, and movement of the body. Bicuspid-like valves within the lymphatic vessels promote unidirectional flow. Because lymphatic vessels are often collapsed in skin and because lymphatic vessels have thinner walls than blood vessels, they are rarely seen on routine histologic section.

Pathologic conditions that involve or highlight the function of lymphatic vessels include lymphedema, lymphangioma circumscriptum (clustered, deep vesicles on the skin resulting from lymphatic dilation and

malformation), and stasis dermatitis. Lymphatics are also important for the progression and spread of cancer. For example, melanoma cells destroy the endothelial cells of the local lymphatics to gain entry to the lymphatic circulation, and tumors themselves can promote lymphangiogenesis as part of their process of metastasis.

CUTANEOUS NERVES AND RECEPTORS

The nerve networks of the skin contain somatic sensory and sympathetic autonomic fibers. The sensory fibers alone (free nerve endings) or in conjunction with specialized structures (corpuscular receptors) function as receptors of touch, pain, temperature, itch, and mechanical stimuli. The differing density and types of receptors in different body regions account for the variation in sensory acuity at different body sites. Receptors are particularly dense in hairless areas such as the areola, labia, and glans penis. Sympathetic motor fibers run with the sensory nerves in the dermis until they branch to innervate the sweat glands, vascular smooth muscle, the arrector pili muscle of hair follicles, and sebaceous glands.

The nerves of skin branch from musculocutaneous nerves that arise segmentally from spinal nerves. The pattern of nerve fibers in skin is similar to the vascular patterns—nerve fibers form a deep plexus, then ascend to a superficial, subpapillary plexus.

Free nerve endings, which are the most widespread sensory receptors in skin, are particularly common in the papillary dermis. The penicillate fibers, which are the primary nerve fibers found subepidermally in haired skin, are rapidly adapting receptors that function in the perception of touch, temperature, pain, and itch. Papillary nerve endings are found at the orifice of a follicle and are thought to be particularly receptive to cold sensation.

Corpuscular receptors, which contain a capsule and inner core, are composed of both neural and non-neural components. Meissner corpuscles are elongated or ovoid mechanoreceptors that are located in the dermal papillae of digital skin and oriented vertically toward the epidermal surface. Pacinian corpuscles lie in the deep dermis and subcutaneous tissue of skin that covers weight-bearing surfaces of the body; they have a characteristic capsule and lamellar wrappings and serve as rapidly adapting mechanoreceptors that respond to vibrational stimuli.

Pathophysiology of Pruritus

Pruritus (itching) is mediated by unmyelinated C fibers, the same fibers that are responsible for the transmission of pain.[9] The receptors for these fibers are probably the free nerve endings in the dermis and epidermis. Stimuli that trigger these nerve fibers result in the transmission of signals along peripheral nerves to the dorsal root ganglion, spinal cord, and finally to the thalamus and other parts of the brain.

Pruritus, which can be subdivided into clinical categories based on the presumptive mechanism (Table 435-1),[10] is associated with a number of systemic as well as skin-specific diseases (Table 435-2). Antihistamines, although commonly prescribed, are ineffective for many causes of pruritus—with the exception of urticaria—because they primarily cause sedation. Depending on the suspected mechanism of pruritus, classes of medication as diverse as the opiate antagonists (e.g., naltrexone), antidepressants (e.g., mirtazapine), anticonvulsants (e.g., gabapentin), and substance P antagonists (e.g., aprepitant) have proved to be useful (Tables 435-3 and 435-4). Although the precise targets of these classes of medications are poorly understood in pruritus, the clinical effectiveness of these agents may offer insight regarding the molecular and cellular pathways involved in these conditions.[11] Ultraviolet

TABLE 435-1 PATHOPHYSIOLOGY OF PRURITUS		
PRURITUS CATEGORY	PRURITUS MEDIATOR	CLINICAL EXAMPLES
Pruritoceptive	Generated in skin, usually inflammatory	Atopic dermatitis, allergic contact dermatitis, lichen planus
Neurogenic (systemic)	Generated in central nervous system but without any neural pathology	Renal failure, liver disease, lymphoproliferative disorders, malignancy
Neuropathic	Neuronal pathology along afferent pathway	Brachioradial pruritus, notalgia paresthetica
Psychogenic	Caused by psychological disorder	Delusions of parasitosis

TABLE 435-2 TERMINOLOGY TO DESCRIBE THE MORPHOLOGY OF INDIVIDUAL SKIN LESIONS

TERM	DEFINITION	EXAMPLE
PRIMARY SKIN LESIONS: INITIAL PATHOLOGIC CHANGE		
Macule	Circumscribed change in skin color that is flush with the surrounding skin. Lesion is <1 cm in diameter	Solar lentigo Traumatic purpura
Patch	Circumscribed change in skin color that is flush with the surrounding skin. Lesion is ≥1 cm in diameter	Café au lait spot Vitiligo
Papule	A solid or cystic elevation <1 cm in diameter	Acne Eruptive xanthoma
Nodule	A solid or cystic elevation >1 cm but <2 cm in diameter	Dermatofibroma
Tumor	A solid or cystic elevation >2 cm in diameter	Follicular cyst
Plaque	An elevated lesion that is >1 cm in diameter	Psoriasis
Scale	Desiccated, thin plates of cornified epidermal cells that form flakes on the skin surface	Ichthyosis
Wheal	Circumscribed, flat-topped, firm elevation of skin with a well-demarcated and palpable margin	Urticaria
Vesicle	Circumscribed, elevated lesion containing clear serous or hemorrhagic fluid that is <1 cm in diameter	Contact dermatitis Herpes simplex
Bulla	Circumscribed, elevated lesion containing clear serous or hemorrhagic fluid that is >2 cm in diameter	Bullous pemphigoid
Pustule	A vesicle containing purulent exudate	Folliculitis
Atrophy	A depression from the surface of the skin with underlying loss of epidermal or dermal substance	Lichen sclerosis et atrophicus
Erosion	A depression from the surface of the skin with a loss of all or part of the epidermis Can be a secondary lesion	Burn Ruptured bulla
Ulceration	A depression from the surface of the skin with a loss of the entire epidermis and at least some of the dermis Can be a secondary lesion	Ecthyma Excoriation of acne papule
SECONDARY SKIN LESIONS: RESULT FROM EXTERNAL FORCES SUCH AS SCRATCHING, PICKING, INFECTION, OR HEALING OF PRIMARY LESIONS		
Lichenification	Dry, leathery thickening of the skin with exaggerated skin markings	Chronic eczema
Scar	An elevated or depressed area of fibrosis of the dermis or subcutaneous tissue resulting from an antecedent destructive process	Healing wound
Fissure	A deep linear split in the skin extending through the epidermis	Traumatized eczema
Crust	Dried exudates of serum, blood, sebum, or purulent material on the surface of the skin	Impetigo

Modified from Armstrong CA. Examination of the skin and approach to diagnosing skin diseases. In: Goldman L, Schafer AI, eds. *Goldman's Cecil Medicine.* 24th ed. Philadelphia: Saunders; 2012: Table 444-1.

TABLE 435-3 TOPICAL TREATMENTS FOR PRURITUS

MEDICATION	DOSE	COMMENTS
Emollients	Variable	For skin barrier damage, dry skin itch
Corticosteroids	Variable	Useful in pruritus due to inflammatory skin dermatitides. Low-potency agents safest for use in children and on face and in skin folds
Calcineurin inhibitors	Tacrolimus 0.03 and 0.1% ointment Pimecrolimus 1% cream	For use in atopic dermatitis and contact dermatitis. Particularly useful in facial or anogenital pruritus. May cause transient burning and stinging
Doxepin	5% cream	Topical formulation of tricyclic antidepressant; 20-25% risk for sedation owing to systemic absorption
Menthol	1-5% cream	Useful in patients who report cooling as an alleviating factor. Higher concentrations can cause hypersensitivity reactions and burning sensation
Anesthetic agents		
Lidocaine/prilocaine	2.5-5%	Useful for neuropathic and postburn itch. Risk for methemoglobinemia
Capsaicin	0.025-0.1% cream	Particularly useful in neuropathic itch and itch caused by chronic kidney disease. May cause transient burning
Pramoxine	1-2.5%	Useful on face and genitals, for chronic kidney disease, and for neuropathic itch

Data from Yosipovitch G, Bernhard JD. Chronic pruritus. *N Engl J Med.* 2013;368:1625-1634.

TABLE 435-4 SYSTEMIC TREATMENTS FOR PRURITUS

MEDICATION	DOSE	COMMENTS
Antihistamines	Hydroxyzine 10-50 mg four times daily Cetirizine 10 mg/day Fexofenadine 60-180 mg/day	Sedating, but no direct effect on pruritus, except in urticaria
Antidepressants		
Tricyclic antidepressants	Amitriptyline 25-150 mg/day	Neuropathic itch. May cause drowsiness, dizziness, constipation, urinary retention, blurred vision, palpitations, low blood pressure
Noradrenergic and specific serotonergic antidepressants	Mirtazapine 7.5-15 mg PO at bedtime	Nocturnal pruritus. May increase appetite and weight
Selective serotonin reuptake inhibitors	Paroxetine 10-40 mg/day PO Fluvoxamine 25-150 mg/day PO Sertraline 50-200 mg/day PO	Psychiatric patients and paraneoplastic pruritus Psychiatric patients and paraneoplastic pruritus Cholestatic pruritus
Opioids		
μ Antagonist	Naltrexone 25-50 mg/day PO	Pruritus associated with cholestatic or chronic kidney disease. Can cause nausea, vomiting, and drowsiness
κ Agonist and μ antagonist	Butorphanol, 1-4 mg inhaled at bedtime	Intractable itch. May cause nausea, vomiting, and drowsiness
Anticonvulsants	Gabapentin 100-1200 mg PO three times per day Pregabalin 25-200 mg PO twice per day	Neuropathic itch and pruritus from chronic kidney disease. Can cause drowsiness, weight gain, and leg swelling
Substance P antagonist	Aprepitant 80 mg/day PO	Sézary syndrome
Immunosuppressants	Cyclosporin 2.5-5 mg/kg/day PO Azathioprine 2.5 mg/kg/day PO	Short-term use for refractory atopic dermatitis. Monitor blood pressure and renal function Refractory atopic dermatitis. Monitor for myelosuppression
Ultraviolet B radiation (broad and narrow band)	Three times per week	Atopic dermatitis, psoriasis, pruritus from chronic kidney disease

Data from Yosipovitch G, Bernhard JD. Chronic pruritus. *N Engl J Med.* 2013;368:1625-1634.
PO = orally.

phototherapy is also effective for multiple forms of pruritus, including pruritus that results from chronic kidney disease, as well as more inflammatory conditions such as psoriasis and atopic dermatitis; however, the mechanism underlying the resulting improvement is poorly understood.

GENERAL REFERENCES

For the General References and other additional features, please visit Expert Consult at https://expertconsult.inkling.com.

436

EXAMINATION OF THE SKIN AND AN APPROACH TO DIAGNOSING SKIN DISEASES

JAMES C. SHAW

Dermatology encompasses well over a thousand disease entities, many of which expand further into multiple subclassifications, variants, and etiologies. The first goal of a clinician is quickly to recognize the few skin diseases that can rapidly cause severe morbidity or even kill the patient. For the remaining hundreds of non–life-threatening dermatoses, a careful history and physical examination, which is often performed before or simultaneously with the history, can help the clinician make an accurate diagnosis or obtain expert dermatologic referral for doing so.[1]

THE SKIN EXAMINATION

The basic requirements for good examination of the skin are lighting and magnification. The best lighting is natural daylight or window light, but bright fluorescent ceiling lights, surgical lamps, or specialized magnifying lights all suffice. For simple magnification, a 4× hand lens is highly effective, but a 10× handheld polarized dermatoscope is even better, especially for diagnosing melanoma[2] and basal cell carcinoma.

Color

Attention to the color of the skin lesions can be key to making a correct diagnosis (Table 436-1). The color of the adjacent normal skin also can influence the appearance of dermatoses. Subtle colors such as violaceous or yellow or even simple erythema can be more difficult to appreciate in darker skin types than in light-colored skin (Fig. 436-1). The lighter an individual's skin, the higher the risk is for developing sun-induced skin cancer (Chapter 203).

Palpation

Palpation with an ungloved hand is often important in dermatologic diagnosis. Examples include the skin fibrosis and sclerosis of scleroderma (Chapter 267), the induration and firmness of cellulitis (Chapter 290), the roughness of subtle actinic keratoses (Chapter 440), the firmness of a dermatofibroma (Chapter 440), the palpable purpura of leukocytoclastic vasculitis (Chapter 439), and the difference between a lipoma (soft, subcutaneous) and an epidermoid cyst (firmer, intradermal) or between a dermal nevus (somewhat firm) and a solitary neurofibroma (rubbery soft).

A glove should be worn for protection when examining patients who may have blood-borne diseases, such as hepatitis B (Chapters 148 and 149) and human immunodeficiency virus (HIV) infections, or patients who may have secondary syphilis (Chapter 319) or herpes simplex (Chapter 374). Gloves are also essential when the clinician wishes to examine mucosae, denuded skin, blood, or exudates. Routine skin infections such as scabies (Chapter 441), human papillomavirus infection (Chapter 373), and superficial fungal infections (Chapter 438) are not highly contagious, but handwashing after contact is important to prevent transmission.

Another clue to diagnosis is determining the depth of the lesion (Chapter 435) and whether it involves the epidermis, the dermis, the fat layer below the dermis, or more than one layer (Table 436-2). Epidermal pathology includes the disorderly yet benign growth of keratinocytes resulting in flaking (scaling) and a thickened epidermis (psoriasis); the presence of microvesiculation (histologic term: spongiosis) that leads to oozing of serum (contact dermatitis); and hyperplasia of the epidermis in benign lesions (seborrheic keratoses), infections (warts), or malignancies (basal cell carcinomas and squamous cell carcinomas).

Dermal pathology often leads to inflammation because of the recruitment of lymphocytes, neutrophils, and histiocytes, as well as infiltration of malignant cells (lymphoma), antibody deposition (lupus erythematosus, autoimmune blistering diseases, drug eruptions), infections, or vascular damage. Erythema, which is caused by vasodilation of vasculature, is the most common dermal finding, even in diseases that are primarily epidermal. Abnormalities are less common in the subcutaneous fat than in the epidermis or dermis, but benign hyperplasia of the fat layer results in benign lipomas. Vasculitis of midsize vessels will often extend into the fat layer in polyarteritis nodosa (Chapter 270), and several panniculitides (e.g., erythema nodosum) also involve the fat.

HISTORY

The two most important facts to establish immediately from the history are whether the problem is acute (new onset within the last few days or hours) and whether the patient is systemically ill. Key clues to the diagnosis come from whether the lesions are associated with pruritus or pain, and what medications, especially new medications, the patient is taking (Table 436-3). For example, the absence of pruritus makes the diagnosis of allergic contact dermatitis (Chapter 440) highly unlikely. In the setting of unilateral acute severe pain, burning, and itching, herpes zoster (Chapter 439) should always be considered, even in the absence of skin findings.

DIFFERENTIAL DIAGNOSIS

Morphology

In the ambulatory outpatient who does not have a life-threatening skin problem, lesions are commonly classified as macules, patches, papules, plaques, nodules, tumors, vesicles, bullae, or pustules (Table 436-4). However, plain language can be just as effective in arriving at an accurate diagnosis. For example, a description of "small, raised solid bumps 0.4 cm in diameter" is as clear as "multiple papules." Furthermore, if dermatologic terms are used incorrectly, clinicians may be misled toward an incorrect diagnosis. Although primary lesions (which develop de novo) are most helpful in leading to a correct diagnosis, secondary features (which are altered by superinfection, manipulation, healing, etc.) are also important.

Text continued on p. 2644

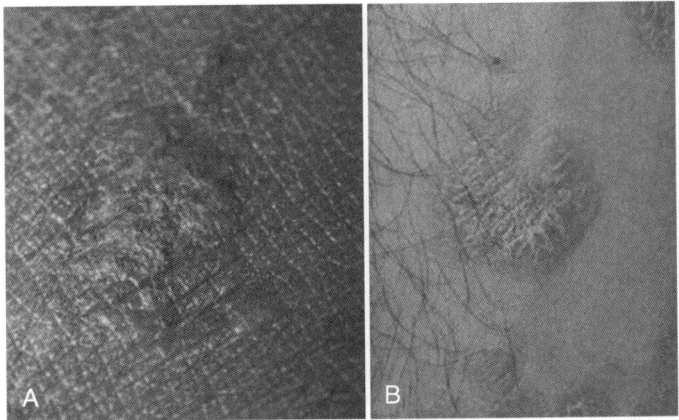

FIGURE 436-1. Skin pigmentation. Lichen planus presents differently in darkly pigmented (**A**) versus lightly pigmented (**B**) skin. The violaceous hue seen in **B** is more muted in **A**, and these lesions appear brown-black in color. Wickham striae (lacy white pattern) are more easily seen in **B**. (From Bolognia JL, Jorizzo JL, Schaffer JV. *Dermatology,* 3rd ed. Philadelphia: Saunders; 2012:8.)

TABLE 436-1 COLOR CLUES IN DIAGNOSING SKIN DISEASE

COLOR	CLINICAL EXAMPLE

Erythema: Pink

Pink is a common finding when vasodilation (with minimal cellular infiltrate) is the primary dermal pathology.

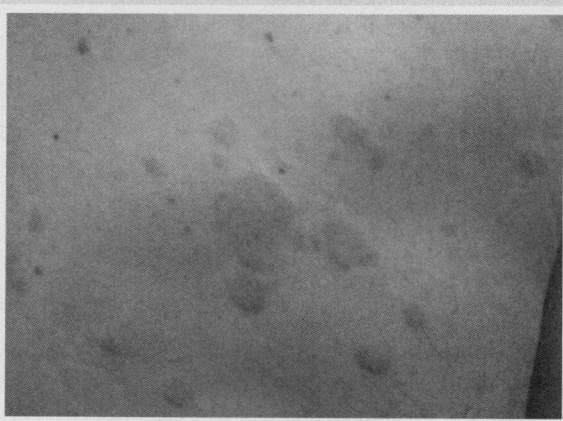

FIGURE 436-2. Urticaria (Chapter 440).

Erythema: Pink-Red

Although many dermatoses can be pink-red, pityriasis rosea is classic.

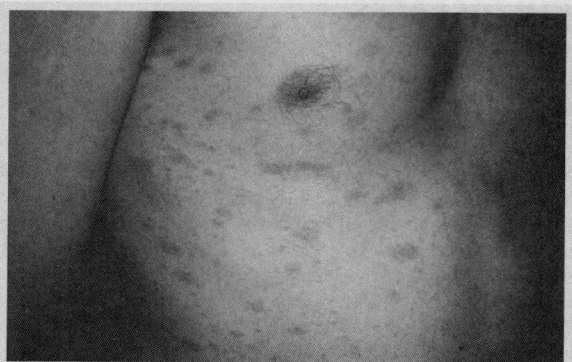

FIGURE 436-3. Pityriasis rosea (Chapter 438).

Erythema: Orange-Red (with Scale)

Color in psoriasis ranges from orange-red to purple-red. A related condition, pityriasis rubra pilaris, also is orange-red.

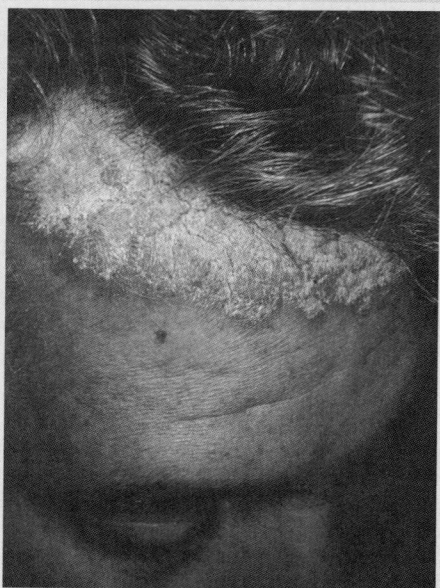

FIGURE 436-4. Psoriasis (Chapter 438).

TABLE 436-1   COLOR CLUES IN DIAGNOSING SKIN DISEASE—cont'd

COLOR	CLINICAL EXAMPLE

Erythema: Red-Orange-Pink
A mixture of erythematous hues is common and makes diagnosis difficult by color alone.

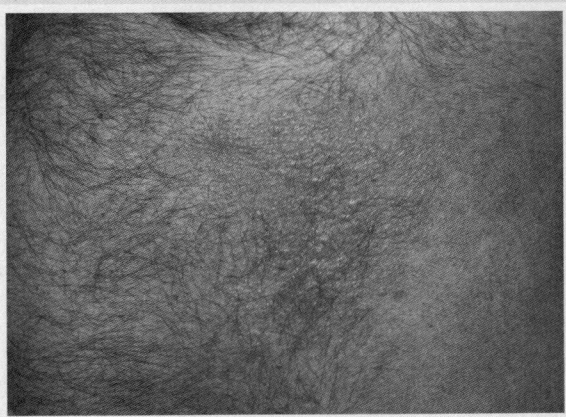

FIGURE 436-5. Allergic contact dermatitis (Chapter 438).

Erythema: Copper-Red
Mixed cellular infiltrates with plasma cells, classically seen in syphilis.

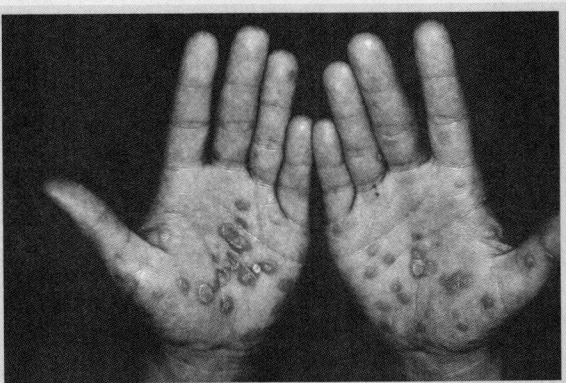

FIGURE 436-6. Secondary syphilis (Chapter 319).

Erythema: Red-Brown
The color of histiocytic infiltrates, seen commonly in granulomatous diseases (e.g., cutaneous tuberculosis, deep fungal infections, atypical mycobacteria, sarcoidosis, granuloma annulare, leprosy, necrobiosis lipoidica) depends on depth of the infiltrates.

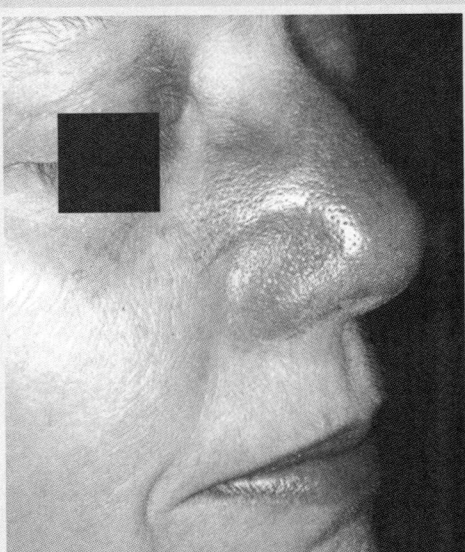

FIGURE 436-7. Sarcoidosis (Chapter 95).

TABLE 436-1   COLOR CLUES IN DIAGNOSING SKIN DISEASE—cont'd

COLOR	CLINICAL EXAMPLE

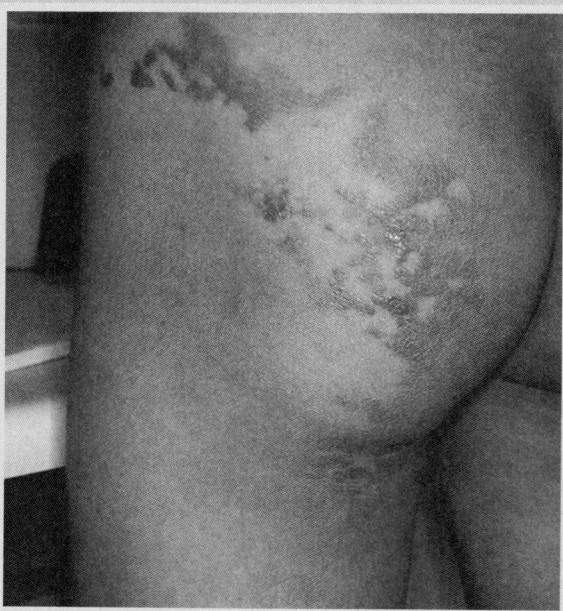

FIGURE 436-8. Leprosy (Chapter 326).

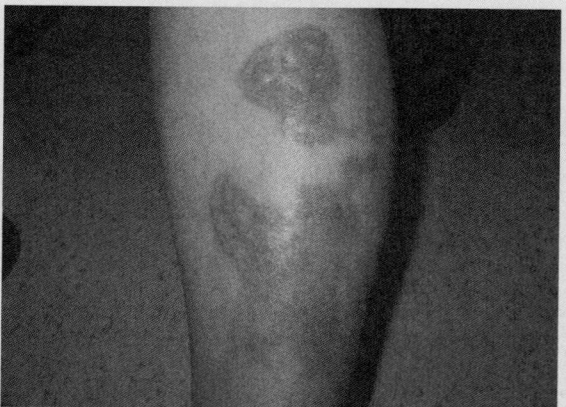

FIGURE 436-9. Necrobiosis lipoidica (note the characteristic slight yellow tinge; Chapter 440).

Violaceous: Purple
Lymphocytes in the dermis impart a violaceous color in lichen planus, lupus erythematosus, lymphoma cutis, and pseudolymphoma.

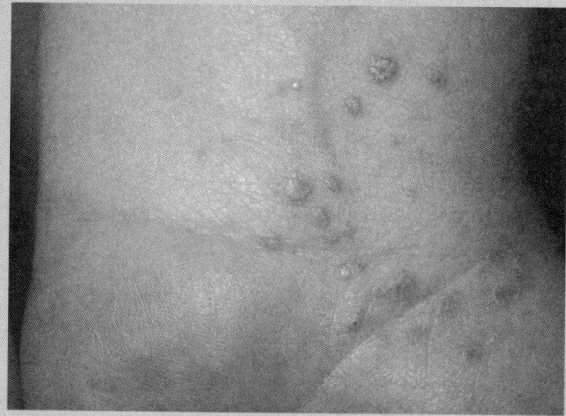

FIGURE 436-10. Lichen planus (pruritic purple polygonal papules; Chapter 438).

TABLE 436-1 COLOR CLUES IN DIAGNOSING SKIN DISEASE—cont'd

COLOR	CLINICAL EXAMPLE

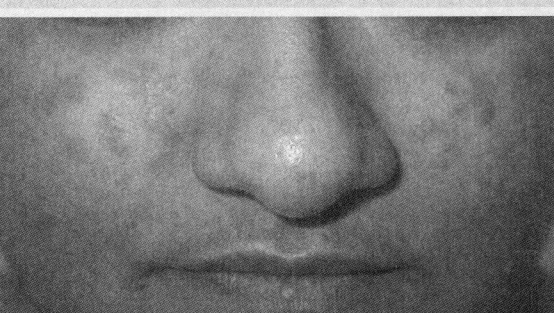

FIGURE 436-11. Lupus erythematosus on sun-exposed surface (the "butterfly" rash when more confluent; Chapter 266).

Violaceous: Purple to Black
Blood in the dermis (e.g., ecchymoses, vasculitis, subungual hemorrhage) leads to a dark purple color with blue and black overtones. Unlike blood in vessels, lesions do not blanch with pressure.

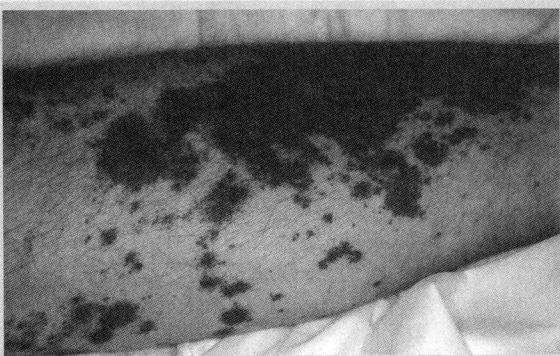

FIGURE 436-12. Purpura. Small vessel vasculitis with small lesions coalescing into larger plaque (Chapter 439).

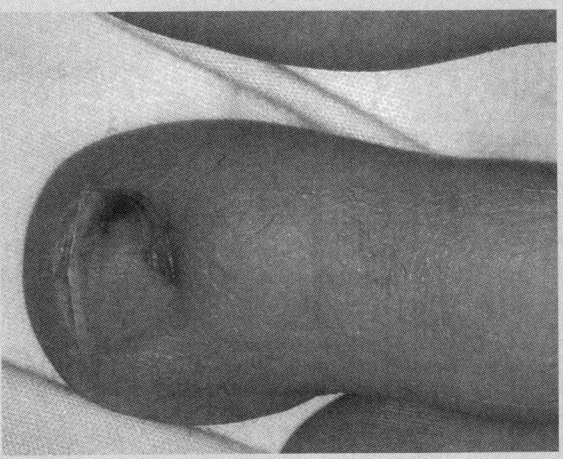

FIGURE 436-13. Subungual hemorrhage can mimic melanoma.

TABLE 436-1 COLOR CLUES IN DIAGNOSING SKIN DISEASE—cont'd

COLOR	CLINICAL EXAMPLE

Gray

Necrotic keratinocytes (e.g., center of target lesions of erythema multiforme and the border of pyoderma gangrenosum) impart a grayish color. Gray color also is seen with melanin in the dermis (e.g., postinflammatory pigmentary change).

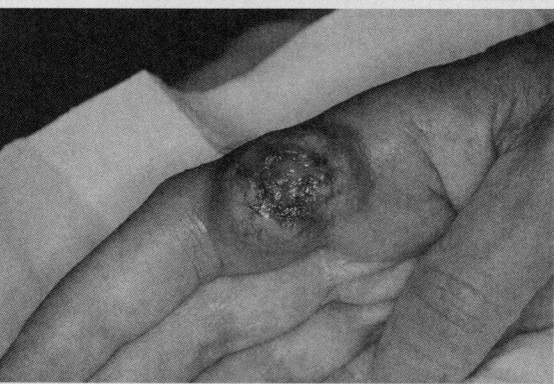

FIGURE 436-14. Border of pyoderma gangrenosum (Chapter 440); note gray representing keratinocyte necrosis.

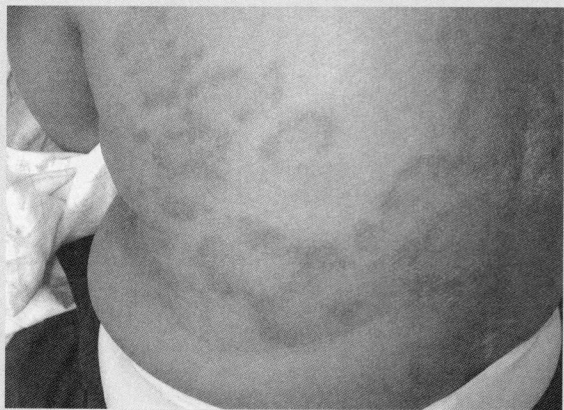

FIGURE 436-15. Postinflammatory gray centrally in subacute cutaneous lupus (Chapter 266) in person with olive skin.

Black

Black is a sign of dermal and epidermal necrosis (e.g., polyarteritis nodosa, antiphospholipid antibody syndrome, warfarin necrosis, heparin necrosis, calciphylaxis, ANCA-positive vasculitis) from vascular compromise, infection (e.g., mucormycosis, aspergillosis, anthrax, DIC from meningococcemia), or from melanin (the more superficial the melanin, the darker the color).

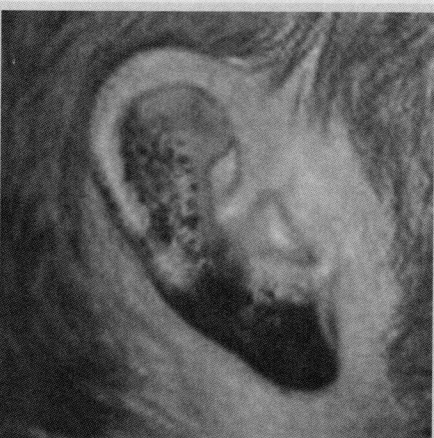

FIGURE 436-16. Ischemic necrosis secondary to vasculopathy from levamisole-contaminated cocaine. (From Bolognia JL, Jorizzo JL, Schaffer JV. *Dermatology,* 3rd ed. Philadelphia: Saunders; 2012: Table 0.4.)

TABLE 436-1 COLOR CLUES IN DIAGNOSING SKIN DISEASE—cont'd

COLOR	CLINICAL EXAMPLE
	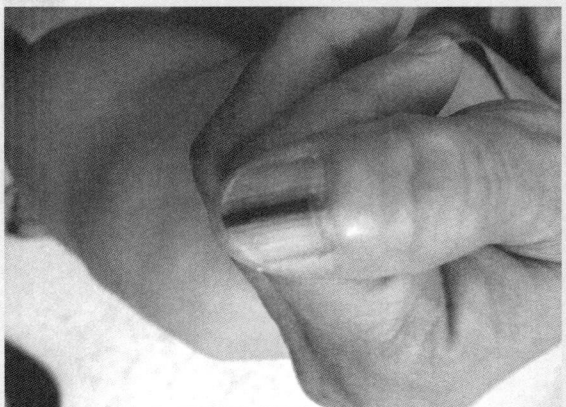

FIGURE 436-17. Melanoma (Chapter 203) demonstrating superficial deposition of melanin in the nail plate.

Brown
Brown is a result of pathologic pigments (e.g., hemosiderin; hemochromatosis; drug induced) in the dermis or normal epidermal melanin in individuals of color.

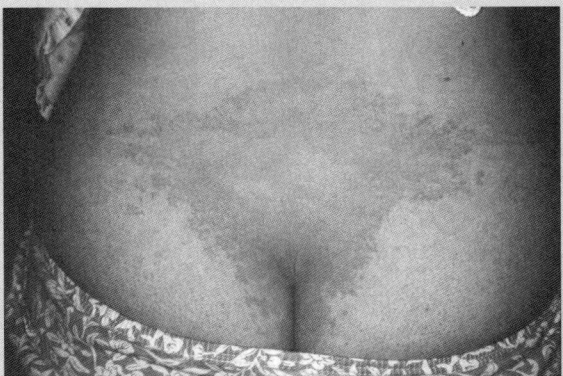

FIGURE 436-18. Tinea versicolor (Chapter 438); note bran-colored scaling.

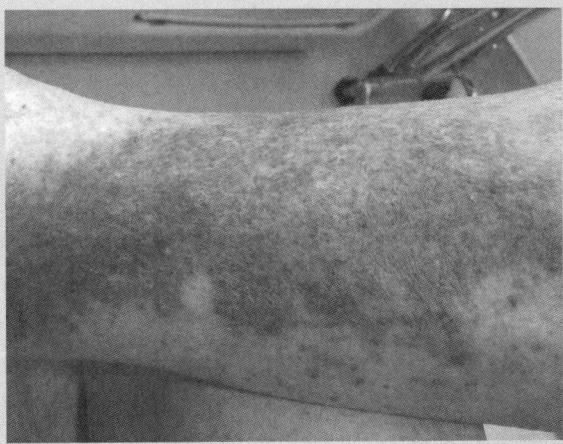

FIGURE 436-19. Stasis dermatitis (Chapter 440); note brown superiorly from hemosiderin.

TABLE 436-1   COLOR CLUES IN DIAGNOSING SKIN DISEASE—cont'd

COLOR	CLINICAL EXAMPLE
White White can be seen in hyperplastic mucosal epithelium, sclerosis of dermis, scar tissue, loss of pigmentation, or small epidermal cysts.	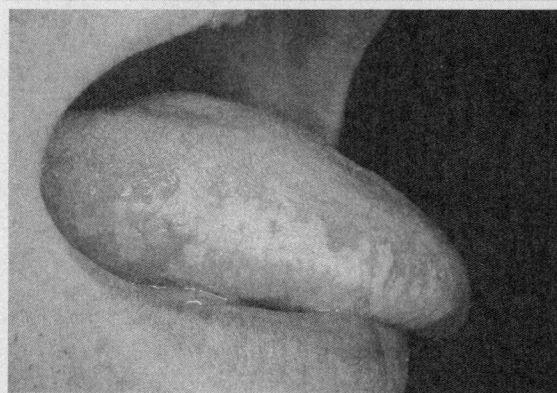 **FIGURE 436-20.** Oral hairy leukoplakia (Chapter 425). 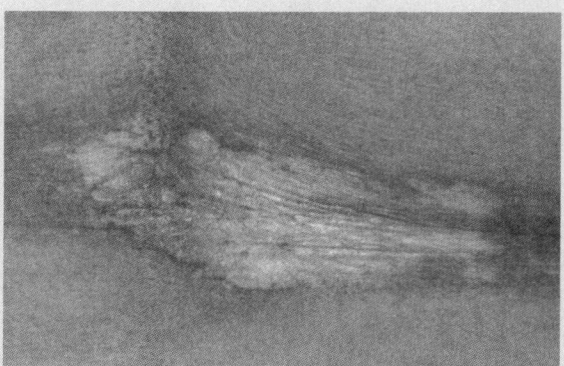 **FIGURE 436-21.** Lichen sclerosis (Chapter 440) (From Bolognia JL, Jorizzo JL, Schaffer JV. *Dermatology,* 3rd ed. Philadelphia: Saunders; 2012: Fig. 44-12).

ANCA = antineutrophil cytoplasmic antibodies; DIC = disseminated intravascular coagulation.

Purpura refers to the appearance of skin into which red blood cells have extravasated, thereby producing a bluish to dark purple to black color. Purpura is macular in cases of tiny petechiae and ecchymoses from minor trauma. In small vessel leukocytoclastic vasculitis, purpura becomes palpable, usually as small papules. In deeper vasculopathies, purpura can be nodular, linear, stellate or associated with ulceration because of damage to vascular structures in the dermis or subcutaneous fat.

Scaling, which is a manifestation of abnormal production of stratum corneum, is frequently an important clue to the correct diagnosis. It is commonly seen as a primary component of conditions such as psoriasis, tinea, and pityriasis rosea.

Secondary characteristics include crusting, fissures, erosion, ulceration, excoriation, atrophy, and lichenification (Table 436-5). Each may be helpful in diagnosing a skin disorder depending on whether the finding represents a normal evolution of the disease, such as ulcer formation in pyoderma gangrenosum, or an extraneous influence, such as lichenification from scratching in a patient with atopic dermatitis.

Distribution

Some dermatologic diseases can be recognized by where they manifest on the body (Table 436-6). Prime examples include herpes zoster (unilateral dermatomal distribution of vesicles), dermatitis herpetiformis (pruritic vesicles over extensor areas of elbows, knees, and sacral skin), and hidradenitis suppurativa (inflammatory acne-like nodules and cysts in the axillae, inguinal, and intergluteal areas). Other sites manifestation include sun-exposed skin for lupus erythematosus and dermatomyositis, facial distribution for acne vulgaris and rosacea, and penile involvement for psoriasis and lichen planus.

Sun-exacerbated diseases spare areas under the nose and chin, inner arms, intertriginous regions, the mid and distal phalanges, and clothed areas. In a patient with bilateral erythema and swelling of the legs with dermatitis, the odds of cellulitis are extremely low, because cellulitis of the extremities is a unilateral disease.[A1]

Life-Threatening Emergencies

In the acutely ill patient with a dermatosis, a clinician must determine whether the patient has a potentially rapidly fatal skin disease—typically a systemic infection or severe drug reaction—and if so, what treatment to initiate urgently. The most common rapidly fatal diseases with skin involvement are disseminated herpes zoster infection[3] (mortality up to 30%, Chapter 375); disseminated herpes simplex infection (mortality up to 80% in the presence of encephalitis, Chapter 374); toxic epidermal necrolysis[4] or its variant Stevens-Johnson syndrome (mortality up to 20% for toxic epidermal necrolysis Chapter 440); meningococcemia (mortality up to 35%, Chapter 298); toxic shock syndrome (mortality up to 30%, Chapters 288 and 290); necrotizing fasciitis (mortality 20 to 40%, Chapters 288 and 290); and disseminated fungal diseases including candidiasis (Chapter 338), histoplasmosis (Chapter 332), cryptococcosis (Chapter 336).

In the acutely ill patient, physical findings that can often help make the correct diagnosis include the following:

- Multiple small, discrete lesions (10 to several hundred; <1 cm diameter) scattered over the body that do not become confluent into large sheets imply a hematogenously spread infectious disease, such as seen in

Text continued on p. 2654

TABLE 436-2 REPRESENTATIVE DIAGNOSES BASED ON DEPTH OF PATHOLOGY IN THE SKIN

DEPTH	CHARACTERISTICS	DISORDERS		CLINICAL EXAMPLE
Epidermal	Distinct, even sharp margins Scaling Epidermal thickening Absence of induration May have mild erythema as well (some dermal involvement)	Seborrheic keratosis Warts In situ squamous cell carcinoma (Bowen's disease) Ichthyosis Bullous impetigo Superficial basal cell carcinoma Acanthosis nigricans	Seborrheic dermatitis Thin-plaque psoriasis Mild contact dermatitis Pityriasis rosea Tinea versicolor Tinea corporis Actinic keratosis Patch stage mycosis fungoides	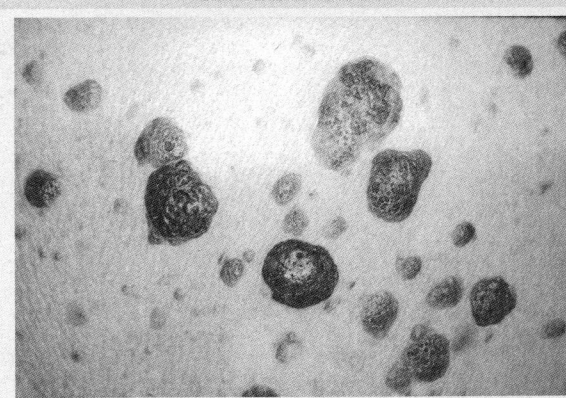 **FIGURE 436-22.** Seborrheic keratosis (Chapter 440).
Epidermal and dermal Most skin diseases will have some degree of dermal and epidermal involvement	Margins moderately well defined Scale can be present Inflammation (erythema) Usually palpable lesions (raised)	Lichen planus Systemic lupus erythematosus Chronic cutaneous lupus Nummular (discoid) dermatitis Plaque-stage mycosis fungoides Pyoderma gangrenosum	Atopic dermatitis Small vessel vasculitis Secondary syphilis Cellulitis/erysipelas Nodular basal cell carcinoma Squamous cell carcinoma Melanoma Most vesiculobullous diseases (HSV, autoimmune)	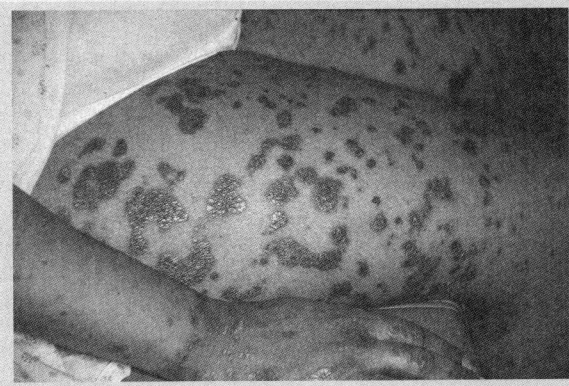 **FIGURE 436-23.** Lichen planus (Chapter 438).
Dermal Diseases with only dermal involvement usually consist of infiltrates with inflammatory or malignant cells that do not influence epidermal function	Margins moderately defined No scale Smooth surface No ulcer Variable inflammation Usually palpable	Urticaria Sarcoidosis Granuloma annulare Leprosy Necrobiosis lipoidica Morphea Scleroderma Plaque- or tumor-stage mycosis fungoides	Cutaneous metastases Most cysts Dermatofibromas Dermal melanocytic nevi Pretibial myxedema Other cutaneous lymphomas	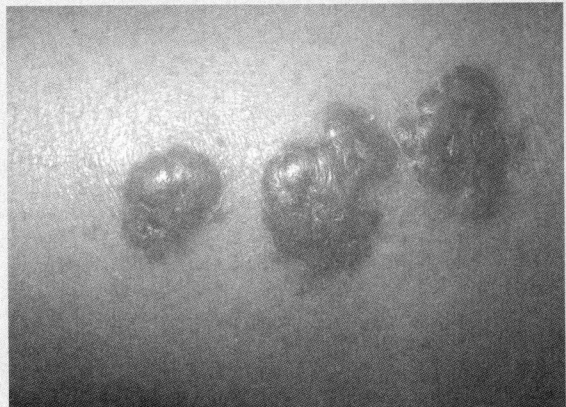 **FIGURE 436-24.** Sarcoidosis: Histiocyte collections in the upper dermis (Chapter 95).

TABLE 436-2 REPRESENTATIVE DIAGNOSES BASED ON DEPTH OF PATHOLOGY IN THE SKIN—cont'd

DEPTH	CHARACTERISTICS	DISORDERS	CLINICAL EXAMPLE
Subcutaneous fat	Margins rounded and/ or poorly defined Variable inflammation Smooth overlying skin	Large cysts, lipoma Erythema nodosum Panniculitis of any etiology Some lymphomas Medium-vessel vasculitis (polyarteritis nodosa)	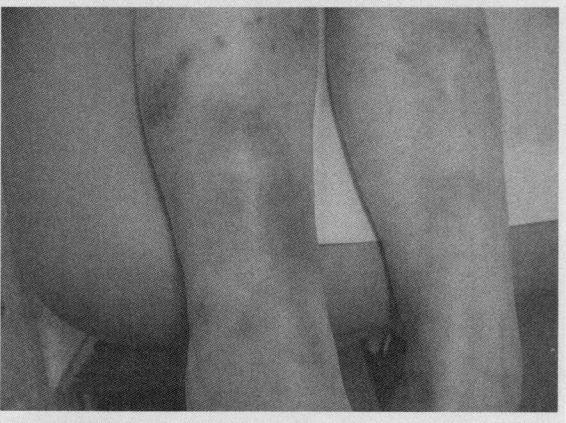 **FIGURE 436-25.** Erythema nodosum (Chapter 440).

HSV = herpes simplex virus.

TABLE 436-3 IMPORTANT CLUES FROM THE HISTORY AND GENERAL HEALTH STATUS

CLUES	POSSIBLE DIAGNOSES	
Pruritus (itch)	Atopic dermatitis (eczema) Allergic contact dermatitis Urticaria Scabies	Bullous pemphigoid Lichen planus Dermatitis herpetiformis Inflammatory tinea pedis
Absence of pruritus	Acne vulgaris Rosacea Syphilis	Skin malignancies Lupus Pemphigus vulgaris Erythema multiforme
Pain	Herpes zoster Ischemic necrosis from all causes Cellulitis Furunculosis	Carbuncles Pyoderma gangrenosum Severe systemic illnesses
Medications (especially new)	Severe drug eruptions Fixed drug eruptions Morbilliform drug eruptions Immunosuppression	Subacute cutaneous lupus Psoriasis exacerbation Urticaria Drug induced hair loss
Cachexia/ malnourished	Paraneoplastic dermatoses Skin malignancy Alcohol exacerbated psoriasis	Nutritional deficiencies Metastatic disease Eating disorders leading to nutritional deficiencies
Obesity or weight gain	Dermatoses of diabetes Thyroid disease Cushing's disease Polycystic ovarian syndrome Acne	Hirsutism Striae Acanthosis nigricans Eruptive xanthomas
Poor hygiene	Bacterial skin infections Infestations	Substance abuse
Psychiatric illness	Self-inflicted skin disease	Drug-induced dermatoses

TABLE 436-4 MORPHOLOGIC TERMS FOR PRIMARY LESIONS

TERMS	ILLUSTRATIONS
Macule: Flat, nonpalpable, <1 cm diameter	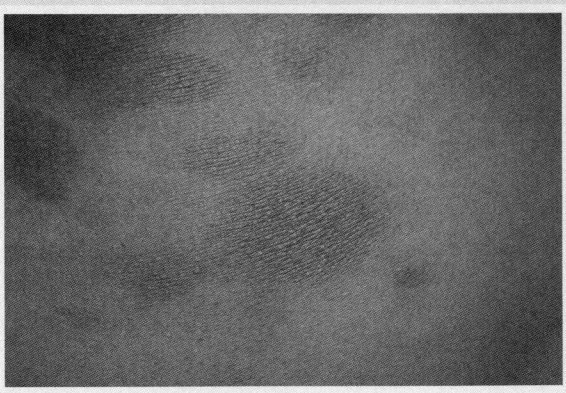 **FIGURE 436-26.** Fixed drug eruption (Chapter 440). 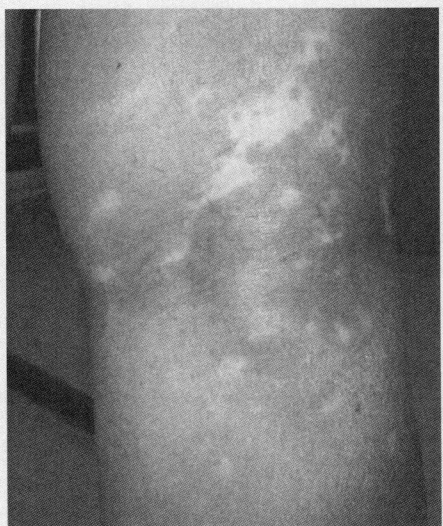 **FIGURE 436-27.** Vitiligo (Chapter 441).
Patch: Large macules >1 cm diameter	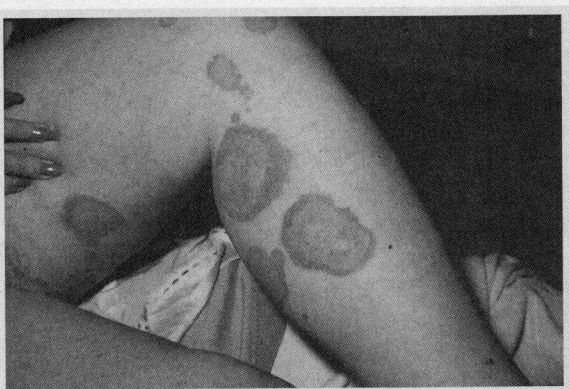 **FIGURE 436-28.** Erythema multiforme (Chapter 439).

TABLE 436-4   MORPHOLOGIC TERMS FOR PRIMARY LESIONS—cont'd

TERMS	ILLUSTRATIONS

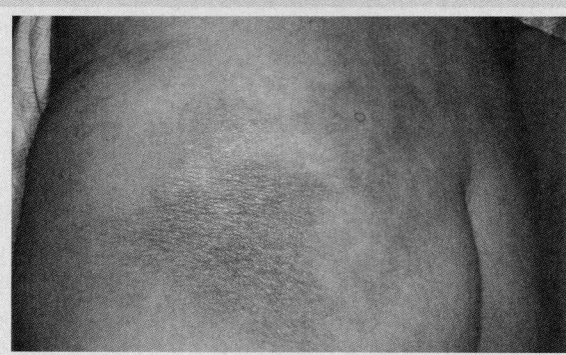

FIGURE 436-29. Mycosis fungoides (cutaneous T-cell lymphoma [CTCL]; Chapter 185).

Papule: Superficial, raised, palpable, <1 cm diameter

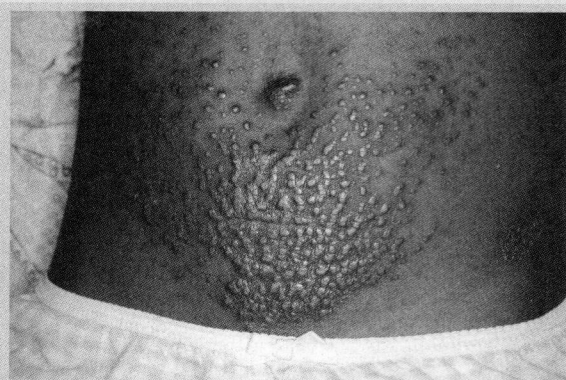

FIGURE 436-30. Atopic dermatitis with follicular accentuation (Chapter 438).

Plaque: Raised, palpable, >1 cm diameter

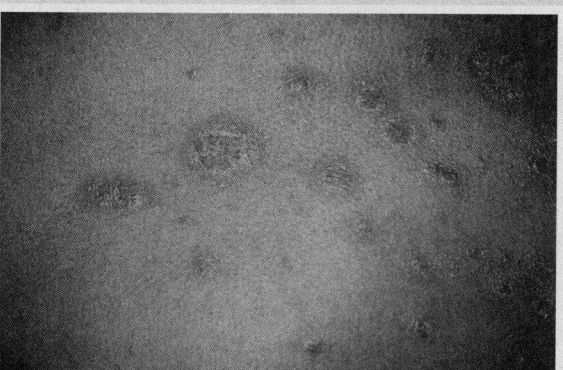

FIGURE 436-31. Psoriasis (Chapter 438).

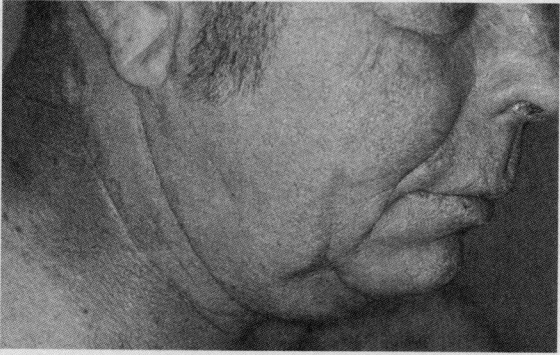

FIGURE 436-32. Discoid lupus (Chapter 266).

TABLE 436-4 MORPHOLOGIC TERMS FOR PRIMARY LESIONS—cont'd

TERMS	ILLUSTRATIONS
Nodule: Deeper than a papule, usually <1 cm diameter	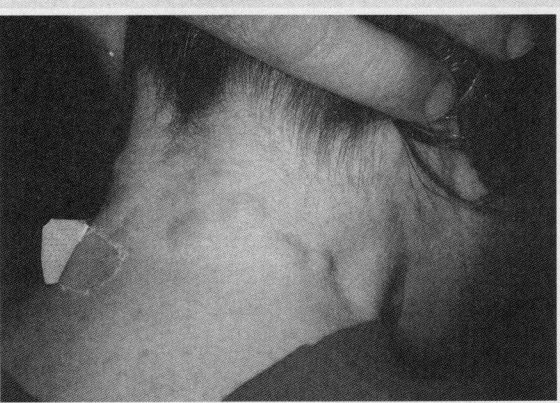 **FIGURE 436-33.** Metastatic breast carcinoma (Chapter 198).
Tumor: Large nodule, >1 cm diameter	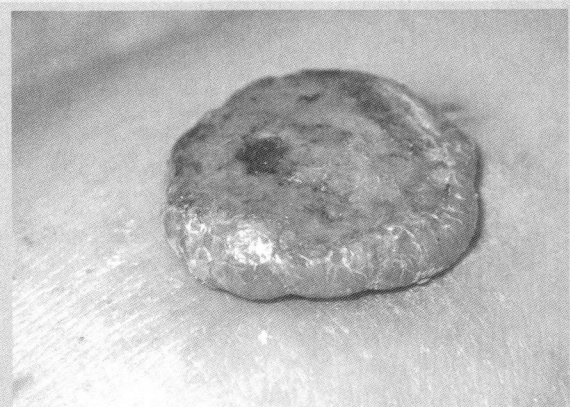 **FIGURE 436-34.** Amelanotic melanoma (Chapter 203). 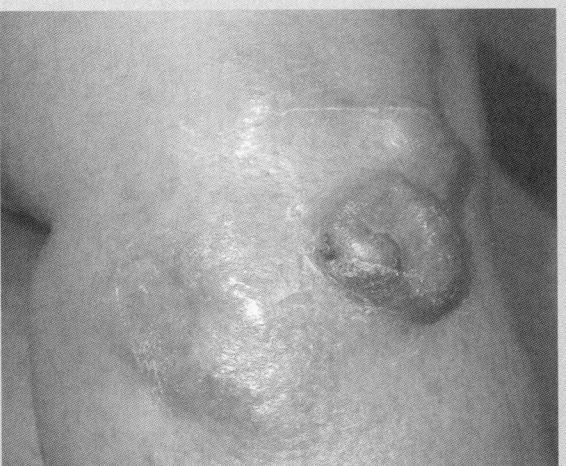 **FIGURE 436-35.** Post-transplant lymphoproliferative disorder (Chapter 185).

TABLE 436-4 MORPHOLOGIC TERMS FOR PRIMARY LESIONS—cont'd

TERMS	ILLUSTRATIONS
Vesicle: <1cm fluid-filled, may be umbilicated or contain pus or blood	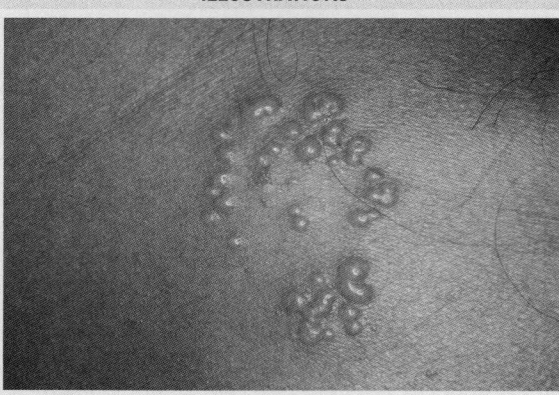 FIGURE 436-36. Herpes simplex (Chapter 374).
Bulla: >1-2 cm, filled with clear fluid, pus, or blood	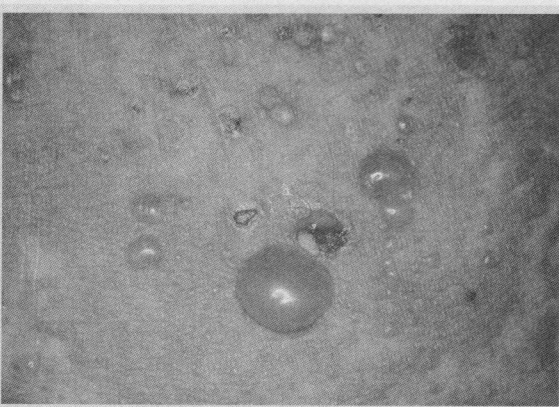 FIGURE 436-37. Bullous pemphigoid with small and larger bullae (Chapter 439).
Pustule: White, pus-filled, small, raised, <1 cm diameter	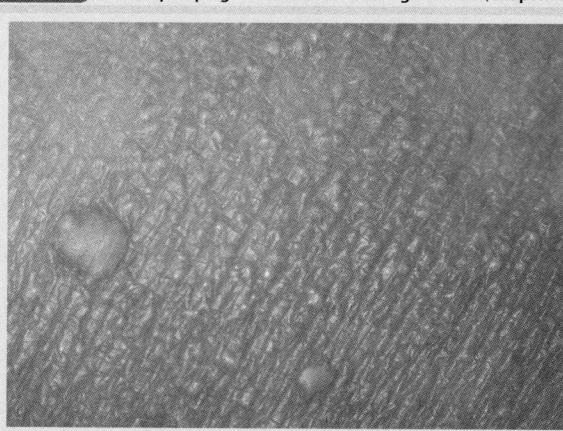 FIGURE 436-38. Acute generalized exanthematous pustulosis (Chapter 439).

TABLE 436-4 MORPHOLOGIC TERMS FOR PRIMARY LESIONS—cont'd

TERMS	ILLUSTRATIONS
Scale: White keratinous flakes of retained stratum corneum	

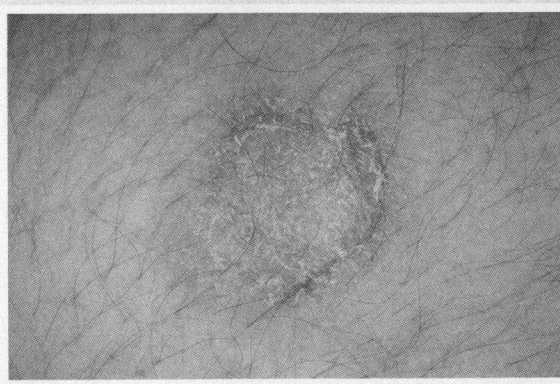

FIGURE 436-39. Nummular dermatitis (Chapter 438).

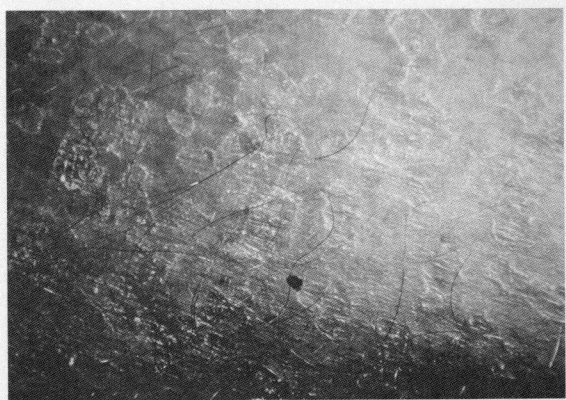

FIGURE 436-40. Disseminated superficial actinic porokeratosis (Chapter 440).

TABLE 436-5 MORPHOLOGIC TERMS FOR SECONDARY FEATURES

Crust: Dried serum, yellow to hemorrhagic depending on number of cells in exudate

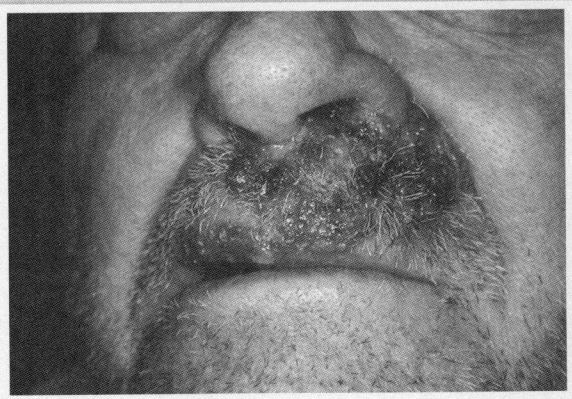

FIGURE 436-41. Impetigo (Chapter 441).

TABLE 436-5 MORPHOLOGIC TERMS FOR SECONDARY FEATURES—cont'd

Fissure: Small linear splits in skin, usually superficial

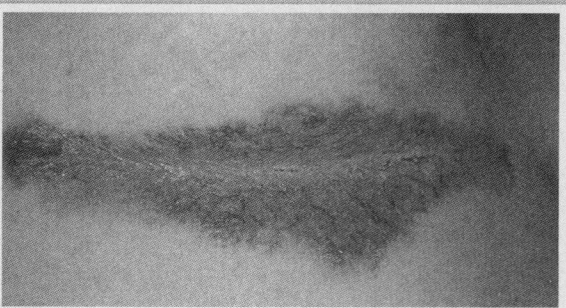

FIGURE 436-42. Hailey-Hailey disease.

Erosion: Loss of part or all of epidermis into upper dermis at most

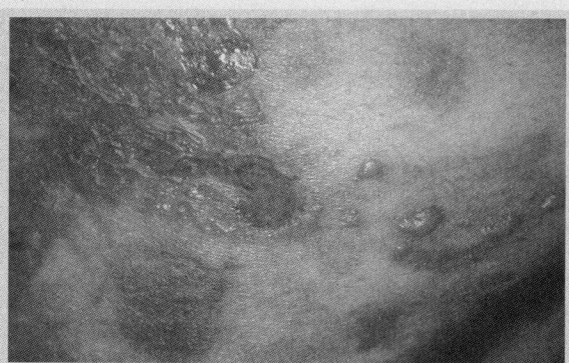

FIGURE 436-43. Pemphigus vulgaris (Chapter 439).

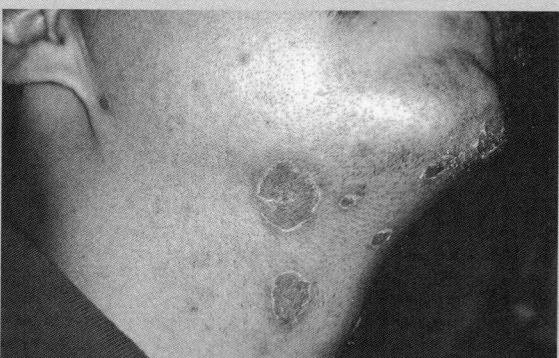

FIGURE 436-44. Staphylococcal bullous impetigo (Chapter 441).

Ulceration: Loss of epidermis into deep dermis or fat

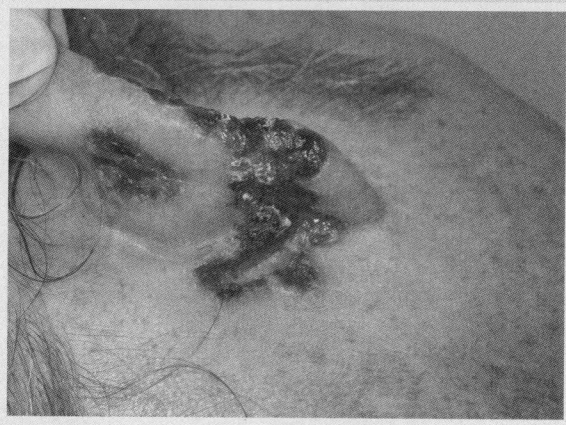

FIGURE 436-45. Chronic erosive herpes simplex (Chapter 374).

TABLE 436-5 MORPHOLOGIC TERMS FOR SECONDARY FEATURES—cont'd

Excoriation: Self-inflicted erosion or ulcer

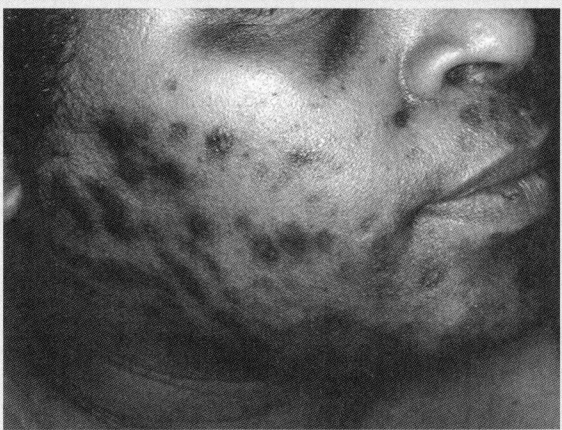

FIGURE 436-46. Factitial dermatitis (dermatitis artefacta).

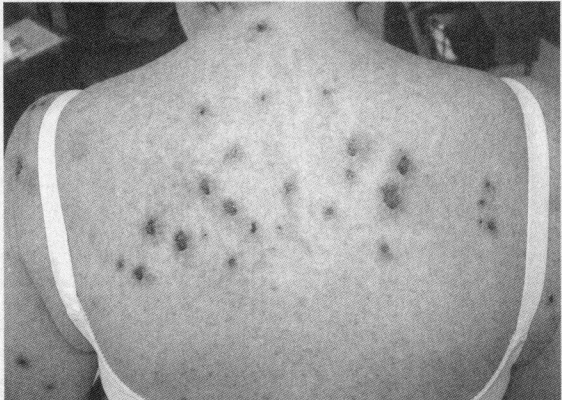

FIGURE 436-47. Neurodermatitis; note inferior cutoff where patient cannot reach.

Atrophy: Thinning or loss of dermal structures or fat usually; may apply to any tissue

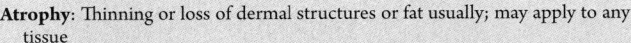

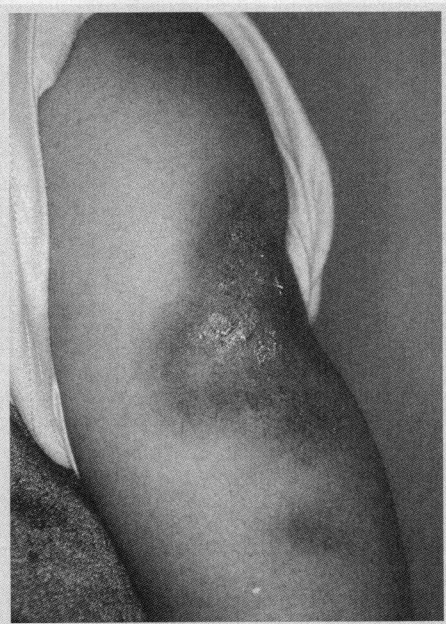

FIGURE 436-48. Fat atrophy: Lupus panniculitis.

TABLE 436-5 MORPHOLOGIC TERMS FOR SECONDARY FEATURES—cont'd

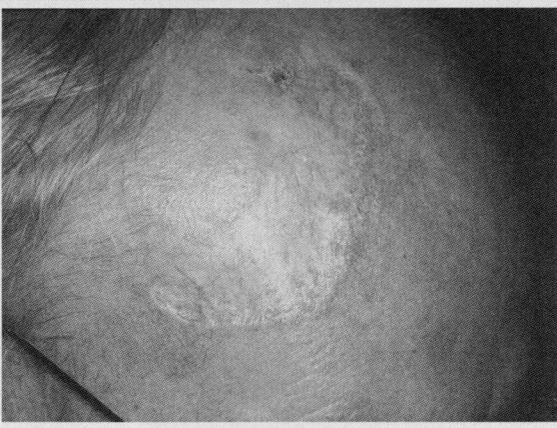

FIGURE 436-49. Central atrophy: Annular elastotic giant cell granuloma.

Lichenification: Thickened skin from chronic rubbing. Poorly demarcated, skin lines accentuated.

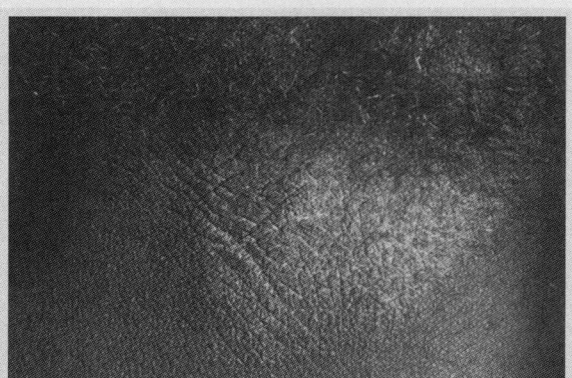

FIGURE 436-50. Lichen simplex chronicus.

TABLE 436-6 LOCATION OF SKIN LESIONS AS A DIAGNOSTIC CLUE

LOCATION	POSSIBLE DIAGNOSES	
Unilateral	Herpes zoster Herpes simplex Deep vein thrombosis Embolic disease	Contact dermatitis where exposed Cellulitis Necrotizing fasciitis Solitary skin malignancies
Bilateral, widespread	Hematogenously spread process Severe drug eruption Disseminated viral, bacterial, or fungal infection Vasculitis Autoimmune disease	Psoriasis Cutaneous T-cell lymphoma Scabies Urticaria Atopic dermatitis (eczema) Other drug eruptions
Bilateral, limited sites	Stasis dermatitis Contact dermatitis	Vasculitis Erythema multiforme

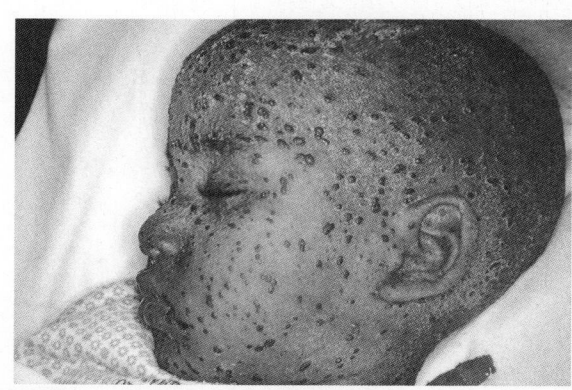

FIGURE 436-51. Chickenpox (Chapter 375). Multiple small vesicles that do not coalesce into larger bullae. Several lesions demonstrate central umbilication.

chickenpox (Fig. 436-51), disseminated herpes zoster (herpes simplex virus) (Fig. 436-52), disseminated fungal disease (Fig. 436-53), or a vascular immune process, such as autoimmune vasculitis (Fig. 436-54).
- Confluence of individual red lesions into sheets of erythema, especially in the presence of skin detachment or fluid-filled bullae, suggests a severe drug eruption such as toxic epidermal necrolysis or Stevens-Johnson syndrome (Fig. 436-55; Chapter 440).
- Mucositis, which is inflammation and erosions of conjunctivae or of the oral or anogenital mucosae, in the acutely ill patient also strongly suggests toxic epidermal necrolysis or Stevens-Johnson syndrome (Chapter 440).

Although some viral infections, such as herpesvirus and coxsackievirus, can cause multiple discrete mucosal lesions, severe mucositis is rarely a presenting finding in patients with disseminated viral, fungal, or bacterial infections.
- Widespread vesicles (Fig. 436-56) suggest disseminated herpesvirus infection, either varicella (Chapter 375) or simplex (Chapter 374). The vesicles often become hemorrhagic or pustular 2 to 5 days later when red blood cells or neutrophils infiltrate them.
- Widespread bullae (Fig. 436-57) with and without skin detachment suggest severe drug eruptions, as in toxic epidermal necrolysis and the

Stevens-Johnson syndrome (Chapter 440). By comparison, bullae accompanied by intense pruritus suggest autoimmune bullous pemphigoid (Fig. 436-58; Chapter 439) or severe allergic contact dermatitis (Fig. 436-59; Chapter 438).

- Widespread purpura (see Fig. 436-12) in an acutely ill patient may be a sign of disseminated intravascular coagulation (Chapter 174), which is seen in severe systemic infections, such as meningococcemia (Chapter 298). In less urgent settings, purpura can be caused by localized coagulation disorders (reactions to warfarin or heparin) or can be palpable and a sign of small vessel leukocytoclastic vasculitis[5] (Chapter 270). Purpura above the waist or on mucosal surfaces strongly implies systemic vasculitis or coagulation disorder, whereas purpura below the waist, especially below the knees, can be caused by the extravasation of red blood cells owing to increased hydrostatic pressure in association with any cause of tissue inflammation.

- Acute erythema of the hands, feet, and pelvic groin region (Fig. 436-60) associated with systemic illness can suggest a bacterial exotoxin as seen in toxic shock syndrome (Chapters 288 and 290). Peeling of palmar and plantar skin is not seen until 2 weeks later, so early diagnosis and treatment during the erythematous phase is critical. By comparison, erythroderma, which is confluent erythema without individual lesions, usually is not immediately life-threatening and can be seen in severe forms of psoriasis (Chapter 438), cutaneous T-cell lymphoma (mycosis fungoides, Chapter 185), and erythrodermic drug eruptions (Chapter 440).

Diagnostic Tests

Diascopy is merely pressing carefully on the skin with something transparent to look at the vasculature. Options include a clear plastic diascope, a glass slide, or any other lens. Vascular malformations and small hemangiomas can be diagnosed this way, and careful examination may reveal pulsations in spider telangiectasias.

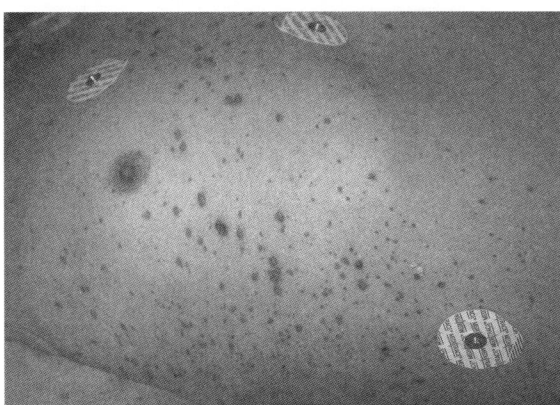

FIGURE 436-52. Disseminated varicella-zoster virus. Widespread, individual papules and vesicles, many with hemorrhage. Note the absence of coalescence into larger bullae.

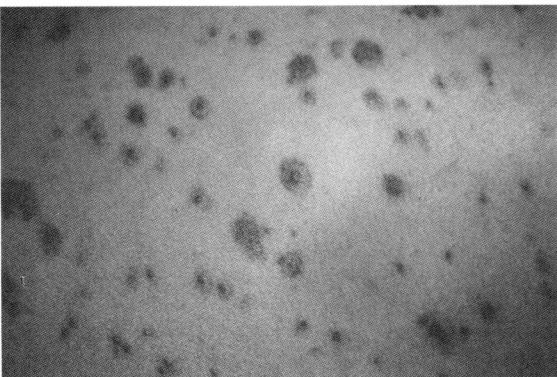

FIGURE 436-53. Disseminated candidiasis. Multiple individual small lesions, papules mostly, some with surrounding purpura, consistent with hematogenously spread disease.

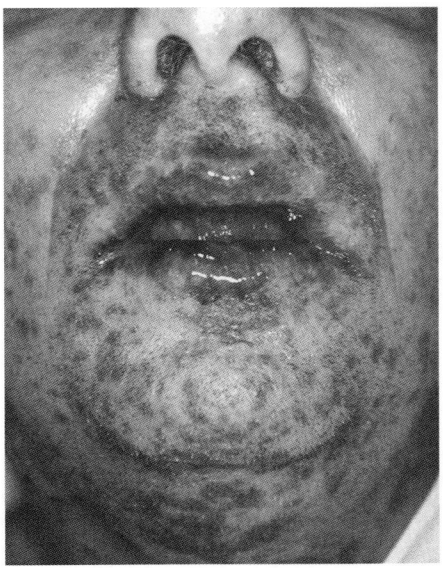

FIGURE 436-55. Mucositis (Stevens-Johnson syndrome). Extensive erosive changes on lips and oral mucosa are highly suggestive of a severe drug eruption such as Stevens-Johnson syndrome or toxic epidermal necrolysis.

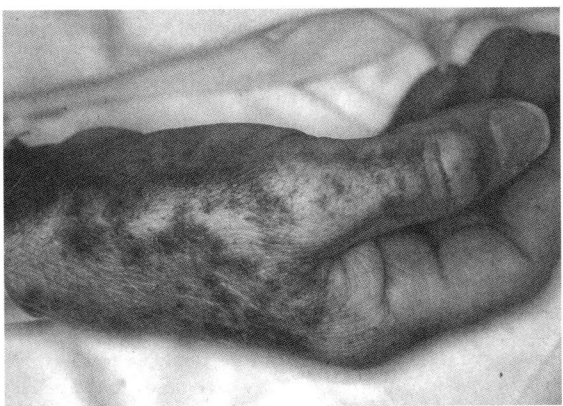

FIGURE 436-54. Autoimmune vasculitis. Purpura with individual small petechiae and coalescence into linear purpura.

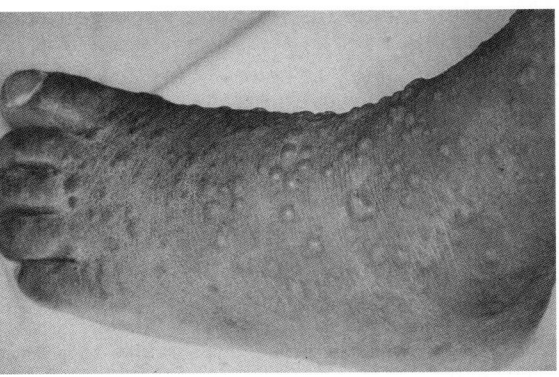

FIGURE 436-56. Varicella-zoster virus. Multiple vesicles characteristic of severe varicella (chickenpox).

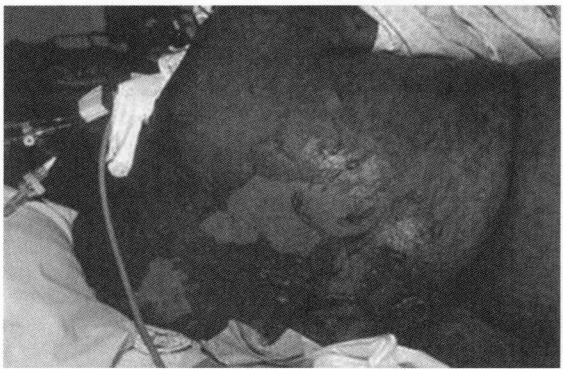

FIGURE 436-57. Bullae (toxic epidermal necrolysis). Detachment of large sheets of necrolytic epidermis (>30% body, surface area), leading to extensive areas of denuded skin. A few intact bullae are still present. (From Bolognia JL, Jorizzo JL, Schaffer JV. *Dermatology*, 3rd ed. Philadelphia: Saunders; 2012:328, Fig. 20.10A.)

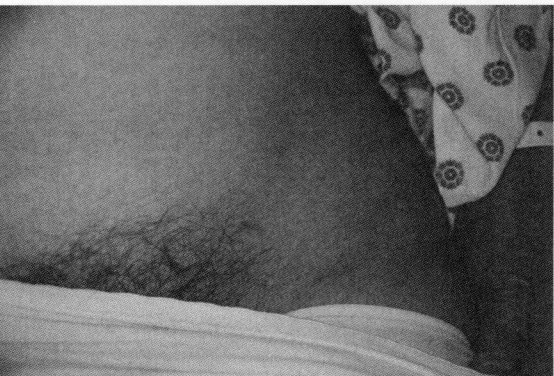

FIGURE 436-60. Toxic shock syndrome. Acute erythema in a swim-trunk distribution can be an early sign of toxic shock syndrome. Similar erythema occurs on dorsal hands and feet.

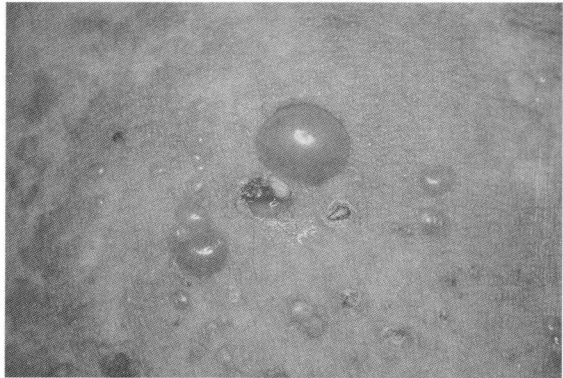

FIGURE 436-58. Vesicles and bullae (bullous pemphigoid). Large bullae as well as smaller bullae and vesicles on a background of urticarial-like erythema.

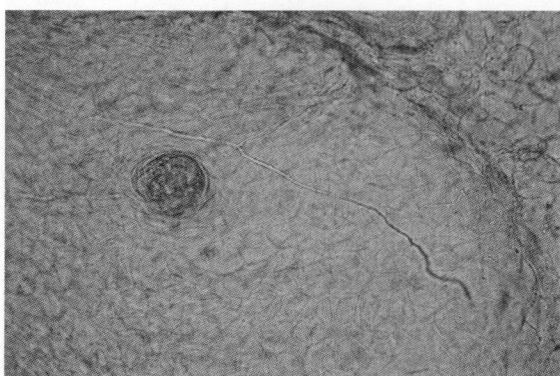

FIGURE 436-61. Potassium hydroxide examination at 40× demonstrating linear fungal hyphae.

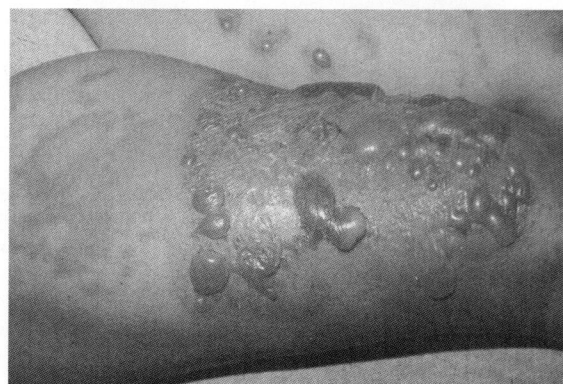

FIGURE 436-59. Severe allergic contact dermatitis. Bullae and vesicles on a background of erythema. Severe cases such as this can be mistaken for the autoimmune disease bullous pemphigoid.

Dermoscopy, also known as dermatoscopy, uses a polarized magnification light source to reveal otherwise nonvisible features of skin lesions. Dermoscopy requires specialized training not usually available to the nondermatologist.

The scaly portion of a lesion can be scraped with a scalpel blade, held perpendicular to the skin to avoid lacerations, to obtain a specimen to be analyzed using 10% solution potassium hydroxide (KOH), which dissolves keratin, thereby exposing microscopic nonkeratinized structures (primarily fungal hyphae). The scales should be placed on a glass slide, and the KOH solution should then be applied and covered with a coverslip. The slide is exposed briefly to flame heat (a Bunsen or alcohol burner are best) while applying gentle pressure. The specimen is then examined under low and medium power (Fig. 436-61). Finding and interpreting fungal elements requires some training. The same approach is also highly effective for identifying scabies mites (Fig. 436-62) and eggs, although mineral oil can be used instead of KOH.

The Tzanck smear, which is a time-honored test for herpes zoster and herpes simplex, does not differentiate between the two. Other methods for detecting herpesvirus include viral culture (best for herpes simplex), direct fluorescent antibody staining, polymerase chain reaction testing, and electron microscopy. The preferred method usually depends on local availability.

For the Tzanck smear, any nuclear stain (methylene blue, alanine, hematoxylin, etc.) can be used to identify the pathognomonic multinucleated keratinocytes, often called giant cells (Fig. 436-63). To obtain the specimen, the clinician should unroof and scrape the base of a vesicle, fix the smeared material to the slide with mild heat, place several drops of stain, rinse with water after a few seconds, lightly blot the slide dry, and examine it under medium power. Immersion oil is necessary for good optics, with or without coverslip. To perform a Gram stain to look for bacteria or fungal forms, the clinician should fix the material onto the slide, apply each stain (crystal violet, iodine, alcohol, safranin) in order for a few seconds, rinse, gently blot dry, mount under immersion or mineral oil, and examine under high power.

A skin biopsy can add valuable information but does not always provide a definitive diagnosis. The vast majority of skin lesions should be biopsied at the site of the most obvious pathologic process, not at the periphery. The biopsy should be performed on the periphery only of a lesion in the setting of an ulcer, where the center may show only nondiagnostic granulation

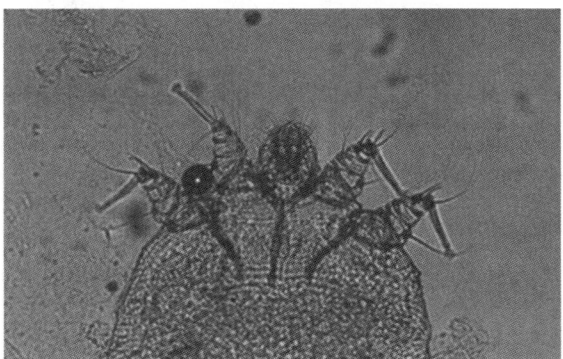

FIGURE 436-62. A scabies mite is seen on this microscopic examination of an oil mount of a scraping taken from the end of a small burrow on the wrist.

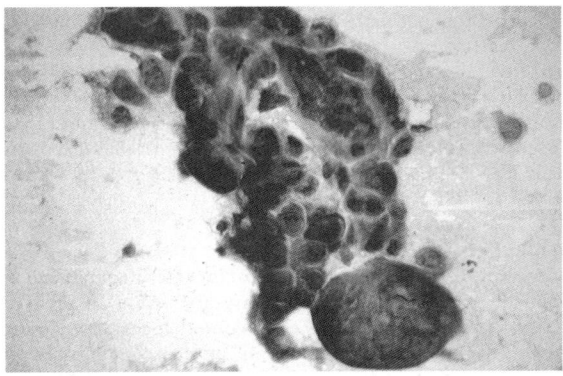

FIGURE 436-63. Multinucleated keratinocytes in a Tzanck preparation for herpes simplex, zoster, or varicella. Sample taken from the base of a vesicle (40×).

tissue[6]; for bullae, in which the edge at the junction of a bulla and normal skin is preferable; and when obtaining perilesional normal skin for immunofluorescence studies. Otherwise, there is no need to have normal skin in a biopsy specimen.

A skin biopsy is most commonly performed as a punch biopsy, which cuts a circular piece of skin or drills a core of skin down to subcutaneous fat. Biopsy specimens range from 2 to 8 mm in diameter. Infiltration of the soft tissue with lidocaine plus epinephrine 5 to 10 minutes before the procedure can minimize bleeding. For biopsies of 4 mm and greater, sutures control bleeding and speed healing.

When the diagnosis is probable melanoma, excision, not punch biopsy, should be performed by a dermatologist or surgeon. If the depth of involvement is not essential for diagnosis or treatment decisions, shave biopsies are useful for removing small raised lesions at the skin surface. The snip excision/biopsy can be particularly useful on the flaccid skin of eyelids or genitalia.

WHEN TO REFER

Most physicians know when a medical problem goes beyond their level of expertise or knowledge. Because cutaneous manifestations of life-threatening disease must be diagnosed quickly, an urgent consultation is appropriate for inpatients who develop new skin lesions or outpatients with severe underlying illnesses. Early referral also is indicated when a malignancy, especially melanoma, is suspected.

Grade A Reference

A1. Arakaki RY, Strazzula L, Woo E, et al. The impact of dermatology consultation on diagnostic accuracy and antibiotic use among patients with suspected cellulitis seen at outpatient internal medicine offices: a randomized clinical trial. *JAMA Dermatol.* 2014;150:1056-1061.

GENERAL REFERENCES

For the General References and other additional features, please visit Expert Consult at https://expertconsult.inkling.com.

The goal of therapy is to improve a skin condition with the least toxic and most specific approach. Because many treatments or medications can be applied directly to the skin, the option for topical therapy is attractive for treating many dermatologic diseases. However, many diseases require systemic therapy, particularly when patients have widespread involvement of the skin or a disease that cannot be improved with topical therapy. Therapies work by improving barrier function, removing scale, and altering inflammation in the skin, altering blood flow, providing antimicrobial effects, or affecting proliferating cells. Recent advances in the understanding of cutaneous biology have not been routinely accompanied by evidence-based documentation of the benefits of many specific therapies.

PRINCIPLES OF TOPICAL THERAPY

Soaks and Dressings

Water or saline applied by soaks and wet dressings can be beneficial for many skin conditions, including ulcers, by promoting healing of the epidermis and débridement of crusts. Soaked gauze is applied to involved areas for 15 to 30 minutes several times per day, and care should be taken not to allow the gauze to dry and adhere. If adherence occurs, the gauze should be soaked before the dressing is removed. Use of strong antiseptic solutions, including hydrogen peroxide, is not recommended because of toxicity to cells. Whirlpool action can enhance débridement. When large areas of skin are involved, baths are a convenient way to treat the skin with medications that reduce itching and inflammation. The best time to apply moisturizers that help trap water in the upper layers of skin is immediately after a bath or shower.

Wet-to-dry dressings are rarely used, except when initial vigorous wound débridement is necessary. Continued use after wounds are débrided traumatizes wounds and delays healing. Moist wound healing, which is often ideal, can be accomplished with a topical antibiotic such as a combination of polymyxin B and bacitracin (Polypore) or mupirocin (Bactrian), gauze impregnated with petrolatum (Vaseline), or an occlusive hydrocolloid dressing. Little evidence indicates that débriding enzymes are beneficial. Compression with an Unna or multilayered boot, which includes an elastic dressing such as Coban, can decrease local edema and facilitate wound healing. Polysporin/petrolatum gauze or occlusive dressings are placed underneath, an approach that is helpful for chronic venous, diabetic, and pressure ulcers, as well as for acute wounds. Closed wet dressings, in which gauze is soaked and then covered with an impervious material, can help when maceration and heat retention are needed. Biologic dressings with skin substitutes or keratinocytes can be beneficial for wounds that are resistant to healing. Skin grafts also can facilitate healing of otherwise nonhealing wounds. Platelet-derived growth factor, which is approved for use on diabetic ulcers, can modestly improve wound healing.

Topical Medications

Topical medications mix an active drug with preservatives, emulsifying agents, and an appropriate base or vehicle. Systemic absorption varies among patients, sites, and vehicles. Topically applied drugs are absorbed more readily through inflamed, thin skin. The base can be any of the following: a *powder,* which promotes dryness and is used to reduce maceration in intertriginous areas; a *lotion,* which is a suspension of oil in water; *solutions,* which include water, alcohol, and propylene glycol, but not oil; *gels,* which are solid at room temperature but melt on contact with the skin; a *cream,* which is an emulsion of oil in water that leaves a thin oil coating as the water evaporates; an *ointment,* which combines oils, such as petrolatum (Vaseline), with small amounts of water and which is more occlusive and hence increases the absorption of medication but also results in a greasier appearance; a *paste,* which is a mixture of powder and ointment; or a *spray.* Lotions, solutions, and gels provide less penetration than ointments do, but they are especially useful for the treatment of hair-bearing areas such as the scalp, where greasiness is displeasing. Creams are less greasy than ointments and are useful for the face, groin, and intertriginous areas. Ointments are often more effective for dry, scaly conditions such as eczema and psoriasis and are helpful in areas that have thick skin, such as the palms and soles, but they should be avoided in infected or intertriginous areas. The choice of base is determined by the skin condition and location. Impregnated tapes are another delivery method to provide occlusion and protect the skin from manipulation.

● ANTI-INFLAMMATORY AGENTS

Glucocorticoids

Topical glucocorticoids work because of their effects on vasoconstriction, proliferation, immunosuppression, and inflammation. Assays related to the ability to vasoconstrict and clinical trials of efficacy have allowed glucocorticoids to be divided into various classes based on potency (Table 437-1). These medications are typically used twice per day. Side effects include atrophy of the skin, telangiectases, purpura, striae, local skin infections (e.g., folliculitis, tinea, and candidiasis), hypopigmentation, hypertrichosis, systemic adrenal suppression when these agents are used on as little as 20% of the skin's surface area, and glaucoma when they are used around the eye. Side effects are especially prevalent when fluorinated steroids are used on thin skin (e.g., face, groin, or scrotum), and prolonged use on the face can result in facial dermatitis, acne, and an eruption resembling acne rosacea that is often exacerbated when use of the steroid is terminated. Certain conditions are more responsive to steroids, and the potency of the steroid chosen must be based on the condition and its location (Table 437-2). The superpotent class I agents should be restricted to patients with severe dermatoses, and their use normally should not exceed 2 weeks. Patients who receive these potent agents require frequent follow-up and must be carefully evaluated for the need to continue strong topical steroids. Use of any fluorinated steroid on the face requires an exact diagnosis and should be limited in the extent of application and duration of use. Intralesional glucocorticoids can be injected into individual lesions to improve delivery of the medication, and this method is commonly used to treat patients with acne cysts, hypertrophic scars, keloids, alopecia areata, granuloma annulare, discoid and panniculitic lupus erythematosus (Chapter 266), psoriasis, and lichen simplex chronicus. Triamcinolone acetonide is most frequently used, followed by the longer acting triamcinolone hexacetonide. It is important to use proper

---

TABLE 437-1   RANKING OF SOME COMMONLY USED TOPICAL STEROIDS BY POTENCY

Super potency	Clobetasol propionate (Temovate ointment and cream), betamethasone dipropionate (Diprolene cream and ointment), diflorasone diacetate (Psorcon E ointment), halobetasol propionate (Ultravate ointment)
High potency	Amcinonide, mometasone furoate ointment, diflorasone diacetate (Florone ointment), halcinonide 0.1% cream, fluocinonide, desoximetasone, triamcinolone acetonide, diflorasone diacetate ointment and cream, betamethasone dipropionate (Diprosone), betamethasone benzoate and valerate
Medium potency	Fluticasone propionate; mometasone furoate cream; halcinonide 0.25% ointment; triamcinolone acetonide 0.1% cream and lotion; fluocinolone acetonide 0.2%, 0.25%, and 0.1% cream and 0.25% ointment and 0.5% solution; hydrocortisone valerate 0.2% ointment and cream; alclometasone dipropionate 0.5% ointment; betamethasone dipropionate 0.5% lotion; hydrocortisone butyrate 0.1% cream; betamethasone benzoate 0.25% cream; betamethasone valerate 0.1% cream and 0.5% lotion; flumethasone pivalate 0.3% cream; desonide 0.5% cream
Low potency	Hydrocortisone 1% cream

TABLE 437-2   CLINICAL APPLICATION OF TOPICAL GLUCOCORTICOIDS

Super potency and high potency	Plaque and palmoplantar psoriasis, lichen planus, dyshidrotic eczema, lichen simplex chronicus, granuloma annulare, sarcoidosis
Medium potency	Dermatitis: allergic contact, atopic, neurodermatitis
Low potency	Intertrigo, pruritus ani, seborrheic dermatitis

---

dilutions, such as 2.5 mg/mL on the face and 5 mg/mL elsewhere, to avoid local skin atrophy.

Systemic glucocorticoids are used for acute and chronic conditions in dermatology, but they should be avoided, if possible, or minimized because of their well-known side effects (Chapter 35). Acute conditions that commonly require systemic steroids include severe contact dermatitis such as poison ivy, photodermatitis, severe atopic dermatitis, and acute urticaria. Many skin conditions such as psoriasis and eczema become exacerbated when use of the steroids is tapered, so steroids should be avoided when possible in these conditions. The dose of steroid must be individualized to the condition and its severity. Steroid-sparing drugs, such as immunosuppressive agents, can be used to minimize the long-term use of steroids for selected conditions.

Nonsteroidal Anti-Inflammatory Agents

Psoriasis Therapies

Tars and anthralin are used for psoriasis (Chapter 438). Tars are most commonly used in conjunction with ultraviolet B (UVB) light. Tars also are used in shampoos and bath oils to treat seborrhea and psoriasis. Anthralin is a synthetic hydroxyanthrone that inhibits keratinocyte proliferation; it stains and can be irritating, but it can be effective therapy[A1] (Chapter 438).

Calcipotriol

Calcipotriol is a vitamin D derivative that has antiproliferative and immunomodulatory effects on skin. Hypercalcemia can occur if more than 100 g/week is used, so this agent cannot be used for widespread disease. It is applied twice daily, can be irritating on thin skin, and takes 6 to 8 weeks to be effective.

Retinoids

The retinoids are a group of compounds that include vitamin A and its derivatives. Their effects are mediated through several different classes of receptors, and the receptor-drug complex has effects on other regulatory proteins that affect growth factors, oncogenes, keratins, or transglutaminases. Retinoids affect cell growth, differentiation, and morphogenesis; inhibit tumor promotion and malignant cell growth; have immunomodulatory effects; and alter cell cohesion.

Topical retinoids include all-*trans*-retinoic acid (tretinoin), which is approved for acne (Retin-A) and photoaging (Renova 0.05% cream) and is also useful for hyperpigmentation, steroid-induced atrophy, and early stretch marks. Tretinoin is available as a cream (0.025%, 0.05%, 0.1%), a gel (0.01%, 0.025%), and a solution (0.05%). Adapalene (Differin 0.1% gel) and tazarotene (Tazorac) are used for acne (Chapter 439). Tazarotene is also used for psoriasis, often in combination with topical steroids to minimize irritation and chronic photodamage. Bexarotene (Targretin) 1% gel is used for the topical treatment of cutaneous lesions in patients who have refractory or persistent stage IA or IB cutaneous T-cell lymphoma. Topical retinoids can be irritating and frequently cause an exacerbation before improvement. However, they should be used regularly on lesion-prone skin to produce improvement. Moisturizers may be needed to minimize drying effects.

Systemic retinoids commonly used for the skin include isotretinoin, acitretin, and bexarotene (Targretin). They have many applications, but most frequently isotretinoin (Accutane) is used for cystic and conglobate acne, acitretin for severe psoriasis (especially the erythrodermic and pustular forms), and bexarotene for cutaneous T-cell lymphoma. Isotretinoin and acitretin also have been used to treat several forms of ichthyosis and lupus erythematosus and for the chemoprevention of skin cancers, particularly in immunosuppressed transplant recipients. The many side effects of systemic retinoids include teratogenicity, cheilitis, hair loss, headaches, hyperlipidemia, abnormal liver enzyme levels, vertebral hyperostosis, tendon and ligament calcification, osteoporosis, and central hypothyroidism with bexarotene.[1] Pregnancy must be avoided, and the use of retinoids in women of childbearing age therefore requires careful monitoring. Treatment of acne is reserved for cases of cystic acne not responding to less toxic therapies; in this setting, a 4- to 5-month course of Accutane, 0.5 to 1 mg/kg/day, is curative in 85 to 90% of patients.

Brimonidine

This selective α_2-adrenergic receptor agonist with vasoconstrictive activity is used in rosacea.[A2]

Antimalarial Drugs

Aminoquinolines include hydroxychloroquine, quinacrine, and chloroquine. These agents have inhibitory effects on pro-inflammatory cytokine production, DNA replication, and chemotaxis. They are useful in patients with connective tissue diseases, polymorphous light eruption, sarcoidosis (Chapter 95), porphyria cutanea tarda (Chapters 210 and 439), sclerosing conditions, and vasculitis. Side effects include diarrhea, headache, irritability, psychosis, skin dyspigmentation, and, rarely, retinopathy. Retinopathy is rare if doses of chloroquine are 3.5 mg/kg/day or less and doses of hydroxychloroquine are 6.5 mg/kg/day or less. Combinations of hydroxychloroquine or chloroquine with quinacrine are frequently helpful when a solitary agent is inadequate.[2] The combination of hydroxychloroquine and chloroquine should not be used because of the additive risk for retinopathy.

Dapsone

Dapsone is a sulfone that inhibits the response of neutrophils and possibly eosinophils to chemotactic stimuli. It is useful for dermatitis herpetiformis (Chapter 439), cutaneous vasculitis (Chapter 440), pyoderma gangrenosum (Chapter 440), bullous lupus erythematosus (Chapter 266), Behçet's disease (Chapter 270), and autoimmune bullous diseases (Chapter 439). Topical 5% gel is approved for use in acne. Systemic use can be associated with side effects that include hemolysis, methemoglobinemia, peripheral neuropathy, agranulocytosis, and, rarely, a hypersensitivity syndrome with hepatitis, fevers, and rash. The glucose-6-dehydrogenase level should be checked before starting the drug, and it is common for patients with a normal glucose-6-dehydrogenase level to experience a 2-g/dL decrease in hemoglobin after achieving therapeutic doses of 100 to 200 mg/day.

Thalidomide

Thalidomide has potent anti-inflammatory effects, probably resulting from inhibition of tumor necrosis factor-α (TNF-α). It also modifies adhesion molecules on circulating leukocytes. Thalidomide is a serious teratogen, and patients must comply with strict birth control and monitoring. It is effective at a dose of 50 to 100 mg/day, with improvement beginning in 2 weeks and a full clinical response seen in 2 to 3 months in patients with severe cutaneous lupus erythematosus (Chapter 266), erythema nodosum leprosum (Chapter 438), aphthae, Behçet's disease (Chapter 270), scleromyxedema, actinic prurigo, chronic graft-versus-host disease (Chapter 178), multiple myeloma (Chapter 187), and numerous other inflammatory dermatoses. Besides teratogenesis, the main side effects include peripheral neuropathy, constipation, sedation, and, rarely, amenorrhea.

Colchicine

Colchicine, usually at a dose of 0.6 mg twice daily, is used for leukocytoclastic vasculitis (Chapter 439) and Behçet's disease, as well as some patients with epidermolysis bullosa acquisita. The main side effect of this low oral dose is diarrhea.

● ANTIMICROBIAL AGENTS
Antibacterials

Topical antibiotics are used to treat superficial skin diseases, such as acne and folliculitis, as well as skin wounds and ulcers. They may work by decreasing neutrophil chemotaxis and other anti-inflammatory mechanisms. Topical solutions, gels, pledgets, and ointments are available, depending on the agent, and antibiotics include erythromycin, clindamycin, tetracycline, and metronidazole.[3,4] Benzoyl peroxide also has antibacterial properties and is quite effective for mild-to-moderate acne, while also minimizing bacterial resistance when topical antibiotics are also used (Chapter 439). Bacitracin and Polysporin ointments are typically used for wounds, but they can cause contact hypersensitivity; neomycin should be avoided because of the high incidence of allergic reactions. Mupirocin is particularly effective against *Staphylococcus* and *Streptococcus* spp., and it can be used in the nose for carriers of staphylococci. Systemic antibiotics such as penicillins, cephalosporins, and erythromycin are used in patients with soft tissue infections such as impetigo, folliculitis, furuncles, carbuncles, cellulitis, ecthyma, erysipelas, postoperative wound infections, and necrotizing fasciitis. Tetracycline, doxycycline, and minocycline are used for acne, rosacea, and perioral dermatitis.[5] Fluoroquinolones such as ciprofloxacin are useful for the treatment of gram-negative soft tissue infections.

Antifungals

Topical antifungal agents are used in patients with limited superficial fungal infections of the skin (Chapter 438). The numerous topical antifungal drugs available include the azoles (clotrimazole, econazole, ketoconazole, oxiconazole, and miconazole), which are available as creams and lotions applied once or twice daily. The creams tend to be more effective. Topical agents used for dermatophytes, but not *Candida*, are haloprogin and tolnaftate. The newer allylamine antifungals naftifine and terbinafine have fungicidal effects. Ciclopirox 8% topical solution was recently approved for use in treating and preventing relapses of onychomycosis. Nystatin creams, oral suspensions, and vaginal tablets are effective for the treatment of *Candida* infections. The combination of antifungals with potent topical steroids such as betamethasone dipropionate is not advised because of increased side effects from the steroid and decreased efficacy of the antifungal as a result of the concomitant steroid.

Systemic antifungal agents include griseofulvin, terbinafine (allylamine), ketoconazole (imidazole), itraconazole, and fluconazole. These agents are used for extensive or severe superficial skin fungal infections (Chapter 438) caused by dermatophytes, *Candida*, or *Malassezia furfur* or for local infections not responsive to topical drugs, such as those found in the nails and scalp. Itraconazole and terbinafine are the only oral antifungals approved in the United States for the treatment of onychomycosis,[6] and griseofulvin is the only oral agent approved for tinea capitis. Griseofulvin is best taken with a fatty meal to improve absorption and is the only antifungal drug not requiring regular monitoring of liver enzymes. Griseofulvin shows weak affinity for keratin, and thus it must be used for 18 months for onychomycosis of the toenails and 6 months for the fingernails to achieve even relatively poor cure rates. Terbinafine is the only fungicidal drug; the rest are fungistatic. The number of interactions with medications is lower with terbinafine than with the triazole antifungals and ketoconazole because terbinafine does not inhibit or induce hepatic isoenzyme cytochrome P (CYP3A4) (Chapter 29). However, terbinafine affects CYP2D6, another hepatic isoenzyme, so it is relatively contraindicated in patients who are taking cyclosporine or rifampin. Itraconazole and fluconazole have been used in pulse-dosing regimens for the treatment of onychomycosis. Fluconazole and terbinafine are not dependent on gastric acidity for optimal gastrointestinal absorption. Overall, the side effects of the systemic antifungal agents are similar and include headache and gastrointestinal symptoms (griseofulvin, terbinafine), nausea and vomiting (itraconazole, fluconazole, ketoconazole), hepatitis, and lupus-like syndromes (terbinafine).

Antivirals

Verrucae are treated with various destructive modalities, including 50 to 80% dichloroacetic acid and trichloroacetic acid solutions, podophyllin resin, and podofilox. Topical antiviral creams such as penciclovir and acyclovir do not significantly shorten the course of herpes simplex. Systemic antiviral drugs include acyclovir, valacyclovir, famciclovir, and foscarnet, which are used to treat primary and recurrent herpes simplex (Chapter 374) and herpes zoster (Chapter 375), although only acyclovir is approved for treatment of herpes zoster. These agents specifically block the function of herpesvirus DNA polymerase. Valacyclovir and famciclovir are available only orally in the United States, but their prolonged intracellular half-life allows less frequent dosing than with acyclovir. Patients with herpes zoster require higher doses than do patients with herpes simplex. Side effects include nausea and headaches. The varicella-zoster vaccine has significantly decreased the incidence of herpes zoster in individuals older than 50 years of age, and current recommendation is for vaccination after the age of 60 (Chapter 18). If possible, it should be administered before starting oral immunosuppressive agents.

Antiparasitics

Topical antiparasitic medications are used to treat pediculosis capitis, pediculosis pubis, and scabies. In addition, topical metronidazole has anti-inflammatory properties and is used to treat rosacea. For pediculosis and scabies, clothing and bedding must be washed and all family members must be treated. Effective treatment includes 1% γ-benzene hexachloride (lindane), a chlorinated hydrocarbon pesticide that should not be used on young children or on pregnant or lactating women. It is ineffective against nits and thus must be reapplied after 1 week. Permethrin 5% cream (Elimite) for scabies or 1% cream rinse is particularly effective for head lice and requires just one application; 10% crotamiton (Eurax) and 5% topical sulfur ointments are less effective. Malathion is a moderately toxic organophosphate insecticide, but it must be applied overnight to treat lice. Pyrethrins (RID, Nix) are best used twice, 1 week apart, to treat head lice and nits.

● ANTIPRURITIC OR ANESTHETIC AGENTS
Topical Analgesics

Capsaicin, an active ingredient of cayenne peppers and other plants of the genus *Capsicum* is used for postherpetic neuralgia and other painful nerve-related conditions. It causes excitation of neural afferent C fibers and reduces substance P levels. Capsaicin causes a burning sensation and is applied four or five times daily for 5 to 6 weeks. Eutectic mixture of local anesthetic (EMLA) is a mixture of lidocaine and prilocaine that is used under occlusion to induce cutaneous anesthesia before a procedure. Lidocaine can be used as a topical anesthetic, but benzocaine should be avoided because it is a sensitizer.

Antipruritic Agents

Doxepin 5% cream is used for localized pruritus. Menthol is a cyclic terpene plant alcohol used for non–histamine-related itching. Pramoxine hydrochloride is a topical anesthetic used for mild-to-moderate itching. Oral antihistamines play an important role in controlling pruritus in many skin conditions (Table 437-3), especially those mediated by histamine, such as urticaria,[7] angioedema, and urticaria pigmentosa. The sedating and anticholinergic properties of many H_1-receptor antihistamines probably account for some of their efficacy. H_1-receptor antihistamines are the cornerstones of routine therapy, and if an agent from one group of H_1-receptor antihistamines is ineffective, an agent from a different class should be administered or combined. Second-generation H_1-receptor antihistamines are less sedating and are used if patients cannot tolerate or do not improve after taking first-generation agents. The combination of two different H_1-receptor antihistamines can be used when a solitary agent does not work; in particular, use of a sedating antihistamine at night and a second-generation antihistamine during the day can be helpful. The skin contains both H_1- and H_2-receptors, and occasionally combining H_1- and H_2-receptor antagonists can be beneficial. Usually, first-generation agents (e.g., hydroxyzine, 10 to 25 mg every 6 hours) are started at low doses and increased as tolerated, and regular continuous dosing is recommended. The tricyclic antidepressant doxepin, normally started at 10 to 25 mg at bedtime, has both anti–H_1- and H_2-receptor activity, but it interacts with drugs metabolized by the CYP450 pathway. Side effects of commonly used first-generation antihistamines include sedation, dry mouth, blurred vision, constipation, and urinary retention, and lower doses may be required in elderly patients. The recommended dose for second-generation antihistamines (e.g., fexofenadine, 60 mg twice daily) should not be exceeded.

● AGENTS THAT IMPROVE SURFACE FUNCTIONS (LUBRICATION, SCALE)

Moisturizers

Moisturizers improve skin by diminishing scale and increasing water content. They usually contain mixtures of water and fatty substances such as petrolatum, lanolin, lanolin derivatives, and fatty alcohols. Greasy moisturizers tend to function better, but they are less acceptable cosmetically.

Keratolytics

α-Hydroxy acids (lactic acid, glycolic acid, citric acid, glucuronic acid, pyruvic acid) are extremely effective keratolytics. They are helpful in treating disorders of keratinization and photoaging, as well as acne. Propylene glycol, used in 40 to 60% aqueous solutions, can decrease scaling. Salicylic acid, which works by decreasing keratinocyte adhesion and hydrating keratins, is used in a range of concentrations with many different bases to remove scale, to soften the stratum corneum, or as destructive therapy to remove warts and calluses. Urea is used in varying concentrations to treat scaling.

● IMMUNE THERAPIES

Hormonal Therapies

Systemic therapies to modulate androgen production can be beneficial in patients with acne and hidradenitis suppurativa. Such treatments for moderate acne include spironolactone and, in women, U.S. Food and Drug Administration (FDA)-approved combination oral contraceptives, such as Ortho Tri-Cyclen (norgestimate and ethinyl estradiol), Estrostep (norethindrone acetate and ethinyl estradiol), and Yaz (drospirenone and ethinyl estradiol), as they would be prescribed for contraception (Chapter 238). [A4]

Immunosuppressive Agents

Topical cytotoxic drugs include 5-fluorouracil, mechlorethamine (nitrogen mustard), carmustine (BCNU), bleomycin, and the calcineurin inhibitors tacrolimus and pimecrolimus. [A5] Topical 5-fluorouracil interferes with pyrimidine metabolism and action and blocks DNA synthesis. It is used to treat actinic keratosis, [A6] superficial basal cell cancer, Bowen's disease, bowenoid papulosis, actinic cheilitis, and warts. Topical use does not cause systemic toxicity, but expected side effects include local irritation, erythema, and pain. Nitrogen mustard and BCNU, which have alkylating agents that inhibit DNA, RNA, and protein synthesis, are used to treat cutaneous T-cell lymphoma (Chapter 185); they can cause cutaneous reactions and myelosuppression, and nitrogen mustard commonly causes a cutaneous hypersensitivity reaction.

Intralesional bleomycin, which disrupts DNA synthesis, has been used to treat warts. Topical tacrolimus (Prograf) and pimecrolimus, immunosuppressive macrolides that act on T lymphocytes to inhibit interleukin-2 (IL-2) transcription, are used for atopic dermatitis, allergic contact dermatitis, psoriasis, and several other inflammatory skin conditions. They frequently cause a burning sensation in the skin; although systemic absorption is minimal, ongoing studies are assessing whether the risk for cancer is increased by their topical use. Systemic immunosuppressives such as methotrexate, azathioprine, thioguanine, hydroxyurea, mycophenolate (CellCept), cyclophosphamide, chlorambucil, rapamycin, and cyclosporine are used for numerous inflammatory or immunologically mediated skin conditions, particularly for widespread psoriasis (Chapter 438) and as glucocorticoid-sparing agents for autoimmune blistering diseases.

Immunomodulatory Therapies

Imiquimod, available as a 5% cream, is an imidazoquinolinamine that has antitumor and antiviral activity. It induces local production of interferon-γ and is used to treat warts and superficial skin cancers. Topical 3% diclofenac in hyaluronic acid, which blocks the induced cyclooxygenase-2 found in precancerous lesions, is approved to treat actinic keratosis. Many systemic immunomodulatory drugs are currently used in dermatology. These include interferons and TNF-α inhibitors such as etanercept, adalimumab, and infliximab (Remicade). [8] Anti-IL-12/23 therapy and anti-IL-17 therapy are effective for psoriasis. Ipilimumab, an antibody against T-lymphocyte-associated antigen 4 is effective for advanced melanoma. Anti-CD20 antibodies have been effective in the treatment of autoimmune skin-blistering diseases. Interferon alfa-2b is used both intralesionally and subcutaneously to treat genital warts, high-risk

TABLE 437-3   OVERVIEW OF ANTIHISTAMINES

ANTIHISTAMINE GROUP	GENERIC NAME	AVERAGE ORAL ADULT DOSES
FIRST-GENERATION H₁-TYPE ANTIHISTAMINES		
Alkylamine	Brompheniramine (Dimetapp)	4 mg q4-6h
	Chlorpheniramine (Chlor-Trimeton)	4 mg q4-6h (short acting); 8-12 mg q8-12h (long acting)
Amino alkyl ether (ethanolamine)	Clemastine fumarate	1.34 mg bid or 2.68 mg qd-tid
	Diphenhydramine (Benadryl)	25-50 mg q4-6h
Ethylenediamine	Pyrilamine (Triaminic)	30 mg bid
Phenothiazine	Promethazine (Phenergan)	10-12.5 mg qid
	Trimeprazine (Temaril)	2.5 mg q6h
Piperidine	Azatadine	1-2 mg q8-12h
	Cyproheptadine	4 mg q8h
	Diphenylpyraline	2 mg tid-qid
Piperazine	Hydroxyzine (Atarax)	25-100 mg tid-qid
SECOND-GENERATION H₁-TYPE ANTIHISTAMINES		
Alkylamine	Acrivastine (combined with pseudoephedrine in allergy medication)	8 mg qid
Piperidine	Astemizole (Hismanal)	10 mg qd
	Loratadine (Claritin)	10 mg qd
	Fexofenadine (Allegra)	60 mg bid or 180 mg qd
Piperazine	Cetirizine (Zyrtec)	5-10 mg/day
H₂-TYPE ANTIHISTAMINES		
	Cimetidine (Tagamet)	400 mg bid
	Ranitidine (Zantac)	150 mg bid
	Famotidine	10 mg bid
	Nizatidine	300 mg hs
H₁- AND H₂-TYPE ANTIHISTAMINES		
	Doxepin (Sinequan)	10-25 mg hs

bid = twice daily; hs = at bedtime; qd = once daily; qid = four times daily; tid = three times daily.

melanoma, Kaposi's sarcoma, hemangiomas, cutaneous T-cell lymphoma, keloids, Behçet's disease, cryoglobulinemia and vasculitis from hepatitis C (Chapter 149), and perhaps basal cell and squamous cell carcinoma. Total interferon doses are generally 3 million IU or less per session, and systemic doses are usually administered 3 days per week. Side effects include flulike symptoms, leukopenia, anemia, and hepatitis. Denileukin diftitox is a fusion protein consisting of a fragment of diphtheria toxin genetically fused to IL-2. It targets IL-2 receptors on the surface of malignant cells and is approved for use in patients with resistant or recurrent cutaneous T-cell lymphoma. Alefacept, which is used to treat psoriasis, affects T cells by blockade of costimulatory signals. Intravenous immunoglobulin, which is used to treat certain autoimmune skin diseases, including pemphigus vulgaris, cicatricial pemphigoid, and dermatomyositis, probably works through Fc receptor modulation and anti-idiotype interactions. Antibodies against the programmed cell death 1 (PD-1) receptor are effective in advanced melanoma.[A7]

Histone deacetylase inhibition increases acetylation of lysine residues that form the octomeric histone core of chromatin, thereby decreasing the ability of the histones to bind to DNA. This decreased binding allows chromatin expansion, permitting transcription of the tumor suppressor genes. However, histone deacetylase inhibitors affect acetylation globally and may have wider effects on various cellular functions. Two novel inhibitors (vorinostat and romidepsin) are approved by the FDA for use in patients with cutaneous T-cell lymphoma.[9]

Extracorporeal photochemotherapy (photopheresis), which combines 8-methoxypsoralen and ultraviolet A (UVA) irradiation of lymphocytes, is used for Sézary's syndrome, the leukemic form of cutaneous T-cell lymphoma (Chapter 185). Plasmapheresis, used in combination with other immunosuppressive therapies, can remove autoantibodies and immune complexes in patients in whom autoimmune disease or cryoglobulinemia is resistant to other therapies.

TARGETED PATHWAYS FOR CANCER TREATMENT

Hedgehog Signaling Pathway Inhibition
The hedgehog pathway is activated in most basal cell carcinomas. The central component of the hedgehog signaling pathway is smoothened (SMO), a transmembrane protein that initiates a signaling cascade. Vismodegib, an antismoothen inhibitor, has been approved for treatment of patients with advanced basal cell carcinomas.[A8]

BRAF Kinase Inhibition
Vemurafenib is a potent inhibitor of mutated BRAF. It has antitumor effects against the BRAF V600E mutation, and is used for advanced melanoma.[A9]

Other Therapies

Phototherapy and Laser
Ultraviolet treatments are given with different wavelengths, depending on the condition and the response to treatment. Currently, clinicians use broadband UVB (290 to 320 nm), narrow-band 311-nm UVB, PUVA (psoralen with 320- to 400-nm UVA), and UVA1 (340 to 400 nm). Both forms of UVB and PUVA are used for psoriasis and vitiligo, but other conditions such as nummular and atopic dermatitis, pruritus resulting from uremia, and cutaneous T-cell lymphoma are treated in this way. High-dose UVA1 is used, mainly in Europe, to treat atopic dermatitis, localized scleroderma, and mastocytosis. PUVA is associated with increased risk for skin cancers, including melanoma. The risks related to long-term UVA therapy are currently unknown, but photoaging is associated with UVA and there have been reports of an increase in melanoma associated with use of suntanning beds, in which much of the exposure is to UVA. Laser therapy is used to treat vascular lesions such as port-wine stains, tattoos, psoriasis, benign skin tumors, and photodamage, as well as to remove hair. Photodynamic therapy involves activation of a photosensitizer by illumination with visible light, which leads to photochemical tissue destruction or immunomodulation. Photodynamic therapy can be used to treat actinic keratosis, Bowen's disease, and superficial basal cell carcinoma by causing selective tissue necrosis and tumor destruction. Fractional lasers have been successfully used for treatment of actinic keratoses,[A10] photodamage, and scars.

Dermatologic Surgery
Although approaches such as desiccation and curettage can be used for some skin tumors, others require excisional surgery or Mohs' microscopic controlled surgery to ensure complete removal of lesions. If the tumors are recurrent, of a pathologic type that increases the likelihood for recurrence, or large and requiring clearance of the tumor before repair, the Mohs approach can provide rapid documentation of full removal while sparing as much normal tissue as possible. After the margins have been cleared of tumor, flaps and grafts can be used immediately for repair of the resultant defects.

Patients with extensive actinic damage resulting in either large numbers of actinic keratoses or photodamage can be treated with various ablative approaches that use either chemical peels or laser resurfacing with the carbon dioxide laser. Chemical peels can be performed at different depths and intensities, and agents can include glycolic acid, acetic acid, or even phenol. Lasers used to remove sun-induced lentigines include Q-switched lasers such as the neodymium:yttrium-aluminum-garnet, ruby, and alexandrite lasers. Many patients seek treatment of wrinkles with soft tissue augmentation that uses human-derived collagen and hyaluronic acid or with a muscle relaxer, botulinum type A exotoxin.

Hair transplants are a surgical approach to the problem of hair loss. The process includes harvesting hair grafts from the posterior of the scalp and placing the grafts in areas of alopecia.

Sunscreen
Transparent sunscreens absorb photons of light. They are rated by the sun protection factor (SPF), which is determined by the ratio of ultraviolet exposure needed to cause erythema in protected versus unprotected skin. Most sunscreens work in the UVB range or shorter UVA wavelengths. Examples of UVB-absorptive compounds include aminobenzoates, cinnamates, salicylates, and benzophenones. Short-wavelength UVA-absorptive compounds include benzophenones and anthranilates. The best UVA blocking agent in the United States is avobenzone (Parsol 1789), which can be combined with UVB screens.[10] Some sunscreens are water resistant or waterproof, as determined by the substantivity of the sunscreen, and these agents provide continued protection after sweating or swimming. Sunscreens can cause irritation and, rarely, contact allergic reactions. Physical sunscreens, such as zinc oxide and titanium dioxide, reflect light from the skin and include newer micronized reflecting powders that provide broad-spectrum (UVB and UVA) protection. Sunscreens decrease skin cancers and photodamage. UVB is partially reflected by clothing, and sun-protective clothing can provide substantial protection (Solumbra, SPF of 30).

Cosmetics: Camouflage, Bleaching, and Hair Loss
Patients with numerous skin conditions benefit from camouflage cosmetics, which can also cause contact hypersensitivity. Products such as Dermablend can be blended to match skin colors, are thicker, can cover disfiguring lesions, and can be fixed with powder. Hydroquinones, topical retinoic acid, and azelaic acid (inhibits tyrosinase) are used to treat hyperpigmented conditions such as melasma and lentigines; these agents can be irritating and cause dyspigmentation. Topical minoxidil, 2% (available over the counter) and 5% solutions, are used for androgenic alopecia and alopecia areata. Finasteride, a 5α-reductase inhibitor, is effective in men with androgenic alopecia.

Grade A References

A1. Mason AR, Mason J, Cork M, et al. Topical treatments for chronic plaque psoriasis. *Cochrane Database Syst Rev.* 2013;3:CD005028.

A2. Jackson JM, Fowler J, Moore A, et al. Improvement in facial erythema within 30 minutes of initial application of brimonidine tartrate in patients with rosacea. *J Drugs Dermatol.* 2014;13:699-704.

A3. El-Gohary M, van Zuuren EJ, Fedorowicz Z, et al. Topical antifungal treatments for tinea cruris and tinea corporis. *Cochrane Database Syst Rev.* 2014;8:CD009992.

A4. Arowojolu AO, Gallo MF, Lopez LM, et al. Combined oral contraceptive pills for treatment of acne. *Cochrane Database Syst Rev.* 2012;7:CD004425.

A5. Lessin SR, Duvic M, Guitart J, et al. Topical chemotherapy in cutaneous T-cell lymphoma: positive results of a randomized, controlled, multicenter trial testing the efficacy and safety of a novel mechlorethamine, 0.02%, gel in mycosis fungoides. *JAMA Dermatol.* 2013;149:25-32.

A6. Gupta AK, Paquet M, Villanueva E, et al. Interventions for actinic keratoses. *Cochrane Database Syst Rev.* 2012;12:CD004415.

A7. Robert C, Long GV, Brady B, et al. Nivolumab in previously untreated melanoma without BRAF mutation. *N Engl J Med.* 2015;372:320-330.

A8. Sekulic A, Migden MR, Oro AE, et al. Efficacy and safety of vismodegib in advanced basal-cell carcinoma. *N Engl J Med.* 2012;366:2171-2179.

A9. Chapman PB, Hauschild A, Robert C, et al. Improved survival with vemurafenib in melanoma with BRAF V600E mutation. *N Engl J Med.* 2011;364:2507-2516.

A10. Togsverd-Bo K, Haak CS, Thaysen-Petersen D, et al. Intensified photodynamic therapy of actinic keratoses with fractional CO2 laser: a randomized clinical trial. *Br J Dermatol.* 2012;166:1262-1269.

GENERAL REFERENCES

For the General References and other additional features, please visit Expert Consult at https://expertconsult.inkling.com.

438

ECZEMAS, PHOTODERMATOSES, PAPULOSQUAMOUS (INCLUDING FUNGAL) DISEASES, AND FIGURATE ERYTHEMAS

HENRY W. LIM

ECZEMA

The more commonly encountered eczemas (Table 438-1) share similar histologic characteristics. However, they have varying degrees of edema within the epidermis (spongiosis) and of infiltration with lymphocytes and macrophages in the superficial dermis.

Nummular Dermatitis

Nummular dermatitis occurs most frequently in patients who are in their 50s to 60s. Both sexes are affected; in temperate climates, this condition is most frequently seen in the winter. The condition appears to be more frequent and severe among Asians. The pathogenesis is unclear, although xerosis plays a significant role.

Patients usually present with pruritic, coin-shaped, erythematous patches with some scales and occasionally with pinhead-sized vesicles (Figs. 438-1 and 438-2). Lesions may be excoriated and lichenified (i.e., thickened skin with accentuation of skin markings). Legs and arms are commonly affected, and less so on the trunk; facial involvement is uncommon. All patients should be educated about the care of dry skin, such as the use of emollients and moisturizing soaps, and avoidance of long, hot showers. Topical corticosteroid ointments (e.g., triamcinolone ointment, 0.1% twice daily for 1 to 2 weeks) are helpful for active lesions, and oral antihistamines (e.g., fexofenadine, 180 mg every morning, and hydroxyzine, 25 to 50 mg at bedtime, as needed) are useful for pruritus. In severe cases, narrow-band ultraviolet B

TABLE 438-1	ECZEMAS
Nummular dermatitis	
Dyshidrosis	
Atopic dermatitis	
Seborrheic dermatitis	
Allergic contact dermatitis	
Irritant contact dermatitis	

(NB-UVB) phototherapy, a short course of oral corticosteroids (prednisone, 0.5 to 1 mg/kg/day, with a maximal dose of 60 mg/day, for 1 to 2 weeks, then taper in 10 to 14 days) or day hospitalization for intensive topical and NB-UVB therapy is beneficial.

Dyshidrosis

Dyshidrosis manifests as deep-seated, pinhead-sized vesicles, most commonly along the sides of the fingers (Figs. 438-3 and 438-4). In severe cases, the palms and soles also may be involved. Lesions are usually pruritic, associated with xerosis, scaliness, and fissures. Dyshidrosis is seen in individuals who wash their hands frequently, such as restaurant workers and mothers of young infants. With the widespread use of hand sanitizers, dyshidrosis has become less common in health care workers. Treatment follows a sequential

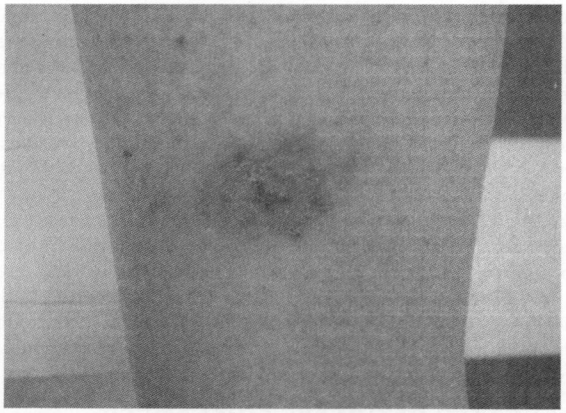

FIGURE 438-2. Nummular dermatitis. Coin-shaped erythematous patch.

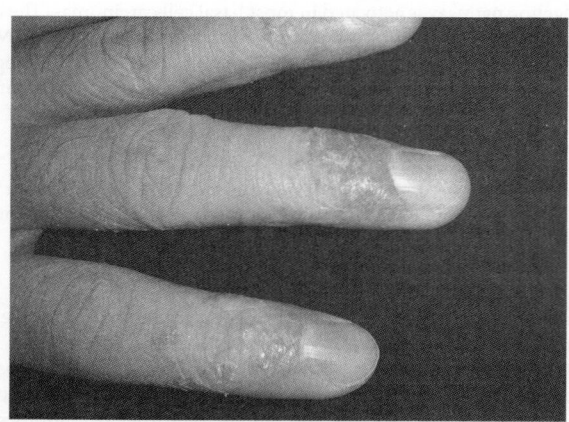

FIGURE 438-3. Dyshidrosis. Deep-seated vesicles and scaliness on fingers.

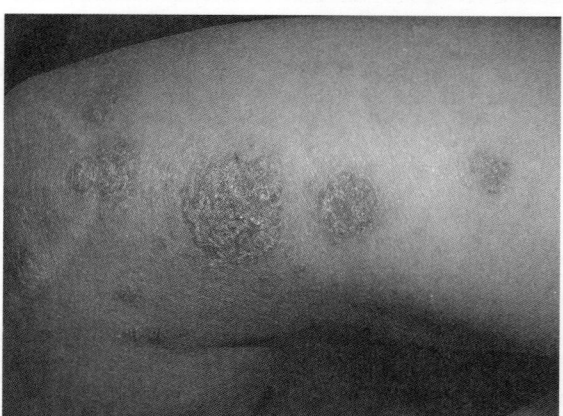

FIGURE 438-1. Nummular dermatitis. Coin-shaped erythematous patches.

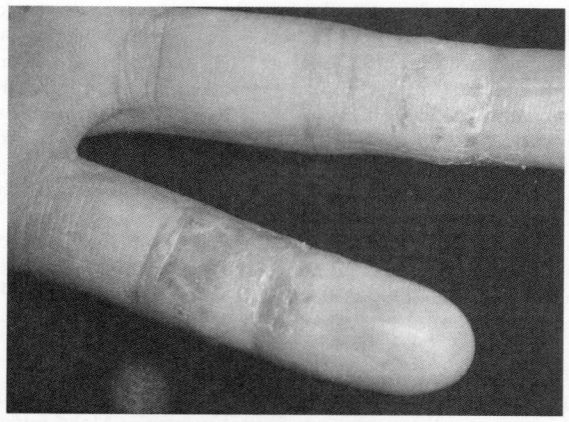

FIGURE 438-4. Dyshidrosis. Deep-seated vesicles and scaliness on fingers.

order: (1) replacing soap-and-water handwashing with the use of hand sanitizers, (2) liberal use of emollients, (3) topical corticosteroid ointments (e.g., fluocinonide ointment, 0.05% twice daily for 2 weeks), and (4) oral antihistamines (e.g., fexofenadine, 180 mg every morning, and hydroxyzine, 25 to 50 mg at bedtime, as needed).

Atopic Dermatitis

Atopic dermatitis is most commonly seen among young children, but severe cases persist into adulthood. In 90% of patients, the disease starts before the age of 5 years. The prevalence has been estimated at between 15 and 23%. Patients usually present with xerosis, erythematous scaly patches, small vesicles, excoriations, crusting, and, not infrequently, impetiginization (Fig. 438-5). In dark-skinned patients, a papular variant is commonly seen (Fig. 438-6). With chronic scratching and rubbing, hyperpigmentation and lichenification occur. Commonly affected sites include the periorbital area and flexor areas such as the neck, antecubital fossa, and popliteal fossa. In severe cases, the entire skin surface may be involved. Diagnosis is made by the typical morphology, the distribution of lesions, and family and personal history of atopy. The therapeutic ladder consists of (1) emollients; (2) topical corticosteroid ointments (e.g., triamcinolone ointment, 0.1% twice daily for 1 to 2 weeks), or topical calcineurin inhibitors (tacrolimus ointment, 0.1% for 3 to 4 weeks, or pimecrolimus cream, 1% for 3 to 4 weeks)[A1]; (3) oral antihistamines (e.g., fexofenadine, 180 mg every morning, and hydroxyzine, 25 to 50 mg at

bedtime, as needed); and (4) NB-UVB phototherapy. Although topical tacrolimus and pimecrolimus have "black box" warnings from the U.S. Food and Drug Administration for their potential association with the development of malignancy, a safety study of tacrolimus ointment for up to 4 years in patients with pediatric atopic dermatitis showed no immunosuppressive side effects. In patients with recalcitrant cases, day hospitalization, oral prednisone (0.5 to 1 mg/kg/day), cyclosporine (3 to 5 mg/kg/day), mycophenolate mofetil (1 to 2 g/day), and dupilumab (an interleukin-4 and -13 blocker at 300 mg subcutaneously weekly)[A2] have been successful.

Seborrheic Dermatitis

Seborrheic dermatitis is a common condition that occurs as erythematous patches with fine, greasy-appearing scales, most commonly on the malar area, midforehead, midchest, and scalp (Fig. 438-7). In dark-skinned individuals, lesions may be hypopigmented (Fig. 438-8). The pathogenesis is unknown, although *Pityrosporum ovale* is believed to play a role. Lesions are common in patients with human immunodeficiency virus (HIV) infection (Chapter 392). The diagnosis is made clinically. Topical corticosteroids (e.g., hydrocortisone cream 2.5%, twice daily for 1 to 2 weeks for facial lesions, fluocinolone acetonide 0.01% solution for the scalp, twice daily for 3 to 4 weeks) can rapidly reduce the inflammation; then topical ketoconazole cream, 2% twice daily, as needed (or shampoo 2% daily or every other day for the scalp), is safe for long-term treatment.

Allergic Contact Dermatitis and Irritant Contact Dermatitis

Allergic contact dermatitis and irritant contact dermatitis are induced by exogenous agents. Allergic contact dermatitis is a delayed hypersensitivity response to external allergens, whereas irritant contact dermatitis is a nonspecific toxic response to contact irritants. In both conditions, lesions occur in the exposed area. In severe cases, however, nonexposed areas may be less intensely involved. Patients with allergic contact dermatitis present with

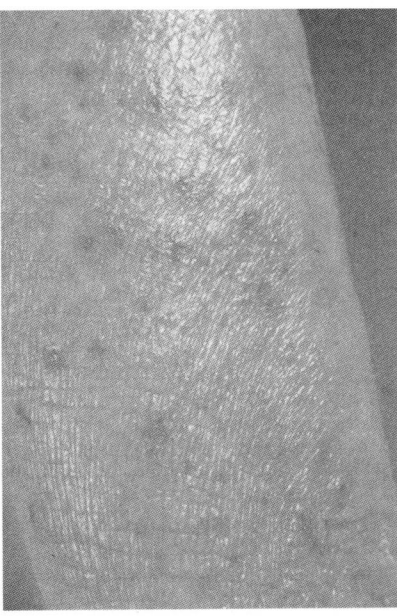

FIGURE 438-5. Atopic dermatitis. Note the erythema, excoriation, and lichenification.

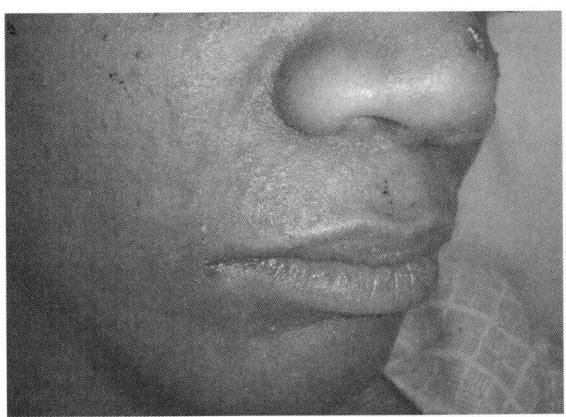

FIGURE 438-7. Seborrheic dermatitis presenting as erythematous patches and plaques with fine scales on the malar area of an HIV-positive patient.

FIGURE 438-6. Atopic dermatitis in a dark-skinned patient. Note the typical papular variant commonly seen in dark-skinned individuals.

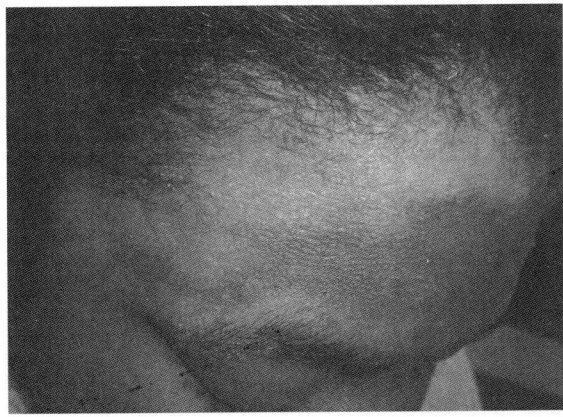

FIGURE 438-8. Seborrheic dermatitis. Hypopigmentation with fine scales on the forehead and scalp.

erythematous pruritic papules and vesicles. Lesions resolve with fine scales. Postinflammatory hyperpigmentation may be observed, especially in dark-skinned individuals. Histologically, epidermal edema and dermal histiocytic infiltrates are observed. Irritant contact dermatitis manifests with lesions morphologically similar to those of allergic contact dermatitis. However, irritant contact dermatitis is usually associated with a burning sensation rather than with pruritus. Postinflammatory hyperpigmentation is frequently observed. Histologic changes consist of necrotic keratinocytes, epidermal necrosis, and neutrophilic infiltrates. Management includes identification and removal of the offending agent, as well as symptomatic treatments such as topical corticosteroids and oral antihistamines.

● PHOTODERMATOSES

Photodermatoses are cutaneous eruptions secondary to exposure to sunlight (Table 438-2). By convention, electromagnetic radiation in the UV region is divided into UVC (200 to 290 nm), UVB (290 to 320 nm), UVA-2 (320 to 340 nm), and UVA-1 (340 to 400 nm). Visible light extends from 400 to 760 nm. Because UVC emitted by the sun is absorbed by ozone in the stratosphere, UVC does not reach the Earth's surface. UVB, UVA, and less frequently, visible light are the relevant spectra in photodermatoses.

Polymorphic Light Eruption

Polymorphic light eruption, the most common immunologically mediated photodermatosis, occurs in 10 to 20% of the general population. It usually occurs in young adults, has a slight female predominance, and is seen worldwide.[1] Affected individuals are less susceptible to cutaneous photoimmunosuppression and hence have an enhanced response to UV-induced neoantigens in the skin. Lesions usually occur in early spring, within a few hours of exposure to sunlight. Lesions can manifest as pinhead papules (common among dark-skinned patients), papules, papulovesicles, or, less commonly, vesicles (Fig. 438-9); they can also be pruritic. Usually, lesions persist for several days and resolve spontaneously. The condition tends to improve as the sunny season progresses, a phenomenon known as hardening.

The course is chronic; only 11% of patients have complete resolution of the disease in 16 years and 24% in 32 years. Diagnosis is based on the typical history and morphologic features of the lesion; the diagnosis can be confirmed by the induction of lesions with provocative phototesting. When lesions occur primarily on the face, a diagnosis of lupus must be excluded. Management consists of sun avoidance and the use of broad-spectrum sunscreens, topical corticosteroids, and oral antihistamines. In severe cases, desensitization treatment using NB-UVB has been successful. Desensitization is usually performed in early spring by exposing patients to increasing doses of NB-UVB three times weekly for 15 treatments.

Chronic Actinic Dermatitis

Chronic actinic dermatitis is a chronic photodermatosis that occurs most commonly in men in their 60s and 70s. It occurs in patients of all ethnic groups, but in the United States it is more commonly seen in dark-skinned individuals. It is seen in 5 to 17% of patients referred for evaluation of photosensitivity. Chronic actinic dermatitis can evolve from photoallergic contact dermatitis, allergic contact dermatitis, or exposure to a known photosensitizing agent; however, it also can arise de novo. Investigators have postulated that this condition represents a delayed hypersensitivity response to an unidentified antigen.

Patients present with lichenified plaques on sun-exposed areas (Figs. 438-10 and 438-11). Typically, sun-protected areas, such as the postauricular area, the area underneath the chin, the area above the eyes, and the trunk, are spared. Histologically, a dermal lymphohistiocytic infiltrate is seen and atypical mononuclear cells may be observed. On phototesting, patients have increased sensitivity to UVA, UVB, or visible light or a combination of these. In a study of 178 cases, 10% resolved in 5 years and 50% in 15 years. An association with HIV infection (Chapter 392) has been reported.

The diagnosis is based on the patient's history and on the morphologic features and distribution of the lesions. It is confirmed by phototesting.

Management is challenging. During the sunny season, it is critical that patients practice maximal photoprotection, consisting of staying in the shade, using broad-spectrum sunscreens with high sun protection factor, wearing

TABLE 438-2	SELECTED PHOTODERMATOSES
	Polymorphic light eruption
	Chronic actinic dermatitis
	Phototoxicity and photoallergy
	Porphyrias

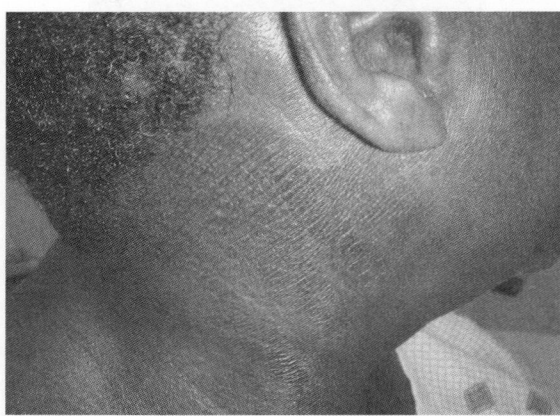

FIGURE 438-10. Chronic actinic dermatitis. Hyperpigmentation and lichenification; note sparing of the sun-protected areas of the neck and infra-auricular area.

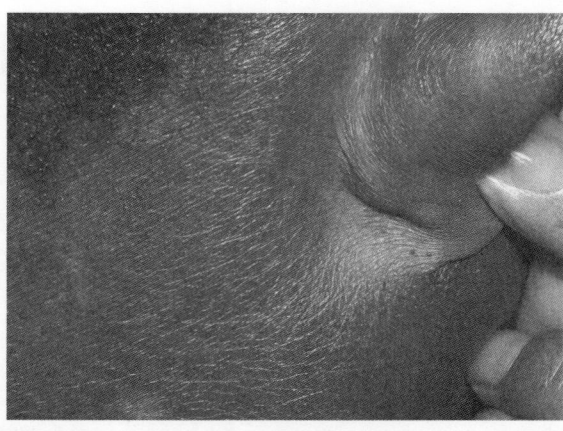

FIGURE 438-11. Hyperpigmentation and lichenification in a patient with chronic actinic dermatitis. Note sparing of the sun-protected postauricular area.

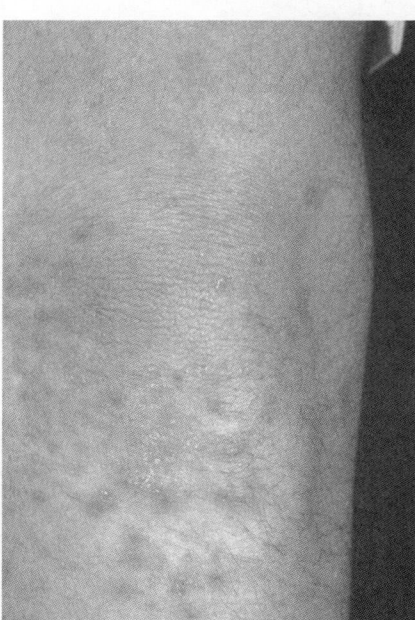

FIGURE 438-9. Polymorphic light eruption. Erythematous papules a few hours after exposure to sunlight.

appropriate clothing, and wearing a wide-brimmed hat. Other treatment modalities, in approximate sequential order, are topical corticosteroids (fluocinonide ointment 0.05% twice daily), tacrolimus ointment (0.1% twice daily), oral mycophenolate mofetil (1 to 2 g/day), oral cyclosporine (3 to 5 mg/kg/day), and azathioprine (up to 2 to 2.5 mg/kg/day). Treatment with oral corticosteroids (e.g., prednisone, 1 mg/kg/day) may be needed for acute flare. In recalcitrant cases, the following may be used: PUVA in conjunction with oral corticosteroids or a combination of mycophenolate mofetil, PUVA, and oral corticosteroids.

Phototoxicity and Photoallergy

The terms *phototoxicity* and *photoallergy* refer to the development of skin lesions after combined exposure to an oral or topical photosensitizer and electromagnetic radiation. Phototoxicity is a nonspecific cutaneous toxic reaction, whereas photoallergy is a delayed hypersensitivity response. For most photosensitizers, the action spectrum for both lies in the UVA range (Table 438-3).

Porphyrias

The most common cutaneous porphyria is porphyria cutanea tarda, in which patients present with skin fragility and blister formation on sun-exposed areas, most commonly the dorsum of the hands and the forearms (Fig. 438-12; Chapter 210). Patients usually have periorbital hypertrichosis and, less frequently, periorbital mottled hyperpigmentation and hypopigmentation. Sclerodermoid skin changes can occur in both sun-exposed and sun-protected areas. The defective enzyme is uroporphyrinogen decarboxylase. Porphyria cutanea tarda is associated with excessive alcohol intake, exposure to estrogens, hepatitis C infection (Chapter 149), HIV infection (Chapter 392), and hemochromatosis (Chapter 212). Patients invariably have an elevated level of ferritin and frequently have elevated liver enzyme values.

The diagnosis is suggested by the typical clinical appearance and is confirmed by the characteristic porphyrin profile (elevated levels of 8-, 7-, 6-, 5-, and 4-carboxyl porphyrins in the urine and isocoproporphyrin in feces; Chapter 210). Management consists of avoidance of precipitating factors (alcohol, iron-containing vitamins, estrogen-containing birth control pills) and weekly phlebotomy. In patients who are anemic (e.g., those with HIV infection), low-dose hydroxychloroquine (200 mg/week) is beneficial.

TABLE 438-3	PHOTOTOXICITY AND PHOTOALLERGY	
FEATURES	PHOTOTOXICITY	PHOTOALLERGY
Lesions after first exposure	Yes	No
Onset	Minutes after sun exposure	Delayed (24-48 hr after sun exposure)
Common offending agents	Systemic medications	Sunscreen agents
Morphology	Vesicles, bulla, hyperpigmentation	Eczematous (erythema, scaliness)
Management	Symptomatic (topical corticosteroids, antihistamine) Removal of the offending agent	

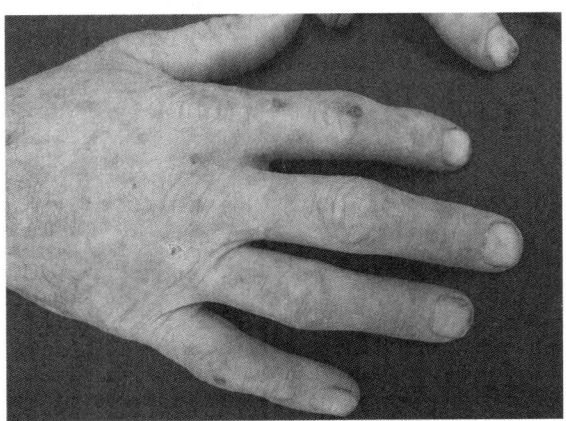

FIGURE 438-12. Erosion, crusting, and vesicles on the dorsum of the hand of a patient with porphyria cutanea tarda.

PAPULOSQUAMOUS (INCLUDING FUNGAL) DISEASES

Common papulosquamous diseases are listed in Table 438-4.

Psoriasis

EPIDEMIOLOGY

Psoriasis is the most commonly recognized papulosquamous disease. It occurs in 2 to 3% of the general population, with considerable variation in different parts of the world. It affects male and female patients equally. Approximately one third of the patients have a positive family history. Psoriasis has a bimodal peak of onset, at 22.5 years of age and again at age 55 years. The onset of psoriasis before the age of 15 years is associated with a higher prevalence of positive family history of psoriasis and with more severe disease.

PATHOBIOLOGY

Psoriasis involves the innate and adaptive immune systems, with abnormal keratinocyte proliferation. Factors playing a role in the pathogenesis include activation of antigen-presenting cells and development of T_H1 and T_H17 cells. Mediators include interleukin-12 (IL-12), IL-23, tumor necrosis factor-α (TNF-α), and interferon-γ.[2] In genetically susceptible individuals, exposure to precipitating factors such as infections (e.g., streptococcal or HIV infections), stress, or physical injury may activate T cells and stimulate the influx of neutrophils and the subsequent release of inflammatory mediators, which lead to the development of cutaneous lesions.

Psoriasis has a complex, polygenetic inheritance.[3] Cutaneous psoriasis is strongly associated with human leukocyte antigen–Cw6 (HLA-Cw6), whereas psoriatic arthritis can be associated with HLA-Cw6, HLA-B38/39, or HLA-B27.[4] Approximately 40 non–major histocompatibility complex loci have been reported by genome-wide studies to increase the risk for psoriasis, with the number expected to increase as larger cohorts are studied. Many of these loci contain genes involved in signaling pathways targeted by highly effective biologic therapies. Psoriasis also is associated with ulcerative colitis, lymphoma, the metabolic syndrome, heart disease, depression, smoking, and alcohol consumption.[5,6]

CLINICAL MANIFESTATIONS

Psoriasis can involve the skin, scalp, and nails. Skin lesions are characterized by erythematous macules, papules, or plaques that are usually covered with silvery scales (Fig. 438-13). On removal of the scales, pinpoint bleeding may be observed (the Auspitz sign), a finding reflecting the proliferation of blood vessels in the superficial dermis. Nail involvement includes pittings, yellowish macules underneath the nail plate ("oil drop" sign), and thickening of the nail (onychodystrophy) (Fig. 438-14). Minor injury to the skin can result in the development of psoriatic lesions (Koebner phenomenon). The association of psoriasis with HIV infection (Chapter 392) has been well documented.

Several distinct forms of psoriasis are recognized. *Psoriasis vulgaris*, the most common type, appears as a persistent erythematous scaly papule and plaque most commonly on elbows, knees, and scalp, where it can be associated with erythematous patches with pustules (Fig. 438-15). *Guttate psoriasis* usually occurs after viral or bacterial (most commonly streptococcal) infection; it appears as small, erythematous, scaly papules scattered over a large area of the body in a raindrop distribution (*guttate* means "droplike"). *Inverse psoriasis* refers to psoriasis that occurs in skin-fold areas such as the groin, axilla, and inframammary folds. It appears as an erythematous, somewhat shiny patch; because of the constant friction in the involved areas, scales are usually absent. *Erythrodermic psoriasis* appears as widespread erythroderma

TABLE 438-4	PAPULOSQUAMOUS DISEASES
Psoriasis	
Pityriasis rubra pilaris	
Pityriasis rosea	
Lichen planus	
Lichen nitidus	
Secondary syphilis	
Pityriasis lichenoides	
Parapsoriasis	
Mycosis fungoides	
Acrokeratosis paraneoplastica of Bazex	
Necrolytic acral erythema	
Dermatophytosis	
Tinea versicolor	

with fine silvery scales. *Palmoplantar psoriasis* manifests as keratotic scaly patches and plaques on the palms and soles, very frequently with accompanying fissures. *Pustular psoriasis of von Zumbusch* is a rare variant of psoriasis occurring with generalized pustules that are 2 to 3 mm in diameter and associated with the onset of fever.

Of patients with psoriasis, 5 to 30% also may have psoriatic arthritis, which may precede the appearance of cutaneous lesions (Chapter 265). Approximately 95% of these patients present with peripheral asymmetrical oligoar-

thritis involving the interphalangeal joints of the hands and feet, whereas 5% have exclusively axial or skeletal disease.

DIAGNOSIS

In most cases, the diagnosis of psoriasis can be made based on the history and physical examination alone. However, in patients with erythrodermic psoriasis, skin biopsy is needed to exclude other causes of generalized erythroderma, such as drug eruption, cutaneous T-cell lymphoma (Chapter 185), and pityriasis rubra pilaris.

TREATMENT   Rx

Sequential treatment modalities (Table 438-5)[A3-A9] start with topical therapy, UV-based therapy, and then traditional systemic therapy, biologics, or an oral phosphodiesterase inhibitor.[7] For recalcitrant cases, combination therapy is frequently used. Oral corticosteroids should not be used because psoriasis may worsen when they are discontinued.

Pityriasis Rubra Pilaris

EPIDEMIOLOGY

Pityriasis rubra pilaris occurs equally in men and women; the incidence ranges from 1 in 5000 new dermatology patients in Great Britain to 1 in 50,000 in India. This disease most frequently occurs as the acquired form, although a familial form (autosomal dominant with variable expression) occasionally has been reported. Abnormal vitamin A metabolism and autoimmunity have been postulated as possible precipitants.

CLINICAL MANIFESTATIONS

The most common form of pityriasis rubra pilaris is type I, which is characterized by widespread salmon-colored plaques with fine scales, islands of sparing, scaliness on the scalp, waxy keratoderma of the palms and soles, and follicular hyperkeratosis (Figs. 438-16 and 438-17). In adult patients, the condition typically starts on the face and moves to the lower extremities; in the juvenile form, it usually starts in the lower half of the body. Ectropion and pruritus may occur. Atypical adult pityriasis rubra pilaris can manifest with palmar plantar keratoderma with coarse scales and alopecia.

DIAGNOSIS

Diagnosis is based on the clinical presentations and by the characteristic histologic findings of alternating vertical and horizontal parakeratosis in the stratum corneum.

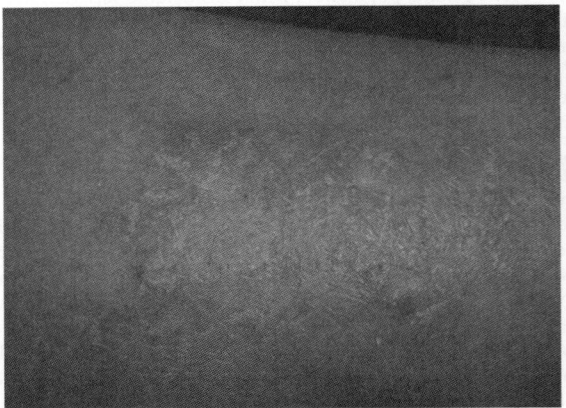

FIGURE 438-13. Psoriasis. Erythematous plaques with silvery scales.

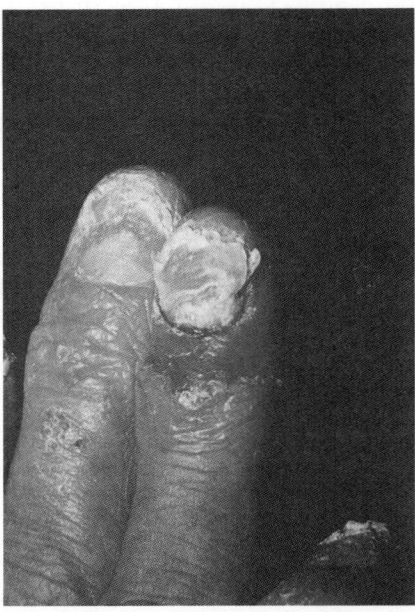

FIGURE 438-14. Psoriasis. Thickening and crumbling of the nail plate (onychodystrophy). Note the erythematous patches with silvery scales in the periungual area.

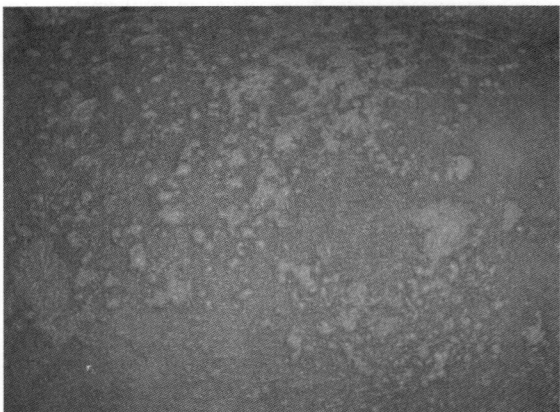

FIGURE 438-15. Psoriasis. Erythematous patch with pustules in a patient with active disease.

TABLE 438-5	SEQUENTIAL THERAPEUTIC APPROACH IN PSORIASIS
Topical agents	Corticosteroids (e.g., triamcinolone ointment 0.1%) Vitamin D analogues (e.g., calcinotriene cream 0.005%) Retinoids (e.g., tazarotene cream 0.1%)
Phototherapy	Narrow band ultraviolet B (three times/wk) PUVA (psoralen and ultraviolet A, three times/wk)
Traditional systemic therapy	Methotrexate (10-20 mg/wk) Cyclosporine (3-5 mg/kg/day) Mycophenolate mofetil (1.5-2 g/day) Acitretin (25-50 mg/day)
Biologics	TNF-α inhibitors • Etanercept (50 mg/wk SC)[A3] • Adalimumab (40 mg every 2 wk SC) • Infliximab (5-10 mg/kg every 8 wk IV) Anti–IL-12/23 • Ustekinumab (45-90 mg every 12 wk SC)[A4]
Oral phosphodiesterase-4 inhibitor	Apremilast (30 mg twice/day)[A5]
Potential future treatments*	Anti–IL-17 receptor antibody • Brodalumab[A6] Anti–IL-17 antibody • Secukinumab[A7] • Ixekizumab[A8] Oral Janus kinase inhibitor • Tofacitinib[A9]

IL = interleukin; IV = intravenously; SC = subcutaneously; TNF = tumor necrosis factor.
*Doses may change if and when FDA approved.

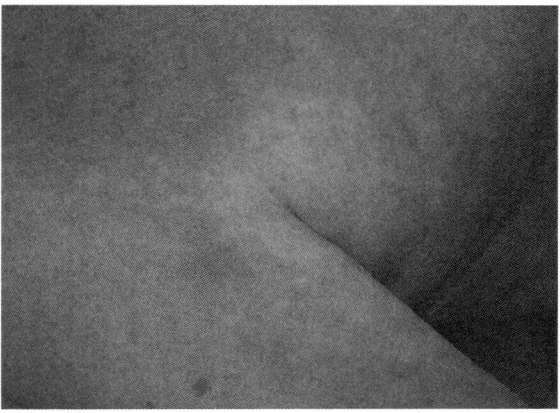

FIGURE 438-16. Pityriasis rubra pilaris. Note the erythematous orange plaques with islands of sparing.

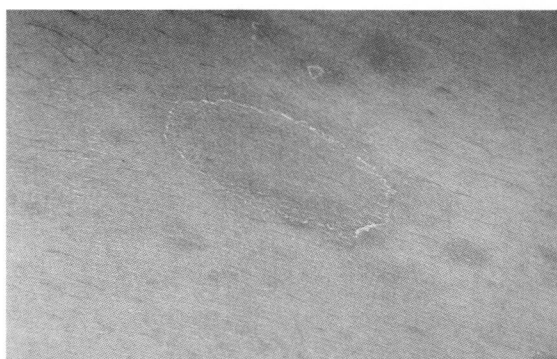

FIGURE 438-18. Pityriasis rosea. Large erythematous oval patch (herald patch) accompanied by smaller erythematous patches.

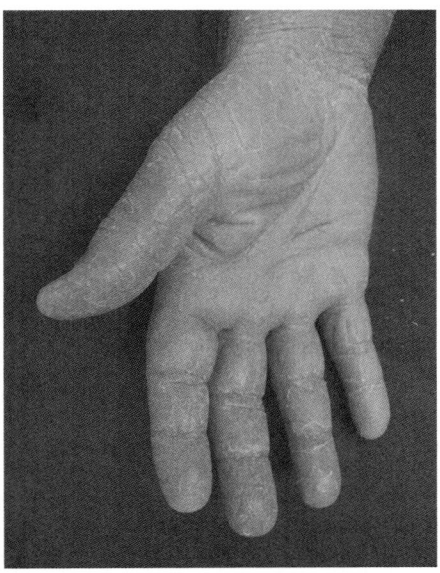

FIGURE 438-17. Pityriasis rubra pilaris. Palmar hyperkeratosis with waxy scales.

TREATMENT Rx

The most effective treatment is with oral retinoids (acitretin, 25 to 50 mg/day for 2 to 4 months). Some patients benefit from methotrexate (7.5 to 15 mg/week) or cyclosporine (3 to 5 mg/kg/day). TNF antagonists, used at the same doses as for psoriasis, are helpful for patients with recalcitrant type I disease.[A10] Topical keratolytic agents, such as ammonium lactate lotion 12%, twice daily, are helpful as adjunctive therapy.

Pityriasis Rosea
EPIDEMIOLOGY AND PATHOBIOLOGY

The incidence of pityriasis rosea has been reported as 3 to 30 per 1000 patients. It occurs in all ethnic groups, most commonly in the third and fourth decades of life, with a slight female predominance. The cause is not known, and a possible association with human herpesvirus types 6 and 7 has been reported.[8]

CLINICAL MANIFESTATIONS

In 50 to 90% of patients, pityriasis rosea starts with a primary lesion (herald patch), which is an erythematous, scaly, oval patch a few centimeters in diameter (Fig. 438-18). This lesion is usually followed within a few days by smaller, minimally pruritic, erythematous scaly patches on the trunk, less commonly on the proximal extremities. As a rule, the palms and soles are spared. The distribution of the eruption, especially on the back, tends to follow the lines of cleavage of the skin, with a resulting "Christmas tree" distribution. The eruption is self-limited and resolves within 6 to 8 weeks. In rare instances, lesions may persist.

DIAGNOSIS

The diagnosis usually can be made clinically. The most important differential diagnosis is secondary syphilis, which, in contrast to pityriasis rosea, usually involves the palms and soles. Serology testing to exclude syphilis (Chapter 319) is advisable.

TREATMENT Rx

Treatment is primarily symptomatic, including topical corticosteroids and oral antihistamines. NB-UVB phototherapy should be reserved for severe, recalcitrant cases.

Lichen Planus
EPIDEMIOLOGY

Lichen planus occurs most commonly in patients between 30 and 60 years of age. Women are affected more frequently than men and tend to be somewhat older at the onset of disease. The prevalence in the general population is approximately 1%.

PATHOBIOLOGY

Histologically, lichen planus is characterized by dense lymphocytic infiltrate at the dermal-epidermal junction. The infiltrates consist of predominantly T cells, a finding suggesting the pathogenic role of cell-mediated immunity. Because lichen planus or lichen planus–like eruptions can occur after exposure to drugs or chemicals (e.g., color film developer), the role of drugs and chemicals in inducing a T-cell–mediated response against the epidermis has been postulated. Lichen planus may be associated with hepatitis C infection (Chapter 149).

CLINICAL MANIFESTATIONS

Patients present with erythematous-to-violaceous flat-topped papules, often with white lacy lines (Wickham striae) on the wrists, forearms, and genitalia (Fig. 438-19).[9] *Oral lichen planus* occurs as white papules and plaques with a reticulated appearance, most commonly along the bite line on the buccal mucosa. Similar lesions can be seen on the tongue (Fig. 438-20) and genital mucosa. Painful erosion may occur. *Hypertrophic lichen planus* usually occurs on the lower extremities as lichenified, violaceous plaques, probably secondary to chronic rubbing and scratching of the lichen planus lesions.

DIAGNOSIS

The diagnosis is made clinically and is confirmed by the characteristic histologic findings of infiltration by the lichenoid infiltrate of lymphocytes at the dermal-epidermal junction.

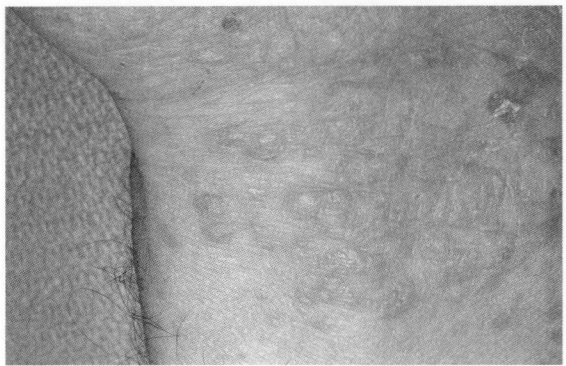

FIGURE 438-19. Lichen planus. Erythematous flat-topped papules on the wrist.

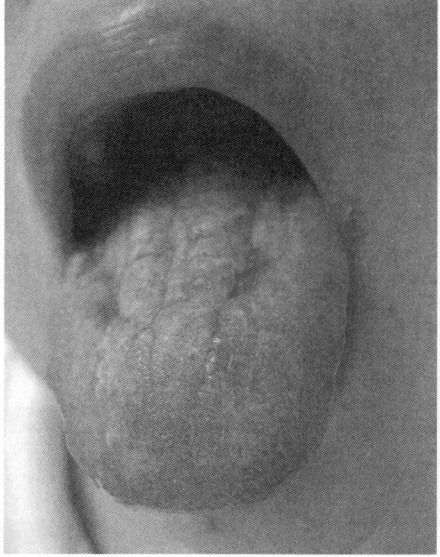

FIGURE 438-20. Lichen planus of the tongue. Note white plaques on dorsal surface of the tongue, with reticulated white line on the distal aspect of the tongue.

TABLE 438-6 THERAPEUTIC OPTIONS FOR LICHEN PLANUS

CUTANEOUS LESIONS

Topical corticosteroids (triamcinolone ointment 0.1% twice/day)

HYPERTROPHIC LESIONS

Intralesional corticosteroids (triamcinolone suspension 3-5 mg/mL)

ORAL LESIONS

Corticosteroid paste (triamcinolone 0.1% paste twice/day) or cyclosporine solution (100 mg/mL, 2 mL, twice/day, swish and spit).

GENERALIZED LICHEN PLANUS, PAINFUL ORAL/GENITAL EROSIONS, RECALCITRANT DISEASE

Narrow band UVB phototherapy (2-3 times/wk)
Oral prednisone (0.5-1 mg/kg, taper in 6-8 wk)
Mycophenolate mofetil (1-2 g/day)
Cyclosporin (3-5 mg/kg)
Tumor necrosis factor-α inhibitors (see Table 438-5)

TREATMENT   Rx

Therapeutic options depend on the location of lesions (Table 438-6). Without treatment, cutaneous lesions usually resolve in approximately 1 year, whereas oral and hypertrophic lesions tend to be much more chronic, persisting for an average of 4.5 years and 8.5 years, respectively.

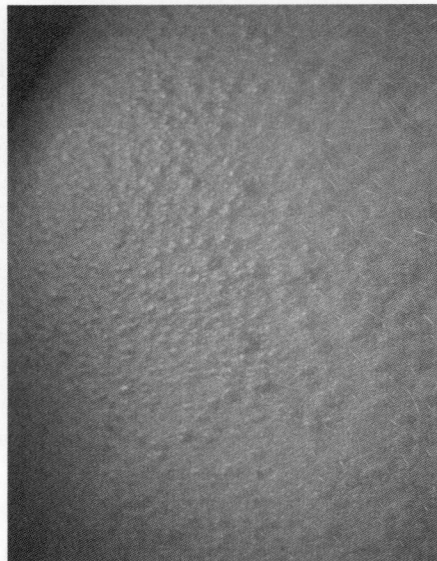

FIGURE 438-21. Lichen nitidus. Note skin-colored fine papules on the upper back.

Lichen Nitidus

Lichen nitidus is a rather uncommon condition that usually occurs in children or young adults. The incidence has been estimated to be 3.4 cases per 10,000 persons. It is more commonly observed in dark-skinned individuals. The cause is unclear.

The lesions are asymptomatic, 1- to 2-mm, shiny, skin-colored discrete papules, sometimes with fine scales on their surface, occurring most commonly on the genitalia or forearms and occasionally on the trunk (Fig. 438-21). A generalized form has rarely been reported. Histologically, a dense lymphocytic infiltrate can be seen in the superficial dermis and at the dermal-epidermal junction. In contrast to lichen planus, in which the infiltrate tends to involve the entire dermal-epidermal junction, the infiltrate in lichen nitidus tends to be much more focal.

The diagnosis can be confirmed from the typical clinical appearance and the characteristic histologic changes. The condition tends to remit spontaneously in a few years, so therapy, with topical corticosteroids (e.g., triamcinolone ointment, 0.1% twice daily for 2 weeks) and oral antihistamines (e.g., fexofenadine, 180 mg every morning, and hydroxyzine, 25 to 50 mg at bedtime, as needed), should be reserved for symptomatic cases only.

Secondary Syphilis

Lesions typically occur 1 to 2 months after the development of a primary chancre lesion (Chapter 319). However, up to 25% of patients may not remember having a chancre. Once the eruption occurs, it lasts for 1 to 3 months.

Clinically, secondary syphilis may appear as erythematous macules (roseola syphilitica), erythematous-to-hyperpigmented oval or circular papules and plaques covered with scales, or a maculopapular eruption (Fig. 438-22). Nodular eruption also may occur occasionally. The lesions tend to be widespread, and the palms and soles are very frequently involved (Fig. 438-23). The diagnosis is made based on the history, physical examination, and a positive serology. Skin biopsy shows the proliferation of endothelial cells in the dermis and a dense dermal infiltrate containing many plasma cells. Intramuscular benzathine penicillin G (2.4 million U intramuscularly in a single dose) is currently the recommended treatment.

Pityriasis Lichenoides

Pityriasis lichenoides occurs as erythematous papules that may be minimally pruritic and covered with scales, scattered on all parts of the body. In the acute form (pityriasis lichenoides et varioliformis acuta [PLEVA]), the central part of the lesions develops vesicles, pustules, and hemorrhages, with eventual crusting of the lesions. The patient may have mild constitutional symptoms of fever and malaise. The chronic form (pityriasis lichenoides chronica [PLC]) occurs as asymptomatic erythematous-to-hyperpigmented papules and plaques covered with fine scales; the trunk and extremities are common

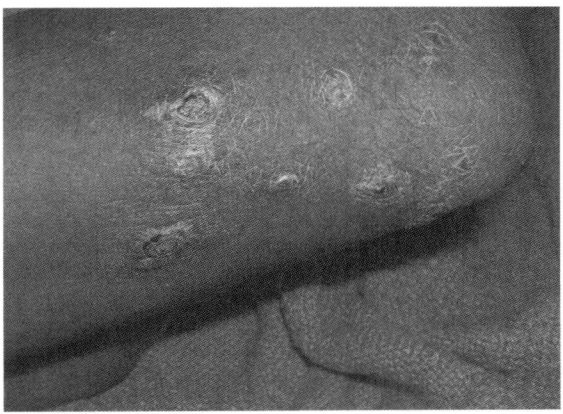

FIGURE 438-22. Secondary syphilis. Papules with crust on elbow.

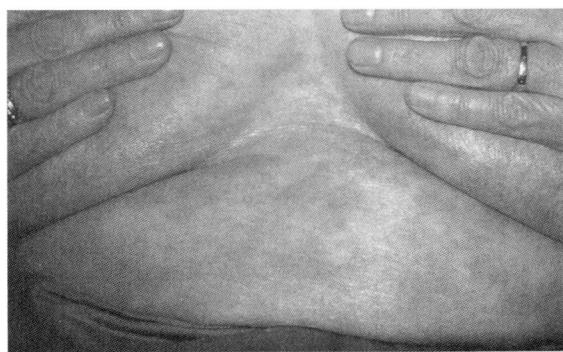

FIGURE 438-24. Large plaque parapsoriasis. Erythematous patches with fine scales.

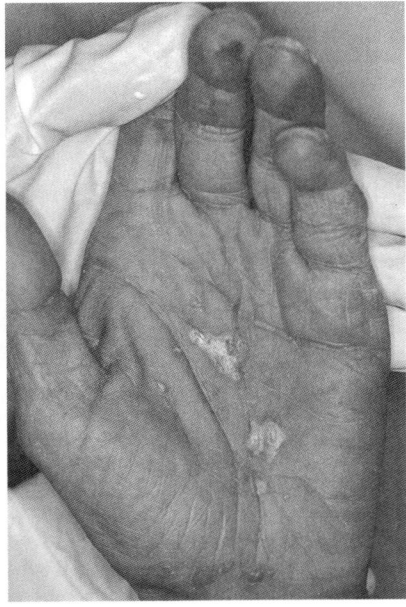

FIGURE 438-23. Secondary syphilis. Scaly papules and plaques on the palm.

FIGURE 438-25. Mycosis fungoides. Hypopigmented patches in a dark-skinned patient.

sites. Histologically, both PLEVA and PLC are characterized by dense lymphocytic infiltrates in the dermis, with CD8 lymphocytes predominating in PLEVA and CD4 lymphocytes in PLC.

PLEVA usually resolves in a few months, although it can persist. PLC usually lasts for a few years. Both disorders affect patients of all ages, with a slight male predominance.

Treatment generally follows a sequential order: (1) topical corticosteroids (e.g., triamcinolone ointment, 0.1% twice daily for 1 to 2 weeks) and antihistamines, (2) doxycycline (100 mg twice daily) or erythromycin (1 to 2 g/day), (3) NB-UVB phototherapy (three times weekly for 8 to 10 weeks with increasing doses of NB-UVB), and (4) methotrexate (7.5 to 15 mg/week).

Parapsoriasis

The two common variants of parapsoriasis are large plaque parapsoriasis and small plaque parapsoriasis. The peak incidence is in the fifth decade, although rare cases may begin in childhood. Large plaque parapsoriasis appears as minimally pruritic, oval-to-circular, erythematous-to-hyperpigmented macules and patches with fine scales and superficial atrophy (crinkling atrophy) scattered on all parts of the body (Fig. 438-24). These lesions are usually larger than 5 cm. Large plaque parapsoriasis is considered by some to be a less aggressive variant of mycosis fungoides (see later). Small plaque parapsoriasis appears as circular-to-oval, erythematous-to-hyperpigmented

patches or minimally elevated plaques, with lesions smaller than 5 cm in diameter and usually covered with fine scales. Digitate dermatosis is a distinct variant of small plaque parapsoriasis in which lesions appear along the lines of cleavage, usually on the lateral aspect of the trunk in the shape of fingerprints. Histologically, large plaque parapsoriasis is characterized by a dermal lymphocytic infiltrate, which may extend into the epidermis whereas small plaque parapsoriasis is characterized by spongiotic dermatitis, with a mild superficial lymphocytic infiltrate in the dermis. In up to one third of patients, large plaque parapsoriasis may evolve into mycosis fungoides. As a result, treatment of large plaque parapsoriasis is similar to that of early-stage mycosis fungoides: high-potency topical corticosteroids, topical nitrogen mustard, NB-UVB phototherapy, and psoralen and UVA (PUVA). By comparison, patients with small plaque parapsoriasis have a benign course and management should be symptomatic only, with emollients, topical corticosteroids, and NB-UVB phototherapy.

Mycosis Fungoides

Mycosis fungoides is the most common variant of cutaneous T-cell lymphoma (Chapter 185). The four types of cutaneous manifestations are patch, plaque, tumor, and erythrodermic. Patch-stage disease manifests as skin-colored or minimally erythematous patches with fine "cigarette paper" wrinkling of the epidermis; hyperpigmented or hypopigmented lesions are frequently seen in dark-skinned patients. The patches can vary from a few millimeters to a few centimeters in diameter; they are more common on sun-protected areas such as the buttocks (Fig. 438-25). The patches are usually asymptomatic, although they occasionally may be mildly pruritic. Lesions may be present for years. As the disease progresses, some of the patches may become more indurated and may evolve into plaques (Fig. 438-26). Nodular lesions may occur in patients without any patch or plaque lesions, although more commonly these lesions occur in conjunction with patches and plaques. Erythrodermic mycosis fungoides occurs as a generalized erythroderma with significant scaling and pruritus. Hyperkeratosis of the palms and soles, as well as fissuring of hands and feet, are quite common.

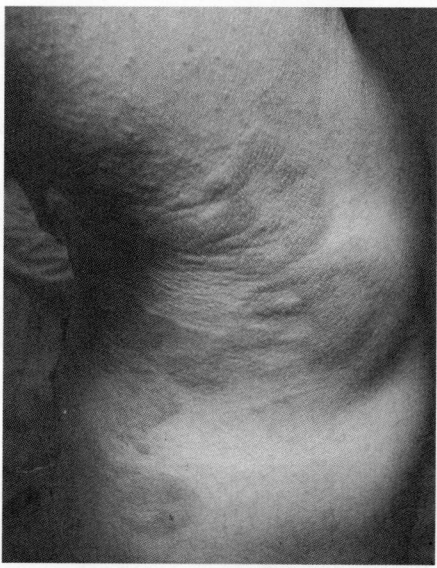

FIGURE 438-26. Mycosis fungoides. Plaque-stage disease.

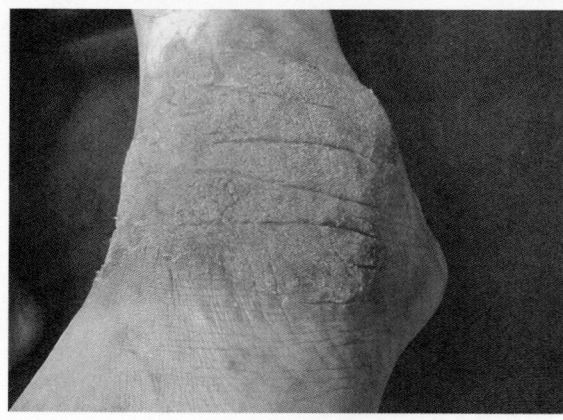

FIGURE 438-27. Necrolytic acral erythema. Lichenified plaques with fine scales on anterior lateral ankle.

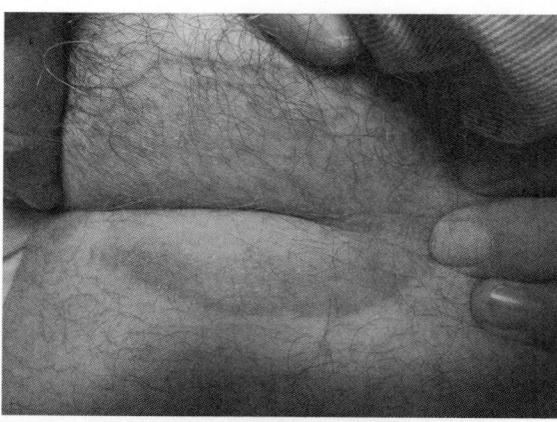

FIGURE 438-28. Tinea cruris. Erythematous patch with erythematous papules and scales at the periphery.

TABLE 438-7	TREATMENT FOR MYCOSIS FUNGOIDES
CLINICAL TYPE	**TREATMENT**
Patch and localized plaque	Topical corticosteroids (e.g., triamcinolone ointment 0.1% q12h)
	Topical nitrogen mustard (mechlorethamine 0.01% in aquaphor, qd)
	Topical retinoids (e.g., bexarotene gel 1%, 1-4 times/day)
	Narrow band UVB (2-3 times/wk)
Extensive plaques and Tumors	Psoralen and UVA (PUVA; 2-3 times/wk)
	Oral bexarotene (300 mg/m²/day)
	Methotrexate (10-15 mg/wk)
	Interferon-α (1-5 million U 3-5 times/wk SC)
	Total skin electron beam therapy
	Histone deacetylase inhibitors: Vorinostat (400 mg/day PO); romidepsin (14 mg/m² IV on days 1, 8, and 15 of a 28-day cycle)
	Anti-CD52 antibody: Alemtuzumab (10-15 mg three times/wk SC)
	Denileukin diftitox (9 or 18 μg/kg/day IV for 5 consecutive days every 21 days for 8 cycles
	Radiation therapy for localized tumors
Erythrodermic	Extracorporeal photopheresis (2 consecutive days every 2-4 wk)

IV = intravenously; PO = orally; qd = daily; UVA = ultraviolet A; UVB = ultraviolet B.

The diagnosis is confirmed by histologic demonstration of atypical mononuclear cells both in the epidermis and in the dermis, as well as immunophenotypic markers showing predominance of CD4 cells in the infiltrate.[10] Treatment options are summarized in Table 438-7.

Bazex Syndrome and Necrolytic Acral Erythema

Patients with Bazex syndrome (acrokeratosis neoplastica) present with symmetrical, scaly, erythematous-to-violaceous hyperkeratotic plaques on acral areas, such as digits, palms, soles, nose, and ears. Almost all have involvement of the ears and ridging of the nails.[11] Bazex syndrome is associated with malignancy, especially of lips, tongue, larynx, pharynx, and esophagus, perhaps because of cross reactivity between tumor antigens and normal keratinocytic antigens.

Necrolytic acral erythema is a marker of chronic hepatitis C infection (Chapter 149).[12] It manifests with well-defined hyperkeratotic, lichenified plaques on dorsum of hands and feet (Fig 438-27). Low serum zinc levels have been reported in some patients whose disease improved following oral zinc therapy.

Dermatophytoses

Fungal infections that occur as papulosquamous eruptions include tinea corporis, tinea manuum, tinea cruris, and tinea pedis. *Tinea corporis* manifests as a polycyclic erythematous scaly patch that has elevated borders and consists of papules and sometimes pustules. As the lesion progresses, the border advances centrifugally. The trunk is the most common site. *Tinea cruris* has similar morphology, except it is located in the inguinal folds (Fig. 438-28). *Tinea manuum* presents as an erythematous scaly patch with an advancing active border, usually located on the dorsum of the hands, or it may occur as diffuse scaly patches with mild hyperkeratosis involving part or the entire surface of the palm and palmar aspect of the fingers. *Tinea pedis* has two clinical manifestations: it can occur as scaly macerated lesions with erythema in the toe webs or as patchy or diffuse scaliness on the sole extending to the medial and lateral aspect of the foot (moccasin distribution). The latter presentation can be associated with diffuse scaliness of one but not both palms, a condition known as the "one-hand, two-feet syndrome." The diagnosis can be confirmed by examination of skin scrapings using 10% potassium hydroxide preparation or by fungal culture. Treatment consists of topical or oral antifungal medications (e.g., clotrimazole cream, 1%, twice daily for 2 to 4 weeks, or terbinafine, 250 mg for 2 to 12 weeks), depending on the site involved.

TINEA VERSICOLOR

Tinea versicolor is a fungal infection of the skin caused by *Malassezia furfur*. It occurs in otherwise healthy young individuals, especially in warm and moist environments during the summer. The prevalence is estimated to be 2 to 8% in the United States and up to 50% in the tropical countries. Clinically, it appears as macules and patches with very fine scales; the color can be hypopigmented, skin colored, minimally erythematous, or light brown (Fig. 438-29). The patches start as perifollicular macules, with the midchest and midback the most common sites. As the lesions progress, hypopigmentation of the skin also may occur. The lesion usually is asymptomatic. The diagnosis

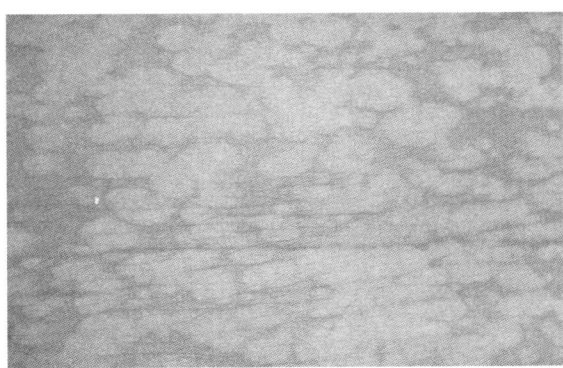

FIGURE 438-29. Tinea versicolor. Hypopigmented patches on the trunk.

GENERAL REFERENCES

For the General References and other additional features, please visit Expert Consult at https://expertconsult.inkling.com.

439

MACULAR, PAPULAR, VESICULOBULLOUS, AND PUSTULAR DISEASES

NEIL J. KORMAN

is confirmed by the characteristic appearance of the fungal elements on a 10% potassium hydroxide preparation—grapelike clusters of yeast and short, septate branching hyphae ("spaghetti and meatballs" appearance).[13] Treatment is with 2.5% selenium sulfide shampoo (applied for 10 minutes then wash off, 5 times weekly for 4 to 6 weeks), topical antifungal preparations (e.g., clotrimazole cream, 1% twice daily for 4 weeks), or a 1- to 3-day course of oral ketoconazole (200 mg/day).

FIGURATE ERYTHEMIAS
The figurative erythemas (which include erythema annulare centrifugum, erythema gyratum repens, and erythema chronicum migrans) appear as erythematous circular or polycyclic plaques with central clearing and, frequently, a centrifugally migrating border. Occasionally, fine scaling also may be observed. The extremities are the most common sites. The diagnosis frequently can be made by the typical history and morphologic features.

Erythema annulare centrifugum is most commonly idiopathic; however, it also can be a manifestation of a hypersensitivity response to medications. Management includes identification of a precipitating agent (if possible) and treatment with topical or systemic corticosteroids. *Erythema gyratum repens* occurs as concentric erythematous plaques with fine scales, resembling a wood-grain pattern. This unusual form of figurate erythema has been associated with malignant hematologic diseases and with carcinomas of the breast, lung, gastrointestinal tract, prostate, and cervix. Treatment of the underlying malignant disease results in the resolution of the skin lesion in a few months. *Erythema chronicum migrans,* which is a cutaneous manifestation of Lyme disease and is caused by the spirochete *Borrelia burgdorferi* (Chapter 321), appears as a concentric ring of erythema that progresses centrifugally from the site of a tick bite. Occasionally, it may appear as a circular erythematous patch. The diagnosis is made by a history of a tick bite, the characteristic cutaneous lesion, or elevated serum antibodies to *B. burgdorferi.* Management is the same as for Lyme disease.

Grade A References

A1. Paller AS, Lebwohl M, Fleischer AB Jr, et al. Tacrolimus ointment is more effective than pimecrolimus cream with a similar safety profile in the treatment of atopic dermatitis: results from 3 randomized, comparative studies. *J Am Acad Dermatol.* 2005;52:810-822.
A2. Beck LA, Thaci D, Hamilton JD, et al. Dupilumab treatment in adults with moderate-to-severe atopic dermatitis. *N Engl J Med.* 2014;371:130-139.
A3. Ohtsuki M, Terui T, Ozawa A, et al. Japanese guidance for use of biologics for psoriasis (the 2013 version). *J Dermatol.* 2013;40:683-695.
A4. McInnes IB, Kavanaugh A, Gottlieb AB, et al. Efficacy and safety of ustekinumab in patients with active psoriatic arthritis: 1 year results of the phase 3, multicentre, double-blind, placebo-controlled PSUMMIT 1 trial. *Lancet.* 2013;382:780-789.
A5. Papp K, Cather JC, Rosoph L, et al. Efficacy of apremilast in the treatment of moderate to severe psoriasis: a randomised controlled trial. *Lancet.* 2012;380:738-746.
A6. Papp KA, Leonardi C, Menter A, et al. Brodalumab, an anti-interleukin-17-receptor antibody for psoriasis. *N Engl J Med.* 2012;366:1181-1189.
A7. Langley RG, Elewski BE, Lebwohl M, et al. Secukinumab in plaque psoriasis—results of two phase 3 trials. *N Engl J Med.* 2014;371:326-338.
A8. Leonardi C, Matheson R, Zachariae C, et al. Anti-interleukin-17 monoclonal antibody ixekizumab in chronic plaque psoriasis. *N Engl J Med.* 2012;366:1190-1199.
A9. Menter A, Papp KA, Tan H, et al. Efficacy of tofacitinib, an oral janus kinase inhibitor, on clinical signs of moderate-to-severe plaque psoriasis in different body regions. *J Drugs Dermatol.* 2014;13:252-256.
A10. Petrof G, Almaani N, Archer CB, et al. A systematic review of the literature on the treatment of pityriasis rubra pilaris type 1 with TNF-antagonists. *J Eur Acad Dermatol Venereol.* 2013;27:e131-e135.

MACULAR AND PAPULAR EXANTHEMS
An exanthem is an acute generalized eruption of the skin, and there are two major types, scarlatiniform eruptions and morbilliform eruptions. Scarlatiniform eruptions consist of confluent blanching erythema; their name was derived from their similarity to the eruption of scarlet fever (Table 439-1). Morbilliform eruptions consist of erythematous macules and papules; they are named for their resemblance to the measles eruption. Morbilliform eruptions can be caused by exposure to medications (Chapter 440) or viral infections.

Scarlatiniform Eruptions
SCARLET FEVER
Scarlet fever is caused by infection of the ears, nose, throat, and skin with toxin-producing β-hemolytic streptococci (Chapter 290). It most commonly occurs in children after streptococcal wound infections, burns, and upper respiratory tract infections. Occasional cases of scarlet fever can also be caused by infection with *Staphylococcus aureus* (Chapter 288), *Haemophilus influenzae* (Chapter 300), and *Clostridium* spp. (Chapter 296). The rash is caused by a circulating toxin that induces local production of inflammatory mediators and alteration of cutaneous cytokines. Patients may have an abrupt onset of fever, headache, vomiting, malaise, chills, and sore throat. The mucous membranes are usually erythematous with petechiae, and the tongue commonly has a white membrane. Red, exudative tonsils are present with pharyngeal infections. The skin eruption appears after the fever and is characterized by fine erythematous papules, first on the upper part of the trunk and then in a more general distribution. The face is flushed, and circumoral pallor is seen. This eruption lasts 4 to 5 days followed by fine desquamation, the extent and duration of which are related to the severity of the eruption. Treatment is 1.2 million units of benzathine penicillin G given intramuscularly or oral penicillin VK, 1000 mg twice daily for 10 days. Most patients recover after 4 to 5 days, and the rash usually resolves completely over a period of several weeks.

TABLE 439-1 MACULAR AND PAPULAR ERUPTIONS

SCARLATINIFORM ERUPTIONS

Scarlet fever
Toxic shock syndrome
Kawasaki disease

MORBILLIFORM ERUPTIONS

Measles
Rubella
Erythema infectiosum
Roseola

PAPULAR ERUPTIONS

Molluscum contagiosum
Warts

TOXIC SHOCK SYNDROME

DEFINITION

Toxic shock syndrome is an acute febrile illness caused by toxin-producing strains of *S. aureus* (Chapter 288) or, less commonly, *Streptococcus* spp. (toxic shock–like syndrome [Chapter 290]).

PATHOBIOLOGY

Most cases of staphylococcal toxic shock syndrome or streptococcal toxic shock–like syndrome occur in young healthy persons age 20 to 50 years. These toxins cause massive release of tumor necrosis factor-α and interleukin-1, cytokines that mediate fever, rash, hypotension, tissue injury, and shock.

CLINICAL MANIFESTATIONS

The hallmarks of the disease are fever, rash (Fig. 436-12 in Chapter 436), hypotension, and involvement of multiple organs, including the lungs, kidneys, liver, and gastrointestinal tract. Desquamation of the palms and soles follows onset of the illness by 1 to 2 weeks. There is diffuse macular erythema with flexural accentuation, mucous membrane erythema, and severe conjunctival involvement. Blood cultures are positive in 5% to 15% of patients with staphylococcal toxic shock syndrome and approximately 50% of those with streptococcal toxic shock–like syndrome.

TREATMENT Rx

Treatment is supportive and includes hydration, vasopressors, appropriate antibiotics, and drainage of infected sites. Patients with staphylococcal toxic shock should be treated with intravenous (IV) vancomycin to cover methicillin-resistant staphylococci, 1 g every 12 hours for 10 to 15 days, with dose adjustment based on creatinine clearance. Patients with streptococcal toxic shock should be treated with both IV penicillin G, 3 to 4 million units every 4 hours, and IV clindamycin, 600 to 900 mg every 8 hours for 10 to 15 days, followed by oral therapy. Double antibiotic coverage is the standard of care for streptococcal toxic shock syndrome because this infection is characterized by extremely large numbers of stationary bacteria and penicillin alone is not effective in this scenario inasmuch as penicillin-binding proteins are not expressed during the stationary group phase of streptococci. Silver sulfadiazine cream may lead to increased toxin production; therefore, mupirocin ointment should be used for infected sites.

PROGNOSIS

The mortality rate in patients with staphylococcal toxic shock syndrome is 5% to 15%; that for streptococcal toxic shock–like syndrome may be five times higher.

KAWASAKI DISEASE

EPIDEMIOLOGY

Kawasaki disease, a systemic vasculitis of unknown etiology, occurs in children of all races but is up to 20 times more common in North East Asians than in whites. Although primarily an illness of children younger than 5 years, Kawasaki disease also occurs in adults. Its epidemiologic and clinical manifestations imply that an infection is the cause, but bacterial, viral, and serologic studies have yet to confirm such an etiology.

CLINICAL MANIFESTATIONS

The clinical hallmarks are fever lasting up to 2 weeks, with spikes to 40°C (104°F), and a toxic-appearing patient.[1] During the acute phase, the polymorphic eruption may be scarlatiniform, urticarial, morbilliform, or targetoid. Desquamation occurs in the perianal area 2 days after the onset of fever and on the extremities 2 to 3 weeks later. Patients often have hemorrhagic, dry fissured lips; conjunctival injection; a "strawberry tongue;" and cervical lymphadenitis. Myocarditis and coronary artery aneurysms may develop in untreated patients, so prompt diagnosis is critical. Other findings include arthralgias and arthritis, urethritis, aseptic meningitis, pneumonitis, and diarrhea.

DIAGNOSIS

Despite the lack of specific diagnostic tests for this syndrome, the typical skin eruption accompanied by myocarditis is characteristic.

TREATMENT

Recommended therapy in the acute phase of Kawasaki disease is a single infusion of 2 g/kg of IV gamma globulin. When this therapy is given within 5 to 10 days after the onset of fever, 85% to 90% of patients will become afebrile within 36 hours, and the risk of developing coronary artery aneurysms is significantly reduced.[A1] The addition of prednisolone (2 mg/kg/day for 15 days after the C-reactive protein normalizes) further reduces the risk of developing coronary artery abnormalities.[A2] During the subacute and convalescent phase, acetylsalicylic acid is usually given at 3 to 8 mg/kg for 6 to 8 weeks. The optimal salicylate regimen for Kawasaki disease remains uncertain, and there are no controlled trials to prove that aspirin reduces coronary artery aneurysms.

Morbilliform Eruptions

MEASLES

Measles is caused by a paramyxovirus (Chapter 367) that infects respiratory epithelium and is highly transmissible. The incubation period is 7 to 14 days. The prodrome consists of cough, coryza, and conjunctivitis. The enanthem, or Koplik spots (Fig. 367-1 in Chapter 367), predates the exanthem by 1 to 2 days and lasts 2 to 4 days. These blue-white spots surrounded by a red halo appear on the buccal mucosa and are pathognomonic for measles. The exanthem (Fig. 367-2 in Chapter 367) begins on the fourth or fifth day as papules on the face and behind the ears; it then spreads to the trunk and extremities. Measles is diagnosed on clinical grounds. Active immunization with live attenuated virus has dramatically reduced the incidence of measles infection (Chapter 18) and is the most important preventive measure. Treatment consists of supportive care, with attention to maintaining good hydration.

RUBELLA

Rubella is an RNA virus of the Togaviridae family (Chapter 368). Infection with this virus leads to an illness involving the skin, lymph nodes, and occasionally the joints, primarily in young children. The disease is spread by nasal droplet infection and has an incubation period of 14 to 21 days. Patients are most contagious when the rash is erupting. In children, there may be no prodrome; in adults, however, fever, sore throat, and rhinitis may be present. The exanthem (Fig. 368-1 in Chapter 368) begins as pink macules and papules on the face that spread to the trunk and extremities; it lasts 1 to 3 days. Generalized tender lymphadenopathy, especially the suboccipital, post-auricular, and cervical nodes, is the hallmark of rubella. In normal children and adolescents, the diagnosis is made clinically, and laboratory work is unnecessary. If the diagnosis is questioned, a rising immunoglobulin M (IgM) antibody titer over a 2-week period indicates recent infection. No treatment exists, and the disease is usually self-limited. Rest and fluids are appropriate. The best protection is vaccination given with measles and mumps vaccine (i.e., measles, mumps, and rubella) at 12 to 15 months and again at 4 to 6 years (Chapter 18).

ERYTHEMA INFECTIOSUM

Erythema infectiosum is an exanthem caused by human parvovirus B19 (Chapter 371). It has a 4- to 14-day incubation period and is spread by aerosolized respiratory droplets. Acute infection leads to the production of IgM antibodies and the formation of immune complexes, which are deposited in the skin and joints. Bright red erythema appears abruptly over the cheeks (Fig. 371-1 in Chapter 371). Within 1 to 4 days, an erythematous morbilliform eruption occurs on the extremities; it fades within several days to a reticulate pattern (Fig. 439-1). There may also be malar erythema or a reticulate eruption on the extremities. Exposure of adults to parvovirus B19 leads to an acute polyarthropathy of the hands, wrists, knees, and ankles. Parvovirus B19 can interfere with erythropoiesis (Chapter 165) and can cause aplastic crisis in patients with sickle cell disease (Chapter 163). The diagnosis is clinical, and further testing is not generally necessary. Erythema infectiosum is usually a benign, self-limited disease.

ROSEOLA

Roseola (exanthem subitum) is caused by human herpesvirus 6 (Chapter 374). Virus replication occurs in leukocytes and salivary glands. Early invasion of the central nervous system (CNS) may lead to seizures. The classic patient is a healthy 9- to 12-month-old infant with an abrupt onset of high fever (40°C [104°F]) lasting 3 days. Febrile seizures occur in 15% of cases. Its rapid defervescence is striking, with the onset of a generalized pink mor-

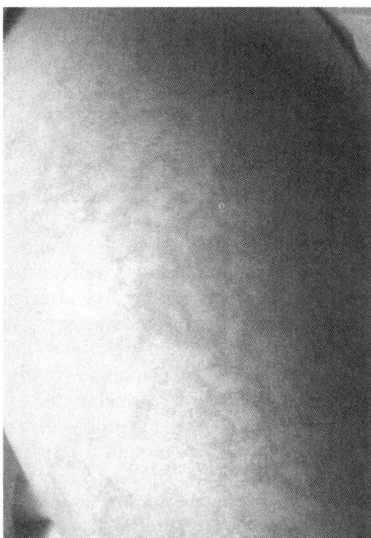

FIGURE 439-1. Reticulate macular erythema on the thigh of a patient with erythema infectiosum.

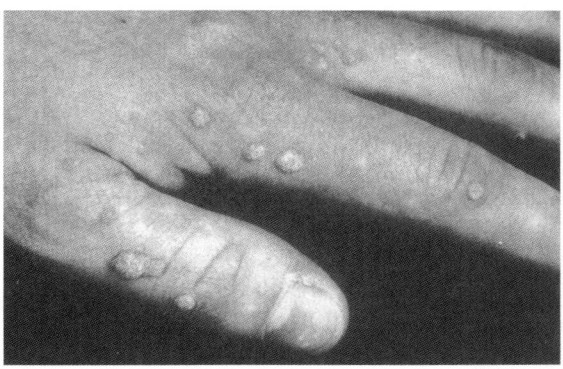

FIGURE 439-2. Hand of a patient with verruca vulgaris revealing many verrucous papules.

billiform exanthem. The eruption lasts 2 days and consists of pink papules or blanchable macular erythema. The lack of symptoms during the febrile phase and appearance of the exanthem as the fever subsides help with the diagnosis, but rubella and measles must also be considered. In an immunocompromised child or adult, there is usually an abrupt onset of fever, malaise, and sometimes CNS involvement. Virus isolation, seroconversion (IgM), or detection of viral DNA sequences in peripheral blood mononuclear cells can confirm the diagnosis. No antiviral therapy is available for roseola, and treatment is supportive. Practically all immunocompetent patients recover from roseola without sequelae, but chronic infection with multisystem complications may develop in immunocompromised patients.

Papular Eruptions
MOLLUSCUM CONTAGIOSUM
Molluscum contagiosum is a cutaneous infection caused by a large DNA poxvirus (Chapter 372) that affects both children and adults. Firm, smooth, umbilicated papules, usually 2 to 6 mm in diameter, are present in groups or widely disseminated on the skin and mucosal surfaces. Patients infected with human immunodeficiency virus (HIV) may have hundreds of lesions, and some lesions can be larger than 15 mm (Chapter 392). The diagnosis is made on clinical grounds. Molluscum contagiosum is self-limited, with the goal of treatment being destruction of the lesions. Commonly used treatments are all topical and include cryotherapy with liquid nitrogen, curettage, cantharidin, podophyllin, and tretinoin.

WARTS
Warts are benign proliferations of skin and mucosa caused by human papillomaviruses (HPVs) (Chapter 373). More than 150 types of HPV have been identified. Certain types of HPV occur at particular anatomic sites; however, warts of any HPV type may be found at any site. Variants include common warts, genital warts, flat warts, and deep palmoplantar warts. Common warts, known as verruca vulgaris, are hard papules that range in size from 1 mm to more than 1 cm with a rough scaly surface (Fig. 439-2) and can occur anywhere on the body. Warts are transmitted by direct contact, and disruption of the epithelial barrier is a predisposing factor. HPV subtypes 6, 11, 16, 18, 31, and 35 may be associated with malignancies (Chapter 373). Malignant transformation, although uncommon, can occur in patients with genital warts or in immunocompromised patients. Infection is confined to the epithelium and does not result in systemic viral dissemination. The diagnosis is made on clinical grounds. Viral DNA identification by Southern blot hybridization is used to identify specific HPV subtypes. All therapies are methods of physical destruction of the skin where the virus is located because there are no specific anti-HPV medications. Common topical therapies include in-office treatment with liquid nitrogen, cantharidin, or podophyllin, as well as prescription-strength tretinoin or imiquimod. Over-the-counter liquid nitrogen is neither as cold nor as effective as in-office treatment.

TABLE 439-2	PURPURIC ERUPTIONS

NONPALPABLE PURPURA

Cutaneous Disorders

Solar purpura
Steroid purpura
Pigmented purpuric dermatosis

Systemic Disorders

Idiopathic thrombocytopenic purpura
Abnormal platelet function in renal or hepatic disease
Thrombocytosis in myeloproliferative neoplasms
Clotting factor abnormalities
Ehlers-Danlos syndrome
Scurvy
Amyloidosis
Disseminated intravascular coagulation
Thrombotic thrombocytopenic purpura
Monoclonal cryoglobulinemia
Warfarin necrosis
Emboli
    Cholesterol emboli
    Fat emboli
    Tumor emboli from atrial myxomas
    Emboli from endocarditis

PALPABLE PURPURA

Vasculitis

Leukocytoclastic vasculitis
Henoch-Schönlein purpura
Urticarial vasculitis
Polyarteritis nodosa

Infectious Emboli

Meningococcemia
Gonococcemia
Rocky Mountain spotted fever
Ecthyma gangrenosum

Purpuric Eruptions
Purpura occurs when red blood cell extravasation leads to visible hemorrhage in the skin (Table 439-2). Petechiae (<3 mm) and purpura (>3 mm) may be nonpalpable or palpable. When the condition is severe, petechiae and purpuric lesions may become confluent and form ecchymoses larger than 1 cm.

NONPALPABLE PURPURA
Dermal Causes
Frequent causes of nonpalpable purpura (Fig. 436-11 in Chapter 436) include solar purpura, steroid purpura, and Schamberg disease. Solar purpura, caused by chronic sun exposure and aging, is usually found on the forearms. Steroid purpura, which is caused by prolonged use of topical or systemic steroids, can occur in any location (Chapter 35). Both conditions are caused by changes in the dermal connective tissue surrounding blood vessels. Schamberg disease, or pigmented purpuric dermatosis, is a capillaritis with yellow-brown macules and petechiae on the lower part of the legs. This capillaritis occurs as a result of red blood cell extravasation secondary to perivascular lymphocyte inflammation.

Systemic Causes

Systemic causes of nonpalpable purpura include idiopathic thrombocytopenic purpura (Chapter 172), abnormal platelet function as a result of renal or hepatic insufficiency (Chapters 130 and 153) or thrombocytosis as seen in myeloproliferative diseases (Chapter 166), and clotting factor abnormalities (Chapter 174). Fragility of the blood vessels, especially the capillaries, is found in Ehlers-Danlos syndrome (Chapter 260), scurvy (Chapter 213), and systemic amyloidosis (Chapter 188).

Thrombi

Thrombus formation within skin blood vessels also leads to purpura in patients with disseminated intravascular coagulation (DIC) (Chapter 175), thrombotic thrombocytopenic purpura (Chapter 172), monoclonal cryoglobulinemia (Chapter 187), and drug reactions to warfarin (Chapter 38). DIC may be caused by infectious agents (bacterial, particularly meningococcemia, viral, or rickettsial) and by malignancies such as leukemia (Chapter 175). Purpura fulminans is a type of DIC associated with fever and hypotension; it is usually found in children after a bacterial or viral infection. Widespread purpura and hemorrhagic bullae can be seen in DIC and purpura fulminans (Fig. 439-3). Thrombotic thrombocytopenic purpura (Chapter 172) is manifested as fever, purpura, renal failure, microangiopathic hemolytic anemia, and neurologic disease. Monoclonal cryoglobulinemia may be associated with leukemia, lymphoma, multiple myeloma, and Waldenström macroglobulinemia. Mixed cryoglobulinemia is frequently associated with hepatitis C infection (Chapter 149). Widespread purpura, along with ulcerations limited to the lower extremities or fingers and toes, can occur. Skin biopsy specimens may reveal intracapillary deposits of precipitated cryoglobulins. Disease can be worsened by exposure to cold. The vessels of the lungs, brain, and kidneys may be involved. Warfarin necrosis of the skin (Chapter 38) is an uncommon reaction that occurs between the third and tenth day of therapy and is characterized by painful erythematous to purpuric plaques in which hemorrhagic bullae develop. The most common sites include the breasts, thighs, and buttocks. The onset of disease is unrelated to the dose of warfarin, and continued warfarin therapy does not alter the course of the disease.

Emboli

Cholesterol emboli are found in the lower extremities of patients with severe atherosclerosis as a result of occlusion of small- and medium-caliber arteries by cholesterol crystals (Chapters 80 and 125). Cholesterol emboli are triggered by vascular procedures or thrombolytic therapy, but they can also occur spontaneously. Other sources of emboli that may cause petechiae or purpura include fat emboli occurring after major injury (Chapters 98 and 111), tumor emboli from atrial myxomas (Chapter 60), emboli from infective endocarditis (Chapter 76), or nonbacterial thrombotic endocarditis (Chapters 60 and 179).

PALPABLE PURPURA

Vasculitis

Palpable purpura results from inflammatory damage to cutaneous blood vessels.[2] Leukocytoclastic vasculitis, which is manifested as palpable purpura (Fig. 439-4), may be idiopathic or associated with sepsis, drug reactions, connective tissue diseases, cryoglobulinemia, hepatitis B or C infection, or underlying malignancies. Evaluation of patients with palpable purpura should always include histopathologic evaluation to confirm the diagnosis. Skin biopsy specimens from patients with leukocytoclastic vasculitis reveal angiocentric inflammation with endothelial cell swelling, fibrinoid necrosis of blood vessel walls, a neutrophilic cellular infiltrate with fragmentation of nuclei (karyorrhexis or leukocytoclasia) around and within blood vessel walls, and extravasated red blood cells (Fig. 439-5). Fresh skin biopsy specimens processed for direct immunofluorescence reveal deposits of immunoglobulins and complement in blood vessel walls. After the diagnosis is confirmed, renal and liver function testing and urinalysis should be performed in all patients, but specialized tests should be targeted to specific patients with suggestive findings. If an etiologic agent can be identified and treated, the vasculitis will often resolve. Patients with idiopathic leukocytoclastic vasculitis can be treated with oral colchicine (0.6 mg twice daily); oral dapsone (up to 200 mg once daily); or in the most severe cases, immunosuppressive agents such as mycophenolate mofetil (up to 45 mg/kg for as long as the disease is active), azathioprine (up to 2.5 mg/kg for as long as the disease is active, as guided by the thiopurine methyltransferase level), or cyclophosphamide (up to 2.5 mg/kg for as long as the disease is active).

Henoch-Schönlein purpura is an IgA mediated leukocytoclastic vasculitis that affects children and young adults; it is often preceded by an upper respiratory infection with associated fever, arthralgias, abdominal pain, and renal vasculitis (Chapter 121).

Urticarial or hypocomplementemic vasculitis (Chapter 270) is characterized by urticarial lesions that last longer than 24 hours; arthritis, facial, and laryngeal edema; and low serum complement levels. In some patients, systemic lupus erythematosus (Chapter 266) may develop. In polyarteritis nodosa (Chapter 270), vasculitis of the arterial blood vessels leads to ischemia of the skin. Skin lesions usually include ulcerated nodules and ecchymoses.

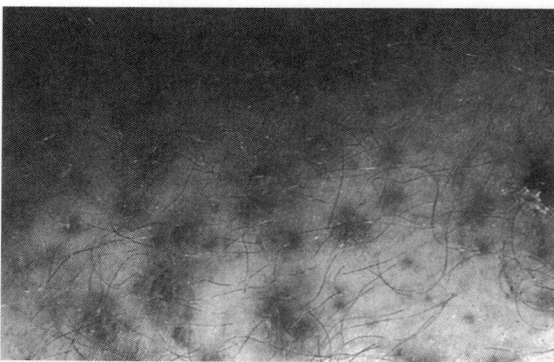

FIGURE 439-4. Palpable purpura. Leukocytoclastic vasculitis commonly causes raised purpuric and ulcerated lesions on the legs.

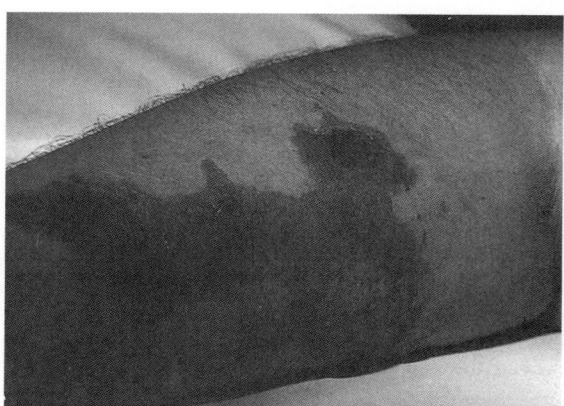

FIGURE 439-3. Purpura fulminans. Purpura and hemorrhagic blisters are seen on the arm of this patient.

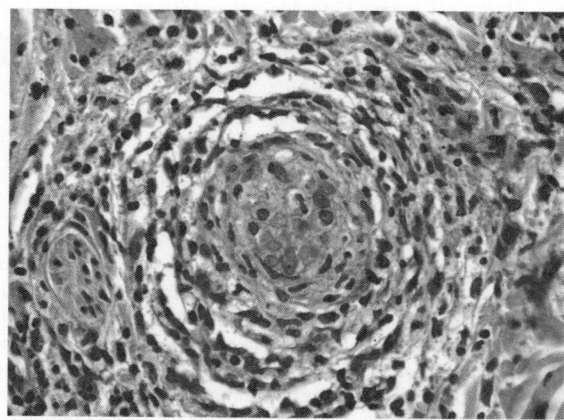

FIGURE 439-5. Leukocytoclastic vasculitis. Histologic evaluation reveals a smudged blood vessel in the dermis with neutrophils, neutrophilic dust, and red blood cells.

Cutaneous Emboli

In addition to vasculitis, cutaneous emboli can also lead to the development of palpable purpura. Infectious emboli (Chapter 76) can be caused by gram-negative cocci, gram-negative rods, *Rickettsia* spp., and in immunocompromised patients, *Candida* spp. and opportunistic fungi. Acute meningococcemia (Chapter 298) occurs after an upper respiratory tract infection and is associated with headache, fever, meningitis, hypotension, and DIC. The embolic lesions, which are found on the trunk and lower extremities, can range from 1 mm up to several centimeters. Disseminated gonococcal infection (Chapter 299) is accompanied by fever, arthralgias, tenosynovitis, and a small number of vesiculopustules with purpura or hemorrhagic necrosis over the distal ends of the extremities. Rocky Mountain spotted fever (Chapter 327) is a tick-borne disease characterized by headache, fever, chills, photophobia, and myalgias. The cutaneous eruption starts acrally and spreads centripetally as small, erythematous, blanchable macules that evolve into petechiae, palpable purpura, and ecchymoses. Ecthyma gangrenosum is manifested as erythematous papules and plaques in which central purpura and hemorrhagic necrosis develop; *Pseudomonas aeruginosa* (Chapter 306) is the most common organism, but *Klebsiella* spp. (Chapter 305), *Escherichia coli* (Chapter 304), and *Serratia* spp. (Chapter 305) have also been implicated. In immunocompromised patients, ecthyma gangrenosum may develop as a result of infection with *Candida* spp. or opportunistic fungi.

● VESICULOBULLOUS DISEASES

Vesicles are clear, fluid-filled lesions measuring smaller than 5 mm; bullae or blisters are clear, fluid-filled lesions larger than 5 mm. Vesiculobullous lesions in the skin may be caused by immunologically mediated mechanisms, hypersensitivity reactions, metabolic disorders, inherited genetic defects, and infections (Table 439-3).

Immunologically Mediated Blistering Diseases
BULLOUS PEMPHIGOID

DEFINITION

Bullous pemphigoid is an autoimmune blistering disease that occurs in elderly adults.[3] Tense blisters and urticarial plaques occur on the flexor surfaces of the arms and legs, axilla, groin, and abdomen (Fig. 439-6). The incidence is 162 cases per million per year.

TABLE 439-3 VESICULOBULLOUS DISEASES

IMMUNOLOGICALLY MEDIATED DISEASES

Bullous pemphigoid
Herpes gestationis
Mucous membrane pemphigoid
Epidermolysis bullosa acquisita
Dermatitis herpetiformis
Linear immunoglobulin A bullous dermatosis
Pemphigus
    Vulgaris
    Foliaceus
    Paraneoplastic

HYPERSENSITIVITY DISEASES

Erythema multiforme minor
Erythema multiforme major (Stevens-Johnson syndrome)
Toxic epidermal necrolysis

METABOLIC DISEASES

Porphyria cutanea tarda
Pseudoporphyria
Diabetic blisters

INHERITED GENETIC DISORDERS

Epidermolysis bullosa
    Simplex
    Junctional
    Dystrophic

INFECTIOUS DISEASES

Impetigo
Staphylococcal scalded skin syndrome
Herpes simplex
Varicella
Herpes zoster

PATHOBIOLOGY AND DIAGNOSIS

IgG autoantibodies bind to the epidermal basement membrane and activate complement, which attracts inflammatory cells. These inflammatory cells release proteases that degrade basement membrane proteins and lead to blister formation. Histology reveals a subepidermal blister with an eosinophilic infiltrate. Direct immunofluorescence shows linear deposits of IgG and C3 at the basement membrane. Indirect immunofluorescence studies using salt-split skin demonstrate circulating IgG antibodies that bind to the epidermal side.[4]

TREATMENT   Rx

Treatment is dictated by the degree of involvement and the rate of progression of the disease. The ultrapotent topical steroid clobetasol (10-30 g/day), applied to the skin of patients with bullous pemphigoid until 15 days after disease control is obtained and then tapered over 4 months, is effective, superior to oral corticosteroid treatment, and is associated with fewer side effects than higher dose clobetasol in patients with both moderate and severe disease.[A3] Nevertheless, the practicality of such potent topical steroids is controversial, and many experts use oral prednisone, 1 mg/kg in an early morning daily dose, as a foundation of therapy for patients with generalized disease. Other treatments include dapsone (up to 200 mg/day), azathioprine (up to 2.5 mg/kg as guided by the thiopurine methyltransferase level), methotrexate (up to 15 mg weekly), mycophenolate mofetil (35-45 mg/kg divided into two daily doses), and cyclophosphamide (up to about 2.5 mg/kg). The duration of therapy with these medications varies, depending on the activity of the disease. Left untreated, bullous pemphigoid generally persists for months to years. Spontaneous remissions and exacerbations occur. The 1-year mortality rate is about six times worse than for the general population.

Herpes Gestationis

Herpes gestationis is a rare autoimmune dermatosis of pregnancy. Despite the name, herpes gestationis has no relationship to herpesvirus infection. Most patients have intense pruritus. Periumbilical urticarial plaques progress to vesicles and blisters. The eruption spreads peripherally (Fig. 439-7), typically sparing the face, palms, soles, and mucous membranes. IgG autoantibodies are produced against bullous pemphigoid antigen II, which is critical in epidermal-dermal adhesion. Antibody binding triggers an immune response leading to blister formation. Histology reveals a subepidermal blister, and direct immunofluorescence shows linear C3 deposits at the basement membrane.

Corticosteroids are the mainstay of therapy. Patients with mild disease are treated with moderate- to high-potency topical corticosteroids, such as 0.05% fluocinonide ointment applied twice daily to affected areas, but patients with extensive disease require systemic corticosteroids, such as prednisone, 1 mg/kg given once daily as an early morning dose. Disease clears within 1 to 2 weeks after initiation of treatment. There is an increased risk for premature delivery and birth of infants who are small for gestational age, suggesting that these women should be managed by obstetricians experienced in high-risk pregnancies.

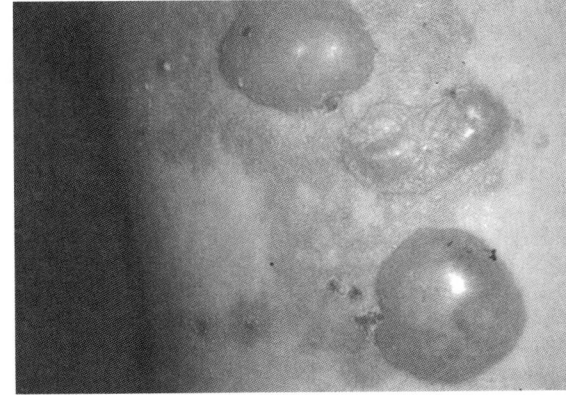

FIGURE 439-6. Bullous pemphigoid. Tense subepidermal bullae are seen on an erythematous base.

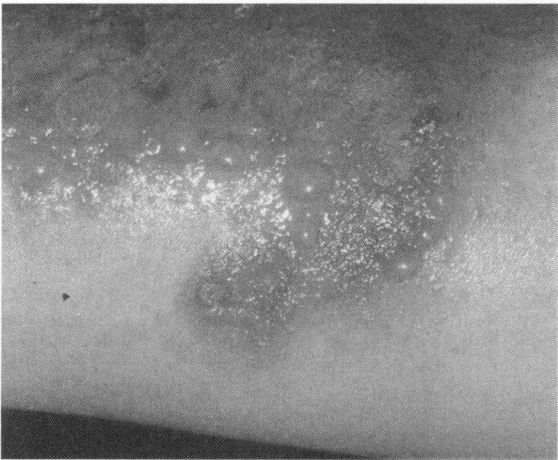

FIGURE 439-7. Herpes gestationis. Multiple tense blisters and erosions on an erythematous base are present.

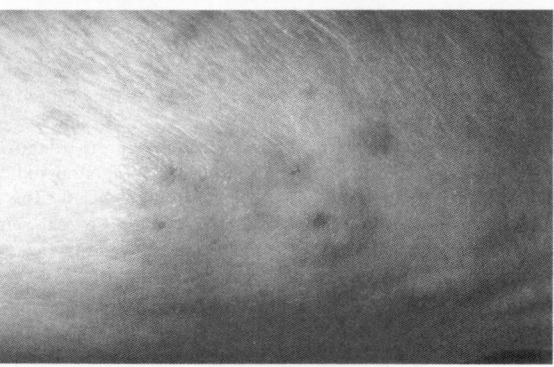

FIGURE 439-8. Dermatitis herpetiformis. The elbow of a patient has eroded erythematous papules and papulovesicles.

Mucous Membrane Pemphigoid

DEFINITION
Mucous membrane pemphigoid, previously called cicatricial pemphigoid, is a group of subepithelial blistering diseases that involve the mucosal surfaces. Patients have blisters of the oral, ocular, nasopharyngeal, laryngeal, anogenital, and esophageal mucosa that heal with scarring, which causes the major morbidity associated with the disease.

PATHOBIOLOGY
There are several subgroups of mucous membrane pemphigoid. Some patients have circulating IgG autoantibodies that bind to the dermal side of salt-split skin and recognize laminin 332. A second subgroup includes patients who have pure ocular disease and IgG antibodies directed against β_4 integrin. A third subgroup has mucosal disease and skin lesions. The fourth variant includes patients with oral disease but without skin disease. Histology reveals a subepidermal blister with an inflammatory cell infiltrate. Direct immunofluorescence shows linear IgG, IgA, and C3 deposits at the basement membrane. Indirect immunofluorescence reveals circulating IgG or IgA antibodies, or both.

TREATMENT   Rx
Treatment is dictated by the extent, severity, and location of disease; it ranges from topical corticosteroids, such as 0.05% fluocinonide ointment applied twice daily to affected areas under occlusion in patients with only oral disease; to prednisone, 1 mg/kg given once daily as an early morning dose; and cyclophosphamide, up to 2.5 mg/kg given as an early morning dose for up to 2 years, for severe ocular disease. Management teams should include ophthalmologists, otolaryngologists, dermatologists, and internists for patients with severe disease. Patients with both circulating IgG and IgA antibodies tend to have more severe disease.

PROGNOSIS
Mucous membrane pemphigoid is a chronic disease. Untreated ocular disease can result in blindness.

EPIDERMOLYSIS BULLOSA ACQUISITA
Epidermolysis bullosa acquisita is an acquired autoimmune blistering disease that generally occurs in middle age.[5] There are two types of skin lesions, noninflammatory acral blisters that heal with scarring and milia formation and widespread inflammatory vesiculobullous disease.

PATHOBIOLOGY
Epidermolysis bullosa acquisita is characterized by IgG autoantibodies that target collagen VII, the major protein of anchoring fibrils. These autoantibod-

ies alter dermal-epidermal adhesion and lead to blister formation. Histology reveals a subepidermal blister containing few inflammatory cells when mechanobullous lesions are sampled or a neutrophil-rich infiltrate when inflammatory blisters are sampled. Direct immunofluorescence reveals linear IgG deposits at the basement membrane. Indirect immunofluorescence shows circulating IgG autoantibodies that bind the dermal side of salt-split skin.

TREATMENT   Rx
Epidermolysis bullosa acquisita is a chronic disease that is very difficult to treat. Dapsone (at doses up to 200 mg/day), colchicine (0.6 mg twice daily), azathioprine (up to 2.5 mg/kg as guided by the thiopurine methyltransferase level), or cyclophosphamide (2.5 mg/kg given as an early morning dosage) alone or along with prednisone (60 mg given once daily as an early morning dose) is only occasionally successful. Cyclosporine at doses of up to 5 mg/kg, extracorporeal photopheresis, and IV immunoglobulin (at doses of 2 gm/kg given monthly) have been used successfully in patients with severe disease. Because of nephrotoxicity, cyclosporine should be reserved for crisis management of patients who have severe disease and are experiencing a major flare.

DERMATITIS HERPETIFORMIS
Dermatitis herpetiformis is an immune-mediated vesicular disease that occurs in young to middle-aged patients.[6] Skin lesions are extremely pruritic; grouped vesicles and erosions located on the scalp; posterior of the neck; and extensor surfaces of the elbows, knees, and buttocks (Fig. 439-8). Most patients have a subclinical gluten-sensitive enteropathy (Chapter 140) that is reversible with a gluten-free diet. Diet alone can sometimes control the skin disease, with clearance of the cutaneous granular IgA deposits at the basement membrane. Biopsy specimens of skin lesions reveal dermal papillary neutrophilic microabscesses. Direct immunofluorescence shows dermal papillary granular IgA deposits. Most patients with dermatitis herpetiformis have circulating IgA antibodies directed against tissue transglutaminase. Dermatitis herpetiformis can be treated with dapsone, up to 200 mg/day given chronically. Dermatitis herpetiformis is a lifelong disease.

LINEAR IMMUNOGLOBULIN A BULLOUS DERMATOSIS
Linear IgA bullous dermatosis is an acquired autoimmune blistering disease. Primary lesions are papulovesicles, and involvement of the oral mucous membranes is common. The disease occurs throughout adulthood. Deposition of IgA antibody specific for a portion of bullous pemphigoid antigen II leads to complement activation and neutrophil chemotaxis. Proteolytic enzymes are released, destroy the dermal-epidermal junction, and cause blister formation. Histology reveals a subepidermal vesicle with neutrophil predominance. Direct immunofluorescence shows linear deposits of IgA at the basement membrane. Indirect immunofluorescence demonstrates circulating IgA antibodies. Most patients respond to dapsone, up to 200 mg/day, given chronically. Patients whose disease is not controlled with dapsone may benefit from the addition of oral prednisone, 1 mg/kg once daily as an early morning dose. The disease tends to be chronic in adults, but the childhood version (called chronic bullous disease of childhood) may run a several-year course and then remit.

PEMPHIGUS

DEFINITION

Pemphigus refers to a group of autoimmune blistering intraepidermal diseases of the skin and mucous membranes that are most common in middle age.[7]

PATHOBIOLOGY

Autoantibodies in pemphigus vulgaris target desmoglein III, and autoantibodies in pemphigus foliaceus target desmoglein I. Circulating antibodies in paraneoplastic pemphigus recognize a complex of proteins, including desmoplakin I and II, bullous pemphigoid antigen I, envoplakin, periplakin, and desmoglein I and III.

CLINICAL MANIFESTATIONS

Patients with pemphigus vulgaris have flaccid blisters and erosions in the oropharynx (Fig. 439-9), trunk, head, neck, and intertriginous areas. Pemphigus foliaceus is accompanied by erythema, scaling, and crusting of the face, scalp, and upper part of the trunk. Patients with paraneoplastic pemphigus have ocular and oral blisters and erosions along with skin lesions resembling erythema multiforme and an associated underlying malignancy that is generally lymphoreticular in origin (Chapter 179).

DIAGNOSIS

Skin biopsy specimens from patients with pemphigus vulgaris reveal suprabasilar acantholysis, but pemphigus foliaceus biopsy specimens demonstrate subcorneal acantholysis. Biopsy specimens of paraneoplastic pemphigus show suprabasilar acantholysis and dyskeratotic keratinocytes with basal cell vacuolization.

Whereas direct immunofluorescence demonstrates cell surface deposits of IgG in patients with pemphigus vulgaris and foliaceus, indirect immunofluorescence reveals circulating IgG antibodies that recognize molecules on the epidermal cell surface. Patients with paraneoplastic pemphigus have circulating and tissue-bound IgG antibodies that are indistinguishable from those in pemphigus vulgaris and that also recognize the cell surface of simple epithelia, including the liver and heart.

TREATMENT   Rx

Treatment regimens depend on the patient's age, the degree of involvement, the rate of disease progression, and the subtype of pemphigus.[8] Whereas systemic corticosteroids (e.g., oral prednisone, 1 mg/kg once daily as an early morning dose) are required for the treatment of patients with pemphigus vulgaris, topical corticosteroids (e.g., 0.05% fluocinonide ointment applied twice daily to affected areas) may occasionally control pemphigus foliaceus. One course of IV immunoglobulin (400 mg/kg/day for 5 days) appears to be a safe and effective treatment for patients whose disease is resistant to steroids.[A4] Other agents include dapsone (up to 200 mg/day), hydroxychloroquine (administered at less than 6 mg/kg of lean body mass divided into two daily doses), mycophenolate mofetil (35-45 mg/kg/day divided into two daily doses), azathioprine (up to 2.5 mg/kg as guided by the thiopurine methyltransferase level), cyclophosphamide (up to 2.5 mg/kg given as an early morning dose), and rituximab (four weekly doses of 375 mg/m²). The duration of therapy with each of these medications varies according to the level of disease activity. Although the use of steroid-sparing agents is supported by clinical experience, few controlled studies have demonstrated their benefit. For paraneoplastic pemphigus caused by benign tumors such as Castleman disease (Chapter 185), tumor removal is often curative. Patients with associated malignant tumors have recalcitrant disease, although there are occasional successes with pulse corticosteroids (methylprednisolone, 1000 mg given daily for 3 consecutive days), pulse cyclophosphamide (500-1000 mg given monthly for 6 months to 1 year, often along with varying doses of prednisone), immunoapheresis, immunoablative high-dose cyclophosphamide (50 mg/kg/day for 4 days), and rituximab (four weekly doses of 375 mg/m²).

PROGNOSIS

Before the availability of corticosteroids, 60% to 90% of patients with pemphigus vulgaris died; the mortality rate has now decreased to the 5% to 10% range. Overall, however, the mortality rate is about twice that of the general population. The prognosis of patients with paraneoplastic pemphigus is related to the type of associated neoplasm. Patients with benign tumors usually experience clearance of their lesions after tumor resection, but those with malignant tumors generally have a poor prognosis.

Hypersensitivity Reactions That Cause Blisters
ERYTHEMA MULTIFORME

DEFINITION

Erythema multiforme is an acute blistering eruption that occurs in all age groups.[9] Erythema multiforme minor is localized, with minimal or no mucosal involvement. Erythema multiforme major, also known as Stevens-Johnson syndrome, is a more severe mucosal and skin disease characterized by signs and symptoms reminiscent of serum sickness (Chapter 47).

CLINICAL MANIFESTATIONS

Toxic epidermal necrolysis is at the most severe end of the erythema multiforme spectrum. The primary lesions of erythema multiforme minor are erythematous macules and edematous papules with vesicular centers that become dusky violet. Target lesions are found on extensor surfaces of the extremities and spread centripetally (Fig. 439-10). The skin lesions of Stevens-Johnson syndrome resemble those of erythema multiforme minor but are likely to be generalized and show confluent erythema with urticarial and purpuric lesions. Erosions of two or more mucosal surfaces occur in Stevens-Johnson syndrome and may include hemorrhagic crusting of the lips, ulceration of the ocular mucosa, and genital involvement. Patients with erythema multiforme major have a 1- to 14-day prodrome that includes fever, cough, sore throat, vomiting, and diarrhea. Patients with toxic epidermal necrolysis may have a similar prodrome, rapidly followed by generalized macular erythema that progresses to confluent erythema with skin tenderness. Large blisters follow soon afterward, and then skin sloughing occurs as the large blisters break and leave denuded skin.

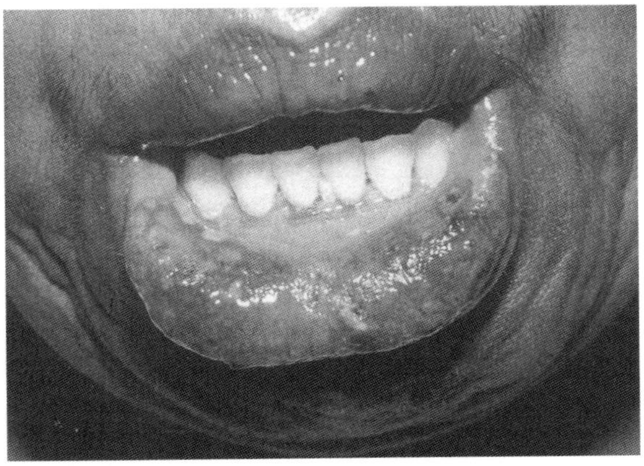

FIGURE 439-9. Pemphigus vulgaris. The lower lip of a patient has confluent erosions with scattered crusting.

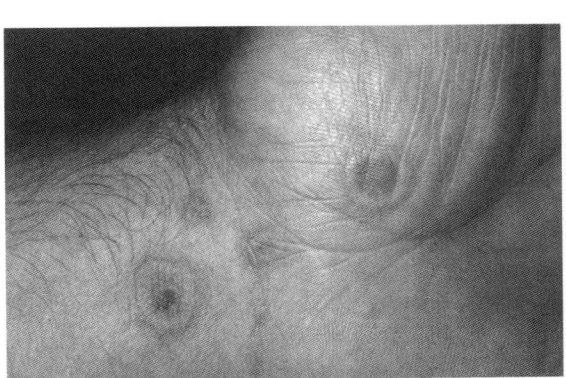

FIGURE 439-10. Erythema multiforme. Target or "bull's-eye" annular lesions with central vesicles and bullae are characteristic of erythema multiforme.

PATHOBIOLOGY

Common etiologic associations of erythema multiforme include infections such as herpes simplex (Chapter 374) (especially recurrent erythema multiforme minor), *Mycoplasma pneumoniae* (Chapter 317), and drug reactions (Chapter 254). Sulfonamides, penicillins, barbiturates, carbamazepine, phenytoin, allopurinol, and nonsteroidal anti-inflammatory drugs (NSAIDs) are the most common drugs implicated in Stevens-Johnson syndrome and toxic epidermal necrolysis.

DIAGNOSIS

The diagnosis of erythema multiforme is clinical.

TREATMENT   Rx

Chronic antiviral treatment with acyclovir (400 mg twice daily for 6 months) decreases outbreaks in a subset of patients with recurrent erythema multiforme minor. Treatment of erythema multiforme major is otherwise nonspecific, with attention to fluid and electrolyte balance and eye disease being critical. If a drug is suspected, it must be withdrawn. Systemic corticosteroid treatment is contraindicated in Stevens-Johnson syndrome. Treatment of toxic epidermal necrolysis is very difficult, but uncontrolled studies suggest that IV immune globulin (2-3 g/kg over a period of 2-5 days) may improve the prognosis.

PROGNOSIS

Erythema multiforme minor usually subsides within 2 to 3 weeks. Erythema multiforme major takes 3 to 6 weeks to clear and has less than a 5% mortality rate. Toxic epidermal necrolysis has a mortality rate approaching 30%, and patients are best managed in an intensive care or burn unit.

Metabolic Disorders That Cause Blisters
PORPHYRIA CUTANEA TARDA

Porphyria cutanea tarda is caused by deficient activity of the heme synthetic enzyme uroporphyrinogen decarboxylase (Chapter 210).[10] The fragility of sun-exposed skin leads to erosions and bullae, which are worst on the dorsal surface of the hands (Fig. 439-11), forearms, and face. Healing of crusted erosions and blisters leaves scars, milia, and hyperpigmented and hypopigmented atrophic patches. Hypertrichosis is common and most florid over the temporal and malar areas. Urinary porphyrin levels are abnormally high. Histology reveals a subepidermal blister with minimal dermal infiltrate, and direct immunofluorescence demonstrates immunoglobulin and complement deposition in dermal capillaries and at the basement membrane. Phlebotomy is the standard treatment, and the goal is to reduce serum ferritin to the lower limit of the normal range. Another treatment option is oral hydroxychloroquine at a dose (200 mg twice weekly until the disease is under control) that is much lower than that used for photoprotective indications. Alcohol and estrogen use should be discontinued because they can cause the disease to flare.

PSEUDOPORPHYRIA

Pseudoporphyria is a bullous eruption that mimics porphyria cutanea tarda clinically and histologically without porphyrin abnormalities. Many medications can cause pseudoporphyria, including propionic acid–derivative NSAIDs (e.g., naproxen, diflunisal, ketoprofen, nabumetone, oxaprozin, and mefenamic acid), furosemide, tetracycline, fluoroquinolones, amiodarone, cyclosporine, dapsone, etretinate, and flutamide. The prognosis is good for patients with pseudoporphyria after the offending agent has been discontinued. However, resolution of the disease may take several months. In patients with chronic renal failure treated by hemodialysis, true porphyria cutanea tarda or pseudoporphyria may develop and is very difficult to treat.

DIABETES MELLITUS

Distal extremity blisters may occasionally develop in patients with diabetes mellitus (Chapter 229). There is no correlation between the development of blisters and the severity, duration, or complications of diabetes. The mechanism of blister formation is not understood.

Inherited Genetic Disorders That Cause Blisters

Epidermolysis bullosa is a group of inherited bullous disorders characterized by blister formation in response to mechanical trauma. Subtypes include epidermolysis bullosa simplex (intraepidermal skin separation) (Fig. 439-12), junctional epidermolysis bullosa (skin separation in the lamina lucida), and dystrophic epidermolysis bullosa (sublamina densa separation). Infancy is an especially difficult time, and epidermolysis bullosa may be accompanied by blistering that is complicated by infection and sepsis. Many patients with junctional epidermolysis bullosa have severe disease that can lead to death, usually secondary to infection, and metastatic squamous cell carcinoma may develop in some patients with recessive dystrophic epidermolysis bullosa and can also lead to death. In contrast, epidermolysis bullosa simplex, milder forms of junctional epidermolysis bullosa, and dominant dystrophic epidermolysis bullosa do not usually affect life expectancy. Epidermolysis bullosa simplex is caused by mutations of the genes coding for keratins 5 and 14. Junctional epidermolysis bullosa has a variable molecular etiology, and mutations in genes coding for laminin 5 subunits, bullous pemphigoid antigen I, α_6 integrin, and β_4 integrin have been demonstrated. Dystrophic epidermolysis bullosa is caused by mutations of the type VII collagen gene. Epidermolysis bullosa is a lifelong disease. Some subtypes, especially the milder forms, improve with age. No medications are known to correct the underlying molecular defects, but gene therapy is being actively pursued.

Infectious Diseases That Cause Blisters
IMPETIGO

Impetigo is a bacterial infection of the superficial layers of the epidermis. Bullous impetigo is caused by *S. aureus* (Chapter 288), and nonbullous impetigo is caused by group A β-hemolytic streptococci (Chapter 290). Bullous impetigo is manifested as vesicles and bulla (Fig. 439-13). Lesions are common on the face but may appear anywhere. Nonbullous impetigo is characterized by fragile vesicles or pustules that rupture and leave honey-colored crusted papules or plaques, especially near the nose and mouth and on the extremities. Lesions develop on normal or traumatized skin or are superimposed on preexisting conditions, including scabies, varicella, or atopic dermatitis. The causative agent of bullous impetigo is coagulase-positive *S. aureus*,

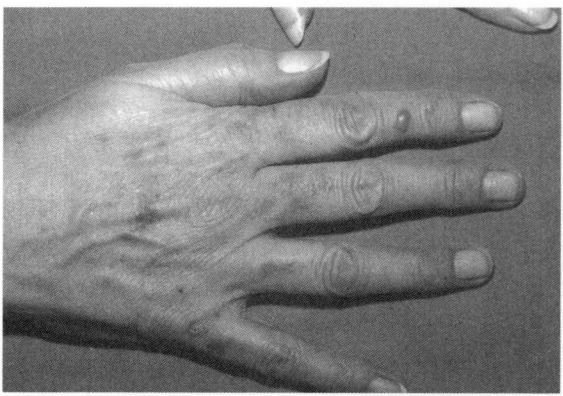

FIGURE 439-11. Porphyria cutanea tarda. A blister and erosions are present on the dorsal surface of the hand.

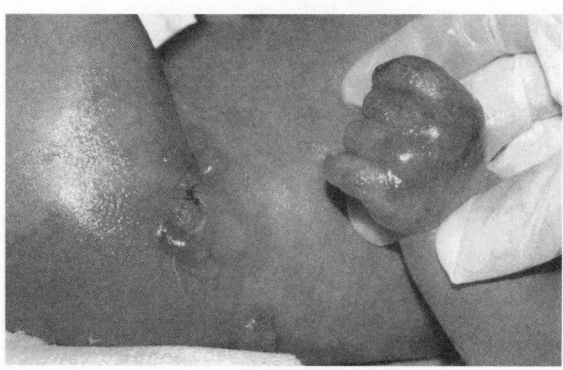

FIGURE 439-12. Epidermolysis bullosa simplex. Tense blisters and erosions are present on the trunk and extremities of a newborn.

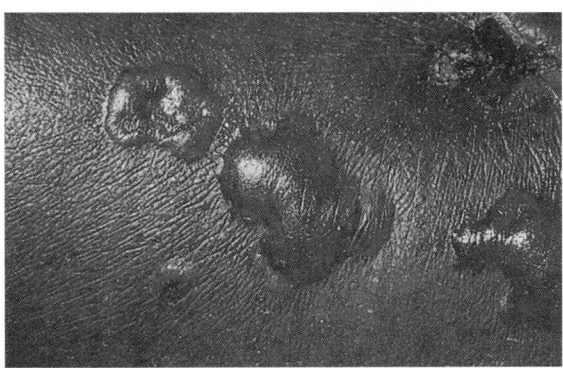

FIGURE 439-13. Bullous impetigo. Multiple blisters are present on the trunk of this patient.

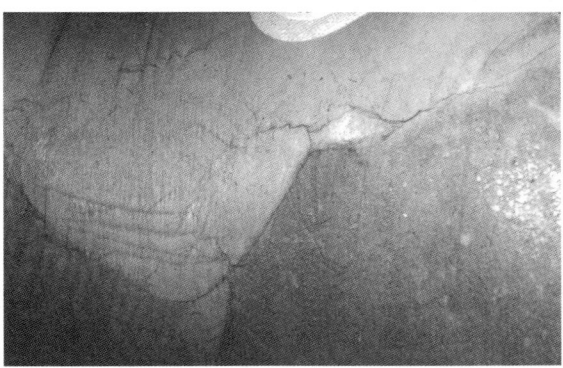

FIGURE 439-14. Staphylococcal scalded skin syndrome. Confluent erythema with exfoliation of skin is seen on the trunk.

which produces exfoliatins A and B. The toxins cause cleavage within or below the stratum granulosum. Impetigo is diagnosed clinically. Culture and sensitivity studies are recommended if topical or oral treatment is ineffective. Oral antibiotics, including dicloxacillin (500 mg four times daily for 7 days) or cephalexin (500 mg three times daily for 7 days), are used for extensive disease or in patients refractory to topical mupirocin. Gentle débridement of crusts is recommended. Lesions resolve after 7 to 10 days of treatment. Acute glomerulonephritis (Chapter 121) develops in 2% to 5% of young children with nonbullous impetigo, usually within 10 days after the skin lesions appear.

STAPHYLOCOCCAL SCALDED SKIN SYNDROME

Staphylococcal scalded skin syndrome is a blistering disease caused by an exotoxin produced by *S. aureus* (Chapter 288). It is most common in young children but may occur in adults who have renal insufficiency or are immunocompromised. The site of the staphylococcal infection is usually extracutaneous. Staphylococcal scalded skin syndrome is manifested as a sudden onset of fever and tender, blanchable erythema. It starts on the central part of the face, neck, and intertriginous areas and rapidly generalizes. The palms, soles, and mucous membranes are spared. Flaccid blisters occur within 1 to 2 days and soon exfoliate in large sheets, with superficially denuded skin remaining (Fig. 439-14). The disease must be distinguished from toxic epidermal necrolysis by skin biopsy. Whereas in staphylococcal scalded skin syndrome, there is an upper epidermal blister, toxic epidermal necrolysis causes a dermal-epidermal blister. Patients with the most severe staphylococcal scalded skin syndrome should be treated with IV nafcillin or oxacillin, 2 g every 4 to 6 hours for 10 to 14 days. If the patient is found to have methicillin-resistant staphylococci, vancomycin, 1 g every 12 hours (with dose adjustment based on creatinine clearance), should be given for 10 to 14 days. Patients with mild disease may be treated with oral dicloxacillin, 500 mg four times daily for 10 to 14 days, unless the staphylococcal isolate is methicillin resistant, in which case the choice of antibiotics should be guided by the results of sensitivity testing. For severe methicillin-resistant gram-positive skin infections, one dose of intravenous oritavancin (1200 mg)[A5] or two doses of intravenous dalbavancin (1 g on day 1, 500 mg on day 8) is as efficacious as twice daily intravenous vancomycin for up to 7-10 days.[A6]

HERPES SIMPLEX VIRUS INFECTION

PATHOBIOLOGY

Herpes simplex virus (HSV) infection (Chapter 374) may be caused by type 1 or type 2 HSV. The hallmark of HSV infection is its ability to establish latent infection. Disease commonly occurs as a recurrent vesicular eruption of the oral, perioral (typically HSV-1), or genital (typically HSV-2) regions, although primary gingivostomatitis (typically in children and young adults and caused by HSV-1) and primary genital herpes (typically HSV-2) are less common.

CLINICAL MANIFESTATIONS

Patients with primary gingivostomatitis have high fever, regional lymphadenopathy, and malaise. Patients with primary genital herpes have fever, flulike symptoms, tender inguinal adenopathy, and aseptic meningitis. These infections all reveal grouped vesicles on an erythematous base. Recurrent eruptions can be triggered by skin trauma, cold or heat, concurrent infection, and

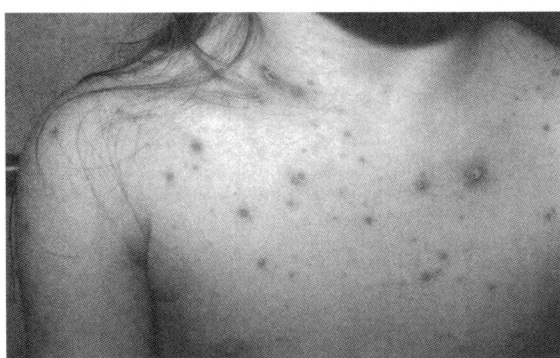

FIGURE 439-15. Erythematous macules and vesicles with crusted erosions on the chest of a patient with varicella.

menstruation. Chronic erosive ulcers of the face and anogenital areas may develop in immunocompromised patients.

DIAGNOSIS

Tzanck smear of fluid from the roof of a vesicle can be helpful in confirming the diagnosis (see Fig. 436-15 in Chapter 436), but viral culture is the diagnostic "gold standard." The direct fluorescent antibody test is an antigen-based technique that not only yields same-day results but can also distinguish HSV from varicella-zoster virus (VZV) and is becoming widely used.

TREATMENT

In healthy individuals, HSV infection is self-limited. The goal of treatment is to shorten the current attack and prevent recurrences. Acyclovir is effective in the treatment of HSV infections; valacyclovir and famciclovir are closely related, effective medications with improved oral bioavailability. The doses and duration of therapy vary depending on whether the infection is limited to the oral or genital mucous membranes or is disseminated and on whether it is primary or recurrent disease (Chapter 374).

CHICKENPOX

Chickenpox is caused by VZV (Chapter 375). It is usually a childhood disease, but affected adults have more morbidity. Skin lesions occur 10 to 21 days after exposure to VZV. Erythematous macules appear on the scalp, face, trunk, and proximal ends of the limbs, with rapid progression to papules, vesicles, pustules, and crusting (Fig. 439-15). Adults may experience a more widespread eruption, prolonged fever, and pneumonia. The diagnosis is usually made clinically, but direct fluorescent antibody or culture confirmation is sometimes needed. Treatment of healthy children is unnecessary because the disease is self-limited. Adults should be treated with oral acyclovir, 800 mg five times a day for 7 days. The varicella vaccine given once to

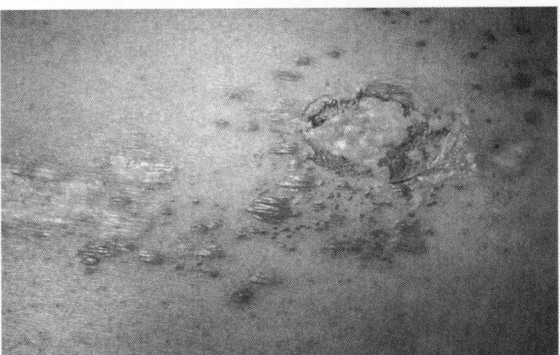

FIGURE 439-16. Herpes zoster. Necrotic blisters and erosions in a dermatomal pattern are seen on the trunk of this patient.

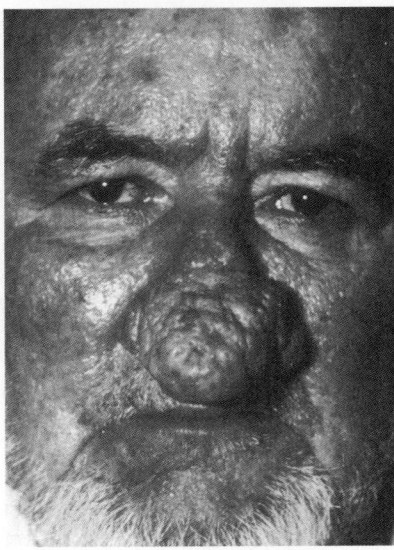

FIGURE 439-17. Sebaceous gland hyperplasia. A large red bulbous nose known as rhinophyma is characteristic of late-stage rosacea.

healthy children 12 to 18 months of age and twice, in a 4- to 8-week interval, to susceptible persons older than 13 years (Chapter 18) is highly effective.

HERPES ZOSTER

PATHOBIOLOGY

Herpes zoster (Chapter 375) is caused by reactivation of VZV from a previous chickenpox infection. The disease is more common in older and immunocompromised patients.

CLINICAL MANIFESTATIONS

The typical manifestation is painful grouped herpetiform vesicles on an erythematous base confined to cutaneous surfaces innervated by one sensory nerve and preceded by radicular pain (Fig. 439-16). The major morbidity, which is pain within the affected dermatome, can be severe and persist after the skin lesions have resolved (postherpetic neuralgia). Immunocompromised patients have an increased risk for cutaneous dissemination and visceral involvement of the bladder, lungs, and CNS.

TREATMENT   Rx

Acyclovir (800 mg orally five times daily for 7 days) and its derivatives valacyclovir (500 mg orally three times daily for 7 days) and famciclovir (500 mg orally three times daily for 7 days) are safe and effective in the treatment of active disease and prevention of postherpetic neuralgia. In an immunocompromised patient, acyclovir should be given intravenously (10 mg/kg every 8 hours for 7-10 days). The earlier antiviral medications are started, the more effective they are in shortening the duration of herpes zoster and in preventing or decreasing the severity of postherpetic neuralgia. Oral steroids are not effective in reducing the incidence of acute pain or postherpetic neuralgia. Patients with postherpetic neuralgia of more than 3 months' duration benefit from the use of gabapentin, 1600 or 2400 mg/day, with a significant reduction in pain. VZV vaccine markedly reduces both the morbidity from herpes zoster and postherpetic neuralgia in healthy adults older than 60 years (Chapter 375).

PUSTULAR ERUPTIONS
Acne Vulgaris
DEFINITION

Acne vulgaris is the most common pustular skin condition. Teenagers are usually affected, but the disease may persist into adulthood. The comedo, which is the primary lesion, can be either closed (whitehead) or open (blackhead).

PATHOBIOLOGY

Androgen production after puberty stimulates the release of sebum by sebaceous glands. Sebum flow is impeded because of abnormal keratinization within the pilosebaceous canal, a process that leads to the formation of comedones. Bacterial (*Propionibacterium acnes*) proliferation within the comedo predisposes to rupture of the pilosebaceous unit with extravasation into the surrounding dermis, which results in papules, pustules, and cysts.

TREATMENT   Rx

Patients with mild disease are treated topically with benzoyl peroxide, tretinoin, adapalene, or tazarotene, which normalize follicular keratinization. In patients with mild to moderate disease, treatment with benzoyl peroxide is the most cost-effective therapy.[A7] The addition of topical antibiotics helps control inflammatory papules and pustules. More significant disease is often treated with oral tetracycline (250-1000 mg/day), doxycycline (200 mg/day), or minocycline (200 mg/day). Dapsone gel (5%) is safe and effective.[A8] Another approach is oral contraceptives containing either ethinyl estradiol and norgestimate or ethinyl estradiol and drospirenone, both of which are superior to placebo in the treatment of acne in women.[A9] Isotretinoin (1 mg/kg given for 5 months), which decreases sebaceous gland size and sebum production, is reserved for severe cystic disease because of its teratogenicity, possible associated risk for depression, and other significant side effects. Acne may be exacerbated by the use of oil-based cosmetics or hair preparations. Androgenic hormones, systemic corticosteroids, lithium, phenytoin, phenobarbital, isoniazid, and endocrinologic conditions such as polycystic ovary disease and adrenal or ovarian tumors may produce acneiform eruptions or aggravate preexisting acne.

ROSACEA

Rosacea, which is a chronic inflammatory disease of the face, affects the pilosebaceous units and blood vessels and generally occurs in middle age. Erythema, telangiectases, erythematous papules, and pustules occur on the central part of the face. Ocular rosacea can lead to keratitis, iritis, blepharitis, and recurrent chalazion; it should be managed by an ophthalmologist. In its most severe form, rosacea can cause sebaceous gland hyperplasia leading to a large red bulbous nose known as rhinophyma (Fig. 439-17). Rosacea is more likely to develop in patients with a tendency toward facial flushing. Flushing[11] can be caused by heat, spicy foods, hot drinks, alcohol, or emotional stimuli. With time, the flushing reaction lasts longer and longer until it persists. Topical antibiotics, including 0.75% to 1% metronidazole, are helpful in mild disease, and the combination of a subantimicrobial dose (20 mg twice daily) of doxycycline plus topical 0.75% metronidazole is more efficacious than topical metronidazole alone.[A10] Patients with more severe disease require oral tetracycline 500 mg twice daily for 3 to 4 months, oral doxycycline 100 mg twice daily, oral minocycline 100 mg twice daily, or low-dose isotretinoin 0.3 mg/kg.[A11] Topical azelaic acid gel (15%) can significantly improve papulopustular rosacea.

PERIORAL DERMATITIS

Perioral dermatitis is characterized by erythematous papules and pustules as well as scaling patches around the mouth and eyes (Fig. 439-18). Most

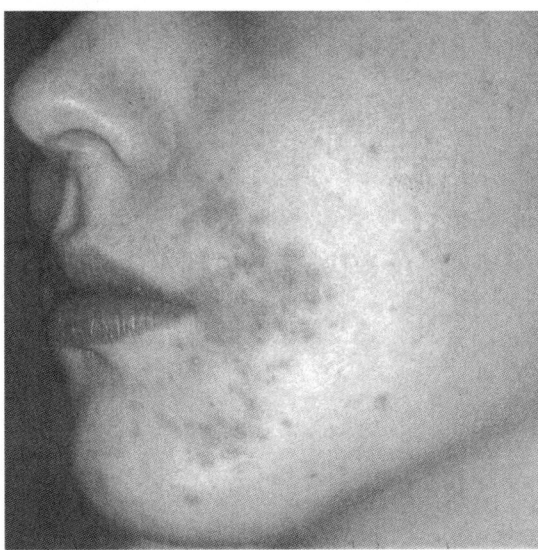

FIGURE 439-18. Perioral dermatitis. Erythematous papules and pinpoint pustules are evident around the mouth.

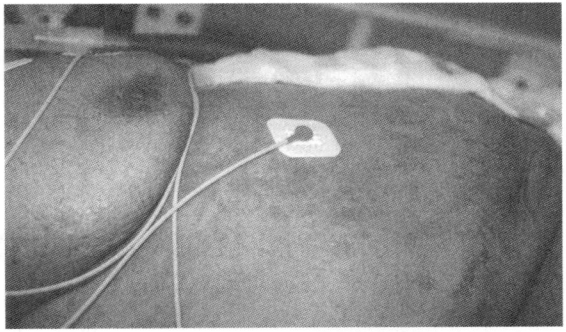

FIGURE 439-19. Acute generalized exanthematous pustulosis. Erythematous macules and numerous superficial pustules are present on the trunk of this patient.

patients have used potent topical corticosteroids inappropriately for long periods. The eruption generally clears after stopping the corticosteroid and using tetracycline, 250 mg orally twice daily for 6 weeks.

ACUTE GENERALIZED EXANTHEMATOUS PUSTULOSIS

Acute exanthematous pustulosis is a generalized pustular eruption that is associated with fever and frequently caused by antibiotics. Pustules develop within 2 days of drug administration, start on the face or in flexural areas, and rapidly disseminate (Fig. 439-19). Spontaneous resolution occurs in less than 2 weeks.

PUSTULAR PSORIASIS

Pustular psoriasis is a variant of psoriasis (Chapter 438) that localizes to the palms and soles or generalizes over the entire body. Patients with generalized disease have fever and leukocytosis and require systemic therapy. Pustules can also be seen in patients with septic emboli of bacterial or fungal origin, including gonococcemia and systemic candidiasis (see Purpuric Eruptions).

FOLLICULITIS

Folliculitis is inflammation of the hair follicles caused by infection with staphylococci. It is caused by obstruction of individual hair follicles and associated pilosebaceous units. Folliculitis is more common in patients with diabetes mellitus, obesity, or immunocompromised states. The primary lesion is a pustule with a central hair. Typical affected sites are the scalp, thighs, trunk, axilla, and inguinal area. Sometimes the infection can extend deeper into the

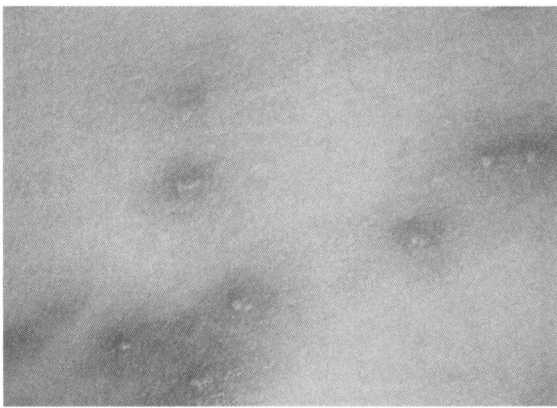

FIGURE 439-20. *Pseudomonas* species folliculitis. The trunk of this patient has numerous pustules on an erythematous base.

dermis and form larger erythematous nodules from one (furuncle) or more (carbuncle) follicles. Treatment with oral antibiotics such as cephalexin, 500 mg twice daily for 14 days, clears extensive infections, but topical antibiotics (e.g., clindamycin solution applied twice daily for 2 weeks or longer) and antibacterial soaps (e.g., Dial or Lever 2000) help in milder disease.

Pseudomonas Folliculitis

Pseudomonas folliculitis is acquired from hot tubs contaminated with *P. aeruginosa* (Chapter 306). The typical finding is papules and pustules in areas of skin occluded by a bathing suit (Fig. 439-20). Treatment with ciprofloxacin, 500 mg twice daily for 10 to 14 days, is usually curative.

Pityrosporum folliculitis is a pruritic, acne-like eruption that occurs on the upper part of the back and the chest, arms, and face and is caused by *Pityrosporum ovale*. Treatment is with oral itraconazole, 200 mg/day for 1 week, and 2% ketoconazole shampoo applied to the affected area daily for 1 month.

Eosinophilic Pustular Folliculitis

Eosinophilic pustular folliculitis is a sterile, intensely pruritic folliculitis usually found on the faces, chests, and backs of patients who are positive for HIV (Chapter 392). Skin biopsy is needed to confirm the diagnosis. Treatment is difficult, but options include potent topical corticosteroids, such as 0.1% triamcinolone ointment applied twice daily for several months (although this class 4 topical corticosteroid should not be used on the face); tacrolimus ointment 0.1% is another topical option that is safe for facial use. Systemic options include antihistamines, such as hydroxyzine, 25 mg every 8 hours as needed, and ultraviolet light therapy.

⬤ HIDRADENITIS SUPPURITIVA

Hidradenitis suppurativa is a chronic recurring inflammatory disease that occurs in skin-bearing apocrine glands and is characterized by painful deep-seated nodules and abscesses.

EPIDEMIOLOGY AND PATHOBIOLOGY

Hidradenitis most commonly occurs in the early 20s, and its incidence declines after age 50 years. There is a 3:1 predominance of women to men. Cigarette smoking and obesity are risk factors that also correlate with the severity of disease.

The pathogenesis of hidradenitis remains poorly understood. Histologic studies suggest a multifocal nature, with early atrophy of the sebaceous glands followed by lymphocytic inflammation of the pilosebaceous unit and later by destruction of the hair follicles and the formation of granulomas. More recent evidence supports the concept that hidradenitis suppurativa is an inflammatory or immune disease.

CLINICAL MANIFESTATIONS AND DIAGNOSIS

Hidradenitis is characterized by its chronicity, with periods of flares and remissions. Although the typical presentation is with a painful, inflamed nodule in the axilla or the groin, lesions also are often found in the inframammary, genital, and perineal regions. The initial inflamed nodule may either resolve or develop into a persisting painless nodule that intermittently flares (often related to menses) or into a discharging abscess with substantial pain.

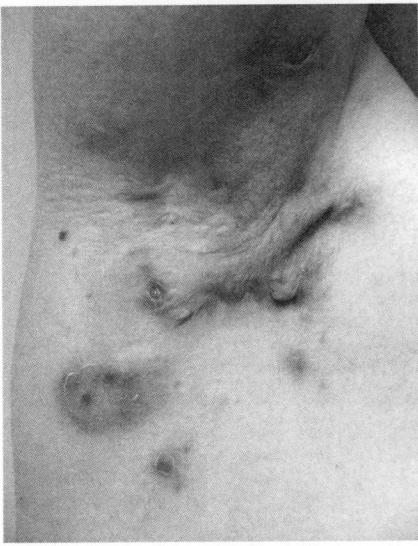

FIGURE 439-21. Hidradenitis suppurativa. The axilla of this patient has several erythematous nodules with draining sinus tracts

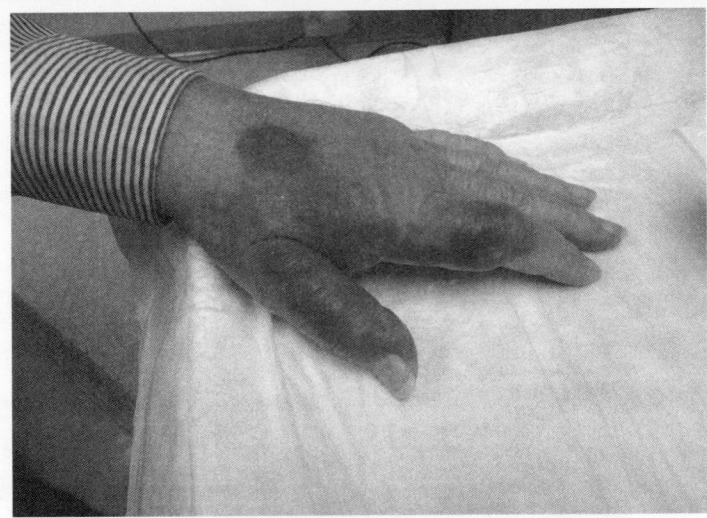

FIGURE 439-22. Sweet syndrome. The distal extremity of this patient has very large edematous indurated plaques and nodules

Lesions typically recur at the same sites or very nearby despite treatment by incision and drainage as well as with antibiotics. Over time, more sites may become affected, and patients sometimes develop sinus tracts and cordlike scarring (Fig 439-21).

TREATMENT   Rx

Treatment is determined by the staging of disease. Localized (Hurley stage 1) disease should be managed with topical clindamycin (1% solution) used twice daily or intralesional triamcinolone (5-10 mg/cc). Patients with Hurley stage 2 (which is defined by the presence of one or more widely separated recurrent abscesses with tract formation and scars) and Hurley stage 3 (which is defined by the presence of multiple interconnected tracts and abscesses throughout an entire area) require more aggressive treatment. A variety of oral antibiotics, systemic corticosteroids, antiandrogens, retinoids, dapsone, and cyclosporine have been used but with minimal evidence to support their efficacy. Recent studies demonstrate improvement with the tumor necrosis factor inhibitors adalimumab or infliximab.[A12][A13]

SWEET SYNDROME

Sweet syndrome (also known as acute febrile neutrophilic dermatosis) is characterized by fever; peripheral neutrophilia; and painful papules, nodules, or plaques with a dense neutrophilic infiltrate but without any frank vasculitis[12] Although the pathogenesis of this syndrome is unknown, it may represent a hypersensitivity reaction occurring in response to either underlying systemic disease or antigenic stimulation

CLINICAL MANIFESTATIONS

Sweet syndrome may be subdivided into three distinct subtypes: classic or idiopathic, paraneoplastic, and drug-induced. Classic Sweet is more common in women, especially between the ages 30 and 60 years. It is often preceded by a flulike (respiratory or gastrointestinal) syndrome and then presents as multiple firm, tender, deeply erythematous papules or nodules, which may turn into edematous plaques. Common locations include the head, neck, and upper and lower extremities (Fig. 439-22 and Fig. 440-23 in Chapter 440) Patients may have fever, arthralgias, arthritis, and myalgias when the disease is active.

Sweet syndrome can be the presenting manifestation of a malignancy, and recurrent episodes of the syndrome can be a sign of recurrent cancer. Malignancy associated Sweet syndrome affects men and women equally. Hematologic malignancies are the most common paraneoplastic association, and acute myelogenous leukemia accounts for the majority of these cases. Drug-induced Sweet syndrome most typically occurs in patients receiving granulocyte colony-stimulating factor.

TREATMENT   Rx

Oral corticosteroids (e.g., prednisone, 1 mg/kg/day given over a 4- to 6-week period with tapering at that time) are the standard and most effective therapy for Sweet syndrome, but some patients may require longer low-dose prednisone to prevent recurrences. The two other most effective therapies are potassium iodide (300 mg three times daily) and colchicine (0.6 mg three times daily).

Grade A References

A1. Oates-Whitehead RM, Baumer JH, Haines L, et al. Intravenous immunoglobulin for the treatment of Kawasaki disease in children. *Cochrane Database Syst Rev.* 2003;4:CD004000.

A2. Kobayashi T, Saji T, Otani T, et al. Efficacy of immunoglobulin plus prednisolone for prevention of coronary artery abnormalities in severe Kawasaki disease (RAISE study): a randomised, open-label, blinded-endpoints trial. *Lancet.* 2012;379:1613-1620.

A3. Kirtschig G, Middleton P, Bennett C, et al. Interventions for bullous pemphigoid. *Cochrane Database Syst Rev.* 2010;10:CD002292.

A4. Amagai M, Ikeda S, Shimizu H, et al. A randomized double-blind trial of intravenous immunoglobulin for pemphigus. *J Am Acad Dermatol.* 2009;60:595-603.

A5. Corey GR, Kabler H, Mehra P, et al. Single-dose oritavancin in the treatment of acute bacterial skin infections. *N Engl J Med.* 2014;370:2180-2190.

A6. Boucher HW, Wilcox M, Talbot GH, et al. Once-weekly dalbavancin versus daily conventional therapy for skin infection. *N Engl J Med.* 2014;370:2169-2179.

A7. Ozolins M, Eady EA, Avery AJ, et al. Comparison of five antimicrobial regimens for the treatment of mild to moderate inflammatory facial acne vulgaris in the community: randomized controlled trial. *Lancet.* 2004;364:2188-2195.

A8. Draelos ZD, Carter E, Maloney JM, et al. Two randomized studies demonstrate the efficacy and safety of dapsone gel 5% for the treatment of acne vulgaris. *J Am Acad Dermatol.* 2007;56:439.

A9. Koltun W, Lucky AW, Thiboutot D, et al. Efficacy and safety of 3 mg drospirenone/20 mcg ethinylestradiol oral contraceptive administered in 24/4 regimen in the treatment of acne vulgaris: a randomized double-blind, placebo-controlled trial. *Contraception.* 2008;77:249-256.

A10. Sanchez J, Somolinos AL, Almodovar PI, et al. A randomized, double-blind, placebo-controlled trial of the combined effect of doxycycline hyclate 20-mg tablets and metronidazole 0.75% topical lotion in the treatment of rosacea. *J Am Acad Dermatol.* 2005;53:791-797.

A11. Gollnick H, Blume-Peytavi U, Szabo EL, et al. Systemic isotretinoin in the treatment of rosacea-doxycycline- and placebo-controlled, randomized clinical study. *J Dtsch Dermatol Ges.* 2010;8:505-515.

A12. Kimball AB, Kerdel F, Adams D, et al. Adalimumab for the treatment of moderate to severe hidradenitis suppurativa: a parallel randomized trial. *Ann Intern Med.* 2012;157:846-855.

A13. Grant A, Gonzalez T, Montgomery MO, et al. Infliximab therapy for patients with moderate to severe hidradenitis suppurativa: a randomized, double-blind, placebo-controlled crossover trial. *J Am Acad Dermatol.* 2010;62:205-217.

GENERAL REFERENCES

For the General References and other additional features, please visit Expert Consult at https://expertconsult.inkling.com.

440

URTICARIA, DRUG HYPERSENSITIVITY RASHES, NODULES AND TUMORS, AND ATROPHIC DISEASES

MADELEINE DUVIC

URTICARIA

DEFINITION AND EPIDEMIOLOGY

Urticaria, also known as hives, is one of the most common cutaneous reaction patterns (Fig. 440-1). It is triggered by a wide variety of antigens or by physical stimuli, including cold, pressure, and sunlight (Table 440-1). The term *urticaria* refers to a disease spectrum ranging from simple wheals to angioedema. Clinical distinction between acute and chronic urticaria is important for diagnosis and treatment. Chronic urticaria, defined as urticaria that recurs over a period of 6 weeks or more, is often of unknown cause.

Urticaria is common worldwide in persons of all ages, although certain types of urticaria have a predilection for certain age groups. For example, whereas acute urticaria is often seen in children with atopic dermatitis, chronic urticaria peaks in the fourth decade.

PATHOBIOLOGY

Urticaria can be caused by immunologic (autoimmune, immunoglobulin E [IgE] –dependent, immune complex–mediated, complement-kinin dependent) or nonimmunologic (direct mast cell–releasing agents, vasoactive stimuli, drugs) reactions. Local degranulation of mast cells with the release of histamine and other factors, such as slow-reacting substance of anaphylaxis, precipitates urticaria. Functional IgG autoantibodies, which release histamine from mast cells and basophils, are commonly found in the blood of patients with chronic urticaria. Additionally, basophils are recruited into the wheals, where they sustain the response by releasing histamine. Eosinophils also contribute through leukotriene C_4 (LTC$_4$), leukotriene D_4 (LTD$_4$), leukotriene E_4 (LTE$_4$), and major basic protein. Urticaria is typically transient and self-limited, without leakage of blood cells into the skin or damage to the blood vessels. Leakage of plasma into the dermis from capillaries and small postcapillary venules correlates clinically with development of a demarcated, pink, raised lesion (hive).

CLINICAL MANIFESTATIONS

Urticarial lesions are pink to light red, blanch with pressure, and are raised above the surface of the skin. The center of the lesions may be paler than the leading edge. By definition, individual wheals come and go within 24 hours. A mosquito bite (Chapter 253) is the archetypal urticarial lesion. Individual hives can coalesce into giant plaques or annular rings called giant urticaria as is seen in serum sickness, in which they are accompanied by arthralgias and fever. Confluent urticaria may also be accompanied by swelling of the underlying soft tissue or the mucous membranes (angioedema) as well as by anaphylaxis with laryngeal edema, a life-threatening emergency. In otherwise normal individuals, pressure or writing on the skin will cause spontaneous local release of histamine, which induces a wheal-and-flare reaction known as dermatographism. Deep swelling develops at the site of sustained pressure and may remain for days in a condition known as delayed pressure urticaria. Affected individuals may develop lesions from tight-fitting clothing, shoes, socks, or sexual intercourse.

Other physical stimuli such as cold, heat, sun, or exercise may induce urticaria. Cold urticaria may be precipitated by putting an ice cube on the skin; the interval until hives develop and the duration of the hives correlate with the severity of the condition, which can be life threatening if the patient is suddenly immersed in cold water. Heat, exercise, or exertion may be accompanied by small, 2- to 3-mm urticarial lesions in a condition called cholinergic urticaria. Exercise-induced anaphylaxis may be hereditary, but the defect is unknown. Patients with vibratory angioedema develop swelling and erythema within a few minutes of exposure to a vibratory stimulus. Lesions persist for about 30 minutes. Other forms of physically induced urticaria include solar urticaria and aquagenic urticaria (urticarial lesions caused by exposure to sun and water, respectively).

Food and exercise–induced anaphylaxis is a syndrome in which a few minutes of exercise after ingestion of specific foods results in angioedema or anaphylaxis. The cause of this syndrome is still controversial, but reduced gastric acid secretion may be involved in food and exercise-induced anaphylaxis.

DIAGNOSIS

A detailed history (duration, occupation, medications, frequency of episodes, associated illness) is critical. Urticaria typically results from exposure to antigen only minutes to a few hours before the onset of the lesions. In many cases, pruritus may precede onset of the rash. The most common triggers of IgE-mediated allergic urticarial reactions are drugs (especially penicillin, sulfa drugs, antibiotics, and contrast dye), foods (shellfish, salicylates in berries, tomatoes, yeast, and penicillin in blue cheese), food additives (sodium benzoate), nuts (especially peanuts), latex, and insect bites.

TABLE 440-1 COMMON CAUSES OF URTICARIA
URTICARIA MAY BE ACCOMPANIED BY ANGIOEDEMA AND ANAPHYLAXIS
Blood products: red blood cells, platelets, gamma globulin
Drugs
Antibiotics: penicillins, cephalosporins, sulfonamides, isoniazid
Aspirin: salicylates, benzoates, phenylbutazone
Anticonvulsants: hydantoin
Chemotherapy: doxorubicin, daunorubicin, L-asparaginase, chlorambucil, cyclophosphamide, melphalan, methotrexate, nitrogen mustard, procarbazine
Dextran
Nonsteroidal anti-inflammatory drugs
Opiates
Quinidine
Radiocontrast dyes, iodine
Environmental: animal dander or proteins, formaldehyde, pollen, mold, plants, latex, plastic tubing, exercise, heat, cold, sunlight
Foods: berries, eggs, milk, nuts, tomatoes, shellfish, soy
Food additives: sodium benzoate, tartrazine (yellow dye #5)
Hormones
Infections: streptococcal, staphylococcal, sinusitis or abscesses, viral hepatitis, Epstein-Barr virus mononucleosis, *Candida* spp.
Insect bites or venom: Hymenoptera, mosquitoes, mites, scabies
Mechanical stimuli (dermographism, vibratory angioedema, delayed-pressure urticaria)
Vaccines
URTICARIA-LIKE ERUPTIONS AND REACTIVE ERYTHEMAS
Erythema multiforme: herpes simplex, DNA viruses, *Mycoplasma pneumoniae*, drugs
Erythema marginatum: streptococcal rheumatic fever
Juvenile rheumatoid arthritis
Erythema chronicum migrans: *Borrelia* spp. infections
Erythema annulare centrifugum: tinea, drugs
Figurate erythemas: erythema repens (often with underlying carcinoma)
Urticaria pigmentosa (mastocytosis)

FIGURE 440-1. Urticaria. (From DermNet. Urticaria; 2014. http://www.dermnetnz.org/reactions/urticaria.html. Accessed October 23, 2014.)

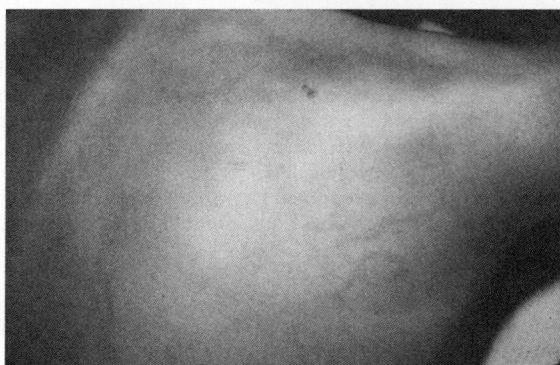

FIGURE 440-2. Erythema marginatum. (From Medscape. Urticaria; n.d.. http://www.medscape.com/content/1998/00/41/73/417394/art-m5649.fig2.jpg. http://www.dermnetnz.org/reactions/urticaria.html. Accessed October 23, 2014.)

Nonimmunologic mediators of urticaria include aspirin and opiates as well as physical agents that work through the prostaglandin pathway or degranulate mast cells.

Acute urticaria can also be triggered by skin contact with an antigen, such as latex, and can progress to anaphylaxis. In addition, urticaria can be a sign or prodrome of a latent infection, especially streptococcal pharyngitis in children or viral hepatitis in adults. The migratory urticarial rash accompanying rheumatic fever, erythema marginatum (Fig. 440-2), is characterized by evanescent, scalloped lesions that change location over the course of hours.

When urticarial lesions are present for more than 24 hours, underlying urticarial vasculitis should be suspected. A skin biopsy is required to distinguish urticarial vasculitis from urticaria in which no damage to the blood vessels is evident. When vascular damage is present, the lesion is termed *leukocytoclastic vasculitis,* the most severe expression of hypersensitivity reactions involving cutaneous blood vessels.

Chronic urticaria can be caused by occult infections (sinusitis, gallbladder disease, *Helicobacter pylori,* yeast infections, tooth abscesses, or silent hepatitis) as well as by collagen vascular diseases and tumors, especially Hodgkin lymphoma. Deficiency of the C1 esterase inhibitor can be manifested as chronic urticaria with angioedema. Allergy testing is recommended if the history is unrevealing. If lesions persist for more than 24 hours, skin biopsy is indicated to determine whether vasculitis or mastocytosis is present. If infection, collagen vascular disease, or a tumor is suspected, a full serologic evaluation should be undertaken. Although a thorough medical evaluation may aid in diagnosis, the cause of chronic urticaria may remain uncertain. In the absence of a known antigen, stress is often invoked as the underlying cause of chronic recurrent idiopathic urticaria.

Systemic mastocytosis (Chapter 255) may be accompanied by urticarial lesions and gastrointestinal symptoms. In the form of mastocytosis known as *urticaria pigmentosa,* stroking the lesions produces urticaria, known as *Darier sign.* A skin biopsy shows an increased number of dermal mast cells. Serum tryptase and histamine levels may be elevated during an attack.

TREATMENT   Rx

Management of urticaria depends on its severity and the duration of the problem (Chapter 252). For mild urticaria limited to the skin, traditional antihistamines (diphenhydramine) or the newer nonsedating agents (terfenadine, cetirizine, loratadine)[A1] can be administered by mouth intermittently as needed (Table 440-2). Acute urticaria is often treated with diphenhydramine orally. If the urticaria is severe, short-term corticosteroids, up to 1 mg/kg, can be used. For urticaria associated with wheezing or anaphylaxis, subcutaneous epinephrine, intravenous (IV) corticosteroids, and oxygen should be administered immediately. For chronic urticaria that persists despite antihistamines, cyclosporine at doses of 3 mg/kg or higher for 8 to 16 weeks may be helpful.[A2] More recently, omalizumab, an anti-IgE monoclonal antibody, has been shown to significantly reduce symptoms when given as three doses of 150 or 300 mg at 4-week intervals in patients with moderate to severe chronic urticaria.[A3] Finding the cause and removing the antigen of chronic recurrent urticaria is highly preferable to chronic administration of corticosteroids or antihistamines.[1] The patient should avoid aspirin compounds and other drugs that could be the cause.

TABLE 440-2 TREATMENT OF URTICARIA

1. Avoid the inciting agent!
2. Medications based on severity
    A. Mild to moderate, acute urticaria
        Oral antihistamines, e.g., diphenhydramine (Benadryl), 10-50 mg PO q12h, or hydroxyzine, 10-25 mg PO q8h; nonsedating alternatives include cetirizine (Zyrtec), 5-10 mg, or loratadine (Claritin), 10 mg/day
    B. Severe urticaria with or without angioedema
        Antihistamines, e.g., diphenhydramine (Benadryl), 25-50 mg PO q6-8h or 10-50 mg IV q2-4h, not to exceed 400 mg/24 hr
        Corticosteroids, e.g., prednisone, 10-60 mg PO every morning with tapering over a 2-wk period; triamcinolone (Kenalog), 40 mg IM for one dose; or dexamethasone, 0.6-0.75 mg/m²/day IV in divided doses q6-12h, depending on severity
    C. Anaphylaxis
        A—Airway (intubation)
        B—Breathing (oxygen)
        C—Circulation: parenteral aqueous epinephrine, 1 : 1000 IV, saline or volume expanders
        IV corticosteroids (e.g., methylprednisolone, 125 mg)
        Histamine H₁- and H₂-antagonists (50 mg each of diphenhydramine and ranitidine)
    D. Chronic idiopathic urticaria—combination therapy
        Nonsedating antihistamine: cetirizine, 10 mg/day, or fexofenadine, 30-180 mg twice daily, alone or with montelukast, 10 mg/day, or H₁ and H₂ antagonists (50 mg each of diphenhydramine and ranitidine) and/or low-dose corticosteroids (if unavoidable)

IV, Intravenous; *PO,* oral; *q,* every.

DRUG RASHES

DEFINITION

Drugs have been associated with every type of cutaneous reaction pattern ranging from mild and self-limited to severe and life threatening. Urticaria and exanthematous eruptions are common manifestations of cutaneous drug reactions. Less commonly seen are fixed drug, lichenoid, pustular, phototoxic, bullous, or vasculitic reactions, as well as Stevens-Johnson syndrome and toxic epidermal necrolysis.

PATHOBIOLOGY

Drug rashes, which result from drug toxicity, overdose, drug–drug interactions, or products of metabolism, may be caused by immunologic or nonimmunologic mechanisms. Drugs or their metabolites can act as haptens and induce cell-mediated or humoral responses. Mechanisms include IgE-dependent anaphylaxis and urticaria, cytotoxic reactions resulting in thrombocytopenia and resultant petechiae, immune complex–mediated serum sickness, and delayed-type hypersensitivity resulting in exanthematous or fixed drug eruptions or Stevens-Johnson syndrome.

CLINICAL MANIFESTATIONS AND DIAGNOSIS

Most drug rashes are either immediate (urticaria) or delayed hypersensitivity reactions (exanthems). Immediate reactions such as pruritus, hives, angioedema, and anaphylaxis occur within minutes to a few hours after the drug is taken. The most common drug-related rash (Table 440-3) is a T cell–mediated hypersensitivity reaction manifested as a macular, bright pink to salmon-colored exanthem that appears as early as 7 to 10 days and as late as 14 days after a drug is first administered. Delayed hypersensitivity reactions can be macular or papular exanthems (or both), morbilliform eruptions, annular erythema, or confluent erythema (Fig. 440-3). After sensitization to a particular drug has occurred, readministration of the same drug may trigger an eruption within 24 to 72 hours. Drug hypersensitivity reactions are typically symmetrical. They characteristically begin on the face and upper trunk and progress to the lower extremities, where they may become purpuric. Exanthems secondary to drugs most often become confluent erythematous patches after several days.

Pruritus is the most common symptom. The differential diagnosis for drug rashes includes viral exanthems (Chapter 439), graft-versus-host disease or the leukocyte recovery rash after allogeneic bone marrow transplantation, erythematous exanthems that accompany streptococcal (scarlet fever

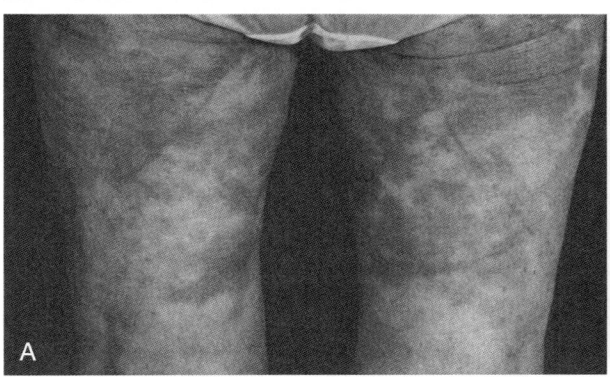
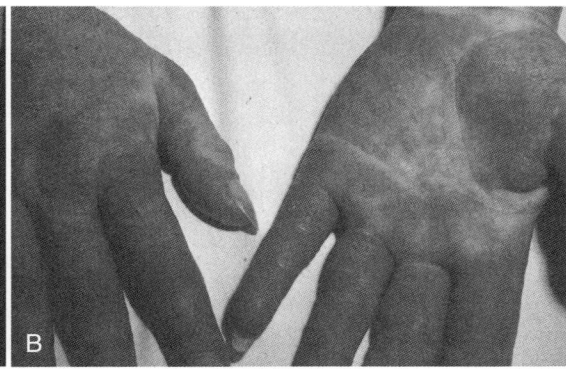

FIGURE 440-3. Delayed hypersensitivity reaction. **A,** Drug reaction. **B,** Acral erythema.

TABLE 440-3 DELAYED HYPERSENSITIVITY DRUG RASHES BY CATEGORY

MACULOPAPULAR EXANTHEMS—ANY DRUG CAN PRODUCE A RASH 7-10 DAYS AFTER THE FIRST DOSE

Allopurinol
Antibiotics: penicillin, sulfonamides
Antiepileptics: phenytoin, phenobarbital
Antihypertensives: captopril, thiazide diuretics
Contrast dye: iodine
Gold salts
Hypoglycemic drugs
Meprobamate
Phenothiazines
Quinine

DRUG RASH WITH EOSINOPHILIA AND SYSTEMIC SYMPTOMS (DRESS)

Anticonvulsants: phenytoin, phenobarbital, valproate, lamotrigine
Antibiotics: sulfonamides, minocycline, dapsone, ampicillin, ethambutol, isoniazid, linezolid, metronidazole, rifampin, streptomycin, vancomycin
Antihypertensives: amlodipine, captopril
Antidepressants: bupropion, fluoxetine
Allopurinol
Celecoxib
Ibuprofen
Phenothiazines

ERYTHEMA MULTIFORME/STEVENS-JOHNSON SYNDROME

Sulfonamides, phenytoin, barbiturates, carbamazepine, allopurinol, amikacin, phenothiazines
Toxic epidermal necrolysis: same as for erythema multiforme but also acetazolamide, gold, nitrofurantoin, pentazocine, tetracycline, quinidine

ACUTE GENERALIZED EXANTHEMIC PUSTULOSIS

Antibiotics: penicillins, macrolides, cephalosporins, clindamycin, imipenem, fluoroquinolones, isoniazid, vancomycin, minocycline, doxycycline, linezolid
Antimalarials: chloroquine, hydroxychloroquine
Antifungals: terbinafine, nystatin
Anticonvulsants: carbamazepine
Calcium-channel blockers
Furosemide
Systemic corticosteroids
Protease inhibitors

COLLAGEN VASCULAR OR LUPUS-LIKE REACTIONS

Procainamide, hydralazine, phenytoin, penicillamine, trimethadione, methyldopa, carbamazepine, griseofulvin, nalidixic acid, oral contraceptives, propranolol

ERYTHEMA NODOSUM

Oral contraceptives, penicillin, sulfonamides, diuretics, gold, clonidine, propranolol, opiates
Fixed drug reactions: phenolphthalein, barbiturates, gold, sulfonamides, meprobamate, penicillin, tetracycline, analgesics

[Chapter 290]) or staphylococcal (toxic shock syndrome [Chapter 288]) infections, and the acute manifestation of collagen vascular diseases.[2] A similar exanthem occurs when ampicillin is administered to patients who have infectious mononucleosis. A careful drug history is critical in diagnosis and treatment.

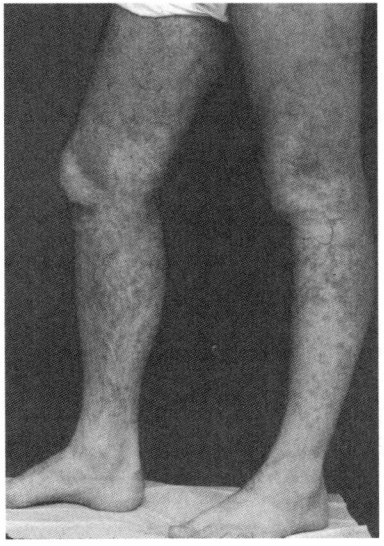

FIGURE 440-4. Hypersensitivity drug rash caused by phenytoin.

TREATMENT AND PROGNOSIS Rx

After the offending drug is discontinued, delayed hypersensitivity reactions resolve in about 1 week. Therapy is mostly supportive. Corticosteroids, such as 0.01% triamcinolone cream, applied several times per day to the affected area and antihistamines given orally three to four times daily are helpful in reducing the itching and shortening the course.

Specific Syndromes

DRUG RASH WITH EOSINOPHILIA AND SYSTEMIC SYMPTOMS

An especially severe hypersensitivity *drug rash with eosinophilia and systemic symptoms* (DRESS) is most frequently seen with sulfonamides and anticonvulsants (Fig. 440-4). This condition is thought to be caused by an alteration in drug metabolism. Activated T lymphocytes release interleukin-5 (IL-5), leading to characteristic eosinophilia. DRESS may be delayed in onset by 2 to 6 weeks, persists longer than classic drug-induced eruptions, and becomes generalized and severe even when use of the agent is discontinued. It typically begins as a morbilliform eruption, which later evolves into an edematous pustular eruption with erythroderma and purpura. The rash begins on the face, upper trunk, and extremities and later becomes generalized.[3] Continued administration of the drug can result in exfoliative erythroderma; toxic necrolysis; and systemic hypersensitivity, including hepatitis (50%), nephritis (10%); or atypical lymphocytosis and lymphadenopathy mimicking mononucleosis or T-cell lymphoma. Less commonly seen are pneumonitis,

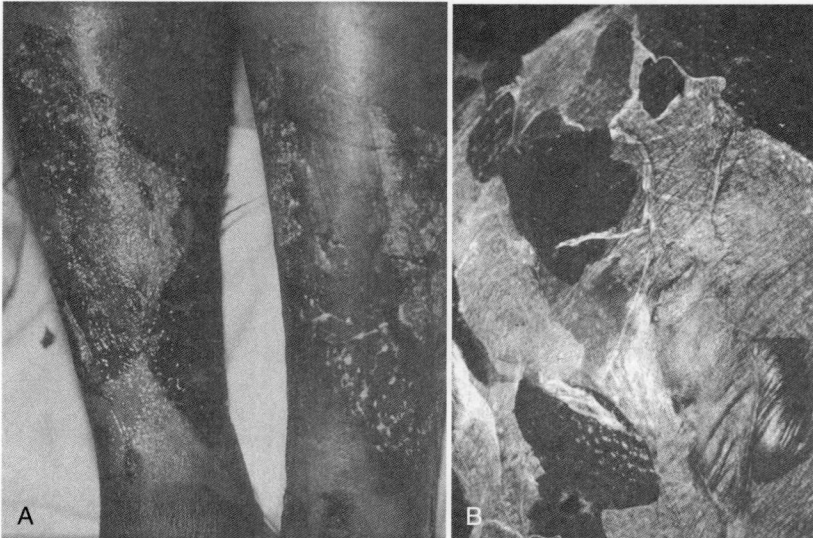

FIGURE 440-5. Toxic epidermal necrolysis. A, Clinical appearance. B, Close-up appearance of epidermal sheets.

myocarditis, and pericarditis. With visceral involvement, there is a 10% mortality rate, usually from hepatic failure. The initial step in management is the immediate withdrawal of the suspected drug. Systemic corticosteroids (e.g., oral prednisone at 1.0 mg/kg/day and tapered over 3 to 6 months or IV methylprednisolone at 30 mg/kg for 3 days) should be started as early as possible. For patients who develop exfoliative dermatitis, admission to a specialized unit such as a burn unit or intensive care unit is critical.

ERYTHEMA MULTIFORME, STEVENS-JOHNSON SYNDROME, AND TOXIC EPIDERMAL NECROLYSIS

Stevens-Johnson syndrome and toxic epidermal necrolysis represent a spectrum of the same disease, of which erythema multiforme (see Fig. 439-10 in Chapter 439) is the least severe. Stevens-Johnson syndrome is defined as less than 10% body surface area involvement, and toxic epidermal necrolysis is defined as greater than 30% body surface area involvement. Erythema multiforme, a hybrid of urticaria and vasculitis, consists of symmetrically distributed red macules or papules that evolve into classic target or bull's-eye lesions with deep red centers and pink urticarial rims. It is commonly precipitated by herpes simplex infections, other DNA viruses, or drugs. Stevens-Johnson syndrome is characterized by severe mucosal involvement with purpuric lesions. Widespread epidermal necrosis resulting from cell apoptosis is seen in toxic epidermal necrolysis.[4] Drugs are almost always implicated when Stevens-Johnson syndrome or toxic epidermal necrolysis develops in adults (Fig. 440-5). Commonly implicated medications include nonsteroidal anti-inflammatory drugs (NSAIDs), acetaminophen, allopurinol, phenytoin, and sulfa drugs. Alterations in drug metabolism (i.e., slow acetylators of sulfonamides) are often implicated. Full-thickness keratinocyte necrosis or cell apoptosis leads to separation at the dermal-epidermal junction.

Each of these conditions may start as a morbilliform drug rash and progress. Symptoms include fever, severe pain, or sometimes asthenia. The condition can progress rapidly, so it is critical to determine and discontinue the causative agent immediately. Superinfection and fluid and electrolyte imbalances can lead to death in 5% of cases of Stevens-Johnson syndrome and 30% of cases of toxic epidermal necrolysis.

Management includes supportive care such as fluid and electrolyte replacement, transfer to a burn unit, and ophthalmologic evaluation. The use of corticosteroids in Stevens-Johnson syndrome and toxic epidermal necrolysis remains controversial. In Stevens-Johnson syndrome, corticosteroids (e.g., IV methylprednisolone at 60 mg every 6 hours or 1-2 mg/kg for a short course) are frequently used and may decrease the duration of fever and slow eruptions. In toxic epidermal necrolysis, however, retrospective studies suggest that corticosteroids may increase mortality. IV immunoglobulin and tumor necrosis factor-α inhibitors, such as infliximab, may reduce the severity of toxic epidermal necrolysis, but no randomized control trials have been done to date.

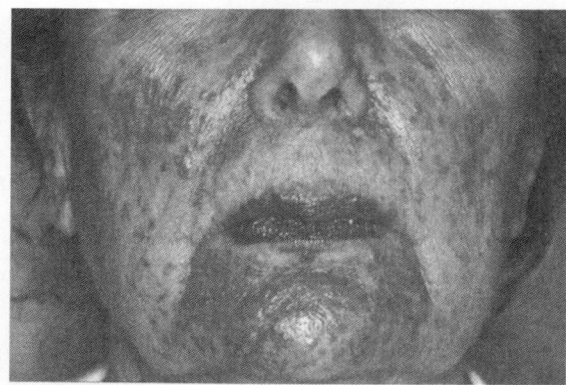

FIGURE 440-6. Epidermal growth factor receptor inhibitor–associated rash.

LEUKOCYTOCLASTIC VASCULITIS

Severe drug reactions can also be manifested as vasculitis, neutrophilic eruptions, and ulcerations. Vasculitis is further categorized by the size of the involved vessel and the nature of the cellular reaction and immune complexes. Leukocytoclastic vasculitis, which is the most common form of vasculitis induced by drugs, is manifested as palpable purpura, usually on the lower extremities (see Figs. 439-4 and 439-5 in Chapter 439).[5]

NEUTROPHILIC DRUG REACTIONS

Neutrophilic drug reactions include iododermas, bromodermas, acute generalized exanthematous pustulosis, and acneiform folliculitis. Sweet syndrome (acute febrile neutrophilic dermatosis; see later) also can be drug related. Epidermal growth factor receptor inhibitors and protein kinase inhibitors cause an acneiform facial or chest eruption that is associated with drugs (Fig. 440-6).

Acute generalized exanthematous pustulosis is characterized by numerous (>100), small (<5 mm), nonfollicular subcorneal pustules that arise on erythematous skin, often beginning in skin creases or on the face. High fever and peripheral neutrophilia may precede or accompany the eruption. The pustules are sterile, present for 5 to 10 days, and followed by desquamation. They usually appear less than 2 days after the administration of the causative drug. Ninety percent of cases are due to drugs, most commonly β-lactam antibiotics, macrolides, and calcium channel blockers. This syndrome has also been called pustular drug rash, pustular psoriasis after corticosteroid withdrawal, and toxic pustuloderma. When severe, it may be confused with toxic epidermal necrolysis, but the mortality rate is only 1% to 2%. Skin patch testing is frequently positive.

TABLE 440-4 DRUGS ASSOCIATED WITH SUN SENSITIVITY

PHOTOTOXIC

Chlorpromazine
Hydralazine
Levaquin
Procainamide
Psoralens
Porphyrins
Sulfonamides
Tetracyclines
Thiazide diuretics

PHOTOALLERGIC

Chlorothiazide
Griseofulvin
Hypoglycemic drugs
Promethazine

TABLE 440-5 TUMORS AND NODULES OF THE SKIN

Benign, nonpigmented tumors and nodules
  Epidermal: warts, acrochordons, tricholemmomas, sebaceous hyperplasia
  Adnexal: epidermal cysts, syringomas, follicular cysts, pilomatricoma, apocrine or
    eccrine adenomas
  Dermal and subcutaneous: lipomas, angiolipomas, neurofibromas, leiomyomas

Benign, pigmented tumors and nodules
  Epidermal: seborrheic keratoses
  Melanocytic compound nevi (junctional nevi are flat)
  Spitz nevus
  Blue nevus
  Dermatofibromas

Malignant, nonpigmented tumors and nodules
  Basal cell carcinoma (nodular, superficial, morpheaform, pigmented)
  Squamous cell carcinoma (actinic keratoses, Bowen disease, keratoacanthomas)
  Cutaneous T- and B-cell lymphomas
  Amelanotic melanomas
  Merkel cell carcinoma
  Adnexal carcinomas of the sebaceous and apocrine glands

Malignant, pigmented tumors and nodules
  Pigmented basal cell carcinoma
  Malignant melanoma: in situ, superficial spreading, nodular, acral lentiginous
  Dermatofibrosarcoma protuberans

Inflammatory nodules over joints
  Gottron papules (dermatomyositis)
  Gouty tophi
  Heberden nodes (osteoarthritis)
  Multicentric reticulohistiocytosis (paraneoplastic syndrome)
  Rheumatoid nodules
  Granuloma annulare

Inflammatory nodules of the lower extremities
  Panniculitis
  Vasculitis: periarteritis nodosa

Metabolic nodules of the skin
  Amyloidosis
  Gouty tophi
  Xanthomas, necrobiotic xanthogranuloma
  Xanthelasma

Vascular lesions
  Benign: nevus flammeus, angiokeratomas, spider hemangiomas, capillary
    hemangiomas, cavernous hemangiomas, blue rubber bleb nevi, pyogenic
    granulomas
  Malignant: Kaposi sarcoma, angiosarcoma

FIXED DRUG ERUPTIONS

A fixed drug reaction appears at the same location 1 to 2 weeks after first drug exposure and within 24 hours of repeat exposure. The lips, hands, face, feet, and genitalia are most commonly involved. The lesion may begin as erythema and then become gray, brown, or violaceous. Trimethoprim–sulfamethoxazole, NSAIDs, tetracyclines, and pseudoephedrine are common causes.

PHOTOSENSITIVITY AND WITHDRAWAL REACTIONS

Light combined with drugs (Table 440-4) can produce photosensitivity reactions that can be quite severe and mimic sunburn. Ultraviolet radiation interacts with a drug or its metabolite to generate reactive oxygen species, leading to cellular damage. Tetracyclines, sulfa drugs, NSAIDs, and fluoroquinolones are often implicated in photosensitivity reactions. Photosensitizing drugs may exacerbate lupus erythematosus (Chapter 266) or porphyria cutanea tarda (Chapter 210).

CONTACT DERMATITIS

Allergic contact dermatitis is a T cell–mediated delayed hypersensitivity reaction that occurs after topical drug application or exposure to poison ivy, oak, or sumac. It is manifested by erythema and microvesiculation and may spread beyond the area of application (id reaction). Common contact sensitizers include Neosporin (polymyxin B, neomycin, and bacitracin), bacitracin, diphenhydramine, doxepin, lidocaine, lanolin, mercury, henna, ethyl cyano-acrylate (eyelash adhesive), nickel, hair dyes, latex, and *p*-aminobenzoic acid.

⬤ BENIGN PAPULES, NODULES, AND TUMORS

The skin is heterogeneous, composed of epidermis, dermis, subcutaneous compartments, and blood vessels. The skin hosts a number of migrating cells (Chapter 435), all of which can give rise to benign or malignant tumors. Lesions that arise from epidermal keratinocytes are usually papules (warts, sebaceous hyperplasia) or plaques (psoriasis, Bowen disease). Nodules are deeper lesions that may be tender or asymptomatic and single or multiple, and they break down to form ulcers. Nodules are classified as inflammatory (granulomas, vasculitis, or panniculitis), infectious, vascular, or metabolic; they can be benign or malignant tumors that arise from skin cells or migrant cells (Table 440-5). Nodules that are smaller and symmetrical are more likely to be benign than lesions that grow rapidly, are larger, or invade surrounding tissue. Any rapidly changing skin nodule should be investigated with an excisional biopsy to the level of fat and sent for histology as well as for bacterial, fungal, and acid-fast cultures.

Benign Epidermal Tumors

The top layer of skin is the avascular epidermis composed of keratinocytes that undergo apoptosis from the stratum corneum. Melanocytes, Langerhans cells, and inflammatory cells may enter the epidermis. Epidermal stem cells form adnexal organs such as hair follicles and sebaceous, eccrine, and apocrine glands that can give rise to tumors.

ACTINIC KERATOSES

Actinic keratoses are pink, scaly macules composed of sun-damaged keratinocytes and are precursors of in situ squamous cell carcinoma (Bowen disease) or invasive squamous carcinomas (Chapter 203). Actinic keratoses are 0.1 cm to 1.0 cm large and are found on sun-exposed areas such as the

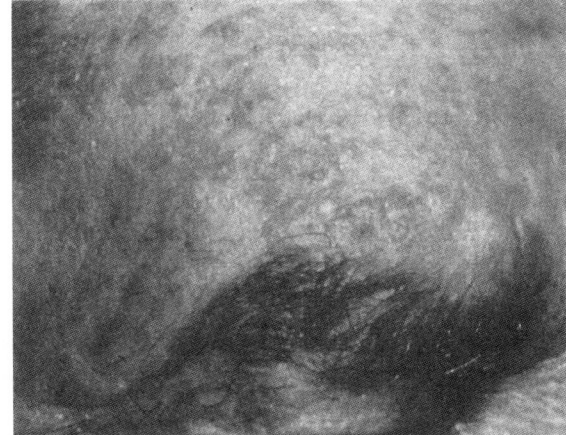

FIGURE 440-7. Actinic keratoses.

forearms, hands, face, and scalp (Fig. 440-7). Lesions with induration, thick crusts, ulceration, or pain are excised for biopsy to exclude invasive squamous cell carcinoma. In randomized studies, ingenol mebutate gel (self-applied to a 25-cm² contiguous field once daily for 3 consecutive days for lesions on the face or scalp or for 2 consecutive days for the trunk or extremities) led to complete clearance in 42% of treated patients versus 4% of control participants on the face and scalp and 34% versus 5% for the trunk and extremities.

Actinic keratoses also can be treated with cryotherapy and topical fluorouracil, retinoids, or imiquimod. To treat and prevent actinic keratoses, sun-exposed areas may be treated topically with 5-fluorouracil cream (5%) applied daily for 2 weeks or twice weekly for 8 weeks.

SEBORRHEIC KERATOSES

Seborrheic keratoses are common verrucous or stuck-on epidermal papules of various colors (Fig. 440-8). They are commonly seen with advancing age but may arise suddenly (sign of Leser-Trélat) in association with internal malignancy. Seborrheic keratoses consist of a single clone of keratinocytes and inherited as an autosomal dominant trait. Seborrheic keratoses have FGFR3, PIK3CA, KRAS, EGFR, HRAS, and AKT mutations but remain clinically benign. Their surface may be friable, and lesions can be scraped off. Seborrheic keratoses spare the palms, soles, and mucosal surfaces. Although benign, seborrheic keratoses must be differentiated from melanocytic nevi, melanomas, and pigmented basal cell carcinoma, usually by the presence of white to yellow horn cysts on their surface, best appreciated with dermoscopy.

WARTY LESIONS

Epidermal papules include common warts (see Fig. 439-2 in Chapter 439) caused by human papillomavirus (HPV). HPV can also be detected in squamous carcinomas arising on the digits and in keratoacanthomas, which are low-grade, well-demarcated, dome-shaped papules or nodules that grow rapidly and spontaneously involute in 6 to 8 weeks. Acrodermatitis verruciformis is characterized by multiple warts with the appearance of seborrheic keratoses on the dorsal extremities and gives rise to squamous cell carcinomas. Molluscum contagiosum (Chapter 439) (Fig. 440-9), caused by a DNA virus, are small, shiny, domed-shaped, 1- to 5-mm papules with a central depression. Molluscum contagiosum lesions are common in children and immunocompromised patients. Treatment with anti-cancer BRAF inhibitors can cause warty papules, keratoacanthomas, and eruptive keratosis pilaris.

Cowden syndrome (Chapter 193), caused by mutations in *PTEN* gene, is associated with warty papules (tricholemmomas; Fig. 440-10); cobblestone papules on the gums and tongue; fibrous papules; and multiple hamartomas involving the breast, thyroid, intestines, ovary, and cerebellum.

ADNEXAL TUMORS

Adnexal tumors arise from hair follicles or glands and are commonly found on the face or scalp. Trichoepitheliomas resemble basal cell carcinomas. Sebaceous hyperplasia consists of small yellow papules with a central depression. Adnexal tumors of sebaceous origin, including sebaceous adenomas and sebaceous carcinomas, can also occur on the face, where they may be markers of the Muir-Torre syndrome of familial breast and colon cancer. Epidermal or sebaceous cysts, which are found in acne or as single firm nodules with a central pore, are filled with sebum or keratin. Epidermoid tumors of the scalp and a family history of colon cancer raises question of a diagnosis of Gardner syndrome (Chapter 193).[6]

DERMATOFIBROMAS AND COLLAGENOMAS

Fibroblasts, the resident cells of the dermis, produce collagen, elastin, and mucopolysaccharides. Accumulation of these products results in sclerosis, papules, or nodules. Fibroblasts in small, dense clusters form firm brown or tan papules known as dermatofibromas. Dermatofibromas are hypertrophic scars that are commonly found on the extremities and that may form after insect bites or trauma. They are firm and well-demarcated papules, and the skin puckers when lateral pressure is applied. Dermatofibromas can be treated, but increased scarring may occur. The malignant counterpart is dermatofibroma sarcoma protuberans, which is a poorly defined, rapidly expanding, dermal, malignant tumor. Overlying erythema or hyperpigmentation is often present.

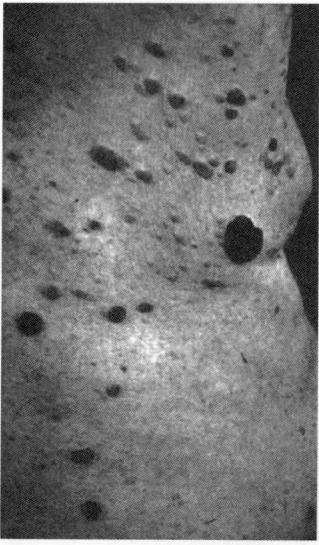

FIGURE 440-8. Seborrheic keratoses.

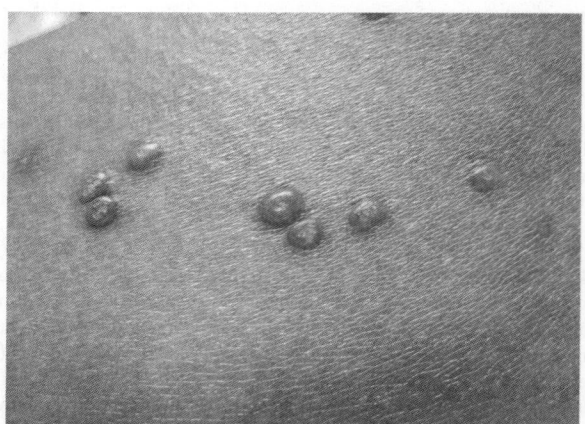

FIGURE 440-9. Molluscum contagiosum.

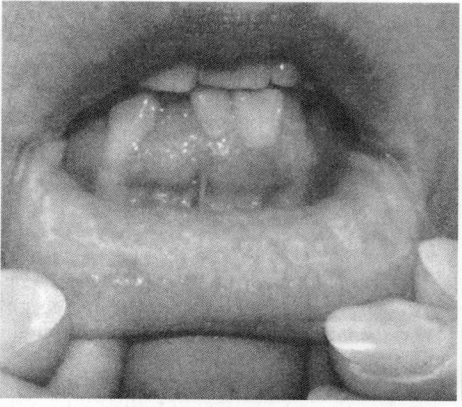 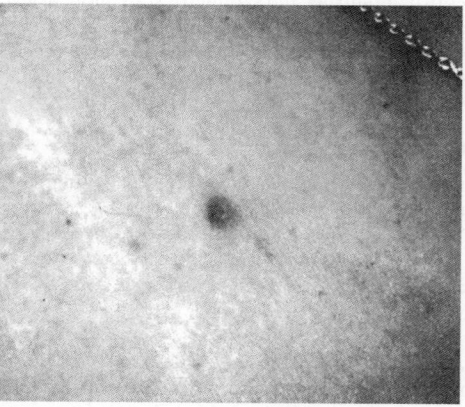

FIGURE 440-10. Cowden syndrome: cobblestone gums *(left)* and tricholemmoma *(right)*.

Some individuals have more pronounced and hypertrophic scar formation known as keloids, with an autosomal dominant or autosomal recessive inheritance pattern. Keloids, which are shiny and firm in appearance, result from an overproduction of collagen. They are especially common on the anterior chest, neck, and earlobes and may require antineoplastic treatment, such as interferon alfa 2b, mitomycin C, bleomycin, and 5-fluorouracil (Chapter 179), and laser therapy.[7]

Collagenomas and elastic tumors with the appearance of small white to yellow papules are found in the skin and bone of patients with Buschke-Ollendorff syndrome. *Pseudoxanthoma elasticum* (Chapter 260), an autosomal recessive disorder, is typically manifested as cutaneous yellow plaques on the neck or antecubital fossa from damaged elastin tissue. Mucin cysts are gray, shiny, well-demarcated, round nodules that generally arise on the mucosa or on the digits, where they may have an underlying connection to the joint space.

NEURAL CREST CELL TUMORS

Benign tumors in the dermis arising from neural crest cells include neurofibromas (soft, flesh-colored papules; Fig. 440-11), schwannomas (larger subcutaneous soft tumors or plaques; Fig. 440-12), and melanocytic lesions. Although solitary neurofibromas may occur, multiple lesions with cafe au lait spots (tan macules) or axillary freckling (Crowe sign) are diagnostic of neurofibromatosis type I, an autosomal dominant disorder caused by mutations in neurofibromin (Chapter 417). Schwannomas can become malignant and

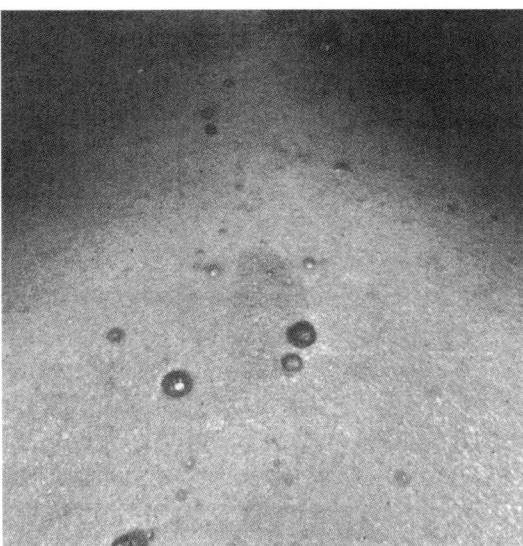

FIGURE 440-11. Neurofibromatosis with cafe au lait spots and neurofibromas.

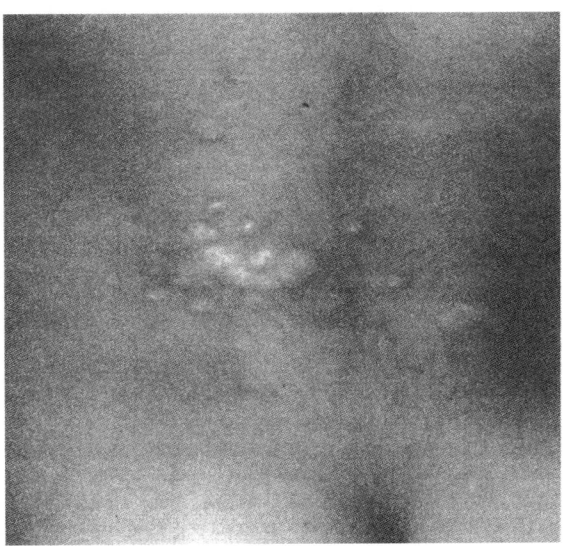

FIGURE 440-12. Schwannoma.

be manifested as dermal nodules. Merkel cell carcinoma, which is a neuroendocrine carcinoma of the skin, is a particularly aggressive small cell tumor arising from the cutaneous nerve endings or Meissner corpuscles. Merkel cell polyomavirus is associated with development of Merkel cell carcinoma.[8] Merkel cell carcinoma may present as a solitary pink to purple dome-shaped papule on the head or neck (Fig. 440-13). Sentinel lymph node biopsy is recommended in all patients with primary Merkel cell carcinoma. Treatment requires full excision, radiation therapy, and often chemotherapy because the cancer tends to recur and metastasize.

Melanocytic Lesions

Benign melanocytic moles or nevi (new) are discrete nests of melanocytes acquired during childhood and young adulthood, stimulated by sun exposure. Nevi are benign and composed of melanocytes (Chapter 203). They regress with age and change in color during pregnancy. Benign melanocytic nevi are formed by nests of melanocytes at the epidermal junction (junctional nevi), in the dermis (intradermal nevi), or in both compartments (compound nevi). Their appearance depends on type and age of the lesion. Junctional nevi (Fig. 440-14) are small, flat, and light to dark brown. Intradermal nevi are soft, flesh-colored to pink papules with smooth regular borders and surface. Compound nevi are globular papules with brown pigmentation. Whereas blue nevi (Fig. 440-15) are flat, grayish blue, and regular. Small congenital nevi are dark brown, dysplastic nevi (Fig. 440-16) have variegated colors and may transform into melanoma. More than 10 large, atypical moles with irregular borders and colors confer higher risk of developing melanoma, especially with a positive family history. Other recognized risk factors for melanoma include having more than 50 small nevi, red or blonde hair, or fair skin that burns and a history of blistering sunburns as a child. Patients with higher risk for melanoma should have surveillance and regular skin examinations.

Langerhans Cell Histiocytosis

Skin surveillance is mediated by antigen-presenting cells: Langerhans cells, dermal dendritic cells, and skin-homing T lymphocytes. Proliferation of Langerhans cells is called histiocytosis. Childhood histiocytosis X is manifested as severe seborrheic dermatitis of the scalp and gluteal areas with

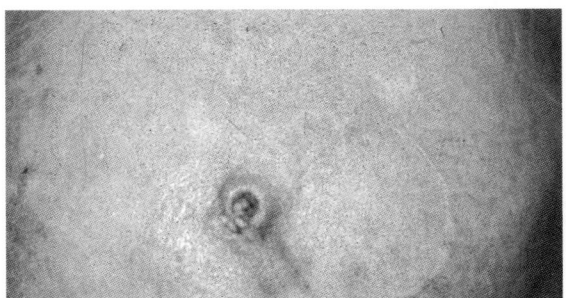

FIGURE 440-13. Merkel cell tumor.

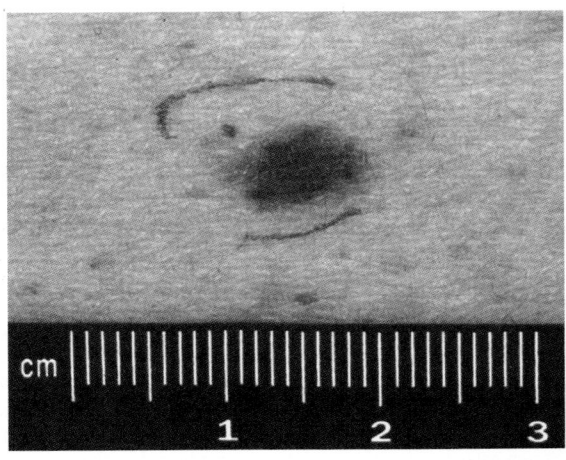

FIGURE 440-14. Junctional nevus.

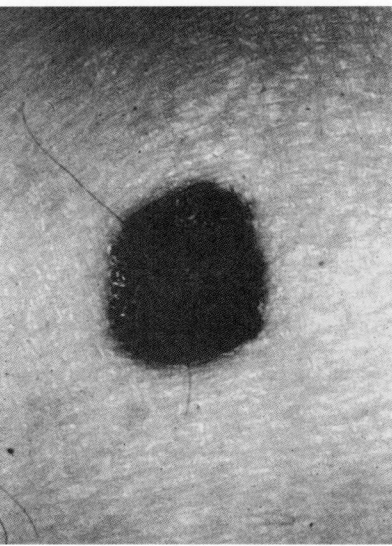

FIGURE 440-15. Benign blue nevus.

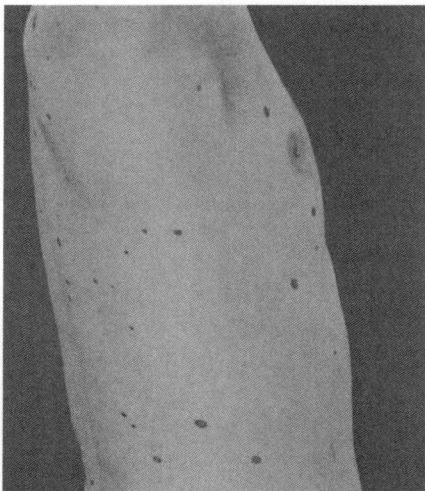

FIGURE 440-16. Dysplastic nevus syndrome.

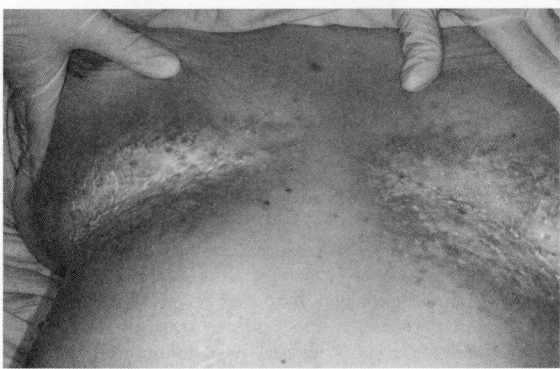

FIGURE 440-17. Histiocytosis X.

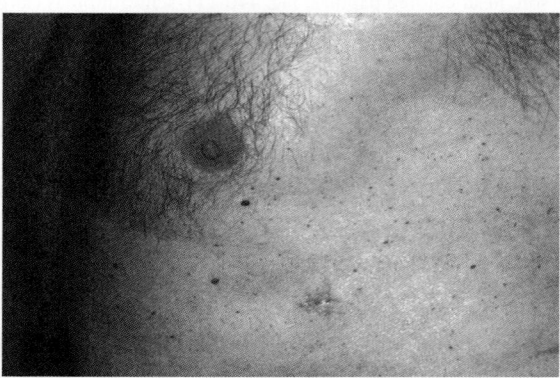

FIGURE 440-18. Benign capillary hemangioma.

underlying purpura and may result in the hemophagocytic syndrome. In adults, lesions appear in the intertriginous areas (Fig. 440-17). Patients with the non–Langerhans cell histiocytosis have lytic bone involvement (eosinophilic granulomas) or diabetes insipidus (Hand-Schüller-Christian syndrome).

Vascular Lesions
HEMANGIOMAS
Benign capillary, or cherry, hemangiomas are bright cherry-red to purple papules, generally less than 5 mm in diameter. They appear on the trunk with aging and may be numerous (Fig. 440-18). Pyogenic granulomas can resemble hemangiomas but contain polymorphonuclear leukocytes, are friable, and bleed easily. Multiple pyogenic granulomas are seen in infectious bacillary angiomatosis in immunocompromised hosts (Chapter 315). Cavernous or strawberry hemangiomas can also appear in the neonatal period as rapidly growing vascular tumors; they may obstruct the eye or the pharynx before regressing. Propranolol 2 mg/kg/day in two or three divided doses for variable duration can decrease the hemangioma's volume, color, and elevation in children younger than 5 years of age.[A5] Corticosteroids, interferon, or antiangiogenic factors also can treat these lesions if propranolol is not successful. Cavernous hemangiomas are deeper and less likely to resolve than smaller lesions. When associated with platelet consumption, Kasabach-Merritt syndrome is present (Chapter 171).

KAPOSI SARCOMA
Kaposi sarcoma (Chapter 392) is a disseminated angiomatosis that arises from viral IL-8 production by herpesvirus 8. Lesions are symmetrical purple, red, gray, or brown patches, papules, nodules, or ulcers (Fig. 440-19). Mucosal involvement is more common in advanced disease. Kaposi sarcoma in young African adults and Kaposi sarcoma associated with human immunodeficiency virus (HIV) infection often have a more aggressive course than Kaposi sarcoma in elderly men of Mediterranean background, whose disease is indolent and often confined to the lower extremities. Treatment of HIV disease with highly active antiretroviral therapy has been associated with a marked decreased incidence and severity of HIV-associated Kaposi sarcoma. Angiosarcomas are malignant purple to red vascular tumor nodules that are more common in elderly individuals or on the extremities of patients with chronic lymphedema.[9] To help distinguish cutaneous angiosarcomas from benign histologic mimics, immunohistochemistry staining for ERG, an Ets family transcription factor, is a specific and sensitive marker for endothelial differentiation.

Inflammatory and Hematopoietic Papules and Tumors
Inflammatory diseases of the skin involve the superficial or dermal vessels or subcutaneous tissue. Inflammatory infiltrates can be mixed or restricted in nature. Lymphocytes, polymorphonuclear leukocytes, histocytes, eosinophils, and plasma cells are involved in the most common inflammatory reactions. Hematologic malignancies can present with secondary skin lesions, including patches, nodules, papules, or vasculitic lesions. Skin-homing CD4$^+$ T cells give rise to cutaneous T-cell lymphomas. Mycosis fungoides (Chapter 185) lesions are pleomorphic pink, white, or brown patches or plaques, alopecia, or diffuse erythroderma with blood involvement (Sézary syndrome). Early patch or plaque mycosis fungoides is indistinguishable from chronic eczematous or psoriasiform dermatitis. Tumors occur late in mycosis fungoides and can transform to a large cell lymphoma phenotype, with or without expression of CD30. Peripheral cutaneous T-cell lymphomas may also be found in subcutaneous tissue as panniculitic lesions. Lymphomatoid papulosis is characterized by crops of red to pink self-regressing papules with

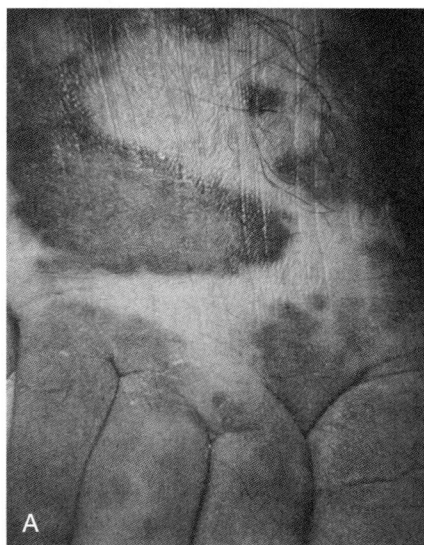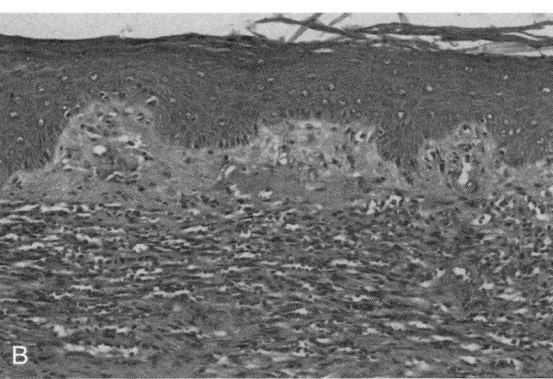

FIGURE 440-19. Kaposi sarcoma. A, Involvement of the lower extremity (Mediterranean Kaposi sarcoma). B, Histology.

histologic findings similar to those of anaplastic large cell lymphoma (Chapter 185), including expression of CD30 antigen. Clinically, lymphomatoid papulosis presents as self-regressing papules, CD3+ anaplastic T-cell lymphomas can present as tumors, and patients with transformed CD30+ mycosis fungoides initially have patch or plaque stage disease before developing tumors. Treatment of lymphomatoid papulosis consists of topical corticosteroids, methotrexate, or bexarotene. For CD30+ anaplastic T-cell lymphoma, therapeutic options include radiation therapy, methotrexate, bexarotene, brentuximab vedotin, and chemotherapy (Chapter 185). Natural killer T-cell lymphomas, immunoblastic lymphomas, and plasmacytoid dendritic cell tumors appear as brown to purple dermal nodules often with purpura.

Cutaneous B-cell lymphomas present as pink, infiltrated, dome-shaped shiny papules or tumors. Whereas follicular B-cell lymphoma is commonly located on the face, scalp, or upper part of the back, mucosa-associated B-cell tumors are more common on the trunk. With the exception of large B-cell lymphoma, follicular and MALT (mucosa-associated lymphoid tissue) B-cell lymphomas of the skin are indolent. Cutaneous MALT lymphomas (Fig. 440-20) have been associated with *Borrelia* spp. infection (Chapter 321), *Helicobacter pylori* infection, and chronic inflammation.[10] Plasmacytomas can arise in the skin, in bone, with multiple myeloma (Chapter 187), or independently. Extramedullary hematopoiesis or endometriosis can be associated with red or brown nodules in the dermis.

Granulomatous Diseases

Sarcoidosis is an inflammatory granulomatous process manifested as ichthyosis, papules, plaques, or tumors with an apple-jelly color (Fig. 440-21). Patients with lepromatous leprosy also can have histiocytic plaques or tumors (Fig. 440-22); treatment of leprosy may induce an inflammatory reaction called erythema nodosum leprosum. Granulomatous mycosis fungoides, which is a variant of cutaneous T-cell lymphoma, is difficult to diagnose and treat. Granulomatous inflammation within the dermis can result in damage to collagen, as seen in granuloma annulare (ringlike pink to red infiltrated lesions, often on the hands or elbows), rheumatoid nodules that occur on the extensor surface of the arms, and necrobiosis lipoidica on the shins of patients with diabetes. All three lesions typically include fibrin deposits within dermal blood vessels. Multicentric reticulohistiocytosis is a rare paraneoplastic syndrome in which histiocytic nodules form over joints with associated arthritis.

Inflammatory Skin Lesions and Nodules

Inflammatory skin nodules arise from inflamed blood vessels (vasculitis) or adipose tissue (panniculitis). Either can arise in response to underlying infection or antigen stimulation with influx of inflammatory cells. Vasculitis is categorized by vessel size and circulating immune complexes. Damage to blood vessels results in leakage of red blood cells with the development of purpura (nonblanching red to purple lesions; Chapter 270).

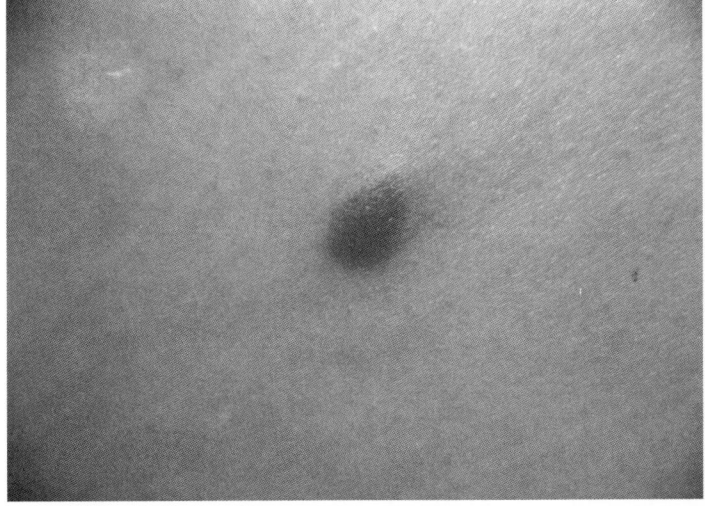

FIGURE 440-20. Cutaneous MALT (mucosa-associated lymphoid tissue) lymphoma.

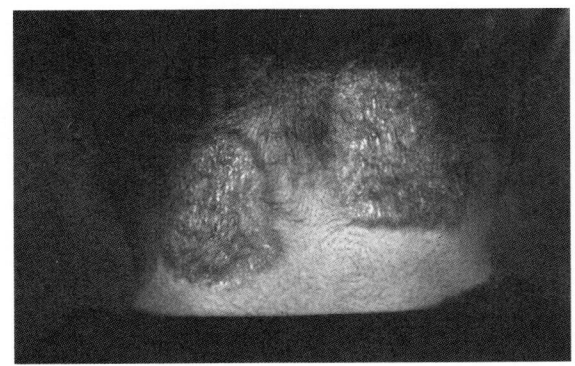

FIGURE 440-21. Cutaneous sarcoidosis.

Sweet syndrome, also called febrile neutrophilic dermatosis (Fig. 440-23), is accompanied by fever, leukocytosis, and tender reddish skin plaques. Some patients also have arthralgia. Biopsy shows sheets of leukocytes filling the upper dermis in the absence of infection. It can be idiopathic; drug induced; or associated with an underlying disease, typically with an underlying streptococcal infection, acute myelogenous leukemia, other malignancies, inflammatory bowel disease, or rheumatoid arthritis.[11] Use of hematopoietic growth factors also can precipitate Sweet syndrome. Sweet syndrome, but not erythema elevatum diutinum, is highly responsive to corticosteroids (oral prednisone 1-2 mg/kg/day gradually tapered over 6 weeks to 3 months) or indomethacin (150 mg per day for 1 week; then 100 mg per day for 2 weeks), but oral dapsone (100-200 mg/day) can improve both conditions.

Erythema elevatum diutinum is manifested as multiple, infiltrated pink, yellow, red, or violaceous nodules or papules that may be painful or asymptomatic. The lesions can coalesce to form gyrate lesions on the dorsum of the hands or extensor surfaces similar to granuloma annulare. Erythema elevatum diutinum is associated with upper respiratory infections (especially *Streptococcus* spp.), HIV infection, and inflammatory bowel disease. Clinically, the lesions look similar to Sweet syndrome, but their underlying histopathology (a necrotizing vasculitis with neutrophils and hyalinization of the vessels) can be distinguished from the neutrophils seen in the upper dermis in Sweet syndrome on biopsy.

Polyarteritis Nodosa and Panniculitis

Polyarteritis nodosa (Chapter 270) arises in larger arterioles and may be associated with hepatitis C infection, mesenteric aneurysms, cryoglobulinemia, cutaneous ulceration, and livedo reticularis. Polyarteritis nodosa is distinct from small vessel leukocytoclastic vasculitis, which is characterized by smaller areas (a few millimeters) of purpura.

In the clinical setting, *panniculitis* occurs more frequently than nodular vasculitis. The diagnosis of vasculitis versus septal or lobular panniculitis requires an excisional biopsy, including fat, with appropriate cultures and stains.

Erythema nodosum (Fig. 440-24) is a septal panniculitis characterized by tender nodules that are 1 to 2 cm in diameter with warm, pink, overlying epidermis. They appear in crops on the extremities. A perivascular inflammatory infiltrate is present around small intralobular vessels without vasculitis.

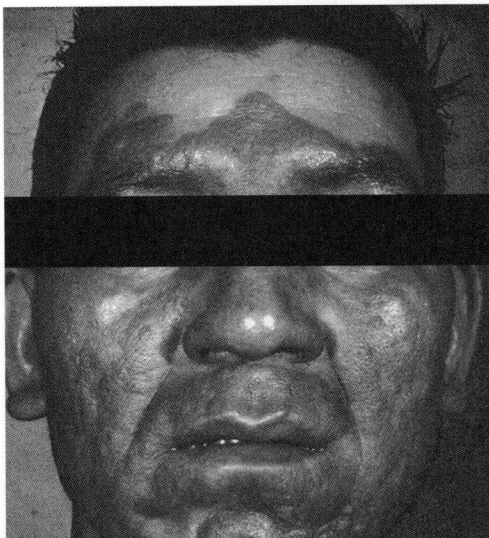

FIGURE 440-22. Leonine facies associated with lepromatous leprosy.

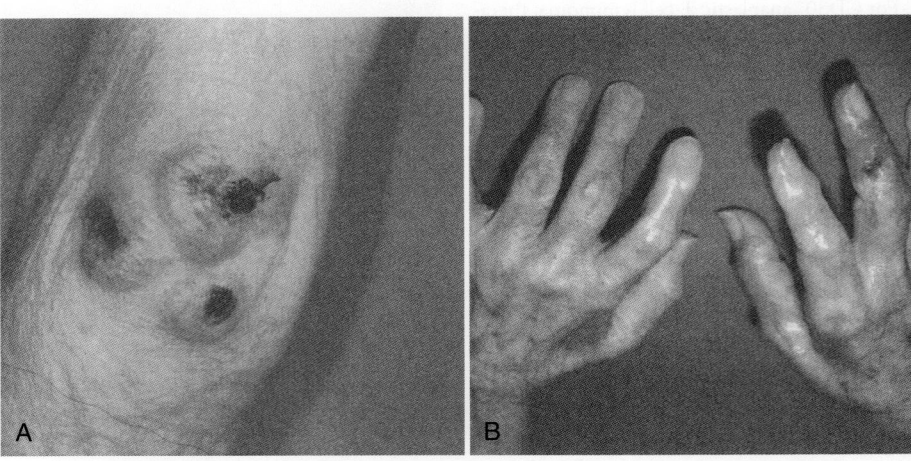

FIGURE 440-23. Sweet syndrome. A and B, Sweet syndrome in patients with leukemia.

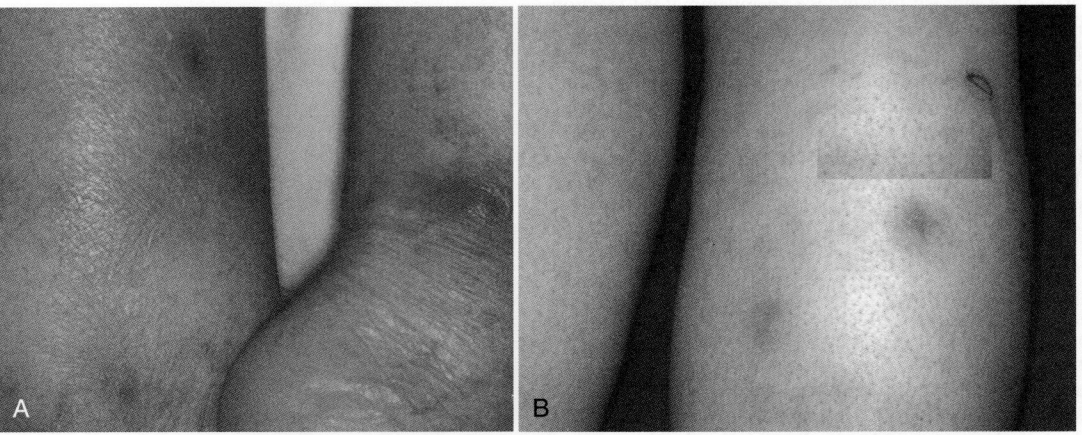

FIGURE 440-24. Erythema nodosum. A and B, Erythema nodosum and septal panniculitis of the lower extremities.

Erythema nodosum arises frequently in response to sarcoidosis (Chapter 95), various infections, inflammatory bowel disease, or drug use and less commonly in patients with azathioprine-induced pancreatitis or primary biliary cirrhosis. Often, however, the underlying cause remains unknown (Table 440-6).

Lobular panniculitis with necrosis and purpura is called nodular vasculitis or erythema induratum. Nodular vasculitis is characterized by painful, chronic recurrent nodules on the shin or thighs that become bluish, ulcerate, and heal with scarring. Erythema induratum (Fig. 440-25) is exacerbated by cold exposure and is sometimes associated with *Mycobacterium tuberculosis* (Chapter 325). True lobular panniculitis, with or without fat necrosis, is more frequent in men with underlying pancreatitis (Chapter 144) and may precede pancreatic cancer (Chapter 194). The lesions have a predilection for the anterior aspect of the shins and may be fluctuant as a result of fat necrosis. *Lupus panniculitis*, or lupus profundus, which involves the fat, is diagnosed by overlying granular immune complex deposition of IgM along the dermal-epidermal junction and is often difficult to distinguish from subcutaneous panniculitic T-cell lymphoma. Subcutaneous panniculitic γ/δ T-cell lymphoma is more aggressive and has a poor prognosis compared with α/β panniculitic T-cell lymphoma. Lupus panniculitis of the breast, which can be mistaken for adenocarcinoma, is treated with antimalarials or corticosteroids. Lobular panniculitis with calcification of the small arterioles, which occurs in the setting of renal failure with hyperparathyroidism, is called calciphylaxis (Chapter 130). Granulomatous lobular panniculitis may also arise in the setting of schistosomiasis (Chapter 355), Sjögren syndrome (Chapter 268), Crohn disease (Chapter 141), sarcoidosis (Chapter 95), ruptured epidermal cysts, atypical mycobacterial infection (Chapter 325), or tuberculosis (Chapter 324).

Fungal Infections

In immunocompromised patients, necrotic or granulomatous lobular panniculitis can be caused by disseminated fungal infections with *Candida* spp., *Sporothrix schenckii*, *Cryptococcus* spp., *Histoplasma* spp., *Nocardia* spp., *Rhizopus* spp., *Aspergillus* spp., *Fusarium* spp., or chromomycosis. Fungal mycelia invade vessel walls, where they produce purpuric and painful lesions that may

ulcerate. Osler nodes, which are tender nodular vasculitic lesions on the extremities, occur in the setting of bacterial endocarditis (Chapter 76). Staphylococcal or streptococcal sepsis may be manifested as pustules, papules, or panniculitic lesions.

● ATROPHIC AND SCLEROTIC LESIONS
Atrophic Lesions

Atrophic lesions result from thinning or loss of the epidermal and dermal layers (Table 440-7). Examples are photoaging caused by loss of epidermal thickness and collagen, discoid lupus, and genetic disorders of collagen production (e.g., Ehlers-Danlos syndrome; Fig. 440-26). Epidermal wrinkling can result in a cigarette paper appearance with prominence of the underlying blood vessels. High-potency topical corticosteroids cause loss of collagen,

TABLE 440-7	ATROPHIC SKIN CONDITIONS WITH SCARRING, ULCERATIONS, OR TELANGIECTASES

ATROPHY

Epidermal: chronic corticosteroid use, photoaging, mycosis fungoides
Dermal elastin: anetoderma, cutis laxa, intrinsic aging
Dermal collagen: Ehlers-Danlos syndrome, aging
Subcutaneous: granulomatous slack skin (a mycosis fungoides variant)
Lipodystrophy (loss of fat)

SCARRING OR ATROPHY WITH TELANGIECTASIAS

Discoid and subacute cutaneous lupus erythematosus
Dermatomyositis
Keloid formation
Large plaque parapsoriasis (poikiloderma vasculare atrophicans variant of mycosis fungoides)
Photoaging
Necrobiosis lipoidica diabeticorum
Radiation dermatitis
Porphyrias
Thermal burns (erythema ab igne)

SCLEROSIS OR INFILTRATIVE PROCESSES

Amyloidosis
Systemic sclerosis, scleroderma
Localized sclerosis, morphea
Lichen sclerosis et atrophicus
Lichen myxedematosus or papular mucinosis (mucopolysaccharide deposition with paraproteinemia)
Myxedema (mucin deposits with anti–thyroid-stimulating hormone receptor antibodies)

ULCERATIONS

Secondary breakdown of any blister or nodule: infectious, inflammatory, tumor, vasculitis
Decubitus or pressure ulcers
Genital ulcers: syphilis, herpes simplex, chancroid, lymphogranuloma venereum, Behçet syndrome
Pyoderma gangrenosum, Sweet syndrome

TABLE 440-6	TRIGGER FACTORS ASSOCIATED WITH ERYTHEMA NODOSUM

Infections
    Bacterial: *Streptococcus* spp., tuberculosis, leprosy, *Mycoplasma* spp., *Yersinia* spp., *Salmonella* spp., leptospirosis, tularemia
    Fungal: coccidioidomycosis, blastomycosis, histoplasmosis, dermatophytosis
    Viruses and *Chlamydia*: paravaccinia, Epstein-Barr virus, lymphogranuloma venereum, cat-scratch disease, psittacosis, hepatitis B

Drugs: sulfonamides, bromides, oral contraceptives

Malignancies: lymphoma, leukemia, carcinoma, after tumor radiation

Inflammatory: ulcerative colitis, Crohn disease, Whipple disease, Behçet syndrome, Sweet syndrome, collagen vascular diseases

Pregnancy

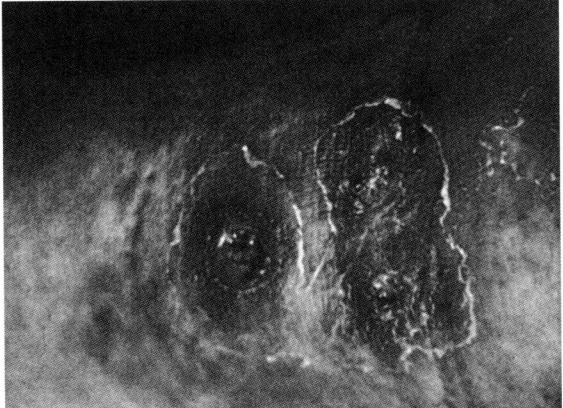

FIGURE 440-25. Erythema induratum.

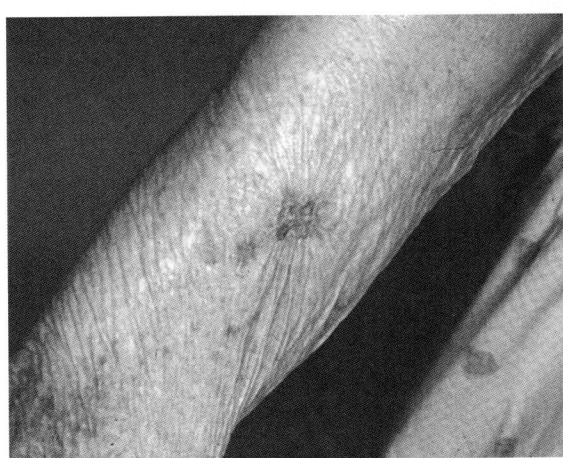

FIGURE 440-26. Atrophic skin in Ehlers-Danlos syndrome type 2.

resulting in atrophy. In Cushing syndrome (Chapter 227), striae appear as red or purple streaks because the underlying dermis can be seen through the epidermis.

Aging skin is most pronounced in sun-exposed areas, but intrinsic aging beginning as early as 30 years of age is characterized by abnormalities in the formation of elastin fibers. Aging of the skin is accompanied by decreased rete ridges and diminished circulation. Sunlight ages the skin by inducing proteolytic enzymes that digest the underlying collagen and elastin (wrinkles). In addition, sun exposure induces pigment incontinence (freckling), increased junctional nevi, and proliferation of benign keratinocyte growths (seborrheic keratoses).

Atrophy can also result from ongoing inflammatory processes that cause scarring, such as collagen vascular disease or mycosis fungoides. The cutaneous and discoid forms of lupus erythematosus (Chapter 266) are manifested as scaly plaques with atrophy or alopecia on sun-exposed areas; the systemic form is characterized by malar rash, urticaria, or vasculitic lesions. Dermatomyositis (Chapter 269) can be associated with collagen vascular disease or malignancy; periorbital suffusion, telangiectasia of the nail beds, and Gottron papules or scaly lesions over the joints are the skin manifestations. Anetodermas are localized sclerotic lesions (Fig. 440-27) with distinctive clinical features from underlying inflammation.

Eosinophilic fasciitis is accompanied by nodules or sclerosis of the lower extremities, myopathy, pulmonary disease, and eosinophilia. This syndrome, which follows the ingestion of L-tryptophan or its contaminants, resembles the panniculitis seen in systemic sclerosis, in which fat lobules are replaced by new collagen formation. Eosinophilic cellulitis, or Wells syndrome, is manifested as nodules, papules, or ulcerative lesions, as well as red plaques in which eosinophils infiltrate the area between collagen fibers.

Sclerotic Lesions

Sclerotic lesions are accompanied by more collagen production, which results in skin with a glossy appearance. Sclerosis may also result from the accumulation of mucopolysaccharides in scleromyxedema (lichen myxedematosus) or from amyloid deposits. Papular mucinosis, lichen myxedematosus (Fig. 440-28), and scleromyxedema are a spectrum of diseases that are caused by deposition of hyaluronic acid. An entity associated with renal failure and gadolinium exposure, nephrogenic fibrosing dermopathy[12] (Fig. 440-29), is also characterized by acral fibrosis and deposition of hyaluronate in the skin. In scleroderma (Chapter 267), increased collagen deposition may be associated with Raynaud syndrome, calcinosis, and telangiectasia. A localized form of scleroderma, termed *morphea,* may occur down the center of the face (coup de sabre) or as plaques on the extremities (Fig. 440-30), after radiation exposure, or with *Borrelia* spp. infection. Lichen sclerosis et atrophicus is a superficial inflammatory morphea characterized by white atrophic patches, especially in the genital region. Widespread systemic sclerosis may also follow bone marrow transplantation in the setting of chronic graft-versus-host disease.

Telangiectasia

Telangiectasia is prominence of skin blood vessels that frequently accompanies atrophic as well as sclerotic processes and is common in photoaged skin and after radiation therapy. Telangiectasia of the mucous membranes is found in Osler-Weber-Rendu syndrome (Chapter 173), and vascular spiders are

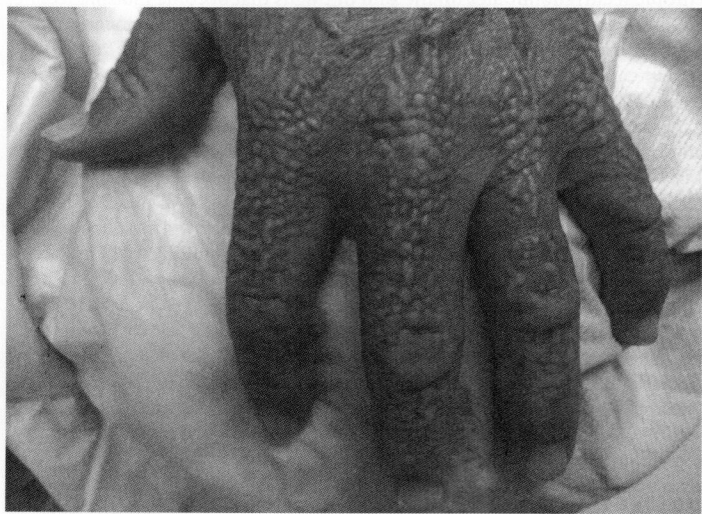

FIGURE 440-28. Lichen myxedematosus.

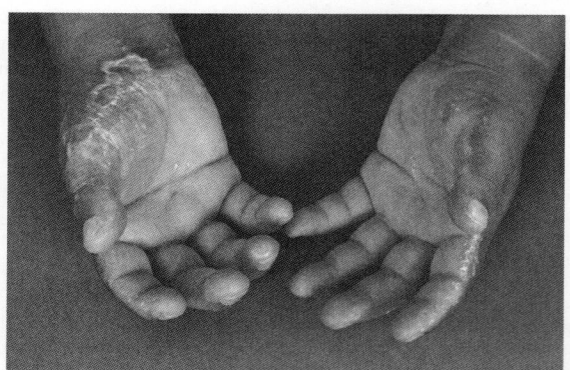

FIGURE 440-29. Nephrogenic fibrosing dermopathy.

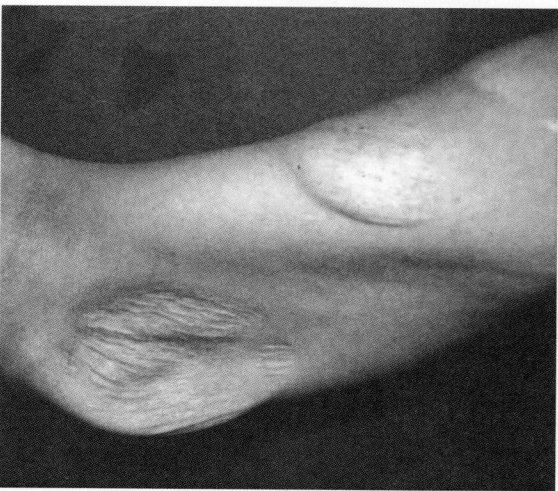

FIGURE 440-27. Anetoderma.

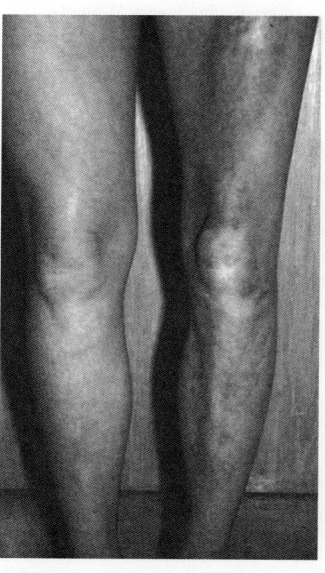

FIGURE 440-30. Linear morphea.

found both in α_1-antitrypsin deficiency and alcoholic liver disease. The presence of telangiectasia, hyperpigmentation, and hypopigmentation (poikiloderma) in sun-shielded areas of the body should alert the clinician to the diagnosis of early mycosis fungoides.

Ulcers

Ulcers are secondary skin lesions that may arise from trauma, loss of proper blood supply, aging, vasculitis, blister formation, infection, or underlying neoplasia. Ulcers may be shallow erosions (loss of the epidermis) or may be deeper and involve the dermis and underlying subcutaneous structures. Ulcers most commonly appear on the lower extremities, where they result from stasis dermatitis and venous insufficiency, arteriolar insufficiency, diabetic neuropathy, or vasculitis. *Pyoderma gangrenosum* is a trauma-induced ulcer that is part of the spectrum of Sweet syndrome, accompanies other conditions, and may require immunosuppressive therapy. Diagnosis requires skin biopsy, cultures, and serologic testing for other associated diseases. In contrast, decubitus ulcers require débridement, elimination of local pressure, and attention to nutrition.

Grade A References

A1. Sharma M, Bennett C, Cohen SN, et al. H1-antihistamines for chronic spontaneous urticaria. *Cochrane Database Syst Rev.* 2014;11:CD006137.
A2. Vena GA, Cassano N, Colombo D, et al. Cyclosporine in chronic idiopathic urticaria: a double-blind, randomized, placebo-controlled trial. *J Am Acad Dermatol.* 2006;55:705-709.
A3. Maurer M, Rosen K, Hsieh H, et al. Omalizumab for the treatment of chronic idiopathic or spontaneous urticaria. *N Engl J Med.* 2013;368:924-935.
A4. Lebwohl M, Swanson N, Anderson LL, et al. Ingenol mebutate gel for actinic keratosis. *N Engl J Med.* 2012;366:1010-1019.
A5. Hogeling M, Adams S, Wargon O. A randomized controlled trial of propranolol for infantile hemangiomas. *Pediatrics.* 2011;128:e259-e266.

GENERAL REFERENCES

For the General References and other additional features, please visit Expert Consult at https://expertconsult.inkling.com.

441

INFECTIONS, HYPERPIGMENTATION AND HYPOPIGMENTATION, REGIONAL DERMATOLOGY, AND DISTINCTIVE LESIONS IN BLACK SKIN

JEAN BOLOGNIA

INFECTIONS, INCLUDING CELLULITIS

Cutaneous infections can be divided into four major categories: bacterial, fungal (Chapter 438), viral, and parasitic (Table 441-1).

Bacterial Infections

Of the cutaneous bacterial infections, impetigo, folliculitis, furuncles, and cellulitis are most commonly encountered.

IMPETIGO

Impetigo, which is caused by *Staphylococcus aureus* or group A β-hemolytic streptococci, is usually seen as honey-colored crusts (Fig. 441-1); less often, subcorneal (superficial) bullae are present. This infection is most commonly found on the face in children, but it can develop at any site where the cutaneous barrier has been disrupted (e.g., areas of dermatitis, sites of trauma, or arthropod bites). A deeper, but less common, bacterial infection of the skin is ecthyma, which is most frequently streptococcal in origin; it is characterized by thick hemorrhagic crusts overlying erosions or ulcerations, usually 0.5 to 1.5 cm in diameter. These lesions favor the extremities, especially in the setting of lymphedema. Ecthyma should not be confused with ecthyma

TABLE 441-1 SKIN INFECTIONS

BACTERIAL DISEASES

Impetigo
Ecthyma
Folliculitis
Furuncle/carbuncle
Abscess
Erysipelas
Cellulitis
Necrotizing fasciitis
Ecthyma gangrenosum
Other
  Gram-negative cocci: Meningococcemia, gonococcemia
  Gram-positive bacilli: Erythrasma, anaerobic cellulitis
  Spirochetes: Lyme disease, syphilis, endemic treponematoses
  Mycobacteria
  Rickettsia

VIRAL DISEASES

Herpes simplex virus: Oral, genital
Human papillomavirus: Common warts, condyloma acuminata
Poxvirus: Molluscum contagiosum
Varicella-zoster virus
Viral exanthems (e.g., enteroviruses, rubeola, rubella, parvovirus, Epstein-Barr virus, adenovirus, dengue virus, human immunodeficiency virus [seroconversion])

FUNGAL DISEASES

Candidiasis
Tinea (dermatophytoses): pedis, corporis, cruris, manuum, capitis
Pityriasis (tinea) versicolor
Emboli (e.g., *Aspergillus, Mucor* spp)

ECTOPARASITES/PARASITES

Scabies
Lice: Scalp, pubic, body
Leishmaniasis
Schistosomiasis, human and animal
Onchocerciasis
Strongyloidiasis
Amebiasis
Trypanosomiasis
Hookworm infections, human and animal
Filariasis
Acanthamoebiasis

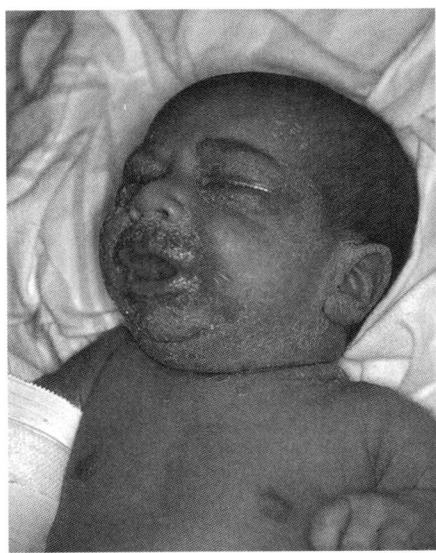

FIGURE 441-1. Impetigo in an infant and marked involvement of the face with honey-colored crusts and superficial erosions. (Courtesy Yale Dermatology Residents' Slide Collection.)

gangrenosum, which represents an embolic phenomenon most often caused by bacteremia with gram-negative bacilli. Although mild cases of impetigo usually respond to topical 2% mupirocin three times daily or 1% retapamulin twice daily, more severe impetigo and ecthyma require oral antibiotics that cover *S. aureus* (e.g., dicloxacillin, 250 mg orally [PO] four times daily, or

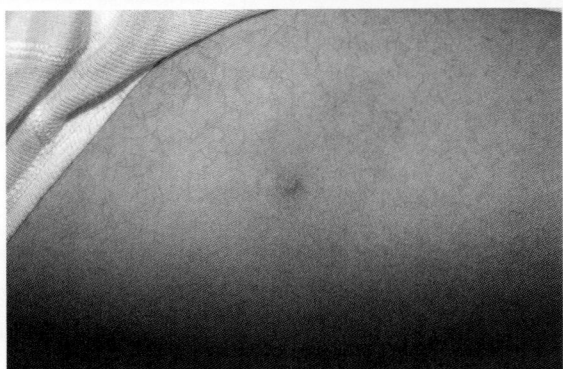

FIGURE 441-2. Furuncle with surrounding cellulitis. This common presentation of methicillin-resistant *Staphylococcus aureus* should be treated with incision and drainage, as well as the administration of systemic antibiotics. (Courtesy Yale Dermatology Residents' Slide Collection.)

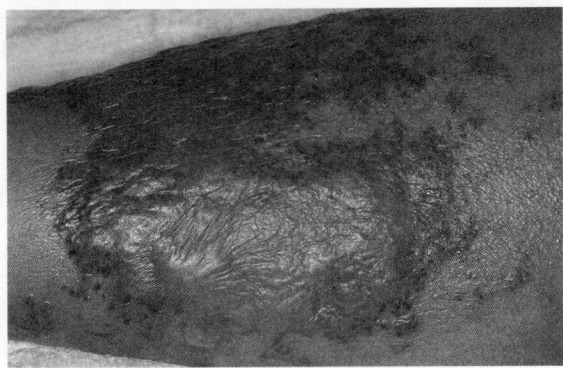

FIGURE 441-3. Bullous and hemorrhagic cellulitis of the shin. (Courtesy University of Southern California Dermatology Residents' Slide Collection.)

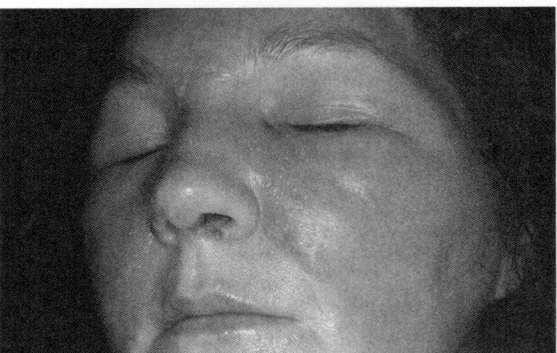

FIGURE 441-4. Erysipelas of the face with well-demarcated erythematous plaques. (Courtesy Yale Dermatology Residents' Slide Collection.)

cephalexin, 250 mg PO four times daily). Compared with furuncles and abscesses, impetigo is less often due to methicillin-resistant *S. aureus* (MRSA).

FOLLICULITIS

The initial lesions of folliculitis are follicular pustules that are often surrounded by a rim of erythema (Chapter 439). *Pseudomonas* folliculitis, which favors the trunk, is usually associated with the use of hot tubs or whirlpools because their higher temperatures (vs. swimming pools) make eradication of *Pseudomonas* more difficult (see Fig. 439-20).

FURUNCLES

Furuncles, also called *boils*, represent *S. aureus* cutaneous infections that are localized primarily within the dermis. In contrast to folliculitis, the lesions are larger and manifest as tender erythematous nodules (Fig. 441-2). A central follicular structure may be noted, as may a central pustule ("pointing"). Because a furuncle is an abscess, the preferred treatment is incision and drainage followed by oral antistaphylococcal antibiotics (e.g., dicloxacillin, 250 mg PO four times daily, or cephalexin, 250 mg PO four times daily); if MRSA is likely (e.g., use of health care facilities such as dialysis units, participation in skin-to-skin contact sports, an elevated prevalence of methicillin-resistant isolates in the local community), the antibiotic should be changed to clindamycin (300 to 600 mg PO three times daily), doxycycline (100 mg PO twice daily), minocycline (100 mg PO twice daily), trimethoprim-sulfamethoxazole (160 mg/800 mg PO twice daily), or linezolid (600 mg PO twice daily), depending on local sensitivity patterns.[1] The duration of therapy is usually 10 to 14 days. Carbuncles, which are larger, more complex, and more extensive versions of furuncles, may be accompanied by systemic symptoms such as fever. In addition to incision and drainage, they may require a more prolonged course of antibiotic therapy.

CELLULITIS

Cellulitis is a fairly common cutaneous infection that occurs most often on the lower extremities. Locally, it manifests as erythema, edema, warmth, and tenderness; systemic findings can include fever, malaise, and leukocytosis. Most cases are bacterial in origin, but some are caused by fungal infections (e.g., *Cryptococcus* spp) or chemical reactions (e.g., extravasated oxacillin or calcium salts). Bacterial cellulitis is most commonly caused by group A β-hemolytic streptococci and *S. aureus*, with the former being associated with the more severe, necrotizing variant. In patients who have diabetes or are immunocompromised, cellulitis can be caused by gram-negative bacilli or atypical mycobacteria. Risk factors include a preceding break in the skin barrier, edema secondary to venous hypertension, lymphedema, and previous bouts of cellulitis.

Although the diagnosis of cellulitis is usually fairly straightforward (Fig. 441-3), it can sometimes be difficult in patients with chronic lower extremity edema, especially in those who are afebrile and have persistent discoloration. One complication of chronic lower extremity edema is lipodermatosclerosis (i.e., inflammation followed by fibrosis of subcutaneous fat), which is seen acutely as erythema, warmth, and tenderness and is easily confused with cellulitis. The skin above the medial malleolus is often the initial site of involvement for lipodermatosclerosis, but the inflammation can extend onto the shin and calf. The chronic phase of lipodermatosclerosis is characterized

by induration, a permanent brown-red to violet discoloration of the skin, and an "inverted wine bottle" appearance of the distal end of the lower extremity. It is important for the clinician to realize that in patients with chronic lipodermatosclerosis and superimposed cellulitis, the skin will never return to the color of uninvolved skin, even after adequate antibiotic therapy.

Unless there is an associated bacteremia, the diagnosis of cellulitis is primarily clinical.[2] In immunocompromised hosts, a saline injection followed by aspiration and culture can be helpful. Histologically, cellulitis is characterized by an infiltrate of neutrophils within the dermis. Skin biopsy can exclude disorders that may be confused with cellulitis, such as contact dermatitis, erythema migrans, inflammatory carcinoma, toxic erythema of chemotherapy, and Wells syndrome (an idiopathic disorder in which eosinophils infiltrate the dermis). Treatment of cellulitis varies from oral cephalexin[A1] (250-500 mg four times daily for 10 to 14 days) to intravenous vancomycin plus intravenous ceftazidime (15 mg/kg twice daily and 0.5 to 1 g three times daily, respectively, until clinical response allows transition to oral medications), depending on the suspected pathogens, the host, and the severity of systemic toxicity. Penicillin (250 mg twice daily) is effective for preventing recurrent cellulitis.[A2]

Cellulitis resides in the middle of a spectrum of soft tissue infections that includes erysipelas (more superficial and more sharply demarcated; Fig. 441-4) at one end and necrotizing fasciitis (deeper, more necrotic, and undermining) at the other. In healthy adults, erysipelas can be treated with oral penicillin (200,000 units four times daily) or, if methicillin-sensitive *S. aureus* (MSSA) is of concern, oral dicloxacillin (500 mg four times daily) for a 10-day course. Necrotizing fasciitis is usually caused by multiple organisms, including anaerobic streptococci; its diagnosis requires a high index of suspicion, and it must be considered when there are areas of painful violaceous induration or a foul-smelling discharge. Prompt surgical débridement and broad-spectrum systemic antibiotics (e.g., a β-lactam/β-lactamase inhibitor such as intravenous piperacillin-tazobactam, 4.5 g every 6 hours for a total of 18 g/day [16 g piperacillin/2 g tazobactam]) for at least 2 weeks, are mandatory; addition of ciprofloxacin (500 mg PO or 400 mg intravenously [IV] twice daily), metronidazole (500 mg IV three times daily), and vancomycin (15 mg/kg IV twice daily) depends on suspected pathogens. Unless only a single organism is seen on Gram stain and isolated on culture, broad-spectrum antibiotic coverage should be continued because of the polymicrobial nature of necrotizing fasciitis and the difficulty of culturing anaerobes.

Although *Clostridium perfringens* can cause anaerobic cellulitis and gas gangrene, the most common cutaneous infection by gram-positive bacilli is erythrasma, which manifests as interdigital toe web maceration with fissures, as well as shiny or scaly brown-red patches in the axillae and groin. The latter is often confused with tinea cruris (Chapter 438) and seborrheic dermatitis. A diagnostic finding is the presence of coral (orange-pink) fluorescence on Wood lamp illumination (ultraviolet A). The responsible organism is *Corynebacterium minutissimum*. Treatment options include topical and oral erythromycin (e.g., 333 mg three times daily for 7 to 14 days).

TOXIC ERYTHEMAS

Eruptions caused by the release of toxins (e.g., exfoliative toxins ET-A and ET-B, erythrogenic toxin) produced by *S. aureus* and streptococci include staphylococcal scalded skin syndrome (Chapters 288 and 439), scarlet fever (Chapter 290), and toxic shock syndrome (Chapter 439). Staphylococcal scalded skin syndrome (see Fig. 439-14) is characterized by large areas of tender erythema in which superficial desquamation (peeling) develops, often with scaling and crusting in a radial array around the mouth. The areas of erythema are sterile; the conjunctivae, nasopharynx, or a distant site on the skin is the usual site of the primary staphylococcal infection. A clue to the diagnosis of scarlet fever is the presence of a strawberry tongue with prominent red papillae. Management involves treatment of the systemic infection (Chapters 288 and 439).

NEISSERIA INFECTIONS

Both gonococcemia (Chapter 299) and meningococcemia (Chapter 298) can manifest with cutaneous lesions. The former gives rise to a small number of vesicopustules on an erythematous base, generally acral in location (Fig. 441-5); these lesions represent septic emboli and are accompanied by fever, arthritis, and tenosynovitis. The earliest lesions of acute meningococcemia may be subtle (macular areas of erythema), but central hemorrhage (petechiae and purpura) and necrosis (gun-metal gray color) soon follow (Fig. 441-6). When accompanied by disseminated intravascular coagulation, large areas of retiform purpura and severe peripheral ischemia may develop. Cutaneous involvement in chronic meningococcemia is a reflection of lymphocytic or leukocytoclastic vasculitis. Management is systemic treatment (Chapters 298 and 299).

PSEUDOMONAS INFECTIONS

Pseudomonas infections of the skin vary from "hot tub" folliculitis (Chapter 439) to soft tissue infections of the external ear. Interdigital toe web infections that begin as simple tinea pedis can be complicated by superimposed *Pseudomonas* infection and result in erythema, swelling, tenderness, and drainage. Depending on its severity, treatment varies from topical antiseptics to oral or intravenous fluoroquinolones (e.g., ciprofloxacin, 500 mg PO twice daily for 7 to 14 days). In immunocompromised hosts, *Pseudomonas* and other gram-negative bacilli can produce cellulitis and secondary septic emboli in the skin. The latter begin as purpura or purpuric bullae in which central necrosis then develops. These lesions, which arise as a result of ischemic infarction of the skin, are termed *ecthyma gangrenosum*. Management is treatment of the systemic pseudomonal disease (Chapter 306).

SPIROCHETES

Spirochetal infections have a wide range of skin findings, from erythema migrans secondary to *Borrelia burgdorferi* (Chapter 321), to endemic treponematoses such as yaws and pinta (Chapter 320), to the cutaneous manifestations of the three stages of syphilis (Chapter 319). Syphilitic lesions include a firm, generally nontender ulceration (chancre) in primary syphilis; a generalized papulosquamous eruption (Chapter 438) plus alopecia, oral ulcers, and condylomata lata in secondary syphilis; and thick plaques and ulcers in tertiary disease. Management involves treatment of the systemic disease.

MYCOBACTERIA INFECTIONS

Infections with *Mycobacterium tuberculosis* and mycobacteria other than *M. tuberculosis* (atypical mycobacteria) are associated with skin lesions, including verrucous or crusted papules, scarring granulomatous plaques, and draining ulcers. In immunocompetent hosts in developed countries, *Mycobacterium marinum* (Chapter 325) is most commonly associated with skin disease, which is usually manifested in a lymphocutaneous (i.e., sporotrichoid) pattern. Lower extremity furunculosis due to atypical mycobacteria can occur following pre-pedicure footbaths, and injection of tattoo ink contaminated with *Mycobacterium chelonae* can lead to erythematous papules.[3] Treatment of cutaneous mycobacterial disease is the same as for systemic disease (Chapters 324 and 325).

Viral Infections

The most common viral infections of the skin are verrucae (warts; see Fig. 439-2), recurrent oral and genital herpes simplex (Chapters 374 and 439), molluscum contagiosum (see Fig. 440-9), and exanthems (Chapter 439). Varicella and herpes zoster are seen less frequently (Chapter 375).

Fungal Infections

A variety of fungal infections involve the skin and nails and are most commonly due to dermatophytes (tinea), *Candida* spp, and *Malassezia* spp (pityriasis versicolor, also referred to as tinea versicolor) (Chapter 438; also see Table 441-1). Although both dermatophyte infections and pityriasis versicolor are associated with scaling, cutaneous candidiasis is characterized by erythema, a more erosive appearance, and satellite pustules. Treatment is described in Chapter 438.

Septic emboli caused by *Candida* or other opportunistic fungi such as *Aspergillus* (Chapter 339) or *Fusarium* often have a clinical appearance similar to that of ecthyma gangrenosum secondary to gram-negative rods such as *Pseudomonas*. The responsible organisms can be detected histologically in biopsy specimens or by bedside examination of dermal scrapings; culture confirms the specific organism. While rare, cutaneous plaques secondary to *Pneumocystis jiroveci* favor the internal ear. Treatment is for the underlying fungal infection.

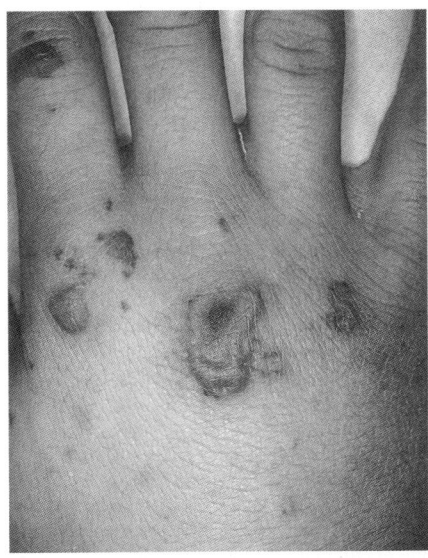

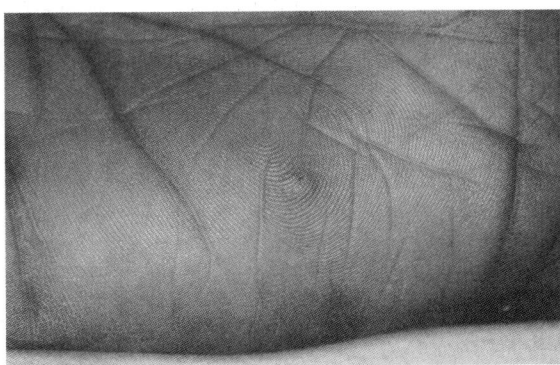

FIGURE 441-5. Disseminated gonococcal infection with an acral pustule on a red-violet base. (Courtesy Yale Dermatology Residents' Slide Collection.)

FIGURE 441-6. Purpuric and necrotic embolic lesions of meningococcemia. (Courtesy Yale Dermatology Residents' Slide Collection.)

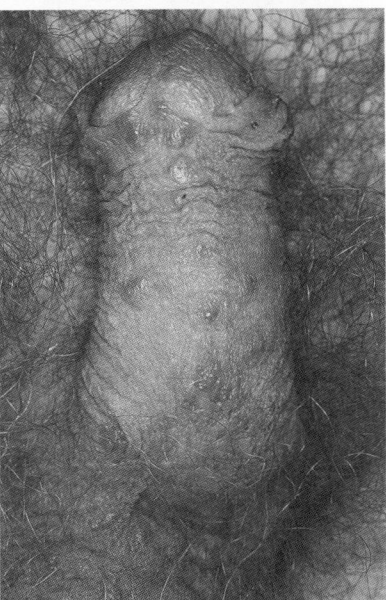

FIGURE 441-7. Scabies with involvement of the penis. (From Bolognia JL, Jorizzo JL, Schaffer JV, eds. *Dermatology*, 3rd ed. London: Elsevier; 2012.)

Ectoparasites and Parasites
ECTOPARASITES: SCABIES AND LICE

The most common ectoparasitic cutaneous infestations are (1) scabies from the human variant of the *Sarcoptes* mite; and (2) lice, of which there are three subtypes: head, body, and pubic. Scabies is characterized by pruritus in association with papules, papulovesicles, and linear burrows, as well as signs of scratching, such as excoriations and areas of dermatitis. Sites of predilection include the wrists, ankles, fingers, and toes (including the web spaces), areolae, and genitalia (especially the penis) (Fig. 441-7). The number of mites living within the stratum corneum is limited in immunocompetent hosts; when scraped and examined microscopically, linear burrows provide the highest yield of mites and eggs. In elderly and immunosuppressed patients, a form of scabies known as crusted (previously Norwegian) scabies manifests as multiple areas of scaling and crusting that are teeming with mites.

Infestations with scalp lice are seen most commonly in children, who may be asymptomatic or have marked pruritus. In addition to the lice, multiple egg casings ("nits") are attached to the proximal portions of scalp hairs. In developed countries, body lice are seen primarily in homeless individuals; patients typically have multiple erythematous papules at the sites of bites, as well as signs of scratching. The lice and their eggs are found in the patient's clothing. Pubic lice are sometimes called "crabs" because their bodies are shorter and broader than those of scalp or body lice and thus resemble the shape of a crab. Because of their leg span, these lice reside primarily on pubic hairs and less often on axillary hairs or eyelashes.

The first-line U.S. Food and Drug Administration–approved treatments for head lice, pubic lice, and routine scabies are topical 0.5% malathion lotion or gel, 5% permethrin cream, and 5% permethrin cream, respectively[4]; each of these topical medications is applied for 8 to 12 hours on days 1 and 8. Recently, topical ivermectin 0.5% lotion was also approved for the treatment of head lice.[5] For crusted scabies, epidemic outbreaks of scabies (e.g., in nursing homes), or difficult-to-treat head lice, oral ivermectin (250 to 400 µg/kg; off-label use) can eradicate the infestation.[A3] Treatment of body lice involves discarding egg- and lice-infested clothing; for head lice, potential sources of reinfection, such as hairbrushes, should be discarded. Sexual and household contacts of patients with pubic lice and scabies, respectively, must be treated similarly to the symptomatic patient.

OTHER PARASITES

Cutaneous lesions are seen in leishmaniasis (Chapter 348), amebiasis (Chapter 352), schistosomiasis (Chapter 355), onchocerciasis (Chapter 358), strongyloidiasis (Chapter 357), and hookworm infections (Chapter 357). Exposure to water infested with the cercariae of animal schistosomes results in multiple erythematous papules, which occur most commonly on the feet and are termed *swimmer's itch*. Dog and cat hookworm infections lead to cutaneous larva migrans, with serpiginous erythematous tracks that correspond to the path of migration of the hookworm larvae in sites where there has been direct contact with infected sand, most commonly the feet. Both of these infections are self-limited because the parasite's life cycle cannot be completed in humans. In immunocompromised hosts, cutaneous plaques can occasionally develop from free-living amebae such as *Acanthamoeba*.

● DISORDERS OF HYPOPIGMENTATION AND HYPERPIGMENTATION

Disorders of pigmentation can be divided into four major categories: diffuse, linear, circumscribed, and either reticulated (in the case of hyperpigmentation) or guttate (in the case of hypopigmentation) (Table 441-2).

Hypopigmentation
ALBINISM

The primary disorder of diffuse hypopigmentation is oculocutaneous albinism, an autosomal recessive disorder in which there is a pigmentary dilution

---

TABLE 441-2 DISORDERS OF PIGMENTATION

HYPOPIGMENTATION

Diffuse (Pigmentary Dilution)

Oculocutaneous albinism
Hermansky-Pudlak syndrome
Chédiak-Higashi syndrome
Generalized (total) vitiligo
Inborn errors of metabolism (e.g., phenylketonuria)

Circumscribed

Decrease in pigment
    Acquired: Postinflammatory hypopigmentation (e.g., atopic dermatitis, sarcoidosis, systemic lupus erythematosus, mycosis fungoides), pityriasis (tinea) versicolor secondary to *Malassezia* spp infection
    Congenital: Nevus depigmentosus, ash-leaf spots of tuberous sclerosis
Absence of pigment
    Acquired: Vitiligo, chemical leukoderma, leukoderma of scleroderma, leukoderma of melanoma
    Congenital: Piebaldism

Linear

Linear nevoid hypopigmentation, segmental nevus depigmentosus

Guttate

Idiopathic guttate hypomelanosis
Confetti macules of tuberous sclerosis

HYPERPIGMENTATION

Diffuse

Drug reactions (e.g., cyclophosphamide, busulfan)
Addison disease
Ectopic adrenocorticotropic hormone production (e.g., small cell lung cancer)
Hemochromatosis
Scleroderma
Primary biliary cirrhosis
Hyperthyroidism
Vitamin B$_{12}$ or folate deficiency
Porphyria cutanea tarda
POEMS syndrome (see Table 441-3)
Melanosis secondary to metastatic melanoma
Argyria (gray hue)

Circumscribed

Postinflammatory hyperpigmentation (e.g., acne vulgaris, arthropod bites, dermatitis, lichen planus)
Melasma
Pityriasis (tinea) versicolor
Mastocytosis
Fixed drug reactions
Deposits of drugs and their metabolites

Linear

Exposure to psoralen-containing plants (e.g., limes) plus ultraviolet A light
Drug reactions (e.g., bleomycin)
Linear nevoid hyperpigmentation
Genodermatoses (e.g., incontinentia pigmenti)

Reticulated

Erythema ab igne
Genodermatoses

of melanin-containing structures (i.e., the eyes, hair, and skin). The phenotype varies from total absence of melanin pigment to a subtle decrease whose recognition requires comparison with first-degree relatives; the density of melanocytes in skin is normal, but their ability to produce pigment is absent or decreased. Ninety percent of patients with oculocutaneous albinism have mutations in the genes that encode either tyrosinase (type I) or P protein (type II). Complications of oculocutaneous albinism include decreased visual acuity, nystagmus, photophobia, and an increase in cutaneous carcinomas, especially squamous cell carcinoma. These signs and symptoms are most severe in those who produce the least pigment and have the greatest amount of cumulative sun exposure. The differential diagnosis includes total vitiligo (absence of melanocytes histologically) and a few inborn errors of metabolism (e.g., phenylketonuria). Treatment consists of longitudinal ophthalmologic care and minimizing sun exposure.

LINEAR HYPOPIGMENTATION

Disorders of linear hypopigmentation consist primarily of nevoid conditions (e.g., linear nevoid hypopigmentation, segmental nevus depigmentosus), in which streaks of hypomelanosis follow the Blaschko lines, or patients have blocklike hypopigmented patches due to mosaicism. A minority of patients have associated central nervous system and musculoskeletal abnormalities (hypomelanosis of Ito).

CIRCUMSCRIBED (PATCHY) HYPOPIGMENTATION
Vitiligo

Vitiligo (Fig. 441-8) is usually slowly progressive and occurs principally in periorificial areas (around the eyes, nose, lips, genitalia) and the hands, feet, flexor surface of the wrists, ankles, elbows, knees, and major body folds. Vitiligo, which is caused by a loss of melanocytes within the skin, is also associated with autoimmune endocrinopathies and alopecia areata. T cells that recognize antigens on the surface of melanocytes (and melanoma cells) are found within the skin and in peripheral blood. Treatment includes topical corticosteroids, topical immunomodulators (e.g., tacrolimus), and phototherapy.[Ad] The differential diagnosis is primarily chemical leukoderma secondary to compounds that are cytotoxic to melanocytes (e.g., catechols, phenols), the leukoderma of melanoma (a good prognostic sign if seen in association with immunotherapy but an indication to exclude metastases if occurs spontaneously), and the leukoderma of scleroderma with retention of perifollicular pigmentation.

Guttate Hypopigmentation

Idiopathic guttate hypomelanosis, in which there are well-demarcated hypopigmented macules usually measuring 2 to 4 mm in diameter, is the most common cause of guttate ("raindrop") leukoderma (Fig. 441-9). The favored sites for this common age-related disorder, which may be related to chronic sun exposure, are the shins and the extensor surface of the forearms.

Other Acquired Causes

Circumscribed hypomelanosis is seen in patients with pityriasis (tinea) versicolor (see Fig. 438-29) and postinflammatory hypopigmentation. Although postinflammatory hypopigmentation is most often associated with atopic

dermatitis, it also can occur with sarcoidosis (Chapter 95), lupus erythematosus (Chapter 266), and mycosis fungoides (Chapter 185).

Congenital Causes

Congenital circumscribed areas of hypomelanosis include *nevus depigmentosus,* a common tan "birthmark" seen in 1 in 50 infants in whom there is a partial decrease in pigment; *piebaldism,* an unusual autosomal dominant disorder with areas of complete absence of pigment caused by mutations in the *KIT* gene; *nevus anemicus,* a localized area of vasoconstriction; and the *ash-leaf spots* of tuberous sclerosis (Chapter 417), with a partial decrease in pigment.

Hyperpigmentation
DIFFUSE HYPERPIGMENTATION

Diffuse hyperpigmentation is most commonly due to drugs (e.g., cyclophosphamide, zidovudine) and endocrinopathies associated with increased circulating levels of adrenocorticotropic hormone (ACTH) (e.g., Addison disease [Chapter 227], ectopic ACTH production by tumors such as small cell lung carcinoma [Chapter 191]). ACTH, as well as melanocyte-stimulating hormone, can bind and activate the melanocortin-1 receptors on melanocytes, thereby leading to increased melanin production. Additional causes include hemochromatosis (Chapter 212), scleroderma (Chapter 267), primary biliary cirrhosis (Chapter 155), POEMS syndrome (*p*olyneuropathy, *o*rganomegaly, *e*ndocrinopathy, *m*onoclonal protein, *s*kin changes (Table 441-3), and hyperthyroidism (Chapter 226). Systemic exposure to silver (argyria; Chapter 22) can lead to a slate-gray color.

TABLE 441-3	CUTANEOUS FINDINGS IN POLYNEUROPATHY, ORGANOMEGALY, ENDOCRINOPATHY, MONOCLONAL (M) PROTEIN, AND SKIN CHANGES (POEMS) SYNDROME

Diffuse hyperpigmentation
Vascular tumors, including glomeruloid hemangiomas
Peripheral edema
Induration (sclerodermoid)
Hypertrichosis
Hyperhidrosis
Acrocyanosis
Clubbing and/or leukonychia
Acquired facial lipoatrophy
Livedo reticularis

POEMS = polyneuropathy, organomegaly, endocrinopathy, monoclonal protein, skin changes.

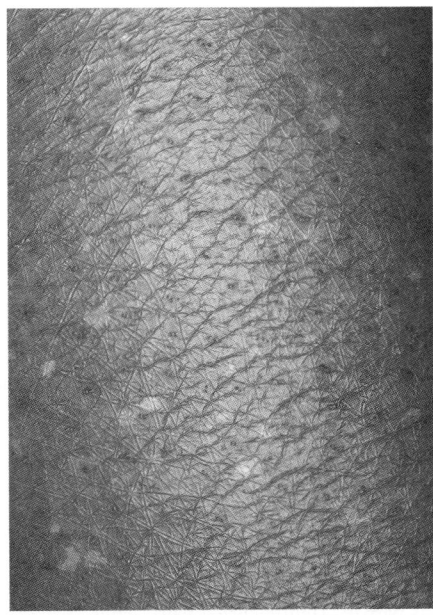

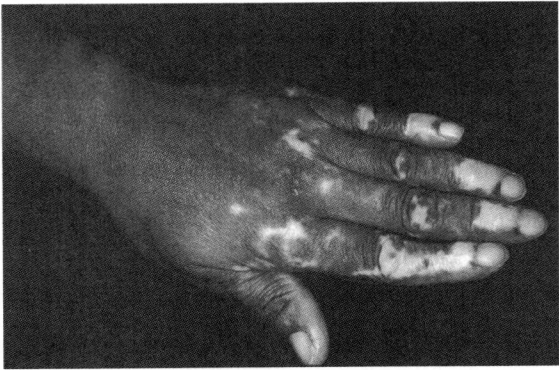

FIGURE 441-8. Striking leukoderma of the hand in a patient with vitiligo. In well-developed lesions, the skin is white, not tan, in color.

FIGURE 441-9. Idiopathic guttate hypomelanosis with small, well-demarcated hypopigmented macules on the shin.

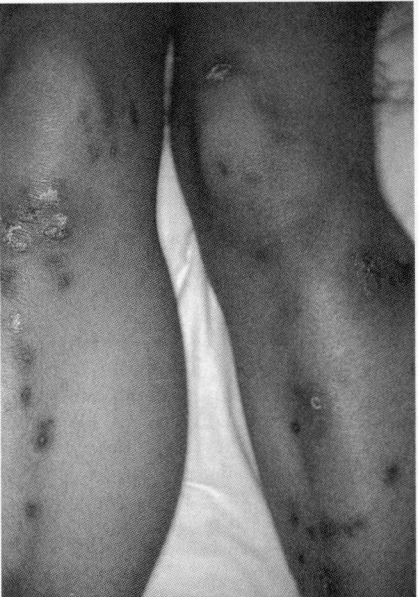

FIGURE 441-10. Postinflammatory hyperpigmentation secondary to arthropod bites. (Courtesy Yale Dermatology Residents' Slide Collection.)

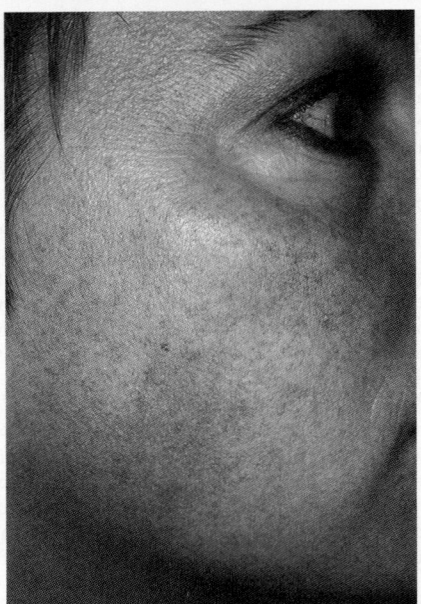

FIGURE 441-11. Hyperpigmented patches on the cheek in a patient with melasma.

LINEAR AND RETICULATED HYPERPIGMENTATION

Linear streaks of hyperpigmentation can be due to nevoid conditions that reflect cutaneous mosaicism, as in linear hypopigmentation (see earlier) and in genodermatoses (e.g., incontinentia pigmenti, which is an X-linked dominant disorder caused by mutations in the gene *NEMO*), or due to exposure to either plant-derived psoralens (e.g., from limes) plus ultraviolet A irradiation or systemic bleomycin (flagellate pigmentation). Reticulated hypermelanosis is also seen in several genodermatoses (e.g., dyskeratosis congenita) and after chronic exposure to heat (erythema ab igne). The latter corresponds to the cutaneous venous plexus and is seen most commonly in the lumbosacral region where heating pads have been applied or on the anterior thighs from laptop computers.

CIRCUMSCRIBED (PATCHY) HYPERPIGMENTATION

The most common causes of circumscribed hypermelanosis are pityriasis (tinea) versicolor (which can present as both hypopigmentation and hyperpigmentation, hence its name), postinflammatory hyperpigmentation, and melasma. Postinflammatory hyperpigmentation (Fig. 441-10) is observed more frequently in darkly pigmented individuals and often follows acne vulgaris,[6] arthropod bites, chronic dermatitis, and lichen planus. Additional causes of circumscribed darkening of the skin are cutaneous mastocytosis (urticaria pigmentosa; Chapter 255), deposits of drugs such as antimalarials and minocycline (blue-gray discoloration), and medications that produce fixed drug reactions, most frequently trimethoprim-sulfamethoxazole and nonsteroidal anti-inflammatory drugs. In melasma (Fig. 441-11), symmetrical hyperpigmented patches are seen on the lateral aspect of the forehead, upper part of the cheek, and mandibular area. At least 90% of patients with melasma are women. The lesions are exacerbated by ultraviolet light and estrogen (oral contraceptives, pregnancy). Melasma is treated with daily broad-spectrum sunscreens plus lightening agents such as hydroquinone (4% cream) and retinoic acid (0.025 to 0.10% cream) for 3 to 4 months, often in combination with mild topical corticosteroids to reduce irritation[7]; if irritation develops, the creams are discontinued temporarily and then restarted at a reduced frequency.

● DISTINCTIVE LESIONS IN BLACK SKIN

Although some diseases are more common in patients of African ancestry (e.g., tinea capitis, pseudofolliculitis barbae, dissecting cellulitis), others are simply more noticeable (e.g., vitiligo and postinflammatory hypopigmentation) (Table 441-4). The explanation for the increased incidence is speculative in most instances, with the exception of curled hairs leading to pseudofolliculitis barbae. Tightly curled hairs, when shaved, are usually cut at an oblique angle, which results in a sharp tip at the distal end of the hair shaft that allows penetration of the skin adjacent to the hair follicle and

TABLE 441-4	DISORDERS SEEN MORE COMMONLY IN PATIENTS OF AFRICAN ANCESTRY
HEAD AND NECK	
Folliculitis decalvans/dissecting cellulitis	
Tinea capitis due to *Trichophyton tonsurans*	
Traction alopecia	
Central centrifugal cicatricial alopecia*	
Acne keloidalis nuchae	
Pseudofolliculitis barbae	
Pomade acne	
Dermatosis papulosa nigra	
Inherited patterned lentiginosis	
Melasma	
Discoid lupus erythematosus	
PALMAR	
Keratosis punctata of the palmar creases	
LOWER EXTREMITIES	
Ulcers secondary to sickle cell anemia	
GENERALIZED	
Keloids	
Cutaneous sarcoidosis	
Papular eczema and follicular-based inflammation	

*Also termed *follicular degeneration syndrome* or *hot comb alopecia*.

subsequent inflammation. Some cutaneous disorders are seen less commonly in black skin (e.g., acne rosacea and scabies).

Another entity seen more commonly in individuals of African descent is keloids (Fig. 441-12). Keloids generally appear at sites of trauma (e.g., ear piercing) but can occasionally develop spontaneously, especially on the trunk. In the former situation, they are thought to represent an exaggerated response to wound healing, with increased formation of collagen not only at the site of the trauma (as in hypertrophic scars) but also in adjacent, previously uninvolved skin. Treatment options include intralesional corticosteroids, intralesional interferon, pulsed dye laser, or excision followed by radiation therapy.[8]

● REGIONAL DERMATOSES

Some common dermatoses have a predilection for particular anatomic sites (Fig. 441-13 and Table 441-5). These locations can help narrow the differential and guide further diagnostic testing and therapy in many patients.

One regional dermatosis is acanthosis nigricans (Fig. 441-14). Because of its potential systemic implications, careful medical evaluation is required (Table 441-6).

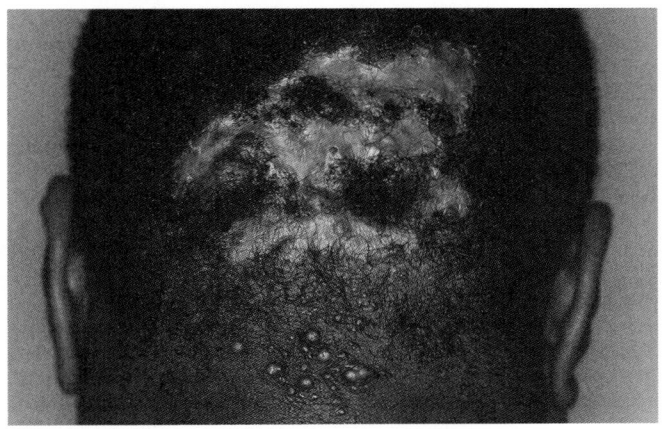

FIGURE 441-12. Acne keloidalis in an African American man. (Courtesy Kalman Watsky, MD.)

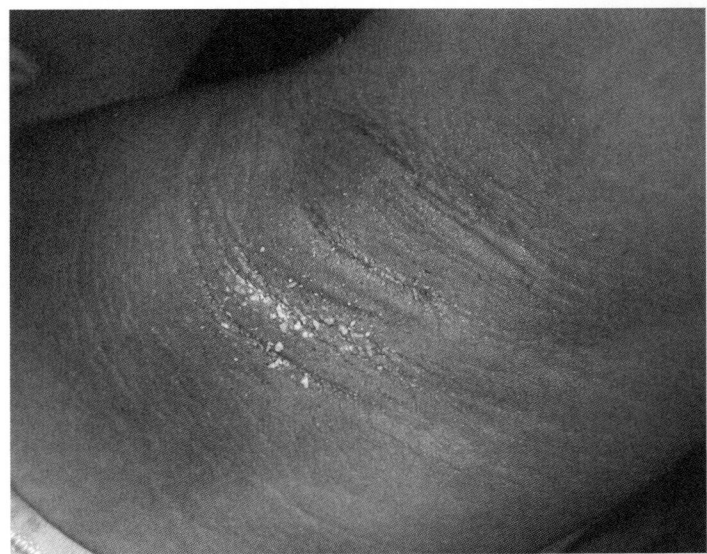

FIGURE 441-14. Acanthosis nigricans of the axilla. Note the velvet-like appearance of the skin. (Courtesy Yale Dermatology Residents' Slide Collection.)

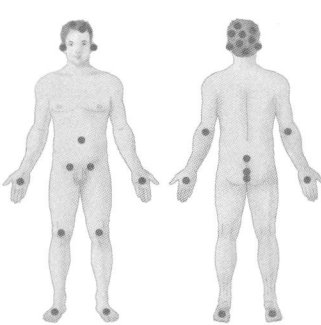

Psoriasis

Scalp, ears, scalpline
Palms, soles
Dorsal hands, feet
Elbows, knees/shins
Presacrum
Intergluteal fold
Nails

Inverse Psoriasis

Submammary
Inguinal fold
Umbilicus

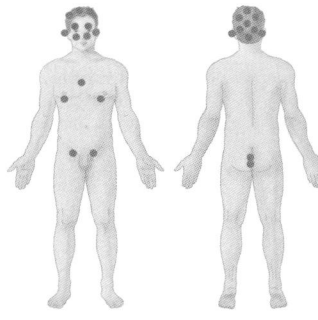

Seborrheic Dermatitis

Scalp, ears, postauricular
Eyebrows
Nasolabial folds
Central chest
Intergluteal fold
Submammary
Inguinal fold

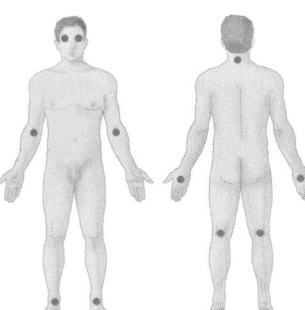

Atopic Dermatitis (adults)

Eyelids
Antecubital fossa
Popliteal fossa
Posterior neck
Ankles
Hands

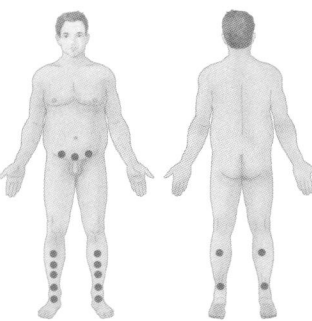

Stasis Dermatitis (adults)

Legs, below knees, but
  greater on shins than
  calves
Lower pannus

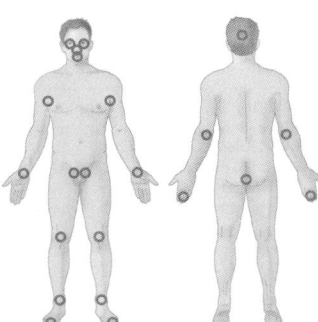

Vitiligo

Loss of color:
Around eyes
Around nose
Around mouth
Axillae, groin
Wrists (flexor)
Poliosis (streak of
  white hairs)
Elbows, knees, ankles
Backs of hands/feet
  (includes digits)
Perianal

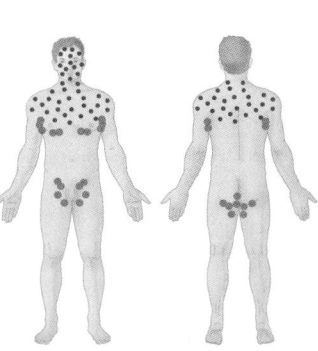

**Acne Vulgaris/
Hidradenitis Suppurativa**

∴ = papulopustules,
      blackheads or
      whiteheads
      Face/neck/upper
      trunk/shoulders

● = nodules of hidradenitis
      suppurativa

FIGURE 441-13. Regional involvement of specific skin diseases.

TABLE 441-5   REGIONAL DERMATOLOGY

REGION OF SKIN	TYPE OF SKIN LESION	DISEASE PROCESS
Scalp	Papulosquamous and eczematous	Seborrheic dermatitis, psoriasis, tinea capitis, eczema (atopic, contact)
	Pustular	Folliculitis, kerion
	Papulonodular	Melanocytic nevi, seborrheic keratoses, pilar cysts, verrucae, hemangiomas, actinic keratoses (bald scalp)
Face	Pustular	Acne, rosacea, folliculitis (beard), tinea
	Papulosquamous and eczematous	Seborrheic dermatitis, psoriasis (hairline), contact dermatitis (e.g., cosmetics), atopic dermatitis, impetigo, systemic lupus erythematosus, photodermatitis
	Vesicular	Herpes simplex, herpes zoster, bullous impetigo
	Papulonodular	Melanocytic nevi, actinic keratoses, seborrheic keratoses, sebaceous hyperplasia, basal cell carcinomas, squamous cell carcinomas, melanomas
	Atrophic and telangiectatic	Discoid lupus erythematosus
Trunk	Papulosquamous and eczematous	Psoriasis, atopic dermatitis, contact dermatitis, tinea versicolor, pityriasis rosea, scabies, secondary syphilis, subacute cutaneous lupus (upper trunk)
	Vesiculobullous	Bullous pemphigoid, pemphigus, erythema multiforme/Stevens-Johnson syndrome, herpes zoster
	Maculopapular	Morbilliform drug reactions, viral exanthems
	Papulonodular	Melanocytic nevi, seborrheic keratoses, angiomas, lipomas, epidermoid inclusion cysts, basal and squamous cell carcinomas, keloids, neurofibromas, melanoma
	Pustular	Acne, folliculitis
	Urticarial	Hives, drug reactions, early herpes zoster
Arms and forearms	Eczematous and papulosquamous	Contact dermatitis (e.g., plants), atopic dermatitis, psoriasis, lichen planus, photodermatitis (drugs, contactants, dermatomyositis, subacute cutaneous lupus)
	Papulonodular	Melanocytic nevi, verrucae, seborrheic keratoses, actinic keratoses, squamous cell carcinomas, polymorphic light eruption, rheumatoid nodules (elbows), xanthomas (elbows)
	Purpuric	Actinic (solar) purpura
	Annular	Granuloma annulare, subacute cutaneous lupus
Legs	Eczematous and papulosquamous	Stasis dermatitis, eczema craquelé (xerotic eczema), contact dermatitis, atopic dermatitis, psoriasis, lichen planus
	Papulonodular	Melanocytic nevi, dermatofibromas, erythema nodosum, melanoma, xanthomas (knees, Achilles tendon), Kaposi sarcoma
	Purpuric	Schamberg disease (capillaritis), vasculitis
	Ulcerative	Stasis ulcers, arterial insufficiency, pyoderma gangrenosum, trauma, livedoid vasculopathy, squamous cell carcinoma, diffuse dermal angiomatosis
Genitalia and groin	Eczematous and papulosquamous	Seborrheic dermatitis, tinea, psoriasis, contact dermatitis, scabies, reactive arthritis (Reiter syndrome), erythrasma, candidiasis, lichen planus, lichen simplex chronicus
	Vesiculobullous	Herpes simplex, Stevens-Johnson syndrome
	Ulcerative	Herpes simplex, syphilis, chancroid, Behçet disease, squamous cell carcinoma, trauma
	Papulonodular	Condyloma acuminata, molluscum contagiosum, angiokeratomas, epidermoid inclusion cysts, hidradenitis suppurativa, squamous cell carcinoma
	Pustular	Folliculitis, candidiasis, hidradenitis suppurativa
Hands	Eczematous and papulosquamous	Irritant and allergic contact dermatitis, atopic dermatitis, tinea, scabies, secondary syphilis
	Vesiculobullous, pustular	Dyshidrotic eczema, erythema multiforme, hand-foot-and-mouth disease (palmar), porphyria cutanea tarda (dorsal), epidermolysis bullosa acquisita, herpetic whitlow, blistering dactylitis, psoriasis (palmar)
	Papulonodular	Warts, actinic keratoses (dorsal), squamous cell carcinomas (dorsal), pyogenic granuloma, granuloma annulare, digital mucous cysts (dorsal fingers)
	Depigmentation	Vitiligo, chemical leukoderma
	Cuticular telangiectases	Scleroderma, dermatomyositis, systemic lupus erythematosus, Osler-Weber-Rendu disease
Feet	Eczematous and papulosquamous	Tinea, psoriasis, contact dermatitis, atopic dermatitis, syphilis (plantar)
	Vesiculobullous	Tinea, arthropod bites, epidermolysis bullosa (inherited and acquired), erythema multiforme, hand-foot-and mouth disease (plantar)
	Papules	Verrucae (plantar), corns, perniosis
	Ulcerative	Neuropathic ulcers (plantar)

TABLE 441-6   CLUES TO UNDERLYING SYSTEMIC CONDITIONS ASSOCIATED WITH ADULT-ONSET ACANTHOSIS NIGRICANS

Polycystic ovary syndrome	Women with acne, hirsutism, and/or menstrual irregularities
Malignancy	Sudden onset, weight loss, inflamed seborrheic keratoses, tripe palms
Endocrinopathy	Consider type 2 diabetes, Cushing syndrome (striae, hypertension, central obesity, buffalo hump), hypothyroidism
Drug-induced	Especially niacin, human growth hormone, oral contraceptive agents, corticosteroids, protease inhibitors

Grade A References

A1. Pallin DJ, Binder WD, Allen MB, et al. Clinical trial: comparative effectiveness of cephalexin plus trimethoprim-sulfamethoxazole versus cephalexin alone for treatment of uncomplicated cellulitis—a randomized controlled trial. *Clin Infect Dis.* 2013;56:1754-1762.

A2. Thomas KS, Crook AM, Nunn AJ, et al. Penicillin to prevent recurrent leg cellulitis. *N Engl J Med.* 2013;368:1695-1703.

A3. Chosidow O, Giraudeau B, Cottrell J, et al. Oral ivermectin versus malathion lotion for difficult-to-treat head lice. *N Engl J Med.* 2010;362:896-905.

A4. Whitton ME, Pinart M, Batchelor J, et al. Interventions for vitiligo. *Cochrane Database Syst Rev.* 2010;1:CD003263.

GENERAL REFERENCES

For the General References and other additional features, please visit Expert Consult at https://expertconsult.inkling.com.

442

DISEASES OF HAIR AND NAILS

ANTONELLA TOSTI

HAIR DISORDERS

Normal Hair

The hair shaft is a fully keratinized structure that is produced by the hair follicle. The entire skin, with the exception of the palms and soles, contains hair follicles. Hair follicles are of two types: terminal follicles and vellus follicles. Terminal follicles, which reach the hypodermis, produce terminal hairs, which are long, thick (60 to 80 μm), and pigmented. Terminal hairs are present since birth on the scalp, eyebrows, and eyelashes and later develop after puberty on the axillae, pubis, and beard region in males. Vellus follicles are small and localized to the superficial dermis and mid-dermis, where they produce vellus hairs, which are thin (<30 μm), short (<2 cm), and not pigmented and cover all the glabrous skin.

The hair follicle is formed by an upper permanent portion and a lower dynamic transient portion that migrates during the hair cycle. The transient portion includes the hair bulb, which is surrounded by the dermal papilla and contains the hair matrix that produces the hair shaft and its sheaths. The anatomic division between the permanent and the transient portion is just below the bulge region, which corresponds to the insertion of the erector pili muscle. The bulge region contains the epithelial stem cells that regenerate the follicle in each hair growth cycle; its damage results in stem cell destruction and cicatricial alopecia.

Hair Cycle

Hair follicles have a cyclic activity, characterized by alternating periods of hair shaft production and periods of resting (anagen, catagen, telogen). During the anagen phase, the follicles produce the hair shaft. Duration of anagen, which in the scalp ranges from 2 to 7 years, determines hair shaft length. Maximal length and growth rate of terminal hair varies in the different body regions. Scalp hair grows approximately 0.4 mm/day and may reach a length of more than 1 m. Maximal hair length decreases with age. During telogen, hair production is absent, even if the shaft remains within the follicle to be shed only when, after 3 months, the follicle reenters the anagen phase.

The hair cycle of adjacent scalp follicles is not synchronized. In normal conditions, approximately 85 to 90% of follicles are in anagen and 10 to 15% in telogen.

Hair Loss and Alopecias

Hair loss distresses most patients, independently from its severity and pattern. In some cases, the decrement in quality of life attributable to hair loss is comparable with that caused by major chronic diseases.

The first diagnostic step is to assess family history, drug intake, systemic illness, and severity and duration of hair loss (Table 442-1).[1] The second step is to establish whether the hair density is normal or decreased. The third step is to evaluate whether the rate of hair shedding is normal or increased. Acute and severe hair loss is typical of diseases that interrupt the mitotic activity of anagen follicles (drugs, alopecia areata). A normal hair density suggests telogen effluvium, which may be acute or chronic. A reduced hair density may involve the whole scalp (diffuse alopecia), may be limited to specific scalp regions (patterned alopecia), or may manifest with bald patches (patchy alopecia). In patchy alopecias, the scalp may show patches of alopecia that are completely devoid of hairs (alopecia areata, cicatricial alopecia) or have short broken hairs (trichotillomania, hair shaft disorders). Dermatoscopy is a rapid, noninvasive technique that greatly improves the clinical diagnosis of alopecias and hair shaft disorders in adults and children (Table 442-2).[2]

TELOGEN EFFLUVIUM

Acute Telogen Effluvium

Acute telogen effluvium results from noxious events that precipitate the entry of a large number of follicles into their resting phase (telogen). Possible causes include systemic diseases, drugs (Table 442-3), fever, stress, weight loss, delivery, iron deficiency, and inflammatory scalp disorders. For drugs, the severity of hair loss depends on the drug, its dosage, and the patient's susceptibility.[3]

Hair loss starts approximately 3 months after the causative event, a time frame that corresponds with the duration of the telogen phase. Telogen hairs are retained within the follicle during telogen, to be shed when the follicle produces a new anagen hair. Hair loss is severe when 100 to 200 hairs are shed daily. The patient usually remembers quite precisely when the increased shedding began. Acute telogen effluvium does not usually produce visible alopecia because approximately 50% of hairs need to be lost before reduction of hair density is evident.

TREATMENT AND PROGNOSIS   Rx

Acute telogen effluvium subsides spontaneously in a few months after removal of the cause. It may, however, unmask or aggravate androgenetic alopecia.

Chronic Telogen Effluvium

Chronic telogen effluvium, which is characterized by increased hair shedding lasting for more than 6 months, mostly affects middle-aged women and frequently remains unexplained. The daily shedding is mild (<100 hairs daily), but patients are distressed and complain of progressive temporal thinning and decreased hair mass. Scalp pain (trichodynia) is frequently reported. Patients who have a high hair density may bring in envelopes of shed hairs to prove the amount of hair loss. There is no effective treatment. Chronic telogen effluvium has a chronic course with periodic exacerbations.

DIFFUSE ALOPECIA

Anagen Effluvium

Acute hair shedding leading to diffuse alopecia is a typical side effect of cancer chemotherapy and scalp radiation. Hair loss is acute and severe and may

TABLE 442-1 CAUSES OF HAIR LOSS

DIFFUSE ALOPECIA

Telogen effluvium (e.g., after illness or stress)
Anagen effluvium (e.g., after chemotherapy or radiation therapy)
Medications (see Table 442-3)
Nutritional deficiency
Hair treatments
Androgenetic alopecia (in women)
Hormonal changes (e.g., menopause, discontinuation of oral contraceptives, hypothyroidism)

PATCHY ALOPECIA

Alopecia areata (probably autoimmune)
Cicatricial (scarring) alopecia (e.g., lichen planopilaris, discoid lupus erythematosus, folliculitis decalvans, central centrifugal cicatricial alopecia)
Traction alopecia (e.g., excessive hair straightening or braiding)
Trichotillomania (hair pulling)
Scalp infection (e.g., ringworm)

TABLE 442-2 DERMATOSCOPIC SIGNS IN HAIR AND SCALP DISORDERS

Alopecia areata	Yellow dots, exclamation mark hairs
Androgenetic alopecia	>20% variability in the hair diameter
Lichen planopilaris/frontal fibrosing alopecia	Peripilar casts; loss of follicular openings
Trichotillomania	Broken hairs, question mark hairs
Tinea capitis	Comma hairs, corkscrew hairs
Traction alopecia	Hair casts
Discoid lupus erythematosus	Red dots, follicular plugs
Folliculitis decalvans	Hair tufts
Scalp psoriasis	Coiled capillaries
Seborrheic dermatitis	Arborizing vessels

TABLE 442-3   DRUGS REPORTED TO INDUCE HAIR LOSS

ACE inhibitors (captopril, enalapril, moexipril, ramipril)	Immunoglobulins
Allopurinol	Indanediones
Amiodarone	Indinavir*
Amphetamines*,†	Interferons*,†
Analgesics, anti-inflammatories (ibuprofen, indomethacin, naproxen)	Isonicotinic acid hydrazide‖
	Leflunomide*
Androgens*,‡	Levodopa
Anticoagulants (coumarin, dextran, heparin/heparinoids)*,†	Lithium*
	Maprotiline
Antiepileptics (carbamazepine, hydantoins, lamotrigine, troxidone, valproic acid, vigabatrin)*,†	Mesalazine
	Methyldopa
	Methysergide
	Metyrapone
Antipsychotics (flupenthixol decanoate, fluphenazine decanoate)	Minoxidil¶
	Nicotinic acid
Antithyroid drugs (carbimazole, iodine, thiouracil)*	Nitrofurantoin
	Octreotide
Appetite suppressants	Olanzapine
Aromatase inhibitors (fadrozole, formestane [4-OHA], vorozole)*,‡	Pentosan polysulfate
	Phenindione
Benzimidazoles (albendazole, mebendazole)	Piroxicam
	Potassium thiocyanate
β-Blockers (levobunolol, metoprolol, nadolol, propranolol, timolol)*	Pyridostigmine
	Radiation (<700 Gy)*,‖
	Retinol (vitamin A)*
Bromocriptine	Retinoids (acitretin, etretinate, isotretinoin)*,†
Buspirone	
Butyrophenones	Risperidone
Cantharidin	Salicylates
Cholestyramine	Serotonin reuptake inhibitors (fluoxetine, fluvoxamine, paroxetine, sertraline)*
Chloramphenicol	
Cidofovir	Sorafenib
Cimetidine	Strontium ranelate*,†
Clonazepam	Sulfasalazine
Clotrimazole	Tamoxifen
Colchicine	Terbinafine
Contraceptives (oral)§	Terfenadine
Danazol	Thiamphenicol
Diclofenac	Thyroxine
Dixyrazine	Tocopherol (vitamin E)
Diazoxide	Trazodone
Ethambutol	Triazoles (fluconazole, itraconazole)
Ethionamide	Tricyclic antidepressants (amitriptyline, desipramine, doxepin, imipramine, maprotiline)
Fibrates (clofibrate, fenofibrate)	
Gentamicin	
Gefitinib‖	
Glatiramer acetate	Trimethadione
Glibenclamide	Triparanol
Gold salts	Vasopressin
Granulocyte-colony stimulating factor	Vismodegib*,†
Haloperidol	Spironolactone

*Established by multiple reports or proved by rechallenge.
†Hair loss usually severe.
‡May produce androgenetic alopecia.
§May produce permanent alopecia.
‖May produce anagen effluvium.
¶May produce telogen effluvium 3 mo after discontinuation.
ACE = angiotensin-converting enzyme inhibitor.

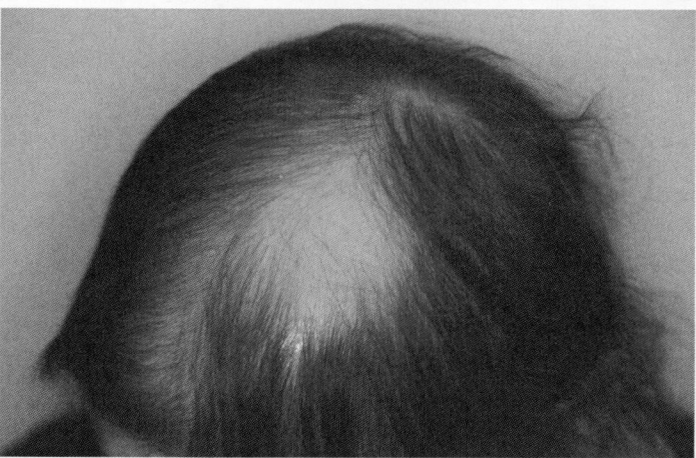

FIGURE 442-1. Alopecia areata: patchy hair loss. The alopecic area is devoid of hairs, and the scalp does not present inflammatory changes. Note diffuse thinning of the scalp surrounding the patch.

effects of the testosterone metabolite dehydrotestosterone (DHT). This sensitivity to DHT, which requires the 5α-reductase enzymes, is genetically determined. In men, androgenetic alopecia involves the frontotemporal areas and the vertex, following a pattern that corresponds to the Hamilton-Norwood scale. In women, androgenetic alopecia produces diffuse thinning of the crown region with maintenance of the frontal hairline (Ludwig pattern), a pattern that can easily be appreciated by making a central parting and comparing hair density at the top with hair density at the occipital region. In premenopausal women, androgenetic alopecia can be a sign of hyperandrogenism, together with hirsutism and acne. In most women, however, it occurs in the absence of biochemical and clinical evidence of androgen excess and may be due to excessive follicular sensitivity to androgens. Recent data show that patients with androgenetic alopecia may be at increased risk for dying from diabetes and heart disease.[4]

Androgenetic alopecia is a progressive disease that tends to worsen with time. Medical treatments include 2% topical minoxidil in women[A2] and 5% topical minoxidil and/or oral finasteride, 1 mg/day, in men.[A3] Clinical improvement is mostly due to thickening of the preexisting hair.

Treatments for androgenetic alopecia should be continued for at least 6 months before assessing efficacy, and regular drug use is mandatory for maintaining results. Interruption of minoxidil produces an acute telogen effluvium, which becomes evident 3 to 4 months after interruption and cannot be prevented by concomitant finasteride treatment. Interruption of finasteride is followed by gradual hair loss, with return to the pretreatment status after 1 year. Hair transplantation is a good option for men with severe androgenetic alopecia, and treatment with finasteride, 1 mg/day, improves the long-term results of surgery. Hair transplantation in women is more complicated because the hair thinning is often diffuse in the parietal and occipital regions, so there is not a good hair donor area.

● PATCHY ALOPECIA
Alopecia Areata

Alopecia areata is a common form of nonscarring, usually patchy hair loss affecting up to 2% of the population.[5] The etiology is unknown, but evidence is consistent with an autoimmune disease to which both a genetic predisposition and environmental factors contribute.[6] In genetically predisposed individuals, various triggering factors cause a predominantly CD8-driven, T_H1-type T-cell autoimmune reaction against the hair follicles, thereby resulting in acute hair loss.

Alopecia areata can start at any age, but severe forms often start during childhood and are more frequent in males. Clinical examination reveals one or multiple well-circumscribed smooth patches of nonscarring absence of hair that enlarge in a centrifugal way (Fig. 442-1). The margins of the patches often show 3-mm-long broken hairs with a pigmented tip (exclamation mark hairs), which indicates disease progression.

Alopecia areata may affect all hairy body areas, including the eyebrows and eyelashes (Fig 442-2). Severe forms involve the entire scalp (alopecia totalis) or all body hair (alopecia universalis). Involvement of the scalp margins

produce loss of most of the scalp hair, eyebrows, and eyelashes; other body hairs are less commonly involved. Hair shedding usually starts 4 to 6 weeks after drug intake with up to 1000 hairs shed daily. Regrowth is usually fast after discontinuation of therapy, but hair shape and color may be different. Permanent alopecia may occur with high-dose radiation and certain drug regimens, such as busulfan and taxanes. Scalp hypothermia prevents or reduces hair loss during chemotherapy except in patients treated with the combined taxotere, doxorubicin (Adriamycin), and cyclophosphamide regimen.[A1] Topical minoxidil accelerates hair regrowth but does not prevent hair loss.

Patterned Alopecia (Androgenetic Alopecia)

Androgenetic alopecia, which is the most common form of hair loss, affects up to 80% of men and 50% of women in the course of their life. Androgenetic alopecia is caused by a progressive reduction in the diameter, length, and pigmentation of the hair. Hair thinning is not diffuse, but rather is limited to the frontal, temporal, and vertex areas, where hair follicles are sensitive to the

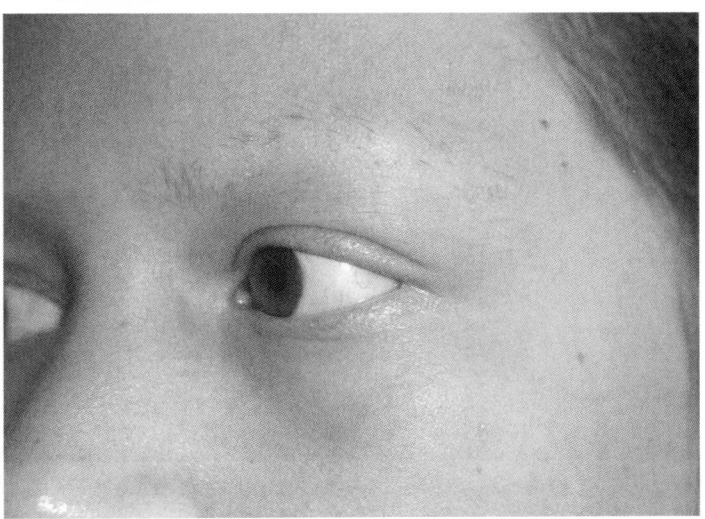

FIGURE 442-2. Alopecia areata: patchy hair loss. Hair loss involves the eyelashes and eyebrows.

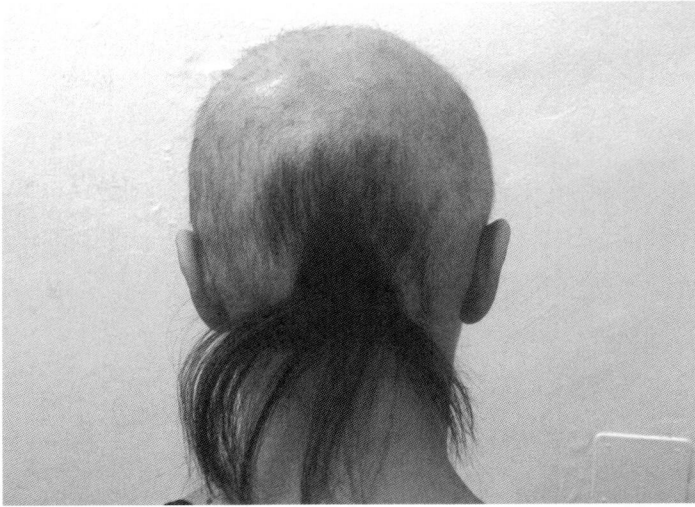

FIGURE 442-3. Trichotillomania: patchy hair loss. The alopecic area presents hairs broken at different lengths.

(ophiasis) is associated with a poor prognosis. Alopecia areata may be associated with other autoimmune diseases, most commonly thyroid diseases (Chapter 226). Other possible associations include celiac disease (Chapter 140), vitiligo (Chapter 441), and atopy (Chapter 438). Nail abnormalities are common, especially in children.

The natural history of alopecia areata is unpredictable. Studies indicate that 34 to 50% of patients will recover within 1 year and 15 to 25% will progress to alopecia totalis/universalis, a condition from which full recovery is only approximately 10%. To date, available treatments may induce temporary hair regrowth but do not change the long-term prognosis.[7]

Relapses occur in a high percentage of patients, even during therapy. High-dose pulse corticosteroid therapy is effective in approximately 60% of patients with acute alopecia areata but is not useful in ophiasis or long-standing alopecia totalis/universalis. Intralesional steroids can be used in localized areas, including the eyebrows. High-potency topical steroids (clobetasol propionate cream 0.05%) under occlusion induce regrowth in approximately 25% of patients with long-standing alopecia totalis/universalis, but relapses are common. Clobetasol propionate 0.05% in foam can be used in patchy alopecia areata. Topical immunotherapy with diphenylcyclopropenone (DPCP) or squaric acid dibutylester (SADBE), which is not approved by the U.S. Food and Drug Administration, induces hair regrowth in approximately 20% of patients with severe alopecia totalis/universalis. Medium- and low-potency topical steroids and topical minoxidil are probably only placebo treatments. Recent data suggest potential benefit from Janus kinase inhibitors, such as ruxolitinib.[8]

Trichotillomania

Trichotillomania is a compulsive disorder that is more common in children. Repetitive hair pulling and plucking produces patches of irregular alopecia. The scalp is not completely bald, but rather shows broken hairs of various lengths (Fig. 442-3). The frontal, parietal, and occipital scalp are most commonly affected, but other terminal hairs can be involved, especially the upper eyelashes.

Occasionally, patients develop the habit of chewing or eating the pulled hairs. Patients with trichotillomania frequently do not admit their habit, and parents of affected children may be recalcitrant to accept the diagnosis. Psychiatric referral is indicated in adults.

Cicatricial Alopecias (Scarring Alopecia)

The hallmark of cicatricial alopecias is loss of follicular ostia. Cicatricial alopecias include diseases that primarily affect the hair follicles and diseases that affect the dermis and secondarily cause follicular destruction.

Primary cicatricial alopecias are classified as lymphocytic or neutrophilic, based on the principal inflammatory cell type seen on pathologic examination. Lymphocytic cicatricial alopecias include lichen planopilaris, frontal fibrosing alopecia, and discoid lupus erythematosus. Neutrophilic cicatricial alopecias include folliculitis decalvans and dissecting cellulitis.

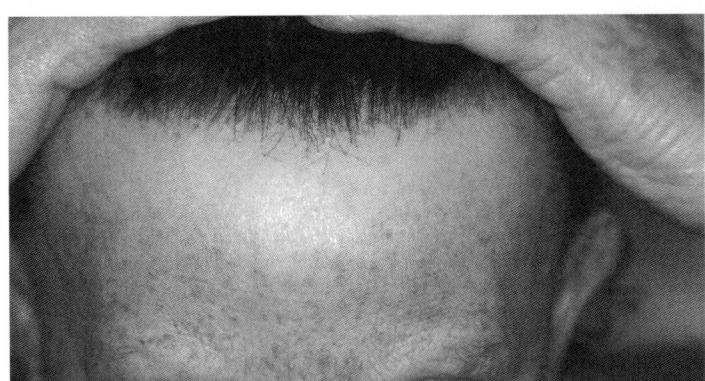

FIGURE 442-4. Frontal fibrosing alopecia. Scarring alopecia of the hair margin with recession of the frontal hairline. The alopecic area can be easily distinguished because it shows no photoaging compared with the normal forehead. Note alopecia of the eyebrows.

Secondary cicatricial alopecias, which result from disorders that cause diffuse scarring of the dermis, including burns, radiation, severe skin infections, localized scleroderma, and scalp tumors. The diagnosis of primary scarring alopecia requires a scalp biopsy, which should be taken from areas with active evidence of inflammation because biopsy of atrophic scalp will typically show only follicular or dermal fibrosis. In scarring alopecias, hair loss is permanent; treatment can prevent progression but not induce hair regrowth.

LICHEN PLANOPILARIS

In lichen planopilaris, which is the most common form of cicatricial alopecia, the hair follicles surrounding the alopecic patches show perifollicular erythema and scaling. The patient usually complains of severe itching. A variant of lichen planopilaris is frontal fibrosing alopecia, which typically affects the frontal hairline of postmenopausal women with a bandlike scarring alopecia, often associated with marked decrease or complete loss of the eyebrows (Fig. 442-4). No therapy is consistently effective, but options include intralesional or systemic steroids, systemic antimalarial agents, and excimer laser treatment.

DISCOID LUPUS ERYTHEMATOSUS

In discoid lupus erythematosus, the alopecic area shows active inflammation with erythema, edema, scaling, and follicular plugging, as well as atrophy with variable degrees of telangiectasia and dyspigmentation (Fig. 442-5).

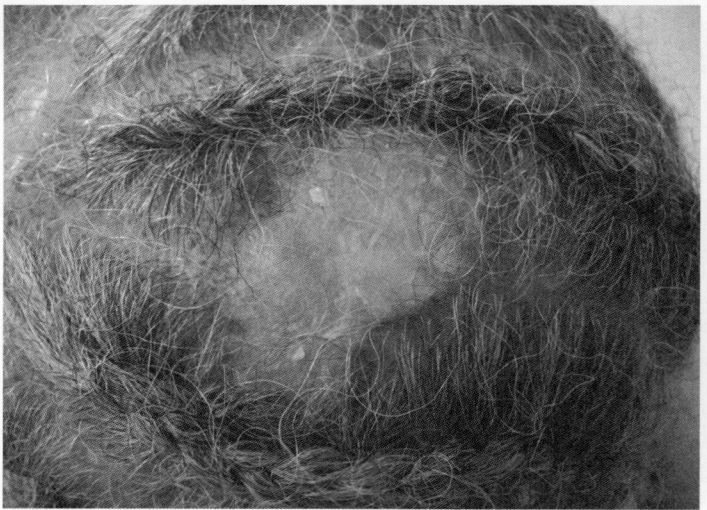

FIGURE 442-5. Discoid lupus erythematosus. The alopecic patch shows erythema, scaling, and depigmentation.

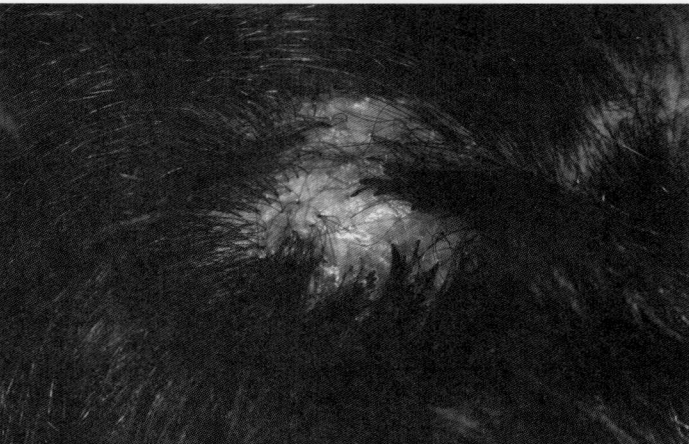

FIGURE 442-6. Folliculitis decalvans. Note alopecia with tufts of six or more hairs emerging together.

The disease is more common in African American women. Approximately 5 to 10% of adults with discoid lupus erythematosus will develop systemic lupus erythematosus (Chapter 266), especially those with widespread discoid lesions. In localized lesions, treatment with high-potency topical steroids (see Table 437-1) is usually effective. Antimalarials are a second-line treatment. Hair regrowth may occur when treatment is promptly started. Therapeutic strategy should include photoprotection of the involved area.

FOLLICULITIS DECALVANS

In folliculitis decalvans, the scalp shows papulopustular lesions that often coalesce to form exudative crusted areas that result in cicatricial alopecia. A typical finding is tufted folliculitis, in which tufts of 6 to 15 hairs emerge together from the scalp (Fig. 442-6). The cause is unknown, but the condition may reflect an abnormal host response to bacterial antigens. *Staphylococcus aureus* often is isolated from active lesions. Folliculitis decalvans responds to oral antibiotics (e.g., trimethoprim-sulfamethoxazole [one tablet, 160 mg/800 mg/day] or clindamycin [300 mg twice daily] with or without rifampin [300 mg twice daily] for 8 to 10 weeks) but usually relapses after interruption of therapy.

DISSECTING CELLULITIS

Dissecting cellulitis of the scalp is a follicular occlusion disorder that may progress to scarring alopecia. Patients typically complain of relapsing multifocal alopecic painful nodules, boggy plaques, and draining tracts. Possible treatments include systemic antibiotics, isotretinoin, and tumor necrosis factor-α inhibitors, but data are limited to small case series.

⬤ HAIR DISORDERS IN CHILDREN

Hereditary and congenital alopecias are present since birth or appear in the first years of life. Aplasia cutis congenita is the most common form of focal alopecia in newborns.

Hereditary hair shaft abnormalities associated with increased hair fragility produce diffuse or patchy alopecia that appears during childhood. The most common hereditary hair shaft disorder is monilethrix, in which hair shaft fragility is associated with follicular hyperkeratosis. The hair is dull and fragile and breaks easily, especially in the nape and occipital areas. Diagnosis is confirmed by finding hair beading on dermoscopy or microscopic examination.

Congenital triangular alopecia is usually noticed by the age of 6 years as an irregularly triangular patch of alopecia with vellus hairs on the frontotemporal region.

The loose anagen hair syndrome is characterized by a defective anchorage of the hair to the follicle, resulting in hairs that are easily and painlessly pulled out from the scalp. The condition is typical of children and may manifest with patchy hair loss due to hair pulling while playing.

Short anagen syndrome is a congenital disease characterized by short (<6 cm) fine hair and increased hair shedding. The condition is due to a decreased duration of the anagen phase.

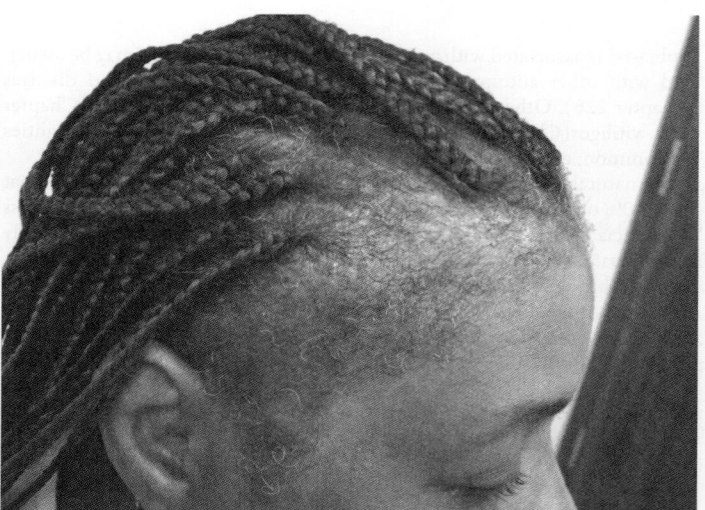

FIGURE 442-7. Traction alopecia. Hair loss involves the temporal scalp. Note presence of remaining hairs along the hairline.

⬤ RACIAL DIFFERENCES

The frequency and clinical aspects of hair disorders vary in different races.[9] Androgenetic alopecia, for instance, is more frequent in whites than in blacks and Asians, whereas black and Asian hair is more susceptible to weathering and fragility.

The black hair shaft is flat, highly twisted, and difficult to manage without strong chemical or hair styling procedures, which often cause considerable damage. Hair straightening and braiding are responsible for traction alopecia, which is common and typically produces cicatricial alopecia of the frontal and lateral margins (Fig 442-7). Central centrifugal cicatricial alopecia is a very common cause of scarring alopecia in black women (Fig 442-8). It manifests as slowly progressive scarring hair loss in the vertex or crown that spreads in a centrifugal pattern.

In Asians, the hair shaft is round, thick, robust, and straight. Asian hair is very difficult to style and dye, and it is often damaged by its treatment with high concentrations or long exposure to chemicals.

⬤ EXCESSIVE HAIR GROWTH

Hirsutism describes excessive terminal hair with male distribution in a female. Hirsutism should be distinguished from hypertrichosis, which is characterized by the presence of an excessive amount of hair in a non–androgen-dependent area.

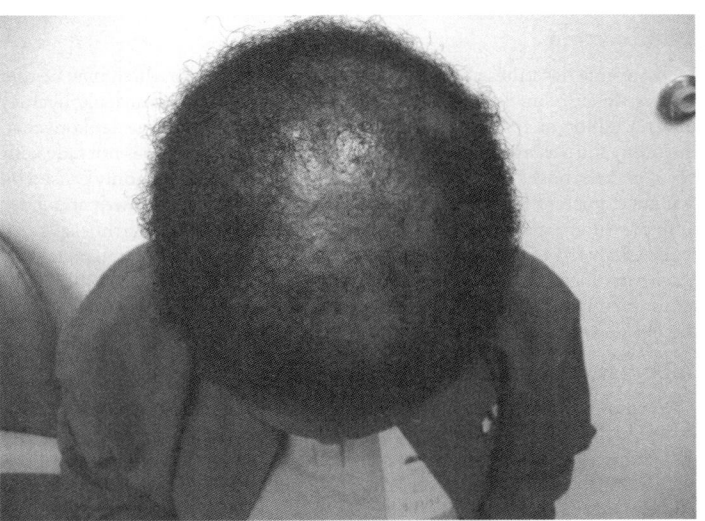

FIGURE 442-8. Central centrifugal cicatricial alopecia. The alopecic area involves the central portion of the scalp and expands centrifugally.

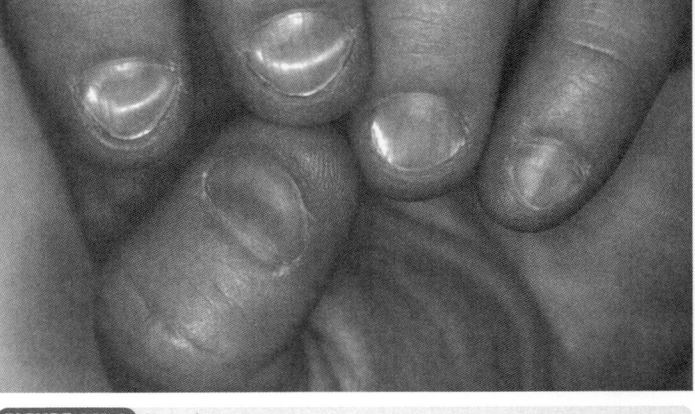

FIGURE 442-9. Spooning.

Hirsutism

Hirsutism is a common condition that affects up to 10% of women and is more frequent in Hispanic and Mediterranean women.[10] Hirsutism may be associated with hyperandrogenism, but it is idiopathic in approximately 15% of cases.

Hypertrichosis

Hypertrichosis results from the presence of terminal hairs in anatomic areas that are normally characterized by vellus hair. Hypertrichoses can be congenital or acquired, localized or generalized. Acquired hypertrichoses are most commonly iatrogenic, metabolic (e.g., Cushing syndrome, porphyria, hyperthyroidism), nutritional (e.g., anorexia nervosa), or paraneoplastic (Chapter 179).

⬤ NAIL DISORDERS

Normal Nail

The nail plate is a keratinized hard structure produced by the nail matrix, which is a specialized epithelium located above the distal phalanx of the finger. In longitudinal sections, the matrix consists of a dorsal, an apical, and a ventral portion. The proximal matrix (dorsal portion and apex) produces the dorsal nail plate (two thirds upper plate), and the distal matrix (ventral portion) produces the ventral plate (one third lower plate). The nail plate is produced continuously throughout life. Nails grow slowly, and the nail plate can reflect illnesses that occurred several months earlier. Complete replacement takes approximately 6 months for fingernails and 12 to 18 months for toenails. Many medications (e.g., anticonvulsants, neuroleptics, antifungals), drugs (e.g., amphetamine, cocaine, doping substances), and poisons (e.g., mercury, arsenic) are retained in the nails, whose fragments (nail clippings) can be used to monitor previous exposure.

⬤ NAIL DISORDERS

Nail abnormalities can be congenital or acquired and may caused by developmental, traumatic, inflammatory, infective, and neoplastic disorders or by medications. The diagnosis of nail dystrophies usually relies on a careful clinical examination and an accurate history, but radiographic or magnetic resonance imaging investigation of the digit and pathology may be required.

Koilonychia (Spoon Nails)

In koilonychia (Fig. 442-9), which is also called spooning of the nails, the nail plate is thin and has a concave appearance. Koilonychia is physiologic in children. In adults, it can be occupational or, more rarely, a sign of iron deficiency (Chapter 159).

Clubbing

Clubbing (Fig. 442-10) develops when enlargement of the soft tissue of the distal digit causes a bulbous digit with an enlarged and overcurved nail plate.

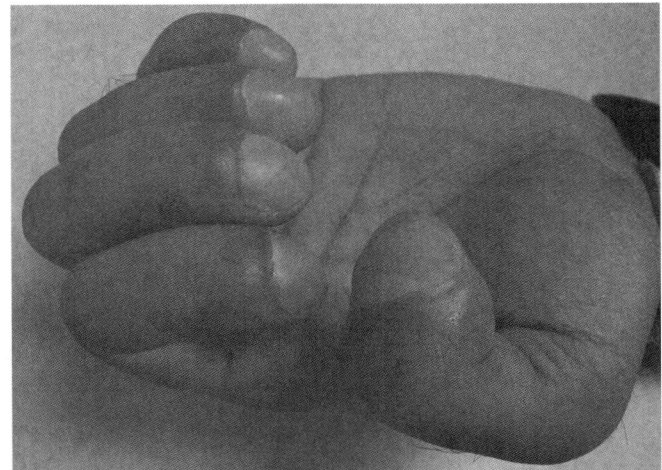

FIGURE 442-10. Clubbing.

The angle between the proximal nail fold and the nail plate (Lovibond angle) is greater than 180 degrees. Clubbing may be congenital (i.e., in congenital heart disease; Chapter 69) or acquired. Other causes of acquired clubbing include intrathoracic (Chapter 191) and gastrointestinal neoplasms (Chapters 192 to 196), chronic intrathoracic suppurative disease (Chapters 90 and 99), inflammatory bowel disease (Chapter 141), and liver disorders.

Beau Lines and Onychomadesis

Beau lines (Fig. 442-11) and onychomadesis are due to a temporary reduction or arrest of nail growth. Beau lines appear as transverse grooves of various depth; onychomadesis as a full-thickness transverse groove of the proximal nail plate. Causes include trauma, skin diseases involving the proximal nail fold and the matrix, drugs, and systemic diseases (Table 442-4). In the latter case, Beau lines or onychomadesis involve all the nails and are localized at the same level.

Pitting

Pitting (Fig. 442-12) appears as punctate depressions of the dorsal nail plate, with variable size and depth. Pitting is caused by inflammatory skin disorders such as psoriasis (Chapter 438), alopecia areata, and eczema (Chapter 438).

Longitudinal Grooves and Striations

Normal nails often show superficial thin longitudinal ridges that increase in number with aging. Deep longitudinal fissures, which indicate damage to the proximal matrix, can be caused by nail lichen planus, vascular insufficiency, trauma, and tumors involving or compressing the matrix.

TABLE 442-4 CAUSES OF BEAU LINES AND ONYCHOMADESIS

SYSTEMIC

Acrodermatitis enteropathica
Severe metabolic stress
High fever
Viral infections (Kawasaki disease, measles, hand-foot-and-mouth syndrome)
Typhus
Stevens-Johnson syndrome
Drugs
Bullous disorders (pemphigus, pemphigoids)
Deep saturation, high altitude
Hemodialysis
Myocardial infarction

LOCAL

Trauma (including manicure)
Paronychia
Congenital malalignment (big toenails)

Leukonychia

Leukonychia describes a whitish discoloration of the nail, which may be due to persistence of nuclei in the cells of the ventral nail plate (true leukonychia) or to a pallor of the nail bed (apparent leukonychia). True leukonychia, including the Mees lines of arsenic exposure (Chapter 22), does not fade with pressure and moves distally with nail growth; it is most commonly caused by trauma. Apparent leukonychia, which does not follow nail growth and fades with pressure, may be a sign of systemic diseases such as liver cirrhosis (Terry nails; Chapter 146), chronic renal diseases (half-and-half nails, characterized by apparent leukonychia of the proximal half of the nail; Chapter 130), hypoalbuminemia (Chapter 121), and systemic chemotherapy (Muehrcke lines; Fig. 442-13).

Yellow Nail Syndrome

The yellow nail syndrome is a chronic nail disorder characterized by an arrest or a reduction of nail growth, resulting in nail thickening and hardening and yellow discoloration.[11] Fingernails and toenails are excessively curved from side to side, and cuticles are absent (Fig. 442-14). Yellow nail syndrome occasionally may be paraneoplastic (Chapter 179). The pathogenesis of yellow nail syndrome is unknown, but a congenital abnormality of the lymphatic vessels may be involved. Typical cases have associated lymphedema or respiratory disturbances. The nail abnormalities improve with treatment of the associated respiratory disorders. Oral vitamin E (1200 mg/day for several months) is useful in some cases.

Splinter Hemorrhages

Splinter hemorrhages (see Fig. 51-11) appear as longitudinal thin red-brown lines of variable length. Splinter hemorrhages are usually localized in the distal nail and are commonly seen in inflammatory diseases, including eczema (Chapter 438), psoriasis (Chapter 438), and onychomycosis. Multiple splinter hemorrhages localized in the proximal nail plate can be a sign of systemic

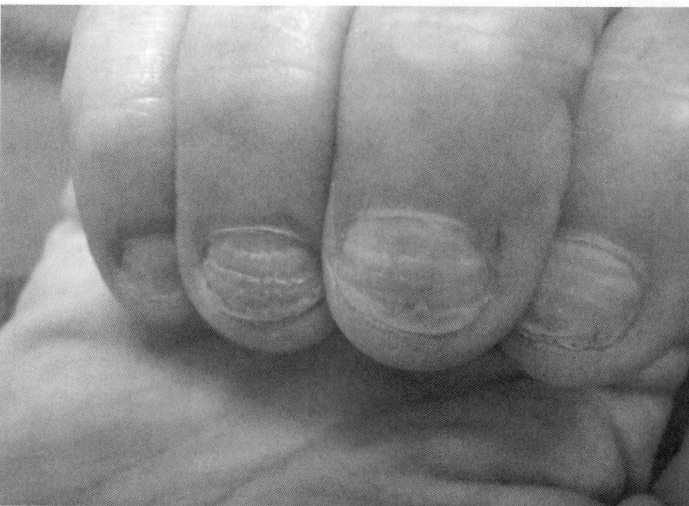

FIGURE 442-11. Beau lines due to chemotherapy. The lines affect all the nails at the same level.

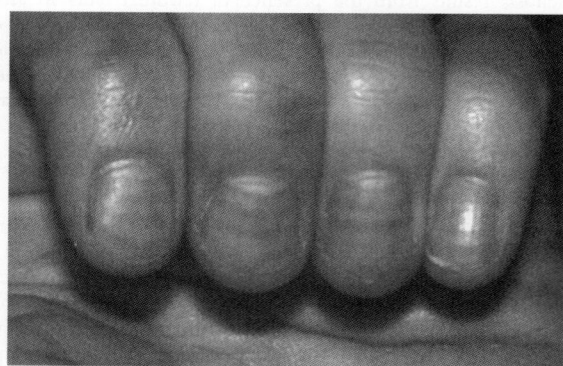

FIGURE 442-13. Muehrcke lines. (From Wikipedia Commons.)

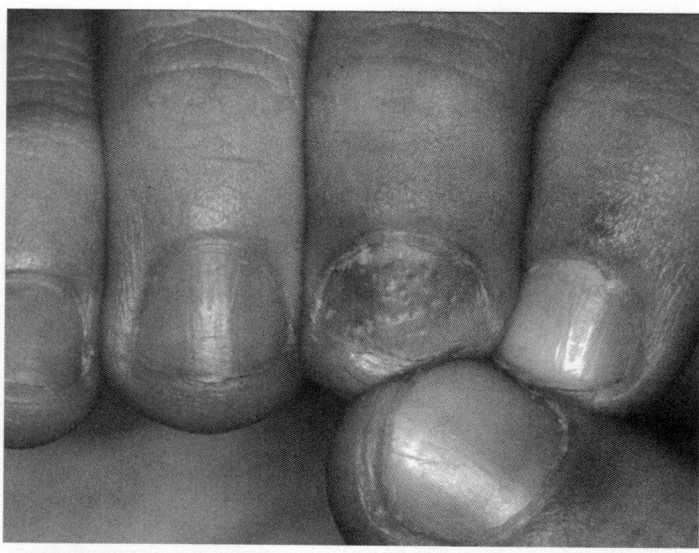

FIGURE 442-12. Pitting. Multiple punctate depressions on the nail plate surface.

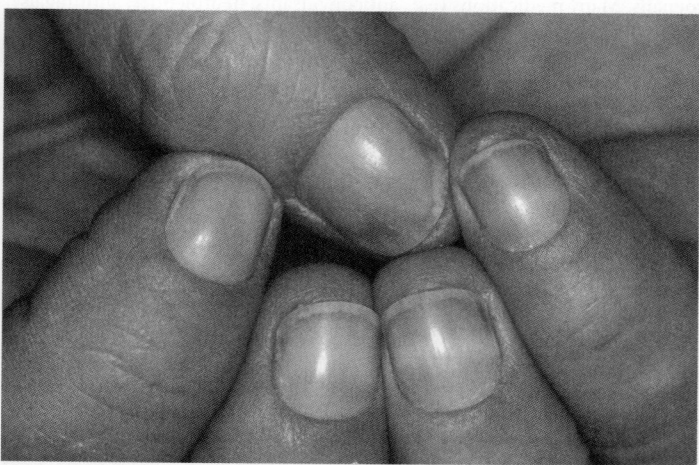

FIGURE 442-14. Yellow nail syndrome. The nails are yellow, overcurved, and do not grow.

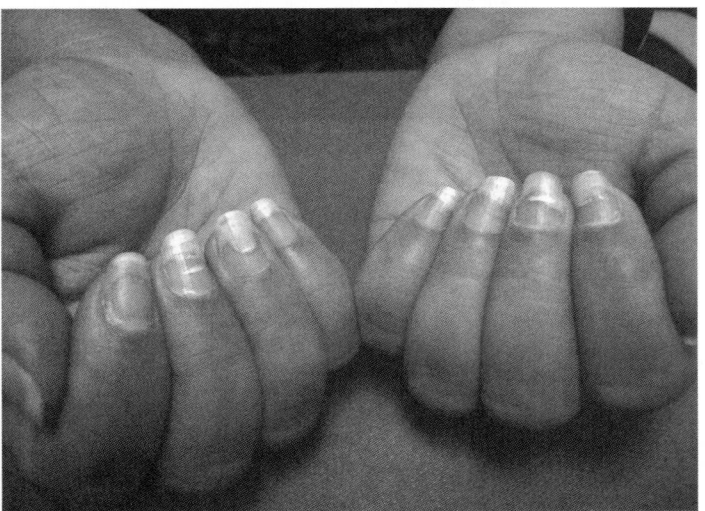

FIGURE 442-15. Onycholysis. The detached nail plate is white in color.

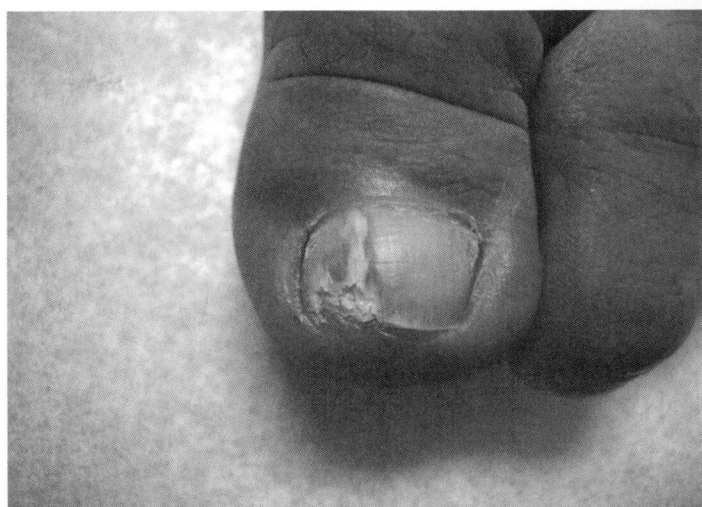

FIGURE 442-16. Distal subungual onychomycosis. The nail shows subungual hyperkeratosis and a yellow streak.

diseases, including infectious or marantic endocarditis (Chapter 76), trichinosis (Chapter 357), and the antiphospholipid syndrome.

Onycholysis

Onycholysis (Fig. 442-15) describes detachment of the nail plate from the bed. The detachment usually occurs at the free lateral margins of the nail. The onycholytic area is white owing to the presence of air, but it may acquire a green-brown color if the space if colonized by bacteria, such as *Pseudomonas aeruginosa*.

Onycholysis of the fingernails is a common sign of nail psoriasis (Chapter 438). It also may be due to prolonged and frequent contact with water, detergents, or irritants (idiopathic onycholysis). Toenail onycholysis is almost exclusively caused by trauma or onychomycosis. When onycholysis is limited to one digit, the possibility of a nail tumor always should be considered.

Paronychia

Paronychia, which describes the acute or chronic inflammation of the proximal and lateral nail folds, is common in the fingernails at any age. In acute paronychia, the affected digit is painful, with erythema, swelling, and pus discharge localized to one corner of the proximal nail fold. Acute paronychia usually follows a trauma to the nail fold, as in children who pick or bite the cuticles or in women after a manicure.

In chronic paronychia, prolonged mechanical or environmental trauma (such as contact with water and irritants) damages the cuticle, allowing penetration of dirt, bacteria, and other particles under the proximal nail fold. The result is an inflammatory reaction of the proximal nail fold and nail matrix, with edema and redness of the fold, absence of the cuticles, Beau lines, and abnormalities of the nail plate surface. Treatment includes protective measures, such as use of cotton and rubber gloves to avoid contact with irritants, as well as topical steroids and topical antimicrobials.

Onychomycosis

Fungal nail infections most commonly affect the toenails of adults. Dermatophytes (particularly *Trichophyton rubrum*) are responsible for most infections. The clinical presentation varies depending on the modality of the nail invasion. In distal subungual onychomycosis, the most common form, fungi spread from plantar skin and invade the nail bed. The affected nail shows subungual hyperkeratosis, onycholysis, and yellow streaks (Fig. 442-16). In white superficial onychomycosis, which only affects toenails, fungi colonize the surface of the nail plate, where they cause multiple white friable patches (Fig. 442-17). Proximal subungual onychomycosis produces a true leukonychia, owing to the presence of fungal hyphae in the deep layers of the plate. Proximal subungual onychomycosis caused by *T. rubrum* is typical in immunosuppressed patients. Diagnosis of onychomycosis must always be confirmed by mycologic examination. Treatment depends on clinical type, number of affected nails, and severity of nail involvement. A systemic treatment is always required for proximal subungual onychomycosis and for distal subungual onychomycosis involving the proximal nail. Terbinafine (250 mg/

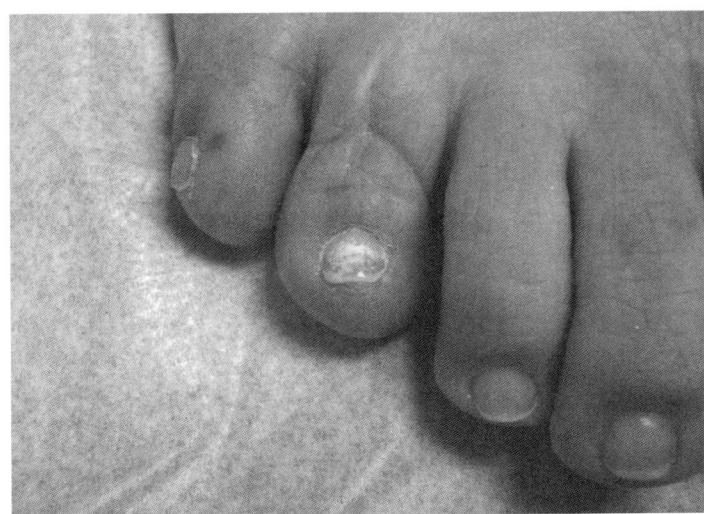

FIGURE 442-17. White superficial onychomycosis. The affected nail shows white superficial patches.

day) for 2 (fingernails) or 3 (toenails) months is the most effective treatment for dermatophyte infections.

Ingrowing Toenails

Ingrown toenails are a common condition, especially in young patients. Nail ingrowing most commonly affects one or both the big toes and is related to genetic factors, hyperhidrosis, and poorly fitting shoes. Ingrowing is usually precipitated by incorrect nail trimming, with formation of a sharp edge (spicule) of the lateral nail plate that penetrates and injures the soft tissues of the lateral nail fold (Fig. 442-18). Depending on severity, treatment varies from simple disembedding of the spicule to chemical destruction of the lateral nail matrix by phenolization.[12]

Nail Pigmentation

Nail pigmentation is usually caused by staining from external agents, such as nicotine or hair dyes. It rarely may be due to drug deposition in the nail plate or into the nail bed (i.e., antimalarials) or systemic diseases (argyria). In these cases, the proximal margin of the pigmentation follows the shape of the lunula.

Melanonychia

Melanonychia is defined by the presence of melanin within the nail plate. It appears more often as a longitudinal brown-black band starting from the matrix and extending to the free edge of the nail plate (Fig. 442-19).

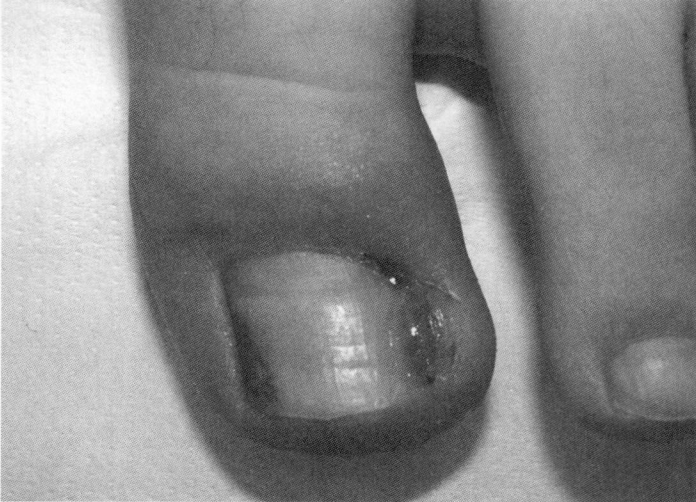

FIGURE 442-18. Ingrowing toenail. Penetration of the nail spicule causes inflammation and granulomatous reaction.

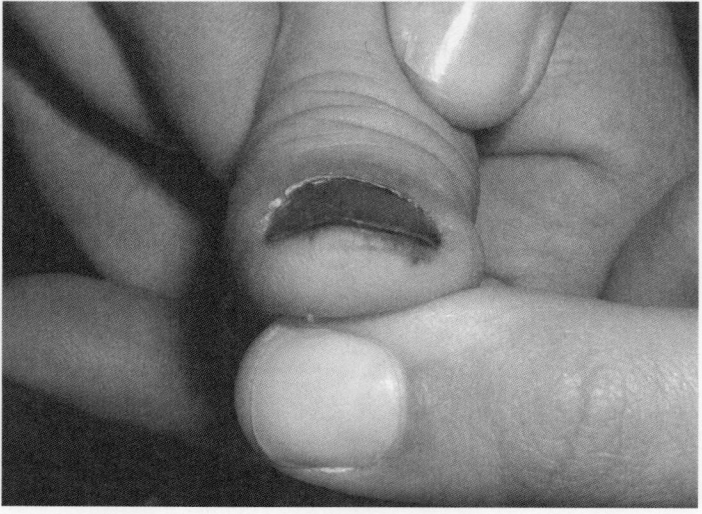

FIGURE 442-20. Nail melanoma. Melanonychia and periungual pigmentation (Hutchinson sign).

Melanonychia results from production of melanin by melanocytes of the nail matrix. Melanonychia has three main causes: simple melanocytic activation, benign melanocyte proliferations (lentigo, nevus), and malignant melanocyte proliferation (melanoma; Chapter 203).

Common causes of longitudinal melanonychia due to melanocytic activation include inflammatory and traumatic nail disorders, drugs (chemotherapy, azidothymidine, antimalarials, psoralen and ultraviolet A [PUVA] therapy), and systemic diseases (acquired immunodeficiency syndrome [Chapter 392]; Addison disease [Chapter 227]).

Nail melanoma is rare and most frequently involves the thumb of middle-aged individuals. Diagnosis is often delayed, and the 5-year survival is only 15%. Hutchinson sign, extension of the pigmentation to the proximal or lateral nail folds, is an important indicator of nail melanoma (Fig. 442-20).

Grade A References

A1. Shin H, Jo SJ, Kim do H, et al. Efficacy of interventions for prevention of chemotherapy-induced alopecia: a systematic review and meta-analysis. *Int J Cancer*. 2015;136:E442-E454.
A2. van Zuuren EJ, Fedorowicz Z, Carter B. Evidence-based treatments for female pattern hair loss: a summary of a Cochrane systematic review. *Br J Dermatol*. 2012;167:995-1010.
A3. Varothai S, Bergfeld WF. Androgenetic alopecia: an evidence-based treatment update. *Am J Clin Dermatol*. 2014;15:217-230.
A4. de Sá DC, Lamas AP, Tosti A. Oral therapy for onychomycosis: an evidence-based review. *Am J Clin Dermatol*. 2014;15:17-36.

GENERAL REFERENCES

For the General References and other additional features, please visit Expert Consult at https://expertconsult.inkling.com.

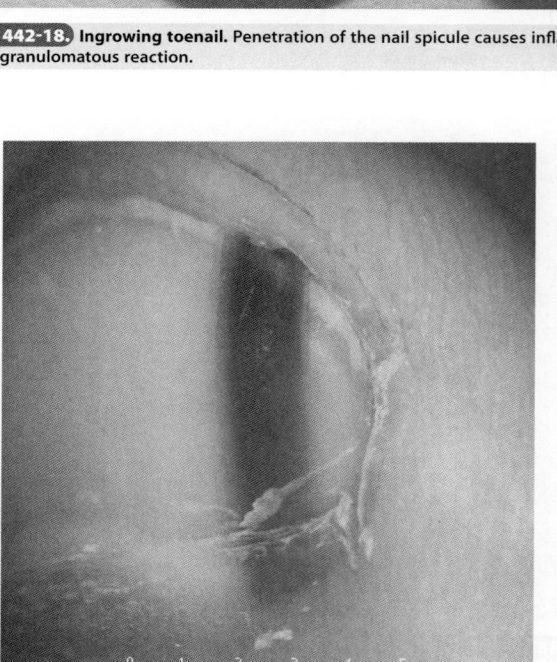

FIGURE 442-19. Longitudinal melanonychia. Black longitudinal pigmented band extending from the proximal nail fold to the free edge.

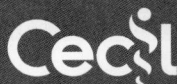

Appendix

§ LABORATORY REFERENCE INTERVALS
AND VALUES

REFERENCE INTERVALS AND LABORATORY VALUES

RONALD J. ELIN

Reference intervals are invaluable guidelines based upon the methodology of the laboratory for the clinician to assess health and disease, but they should not be used as absolute indicators of health and disease. For essentially every test, significant overlap exists between healthy and diseased populations. Many factors may influence the determination of the reference interval. The method and mode of standardization are variables for the reference interval, particularly for immunologic and enzymatic tests. The selection of the "normal" population is also important because factors such as age, gender, race, diet, personal habits (e.g., alcohol consumption, smoking, etc.), and exercise may influence the reference interval for a given analyte. Finally, the statistics chosen to define the reference interval are also a factor. These multiple variables for determining the reference interval indicate why differences exist among institutions for the same analyte.

The values in this appendix are primarily for adults in the fasting state.[1,2] Values for other groups, when included, are clearly identified. Prefixes and abbreviations are listed in Table Appendix-1. Clinical chemistry, toxicology, and serology are summarized in Table Appendix-2; hematology and coagulation in Table Appendix-3; and drugs, therapeutic and toxic, in Table Appendix-4. The lists include reference intervals for the most common tests used in the practice of internal medicine.

All laboratory values are given in conventional and international units. If the value and units for a reference interval are the same for conventional and international units, the interval is listed only in the column for international units. The temperature for all enzyme assays listed is 37° C. The pertinent prefixes denoting the decimal factors and abbreviations are listed in Table Appendix-1.

REFERENCES

1. Burtis CA, Ashwood ER, Bruns DE, eds. *Tietz Textbook of Clinical Chemistry and Molecular Diagnosis.* 5th ed. St. Louis: Elsevier Saunders; 2012. *A comprehensive text of clinical chemistry.*
2. Wu AHB, ed. *Tietz Clinical Guide to Laboratory Tests.* 4th ed. St. Louis: Elsevier Saunders; 2006. *A comprehensive text of reference intervals.*

TABLE APPENDIX-1 PREFIXES AND ABBREVIATIONS

PREFIXES DENOTING DECIMAL FACTORS

PREFIX	SYMBOL	FACTOR
mega	M	10^6
kilo	k	10^3
hecto	h	10^2
deca	da	10^1
deci	d	10^{-1}
centi	c	10^{-2}
milli	m	10^{-3}
micro	μ	10^{-6}
nano	n	10^{-9}
pico	p	10^{-12}
femto	f	10^{-15}

ABBREVIATIONS

AU	Arbitrary units
CSF	Cerebrospinal fluid
EDTA	Ethylenediaminetetraacetic acid
EU	Ehrlich unit
F	Female
Hb	Hemoglobin
hpf	High-power field
IFA	Immunofluorescent assay
IFCC	International Federation of Clinical Chemistry
IU	International unit (of hormone activity)
Kat	Katal
M	Male
Pa	Pascal
RBC	Red blood cell
RID	Radial immunodiffusion
S	Substrate
U	International unit (of enzyme activity)
WBC	White blood cell

TABLE APPENDIX-2 CLINICAL CHEMISTRY, TOXICOLOGY, AND SEROLOGY

TEST	SPECIMEN	REFERENCE INTERVAL (CONVENTIONAL UNITS)	REFERENCE INTERVAL (INTERNATIONAL UNITS)
Acetoacetate Semiquantitative	Serum or plasma (fluoride/oxalate)	Negative (<1 mg/dL)	Negative (<0.1 mmol/L)
Acetone Semiquantitative	Urine Serum or plasma (fluoride or oxalate)	Negative Negative (<1 mg/dL)	Negative Negative (0.17 mmol/L)
Acid phosphatase (S:p-nitrophenylphosphate)	Serum		M: 2.5-11.7 U/L F: 0.3-9.2 U/L
Adrenocorticotropic hormone (ACTH)	Plasma (EDTA)	0800 hr: <120 pg/mL 24-hr, supine: <85 pg/mL	<26 pmol/L <19 pmol/L
Alanine aminotransferase (ALT, SGPT)	Serum	M: <45 U/L F: <34 U/L	<0.77 μKat/L <0.58 μKat/L
Albumin Nephelometric, colorimetric	Serum CSF Urine	3.4-4.8 g/dL 17.7-25.1 mg/dL	34-48 g/L 177-251 mg/L 3.9-24.4 mg/day
Aldolase	Serum	2.5-10.0 U/L	0.04-0.17 μKat/L

Aldosterone	Plasma (heparin EDTA) or serum	Adult, average sodium diet
		  Supine: 3-16 ng/dL
		  Upright: 7-30 ng/dL
			0.8-0.44 nmol/L
			0.19-0.83 nmol/L

TABLE APPENDIX-2 CLINICAL CHEMISTRY, TOXICOLOGY, AND SEROLOGY—cont'd

TEST	SPECIMEN	REFERENCE INTERVAL (CONVENTIONAL UNITS)	REFERENCE INTERVAL (INTERNATIONAL UNITS)
Alkaline phosphatase, IFCC	Serum	M: (>20 yr): 53-128 U/L F: (>20 yr): 42-98 U/L	0.90-2.18 µKat/L 0.71-1.67 µKat/L
Aluminum	Serum	<5.41 µg/L	<0.2 µmol/L
δ-Aminolevulinic acid (δ-ALA)	Serum Urine	15-23 µg/dL 1.5-7.5 mg/day	1.1-8 µmol/L 11.4-57.2 µmol/day
Ammonia nitrogen	Serum or plasma (Na-heparin) Urine, 24-hr	15-45 µg N/dL 140-1500 mg N/day	11-32 µmol/L 10-107 mmol N/day
Amylase, IFCC	Serum Urine, timed specimen	28-100 U/L	0.48-1.70 µKat/L 1-17 U/hr
Angiotensin I	Peripheral venous plasma (EDTA)	<25 pg/mL	<25 ng/L
Angiotensin II	Arterial blood plasma (EDTA)	10-60 pg/mL	10-60 ng/L
α₁-Antitrypsin	Serum	90-200 mg/dL	0.9-2.0 g/L
Anion gap [$Na^+ - (Cl^- + HCO_3^-)$]	Serum or plasma (heparin)	7-16 mEq/L	7-16 mmol/L
Arsenic	Whole blood (heparin)	0.2-2.3 µg/dL Chronic poisoning: 10-50 µg/dL Acute poisoning: 60-930 µg/dL	0.3-0.31 µmol/L 1.33-6.65 µmol/L 7.98-124 µmol/L
Ascorbic acid (see Vitamin C)			
Aspartate aminotransferase (AST, SGOT)	Serum	M: <35 U/L F: <31 U/L	<0.60 µKat/L <0.53 µKat/L
Bicarbonate	Serum	22-29 mEq/L	22-29 mmol/L
Bilirubin, conjugated (direct)	Serum	0-0.2 mg/dL	0-3.4 µmol/L
Bilirubin, total	Serum Urine	0-2.0 mg/dL	0-34 µmol/L Negative
B-type natriuretic peptide (BNP)	Whole blood or plasma (EDTA)	<100 pg/mL	<28.8 pmol/L
Calcium, ionized (iCa)	Serum	4.65-5.28 mg/dL	1.16-1.32 mmol/L
Calcium, total	Serum Urine, 24-hr	8.6-10.2 mg/dL 100-300 mg/day	2.15-2.55 mmol/L 2.5-7.5 mmol/day
Cancer antigen 125 (CA 125)	Serum	<35 U/mL	<35 kU/L
Cancer antigen 15-3 (CA 15-3)	Serum	<30 U/mL	<30 kU/L
Carbohydrate antigen 19-9 (CA 19-9)	Serum	<37 U/mL	<37 kU/L
Carbon dioxide, partial pressure (Pco_2)	Whole blood, arterial (heparin)	M: 35-48 mm Hg F: 32-45 mm Hg	4.66-6.38 kPa 4.26-5.99 kPa
Carbon dioxide, total (Tco_2)	Serum or plasma (heparin)	23-29 mEq/L	23-29 mmol/L
Carcinoembryonic antigen (CEA)	Serum	Nonsmokers: <3 ng/mL	<3 µg/L
β-Carotene	Serum	10-85 µg/dL	0.19-1.58 µmol/L
Catecholamines, total	Urine, 24-hr	<100 µg/day	<5.91 nmol/day
Ceruloplasmin	Serum	20-60 mg/dL	0.2-0.6 g/L
Chloride	Serum or plasma (heparin) Urine, 24-hr	98-107 mEq/L 110-250 mEq/day	98-107 mmol/L 110-250 mmol/day
Cholesterol, total	Serum or plasma (EDTA)	Recommended: <200 mg/dL Moderate risk: 200-239 mg/dL High risk: >239 mg/dL	<5.18 mmol/L 5.18-6.19 mmol/L >6.19 mmol/L
Chorionic gonadotropin, intact	Serum or plasma (EDTA)	M and nonpregnant F:	<5.0 IU/L
Complement C3	Serum	90-180 mg/dL	0.9-1.8 g/L
Complement C4	Serum	10-40 mg/dL	0.1-0.4 g/L
Copper	Serum Urine, 24-hr	M: 70-140 µg/dL F: 80-155 µg/dL <60 µg/day	10.99-21.98 µmol/L 12.56-24.34 µmol/L <1.0 µmol/day
Cortisol, total	Serum or plasma (heparin)	0800 hr: 5-23 µg/dL 1600 hr: 3-16 µg/dL 2000 hr: ≤50% of 0800 hr	138-635 nmol/L 83-441 nmol/L Fraction of 0800 hr: ≤0.50
Cortisol, free	Urine, 24-hr	20-90 µg/day	55-248 nmol/day
C-peptide	Serum	0.78-1.89 ng/mL	0.26-0.62 nmol/L
C-reactive protein (CRP)	Serum	<0.5 mg/dL	<5 mg/L
Creatine kinase (CK) IFCC	Serum	M: 46-171 U/L F: 34-145 U/L	M: 0.78-2.90 µKat/L F: 0.58-2.47 µKat/L

TABLE APPENDIX-2 CLINICAL CHEMISTRY, TOXICOLOGY, AND SEROLOGY—cont'd

TEST	SPECIMEN	REFERENCE INTERVAL (CONVENTIONAL UNITS)	REFERENCE INTERVAL (INTERNATIONAL UNITS)
Creatinine Enzymatic	Serum	M: 0.62-1.10 mg/dL F: 0.45-0.75 mg/dL	55-96 μmol/L 40-66 μmol/L
	Urine, 24-hr	M: 14-26 mg/kg/day F: 11-20 mg/kg/day	124-230 μmol/kg/day 97-177 μmol/kg/day
Creatinine clearance (glomerular filtration rate endogenous)	Serum or plasma, and urine	M: 90-139 mL/min/1.73 m² F: 80-125 mL/min/1.73 m²	0.87-1.34 mL/sec/m² 0.77-1.20 mL/sec/m²
Dehydroepiandrosterone (DHEA), unconjugated	Serum	M: 1.8-12.5 ng/mL F: 1.3-9.8 ng/mL	6.25-43.4 nmol/L 4.51-34.0 nmol/L
11-Deoxycortisol (compound S)	Serum	20-158 ng/dL	0.6-4.6 nmol/L
Erythropoietin	Serum		5-36 U/L

Estradiol	Serum	M: 10-50 pg/mL
		F, cycle:
		  Follicular phase: 20-350 pg/mL
		  Luteal phase: 30-450 pg/mL
		  Postmenopausal: <21 pg/mL
			37-184 pmol/L
			
			73-1285 pmol/L
			110-1652 pmol/L
			<74 pmol/L

Fat, fecal	Feces, 72-hr		<7 g/day
Fatty acids, nonesterified (free)	Serum or plasma (heparin)	8-25 mg/dL	0.28-0.89 mmol/L
Ferritin	Serum	M: 20-250 ng/mL F: 10-120 ng/mL	20-250 μg/L 10-120 μg/L
α₁-Fetoprotein (AFP)	Serum	<15 ng/mL	<15 μg/L
Fibrinogen (see Table Appendix-3)			
Folate	Serum Erythrocytes (EDTA)	2.6-12.2 ng/mL 103-411 ng/mL packed cells	6.0-28.0 nmol/L 237-948 nmol/L packed cells

Follitropin (FSH)	Serum or plasma (heparin)	M: 1.4-15.4 mIU/mL
		F: Follicular phase: 1.4-9.9 mIU/L
		  Luteal phase: 1.1-9.2 mIU/mL
		  Postmenopausal: 19.3-100.6 mIU/mL
			1.4-15.4 IU/L
			1.4-9.9 IU/L
			1.1-9.2 IU/L
			19.3-100.6 IU/L

Fructosamine	Serum		205-285 μmol/L
Gastrin	Serum	25-90 pg/mL	25-90 ng/L
Glucagon	Plasma (heparin or EDTA)		70-180 ng/L
Glucose	Serum, fasting	Adult: 74-100 mg/dL >60 yr: 82-115 mg/dL	4.1-5.6 mmol/L 4.6-6.4 mmol/L
	Whole blood (heparin) CSF	65-95 mg/dL 40-70 mg/dL	3.6-5.3 mmol/L 2.2-3.9 mmol/L
Quantitative, enzymatic Qualitative	Urine Urine	<0.5 g/day	<2.8 mmol/day Negative
Glucose, 2-hr postprandial	Serum	<126 mg/dL	<7.0 mmol/L
γ-Glutamyltransferase (GGT) IFCC	Serum	M: <55 U/L F: <38 U/L	<0.94 μKat/L <0.65 μKat/L
Glycated hemoglobin (HbA₁c)	Whole blood (EDTA or heparin)	Diagnosis: <6.5% total Hb (NGSP)	<6.5 Hb fraction

Growth hormone (hGH, somatotropin)	Serum	Adult, M: 0-4 ng/mL
		  F: 0-18 ng/mL
		>60 yr, M: 1-9 ng/mL
		  F: 1-16 ng/mL
			0-4 μg/L
			0-18 μg/L
			1-9 μg/L
			1-16 μg/L

Haptoglobin (see Table Appendix-3)			
HDL cholesterol (HDLC) (5th percentile from Lipid Research Clinics)	Serum or plasma (EDTA)	M: >29 mg/dL F: >35 mg/dL	>0.75 mmol/L >0.91 mmol/L
5-Hydroxyindole acetic acid (5- HIAA)	Plasma Urine	5.2-13.4 ng/L <16 mg/g creatinine	27-70 nmol/L <13 mmol/mol creatinine

17-Hydroxyprogesterone (17-OHP)	Serum	M: 27-199 ng/dL
		F, Follicular: 15-70 ng/dL
		  Luteal: 35-290 ng/dL
		  Postmenopausal: ≤0.70 ng/dL
			0.8-6.0 nmol/L
			0.4-2.1 nmol/L
			1.0-8.7 nmol/L
			≤2.1 nmol/L

Immunoglobulin A (IgA)	Serum	90-410 mg/dL	0.9-4.1 g/L
Immunoglobulin D (IgD)	Serum	0-384 ng/mL	0-384 μg/L

Glucose tolerance test (GTT), oral — Serum

	mg/dL Normal	Diabetic	mmol/L Normal	Diabetic
Fasting:	70-105	>140	3.9-5.8	>7.8
60 min:	120-170	≥200	6.7-9.4	≥11
90 min:	100-140	≥200	5.6-7.8	≥11
120 min:	70-120	≥140	3.9-6.7	≥7.8

TABLE APPENDIX-2 CLINICAL CHEMISTRY, TOXICOLOGY, AND SEROLOGY—cont'd

TEST	SPECIMEN	REFERENCE INTERVAL (CONVENTIONAL UNITS)	REFERENCE INTERVAL (INTERNATIONAL UNITS)
Immunoglobulin E (IgE)	Serum	0-160 kIU/L	0-380 µg/L
Immunoglobulin G (IgG)	Serum	700-1,600 mg/dL	7.0-16 g/L
	CSF	0-5.5 mg/dL	0-55 mg/L
Immunoglobulin M (IgM)	Serum	40-230 mg/dL	0.4-2.3 g/L
Insulin	Serum	2-25 µIU/mL	12-150 pmol/L
Intrinsic factor (see Vitamin B$_{12}$)			
Iron	Serum	M: 65-175 µg/dL	11.6-31.3 µmol/L
		F: 50-170 µg/dL	9.0-30.4 µmol/L
Iron-binding capacity, total (TIBC)	Serum	250-450 µg/dL	44.8-80.6 µmol/L
Iron saturation	Serum		Fraction of iron saturation:
		M: 20-50	0.20-0.50
		F: 15-50	0.15-0.50
Ketone bodies			
Qualitative	Serum	Negative	Negative
	Urine, random		Negative
L-Lactate	Whole blood (heparin)	Venous: 3-7 mg/dL	0.36-0.75 mmol/L
		Arterial: 16-17 mg/dL	1.78-1.88 mmol/L
Lactate dehydrogenase (LDH) IFCC	Serum	125-220 U/L	2.1-3.7 µKat/L
Lead	Whole blood (heparin)	<25 µg/dL	<1.21 µmol/L
		Toxic: ≥100 µg/dL	≥4.83 µmol/L
	Urine	<80 µg/dL	<0.39 µmol/L
Lipase	Serum	<38 U/L	<0.65 µKat/L
Low-density lipoprotein cholesterol (LDLC)	Serum or plasma (EDTA)	Recommended: <100 mg/dL	<2.59 mmol/L
		Mild risk: 100-129 mg/dL	2.59-3.34 mmol/L
		Moderate risk: 130-159 mg/dL	3.37-4.12 mmol/L
		High risk: ≥160 mg/dL	≥4.14 mmol/L
Luteinizing hormone (LH)	Serum or plasma (heparin)	M: 1.2-7.8 mIU/mL	1.2-7.8 IU/L
		F, Follicular phase: 1.7-15.0 mIU/mL	1.7-15.0 IU/L
		Midcycle: 21.9-56.5 mIU/mL	21.9-56.6 IU/L
		Luteal: 0.6-16.3 mIU/mL	0.6-16.3 IU/L
		Postmenopausal: 14.2-52.3 mIU/mL	14.2-52.3 IU/L
Magnesium AAS	Serum	1.6-2.6 mg/dL	0.66-1.07 mmol/L
	Urine, 24-hr	6.0-10.0 mEq/day	3.00-5.00 mmol/day
Magnesium, free	Serum		0.45-0.60 mmol/L
Manganese	Whole blood (heparin)	5-15 µg/L	90-270 nmol/L
	Serum	0.5-1.3 µg/L	9-24 nmol/L
	Urine	0.5-9.8 µg/L	9-178 nmol/L
Mercury	Whole blood (EDTA)	<5.0 µg/dL	<0.25 µmol/L
	Urine, 24-hr	<20 µg/L	<0.1 µmol/L
		Toxic: >150 µg/L	>0.75 µmol/L
Nickel	Whole blood	1-28 µg/L	17-476 nmol/L
	Serum	0.14-1.0 µg/L	2.4-17.0 nmol/L
	Urine, 24-hr	0.1-10 µg/day	2-170 nmol/day
Osmolality	Serum		275-295 mOsmol/kg
Oxalate	Serum	1-2.4 µg/mL	11-27 µmol/L
		Ethylene glycol poisoning:	Ethylene glycol poisoning:
		>20 µg/mL	>228 µmol/L
Oxygen (Po$_2$)	Whole blood, arterial (heparin)	83-108 mm Hg	11-14.4 kPa
Oxygen saturation	Whole blood, arterial (heparin)	94-98%	Fraction saturated: 0.94-0.98
Parathyroid hormone, intact	Serum	10-65 pg/mL	10-65 ng/L
Parathyroid hormone, (1-84)	Serum	6-40 pg/mL	6-40 ng/L
pH (37° C)	Whole blood, arterial (heparin)		7.35-7.45
	Serum	2.5-4.5 mg/dL	0.81-1.45 nmol/L
Phosphate			
	Urine, 24-hr	0.4-1.3 g/day	13-42 mmol/day
Porphobilinogen (PBG)			0-8.8 µmol/day
Quantitative	Urine, 24-hr	0-2.0 mg/day	0-8.8 µmol/day
Qualitative	Urine, fresh random		Negative
Potassium	Serum	3.5-5.1 mEq/L	3.5-5.1 mmol/L
	Plasma (heparin)	3.5-4.5 mEq/L	3.5-4.5 mmol/L
	Urine, 24-hr	25-125 mEq/day	25-125 mmol/day

TABLE APPENDIX-2 CLINICAL CHEMISTRY, TOXICOLOGY, AND SEROLOGY—cont'd

TEST	SPECIMEN	REFERENCE INTERVAL (CONVENTIONAL UNITS)	REFERENCE INTERVAL (INTERNATIONAL UNITS)
Proinsulin	Serum		1.1-6.9 pmol/L
Prolactin	Serum	M: 3.0-14.7 ng/mL	3.0-14.7 µg/L
Prostate-specific antigen (PSA)	Serum	F: 3.8-23.2 ng/mL	3.8-23.2 µg/L
		M: 40-49 yr 0-2.5 ng/mL	0-2.5 µg/L
		50-59 yr 0-3.5 ng/mL	0-3.5 µg/L
		60-69 yr 0-4.5 ng/mL	0-4.5 µg/L
		70-79 yr 0-6.5 ng/mL	0-6.5 µg/L
Protein			
Total	Serum	6.4-8.3 g/dL	64.0-83.0 g/L
Electrophoresis (cellulose acetate)	Serum	Albumin: 3.5-5.0 g/dL	35-50 g/L
		α_1-Globulin: 0.1-0.3 g/dL	1-3 g/L
		α_2-Globulin: 0.6-1.0 g/dL	6-10 g/L
		β-Globulin: 0.7-1.1 g/dL	7-11 g/L
		γ-Globulin: 0.8-1.6 g/dL	8-16 g/L
Total	Urine, 24-hr	<100 mg/day	<0.1g/day
Total	CSF	Lumbar: 15-25 mg/dL	150-250 mg/L
Pyruvic acid	Whole blood (heparin)	0.3-0.9 mg/dL	0.03-0.10 mmol/L
Renin (normal diet)	Plasma (EDTA)	Supine: 0.2-1.6 ng/mL/hr	0.2-1.6 µg/L/hr
		Standing: 0.7-3.3 ng/mL/hr	0.7-3.3 µg/L/hr
Riboflavin (see Vitamin B$_2$)			
Sediment	Urine, fresh, random		Hyaline: occasional(0-1) casts/hpf
Casts			RBC: not seen
			WBC: not seen
			Tubular epithelial: not seen
			Transitional and squamous epithelial: not seen
Cells			RBC: 0-2/hpf
			WBC: M: 0-3/hpf
			F: 0-5/hpf
			Epithelial: few
			Bacteria:
			Unspun: no organisms/oil immersion field
			Spun: <20 organisms/hpf
Selenium	Serum	63-160 µg/L	0.8-2.0 µmol/L
	Whole blood	58-234 µg/L	0.74-2.97 µmol/L
	Urine, 24-hr	7-160 µg/L	0.09-2.03 µmol/L
Sodium	Serum or plasma (heparin)	136-145 mEq/L	136-145 mmol/L
	Urine, 24-hr	40-220 mEq/day	40-220 mmol/day
Specific gravity	Urine, random		1.002-1.030
	Urine, 24-hr		1.015-1.025
Testosterone, free	Serum	M: 50-210 pg/mL	174-729 pmol/L
		F: 1.0-8.5 pg/mL	3.5-29.5 pmol/L
Testosterone, total	Serum	M: 260-1000 ng/dL	9.0-34.7 nmol/L
		F: 15-70 ng/dL	0.5-2.4 nmol/L
Thiamine (see Vitamin B$_1$)			
Thyroglobulin (Tg)	Serum	3-42 ng/mL	3-42 µg/L
Thyroglobulin antibodies	Serum		<1:10
Thyroid microsomal antibodies	Serum		Nondetectable
Thyrotropin (hTSH)	Serum or plasma	0.4-4.2 µU/mL	0.4-4.2 mU/L
Thyrotropin-releasing hormone	Plasma	5-60 pg/mL	5-60 ng/L
Thyroxine, free (FT$_4$)	Serum	0.8-2.7 ng/dL	10.3-34.7 pmol/L
Thyroxine (T$_4$), total	Serum	M: 4.6-10.5 µg/dL	59-135 nmol/L
		F: 5.5-11.0 µg/dL	71-142 nmol/L
Thyroxine-binding globulin (TBG)	Serum	15.0-34.0 µg/mL	15.0-34.0 mg/L
Thyroxine index, free	Serum	4.2-13.0 µg/dL	54-168 nmol/L
Transcortin	Serum	M: 18.8-25.2 mg/L	323-433 nmol/L
Transferrin	Serum	F: 14.9-22.9 mg/L	256-393 nmol/L
		200-360 mg/dL	2.0-3.6 g/L
		>60 yr: 160-340 mg/dL	1.6-3.4 g/L
Transthyretin (prealbumin)	Serum	20-40 mg/dL	200-400 mg/L
Triglycerides (TG)	Serum, after ≥ 12-hr fast	Recommended: <150 mg/dL	1.7 mmol/L
Triiodothyronine, free	Serum	210-440 pg/dL	3.2-6.8 pmol/L
Triiodothyronine, total (T$_3$)	Serum	70-204 ng/dL	1.08-3.14 mmol/L
Troponin-I	Serum		<10 µg/L

TABLE APPENDIX-2 CLINICAL CHEMISTRY, TOXICOLOGY, AND SEROLOGY—cont'd

TEST	SPECIMEN	REFERENCE INTERVAL (CONVENTIONAL UNITS)	REFERENCE INTERVAL (INTERNATIONAL UNITS)
Troponin-T	Serum		0-0.1 µg/L
Urea nitrogen	Serum or plasma	6-20 mg/dL	2.1-7.1 mmol/L
	Urine, 24-hr	12-20 g/day	0.43-0.71 mol/day
Urea nitrogen/creatinine ratio	Serum		12/1-20/1
Uric acid (uricase)	Serum	M: 3.5-7.2 mg/dL	0.21-0.42 mmol/L
		F: 2.6-6.0 mg/dL	0.15-0.35 mmol/L
	Urine, 24-hr	250-750 mg/day	1.48-4.43 mmol/day
Urinary sediment (see Sediment)			
Vanillylmandelic acid (VMA)	Urine, 24-hr	2-7 mg/day	10.1-35.4 µmol/L
Viscosity	Serum		1.10-1.22 centipoise
Vitamin A	Serum	30-80 µg/dL	1.05-2.8 µmol/L
Vitamin B_1 (thiamine)	Whole blood		90-140 nmol/L
Vitamin B_2 (riboflavin)	Serum	4-24 µg/dL	106-638 nmol/L
Vitamin B_6	Plasma (EDTA)	5-30 ng/mL	20-121 nmol/L
Vitamin B_{12}	Serum	206-678 pg/mL	151-497 pmol/L
Vitamin C	Serum	0.4-1.5 mg/dL	23-85 µmol/L
Vitamin D_3, 1,25-dihydroxy	Serum	15-60 pg/mL	36-144 pmol/L
Vitamin D_3, 25-hydroxy	Serum	10-65 ng/mL	25-162 nmol/L
Vitamin E	Serum	5.0-18.0 µg/mL	12-42 µmol/L
Zinc	Serum	80-120 µg/dL	12-18 µmol/L

TABLE APPENDIX-3 HEMATOLOGY AND COAGULATION

TEST	SPECIMEN	REFERENCE INTERVAL (CONVENTIONAL UNITS)	REFERENCE INTERVAL (INTERNATIONAL UNITS)
Activated partial thromboplastin time (APTT)	Plasma (Na citrate)		25-35 sec
Antithrombin III	Plasma (Na citrate)	85-115% of normal human plasma	0.85-1.15
Bleeding time (BT) Ivy Simplate (G-D)	Blood from skin		Normal: 2-7 min Borderline: 7-11 min 2.75-8 min
Blood volume	Whole blood (heparin)		M: 52-83 mL/kg F: 50-75 mL/kg
Bone marrow	Bone marrow aspirate	% (mean)	Number fraction (mean)
Differential count			
Myeloblasts		0.3-5.0 (2.0)	0.003-0.05 (0.02)
Promyelocytes		1.0-8.0 (5.0)	0.01-0.08 (0.05)
Myelocytes			
Neutrophilic		5.0-19.0 (12.0)	0.05-0.19 (0.12)
Eosinophilic		0.5-3.0 (1.5)	0.005-0.03 (0.015)
Basophilic		0.0-0.5 (0.3)	0.00-0.005 (0.003)
Metamyelocytes		13.0-32.0 (22.0)	0.13-0.32 (0.22)
Polymorphonuclear neutrophils		0.7-3.0 (2.0)	0.007-0.03 (0.02)
Polymorphonuclear eosinophils		0.5-4.0 (2.0)	0.005-0.04 (0.02)
Polymorphonuclear basophils		0.0-0.7 (0.2)	0.0-0.007 (0.002)
Lymphocytes		3.0-17.0 (10.0)	0.03-0.17 (0.10)
Plasma cells		0.0-2.0 (0.4)	0.00-0.02 (0.004)
Monocytes		0.5-5.0 (2.0)	0.005-0.05 (0.02)
Reticulocytes		0.1-2.0 (0.2)	0.001-0.02 (0.002)
Megakaryocytes		0.3-3.0 (1.0)	0.003-0.03 (0.01)
Pronormoblasts		1.0-8.0 (4.0)	0.01-0.08 (0.04)
Normoblasts		7.0-32.0 (18.0)	0.07-0.32 (0.18)
Clot lysis, 37° C	Whole clotted blood		47-72 hr
Clot retraction screen	Whole blood (no anticoagulant)		Retraction begins at 1 hr maximum at 24 hr
Clotting time, Lee-White, 37° C	Whole blood (no anticoagulant)		5-8 min
Differential count (see bone marrow differential count or leukocyte differential count)			
Eosinophil count	Whole blood (EDTA); capillary blood	50-400 cells/µL (mm³)	$50\text{-}400 \times 10^6$ cells/L
Erythrocyte count (RBC count)	Whole blood (EDTA)	$\times 10^6$ cells/µL M: 4.3-5.7 F: 3.8-5.1	$\times 10^{12}$ cells/L 4.3-5.7 3.8-5.1

TABLE APPENDIX-3 HEMATOLOGY AND COAGULATION—cont'd

TEST	SPECIMEN	REFERENCE INTERVAL (CONVENTIONAL UNITS)		REFERENCE INTERVAL (INTERNATIONAL UNITS)	
Erythrocyte sedimentation rate (ESR), Wintrobe				M: 0-15 mm/hr F: 0-20 mm/hr	
Ferritin (see Table Appendix-2)					
Fibrin degradation products (agglutination, Thrombo-Wellco test)	Whole blood: special tube containing thrombin and proteolytic inhibitor	<10 µg/mL		<10 mg/L	
Fibrinogen	Plasma (Na citrate)	200-400 mg/dL		2.00-4.00 g/L	
Glucose-6-phosphate dehydrogenase (G6PD) in erythrocytes	Whole blood (ACD, EDTA, or heparin)	12.1 ± 2.09 U/g Hb (1 SD)		0.78 ± 0.13 MU/mol Hb (1 SD)	
Haptoglobin (Hp)	Serum; avoid hemolysis	26-85 mg/dL		260-850 mg/L	
Hematocrit (HCT, Hct)	Whole blood (EDTA)				
Calculated from MCV and RBC (electronic displacement or laser)		M: 39-49% F: 35-45%		0.39-0.49 volume fraction 0.35-0.45 volume fraction	
Hemoglobin (Hb)	Whole blood (EDTA) Plasma (heparin, ACD) Urine, fresh, random	M: 13.5-17.5 g/dL F: 12.0-16.0 g/dL <3 mg/dL		2.09-2.71 mmol/L 1.86-2.48 mmol/L <0.47 mmol/L Negative	
Hemoglobin electrophoresis	Whole blood (EDTA, citrate, or heparin)	HbA: >95% HbA₂: 1.5-3.5% HbF: <2%		Mass function >0.95 0.015-0.035 <0.02	
Leukocyte count (WBC count)	Whole blood (EDTA) CSF	4.5-11.0 × 10³ cells/µL (mm³) 0.5 mononuclear cells/µL		4.5-11.0 × 10⁹ cells/L 0.5 × 10⁶ cells/L	
Leukocyte Differential count Myelocytes Neutrophils—bands Neutrophils—segmented Lymphocytes Monocytes Eosinophils Basophils	Whole blood (EDTA)	% Cells/µL (mm³) 0 3-5 54-62 23-33 3-7 1-3 0-0.75	0 150-400 3000-5800 1500-3000 285-500 50-250 15-50	Number fraction cells × 10⁶/L 0 0.03-0.05 0.54-0.62 0.23-0.33 0.03-0.07 0.01-0.03 0-0.0075	0 150-400 3000-5800 1500-3000 285-500 50-250 15-50
Leukocyte Differential count Lymphocytes Monocytes (includes pia- arachnoid mesothelial cells) Neutrophils Histiocytes Ependymal cells Eosinophils	CSF	% 62 ± 34 36 ± 20 2 ± 5		Number fraction 0.62 ± 0.34 0.36 ± 0.20 0.02 ± 0.05 Rare Rare Rare	
Mean corpuscular hemoglobin (MCH)	Whole blood (EDTA)	26-34 pg/cell		0.40-0.53 fmol/cell	
Mean corpuscular hemoglobin centration (MCHC)	Whole blood (EDTA)	31-37% Hb/cell or g Hb/dL RBC		4.81-5.74 mmol Hb/L RBC	
Mean corpuscular volume (MCV)	Whole blood (EDTA)			80-100 fL	
Methemoglobin (MetHb)	Whole blood (EDTA, heparin, or ACD)	0.06-0.24 g/dL		9.3-37.2 mmol/L	
Plasma volume	Plasma (heparin)	M: 25-43 mL/kg F: 28-45 mL/kg		0.025-0.043 L/kg 0.028-0.045 L/kg	
Platelet count (thrombocyte count)	Whole blood (EDTA)	150-450 × 10³/µL (mm³)		150-450 × 10⁹/L	
Prothrombin time, one-stage	Plasma (Na citrate)	Reference values will vary with the type of thromboplastin		In general: 11-16 sec	
International normalized ratio (INR)		Relevant only in patients on warfarin $INR = \left[\dfrac{Patient\ PT}{Normal\ mean\ PT}\right]^{ISI}$ ISI = International Sensitivity Index of thromboplastin		INR 2.0-3.0 (for most indications)	
Red cell volume	Whole blood (heparin)	M: 20-36 mL/kg F: 19-31 mL/kg		M: 0.020-0.036 L/kg F: 0.019-0.031 L/kg	
Reticulocyte count	Whole blood (EDTA, heparin, or oxalate)	0.5-1.5% of erythrocytes		0.005-0.015 (number fraction)	
Sulfhemoglobin	Whole blood (EDTA, heparin)	≤1.0% of total Hb		<0.010 of total Hb (mass fraction)	
Thrombin time	Whole blood (Na citrate)			Time of control ±25 when control is <22 sec	

TABLE APPENDIX-4 DRUGS: THERAPEUTIC AND TOXIC

DRUG	SPECIMEN	REFERENCE INTERVAL (CONVENTIONAL UNITS)		REFERENCE INTERVAL (INTERNATIONAL UNITS)
Acetaminophen	Serum or plasma (heparin or EDTA)	Therapeutic:	10-30 µg/mL	66-199 µmol/L
		Toxic:	>200 µg/mL	>1324 µmol/L
Amikacin	Serum or plasma (EDTA)	Therapeutic:		
		Peak	25-35 µg/mL	43-60 µmol/L
		Trough (severe infection)	4-8 µg/mL	6.8-13.7 µmol/L
		Toxic:	>40 µg/mL	>68 µmol/L
		Peak	>10 µg/mL	>17 µmol/L
		Trough		
ε-Aminocaproic acid	Serum or plasma (heparin or EDTA); trough	Therapeutic:	100-400 µg/mL	0.76-3.05 mmol/L
Amitriptyline + nortriptyline	Serum or plasma (heparin or EDTA); trough (>12 hr after dose)	Therapeutic:	80-200 ng/mL	289-722 nmol/L
		Toxic:	>500 ng/mL	>1805 nmol/L
Amobarbital	Serum	Therapeutic:	1-5 µg/mL	4-22 µmol/L
		Toxic:	>10 µg/mL	>44 µmol/L
Amphetamine	Serum or plasma (heparin or EDTA)	Therapeutic:	20-30 ng/mL	148-222 nmol/L
		Toxic:	>200 ng/mL	>1480 nmol/L
Bromide	Serum	Toxic:	>1250 µg/mL	>15.6 µmol/L
Caffeine	Serum or plasma (heparin or EDTA)	Therapeutic:	8-20 µg/mL	41-103 µmol/L
		Toxic:	>20 µg/mL	>103 µmol/L
Carbamazepine	Serum or plasma (heparin or EDTA); trough	Therapeutic:	4-12 µg/mL	17-51 µmol/L
		Toxic:	>15 µg/mL	>63 µmol/L
Carbenicillin	Serum or plasma	Therapeutic:	Dependent on inhibitory concentration of specific organism	Same
		Toxic:	>250 µg/mL	>660 µmol/L
Chloramphenicol	Serum or plasma (heparin or EDTA); trough	Therapeutic:	10-25 µg/L	31-77 µmol/L
		Toxic:	>25 µg/mL	>77 µmol/L
Chlordiazepoxide	Serum or plasma (heparin or EDTA); trough	Therapeutic:	700-1000 ng/mL	2.34-3.34 µmol/L
		Toxic:	>5000 ng/mL	>16.7 µmol/L
Chlorpromazine	Serum or plasma (heparin or EDTA); trough	Therapeutic:	30-300 ng/mL	94-942 nmol/L
		Toxic:	>750 ng/mL	>2355 nmol/L
Cimetidine	Serum or plasma (heparin or EDTA); trough	Therapeutic:	0.5-1.2 µg/mL	2-5 µmol/L
Ciprofloxacin	Serum	Therapeutic (oral):	0.5-1.5 µg/mL	2-5 µmol/L
		Toxic:	>5.0 µg/mL	>15 µmol/mL
Clonazepam	Serum or plasma (heparin or EDTA); trough	Therapeutic:	20-70 ng/mL	63-222 nmol/L
		Toxic:	>80 ng/mL	>254 nmol/L
Clonidine	Serum or plasma (heparin or EDTA)	Therapeutic:	1.0-2.0 ng/mL	4.4-8.7 nmol/L
Cocaine	Serum or plasma (heparin or EDTA) on ice	Therapeutic:	100-500 ng/mL	330-1650 nmol/L
		Toxic:	>1000 ng/mL	>3300 nmol/L
Codeine	Serum	Therapeutic:	10-100 ng/mL	33-334 nmol/L
		Toxic:	>1100 ng/mL	>3340 nmol/L
Cyclosporine A	Serum (12-hr after dose)	Therapeutic:	50-350 ng/mL	42-291 nmol/L
		Toxic:	>350 ng/mL	>291 nmol/L
Desipramine	Serum or plasma (heparin or EDTA); trough (>12 hr after dose)	Therapeutic:	100-300 ng/mL	375-1125 nmol/L
		Toxic:	>400 ng/mL	>1500 nmol/L
Diazepam	Serum or plasma (heparin or EDTA); trough	Therapeutic:	100-1000 ng/mL	0.35-3.51 µmol/L
		Toxic:	>5000 ng/mL	>17.55 µmol/L
Digitoxin	Serum or plasma (heparin or EDTA) >6 hr after dose	Therapeutic:	10-30 ng/mL	13-39 nmol/L
		Toxic:	>45 ng/mL	>59 nmol/L
Digoxin	Serum or plasma (heparin or EDTA) trough (>12 hr after dose)	Therapeutic:	0.5-2.0 ng/mL	0.6-3.0 nmol/L
		Toxic:	>1.5 ng/mL	>2 nmol/L
Diphenylhydantoin (see Phenytoin)				
Disopyramide	Serum or plasma (heparin or EDTA); trough	Therapeutic:	2.8-7.5 µg/mL	8-22 µmol/L
		Toxic:	>5 µg/mL	15 µmol/L
Doxepin	Serum or plasma (heparin or EDTA); trough (>12 hr after dose)	Therapeutic:	50-150 ng/mL	179-537 nmol/L
		Toxic:	>500 ng/mL	>1790 nmol/L
Ephedrine	Serum	Therapeutic:	0.05-0.10 µg/mL	0.30-0.61 µmol/L
		Toxic:	>2 µg/mL	>12.1 µmol/L
Ethchlorvynol	Serum or plasma (heparin or EDTA)	Therapeutic:	2-8 µg/mL	14-55 µmol/L
		Toxic:	>20 µg/mL	>138 µmol/L
Ethosuximide	Serum or plasma (heparin or EDTA); trough	Therapeutic:	40-100 µg/mL	283-708 µmol/L
		Toxic:	>150 µg/mL	>1062 µmol/L

TABLE APPENDIX-4 DRUGS: THERAPEUTIC AND TOXIC—cont'd

DRUG	SPECIMEN	REFERENCE INTERVAL (CONVENTIONAL UNITS)		REFERENCE INTERVAL (INTERNATIONAL UNITS)
Everolimus	Whole blood	Therapeutic: Toxic:	3-15 ng/mL >15 ng/mL	3-16 nmol/L >16 nmol/L
Fenoprofen	Plasma (EDTA)	Therapeutic:	20-65 µg/mL	82-268 µmol/L
Flecainide	Serum or plasma (heparin or EDTA); trough	Therapeutic: Toxic:	0.2-1.0 µg/mL >1.0 µg/mL	0.5-2.4 µmol/L >2.4 µmol/L
Fluoxetine	Serum or plasma	Therapeutic: Toxic:	120-300 ng/mL >1000 ng/mL	388-969 nmol/L >3230 nmol/L
Flurazepam	Serum or plasma (EDTA)	Therapeutic: Toxic:	Not well defined >0.2 µg/mL	 >0.5 µmol/L
Gabapentin	Serum or plasma	Therapeutic: Toxic:	2-20 µg/mL >12 µg/mL	12-117 µmol/L >70 µmol/L
Gentamicin	Serum or plasma (EDTA)	Therapeutic: Peak (severe infection) Trough (severe infection) Toxic: Peak Trough	 8-10 µg/mL <4 µg/mL >10 µg/mL >2 µg/mL	 16.7-20.9 µmol/L <8 µmol/L >21 µmol/L >4 µmol/L
Glutethimide	Serum	Therapeutic: Toxic:	2-6 µg/mL >5 µg/mL	9-28 µmol/L >23 µmol/L
Haloperidol	Serum or plasma (heparin or EDTA)	Therapeutic: Toxic:	5-17 ng/mL >42 ng/mL	13-45 nmol/L >112 nmol/L
Ibuprofen	Serum or plasma (heparin or EDTA)	Therapeutic: Toxic:	10-50 µg/mL >200 µg/mL	49-243 µmol/L >970 µmol/L
Imipramine + desipramine	Serum or plasma (heparin or EDTA); trough (>12 hr after dose)	Therapeutic: Toxic:	150-300 ng/mL >400 ng/mL	536-1071 nmol/L >1428 nmol/L
Isoniazid	Serum or plasma (heparin or EDTA)	Therapeutic: Toxic:	1-7 µg/mL >20 µg/mL	7-51 µmol/L >146 µmol/L
Itraconazole	Serum or plasma	Therapeutic:	>1.5 µg/mL	>2 µmol/L
Kanamycin	Serum or plasma (EDTA)	Therapeutic: Peak Trough (severe infection) Toxic: Peak Trough	 25-35 µg/mL 4-8 µg/mL >35 µg/mL >10 µg/mL	 52-72 µmol/L 8-16 µmol/L >72 µmol/L >21 µmol/L
Lidocaine	Serum or plasma (heparin or EDTA); >45 min following bolus dose	Therapeutic: Toxic:	1.5-5 µg/mL >6 µg/mL	6-21 µmol/L >26 µmol/L
Lithium	Serum or plasma (heparin or EDTA); >12 hr after last dose	Therapeutic: Toxic:	0.5-1.2 mEq/L >2 mEq/L	0.5-1 nmol/L >2 µmol/L
Lorazepam	Serum or plasma (heparin or EDTA)	Therapeutic:	50-240 ng/mL	156-746 nmol/L
Meperidine	Serum or plasma (heparin or EDTA)	Therapeutic: Toxic:	70-500 ng/mL >1 µg/mL	283-2020 nmol/L >4040 nmol/L
Meprobamate	Serum	Therapeutic: Toxic:	6-12 µg/mL >60 µg/mL	28-55 µmol/L >275 µmol/L
Methadone	Serum or plasma (heparin or EDTA)	Therapeutic: Toxic:	100-400 ng/mL >2000 ng/mL	0.32-1.29 µmol/L >6.46 µmol/L
Methamphetamine	Serum	Therapeutic: Toxic:	0.01-0.05 µg/mL >0.5 µg/mL	0.07-0.34 µmol/L >3.35 µmol/L
Methaqualone	Serum or plasma (heparin or EDTA)	Therapeutic: Toxic:	2-3 µg/mL >10 µg/mL	8-12 µmol/L >40 µmol/L
Methsuximide (N-desmethyl methsuximide)	Serum	Therapeutic: Toxic:	10-40 µg/mL >40 µg/mL	53-212 µmol/L >212 µmol/L
Methyldopa	Plasma (EDTA)	Therapeutic: Toxic:	1-5 µg/mL >7 µg/mL	4.7-23.7 µmol/L >33 µmol/L
Methyprylon	Serum	Therapeutic: Toxic:	8-10 µg/mL >50 µg/mL	43-55 µmol/L >273 µmol/L
Morphine	Serum or plasma (heparin or EDTA)	Therapeutic: Toxic:	10-80 ng/mL >200 ng/mL	35-280 nmol/L >700 nmol/L
Netilmicin	Serum or plasma (EDTA)	Therapeutic: Peak (severe infection) Trough (severe infection) Toxic: Peak Trough	 8-10 µg/mL <4 µg/mL >10 µg/mL >2 µg/mL	 17-21 µmol/L <8 µmol/L >21 µmol/L >4 µmol/L

TABLE APPENDIX-4 DRUGS: THERAPEUTIC AND TOXIC—cont'd

DRUG	SPECIMEN	REFERENCE INTERVAL (CONVENTIONAL UNITS)		REFERENCE INTERVAL (INTERNATIONAL UNITS)
Nortriptyline	Serum or plasma (heparin or EDTA); trough (>12 hr after dose)	Therapeutic: Toxic:	70-170 ng/mL >500 ng/mL	266-646 nmol/L >1900 nmol/L
Oxazepam	Serum or plasma (heparin or EDTA)	Therapeutic:	0.2-1.4 µg/mL	0.70-4.9 µmol/L
Oxycodone	Serum	Therapeutic: Toxic:	10-100 ng/mL >200 ng/mL	32-317 nmol/L >634 nmol/L
Paroxetine	Serum or plasma	Therapeutic:	70-120 ng/mL	213-365 nmol/L
Pentazocine	Serum or plasma (EDTA)	Therapeutic: Toxic:	0.05-0.2 µg/mL >1 µg/mL	0.2-0.7 µmol/L >3.5 µmol/L
Pentobarbital	Serum or plasma (heparin or EDTA); trough	Therapeutic, hypnotic: Therapeutic, coma: Toxic:	1-5 µg/mL 20-50 µg/mL >10 µg/mL	4-22 µmol/L 88-221 µmol/L >44 µmol/L
Phenacetin	Plasma (EDTA)	Therapeutic: Toxic:	1-30 µg/mL 50-250 µg/mL	6-167 µmol/L 279-1395 µmol/L

Phenobarbital	Serum or plasma (heparin or EDTA); trough	Therapeutic:
		Toxic:
		  Slowness, ataxia, nystagmus
		  Coma with reflexes
		  Coma without reflexes
			10-40 µg/mL
			
			35-80 µg/mL
			65-117 µg/mL
			>100 µg/mL
				43-173 µmol/L
				
				151-345 µmol/L
				280-504 µmol/L
				>430 µmol/L

Phensuximide + norphensuximide	Serum or plasma (heparin or EDTA)	Therapeutic:	40-60 µg/mL	212-317 µmol/L
Phenylbutazone	Plasma (EDTA)	Therapeutic: Toxic:	50-100 µg/mL >100 µg/mL	162-324 µmol/L >324 µmol/mL
Phenytoin	Serum or plasma (heparin or EDTA); trough	Therapeutic: Toxic:	10-20 µg/mL >20 µg/mL	40-79 µmol/L >79 µmol/L
Primidone + phenobarbital	Serum or plasma (heparin or EDTA); trough	Therapeutic: Toxic:	5-10 µg/mL >15 µg/mL	23-46 µmol/L >69 µmol/L
Procainamide	Serum or plasma (heparin or EDTA); trough	Therapeutic: Toxic:	4-10 µg/mL >12 µg/mL	17-42 µmol/L >51 µmol/L
Propoxyphene	Plasma (EDTA)	Therapeutic: Toxic:	0.1-0.4 µg/mL >0.5 µg/mL	0.3-1.2 µmol/L >1.5 µmol/L
Propranolol	Serum or plasma (heparin or EDTA); trough	Therapeutic:	20-100 ng/mL	77-386 nmol/L
Protriptyline	Serum or plasma (heparin or EDTA); trough (>12 hr after dose)	Therapeutic: Toxic:	70-260 ng/mL >500 ng/mL	266-988 nmol/L >1900 nmol/L
Quinidine	Serum or plasma (heparin or EDTA); trough	Therapeutic: Toxic:	2-5 µg/mL >6 µg/mL	6-15 µmol/L >19 µmol/L
Risperidone + 9-hydroxyrisperidone	Serum or plasma	Therapeutic:	20-60 ng/mL	49-146 nmol/L
Salicylates	Serum or plasma (heparin or EDTA); trough	Therapeutic: Toxic:	150-300 µg/mL >300 µg/mL	1086-2172 µmol/L >2172 µmol/L
Secobarbital	Serum	Therapeutic: Toxic:	1-2 µg/mL >5 µg/mL	4.2-8.4 µmol/L >21.0 µmol/L
Sirolimus	Whole blood	Therapeutic: Toxic:	4-20 ng/mL >20 ng/mL	4-22 nmol/L >22 nmol/L
Sulfonamides as sulfanilamide	Serum or plasma	Therapeutic: Toxic:	5-15 mg/mL >20 mg/mL	29-87 mmol/L >116 mmol/L
Theophylline	Serum or plasma (heparin or EDTA)	Therapeutic: Toxic:	8-20 µg/mL >20 µg/mL	44-111 µmol/L >111 µmol/L
Thiopental	Serum or plasma (heparin or EDTA); trough	Hypnotic: Coma: Anesthesia: Toxic:	1-5 µg/mL 30-100 µg/mL 7-130 µg/mL >10 µg/mL	4.1-20.7 µmol/L 124-413 µmol/L 29-536 µmol/L >41 µmol/L
Thioridazine	Serum or plasma (heparin or EDTA)	Therapeutic: Toxic:	0.2-2.0 µg/mL >10 µg/mL	0.5-5 µmol/L >27 µmol/L

Tobramycin	Serum or plasma (heparin or EDTA)	Therapeutic:
		  Peak (severe infection)
		  Trough (severe infection)
		Toxic:
		  Peak
		  Trough
			
			8-10 µg/mL
			<4 µg/mL
			
			>10 µg/mL
			>2 µg/mL
				
				17-21 µmol/L
				<9 µmol/L
				
				>21 µmol/L
				>4 µmol/L

TABLE APPENDIX-4 DRUGS: THERAPEUTIC AND TOXIC—cont'd

DRUG	SPECIMEN	REFERENCE INTERVAL (CONVENTIONAL UNITS)		REFERENCE INTERVAL (INTERNATIONAL UNITS)
Tocainide	Serum or plasma (heparin or EDTA)	Therapeutic: Toxic:	6-15 µg/mL >15 µg/mL	31-78 µmol/L >78 µmol/L
Tolbutamide	Serum	Therapeutic: Toxic:	90-240 µg/mL >640 µg/mL	333-888 µmol/L >2368 µmol/L
Valproic acid	Serum or plasma (heparin or EDTA); trough	Therapeutic: Toxic:	50-100 µg/mL >100 µg/mL	347-693 µmol/L >693 µmol/L
Vancomycin	Serum or plasma (heparin or EDTA); trough	Therapeutic: Peak: Trough: Toxic: (not well established)	 20-40 µg/mL >10 µg/mL >80 µg/mL	 14-28 µmol/L >7 µmol/L >55µmol/L
Warfarin	Serum or plasma (heparin or EDTA)	Therapeutic: Toxic:	1-10 µg/mL >10 µg/mL	3-32 µmol/L >32 µmol/L
Zidovudine	Serum or plasma	Therapeutic:	>0.2 µg/mL	>0.8 µmol/L

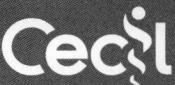

INDEX

Page numbers followed by "*f*" indicate figures, "*t*" indicate tables, and "*b*" indicate boxes.

A

A blood group antigens, 238
A disintegrin-like and MMPs with thrombospondin type 1 repeats (ADAMTS), 1732-1733
AADLs. *See* Advanced activities of daily living
Abacavir, 2288*t*
  CSF-to-plasma ratios, 2331*t*
  fixed-dose combinations, 2289, 2290*t*
  for HIV/AIDS, 2290*t*
  side effects of, 2289
Abatacept (Orencia), 171, 1762
Abciximab (ReoPro), 180, 438*t*-439*t*, 448
Abdomen: acute emergencies of, 2252*t*-2253*t*
Abdominal actinomycosis, 2061
Abdominal aortic aneurysm
  CT findings, 493, 493*f*
  epidemiology of, 492, 492*f*
  risk factors for, 492
  screening for, 55-56
  treatment of, 493
Abdominal compartment syndrome, 715
Abdominal examination, 27, 851
  in cardiovascular disease, 254
  in heart failure, 303
  in liver disease, 978
Abdominal imaging
  in acute pancreatitis, 962
  in gallstones, 1040, 1040*f*
  in liver disease, 980
Abdominal injury, 714, 714*f*
Abdominal pain, 854-859
  acute, 854-858
    approach to, 859*f*
    clinical manifestations of, 855*t*-858*t*
    physical findings, 854-858
  approach to, 852*t*, 979*t*
  chronic, 859
    approach to, 860*f*
    clinical manifestations of, 855*t*-857*t*
  in chronic pancreatitis, 965
  differential diagnosis of, 857*f*
  in HIV infection, 2303*t*
  in hospital, 858
  location of, 854, 857*f*
  pathobiology of, 854
Abdominal tuberculosis, 2034-2035
Abetalipoproteinemia, 929
Abiraterone acetate (Zytiga), 1211*t*-1216*t*, 1369
Ablation techniques, 295
Abnormal automaticity, 342
Abnormal movements, 2469
Abnormal vision, chronic, 2558
Abortion
  HgbA₁c and, 1620, 1620*f*
  infection associated with, 1926
  septic, 2252*t*-2253*t*
Abrasion, corneal, 2563
Abraxane, 1211*t*-1216*t*
Abscesses
  Bezold's, 2489
  brain, 2495-2497
  brain stem, 2496, 2497*f*
  cold, 2035
  in Crohn's disease, 942
  deep neck, 2603
  eyelid, 2564, 2564*f*
  liver
    amebic, 1011*t*, 1013, 2140, 2141*t*
    bacterial, 1011*t*
    pyogenic, 1011-1012, 1011*f*

Abscesses *(Continued)*
  perianal, 969
  peritonsillar, 2602*t*, 2603, 2603*f*
  spinal epidural, 2497-2498, 2498*f*
  subdural, 2498, 2498*f*
  visceral, 790
Absence seizures
  atypical, 2402
  childhood, 2404-2405
  clinical manifestations of, 2401*t*, 2402
  drugs for, 2407*t*
  EEG findings, 2342, 2343*f*
Absolute measures, 33
Absolute refractoriness, 341
Absolute risk reduction (ARR), 33
Abstainers, 149
Abstinence, 1880
Abuse. *See also* Substance abuse
  alcohol use disorders, 149-156
  drugs of, 156-162
  intimate partner violence, 1629-1633
  physical, 1629-1633, 2339
Acamprosate, 155*t*, 156, 1021
Acanthamoeba, 2142, 2142*t*
Acanthamoeba keratitis, 2566
Acanthocytes, 1059*t*
Acanthophis (death adders), 720
Acanthosis nigricans, 2700, 2701*f*, 2702*t*
Acarbose, 1537
Access to health care, 15
  access to AIDS therapy, 2272
  access to dialysis, 842
  disparities in, 15-16
  organizational barriers and interventions, 16
Accessory pathway tachycardia, 360-361, 364-365
Accidental infection, 2217
Accidental trauma, ocular, 2563
Accidents
  radiologic, 82-83, 83*t*, 85
  Swiss cheese model of, 45
Accutane (isotretinoin), 2658
Acebutolol, 388*t*, 430*t*
Acetaminophen
  dose-response effects, 1007, 1008*t*
  for headache, 2357*b*, 2358, 2360
  metabolism of, 1007-1009, 1007.*e*1*f*
  for spinal stenosis, 2377
  toxicity, 699*t*-703*t*, 703, 706*t*-710*t*, 1008-1009
  for venomous fish and stingray injuries, 721*b*
Acetazolamide
  for altitude sickness, 596-597, 597*t*, 1884-1885
  for calcium channelopathies, 2544
  for hyperkalemia, 761
  for hyperkalemic periodic paralysis, 762
  for hypokalemic periodic paralysis, 762
  for intracranial hypertension, 2362
  for myoclonus, 2466-2467
  for perimenstrual seizures, 2408
  for seizures, 2407*t*
  for sodium channelopathies, 2544
Acetazolamide-responsive myotonia, 2542*t*
Acetest, 1540
Acetowhitening, 2221
Acetyl sulfisoxazole (Gantrisin), 1088*t*
Acetylcholine, 549
Acetylcholine esterase deficiency, 2548*t*
Acetylcholine receptor antibodies, 2550
Acetylcholine receptor deficiency, 2548*t*, 2549, 2549*f*

Acetylcholine receptor kinetic abnormalities, 2548*t*
N-Acetylcysteine, 706*t*-710*t*, 1009, 1021
Acetylsalicylic acid. *See* Aspirin
N-Acetyltransferase, 189*t*
Achalasia, 903-904
  clinical manifestations of, 903
  diagnosis of, 903
  epidemiology of, 903
  pathobiology of, 903
  prevalence of, 903
  prognosis for, 904
  radiographic findings, 903, 903*f*
  treatment of, 903*b*-904*b*
Achilles reflex, 2372*t*
Achilles tendinitis, 1754
Achilles tendon rupture, 1754
Achlorhydria, 1335*t*, 1337
Achondroplasia, 1672
Acid excretion
  absent secretion, 1107
  net (NAE), 766
Acid maltase deficiency, 2545
Acid peptic disease, 908-918
  acute, 914
  clinical manifestations of, 912, 912*t*, 914
  complications of, 915-917
  definitions, 908
  diagnosis of, 912-914
  differential diagnosis of, 914
  epidemiology of, 909
  H. pylori–negative, non-NSAID, 910
  idiopathic, 910
  pathobiology of, 909-912
  physical findings, 912
  prevention of, 915-917
  prognosis for, 917
  treatment of, 914*b*-915*b*
Acid-base balance, 763
  in hypovolemia, 745
  renal mechanisms, 763, 763.*e*1*f*
Acid-base disorders, 762-774
  clinical manifestations of, 764-766
  compensatory changes in, 765-766, 765*t*
  definition of, 762
  diagnosis of, 764-766
  epidemiology of, 762
  identification of, 764, 765*t*
  pathobiology of, 762-764
Acidemia, 762, 765*f*
Acidity, 652
Acidosis
  definition of, 762
  distal renal tubular, 770, 770*t*, 824
  hyperchloremic, 762, 762*t*, 769-771
  hyperkalemic renal tubular, 770*t*
  hypochlorhydric, 769
  lactic, 767
    in HIV infection, 2303*t*
    mitochondrial encephalomyopathy with lactic acidosis and strokelike episodes (MELAS), 1652*t*, 1660-1661, 2546
  life-threatening, 661
  metabolic, 766-771
    anion gap, 766-769
    of chronic kidney disease, 840
  proximal renal tubular, 823*t*-824*t*
  respiratory, 773
  in shock, 675
  uremic, 767
Acids
  carbonic, 763
  endogenous, 767-769

Acids *(Continued)*
  nonvolatile or fixed, 763
  production and excretion by kidney, 763
  urinary secretion of, 764
  volatile, 763
Acinetobacter baumannii infections, 1863*t*, 1864, 1968
Acinetobacter baumannii-calcoaceticus complex, 1968
Acinetobacter meningitis, 1969
Acinetobacter species, 1968-1970
  extremely drug-resistant, 1968, 1970
  identification of, 1968.*e*3*t*
  members, 1968.*e*3*t*
  methods of typing, 1968.*e*3*t*
  multidrug-resistant, 1970
Acinetobacter species infections
  clinical manifestations of, 1968-1969
  epidemiology of, 1968
  prevention of, 1970
  prognosis for, 1970
  treatment of, 1969*b*-1970*b*
Acitretin, 2658, 2666*t*, 2667
Aclidinium, 560*t*
ACLS. *See* Advanced cardiac life support
Acne
  preferred medications for women, 1602*t*
  pyogenic arthritis with pyoderma gangrenosum and, 1740*t*, 1743
Acne keloidalis, 2700, 2701*f*
Acne vulgaris, 2680-2681
  definition of, 2680
  pathobiology of, 2680
  regional involvement, 2701*f*
  treatment of, 2680*b*
Acoustic neuroma, 1291, 1292*f*, 2595
Acquired idiopathic aplastic anemia, 1118*t*, 1121
Acquired immunodeficiency syndrome (AIDS), 1837, 2272-2278
  access to therapy, 2272
  AIDS-defining malignancy, 2322-2323, 2323*f*, 2323*t*
  antiretroviral therapy for, 2287-2292, 2294
  CMV infection in, 2230
  definition of, 2323
  demographic impact, 2272
  diagnosis of, 2276-2278
  diarrhea in, 926
  distinguishing characteristics of, 2252*t*-2253*t*
  economic impact, 2272
  gastrointestinal manifestations of, 2302-2305
  global response, 2272
  global statistics, 2272, 2273*t*
  historical perspective on, 2272.*e*1
  Hodgkin's lymphoma in, 1273
  immune reconstitution inflammatory syndrome in, 2332-2335
  infectious complications of, 2292-2295
    clinical manifestations of, 2293-2294
    diagnosis of, 2294
    empirical management of, 2294
    pathobiology of, 2293
    treatment of, 2294*b*
  likelihood for development of, 2293, 2293*f*
  lymphoma in, 1267
  malabsorption in, 931-932
  metabolic disorders in, 2295-2302
  opportunistic infection in, 2291, 2297*t*-2301*t*
  prophylaxis in, 2068
  pulmonary manifestations of, 2305-2318

Coats' disease, 2560
Cobalamin. *See* Vitamin B$_{12}$
Cobalamin-processing (CblC) defect, 1405
    clinical features of, 1406, 1406*t*
    diagnosis of, 1406
    pathobiology of, 1404*f*, 1405
    prognosis for, 1407
    treatment of, 1407
Cobalt toxicity, 93*t*, 96-97
Cobb angle, 629, 630*f*
Cobicistat
    fixed-dose combinations, 2289, 2290*t*
    for HIV/AIDS, 2290*t*
    side effects of, 2289
Cobra venom factor, 246
Cobras, 719
Coca-Cola, 160
Cocaine, 160, 1008*t*
Cocaine use
    cardiomyopathy due to, 330
    clinical manifestations of, 160
    epidemiology of, 160
    pathobiology of, 160
    recommended treatment of, 395*t*
    screening for, 699-702, 702*t*
Coccidia, 2146, 2146*f*
Coccidian enteritis, 2146-2147
    clinical manifestations of, 2146
    diagnosis of, 2146
    epidemiology of, 2146
    pathobiology of, 2146
    prevention of, 2147
    prognosis for, 2147
    treatment of, 2147*b*
Coccidioides, 2072
Coccidioidomycosis, 2072-2073
    clinical characteristics of, 2072*t*
    clinical manifestations of, 2072-2073
    definition of, 2072
    diagnosis of, 2073
    epidemiology of, 2072
    extrapulmonary dissemination, 2073
    incidence of, 2072
    oral ulcers, 2580*t*
    pathobiology of, 2072
    prevalence of, 2072
    prognosis for, 2073
    pulmonary infection, 2072-2073, 2073*f*
    treatment of, 2073*b*
Coccidioidomycosis pneumonia, 532.e1*f*
Coccydynia, 1753
Cochlear damage, 2595
Cockcroft-Gault equations, 728, 730*t*
Code blue teams, 2608
Codeine
    formulations, dosages, and pharmacologic
        information, 139*t*-140*t*
    for migraine headache, 2358
    for restless legs syndrome, 2468-2469
    toxicity, 699*t*-702*t*
Codfish vertebrae, 1824
Coenurosis, 2153
Coenzyme Q10 (ubiquinone) deficiency,
        primary, 2546
    diagnosis of, 2546
    prognosis for, 2546
    treatment of, 2546
Coenzyme Q10 (ubiquinone) supplements,
        2546
Coffee, 387
Cogan's syndrome, 1799
    clinical manifestations of, 1799
    treatment of, 1799
Cognitive assessment, geriatric, 104
Cognitive dysfunction
    executive, 2386-2388
    in fibromyalgia, 1818
    in heart failure, 302
Cognitive impairment, 2382
    definition of, 2389
    mild, 2389-2390
Cognitive therapy, 2348*t*, 2421*t*
Cognitive-behavioral therapy
    for bulimia nervosa, 1457
    for executive cognitive dysfunction,
        2388
    for insomnia, 2421*t*
    for smoking, 147, 147*t*
Coitus interruptus, 1606
Colazal (balsalazide), 939*t*

Colchicine, 2659
    for acute gout, 1814-1815
    for acute pericarditis, 486
    for epidermolysis bullosa acquisita, 2676
    for familial Mediterranean fever, 1148, 1741
    for pericardial constriction, 490
    for Sweet's syndrome, 2682
Cold: disorders due to, 691-695
Cold, common. *See* Common cold
Cold abscesses, 2035
Cold agglutinin disease
    chronic, 1076-1077
    epidemiology of, 1073-1074
Cold agglutinin phenomenon, 2006
Cold agglutinin syndrome, 1075*t*
Cold agglutinins, 1075
Cold autoimmune hemolytic anemia,
        1075-1076, 1077*f*
Cold autoinflammatory disease, familial, 231
Cold autoinflammatory syndrome, familial,
        1740*t*-1741*t*, 1742
Cold hemoglobinuria, paroxysmal
    characteristics of, 1075*t*
    classification of, 1075
    epidemiology of, 1073-1074
Cold injury, 693-695
    clinical manifestations of, 694
    definition of, 693
    diagnosis of, 694
    epidemiology of, 693-694
    factors predisposing to, 694*t*
    pathobiology of, 694
    peripheral, 693
    prevention of, 694
    prognosis for, 695
    treatment of, 694*b*-695*b*
Cold urticaria, familial, 1131, 1742
Colesevelam
    for diarrhea, 933
    for lipid disorders, 1396*t*
    for small bowel rapid transit dysmotility,
        888
    for type 2 diabetes, 1536
Colestipol, 1396*t*
Colic, 854
Colistimethate sodium (colistin)
    for *Acinetobacter* species infections,
        1969-1970
    for *P. aeruginosa* bacteremia, 1966
    for *Pseudomonas* infection, 1967
Colitis
    amebic, 2139-2140, 2141*t*
    Crohn's, 943
    cytomegalovirus, 1861, 2181*t*,
        2297*t*-2301*t*
    differential diagnosis of, 937*t*
    extensive, 941-942
    indeterminate, 935
    ischemic, 953*f*, 955-956
    medical management of, 941-942
    microscopic, 934
    neutropenic, 948, 948.e1*f*
    ulcerative, 1768, 1768*t*
Collagen, 1737, 2634
Collagen vascular disease, 1720
    in immunocompromised patients, 1855*t*
    pleural fluid characteristics, 634*t*
    in pregnancy, 1614*t*
Collagen vascular reactions, 2685*t*
Collagenases, 233*t*
Collagenomas, 2688-2689
Collagenous colitis, 934
Collagens, 1731
Collecting duct carcinoma, 1346*t*
Collecting duct natriuretics, 749
Collecting ducts
    acid secretion in, 739, 740*f*
    functional disorders of, 823*t*, 824
Colles fracture, 1637
Colloids
    burn resuscitation formula, 714.e1*t*
    for shock, 676
    solutions containing, 746
Colon. *See also* Rectum; Small bowel
    diverticulitis of, 946-947
    inflammation of, 945-948
    polyps of, 1325-1327
Colon adenoma
    saline lift polypectomy of, 1327.e1
    snare polypectomy of, 1326, 1326.e1

Colon cancer profile, 1380
Colonic diverticula, 946-947, 947.e1*f*
Colonic microbiome
    and colorectal cancer, 1842
    and inflammatory bowel disease, 1842
Colonic motility, 885
Colonic motility disorders, 888-890
Colonization pressure, 1915
Colonography, CT, 869-870, 869*f*, 876
Colonoscopy, 1329
    applications, 873*t*
    surveillance, 942-943
    surveillance intervals, 1326*t*
    virtual, 869-870, 869*f*, 1329
Color, 2637, 2638*t*-2644*t*
Color flow Doppler imaging, 276, 1726
Color vision change, 2558
Colorado tick fever, 2256-2257
    clinical manifestations of, 2257
    definition of, 2256-2257
    diagnosis of, 2257
    epidemiology of, 2257
    pathobiology of, 2257
    prognosis for, 2257
    treatment of, 2257*b*
Colorado tick fever virus, 2257
Colorectal cancer, 1322-1331
    chemoprevention of, 1329
    clinical manifestations of, 1327-1328
    colonic microbiota and, 1842
    combination therapy for, 1330
    development of, 1226, 1226*f*
    diagnosis of, 1328-1329
    dietary prevention of, 1329-1330
    endoscopy in, 876
    epidemiology of, 1322
    general features of, 1323*t*
    genetic changes associated with, 1226,
        1226*f*
    genetic syndromes, 1325
    hereditary nonpolyposis, 1324
    in inflammatory bowel disease, 942-943
    inherited syndromes, 1323*t*
    metastatic
        locally directed treatment of, 1331
        treatment of, 1331
    molecular basis, 1327, 1327*f*
    molecularly guided therapeutics for,
        202.e1*t*
    nutritional influences, 1429
    pathobiology of, 1322-1323, 1327
    predisposing conditions, 1322-1323
    prognosis for, 1331
    radiation therapy for, 1330
    screening for, 56, 1328-1329, 1328*t*
    staging, 1329-1330, 1329*t*
    surveillance of, 1331
    systemic therapy for, 1330
    targeted therapy for, 202, 202*t*
    treatment of, 1329*b*-1331*b*
Colorectal polyps, 878-879, 878*f*
Colubridae, 717
Coma, 2409-2413, 2410*f*
    causes of, 2410, 2410*t*-2411*t*
    clinical manifestations of, 2411
    diagnosis of, 2411-2412, 2411*t*
    emergency management of, 2412, 2413*t*
    epidemiology of, 2410
    FOUR Score assessment of, 2411, 2411*t*
    likelihood for recovery of awareness, 2413
    neurologic examination in, 2339
    pathobiology of, 2410-2411
    pharmacologic, 2368
    prognosis for, 2413
    treatment of, 2412*b*-2413*b*
Comanagement, 2610
Combination therapy, 1208-1209, 1209*t*
Combined hyperlipidemia, familial, 1393
Comet sign, 593
Cometriq (carbozantinib), 1211*t*-1216*t*
Comfort care, 10
Common cold, 2185-2187, 2241*t*
    clinical manifestations of, 2185-2186
    definition of, 2185
    diagnosis of, 2186
    epidemiology of, 2185
    pain-related symptoms, 2186
    pathobiology of, 2185
    pathogens, 2185
    prevention of, 2186

Common cold (*Continued*)
    prognosis for, 2186
    remedies for, 2186
    treatment of, 2186*b*, 2186*t*
    viruses associated with, 2185*t*
Common couple violence, 1629-1630
Common variable immune deficiency, 1679,
        1680*t*
Commonwealth Foundation, 43.e1*t*
Communication
    core skills for, 14*t*
    model for discussing palliative care topics,
        14*t*
    nonverbal empathy, 14*t*
    verbal empathy, 14*t*
Community disturbance, 1839-1840
Community health centers, 16
Community health workers, 16-17
Community resources, 49
Community-acquired pneumonia, 1902
    due to *L. feeleii*, 1995, 1995*f*
    due to *L. pneumophila*, 1995, 1995*f*-1996*f*
    incidence of, 610.e1*f*
    indications for diagnostic testing, 1904,
        1904*t*
    staphylococcal, 1899
    treatment of, 1905
        antibiotic regimens for, 689*t*
        duration of therapy, 1896
        empirical, 616*t*, 1905
Comparative genomic hybridization, 195
Compartment syndrome, 726, 1174
Compazine, 2573*t*
Compensated cirrhosis, 1026-1027, 1029*f*
Compensatory responses, 672, 765-766,
        765*t*
Complement, 231, 1722
    activation of, 241-246, 245*f*
        alternative pathway, 241-244
        classical pathway, 241-242
        lectin pathway, 242
        pathologic conditions associated with,
            241*t*
        pathways of, 241, 242*f*
        regulators of, 241, 244, 246*f*
        tissue injury or degeneration and, 241,
            242*t*
    in glomerular disorders, 785*t*
    in glomerular syndromes, 734
    in systemic lupus erythematosus,
        1770-1771
Complement C1 inhibitor, 243*t*
Complement C1 inhibitor concentrate
        (Berinert, Cinryze), 1697
Complement C1 inhibitor deficiency, 1682,
        1682*b*
Complement C3 convertase, 244
Complement C3a, 245
Complement C3a receptor, 245
Complement C3d receptor, 2232
Complement C4 binding protein (C4bp),
        243*t*
Complement C4b/C3b receptor (CR1,
        CD35), 243*t*
Complement C5, 243*f*, 246
Complement C5 convertase, 244
Complement C5a, 245
Complement C5a receptor (C5aR [CD88]),
        245
Complement C5b-9, soluble, 245
Complement defects, 1681*f*
Complement deficiency, 1677*t*
Complement disorders, 1681-1682, 1682*b*,
        1740*t*
Complement factor H gene (*CFH*), 2574
Complement inhibitors, 246
Complement receptors, 217-218, 246, 1146
Complement regulating complement, 243*t*
Complement system
    in disease, 240-246, 241*t*
    features of, 241, 241*t*
    function of, 240, 240*f*
    in host defense, 240, 241*t*
Complementary and alternative medicine
        (CAM), 181-184
    definition of, 181
    for osteoarthritis, 1749
    for pain, 142
    use of, 182*t*
Complementary health approaches, 181

Doxycycline (Continued)
for COPD exacerbations, 562
for cystitis, 1875t
for ehrlichiosis, 2053
for furuncles, 2696
for gastroparesis and pseudo-obstruction, 888
for gonorrhea, 1945t, 2603
for granuloma inguinale, 2002
for *H. pylori* eradication, 915t
for infectious rhinosinusitis, 2588
for legionnaires' disease, 1996t
for leptospirosis, 2030
for leptospirosis prophylaxis, 2030
for Lyme disease, 2025t, 2026
for lymphatic filariasis, 2168
for malaria, 1883, 2105, 2111t-2112t
for MRSA infection, 1901
for *Mycoplasma* pneumonia, 2006
for nematodes, 2165t
for onchocerciasis, 2170
for peliosis hepatis, 2001
for pelvic inflammatory disease, 1945
for pityriasis lichenoides, 2669
for plague, 89b, 1989t
for pneumonia, 616t
for prophylaxis in HIV infection, 2295t
for psittacosis, 2012
for Q fever, 2056
recommended doses and schedules, 1891t-1892t
for Rocky Mountain spotted fever, 2049
for rosacea, 2680
for *S. pneumoniae* infection, 1905t
for scrub typhus, 2052
for syphilis, 2018
for tick bites, 2174
for tick-borne rickettsioses, 2051
for travel-related health problems, 1884
for trench fever, 2000
for tularemia, 90b, 1983
for typhus, 2052b
for urethritis, 1878t
for *Vibrio* infections, 1953
Dracunculiasis, 2165t, 2171
Dracunculus medinensis, 2159, 2171
Dravet's disease, 2404
DRESS syndrome (drug reaction or rash with eosinophilia and systemic symptoms), 1153
Dressings, 2657
Dressler's syndrome, 491, 635
Drinking
at-risk
criteria for, 150t
definition of, 149-150
treatment of, 154
binge, 149-150
heavy, 149-150
moderate, 149
problem
behavioral interventions for, 57
prevalence of, 150
Driving
with arrhythmias, 351t
with heart failure, 315-316
Dronabinol, 865t
Dronedarone, 363t-364t, 366
Droopy eyelid (ptosis), 2560, 2560f
Droperidol, 865t
Drospirenone and ethinyl estradiol (Yaz), 2660
Drowning, 595-596
clinical manifestations of, 595
definition of, 595
diagnosis of, 595
epidemiology of, 595
near-drowning, 595
pathobiology of, 595
prevention of, 595
prognosis for, 596
treatment of, 595b-596b
Droxidopa, 2521
Drug(s). See also specific drugs
absorption of, 124
decreased, 130
increased, 130-131
of abuse, 156-162
addictive, 143, 144t, 145
administration of, 124

Drug(s) (Continued)
adverse reactions to, 131-132
for alcohol dependence, 155t
allergic reactions to, 1703t
for amebiasis, 2141t
antianxiety, 2352t
antiarrhythmic, 354-355, 363t-364t, 366
antidepressant, 2347-2348, 2349t
antidiabetic, 1537
antiepileptic, 2407-2408, 2407t-2408t
antihypertensive, 387-391
antipsychotic, 2353, 2354t
antithrombotic, 175-181
and aplastic anemia, 1118
associated toxidromes, 696, 696t
associated with acute interstitial nephritis, 779, 779t
associated with aplastic anemia, 1115, 1115t
associated with ischemic colitis, 955, 956t
associated with photoallergy, 2687t
associated with photosensitivity, 2687
associated with sun sensitivity, 2687t
for benign prostatic hyperplasia, 830, 830t
bioavailability of, 124
for bloating, 894
for bowel habit abnormalities, 894
for cancer, 1211t-1216t
for chronic neuropathic pain, 137t
clearance of, 124-125
dose adjustments by, 128
tests based on, 990
total, 124
decreasing levels, 127
delivery of, 1208
determination of accumulation of, 126, 126f-127f
and dietary requirements, 1445t, 1453
discharge medication checklist, 454t
disease-modifying antirheumatic, 1723, 1760-1762
disease-modifying osteoarthritis, 1749
for disseminated intravascular coagulation, 1183, 1183t
distribution of, 124
altered, 130
volume of, 124
dose-response effects, 1007, 1008t
dosing, 128-129, 1208
elimination of, 124-125, 127, 127f
decreased, 131
effects of dose increases on, 127, 127f
for erectile dysfunction, 1578-1579
for esophageal disorders, 900t
first-pass effects of, 124
and folate deficiency, 1108
future, 142-143
genetic polymorphisms that affect, 189t
genetic testing for, 188-191
germline genetic variants and, 202
half-life of, 125
for heart failure with reduced left ventricular ejection fraction, 309-314
for human African trypanosomiasis, 2115t
for hyperphosphatemia, 778t
hypnotic, 2352t
idiosyncratic responses to, 1118
immunosuppressive, 162-169, 1037-1038, 1037t
for incontinence, 114
for inflammatory bowel disease, 939t
for influenza, 2441
for insomnia, 2421, 2421t
for irritable bowel syndrome, 893t, 894
for ischemic heart disease, 428, 429f
laboratory values, 2717t-2718t
and leukemia, 1240
for lipid disorders, 1396t
loading dose, 125-126
formula for, 125
in renal insufficiency, 128
maintenance dose, 126-127
maternal exposure to, 1564
metabolism of, 1007, 1007t
decreased, 130
genetic polymorphisms that affect, 189t
increased, 130
and micronutrient status, 1453, 1453t
mydriatic, 2576

Drug(s) (Continued)
for myeloproliferative neoplasms, 1128
for myofascial trigger points, 1822
neurotoxic effects of, 2548t
ocular effects of, 2572-2573, 2573t
off-label, 149
for older adults, 116-117, 117t
for osteoarthritis, 1748-1749
for osteoporosis, 1642-1644, 1643t
over-the-counter, 117t
for pain, 136-138, 142-143
and pancreatitis, 960-961, 960t
for Parkinson's disease, 2456-2460, 2457t-2459t
perioperative, 2611-2612, 2613t
for *Pneumocystis* pneumonia, 2096t
preventive of headache, 2357, 2358t
preventive of *Pneumocystis* pneumonia, 2098, 2098t
preventive of relapse to alcohol use, 155-156
preventive of toxicity, 1218
principles of, 124-133, 125f
psychoactive effects of, 116, 117t
psychotropic, 2626, 2626t
to reduce angina and ischemia, 429
reference intervals, 2719t-2722t
and rheumatic disease, 1717
for septic shock, 690
side effects of, 2302
sideroblastic anemia due to exposure to, 1072
skin diseases due to, 2646t
stem cell-derived platforms for, 210
stroke due to, 2443
targeting, 202
testicular hypogonadism due to, 1573
that affect sweating, 2520, 2520t
that alter lipid metabolism, 428
that cause dry eye, 2570t
that cause hair loss, 2704t
that cause hearing loss, 2595
that cause hypercalcemia, 1658
that induce autonomic neuropathy, 2520
that promote weight gain, 1461, 1462t
for thyrotoxicosis, 1508
for tobacco dependence, 147-149, 147t
topical, 2657-2658
for type 2 diabetes, 1535-1536, 1537f
to use with caution in heart failure, 314
for vasomotor symptoms, 1627
and weight gain, 1461, 1462t
for weight loss, 1465-1466
for women of reproductive potential, 1602t
Drug abuse, 143, 162, 2339. See also Substance abuse
in adolescents, 65t
CRAFFT screening tool for, 65t
in elderly, 129-130
epidemiology of, 157
injection drug use, 1926
pathobiology of, 157
Drug addiction, 143
Drug Addiction Act, 159
Drug adherence, 315
Drug allergy, 1703-1705
clinical manifestations of, 1704
definition of, 1703
diagnosis of, 1704-1705
differential diagnosis of, 1704-1705
epidemiology of, 1703
future directions, 1705
pathobiology of, 1704
prevention of, 1705
prognosis for, 1705
risk factors for, 1703
treatment of, 1705b
evidence-based, 1705
guidelines for, 1705f
Drug concentrations
interpreting, 127-128
therapeutic window, 127
Drug counseling, 315t
Drug Database for Porphyria, 1415
Drug eruptions, 2647f
fixed, 2687
in immunocompromised patients, 1858-1859

Drug interactions, 130-131
with antimicrobial therapy, 1846
cancer drugs, 1208
diagnosis of, 131
drugs at risk for, 131t
pharmacodynamic, 131
pharmacokinetic, 130-131
prevention of, 131
types of, 130
Drug monitoring, 127-128
Drug overdose
approach to, 129
distinguishing characteristics of, 2252t-2253t
Drug paraphernalia, 158
Drug rashes, 2684-2687
clinical manifestations of, 2684-2685
definition of, 2684
delayed hypersensitivity reactions, 2684, 2685f, 2685t
diagnosis of, 2684-2685
EGFR inhibitor–associated, 2686, 2686f
with eosinophilia and systemic symptoms, 2685-2686, 2685t
pathobiology of, 2684
prognosis for, 2685b
treatment of, 2685b
Drug reaction with eosinophilia and systemic symptoms (DRESS) syndrome, 1004
Drug reactions, 1010, 1018t, 2617-2618
cholestatic, 1009
differential diagnosis of, 1010
hepatocellular, 1008-1009
hypersensitivity reactions, 2684, 2685f, 2685t
idiosyncratic reactions, 1008
immunoallergic, 1009
neutrophilic, 2686
oral ulcers, 2580t
prevention of, 1010
types of, 1008-1010, 1008t
Drug resistance
chromosomally encoded, 1964
emergence of, 1887-1888
in health care–associated infections, 1863, 1863t
prevention of, 1847
suppression of, 1888
Drug screens, 702t
Drug sensitivity, 2252t-2253t
Drug testing, 699-702, 702t
Drug toxicity, 702-703, 703t
measurement of, 127, 128f
predictable responses, 131-132
reduction of, 1846
stem cell, 1116
unpredictable responses, 132
Drug use disorders
clinical manifestations of, 157-158
epidemiology of, 157
medical complications related to, 157-158
pathobiology of, 157
treatment of, 158, 158b
Drug-induced aplastic anemia, 1115, 1115t
Drug-induced fever, 1853, 1853t
Drug-induced gingival hyperplasia, 2583, 2584f
Drug-induced hypersensitivity, 1859
Drug-induced immune hemolytic anemia, 1078
Drug-induced interstitial lung disease, 576-577, 577t, 586
Drug-induced liver disease, 1006-1010, 1018t
clinical manifestations of, 1008
definition of, 1006
diagnosis of, 1000t, 1008-1010
differential diagnosis of, 1010
epidemiology of, 1006
future directions, 1010
genetics of, 1007
idiosyncratic reactions, 1008
mechanisms of, 1007-1008, 1008.e1f
pathobiology of, 1006-1008
pathogenesis of, 1007
prevention of, 1010
treatment of, 1010b
Drug-Induced Liver Injury Network, 1010
Drug-induced neutropenia, 1135, 1135f
Drug-induced neutrophilia, 1130